Essentials of **Neonatal Emergencies** and Clinical Guidelines

THE EVALUATION-DECISION-ACTION-PLAN/ALGORITHM FOR MANAGING *NEONATAL RESUSCITATION*

SUBJECTIVE FINDINGS

* *Anticipate* the need for resuscitation of a depressed baby in a high-risk delivery * *Adequately prepare* the necessary equipment upon arrival in the delivery room and *ensure* that an advanced resuscitator/a senior consultant is available in case of difficult situations.* *Check* that the oxygen source is adequate & ensure the supplies of essential medications * *Observe* universal sterile precautions by wearing caps, glasses, gloves & gowns.

OBJECTIVE FINDINGS

* *Assess* the infant's breathing- whether the infant is crying vigorously/breathing irregularly & slowly/apneic

* *Assess* the baby's heart rate - whether the heart beat is >100bpm/ <100bpm/<60bpm or absent

* *Assess* the baby's color (trunk & tongue) - pink/blue/pale or white

* *Do not delay assessing the baby`s condition until the end of the first minute!*

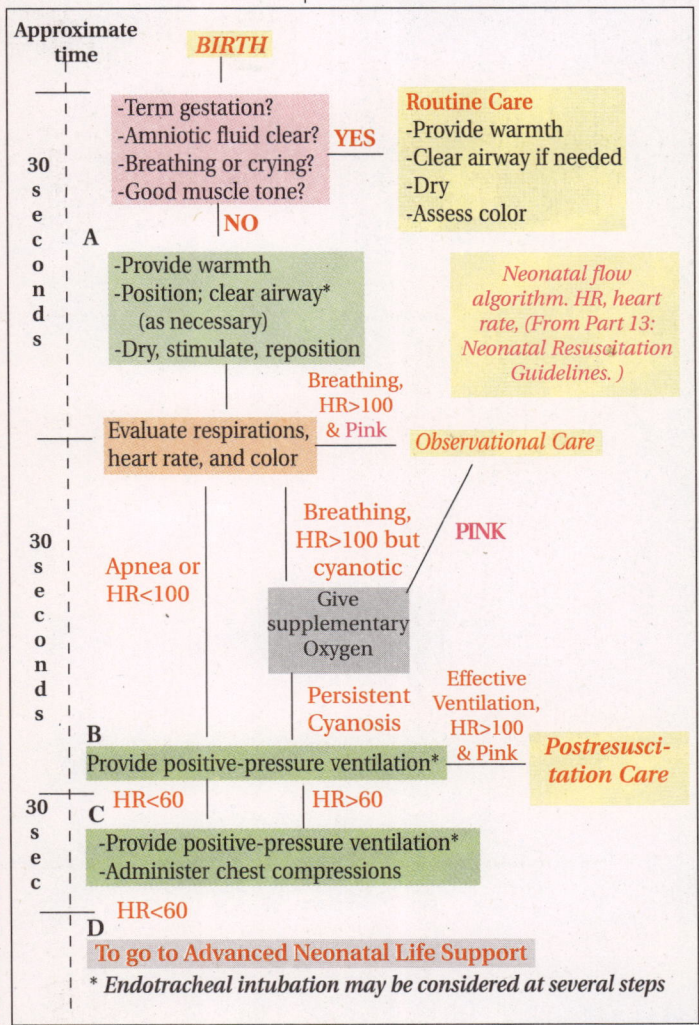

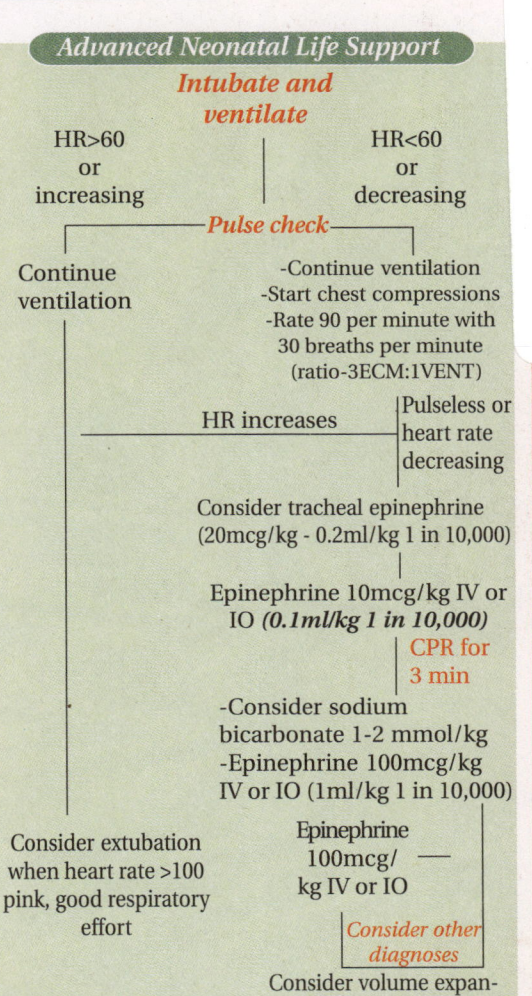

Approximate time

BIRTH

-Term gestation?
-Amniotic fluid clear?
-Breathing or crying?
-Good muscle tone?

YES

Routine Care
-Provide warmth
-Clear airway if needed
-Dry
-Assess color

NO

30 seconds **A**

-Provide warmth
-Position; clear airway* (as necessary)
-Dry, stimulate, reposition

Neonatal flow algorithm. HR, heart rate, (From Part 13: Neonatal Resuscitation Guidelines.)

Evaluate respirations, heart rate, and color

Breathing, HR>100 & Pink

Observational Care

30 seconds

Apnea or HR<100

Breathing, HR>100 but cyanotic

PINK

Give supplementary Oxygen

Persistent Cyanosis

Effective Ventilation, HR>100 & Pink

Postresuscitation Care

B Provide positive-pressure ventilation*

30 sec **C** HR<60 / HR>60

-Provide positive-pressure ventilation*
-Administer chest compressions

D HR<60

To go to Advanced Neonatal Life Support

* *Endotracheal intubation may be considered at several steps*

Advanced Neonatal Life Support

Intubate and ventilate

HR>60 or increasing

HR<60 or decreasing

Pulse check

Continue ventilation

-Continue ventilation
-Start chest compressions
-Rate 90 per minute with 30 breaths per minute (ratio-3ECM:1VENT)

HR increases | Pulseless or heart rate decreasing

Consider tracheal epinephrine (20mcg/kg - 0.2ml/kg 1 in 10,000)

Epinephrine 10mcg/kg IV or IO *(0.1ml/kg 1 in 10,000)*

CPR for 3 min

-Consider sodium bicarbonate 1-2 mmol/kg
-Epinephrine 100mcg/kg IV or IO (1ml/kg 1 in 10,000)

Epinephrine 100mcg/ kg IV or IO

Consider extubation when heart rate >100 pink, good respiratory effort

Consider other diagnoses

Consider volume expansion 20ml/kg NS

ID = Internal Diameter, Adapted from circulation from 1999 : 1927-38, American Heart Association, Inc

Guidelines for Tracheal Tube Size and Depth of Insertion

Tube Insertion (mm ID)	Depth of from Upper Lip (cm)	Weight (g)	Gestation (wk) Size
2.5	6.5-7	< 1,000	<28
3	7-8	1,000-2,000	28-34
3/3.5	8-9	2,000-3,000	34- 38
3.5/4.0	≥9	>3,000	> 38

1. All drugs should be followed by a 0.5-1.0 mL flush of 0.9% saline.

2. If there is likely to be a delay in establishing IV access, then epinephrine (adrenaline) should be given via the ETT. This should be given rapidly down a catheter placed to lie just beyond the end of the ETT and followed by a 0.5-1.0mL normal saline flush and five rapid inflations. This route should only be used whilst IV access is being established. It must not be used in preference to IV access.

3. The dose of sodium bicarbonate is not intended to correct the metabolic acidosis but to increase the pH within the coronary arteries and hopefully increase the action of the subsequent epinephrine (adrenaline). IV sodium bicarbonate 1-2 mmol/kg (2-4 ml/kg 4.2% solution)

4. During the process of prolonged resuscitation, hypoglycemia (i.e. whole BG <45mg/dL) should be sought and treated, if present, with 10% glucose 5 mL/kg IV.

* *Pearl/Peril/Pitfall: Delaying delivery for prolonged suctioning and/or suctioning vigorously enough to cause vagally-mediated bradycardia is not indicated whether or not meconium is present.*

Essentials of
Neonatal Emergencies and Clinical Guidelines

MEDICATIONS FOR NEONATAL RESUSCITATION

Medication	Dose	Route	Rate /Precautions	Important clinical notes
1. Adrenaline 1 in 10,000	0.1–0.3 ml/kg	IV or ET	Give rapidly. Dilute with NS to 1–2 ml if giving ET	Try further doses 1ml/kg at 3–5 minute intervals, if there is no response.
2. Volume Expander (O-ve blood, NS, RL)	10 ml/kg	IV	Give over 5–10 minutes	Useful in hypovolemia due to blood loss or to loss of vascular tone following asphyxia.
3. Sodium Bicarbonate (4.2%)	2–4 ml/kg	IV	Give slowly, over at least 2 minutes	Give only if infant is effectively ventilated; useful to improve the myocardial performance and to enhance the effects of O_2 and Adrenaline.
4. Dextrose 10%	2 ml/kg	IV	Mix with Sodium Bicarbonate at 1:1 dilution	Hypoglycemia is a potential problem for all stressed or asphyxiated babies. Glucostix are not reliable in Neonates when reading <90mgs/dL.
5. Naloxone 1ml = 400mcg	100 mcg/kg or 0.25 ml/kg	IV or ET	Give rapidly. IM / SC acceptable	Useful if the mother had opiate analgesia < 4 hours before delivery. Don't give it if there is history / suspicion of maternal drug abuse as it may initiate Neonatal withdrawal.

6. Atropine & Calcium gluconate have no place in the acute care of Neonatal resuscitation.

CAUSES OF POOR RESPONSE TO ADEQUATE RESUSCITATION

Infant doesn't respond to IPPV and CPR + Drugs at 5–10 minutes of age

The baby remains *cyanosed and bradycardic*
* Technical errors
  - ET tube; displaced/ obstructed
  - Inadequate inflation pressure
  - Too small an ET tube (2.5 mm ID)
  - Oxygen supply disconnected
* Pneumothorax * Congenital malformations that prevent oxygenation - CDH
* Serious evolving lung disease - Meconium aspiration syndrome- Congenital pneumonia - Severe RDS

The infant becomes active, vigorous, makes good respiratory efforts, *yet fails to go pink*
* Unasphyxiated baby with a serious malformations in his respiratory tract or CVS
* Persistent pulmonary hypertension (PPHN) with right-to-left shunting of blood through the PFO and PDA

The infant remains apneic or with very feeble respiratory efforts, hypotonic but *shows good heart rate and perfusion*
* Narcotic administration to mother within 4–6 hours of delivery of the baby
* CNS malformations
* Primary neuromuscular disease
* Severe antenatal brain damage

Do always follow the Ten recommendations to avoid the common pitfalls of newborn resuscitations-Refer to Page 710

IMPORTANT RULES OF RESUSCITATION

1. *Do not panic if an endotracheal tube cannot be placed immediately.* Concentrate on bag-and-mask ventilation and *call for help.* Do not assume that medication is a substitute for ventilation.

2. *Do not perform excessive suctioning of clear fluid from the infant's nasopharynx.* Fluid is normally absorbed into the lungs.

3. *Do not use excessive oxygen concentrations to resuscitate the premature infant unless the infant clearly requires it. The* minimal concentration of oxygen needed should always be used. Babies > 32 weeks gestation should be initiated with FiO2 (inspiratory fraction of oxygen) of 21% and babies <32 weeks gestation with FiO_2 of 21-30% . Further adjustments should be carried out according to the response in heart rate and oxygen saturation.

4. *Do not use too much ventilatory pressure to expand the infant's lungs.* The required initial pressure for expanding the lung may be briefly higher right after birth than it is within just 15 to 30 minutes after birth. *Use good clinical judgment.* Watch the infant's chest and listen to breath sounds. Try reducing ventilation with hand ventilation to ensure that the lowest pressure necessary is being used. Excessive pressure on lungs that are normalizing may decrease venous return to the heart and decrease cardiac output and cause injury to lung tissue.

5. *Avoid hypocapnia.* There is evidence that even brief overdistention of the lung may raise the risk of bronchopulmonary dysplasia (BPD)

6. *Do not give volume replacement or sodium bicarbonate automatically.* Each of these agents has been associated with production of intracranial hemorrhage in animal models.

7. *Do not focus or rely too heavily on cardiac resuscitation,* because, the most likely problem by far in Neonatal resuscitation is the need for ventilatory support.

8. *Maintain normoxia in the term or post-term infant with meconium aspiration or asphyxia,* because such an infant may have reactive pulmonary blood vessels, and pulmonary vasoconstriction may develop if hypoxia persists.

9. *If adequate ventilation is not achievable, consider* * Displaced tube (often in esophagus or right main bronchus) *O*bstructed tube (especially meconium) *P*neumothorax or other patient problems - lung immaturity / respiratory distress syndrome, diaphragmatic hernia, pleural effusion - shock from blood loss - upper airway obstruction, e.g. choanal atresia * Equipment failure, e.g. exhausted gas supply.

10. *Use the "mnemonic* ": "1-2-3 . . . 7-8-9" to determine the placement of the orotracheal ET tube . For a 1-kg newborn, the tube placement should be 7 cm at the lip level. For a 2-kg newborn, placement should be 8 cm at the lip level; for a 3-kg newborn, placement should be 9 cm at the lips.

Essentials of
Neonatal
Emergencies
and Clinical Guidelines

for the Improved Survival of the Sick Newborn

Compiled and Edited by

Nageswara Prasad Vunnava
MD, DCH, MRCP (UK), MRCPCH (London)

Chief Neonatal and Pediatric Intensivist
Apple Excel Tertiary Plus Criticare Hospital for sick newborn and children
forthcoming beside NH16 (Guntur–Vijayawada), Andhra Pradesh, India

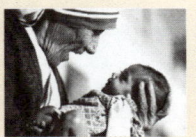

"The level of civilization attained by any society will be determined by the attention it has paid to the welfare of its newborn and children."
— Billy F. Andrews, The Children's Bill of Rights, May 19, 1968

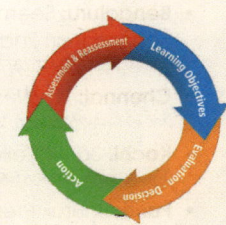

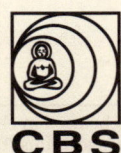

CBS Publishers & Distributors Pvt Ltd
New Delhi • Bengaluru • Chennai • Kochi • Pune
Hyderabad • Kolkata • Mumbai • Nagpur • Patna

Disclaimer

Science and technology are constantly changing fields. New research and experience broaden the scope of information and knowledge. The editor has tried his best in giving information available to him while preparing the material for this book. Although all efforts have been made to ensure optimum accuracy of the material, yet it is quite possible some errors might have been left uncorrected. The publisher, printer and the editor will not be held responsible for any inadvertent errors or inaccuracies.

Essentials of
Neonatal Emergencies
and Clinical Guidelines

ISBN: 978-81-239-2326-0

First Edition: 2013

Published by Satish Kumar Jain for
CBS Publishers & Distributors Pvt Ltd
4819/XI Prahlad Street, 24 Ansari Road, Daryaganj, New Delhi 110 002, India.
Ph: 23289259, 23266861, 23266867 Fax: 011-23243014 Website: www.cbspd.com
e-mail: delhi@cbspd.com; cbspubs@airtelmail.in

Corporate Office: 204 FIE, Industrial Area, Patparganj, Delhi 110 092
Ph: 4934 4934 Fax: 4934 4935 e-mail: publishing@cbspd.com; publicity@cbspd.com

Branches

- **Bengaluru:** Seema House 2975, 17th Cross, K.R. Road, Banasankari 2nd Stage, Bengaluru 560 070, Karnataka
  Ph: +91-80-26771678/79 Fax: +91-80-26771680 e-mail: bangalore@cbspd.com
- **Chennai:** 20, West Park Road, Shenoy Nagar, Chennai 600 030, Tamil Nadu
  Ph: +91-44-26260666, 26208620 Fax: +91-44-42032115 e-mail: chennai@cbspd.com
- **Kochi:** 36/14 Kalluvilakam, Lissie Hospital Road, Kochi 682 018, Kerala
  Ph: +91-484-4059061-65 Fax: +91-484-4059065 e-mail: kochi@cbspd.com
- **Pune:** Bhuruk Prestige, Sr. No. 52/12/2+1+3/2 Narhe, Haveli (Near Katraj-Dehu Road Bypass), Pune 411 041, Maharashtra
  Ph: +91-20-64704058, 64704059, 32392277 Fax: +91-20-24300160 e-mail: pune@cbspd.com

Representatives

- **Hyderabad** 0-9885175004
- **Kolkata** 0-9831437309, 0-9051152362
- **Mumbai** 0-9833017933
- **Nagpur** 0-9021734563
- **Patna** 0-9334159340

Printed at Paras Offset Pvt. Ltd., New Delhi

Editor's Note: The Information provided in this book should only be used in clinical practice if the reader-user has substantial reason to believe that the clinical advice contained in the Flowcharts/Care Plans/Algorithms/Tables/Figures/Overviews is valid and accurate. The Flowcharts/Care Plans/Algorithms are not meant to be "authoritative" . Variations, taking into account individual circumstances, may be appropriate and in case of any doubt/uncertainty the reader-user should consult standard Pediatric/Neonatal textbooks and expert opinion articles/guidelines for more authoritative advice. All of those are intended to supplement, rather than substitute for, professional judgment and may be changed depending upon a Neonate's individual needs. Failure to comply with the pathways does not represent a breach of the standard of care. The reader-user should particularly confirm all drug doses, their indications and contra-indications, prior to their use. Neither the Editor nor the Publishers assume any liability for any injury and/or damage to persons or property arising from this Publication. Finally, please contact us, if any author has any objections to adapting his or her scientific work into this book and I will remove it, from the next edition, unconditionally.

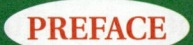

PREFACE

"A baby is God's way of saying the world should go on."
Doris Smith

"Although the world is full of suffering, it is also full of the overcoming of it". Helen Keller

Survival skills are techniques a person may use for an indefinite duration to survive a dangerous situation. Generally speaking, these techniques are meant to provide the basic (bare) necessities for human life: fire, water, food, shelter, habitat, and the need to *think straight*, *to signal for help*, to *navigate safely*, to *avoid unpleasant interactions with animals and plants, and for first aid*. In addition, survival skills are often basic ideas and abilities that ancient humans had to use for thousands of years, so these skills are partially a reenactment of history. *In a similar way Neonatal Intensive Care Unit demands the Staff to fulfil the neonate's basic necessities for improving the survival of the sickest of the Newborn babies by safely navigating them out of the worst of Neonatal Emergencies.*

We're not satisfied delivering good care. We want to deliver the best care. "To live through an impossible situation, you do not need the reflexes of a Grand Prix driver, the muscles of a Hercules, the mind of an Einstein. You simply need to know what to do." -Anthony Greenbank.

To reach our goal, we should continually assess quality and look for ways to improve. "We should love what we do, we should work as a team and we would smile more than we frown." As you all know, *"Chance favors the prepared mind"* ; therefore the NICU Staff should prepare themselves physically, mentally, and with great team spirit to deal with *anticipated and/or Tsunami like chaotic emergencies in Neonates.*

"Good judgement comes from experience but experience comes from bad judgement"- Senior experienced NICU specialists can often tell you how they learned the lessons that made their practice safe. If any practising pediatrician does not have that facility, it is important to share one's experiences with colleagues, to serve the needy and totally dependent Neonates. To work in a NICU/PICU you do need to keep your wits about you and keep your clinical skills as well as your knowledge of physiology and technology. The work includes many urgent and emergency clinical situations but should not be considered stressful. *The diversity of the clinical case load and high quality results mean that professional satisfaction and the psychological and emotional rewards of a career in NICU/PICU are high-*Gale Pearson.

The most favorable outcomes for acutely ill Neonates are the result of a finely tuned collaboration between diverse disciplines and institutions, working together to ensure the best chance of survival and the best long term outcomes. Neonatal Nursing is the protection, promotion, and optimization of health and abilities, prevention of illness and injury, alleviation of suffering through the diagnosis and treatment of human response, and advocacy in the care of individuals, families, communities, and populations. The NICU staff should ensure to follow the key aspects of Neonatal care including: *Communication with doctors *Communication with nurses *Responsiveness of hospital staff *Pain management *Communication about medications *Discharge information *Quietness of the hospital environment *Cleanliness of patient rooms.

Huxley once wrote, *"Logical consequences are the scare crows of fools and the beacons of wise men".* One such beacon is the notion that the best outcomes result when the needs of the patients are matched to the skill, knowledge and experience of caregivers; the most advanced technology is to be employed; and the most appropriate support services are to be provided. *Neonatal care is no different.*

I compiled & edited this Essentials of Neonatal Emergencies & Clinical Guidelines with utmost care, commitment, and an intense passion for the Care of Newborn. This first edition covers 108 *Problem-Oriented Neonatal Emergencies* and about 100 of Clinical Guidelines about *essential but mostly elective topics* in Neonatology. I hope you will find this compilation helpful in your fight for the survival while facing many of the *NICU trials and tribulations*. I request you to let me know the *errors of omission and commission* in this book, if any found, so that a much better 2nd edition of this book will be a natural consequence in a couple of years.

"Never doubt that a small group of thoughtful, committed people can change the world. Indeed it is the only thing that ever has." - **Margaret Mead.** *I am deeply indebted to* such committed Senior Consultant Pediatricians *Dr Andrew Porter*, Ashford, SE Kent, UK, *Dr Surya Hanumara,* Boston, UK, *Dr David Field*, Leicester, UK, *Dr A Campbell*, Preston UK, & *Dr John Owen*, Preston, UK for all their help during my training period in the UK. I am ever grateful to *Dr ML Kulkarni*, Professor and Head, Department of Pediatrics, JJM Medical college, Davangere, Karnataka, India for his excellent teaching and guidance.

I am thankful to many great authors whose exceptional scientific work has been adapted into this book. Their experience and expertise enhance the authenticity of the book. I am extremely indebted to Dr *Alan R. Spitzer, MD* for his great instructive Case Studies adapted into few chapters here and there as well as for his timeless laws of Neonatology.

I am thankful to ...my learned colleagues for their encouragement and support in my profession: Dr Niranjan Reddy (Ongole), Dr Chandrasekhar, Dr Vijaya Lakshmi, Dr Dhanamjaya Rao, Dr Surendra Kumar, Dr Pratap Kumar, Dr Peraiah Chetty, Dr Peraiah, Dr Ram Murthy, Dr Ala Venkateswarlu, Dr Chandrasekhar Reddy, Dr TV Subrahmanya Sastri , Dr Venkata Subbamma, Dr Raja, Dr Ram Prasad, Dr Raghuram Reddy, Dr A Srinivasa Rao, Dr Asha (Chirala), Dr Hanumantha Rao (Chirala), Dr Ravi (Huzur Nagar), Dr Ramesh Kancharla (Rainbow Hosp. Hyderabad), Dr PVT Ramesh (Vijayawada), Dr M Srilatha (Ponnur), Dr K Mohan (Gullapalli), Dr Gavini Venkateswara Rao, Dr Chakravarthy (Tenali), Dr Rama Tharaknadh, Neurophysician, Dr KS Varaprasad, Neurosurgeon, Dr Manohara Rao, Cardiologist, Dr Srinivasa Reddy, Cardiologist, Dr Seetharamanjaneyulu, Orthopedecian, Dr Y Nayudamma, Senior Ped. surgeon, Dr Rajendra Prasad, ENT surgeon, Dr K Rajanikanth, Ped. surgeon, and to many other pediatricians and obstetricians.

I gratefully acknowledge the experience & expertise of

CBS Publishers & Distributors for their excellent print work of this book

Mr Srinivas (Suchitra Graphics) for his Graphical magic

Mrs Lavanya and **Mr Siva Sankar** for their good Pagemaking skills

Mr Bhaskar, Biomedical engineer for his great professionalism in maintaining the NICU equipment

Mr Muralidhar J, Advocate for his excellent Medicolegal help.

Special thanks goes to my wife **Mrs Padma** and to my beloved children **Raga Rachana** and **Sravan** for their cooperation. I am also thankful to My mother **Mrs. Rajeswari** & my loving brothers **Seetharamaiah and Srihari babu** for their continuous support and encouragement.

I would like to dedicate this book to my beloved late father **Sri Krishna Rao** who always thought of my well-being and progress in my personal and professional life and to my loving late brother **Raghunath ,** who recently reached the Heaven untimely, leaving all of us shattered and shell-shocked.

Finally , I think anyone who has lived through a NICU experience would agree that *NICU Parents and their families are the real heroes.* These are ordinary people who have been challenged with an extraordinary event (the sudden NICU hospitalization of a Newborn) and yet despite this obstacle, somehow find the courage, the strength and the will to persevere despite the challenge. *" To cure sometimes, to relieve often, to comfort always"* is a reminder that our role as comforter must provide the basis for our care regardless of whether we can relieve suffering or cure disease.

Yours sincerely

Nageswara Prasad Vunnava

Greatest Quotations
to inspire all of us to save little Angels with the best of Care, Concern and Compassion!

@ *"From inability to let well alone; from too much zeal for the new and contempt for what is old; from putting knowledge before wisdom, science before art, and cleverness before common sense, from treating patients as cases, and from making the cure of the disease more grievous than the endurance of the same, Good Lord, deliver us"*- **Sir Robert Hutchison.** BMJ 1:671, 1953 - Universally Applicable to all the medical and surgical specialities, every time and everywhere!!

@ *"By failing to prepare, you are preparing to fail"*- **B. Franklin** - Best applicable to Neonatal Resuscitation! Before ensuring adequate preparation, anticipate the delivery of a High-Risk Neonate in advance!

@ *"Not everything that counts can be counted, and not everything that can be counted counts"*- **Einstein**- Observe the baby, not the electronic monitoring gadget attached to him/her! It is for good reason that experienced clinicians respond to trends in preference to isolated values. Use your clinical skills and resist the urge to treat numbers in isolation. Treat causes in preference to the effects and avoid generating chaos!

@ *"The patient is first, last and always"* and *"Give every patient your best effort."*-Colonel Ogden C. Bruton, discoverer of agammaglobulinemia.

@ *"Medical care should be humane, and painless; ideally promotive, preferably preventive, desirably curative, at times rehabilitative and always reassuring and consoling"*- **ML Kulkarni** (c/f *To cure sometimes, to relieve often, to comfort (communicate) always* - Trudeau) - The Core philosophy of Neonatal/Pediatric medical services!

@ *"I have yet to see a problem, however complicated, that when you look at it the right way does not become more complicated."* - **Paul Aldeston**- Think it over, when you come across a baby with a life-threatening condition!

@ *"Insanity is doing the same things over and over again and expecting the different results"*- **Einstein** - Do practice Evidence-Based Neonatology where Conclusive clinical guidelines (e.g. Cochrane data base) are available! Otherwise, Be wise to follow good old time-tested practice with common sense approach!

@ *"A smart mother makes often a better diagnosis than a poor doctor."*-**Auguste Bier:** In reality, of course, any mother is likely to make a better diagnosis than a "poor" doctor. About 70 to 80% of pediatric diagnoses are based largely on history. It is essential that students ask the mother what her worries are.

@ *"Success is the natural consequence of constantly applying the conceptual basics and fundamentals, in the worst of the clinical scenario, while hoping for the best and preparing for the worst"*- **Anonymous** - Modern NICU philosophy that truly reduces the Neonatal morbidity and mortality.

@*"Thinking without action is a Daydream; action without thinking is a nightmare"* -*We have to do our best to understand what we are doing. The more we understand, the more we can do….To prevent too much harm before it happen .,* Anonymous- Our errors of commission are more harmful than our errors of omission, most of the times. Ignorance is bliss; may be *? blissful crime,* when it is vital to the diagnosis and management.

@*"Life is like riding a bicycle. To keep your balance you must keep moving"*- **Einstein** - Our postgraduate qualifications should be viewed as just the beginning of our learning; Continuing Medical Education and updating our knowledge with bed side application must be ensured. Change yourself to meet the new challenges, or hang your stethoscope & proclaim yourself as illiterate pediatrician of 21st century, who cannot learn, unlearn & relearn. *"We are what we repeatedly do. Excellence then, is not an act, but a habit."*- **Aristotle .**

@*"HIT(History, Interpretation, Investigation and then Treatment) should replace MISS pattern (Manage first without diagnosis, if not improved, they Investigate next & if no diagnosis is reached, they enquire about Symptoms & Signs) of practice"* -**Y.K. Amdekar**- But, Critically ill Neonates often demand emergent stabilization of ABCDs, and rapid investigations at the time of admission; however, *soon after the Golden hour management,* one should follow 'HIT PLAN' to avoid the medical and legal pitfalls.

@*"Nothing is new except that which is forgotten"*- **Deborah J Tuttle** - Concept based learning lasts much longer than Content based rote learning. The golden way of learning without taxing our rigid memory. "A fool takes in all the lumber of every sort that he comes across, so that the knowledge which might be useful to him gets crowded out, or at best is jumbled up with a lot of other things, so that he has a difficulty in laying his hands upon it. Now the skilful workman is very careful indeed as to what he takes into his brain-attic. He will have nothing but the tools which may help him in doing his work, but of these he has a large assortment, and all in the most perfect order. It is a mistake to think that little room has elastic walls and can distend to any extent "-**Sherlock Holmes (Sir AC Doyle).**

A Newborn's Conversation with God

A baby asked God, "They tell me you are sending me to earth tomorrow, but how am I going to live there being so small and helpless?" God said, "Your angel will be waiting for you and will take care of you."

The child further inquired, "But tell me, here in heaven I don't have to do anything but sing and smile to be happy." God said, "Your angel will sing for you and will also smile for you. And you will feel your angel's love and be very happy."

Again the small child asked, "And how am I going to be able to understand when people talk to me if I don't know the language?" God said, "Your angel will tell you the most beautiful and sweet words you will ever hear, and with much patience and care, your angel will teach you how to speak."

"And what am I going to do when I want to talk to you?" God said, "Your angel will place your hands together and will teach you how to pray."

"Who will protect me?" God said, "Your angel will defend you even if it means risking its life."

"But I will always be sad because I will not see you anymore." God said, "Your angel will always talk to you about Me and will teach you the way to come back to Me, even though I will always be next to you."

At that moment there was much peace in Heaven, but voices from Earth could be heard and the child hurriedly asked, "God, if I am to leave now, please tell me my angel's name."

God said, You will simply call her, " **Mom .**"

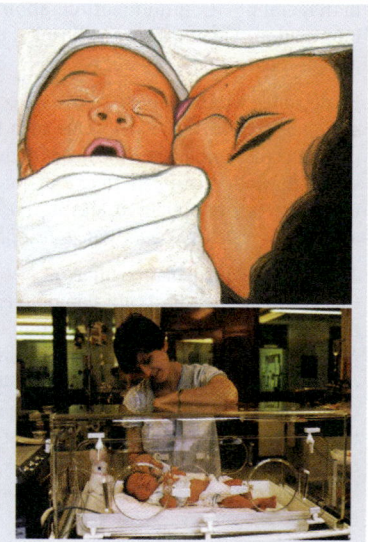

HOW TO USE THIS BOOK?

Essentials of Neonatal Emergencies & Clinical Guidelines, First Edition has been edited to bring **the State-of-the Art** developments in delivering the best of the Neonatal Intensive & Elective Care to improve the survival of the sickest of Newborn Infants. This book contains the *following sections:*

1. Essentials of Neonatal Emergencies

2. Essential Neonatal Clinical Guidelines

3. Essential Neonatal Procedures

4. Quintessential Quick Reference Tables/Figures/Nomograms

5. Essential Neonatal Drug Formulary

6. Back to Neonatal Basics : Self-assessment review in clinical photographs and data.

Essential Neonatal Emergencies: Each of the topics is covered in a Standard Format, which describes the essential aspects of diagnosis and management; contains the following **broad divisions** to enhance the **Reader-User's** understanding and practical application of the Clinical Problems:

A) At the Outset *"An Illustrated Visual Window"* to highlight the essence of the problem in a pictorial way.

B) *Bird's Eye view/Overview/Synopsis* outlines the topic to help the reader-user in having an overall background understanding of the problem, i.e. an aerial view of the topic.

C) *Evaluation-Decision-Action Plan/Algorithm* for the Diagnosis and Management of the Problem: *The Breath and Soul of this Book!* It incorporates the Time tested "SOAP" Approach, i.e. **S**ubjective (History), **O**bjective (Physical Examination), **A**ssessment of the Clinical problem with relevant Investigations, and **P**lan of Management in *a Flowchart or Decision making Tables* whichever is appropriate & relevant.

D) Reference Tables/Figures/Charts/Imaging Pictures to complement the Text and Flowchart.

E) *Key Points For Clinical Practice:* Highlights/Repeats the most important of the various features of the problem useful to improve the existing Clinical Practice.

F) *References and Further Reading* for those who desire to dig deeper to grasp the root value of the problem.

Besides, I included **two more Boxes** just below the Illustrated Visual Window; one is for the *Review of Clinical Problems* for the Self-Assessment and another for *Learning Objectives* of the Chapter with a purpose to improve the current Neonatal Practice. *Review of Clinical Problems* can be done before (easy for the veterans) or after (ideal for the beginners) reading through the Chapter. The readers-users may/will be able to achieve the *Learning Objectives* enlisted in the adjacent box.

Essential Neonatal Clinical Guidelines: Modern clinical guidelines briefly identify, summarize and evaluate the best evidence and most current data about prevention, diagnosis, prognosis, therapy including dosage of medications, risk/benefit and cost-effectiveness. Mostly I selected the elective Neonatal problems common to all levels of Neonatal Care(NICU/SCBU/ High Dependency Unit/Postnatal ward/ Parents In Nursery/ Home). The Essential Clinical Guidelines are *intended to cover common situations* and are not meant to be encyclopedic.

Essential Neonatal Procedures: Covers commonly performed procedures, such as peripheral and umbilical line placement, endotracheal intubation, radial artery cannulation, peritoneal dialysis, tracheostomy, long line insertion (PICC), IO access, drainage of pneumothorax, subdural taps, paracentesis, etc.

Quintessential Quick Reference Tables/Figures/Nomograms: Include the most sought after References to guide the diagnosis and management of Neonatal Emergencies especially, when time does not permit us to browse through the nook and corner of the book.

Essential Neonatal Drug Formulary: Enlists the essential aspects of neonatal drugs and medications, dosage, route, indications, adverse effects, and contraindications.

Finally, **Back to Neonatal Basics** incorporates Newborn clinical photographs and data for a self assessment review with a full complement of relevant answers in the end.

I sincerely hope, you get the best out of this Edition, if you follow the points mentioned above. I wish you will find this book helpful, in your Decision Making about the Critically ill Neonates.

It supplements many Classic Neonatology textbooks brought to us by great authors with international reputation.

PROFESSIONALISM is the Ultimate Purpose of this Book!
Throughout NICU career, let us demonstrate professionalism by showing the following **CHARACTER** attributes:

1. **C**ompassion (empathy; awareness of other's feelings and experiences)

2. **H**onesty (truthfulness, including admission of mistakes)

3. **A**ltruism (unselfish concern for the welfare of others)

4. **R**esponsibility (for conduct, work obligations, and self-improvement)

5. **A**iming for excellence (in self, others, and the system of healthcare)

6. **C**onfidentiality

7. **T**eam player

8. **E**thical approach

9. **R**espect to patients/families, colleagues, team members and faculty (including respect and sensitivity for diversity)

Yours Sincerely

N P Vunnava

Nageswara Prasad Vunnava

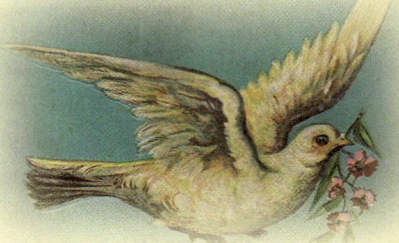
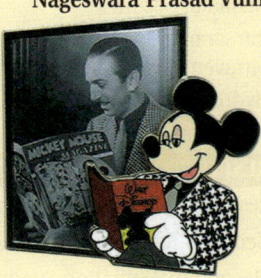

CONTENTS

INFECTIOUS EMERGENCIES

NEONATE-INFANT TRANSITIONAL EMERGENCIES

NEONATAL SURGICAL EMERGENCIES

Section II

Section III

Section IV

Section V

Section VI

Section VII

Index

NEONATAL EMERGENCY: HOW TO DEAL WITH IT EFFICIENTLY & EVERY TIME?

*A **Neonatal Emergency** is a situation that poses an *immediate risk to the infant* that threatens Neonate's life, limb, sight, hearing, or neurodevelopment on long-term follow-up. Most emergencies require urgent intervention to prevent a worsening of the situation, although in some situations, mitigation may not be possible.

*Some emergencies are not immediately threatening to life, but might have serious implications for the continued health and well-being of a Neonate (although a Neonatal emergency can subsequently escalate to be threatening to life).

*The process of emergency management involves **four** phases: mitigation, preparedness, response, and recovery.*

a) Mitigation efforts attempt to prevent hazards from developing into disasters altogether, or to reduce the effects of disasters when they occur. The mitigation phase differs from the other phases because it focuses on long-term measures for reducing or eliminating risk.

b) Preparedness is a continuous cycle of planning, organizing, training, equipping, exercising, evaluation and improvement activities to ensure effective coordination and the enhancement of capabilities to prevent, protect against, respond to, recover from, and mitigate against Neonatal Emergency Disasters.

c) Response Phase includes the mobilization of the necessary emergency services and first responders in the Neonatal Emergency Triage area. A well rehearsed emergency plan (Mock Resuscitation Codes) developed as part of the preparedness phase enables efficient coordination of the emergency care interventions. There is a need for both discipline (structure, doctrine, process) and agility (creativity, improvisation, adaptability) in responding to a Neonatal emergency.

d) During Recovery Phase following an emergency, the NICU Staff should assist the parents involved overcome their mental trauma due to their beloved little baby's separation from them (either NICU admission or death).

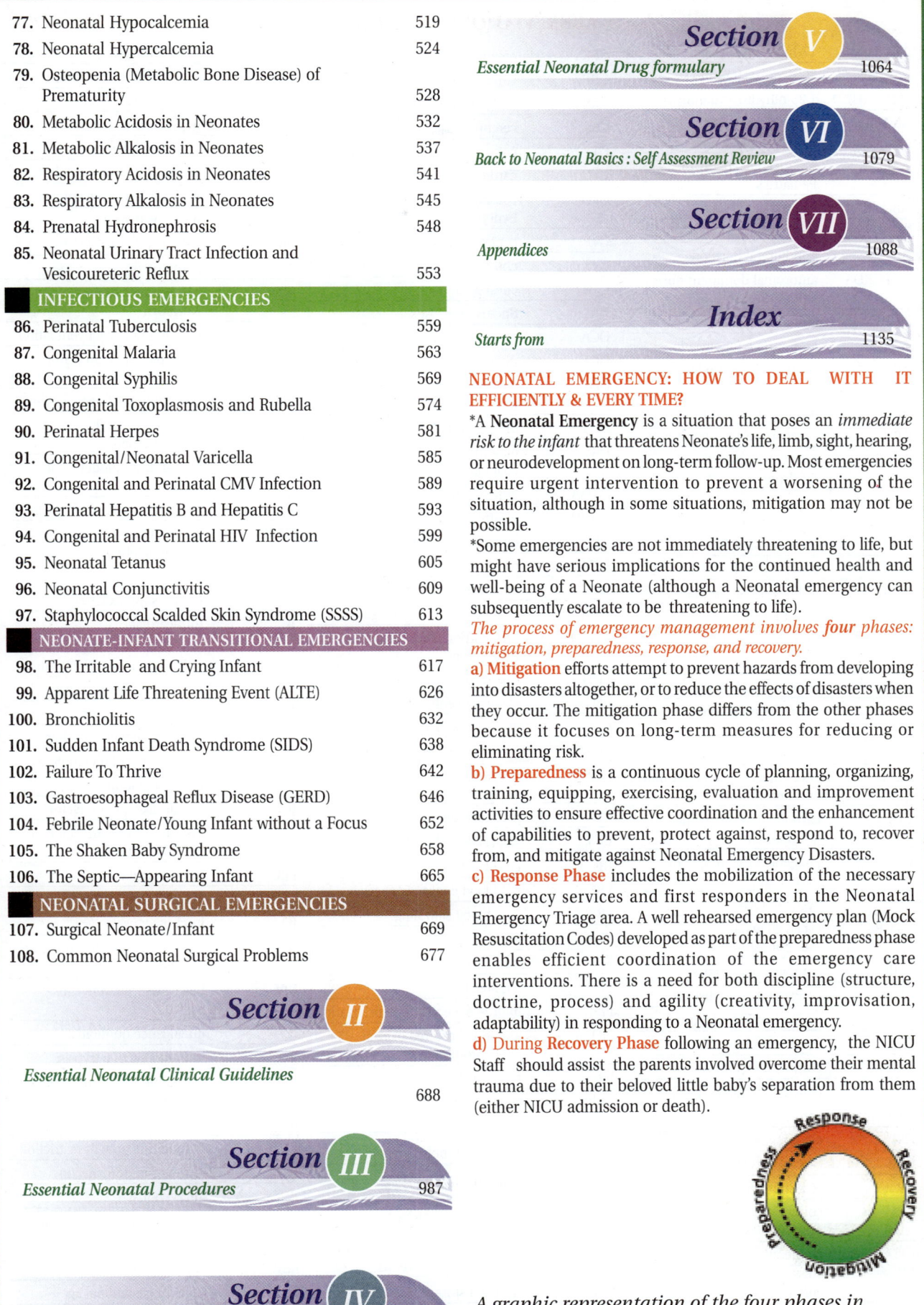

A graphic representation of the four phases in emergency management

ABBREVIATIONS IN THE BOOK

17-OHP	17-hydroxyprogesterone
25-OHD	25-hydroxyvitamin D
1,25-(OH)$_2$D	1,25-dihydroxyvitamin D
3b-HSD	3b-hydroxysteroid dehydrogenase
AAP	American Academy of Pediatrics
ABG	Arterial Blood Gas
ACE	angiotensin-converting enzyme
ADH	antidiuretic hormone
ADPCKD	autosomal dominant polycystic kidney disease
AFP	alpha-fetoprotein
AGA	appropriate for gestational age
AIDS	acquired immunodeficiency syndrome
ALT	alanine aminotransferase
APH	antepartum hemorrhage
ARDS	acute respiratory distress syndrome
ARPCKD	autosomal recessive polycystic kidney disease
ASD	atrial septal defect
AST	aspartate aminotransferase
AVSD	atrioventricular septal defect
BP	blood pressure
BPD	bronchopulmonary dysplasia
BT	bleeding time
CAH	congenital adrenal hyperplasia
CAM	cystic adenomatoid malformation
CBF	cerebral blood flow
CDC	US Centers for Disease Control and Prevention
CDG	carbohydrate-deficient glycoprotein
CDH	congenital diaphragmatic hernia
CF	cystic fibrosis
cGMP	cyclic guanylate monophosphate
CHB	complete heart block
CHD	congenital heart disease
CHF	congestive heart failure
CI	confidence interval
CLD	chronic lung disease
CM	conventional management
CMD	congenital muscular dystrophy
CMV	cytomegalovirus
CNS	central nervous system
CP	cerebral palsy
CPAP	continuous positive airway pressure
CPD	citrate, phosphate, dextrose
CPDA	citrate, phosphate, dextrose and adenine
CPK	creatine phosphokinase
CRP	C-reactive protein
CRS	congenital rubella syndrome
CSF	cerebrospinal fluid
CT	computerized tomography
CTG	cardiotocograph
CVH	combined ventricular hypertrophy
CVP	central venous pressure
CVS	chorionic villus sampling
CXR	chest X-ray
DA	ductus arteriosus
DCA	dichloroacetate
DCT	direct Coomb`s test
DDH	developmental dysplasia of the hip
DHT	dihydrotestosterone
DIC	disseminated intravascular coagulation
DMSA	dimercaptosuccinic acid
DNPH	dinitrophenylhydrazine
DPPC	dipalmitoyl phosphatidylcholine
EBM	expressed breast milk
ECG	electrocardiogram
ECM	external cardiac massage
ECMO	extracorporeal membrane oxygenation
EDD	expected date of delivery
EEG	electroencephalogram
EFA	essential fatty acid
ELBW	extremely low birth weight
ELISA	enzyme-linked immunosorbent assay
EMG	electromyogram
ENT	ear, nose, and throat
ET	endotracheal
FBC	full blood count
FBS	fetal blood sampling
FDP	fibrin-degradation products
FFP	fresh-frozen plasma
FHR	fetal heart rate
FISH	fluorescence in situ hybridization
FiO$_2$	fractional inspired oxygen concentration
FRC	functional residual capacity
G6PD	glucose-6-phosphate dehydrogenase
GABA	gamma-aminobutyric acid
GBS	group B streptococcus
GFR	glomerular filtration rate
GH	growth hormone
GER	gastroesophageal reflux
GSD	glycogen storage disease
GU	genito urinary
HAS	human albumin solution
Hb	hemoglobin
HBeAg	hepatitis B 'e' antigen
HBF	fetal hemoglobin
HBIG	hepatitis B immunoglobulin
HBsAg	hepatitis B surface antigen
HBV	hepatitis B virus
HCV	hepatitis C virus
Hct	hematocrit
HDN	hemorrhagic disease of the Newborn
HFJV	high-frequency jet ventilation
HFOV	high-frequency oscillatory ventilation
Hib	hemophilus influenzae type b
HIE	hypoxic-ischemic encephalopathy
HIV	human immunodeficiency virus
HLHS	hypoplastic left heart syndrome
HNIG	human normal immunoglobulin
HR	heart rate
HSV	herpes simplex virus
IC	intracardiac
ICROP	International Classification of Retinopathy of Prematurity
ICH	intracranial hemorrhage
ICP	intracranial pressure
IDM	infant of diabetic mother
IEM	inborn error of metabolism
Ig	immunoglobulin
IGF	insulin-like growth factor
IGFBP	insulin-like growth factor binding protein
i.m.	intramuscular
INO	inhaled nitric oxide
IO	intra osseous
IPPV	intermittent positive pressure ventilation
IPV	inactivated poliomyelitis vaccine
IQ	intelligence quotient
IRT	immunoreactive trypsin
ITP	idiopathic thrombocytopenic purpura
IU	international units
IUGR	intrauterine growth restriction
IUT	intrauterine transfusion
IV	intravenous
IVH	intraventricular hemorrhage
IVIG	intravenous immunoglobulin
LBW	low birth weight
LGA	large for gestational age

ABBREVIATIONS IN THE BOOK

LP	lumbar puncture	PFC	persistent fetal circulation	SVT	supraventricular tachycardia
LV	left ventricle	PFO	patent foramen ovale	TA-GVHD	transfusion-associated graft versus host disease
LVH	left ventricular hypertrophy	PG	prostaglandin	TAPVD	total anomalous pulmonary venous drainage
MAG-3	mercapto-acetyl- triglycerine-3	PHH	post-hemorrhagic hydrocephalus	TAR	thrombocytopenia with absent radius
MAP	mean airway pressure	PI	protease inhibitor		
MAS	meconium aspiration syndrome	PIE	pulmonary interstitial emphysema	TB	tuberculosis
MCUG	micturating cystourethrogram	PIP	peak inspiratory pressure	TDF	testis-determining factor
MEF	minimal enteral feeding	PKU	phenylketonuria	Te	expiratory time
mIU	milli international units	p1^{A1}	platelet A1 antigen	TGA	transposition of great arteries
MIS	Mullerian inhibitor substance	PLH	pulmonary lymphoid hyperplasia	THAM	tris-hydroxymethyl aminomethane
MRI	magnetic resonance imaging	PM	post-mortem		
MRSA	methicillin-resistant *Staphylococcus aureus*	PMA	postmenstrual age	Ti	inspiratory time
		PNDM	permanent neonatal diabetes mellitus	TMI	transient myocardial ischemia
MSUD	maple syrup urine disease			TNDM	transient neonatal diabetes mellitus
mU	milli units	p.o.	by mouth		
NAS	neonatal abstinence syndrome	PPHN	persistent pulmonary hypertension of the newborn	TEF	tracheo-esophageal fistula
NEC	necrotizing enterocolitis	PROM	premature rupture of membranes	TOF	tetralogy of Fallot
NICE	National Inst. of Clinical Excellence	PS	pulmonary stenosis	TORSCH	toxoplasmosis, other (particularly syphilis), rubella, cytomegalovirus, herpes
		PT	prothrombin time		
NICHD	National Institute of Child Health and Human Development	PTH	parathormone	TPHA	Treponema pallidum hemagglutination assay
		PTT	partial thromboplastin time	TPN	total parenteral nutrition
		PTV	patient-triggered ventilation		
NICU	neonatal intensive care unit	PUJ	pelvi-ureteric junction	TRH	thyroid-releasing hormone
NIPS	neonatal infant pain score	PVH	periventricular hemorrhage	TSH	thyroid-stimulating hormone
NKH	non-ketotic hyperglycinemia	PVL	periventricular leucomalacia	TT	thrombin time
NNU	neonatal unit	PVR	pulmonary vascular resistance	TTN	transient tachypnea of newborn
NO	nitric oxide	RDS	respiratory distress syndrome		
NO$_2$	nitrogen dioxide	rHuEPO	recombinant human erythropoietin	U and E	urea and electrolytes
NOS	nitric oxide synthase			UAC	umbilical artery catheter
NTD	neural tube defect	ROP	retinopathy of prematurity	UDCA	ursodeoxycholic acid
nvCJD	new variant Creutzfeldt- Jakob disease	RSV	respiratory syncytial virus	UDPGT	uridine diphosphate glucuronyl transferase
		RSVIG	respiratory syncytial virus immunoglobulin		
OI	oxygenation index			UTI	urinary tract infection
OPV	oral poliomyelitis vaccine	RT	reptilase time	UVC	umbilical venous catheter
OR	odds ratio	RTA	renal tubular acidosis	VCV	volume-controlled ventilation
PA	pulmonary artery	RVH	right ventricular hypertrophy	VDRL	Venereal Disease Research Laboratory
PaCO$_2$	arterial carbon dioxide tension	SaO$_2$	oxygen saturation		
PaO$_2$	arterial oxygen tension	SBR	serum bilirubin	VKDB	vitamin K deficiency bleeding
PAS	periodic acid-Schiff reaction	s.c.	subcutaneous	VLBW	very low birthweight
PBF	pulmonary blood flow	SCID	severe combined immunodeficiency	VSD	ventricular septal defect
PCA	postconceptional age			VT	ventricular tachycardia
PCKD	polycystic kidney disease	SGA	small for gestational age	VUR	vesico-ureteric reflux
PCP	Pneumocystis carinii pneumonia	SIADH	syndrome of inappropriate antidiuretic hormone	VZV	varicella-zoster virus
				VZIG	varicella-zoster immunoglobulin
PCR	polymerase chain reaction	SIDS	sudden infant death syndrome		
PCV	packed cell volume	SIMV	synchronized IMV	WBC	white blood cell
PDA	patent ductus arteriosus	SLE	systemic lupus erythematosus	WPW	Woolf-Parkinson-White syndrome
PE	pre-eclampsia	SMA	spinal muscular atrophy		
PEEP	positive end-expiratory pressure	sPDA	symptomatic patent ductus arteriosus	ZDV	zidovudine
PET	pre-eclamptic toxemia	SRY	sex determining region Y	ZIG	zoster immune globulin

IMPROVING NEONATAL SURVIVAL : MILES TO GO BEFORE WE CAN SLEEP!

Each year, around 4 million children die within the first 28 days of life—the newborn (neonatal) period. Given that these newborn deaths account for 37 per cent of all under-five deaths, improving neonatal survival is essential.

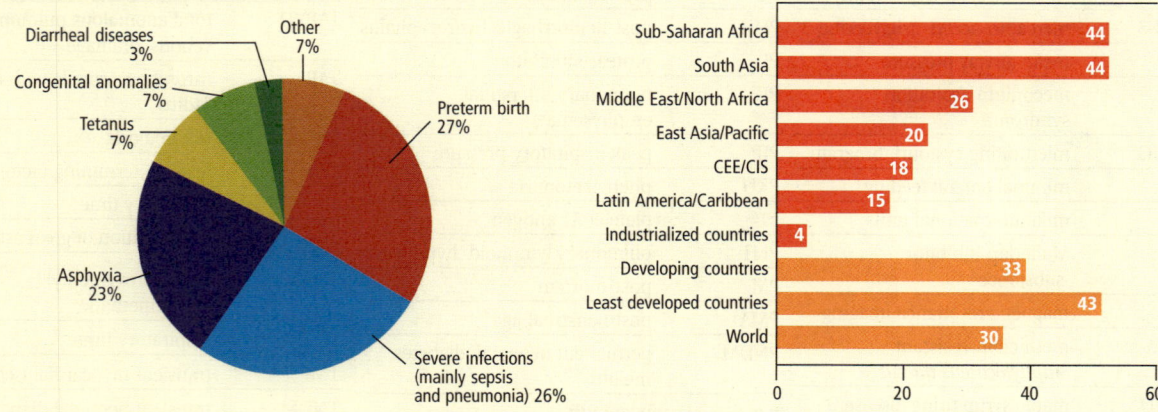

EACH YEAR, AROUND 4 MILLION NEWBORNS PERISH IN THE FIRST 28 DAYS OF LIFE-Global distribution of neonatal deaths by cause (2000)

NEWBORNS IN DEVELOPING COUNTRIES ARE EIGHT TIMES MORE LIKELY TO DIE THAN NEWBORNS IN INDUSTRIALIZED COUNTRIES–Neonatal mortality rate (per 1,000 live births), by region (2000)

Reducing neonatal deaths requires improving women's health during pregnancy, providing appropriate care for both mother and newborn during and immediately after birth, and caring for the baby during the first weeks of life. Cost-effective, feasible interventions include initiating breast feeding within one hour of birth, ensuring proper cord care, keeping the baby warm, recognizing danger signs and seeking care, and giving special care to infants with low birthweight. A continuum of care from pregnancy to early childhood should link community-based programmes to strengthened health systems. Efforts to develop a core set of indicators to monitor newborn care interventions are under way. But more work is needed to finalize these indicators for inclusion in household surveys. Note: Coverage of many interventions to improve neonatal survival is analysed elsewhere in this statistical review. For nutritional interventions such as exclusive breast feeding for the first six months of life; for interventions during pregnancy and childbirth; for preventing mother-to-child transmission of HIV.

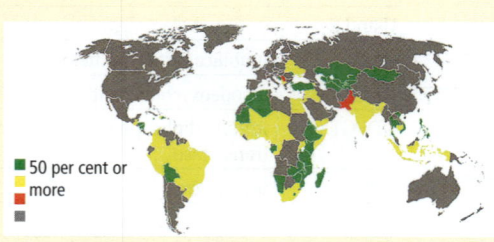

INITIATION OF BREAST-FEEDING WITHIN ONE HOUR OF BIRTH IS CRITICAL FOR NEWBORN HEALTH AND WELL-BEING- Percentage of women aged 15-49 who breastfed their infants within the first hour after birth (1990-2006)

COVERAGE OF KEY NEONATAL SURVIVAL INTERVENTIONS IN THE DEVELOPING WORLD

Pre-conception	Folic acid supplementation
Antenatal	Syphilis screening and treatment
	Pre-eclampsia and eclampsia prevention
	Tetanus toxoid immunization
	Intermittent preventive treatment for malaria
	Detection and treatment of asymptomatic bacteriuria
Intrapartum (birth)	Antibiotics for preterm rupture of membranes
	Corticosteroids for preterm labor
	Detection and management of breech
	Labor surveillance for early diagnosis of complications
	Clean delivery practices
Postnatal	Resuscitation of newborn baby
	Breast-feeding
	Prevention and management of hypothermia
	Kangaroo mother care (for infants with low birth weight) in health facilities
	Community-based case management of pneumonia

Essential Components of Newborn Care

1. Care at birth—aseptic techniques at delivery time
2. Prevention and management of hypothermia— ensuring maintenance of warmth for the infant
3. Resuscitation of infant not crying—identification and referral of at-risk neonates
4. Physical examination of infant and identification of risk—identifying infants with low birthweight for home care; identifying infants with low birthweight who need referral
5. Ensuring early and successful breast feeding and breast milk feeding by spoon—ability to identify feeding problems; successfully initiating breast feeding soon after birth
6. Identifying signs of illness—providing essential newborn care
7. Grading severity of illness

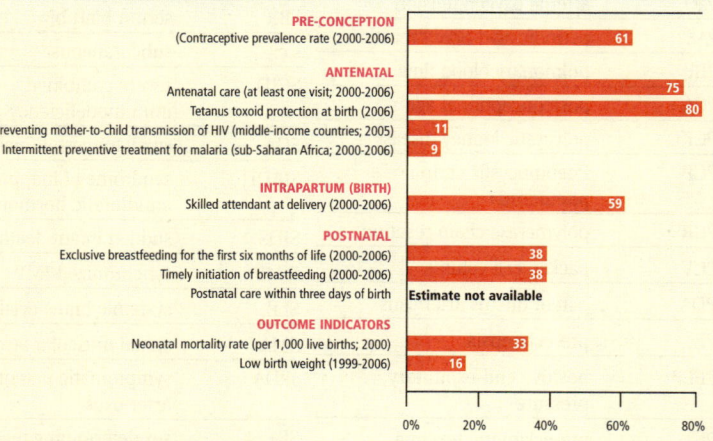

KEY INTERVENTIONS FOR REDUCING NEONATAL MORTALITY AND MORBIDITY

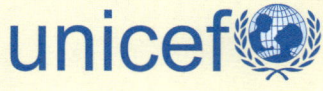

IMPROVING UNDER-5S` SURVIVAL: MANY MORE MILES TO GO BEFORE WE CAN SLEEP!

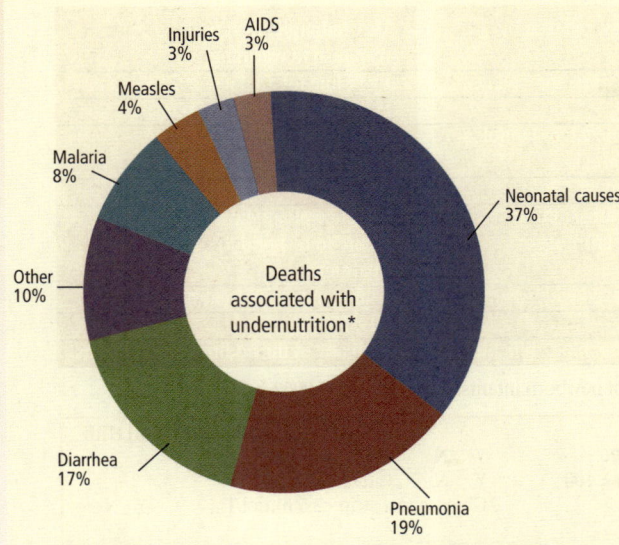

MAJOR CAUSES OF CHILD MORTALITY-Global distribution of under-five deaths by cause (2000–2003)

* Undernutrition has been estimated to be an underlying cause in up to half of all under-five deaths.

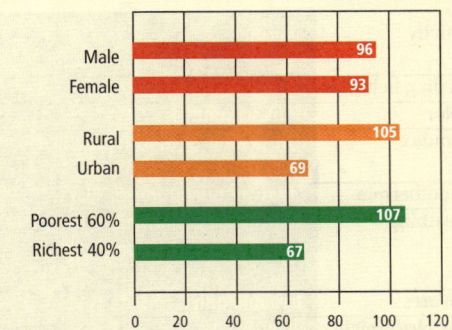

CHILD MORTALITY IS HIGHER AMONG CHILDREN LIVING IN RURAL AREAS AND IN THE POOREST HOUSEHOLDS
Under-five mortality rate (per 1,000 live births) by background characteristics (1998–2006)

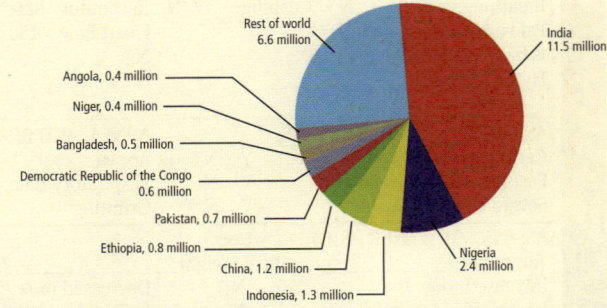

OF THE WORLD'S 26 MILLION CHILDREN NOT IMMUNIZED WITH DPT3, 20 MILLION LIVE IN 10 COUNTRIES-Number of children not immunized with DPT3 (2006)

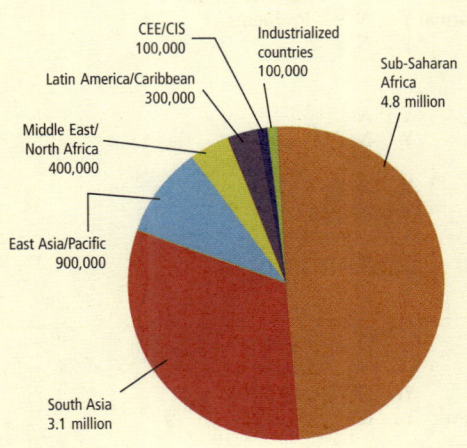

9.7 MILLION CHILDREN DIED IN 2006 BEFORE THEY REACHED THEIR FIFTH BIRTHDAY

Estimated number of under-five deaths, by region (2006)

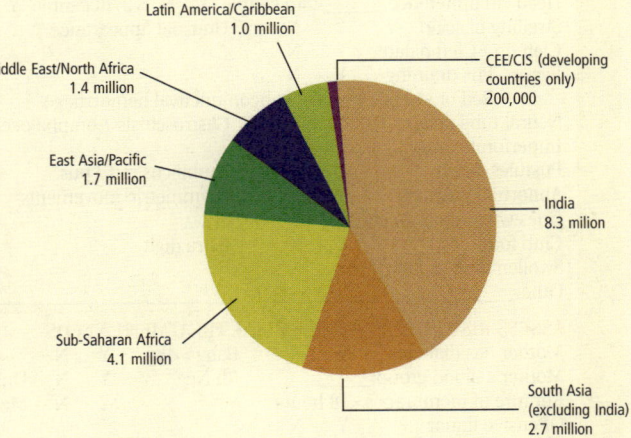

MORE THAN 19 MILLION INFANTS IN THE DEVELOPING WORLD HAVE LOW BIRTHWEIGHT

More than half are in South Asia; 8.3 million are in India
Number of infants weighing less than 2,500 grams at birth, by region

The Challenge of Newborn Care in India

Meeting the commitment to reach the Millennium Developmental Goal of reducing infant mortality rate to less than 30 in India is only possible through improved neonatal survival. The formidable hurdles that contribute to the high neonatal mortality include domiciliary births aided by unskilled birth attendants, low exclusive breastfeeding rates, high burden of low-birthweight infants, poor care-seeking practices for sick children (with female infants receiving less care), and high cost of care for sick newborns compared with family incomes. Creating models of community and domiciliary newborn care and establishing low-cost newborn care units at district health facilities have reduced neonatal mortality significantly. Taking these experiments to scale appears to be the road map for India to reduce its burden of neonatal deaths. (**Siddarth Ramji, MD** Professor, Department of Neonatology, Maulana Azad Medical College, New Delhi, India).

Source for figures : UNICEF global databases, 2007. Global distribution of neonatal deaths by cause: Lawn, Joy E., Simon Cousens and Jelka Zupans, '4 million neonatal deaths: When? Where? Why?' The Lancet, vol. 365, no. 9462, 3 March 2005, pp. 891–900. Key interventions: Darmstadt, G.L., et al., 'Evidence-based, cost-effective interventions: How many newborns can we save?' The Lancet, vol. 365, no. 9463, 12 March 2005, pp. 977–988. ,UNICEF global databases, 2007. Measles and DPT3: WHO/UNICEF Joint Working Group on Immunization, 2007.

Grading Severity of Illness in a Newborn: Neonatal Care in Developing Countries

	Mild	Moderate	Severe
Activity	Normal	Mild lethargy, relieved by feeding	Very lethargic, with poor response to warming
Feeding behavior	Poor feeding by spoon	By tube or IV line for <3 days	By IV line for >3 days
Color	Pink without O_2	Pink with O_2	Poor response to O_2 or signs
Jaundice	Onset after 24 h, with jaundice over trunk and up to face	Onset within 24 h or jaundice up to arms and legs	Jaundice over palms and soles, or infant symptomatic
Hypothermia	Body temperature 35–36.5°C	Temperature 32–35°C	Temperature ≤32°C
Breathing	Rate 60–80 breaths/min; no grunting or retractions	Rate .80 breaths/min or presence of grunting or retractions	Presence of apneic attacks or failure to respond to treatment
Seizures	Irritable only	Seizure relieved with treatment	Poor response to treatment
Low birthweight	2000–2500 g	1500–2000 g	All ≤ 1500 g
	Weak sucking, color pale	Weak sucking, blue, difficulty	With any of the additional symptoms,

Courtesy: Bhakoo ON et al: Facilities required for primary care (level 1) of newborn infants, *J Neonatol* 16:9, 2002.

ASSESS NEED FOR EMERGENCY CARE   RESPIRATORY FAILURE
Breathing well?   Y N   Gasping? Y N   Respiratory Rate <20   Y N   Yes___ No___
Pale or cold?   Y N   Heart Rate > 180 or < 100   Y N   Circulatory failure
Is baby extremely lethargic?   Y N   Glucose test strip <2.5 mmol/l   Y N
Hypoglycemia
                                                                                          Yes   N

ASSESS FOR PRIORITY SIGNS: **APNEA AND RESPIRATORY DISTRESS**   Classify for apnea
Central cyanosis   Y N   Apnea   Y N   and respiratory
Fast breathing   Y N   Respiratory Rate_____   distress
Severe chest indrawing   Y N   Grunting   Y N

ASSESS FOR OTHER PRIORITY SIGNS :   Classify for priority
Temperature_____Birth Weight_____Jaundice Y N   Signs
Increased tone   Y N   Decreased tone / floppy   Y N
Irregular jerky movements Y N   Reduced activity   Y N
Lethargic or unconscious   Y N   Bulging fontanel   Y N
Abnormal distension   Y N   Bile stained vomiting   Y N

ASSESS FOR BIRTH INJURIES, MALFORMATIONS, LOCAL INFECTIONS   Classify for all
Head circumference_____<3rd centile Y N >97th centile Y N Normal Y N   Problems
Swelling of scalp   Y N   Unusual appearance   Y N
Cleft lip / Cleft palate   Y N
Eyes : Pus draining   Y N
              Red or swollen eyelid / Subconjunctival hemorrhage   Y N
Neural tube defect   Y N   Gastroschisis / omphalocele   Y N
Imperforate anus   Y N
Pustules / rash   Y N   Umbilicus red / pus   Y N
Abnormal position   Y N   Asymmetric movements   Y N
Cries when limb touched   Y   N
Club foot   Y N   Extra digit   Y N
Swollen limb or joint   Y N
Other_____

ASSESS RISK FACTORS AND SPECIAL TREATMENT NEEDS   Classify for all risk
Mother has diabetes   Y N   Baby > 4kg   Y N   factors
Mother's blood group:_____ Rh Neg   Y N   Unknown   Y N
Rupture of membranes> 18 hours   Y N   Maternal fever Y N
Offensive liquor   Y   N
Apgar < 7 at 5 minutes   Y   N
Mother's RPR :_____ ☐ Positive ☐ Partially treated ☐ Unknown
Mother HIV status: ☐ Positive ☐ Negative ☐ Unknown
Mother has TB, or has been on TB treatment within the last 6 months   Y N

Baby can be discharged home: Safe *transitioning of high-risk infants from hospital to home requires these essential elements: (1) a thorough understanding and adherence to infant-identified discharge criteria; * A sustained pattern of weight gain of sufficient duration; * Adequate maintenance of normal body temperature with the infant fully clothed in an open bed with normal ambient temperature (24°C to 25°C); * Competent suckle feeding, breast or bottle, without cardiorespiratory compromise; and * Physiologically mature and stable cardiorespiratory function of sufficient duration. In addition, *Appropriate immunizations have been administered; * Appropriate metabolic screening has been performed; * Hematologic status has been assessed and appropriate therapy instituted as indicated; * Nutritional risks have been assessed and therapy and dietary modification instituted as indicated; * Sensorineural assessments, hearing and funduscopy, have been completed as indicated; * Review of hospital course has been completed, unresolved medical problems identified, and plans for treatment instituted as indicated. (2) the coordination and progression of educational activities that prepare families for care at home; (3) the appropriate identification and utilization of referral services, both during hospitalization and in the community; (4) the involvement of community healthcare providers well versed in the care and follow-up of infants born ill or prematurely; (5) the psychosocial adaptations parents make as they accept their role as independent caregiver. A family Social assessment, Advocacy by all healthcare team members for the safety and well-being of the infant, strong Family involvement, and accessible Environmental resources contribute to the success of a SAFE discharge.*

THE EVOLUTION & REVOLUTION OF NEONATOLOGY

The Evolution & Revolution : The past 150 years have produced dramatic changes in Neonatal and Infant mortality and morbidity; the latter half of the 20th century in particular saw an explosion of new concepts and technology in perinatology and Neonatology. The current practice of Newborn medicine has been sculpted by significant recent accomplishments as well as by well-intentioned medical misadventures. In 1960, the terms "Neonatology" and "Neonatologist" were introduced. Thereafter, an increasing number of pediatricians devoted themselves to full-time neonatology. One of the most important factors that improved the care of the Neonate was the miniaturization of blood samples needed to determine blood gases, serum electrolytes, glucose, calcium, bilirubin, and other biochemical measurements. Another factor was the ability to provide nutrition intravenously, and the third was the maintenance of normal body temperature. The management of respiratory distress syndrome improved with IV glucose and correction of metabolic acidosis, followed by assisted ventilation, continuous positive airway pressure, antenatal corticosteroid administration, and the introduction of exogenous surfactant. Pharmacologic manipulation of the ductus arteriosus, support of blood pressure, echocardiography, and changes in the management of persistent pulmonary hypertension, including the use of nitric oxide and extracorporeal membrane oxygenation, all have influenced the cardiopulmonary management of the Neonate. Regionalization of Neonatal care; changes in parent–infant interaction; and technological changes such as phototherapy, oxygen saturation monitors, and brain imaging techniques are among the important advances. Most remarkable, a 1-kg infant who was born in 1960 had a mortality risk of 95% but had a 95% probability of survival by 2000. However, errors in Neonatology are to be acknowledged, and potential directions for the future may be explored.

TOP 10 NEONATAL ADVANCES OF THE 20th CENTURY & the NEW MILLENNIUM:

1) **THERMOREGULATION: a)** Servo-Controlled Radiant Warmer/Incubator both in the delivery room and in premature nurseries, **b)** Kangaroo Mother Care (KMC), **c)** Parent–Infant Interaction.

2) **NUTRITION: a)** "Breast" is best", **b)** Early Gut Priming or Trophic Feeding(Minimal Enteral Nutrition) for the very immature infant, **c)** TPN-Total Parenteral Nutrition (with the microinfusion pumps, now able to deliver increments as small as 0.1 mL/h. This facilitated the accurate administration of i.v. fluids to extremely preterm infants.)

3) **RESPIRATORY SUPPORT: a)** Controlled Oxygen Therapy (with the help of Technology-Pulse Oximetry, Transcutaneous Pa O_2 monitoring, & ABG Analysis), **b)** Controlled Ventilation (Capnography & ABG Analysis), **c)** Efficient & Timely Neonatal Resuscitation in the delivery room (NRP Programme) **d)** Assisted ventilation: CPAP, Mechanical Ventilation-Conventional, High Frequency Oscillatory Ventilation, High Frequency Jet Ventilation, liquid ventilation with perfluorocarbons, **e)** Exogenous Surfactant Therapy.

4) **CARDIOPULMONARY SUPPORT a)** Patent ductus arteriosus management, **b)** Blood pressure support, **c)** Persistent pulmonary hypertension management- 1) inhaled nitric oxide (iNO) and 2) extracorporeal membrane oxygenation (ECMO), **d)** Echocardiography.

5) **NEONATAL INFECTION: a)** Thorough Hand Washing Techniques, **b)** Sterilization and Disinfection of NICU Equipment, **c)** Isolation of Suspected/Proven Infected Neonates, **d)** Newer Antibiotics/Antifungals/Antivirals.

6) **JAUNDICE : a)** Phototherapy **b)** Exchange Transfusion.

7) **NEONATAL SURGERY: Advances** in Neonatal surgery are closely tied to parallel advances in Neonatology; also closely allied to advances in the field of Pediatric anesthesiology.

8) **NEONATAL SCREENING** for **ROP** (Retinopathy Of Prematurity), Hearing Screening and Management along with METABOLIC screening for IEM.

9) **REGIONALIZATION and/or Centralization of Perinatal care with** a multidisciplinary team approach & Transport of Sick Neonates from distant primary care hospitals.

10) **TELENEOMEDICINE, and** Evidence-based medicine, systematic reviews

Although it would be comforting to think that modern Neonatal care evolved seamlessly in a series of logical steps, there were many missteps along the way.

ERRORS IN NEONATOLOGY

Event	Result	Years
I. The "Hands -Off" years		
Lowered thermal environment	increased mortality	1900–1964
Supplemental oxygen	RLF	1941–1954
Initial thirsting and starving	? neurological deficits	1945–1970
Synthetic vitamin K	kernicterus	1945–1961
SMA formula	seizures	1951–?1952
Diaper markings	methemoglobinemia	1886–1995
II. The "Heroic" years		
Bloxsom Air - Lock	? delayed resuscitation	1950–1956
Sulfisoxazole	kernicterus	1953–1956
Chloramphenicol	"gray baby" syndrome	1956–1960
Novobiocin	jaundice	1957–1962
Hexachlorophene	brain lesions	1952–1971
Epsom salts enemas	magnesium intoxication	1964–1965
Feeding gastrostomy	increased mortality	1963–1969
Diaper laundering	"sweating" syndrome	1969
Equipment cleaning	jaundice	1972–1975
III. The "Experienced" years		
Neo - Mul - Soy formula	metabolic alkalosis	1978–1979
Premature infant formulas	lactobezoars	1977–1980
Erythromycin	pyloric stenosis	1976–1999
Propylene glycol	hyperosmolality, seizures	1981–1983
Benzyl alcohol	"gasping" syndrome ????–	1982
Intravenous vitamin E	multiorgan damage	1983–1984
Steroids	? cerebral palsy	1985–2001

WHAT DOES THE FUTURE HOLD?

Courtesy: ALISTAIR G.S. PHILIP, *Department of Pediatrics, Division of Neonatal and Developmental Medicine, Stanford University School of Medicine, Palo Alto, CA 94304*

Simulation techniques: A simulated delivery room in which realistic maternal and infant mannequins can have their vital signs manipulated so that students, residents, nurses, etc. can practice resuscitation and other emergency responses while being videotaped. Such simulation activity allows people to become proficient and respond appropriately, before being subjected to a real, live, situation. There is also simulation for responding to emergencies in an infant who is on ECMO (http://cape.lpch. org). Other centers are likely to adopt these approaches, and in the future, they may evolve into the use of virtual reality techniques.

Multidisciplinary/multicenter studies: To answer questions about clinical medicine by developing research protocols that can be used in a large number of centers to answer those questions in a much shorter time frame than would have been possible several years ago. It seems likely that these initiatives will expand even further in the future and will allow the best practices to be identified and endorsed.

Gene therapy: It seems likely that the difficulties associated with this technique will be overcome in the future. After identifying a single genetic defect as the cause of a problem in a Neonate, it will be possible to replace the defective gene.

Biologic reporters: Light-emitting enzymes, luciferases, can label genes and cells. These internal light sources can be detected externally and become biologic indicators or reporters. This bioluminescent imaging has been used with target and therapeutic genes in living laboratory animals to analyze gene delivery and to monitor gene expression and immune therapies. Extension of these techniques to human newborn infants seems likely.

Artificial placenta: Futuristic idea remains just that, and I doubt that hooking up an infant to an artificial placenta will occur any time soon.

The changing role of pediatricians: Today's pediatric residents are not as well prepared to deal with unusual findings or neonatal emergencies. This has resulted in increasing reliance on neonatologists to provide consultations in well-infant nurseries, with further erosion of the general pediatrician's skills with the neonate.

Rapid identification of infectious disease: In the future, it seems likely that specimens will be screened with PCR to detect a battery of pathogenic organisms, and more judicious use of antibiotics will be needed to prevent the emergence of resistant organisms.

New vaccines: Considerable progress has been made in developing GBS vaccines to individual subtypes. In the future, a polyvalent vaccine should be available as well as vaccine against HIV.

Blood substitutes: Although each transfusion of blood in the neonate is comparatively small, NICUs are among the heaviest users of blood banks. Despite all of the safeguards to keep the blood supply free from contamination, it still seems worthwhile to seek blood substitutes.

Technological advances: It is already possible to gain access to fetal cells and to grow them selectively. This offers therapeutic potential, and such tissue engineering has already occurred. There has been a recent surge of interest in harvesting blood from the placenta to provide autologous blood transfusion in preterm infants, which minimizes demands for donor blood and its attendant risks. Newer imaging techniques have been described in animal or experimental models. These are likely to reach the bedside soon along with skin surface electrodes that can measure glucose, electrolytes, and other biochemical determinations.

Better understanding: There are many areas that still require elucidation and may yield answers with practical applications. Examples are *1)* a better understanding of thrombophilia, which on the maternal side may be implicated in preeclampsia and IUGR and in the neonate may influence thrombotic complications; *2)* a better understanding of organ damage and repair; and *3)* an improved recognition and treatment of genetic disorders. Perhaps most important of all would be a better understanding of how to prevent prematurity.

A short history of Baby Care.

"Oh Doctor, how should I look after my baby?"

BC 2000	"Just carry it next to your skin. Breastfeed it whenever it is hungry."
AD 1660	"Breastfeeding is undignified. Hand it over to a wet-nurse."
AD 1850	"Wet-nurses are low class and have an undesirable influence on the child. Get a good experienced nanny to bottle feed it cow's milk, and wean it on to a cup as soon as possible."
AD 1930	"Cow's milk is unsuitable for babies. It must be bottle fed on a special infant formula."
AD 1950	"Bottle feeding at all hours is bad for the baby. Follow a strict routine, let it sleep in its own room and ignore it when it cries at other times."
AD 2000	"Bottle feeding is unsuitable, a strict time-table is nonsense, babies don't like being alone, and crying is stressful. Just carry it next to your skin. Breastfeed it whenever it is hungry."

(Courtesy: Joan Norton, 2001)

Key Concepts Underlying Ethical Care in the Neonatal Intensive Care Unit

* Respecting parental authority/autonomy
* Applying the best interests of the infant standard of judgment
* Minimizing harm to the newborn
* Developing sound parent–physician relationships
* Empowering and informing parents
* Applying family-centered care principles
* Respecting parents' values and cultural and religious beliefs
* Sharing decision making
* Developing respectful interprofessional (moral) teamwork

Common Malpractice Suits in Neonatology

DELIVERY ROOM MANAGEMENT OR RESUSCITATION
Poor neurologic outcome
Cerebral palsy: neonatologist named as codefendant with obstetrician-perinatologist
Asphyxia: plaintiff alleges some component of injury occurred postnatally

LINE COMPLICATIONS
Vascular accidents related to central venous lines
Loss of fingers or toes associated with central lines
Thrombus and complications from thrombus

DELAY IN DIAGNOSIS OR TREATMENT
Poor blood gases, prolonged hypotension (see also poor neurologic outcome)
Delay in antibiotic administration
Congenital hip dislocation
Congenital heart disease

TRANSPORT TEAM
Medications or care provided by transport team (e.g., excessive heparin given)

FAILURE TO MONITOR ADEQUATELY
Blood glucose
Blood oxygen: either hypoxia (brain damage) or hyperoxia (retinopathy of prematurity)
Seizure

Ethical Responsibilities of Neonatal Physicians

To neonatal patients—"right and good" action in their best interests

To parents—constructive, respectful relationship

To NICU team—leadership, direction with open, questioning culture

To trainees—educational experience

To institution—in accord with mission, maintenance of data, review of practice

To society—trust in profession, technical competence, and moral discretion in resource use

To self—moral conscience

Key Behavioral Skills in NICU:
Know your environment. *Anticipate and plan. Assume* the leadership role. *Communicate* effectively. *Delegate* workload optimally. *Allocate* attention wisely. *Use* all available information. *Use* all available resources as well as your own senses. *Call for help* when needed. *Maintain* professionalism.

Neonatal Resuscitation

1

@ *"Time is of the utmost importance. Delay is damaging to the infant. Act promptly, accurately and gently"*-Virginia Apgar. *Nevertheless, recent NRP Changes instruct us "Do not delay the resuscitative efforts to obtain an Apgar Score". !*

1. **Anticipation**
2. **Adequate Preparation**
3. **Timely Recognition**
4. **Quick and correct action**
are critical for the success of resuscitation

Bag & Mask is the most important of the Neonatal Resuscitation Equipment.

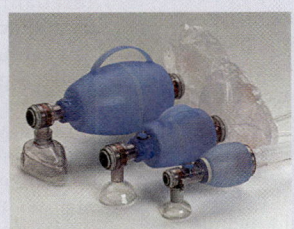

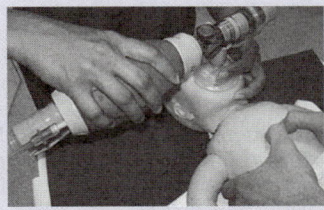

Bag-and-mask ventilation.
Caveat: The middle finger should be placed on the jaw without putting pressure on the floor of the mouth.

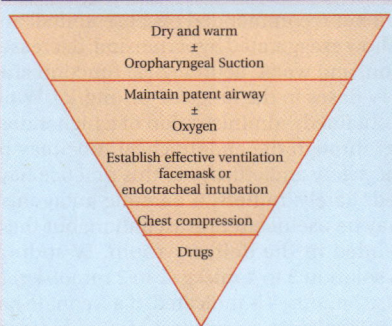

| Dry and warm ± Oropharyngeal Suction |
| Maintain patent airway ± Oxygen |
| Establish effective ventilation facemask or endotracheal intubation |
| Chest compression |
| Drugs |

The *"inverted triangle"* shows how commonly certain interventions are needed.

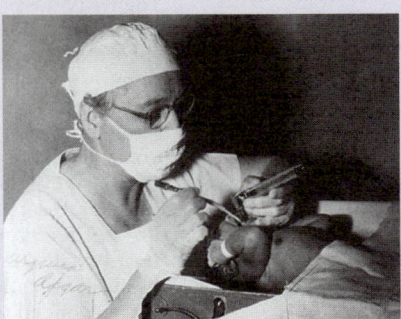

Virginia Apgar (1909-1974)
intubating an asphyxiated Neonate.

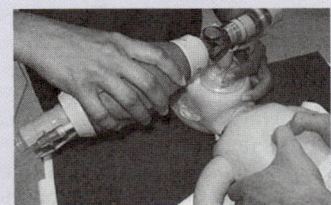

Chest compressions (compression phase).
Caveat: Apply sufficient pressure in order to reduce the anteroposterior thoracic diameter by a third.

REVIEW OF CLINICAL PROBLEMS

1. Mention the Precise indications for positive pressure ventilation (PPV), chest compressions and endotracheal intubation during Neonatal resuscitation.
Ans: Refer to Table 2 of the Chapter.

2. Mention the major changes in Resuscitation Guidelines for Newborn Resuscitation from 2005 to 2010.
Ans: Refer to Table AHA/AAP Neonatal Resuscitation Guidelines 2010.

3. What are the factors responsible for the poor response to / failure of Neonatal resuscitation ?
Ans: Refer to No. 6 of "Bird`s eye view/overview/Synopsis.

4. Mention the size of the endotracheal tube and the depth of insertion for a 2 kg Neonate, when ET intubation is indicated during Neonatal resuscitation.
Ans: Refer to the Table given in the Evaluation -Decision making -Action Plan/Algorithm for Neonatal resuscitation.

5. When do you consider to stop/abandon the resuscitation ? *Ans:* Refer to Table AHA/AAP Neonatal Resuscitation Guidelines 2010.

LEARNING OBJECTIVES

After completing this article, readers will be able to:

1. Recognize normal and abnormal cardio-pulmonary transition of the Newborn baby.

2. Provide resuscitation and transitional needs required by healthy and sick Newborns. Understand to implement the recent NRP Guidelines (2010).

3. Anticipate, diagnose, and treat common factors responsible for poor response to resuscitation.

4. Ensure availability of adequate staffing and equipment prepared when anticipated or unexpected resuscitation needs arise.

5. Collaborate with the family with all decision making, especially with *withholding* or *discontinuing* resuscitative efforts.

*** Pearl/Peril/Pitfall:** The goals of resuscitation are to assist with the initiation and maintenance of adequate ventilation and oxygenation, adequate cardiac output and tissue perfusion, and normal core temperature and serum glucose.*

BIRD'S EYE VIEW/OVERVIEW/SYNOPSIS

1. *Do anticipate* the delivery of a depressed baby and the need for resuscitation on the basis of the antepartum and intrapartum histories ; Keep these factors well in mind, as they will alert you about the potential problems. It is estimated that about 10% of neonates require some assistance at birth for normal transition.

   CONDITIONS COMMONLY ASSOCIATED WITH ANTICIPATED MODERATE-RISK AND HIGH-RISK DELIVERIES

   A. Prematurity (<37 WEEKS) **B.** Cesarean section (except for repeat elective c/s). **C.** Pregnancy induced hypertension. **D.** Multiple gestation **E.** Intrauterine growth restriction (IUGR). **F.** Oligo/poly hydramnios. **G.** Significant vaginal bleeding. **H.** Post-term gestation **I.** Meconium staining **J.** Abnormal fetal heart monitoring pattern **K.** Administration of narcotics within 4 hours of delivery **L.** Abnormal presentation **M.** Maternal diabetes **N.** In-utero drug /alcohol abuse **O.** Rh sensitization **P.** Prolonged labor /rupture of membranes (ROM) >24 hr or Maternal fever/chorioamnionitis

2. *Adequate preparation for any delivery* should include *a radiant warmer, heated, and ready for use *all resuscitation equipment immediately available and in working order *at least one person skilled in a Neonatal Resuscitation in the delivery room and 1 or 2 other persons available to assist with the resuscitation of a depressed infant. *In a multiple gestation, a full complement of equipment and staff must be available for each infant.*

3. *Do remember the steps in resuscitating Newborn infants*, which follow the well-known ABCs of resuscitation. The goals of Neonatal Resuscitation are to prevent morbidity and mortality associated with hypoxic-ischemic tissue (Brain, Heart, Kidney) injury and to reestablish adequate spontaneous respiration and cardiac output.

   A- Establish an open airway **B**-Initiate breathing **C**-Maintain circulation

   The components of the Neonatal resuscitation procedure related to the ABCs of resuscitation are shown here:

   A- Establish an open airway : * Position the infant * Suction the mouth, nose, and in some instances the trachea; it is recommended that suctioning immediately following birth (including suctioning with a bulb syringe) should be reserved for babies who have obvious obstruction to spontaneous breathing or who require positive-pressure ventilation *If necessary, insert an ET tube to ensure an open airway. **B- Initiate breathing** : *Use tactile stimulation to initiate respirations *Use IPPV when necessary, (If the infant remains apneic or gasping, or if the heart rate remains 100 per minute after administering the initial steps, start PPV) using either - Bag and mask or - Bag and ET tube. **Term babies** (≥ 37 **weeks)** • Start with room air (21%) • No improvement in heart rate or oxygenation as assessed by pulse oximetry- use higher concentration by graded increase up to 100% to attain target saturations • Use blender for graded increased in delivered oxygen concentrations. **Preterm** (<32weeks) • Initiate resuscitation using O_2 concentration between 30-90% • Titrate O2 concentration to attain SPO2 values recommended at different time points • Uses blended air oxygen mixture judiciously guided by pulse oximetry, If the baby is bradycardic (HR 60 per minute) after 90 seconds of resuscitation with a lower concentration of oxygen, oxygen concentration should be increased to 100% until recovery of a normal heart rate. It is recommended that the goal in babies being resuscitated at birth, whether born at term or preterm, should be an oxygen saturation value in the interquartile range of preductal saturations measured in healthy term babies following vaginal birth at sea level. These targets may be achieved by initiating resuscitation with air or a blended oxygen and titrating the oxygen concentration to achieve an SpO_2 in the target range as described in the *Evaluation-Decision-Action-Plan/Algorithm* using pulse oximetry. **C- Maintain circulation**: *Stimulate and maintain the circulation of blood with - Chest compressions - Medications. Drugs are rarely indicated in resuscitation of the newly born infant. Bradycardia in the newborn infant is usually the result of inadequate lung inflation or profound hypoxemia, and establishing adequate ventilation is the most important step toward correcting it. However, if the heart rate remains 60 per minute despite adequate ventilation (usually with endotracheal intubation) with 100% oxygen and chest compressions, administration of Adrenaline or volume expansion using an isotonic crystalloid solution or blood, or both, may be indicated. When resuscitating premature infants, care should be taken to avoid giving volume expanders rapidly, because rapid infusions of large volumes have been associated with intraventricular hemorrhage. *If the heart rate remains <60 bpm despite 30 seconds of positive - pressure ventilation with 100 % oxygen and chest compressions, medications should be given.* IV Adrenaline 1:10, 000 solution 0.1 to 0.3 ml/kg (0.01 to 0.03 mg/kg) every 3 to 5 minutes is the drug of choice. Higher IV doses are not recommended because animal and pediatric studies show exaggerated hypertension, decreased myocardial function, and worse neurological function after administration of IV doses in the range of 0.1 mg/kg. While IV access is being obtained, administration of a higher dose (0.05 to 0.1 mg/kg) through the endotracheal tube may be considered, but the safety and efficacy of this practice have not been evaluated. Rarely, buffers, a narcotic antagonist, or vasopressors may be useful after resuscitation, but these are not recommended in the delivery room. IV sodium bicarbonate 4.2 % solution 2 to 4 ml/kg (1 to 2 mmol/kg) to be given over atleast 2 minutes is indicated, if a Neonate has not responded to epinephrine, or external cardiac massage despite adequate IPPV and has persisting bradycardia. Naloxone IV/IM/SC/IT 100 microgram/kg is recommended for Newborns with respiratory depression whose mothers received narcotics within 4 to 6 hours of delivery. Recent NRP guidelines state, that Naloxone is not indicated in delivery room, giving more emphasis on establishing ventilation, rather than depending on the drugs without established safety.

4. *The Evaluation-Decision-Action-Plan/Algorithm* describes the essential aspects of Neonatal resuscitation of a depressed baby.First,assess whether the infant is **breathing spontaneously.** Next assess whether the **heart rate is >100 bpm.** Finally, evaluate the infant's oxygenation status with pulse oximetry. If any of these three features is abnormal, take immediate steps to correct the deficiency, & reevaluate every 15-30 seconds until all features are present & stable. *Always call for the help of an advanced resuscitator, if the baby needs E.T intubation.*

5. **Monitor the response to resuscitation : A).** Resuscitation does not end with the baby achieving, a good heart rate and spontaneous breathing. **B).** Observations should continue and a decision made as to whether it is safe for the baby to remain with the mother or whether he/she should be admitted to the nursery for further observation in SCBU/ NICU. **C).** Any baby who has required resuscitation should have early glucose screening & ABG analysis until stable. Very low-birth-weight (1500 g) preterm babies are likely to become hypothermic despite the use of traditional techniques for decreasing heat loss. For this reason additional warming techniques are recommended (e.g., prewarming the delivery room to 26°C, covering the baby in plastic wrapping (food or medical grade, heat-resistant plastic), placing the baby on an exothermic mattress, and placing the baby under radiant heat. The infant's temperature must be monitored closely because of the slight, but described risk of hyperthermia when these techniques are used in combination.

6. *Beware of the factors responsible for the poor response to / failure of resuscitation* : Inadequate mask ventilation due to poor technique/lack of O_2: Tracheal tube in oesophagus or down a bronchus or blocked with secretions or meconium : Birth asphyxia / trauma : Lung disorders ; lung immaturity /respiratory distress syndrome; pneumothorax ; diaphragmatic hernia ; lung hypoplasia ; pleural effusion ; Shock from blood loss : Upper airways obstruction-choanal atresia: Congenital heart disease (duct dependent malformation / PPHN) *(Refer to "Chapter 3" for a detailed discussion of resuscitation problems in difficult/special situations).*

7. Successful resuscitation of a newborn infant involves not only interrupting the cycle of hypoxia and acidemia and bringing the infant back toward the physiologic norm but also avoiding iatrogenic damage. *(Refer to important "rules" of resuscitation -Table 2)*

8. Endotracheal intubation may be indicated at several points during neonatal resuscitation: *Initial endotracheal suctioning of nonvigorous meconium-stained newborns *If bag-mask ventilation is ineffective or prolonged * When chest compressions are performed *For special resuscitation circumstances, such as congenital diaphragmatic hernia or extremely low birth weight. After endotracheal intubation and administration of intermittent positive pressure, a prompt increase in heart rate is the best indicator that the tube is in the tracheobronchial tree and providing effective ventilation. Exhaled CO_2 detection is effective for confirmation of endotracheal tube placement in infants, including very low birth-weight infants. A positive test result (detection of exhaled CO2) in patients with adequate cardiac output confirms placement of the endotracheal tube within the trachea, whereas a negative test result (i.e., no CO2 detected) strongly suggests esophageal intubation. However, it should be noted that poor or absent pulmonary blood flow may give false negative results (i.e., no CO2 detected despite tube placement in the trachea). A false-negative result may thus lead to unnecessary extubation and reintubation of critically ill infants with poor cardiac output.

9. The current NRP guidelines state that "if there is no heart rate after 10 minutes of complete and adequate resuscitation efforts, and there is no evidence of other causes of newborn compromise, discontinuation of resuscitation efforts may be appropriate. Current data indicate that, after 10 minutes of asystole, newborns are very unlikely to survive, or the rare survivor is likely to survive with severe disability."

10. *Ensure good record keeping :* A) Condition at birth, color / tone / respiration B) Time to first gasp, time to regular respiration, cry C) Heart rate at the start and at intervals : time when heart rate rose above 100 bpm D) Apgar scores at 1 & 5 minute intervals to supplement the above (but not to replace these observations) E) Time commencing bag and mask ventilation, duration F) Time at tracheal intubation, duration of intubation G) Umbilical cord pH (specify whether arterial or venous) H) Drugs given, dose, route, and time I) Names and designations of personnel ; time of their arrival J) Reasons for any delay K) Information given to the parents. *Ensure* POSTRESUSCITATION CARE of those babies who require resuscitation by providing close monitoring and anticipatory care.

Major Changes in International Liaison Committee on Resuscitation Guidelines for Newborn Resuscitation from 2005 to 2010

The summary of key changes is based on the 2010 ILCOR and American Heart Association guidelines .

* Progression to the next step following an initial evaluation is now defined by simultaneous evaluation of HR and respirations.

* Pulse oximetry should be used for evaluation of oxygenation because color assessment is unreliable. Target saturation (preductal): Target SpO_2 ranges provided as a part of algorithm (1min- 60-65% 2 min- 65-70% 3min- 70-75% 4min- 75-80% 5min- 80-85% 10min- 85-95% (same for both term and preterm). Color has been removed from the signs of assessment. Precordial auscultation better than umbilical cord palpation for detection of heart rate. Increase in HR most sensitive indicator of resuscitation efficacy.

* **Initial oxygen concentration for resuscitation in case of PPV: Term babies ($\geq$ 37 weeks)** • Start with room air (21%) • No improvement in heart rate or oxygenation as assessed by pulse oximetry- use higher concentration by graded increase up to 100% to attain target saturations • Use blender for graded increased in delivered oxygen concentrations. **Preterm(<32weeks)** • Initiate resuscitation using O2 concentration between 30-90% • Titrate O2 concentration to attain SPO2 values recommended at different time points • Uses blended air oxygen mixture judiciously guided by pulse oximetry

* No routine oropharyngeal and nasopharyngeal suction required. Available evidence does not support or refute routine endotracheal suctioning of infants born through MSAF, even when depressed. Until further information is available, endotracheal suctioning of nonvigorous babies should be performed.

* The chest compression-ventilation ratio remains at 3:1. A higher ratio might be considered if an arrest is of cardiac etiology, where ratio of 15:2 may be considered. Two thumb technique better than two finger technique • The compression is applied at the lower one third of sternum • The depth of compression should be one-third of the antero-posterior diameter of the chest.

* Naloxone is not recommended as part of initial resuscitation in babies with respiratory depression. Focus needs to be on effective ventilation. Naloxone is not indicated in delivery room.

* Therapeutic hypothermia should be considered within 6 h for infants born at term or late preterm gestation with evolving moderate-severe hypoxic ischemic encephalopathy (with protocol and follow-up through a regional perinatal system).

* It is appropriate to consider discontinuing resuscitative efforts after there has been no detectable heart rate for 10 min.

* Cord clamping should be delayed for at least 1 min in babies not requiring resuscitation. There is insufficient evidence to recommend a time for clamping in babies who require resuscitation.

* Simulation should be used as a teaching methodology in resuscitation education, but the most effective methods of teaching and evaluation remain to be defined.

* It is reasonable to recommend the use of briefings and debriefings during learning activities both in simulation and in clinical activities.

Newborn resuscitation Current challenges

• Optimal heart rate response not established
• Ratio ventilation : chest compression not established
• Sustained inflation?
• Optimal PEEP not established
• Optimal pCO_2 not established
• Optimal adrenaline dose not established
• Optimal FiO_2 and other procedures for ELGANS not established
• Better biochemical asphyxia indicators needed
• Time for a revised Apgar Score?

* *Pearl/Peril/Pitfall: It is important that all the resuscitation equipment is kept clean and in good working order. After a resuscitation all the equipment must be cleaned to prevent the spread of infection. The masks and mucus extractors must be washed with water and soap or detergent and rinsed. The self-inflating bags, e.g. Laerdal, Ambu and Penlon must be sterilized.*

The Evaluation-Decision-Action-Plan /Algorithm for managing *Neonatal Resuscitation*

SUBJECTIVE FINDINGS

* *Anticipate* the need for resuscitation of a depressed baby in a high-risk delivery *Adequately prepare* the necessary equipment (refer to Table No.1) upon arrival in the delivery room and *ensure* that an advanced resuscitator/a senior consultant is available in case of difficult situations.*Check* that the oxygen source is adequate & ensure the supplies of essential medications *Observe* universal sterile precautions by wearing caps, glasses, gloves & gowns. *Do not delay assessing the baby's condition until the end of the first minute!*

OBJECTIVE FINDINGS

Initially-rapidly *Assess* 3 characteristics: *Term gestation? * Crying or breathing? *Good muscle tone?

Midway-after 60 seconds ("the Golden Minute")- *Assess* the infant's breathing- (apnea, gasping, or labored or unlabored breathing) * *Assess* the baby's heart rate by intermittently auscultating the precordial pulse. - whether the heart beat is >100bpm /<100bpm/ <60bpm or absent. *Assessment of skin color is a very poor indicator of oxyhemoglobin saturation during the immediate neonatal period.*

Once positive pressure ventilation or supplementary oxygen administration is begun-assessment should consist of simultaneous evaluation of 3 vital characteristics: heart rate, respirations, and the state of oxygenation, the latter optimally determined by a pulse oximeter.

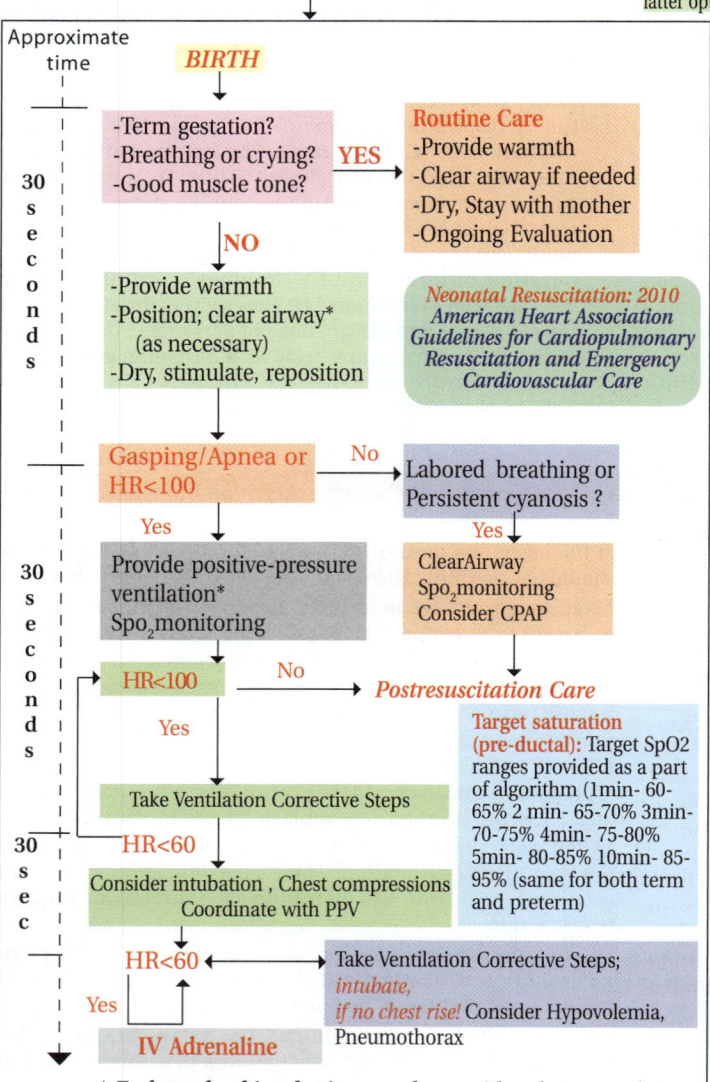

Advanced Neonatal Life Support

Intubate and ventilate

HR>60 or increasing | HR<60 or decreasing

Pulse check

Continue ventilation (HR>60)

HR<60:
-Continue ventilation
-Start chest compressions
-Rate 90 per minute with 30 breaths per minute (ratio-3ECM:1VENT)

HR increases | Pulseless or heart rate decreasing

Consider extubation when heart rate >100, good respiratory effort, and >Target Pulse oximetry readings

Consider tracheal **Adrenaline** (50-100 mcg/kg i.e., 0.5-0.1ml/kg 1 in 10,000)

Prefer IV or IO **Adrenaline** 10-30 mcg/kg (0.1 to 0.3 ml/kg *1 in 10,000)*

CPR for 3 min

Consider Volume expansion NS/O-negative blood cross-matched with the mother 10ml/kg over 5-10 minutes; the solution may be infused more cautiously in extremely preterm infants.

Adrenaline 10-30 mcg/kg IV or IO (0.1 to 0.3 ml/kg *1 in 10,000)*

Do not give high doses of i.e., 100mcg/kg intravenous Adrenaline! (Causes exaggerated hypertension, decreased myocardial function, and worse neurological function)

Consider other diagnoses

Consider volume expansion 10ml/kg

Instructions To Follow:
1. All drugs should be followed by a 0.5-1.0 mL flush of 0.9% saline.
2. If there is likely to be a delay in establishing IV access, then epinephrine (adrenaline) should be given via the ETT. This should be given rapidly down a catheter placed to lie just beyond the end of the ETT and followed by a 0.5-1.0mL normal saline flush and five rapid inflations. This route should only be used whilst IV access is being established. It must not be used in preference to IV access.
3. Consider sodium bicarbonate 1-2 mmol/kg in cases of prolonged arrest after adequate ventilation is established.} The dose of sodium bicarbonate is not intended to correct the metabolic acidosis but to increase the pH within the coronary arteries and hopefully increase the action of the subsequent epinephrine (adrenaline). IV sodium bicarbonate 1-2 mmol/kg (2-4 ml/kg 4.2% solution) .Use of sodium bicarbonate in the delivery room has been associated with an increased incidence of intraventricular hemorrhage in very low birth weight infants. However, studies show that 0.9% saline provides better cardiac and blood pressure support to correct both the metabolic acidosis itself and the underlying cause of the acidosis.
4. During the process of prolonged resuscitation, hypoglycemia (i.e. whole BG <45mg/dL) should be sought and treated, if present, with 10% glucose 5 mL/kg IV. Administration of naloxone is not recommended as part of initial resuscitative efforts in the delivery room for newborns with respiratory depression.
5. All drugs should be checked before giving and a record of drug administration kept.

ID = Internal Diameter, Adapted from circulation from 1999 : 1927-38, American Heart Association, Inc

Guidelines for tracheal tube size and depth of insertion

Tube Insertion (mm ID)	Depth of from Upper Lip (cm)	Weight (g)	Gestation (wk) Size
2.5	6.5-7	< 1,000	<28
3	7-8	1,000-2,000	28-34
3/3.5	8-9	2,000-3,000	34- 38
3.5/4.0	≥9	>3,000	> 38

* Pearl/Peril/Pitfall: Delaying delivery for prolonged suctioning and/ or suctioning vigorously enough to cause vagally-mediated bradycardia is not indicated whether or not meconium is present.

TABLE 1 — Equipment for neonatal resuscitation

Thermoregulation	Radiant heat source with platform, mattress covered with warm sterile blankets, servo-control heating, temperature probe
Airway management	Suction : Bulb suction, mechanical suction with sterile catheters (6F, 8F, 10F), meconium aspirator
	Ventilation : Manual infant resuscitation bag connected to manometer or with a pressure-release valve capable of delivering 100% oxygen, appropriate masks for term and preterm infants, oral airways, stethoscope , CO2 detector (e.g.. Pedicap®)
	Intubation : Neonatal laryngoscope with No. 0 and No. 1 blades ; endotracheal tubes (2.5, 3.0, 3.5 mm internal diameter with stylet) : extra bulbs and batteries for laryngoscope ; scissors, adhesive tape, gloves
Gastric decompression	Nasogastric tube:8F with 20-mL syringe
Administration of drugs and volume replacement	Sterile umbilical catheterization tray, umbilical catheters (3.5F and 5F), volume expanders (Ringer's lactate, 5% albumin or normal saline), drug box (*Epinephrine 1:10,000 ; Naloxone hydrochloride 0.4 mg./ ml, Sodium bicarbonate 4.2% (5mEq / 10 mL) ; 10% dextrose.* with appropriate neonatal vials and dilutions, sterile syringes, needles, and alcohol sponges
Transport	Warmed transport isolette with oxygen source
Resuscitation within theTimeframe	Stop Clock

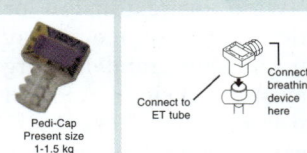

Pedi-Cap
Present size
1-1.5 kg

Connect to
ET tube

Connect
breathing
device
here

TABLE 2 — Indications for CPR & ET Intubation

Indications for positive - pressure ventilation

* Apnea or gasping respirations unresponsive to gentle tactile stimulation
* Bradycardia (heart rate <100 beats/min) even when breathing
* Persistent central cyanosis despite 100% free-flow oxygen

Indications for chest compressions

* Heart rate <60 beats/min despite 30 seconds of positive pressure ventilation
* Absence of known congenital heart block

Indications for Endotracheal intubation and laryngeal mask airway

Endotracheal intubation

* Suctioning meconium from trachea if meconium - stained skin or amniotic fluid *in a nonvigorous depressed baby only* and
* Absent/depressed respiratory efforts, hypotonia, or heart rate <100 beats/min
* Ineffective or prolonged (several minutes) bag-mask ventilation
* When chest compressions are performed (Improved coordination of positive pressure ventilation and chest compressions)
* Epinephrine administration
* *Special situations:* extreme prematurity, surfactant administration, congenital diaphragmatic hernia, apnea unresponsive to bag mask ventilation, severe hydrops fetalis, hyaline membrane disease, pulmonary hypoplasia

Laryngeal mask airway: A laryngeal mask should be considered during resuscitation if facemask ventilation is unsuccessful and tracheal intubation is unsuccessful or not feasible. Shown to be effective for ventilating newborns weighing more than 2000 g or delivered ≥34 weeks gestation. There are limited data on the use of these devices in small preterm infants, ie, <2000 g or <34 weeks .)

TABLE 3 — Important Rules of Resuscitation

1. *Do not panic if an endotracheal tube cannot be placed immediately.* Concentrate on bag-and-mask ventilation and *call for help.* Do not assume that medication is a substitute for ventilation.

2. *Do not perform excessive suctioning of clear fluid from the infant's nasopharynx.* Fluid is normally absorbed into the lungs.

3. *Do not use excessive oxygen concentrations to resuscitate the premature infant unless the infant clearly requires it.* The minimal concentration of oxygen needed should always be used. Babies > 32 weeks gestation should be initiated with FiO2 (inspiratory fraction of oxygen) of 21% and babies <32 weeks gestation with FiO2 of 21-30% . Further adjustments should be carried out according to the response in heart rate and oxygen saturation.

4. *Do not use too much ventilatory pressure to expand the infant's lungs.* The required initial pressure for expanding the lung may be briefly higher right after birth than it is within just 15 to 30 minutes after birth. *Use good clinical judgment.* Watch the infant's chest and listen to breath sounds. Try reducing ventilation with hand ventilation to ensure that the lowest pressure necessary is being used. Excessive pressure on lungs that are normalizing may decrease venous return to the heart and decrease cardiac output and cause injury to lung tissue.

5. *Avoid hypocapnia.* There is evidence that even brief overdistention of the lung may raise the risk of bronchopulmonary dysplasia (BPD)

6. *Do not give volume replacement or sodium bicarbonate automatically.* Each of these agents has been associated with production of intracranial hemorrhage in animal models.

7. *Do not focus or rely too heavily on cardiac resuscitation,* because, the most likely problem by far in Neonatal resuscitation is the need for ventilatory support.

8. *Maintain normoxia in the term or post-term infant with meconium aspiration or asphyxia,* because such an infant may have reactive pulmonary blood vessels, and pulmonary vasoconstriction may develop if hypoxia persists.

9. *If adequate ventilation is not achievable, consider* *Displaced tube (often in esophagus or right main bronchus) *Obstructed tube (especially meconium) *Pneumothorax or other patient problems - lung immaturity / respiratory distress syndrome, diaphragmatic hernia, pleural effusion - shock from blood loss - upper airway obstruction e.g. choanal atresia * Equipment failure, e.g. exhausted gas supply.

---

* *Pearl/Peril/Pitfall:* Obtaining vascular access should take priority over drawing up and administering multiple doses of epinephrine via the endotracheal tube as it is unlikely that subsequent doses will have any effect if there was no response to the initial dose.

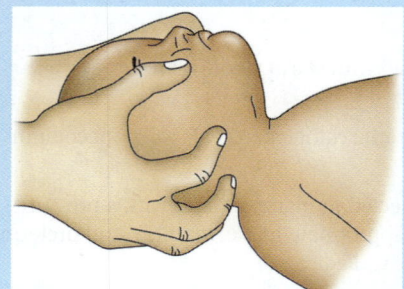

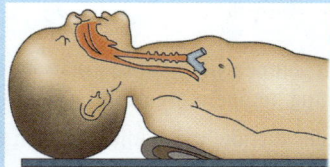

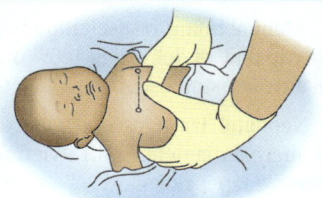

Correct position of the head for ventilation-Position the infant supine or on his or her side with the neck either in a neutral position or slightly extended. Avoid overextension or flexion which may produce airway obstruction. A slight Trendelenburg position may also be helpful. A folded towel (approximately 2.5 cm thick) placed under the infant's shoulders may be useful if the infant has a large occiput.

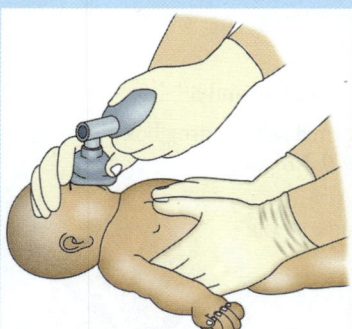

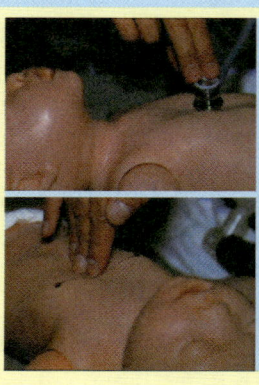

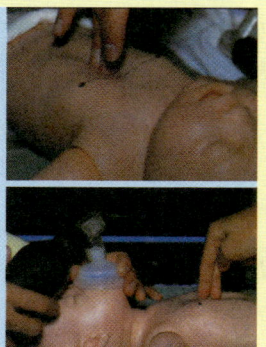

Chest Compressions- Location: Pressure should be applied to the lower third of the sternum , just below an imaginary line drawn between the nipples. Take care not to apply pressure to the xiphoid. *Thumb Method:* Encircle the torso with both hands and compress the sternum with both thumbs side-by-side while the fingers support the back. In very small neonates the thumbs may have to be superimposed. Use just the tips of the thumbs to compress to avoid squeezing the whole chest wall and fracturing ribs. *Two-finger Method:* This method is used if the resuscitator's hands are too small to encircle the chest properly or if access to the umbilicus is necessary for medications. The middle and ring fingers of one hand are held perpendicular to the chest and the tips apply pressure to the sternum while the other hand is used to support the back from below. *Because the 2 thumb–encircling hands technique may generate higher peak systolic and coronary perfusion pressure than the 2-finger technique, the 2 thumb–encircling hands technique is recommended for performing chest compressions in newly born infants. Pressure*: Use just enough pressure to a depth of approximately one third of the anterior-posterior diameter of the chest , then release the pressure to allow the heart to fill. One compression consists of the downward stroke plus the release. *Rate*: There should be a 3:1 ratio of compressions to ventilations with 90 compressions and 30 breaths to achieve approximately 120 events per minute to maximize ventilation at an achievable rate. Thus each event will be allotted approximately 1/2 second, with exhalation occurring during the first compression after each ventilation

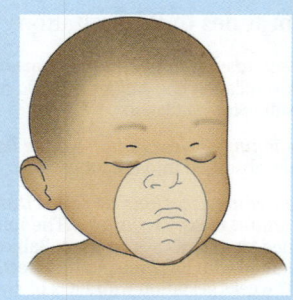

Cautions: Do not remove the tips of your fingers from the chest. You may waste time relocating the compression site or end up compressing the wrong area, producing broken ribs with the possibility of pneumothorax or a lacerated liver. To make sure the circulation produced by the chest compressions is adequate, the rate and the depth of the compressions must be consistent. Respirations, heart rate, and oxygenation should be reassessed periodically, and coordinated chest compressions and ventilations should continue until the spontaneous heart rate is 60 per minute.

Fitting the face mask-Face Masks: Every delivery room should have a variety of sizes: preterm, term and large newborn. (i.e, sizes 0, 1 and 2). Anatomically shaped face masks with cushioned rims are recommended because of better fit and tighter seal. A properly fitting mask should cover the chin, mouth and nose and not put pressure on the infant's eyes.

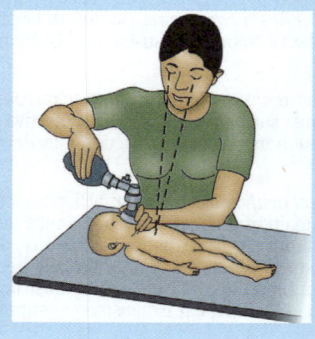

Ventilation with bag and mask-Adequate ventilation is assessed by observing chest wall motion and hearing breath sounds bilaterally. If chest expansion is inadequate, the following steps should be followed in sequence: *reapply the face mask to rule out a poor seal *reposition the head - extend the head a bit further - reposition the shoulder towel *check for secretions - suction if necessary *try ventilating with the infant's mouth slightly open - perhaps with an oral airway *increase pressure to 20-40 cm H2O *abandon bag and mask - intubate trachea

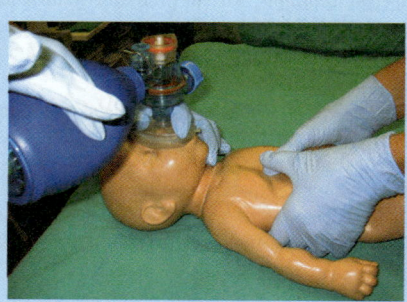

* *Pearl/Peril/Pitfall : No evidence is available to support a recommendation for using a specific oxygen concentration between 21% and 100% at present. If an oxygen concentration <100% is used to initiate resuscitation, crossover to 100% oxygen is recommended if there is no improvement in 90 seconds.*

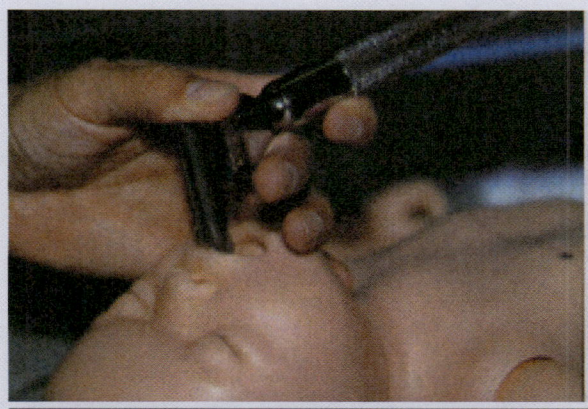

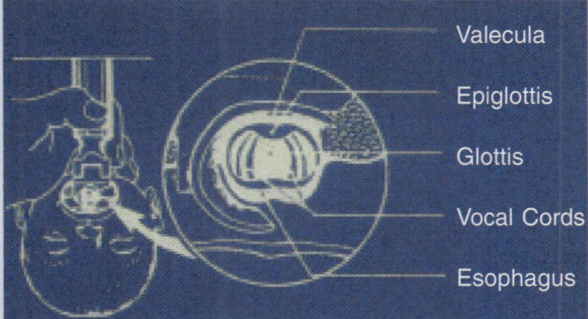

Valecula

Epiglottis

Glottis

Vocal Cords

Esophagus

Correct   Incorrect

Epiglottis

Base of the tongue

Vocal Cords

Arytenoids

Vestibular fold

Larynx

Esophagus

View of the glottic area via direct laryngoscopy

@ *Exhaled CO2 detection is effective for confirmation of endotracheal tube placement in infants, including very low birth weight infants . A positive test result (detection of exhaled CO2) in patients with adequate cardiac output confirms placement of the endotracheal tube within the trachea, whereas a negative test result (i.e., no CO2 detected) strongly suggests esophageal intubation .Poor or absent pulmonary blood flow may give false-negative results (i.e., no CO2 detected despite tube placement in the trachea), but endotracheal tube placement is correctly identified in nearly all patients who are not in cardiac arrest. A false-negative result may also lead to unnecessary extubation in critically ill infants with poor cardiac output.*

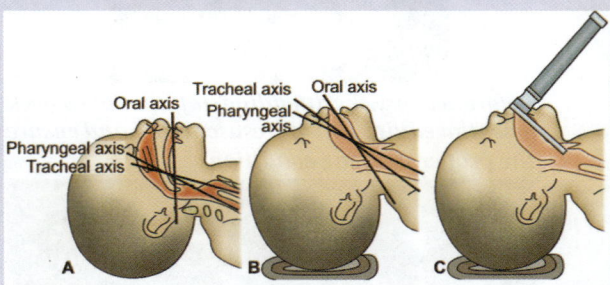

Oral axis Tracheal axis Oral axis

Pharyngeal axis Pharyngeal axis

Pharyngeal axis Tracheal axis

A) Illustration of the axes (oral pharyngeal and tracheal); **B)** alignment of these axes with correct positioning; **C)** viewing the glottic fold with a straight blade

Skills Necessary for Successful Intubation

Cognitive Skills : Know the indications for intubation of the newborn, Know how to recognize these indications when present, Know what equipment (e.g., size of endotracheal tube, laryngoscope blade) to use to accomplish intubation, Know the indications of a successful intubation.

Technical Skills: Know how to assemble the laryngoscope, Know how to hold the laryngoscope, Know how to use the equipment to expose the airway to view, Know how to insert the endotracheal tube into the airway, Know how to assess for proper placement of the endotracheal tube in the airway, Know how to secure the endotracheal tube in the airway.

Behavioral Skills: Communicate effectively with team members regarding the need for intubation, specific pieces of equipment, and the like , Distribute the workload so that specific tasks are assigned to the team members most likely to carry them out successfully, Delegate responsibility and supervise appropriately, Call for help when necessary.

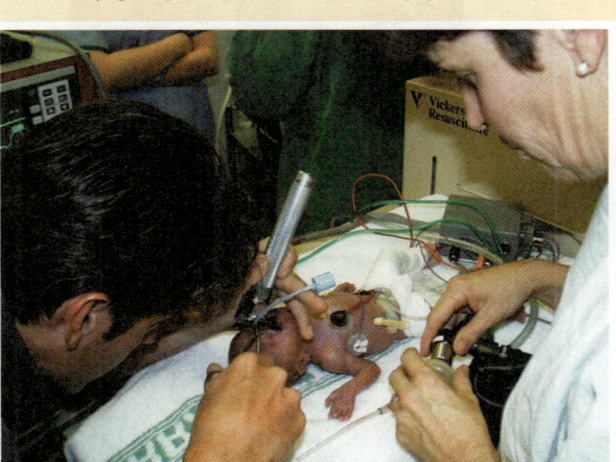

ENDOTRACHEAL TUBE PLACEMENT

Endotracheal intubation may be indicated at several points during neonatal resuscitation:

* When tracheal suctioning for meconium is required
* If bag-mask ventilation is ineffective or prolonged
* When chest compressions are performed
* When endotracheal administration of medications is desired
* For special resuscitation circumstances, such as congenital diaphragmatic hernia or extremely low birth weight (1000 g)

The timing of endotracheal intubation may also depend on the skill and experience of the available providers.

Refer to Section 3-Essential Neonatal Procedures for the details of ET Intubation.

DOCUMENTING RESUSCITATION

Records : All health care institutions should keep records/logbooks with basic information on every birth. This basic information should include some important details about the condition of the newborn at birth and about resuscitation if this is done. The information should also be recorded in home-based records. Documenting conditions and procedures at birth is important for several reasons. There are, for instance, medicolegal implications. If any problems arise later thorough documentation can help in understanding the circumstances at the birth. Case reviews also provide a basis for further education and the improvement of practice. Details of resuscitation to be recorded are: - identification of the newborn; - condition at birth; - procedures necessary to initiate breathing; time from birth to initiation of spontaneous breathing; - clinical observations during and after resuscitation; - outcome of resuscitation; - in case of failed resuscitation, possible reasons for failure; - names of health care providers involved. An example of a record of newborn resuscitation is shown in Table given below.. This is the record of the resuscitation only and does not replace the record of delivery/birth.

Neonatal resuscitation record

Newborn
Name:...

Date of birth: .... Time of birth:...............................

Condition at birth:..

Immediate cry/breathing...

Delayed cry/breath-
ing...

Resuscitation not attempted..

Explain why not:...
Resuscitation initiated.

* Describe Procedures:...

* When did spontaneous breathing begin?

* For how long (minutes) was ventilation needed?

* How was the condition (breathing, body temperature, suckling) of the newborn 30-60 min after resuscitation?

* If no spontaneous breathing, when did ventilation stop?

How would you describe the outcome?

 a) Liveborn infant, resuscitation successful.

 b) Liveborn infant, resuscitation not successful, the newborn died.

 c) Stillborn, resuscitation not successful.

 d) Stillborn, resuscitation not attempted.

The **New guidelines** from the International Liaison Committee on Resuscitation and American Heart Association/American Academy of Pediatrics for newborn resuscitation underline that efficient ventilation is the key to a successful resuscitation of the newly born infant. Compared with the former guidelines published in 1999, the major changes are (i) less emphasis on using supplemental oxygen when initiating resuscitation, (ii) no need for routine intrapartum oropharyngeal and nasopharyngeal suctioning for vigorous infants born to mothers with meconium staining of amniotic fluid, (iii) occlusive wrapping of very low birth weight infants <28 weeks to reduce heat loss is recommended, (iv) preference for the intravenous versus endotracheal route for adrenaline and (v) more emphasis on parental autonomy at the threshold of viability.

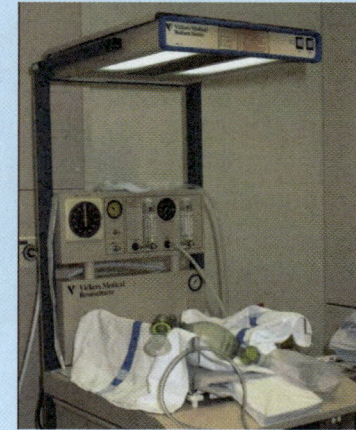

Before delivery, the attending staff should recheck essential equipment for resuscitation and ensure the proper working condition.

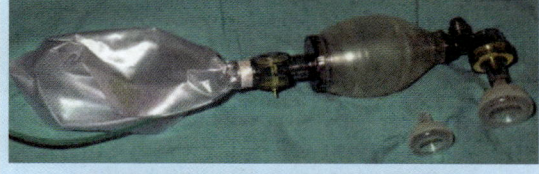

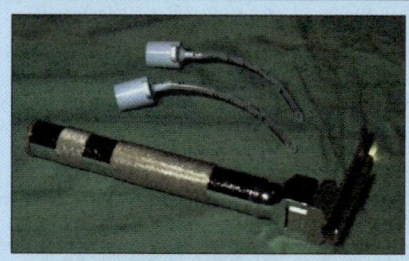

Withholding Resuscitation: It is possible to identify conditions associated with high mortality and poor outcome in which withholding resuscitative efforts may be considered reasonable, particularly when there has been the opportunity for parental agreement A consistent and coordinated approach to individual cases by the obstetric and neonatal teams and the parents is an important goal. Noninitiation of resuscitation and discontinuation of life-sustaining treatment during or after resuscitation are ethically equivalent, and clinicians should not hesitate to withdraw support when functional survival is highly unlikely.

The following guidelines must be interpreted according to current regional outcomes:

*When gestation, birth weight, or congenital anomalies are associated with almost certain early death and when unacceptably high morbidity is likely among the rare survivors, resuscitation is not indicated Examples may include extreme prematurity (gestational age <23 weeks or birth weight <400 g), anencephaly, and chromosomal abnormalities incompatible with life, such as trisomy 13.

*In conditions associated with a high rate of survival and acceptable morbidity, resuscitation is nearly always indicated (Class IIa). This will generally include babies with gestational age 25 weeks (unless there is evidence of fetal compromise such as intrauterine infection or hypoxia-ischemia) and those with most congenital malformations. ·In conditions associated with uncertain prognosis in which survival is borderline, the morbidity rate is relatively high, and the anticipated burden to the child is high, parental desires concerning initiation of resuscitation should be supported.

Discontinuing Resuscitative Efforts: Infants without signs of life (no heart beat and no respiratory effort) after 10 minutes of resuscitation show either a high mortality or severe neurodevelopmental disability. After 10 minutes of continuous and adequate resuscitative efforts, discontinuation of resuscitation may be justified if there are no signs of life.

* *Pearl/Peril/Pitfall: Discontinuing resuscitation may be justified in infants who have not responded to continuous and appropriate resuscitation for a full 10 minutes and who have no heart rate or respiratory effort (no signs of life).*

Figure 1 Preparation for Neonatal Resuscitation

* All health professionals dealing with Newborn infants should be proficient in basic resuscitation, i.e. **A**irway, **B**reathing with mask ventilation, **C**irculation with cardiac compressions.
* Additional skilled assistance is needed if the baby does not respond rapidly and should be called without delay.
* A person proficient in advanced resuscitation (**A**irway, **B**reathing via tracheal ventilation, **C**irculation, **D**rugs) should be available at short notice in a maternity unit at all times.
* The need for resuscitation can usually be anticipated and a person proficient in advanced resuscitation should be in attendance at all high-risk deliveries.
* A **clock** should be started at birth for accurate timing of changes in the infant's condition and for determining the Modified Apgar Scores.
* Babies should be prevented from becoming cold.

Keep warm and dry
Position, suction, stimulate, Oxygen
Establish effective ventilation
*mask ventilation
* endotracheal ventilation
Chest Compressions
Drugs

Always needed

Rarely needed

The *inverted pyramid* showing the relative frequency of procedures in Neonatal resuscitation. (Adapted from *Pediatric Advanced Life Support*, American Heart Association)

TABLE 4	The APGAR Score		
	Score		
	0	**1**	**2**
Heart rate	Absent	<100 bpm	>100bpm
Respiratory effort	Absent	Gasping or irregular	Regular, strong cry
Muscle tone	Flaccid	Some flexion of limbs	Well flexed, active
Reflex irritability	None	Grimace	Cry, cough
Color	Pale/blue	Body pink, extremities blue	Pink

* APGAR Scores 8-9 at 1 & 5 minutes =normal cardiopulmonary adaptation.

* APGAR Scores of 4-7 warrant close attention.

* APGAR Score of 0-3 indicates cardiopulmonary arrest or CNS depression.

The ABCDs of Neonatal Resuscitation

A. Establish an open airway *Position the infant supine with the head neutral position * Gently suction the mouth, nose and in some instances the trachea (avoid blind deep suction which can cause bradycardia and laryngospasm) * Don't suction for > 5 seconds at a time *If necessary insert an ET tube to ensure an open airway.

B. Initiate breathing *Use tactile stimulation to initiate respirations (flick the soles and rub the back but don't batter the baby). *Use positive pressure ventilation with 100% oxygen/room air if oxygen is not available when the baby don't commence respirations within 20 seconds, or remain irregular, or if the heart rate is below 100/mt using **BAG AND MASK WITH GOOD SEAL** over mouth and nose (give 5 inflation breaths, each 2-3 seconds duration and confirm a response - *visible chest movement or increasing in heart rate*). Continue with ventilation breaths at 30–40 bpm with no spontaneous breathing. Reassess every 30 seconds if not responding, **check** mask position, head position, and circuit. *Decompress the stomach through NG tube, if the baby needs bag and mask ventilation for > 2 minutes.*

The pressure given should be enough to move the chest wall; about 20 Cms H_2O, although the first few breaths may need to be 30–40 cm of H_2O pressure. *Successful ventilation is determined by adequate chest rise, symmetric breath sounds, improved pink color, heart rate > 100 bpm, spontaneous respirations and improved muscle tone.*

ENDOTRACHEAL INTUBATION AND ARTIFICIAL VENTILATION: *To be started if effective mask ventilation is not established or if the baby is depressed because of meconium aspiration or apneic, pulseless, cyanotic and limp at birth.* Early intubation is recommended for extremely low birth weight preterm infants.

If adequate ventilation still not achieved, consider * **D**isplaced tube (often in esophagus or right main bronchus) *O**bstructed tube (especially meconium) *P**neumothorax or other patient problems - lung immaturity / respiratory distress syndrome, diaphragmatic hernia, pleural effusion - shock from blood loss - upper airway obstruction e.g. choanal atresia * **E**quipment failure, e.g. exhausted gas supply.(*Refer to* the Chapter No. 3 "Neonatal Resuscitation in Special Circumstances".)

C. Maintain circulation Stimulate and maintain the circulation of the blood with external cardiac compressions, if the heart rate < 60 bpm or 80 bpm but not rising or pulse absent, after 15-30 seconds of effective bag and mask / endotracheal ventilation ; compress the chest briskly, by 1/3 rd of its depth, with the both thumbs are apposed at the lower one third of sternum (at a ratio of cardiac compression : lung inflation of 3:1 @rate of 90 compressions : 30 breaths /mt). (After 15-30 seconds of effective ventilation, the heart rate of the neonate should be evaluated. To save valuable time, the heart rate over a 6 second period is counted and multiplied by 10 to give an approximation of the 1-minute heart rate. (e.g. 8 beats in 6 seconds = 80 bpm)

D. Administer drugs Consider drugs if the heart rate is not rising in spite of an appropriate *cardiopulmonary combined resuscitation* being done for > 30 seconds or during asystole.

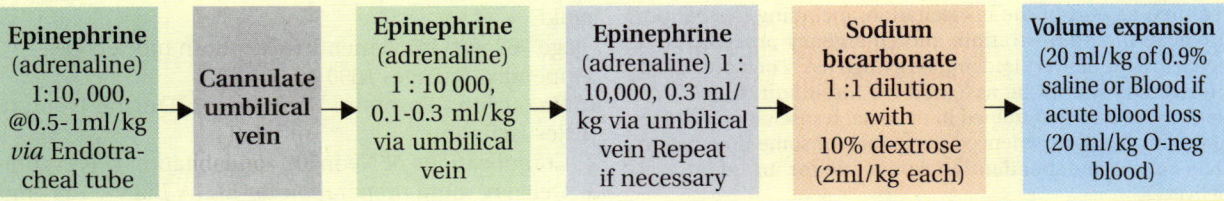

| Epinephrine (adrenaline) 1:10, 000, @0.5-1ml/kg *via* Endotracheal tube | → | Cannulate umbilical vein | → | Epinephrine (adrenaline) 1 : 10 000, 0.1-0.3 ml/kg via umbilical vein | → | Epinephrine (adrenaline) 1 : 10,000, 0.3 ml/ kg via umbilical vein Repeat if necessary | → | Sodium bicarbonate 1 :1 dilution with 10% dextrose (2ml/kg each) | → | Volume expansion (20 ml/kg of 0.9% saline or Blood if acute blood loss (20 ml/kg O-neg blood) |

* **Pearl/Peril/Pitfall:** *All infants with Asphyxia, or a 1 minute APGAR score below 7, require resuscitation. Any infant can have ASPHYXIA at birth without warning signs during labor and delivery. It is not necessary to routinely suction and the mouth and nose of infants after delivery. Resuscitation involves knowing much more than an ordered list of skills and having a resuscitation team; it requires excellent assessment skills and a grounded understanding of physiology.*

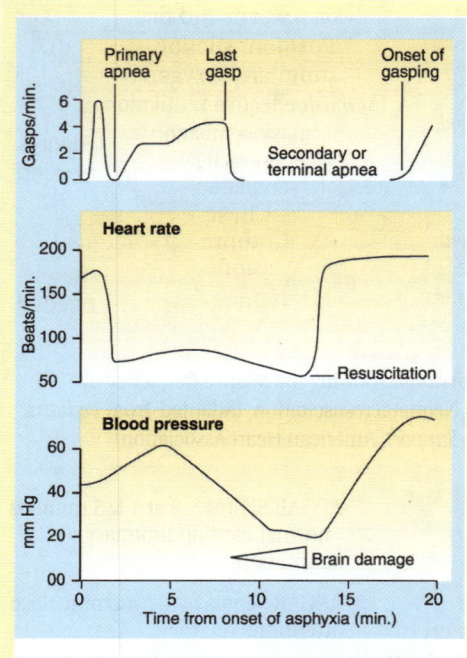

(Adapted from Birth asphyxia, resuscitation, and brain damage. In Dawes GS: Foetal and Neonatal Physiology. Chicago,Year Book Medical Publishers, 1968, p 141.)

Pathophysiological changes during resuscitation of a newborn monkey (Adapted from Dawes et al., 1963) When an acute asphyxia is induced in the newborn monkeys before the onset of breathing by sealing their heads in a bag of saline, after a few shallow breaths without achieving any gas exchange the animals stop breathing. This period of primary apnea may last 10 minutes. However, after 1-2 minutes in primary apnea most animals start to gasp with increasing frequency and vigor, and then decreasing frequency and vigor until literally reach the last gasp. Gasping lasts for 5-10 minutes after which the animal again apneic. The heart rate falls rapidly after birth, rises slightly in primary apnea and early in the phase of gasping, but then slows. Cardiac activity continues for 10 minutes or more after the last gasp. The period between the last gasp, and cardiac arrest, is known as secondary or terminal apnea. To resuscitate an animal in terminal apnea, positive pressure ventilation must be used. If the heart rate is very slow or has stopped, external cardiac massage will be necessary. *Similarly, a Newborn baby in Primary apnea can be resuscitated with appropriate sensory stimuli while a newborn in terminal apnea cannot be resuscitated without positive pressure ventilation. Primary apnea is more likely, if the baby is cyanosed, with good muscle tone, heart rate around 100 bpm and he gasps before becoming pink on resuscitation; In Terminal apnea, the baby is pale, flaccid, with heart rate 60 bpm and he turns pink before gasping on resuscitation. However, this differentiation is usually made in retrospect and is generally not useful in determining the need for active resuscitation in a given baby.* • ASSUME NEWBORN IS IN SECONDARY APNEA UNTIL PROVEN OTHERWISE! • DELAY IN INITIATING ASSISTED VENTILATION CAN RESULT IN LONG DELAY IN ESTABLISHING SPONTANEOUS RESPIRATIONS

WHO IS WHO? AMONG PROFESSIONALS RESPONSIBLE FOR RESUSCITATION OF BABIES AT BIRTH

Whether birth takes place in hospital or at home, the professionals present must be trained and experienced in the systematic application of resuscitation techniques.

Novices
Students and those transferring to work in delivery suites, but not expected to be primarily responsible for resuscitation

• Background reading is essential and should be readily available • Attendance at seminars covering the physiology and biochemistry of the adaptation to extra-uterine life • Attendance at training sessions using simulations and manikins • Training in effective airway positioning, bag, valve-, mask-ventilation and external chest compression• Observation of resuscitation procedures carried out by trained instructors • Knowledge of unit guidelines and protocols

Trainees
Qualified staff in junior positions who will work in departments where they always have more experienced staff immediately available • Revision with supervised practice of all aspects applicable to novices • Participation as assistants in resuscitation procedures - formalized and documented • Review of specific needs in relation to their post and expected responsibilities

Staff with responsibility for resuscitation

Midwives in hospitals and community units, those responsible for home deliveries including general practitioners, senior house officers and specialist registrars in obstetrics, paediatrics and anesthetics, neonatal nurses and practitioners • Revision and appraisal of all skills previously acquired • Training with supervised practice • Regular audit of skills and training and dissemination of information

Experienced staff
Specialist registrars in paediatrics and neonatology, staff grade and consultant pediatricians, and others working in hospitals such as obstetricians, anesthetists, midwives, neonatal nurses and practitioners who have positions of responsibility for resuscitation should undertake

• Regular revision of skills • Training in tracheal intubation with practice and supervision • Training in umbilical venous catheterization • Training in appropriate drug therapy • Supervision of novices, trainees, and staff with responsibilities • Participation in teaching and training courses • Responsibility for organization and audit of skills and training.

The most important action to be taken is earlier paging for the assistance of skilled personnel in cases of complicated deliveries and in cases of unexpectedly depressed infants.

AS RECOMMENDED BY ROYAL COLLEGE OF PEDIATRICS AND CHILD HEALTH & ROYAL COLLEGE OF OBSTETRICIANS AND GYNECOLOGISTS, UK

Trained Personnel: For all deliveries, at least one person should be present who is skilled in neonatal resuscitation and has responsibility for only the infant. This person must be skilled in initiation of resuscitation, use of bag mask ventilation, and performance of chest compressions. Additional personnel should be immediately available to assist in tasks that may be required as part of the resuscitation, including intubation, medication administration, and emergency procedures, if needed. If the delivery is identified as high risk, 2 or more skilled individuals should be assigned for the infant at delivery. Remember that staff trained in neonatal resuscitation need to apprentice with experienced personnel for some time before they can be independently responsible for an infant at a delivery.

Refer to :
*Chapter 2, Page- 15, "Neonatal Post Resuscitation Care" for Post Resuscitation Considerations
*Page -710, for Pitfalls of Neonatal Resuscitation : How to avoid?
*Page 762, for Implementing Newborn mock codes
*Appendix -B: Page- 1090 for
1. Hazardous Forms of Stimulation During Neonatal Resuscitation
2. Complications of Neonatal Resuscitation & Prevention
3. Delivery room preparation for ELBW Baby < 750 gms.

* Pearl/Peril/Pitfall: *Narcan will not help resuscitate an infant if the mother has not received a narcotic analgesic during labor, or has received a non-opioid general anaesthetic, barbiturates or other sedatives.*

TABLE 5   Medications for neonatal resuscitation

Medication	Dose	Route	Rate /Precautions	Important clinical notes
1. Adrenaline 1 in 10,000	0.1-0.3 ml/kg	IV or ET	Give rapidly. Dilute with NS to 1-2ml if giving ET	Try further doses 1ml/kg at 3-5 minute intervals, if there is no response.ET: 0.3–1 ml/kg
2. Volume Expander (O-ve blood, NS, RL)	10ml/kg	IV	Give over 5-10 minutes	Useful in Hypovolemia due to blood loss or to loss of vascular tone following asphyxia.
3. Sodium Bicarbonate (4.2%)	2-4ml/kg	IV	Give slowly, over at least 2 minutes	Give only if infant is effectively ventilated useful to improve the myocardial performance and to enhance the effects of O_2 and Adrenaline.
4. Dextrose 10%	2ml/kg	IV	Mix with Sodium Bicarbonate at 1:1 dilution	Hypoglycemia is a potential problem for all stressed or asphyxiated babies. Glucostix are not reliable in Neonates when reading <90mgs/dL.
5. Naloxone 1ml = 400mcg	100mcg/kg or 0.25ml/kg	IV or ET	Give rapidly. IM / SC acceptable	Useful if the mother had opiate analgesia < 4 hours before delivery. Don't give it if there is history / suspicion of maternal drug abuse as it may initiate Neonatal withdrawal

6. **Atropine & Calcium gluconate have no place in the acute care of Neonatal resuscitation**

ALGORITHM FOR THE USE OF MEDICATIONS DURING NEONATAL RESUSCITATION

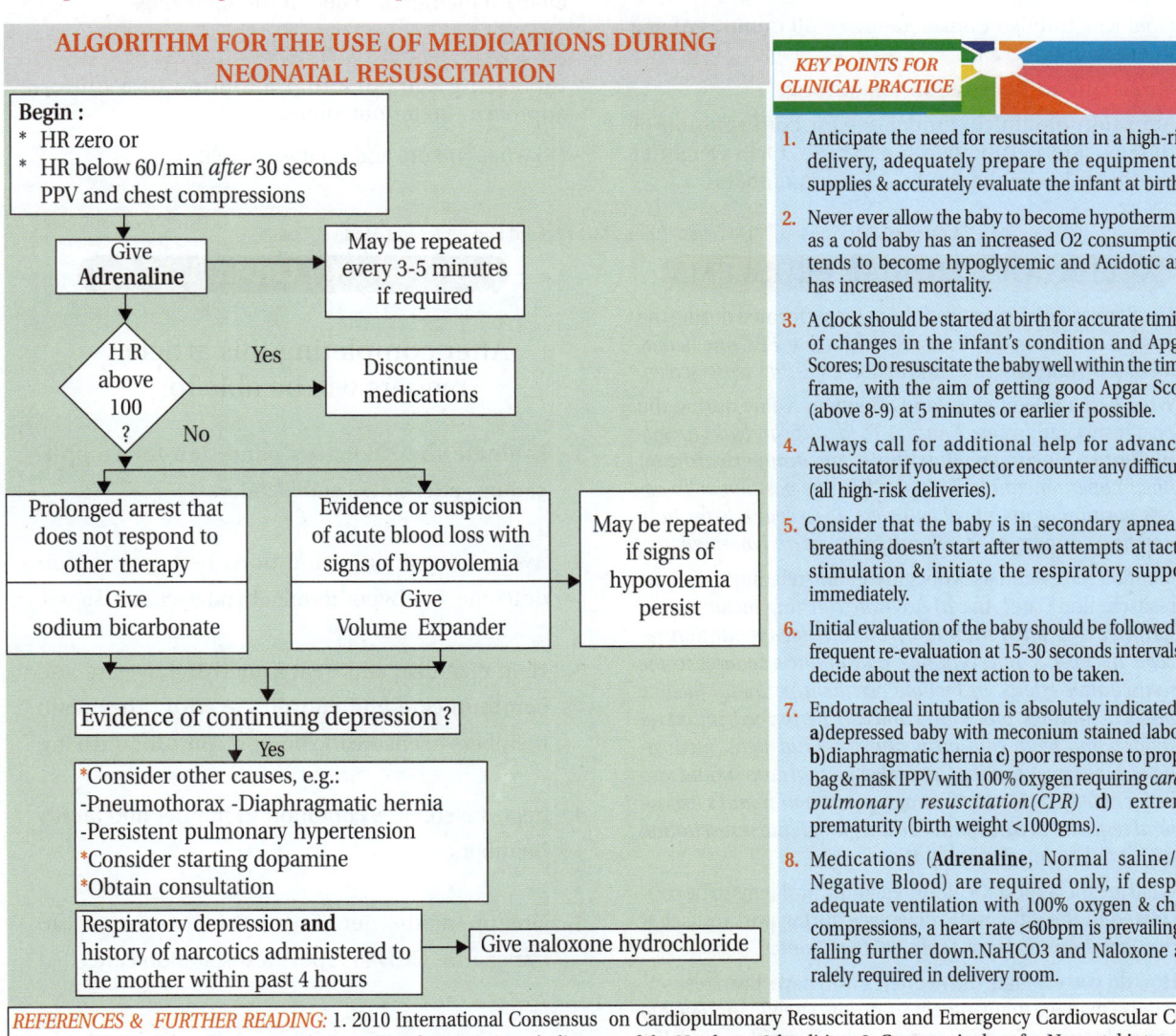

KEY POINTS FOR CLINICAL PRACTICE

1. Anticipate the need for resuscitation in a high-risk delivery, adequately prepare the equipment & supplies & accurately evaluate the infant at birth.

2. Never ever allow the baby to become hypothermic- as a cold baby has an increased O2 consumption, tends to become hypoglycemic and Acidotic and has increased mortality.

3. A clock should be started at birth for accurate timing of changes in the infant's condition and Apgar Scores; Do resuscitate the baby well within the time-frame, with the aim of getting good Apgar Score (above 8-9) at 5 minutes or earlier if possible.

4. Always call for additional help for advanced resuscitator if you expect or encounter any difficulty (all high-risk deliveries).

5. Consider that the baby is in secondary apnea, if breathing doesn't start after two attempts at tactile stimulation & initiate the respiratory support immediately.

6. Initial evaluation of the baby should be followed by frequent re-evaluation at 15-30 seconds intervals & decide about the next action to be taken.

7. Endotracheal intubation is absolutely indicated in **a)** depressed baby with meconium stained labour **b)** diaphragmatic hernia **c)** poor response to proper bag & mask IPPV with 100% oxygen requiring *cardio pulmonary resuscitation(CPR)* **d)** extreme prematurity (birth weight <1000gms).

8. Medications (**Adrenaline**, Normal saline/O-Negative Blood) are required only, if despite adequate ventilation with 100% oxygen & chest compressions, a heart rate <60bpm is prevailing & falling further down.NaHCO3 and Naloxone are ralely required in delivery room.

REFERENCES & FURTHER READING: 1. 2010 International Consensus on Cardiopulmonary Resuscitation and Emergency Cardiovascular Care Science with Treatment Recommendations. *Circulation.* 2. Avery's diseases of the Newborn, 8th edition. 3. Core curriculum for Neonatal intensive care nursing, 3rd edition. 4. Klaus & Fanaroff Care of the high-risk Neonate, 5th edition. 5. Roberton's text book of Neonatology, 4th edition.

* *Pearl/Peril/Pitfall: Although not essential for basic resuscitation, it is very useful to have an infant laryngoscope and endotracheal tubes so that infants with severe asphyxia can be intubated, if bag and mask ventilation is not adequate. If possible, everyone who regularly resuscitates newborn infants should learn how to intubate them.*

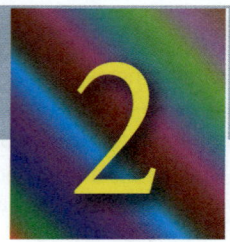

Neonatal Post-Resuscitation Care ("Golden Hour Management")

@ *"Good communication between obstetric and pediatric teams allows preparation to be made for an admission and prevents potentially life-threatening delays while appropriate staff and equipment are found."*

What is "The Golden Hour?"

* A Protocolized, scripted, multidisciplinary approach to the initial respiratory management of the Premature infant/ any critically ill Newborn.

* Developed to improve outcomes and facilitate communication and teamwork among team members

* Uniform, controlled Resuscitation = Safer Resuscitation

Pieces of the Puzzle

* Scripting
* Team cooperation, communication
* Tidal volume monitoring, gentle ventilation
* Early surfactant administration
* Protocolized initial ventilation
* Early attention to thermoregulation, developmentally supportive care

Early Surfactant administration

* Strong evidence to suggest benefits of early prophylactic surfactant administration

* Goal to administer Surfactant in < 30 minutes of age in every infant

* Surfactant administration first priority

* Adoption of clinical guidelines for confirmation of tube position (Tube depth at 6 cm + birth weight at the lip and Auscultation by 2 Team members)

Protocols

* Although viewed negatively by some, protocols allow all team members to be "on the same page"

* Allows for continuous feedback

* Increasing evidence that adoption of a uniform approach- better outcomes

* Do what you do, and do it very well!

Courtesy: NickMickas, MD William Rhine, MD Packard and John Muir Medical Center

REVIEW OF CLINICAL PROBLEMS

1. List five essential investigations to be performed during the post resuscitation care ? *Ans: Blood glucose, FBC and hematocrit, ABG analysis, chest and abdomen X-Ray, sepsis screen.*

2. What is the role of chest and abdomen X-Ray during the post resuscitation care ? *Ans: a) To identify air leaks (pneumothorax, pneumomediastinum, pneumopericardium, pneumoperitoneum b) To assess ET tube position c) To assess position of umbilical catheters d) To evaluate for lung and heart disease. e) To rule out fractures and anomalies.*

3. Mention the essentials of documentation relating to the Post resuscitation Care? *Ans: a) Accurate charting including descriptive and often minute-by-minute documentation reveals the events, interventions, and infant responses to the resuscitative efforts. b) Include pertinent perinatal factors, physical findings, procedures and care performed, infant response, and team communication. c) Vital signs, medications, laboratory findings and other factual data should also be included. d) Developmental support and infant's behavioral response to care should be integrated into resuscitation and stabilization documentation.*

4. What are the important life-threatening problems to be considered in the differential diagnosis during post resuscitation care ? *Ans: Refer to Table 2 of the Chapter.*

5. How do you evaluate the neonates who have been resuscitated & manage them timely & appropriately? *Ans: Refer to the evaluation - decision - action - plan/algorithm for delivering the post resuscitation care.*

LEARNING OBJECTIVES

After completing this article, readers will be able to:

1. Evaluate the Neonate's condition for complications, after initial stabilization.

2. Avoid intensifying conditions that may impair outcome, e.g. hypothermia, hypoglycemia, sepsis.

3. Help diagnose and treat underlying disease and communicate and coordinate with other team members to ensure the best outcome for the baby.

4. Report Neonate's condition to mother and family members.

5. Document the details of initial resuscitation, transfer to NICU and post resuscitation care.

* *Pearl/Peril/Pitfall: All infants that require resuscitation must be carefully observed for at least 12 hours. Their temperature, pulse and respiratory rate, colour and activity should be recorded and their blood glucose concentration measured. Keep these infants warm and provide fluid and energy, either intravenously or orally.*

1. Neonates who require initial resuscitation may have an underlying illness, congenital anomaly, prematurity, or asphyxia. Discontinuation of resuscitative efforts is reasonable if there is no heart rate after 15 minutes of complete and adequate resuscitation (APGAR score of 0). But continued resuscitative efforts are warranted for depressed infants who show signs of recovery.

2. Babies who required extensive resuscitation should have ongoing assessment for at least 12–24 hours after birth. Even those who have responded appropriately to resuscitation may need further intervention to support breathing, achieve adequate oxygenation, avoid hyperthermia, and maintain glucose and fluid balance. Many of the gains from successful neonatal resuscitation can be lost by poor aftercare and not attending to potential complications.Limited studies indicate that long-term neurological outcomes may be modified by corrective responses to clinically important issues, such as thermal balance, serum glucose levels, oxygen use, seizure control, and medication dosing. Management of neonatal encephalopathy is not feasible in community settings, and requires referral to a district- or tertiary-level facility. Table 1 outlines *"indications"* f or admitting a baby to the NICU; these will vary between hospitals depending on the transitional care facilities available.

3. Good communication between obstetric and pediatric teams allows preparation to be made for an admission and prevents potentially life-threatening delays while appropriate staff and equipment are found. The neonatal resident responsible for resuscitation must accompany the baby from the labor ward with a trained neonatal staff who will ensure the baby is labelled properly. Always have a copy of the maternal notes or a good history is vital for not missing an important diagnosis such as maternal HIV or Hepatitis infection for which immediate treatment is required.

4. After resuscitation, any baby who requires admission to NICU *must not* be allowed to become *hypothermic, hypoxic & hypoglycemic* while being transferred from the labor ward to the NICU. Always recheck the effectiveness of ventilation, chest compressions, medications, and, if not previously performed, endotracheal intubation after the initial resuscitative measures. It is sensible to keep a resuscitated baby (by IPPV) intubated & ventilated during transport & until baseline blood gases have been obtained after admission to the NICU. **Therapeutic hypothermia •** Hypothermia may reduce the extent of brain injury following hypoxia-ischemia. Currently, routine anticonvulsant therapy for term newborns in the period immediately following intrapartum-related hypoxia cannot be recommended. The use of higher thermal control set points or an uncontrolled warming device should be avoided in babies with neonatal encephalopathy. Carefully controlled environmental temperature or skin-to-skin care may offer safer alternatives.• *Refer to Page 1123: Neonatal Pearls of Wisdom to Remember:* 94.Hypoxic Ischemic Encephalopathy and Hypothermic Intervention for Neonates.While therapeutic hypothermia is a high technology intervention, modifications have been developed for application in low-resource settings, including use of water bottles and servo-controlled fans. However, the effectiveness may not be equivalent given different methods and settings, and randomized controlled trials are required and presently being conducted. (*From Neonatal resuscitation in low-resource settings: What, who, and how to overcome challenges to scale up? Stephen N. Wall et al, http:// www.ncbi.nlm.nih.gov/pmc/articles/PMC2875104/*)

5. If the baby doesn't show good response to proper intubation and ventilation, consider hypovolemia & acidosis and manage appropriately. If hypotension doesn't respond adequately to volume expansion, consider dopamine infusion. Occasionally, hypotension is a complication of pneumothorax or other intrathoracic air leak.

In this situation thoracentesis may be life saving. A frequent misconception is that delay/depression of respiration at birth is always the result of intrapartum asphyxia, but one should consider many additional factors which can delay the onset of respiration as well (refer to Table 4)

6. Good first-hour care is of particular importance in the premature baby at risk from RDS, in whom failure to control clinical, biochemical and physiological abnormalities results in severe surfactant depletion and RDS because of hypoxemia, hypotension, acidemia, hypothermia, & hypoventilation. *In other words neglected first-hour care can convert mild RDS into severe, or fatal RDS, or a treatable case of septicemia into a fatal one.* All babies with low APGAR scores may not have suffered *in utero* hypoxia, but some will develop hypoxic—ischemic encephalopathy requiring close monitoring; others need investigation to exclude sepsis, peripheral neuromuscular disease or some other pre-existing CNS disorder.

7. *The Evaluation-Decision-Action-Plan/Algorithm* to evaluate the post resuscitated babies and to manage them timely & appropriately describes the essential aspects of *golden hour* management. Refer to respiratory care map for 'Care Protocol' for babies ≤ 1,000 gm.

8. On admission to the Neonatal unit, weigh the baby, transfer to incubator/radiant heater & attach to ventilator if intubated. Allow nursing staff 5 minutes to take baby's temperature, attach temperature probe, cardiac, respiratory and transcutaneous oxygen & carbon dioxide monitors and give vitamin-K 1mg IM if the baby weighs >1.5kg and 0.5mg IM if <1.5kg. Take digital photographs for parents.

9. All ill babies admitted directly from the delivery suite should have the following investigations set in train within 30 minutes of admission: **1.**arterial blood gases; **2.**blood glucose; **3.**Hemoglobin (PCV), full blood count with differential WBC; **4.** swabs from ear and throat; **5.** blood culture; **6.** group and crossmatch; **7.** electrolytes, urea, creatinine. A chest X-ray will be required but can wait, especially if arterial lines are to be inserted. Coagulation studies may be indicated. Think about collecting blood for chromosomes if you need to give a blood transfusion urgently, as per the clinical situation.

10. On the basis of the initial investigations, make a working differential diagnosis & start appropriate treatment without delay. Give surfactant for RDS, correct acidosis & hypotension, treat anemia with packed RBC transfusion, polycythemia with partial exchange transfusion, DIC with platelet or FFP transfusion. Blood gas values help guide adjustments in ventilation and the decision to treat metabolic acidosis with sodium bicarbonate; *perfusion & adequate ventilation must be acceptable before giving sodium bicarbonate.* Base deficits of 10-20 mmol/L usually correct spontaneously and rapidly and there is no need to give otherwise asymptomatic acidemic term babies IV bicarbonate/THAM. Hypoglycemia usually responds to initiation of IV glucose 2ml/kg 10% dextrose followed by an infusion of 4-7mg/kg/minute or 10% dextrose 100ml/kg/day & serial glucose measurements. Calcium is not indicated during the acute phase of neonatal resuscitation but during post resuscitation if the ionized calcium levels are low (normal range 1.1-1.4mmol/L or 4.5-5.6mg/dL), give calcium gluconate 1-2ml/kg or calcium chloride 0.35-0.7ml/kg by IV infusion over 10-30 minutes, carefully weighing the risks such as bradycardia, subcutaneous necrosis against the benefits of calcium infusion. Table-2 describes life-threatening problems and care considerations for the newborn after initial resuscitation. Table-3 enlists non life-threatening problems and care considerations for the newborn after initial resuscitation. Parents and their families need to be involved in the discussions and exchange of information regarding their ill newborn. Give the family as much information as possible about the infant's condition and arrange for contact with the baby before transport.

Pearl/Peril/Pitfall: Hyperthermia may worsen the extent of brain injury following hypoxia-ischemia. The goal should be to achieve normothermia and to avoid iatrogenic hyperthermia in resuscitated Newborns.

THE EVALUATION-DECISION-ACTION-PLAN/ALGORITHM TO DELIVER
POST RESUSCITATION CARE OF THE NEWBORN ("GOLDEN HOUR MANAGEMENT")

SUBJECTIVE FINDINGS

Obtain resuscitation details, APGAR scores at 1 minute, 5 minutes & 10 minutes

Note the indications for NICU admission

Hx of high-risk delivery - maternal, fetal & placental factors

Communicate with obstetrician/ referring physician to know the important aspects of maternal problems. *After resuscitation,* explain to the mother and family what has happened and how the baby is now.

OBJECTIVE FINDINGS

Assess ABCDs & monitor CRT, O_2 saturations, BP, vitals, central & peripheral pulses - ; reassess @ 5-10 minutes for any deterioration

Attach to various monitoring devices- pulse oximetry, transcutaneous O_2 & CO_2 monitoring

Look for life-threatening symptoms - central apnea, obstructive apnea, respiratory distress, poor perfusion & bradycardia, pallor and diminished pulses, jitteriness associated with seizures. *Identify* obvious congenital anomalies!

INVESTIGATIONS

Blood-Hb, hematocrit, FBC with differential count, platelets

Blood glucose, Electrolytes (baseline), BUN, creatinine

Blood group & type and crossmatch

Arterial Blood gas analysis

Blood cultures & *take swabs from ear and throat*

Chest X-ray, Abdomen X-ray

Echocardiogram to identify PPHN and duct dependent cardiac malformations

Coagulation studies, chromosomal studies optional at the time of admission.

POST RESUSCITATION CARE OF THE NEWBORN IN THE GOLDEN HOUR

Weigh the baby, *Ensure* ABCs, pulse oximetry, IV access, monitor BP & CRT, *Administer* oxygen to maintain the saturation between 90 and 93%. *Consider* ET intubation & *Assist* ventilation in neonates with respiratory insufficiency,

Treat shock with 20ml/kg NS IV bolus, repeat PRN &

Consider packed RBC transfusion 15ml/kg, to maintain hematocrit >40%.

Correct and maintain hypoglycemia, hypothermia & hypocalcemia

Start IV broadspectrum antibiotics to cover for sepsis, after blood cultures.

Give vitamin-K 1mg IM if the baby weighs >1.5kg and 0.5mg IM if <1.5kg

Take digital photographs for parents

Review systems @frequent intervals, following the Table "Neonatal Postresuscitation Considerations" (see next page)

ATTACH TO VENTILATOR IF INTUBATED AT THE TIME OF ADMISSION

Initial ventilator settings

	Non-compliant stiff lungs	Compliant normal lungs
Rate	60/min	40/min
Ti	0.4s	0.3–0.4s
PIP	Increase from 18 cmH_2O until adequate chest wall movement	14 cm H_2O
PEEP	4 cm H_2O	3 cmH_2O
FiO2	As required to maintain oxygenation	As required to maintain oxygenation

Essential Components of Post resuscitation Care

1. Assess oxygenation, ventilation, perfusion and acid-base balance
2. Monitor glucose concentrations to ensure normoglycemia
3. Volume (Maintain Hct> 40%) & electrolyte support
4. Chest and abdominal X-ray for air leaks
5. Monitor vital signs including BP and for seizure activity
6. Screen for infection
7. Support family
8. Documentation
9. Ethical decisions about non initiation or discontinuation of intensive care

PRETERM INFANT VENTILATED FOR RESPIRATORY DISTRESS

* Give surfactant -observe clinical effect and adjust ventilator setting accordingly.
* Obtain venous access either peripherally or, in the extremely preterm baby <26 weeks, via a UVC. Obtain a blood glucose (BG) reading and send blood for FBC, blood group, DCT and blood culture.
* Commence IV fluids of 10% dextrose @ 60mL/kg.
* Give IV antibiotics where indicated (to all babies with respiratory distress for 48 h until blood cultures are known to be negative.)
* Commence pain relief/sedation with either morphine or diamorphine.
* If the baby is requiring > 40 % oxygen obtain, arterial access preferably via the umbilical artery. In infants > 30 weeks gestation where early enteral feeding is likely, some neonatologists prefer peripheral arterial access.
* Complete examination of baby. This should include gestational assessment if there is any doubt of the baby's gestational age.
* CXR at 4 h. include AXR if either UAC or UVC inserted.

Adapted from "Pocket Neonatology" by Terence Stephenson, 2000

---

* *Pearl/Peril/Pitfall:* Post resuscitation care may include: *arterial pH and blood gas determinations *correction of documented metabolic acidosis *use of volume expanders and/or pressors if hypotension persists *appropriate fluid therapy *treatment of seizures *screening for hypoglycemia and hypocalcemia *chest X-rays for diagnostic purposes and ET tube position checks.

Respiratory care map for infants ≤ 1000 grams

Courtesy: NickMickas, MD William Rhine, MD Packard and John Muir Medical Center

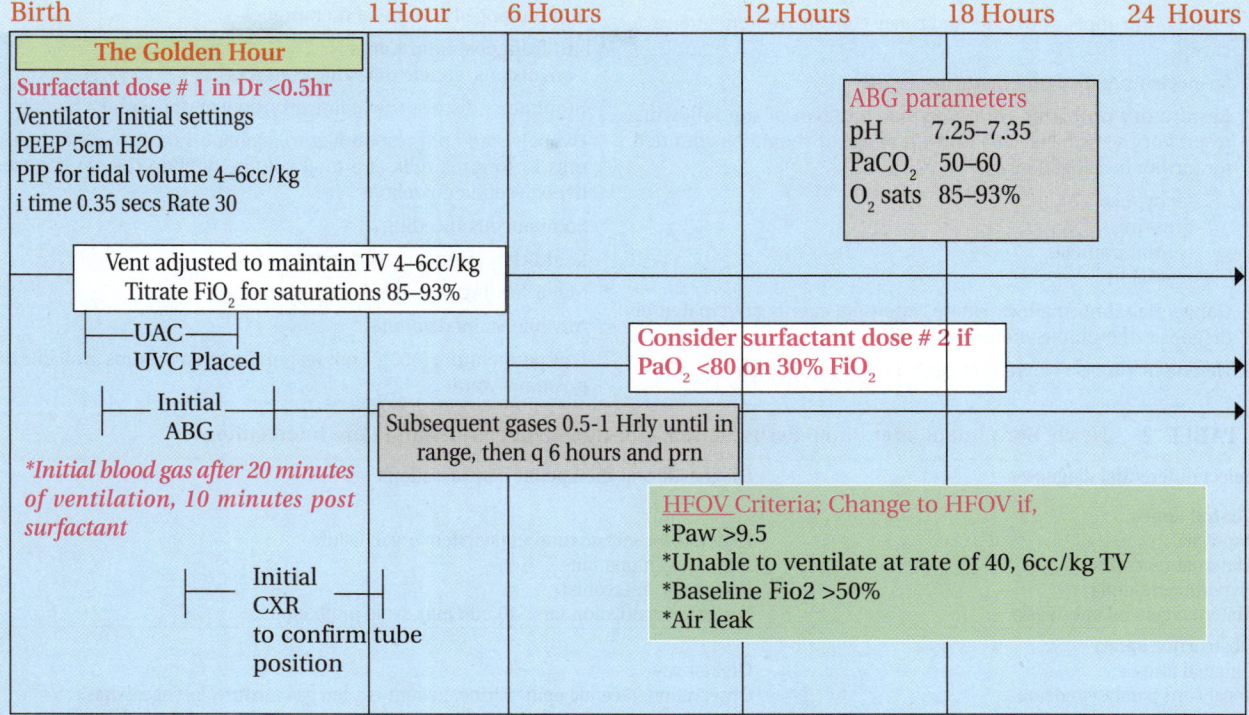

| Birth | 1 Hour | 6 Hours | 12 Hours | 18 Hours | 24 Hours |

The Golden Hour

Surfactant dose # 1 in Dr <0.5hr
Ventilator Initial settings
PEEP 5cm H2O
PIP for tidal volume 4–6cc/kg
i time 0.35 secs Rate 30

ABG parameters
pH   7.25–7.35
$PaCO_2$ 50–60
O_2 sats   85–93%

Vent adjusted to maintain TV 4–6cc/kg
Titrate FiO_2 for saturations 85–93%

UAC
UVC Placed

Consider surfactant dose # 2 if PaO_2 <80 on 30% FiO_2

Initial ABG

Subsequent gases 0.5-1 Hrly until in range, then q 6 hours and prn

Initial blood gas after 20 minutes of ventilation, 10 minutes post surfactant

HFOV Criteria; Change to HFOV if,
*Paw >9.5
*Unable to ventilate at rate of 40, 6cc/kg TV
*Baseline Fio2 >50%
*Air leak

Initial
CXR
to confirm tube position

Neonatal postresuscitation considerations

Organ system	Potential complication	Postresuscitation action
Brain	Apnea Seizures	Monitor for apnea. Support ventilation as needed. Monitor glucose and electrolytes. Avoid hyperthermia. Consider anticonvulsant therapy.
Lungs	Pulmonary hypertension Pneumonia Pneumothorax Transient tachypnea Meconium aspiration syndrome Surfactant deficiency	Maintain adequate oxygenation and ventilation. Consider antibiotics. Obtain radiograph if respiratory distress is present. Consider surfactant therapy. Delay feedings if respiratory distress is present.
Cardiovascular	Hypotension	Monitor blood pressure and heart rate. Consider inotrope (e.g., dopamine) and/or volume replacement.
Kidneys	Acute tubular necrosis	Monitor urine output. Restrict fl uids if oliguric volume and vascular volume are adequate. Monitor serum electrolytes.
Gastrointestinal	Ileus Necrotizing enterocolitis	Delay initiation of feedings. Give intravenous fl uids. Consider parenteral nutrition.
Metabolic/Hematologic	Hypoglycemia Hypocalcemia; hyponatremia Anemia Thrombocytopenia	Monitor blood sugar Monitor electrolytes Monitor hematocrit Monitor platelets

Pearl/Peril/Pitfall: *Researchers also suggest that all infants delivered earlier than 30 weeks' gestation receive their first dose of surfactant in the delivery room within a few minutes of life, following cardiopulmonary stabilization. Infants born later than 30 weeks' gestation should receive rescue therapy as soon as they show clinical signs of RDS. Infants born at 30-36 weeks' gestation may benefit from surfactant with rapid extubation to CPAP.*

TABLE 1   Justifiable Indications for admitting a baby to the NICU

Babies requiring immediate admission to the neonatal unit from the labor suite or immediately after delivery elsewhere

* Infants <1800 g or <34 weeks gestation
* Infants who appear unstable and cause concern/require intensive care
* Suspected significant perinatal asphyxia
* Respiratory problems--if a baby has any two of the following respiratory signs between 1 and 4 h of age, it should be admitted for further investigation:

    -tachypnea >70 bpm
    -grunting
    -central cyanosis
    -recession

* Congenital abnormalities-where intensive care is anticipated or diagnosis of multiple anomalies is in doubt
* Hemolytic disease where exchange transfusion is likely*

Consider admitting where there is unexplained death of sibling in first week of life

* Chorioamnionitis, i.e. presence of maternal pyrexia, purulent liquor and prolonged rupture of membranes

Admit from postnatal wards

* Convulsions, apneic or cyanotic attacks
* Respiratory distress (including grunting) at or beyond 4 h of age
* Hypoglycemia not responding to regular 3-hourly feeds of breast milk or formula milk at a total volume of 90mL/kg per day (see hypoglycemia guideline)
* Spontaneous bleeding
* Jaundice requiring exchange transfusion
* Major feeding problem and/or vomiting
* Any bile-stained vomit
* Low temperature (<36⁰C) not responding to measures available on postnatal ward

TABLE 2   Newly Born Infant after initial Resuscitation: Life-threatening Issues and Care Interventions

Select differential diagnoses	Diagnostic and therapeutic considerations
Central apnea	
Asphyxia	High risk for seizures and multisystem organ failure
Maternal narcotics	Naloxone, intubation
Hypermagnesemia	No specific antagonist
Maternal general anesthesia	Bag-mask ventilation for 5–10 min may avoid intubation
Obstructive apnea	
Choanal atresia	Oral airway
Vocal cord paralysis/edema	Observation, racemic epinephrine, helium-oxygen gas mixture, laryngeal mask airway
Upper airway anomaly	Laryngeal mask airway, tracheostomy
Micrognathia	Prone position, oral airway, laryngeal mask airway
Respiratory Disease	
Pneumothorax	Thoracentesis, nitrogen washout, high-frequency ventilation
Congenital diaphragmatic hernia	Immediate intubation, orogastric tube, high risk for persistent pulmonary hypertension, and pneumothorax, consider surfactant
Pulmonary hypoplasia	Low threshold for intubation, high risk for pneumothorax, high-frequency ventilation
Hyaline membrane disease	Continuous positive airway pressure, surfactant
Transient tachypnea	Supportive therapy, increased risk after cesarean birth
Pneumonia/sepsis	Antibiotics, volume resuscitation
Persistent pulmonary hypertension	Oxygen lability, pre/postductal difference in oxygen saturation, hyperventilation, consider surfactant and inhaled nitric oxide
Meconium aspiration	Tracheal suctioning, consider surfactant
Congenital heart disease	Cyanosis unresponsive to oxygen, pulmonary compliance often normal, prostaglandin infusion
Hydrops/anasarca	Thoracentesis, paracentesis, pericardiocentesis, pulmonary hypoplasia, pleural effusions, high-frequency ventilation
Diminished pulses, pallor, poor perfusion, bradycardia	
Asphyxia	Volume resuscitation, dopamine
Acute blood loss	Volume resuscitation, emergency red blood cell transfusion
Sepsis	Volume resuscitation and antibiotics
Hypoplastic left heart syndrome, aortic atresia/stenosis, severe coarctation of the aorta	Widely patent ductus arteriosus may allow cardiovascular compensation for days to weeks, prostaglandin E1, dopamine judicious volume expansion
Congenital diaphragmatic hernia	Cardiovascular compromise with mediastinal shift and/or complicating pneumothorax; see Respiratory Distress above
Tension pneumothorax	See Respiratory Distress above
Hypertrophic cardiomyopathy	Vasopressors may worsen left ventricular outflow tract obstruction, infant of diabetic mother
Congenital heart block	Often asymptomatic, maternal collagen disease
Hypothermia	Overhead warmer, warmed blankets, kangaroo care
Seizures	
Hypoxic-ischemic encephalopathy; Metabolic disturbances.	Phenobarbital, intravenous glucose or calcium

Pearl/Peril/Pitfall: *Because radiant warmers are used routinely at deliveries because of a need for maximal patient access, infants less than 1000 g should have a plastic blanket or other barrier applied to decrease evaporative water loss until they can be placed in a humidified environment.*

TABLE 3 Newly born infant after initial Resuscitation: Nonlife-threatening Issues and Care Interventions

Select differential diagnoses	Diagnostic and therapeutic considerations
Bilious and/or copious gastric secretions, abdominal distention, excessive oral secretions	
Esophageal atresia	Inability to pass orogastric tube, urgent surgical gastric decompression
Bowel obstruction or ileus	Orogastric decompression
Renal mass	Risk for pulmonary hypoplasia, pneumothorax, flattened facies, low-set ears, clubfeet (Potter syndrome)
Meconium ileus	Risk for cystic fibrosis, surgical consultation
Bowel perforation	Paracentesis, surgical consultation
Hepatosplenomegaly	Hemolytic anemia, congenital infection
Gaseous distention/perforation	Positive-pressure ventilation
Congenital anomalies	
Gastroschisis, omphalocele	Sterile "bowel bag," volume expansion, positioning, latex precautions, midline anomaly evaluation, temperature control
Meningomyelocele	Latex precautions, sterile occlusive dressing and/or sterile bowel bag
Multiple congenital anomalies	Multisystem evaluation
Ambiguous genitalia	Multisystem evaluation, family support, postpone choice of first name or choose gender-neutral name
Bladder or cloacal extrophy	Sterile bowel bag, saline dressing, latex precautions
Congenital anomalies	
Patent ductus arteriosus	Murmur present after fall in pulmonary vascular resistance, often after leaving delivery room
Congenital heart disease	Heart murmurs unusual immediately after birth, high index of suspicion for congenital heart disease, prostaglandin, chest radiograph, echocardiogram
Jitteriness	
Hypothermia	Radiant warmer, warm blankets, kangaroo care
Hypoglycemia	Early feeding and/or intravenous glucose
Hypocalcemia	Intravenous calcium
Jaundice, yellow skin discoloration	
Isoimmune hyperbilirubinemia	Evaluation recommended if jaundice present before 24hr of age, anemia, phototherapy, Hydrops/Anasarca
Meconium staining	Risk for asphyxia and meconium aspiration

TABLE 4 Factors other than asphyxia that may delay the onset of respiration after delivery

* Central nervous system injury or abnormality present prior to labor
* Drugs depressing the central nervous system
* Maternal hypocapnia
* Trauma, especially to the central nervous system
* Prematurity, in particular surfactant - deficient, stiff lungs
* Sepsis, especially group B streptococci
* Muscle weakness due to prematurity or primary muscle disease
* Anemia, hypovolemia
* Congenital malformations
  - Obstructing the airway or preventing lung expansion
  - Neurological, impairing respiratory control

KEY POINTS FOR CLINICAL PRACTICE

1. All the Newborn babies resuscitated for apnea/gasping, unless they are pink, vigorous and neurologically normal by 5–10 minutes of age, should be admitted to NICU for further care and evaluation. When presenting the golden hour of care in critically ill neonates, we are specifically referring to the initiation of treatments in a systematic, efficient manner in an effort to rapidly stabilize the patient, lessen the progression of illness, and prevent harm.

2. It is important to examine him/her, while monitoring oxygenation, ventilation, perfusion, BP and vital signs, blood glucose, hematocrit, calcium and acid-base balance.

3. Anemia, polycythemia, and DIC may need to be treated with RBC transfusion, partial exchange transfusion, or platelet and fresh frozen plasma transfusion, respectively.

4. It is useful to perform a chest X-Ray and an abdominal X-Ray to recognize air leaks and to assess ET tube position, UAC position, and lung and heart disease.

5. Collaboration with the family is essential with all decision making. The promise of the golden hour in neonatal care lies not only in evidence-based treatment but also in team structure, communication, and proficiency.

REFERENCES & FURTHER READING

1. Neonatal resuscitation in low-resource settings: What, who, and how to overcome challenges to scale up? Stephen N. Wall et al http://www.ncbi.nlm.nih.gov/pmc/articles/PMC2875104/ **2.** Core curriculum for Neonatal intensive care nursing, 3rd edition **3.** Avery's diseases of the Newborn 8th edition. **4.** Current diagnosis & Treatment Pediatrics 19th edition

Pearl/Peril/Pitfall: When administering hyperosmolar medications (e.g. sodium bicarbonate), slow administration is important. Mechanical ventilation may lead to harmful fluctuations in cerebral blood flow, especially when pCO_2 and pH are rapidly altered. Rapid alterations in pCO_2 and pH result in acute fluctuations in the cerebral blood flow of the premature infant with immature cerebral vascular autoregulation.

Neonatal Resuscitation in Special Circumstances

3

@ *"If all the steps in Neonatal resuscitation have been carried out, but the heart rate remains <60bpm, efforts should be redoubled to check several points".*

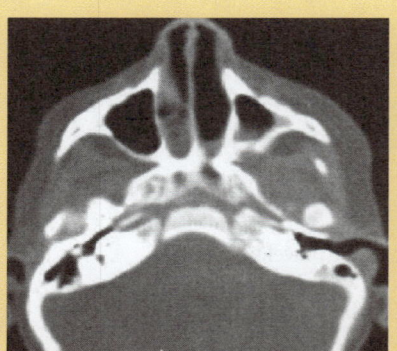

Choanal atresia.
CT SCAN is the choice in evaluating it

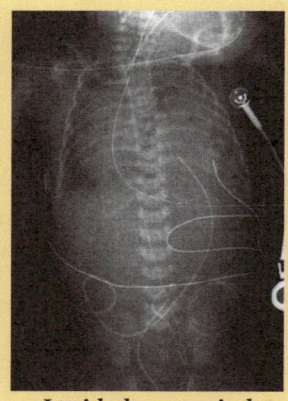

Lt sided congenital diaphragmatic hernia

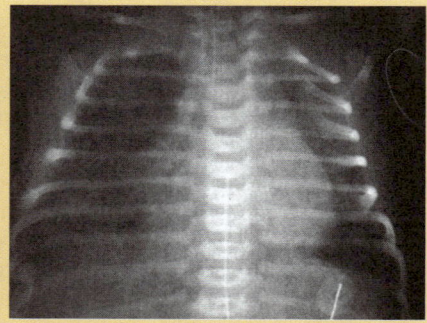

Meconium aspiration Syndrome:
Air trapping and hyperexpansion from airway obstruction

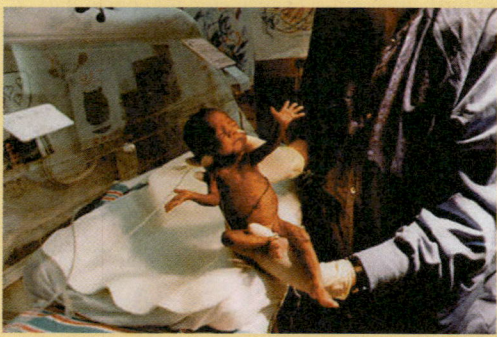

Extreme prematurity

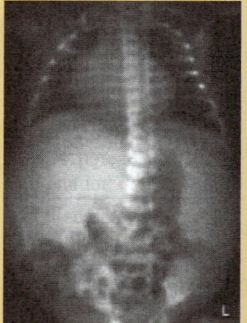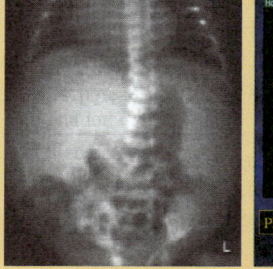

Hydrops fetalis /fetal hydrops

REVIEW OF CLINICAL PROBLEMS

1. What reasons should you consider, if the baby remains cyanosed and bradycardic, inspite of adequate Neonatal resuscitation for 5 to 10 minutes?
   Ans: Refer to Table 2 of the Chapter.

2. Mention the important underlying causes, if the baby remains apneic or with very feeble respiratory efforts and hypotonic but with a good cardiovascular response ?
   Ans: Refer to Table 2 of the Chapter.

3. Mention four possible causes that can result in obstructive apnea in the Newlyborn distressed baby?
   Ans: 1. Choanal atresia 2. Vocal cord paralysis/edema 3. Upper airway anomaly 4. Micrognathia.

4. When should you carry out tracheal suctioning, in babies born through meconium-stained amniotic fluid ?
   Ans: Refer to Table 1 of the Chapter.

5. How do you decide whether to resuscitate or not, when a mother is likely to deliver at or before the limits of viability (23 weeks gestational age) ?
   Ans: Refer to Table 1 of the Chapter.

LEARNING OBJECTIVES

After completing this article, readers will be able to:

1. Identify complications and conditions that can interfere with expected response to resuscitation.

2. Modify the resuscitation process, appropriate to the needs of the baby in special circumstances.

3. Gather more information and plan and consult with parents and senior Neonatalogists regarding further intervention.

4. Determine when to resort to Non-Initiation/ Discontinuation of Neonatal Resuscitation

5. Provide good parental support and communication regarding prognosis and further NICU Care.

---

* ***Pearl/Peril/Pitfall:*** *Premature infants have special needs that must be considered during the critical period immediately following delivery if mortality and morbidity are to be decreased in this group. This population of infants is at increased risk for respiratory failure, insensible water losses, hypoglycemia, and intraventricular hemorrhages.*

1. **Neonatal Resuscitation Program (NRP)** of the AAP (American Academy of Pediatrics) ensures that everybody employes a consistent approach to resuscitation that is successful in a very high percentage of cases & aids pediatricians in more rapidly identifying special or unusual circumstances in which specialized interventions may be required. If all the steps in neonatal resuscitation have been carried out (airway opening, suction, bag & mask ventilation, endotracheal intubation, cardiopulmonary resuscitation, UVC insertion & medications), but the heart rate remains <60bpm, efforts should be redoubled to check several points, i.e. **If mask ventilation is being performed:** *Is the face mask of the correct size? *Is there a good seal? *Is the neck position correct? *Are oral secretions present? **If baby is intubated and there is poor or absent chest movement:** *Is the ETT in the esophagus? Air entry will be better over the stomach than over the lung fields. *Is the ETT down the right main bronchus? Consider this if there is asymmetry of breath sounds and chest wall movement. Inflation and air entry will improve as the tube is withdrawn. *Is the inflation pressure adequate? If the ETT appears to be in the correct position. i.e. breath sounds present and symmetrical but poor chest wall movement, then the most likely problem is that the baby is receiving insufficient pressure to open up the lungs. Therefore: - Check the PIP on the pressure manometer and increase to 30–40 cmH$_2$O. -Check oxygen flow rate. This should be set on the resuscitaire at 5–8 L/min for mask ventilation, and 3-5 L/min for ET IPPV. -If , on increasing inspiratory pressure, there is still poor or absent chest movement, consider increasing the inspiratory time.*Does the baby have lung pathology? For example: - Pneumothorax -Diaphragmatic hernia (Is there a scaphoid abdomen? Is the apex beat displaced?) -Hypoplastic lungs (Does the child have signs of Potter's syndrome?) -Pleural effusions -Evolving lung disease such as severe respiratory distress syndrome -Thoracic dystrophy (the baby may benefit from having the peak inspiratory pressure reduced.) **If in any doubt, reintubate.**

2. **If there is good chest movement:** *Has there been fetal haemorrhage? Suspect if mother has had large antepartum haemorrhage or abruption. If hypovolemia due to fetal blood loss is suspected, then plasma, uncross-matched 'O'-negative blood or blood cross-matched against mother should be given in a volume of 10-20 mL/kg, repeated as necessary. *Is there severe birth asphyxia? *Does the baby have severe cyanotic congenital heart disease? or PPHN.

3. **The Evaluation-Decision-Action-Plan/Algorithm** helps to evaluate the underlying cause for poor response to resuscitation & to take remedial action to correct the problem. *Always call for senior help* to co-ordinate the decisions concerning the progress of difficult resuscitations.

4. Attempts to aspirate meconium from the nose and mouth of the unborn baby, while the head is still on the perineum, are not recommended. If presented with a floppy, apnoeic baby born through meconium it is reasonable to rapidly inspect the oropharynx to remove potential obstructions. If appropriate expertise is available, tracheal intubation and suction may be useful. However, if attempted intubation is prolonged or unsuccessful, start mask ventilation, particularly if there is persistent bradycardia. Vigorous infants (strong respiratory effort, heart rate >100bpm and good muscle tone) dont require ET suctioning. But if the baby is born through meconium & has depression of respiratory drive, decreased tone and a heart rate <100bpm, direct suctioning of the trachea soon after delivery is indicated. If any time heart rate is <60 bpm, don't do further ET suctions & proceed with IPPV resuscitation. These babies always require post resuscitation care under the supervision of NICU personnel to provide adequate oxygen & prevent even transient hypoxemia.

5. If the diagnosis of congenital diaphragmatic hernia is being considered, avoid bag and mask ventilation always in favour of IPPV through an endotracheal intubation. Decompression of the stomach with a large bore nasogastric tube should be instituted as soon as possible. Sedation or paralysis is helpful during ventilation of these babies. Support of the cardiac output with vasoactive agents and measures to achieve pulmonary vasodilatation are often required.

6. If the mother has received opiate analgesia more frequently than 3hrly or within 4hrs pre-delivery and if with mask resuscitation the baby becomes pink and has a good heart rate but doesn't breathe spontaneously give naloxone 100mcg/kg IV or ET and repeat 2 or 3 times if needed. Always ensure ventilation before and during administration. Naloxone must not be given to the infant of an opiate dependent mother as it can cause severe & acute withdrawl symptoms.

7. Significantly preterm babies, particularly those born below 30 weeks gestation, are a different matter. Most babies in this group are healthy at the time of delivery and yet all can be expected to benefit from help in making the transition. Intervention in this situation is usually limited to maintaining a baby healthy during this transition and is more appropriately called stabilisation. Premature & VLBW (<1000 gms) infants require additional special care like prevention of heat loss with plastic wraps, endotracheal intubation & surfactant administration as early as possible and correction of problems like hypotension, hypoglycemia and respiratory insufficiency. Always consider the possibility of airleak syndromes (tension pneumothorax & pneumopericardium) if an infant fails to respond full & proper resuscitation efforts & should be ruled out by transillumination or diagnostic thoracentesis.

8. **Shock** due to hypovolemia (intrapartal blood loss), sepsis, hypoxemia due to any cause & acidosis require immediate transfusion with 'O' - negative packed RBC 20ml/kg over 5 minutes through an umbilical venous catheter & IV Dopamine or Dobutamine to support the cardiac output. These babies always require effective ventilatory support during & after resuscitation.

9. **Infant with hydrops** demands establishment an airway & adequate respiratory support, surfactant administration, packed cells by isovolumic exchange transfusion for severe anemia, paracentesis & thoracentesis of excessive fluid in the abdomen & thorax (USG scan evaluation is necessary) & continued mechanical ventilation in NICU.

10. **Airway obstruction** is a frightening prospect in the newborn requiring resuscitation. Here bag & mask ventilation, oropharyngeal airway insertion or laryngeal mask airway can be life saving. Refer to table -1 for detailed discussion of above special situations. The LMA should be considered during resuscitation of the newborn if face mask ventilation is unsuccessful and tracheal intubation is unsuccessful or not feasible. The LMA may be considered as an alternative to a face mask for positive pressure ventilation among newborns weighing more than 2000 g or delivered ≥34 weeks gestation. There is limited evidence, however, to evaluate its use for newborns weighing < 2000 g or delivered < 34 weeks gestation. The LMA may be considered as an alternative to tracheal intubation as a secondary airway for resuscitation among newborns weighing more than 2000 g or delivered ≥34 weeks gestation. The LMA has not been evaluated in the setting of meconium stained fluid, during chest compressions, or for the administration of emergency intra-tracheal medications.

Non-initiation and discontinuation of resuscitation
Ethical considerations may cause a provider to contemplate non-initiation of resuscitation in extremely premature infants and infants with severe congenital abnormalities. For infants with confirmed gestation less than 23 weeks or birth weight less than 400 grams or in cases of anencephaly or confirmed trisomy 13 or 18, for example, resuscitation is very unlikely to result in survival, and high morbidity is likely among the rare survivors. In such cases, resuscitation is not indicated, although exceptions may be reasonable to comply with parental wishes. In conditions with uncertain prognosis in which survival is borderline, the morbidity rate is relatively high, and the anticipated burden to the child is high, parental desires concerning initiation of resuscitation should be supported. Discontinuation of resuscitation may be justified if after 10 minutes of complete and adequate resuscitative efforts, there is no heart beat and no respiratory effort. After 10 minutes of asystole, resuscitation is very unlikely to result in survival, or survival without severe disability.

Pearl/Peril/Pitfall: *Choanal atresia —Complete bilateral stenosis usually results in a Neonatal respiratory emergency at birth because infants generally are obligate nasal breathers during the first 6–8 weeks of life. At rest, these infants usually manifest severe apnea, retractions, and respiratory distress that may be relieved with crying.*

THE EVALUATION-DECISION-ACTION-PLAN/ALGORITHM IN THE EVENT OF
POOR INITIAL RESPONSE TO NEONATAL RESUSCITATION

EVALUATION			DECISION	ACTION
CHECK AIRWAY → Inadequate	- Dimished breath sounds little chest wall movement		a. Compression of airway	• Apply upward force to mandible to counteract downward force holding face mask in place ; tilt head backward
Adequate			b. Blocked ET tube	• Replace it
			c. Displaced ET tube	• Reinsert it and check for equal breath sounds in the axillae
CHECK BREA-THING → Inadequate	- Dimished breath sounds little chest wall movement		a. Inadequate face mask and seal	• Readjust face mask and seal tightly
			b. Improper face mask ventilation	• Increase insufflation pressure until breath sounds are audible and chest movement seen
			c. Insufficient insufflation pressure	
			d. Maternal opiates related CNS depression	• Give Naloxone 100mcg/kg IV or ET
Adequate	- Asymmetry of breath sounds ; transillu-mination and chest X-ray		e. Pneumothorax	• Decompress tension Pneumotho-rax with a 21 G butterfly needle through the second ICS in the midclavicular line ; follow with proper chest drain with under-water seal
CHECK CIRCU-LATION → Inadequate	- Poor Capillary Refill Time, Cyanosis, Bradycardia/Tachy-cardia		a. Hypothermia	• Dry off infant
			b. Congenital heart disease	• Arrange Echocardiogram to eva-luate the cardiac structure and function
			c. Persistent Pulmonary hypertension	
Adequate			d. Severe Anemia or Hypovolemia	• Give 20 ml/kg O Negative blood or volume expander
			e. Sepsis	• Give IV antibiotics + Inotropes
CHECK DEX-TROSE → Inadequate	- Cyanosis and poor perfusion		a. Hypoglycemia	• Give 2ml/kg 10% Dextrose bolus ; always to be followed by continuous IV infusion of 10% Dextrose
Adequate				
CHECK EQUIP-MENT → Inadequate	- Cyanosis, brady-cardia poor perfusion		a. Inadequate FiO$_2$	• Give 100% O$_2$
			b. Empty O$_2$ Cylinder	• Start new O$_2$ cylinder
			c. Disconnected O$_2$ line	• Reconnect line
			d. Disconnected IV line	• Reestablish IV line

Adequate

CONTINUE FULL RESUSCITATION IF NO CARDIAC OUTPUT AFTER 10 MINUTES OF FULL RESUSCITATION

Abandon resuscitation after discussing with the senior Neonatologist.

If the baby has a heart beat but is not making respiratory effort, artificial ventilation should continue while further information is sought.

Pearl/Peril/Pitfall: *Pierre Robin syndrome—Respiratory distress and cyanosis are caused by the obstruction of the up-per airway. In the delivery room, the infant should be given supplemental oxygen and placed in a prone position in an attempt to have the tongue move forward in a dependent fashion from the posterior pharynx, relieving the airway obstruction. If the infant continues to have persistent respiratory distress, an oral airway may be placed.*

Difficult Neonatal Airways *Must always be prepared for something abnormal*Increasing awareness of problems beforehand because of Neonatal ultrasound *Congenital malformations: <u>*"Things you can see" versus "Things you may find"*</u>

<u>"Things you can see"*</u>- Laryngomalacia, Hemangioma, or Lymphangioma, Tracheal web, Laryngeal atresia, Subglotic stenosis (illustrated v.i)

***Predictable from looking at the patient:**Cleft lip and palate *Pierre Robin syndrome *Treacher Collins syndrome *Goldenhar syndrome *Apert and Crouzon Syndrome (Photographs arranged in the respective sequence)

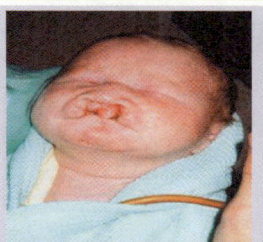 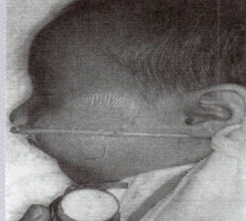 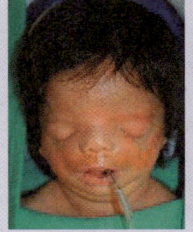 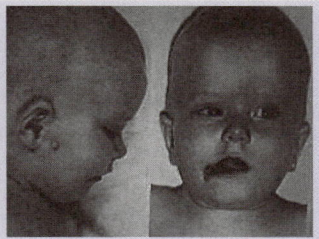

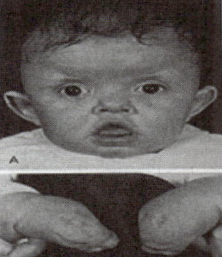 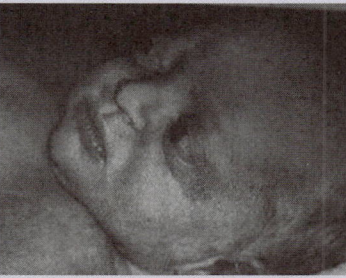 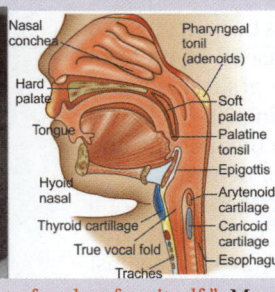

The Neonatal Airway

Compared to adults, structures are…
* Smaller
* More anterior
* Epiglottis is floppier
* Larger tongue
* Larger occiput
* Narrowest portion of airway is the cricoid

@Fear and Fumbling {Valuable Maxims}: "There is nothing to fear but fear itself." Most airway problems, even extreme, can be worked as an algorithmic sequence of steps. The best that can be done, under the circumstances, is to be done. If help can be called, do so early before the situation has utterly deteriorated. Even a small partial airway may be sufficient to stave off cerebral death until help arrives. Fall back to a simple method if it will at least temporize. Even a modest plan may be successful if continued firmly. Use *any* method in which one has confidence and experience, yet, if need be, pursue a method that seems applicable despite only textbook knowledge without experience.

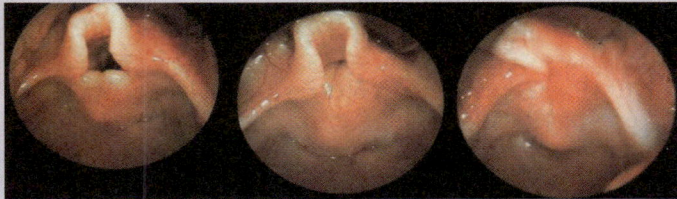

*Laryngomalacia -A sequence between fully formed to atresia

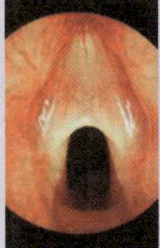 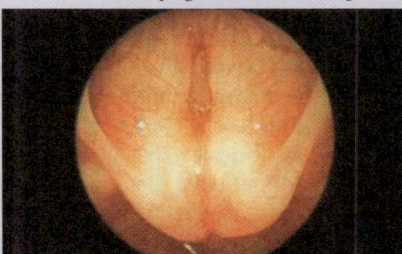 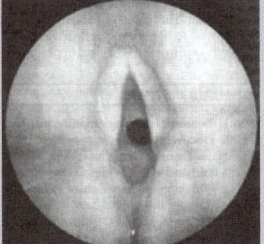 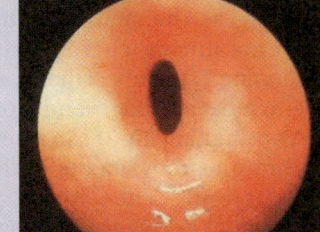

Laryngeal Web   *Tracheal atresia—Survive only   Subglottic stenosis
                  if tracheoesophageal fistula or emergent tracheostomy

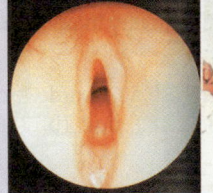 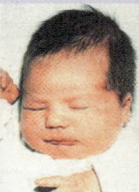 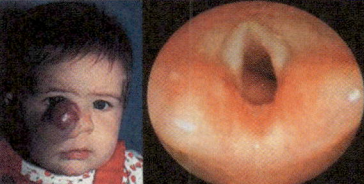

* Hemangioma or lymphangioma-only about 30% present at birth

Courtesy: Matthew L. Paden, MD Pediatric Critical Care Fellow Emory, University Children's Healthcare of Atlanta

* *Pearl/Peril/Pitfall: CDH- Delivery room management includes immediate intubation and passage of a large catheter for gastric decompression. Intubation prevents distention of the stomach and bowel contents because of crying or bag-valve-mask ventilation. The gastric decompression should be achieved with a Replogle or Salem pump suction catheter connected to a low continuous drain.*

The Laryngeal Mask Airway (LMA) offers many advantages over the face mask. Its use does not require manipulation of the patient's head, neck, and jaw. It also avoids compression of facial nerves. After positioning, the LMA is quite stable and frees the operator's hands for other important tasks. A better airtight seal is achieved with the LMA, providing more effective PPV. Its insertion technique, stable positioning, and function is not influenced by anatomical factors that may make face mask ventilation difficult, *especially in cases of congenital pathologies such as Pierre-Robin and Treacher Collins syndrome.* Less skill is required to achieve and maintain effective PPV with the LMA compared with the face mask. For proper positioning of the LMA in infants, the following steps must be followed. (1) Use the correct size of LMA for the patient. Size 1 is suitable for neonates weighing 2.5–5 kg. It has been postulated that a smaller size (0.5) could be useful in preterm newborns. However, there are reports of successful use of size 1 in preterm neonates weighing 0.8–1.5 kg. (2) Fully deflate the cuff as described in the manual, and lubricate the back of the mask tip (for neonates in the labor ward, lubrication may not be necessary, as oral and pharyngeal secretions may reproduce this function). (3) Press (flatten) the tip of the LMA against the hard palate. During this manoeuvre, the operator should grasp the LMA like a pen with the index finger at the junction between the mask and the distal end of the airway tube. (4) Gently advance the LMA with one single movement, applying continuous pressure against the palatopharyngeal curvature with the index finger. The vector of the force applied must be directed cranially and not caudally. (5) Continue pushing the LMA against the soft palate so that the cuff passes along the posterior pharyngeal wall and the tip locates itself in the hypopharynx—that is, it cannot be pushed further inwards. (6) Inflate the mask to the minimum air volume necessary to establish an adequate seal. The maximum recommended volume for each size is rarely required. Do not hold the shaft of the LMA during cuff inflation, as the shaft may be observed to move outwards during cuff inflation allowing correct positioning. (7) Connect the proximal end of the airway tube to a device (bag, ventilator) for PPV. (8) Correct LMA positioning (fig 2) can be evaluated by observing synchronous movements of the chest and by neck auscultation. The most common problem encountered during this manoeuvre is obstruction at the base of the tongue. In this case, the mask must be removed and the procedure reviewed in all its phases. Failure to follow the recommended insertion technique strictly may result in malposition of the LMA. Specifically, the epiglottis may be "downfolded", the mask lumen may not be correctly aligned with the laryngeal inlet, or the cuff may fold inwards or lie too high in the pharynx.

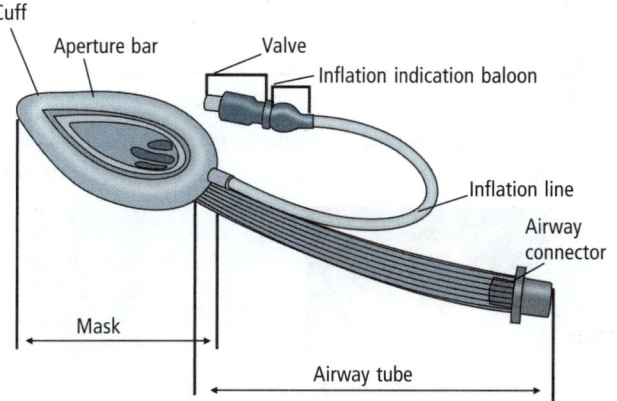

Figure 1 Basic laryngeal mask airway design. Reproduced by permission from Dr A I J Brain. Laryngeal mask instructor manual, 2000. Courtesy of The Laryngeal Mask Company Limited.

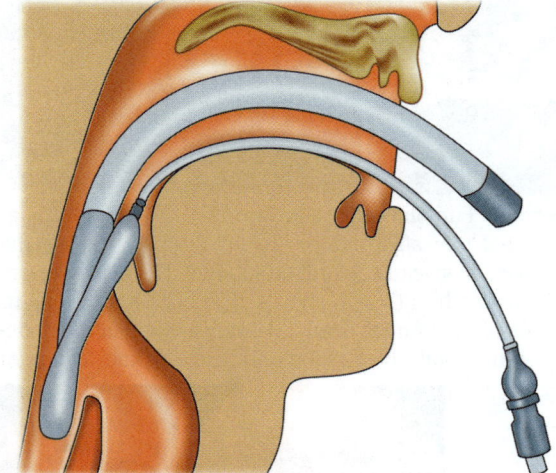

Figure 2 Demonstration of correct anatomical positioning of the laryngeal mask airway cuff around laryngeal inlet, Reproduced by permission from Dr A I J Brain, Laryngeal mask instructor manual, 2000, Courtesy of The Laryngeal Mask Company Limited.

Potential disadvantages of LMA: Gastric insufflation and aspiration, Inadequate alveolar ventilation, Impossibility of suctioning the airway or administering drugs endotracheally. Features of more recent LMA versions appear to overcome the limits of the classic device, thus producing optimal conditions for use in neonatal patients. There are currently no randomized, controlled trials on the use of the LMA during neonatal resuscitation. Although this device cannot be considered a substitute for the tracheal tube, it could, at least theoretically, play an ancillary role, particularly in situations where assistance to the asphyxiated neonate is offered by paramedical staff or doctors who, because of the rarity of the event, may have difficulty maintaining a high level of skill.

Courtesy: D Trevisanuto, M Micaglio, P Ferrarese, V Zanardo Arch Dis Child Fetal Neonatal Ed 2004;89:F485–F489. doi: 10.1136/adc.2003.038430

---

* *Pearl/Peril/Pitfall: Transillumination of the chest may be used for the rapid diagnosis of severe tension pneumothorax. In cases where the clinical situation allows, radiography should be performed to make or confirm the diagnosis. Infants in acute distress should have a needle aspiration performed to evacuate the extrapulmonary air while preparation is made to place a chest tube.*

TABLE 1 Neonatal resuscitation in specific emergencies in the delivery room

A. TERM INFANT WITH MECONIUM STAINING: Attempts to aspirate meconium from the nose and mouth of the unborn baby, while the head is still on the perineum, are not recommended. The current guidelines (American Academy of Pediatrics Neonatal Resuscitation Program Steering Committee -2010) are as follows: * If the baby is not vigorous (defined as depressed respiratory effort, poor muscle tone, and/or heart rate < 100 beats/min): Use direct laryngoscopy, intubate, and suction the trachea immediately after delivery. Suction for no longer than 5 seconds. If no meconium is retrieved, do not repeat intubation and suction. If meconium is retrieved and no bradycardia is present, reintubate and suction. If the heart rate is low, administer positive pressure ventilation and consider suctioning again later. * If the baby is vigorous (defined as normal respiratory effort, normal muscle tone, and heart rate >100 beats/min): Do not electively intubate. Clear secretions and meconium from the mouth and nose with a bulb syringe or a large-bore suction catheter. * In both cases, the remainder of the initial resuscitation steps should ensue, including drying, stimulating, repositioning, and administering oxygen as necessary.

B. TERM INFANT WITH PERINATAL ASPHYXIA: *Expand lungs immediately by proper bag and mask ventilation with 100% O_2 *Go for endotracheal intubation and ventilation, if bag and mask ventilation is ineffective or if prolonged positive pressure ventilation is necessary. *Extubate the infant, if effective spontaneous respiratory effort results and closely observe while breathing supplemental O_2 . * External cardiac massage, correction of acidosis, and circulatory support with drugs are important adjuncts to ventilation. Newly born infants born at term or near-term with evolving moderate to severe hypoxic–ischaemic encephalopathy should, where possible, be treated with therapeutic hypothermia.Treatment should be consistent with the protocols used in the randomised clinical trials, i.e. commence within 6 h, continue for 72 h and re-warm over at least 4 h. This does not affect immediate resuscitation but is important for postresuscitation care.

C. POST TERM INFANT: Postmaturity is when a baby has not yet been born after 42 weeks of gestation. Post-term, postmaturity, prolonged pregnancy, and post-dates pregnancy all refer to **post mature birth.** Post-mature births do not have any harmful effects on the mother, but the fetus, however, can begin to suffer from malnutrition. After the 42nd week of gestation, the placenta, which supplies the baby with nutrients and oxygen from the mother, starts aging and will eventually fail. Most post term infants are normal appearing; in some the most common symptoms are dry skin, overgrown nails, creases on the baby's palms and soles of their feet, minimal fat, a lot of hair on their head, and either a brown, green, or yellow discoloration of their skin. *Post term gestation infants represent about 10% of the newborn population and, as compared to term gestation infants, have an increased incidence of perinatal and neonatal problems. *Fetal distress–a sign the baby may be having problems *Macrosomia–a condition in which the baby may grow too large to pass safely through the birth canal *Meconium aspiration–a condition in which the baby passes meconium (a greenish-black waste product found in the baby's bowels) into the amniotic fluid and it gets into the baby's lungs *An increased risk of Caesarean section, which may place the mother at higher risk than having a vaginal delivery. A smaller number experience the onset of fetal wasting late in gestation and appear dysmature (post mature) at birth. The incidence of infants with dysmaturity increases as post term gestation continues; however, the prevalence of dysmaturity is greater in term infants. *The most significant neonatal problems in the post term gestation infant are the result of fetal distress and perinatal asphyxia. Those infants affected most severely may have hypoxic encephalopathy, seizures and meconium aspiration syndrome. *Other problems are birth trauma (due to the large size of some post term infants) and polycythemia. Anencephaly is associated with post term gestation. *The later intellectual development of post term gestation infants appears normal except for those with perinatal asphyxia or severe neonatal problems. *The long-term somatic growth is normal, even in dysmature-appearing infants. Post term infants are at increased risk for perinatal asphyxia; however, with careful obstetric management, most neonatal problems can be prevented. During the weeks after a baby's due date, specific tests may be performed to determine the baby's health. These may included a fetal kick count, a nonstress test or a biophysical profile. If the baby seems active and healthy, and if the amniotic fluid volume seems normal, the pregnancy may continue with the woman and baby being monitored on a regular basis. If the baby appears to be in danger, the baby should be delivered, either by inducing labor or by Caesarean birth. Labor can be induced by giving a drug to bring on labor contractions.

D. PRETERM INFANT: *Anticipate that the babies born before 32 weeks or < 1200gms may need help to establish prompt aeration and ventilation. *Go for ET intubation directly if the medical situation warrants it. *Give higher inflating pressures (25-30cms of water initially but increase this if there is no heart response and chest movement is inadequate after initial breaths. *Decrease the pressure to as low as 10-15cms water by the end of the resuscitation if the clinical course permits. *Administer surfactant intratracheally as prophylaxis for hyaline membrane disease (give it only to a stable neonate and surfactant is not a resuscitative medication). *Start Nasal CPAP @5 cm H_2O, in the delivery suite, after the initial elective intubation and surfactant administration permit a plan for early extubation,to reduce the need for reintubation, mechanical ventilation and BPD.

E. CHOANAL ATRESIA/UPPER AIRWAY OBSTRUCTION: *Suspect it if respiratory movements are made with the mouth closed but the infant fails to move air in and out of the lungs. *Open the mouth and clear the mouth and posterior of the pharynx of secretions by gentle suction . *Keep the baby in prone position and insert an oropharyngeal airway and seek the source of the obstruction immediately. *Do laryngoscopy, if effective respiratory flow is not produced by opening the infant's mouth and clearing the airway. *Insert an ET tube, with obstructive malformations of the mandible, epiglottis, larynx, or trachea.

F. DIAPHRAGMATIC HERNIA/EVENTRATION: (If diagnosed antenatally/suspected soon after delivery by a barrel chest and scaphoid abdomen) *Avoid gaseous distension of the gut. a) Paralyze, intubate, and ventilate as soon as possible (i.e. in the delivery room). Do not use positive pressure ventilation via mask or airway ; this will cause gaseous distension of the gut. b) Pass a wide bore nasogastric tube in the delivery room, ensure it is left on free drainage—aspirate every 30 minutes. Alternatively, insert a Replogle tube and use continuous suction. * Minimize factors that could precipitate pulmonary hypertension. a) Use adequate sedation b) Try to ensure adequate but gentle ventilation with low tidal volumes.

G. NARCOSIS: * Avoid narcosis by using appropriate analgesic and anesthetic practices. * Stimulate physically and secure a patent airway. * Initiate bag and mask ventilation and administer Naloxone 100mcg/kg by IV or ET and repeat 2-3 times if needed . *Ventilation is essential before and during administration of this antidote. *Continue artificial respiration until the infant is able to sustain ventilation. * Don't use CNS stimulant drugs because they are ineffective and harmful.

H. SHOCK: *Anticipate shock at birth as a result of severe asphyxia or hemorrhage during gestation, labor or delivery or from overwhelming infection. *Look for respiratory distress, cyanosis, pallor, flaccidity, cold, mottled skin, tachycardia or bradycardia, hepatosplenomegaly, and rarely, convulsions - indicative of shock . *Give O Negative blood or normal saline 20ml/kg over 5 minutes and start Dopamine / Dobutamine infusion to support cardiac output and blood pressure. *Give O_2 and correct acidosis after establishing effective ventilation. *Give appropriate antibiotics always to cover for sepsis. *Establish a specific diagnosis after the stabilization and institute appropriate continuing treatment.

I. HYDROPS FETALIS: *Ensure airway by endotracheal intubation and positive pressure mechanical ventilation. *Perform therapeutic thoracentesis /abdominocentesis to remove fluid that may further compromise respiratory effort. *Give packed cells 10ml/kg and fresh frozen plasma containing high molecular weight proteins (don't give albumin). *Start Dopamine or Dobutamine infusion and give furosemide for pulmonary edema. *Perform ECG and Echocardiography to determine the presence of cardiac abnormalities. *Perform isovolumetric partial exchange transfusion with O negative packed RBC to raise the hematocrit and improve the O_2 carrying capacity. *Monitor arterial Blood Gases, Fluid and Electrolytes, renal and hepatic function and the blood pressure + Central Venous Pressure.

J. Resuscitating at the limit of viability - *Don't resuscitate the babies born at a gestational age of <23 weeks *If there is any doubt about the gestation of the baby, resuscitation should be commenced and advice on whether to continue should be sought from a senior colleague. *Discuss the plan of management with the parents and record in the mother's notes.

*Pearl/Peril/Pitfall: Hydrops-When preparing for the resuscitation of a hydropic infant, a sufficient number of skilled personnel must be in the delivery room to ensure that the multiple needs of this significantly compromised neonate can be met.

TABLE 2	Causes of poor response to adequate resuscitation

Infant doesn't respond to IPPV and CPR + drugs at 5–10 minutes of age

The baby remains cyanosed and bradycardic

* **Technical errors**
  - ET tube; displaced/ obstructed
  - Inadequate inflation pressure
  - Too small an ET tube (2.5 mm ID)
  - Oxygen supply disconnected

* **Pneumothorax**

* **Congenital malformations that prevent oxygenation** (refer to Table 3)

* **Serious evolving lung disease**
  - Meconium aspiration syndrome
  - Congenital pneumonia
  - Severe RDS

The infant becomes active, vigorous, makes good respiratory efforts, yet fails to go pink

* Unasphyxiated baby with a serious malformations in his respiratory tract or CVS

* Persistent pulmonary hypertension with right -to-left shunting of blood through the PFO and PDA

The infant remains apneic or with very feeble respiratory efforts, hypotonic but shows good heart rate and perfusion

* Narcotic administration to mother within 4–6 hours of delivery of the baby

* CNS malformations

* Primary neuromuscular disease

* Severe antenatal brain damage

TABLE 3	Malformations causing persistent cyanosis or dyspnea after delivery

Upper respiratory tract: *Choanal atresia *Pierre Robin's syndrome *Laryngeal and tracheal malformations -Atresia - Webs-Luminal tumors - Clefts

Lung : *Pulmonary hypoplasia -Potter's syndrome -Prolonged membranes rupture -Idiopathic *Pleural effusions with or without hydrops *Congenital cystic adenomatoid malformation *Congenital lobar emphysema *Pulmonary lymphangiectasia

Extrapulmonary : * Diaphragmatic hernia * Diaphragmatic space-occupying tumors *Gross abdominal distention splinting the diaphragm-Tumors-Hepatosplenomegaly-Ascites-Dilated renal tract *Small chest -Asphyxiating thoracic dystrophy-Thanatophoric dwarfism

Infant with unexpected Congenital anomalies- Resuscitation: Unless there has been prior discussion and the development of a care plan with the parents, usually all infants should receive a complete and thorough resuscitation. Those infants with life-limiting Congenital anomalies are often best evaluated in the NICU after resuscitation when more information will be available and the parents can be part of management discussions and decision making. *It is a prerequisite that the decision not to initiate resuscitation is the consensus of all those involved. In the*

KEY POINTS FOR CLINICAL PRACTICE

1. It is useful to identify whether the depressed baby remains "cyanosed and bradycardic" or "apneic and hypotonic" but showing good cardiovascular response.

2. One should consider hypovolemia due to blood loss, severe birth asphyxia, severe cyanotic CHD, PPHN, if the poorly responsive cyanosed baby shows good chest movement.

3. Tracheal suctioning should be carried out under direct laryngoscopy, if the meconium stained baby has depressed respiration, hypotonia and a heart rate <100bpm. Suction should be limited to 3 seconds and can be repeated if meconium is aspirated and the heart rate remains >60bpm.

4. Never give Naloxone to an apneic unventilated infant and to the infant of an opiate dependent mother as it can cause acute drug withdrawal symptoms.

5. One should be as gentle as possible with the ELBW babies (i.e., drying, ventilating, and CPR)

REFERENCES & FURTHER READING: 1) *Neonatal Resuscitation Text Book, 4th edition 2000 (AHA+AAP). 2) Resuscitation of babies at birth, BMJ 1997 (RCPCH + RCOG). 3) Manual of Neonatal Respiratory Care by Dr. Sunil K. Sinha 2000. 4) Neonatology by TL Gomella (Lange-1999). 5) Nelson Text Book of Pediatrics 18th edtion 6) Illustrated Text Book of Pediatrics - 2nd edition, 2001.*

* *Pearl/Peril/Pitfall:* Severe malformations observed in the delivery room should not change the resuscitative management unless skilled and experienced care providers are able to determine that the condition is incompatible with life. The family should be involved in any decision in which no resuscitation is to occur. Infants with severe malformations should be resuscitated and stabilized until an accurate diagnosis can be made.

Sick Neonate—A Rapid Evaluation, Decision Making and Action Plan

4

@ *To cure sometimes, to relieve often, to comfort (communicate) always - Trudeau*

OBSERVE-ASSESS-DECIDE-PRIORITIZE- AND ACT EARLY, WITHIN THE TIME FRAME !

DANGER SIGNS IN A SICK NEONATE

1. Not feeding well
2. Less active than before
3. Fast breathing >60 breaths per minute
4. Slow breathing <20–30 breaths per minute/Apneas-Bradys
5. Moderate or severe chest indrawing
6. Grunting or Moaning
7. Convulsions
8. Floppy or Stiff
9. Fever (Temperature>37.5°C)
10. Cold to touch (Temperature <35.5°C or not rising after re-warming)
11. Umbilicus draining pus or Umbilical redness extending to the surrounding skin
12. More than 10 Skin pustules or bullae, or swelling, redness, or hardness of skin
13. Bleeding from umbilical stump/GIT/Urine/Airways
14. Pallor/Plethora/Central Cyanosis/Petechiae/Purpura/Poor pulses
15. Jaundice on day 1 of life

DO REMEMBER THAT...

* **No Neonate, even one on a Ventilator, is too ill for the parents to see and touch.**

* **Intensive parental support is essential, with as many counseling sessions as are needed for parents to understand their infant's condition and recommended treatment and to accept the infant psychologically.**

Indications for additional testing of sick neonates

Clinical signs	Commonly used diagnostic aids
No stool for 24 hours	Abdominal radiograph
Cyanosis, tachypnea	Arterial blood gases, CXR
Cyanosis (cardiac cause suspected)	Four-limb blood pressure and pulse oximetry, hyperoxia test, electrocardiography/ECHO
Risk factors for sepsis	Complete blood count with neutrophil differential, blood C/S
Jaundice (nonphysiologic)	ABO and D(Rh) blood-type matching (infant and mother), peripheral blood smear, direct Coomb's test.

REVIEW OF CLINICAL PROBLEMS

1. How do you recognize that a "Sick neonate" is in a state of preterminal (pre arrest) condition?

   Ans: Refer to the "No. 3" of the "BIRD'S EYE VIEW/OVERVIEW/SYNOPSIS' of the Chapter.

2. What are the signs of illness in the Newborn during first 30 to 45 minutes of life?

   Ans: Refer to the "Table 3" of the Chapter.

3. What do you consider the relevant differential diagnoses, when a previously well baby later demonstrates a rapid deterioration of his/her condition ?

   Ans: Refer to the "Table 4" of the Chapter.

4. How do you recognize and manage a "Sick Neonate" promptly and effectively ?

   Ans: Refer to the EVALUATION-DECISION-ACTION-PLAN/ALGORITHM FOR THE DIAGNOSIS AND MANAGEMENT OF "THE SICK NEONATE".

5. When do you consider "Endotracheal intubation and Mechanical ventilation", in a Sick Neonate ?

   Ans: Refer to the EVALUATION-DECISION-ACTION-PLAN/ALGORITHM FOR THE DIAGNOSIS AND MANAGEMENT OF "THE SICK NEONATE".

LEARNING OBJECTIVES

After completing this article, readers will be able to

1. Recognize conditions that put Newborns at risk for becoming ill, and provide appropriate monitoring.

2. Recognize ill Newborns.

3. Stabilize ill Newborns, and provide acute treatment.

4. Triage care of ill Newborns appropriately.

5. Arrange transport for ill Newborns when care needed is greater than the level provided at the center of birth.

Pearl/Peril/Pitfall: The practical nurse performs a vital role in caring for the sick neonate. Constant attention must be directed to the accurate observation of the neonate so that significant changes may be reported immediately. Their survival, and perhaps their quality of life, is entrusted to the knowledge, skill, and expertise of the health care team.

BIRD'S EYE VIEW/OVERVIEW/SYNOPSIS

1. A 'Sick Neonate' whether brought to the health care facility from home, transferred from another institution or postnatal ward, or brought from the delivery room as a result of a complicated birth demands a *rapid and effective* Evaluation - Decision - Action clinical planning. This is a crucial assessment skill that must be exercised by the pediatrician/neonatologist, because of the rapidity of deterioration and the subtlety of the changes shown by the Newborn baby. *Missing subtle changes in the immediate postnatal period leads to serious morbidity and/or mortality.*

2. A *rapid and effective* evaluation of a potentially sick Newborn baby demands **a)** anticipation of problems in a high-risk neonate **b)** Primary assessment of airway, breathing, circulation, disability, exposure and evaluate further with speed and skill **c)** secondary and serial assessment of ongoing/new problems **d)** decision making appropriate to the most probable diagnosis and differential diagnosis **e)** provision of immediate and essential management to reduce morbidity and/or mortality.

3. The caring physician should always pay prompt attention to identify *preterminal illness* manifested as **a)** Apneic baby, gasping and with respiratory rate <20 bpm **b)** Shock (pallor, cold to touch, CRT >5 sec, heart rate <100bpm / > 180bpm, extremely lethargic or unconscious) **c)** Bleeding and/or unresponsive baby and intervene with appropriate resuscitation of ABCDs promptly.

4. One should be aware of the fact that recognizing disease in the Newborn infants depends on the knowledge of the disorder and evaluation of a limited number of relatively 'nonspecific' clinical signs and symptoms for e.g.: Central cyanosis has respiratory, cardiac, CNS, hematologic, and metabolic causes while acute renal failure can be a complication of a preexisting cardiac, respiratory failure or NEC with third space losses, in addition to intrinsic causes.

5. One should anticipate disease in the Newborn baby from **a)** Common prenatal warning signs for illness (listed in Table 1) **b)** Failure of the baby to follow the expected postnatal *transitional period* (refer to Table 3) and **c)** Infant's postnatal age at the time the abnormal findings are first recognized. The mother who is constantly with the baby may notice subtle changes in the baby's condition. Listen to her comments and reexamine the baby at any time if there is concern. Nursing and pediatric providers must be aware of the pattern and progression of infant's symptoms and signs and establish nursery protocols and flow sheets that allow for early recognition of abnormalities.

6. Neonatal problems can be identified early either by failure of normal postnatal pattern to be seen immediately after birth or by failure of this pattern to disappear by 45 to 60 minutes of life (refer to Table 2 and Table 3).

7. Tables 1 and 5 provide the information about the myriad of possible findings on both the history and physical examination of the Newborn baby. These findings suggest the range of those that require parental reassurance at most, to those suggesting genuine alarm that the neonate is sick mostly. Alarming findings on history and physical examination should make the physician to identify the clinical indications for admitting a Newborn baby to the NICU. (Refer to Table 6 for the clinical indications). The most important manifestations of a "Sick Neonate" include a) apnea b) tachypnea c) grunting d) bradycardia e) central cyanosis f) hypotonia g) decreased breath sounds h) heart murmurs i) organomegaly j) pallor or plethora k) jaundice l) diffuse petechiae m) evident anomalies other than of ears and digits.

8. Decision making should start from the first impression (appearance - breathing - circulation) of the Neonate and if a problem is identified, perform necessary interventions - *"treat as you find."* Decision making is a dynamic process, which depends on the ongoing assessment of ABCDs. The *Evaluation - Decision - Action Plan / Algorithm* describes the essential aspects of recognizing the Sick Neonate and appropriate management promptly and effectively to prevent mortality and morbidity. *If poor oxygen saturation despite supplemental oxygen >0.6 to 0.7 FiO$_2$ irregular respirations, or apnea is seen, the Neonate needs immediate intubation and IPPV. Then treat shock as per NALS guidelines (volume expansion with NS, 5% albumin, vasopressors and corticosteroids) and correct hypoglycemia (IV 10% dextrose 2ml/kg bolus, to be followed by an IVI of 10% dextrose @ 6–8 mg/kg/minute), hypothermia, anemia, convulsions and administer IV antibiotics to cover for possible sepsis.* After this, one should continue to reassess the baby for ongoing problems to categorize the findings and to treat priority findings first. Avoid excessive handling and unnecessary stimulation of an already stressed infant and provide a neutral thermal environment and always observe infant for apnea and hypotension during warming.

9. Many babies, initially appear well, but deteriorate suddenly ('crash' or 'crump') because of various causes which are listed in Table 4. Always look for signs of a Tension Pneumothorax such as *shift of cardiac apical impulse *decreased breath sounds on the affected side *asymmetric subcostal retractions and chest wall movement *ballooning of the chest on the affected side * increased halo of light with transillumination *cardiovascular changes: hypotension, narrow pulse pressure, bradycardia, tachycardia. Although murmurs are present in a large percentage of healthy Newborns during the first day of life secondary to the closing ductus arteriosus, *a murmur in the presence of cyanosis, poor perfusion, or poor pulses is often associated with cardiac disease.* A complete physical examination, FBC, ABG analysis, CXR, AXR, ultrasound of suspected parts and ECG will indicate the need and direction for further investigation and management.

10. The outcome of an ill newborn depends on the underlying condition, the promptness with which it is recognized, and timely institution of treatment. The generalist must be able to distinguish symptoms of illness and meticulously follow a careful, logical approach to the initial evaluation and stabilization of ill Newborns, with appropriate triage to other providers and facilities that are appropriate to the level of care needed.

---

* ***Pearl/Peril/Pitfall:*** *When an infant has a birth defect, the parents should see the infant as soon after birth as possible, regardless of the medical condition. Otherwise, they may imagine the appearance and condition to be much worse than the reality.*

THE EVALUATION-DECISION-ACTION-PLAN/ALGORITHM FOR THE DIAGNOSIS AND MANAGEMENT OF *"THE SICK NEONATE"*.

SUBJECTIVE FINDINGS

Hx of presenting symptoms - determine the onset, duration, progression and severity.

Hx of delivery details such as gestational age, birth weight, mode of delivery/assisted ?, prolonged 2nd stage, APGAR scores, PROM, resuscitation details, maternal medications and illnesses.

Hx of antenatal period - maternal and fetal status (clinical, biochemical and biophysical) and review for high-risk problems.

Listen to mother's comments about the baby's symptoms. Always, as she may notice subtle changes in the baby's condition and re-examine the baby at any time if there is concern.

Review: the nursing observations such as O_2 sats., TPR chart, blood sugars, bowels open?, passing urine ? etc.

OBJECTIVE FINDINGS

Assess ABCDs and monitor CRT, O_2 sats, BP, core-peripheral temperature difference, RR, HR, central and peripheral pulses, urine output.

Determine whether the baby is in preterminal ("pre arrest") conditions such as apnea, gasping or RR <20 bpm, shock, extremely lethargic or unresponsive limpy baby, bleeding, etc. and intervene with appropriate resuscitation of ABCDs promptly.

Note the other alarming signs such as convulsions, irritability, pallor, central cyanosis, hypothermia, abdominal distention, bilious vomiting, petechiae and ecchymoses, vesicles, etc.

Note: dysmorphic features (facies), obvious congenital malformations/evidence for birth trauma/stigmata of congenital infections

Perform: systemic examination quickly to identify the problems which require emergent life saving procedures such as pneumothorax, upper airway obstruction, bowel obstruction, PDA, etc.

INVESTIGATIONS

Blood FBC, differential, platelets, *hematocrit*, reticulocyte count, Group and type and cross match, Smear, coagulation screen (PT, APTT, fibrinogen, thrombin time, bleeding time and clotting time), blood cultures, ABG analysis, *Blood sugar*, BUN, creatinine, electrolytes, Ca^{++} Mg^{++}, LTFs, drug screen

Urine analysis

Imaging CXR, plain abdominal x-ray, USG scan/CT scan of head,

Perform partial sepsis screen (**defer LP**)-FBC, CRP, blood and urine cultures, CXR, etc.

Consider ECG, 2D ECHO, MRI brain scan, USG Abdomen, metabolic screen, *when clinical course demands.*

SICK NEONATE

Provide: Supplemental oxygen by oxyhood to maintain oxygen saturation between 88–95% range; consider CPAP up to 8 cm H_2O, if >60% FiO_2 is required to keep O_2 sat >90%.

Intubate and ventilate if: a) Severe respiratory distress causing exhaustion or depression leading to apneas b) Failure of CPAP with >60% FiO_2 in a preterm baby or >70–80% FiO_2 in a term baby c) Unresponsive and limpy baby d) shock and hypotension e) bleeding from airways, etc.

Start: IV broadspectrum antibiotics to cover for possible sepsis in any sick Neonate, after partial sepsis screen done

Call for additional help: to perform essential medical procedures such as, a) venous access and UAC insertion b) monitoring (BP, ECG, and respiratory) c) organization of relevant investigations, etc.

Review : The list of differential diagnoses again after receiving the results of the initial investigations(e.g. blood glucose) and after observing the baby's response to initial treatment. Make any changes in treatment that may be necessary.

Explain to both parents: The reason for admission and the care the baby is receiving and *inform* consultant of all high-risk admissions or where there is a major congenital malformation.

Document all information when time permits: including the findings of the history, examination, and laboratory investigations, treatment given, changes in baby's condition.

Listen to the parents: allow them to express their reactions as they compare their "dream" infant with the real infant they now have (sick, too tiny, not the right sex, deformed, premature)

Perform appropriate triage care of sick Newborns and arrange transport to the higher center where and when necessary

Ensure ABCs- CR and apnea monitor, supplemental O_2 Pulse oximetry, monitor BP, CRT, temperature and blood sugar.

Treat Shock as per NALS guidelines (fluids, FFP, and inotropes)

Correct hypothermia, acid-base and electrolyte disturbances and control seizures if any.

Correct hypoglycemia with IV 10% dextrose 2ml/kg (4ml/kg in the presence of convulsions) bolus, to be followed by an IVI of 10% dextrose @ 8mg/kg/minute to 12mg/kg/minute.

Treat Anemia due to blood loss with PRBC 15–20 mL/Kg and maintain the hematocrit >40%.

Treat a Neonate with upper GIT bleeding with IV inj. Vitamin K 2mg along with FFP 10 ml/kg every 12–24 hr, IV inj. Ranitidine 1mg/kg every 12 hr and monitor PT, PTT, platelets and fibrinogen levels.

If an acute abdomen is suspected put the baby on nil oral, NG tube decompression continuously and reliably, IV fluids + inotropes + IV antibiotics and *consult* Pediatric surgeon.

Perform focused examination and search for , findout and treat the treatable/reversible causes.

Identify life-threatening underlying conditions such as Pneumothorax, duct-dependent cardiac lesions, diaphragmatic hernia, tracheoesophageal fistula etc., and manage them accordingly! (*refer to the individual chapters for details*)

Avoid excessive handling organize care and interventions to avoid frequent, unnecessary stimulation of an already stressed infant.

Perform an ongoing assessment (Monitor and reassess and document)
* airway patency, oxygen saturation, *vital signs.
* breathing effectiveness. *pulse rate and quality, perfusion status, cardiac rhythm. *capillary refill.
* mental status and activity level.
* emergency care interventions.

Pearl/Peril/Pitfall: Neonatal Alteration of Sensorium and DD: **Traumatic:** Nonaccidental injury (e.g. shaken baby)– Accidental injury, **Non-traumatic:***Infection*– Inborn errors of metabolism– Metabolic disorders– Status epilepticus– Congenital heart disease– Hypertensive encephalopathy– Kernicterus– Brain malformations– Hypoxic-ischemic injury– Exogenous toxins.

TABLE 1	Common prenatal warning signs for illness in newborns
Sign	**Conditions in newborn**
Oligohydramnios	Severe placental insufficiency, congenital renal aplasia or dysplasia, pulmonary dysplasia
Polyhydramnios	Spina bifida, high intestinal obstruction, severe neurologic lesion impairing fetal swallowing
Membrane rupture before labor	Infection, large amniotic fluid volume, placental abruption, Fetal infection, Fetal anemia
Fetal tachycardia	Maternal drug injections, maternal fever
Absent, diminished Fetal movements	Fetal neurologic injury, neuromuscular defect, hypoxemia
Maternal diabetes	Fetal anomalies, hypoglycemia, polycythemia, macrosomia with birth injury
Maternal bleeding	Abruptio placentae, placenta previa, and vasa previa or cord traction injury may have associated fetal anemia or hypovolemic shock
Maternal smoking	Small-for-gestational-age infant with hypoglycemia, polycythemia
Maternal drug (cocaine) use	Fetal and neonatal strokes
Forceps delivery	Mechanical injuries, skull fractures, brain lacerations, subarachnoid and subdural bleeding
Vacuum extractor	Bruising and bleeding of the scalp ("chignon"), sub galeal hemorrhage
Oxytocin	Hyperstimulation of the uterus with fetal hypoxia, uterine rupture

TABLE 2	Normal patterns of activity during postnatal period in a healthy infant - 3 transitional levels

A. First 15 to 30 minutes
1. Immediate tachycardia to 160 to 180 beats per minute, with a gradual drop to 100 to 120 beasts per minute.
2. Irregular respirations, tachypnea to 60 to 80 respirations per minute, brief moments of apnea.
3. Moist-sounding lung fields, transient grunting and retraction.
4. Awake, moving, alert, easily, startled, crying, transient tremors.

B. Next 60 to 90 minutes
1. Sleepy or sleeping, somewhat unresponsive.
2. Heart rate 100 to 120 beats per minute, transient tachycardia.
3. Respiratory rate 50 to 60 respirations per minute, transient tachypnea.
4. Usually, passage of meconium.

C. Next 10 to several minutes
   Again, awake, alert, easily startled, crying, easily stimulated, and reactive.

D. At last, behaving like a baby
   "over" being born, eager for feeding and the world, and eager, at times, for sleep.

TABLE 3	Signs of illness in the Newborn during first 30 to 45 Minutes of Life
Sign	**Illness**
Decreased activity, quiet, poorly reactive	***with low respiratory and heart rate:*** maternal medications, prenatal neurologic impairment traumatic brain injury during delivery ***with tachypnea and tachycardia:*** fetal infection with septic shock, fetal anemia and hypovolemic shock
Cardiogenic shock (rare)	diminished or absent pulmonary blood flow combined with an absence of available shunts (e.g. pulmonary atresia with intact septum)
Respiratory distress	lung lesion ***present at birth,*** including: pulmonary hypoplasia, congenital diaphragmatic hernia cystic adenomatoid malformation ***condition initiated at or immediately before birth:*** clear amniotic fluid, blood, or meconium aspiration

Pearl/Peril/Pitfall: PPHN must be considered whenever a late preterm, term, or postdated neonate presents with hypoxia. Indicators of intrauterine or perinatal stress, such as the presence of meconium, acidosis, respiratory depression at birth, and signs or symptoms indicative of infection, are important findings.

| TABLE 4 | Neonates who present with sudden deterioration (Acute Collapse) |

A. Baby on Mechanical Ventilator

Consider the following possibilities

    i. Hypo/Single Lung ventilation due to blockage of an endotracheal tube, displacement, disconnected ventilator, etc.

    ii. Large Air leak-Pneumothorax/Pneumomediastinum which is detected by transillumination or radiograph.

    iii. Intracranial hemorrhage which is detected by full fontanel, falling hematocrit, metabolic acidosis, cranial ultrasound, etc.

    iv. Pneumonia/Sepsis / Meningitis/Worsening RDS

B. Baby Breathing Spontaneously

Consider the following possibilities

    i. Overwhelming infection either bacterial or viral

    ii. Massive hemorrhage, e.g. subcapsular hematoma of liver, pulmonary hemorrhage, IVH, Adrenal hemorrhage, etc.

    iii. Congenital heart disease which is precipitated by the closure of ductus arteriosus

    iv. Necrotizing enterocolitis (NEC)

    v. Metabolic problems, e.g. hyperammonemia, hypoglycemia, hypocalcemia, CAH, etc.

| TABLE 5 | Levels of surveillance of the newborn based on examination findings |

LEVEL OF SURVEILLANCE

Characteristic	Normal	Alert	Alarm
Respiration		Paradoxical, periodic, or retractions	Apnea, expiratory grunt flaring alae nasi
Circulation	Acrocyanosis, heart rate 110–165 beats/min	Tachycardia, or Cardiac murmur	Central cyanosis, pallor Hypertension, Bradycardia Hypotension, enlarged heart
Behavior	*Awake*:crying, active quiet alert *asleep*:active, indeterminate quiet	Hyperalert, lethargic	Stupor, coma
Tone	Obtuse popliteal angle	Limp in upright suspension	Limp in ventral suspension
Posture	Flexor, symmetrical	Extensor, asymmetrical	Obligatory, decerebrate
Movement	All extremities, non-repetitive, random symmetrical	Jitteriness, tremor	Seizures
Reflexes	Active, symmetrical	Asymmetrical	Absent
Sensory	Pinprick response slow	Equivocal	No response
Metabolism	body temperature of 95.9°F to 99.5°F (36.5°C - 37.5°C)	Hyperthermia	Hypothermia
Digestion	Drooling or transitional stools	Spitting	Vomiting or diarrhea
Excretion		No voiding(>24 hr) and no stooling(>24 hr)	Dribbling stream
Jaundice	>24 hr	18 to 24 hr	<18 hr
Skin pustules	Erythema toxicum		Large and dermal
Vesicles			Any
Nodules		Subcutaneous fat necrosis	Sclerema
Desquamation	Delicate scaling > 2 days	peeling < 2 days	Denuded sheets any time
Hemorrhage	Petechiae(head or upper body)	petechiae(elsewhere)	Ecchymoses and purpura
Liver	Smooth edge		Enlarged
Spleen	Nonpalpable	Palpable	Enlarged
Kidneys	Lobulated or palpable (lower poles)	Horseshoe	Enlarged

Pearl/Peril/Pitfall: Noninvasive diagnostic testing, such as chest radiography, and basic laboratory evaluation, such as blood gas analysis and complete blood count, can also guide therapy and direct the urgency of interventions IN A SICK NEONATE. It is essential that these early pieces of information are obtained in the most accurate manner possible.

| TABLE 6 | Indications for admitting a baby to the NICU |

Babies requiring immediate admission to the Neonatal unit from the labor suite or immediately after delivery elsewhere
- Infants <1800 g or <34 weeks gestation
- Infants who appear unstable and cause concern/require intensive care
- Suspected significant perinatal asphyxia
- Respiratory problems—if a baby has any two of the following respiratory signs between 1 and 4 h of age, it should be admitted for further investigation
  * tachypnea>70 bpm
  * grunting
  * central cyanosis
  * recession
- Congenital abnormalities - where intensive care is anticipated or diagnosis of multiple anomalies is in doubt.
- Hemolytic disease where exchange transfusion is likely.
- Consider admitting where there is unexplained death of sibling in first week of life
- Chorioamnionitis, i.e. presence of maternal pyrexia, purulent liquor and prolonged rupture of membranes

Admit from postnatal wards
- Convulsions, apneic or cyanotic attacks • Respiratory distress (including grunting) at or beyond 4 h of age
- Hypoglycemia not responding to regular 3-hourly feeds of breast milk or formula milk at a total volume of 90 ml/kg per day • Spontaneous bleeding • Jaundice requiring exchange transfusion • Major feeding problem and/or vomiting • Any bile - stained vomit • Low temperature (<36° C) not responding to measures available on postnatal ward

---

Common differential diagnoses for the alarming symptoms in the sick neonate

1. **Pallor:** anemia, acute hemorrhage, hypoxia, asphyxia, hypoglycemia, sepsis, shock, or adrenal failure

2. **Central cyanosis:** pulmonary conditions, CNS depression, cyanotic CHD or methemoglobinemia, PPHN, hypoglycemia, sepsis and shock

3. **Apnea:** respiratory distress, sepsis, hypoglycemia, pulmonary/CNS bleed, cardiac failure, hypo/hyper natremia, hypothermia, drug induced, GE reflux, idiopathic.

4. **Hypotension:** shock from hypovolemia, SIRS (sepsis, IU infection), cardiac dysfunction, pneumothorax, pericardial effusion, hypoglycemia, salt - losing CAH

5. **Lethargy :** infection, asphyxia, hypoglycemia, hypercapnia, sedation, cerebral defect, any severe disease including inborn errors of metabolism

6. **Irritability:** meningeal irritation, acute abdomen, drug withdrawal, infections, congenital glaucoma, hypoxia, hypoglycemia, hypocalcemia, CNS damage, GE reflux, cold exposure.

7. **Convulsions:** CNS disorder, hypoglycemia, hypocalcemia, drug withdrawal, hypo/hyper natremia, pyridoxine dependence, inborn errors of metabolism.

8. **Jaundice:** physiologic, septicemia, TORCH, hemolytic anemia, galactosemia, EHBA, etc.

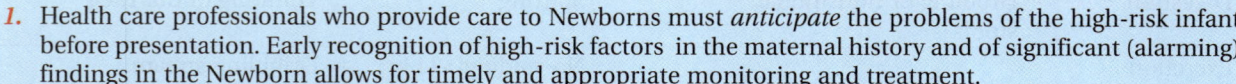

KEY POINTS FOR CLINICAL PRACTICE

1. Health care professionals who provide care to Newborns must *anticipate* the problems of the high-risk infant before presentation. Early recognition of high-risk factors in the maternal history and of significant (alarming) findings in the Newborn allows for timely and appropriate monitoring and treatment.

2. The goal of active anticipation and intervention is to prevent the development or progression of more serious illness and to minimize the risk of both morbidity and mortality in the high-risk Newborn.

3. If an infant is critically ill, it is essential to intervene rapidly and effectively in order to stabilize the infant, following the standard ABCDs {Airway - Breathing - Circulation - Disability (don't ever forget dextrose)}. Once stabilized, it is important to reassess the baby's condition serially and manage the ongoing problems.

4. It is useful to follow a single system of evaluation and stabilization that is acceptable in most infants. However in some special conditions, special therapies apply (e.g., IVI Prostin therapy for a duct dependent cardiac malformation).

5. It is extremely important to communicate with the parents about the baby's condition, management plan, and the arrangements for the transport of ill Newborn to a higher Neonatal center, if necessary.

REFERENCES AND FURTHER READING: 1) Core curriculum for Neonatal intensive care nursing , 3rd edition. 2) Klaus and Fanaroff Care of the high-risk Neonate. 3) Primary care of the Newborn, 4th edition. 4) Wong's essentials of pediatric nursing, 7th edition.

Pearl/Peril/Pitfall: Nursing assessment of the newborn with cyanosis or hypoxia should initially include as many noninvasive assessments as possible, including a full evaluation of all systems, and careful acquisition of vital signs and pulse oximeter readings. These assessments not only guide diagnosis but also direct the urgency of medical interventions.

Stabilization and Transport of Critically Ill Newborns

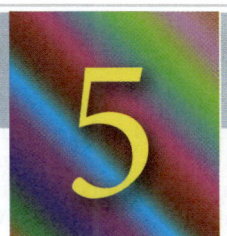

@ *Safe and expedient transport is a key component of an effective system for neonatal critical care. The best outcomes are thought to be dependent on four inter-related mechanisms: the ability of clinicians to discern when delivery is imminent to ensure in-utero transport; the ability of clinicians to stabilize and sustain the neonate until the transport team arrives; the rapid response of the team itself; and the skill and expertise of the transport team members. When these components are effectively organized, the highest level of support and care can be provided while the neonate travels to the NICU.*

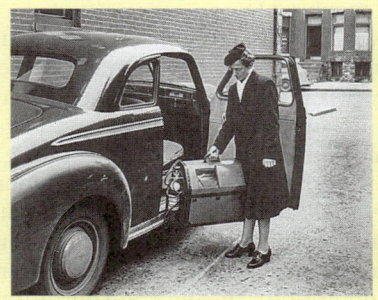

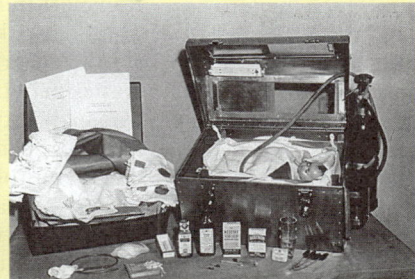

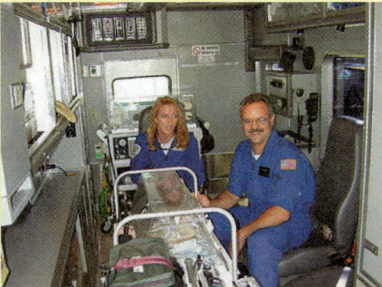

Early Neonatal Transport Technology; Typically, these incubators were hand-carried, and were moved from home to hospital by car or train

Interior of an ambulance configured for neonatal ground transport.Note the excellent patient access and equipment availability.

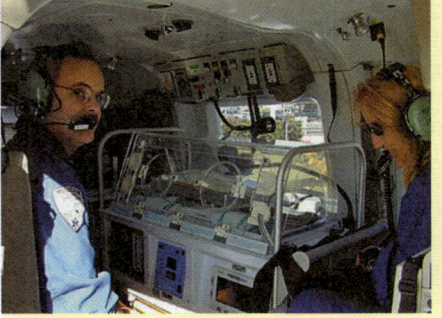

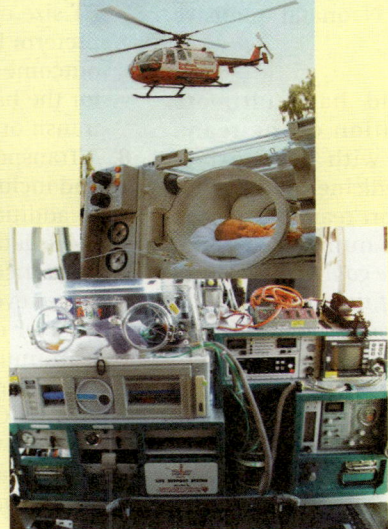

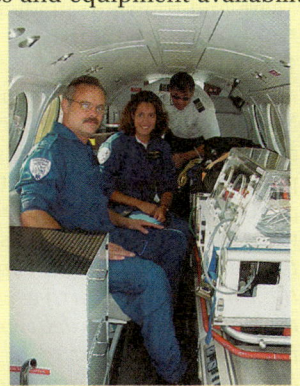

Interior of a rotor-wing aircraft (helicopter) configured for neonatal transport. A flight incubator and 2 crew members are on board.

Interior of a fixed-wing aircraft configured for neonatal transport. A flight incubator and 2 crew members are on board.

REVIEW OF CLINICAL PROBLEMS

1. What are the contraindications for "in-utero transfer" to the tertiary center ?
   Ans: Refer to the Table 6 of the Chapter.

2. Describe the responsibilities of the doctor in the referring hospital.
   Ans: Refer to the Table 8 of the Chapter.

3. What precautions should you take while transporting a Neonate born, with either exomphalos/ gastroschisis /myelomeningocele ?
   Ans: Refer to the Table 4 of the Chapter.

4. How do you ensure the safe transport for infants under 1,000g birth weight ?
   Ans: Refer to the 7 of the "BIRD'S EYE VIEW/ OVERVIEW/SYNOPSIS"of the Chapter.

5. Mention the principles of stabilization of the sick Neonate, before transporting to the higher center.
   Ans: Refer to the Tables 1 and 2 of the Chapter.

LEARNING OBJECTIVES

After completing this article, readers will be able to:

1. Understand the responsibilities of the referring hospital and its personnel during the transport of a Neonate and prepare the hospital to fulfill these responsibilities.

2. Provide high-quality, short-term care of a Neonate before transport.

3. Support the emotional needs of the family of a transported Neonate.

4. Manage convalescing Neonates after back transport.

5. Support the education and training of nursery staff to stabilize infants optimally in preparation for transport.

* *Pearl/Peril/Pitfall: For infants expected to require treatment in a level 2 or level 3 institution, maternal transfer prior to delivery is usually wiser than a postnatal transfer exceptions apply where the pregnancy complication is of such a severe degree that any delay in delivery would jeopardize the survival or quality of survival of the infant or mother, or where delivery might occur during the transfer.*

BIRD'S EYE VIEW/OVERVIEW/SYNOPSIS

1. Ideally, high-risk mothers should be transported to and their babies delivered at centers where specialized Neonatal intensive care facilities are available. With few exceptions the best portable incubator for the high - risk fetus is the uterus, with delivery of the infant where support and expertise are readily available. The indications for antenatal (in utero) transfer are listed in table 5, and the clinical situations in which in utero transfer is undesirable are included in table 6.

2. However, consideration should be given to the postnatal transfer of the high-risk Neonates born at a base hospital not having special care/intensive care facilities (refer to table 7 for the high-risk categories of Neonates needing specialized transport).

3. Transport of sick, newborn infants is a hazardous procedure and should not be left to the most junior member of the team. The transport team should consist of :
   * a transport co-ordinator (who may be either a senior doctor or nurse);
   * a doctor who is experienced in Neonatal intensive care and transport medicine;
   * an experienced nurse.
   Transport coordinators should have ultimate responsibility for the composition of the team. Neonatal nurse practitioners, with appropriate additional training in transport medicine, may take the place of doctors on some transport teams. If special problems are anticipated, the number of team members should be increased. *The goal of a transport team is to provide total support of the Newborn from the time the team arrives at the referring hospital to the time the infant is delivered to the receiving hospital. In fact, the transport team should be an extension of the intensive care nursery, and at no time should the infant be compromised by the transport process itself.*

4. Communication is the most important principle of transporting the sick newborn.
   * Never either directly or by implication criticize the referring doctor's management.
   * The transport team must introduce themselves to parents and explain the nature of the transport, treatment and likely prognosis ; encourage parents to touch their baby and offer them a digital photograph if possible.
   * The retrieval staff must be sensitive to needs of the parents during this stressful period and in relating to referral hospital personnel.
   * A debriefing with referring staff is an essential component of quality management.
   * Smooth communication and relationship between referring and receiving units are essential for effective regionalization of care.

5. The responsibilities of the doctor in referring hospital and those of Neonatal transport team are listed in the table 8.

6. Equipment and drugs for transport teams should be kept in state of readiness and should be regularly checked to ensure that electrical equipment is charged, gas supplies are adequate and drugs are not out of date. A comprehensive range of equipment and drugs should be taken to ensure that full intensive care is available to the infant during transport (refer to table 11).

7. The high-risk Neonate should be resuscitated and stabilized prior to transport. The preparation for transport, the principles of stabilization and transportation are summarized on the next page. Most of the infants under 1000g birth weight have a greater morbidity, and mortality, their safe transport requires greater vigilance and proficiency of the transporting team. Most of these infants will require assisted ventilation during transfer, and they are more likely to deteriorate during transportation. They are more vulnerable to cold stress, hypoglycemia, and ET tube blockage (due to narrow ET size of 2–2.5mm). For the transfer of extremely preterm infants (22–24 weeks' gestation) when the outcome appears unfavorable, it may be preferable for the baby to stay with its parents and not die in transit or in a distant hospital away from them.

8. A Transport Log should be kept by the receiving unit and include the information given in the table 12 . In addition to acting as a record of the transport, these data can be used for internal audit and quality assurance measures.

9. Never ever neglect parents during the heat of the transfer of their high-risk Neonate. The transport team must be able to lucidly explain the infant's condition, prognosis, and treatment plans to the parents. Clearly, communication before, during, and after the transport are of paramount importance.
   * Have plans for transfer been discussed with parents?
   * Have parents been given written information which
     includes contact numbers for the referral unit ?
   * Do parents have digital photographs of their baby?
   * Has a contact number for parents been obtained ?
   * Has surgical consent been obtained if required ?
   * Has a sample of maternal blood been obtained to cross-match blood for the baby at the receiving unit?

10. Transporting babies with special problems require specific interventions in addition to the general intensive care that is necessarily to be provided. The special problems include a) diaphragmatic hernia b) esophageal atresia with TE fistula c) exomphalos/gastroschisis/myelomeningocele d) bowel obstruction e) Pierre Robin sequence/ Choanal atresia (refer to the next page for details).

Pearl/Peril/Pitfall: Ventilation is individualized to the Newborn aiming for adequate, though not excessive, chest movement and normal arterial blood gases. Again, talk to the retrieval service if in doubt. If you have an infant ventilator available you could start with an inspiratory pressure of 20 cm of H2O and end expiratory pressure set at 5 cm of H_2O with a rate of 30/min (term newborn) or 60/min (preterm newborn). Inspiratory pressure should be titrated to chest movement, oxygenation and $PaCO_2$.

THE PRINCIPLES AND PRACTICE OF THE TRANSPORT OF HIGH-RISK NEONATE

TABLE 1   Preparation for transport

The infant should be resuscitated and his condition stabilized prior to transport. While awaiting transfer the referring hospital should provide the following care :

1. The infant is kept warm (ideally servo-controlled to a skin temperature of 36.5°C). Bubble plastic may help to reduce heat loss;
2. The infant is given sufficient oxygen to maintain a pink color (cyanotic threshold test is useful). If blood-gas analysis is available, the arterial oxygen tension should be maintained at 50-80 mmHg (6.7-9.7 kPa). Oxygen saturation should be maintained > 90%.
3. Ensure a clear airway by adequate suction;
4. Ensure adequate respiration;
5. Frequent observations of temperature, heart rate, respiratory rate, blood pressure and blood sugar by reagent stick ;
6. Procedures for surgical patients :
   a. attention to fluids and electrolytes ;
   b. intravascular volume ;
   c. special requirements ; *vide infra*
7. Intravenous dextrose with maintenance of blood glucose > 45mg/dL
8. Prostaglandin E (PGE) infusion, if possibility of duct-dependent cyanotic heart disease.

TABLE 2   Principles of stabilization

* Don't waste time, power, O_2 or air.

* Be aware of the difficulties of detecting and correcting problems in transit and ensure appropriate stabilization before transport.

* Before leaving, the referring hospital should provide the following :

1. perinatal history sheet, completed in detail ;

2. signed parental consent for the infant's transfer and treatment

3. copies of relevant records and results of tests, including X-rays;

4. 10 ml of clotted blood from the mother to allow accurate cross-matching prior to surgery or exchange transfusion;

5. cord blood if available ;

6. placenta if available

TABLE 3   Principles of transportation

1. ensure complete resuscitation and stabilization of the infant prior to transport ;
2. procedures such as insertion of an intravenous line or umbilical artery catheter, intubation, mechanical ventilation and digital photography of the baby for the mother are performed prior to transport if indicated ;
3. the baby is not fed during transport and the stomach is aspirated prior to leaving the referring hospital. Gastric tube remains *in situ* ;
4. frequent gastric and pharyngeal suction is necessary to prevent aspiration ;
5. an intravenous (i.v.) line with 10% dextrose is set up prior to transfer to prevent hypoglycemia ;
6. if oxygen is necessary, it should ideally be warmed

and humidified ; drain Pneumothorax if significant clinically.
7. the percentage of inspired oxygen should be measured with an oxygen analyser ;
8. a head box should be used if greater than 30% inspired oxygen is necessary ;
9. oxygenation should be monitored continuously by either pulse oximetry or transcutaneous PO_2 especially in a premature baby
10. monitoring of temperature, heart rate and respiratory rate is essential, and monitoring of blood pressure is desirable.
11. check blood gases, correct metabolic abnormalities, remedy hypotension with plasma expanders or DOPAMINE and control infusions.

TABLE 4   Transporting babies with special problems

1. *Diaphragmatic hernia:*Never give bag and mask ventilation. Pass NG tube and aspirate frequently to decompress stomach contents. If possible, very high ambient oxygen environments are preferable to ventilation because of the risk of Pneumothorax. *If mechanical ventilation is necessary, it should be through a carefully positioned ET tube. Correct acidosis before departure and consider paralysis if hypoxic.*

2. *Esophageal atresia with TE fistula:* Never feed the baby and empty the blind - ending of the upper pouch by an indwelling nasopharyngeal tube. Use pacifier to limit crying. Nurse the infant prone with body elevated to 30° from the horizontal.

3. *Exomphalos / gastroschisis / myelomeningocoele:* Wrap the eviscerated lesions in a sterile plastic bag to prevent heat and fluid losses from evaporation and excessive cooling. Nurse the infant on the surface opposite to the lesion. Reposition the bowel if it appears to have impaired blood supply. Assess perfusion and give colloid if necessary. Pass NG tube and aspirate intermittently. An IV infusion is desirable. Moist packs are contraindicated as they quickly become cold and lead to hypothermia.

4. *Bowel obstruction:* Correct F and E disturbances prior to transport and maintain continuous NG suction throughout. Nurse the infant prone with the head-up.

5. *Pierre robin sequence/choanal atresia:* Establish adequate airway for the infant, both while awake and when asleep. Nurse the infant prone and strap an oropharyngeal airway in place. Consider a long nasopharyngeal tube positioned just above the epiglottis in some cases. Observe respiratory pattern, skin colour, oxygen sats. continuously.

Pearl/Peril/Pitfall: Maintain in the neutral position and ensure patency. Remember a crying baby has a patent airway. Gentle suction may be necessary. If obstruction is noted and airway positioning has not helped, try an oropharyngeal or nasopharyngeal airway. A nasopharyngeal airway is simply an appropriately sized endotracheal tube inserted to the level of the pharynx (measure from the nasal philtrum to the tragus of the ear and insert this far). Assess the nares for patency with passage of a 5 Fr gauge feeding tube. If obstruction remains a problem, expert help may be needed.

TABLE 5	Indications for antenatal (in utero) transfer

1. Obstetric assessment of the high-risk fetus where urgent delivery is likely (e.g. IUGR, fetal cardiac rhythm disorders)
2. The severely ill mother (e.g. with pregnancy-associated hypertension) at an early stage of pregnancy with a potentially viable fetus
3. Early preterm labor where the referring hospital has inadequate facilities
4. Hemolytic disease with a severely affected fetus
5. Fetal malformation needing postnatal surgery
6. Prolonged and preterm rupture of the fetal membranes with resulting oligohydramnios
7. Any other situation where advanced neonatal resuscitation is anticipated.

TABLE 6	Contraindications for in utero transfer

* Where there is a risk to the woman's life (e.g. severe preeclampsia where there is a risk of eclampsia)

* Where either woman or fetus is placed at risk (e.g. antepartum haemorrhage which poses threat to mother and child)

* Scenarios where the fetus may deliver *en route* (established preterm labour) - it is never necessary for neonatal staff to accompany an in utero transfer, which places mother, fetus and the neonatal team at risk.

TABLE 7	High-risk Neonates requiring specialized transport to a NICU

1. birth weight less than 1750 g ; and Gestational age <32 weeks
2. respiratory distress of early onset or persisting more than 4-6 h;
3. oxygen requirement > 50% or associated apnea, meconium aspiration or suspected pneumonia;
4. apneic episodes;
5. convulsions;
6. depression following birth asphyxia;
7. jaundiced infants in need of exchange transfusion;
8. bleeding;
9. surgical conditions;
10. congenital heart disease;
11. severe or multiple congenital abnormalities ;
12. need for special diagnostic or therapeutic services ;
13. 'unwell' infants with lethargy, poor perfusion, oliguria, etc.

TABLE 8	The responsibilities of the doctor in referring hospital and those of Neonatal transport team

a. *Doctor in referring hospital should*
Request transfer of sick infants early, and give a clear history to the staff at the referral centre
Ask for telephone advice if needed before the arrival of the transport team
Prevent cold stress, hypoxia and hypoglycemia in the infant until the transport team arrive
Take appropriate samples for culture and commence antibiotics if sepsis seems likely
Explain to the parents what is happening
Ensure notes, X-rays and a sample of mother's blood (plus cord blood if possible) are available for the transport team
Obtain written consent from parents for any planned surgical procedure.

b. *Neonatal transport team (an experienced doctor and experienced nurse) should*
Travel to the referring hospital as quickly as possible
Be fully equipped to institute and to maintain intensive care of sick infants during transport
Spend as long as necessary (sometimes several hours) at the referring hospital stabilizing the infant's condition
Give a full explanation to the infant's parents, show them the infant, leave a digital photograph, and ensure they know the telephone number of the referral centre
Obtain notes, X-rays, consent forms and a sample of mother's blood
Explain to the ambulance crew the need for the above procedures, and ensure the ambulance is warm (25°C) and has windows closed
Ensure details on baby's identification band are correct
Travel back to the referral centre smoothy rather than rapidly

TABLE 9	Sedation for airway management and transport of infants
Morphine	0.05–0.1 mg/kg i.v. or s.c. infusion 5–20 mcg/kg/hour
Midazolam	150 mcg/kg i.v. infusion 60 mcg/kg/hour
Atracurium	0.4 mg/kg, i.v. bolus (may be repeated) 2–10 mcg/kg/mt as i.v. infusion
Vecuronium	0.1 mg/kg, i.v. infusion 50–150 mcg/kg/hour

TABLE 10	Special considerations in air transport

* increase FiO_2 to result in an adequate PaO_2, because of a decrease in oxygen tension (PaO_2) at high altitude : monitor and adjust FiO_2 using transcutaneous monitoring techniques.
* anticipate problems (e.g. a small pneumothorax or normal gaseous distention of the intestinal tract may become clinically significant because of dysbarism i.e., imbalance between air pressure in the atmosphere and the pressure of gases within the body) and put a drain or vent (NG tube) before transport.
* because BP varies with changing gravitational course, fluctuations noted during climbing or descent should not be cause for alarm.

Pearl/Peril/Pitfall: Inspired oxygen concentrations, oxygen saturations, BP, pulse, capillary refill, effort of breathing and temperature should be monitored every 30 minutes. Blood glucose levels should be monitored every 2 hours if stable on intravenous dextrose. Arterial blood gas monitoring will depend on the emerging clinical situation.

Referral: Information required at initial contact between referring and receiving center/providers to facilitate transport.

T.1 Transport type ☐ DR Attendance Requested ☐ ASAP Neonatal ☐ Scheduled Neonatal / Other
_____

T.2 Indication c Medical Dx/Rx Services ☐ Growth/Discharge Planning ☐ Surgery
☐ Chronic Care ☐ Insurance

T.3 Date/Time(D/T) Referral: @   **T.4** Acceptance   @

T.5 Maternal Admission to Labor and Delivery/Hospital Date/Time   @

Patient Identification/History: Information to be obtained prior to transport.

Infant's Name_____ ☐ Singleton c Multiple __of __

T.6 Birth D/T _____ @_____Ins. _____

T.7 Birth wt. _ _ _ _ gms   Current wt. _ _ _ _ gms   **T.8** Gestational Age _ _wks_ days
T.9 ☐ M ☐ F cUnk

T.10 Prenatally Diagnosed Congenital Anomalies ☐ Y ☐ N ☐ Unk Describe

Mother's Name   Birth Date   Age _ _ yrs

Med Rec#

T.11 G _ P ☐ AB ☐ L ☐ ROM Date/Time   @   Duration _ _ hrs Fluid ☐ Clear ☐
Meconium

Antenatal Conditions

☐ None   ☐ Unknown
☐ Hypertension   ☐ Diabetes
☐ Infection   c Preterm Labor
☐ Bleeding/Abrupt/Previa
☐ Other: _____   Significant Antepartum/Intrapartum Issues: Delivery
☐ Spont. Vag
☐ Op. Vag
    ☐ Vacuum
    ☐ Forceps
☐ Cesarean
    ☐ Primary
    ☐ Repeat

Apgar Scores

Score	N/D	Unk
1	_ _ ☐	☐
5	_ _ ☐	☐
10	_ _ ☐	☐
15	_ _ ☐	☐

_____

_____

Antibiotics Y Specify_____ N / Unknown

T.12 Steroids Y / N (last dose)   @

Pearl/Peril/Pitfall: Data collection increases the efficiency of a transport service. Monitoring the hour of transport requests, length of transport time, length of time at bedside, incidence of delayed calls, and incidence of overtime is useful in altering schedules or timing of elective reverse transports.

@ The modified transport risk index of physiologic stability *(TRIPS) Score contained in the Infant Condition Section will provide uniform assess of patient status and stability @Obtained three times: *Within 15 minutes of the time of referral by referring hospital staff *Within 15 minutes of transport team arrival at referring facility by transport team *Within 15 minutes of team return to receiving NICU by receiving hospital staff*

Modified TRIPS Score.to be recorded on referral, within 15 minutes of arrival at referring hospital and admit to NICU			Referral a	Initial TTEvalu. b	NICU Admit c
Time (24 hour)					
T.13 Responsiveness ✦					
T.14 Respiratory	Rate				
	O$_2$ Saturation				
	Status ✱				
	Oxygen Index *	MAP			
		FiO$_2$			
		PAO$_2$			
T.15 Vital Signs	HR				
	BP Sys/Dia, Mean				
	Pressors		□ Y □ N	□ Y □ N	□ Y □ N
	Temp. C°				
T.16 Blood Glucose					
T.17 Bld. Gas	Resp. Support ★				
	pH				
	pCO$_2$				
	BE				

✦ Responsiveness : 0 = Death, 1 = None, Seizure, Muscle Relaxant 2 = Lethargic. no cry 3 = Vigorously withdraws. cry.
★ Resp Support : None, Hood/NC. NCPAP. E.T.T.
✱ Respiratory Status : 1 = Respirator, 2 = Severe (apnea, gasping, intubated but not on respirator), 3 = Other
* Oxygen Index completed if pt. is on vent.

@ Each neonatal patient undergoes a careful assessment (e.g. vital signs), a rapid blood glucose determination, and establishment of intravenous access. Because respiratory distress is such a frequent problem with a large proportion of critically ill neonates, special effort should be paid to assessing the airway and the competence of oxygenation and ventilation.

@ Following this initial rapid assessment, most neonates who are not stable or are deteriorating rapidly are stabilized quickly and then expediently transferred. Alternatively, some clinical situations require more extensive and immediate interventions in the field, including artificial surfactant administration for extreme respiratory failure, and evacuation of a pneumothorax, among others.

Skills required for neonatal transport

* Airway

* Most critically ill neonates who require transfer to a neonatal ICU (NICU) have existing or impending *respiratory failure,* either as a primary diagnosis or secondary to their primary disease process. For this reason, transport teams commonly include respiratory therapists. Competence in airway management for resident physicians widely vary, depending on the level of experience of the resident and the skill level attained.

Because competence in airway management must be dependable and consistent, this issue dictates the extent of resident participation in neonatal transport.

* Team competence in neonatal airway management is imperative. The team should be capable of (1) recognizing impending respiratory failure, (2) performing effective bag-valve-mask ventilation, (3) performing atraumatic intubation with appropriate endotracheal tubes, (4) instillation of artificial surfactant, and (4) management of ventilator settings.

* Intravenous access: Nearly all ill neonates require peripheral or central intravascular access during transport. The team must have the necessary equipment and skills for routinely and reliably securing intravenous (IV) access in these tiny and challenging patients.

* Advanced procedures: Staff competency also ideally includes training in other unusual invasive procedures, such as percutaneous needle aspiration of the chest, chest tube insertion, umbilical catheter insertion, and intraosseous vascular access.

* Other important skills
* Independent thought and action
* Extensive experience in the rapid performance of advanced clinical skills under less-than-ideal conditions
* Experience in other areas of patient care

Pearl/Peril/Pitfall: With careful planning, attention to detail, and maintenance of clinical skills and equipment, Newborn intensive care can be provided in most hospitals for brief periods while awaiting the arrival of the retrieval team.

Care of the Neonate in the Transport Environment

Thermal control

The critically ill neonate often may be an extremely premature infant who may have a birthweight of less than 1 kg and markedly immature skin that is prone to massive insensible fluid losses. The low fat stores render this patient vulnerable to hypothermia.

In the neonatal ICU (NICU), infants are managed with specially designed neonatal radiant warmers or incubators, which decrease and/or compensate for these fluid and heat losses. During transport, thermal control becomes very difficult due to environmental conditions which may include cold weather, high winds, high elevations, travel over a long period of time, and less efficient equipment. Polyethylene bags or sheets placed over the infant may help maintain body temperature during resuscitation and/or transport of very low-birthweight infants. A hypothermic neonate should be rewarmed in a highly controlled fashion (approximately 1°C/h), which is extremely difficult to accomplish during transport. Rapid rewarming of hypothermic neonates is associated with increased mortality and increased severe morbidities.

Ventilation and airway management

In those patients who require positive pressure ventilatory assistance, the first level of intervention is bag-valve-mask ventilation, although it is unacceptable for prolonged airway management during transport.

Intubation in the neonate requires an uncuffed endotracheal tube of appropriate size, varying from 2.5-4 French external diameter. The neonatal transport team must know how to perform rapid, atraumatic intubation, with subsequent tube positioning and security.

Positive pressure ventilation can be accomplished by hand-bag ventilation for transports of short duration, but transport ventilators are generally used for most transports. Transport ventilators are often different from those models used in the receiving NICU; therefore, the transport personnel must be experienced in the setup and use of these ventilators. Due to limitations in current technology, transport ventilators are not currently capable of patient synchronization, patient-triggered ventilation modes, heated ventilation circuits, or high-frequency ventilation modes.

Monitoring issues

Routine NICU care involves patient monitoring with cardiorespiratory monitors that use adhesive chest leads and pulse oximetry monitors that use pulse-detecting extremity probes. Continuous monitoring of blood pressure requires the use of transducers that are in line with indwelling central lines (e.g. umbilical catheters). The increased vibration and electromechanical interference associated with transport environment frequently interferes with or precludes such monitoring.

The premature neonate's small size and small signals complicate electronic interference issues. These interference problems are greatest during aircraft takeoff and landing. During this time, the crew may be distracted by required flight protocols, are restrained for safety reasons, and may be unable to accurately assess the patient. The highest probability of monitoring failure, therefore, occurs during the periods when the patient is most likely to become destabilized and require intervention.

Reverse Transport of the Convalescent Neonate

Patient Issues

* Does the convalescing newborn's medical condition require care that can be provided at the proposed accepting hospital? In other words, is the accepting hospital capable of providing the care required by the recovering neonate?
* Can the predictable future needs of the infant be met by the institution (e.g., subspecialty medical or surgical consultations)?
* Have the parent(s) granted permission for the infant to be transported?
* Does the remaining estimated length-of-stay balance the costs and risks of reverse transport?
* Have any social factors that may affect the choice of convalescing hospital been identified?
* Does the third-party payer (e.g., insurance company) "approve" the transfer? Will the costs of the transport and subsequent hospitalization be approved by or be acceptable to the parents?
* Do the physicians and hospitals at both facilities agree the transfer is in the baby's and family's best interests?
* Will the ultimate follow-up physician provide care at the receiving hospital, thereby facilitating continuity of care?

Administration issues

* Are adequate Level I and II nursery personnel available who are sufficiently experienced in caring for the infant population?
* Are enough Level II beds available at the tertiary center?
* Is a well-functioning working relationship noted between the tertiary and Level I and II hospitals, relative to physicians, staff, and administration?
* What motivates the Level I and II hospitals to participate in the perinatal system as full partners, rather than be resigned to a role such as "patient donors" or competitors to the tertiary hospital?

Team configuration issues

* The triage of personnel for a reverse transport is generally easier because the infant is more stable and the medical condition is known. This allows matching the transport team configuration to the infant's medical needs. For example, if the infant has stable respiratory status (i.e. no oxygen requirement), then the presence of a physician or respiratory therapist is less important.
* These considerations reduce costs and maintain the availability of the primary team for incoming calls.

Pearl/Peril/Pitfall: *Transport teams need to be open to new technology that facilitates collaboration. Hence, investment in computerised infrastructure is essential. For instance, telemedicine is a valuable resource that allows patient triage through video conferencing, or consultation and advice when healthcare providers are not close by. Advanced methods of communication are likely to allow a more appropriate allocation of team resources. Transport teams need to develop audit and research through partnership with universities and other networks. Constructive engagement will be crucial, as will be the creation of a platform for dialogue and consensus.*

TABLE 11 Necessary equipment for the transport of sick newborn infants

Transport incubator	Internal and AC/DC power capability Heater Oxygen cylinder and air cylinder (or compressor) Thermometer
Transport ventilator	Able to work on internal power supply and AC/DC supply Compatible with portable gases/compressor and ambulance gas supply Adjustable FiO_2 and integral O_2 analyser Facilities for CPAP, IPPV, PEEP and IMV
Monitors	ECG monitor with leads Thermometer (low reading) plus two thermocouple probes Transcutaneous PO_2 (and spare membranes) Pressure monitor and transducers Non-invasive blood pressure monitor and cuffs Stethoscopes
Airway	Self-inflating bag and masks (all sizes) Endotracheal tubes (all sizes) Two laryngoscopes plus spare bulbs/batteries Magill forceps Oxygen cylinders (take three times estimated requirement) Suction catheters and portable suction device Nasogastric tubes (all sizes) Chest drains (all sizes) Heimlich flutter valves for chest drains
Circulation	Intravenous syringe pumps (minimum of three) i.v. catheters, tubing and connectors i.v. solutions Umbilical catheters Central venous catheters Needles/butterflies (all sizes) Syringes (all sizes) Three-way taps
Other	Sterile gloves, cleaning solutions i.v. cut-down pack, suture materials Lumbar puncture needles Specimen containers (clotted blood, cultures, etc.) Sterile water/saline Adhesive tape, splints Space blanket and spare blankets for incubator Digital camera, Spare batteries, Travel sickness tablets for staff

Drugs **Resuscitation drugs**
Adrenaline 1:10,000
Calcium gluconate 10% solution
Dextrose 10% solution (500mL)
Dextrose 50%
Naloxone
Phenobarbitone
Phenytoin
Dopamine
Human albumin solution 4.5%
Dried salt-poor albumin

Cardiovascular drugs
Digoxin
Adenosine
Lignocaine
Dobutamine
Frusemide
Prostaglandin E_2

Antibiotics
Penicillin G
Gentamicin or netilmicin
Cefotaxime
Metronidazole

Sedatives/muscle relaxants
Morphine
Midazolam
Pancuronium
Vecuronium

Others
Vitamin K_1
Heparinized saline (10 units/mL)

TABLE 12 Information needed by receiving hospital—the transfer log

From referring hospital
* Baby's name
* Gestation
* Birth weight
* Date and time of birth
* Date and time of transfer request
* Doctor requesting transfer
* Baby's pediatric consultant
* Name of referring hospital
* Contact number
* Provisional diagnosis/reason for transfer
* Respiratory
  – oxygen/CPAP/IPPV; FiO_2, PIP, PEEP/CPAP, rate, inspiratory time
  – blood gas art/cap : pH, P_aO_2, P_aCO_2 base excess

* Circulation—BP, perfusion, plasma/inotropes
* Temperature
* Blood sugar
* Drugs and infusions
* Other information

From own neonatal unit
* Number of intensive care cots available
* Number of nursing staff available
* Predicted demand 'in house' for intensive care cots in next few hours
* Always consider the baby's potential needs before leaving the base unit and confirm that all drugs and equipment which may be necessary for the baby are available, e.g. sedating and paralysing agents, sufficient infusion pumps.

KEY POINTS FOR CLINICAL PRACTICE

1) Neonatal transportation is a serious undertaking and its success requires skilled personnel, appropriate equipment, and good communication and organization. *2)* The transport team must be able to lucidly explain the infant's condition, prognosis, and treatment plans to the Parents.

REFERENCES and FURTHER READING:*1) Field D (ed.) Neonatal transport. Seminars in Neonatology (1999) 2) Mir NA (ed) . Manual of Neonatal Transport. Manchester:E Petch printers, 1997.3)Leslie A, Stephenson T. Neonatal transfers by advanced neonatal nurse practitioners and paediatric registrars. Arch Dis Child Fetal Neonatal Ed 2003;88:F509–12.*

Pearl/Peril/Pitfall: Early contact with the retrieval service and ongoing consultation during the process will help rural and regional centres to provide optimal care and outcomes.

6

Daily Assessment and Monitoring of the High-risk Sick Neonate

@ *"An experienced and alert nurse can observe subtle but important deviations in the infant that no monitor can detect." Dr. Nicholas Nelson once asked, "Who shall monitor the monitor?" This is a highly pertinent question in present day technology. Since there is a multitude of electronic equipment surrounding the critically ill, tiny, premature infant, it is virtually impossible for a nurse or a physician to watch the monitors or for that matter follow the monitors closely. In order to instill some reasoning and logic, it is essential that we develop computer assisted systems to monitor the monitors. This is not a far cry from reality. Several methods of innovative desk top and commercial computer systems are being introduced into neonatal management systems. These will soon provide some form of order and logic for the clinicians to monitor the monitors.*

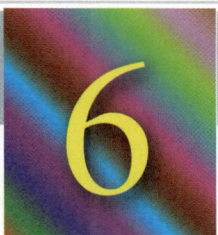
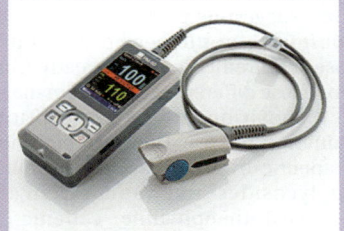
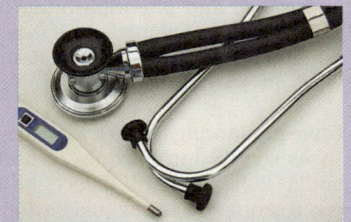
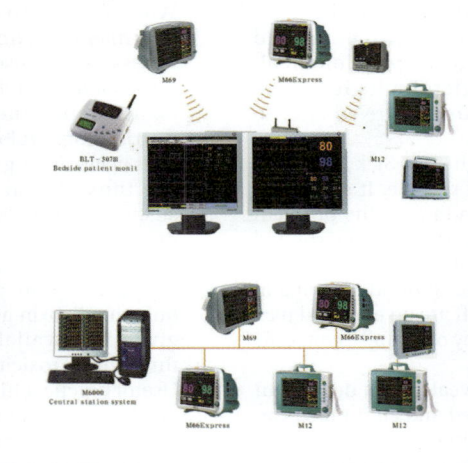
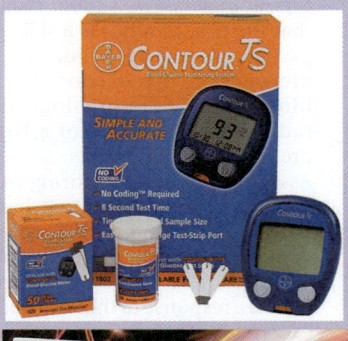
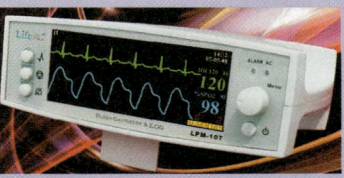
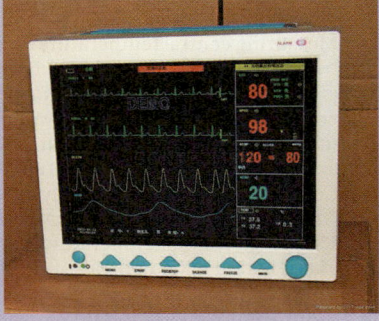
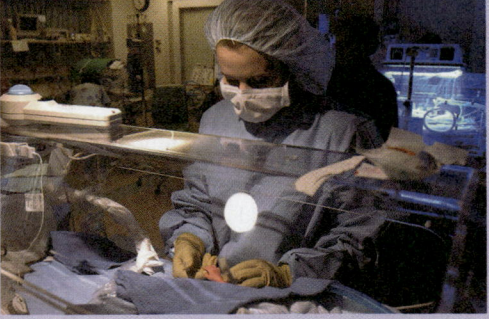

REVIEW OF CLINICAL PROBLEMS

1. How do you perform "daily assessment and monitoring" of the High-Risk Sick Neonate ?
   Ans: Refer to the "NICU DAILY ASSESSMENT and MONITORING OF HIGH-RISK SICK NEONATE.

2. How often should a Sick Neonate be monitored by various methods ?
   Ans: Refer to the Table 2 of the Chapter.

3. Which of the Neonatal medications require Therapeutic Drug Monitoring?.
   Ans: Refer to the "No.9" of the "BIRD'S EYE VIEW/ OVERVIEW/SYNOPSIS" of the Chapter.

4. How do you monitor Fluid balance in a Neonate?
   Ans: Refer to the "No.9" of the "BIRD'S EYE VIEW/ OVERVIEW/SYNOPSIS" of the Chapter.

5. Describe the significant deviations from the Normal Neonatal Observations.
   Ans: Refer to the Table 1 of the Chapter.

LEARNING OBJECTIVES

After completing this article, readers will be able to

1. Understand the priorities of daily assessment and monitoring of the high-risk Neonate

2. Learn that electronic monitoring is an adjunct but not a substitute to good clinical assessment.

3. Follow the continuous trend monitoring rather than simply looking at the values (by monitors or blood tests) at a single moment.

4. Ensure electrical safety, with the large number of devices attached to babies.

5. Screen the babies for infection, whenever there is a clinical indication of suspected sepsis.

Pearl/Peril/Pitfall: Catecholamine-mediated mobilization of glycogen stores can result in marked hyperglycemia in association with stress . Premature infants are at risk for hyperglycemia with exogenous glucose infusion because they secrete insulin sluggishly in response to rising serum glucose concentrations.

BIRD'S EYE VIEW/OVERVIEW/SYNOPSIS

1. All members of the Neonatal team caring for the High-Risk Sick Neonate must be able to assess changes in condition promptly and to provide appropriate care (refer to next page for comprehensive assessment of High-Risk Sick Neonates). They need to have specialized knowledge concerning the physiology, characteristics, and pathophysiology of these infants.

2. In spite of advanced electronic Neonatal monitoring (e.g. pulse oximetry, doppler BP monitor, cardiorespiratory monitor, transcutaneous O_2 and CO_2 monitoring, digital thermometers), we should remember the GOLDEN FACT that the best monitor is a skilled and experienced nurse / pediatrician who is looking, listening, feeling and identifying the trends in clinical, physiological, biochemical, hematological, microbiological and radiological variables of a High-Risk Sick Neonate, to prevent untoward events.

3. Assessment and monitoring of High-Risk Sick Neonates should not be merely a mechanical routine. It should be individualized and prioritized depending on the problem of the Sick Neonate. The electronic data must be interpreted in the context of the history, repetitive physical examinations, response to therapy, and a background of Neonatal experience. Experienced nursing staff are an essential part of the monitoring of the baby and they often raise concerns about potential problems.

4. Although electronic monitors can reveal a great deal about a Neonate's condition, an experienced and alert nurse can observe subtle but important deviations in the infant that no monitor can detect (refer to Table 1 of the Chapter for the significant observations indicating deviations from normal in nursing assessment of Neonate).

5. The nurse who is responsible for assessing the Sick Neonate does so systematically and at regular and frequent intervals (refer to table 2), unless by so doing the infant is unnecessarily disturbed and can not get adequate rest. Continuous trend monitoring either by devices or by blood tests facilitates detection of abnormalities and allows earlier interventions.

6. All the Neonatal team members, should never fail to wash their hands meticulously and thoroughly between handling of different Sick Neonates for assessment. In general, the hands should be washed for at least 2 minutes to above the elbows when first entering the nursery. Washing for at least 15 seconds should also be done between assessing and caring for different infants.

7. If a problem of malfunctioning or an electrical hazard arise with the monitoring equipment, and can not be resolved by the staff, immediate reporting and recording of the observation is mandatory so that proper action can be taken.

8. Monitor respiration (apnea), heart rate (ECG), BP, and arterial blood gases continuously in critically ill neonates on mechanical ventilation. Arterial PO_2 is the only acceptable and safe way to avoid hyperoxemia and minimize the risk of ROP; capillary samples and intermittent arterial puncture are useless.

9. Monitor the fluid balance by daily weighing, continuous records of fluid input and output and frequent estimations of serum electrolytes and creatinine. In VLBW babies in intensive care blood electrolytes, creatinine, and full blood count should be monitored daily with more frequent estimations in ELBW. Consider daily chest X-ray until a baby is stable on ventilation with <30% of inspired oxygen. This helps to detect the development of pneumonia, small pneumothoraces and in particular pulmonary interstitial emphysema (PIE), and misplaced ET tubes which help immediate alterations in therapy. It is essential to maintain close liaison with the microbiology department with frequent monitoring of blood cultures, tracheal aspirates and surface swabs. Such surveillance enables identification of colonization of the respiratory tract with serious pathogens, and can help to target therapy, if ill babies develop a deteriorating chest X-ray, a rise in CRP and/or WBC, or other symptoms suggesting pneumonia.

Therapeutic drug monitoring in the newborn infant is necessary because dose requirements differ greatly from those for older children. These differences stem from major changes in kinetic disposition at the absorption, distribution, and elimination phases. The most common tests necessitating therapeutic drug monitoring in neonates are those for aminoglycosides and vancomycin (in suspected or proven sepsis), theophylline/ caffeine (in neonatal apneas), digoxin (in congestive heart failure and supraventricular arrhythmias), and phenobarbital (in neonatal seizures and ischemic encephalopathy). Of these, only the digoxin assay should be available on a stat basis, given the availability of an antidote in case of life-threatening toxicity.

10. Useful practical hints while monitoring the sick Neonate:
   a. Apnea monitor misses significant episodes of both apnea and bradycardia. Pulse oximetry detects both bradycardia and oxygen saturation and should be done if there are true concerns about the baby's respiratory status.
   b. Measuring central temperature (core) in the axilla, or in between the scapulae is important; rectal temperature is unreliable and can cause damage to the mucosa. The continuous measurement and display of a central (abdominal, axilla or zero heat flux between scapulae) and a peripheral (foot) temperature detects cold stress. Central temperature is usually between 36.8°C–37.3°C with a central - peripheral temperature gap of around 1°C. A high central temperature, particularly if unstable, along with a wide central—peripheral gap is seen in septic babies.
   c. Input/output charts should be used to help assess fluid balance, but it is important to measure all fluids given to the baby, including drugs and flushes for catheters.
   d. Blood losses from sampling should be recorded and the sick ventilated baby must have a hemoglobin and hematocrit measured daily. Daily WBC count and the differential, can give an indication of developing sepsis.
   e. Flow charts and plotting results on graphs are useful as they show trends in biochemical and hematological data.
   f. Close observation of the IV infusion site at regular intervals, stopping the infusion at the first sign of swelling or redness, is all that is available to detect fluid extravasation and hopefully prevent or minimise subsequent tissue damage.
   g. Whatever method is used to monitor blood gases, users must have a good understanding of how the values are obtained and the pitfalls in their interpretation.
   h. Mobile phones can interfere with monitoring systems and should not be used within intensive care areas.

Pearl/Peril/Pitfall: *Plasma creatinine concentration is of limited value in assessing renal function in the first week of life. First, plasma creatinine concentration in cord blood is a function of maternal renal function and is almost identical to the maternal concentration. Second, abrupt changes in extracellular volume and glomerular filtration rate (GFR) after birth result in non-steady-state conditions in the first few days of life.*

THE NICU DAILY ASSESSMENT AND MONITORING OF HIGH-RISK SICK NEONATE

DAY	Problems		
DATE	1.	3.	5.
TIME	2.	4.	6.

VENTILATION

Self Ventilating ☐	In Air ☐		How much O_2 ?	Current SaO_2
	In O_2 ☐		TcO_2	$TcCO_2$
If on Mechanical ventilator	Mode-CMV/SIMV/PTV/CPAP			Tidal Volume
Ratio	PIP-		PEEP-	MAP- I:E
	RATE :		FiO_2	
Recent CBG/ABG : pH	PaO_2		$PaCO_2$	HCO_3 BE

FLUIDS

Type of fluid   Volume (ml/kg/d)   Route — IV / Oral / TPN (Long Line)

Additives if any   IV -   Oral -
Urine output
NG tube losses
*Recent renal functions   Na   K   BUN   Cr   Ca   24 hours Balance

*Wt changes (Last 12/24 hrs): ☐ Appropriate   ☐ Inappropriate — Excess ☐ / Less ☐

MEDICATIONS

Antibiotics		Others:	Therapeutic Drug Levels:	
1).	Day -	a)		d)
2).	Day -	b)		e)
3).	Day -	c)		f)

IM VIT 'K' given ?   MV Drops   Vit A/D/E Supplements

OBSERVATIONS

1. TPR fluctuations   2. BP Abnormalities   3. Apneas, Brady's and Desat's
4. Bowels open ?   5. Passed Urine ?
6. *Any recent change from the previous day such as the following*
a) Pallor   b) Jaundice   c) Central Cyanosis
d) Jitteriness/Convulsions   e) High Pitched cry   f) Bleeding
g) Resp. Distress   h) Abdominal distention + gastric aspirates   i) Others

RECENT LABORATORY PARAMETERS

HB %	Hematocrit	* Recent Blood /Urine/CSF/ET Secretions C / S-
		* Radiological / Imaging changes - CXR, AXR,
Neutropenia ?		USG head and kidneys scan, Echo,MRI /CT etc
Low Platelets ?	SBR-Total	Direct Indirect

PARENTAL COMMUNICATION

☐ Explained /Not   ☐ "DIAGNOSIS"   ☐ 'TREATMENT'   ☐ 'PROGNOSIS"

CURRENT EXAMINATION FINDINGS

Cry-	Color	Activity	Any other notable features
Spontaneous	Dysmorphic Features:		
Limb Movements	Deformities -		
Anemia ?	Jaundice		
Central Cyanosis ?	Edematous ?		
Respiratory Distress ?	Abdominal Distention ?	Umbilicus	
IV Sites Checked ?	Eyes ?	AF	
Nappy Area ?	Oral Thrush ?		

RESPIRATORY

Chest expansion -   Air entry -
Adventitious sounds -

CVS

Perfusion - CRT < 2 Sec / > 2 Sec
Femorals -   S1 - S2 - S3   HEART MURMURS

ABDOMEN

Soft ?	Distended ?	Tender ?	Organs/masses felt ?
Bowel sounds ?	Hernial sites	Genitalia	HIP joints -

CNS

a) Handles well ?   b) Red reflexes   c) Focal Signs   d) Neonatal reflexes

FINAL ASSESSMENT

MANAGEMENT PLAN

1)   2)   3)   4)
5)   6)

Doctor's Signature

Pearl/Peril/Pitfall : Delivery of drugs to neonates should utilize pumps calibrated to accurately deliver very small volumes. If desired, these small volumes can then be infused at a rate much higher than the maintenance infusion rate, thus guaranteeing rapid delivery in only a small volume of fluid.

Area of assessment	Observation	Area of assessment	Observation
TABLE 1	**Significant observations indicating deviations from normal in nursing assessment of neonate**		
Temperature	Higher or lower than normal axillary temperature in relationship to environmental temperature	CVS	(a mediastinal shift may be evidenced by a change in PMI); blood pressure (extremity used); peripheral pulses; central venous pressure if in use
Color	Pallor, florid, jaundice, cyanosis	Abdomen	Distention; presence or absence of bowel sounds Cord Inflammation, bleeding, discharge
Skin	Texture, turgor, edema, discolorations, irritations, rashes, signs of infiltration of intravenous infusion	Stools	Frequency, characteristics, presence of occult blood
Mucous membranes	Bleeding / thrush	Urinary	Frequency, amount, characteristics (color and specific gravity)
Fontanels	Bulging or sunken	Activity	Decrease or increase in motor activity " lethargy,
Eyes	Irritation, discharge	level	hyperactivity, twitching or seizures ; presence of reflexes; characteristics of cry: quality, frequency
Respiratory	Rate : rhythm ; quality of breath sounds (rales, rhonchi, wheezing or absence of sounds) ; retractions : subclavicular, sternal, or intercostal :flaring of ala nasi ; labored : grunting ; need for suctioning	Oral feeding	Quality of sucking ability, acceptance of oral feedings ; vomiting ; regurgitation ; characteristics of emesis ; whether satisfied after feeding or not
Cardio-vascular	Heart rate and rhythm ; quality of heart sounds ; point of maximal intensity (PMI), where the heart sounds are loudest	Parenteral infusion	Kind, amount, rate of flow
		Weight gain	Slower or more rapid than expected

TABLE 2   Routine monitoring of the ill neonate

CXR
-3 times per week
Albumin
ETT aspirate culture
CRP
Weekly
Liver enzyme (when on TPN)
Triglycerides (when on TPN)
Alkaline phosphatase (for osteopenia)
Reticulocytes (for anemia of prematurity)

* *in babies with appropriate diagnoses. In stable babies glucose need only be checked daily. Bilirubin need not be measured in the absence of clinical jaundice.*

^ *Electrolytes should be measured 2-3 times per day in all babies <1 kg in the first 3-4 days until fluid balance stabilizes.*

TABLE 3   Suggested protocol for clinically monitoring the sick neonate

A. At birth and during resuscitation: *Clinical* - monitoring of HR, respiration, colour and perfusion
Equipment - SpO$_2$ by pulse oximetry

B. During transport of the sick neonate: *Clinical* - as above, *Equipment* - SpO$_2$, ECG and temperature monitors to be used.

C. Monitoring a baby with/without respiratory distress in a level II setup or level II NICU: *Clinical* - TPR, urine output, BP (non invasive), abdominal girth, stool output, intake-output charting, respiratory distress scoring (Downe's scoring), weight checks. *Equipment* - SpO$_2$, ECG, apnea alarm, continuous temperature, non invasive BP monitoring, arterial blood gases, FiO$_2$ or percentage of oxygen delivered. preferably indwelling continuous arterial catheter with invasive BP recording and also TcPO$_2$/ TcPCO$_2$ monitoring, CVP monitoring (in multiorgan dysfunction).

KEY POINTS FOR CLINICAL PRACTICE

1) It is essential to monitor the progress of a high-risk Neonate clinically, biophysically, biochemically, hematologically, bacteriologically and by imaging. What needs to be monitored will always depends on the clinical condition of the baby. *2)* Monitoring is not just about reading values from machines. It is the ability to integrate a whole range of data, including the observation of the whole baby, into meaningful information. *3)* It is important to know the limitations of the electronic monitoring devices and the circumstances in which they become unreliable. *4)* Continuous trend monitoring allows trends to be visualized, hopefully facilitating detection of abnormalities and allowing earlier interventions. *5)* The most common tests necessitating therapeutic drug monitoring in neonates are those for aminoglycosides and vancomycin (in suspected or proven sepsis), theophylline/ caffeine (in neonatal apneas), digoxin (in congestive heart failure and supraventricular arrhythmias), and phenobarbital (in neonatal seizures and ischemic encephalopathy).

REFERENCES AND FURTHER READING: 1) Text book of Pediatric nursing, 6th edition, Dorothy R.Marlow 2) Rennie. J.M. and Roberton N.R.C. (2004) a manual of neonatal intensive care. Fifth edition. 3) Aranda JV, Cohen S, Neims AH. Drug utilization in a newborn intensive care unit. Pediatr J 1976;89:315–7.4)Wilkins BH. Renal function in sick very low birth weight infants: 2. Urea and creatinine excretion. Arch Dis Child 1992;67:1145–53.

Pearl/Peril/Pitfall: Blood transfusion in a critically ill newborn may be required when >10% of blood volume (80 mL/kg body weight in the full term; 100 mL/kg body weight in the preterm) is withdrawn over , 2–3 days. Thus, for a 750 g infant, withdrawal of as little as 8 mL of blood over a short period may necessitate blood transfusion.

7 Rapid yet Complete Assessment of the Newborn Infant

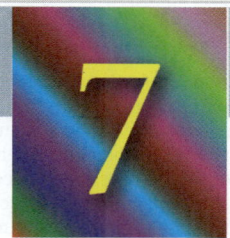

@*"Examining a Newborn requires patience, gentleness and procedural flexibility and involves all of the Special Senses."*

Rennie, JM. states that the Newborn examination "gives healthcare advice, to ensure that plans made regarding antenatal diagnosed abnormalities are implemented, and to provide reassurance about minor medically unimportant deviations from normal which worry parents".

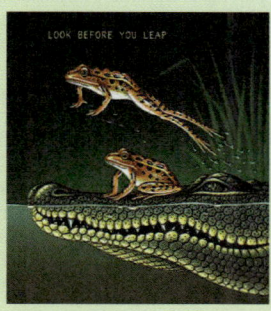
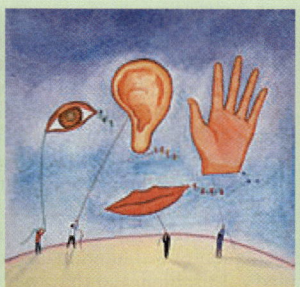
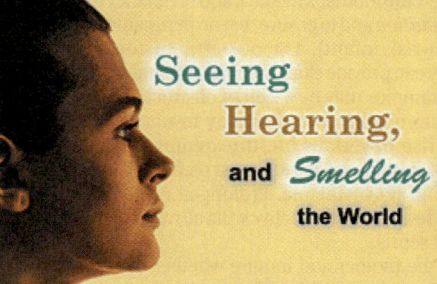
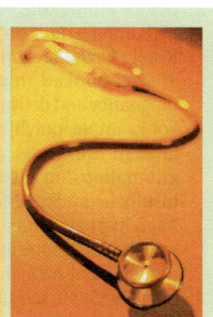

"Look before you leap" start with observation-*(one should be careful not to "miss the forest for the trees" during the examination of the Newborn)* then auscultation of the chest and then palpation of the abdomen.

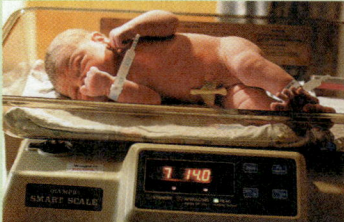
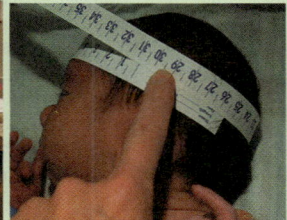
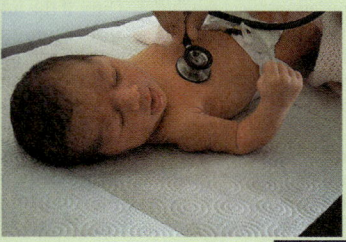

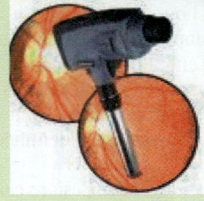

Examination of the Eyes, Ears, Throat and Hips should be done last, since these maneuvers are most disturbing to the infant. Remember look, listen, feel {touch}, smell the baby in that order to make most out of your quick assessment of the baby.

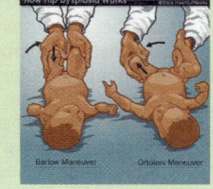

REVIEW OF CLINICAL PROBLEMS

1. How do you perform rapid yet complete assessment of the Newborn infant?
   Ans: Refer to the Evaluation-Decision-Action plan to assess the Newborn baby.

2. What clinical manifestations in the Newborn are suspicious about abnormal postnatal transition?
   Ans: Refer to the Table 2 of the Chapter.

3. Mention the suspicious Neurological signs in the Newborn which need careful follow-up?
   Ans: Refer to the Table 3 of the Chapter.

4. What additional points should you note, while performing the "discharge examination" of the Newborn baby?
   Ans: Refer to the Table 6 of the Chapter.

5. How do you assess the gestational age, growth and maturity of the Newborn baby?
   Ans: Refer to the "Quintessential Quick References" Section of the book.

LEARNING OBJECTIVES

After completing this article, readers will be able to

1. Review and Document any problems arising or suspected from antenatal screening, family history or the events of labor.

2. Diagnose congenital malformations and common Neonatal problems, and give advice about management.

3. Ascertain whether or not the family have any worries about the baby and to try to address them.

4. Promote bonding between Newborn and mother.

5. Refer when appropriate to specialists for assistance in evaluation and management.

Pearl/Peril/Pitfall: Inspection without contact- A considerable amount of information is available by simply looking at an infant. When first approaching the infant, the examiner should not abruptly place a stethoscope on the infant's chest before doing anything else.

BIRD'S EYE VIEW/OVERVIEW/SYNOPSIS

1. Within 24 hours of birth, every baby should have a full and thorough medical examination to **a)** Detect congenital abnormalities not already identified at birth **E.g.:** - Congenital Heart Disease, Congenital Dislocation of the HIP **b)** Check whether the infant has made a successful transition from fetal life to air breathing **c)** Check for potential problems arising from maternal disease or familial disorders (Check for any sign of infection or metabolic disease) **d)** Provide an opportunity for the parents to discuss any questions about their baby.

2. Before embarking on the physical examination of the infant, the pediatrician must review the mother's medical and pregnancy history to help *focus the examination* and to ensure that no pertinent findings are overlooked (high-risk infant). The obstetric history of the pregnancy and delivery can provide clues to some neonatal problems. For example, polyhydramnios may be a sign of obstruction at some level in the bowel, and oligohydramnios may result from renal anomalies and give rise to serious life-threatening pulmonary insufficiency. Small-for-gestational age and post mature infants may have hypoglycemia and polycythemia. Prolonged rupture of the membranes, maternal fever, and fetal tachycardia all raise the serious possibility of neonatal sepsis.

3. Introduce yourself to the mother and inquire whether she has any specific concerns or questions. Always do examine the baby fully naked in the presence of his mother or ideally both parents present ; ensure that the naked baby must not be cold stressed or unnecessarily separated from his parents. *Examining a Newborn requires patience, gentleness and procedural flexibility.* Thus, if the infant is quiet and relaxed at the beginning of the examination, palpation of the abdomen or auscultation of the heart should be performed first before other, more disturbing manipulations are attempted. Observe the infants appearance, posture, and state of consciousness before proceeding with the formal aspects of palpation and auscultation. *"Look before you leap"* - start with observation-*(one should be careful not to "miss the forest for the trees" during the examination of the Newborn)* then auscultation of the chest and then palpation of the abdomen. Examination of the Eyes, Ears, Throat & Hips should be done last, since these maneuvers are most disturbing to the infant. Remember *look, listen, feel {touch}, smell the baby in that order* to make most out of your quick assessment of the baby.

4. If any anomaly is found, look carefully for others, because they often coexist. Constellations of physical findings may indicate the presence of a syndrome. For example, if the physical features of Down syndrome are found, confirmatory chromosomal analysis is required. Signs of trauma that occurred during the birth should be noted. This is particularly common in large infants or after difficult deliveries by the breech or when forceps have been used. Evidence of trauma in one part of the baby should lead to a search for trauma in other areas.

5. You should take no more than 5 to 10 minutes to examine the Newborn baby thoroughly without causing cold stress, light and noise stress and cross infection. If a satisfactory ambient temperature cannot be guaranteed, examine the infant under a servo-controlled radiant warmer alternatively. Thorough hand washing before and after handling each infant is essential to prevent the spread of pathogenic organisms.

6. The extent and focus of the Newborn examination varies with circumstances. There are typically 3 distinct periods of time during which the infant is examined : *1) a* brief examination immediately after birth in the delivery room *2)* a complete examination in the Newborn nursery or mother's room 12 to 18 hours after birth and 3) a focused examination before discharge. If any abnormalities are detected at any time of examination, more frequent examination should occur, and a plan made for investigation and initial therapy.

7. The examiner, throughout the history and physical examination, seeks answers whether there are any problems with regard to the following aspects of the Neonate: * Whether the infant is acutely ill *Any specific organ system * Infection *Inadequate oxygen or Nutrients (acute or chronic)* Abnormal in utero environment *Growth *Anomalies or genetic disease *Trauma *Maturity *Transition from in utero existence *Home environment. The history, physical examination, and laboratory evaluations are never complete for sick infants in an intensive care setting. Information is constantly being compiled from diagnostic studies, physicians, nurses and family members. Integration of these data with clear and appropriate communication in interviews with parents is extremely important.

8. The use of careful, succinct, system-or problem-oriented, dated, and timed notes in the Neonate's hospital chart, including information about what has been told to the parents as well as their concerns.

9. Should there be any uncertainty about the baby's sex, it is best not to guess but to explain to the parents that further tests are necessary, and guide them not to name the child until the final decision, to be made after thorough investigations.

10. Always perform the newborn examination with a purpose so that, the initial evaluation, assessment and management of a newborn must be directed toward promoting and facilitating normal adaptation to extrauterine life and early detection of significant medical problems so that they can be evaluated and treated appropriately.

Some significant abnormalities will not be identified because of the limitations of the examination. Sometimes this is due to inexperience of the examiner or the difficulty of performing a satisfactory examination in an uncooperative newborn (e.g., getting a good view of the eyes and red reflex, hearing a heart murmur, or testing for DDH). Parents need to be made aware that not all abnormalities can be detected at the initial examination. This situation also stresses the importance of clear documentation of the routine examination for future reference.

Identification of syndromes: Some syndromes can be difficult or impossible to identify in the immediate neonatal period but become apparent as the child grows older.

Jaundice: Jaundice usually develops after 24 hours of age, unless it is due to hemolysis. Significant jaundice can develop at several days of age even though the infant was apparently normal only 1 or 2 days earlier.

Eye Abnormalities: Vision is better if surgery for congenital cataracts is performed before 8 weeks of age. However, a survey in the United Kingdom revealed that only 35% of congenital cataracts were identified on the routine examination.

Congenital Heart Disease: Infants with ductus-dependent lesions can present clinically with heart failure, shock, cyanosis, or death just days or weeks after a normal routine examination. A ventricular septal defect (the most common congenital heart lesion) or other heart lesions might not have a heart murmur at the routine examination because the pressure difference between the left and right sides of the heart will be insufficient to generate turbulent flow at this stage. An additional limitation is that a heart murmur may be heard but because most are innocent, those from significant heart lesions are not always identified. Pulse oximetry screening has been advocated to assist the detection of ductal dependent lesions.

Developmental dysplasia of hip: An examiner might fail to identify DDH at the initial examination because the examiner is inexperienced or because the examination is suboptimal when the infant is not relaxed. In some infants with a flat acetabular shelf, the clinical examination may be normal in the neonatal period, but the dysplasia progresses with age. Also, the irreducible dislocated hip is easily missed on examination. Ultrasound will identify DDH, including a shallow acetabular shelf. However, ultrasound has a high false positive rate, and it is only helpful in the first 5 months of life.

---

* Pearl/Peril/Pitfall: Spontaneous movements can be evaluated only if the infant is undisturbed. At rest, sporadic, well-coordinated movements are the rule, but they are not symmetrical. Bilaterally identical, repetitive movements of the extremities are suggestive of seizure activity. Facial and eyelid twitches are also suggestive of convulsions. The infant who moves little or not at all is usually flaccid as well. Absent or diminished movement of one extremity when the others are used normally is indicative of paresis or paralysis. Information about respiration is first obtainable by simple inspection. Retractions are obvious, and grunting and stridor are audible to the naked ear. Increased anteroposterior diameter of the chest (barrel chest) usually indicates an overexpanded lungs, which may be due to meconium aspiration or respiratory distress syndrome type 2. If one side of the chest appears larger than the other, pneumothorax, chylothorax, or diaphragmatic hernia is suggested. If the left side of the chest is larger, cardiomegaly associated with congenital heart disease is an additional possibility.

SUBJECTIVE FINDINGS

Obtain important aspects of maternal and perinatal history—**family history** of inherited diseases, **maternal history**—chronic medical illness, previous pregnancies, current pregnancy, labor and delivery details, drugs, age, blood type & sensitization

Neonatal history: Passage of urine & meconium, concerns with feeding & breathing

OBJECTIVE FINDINGS

Activate your special senses i.e. visual observation, hearing acumen, fine touch & smell to get the most out of your examination of the newborn.

Always try to identify the life-threatening symptoms and signs - central cyanosis, apneas, seizures, focal neurological deficits, pallor and ashen grey + mottling, dysmorphism, obvious congenital anomalies

Perform the disturbing aspects of examination in the end only, i.e. eyes, hips, head circumference, femoral pulses etc.

INVESTIGATIONS

Observe nursing chart for weight, vitals, known congenital anomalies to the staff, blood sugars, etc.,

RAPID YET COMPLETE ASSESSMENT OF THE NEWBORN

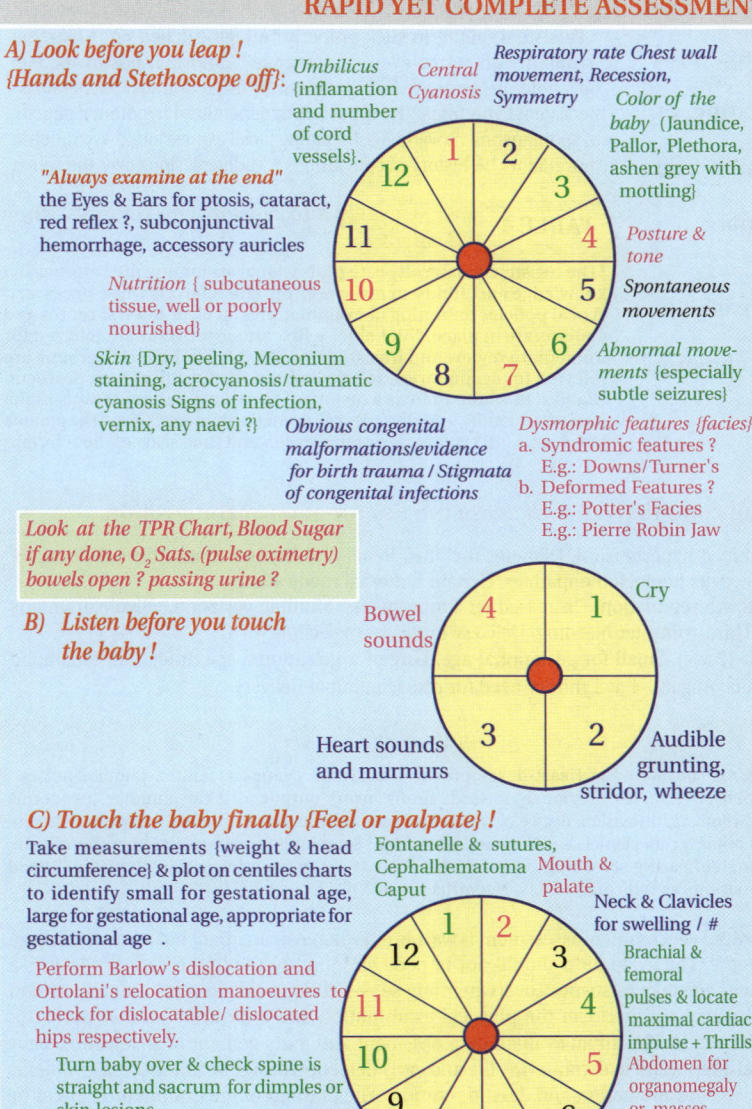

A) Look before you leap ! {Hands and Stethoscope off}:

"Always examine at the end" the Eyes & Ears for ptosis, cataract, red reflex ?, subconjunctival hemorrhage, accessory auricles

Nutrition { subcutaneous tissue, well or poorly nourished}

Skin {Dry, peeling, Meconium staining, acrocyanosis/traumatic cyanosis Signs of infection, vernix, any naevi ?}

Umbilicus {inflamation and number of cord vessels}.

Central Cyanosis

Respiratory rate Chest wall movement, Recession, Symmetry

Color of the baby {Jaundice, Pallor, Plethora, ashen grey with mottling}

Posture & tone — Spontaneous movements

Abnormal movements {especially subtle seizures}

Obvious congenital malformations/evidence for birth trauma / Stigmata of congenital infections

Dysmorphic features {facies}
a. Syndromic features ?
E.g.: Downs/Turner's
b. Deformed Features ?
E.g.: Potter's Facies
E.g.: Pierre Robin Jaw

Look at the TPR Chart, Blood Sugar if any done, O_2 Sats. (pulse oximetry) bowels open ? passing urine ?

B) Listen before you touch the baby !

Circle (clockwise): 1 Cry, 2 Audible grunting, stridor, wheeze, 3 Heart sounds and murmurs, 4 Bowel sounds

C) Touch the baby finally {Feel or palpate} !

Take measurements {weight & head circumference} & plot on centiles charts to identify small for gestational age, large for gestational age, appropriate for gestational age .

Perform Barlow's dislocation and Ortolani's relocation manoeuvres to check for dislocatable/ dislocated hips respectively.

Turn baby over & check spine is straight and sacrum for dimples or skin lesions

Assess tone & neonatal reflexes

Check equal leg length & foot position

Check anus for patency and position

Circle labels: 1, 2 Fontanelle & sutures, Cephalhematoma Caput; Mouth & palate; 3 Neck & Clavicles for swelling / #; 4 Brachial & femoral pulses & locate maximal cardiac impulse + Thrills; 5 Abdomen for organomegaly or masses; 6 Testes in boys & examine introitus in girls

D) Don't ever forget to smell the baby !-
E.g.. Inborn errors of metabolism

Ensure the following things while assessing the Newborn baby!

1. Introduce yourself to the mother with an explanation about what you are doing.

2. Observe the mother's attitude to her baby, and whether she is confident and happy or tense and withdrawn.

3. Check the maternal medical, obstetric and social history from the notes, the mother and the nursing staff.

4. Always ask the mother whether she has any specific worries, when she is expecting to be discharged and what support she has at home.

5. Observe the baby, noting color, facies, breathing pattern, posture and movements before trying to touch the baby.

6. After examining the baby fully with flexibility, make sure you have not omitted anything and check you have paid attention to any concerns expressed by the mother.

7. Give advice and information, arrange follow-up and provide reassurance where appropriate.

8. Review the maternal, obstetric, and Neonatal conditions that increase the risk for abnormal transition (refer to the Table No. 4 of the chapter)

9. Look for the clinical manifestations in the Newborn signaling abnormal transition (refer to the Table No. 2 of the Chapter)

10. Ask for another opinion and to follow-up, if the significance of a finding is in doubt.

11. Ascertain that the infant has received vitamin K prophylaxis, BCG and hepatitis B vaccinations.

12. At discharge, reexamine the baby and note the additional points mentioned in the Table No. 5 of the Chapter.

13. On completing the examination the baby is redressed and offered to the parents for a cuddle, or left comfortable in the cot while the examiner completes the documentation.

14. When you have completed the examination, reassure the mother about your findings and record them accurately in the clinical notes, remembering to sign and date the entry.

---

* Pearl/Peril/Pitfall: *The baby's posture is also informative. Normal flexion of the extremities indicates good muscle tone. Lack of flexion is associated with hypotonicity, whereas excessive flexion usually suggests hypertonicity. If only one arm is consistently straight and the infant does not flex that extremity, brachial plexus injury must be considered. Breech presentations are often identified by the characteristic positions of the lower extremities .*

TABLE 1 Common findings in the neonate that are of little clinical significance

Head	Caput succedaneum, cephalhematoma, asymmetries, bony protrusions, molding
Ears	Skin tags
Eyes	Position (close-set), conjunctival hemorrhage
Nose	asymmetric nares
Mouth	Ranula, sucking calluses, epulis, frenulum, natal teeth, Epstein pearls
Face	Unusual features not consistent with known syndromes
Skin	Sparse petechiae on the head, erythema toxicum, mongolian spot, nevus flammus, telangiectasia, nevi, inclusion cysts, bruises, prominent lanugo or vernix, milia, miliaria, dark pigmentation over genital skin, skin tags sacrococcygeal dimple, **Harlequin color change** (infant is pale on one side and flushed on the contralateral side with a distinct border in the midline)
Neck	Relative absence
Chest	Nipple spacing, extra nipples, breast hypertrophy, witch's milk
Umbilicus	Erythema or umbilicus cutis
Abdomen	Evanescent masses
Heart	Evanescent murmurs and adventitious sounds
Genitalia	Mild hypospadias, prominent labia, mucous secretion, transient vaginal blood, phimosis Extremities Extra digits, syndactyly, hips tight on abduction, neck in extension after breech delivery .
Neurologic	Transient tone asymmetries or abnormality, jitters, sudden jerky movements

TABLE 2 Neonatal clinical manifestations signalling abnormal transition

* Persistent tachypnea, flaring, grunting, and retractions; fixed bradycardia
* Diffuse and persistent rales, retractions, flaring, or grunting
* Persistent cyanosis and prolonged apnea and bradycardia
* Episodes of prolonged apnea and bradycarda
* Marked pallor or ruddiness
* Temperature instability
* Poor capillary filling and blood pressure instability
* Unusual neurologic behavior
* Excessive oral secretions, drooling, and choking spells

TABLE 3 Suspicious neurological signs

* Persistent failure to suck properly *A high-pitched cry * Extreme irritability or 'starey-eyed' appearance *Abnormal posturing, e.g. opisthotonus, excessive fisting, constantly fisted thumbs *Generalized persistent hypertonia *'Frog' posture or generalized hypotonia; paucity of spontaneous movements, including facial expressions * Asymmetric movements * A history of convulsions * Midline lesions over the spine.

TABLE 4 Ensure timely and appropriate referrals when indicated!

*The registered maternity care professional examining the baby has the knowledge and ability to make appropriate referrals when necessary. *Local policies on timing of examination and clear referral routes and systems are in place. *All babies with cardiac murmur are referred for immediate review and investigation. *Babies in high risk groups are referred for secondary screening within the locally agreed protocol. *Babies, in whom there is a history of hereditary eye conditions in the immediate family, are referred for examination by a specialist. *The parents are given a full explanation of the reason and time scale of the referral.

TABLE 5 Maternal, obstetric, and neonatal conditions that increase the risk for abnormal transition

Maternal factors: Chronic hypertension, Pregnancy-induced hypertension, Diabetes mellitus, Renal disease, Infection, Abuse of tobacco, alcohol, or illicit drugs, Collagen vascular disease, Hemizygous hemoglobinopathies, Certain maternal medications.
Obstetric factors: Rh or other isoimmunization, Fetal growth retardation, Decreased fetal movements, Multiple gestation, Oligohydramnios or polyhydramnios, Premature rupture of membranes, Third-trimester bleeding, Delivery by cesarean section.
Neonatal factors: Prematurity (<37 wk), Postmaturity (>42 wk), Small for gestational age, Large for gestational age, Infection, Metabolic abnormalities, Birth trauma, Major malformations, Anemia, Apgar 0-4 at 1 min or need for resuscitation at delivery.

TABLE 6 Discharge examination

* *The infant should be reexamined with the following points considered* a) Heart-development of murmur, cyanosis, failure, femoral pulses . b) CNS-fullness of fontanelles, sutures, activity c) Abdomen-any masses previously missed, stools, urine output. d) Skin-jaundice, pyoderma e) Cord-infection f) Infection-signs of sepsis. g) Feeding-spitting, vomiting, distension, degree of weight loss/gain, dehydration. h) Parental competence to provide adequate care i) Follow-up arrangements made with infant's primary care physician. j) **Neonatal screening:** Screening for congenital hypothyroidism, phenylketonuria and cystic fibrosis and the universal Neonatal hearing screening is performed. Parents are given information about the 'blood spot screening' and hearing test. k) Ensure the initial vaccinations as indicated (BCG, Hepatitis B, and OPV).

KEY POINTS FOR CLINICAL PRACTICE *1)* A rapid yet complete assessment is warranted whenever an infant has an acute change in status. The evaluation should not impede attention to the immediate needs. It is a novice's mistake to suspect overwhelming sepsis, then to take several hours to obtain the history and perform the physical examination and a leisurely lumbar puncture before ensuring that antibiotics have been given to the infant. *2)* The initial evaluation, assessment and management of a Newborn baby must be directed toward promoting and facilitating normal adaptation to extrauterine life and early detection of significant medical problems so that they can be evaluated and treated appropriate ly. *3)* Communication and documentation: The findings of the examination are to be discussed with the parents and any questions/queries answered. The findings of the examination must be appropriately and accurately recorded. Relevant information relating to the baby should be provided to those involved in the future health care of the baby.

REFERENCES and FURTHER READING 1) Avery's diseases of the Newborn, 8th edition 2)Roberton's text book of Neonatology, 4th edition 3)Nelson text book of pediatrics, 18th edition

Pearl/Peril/Pitfall: Pallor usually accompanies other signs of distress except in anemic infants in whom there has been a fetomaternal hemorrhage across the placenta over a protracted period of time (chronic abruption). Such infants are in no obvious distress even though their pallor may be extreme. Pallor is more commonly a sign of acute blood loss, hypoxia, or poor peripheral perfusion due to hypotension. Subcutaneous edema may mimic pallor.

Significant Neonatal Problems which require further evaluation and management

Significant neonatal problem	Diagnostic features	Differential diagnosis	Clinical significance
1) *CEPHALHEMATOMA*	a) Localized {confined within the margins of the skull sutures} collection of blood beneath the Periosteum of one or both parietal bones b) On palpation, the border feels elevated and the center depressed c) Occasionally accompanied by a linear skull fracture.	In contrast Caput Succedaneum is bruising and oedema of the presenting part extending beyond the margins of the skull bones, resolves in a few days.	Mostly uncomplicated course with slow resolution over 1 or more months, with possible calcification. Occasional complications 1) Indirect hyperbilirubinemia 2) Secondary anemia 3) Depressed under lying skull fracture 4) Infection when the integrity of the overlying skin is broken {needle aspiration is contraindicated for the same reason}.
2) *PORTWINE STAIN (NAEVUS FLAMMEUS)*	a) Vascular malformation of the capillaries in the dermis, most commonly located unilaterally on the face. Present from birth and usually grows with the infant.	Unlike hemangiomas portwine stains remain flat.	Portwine stain involving the Ophthalmic branch of the 5th cranial nerve, can be associated with *STURGE - WEBER SYNDROME* {seizures, mental retardation, hemiplegia, and glaucoma}. If it involves an extremity it may lead to hemihypertrophy, a phenomenon called the *Klippel-Trenaunay- Weber syndrome*. Disfiguring lesions can now be improved with laser therapy.
3) *STRAWBERRY NAEVUS {CAVERNOUS HEMANGIOMIA}*	a) Not present at birth usually, but appears in the first month of life and increased in size until 3 to 9 months old, then gradually regresses b) More common in preterm infants c) Soft, compressible and usually range in size from a few millimeters to 5 cm, although some can be much larger.	Deep Hemangiomias appear bluish in colour and can mimic lymphangiomas. When placed in a dependent position, dependent deep hemangiomias enlarge as they fill with blood- a finding that helps differentiate them clinically from lymphangiomas.	No treatment is indicated unless the lesion interferes with vision or the airway. Ulceration can be treated with wet compresses, topical antibiotics and pulsed dye laser therapy. Steroids, interferon or surgical intervention may be indicated if the lesion is life - threatening {airway} for interfering vital functions {vision}. *Kasabach-Merritt Syndrome* - Thrombocytopenia associated with a rapidly expanding hemangioma
4) *FACIAL NERVE PALSY*	a) Facial asymmetry with crying: the corner of the mouth droops and the nasolabial fold is absent in the parlized side.	1) Mobius syndrome (usually bilateral) 2) Absence of the depressor anguli oris muscle (absence of involvement of the forehead, eyelid, or nasolabial area)	Excellent prognosis, with resolution within the first month if the palsy is secondary to trauma (from forceps or from compression of the nerve against sacral promontory while the head is in the birth canal) In the meantime, prevention of corneal drying is essential. Surgery is reserved for cases which clear-cut severing of the facial nerve has occurred. If the palsy persists, then absence of the nerve should be ruled out.
5) *ERB-DUCHENNE PARALYSIS (C5, C6)*	a) Adduction and internal rotation of the arm b) Pronation of the forearm, with the power of extension retained. c) Wrist is flexed.	*Klumpke's paralysis (C$_7$, C$_8$ and T1)* The hand is flaccid with little or no control..The distinction may not be clear-cut in some cases. If the sympathetic fibers of the T1 are injured, Ipsilateral ptosis and miosis can occur.	Treatment is deferred for at least 7–10 days ; then specific physical therapy and splinting should be undertaken. Most infants with brachial plexus palsies demonstrate complete recovery in first few months of life. EMG is indicated to assess the severity of the injury and to determine the prognosis in patients not showing improvement after 6-8 weeks. The earlier the onset of recovery, the better the long-term prognosis.
6) *STERNO CLEIDO MASTOID MUSCLE TUMOR*	a) Transient torticollis after birth due to SCM injury b) A well circumscribed, immobile mass in the mid portion of the SCM, that enlarges, regresses and disappears. c) The head tilts toward the involved side, the chin is elevated and rotated, and the patient can not move her head into normal position.	The differential diagnosis of Torticollis is extensive. It is a sign, not a disease. In neonatal period it may be the result of in utero positional (postural) effects or traumatic lesions of the sterno Cleido Mastoid Muscle or of congenital abnormalities of the cervical spine.	Conservative therapy should be initiated as soon as possible. Most recover with conservative management. If not, surgery should be considered. Instruct the parents to rotate the chin gently toward the side of the head tilt, while simultaneously bringing the head to the upright position. As the range of motion improves, the chin can be rotated past neutral and the head tilted toward the opposite side (gentle passive stretching exercises + stimulation).
7) *NATAL TEETH*	a) Natal teeth are present at birth, where as neonatal teeth erupt in the first month of life. Usually there are two in the position of the mandibular central incisors. b) Attachment of natal/neonatal teeth is generally limited to the gingival margin, with little root formation or bony support. c) They may be a supernumerary or a prematurely erupted primary tooth.	* A radiograph can easily differentiate between natal teeth and primary teeth. * Natal teeth are associated with cleft - palate, Pierre - Robin syndrome, - Ellis - Van Creveld syndrome, Hallermann - Streiff Syndrome etc. * A family history of natal teeth or premature eruption is present in 15–20% of affected children.	Extract natal teeth because of risk of detachment with aspiration, maternal discomfort because of abrasion or biting of the nipple during nursing. Decisions regarding extraction of prematurely erupted primary teeth must be made on an individual basis.
8) *CONGENITAL DISLOCATION OF THE HIP JOINT*	a) 6 times more common in females than in males with an overall incidence of 1.5 in 1000 live births. b) Associated factors include breech presentation, oligohydramnios and first - born infants. c) The pathologic anatomy involves superior capsular laxity and a shallow acetabulum due to limited concen tric contact with the femoral head.	* The key diagnostic sign on physical examination of the newborn is hip instability with the capacity for Hip dislocation *(Barlow manoeuvre)* and subsequent relocation back into the acetabulum *(Ortolani manoeuvre)* * Only 1 Hip should be examined at a time * Ultrasound examination of the Hip joint can identify the CDH between 2–6 weeks of age. (False positives are more common before 2 weeks of age).	Ideally orthopedic consultation for treatment should be obtained within the first 6 months of life. Early recognition of CDH is important as it reduces long term morbidity.

Obvious significant problems include 1. Skin and mucous membranes - Central Cyanosis, Severe Pallor, Jaundice noticed within 1st 24 hours, Sclerema 2. Vitals - Tachypnea, dyspnea, apnea, tachycardia, prolonged capillary refill time, low BP, Hypothermia / Hyperthermia 3. Significant heart murmurs and absent femoral pulses. 4. Abdominal distention 5. Bilious aspirates 6. Seizures 7. Poor feeding and lethargy. 8. Oliguria and / or anuria 9. Generalized edema. 10. Large and tense AF 11. Cataracts 12. Dysmorphic features 13. Abdominal masses/wall defects 14. Ambiguous genitalia and hydrometrocolpos due to imperforate hymen 15. Talipes equino varus / arthrogryposis 16. Hypotonia. 17. Bleeding tendency 18. Excessive salivation, gagging and cyanosis. 19. Not passing meconium < 36 hours, and urine within 48 hours.

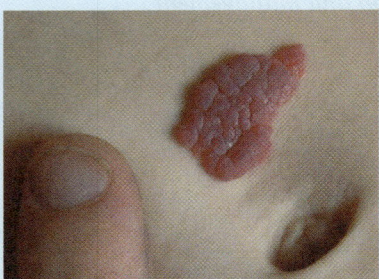 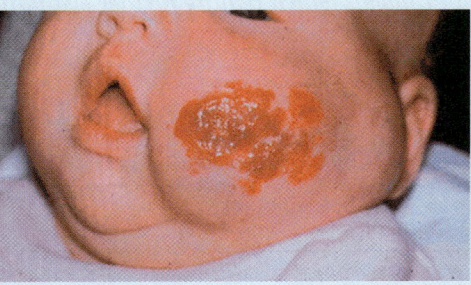 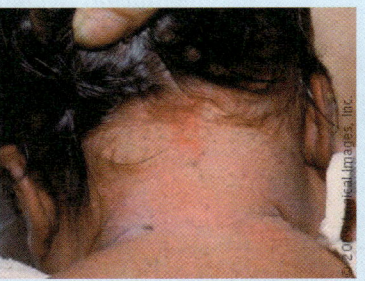

Strawberry hemangiomas: Because infantile hemangiomas are likely to improve or regress completely with time, there is no need for specific treatment in most cases. Treatment should be considered in the following circumstances. ·Very large and unsightly lesions ·Ulcerating hemangiomas (up to 5–25% of lesions) ·Lesions that impair vision, hearing, breathing or feeding ·If they fail to resolve by school age.

Salmon patch (Stork bite mark) these lesions become less intense with time, but are frequently visible into adulthood.

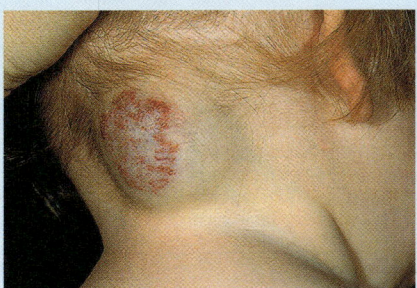
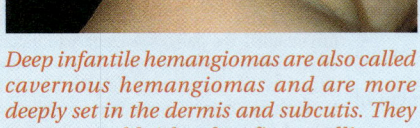
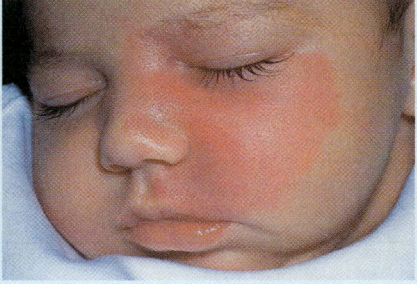 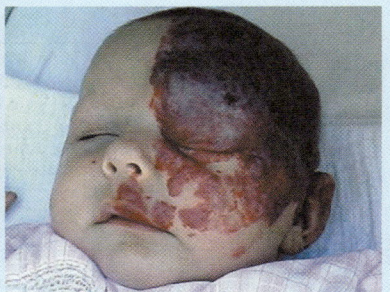

Deep infantile hemangiomas are also called cavernous hemangiomas and are more deeply set in the dermis and subcutis. They appear as a bluish soft to firm swelling.

Portwine stains maxillary and ophthalmic divisions of Vth cranial nerve: Port-wine stains affecting the entire V1 (ophthalmic) distribution predict strongly for underlying neurological and/or ocular disorders that require on-going ophthalmological surveillance and/or neurological management. Although the classical Sturge-Weber syndrome encompasses a triad of clinical manifestations (glaucoma, seizures, and port-wine stain, and it involves angiomas of the brain and meninges), incomplete forms are not uncommon. This neurooculo-cutaneous syndrome is believed to be a result of vascular malformations of associated structures derived from the neuroectoderm (facial skin, eye, and parieto-occipital region of the brain and leptomeninges) during the first trimester. However, the pathogenesis of port-wine stains and Sturge-Weber syndrome remains unclear.

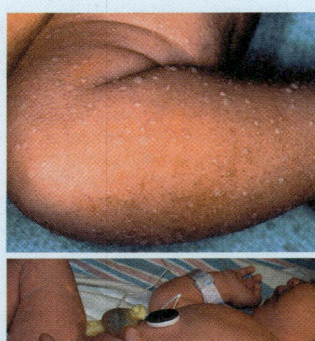
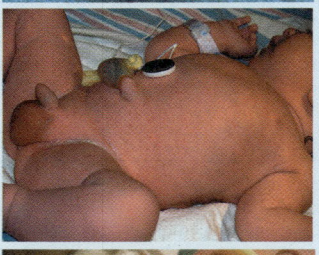
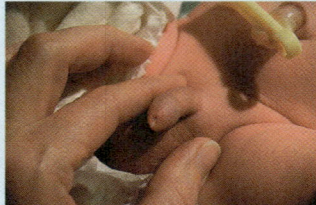

Transient neonatal pustular melanosis: All the lesions seen here are consistent with this diagnosis. The hallmark of this rash is the hyperpigmented spots that remain (seen here on the chest) after the fragile pustules (seen on the scrotum and thigh) have resolved. Because the rash starts in utero, lesions may be in any stage at birth. Despite the anxiety-provoking appearance of a newborn covered in pustules in the delivery room, no evaluation is needed when non-inflammatory pustules occur in combination with hyperpigmented macules in an otherwise well infant.

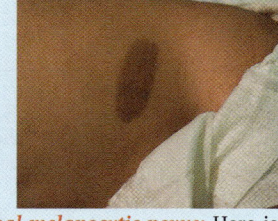

Junctional melanocytic nevus: Here is a typical appearance of a junctional melanocytic nevus. The lesion is completely flat and is medium to dark brown in color. It may be present at birth, as it was in this infant. It may become slightly raised as the infant grows and may become a compound nevus if intradermal melanocytes develop. It is considered a benign lesion.

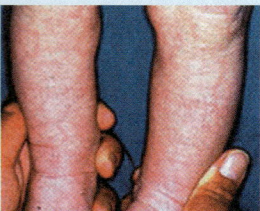
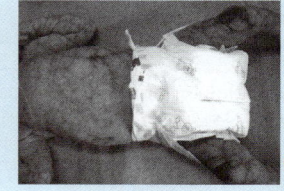

Penile Pearl: Pearls" may be found in a variety of locations in the newborn. In the mouth, they are referred to as "Epstein Pearls". The tip of the foreskin is another relatively common location. The pearl is a small, firm, white nodule that contains keratin. It will spontaneously exfoliate and resolve with time. It is a normal finding and is not a contraindication to circumcision, if desired.

Mottling (Cutis Marmorata): The lacy erythema present on the thigh of this newborn is mottling. Not to be confused with cutis marmorata telangiectasia congenita, cutis marmorata (mottling) is a transient and common finding in newborns. It is particular visible when the infant is cold and disappears with warming.

Cutis marmorata telangiectatica congenita: a rare benign sporadic congenital vascular anomaly characterised by persistent cutis marmorata, telangiectasia, and phlebectasia and often associated with skin atrophy and ulceration. The cutaneous lesions commonly occur on the legs, arms, and trunk and rarely involve the face and scalp. Associated abnormalities such as body asymmetry, vascular and neurological anomalies, glaucoma, macrocephaly, and psychomotor retardation occur in many patients. The diagnosis is mainly clinical, and prognosis is generally good, with cutaneous lesions improving during infancy. There is no specific treatment, and long term follow up is indicated with associated abnormalities.

Courtesy: P Manikoth, P A K Nair, M G Pai, M A A Ajmi Special Care Baby Unit, Royal Hospital, Muscat, Oman; manikoth@omantel.net.com

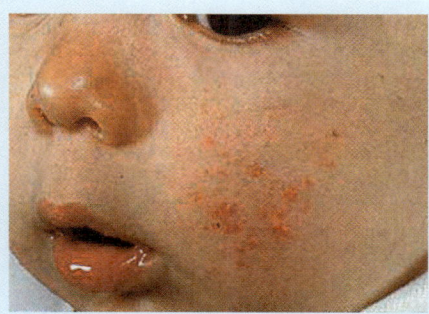

Acne neonatorum occurs in up to 20 percent of newborns. It typically consists of closed comedones on the forehead, nose, and cheeks, although other locations are possible. Open comedones, inflammatory papules, and pustules can also develop. Neonatal acne is thought to result from stimulation of sebaceous glands by maternal or infant androgens. Parents should be counseled that lesions usually resolve spontaneously within four months without scarring. Treatment generally is not indicated, but infants can be treated with a 2.5% benzoyl peroxide lotion if lesions are extensive and persist for several months. Parents should apply a small amount of benzoyl peroxide to the antecubital fossa to test for local reaction before widespread or facial application. Severe, unrelenting neonatal acne accompanied by other signs of hyperandrogenism should prompt an investigation for adrenal cortical hyperplasia, virilizing tumors, or underlying endocrinopathies.

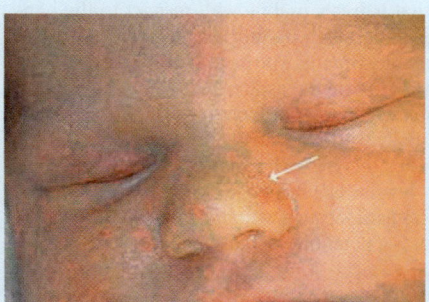

Milia: The white papules on this baby's chin and cheeks are milia. Milia are keratin filled epithelial cysts which occur in up to 40% of newborns. Spontaneous exfoliation and resolution is expected within a few weeks. Parents will occasionally mistake these lesion for neonatal acne, but milia are present at birth and have no inflammatory component. Acne, even though caused by maternal hormones, does not generally appear until *after* 2 weeks of age

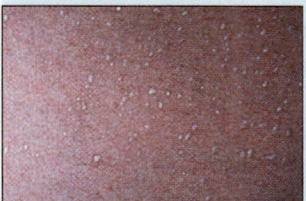

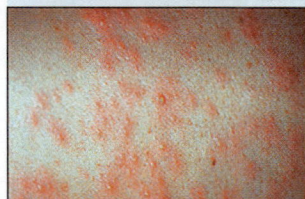

Miliaria Miliaria results from sweat retention caused by partial closure of eccrine structures. Both milia and miliaria result from immaturity of skin structures, but they are clinically distinct entities. Miliaria affects up to 40 percent of infants and usually appears during the first month of life. Several clinically distinguishable subtypes exist; miliaria crystallina and miliaria rubra are the most common. **Miliaria crystallina** (Figure on top) is caused by superficial eccrine duct closure. It consists of 1- to 2-mm vesicles without surrounding erythema, most commonly on the head, neck, and trunk. Each vesicle evolves, with rupture followed by desquamation, and may persist for hours to days. **Miliaria rubra,**(Figure on bottom) also known as heat rash, is caused by a deeper level of sweat gland obstruction. Its lesions are small erythematous papules and vesicles, usually occurring on covered portions of the skin. Miliaria crystallina and miliaria rubra are benign. Avoidance of overheating, removal of excess clothing, cooling baths, and air conditioning are recommended for management and prevention of these disorders.

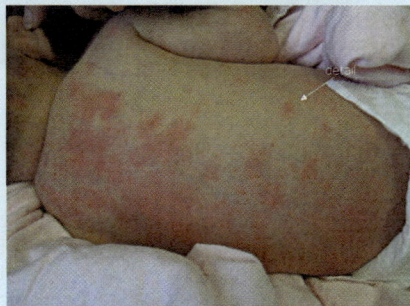 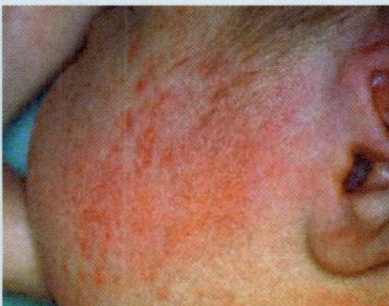 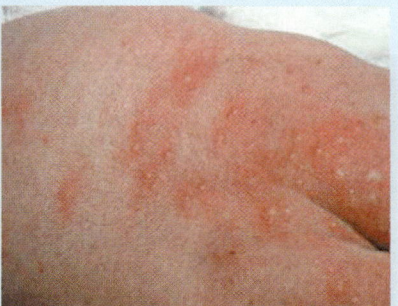

Erythema Toxicum Neonatorum: Erythema toxicum neonatorum is the most common pustular eruption in newborns. Estimates of incidence vary between 40 and 70 percent. It is most common in infants born at term and weighing more than 2,500 g (5.5 lb). Erythema toxicum neonatorum may be present at birth but more often appears during the second or third day of life. Typical lesions consist of erythematous, 2- to 3-mm macules and papules that evolve into pustules. Each pustule is surrounded by a blotchy area of erythema, leading to what is classically described as a "flea-bitten" appearance. Lesions usually occur on the face, trunk, and proximal extremities. Palms and soles are not involved. Several infections (e.g., herpes simplex, Candida, and Staphylococcus infections) also may present with vesiculopustular rashes in the neonatal period; infants who appear sick or who have an atypical rash should be tested for these infections. In healthy infants, the diagnosis of erythema toxicum neonatorum is made clinically and can be confirmed by cytologic examination of a pustular smear, which will show eosinophilia with Gram, Wright, or Giemsa staining. Peripheral eosinophilia may also be present. The etiology of erythema toxicum neonatorum is not known. Lesions generally fade over five to seven days, but they may recur for several weeks. No treatment is needed, and the condition is not associated with any systemic abnormality.

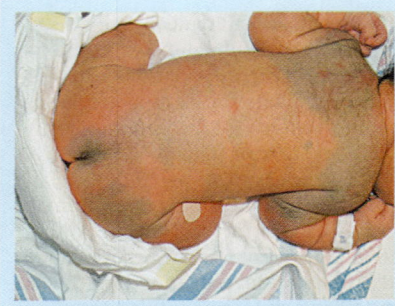

DERMAL MELANOSIS/MONGOLIAN BLUE SPOTS/SLATE GREY PATCHES:
Dermal melanosis is another type of pigmented birthmark. Commonly known as "mongolian spots," these flat bluish-gray or brown lesions arise when melanocytes are trapped deep in the skin. These lesions most often occur on the back or buttocks and may easily be mistaken for bruises. The incidence of dermal melanosis varies widely among racial and ethnic groups; they are more common in black, Native American, Asian, and Hispanic populations. Because the "bruise" appearance may raise suspicion for child abuse in some settings, dermal melanosis should be documented in the medical record. They can be easily differentiated from bruises by the absence of other colors associated with bruises — red, purple, green, brown or yellow. Most lesions fade by two years of age and do not require treatment.

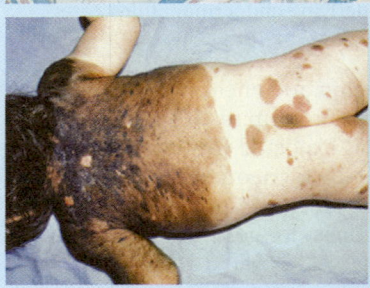
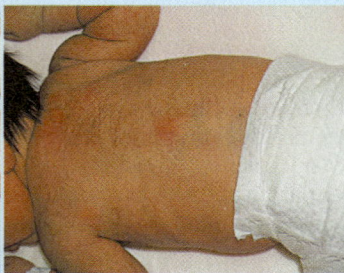

Subcutaneous Fat Necrosis: On palpation, there is a firm nodule in the subcutaneous tissue under the area of redness that is freely mobile with respect to the bony structures underneath it. Subcutaneous fat necrosis is more common in infants who have had difficult deliveries, cold stress, or perinatal asphyxia. Lesions are typically asymptomatic and resolve spontaneously within several weeks, usually without scarring or atropy. Infants with extensive lesions or with renal disease should have calcium levels followed once or twice weekly. Hypercalcemia associated with subcutaneous fat necrosis is rare, but is a potentially lethal complication.

Congenital Giant melanocytic nevi: (i.e. "garment nevi") are larger than 40 cm in adulthood and carry the highest risk of malignancy. Large lesions (20 to 40 cm in adulthood) occur in 0.025 percent of newborns and carry a 4 to 6 percent lifetime risk of malignancy. Greater numbers of satellite nevi near a large lesion also increase risk. Smaller nevi are not well studied, but lesions that are projected to grow to less than 1.5 cm in adulthood rarely progress to melanoma.

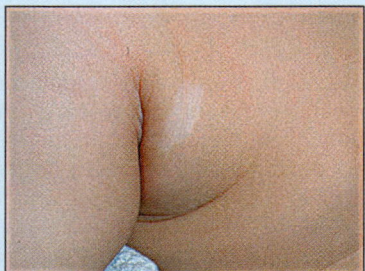

Hypopigmented macules, also known as "ash-leaf spots," can be present at birth and are most common on the trunk and lower extremities. They appear in 80 percent of persons with tuberous sclerosis by one year of age. Thus, they are the earliest indicator of this disorder. Affected patients also may have had a white tuft of scalp hair since birth. A Wood's lamp examination helps identify hypopigmented lesions because areas with reduced or absent melanin do not absorb the light and appear lighter than normal skin.

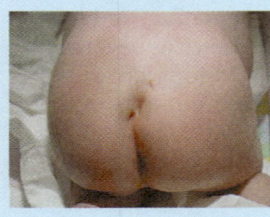

Sacral dimples are relatively common, occurring in 2-4% of newborn infants. They may be associated with a tuft of hair. Almost always, if the dimple is within the gluteal crease, there is no underlying spinal abnormality and no investigation is necessary. Dimples that may require further investigation are those that are large (>5mm), deep (may represent dermal sinuses and may communicate with the underlying spinal canal), those above the gluteal crease, or those associated with other cutaneous markers of spinal dysraphism. The deeper lesions may be prone to infections secondary to trapped debris and hair etc. The parents should be advised to maintain local hygiene and to teach the child the same at a later stage. In the neonatal period, an ultrasound may give pictures which demonstrate any communication with the cutaneous abnormality. The lower image to the left shows a normal spinal cord as imaged above the lesion; no communication is normal, and the spinal cord is seen tapering.

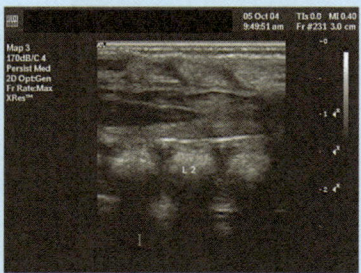

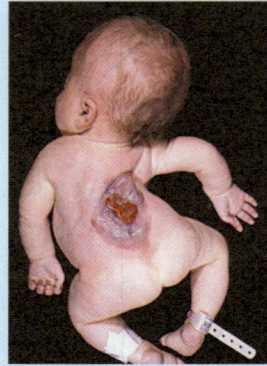

Myelomeningocele: ·Occurs in 80-90% of spina bifida cystica cases. ·80% are lumbosacral consisting of a sac covered with a thin membrane that may leak CSF. ·Level of lesion is best assessed by determining upper limit of sensory loss but at all levels there is disturbance of bladder and bowel control. ·Higher lesions are associated with bladder outlet obstruction with consequent dilatation of the upper urinary tract and ·chronic pyelonephritis. ·Hydrocephalus occurs in approximately 90% of cases at birth even with normal head circumference. ·Usually associated with Chiari II malformation but may also be due to aqueduct stenosis or have no clear cause. ·Usually detected by ultrasound. ·If signs of progressive ventricular dilatation or ·rising intracranial pressure, usually needs insertion of a ventriculoperitoneal shunt.

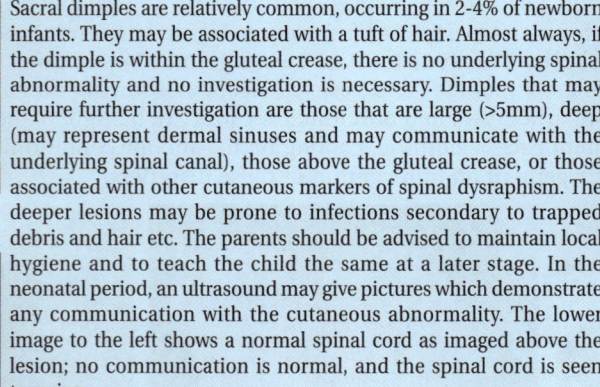

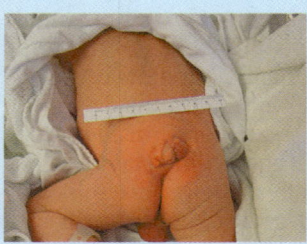
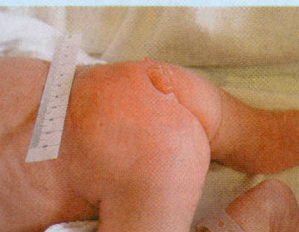
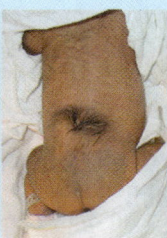

Any lesion (Tuft of Hair/Lipoma) from the lower lumbar region to the upper cervical region that covers the midline should be treated with respect. Consider the possibility of an underlying spinal anomaly until proven otherwise and obtain the necessary investigations: plain films and ultrasound. *If any doubt remains, MRI is the study of choice for imaging neural tissue and for identifying contents of the defect in the newborn.*

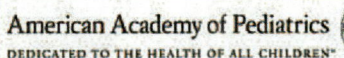
American Academy of Pediatrics
DEDICATED TO THE HEALTH OF ALL CHILDREN®

Section on Ophthalmology

See RED

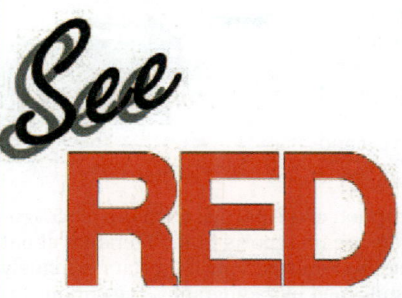

Red reflexes from the retinas can be used by the physician to great advantage. The illustration shown here depicts the inequality of the red reflection or the interference with the red reflections in various conditions. The white dots represent corneal light reflexes.

Techniques: Set the ophthalmoscope (preferably one with a halogen light source*) on zero or close to zero, stand a few feet away from the child seated in the parent's lap, attract the child with voice or noise encouraging the child to look at the light, compare the red reflection from each pupil. Both red reflections should be viewed simultaneously and alternately. An expanded observation is the position of the white reflection, the corneal light reflex.

The beauty of this test is that it can be done with a "hands-off" approach; it can furnish accurate information without dilatation of the pupils. As a screening device it is very cost effective. We encourage you to work with this technique. It is useful far beyond all other manual inspection tests for assessments of vision, refraction, motility, alignment, injury evaluations, and eyelid-pupil relationships.

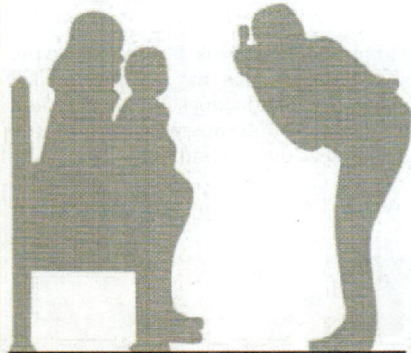

REFERENCE
Tongue AC, Cibis CW: Bruckner test. Ophthalmology. 1981;88:1041–1044.
*Welch Allyn Ophthalmoscope # 11720

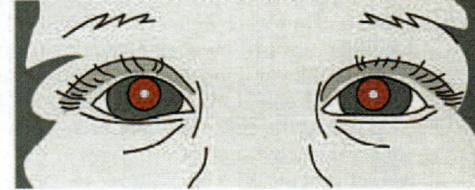
↓ **NORMAL**—Child looks at light. Both red reflections are equal.

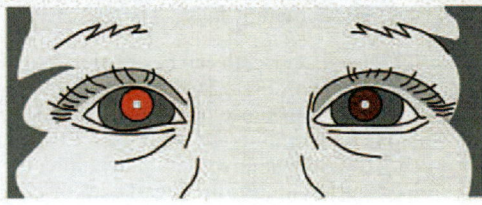
↓ **UNEQUAL REFRACTION**—One red reflection is brighter than the other.

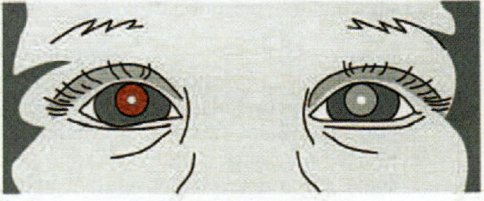
↓ **NO REFLEX (CATARACT)**—The presence of lens or other media opacities blocks the red reflection or diminishes it.

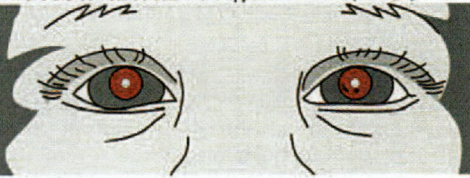
↓ **FOREIGN BODY/ABRASION (LEFT CORNEA)**—The red reflection from the pupil will back-light corneal defects or foreign bodies. Movement of the examiner's head in one direction will appear to move the corneal defects in the opposite direction. (Parallax)

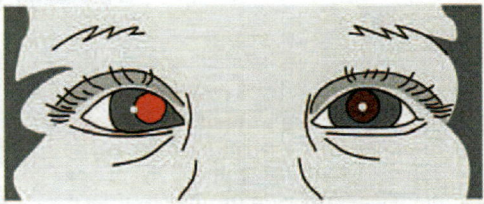

↓ **STRABISMUS**—The red reflection is more intense from the deviated eye.

Copyright © 1991, Alfred G. Smith, MD, Miami, FL

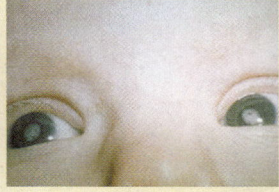

Congenital Cataract: With a closer view, cloudiness within the pupil is clearly seen. Congenital cataracts require early intervention to preserve sight, so immediate referral to a pediatric ophthalmologist is indicated. It is important to remember that cataracts that are less dense may not be visibly cloudy, so any time red reflexes cannot be obtained on exam, even if the eye appears grossly normal, referral is required.

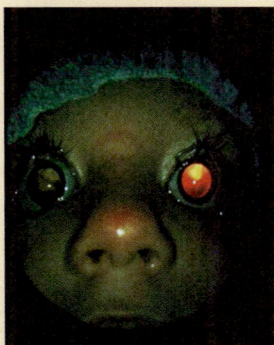

The red reflex: should be assessed as soon as possible after birth although this may be difficult with swollen or edematous lids in the newborn. The six week check is an ideal time to assess the red reflex. It is best done in a dimly lit room, with a direct ophthalmoscope set a +4.00 diopters and a working distance of 12 to 18 inches to illuminate both pupils simultaneously. The reflex should be identical in each eye and if it is not immediate referral is indicated. Infants and children with ocular opacities often present with leucocoria (a white pupillary reflex).

AAP Recommendations: All neonates, infants, and children should have an examination of the red reflex of the eyes performed by a pediatrician or other primary care clinician trained in this examination technique before discharge from the neonatal nursery and during all subsequent routine health supervision visits. *The result of the red reflex examination is to be rated as normal when the reflections of the 2 eyes viewed both individually and simultaneously are equivalent in color, intensity, and clarity and there are no opacities or white spots (leukokoria) within the area of either or both red reflexes. *All infants or children with an abnormal Bruckner reflex or absent red reflex should be referred immediately to an ophthalmologist who is skilled in pediatric examinations. *It is essential that the referring practitioner communicate the abnormal findings directly to the ophthalmologist and receive confirmation back from the ophthalmologist that proper follow-up consultation was performed. *Infants or children in high-risk categories, including relatives of patients with retinoblastoma, infantile or juvenile cataracts, retinal dysplasia, glaucoma, or other vision-threatening ocular disorders that can present in infancy, should not only have red reflex testing performed in the nursery but also be referred to an ophthalmologist who is experienced in examining children for a complete eye examination regardless of the findings of the red reflex testing by the pediatrician. *Infants or children in whom parents or other observers describe a history suspicious for the presence of leukokoria (a white pupil reflex) in 1 or both eyes should be examined by an ophthalmologist who is experienced in the examination of children, because small retinoblastoma tumors or other serious lesions may present in a subtle fashion.

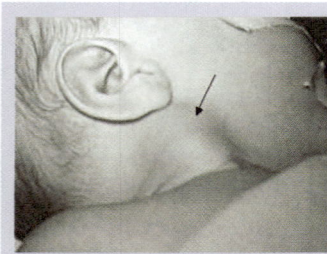

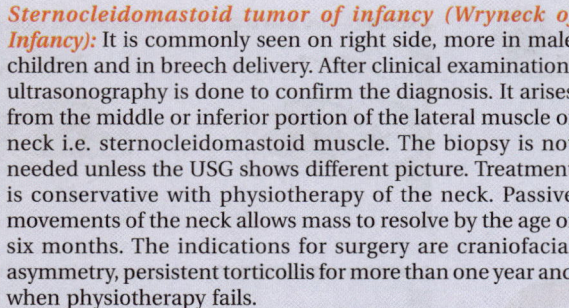

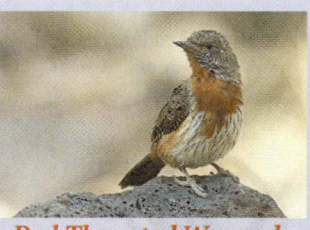

Sternocleidomastoid tumor of infancy (Wryneck of Infancy): It is commonly seen on right side, more in male children and in breech delivery. After clinical examination, ultrasonography is done to confirm the diagnosis. It arises from the middle or inferior portion of the lateral muscle of neck i.e. sternocleidomastoid muscle. The biopsy is not needed unless the USG shows different picture. Treatment is conservative with physiotherapy of the neck. Passive movements of the neck allows mass to resolve by the age of six months. The indications for surgery are craniofacial asymmetry, persistent torticollis for more than one year and when physiotherapy fails.

Red Throated Wryneck

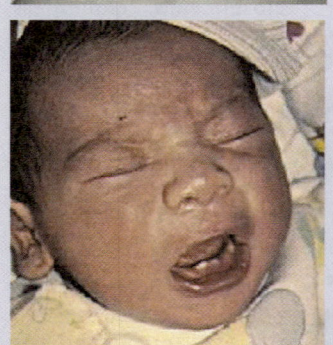

Natal teeth: The teeth can be either a premature eruption of the normal teeth (up to 95%) or supernumerary (5%). The cause is not known. There are no reports in the literature about the actual occurrence of aspiration. Natal teeth may be removed only if they are extremely mobile. Supernumerary teeth need extraction if confirmed by radiography. Indications for extraction include hypermobility, difficulties during breast-feeding, traumatic ulcerations on tongue/frenulum/lip (Riga-Fede's disease), inflammation, etc. Some authors recommend splinting or disking of the affected teeth to prevent traumatic injuries. Although no case is reported in the literature, there is usually great concern about possible aspiration or swallowing of hypermobile.

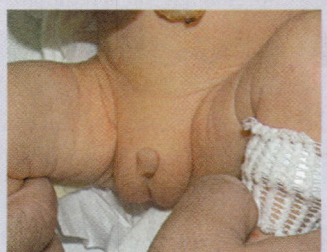

Ambiguous Genitalia: In any case where the genitalia are ambiguous, a work-up to determine gender and the underlying cause of the ambiguity should begin immediately. These infants should be initially observed in the NICU so that any electrolyte abnormalities can be identified and treated rapidly, and appropriate specialists involved (e.g. endocrine, genetics, urology). Circumcision is absolutely contraindicated when genital ambiguity exists. This particular infant was an under-virilized male with hypospadias, micropenis, and bifid scrotum (testes were present bilaterally).

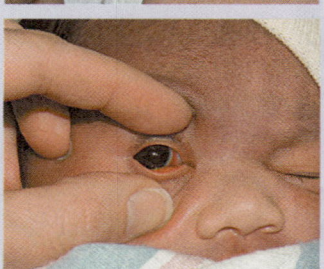

Subconjunctival hemorrhage is a frequent finding in normal newborns. It results from the breakage of small vessels during the pressure of delivery. The red area may be large or small but is always confined to the limits of the sclera. It is asymptomatic, does not affect vision, and spontaneously resolves in several days. Note also the numerous petechiae on the forehead. This infant had significant facial bruising as well as the eye finding.

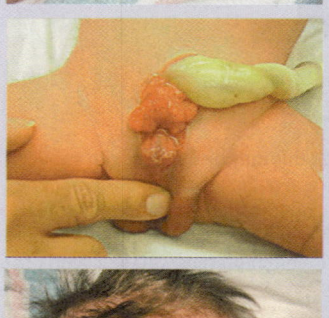

This is an example of ***severe epispadias and bladder exstrophy.*** The penis appears to be nearly completely splayed open lengthwise on the dorsal surface, and actually has a dorsal curvature which is minimized by the downward pressure applied to the scrotum. The red tissue inferior to the umbilical cord is the inner (posterior) wall of the bladder which is also splayed apart and protruding through a defect in the anterior pelvic wall. Surgical correction is required.

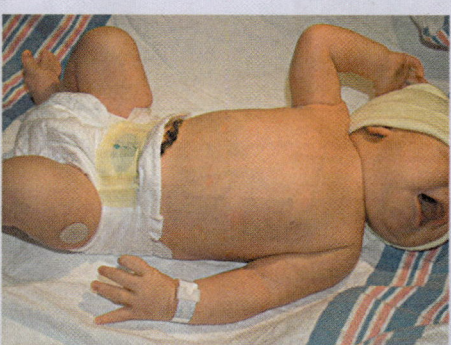

Erb's Palsy: When shoulder dystocia occurs during the birth, injury to the brachial plexus can occur. This photo shows how the posture of the arms is asymmetric: the left arm is at the side and the hand is medially rotated at a time when the other arm is flexed with crying. Testing the Moro (startle) reflex in this infant produces a similar result as the left arm does not raise as high as the right. Most brachial plexus injuries of this type resolve spontaneously. Improvement in movement can often be noted within the first 24 hours. If improvement does not occur, referral to a pediatric neurologist, and possibly a physical therapist, is warranted.

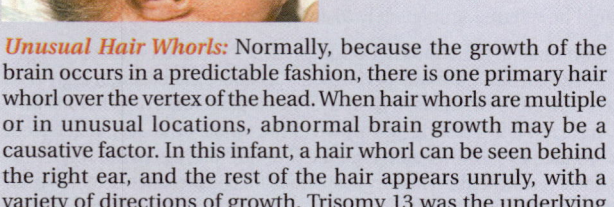

Unusual Hair Whorls: Normally, because the growth of the brain occurs in a predictable fashion, there is one primary hair whorl over the vertex of the head. When hair whorls are multiple or in unusual locations, abnormal brain growth may be a causative factor. In this infant, a hair whorl can be seen behind the right ear, and the rest of the hair appears unruly, with a variety of directions of growth. Trisomy 13 was the underlying diagnosis.

"From a drop of water," said the writer, "a logician could infer the possibility of an Atlantic or a Niagara without having seen or heard of one or the other. So all life is a great chain, the nature of which is known whenever we are shown a single link of it. Like all other arts, the Science of Deduction and Analysis is one which can only be acquired by long and patient study nor is life long enough to allow any mortal to attain the highest possible perfection in it. Before turning to those moral and mental aspects of the matter which present the greatest difficulties, let the inquirer begin by mastering more elementary problems. Let him, on meeting a fellow-mortal, learn at a glance to distinguish the history of the man, and the trade or profession to which he belongs. Puerile as such an exercise may seem, it sharpens the faculties of observation, and teaches one where to look and what to look for. By a man's finger nails, by his coat-sleeve, by his boot, by his trouser knees, by the callosities of his forefinger and thumb, by his expression, by his shirt cuffs — by each of these things a man's calling is plainly revealed. That all united should fail to enlighten the competent inquirer in any case is almost inconceivable."
From "The Book of Life", an article by Holmes quoted in "A Study in Scarlet"

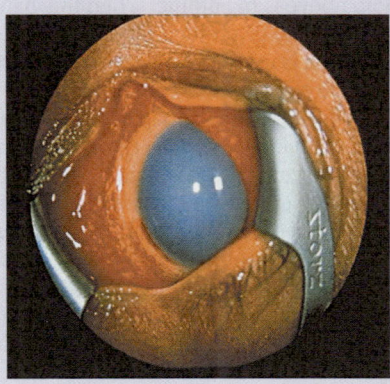 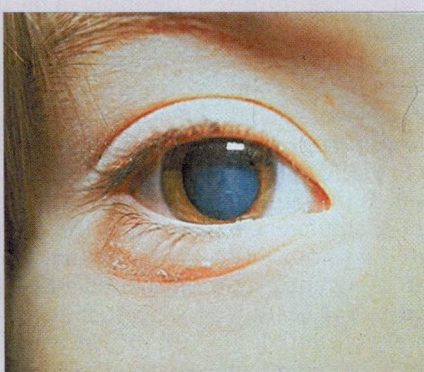

Absent Red Reflex is common to both - but two different Ophthalmic Emergencies!

Deviation of Angle of Mouth common to both-but two different conditions of Facial Asymmetry!

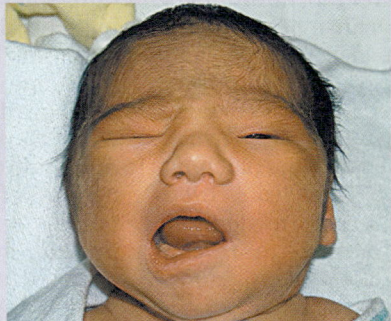 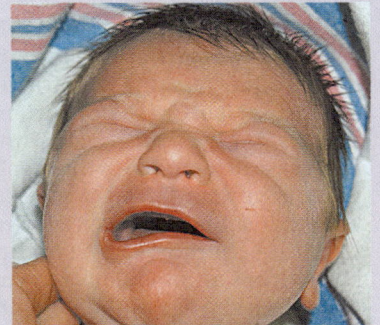

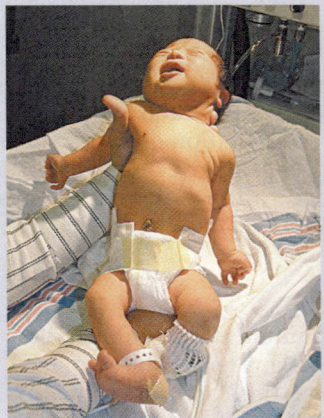 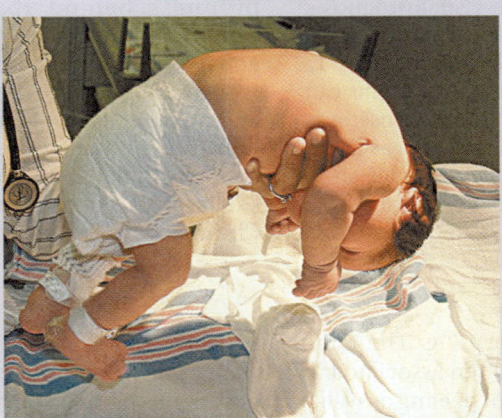

Floppy infant syndrome- outline the differential diagnosis

What is the most likely underlying diagnosis ?

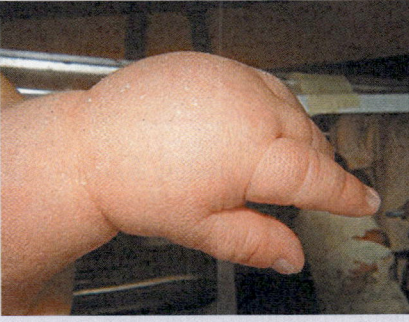 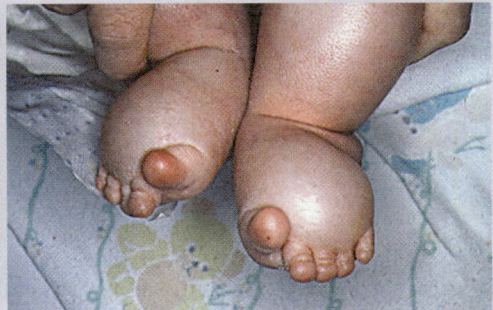

1. Congenital glaucoma (Photo on Lt side) may be sporadic or inherited as an autosomal dominant. Characteristically the children are described as having "large beautiful eyes" and this should signal an alarm, particularly if the eyes are of obviously different size. These children present with constant tearing and photophobia and are intolerant even of ordinary room illumination. The increased intraocular pressure drives aqueous humor through the cornea into the corneal epithelium which breaks down causing significant pain and discomfort. The disease is most often bilateral and as the pressure increases the normally clear cornea takes on a white or bluish appearance, beginning centrally. Eventually the cornea becomes completely opaque. The disease is more common in children with Down's syndrome. even if treated successfully the resultant enlarged eye changes the refractive error and often leads to significant amblyopia. Congenital cataract (Photo on Rt side) : In contrast to the first photo, the opacity here occur behind the pupil, as the pupil is easily and clearly seen along its entire circumference. Again, the opacity can be appreciated without any special equipment (a good reminder to assess the eyes visually even if an ophthalmoscope is not readily available). Whenever this finding is encountered, a workup for an underlying etiology should be sought as a long list of metabolic, infectious, and genetic disorders are associated with cataracts. Because of the rapid growth of the eye during the first two years of life, and the resultant change in refractive power of the eye, intraocular lenses are not currently recommended for infants. Aggressive occlusion therapy is always necessary to force use of the involved eye, and patching is frequently continued to the age of eight years. Even with early surgery and aggressive optical correction and patching therapy, the visual prognosis in an eye harbouring a uniocular congenital cataract is quite poor. Past the age of three months cataract surgery is not recommended at all because the visual prognosis is so grim from the resultant deprivational amblyopia.

2. This infant has a facial nerve palsy on the left (Photo on Lt side). Here, both the abnormal lip and eyelid positions can be seen. When the eyelid does not completely close, it is important to protect the eye with a lubricant, such as Lacri-Lube, to prevent corneal abrasions. An infant (Photos on Rt side) whose face appears symmetrical at rest and whose mouth is pulled downward to one side when crying is said to have an "asymmetric crying facies". The cause of the facial asymmetry in this disorder is congenital absence or hypoplasia of the depressor anguli oris muscle at the corner of the mouth. Asymmetric crying facies may be isolated or it may be associated with various anomalies related to cardiovascular, musculoskeletal, respiratory, gastrointestinal, central nervous system or genitourinary systems.

3. *Neonatal hypotonia:* The assessment of tone can be made both from observing the posture and activity of the infant when undisturbed and also by handling the baby. Infants with normal tone will not feel "floppy" when held by the examiner. The infant in the photo above is hypotonic. When this baby was lifted, the examiner had to give much more support to the head and shoulders than is usual to keep the infant from sliding our of her hands. Notice how the both arms fall back (instead of being held in flexion), and the baby's chest seems to drape over the physician's hand. *Neonatal Hypotonia:* Here is the same infant held in ventral suspension. Normally newborns do have a convex curvature of the spine in this position, but not to this degree. Here the head drops much lower than one would expect, and the examiner has the sense that the infant could easily slip out of her hand without extra support. In this case, the hypotonia was caused by trisomy 21. For Differential Diagnosis Refer to The Chapter "Neonatal Hypotonia-Floppy Infant Syndrome".

4. Congenital lymphedema is a frequent finding in those patients who are subsequently diagnosed with Turner's syndrome. Although not all edema is related to Turner's syndrome, the diagnosis should be considered in infants who have this finding. Other physical findings associated with this disorder include short stature, short fourth metacarpal, webbed neck, high palate and nail dysplasia. In the photo on Lt side, the edema of the hand is striking. In this case, Turner's syndrome was the underlying diagnosis. Here is an example of lymphedema of the feet (photo on Rt side) as a result of Turner's syndrome. From this angle, the excessive puffiness behind the toes can be easily seen. Lymphedema: Lymphedema may be present at any age and is one finding that can suggest Turner syndrome on fetal ultrasonography. Lymphedema is the cause of other anomalies, such as the webbed neck and low posterior hairline. In infants, the combination of dysplastic or hypoplastic nails and lymphedema gives a characteristic sausage like appearance to the fingers and toes. Chromosomal testing confirmed the clinical diagnosis.

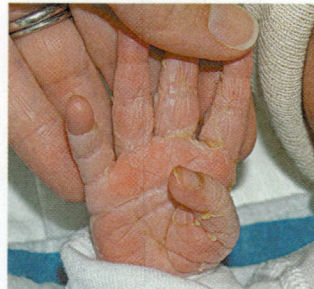

Normal peeling: The hands and feet are especially common places to observe peeling. Often associated with infants who are post dates, many term babies exhibit this kind of peeling as well. In this patient, the skin and nails (look at the thumbnail) are stained yellow from the presence of meconium in utero. This photo was taken a few hours after birth, so the moist appearance of the skin is still visible. By the following day, the skin was more dry and the difference between the peeled and non-peeled areas of the hand was less visible.

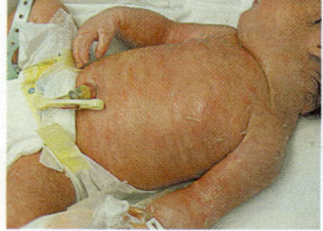

Icthyosis: In contrast, this type of peeling is not normal. Notice how the skin under the peeled areas is red and fissured and how the fingers on the right hand appear edematous. This newborn had an uncomplicated pregnancy and delivery, but this skin appearance in the delivery room prompted transfer to the NICU for further evaluation. For this baby, Aquaphor was liberally applied to the skin, and the infant was kept in an isolette to minimize fluid losses.

Routine neonatal examination

Known colloquially as 'the baby check', this examination should be carried out by a member of the paediatric team where the baby is still in hospital, or by the GP and primary care team following home births. Ensure the aims of the examination are fully explained to the parent(s) before it is conducted. The findings should be shared with the parent(s) and recorded in the postnatal care plan and the personal child health record. The examination should be carried out within 72 hours of birth and incorporate: *A review of parental concerns and the baby's medical history *Family, maternal, antenatal and perinatal history *Fetal, neonatal and infant history including any previously plotted birth-weight and ● head circumference *Whether the baby has passed meconium and urine (and urinary stream in a boy) *Other screening tests as recommended by the IAP/UK National Screening Committee/AAP should also be carried out or arranged at this time. ● **The examination is best conducted in a well-lit, warm, private room with the mother in attendance and able to see and help with what is being done.**

Suggested schema for screening neonatal examination

First wash your hands thoroughly to reduce the risk of cross-infection. Then:

* **Listen and observe**
  * *Assess overall appearance.* Note general tone, sleepiness and rousability. Observe general condition, proportions and maturity.
  * *Look* carefully for evidence of jaundice (preferably in bright, natural light). Are there any · birthmarks, rashes or other skin abnormalities?
  * *Listen* to the baby's cry and note its sound.
  * *Weigh* the baby and plot this reading on its · growth chart.

* **Perform a systematic 'head-to-toes' examination**
  This should be done carefully and in good light to detect abnormalities:

* **Head**
  * Shape, presence of · fontanelle and whether normal, sunken or bulging
  * Measure and record head circumference on growth chart
  * Assess facial appearance and eye position
  * Look for any asymmetry or abnormality of facial form

* ***Eyes**
  * Normal shape and appearance?
  * Check for presence of · red reflex
  * Look for obvious cataracts or signs of · ophthalmic infection

* ***Ears**
  * Shape and size
  * Are they set at the normal level or 'low set'?
  * Check patency of external auditory meatus

* ***Mouth**
  * Color of mucous membrane, observe the palate
  * Check suckling reflex by inserting a **clean** little finger gently inside baby's mouth

* ***Arms and hands**
  * Are they of normal shape and moving normally?
  * Look for evidence of traction birth injury (e.g. · Erb's palsy) by checking neck, shoulders and clavicles
  * Count fingers and observe their shape – is there any evidence of · clinodactyly (incurving of fingers)?
  * Check palmar creases – are they multiple or single? A single palmar crease may be normal, but can be a sign of · Down's syndrome.

* ***Peripheral pulses**
  * Check brachial, radial and femoral pulses for rate, rhythm and volume
  * A hyperdynamic pulse may suggest · persistent ductus arteriosus
  * A weak pulse may occur with a congenital cardiac anomaly (impairing cardiac output and in conjunction with other signs from the examination)
  * Check for radio-femoral delay (·aortic coarctation)

*Heart
  * Check cardiac position by palpation and feel for any thrill or heave
  * Listen to the ·heart sounds carefully and for any added sounds or ·murmurs
  * Suspected abnormalities require further examination (and often more expert opinion and investigation)

*Lungs:
  * Watch respiratory pattern, rate and depth for a few seconds
  * Look for any evidence of · intercostal recession
  * Listen for ·stridor
  * Auscultate lung fields for added sounds

*Abdomen
  * Look at abdominal girth and shape
  * Carefully check the umbilical stump for infection or surrounding · hernia
  * Palpate gently for organs, masses or herniae
  * It is common to be able to feel the liver and/or spleen in healthy newborns
  * Check the external genitalia carefully (see · Ambiguous Genitalia)
  * Palpate for testicles in boys
  * Inspect the anus (has meconium been passed?)

*Back
  * Look carefully at skin over back and at spinal curvature/ symmetry · Is there any evidence of · spina bifida occulta or pilonidal sinus hidden by flesh creases or dimples?
  * Palpate the spine gently

*Hips
  * Specifically test for · congenital dislocation of the hip (a.k.a. congenital hip dysplasia) using combination of Barlow and Ortolani maneuvers (follow link for more detail)

*Legs
  * Watch movements at each joint
  * Check for any evidence of · talipes equinovarus
  * Count toes and check shape

*CNS
  * Observe tone, behavioral, movements and posture
  * Elicit newborn reflexes only if there is cause for concern
  * Further examination should be conducted as necessary according to any abnormalities that are detected, or suspicions of undetected illness in the baby.

*Record findings
  * Always document the findings of the examination in the postnatal care plan and personal child health record. A proforma for the examination, kept within the notes, can save time and act as a prompt to ensure that no element of the examination is missed.

Late examination At the end of the first w -10 days) the check should include the following: ● Weight (relate to birth weight) ● Head circumference (relate to birth head circumference) ● Length (relate to birth length) ● Feeding ● Meconium passage in first day ● Vomiting (especially bile stained) ● Colour, especially Cyanosis and Jaundice ● Respiratory distress (including respiratory rate) ● Heart murmur ● Femoral pulses ● Eye check: Eyes open; Pupil size, shape, equal and Cornea clear, Red reflex. ● Hips ● Cord ● Tone and activity· Newborn screening done

Pearl/Peril/Pitfall: *Cataracts, if present, should be identified at the time of the first nursery examination. Cataracts vary in size from pinpoint to involvement of the entire lens. Occasionally they can develop several days or weeks after birth. If the entire lens is affected, cataracts are easily seen by shining a light tangentially into the eye by the light source being held to one side. If the opacity is small, it can be identified only with an ophthalmoscope. White pupils may also be seen in the presence of lesions deeper in the eye, such as retinoblastoma. Cataracts are usually bilateral. They are a major manifestation of intrauterine rubella infection and are occasionally seen in cytomegalovirus infection. They may be transmitted as a dominant trait from an affected parent. In congenital galactosemia, cataracts sometimes appear several weeks after birth.*

Acute Collapse in a Neonate

8

@ *"ACUTE COLLAPSE in an apparently well baby is often the most demanding of crises that would happen in any SCBU/NICU. The parents tend to think that "it must be somebody's fault" understandably, and a painful one for the dedicated staff to cope with."*

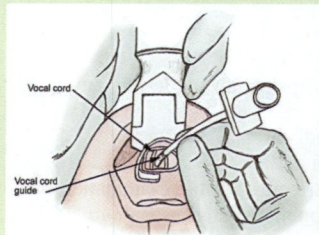

Ensure ABCs by changing a blocked/displaced ET Tube!

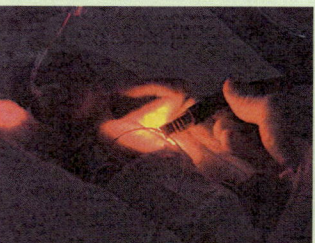

Transilluminate the Chest/Emergent CXR to identify Pneumothoraces!

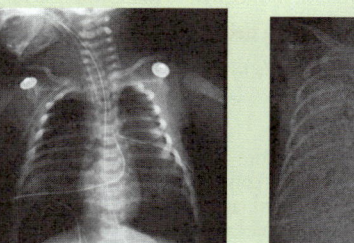

Visualize the Vocal cords for oozing of Pulmonary Bleed!

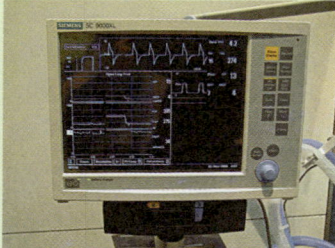

Check the Ventilator, the Circuit and Oxygen resource + Compressor!

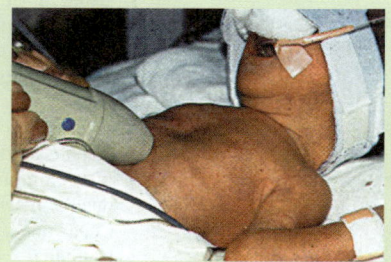

Organize an ECHOCARDIOGRAM to exclude a Ductus-dependent cardiac malformation!

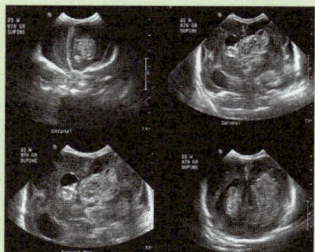

Perform an urgent USG Scan of Head to confirm/exclude IVH in a Premature baby!

REVIEW OF CLINICAL PROBLEMS

1. How does an "Acute Collapse" in a Neonate present clinically ?
   Ans: Refer to the "No. 2" of the "BIRD'S EYE VIEW OVERVIEW/ SYNOPSIS" of the Chapter, and to the Table 1 of the Chapter.
2. How do you manage an acutely collapsed Neonate, who has been *breathing spontaneously* until the event happened?
   Ans: Refer to the "No. 3" of the "BIRD'S EYE VIEW/ OVERVIEW/SYNOPSIS" of the Chapter.
3. How do you manage an acutely collapsed Neonate, who has been *on a mechanical ventilator* until the event happened?.
   Ans: Refer to the "No. 5" of the "BIRD'S EYE VIEW/ OVERVIEW/SYNOPSIS" of the Chapter.
4. What are the essential aspects of counseling the parents, when their baby has shown sudden deterioration/collapse?
   Ans: Refer to the "No. 8" and "No. 10" of the "BIRD'S EYE VIEW/OVERVIEW/SYNOPSIS" of the Chapter.
5. Mention the important investigations you may have to do, after stabilizing an acutely collapsed Neonate?
   Ans: Refer to the Evaluation-Decision-Action Plan/ Algorithm to diagnose and manage a Neonate with an acute collapse.

LEARNING OBJECTIVES

After completing this article, readers will be able to

1. Assess the *Neonate's ABCDs rapidly*, when collapses suddenly.
2. Resuscitate the dying infant effectively and timely by *supporting, stabilizing and maintaining ABCDs.*
3. Treat the *treatable conditions* such as, pneumothorax, ET tube block/displacement, ventilator malfunction, sepsis, pneumonia, metabolic problems, anemia, pulmonary hemorrhage, GE reflux with aspiration, etc.
4. *Search for* GMH-IVH in a preterm, duct-dependent cardiac malformation, intraabdominal hemorrhage, inborn errors of metabolism and endocrine disorders (salt-losing Congenital Adrenal Hyperplasia).
5. *Counsel the parents (and "to listen to them") about the event*, its ongoing management and diagnostic evaluation, and the guarded prognosis of the catastrophic situation.

Pearl/Peril/Pitfall: Diminished pulses in all extremities indicate poor cardiac output or peripheral vasoconstriction. Absent or diminished femoral pulses suggest the presence of ductal-dependent cardiac lesions (e.g. coarctation of the aorta). In Newborns, a murmur does not always signify the presence of heart disease, nor does the absence of a murmur provide reassurance of normalcy. @ *Irrespective of the underlying cause, the major objectives should be to re-establish adequate gas exchange and maintain the cardiovascular circulation.*

1. *Acute collapse* in a previously well or already an unwell Neonate is a medical emergency where swift and appropriate response can make the difference to outcome. *Irrespective of the underlying cause, the major objectives should be to re-establish adequate gas exchange and maintain the cardiovascular circulation and perfusion.*

2. **Clinical presentation:** Suddenly there is an acute deterioration of a previously *well/unwell, ventilated/ spontaneously breathing baby,* especially, when the staff and the parents have relaxed, and believe that their infant is *"out of the woods"*. It presents with an acute onset of *any or a combination of-* pallor or cyanosis, bradycardia, hypotension, apnea or labored respiratory effort, cool mottled skin, marked hypotonia, ill-look, seizures, abdominal distention, bloody vomitus/diarrhea, bilious NG aspirates etc. *Refer to the Table 1 of the Chapter* for a list of essential signs to look for, when encountered with an acutely collapsed Neonate.

3. *If a spontaneously breathing Neonate suddenly collapses, the immediate priority should be to ensure ABCDs,* i.e. clearance of oropharynx, visualization of vocal cords for any pulmonary bleed oozing out of them, intubation, IPPV with 100% oxygen, External cardiac massage, fluid resuscitation, IV/ET Adrenaline, 10% Dextrose and /or base *as required.* Then the Cardiorespiratory support should be continued via Mechanical ventilation, and IVI of inotropes. *Concurrently, one should perform the following essential diagnostic/therapeutic interventions such as: a)* Transillumination of the chest to exclude a tension pneumothorax (if present, needle aspiration to be followed by proper Intercostal Tube Drainage), *b)* ABG Analysis and electrolytes, Hematocrit, Group and Cross match, Blood sugar *c)* Ultrasound head scan to exclude a large IVH in a preterm, and USG scan of abdomen to exclude subcapsular hematoma of liver *d)* Checking clotting and administering FFP/CRYOPRECIPITATE (if fibrinogen <1g/L) and IV vitamin K, if a hemorrhage has occurred, *e)* IV Broadspectrum antibiotics to cover for fulminant sepsis after sepsis screen (defer LP), *f)* Correction of anemia, hypoglycemia, hypocalcemia, acidosis, hypothermia, etc. *g)* Echocardiogram to exclude a duct-dependent cardiac malformation (if present, maintain ductal patency by IV Prostin infusion). *h)* suspecting adrenal insufficiency if dehydration, low sodium (<130 mEq/L) and high potassium (>5 mEq/L) and with/without hypoglycemia (if so, give IV Hydrocortisone) *i)* Metabolic screen(Ammonia, Urine aminoacids and organic acids, plasma amino acids, urinary + serum ketones) if Inborn Errors of Metabolism are suspected *j)* Gastroesophageal Reflux and aspiration sometimes can present with an *"unexplained"* deterioration in respiratory status. needs a CXR, Barium swallow, 24 hour esophageal pH monitoring and endoscopy to exclude. *Refer to the Table 2 of the Chapter for the common causes of Neonatal Acute Collapse.*

4. If the infant remains unresponsive to full cardio-pulmonary resuscitation for 4–5 minutes, give 1:1000 adrenaline 0.4–1 ml IV and consider giving base if the resuscitation efforts are still unsuccessful by 10 minutes (3–5 mEq of 4.2% NaHCO3). Needle both sides of the chest in case bilateral pneumothoraces are present. Continue with resuscitation efforts for at least 20 minutes.

5. *Sudden deterioration in a baby on assisted ventilation may be due to: (a)* Mechanical problems such as a displaced/obstructed ET tube, a leak around the ET tube, or Ventilatory failure-Check all machinary for leaks, try hand-ventilating with a bag and mask and insert a larger ET tube, *(b)* An air leak, usually a tension pneumo-thorax—consider chest aspiration after confirming it either by a transillumination or by a CXR, *(c)* Sudden development of a large GMH-IVH-*confirm it by an urgent USG SCAN of head, (d)* The baby may have only moderately severe RDS but has uncorrected acidosis, hypotension, or hypoglycemia-check pH, BP, Hct, glucose and treat accordingly, *(e)* There may have been *an incorrect diagnosis, or a complication of RDS* may have developed; pulmonary hemorrhage, PPHN, pneumonia and fulminant sepsis, pulmonary edema / fluid overload/ a large, hemodynamically significant PDA or congenital heart disease. *Cardiac conditions which may present with collapse are listed in the Tables 3 and 4 of the Chapter.* Differentiating cardiac from non-cardiac causes is usually not difficult although conditions with duct-dependent circulation can, *mimic septicemia and primary metabolic disorders, when ductal closure occurs.*

6. In contrast, *a gradual deterioration in a ventilated baby* may be due to: (a) worsening of RDS over the first 24–48 hours, (b) pneumonia, (c) a GMH-IVH, (d) anemia/hypo-tension/ an air leak/ pulmonary edema, (e) partial blockage of the ET tube and, (f) progression to chronic lung disease.

7. *The Evaluation-Decision-Action- Plan/Algorithm* describes the essential aspects of diagnosis and mana-gement of a *Neonate with an Acute collapse* whether he/ she is spontaneously breathing or on mechanical ventilator. *Near normal gas exchange, adequate tissue perfusion, and normal blood pressure should be re-established and maintained as rapidly as possible.*

8. *ACUTE COLLAPSE* in an apparently well baby is often the most demanding of crises that would happen in any SCBU/NICU. The parents tend to think that *"it must be somebody's fault"* understandably, and a painful one for dedicated staff to cope with. *In such circumstances, honesty is the best policy.* The physician should be very candid but also emphasise the positive aspects of care. He/She should counsel parents that their baby has to be kept back on the ventilator, being treated for an infection, and is to be urgently investigated further, with the help of a specialist/ cardiologist. They should be reassured that their baby has been getting the best possible intensive care until a complete diagnosis is known, to discuss further plans and the prognosis.

9. With an unsuccessful resuscitation, always try to obtain parental consent for an autopsy. Where inherited metabolic disease is a possibility, obtain urine/blood/ skin-liver-muscle biopsies, and store them appropriately before transporting them at the earliest opportunity.

10. Staff need to be articulate, thoughtful, sensitive and above all, excellent at listening to both the parents in times of crisis. Counseling and support for parents cannot adequately be achieved in one meeting and takes great patience and tact.

Pearl/Peril/Pitfall: Assess for the Important Clinical features of neurologic impairment in Newborns with an acute Collapse: hypotonia (less frequently, hypertonia), weakness (decreased strength), asymmetry of muscle tone and/or movement, alterations in level of consciousness, seizures, single or multiple cranial nerve involvement, fasciculations.

THE EVALUATION-DECISION-ACTION- PLAN/ALGORITHM FOR THE DIAGNOSIS AND MANAGEMENT OF *AN ACUTE COLLAPSE IN A NEONATE*

SUBJECTIVE FINDINGS

*Do not waste time in taking history, when a Neonate has acutely collapsed; first of all try to save the infant`s life by rapidly assessing ABCDs within a minute of arrival and by stabilizing them underlined *emergently!* *Then only assess the history of relevant factors that have led to an acute collapse, when time permits. *Keep yourself & the staff cool and composed to meet the crisis; *omit nothing necessary and add nothing superfluous!*

OBJECTIVE FINDINGS

Assess ABCDs and monitor CRT, O_2 sats, BP, core-peripheral temperature difference, RR, HR, central & peripheral pulses, urine output.

Determine whether the baby is in preterminal ("pre arrest") conditions such as apnea, gasping or RR <20 bpm, shock, extremely lethargic or unresponsive limpy baby, bleeding etc.. and *intervene with appropriate resuscitation of ABCDs promptly.*

Note the other alarming signs such as convulsions, irritability, pallor, central cyanosis, hypothermia, abdominal distention, bilious vomiting, petechiae and ecchymoses, vesicles, etc..

Note-dysmorphic features (facies), obvious congenital malformations/evidence for birth trauma/stigmata of congenital infections

Perform systemic examination quickly to identify the problems which require *emergent life saving procedures* such as pneumothorax, upper airway obstruction, bowel obstruction, PDA etc....

INVESTIGATIONS

Blood FBC, TC, DC, **Hct**, Platelets, CRP, Blood cultures, **ABG analysis, electrolytes,** calcium & magnesium, **blood sugar,** creatinine, BUN, coagulation profile, LFTs.

CXR for respiratory infections/air leaks

LP after stabilization only for CNS infection/hemorrhage

Urine analysis and culture

Imaging USG scan Head/Abdomen

Consider ECG and Echocardiogram

Observe **nursing charts** for episodes of apnea, bradys, desaturations, hypoglycemia, and interventions to maintain the baby's temperature (a record of both environmental and core temperature, along with observation for other signs of sepsis)

ACUTE COLLAPSE IN A NEONATE-SPONTANEOUSLY BREATHING

Transilluminate the chest to exclude a tension pneumothorax-if so, perform needle decompression, to be followed by ICTD with an underwater seal.

Perform Ultrasound head scan to exclude a large IVH in a preterm, and USG scan of abdomen to exclude subcapsular hematoma of liver.

Consult a Pediatric Cardiologist to perform a Echocardiogram to exclude a duct-dependent cardiac malformation (if present or even if cardiologist opinion not available, maintain ductal patency by IV Prostin infusion).

Perform Metabolic screen(Ammonia, Urine aminoacids and organic acids, plasma amino acids, urinary + serum ketones), if Inborn Errors of Metabolism are suspected

Suspect adrenal insufficiency if dehydration, low sodium (<130 mEq/L) and high potassium (>5(>5 mEq/L) and with/without hypoglycemia (if so, give IV Hydrocortisone)

Ensure ABCs, O_2 saturations, BP, CR monitor

Intubate & ventilate for apnea, severe respiratory distress, pulmonary hemorrhage, unresponsive shock, underlying severe sepsis/meningitis, CNS dysfunction, etc.

Correct shock with 20ml/kg NS over 5 minutes, (with CPR + IV Adrenaline + IV NaHCO₃, if necessary) and IVI of Dopamine &/or Dobutamine; *Correct* Hypoxia, Hypothermia, Hypoglycemia, Hypocalcemia, Anemia, Electrolyte disturbances etc.,

Administer IV Broadspectrum Antibiotics to cover for fulminant sepsis/meningitis, after sepsis screen (defer LP)

Check coagulation, and give FFP/PLATELETS/CRYOPRECIPITATE/Vitamin K, as necessary

---

ACUTE COLLAPSE IN A NEONATE-ON A MECHANICAL VENTILATOR

1. *On arrival, check whether:* a) infant`s chest is moving with ventilator b) breathing is in phase with ventilator

2. *If the infant is not ventilating* disconnect from ventilator and hand ventilate with 100% oxygen by bag and mask; a) *if there is an improvement,* consider a leaky ventilator circuit; remedy this and also consider deteriorating disease with very stiff lungs and inadequate IPPV pressure; increase ventilation. b) *if no improvement* consider a

blocked/displaced ET tube and insert a larger ET tube.

3. *If the infant is ventilating-* increase pressure by 5 cm, rate by 20/min and O2 by 20% (if possible) to try to bring into phase with ventilator and paralyse the infant, if still fighting against the ventilator.

4. *If the infant is ventilating and in phase with ventilator, but not improving* consider other pathology as discussed above and manage accordingly!

EMERGENCY MEDICINES IN ACUTE COLLAPSE : *1)* In the presence of profound unresponsive bradycardia or cardiac arrest, despite 30 seconds of effective CPR +INTUBATION AND VENTILATION, Give *IV/ET Adrenaline 1:10,000 rapidly,* initially @ 0.1-0.3 ml/kg and subsequently 1:1,000 undiluted *IV Adrenaline@0.3-1ml/kg* may be tried at 3-5 minute intervals if there is no response. *2)* Volume expansion with *NS @10ml/kg IV over 5–10 minutes* is to be given, if peripheral circulation is inadequate; if necessary, follow this by *IVI of DOPAMINE and/or DOBUTAMINE @5–20 microgram/kg/min.* *3)* If the infant remains unresponsive to full CPR and effective ventilation for 10 minutes, give *IV NaHCO₃ @2–4 ml/kg of 4.2% solution(1–2 mEq/kg) slowly over at least 2 minutes,* to treat profound acidosis, unresponsive bradycardia. *4)* If hypoglycemia is documented, give 10% Dextrose 5ml/kg IV *5)* Pressor resistant Hypotension (refractory)- start *IV Hydrocortisone 1mg/kg/dose-*

*repeat every 8–12 hrs for 3 days–*to treat transient adrenal insufficiency, salt losing variety of congenital adrenal hyperplasia & babies who are otherwise cortisol deficient (serum cortisol <15mcg/dl). In such cases an increase in BP is expected within 2 hrs of the first dose. Keep in mind the common adverse effects of hydrocortisone such as hyperglycemia, salt and water retention, GI perforations, disseminated fungal infection. *6)* If a duct-dependent cardiac malformation is confirmed by an ECHOCARDIOGRAM, start *IVI PROSTAGLANDIN E2 @0.005–0.05 micrograms/kg/min* to maintain the ductal patency until some palliative surgery is done as soon as possible; at a low dose initially and increase at 15-30 minute intervals if no response. (500 micrograms in 500 ml of 5% dextrose, that is 1 microgram/ml. Starting dose-0.3 ml/kg/hr=0.005micrograms/kg/min. Double the dose in 20 minutes if SaO_2 is unchanged.)

Pearl/Peril/Pitfall: CLUES TO CONGENITAL HEART DISEASE—BLUE: Cyanotic heart disease with right to left shunting MOTTLED or GRAY ‹ outflow obstruction with systemic hypoperfusion and shock PINK: congestive heart failure with left to right shunting AGE OF PRESENTATION Ductus-dependent lesions - cyanotic or shock-producing cardiac lesions- usually have sudden onset and usually present in first week of life CHF lesions - usually have slower onset and present in late neonatal or early infancy period .

TABLE 1 Signs of emergencies in neonates, to look for when they collapse suddenly

SIGNS	CAUSES/IMPLICATIONS	COMMON EXAMPLE OF SERIOUS CAUSES
Apnea (and decreased breathing effort)	CNS depression	Intra-ventricular hemorrhage, excess narcotic administration
Increased respiratory effort (and tachypnea)	Airway obstruction, restrictive lung, or chest wall disease	Blocked/Displaced ET tube, Choanal atresia, Hyaline membrane disease, or diaphragmatic hernia
Cyanosis	Deoxygenated arterial or capillary blood	Transposition of Great Arteries, right heart obstruction, Pneumothorax, Poor peripheral perfusion
Hypotension, mottling, poor peripheral perfusion *Tachycardia or bradycardia*	Inadequate heart function, decreased vascular tone, vasoconstriction of the skin. Decreased cardiac output (sinus tachycardia or tachyarrhythmia; autonomic dysfunction or bradyarrhythmia	Left heart obstruction, Sepsis, Hypovolemic shock, Adrenocortical failure. Hypovolemic shock, Supraventricular tachy cardia; Asphyxia
Abnormal repetitive movements	Seizures	Hypoglycemia, Hypoxic-ischemic encephalopathy, Meningitis
Abdominal distention ± bilious vomiting	Bowel obstruction or ileus	Volvulus and Peritonitis, Perforation of viscus (NEC)
Bleeding	Reduced clotting factors, trauma	Disseminated intravascular coagulation, thrombocytopenia, vascular laceration Pulmonary hemorrhage
Impaired temperature regulation	Diminished hypothalamic function, nonneutral thermal environment	Infection

TABLE 2 Neonates who present with sudden deterioration (Acute Collapse)

A. Baby on Mechanical Ventilator

Consider the following possibilities:

i. Hypo/Single Lung ventilation due to blockage of an endotracheal tube, displacement, disconnected ventilator, etc.

ii. Large Air leak-Tension Pneumothorax/ Pneumomediastinum which is detected by transillumination or radiograph.

iii. Intracranial hemorrhage which is detected by full fontanel, falling hematocrit, metabolic acidosis, cranial ultrasound, etc.

iv. Pneumonia/Sepsis / Meningitis/Worsening RDS

B. Baby Breathing Spontaneously

Consider the following possibilities:

i. Overwhelming infection either bacterial or viral

ii. Massive hemorrhage, e.g. subcapsular hematoma of liver, pulmonary hemorrhage, IVH, Adrenal hemorrhage, etc.

iii. Congenital heart disease which is precipitated by the closure of ductus arteriosus

iv. Necrotizing enterocolitis (NEC)

v. Metabolic problems, e.g. hyperammonemia, hypoglycemia, hypocalcemia, CAH, etc.

TABLE 3 Structural lesions presenting with respiratory distress or collapse in the early Newborn period. All may have cyanosis if PPHN or shocked; all have cardiomegaly with congested lung fields on chest X-ray

Condition	Pulses	Cyanosis	Precordium	Auscultation	ECG	Extracardiac associations
Hypoplastic left heart	Weak, femoral stronger if DA open	Mild	Active	Gallop	Small LV voltages	Uncommon
Aortic arch interruption	Strong Proximal to lesion	None	Active	Gallop LVOT, systolic murmur	LV/RV+ T↓ V_{5-6}	Common (DiGeorge)
Coarctation	Weak femorals	None	Active	Gallop, EC, LVOT, systolic murmur Murmur between scapulae	RA+ RV+ T↓ V_{5-6}	Uncommon (Turner)
Critical aortic stenosis	Weak	None	Active	Gallop, EC, LVOT, systolic murmur	LV+ ST↓ , T↓V_{5-6}	Uncommon

Pearl/Peril/Pitfall: COMMON CAUSES OF A CRASHING NEONATE (term infant, with usually normal Apgars, who suddenly deteriorates in the first 1–2 weeks of life after a well interval at home—> presents to the ED in extremis) -S – Sepsis Viral (Herpes, Enterovirus) Bacterial (E.coli, Strep, Listeria) S - Seizures I - Inborn Errors of Metabolism or other metabolic derangements C - Congenital cardiac disease Ductus-dependent left-outflow obstruction lesions Large left-to-right shunts Cardiomyopathies Dysrhythmias, e.g. SVT C - Congenital Adrenal Hyperplasia (CAH) C-CNS hemorrhages AV malformation Child abuse Vitamin K deficiency (Hemorrhagic Disease of the Newborn) F - Formulas mix-ups I - Intestinal disasters Volvulus Necrotizing enterocolitis Incarcerated hernias T - Toxins and other home remedies.

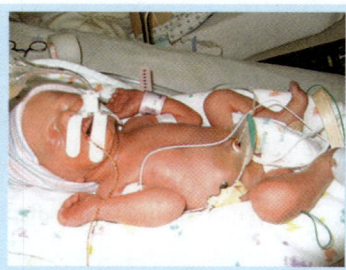

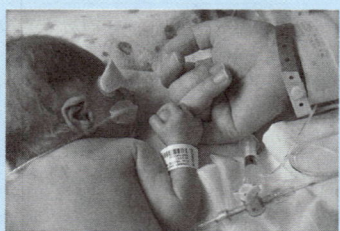

Technology should meet care, concern and compassion of the NICU Staff to improve the survival rates of the Sick Neonates with Life-Threatening Illnesses.

"It is as natural to die as to be born; and to a little infant, perhaps, the one is as painful as the other."
— **Francis Bacon,** 1597–1625, in "Of Death," Essays

TABLE 4	Cardiac conditions which may present with collapse

Arrhythmias primary or secondary

Duct-dependent circulation

Transposition ASD, VSD, PDA

Pulmonary Pulmonary atresia—without collaterals, Tricuspid atresia - with restrictive VSD

Systemic Hypoplastic left heart, Aortic atresia, Critical aortic stenosis, Interrupted arch, Coarctation

Critically ill Newborn patients can be challenging for the emergency physician; these small mute beings are a frightening enigma to the unprepared. An organized diagnostic approach is essential for accurate and timely intervention, and the mnemonic "THE MISFITS" can assist in this endeavor. *The following may cause an acute collapse in a Neonate recently discharged home.*

Causes of Shock/Severe Illness In

The Newborn: THE MISFITS. T-Trauma/non-accidental trauma **H** -Heart disease (congenital/hypovolemia/hypoxia/respiratory complaints) **E**-Endocrine (congenital adrenal hyperplasia, thyrotoxicosis) **M**-Metabolic disturbances (hypoglycemia, hyponatremia) **I**-Inborn errors of metabolism **S**-Sepsis **F**-Formula dilution or over-concentration **I**-Intestinal catastrophes **T**-Toxins (home remedies) **S** -Seizures.

The history and physical examination should address the most common concerns, including sepsis and meningitis. A feeding history is important, as sweating with feeds can be associated with congenital heart defects. If the infant has been vomiting, ask if the vomitus is bilious or projectile; bilious vomiting requires surgical consultation, while projectile vomiting mandates an evaluation for hypertrophic pyloric stenosis. If the patient is formula-fed, it is imperative to ask exactly how the caregiver is mixing the formula, as improper preparation can lead to electrolyte abnormalities, especially hypernatremia. Laboratory and radiographic studies can provide clues to less common conditions, such as inborn errors of metabolism and other congenital problems. *The need to treat may be more pressing than the ability to diagnose.* Certain conditions may require empiric therapy— in particular, suspected sepsis and possible ductal-dependent cardiac lesions.

KEY POINTS FOR CLINICAL PRACTICE

1. Acute collapse in a previously well or already an unwell Neonate is a medical emergency where swift and appropriate response can make the difference to outcome. *Irrespective of the underlying cause, the major objectives should be to re-establish adequate gas exchange and maintain the cardiovascular circulation and perfusion.*

2. It presents with an acute onset of *any or a combination of* pallor or cyanosis, bradycardia, hypotension, apnea or labored respiratory effort, cool mottled skin, marked hypotonia, ill-look, seizures, abdominal distention, bloody vomitus/diarrhea, bilious NG aspirates etc.,

3. *If a Neonate whether spontaneously breathing or on assisted ventilation suddenly collapses, the immediate* *priority should be to ensure ABCDs; Concurrently, one should perform the essential diagnostic/therapeutic interventions to treat the treatable.*

4. *ACUTE COLLAPSE* in an apparently well baby is often the most demanding of crises. The parents tend to think that *"it must be somebody`s fault"* understandably, and a painful one for dedicated staff to cope with. In such circumstances, *honesty is the best policy* in communicating with the anxious parents, who tend to blame the NICU Staff.

5. Staff need to be *articulate, thoughtful, sensitive and above all, excellent at listening to both the parents in times of crisis.* Counseling and support for parents cannot adequately be achieved in one meeting and takes great patience and tact.

REFERENCES AND FURTHER READING : **1)**Roberton's Text Book of Neonatology ,4th Edition. **2)** Black JA. Neonatal Emergencies: Early Detection and Management, 2nd edin. Oxford:Butterworth-Heinemann, 1991. **3)** Nelson Text Book of Pediatrics, 18th edition **4)**Burchfield DJ. Medication use in neonatal resuscitation. Clinics in Perinatology 1999 26:683-91. **5)**Willett LD et al. Outcome of CPR in the NICU. Critical Care Medicine (1986) 14:773-6

Pearl/Peril/Pitfall: An infant who continues to bleed after lab draws or venipuncture should raise suspicion. Hemorrhage can range from oozing of a wound to frank blood in the mouth, nose, or orogastric or endotracheal tube indicating a major gastrointestinal or pulmonary bleed, the latter almost always associated with some degree of hypotension or shock.

Neonatal Shock and Hypotension

9

@ *Most preterm infants, even at 24-26 weeks' gestation, have a mean blood pressure of 30 mm Hg or greater by the third day of life. The systolic blood pressure correlates with the gestational age reference range 4-24 hours after birth; only 3% of babies with normal long-term outcome have systolic blood pressures below the reference range for the gestational age.*

Shock is a progressive disorder but can generally be divided into 3 phases: compensated, uncompensated, and irreversible. Each phase has characteristic clinicopathologic manifestations and outcomes; however, in the Neonatal setting, distinguishing them may be impossible. Initiate aggressive treatment in all cases where shock is suspected.

*Compensated shock *In compensated shock, perfusion to vital organs, such as the brain, heart, and adrenal glands, is preserved by sympathetic reflexes, which increase systemic arterial resistance. *Derangement of vital signs, such as heart rate, respiratory rate, blood pressure, and temperature, is absent or minimal. *Increased secretion of angiotensin and vasopressin allows the kidneys to conserve water and salt. The release of catecholamines enhances myocardial contractility, and decreased spontaneous activity reduces oxygen consumption. *Clinical signs at this time include pallor, tachycardia, cool peripheral skin, and prolonged capillary refill time. As these homeostatic mechanisms are exhausted or become inadequate to meet the metabolic demands of the tissues, the uncompensated stage ensues.

*Uncompensated shock *During uncompensated shock, delivery of oxygen and nutrients to tissues becomes marginal or insufficient to meet demands. Anaerobic metabolism becomes the major source of energy production, and lactic acid production is excessive, which leads to systemic metabolic acidosis. Acidosis reduces myocardial contractility and impairs its response to catecholamines.

*Numerous chemical mediators, enzymes, and other substances are released, including histamine, cytokines (especially tumor necrosis factor and interleukin-1), xanthine oxidase (which generates oxygen free radicals), platelet-aggregating factor, and bacterial toxins (in the case of septic shock). This cascade of metabolic changes further reduces tissue perfusion and oxidative phosphorylation. *A further result of anaerobic metabolism is the failure of the energy-dependent sodium-potassium pump, which maintains the normal homeostatic environment in which cells function. The integrity of the capillary endothelium is disrupted, and plasma proteins leak, with the resultant loss of oncotic pressure and extravasation of intravascular fluids into the extravascular space. *Sluggish flow of blood and chemical changes in small blood vessels lead to platelet adhesion and activation of the coagulation cascade, which may eventually produce a bleeding tendency and further deplete blood volume.

*Clinically, patients with uncompensated shock present with falling blood pressure, very prolonged capillary refill time, tachycardia, cold skin, rapid breathing (to compensate for the metabolic acidosis), and reduced or absent urine output. If effective intervention is not promptly instituted, progression to irreversible shock follows.

*Irreversible shock: A diagnosis of irreversible shock is actually retrospective. Major vital organs, such as the heart and brain, are so extensively damaged that death occurs despite adequate restoration of the circulation. Early recognition and effective treatment of shock are crucial to prevent inevitable progression to this stage.

REVIEW OF CLINICAL PROBLEMS

1. What are the common causes of Neonatal Shock and Hypotension?
   Ans: Refer to the "No. 1" and "No. 2" of the "BIRD`S EYE VIEW/OVERVIEW/SYNOPSIS" of the Chapter.
2. How do you monitor the patient, while managing Neonatal Shock and Hypotension ?
   Ans: Refer to the "No. 5" of the "BIRD'S EYE VIEW/OVERVIEW/SYNOPSIS" of the Chapter.
3. What are the 3 stages of Shock and their differentiating features ?
   Ans: Refer to the "No. 6" of the "BIRD'S EYE VIEW/OVERVIEW/SYNOPSIS" of the Chapter and to the Table 2 of the Chapter.
4. How do you manage neonatal shock and Hypotension?
   Ans: Refer to the Evaluation-Decision-Action Plan/Algorithm to diagnose and manage a Neonate with shock and hypotension.
5. Mention the therapeutic endpoints for vasoactive drugs, in treating Neonatal Shock and Hypotension?
   Ans: Refer to the "No. 7" of the "BIRD'S EYE VIEW/OVERVIEW/SYNOPSIS" of the Chapter.

LEARNING OBJECTIVES

After completing this article, readers will be able to:

1. Recognize the various clinical manifestations of Neonatal Shock and Hypotension.

2. Develop a rational approach in the diagnosis and management of Neonatal Shock and Hypotension.

3. Apply appropriate general and specific measures in the management of Neonatal Shock and Hypotension.

4. Understand the indications and risks of using vasoactive drugs in the management of Neonatal Shock and Hypotension.

5. Monitor for the clinical and laboratory response while managing Neonatal Shock and Hypotension.

Pearl/Peril/Pitfall: The priority is to establish whether hypotension is symptomatic of another problem. Conditions to consider include: Patent ductus arteriosus. Hypovolemia or blood loss. Pneumothorax. ·Sepsis (particularly in persistent or late hypotension). Adrenocortical insufficiency in extreme prematurity. High mean airway pressure on mechanical ventilation.

BIRD'S EYE VIEW/OVERVIEW/SYNOPSIS

1. *NEONATAL SHOCK is defined as a state of circulatory dysfunction leading to inadequate cellular perfusion and tissue hypoxia due to either an increase in metabolic demands and/or a decrease in the metabolic supply (oxygen delivery).* **Hypotension is not synonymous with shock, but it may be associated with the later stages of shock.** Blood pressure (blood flow x peripheral resistance) correlates only weakly with cardiac output and babies can have low BP and normal cardiac output and normal BP and low cardiac output. In addition to hypotension and tachycardia (increased heart rate is not always present in very premature infants), shock is manifested principally by a) pallor + poor skin perfusion b) cool extremities c) CNS signs of lethargy d) decreased urine output. In preterm infants shock and hypotension predispose to intraventricular hemorrhage and periventricular leukomalacia due to decrease in brain blood flow and oxygen supply. In ELBW infants ischemic brain damage may occur due to vasoconstriction of cerebral cortex because of myocardial dysfunction/shock.

2. **NEONATAL SHOCK** is a final common pathway of impaired tissue perfusion resulting from different causes namely *a)* Hypovolemic shock e.g. blood loss or fluid loss *b)* Cardiogenic shock e.g. asphyxia, PDA, HLHS, obstructed TAPVR, ALCAPA, myocarditis, sepsis, hypoglycemia *c)* Distributive shock e.g. sepsis, HIE, muscle relaxants, adrenal insufficiency, vasodilators *d)* Septic shock, e.g. sepsis *e)* Obstructive shock e.g. tension pneumothorax, PIE, diaphragmatic hernia and *f)* Dissociative shock, e.g. profound anemia, methemoglobinemia. The hemodynamic variables are affected in different manner in the various forms of shock. *Refer to Table No-1 of the Chapter.*

3. *Anticipate the common causes of Neonatal shock and have a high index of suspicion and monitor continuously in those situations a)* Hypovolemic shock - antepartum loss due to placenta previa, abruptio placentae, twin - twin transfusion, fetomaternal hemorrhage, postpartum loss due to coagulation disorders, vitamin K deficiency, birth trauma *b)* Septic shock -Esch.coli, Klebsiella Spe. , Staph.aureus, etc. *c)* Cardiogenic shock due to birth asphyxia, metabolic problems (hypoglycemia, hyponatremia, hypocalcemia), congenital heart disease (HLHS or critical Aortic stenosis), cardiac arrhythmias *d)* Obstructive due to tension pneumothorax *e)* Drug induced - tolazoline, sedatives, magnesium sulphate, digitalis, and barbiturates.

4. *Rapidly do assess the infant and determine what is causing the hypotension and/or shock, in order to direct treatment accordingly.* The basic decision is whether the infant requires volume replacement or administration of inotropic agents. *4 parameters are useful in making this decision : a)* History (to rule out birth asphyxia, blood loss {antepartum or postpartum}, drug infusion and birth trauma {adrenal hemorrhage or liver injury} *b)* Physical examination (to reveal which organ systems are involved) *c)* Chest X-ray - a small heart is seen in volume depletion : a large heart is seen in cardiac disease *d)* Central venous pressure (if it is below 4mmHg the infant is volume depleted and if it is above 6mmHg the infant probably has cardiogenic shock).

5. *Monitoring of Sick Neonate in shock includes* a) Heart Rate, Respiratory Rate, Temperature, Color, O_2 Saturations, sensorium, Capillary Refill Time + Peripheral Pulses, Daily Weights, and Urine Output b) ABG analysis and invasive BP monitoring and CVP monitoring.
Lab investigations should include - FBC, CRP, blood culture, serum electrolytes, blood sugar, creatinine and BUN, calcium, ECG, CXR, Echocardiogram, coagulation profiles, ultrasound head and adrenals and others depending on the clinical presentation.

6. The progression of Neonatal shock is categorized into three stages, i.e. 1)early compensated shock 2)late decompensated shock 3)terminal irreversible shock. It is very difficult to differentiate the three stages in Neonate. From management point of view, prolonged CRT (>3 seconds) should initiate aggressive management. *Refer to Table 2 for differentiating the three stages of shock.*

7. *Shock is an emergency where intervention and search for the cause should happen concurrently.* The management options of Neonatal shock include *a)* Stabilization of ABCs (mechanical ventilation if necessary) *b)* Volume replacement (10ml/kg upto 60ml/kg in case of septic shock) with blood or 5% Albumin or normal saline *c)* Inotropic support (Dopamine + Dobutamine infusion) *d)* Vasopressor support (Noradrenaline and Adrenaline) *e)* Vasodilators *f)* Correction of hypoglycemia, hypocalcemia, and severe metabolic acidosis *g)* Steroids in critically ill preterm babies with pressor resistant hypotension *h)* Broad-spectrum IV antibiotics to cover for Sepsis *i)* Treating associated primary pulmonary hypertension (PPHN) *j)* Treating cardiac arrhythmias if any associated. *The therapeutic end points for vasoactive drugs* are 1)Normalization of blood pressure (mean arterial pressures are the most important); 2)Normalization of organ and tissue prefusion as evidenced by-a)Normal urine output (>1ml/kg/hr), b)Normal sensorium, c)Capillary refill <3sec d)Normalization of arterial lactate levels (serial measurements and trends offer a good indication).

8. *The Evaluation-Decision-Action-Plan/Algorithm* describes the essential practical aspects of diagnosis and management of Neonatal shock. The lower limit of mean arterial pressure during the first post-natal day roughly equals the gestational age of the infant. However, by the third day, >90 of preterm infants <26 weeks' gestation have a mean arterial BP >30 mmHg. Morethan 90% of term infants have a mean BP of >45 mmHg immediately after birth with a rise to >50 mm Hg by the third postnatal day.

9. If CVP/IBP monitor available: *Maintain a CVP of 5-8cm H_2O. In many infants, maintaining CVP at 5 to 8 mm Hg with volume infusions is associated with improved cardiac output. If CVP exceeds 5 to 8 mm Hg, additional volume will usually not be helpful. CVP is influenced by noncardiac factors such as ventilator pressures and by cardiac factors such as tricuspid valve function. Both types of factors may affect the interpretation and usefulness of CVP measurements. *The best parameter to see response to management of shock is improvement in CVP and BP.*

10. *Vasopressor resistant hypotention-* a proportion of VLBW infants become dependent on medium to high doses of vasopressors beyond the first postnatal days, due to relative cortisol deficiency, adrenal insufficiency, and downregulation of adrenergic receptors. Consider IV hydrocortisone 1 mg/kg/dose - repeat every 8-12hrs for 3 days, as it results in a rapid increase in intracellular calcium availability which enhances the responsiveness to adrenergic agents. It raises BP within 2 hrs of administration, but the long term neurologic effects of this treatment on the VLBW infant are under investigation. Role of high-dose steroids in sepsis is controversial. Vasopressin is not routinely used to treat shock in the Neonate but may be a therapeutic option to consider in the setting of abnormal peripheral vasoregulation as occurs in sepsis.

Pearl/Peril/Pitfall: Neonatal Shock; when to intervene : *In any baby with clinical or laboratory evidence of poor perfusion including pallor, metabolic acidosis, rising potassium and urine output <0.5 ml/kg/hr together with echocardiographic evidence of low systemic blood flow. And/ or Mean BP persistently below gestation in weeks.*

THE EVALUATION -DECISION-ACTION-PLAN/ALGORITHM FOR THE DIAGNOSIS AND MANAGEMENT OF *NEONATAL SHOCK AND HYPOTENSION*

SUBJECTIVE FINDINGS

Assess the *risk factors* for neonatal shock - history suggestive of:

* Blood loss - antepartum/postpartum
* Septic factors
* Birth asphyxia
* Congenital heart disease/ arrhythmias
* Birth trauma and intracranial hemorrhage
* Inborn errors of metabolism
* Drugs

OBJECTIVE FINDINGS

Assess ABCDs - vitals, BP, CRT, core-peripheral temperature difference, O_2 sats, Urine output, Pulses, skin rashes including petechiae, sensorium, seizures and focal neurological signs

Attempt to differentiate the three stages of shock, though it is very difficult - Refer to Table 2

Look for diminished femoral pulses, tachy/brady-cardia, heart murmur, gallop (to identify serious cardiac problems)

Search for multiorgan dysfunction acute renal failure, liver failure, bleeding diathesis, NEC, respiratory failure and CNS hemorrhage and ischemia

INVESTIGATIONS

Blood Hb, Haematocrit, TC and DC, Platelets., *ABG Analysis*, Electrolytes, *Glucose*, Calcium ++, P, BUN, Creatinine, PT, PTT, Lactic acid, Coomb's test, reti.count, LFTs, Group, type, and crossmatch, cultures.

Urine Output, analysis, C/S.

Imaging CXR, ECG and *Echo-cardiogram*, CT/USG Head Scan

CVP and IBP measurements

| 0 min 5 min | Recognize decreased perfusion, cyanosis, RDS. Maintain airway and establish IV/IO access according to NRP guidelines |

Push 10cc/kg isotonic crystalloid or colloid boluses upto 60 cc/kg, Correct hypoglycemia, and hypocalcemia. Begin Prostaglandin infusion until echocardiogram shows no ductal-dependent lesion

15 min

Fluid responsive → Observe in NICU

Fluid-refractory shock
Establish central venous and arterial access
Titrate Dopamine and Dobutamine

Fluid-refractory-dopamine resistant shock
Titrate epinephrine
Systemic alkalinization if PPHN and acidosis is present

Catecholamine-resistant shock

60 min
Direct therapies using echocardiogram and arterial and CVP monitoring

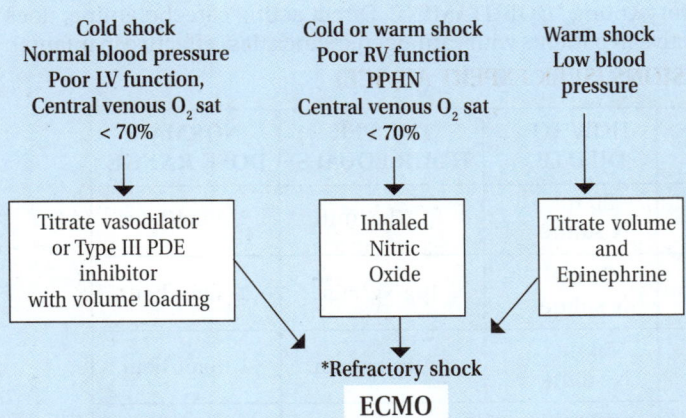

Cold shock
Normal blood pressure
Poor LV function,
Central venous O_2 sat < 70% → Titrate vasodilator or Type III PDE inhibitor with volume loading

Cold or warm shock
Poor RV function
PPHN
Central venous O_2 sat < 70% → Inhaled Nitric Oxide

Warm shock
Low blood pressure → Titrate volume and Epinephrine

*Refractory shock

ECMO

RDS= Respiratory Distress Syndrome, **NRP** = Neonatal Resuscitation Program, **NICU** = Neonatal Intensive Care Unit, **PPHN** - Persistent Pulmonary Hypertension, **PDE** = Phosphodiesterase, **ECMO** = Extra Corporeal Membrane Oxygenation

* **Pressor resistant Hypotension** *(refractory)*- start IV hydrocortisone 1mg/kg/ dose - repeat every 8–12 hrs for 3 days to treat transient adrenal insufficiency, salt losing variety of congenital adrenal hyperplasia and babies who are otherwise cortisol deficient (serum cortisol <15mcg/dl). In such cases an increase in BP is expected within 2 hrs of the first dose. Keep in mind the common adverse effects of hydrocortisone such as hyperglycemia, salt and water retention, GI perforations, disseminated fungal infection, etc.

---

* Early use of mechanical ventilation, in Neonatal Shock (especially in septic shock) removes work of breathing and allows for redistribution of limited cardiac output to vital organs. It with PEEP may improve oxygenation and decreases PVR and LV afterload.

* Correct negative inotropic factors, such as, hypoxia, acidosis, hypoglycemia, hypothermia, hypocalcemia and hypo-magnesemia.

* Beware of the causes of persistent low blood pressure such as, a) inadequate dose, compliance, IV patency for inotropes b) iatrogenic causes such as drugs/overventilation/air leak c) PPHN d) adrenal insufficiency/hemorrhage e) neurogenic shock f) pneumothorax/pericardium. Always search for such underlying cause when response to treatment is inadequate.

* Maintain CVP between 5–8 cm of water: if CVP < 5, push isotonic fluids and if CVP >8 restrict fluids. If CVP is normal but BP low increase vasopressor dose.

* In the absence of CVP, improvement during management of shock is judged by - improvement in CRT, decrease in heart rate by atleast 10 bpm, increase in urine output, increase in MAP by 5mmHg if NIBP monitor is on and fall in base deficit by 5 on ABG.

* When CVP/BP monitoring not possible - check color, tone, temperature (peripheral-core difference), CRT, respiration, zheart rate, activity, arousal state, AF, skin turgor. If improving continue monitoring and reassessing and treating accordingly. If not improving - refer to a level -3 NICU.

* Shock in VLBW neonate - dopamine is the recommended therapy with judicious use of volume if hypovolemia is suspected. Don't give large volume infusions to prevent increased risk of BPD.

* Shock in preterm/term baby due to perinatal depression - dopamine with dobutamine upto 10 microgram/kg/minute is recommended. Milrinone can be used to provide afterload reduction and inotropy. Inhaled NO is warranted in cases associated with pulmonary hypertension.

* Preterm baby with PDA - avoid high dose dopamine (>10 mcg/ kg/minute), to prevent further increase in left to right shunting. Use dobutamine or milrinone to enhance inotropy. Ventilate with PEEP, maintaining permissive hypercarbia and avoiding hyperoxygenation.

* Start IV Broad spectrum antibiotics to cover for septic shock (IV Ampicillin + Cephaperazone + Gentamicin/Netilmicin.

* Provide supportive management for associated multiorgan dysfunction-renal failure, coagulation problems, dyselectrolytemia, anemia and metabolic problems.

Pearl/Peril/Pitfall: BP is used in neonatology as a marker of systemic perfusion. However BP correlates only weakly with cardiac output and babies can have low BP and normal cardiac output and normal BP and low cardiac output. Therefore BP should not be the only criteria by which systemic perfusion is assessed. *The first priority is to confirm the BP reading is accurate and that the transducer has been calibrated and positioned correctly.

INOTROPIC DRUGS

Drug	Dosing range	Receptors	Use	Risk
Dopamine	2-20mcg/kg/min	D1/D2 >β >α	Renal effects, early inotropy needs, septic shock	Peripheral vasoconstriction
Dobutamine	3-20mcg/kg/min	$\beta_1 > \beta_2 > \alpha$	Contractility vasodilation	Tachycardia,
Epinephrine	0.01-2mcg/kg/min	$\beta_1 = \beta_2 > \alpha$	Contractility, vasoconstriction (higher doses)	Tachycardia, Vasoconstriction
Milrinone	0.3-0.7mcg/kg/min	Phosphodiesterase Inhibitor	Inotropy, vasodilation	Tachycardia, vasodilation
Amrinone	5-10mcg/kg/min	Phosphodiesterase Inhibitor	Inotropy, vasodilation	Tachycardia, vasodilation

VASODILATOR AGENTS

Drug	Dosing range	Site of action	Use	Risk(similar for both)
Nitroprusside	0.3-7mcg/kg/min	Arteries > veins	Afterload reduction	Cyanide toxicity, hypotension
Nitroglycerin	0.5-5mcg/kg/min	Veins > Arteries	Preload and afterload reduction	Hypotension, Methemoglobinemia

VASOCONSTRICTIVE AGENTS

Drug	Dose range	Receptor activity	Use	Risk
Epinephrine	0.01–2mcg/kg/min*	$\beta_1 = \beta_2 > \alpha$	anaphylaxis, cardiogenic shock, septic shock	Ischemia, hypertension
Norepinephrine	0.05–1mcg/kg/min	$\beta_1 > \alpha > \beta_2$	Severe vasodilation, hypotension	Acidosis from poor perfusion, ischemic injury
Phenylephrine	0.1–0.5mcg/kg/min	α selective	Severe hypotension Tetralogy spells	Acidosis, ischemic injury

* Vasoconstrictive dose is > 0.2 mcg/kg/mt

INOTROPES—PRACTICAL POINTS

*Can cause Tachyarrhythmias *Extravasation can result in severe tissue damage *May be diluted in saline/Dextrose solutions *Inactivated by $NaHCO_3$ *Never interrupt the infusion-as the half life is very short *Never flush through an IV cannula; rapid treatment could be fatal *Accurately label all IVI with the name, concentration, diluent and rate ***DOPAMINE**-dependent on the patient's noradrenaline stores for part of its action so it may be ineffectual in children with chronic cardiac conditions and the very young ***DOBUTAMINE** :Direct acting catecholamine, does not depend on endogenous adrenaline so more effective in patients with cardiogenic shock (less effective in infants).

INOTROPE INFUSIONS (SEEK EXPERT ADVICE)

INOTROPE	HOW MUCH INOTROPE IN mg	HOW TO DILUTE	1ML PER HOUR EQUALS	NORMAL DOSE RANGE
Dopamine	3 × body weight (kg)	50 ml N saline	1μg/kg/min	1–10ml/hour
Dobutamine	3 × body weight (kg)	50 ml N saline	1μg/kg/min	1–10ml/hour
Adrenaline	0.3 × body weight (kg)	50 ml N saline	0.1μg/kg/min	1–10ml/hour
Nor-adrenaline	0.3 × body weight (kg)	50 ml N saline	0.1μg/kg/min	1–10ml/hour

1. These can be double strength for fluid restricted patients or patients under age 10. The rate is halved if the strength is doubled.
2. Low dose of Dopamine is 2–5mcg/kg/min: increase renal perfusion, no effect on cardiac output. High dose of Dopamine is >20 mcg/kg/min: increases cardiac output, decreases renal perfusion.
3. Dobutamine and Dopamine are inactivated by alkaline drugs.
4. Dopamine ampoule 1 ml = 40 mgs ; Dobutamine 1 ml = 25 mgs (Varies with the pharma brand name; Check with drug information sheet)

Pearl/Peril/Pitfall: *Volume replacement. As a group, hypotensive babies are not hypovolemic and volume replacement improves BP in slightly less than half of preterm babies. However, since hypovolemia does occur, and is difficult to diagnose clinically, small amounts of volume replacement are unlikley to be harmful and inotropes will not help if a baby is hypovolemic. We would therefore commence circulatory support with 10 mls/kg of NS over 20-30 minutes.*

DETERMINANTS OF CARDIAC OUTPUT AND ARTERIAL BLOOD PRESSURES

Sympathetic nervous system endogenous catecholamines

Intravascular volume

Venous capacitance

Systemic vascular resistance

Preload

Contractility

Afterload

Heart rate

Stroke volume

Cardiac output

Systemic vascular resistance

Arterial blood pressure

SEQUENCE OF PATHOPHYSIOLOGIC EVENTS IN THE CLINICAL SHOCK STATE. HR, HEART RATE

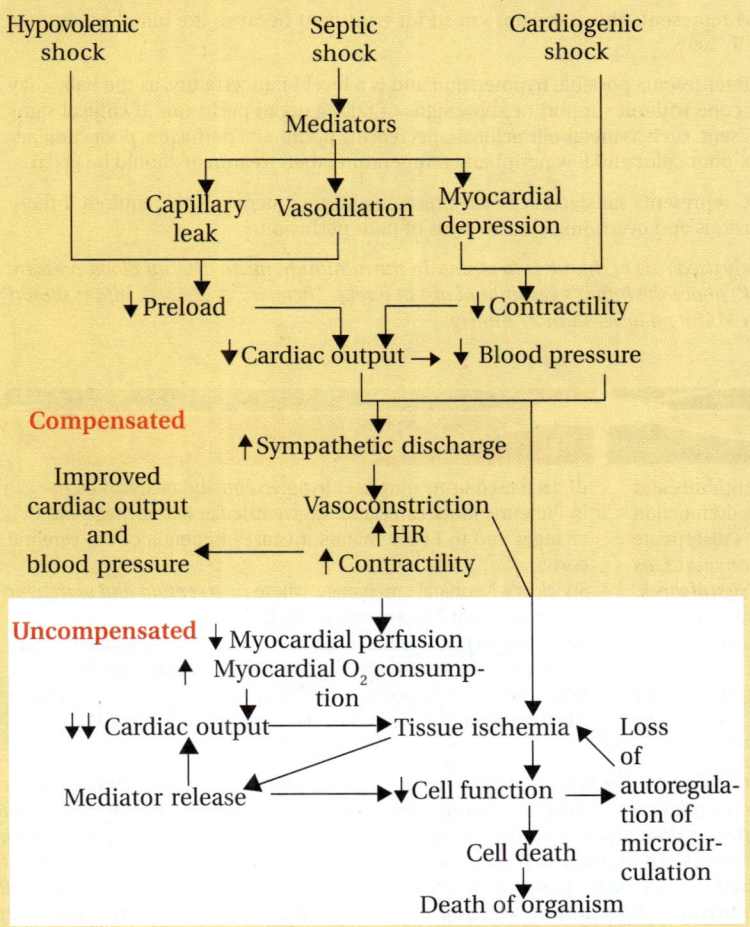

Hypovolemic shock

Septic shock

Cardiogenic shock

Mediators

Capillary leak

Vasodilation

Myocardial depression

↓Preload

↓Contractility

↓Cardiac output → ↓Blood pressure

Compensated

↑Sympathetic discharge

Improved cardiac output and blood pressure

Vasoconstriction

↑HR

↑Contractility

Uncompensated

↓Myocardial perfusion

↑Myocardial O_2 consumption

↓↓Cardiac output

Tissue ischemia

Loss of autoregulation of microcirculation

Mediator release

↓Cell function

Cell death

Death of organism

ESSENTIAL ASPECTS OF NEONATAL SHOCK AND HYPOTENSION

*Hypovolemia is a relatively uncommon primary cause of circulatory compromise, especially during the first postnatal days.

*Indeed, it is only when Mean BP is >40 mm Hg during the 1st postnatal day in the preterm neonate born before 30 weeks' gestation that the systemic blood flow can definitely assumed to be normal. This is due to their unique circulatory vulnerability in the 1st 12–24 hours, because of transitional circulatory changes making preterm infant`s adaptation difficult.

*The circulation of the very preterm infant exists in a state of precarious balance. The peripheral circulation is balanced between overconstriction, which may compromise systemic blood flow, and overdilation, which may result in vasodilatory shock. Data now suggest that the former situation dominates in the 1st 24 hours and the latter becomes increasingly important after that time. This creates a therapeutic dilemma. Therefore, accurate diagnosis of the type of the circulatory failure is imperative.

*In clinical practice, tissue perfusion is routinely assessed by monitoring heart rate, blood pressure, capillary refilling time, acid-base status, and urine output. However, none of these parameters has sufficient accuracy to be used on its own to evaluate systemic blood flow and tissue perfusion. Therefore, the addition of echocardiographic hemodynamic assessment to BP monitoring and thorough continuous clinical evaluation of the infant are necessary to better understand changes in organ blood flow and tissue perfusion, especially in preterm neonates during vulnerable period of immediate transition to extrauterine life.

REFERENCES AND FURTHER READING

1) Seri I, Noori S. Diagnosis and treatment of neonatal hypotension outside the transitional period. *Early Hum Dev*. May 2005;81(5):405–11. 2) Northern Neonatal Nursing Initiative. Systolic blood pressure in babies of less than 32 weeks gestation in the first year of life. *Arch Dis Child Fetal Neonatal Ed*. Jan 1999;80(1):F38-42. 3) Subhedar NV. Treatment of hypotension in newborns. *Semin Neonatol*.4) Dec 2003;8(6):413–23. 4) Seri I, Evans J. Controversies in the diagnosis and management of hypotension in the newborn infant. *Curr Opin Pediatr*. Apr 2001;13(2):116–23. 5) Zubrow AB, Hulman S, Kushner H, et al. Determinants of blood pressure in infants admitted to neonatal intensive care units: a prospective multicenter study. Philadelphia Neonatal Blood Pressure Study Group. *J Perinatol*. Nov-Dec 1995;15(6):470-9.

Pearl/Peril/Pitfall: *Hydrocortisone: Some very preterm babies have an immature corticosteroid stress response. Bouchier et al showed hydrocortisone 2.5 mg/kg in two doses 4 hours apart increased blood pressure in 81% of babies. However we do not know whether this effect is mediated by increased flow or resistance and we do not know effects on long term outcomes.*

TABLE 1 Hemodynamic variables in different types of shock

Etiology	Preload	Afterload	Myocardial contractility
Hypovolemic shock	decreased	increased	normal
Distributive shock	decreased	decreased	increased
Septic shock, early stage	decreased	decreased	increased
Septic shock, late stage	increased	increased	decreased
Cardiogenic shock	increased	increased	decreased

TABLE 2 Clinical stages of shock

Clinical feature	Compensated shock	Decompensated shock	Irreversible shock
Heart rate	Tachycardia	Marked tachycardia	Severe tachycardia/bradycardia
Peripheral pulses	Bounding	Feeble	Imperceptible
Respiratory rate	Normal or slightly high	Tachypnea	Tachycardia/apnea
Skin	Cold/flushed and warm	Mottled	Cold and cyanotic
B.P.	Normal	Hypotension	Gross hypotension
Pulse pressure	Normal/wide	Low	Remarkably low
Capillary refill time	Increased (> 3 seconds)	Increased	Remarkably increased
Peripheral core temp. gradient	Over 2^{0}C	Over 5^{0}C	
Mental status	Irritable	Lethargic	Comatose
Urine output	Normal or reduced	Oliguria	Anuria

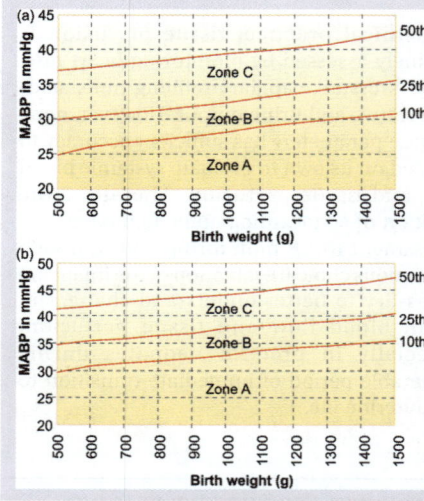

Normal range Blood pressure varies normally with gestational age and postnatal age, and both may need to be considered when deciding whether a baby needs treatment for low blood pressure. The normal range for blood pressure is shown in the figure on left. *Top Figure: VLBW infants <36 hrs old *Bottom Figure: VLBW infants >36 hrs old,*

Zone A represents the mandatory need for treatment because the blood pressure is critically low.

Zone B represents possible hypotension and is a level of uncertainty, as the baby may either cope without support or show signs of failing organ perfusion. If clinical signs are present, such as metabolic acidosis, decreasing peripheral perfusion, poor capillary return, poor color and low peripheral temperature, then treatment should be given.

Zone C represents satisfactory blood pressure and treatment is only required if there are obvious and overriding clinical signs of poor perfusion.

A widely used rule of thumb is to maintain the minimum mean arterial blood pressure (MABP) above the infant's gestational age in weeks. Therefore, a 27-week infant should have a MABP no lower than 27 mmHg.

KEY POINTS FOR CLINICAL PRACTICE

1. Neonatal shock remains a major cause of Neonatal morbidity and mortality and it is an acute complex state of circulatory dysfunction resulting in insufficient oxygen and nutrient delivery to satisfy tissue requirements. *Shock and hypotension are not synonymous, as hypotension is a late, decompensated and preterminal sign of shock.* Risk factors for hypotension and poor perfusion • Short gestational age • Lack of antenatal steroids • Positive pressure ventilation • Patent ductus arteriosus • Perinatal asphyxia • Systemic infection

2. *Shock is a clinical diagnosis* manifested principally by a) pallor and poor skin perfusion b) cool extremities c) CNS lethargy d) decreased urine output e) hypotension and tachycardia.

3. In Preterms shock can cause intraventricular hemorrhage and PVL changes and in ELBW infants it causes ischemia of the cerebral cortex.

4. Shock is a Neonatal emergency, where *intervention and search for the cause could happen concurrently.*

5. *Restoring perfusion is the cornerstone in shock management.* There is no ideal drug/dose for management of shock; modify as per assessment and response. Ventilatory support may be needed in which case the baby must be referred to a level III NICU.

Pearl/Peril/Pitfall: Inotropes: Dopamine and dobutamine are the most widely used inotropes in neonatology. Dopamine is better than dobutamine at improving blood pressure, however while the central actions of these drugs is similar, peripherally dopamine vasoconstricts while dobutamine vasodilates. This effect is dose dependent, Roze et al in the only study to date which has looked at flow, demonstrated that dopamine, at doses above 10 mcg/kg/min. increased vascular resistance and reduced cardiac output while dobutamine reduced vascular resistance and increased cardiac output. Seri et al showed improvements in renal blood flow with dopamine at 4 mcg/kg/min. Therefore: First line inotrope: Dobutamine starting at 10 micrograms/kg/min increasing to 20 micrograms/kg/min depending on response. Second line inotrope: Dopamine starting at 5 micrograms/kg/min increasing to 10 micrograms/kg/min depending on response. Doses above 10 mcg/kg/min should be avoided. Third line inotrope: Adrenaline starting at 0.05 micrograms/kg/min increasing to 1 micrograms/kg/min depending on response. Adrenaline markedly increases vascular resistance and should only be given after echocardiographic assessment and consultation at a senior level.

10 Early Onset Neonatal Sepsis (EOS)

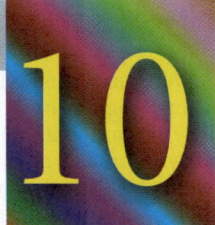

@ *"Consider other diagnoses such as TTN, MAS, duct dependent cardiac malformation, bowel obstruction, viral sepsis, NEC, inborn errors of metabolism in the differential diagnosis of early onset sepsis".*

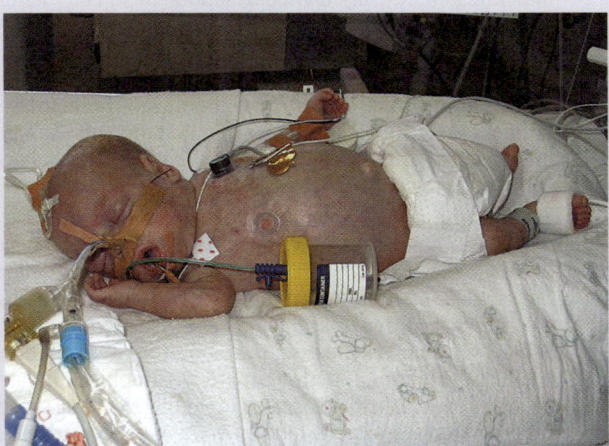

*A large WHO study published in 2003 identified nine clinical features which predict severe bacterial illness in young infants 1. Feeding ability reduced 2. No spontaneous movement 3. Temperature >38 C 4. Prolonged capillary refill time 5. Lower chest wall in drawing 6. Resp rate > 60/minute 7. Grunting 8. Cyanosis 9. H/O of convulsions .

*When Neonatal sepsis is suspected, treatment should be initiated immediately because of the Neonate's relative immunosuppression. Begin antibiotics as soon as diagnostic tests are performed. Additional therapies have been investigated for the treatment of Neonatal sepsis; however, no substantial clinical trials have shown that these treatments are beneficial. These additional therapies include granulocyte transfusion, intravenous immune globulin (IVIG) replacement, exchange transfusion, and the use of recombinant cytokines.

Transfer: *The infant may require transfer to a level III perinatal center, especially if he or she requires cardiopulmonary support, parenteral nutrition, or prolonged intravenous access. (like the one in the picture) *Multidisciplinary services available at larger centers may be necessary when treating an acutely compromised Neonate.

Sepsis screen (Screen positive if ≥ 2 points)

Test	Point value
Absolute neutrophil count < 1750/mm³	1 point
Total white blood count < 7500/mm³ or > 40,000/mm³	1 point
Immature/total neutrophil ratio (≥ 0.20)	1 point
Immature/total neutrophil ratio (≥ 0.40)	2 points
CRP + (≥ 1 mg/dL)	1 point
CRP + (≥ 5 mg/dL)	2 points

REVIEW OF CLINICAL PROBLEMS

1. What are the common risk factors for Neonatal Sepsis?
Ans: Refer to Table 1 of the Chapter.

2. How do you evaluate neonatal sepsis?
Ans: Refer to Table 3 of the chapter.

3. Mention the differential diagnoses of neonatal sepsis.
Ans: Refer to Table 4 of the Chapter.

4. What are the supportive measures for neonatal sepsis?
Ans: Refer to Table 11 of the Chapter.

5. How do you monitor the patient, while managing neonatal sepsis ?
Ans: Refer to Table 12 of the Chapter.

LEARNING OBJECTIVES

After completing this article, readers will be able to

1. Suspect sepsis in any ill Neonate with varied clinical symptoms and signs.

2. Develop a rational approach in the diagnosis and management of Early Neonatal Sepsis.

3. Apply appropriate general and specific measures in the management of Early Neonatal Sepsis.

4. Understand the MODS associated with Sepsis and deal with it intensively.

5. Monitor for the clinical and laboratory response while managing Early Neonatal Sepsis.

Pearl/Peril/Pitfall: *In thrombocytopenic VLBW babies with sepsis, organism-specific platelet response is seen. In addition, persistent bacteremia, multiorgan failure and death are more in these babies, and survival decreases with the increased severity and duration of thrombocytopenia, with prolonged ventilation and increased need for platelet transfusions.*

BIRD'S EYE VIEW/OVERVIEW/SYNOPSIS

1. **Neonatal sepsis:** (symptomatic and systemic bacteremia) A frequent and serious illness with serious implications in terms of mortality and morbidity, more so in preterm, which if not recognized early, can lead to **Septic shock, multiple organ dysfunction (MODS) and Death.** Early onset sepsis (EOS) is caused by infections acquired before or during delivery due to vertical transmission from the mother. The most common bacteria are Group-B streptococcus, Esch.coli, Listeria, Gonococci. The age at onset depends on the timing of vertical transmission & the virulence of the infecting organism. EOS is usually apparent in the first hours of life; 90% of infants are symptomatic by 24hrs of age. It can be manifested upto 7 days after birth. *In India Klebsiella pneumoniae (30.0%). Staph aureus (13%) and E. coli (12.2%) are main organisms responsible for Neonatal Sepsis.*

2. *Major risk factors for EOS include* *Maternal intrapartum fever, >100.4^{0}F/38^{0}C *Rupture of membranes > 24hours *Chorioamnionitis *Sustained fetal heart rate >160/mt. *Minor risk factors for EOS include* *Rupture of membranes >12 hrs *Maternal intrapartum fever, >99.5^{0}F *Maternal WBC count, >15,000/cmm *Preterm labor, <37weeks, *Low Apgar score, <5 at 1 min, <7 at 5 min *Multiple gestation *Foul lochia *Maternal GBS colonization. *Infants with 1 major or 2 minor risk factors should have a sepsis screening done.* Refer to Table No -1 for various risk factors for EOS. Late Onset Sepsis (LOS) occurs usually after 7 days of life (but can occur after 72hrs of life) up to 90 days of life. It is divided into two distinct entities: disease occurring in premature babies >72hrs of life in NICU & disease occurring in healthy term infants in the community after 7 days of life. The late onset sepsis is discussed in a separate chapter (refer to Chapter 11).

3. **Prematurity:** *Preterm infants are more likely to require invasive procedures, such as umbilical catheterization and intubation. *Prematurity is associated with infection from cytomegalovirus (CMV), herpes simplex virus (HSV), hepatitis B, toxoplasmosis, *Mycobacterium tuberculosis, Campylobacter fetus,* and *Listeria* species. *Intrauterine growth retardation and low birth weight are also observed in CMV and toxoplasmosis infections. *Premature infants have less immunologic ability to resist and combat infection. This leads to infection with common organisms such as coagulase-negative staphylococci, an organism usually not associated with severe sepsis.

4. **Diagnosis of neonatal sepsis** is often hard as signs of SEPSIS may be minimal and nonspecific and cultures take time - **and time is most definitely not on your side.** A high index of suspicion is required for early detection of cases. Signs include : * Unusual crying *Sleepiness * Listlessness * Shock *Fits/apnea * Hypotonia * Vomiting *Rashes *T^0 ↓↓ or ↓ *Bradycardia. Also : feeding difficulty, abdominal wall reddening (omphalitis) ; grunting, rib recession, ↑↑ use of respiratory muscles, tachypnea, cyanosis, cool peripheries; delayed capillary return on pressing the skin. Refer to Table No -2 for the common signs & symptoms of Early Onset Sepsis. Specific *signs of an infected organ may pinpoint the primary site or a metastatic site.* * Most neonates with early-onset GBS (and many with L. monocytogenes) infection present with respiratory distress that is difficult to distinguish from respiratory distress syndrome.* Periumbilical erythema, discharge, or bleeding without a hemorrhagic diathesis suggests omphalitis (infection prevents obliteration of the umbilical vessels). * Coma, seizures, opisthotonos, or a bulging fontanelle suggests meningitis, encephalitis, or brain abscess. * Decreased spontaneous movement of an extremity and swelling, warmth, erythema, or tenderness over a joint indicates osteomyelitis or pyogenic arthritis. * Unexplained abdominal distention may indicate peritonitis or necrotizing enterocolitis (particularly when accompanied by bloody diarrhea and fecal leukocytes). * Cutaneous vesicles, mouth ulcers, and hepatosplenomegaly (particularly with disseminated intravascular coagulation [DIC]) can identify disseminated herpes simplex. <u>SCLEREMA NEONATORUM</u> is a diffuse spreading waxy hardness of the skin and subcutaneous tissue, which seems to bound to underlying muscle and bone. It is observed commonly in thighs, buttocks, and trunk. Sclerema is a manifestation of shock and insufficiency of the peripheral circulation and associated with poor prognosis.

5. *The Evaluation-Decision-Action-Plan/Algorithm* to diagnose & manage the EOS describes the essential aspects of Early Onset Sepsis in the Neonates. *(Always do resuscitate the septic baby if ABC's are compromised as per the NALS guidelines before evaluation and definitive management!).* **Table 3 summarizes the essential laboratory investigations useful in evaluating a septic Neonate;** Neutrophil ratios have been more useful in diagnosing or excluding Neonatal sepsis; the immature-to-total (I/T) ratio is the most sensitive. All immature neutrophil forms are counted, and the maximum acceptable ratio for excluding sepsis during the first 24 hours is 0.16. In most healthy, nonseptic Newborns, the ratio falls to 0.12 within 60 hours of life. The sensitivity of the I/T ratio has ranged from 60-90%, and elevations may be observed with other physiological events, limiting the positive predictive value of these ratios; therefore, when diagnosing sepsis, the elevated I/T ratio should be used in combination with other signs.

6. **After stabilizing ABCD's give antibiotics on clinical suspicion as blood and other cultures though definitive but take 48-72 hours ; try Ampicillin + Ceftazidime + Amikacin for early onset SEPSIS (<3days) . Duration of IV antibiotic therapy depends on CSF Analysis ; treat for 14 days for suspected or proven bacteremia and for 21 days for Meningitis (common in late onset NEONATAL SEPSIS) ;** *always modify* the antibiotic choice depending on culture sensitivity results.

7. *Consider other serious systemic illness in Newborns as important* Differential Diagnosis of NEONATAL SEPSIS! A) Perinatal Asphyxia B) Aspiration Pneumonia C) Congenital Heart Disease D) Metabolic (Hypoglycemia, Adrenal Insufficiency, Organic Acidosis, Urea Cycle Disorders) E) Neurologic (Intracranial Hemorrhage) F) Hematological (Neonatal Purpura Fulminans, Severe Anemia, Congenital Leukemia)

8. **Therapy for neonatal sepsis** Consists of A) Temperature Regulation B) Fluid & Electrolyte Balance C) Use of Inotropes D) Assisted Ventilation when Required E) Bacterial Eradication F) Exchange Transfusion G)New Modalities (IV Immunoglobulin, Granulocyte Transfusion, G-CSF) which are inconclusive and not recommended routinely.

9. **Single Volume Exchange Transfusion (85 ml/kg)** is to be considered in NEONATAL SEPSIS if complicated by A) Sclerema B) Respiratory Distress Syndrome C) DIC D) Neutropenia. E) Hyperbilirubinemia.

10. The mortality rate in Neonatal sepsis varies between 45–60% in India; early sepsis screen, judicious and early antibiotics, close monitoring of vital signs and intensive care support are the most crucial factors responsible for a better outcome.

Pearl/Peril/Pitfall: Rupture of membranes without other complications for more than 24 hours prior to delivery is associated with a 1% increase in the incidence of Neonatal sepsis; however, when chorioamnionitis accompanies the rupture of membranes, the incidence of Neonatal infection is quadrupled.

THE EVALUATION-DECISION-ACTION-PLAN/ALGORITHM FOR THE DIAGNOSIS AND MANAGEMENT OF *A NEONATE WITH EARLY ONSET SEPSIS (EOS)*

SUBJECTIVE FINDINGS

Assess the presence of various risk factors for Early Onset Sepsis - Refer to Table 1

Assess the symptoms of early sepsis, with a high index of suspicion - Refer to Table 2

OBJECTIVE FINDINGS

Assess ABCDs -vitals, BP, CRT, O_2 sats, Urine output, Pulses, skin rashes including petechiae, sensorium, seizures and focal neurological signs.

Look for various signs pointing toward EOS - respiratory distress, jaundice, poor Neonatal reflexes/feeding, shock and mottling of skin, scleredema

Perform complete systemic examination - to identify localization such as pneumonia, cellulitis, mastitis, omphalitis, subcutaneous abscesses, ecthyma gangrenosum (Pseudomonas), vesicular rash (Herpes virus)

Assess for multiorgan dysfunction—cardiac failure, renal failure, pulmonary hypertension, cerebral edema/thrombosis, adrenal hemorrhage/insufficiency, bone marrow dysfunction and DIC

INVESTIGATIONS

Perform partial septic screen - FBC, TC, DC, Immature-to-Total neutrophil ratio, micro ESR, CRP, blood cultures, urine complete examination with cultures, chest X-ray. Buffy coat examination of leukocytes with Gram stain and methylene blue stain - to identify intracellular bacteria.

Perform LP and complete CSF analysis along with the above screen (complete septic screen)- only on a) infants with positive blood cultures b) symptomatic infants with negative blood cultures who are treated empirically for the clinical diagnosis of sepsis.

A NEONATE WITH EARLY ONSET SEPSIS

Infant with symptoms of sepsis and of mothers with chorioamnionitis

Diagnostics
Serial WBC/differential and CRP Blood Culture Chest X-ray if signs of distress Lumbar puncture

Begin antibiotics

* Ensure ABCs, Pulse Oximetry, CR monitor, BP, urine output. *ABG analysis and electrolytes, blood sugar,serum creatinine, coagulation studies and echocardiogram if necessary.

Results
Culture positive (or presence of focal disease) or sepsis score ≥ 2 or LP abnormal or symptoms persist for > 24 hr and clinical course is consistent with sepsis

If there are no risk factors for sepsis and cultures are negative and sepsis score < 2 and symptoms resolve by 24 hr or symptoms and clinical course are consistent with a noninfectious condition

Management
Treat for 7-10 days for suspected or proven bacteremia and 14-21 days for meningitis

Treat for 48 hr and send home if appropriate

Asymptomatic infants of at least 35 wks GA with 1 or more risk factors for Sepsis

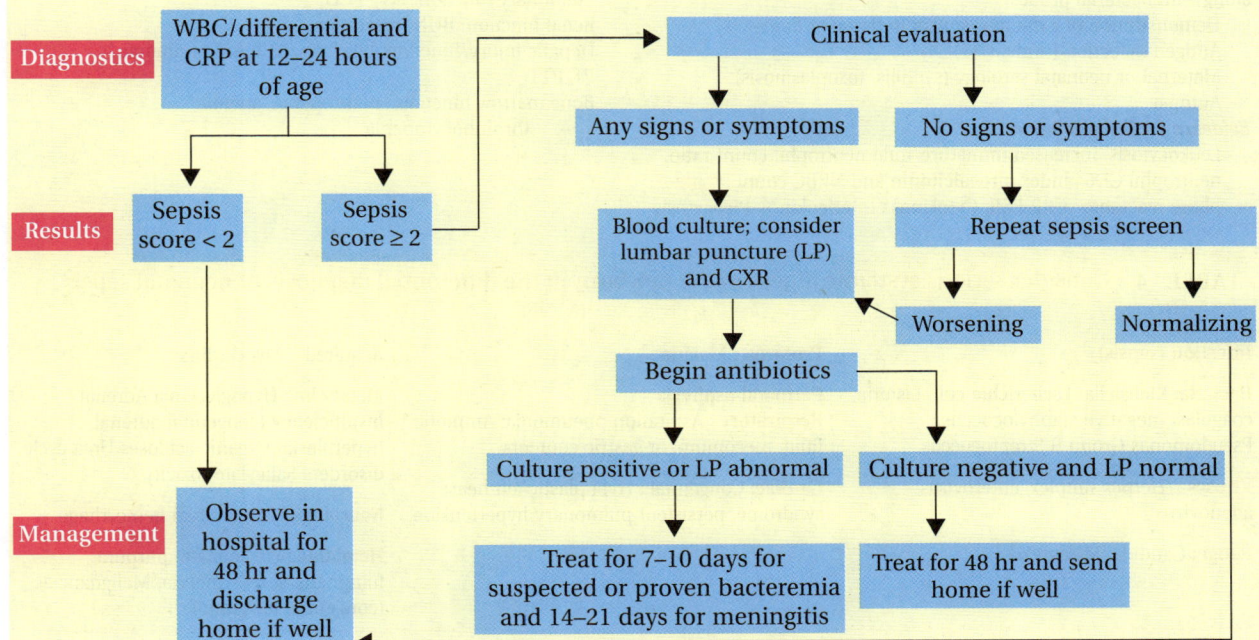

Diagnostics
WBC/differential and CRP at 12–24 hours of age

Clinical evaluation

Any signs or symptoms

No signs or symptoms

Results
Sepsis score < 2

Sepsis score ≥ 2

Blood culture; consider lumbar puncture (LP) and CXR

Repeat sepsis screen

Worsening

Normalizing

Begin antibiotics

Culture positive or LP abnormal

Culture negative and LP normal

Management
Observe in hospital for 48 hr and discharge home if well

Treat for 7–10 days for suspected or proven bacteremia and 14–21 days for meningitis

Treat for 48 hr and send home if well

Pearl/Peril/Pitfall: Recent data in large numbers of patients show a 38% rate of culture-positive meningitis in neonates with negative blood culture results and suspected sepsis. Therefore, a lumbar puncture should be part of the evaluation of an infant with suspected sepsis.

TABLE 1   The risk factors for sepsis !

History (specific risk factors)

Maternal infection during gestation or at parturition (type and duration of antimicrobial therapy)

Urinary tract infection (Maternal intrapartal fever > 100.4ºF

Chorioamnionitis or 38ºC)

Maternal colonization with GBS, *Neisseria gonorrhoeae*, herpes simplex

Gestational age/birth weight

Multiple birth

Duration of membrane rupture (>18hrs)

Complicated delivery

Fetal tachycardia (distress) (Fetal heart rate >160)

Age at onset (in utero, birth, early postnatal, late)

Medical intervention

Vascular access
Endotracheal intubation
Parenteral nutrition
Surgery

Evidence for Other Disease*

Congenital malformations (heart disease, neural tube defect)
Respiratory tract disease (HMD, aspiration)
Necrotizing enterocolitis
Metabolic disease, e.g., galactosemia

Evidence for Focal or Systemic Disease

General appearance, neurologic status
Abnormal vital signs
Organ system disease
Feeding, Stools, urine output

TABLE 2   Clinical signs and symptoms of neonatal sepsis

SUSPECT SEPSIS—with a **high index** in any sick looking Newborn baby, as clinical signs of SEPSIS are *nonspecific and often subtle and overlap* with the signs and symptoms of many other disorders (eg : Respiratory, Cardiac or Hematologic, Inborn errors of Metabolism, Bowel Perforation, NEC and Viral / Fungal SEPSIS in Preterm Babies).

General
Fever, temperature instability, "Not doing well", Poor feeding Edema

Gastrointestinal system
Abdominal distention, vomiting, diarrhea, hepatomegaly !

Respiratory system

Apnea, dyspnea, tachypnea, retraction, flaring, grunting, cyanosis

Renal System
Oliguria

Cardiovascular system
Pallor ; mottling ; cold, clammy skin tachycardia, hypotension, bradycardia

Central nervous system
Irritability, lethargy, tremors, seizures

Hyporeflexia, hypotonia, abnormal moro reflex, irregular respirations, full fontanel, high-pitched cry

Hematologic System
Jaundice, splenomegaly, pallor, petechiae, purpura, bleeding

TABLE 3   Laboratory evaluation of the septic newborn for the evidence of infection, inflammation and for multi organ system disease !

Laboratory Studies
Evidence for Infection

Culture from a normally sterile site (blood, CSF, other) (conventional and automated), PCR of 16s rRNA gene along with bacterial probes

Demonstration of a microorganism in tissue or fluid
Antigen detection (urine, CSF)
Maternal or neonatal serology (syphilis, toxoplasmosis)
Autopsy

Evidence for Inflammation

Leukocytosis, increased immature/total neutrophil count ratio, neutrophil CD64 index, **procalcitonin** and NRBC count, Acute-phase reactants : CRP, ESR, Cytokines : Interleukin-6, Pleocytosis

in CSF, synovial, or pleural fluid
Disseminated intravascular coagulation : fibrin split products

Evidence for Multiorgan System Disease

Metabolic acidosis: pH, PCO_2
Pulmonary function: PO_2, PCO_2
Renal function: BUN, creatinine
Hepatic injury/function: bilirubin, ALT, AST, ammonia, PT, PTT
Bone marrow function : neutropenia, anemia, thrombocytopenia

TABLE 4   Consider serious systemic illness in the newborn in the differential diagnosis of neonatal sepsis !

Infection (sepsis)

Bacteria: Klebsiella, Escherichia coli, Listeria, coagulase-negative staphylococcus, Pseudomonas Group B Streptococcus

Viruses : Herpes simplex, enterovirus, adenovirus

Fungi : Candida, Malassezia

Protozoa : Malaria

Perinatal asphyxia
Respiratory : Aspiration pneumonia: Amniotic fluid, meconium, or gastric contents

Cardiac: Congenital : Hypoplastic left heart syndrome, persistent pulmonary hypertension

Acquired: Myocarditis

Metabolic : Hypoglycemia Adrenal insufficiency (congenital adrenal hyperplasia) Organic acidoses Urea cycle disorders Salicylate toxicity

Neurologic: Intracranial hemorrhage

Hematologic: Neonatal purpura fulminans Severe anemia, Malignancies (congenital leukemia)

Pearl/Peril/Pitfall: Blood, cerebrospinal fluid (CSF), and urine cultures · Aerobic and anaerobic cultures are appropriate for most of the bacterial etiologies associated with Neonatal sepsis. Anaerobic cultures are especially important in Neonates with abscess formation, processes with bowel involvement, massive hemolysis, and refractory pneumonia.

BEWARE OF THE NATURAL COURSE OF SEPSIS IN NEWBORN !

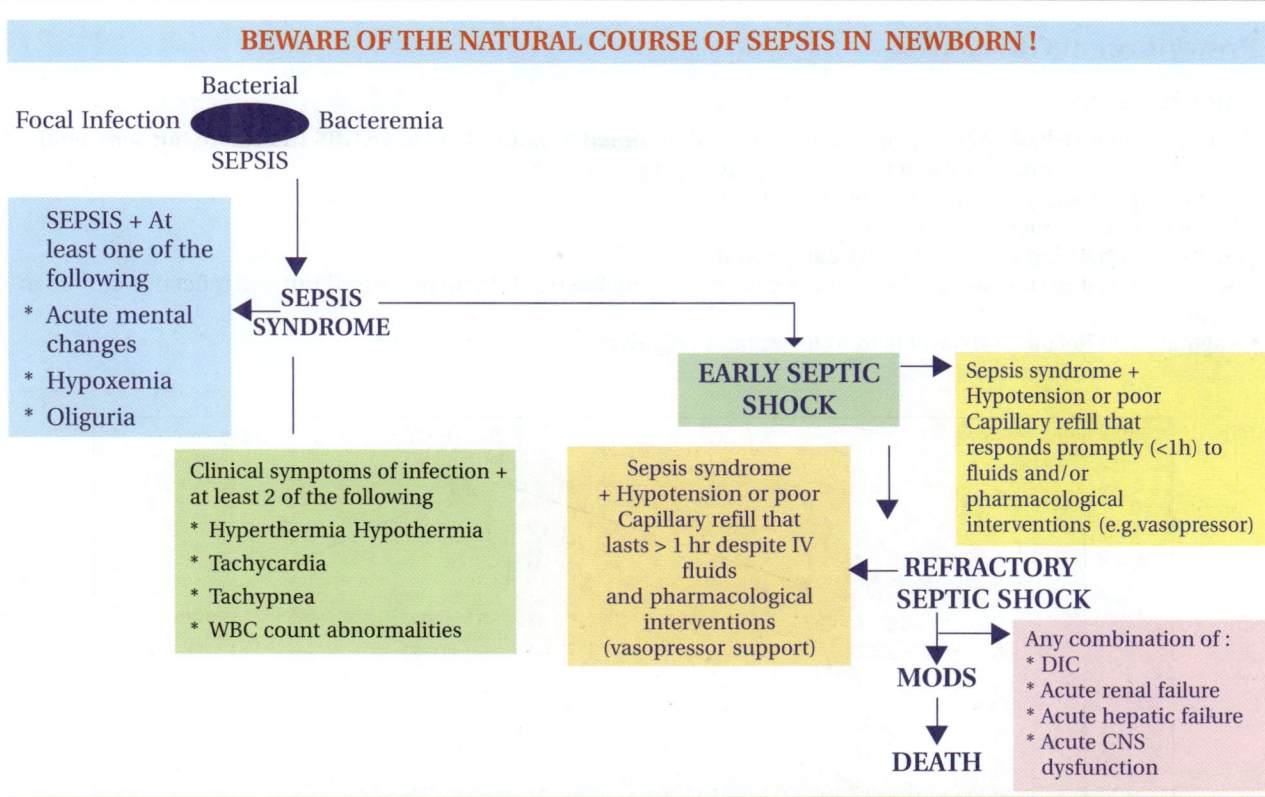

Focal Infection — Bacterial SEPSIS — Bacteremia

SEPSIS SYNDROME

SEPSIS + At least one of the following
* Acute mental changes
* Hypoxemia
* Oliguria

Clinical symptoms of infection + at least 2 of the following
* Hyperthermia Hypothermia
* Tachycardia
* Tachypnea
* WBC count abnormalities

EARLY SEPTIC SHOCK

Sepsis syndrome + Hypotension or poor Capillary refill that responds promptly (<1h) to fluids and/or pharmacological interventions (e.g.vasopressor)

Sepsis syndrome + Hypotension or poor Capillary refill that lasts > 1 hr despite IV fluids and pharmacological interventions (vasopressor support)

REFRACTORY SEPTIC SHOCK

MODS

Any combination of :
* DIC
* Acute renal failure
* Acute hepatic failure
* Acute CNS dysfunction

DEATH

TABLE 5   Normal ranges for WBC indices at 4 hours of age

	Mean	± SD	10%–90% range
Total WBC ($\times 10^9$/L)	24.06	6.11	16.20–31.50
ANC ($\times 10^9$/L)	15.62	4.69	9.50–21.50
I/T ratio	0.16	0.10	0.05–0.27

TABLE 6   NEED TO KNOW PRACTICAL ASPECTS ABOUT THE LAB DIAGNOSIS OF THE SEPSIS IN THE NEWBORN !

A). *Indications for SEPSIS Screen -*
At birth

* Rupture of membranes > 24 hr
* Maternal intrapartum fever > 100.4°F
* Chorioamnionitis

Minor risk factors:

* Rupture of membrane > 12 hour
* Maternal intrapartum fever > 99.5°F
* Maternal WBC > 15,000/ml
* Low Apgar score (<5 at 1 min, < 7 at 5 min)
* LBW (<1500g)
* Preterm labour (<37 weeks) is present in 39%, if 2 SEPSIS screen panel results are positive.

Clinically useful tests to suggest / detect

SEPSIS and to monitor the response to treatment:
An immature (band) to total neutrophil ratio of > 0.2, neutropenia < 1,000, thrombocytopenia <1,00,000, chest X-ray infiltrations, negative CRP (excludes infection), (The micro-ESR may be elevated with sepsis and fall of > 15 mm during first hour indicates infection.) culture sensitivity tests of body fluids (blood, urine and CSF) - a gold standard in the diagnosis of NEONATAL SEPSIS and MENINGITIS.

After Birth
If baby develops respiratory distress or nonspecific features of NEONATAL SEPSIS it is an indication for SEPSIS screen. SEPSIS screen panel consists of TLC, I/T ratio, CRP, haptoglobin and micro ESR. An abnormality in any two or more of these items is considered to be a positive screen and in one or none is considered as negative screen. Probability that serious bacterial infection frequency of both RDS and advanced items are positive. A study has shown that two sepsis screens performed 12-24 hour apart has 100% negative predictive value. *When the evidence obtained by history or physical examination conflicts with a negative screen, antibiotics should be started. Thus clinical signs of SEPSIS remain the most important criteria for use of antibiotics.*

Antenatal
Mothers having one or more risk factors associated with development of Neonatal SEPSIS are given intrapartum antibiotic chemoprophylaxis. Neonatal morbidity improves in mothers with preterm premature rupture of membranes treated with different antibiotic regimens. Single course of steroid administered antenataly to decrease grades of IVH in mothers with pre-term deliveries even with preterm premature rupture of membranes is not associated with any increase in perinatal infections morbidity.

---

* *Pearl/Peril/Pitfall :* The CRP level is not recommended as a sole indicator of neonatal sepsis but may be used as part of a sepsis workup or as a serial study during infection to determine response to antibiotics, duration of therapy, and/or relapse of infection.

Prevention of GBS sepsis

Antenatal strategies

Women at high risk of GBS carriage at delivery and assumed to potentially have GBS (therefore not screened)
- GBS grown from urine or vaginal swabs in current pregnancy
- Previous pregnancy with a GBS infected neonate
- Previous GBS carriage

Screen all remaining women for GBS carrier status
- Screening best performed at 35–37 weeks gestation to enable result to be processed but still reflective of flora at term
- Vaginal AND Rectal swabs will lead to fewer false negatives

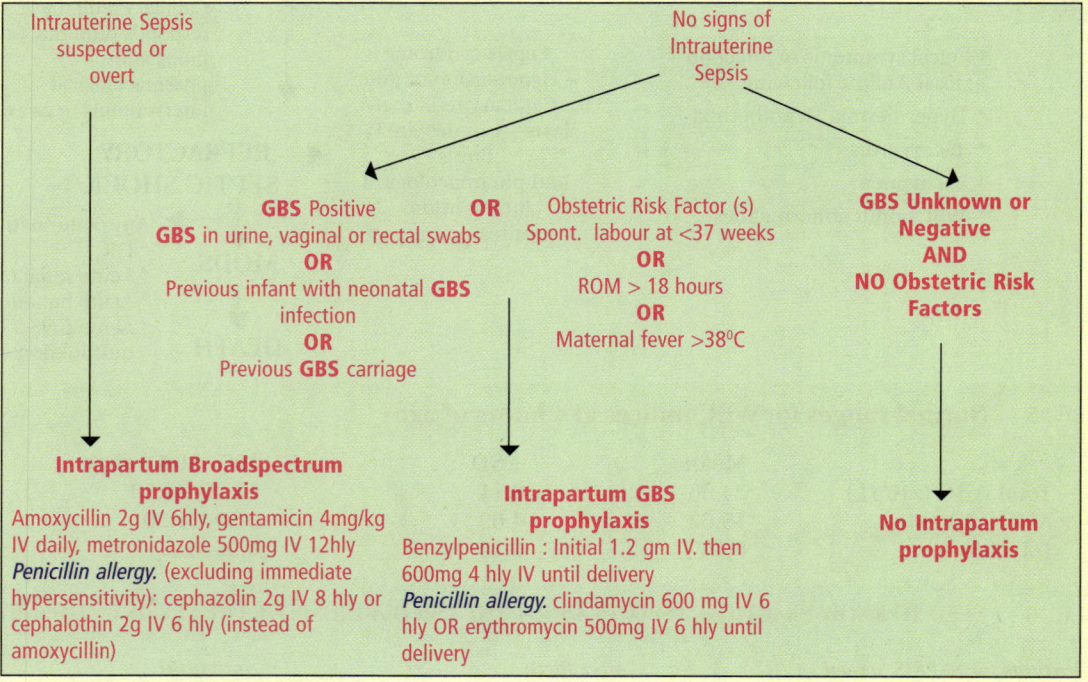

Intrauterine Sepsis suspected or overt

No signs of Intrauterine Sepsis

GBS Positive
GBS in urine, vaginal or rectal swabs
OR
Previous infant with neonatal **GBS** infection
OR
Previous **GBS** carriage

OR

Obstetric Risk Factor (s)
Spont. labour at <37 weeks
OR
ROM > 18 hours
OR
Maternal fever >38⁰C

GBS Unknown or Negative
AND
NO Obstetric Risk Factors

Intrapartum Broadspectrum prophylaxis
Amoxycillin 2g IV 6hly, gentamicin 4mg/kg IV daily, metronidazole 500mg IV 12hly
Penicillin allergy. (excluding immediate hypersensitivity): cephazolin 2g IV 8 hly or cephalothin 2g IV 6 hly (instead of amoxycillin)

Intrapartum GBS prophylaxis
Benzylpenicillin : Initial 1.2 gm IV. then 600mg 4 hly IV until delivery
Penicillin allergy. clindamycin 600 mg IV 6 hly OR erythromycin 500mg IV 6 hly until delivery

No Intrapartum prophylaxis

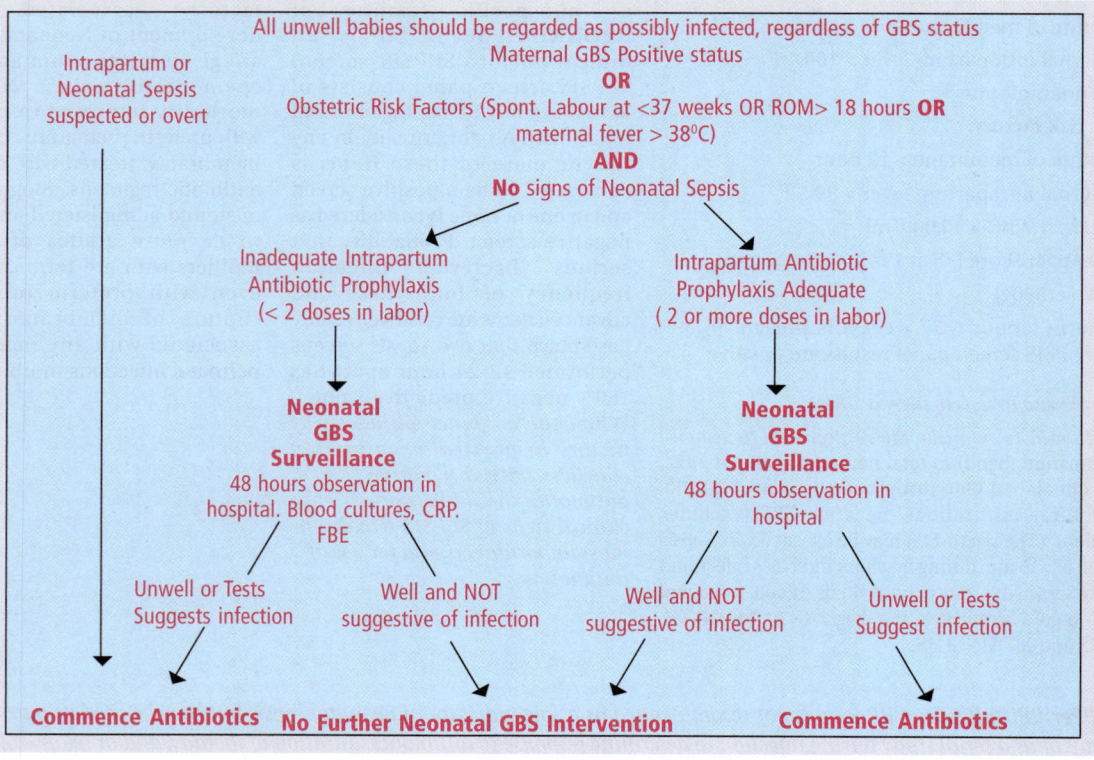

All unwell babies should be regarded as possibly infected, regardless of GBS status
Maternal GBS Positive status
OR
Obstetric Risk Factors (Spont. Labour at <37 weeks OR ROM> 18 hours **OR** maternal fever > 38⁰C)
AND
No signs of Neonatal Sepsis

Intrapartum or Neonatal Sepsis suspected or overt

Inadequate Intrapartum Antibiotic Prophylaxis (< 2 doses in labor)

Intrapartum Antibiotic Prophylaxis Adequate (2 or more doses in labor)

Neonatal GBS Surveillance
48 hours observation in hospital. Blood cultures, CRP. FBE

Neonatal GBS Surveillance
48 hours observation in hospital

Unwell or Tests Suggests infection

Well and NOT suggestive of infection

Well and NOT suggestive of infection

Unwell or Tests Suggest infection

Commence Antibiotics

No Further Neonatal GBS Intervention

Commence Antibiotics

TABLE 7	Practical sepsis screen

Components	Abnormal value
Total Leukocyte count	< 5000 / mm³
Absolute Neutrophil count	Low counts as per Manroe chart for term and Mouzinho's chart for VLBW Infants
Immature / total Neutrophil	> 0.2
Micro—ESR	> 15 mm in 1st hour
C reactive protein (CRP)	> 1 mg /dL

TABLE 8	Duration of antibiotic therapy in neonatal sepsis

Diagnosis	Duration
Meningitis (with or without positive blood / CSF culture)	21 days
Blood culture positive but no meningitis	14 days
Culture negative, but sepsis screen positive and clinical course consistent with sepsis	7–10 days
Culture and sepsis screen negative, but clinical course compatible with sepsis	5–7 days

TABLE 9	Empirical choice of antibiotics for treatment of neonatal sepsis

Clinical situation	Septicemia and pneumonia	Meningitis
FIRST LINE Community - acquired (Resistant strains are unlikely)	Penicillin or Ampicillin and Gentamicin	Add Cefotaxime/Cefaperazone
SECOND LINE Hospital-acquired (some strains are likely to be resistant)	Ampicillin or Cloxacillin and Gentamicin or Amikacin	Add Cefotaxime/Cefaperazone
THIRD LINE Hospital-acquired sepsis (Most strains are likely to be resistant)	Cefotaxime or Piperacillin-Tazobactam or Ciprofloxacin and Amikacin;	Same (Avoid Ciprofloxacin)

TABLE 10	Common antibiotics: drugs, route of administration and doses

Drug	Route	Birth weight ≤ 2000g		Birth Weight > 2000g	
		0–7 d	> 7days	0–7 days	> 7days
Amikacin	I/V, I/M	7.5 q12h	7.5 q8h	10 q12h	10 q8h
Ampicillin					
Meningitis	I/V	100 q12h	100 q8h	100 q 8h	100 q6h
Others	I/V, I/M	25 q12h	25 q8h	25 q8h	25 q6h
Cefotaxime					
Meningitis	I/V	50 q6h	50 q6h	50 q6h	50 q6h
Others	I/M, I/V	50 q12h	50 q8h	50 q12h	50 q8h
Piperacillin+ Tazobactam	I/V	50–100 q12h	50–100 q8h	50–100 q12h	50–100 q12h
Ceftriaxone	I/M, I/V	50 q24h	50 q24h	50 q24h	75 q24h
Ciprofloxacin	I/V, PO	10–20 q24h	10–20 q24h	10–20 q12h	10-20 q12h
Cloxacillin					
Meningitis	I/V	50 q12h	50 q8h	50 q8h	50 q6h
Others	I/V	25 q12h	25 q8h	25 q8h	25 q6h
Gentamicin					
Conventional	I/V, I/M	2.5 q12h	2.5 q8h	2.5 q12h	2.5 q8h
Single dose	I/M	4 q24h	4 q24 hr	5 q24h	5 q24h
Netilmicin	I/V, I/M	2.5 q12h	2.5 q8h	2.5 q12h	2.5 q8h
Penicillin G		(units/kg/dose)			
Meningitis	I/V	75,000 q12h -1,00,000	75,000 q8h -1,00,000	75,000 q8h -1,00,000	75,000 q6h -1,00,000
Others	I/V, I/M	25,000 q12h	25,000 q8h	25,000 q8h	25,000 q6h
Vancomycin	I/V	15 q12h	15 q8h	15 q12h	15 q8h

*All doses are in mg/kg/dose

Pearl/Peril/Pitfall: The Joint Commission on Infant Hearing of the AAP recommends that infants who received aminoglycosides should have audiology screening before discharge. Screen these infants again at 3 months, but no later than 6 months, to determine whether damage has occurred.

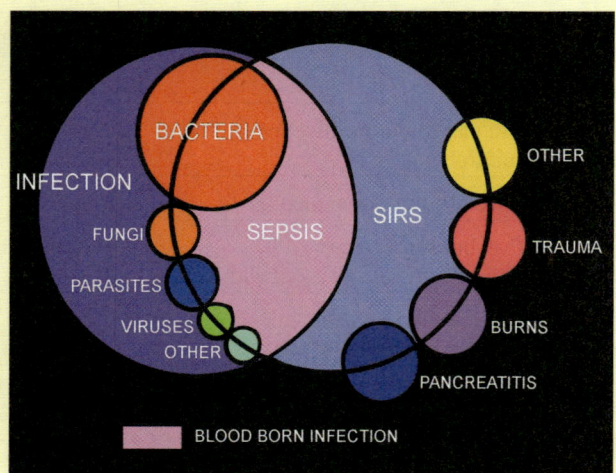

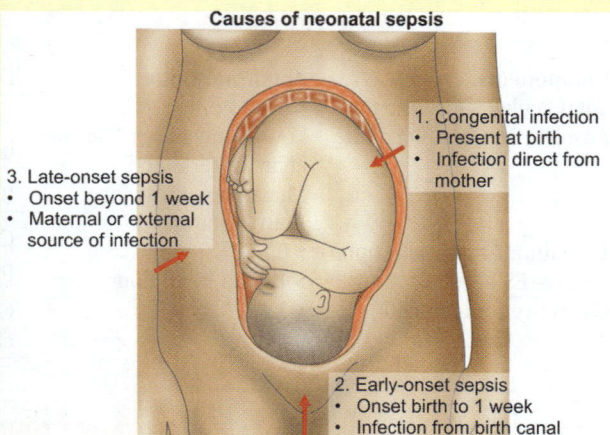

Causes of neonatal sepsis

1. Congenital infection
• Present at birth
• Infection direct from mother

2. Early-onset sepsis
• Onset birth to 1 week
• Infection from birth canal

3. Late-onset sepsis
• Onset beyond 1 week
• Maternal or external source of infection

Despite similar clinical presentations, the molecular and cellular processes that elicit the sepsis response differ depending on whether the organism is gram-negative, gram-positive, fungal, or viral in nature. The steps in this response are the same, independent of the initiating organism. The sepsis response to a gram-negative organism begins with the release of lipopolysaccharide (LPS), an endotoxin from within the cell wall of the gram-negative bacteria, which is released during lysis. Gram-positive, fungal, and viral organisms, however, initiate a sepsis response that begins with the release of exotoxins and cellular antigenic components.

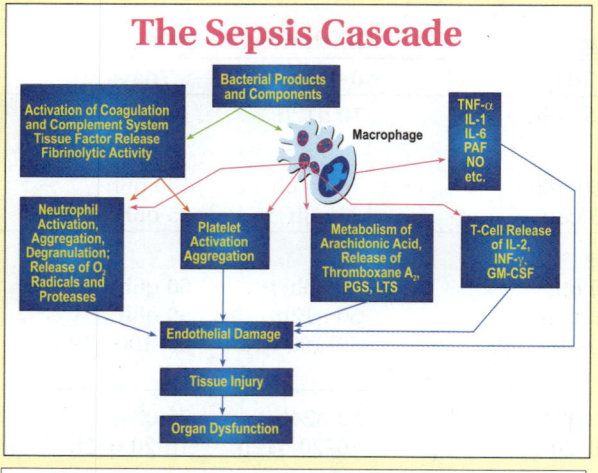

The Sepsis Cascade

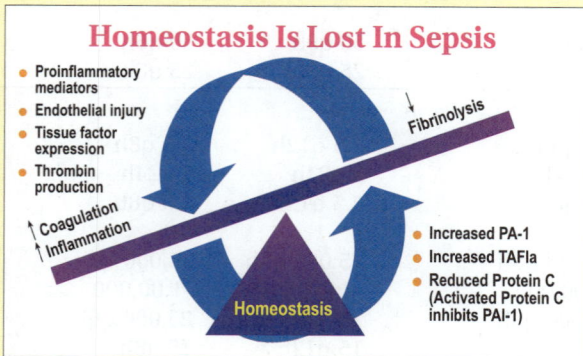

Homeostasis Is Lost In Sepsis

- Proinflammatory mediators
- Endothelial injury
- Tissue factor expression
- Thrombin production

↑ Coagulation
↑ Inflammation

↓ Fibrinolysis

Homeostasis

- Increased PA-1
- Increased TAFIa
- Reduced Protein C (Activated Protein C inhibits PAI-1)

Neonatal sepsis indian scenario

At the XXIV Annual Meeting of the National Neonatology Forum (2005), a number of papers were presented, on the incidence and outcome of sepsis, the organisms causing neonatal sepsis, and their sensitivity to antibiotics. The common themes that emerged from these papers: (*a*) the organisms causing early onset sepsis are very similar to those causing late onset sepsis, (*b*) the commonest organisms causing early and late onset sepsis are Gram negative bacilli, particularly Klebsiella, Enterobactor and *Escherichia coli. Staphylococcus aureus* is the commonest Gram positive organism. Group B streptococcus is virtually never isolated, (*c*) there was a high incidence of fungal infection causing late onset sepsis, and anecdotally many of the infected babies weighed >1500g at birth, and some were even full term.

Most worrying was that there are exceedingly high rates of resistance of Gram negative bacilli to almost all antibiotics. Resistance to aminoglycosides is about 50% for amikacin, higher for netilmicin and over 75% for gentamicin. Resistance to third generation cephalosporins is 80% plus. Bacteria are less resistant (30-46%) to piperacillin-tazobactam. Imipenem resistance is already appearing (about 20%).

It appeared that the major reason for these frightening data were that Doctors often do not take blood cultures before starting antibiotics, if blood cultures are performed and are negative, antibiotics are almost always continued, if the baby remains "sick", more and more potent broad spectrum antibiotics are used, and the belief that a raised serum C-reactive protein (CRP) is proof of sepsis, even if blood cultures are negative. -**David Isaacs,** *Clinical Professor, University of Sydney, NSW,2006*

The pathophysiology of the sepsis cascade: In response to microbial invasion, macrophages release primary inflammatory mediators that result in endothelial damage. The clinical result of the endothelial damage is capillary leak, vasodilation, and formation of microthrombi resulting in organ dysfunction. (Adapted from Bone RC. The pathogenesis of sepsis. Ann Intern Med. 1991;115:457-469.)

The loss of homeostasis in sepsis: The pathophysiology of sepsis includes the activation of inflammation, the activation of coagulation, and impairment of fibrinolysis. This creates an imbalance in normal homeostasis between procoagulant and anticoagulant mechanisms. PAI-1, plasminogen activator inhibitor-1; TAFIa, thrombin activatable fibrinolysis inhibitor. Multiorgan Dysfunction Syndrome (MODS) may develop when shock, capillary leak, and vasodilation are not stabilized, and may result in death.

Pearl/Peril/Pitfall: The primary care provider (PCP) should evaluate the infant with neonatal sepsis within one week of discharge from the hospital. The infant can be evaluated for superinfection and bacterial colonization associated with antibiotic therapy, especially if the therapy was prolonged. The PCP should evaluate growth and determine if the feeding regimen and activity have returned to normal.

TABLE 11 — Do provide supportive therapy where appropriate !

1) Support ABC's Mechanically Ventilate for respiratory failure caused by congenital pneumonia, persistent fetal circulation or ARDS (shock lung) and give Surfactant for ARDS. Identify shock, hypoxia and metabolic acidosis and manage with Inotropes, fluid resuscitation and mechanical ventilation *2) Monitor carefully the fluids, electrolytes and glucose levels with correction of* - hypovolemia, hyponatremia, hypocalcemia and hypoglycemia and limitation of fluids if there is SIADH. *3) Administer Cortico Steroids for adrenal insufficiency* (IV Hydrocortisone 1mg/kg/dose 6 hourly until stable haemodynamic status achieved [5–7 days]) *4) Monitor* *hyperbilirubinemia and treat with exchange transfusion* because the risk of kernicterus increases in the presence of SEPSIS and meningitis *5) Monitor DIC (Platelet counts, Hb, PCV, PT, PTT and fibrin split products)* and treat with FFP, platelet transfusions or whole fresh blood and single volume exchange transfusion (85ml/kg) *6) Consider intravenous (through long line) hyperalimentation for infants who can not sustain enteral feedings 7) Remember that non bacterial infectious agents (HSV infection and systemic candidiasis) can produce the syndrome of NEONATAL SEPSIS and treat with IV Acyclovir / IV Fluconazole or IV Liposomal Amphotericin if available.*

TABLE 12 — Monitor (clinically and lab wise) the septic baby concurrently, closely and diligently while treating him / her !

Clinically : a) Core Temperature (Axilla) and Peripheral Temperature (Skin of Shin /Big toe) continuously b) Cardio Respiratory Monitoring (Heart Rate alarm limits set at 90-100 [low alarm] and 160-180 [high alarm] continuously) c) Apnea Monitoring continuously (set the delay to 20 seconds and ensure the monitor is 'triggering' with each breath d) Continuous Pulse Oximetry for O_2 Sats and transcutaneous ($TcPO_2$) monitoring to maintain O_2 Sats above 94% and $TcPO_2$ above 50-70mmHg e) Measure BP (with doppler device) 2-6 hourly or from indwelling arterial cannula f) Check Capillary Blood Glucose (Glucostixs 4 hourly and maintain blood glucose between 45-125mg/dL g) Weigh the infant twice daily to maintain the fluid balance (but remember minimal handling) *Lab. wise:* a) Check arterial Blood Gases 4-6 hourly in all infants against PO_2 measured on arterial samples of blood b) Check Urea, Creatinine, Sodium, Potassium, Chlorides, Ionized Calcium, Bilirubin, Hemoglobin, Hematocrit, WBC, Platelets once or twice daily for the first 5 days at least c) Check Urine for Blood, Protein, Sugar daily and Monitor Urine output and measure specific gravity every 6-24 hours d) Surveillance for infection—send body fluids (Blood, Urine, CSF, Nasal—Endotracheal secretions, etc.) and Rectal and Umbilical Swabs for culture at the time of admission and then if there is any suspicion of SEPSIS.

TABLE 13 — Principles and practice of management of neonatal sepsis !

A) *Stabilize Hemodynamics and tissue oxygenation* B) *Eradicate Bacteria by administering IV antibiotics* depending on the likely etiological agent, the microbial susceptibility pattern in the nursery, tissue penetration, toxicity, cost and availability. C) *Do an Exchange Transfusion when indicated* - in *NEONATAL SEPSIS* with sclerema, respiratory distress syndrome, disseminated intravascular coagulation and neutropenia. D) *Give IV Immunoglobulin to premature LBW Newborns (250-1000mgs/kg/day/one dose only),* as it was shown *(META ANALYSIS)* that addition of IVIG to standard therapies is of minimal but demonstrable benefit in preventing SEPSIS and of unequivocal benefit in prevention of death when administered therapeutically for early onset SEPSIS E) *Granulocyte Transfusion can be given to Neonates with fulminant bacterial infection with neutropenia* (<3 x $10^9/1$ in 1st week of life, < 1 x $10^9/1$ thereafter) and severely diminished neutrophil bone marrow storage pool (< 10% of nucleated marrow cells being post mitotic neutrophils). F) *Colony Stimulating factors (G-CSF, GM-CSF)* These colony stimulating factors enhance production and functional capabilities of granulocytes, increase bone marrow granulocyte pool by proliferation of progenitor cells. Various studies have been performed to evaluate the efficacy of G-CSF in reducing mortality of neutropenic Newborns. *However, results of these studies are inconclusive.* G) *Anticipate and manage the complications of SEPSIS* - Endocarditis, Septic Emboli, Abscess Formation, Septic Joints with residual disability and osteomyelitis and bone destruction *and those of meningitis* - Ventriculitis, Cerebritis, Brain abscess, Hearing loss, abnormal behaviour, developmental delay, cerebral palsy, focal motor disability, seizure disorders and hydrocephalus H) *Never ever forget to explain the prognosis to the parents.*

KEY POINTS FOR CLINICAL PRACTICE

1. Early Onset Sepsis (EOS) in Neonates can manifest as asymptomatic bacteremia, generalized sepsis, pneumonia, and/or meningitis. The clinical signs of EOS are usually apparent in the 1st hours of life; 90% of infants are symptomatic by 24hrs of age. Respiratory distress is the most common presenting symptom.

2. One should consider the other diagnoses, such as TTN of the Newborn, meconium aspiration syndrome, intracranial hemorrhage, congenital viral disease, cyanotic congenital heart disease, duct-dependent cardiac anomaly (critical coarctation of the aorta and hypoplastic left heart syndrome), NEC, bowel obstruction and inborn errors of metabolism- in the differential diagnosis of sepsis.

3. Early clinical signs of EOS often are subtle and nonspecific. Clinicians must remain extremely vigilant to make a prompt diagnosis and institute effective therapy.

4. An infant who "looks septic" is poorly perfused, mottled, lethargic, and sick appearing. If treatment is delayed until this late stage, the infant may not survive. All infants with this clinical presentation require rapid stabilization of ABCs and appropriate IV antibiotics after blood cultures and immediate transfer to a tertiary center.

5. Prevent Neonatal sepsis by aggressively managing maternal infections like chorioamnionitis and UTI, rapid delivery of at risk infant, and strict infection control measures in the hospital.

REFERENCES AND FURTHER READING: 1)Klein JO, Marcy SM. *Bacterial Sepsis and Meningitis. Infectious Diseases of the Fetus and Newborn Infant.* 4th ed. 1995:835-78. 2) Ng PC, Lam HS. Diagnostic markers for neonatal sepsis. *Curr Opin Pediatr.* Apr 2006;18(2):125-31. 3) Tausch WH, Ballard RA, Avery. *Schaffer and Avery's Diseases of the Newborn.* 7th ed. 1998:435-52, 490-512. 4) Hawk M. C-reactive protein in neonatal sepsis. *Neonatal Netw.* Mar-Apr 2008;27(2):117-20. 5)Arnon S, Litmanovitz I. Diagnostic tests in neonatal sepsis. *Curr Opin Infect Dis.* Jun 2008;21(3):223-7.

Pearl/Peril/Pitfall: Intrapartum antibiotic prophylaxis is indicated for all of the following: Previous infant with GBS disease, GBS bacteriuria in the current pregnancy, Positive GBS screening culture results during the current pregnancy (unless a planned cesarean delivery, in the absence of labor or amniotic membrane rupture, is performed), Unknown GBS status (culture not done, or results unknown) and any of the following: Delivery earlier than 37 weeks' gestation, Amniotic membrane rupture at 18 hours or later, Intrapartum temperature of 100.4°F or higher (≥38°C). In India, Gram negative and Fungal sepsis is much more common than GBS.

11 Late Onset Neonatal Sepsis (LOS)

@ *"In the late onset sepsis, meningitis and urinary tract infections are more common than in the early onset sepsis, making LP and urine culture the mandatory investigations to be done"*

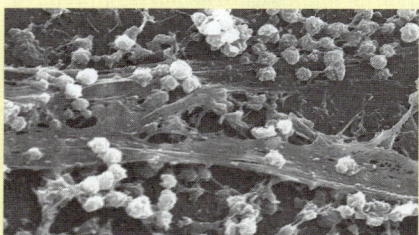

Coagulase negative *staph.aureus* central vascular catheter infection

Scanning electron micrograph of a Staphylococcus biofilm on the inner surface of a needleless connector. A distinguishing characteristic of biofilms is the presence of extracellular polymeric substances, primarily polysaccharides, surrounding and encasing the cells. Here, these polysaccharides have been visualized by scanning electron microscopy.

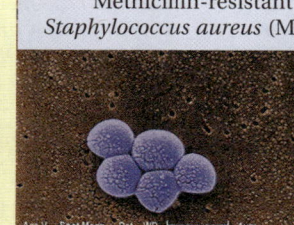

Methicillin-resistant *Staphylococcus aureus* (MRSA)

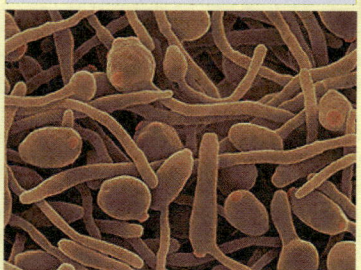

Escherichia coli

Methicillin-resistant Staphylococcus aureus (MRSA) are bacteria that are resistant to penicillinase stable semisynthetic penicillins such as Methicillin, Nafcillin, Oxacillin and Cloxacillin. The mecA gene encodes this type of resistance and expression of this gene results in production of a penicillin binding protein (PBP2a). This binding protein has low affinity to methicillin making bacteria that produce it resistant to all -lactam antibiotics, and even to other antibiotics from other classes, including tetracyclines, macrolides, flouroquinolones.

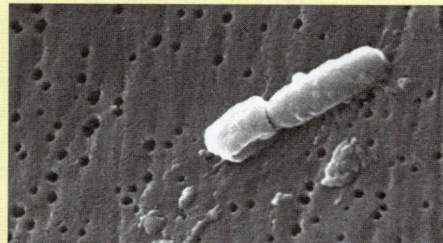

Klebsiella pneumoniae

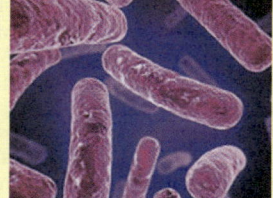

Mycobacterium tuberculosis

Pseudomonas aeruginosa

Candida albicans - yeast and hyphae stages

@ *Although late onset neonatal sepsis is commonly caused by the above illustrated bacteria and fungi, except for Listeria, the organisms responsible for early-onset sepsis also cause later onset disease.*

REVIEW OF CLINICAL PROBLEMS

1. Name the risk factors associated with increased incidence of Late-Onset Sepsis in Neonates.
   Ans: Refer to the "No.2 " of the "BIRD'S EYE VIEW/OVERVIEW/ SYNOPSIS" of the Chapter.

2. How do you evaluate a Neonate suspected to have Fungal Sepsis?
   Ans: Refer to the Section "Workup and evaluation When Fungal Sepsis is Suspected".

3. What are the Focal infections associated with LOS ?
   Ans: Refer to the Evaluation-Decision-Action Plan/Algorithm to diagnose and manage LOS in a Neonate.

4. How do you manage a Neonate with Generalized Late-Onset Neonatal Sepsis?
   Ans: Refer to the Evaluation-Decision-Action Plan/Algorithm to diagnose and manage LOS in a Neonate.

5. Mention the essential aspects of Coagulase Negative Staph. proven LOS.
   Ans: Refer to the "No.1" of the "BIRD'S EYE VIEW/OVERVIEW/ SYNOPSIS" of the Chapter.

LEARNING OBJECTIVES

After completing this article, readers will be able to

1. Develop a systematic approach to the diagnosis of Late-Onset Neonatal sepsis which will result in accurate diagnosis of all cases and minimize duration of therapy.

2. Understand methods for determining whether various symptoms in a Neonate are the result of sepsis or of another neonatal condition.

3. Assess the rationale for when to perform a lumbar puncture in a Neonate.

4. Understand the use of adjunctive tests to aid in diagnosis.

5. Acquire expertise in providing antimicrobial therapy and supportive care for the septic neonate.

Pearl/Peril/Pitfall: Late onset sepsis is associated with the following risk factors: prematurity, central venous catheterization (duration of >10 d), nasal cannula or continuous positive airway pressure (CPAP) use, H2 blocker/ proton pump inhibitor use, and gastrointestinal tract pathology.

BIRD'S EYE VIEW/OVERVIEW/SYNOPSIS

1. *Late Onset neonatal Sepsis (LOS)* occurs between 8-90 days of life and it consists of two distinct entities a)disease occurring in premature infants and VLBW infants in the NICU at >72hrs of life but before 7 days b)disease affecting otherwise healthy term infants in the community. The most common organisms responsible for late-onset sepsis are coagulase-negative staphylococci. Other common invaders include gram-negative organisms (E. coli, Klebsiella, Enterobacter, Pseudomonas, Stenotrophomonas), enterococcus, Staphylococcus pyogenes, and fungi such as Candida. Except for Listeria, the organisms responsible for early-onset sepsis also cause later onset disease. Viral causes include respiratory viruses, Cytomegalovirus, and enteroviruses. These viruses can be acquired from family members or infected caregivers. Nursery-acquired herpes virus infections are rare. Community-acquired pathogens such as Strep. pneumoniae may also cause infection in Newborn infants after discharge from the hospital. Fungi are responsible for an increasing number of systemic infections acquired during prolonged hospitalization of preterm neonates. Coagulase-Negative Staphylococcus (CONS) infection is the most common blood stream infection treated in Neonatal and Pediatric intensive care units and significantly impacts patient mortality and morbidity. Staphylococcus epidermidis is the most common CONS species isolated clinically and investigated for its pathogenicity and virulence. Difficulties exist in the differentiation of CONS infection from culture contamination in clinical specimens, as CONS is a common skin commensal. Most CONS isolates have the mecA gene and exhibit beta-lactam resistance. The glycopeptide antibiotics, such as vancomycin, are the mainstay in therapy, although resistance has been reported. Arbekacin, linezolid, and streptogramins are newer antibiotics being evaluated as alternatives to glycopeptides. Monoclonal and polyclonal antibodies have been developed against the cell-wall components of staphylococcus and may hold promise for immune prophylaxis and treatment of CONS infection.

2. A number of clinical risk factors are associated with an increased incidence of late onset sepsis. The incidence is inversely related to birth weight: Risk Factors for Late-onset Sepsis in Infants with Birth Weight Less Than 1,500 g and Birth weight <750g: Presence of central venous catheters (umbilical, percutaneous, and tunneled), Delayed enteral feeding, Prolonged hyperalimentation, Mechanical ventilation, Complications of prematurity:
   • Patent ductus arteriosus
   • Bronchopulmonary dysplasia
   • Necrotizing enterocolitis

3. Nosocomial infections occur in preterm or term infants who require intensive care. Risk factors include prematurity, LBW, invasive procedures, indwelling vascular catheters, parenteral nutrition with lipid emulsions, endotracheal tubes, ventricular shunts, alterations in the skin and/or mucous membrane barriers, frequent use of broad-spectrum antibiotics, and prolonged hospital stay. Most nosocomial infections are bloodstream infections associated with an intravascular catheter. Other serious infections include pneumonia, meningitis, omphalitis, and necrotizing enterocolitis.

4. Systemic candidiasis is a serious form of nosocomial infection in VLBW infants, causing mortality in 1/3rd of affected infants and is associated with overall poor neurodevelopmental outcome and higher rates of ROP (Retinopathy of Prematurity). Most cases of systemic candidiasis present as LOS in VLBW infants after the 3rd week of life with nonspecific clinical features. The clinical picture is initially difficult to distinguish from sepsis caused by CONS (Coagulase Negative Staphylococci) infections, and contrasts with the abrupt onset of septic shock that often accompanies LOS caused by gram-negative organisms. Candidemia can be complicated by meningitis and brain abscess, as well as end-organ involvement of the kidneys, heart, joints, and eyes (endophthalmitis). The fatality rate of disseminated candidiasis is high relative to that found in CONS infections, and increase in the presence of CNS involvement.

5. Neonatally acquired Herpes Simplex Virus (HSV) infections typically present at 3–5 days of life and often mimic bacterial sepsis. During the first 2 weeks of life, specimens from the eye, nasopharynx, and rectum should be sent for HSV PCR or culture or both. In this age group, empirical antibiotic coverage should include antiherpetic therapy (IV acyclovir).

6. As with early onset disease, a high index of suspicion and prompt use of diagnostic tests are important; serial tests are more useful. Besides peripheral venous/arterial specimens, blood cultures should be obtained from indwelling vascular catheters.

7. In the late onset sepsis, meningitis and urinary tract infections are more common than in the early onset sepsis, so the initial diagnostic assessment should include a lumbar puncture with complete CSF analysis and urine culture obtained by bladder tap or aseptically obtained catheter specimens.

8. *The Evaluation-Decision-Action-Plan/Algorithm* to diagnose and manage the late onset sepsis describes essential aspects of presentation, diagnostic evaluation and appropriate management. The infant may require transfer to a level III perinatal center, especially if he or she requires cardiopulmonary support, parenteral nutrition, or prolonged intravenous access. Multidisciplinary services available at larger centers may be necessary when treating an acutely compromised Neonate.

9. Initial empirical antibiotic therapy is directed toward the expected multiple resistant organisms and should be tailored to local epidemiologic data. Culture results direct more focused therapy. A pencillinase-resistant penicillin with an aminoglycoside/Vancomycin is essential to cover potential resistant staphylococci and enterococci. Data suggest that gram-positive bacterial infections of indwelling venous lines, particularly Coagulase-Negative Staphylococci, can be treated effectively through the line if removal is not practical. In contrast, gram-negative bacterial or fungal sepsis mandates removal of infected catheters because these infections do not seem to clear if the catheters are left in place.

10. Improved use of universal precautions, in particular, careful attention to hand washing between patient contacts, reduces the spread of pathogens in nurseries. Prophylactic antibiotic usage does not reduce the risk of nosocomial sepsis. Routine rotation of the initial antibiotics used to treat infants with presumed sepsis does not reduce the risk of infection with resistant organisms.

Pearl/Peril/Pitfall: The clinical manifestations of Late-Onset Sepsis may be acute physiological deterioration or manifestations of a more localized infection that has progressed to sepsis. Acquired infections have slower onsets and have a decreased mortality rate of around 10% to 20%. Common pathogens responsible for late onset infections include Candida Albicans, Coagulase Negative Staphylococci, Serratia, GBS, and Pseudomonas.

THE EVALUATION-DECISION-ACTION-PLAN/ALGORITHM TO *ASSESS AND MANAGE LATE ONSET NEONATAL SEPSIS (LOS)*

SUBJECTIVE FINDINGS

Assess the various risk factors associated with late onset sepsis- *birth weight <1500gm, in situ central venous catheters, delayed enteral feeding, prolonged TPN, mechanical ventilation, complications of prematurity, such as PDA, BPD, NEC

Assess the symptoms of late onset sepsis—lethargy, poor feeding, hypo/hyperthermia, apneic spells, jaundice and breathing problems

OBJECTIVE FINDINGS

Assess ABCDs - vitals, BP, CRT, O$_2$ sats, Urine output, Pulses, skin rashes including petechiae, sensorium, seizures and focal neurological signs.

Look for various signs pointing toward LOS - lethargy, apneic spells, temperature instability, bilious gastric aspirates, respiratory distress, jaundice, poor neonatal reflexes/feeding, shock and mottling of skin, scleredema.

Look for vesicular lesions (?herpes simplex), mucocutaneous candidiasis, conjunctivitis, omphalitis, bone and joint dysfunction and urine stream observation especially in male infants.

Assess for multiorgan dysfunction - cardiac failure, renal failure, pulmonary hypertension, cerebral edema/thrombosis, adrenal hemorrhage/insufficiency, bone marrow dysfunction and DIC.

INVESTIGATIONS

Perform full septic screen i.e. FBC, TC, DC, platelets, CRP, Blood, urine and CSF cultures, urine and CSF complete analysis, chest x-ray,

Perform both fungal culture and fungal staining (KOH preparation), suprapubic aspirated urine specimen - to diagnose systemic candidiasis: also obtain CSF for cell count and fungal culture before starting antifungal therapy.

When HSV is suspected - perform tissue scrapes from the vesicles to identify virus directly and by direct fluorescent antibody (DFA) technique and MRI brain scan for HSV encephalitis and EEG.

A NEONATE WITH LATE ONSET SEPSIS

*When HSV infection is suspected, give IV acyclovir 20mg/kg/dose every 8hrs for 14 days for disseminated HSV infection and for 21 days for CNS disease

Ensure ABCs, supplemental oxygen, pulse oximetry, monitor BP, IV/IO access

Intubate if necessary
* If the indications exist, such as severe respiratory distress/depression, shock, coma and seizures, bleeding from the airways, renal failure with pulmonary edema

Check for hypoglycemia, ABG analysis and electrolytes

Generalized sepsis without any localization

* *Start* broad spectrum IV antibiotics, after obtaining full septic screen to cover the organisms known to cause Late onset sepsis (LOS)—**Staphylococcus aureus—both methicillin—sensitive (MSSA) and methicillin—resistant (MRSA) strains, enterococci, pseudomonas aeruginosa, enterobacter, E.coli, Klebsiella, Serratia and Coagulase Negative Staph. epidermidis (CONS)** *Piperacillin/Tazobactam + Tobramicin or Gentamicin + Vancomycin should cover all the bacteria mentioned above.*
* *Be aware of* local variation in the microbiology of LOS, in choosing empiric antibiotic therapy for the acutely ill infant in whom LOS is suspected
* *Modify* the antibiotic coverage guided by isolate antibiotic sensitivity testing.
* *Remove* the central vascular catheters, especially when gram negative and fungal sepsis is suspected and/or evident. Gram positive infections also may require the removal of central lines to reduce the complications.
* *Institute* supportive management for multiorgan dysfunction-
  a. Mechanical ventilation for respiratory failure caused by sepsis, pneumonia, pulmonary hypertension, or ARDS.
  b. Fluid resuscitation and inotropic agent for shock and metabolic acidosis.
  c. FFP, platelet transfusions, or whole blood for DIC.
  d. Phototherapy and/or exchange transfusion for hyperbilirubinemia, because the risk of kernicterus increases in the presence of sepsis and meningitis.
  e. Anticonvulsants for seizures.
  f. TPN for any Neonate who cannot tolerate enteral feeding.
  g. Corticosteroids for documented adrenal sufficiency (*hyperkalemia, hyponatremia, metabolic acidosis, hypoglycemia, shock*).
  h. Monitor, correct and maintain - hypovolemia, hyponatremia, hypocalcemia, and hypoglycemia.
* *Consider* anaerobes (B.fragilis, Peptostreptococcus, and Clostridia perfringens) in generalized as well as focal LOS—treat with ampicillin, gentamicin and clindamycin or imipenem and metronidazole.

Identify focal infections (localized) of late onset sepsis such as

*PNEUMONIA
*MENINGITIS
*URINARY TRACT INFECTION
*OSTEOMYELITIS
*SEPTIC ARTHRITIS
*OPHTHALMIA NEONATORUM
*OMPHALITIS

Refer to individual chapters for detailed discussion!

* *Consider* systemic candidiasis in VLBW infants with the risk factors such as a) delay in enteral feeding b) exposure to third generation cephalosporins c) prolonged intubation d) prolonged presence of central venous catheters for TPN and intralipid infusions e) use of H$_2$-blockers and systemic steroids. *Suspect* late-onset invasive candidiasis by the presence of non specific symptoms-lethargy, increased apnea, or need for increased ventilatory support, poor perfusion, feeding intolerance and hyperglycemia. Hyperthermia, an unusual sign of sepsis in LBW infant can be present. Thrombocytopenia is a consistent feature, but the TC and DC can be normal early in the course of infection. It mimics CONS infection initially but contrasts with the abrupt onset of septic shock caused by LOS due to gram negative organisms. *Diagnose* by obtaining blood culture, urine culture and CSF culture for candida. *Treat* with IV liposomal amphotericin B 5mg/kg/day for 7–14 days after a documented negative blood culture. Add fluconazole (6mg/kg/day) or 5-fluorocytosine (100–150 mg/kg/day) if CNS disease is confirmed. Always remove the central catheters. *Perform* renal and brain ultrasonography to rule out fungal abscess formation and ophthalmic examination to rule out enopthalmitis and an Echocardiogram to rule out endocarditis or vegetation formation.

Pearl/Peril/Pitfall: Recent data in large numbers of patients show a 38% rate of culture-positive meningitis in neonates with negative blood culture results and suspected sepsis. Therefore, a lumbar puncture should be part of the evaluation of an infant with suspected sepsis.

SCALP RASH IN A NEWBORN

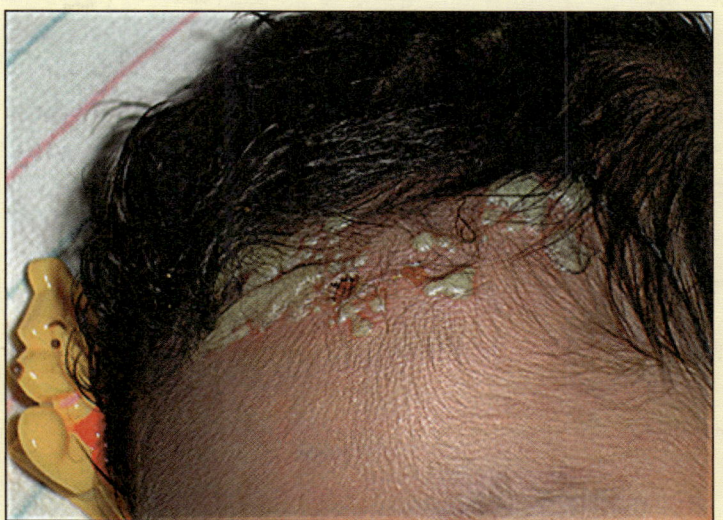

An otherwise healthy, full-term newborn presented with a rash on her scalp. The mother had no history of sexually transmitted infections, no genital rashes or lesions immediately before delivery, and no complications during pregnancy. The infant was delivered by cesarean because of arrest of descent. She was afebrile and showed no signs of toxicity after delivery. No rash was present on the initial physical examination. However, on the second day of life, physical examination showed a papulopustular rash confined to the intrapartum presenting area of the scalp. No lymphadenopathy, vesicles, or other pathologic findings were noted. Results of a complete blood count with differential were unremarkable. A potassium hydroxide preparation showed no fungal elements. Tzanck test and viral culture results were also unremarkable. Clusters of gram-positive cocci were present.

Based on the patient's history, physical examination, and laboratory studies, which one of the following is the most likely diagnosis?

- A. Cutaneous candidiasis.
- B. Erythema toxicum neonatorum.
- C. Herpes simplex virus (HSV) infection.
- D. Methicillin-resistant Staphylococcus aureus (MRSA) pustulosis.
- E. Neonatal acne.
- F. Transient neonatal pustular melanosis.

Discussion

The answer is D: MRSA pustulosis. MRSA infections have been associated with patients in heath care facilities and in infants in neonatal intensive care units (i.e., because of premature birth, low birth weight, prolonged hospitalization, or indwelling catheters). However, the incidence of community-associated infections in full-term, otherwise healthy newborns is increasing. In full-term newborns, MRSA infection usually first appears as a skin and soft tissue infection, but may rapidly progress

to osteomyelitis, pneumonia, and sepsis. Staphylococcal pustulosis manifests on any area of skin as a papulopustular rash that may coalesce and form bullae. Physicians should obtain a Gram stain and culture of any pustular lesions in a newborn. Culture is the first-line test for diagnosis of staphylococcal pustulosis. In one study, 44 percent of culture-positive patients had a negative Gram stain result. Patients with severe pustulosis or systemic symptoms may require blood, urine, and cerebrospinal fluid cultures to rule out systemic infection.

Cutaneous candidiasis is uncommon in newborns but is thought to be acquired from maternal vaginal colonization. The condition may appear as an erythematous, papulopustular rash on any area of the skin, usually with crusting and desquamation. Systemic infection is rare in fullterm infants.

Erythema toxicum neonatorum is one of the most common benign rashes in the neonatal period. It is characterized by erythematous macules, often with a central pustule or vesicle. The macules may appear on the face, trunk, and extremities. The rash usually resolves spontaneously within a week.

HSV infection is a potentially devastating infection in newborns. It initially manifests as vesicles or pustules grouped on an erythematous base, and can lead to significant systemic disease. It may appear on the face and scalp. A maternal history of HSV infection can assist in the diagnosis, but most cases of neonatal HSV infection develop after delivery by an asymptomatic mother.

Neonatal acne is characterized by an inflammatory, erythematous, papulopustular rash on the face and scalp. Although it may appear at birth, this condition usually occurs after two weeks of life and resolves spontaneously during the first few months of life.

Transient neonatal pustular melanosis is a benign skin condition of unknown etiology. It may appear at birth, usually on the chin, forehead, chest, or back. The condition is present in up to 5 percent of black newborns and in less than 1 percent of white newborns. It is characterized by nonerythematous vesicles filled with a milky fluid, superficial pustules, and pigmented macules that are usually 2 to 10 mm in size. If diagnosis is required, Wright stain of the pustular fluid would reveal neutrophils with few eosinophils. This condition usually resolves within 48 hours, although hyperpigmented macules may remain for several months.

Summary (Condition—Characteristics)

Cutaneous candidiasis-Erythematous, papulopustular rash on any area of skin, usually with crusting and desquamation; uncommon in newborns *Erythema toxicum neonatorum*-Erythematous macules, usually with small, central vesicles or pustules; may appear on the face, trunk, and extremities *Herpes simplex virus infection*- Vesiculopustular rash, grouped on an erythematous base, on the face and scalp *Staphylococcal pustulosis*- Papulopustular rash that may coalesce and form bullae; may appear on any area of skin *Neonatal acne*- Inflammatory, erythematous, papulopustular rash on the face and scalp; usually appears after two weeks of life, although it may be present at birth *Transient neonatal pustular melanosis*- Nonerythematous vesicles filled with a milky fluid, superficial pustules, and pigmented macules that are usually 2 to 10 mm in size; appears on the chin, forehead, chest, or back; more common in black newborns than in white newborns

Courtesy: DAVID D. ORTIZ, MD, Christus Santa Rosa Family Medicine Residency Program, San Antonio, Texas Reference : Centers for Disease Control and Prevention. Community-associated methicillin-resistant Staphylococcus aureus infection among healthy newborns—Chicago and Los Angeles County, 2004. *MMWR Morb Mortal Wkly Rep.* 2006;55(12):329–332.

Pearl/Peril/Pitfall: *The CSF findings in infectious neonatal meningitis are an elevated WBC count (predominately PMNs), an elevated protein level, a depressed glucose level, and positive culture results. The decrease in glucose is not reflective of serum hypoglycemia. The CSF abnormalities are more severe in late onset and with gram-negative organisms.*

Pathogenesis and invasive fungal infections in very low birth weight infants. From Kaufman and Fairchild 2004, with permission.

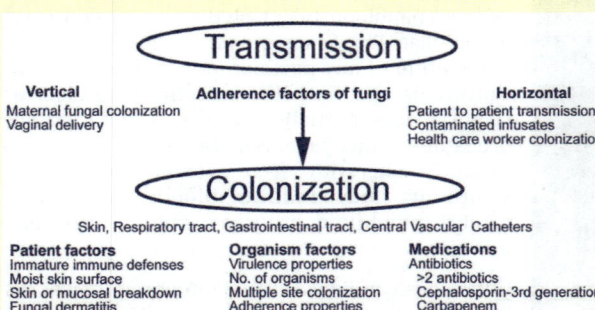

Transmission

Vertical
Maternal fungal colonization
Vaginal delivery

Adherence factors of fungi

Horizontal
Patient to patient transmission
Contaminated infusates
Health care worker colonization

Colonization

Skin, Respiratory tract, Gastrointestinal tract, Central Vascular Catheters

Patient factors
Immature immune defenses
Moist skin surface
Skin or mucosal breakdown
Fungal dermatitis
Necrotizing enterocolitis
Intestinal perforation
Abdominal Surgery
Hyperglycemia
Invasive catheters, tubes
   Central vascular catheter
   Endotracheal tube

Organism factors
Virulence properties
No. of organisms
Multiple site colonization
Adherence properties

Medications
Antibiotics
   >2 antibiotics
   Cephalosporin-3rd generation
   Carbapenem
H2 antagonists
Postnatal steroids

Infusates
Parenteral Nutrition
Lipid emulsions

Infection

Blood, Urine, Cerebrospinal fluid, Peritoneal fluid

Immature immune defenses
Tissue or valve injury
Co-infection

Adherence properties

Persistent fungemia
Delayed vascular catheter removal
Delayed diagnosis
Inadequate antifungal dosing

End-Organ Dissemination

Endocarditis
Renal or bladder abscess
Central nervous system
   Meningitis, Encephalitis, abscess
Endophthalmitis

Liver abscess
Splenic abscess
Cutaneous abscess
Osteomyelitis
Septic arthritis

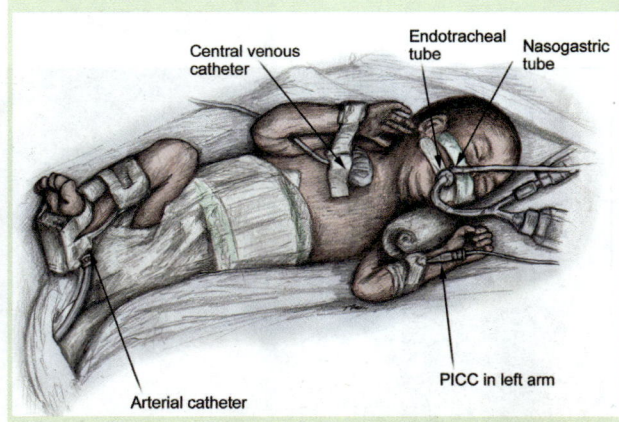

Labels: Central venous catheter, Endotracheal tube, Nasogastric tube, PICC in left arm, Arterial catheter

Risk factors

Invasive therapies
Central vascular catheters
Endrotracheal tube

Patient factors
Immature skin
Dermatitits
Colonization
Necrotizing enterocolitis
Focal bowel perforation
Cholestasis

Infusates
Parenteral nutrition
Lipid emulsions

Medications
Postnatal steroids
Broad-spectrum antibiotics
H2 antagonists

Fungal Infection
Sepsis
Urinary tract infection
Meningitis

End-Organ Dissemination
Endocarditis
Abscess formation
(kidneys, liver, brain,skin)
Endophthalmitis
Bone and joints

Risk factors for Candidemia. PICC = Peripherally Inserted Central Catheter.

Percutaneous intravenous central catheter and fungal biofilm formation

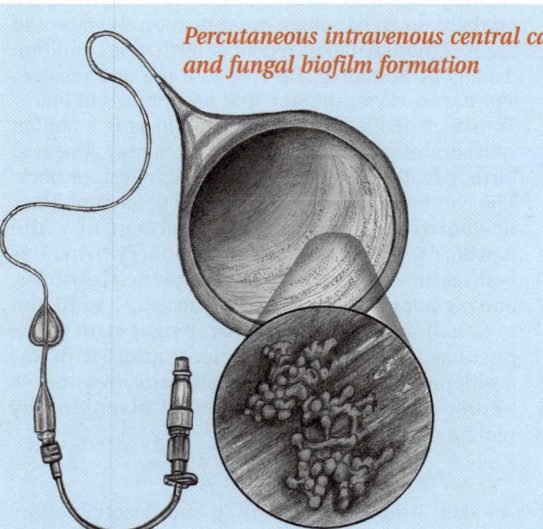

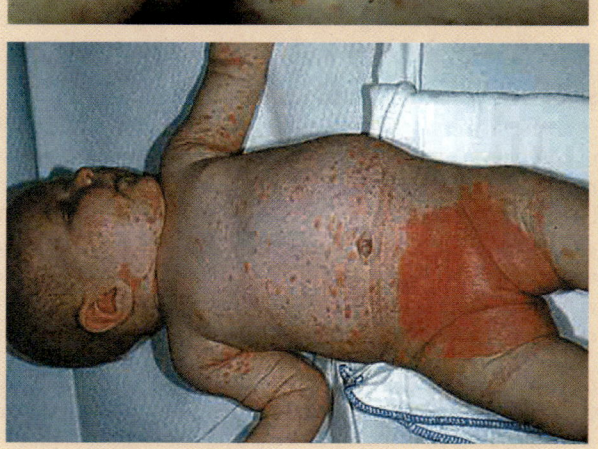

Main organisms causing late onset systemic (LOS) infection in very low birthweight infants (VLBW)

Gram positive organisms

* Coagulase Negative Staphylococci

* *Staphylococcus aureus*

* Enterococci

Fungi

* Mainly *Candida* spp

Gram negative organisms

* *E. coli*

* *Klebsiella* spp

* *Pseudomonas* spp

Pearl/Peril/Pitfall: The emergence of Gram positive organisms which are resistant to vancomycin, and for which there is no effective antibiotic, is of deep concern. The first were the vancomycin resistant enterococci (VRE), but the emergence of strains of vancomycin insensitive Staphylococcus aureus (VISA) is even more worrying.

Renal fungal ball: Preterm infants are prone to fungal infections because of immaturity of their host defence systems (immunology and skin). Other risk factors include multiple antibiotic therapy, prolonged use of umbilical or percutaneous catheters, total parenteral nutrition, colonization and/or past mucocutaneous candidiasis, low birth weight, endotracheal tube placement, and congenital malformation. Common sites for invasive candidiasis are the renal system, eyes, brain, and heart. Diagnostic tests should include blood and urine cultures, renal ultrasound, ophthalmological assessment, cardiac ultrasound, and examination of cerebrospinal fluid. Candiduria may indicate colonization, but the presence of other clinical signs increases the risk of invasive candidiasis. Fungal ball is the commonest presentation of renal fungal disease. The standard principles of intervention and removal of the bezoar may not be possible in the Neonate, because placement of a percutaneous irrigating catheter is not always feasible or appropriate in this patient population. Amphotericin B is an ideal antifungal for percutaneous irrigation for fungal renal bezoars but not as effective as systemic treatment for renal bezoars. Flucytosine is an excellent antifungal agent for urinary fungal infections and is synergistic with amphotericin B. The concomitant use of amphotericin B and flucytosine reduces the toxic side effects of both antifungal agents as well as increases their efficacy. Fluconazole is administered as a third line of treatment because of its low side-effect profile and rapid oral absorption and renal excretion, which makes it ideal as a long-term oral medication.

@Risk factors for invasive fungal infection in very low birthweight infants
* Fungal colonization
* Severe illness at birth
* Use of multiple courses of antibiotics, especially, third generation cephalosporins
* Use of parenteral nutrition
* Presence of a central venous catheter
* Use of H2 receptor antagonists

@Antifungal treatments for preterm infants
* Amphotericin B
* Lipid complex amphotericin B
* 5-Fluorocytosine (flucytosine)
* Triazoles (fluconazole, itraconazole)
* Imidazoles (miconazole, ketoconazole)

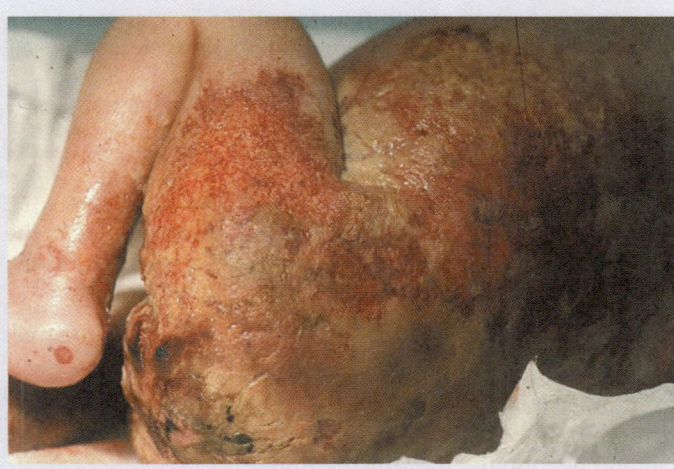

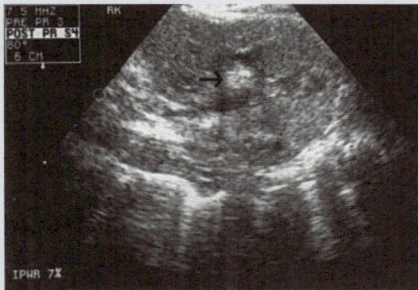

Renal ultrasonography is the method of choice for evaluating the upper tracts for obstruction or renal bezoar. In addition, voiding cystourethrography should be performed to rule out vesicoureteral reflux. Furthermore, evaluation including blood cultures and cardiac sonography should be done when indicated.

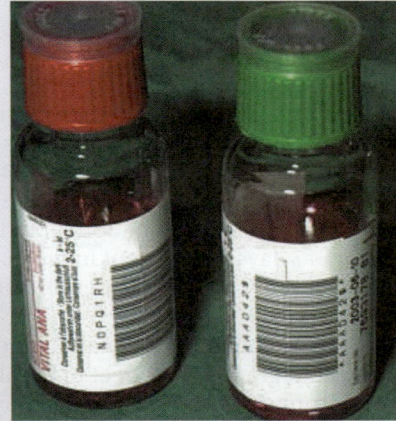

Coagulase negative staphylococci are skin commensals and may contaminate samples that have been taken inappropriately. Conversely, blood samples that are of insufficient volume may give falsely reassuring negative results on culture. Blood samples for microbial culture (ideally, at least 1 ml) should be obtained from peripheral sites rather than indwelling cannulas. Urine should be obtained by suprapubic aspiration or "in out" aseptic catheterization of the bladder.

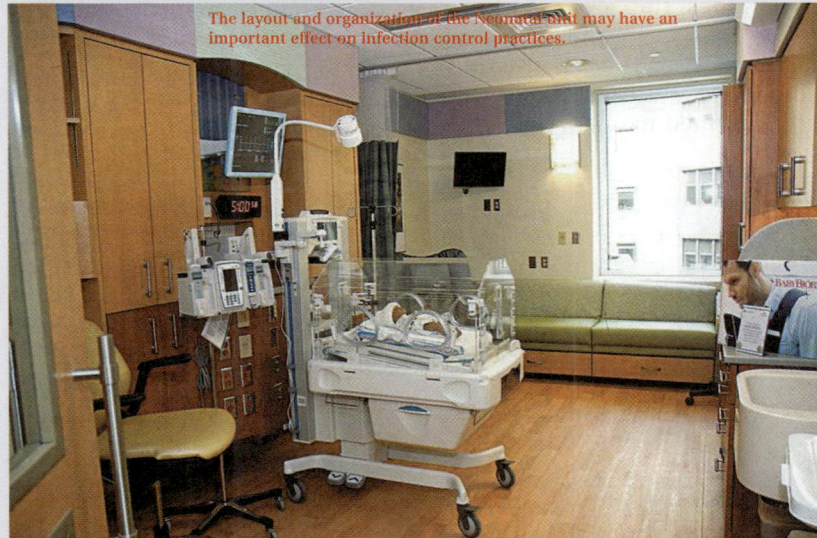

The layout and organization of the Neonatal unit may have an important effect on infection control practices.

Pearl/Peril/Pitfall: *In developing countries, further obstacles to the implementation of hand washing include the lack of water, soap, and sinks in the nurseries, low level of staffing and consequently low morale and overcrowding. Bedside dust is ubiquitous and difficult to deal with.*

WORKUP AND EVALUATION WHEN FUNGAL SEPSIS IS SUSPECTED:

Workup and evaluation for fungal infections in preterm infants includes the following tests: blood, urine, and CSF cultures. Clearance of blood stream infection should be documented with 3 or more negative blood culture results. Each negative culture result should be obtained at least 24 hours apart.

Laboratory studies at presentation

- Obtain a CBC count with manual differential and platelet count.
- To assess liver function, measure total and direct bilirubin levels. Also measure the levels of the liver enzymes aspartate amino transferase (AST), alanine aminotransferase (ALT), gamma-glutamyltransferase (GGT), and alkaline phosphatase.
- Measure BUN and creatinine levels to assess renal function.

Laboratory studies during the infection

- Thrombocytopenia is extremely common and can persist until clearance of *Candida* infection and should be closely monitored during treatment until resolution.
- Liver and renal function should be evaluated at the time of diagnosis (or if candidemia is persistent) because they may suggest liver or renal dissemination and the need for ultrasonography.
- Antifungal treatment can affect serum electrolytes and the hematologic, hepatic, and renal systems and should be monitored during treatment.

Screening tests for dissemination

- Screening for end-organ dissemination should be performed at the time of diagnosis in all sepsis cases and repeated if fungemia persists for longer than 5 days. Dissemination affects length of treatment.
- The optimal timing of surveillance is not well defined, but persistent fungemia (>5 d) is associated with increased dissemination (Chapman, 2000; Noyola, 2001). Consequently, appropriate cultures and surveillance for end-organ dissemination should occur at onset and after 5–7 days if persistent fungemia is present.
- The screening for dissemination includes the following:
  #Echocardiography #Renal ultrasonography #Head ultrasonography #Indirect ophthalmoscopy #Peritoneal cultures if laparotomy is performed to manage NEC or FBP

Laboratory testing in patients with persistent candidemia

- In patients with persistent candidemia that lasts more than 2 days, central catheters should be removed if they still remain (central catheters should be removed when bloodstream infection is diagnosed).
- In patients with persistent candidemia of longer than 5 days, repeat screening tests for vegetation or abscess, including the following: *Echocardiography and renal and head ultrasonography *Liver and spleen ultrasonography *Lumbar puncture
- Bone scan or joint aspiration (if clinical symptoms warrant)
- Ultrasonography or laparotomy of the abdomen (in patients with a history of abdominal surgery, NEC, or FBP, to evaluate for abscesses) *Ultrasonography, venography, or magnetic resonance venography (MRV) of the previous location of the catheter tip (if the patient had any vascular catheters prior to or at the time of diagnosis, to evaluate for a thrombus)

Future diagnostic tests

Investigators are studying molecular techniques to identify fungi and other microorganisms and to reveal the diagnosis more rapidly and with higher sensitivity than with blood cultures. Examples include polymerase chain reaction (PCR) and DNA microarray technology. These techniques will hopefully allow for the rapid detection of small numbers of organisms in minute volumes of blood, even after antimicrobial treatment is started. Fungal PCR to detect the gene for 18S ribosomal RNA (rRNA) in VLBW infants has yielded promising results but requires additional study (Scheffler, 2003). PCR results are positive not only in patients with candidemia but also in those with *Candida* peritonitis and those with candiduria (Tirodker, 2003). In addition, investigators are examining the role of monitoring markers of fungal disease to diagnose and evaluate responses to antifungal therapy. These markers include beta-glucan of the cell wall, anti-*Candida* antibodies, D-arabinitol (candidal metabolite), and fungal chitin synthase (assessed with PCR). Microarray technology and gene chips are being studied to rapidly determine susceptibility and resistance patterns at the time.

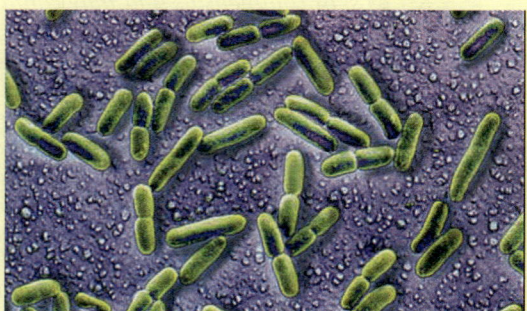

Gram negative bacilli, particularly *E. coli*, are an increasingly common cause of early onset infection in very low birthweight infants.

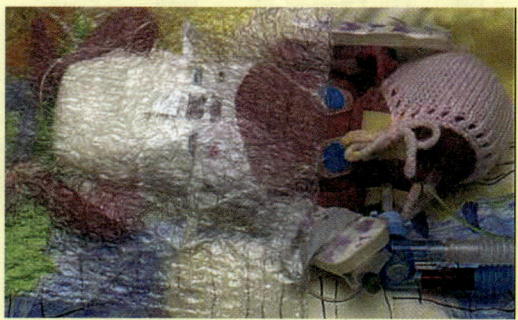

A **preterm infant** may need invasive interventions, such as ventilation and vascular access, which may increase the risk of infection

Pearl/Peril/Pitfall: The most commonly used neonatal definitions for CONS infection involve one positive culture with clinical signs or symptoms of infection or one positive culture with elevated inflammatory markers, or treatment with antibiotics for 5 days or more (a surrogate for the clinician's impression of sepsis).

TABLE 1	Neonatal Infection by Age of Onset		
Characteristics	**Early onset**	**Late onset**	**Late,late (Nosocomial)**
Age at onset	Birth to 7 days usually <72hr	7 to 30 days	>30 days
Maternal obstetric complications	Common	Uncommon	Varies
Prematurity	Frequent	Varies	Usual
Organism source	Maternal genital tract	Maternal genital tract/environment	Environment/community
Manifestation	Multisystem	Multisystem or focal	Multisystem or focal
Site	Normal nursery, NICU, community	NICU, community	NICU, community

Focal-Meningitis, UTI, Pneumonia, Septic arthritis

ANTIBIOTICS AND ANTIBACTERIALS FOR LATE ONSET SEPSIS (LOS)

Recommended antibiotic regimens for empiric treatment of suspected late onset sepsis (with normal CSF)
Situation and Antibiotic regimen : No MRSA on unit- Flucloxacillin and gentamicin.
Risk of MRSA— Vancomycin and gentamicin. ESBL outbreak- Imipenem or meropenem

Conclusions

* Rational antibiotic use involves rationing antibiotic use.
* Use narrow spectrum antibiotics whenever possible.
* Keep potent broad spectrum antibiotics in reserve.
* Stop antibiotics early, after 2 to 3 days, if systemic cultures are negative.
* Treat sepsis, not colonisation.
* Do not use prophylactic antibiotics without evidence of their efficacy.

TABLE 2	Normal cerebrospinal fluid examination in neonates
CSF Components	**Normal range**
Cells / mm3	8 (0–30 cells)
PMN (%)	60%
CSF protein (mg/dL)	90 (20–170)
CSF glucose (mg/dL)	52 (34–119)
CSF/blood glucose (%)	51 (44–248)

KEY POINTS FOR CLINICAL PRACTICE

1. Late Onset Sepsis occurs after 72 hrs of life in VLBW infants in the NICU and after 7 days in term babies in the community. Mostly LOS presents with nonspecific symptoms and signs, demanding a high index of suspicion and prompt use of diagnostic tests.

2. Meningitis and urinary tract infections are more common in the LOS than in the immediate neonatal period, so the initial diagnostic assessment should include a lumbar puncture and urine culture obtained by suprapubic bladder aspiration under ultrasound guidance.

3. CONS (Coagulase Negative Staph) account for 50% of LOS infections; Staph aureus, Pseudomonas aeruginosa, Klebsiella spe, enterococci, E.coli are other organisms responsible for LOS. Viral causes of LOS include HSV, RSV, CMV and enteroviruses. Candidiasis can mimic CONS infection in VLBW infants with risk factors. Infants with prolonged duration of central catheters and parenteral hyperalimentation, those with delayed initiation of enteral feedings, and those with a prolonged period to reach full enteral feedings or to regain their birth weight are all at substantially increased risk of late-onset sepsis.

4. Antibiotic coverage should be empirically broad enough to cover the responsible bacteria, and it should be modified by the culture sensitivity reports; consider IV acyclovir therapy for suspected HSV infection and IV liposomal amphotericin B. for systemic candidiasis.

5. CONS infection of indwelling venous lines, can be treated effectively through the line if removal is not practical. In contrast, gram-negative bacterial or fungal sepsis mandates removal of infected catheters because these infections do not seem to clear if the catheters are left in place.

REFERENCES AND FURTHER READING: 1)Bellig, L. (2004, June 23). Neonatal sepsis. Emedicine. Retrieved July 12, 2004 from http://www.emedicine.com/ped.topic2630.htm 2)Byington CL, Enriquez FR, Hoff C. Serious bacterial infections in febrile infants 1 to 90 days old with and without viral infections. Pediatrics. Jun 2004;113(6):1662-6. 3)Graham PL, Begg MD, Larson E. Risk factors for late onset gram-negative sepsis in low birth weight infants hospitalized in the neonatal intensive care unit. Pediatr Infect Dis J. Feb 2006;25(2):113-7. 4)Khashu M, Osiovich H, Henry D. Persistent bacteremia and severe thrombocytopenia caused by coagulase-negative Staphylococcus in a neonatal intensive care unit. Pediatrics. Feb 2006;117(2):340-8. 5)Guerina NG. Bacterial and fungal infections In: Cloherty JP, Stark AR, eds. Manual of Neonatal Care. 4th ed. New York:. Lippincott-Raven;1998:271-291.6)Coagulase-Negative Staphylococcal Infections in the Neonate and Child: An Update Mohan P. Venkatesh, MD, Frank Placencia, MD, and Leonard E. Weisman, MDSemin Pediatr Infect Dis 17:120-127 © 2006 Elsevier Inc.

Pearl/Peril/Pitfall: In Neonates with a CVC and CONS bacteremia, an attempt to salvage the line with antibiotics can be undertaken, but more than three positive blood cultures warrants removal to reduce the risk of death and end organ damage.

Neonatal Meningitis

12

@ *Bacterial or viral meningitis always should be considered among disorders that cause shock, DIC, or hepatic failure in Neonates; however, by the time these conditions develop, the opportunity for successful intervention may have passed. Therefore, consideration of meningitis remains prudent whenever a Neonate demonstrates even slight lethargy or irritability.*

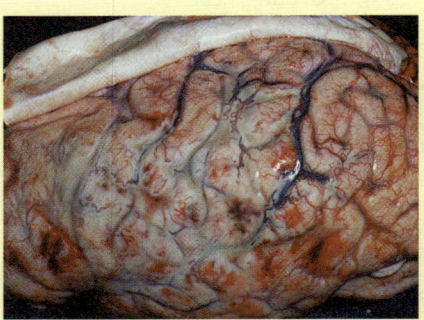

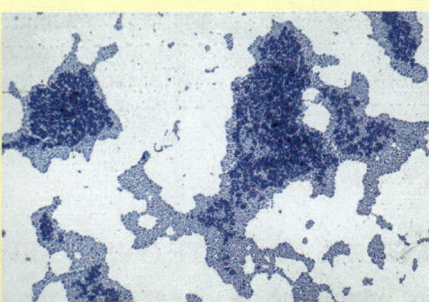

Bacteria in the CSF: DIAGNOSIS AND PATHOLOGY. The cornerstone in the diagnosis of bacterial meningitis is CSF examination. The CSF in meningitis shows hundreds, even thousands of neutrophils and is teeming with organisms. CSF protein is elevated and glucose is low (because it is consumed by inflammatory cells).

Meningitis-purulent exudate purulent exudate covers the cerebral hemispheres and settles along the base of the brain, around cranial nerves and the openings of the fourth ventricle.

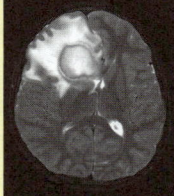

Brain abscess causes loss of neurological function due to destruction of brain tissue. More important, it causes increased intracranial pressure. Its mass effect is due to the collection of pus and to **cerebral edema** around the abscess. Since the infection is contained within brain tissue, the CSF usually shows only a few mononuclear cells with normal protein and glucose.

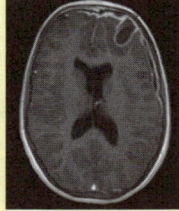

Subdural empyema and brain abscess : Locally, neutrophils destroy tissues with their enzymes. This damage is followed by formation, in the subdural space, of a vascularized inflamed connective tissue and then a fibrous scar. Histologically, acute subdural empyema shows a layer of neutrophils overlying the arachnoid membrane. The inflammatory cells may infiltrate the arachnoid membrane and extend into the subarachnoid space.

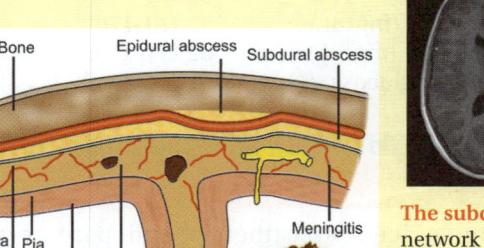

The subdural space is traversed by bridging arteries and veins but has no vascular network of its own. Therefore, antibiotics have no access to this space. Treatment of the subdural abscess consists of evacuation plus intravenous antibiotics. Epidural and subdural abscesses are collections of pus. If they are large enough, they compress the brain and spinal cord, resulting in loss of function and increased intracranial pressure.

REVIEW OF CLINICAL PROBLEMS

1. Mention the complications of Neonatal Meningitis.
   Ans: Refer to the Section "Complications of Neonatal Meningitis".

2. Mention the role of corticosteroids in Neonatal Meningitis.
   Ans: Refer to Table 8 of the Chapter.

3. Discuss the role of Imaging studies in the management of Neonatal Meningitis.
   Ans: Refer to the Section "Imaging studies in Neonatal Meningitis".

4. How do you determine the duration of IV Antibiotic therapy in treating Neonatal Meningitis ?
   Ans: Refer to Table 7 of the Chapter.

5. How do you explain the Prognosis of Neonatal Meningitis to the parents ?
   Ans: Refer to the Section "Prognosis in Neonatal Meningitis".

LEARNING OBJECTIVES

After completing this article, readers will be able to:

1. Consider performing a lumbar puncture if any signs of sepsis in a Neonate and to repeat lumbar puncture at 24–48 hours.

2. Reassess therapy based on culture and antibiotic susceptibility results.

3. Continue antibiotic therapy (intravenously) for at least two weeks (GBS and Listeria) or three weeks (Gram negative bacteria) after sterilization of CSF cultures.

4. Consider longer duration of therapy if focal neurological signs persist at two weeks, if >72 hours required to sterilize CSF, or if obstructive ventriculitis, infarcts, encephalomalacia, or brain abscesses are found by neuroimaging studies.

5. Ensure Follow-up of survivors for various CNS sequelae.

Pearl/Peril/Pitfall: There are few contraindications to performing a LP in a Neonate. Cardiorespiratory compromise during the procedure can be minimised using a modified left lateral position (hip flexion at 90° without flexion or extension of the neck). In an unstable Neonate the procedure can be deferred until stabilisation is achieved.

1. Neonatal meningitis contributes substantially to neurological disability worldwide, despite development of effective vaccines, tools for rapid identification of pathogens, and potent antimicrobial drugs. The absence of specific clinical findings makes diagnosis of meningitis more difficult in Neonates than in older children and adults. Moreover, a wide variety of pathogens are seen in infants because of immaturity of their immune systems and intimate exposure to possible infection from their mothers. This Chapter focuses on common presentations of treatable bacterial meningitis in the Neonatal period, defined as birth to 44 weeks postconceptional age; meningitides caused by HSV,VZV, HIV and fungi as well as other organisms implicated in congenital CNS damage (e.g. cytomegalovirus, toxoplasmosis) are discussed elsewhere.

2. Neonates are at greater risk of sepsis and meningitis than other age groups because of deficiencies in humoral and cellular immunity and in phagocytic function. Infants younger than 32 weeks' gestation receive little of the maternal immunoglobulin received by full-term infants. Inefficiency in the neonates' alternative complement pathway compromises their defense against encapsulated bacteria. T-cell defense and mediation of B-cell activity also are compromised. Finally, deficient migration and phagocytosis by neutrophils contribute to neonatal vulnerability to pathogens of even low virulence.

3. Neonatal meningitis occurs in roughly 0.3 per 1000 live births; it is closely associated with sepsis, which is 5 times as common. Regardless of the specific pathogen involved, neonatal meningitis is most often caused by vertical transmission during labor and delivery. It occurs most frequently in the days following birth and is more common in premature infants than term infants. When evaluating a neonate for meningitis, consider these 3 key points: (1) be vigilant for maternal infection "set-ups," including prolonged rupture of membranes, fever, and chorioamnionitis, remembering that asymptomatic maternal infection is always a possibility even with screening; (2) early-onset and late-onset bacterial infections have distinctive clinical courses, as detailed below; and (3) in HSV and VZV infections, the presence of skin lesions in a meningitic neonate are the exception more than the rule.

4. **Bacterial meningitis, *early onset*** *Symptoms appearing in the first 48 hours of life are referable primarily to systemic illness rather than meningitis. These include temperature instability, episodes of apnea or bradycardia, hypotension, feeding difficulty, hepatic dysfunction, and irritability alternating with lethargy. *Respiratory symptoms can become prominent within hours of birth in GBS infection; however, the symptom complex also is seen with infection by *E coli* or *Listeria* species.**Bacterial meningitis, *late onset*** *Late-onset bacterial sepsis is more likely to be associated with neurologic symptoms. Most commonly seen are stupor and irritability, which Volpe describes in more than 75% of affected neonates. *Between 25% and 50% of neonates will exhibit the following neurological signs: seizures; bulging anterior fontanel; extensor posturing/ opisthotonus; focal cerebral signs including gaze deviation and hemiparesis; cranial nerve palsies. Nuchal rigidity per se is the least common neurologic sign in neonatal bacterial meningitis, occurring in fewer than 25% of affected neonates (Volpe, 2001).

5. Bacterial meningitis in Neonates almost always occurs with sepsis but is difficult to distinguish clinically from sepsis alone, as both present with a constellation of symptoms that indicate systemic illness. Therefore, treatment is started on the basis of presumed infection rather than proven infection. Because the goal in the Neonate is to manage any life-threatening condition responsive to intervention, the differential diagnosis includes disorders of cardiac, pulmonary, and metabolic functions.

6. Bacterial or viral meningitis always should be considered among disorders that cause shock, DIC, or hepatic failure in neonates; however, by the time these conditions develop, the opportunity for successful intervention may have passed. Therefore, consideration of meningitis remains prudent whenever a neonate demonstrates even slight lethargy or irritability. Other CNS problems may present in a manner that simulates meningitis. These include hemorrhage and stroke, the latter of which has also been reported in the context of VZV intracranial arteriopathy. Also, hypoxic-ischemic encephalopathy or cerebral edema associated with nonhemorrhagic trauma may present a confounding picture. Additional considerations should include drug withdrawal, inborn errors of metabolism (including aminoacidopathies, organic acidurias, urea cycle disorders, and mitochondrial disease), and GI problems such as necrotizing enterocolitis or perforated bowel.

7. ***The Evaluation-Decision-Action-Plan/Algorithm*** describes the essential aspects of diagnosis and management of Neonatal Meningitis. Neonatal meningitis occurs in the absence of bacteremia and in the presence of normal CSF values. No single CSF value can be used to exclude meningitis, and peripheral WBC counts are also poor predictors of Neonatal meningitis. The CSF culture is critical to the diagnosis, regardless of other laboratory results.

8. Early initiation of antimicrobial drugs is essential; a confirmed diagnosis of meningitis seldom is established before treatment is started. Dexamethasone is not recommended for neonates with meningitis (Chaudhuri, 2004). Supportive care is focused on supporting blood pressure to maintain adequate cerebral perfusion and on preventing secondary brain injury. Meticulous fluid management is important to minimize cerebral edema and to respond to inappropriate antidiuretic hormone (ADH) secretion. Neither steroids nor hyperosmolar agents have been proven to be helpful. The syndrome of inappropriate ADH secretion may cause hyponatremia and hypo-osmolality, which may increase lethargy and seizures while further increasing intracranial pressure.

9. Management of seizures is a common challenge in Neonates with meningitis. Phenobarbital and phenytoin remain the current drugs of choice, with benzodiazepines utilized as adjunctive therapy. Respiratory dysfunction, DIC, and nutritional deficiencies require management by experienced neonatologists. Lumbar puncture, especially for CSF culture and sensitivity, should be repeated 24–36 hours after the initial study to monitor the course of the infection and guide further treatment decisions. With persistent infection in the lumbar CSF or with clinical deterioration not explained by other complications, a diagnostic tap of the lateral ventricle should be performed to determine the presence of ventriculitis. This may occur, especially with gram-negative bacteria, in the absence of pleocytosis in the lumbar CSF or with sterile CSF. Ventriculostomy with external drainage may be required with the development of acute hydrocephalus secondary to obstruction of CSF flow. Ventriculostomy with intermittent administration of intraventricular antibiotic may be required for the management of ventriculitis.

10. The complications and Prognosis of Neonatal Meningitis are summarized elsewhere in the Chapter.

Pearl/Peril/Pitfall: Examination of cerebrospinal fluid (CSF) via lumbar puncture (LP) is the only way to confirm meningitis as clinical signs are nonspecific and unreliable and blood cultures may be negative in 15–55% of cases.

THE EVALUATION-DECISION-ACTION-PLAN/ALGORITHM FOR THE DIAGNOSIS AND MANAGEMENT OF *NEONATAL MENINGITIS*

SUBJECTIVE FINDINGS

Hx of onset, duration, and details regarding fever, headache, and neck stiffness

Hx of feeding, nausea, vomiting, responsiveness, irritability, lethargy, and inconsolable crying in a child < 3 months

Hx of prior antibiotic use (onset, route, duration, dosage,) travel, insect or animal bites

Hx of close contact with sick individuals or animals, and recent immunizations

Hx of focus of infection CSOM, pneumonia, gastroenteritis, UTI, skin lesions - pustules / herpetic vesicles

Hx of head trauma with CSF leaks

OBJECTIVE FINDINGS

Assess ABCs Respiratory distress/depression, shock, purpura, or DIC

Assess disability Coma scale and convulsions and focal neurodeficits

Assess fundi (Papilledema is uncommon in uncomplicated meningitis and should suggest a more chronic process, such as subdural empyema, brain abscess or occlusion of a dural venous sinus)

Look for bulging fontanelle, widening of sutures and for signs of meningeal irritation like nuchal rigidity, Kernig sign, and Brudzinski sign *(not consistently present in children < 12-18 months)*

INVESTIGATIONS

Blood CBC with differential, glucose, ABG, calcium, phosphate, electrolytes, urea and creatinine, osmolality, cultures, consider specific antibody titers. *Save serum for serology.* Consider PT and PTT

Urine Culture, specific gravity, osmolality,

CSF Gram's stain, cell count with differential, glucose, protein, bacterial antigen, culture PCR (specific). *Save CSF for future studies*

Neuroimaging CT or MRI head scan

CXR

Strict intake and output monitoring

Neonate with suspected meningitis

Note: Keep patients in respiratory droplet isolation until culture results are known or after 24 hours of antibiotics

Ensure ABCs
Pulse oximetry
CR monitor
Frequent BP determination
IV access, draw blood work

Is patient stable ?

No → ↑ICP / SHOCK / Seizures / SIADH / Coma / DIC

Yes

If suspecting HSV meningitis begin ACYCLOVIR
< 2 months of age 60mgs/kg/day IV div q 8 h
> 2 months of age 30mgs/kg/day IV div q 8 h

* *Administer first dose of antibiotics*
* If possible, obtain blood culture prior to antibiotics
* If focal signs, obtain head imaging studies
* Perform lumbar puncture once stable

* Perform lumbar puncture
* Obtain other diagnostic tests especially cultures
* Administer broad spectrum antibiotics
* Monitor fluid status and electrolytes
* Serial head circumference
* Serial neurological examination
* Supportive management

CSF Gram stain or culture or antigen test positive ?

No

ASEPTIC MENINGITIS
* Consider stopping antibiotics after 48–72 h if patient is clinically stable and cultures remain negative.
* Consider repeat lumbar puncture after 24–48 h if the patient remains symptomatic
* Consider other diagnostic tests : viral specific CSF for, e.g., HSV, Enterovirus, fungal studies.
* Continue supportive management

If patient is 2 months of age and has not received Hib vaccine or if CSF shows Gram (-) coccobacilli, (*H.influenzae*) administer dexamethasone prior to first dose of antibiotics *0.15 mg/kg/dose IV q 6 h × 2 d: <u>Not recommended in Neonatal Meningitis</u>

* *Neuroimaging should be performed prior to LP if there is* 1) Suspicion of a mass 2) Patients with depressed sensorium 3) Papilledema 4) Presence of focal neurologic signs.

* *Contraindications to lumbar puncture:* 1) increased ICP 2) Bleeding diathesis/ disorders 3) Cardiorespiratory instability 4) DIC 5) Thrombocytopenia (<50,000/cumm) or infection over puncture site.

Yes

* Change antibiotic overage based on Gram stain, culture and susceptibility results.
* Consider repeat lumbar puncture after 24-48 hours to document sterilization of the CSF.
* Continue supportive management.
* Observe for development of complications.

Pearl/Peril/Pitfall: L monocytogenes is not susceptible to cephalosporins. Ampicillin is the mainstay of therapy, and the combination of ampicillin and gentamicin is synergistic in vitro and provides more rapid bacterial clearance in animal models of infection.

TABLE 1   Cerebrospinal Fluid (CSF) Findings in Various Central Nervous System Disorders

Condition	Pressure	Leukocytes (/mm)	Protein (mg/dL)	Glucose (mg/dL)	Comments
Normal	50–180 mmH₂O	<4;60–70% lymphocytes 30-40% monocytes, 1-3% neutrophils	20–45	>50 or 75% blood glucose	
Acute bacterial meningitis	Usually elevated	100–60,000+ ; usually a few thousand ; PMNs predominate	100–500	Depressed compared with blood glucose ; usually < 40	Organism may be seen on Gram stain and recovered by culture
Partially treated bacterial meningitis	Normal or elevated	1-10,000 PMNs usual but monocuclear cells may predominate if pretreated for extended	100+	Depressed or normal	Organisms may be seen ; pretreatment may render CSF sterile in pneumococcal and meningococcal disease, but antigen may be detected
Tuberculous meningitis	Usually elevated ; may be low because of block in advanced stages	10–500; PMNs early but lymphocytes and monocytes predominate later	100–500 ; may be higher in presence of block	<50 usual; decreases with time if treatment not provided	Acid-fast organisms may be seen on smear; organism can be recovered in culture or by PCR, PPD, chest X-ray positive
Fungal	Usually elevated	25-500 ; PMNs early ; mononuclear cells predominate later	20–500	<50;decreased with time if treatment not provided	Budding yeast may be seen ; organisms may be recovered in culture; India ink preparation or antigen may be positive in cryptococcal disease
Viral meningitis or meningoencephalitis	Normal or slightly elevated	PMNs early ; mononuclear cells predominate later, rarely more than 1000 cells except in eastern equine	20–100	Generally normal ; may be depressed to 40 in some viral disease (15-20% of mumps)	Enteroviruses may be recovered from CSF by appropriate viral cultures or PCR;HSV by PCR
Abscess (parameningeal infection)	Normal or elevated	0-100 PMNs unless rupture into CSF	20–200	Normal	Profile may be completely normal
Syphilis (acute and leptospirosis)	Usually elevated	1,000-10,000 or more ; PMNs predominate	50–200	Usually normal	Positive CSF serology. Spirochetes not demonstrable by usual techniques of smear or culture ; darkfield examination may be positive
Amebic (Naegleria) meningoencephalitis	Elevated	1,000-10,000 or more ; PMNs predominate	50–500	Normal or slightly decreased	Mobile amebae may be seen by hanging-drop examination of CSF at room temperature
Tumor, leukemia	Slightly elevated to very high	0-100 or more ; mononu clear or blast cells	50–1,000	Normal to decreased (20–40)	Cytology may be positive

TABLE 2   Normal CSF Parameters by Age Group

Age	WBC/ mm³	PMN/ mm³	Glucose (mg/dL)	Protein (mg/dL)	RBC/ mm³
≤ 1 wk (preterm (term)	≤ 25	≤ 25 ≤ 15	> 30	< 150 < 170	> 1000 < 800
≥ 1 week ≤1month	≤ 7	≤ 5	> 60	< 170	< 50
≥ 1 month ≤ 1 year	≤ 5	< 1	> 60	< 40 (lumbar) < 25 (cisternal) < 15 (ventricular)	< 5
≥ 1 year	≤ 5	< 1	> 40		

DNA, Deoxyribonucleic acid ; HSV, herpes simplex virus ; PCR, polymerase chain reaction; PMN, polymorphonuclear leukocyte;PPD, purified protein derivative of tuberculin

Pearl/Peril/Pitfall : Intensive care support: The appropriate and early use of supportive care, including fluid management, inotropes, anticonvulsants, and ventilation appear to be a critical part of Neonatal Meningitis management. There are no clinical trials, however, which address this.

TABLE 3 — Etiology of bacterial meningitis

I. Etiology. The etiologies vary by age

A. *Infants* The most common bacterial etiologies during the first two months of life are group B *Streptococcus, Escherichia coli, Listeria,* and other gram-negative enteric bacilli.

B. *Children and adolescents:* The introduction of the conjugated vaccine against *H. influenzae* type b in 1988 has virtually eliminated this as a pathogen in developed countries. The principal causes of bacterial meningitis in this age group are *N. meningitidis* and *Streptococcus pneumoniae.*

C. *Immunocompromised: C. neoformans* and *Listeria monocytogenes* should be considered in immuno compromised patients.

D. *Trauma::* Direct inoculation of the cerebrospinal fluid (CSF) occurs in children after penetrating injuries and neurosurgical procedures where skin flora, including *Staphylococcus aureus* and *Staphylococcus epidermidis,* is the most common cause of meningitis.

E. *Extension from preexisting source:* Sinus and middle ear disease can also lead to contiguous spread to the meninges. *S. pneumoniae* is the pathogen in most of these cases.

TABLE 4 — Laboratory diagnosis

Gram stain:

Gram-positive diplococci: *Streptococcus pneumoniae*

Gram-positive cocci in pairs and chains: *Streptococcus pyogenes*

Gram-positive rods: *Listeria monocyogenes*

Gram-negative enteric rods: Gram-negative aerobic organisms

Gram-negative diplococci: *Neisseria meningitidis*

Gram-negative pleomorphic rods: *Haemophilus influenzae* type B

Latex agglutination:

No more sensitive than CSF Gram stain; should not be used except in cases where the Gram stain is negative and antibiotics have been given prior to lumbar puncture; the impact of oral antibiotics on CSF Gram stain and culture is small.

AFB stain: *Mycobacterium tuberculosis*
Cryptococcal antigen: *Cryptococcus neoformans*
CSF-PCR for HSV: Herpes simplex virus

Amebic meningoencephalitis:

Motile trophozoites on a wet mount centrifuged CSF : *Naegleria fowleri*

TABLE 5 — Signs and symptoms of meningitis

Age (mo)	Symptom	Signs	
		Early	Late
0–3	Paradoxical irritability Altered sleep pattern Vomiting Lethargy	Lethargy Irritability Fever (±) Hypothermia (<1mo)	Bulging fontanelle Shock
4–24	Irritability Altered sleep pattern Lethargy	Fever Irritability	Nuchal rigidity Coma Shock
>24	Headache Neck pain Lethargy	Fever Nuchal rigidity Irritability	Coma Shock

TABLE 6 — Empiric antibiotic coverage

> 1 week to < 1 month of age : *Group B Streptococcus, Listeria monocytogenes, Escherichia coli*
Ampicillin IV 200mgs/kg/24 hours, given every 6 hour
+
Cefotaxime IV 150mgs/kg/day, given every 8 hour
+
Gentamicin IV 7.5mgs/kg/day, given every 8 hour
1-3 months of age : *same as above plus Streptococcus pneumoniae*, *Neisseria meningitidis, Haemophilus influenzae*
Ceftriaxone IV 100mgs/kg/day, given once a day
+
Ampicillin IV 200mgs/kg/day, given every 6 hour
+ If the patient is immunocompromised and gram negative bacterial meningitis is suspected, initial therapy might include Ceftazidime and an aminoglycoside.
> 3 months of age : *Streptococcus pneumoniae, Neisseria meningitidis, Haemophilus influenzae*
Vancomycin IV 60mgs/kg/24 hours, given every 6 hour
+ Ceftriaxone IV 100mgs/24 hours, given once a day

TABLE 7 — Duration of the antibiotic therapy

1. H. influenzae meningitis — 10 days

2. Strep. pneumoniae meningitis — 14 days

3. Neisseria meningitidis meningitis — 7 days

4. Listeria monocytogenes meningitis — 14–21 days

5. Meningitis due to Esch. Coli and Pseudomonas aeruginosa — 21 days

Gram negative bacillary meningitis should be treated for 3 weeks or for at least 2 weeks after CSF sterilization, which may occur after 2–10 days of treatment

TABLE 8 — Role of corticosteroids in meningitis

Data support the use of IV Dexamethasone, 0.15mg/kg/dose given every 6 hour for 2 days, in the treatment of children > 6 weeks with an acute bacterial meningitis caused by *H.influenzae type B*. Give the first dose of Dexamethasone prior to the first dose of antibiotics. This reduces fever, CSF protein, and lactate levels and a reduction in permanent auditory nerve damage. It may be considered for use in suspected Strep. pneumoniae meningitis. ***Not recommended in Neonates.***

*** Pearl/Peril/Pitfall :** A repeat lumbar puncture 24–48 hours into antibiotic therapy is recommended to document CSF sterilisation. Persistence of infection may indicate a focus, such as obstructive ventriculitis, subdural empyema, or multiple small vessel thrombi.*

Laboratory studies

*CSF and blood cultures
*Suspected bacterial infection is confirmed often, but not uniformly, by positive results of cultures of CSF or blood. CSF cultures should be obtained in all symptomatic infants; despite the close relationship between bacterial sepsis and meningitis, it has been estimated that 15-30% of infants with CSF-proven meningitis will have negative blood cultures (Malbon, 2006). *A recent study from Duke emphasized that no single CSF value can be relied upon to exclude neonatal meningitis except CSF culture (Garges, 2006). *The onus is on the clinician to justify initiation of antimicrobial and antiviral therapy regardless of the CSF values. *Polymerase chain reaction: Polymerase chain reaction (PCR) assay is a powerful diagnostic tool with excellent sensitivity and specificity. It permits identification of GBS antigen in urine or in cerebrospinal fluid, and it is the criterion standard for identification of HSV and enteroviral infection in CSF. *Latex particle agglutination: Rapid screening is available with latex particle agglutination (LGA) test of urine, which can be performed for GBS, *E coli,* and *Streptococcus pneumoniae.* Unfortunately, the presence of GBS antigen does not prove invasive disease. *Fluid culture of cutaneous lesions: If vesicles are present on the skin, evaluation for HSV or VZV infection should include cultures of fluid from vesicles on the skin. Swabs of the nasopharynx, conjunctiva, and rectum have also been used to identify these agents. DNA from HSV, VZV, or enteroviruses can be identified from either vesicles or CSF using PCR. *CSF analysis -Lumbar puncture is indicated to evaluate CSF in all neonates suspected of having sepsis or meningitis, even in the absence of neurological signs. Many clinicians are reluctant to perform a tap on a critically ill infant. Although the theoretical complications of lumbar puncture include trauma, brain-stem herniation, introduction of infection, and hypoxic stress, none of these occurred in a Neonate. *Interpretation of CSF findings is more difficult in neonates than in older children, especially in premature infants whose more permeable blood-brain barrier causes higher levels of glucose and protein. *The classic finding of decreased CSF glucose, elevated CSF protein, and pleocytosis is seen more with gram-negative meningitis and with late gram-positive meningitis; this combination also is suggestive of viral meningitis, especially HSV. *Only if all 3 parameters are normal does the lumbar puncture provide evidence against infection; no single CSF parameter exists that can reliably exclude the presence of meningitis in a neonate (Garges, 2006). *Bacterial meningitis commonly causes CSF pleocytosis greater than 100 WBC/µL, with predominantly polymorphonuclear leukocytes gradually evolving to lymphocytes. *In neonates with viral meningitis, the picture may be similar but with a less dramatic pleocytosis. HSV meningitis, particularly, may be associated with a large number of RBCs in the CSF. *Maternal investigation: Particularly if a mother is symptomatic, bacterial or viral cultures can provide valuable adjunctive information.

Imaging Studies

*Brain MRI *MRI is the neuroimaging modality of choice to identify focal areas of infection, infarction, secondary hemorrhage, cerebral edema, hydrocephalus, or, rarely, abscess formation. It should be considered in the context of focal neurological abnormalities, persistent infection, or clinical deterioration. Sinovenous occlusions, ventriculitis, and subdural collections are best discussed with MRI.

*Follow-up MRI scans are useful in following the resolution of the infection as well as in contributing to prognostication. If available, MR spectroscopy can add important information on the metabolic function of the neonatal brain.

*CT scan - *Although CT carries the risk of exposing the neonatal brain to radiation, the rapidity and ease with which it can be obtained makes it useful in decision-making for potential neurosurgical interventions, such as ventriculostomy for hydrocephalus or surgical drainage of empyema or abscess.

*Cranial ultrasonography: Cranial ultrasonography provides an alternative imaging modality for critically ill neonates, but it does not provide optimal detail in all circumstances. However, it is low risk and thus useful for monitoring ventricular size for hydrocephalus during the acute phase of meningitis.

*Chest radiography: Chest radiograph provides important information about the lung parenchyma and cardiac silhouette. Meningitis or sepsis may occur with pneumonia but may be distinguishable from surfactant deficiency, pulmonary hypertension, and obstructive cardiac disease.

Other Tests

*Electroencephalography (EEG) -EEG is not an essential part of the initial diagnostic process; however, in neonates who are unresponsive or have seizures presenting as episodes of apnea, bradycardia, or rhythmic focal movements, EEG monitoring provides useful information to guide treatment with anticonvulsant drugs. -Not surprisingly, infants with normal or mildly abnormal EEGs had better outcomes, while those with moderate-to-markedly abnormal EEGs were more likely to die or to suffer adverse outcomes (Klinger, 2001).

---

* *Pearl/Peril/Pitfall :* Neuroimaging is recommended to detect the complications of meningitis. Complications should be suspected when the clinical course is characterized by shock, respiratory failure, focal neurological deficits, a positive CSF culture after 48–72 hours of appropriate antibiotic therapy, or infection with certain organisms. Citrobacter koseri and Enterobacter sakazakii meningitis, for example, are frequently associated with the development of brain abscesses, even in infants who have a benign clinical course. The most useful and non-invasive method early in the course is ultrasonography, which will provide information regarding ventricular size and the presence of hemorrhage. Computed tomography will be useful in detecting cerebral abscesses and later in the treatment course in identifying areas of encephalomalacia that may dictate prolonged therapy.

Complications *Regardless of etiology, meningitis in neonates can progress rapidly to serious complications. These include cerebral edema; hydrocephalus; hemorrhage; ventriculitis, especially with bacterial infection; and cerebral infarction. Cerebral edema, hydrocephalus, and hemorrhage each may cause increased intracranial pressure, with potential for secondary ischemic injury to the brain because of decreased brain perfusion. *Cerebral edema results from vasogenic changes, cytotoxic cell injury, and, at times, inappropriate antidiuretic hormone (ADH) secretion. *Hydrocephalus develops as a result of debris obstructing CSF flow through the ventricular system or dysfunction of arachnoid villi. *Hemorrhage occurs in regions of infarction or necrosis and should be suspected in a neonate with new focal neurological findings or clinical deterioration. *Ventriculitis results in sequestration of infection to areas poorly accessible to systemic antimicrobial drugs. Inflammation of the ependymal lining of ventricles often obstructs CSF flow. Thus, all of these complications are interactive, making effective management difficult. *Cerebral infarction, both focal (arterial) and diffuse (venous), may complicate recovery. *Necrotizing lesions secondary to HSV meningitis can be deleterious to the developing brain.

Prognosis *Survivors of neonatal meningitis are not only more likely to have moderate-to-severe disabilities than children who had meningitis after one month of age, they are also more likely to have subtle problems, including visual deficits, middle-ear disease, and behavioral problems. *Poor prognostic indicators include low birth weight, significant leukopenia or neutropenia, high CSF protein, and coma. *In addition to coma and leukopenia, seizures lasting longer than 72 hours and the need for inotropes predict moderate/severe disability or death with 88% sensitivity and 99% specificity . *Brain MRI, both in the acute and convalescent phases of illness, is a good modality to assist in determining prognosis. *Although neonatal meningitis is an acute infectious process, significant complications may result. These include residual epilepsy, cognitive impairment, hearing loss, visual impairment, spastic paresis, and, occasionally, microcephaly. Some of these disorders may be difficult to detect during infancy. *Hearing, for example, is difficult to evaluate without the child's cooperation, and then assessment may be limited to behavioral response to sounds. Brainstem auditory evoked response (BAER) testing does not evaluate all dimensions of hearing, but this test, which can be performed reliably in sedated infants, only slightly overestimates hearing loss, which occurs in 30% of survivors of bacterial meningitis and 14% of survivors of nonbacterial meningitis. Subtle impairment of sound discrimination may not be readily apparent.*Similarly, cognitive impairment may not be apparent until the child has started school or advanced into higher grades when more complex analysis of information is necessary. Careful screening for neurological deficits must be conducted as part of routine pediatric care over the period of many years, and the responsible physician should be attentive to possible problems with perception, learning, or behavior that may result from neonatal infection.

KEY POINTS FOR CLINICAL PRACTICE

1. When evaluating a neonate for meningitis, consider these 3 key points: (1) be vigilant for maternal infection "setups," including prolonged rupture of membranes, fever, and chorioamnionitis, remembering that asymptomatic maternal infection is always a possibility even with screening; (2) early-onset and late-onset bacterial infections have distinctive clinical courses, and (3) in HSV and VZV infections, the presence of skin lesions in a meningitic neonate are the exception more than the rule.

2. Aggressive antimicrobial intervention is lifesaving in Neonates with suspected meningitis. Because distinguishing viral from bacterial meningitis is difficult early in the clinical course, a combination of agents is often necessary, providing coverage for both types of infection.

3. Delays in diagnosis and initiation of treatment are the most critical pitfalls. Failure to perform a lumbar puncture and detect infection in a neonate with mild fever and minimal, nonspecific clinical findings is problematic; all neonates in whom meningitis might be the cause of symptoms should undergo CSF examination. Delay in treatment because of equivocal laboratory screening tests or because findings are altered by prior partial treatment may cause significant harm.

4. Brainstem auditory evoked response testing: Because of the potential for hearing loss, neonates with meningitis should undergo brainstem auditory evoked response (BAER) testing at 4-6 weeks after discharge.

5. Although Neonatal meningitis is an acute infectious process, significant complications may result. These include residual epilepsy, cognitive impairment, hearing loss, visual impairment, spastic paresis, and, occasionally, microcephaly. Some of these disorders may be difficult to detect during infancy.

REFERENCES AND FURTHER READING: 1) Malbon K, Mohan R, Nicholl R. Should a neonate with possible late onset infection always have a lumbar puncture?. *Arch Dis Child.* Jan 2006;91(1):75-6. 2) Heath PT, Nik Yusoff NK, Baker CJ. Neonatal meningitis. *Arch Dis Child Fetal Neonatal Ed.* May 2003;88(3):F173-8. 3)Stevens JP, Eames M, Kent A, et al. Long term outcome of neonatal meningitis. *Arch Dis Child Fetal Neonatal Ed.* 2003;88:F179-184. 4) Chaudhuri A. Adjunctive dexamethasone treatment in acute bacterial meningitis. *Lancet Neurol.* Jan 2004;3(1):54-62. 5) Garges HP, Moody MA, Cotten CM, et al. Neonatal meningitis: what is the correlation among cerebrospinal fluid cultures, blood cultures, and cerebrospinal fluid parameters?. *Pediatrics.* Apr 2006;117(4):1094-100.

Pearl/Peril/Pitfall: *Judicious antibiotic use, including the use of narrow spectrum antibiotics, stopping antibiotics when cultures are negative, and not using antibiotics to treat colonization or as prophylaxis, as well as enforcement of hand hygiene policies, are obvious prevention strategies for neonates remaining in the hospital.*

13 Neonatal Hypothermia and Cold Injury

@ *Evaluate* the Neonate with cold injury for infection, bleeding, or injury and metabolic disturbances. *Rewarm* the infant under radiant warmer by setting skin temperature at 37°C in skin servo mode/ setting air temperature at 35–36°C in air servo mode and *carefully watch for* apnea, hypoxia and hypoglycemia during rewarming.

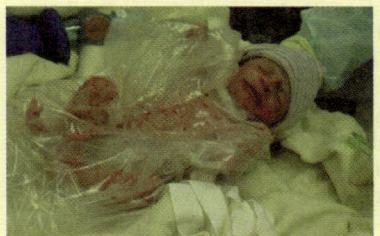

Avoidance of hypothermia/cold stress is paramount; heat loss can be minimised by the following: *infants less than 28 weeks gestation should be placed immediately after birth in a polyethylene bag or wrap and the body completely covered (appropriate size, food grade, heat resistant) *a less satisfactory alternative is to take the following steps *avoid evaporative heat loss — dry the infant *avoid conductive heat loss — ensure that wraps are/remain warm (i.e. replace if necessary) *reduce radiant heat loss — manage baby under a radiant heater *avoid convective heat loss — avoid draughts, keep baby away from air conditioning ducts *N.B. 'blanketing' is ineffective in tiny babies as they are unable to generate enough heat to warm the air between the skin and the blanket; bubble wrap between the baby and the overhead heater is preferable as it allows transmission

Adverse consequences of hypothermia
* High O_2 consumption → hypoxia, bradycardia
* High glucose usage → hypoglycemia / decreased glycogen stores
* High energy expenditure → reduced growth rate, lethargy, hypotonia, poor suck/cry
* Low surfactant production → RDS
* Vasoconstriction → poor perfusion → metabolic acidosis
* Delayed transition from fetal to newborn circulation
* Thermal shock → DIC → death

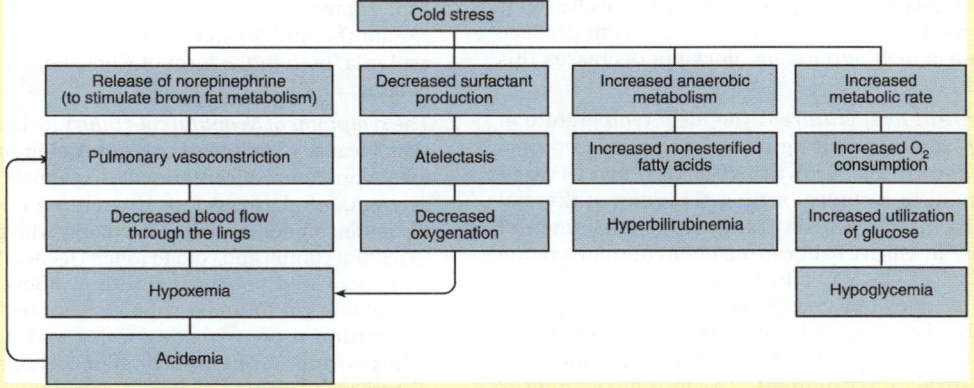

Cold stress chain of events. The hypothermic, or cold-stressed, Newborn attempts to compensate by conserving heat and increasing heat production. These physiologic compensatory mechanisms initiate a series of metabolic events that result in hypoxemia and altered surfactant production, metabolic acidosis, hypoglycemia, and hyperbilirubinemia.

REVIEW OF CLINICAL PROBLEMS

1. How do you assess the severity of Hypothermia ?
   Ans: Refer to the "No. 4" of the "BIRD'S EYE VIEW/ OVERVIEW/SYNOPSIS" of the Chapter.

2. Mention the Risk factors involved in producing Hypothermia in Neonates ?
   Ans: Refer to the "No. 6" of the "BIRD'S EYE VIEW/ OVERVIEW/SYNOPSIS" of the Chapter.

3. What are the Signs and Symptoms of Hypothermia in Neonates ?
   Ans: Refer to the "No. 7" of the "BIRD'S EYE VIEW/ OVERVIEW/SYNOPSIS" of the Chapter.

4. Mention the indications for Intubation and Mechanical ventilation in managing Cold injury in Neonates?
   Ans: Refer to the Evaluation–Decision–Action Plan/ Algorithm to diagnose and manage a Neonate with Hypothermia and Cold injury.

5. How do you Assess—Evaluate and Manage a Neonate with Cold injury ?
   Ans: Refer to the evaluation–decision-action plan/ algorithm to diagnose and manage a neonate with hypothermia and cold injury.

LEARNING OBJECTIVES

After completing this article, readers will be able to

1. Prevent cold stress and cold injury in high-risk Neonates by following the "10 commandments" of warm chain.

2. Identify the clinical symptoms and signs of cold stress and cold injury and to evaluate all hypothermic infants for possible sepsis.

3. Manage hypothermia and its complications promptly and effectively.

4. Watch for hypoxia, hypoglycemia, and poor tissue perfusion during rewarming.

5. Educate the parents/caregivers about keeping the baby away from exposure to cold stress/heat stress.

*Pearl/Peril/Pitfall: WHAT IS THE NORMAL RANGE OF BODY TEMPERATURE? This depends on the site where the temperature is measured: 1. The normal axillary temperature is 36.5–37°C. 2. The normal abdominal skin temperature is 36–36.5°C. All newborn infants have the same range of normal body temperature. *** The normal oral temperature is 37–37.5°C and rectal temperature is 37.5 – 38°C. Neither are used in newborn infants.*

BIRD'S EYE VIEW/OVERVIEW/SYNOPSIS

1. Neonates should be kept in the thermoneutral range, with a core body temperature as close to 37°C as possible. During pregnancy, maternal mechanisms maintain intrauterine temperature. After birth, newborn must adapt to their relatively cold environment by the metabolic production of heat because they are not able to generate an adequate shivering response. Premature infants have special problems in temperature maintenance, when compared with term infants which include: 1) A higher ratio of skin surface area to weight. 2) Highly permeable skin leads to increased transepidermal water loss. 3) Decreased subcutaneous fat, with less insulative capacity. 4) Less-developed stores of brown fat. 5)The inability to take in enough calories to provide nutrients for thermogenesis and growth. 6)Limitation of oxygen consumption in some preterm infants because of pulmonary problems.

2. Term newborns have a source for thermogenesis in brown fat, which is highly vascularized and innervated by sympathetic neurons. When these infants face cold stress, norepinephrine levels increase and act in the brown-fat tissue to stimulate lipolysis. Most of the Free Fatty Acids (FFAs) are re-esterified or oxidized; both reactions produce heat. Hypoxia or b-adrenergic blockade decreases this response.

3. *Thermoneutral temperature* is the ideal temperature at which the babies should be nursed to achieve optimal somatic and brain growth with minimal oxygen consumption. In a clinical setting this zone of thermal comfort is in the narrow range of environmental temperature in which a baby can maintain core temperature between 36.7°C–37.3°C and his mean core and skin temperature does not change >0.2°C and 0.3°C per hr respectively when recorded continuously by an electronic thermometer. Sick/Premature infants require a thermoneutral environment to minimize energy expenditure; the incubator should be kept at an appropriate temperature on air mode, if a skin probe cannot be used because of potential damage to skin in small premature infants. Alternatively, skin mode or servocontrol can be set so that the incubator's internal thermostat responds to changes in the infant's skin temperature to ensure a normal temperature despite any environmental fluctuation (Refer to Table No-1 for appropriate neutral thermal environmental temperatures).

4. Hypothermia in a Newborn baby is defined as a skin temperature of <35.5°C or core temperature of <36°C. The babies in cold stress have a core temperature between 36–36.5°C. The difference between the core and peripheral temperature is likely to be >1.5°C and extremities are cold and pale. Premature babies are unable to gain weight because of caloric loss from unrecognized chronic cold stress, resulting in excess oxygen consumption. Moderate hypothermia is diagnosed when core temperature ranges between 32°C–35.9°C *while a core temperature of <32°C is designated as severe hypothermia or Neonatal cold injury.It is important that a low reading thermometer is used, not the standard thermometer with a minimum reading of 35°C.*

5. Neonates become cold because of four means of heat loss: a)by *radiation* to a colder object in the environment b)by *convection* from the moving cold draughts c)by *evaporation* from the wet skin d)by *conduction* to the surface and which he or she lies. This heat transfer is complex, and the contribution of each component depends on the temperature of the surroundings (air and walls), air speed, and water vapor pressure.

6. *Neonatal cold injury* (core temperature is <32.2°C) occurs in LBW infants, premature babies and term infants with CNS disorders such as asphyxia and drugs. It occurs more often in home deliveries/emergency deliveries/settings (surgery) where inadequate attention is paid to the thermal environmental and heat loss. Premature infants respond with peripheral vasoconstriction, causing anaerobic metabolism and metabolic acidosis, which can cause pulmonary vasoconstriction, leading to further hypoxemia, anaerobic metabolism, and acidosis. Hypoxemia further compromises the infant's response to cold. Intentional hypothermia is used as an adjunct to cardiopulmonary bypass when newborn infants have major heart surgery-body temperature is lowered to about 28°C by surface cooling with ice to reduce the metabolic demands of the brain. The infants tolerate this brief, acute severe hypothermia well. Similar hypothermia appears to be an effective method for preventing brain damage in asphyxiated animals.It is currently undergoing trials as rescue therapy for newborn infants with severe birth asphyxia, both in the form of whole body and local head cooling.

7. The *symptoms of Neonatal cold injury* include a)bright red skin because of failure of oxyhemoglobin to dissociate at low temperature b)central pallor/cyanosis c)edema and sclerema of skin and face d)vomiting and abdominal distention e)poor feeding and lethargy with poor response to painful stimuli and cold to touch f)generalized bleeding and shock and poor urine output. *Signs may include* a)hypotension b)bradycardia c)slow, shallow, irregular respiration d)poor sucking reflex and poor neonatal reflexes and e)pulmonary hemorrhage. Metabolic disturbances include, hypoglycemia, metabolic acidosis, hyperkalemia, azotemia.

8. *The Evaluation-Decision-Action-Plan/Algorithm* describes the essential aspects of diagnosis and management of Neonatal cold injury and its complications. It also highlights the routine postnatal precautions to be taken to prevent hypothermia and cold injury in the Neonates. It is uncertain whether warming should be rapid or slow. Setting the abdominal skin temperature 1°C higher than the core temperature in a radiant warmer will produce slow rewarming and setting it to 36.5°C will also result in slow rewarming. One should correct shock with 10–20ml/kg NS and metabolic acidosis with sodium bicarbonate/FFP and evaluate the Neonate with cold injury for infection, bleeding, or injury and treat appropriately.

9. In addition to rewarming, oxygen is administered, blood sugar monitored closely and carefully, and antibiotics are administered only when infection is suspected or documented. The infant should be fed only by IV infusion or gavage of dextrose solution until the temperature is 35°C. Hypothermic infants should not be permitted to feed by nipple.

10. Servocontrol temperature may mask the hypothermia/ hyperthermia associated with infection. A record of both environmental and core temperatures, along with observation for other signs of sepsis, will help detect this problem. Hypothermia is an important symptom of septicemia in preterm babies and hypothermia can predispose babies to severe bacterial infection.

Pearl/Peril/Pitfall: PROVIDE OXYGEN. Although centrally pink, cold infants are often hypoxic. Therefore, give 30% oxygen (FiO² 0.3) while the infant is being warmed. A normal oxygen saturation in a cold infant does to exclude tissue hypoxia.

THE EVALUATION-DECISION-ACTION-PLAN/ALGORITHM FOR THE DIAGNOSIS AND MANAGEMENT OF *NEONATAL HYPOTHERMIA and COLD INJURY*

SUBJECTIVE FINDINGS

Hx of risk factors for hypothermia such as **a)** prematurity and IUGR **b)** home deliveries **c)** emergency deliveries **d)** term babies with CNS depression due to asphyxia, drugs **e)** exposure to cold stress in the delivery room **f)** wet baby with poor nursing care **g)** exposure to cold draught **h)** surgery, etc.

Hx of symptoms of cold injury such as poor feeding, lethargy, feel cold to the touch, bright red color (due to the failure of dissociation of oxyhemoglobin at low temperatures,) central cyanosis/pallor, feeble cry, abdominal distention and vomiting, minimal reaction to painful stimuli, edema of extremities and face/sclerema, shallow and irregular respirations, shock and bleeding.

OBJECTIVE FINDINGS

Assess airway, breathing, circulation and disability by observing the vitals, BP, O$_2$ sats, color, CRT, pulses, sensorium, focal neurologic deficits, seizures, abnormal movements, tone and reflexes, etc.

Obtain core temperature (often <32.2°C/90°F)
Look for signs of cold injury such as hypotension, bradycardia, slow, shallow, irregular respirations, poor sucking reflex, decreased neonatal reflexes, decreased activity and response to stimulus, generalized bleeding, including pulmonary hemorrhage.

Assess for metabolic derangements such as metabolic acidosis, hypoglycemia, hyperkalemia, azotemia, and oliguria.

INVESTIGATIONS

Blood FBC, TC, DC, Platelets, CRP, Blood cultures, ABG analysis, electrolytes, calcium and magnesium, blood sugar, creatinine, BUN, coagulation profile.

CXR for respiratory infections

LP after stabilization only for CNS infection/hemorrhage

Urine analysis and culture

Observe nursing charts for interventions to maintain the baby's temperature (a record of both environmental and core temperature, along with observation for other signs of sepsis)

NEONATAL HYPOTHERMIA and COLD INJURY

Evaluate the neonate with cold injury for infection, bleeding, or injury and metabolic disturbances

Correct shock with 20ml/kg NS over 5 minutes and IVI of Dopamine and/or Dobutamine; *Correct* hypoxia and hypoglycemia; *Keep the infant on NPO*, until a normal body temperature is achieved

Intubate and ventilate for complications of cold injury such as apnea, pulmonary hemorrhage, CNS dysfunction, unresponsive shock, underlying severe sepsis/meningitis etc.

Mild hypothermia or cold stress **Supervised Kangaroo Mother Care (KMC) and skin-to-skin contact** is the best method to rewarm a baby; remove cold clothes from the baby and ensure the room should be warm (28–32°C) and draught free and continue breast feeding

Ensure ABCs, O$_2$ saturations, BP, CR monitor

Measure core (Axilla/Rectal) body temperature and categorize the severity of hypothermia (Cold stress = 36–36.5°C/Moderate hypothermia = 32–35.9°C/Severe hypothermia = <32°C)

Administer IV broadspectrum antibiotics, only when infection is suspected or documented

Give Vitamin-K IM 0.5–1mg in the event of hemorrhagic manifestations and *perform* exchange transfusion for DIC and sclerema

Rewarm the infant under radiant warmer by setting skin temperature at 37°C in skin servo mode/ setting air temperature at 35–36°C in air servo mode and *carefully watch for* apnea, hypoxia and hypoglycemia during rewarming

Do Follow the routine practices to keep the core body temperature as close to 37°C as possible!

1. *Keep labor wards as warm and as draught-free as possible, and make special efforts when a premature baby is being delivered. Ideally the room should be warmed to 28–32°C. The resuscitation area must be draught-free, away from windows and air conditioning, and the resuscitation carried out under an overhead radiant heater.*
2. *Dry all babies after delivery with a warm towel, and thereafter keep them either wrapped up, or under the radiant heat source.*
3. *Avoid bathing babies on the labor ward.*
4. *Keep nurseries and NNUs hot enough (28–32°C) to minimize radiant heat loss.*
5. *Nurse babies in incubators set at the temperatures given in the Table 1.*
6. *Minimize radiant heat loss in incubators by:*
   a. *using double-glazed incubators;*
   b. *covering the baby with a radiant heat shield;*
   c. *covering the baby with an insulating fabric (silver swaddlers, bubble-wrap, clingfilm);*

d. *using hats and bootees/leggings even in neonates requiring intensive care;*
   e. *dressing babies once they no longer require intensive care and meticulous observation.*
7. *Minimize evaporative heat loss by:*
   a. *avoiding very dry environments. Put water in the incubator humidifier for babies of less than 30 weeks gestation who are having any problem maintaining their temperature; b) covering the baby with clingfilm or an insulating fabric to create a humid microenvironment. Clothing has a similar effect; c) avoiding overhead radiant heaters for thin skinned ELBW babies in the first week.*
8. *Avoid convective heat loss by:*
   a. *wrapping the babies in clingfilm or dressing them (v.s.);*
   b. *blocking off one end of a radiant heat shield with clingfilm to prevent a wind tunnel effect.*
9. *Warm and humidify all medical gases administered to babies.*
10. *Warm up operating theatres and anesthetic rooms before the baby arrives.*

Pearl/Peril/Pitfall : Hypothermic infants present with the following signs: 1. They are cold to the touch. 2. They are lethargic, hypotonic, feed poorly and have a feeble cry. 3. Their hands and feet are usually pale or blue, but their tongue and cheeks are pink. Note that they are not centrally cyanosed. The pink cheeks may incorrectly suggest that the infant is well. 4. Peripheral edema or sclerema (a woody or plastic feel to the skin). 5. Shallow, slow respiration or signs of respiratory distress. 6. Bleeding from the mouth, nose or needle punctures. Hypothermic infants often die of massive pulmonary hemorrhage.

TABLE 1 @Neutral thermal environmental temperatures

Age and weight	Range of temperature (°C)	Age and weight	Range of temperature (°C)
0–6 h		**72–96 h**	
< 1200 g	34.0–35.0	< 1200 g	34.0–35.0
1200–1500 g	33.9–34.4	1200–1500 g	33.0–34.0
1501–2500 g	32.8–33.8	1501–2500 g	31.1–33.2
>2500 g (and >36 wk)	32.0–33.8	>2500 g (and >36 wk)	29.8–32.8
6–12 h		**4–12 d**	
< 1200 g	34.0–35.4	<1500 g	33.0–34.0
1200–1500 h	33.5–34.4	1501–2500 g	31.0–33.2
1501–2500 g	32.2–33.8	>2500 g (and >36 wk)	
>2500 g (and > 36 wk)	31.4–33.8	4–5 d	29.5–32.6
12–24 h		5–6 d	29.4–32.3
< 1200 g	34.0–35.4	6–8 d	29.0–32.2
1200–1500 g	33.3–34.3	8–10 d	29.0–31.8
1501–2500 g	31.8–33.8	10–12 d	29.0–31.4
>2500 g (and >36 wk)	31.0–33.7	**12–14 d**	
24–36 h		< 1500 g	32.0–34.0
< 1200 g	34.0–35.0	1501–2500 g	31.0–33.2
1200–1500 g	33.1–34.2	>2500 g (and >36 wk)	29.0–30.8
1501–2500 g	31.6–33.6	**2–3 wk**	
>2500 g (and >36 wk)	30.7–33.5	< 1500 g	32.2–34.0
36–48 h		1501–2500 g	30.5–33.0
< 1200 g	34.0–35.0	**3–4 wk**	
1200–1500 g	33.0–34.1	< 1500 g	31.6–33.6
1501–2500 g	31.4–33.5	1501–2500 g	30.0–32.7
>2500 g (and >36 wk)	30.5–33.3	**4–5 wk**	
48–72 h		< 1500 g	31.2–33.0
< 1200 g	34.0–35.0	1501–2500 g	29.5–32.2
1200–1500 g	33.0–34.0	**5–6 wk**	
1501–2500 g	31.2–33.4	< 1500 g	30.6–32.3
>2500 g (and >36 wk)	30.1–33.2	1501–2500 g	29.0–31.8

@The neutral thermal environment (best room or incubator temperature) is that environmental temperature at which the skin temperature is normal and the infant's metabolic rate is at its lowest. In this state the infant uses the least amount of oxygen and the energy. The energy in feeds, therefore, can be used for growth rather than for generating heat. It is important to ensure that all infants are nursed as close as possible to their own neutral thermal environment.

Generally speaking, the smaller infants in each weight group require a temperature in the higher portion of the temperature range. Within each time range, the younger the infant, the higher the temperature required. Adapted from Scopes J, Ahmed l: Dis Child 41:417, 1996. For their table, Scopes and Ahmed had the walls of the incubator 1°C to 2°C warmer than the ambient air temperatures.

ESSENTIAL FACTS OF THERMOREGULATION IN NEONATES

***10 COMMANDMENTS OF WARM CHAIN TO MINIMIZE HYPOTHERMIA IN NEONATES:** 1)Warm delivery room(28–32°C) 2)Warm resuscitation (under a preheated warmer) 3) Immediate drying (not ignoring head, axillae, and groin) 4) Skin to skin contact between mother and baby 5) Breast feeding (start within 30 minutes to 1 hr after birth) 6) Bathing and weighing postponed 7) Appropriate clothing and bedding 8) Mother and baby together (Room–In) 9) Warm transportation 10) Training and awareness of health care providers

***NORMAL TEMPERATURE AT DIFFERENT SITES:** 1) Axillary- 36.5°C–37.5°C 2) Rectal- 36.5°C–37°C 3) Abdominal skin- 36.5°C–37°C 4) Deltoid

skin- 36°C–36.5°C 5) Toe- 35°C–36°C (Rectal temperature is not recommended for routine monitoring because there is a risk of injury and infection.)

***SUGGESTED ABDOMINAL SKIN TEMPERATURE SETTINGS FOR INFANTS NURSED IN SERVO MODE INCUBATORS OR UNDER RADIANT WARMERS:** 1) Birth weight <1kg-36.9°C 2) Birth weight 1–1.5kg-36.7°C 3) Birth weight 1.5–2 kg-36.5°C 4) Birth weight 2-2.5kg-36.3°C 5) Birth weight >2.5kg-36°C

***KANGAROO-MOTHER CARE:** Refer to Essential Clinical Guidelines Section for the Practical Details of KMC.

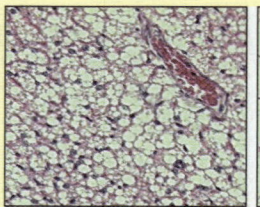 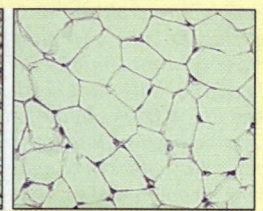

Examination of sections of white and **brown fat** at low magnification reveal dramatic differences in structure, as seen below in images of mouse tissues. · White adipocytes (*right panel*) have a scant ring of cytoplasm surrounding a single large lipid droplet. Their nuclei are flattened and eccentric within the cell. · Brown adipocytes (*left panel*) are polygonal in shape, have a considerable volume of cytoplasm and contain multiple lipid droplets of varying size. Their nuclei are round and almost centrally located.

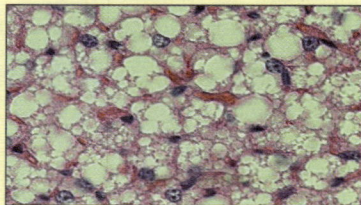

These features of **brown fat** are seen at a higher magnification in the image below (HandE stain). Note the abundance of blood-filled capillaries and variable size of lipid droplets. Electron micrographs of brown fat cells reveal one of their hallmarks: an extraordinary number of mitochondria, are involved in heat generation. The mitochondria are typically round, with cristae across their entire width.

Pearl/Peril/Pitfall: Infants who produce too little heat or lose too much heat are at the greatest risk. These high risk infants are: 1. Preterm infants. 2. Underweight for gestational age infants. 3. Wasted infants. 4. Infants who have not been fed. 5. Infected infants. 6. Hypoxic infants. 7. Wet infants. 8. Infants exposed to a cold environment. 9. Infants who are nursed naked and not covered. 10. Infants nursed close to a cold window.

Heat and fluid loss

Preterm infants are susceptible to heat and fluid loss because
- High surface area to volume ratio
- Thin non-keratinized skin
- Lack of insulating subcutaneous fat
- Lack of thermogenic brown fat
- Inability to shiver

Potential adverse consequences of hypothermia
- High oxygen consumption can lead to hypoxia
- High use of glucose can lead to hypoglycemia
- High energy expenditure can cause reduced rate of growth
- Low surfactant production can cause respiratory distress
- Vasoconstriction may cause poor perfusion or metabolic acidosis
- Delayed adjustment from fetal to newborn circulation

Monitor the Variables that should be monitored in the very preterm infant
- Temperature: core and peripheral
- Heart rate
- Respiratory rate
- Peripheral oxygen saturation
- Blood pressure
- Urine output
- Partial pressure of oxygen and carbon dioxide
- Acid-base status
- Electrolyte balance
- Weight gain or loss

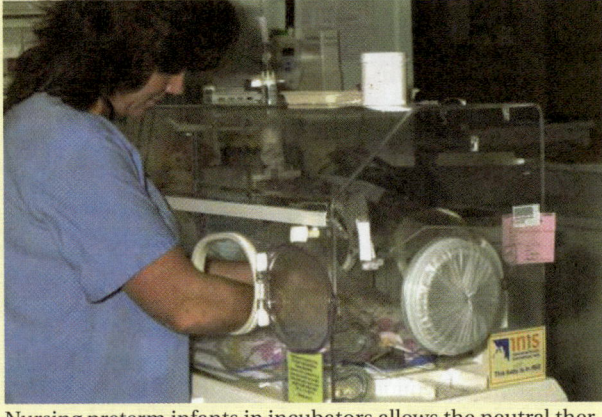

Nursing preterm infants in incubators allows the neutral thermal environment, noise, and light to be controlled effectively. Ports allow access to the infant

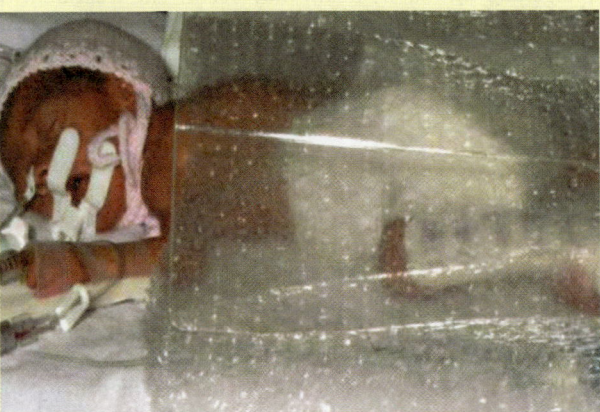

Covering the preterm infant with a polythene blanket reduces heat and fluid loss
Courtesy: William McGuire, Peter McEwan, Peter W Fowlie

KEY POINTS FOR CLINICAL PRACTICE

1. BEWARE OF THE *DELETERIOUS EFFECTS OF COLD INJURY* ON LOW BIRTH WEIGHT BABIES SUCH AS - A) Decreased surfactant synthesis and efficacy B) Metabolic acidosis C) Hypoxia D) Hypoglycemia E) Increased oxygen consumption F) Diversion of cardiac output to brown fat G) Increased postnatal weight loss and Decreased weight gain H) Sclerema I) Coagulation failure and J) Increased neonatal mortality.

2. Hypothermia in a Newborn baby is defined as a skin temperature of <35.5˚C or core temperature of <36˚C. Moderate hypothermia is diagnosed when core temperature ranges between 32˚C–35.9˚C while a **core temperature of <32˚C is designated as severe hypothermia or Neonatal cold injury.** *It is important that a low reading thermometer is used, not the standard thermometer with a minimum reading of 35˚C.*

3. Neonatal cold injury (core temperature is <32.2˚C) occurs in LBW infants, premature babies and term infants with CNS disorders such as asphyxia and drugs. It occurs more often in home deliveries/emergency deliveries / settings (surgery) where inadequate attention is paid to the thermal environmental and heat loss.

4. Warm chain (Refer to the 10 "Commandments" of it) should be maintained for minimizing the likelihood of hypothermia in all Newborns.

5. Rewarm the infant under radiant warmer by setting skin temperature at 37˚C in skin servo mode/ setting air temperature at 35–36˚C in air servo mode and *carefully watch for* apnea, hypoxia and hypoglycemia during rewarming.

REFERENCES AND FURTHER READING : 1) Klaus MA, Martin RJ, Fanaroff AA, eds. The physical environment. In: *Care of the high risk neonate*, 5th ed. Philadelphia: WB Saunders, 2001. 2) Sherman T. Optimizing the neonatal thermal environment. *Neonatal Netw* 2006;25(4): 251–258 3) Sinclair JC. Servo-control for maintaining abdominal skin temperature at 36˚C in low-birth-weight infants. *Cochrane Database Syst Rev* 2002;1:CD001074. 4)McCall, E.M. "Interventions to prevent hypothermia at birth in preterm and/or low birthweight babies." Cochrane Database of Systematic Reviews. Vol (3), 2007.5)Watkinson, M.A. "Temperature Control of Premature Infants in the Delivery Room." Clin Perinaol 33 (2006) 43–53.

Pearl/Peril/Pitfall : WHICH INFANTS PRODUCE TOO LITTLE HEAT? The following infants are often unable to produce enough heat to maintain a normal body temperature: 1. PRETERM INFANTS. They are born before adequate stores of brown fat have been deposited. 2. UNDERWEIGHT FOR GESTATIONAL AGE or WASTED INFANTS. They have used up their stores of brown fat before delivery. 3. INFECTED OR HYPOXIC INFANTS. Generalized infection or severe hypoxia prevents the normal break down of brown fat and, thereby, decreases the production of heat. Infected and hypoxic infants, therefore, commonly present with a drop rather than a rise in body temperature.

Neonatal Hyperthermia

@All Neonates with fever should be evaluated for hydration, weight loss, & foci of infection such as cellulitis, septic arthritis/osteomyelitis, omphalitis, & presence of colonized foreign bodies e.g., in a central venous line.

Hyperthermia is usually secondary to overheating due to an external source; however it can be secondary to other factors including sepsis, hypermetabolism, neonatal abstinence syndrome, and maternal hyperthermia at delivery. Clinically hyperthermia may present with irritability, poor feeding, flushing, hypotension, tachypnoea or apnoea, lethargy and abnormal posturing, in addition to an elevated peripheral or core temperature. If untreated then seizures, coma, neurological damage and ultimately death may occur. The treatment of hyperthermia requires the same close monitoring and observation for signs of deterioration as described for the management of neonatal hypothermia. Rapid reduction in temperature is associated with the potential for cold stress shock.

Infection should always be suspected first, unless there are very obvious external reasons for the baby becoming overheated. Febrile neonates younger than 4 weeks old should have a full evaluation for sepsis. A full evaluation for sepsis consists of a complete blood cell count (CBC) with differential, blood culture, enhanced urinalysis (UA), urine culture, and a lumbar puncture (LP) to collect cerebrospinal fluid (CSF). CSF should be analyzed for cell counts, protein, glucose, and culture. A full evaluation for sepsis in febrile neonates is warranted because their risk for serious bacterial infection (SBI) is relatively high; even among those who otherwise meet low risk criteria, the rates of SBI are about 5%. Similarly, about 10% of febrile neonates who have documented respiratory syncytial virus or clinical bronchiolitis have SBI. This infection rate is about the same as for those without documented respiratory syncytial virus or clinical bronchiolitis; therefore, a full evaluation for sepsis should be performed for these patients. Evaluating febrile neonates for herpes simplex infection should be considered when the following risk factors are present: age younger than 3 weeks, vesicles, seizure, toxic or ill-appearing, CSF pleocytosis or red blood cells, or maternal history of herpes. Laboratory studies to screen for herpes infection may include vesicle fluid for culture and direct fluorescent antibody, swabbing nasopharynx, conjunctiva, and rectum for culture, or CSF for polymerase chain reaction testing and culture. One study determined that evaluating CSF for enterovirus by polymerase chain reaction testing reduced the duration of hospitalization and antibiotic use for young infants.

Medicolegal Pitfalls *Failure to recognize/suspect occult bacteremia, serious bacterial infection (SBI), and/or sepsis *Failure to properly workup or treat fever or unknown source (FUS) *Failure to transfer/admit a child to the hospital for further testing and treatment when it is indicated *Failure to administer antibiotics and/or antiviral when it is indicated *Failure to ask about a child's immunization status *Failure to consult a pediatrician when it is indicated.

Special Concerns *Immunocompromised patients *Lack of reliable caretakers or safe home environment *Lack of reliable outpatient follow-up *History of abuse or neglect *Immunizations are not up to date for age.

REVIEW OF CLINICAL PROBLEMS

1. How do you differentiate between a healthy infant who is overheated from a febrile infant with a raised set-point ?
   Ans: Refer to the "No. 2" of the "BIRD'S EYE VIEW/ OVERVIEW/SYNOPSIS" of the Chapter.

2. How do you assess and evaluate a febrile Neonate ?
   Ans: Refer to the "No. 8" of the "BIRD'S EYE VIEW/ OVERVIEW/SYNOPSIS" of the Chapter. and to the Evaluation-Decision-Action Plan/Algorithm to diagnose & manage a Neonate with Hyperthermia.

3. What are the complications of Hyperpyrexia from Overheating?
   Ans: Refer to the "No. 2" of the "BIRD'S EYE VIEW/ OVERVIEW/SYNOPSIS" of the Chapter.

4. How do you manage Neonatal Hyperthermia?
   Ans: Refer to the Evaluation-Decision-Action Plan/ Algorithm to diagnose & manage a Neonate with Hyperthermia.

5. Describe Dehydration fever.
   Ans: Refer to the "No. 3" of the "BIRD'S EYE VIEW/ OVERVIEW/SYNOPSIS" of the Chapter.

LEARNING OBJECTIVES

After completing this article, readers will be able to

1. Learn the clinical differences between a healthy infant who is overheated and a febrile infant with a raised set-point and to avoid unnecessary septic evaluations in the former infant.

2. Examine the infant's environment for overheating and to avoid iatrogenic hyperpyrexia.

3. Understand that the LBW premature infant is extremely vulnerable to harsh fluctuations in physical environment.

4. M*onitor* body weight and input + output chart closely in infants cared for on radiant warmers.

5. Assess and evaluate the febrile infants for sepsis, especially those with temperature elevations exceeding 38°C–39°C.

---

* **Pearl/Peril/Pitfall:** *Pyrexia (high body temperature) is defined as an abdominal skin temperature of 37°C or more, or an axillary temperature of 37.5°C or more. As newborn infants can only sweat a little, they are unable to cool themselves and, therefore, easily become too hot.*

BIRD'S EYE VIEW/OVERVIEW/SYNOPSIS

1. Hyperthermia/Neonatal pyrexia is defined as a rectal (core body) temperature >37.4°C (Craig); some investigators accept normal temperatures upto 37.8°C. Between 1% to 2.5% of all Newborns admitted to the normal nursery have fever as judged from rectal/axillary temperatures and depending on the limits chosen. *Fever is an inconsistent and uncommon sign of sepsis (<10% of febrile Neonates have culture proven sepsis); paradoxically, septic Neonates more commonly present with hypothermia.*

2. The most common cause of Neonatal Hyperthermia is inappropriate incubation (high ambient air temperature and humidity). Hyperthermia may be caused by a relatively hot environment in tiny premature infant as a complication of the improper use of shielding devices either in convection-warmed incubators or under radiant warmers. When incubated, babies should always have a strictly monitored and controlled source of heat. Fever secondary to overheating particularly in association with incubators is more common in tropical countries. *If environmental temperature is the cause of hyperthermia, the trunk and extremities are of the same temperature or <1°C and the infant appears vasodilated. In contrast, infants with sepsis are often vasoconstricted & the extremities are 2°C-3°C colder than the trunk. The overheated baby needs a cooler environment, not a series of painful investigations to find an infective cause for fever.* Placing Newborns in sunlight to control bilirubin is hazardous and may be associated with significant hyperthermia. The American Academy of Pediatrics has published the following warning statement: "*The use of infant radiant warmers poses a hazard of Neonatal Hyperthermia. Serious overheating can result from mechanical failure of the controls, from dislodgment of the sensor probe, or from manual operation without careful monitoring. Deaths have been associated with hyperthermia induced by radiant warmers.*" Mild overheating is not dangerous though it may be associated with an increase in apnea of prematurity. However, hyperpyrexia from overheating can cause shock, protracted fits, diarrhea, DIC, renal and hepatic failure. Few infants who have died from overheating have done so suddenly, without prior symptoms. Sudden death in infancy has been linked with overheating, and is described in families with a history of malignant hyperpyrexia and anhidrotic ectodermal dysplasia.

3. Dehydration occurring in healthy term infants between the 3rd and 4th days of life, probably due to an inadequate intake of milk is an uncommonly recognized cause of fever in the Newborn period. Temperature may be anywhere between 37.8°C and 40°C. Rehydration leads to resolution of fever and is key to the diagnosis of this entity.

4. Sepsis is an uncommon cause of fever in Neonates; however, sepsis is probably the most treatable life-threatening illness occurring in febrile newborn infants, especially those with temperature elevations exceeding 38°C–39°C, who are more likely to have bacteremia, purulent meningitis, and pneumonia. Most neonatal febrile episodes are noted in the first day of life; however, any fever occurring on the third day of life and fever above 39°C have both correlated with a significantly higher chance of bacterial disease. *Severe temperature elevation is also associated with viral disease, particularly herpes simplex encephalitis, so septic evaluations in these infants should include a lumbar puncture.*

5. Hyperpyrexia is seen in a baby born to a pyrexial mother, regardless of whether the baby is infected. A baby's temperature at birth reflects maternal temperature and is usually about 0.5°C higher. With the growing use of epidural analgesia during labor, the recognition of epidural neonatal (mechanism is unknown) fever is an important consideration in the evaluation of the febrile neonate.

6. Neonatal Typhoid fever and Congenital Malaria should be considered in 3rd world countries, in the differential diagnosis of Neonatal fever. An increase in unexplained neonatal fevers was associated with the introduction of routine hepatitis B vaccination. In addition, temperature elevations may be seen with hypothalamic/other CNS malformations or masses. Subarachnoid or other intracranial hemorrhages may also be associated with temperature elevation. Rarely, acute myelopathy due to neonatal spinal neurenteric cysts is associated with persistent fever during infancy (>3 wks in duration). Temperature elevation may also occur with increased infant metabolic rate, such as that seen with skeletal muscle rigidity and status epilepticus. *Crisponi syndrome* is characterized by marked muscular contraction facial grimace in response to tactile external stimuli/during crying, with trismus, opisthotonos and abundant salivation as in a myotonic tetany; clinical course is characterized by the appearance of fever at about 38°C, with peaks of 42°C. It is evident at birth, in Italian families, probably transmitted as autosomal recessive trait and death occurs in the first few months and coincides with a fever of about 42°C.

7. The mechanisms reducing Neonatal fever are incompletely understood. They result from disturbances in the complex interactions between heat conservation anf heat dissipation mechanisms. Fever may occur when immunogenic pyrogens commonly prostaglandin E_2 lead to upward displacement of the normal thermal set point in the hypothalamus, leading to activation of heat conservation and heat generation physiologic responses.

8. *The Evaluation-Decision-Action-Plan / Algorithm* describes the essential aspects of diagnosis and management of Neonatal hyperthermia/pyrexia. The relevant perinatal history should be evaluated for risk factors so as to mitigate a laboratory evaluation or presumptive treatment for infection. Signs of sepsis such as diminished activity, irritability, seizures should be considered. *All Neonates with fever should be evaluated for hydration, weight loss, and foci of infection such as Cellulitis, Septic arthritis/Osteomyelitis, Omphalitis, and presence of colonized foreign bodies e.g. in a central venous line.*

9. An infant's environment should be examined for overheating, and in breast-feeding infants with fever at 3 to 4 days of life and excessive weight loss, dehydration fever should be considered and treated to establish this diagnosis. Mothers receiving epidural analgesia often manifest shivering with their temperature rise, and they experience a rapid defervescence after discontinuation of the epidural infusion; recognition of this pattern may avoid unnecessary sepsis evaluations in neonates with early fever.

10. The LBW premature newborn is extremely vulnerable to harsh fluctuations in physical environment. These infants require frequent assessments of skin, core, and air temperatures and relative humidity so that an optimal strategy may be designed for thermal regulation. In the care of smaller babies, heat replacement is often required, and refinement of techniques to accomplish heat replacement without inducing hyperthermia is needed.

---

* *Pearl/Peril/Pitfall: IS PYREXIA DANGEROUS? Yes. Pyrexia is an important cause of recurrent apnoea which can result in death if the infant is not cooled. Prolonged pyrexia can also lead to dehydration and increases the body's oxygen and energy needs.*

THE EVALUATION-DECISION-ACTION-PLAN / ALGORITHM FOR THE DIAGNOSIS AND MANAGEMENT OF *NEONATAL HYPERTHERMIA*

SUBJECTIVE FINDINGS

Hx of predisposing factors exposed to hot environment, LBW premature babies, inadequate intake of milk in healthy term infants, radiant warmer/incubator with improper use of shielding devices, maternal epidural analgesia, CNS dysfunction, or medications, phototherapy etc.

Observe the nursing charts For episodes of hyperthermia (core temperature >37.8°C). *Any fever occurring on the third day of life and fever above 39°C correlate with a significantly higher chance of sepsis or herpes simplex encephalitis.*

Hx of other coexisting symptoms suggestive of sepsis Poor feeding, lethargy, jaundice, respiratory distress, seizures, shock, etc.

OBJECTIVE FINDINGS

Assess airway, breathing, circulation & disability by observing the vitals, BP, O_2 sats, color, CRT, pulses, urine output, sensorium, focal neurologic deficits, seizures, abnormal movements, tone and reflexes etc.

Obtain Peripheral (TOES) and Core (AXILLA/RECTAL) body temperature If environmental temperature is the cause of hyperthermia, the trunk and extremities are the same temperature & the infant appears healthy & vasodilated (pink). In contrast, infants with sepsis are often vasoconstricted (pale) & the extremities are 2°C-3°C colder than the trunk and look unwell.

Perform complete physical examination for foci of infection such as cellulitis, septic arthritis, osteomyelitis, omphalitis, colonized central venous lines.

Evaluate for hydration status & weight loss

INVESTIGATIONS

Examine the infant's environment for over heating.

Consider dehydration fever in breast-feeding infants with fever at 3-4 days of life and excessive weight loss.

Perform full septic screen (blood/urine/CSF C/S, CXR, CRP, FBC & DIFFERENTIAL, AND I:T RATIO, PB Smear) including lumbar puncture in febrile Newborn infants, especially those with temperature elevations exceeding 38°C–39°C.

Observe mothers receiving epidural analgesia for shivering with temperature rise, with rapid defervescence after discontinuation of epidural infusion.

NEONATAL HYPERTHERMIA

Design an optimal strategy for thermal regulations by performing frequent assessments of skin, core, and air temperatures & relative humidity, especially for premature LBW newborn.

Monitor body weight and input + output closely in infants cared for on radiant warmers.

Rehydrate the infant with "dehydration fever" (either by IV fluids or by enteral feeds); resolution of fever after proper hydration is the key to the diagnosis of this entity.

Ensure ABCs, O2 sats, CR monitor & BP.

Correct dehydration with IV fluids & enteral feeds where appropriate.

Give IV broadspectrum antibiotics, in febrile Newborns with temperature elevations >38°C-39°C after performing septic screen. (*especially to those with subtle signs of sepsis, such as fever with flexed posturing, temperature and color fluctuations, peripheral-core temperature difference >2.5°C, unexplained tachycardia, hyperglycemia, metabolic acidosis on ABG analysis, thrombocytopenia, and direct hyperbilirubinemia etc.,*)

Cooling a Neonate with fever should be accomplished by unswaddling the over wrapped infant and returning him/her to an appropriately thermal neutral environment (in an incubator only after the equipment has been checked. Do not use any acetaminophen or other pyrolytic agents during the neonatal period. Except in the setting of hypoxic-ischemic encephalopathy, do not use a cooling device specifically. Surface cooling is passive, rapid, and safe.

KEY POINTS FOR CLINICAL PRACTICE:

1. Sepsis is an uncommon cause of fever in the Neonates; paradoxically, septic Neonates more commonly present with hypothermia. However, if the core body temperature exceeds > 38°C - 39°C & any fever occurring on the 3rd day of life have been correlated with a significantly higher chance of bacterial disease.

2. Dehydration fever occurring in healthy term infants between the 3rd and 4th days of life, because of inadequate breast milk & exposure to hot summer months in the tropical areas is an uncommonly recognized cause of fever. Rehydration leads to resolution of fever and is key to the diagnosis.

3. The LBW premature infant is extremely vulnerable to harsh fluctuations in physical environment. In the care of smaller babies, heat replacement should be accomplished without inducing hyperthermia.

4. All Neonates with fever should be evaluated for hydration, weight loss, & foci of infection (cellulitis, septic arthritis/osteomyelitis, omphalitis, & herpes simplex encephalitis & colonized central venous lines.

5. Congenital malaria & Neonatal typhoid fever should be considered in the differential diagnosis of Neonatal fever, in third world countries.

REFERENCES AND FURTHER READING : 1) Klaus MA, Martin RJ, Fanaroff AA, eds. The physical environment. In: *Care of the high risk neonate*, 5th ed. Philadelphia: WB Saunders, 2001. 2) Sherman T. Optimizing the neonatal thermal environment. *Neonatal Netw* 2006;25(4): 251-258 3) Sinclair JC. Servo-control for maintaining abdominal skin temperature at 36°C in low-birth-weight infants. *Cochrane Database Syst Rev* 2002;1:CD001074. 4)McCall, E.M. "Interventions to prevent hypothermia at birth in preterm and/or low birthweight babies." Cochrane Database of Systematic Reviews. Vol (3), 2007.5)Watkinson, M.A. "Temperature Control of Premature Infants in the Delivery Room." Clin Perinaol 33 (2006) 43–53.

* *Pearl/Peril/Pitfall:* Pyrexia may be caused by: *1. A HIGH ENVIRONMENTAL TEMPERATURE. This is usually due to the incubator or room being too hot for the infant's needs, or the infant being placed in the sun or too close to a heater. 2. INFECTION. However, most infants become hypothermic when infected.*

15 Infant of Diabetic Mother (IDM)

@Anticipate the effects maternal diabetes on the Newborn, such as macrosomia, acute metabolic complications and congenital malformations and monitor closely for alarming symptoms and manage promptly and appropriately."

Which of the following two babies could have been born to a Diabetic Mother ?

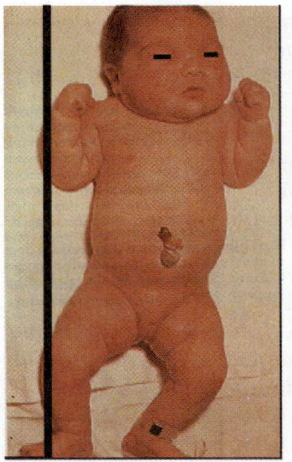 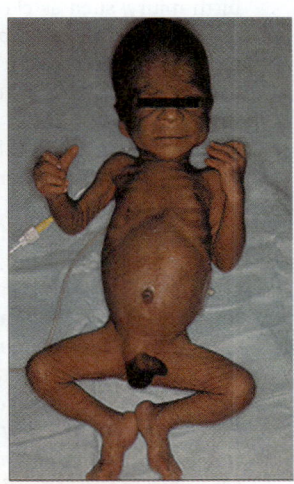

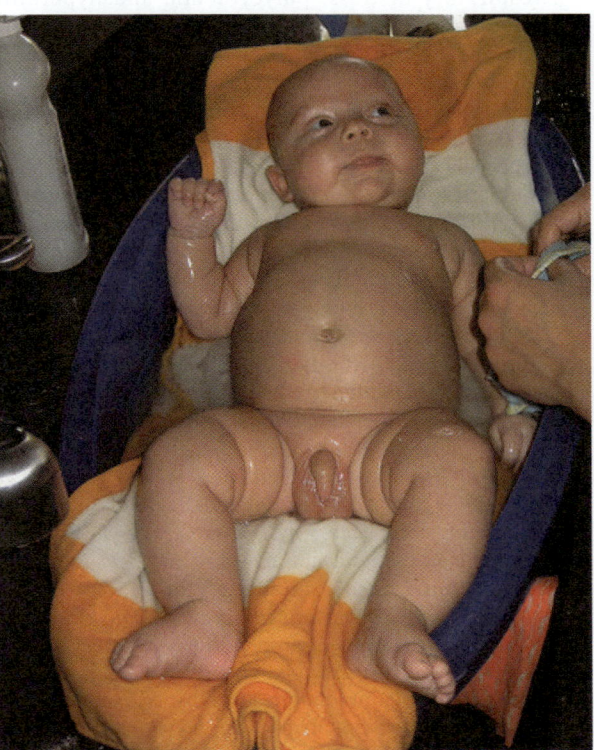

Big baby boy weighs in at 19-pounds at birth in North Sumatra

Sep 24, 2009 ... A woman in Indonesia has given birth to a **19-pound (8.5 kg) baby boy,** the heaviest birth ever recorded in the country.

REVIEW OF CLINICAL PROBLEMS

1. A Newborn infant of a diabetic mother, born at 37 weeks by an elective C/S with good APGARs and birth weight 4.25kg. developed tachypnea and cyanosis at 2 hrs of life. In addition to respiratory distress syndrome, what other possible causes should you consider in the differential diagnosis and investigate further? *Ans:Refer to "No. 7" of the "BIRD'S EYE VIEW/OVERVIEW/SYNOPSIS" of the Chapter.*

2. How often should you measure blood glucose levels in a Neonatal infant of diabetic mother, even if he is asymptomatic? When should you start IV glucose administration, instead of oral/gavage feedings? *Ans:refer to The E-D-A Plan/Algorithm to diagnose and manage a IDM with hypoglycemia)*

3. A neonatal infant of diabetic mother (IDM) developed "seizures" at 10hrs of age; in spite of correction and maintenance of hypoglycemia, hypocalcemia and hypo-magnesemia, the Neonate continued to have seizures. What could be the other possible underlying causes of his seizure activity? *Ans: Refer to "No. 8" of the "BIRD'S EYE VIEW/OVERVIEW/SYNOPSIS" of the Chapter.*

4. A Neonatal Infant of a Diabetic Mother (IDM) developed hematuria, hypertension, thrombocytopenia and abdominal distention on day 2 of life. What complication have occurred and what is the investigation of choice? *Ans:Refer to the "No. 9" of the "BIRD'S EYE VIEW/ OVERVIEW/SYNOPSIS" of the Chapter.*

5. What is the differential diagnosis of myocardial dysfunction that is due to diabetic cardiomyopathy of the Newborn? *Ans: Refer to the "No. 7" of the "BIRD'S EYE VIEW/ OVERVIEW/SYNOPSIS" of the Chapter.)*

LEARNING OBJECTIVES

After completing this article, readers will be able to:

1. Recognize adverse effects of maternal gestational diabetes on Neonatal infants.

2. Diagnose complications of gestational diabetes in Neonates.

3. Treat acute complications such as hypoglycemia, hypocalcemia, hypomagnesemia, mild to moderate respiratory distress and hyperbilirubinemia.

4. Anticipate severe complications such as severe respiratory distress enough to warrant CPAP, endotracheal intubation, surfactant replacement, and mechanical ventilation and to refer to the appropriate specialist center for further management.

5. Identify congenital abnormalities of the renal, cardiac, GIT and musculoskeletal system for referral to the higher center for specialist's advice.

*Pearl/Peril/Pitfall: Major causes of morbidity in an Infant of Diabetic Mother include the following: *Abnormalities in fetal growth (either overgrowth or undergrowth) *Hypoglycemia *Prematurity *Respiratory distress syndrome *Intrapartum asphyxia. Prior to birth, elevated insulin levels may inhibit the maturational effect of cortisol on the lung, including the production of surfactant from type 2 pneumocytes. This puts the fetus at risk for developing respiratory distress syndrome after birth at a gestational age normal lung function is expected.*

BIRD'S EYE VIEW/OVERVIEW/SYNOPSIS

1.' *Neonatal Infant of a Diabetic Mother (IDM)* is at significant risk for neonatal morbidity and mortality, when maternal blood glucose levels are not controlled adequately during pregnancy and periconceptional periods. Birth trauma and asphyxia from macrosomia, hypoglycemia, respiratory distress, polycythemia and hyperbilirubinemia and congenital anomalies are the common complications of IDM. Diabetic mothers have a high incidence of polyhydramnios, preeclampsia, pyelonephritis, preterm labor and chronic hypertension; their fetal mortality rate, which is high at all gestational ages, especially after 32 week, is greater than that of nondiabetic mothers. *Fetal loss throughout pregnancy is associated with poorly controlled maternal diabetes (especially ketoacidosis) and congenital anomalies.*

2. Gestational diabetes mellitus (accounts for 80-90% of cases), the mildest form of maternal diabetes that has its onset during the pregnancy, also increase the risk of perinatal loss. Although improved maternal care has reduced the incidence of this complication, *infants of women with gestational diabetes remain at increased risk of all of the morbidities except for congenital anomalies, subsequent obesity, and diabetes mellitus late in life.* Pregnancy in the insulin-dependent diabetic mother is commonly complicated by 1 or more of a wide variety of problems in the fetus and newborn *(Refer to Table No-1).*

3. Most infants born to diabetic mothers are large for gestational age. *If the diabetes is complicated by vascular disease, infants may be growth restricted, especially those born after 37 week gestation.* The neonatal mortality rate is over 5 times that of infants of nondiabetic mothers and is higher in all gestational ages and in every birth weight for gestational age category. Congenital anomalies in an infant of diabetic mother correlate with poor metabolic control during the periconception and organogenesis periods and may be due to hyperglycemia induced teratogenesis. Tight glucose control is paramount during the periconceptional period and throughout pregnancy, which requires coordinated care between endocrinologists, maternal-fetal medicine specialists, diabetes nurse educators, nutritionists. Treatment of infants of diabetic mothers should be initiated before birth by frequent prenatal evaluation of fetal maturity, by biophysical profile, by Doppler velocimetry, and by planning the delivery of these infants in hospitals where expert. Obstetric, and pediatric care is continuously available. *Periconception glucose control reduces the risk of anomalies, and glucose control during labor reduces the incidence of Neonatal hypoglycemia. (Refer to Table* 2 for managing a diabetic mom from periconception to peripartum).

4. *Refer to Figure 1,* for the proposed pathophysiology of development of abnormalities in the Neonatal Infant of a Diabetic Mother. Maternal hyperglycemia causes fetal hyperglycemia leading to fetal pancreatic islet beta cell hypertrophy and hyperplasia causing fetal hyperinsulinemia. Hyperinsulinism and Hyperglycemia produce fetal acidosis and may result in an increased rate of still birth. All the fetal and neonatal complications of diabetic pregnancy are the consequences of metabolic disturbances in the mother due to lack of insulin.

5. *One should anticipate the complications of IDM and monitor the Neonates who are depressed at birth closely for signs of perinatal injury and respiratory distress.* IDMs should be examined carefully for congenital anomalies with special attention to the respiratory, cardiac, renal, GIT and musculoskeletal systems. Seek after the signs birth injury, such as clavicular fractures and Erb's palsy. *IDM should be screened for hypoglycemia and polycythemia within 2 hrs of delivery or at the onset of symptoms.* Follow-up testing is dictated by the initial results and intervention applied.

6. Regardless of size, all infants of diabetic mothers should initially receive intensive observation and care. Asymptomatic infants should have a blood glucose determination within 1hr of birth and then every hour for the next 6-8 hours; if clinically well and normoglycemic, oral or gavage feeding with breast milk or formula should be started as soon as possible and continued at 3 hour intervals. *If any question arises about an infant's ability to tolerate oral feeding, the feeding should be discontinued and glucose given by IV infusion at a rate of 6-8 mgs/kg/mt (10% dextrose @ 80–120 ml/kg/day). (Refer to The E-D-A Plan/Algorithm).* Hyperbilirubinemia, birth asphyxia, polycythemia, RDS, IUGR, hypocalcemia, hypomagnesemia are often coexisting in infants of diabetic mothers and *need prompt evaluation and management.*

7. *Besides RDS, causes of respiratory distress and cyanosis in a IDM include* **a)**TTN by exclusion of other diagnoses **b)**Hypoglycemia **c)**Hypothermia **d)**Polycythemia **e)**Cardiac failure **f)**Pneumonia **g)** Pneumothorax **h)** Phrenic nerve palsy (associated usually with Erb's palsy) **i)**Cerebral edema from birth trauma or asphyxia. *Consider the following* in the differential diagnosis of myocardial dysfunction in an IDM **a)**Postasphyxial cardiomyopathy **b)** Myocarditis **c)** Endocardial fibroelastosis **d)** Glycogen storage disease of the heart **e)** ALCAPA (aberrant left coronary artery coming off the pulmonary artery).

8. Hypocalcemia, Hypomagnesemia, Hypoxic-ischemic encephalopathy due to birth trauma secondary to macrosomia and cerebral venous thrombosis secondary to polycythemia can cause seizures in an IDM.

9. *Renal vein thrombosis* presents with flank mass, hematuria, hypertension, abdominal distention and thrombocytopenia and it may occur *in utero* or after birth in male infants more often than females. Associated risk factors in addition to diabetic mother include; perinatal asphyxia, hypotension, polycythemia, increased blood viscosity and cyanotic congenital heart disease. Ultrasonography of abdomen is the investigation of choice. Management is conservative usually.

10. IDM requires close surveillance and interdisciplinary collaboration among obstetricians, nutritionists, perinatologists, pediatricians and sometimes endocrinologists. The closer to physiologic range of mother's blood glucose is maintained, the better the neonatal outcome.

Pearl/Peril/Pitfall: Infants with feeding intolerance, abdominal distention, nonbilious emesis, or poor passage of meconium may require a barium enema. Congenital anomalies of the GI tract are more common in infants of diabetic mothers. These infants may have "small left colon syndrome," also known as "lazy colon."

THE EVALUATION-DECISION-ACTION-PLAN/ALGORITHM FOR THE DIAGNOSIS AND MANAGEMENT OF *A NEONATAL INFANT OF DIABETIC MOTHER (IDM)*

SUBJECTIVE FINDINGS

Take details of **current pregnancy**- severity of maternal diabetes, level of glycemic control (blood glucose and HbA$_{1c}$) mothers retinal and renal health and medications (antihypertensive and thyroid), fetal maturity assessments by biophysical profile and doppler velocimetry. **Delivery details**- mode of delivery, APGAR scores and resuscitation details. **Neonatal presentation** -respiratory distress, cyanosis, poor feeding, convulsions, tremors, lethargy, apathy, apnea, abnormal cry, cardiac arrest etc.

Details of previous pregnancies and outcome-

OBJECTIVE FINDINGS

Assess ABCs, vital signs, O$_2$ sats, work of breathing, central cyanosis, CRT, urine output, signs suggestive of sepsis, birth asphyxia and CCF.

Look for a typical plump, plethoric and large infant of a diabetic mother and *examine him* for obvious and occult congenital malformations *(Refer to Table 1)* *Assess* cardiac impulse, heart sounds, gallop, murmurs, breath sounds, rales, hepatomegaly. *Assess for* symptoms and signs of hypoglycemia, hypocalcemia and/or hypomagnesemia-jumpy, tremulous, hyperexcitable, hypotonic, lethargic with poor suck. *Perform* complete systemic examination to identify signs and symptoms of birth trauma, asphyxia, renal, hematological and neurological complications of IDM

INVESTIGATIONS

Blood FBC with hematocrit and platelets, ABG analysis with electrolytes, calcium^{++}, Mg^{++}, BUN and creatinine, urine analysis and culture, blood culture if infection is suspected, *Blood glucose serial monitoring protocol.*

Imaging Chest X-ray for RDS, Echocardiogram for HOCM or a cardiac anomaly (along with ECG), renal ultrasound examination for suspected renal vein thrombosis, contrast enema studies for suspected small left colon syndrome, abdominal x-ray for duodenal atresia, MRI brain scanning for HIE and cerebral venous thrombosis, MRI spine for neural tube defects.

NEONATAL INFANT OF DIABETIC MOTHER (IDM)

Perform IV access and correct hypoglycemia, hypocalcemia, hypomagnesemia and *maintain* normothermia and electrolytes

Apply CPAP and if necessary *intubate and ventilate* along with *surfactant administration*, in any IDM manifested as severe respiratory distress

Identify signs of perinatal trauma and asphyxia and evaluate and manage further (Refer to the chapters on birth trauma and birth asphyxia) (HIE)

Ensure ABCs, give supplemental oxygen, pulse oximetry, CR monitor and BP.

Catheterize the bladder to monitor urine output in any sick IDM.

Give IV broadspectrum antibiotics to cover for sepsis

Identify the obvious congenital anomalies and *organize* appropriate *referrals* to the concerned specialists

---

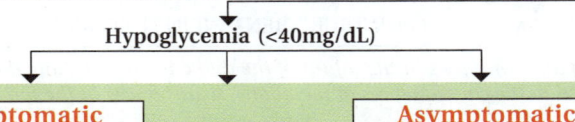

Hypoglycemia (<40mg/dL)

Anticipate the other complications of IDM and *Manage* accordingly!

Asymptomatic normal dextrostix	* **Symptomatic** ** **Sick** * **Bwt. < 2 kg** * **Blood Glucose <**	Asymptomatic BS < 40 mg/dL

Asymptomatic normal dextrostix

* Feed
* Do Dstix
1 Feed at or before 1 hour, by 10% Dextrose 5ml/kg by bottle or gavage

2 Give hourly formula feeds for 3–4 feeds

3 If Dstix WNL feed 2 hourly and later 3 hourly and ↑Volume of feed

* **Symptomatic**
** **Sick**
* **Bwt. < 2 kg**
* **Blood Glucose < 40 mg/dL after enteral feeds for two hours**
* **Not retaining feed -Vomiting**

Start Parenteral Rx | If | no → Seizures

Seizures + RDS

25% Dextrose Push 2–4 ml/kg @ 1ml/ mt

Dextrose IVI 6–8 mg/kg/ min (10% D/W at 80–120 ml/kg/day)

Asymptomatic BS < 40 mg/dL

No bolus but Push 5–10 ml of 10% Dextrose at 1 ml/ min, followed by

Dextrose IVI @ 4–8mg/kg/min (10% D/ W @ 60-120ml/kg/day)

10% Dextrose Push (2ml/kg over 2–3 mts)

Give IM hydrocortisone 5 mg/kg/ day in 2 divided doses in difficult cases!

* Check capillary blood glucose levels at 1,2,3,6,12,24, and 48 hrs. * Readings below 40mg/dL on Dextrostix should be verified by serum glucose measurements. * Other drugs like Epinephrine, diazoxide, or growth hormone are rarely required, apart from hydrocortisone. * If IV access is difficult, IM/SC crystalline Glucagon 300mcg/kg to a maximum dose of 1mg can cause rapid rise in blood levels which may last 2-3hrs and is useful until IV glucose can be started * Consider other causes of hypoglycemia, such as islet-cell hyperplasia, Beckwith-Wiedemann syndrome, hypopituitarism, and hereditary congenital metabolic disorders, if infants fail to respond to conventional therapy for hypoglycemia.

1. *Polycythemia - defined as a central venous hematocrit more ≥ 65% with/without signs, such as plethora, lethargy, feed intolerance, apnea, respiratory distress and CNS symptoms. Consider symptomatic infants or asymptomatic infants with >70% hematocrit for partial exchange transfusion with normal saline (30ml/kg) to decrease the hematocrit to about 50%.*

2. *Hyperbilirubinemia (>15mg/dL) - due to polycythemia, prematurity, impaired hepatic conjugation, poor feeding with increased enterohepatic circulation of bilirubin, requires phototherapy or rarely double volume exchange transfusion (170ml/kg).*

3. *Hypocalcemia (ionized calcium <3mg/dL) and Hypomagnesemia (serum Mg <1.5mg/dL) - present with lethargy, poor feeding, irritability, jitteriness, tetany, and seizures. Give IV 10% Calcium gluconate 0.5-1ml/kg diluted 1:4 with 10% dextrose with continuous cardiac monitoring over 10–15 minutes or until seizures cease. Give Magnesium Sulphate 50% 0.2ml/kg IV or IM as a single dose or every 6hrs until normalization of Magnesium levels to correct hypomagnesemia accompanying hypocalcemia. Both are transient and do not warrant aggressive correction in asymptomatic infants.*

4. *Hypertrophic Obstructive Cardiomyopathy (HOCM - diagnosed by Echocardiogram) - rarely requires specific therapy (propranolol) and usually resolves spontaneously by 2–12 weeks. Inotropic drugs are contraindicated.*

5. *Renal vein thrombosis (diagnosed by ultrasonography of the abdomen) - presents with flank mass, hypertension, hematuria, abdominal distention and thrombocytopenia. Management is conservative in approach, but bilateral RVT + inferior vena caval extension, with renal dysfunction requires anticoagulation with heparin.*

---

* **Pearl/Peril/Pitfall:** *A suggestion of operational thresholds for Hypoglycemia in an Infant of Diabetic Mom was proposed by Cornblath et al. Their suggestion in an infant with compromised metabolic adaptation (i.e. infant of diabetic mother) should include blood glucose measurements (1) as soon as possible after birth, (2) within 2–3 hours after birth and before feeding, and (3) at any time abnormal clinical signs are observed.*

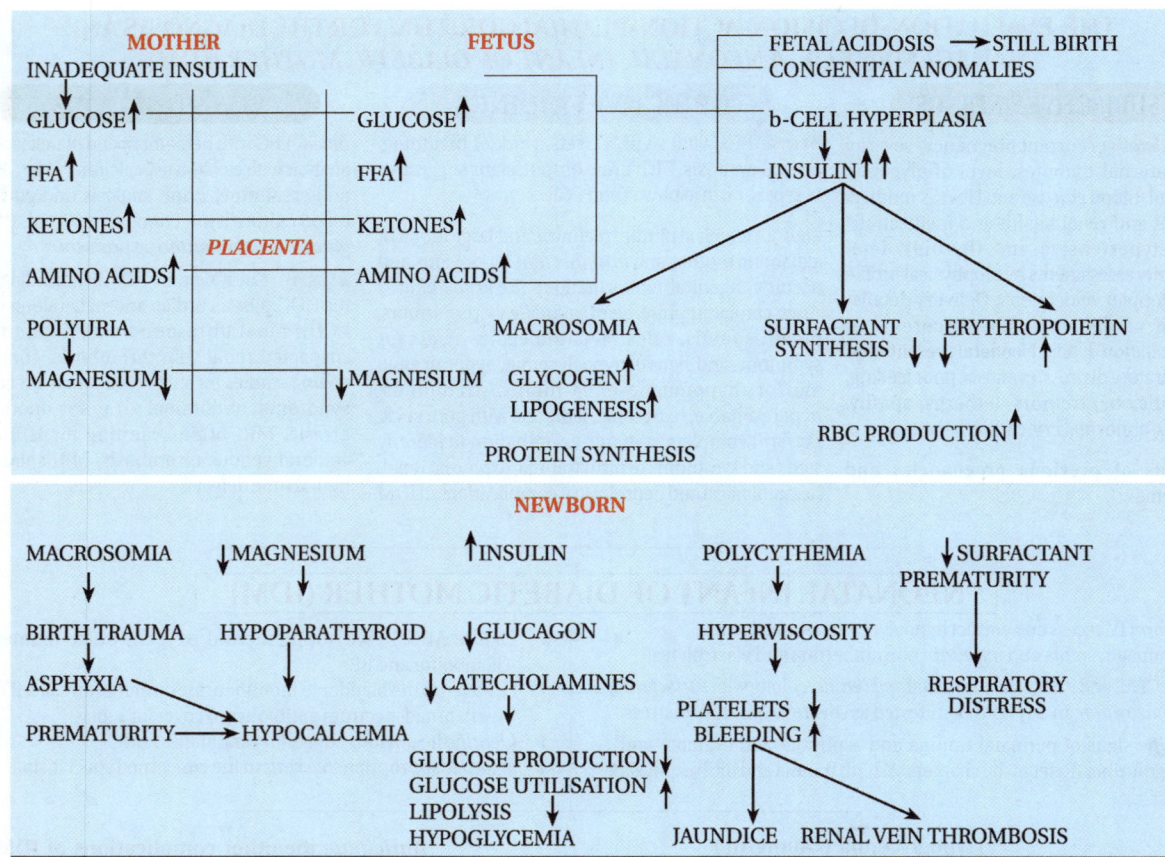

Fig. 1: *Proposed pathophysiology of development of abnormalities in the infant of the diabetic mother. Note that all the fetal and neonatal complications are attributed to the consequences of metabolic disturbances in the mother following inadequate insulin.*

TABLE 1	Common problems in the fetus and newborn due to poorly/inadequately controlled insulin dependent maternal diabetes

- Sudden fetal death late in the 3rd trimester
- Premature birth from early induction of labor to avoid 3rd trimester fetal death
- Macrosomia (large, plump with puffy and plethoric facies)
- Birth trauma as result of macrosomia
- Intrapartum asphyxia
- C/S delivery to avoid birth trauma and intrapartum asphyxia
- Intrauterine growth retardation (if delivered term or the mother has associated vascular disease)
- Neonatal respiratory distress syndrome (Tachypnea develops in many infants of diabetic mothers during the first 2 days of life and may be a manifestation of hypoglycemia, hypothermia, polycythemia, cardiac failure, transient tachypnea, or cerebral edema from birth trauma or asphyxia)
- Hypoglycemia (25–50% of infants of diabetic mothers and 15–25% of infants of mothers with gestational diabetes)

- Hypocalcemia and Hypomagnesemia
- Hyperbilirubinemia
- Hyperviscosity (polycythemia) syndrome
- Renal vein thrombosis (flank mass, hematuria and thrombocytopenia)
- Cardiomyopathy -(Cardiomegaly 30% , heart failure 5-10%) Asymmetric septal hypertrophy (mimics IHSS)
- Congenital anomalies (3 fold increase)
- Cardiac—VSD, ASD,TGA, Truncus, double outlet right ventricle, Coarctation of aorta
- Lumbosacral agenesis, Neural tube defects
- Renal - Agenesis, dysplasia, double ureter
- GIT - Duodenal or anorectal atresia, small left colon syndrome
- CNS- Holoprosencephaly
- Increased risk of obesity and of diabetes mellitus in later life

TABLE 2	Maternal diabets affecting fetus and newborn—monitoring, management and follow-up

Periconception period: Counsel the diabetic mom about the level of glycemic control, current status of the patient's retinal and renal health, any medications being taken (e.g., antihypertensive or thyroid medications) and risk of complications. *Establish* a regimen of frequent, regular monitoring of capillary glucose levels. *Adopt* an insulin dosing regimen to ensure a smooth interprandial glucose profile (fasting glucose 80-100mg/dL, 2- hour postprandial glucose< 120 mg /dL, no reactions between meals or at night). *Bring* Hb A$_{1c}$ level into the normal range. *Develop* family, financial, and personal resources to assist the patient

should pregnancy complications necessitate lost time from job or bed rest.

Antenatal Period: The goals of glycemic monitoring, dietary regulation and insulin therapy in diabetic pregnancy are to prevent the postnatal sequelae of the diabetes in the Newborn *(refer to table 1). Institute* these measures early and aggressively if they are to be effective. *Diet* should contain 50-60% carbohydrate, 12-20% protein, <10% saturated fatty acids, and upto 10% PUFA. *3 major* meals and 3 snacks are preferred and always

* Pearl/Peril/Pitfall: *Communication between members of the perinatal team is of crucial importance to identify infants who are at highest risk of complications from maternal diabetes.*

avoid single, large meals and foods with a large percentage of simple carbohydrates. *any* insulin regimen for pregnant women must be designed to avoid excessive unopposed insulin action during the fasting state. *Use* of regular insulin before each major meal helps limit postprandial hyperglycemia. *To provide* basal insulin levels between feedings, a longer- acting preparation is necessary, such as NPH or lente. *Typical* dose ratios are 2:3 of total insulin in the morning, with 2:3 intermediate acting insulin and 1:3 regular insulin.

Prenatal obstetric management: Perform periodic fetal biophysical testing *(fetal movement counting, nonstress test, contraction stress test, and ultrasound biophysical profile)* at frequent intervals staring from 28 weeks of gestational age. In lower risk patients, one can start fetal testing by 34 weeks. *Plot* fetal growth parameters serially (typically every 1.5–3 weeks). *Select* the timing of delivery, to minimize maternal and neonatal morbidity and mortality. *An optimal* time for delivery of most diabetic pregnancies is between 38.5 and 40 weeks *(traditionally, delivery was at 36–38 weeks to avoid still birth). Verify* the fetal lung maturity (>3% phosphotidyl glycerol in amniotic fluid specimen), if the delivery should be performed before 38.5 weeks. *In patients* with gestational diabetes and superb glycemic control, continued fetal testing and expectant management can be considered until 41 weeks. *Deliver* the baby where there are good neonatal facilities.

Intrapartal glycemic management: Maintain intrapartum euglycemia, to avoid fetal hypoxemia and to promote a smooth postnatal infant transition. *Monitor* capillary blood glucose levels hourly and use a combination of insulin and glucose infusion during labor to maintain blood glucose between 80-120mg/dL(typical infusion rate for 5% Dextrose in Ringer Lactate is 100ml/hr and for regular insulin at 0.5–1 unit /hr). *Beware* of shoulder dystocia with macrosomic babies and arrange C/S if labor is prolonged. *Return* to pre-pregnancy insulin levels, 24 hrs postpartum. *Liaise* with pediatricians, who are skilled at resuscitation and about the neonatal management of various problems in the Newborn secondary to maternal diabetes.

Postnatal management: If breast feeding, oral hypoglycemics are contraindicated. *Encourage* pre-pregnancy counseling before next pregnancy to transfer to insulin. *Do* a postpartum glucose tolerance test (5% of those with gestational diabetes will be insulin dependent in < 5 years and 50% develop NIDDM in < 10years). *Advising* exercise and *avoiding* obesity and smoking lower this risk.

Neonatal management: Anticipate birth asphyxia and birth trauma and resuscitate appropriately. *Monitor* and manage hypoglycemia as per the protocol. Correct hypocalcemia, hypomagnesemia, hyperviscosity, and polycythemia (hematocrit > 65%), hyperbilirubinemia, CCF due to hypertropic/congestive cardiomyopathy and manage respiratory distress syndrome as per the standard protocol depending on its severity.

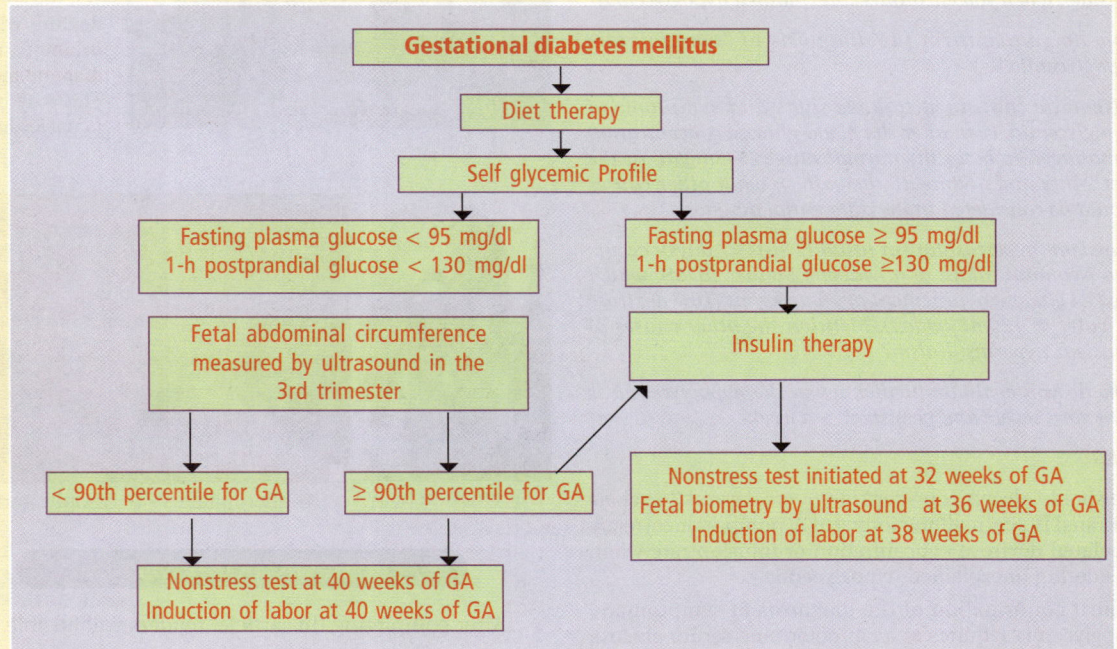

Gestational diabetes mellitus

Diet therapy

Self glycemic Profile

Fasting plasma glucose < 95 mg/dl
1-h postprandial glucose < 130 mg/dl

Fasting plasma glucose ≥ 95 mg/dl
1-h postprandial glucose ≥130 mg/dl

Fetal abdominal circumference measured by ultrasound in the 3rd trimester

Insulin therapy

< 90th percentile for GA

≥ 90th percentile for GA

Nonstress test initiated at 32 weeks of GA
Fetal biometry by ultrasound at 36 weeks of GA
Induction of labor at 38 weeks of GA

Nonstress test at 40 weeks of GA
Induction of labor at 40 weeks of GA

KEY POINTS FOR CLINICAL PRACTICE

1. Most of the complications in IDM are preventable; others could be anticipated and managed appropriately to ensure uneventful transition to extrauterine life; periconception glucose control of a diabetic mother reduces the risk of congenital anomalies and peripartal glucose control reduces the incidence of neonatal hypoglycemia.

2. IDMs are usually large for gestational age, but they may also be of normal or low birth weight, particularly if delivered before term or the mother has associated vascular disease which causes IUGR.

3. All IDMs should have proper resuscitation care and intensive observation for hypoglycemia, respiratory distress, hypocalcemia + hypomagnesemia, polycythemia + hyperbilirubinemia and birth asphyxia and trauma need prompt evaluation and management.

4. IDM requires close surveillance and interdisciplinary collaboration among obstetricians, nutritionists, perinatologists, pediatricians and sometimes endocrinologists.

5. IDMs should be examined carefully for congenital anomalies with special attention to the respiratory, cardiac, renal, GIT, and musculoskeletal systems and should be evaluated accordingly at a tertiary neonatal center.

REFERENCES AND FURTHER READING: (1)Nold JL, Georgieff MK: Infants of diabetic mothers. PCNA 2004 (2)Persson B, Hanson U: Neonatal morbidities in gestational diabetes. Diabetes Care 1998 3)Cowett RM: The infant of the diabetic mother 1991 4)Nelson Text Book of Pediatrics 18th edition 2008. (5)Manual of Neonatal Care by Cloherty 6th ed 2008

*Pearl/Peril/Pitfall: If the infant requires a dextrose concentration more than D12.5 through a peripheral vein at 80-100 mL/kg/d, placement of a central venous catheter may be considered to avoid venous sclerosis. Continued enteral feedings hasten improvement in glucose control because of the presence of protein and fat in the formula. Hydrocortisone therapy may be required for ongoing hypoglycemia.

Neonatal Hypoglycemia

16

@ *"It is important to anticipate hypoglycemia and prevent it in high risk Newborn babies, since it is easily treatable and can occur in infants who appear well, which can lead to neurodevelopmental sequelae "*

Hypoglycemia is common to these 4 different Neonatal Problems.

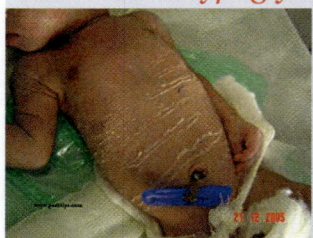 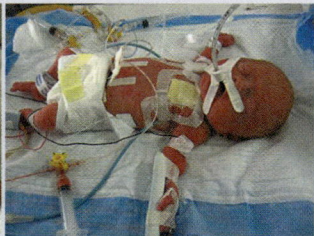

REVIEW OF CLINICAL PROBLEMS

1. *What sort of "mechanical errors" (iatrogenic), should you consider, when you encounter unexplained hypoglycemia?*

2. *How do you confirm the diagnosis of "symptomatic hypoglycemia"?*

3. *A Neonate continued to have signs and symptoms of hypoglycemia, even after the blood glucose concentration is managed to be in the normal range (>45mg/dL in the first 24hrs and >50mg/dL thereafter); what other causes should be considered in the differential diagnosis?*

4. *Transient hyperinsulinism (usually lasts <7 days) occurs in a Neonatal Infant of a Diabetic Mother (IDM), which needs a glucose requirement of >8mg/kg/mt (10% dextrose in water @ 120ml/kg/day). Mention the other causes of transient hyperinsulinism?*

5. *How do you evaluate further, when the hypoglycemia is refractory, severe and persistent > a week?*

ANSWERS

1. One should always consider "*mechanical errors*" such as infiltrated IV site, malfunctioning of IV pump, or incorrectly calculated dextrose concentration or infusion rate when considering unexplained hypoglycemia.

2. Clinical confirmation of the diagnosis of symptomatic hypoglycemia requires a) a lab-determine serum glucose level of <40mg/dL at the time of symptoms and b) prompt resolution of the symptoms with the administration of IV glucose and correction of the hypoglycemia.

3. In this situation, one should consider a) sepsis b) CNS disease c) adrenal insufficiency d) metabolic abnormalities, such as hypocalcemia, hypomagnesemia, hypo/hyper natremia, pyridoxine deficiency e) heart failure f) renal failure g) liver failure h) toxic exposure.

4. *"Transient hyperinsulinism"* occurs in infants a) with IUGR b) erythroblastosis fetalis c) maternal drug exposure (beta-blockers, chlorpropamide, beta-mimetics and oral hypoglycemics) d) improper position of umbilical artery catheter located near T11-T12 and e) Neonatal Infant of Diabetic Mother (IDM).

5. *Refer to Tables 1 and 2* for lab studies and interpretation in the evaluation of refractory and persistent hypoglycemia.

1) Newborn babies with **IUGR** often appear thin, pale, and have loose, dry skin. The umbilical cord is often thin and dull-looking rather than shiny and fat. Babies with IUGR sometimes have a wide-eyed look. Some babies do not have this malnourished appearance but are small allover.

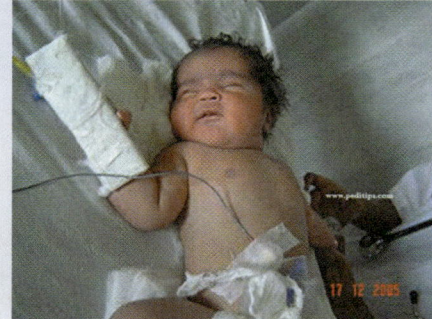

2) The plethora on the face, and the yellowish hue to the pink cherubic cheeks, in a newborn who is little overweight; yes; you are surely dealing with an **infant of a diabetic mother**. This may be due to polycythemia.

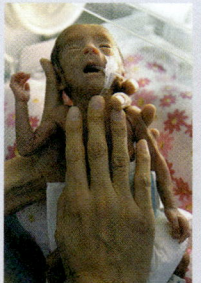 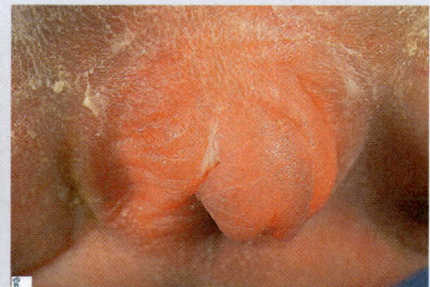

3) Premature baby

4) Microphallus - ? Hypopituitarism

LEARNING OBJECTIVES

After completing this article, readers will be able to

1. Anticipate hypoglycemia in high risk Neonates and to identify the nonspecific symptoms and signs of hypoglycemia with a high index of suspicion.
2. Make a reliable measurement of low blood glucose level and to ensure resolution of signs and symptoms after blood glucose level is restored to normal range.
3. Understand the importance of preventing hypoglycemia in high risk Neonates and to initiate IV glucose therapy if hypoglycemia is symptomatic.
4. Consider other causes, such as sepsis, CNS disease, other metabolic problems, adrenal insufficiency, heart failure, renal failure and liver failure in the differential diagnosis of hypoglycemia.
5. Diagnose and Manage Hyperinsulinism related Hypoglycemia.

Pearl/Peril/Pitfall: *Take 5 ml of blood from these infants for glucose and insulin estimation before giving the hydrocortisone. This is very important in identifying the correct cause of the hypoglycemia. Glucagon 0,3 mg/kg IM or IV can be used if hydrocortisone fails to correct the blood glucose concentration.*

1. Neonatal hypoglycemia, i.e. a serum glucose level < 40mg/dL at any time, in any Newborn deserves evaluation and treatment with a goal to maintain the glucose level > 40mg/dL in the first day and > 40-50mg/dL thereafter. Serum glucose levels decline after birth until 1–3 hr of age, when levels spontaneously increase in normal infant. Both premature and fullterm infants are at risk for serious neurodevelopmental deficits from equally low glucose levels. This risk is related to depth and duration of the hypoglycemia. The absence of overt symptoms at low glucose levels doesn't rule out CNS injury. There is no evidence indicating that the premature or young infant is being protected from the effects of inadequate glucose delivery to the CNS.

2. Confirmation of the diagnosis of symptomatic hypoglycemia requires both of the following : 1) a lab-determined serum glucose level of < 40mg/dL at the time symptoms are present such as lethargy, apathy, limpness, apnea, cyanosis, weak or high - pitched cry, seizures, coma, poor feeding and vomiting, tremors, jitteriness, or irritability. 2) prompt resolution of the symptoms with the administration of IV glucose 10%, 4ml/kg (if seizures present) or 2ml/kg (if symptoms, other than seizures present) and correction of the hypoglycemia.

3. Many Neonates with low serum glucose levels are asymptomatic but are at increased risk for neuro-developmental sequelae, whereas normoglycemic infants may have nonspecific signs of hypoglycemia. It is important to anticipate hypoglycemia in both the Newborn nursery and the NICU and evaluate babies with either risk factors for hypoglycemia (refer to tables 3 and 4) or symptoms, because hypoglycemia is usually easily treatable and can occur in infant who appear well.

4. Infants at increased risk for hypoglycemia should have their serum glucose measured within 1 hr of birth, every 1–2 hr for the 1st 6-8 hr, and then every 4–6 hr until 24 hr of life. Normoglycemic high-risk infants should receive oral or gavage feeding with human milk or formula started at 1–3 hr of age and continued at 2–3 hr intervals for 24–48 hr. Initial bolus of 10% Dextrose 2–4ml/kg always is to be followed by an intravenous infusion of glucose at the rate of 4–8 mg/kg/min, to prevent rebound hyper/hypoglycemia (10% Dextrose at a rate of 110ml/kg/day or 4.6ml/kg/hr gives 8mg/kg/mt of glucose) should be provided if oral feedings are poorly tolerated or if asymptomatic transient neonatal hypoglycemia develops. Recheck glucose level after 20–30 minutes and hourly until stable, to determine if additional therapy is needed.

5. *The Evaluation-Decision-Action-Plan/Algorithm* to diagnose and manage Neonatal hypoglycemia summarizes the essential aspects of history, physical examination, relevant investigations and emergent management. If a reagent strip reveals a concentration < 40mgs/dL blood glucose, treatment should not be delayed while one is awaiting confirmation of hypoglycemia by laboratory analysis of serum glucose which is about 15% higher than blood glucose measured by the reagent strip. Treatment should be initiated immediately after the confirmatory lab. Blood sample is obtained.

6. The differential diagnosis of Neonatal Hypoglycemia includes many other causes with or without associated hypoglycemia. If symptoms persist after the glucose concentration is in the normal range, one should consider other etiologies such as a)adrenal insufficiency b) maternal drug use c) heart disease d) renal failure e) liver failure f) CNS disease g) metabolic abnormalities like hypocalcemia, hypo/hypernatremia, hypo-magnesemia, and pyridoxine deficiency h) sepsis i) asphyxia.

7. Persisting /recurring hypoglycemia over a period of > 7 days needs further studies to help differentiate a metabolic defect, hypopituitarism and hyper-insulinism (refer to tables 1 and 2).

8. In cases of persistent hypoglycemia, consult a Pediatric endocrinologist and continue to increase the rate of IV glucose administration to 16–20mg/kg/mt (9.2–11.5ml/kg/mt of 10% Dextrose). Consider a trial of IV hydrocortisone 5mg/kg/day every 12 hr, or Prednisone 2mg/kg/day orally daily. If hypoglycemia persists, consider adding the following drugs to the IV hydrocortisone. a) Human Growth Hormone - 0.1unit/day IM b) Diazoxide IV 3-5mg/kg/dose; repeat in 20 minutes if no effect c) Somato-statin (octreotide) 2–10 mcg/kg/day subcuta-neously divided every 6–8 hr, or by continuous IV infusion (maximum dose 40mcg/kg/day) d) glucagon 0.3mg/kg/dose SC /IM ; may repeat in 20 minutes prn e) susphrine 0.005–0.01ml/kg/dose S/C, given every 6 hour) subtotal pancreatectomy may be necessary for insulin secreting tumours.

9. Glucose rate calculator (Refer to Quintessential Quick Reference Section) helps to determine the rate of glucose infusion being given and to modify the concentration of IV glucose and volume of the IV fluid to be given in a day, in relation to the frequently monitored serum glucose levels in high risk babies. If > 12.5% IV glucose solution is required, a central venous catheter will have to be placed.

10. Most hypoglycemias will resolve in 2–3 days. A requirement of > 8mgs of glucose/kg/minute (>4.6ml/kg/hr of 10% Dextrose) suggests increased utilization due to hyperinsulinism. This is usually transient in infants of diabetic mothers. If it lasts > 7 days, endocrine evaluation may be necessary to rule out excess insulin secretion from an insulin secreting tumor or other causes listed in the Table 4. The prognosis for normal intellectual function must be guarded because prolonged, recurrent, and severe symptomatic infants with hypoglycemia (particularly LBW infants, persistent hyper-insulinism states and infants of diabetic mother) is associated with neurologic sequelae.

Pearl/Peril/Pitfall: In an emergency, if you are unable to give intravenous dextrose, give the infant 10 ml/kg breast milk or formula (or cow's milk if neither is available) by mouth or via a nasogastric tube. You can add 5 ml (a teaspoon) of sugar, or 5 ml of 50% dextrose, per 10 ml feed to increase the glucose concentration. Do not give pure 50% dextrose as it will cause vomiting.

THE EVALUATION-DECISION-ACTION-PLAN/ALGORITHM FOR THE DIAGNOSIS AND MANAGEMENT OF *NEONATAL HYPOGLYCEMIA*

SUBJECTIVE FINDINGS

Hx of nonspecific symptoms lethargy, apathy, limpness, weak or high - pitched cry, cyanosis, seizures, coma, poor feeding, vomiting, tremors, jitteriness, irritability, temperature instability.

Hx of asymptomatic hypoglycemia on careful observation and random screening for repeated low glucose concentrations in high risk babies *(refer to table 4)*.

Hx suggestive of sepsis, asphyxia, hypothermia, infant of diabetic mother, IUGR/premature babies, abrupt cessation of high-glucose infusions (iatrogenic), maternal drugs.

OBJECTIVE FINDINGS

Assess ABCDs, O_2 sats, CRT, urine output, hypo/hyperthermia and signs suggestive of sepsis, asphyxia, IUGR/large for dates and prematurity.

Look for jitteriness, tremors, seizures, apnea, coma and cyanosis.

Look for features suggestive of Beckwith-Weidemann syndrome (macroglossia, omphalocele, macrosomia, mild microcephaly, visceromegaly + hypoglycemia).

Identify hypothyroidism, hypopituitarism, adrenal insufficiency, infant of diabetic mother, glycogen storage disease, CHD etc.,

INVESTIGATIONS

FBC with differential, blood cultures, CRP to evaluate for sepsis and to rule out polycythemia.

A serum glucose level should be obtained to confirm the bedside reagent determination, *hypoglycemia is defined as a serum glucose value < 40mg/dL and a blood glucose (reagent) value < 35 mg/dL.*

In cases of persistent hypoglycemia - for follow-up studies and interpretation, *refer to Tables 1 and 2.*

A neonate with hypoglycemia (high risk or symptomatic Neonate)

Ensure ABCs, pulse oximetry, CR monitoring, *intubate and ventilate* if apneic and cyanosed. *Check* blood glucose (dextrostix) and *send* sample to the lab. for serum glucose

Ensure recommended screening for hypoglycemia

Baby diagnosis	Glucose sample timing
SFD	2, 6, 12, 24, 36, 48 hours prefeed.
Preterm	2 hours and 6–12 hourly until levels reliably above 45mg/dL and tolerating feeds.
HIE	On admission; 2, 6, 12, 24 hours or regularly during IPPV as for serious illness
Serious illness	6–12 hourly during illness
IDM	On admission and at 2, 6, 12, 24 hours or until two consecutive samples are above 45mg/dL
Hemolytic disease	1,2 and 4 hours after an exchange transfusion of the Newborn
Fitting or excessive jittering	Immediately

HIGH RISK OR SYMPTOMATIC NEONATE

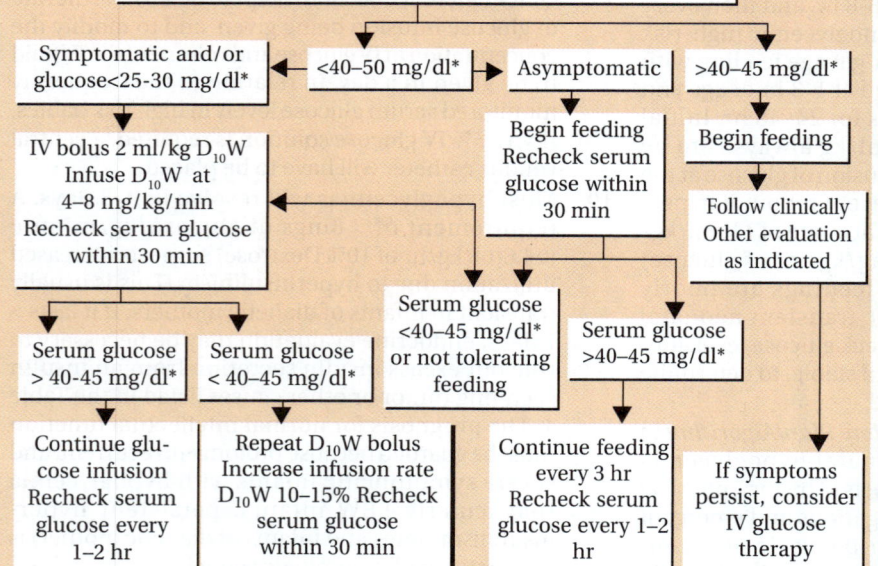

Adjunct therapies for persistent neonatal hypoglycemia

Corticosteroids
Decreases peripheral glucose utilization—Hydrocortisone 5–15 mg/kg/d or Prednisone 2mg/kg/d

Glucagon
Stimulates glycogenolysis - 30μg/kg with normal insulin, 300μg/kg with hyperinsulinemia

Diazoxide
Inhibits insulin secretion 2–5mg/kg/dose orally q8hr

Somatostatin (long acting octreotide)
Inhibits insulin and growth hormone release 5–10μg/kg every 6-8hour

Subtotal pancreatectomy
Decreases insulin secretion causes diabetes and pancreatic insufficiency

---

***Pearl/Peril/Pitfall:** Infants with severe hypoglycemia(Blood Glucose <25mg/dL) should have their blood glucose concentration measured every 15 minutes until it has increased above 25mg/dL. Then measure the blood glucose concentration hourly for 3 hours and then 3 hourly until 100 ml/kg milk feeds are established.*

TABLE 1 Follow-up studies in case of persisting /recurring hypoglycemia over a period of > 7 days

Mandatory
- Laboratory blood sugar*
- Plasma cortisol*
- Plasma insulin*

Consider
- Investigations for IEM:
  - Plasma lactate, free fatty acids, hydroxybutyrate (1.5mL blood in fluoride oxalate bottle)*
  - Urinary organic acids and amino acids*

- Urine-reducing sugars * or RBC galactose-1 phosphate uridyl transferase level
- plasma triglyceride and urate*
- infection screen including LP
- Investigations for hypopituitarism (especially if unstable temperature or small penis):
  - cerebral USS (+/- MRI or CT scan)
  - random GH, thyroid function tests - synacthen test
- Abdominal USS for hyperinsulinemic hypoglycemia

* These samples must be taken when the child is hypoglycemic. Take : 1-2 mL in lithium heparin bottle ; 1–2 mL in fluoride oxalate bottle ; 6–10 mL of urine. Detailed investigation can subsequently be agreed with the metabolic laboratory.

TABLE 2 Diagnosis of persistent hypoglycemia before and after parenteral glucagon administration

Variable	Hyperinsulinism Before	After	Hypopituitarism Before	After	Metabolic defect Before	After
Glucose	↓	↑↑↑	↓	↑ / N	↓	↓ /N
Ketones	↓	↓	N/ ↓	N	↑	↑
Free fatty acids	↓	↑	N/ ↓	N	↑	↑
Lactate	N	N	N	N	↑	↑↑
Alanine	N	?	N	N	↑	↑↑
Uric acid	N	N	N	N	↑	↑↑
Insulin	↑↑	↑↑↑	N/↓	↑	N	↑
Growth hormone	↑	↓	↓	↓	↑	↑
Cortisol	↑	↓	↓a	↓a	↑	↑
TSH and T$_4$	N	N	↓a	↓a	N	N

N, normal or no change ; ↑, elevated ; ↓, lowered ; ?, unknown ; TSH, thyroid-stimulating hormone ; T$_4$, thyroxine, [a]Response may vary depending on the degree of hypopituitarism. *Courtesy of Marcin Cornblath, MD, Baltimore, Maryland.*

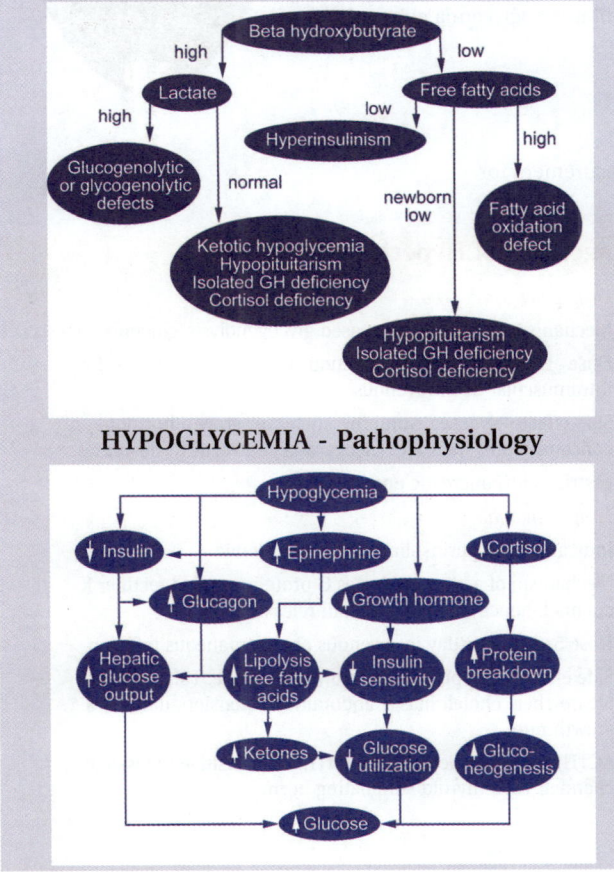

HYPOGLYCEMIA - Pathophysiology

TABLE 3 Neonatal hypoglycemia : etiologies and time course

Mechanism	Clinical setting	Expected duration
Decreased substrate availability	Intrauterine growth restriction	Transient
	Prematurity	Transient
	Glycogen storage disease	Prolonged
	Inborn errors eg, fructose intolerance)	Prolonged
Endocrine disturbances		
Hyperinsulinemia	Infant of diabetic mother	Transient
	Beckwith-Wiedemann syndrome	Prolonged
	Erythroblastosis fetalis	Transient
	Exchange transfusion	Transient
	Islet cell dysplasias	Prolonged
	Maternal β-agonist tocolytics	Transient
	Improperly placed umbilical artery catheter	Transient
Other endocrine disorders	Hypopituitarism	Prolonged
	Hypothyroidism	Prolonged
	Adrenal insufficiency	Prolonged
Increased utilization	Perinatal asphyxia	Transient
	Hypothermia	Transient
Miscellaneous/ Multiple mechanisms	Sepsis	Transient
	Congenital heart disease	Transient
	CNS abnormalities	Prolonged

Pearl/Peril/Pitfall: *Infants with mild hypoglycemia(Blood Glucose 25-35 mg/dL) should be monitored every 30 minutes until the blood glucose concentration has returned to the normal range. Readings should then be made hourly for 3 hours to ensure that the blood glucose concentration does not fall again. Thereafter, measure the blood glucose concentration 3 hourly until milk feeds are established.*

The diagnostic criteria for hyperinsulinism

- Glucose requirements > 6–8 mg/kg/min to maintain blood glucose above 2.6–3 mmol/litre (1mmol/L= 18mg/dL)
- Laboratory blood glucose < 2.6 mmol/litre
- Detectable insulin at the point of hypoglycemia with raised C peptide
- Inappropriately low blood free fatty acid and ketone body concentrations at the time of hypoglycemia
- Glycemic response after the administration of glucagon when hypoglycemic
- Absence of ketonuria

Courtesy: A Aynsley-Green, K Hussain, J Hall, J M Saudubray, C Nihoul-Fékété,

P De Lonlay-Debeney, F Brunelle, T Otonkoski, P Thornton, K J Lindley

Arch Dis Child Fetal Neonatal Ed 2000;**82**:F98–F107

Recommended guidelines to referring hospitals for transfer of babies with hyperinsulinism (transfer of babies/ children with hypoglycemia, regardless of etiology)

1. Before transfer discuss the case with the endocrine registrar/consultant on call

2. Must have secure intravenous access at all times before transfer (even if not requiring intravenous fluids at time of transfer)

3. Baby/child must be transferred with nurse and doctor escort

4. Before transfer ensure you have : 10% dextrose (preferably 500 ml bag), Hypostop/sugary drink, Glucagon intramuscular/intravenous 0.1 mg/kg up to 1 mg maximum, Blood glucose monitoring equipment

5. Monitoring:- Check blood glucose before leaving, then hourly if stable, or 15–30 minutes if unstable Aim to keep blood glucose above 3.0 mmol/litre (54mg/dl)

6. Hypoglycemic event during journey (blood glucose < 2.6 mmol/litre) Recommendations: 2 ml/kg of 10% dextrose bolus over three minutes, start maintenance infusion 6–8 mg/kg/min, which approximately equals 5 ml/kg/hour of 10% dextrose, Recheck blood glucose 15 minutes later. If still low increase infusion by 1 mg/kg/min until normoglycemia attained

If intravenous access lost give:

(a) Hypostop and repeat blood glucose in children > 2 years

(b) Give one dose of glucagon and repeat blood glucose measurement for infants.

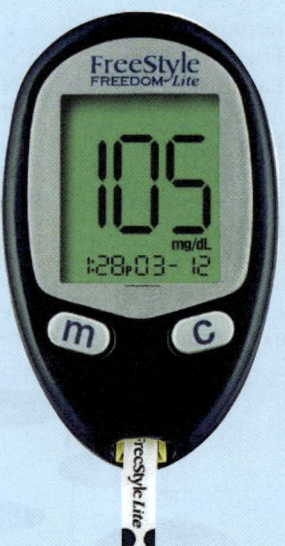

Drugs used in the Medical management of Hyperinsulinism

Drug diazoxide

Indication— Hyperinsulinemic hypoglycemia

Mechanism of action- Opens KATP channels, increases adrenaline (epinephrine) secretion, increases gluconeogenesis

Dose 5–20 mg/kg/day orally 8 hourly

Side effects- Fluid retention (chlorothiazide + diazoxide used together), hypertrichosis, hyperuricemia, facial changes,

hypotension, rarely leucopenia, thrombocytopenia

Drug Chlorothiazide (act synergistically with diazoxide by activating non-KATP channels)

Dose 7–10 mg/kg/day in 2 divided doses

Side effects- Hyponatremia, hypokalemia

Drug nifedipine (slow release preparation)

Indication: Hyperinsulinemic hypoglycemia
Mechanism of action- Calcium channel antagonist, inhibits insulin release
Dose: 0.25–2.5mg/kg/day orally 8 hourly
Response rate—Limited experience
Side effects—Hypotension

Drug glucagon

Mechanism of action—Increased glycogenolysis/gluconeogenesis

Dose- 1–10 µg/kg/hour intravenous infusion, 1 mg bolus dose intramuscular or intravenous

Side effects—Nausea, vomiting, increases growth hormone concentrations, increases myocardial contractility, decreases gastric acid/pancreatic enzymes

Drug octreotide

Indication—Hyperinsulinemic hypoglycemia

Mechanism of action- Activates G protein coupled rectifier K channel, hence inhibiting insulin release

Dose 5–20 µg/kg/day intravenous or subcutaneous infusion

Side effects—Suppression of growth hormone, TSH, ACTH. Steatorrhea, cholelithiasis, abdominal distension, decreases growth rate

ACTH, adrenocorticotrophin; KATP, ATP sensitive potassium channel; TSH, thyroid stimulating hormone.

Pearl/Peril/Pitfall: Never suddenly withdraw intravenous dextrose as this may precipitate hypoglycemia, as commonly happens if the drip infiltrates the tissues. Reduce the drip rate gradually when oral feeds are introduced.

TABLE 4 Etiology of neonatal hypoglycemia

1. *Increased utilization of glucose: hyperinsulinism*

   a. Diabetic mothers

   b. Erythroblastosis (hyperplastic islets of Langerhans)

   c. Islet-cell hyperplasia or hyperfunction

   d. Beckwith-Weidemann syndrome (macrosomia, mild microcephaly, omphalocele, macroglossia, hypoglycemia, and visceromegaly)

   e. Insulin-producing tumors (nesidioblastosis, islet-cell adenoma, or islet-cell dysmaturity)

   f. Maternal tocolytic therapy with beta-sympatho-mimetic agents (terbutaline, isoxsuprine, albuterol [salbutamol])

   g. Maternal chlopropamide therapy (Diabinase) ; possibly maternal benzothiadiazides (chlorothiazide)

   h. Malpositioned umbilical artery catheter used to infuse glucose in high concentration into the celiac and superior mesenteric arteries T11-12, stimulating insulin release from the pancreas

   i. Abrupt cessation of high-glucose infusions

   j. After exchange transfusion with blood containing a high glucose concentration

2. *Decreased production/stores*

   a. Prematurity. Incidence : premature SGA, 67%, premature LGA, 38% b. Intrauterine growth retardation (IUGR). Incidence : premature SGA, 67%, postterm SGA, 18% c. Inadequate caloric intake

3. *Increased utilization and/or decreased production or other causes*

   Any baby with one of the following conditions should be evaluated for hypoglycemia ; parenteral glucose may be necessary for the management of these infants.

   a. Perinatal stress

   (1) Sepsis (2) Shock (3) Asphyxia (4) Hypothermia (increased utilization)

   b. Exchange transfusion with heparinized blood that has a low glucose level in the absence of a glucose infusion ; reactive hypoglycemia after exchange with relatively hyperglycemic citrate-phosphate-dextrose (CPD) blood

   c. Defects in carbohydrate metabolism

   (1) Glycogen storage disease
   (2) Fructose intolerance
   (3) Galactosemia

   d. Endocrine deficiency

   (1) Adrenal insufficiency
   (2) Hypothalamic deficiency
   (3) Congenital hypopituitarism
   (4) Glucagon deficiency
   (5) Epinephrine deficiency

   e. Defects in amino acid metabolism

   (1) Maple syrup urine disease
   (2) Propionic acidemia
   (3) Methylmalonic acidemia
   (4) Tyrosinemia
   (5) Glutaric acidemia type II
   (6) Ethylmalonic adipic aciduria
   (7) Glutaricidemia

   f. Polycythemia (possibly due to glucose utilization by the increased mass of red blood cells. The decreased amount of serum per drop of blood may cause a reading consistent with hypoglycemia on whole blood measurements, but may yield a normal glucose level on laboratory analysis of serum.)

   g. Maternal therapy with propranolol. Possible mechanisms include the following :

   (1) Prevention of sympathetic stimulation of glycogenolysis
   (2) Prevention of recovery from insulin-induced decreases in free fatty acids and glycerol
   (3) Inhibition of epinephrine-induced increases in free fatty acids and lactate after exercise

KEY POINTS FOR CLINICAL PRACTICE

1. Most cases of Neonatal hypoglycemia are transient, respond readily to treatment, and are associated with an excellent prognosis.

2. Symptomatic infants with hypoglycemia, particularly LBW infants, those with persistent hyperinsulinism states, and infants of diabetic mothers, have a poorer prognosis for subsequent normal intellectual development than asymptomatic infants do.

3. Hypoglycemia recurs in 10–15% of infants after adequate treatment; recurrence is more common if IV fluids are extra vasated or discontinued too rapidly before oral feedings are well tolerated.

4. Infants at increased risk for hypoglycemia should have their serum glucose measured within 1hr of birth, every 1–2 hr for the first 6–8 hr, and then every 4–6 hr until 24 hr of life. An IV infusion of glucose at 4–6mg/kg/mt (10% dextrose in water @ 60–80ml/kg/day) should be provided in sick and LBW infants and if oral feedings are poorly tolerated or if asymptomatic transient neonatal hypoglycemia develops.

5. Consider all cases of persistent (>7 days), recurrent and severe (glucose requirements >10 mg/kg/mt) hypoglycemia for further evaluation which requires drawing blood for insulin, cortisol, and aminoacids at a time when the glucose level is below 40mg/dL.

REFERENCES AND FURTHER READING 1) Nelson text book of Pediatrics - 18th edition 2) Manual of Neonatal Intensive Care - NRC Roberton - 5th edition 3) Manual of Neonatal care - Cloherty - 6th edition 4) Sperling MA et all - Differential Diagnosis and Management of Neonatal Hypoglycemia -PCNA 2004

Pearl/Peril/Pitfall : The risk of brain damage depends on the severity, duration and number of hypoglycemic attacks. The prognosis is worst if the hypoglycemia has produced clinical signs, especially convulsions. The risk of permanent brain damage is probably low if the hypoglycemia is asymptomatic. However, asymptomatic hypoglycemia remains dangerous and must be treated urgently as clinical signs may suddenly develop.

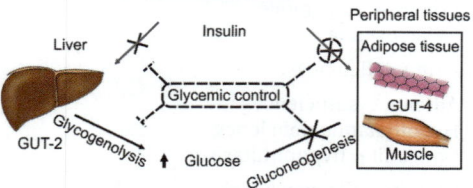

Neonatal Hyperglycemia

@ "*There are no specific symptoms associated with Neonatal hyperglycemia, but the major clinical problems associated with hyperglycemia are hyperosmolarity & osmotic diuresis.*"

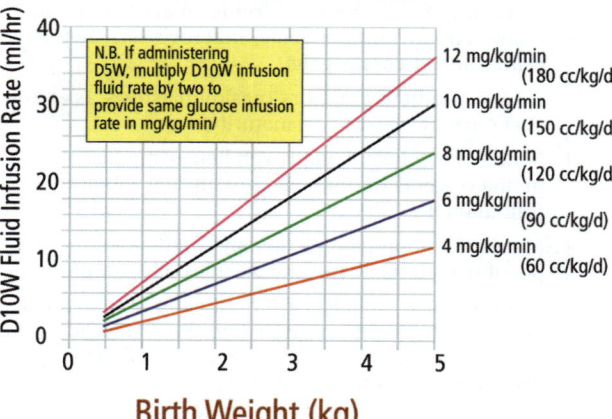

Figure: Mechanism of stress-induced hyperglycemia. Changes occuring during stress (dark solid lines) cause insulin resistance (x) in the liver (stimulating glycogenolysis) and in peripheral tissues (reducing glucose uptake and stimulating gluconeogenesis). Insulin therapy (dashed lines) reverses peripheral but not heptic insulin resistance

* *Hyperglycemia in a Neonate warrants a full septic screen, especially in a baby who has been maintaining euglycemia previously. In addition to sepsis, other stress factors such as surgery, hypoxia, painful stimuli & mechanical ventilation can induce hyperglycemia due to increased secretion of catecholamines; these decrease insulin secretion and interfere with peripheral insulin action.*

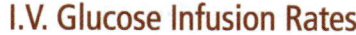

I.V. Glucose Infusion Rates

N.B. If administering D5W, multiply D10W infusion fluid rate by two to provide same glucose infusion rate in mg/kg/min/

- 12 mg/kg/min (180 cc/kg/d)
- 10 mg/kg/min (150 cc/kg/d)
- 8 mg/kg/min (120 cc/kg/d)
- 6 mg/kg/min (90 cc/kg/d)
- 4 mg/kg/min (60 cc/kg/d)

Birth Weight (kg)

This graph may be used in your management of Neonates as an aid for determining: the IV rate needed to achieve a desired glucose infusion rate, i.e., in mg/kg/min as is needed for writing orders; or determining the glucose infusion rate of an existing i.v. to determine an infant's caloric intake. As an example, a 2.5 kg infant whom you would like to have receive 6 mg/kg/min of glucose should be receiving 9.5 cc/hr of D10W (equivalent to 90 cc/kg of i.v. fluid).

Guidelines for monitoring plasma glucose in hyperglycemic infants:
Plasma glucose measurements should be determined every 1 to 4 hours depending on the degree of hyperglycemia, with therapy adjusted according to plasma plasma glucose results. Glucose determinations should be done on capillary blood from an extremity, or from a non-glucose-containing indwelling catheter.
Courtesy: John A. Widness, MD Iowa Neonatology Handbook.

REVIEW OF CLINICAL PROBLEMS

1. *Mention the 4 important clinical factors, in anticipating Hyperglycemia in the Neonates?*

   Ans: The 4 paramount factors in anticipating hyperglycemia are a) Immaturity: infant almost always less than 30 weeks' gestation and 1.0 kg birth weight b) Age: usually less than 3 days, most often 24hours c) Glucose infusion rates: exceed 8 mg/kg/min (equivalent to 10% glucose at 100mg/kg/24h) d) Septicemia: bacterial and fungal.

2. *Name the 2 most serious secondary problems consequent upon Neonatal Hyperglycemia?*

   Ans: Neonatal Hyperglycemia causes a) osmotic diuresis leading to dehydration & electrolyte disturbances rapidly in small premature infants with large insensible fluid losses b) intraventricular hemorrhage because of osmotic fluid shift from the intracellular compartment to the extracellular compartment secondary to hyperosmolal state induced by Hyperglycemia (an increase of 25–40 mOsm with a glucose level of >450–720mg/dL)

3. *Mention 5 drugs that can cause Neonatal Hyperglycemia?*
   Ans: Refer to the "No.3" of the "BIRD`S EYE VIEW/OVERVIEW/SYNOPSIS"of the Chapter.

4. *Name 5 common causes of Neonatal Hyperglycemia, other than drugs?*

   Ans: a) ELBW (<1000 gms) infants b) Sepsis c) "Stressed" premature infant (mechanical ventilation, surgery, hypoxia acting as painful stimuli) d) TPN with lipid infusion (FFA) e) Ingestion of hyperosmolar formula due to inappropriate dilution.

5. *How do you elicit the history, examine the baby and investigate accordingly in a Neonate with Hyperglycemia?*
   Ans: Refer to the E-D-A Algorithm to diagnose & manage a Neonate with Hyperglycemia.

LEARNING OBJECTIVES

After completing this article, readers will be able to:

1. Anticipate hyperglycemia in high risk Neonates & to diagnose it rapidly before serious problems like dehydration & IVH supervene in small premature babies.

2. Investigate for "sepsis" - a must especially in a baby who has been maintaining euglycemia previously.

3. Keep in mind about "Transient Neonatal Diabetes Mellitus", when no other cause of Neonatal Hyperglycemia is forthcoming.

4. Prevent hyperglycemia, by regular glucose monitoring in high-risk groups, by giving no more than 5% dextrose infusions to ELBW infants & early enteral feeds as soon as possible.

5. Consult a "specialist" at higher Neonatal center, if hyperglycemia is severe (>300mg/dL) and persistent despite reducing the glucose infusion rate to < 3–4mg/kg/mt (@ 10% dextrose in water IV 50–60ml/kg/day) for starting insulin therapy.

* **Pearl/Peril/Pitfall:** *Hyperglycemia (hyper = high; glycemia = blood glucose) is defined as a blood glucose concentration above 7.0 mmol/l (120 mg/dL). Usually hyperglycemia does not cause problems until the blood glucose concentration increases above 10 mmol/l.*

BIRD'S EYE VIEW/OVERVIEW/SYNOPSIS

1. *Hyperglycemia is defined as the whole-blood glucose concentration of > 125mg/dL (or laboratory plasma concentration > 145mg/dL), regardless of gestational age, birth weight, or postnatal age.* The incidence of hyperglycemia is inversely proportional to the birth weight in the preterm infant, ranging from about 2% in infants who weigh > 2,000 gms to about 45% in those weigh < 1,000 gms, and upto 80% in ELBW infants weighing < 750gms.

2. The Neonate with hyperglycemia is usually asymptomatic, or have signs of associated disease processes. Recognizable signs associated with hyperglycemia *include* dehydration from osmotic diuresis, weight loss, fever, glycosuria, ketosis, and metabolic acidosis. The last three signs are common among infants who have transient or permanent Neonatal diabetes mellitus. *Hyperglycemia in very premature infants has been associated with an increased mortality, increased incidence of intracranial hemorrhage due to hyperosmolarity (Note:* each 18mg/dL rise in blood glucose causes an increase in serum osmolarity of 1mOsm/lt. Normal osmolarity is 280–300mOsm/lt) *and developmental delay.*

3. Hyperglycemia is caused by excessive rates of IV glucose infusion in the presence of physiological and biochemical mechanisms that lead to excess glucose production, insulin resistance and glucose intolerance. *In an infant who has normal glucose levels and then becomes hyperglycemic without an excess glucose load, sepsis should be the prime consideration :* in sepsis stress hormones such as cortisol and catecholamines are elevated and the glucose utilization is decreased due to depressed insulin release, cytokines, or endotoxin. Various drugs such as *corticosteroids,* caffeine, theophylline, phenytoin, maternal diazoxide & prostaglandin E1 infusion can cause Neonatal hyperglycemia.

4. *The Evaluation-Decision-Action-Plan/Algorithm to diagnose and manage a Neonate with hyperglycemia summarizes the essential aspects of history taking, physical examination and relevant investigations, differential diagnosis and management.*

5. *Transient Neonatal diabetes mellitus :* a rare disorder, seen characteristically, in term small for gestational age infants, usually before the age of 15 days (range 2 days to 6 weeks) and presents with marked glycosuria, hyperglycemia (240-2,300mg/dL), polyuria, severe dehydration, acidosis, mild or absent ketonuria, reduced subcutaneous fat, and failure to thrive. Insulin values are either absolutely or relatively low for the corresponding blood glucose elevation. Treatment consists of rehydration, and the majority require Insulin (intermediate acting insulin 2 units/kg/day SC divided q 12 hour). Monitor serum electrolytes, glucose, and acid-base balance. Repeated plasma insulin values are necessary to distinguish transient from permanent diabetes mellitus. Attempts at gradually reducing the dose of insulin may be made as soon as recurrent hypoglycemia becomes manifested or after 2 months of age. The average length for insulin treatment is 65 days (range 3 days to 18 months). 50% of the cases are transient. Some transient cases will have a later recurrence. Some cases are permanent. Cases presenting after 3 weeks and in infants with HLA - DR3 + DR4 haplotypes have a higher incidence of permanent diabetes. Diabetes mellitus in the Newborn may be permanent due to rare syndrome of pancreatic agenesis. *The majority of all these infants are small at birth.* Long term follow-up of a cohort of patients with Neonatal diabetes revealed that almost 50% had permanent diabetes, 1/3rd had transient diabetes, and about 1/4th had transient diabetes that recurred when they were 7–20 year old.

6. *A history of hyperosmolar formula feed causing glycosuria, hyperglycemia and dehydration is the key for diagnosing transient hyperglycemia associated with ingestion of inappropriate formula.* Treatment consists of rehydration, discontinuation of hyperosmolar formula, and appropriate instructions for mixing powder formula. Insulin has been used briefly but cautiously.

7. *Treatment of Neonatal hyperglycemia must include simultaneous treatment of underlying conditions.* With modest hyperglycemia (plasma glucose concentration < 300 mg/dL), reducing exogenous glucose (Dextrose) infusion rates usually is sufficient to resolve the hyperglycemia. The rate of infusion should be decreased gradually by 1–2mg/kg/mt every 2–4 hrs, with frequent measurement of blood glucose concentrations until normoglycemia is achieved.

8. IV infusion (0.01–0.1 unit/kg/hr) or subcutaneous boluses (0.1–0.2 unit/kg/dose every 6 hours) of regular insulin should be reserved for infants who have severe hyperglycemia (>300mg/dL) that persists despite reducing the glucose infusion rate to < 3–4 mg/kg/mt. Monitor glucose level on hourly basis and the potassium level. *Prevent hypokalemia by addition of potassium to IV solutions during the insulin infusion.* Small IV infusions of potassium (0.1mEq/kg potassium as KCl or Kacetate) can be added every 1–2 hrs if hypokalemia is significant and persistent.

9. *VLBW infants (< 800 gms) should start with an IV dextrose concentration no higher than 5%.* If hyperglycemia is documented, parenteral glucose intake is reduced to 4-6 mg/kg/mt by reducing the concentration or the rate (or both) of glucose infusion and monitoring the falling blood glucose level. Avoid hypotonic fluids with dextrose < 5%, to prevent hemolysis, with resulting hyperkalemia.

10. Enteral feeding promotes the secretion of insulin by inducing gut production of "enteroinsular hormones" (incretins), including gastric inhibitory polypeptide and pancreatic polypeptide and prevents / ameliorates hyperglycemia, unless the infant is very ill or there are clear signs of feeding intolerance. Even minimal amounts, such as in "minimal enteral feeding" regimens, induces the gut production of "enteroinsular hormones," These hormones increase insulin secretion by direct actions on the pancreatic beta cells. Such observations warrant efforts to feed preterm infants who have hyperglycemia, even if full enteral feedings cannot or should not be attempted.

Summary of Recommendations for Prevention and Management of Neonatal Hyperglycemia

* Improved physiologic control
* Early and increased parenteral nutrition with amino acids
* Early initiation of enteral feedings
* Limited intravenous glucose infusion rates during hyperglycemia to what is required for achieving normal glucose concentrations
* Limited intravenous lipid infusions during hyperglycemia
* Reservation of insulin therapy only for severe hyperglycemia with associated clinical signs and complications.

Pearl/Peril/Pitfall: Hyperglycemia is usually due to a 10% dextrose or Neonatalyte infusion given to a preterm infant during the first few days of life. Some immature infants are not able to remove glucose fast enough from the blood stream. Hyperglycemia may be caused by a severe intraventricular hemorrhage.

THE EVALUATION-DECISION-ACTION-PLAN/ALGORITHM FOR THE DIAGNOSIS AND MANAGEMENT OF *A NEONATE WITH HYPERGLYCEMIA*

SUBJECTIVE FINDINGS

Hx of excessive glucose administration to ELBW/extreme premature babies.

Hx of sepsis, e.g. temperature instability, increasing gastric aspirates/feed- intolerance, changes in perfusion, respiratory distress etc.

Hx of familial diabetes mellitus in previous siblings/family members.

Determine maternal and infant medications known to cause hyperglycemia, e.g. maternal diazoxide, steroids, theophylline, caffeine, phenytoin, prostaglandin IVI.

Hx of "stress" like surgical intervention, mechanical ventilation in premature babies.

OBJECTIVE FINDINGS

Assess ABCDs, hydration status, O_2 sats, CRT, BP, urine output.

Look for signs suggestive of underlying disorders IUGR, ELBW babies, sepsis, hypoxia, surgical intervention.

Recognize Signs associated with hyperglycemia like dehydration from osmotic diuresis, weight loss, fever, glycosuria, ketosis & metabolic acidosis.

Perform A complete physical examination.

INVESTIGATIONS

FBC with differential, blood cultures, CRP as a screening for sepsis.

Serum glucose level, electrolytes, ABG analysis (to confirm hyperglycemia, losses of electrolytes due to osmotic diuresis, metabolic acidosis respectively).

Urine cultures and Dipstick testing for UTI & glycosuria respectively.

Serum insulin level usually low in cases of rare transient Neonatal diabetes mellitus.

Serum or urine C-Peptide levels will be low to absent in insulin dependent diabetes mellitus.

Always treat underlying conditions of Neonatal hyperglycemia e.g. reduce the concentration of Dextrose to 5% and to rate of 4-6mg/kg/mt in cases of excess glucose administration especially in VLBW premature infants (< 800gms), broadspectrum antibiotics for sepsis, proper dilution of the formula feed in cases associated with ingestion of hyperosmolar formula, discontinuation of medications causing hyperglycemia like caffeine, phenytoin, steroids, theophylline

A Neonate with Hyperglycemia

Ensure ABCs, *treat* shock (10ml/kg NS IV bolus), *correct* dehydration and *monitor* serum electrolytes, glucose and acid-base balance and pulse oximetry.

Intubate & ventilate if the baby collapses due to hypovolemic shock consequent upon unrecognized severe hyperglycemia and osmotic diuresis.

Excess glucose administration

Causes : 1) Exogenous IV glucose administration > 6mg/kg/mt in term infants & > 6.6mg/kg/mt in preterm infants (< 1,100gm) 2) IV 10% Dextrose with 200ml/kg/day in VLBW babies (<1,000 gm) 3) Ingestion of hyperosmolar formula 4) Hypoxia (increases glucose production in the absence of a change in peripheral utilization.

Management :

* *Decrease* the rate of infusion gradually 1-2mg/kg/mt every 2-4 hrs (to 4-6mg/kg/mt), with frequent measurement of glucose concentrations until normoglycemia is achieved.

* *Reduce* the concentration of IV dextrose to 5% ; avoid giving hypotonic IV solutions (< 4.7%) to prevent hemolysis, with resulting hyperkalemia.

* If the urine glucose level is negative, it is acceptable to have a higher serum glucose level, if glucose is being given to increase the caloric intake : perform dextrostix and urinary glucose testing every 4-6 hr.

Inability to metabolize glucose

Causes : 1. Sepsis
2. Stress like mechanical ventilation in premature babies
3. Surgical procedures

Management

* *Reduce* the concentration or the rate (or both) of glucose infusion and monitor the falling blood glucose level as mentioned previously.

* *Use* insulin in infants with severe hyperglycemia (>300mg/dL) that persists despite reducing the glucose infusion rate to < 3-4mg/kg/mt).

* *Regular Insulin* can be given as continuous IVI 0.02-0.1 unit/kg/hr, monitoring for hypokalemia and hypoglycemia. Prevent hypokalemia by adding KCl 0.1mEq/kg every 1-2 hours if hypokalemia is significant and persistent. Monitor for rebound hyperglycemia. Flush the IV tubing with insulin solution to saturate binding sites.

* *Regular Insulin* can be given subcutaneously, 0.05-0.1 unit/kg/dose, every 6 hour. with frequent blood glucose monitoring at 1,2 and 4 hours & potassium level monitoring every 6 hours initially.

Transient Neonatal D.mellitus

Causes : 1) Functional delay in beta cell maturation
2) Chromosome 6 abnormalities with HLA - DR3 / DR4 haplotypes
3) Familial

Management :

* *Correct* dehydration & monitor electrolytes, glucose, and acid-base balance as mentioned above.

* *Start intermediate acting insulin* 2 units/kg/day, subcutaneously divided q 12 hr.

* *Repeat* plasma insulin values to distinguish transient from permanent diabetes mellitus.

* *Consult* a Pediatric endocrinologist and *arrange* regular follow-ups to monitor the need for insulin requirement.

* *Attempt at* gradually reducing the dose of insulin, as soon as recurrent hypoglycemia becomes manifested or after 2 months of age.

---

* *Pearl/Peril/Pitfall: The raised blood glucose concentration usually can be lowered into the normal range by simply changing the intravenous solution from Neonatalyte or 10% dextrose to a 5% dextrose solution. Once milk feeds are established, hyperglycemia usually returns to normal.*

Role of insulin therapy in neonatal hyperglycemia: If severe hyperglycemia persists, exogenous insulin administration may be warranted. Guidelines about when to use insulin treatment and how to provide this form of therapy remain highly controversial and vary widely among clinicians and institutions. Many consider insulin treatment unnecessary, others use it sparingly if at all, and many use it according to fairly liberal guidelines, considering that it also might provide a positive protein balance, improve nutrition, and control glucose concentration. Reasonable guidelines indicate that insulin treatment should be reserved until plasma glucose concentrations exceed 16.7 to 22.2 mmol/L (300 to 400 mg/dL) despite reducing the glucose infusion rate to less than 3 to 4 mg/kg per minute. The usual method of insulin administration involves a continuous infusion, beginning at 0.02 to 0.05 U/kg per hour. Although higher infusion rates have been used, they usually are not necessary and increase the risks of hypokalemia and subsequent hypoglycemia. Hypokalemia can be prevented by the addition of potassium to IV solutions during the infusion. Normal infusion rates of potassium usually are sufficient, but during insulin treatment, frequent monitoring of serum potassium concentrations is warranted. Small IV boluses of potassium (0.1 mEq potassium as potassium chloride or potassium acetate) can be added every 1 to 2 hours if hypokalemia is significant and persistent. Urine flow rates should be good before repeating potassium doses. Hypoglycemia is a potentially severe problem if insulin is administered through a single IV line. If it becomes disconnected, the infused insulin lasts much longer in the circulation than the infused glucose or endogenously produced glucose, leading to potentially severe hypoglycemia. Although this has been an infrequent complication of insulin treatment, it remains a serious potential risk. Obviously, blood glucose concentration should be measured repetitively and frequently (every 1 to 2 hours or whenever signs of possible hypoglycemia develop) during the administration of insulin to the neonate. VLBW infants younger than 30 weeks' gestational age can increase glucose tolerance using insulin infusion therapy. After one treatment of 3 to 6 hours in duration, such infants have been shown to increase glucose tolerance by 50% to 300% and were able to maintain normoglycemia thereafter. ELBW very preterm infants may not demonstrate such dramatic improvement in glucose tolerance, although reports have noted that observations were made on much sicker infants who probably had much higher concentrations of counterregulatory hormones. Other factors may contribute to persistent glucose intolerance, including insulin resistance. A few infants who initially responded to insulin therapy have developed resistance to insulin within hours to days. Despite increasing insulin infusion rates to as high as 16 U/kg per hour, resistance persisted. None of these neonates was septic, but all were receiving antibiotic therapy for other conditions as well as ventilator support. One major caveat regarding continuous insulin infusion is the variable delivery of insulin due to its adsorption to the walls of plastic tubing in the IV pump. An infant may require initially increased rates of insulin infusion to overcome this loss. This increased rate can lead to hypoglycemia as the infusion continues and the rate of adsorption slows markedly. One approach to prevent or limit this problem is to flush the insulin delivery system with diluted insulin 2 hours before beginning therapy. Others have mixed the insulin infusion with albumin at a concentration of 0.3 g/100 mL of solution to decrease adsorption.

Interventions for treatment of neonatal hyperglycemia in very low birth weight infants: Higher-than-normal blood sugar levels are frequently seen in babies born very early (before 32 weeks gestation) or with very low birth weight (< 1500 grams) and who are fed totally or partially by vein. Several types of adverse outcomes have been associated with high blood sugar levels, including increased risks for death, infections, eye problems, and bleeding into the brain. It is not known if treatment to lower the baby's blood sugar helps to prevent those complications and, if so, which treatment is best. These treatment options include decreasing the amount of sugar delivered by vein to nourish the baby or administration of insulin. This review of trials found no evidence of significant effects of these treatments on the risks of death or major complications. However, the studies reviewed were very small. There is a need for larger trials to answer these questions. This is a Cochrane review abstract and plain language summary, prepared and maintained by The Cochrane Collaboration, currently published in The Cochrane Database of Systematic Reviews 2010 Issue 2, Copyright © 2010 The Cochrane Collaboration. Published by John Wiley and Sons, Ltd.

Risks for Hyperglycemia in Newborn Infants
*Preterm birth
* Intrauterine growth restriction (IUGR)
* Increased stress hormones
–Increased catecholamine infusions and plasma concentrations
–Increased glucocorticoid concentrations (from use of antenatal steroids, postnatal glucocorticoid administration, and stress)
–Increased glucagon concentrations
*Early and high rates of intravenous (IV) lipid infusion
*Higher-than-needed rates of IV glucose infusion
*Insufficient pancreatic insulin secretion (preterm and IUGR)
*Absence of enteral feedings, leading to diminished "incretin" secretion and action, limiting their potential to promote insulin secretion

Complications of Hyperglycemia or Conditions Associated With Hyperglycemia : *Increased morbidity and mortality *Impaired immunity *Increased infection *Poor wound healing *Loss of skeletal and cardiac muscle

KEY POINTS FOR CLINICAL PRACTICE:

1. ELBW infants (<1000gm) with a high glucose infusion rate of >6mg/kg/mt is the most common cause of Neonatal Hyperglycemia, seen in 68% of such babies, due to variable insulin release and a relative insulin resistance and immature development of glucose transport proteins like GLUT 4.

2. Hyperglycemia in a Neonate warrants a *full septic screen*, especially in a baby who has been maintaining euglycemia previously. In addition to sepsis, other stress factors such as surgery, hypoxia, painful stimuli and mechanical ventilation can induce hyperglycemia due to increased secretion of catecholamines; these decrease insulin secretion and interfere with peripheral insulin action.

3. The two most serious problems secondary to Neonatal Hyperglycemia, such as dehydration + electrolyte losses due to osmotic diuresis and intraventricular hemorrhage due to hyperosmolarity are common in small premature babies.

4. Although rarely seen in the first months of life, diabetes mellitus, can present with severe clinical symptoms including polyuria, dehydration, and ketoacidosis that require prompt treatment.

5. The primary goal of management of Neonatal Hyperglycemia is prevention and early detection of hyperglycemia by carefully adjusting glucose infusion rates, and frequently monitoring blood glucose levels and urine for glycosuria. If present, evaluation and possible intervention are indicated.

REFERENCES AND FURTHER READING : 1) Neonatal Hyperglycemia by Hemachandra AH & Cowett RA - Pediatric Review -1999 2) Transient & Permanent Neonatal Diabetes- Fosel S. Eur J Pediatrics - 1995 3) Manual of Neonatal Care by Cloherty - 6 th edition 4) Nelson Text Book of Pediatrics - 18th edition

* **Pearl/Peril/Pitfall :** *Various drugs such as corticosteroids, caffeine, theophyllin, phenytoin, maternal diazoxide & prostaglandin E1 infusion can cause Neonatal hyperglycemia.*

18 Nosocomial Infections in the NICU

@ *Healthcare-associated infection is a serious but preventable problem for hospitalized neonates and demands not only individual accountability and a culture of safety, but also the hospital infrastructure to support employees in their efforts to prevent infections. Without this support, the gap between knowledge and practice in the prevention of healthcare-associated infection will persist.*

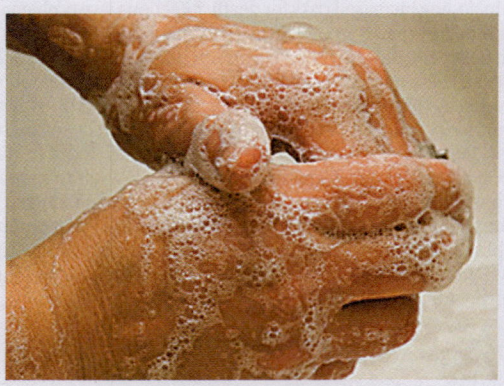

No factor is more important in preventing Nosocomial infections than hand hygiene. Yes, we've heard it all before, but knowledge is not always translated into practice . Observational studies reveal that clinicians wash their hands only 40% of the time that they should. Hand hygiene education can temporarily improve handwashing rates, but over time, compliance tends to deteriorate. Hand hygiene compliance was independently associated with a 60% decrease in the risk of healthcare-associated infection among VLBW neonates. Furthermore, hand hygiene doesn't entirely prevent nurses from becoming colonized with resistant microbial flora. Within a few months of starting work in the NICU, similar patterns of methicillin-resistant, coagulase-negative staphylococcus can be isolated from the hands of new graduates as from the hands of experienced NICU nurses. Colonization of the nurses' hands occurred in spite of adherence to hand hygiene practices.

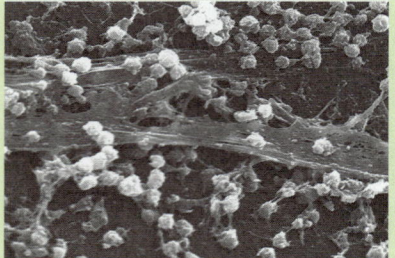

Catheter biofilm. Electron micrograph depicting numbers of *Staphylococcus aureus* bacteria, which were found on the luminal surface of an indwelling catheter. A red blood cell is present with its biconcave cytomorphology. The sticky-looking substance woven among the round cocci bacteria, composed of polysaccharides, is known as "biofilm." This bacteria-secreted substance protects the bacteria from attacks by antimicrobial agents.

Petri dish culture of nurse's hands before (left) and after (right) handwashing.

REVIEW OF CLINICAL PROBLEMS

1. Name the risk factors that increase the incidence of Nosocomial Infections in the NICU. *Ans: Refer to the Evaluation-Decision-Action Plan/Algorithm to diagnose and manage Nosocomial Infections in the NICU.*

2. Mention the Recommendations for good Hand Hygiene Practice in the NICU. *Ans: Refer to the Evaluation-Decision-Action Plan/Algorithm to diagnose and manage Nosocomial Infections in the NICU.*

3. What are the general principles for preventing Nosocomial Infections in the NICU ? *Ans: Refer to the"No.1" of the "BIRD`S EYE VIEW/OVERVIEW/SYNOPSIS" of the Chapter.*

4. Discuss the 10-Point Plan on the Antibiotic use in the NICUs. *Ans: Refer to Section "The 10-Point Plan on the Antibiotic use" of the Chapter.*

5. What are other important Measures to Prevent/Reduce NICU Nosocomial Infections? *Ans: Refer to the Evaluation-Decision-Action Plan/Algorithm to diagnose and manage Nosocomial Infections in the NICU.*

LEARNING OBJECTIVES

After completing this article, readers will be able to

1. Practise thorough Hand Washing technique in the NICU and observe Good Compliance with it.

2. Protect the immature skin of ELBW infants by reducing the number of heelsticks and by using hydrogel electrodes to monitor.

3. Perform continuous monitoring and surveillance of Nosocomial infection rates in the NICU.

4. Provide education and feedback for nursery personnel.

5. Minimize risk of contamination of central venous catheters (CVCs).

Pearl/Peril/Pitfall: Strategies to reduce or prevent catheter-related BSIs have included the use of antibiotic-coated catheters and prophylactic administration of systemic antibiotics. Such strategies may contribute to antibiotic resistance and toxicity. The implementation of the closed medication system and associated policies is associated with a significant decrease in the nosocomial infection rate.

BIRD'S EYE VIEW/OVERVIEW/SYNOPSIS

1. Nosocomial infections in the NICU are one of the leading causes of Neonatal mortality in developing countries and most of them are preventable if strict asepsis is maintained in the NICU. Principles for the prevention of nosocomial infection include: **a)** adherence to universal precautions with all patient contact, **b)** avoiding nursery crowding and limiting nurse-to-patient ratios **c)** strict compliance with hand-washing, **d)** minimizing the risk of catheter contamination, **e)** meticulous skin care, **f)** encouraging early and appropriate advancement of enteral feedings, **g)** education and feed back for nursery personnel and parents, **h)** continuous monitoring and surveillance of nosocomial infection rates in the NICU.

2. Handwashing remains the most important and effective means of reducing nosocomial infections. A thorough two-minute hand washing is mandatory before entering the nursery, before performing an invasive procedure and after providing care to an infected baby. A half-minute hand wash is recommended for in-between touching the babies. Soapy antiseptic preparations containing povidone-iodine or chlorhexidine are ideal for handwashing and alcohol-based antiseptic solutions like sterillium (ethyl-hexadecyl-dimethyle ammonium- ethyl sulfate in propanol) are useful before touching any baby during the round. The hands should be dried with autoclaved napkins, disposable sterile paper napkins or allow them to dry spontaneously.

3. VLBW infants are born with an ineffective epidermal barrier that results in increased transepidermal water loss and an increased risk for infection. Efforts to reduce traumatic injury to this immature skin are important, including a reduction in the number of heelsticks.

4. Most nosocomial infections in the NICU are bloodstream infections associated with an intravascular catheter (peripheral or central). Efforts to reduce catheter-related infections include proper antisepsis of the skin before insertion of the catheter, sterile precautions during catheter insertion, aseptic technique when entering the line, minimizing repeated entry into the line for blood sampling, sterile preparation of fluids to be used with a central venous catheter, and, finally, minimizing the number of catheter days.

5. While performing any procedure in the NICU, apart from thorough handwashing, sterile gloves should be worn for obtaining blood culture samples, endotracheal suction, and emergency drainage of tension pneumothorax. Mask and sterile gloves should be worn for performing lumbar puncture and suprapubic aspiration of bladder. Sterile gloves and gown and mask should be worn while performing more invasive procedures like umbilical vessel catheterization, exchange blood transfusion, insertion of intercostal tube and establishing TPN lines, etc.

6. Rigorous house keeping routines should be enforced to control the heavily contaminated environment of the NICU. It is preferable to use vaccum cleaners to clear the dust from floor, walls and equipment and to wet mop the floors with soap and water containing 3% phenol at least thrice daily, and to wipe the walls with 2% bacillocide once a week. The sinks should be washed with 3% phenol or 5% lysol once a day and the fomites like files, x-ray film, pen, torch etc., should not be kept on the baby cot. Adequate provision of foot-operated bins (with plastic bags kept as hampers) adjacent to each baby unit for disposal of used material and soiled linen must be in place and they should be mopped with 3% phenol every day.

7. *Disinfection and/or sterilization (killing of spores as well) of equipment* is the most essential aspect of prevention and control of nosocomial infections in the NICU.

8. Ongoing education of staff regarding practices that are likely to reduce nosocomial infections and active surveillance of infection rates are important components of nosocomial infection control procedures to be followed if an epidemic is suspected or proved. Appropriate hospital infection control officers are to be informed of the situation. Hands, nasal and throat swabs of personnel and nursery air should be cultured as and when necessary.

9. *Screening of admissions and isolation of infected babies* with gastroenteritis, skin infections like staphylococcal, herpes etc., are important and they should be managed by different nurses. The mother should be taught general principles of hygiene and importance of handwashing for prevention of spread of infection. The use of a surgical mask while feeding will reduce the chances of droplet infection.

10. *The Evaluation-Decision-Action-Plan/Algorithm* describes the essential aspects of the prevention and control of nosocomial infections in the NICU. Babies with cytomegalovirus (CMV) infection, rubella, syphilis and chicken pox are highly infectious. Depending upon the nature of infection, they may continue to discharge infecting agent in the nasopharynx, mucous membranes, urine and skin, sometimes for several weeks and months. Female health care personnel working in the NICU are at great risk. These Neonates should be isolated and looked after in a separate room. The use of sterile gloves and thorough hand washing is essential while nursing these babies.

Pearl/Peril/Pitfall: Evidence indicates that a minimum volume of 1 mL of blood is required to detect bloodstream infections. The volume of blood drawn should be documented. Blood cultures should be obtained from 2 peripheral skin punctures or a peripheral skin puncture and a central catheter hub. The use of blood cultures from central catheters is helpful in that it avoids a skin puncture and often helps to determine whether there is a central line infection.

THE EVALUATION-DECISION-ACTION-PLAN/ALGORITHM FOR THE DIAGNOSIS AND MANAGEMENT OF *NOSOCOMIAL NICU INFECTIONS*

Assess the risk factors for acquiring nosocomial infection in the neonatal intensive care unit!

Low birth weight, invasive device, intravascular device (PIVC, umbilical catheter, PICC, CVC,), Mechanical ventilator, Urinary catheter, Ventriculoperitoneal shunt, Medications, Histamine2-blocking agents, Steroids, Others, Prolonged administration of hyperalimentation, Intralipid administration, Delayed enteral feedings, Feeding with formula rather than human milk, Inadequate nursery staffing and overcrowding, Poor compliance with handwashing.

(CVC, central venous catheter; PIVC, percutaneous intravenous catheter; PICC, peripherally inserted central catheter.)

Do follow the principles and practice for the prevention of nosocomial infection in the NICU

* Observe recommendations for standard precautions with all patient contact
* Observe recommendations for transmission-based precautions as indicated:
  Gowns, Gloves, Masks, Isolation
* Use good nursery design/engineering:
  Appropriate nursing-to-patient ratio
  Avoidance of overcrowding and excessive workload
  Readily accessible sinks, antiseptic solutions, soaps, and paper towels
* Maintain hand-washing practices:
  Improving hand-washing compliance
  Washing of hands before and after each patient encounter
  Appropriate use of soap, alcohol-based preparations, or antiseptic solutions
  Alcohol-based antiseptic solution at each patients bedside

  Emollients provided for nursery staff
* Minimize risk of contamination of central venous catheters (CVCs)
  Maximal sterile barrier precautions during CVC insertion
  Local antisepsis with chlorhexidine gluconate
  Minimal entries into the line for laboratory tests
  Aseptic technique when entering the line
  Minimal CVC days
  Sterile preparation of all fluids to be administered via a CVC
* Provide meticulous skin care
* Encourage early and appropriate advancement of enteral feedings
* Provide education and feedback for nursery personnel
* Perform continuous monitoring and surveillance of nosocomial infection rates in the NICU

RECOMMENDATIONS FOR HAND HYGIENE PRACTICES IN THE NICU*

Indications for handwashing
* Wash hands with a non-antimicrobial soap or an antimicrobial soap and water when hands are visibly soiled or contaminated with proteinaceous material.
* If the hands are not visibly soiled, alcohol-based waterless antiseptic agents are strongly preferred for routine decontamination of hands in all other clinical situations.
* Alcohol-based waterless antiseptic agents should be available at each patient area and other convenient locations, and in individual pocket-sized containers for health care providers.
* Antimicrobial soaps may be considered in settings with few time constraints and easy access to hand hygiene facilities.
* Decontaminate hands after contact with intact patient skin (i.e., checking pulse or lifting).
* Decontaminate hands after contact with body fluids or excretions, mucous membranes, non-intact skin, or wounds.
* Decontaminate hands before applying sterile gloves or inserting a central intravascular catheter.

* Decontaminate hands before inserting indwelling urinary catheters or other invasive devices not requiring surgical procedures.
* Decontaminate hands after removing gloves.
* Decontaminate hands before caring for patients with severe neutropenia or severe immunosuppression.
* Decontaminate hands after contact with inanimate objects in the immediate vicinity of the patient.

Recommended techniques for hand hygiene:
* When using a waterless antiseptic agent, apply enough of the product to cover all surfaces of the hands and fingers, and rub hands together until they are dry. Each manufacturer has guidelines for the volume to be used; in general, however, enough should be applied such that it takes 15 to 25 seconds to dry.
* When using a non-antimicrobial or antimicrobial soap, wet hands, apply 3 to 5 mL of solution to the hands, and rub for at least 15 seconds. Be sure to cover all surfaces of the hands and fingers. Rinse hands with warm water, and dry thoroughly. Foot pedals or towels should be used to turn off the water.

Other Important Measures to Prevent/Reduce NICU Nosocomial Infections

1. Limit the number of days that percutaneous deep lines are in place to <21: Most VLBW infants will be close to full enteral calories by 21 days of age, so this target of 21 days is feasible. Other important strategies are necessary to achieve this target, such as early introduction of trophic feeds with breast milk, consistent advancing of feeding volumes, and removal of the deep lines in some infants before full enteral calories are actually reached.

2. Reduce the duration of IV lipid use: Several animal studies suggest that IV lipids are immunosuppressive, are easily contaminated, and support the growth of fungi and bacteria. There are also reports of epidemics and isolated cases related to contamination in human patients. Because lipids are a critical part of parenteral nutrition in premature infants, they remain an essential part of early management. Clinicians must balance the risk of infection against the benefit of enhanced caloric intake when deciding how early to curtail the use of IV lipids.

3. Decrease the number of skin punctures: Venipunctures, arterial punctures, IV line starts, and heel sticks provide opportunities for

microflora colonizing the skin to be introduced into the bloodstream. It follows that reducing the number of skin punctures should reduce these opportunities. One unpublished retrospective study showed a positive correlation between >5 peripheral IV stick attempts in a 48-hour period and the incidence of bacteremia.

4. Selected use of topical application of preservative-free ointment in preterm infants: The rationale for this practice is that topical emollient therapy decreases dermatitis and fissuring, thus decreasing the entry of bacteria into the bloodstream. Emollients have a place in maintaining skin integrity, but routine application for intact skin is unnecessary and the risks may outweigh the benefits. The practice of routine ointment application remains controversial because a third, more recent randomized trial demonstrated an increase in CONS in preterm infants who received twice-daily petrolatum ointment application. The routine application of emollients may actually increase colonization, with no added benefit for patients who have intact skin.

5. Use maximal barrier precautions for insertion of central catheters: Maximal barrier precautions require the use of sterile cap, mask, gown, gloves, and drape. The rationale for this practice is the reduction of contamination during insertion of an indwelling catheter.

Pearl/Peril/Pitfall: Hands must be washed before and after contact with the patient, any equipment that comes in contact with the patient, or any contaminated objects in the environment. If gloves have been used, hands should be washed on their removal. Hands should be washed by rigorously rubbing together for at least 10 to 15 seconds with either chlorhexidine gluconate or triclosan handwashing agents. These 2 agents are relatively fast acting and have broad Gram-negative and Gram-positive spectra. Chlorhexidine gluconate has particularly effective residual antimicrobial activity.

UNIVERSAL PRECAUTIONS IN THE CARE OF ALL PATIENTS TO PREVENT POSSIBLE CONTAGION

Because persons of all ages and backgrounds may be sources of infection for the examiner, it is important to take proper precautions when working with blood and body fluids from all patients. Examples of sources of infection are tuberculosis, acquired immunodeficiency syndrome, or any potentially infected body fluid or discharge.

- Use gloves when the possibility exists of contact with a patient's blood or potentially infectious body secretions or excretions.

  Examples : starting intravenous lines, drawing blood, doing cardiopulmonary resuscitation (CPR) or other emergency procedures, and handling soiled linen and waste.

- Wash hands after removing gloves (do not wash gloves), and use clean gloves with each patient.

- Do not wear gloves or protective clothing when contact with the patient is unlikely to result in exposure to blood or potentially infectious body secretions or excretions. **Examples:** Shaking hands, delivering supplies and medications, removing trays and holding infants.

- Wear gown, mask, and protective eyewear in addition to gloves during procedures in which spattering of blood or body fluids may occur. **Examples:** arterial punctures, endoscopies, insertion of arterial lines, hemapheresis, and hemodialysis.

- Always be cautious when working with needles, scalpels, or other sharp instruments.

- Always dispose of needles and sharp instruments in the impervious containers readily available in health care facilities. Do not recap, clip or bend needles or throw them in the trash.

- Use the accompanying chart as a guide in identifying precautions that should be taken in specific situations.

UNIVERSAL PRECAUTIONS IN THE CARE OF ALL PATIENTS TO PREVENT POSSIBLE CONTAGION

Procedure	Guidelines				
	Wash Hands	Gloves	Gown	Mask	Eyewear
Talking with patients	—	—	—	—	—
Adjusting IV fluid rate or noninvasive equipment	—	—	—	—	—
Examining patient without touching blood, body fluids, mucous membranes	X	—	—	—	—
Examining patient with significant cough	X	X	—	—	—
Examining patient including contact with blood, body fluids, mucous membranes, drainage	X	X	—	—	—
Drawing blood	X	X	—	—	—
inserting venous access	X	X	—	—	—
Suctioning	X	X	Use gown, mask and eyewear if bloody body fluid spattering is likely.		
Inserting body or face catheters	X	X	Use gown, mask and eyewear if bloody body fluid spattering is likely.		
Handing solid waste, linen, other materials	X	X	Use gown, mask, and eyewear only if waste or linen is extensively contaminated and spattering is likely.		
Intubation	X	X	X	X	X
Inserting arterial access	X	X	X	X	X
Endoscopy, bronchoscopy	X	X	X	X	X
Operative and other procedures that produce extensive spattering of blood or body fluids and are likely to soil clothes	X	X	X	X	X

Data from the Centers for Disease Control and Prevention : MMWR 36 (suppl 25) : 3, 1987

The ten point plan on antibiotic use

1. Always take cultures of blood (and perhaps CSF and/or urine) before starting antibiotics.

2. Use the narrowest spectrum antibiotics possible, almost always a penicillin (e.g. piperacillin-tazobactam) and an aminoglycoside (e.g. amikacin).

3. Do not start treatment, as a general rule, with a third generation cephalosporin (e.g. cefotaxime, ceftazidime) or a carbapenem (e.g. imipenem, meropenem).

4. Develop local and national antibiotic policies to restrict the use of expensive, broadspectrum antibiotics like imipenem for emergency treatment.

5. Trust the microbiology laboratory: rely on the blood culture results.

6. Stop believing that a raised CRP means the baby is definitely septic.

7. If blood cultures are negative at 2–3 days, it is almost always safe and appropriate to stop antibiotics.

8. Try not to use antibiotics for long periods.

9. Treat sepsis but not colonization.

10. Do your best to prevent nosocomial infection, by reinforcing infection control, particularly hand washing.

Courtesy: **David Isaacs,** *Clinical Professor, University of Sydney, NSW,2006*

Pearl/Peril/Pitfall: When preparing for blood culture, the site should be cleaned to remove soiling, and the remaining microorganisms on the skin should be chemically killed. Skin preparation may be a 1- or 2-stage procedure involving 10- to 30-second swabbing of skin and allowing the agents to dry. Alcohol, povidone iodine, tincture of iodine, and chlorhexidine have been shown to be effective. The quality of skin preparation is believed to be important in reducing contamination of blood cultures.

STOP! HAVE YOU WASHED YOUR HANDS?

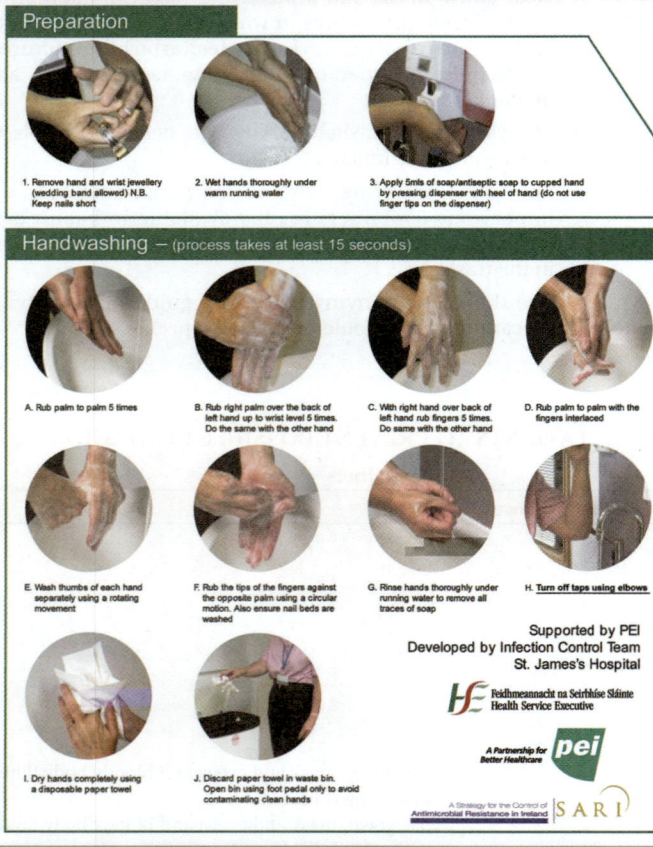

Handwashing Technique

Preparation

1. Remove hand and wrist jewellery (wedding band allowed) N.B. Keep nails short
2. Wet hands thoroughly under warm running water
3. Apply 5mls of soap/antiseptic soap to cupped hand by pressing dispenser with heel of hand (do not use finger tips on the dispenser)

Handwashing – (process takes at least 15 seconds)

A. Rub palm to palm 5 times
B. Rub right palm over the back of left hand up to wrist level 5 times. Do the same with the other hand
C. With right hand over back of left hand rub fingers 5 times. Do same with the other hand
D. Rub palm to palm with the fingers interlaced
E. Wash thumbs of each hand separately using a rotating movement
F. Rub the tips of the fingers against the opposite palm using a circular motion. Also ensure nail beds are washed
G. Rinse hands thoroughly under running water to remove all traces of soap
H. **Turn off taps using elbows**
I. Dry hands completely using a disposable paper towel
J. Discard paper towel in waste bin. Open bin using foot pedal only to avoid contaminating clean hands

Supported by PEI
Developed by Infection Control Team
St. James's Hospital

HSE Feidhmeannacht na Seirbhíse Sláinte Health Service Executive

A Partnership for Better Healthcare **pei**

A Strategy for the Control of Antimicrobial Resistance in Ireland SARI

Clean your hands
Say no to infection

How to wash your hands ?

Studies show that health care staff frequently use poor hand washing techniques and the most commonly neglected areas are the tips of the fingers, palm of the hand and the thumb. It is important that hand washing is carried out correctly to prevent the spread of infection Washing with liquid soap and water removes the majority of transient organisms. This is adequate for most purposes. An alcohol rub is a useful alternative when hand washing facilities are not available. This technique is only suitable if hands are not visibly soiled.

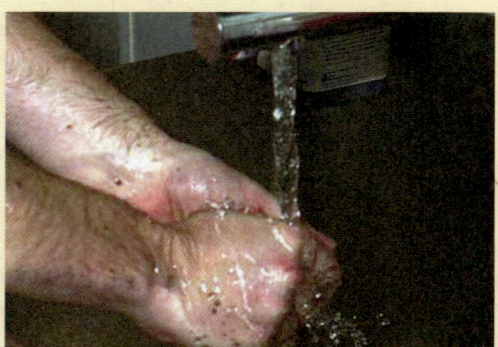

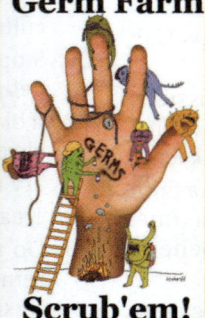

Germ Farm

GERMS

Scrub'em!

Hand washing is a cornerstone of infection control !

Equipment needed for effective handwashing:

* hands free wash basin *liquid soap *disposable paper towls (autoclaved, if possible) *foot operated pedal bin

Method of applying an alcohol handrub:

* When using an alcohol rub, the preparation should be rubbed into all areas of the hands, again paying attention to the thumbs, fingertips, between the fingers and the backs of the hands (see diagram 1) until the hands feel dry. Sufficient must be used to cover all areas of the hands.

Hand Washing is the most important single method of controlling infection:

The hands normally have a "resident" population of micro-organisms. Other organisms (germs) are picked up during everyday activities and these are termed "transient" organisms. Many infection control problems are caused by these transient organisms. Hand washing removes these transient organisms before they are transferred to another individual, or to a susceptible area on the same person. The potential chain of infection is broken by effective hand hygiene.

Good practice

*Fingernails should be kept clean, nail varnish free and short. *Jewellery should not be worn, except a plain band. *Breaks anywhere on the skin should be covered with a waterproof dressing. *Medical advice should be sought for skin damage by other agencies e.g. eczema.

Hands must be washed before and after each care activity or client contact for example:-

• Before handling food
• When the hands are visibly soiled
• Before a clean procedure
• After a dirty procedure, even if gloves were worn
• Between care episodes for one person
• Between different individuals

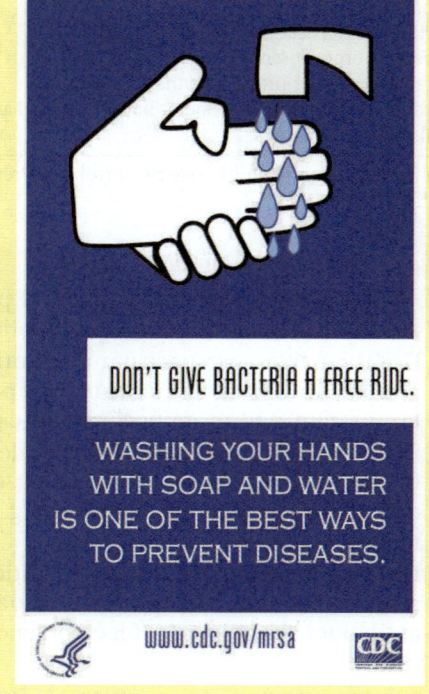

DON'T GIVE BACTERIA A FREE RIDE.

WASHING YOUR HANDS WITH SOAP AND WATER IS ONE OF THE BEST WAYS TO PREVENT DISEASES.

www.cdc.gov/mrsa CDC

Pearl/Peril/Pitfall: Continuing education, monitoring, reporting, and feedback to staff on behavior and infection surveillance data will improve compliance and effectiveness of handwashing practices. Continual vigilance in reminding staff to wash their hands is necessary. Reminders can be education programs, clever signs throughout the nursery, and individual prompting.

Practices that may decrease late-onset sepsis and limit vancomycin use include 1) use of full barrier precautions when placing central venous catheters, 2) use of optimal skin and catheter surface disinfection before obtaining blood for culture and changing tubing, 3) routinely obtaining 2 blood cultures from neonates with suspected sepsis and generally interpreting isolation of CoNS from a single culture as a contaminant, 4) restricting the prescribing of vancomycin for empiric therapy of neonates with suspected sepsis, 5) routine use of tests (e.g., CRP and semiquantitative blood cultures and/or the time to culture positivity) and identification of CoNS to the species level to aid in interpretation of the significance of a CoNS blood culture isolate, 6) discontinuation of empiric antimicrobials after 48 hours when cultures remain negative, and 7) limitation of the duration of antibiotic treatment of CoNS sepsis to 7 to 10 days. Use of such measures is likely to have an important impact on decreasing the use of vancomycin and other antimicrobials in neonates and in improving patient outcomes.

The most common clinical symptoms associated with VAP(Ventilator-Associated Pneumonia in ELBW Preterms)-included hypothermia and tachypnea, whereas purulent tracheal aspirates (>25 white blood cells/high-powered field on tracheal aspirate Gram stain) was the most common laboratory finding. Microorganisms associated with purulent tracheal aspirates in extremely preterm neonates include *Pseudomonas* species, *Enterobacter* species, *Klebsiella* species, and *Staphylococcus aureus*. Multiple organisms were isolated from respiratory secretions in 11 episodes (11 of 19 [58%]) of VAP. Gram-negative bacteria were isolated from respiratory secretions in 18 (18 of 19 [94%]) VAP episodes. Low birth weight, the presence of central venous or arterial catheters, indomethacin for treatment of patent ductus arteriosus, broad-spectrum antibiotic therapy, and total parenteral nutrition with lipid emulsions all have been shown to be associated with nosocomial infections in NICU patients. However, data on risk factors for VAP in this population are scarce.

VAP occurred at high rates in extremely preterm neonates in the NICU and was associated with previous BSI and with prolonged duration of endotracheal intubation. Patients with VAP were more likely to die and had significantly prolonged NICU LOS. Systematic surveillance programs to identify VAP rates in NICU patients may be helpful in guiding daily practice and as a measure of quality improvement. Interventions to prevent BSIs and reduce the duration of endotracheal intubation may help to prevent VAP in NICU patients. Additional studies of rates, risk factors, and outcomes as well as studies to determine the attributable LOS and mortality as a result of VAP in NICU patients are needed. PEDIATRICS Vol. 110 No. 4 October 2002, pp. e42.

KEY POINTS FOR CLINICAL PRACTICE

1. Handwashing (mechanical removal of organisms from hands) is considered a key aspect of hand hygiene (elimination of organisms from hands). The importance of vigorously washing hands 15 to 30 seconds before and after all patient contacts, after using gloves during patient care, and when in contact with patient equipment should be followed strictly by the NICU Staff. Barriers to compliance included skin breakdown from repeated friction and application of antisepsis agents, lack of time, involvement of multiple disciplines, and human nature. Strategies to overcome these barriers included introduction of new antisepsis agents: 2% chlorhexidine instead of 4% chlorhexidine, the addition of 3% triclosan at the sinks for staff with chlorhexidine-sensitive skin, and use of lotions that were compatible with the antibacterial agents. Continuing education, monitoring, reporting, and feedback to staff on behaviour and infection surveillance data will improve compliance and effectiveness of handwashing practices.

2. Reducing the duration of endotracheal tube use, adhering to sterile precautions with ventilator tubing and during tracheal suctioning, and addressing factors that inhibit pulmonary toilet (sedation, immobilization) are important in preventing respiratory infections.

3. Despite numerous published guidelines on the appropriate use of antibiotics and repeated warnings about the dangers of antibiotic resistance, physicians continue to use antibiotics both inappropriately and excessively. Neonatologists must promote the rational use of antibiotics including optimal choice of drug (narrow spectrum when possible; broad spectrum in selected patients) and optimal duration of therapy (2–3 days in patients whose blood or other systemic cultures are negative; longer in patients with proven infection).

4. *Screening of admissions and isolation of infected babies* with gastroenteritis, skin infections like staphylococcal, herpes etc., are important and they should be managed by different nurses. The mother should be taught general principles of hygiene and importance of handwashing for prevention of spread of infection. The use of a surgical mask while feeding will reduce the chances of droplet infection.

5. Most nosocomial infections in the NICU are bloodstream infections associated with an intravascular catheter (peripheral or central). Efforts to reduce catheter-related infections include proper antisepsis of the skin before insertion of the catheter, sterile precautions during catheter insertion, aseptic technique when entering the line, minimizing repeated entry into the line for blood sampling, sterile preparation of fluids to be used with a central venous catheter, and, finally, minimizing the number of catheter days.

REFERENCES AND FURTHER READING: 1) Risk factors for nosocomial sepsis in newborn intensive and intermediate care units Journal European Journal of Pediatrics Publisher Springer Berlin / Heidelberg ISSN 0340-6199 (Print) 1432–1076 Volume 155, Number 4 / April, 1996 2) P. Manzoni, D. Farina, M. Leonessa, E. A. d'Oulx, P. Galletto, M. Mostert, R. Miniero, and G. Gomirato Risk Factors for Progression to Invasive Fungal Infection in Preterm Neonates With Fungal Colonization Pediatrics, December 1, 2006; 118(6): 2359–2364. 3) C. Gomez-Gonzalez, C. Alba, J. R. Otero, F. Sanz, and F. Chaves Long Persistence of Methicillin-Susceptible Strains of Staphylococcus aureus Causing Sepsis in a Neonatal Intensive Care Unit J. Clin. Microbiol., July 1, 2007; 45(7): 2301–2304. 4) D. B Bartels, F. Schwab, C. Geffers, C. F Poets, and P. Gastmeier Nosocomial infection in small for gestational age newborns with birth weight <1500 g: a multicentre analysis Arch. Dis. Child. Fetal Neonatal Ed., November 1, 2007; 92(6): F449–F453. 5) J A Walsh, M E Walsh, S J Knowles, and C P F O'Donnell Bacterial colonisation of previously prepared neonatal endotracheal tubes in the delivery room Arch. Dis. Child. Fetal Neonatal Ed., November 1, 2008; 93(6): F475–F476.

*Pearl/Peril/Pitfall: Several host factors and invasive procedures are independently associated with an increased risk of Nosocomial sepsis. After adjustment for clinical severity, intravascular catheterization and assisted ventilation were found to be responsible for a considerable proportion of observed sepsis. They should therefore be considered as priorities for interventions, aimed both at reducing unnecessary use and promoting more strict compliance with aseptic practices.

Twins and Multiple Births

19

@ *"Intertwin transfusion is a normal event, since all monochorionic placentas have vascular anastomoses between the 2 fetal circulations. It is only when this transfusion becomes unbalanced TTTS happens".*

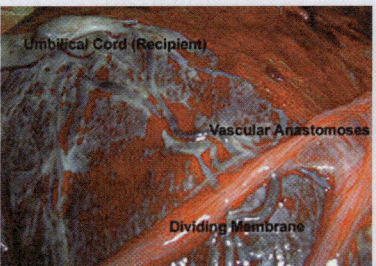
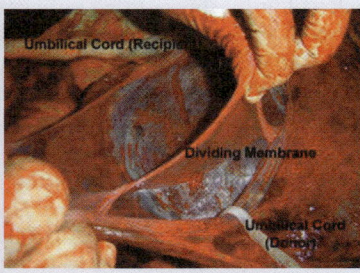

Fetal surface of the placenta showing two sacs, a dividing membrane and the vascular anastomoses

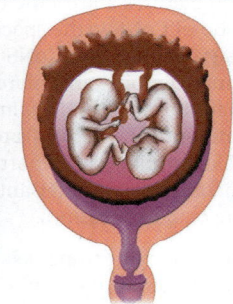

Twin to twin transfusion complicates about 15% of monochorial twin gestations and is responsible for 17% of the perinatal mortality in multiple pregnancies.

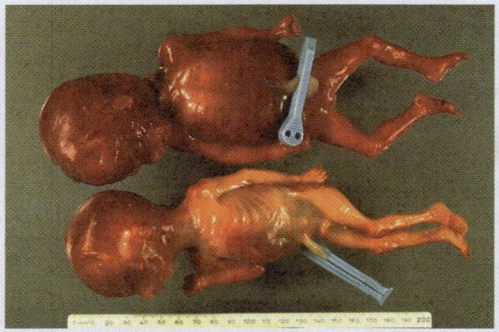

Twins are more than twice the trouble-The newborns with Twin-to-twin-Transfusion Syndrome: the upper one is bigger and plethoric; the lower one is smaller and anemic.

@Ultrasonographic criteria for the diagnosis of twin to twin transfusion syndrome include monochorionic placentation, with visualization of a separating membrane, fetus of the same sex, mid-pregnancy polyhydramnios-oligohydramnios sequence (polyhydramnios at the recipient's sac and oligohydramnios at the donor's sac), in the absence of other causes of abnormal amniotic fluid volume, and marked growth discordance. Significant weight discordance is considered a difference between the twin's size equal or over 20%. Other findings that might be observed include non visualization of the donor's bladder with enlarged recipient's bladder, abnormal Doppler S/D ratio at the umbilical cord, hydrops or evidence of congestive heart failure of either twin (more commonly found at the recipient twin). Milder forms of the disease are more difficult to diagnose due to the lack of uniform criteria, however, one should suspect twin to twin transfusion in the presence of amniotic fluid discrepancy between the cavities.

REVIEW OF CLINICAL PROBLEMS

1. What are the Maternal and fetal risks associated with multiple births?
   Ans: Refer to the Table "1" and "2" of the Chapter.
2. How do you determine the "Zygosity" in twins and multiple births ?
   Ans: Refer to the "No.3" of the "BIRD'S EYE VIEW/ OVERVIEW/SYNOPSIS" of the Chapter and to the Figure No "1" of the Chapter.
3. What are the essential aspects of Twin-To-Twin Transfusion Syndrome (TTTS)?
   Ans: Refer to the "No.4" of the "BIRD'S EYE VIEW/ OVERVIEW/SYNOPSIS" of the Chapter and to the Evaluation-Decision-Action Plan/Algorithm to diagnose and manage Twins and Multiple births.
4. How do you prepare for the resuscitation of a Twin delivery?
   Ans: Refer to the Evaluation-Decision-Action Plan/ Algorithm to diagnose and manage Twins and Multiple births.
5. Specify the essentials of postnatal care to be provided to the surviving twins and multiple births ?
   Ans: Refer to the Table 5 of the Chapter.

LEARNING OBJECTIVES

After completing this article, readers will be able to

1. Anticipate the risks associated with twins and multiple births and to act in coordination with the obstetric team involved in the management.
2. Observe closely during labor and in the immediate neonatal period, so that prompt treatment of asphyxia or TTTS (Twin-To-Twin Transfusion Syndrome) can be initiated.
3. Judge clinically and decide to perform an immediate blood transfusion in a severely anemic "donor" twin or to perform a partial exchange transfusion of a polycythemic "recipient" twin.
4. Determine the zygosity of the multiple births, for a prognostic purpose to counsel the parents
5. Ensure adequate postnatal care and follow-up of the surviving infants from multiple births.

*Pearl/Peril/Pitfall: Imaging Studies useful in Multifetal Pregnancies- ●Obstetrical: Prenatal ultrasonography is used to confirm multifetal pregnancy and to monitor intrauterine fetal growth. ● Fetal echocardiography : This is used to screen for congenital heart disease in neonates. ● Fetal MRI: This is used to screen for fetal anomalies. ● Neonatal : Chest radiography is used to evaluate respiratory distress. ● Ultrasonography : This is used to screen for intraventricular hemorrhage, periventricular leukomalacia, and abdominal abnormalities. ● Echocardiography : This is used to screen for congenital heart disease.

1. Twin and higher order multiple births (triplets, quadruplets or more) are becoming more common as a result of the more frequent use of ovulation induction and assisted reproduction techniques. The risk of prematurity is very high and the impact on NICU occupation by preterm birth in Multiple -Fetus - Pregnancies can stretch neonatal resources to the limit. Twins account for only 2% of births, but 9% of all perinatal deaths due to their prematurity and low birth weight. The prevalence rate of twin births varies from 6.7/1000 deliveries in Japan to 40/1000 deliveries in Nigeria. This is largely due to variations in dizygotic twinning, as the prevalence of monozygotic twinning is relatively constant worldwide at 3.5/1000 births. Approximately 25% of twins are born preterm. The mean gestational age at delivery for triplets is 33 weeks (with 85-90% delivering <37 wks and 20-30% <32 wks). Almost all quadruplets experience preterm delivery; 50% before 32 wks' gestation. Both mother and fetuses are at increased risks for morbidity and mortality because every complication of pregnancy occurs more commonly. *(Refer Table 1 and 2)*

2. Dizygotic (DZ) twins (*Fraternal*) arise when 2 ova are released and fertilized in one menstrual cycle, whereas Monozygotic (MZ) (*Identical*) twins arise when 1 ovum is fertilized and the resulting zygote divides into two.DZ twins always have 2 placentas with 2 chorions and 2 amnions (dichorionic diamniotic) ;placentas may be fused and *vascular connections do not occur.* MZ twins commonly have 1 placenta with 1 chorion and 2 amnions (monochorionic diamniotic)-*when the zygote splits at 4-8 days* or rarely, 1 placenta with 1 chorion and 1 amnion-*when the zygote splits at 9-12 days* (monochorionic monoamniotic).Splitting even later at day 14 and thereafter produces Conjoined twins.*Vascular anastomoses between two circulations are almost invariable in MZ twins* except when they are dichorionic, which is also possible with early division of zygote within Ist 3 days.

3. *Determination of zygosity* is important not only for epidemiological, genetic, obstetric, and pediatric reasons but also because of the difference in prognosis between MZ and DZ sets (worse in MZ, due to single placenta) .Twins of different sex are obviously DZ (1/3rd of DZ), but 2/3rds of DZ TWINS born will be of same sex.MZ twins must be of the same sex with some identical features and their anthropometric values must show close agreement.Monozygosity can be proven on the basis of a monochorionic placenta.However, MZ twins with dichorionic placentas can only be distinguished reliably from like-sex DZ twins by DNA Analysis using minisatellite probes.Prenatally, DNA can be obtained by CVP (Chorionic Villus Sampling) or amniocentesis. Postnatally, DNA typing should optimally be performed on umbilical cord tissue, buccal smear, or a skin biopsy specimen instead of blood.*Refer to the Figure No "1" of the Chapter for the flow chart to determine zygosity.*

4. *Twin-To-Twin Transfusion Syndrome* (TTTS) occurs only in monochorionic twins and complicates 20-30% of such pregnancies. Intertwin transfusion is a normal event, since all monochorionic placentas have vascular anastomoses between the 2 fetal circulations.It is only when this transfusion becomes unbalanced, TTTS happens.Acute TTTS results from an acute hemodynamic imbalance across the superficial arterioarterial/ venovenous anastomoses.It most commonly occurs during labour and may cause severe hypovolemia in one twin and hypervolemia in the other. It may also occur following the intrauterine death of one twin. Chronic TTTS results from a hemodynamic imbalance in the parenchymatous AV network and there is a conspicuous absence of superficial anastomoses.It complicates up to a third of monochorionic pregnancies and is the cause of up to 20% of perinatal mortality in twins.It may begin as early as 13 weeks and is well developed by 20–22 weeks.Mortality may be as high as 80-100% for twins presenting acutely at 18–26 weeks` gestation. Recipient fetus shows severe polyhydramnios, venous overload, cardiac hypertrophy, tricuspid regurgitation, hydrops and for the Donor fetus oligo hydramnios, IUGR, and sometimes a "stuck twin" are the usual problems.Although the donor is initially stressed, the recipient is always decompensated and dies first.This leads to exsanguination of the surviving twin into the demised fetus leading to multiorgan infarctions in survivor.*Fetal treatment interventions* include serial amnioreduction, microseptostomy of the intertwin membrane, fetoscopic laser photocoagulation, selective feticide(with transabdominal intrathoracic fetal injection of KCL), transfusion of the donor with exsanguination of the recipient. Amnioreduction results in higher survival rates than laser ablation in the less severe cases, whereas laser ablation appears to be more successful than amnio-reduction in the most severe. *In the Newborn, the recipient twin is* heavier,polycythemic (a Hb difference of at least 5 g/dL is noted between the twins) and faces the complications of high blood viscosity, such as cardiac failure, hyperbilirubinemia and intravascular thromboses, whereas *the donor* shows signs of IUGR, anemia and hypoproteinemia. Renal failure and/or renal tubular dysgenesis due to chronic renal hypoperfusion in utero may also occur. Neonatal management is similar to that of the polycythemic/to that of the anemic singletons. *Refer to the Evaluation-Decision-Action Plan/Algorithm for the details of resuscitation in twins and multiple births.*

5. *The Evaluation-Decision-Action Plan/Algorithm* describes the essential aspects of the diagnosis and management of TTTS and other specific problems associated with multiple births.

6. *Fetal nutrition and iu growth:* Fetal growth in twins is similar to that of singletons until 26 weeks of GA, and thereafter, body weight falls disproportionately more than head growth.The average birth weight of a newborn twin is 500 g < that of a singleton. Dichorionic twins tend to be heavier than monochorionic but DZ twins are heavier than both di- and monochorionic MZ twins.

7. **Congenital malformations:** Occur in ~6% of twin pregnancies, or 3% of individual twins.The risk in MZ twins is ~2.5 fold > in DZ twins or singletons.*Refer to the Table "3" of the Chapter for the common Congenital anomalies seen in twins and multiple births.*

8. **Resuscitation and birth preparedness:** At the delivery one resuscitaire and one trained member of the neonatal staff should be available for each baby, and supported by an assistant. A consultant should be designated coordinator and act as backup for the difficult resuscitation.*Refer to the Evaluation-Decision-Action Plan/Algorithm for the details of resuscitation in twins and multiple births.*

9. **Postnatal care of multiple births:** *Refer to the Table 5 of the Chapter for the details.*

10. **Death of a cotwin:** Occurs in 0.5–6.8% of twin pregnancies, after the 1st trimester.The emboli and debris from the dead fetus may enter the circulation of the surviving monochorionic twin producing multiple infarcts in brain, GIT,and kidneys.(Refer to *Table No "4" of the Chapter .*) In contrast, surviving dichorionic twins have a good prognosis. Female fetuses fare better than males, regardless of their zygosity.Second born monochorionic twin is at greater risk of mortality and morbidity, because of abnormal presentation of itself, loss of uterine tone and closure of cervix, and placental separation after the 1st twin`s delivery.

Pearl/Peril/Pitfall: Twin-to-twin transfusion syndrome (TTTS) syndrome: This syndrome occurs in monochorionic/monoamniotic or monochorionic/diamniotic twins. Vascular anastomoses in the monochorionic placenta may result in net transfusion of blood from one twin (i.e. the donor) to the other twin (i.e. the recipient). Polyhydramnios develops in the sac of the recipient twin because of the volume overload and increased fetal urine output. Oligohydramnios develops in the sac of the donor twin because of the hypovolemia and decreased urine output. Severe oligohydramnios can result in the stuck twin phenomena, in which the twin appears in a fixed position against the uterine wall.

THE EVALUATION-DECISION-ACTION-PLAN/ALGORITHM FOR THE DIAGNOSIS AND MANAGEMENT OF *TWINS and MULTIPLE BIRTHS.*

SUBJECTIVE FINDINGS

Hx of
- antenatal events such as prenatal diagnosis of twin pregnancy,intrauterine growth, chorionicity of placenta, zygosity by DNA analysis,maternal complications, 1st trimester USG scan to assess for nuchal translucency to screen for chromosomal abnormalities, 2nd trimester USG scan to assess for anatomic defects,fetal TTTS, Steroids given for inducing lung maturity, etc.
- natal events such as premature labor, delayed delivery of 2nd twin, APGAR scores and resuscitation details, for each twin, features of TTTS,placental examination findings if any?
- postnatal problems such as RDS,IUGR, hydrops,congenital anomalies etc.,

OBJECTIVE FINDINGS

Assess ABCDs and monitor CRT, O_2 sats, BP, core-peripheral temperature difference, RR, HR, central and peripheral pulses, urine output, and *look for* the features of TTTS(*Anemic* donor twin and *Plethoric* recipient twin)

Assess for IUGR and HYPOGLYCEMIA in the donor twin, signs of CHF in the recipient twin

Assess for congenital malformations, prematurity, RDS, Shock, DIC, postresuscitation care, need for NICU admission etc.,

INVESTIGATIONS

Blood FBC, differential, platelets, *hematocrit*, reticulocyte count, Group and type and cross match, Smear, coagulation screen (PT, APTT, fibrinogen, thrombin time, bleeding time and clotting time), blood cultures, ABG analysis, *Blood sugar*, BUN, creatinine, electrolytes, Ca^{++} Mg^{++}, LTFs, drug screen

Urine analysis
Imaging CXR, plain abdominal x-ray, USG scan/CT scan of head,

Perform partial sepsis screen (**defer LP**)-FBC, CRP, blood and urine cultures, CXR, etc.

Consider ECG, 2D ECHO, MRI brain scan metabolic screen, karyotyping when clinical course demands.

TWINS and MULTIPLE BIRTHS

If both the twins are born in good condition, near-term with AGA and are stable- provide routine postnatal care of any singleton!

Admit to SCBU/NICU, If there is an indication such as-RDS,Prematurity,IUGR,Life-Threatening Congenital malformations, shock, bleeding, hydrops etc.,

Ensure adequate preparation for proper Resuscitation !

*Each twin needs a full complement of resuscitation equipment, personnel, and expertise *Anticipate a high-risk preterm, asphyxiated, anemic/hydropic/malformed infant and prepare for an ET intubation, if necessary *Pay more attention to the 2nd born twin, as he/she is at higher risk for asphyxia, bleeding, RDS, and ICH

Judge clinically, whether there is TTTS!

*Cord blood Hb difference of >5g %/Hct of >15% suggests TTTS
*Weight difference of >25% suggests discordant growth

IF POSITIVE FOR TTTS

Anticipate the following problems and manage accordingly!

ARTERIAL SIDE-DONOR TWIN
Prematurity
Oligohydramnios
Small premature
Malnourished
Pale
Anemic
Hypovolemia
Hypoglycemia
Microcardia
Glomeruli small or normal
Arterioles thin walled

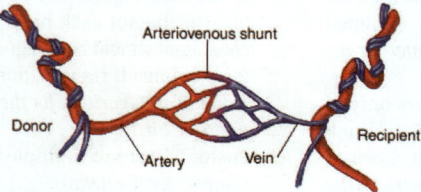

VENOUS SIDE-RECIPIENT TWIN
Prematurity
Polyhydramnios
Hydrops
Large premature
Well nourished
Plethoric
Polycythemic
Hypervolemic
Cardiac hypertrophy
Myocardial dysfunction
Tricuspid valve regurgitation
Right venticular outflow obstruction
Glomeruli large
Arterioles thick walled

Ensure adequate resuscitation at birth and continue ventilatory + cardiovascular support *Establish* rapid intravascular access for volume expansion to treat hypotension,correct hypoglycemia, and transfuse Packed RBCs to treat anemia in the donor twin, partial exchange transfusion in the recipient twin to treat significant polycythemia *Perform* neuroimaging to detect CNS injury.

Pearl/Peril/Pitfall: Conjoined twins ·Incomplete late division of monozygotic twins produces conjoined twins. · Conjoined twins are connected at identical points and are classified according to site of union; as follows :·Thoracopagus – Joined at chest (40%) ·Xiphopagus/ omphalopagus – Joined at abdomen (34%)· Pygopagus – Joined at buttocks (18%) ·Ischiopagus – Joined at ischium (6%)· Craniopagus – Joined at head (2%).

TABLE 1 — Maternal risks associated with multiple pregnancy

- Increased symptoms of early pregnancy (such as nausea and vomiting)
- Increased risk of miscarriage
- The vanishing twin syndrome
- Preterm labor and delivery
- Hypertension (pre-eclampsia and eclampsia)
- Antepartum hemorrhage
- Hydramnios (in up to 12% of multiple pregnancies)
- Possible need for prenatal hospitalization for prolonged periods
- Antepartum fetal death (risk of DIC in up to 25%)
- Risk of operative delivery (increased risk of trauma and infection)
- Increased likelihood of caesarean delivery
- Postpartum hemorrhage
- Postnatal problems (such as increased risk of depression)

TABLE 2 — Fetal risks associated with multiple pregnancy

- Congenital abnormalities (twice common as with singletons)
- IUGR (25–33% have birth weight <10th percentile)
- Preterm labor and delivery (rates of 30–50%)
- Twin-to-twin transfusion
- Death of cotwin
- Hydramnios (malpresentation)
- Operative vaginal delivery
- Cord accidents (carry perinatal mortality of up to 50%)
- Risk of asphyxia (mortality risk from asphyxia for twins is four to five times that of a singleton)
- Stillbirth or neonatal death (perinatal mortality rate of twins is up to ten times that of singletons)
- The 'stuck' twin phenomenon (occurs in 8% of twin pregnancies but mortality is over 80% for both twins)
- Twin entrapment (rate, typically occurring in monoamniotic twins; incidence of one in 800, and high risk of fetal death).

Fig. 1: Flowchart for determining zygosity

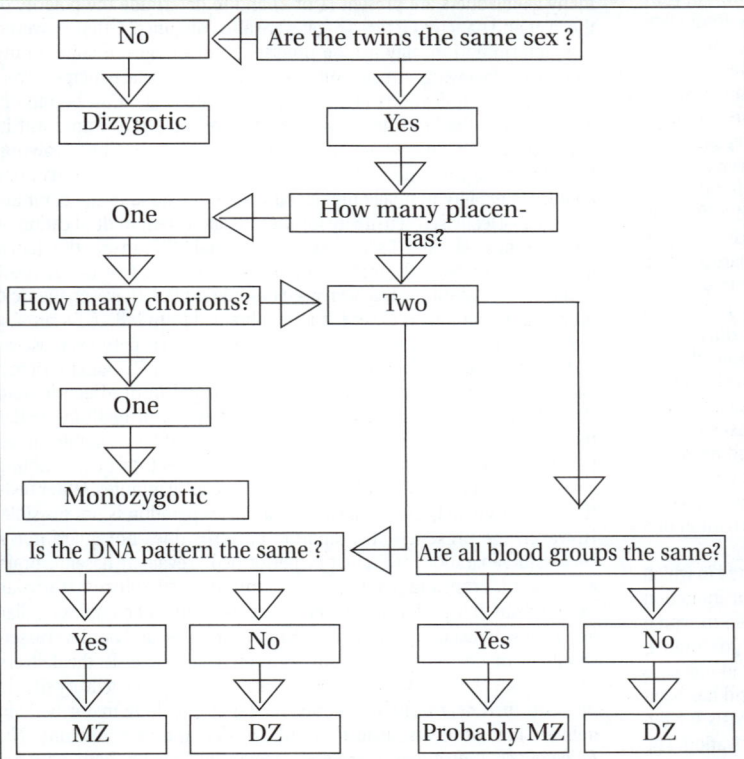

TABLE 3 — Congenital malformations in multiple births

1. Early structural defects

a) Caudal malformations (sirenomelia, sacro-coccygeal teratoma), b) Urological malformations (cloacal or bladder exstrophy) c) The VATER spectrum (vertebral anomalies, anal atresia, tracheoesophageal fistula, renal agenesis, cardiac defects) d) Neural tube defects (anencephaly, encephalocele, or holoprosencephaly) e) defects of laterality (situs inversus, polysplenia, or asplenia).

2. Vascular disruption syndromes

a. Early—acardia

b. Late—Cutis aplasia, limb interruption, intestinal atresia, gastroschisis, anorchia or gonadal dysgenesis, hemifacial microsomia, Goldenhar syndrome (facioauriculovertebral defects), or Poland sequence. Cranial abnormalities include porencephalic cysts, hydranencephaly, microcephaly, and hydrocephalus.

3. Deformations

Clubfoot, dislocated hips, and cranial synostosis.

TABLE 4 — Intrauterine fetal demise/death of a cotwin

*Death of 1 twin after 20 wks' gestation but before delivery occurs in 9% of multiple pregnancies *4–6 times more common in MZ pregnancies *Surviving twin is at a 20–40% significant risk of neurological injury (multicystic encephalomalacia) as a result of associated severe hypotension or thromboembolic events upon death of the cotwin *The death of one DZ twin has minimal adverse effect on the surviving twin, due to lack of a shared circulation (the dead fetus is either completely resorbed or compressed between the amniotic sac of its cotwin and the uterine wall i.e.,fetus papyraceous) *DIC is a complication in 25% of women who retain dead fetus for >3 weeks; monitor maternal coagulation profiles and consider delivery within this time frame *Other complications in the surviving twin; stillbirth, preterm delivery, placental abruption, and chorioamnionitis.

Pearl/Peril/Pitfall: Monochorionic/monoamniotic twins are rare; only 1% of monozygotic twins have this form of placentation. Monochorionic/monoamniotic twins have a common placenta, with vascular communications between the 2 circulations. These twins can develop twin-to-twin transfusion syndrome (TTTS). If twinning occurs more than 12 days after fertilization, then the monozygotic fertilized ovum only partially splits resulting in conjoined twins.

Pearl/Peril/Pitfall: Acardia is a rare anomaly unique to multifetal pregnancy. In this condition, one twin has an absent or rudimentary heart. TRAP sequence occurs when an acardiac twin receives all of the blood supply from the normal "pump" twin. This only occurs in monochorionic twins. Blood enters the acardiac twin in a reversed perfusion manner. Blood enters the fetus via an umbilical artery and exits via the umbilical vein. The excessive demands on the normal "pump" twin can cause cardiac failure in that twin.

CONJOINED TWINS

- Twinning occurs in approximately 1 of every 87 live births. Monozygotic twins account for one third of twin births. Conjoined twins account for 1% of monozygotic twins. Conjoined twins are identical twins whose bodies are joined in utero. It is a rare phenomenon; it is estimated to range from 1 in 50,000 births to 1 in 200,000 births, with a somewhat higher incidence in Southwest Asia, India and Africa.Exact epidemiology across different races and nations is not known because of underreporting and lack of facilities for prenatal diagnosis. Approximately half are stillborn, and a smaller fraction of pairs born alive have abnormalities incompatible with life. The overall survival rate for conjoined twins is approximately 25%.When born live, females are affected more often than males, with a female-to-male ratio of 3:1 or greater.

    Perhaps the most famous pair of conjoined twins was Chang and Eng Bunker (1811–1874), Chinese brothers born in Siam, now Thailand. They traveled with P.T. Barnum's circus for many years and were billed as the **Siamese Twins**; due to their fame and the rarity of the condition, the term came to be used as a synonym for conjoined twins, although in recent years the term has fallen out of favor and is considered a pejorative term.*The term Siamese twins is no longer considered appropriate.* Conjoined twins aren't limited to any racial or ethnic group and indeed have been born all over the world. Chang and Eng were joined by a band of flesh, cartilage, and their fused livers at the torso. In modern times, they could have been easily separated.

- Conjoined twins show characteristic points of attachment. They are classified according to the site of union, with the following frequency: *Thoracoomphalopagus (i.e., joined at the chest, abdomen, or both) - 74% *Thoracopagus or xiphopagus (i.e., joined at the chest) - 40% *Omphalopagus (i.e., joined at the abdomen) - 34% *Pygopagus (i.e., joined at the buttocks) - 18% *Ischiopagus (i.e., joined at the ischium) - 6% *Craniopagus (i.e., joined at the head) - 2%. **Cephalopagus:** Heads fused, bodies separated. These twins generally cannot survive due to severe malformations of the brain. Also known as janiceps (after the two-faced god Janus) or syncephalus. **Cephalothoracopagus:** Bodies fused in the head and thorax. In this type of twins, there are two faces facing in opposite directions, or sometimes a single face and an enlarged skull. These twins also generally cannot survive. (Also known as epholothoracopagus or craniothoracopagus.). **Dicephalus:** Two heads, one body with two legs and two, three, or four arms (*dibrachius, tribrachius* or *tetrabrachius,* respectively.) **Heteropagus:** Conjoined twins joined unequally usually resulting in a parasitic twin. **Ischio-omphalopagus:**The Twins are conjoined with spines in a Y-shape. They have four arms and usually two or three legs. These cases can be challenging because the twins often share reproductive and excretory systems. **Parapagus:** lateral union of the lower half extending variable distances upward, with the heart sometimes involved (5% of cases). **Diprosopus:** One head, with two faces side by side. A malformation of a single embryo, not true conjoined twinning.

- **Etiopathogenesis:** Seven cases (2 published) have been reported in which conjoined twinning occurred with the use of clomiphene for induction of ovulation. Two cases of thoracopagus have been reported in which conjoined twinning occurred with periconceptional maternal griseofulvin intake. Spina bifida is associated with conjoined twinning, and one case of conjoined twinning after maternal exposure to valproic acid has been reported. No gene mapping or linkage analysis currently exists for the malformation. Some investigators implicate abnormal X inactivation. The latter may be related to the increased incidence in female twins. Other studies refute abnormal X-chromosome inactivation.Pathophysiology- The morula becomes a blastocyst on day 6 after the ovum is fertilized. An inner cell mass develops at one end within this vesicle. The inner cell mass can form a whole fetus. Conjoined twins are produced when this inner cell mass, derived from a single zygote, incompletely splits late, after the 12th day of gestational life. Two contradicting theories exist to explain the origins of conjoined twins. The older and most generally accepted theory is *fission*, in which the fertilized egg splits partially. The second theory is fusion, in which a fertilized egg completely separates, but stem cells (which search for similar cells) find like-stem cells on the other twin and fuse the twins together.

- **Investigations:** *Chromosomal studies are inconclusive. An abnormal X-chromosome inactivation has been proposed, but this has not been proven. *Amniocentesis with an estimation of the lecithin-sphingomyelin ratio is performed to assess fetal lung maturity and to determine the optimal time for a cesarean delivery. *Imaging Studies *Prenatal ultrasonography can reveal conjoined twinning as early as 8 weeks' gestation. Conversely, twins with extreme fusion may be mistaken for a singleton. The twin fetuses do not move apart with fetal movement.

Polyhydramnios is frequent (75%). A monoamniotic cavity is present, and more than 3 umbilical vessels may be observed. Fusion sites include the thorax (thoracopagus), abdomen (omphalopagus), pelvis (ischiopagus), sacrum (pygopagus), or skull (craniopagus). Extensive zones of fusion may be named by the prefix di- (meaning 2), followed by the portion of the twins that is unfused. Examples include dicephalus (2 heads on one body), and dipygus (double buttocks; single head and torso with separate pelves and 4 legs). Serial scans may be required to monitor for hydrops. *Prenatal echocardiography has better yield than postnatal echocardiography in thoracopagus twins, because surface scanning may be difficult. *MRI of the brain is performed along with magnetic resonance angiography and magnetic resonance venography to delineate structures and blood supply in the craniopagus variety. *Radionuclide angiography is performed to calculate the extent of cross-circulation. Selective angiography is usually not necessary in twins with a shared liver. *Sonography allows for a complete anatomic examination and search for associated lethal malformations. A detailed ultrasound examination to exclude the possibility of conjoined twins is mandatory in all multiple pregnancies. Two-dimensional ultrasonography is instrumental in prenatally diagnosing conjoined twins, but precise classification is difficult because of 3-dimensional structures. Three-dimensional ultrasound has shown promise in improving the visualization of complex anatomic spatial relationships. Abdominal ultrasonography is performed to determine how many gallbladders are present (1 or 2) and to determine the polarity of the liver and pancreas if these organs are also conjoined. Often, however, this determination may not be precise. *Advantages of sonography include the following: -Images other structures (eg, aorta, pancreas, liver) -Identifies complications (eg, stenosis, obstruction) -Can be rapidly performed at the bedside -Does not involve radiation (important in pregnancy) -Disadvantages of sonography include the following: Dependent on the type and extent of fusion, as well as the operator's abilities—Inability to image the ductal system proximal to the common bile duct—Decreased sensitivity for the site and extent of duplication or fusion compared with CT scanning or MRI. -Fetal MRI can identify shared anatomy of twins with precise detail. However, this test is not 100% accurate.—CT scanning has been used in some studies. However, the yield for complex anatomy is lower than that obtained from MRI. CT scanning may be helpful in shared bony pelvis and shared pelvic perineal muscles. -Contrast studies are performed to evaluate the extent of GI ,genitourinary, and reproductive system fusions.· Diisopropyl iminodiacetic acid (DISIDA) scanning is a nuclear medicine study performed to visualize the biliary tract. Technetium-labeled analogue of DISIDA is administered intravenously (IV) and is secreted by hepatocytes into bile, enabling visualization of the gall bladder and biliary tree in 30 minutes. **Other tests** *On ECG, a single QRS indicates that cardiac separation is not possible. However, the presence of 2 separate patterns does not guarantee a successful separation. *EEG may be performed to evaluate baseline brain activity in craniopagus twins. Diagnostic procedures *Cardiac catheterization is performed to determine the nature of complex cardiac anomalies. An accurate estimation of all major inflow and outflow vessels should be made. *Surgical therapy: With prenatal diagnosis, the delivery should always be by cesarean section. An elective cesarean delivery should be performed near term after confirmation of fetal lung maturity. Twin delivery may otherwise lead to overdistension and uterine atony. *The following are indications for emergent separation:* *One or both twins are in a life-threatening situation. *A correctable, life-threatening associated congenital anomaly (e.g. intestinal atresia, malrotation with midgut volvulus, ruptured exomphalos, anorectal agenesis) is present. If the condition of the twins is stable and early separation is not indicated, the surgery is usually delayed until age 6–12 months. At that age, the twins are larger and better able to tolerate surgery. Rapid expansion of the body wall can occur to close substantial defects. The anatomy of the junction and the shared organs and structures dictate the technical details of the procedure.Once the diagnosis has been confirmed, the parents should be counseled on the possible outcomes. The team that will attempt the possible separation should provide this advice. The management of conjoined twins can be divided into 2 time points: prenatal and postnatal. Prenatally, elective termination is recommended where there is cardiac or cerebral fusion. There have been only 2 successful separations of conjoined hearts. The parents may elect interruption of the pregnancy particularly when the anticipated severity of deformity following separation would be unacceptable. If the pregnancy is allowed to continue, elective cesarean delivery should be planned for 36 to 38 weeks' gestation pending confirmation of satisfactory lung maturation.

The delivery should take place in or close to the pediatric surgical center where separation is planned to occur. Recently, prenatal magnetic resonance imaging scan has been found to be of value in planning for an extrauterine intrapartum procedure and immediate separation. Postnatal management rests on 3 possible situations: nonoperative care, emergency separation, or elective separation. Nonoperative care is indicated when no attempt at surgical separation should be considered in the presence of complex cardiac fusion or where there would be severe unacceptable deformity following separation. Emergency separation is undertaken when 1 twin is dead or dying and threatening the survival of the remaining twin, or where a life-threatening correctable congenital abnormality (e.g., intestinal atresia, malrotation with or without volvulus, ruptured omphalocele, or anorectal agenesis) is present in 1 or both twins. Under these circumstances the only chance of saving 1 or both infants lies in immediate separation. Emergency separation carries a significantly higher mortality rate (70%-80%) compared with elective procedures. Elective separation will normally take place between 2 to 4 months of age. It allows the twins to stabilize and thrive and provides time to carry out detailed investigations to define the nature and the extent of union. It also allows the application of methods to be carried out to achieve primary closure of the wound such as tissue expansion. Detailed planning of the operative procedure with all members of the operating team should take place before the separation. The survival rate for elective separation approximates 80%.

Anesthetic management: Two sets of anesthesiologists, one for each infant, are essential, as each infant has to be separately monitored throughout the procedure. Essential monitoring consists of arterial and central venous catheters, electrocardiogram, pulse oximetry, capnography, and urinary output. Regular blood gas analyses are undertaken throughout the procedure. All drugs and intravenous fluids are calculated on a total weight basis with half being delivered to each twin. Because of the cross-circulation, drugs given intravenously may have an unpredictable effect. Thus, particular care is essential when administering drugs such as opioids, which should be given incrementally.

Principles of the operative procedure: The infants are initially positioned on the side opposite to the preferred approach, and the skin and deep fascia are incised to a convenient depth. A swab is left in the wound and the skin incision is closed with a continuous suture. This step provides a predetermined site to work toward in the final stages of separation. The infants are then carefully turned to the operative side, ensuring that all tubes and lines are securely attached. The operation then proceeds according to the plan based on imaging investigations; however, unexpected findings are not uncommon and the operative plan may have to be varied accordingly. Blood loss during division of the liver can be minimized by the use of the ultrasonic dissector and bipolar coagulation and by applying fibrin sealant to the raw surface. Assignment of organs, such as intestine, will be equal unless 1 twin is nonviable. In ischiopagus, parapagus, and pygopagus twins, urological anatomy is often complex with 1 ureter from each twin frequently crossing to enter the contralateral bladder. Achieving body wall closure may be another problem despite the use of preoperative tissue expansion. We have a preference for inserting polypropylene mesh securely sutured to the edges of the defect. The mesh is progressively plicated postoperatively aiming at full closure 2 to 3 weeks postoperatively.

Postoperative management: Following prolonged operative procedures, it is necessary to electively paralyze and mechanically ventilate the infants for 48 to 72 hours postoperatively. The infants require meticulous monitoring in the intensive care unit, paying particular attention to cardiac underperformance (poor cardiac output). Fluid and electrolyte replacement should be accurately administered as there will be huge losses when large prosthetic closure has been used. Strict infectious precautions must be exercised to avoid sepsis, particularly where there are large skin defects. **Complications** are common and may include the following: *Congestive cardiac failure: This is observed when a conjoined heart is divided. *Inadequate or incomplete organ systems: This complication occurs when the twins have unequal distribution of their organs (e.g. one shared biliary tract).

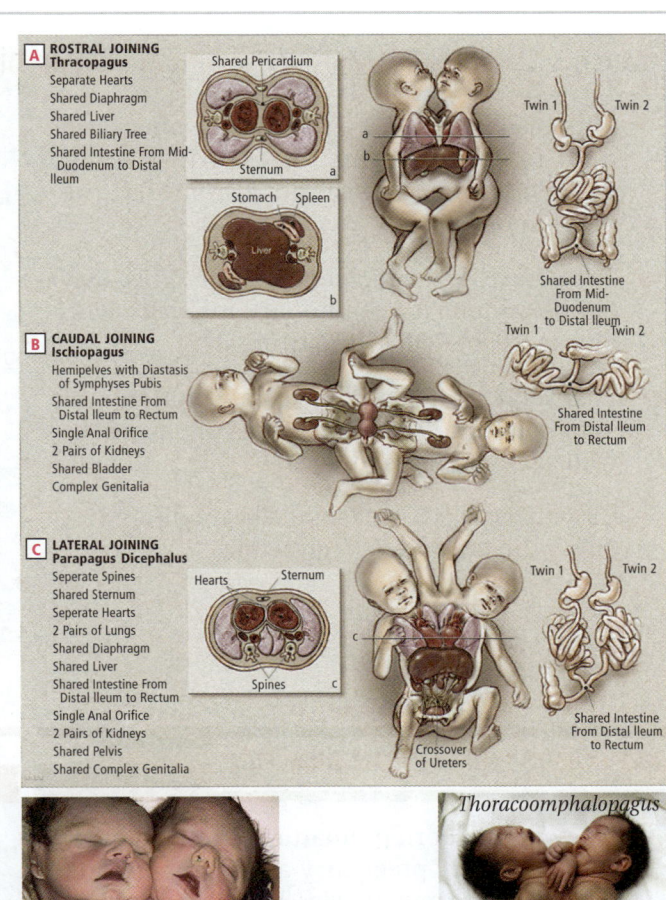

A ROSTRAL JOINING
Thoracopagus
Separate Hearts
Shared Diaphragm
Shared Liver
Shared Biliary Tree
Shared Intestine From Mid-Duodenum to Distal Ileum

Shared Pericardium
Sternum
Stomach   Spleen
Liver
Twin 1   Twin 2
Shared Intestine From Mid-Duodenum to Distal Ileum

B CAUDAL JOINING
Ischiopagus
Hemipelves with Diastasis of Symphyses Pubis
Shared Intestine From Distal Ileum to Rectum
Single Anal Orifice
2 Pairs of Kidneys
Shared Bladder
Complex Genitalia

Twin 1   Twin 2
Shared Intestine From Distal Ileum to Rectum

C LATERAL JOINING
Parapagus Dicephalus
Seperate Spines
Shared Sternum
Seperate Hearts
2 Pairs of Lungs
Shared Diaphragm
Shared Liver
Shared Intestine From Distal Ileum to Rectum
Single Anal Orifice
2 Pairs of Kidneys
Shared Pelvis
Shared Complex Genitalia

Hearts   Sternum
Spines
Crossover of Ureters
Twin 1   Twin 2
Shared Intestine From Distal Ileum to Rectum

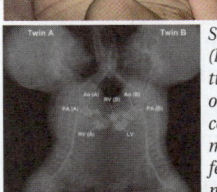

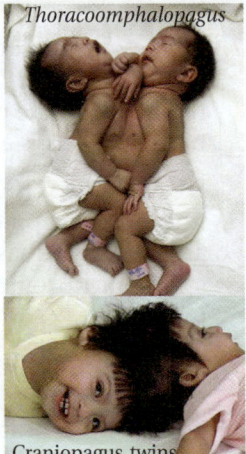

Thoracoomphalopagus

Stillborn double-headed (bicephalus) conjoined twins, a rare occurrence. Even though conjoined twinning is more common in female fetuses (75% of cases), most stillborn conjoined twins are male. A single penis and 2 testes were present in this case.

Craniopagus twins.

Thoracopagus is the most common form of conjoined twins, with fusion from the anterior thorax to the umbilicus. A common pericardial sac is present in 90% of thoracopagus twins, and conjoined hearts are seen in 75%. Postmortem angiography demonstrated conjoined hearts with a left ventricle common to both twins (Figure on left). At autopsy, the cardiac anatomy for both hearts was found to be an unbalanced complete atrioventricular canal defect with a common left ventricle. **Courtesy:** R. Thomas Collins, II, MD; Tricia R. Bhatti, MD; Dale S. Huff, MD; Paul M. Weinberg, MD, **Images in Cardiovascular Medicine,** *Circulation* 2008;118;1496

Adequate preplanning in these cases is essential. *Enormous skin defect: This may result following separation of a large bridge and can often be avoided by delaying the surgery until age 1 year. Preseparation tissue expanders may be useful to avoid this problem. The expanders are essentially pouches, which are gradually filled with saline solution. This stretches the skin, allowing the surgeons to close the wounds after separation surgery. *Infection: Strict infectious precautions are required for 2 days following the surgical procedure, and patients are kept in the ICU. If they do well, routine precautions are adequate for follow-up care. *Hemorrhage: Life-threatening exsanguination can result, especially in craniopagus twins who have a large communicating venous sinus.

Conclusion: Success in the management of conjoined twins is dependent on the experience of the team and the full range of resources, medical and nursing, at the tertiary referral center. Advances in imaging modalities, preoperative and postoperative management, and anesthetic care have been major factors in improving the outcome.

REFERENCE: Lewis Spitz, MD, PhD, FRCS; Edward M. Kiely, FRCS *JAMA.* 2003;289:1307–1310.

TABLE 5 Postnatal care of survivors from multiple births

- Multiple births require special care after birth due to prematurity, low birth-weight, congenital anomalies and respiratory and neuro morbidity.

- Twins have higher incidence of RDS. They may be discordant for pulmonary maturity with higher risk of RDS in 2nd twin.

- Postnatal management of polycythemic or anemic twins is similar to that of singletons with same problem.

- Growth retarded twins should be monitored for polycythemia and hypoglycemia.

- Twins have higher incidence of neuro morbidity due to prematurity, growth retardation, birth trauma and birth asphyxia.

- One should screen for coagulopathy if there was history of intrauterine demise of a co-twin.

- Counseling for parenting, and family adjustment for support and care of low birth-weight twins must be done.

- Help promote, initiate and family adjustment for support and care of low birth-weight twins must be done.

- Breast-feeding in twins is a challenging task and requires great motivation and support.

KEY POINTS FOR CLINICAL PRACTICE

1. Most twins are born **premardy,** and maternal complications of pregnancy are more common than with single pregnancies. The perinatal mortality of twins is about 4 times that of singletons.

2. **DETERMINATION OF ZYGOSITY** is important not only for epidemiological, genetic, obstetric, and pediatric reasons but also because of the difference in prognosis between MZ and DZ sets (worse in MZ, due to single placenta)

3. **Second born monochorionic twin is at greater risk of mortality and morbidity,** because of abnormal presentation of itself, loss of uterine tone and closure of cervix, and placental separation after the 1st twin's delivery.

4. *TWIN-TO TWIN TRANSFUSION SYNDROME: In the Newborn,* the recipient twin is heavier, polycythemic (a Hb difference of at least 5 g/dL and Hematocrit >15% is noted between the twins) and faces the complications of high blood viscosity, such as cardiac failure, hyperbilirubinemia and intravascular thromboses, whereas *the donor* shows signs of IUGR, anemia and hypoproteinemia. Renal failure and/or renal tubular dysgenesis due to chronic renal hypoperfusion in utero may also occur.

5. **RESUSCITATION AND BIRTH PREPAREDNESS:** At the delivery one resuscitaire and one trained member of the neonatal staff should be available for each baby, and supported by an assistant. A consultant should be designated coordinator and act as backup for the difficult resuscitation.

REFERENCES AND FURTHER READING: 1) Pietrantoni M, et al. Mortality conference: twin-to-twin transfusion. J Pediatr. 1998 Jun; 132(6): 1071-1076. 2) Ville Y, et al. Endoscopic laser coagulation in the management of severe twin-to-twin transfusion syndrome. Br J Obstet Gynaecol. 1998 Apr; 105(4): 446-453. 3) Howarth GR, et al. Management of early onset severe twin-twin transfusion syndrome in the absence of fetoscopic equipment by exteriorisation, ligation and replacement of the umbilical cord of the sacrificed twin. S Afr Med J. 1998 Mar; 88(3): 286. 4) van Gemert MJ, et al. Placental anatomy, fetal demise and therapeutic intervention in monochorionic twins and the transfusion syndrome: new hypotheses. Eur J Obstet Gynecol Reprod Biol. 1998 May; 78(1): 53-62. 5) Feldman DM, et al. Iatrogenic monoamniotic twins as a complication of therapeutic amniocentesis. Obstet Gynecol. 1998 May; 91(5 Pt 2): 815-816.

Pearl/Peril/Pitfall : Dizygotic twins develop when 2 ovum are fertilized. Dizygotic twins have separate amnions, chorions, and placentas. The placentas in dizygotic twins may fuse if the implantation sites are proximate. The fused placentas can be easily separated after birth. Monozygotic twins develop when a single fertilized ovum splits after conception. An early splitting (i.e. within 2 d after fertilization) of monozygotic twins produces separate chorions and amnions. These dichorionic twins have different placentas that can be separate or fused. Approximately 30% of monozygotic twins have dichorionic/diamniotic placentas. Later splitting (i.e. 3–8 d after fertilization) results in monochorionic/diamniotic placentation.

20 Extremely (Preterm) Low Birth Weight Infant "Micro premie" (< 1000g)

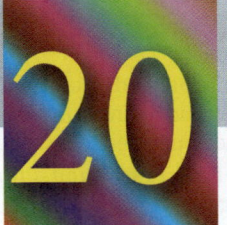

@ *The best practice of the management of the ELBW is to formulate decisions in concert with parents, after providing them with clear, realistic, and factual information about the possibilities for success of therapy and its long-term outcome.*

Small for gestational age (SGA) babies are those whose birth weight lies below the 10th percentile for that gestational age. Low birth weight (LBW), is sometimes used to define a baby that weighs less than 5 lb 8 oz (2,500 g) regardless of gestational age. One third of babies born with a low birth weight are also small for gestational age. Other definitions include *Very Low Birth Weight* (VLBW) which is less than 3 lb 5 oz (1,500 g) and *Extremely Low Birth Weight* (ELBW) which is less than 2 lb 3 oz (1,000 g).

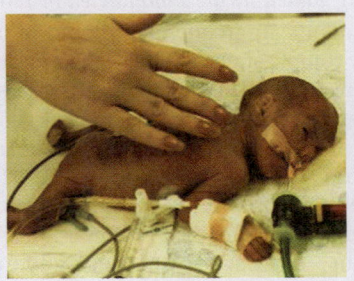

4 factors *should be considered in addition to gestational age when determining the likelihood of favorable outcome of ELBW babies with intensive care:*

* *Sex: Female sex has the more favorable outcome.*

* *Exposure to antenatal corticosteroids (with favorable effect)*

* *Single or multiple birth: Single birth has a favorable effect.*

* *Birth weight: Increasing increments of 100 g each week add to favorable outcome potential.*

The main causes for low birth weight

The two main causes of LBW are early delivery, also known as preterm birth, and poor fetal growth. About 70% of all LBW babies are born preterm - before 37 completed weeks of pregnancy. The remaining 30% of low birth weight babies are born at full term, but did not grow properly in the womb. Most extremely low birth weight infants are also the youngest of premature newborns, "micro premies", usually born at 27 weeks' gestational age or younger.

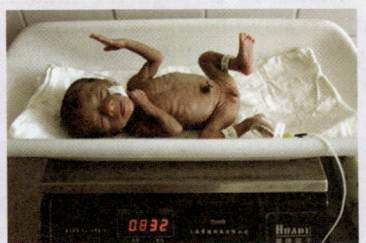

Infants with extremely low birth weights (ELBWs) are more susceptible to all of the possible complications of premature birth, both in the immediate neonatal period and after discharge from the nursery. Although the mortality rate has diminished with the use of surfactants, the proportion of surviving infants with severe sequelae, such as chronic lung disease, cognitive delays, cerebral palsy, and neurosensory deficits (i.e. deafness and blindness), has not. Although improved neurodevelopmental outcomes have been reported in a few small studies, such improvement has not been seen on a global scale.

REVIEW OF CLINICAL PROBLEMS

1. Discuss the Major problems of an ELBW Infant.
   Ans: Refer to Table 1 of the Chapter.

2. Outline the treatment guidelines for an initial management of an ELBW Infant.
   Ans: Refer to Table 2 of the Chapter.

3. What are the investigations to be done while managing an ELBW Infant?
   Ans: Refer to the Evaluation-Decision-Action Plan/ Algorithm to diagnose and manage an ELBW Infant.

4. What are the late sequelae of LBW Infants ?
   Ans: Refer to Section "Late Sequelae of LBW Infants" of the Chapter.

5. Outline the recommended Screening procedure for Follow-up of the common complications of ELBW Infants.
   Ans: Refer to Table 5 of the Chapter.

LEARNING OBJECTIVES

After completing this article, readers will be able to

1. Formulate decisions in concert with parents, at the time of delivery after providing them with clear, realistic, and factual information about the possibilities for success of therapy and its long-term outcome.

2. Ensure proper Golden Hour management and ongoing NICU Care necessary for the better outcome of ELBW Infants.

3. Anticipate the common complications of ELBW Infants and screen for them promptly and manage them appropriately.

4. Ensure the recommended Follow-up Care for these ELBW Infants with possible long-term sequelae.

5. Counsel the parents about the prognosis and educate them about the Follow-up visits.

Pearl/Peril/Pitfall: *For transport to the neonatal ICU (NICU) from the delivery room, the ELBW infant should be covered with either warmed blankets or cellophane wrap. For transport of more than very short distances, the infant should be placed in a double-walled, heated incubator. The delivery room and NICU should be kept warm to aid in the prevention of hypothermia in the preterm infant.*

BIRD'S EYE VIEW/OVERVIEW/SYNOPSIS

1. Extremely Low-Birth-Weight Infants (birth weight <1,000g) are physiologically immature, and they are extremely sensitive to small changes in respiratory management, blood pressure, fluid administration, nutrition and other aspects of neonatal care. These infants ("micro premies") present one of the greatest medical and ethical challenges, because they often are the most critically ill and at the highest risk for mortality and long-term morbidity of any NICU patient. These infants should be delivered in a facility with a high-risk obstetrical service and a level-III NICU. The safety of in utero transfer must be weighed against the risks of infant transport. Prenatal administration of beta- or dexamethasone, 2 doses of 12mg 12hr apart produces measurable benefit for the ELBW infant born between 12hr and 7 days later, producing a 40% reduction in mortality and similarly reduced rates and severity of respiratory distress syndrome, through the induction of lung surfactant and antioxident production.

2. If the delivery of an ELBW infant is threatened, the neonatologist and the obstetrician should consult with parents and discuss certain important issues such as **a)**survival chances (<23 wks' gestational age = 0, and at 23, 24 and 25 wks it would be 15%, 55%, and 79% respectively) **(b)** delivery room management and resuscitation of the baby **(c)** potential risks of both the extent of prematurity and the proposed therapeutic interventions **(d)** short-term and long-term morbidity. The best practice is to formulate decisions in concert with parents, after providing them with clear, realistic, and factual information about the possibilities for success of therapy and its long-term outcome.

3. *Delivery room care of ELBW infant* (a)ensure good thermoregulation (preheated warmer, quick drying the baby, removal of wet toweling etc.) (b)"gentle" ventilation with low tidal volume strategy avoiding hyperventilation and hyperoxia and early surfactant therapy once correct Endotracheal Tube position has been confirmed clinically c)transport of the ELBW infant to the NICU in a prewarmed transport incubator/radiant warmer combination unit (Giraffe Bed, Ohmeda Medical).

4. *Care of ELBW infant in the NICU-Refer to Table 1* for an outline of management of ELBW infant. Careful attention to detail and frequent monitoring are the basic components of care of the ELBW infant, because critical changes can occur rapidly. Delicate pulmonary status, large fluid losses, balances between fluid intake and blood glucose levels, and the immaturity and increased sensitivity of several organ systems all require close monitoring. Monitoring itself, however, may cause increased risks because of small blood volumes, tiny blood vessels, and limited skin integrity. (*Refer to Table 4* for practical guidelines for skin care of ELBW infants).

5. The first 24-48hrs are the most critical period for survival of ELBW infants. Infants who require significant respiratory, cardiovascular, and/or fluid support are assessed continuously, and their chances for survival are estimated. If the death is imminent, continued treatment is futile, or treatment is likely to result in survival of a neurologically compromised infant, withdrawal of intensive care support and redirection of care to comfort measures only can be done after counseling the parents.

6. *The Evaluation-Decision-Action-Plan/Algorithm* outlines the management of the ELBW infants. The essential components of the management include a)respiratory support (conventional/HFOV ventilation, surfactant therapy, vitamin-A supplementation and caffeine citrate) b)fluids and electrolyte management c)skin care d)cardiovascular support e)PDA management f)blood transfusions as appropriate g)infection control and h)nutritional support (total parenteral nutrition + trophic feeding with breast milk).

7. *The ELBW infants should be screened for common complications such as IVH, ROP and hearing screen. The screening guidelines are summarized in* Table 5.

8. ELBW infants are frequently exposed to perinatal and delivery complications that raise their risk of early-onset infections. The need for prolonged IV access, exposure to parenteral nutrition and mechanical ventilation also subject the ELBW infant to a high risk of late-onset (> 7 days) nosocomial infections. Immaturity of both humoral and cellular immunity in the ELBW population contributes to the frequent infections. In addition to the judicious use of antibiotics and antifungals, environmental controls, nursery surveillance, and modulation of the immature immune response have been proposed as possible interventions to prevent infections in extremely premature infants.

9. Total Parenteral Nutrition (TPN) has been life saving for ELBW infants and is begun shortly after birth using a standard solution administered at a rate of 60ml/kg/day, resulting in protein administration of 1.5g/kg/day. On subsequent days, customized parenteral solutions are formulated to increase the protein administration rate by 1g/kg/day upto a maximum of 3.5g/kg/day. IV lipids are begun on day 2, @ 0.5g/kg/day and advanced each day to a maximum of 3g/kg/day. Enteral feeding is begun as soon as the baby is clinically stable, and is not receiving indomethacin or pressor therapy. The safe initiation of enteral feeds begins with the introduction of small trophic amounts of breast milk (@ 10–20ml/kg/day), with the goal of priming the gut by inducing local factors necessary for normal gut function. This amount may be started even in the presence of an umbilical arterial line, and or continued for 3–4 days without a change in volume. Feedings of 20cal/30ml breast milk or formula are then slowly advanced (10–20 ml/kg/day) while monitoring for signs of feeding intolerance such as abdominal distention, vomiting (rare), and increased gastric residuals.

10. It is the responsibility of neonatologists to stay abreast of clinical improvements and the short-term and long-term consequences of established and newly proposed medical interventions so as to provide the best care for these vulnerable ELBW infants and to keep parents informed and involved.

Pearl/Peril/Pitfall: Because symptoms of hypoglycemia (seizures, jitteriness, lethargy, apnea, poor feeding) may be less obvious in preterm infants, hypoglycemia may only be detected on routine sampling. One form of accepted treatment consists of an immediate intravenous dextrose infusion of 2 mL/kg of 10% dextrose-in-water solution (200 mg/kg) followed by a continuous intravenous infusion of dextrose at 6–8 mg/kg/min to maintain a constant supply of glucose for metabolic needs and to avoid further hypoglycemia.

THE EVALUATION-DECISION-ACTION-PLAN/ALGORITHM FOR THE DIAGNOSIS AND MANAGEMENT OF *EXTREMELY LOW-BIRTH-WEIGHT INFANTS*

SUBJECTIVE FINDINGS

Counsel parents: about a)survival chances of ELBW soon-to-be born baby b)parental desires for attempting/withholding resuscitation at very low gestational ages (23-24 wks) c)short-term complications in NICU d)long-term morbidity on follow-up.

Ensure adequate delivery room care: a) define limits of resuscitative efforts b)respiratory support with low tidal volume ventilation strategy c)prevention of heat and water loss d)early surfactant therapy.

Provide proper care after resuscitation: a)plastic-wrap the infant b)place the infant in a prewarmed transport incubator c)monitor for ABCs and recheck the infant's temperature to prevent hypothermia.

OBJECTIVE FINDINGS

Assess ABCs, vitals, BP, O$_2$ sats, work of breathing, central cyanosis, CRT, pulses, Urine output, signs suggestive of sepsis/birth asphyxia/CCF. *Anticipate the short-term complications, such as* respiratory distress syndrome, air leaks, apnea of prematurity, bronchopulmonary dysplasia, hypotension, PDA, water/electrolyte imbalance + acid-base disturbances, intraventricular hemorrhage and periventricular leukomalacia, nosocomial infections and immune deficiency, feeding intolerance and NEC, iatrogenic anemia, ROP etc. (*Refer to Table 1*). *Ensure frequent reassessment of the ELBW baby to avoid* hyperoxia, hypocarbia, hypotension, acidosis, hypothermia, excess weight gain, hyperglycemia with osmotic diuresis, electrolyte + acid-base disturbances, anemia, infections, skin breakdown, oliguria, dehydration/over hydration, bleeding tendency including pulmonary hemorrhage, poor nutrition and excess catabolism, etc.

INVESTIGATIONS

Monitor the following parameters a) *4 hrly* TPR, glucose, bilirubin and ABG analysis. b) *daily* weight (twice a day), hemoglobin, PCV, WBC, Platelets and electrolytes (2 or 3 times/day in the first 3–4 days until fluid balance stabilizes), calcium, phosphate, glucose and creatinine and chest X-ray. c) *2 or 3 times/week* - albumin, ET tube aspirate culture, CRP. d) *weekly* liver enzymes (when on TPN), triglycerides (when on TPN), alkaline phosphatase for osteopenia and reticulocytes for anemia of prematurity. e) *partial/full septic screen* (culture - blood ± CSF ± Urine) and coagulation screen where appropriate f) *screen for common complications of ELBW: Refer to Table 5* for recommended screening.

EXTREMELY LOW-BIRTH-WEIGHT INFANTS (Birth Weight <1,000 g)

Screen for early-onset sepsis immediately after birth and treat with prophylactic antibiotics (Ampicillin and gentamicin) pending culture results: Always screen for nosocomial infections/late-onset infections with coagulase-negative staph. , gram negative organisms and fungi, especially with risk factors like prolonged mechanical ventilation, umbilical and central venous lines, and parenteral nutrition support.

Prevent/reduce the incidence of nosocomial infections: strict and meticulous handwashing techniques, standardized protocol for skin care (*Refer to Table No-4*), use of TPN solutions, prepared under laminar flow only, early introduction of human milk feedings, minimal usage of central lines and mechanical ventilation, skin punctures and patient handling.

Start "Trophic Gut Priming" with breast milk: initiate with 10-20ml/kg/day and continue for 3-4 days without a change in volume. Then slowly advance the breast milk or formula @ 10-20ml/kg/day while monitoring for signs of feeding intolerance such as abdominal distention, vomiting (rare), and increased gastric residuals. Always suspect early NEC and manage it appropriately (*Refer to the Chapter on Neonatal NEC*). Once successful tolerance of feedings is established at 90–100ml/kg/day, caloric density is advanced to 24calories/30ml and then the volume is advanced. Advance the density of feedings by 2 calories/30ml/day upto a maximum of 30-32 calories/30ml, once full feedings of 24calories/30ml is established. Restrict total fluids 130-140ml/kg/day to minimize the problems with fluid excess while still providing adequate caloric intake.

Monitor for anemia and administer packed cells support as indicated employing strict uniform criteria for transfusion: each unit can be split to provide as many as 8 transfusions for a single patient over a period of 21 days with only a single donor exposure. Erythropoietin therapy in conjunction with adequate iron therapy may be useful in accelerating erythropoiesis, but not routinely used in these patients.

Following discharge* Specialist community nursing support helpful, if available *Increased risk of respiratory infection and wheezing—especially from bronchiolitis (caused by respiratory syncitial virus, RSV) and pertussis; may need intensive care * Consider prophylaxis against RSV infection *Increased rehospitalization—respiratory disorders, inguinal hernias * Monitor growth, development (for learning disorders, coordination, cerebral palsy), behavior, attention, vision, hearing-increased risk of impairment.

Ensure respiratory support, when required (75%) - early surfactant therapy + nasal CPAP (65%) + mechanical ventilation (70%), avoiding hyperventilation, hyperoxia and hypocarbia + IM vitamin A 5,000 IU/dose, 3 times a week for the first 4 wks to reduce the incidence of chronic lung disease + Caffeine Citrate 20mg/kg IV loading dose (infuse over 30 minutes) followed by 5–12 mg/kg IV or orally daily, starting 24hrs after loading dose - to be administered within the first 10 days after birth.

Monitor blood pressure (accept mean blood pressure of 26–28 mmHg for infant of 24–26 wks GA) treat early hypotension with 10–20 ml/kg fluid bolus (NS) and IVI dopamine @ 2.5-25mcg/kg/minute. Begin dopamine IVI at a low dose and titrate to obtain desired mean arterial pressure. Central venous access preferred. Do not administer vasopressors through UAC. Stress dose hydrocortisone (1mg/kg/dose q12 hr for 2 doses) may be useful in infants with hypotension refractory to the above measures. *Maintain vigilance for the symptomatic PDA complication, and suspect it by an increasing need for ventilatory support or an increase in oxygen requirements* occurs in 70% of ELBW infants and now commonly occurs between 24 and 48 hrs after birth, because the natural timing of presentation has been accelerated by surfactant therapy. Confirm it by echocardiogram before starting medical therapy (Ibuprofen/indomethacin) and surgical ligation for recurrent/persistent confirmed PDA, after treatment with a second course of medical therapy.

Monitor for bilirubin and give phototherapy as indicated (low treatment threshold)

Fluids and electrolytes management (Refer to Table 3 for details)

* Insert an umbilical arterial line and a double-lumen umbilical venous line shortly after birth: maintain these lines for 7–10 days and then replace them by peripheral arterial line and Percutaneously Inserted Central venous Catheters (PICC).
* Initial rates of fluid administration depend on gestational age and birth weight.
* Start with 5–7.5% dextrose IV solutions @ 4-10mg glucose/kg/minute.
* If hyperglycemia (>180mg/dl) persists, with 5% IV dextrose—Start insulin infusion @ 0.05 to 0.1 unit/kg/hr and adjust as required.
* Begin Total Parenteral Nutrition (TPN) as per the protocol (Refer to the Chapter on TPN for details of administration—Essential clinical guidelines.)
* Monitor weight, blood pressure, urine output, and serum electrolyte levels frequently
* Adjust fluid rate to avoid dehydration or hypernatremia.
* Anticipate marked diuresis and natriuresis and assess frequently and adjust fluids and electrolytes.

*Pearl/Peril/Pitfall: The goals of the ELBW Neonatal follow-up clinic are early identification of developmental disability; parental counseling; identification and treatment of medical complications; and provision of feedback for neonatologists, pediatricians, obstetricians, and other providers. Specific evaluations of cognitive development, vision and hearing ability, and neurodevelopmental progress is extremely important.

TABLE 1   Major problems of extremely low-birth-weight infants

	Short-term problems	Long-term problems
Respiratory	Respiratory distress syndrome Air leaks Bronchopulmonary dysplasia Apnea of prematurity	Chronic lung disease Reactive airway disease
Cardiovascular	Hypotension Patent ductus arteriosus	
Hematologic	Iatrogenic anemia Frequent transfusions Anemia of prematurity	
Renal	Water/electrolyte imbalance Acid-base disturbances	
Immunologic/infection	Immune deficiency Perinatal infection Nosocomial infection	Respiratory syncytial virus
Ophthalmologic	Retinopathy of prematurity	Blindness, retinal detachment Myopia Strabismus
Gastrointestinal/nutritional	Feeding intolerance Necrotizing enterocolitis Growth failure	Growth failure Failure to thrive Inguinal hernias
Endocrine	Transient hypothyroxinemia ?Cortisol deficiency	
Central nervous system	Intraventricular hemorrhage Periventricular white matter disease Hearing loss	Cerebral palsy Neurodevelopmental delay

TABLE 2   Treatment guidelines for initial management of extremely low-birth-weight infants

Delivery room	Ensure good thermoregulation, "Gentle" ventilation as required, Avoid hyperventilation and hyperoxia, Administer surfactant if prophylaxis approach)
NICU admission	Obtain weight, Administer surfactant within first hour (if rescue approach), Establish vascular access:, Peripheral intravenous catheter, Umbilical arterial catheter, Umbilical venous catheter (central, double-lumen), Start intravenous fluids as soon as possible with dextrose solution, Limit evaporative water losses (humidified incubator), Minimize stimulation, Avoid hyperventilation and hyperoxia, Obtain specimens for complete blood count with differential, blood culture, blood glucose measurement, Give antibiotics as indicated, Give parents information about their child

First 24 to 48 hours

Cardiovascular	Monitor blood pressure; give vasopressors as required, Maintain vigilance for presence of patent ductus arteriosus, Obtain echocardiogram as indicated
Respiratory	Give additional surfactant doses as indicated, Maintain low tidal volume ventilation, Avoid hyperventilation and hyperoxia, Extubate infant and start on continuous positive airway pressure when possible
Fluid Management	Obtain weight every 12 to 24 hours, Monitor serum electrolyte, blood glucose, and calcium concentrations every 4 to 8 hrs, Limit evaporative water losses, Administer skin care
Hematologic	Obtain second blood count, Administer transfusion support as indicated, Monitor bilirubin; give phototherapy as indicated
Infection	Consider discontinuing antibiotics if blood culture results negative at 48 hrs
Nutrition	Start amino acid solution/parenteral nutrition
Neurologic	Minimize stimulation, Perform screening head ultrasonography
Social	Arrange to meet with family

TABLE 3   Fluid administration rates for the first 2 days of life for infants on radiant warmers*

Birth weight (g) Gestational age (wk)	Fluid rate (mL/kg/d)	Frequency of electrolyte testing
500–600/23wk GA	140–200	q6h
601–800/24wk GA	120–130	q8h
801–1,000/25-26wk GA	90–110	q12h

* Rates should be 20%–30% lower when a humidified incubator is used. Urine output and serum electrolytes should be monitored to determine the best rates.

Pearl/Peril/Pitfall: Compared with fullterm newborns, infants with extremely low birth weights have proportionally more fluid in the extracellular fluid compartment than the intracellular compartment, and a larger proportion of their body weight is attributable to water. During the first days after birth, diuresis may result in a 10-20% weight loss, which can be exacerbated by iatrogenic causes (e.g., radiant warmers, phototherapy).

ELBW : Delivery room care and Golden hour care

LandD staff places call to NICU for 23 to 32-week gestation delivery

23-27 weeks gestation   28-32 weeks gestation

↓   ↓

OR for delivery   OR/LDR for delivery

↓

NICU unit assistant activities NICU team via cell phone with OR/ LDR # of delivery

NICU team (NNP/MD, RN, RT) responds to cell phone notification; reports to appropriate OR/LDR.

↓

LandD team ensures that the room is set as close to 80 degrees as possible. NICU team verifies.

↓

1. Preheat warmer (37^0C)
2. Ensure transport ventilator is securely mounted and tank is full
3. Activate chemical warming mattress and place in warmer
4. Place 2 infant hats under chemical mattress
5. Obtain warm blankets from warmer
6. Place warm blanket and warm blanket roll/nest on chemical mattress
7. Check/prepare resuscitation equipment
8. Set blender at 40% (adjust per O_2 saturation : 85–92)
9. Set up T-piece resuscitator (Neopuff) to blender – preset desired settings
10. Cut hydrocolloid barrier

↓

1. Receive infant from OB in warm blanket
2. Place infant under pre heated radiant warmer
3. Dry infant thoroughly and remove wet linen
4. Apply pulse oximeter probe and temp probe and place on servo control

↓

1. Intubate, if indicated, Insert ETT to cm marking that equals 6+ estimated weight in kg.
2. Weigh infant on bed scale (if in resuscitation room)
3. Attach T-piece resuscitator (Neopuff) to ETT and begin ventilation, generally at a rate of 40
4. Wean FiO_2 for oxygen saturation (85–92)
5. Use visual signal for heart rate
6. Place hydrocolloid barrier on cheeks prior to securing ETT
7. Verify equal breath sounds
8. Place fresh, warm blanket on warmer
9. Place 2 caps (layered effect) on infant's head

↓

1. Set transport ventilator settings
2. Place infant prewarmed transport incubator
3. Close incubator and close all portholes
4. Complete Golden Hour tracking form for internal quality improvement
6. Place completed form in "mail safe" in the NICU

↓

Monitor Outcome Measurement/Process Assessment

1. CO_2 40–60 mmHg
2. Oxygen saturation 85–92%
3. Admission temperature 97–99^{0}F
4. Surfactant administration within 1 hour
   Administer surfactant if infant is <27 weeks gestation when HR>100 beats per minute
   Instill surfactant in a quick, steady bolus
   Split the dose in half; administer by tilting infant to each side
5. Decreased incidence of Grade 3 or Grade 4 IVH

FEEDING CARE MAP FOR ELBW INFANTS

Days of Life	0	7	14	21	28	35	42	49	56	63	70	77	84	91	98	105	112
Weeks of Life	0	1	2	3	4	5	6	7	8	9	10	11	12	13	14	15	16
Corrected GA	<25	26	27	28	29	30	31	32	33	34	35	36	37	38	39	40	41

Non-Nutritive Suck

Kangaroo Care

Breast Pumping: Initiation Phase — Maintenance Phase — Discharge Phase

Tube to Breast: NGT/OGT — NGT/OGT & Breast — NGT/OGT & Breast + Bottle — Breast + Bottle

Breastfeeding Phases: KC Phase 1 — Lick & Sniff Phase 2 — Nibble & Swallow Phase 3 — Milk Transfer Matures Phase 4 — All Breastfeeding Phase 5

Nutritive Suck Development: Beginning of SS Coordination — Maturing SSB Coordination

Positioning: Upright or Diagonal with Viewing Mirror — 'En Face' in Football — Cross-Cradle

Test Weights Nipple Shield: Test Weights → / Nipple Shield → Begin to Assess

Supplemental Bottle Feed

Rooming-In Cue Based Feeds: Rooming-In → / Cue-Based Feeds →

State Regulation: States Difficult to Identify — States Begin to Emerge — States Become Organized & Defined

Muscle Tone Development: No Tone in Upper and Lower Extremities — Flexor Tone Begins in Lower Extremities — Flexor Tone Begins in Upper and Increases in Lower Extremities — Arms and Legs Flexed; Makes Attempt to pull to Midline

Respiratory Support: Maximum Support — Moderate Support — Minimal or No Support — BPD may alter or delay timelines

Key : BPD : bronchopulmonary dysplasia, NGT nasogastric tube, OGT : orogastric tube, SS : suck-swallow, SSB : suck-swallow-breathe

Pearl/Peril/Pitfall: Periventricular leukomalacia (PVL) is defined as damage to cerebral white matter that can result in severe motor and cognitive deficits in infants with extremely low birth weight who survive; it occurs in 10-15% of these infants. PVL most often occurs at the site of the occipital radiation at the trigone of the lateral ventricles and around the foramen of Monro. The origin of PVL is believed to be multifactorial; the injury possibly results from episodes of fluctuating cerebral blood flow, which are caused by prolonged episodes of systemic hypertension or hypotension. PVL has also been linked to periods of hypocarbic alkalosis and chorioamnionitis.

TABLE 4   Practical guidelines for skin care of extremely low-birth-weight infants

Interventions	Guidelines
Adhesive application	Increase adhesive track by applying to dry, clean skin surface
	Avoid alcohol for skin cleansing
	Use smallest amount of tape possible
	Use a hydrocolloid or pectin-based layer on the skin, before application of heavy adhesive
	Avoid using adhesive over areas of skin breakdown
	Avoid adhesive bonding agents (e.g. benzoin)
	Use hydrophilic gel or pectin-based adhesives preferentially
Adhesive removal	Avoid adhesive removes and solvents
	Use warm, wet cotton ball to periodically saturate hydrogel adhesives (avoid over-drying and over-saturation)
	Facilitate removal of adhesive with mineral oil, petrolatum, and emollients if reapplication is not necessary
Emollient application	Infants born at <27 weeks may benefit from emollient use
	Avoid multidose containers (e.g. large jars)
	Use non-perfumed, nonirritating hydrophilic emollients
	Recognize potential for emollients to interfere with adhesive and conductive properties of monitoring devices
Emollient removal	Wipe off gently with a soft cloth/gauze if site is contaminated
	Avoid repeated attempts to thoroughly cleanse the skin (undesired friction effect)
	Remove emollients before attaching thermistors or other monitoring devices

Data from Hoath S, Narendran V: Adhesives and emollients in the preterm infant. Semin Neonataol 5:289-296, 2000.

TABLE 5   Recommended screening for common complications of extremely low-birth-weight infants

Intraventricular hemorrhage (IVH):	Head ultrasonography (HUS) on day 1–3 repeat on day 7–10
Germinal matrix hemorrhage	Repeat HUS weekly until findings normal
Intraventricular hemorrhage	Repeat HUS every 3 to 7 days until stable/resolved
IVH with ventricular dilation or	Repeat HUS every 3 to 7 days until stable/resolved
intraparenchymal bleeding	Consider measurement of resistive indices for progressive ventricular dilatation
Periventricular white matter disease	HUS at day 30; repeat at 36 weeks of postmenstrual age or at discharge
	Consider magnetic resonance imaging if HUS findings equivocal
Retinopathy of prematurity (ROP) :	Perform ophthalmologic examination (OE) exam at 4 to 6 weeks of postnatal age
	Repeat every 2 weeks if no ROP
	Repeat weekly if ROP present
	Repeat twice weekly for pre-threshold disease or rapidly progressive ROP
Absence of ROP	Repeat OE every 2 weeks
Presence of ROP	Repeat OE weekly
Presence of prethreshold disease or rapidly progressive ROP	Repeat OE twice weekly
Audiology screening	Hearing screen no earlier than 34 weeks of postmenstrual age but prior to discharge home

Late sequelae of low birthweight

1. Mental retardation, spastic diplegia, microcephaly, seizures, poor school performance.

2. Mental retardation, spasticity, seizures, hydrocephalus

3. Hearing, Visual impairment, retinopathy of prematurity, strabismus, myopia.

4. Bronchopulmonary dysplasia, cor pulmonale, bronchospasm, malnutrition, subglottic stenosis, iatrogenic cleft palate, recurrent pneumonia.

5. Short-bowel syndrome, malabsorption, malnutrition, infectious diarrhea

6. Cirrhosis, hepatic failure, carcinoma, malnutrition

7. Osteopenia, fractures, anemia, vitamin E, growth failure

8. Child abuse or neglect, failure to thrive, divorce

9. Sudden infant death syndrome, infections, inguinal hernia,

cutaneous scars (chest tube, patent ductus arteriosus ligation, intravenous infiltration), gastroesophageal reflux, hypertension, craniosynostosis, cholelithiasis, nephrocalcinosis, cutaneous hemangiomas

Prevalence of neuromotor and sensory findings at 18 months in extremely low birthweight infants

* **Abnormal neurological examination—25%**

* Cerebral palsy—17% *Seizure disorder—5% *Hydrocephalus with shunt—4%

Any vision impairment—9%

* Unilateral blindness—1% *Bilateral blindness—2%

Hearing impairment—11%

* Wears hearing aids—3% *Adapted from Vohr BR et al. *Paediatrics* 2000;105:1216-26

***Pearl/Peril/Pitfall:** Signs of infection in ELBW infants are myriad, may be nonspecific, and include temperature instability (hypothermia or hyperthermia), tachycardia, decreased activity, poor perfusion, apnea, bradycardia, feeding intolerance, increased need for oxygen or higher ventilatory settings, and metabolic acidosis. Laboratory studies may include CBC count with differential, blood culture, cerebrospinal fluid culture, urine culture, and cultures from indwelling foreign bodies, such as central lines or endotracheal tubes.*

STABILIZING THE PRETERM OR SICK INFANT: AN OVERVIEW FOR A QUICK RECAP

Additional oxygen and artificial ventilation

Many infants with respiratory distress require additional inspiratory oxygen and ventilatory support. In preterm infants this is often for respiratory distress syndrome, but even in the absence of this disorder, many infants <30 week's gestation require artificial ventilation because of lung immaturity or to avoid recurrent apnea.

Circulatory support

Circulatory support with colloid infusion and inotropic drugs is required to treat hypotension, if peripheral perfusion appears inadequate. Echocardiography can provide information on ventricular function.

Monitoring

The heart rate, respiratory rate and temperature are monitored continuously. Oxygenation is measured indirectly by pulse oximetry for oxygen saturation and with a transcutaneous electrode for oxygen tension. The arterial CO_2 tension can also be measured transcutaneously. Blood gas analysis is performed on arterial samples from a peripheral or umbilical artery catheter. The arterial oxygen tension is maintained at 8–12 kpa (60–90 mmHg) and the CO_2 tension at 4.5–6.5kpa (35–50 mmHg).

A chest X-ray is required to help diagnose respiratory disorders and confirm the position of the tracheal tube and umbilical artery catheter.

Avoiding hypothermia

Hypothermia increases mortality and should be prevented by placing the baby under a radiant warmer or in an incubator.

Antibiotics

Infants requiring intensive care are often given broad-spectrum antibiotics. Infection with the Group B streptococcus and other organisms can mimic respiratory distress syndrome.

Metabolic disturbance

Blood glucose is checked regularly and IV dextrose given to prevent hypoglycemia. Fluid requirements are very variable ad must be closely monitored.

Minimal handling

All procedures, especially painful ones, adversely affect oxygenation and the circulation. Sedation and analgesia, e.g. an iv infusion of morphine, are given as required. Handling is kept to a minimum and done as rapidly and efficiently as possible.

Parents

Although medical and nursing staff are usually fully occupied stabilizing the baby, time must be found for parents to allow them to see and touch their baby to be kept fully informed.

History relevant to preterm delivery

* Maternal medical and obstetric history
* Estimated gestation
* Singleton or multifetal pregnancy?
* Assessments of fetal growth and well-being
* Details of suspected congenital anomalies
* Risk of fetal-maternal infection and chorioamnionitis
* Course of labor, if laboring
* Intrapartum monitoring results
* Antenatal interventions, tocolytic drugs, steroids, antibiotics
* Use of opiates and anesthetic drugs

> *Stabilizing a Preterm/Sick infants is extremely important to prevent complications. This preterm infant has leads on his limbs and trunk for Monitoring of the Vital functions and O2 saturations. There are Umbilical arterial and venous catheters, ET Tube and IV cannulae indicated for intensive care of these High-Risk Neonates.*

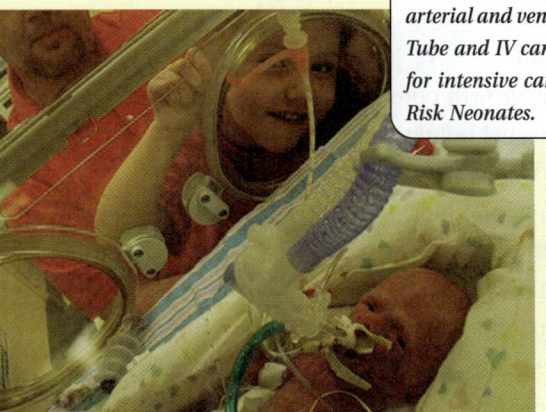

NEONATAL PROBLEMS ASSOCIATED WITH PREMATURE INFANTS *Refer to the individual Chapters for the details of Diagnosis and Management!*

Respiratory

Respiratory distress syndrome (hyaline membrane disease)*

Bronchopulmonary dysplasia

Pneumothorax, Pneumomediastinum; interstitial emphysema

Congenital pneumonia

Pulmonary hypoplasia

Pulmonary hemorrhages

Apnea*

Cardiovascular

Patent ductus arteriosus*

Hypotension

Hypertension

Bradycardia (with apnea)*

Congenital malformations

Hematologic

Anemia (early or late onset)

Hyperbilirubinemia-indirect*

Subcutaneous, organ (liver, adrenal) hemorrhage*

Disseminated intravascular coagulopathy

Vitamin K deficiency

Hydrops-immune or nonimmune

Gastrointestinal

Poor gastrointestinal function - poor motility*

Necrotizing enterocolitis

Hyperbilirubinemia-direct and indirect

Congenital anomalies producing polyhydramnios

Spontaneous gastrointestinal isolated perforation

Metabolic - Endocrine

Hypocalcemia*

Hypoglycemia*

Hyperglycemia*

Late metabolic acidosis

Hypothermia*

Euthyroid but low-thyroxin status

Central Nervous system

Intraventricular hemorrhage*

Periventricular leukomalacia

Hypoxic—ischemic encephalopathy

Seizures

Retinopathy of prematurity

Deafness

Congenital malformations

Kernicterus (bilirubin encephalopathy)

Drug (narcotic) withdrawal

Renal

Hyponatremia* Hypernatremia* Hyperkalemia*

Renal tubular acidosis, Renal glycosuria, Edema

Other

Infections* (congenital, perinatal, nosocomial: bacterial, viral, fungal, protozoal)

*Common.

Ages at which disabilities become evident in VLBW infants

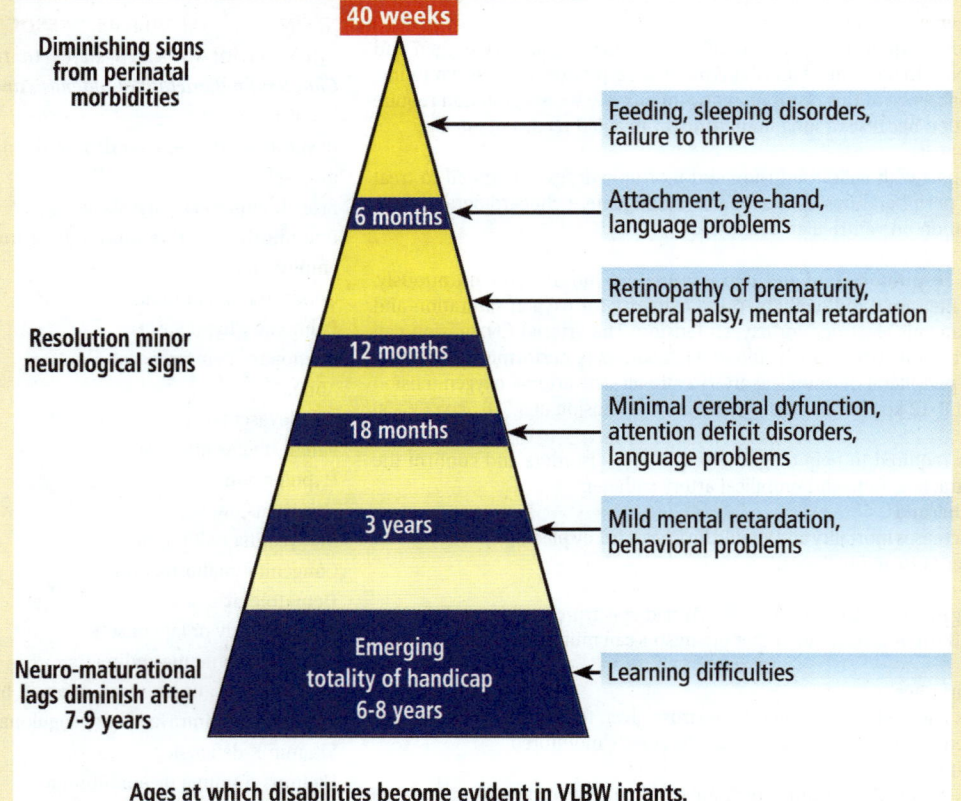

Ages at which disabilities become evident in VLBW infants.

Courtesy : Malcolm I. Levene

Complications in the first year of life in preterm infants

MEDICAL	
Respiratory	Nasal congestion
	Exacerbation of bronchopulmonary dysplasia
	Recurrent wheezing
	SIDS
Cardiac	Patent ductus arteriosus
	Ventricular septal defect
Ophthalmic	Retinopathy of prematurity
	Strabismus
	Myopia
Auditory	Sensorineural hearing loss
	Conductive dysfunction
Growth	Failure to achieve genetic growth potential
Gastrointestinal	Vomiting, gastro-oesophageal reflux, constipation, colic
NEUROLOGICAL	
Major	Spastic diplegia, hypotonia, hemiplegia, quadriplegia, hydrocephalus, microcephaly, mental retardation
Minor	Ataxia, incoordination and clumsiness, specific learning difficulties, attention deficit disorders, mild to moderate cognitive impairment
Surgical	Inguinal hernia, umbilical hernia, undescended testes, hydrocoele
Miscellaneous	Child abuse, neglect, deprivation, behavioral disturbances, emotional disturbances, failure to thrive.

Respiratory care map for infants ≤ 1000 grams

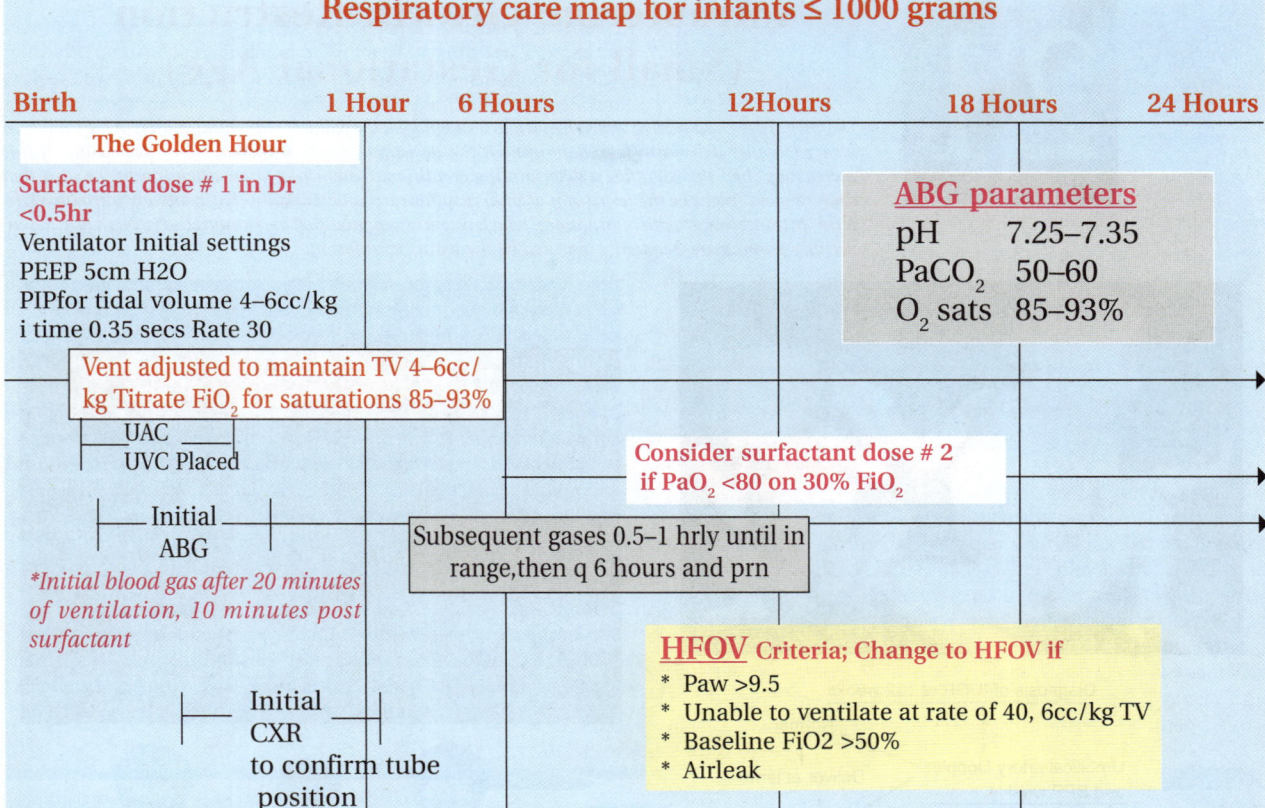

| Birth | 1 Hour | 6 Hours | 12 Hours | 18 Hours | 24 Hours |

The Golden Hour

Surfactant dose # 1 in Dr <0.5hr
Ventilator Initial settings
PEEP 5cm H2O
PIPfor tidal volume 4–6cc/kg
i time 0.35 secs Rate 30

ABG parameters
pH   7.25–7.35
PaCO$_2$ 50–60
O$_2$ sats 85–93%

Vent adjusted to maintain TV 4–6cc/kg Titrate FiO$_2$ for saturations 85–93%

UAC
UVC Placed

Consider surfactant dose # 2 if PaO$_2$ <80 on 30% FiO$_2$

Initial
ABG

Subsequent gases 0.5–1 hrly until in range, then q 6 hours and prn

Initial blood gas after 20 minutes of ventilation, 10 minutes post surfactant

HFOV Criteria; Change to HFOV if
* Paw >9.5
* Unable to ventilate at rate of 40, 6cc/kg TV
* Baseline FiO2 >50%
* Airleak

Initial
CXR
to confirm tube position

KEY POINTS FOR CLINICAL PRACTICE

1. Extremely low birth weight (ELBW) is defined as a birth weight less than 1000 g (2 lb, 3 oz). Most extremely low birth weight infants are also the youngest of premature newborns, usually born at 27 weeks' gestational age or younger. Infants born at less than 1500 g are termed very low birth weight (VLBW).

2. If the delivery of an ELBW infant is threatened, the neonatologist and the obstetrician should consult with parents and discuss certain important issues such as a)survival chances (<23 wks' gestational age = 0, and at 23, 24 and 25 wks it would be 15%, 55%, and 79% respectively) b)delivery room management and resuscitation of the baby c)potential risks of both the extent of prematurity and the proposed therapeutic interventions d)short-term and long-term morbidity.

3. *Delivery room care of ELBW infant* a)ensure good thermoregulation (preheated warmer, quick drying the baby, removal of wet toweling etc.) b)"gentle" ventilation with low tidal volume strategy avoiding hyperventilation and hyperoxia and early surfactant therapy once correct Endotracheal Tube position has been confirmed clinically c)transport of the ELBW infant to the NICU in a prewarmed transport incubator/radiant warmer combination unit (Giraffe Bed, Ohmeda Medical).

4. Careful attention to detail and frequent monitoring are the basic components of care of the ELBW infant, because critical changes can occur rapidly. Delicate pulmonary status, large fluid losses, balances between fluid intake and blood glucose levels, and the immaturity and increased sensitivity of several organ systems all require close monitoring. Monitoring itself, however, may cause increased risks because of small blood volumes, tiny blood vessels, and limited skin integrity.

5. Although the mortality rate has diminished with the use of surfactants, the proportion of surviving infants with severe sequelae, such as chronic lung disease, cognitive delays, cerebral palsy, and neurosensory deficits (i.e., deafness and blindness), has not. Although improved neurodevelopmental outcomes have been reported in a few small studies, such improvement has not been seen on a global scale.

REFERENCES AND FURTHER READING 1)Blaymore-Bier J, Pezzullo J, Kim E, et al. Outcome of extremely low-birth-weight infants: 1980–1990. *Acta Paediatr.* Dec 1994;83(12):1244–8.2) Dollberg S, Hoath S. Temperature regulation in preterm infants: role of the skin-environment interface. *NeoReviews.* 2001;2(12):e282–291. 3) Ziegler EE, Thureen PJ, Carlson SJ. Aggressive nutrition of the very low birthweight infant. *Clin Perinatol.* Jun 2002;29(2):225–44. 4) Kilbride HW. Effectiveness of neonatal intensive care for extremely low birth weight infants. *Pediatrics.* Nov 2004;114(5):1374; author reply 1374–5. 5) Guideline] National Institute of Child Health and Development (NICHD). Follow-up care of high-risk infants. *Pediatrics.* 2004;114(5):1377–1397.

Pearl/Peril/Pitfall: Despite its many immunologic and nutritional advantages, an exclusive diet of unfortified breast milk may provide insufficient quantities of energy, protein, calcium, and phosphorous to support the goals of intrauterine bone mineralization and growth rates in small premature infants. To facilitate this, breast milk must be fortified to provide additional calories, protein, and minerals to promote proper growth. Failure to provide adequate amounts of these essential nutrients, especially calcium and phosphorus, may result in protein malnutrition, hyponatremia, osteopenia of prematurity, or rickets.

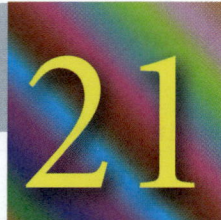

21 Intrauterine Growth Restriction (Small for Gestational Age)

@ *Doppler of the Umbilical Artery: When IUGR is diagnosed, the value of sequential studies of the umbilical artery Doppler waveform is to determine if the Resistance Index is increasing or decreasing. If it is increasing, then this signifies a deteriorating condition. Gruenwald drew attention to the idea that undergrowth might be the result of placental insufficiency, and Warkany et al. probably introduced the term "intrauterine growth retardation," which recently was modified as "intrauterine growth restriction" because parents are frequently alarmed by the word "retardation."*

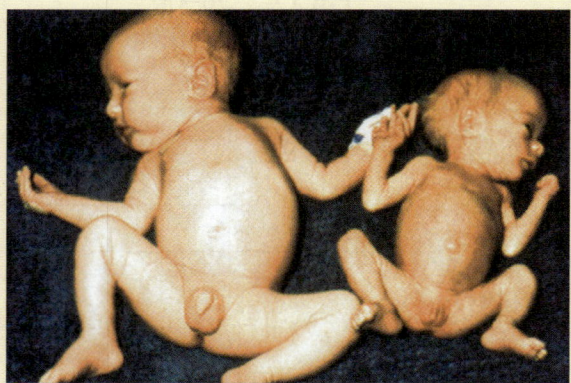

Fetal factors	Maternal factors	Maternal drugs
Abnormal Chromosomes Genetic Diseases Serious Birth Defects Multiple Fetuses (twins, Triplets, etc.)	Poor nutrition Anemia Hypoxia (Asthma, lung disease, high altitude, etc.) Antiphospholipid syndrome Previous delivery of a child with IUGR Maternal fatigue	Tobacco Alcohol Cocaine Narcotics Anticonvulsants Warfarin Aminopterin Angiotensin converting enzyme inhibitors Beta blockers

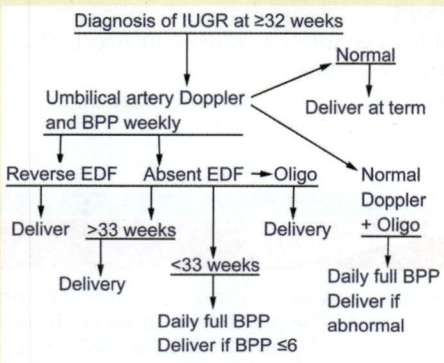

Intrauterine Growth Restriction (IUGR)

REVIEW OF CLINICAL PROBLEMS

1. Name the differences between Symmetric and Asymmetric types of IUGR.
   Ans: Refer to the Table of "Differences between Symmetric and Asymmetric IUGR Babies" of the Chapter.
2. How do you evaluate and investigate an IUGR Baby?
   Ans: Refer to the Evaluation-Decision-Action Plan/Algorithm to diagnose and manage an IUGR/SGA Neonate.
3. What are the Clinical problems of IUGR Babies and How do you manage them ?
   Ans: Refer to the Evaluation-Decision-Action Plan/Algorithm to diagnose and manage an IUGR/SGA Neonate.
4. Describe the essential clinical features of Silver-Russel Syndrome (SRS).
   Ans: Refer to the Section on SRS of the Chapter.
5. What are the common indications for Doppler flow Velocimetry during pregnancy ?
   Ans: Refer to the Section on Doppler flow studies during pregnancy.

LEARNING OBJECTIVES

After completing this article, readers will be able to

1. Identify IUGR Babies and differentiate between Symmetric and Asymmetric Types of IUGR.

2. Provide proper care for the acute complications related to IUGR, including resuscitation at birth.

3. Ensure early initiation of enteral nutrition by promoting breast feeding and/or assisted feeding.

4. Follow-up for long-term Growth and Neurodevelopmental sequelae of IUGR

5. Counsel parents about the prognosis for their IUGR babies.

Pearl/Peril/Pitfall: SYMMETRICAL IUGR-This is characterized by inadequate growth of the head, body and extremities and occurs in 25% of IUGR fetuses. The growth problem is the result of a decrease in the rate of cell reproduction, resulting in fewer cells. This usually has its onset prior to 32 weeks of pregnancy and has a 25% risk for chromosomal abnormalities (Down syndrome, trisomy 13, trisomy 18) ASYMMETRICAL IUGR This usually occurs early in the third trimester and is associated with impaired growth of the body, with normal growth of the head and extremities. This is the result of failure of the cells to increase in size resulting in less fat and smaller abdominal organs. These fetuses often appear to be "long and skinny."

BIRD'S EYE VIEW/OVERVIEW/SYNOPSIS

1. **IUGR/Small-for-gestational age (SGA):** Birth weight< 10th centile of a population-specific birth weight versus gestational age relationship.IUGR: defined as a rate of fetal growth that is less than normal for the population and for the growth potential of a specific infant. IUGR, therefore, produces infants who are SGA. Although most IUGR infants would also be SGA, it is possible that a small minority of IUGR infants may have birth weights > 10th centile. But they are clinically identified by the signs of malnutrition, such as loose skin folds on the face and in the gluteal region, absence of subcutaneous fat and peeling of skin. The management issues are along the same lines as SGA Infants.

2. LBW Baby weighs <2,500 gm at birth (2/3rds of LBW babies are due to IUGR and 1/3rd of them are due to Prematurity (born <37 weeks GA).IUGR Babies are further classified into Symmetric(with head circumference, length, and weight equally affected) or Asymmetric (with head circumference spared and it is relatively at a higher centile than the length or weight.); Symmetric IUGR babies tend to have intrinsic(chromosomal, genetic, teratogenic, TORSCH infections, etc.,) abnormalities in the fetus which begin early in fetal life, whereas the onset of extrinsic adverse factors, such as undernutrition or hypoxia from placental insufficiency, which usually cause asymmetric growth, develop at variable times during gestation.Refer to Table 1 of the Chapter for the etiology of IUGR/SGA.

3. SGA/IUGR babies are more prone to suffer from complications such as birth asphyxia, hypothermia, hypoglycemia, polycythemia, PPHN, Meconium aspiration syndrome,and lethal congenital anomalies. These morbidities are more common in severe IUGR (<3RD Centile) babies. Even after recovering from Neonatal complications, they remain more prone to poor physical growth, poor neuro-developmental outcome, recurrent infection and chronic diseases like hypertension, hyperlipidemia, diabetes mellitus, coronary heart disease later in life. Neurologic disorders occur 5–10 times more often in SGA than in AGA infants. They include hyperactivity, short attention span, and learning disabilities, associated with substandard school performance. Many of these infants even those with normal intelligence, also have subtle neurologic and behavioral problems, including fine motor incoordination, hyperreflexia, speech problems, and diffuse EEG abnormalities. Relative Microcephaly at birth is especially to be associated with poor developmental outcome in severely SGA infants.

4. Physical examination of the SGA infant must include a detailed search for associated abnormalities. • dysmorphic features "unusual" facies • abnormal hands and feet • abnormal palmar creases • in addition to gross anomalies • ocular disorders, such as • cataracts • cloudy cornea • chorioretinitis • features of intrauterine infection • hepatosplenomegaly • jaundice • blueberry-muffin rash.

5. **Investigations:** Investigations are required to • screen for • hypoglycemia·assess the infant according to clinical signs • polycythemia and • hypocalcemia are more common. • if respiratory distress present, ABG and Chest X-ray. • establish the cause of growth restriction • intrauterine infection suspected; check maternal TORCH serology and screen infant urine and saliva for CMV (further investigation will be required if suspicion confirmed). • if dysmorphic; genetic consultation and chromosome studies • if showing signs of withdrawal, urine for drug screen. • ultrasonography and echocardiography, if clinically indicated.

6. *The Evaluation-Decision-Action Plan/Algorithm* describes the essential aspects of the diagnosis and management of common problems associated with IUGR/SGA Babies.At Delivery: Place promptly under a radiant warmer and dry. Infants with severe SGA, particularly in association with fetal distress, are at risk of aspiration of meconium, hypoxemia, hypotension, mixed metabolic and respiratory acidosis and persistent pulmonary hypertension. Hypothermia: Nurse in a thermoneutral environment. Hypoglycemia: Monitor blood glucose and commence early enteral feeds or intravenous glucose infusion. Necrotizing enterocolitis: Infants, particularly preterm SGA, found to have placental insufficiency and abnormal umbilical artery Doppler studies may be at particular risk of developing NEC or gastrointestinal perforation. Enteral feeding should be increased gradually. Polycythemia: Partial volume exchange may be required for symptomatic infants.

7. **Outcome**-Principally determined by the cause. **Postnatal physical growth:** Symmetric SGA - smaller and relatively under weight throughout life. Asymmetric SGA - accelerated velocity of growth ("catch up growth") in first 6 months and normal development. **Neurodevelopmental outcome:** Term SGA - no increase risk of severe neurologic morbidity compared to term AGA infants. However increased hyperactivity, short attention span and learning problems Preterm SGA - Minor neurologic abnormalities more common than in preterm AGA infants.Each case is unique. Some infants who have IUGR develop normally, while others have complications of the nervous system or intellectual problems such as **learning disorders**. If IUGR is related to a disease or a genetic defect, the future of the infant is related to the severity and the nature of that disorder.

8. Nutritional Management of IUGR Babies is summarized in the Table 2 of the Chapter.

9. The diagnosis of severe IUGR before 32 weeks' gestation is associated with a poor prognosis, and therapy must be highly individualized. Once a decision has been made to effect delivery, the mode of delivery is governed by evidence of acidemia, gestational age, and Bishop score. Cesarean delivery without a trial of labor is appropriate (1) in the presence of evidence of fetal distress by nonstress testing or reversed diastolic flow or (2) for traditional obstetrical indications for cesarean delivery (i.e., malpresentation, prior cesarean delivery).

10. The goal in the management of IUGR, because no effective treatments are known, is to deliver the most mature fetus in the best physiological condition possible while minimizing the risk to the mother. Such a goal requires the use of antenatal testing with the hope of identifying the fetus with IUGR before it becomes acidotic. Developing a testing scheme, following it, and having a high index of suspicion in this population when results of testing are abnormal is important. The positive predictive value of an abnormal antenatal test result in fetuses with IUGR is relatively high because the prevalence of acidemia and chronic hypoxemia is relatively high.Maternal bed rest is the initial approach for the treatment of IUGR.The benefit of bed rest is that it results in increased blood flow to the uterus. Studies on the efficacy of bed rest have been inconclusive, although in the early 2000s it is still used in combination with intravenous fluid therapy and oxygen therapy. The use of baby aspirin therapy remains controversial but theoretically it serves to preserve or improve blood flow to the placenta. If the baby does not grow well in utero after conservative treatment, an obstetrician may suggest inducing labor in the mother a few weeks early, or delivering the baby by **cesarean section.**

Pearl/Peril/Pitfall: Of all fetuses at or below the 10th percentile for growth, only approximately 40% are at high risk of potentially preventable perinatal death. Another 40% of these fetuses are constitutionally small. Because this diagnosis may be made with certainty only in neonates, a significant number of fetuses that are healthy but SGA will be subjected to high-risk protocols and, potentially, iatrogenic prematurity.

THE EVALUATION-DECISION-ACTION-PLAN/ALGORITHM FOR THE DIAGNOSIS AND MANAGEMENT OF *IUGR/SGA NEONATE*

SUBJECTIVE FINDINGS

Hx of birth and resuscitation details, Doppler velocimetry assessment of uterine, placental, and fetal circulations antenatally (the most severely affected IUGR fetuses with the greatest risk of death demonstrate absent or reversed diastolic blood flow in their systemic arteries, with increased umbilical venous pulsation, and reversed blood flow in abdominal vena cava.)

Hx of Maternal /fetal/placental factors known to cause IUGR/SGA such as Chromosomal/genetic causes, IU infections, Maternal drug/smoking/alcohol abuse, dwarf syndromes, placenta previa, synsytial knots, partial molar pregnancy, multiple gestation, abruption (chronic, partial), circumvallate/velamentous insertion, chronic hypertension, pre-eclampsia, etc.

OBJECTIVE FINDINGS

Assess ABCs, vitals, BP, O_2 sats, work of breathing, central cyanosis, CRT, pulses, Urine output, signs suggestive of sepsis/birth asphyxia/CCF.

Look for typical IUGR features loose dry skin with peeling, shrunken or 'wizened" facies, widened/ overriding cranial sutures, larger than expected AF, thinner and often meconium stained umbilical cord, disproportionately larger head with undergrown trunk and extremities, decreased subcutaneous fat and skeletal muscle, and scaphoid abdomen (Dd from Congenital Diaphragmatic Hernia).

Anticipate the short-term complications, such as Hypoglycemia, Hypothermia, Polycythemia, Hyperglycemia, Renal insufficiency, and PPHN *Identify* Congenital anomalies and *Prevent* infections.

INVESTIGATIONS

Blood FBC, TC, DC, Hct Platelets, peripheral blood smear, Group/Type and Crossmatch, CRP, Blood cultures and full septic screen, ABG analysis, electrolytes, calcium and magnesium, blood sugar, creatinine, BUN, coagulation profile as clinically indicated.
Ensure frequent reassessment of the IUGR/ SGA baby to avoid the complications blood sugar (asymptomatic Hypoglycemias, osmotic diuresis and prerenal shutdown due to hyperglycemia), hypoxia due to PPHN, Urine output to identify renal failure, Hematocrit to manage Polycythemia-Hyperviscosity if severe and symptomatic, temperature to prevent /treat cold stress/ hypothermia

Measure Wt, Length, and HC and Plot them on IUGR Growth Charts!

Clinical problems of the IUGR/SGA neonate and management

Problem	Pathogenesis/pathophysiology	Prevention/treatment
Intrauterine death	Chronic hypoxia Placental insufficiency Growth failure Malformation Infection Infarction/abruption Preeclampsia	Antenatal surveillance Fetal growth by ultrasound Doppler velocimetry Maternal treatment: ? bed rest,? O_2 Delivery for severe or worsening fetal distress
Asphyxia	Acute hypoxia/abruption Chronic hypoxia Placental insufficiency/preeclampsia Acidosis Glycogen depletion	Antepartum/intrapartum monitoring Adequate neonatal resuscitation
Meconium aspiration	Hypoxia severe aspiration	Resuscitation including tracheal suctioning for definite
Hypothermia	Cold stress Hypoxia Hypoglycemia Decreased fat stores Decreased subcutaneous insulation Increased surface area Catecholamine depletion	Protect against increased heat loss Dry infant Radiant warmer Hat Thermoneutral environment Nutritional support
Persistent pulmonary hypertension	Chronic hypoxia	Cardiovascular support Mechanical ventilation, nitric oxide
Hypoglycemia	Decreased hepatic/muscle glycogen Decreased alternative energy sources Heat loss Hypoxia Decreased gluconeogenesis Decreased counterregulatory hormones Increased insulin sensitivity	Frequent measurement of blood glucose Early intravenous glucose support
Hyperglycemia	Low insulin secretion rate Excessive glucose delivery Increased catecholamine and glucagon effects	Glucose monitoring Decrease glucose infusion to <8 mg/min/kg ?Intravenous insulin administration for severe cases
Polycythemia-hyperviscosity	Chronic hypoxia Maternal-fetal transfusion Increased erythropoiesis	Intravenous glucose, oxygen Partial volume exchange transfusion for severe, symptomatic cases
Gastrointestinal perforation	Focal ischemia Hypoperistalsis	Cautious enteral support
Acute renal failure	Hypoxia/ischemia	Cardiovascular support
Immunodeficiency	Malnutrition Congenital infection	Early, optimal nutrition Specific antibiotic and immune therapy

Pearl/Peril/Pitfall: Infants whose weight is greater than the 10th percentile but who are thin relative to their length and head circumference are at similar risk of Neonatal complications as SGA infants. They should be considered "relatively" SGA (Clifford syndrome). The weight/length ratio (or the Ponderal Index = [weight (g)]/[length (cm)]3) is less than normal for such infants. However, unless great care is taken with the measurement of length the calculated index can be misleading.

TABLE 1   Etiology of IUGR/SGA babies

Fetal
- chromosome disorders (e.g. Trisomy 21, Trisomy 18)
- chronic fetal infection (e.g. CMV, Rubella, Syphilis, Toxoplasmosis)
- congenital malformations: including congenital heart disease, diaphragmatic hernia, tracheo-oesophageal fistula
- syndrome complex
- radiation
- multiple gestation relates more to placental limitation rather than intrinsic baby problem

Mother
- pregnancy induced hypertension
- hypertension or renal disease or both
- hypoxemia (high altitude, cyanotic cardiac or pulmonary disease)
- malnutrition or chronic illness
- drugs (narcotics, alcohol, cigarettes, cocaine, antimetabolites)

Placental
- decreased placental weight or cellularity or both
- decrease in surface area, infarction
- villous placentitis (bacterial, viral, parasitic)
- tumour (chorioangioma, hydatiform mole)
- placental separation
- twin to twin transfusion syndrome

Constitutional
- familial and racial background

TABLE 2   Overview of management of IUGR/SGA neonates

Criteria for admission to Nursery
- All SGA infants <2 SD (3rd percentile)
- Infants with gestational age < 35 wks
- Infants with birth asphyxia, respiratory distress etc.

Care of SGA infants with mothers (birth weight between 3rd and 10th percentile, gestation >35 wks)
- Early initiation of breast feeding (within 1 hour)
- Skin-to-skin care to maintain temperature, monitoring of cold stress by mother and health professionals.
- Monitor blood sugar, hematocrit
- Prevent infections

Care of SGA infants in Nursery (birth weight <3rd percentile or gestation <35 wks)
- Nurse in thermo neutral environment
- It stable, early initiation of feeds (EBM).
- Feed by orogastric tube or katori-spoon / paladai if gestation ≥ 32 wks
- Initial intravenous fluids followed by orogastric or katori spoon / paladai if gestation <32 wks
- Monitor blood sugar, hematocrit

Care of SGA infants with absent or reversed end-diastolic blood flow
- At higher risk of development of NEC
- If preterm (gestation < 32 weeks): Nil per oral or on minimal enteral nutrition for first 48–72 h of life followed by gradual advancement of feed volume.

Courtesy: AIIMS protocol

Pearl/Peril/Pitfall: The goal in the management of IUGR, because no effective treatments are known, is to deliver the most mature fetus in the best physiological condition possible while minimizing the risk to the mother. Such a goal requires the use of antenatal testing with the hope of identifying the fetus with IUGR before it becomes acid.

Pearl/Peril/Pitfall: Despite the theoretical benefit of aspirin in many studies, the role of aspirin, if any, in the prevention of IUGR is still unclear. A large randomized controlled trial using a standardized high-risk population with a standardized treatment regimen could serve to better answer this question.

TABLE 3   Antenatal management of IUGR fetus

Fetal surveillance: Unless delivery occurs, once treatment begins the fetus must undergo surveillance. The purpose of this is to identify further progression of the disease process that would jeopardize the fetus to a point that it would be better to be delivered than to remain in utero. There are four testing modalities, each of which addresses different aspects of surveillance, which are helpful. Most physicians agree that a combination of tests are better than an isolated test. **Non-stress test-**This is one of the first tests used in the surveillance of IUGR fetuses and the simplest to perform. The physician uses a heart rate monitor to determine changes in the fetal heart rate with fetal movement. If the heart rate increases more than 15 beats for more than 15 seconds, this is considered to be a reactive test. If the heart rate does not accelerate, remains flat, or decreases, then this is an abnormal test. The problem with this test is that it changes late in the course of the disease and does not identify a fetus with IUGR. When patients are diagnosed with IUGR and require continuous monitoring, the fetal heart rate tracing may be useful in detecting fetal distress. **Amniotic fluid Index:** The physician measures the vertical depth of four pockets of amniotic fluid to obtain a total amniotic fluid index. This method allows for comparison of changes in amniotic fluid with time. In the normal fetus the amniotic fluid index remains relatively constant. In the fetus with IUGR, it may decrease slowly, or decrease abruptly with time. A decrease in amniotic fluid may occur before there are changes in the non-stress test. The current recommendations are that if the amniotic fluid index decreases below 8 after 35 weeks, then delivery should be considered. The following is an example of a fetus at risk for IUGR in which the amniotic fluid index was measured but the nurses and physician did not understand the principles of an abnormal reading. The fetus was allowed to remain in utero and developed cerebral palsy from oxygen deprivation. The family sued the hospital and the physician and was awarded 9.7 million dollars which was the largest malpractice award in the state of Utah.

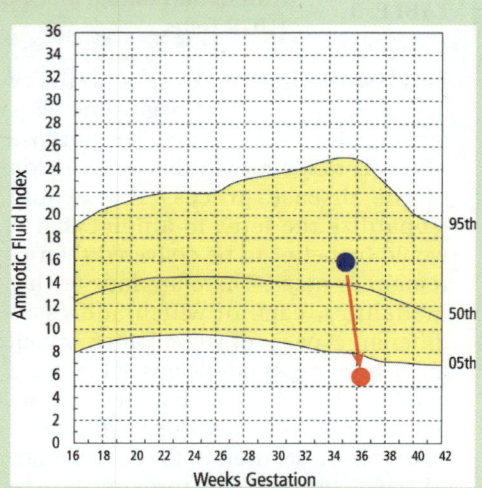

This is the amniotic fluid index in the above case. The blue represents the normal range. At 35 weeks the fluid measurement was 16. Four days later it dropped to 6.3. This sudden drop was ignored by the nurses and physician caring for the patient. A few days later the fetus was damaged because the umbilical cord was compressed, resulting in cerebral palsy.

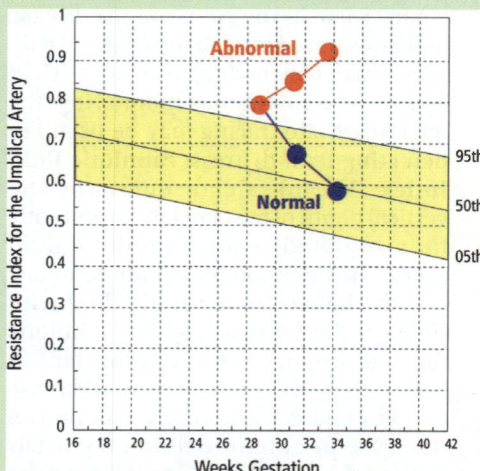

Doppler of the Umbilical Artery. When IUGR is diagnosed, the value of sequential studies of the umbilical artery Doppler waveform is to determine if the Resistance Index is increasing or decreasing. If it is increasing, then this signifies a deteriorating condition. The above graph illustrates these principles. This is a graphical display of the Resistance Index measurement of the umbilical artery Doppler waveform If the measurement increases, this indicates the fetus is at increased risk for adverse outcome.

Biophysical Profile: This test combines the non-stress test and the amniotic fluid index with fetal movement, breathing, and muscle tone. If each of the tests are normal they are given a score of 2. If abnormal, a score of 0. If the score is 6 or less, this suggests the fetus is at risk for adverse outcome. While the biophysical profile is a useful test, when it becomes abnormal the fetus may have already suffered some damage.

Silver-Russell syndrome (SRS)

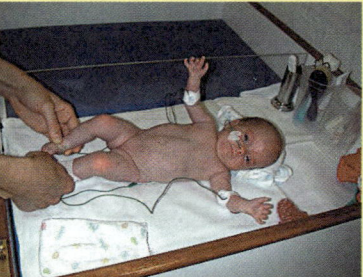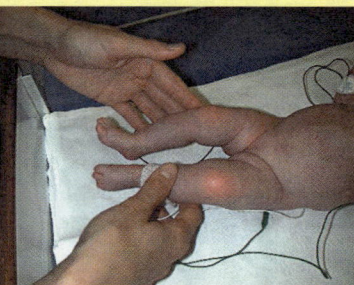

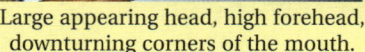

Large appearing head, high forehead, downturning corners of the mouth.

Asymmetry of the legs.

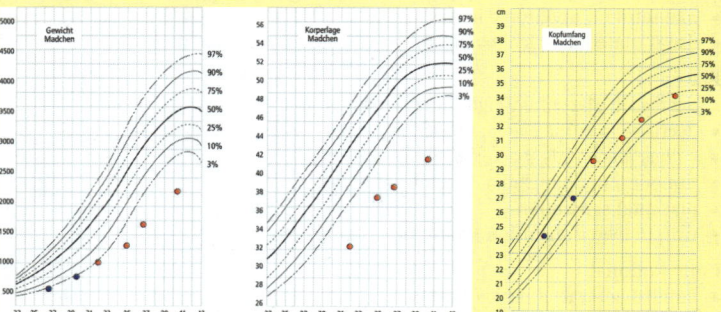

Weight and height (blue: prenatal; red: postnatal) Head circumference (blue: prenatal; red: postnatal)

Silver-Russell syndrome (SRS) was originally described by Silver and colleagues in 1953 and little later by Russell in 1954 . They described children with characteristic facies, low birthweight, body asymmetry and growth retardation. Today SRS is seen as a clinically and genetically heterogeneous disorder involving intrauterine and postnatal growth retardation with a wide spectrum of additional dysmorphic features . Because the syndrome is not only clinically but also genetically heterogeneous , diagnosis is not always easy to confirm. Only about 10% of affected individuals have maternal uniparental disomy (UPD) of chromosome 7 (inheriting 2 copies of maternal chromosome 7, with no paternal contribution) ; a defect which may be documented by molecular analysis. If no UPD can be found, like in our case, the diagnosis remains based solely on clinical criteria. In 1999 Price proposed such diagnostic criteria for SRS : 1) birth weight more or equal to 2 SD below the mean 2) poor postnatal growth more or equal to 2 SD below the mean at diagnosis 3) preservation of occipitofrontal head circumference 4) classic facial phenotype (small triangular face) 5) asymmetry (especially of the limbs).

Growth failure is the primary abnormality . Infants present with intrauterine growth retardation, feeding difficulty, failure to thrive, excessive sweating, tendency towards fasting hypoglycemia or postnatal growth retardation. Older children and adults do not manifest clinical features as clearly as infants or young children. Intelligence may be normal or there may be learning disabilities . Although growth hormone (GH) levels usually are normal in affected individuals, children with SRS exhibit abnormalities of pulsatile growth hormone action and GH treatment may have a positive effect on the growth pattern . Long-term studies have not yet been performed on a large number of patients. The eventual outcome and possible adverse effects of GH treatment therefore have to be further investigated before GH therapy can be introduced as standard treatment in SRS.

References: 1. Silver HK, Kiyasu W, George J. Syndrome of congenital hemihypertrophy, shortness of stature and elevated urinary gonadotropins. Pediatrics 1953;12:368-75 (no abstract available) 2. Russell A. A syndrome of "intrauterine dwarfism" recognizable at birth with craniofacial dysostosis, disproportionately short arms and other abnormalities (5 examples). Proc Royal Soc Med 1954;47:1040-4 (no abstract available) 3. Preece MA. The Genetics of the Silver-Russell Syndrome. Reviews in Endocrine and Metabolic Disorders 2002;3:369–379 (no abstract available) 4. Wakeling EL, Abu-Amero S, Price SM, et al. Genetics of Silver-Russell syndrome. Horm Res 1998;49:32-6 (Abstract)5. Monk D, Bentley L, Hitchins M, et al. Chromosome 7p disruptions in Silver Russell syndrome: delineating an imprinted candidate gene region. Hum Genet 2002;111:376-387 (Abstract)6. Price SM, Stanhope R, Garrett C, et al. The spectrum of Silver-Russell syndrome: a clinical and molecular genetic study and new diagnostic criteria. J Med Genet 1999;36:837-42 (Abstract)

Courtesy: Swiss Society of Neonatology.

Physical findings of intrauterine growth restriction: On first inspection of many small-for-dates infants, several obvious physical characteristics immediately suggest the presence of impaired intrauterine growth. In asymmetric growth retardation, one is immediately impressed by the seemingly large head, but head circumference is actually normal or nearly so; it is the chest and especially the abdominal circumferences that are reduced. The head merely appears large for the body. The brain is spared or less affected by the intrauterine insult, which probably had its inception relatively late in pregnancy. Because the ratio of brain mass to liver mass is high, hypoglycemia is likely to be present in such infants. Diminution of subcutaneous fat and loose, dry skin are prominent. Even though their skin appears pale, many of these infants are polycythemic; their venous hematocrit may be greater than 60. In the extreme, muscle mass over the buttocks, thighs, and cheeks is also diminished. Since body length is not as diminished as subcutaneous fat, these infants often appear thin and long. Longitudinal skin creases in the thighs indicate severe subcutaneous fat depletion, in contrast to the horizontal thigh creases of the larger infant, whose nutritional state is far better. The baby is wide-eyed, presumably as a result of chronic hypoxia *in utero*. The abdomen is flat or sunken (scaphoid), rather than rounded as in the better-nourished infant. At birth, the umbilical cord is commonly thin, in contrast to the normal cords, which are rotund, gray, glistening, and moist. Because all cords wither progressively after birth, their condition after 24 hours of age is of little diagnostic significance. Scalp hair is typically sparse. Skull sutures are frequently wide as a result of impaired bone growth. The anterior fontanel, although large, is soft or sunken, thereby ruling out increased intracranial pressure as a cause of the widened sutures. Most of these infants are more active than expected for their low birth weight. The vigor of their cry may be particularly impressive. Often, an alert, wide-eyed facial expression is combined with repetitive tongue thrusts that stimulate a sucking motion. The overall impression of vigor and well-being is misguided, for these are the result of stress caused by chronic hypoxia *in utero*. Many of these infants convulse 6–18 hours later, particularly those whose anterior fontanel is firm owing to cerebral edema from intrauterine hypoxia. In contrast, when perinatal asphyxia is severe, the infant is depressed, appearing flaccid and lethargic. Another type of growth restriction, symmetric growth restriction, is seen in small-for-dates infants whose appearance is quite different from that described above. These infants, whose insult probably occurred early, do not appear wasted. They are diminutive, but the head and body are of proportionate size. The skin is not redundant, but it is thicker (the subcutaneous vascular patter is obscure or absent) than expected for infants of the same size who are appropriately grown for their gestational age. They are generally quite vigorous and are much less likely to be hypoglycemic or polycythemic. These are hypoplastic babies in whom major malformations can be present or in whom an early intrauterine infection occurred (rubella or cytomegalic inclusion disease). Two general types of fetal undergrowth are identifiable by body measurement and by reference to intrauterine growth curves. In asymmetric growth restriction, which is more common than symmetric growth restriction, the insult seems to begin during the last trimester. These babies have a head circumference and body length within the normal percentiles, generally between the 25th and 50th, but their body weight is below the 10th percentile. Associated maternal factors most frequently include toxemia, chronic hypertension, and chronic renal disease. The second type which is symmetric growth restriction probably begins early in pregnancy. It is characterized by equally distributed reduction in head circumference, body length, and weight. All these measurements fall below the 10th percentile . Associated factors include intrauterine viral infection, chromosomal disorders, major congenital malformations, genetically small but otherwise well infants, and possibly maternal malnutrition.

Clinical differences between two types of intrauterine growth restriction

Symmetric	Asymmetric
Universal, proportionate diminution in size and weight; percentiles of head, length, and weight are similar	Selective, disproportionate diminution in size and weight; percentiles of head and length normal but weight below 10th percentile
Subcutaneous fat appropriate for size; skin taut	Subcutaneous fat diminished for size; skin redundant
Congenital malformation frequent	Congenital malformation infrequent
Intrauterine nonbacterial infection frequent	Intrauterine, nonbacterial infection rare
Hematocrit usually normal	Hematocrit often elevated
Hypoglycemia and hypoproteinemia uncommon	Hypoglycemia, hypoproteinemia common

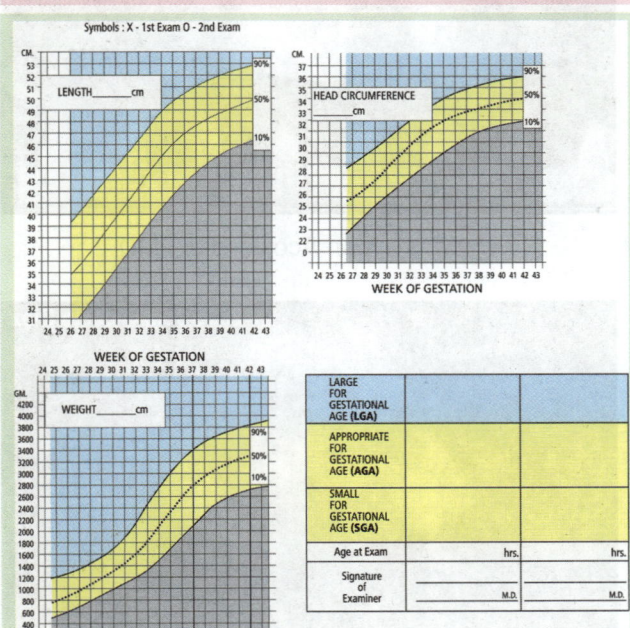

Newborn classification based on maturity and intrauterine growth

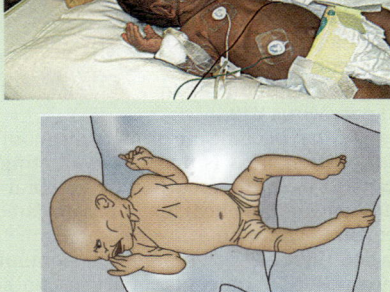

Characteristics of the SGA infant are as follows: a) The infant appears thin and wasted; their skin is loose and dry. (b) There is little subcutaneous fat; their face appears shrunken and wrinkled. (c) The length and head size may be normal but the head looks really big in comparison to the rest of the body.

Pearl/Peril/Pitfall: *IUGR causes a spectrum of perinatal complications, including fetal morbidity and mortality, iatrogenic prematurity, fetal compromise in labor, need for induction of labor, and cesarean delivery.*

Indications for Doppler flow velocimetry during pregnancy

Doppler flow velocimetry (DFV) is a *noninvasive* method to assess *resistance* to, and *velocity* of, blood flow using ultrasound technology. In pregnancy, it has been proven to be a valuable adjunct to fetal assessment because often DFV abnormalities will *precede* detectable fetal abnormalities of growth, amniotic fluid, and placental insufficiency and can help assess the severity of fetal compromise when these abnormalities are suspected.

The principles underlying the most common indications for DFV are as follows: Under *normal* conditions, the placenta offers little resistance to fetal and maternal blood flow, even during diastole (i.e. between heart beats); and, there is no preferential blood flow to the brain as reflected in normally high resistance, especially from late midtrimester on, at the expense of perfusion of other organs. Under *abnormal* conditions, blood flow to the placenta may be reduced and accompanied by increased resistance to perfusion (fetal and/or maternal) and/or there is preferential blood flow to preserve 'essential' organs such as the brain ('brain-sparing effect') as manifested by low resistance Doppler patterns to these organs and eventually reduced perfusion (fetal blood flow redistribution) of 'nonessential' organs such as the kidneys. Some factors that lead to aberrations in DFV patterns include:

- Abnormalities in placentation or of the umbilical cord
- 'Placental insufficiency' regardless of fetal size
- Fetal anemia resulting from maternal isoimmunization, viral infection (e.g. parvovirus B19 and CMV), twin-twin transfusion syndrome, fetal-maternal hemorrhage…
- Chromosomal abnormalities
- Cardiac and intracranial malformations

When indicated, DFV evaluation of the following may contribute valuable information with regard evaluation of the pregnancy, but should be performed by individuals trained and experienced in the performance and interpretation of the results:

Maternal: Uterine arteries
Fetal: Umbilical arteries, Middle cerebral arteries, ductus venosus, Umbilical vein

Common indications for Doppler flow velocimetry studies include:

- Abnormalities of growth (both intrauterine growth restriction(IUGR) and excessive fetal growth (macrosomia)
- Fetal anomalies (e.g. cystic hygromas, cardiac, thoracic, diaphragmatic, neural tube, renal, and abdominal wall)
- Fetal hydrops
- Oligohydramnios (decreased fluid) and polyhydramnios (increased fluid)
- Poor OB history (e.g. preeclampsia, IUGR, previous stillborn…)
- Known maternal risk factors: hypertension, preeclampsia, diabetes, autoimmune disorders (overt and subclinical), thrombophilias (acquired and genetic)
- Abnormal maternal serum screening (e.g. elevated MSAFP and/or increased risk for fetal chromosomal abnormality)
- Multiple gestation
- Maternal trauma (fetal-maternal hemorrhage)
- Suspected placental abruption
- Known maternal isoimmunization
- Exposure to parvovirus B19

In recent years, DFV has become the primary means of screening related to *fetal anemia*. This is done by evaluating the peak systolic velocity (PSV) in the fetal middle cerebral artery. Its *negative predictive value* is so high that it has obviated the need for, and the expense of, repetitive invasive.

procedures when there is known maternal isoimmunization, Parvovirus B19 exposure, or other potential causes of severe fetal anemia such as trauma or placental abruption or placenta previa that might lead to fetal-maternal hemorrhage or fetal blood loss. It is also the primary means of ruling out fetal anemia as a cause of *hydrops fetalis* and it is the mainstay in the assessment of multiple gestations as a means of screening and staging possible *twin-to-twin transfusion syndrome*. DFV of the fetal ductus venosus in early pregnancy has also proven useful in the identification of fetuses at risk for chromosomal abnormalities and major congenital heart defects. DFV of the branch pulmonary arteries can help predict the risk of fetal pulmonary hypoplasia in cases of premature and prolonged rupture of membranes.

DFV is no longer considered 'experimental' and it has become a 'standard of care' in the hands of specialist in Maternal-Fetal Medicine for the evaluation and management of complicated pregnancies.

This is a fetus with intrauterine growth restriction. Note the absent diastolic flow at the umbilical artery and the middle cerebral dilatation.

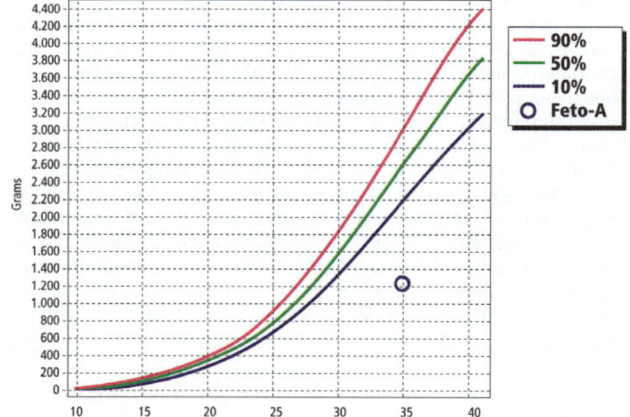

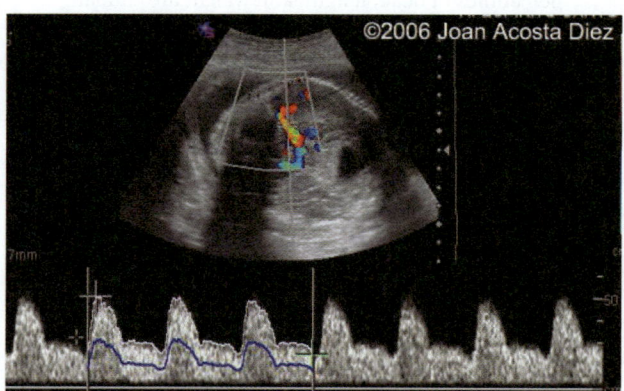

*Courtesy:*Joan Acosta Diez, MD

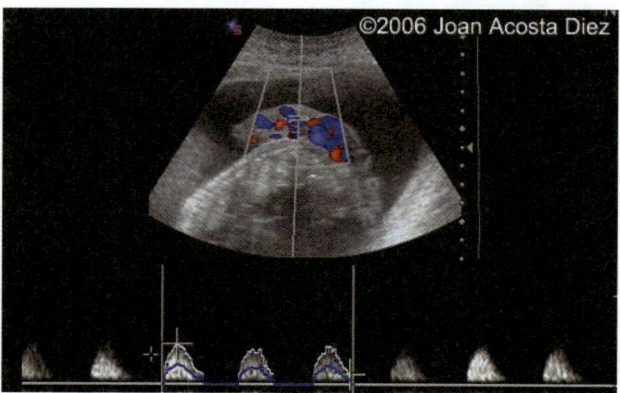

---

*Pearl/Peril/Pitfall: The clinician's challenge is to identify IUGR fetuses whose health is endangered in utero because of a hostile intrauterine environment and to monitor and intervene appropriately. This challenge also includes identifying small but healthy fetuses and avoiding iatrogenic harm to them or their mothers.

Small for gestational age babies: Indian scene: Intrauterine growth retardation (IUGR) is an important determinant of neonatal mortality, morbidity and poor neurologic outcome. The study was aimed to evaluate the magnitude of perinatal risk factors in causation and the neonatal outcome of small for gestational age (SGA) babies. One hundred and three SGA babies born over a period of one year were retrospectively analyzed during their hospital stay. 3.53 per cent of the babies were SGA with mean birth weight of 1657±SD 354 gm (range 600–2200 gm). 68.9 per cent were term babies and 51.5 per cent were females. Toxemia of pregnancy (30.09%), hypertensive diseases of pregnancy (HDP) excluding toxemia (5.8%), diabetes mellitus (1.94%), medical disorders including renal and cardiac (3.88%), anemia (Hb<8 gm%) and IU infection (0.97%) were the main conditions responsible for SGA. In 56.3% pregnancies, no cause could be ascertained. The common perinatal problems were infections in 27 (26.2%), birth asphyxia in 22 (21.36%), polycythemia in 25 (24.3%), jaundice in 22 (21.36%) and hypoglycemia in 7 (6.8%). Congenital malformations in 2 (1.94%) and Hyaline membrane disease in 1 (0.97%) were uncommon problems. 5.8 per cent babies died due to various perinatal problems. Based on these findings it was concluded that idiopathic (? Constitutional) intrauterine growth retardation was the commonest cause of SGA in Indian babies. 58.3 per cent babies had neonatal problems and they had a better survival compared to their western counterparts.

Courtesy: Anil Narang, Mrinal Kanti Chaudhuri and Praveen Kumar. Division of Neonatology, Department of Pediatrics, Postgraduate Institute of Medical Education and Research, Sector 12, 160012 Chandigarh.Indian Journal of Pediatrics Volume 64, Number 2 / March, 1997

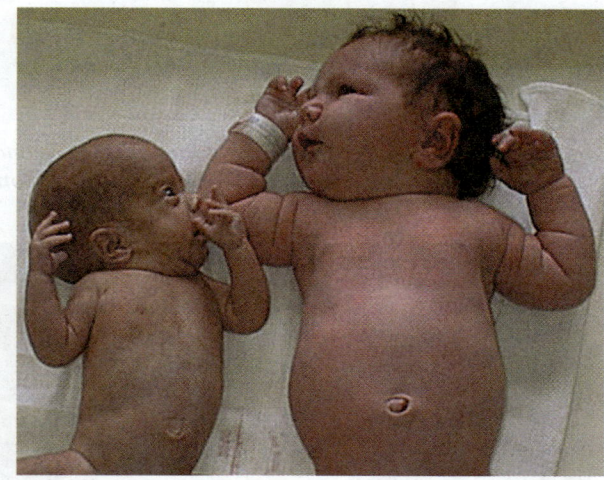

Because they have decreased glycogen and fat stores, small for gestational age (SGA) babies are particularly prone to hypoglycemia after birth; routine glucose measurements during the first few hours of life are recommended. Polycythemia is also common, and is related to the increased erythropoietin levels produced by a relatively hypoxic uterine environment. Fetal growth is influenced by many factors, but decreased uteroplacental function related to pregnancy induced hypertension (PIH) is a fairly common etiology. This baby was mildly SGA with a birth weight of about 5 1/2 pounds. Relatively thin extremities and torso give this baby a typical SGA appearance.

KEY POINTS FOR CLINICAL PRACTICE

1. Intrauterine growth restriction (IUGR) refers to a condition in which a fetus is unable to achieve its genetically determined potential size. This functional definition seeks to identify a population of fetuses at risk for modifiable but otherwise poor outcomes. This definition intentionally excludes of fetuses that are small for gestational age (SGA) but are not pathologically small. SGA is defined as growth at the 10th or less percentile for weight of all fetuses at that gestational age.

2. 20% of fetuses that are SGA are intrinsically small secondary to a chromosomal or environmental etiology. Examples include fetuses with trisomy 18, cytomegalovirus infection, or fetal alcohol syndrome. These fetuses are unlikely to benefit from prenatal intervention, and their prognosis is most closely related to the underlying etiology.

3. The diagnosis of severe IUGR before 32 weeks' gestation is associated with a poor prognosis, and therapy must be highly individualized. Once a decision has been made to effect delivery, the mode of delivery is governed by evidence of acidemia, gestational age, and Bishop score. Cesarean delivery without a trial of labor is appropriate (1) in the presence of evidence of fetal distress by nonstress testing or reversed diastolic flow or (2) for traditional obstetrical indications for cesarean delivery (i.e. malpresentation, prior cesarean delivery).

4. Once IUGR has been detected, the management of the pregnancy should depend on a surveillance plan that maximizes gestational age while minimizing the risks of neonatal morbidity and mortality. Doppler flow velocimetry (DFV) is a *noninvasive* method to assess *resistance* to, and *velocity* of, blood flow using ultrasound technology. In pregnancy, it has been proven to be a valuable adjunct to fetal assessment because often DFV abnormalities will *precede* detectable fetal abnormalities of growth, amniotic fluid, and placental insufficiency and can help assess the severity of fetal compromise when these abnormalities are suspected.

5. The current therapeutic goals are to optimize the timing of delivery to minimize hypoxemia and maximize gestational age and maternal outcome. Further study may elucidate preventive or treatment strategies to assist the growth-restricted fetus.

REFERENCES AND FURTHER READING 1) Dashe JS, McIntire DD, Lucas MJ, Leveno KJ. Effects of symmetric and asymmetric fetal growth on pregnancy outcomes. *Obstet Gynecol.* Sep 2000;96(3):321-7.2) Madazli R. Prognostic factors for survival of growth-restricted fetuses with absent end-diastolic velocity in the umbilical artery. *J Perinatol.* Jun 2002;22(4):286-90. 3) Fong KW, Ohlsson A, Hannah ME, et al. Prediction of perinatal outcome in fetuses suspected to have intrauterine growth restriction: Doppler US study of fetal cerebral, renal, and umbilical arteries. *Radiology.* Dec 1999;213(3):681-9. 4) Pollack RN, Yaffe H, Divon MY. Therapy for intrauterine growth restriction: current options and future directions. *Clin Obstet Gynecol.* Dec 1997;40(4):824-42. 5) Baschat AA, Gembruch U, Reiss I, et al. Absent umbilical artery end-diastolic velocity in growth-restricted fetuses: a risk factor for neonatal thrombocytopenia. *Obstet Gynecol.* Aug 2000;96(2):162-6.

Pearl/Peril/Pitfall: Not all fetuses that are SGA are pathologically growth restricted and, in fact, may be constitutionally small. Similarly, not all fetuses that have not met their genetic growth potential are in less than the 10th percentile for estimated fetal weight (EFW).

Pearl/Peril/Pitfall: IUGR occurs when gas exchange and nutrient delivery to the fetus are not sufficient to allow it to thrive in utero. This process can occur primarily because of maternal disease causing decreased oxygen-carrying capacity (e.g., cyanotic heart disease, smoking, hemoglobinopathy), a dysfunctional oxygen delivery system secondary to maternal vascular disease (e.g., diabetes with vascular disease, hypertension, autoimmune disease affecting the vessels leading to the placenta), or placental damage resulting from maternal disease (e.g., smoking, thrombophilia, various autoimmune diseases). Evaluation of causative factors for intrinsic disorders leading to poor growth may include a fetal karyotype, maternal serology for infectious processes, and an environmental exposure history.

22

Large for Gestational Age Infant (LGA)

@ *Preterm LGA Neonates are at risk for respiratory distress syndrome (RDS), whereas the term LGA Neonate is at risk for meconium aspiration syndrome (MAS).*

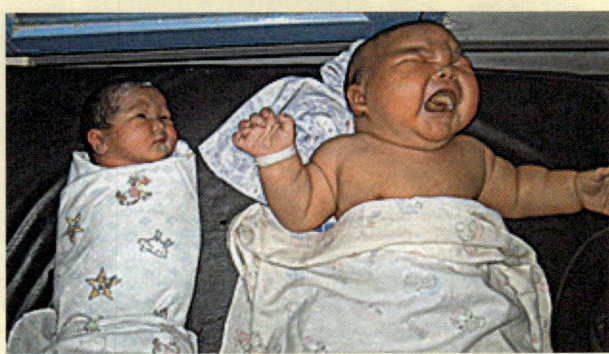

Infant of diabetic mother

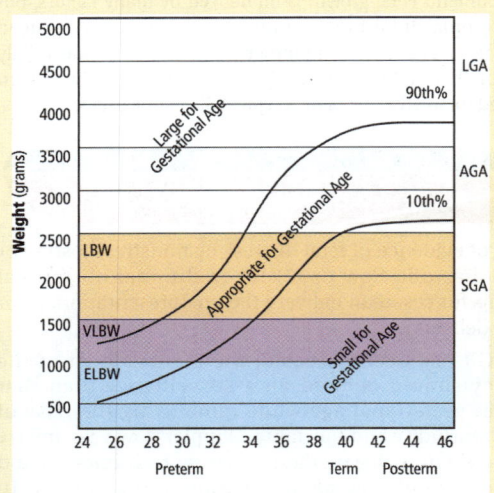

Neonate with **Beckwith-Wiedemann Syndrome (BWS):** Note the large eyes, tongue, stork bite over the eyelids, and creases in the earlobe.

Prevention

- Although no intervention has been proven to significantly reduce the risk of macrosomia, several potentially useful strategies may be helpful.
- In diabetic patients, tight glucose control before pregnancy can reduce the risk of congenital malformation. In both diabetic mothers and in those with gestational diabetes, tight control during pregnancy with the use of diet and insulin can reduce the frequency of macrosomia. The association between postmeal glucose levels and fetal macrosomia was studied and illustrated in 1991.
- Prevention of maternal obesity before pregnancy may reduce the frequency of macrosomia. However, no clinical randomized trials have validated this hypothesis. Obesity is also associated with other morbidities in pregnancy, including higher rates of preeclampsia and cesarean delivery.

REVIEW OF CLINICAL PROBLEMS

1. Mention the effects of Macrosomia on the mother, fetus, and Neonate.
   Ans: Refer to the Table "1" of the Chapter.
2. What are the "Common complications" of LGA Neonates?
   Ans: Refer to the "No. 6" of the "BIRD'S EYE VIEW/ OVERVIEW/SYNOPSIS" of the Chapter.
3. What are the essentials of management of the LGA infants` common complications ?
   Ans: Refer to the Evaluation-Decision-Action Plan/ Algorithm to diagnose and manage a Neonate LGA.
4. How do you organize the Nursing Care of LGA Neonates?
   Ans: Refer to the "NURSING CARE OF THE LARGE FOR-GESTATIONAL-AGE NEONATE" of the Chapter.
5. Mention the essentials of Antenatal management of LGA Fetuses.
   Ans: Refer to the ANTENATAL MANAGEMENT of LGA FETUSES of the Chapter.

LEARNING OBJECTIVES

After completing this article, readers will be able to

1. Anticipate the fetal and Neonatal effects of Macrosomia and Adequately manage them.
2. Perform the Focused Physical assessment of the LGA infant and identify the obvious and occult complications associated with LGA Neonates.
3. Provide appropriate Nursing Care for these LGA Neonates with multitude of clinical problems.
4. Provide appropriate Neonatal delivery room support and family education and guidance.
5. Follow-up those LGA Neonates with long-term Neurodevelopmental/ Rehabilitative needs.

Pearl/Peril/Pitfall: Neonatal: Macrosomic neonates are at risk for shoulder dystocia and birth trauma. This risk is directly related to neonatal birth weight and begins to increase substantially when birth weight exceeds 4500 g and particularly when it exceeds 5000 g.

BIRD'S EYE VIEW/OVERVIEW/SYNOPSIS

1. The prospective physical size of a Neonate is determined by genetic potential from each parent; however, it is affected by a multitude of pregnancy and environmental factors. The designation of LGA or macrosomia is used as both a diagnostic tool and a prognostic marker. The outcome of a macrosomic Neonate is based on *if* an insult occurred during the pregnancy or delivery process, the *type* and *extent* of that insult. The uterine environment is typically monitored throughout pregnancy to ensure fetal well-being. Fetal death rates are increased when the birth weight is greater than or equal to 4250 g in nondiabetic patients and greater than or equal to 4000 g in diabetic patients. Assessing fetal well-being with routine ultrasounds and providing appropriate maternal counseling when concerns for glucose control or excessive weight gain arise is imperative. Monitoring, correcting, and improving fetal well-being is the challenge faced by obstetric nursing and medical staff. Neonatal developmental outcomes can be improved if prenatal problems with excessive growth are identified early in the pregnancy and monitored frequently throughout the pregnancy. The ultimate goal is to optimize the Neonate's chances to survive and thrive.

2. Large-for-gestational-age (LGA) Neonates are defined as having a mean weight 2 standard deviations above the *weight* for the gestational age or above the 90th percentile on the growth charts. This allows for preterm, term, and postterm Neonates to be designated LGA. Another common definition is a birth weight of 4000 to 4500 g (8 lb 13 oz-9 lb 15 oz) or greater than 90% for gestational age after correcting for Neonatal sex and ethnicity. Term LGA Neonates weighing more than 4000 g can be described as macrosomic. Based on this information, LGA affects 1% to 10% of all pregnancies.

3. **Understanding factors that influence fetal growth:** Many factors influence the growth and development of Neonates. Parents of large stature (weight or height) are more likely to reproduce larger neonates. Even when socioeconomic factors and diabetes are controlled for, racial differences are also observed. Hispanic women have a higher incidence of LGA Neonates than do white, African-American, or Asian women. Male Newborns tend to weigh more than female Newborns and comprise the greater proportion of Neonates with birth weights greater than 4500 g at any gestational age. A pregnancy complicated by maternal diabetes carries one of the strongest risk factors for producing an LGA Neonate. Obese women are more likely to produce larger Neonates. Maternal obesity is an additional risk factor for macrosomia in pregnancies complicated by gestational diabetes. Multiparity, grand multiparity, or having a history of a macrosomic Neonate increases the tendency toward LGA with subsequent pregnancies.

4. **Antenatal management:** Refer to the **"ANTENATAL MANAGEMENT of LGA FETUSES"** of the Chapter for the details of antenatal investigation and management of LGA fetuses. Prenatal management is aimed at determining the ideal time and mode of delivery depending on potential complications associated with delivery of a macrosomic neonate. Macrosomia is associated with higher rates of cesarean birth, chorioamnionitis, shoulder dystocia, fourth-degree perineal lacerations, postpartum hemorrhage, and prolonged hospital stays.

5. **Focused physical assessment of the lga neonate:** Anticipate that the appearance of an LGA Neonate will be that of a plump, well-nourished Neonate. Observe and compare the relative size of the head to the body. The Neonate will appear generously proportioned from head to toe. Measure the OFC and compare it to the weight. If the OFC measures greater than the 90th percentile for the gestational age with a normal weight, macrocephaly is present. *The Evaluation-Decision-Action-Plan/Algorithm* describes the essential aspects of diagnosis and management of the common problems of a Neonate Large for Gestational Age.

6. Observe for signs and symptoms of respiratory distress (nasal flaring, grunting, and retractions). Assess the respiratory effort and depth of respirations. *Preterm LGA neonates are at risk for respiratory distress syndrome (RDS), whereas the term LGA neonate is at risk for meconium aspiration syndrome (MAS).* The term LGA Neonate is at risk for perinatal asphyxia, persistent pulmonary hypertension, respiratory distress, meconium aspiration, hypothermia, hypoglycemia, hyperglycemia, hypocalcemia, hyperviscosity, polycythemia, and decreased immunity. Respiratory distress may present in macrosomic Neonates with phrenic nerve damage as asymmetrical chest movement and be confirmed by an elevated diaphragm on X-ray.

7. Assess for clavicle and humerus fractures by bilaterally palpating the clavicles and humerus for crepitus, swelling, tenderness, or bruising, especially after a shoulder dystocia delivery. Note any decreased upper extremity movement. Radiological assessment of the clavicle or humerus will confirm any suspicions of fractures. A weak or limp arm or hand may indicate a brachial plexus injury (Erb's or Klumpke palsy).

8. LGA Neonates continue to grow longer, heavier, and have larger head circumferences after birth. Simple fractures generally heal without complications. Nine of 10 Neonates with brachial plexus palsy recover on their own, depending on the degree of damage. Traumatic facial nerve palsy may improve within days, with full recovery potentially taking months, possibly even years, depending on the severity. The most dismal prognosis associated with LGA Neonates is a spinal cord injury. The survival rates are 13% to 30%, and such Neonates may even require withdrawal of treatment.

9. Understanding the complications and risks associated with the LGA Neonate allows the healthcare team to meet individual needs by *anticipating* and providing the appropriate neonatal delivery room support and family education and guidance.

10. A focused physical assessment with accurate measurements and plotting Neonates on the appropriate growth charts provides valuable information to guide caregivers in the promotion of health and wellness of the Neonate. Providing adequate Neonatal development support for birth injuries remains a challenge postnatally. The use of ancillary support services such as physical therapy is vital to the rehabilitation of Neonates with birth trauma.

Pearl/Peril/Pitfall : Gestational age is associated with macrosomia. Birth weight increases as gestational age increases. Prolonged pregnancies (>41 wk) are associated with an increased incidence of macrosomia. Macrosomic infants account for about 1% of term deliveries and 3-10% of postterm deliveries.

THE EVALUATION-DECISION-ACTION-PLAN/ALGORITHM FOR THE DIAGNOSIS AND MANAGEMENT OF *A NEONATE LARGE FOR GESTATIONAL AGE*

SUBJECTIVE FINDINGS

Hx of symptoms suggestive of common complications of LGA Neonates

Hx of antenatal/natal/ immediate postnatal periods- maternal - fetal - neonatal effects of MACROSOMIA (Refer to the Table 1 of the Chapter)

Risk Factors for Fetal Macrosomia Maternal diabetes, Excessive weight gain, Maternal impaired glucose intolerance, Male fetus, Multiparity,Parental stature, Previous macrosomic infant, Need for labor augmentation, Prolonged gestation, Prolonged second stage, Maternal obesity.

OBJECTIVE FINDINGS

Assess airway, breathing, circulation and disability by observing the vitals, BP, O_2 sats, color, CRT, pulses, sensorium, focal neurologic deficits(facial brachial palsies), seizures, abnormal movements, tone and reflexes etc. *Plot* the weight, length, and occipital-frontal circumference (OFC) on a Growth chart according to the gestational age of the Neonate. *Assess* the skull for indications of birth trauma-Caput succedaneum, cephalhematoma, subgaleal hemorrhage, and skull, humeral and clavicular fractures

Perform complete systemic examination- anticipating the common complications associated with Large For Gestational Neonates- vide infra

(Refer to: Focused physical assessment of the LGA neonate)

INVESTIGATIONS

Blood FBC with hematocrit and platelets, ABG analysis with electrolytes, calcium++, Mg++, BUN and creatinine, urine analysis and culture, blood culture if infection is suspected, Blood glucose.

Other Investigations are to be planned according to the Clinical problems and complications summarized below!

A NEONATE LARGE FOR GESTATIONAL AGE

Clinical problem	Pathophysiology	Nursing management
Asphyxia	Intrauterine hypoxia caused by abruption, placental insufficiency, preeclampsia, shoulder dystocia	Antepartum/intrapartum fetal monitoring Adequate Neonatal resuscitation measures at birth
Beckwith-Wiedemann syndrome	Chromosomal alteration that allows doubling of the insulin-like growth factor (IGF-II) in the fetus	Monitor for development of Wilm's tumors
Birth injury	Macrosomia leads to shoulder dystocia at birth	Monitor for clavicular, humerus fractures, Erb's palsy or central nervous system injury
Cardiomyopathy	Increased fat and glycogen deposition in the myocardium of the Neonate possibly leading to congestive heart failure	Monitor for cardiac murmurs, discrepancies in blood pressures and perfusion
Congenital Malformations (renal agenesis, small left colon syndrome, anencephaly, meningocele, hemivertebrae)	Poor diabetic control in the first trimester	Supportive care and management according to the problem.
Hyperbilirubinemia	Increased bilirubin production secondary to macrosomia, hypoglycemia, and polycythemia	Adequate hydration Monitor serum bilirubin levels Type and Coombs on at risk infants
Hypocalcemia	Maternal diabetes causing decreased function of the parathyroid glands	Monitoring of serum calcium levels Calcium replacement in IV fluids or bolus form
Hypoglycemia	Termination of maternal glucose supply Elevated Neonatal plasma insulin levels	Frequent glucose monitoring Early IV glucose support Prevent hypothermia
Meconium Aspiration	Hypoxia	Appropriate resuscitation measures at birth
Persistent pulmonary Hypertension	Chronic hypoxia	Cardiovascular support Ventilatory support, Nitric Oxide
Polycythemia/ Hyperviscosity	Chronic hypoxia, maternal-fetal transfusion Increased red blood cell production	Monitor oxygen, glucose Partial volume exchange transfusion
Renal Venous Thrombosis	Hyperviscosity, hypotension, disseminated intravascular coagulation	Monitor for hematuria and an abdominal mass
Respiratory distress syndrome	Delayed maturation of pulmonary surfactant production in the fetus	Monitor oxygen saturations, provide oxygen support, surfactant replacement therapy

Pearl/Peril/Pitfall : Morbidity and mortality associated with macrosomia can be divided into maternal, fetal, and neonatal categories. A recent study investigating the effects of birth weight on fetal mortality shows that higher fetal mortality rates are associated with a birth weight of greater than 4250 g in nondiabetic mothers and a birth weight of 4000 g in diabetic mothers.

ANTENATAL MANAGEMENT OF LGA FETUSES

Causative factors for LGA neonates should be investigated antenatally. Fetal well-being is commonly assessed through the use of maternal glucose tolerance testing, nonstress testing, and biophysical profiles. Weight gain is monitored because excessive weight gain is associated with macrosomia and undesirable fetal outcomes. Metabolic syndrome or high serum insulin, non-high density lipoprotein (HDL) cholesterol and low serum HDL cholesterol were associated with an increased risk of macrosomia independent of body mass index, weight gain, placental weight, and gestational diabetes.First trimester fetal ultrasound provides the most accurate estimation of gestational age because it estimates the gestational age at 7 days of true gestational age. The estimated date of confinement (EDC) and the neonate's gestational age is calculated based on the crown-rump length as measured during ultrasound. Follow-up ultrasounds are done based on maternal risk factors and if fundal height measurements are 3 to 4 cm greater than the current gestational age. Ultrasonography has shown to be an accurate screening tool for estimating birth weight. If an ultrasound is done at ≤"38 weeks' gestation and shows an abdominal circumference of 35 cm or larger, this should alert the provider to anticipate a birth weight greater than 4000 g. Research has shown that the abdominal circumference measurement has approximately 90% sensitivity, specificity, and positive and negative predictive values, if obtained 1 to 2 weeks before delivery. However, if an ultrasound is done later between 40 to 41 weeks' gestation, the tendency to overdiagnose macrosomia was increased because none of the ultrasound formulas used provide an accurate weight after 40 weeks' gestation. Identification and evaluation of neonates at risk for LGA should begin during the pregnancy, and such neonates should be followed up postnatally. Obtain a thorough family and pregnancy history to provide appropriate anticipatory care for the neonate at risk for complications. Cesarean birth is often recommended for delivery of infants of diabetic mothers with birth weights estimated at more than 4500 g.

TABLE 1	Maternal, fetal and neonatal effects of macrosomia

A) Maternal—Vaginal Delivery: Cervical lacerations, Perineal lacerations, Vaginal lacerations
B) Maternal—Cesarean Delivery: Major abdominal surgery, Bleeding, Complications associated with regional or general anesthesia, Damage to adjacent organs (bladder, uterus, fallopian tubes, ovaries, intestines, ureter), Infection
C) Fetal: Birth trauma, Brachial plexus injuries (Erb's palsy, phrenic nerve damage), Cardiomyopathy, Congenital malformations, Death, Fractures (clavicular, humerus), Shoulder dystocia
D) Neonatal: Asphyxia, Electrolyte disturbances (hypocalcemia), Hypoglycemia, Hematological disturbances (polycythemia), Meconium aspiration syndrome, Persistent pulmonary hypertension, Renal vein thrombosis, Respiratory distress syndrome

FOCUSED PHYSICAL ASSESSMENT OF THE LGA NEONATE

*Anticipate that the appearance of an LGA neonate will be that of a plump, well-nourished Neonate. *Observe and compare the relative size of the head to the body. The Neonate will appear generously proportioned from head to toe. *Measure the OFC and compare it to the weight. If the OFC measures greater than the 90th percentile for the gestational age with a normal weight, macrocephaly is present. *Palpate the anterior fontanelle; it may be smaller than expected because of overlapping sutures associated with the molding process that occurs as the LGA neonate progresses through the birth canal. With Beckwith-Wiedemann syndrome (BWS), the anterior fontanelle may also be enlarged. There can be a metopic ridge or a ridge in the forehead caused by premature closure of the cranial suture in front of the anterior fontanelle associated with BWS. *Assess the skull for indications of birth trauma. Caput succedaneum, cephalohematoma, subgaleal hemorrhage, and skull fractures may have occurred during the birth process. Caput succedaneum and cephalhematoma are the most common types of birth trauma. Cephalhematomas, subgaleal, or subaponeurotic hemorrhages may occur with the use of vacuum extractions.Bruises and abrasions of the face may occur with a forceps-assisted delivery. *Evaluate the face looking for an obliterated nasolabial fold, a drooping mouth, and a perpetually open eye on the affected side, all of which are indications of facial nerve paralysis. *Utilize an ophthalmoscope to examine the eyes for conjunctival hemorrhages or any obvious corneal damage. The eyes may appear large and prominent in BWS.*Assess the nasal structure for septal deviations that may compromise breathing. Evaluate the ear lobes for creases, pinna abnormalities, or low-set ears, another common finding in BWS.Congenital hairy ears may be seen in neonates born to diabetic mothers regardless of maternal diabetic control. *Observe the size of the tongue. Macroglossia (large tongue) is associated with BWS. *Listen to the Neonate's cry; a high-pitched cry, inspiratory stridor, dysphonia (difficulty crying), or dysphagia (difficulty swallowing) can indicate unilateral or bilateral vocal cord paralysis from overstretching of the laryngeal nerves during delivery. *Scrutinize the skin on the trunk, thighs, or extremities for loose folds. This may indicate weight loss associated with the LGA postterm neonate. *Evaluate the Neonate for increased subcutaneous fat or increased skeletal muscle mass. The skin on the hands and feet may also be dry, cracked, or peeling in the LGA postterm neonate as compared with the smooth and plump term LGA skin appearance. Meconium staining representing fetal distress may also be present in the nail beds, umbilical cord, and peeling skin.The skin may be jaundiced because of adrenal hemorrhage. Neonates with BWS present with organomegaly, specifically enlarged kidneys, liver, and spleen, which puts them at risk for adrenal hemorrhage causing lethargy, jaundice, irritability, and shock. Pallor and decreased capillary refill time may be noted after a nuchal cord or shoulder dystocia delivery of an LGA neonate. *Inspect and measure the abdomen. Palpate the abdomen for organomegaly and any palpable masses that may indicate adrenal hemorrhage or liver trauma with the possible formation of a subcapsular hematoma. Examine the umbilical cord for Wharton's jelly and note the number of umbilical arteries. A thick cord is often seen in LGA neonates and is indicative of good nutrition and oxygenation of the fetus during the pregnancy. Umbilical cord oxygenation values and birth-to-placental weight ratio studies have shown that LGA neonates had a higher umbilical vein $pO2$ and oxygen saturation values. These values were proportionally higher than the values for Neonates in the appropriate for gestational age (AGA) group, with the conclusion that fetal oxygenation is related to size at birth across the entire range of birth weights. The birth weight was also proportional to the placental weight for Neonates in the LGA group when compared with the AGA group. A single umbilical artery is associated with increased incidence of fetal cardiovascular, gastrointestinal, or genitourinary anomalies. A pregnancy complicated by diabetes increases the risk of a single umbilical artery significantly. Umbilical hernias, omphalocele and diastasis recti (separated abdominal muscles) may be present with BWS. Examine the groin and scrotum carefully. Males with BWS commonly have inguinal hernias and cryptorchism (undescended testicles). Females with BWS may present with clitoromegaly. *Evaluate the Neonate's tone and presence of a complete Moro reflex. During a difficult delivery of a macrosomic Neonate, the longitudinal traction and significant flexion of the spinal cord may cause spinal cord injury. The Neonate may present in the delivery room with hypotonia, apnea, or areflexia (absence of neurological reflexes). Macrosomic Neonates are at risk for perinatal asphyxia caused by intrauterine hypoxia, and it may be difficult to differentiate between perineal asphyxia and a spinal cord injury presentation in the delivery room. *Assess the suck and the grasp reflex. Monitor for jitteriness or lethargy related to hypoglycemia or hypocalcemia.

*Pearl/Peril/Pitfall: Neonatal evaluation for hypoglycemia, polycythemia, hyperbilirubinemia, and electrolyte abnormalities is indicated in all macrosomic newborns because maternal hyperglycemia is the most common cause and sometimes this diagnosis is not made in the mother prior to delivery of her child.

Nursing care of the large for- gestational-age neonate: Early complications in the delivery room, such as shoulder dystocia and hypoglycemia, must be anticipated. At least one person capable of neonatal resuscitation should be present at all high-risk deliveries, such as for macrosomic neonates. Provide a neutral thermal environment by placing the newborn on a preheated radiant warmer. Thoroughly dry the neonate, use warm blankets or towels, and place a hat on the head. Next obtain a baseline axillary temperature and if stable (between 97.7°F and 99.5°F or 36.5°C and 37.5°C), bundle the neonate in prewarmed blankets before giving to the parents for bonding. Encourage skin-to-skin contact and breastfeeding once the mother is handed the neonate. If the temperature is less than 97.7°F, encourage the parents to touch and bond while the neonate is on the radiant warmer set on servo mode with the skin probe attached to the skin with a reflective probe cover. Delay bathing or placing the neonate in a crib until the temperature is stable. Traumatic facial nerve palsy may impair the neonate's suck, swallow ability, and gavage feedings may be indicated to ensure adequate nutrition and hydration. Patching the affected eye and using lubricating eye drops is indicated with facial nerve palsy. Facial nerve palsy generally improves within days after birth, but full recovery may take weeks to months. In the absence of a full spontaneous recovery, surgery may be indicated to avoid facial disfigurement. If problems such as clavicular or humerus fractures are identified, a plan of protection of the injured limb needs to be established, taught to the parents and staff, and identified on the neonate's crib so the injury is not inadvertently aggravated. Simple immobilization slings may be created for neonates with clavicular fractures by simply carefully placing a side-snap t-shirt on the neonate (affected arm first) and safety-pinning the shirt sleeve of the affected arm to the t-shirt.Ensure that the parents do not grab the neonate or attempt to pick him up by the affected limb. Pain assessment should be a component of the routine nursing evaluation after birth. Acetaminophen can be administered for pain control. Many fractures require no special treatment other than the simple precaution measures described. However, brachial plexus injuries (BPI) require more intensive treatment. Consultations with members of the orthopedic team and physical therapy should be considered depending on the severity of the injury. Protect the affected arm of a neonate with BPI from dangling when moving or holding the neonate and do not lift the neonate under the axillae. Physical therapy may be initiated with passive range-of-motion exercises at 1 week of age and no later than 3 weeks of age. Surgery may be necessary after 3 months if there is extensive damage to the nerve. Evaluate state presentation (lethargy, apnea, jitteriness, and poor feeding) after delivery to prevent or identify issues with electrolyte imbalances or hypoglycemia. Carefully monitor blood glucose levels per hospital protocol. Glucose sampling is usually accomplished during the first 2 to 4 hours after birth, depending on the size of the neonate and stability of the glucose levels as related to feeding patterns. The LGA neonate may require more frequent glucose assessment even after feedings are established to ensure that glucose needs are being met adequately. Intravenous therapy with 10% or higher dextrose concentrations may be necessary in the infant of a diabetic mother to assist in stabilizing the blood glucose levels because of hyperinsulinism secretion. If the dextrose concentration needs to be higher than 12.5%, a central line (umbilical venous or percutaneous venous line) will be necessary. Ensure that the appropriate informed consents are signed by one of the parents and on the neonate's chart before the initiation of any invasive procedure. Transient mild hypoglycemia in healthy, term LGA neonates does not appear to be harmful to psychomotor development at 4 years of age. Assess the neonate's tolerance of handling and the provision of routine care. If the infant is intolerant of handling, as evidenced by color changes or desaturation episodes, cluster nursing care to prevent overstimulation and stress in the neonate. Provide parents with information about their neonate and include them in the plan of care. Demonstrate correct handling and care of the neonate to the parents, and teach them to recognize neonatal stress clues to facilitate positive bonding.

KEY POINTS FOR CLINICAL PRACTICE

1. The term LGA Neonate is at risk for perinatal asphyxia, persistent pulmonary hypertension, respiratory distress, meconium aspiration, hypothermia, hypoglycemia, hyperglycemia, hypocalcemia, hyperviscosity, polycythemia, and decreased immunity.

2. Prenatal management is aimed at determining the ideal time and mode of delivery depending on potential complications associated with delivery of a macrosomic Neonate.

3. *Preterm LGA Neonates are at risk for respiratory distress syndrome (RDS), whereas the term LGA neonate is at risk for meconium aspiration syndrome (MAS).*

4. Understanding the complications and risks associated with the LGA Neonate allows the healthcare team to meet individual needs by *anticipating* and providing the appropriate Neonatal delivery room support and family education and guidance.

5. A focused physical assessment with accurate measurements and plotting Neonates on the appropriate growth charts provides valuable information to guide caregivers in the promotion of health and wellness of the Neonate. Providing adequate Neonatal development support for birth injuries remains a challenge postnatally.

REFERENCES AND FURTHER READING : **1)** Gregory KD, Henry OA, Ramicone E, Chan LS, Platt LD. Maternal and infant complications in high and normal weight infants by method of delivery. *Obstet Gynecol.* 1998;92:507–13. **2)** Berard J, Dufour P, Vinatier D, Subtil D, Vander-stichele S, Monnier JC, et al. Fetal macrosomia: risk factors and outcome. A study of the outcome concerning 100 cases >4500 g. *Eur J Obstet Gynecol Reprod Biol.* 1998;77:51–9. **3)** Heiskanen N, Raatikainen K, Heinonen S. 2006. Fetal macrosomia - a continuing obstetric challenge. *Biol Neonate.* 90(2):98-103. **4)**RCOG. 2005. *Shoulder dystocia.* Royal College of Obstetricians and Gynaecologists (RCOG) Guideline No. 42. London: RCOG Press. www.rcog.org.uk (pdf file 237 KB opens in a new window) [Accessed September 2007] **5)**Walsh CA, Mahony RT, Foley ME, Daly L, O'Herlihy C. 2007. Recurrence of fetal macrosomia in non-diabetic pregnancies. *J Obstet Gynaecol.* 27(4):374-8.

Pearl/Peril/Pitfall: A history of macrosomia can influence future pregnancies. Women who previously delivered a macrosomic fetus are 5-10 times more likely than women without such a history to deliver a baby considered large for gestational age the next time they become pregnant.

23 Hydrops Fetalis

@ *"Mechanical ventilation is necessary in almost all of the hydropic neonates because of pleural and peritoneal effusions, pulmonary hypoplasia, surfactant deficiency, pulmonary edema, poor chest wall compliance due to edema, or PPHN of the newborn.".*

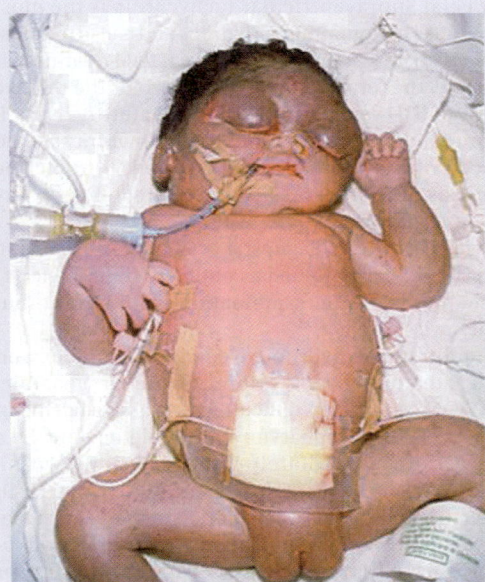

In 22–24% of hydrops cases the etiology is not determined. Cardiac, chromosomal abnormalities, thoracic lesions, twin transfusion and anemia (for example a thalassemia) account for the majority of cases of non-immune hydrops. In the case pictured here these causes could be excluded. Chorioangiomas, which are relatively common benign tumors of the placenta, have been associated with hydrops, polyhydramnios growth retardation and fetal anemia. The pathophysiologic mechanism may be related to arteriovenous shunts or vascular shunts within the chorioangioma, leading to circulatory overload and fetal congestive cardiac failure. In the absence of other causes it is likely that the chorioangiomas, which involved more than 50% of the placenta surface, were the cause for the hydrops in this case.

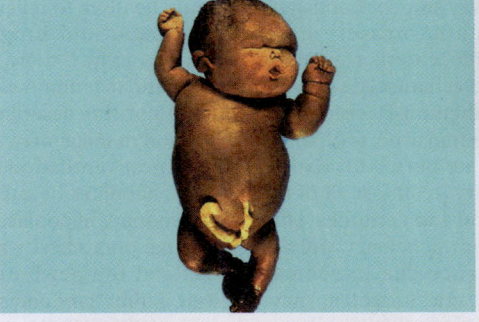

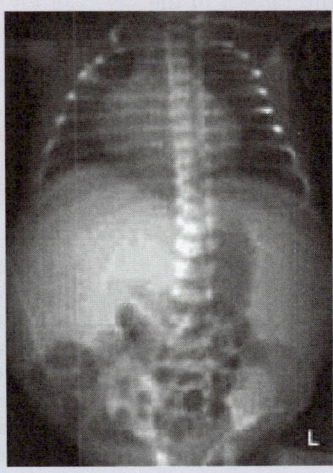

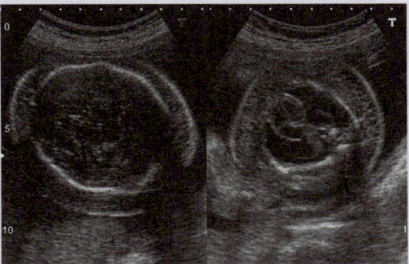

Transverse ultrasonographic sections of the head (*left*) and chest (*right*) of a fetus with hydrops fetalis. Note the halo around the head; this is due to edema. Compare the halo with pseudoedema due to fetal hair. The chest shows gross skin edema and a large, bilateral pleural collection.

Plain radiograph of the chest and abdomen of a Neonate. This image shows a markedly distended abdomen with centrally located bowel loops that are suggestive of ascites. The soft tissues are edematous although the lung fields are clear.

REVIEW OF CLINICAL PROBLEMS

1. Name the few conditions causing Hydrops Fetalis, which are currently amenable to fetal therapy?
   Ans: Refer to the "No. 6" of the "BIRD'S EYE VIEW/OVERVIEW/ SYNOPSIS" of the Chapter.

2. How do you investigate antenatally diagnosed Hydrops Fetalis?
   Ans: Refer to the "No. 4" of the "BIRD'S EYE VIEW/OVERVIEW/ SYNOPSIS" of the Chapter and to the Table 2 of the Chapter.

3. What are the essential aspects of resuscitation, when a Neonatal Hydrops is being delivered?
   Ans: Refer to the "No.8" of the "BIRD'S EYE VIEW/OVERVIEW/ SYNOPSIS" of the Chapter.

4. How do you investigate a Neonatal Hydropic infant, while managing him/her further?
   Ans: Refer to the Table 4 of the Chapter.

5. Describe the essential practical aspects of Neonatal management of Hydrops Fetalis, subsequent to initial resuscitation.
   Ans: Refer to the Evaluation-Decision-Action Plan/Algorithm to diagnose and manage a Neonate with Hydrops Fetalis.

LEARNING OBJECTIVES

After completing this article, readers will be able to

1. Understand that Hydrops Fetalis is not a diagnosis, but an ominous sign of underlying fetal abnormality or disease.

2. Refer all antenatally identified women with Hydrops to a tertiary care unit for assessment, investigation, counseling, and management.

3. Inform parents about the working diagnosis, prognosis, and the risks and benefits of available management options, when fetal therapy is an option at gestations after viability.

4. Expect a depressed Neonatal Hydrops and adequately prepare for an effective resuscitation.

5. Ensure timely and appropriate NICU care of Hydropic Neonates.

*Pearl/Peril/Pitfall: The keystone of management of hydrops fetalis is developing parental knowledge and understanding of all choices to obtain truly informed consent. Because the fetal condition is always urgent and time is short, development of this parental knowledge and understanding may represent a considerable challenge.

BIRD'S EYE VIEW/OVERVIEW/SYNOPSIS

1. *Hydrops fetalis* (referred to simply as hydrops) is a pathologic accumulation of excess body water in the fetus and results in generalized subcutaneous edema and is usually accompanied by ascites and often by pleural and/or pericardial effusions. Immune Hydrops, due to Hemolytic disease of the Newborn-Rh disease(anti-D antibodies) was the major cause of both fetal and neonatal hydrops. Because of the routine use of passive immunization with Rh immunoglobulin in the management of women who are RhD negative, Nonimmune conditions are now the major cause of Hydrops.

2. Nonimmune Hydrops is ~ 10 fold more frequent than Immune Hydrops and occurs at a rate of ~1 in 2000-3000 deliveries with 50%-90% perinatal mortality rate.Severely hydropic fetuses may die in utero; if delivered alive, they may die in the neonatal period from the severity of their underlying disease or from severe cardiorespiratory failure. More than 100 conditions (Refer to the Table 1 of the chapter)are referred to as "causing" Hydrops, but in only a limited number of these conditions can an understandable pathophysiologic link be found between the associated condition and the development of Hydrops.In many of these conditions, edema formation results from one of the processes: *Elevated central venous pressure, in which the cardiac output is <the rate of venous return *Anemia, resulting in high-output failure *Decreased lymphatic flow *Increased capillary leak.

3. The most common causes of Nonimmune Hydrops are chromosomal, cardiovascular, thoracic, infectious, and related to twinning.In about 20% of the Nonimmune Hydrops, an associated condition is not found despite thorough investigation (Idiopathic).

4. A pregnant woman with polyhydramnios, severe anemia, toxemia, or isoimmune disease should undergo ultrasonic examination of the fetus.If the fetus is hydropic, referral to a tertiary care unit for assessment, investigation, counselling, and management is required.A careful search by ultrasonography and real-time fetal echocardiography may reveal a cause and may guide fetal treatment.*Further and rapid* evaluation is directed at identifying possible causes and to determine whether intervention is possible and to estimate the prognosis for the fetus. Antenatal investigation of Fetal Hydrops is outlined in the Table "2" of the chapter.

5. Only a limited number of causes of Nonimmune Hydrops are amenable to specific antenatal therapy, and of these, only some will be successful. In diagnoses in which therapy is futile, the goal is to avoid unnecessary invasive testing and cesarean section.The prognosis should be discussed with the parents, who should be given the option of terminating the pregnancy. If this choice is made, or if the pregnancy results in a stillbirth or neonatal death, then autopsy of the fetus is strongly recommended to verify etiology(refer to the Table 3 of the chapter for the investigation of a stillbirth or a neonatal death with Hydrops Fetalis). This information plays a critical role in counselling the parents for future pregnancies.The recurrence risk is low, unlike isoimmune hydrops fetalis.

6. Intrauterine treatment is well established for Immune Hydrops and consists of intravascular or intraperitoneal packed RBC to correct anemia. The degree of anemia that is associated with hydrops is variable; hydrops is present when fetal hemoglobin is <5 g/dL, frequent when <7 g/dL, and variable between 7 and 9 g/dL.PUBS(Percutaneous Umbilical Blood Sampling) is the standard approach to assess the fetus, if Doppler and Real Time ultrasonography suggest an affected fetus. PUBS is performed to determine fetal hemoglobin levels and to transfuse packed RBC in those with serious fetal anemia(Hct of 25%). Parvovirus BI9 and fetal-maternal hemorrhage are also amenable to this therapy.Fetal Supraventricular tachycardia is the most common cause of Nonimmune Hydrops and is also the most amenable to maternal digitalis therapy. If fetal treatment is not possible, the fetus must be evaluated for the relative possibility of IUD versus the risks of premature delivery. If premature delivery is planned, pulmonary maturity should be induced with steroids if it is not present.Intrauterine paracentesis or thoracentesis just before delivery may facilitate subsequent newborn resuscitation.

7. Following delivery, the diagnostic evaluation of Neonatal Hydrops should be continued as outlined in the Table "4" of the chapter.Placental examination is important, but frequently overlooked.

8. Resuscitation of the hydropic Neonate is complex and requires advance preparation whenever feasible. INTUBATION can be very difficult with massive edema of the head, neck, and oropharynx and should be done by a skilled operator immediately after birth.IPPV with a prolonged initial breath at fairly high pressure (25 cm H2O) for 1–4 seconds may help to establish a functional residual capacity, following which ventilation at rapid rates of 80-120 bpm is usually most effective. Paracentesis and/or thoracentesis with an 18 or 20 gauge angiocatheter attached to a 3-way stopcock and syringe should be done to relieve hydrostatic pressure on the diaphragm and lungs. Pericardiocentesis may also be required rarely, if there is electromechanical dissociation due to cardiac tamponade.

9. **The Evaluation-Decision-Action Plan/Algorithm** describes the essential aspects of the diagnosis and management of a Neonate born with Hydrops.Mechanical ventilation is necessary in almost all of the hydropic neonates because of pleural and peritoneal effusions,pulmonary hypoplasia, surfactant deficiency, pulmonary edema, poor chest wall compliance due to edema, or PPHN of the newborn. Prophylactic Surfactant may be given. Pulmonary edema may improve with diuretics and increased PEEP. HFOV with INO (Inhaled Nitric Oxide) reduces the need for ECMO (Extracorporeal Membranous Oxygenation) in near-term infants with respiratory failure.

10. Meticulous attention must be paid to evaluation of electrolytes, LFTs, and blood glucose. Circulatory support with inotropic agents (Dopamine early and Dobutamine later) is often necessary to maintain blood pressure and urine output.Central venous and arterial lines are needed for monitoring pressures, blood gases and acid-base balance. FFP may help, if a low serum albumin level is contributing to hydrops.Care must be taken not to volume overload an already failing heart, and infusions of colloid may need to be followed by a diuretic.If the hematocrit is <30%, a partial exchange transfusion with 50-80 ml/kg Packed RBCs (Hct 70%) should be performed to raise the hematocrit and increase the oxygen-carrying capacity. With Rh isoimmunization, O Rh negative cells and AB serum cross-matched against mother can be used. An isovolumetric exchange (simultaneous removal of blood from the umbilical artery while blood is transfused in the umbilical vein @2-4 ml/kg/minute)may be better tolerated in infants with compromised cardiorespiratory function.

Pearl/Peril/Pitfall: Anticipate and promptly correct metabolic derangements such as acidosis and hypoglycemia. Surfactant deficiency and hypoplastic lungs may be associated with hydrops and are managed accordingly. Drainage of the pleural cavity and abdominal cavities of pleural and acidic fluid may be necessary to adequately ventilate the infant.

THE EVALUATION-DECISION-ACTION-PLAN/ALGORITHM FOR THE DIAGNOSIS AND MANAGEMENT OF *HYDROPS FETALIS*

SUBJECTIVE FINDINGS

Take the following Hx!

Maternal history Ethnicity: *a*-thalassemia, storage diseases, Diabetes, lupus, preeclampsia/hypertension, Consanguinity.

Past obstetric history Previously affected sibling, Spontaneous abortions.

Pregnancy history Gravida/parity, Gestational age, Multiple gestations, Size-date discrepancy, Polyhydramnios, Infections: erythema infectiosum, syphilis.

OBJECTIVE FINDINGS

Assess ABCDs and monitor CRT, O_2 sats, BP, core-peripheral temperature difference, RR, HR, central and peripheral pulses, urine output, and need for immediate intubation, paracentesis and/or thoracentesis

Assess for Congenital malformations, pleural/peritoneal effusions , signs of CHF such as cardiomegaly, hepatomegaly and pulmonary edema on CXR, SVT on ECG.

INVESTIGATIONS

ANTENATAL INVESTIGATIONS Refer to the Table 2 of the Chapter.

POSTNATAL INVESTIGATIONS Refer to the Table 4 of the Chapter.

HYDROPS FETALIS

Refer to a Tertiary Center for assessment, investigation, counseling, and management (fetal therapy possible? e.g.-IU Exchange Transfusion for Isoimmune Hemolytic anemia and Maternal digitalis therapy for fetal SVT).

STILL BIRTH/TERMINATED, IF FETAL THERAPY IS FUTILE/NEONATAL DEATH

Investigate as outlined in the Table "3" of the Chapter

NEONATAL HYDROPS

If premature delivery is planned, *induce* lung maturity with A/N Steroids, *plan for* Intrauterine paracentesis or thoracentesis just before delivery *to facilitate* subsequent neonatal resuscitation.

Resuscitate *effectively!*

*Endotracheal Intubation is almost always required *A skilled operator should attempt it, because of the difficulty of procedure, due to edema of the face and oropharynx *Maintain ventilation with high pressures up to 30 cm H2O and at a rapid rate of 80–120 bpm *Give Prophylactic Surfactant and prevent Hypothermia *Prepare for possible immediate abdominal paracentesis,thoracentesis and rarely, pericardiocentesis *Treat severe anemia with an exchange transfusion (isovolumetric) as soon as possible after birth to increase oxygen carrying capacity of blood.

Investigate for an underlying cause, after admitting to the NICU-Refer to the Table 4 of the Chapter.

NICU MANAGEMENT

*Mechanical ventilation:*Ventilate initially* with high pressures (PIP of 30 cm H2O and PEEP of 5–6 cm H_2O), Monitor frequently for breath sounds, chest movement, ABG Analysis, and radiographs, so that ventilator support can be reduced in response to improvements in lung compliance and water clearance, Assess for complications of prolonged ventilation-air leaks, pulmonary interstitial edema,and chronic lung changes. HFOV along with Inhaled Nitric Oxide reduces the need for ECMO.

Cardiovascular support: Insert umbilical arterial and venous lines for monitoring invasive BP, CVP, ABGs, fluid resuscitation,and for exchange transfusion,Monitor peripheral perfusion, heart rate, BP, pulses and acid-base balance carefully,Correct metabolic acidosis cautiously and replace volume with blood/colloid depending on hematocrit, or undertake an exchange transfusion for severe anemia (Hct <25%) as indicated using CVP as a guide.Give FFP to institute volume expansion, to treat hypoalbuminemia, and to manage the frequently associated DIC. Administer an IVI of Dopamine initially, later an IVI of Dobutamine to maintain BP and urine output.

Fluid and electrolyte management Moderate fluid restriction(60–80 ml/kd/d) and the use of Furosemide @1mg/ kg/dose help to promote a diuresis and the resolution of edema.Meticulous attention must be paid to evaluation of electrolytes, creatinine, LFTs, and Blood Glucose. Initial maintenance fluids should not contain sodium. Serum sodium and Urine sodium levels, urine volume, and daily weights should be monitored carefully.*Monitor for bacterial,viral, and fungal sepsis- control as appropriate!*

Exchange transfusion: If the *Hematocrit is <30%* a partial exchange transfusion with 50-80 ml/kg Packed RBCs (Hct 70%) should be performed to raise the hematocrit and increase the oxygen-carrying capacity. With Rh isoimmunization, O Rh negative cells and AB serum cross-matched against mother can be used. An isovolumetric exchange (simultaneous removal of blood from the umbilical artery while blood is transfused in the umbilical vein @2–4 ml/kg/minute)may be better tolerated in infants with compromised cardiorespiratory function.If the CVP is >12mmHg(>16cm H2O), it may be necessary to complete the transfusion with a volume deficit. Aim for controlled reduction of CVP to 6 mm Hg after ensuring the tip of the UVC is above the diaphragm on CXR.

Pearl/Peril/Pitfall: After establishing the infant's airway and ventilation, place umbilical arterial and venous catheters to monitor arterial pressure, blood gases, and venous pressure. Packed erythrocytes or whole blood crossmatched with the mother's blood should be available for partial exchange transfusion to correct severe anemia, even when due to nonimmune causes.

TABLE 1 Selected disease categories associated with hydrops and specific examples within each category

Immune hydrops

Immune-mediated hemolytic anemia
Rh disease (anti-D antibodies), Other alloimmune hemolytic antibodies (e.g. anti-kell)

Nonimmune hydrops

Idiopathic (20%)

Chromosomal/syndromic/genetic Abnormalities (10%)

Trisomy 21,18,13, Turner's Syndrome, Chromosomal deletions/rearrangements, Noonan's syndrome, Arthrogryposis, Multiple pterygium syndrome, Myotonic dystrophy, Tuberous sclerosis

Nonimmune anemias (10% including Immune causes)

Homozygous α thalassemia (Hb Bart`s hydrops), Erythrocyte enzyme abnormalities, Erythrocyte membrane abnormalities, Fetal hemorrhage, Fetal-maternal hemorrhage, Twin-twin transfusion sequence (donor or recipient), Parvovirus B19 infection, Diamond-Blackfan red cell aplasia.

Cardiovascular abnormalities (20%)

Arrhythmias (congenital heart block and supra-ventricular tachycardias), Structural heart disease, Intracardiac tumors.

Chest masses (5%)

Congenital cystic adenomatoid malformation, Congenital lymphangiectasis, Sequestration, Bronchogenic cyst.

Gastrointestinal abnormalities (5%)

Diaphragmatic hernia, Meconium peritonitis, Intestinal atresia, Volvulus.

Urinary tract abnormalities (5%)

Kidney dysplasia, Urinary tract malformations and obstructions

Intracranial abnormalities

Developmental brain malformations, Intracranial hemorrhage, Arterial or venous intracranial malformations

Lymphatic and vascular abnormalities

Intravascular thrombosis, Arteriovenous malformations, Arterial calcification, Chylothorax, Cystic hygroma

Placental or umbilical cord abnormalities

Chorioangioma, Umbilical cord angioma

Fetal tumors

Rhabdomyosarcoma, Sacrococcygeal teratoma, Neuroblastoma

Infections (8%)

Parvovirus B19, TORCH infections, Enteroviruses

Metabolic abnormalities

Storage diseases, Skeletal dysplasias

Maternal specific associations (5%)

Antepartum indomethacin, Diabetes mellitus,Toxemia, Thyrotoxicosis.

TABLE 2 Antenatal investigation of fetal hydrops

Maternal
* History, including, age, parity, gestation, Medical and family histories, recent illnesses or exposures *Medications *Complete blood count and indices, *Blood typing and indirect Coombs antibody screening *Hemoglobin electrophoresis *Kleihauer-Betke stain of peripheral blood *Syphilis, TORCH (toxoplasmosis, other infections, rubella, cytomegalovirus, and herpes simplex), and parvovirus B 19 titers * Anti-Ro and anti-La, Systemic lupus erythematosus preparation *Oral glucose tolerance test *Glucose-6-phosphate dehydrogenase, Pyruvate kinase deficiency Screening.

Fetal
* Serial ultrasound evaluations limb length, fetal movement *Echocardiography.

Amniocentesis
* Karyotype *Alpha-fetoprotein *Viral cultures; polymerase chain reaction, analysis for toxoplasmosis, Parvovirus 19 *Establishment of culture for appropriate metabolic or DNA testing *Lecithin-to-sphingomyelin ratio to assess lung maturity.

Fetal blood sampling
* Karyotype *Complete blood count *Hemoglobin analysis *Immunoglobulin M test; specific cultures *Albumin and total protein measurements *Measurement of umbilical venous pressure *Metabolic testing.

TABLE 3 Investigation of a stillbirth or neonatal death with hydrops fetalis

Detailed placental examination, Detailed postmortem examination, Skin biopsy for fibroblast culture, karyotype, Liver biopsy for histopathology, Tissue (liver, kidney, spleen) for B 19 DNA , X-rays, Photograph.

*Pearl/Peril/Pitfall: The keystone of management of hydrops fetalis is developing parental knowledge and understanding of all choices to obtain truly informed consent. Because the fetal condition is always urgent and time is short, development of this parental knowledge and understanding may represent a considerable challenge. ·Medications given to the mother place her at risk; however, the same medications may ultimately reach the fetus in concentrations too low to be effective. In addition, a standard therapy has yet to be established. ·The option of direct fetal access for drug administration has often been used; however, the invasive methods used inevitably place both mother and fetus at increased risk.

TABLE 4 Diagnostic evaluation of newborns with nonimmune hydrops

System	Type of evaluation
Cardiovascular	Echocardiogram, electrocardiogram
Pulmonary	Chest radiograph, pleural fluid examination
Hematologic	Complete blood cell count, Differential, platelet count, blood type and Coombs test, Blood smear for morphologic analysis
Gastrointestinal	Abdominal radiograph, Abdominal ultrasonography, liver function tests, peritoneal fluid examination, total protein and albumin levels
Renal	Urinalysis, blood urea nitrogen and creatinine measurements
Genetic	Chromosomal analysis, skeletal radiographs, genetic consultation
Congenital infections	Viral cultures or serologic testing, including TORCH (toxoplasmosis, other infections, rubella, cytomegalovirus, and herpes simplex) agents and parvo virus
Pathologic	Complete autopsy, placental examination

KEY POINTS FOR CLINICAL PRACTICE

1. In-Utero diagnosis of fetal hydrops identifies a clinical entity which has a myriad of underlying etiologies and associations and it also implies that the fetus is significantly compromised and at imminent risk for serious morbidity or mortality.

2. With the institution of passive maternal immunization with Rh immunoglobulin and fetal intrauterine transfusion over the last few decades, Nonimmune Hydrops has become more prevalent. The most common causes of Nonimmune Hydrops are chromosomal, cardiovascular, thoracic, infectious, and related to twinning. In about 20% of the Nonimmune Hydrops, an associated condition is not found despite thorough investigation (Idiopathic).

3. A pregnant woman with polyhydramnios, severe anemia, toxemia, or isoimmune disease should undergo ultrasonic examination of the fetus. If the fetus is hydropic, referral to a tertiary care unit for assessment, investigation, counseling, and management is required.

4. In diagnoses in which therapy is futile, the goal is to avoid unnecessary invasive testing and cesarean section. The prognosis should be discussed with the parents, who should be given the option of terminating the pregnancy. If this choice is made, or if the pregnancy results in a stillbirth or neonatal death, then autopsy of the fetus is strongly recommended to verify etiology.

5. Resuscitation of the hydropic neonate is complex and requires advance preparation whenever feasible. Intubation (*Bag and Mask IPPV is contraindicated*) can be very difficult with massive edema of the head, neck, and oropharynx and should be done by a skilled operator immediately after birth. Paracentesis and/or thoracentesis with an 18 or 20 gauge angiocatheter attached to a 3-way stopcock and syringe should be done to relieve hydrostatic pressure on the diaphragm and lungs.

When preparing for the resuscitation of a hydropic infant, a sufficient number of skilled personnel must be in the delivery room to ensure that the multiple needs of this significantly compromised neonate can be met. Equipment should be prepared before the delivery, and all personnel in the room should be assigned specific procedures, such as a paracentesis or thoracentesis, if required. These procedures may need to be performed immediately if the fluid accumulation is causing difficulties in ventilation. If the hydrops is caused by anemia, blood for transfusion should be available in the delivery room. Because of the excess fluid in the lungs, often using high pressures and oxygen are necessary initially. Artificial surfactant administration also has been attempted in the delivery room to treat any surfactant deficiency in an attempt to improve pulmonary function. Umbilical venous and arterial lines should be placed and central venous pressures monitored.

From Neonatal Resuscitation in eMedicine by Robin L Bissinger, NNP, MSN, RNC, PhD, Neonatal Nurse Practitioner Coordinator, Assistant Professor, Nursing, Medical University of South Carolina College of Nursing

REFERENCES AND FURTHER READING 1)Avery's diseases of the Newborn, 8th edition 2)Gellis and Kagan's Current Pediatric Therapy, 17th edition. 3)Nelson Text Book of Pediatrics, 18th edition 4)Manual of Neonatal Care, John P. Cloherty, 6th edition. 5)Knight DB Treatment of PDA in Preterm infants Seminars in Neonatology 2001 6;63-73.

Pearl/Peril/Pitfall: The success of intrauterine intraperitoneal fetal transfusion with packed RBCs in the treatment of the severely anemic fetus of the isoimmunized pregnancy has been a modern success story for perinatal medicine. Unfortunately, historic controls form the basis for this conclusion, and definitive evidence from randomized clinical trials will probably never be available. Nevertheless, fetal transfusion using the intraperitoneal route has apparently become accepted as the standard of care for the fetus with severe anemia.

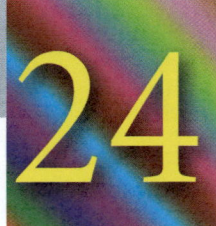

Neonatal Drug Withdrawal (Abstinence) Syndrome

@ *"These infants should be followed-up properly, because of potential problems like a) inadequate parenting b) chaotic lifestyles of parents c) maternal diseases like HIV, Tuberculosis and Hepatitis d) high incidence of child abuse."*.

The WITHDRAWAL mnemonic is a useful aid to recognizing and remembering the clinical symptoms of withdrawal.

W ithdrawal
I rritability
T remors
H yperactive, high pitched cry, hypotonia
D iarrhea, disorganized suck
R espiratory distress, rhinorrhea
A pneic attacks
W eight loss
A lkalosis – respiratory
L acrimation

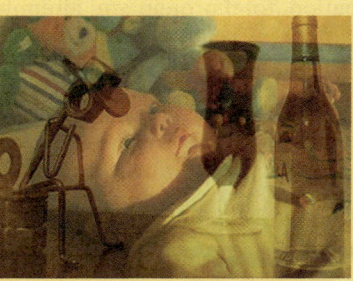

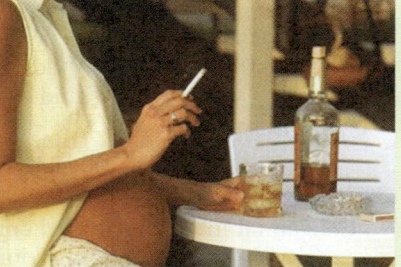

Drug exposed Neonates may experience uncoordinated movements and bizarre postures. Heavy doses of the drug can cause convulsions and coma.

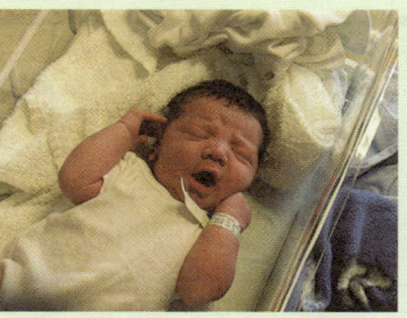

Drug withdrawal should be considered as a diagnosis in infants in whom compatible signs develop. Physicians should be aware of other potential diagnoses that should be evaluated and treated, if confirmed. Drug withdrawal should be scored using an appropriate scoring tool. Infants with confirmed drug exposure who are asymptomatic or minimally symptomatic do not require pharmacologic therapy. Consistent scoring of signs of withdrawal enables decisions about the institution of pharmacologic therapy to be more objective and allows a quantitative approach to increasing or decreasing dosing. Studies of drug withdrawal, including therapeutic approaches and outcomes, must ensure comparability of experimental groups by pretreatment and subsequent withdrawal severity scoring. Pharmacologic therapy of withdrawal-associated seizures is indicated. Other causes of neonatal seizures also must be evaluated. Vomiting, diarrhea, or both, associated with dehydration and poor weight gain, in the absence of other diagnoses, are relative indications for treatment, even in the absence of high total withdrawal scores. Drug selection should match the type of agent causing withdrawal. Thus, for opioid withdrawal, tincture of opium is the preferred drug; for sedative-hypnotic withdrawal, phenobarbital is the agent of choice. Physicians should be aware that the severity of withdrawal signs, including seizures, has not been proven to be associated with differences in long-term outcome after intrauterine drug exposure. Furthermore, treatment of drug withdrawal may not alter the long-term outcome. The use of naloxone in the delivery room is contraindicated in infants whose mothers are known to be opioid-dependent. However, in the absence of a specific history of opioid abuse, naloxone treatment remains a reasonable option in the delivery room management of a depressed infant whose mother recently received a narcotic.

REVIEW OF CLINICAL PROBLEMS

1. What are the indicators of possible drug abuse in pregnancy?
   Ans: Refer to the Table 3 of the Chapter.

2. Describe the Neonatal presentation of Maternal drug abuse?
   Ans: Refer to the Table 1 of the Chapter.

3. How do you assess -evaluate Neonatal Drug Withdrawal syndrome?
   Ans: Refer to the Evaluation-Decision-Action Plan/Algorithm to diagnose and manage NEONATAL DRUG WITHDRAWAL (ABSTINENCE) SYNDROME.

4. How do you manage Neonatal Drug Withdrawal syndrome?
   Ans: Refer to the Evaluation-Decision-Action Plan/Algorithm to diagnose and manage NEONATAL DRUG WITHDRAWAL (ABSTINENCE) SYNDROME.

5. Specify the Guidelines for the use of Neonatal abstinence scoring system: ?
   Ans: Refer to the Figure 1 of the Chapter.

LEARNING OBJECTIVES

After completing this article, readers will be able to

1. Have a high index of suspicion about Neonatal drug withdrawal syndrome in the presence of factors that are known to be associated with maternal drug use.

2. Assess infants with symptoms of drug withdrawal using a Neonatal abstinence scoring system.

3. Provide symptomatic and supportive treatment initially, and to initiate pharmacotherapy later, if necessary.

4. Screen the mother and her partner for sexually transmitted diseases, tuberculosis, hepatitis B and C, HIV as a drug-addicted mother is at an increased risk for developing these diseases.

5. Ensure adequate postdischarge care and follow-up of these infants by proper disposition through coordination of plans with social service agencies, drug treatment centers, and the courts, when necessary.

*Pearl/Peril/Pitfall: Neonatal abstinence syndrome is often a multisystem disorder that frequently involves the CNS, GI system, autonomic system, and respiratory system. Manifestations of neonatal abstinence syndrome depend on various factors, including the drug used, its dose, frequency of use, and the infant's own metabolism and excretion of the active compound or compounds. In addition, prenatal neonatal abstinence syndrome depends on the infant's last intrauterine drug exposure and the mother's drug metabolism and excretion. Withdrawal is generally a function of the drug's half-life; the longer the half-life, the later the onset of withdrawal. A longer half-life is also associated with a decreased likelihood of neonatal abstinence syndrome in the infant.

1. Substance abuse during pregnancy is a serious problem for both the mother and her Newborn. The pregnant women who use illegal drugs or alcohol are at high risk, because of inadequate prenatal care and have a higher incidence of sexually transmitted infections such as Syphilis, HIV, Hepatitis, Gonorrhea and Tuberculosis. *Effects on the fetus and newborn include chronic or intermittent drug exposure,* <u>acute withdrawal syndrome</u> *shortly after birth, poor maternal nutrition, and long-term effects on physical growth and neurodevelopment.* In addition, the risk of preterm labor, IUGR, PROM, and perinatal morbidity and mortality is higher.

2. Physiologic addiction to narcotics occurs in most infants born to actively addicted mothers because opiates cross the placenta. Withdrawal may be manifested even before birth by increased activity of the fetus when the mother feels a need for the drug or withdrawal symptoms develop. Heroin and Methadone are the drugs most frequently associated with withdrawal syndromes. Such syndromes may also occur with alcohol, codeine, phenobarbital, nicotine, amphetamines, neuroleptics, antidepressants and benzodiazepines.

3. The onset of symptoms for acute narcotic withdrawal varies from shortly after birth to 2 weeks of age, but symptoms usually begin in 24–48 hrs, depending on the type of drug and when the mother took the last dose (*Refer Table 2*). The severity of the withdrawal depends on the drugs used. Withdrawal from polydrug use is more severe than that from Methadone, which is more severe than that from opiates alone or cocaine alone.

4. Heroin addiction results in withdrawal manifestations in 50-70% of the newborn infants, usually beginning in the first 48hr, depending on the daily maternal dose (<6mg/day is associated with no/mild symptoms), the duration of addiction (>1yr has a >70% incidence of withdrawal), and the time of last maternal dose (higher incidence, if the last dose was taken within 24 hr of birth). Rarely symptoms may appear as late as 4-6 wk of age. The incidence of RDS and Hyperbilirubinemia may be decreased in preterm infants of Heroin users, because of the accelerated production of Surfactant and induction of hepatic glucuronyl transferase activity respectively. *Refer to Table 1* for the most prominent symptoms of withdrawal from Heroin addiction. Tremors and Hyperirritability are the most prominent symptoms. The typical baby is intensely irritable and miserable with jitteriness, poor sleeping, crying, snuffles and feeding problems. These babies frantically suck at their hands, and are excessively alert and agitated. Despite all the sucking they are not good at coordinating swallowing, and vomiting and diarrhea are frequent. The risk of sudden infant death syndrome is increased. Examining the urine for opiates may reveal only low levels during withdrawal, but quinine, which is often mixed with heroin, may be present in higher concentrations. The diagnosis is generally established by the history and clinical findings. Meconium testing by RIA is more accurate than neonatal urine drug testing, but is an expensive test. *One should consider hypoglycemia, hypocalcemia, hypomagnesemia, sepsis, and meningitis in the differential diagnosis of neonatal drug withdrawal syndrome, even if the diagnosis of drug-addicted mother is certain.*

5. Methadone can cause withdrawal in 75%-90% of infants exposed *in utero*. Methadone because of its ability to block the euphoric effects of heroin, is used in pregnancy to treat heroin addiction. The clinical manifestations are similar to heroin withdrawal but Methadone withdrawal has a higher incidence of seizures (10-20%) and the late onset (2-6 wk of age) of withdrawal. Mothers taking Methadone usually have better prenatal care than those taking heroin; but have a high incidence of polysubstance abuse, including alcohol, barbiturates, and tranquilizers, and they are often heavy smokers.

6. *The Evaluation-Decision-Action-Plan/Algorithm* describes the essential aspects of history taking, physical examination, relevant investigations and management of neonatal drug withdrawal symptoms. *Infants with symptoms of withdrawal should be assessed using a Neonatal withdrawal (abstinence) scoring system.* It can be helpful in assessing the need for and response to drug therapy (*Refer to Figure 1*).

7. The goal of medical management of opiate withdrawal is to maintain infant comfort while enabling the infant to feed, sleep, and gain weight in an appropriate manner. Standard medical practice is to combine both developmental and behavioral methods with pharmacologic interventions as necessary to soothe the infant. *Never give Naloxone to these infants nor to one whose mother was on Methadone; it may precipitate immediate withdrawal symptoms and seizures.*

8. 40% of the Neonates with drug withdrawal symptoms don't require medications; these respond to symptomatic care such as tight swaddling, holding, rocking, placing in a slightly darkened quiet area, and hypercaloric (24calories/1oz) as needed. Infants unresponsive to symptomatic treatment require dilute Tincture of Opium, Paregoric, Phenobarbital and Diazepam either alone are in combination. *Refer to Table 3* for various therapeutic agents used for Neonatal withdrawal syndrome.

9. A total withdrawal score of 8 or higher for 3 consecutive scorings indicates a need for pharmacologic intervention. Once the infant scores 8 or higher, decrease the scoring interval from 4- to 2- hr intervals. Once the desired effect has been obtained for 72hrs, slowly taper the dose until it is discontinued. Observe the infant for 2-3 days before discharge.

10. These infants should be followed-up properly, because of potential problems like a)inadequate parenting b)chaotic lifestyles of parents c)maternal diseases like HIV, Tuberculosis and Hepatitis d)high incidence of child abuse. These factors may be more important to the outcome of the child than the drug abuse .

Pearl/Peril/Pitfall : Evidence of maternal substance abuse should alert the infant's medical caretaker that the mother may have medical, psychological, or behavioral problems that could have an impact on the infant's long-term health and welfare. Testing the mother, infant, or both, with informed consent, is useful in some clinical situations, even when drug use is not suspected.

THE EVALUATION-DECISION-ACTION-PLAN/ALGORITHM FOR THE DIAGNOSIS AND MANAGEMENT OF *NEONATAL DRUG WITHDRAWAL (ABSTINENCE) SYNDROME*

SUBJECTIVE FINDINGS

Hx of Maternal associations with drug abuse such as a)poor or no prenatal care b)preterm labor c)placental rupture d)precipitous delivery e)frequent demands for large doses of pain medications.

Hx of symptoms suggestive of Neonatal Withdrawal Syndrome (Refer to Table 1).

Review medical history of drug-addicted mother for - Hepatitis B and C, AIDS, Tuberculosis etc.

Review psychosocial history of drug addicted mother for - psychotropic medications, chaotic lifestyles, inadequate parenting, social/ organizational services.

OBJECTIVE FINDINGS

Look for signs of maternal drug abuse in the infant such as a)small for gestational age b)microcephaly c)neonatal stroke or any arterial infarction d) malformations e)any of the signs or symptoms listed in Table 1.

Assess ABCDs, vitals, BP, urine output, O_2 sats.

Consider the differential diagnoses such as, hypoglycemia, hypocalcemia, hypo-magnesemia, sepsis and meningitis (even if the diagnosis of drug-addicted mother is certain).

Perform complete systemic examination to exclude other mimicking diagnoses.

INVESTIGATIONS

Blood FBC with hematocrit and platelets, ABG analysis with electrolytes, calcium $^{++}$, Mg^{++}, BUN and creatinine, urine analysis and culture, blood culture if infection is suspected, Blood glucose. *Urine* for toxicologic screen for illicit substances.

Meconium analysis by RIA - expensive test.

Serial assessment by neonatal drug withdrawal scoring system (Refer to Figure 1).

Cranial and Renal Ultrasound, based on clinical indications.

Plot growth parameters on standard growth charts

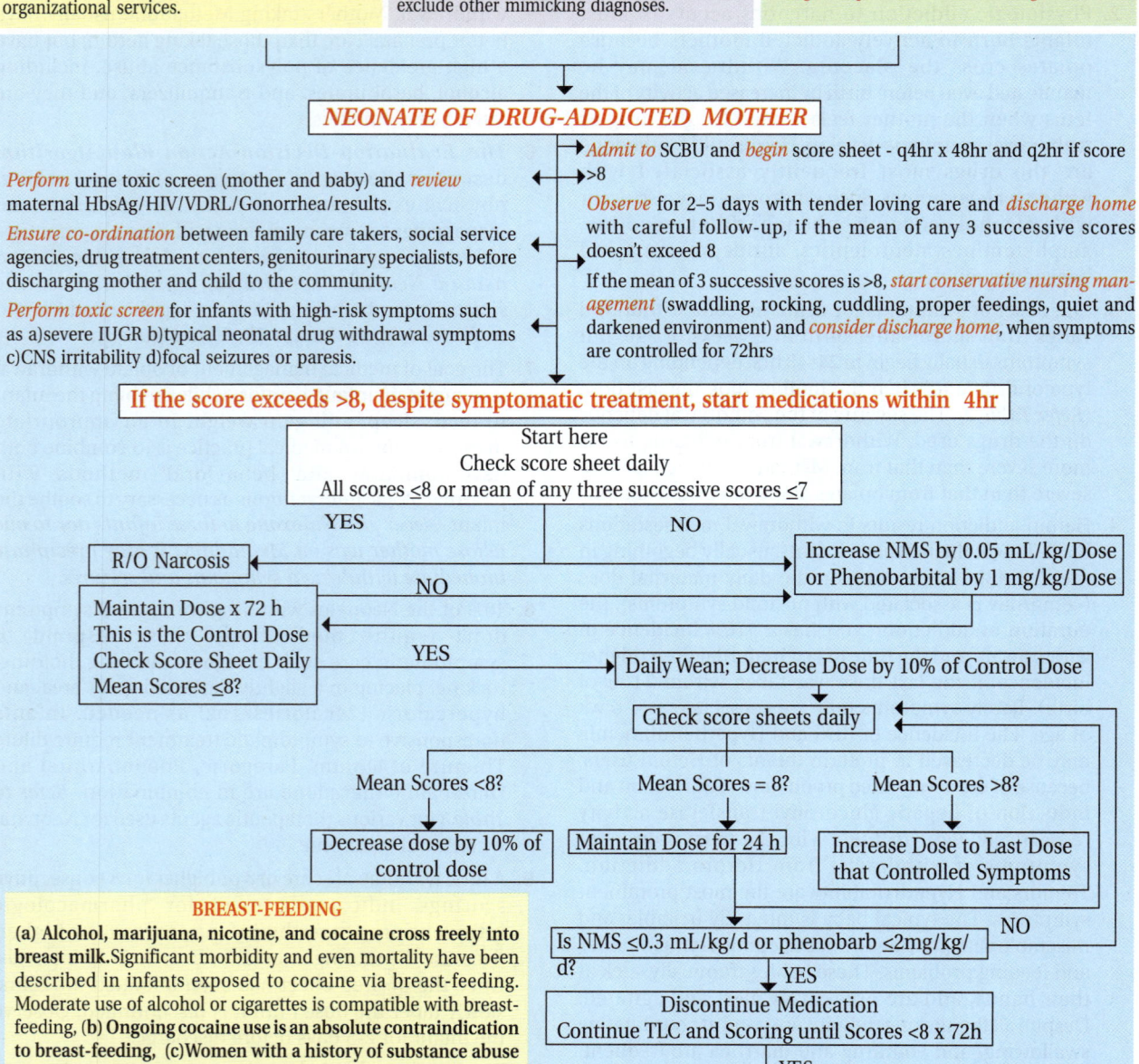

NEONATE OF DRUG-ADDICTED MOTHER

Perform urine toxic screen (mother and baby) and *review* maternal HbsAg/HIV/VDRL/Gonorrhea/results.

Ensure co-ordination between family care takers, social service agencies, drug treatment centers, genitourinary specialists, before discharging mother and child to the community.

Perform toxic screen for infants with high-risk symptoms such as a)severe IUGR b)typical neonatal drug withdrawal symptoms c)CNS irritability d)focal seizures or paresis.

Admit to SCBU and *begin* score sheet - q4hr x 48hr and q2hr if score >8

Observe for 2–5 days with tender loving care and *discharge home* with careful follow-up, if the mean of any 3 successive scores doesn't exceed 8

If the mean of 3 successive scores is >8, *start conservative nursing management* (swaddling, rocking, cuddling, proper feedings, quiet and darkened environment) and *consider discharge home*, when symptoms are controlled for 72hrs

If the score exceeds >8, despite symptomatic treatment, start medications within 4hr

Start here
Check score sheet daily
All scores ≤8 or mean of any three successive scores ≤7

YES — NO

Increase NMS by 0.05 mL/kg/Dose or Phenobarbital by 1 mg/kg/Dose

R/O Narcosis

Maintain Dose x 72 h
This is the Control Dose
Check Score Sheet Daily
Mean Scores ≤8?

NO

YES — Daily Wean; Decrease Dose by 10% of Control Dose

Check score sheets daily

Mean Scores <8? — Mean Scores = 8? — Mean Scores >8?

Decrease dose by 10% of control dose — Maintain Dose for 24 h — Increase Dose to Last Dose that Controlled Symptoms

Is NMS ≤0.3 mL/kg/d or phenobarb ≤2mg/kg/d?

NO

YES

Discontinue Medication
Continue TLC and Scoring until Scores <8 x 72h

YES

Discharge with Careful Follow-up of medical and neurodevelopmental status

BREAST-FEEDING

(a) Alcohol, marijuana, nicotine, and cocaine cross freely into breast milk. Significant morbidity and even mortality have been described in infants exposed to cocaine via breast-feeding. Moderate use of alcohol or cigarettes is compatible with breast-feeding, (b) Ongoing cocaine use is an absolute contraindication to breast-feeding, (c)Women with a history of substance abuse may breast-feed if they remain drug free as demonstrated by regular urine toxicology testing. d) Women on methadone and buprenorphine maintenance may breast-feed as long as no illicit drug use occurs.

Maintenance drugs should be taken just after breast-feeding.

Pearl/Peril/Pitfall: Long-term problems of children exposed to illicit drugs in utero include adverse neurodevelopmental outcomes. Lower intelligence quotient scores have been reported in children with in utero exposure to cocaine or methadone. Speech, perceptual, and cognitive disturbances have been reported in toddlers who were exposed to opiates. Difficulties with expressive language articulation have been reported in children of mothers who abused cocaine.

TABLE 1	Clinical signs of neonatal withdrawal syndrome
Central nervous system dysfunction	Irritability, excessive crying Jitteriness, tremulousness Hyperactive reflexes Increased tone Sleep disturbance Seizures
Autonomic dysfunction	Excessive sweating Mottling Hyperthermia Hypertension
Respiratory symptoms	Tachypnea Nasal stuffiness Diarrhea
Gastrointestinal and feeding disturbances	Excessive sucking Hyperphagia

TABLE 2 — Drugs described as being associated with a neonatal withdrawal syndrome

Drug	Time of onset of withdrawal
Heroin	0–96 hours (peak 12–24 hours)
Methadone	12–72 hours (peak 24–48 hours); can be up to 2 weeks
Short acting barbiturates	0–24 hours
Longer acting barbiturates	>7 days
Diazepam	2–6 hours
Chlordiazepoxide	3 weeks
Tricyclic antidepressants	0–12 hours
Propoxyphene	< 24 hours
Pentazocine	< 24 hours
Codeine	< 24 hours
Dihydrocodeine (DF 118)	< 48 hours
Alcohol	< 24 hours

TABLE 3 — Indicators of possible drug abuse in pregnancy

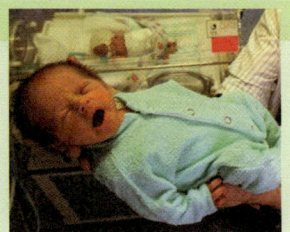

Medical
- Self-admission of use
- Stillbirth or birth of infant with anomalies
- Sporadic or no prenatal care before delivery
- Preterm labor and delivery or abruptio placentae.

Social
- Imprisonment
- Family violence
- Past drug or alcohol abuse
- Removal of other children from the home
- Frequent changes of residence or employment.

TABLE 4 — Medications for neonatal drug withdrawal syndrome

1) Neonatal Morphine Solution-NMS: The treatment of choice for neonatal drug withdrawal syndrome. Contains Morphine sulfate in a concentration of 0.4 mg/ml and the dosing scheme depends on the abstinence score as follows;

Score	NMS DOSE
8-10	0.8 mL/kg/d divided q4h
11-13	1.2 mL/kg/d divided q4h
14-16	1.6 mL/kg/d divided q4h
17 or greater	2.0 mL/kg/d divided q4h; increase by 0.4 mL increments until controlled

Effects of overdosage sleepiness, constipation, poor suck, hypothermia, respiratory depression, apnea, bradycardia, and ultimately profound narcosis with obtundation. If these symptoms occur, stop the medication until the abstinence scores are over 8. Use docusate.

1. If the infant is irritable, despite the dose of NMS is >2 ml/kg/day, add phenobarbital. Once an adequate dose has been found, and the infant scores have been <8 for 72 hrs, wean by 10% of total dose daily. If weaning results in scores >8, restart the last effective dose. Discontinue NMS when the daily dose is <0.3 ml/kg/day. The goal of tapering is to allow the infant to acclimate to a new and lower dose of medication while ensuing that he /she is comfortable, and is able to sleep, eat, and gain weight appropriately. If the scores are low, make sure that the infant is not overdosed.

2. **Phenobarbital** is given at a loading dose of 20 mg/kg (up to a total loading dose of 40 mg/kg), followed by a maintenance dose of 5mg/kg/day in 2 divided doses or q24h. It does not, however, reduce significant physiologic signs of opiate withdrawal such as diarrhea and seizures. Sedation and poor sucking are the side effects and the drug levels must be monitored. It is the drug of choice if the infant is thought to be withdrawing from a nonnarcotic drug or from multiple drug use.

3. **Morphine + Phenobarbital:** It can be initiated together for infants withdrawing from multiple drugs with better results compared with single medical therapy. If the infant improves, Morphine should be withdrawn first and the infant observed for 2–3 days off Morphine and on Phenobarbital alone. The infant can be discharged home on Phenobarbital on maintenance dose and can be allowed to outgrow the dose at home.

4. **Paregoric:** It contains opium 0.4%, equivalent to morphine 0.04% or 0.4 mg/ml. It also contains anise oil, benzoic acid, camphor, and glycerin in an alcohol base. Associated with adverse effects in preterms such as acidosis, CNS depression, respiratory distress, hypotension, renal failure, seizures, and death. Not being used currently.

5. **Methadone** not been studied in neonates, especially in preterms; can be tried in older infants and children at a dose of 0.05-0.1 mg/kg given 6-12q, with increases of 0.05mg/kg until symptoms are controlled.

6. **Chlorpromazine** is no longer used because of its unacceptable side effects, including tardive dyskinesia.

7. **Lorazepam** is often used for sedation either alone or with morphine solution at a dose of 0.05-0.1 mg/kg IV per dose Diazepam, because of respiratory depression is not recommended.

8. **Clonidine** has also been evaluated both as an additive and alternative option for the treatment of opioid withdrawal symptoms. Data evaluating the use of clonidine for the treatment of NAS are limited; only six studies have been published. The β2 adrenergic receptor agonist clonidine is believed to reduce the excessive noradrenergic activity that results from opioid withdrawal. Clonidine has the potential to serve as an attractive option to treat NAS because it possesses a favorable adverse effect profile, is easy to administer, and does not require a long tapering period, unlike other agents currently used to treat NAS. Blood pressure and heart rate must be monitored with clonidine use.

---

* *Pearl/Peril/Pitfall : Breastfeeding confers immunologic benefits to the neonate, and bonding benefits the mother. Advise breastfeeding for the mother who is receiving maintenance doses of methadone if she receives no more than 20 mg of methadone per 24 hours and is not abusing other drugs. Only small amounts of methadone are detected in breast milk.*

	Fig. 1: A scoring system for evaluation and treatment of neonatal abstinence syndrome			
SYSTEM	**SIGNS AND SYMPTOMS**	**SCORE**	**AM**	**PM**
CENTRAL NERVOUS SYSTEM DISTURBANCES	Excessive High-pitched (or other) Cry	2		
	Continuous High-pitched (or other) Cry	3		
	Sleeps < 1 hour after feeding	3		
	Sleeps < 2 hours after feeding	2		
	Sleeps < 3 hours after feeding	1		
	Hyperactive Moro Reflex	2		
	Markedly Hyperactive Moro Reflex	3		
	Mild Tremors Disturbed	1		
	Moderate-Severe Tremors Disturbed	2		
	Mild Tremors Undisturbed	3		
	Moderate-Severe Tremors Undisturbed	4		
	Increased Muscle Tone	2		
	Excoriation (Specify area)	1		
	Myoclonic Jerks	3		
	Generalized Convulsions	5		
METABOLIC/VASOMOTOR/ RESPIRATORY DISTURBANCES	Sweating	1		
	Fever < 101 (99-100.8°F/37.2–38.2°C)	1		
	Fever > 101 (38.4°C. and Higher)	2		
	Frequent Yawning (> 3-4 times/interval)	1		
	Mottling	1		
	Nasal Stuffiness	1		
	Sneezing (> 3–4 times/interval)	1		
	Nasal Flaring	2		
	Respiratory rate >60/Min.	1		
	Respiratory rate > 50/Min. with retractions	2		
GASTROINTESTINAL DISTURBANCES	Excessive sucking	1		
	Poor feeding	2		
	Regurgitation	2		
	Projectile vomiting	3		
	Loose stools	2		
	Watery stools	3		

Guidelines for the use of Neonatal abstinence scoring system:
1)Record time of scoring (end of observation interval). 2)Give points for all behaviors or symptoms observed during the scoring interval, even though they may not be present at the time of recording. (For example, if the baby was diaphoretic at 11 A.M. and is "scored" at noon, when he or she is not, the baby still gets the "sweating" point.) 3)Awaken the baby to test reflexes. Calm before assessing muscle tone, respirations, or More reflex. Many of the signs of hunger can appear the same as withdrawal. Appearance after feeding gives a good idea of muscle activity. 4)Count respirations for a full minute. Always take temperature at the same site. The temperatures on the sheet are *rectal* levels; an axillary temperature that is 2 degrees cooler may also indicate withdrawal. 5)Do not give points for perspiration if it occurs due to swaddling. 6)A startle reflex should not be substituted for the Moro reflex. 7)Record doses administered (dose/time/initials) on sheet. One hour leeway is acceptable

KEY POINTS FOR CLINICAL PRACTICE

1. Effects of maternal substance abuse on the fetus and newborn include chronic or intermittent drug exposure, acute withdrawal syndrome shortly after birth, poor maternal nutrition, and long-term effects on physical growth and neurodevelopment.

2. Infants with symptoms of withdrawal should be assessed using a Neonatal withdrawal (abstinence) scoring system. It can be helpful in assessing the need for and response to drug therapy.

3. One should consider hypoglycemia, hypocalcemia, hypo-magnesemia, sepsis, and meningitis in the differential diagnosis of Neonatal drug withdrawal syndrome, even if the diagnosis of drug-addicted mother is certain.

4. The goal of medical management of opiate withdrawal is to maintain infant comfort while enabling the infant to feed, sleep, and gain weight in an appropriate manner.

5. Never give Naloxone to these infants nor to one whose mother was on Methadone; it may precipitate immediate withdrawal symptoms and seizures.

REFERENCES AND FURTHER READING : 1)Roberton's Text Book of Neonatology ,4th Edition 2)Avery's diseases of the Newborn, 8th edition 3)Nelson Text Book of Pediatrics, 18th edition 4)Manual of Neonatal Care, John P. Cloherty, 6th edition. 5)Johnson k et al Treatment of Neonatal Abstinence Syndrome. Archives of Disease in Childhood Fetal and Neonatal Edition.

*Pearl/Peril/Pitfall: Radioimmunoassay and enzyme immunoassay : These are the most commonly used drug screens. Both are semi quantitative and highly sensitive, but enzyme immunoassay takes less time to perform and is less expensive. These tests inform the clinician about the presence or absence of substance abuse, rather than quantifying the drug level, as in toxicology screens.

25 Retinopathy of Prematurity (ROP)

@ *ROP is rare in infants born after 32 weeks of gestation, but has occurred in infants who never received supplemental oxygen, term infants with cyanotic CHD, and, rarely, even in stillborn infants. Currently no proven methods are available to prevent ROP.*

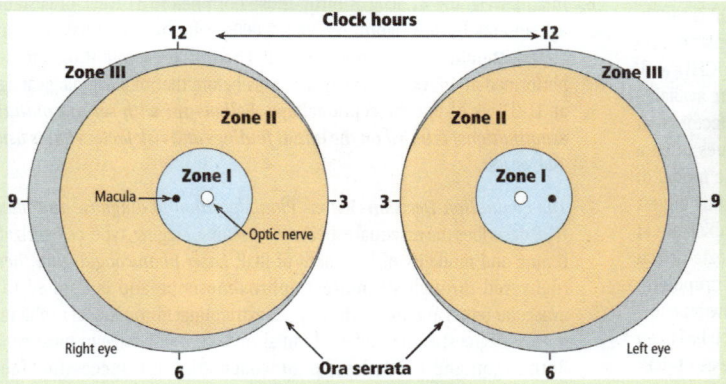

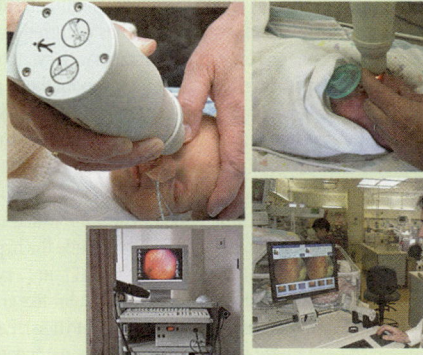

The Present & The Future: ROP Fundus Images being teletransmitted to remote sites for appraisal and feedback .

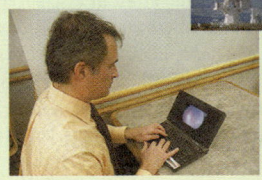

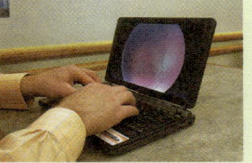

Scheme of retina of the right and left eyes showing borders and clock hours used to describe the location and extent of retinopathy of prematurity. Diagrammatic representation of the potential total area of the premature retina, with zone I (the most posterior) symmetrically surrounding the optic nerve head (the earliest to develop). A larger retinal area is present temporally (laterally) than nasally (medially) (zone III). Only zones I and II are present nasally.

> *"Each Neonatal unit should have a clear protocol so that all infants at risk of severe ROP are identified and screened by an experienced ophthalmologist."*

Retinopathy of prematurity (ROP) is one of the few causes of childhood visual disability which is largely preventable. Many extremely preterm babies will develop some degree of ROP although in the majority this never progresses beyond mild disease which resolves spontaneously without treatment. A small proportion, develop potentially severe ROP which can be detected through retinal screening. If untreated, severe disease can result in serious vision impairment and consequently all babies at risk of sight-threatening ROP should be screened.

REVIEW OF CLINICAL PROBLEMS

1. How do you assess the severity of ROP ?
   Ans: Refer to the Evaluation-Decision-Action Plan/ Algorithm to diagnose & manage Retinopathy of Prematurity.

2. Which high-risk groups of Neonates, should you include for ROP screening and when?
   Ans: Refer to the Evaluation-Decision-Action Plan/ Algorithm to diagnose & manage Retinopathy of Prematurity.

3. How do you organize follow-up examinations for ROP, on the basis of initial retinal findings?
   Ans: Refer to Table 2 of the Chapter.

4. What are the therapeutic options for severe ROP?
   Ans: Refer to the Evaluation-Decision-Action Plan/ Algorithm to diagnose & manage Retinopathy of Prematurity.

5. How do you counsel the parents about the Prognosis of ROP ?
   Ans: Refer to the Table 5 of the Chapter.

LEARNING OBJECTIVES

After completing this article, readers will be able to

1. Provide meticulous Neonatal care to reduce much sight-threatening ROP.

2. Organize ophthalmic screening of high-risk premature and LBW infants born before 31 wks' GA.

3. Communicate with parents and pediatricians and Ophthalmologists at other transferring hospitals about ensuring the *further follow-ups* for ROP.

4. Educate parents about the sequelae of severe ROP and those of laser therapy and/or surgical interventions.

5. Review all infants who develop stage 3 ROP, whether or not they require treatment during early childhood, for visual impairment, strabismus and refractive errors.

---

* *Pearl/Peril/Pitfall : Although oxygen therapy has been blamed for ROP progression in the past, many physicians believe that maximizing the oxygen saturation in these critical babies will induce regression in prethreshold disease. STOP-ROP (Supplemental Therapeutic Oxygen for Prethreshold Retinopathy Of Prematurity), a multicentered national study, found that no benefit was achieved by keeping the oxygen saturation above 95%. However, higher oxygen saturation levels were not found to worsen the disease in prethreshold babies.*

BIRD'S EYE VIEW/OVERVIEW/SYNOPSIS

1. Retinopathy of Prematurity (ROP) is a complex disorder of the developing retinal vasculature in premature infants that increases in incidence with decreasing gestational age; approximately; 65% of infants with a birth weight<1,250g and 80% of those with a birth weight<1,000g, (90% of those<750g birth.wt) will develop some degree of ROP. In >90% of cases, ROP regresses spontaneously, but in <10% progressive disease("threshold ROP") is the leading cause of blindness in preterm infants. ROP is rare in infants born after 32 weeks of gestation, but has occurred in infants who never received supplemental oxygen, term infants with cyanotic CHD, and, rarely,even in stillborn infants.Currently no proven methods are available to prevent ROP. Despite an appreciation for the postnatal risk factors that contribute to the development of ROP, this condition continues to be a major cause of childhood blindness. Studies using the mouse model of oxygen-induced retinopathy (OIR) have identified new therapeutic targets that may be used to guide treatment and determine which babies are at highest risk for ROP development. Such factors include the hypoxia-driven proteins, vascular endothelial growth factor (VEGF) and erythropoietin (EPO) as well as the maternally derived factors insulin-like growth factor-1 (IGF-1) and omega-3 polyunsaturated fatty acids (PUFAs). Each has been demonstrated to have phase-specific effects on the pathogenesis of ROP. (Refer to Pathogenesis-ROP)

2. The onset of Retinopathy Of Prematurity (ROP) consists of 2 stages: **a)** Various insults like hyperoxia, hypoxia, or hypotension etc., cause retinal vascular ischemia, vasoconstriction and arrest in vasculogenesis due to downregulation of the production of growth factors such as vascular endothelial growth factor in a preterm infant. **b)**Neovascularization then occurs i.e., an aberrant retinal vessel growth driven by excess angiogenic factors released by the ischemic relatively hypoxic avascular retina. New vessels grow through the retina into the vitreous.These vessels are permeable and hemorrhage and edema occur. Extensive and severe extraretinal fibrovascular proliferation can lead to retinal detachment and abnormal retinal function. ROP includes all stages of the disease and its sequelae. Retrolental fibroplasia, the previous name for this disease, described only the cicatricial stages.

3. Retinopathy Of Prematurity (ROP) is multifactorial in etiology and has been consistently associated with low gestational age, low birth weight, and prolonged oxygen exposure at high concentrations.Severe ROP develops in the sickest infants, i.e., it correlates with asphyxia, acidosis, sepsis, blood transfusions, IVH, PVL, and CLD. Once the retina is fully vascularized, ROP can no longer develop. Wide variations in arterial oxygen tension may be a greater risk factor than the absolute level of hyperoxia.

4. Retinopathy Of Prematurity (ROP) was classified in 1984, allowing the location, severity, and extent of the disease to be described accurately and it was updated in 1987 to include the sequelae of ROP. (Refer to the International Classification Of ROP (ICROP) given in *The Evaluation-Decision-Action- Plan/Algorithm* for the diagnosis and management of ROP).

5. Each neonatal unit should have a clear protocol so that all infants at risk of severe ROP are identified and screened by *an experienced ophthalmologist*. The pupils should be dilated with cyclopentolate 0.5% and phenylephrine 2.5%, repeated once, if necessary, 30 minutes before examination. The use of a lid speculum, binocular indirect ophthalmoscopy and a scleral depressor permits complete examination of the peripheral retina. The examination can be stressful to fragile preterm infants, and the dilating drops can have untoward side effects; thus discretion must be used in timing the eye examination, and the infants must be carefully monitored during and after the examination The results may then be recorded on a standardised form using the ICROP. Wide-field digital imaging is increasingly used for ROP screening. ROP screening aims to identify infants at risk of severe disease and those who would benefit from the available therapies. Refer to Table 1, for the initial screening of ROP, based on the gestational age of the infant. Table 2 enlists the follow-up examinations, on the basis of the initial retinal findings.

6. Infants weighing <1,500g at birth, those born before 31 week of gestational age, infants born weighing >1,500g-2,000g who have an unstable clinical course should be examined for ROP. The initial examination should be performed at 4-6wk(ROP rarely develops before that)of chronological age or at 31-33 wk of postconceptional age. *Follow-up(with serial ophthalmic examinations) is based on the initial findings and risk factors but is usually 2wk or less.*

7. *The Evaluation-Decision-Action- Plan/Algorithm to diagnose and manage ROP* describes the essential aspects of screening, staging, type-categorization, timing and modality of treatment of ROP. *Laser photocoagulation therapy* (delivered through an indirect ophthalmoscope and is applied to the avascular retina anterior to the ridge of extraretinal fibrovascular proliferation for 360 degrees) is the preferred initial treatment of choice in most centers. Both Argon and Diode laser photocoagulation are successful. Table 3 describes the essentials of preparatiton for Laser photocoagulation therapy. Table 4 outlines the elements of pre and post operative care.

8. *Cryotherapy* (by applying a cryoprobe to the external surface of the sclera and areas peripheral to the ridge of the ROP are frozen until the entire anterior avascular retina has been treated) under local/general anesthesia may be necessary in special cases, such as when there is poor pupillary dilation or vitreous hemorrhage, both of which prevent adequate delivery of laser therapy. The development of cataracts, glaucoma, or anterior segment ischemia following laser therapy or cryotherapy has been reported.

9. Retinal detachment at macula needs **vitrectomy with or without lensectomy, and membrane peeling** if necessary to remove tractional forces causing retinal detachment. A **scleral buckling procedure** may be useful for more peripheral detachments, with drainage of subretinal fluid, for effusional detachments. Reoperations for redetachment of retina are common. The surgical outcome for useful vision in total retinal detachment is poor, but the achievement of even minimal vision can result in a large difference in a child`s overall quality of life.

10. The prognosis of ROP(short-term and long-term) is described in the Table 5 of the Chapter. Infants with stage 2 or 3 ROP that spontaneously regresses or is successfully treated are still at risk for myopia, amblyopia, astigmatism, and late retinal detachment, necessitating careful visual screening and intervention when indicated, throughout childhood.

The conclusion of acute retinal screening examinations should be based on age and retinal ophthalmoscopic findings. Findings that suggest that examinations can be curtailed include the following:
*zone III retinal vascularization attained without previous zone I or II ROP (if there is examiner doubt about the zone or if the postmenstrual age is less than 35 weeks, confirmatory examinations may be warranted);
* postmenstrual age of 45 weeks and no prethreshold disease (defined as stage 3 ROP in zone II, any ROP in zone I) or worse ROP is present; or
* regression of ROP (care must be taken to be sure that there is no abnormal vascular tissue present that is capable of reactivation and progression).
From:Screening Examination of Premature Infants for Retinopathy of Prematurity,*Pediatrics* 2006;117;572

---

* ***Pearl/Peril/Pitfall:*** *Laser surgery (e.g., xenon, argon, diode) has been shown to be as effective as cryotherapy for ROP. The systemic adverse effects are significantly less, the ocular tissues are less traumatized, posterior zone 1 disease is treated easily, general anesthesia is not necessary, and, as many studies show, there is less incidence of late complications. Complications include corneal haze, burns of the iris, cataracts, and intraocular hemorrhages. Scleral buckling surgery and/or vitrectomy is usually performed for stages 4 and 5. Some surgeons recommend surgery for stage 4A, while others do not think surgery should be performed because of the risks and unproven benefit.*

THE EVALUATION-DECISION-ACTION- PLAN/ALGORITHM FOR THE DIAGNOSIS AND MANAGEMENT OF *RETINOPATHY OF PREMATURITY*

Consult an ophthalmologist with expertise in ROP screening to do retinal examination with indirect ophthalmoscope! *Screen* all the following infants for ROP by early and regular retinal examination, because no early clinical signs or symptoms indicate developing ROP *Infants with a birth weight <1,500 g or gestational age <30 weeks. Infants who are born after 30 weeks gestational age may be considered for screening if they have been ill (e.g., those who have had severe respiratory distress syndrome, hypotension requiring pressor support, or surgery in the first several weeks of life). *Because the timing of ROP is related to postnatal age, infants who are born at <26 weeks gestation are examined at the postnatal age of 6 weeks, those born at 27 to 28 weeks at the postnatal age of 5 weeks, those born at 29 to 30 weeks are examined at the postnatal age of 4 weeks, and those born at > 30 weeks at the postnatal age of 3 weeks. *Patients are examined every 2 weeks until the vessels have grown out to the ora serrata and the retina is considered mature. If ROP is diagnosed, the frequency of examination depends on the severity and rapidity of progression of the disease.

Location

refers to how for the developing retinal blood vessels have progressed. The retina is divided into three concentric circles of zones.

a) **Zone 1** Consists of an imaginary circle with the optic nerve at the center and a radius of twice distance from the optic nerve to the macula.

b) **Zone 2** extends from the edge of zone 1 to the equator on the nasal side of the eye and approximately half the distance to the ora serrata on the temporal side.

c) **Zone 3** consists of the outer crescent-shaped area extending from zone 2 out to the ora serrata temporally.

Stage : Severity refers to the stage of disease.

a) **Stage 1.** A demarcation line appears as a thin white line that separates the normal retina from the undeveloped avascular retina.

b) **Stage 2.** A ridge of fibrovascular tissue with height and width replaces the line of stage 1. It extends inward from the plane of the retina.

c) **Stage 3.** The ridge has extraretinal fibrovascular proliferation. Abnormal blood vessels and fibrous tissue develop on the edge of the ridge and extend into the vitreous.

d) **Stage 4.** Partial retinal detachment may result when scar tissue pulls on the retina. **Stage 4 A** is partial detachment outside the macula, so that there is still a chance for good vision. **Stage 4 B** is partial detachment that involves the macula, thereby limiting the likelihood of good vision in that eye.

e) **Stage 5.** complete retinal detachment occurs. The retina assumes a funnel shaped appearance and is described as open or narrow in the anterior and posterior regions.

Plus disease is an additional designation that refers to the presence of vascular dilatation and tortuosity of the posterior retinal vessels in at least two quadrants. This indicates a more severe degree of ROP, and may also be associated with iris vascular engorgement, pupillary rigidity, and vitreous haze. Preplus disease describes vascular abnormalities of the posterior pole (mild venous dilatation or arterial tortuosity) that are present but are insufficient for the diagnosis of plus disease.
Extent refers to the circumferential location of disease and is reported as clock hours in the appropriate zone.

* *Categorize the ROP into the following types!*

1. **Aggressive posterior ROP** (previously referred to as Rush disease) is an uncommon, rapidly progressing, severe form of ROP characterized by its posterior location (usually zone 1), and prominence of plus disease out of proportion to the peripheral retinopathy. Stage 3 ROP may appear as a flat, intraretinal network of neovascularization. When untreated, this type of ROP usually progresses to stage 5.

2. **Threshold ROP** is present if 5 or more contiguous or 8 cumulative clock hours (30-degree sectors) of stage 3 with plus disease in either zone 1 or 2 are present. This is the level

of ROP at which the risk of blindness is predicted to be at least could be reduced to approximately 25%.

3. **Prethreshold ROP** is any of the following; Zone 1 ROP of any stage less than threshold; zone 2 ROP with stage 2 and plus disease; zone 2 ROP with stage 3 with plus disease with fewer than the threshold number of sectors of stage 3. The early treatment for ROP study showed that for eyes with high risk prethreshold ROP, early treatment may reduce the risk of blindness to approximately 15 % .

* *Determine the "Timing" of treatment!*

a) Current recommendations are to consider treatment for "type 1" prethreshold ROP, which includes in zone 1, eyes with any ROP and plus disease or stage 3 with or without plus disease, and in zone 2, stage 2 or 3 with plus disease. Observation is recommended for "type 2" prethreshold ROP, which includes zone 1, stage 1 or 2 ROP without plus disease, or zone 2 stage 3 ROP without plus disease. b) Treatment should be considered for an eye with type 2 ROP when progression to type 1 status or threshold ROP occurs.

LASER PHOTOCOAGULATION (Argon/Xenon or Diode) is the preferred initial treatment in most centers. *CRYOTHERAPY* may be necessary in special cases, such as when there is poor pupillary dilation or vitreous hemorrhage, both of which prevent adequate delivery of laser therapy. *SURGICAL INTERVENTIONS*- vitrectomy, with or without lensectomy, and membrane peeling to remove tractional forces for macular detachment; scleral buckling for more peripheral retinal detachments, drainage of subretinal fluid, for effusional detachments. *SUPPLEMENTAL OXYGEN*- may be beneficial for infants with prethreshold ROP without plus disease. Anti vascular endothelial growth factor (Anti-VEGF) therapy (*Intravitreal Bevacizumab*) has been extensively studied and the studies have demonstrated its promising role early stages of ROP.

* *Pearl/Peril/Pitfall :* A dilated fundus examination with scleral depression is necessary. The instruments used are a Sauer speculum (to keep the eyes gently open), a Flynn scleral depressor (to rotate and depress small eyes), and a 28-diopter lens (for proper identification of zones).

TABLE 1 ROP-initial screening timing based on gestational age at birth

Timing of First Eye Examination Based on Gestational Age at Birth

Gestational Age at Birth wk	Age at Initial Examination, wk Postmenstrual	Age at Initial Examination, wk Chronologic
22a	31	9
23a	31	8
24	31	7
25	31	6
26	31	5
27	31	4
28	32	4
29	33	4
30	34	4
31b	35	4
32b	36	4

Shown is a schedule for detecting prethreshold ROP with 99% confidence, usually well before any required treatment.

aThis guideline should be considered tentative rather than evidence-based for infants with a gestational age of 22 to 23 weeks because of the small number of survivors in these gestational age catagories.

b If necessary

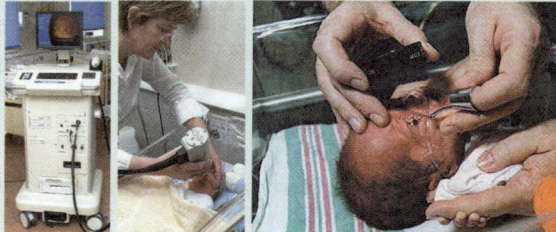

ETROP treatment guidelines.

Zones	Stages 1	Stages 2	Stages 3	Stages 4	Stages 5
I			new		
I w/ plus	new	new			
II					
II w/ plus			new	No min. hours	
III					
III w/ plus				No min. hours	

= Treatment, type 1 ROP   = Observation, type 2 ROP

TABLE 2 Follow-up examinations on the basis of retinal findings-to be determined by the consultant ophthalmologist

- 1-week or less follow-up—Stage 1 or 2 ROP: Zone II, Stage 3 ROP: Zone II
- 1 to 2-week follow-up—Immature vascularization: Zone I-no ROP, Stage 2 ROP: Zone II, Regressing ROP: Zone II
- 2-week follow-up—Stage 1 ROP: Zone II, Regressing ROP: Zone II
- 2-to 3 week follow-up—Immature vascularization: Zone II -noROP, Stage 1 or 2 ROP: Zone III, Regressing ROP : Zone III

Findings that do not warrant further examinations:

- Zone III retinal vascularization attained without previous Zone I or II ROP
- Full retinal vascularization
- Postmenstrual age of 45 weeks and no Prethreshold disease
- Registration of ROP

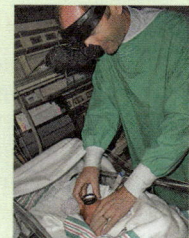

TABLE 3 Preparation for laser photocoagulation therapy

Take consent
Ensure good pupillary dilatation
Nil by mouth 3 h prior to procedure
Start on intravenous fluids
Put on vital sign monitor
Warmer for maintaining temperature
Arrange equipment and check functioning of

Intubation equipment, Endotracheal tubes No. 2.5, 3, 3.5, Resuscitation bag and face masks, Oxygen delivery system, Syringes, Infusion pumps, Ventilator, Arrange drugs, fill syringes in advance with drugs in appropriate dilution and label them: midazolom, normal saline, 10% dextrose, adrenaline.

TABLE 4 Preoperative and postoperative care

Preanesthetic medication: Oral feeds should be discontinued 3 hours prior to the procedure. Baby should be started on intravenous fluids, and put on cardiorespiratory monitor. Dilatation of pupil is done by using 1% tropicamide and 2.5 % phenylephrine.

Anesthesia/Sedation: The procedure can be carried out under sedation supplemented by local anesthesia with topical anesthetic drops.

Procedure : Both the eyes can be treated at the same sitting unless contraindicated by instability of the baby. If baby is not tolerating the procedure, consider abandoning the procedure for the time being. Vital signs and oxygen saturation should be monitored very closely.

Postoperative care

- The baby should be closely monitored. If condition permits, oral feeds can be started shortly after the procedure.
- Premature babies, especially those with chronic lung disease may have increase or reappearance of apneic episodes or an increase in oxygen requirement. Therefore they should carefully be monitored for 48–72 hours after the procedure.
- Antibiotic drops (such as chloramphenicol) should be instilled 6-8 hours for 2–3 days.

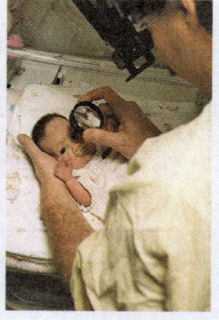

*Pearl/Peril/Pitfall : In obtaining a history for a premature infant, note the following: *Gestational age at birth, especially if younger than 32 weeks' gestation *Birth weight of less than 1500 g, especially less than 1250 grams *Other possible risk factors (e.g. supplemental oxygen, hypoxemia, hypercarbia, concurrent illness).*

RETINOPATHY OF PREMATURITY-STAGING OF SEVERITY

* *Stage 1*: presence of thin white demarcation line separating the vascular from avascular retina.
* *Stage 2*: the line becomes prominent because of lifting of retina to form a ridge having height and width.
* *Stage 3*: presence of extra retinal fibrovascular proliferation with abnormal vessels and fibrous tissue arising from the ridge and extending into vitreous.
* *Stage 4*: partial retinal detachment (4a-not involving macula, 4b-involving macula).
* *Stage 5*: complete retinal detachment.

SCREENING "WINDOW" FOR ROP

*ROP does not develop usually before 2 weeks of postnatal age. *Hardly any ROP is detected before 32 weeks of gestation *The median age for detection of stage 1 ROP is 34 weeks. *Pre-threshold ROP appears at 36 weeks of post-menstrual age and threshold disease at 37 weeks. *Vascularization is complete by 40-44 weeks of gestation. *Therefore the window period for detection of ROP is from 32 weeks to 40 weeks of post-menstrual period. *The critical phase is from 34 weeks to 37 weeks of age during which the progression of the disease takes place and treatment may have to be instituted.

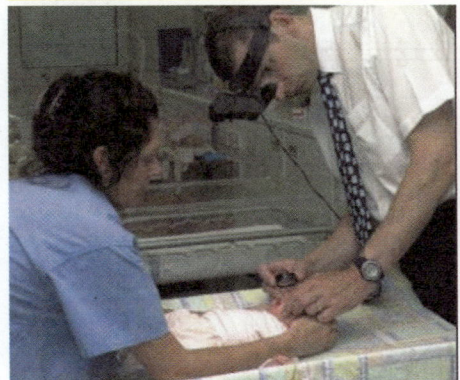

ROP EXAMINATION AND FOLLOW-UP SHOULD BE PERFORMED BY AN OPHTHALMOLOGIST WITH AN EXPERTISE IN ROP SCREENING

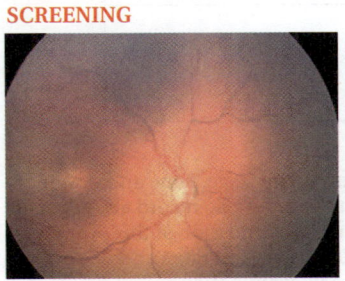

Zone 1 is the most labile *The center of zone 1 is the optic nerve. It extends twice the distance from the optic nerve to the macula in a circle. Using a 28-diopter lens, if any portion of the optic nerve is in the same view as the ridge of ROP, that is considered zone 1. *Any disease in zone 1 (even stage 0, immature) is critical and must be monitored closely. Zone 1 does not follow the ICROP rules. The area is very small and changes can occur very quickly, sometimes within days. The hallmark of the disease worsening is not the presence of neovascularization (as in other zones, as specified by the ICROP) but is by the increasing dilation and tortuosity of the vessels. The vascularized retina seems to rise (like a soufflé) probably because of the increased arteriovenous shunting. *Many ROP experts feel that any disease in zone 1, and certainly any plus disease, requires treatment.*

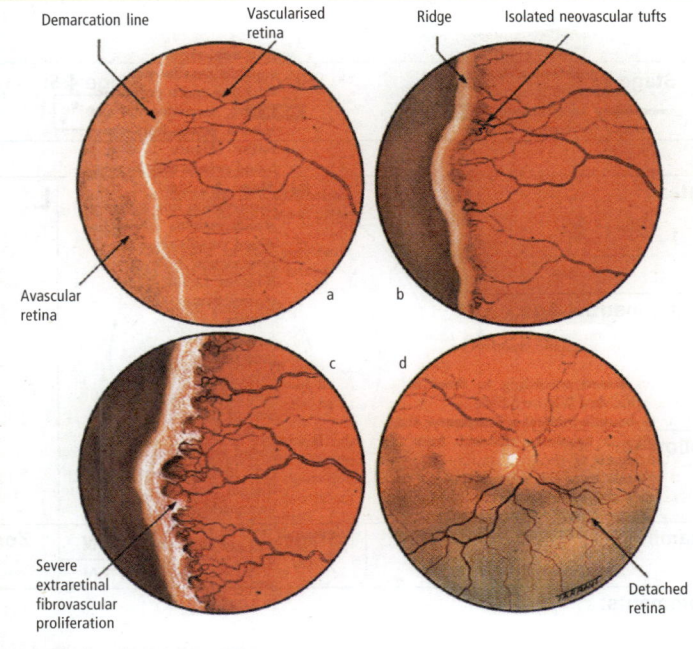

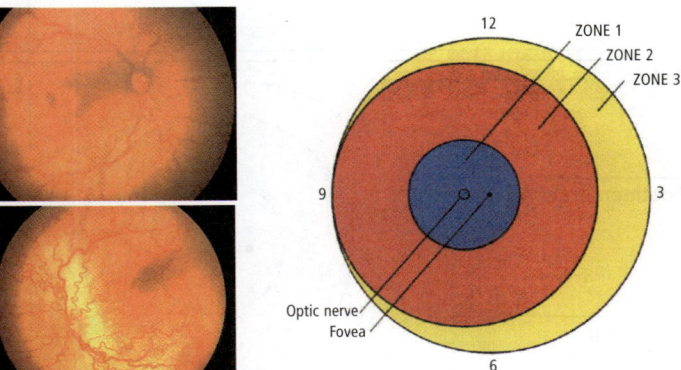

Aggressive Posterior ROP

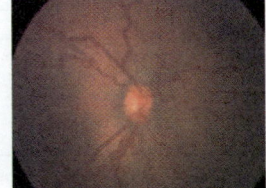

Pre-plus disease: insufficient for the diagnosis of plus disease but posterior retinal vessels demonstrate more arterial tortuosity and more venous dilatation than normal.

Plus disease: Presence of dilatation and tortuosity of posterior retinal vessels. *Plus disease,* has marked dilation and tortuosity of the blood vessels near the optic nerve. It also includes the growth and dilation of abnormal blood vessels on the surface of the iris (*iris hyperemia*), rigidity of the pupil, and vitreous haze, and indicates a more fulminant or rapidly progressive course of ROP.

Pearl/Peril/Pitfall : Patients who are medically monitored must undergo examinations until the retinal vasculature is mature. Ensuring appropriate monitoring of infants is critical if they are discharged from the nursery before retinal vascular maturity is attained. Numerous patients have lost sight due to inappropriate, untimely monitoring. In untreated patients, retinal detachments commonly occur at 38–42 weeks' postmenstrual age.

Neonatal ophthalmology examination record

Name:	Gestation:	Birth Weight:
Hosp. No:		
DoB: __/__/____ Gender: M / F	weeks	grams

Risks:

Stage 1:	Stage 2:	Stage 3:	Stage 4/5:	Laser:	AP-ROP:
▬▬▬	══	▭▭▭▭	• • • •	× × × / × ×	A A A

Date:	R	L
Postmenstrual Age:		
Follow-up:		

Examiner:	Zone:	Stage:	Preplus: Y / N	Zone:	Stage:	Preplus: Y / N
			Plus: Y / N			Plus: Y / N
Comments:						

Date:	R	L
Postmenstrual Age:		
Follow-up:		

Examiner:	Zone:	Stage:	Preplus: Y / N	Zone:	Stage:	Preplus: Y / N
			Plus: Y / N			Plus: Y / N
Comments:						

It is clearly important that accurate records are made for each screening examination in relation to the stage, zone and extent of any ROP and the presence of any pre-plus (as defined by ICROP revisited 6) or plus disease. Notes should also record any adverse events experienced by the baby during the screening. If a further examination is required the need for and time of this examination should be documented. The documentation of clear, easy to interpret information on ROP screening status should form a separate part of the baby's medical record so that it is available if the baby is transferred between examinations.

Courtesy: UK Retinopathy of Prematurity Guideline – May 2008

Algorithm for Ophthalmic Criteria for Screening and Treatment

Observations at each screening examination should determine the appropriate course of action. The ICROP revisited definition of zones of the retina, stage of disease and pre-plus should be used.

Less Severe ———→ More Severe

ROP Observed	NO		YES						More Severe		
ROP Stage	-	-	1 or 2	1 or 2	3	ANY	1	2	ANY	3	3
ROP zone or vessel location	II	I	II or III	II or III	II or III	III	II	II	I	I	II
Plus/ Pre-plus	-	-	None	Pre-plus	None or pre-plus	Plus	Plus	Plus	Plus	None	Plus
Screening Frequency	Every 2 weeks	Every week	Every 2 weeks	Weekly			At least weekly		Treat (see below)		
When to terminate screening	○ Vessels progressed to zone III ○ Infant >36 weeks PMA		When characteristics of regression are observed on **2 successive** examinations: ○ Lack of increase in severity ○ Partial progressing towards complete resolution. Transgression of vessels through demarcation line. ○ Change in color of the ridge from salmon pink to white ○ Commencement of the process of replacement of active ROP lesions by scar tissue.								
When to treat							Consider Treatment		○ Aggressive Posterior ROP - treat within 48 hours ○ Less aggressive ROP but also requiring treatment: treat within 48-72 hours		
Post-treatment							Examination after 5-7 days		Examination after 5-7 days		
Follow up						All stage 3 or requiring treatment – review until at least 5 years of age					

*International Committee for the Classification of Retinopathy of Prematurity. The International Classification of Retinopathy of Prematurity revisited. *Arch Ophthalmol* 2005; 123(7):991-999

Courtesy: UK Retinopathy of Prematurity Guideline – May 2008

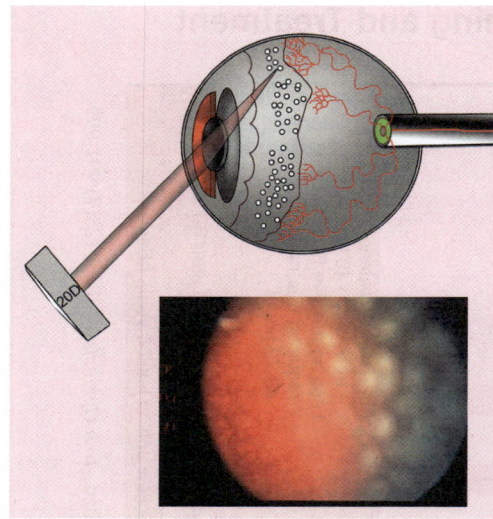

DIODE
LASER PHOTOCOAGULATION THERAPY FOR ROP

* Use diode laser to photocoagulate peripheral, nonvascularized retina.
* Make each laser burn leave a grey-white burn mark 1200-1500 spots per eye
* RPE pigment absorbs the laser energy, transforming it to heat energy.
* Heat energy destroys the surrounding tissue, retina.
* Lightly pigmented eyes require higher laser power to cause a burn ;general anesthesia is not necessary
* Laser photocoagulation is easier and safer than cryotherapy and posterior retina can be reached more readily.
* Complications include corneal haze, burns of the iris, cataracts, and intraocular hemorrhages.

CRYOTHERAPY
PROBE APPLICATION

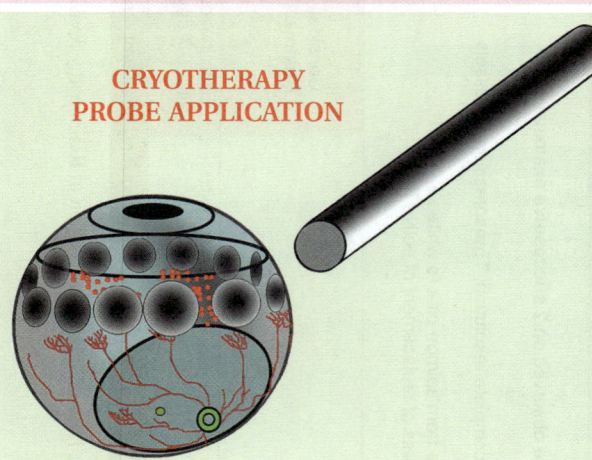

* Cryotherapy involves the application of a probe cooled with liquid nitrogen on the outer aspect of the eye.
* Approximately 35–75 confluent applications are made in each eye to ablate the avascular retina.
* This results in decreased release of the angiogenic factor, which is believed to induce retinal proliferation.
* Cryotherapy is usually done under general anesthesia and is a major procedure with the Neonatal and Ophthalmology teams in full readiness and proper planning.
* Cryotherapy is much more painful than laser therapy, causes substantial lid swelling and conjunctival edema and requires ventilation of the infant during procedure.
* It is difficult to reach posterior retina with Cryotherapy and myopia and retinal detachment are a problem.
* The most common complications include intraocular hemorrhage, conjunctival hematoma, conjunctival laceration, and bradycardia.

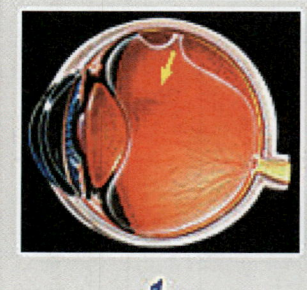 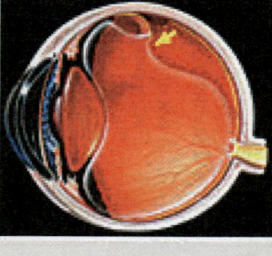 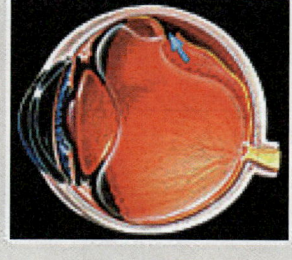 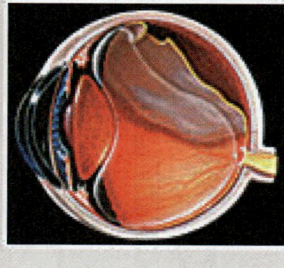

1 **2** **3** **4**

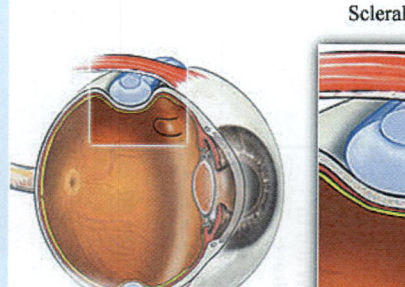

Scleral buckle

Closed tear

Scleral buckling surgery and/or vitrectomy is usually performed for stages 4 and 5. Some surgeons recommend surgery for stage 4A, while others do not think surgery should be performed because of the risks and unproven benefit. Although some surgeons advocate surgery for stage 5, most no longer recommend surgery because of the poor anatomical and visual prognosis.

A scleral buckling procedure may be useful for more peripheral detachments.

* *Pearl/Peril/Pitfall : Rush disease: A very rapidly progressive subtype of ROP is called rush disease. If plus disease is accompanied by vascularization ending in zone 1 or in very posterior zone 2, the risk of rush disease is significant.*

A girl was born prematurely after 25 weeks of gestation, with a body weight of 1 lb 61/2 oz (640 grams). She was treated elsewhere in both eyes with laser and cryotherapy. She also had a scleral buckling in the right eye for retinal detachment. All these procedures failed and she developed bilateral total retinal detachment (advanced stage 5 ROP). When her parents brought the patient to us, she was 5 ½ months old. She had white pupils in both eyes . An ultrasound study showed she had bilateral total retinal detachment with "narrow-narrow" funnels. This shape of retinal detachment makes the prognosis extremely poor. An open-sky vitrectomy was performed in each eye that resulted in complete reattachment of the retina in both eyes . She was followed carefully. Her vision, measured by a special method, showed gradual development. She is now 7 years old. Her vision in the right eye is 20/670 and in the left eye with glasses 20/360. Although vision is low, she attends school with low vision aids.

Courtesy: Schepens Retina Associates Foundation, Cross Street, Suite 109 Fax: (978) 532-4396 Peabody, Massachusetts 01960 USA

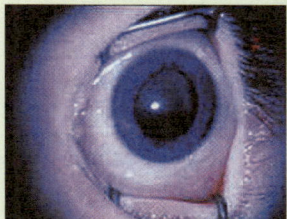 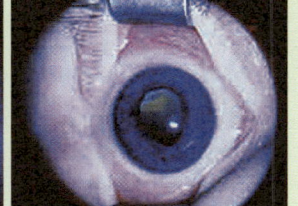

Stage 5 ROP in both eyes, with white pupils.

Right Eye   Left Eye

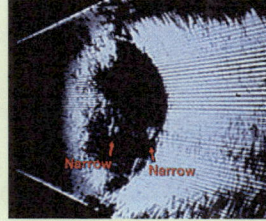 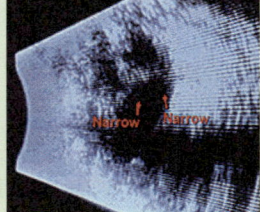 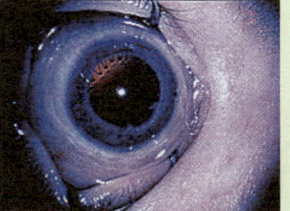

Photograph of right eye after open-sky vitrectomy. Pupil is free from opacities.

Ultrasound picture of both eyes showing total retinal detachments with narrow-narrow funnels.

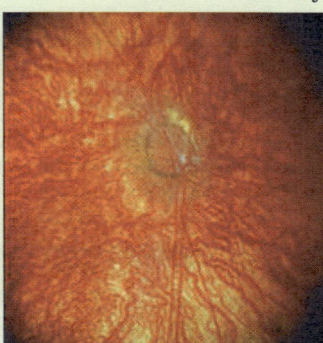 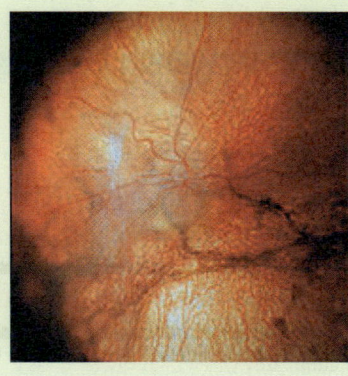

Photographs of the back of the eyes. It shows the retina completely attached in both eyes

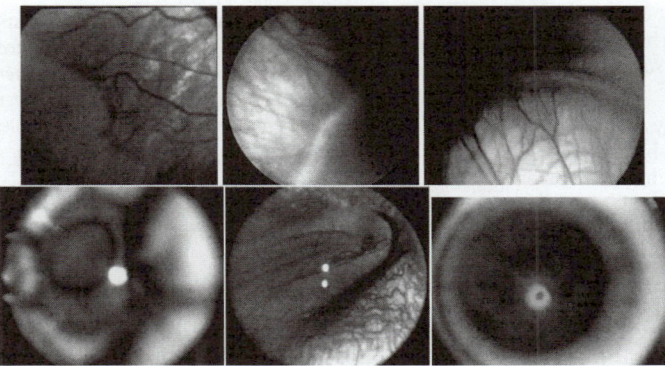 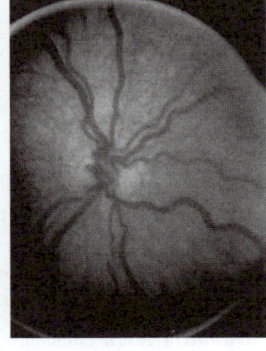

Dilated and tortuous vessels in the posterior pole, which by definition is plus disease.

Stages of retinopathy of prematurity. A. Stage 1, showing a small white line visible between the avascular and vascularized retina. B. Stage 2, with the junction showing a wider white line between avascular and vascularized retina. C. Stage 3, with frank neovascularization extending into the vitreous cavity from the area posterior to the retinal ridge. D. Stage 4A, showing peripheral retinal detachment with the macula attached. E. Stage 4B, with a partial retinal detachment with the macula detached. F. Stage 5, showing total retinal detachment.
Courtesy: MICHAEL T. TRESE and PHILIP J. FERRONE

* *Pearl/Peril/Pitfall : *The timing of examination and follow-up are important factors in the diagnosis and treatment of retinopathy of prematurity (ROP). If a patient misses an examination, it should be performed as soon as possible. *Ensuring that parents are aware of the significance of retinopathy of prematurity and appropriate follow-up is also important. *Patients can be discharged or transferred from the NICU while their retina is still immature. Most follow-up examinations by an ophthalmologist must occur within 2 weeks of discharge.*

ROP-PATHOGENESIS

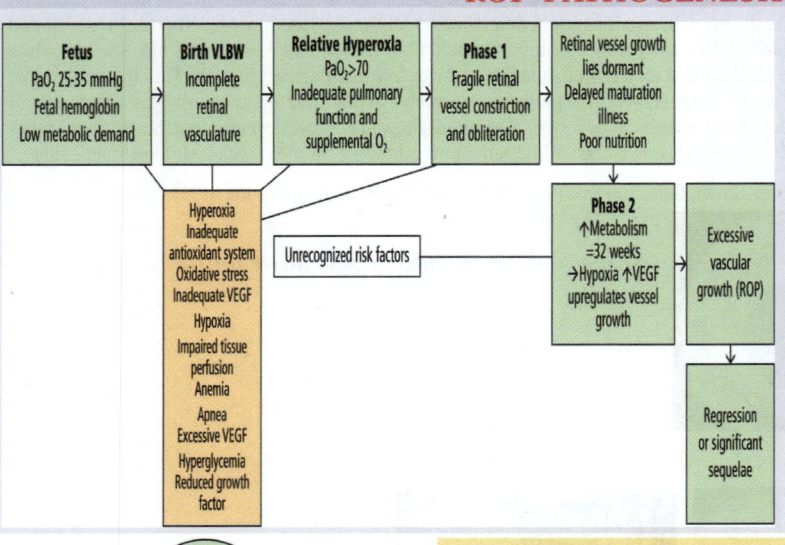

Intravitreal Bevacizumab (Avastin), an angiogenesis inhibitor, is being used as an alternative therapy (as compared with conventional laser therapy), for retinopathy of prematurity (ROP) in some children's hospitals for premature babies. A study by Mintz-Hittner et al examined the use of bevacizumab to treat ROP in 150 infants. The study found that monotherapy with bevacizumab showed a significant treatment benefit in in infants with stage 3+ retinopathy of prematurity in zone I ROP (P=0.003) but not in zone II ROP (P=0.27). However, the study size was too small to assess safety. Long-term studies are still necessary. Development of peripheral retinal vessels continued after treatment with intravitreal bevacizumab, but conventional laser therapy led to permanent destruction of the peripheral retina. This trial was too small to assess safety.

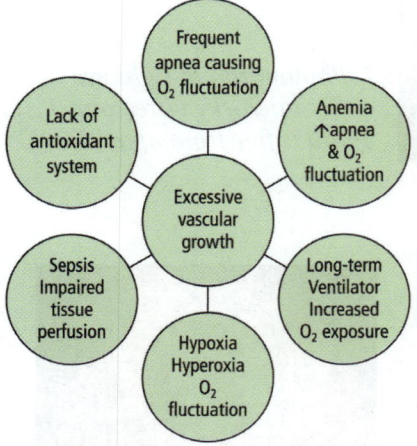

Possible etiological factors of Retinopathy of Prematurity

TABLE 5 ROP PROGNOSIS

A) Short-term Prognosis

*Most infants with stage 1 or 2 ROP will experience spontaneous regression. *Any zone 3 disease has an excellent prognosis for complete recovery *Overall incidence of ROP (CRYO-ROP STUDY) is 66%; stage 1-25%, stage 2-22%, prethreshold ROP-18%, threshold ROP-6%

B) Long-term Prognosis

*With significant ROP, there is an increased risk of high myopia, anisometropia,, strabismus, amblyopia, astigmatism, late retinal detachment,and glaucoma*Cicatricial disease (residual scarring in the retina) may be associated with retinal detachment years later. *The chance for good vision is greater when macula is not involved in the stage 4 ROP. *Once the retina has detached, the prognosis for good vision is poor even with surgical reattachment, although some useful vision may be preserved. *All premature infants who meet screening criteria regardless of the diagnosis of ROP are at increased risk for long-term vision problems, from either ocular or CNS problems. *A follow-up evaluation by an ophthalmologist with expertise in neonatal sequelae at 1 year of age, or sooner is highly recommended, if ocular/visual abnormalities have been noted.

KEY POINTS FOR CLINICAL PRACTICE:

1. Retinopathy Of Prematurity (ROP) is a complex disorder of the developing retinal vasculature in premature infants that increases in incidence with decreasing gestational age; approximately, 65% of infants with a birth weight<1,250g and 80% of those with a birth weight<1,000g, (90% of those<750g birth wt) will develop some degree of ROP.

2. Retinopathy Of Prematurity (ROP) is multifactorial in etiology and has been consistently associated with low gestational age, low birth weight, and prolonged oxygen exposure at high concentrations.Severe ROP develops in the sickest infants, i.e., it correlates with asphyxia, acidosis, sepsis, blood transfusions, IVH, PVL, and CLD.

3. In >90% of cases, ROP regresses spontaneously, but in <10% progressive disease("threshold ROP") is the leading cause of blindness in preterm infants.ROP is rare in infants born after 32 weeks of gestation.

4. Each Neonatal unit should have a clear protocol so that all infants at risk of severe ROP are identified and screened by an *experienced ophthalmologist with expertise in the diagnosis and management of ROP.* ROP screening aims to identify infants at risk of severe disease and those who would benefit from the available therapies.

5. Infants weighing <1,500g at birth, those born before 31 week of gestational age, infants born weighing >1,500g-2,000g who have an unstable clinical course should be examined for ROP. The initial examination should be performed at 4-6wk(ROP rarely develops before that)of chronological age or at 31-33 wk of postconceptional age. *Follow-up(with serial ophthalmic examinations) is based on the initial findings and risk factors but is usually 2wk or less.*

REFERENCES AND FURTHER READING : 1) ICROP Committee:ICROP.Arch Ophthalmol 102:1130-1134,1984 2) ICROP Committee for classification of late stages of ROP:Arch Ophthalmol 105:906-912, 1987 3) AAP.Screening examination of Premature infants for ROP. Pediatrics 2006;117;572-576 4) Retinopathy of Prematurity: Deepak Chawla, Ramesh Agarwal, Ashok K. Deorari and Vinod K. Paul. AIIMS PROTOCOLS IN NEONATOLOGY Indian Journal of Peediatrics: 75;Jan 2008 73-76.5) Early Treatment For Retinopathy Of Prematurity Cooperative Group. Revised indications for the treatment of retinopathy of prematurity: results of the early treatment for retinopathy of prematurity randomized trial. *Arch Ophthalmol.* Dec 2003;121(12):1684-94.6) Retinopathy of Prematurity –Promising Newer Modalities of Treatment, HS NIRANJAN et al, INDIAN PEDIATRICS, VOLUME 49__FEBRUARY 16, 2012.

Pearl/Peril/Pitfall : The prognosis of ROP is always guarded. The development of the visual system may be affected in many ways, even after the ROP has resolved. There may be macular dragging, glaucoma, strabismus, refractive errors, and amblyopia that may, even after aggressive treatment, lead to visual loss. It is important that the parents are advised repeatedly of this guarded prognosis, so that their expectations are realistic, especially in severely affected children. Many children still lose vision, even under the best circumstances.

26 Hearing Screening in the Neonate

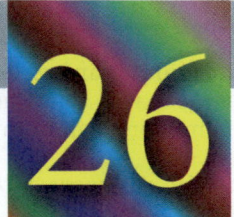

@ *"Since screening Neonates based on the several risk factors for hearing loss misses 50% of hearing impaired infants, AAP STATEMENT-2000 recommends early identification of hearing loss in 100% of babies i.e., Universal hearing screening and appropriate intervention within 6 months of life."*

Age appropriate hearing tests in neonates and children

Test	Description	Type	Youngest Age
Otoacoustic emission (OAE)	Tests sound detection at the level of the cochlea at different frequencies	Screening	1 day (including preterm infants)
Auditory brainstem response (ABR), also called brainstem auditory evoked response (BAER)	Tests sound detection to the level of the midbrain at different frequencies	Screening or diagnostic	1 day (including preterm infants)
Visual reinforcement audiometry	Observe a child's response to sounds (response to sound is rewarded by a visual reinforcer)	Diagnostic	6 months
Conditioned play audiometry	A child is taught to "play" (e.g. drop a block into a box) in response to tones of different frequency and loudness	Diagnostic	2 yr
Speech audiometry	Test provides information about communicative abilities, can be presented in an open-set or closed-set (e.g. picture pointing) format	Diagnostic	3–3.5 yr
Pure-tone audiometry	A child is taught to raise a hand response to tones of different frequency and loudness	Screening or Diagnostic	4–5 yr

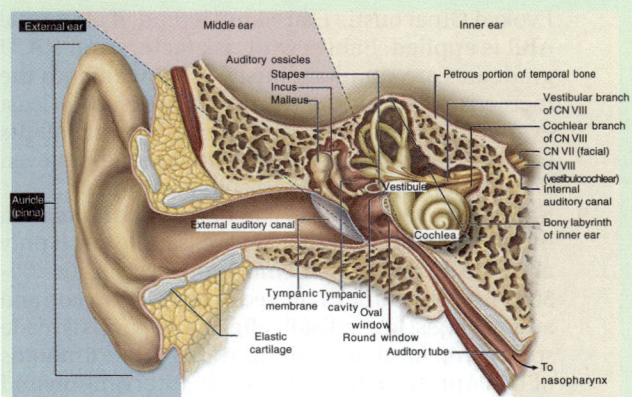

Risk indicators associated with hearing loss for neonates (Birth through 28 days)

1. An illness or condition requiring admission of $\geq$ 48 hours to the Neonatal Intensive Care Unit.
2. Stigmata or other finding associated with a syndrome known to include a sensorineural or conductive hearing loss.
3. Family history of permanent sensorineural hearing loss.
4. Craniofacial anomalies, including anomalies with morphologic abnormalities of the pinna and ear canal.
5. In utero infection, such as cytomegalovirus, herpes, toxoplasmosis, or rubella.

* Even if ABR or OAE test results are normal, hearing cannot be definitively considered normal until a reliable behavioral audiogram can be obtained. Behavioral pure tone audiometry remains the standard for hearing evaluation. It can determine hearing thresholds at specific frequencies as well as the degree of hearing impairment.

REVIEW OF CLINICAL PROBLEMS

1. How do you categorize the "type" and "severity" of Hearing loss in Neonates ?
   Ans : Refer to the Evaluation-Decision-Action Plan/Algorithm to diagnose and manage Hearing Screening in the Neonate.
2. What are the risk factors for hearing loss in Neonates and Infants?
   Ans : Refer to the Table 1 of the Chapter.
3. Mention the common genetic syndromes associated with hearing loss in Neonates?
   Ans: Refer to the Evaluation-Decision-Action Plan/Algorithm to diagnose and manage Hearing Screening in the Neonate.
4. What are the Current objective physiologic measures used in the Universal Newborn Screening programs for detecting hearing loss?
   Ans : Refer to the 5 of the "BIRD'S EYE VIEW/OVERVIEW/SYNOPSIS"and Table 2 of the Chapter.
5. How do you manage a Neonate with confirmed hearing loss?
   Ans : Refer to the Evaluation-Decision-Action Plan/Algorithm to diagnose and manage Hearing Screening in the Neonate.

LEARNING OBJECTIVES

After completing this article, readers will be able to

1. Organize screening of NICU graduates for hearing loss as early as possible, ideally before discharge.
2. Establish protocols to retest Neonates with positive or borderline hearing test results.
3. Diagnose treatable conditions that can lead to hearing loss, such as sepsis, meningitis, prolonged exposure to ototoxic medications and significant hyperbilirubinemia, etc.
4. Diagnose genetic hearing loss in all affected Neonates with the input from a clinical geneticist.
5. Provide parents with available resources for infants with hearing loss and appropriate follow-up.

*Pearl/Peril/Pitfall : A thorough physical examination is essential in the evaluation of a child for hearing loss. Findings on head and neck examination associated with hearing impairment include heterochromia of the irises, malformation of the auricle or ear canal, abnormalities of the eardrum, dimpling or skin tags around the auricle, cleft lip or palate, asymmetry of the facial structures, and microcephaly. Hypertelorism and abnormal pigmentation of the skin, hair, or eyes, which is seen in Waardenburg's syndrome, also may be associated with hearing loss.

BIRD'S EYE VIEW/OVERVIEW/SYNOPSIS

1. Hearing loss in the Newborn population is estimated to occur at a rate of between 1–6 in 1,000 live births. NICU graduates are at high risk of developing hearing loss (20–40 infants per 1,000 survivors of NICU admission can have some degree of sensorineural hearing loss). When undetected, hearing loss can result in delays in language communication, and cognitive development.

2. Hearing loss is categorized into 5 types; a) Sensorineural loss b) Conductive loss c) Mixed (a+b) d) Auditory dyssynchrony or Auditory neuropathy e) Central hearing loss (Refer to the Evaluation-Decision-Action Plan/Algorithm to manage Hearing Screening in a Neonate for a description of these 5 categories of Hearing loss).

3. About 50% of congenital hearing loss is genetic in origin. 25% of childhood hearing loss is due to a nongenetic acquired (intrapartal-perinatal) cause, such as infection (CMV), hypoxia-ischemia, metabolic disease, ototoxic medication, or hyperbilirubinemia. 25% of hearing loss is idiopathic. Among genetic causes of hearing loss, 70% Autosomal recessive, 15% Autosomal dominant and 15% sex-linked in type. About 30% of infants with hearing loss have other medical problems that are part of a Syndrome. (Refer to the Evaluation-Decision-Action Plan/Algorithm to manage Hearing Screening in a Neonate for a brief introduction of common Syndromes).

4. *Newborn hearing screening*—Since screening neonates based on the SEVERAL RISK FACTORS FOR HEARING LOSS (Refer to the Table No 1 of the Chapter) misses 50% of hearing impaired infants, AAP STATEMENT-2000 recommends early identification of hearing loss in 100% of babies and appropriate intervention within 6 months of life. The Joint Committee on Infant Hearing defines the targeted hearing loss for Universal Newborn hearing loss as permanent bilateral, or unilateral, sensory or conductive hearing loss, averaging 35 dB or more in the frequency range important for speech recognition. (approximately 500-4000Hz).

5. *Current objective physiologic measures* used in Universal Newborn Screening programs for detecting hearing loss are a) Evoked otoacoustic emissions (EOAE)-Physiologic test measuring cochlear response to a stimulus b) Auditory brainstem response (ABR)-Electrophysiologic measurement of activity in auditory nerve and brainstem pathway. ABR is the preferred method to screen hearing loss in the NICU graduate. (Refer to the Table 2 of the chapter for details of these 2 methods of hearing screening.)

6. *Ensure* follow-up testing for infants with abnormal screening ABRs: (a) within 2 weeks of their initial test in infants who are abnormal in both ears and (b) within 3 months in infants with unilateral abnormal results *Testing should include a full diagnostic frequency-specific ABR to measure hearing threshold *Evaluate* middle ear function, *Observe* infant's behavioral response to sound and *Note* the parental report of emerging communication and auditory behaviours.

7. *Management goals for newborns with suspected hearing loss*
   a. Prevent unnecessary delays in the detection of hearing loss by testing all neonates before discharge.
   b. Establish protocols to retest neonates with positive or borderline hearing test results.
   c. Minimize prolonged exposure to ototoxic medications and other conditions that may contribute further to hearing loss, such as significant hyperbilirubinemia.
   d. Diagnose treatable conditions that can lead to hearing loss, such as sepsis and meningitis.
   e. Provide parents with available resources for infants with hearing loss and appropriate follow-up

8. *The Evaluation-Decision-Action- Plan/Algorithm* describes the essential aspects of Hearing Screening in a Neonate. Well babies are initially screened with Evoked Otoacoustic Emission Method; if abnormal ABR is applied. Babies with risk factors and NICU graduates are simultaneously tested with both the methods. *Continue* the Hearing Surveillance (at least every 6 months for the 1st 3 years of age) of infants who have risk factors for progressive hearing loss, even if the initial ABR screening results are normal.

9. Short-term hearing loss can occur in infants with middle ear effusion, but in most cases the loss is only about 20 dB. Infants with moderate hearing loss (30-50dB loss) should be evaluated by an ENT surgeon and an audiologist immediately after the diagnosis is made so that amplification can be provided before 6 months of life. Appropriate early speech intervention and education services are important for young infants from birth through 36 months of life. Severe -to-Profound hearing loss requires a multidisciplinary team approach consisting of the primary care provider, ENT surgeon, audiologist, and speech therapist.

10. The outcome for infants and young children with hearing loss-*depends largely on the extent of hearing loss, as well as on the time of diagnosis and treatment. *the earlier hearing habilitation starts, the better the child's chance of achieving age-appropriate language and communication skills *fitting of hearing aids by the age of 6 months, early cochlear implants by the age of 1 year and initiation of early speech intervention services before 3 months of age have been associated with improved speech and cognitive developmental outcome at 3 years of life. Without adequate opportunities to hear and learn language, infants and young children who are deaf fall behind their peers in language, cognition, and social/emotional development. Long-term consequences of undetected hearing loss may include lower educational and employment levels in adulthood.

Pearl/Peril/Pitfall : Failure to detect children with congenital or acquired hearing loss may result in lifelong deficits in speech and language acquisition, poor academic performance, personal-social maladjustment, and emotional difficulties. Physicians need to be able to recognize children who are at risk of congenital or acquired hearing loss, be prepared to evaluate their hearing and, if needed, arrange for proper referral and treatment.

THE EVALUATION-DECISION-ACTION- PLAN/ALGORITHM FOR THE DIAGNOSIS AND MANAGEMENT OF *HEARING SCREENING IN THE NEONATE*

SUBJECTIVE FINDINGS

Hx of parental concerns like- *"baby" does not* awaken to sound/startle to loud noise/blink or widen eyes in response to noise/quieten to mom's voice

Hx of **Risk factors given in the Table 1 of the Chapter.**

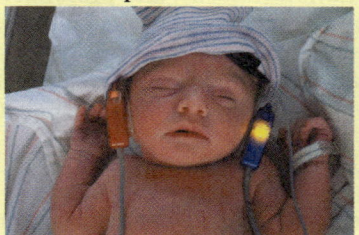

OBJECTIVE FINDINGS

Organize hearing screening Auditory Brainstem Responses- ABR is the preferred method to evaluate hearing loss in the NICU graduate:Evoked Otoacoustic Emissions-EOAE is often combined with automated ABR in a two-step screening system.

Define the degree and severity of Hearing Loss Mild-15-30 dB HL, Moderate-30-50dB HL, Severe-50-70dB HL, Profound-70+dB HL

Define the categories of Hearing loss sensorineural/conductive/mixed/auditory dyssynchrony or neuropathy/central

Arrange additional evaluations, if the infant diagnosed with true hearing loss complete ENT assessment with MRI/CT imaging; Genetic evaluation and counseling, Ophthalmic assessment for associated eye problems, Neuro-Developmental, cardiology and nephrology evaluations as indicated.

INVESTIGATIONS

Imaging MRI/CT head scan
Genetic evaluation if syndromic/familial evidence present *torsch and HIV investigations* as indicated

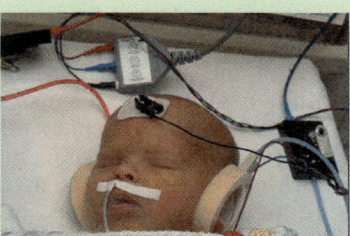

Auditory brainstem responses-ABR

NEONATE WITH A HIGH-RISK FOR HEARING LOSS

* *Ensure* Follow-up Testing for infants with abnormal screening ABRs *a)*within 2 weeks of their initial test in infants who are abnormal in both ears and *b)*within 3 months in infants with unilateral abnormal results

* Testing should include a full diagnostic frequency-specific ABR to measure hearing threshold

* *Evaluate* middle ear function, *Observe* infant`s behavioral response to sound and *Note* the parental report of emerging communication and auditory behaviors

Categorize the Hearing loss into 5 types!

a. *Sensorineural loss:* the result of abnormal development or damage to the cochlear hair cells (sensory end organ) or auditory nerve
b. *Conductive loss:* the result of interference in the transmission of sound from the external auditory canal to the inner ear due to middle ear effusion/canal stenosis/stapes fixation in craniofacial malformations.*c) Mixed*—a combination of conductive and sensorineural hearing loss.
d. *Auditory dyssynchrony or neuropathy*: the inner ear or cochlea receives sounds normally, but the transfer of signal from the cochlea to the auditory nerve is abnormal; severe hyperbilirubinemia, prematurity, hypoxia, immune disorders and genetic predisposition are the risk factors.
e. *Central hearing loss:* an intact auditory canal, inner ear, normal neurosensory pathways but abnormal auditory processing at higher levels of the CNS.

→ *Monitor* infants with mild or unilateral hearing loss closely, as they are at increased risk for both progressive hearing loss and delayed and abnormal development of language and communication skills.

→ *Continue* the Hearing surveillance (at least every 6 months for the 1st 3 years of age) of infants who have risk factors for progressive hearing loss, even if the initial ABR screening results are normal.

→ *Refer* infants with true hearing loss for early intervention services (Personal amplification systems fitted with hearing aids by 6 months of age or Cochlear Implants for profound bilateral hearing loss by the end of 1st year of age) to enhance the child`s acquisition of developmentally appropriate language skills.

→ *Explain* Prognosis to the parents!

*depends largely on the extent of hearing loss, as well as on the time of diagnosis and treatment. *the earlier hearing habilitation starts, the better the child`s chance of achieving age-appropriate language and communication skills and initiation of early speech intervention services before 3 months of age have been associated with improved speech and cognitive developmental outcome at 3 years of life.

Identify the hereditary prenatal causes of sensorineural hearing loss! Consult a clinical geneticist!

* 50% of congenital hearing loss is thought to be of genetic in origin; 70% Autosomal recessive, 15% Autosomal dominant and 15% sex-linked.*30% of these infants have other associated medical problems i.e. Syndromic association.

* *Waardenburg syndrome:* Autosomal dominant disorder with variable expression, comprising some or all of the following traits: unilateral or bilateral perceptive deafness; hypertrichosis of the eyebrows, which meet in the midline; heterochromia of the irises; or a white forelock.

* *Klippel-Feil syndrome:* A short neck which limits head movements with low hairline at back, paralysis of the external rectus muscle in one or both eyes, and perceptive hearing loss, which may be severe.

* *Alport's syndrome:* X- linked dominant affecting boys more severely than girls. There is severe, progressive glomerulonephritis and a pro-

gressive sensorineural loss, which normally manifests after the age of ten years.

* *Pendred's syndrome:* Autosomal recessive. Causes simple goitre at about 4–5 years and severe deafness.

* *Jervell and Lange-Nielsen Syndrome:* Autosomal recessive with cardiac arrhythmia (prolonged QT interval) and severe deafness.

* *Usher's syndrome:* Autosomal recessive. Retinitis pigmentosa with contraction of the visual fields and severe sensorineural deafness, which may be progressive.

* *Refsum's syndrome:* Icthyosis, ataxia, retinitis pigmentosa, mental retardation, and deafness.

Pearl/Peril/Pitfall: About 3% of infants born at < 28 weeks' gestation require hearing aids, though more infants have milder hearing impairment or high-frequency hearing loss.

TABLE 1 Risk factors for hearing loss

1. Parental or caregiver concern regarding hearing, speech, language, or developmental delay.
2. Family history of permanent childhood hearing loss and/or Neurodegenerative disorders, such as Hunter syndrome, or sensory motor neuropathies, such as Friedreich's ataxia and Charcot-Marie-Tooth syndrome.
3. Stigmata or other findings (ear and craniofacial anomalies with morphologic abnormalities of the pinna and ear canal) associated with a syndrome Known to include a sensorineural or conductive hearing loss or eustachian tube dysfunction.
4. Postnatal infections associated with sensorineural hearing loss, including bacterial meningitis.
5. *In utero* infections such as CMV, herpes, rubella, syphilis, human immunodeficiency virus (HIV), and toxoplasmosis.
6. Neonatal indicators: specifically, hyperbilirubinemia at a serum level requiring exchange transfusion (some centers use a level of ≥ 20 mg/dL as a general guideline for risk), hypoxia and ischemia, infection, metabolic disease, persistent pulmonary hypertension of the newborn associated with mechanical ventilation, conditions requiring the use of extracorporeal membrane oxygenation (ECMO), and prolonged treatment with mechanical ventilation (>5 days), ototoxic drugs like aminoglycosides and frusemide.
7. Syndromes associated with progressive hearing loss such as neurofibromatosis, osteopetrosis, and Usher syndrome.
8. Birth weight<1,500g.
9. Birth trauma with fracture of temporal bone.
10. Recurrent/Persistent otitis media with effusion for at least 3 months.

TABLE 2 Hearing screening—methods

Examination of all newborns: The AAP and the Joint Committee on infant Hearing recommend universal hearing screening for all newborns (AAP, 1999; Joint Committee on infant Hearing, 2000). Prompt detection of hearing loss facilitates interventions aimed at preventing speech, language, and cognitive development impairments.
Methodology
   A. **Evoked otoacoustic emissions (EOAE)—Physiologic test measuring cochlear response to a stimulus.**
   1. Measures sound waves generated in the inner ear in response to clicks or tone bursts generated by small microphones placed in the infant's auditory canals.
   2. Advantages: results are specific to each ear; not dependent of the infant's state; short test time(10 minutes).
   3. Disadvantages: Inaccurate in the presence of debris in the ear canal/fluid in the middle ear; infant must be relatively inactive during the test, does not test neural transmission (cortical processing) of sound.
   B. **Auditory brainstem response (ABR)-Electrophysiologic measurement of activity in auditory nerve and brainstem pathway.**
   (1) Using three scalp electrodes, measures brain waves generated in response to mechanically generated ticks. (2) Advantages: ear-specific results; unaffected by ear canal debris. (3) Disadvantages: infant must be in a quite state;does not test neural transmission (cortical processing) of sound.
   C. **Follow-up**
   Hearing screening identifies infants at risk for hearing loss but is not diagnostic. Infants who fail screening tests must be referred for further testing and intervention.

KEY POINTS FOR CLINICAL PRACTICE

1. NICU graduates are at high risk of developing hearing loss(20–40 infants per 1,000 survivors of NICU admission can have some degree of sensorineural hearing loss). When undetected, hearing loss can result in delays in language communication, and cognitive development.
2. Hearing loss is categorized into 5 types; a) Sensorineural loss b) Conductive loss c) Mixed (a+b) d) Auditory dyssynchrony or Auditory neuropathy e) Central hearing loss.
3. *Current objective physiologic measures* used in Universal Newborn Screening programs for detecting hearing loss are a)Evoked otoacoustic emissions (EOAE)-Physiologic test measuring cochlear response to a stimulus b) Auditory brainstem response (ABR)-Electrophysiologic measurement of activity in auditory nerve and brainstem pathway. ABR is the preferred method to screen hearing loss in the NICU graduate.
4. *Ensure:* Follow-up Testing for infants with abnormal screening ABRs-*a)* within 2 weeks of their initial test in infants who are abnormal in both ears and *b)* within 3 months in infants with unilateral abnormal results.
5. Severe-to-Profound hearing loss requires a multidisciplinary team approach consisting of the primary care provider, ENT surgeon, audiologist, and speech therapist.

REFERENCES AND FURTHER READING : 1)AAP Task Force on Newborn Hearing and Infant Screening;Detection and Intervention. Pediatrics 1999;527-530 2)Weichbold V et all.Universal Newborn Hearing screening and postnatal hearing loss. Pediatrics 2006;117(4):e631-e636. 3) Neurodevelopmental outcomes after preterm birth Michael Colvin, William McGuire, Peter W Fowlie,**BMJ** VOLUME 329 11 DECEMBER 2004 bmj.com

Pearl/Peril/Pitfall: Hearing impairment is associated with delayed language development, although very preterm infants with normal hearing may also develop speech and language problems. Early use of hearing aids plus support from audiology services can improve language development in infants with sensorineural hearing loss.

27 Neonatal Birth Injury

@ *"Sensitive counseling of the parents is a most important aspect of management of birth injury"*

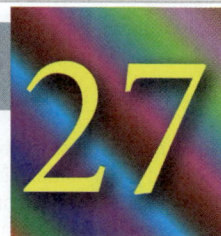
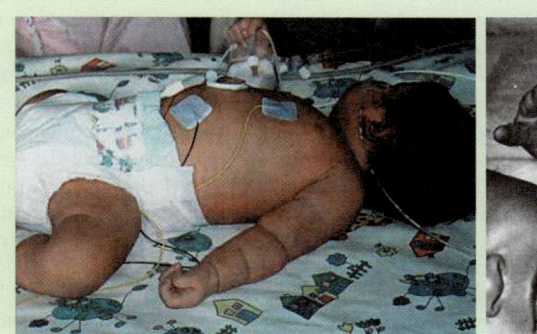
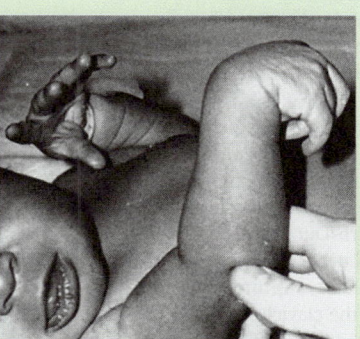
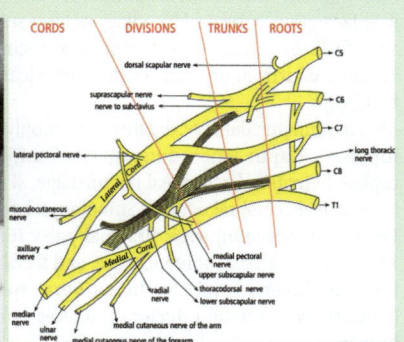

Injury to the Brachial Plexus: Stretch, tear, compression or avulsion of the nerves usually after forceful lateral deviation of the head from the shoulders during delivery. Recent studies suggest intrinsic forces (uterine contractions).

* **Erb's palsy** Restricted active movements and absent Moro and biceps reflexes on affected side; "porter's tip" or "waiter's tip" appearance of upper extremity

* **Klumpke's paralysis** Hand paralysis with possible ptosis, miosis, anhidrosis (Horner syndrome)

* **Fractured clavicle** Crepitus and bony irregularity felt; occasional bruising; possibly restricted active movements with absent Moro reflex on affected side; biceps reflex present

* **Cerebral palsy** Increased upper extremity tone; exaggerated biceps reflex; hyperactive grasp reflex

* **Fractured humerus** Restricted active movements and absent Moro reflex on affected side, biceps reflex present; crepitus may be felt

REVIEW OF CLINICAL PROBLEMS

1. How do you differentiate the Erb's palsy from Klumpke's paralysis ?
   Ans: Refer to the EVALUATION-DECISION-ACTION-PLAN/ALGORITHM TO DIAGNOSE & MANAGE A NEONATE WITH BRACHIAL PLEXUS INJURY.

2. What risk factors should you seek to know the etiology of birth injury?
   Ans: Refer to the Table 1 of the Chapter.

3. When do you refer the Newborn baby who sustained birth injury to a tertiary Neonatal unit?
   Ans: Refer to the EVALUATION-DECISION-ACTION-PLAN/ALGORITHM TO DIAGNOSE & MANAGE A NEONATE WITH BIRTH INJURY.

4. How do you manage a Neonate who developed massive subgaleal bleeding ?
   Ans: Refer to the "SYNOPSIS OF LIFE-THREATENING BIRTH INJURIES".

5. When should you consult a neurosurgeon while managing a Newborn with CNS birth trauma ?
   Ans: Refer to the EVALUATION-DECISION-ACTION-PLAN/ALGORITHM TO DIAGNOSE & MANAGE A NEONATE WITH BIRTH INJURY.

LEARNING OBJECTIVES

After completing this article, readers will be able to

1. Recognize serious traumatic injury and institute early and effective treatment.

2. Recognize subgaleal bleeding and extensive intracranial bleeding, that require emergent treatments, consultation, or referral to a tertiary center.

3. Recognize perinatal conditions that increase risk for traumatic or hypoxic-ischemic injury.

4. Know the outcome and long-term sequelae of traumatic and hypoxic-ischemic birth injury.

5. Coordinate comprehensive follow-up for these sequelae.

Pearl/Peril/Pitfall: SUBCONJUNCTIVAL AND RETINAL HEMORRHAGES- • resulting from increased pressure in the head and neck region during birth • generally disappear within 4 weeks • to induce an infant to open its eyes, gently rock him from an upright to a horizontal position; feed the baby; turn lights off and on.

BIRD'S EYE VIEW/OVERVIEW/SYNOPSIS

1. *Birth injury* is "an impairment of the infant's body function or structure due to adverse influences that occurred at birth". It is a potentially avoidable (unavoidable sometimes) mechanical injury and may occur antenatally, intrapartally, or during resuscitation. Traumatic birth injury resulting from physical trauma during the birth process may occur alone or in combination with hypoxic-ischemic injury & perinatal asphyxia. Most injuries, such as soft tissue trauma, are minor, but others, such as liver laceration, subgaleal bleeding, or large subdural blood collections, are life-threatening & require prompt recognition & intervention. Traumatic birth injury can result in physical & neurodevelopmental handicaps.

   After a traumatic delivery, the most commonly injured systems: **Cranial injuries**: Caput succedaneum, subconjunctival hemorrhage, cephalohematoma, subgaleal hemorrhage, skull fractures, intracranial hemorrhage, cerebral edema **Spinal injuries**: Spinal cord transection **Peripheral nerve injuries**: Brachial palsy (Erb-Duchenne paralysis, Klumpke's paralysis), phrenic nerve, and facial nerve paralysis **Visceral injuries**: Liver rupture or hematoma, splenic rupture, adrenal hemorrhage **Skeletal injuries**: Fractures of the clavicle, femur, and humerus.

2. *Assess the following risk factors which contribute to an increased risk of birth injury*; 1)Primiparity 2)Small maternal stature 3)Maternal pelvic anomalies 4)Prolonged or unusually rapid labor 5)Oligohydramnios 6) Malpresentation of the fetus 7)Use of mid-forceps or vacuum extraction 8)Versions and extraction 9)Very low birth weight or extreme prematurity 10) Fetal macrosomia or large fetal head, 11)Fetal anomalies. (*refer to table-1 for detailed enlisting of risk factors for Neonatal birth injuries*). Traumatic injuries often result from discrepancy between the size or position of the fetus in relation to the birth canal or from an unusually rigid pelvis that has not been adapted gradually to the size of the fetal head.

3. *Evaluate a Newborn at risk for birth injury by thorough examination, including a detailed neurologic evaluation.* Evaluate the Newborns who require resuscitation after birth for an occult injury. Pay particular attention to symmetry of structure & function, cranial nerves, range of motion of individual joints, and integrity of the scalp & skin.

4. *The management of traumatic head injuries consists of recognition, monitoring, & treatment of serious consequences.*Table-2 summarizes common types of injuries. The general pediatrician with careful diagnosis & observation can manage many of the less life-threatening injuries. *Referral or consultation is indicated for* *difficult-to-control seizures *depressed skull fractures *any posterior fossa, subdural, or subgaleal or epidural blood collection *suspected spinal cord injury *Brachial plexus injuries that don't resolve *persistent diaphragmatic paralysis requiring mechanical ventilation *displaced long bone fracture (e.g. any femur fracture).

5. Helpful diagnostic tests to evaluate suspected intracranial bleeding include repeated clinical examinations, serial hematocrits to assess blood loss, and CT brain imaging for epidural, subdural, or subarachnoid blood. A bedside ultrasound examination can miss significant blood collections located in close proximity to the skull. A lumbar puncture can be done in infants without signs of increased intracranial pressure. Xanthochromia, RBCs, and an increased protein level support a diagnosis of intracranial bleeding. Coagulation screen with a prothrombin time, partial thromboplastin time, fibrinogen, and platelet count helps assess congenital coagulation disorders, diffuse intravascular coagulation secondary to shock, and isoimmune thrombocytopenia as causes for the bleeding, *especially in cases without overt history of birth trauma.*

6. *The Evaluation-Decision-Action Plan/Algorithm* to assess, evaluate & manage traumatic birth injury describes the essential aspects of diagnosis and management. Perinatal asphyxia and hypoxic-ischemic encephalopathy are discussed in detail in an exclusively devoted chapter (*refer to Chapter 28*)

7. Acute blood loss and hypovolemia from subgaleal bleeding is a life-threatening emergency that should prompt immediate consultation. The management demands immediate stabilization of circulation, oxygenation & ventilation, correction of coagulation disturbances as well as maintenance of a stable hemodynamic status to ensure adequate organ perfusion. Surgical evacuation of the hematoma is indicated for infants with evidence of cerebral compression. Pressure wrapping of the head is controversial and not generally recommended. Mortality may be as high as 25%.

8. Subarachnoid hemorrhage is the most frequent form of traumatic intracranial bleeding in the term neonate. It is usually of limited degree & rarely of clinical significance. Infants who develop signs of increased intracranial pressure from convexity subdural bleeds or epidural collections & posterior fossa bleeds with evidence of progressive brainstem compression require acute surgical drainage of the blood. Depressed skull fractures can be observed or can be elevated externally (e.g., with an obstetric vaccum). Surgical elevation is rarely indicated.

9. Most nerve palsies resolve spontaneously as swelling around the nerve roots ceases. The essential aspects of Erb's palsy, Klumpke paralysis are described in the *Evaluation - Decision - Action Plan/Algorithm* to assess and manage a Neonate with brachial plexus injury. There are four types of Brachial Plexus Injury: 1. Neuropraxia Brachial Plexus Injury 2. Avulsion Brachial Plexus Injury 3. Rupture Brachial Plexus Injury 4. Neuroma Brachial Plexus Injury Neuropraxia Brachial Plexus Injury, also called Stretch Brachial Plexus Injury, is the most common and results when the nerves are stretched, but not torn. Rupture occurs when the nerve is torn, but not at the spine. Avulsion Brachial Plexus Injury is the most severe since the nerve is torn from the spine. For infants with persistent weakness related to brachial plexus injuries, physical therapy to preserve joint mobility & avoid muscle tightness is indicated, beginning at about 7 to 10 days of age. Infants with diaphragmatic paralysis can be managed symptomatically with oxygen supplementation or mechanical ventilation if needed for respiratory failure. Surgical diaphragm plication should be considered for infants who remain ventilator dependent for 6-8weeks. Though most infants recover from Brachial Plexus Injury within 6 months, those who do not recover require surgery to repair the nerve. The surgery may be a nerve graft or nerve transfer, and may require an extended hospital stay. There may be permanent damage, which will require long term care.Infants with suspected spinal cord injury should be stabilized & referred to a tertiary care centre for further evaluation & management. Seek orthopedic input to manage fractures of the humerus and femur, which may require reduction & immobilization. Fracture clavicle doesn't require any intervention apart from parental reassurance.

   Caput succedaneum, Cephalhematoma, petechiae & bruising are minor injuries and of importance primarily because of an increased risk for hyperbilirubinemia. Subcutaneous fat necrosis can cause symptomatic hypercalcemia at 3-4 weeks of age and presents with vomiting, weight loss, decreased feeding & irritability. It may not be evident at the time of birth.

10. *Educate the parents about the management, outcome & follow-up of the infants with traumatic birth injuries* - care and consideration should be taken when discussing the etiology and outcome of a birth-related injury with parents. Acknowledging that many factors exist which cannot be controlled and that consequences can result from medically necessary interventions is important. Similarly, the obstetrician can be included in the discussion so that parents receive appropriate and accurate information regarding the circumstances of the injury.

Pearl/Peril/Pitfall: CAPUT SUCCEDANEUM • diffuse, edematous swelling of the scalp involving the presenting portion of the head during a vertex delivery • appears in the delivery room • extends across midline, across suture lines • can be ecchymotic • if extensive, can cause anemia and hyperbilirubinemia • should not be routinely aspirated , as this predisposes to infection

THE EVALUATION-DECISION-ACTION-PLAN/ALGORITHM TO DIAGNOSE & MANAGE THE BIRTH INJURY

SUBJECTIVE FINDINGS

Scan through the antenatal history, intrapartal & delivery events to assess the presence of various risk factors responsible for the birth injury - refer to Table 1.

OBJECTIVE FINDINGS

Assess airway, breathing, circulation and disability by observing the vitals, BP, O$_2$ sats, color, CRT, pulses, sensorium, focal neurologic deficits, seizures, abnormal movements, tone and reflexes, etc.

Identify the life—threatening symptoms of birth injury—seizures, hypovolemic shock, raised ICP, brainstem compression, diaphragmatic paralysis, cervical cord injury.

Perform complete physical examination from head to toe including detailed neurological examination.

INVESTIGATIONS

Blood: Hb, hematocrit, WBC, Differential count, platelets,Group/Type and Crossmatch, blood sugar, creatinine, ABG analysis, serum calcium, magnesium, Coagulation studies, serum bilirubin.

Imaging: X-rays of regions where fractures are suspected. Ultrasound abdomen—to identify subcapsular hematoma liver, splenic hematoma, adrenal hemorrhage.

CT/MRI brain imaging in cases of traumatic head injuries.

LP can be done, in infants without signs of raised ICP for xanthochromia, RBC and increased protein.

A NEONATE WITH BIRTH INJURY

Identify Isolated "minor" injuries - like caput succedaneum, cephalhematoma, linear skull fracture, petechiae, bruises, lacerations, abrasions, fat necrosis etc., *Monitor* for infection anemia & Hyperbilirubinemia

Pulse oximetry, CR monitor, BP

Suspect perinatal asphyxia and Hypoxic encephalopathy by the presence of altered sensorium, high-pitched cry, seizures ± multiorgan dysfunction (refer to Chapter No-28 for detailed management)

Institute mechanical ventilation, if airway, breathing and circulation are compromised, *treat* hypovolemia & hypotension due to blood loss energetically with aggressive volume replacement (NS, whole blood ('O' Negative), packed RBC), & vasopressors, *correct* coagulation abnormalities with FFP and platelets, *correct* metabolic acidosis & fluid and electrolyte disturbances, *identify and correct* hypothermia, hypoglycemia and hypocalcemia, *continuously monitor* volume infused and urine output.

Monitor serial hematocrits, coagulation studies, serum bilirubin and head circumference closely.

Treat seizures with IV loading dose of phenobarbitone 10mg/kg/dose- a second 10mg/kg dose can be given for further seizures, but consultation should be sought before any further anticonvulsant administration. *Evaluate* for coagulopathy & myocardial performance, if hypotension continues in spite of 30ml/kg volume replacement along with vasopressors.

Refer to a tertiary neonatal unit, if the following indications exist:
* Traumatic head injury with difficult-to-control seizures
* Posterior fossa subdural bleed; epidural bleed
* Subgaleal bleeding *Depressed skull fracture
* Suspected spinal cord injury * Brachial plexus injuries that do not resolve; persistent diaphragmatic paralysis requiring mechanical ventilation
* Displaced long bone fracture; any femur fracture
* Ophthalmic injury other than subconjunctival hemorrhage, lid ecchymosis, retinal hemorrhage
* Hemoperitoneum secondary to subcapsular hematoma liver, splenic injury *Limb ischemia & gangrene
* Testicular injury especially when torsion cannot be excluded

Do remember the following facts in assessing & managing birth injury & its consequences: 1)Subgaleal (subaponeurotic) hemorrhage may occur together with a caput succedaneum and cephalhematoma 2)an increase of just 2 cms in head circumference might represent 30% of the blood volume of a 3kg infant (240-300ml) and cause irreversible shock 3)it is important to recognize that acute hemorrhage need not cause an immediate change in the hematocrit 4)suspect coagulation defects (both congenital and acquired from shock and DIC) in managing significant bleeding occurring obviously due to birth injury 5)complicated fractures may be painful enough to cause a pseudoparalysis of the arm, mimicking injury to the brachial plexus 6)location of petechiae, birth history, early appearance without development of new lesions and the absence of bleeding from other sites help differentiate petechiae and ecchymoses secondary to birth trauma from those caused by a vasculitis or coagulation disorders. If in doubt rule out coagulopathies and infection 7)monitor for anemia & hyperbilirubinemia even in the presence of minor soft tissue injury like petechiae, ecchymoses, large caput & cephalhematoma etc.

Consult neurosurgeon for a)depressed skull fractures b)posterior fossa bleeds with evidence of progressive brainstem compression c)subdural/epidural bleed in infants who develop signs of raised ICP.

Reassure parents in cases of a)fractures clavicle & humerus b)85% cases of brachial plexus nerve injuries which resolve completely over several days to 4 weeks c)facial nerve injuries d)isolated subarachnoid bleeding & convexity subdural bleeds.

Arrange follow-up for a)monitoring head circumference for developing hydrocephalus b)neurodevelopmental examination for persistent focal neurologic findings and long term sequelae c)anticonvulsant therapy for seizures d)physical and occupational therapy evaluations e)survivors with paralysis after spinal cord injury.

Counsel the parents sensitively, acknowledging that many factors exist in the etiology and outcome of birth related injury, which cannot be controlled and that consequences can result from medically necessary interventions. *Always include* the obstetrician in the discussion so that parents receive appropriate and accurate information regarding the circumstances of the injury.

* *Pearl/Peril/Pitfall: STERNOCLEIDOMASTOID MUSCLE INJURY • result of muscle or fascial sheath injury during hyperextension • associated with breech or forceps births, congenital dislocated hips, and female sex • clinical signs present at birth or in first month - usually right sided , nontender 1 - 2 cm, firm palpable mass in the muscle bed, with shortening or contracture of the muscle, with obligatory head tilt toward affected side, chin away from affected side • treatment - resolves spontaneously in most infants - gentle passive stretching exercises is controversial as to utility.*

THE EVALUATION-DECISION-ACTION-PLAN/ALGORITHM
TO DIAGNOSE and MANAGE A NEONATE WITH BRACHIAL PLEXUS INJURY

SUBJECTIVE FINDINGS

Hx of absent/reduced movement of involved extremity after a prolonged delivery of a macrosomic infant.

Hx of risk factors such as shoulder dystocia, breech delivery, multiparity, prolonged/precipitous 2nd stage labor, instrumentation, fetal macrosomia.

OBJECTIVE FINDINGS

Assess for rapid, shallow breathing and decreased movement of the diaphragm on the affected side (indicative of phrenic nerve paralysis—5% of cases)

Assess for posture of the involved limb (typically adducted, internally rotated at the shoulder, extended and pronated at the elbow, flexed at the wrist and fingers—*waiter's tip* posture), asymmetrical Moro reflex, winging of the scapula, diminished to absent deep tendon reflexes, hypesthesia, *grasp reflex present/absent?* When assessing movement of the extremity, look for movement, function, and strength of all three major joints (shoulder, elbow and wrist) as well as the hand grasp.

Assess for associated findings - birth asphyxia, facial palsy, fractured clavicle and humerus, cephalhematoma, cervical cord injury.

INVESTIGATIONS

X-rays of the clavicle, shoulder, and humerus to diagnose associated injuries

EMG (Electromyography) and Nerve conduction studies to delineate the location and extent of the injury and to assess the degree of recovery

Somatosensory evoked potentials to help to distinguish completed avulsion at the spinal cord from a more distal lesion

MRI scan to demonstrate root avulsion

A NEONATE WITH BRACHIAL PLEXUS INJURY

Look for associated nerve injuries such as facial nerve injury(asymmetric crying facies), recurrent laryngeal nerve injury(hoarseness + inspiratory stridor with crying).

Ensure ABCs—CR and apnea monitor, supplemental O₂, Pulse oximetry, if diaphragmatic paralysis is suspected.

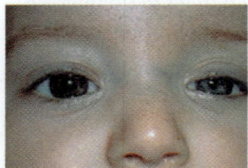

Horner syndrome : Left pupillary miosis, marked hypochromia of the left iris, ipsilateral mild ptosis and left hemifacial anhidrosis

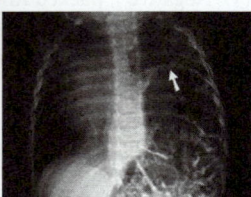

Diaphragmatic Paralysis due to Phrenic Nerve Injury

* Determine whether it is Erb's palsy/Klumpke paralysis/mixed

* Erb's palsy (injury to C5, C6, occasionally C7 nerve roots) - evidenced by the characteristic posture of the limb, absent DTR, intact grasp reflex, asymmetrical & absent Moro on the affected side, sensation variable.

* Klumpke paralysis (injury to C7, C8-T1 nerve roots) -evidenced by the presence of flaccid hand and loss of wrist movement and grasp reflex, ipsilateral Horner syndrome (ptosis, miosis, anhidrosis), loss of sensation on the ulnar side of the forearm and hand

* Total brachial plexus injury is a combination of Erb's palsy & Klumpke paralysis

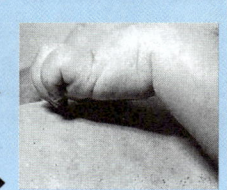

* *Provide* supportive wrapping of the arm against the body (natural position) for 7–10 days to prevent further injury * *Do not* overimmobilize the limb * *Carry out* passive range-of-motion exercises after 10 days * *Try* hand/wrist/digit splints to prevent contractures in Klumpke paralysis * *Avoid* Statue of Liberty splinting to prevent the consequent shoulder contractures * *Explain* the prognosis to the parents - 75%-90% of injuries resolve spontaneously without sequelae which is better for Erb's palsy than for Klumpke or mixed pareses. Most cases recover within 2 weeks to 3 months, but there may be gradual improvement up to 1 year of age. * *Perform* serial neurologic examinations to predict recovery in Erb's palsy . Return to antigravity strength in the biceps, triceps, and deltoid by 6 months of age is predictive of good recovery. There is evidence that if perceptible muscle contractions have not returned to the deltoid and the biceps by the end the third month, the ultimate functional recovery of the shoulder and arm will be suboptimal.

FACIAL NERVE INJURY *The most common Neonatal traumatic nerve injury (1% of live births)* commonly the entire side of face is involved (LMN type) *clinical features include decreased forehead wrinkling, increased eye opening, decreased nasolabial fold, and flattening of the corner of the mouth *often associated with facial bruises or lacerations, hemotympanum, temporal bone fracture, or other birth injuries *usually due to compression of the facial nerve by mid - forceps, maternal sacral promontory or rarely from pressure of a uterine fibroid *nerve compression occurs within the mastoid segment or just outside the stylomastoid foramen * 90% show full recovery within days to weeks, but some may take up to 2 years;10% show only partial or no return of function *nerve conduction studies are helpful when there is no improvement over 4 to 7 days to distinguish partial from complete denervation *differential diagnosis includes Mobius syndrome, hemifacial microsomia and agenesis of depressor anguli oris muscle(which is characterized by an asymmetric cry, with inability to move the affected side of the mouth downward and laterally, other features of facial nerve palsy, such as asymmetric nasolabial folds, inability to wrinkle the forehead, and inability to close the eye, are not present. *protect the eye on the affected side with methyl cellulose eye drops and by patching to prevent corneal injuries *Criteria for surgical exploration of the facial canal and nerve decompression include the following: 1) Unilateral complete paralysis. 2) Hematotympanum and depressed fracture of the petrous bone.3) Absence of voluntary and evoked motor unit responses in all muscles innervated by the facial nerve by 3 to 5 days of life. 4) No return of facial nerve function clinically or electrophysiologically at 5 weeks of age.

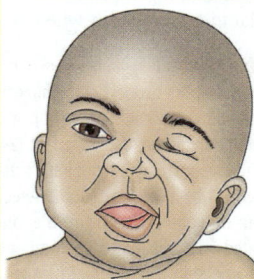

Asymmetry caused by facial nerve paralysis, with inability to close eye, nasolabial fold flattening, and inability to move lips on the affected side. Newborns with facial nerve paralysis have difficulty effecting a seal around the nipple and consequently exhibit drooling of milk or formula from the paralyzed side of the mouth.

TABLE 1 — Risk factors for neonatal birth injuries

A. Maternal factors 1)Diabetes 2)Obesity 3)Undersized pelvis 4)Postmaturity 5)Primiparity **B.Fetal Factors**-1)Macrosomia (associated with multiparity, advanced maternal age, obesity, gestational diabetes, previous macrosomic infant). 2)Increased ratio of chest circumference to head circumference 3)Breech position **C.Obstetric factors** - 1)Shoulder dystocia (major factor in pathogenesis of birth injuries). 2)Forceps (especially midforceps) delivery. 3)Vacuum extraction. 4)Prolonged second stage of labor. 5)Precipitous delivery. **D. Vacuum extraction**-**1)**May be safer than forceps, but complications include the following: a)Cephalhematoma (10%) b)Scalp abrasions and lacerations (1% to 2%) c)Necrosis and avulsion of the scalp d)Subgaleal (subaponeurotic) hemorrhage (0.5% to 1%) e)Skull fractures f)Intracranial bleeding (0.2%) g)Supratentorial hemorrhage; subdural hematoma h)Brachial plexus injury. **2)** No evidence of increased incidence of neurologic sequelae after use of vacuum extraction exists; however, whenever there are clinical signs of neurologic compromise after vacuum extraction, evaluation by computed tomography (CT), magnetic resonance imaging (MRI), or ultrasonography is indicated. **E. Forceps** 1)Complications include the following: a)Facial nerve injury b)Intraventricular hemorrhage c)Brachial plexus injury **2.** Sequential use of vacuum and forceps significantly increases the rates of traumatic complications.

Note:Infants who are large for gestational age (>4500g) and who are delivered vaginally (especially with forceps or vacuum extraction) are at increased risk for fractured clavicle, fractured humerus, brachial plexus injury, asphyxia, hypoglycemia, and cephalhematoma. Newborns >5000g are at increased risk for perinatal mortality.

TABLE 2 — Traumatic Birth Injuries

Types of Injury	*Examples*
Soft tissue injuries	Abrasions, bruising, fat necrosis, lacerations
Extracranial bleeding	Cephalhematoma, subgaleal
Intracranial bleeding	Subarachnoid, epidural, subdural, cerebral, cerebellar
Nerve injuries	Facial, cervical nerve roots (brachial plexus palsies, phrenic), Horner syndrome, recurrent laryngeal
Spinal cord injuries	
Fractures	Clavicle, humerus, femur, skull
Dislocations	
Torticollis*	
Eye injuries	Subconjunctival and retinal hemorrhage
Solid organ injury	Liver, spleen

* Secondary to bleeding in the sternocleidomastoid muscle

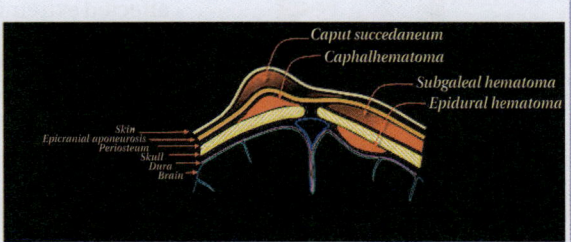

TABLE 3 — Fractures secondary to birth injury

	Specific cause	Potential problem	Treatment	Comment
Skull Linear	1. Forceps pressure 2. Pubic pressure 3. Sacral pressure 4. Ischial spine pressure	Usually none, rarely subdural or extradural hemorrhage		
Depressed	Forceps	Underlying brain injury	1. If asymptomatic, none 2. If symptomatic, elevate	Prevent sustained cortical pressure
Occipital subluxation	Traction on spine in breech deliveries with head fixed in the pelvis	Rupture of underlying venous sinus	Usually fatal from subdural hemorrhage or tentorial tear	
Clavicle (common)	1. Breech-extended arms 2. Difficult shoulder in vertex delivery	Associated brachial plexus injury	1. None - or if pain treat pain 2. Bandage arm to chest with pad in axilla for 10 days	Prognosis excellent
Humerus	Breech-bringing down a displaced arm	Nerve damage	As for clavicle	Prognosis excellent
Femur	Extended breech	Sciatic nerve damage	1. Immobilize leg onto abdomen for 2-4 weeks (the in utero position) 2. Gallows traction	Position unimportant molding will repair
Epiphyseal separation		Callus interferes with joint mobility and bone growth		1. On the upper femur, pain on external rotation 2. Outlook good
Nose	Dislocation of nasal cartilage	Difficulty feeding	1. Insert oral airway 2. Straighten surgically	Nares asymmetrical and nose flat

Pearl/Peril/Pitfall: HEPATIC OR SPLENIC HEMATOMA — *caused by increased abdominal pressure during breech birth — neonate appears normal for 1 - 3 days (up to 1 week), and then may present with nonspecific signs of blood loss such as poor feeding, listlessness, pallor, jaundice, tachypnea, tachycardia — shock and death may result if hematoma ruptures and allows fresh bleeding — exam may show a palpable RUQ mass or "blue" abdomen — ultrasound should diagnose hematoma.*

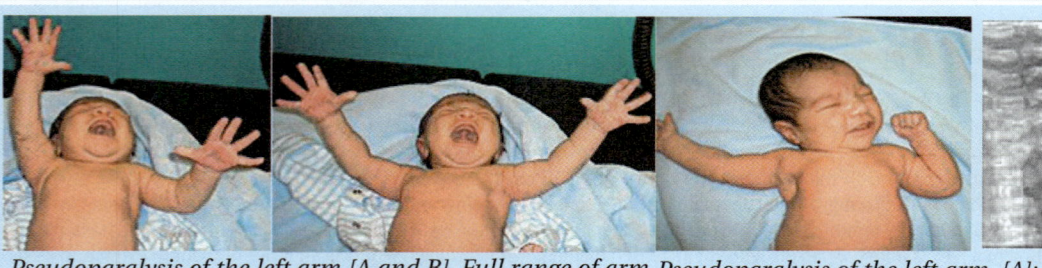

Pseudoparalysis of the left arm [A and B]. Full range of arm movement produced by Moro reflex [B].

Pseudoparalysis of the left arm. [A]: Left arm do not have the typical posture of Erb's palsy or Klumpke palsy. [B]. Clavicular fracture in the same patient.

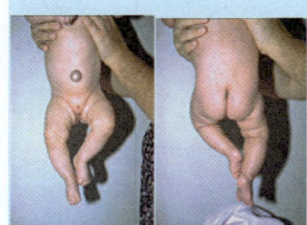

Right leg drop in a patient with septic arthritis of the right hip [A and B].

Pseudoparalysis: Pseudoparalysis occurs with bone fracture or with joint, soft tissue, or bone infections,such as osteomyelitis, pyogenic arthritis and osteomyelitis, osteitis of congenital syphilis(*Parrot`s pseudoparalysis*).Soft tissue inflammation often occurs with osteomyelitis, but occasionally in infancy pseudoparalysis may be the sole sign of infection in bone.Decreased limb movements due to pain are referred to as pseudoparalysis. The neonate with pseudoparalysis cries and grimaces with even minimal attempts to move the affected extremity, but full motion can be elicited by primitive reflexes. Neonates with pseudoparalysis have normal deep tendon reflexes. The painful limbs do not adopt the typical postures that characterize segmental brachial plexus palsy or peripheral nerve lesions. Evidence of trauma or infection in the affected limb supports the diagnosis of pseudoparalysis.

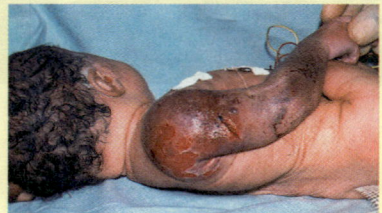

Newborn baby with injuries to its shoulder and arm sustained during birth. Minor bruising is common, but more extensive abrasions and bruises, such as this, can result from the mother having a narrow birth canal or during a complicated birth, for example a breech delivery. Courtesy: DR M.A. Ansary/Science photo library

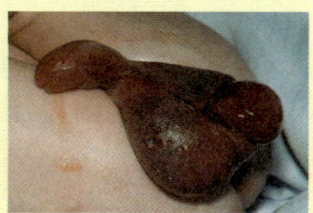

Testicular damage, resulting from birth injury, is extremely rare.The left scrotum had ruptured and the testicle was exposed,following a trail of vaginal breech delivery. Baby was admitted, received fluid, analgesia and had the exposed testicle covered. Local surgeons operated within 3 h of age. The testicle was viable and the scrotum was sutured. Baby recovered well postoperatively.Detailed examination of the scrotum is indicated in all male breech babies. Prompt review, with early surgical input, is essential. The potential for significant long-term damage exists even if testes appear normal on palpation.**Courtesy: R Negrine,W Easter,I Fraser,S Ellis.**Neonatal Unit, University Hospital of Coventry and Warwickshire, Coventry, UK .*Arch Dis Child Fetal Neonatal Ed* 2010;**95**:F193. doi:10.1136/adc.2009.181594

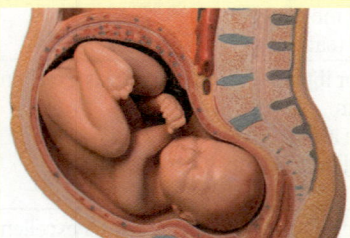

Excessive contractions of the uterus (sometimes called "uterine hyperstimulation" or "tetanic contractions") from labor, or from medicines used to accelerate labor, like pitocin, can cause problems with the baby's oxygen supply. The rapid, powerful contractions of the uterus can prevent maternal oxygen from reaching the baby. If the flow of oxygen to the baby is interrupted, hypoxic or anoxic brain injury can occur. The consequences of this can be severe and may include seizures, brain damage, developmental delay, cerebral palsy, and other problems with motor or cognitive functions.

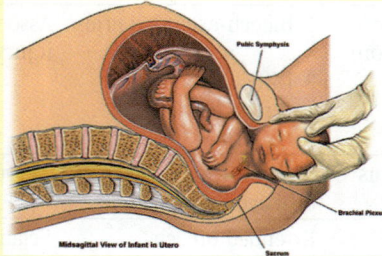

Shoulder Dystocia describes a situation where the fetal head has been delivered, but the shoulders are stuck behind the mother's pelvic bone and cannot be freed. This often results in injury by either blocking the baby's ability to breathe resulting in neurological damage, causing skeletal injury that may fracture the baby's clavicle or humerus, or causing brachial plexus injuries.

Pearl/Peril/Pitfall: SUBCUTANEOUS FAT NECROSIS • *discovered within the 5th - 10th day of life, but as early as day 2 or as late as day 24 • lesions are sharply circumscribed nodules or plaques, hard, and of a dusky reddish-purple hue; surface may be uneven and a sharp margin delineates it from the surrounding normal skin • found in the cheeks, buttocks, back, arms, and thighs; mostly over bony prominences • benign; usually asymptomatic, not hot or tender • occasionally will extensively calcify or drain a liquid material • versus sclerema neonatorum - waxlike diffuse hardening of skin in infants with underlying systemic disease (sepsis, congenital heart disease, dehydration); usually seen in premature or debilitated infants • treatment - avoid warm or hot packs to the area - should be followed by a pediatrician for signs of extensive calcification or drainage - process is usually self-limited and resolves over a few weeks.*

SYNOPSIS OF LIFE-THREATENING BIRTH INJURIES

1. *Subgaleal bleed (subaponeurotic):* Often seen after vacuum-or forceps-assisted deliveries and can result in enormous blood loss which can be life-threatening. A coagulation defect (hemophilia, early hemorrhagic disease due to vitamin-K deficiency in infants born to mothers who are taking anticonvulsants) may complicate the picture. Both the caput succedaneum and subgaleal bleed extend across suture lines, in contrast to a cephalhematoma which is strictly limited by the margins of the individual bones of the skull because of its subperiosteal location. A caput is limited to edema of the skin and subcutaneous tissue; a subgaleal bleed lies beneath the scalp and can often be balloted, with an obvious fluid wave. With massive subgaleal bleeding, the head circumference is symmetrically increased. The hematoma may grow slowly or increase rapidly and result in shock. Management consists of a)Recognition and prompt blood volume replacement b)Surgical drainage only for unremitting clinical deterioration c)Phototherapy for hyperbilirubinemia d)Investigation for a bleeding disorder e)IV antibiotics & drainage for infected because of associated skin abrasions

2. *Depressed skull fracture:* May occur secondary to pressure from forceps, the maternal spine or pelvis, uterine tumors, fetal extremities, or the obstetrician's or midwife's hand. They are usually "ping-pong ball" - type fractures and or secondary to inward buckling of the resilient bone. Surgical elevation is indicated only in symptomatic cases and if the depression is >5mm. The depression may be elevated using the vacuum of a breast pump or an obstetric vacuum extractor.

3. *Phrenic nerve paralysis (C3, 4, or 5):* Risk factors include breech and difficult forceps deliveries which can cause stretch injury due to lateral hyperextension of the neck at birth. 75% of patients also have brachial plexus injury, because injury to the nerve is thought to occur where at crosses the brachial plexus. Infants present with respiratory distress, cyanosis and decreased breath sounds at the lung base and decreased movement of the affected hemithorax. Chest x-ray may show elevation of the affected diaphragm (may not be apparent if the infant is on CPAP or mechanical ventilation. The diagnosis is confirmed by ultrasonography or fluoroscopy that shows paradoxical (upward) movement of the diaphragm with inspiration. The differential diagnosis always includes cardiac, pulmonary, and other neurologic causes of respiratory distress. CPAP or mechanical ventilation may be needed, with careful airway care to avoid atelectasis & pneumonia. Most infants recover in 1–3 months without permanent sequelae. Diaphragmatic plication is necessary in refractory cases. Phrenic nerve pacing is possible for bilateral paralysis.

4. *Spinal cord injury* Associated with midforceps rotations and difficult breech deliveries. Labor with a fetus presenting in the breech position with a hyperextended neck, the so-called "flying fetus", can result in damage to the cervical spinal cord. Elective cesarean section usually avoids this complication. Clinical features include profound hypotonia, absent deep-tendon reflexes, obvious sensory level, flaccid extremities, Horner syndrome, Diaphragmatic paralysis, neurogenic bladder and associated hypoxic-ischemic encephalopathy in 2/3rds of cases. MRI scanning of the cervical & upper thoracic spine is the best diagnostic test and it rules out a potentially treatable lesion, such as an occult dysraphic state. Initial stabilization should include maintenance of adequate oxygenation and perfusion using mechanical ventilation and volume infusions as needed. The bladder should be decompressed with an indwelling catheter, the spine stabilized, and the infant sedated. These patients should be referred to a tertiary care centre for further evaluation & management.

5. *Hemoperitoneum:* Rare and the risk factors include large size, hepatomegaly, breech extraction & forceful manipulation during delivery. Bleeding can occur from the liver, adrenals, spleen, mesentery, umbilical vein, or kidney, but the liver is the most common site. It results from the rupture of a slowly expanding subcapsular hematoma into the free peritoneal cavity. Infants present with pallor, abdominal distention, anemia, and shock without an obvious source of bleeding. A bluish discoloration of the overlying abdominal skin and scrotal ecchymosis and enlargement may be present. Diagnosis is confirmed by paracentesis and laparotomy. Splenic injury requires expectant management with close observation. If laparotomy is necessary, salvage of the spleen is attempted to minimize the risk of sepsis. Adrenal hemorrhage is diagnosed by abdominal ultrasound and the treatment includes blood volume replacement and steroids for adrenal insufficiency. Extensive bleeding that requires surgical intervention is rare.

6. *Bilateral recurrent laryngeal nerve injury:* Bilateral nerve injury is usually due to hypoxia or brain stem hemorrhage or by trauma secondary to excessive traction on the fetal head during breech delivery or lateral traction on the head with forceps. Bilateral paralysis usually results in stridor, severe respiratory distress, and cyanosis. This has variable prognosis and tracheostomy may be required. Always rule out CNS malformations, including Chiari malformation and hydrocephalus. If there is no history of birth trauma, consider CVS anomalies and mediastinal masses. Diagnosis is made by using direct or flexible fiber-optic laryngoscopy. Unilateral nerve injury is asymptomatic at rest, but has hoarseness and inspiratory stridor with crying and it is occasionally associated with hypoglossal nerve injury, and presents with difficulty with feedings and secretions. The left recurrent laryngeal nerve is involved more often because of its longer course. Unilateral injury usually resolves by 6 weeks of age without intervention and treatment. The differential diagnosis for unilateral injury includes congenital laryngeal malformations.

KEY POINTS FOR CLINICAL PRACTICE

1. Care and consideration should be taken when discussing the etiology and outcome of a birth related injury with parents. Acknowledging that many factors exist which cannot be controlled and that consequences can result from medically necessary interventions is important.
2. Birth trauma and asphyxia may occur together, in which cases, prognosis also depends on the degree of the associated hypoxic - ischemic insult suffered perinatally. All infants at risk for Neurodevelopmental sequelae should have close monitoring of developmental milestones.

REFERENCES AND FURTHER READING

1)Manual of Neonatal Care-6th edition by John P.Cloherty - Lippincott 2)Primary Care of the Newborn-4th edition by Henry M. Seidel - Elsevier 3)Pediatrics-First edition by Osborn - Mosby 4)Nelson Text Book of Pediatrics-18th edition- Saunders

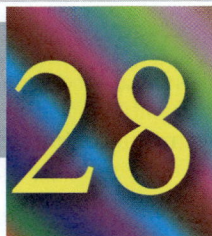

28 Perinatal Asphyxia Including Hypoxic-Ischemic Encephalopathy (HIE)

@ *"The severity of HIE can only be determined retrospectively as the features of HIE take some time to manifest".*

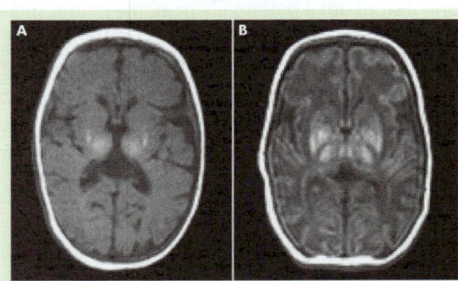

T1 weighted magnetic resonance images of (A) focal injury in an infant with Sarnat stage II neonatal encephalopathy (NE) aged 11 days and (B) global injury in an infant with Sarnat stage III NE aged 12 days. (A) Focal high signal intensity lesions are visible in the lentiform nuclei and thalami, and there is loss of the normal high signal intensity from myelin in the posterior limb of the internal capsule. (B) There are extensive high signal intensity lesions in the lentiform nuclei and thalami, loss of the normal high signal intensity from myelin in the posterior limb of the internal capsule, and abnormal low signal intensity in the white matter with loss of the normal grey/white matter differentiation.

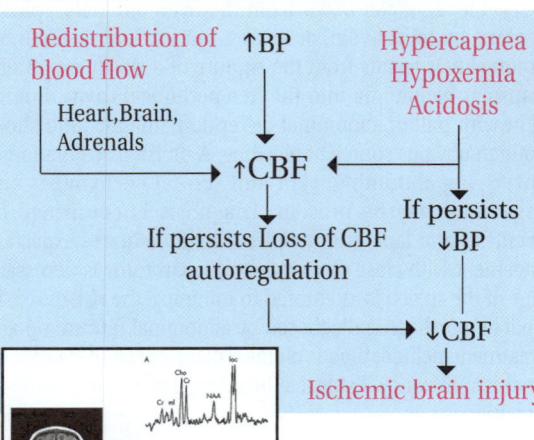

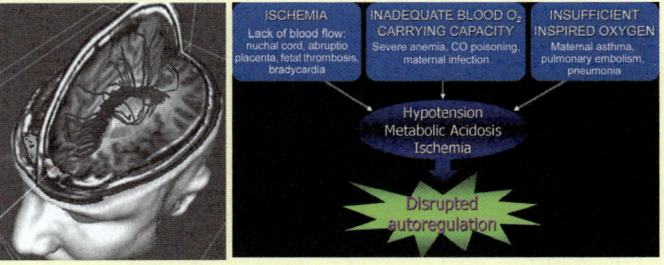

Fibre tracking which in the future may be possible using diffusion tensor imaging. If successful, this technique has huge potential in furthering our understanding of preterm white matter damage.

MR spectroscopy and chemical shift imaging : MR spectroscopy can provide early supplementary prognostic information in Neonatal Encephalopathy (A) H MR spectrum from left basal ganglia showing appreciably raised lactate and reduced N-acetyl aspartate (NAA). (B) P MR spectrum from the whole brain showing severe secondary energy failure with phosphocreatine (PCr) and ATP depletion and increased inorganic phosphate (Pi). The brain pHi was alkaline (7.18). PME, Phosphomonoesters; PDE, phosphodiesters; Cho, choline; Cr, creatine; mI, myo-inositol; lac, lactate.

REVIEW OF CLINICAL PROBLEMS

1. How do you diagnose the Hypoxic-Ischemic encephalopathy syndrome in the Newborn ?
Ans: Refer to No 2 of the "BIRD'S EYE VIEW/OVERVIEW/SYNOPSIS" of the Chapter.

2. How do you assess the severity of the Hypoxic-Ischemic encephalopathy syndrome in the Newborn ?
Ans: Refer to the Tables 4, 5 and 6 of the Chapter.

3. Mention the indications for intubation and ventilation while managing a Newborn with HIE?
Ans: Refer to the Evaluation-Decision-Action Plan/Algorithm to diagnose and manage a Neonate with HIE.

4. What are the prognostic factors to consider to counsel the parents about the Newborn baby with HIE?
Ans: Refer to the Table 7 of the Chapter.

5. How do you monitor for Multi Organ Dysfunction (MODS) Syndrome associated with HIE and manage it ?
Ans: Refer to the Table 2 of the Chapter.

LEARNING OBJECTIVES

After completing this article, readers will be able to

1. Understand that HIE is a multisystem syndromic illness with predominant CNS insult.
2. Assess and manage the ensuing complications of HIE.
3. Recognize perinatal conditions that increase risk for traumatic or hypoxic-ischemic injury.
4. Know the outcome and long-term sequelae of traumatic and hypoxic-ischemic birth injury.
5. Coordinate comprehensive follow-up for these sequelae.

Pearl/Peril/Pitfall : Future strategies to prevent or treat perinatal asphyxia/ HIE will explore the efficacy of multitiered combination therapies, because it is unlikely that a single "magic bullet" agent will effectively inhibit the complex and dynamic cascades of HI injury.

BIRD'S EYE VIEW/OVERVIEW/SYNOPSIS

1. *Perinatal asphyxia* is characterized by a) APGARscore 0–3 at >5 minutes b)Umbilical cord arterial pH <7.0 c)Umbilical cord arterial base deficit >16mmol/L d)Neonatal neurological sequelae including depression, Hypoxic - Ischemic Encephalopathy (HIE), hypoxic-ischemic brain injury e)Evidence of multiorgan system dysfunction in the immediate neonatal period f)Evidence for a prolonged acute hypoxic-ischemic event in labor (refer to Table 1) - 1)evidence of a major 'sentinel' hypoxic event, e.g. a ruptured uterus, antepartum hemorrhage, cord prolapse or amniotic fluid embolism, i.e. something that significantly changes normal fetal oxygenation in labour; 2)evidence of possible fetal compromise ('distress') from the time of the sentinel event, e.g. major changes in the fetal heart rate and/or fetal acidosis on fetal blood sampling; and 3)neonatal ultrasound evidence of recent cerebral edema and/or intracerebral hemorrhage.

2. *Hypoxic-Ischemic Encephalopathy (HIE)* is diagnosed by a)an abnormal neurologic examination on the first day following birth complicated by the perinatal asphyxia suggested by the criteria mentioned above b)seizures within first 24-48hrs after birth (50% of seizures are *not asphyxial*) c)multiorgan dysfunction (refer to Table 2) d)burst-suppression pattern on EEG e)need for positive pressure ventilation for >1minute or first cry delayed > 5minutes f)evidence of HIE changes on MRI brain imaging with Diffusion-Weighted Images (DWI)/MR spectroscopy. g)Exclusion of other causes of encephalopathy, such as septicemia, meningitis, metabolic disturbances, cyanotic congenital heart disease, and structural brain anomalies.

3. Always remember the fact that hypoxia and ischemia can occur postnatally *de novo, and* may be caused by 1)failure of oxygenation as a result of severe forms of cyanotic congenital heart disease or severe pulmonary disease; 2)anemia severe enough to lower the oxygen content of the blood (severe hemorrhage, hemolytic disease); 3)shock severe enough to interfere with the transport of oxygen to vital organs from overwhelming sepsis, massive blood loss, and intracranial or adrenal hemorrhage.

4. Hypoxic-ischemic brain damage is a gradually evolving process, which begins during the insult and extends beyond the resuscitation period, although the initial brain injury is related to hypoxia and ischemia, subsequent reperfusion and generation of free radicals contributes to ongoing injury. The initial hypoxic-ischemic injury results in an area of infarction. the immediate area surrounding this area is termed as penumbra. The penumbra continues to show adverse changes in the form of neuronal necrosis or apoptosis (programmed cell death) even after the hypoxic insult is over. It is possible that these post-hypoxic changes in the penumbra area may be amenable to therapeutic interventions.The mechanisms of neuronal damage in HIE are heterogeneous and include the participation of circulatory factors (dysregulation of the cerebral blood flow), metabolic factors (increased anaerobic metabolism, decreased ATP, hypoglycemia, hyperlactacidemia) and biochemical factors (increased excitatory amino acids, intracellular accumulation of calcium, dysfunction of calcium-binding proteins, activation of nitric oxide synthesis, production of free radicals). These pathogenetic mechanisms of HIE are the basis for the development of new neuroprotective therapies aimed to prevent neuronal damage. Good supportive therapy is essential for the first 48hrs of post-asphyxial period to reduce neuronal injury of the penumbra area, the extent of penumbra and the duration for which these adverse changes continue is variable. The phase may also provide a therapeutic window for newer modes of therapy in asphyxiated neonates.

5. A baby who fails to initiate or sustained respiration needs admission to a SCBU and should be closely monitored to rule out hypoxic-ischemic encephalopathy with an aim to limit secondary damage. In the immediate phase, careful attention to ventilatory status and adequate oxygenation, blood pressure, hemodynamic status, acid-base balance, and possible infection is important. Aggressive treatment of seizures (Refer to Table 3) is critical and may necessitate continuous EEG monitoring. *Prevent secondary hypoxia or hypotension due to complications of HIE.*

6. Infants who have brain injury related to perinatal asphyxia almost uniformly manifest multiorgan injury that must be anticipated, appreciated, and managed vigorously and proactively. (Refer to Table 2) for the features of multiorgan dysfunction and their systemic evaluation. The syndrome evolves gradually over the first 72hrs of life. The syndrome can be mild/moderate/severe and is best categorized by Sarnat's classification (Refer to Table 4). Levene scoring is a simplified scheme to assess HIE routinely Refer to Table 6).

7. Subsequent management of HIE (after 72 hrs) consists of 1)Continuous monitoring to assess metabolic status and homeostasis. 2)Special investigations to evaluate extent of damage: *Imaging-neurosonogram, CT, MRI etc. each has its own limitations. *Functional studies:SPECT, PET etc. *Prognosticating: *Maximum Length Sequence* BERA, S100 proteins levels and *amplitude integrated EEG* etc. (still quite experimental).

8. *The Evaluation-Decision-Action-Plan/Algorithm* to diagnose and manage Perinatal asphyxia and HIE gives detailed practical management of HIE and its acute complications. Newer modes of therapy such as a)induced hypothermia of whole body or of the head b) neuro-protective drugs such as allopurinol, superoxide dismutase, alpha tocopherol, nimodipine, indomethacin, magnesium are not ready for routine use (still experimental). Corticosteroids and mannitol have no role in the management of HIE.The treatment of HIE urgently needs a collective effort to find practical solutions. The goal should be set high: the elimination of perinatal brain damage.

9. Infants with mild encephalopathy all survive, and most are developmentally normal on follow-up. Moderate encephalopathy carries a 5% mortality risk and a 15% chance of late disability. More severe encephalopathy carries a 100% risk of death or disability. Other predictors of a poor outcome include inability to control seizures, a burst suppression pattern on an electroencephalogram not related to anticonvulsants, and selected brain imaging abnormalities.

10. Close neurodevelopmental follow-up for evidence of cerebral palsy (only 5–10% of cases) and cognitive defects is important during the early recovery period from perinatal asphyxia. Appropriate referrals to various specialists such as physical, occupational and speech therapists, orthopedic, ophthalmic and ENT specialists, pediatric neurologist and pediatric surgeon in cases of severe gastroesophageal reflux disease for fundoplication and social support services should be made (*multi-disciplinary team management*).

---

*Pearl/Peril/Pitfall: Management of Perinatal HIE-*Prevention of intrauterine asphyxia *Supportive treatment Maintenance of adequate ventilation, Maintenance of adequate cerebrovascular perfusion, Maintenance of adequate blood glucose levels *Treatment of complications Seizures Cerebral edema *Neuroprotective treatment.*

THE EVALUATION-DECISION-ACTION-PLAN/ALGORITHM TO DIAGNOSE and MANAGE
A NEONATE WITH PERINATAL ASPHYXIA INCLUDING HYPOXIC-ISCHEMIC ENCEPHALOPATHY (HIE)

SUBJECTIVE FINDINGS

Hx of Symptoms suggestive of an encephalopathy, i.e. reduced consciousness, seizures, poor feeding, limpy baby with reduced spontaneous movements *Assess* the various clinical settings involving the risk factors for perinatal asphyxia and HIE - refer to Table 1

Communicate with obstetrician to have a clear idea of the perinatal events, including the details of resuscitation, APGAR scores (<3 at 5 minutes?)

OBJECTIVE FINDINGS

Assess airway, breathing, circulation and disability by observing the vitals, BP, O_2 sats, color, CRT, pulses, sensorium, focal neurologic deficits, seizures, abnormal movements, tone and reflexes, etc.

Identify the multiorgan dysfunction - CNS, cardiac, pulmonary, renal, hematological, metabolic and GI tract signs and symptoms (refer to Table 2)

Perform complete physical examination from head to toe including detailed neurological examination.
Look for an evidence for birth trauma.

INVESTIGATIONS

Blood Hb, hematocrit, WBC, Differential count, platelets,Group/Type and Crossmatch, blood sugar, BUN, creatinine, ABG analysis and electrolytes, serum calcium, magnesium, Coagulation studies, serum bilirubin, LFTs, creatine kinase-BB-(blood and CSF)
Urine Analysis, Sp Gr, osmolality, electrolytes
Imaging-MRI Diffusion-Weighted-Images (DWI) to reveal cytotoxic edema, within hours of the insult; tCT brain scanning - determines the extent of cerebral edema at 2-4days after the insult
Electroencephalography to define burst-suppression, continuous low voltage, or isoelectric patterns

---

Assess the clinical severity at the time of admission and obtain serial recordings 4 times a day (either by Levene scoring or by Sarnat staging).

A Neonate with Perinatal Asphyxia and Hypoxic-Ischemic-Encephalopathy (HIE)

Prevent perinatal asphyxia by applying safe obstetric management of high-risk deliveries and prompt delivery room management of asphyxiated babies

---

Exclude other causes of Neonatal depression and encephalopathy (refer to the Table 1)

Provide Supplemental oxygen to maintain SaO_2 88 to 95% in term and 88 to 92% in preterm

Maintain the airway patent (position the neck in neutral position, suction the naso/oropharynx gently, pass NG tube and aspirate the stomach and put the baby nil oral until seizures are well controlled).

Intubate and ventilate for frequent apneas, hypoventilation secondary to anticonvulsants, associated lung problems like meconium aspiration syndrome, pulmonary hypertension, pneumothorax, hypercarbia(>50 mm Hg) *maintain* pCo_2 at 35-45mm Hg avoiding either hyper or under ventilation so that cerebral vasodilation and relative ischemia are preventable.

Perform sepsis screen (consider LP) and give antibiotics if clinically indicated

Monitor for renal function and manage renal failure conservatively; consider peritoneal dialysis if CNS prognosis is good

Observe for NEC, aspirate gastric contents. *Maintain* caution and patience with enteral feeds. *Monitor* LFTs-ALT, AST, clotting (PT, PTT, fibrinogen), albumin , bilirubin, and ammonia, drug levels where appropriate

Don't try experimental neuroprotective strategies until their efficacy and safety are proven (e.g. allopurinol, superoxide dismutase, magnesium sulfate, vitamin E, indomethacin, nimodipine, etc.). *Induced hypothermia* (selective head or whole body) also cannot be recommended at the moment

Communicate with parents effectively and *give* guarded prognosis and *smear with* godly benevolence and hope in moderate to severe HIE

Withdraw Ventilatory support after discussing with parents, if EEG shows sustained low-voltage states or burst - suppression persisting >6 hours and abnormal Doppler cerebral flow velocities, appearing by 24 hours

Ensure ABCs, Supplemental O_2, IV, UAC,UVC access, , *Monitor* BP, pulses, CRT, CR monitor, Pulse oximetry, temperature, urine output, intake-output chart, ABG analysis, Hypoglycemia

Treat shock and maintain BP and MAP >40mm Hg in term infants (NIBP or IBP) with fluid boluses(10ml/kg NS over 20 minutes) and Inotropes -low dose Dopamine (2 to 5 microgram/kg/min) in combination with Dobutamine (5 to 15 microgram/kg/min) if no response within 30 minutes

Treat hypoglycemia (<45mg/dL) avoiding hyperglycemia (>140 mg/dL, i.e. (maintain Euglycemia(60–100mg/dL)

Treat seizures if frequent (>1/hour), prolonged (one or more minutes), or interfering with respiration or ventilation. IV phenobarbital 20mg/kg as a loading dose is the drug of choice; if seizures continue, give an additional loading dose of 10–20mg/kg IV. Start maintenance dose of 3-5mg/kg/day PO/IV divided BID, 12-24 hours after the loading dose. Consider Phenytoin, midazolam, lorazepam, etc.if necessary (refer to the Table No. 3 for details about anticonvulsants)

Restrict fluids to 20% <maintenance for first 48 hours (anticipating SIADH or renal failure) Monitor fluid balance, infant's weight, serum electrolytes and osmolality, urine specific gravity and urinanalysis. Aim for neutral fluid balance (i.e. replacement of losses)

Identify hypothermia and maintain the environmental temperature in thermoneutral range avoiding hyperthermia

Monitor for hypocalcemia and hypomagnesemia and maintain them within the normal range

Check clotting, give vitamin K. *Treat* DIC with FFP, clotting factors, platelet transfusions, as necessary

Maintain the hematocrit >40% but below 55%; treat polycythemia and bring the hematocrit to <55% by partial exchange transfusion using normal saline.

Treat raised ICP by fluid restriction, adequate ventilation, oxygenation, perfusion, aggressive treatment of seizures, avoiding thermal and metabolic stress: no indications for hyperventilation, corticosteroids, prophylactic anticonvulsants. Role of Mannitol-though not beneficial evidently, in practice it can be used (20% Mannitol IVI 3-5ml/kg q 8hr x 3doses) if the seizures are intractable associated with bulging AF and USG evidence of raised ICP. Avoid Mannitol in preterms

---

Pearl/Peril/Pitfall: No diagnostic tests conclusively prove that a given magnitude of asphyxia has led to a specific neurological injury. Acute perinatal and intrapartum events have been found in only about 20% of children diagnosed as having cerebral palsy. Counseling the parents with realistic explanations about their infant's clinical status and prognosis is always recommended.

TABLE 1	Etiological factors in perinatal asphyxia

A. Factors that increase the risk of perinatal asphyxia include the following:

1. Impairment of maternal oxygenation.
2. Decreased blood flow from mother to placenta
3. Decreased blood flow from placenta to fetus
4. Impaired gas exchange across the placenta or at the fetal tissue level
5. Increased fetal O_2 requirement.

B. Etiologies of perinatal hypoxia-ischemia include the following:

1. Maternal factors: hypertension (acute or chronic), infection, diabetes, hypotension, vascular disease, drug use, and hypoxia due to pulmonary, cardiac or neurologic disease.
2. Placental factors; infarction, fibrosis, abruption, or hydrops.
3. Uterine rupture
4. Umbilical cord accidents: prolapse, entanglement, true knot, compression.
5. Abnormalities of umbilical vessels.
6. Fetal factors: anemia, infection, cardiomyopathy, hydrops, severe cardiac/circulatory insufficiency.
7. Neonatal factors: severe neonatal hypoxia due to cyanotic congenital heart disease, persistent pulmonary hypertension of the newborn (PPHN), cardiomyopathy, other forms of neonatal cardiogenic and/or septic shock

Caveats about Perinatal Asphyxia*

Most of the concepts of HIE have been derived from adult models of stroke. ● In the fetus and newborn, development of brain function becomes an important factor in the manifestation of brain injury. ● The timing of the HI insult becomes especially important in relation to the delivery of the fetus. ● The clinical end point of asphyxia, a metabolic parameter, does not readily translate into a definitive syndrome of brain injury. ● A long latent period is necessary for clinical manifestations of brain deficits. ● The extent of brain injury can be manifested as a spectrum in terms of severity and areas of involvement. ● * Tan S, Parks A. *Clin Perinatol* 1999;26:733-734. HI: hypoxic-ischemic; HIE: hypoxic-ischemic encephalopathy

TABLE 2	Multiorgan dysfunction after perinatal asphyxia - evaluation and management

Organ system	*Manifestation of dysfunction*	*Management*
CNS	Seizures ; apneas ; raised intra-cranial pressure ; intracranial bleeding ; nerve palsies.	Refer to the EDA Algorithm
Respiratory	Respiratory distress due to sur-factant deficiency; ARDS;apnea; PPHN; pulmonary hemorrhage; Meconium aspiration.	Ventilate ; measure--blood gases;correct acidosis;
Cardiovascular	Shock;hypotension;cardiomegaly; heart failure ; ECG evidence of ischemia.	Ventilate; give inotropes ; fluid restriction ; diuretics
Renal	Oliguria; hematuria;proteinuria; myoglobinuria;renal failure	Fluid restriction ; careful monitoring consider dialysis if CNS prognosis good
Hematological	DIC; raised white cell count; raised nucleated red cell count Thrombocytopenia	Vitamin K; fresh frozen plasma; cryoprecipitate;Platelet transfusion cover for infection
Metabolic	Hypoglycemia;hypocal-cemia; hyponatremia	Replace lost ions;careful fluid balance
Gastrointestinal	Ileus; Necrotizing Entero Colitis (NEC)	Start enteral feeds cautiously, treat NEC
Hepatic	Elevated transaminases/ ammonia ; prolonged coagulation times; jaundice DIC-Disseminated Intra-vascular Coagulation	Vitamin K:support coagulation;photo-therapy/exchange| transfusion as indicated

TABLE 3	Anticonvulsants to treat seizures in the newborn

Drug	Loading dose	Maintenance dose	Important clinical notes
a. Phenobarbitone (drug of first choice)	20mg/kg/dose slow IV over 20 minutes	3-5mg/kg/day in 2 d.d start 12 hrs after the loading dose	*If seizures persist after completion of the first loading dose, repeat 10 mg/kg/ dose every 20 minutes till a loading dose of 40mg/kg has been given.
b. Lorazepam	....	0.1 mg/kg IV bolus over 2–5 minutes	*Duration of action 12–24 hrs; less CVS effects when used with Phenobarbitone; may repeat in 10–15 minutes
c. Phenytoin	20mg/kg	5 mg/kg day in 2d.d not recommended	*only to be mixed with normal saline *can cause Arrhythmias and hypotension *Give at a rate of not >1mg/kg/mt under ECG /BP monitoring
d. Midazolam	150*mcg*/kg IV bolus	1–5 *mcg*/kg/mt IV infusion	Ultra short acting Benzodiazepine with half - life 1.5 - 3.5 hours

Pearl/Peril/Pitfall : Potential adverse effects of induced hypothermia (risk increased with depth of hypothermia) include: Increased blood viscosity, mild metabolic acidosis, cardiac arrhythmias, decreased oxygen availability, dysfunction of cellular immunity, coagulation abnormalities and platelet dysfunction, intracellular shift of potassium and choreic syndrome.

Neonatal Encephalopathy: Neonatal Encephalopathy (NE) is "a clinically defined syndrome of disturbed neurological function in the earliest days of life in the term infant, manifested by difficulty with initiating and maintaining respiration, depression of tone and reflexes, sub normal level of consciousness and often seizures". NE occurs in approximately 3.5–6/1000 live births and usually affects the full term infant. The terminology NE is preferred to Hypoxic Ischemic Encephalopathy (HIE) as it is not always possible to document a significant hypoxic-ischemic insult and there are potentially several other etiologies. The differential diagnosis of NE includes *Perinatal hypoxia-ischemia (19–52%) *Infection *Cerebral infarction *Intracranial hemorrhage *Congenital brain malformations *Inborn errors of metabolism *Genetic syndromes. The requirement for investigation to exclude these possibilities will depend on the presentation, history and clinical features of the individual case. Hypoxic-ischemic encephalopathy (HIE) is reserved for the subgroup of term NE who have convincing evidence of intrapartum hypoxia; the criteria of which have been outlined by the International Cerebral Palsy Taskforce. *ESSENTIAL CRITERIA for the diagnosis of HIE, in the neonatal period* *Metabolic acidosis (pH<7, base deficit=12 mmol/L in fetal, cord or early neonatal samples)
* Early onset moderate or severe encephalopathy *SUGGESTIVE CRITERIA* *Sentinel event immediately before or during labor
* Sudden and sustained fetal bradycardia following sentinel event
* Apgar score =6 for longer than 5 minutes *Early evidence of multisystem involvement *Early imaging evidence of abnormality consistent with hypoxia-ischemia.

INSULT

Therapeutic Window :
Hypothermia
Other

Primary energy failure (Minutes)
Na+ overload
Excitotoxicity
Reperfusion

Cerebral metabolism transiently recovers
Ca++ overload
ROS, NO

Secondary phase (Hours to days)
Between 6-72 h after insult
Mitochondrial dysfunction
Caspases activation

Hypoxic ischemic brain injury

IMMEDIATE necrotic cell death

DELAYED apoptotic cell death

Interventions NEED TO BE WITHIN 6 hrs of insult

Pathophysiology of hypoxic-ischemic brain injury in the developing brain. During the initial phase of energy failure, glutamate mediated excitotoxicity and Na+/K+ ATPase failure lead to necrotic cell death. After transient recovery of cerebral energy metabolism, a secondary phase of apoptotic neuronal death occurs. ROS = reactive oxygen species.

Therapeutic hypothermia when applied within 6 hours of birth and maintained for 48–72 hours is a promising therapy for mild-to-moderate cases of hypoxic-ischemic encephalopathy. Many components of its implementation remain to be optimized, including the following:
* Determining optimal timing of initiation of hypothermia therapy: Cooling must begin early, within 1 hour of injury, if possible; however, a favorable outcome may be possible if the cooling begins as long as 6 hours after injury. To this effect, the feasibility and safety of cooling on transport has been described.
* Determining optimal timing of initiation of hypothermia therapy: The greater the severity of the initial injury, the longer the duration of hypothermia needed for optimal neuroprotection. The optimal duration of brain cooling in the human newborn has not been established.
* Determining which method of cooling is best: Two methods have been used in clinical trials: selective head cooling and whole body cooling. In selective head cooling, a cap (CoolCap) with channels for circulating cold water is placed over the infant's head, and a pumping device facilitates continuous circulation of cold water. Nasopharyngeal or rectal temperature is then maintained at 34–35°C for 72 hours. For whole body hypothermia, the infant is placed on a commercially available cooling blanket, through which circulating cold water flows, so that the desired level of hypothermia is reached quickly and maintained for 72 hours. The relative merits and limitations of these 2 methods have not been established.

* Determining optimal rewarming method: In clinical trials, rewarming was carried out gradually, over a 6-8 hour period.
* Improving selection of candidates for hypothermia therapy using EEG and/or aEEG: Predefined subgroup analysis in the CoolCap trial suggested that head cooling had no effect in infants with the most severe aEEG changes but was beneficial only in infants with less severe aEEG changes.
* Establishing long term benefits by providing long term follow-up of all infants undergoing hypothermia therapy

Several meta-analysis have been conducted and indicate that that therapeutic hypothermia is beneficial to term newborns with hypoxic-ischemic encephalopathy.

Pearl/Peril/Pitfall: Continuation of seizure medications should depend on evolving CNS symptoms and EEG findings. In most infants who are developing normally and have a normal EEG before hospital discharge, phenobarbital is discontinued within 3-4 weeks of birth. In those with significant CNS disability with or without persistent episodes of seizures, phenobarbital is continued for 3-6 months; the decision to wean off the drug depends on later changes in EEG and clinical course

HIE and neuroprotective strategies; still experimental!

Strategies	Interventions
Cerebral metabolic rate	Hypothermia
Block NMDA receptor channel	Magnesium
Glutamate release	Adenosine
	Adenosine agonists
	Adenosine uptake inhibitors
Inhibit voltage-sensitive Ca++channels	Free radical scavengers
	Allopurinol
	Vitamin C, E
	Superoxide dismutase (SOD)
Prevent free radical formation	Indomethacin
	Iron chelators
	Allopurinol
	NOS inhibitors
Inflammatory response	Allopurinol
	Inflammatory antagonists
	(blocking 1L-1 and TNF-α, steroids)
Attenuate apoptosis pathway	Caspase inhibitors

Amplitude integrated EEG (aEEG) tracing on cerebral function monitor. Top panel displays raw EEG, bottom panel displays compressed tracing. Note single seizure on compressed tracing. Reproduced with permission of BrainZ Instruments Limited, Mt. Wellington, Auckland, New Zealand.

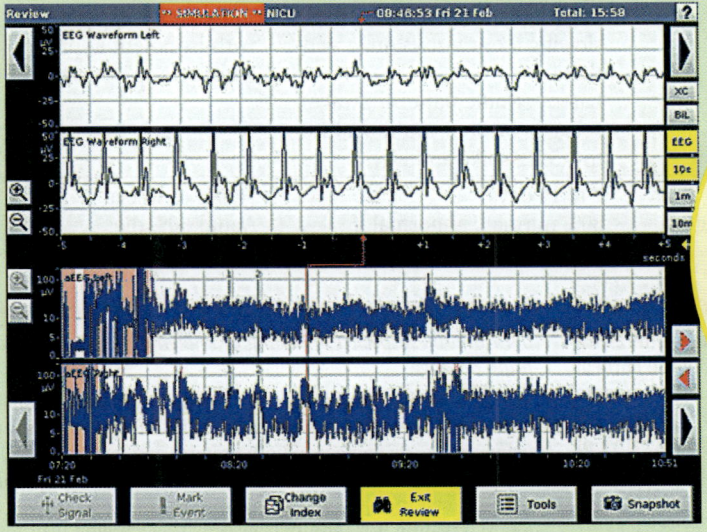 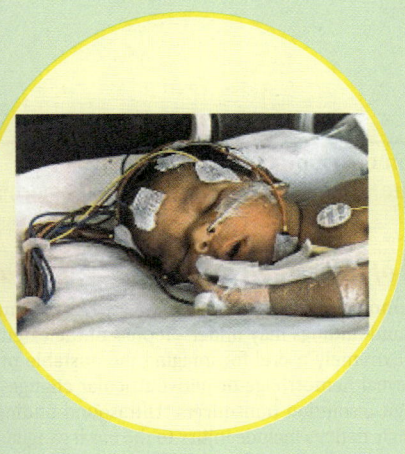

Amplitude Integrated Encephalogram: There is a vital organ in the body of the Neonate that we fail to monitor, and that organ is the brain. We now have a tool that can monitor the brain on a continuous basis, which is complementary to traditional clinical assessment, conventional EEG, and advanced neuroimaging techniques. According to Dr. Terrie Inder, MD, Adjunct Associate Professor, Department of Neurology, at Washington University in St. Louis (Missouri), an amplitude integrated encephalogram (aEEG) is a tool we should be using to advance our understanding of what is happening inside the brain of term and preterm infants, to improve care and to make better decisions regarding treatment of infants with possible brain injury. The clinical tool used is the cerebral function monitor (CFM), a bedside technique for evaluation of functional integrity of the brain by measuring the aEEG. Using a pair of biparietally placed hydrogel electrodes, signals from each brain hemisphere are amplified and filtered. These signals are continuously displayed on the monitor in a time-compressed format. Some monitors also display the continuous raw EEG tracing and allow users to expand events of interest seen on the compressed wave to view the raw EEG and more closely evaluate these events . One possible application of the aEEG is to determine which babies are candidates for hypothermia therapy. Practical experience with CFMs has shown that infants who have suffered hypoxic-ischemic encephalopathy often have seizures that are not detected clinically, but are readily apparent on aEEG. In addition, continuous aEEG monitoring allows the recognition of abnormal background activity, which reflects brain injury.

Pearl/Peril/Pitfall: A pediatric neurologist should help assist in the management of seizures, interpretation of EEG, and overall care of the infant with hypoxic-ischemic encephalopathy. The neurologist should also work with the primary care physician to address long-term disabilities. A developmental specialist can also help plan for long-term assessments and care.

TABLE 4	Sarnat HB, Sarnat MS classification of Hypoxic-Ischemic Encephalopathy		
Stage	**Stage 1 (mild)**	**Stage 2 (moderate)**	**Stage 3 (severe)**
Level of consciousness	Hyperalert ; irritable	Lethargic or obtunded	Stuporous, comatose
Neuromuscular control	Uninhibited, overreactive	Diminished spontaneous movement	Diminished or absent spontaneous movement
Muscle tone	Normal	Mild hypotonia	Flaccid
Posture	Mild distal flexion	Strong distal flexion	Intermittent decerebration
Stretch reflexes	Overactive disinhibited	Decreased or absent	
Segmental myoclonus	Present or absent	Present	Absent
Complex reflexes	Normal	Suppressed	Absent
Suck	Weak	Weak or Absent	Absent
Moro	Strong, low threshold	Weak, incomplete high threshold	Absent
Oculovestibular	Normal	Overactive	Weak or Absent
Tonic neck	Slight	Strong	Absent
Automatic function:	Generalized sympathetic	Generalized parasympathetic	Both systems depressed
Pupils	Mydriasis	Miosis	Mid position, often unequal; Poor light reflex
Respirations	Spontaneous	Spontaneous; occasional apnea	Periodic ; apnea
Heart rate	Tachycardia	Bradycardia	Variable
Bronchial and salivary secretions	Spares	Profuse	Variable
Gastrointestinal motility	Normal or decreased	Increased diarrhea	Variable
Seizures	None	Common focal or multifocal (6 to 24 hours of age)	Uncommon (excluding decerebration)
Electroencephalographic findings	Normal (awake)	Early : generalized low-voltage, slowing (continuous delta and theta) Later:periodic pattern (awake); seizures focal or multifocal;1.0 to 1.5 Hz spike and wave	Early:periodic pattern with isopotential phases Later:totally isopotential
Duration of symptoms	<24 hours	2 to 14 days	Hours to weeks
Outcome	About 100% normal	80% normal ; abnormal if symptoms more than 5 to7days	About 50% die;

Role of Neuroimaging and EEG in the assessment and monitoring of Hypoxic-Ischemic-Encephalopathy

1. **Ultrasonography:** *Insensitive to cortical damage, therefore ultrasound findings may under - represent the extent of the cortical lesion*Extremely useful for imaging the unstable preterm Neonate (may reveal hemorrhage or periventricular changes) if performed with high-resolution transducers *Ultrasound findings suggestive of neurologic deficits include injury to the basal ganglia, periventricular echodensities, and presence of focal/multifocal parenchymal lesions.

2. **CT Brain scan:** *Useful for demonstrating focal ischemic lesions commonly seen in the left middle cerebral artery distribution and to determine the extent of bleeding in an emergency situation when MRI is not available *Often not helpful in making a diagnosis of HIE because it is insensitive to changes in water content.

3. **MRI Brain scan:** *The diagnostic modality of choice particularly when accompanied by diffusion-weighted images (DWI).
*DWI reveals restricted water diffusion not apparent on conventional MRI, by detecting differences in the rates of diffusion of water protons *In the term infant, absence of signal in the posterior limb of the internal capsule is strongly associated with poor neurologic outcome *MRI is more sensitive than ultrasound in identifying PVL changes in a preterm baby. *The combination of T1- and T2-weighted MR imaging and diffusion-weighted imaging is best for the detection of hypoxic-ischemic brain injury in the early neonatal period in term-born infants. FLAIR and contrast-enhanced imaging do not contribute to this. Contrast-enhanced imaging does not seem to be warranted in term-born infants suspected of having or known to have hypoxic-ischemic brain damage.*

4. **Proton magnetic resonance spectroscopy(MRS):** *Useful for depicting age-dependent changes in preterm infant *A powerful tool for diagnosing early damage in both preterm and term infants *Provides a quantitative in vivo measure of brain biochemistry *At long echo times, it can measure resonance intensities for N-acetyl aspartate (NAA), creatine (Cr), and phosphocreatine, choline (Cho), and lactate. *The measure of NAA in reference to baseline Cr or Cho has provided a sensitive indicator of neuronal integrity, where as lactate has indicated the presence of oxidative stress or ongoing injury.*MRS is now being used more extensively to identify areas at risk in perinatal HIE.

5. **EEG (Electroencephalogram):** *Helpful in determining the severity of the insult and in supporting the diagnosis of HIE *Amplitude - integrated EEG is an aid to identify Newborns moderately to severely compromised by hypoxic - ischemic injury *The initial change is a suppression of amplitude and frequency. This followed after 24 hours by a periodic pattern that consists of periods of greater voltage suppression interspersed with bursts of sharp and slow waves. *Subsequently, a "burst suppression" pattern with fever bursts and more severe voltage depression is seen, followed by an isoelectric tracing.

Pearl/Peril/Pitfall: Serum electrolytes—In severe cases, daily assessment of serum electrolytes are valuable until the infant's status improves. Markedly low serum sodium, potassium, and chloride levels in the presence of reduced urine flow and excessive weight gain may indicate acute tubular damage or inappropriate antidiuretic hormone (IADH), particularly during the initial 2-3 days of life. - Similar changes may be seen during recovery; increased urine flow may indicate ongoing tubular damage and excessive sodium loss relative to water loss

TABLE 5	Neonatal morbidity index			
	0	1	2	3
5" Apgar	>6	5–6	3–4	0–2
Base Deficit (mEq/l)	<10	10–14	15–19	>19
FHR Trace	Normal	Variable deceleration	Late	Bradycardia deceleration

(Carter et al Clin.perinatol. June 1993)

NMI score <3: Risk least, MMI score more: Higher risk
* A cluster of abnormal perinatal signs, d epressed APGARs and multiorgan dysfunction, with an encephalopathy, is associated with later neurodevelopmental problems.

TABLE 6	Levene score—a simplified scheme for assessing the clinical severity of the HIE syndrome	
Grade I (mild)	**Grade II (moderate)**	**Grade III (severe)**
Irritability	Lethargy	Coma
Hyperalert	Seizures	Prolonged seizures
Mild hypotonia	Marked abnormalities of tone	Severe hypotonia
Poor sucking	Requirement for tube feeding	Failure to maintain spontaneous respiration

TABLE 7	Poor prognostic indicators in perinatal asphyxia and HIE

1. Severe prolonged asphyxia
2. Sarnat stage 3 of HIE
3. Early onset seizures (<12hrs) that are difficult to control
4. Oliguria in first 36hrs of life (<1ml/kg/hr)
5. Abnormal neurologic signs at discharge
6. Elevated CK-BB (Creatine Kinase-Brain Bound) level
7. Burst suppression pattern on EEG
8. Abnormal MRI

KEY POINTS FOR CLINICAL PRACTICE

1. To diagnose HIE syndrome it is necessary to ascertain positive features, together with excluding alternative conditions that may mimic some of the clinical features.

2. The initial step in management of HIE is early identification of those infants at greatest risk for evolving to the syndrome of Hypoxic—Ischemic Encephalopathy.

3. Ultrasound has limited utility in evaluation of hypoxic injury in the term infant; it is the preferred imaging modality in evaluation of the preterm infant. CT has limited ability to identify cortical injury within the 1st few days of life. Diffusion-weighed MRI is the preferred choice because of its increased sensitivity and specificity early in the process and its ability to outline the topography of the lesion.

4. Current clinically available agents to treat asphyxiated human Newborns include phenobarbital, magnesium sulphate, allopurinol, calcium channel blockers, vitamin C, vitamin E, and hypothermia and are largely supportive and unlikely to directly affect outcome. Future treatments, which hold promise or offer a novel approach to treat hypoxic-ischemia, are monosialog-angliosides, growth factors, gene therapy with anti-apoptotic agents (bcl-2) or calcium binding proteins (calbindin-D28k), and immunization against the NMDA receptor.

5. The prognosis varies depending on whether the metabolic and cardiopulmonary complications (hypoxia, hypoglycemia, shock) are treated, the infant's gestational age (outcome is poorest if the infant is preterm), and the severity of the encephalopathy.

REFERENCES AND FURTHER READING : 1) Sarnat HB, Sarnat MS. Neonatal encephalopathy following fetal distress. Arch Neurol. 1976;33:696–705. **2)**Perlman JM. Brain injury in the term infant. Semin Perinatol. 2004;28:415-424 **3)** de Vries LS, Hellstrom-Westas L. Role of cerebral function monitoring in the newborn. Arch Dis Child Fetal Neonatal Ed. 2005;90:F201-F207 **4)** Rutherford MA, Azzopardi D, Whitelaw A, et al. Mild hypothermia and the distribution of cerebral lesions in neonates with hypoxic ischemic encephalopathy. Pediatrics. 2005;116:1001–1006 **5)**Gluckman PD, Wyatt JS, Azzopardi D, et al. Selective head cooling with mild systemic hypothermia after neonatal encephalopathy: multicentre randomized trial. Lancet. 2005;365:663-670.

Pearl/Peril/Pitfall: ABG: Blood gas monitoring is used to assess acid-base status and to avoid hyperoxia and hypoxia as well as hypercapnia and hypocapnia.

29 Neonatal Seizures

@ *"Not all clinical seizures are correlated with EEG changes and not all seizures shown on EEG recordings are clinically apparent"*

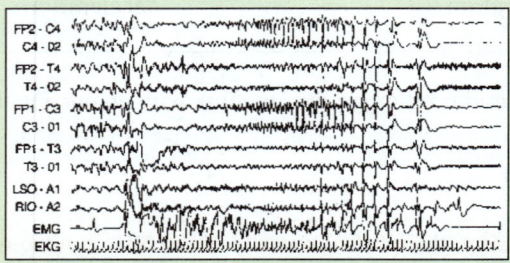

Most electroencephalographic seizures are unilateral and have a restricted electrical field. Seizures with bilateral electroencephalographic onset are rare .

An electroencephalographic seizure. Note generalized high voltage sharp waves followed by a period of depression and a sequence of rhythmic discharges with a well-defined onset, body, offset, and electrical field that do not have the appearance of an artifact or a physiologic activity.

The term electroclinical seizure refers to a clinical paroxysmal event that is associated with an electroencephalographic seizure. The term convulsion refers to an electroclinical seizure characterized by increased motor activity. The term clinically silent electroencephalographic seizure refers to a scalp-recorded electroencephalographic seizure that occurs during the course of normal neonatal activity. In neonates, clinically silent electroencephalographic seizures probably occur more frequently than electroclinical seizures.

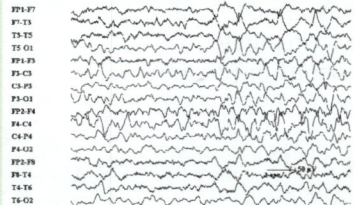

Onset of neonatal seizure demonstrating a focal onset in the right frontal (FP4) region. At this point, the child had head and eye deviation to the left.

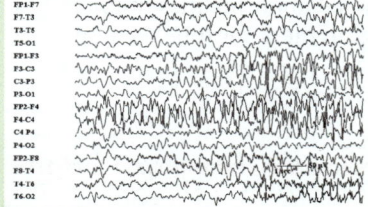

Twenty seconds into a seizure that had focal onset in the right frontal (FP4) region (see Image 1), the seizure shows a rhythmic buildup of activity in the right frontocentral region.

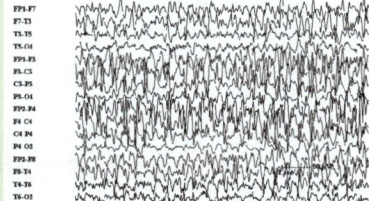

This seizure had focal onset in the right frontal (FP4) region and subsequent buildup of activity in the right frontocentral region (see Images 1 and 2). As the seizure evolves, the EEG shows diffuse involvement of both cerebral hemispheres.

REVIEW OF CLINICAL PROBLEMS

1. How do you differentiate seizures from jitteriness?
   Ans: Refer to the Table 2 of the Chapter.

2. Name the essential aspects of examination of a Newborn baby with seizures?
   Ans: Refer to THE EVALUATION-DECISION-ACTION-PLAN/ALGORITHM TO ASSESS and MANAGE NEONATAL SEIZURES.

3. Mention the first line of investigations in evaluating Neonatal seizures?
   Ans: Refer to THE EVALUATION-DECISION-ACTION-PLAN/ALGORITHM TO ASSESS and MANAGE NEONATAL SEIZURES.

4. How do you manage Neonatal Seizures?
   Ans: Refer to THE EVALUATION-DECISION-ACTION-PLAN/ALGORITHM TO ASSESS and MANAGE NEONATAL SEIZURES.

5. Mention the 7 Caveats in recognizing Neonatal Seizures.
   Ans: Refer to the Table 7 of the Chapter.

LEARNING OBJECTIVES

After completing this article, readers will be able to

1. Recognize seizures in the Newborn promptly and differentiate from the mimicking events.

2. Investigate further the underlying etiology of Neonatal seizures.

3. Identify the epileptic syndromes in the Newborn infant.

4. Monitor respiratory activity and BP when anticonvulsants are being used to treat seizures.

5. Explain the prognosis to the parents according to the underlying cause of Neonatal seizures.

Pearl/Peril/Pitfall: Subtle seizures are more common in fullterm than in premature infants. Video EEG studies have demonstrated that most subtle seizures are not associated with electrographic seizures. Examples of subtle seizures include chewing, pedaling, or ocular movements.

BIRD'S EYE VIEW/OVERVIEW/SYNOPSIS

1. A *seizure* is defined clinically as a paroxysmal alteration in neurologic function, i.e. behavioral, motor, or autonomic function, or all three with or without impairment of consciousness (Volpe 1989). *Five types* of seizures, based on clinical presentation are recognized in the Newborn ; SUBTLE (50%) (sucking, smacking, drooling, swimming, rowing, pedalling movements, apneic spell, eyelid blinking/ fluttering, tonic horizontal deviation of the eyes with or without jerking), CLONIC (25%) (focal /multi focal/ generalized), TONIC (5%) (focal/generalized), MYOCLONIC (20%) (focal/multi focal) and Non-paroxysmal repetitive behaviours. Subtle seizures are the most common subtybe, comprising about 50% of all seizures in term and premature Newborns. They are rarely isolated and are almost always occurring along with other seizure types as well. Most subtle seizures are not associated with EEG seizures and show poor response to conventional anticonvulsants and are considered nonepileptic "brainstem release phenomena". *Refer to* Table 1 which enlists the various disorders likely to cause Neonatal seizures.

2. Neonatal seizures may be difficult to recognize clinically, and seizure mimics like jitteriness, non-nutritive sucking etc. can be confused with Neonatal seizures. True epileptic seizures are rarely stimulus-sensitive. Epileptic seizures cannot be abolished by passive restraint or repositioning of the infant. Epileptic seizures are often associated with autono-mic changes or ocular phenomena. Jitteriness can be differentiated from seizures by the clinical features listed in Table 2. Jitteriness (sparing the face), movements during REM sleep rowing and bicycling movements, decorticate and decerebrate posturing and autonomic dysfunctions *can mimic seizures in the newborn period*, because of poorly developed cerebral cortical organization, synaptogenesis, myelination of cortical efferent pathways with weak propagation to surface electrodes and are fragmentary; advanced limbic system with connections to midbrain and brainstem leads to higher frequency of mouthing, eye deviation and apnoea in Neonates.

3. *Differentiate convulsive apnea from nonconvulsive type*: Heart rate - normal or accelerated for 20 seconds following its onset ; bradycardia occurs subsequently as a result of sustained hypoxemia, *in case of convulsive apnea* and it is often associated with other subtle phenomena mentioned above.
   (C/ F bradycardia at the onset of the episode in case of nonconvulsive apnea)

4. Studies using polygraphic EEG recording with video monitoring have greatly enhanced the char-acterization of Neonatal seizures and their medical management. *Refer to* Table 4 for EEG classification of Neonatal seizures.

5. *Hypoxic—Ischemic Encephalopathy (the most common cause of Neonatal Seizures—nearly 50%), CNS infection, intracranial haemorrhage, cerebral artery infarction, acute metabolic disturbances, constitute > 90% of aetiology of* Neonatal Seizures. Since very few are IDIOPATHIC (2–5%), further investigation and prompt diagnosis of underlying condition is very important. Benign Neonatal Seizures (BFNC–Benign Familial Neonatal Convulsions, BINC – Benign Idiopathic Neonatal Convulsions or 5th day fits, Benign Neonatal Sleep Myoclonus) are the diagnoses by "EXCLUSION"!

6. *The Evaluation-Decision-Action Plan/Algorithm* to diagnose and manage Neonatal seizures describes the essential aspects of assessment, evaluation and therapeutics of various types of Neonatal seizures. Table No 3 helps to consider the differential diagnosis of Neonatal seizures in relation to time of seizure onset. Several caveats useful in the evaluation for suspected Neonatal seizures (*Refer to* the Table 7).

7. Many inborn errors of metabolism cause generalized convulsions in the Neonate. These are often inherited as an autosomal recessive/X-linked recessive fashion. Urea cycle defects, maple syrup urine disease, organic acidopathies, mitochondrial encephalopathies etc. present with Neonatal seizures. *Refer to* the chapter devoted to Inborn Errors of Metabolism for a detailed discussion.

8. *Pyridoxine dependency*—a rare disorder, inherited as an autosomal recessive must be considered when Neonatal seizures are resistant to conventional anticonvulsants, such as phenobarbitone or phenytoin. IV pyridoxine 100–200 mg should be given with EEG recording. The seizures abruptly cease, and the EEG normalizes in the next few hours. Not all cases of pyridoxine dependency respond dramatically to the initial bolus of IV pyridoxine. So, a six week trial of oral pyridoxine (10–20mg/day) or pyridoxal phosphate is recommended for infants with high index of suspicion continues after a negative response to IV pyridoxine. These children require lifelong therapy with oral pyridoxine, 10mg/day. Untreated children have persistent seizures and are uniformly severely mentally retarded.

9. Use anticonvulsants, if there are >2 seizures/hr or if any one seizure lasts for 1 minute or more. Fewer seizures or seizures of shorter duration (despite multiple anticonvulsants) not causing cardio-respiratory compromise may be ignored in certain conditions like HIE stage III as they tend to "burn out" spontaneously. However, in cases where the etiology is not established a trial of inj pyridoxine or other anticonvulsants is warranted, unless EEG is normal during these clinical events. Monitor respiratory activity and BP as many of the Anticonvulsants cause respiratory depression and impair myocardial function. Assisted ventilation may be necessary if polypharmacy is warranted to stop seizures.

10. Explain prognosis to the parents according to the underlying cause— CNS malformations—poor neuro-developmental come ; Infection, HIE and Early Hypoglycemia—30–50% normal; Isolated Hypocalcemia and Benign Neonatal Convulsions – excellent. Effective Parental Communication is as important as the investigation and treatment of Neonatal Seizures.

Pearl/Peril/Pitfall: Jitteriness is not associated with ocular deviation. It is stimulus sensitive (e.g. easily stopped with passive movement of the limb). The movement resembles a tremor, and no autonomic changes are associated with it.

THE EVALUATION-DECISION-ACTION-PLAN/ALGORITHM *TO ASSESS and MANAGE NEONATAL SEIZURES*

SUBJECTIVE FINDINGS

Obtain quick but careful history!

Antenatal: Maternal Infection (PROM) / Medications, ILLICIT Drug use, Maternal Diabetes.

Natal: APGAR SCORE and Resuscitation details. Fetal Monitoring abnormalities Maternal IV fluids (Large, Hypotonic and Dextrose) Maternal Anesthesia (Local Inj.)

Neonatal: Fever, Diarrhoea, Jaundice.

OBJECTIVE FINDINGS

Assess airway, breathing, circulation and disability by observing the vitals, BP, O_2 sats, color, CRT, pulses, sensorium, focal neurologic deficits, seizures, abnormal movements, tone and reflexes etc.

Focus on: DYSMORPHIC Features, Evidence of TRAUMA, STIGMATA of INFECTION, SIGNS of ASPHYXIA

Evaluate: the FONTANELLE Carefully. *Examine* the FUNDI (chorioretinitis - TORCH). AUSCULTATE for CRANIAL BRUIT. EVALUATE ALERTNESS, TONE, REFLEXES between Clinical Seizures to detect obtundation or Coma.

INVESTIGATIONS

Investigate following a neonatal seizure as recommended !
First line Pulse Oximetry, Glucose, Packed cell volume, Serum Calcium (ionized if possible), Sodium, Magnesium, Arterial pH and base deficit , Lumbar Puncture, Blood Cultures, Cranial Ultrasound Scan, EEG.
Second line MRI or CT (Indications: Focal seizures, suspected cerebral infarction, I/C. Hemorrhage, Structural malformations). Maternal and neonatal samples (urine/ hair /meconium) for drugs of abuse. Specimens for virology (Herpes and CMV) and congenital infection (Syphilis and Toxoplasmosis). Serum ammonia, amino acids. Urinary amino acids and organic acids.
Consider therapeutic trial of pyridoxine.
Consider echocardiogram, Video EEG Monitoring , if the clinical situation demands such investigations.

Acute Management of Neonatal Seizures

After each step, evaluate the infant for ongoing seizures. If seizures persist, advance to next step!

Step 1. Stabilize airway, breathing, circulation and maintain the vitals and BP

Step 2. Correct transient metabolic disturbances
a. Hypoglycemia (target blood sugar 70–120mg/dL) 10% dextrose water IV bolus dose 2 mL/kg followed by a continuous infusion at 8 mg/kg/min
b. Hypocalcemia 5% calcium gluconate IV at 4 mL/kg (need cardiac monitoring)
c. Hypomagnesemia 50% magnesium sulfate IM at 0.2 mL/kg

Step 3. Phenobarbital 20mg/kg/IV load
Cardiorespiratory monitoring
5mg/kg IV (may repeat to total dose of 40mg/kg: *limit the total dose to 20mg/kg in severely asphyxiated infants with impaired hepatic and/ or renal functions*)

Consider continuous EEG monitoring, if available
Consider intubation/ventilation for hypoxia and hypercapnea on ABG analysis.

Step 4. Lorazepam 0.05mg/kg IV (may repeat to total dose of 0.1 mg/kg)

Step 5. Phenytoin 20mg/kg slow IV load
(fosphenytoin) 5 mg/kg slow IV (may repeat to total dose of 30mg/kg)

Step 6. Pyridoxine 50-100 mg/kg IV with EEG monitoring

Step 7. Other agents - trial of folinic acid, lidocaine IV infusion with/without loading dose EEG = electroencephalogram

Drug	Loading Dose	Maintenance Dose	Important Clinical Notes
a. Phenobarbitone (drug of first choice)	20mg/kg/dose slow IV over 20 minutes loading dose	3–5mg/kg/day in 2 d.d start 12 hrs after the every 20 minutes	* If seizures persist after completion of the first loading dose, repeat 10mg/kg/dose till a total loading dose of 40mg/kg has been given.
b. Phenytoin	20mg/kg	5mg/kg/day in 2 d.d Not recommended in Neonatal Seizures	* Only to be mixed with Normal Saline. * Can cause Arrhythmias and hypotension * At a rate of not >1mg/kg/mt under ECG/BP Monitoring.
c. Lorazepam	----	0.1mg/kg IV bolus over 2–5 minutes	* Duration of action 12-24 hrs; less CVS effects when used with Phenobarbitone ; may
d. Midazolam	150µg/kg IV bolus	1–5 µg/kg/mt IV infusion	* Ultra short acting Benzodiazepine with half -life 1.5-3.5 hours
e. Pyridoxine	100mg IV with EEG Monitoring if possible	10mg/day oral life long	* IV preparation not available in India * 1ml of neurobion IM injection contains 50mgs of Pyridoxine ; give it in the NICU as Hypotension and Apnoea can occur.

When to withdraw anticonvulsants ? Assess for prognosis at 1 week of age; if normal neurological examination and normal EEG and the seizures are well controlled—withdraw and follow-up closely; if abnormal continue anticonvulsants and follow-up at 6 weeks 3 ,6 ,9 and 12 months.

Pearl/Peril/Pitfall: Metabolic disturbances include hypoglycemia, hypocalcemia, and hypomagnesemia. Less frequent metabolic disorders, such as inborn errors of metabolism, are seen more commonly in infants who are older than 72 hours. Typically, they may be seen after the infant starts feeding.

TABLE 1 Etiologies of neonatal seizures

Etiology	Incidence (%)
1. Cerebral hypoxia-ischemia	-
a. Global (e.g., perinatal asphyxia)	40
b. Focal infarction (arterial or venous)	15
2. Intracranial hemorrhage	15
3. CNS infection	5
4. Metabolic disease	-
a. Transient	5
b. Inborn errors of metabolism	1
5. Cerebral dysgenesis	5
6. Neonatal epileptic syndromes	1
7. Neonatal abstinence syndrome	1
8. Unknown	10

TABLE 2 Jitteriness *vs* seizures

Clinical features	Jitteriness	seizures
Abnormality of gaze or eye movement	0	+
Movements exquisitely stimulus-sensitive	+	0
Predominant movement	*Tremor	**Clonic Jerking
Autonomic changes	0	+
Movements cease with passive flexion	+	0

* Tremor = 6 / Sec with equal Amplitude

** Clonic Jerking = 4 / Sec with slow and fast components

TABLE 3 Major etiologies of neonatal seizures in relation to time of seizure onset and relative frequency

	Time of onset		Relative frequency	
	0–3 days	*>3 days*	*premature*	*Full term*
Hypoxic-ischemic encephalopathy	+		+++	+++
Intracranial hemorrhage	+	+	++	+
Intracranial infection	+	+	++	++
Developmental defects	+	+	++	++
Hypoglycemia	+		+	+
Hypocalcemia	+	+	+	+
Other metabolic	+	+		
Epileptic syndromes	+	+		+

TABLE 4 EEG classification of neonatal seizures

A. *Clinical seizure with a consistent eeg event:* Clinical seizure correlates with EEG recording, clearly epileptic and includes focal clonic, focal tonic, and some myoclonic seizures, likely to respond to an anticonvulsant.

B. *Clinical seizures with inconsistent eeg events:* Clinical seizure doesn't have a corresponding EEG discharge, observed with all generalized tonic seizures and with some myoclonic seizures, likely to be nonepileptic origin and may not require or respond to AEDs. These infants tend to be neurologically depressed or comatose as a result of HIE.

C. *Electrical seizures with absent clinical seizures:* Associated with a markedly abnormal background EEG in comatose patients who are not on AEDs/may persist in patients with focal tonic or clonic seizures without clinical signs after the introduction of an anticonvulsant.

TABLE 5 Dilemmas regarding neonatal seizures

Diagnostic choices-reliance on clinical vs. electroencephalographic criteria

Etiologic explanations-multiple prenatal/neonatal conditions with variable times of onset and duration

Treatment decisions-who, when, how, and for how long?

Prognostic questions-consider mechanisms of injury based on underlying disorder vs.intrinsic vulnerability of the immature brain to prolonged seizures

TABLE 7 Caveats concerning recognition of neonatal seizures

* Stereotypic behaviors occur in association with normal neonatal sleep or waking states, medication effects, and gestational maturity.
* Any abnormal repetitive activity may be a clinical seizure, if out of context for expected neonatal behavior.
* Document coincident electrographic seizures with the suspected clinical event.
* Abnormal behavioral phenomena with inconsistent relationships with coincident electroencephalographic seizures suggest a subcortical seizure focus.*Nonepileptic pathologic movement disorders are independent of the seizure state.

TABLE 6 Paroxysmal disorders of the neonatal period

PAROXYSMAL NONEPILEPTIFORM DISORDERS
Jitteriness
Benign neonatal sleep myoclonus
ACUTE SYMPTOMATIC SEIZURES AND OCCASIONAL SEIZURES
Hypoxic-ischemic encephalopathy
Intraventricular hemorrhage
Acute metabolic disorders
Sepsis-meningitis
EPILEPTIC SYNDROMES
Benign idiopathic neonatal convulsions
Familial
Nonfamilial
Symptomatic focal epilepsy
Brain tumor
Malformations of cortical development
Inherited metabolic disease; mitochondrial disorders
Early-onset generalized epileptic syndromes with encephalopathy
Early myoclonic encephalopathy
Early infantile encephalopathic epilepsy

Pearl/Peril/Pitfall: Benign sleep myoclonus: The clinician should be familiar with this benign condition in which rhythmic movements (which occur only during sleep) mimic seizures. The condition can be alarming and may occur focally during non-rapid eye movement (REM) sleep. Video EEG monitoring shows no electrographic seizures

Neonatal Electroencephalograph

* EEG allows for the diagnosis of neonatal seizures and helps in determining the prognosis for infants with HIE-NE.

* EEG studies of neonates with HIE showed that low-voltage (5- to 15-mV) activity, electrocerebral inactivity (voltage, <5 mV), and burst-suppression patterns are predictive of a poor outcome on follow-up neurodevelopmental examination. Normal EEG activity and maturational delay were not associated with excess morbidity on follow-up. Some data suggest that EEG performed in the first 2 weeks of life may be better than physical-neurologic examination because it increases the specificity for predicting abnormal outcomes.

* One pattern that portends a poor prognosis is the burst-suppression pattern. This pattern contains bursts of high-voltage activity composed of a mixture of delta-theta rhythms and spikes and sharp waves of 1-10 seconds alternating with low amplitude (background suppression) with <5 V. During the bursts, no age-appropriate activity is seen. The burst-suppression pattern is associated with a grim prognosis.

* EEGs may show burst-suppression during sleep but a continuous tracing when the patient wakes up. In these patients, burst-suppression is seen during most of the recording and only vigorous stimulation wakes the patient.

* The outcomes of patients with reactive burst suppression are somewhat better than those of neonates with nonreactive burst suppression. Approximately 20% of patients with reactive burst suppression have severe disability on follow-up, and the rest have mild-to–moderately severe sequelae.

* Nonreactive burst suppression is associated with an 86-100% risk of death or severe sequelae on follow-up. Use caution and serial EEGs in premature infants born at less than 33 weeks' gestational age before confirming the diagnosis of a burst-suppression pattern.

* Besides HIE, the following have been associated with a burst-suppression pattern: -Acquired and congenital infections -Inborn errors of metabolism (e.g. nonketotic hyperglycinemia) -Chromosomal abnormalities -Brain dysgenesis -Intraventricular or periventricular hemorrhage -PVL -Focal cerebral infarcts - Pontosubicular necrosis

* Separating the prognostic value of EEG seizure patterns from the EEG background is difficult. In some studies, EEG seizures had no independent prognostic value above that of the background abnormalities. However, low-frequency (1- to 1.5-Hz) discharges in a suppressed background are correlated with a poor prognosis.

* EEG background patterns of low voltage (<15 mV), burst suppression, and the ominous isoelectric EEG (<2 mV) are associated with a poor outcome in HIE. Neonatal seizures confirmed on EEG are associated with a poor prognosis, especially if the seizures are accompanied by background abnormalities. Normal EEG findings are correlated with a normal neurologic outcome, unless signs of severe brainstem damage are noted after an episode of complete ischemia.

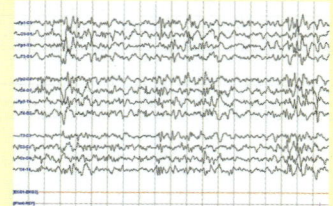

Normal EEG -Term baby 40 wks GA

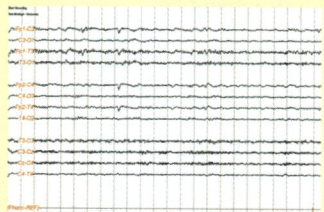

Excessive suppression in HIE -Term baby 40 wks GA

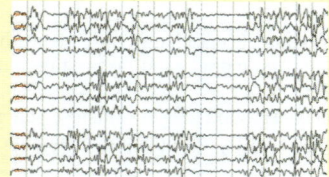

Term baby 40 wks GA-Focal spike discharges

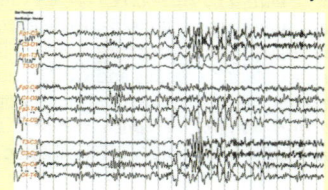

Term baby 40 wks GA-Neonatal Seizures

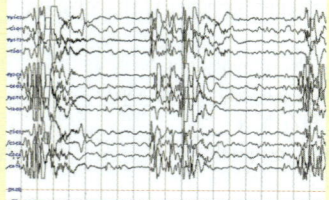

Burst-suppression Pattern in early infantile epileptic encephalopathy

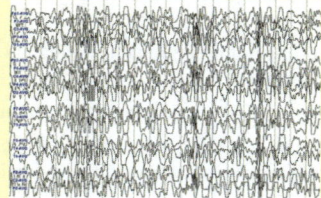

Hypsarrhythmia-Infantile Spasms (West syndrome)

Neonatal seizures and neonatal syndromes
Indicators of prognosis
Indicators of bad prognosis
-- Severe hypoxia–ischaemia
-- Severe congenital malformations of cortical development and meningoencephalitis
-- Subtle and generalized tonic seizures
-- Nearly flat · EEG or of very low voltage and discontinuous · EEG with bursts of high-voltage spikes and slow activity
Indicators of good prognosis
· – Hypocalcaemia (alimentary type) and other transient metabolic changes

· – Extracranial infections with seizures (otitis, pneumonia, gastroenteritis, etc.)
· – Benign familial and non-familial convulsions
· – Clonic seizures that are short and infrequent
· – Normal inter-ictal EEG
Indicators of intermediate or guarded prognosis
· – Moderately severe central nervous system (CNS) infections or malformations
· – Most of the intracranial hemorrhages or infarctions
· – More serious metabolic · CNS disturbances
· EEG persistence of immature patterns
· – Frequent or prolonged clonic seizures and clonic status epilepticus

Pearl/Peril/Pitfall: EEG plays a vital role in properly identifying and differentiating neonatal seizures from nonepileptic events. Video EEG monitoring may be helpful when infrequent neonatal seizures persist.

Neonatal EEG

Neonatal EEG is the measurement of the electrical activity of the newborn brain. It provides a sensitive, real time, continuous measure of cerebral activity and, therefore, brain function. The EEG is capable of detecting changes in oxygenation and blood pressure, detecting electrical signs of seizure and determining the neurodevelopmental outcome of neonates with hypoxic ischemic injury.

The measurement of brain activity via the EEG is performed by attaching several electrodes (or antennae) to the head of the newborn. These electrodes are placed according to the International 10-20 system. The montages are built from recordings of F3, F4, Cz, C3, C4, T3, T4, O1, O2 as shown in Figure 1.

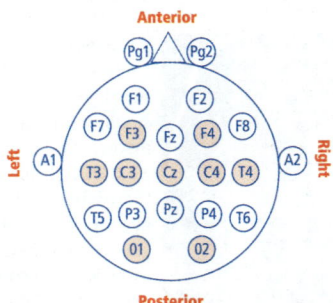

Fig. 1: Electrode placement for measuring Neonatal EEG. This signal that is picked up by each electrode is then amplified, stored and displayed on a monitor. One should measure several other physiological signals in conjunction with the EEG such as the ECG (heart function), respiration (lung function) and EMG (muscle function), as these recordings can influence the EEG.

We then analyze the EEG by visual inspection to assist in the diagnosis and prognosis of the newborn. Our analysis usually involves locating abnormal EEG in a recording. The normal EEG appears to be a random signal without any obvious pattern. The EEG becomes abnormal when certain patterns appear in the EEG and it loses the underlying randomness of a normal recording. The normal EEG pattern and several abnormal EEG patterns are shown in Figure 2

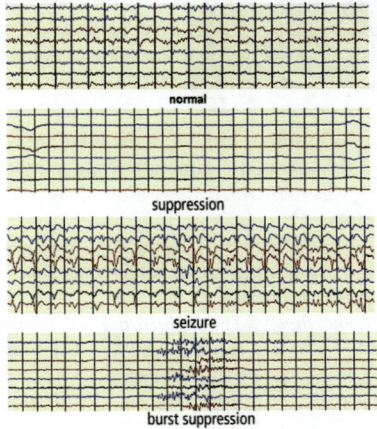

Fig. 2: Examples of normal and abnormal neonatal EEG. In addition to pattern analysis one can also analyze more general characteristics of the EEG such as continuity, amplitude, frequency, synchrony and symmetry as well as more clinical features such as maturational characteristics, sleep state differentiation and reactivity.

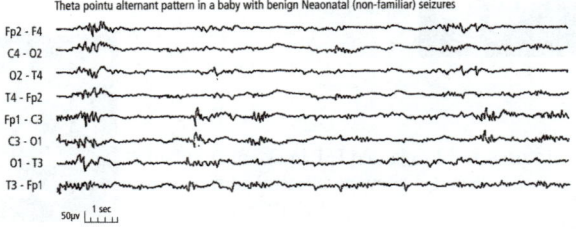

Inter-ictal EEG in a neonate with benign neonatal (non-familial) seizures. The theta pointu alternant pattern is usually associated with a good prognosis.

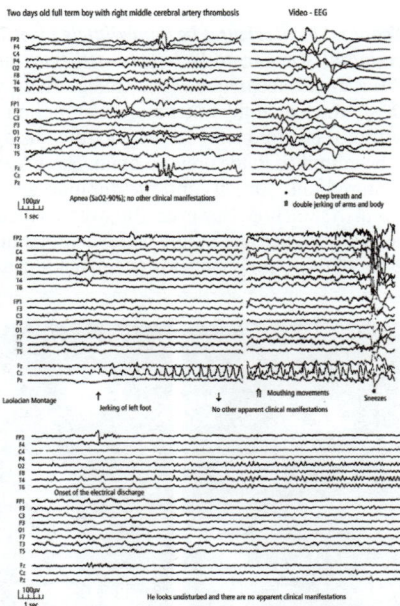

Ictal EEG patterns in a 2-day-old boy with right middle cerebral artery thrombosis. Top and middle: Apnoeic, myoclonic, clonic and subtle seizure of motor automatisms associated with various ictal EEG patterns and locations. Bottom: "Electroclinical dissociation": the electrical discharge is not associated with apparent clinical manifestations.

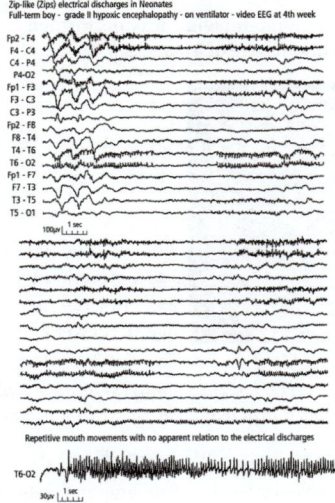

Zip-like electrical discharges

Top and middle: Continuous recording in a neonate with severe brain hypoxia. Zip-like electrical discharges consist of high frequency rapid spikes of accelerating and decelerating speed. They start from various locations, terminating in one while continuing in another. *Bottom:* Amplification of zips with high sensitivity in T6-O2 derivation.

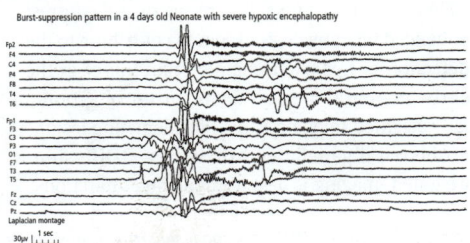

The burst–suppression pattern in a neonate with severe hypoxic encephalopathy

@ *Neonatal focal seizures be immediately investigated by MRI, especially with MR DWI. This image modality provides not only early diagnosis of perinatal ischemic stroke, but also assists to clarify the specific time (prepartum, intrapartum, or postpartum period) of the stroke's occurrence.* (DWI) is an MR technique which studies the Brownian motion of water in tissue and can be used to calculate apparent diffusion coefficients (ADCs), which quantify water molecular motion. Additionally anisotropy,which is a function of the directional dependence of water motion in a restricted environment, can be measured using DWI, and provides an insight into white matter structure. T1 and T2 relaxation values have also been studied in the preterm brain. These MR parameters are associated with cerebral water content, and are raised in pathology and in the immature brain. An EEG and the duration and degree of neonatal encephalopathy provide very useful information on the severity of the cerebral dysfunction. However, MRI, with its high sensitivity and anatomic resolution, contributes important additional information about the time of occurrence and nature of the neuropathology underlying seizure activity. Mortality and neurological morbidity remain a major risk in one out of two term infants with neonatal seizures. MRI yields significant predictive information which is critical to prognosis.

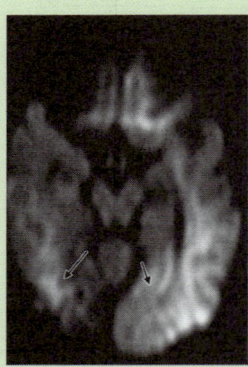 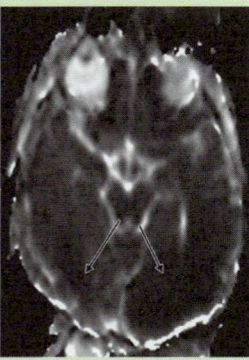

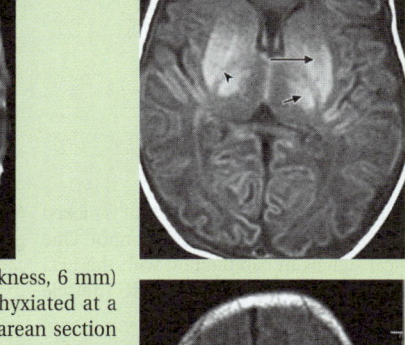

T1-weighted MR image (550/20; section thickness, 4 mm) at level of basal ganglia shows abnormally high signal intensity in basal ganglia (long arrow), thalamus (short arrow), and posterior limb of internal capsule (arrowhead) in infant born at a gestational age of 37 weeks 5 days with severe perinatal asphyxia due to intertwined umbilical cord. Imaging was performed 6 days after birth at a postconceptional age of 38 weeks 4 days.

Diffusion-weighted MR imaging (3447/74; section thickness, 6 mm) at level of occipital poles in infant born severely asphyxiated at a gestational age of 41 weeks 2 days by emergency caesarean section performed because of placenta previa and deterioration of fetal cardiotocographic results. (a) Image obtained at *b* value of 1000 sec/mm2 and (b) ADC image show infarctions (arrows) in left and right occipital regions. Imaging was performed 3 days after birth at a postconceptional age of 41 weeks 5 days.

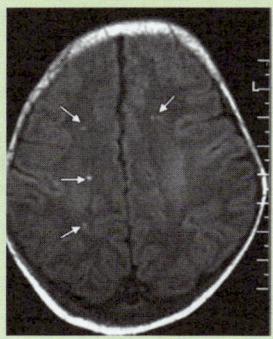

T1-weighted MR image (550/16; section thickness, 4mm)at level of centrum semiovale in infant born at a gestational age of 41 weeks 2 days shows punctate white matter lesions in centrum semiovale (arrows). This infant experienced repetitive intrauterine insults due to umbilical cord problems; meconium aspiration syndrome was also present. Imaging was performed 8 days after birth at a postconceptional age of 42 weeks 3 days.

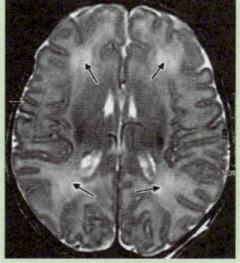

T2-weighted MR image (5406/120; section thickness, 4 mm) at level of body of lateral ventricles in infant born asphyxiated at a gestational age of 39 weeks 1 day shows nonpunctate white matter injury appearing as abnormal high signal intensity (arrows). Imaging was performed 1 day after birth at a postconceptional age of 39 weeks 2 days. Movement artifacts are visible.

MRI patterns (T2-weighted images) in neonatal brain following perinatal asphyxia, according to Baenziger et al14

Pattern A: Diffuse hyperintensity of cerebral hemispheres
Pattern B: Hyperintensity of parasagittal watershed regions
Pattern C: Lesions in basal ganglia or thalamus
Pattern D: Periventricular hyperintensity
Pattern E: Focal parenchymal ischemia or hemorrhage

Association between age of intracranial hemorrhage and changes in T1- and T2 signals after injury

	Age of hemorrhage	T1-weighted images	T2-weighted images
Acute	< 3 days	Iso-to mildly hyperintense	Iso-to hypointense
Subacute	4–14 days	Hyperintense	Hypointense centre, hyperintense periphery
Chronic	>14 days	Hyperintense	Hyperintense

Advances in Knowledge

*The combination of T1- and T2- weighted imaging and diffusion weighted imaging is best for the detection of hypoxic-ischemic brain injury in the early neonatal period in term-born infants.
* Fluid-attenuated inversion recovery and contrast enhanced imaging do not seem to contribute to the detection of hypoxic-ischemic brain injury in the early neonatal period in term-born infants.
*T1-weighted imaging is best for depicting lesions in the basal ganglia and thalamus. *Diffusion-weighted imaging is best for depicting infarctions.

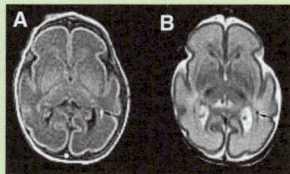

(A) Transverse T1 weighted image of an infant at 29 weeks GA showing a high signal lesion adjacent to the optic radiation on the left (arrow). (B) Transverse T2 weighted FSE image showing the lesion as low signal (arrow).

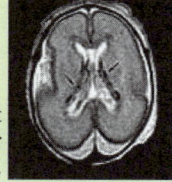

Transverse T2 weighted FSE image of an infant at 27 weeks GA showing bilateral germinal layer hemorrhages (arrows).

Pearl/Peril/Pitfall: MRI is the most sensitive imaging modality to determine etiology for neonatal seizures. Cranial MRI is the most sensitive test in determining the etiology of neonatal seizures, particularly when electrolyte imbalance has been excluded as a cause for seizures. A major disadvantage is that it cannot be performed quickly and, in an unstable infant, it is best deferred until the acute clinical situation resolves.

NEONATAL SEIZURES—ESSENTIAL DIFFERENTIAL DIAGNOSES

1. Benign Familial Neonatal Seizures (BFNS) : *An autosomal dominant condition (2 separate genetic loci at chromosome 20q13.3 and at chromosome 8q24 have been identified in most families, which encodes for a potassium channel (KCNQ2 and KCNQ3 potassium channels) , suggesting an impairment of K⁺-dependent Neuronal depolarization as the basis for the seizures) *Seizures typically begin on the 2nd - 3rd day of life with a frequency of 10–20 for day without obvious risk factors for seizures *May recur for days to weeks, which stop in 1–6 months. *Infants are normal between seizures *Clinically the seizures are tonic-clinic in type (the rare form in the Neonate) which tend to occur mainly during active sleep and may be preceded by brief arousal and the interictal EEG is normal *Investigations fail to pinpoint any underlying etiology *Most cases have a normal long-term Neurodevelopmental outcome and the aggressive anticonvulsant therapy is not indicated. The real puzzle is why this profound abnormality in membrane polarization does not lead to more problems in later life or persistent seizures extending from the neonatal period. This may be evidence that the drive toward homeostasis in the brain is strong, with redundant systems capable of maintaining a seizure-free state until more than one system is affected, or that systems are affected that do not have the redundancy of the voltage-gated potassium channels. Moreover, the normal potassium channels may be up-regulated to accommodate for the deficiency in function of the abnormal channels.Clearly, the immature infant brain is different electrophysiologically during early development. GABA has a seemingly paradoxical excitatory effect. Glutamate synapses are slow to develop, and there is delayed expression of the K⁺/Cl⁻ cotransporter KCC2 and NKCC1. The primary inhibition in the neonatal brain is presynaptic rather than postsynaptic. As the brain matures and expression of postsynaptic inhibitory and excitatory processes develop, the maintenance of neuronal homeostasis as well as postsynaptic EPSPs and IPSPs gradually approach the adult state. Since all of these processes are under development at the same time as neonatal convulsions appear, it is likely that neonatal seizures are affected by the normal developmental sequence of the other neurotransmitter systems.

2. Benign Idiopathic Neonatal Seizures (BINS) : *5th day fits occurs in 5% of seizures in term infants *Multifocal in nature with typical onset between days 4 and 6 of life *Clonic and /or apneic seizures (never tonic like BFNC) *History, physical examination (before and between seizures) and diagnostic testing are normal *Ictal EEG shows brief (1–3 minute) seizures in the rolandic regions but never shows initial voltage attenuation as in BFNS. *The seizure activity is brief usually but intense, with frequent or serial seizures and status epilepticus sometimes *Gradually resolve within 2 weeks of onset *Cause is unknown, may be due to transient zinc deficiency (CSF zinc levels may decrease) * Long-term prognosis is good without any risk for epilepsy (largely determined in retrospect)

3. Neonatal Myoclonic Encephalopathy(NME) : *Typically start as focal motor seizures, and later evolve into typical infantile spasms *Commonly associated with metabolic disorders (especially non ketotic hyperglycemia) *The Ictal EEG shows high-amplitude bursts coinciding with a massive myoclonic seizures and the interictal pattern shows a burst suppression pattern with complex bursts and sharp waves alternating with periods of low-amplitude quiescence *Long-term outcome is poor, with a high mortality in the first year and severe retardation in all survivors.

4. Ohtahara syndrome: *The seizures are typically numerous brief tonic spasms (but not myoclonic) *Associated with structural causes rather than metabolic *Ictal EEG shows a period of EEG suppression without any bursts when tonic spasms occur clinically *The interictal EEG always shows burst suppression pattern *Prognosis is grim like in NME.

5. Migrating partial seizures of infancy (COPPOLA Syndrome): *The seizures are partial clonic and alternate between the 2 sides of the body *Cause is unknown and the condition is refractory to most of the anticonvulsants with severe Neuro-developmental sequelae *EEG shows Multifocal and migratory over both hemispheres.

Idiopathic benign Neonatal seizures (familial and non-familial)
Benign (non-familial) Neonatal seizures versus benign familial Neonatal seizures

	Benign (non-familial) Neonatal seizures	Benign familial Neonatal seizures
Main seizures	Mostly clonic	Tonic-clonic
Onset	Fifth day of life	Second or third day of life
Duration of seizures	Status epilepticus (median 20 hours)	Repetitive isolated seizures
Main causes	Unknown, probably environmental	Autosomal dominant
Subsequent seizures	Practically nil (0.5%)	Relatively high (11%)
Psychomotor deficits	Minor	Practically non-existent
Ictal EEG	Usually localized spikes	Usually generalized flattening
Interictal EEG	Usually theta pointu alternant	Normal or focal abnormalities

KEY POINTS FOR CLINICAL PRACTICE

1. Seizures in Neonates may indicate a serious, life-threatening, and potentially reversible disease, it is essential to carry out timely and organized investigation.

2. The investigations and management should be instituted simultaneously to terminate the seizure and prevent a recurrence, to identify the underlying cause and to institute specific therapy where available.

3. Hypoxic-Ischemic Encephalopathy (the most common cause of Neonatal Seizures-nearly 50%), CNS infection, intracranial hemorrhage, cerebral artery infarction, acute metabolic disturbances, constitute > 90% of etiology of Neonatal Seizures.

4. Not all clinical seizures are correlated with EEG changes and not all seizures shown on EEG recordings are clinically apparent.

5. Monitor respiratory activity and BP as many anticonvulsants cause respiratory depression and impair myocardial function. Assisted ventilation may be necessary if the neonate requires multiple anticonvulsants, to stop seizures.

6. Effectively communicate with parents and explain the prognosis to the parents according to the underlying cause—CNS malformations—poor neuro-developmental outcome; Infection, HIE and Early Hypoglycemia—30–50% normal; Isolated Hypocalcemia and Benign Neonatal Convulsions - excellent.

REFERENCES AND FURTHER READING:1) Evans D, Levene M. Neonatal Seizures. Arch Dis Child. 1998;78:F70-75 **2**) Volpe JJ. Neonatal Seizures, in Neurology of Newborn 4th Edition WB Saunders 2004;178-214 **3**)McBride M.C, Laroia N, Guillet R. Electrographic seizures in neonates correlate with poor neurodevelopmental outcome. Neurology 2000; 55; 506-513. **4**) Holmes G.L. Seizure-induced neuronal injury. Neurology 2002; 59: S3-S6. **5**)Toet MC, Groenendaal F, Osredkar D, van Huffelen AC, de Vries LS. Post neonatal seizures following aEEG detected neonatal seizures. Pediatr Neurol 2005; 32: 241-247.

Pearl/Peril/Pitfall: Antiepileptic medications should be instituted in an orderly and efficient manner (Painter et all 1999). Correct hypoglycemia, if present. Initial treatment with phenobarbital should be considered. If seizures persist, phenytoin should be added. Persistent seizures may require use of an intravenous benzodiazepine such as lorazepam or midazolam.

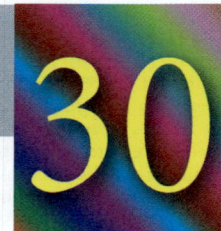

Intracranial Hemorrhage and Intraventricular Hemorrhage

@ *"The pathogenesis, clinical presentation, diagnosis, management, and prognosis of ICH varies according to the ICH location and size, and the infant's GA."*

Intracranial hemorrhage
Classification according to Papile

Grade 1. Hemorrhage limited to subependymal matrix

Grade 2. Hemorrhage extending into ventricular system, < 50%, without acute ventriculomegaly

Grade 3. Hemorrhage extending into ventricular system, with acute dilatation because of flooding of 50% or more of one or both lateral ventricles

Grade 4. Hemorrhage grade 1,2 or 3 with extension into brain tissue

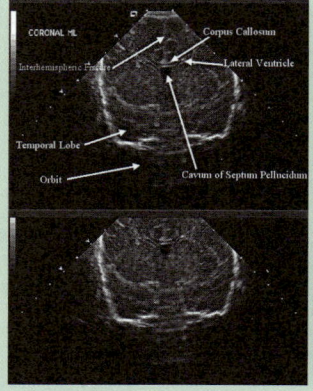

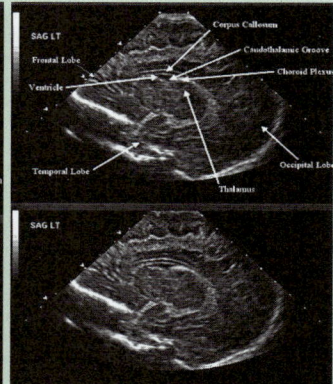

Sonographic appearance of a normal neonatal brain. Image is from a coronal midline scan

Normal neonatal brain shown with left sagittal scan

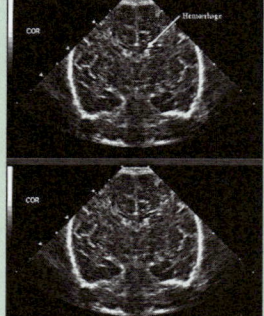

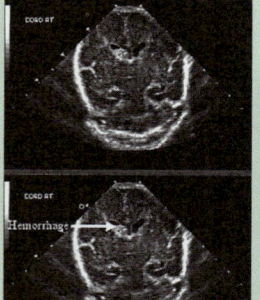

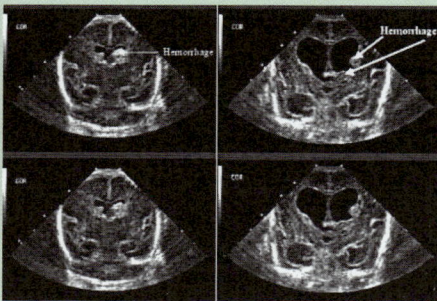

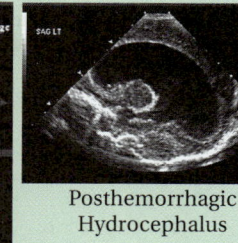

Posthemorrhagic Hydrocephalus

Grade I hemorrhage minimal or grade I periventricular hemorrhage (PVH).

Moderate or grade II hemorrhage (subependymal with no or little ventricular enlargement).

Severe or grade III hemorrhage (subependymal with significant ventricular enlargement).

REVIEW OF CLINICAL PROBLEMS

1. How and when does a GMH-IVH present clinically in a preterm infant?
   Ans: Refer to the Table 2 of the Chapter.

2. How do you assess the severity of GMH-IVH in preterm infants and manage it?
   Ans: Refer to the Evaluation-Decision-Action-plan/algorithm for the diagnosis and management of a preterm baby with intraventricular hemorrhage.

3. What are the preventive strategies to reduce the incidence and/or severity of GMH-IVH in preterm infants?
   Ans: Refer to the Evaluation-Decision-Action-plan/algorithm for the diagnosis and management of a Preterm baby with intraventricular hemorrhage.

4. How do you differentiate various types of ICH in a term baby?
   Ans: Refer to the Table 5 of the Chapter.

5. When should you consult a neurosurgeon for a term infant with subdural hemorrhage?
   Ans: Refer to the Evaluation-Decision-Action-plan/algorithm for the diagnosis and management of a Term baby with ICH.

LEARNING OBJECTIVES

After completing this article, readers will be able to

1. Identify various types of intracranial hemorrhage in preterm or term infants.

2. Understand the multiple risk factors involved in the etiology of ICH and to prevent them if possible.

3. Stabilize the infants with ICH, when ABCDs are compromised.

4. Provide appropriate (conservative and/or neurosurgical) management of ICH, depending on the clinical progression.

5. Monitor for complications of ICH and counsel the parents about the prognosis and outcome.

Pearl/Peril/Pitfall: Although all infants who are born prematurely should be considered at risk for PVH-IVH, neonates delivered at less than 32 weeks' gestation are at significant risk. Beyond approximately 32 weeks' gestation, the germinal matrix has regressed to the point that hemorrhage is significantly less likely. Risk of developing PVH-IVH is inversely proportional to gestational age.

1. Bleeding into the brain and related structures is a very common Neonatal event and is most frequently recognised in premature infants. There are 5 important types of Neonatal intracranial hemorrhage (ICH): a) Subarachnoid b)Subdural c)Intracerebral d) Intracerebellar and e)Intraventricular.The incidence of ICH varies from 2%–30% in Newborns, depending on the gestational age at birth and the type of ICH. Intraventricular hemorrhage (IVH)/Germinal Matrix hemorrhage (GMH) is found principally in the preterm infant (15%–20% in infants <32 weeks' GA), but is uncommon in the term Newborn.The pathogenesis, clinical presentation, diagnosis, management, and prognosis of ICH varies according to the ICH location and size, and the infant's GA.

2. IVH of preterm infants occurs in spontaneous deliveries without apparent trauma. In contrast,Subdural hemorrhage is basically due to trauma to the head and is predisposed by the 1)Rigid birth canal-primipara, elderly multipara, small pelvis.2)Infant with large head.3)Labor-precipitous, prolonged.4) Presentation-breech, foot, face, brow. 5) Delivery-difficult forceps, difficult rotation. Subarachnoid hemorrhage is seen in both premature and fullterm infants and it occurs as a response to hypoxia or trauma.Intracerebral hemorrhage is due to secondary extension of IVH or rebleeding into periventricular ischemic areas of the brain in 80% of such cases. Other causes of primary intracerebral hemorrhage include 1) Coagulation disturbances; 2) Cerebral artery occlusion; 3) TORCH (toxoplasmosis, other, rubella, cytomegalovirus, herpes simplex type II) infection; 4) Thalamic hemorrhage; 5) Arteriovenous malformation (very rare); 6) Tumour (very rare).

3. IVH of preterm infant (GMH/IVH) originates from the fragile involuting vessels of the subependymal germinal matrix, located in the caudothalamic groove. The germinal matrix involutes as the infant approaches fullterm gestation and the tissue's vascular integrity improves,therefore IVH is much less common in the term infant. In the term Newborn, primary IVH typically originates in the choroid plexus or in association with venous and/or sinus thrombosis and thalamic infarction and also in the germinal matrix less commonly. The predisposing factors for IVH include respiratory distress syndrome, hypoxic-ischemic or hypotensive injury, reperfusion injury of damaged vessels, increased or decreased cerebral blood flow, reduced vascular integrity, increased venous pressure, pneumothorax, and hypotension.

4. GMH-IVH in the preterm infant is usually a clinically silent syndrome and is therefore recognized only when a routine ultrasound head scan is performed. The timing and the clinical presentation of GMH-IVH in the preterm are described in the Table No. 2 of the Chapter.

5. The presentation of GMH-IVH ranges from unnoticeable to dramatic with 1)Sudden deterioration. 2)Oxygen desaturation. 3)Bradycardia. 4)Metabolic acidosis. 5)Significant decrease in hematocrit. 6)Hypotonia. 7)Shock. 8)Hyperglycemia. 9)Tense anterior fontanelle.The symptoms of worsening hemorrhage include. 1)Full, tense fontanelle. 2)Increased ventilatory support. 3)Seizure activity. 4)Apnea. 5)Decrease in level of consciousness and/or activity.

6. The diagnostic evaluation of GMH-IVH includes: a) Optimal time to screen: 7days of age because >90% of all hemorrhages have occurred. 1) If test result is normal, there is no need to recheck. 2) If test result is positive for periventricular-intraventricular hemorrhage, repeat test in 2 weeks. b) Serial cranial ultrasonography replaces CT as the principle diagnostic technique. c)Lumbar puncture (CSF studied show elevated red blood cells, increased protein concentration, xanthochromia, and decreased glucose concentration). d) Rule out septic shock or meningitis.

7. *The Evaluation-Decision-Action-Plan/Algorithm* to diagnose and manage a preterm infant with GMH-IVH describes the essential aspects of clinical presentation, assessment of the severity, prevention strategies and therapeutic plans. The prognosis and outcome are enlisted in the Table No. 3 of the Chapter.

8. PVL-Periventricular Leukomalacia i.e., softening of the white matter around the ventricles, now considered as a major risk factor for the subsequent development of cerebral palsy is thought to be due to several major factors. They have been identified to date 1)Vascular anatomic factors, 2) Pressure-passive cerebral circulation, 3) Intrinsic vulnerability of cerebral white matter of the premature Newborn, and 4) Infection/inflammation. PVL is typically a clinically silent lesion, evolving over days to weeks with few or no outward neurologic signs until weeks to months later when spasticity is first detected, or at an even later stage when children present with cognitive difficulties in school. PVL is usually diagnosed in the neonatal period by ultrasound, or less commonly by MRI. Currently, there are no medications or treatments available for the specific treatment of PVL during the Newborn period.

9. In the term Newborn, the ICH can present in various ways i.e., subdural, intraparenchymal, intracerebellar and subarachnoid hemorrhages. The *Evaluation-Decision-Action-Plan/Algorithm* to diagnose and manage ICH in term baby describes the essential aspects of assessment and management. Tables 4, 5 and 6 enlist the various risk factors involved, clinical presentation and diagnostic aspects of ICH in the term infant.

10. In general, although a large ICH is more likely to result in greater morbidity or mortality than a small one, the presence and severity of parenchymal injury, whether due to hemorrhage, infarction, or other neuropathology is usually the best predictor of outcome.

---

* *Pearl/Peril/Pitfall: Postnatally, most hemorrhages occur when the neonate is younger than 72 hours, with 50% of hemorrhages occurring on the first day of life. The extent of hemorrhage is greatest when the neonate is aged approximately 5 days. PVH-IVH can occur when the individual is older than 3 days, especially if a significant life-threatening illness arises. This forms the basis for screening programs and recommendations for screening at age 7 days.*

THE EVALUATION-DECISION-ACTION-PLAN/ALGORITHM TO DIAGNOSE and MANAGE
A PRETERM BABY WITH SUSPECTED IVH

SUBJECTIVE FINDINGS

Hx of Symptoms such as reduced level of consciousness, spontaneous movements, abnormal eye movements, limpy (hypotonic), poor suck, generalized tonic posturing (often thought to be a seizure), muscular twitchings and seizures, pale and apneic baby. *50% present within the first day of life and upto 75 % within the first 3 days of life. A small percentage of infants presents between days 14 and 30.*

Hx of Symptomatic episode intervened with an asymptomatic period or totally silent in 50% of cases. (Grade I and II)

Assess the presence of various risk factors for IVH in a preterm baby. (refer to Table 1)

OBJECTIVE FINDINGS

Assess ABCDs–vitals, BP, CRT, O₂ sats, Urine output, Pulses, skin rashes including petechiae, sensorium, seizures and focal neurological signs + brain stem signs such as apnea, lost extra ocular movements, etc.

Look for bulging AF, pallor, shrill, high-pitched cry respiratory distress, jaundice, poor neonatal reflexes/feeding, shock and mottling of skin, temperature instability, DIC.

Perform complete systemic examination - Often does not reveal any signs, *even with moderate to large hemorrhages sometimes.*

INVESTIGATIONS

Blood FBC, differential, platelets, **hematocrit**, reticulocyte count, Group and type and cross match, Smear, coagulation screen (PT, APTT, fibrinogen, thrombin time, bleeding time and clotting time), blood cultures, ABG analysis, **Blood sugar,** BUN, creatinine, electrolytes, Ca⁺⁺ Mg⁺⁺, LTFs, drug screen

Urine analysis

Imaging CXR, plain abdominal x-ray, **USG scan/CT scan of head,**

Perform partial sepsis screen (**defer LP**)- FBC, CRP, blood and urine cultures, CXR etc.,

Consider ECG, 2D ECHO, MRI brain scan metabolic screen, *when clinical course demands.*

A PRETERM BABY WITH SUSPECTED IVH

Prevent GMH/IVH primarily where could be possible !

* Antenatal corticosteroids (A single course of betamethasone reduces the risk of death, Grade III and IV IVH and PVL, and is recommended in pregnancies 24-34 wk gestation) *Prevention of preterm deliveries by tocolytes *Effective resuscitation at birth *Elective intubation in babies <30 wks to prevent hypoxia, hypercarbia and hypocarbia during ventilation *In utero transport to higher NICU *Optimal management of preterm labor and delivery *Early referral of sick preterms to referral centers *Maintain optimal care (ABCDs) during transport

Ensure the following things at NICU

* Minimal handling and gentle suctioning *Continuous invasive BP monitoring to prevent undue fluctuations *Meticulous fluid and electrolyte balance *Avoidance of bolus administration of colloids or hyperosmolar solutions *Optimal ventilatory strategies to avoid CBF fluctuation (with a sedative or paralytic medication) *Prophylactic administration of low-dose Indomethacin (0.1mg/kg/day for 3days)-reduces the incidence of severe IVH but does not improve the over all long-term developmental outcome.

Assess the severity of IVH

* By ultrasound head scan

Grade I is bleeding confined to the germinal matrix-subependymal region or to <10% of the ventricle (»35% of IVH cases), **Grade II** is intraventricular bleeding with 10-50% filling of the ventricle (» 40% of IVH cases), and **Grade III** is more than 50% involvement with dilated ventricles **ventriculomegaly** is defined as mild (0.5–1cm), moderate (1.0–1.5 cm), or severe (>1.5cm).

* By CT head scan

Grade I hemorrhage represents bleeding isolated to the subependymal area. **Grade II** hemorrhage represents bleeding within the ventricle but without evidence of ventricular dilatation. **Grade III** hemorrhage represents intraventricular hemorrhage with ventricular dilatation. **Grade IV** hemorrhage -hemorrhage grade 1,2 or 3 with extension into brain tissue.

* *Ensure* ABCs, Pulse Oximetry, CR monitor, Invasive BP, urine output.

* ABG analysis and electrolytes, blood sugar, serum creatinine, coagulation studies and echocardiogram if necessary. *(v.s)*

* *DO PROVIDE SUPPORTIVE THERAPY WHERE APPROPRIATE !*

* *Support ABC's* Mechanically Ventilate for respiratory failure, Identify shock, hypoxia and metabolic acidosis and manage with Inotropes, fluid resuscitation and mechanical ventilation and control seizures aggressively with anticonvulsants

* *Avoid events* associated with wide swings in arterial and venous pressures. 1) Seizures.2) Excess motor activity. 3)Apnea. 4)Crying. 5)Pneumothorax

* *Monitor carefully the fluids, electrolytes and glucose levels with correction of* hypovolemia, hyponatremia, hypocalcemia and hypoglycemia and limitation of fluids if there is SIADH.

* *Restore* normal blood volume and hematocrit with packed cell transfusions.

* *Monitor DIC (Platelet counts, Hb, PCV, PT, PTT and fibrin split products)* and treat with FFP, platelet transfusions or whole fresh blood

* *Explain prognosis (short and long-term) to the parents!(refer to the Table 3 of the chapter). Educate and support the parents.*

* *Monitor for the development of post hemorrhagic hydrocephalus-* *By serial head circumference measurements and by USG head scan studies and if is symptomatic (increasing HC, apnea, bradycardia, lethargy, a bulging AF, widely split sutures) and progressive,* a Ventriculo Peritoneal shunt placement is necessary in upto 3-5% of VLBW infants

* Serial LPs, ventricular taps, reservoirs, and externalized ventricular drains -*temporizing measures* but with increased risk of infection and "puncture porencephaly" due to injury to the surrounding parenchyma.

* Acetazolamide and furosemide are carbonic anhydrase inhibitors that can be used to decrease CSF production. However, their combined use often produces electrolyte disturbances and nephrocalcinosis, and may be associated with a worse long term neurologic outcome. For these reasons, the use of acetazolamide and furosemide together has fallen out of favour.

Pearl/Peril/Pitfall: In patients with posthemorrhagic ventricular dilation that regresses, provide close follow-up care because hydrocephalus can recur. Ultrasonography is also the diagnostic tool of choice for the follow-up of individuals with PVH-IVH and posthemorrhagic hydrocephalus. Serial ultrasonography is indicated weekly to follow for progression of hemorrhage and the development of posthemorrhagic hydrocephalus.

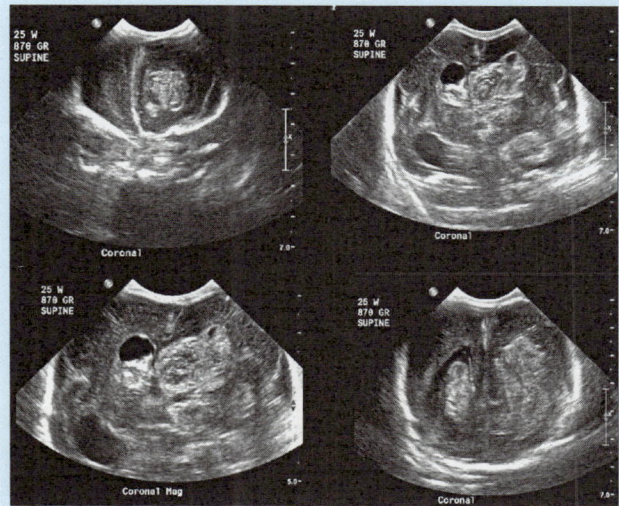

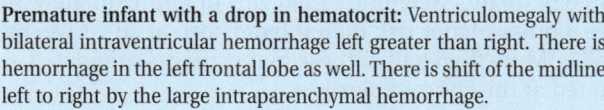

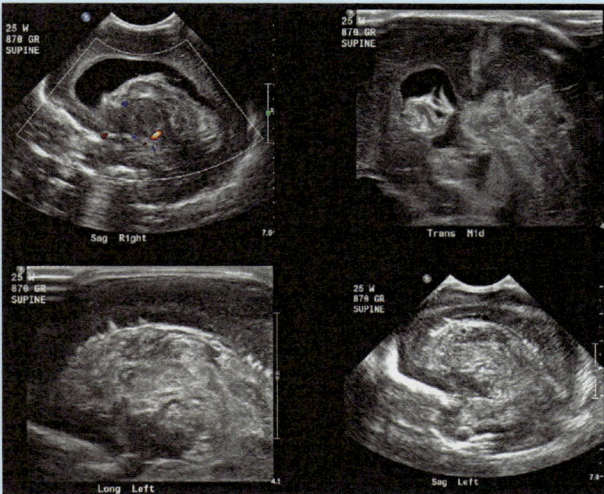

Premature infant with a drop in hematocrit: Ventriculomegaly with bilateral intraventricular hemorrhage left greater than right. There is hemorrhage in the left frontal lobe as well. There is shift of the midline left to right by the large intraparenchymal hemorrhage.

Diagnosis: Grade 4 Neonatal Intracranial Hemorrhage: Cranial sonography (US) is the most widely used neuroimaging procedure in premature infants. US helps in assessing the neurologic status of the child, since clinical examination and symptoms are often nonspecific. It gives information about immediate and long term prognosis. Since it is difficult to predict the presence or absence of neonatal intracranial hemorrhage by clinical criteria, the following schedule is used for routine head ultrasounds for "all" infants d"1500 g birth weight: ·Ultrasound 1. 5–7 day ·Ultrasound 2. 28–30 day or before discharge

·If PVH-IVH is detected on ultrasound, it should be obtained more frequently (weekly) to evaluate progression of ventricular dilatation or cystic change. The timing of the above head ultrasound schedule takes into account that most PVH-IVH occurs in the first week of life. However, the presence of late PVH-IVH does occur and necessitates an ultrasound examination at a month of life. Repeat head ultrasound exams should be done at weekly intervals whenever blood has been identified in the ventricles in order to monitor changes in ventricular size. Discontinuation of ultrasounds must be decided on an individual basis. In addition, consideration should be given to ordering a late head ultrasound exam at about 6 weeks of age in infants born at 26 weeks or less; the purpose of this late exam is to screen for periventricular leukomalacia.

Depending upon the severity of the initial hemorrhage and the clinical presentation, a single CT scan might provide information about cerebral cortical and white matter pathology not available by other means of investigation. If desired for prognostic reasons, the CT scan should be performed near the time of discharge.

At the time an infant with post hemorrhagic hydrocephalus is discharged, arrangements should be made for follow-up in the Neonatology Clinic in four weeks. In some cases a repeat ultrasound may be necessary at that time. The infant who has had a shunt procedure during the hospitalization should also be followed in the Neurosurgery Clinic.

Ultrasound is a fast and bedside examination which makes it ideal for premature infants. Try to get all the information you can. Do not limit yourself to only one transducer or only one acoustic window (figure below). Generally the large fontanel is used as acoustic window. The small fontanel however is a good window to the occipital lobes. This can be useful in patients with borderline hyperechogenicity in these areas. Disadvantages of US are: ·Limited overview in posterior fossa and convexity of the brain ·Absence of US-signs in ischemia in full-terms in first 24 hours ·Difficulty in detecting migration disorders, cortical dysplasia

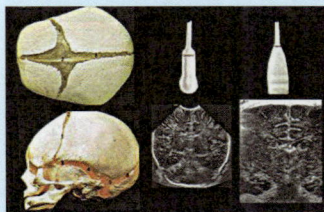

Use both the sector and linear transducer and examine the greater fontanel and if necessary also the lesser and sphenoidal fontanel

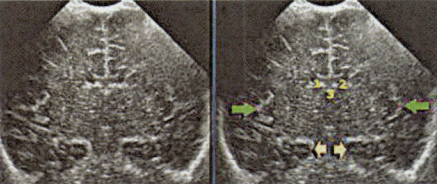

Ventricular measurement: Measurement of the ventricular system should be done in an easy reproducible sonographic plane. Use a coronal section through the lateral ventricles slightly posterior to the foramen of Monro. You will see 3 echogenic dots representing the choroid plexus in the lateral ventricles and in the roof of the third ventricle. Furthermore you should see a symmetrical image of the Sylvian fissure on both sides and the hippocampus (green and orange arrows).

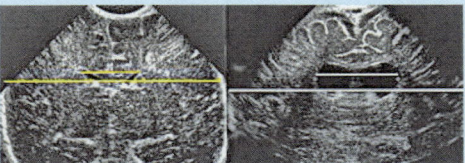

LEFT: Standard measurement of the ventricular index. RIGHT: There is ballooning of the ventricles and the index measurement underestimates the severity of the ventricular widening- **Ventricular index:** The ventricular index is the ratio of the distance between the lateral sides of the ventricles and the biparietal diameter. When using this ratio you have to realize, that when the ventricular system widens, the frontal horns tend to enlarge in the craniocaudal direction more than in the left to right dimension.

* *Pearl/Peril/Pitfall: Grade IV (severe PVH-IVH) IVH with either periventricular hemorrhagic infarction and/or periventricular leukomalacia (PVL): Mortality approaches 80%. A 90% incidence of severe neurological sequelae including cognitive and motor disturbances is noted.*

TABLE 1	Factors associated with an increased risk of GMH-IVH in preterm infants

Prenatal *failure to give antenatal steroids *Maternal aspirin therapy *Maternal smoking *Reason for prematurity other than pre-eclamptic toxemia *Male sex *Breech vaginal delivery (some studies) *Very preterm delivery

At delivery *Birth depression; asphyxia *Birth trauma; bruising

Postnatal *Respiratory distress syndrome, particularly if complicated by pneumothorax *Hypercarbia *Acidosis *Hypoxia *Hypotension, low right ventricular output, low superior vena cava flow *Fluctuating cerebral blood flow *Low cerebral blood flow *Bruising and associated hyperkalemia Coagulation disturbance (prematurity/bruising/sepsis/low platelets) *Tolazoline therapy *Increased illness severity as measured by CRIB, SNAP-II *Patent ductus arteriosus (low blood pressure, cerebral steal) *Postnatal transfer

TABLE 2	Essential clinical features of GMH-IVH in preterm infants

*IVH is rarely present at birth. About 50% occur by 24hrs of age. About 80% occur by 48hrs of age. About 90% occur by 72 hrs of age. By 7 days of age, 99.5% have occurred. A small percentage of infants will have a late hemorrhage between days 14 and 30. IVH is rare after the 1st month of life as a primary event. 20%-40% exhibit progression of the hemorrhage over 3-5days. *GMH-IVH occurs in 30%-40% of infants weighing <1500 gms or approximately 30 weeks' gestation. Infants born at <28 weeks' gestation have 3 times higher risk than infants born at 28-31 weeks' gestation. Only 2%-3% normal term infants have a GMH-IVH. *More than half of these hemorrhages originated at the subependymal germinal matrix. The remainder originated at the choroid plexus.

* IVH can present as: **1)** Crash syndrome: Most dramatic presentation, presenting within few minutes to hours with apnea and seizures, dilated pupils, hypotension, bradycardia and coma. **2)** Saltatory type: symptomatic episode with asymptomatic period intervened. **3)** Silent type: 50% cases (Grade I or II). **4)** Stuttering type: Neonate gradually deteriorates over a few days. Decreased activity, diminished level of consciousness and subtle seizures are due to small to moderate bleeds.*The associated clinical signs of IVH are typically nonspecific or absent;therefore it is recommended that premature infants <34 week's gestation be evaluated with routine real-time cranial ultrasonography through the anterior fontanel to screen for IVH. *Infants <1,000g are at highest risk and should have a cranial ultrasound within the 1st 3-5days of age, when approximately 75% of lesions will be detectable. *Infants weighing 1,001-1,500g should be examined within the 1st 7-14 days of life. *All at risk infants should have a follow-up ultrasound performed at 36-40 wk postmenstrual age to evaluate adequately for PVL, because cystic changes related to perinatal injury may not be visible for at least 2-4 wks. *Approximately 3-5% of VLBW infants will develop posthemorrhagic hydrocephalus and require a ventriculoperitoneal shunt.

TABLE 3	Prognosis and outcome—GMH-IVH in preterm infants

a. Mortality rate is 50% with severe hemorrhage, 15 % with moderate hemorrhage, and 5% with small hemorrhage.

b. These hemorrhages are an important cause of morbidity and death in low birth weight infants.

c. Hemorrhage alone does not account for all neurologic deficits.

d. Approximately 50% premature infants are free of neurologic symptoms Approximately 25% - 30% of very low birth weight infants discharged from a level III Neonatal Intensive Care Unit (NICU) have a periventricular - intraventricular hemorrhage with major neurodevelopmental sequelae.

f. Outcome depends on degree of severity of hemorrhage (Hill and Volpe, 1999; Volpe, 2001.)

   1. Small hemorrhage.

      a. Neurodevelopmental disability similar to that in premature infants without hemorrhage.

      b. Major neurodevelopmental disability in 10%.

   2. Moderate hemorrhage

      a. Major neurodevelopmental disability in 40% during infancy.

      b. Mortality rate 10%, with progressive hydrocephalus in <20%.

   3. Severe hemorrhage.

      a. Major neurodevelopmental disability in 80%

      b. Mortality rate 50%–60%, with hydrocephalus common in survivors.

Pearl/Peril/Pitfall: Pharmacological prophylaxis can be accomplished through the use of indomethacin. Although the mechanism of action is currently unknown, indomethacin has been shown to reduce the incidence of PVH-IVH and, specifically, high-grade hemorrhages.Follow-up of patients enrolled in a multicenter prophylaxis study conducted by Ment et al was less convincing, although sex-related differences favoring treatment in male infants have been postulated. Another large multicenter trial yielded contradictory evidence. With such contradictory evidence of benefit, a lack of a definitive demonstration of improvement in developmental outcomes, and a concern for complications, this therapy is not universally accepted and remains controversial.

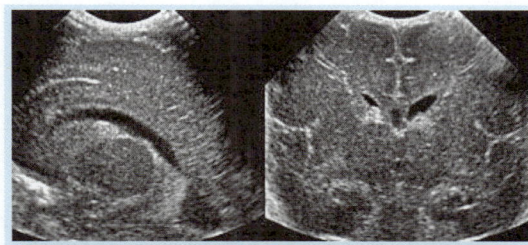

Grade 1 intracranial hemorrhage

On the left an intracranial hemorrhage confined to the caudothalamic groove. It is staged as grade 1 hemorrhage. In the acute phase these bleedings are hyperechoic, changing to iso- and hypo-echoic with time. Sagittal and coronal US of subependymal hemorrhage located in the groove between the thalamus and the nucleus caudatus.

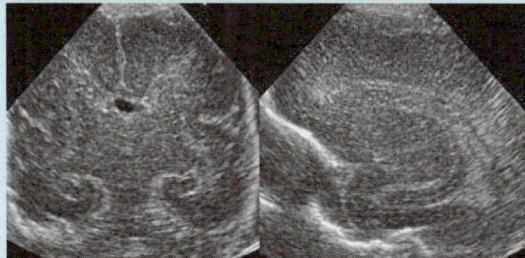

Grade 2 intracranial hemorrhage

On the left a grade 2 intracranial hemorrhage. On the coronal image only the cavum septi pellucidi is seen. Both lateral ventricles are filled with blood, but there is no ventricular dilatation.

Courtesy: *Neonatal Brain US by Erik Beek and Floris Groenendaal*

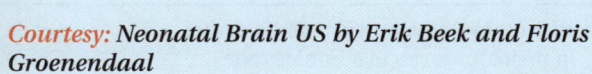

On the left the same patient after 3 days. The ventricles are dilated and clot formation is seen. Secondary hydrocephalus occurring several days after a grade 2 bleed should not be mislabeled as grade 3 hemorrhage.

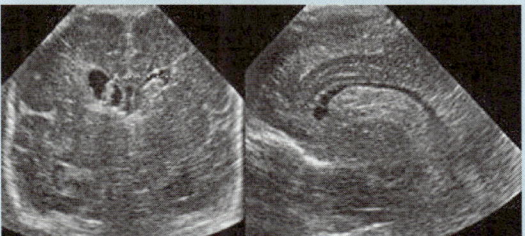

Grade 3 intracranial hemorrhage

On the left a grade 3 intracranial hemorrhage filling the left lateral ventricle. Also note the wedge shaped hyperechoic area on the laterosuperior side of the ventricle. This represents a small venous infarction. LEFT: Coronal image, green arrow indicating grade 3 hemorrhage RIGHT: Sagittal image, yellow arrow indicating venous infarction.

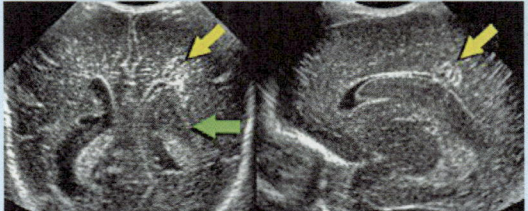

Same patient as above. Two weeks later the venous infarction has developed into a hypoechoic area with cyst formation

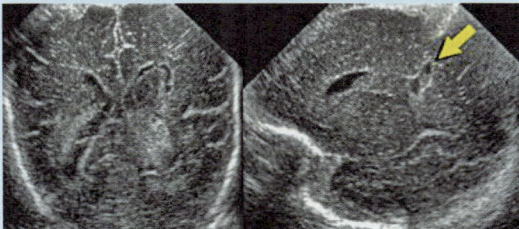

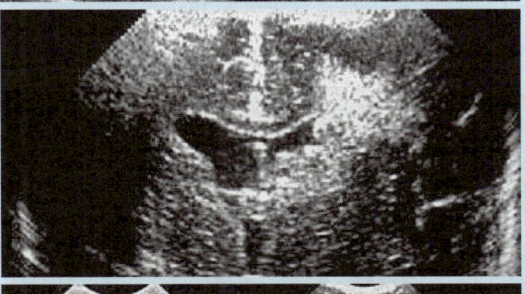

Grade 4 intracranial hemorrhage

Originally these grade 4 hemorrhages were thought to result from subependymal bleeding into the adjacent brain. Today however most regard these grade 4 hemorrhages to be venous hemorrhagic infarctions, which are the result of compression of the outflow of the veins by the subependymal hemorrhage. On the left a grade 4 hemorrhage. There is a large subependymal bleeding but also a large area with increased echogenicity in the brain parenchyma lateral to the ventricle. This is probably the result of a venous infarct.

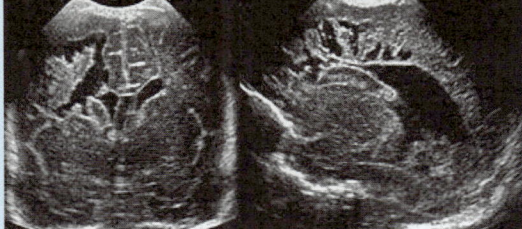

These venous infarctions resolve with cyst formation. These cysts can merge with the lateral ventricle, finally resulting into a **porencephalic cyst**. On the left a different patient with a grade 4 hemorrhage at a later stage with extensive cyst formation. Grade 1 and 2 bleeds generally have a good prognosis. Grade 3 and 4 bleeds have variable long-term deficits, but outcome in grade 3 hemorrhages is usually good when no parenchymal injury has occurred. Hydrocephalus is a common complication and many infants require ventriculoperitoneal shunting. The mechanisms by which hydrocephalus develop include: ***Communicating hydrocephalus**: decreased absorption of cerebral spinal fluid (CSF) secondary to obstruction of arachnoid villi by blood and debris or the development of arachnoiditis ***Obstructive hydrocephalus**: obstruction to CSF circulation.

Pearl/Peril/Pitfall: Although IVH is uncommon in infants who are born at term, the disorder has been reported, especially in association with trauma and asphyxia. The site of hemorrhage in term infants is usually the choroid plexus, a difference from the site of PVH-IVH in infants who are premature.

PVL is also known as Hypoxic-Ischemic Encephalopathy (HIE) of the preterm: It is a white matter disease that affects the periventricular zones. In prematures this white matter zone is a watershed zone between deep and superficial vessels. Until recently ischemia was thought to be the single cause of PVL, but probably other causes (infection, vasculitis) play an additional role. PVL presents as areas of increased periventricular echogenicity. Normally the echogenicity of the periventricular white matter should be less than the echogenicity of the choroid plexus. PVL occurs most commonly in premature infants born at less than 33 weeks gestation (38% PVL) and less than 1500 g birth weight (45% PVL). Detection of PVL is important because a significant percentage of surviving premature infants with PVL develop cerebral palsy, intellectual impairment or visual disturbances. More than 50% of infants with PVL or grade III hemorrhage develop cerebral palsy. Grading PVL: PVL is graded according to the signs as listed in the Table on the left. Regular sonographic examination is mandatory as cysts in PVL can develop as long as 4 weeks after birth (especially in prematures < 32 weeks) and these cysts can resolve in 1-2 weeks. Cranial ultrasonographic findings may be normal in patients who go on to develop clinical and delayed imaging findings of PVL. A good protocol is US-examination at least once a week until discharge and at the age of 40 weeks.

Periventricular leukomalacia
Disorder of the periventricular white matter
In prematures vascular border zone
Combination of Ischemia / Infection
Severe neurological sequelae
-diplegia, quadriplegia
-developmental delay

PVL = Increased Perventricular echogenicity	
Grade 1.	Persisting more than 7 days
Grade 2.	Developing into small periventricular cysts
Grade 3.	Developing into extensive periventricular cysts, occipital and fronto-parietal
Grade 4.	In deep white matter developing into extensive subcortical cysts

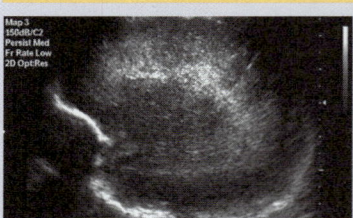
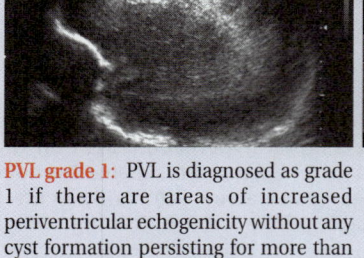
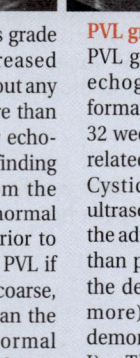
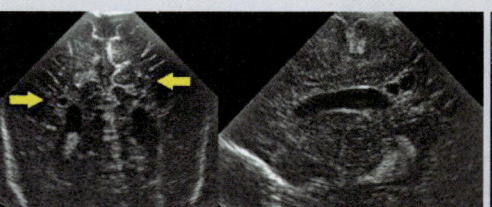
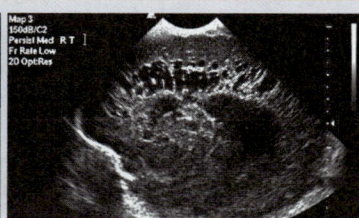

PVL grade 1: PVL is diagnosed as grade 1 if there are areas of increased periventricular echogenicity without any cyst formation persisting for more than 7 days. Increased periventricular echogenicity is however a nonspecific finding that must be differentiated from the normal periventricular halo or normal hyperechoic 'blush' posterosuperior to the ventricular trigones. Suspect PVL if the echogenicity is asymmetric, coarse, globular or more hyperechoic than the choroid plexus. The abnormal periventricular echotexture of PVL usually disappears at 2-3 weeks. PVL can be differentiated from hemorrhages because PVL lacks mass effect.

PVL grade 2: The images on the left demonstrate a PVL grade 2 with small periventricular cysts. The echogenicity has resolved at the time of cyst formation. 2% of the preterm neonates born before 32 weeks develop cystic PVL. The severity of PVL is related to the size and distribution of these cysts. Cystic PVL has been identified on cranial ultrasounds on the first day of life, indicating that the adverse event was at least 2 weeks prenatal rather than perinatal or postnatal. US is highly reliable in the detection of cystic WM injury (PVL grade II or more), but has significant limitations in the demonstration of noncystic WM injury (PVL grade I). This deficiency of neonatal cranial US is important, because noncystic WM injury is considerably more common than cystic WM injury.

PVL grade 3: PVL is diagnosed as grade 3 if there are areas of increased periventricular echogenicity, that develop into extensive periventricular cysts in the occipital and fronto-parietal region.

*Courtesy: **Neonatal Brain US by Erik Beek and Floris Groenendaal***

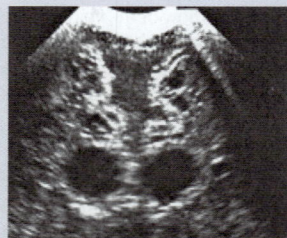
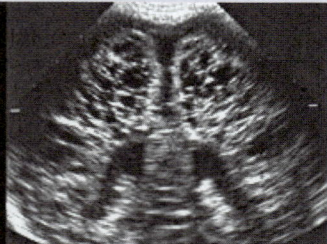
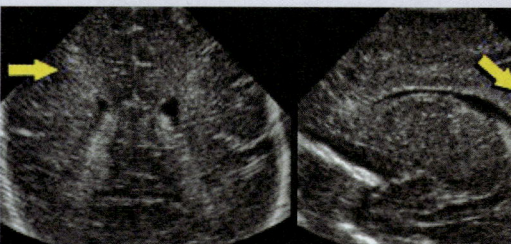

PVL grade 4: PVL is diagnosed as grade 4 if there are areas of increased periventricular echogenicity in the deep white matter developing into extensive subcortical cysts. PVL grade 4 is seen mostly in fullterm neonates as opposed to PVL grade 1-3, which is a disease of the preterm neonate. Flaring persisting beyond the first week of life is by definition PVL garde 1.

The term flaring is used to describe the slightly echogenic periventricular zones, that are seen in many premature infants in the first week of life. During this first week it is not sure if this is a normal variant or a sign of PVL grade 1. Flaring persisting beyond the first week of life is by definition PVL grade 1. Follow up is needed to differentiate flaring from PVL grade I.

Pearl/Peril/Pitfall: PVH-IVH hemorrhage is now thought to be caused by capillary bleeding. Two major factors that contribute to the development of PVH-IVH are (1) loss of cerebral autoregulation and (2) abrupt alterations in cerebral blood flow and pressure.

THE EVALUATION-DECISION-ACTION-PLAN/ALGORITHM FOR THE DIAGNOSIS AND MANAGEMENT OF *A TERM BABY WITH INTRACRANIAL HEMORRHAGE*

SUBJECTIVE FINDINGS

Hx of Symptoms such as irritability, depressed level of consciousness, seizures, hemiparesis or gaze preference, pallor, fever (refer to Table 5 of the Chapter for clinical presentation)

Hx of Risk factors involved in the etiology of intracranial hemorrhage in the term baby(refer to Table No. 4 of the Chapter).

OBJECTIVE FINDINGS

Assess ABCDs—vitals, BP, CRT, O$_2$ sats, Urine output, Pulses, skin rashes including petechiae, sensorium, seizures and focal neurological signs + brain stem signs such as apnea, lost extra ocular movements etc.
Look for bulging AF, pallor, shrill, high-pitched cry respiratory distress, jaundice, poor neonatal reflexes/feeding, shock and mottling of skin, temperature instability, DIC.
Perform complete systemic examination, including detailed neurologic examination for focal signs such as hemiparesis, un-equal pupils, gaze preference and focal seizures.

INVESTIGATIONS

Blood FBC, differential, platelets, **hematocrit**, reticulocyte count, Group and type and cross match, Smear, coagulation screen (PT, APTT, fibrinogen, thrombin time, bleeding time and clotting time), blood cultures, ABG analysis, ***Blood sugar,*** BUN, creatinine, electrolytes, Ca^{++} Mg^{++}, LTFs, drug screen

Urine analysis

Imaging CT head scan/MRI head scan and consider MR Angiography
Perform LP to rule out infection, unless there is increased ICP
Consider Protein C, Protein S, Factor V Leiden if secondary thrombosis is suspected.

A TERM BABY WITH INTRACRANIAL HEMORRHAGE

Manage subdural hemorrhage appropriately !

*Most can be managed with supportive care and treatment of any accompanying seizures *Stabilize infant with rapid evolution of a large infratentorial SDH with volume replacement (fluid and/or blood products), vasopressors, and respiratory support *Consult neurosurgeon if the infant shows signs of progressive brainstem dysfunction(i.e. coma, apnea, cranial nerve dysfunction), Opisthotonus, or tense , bulging AF. *Rule out sepsis, bleeding diathesis with large SDH *Monitor for the development of hydrocephalus, chronic SDH causing increasing OFC *Explain prognosis to the parents that the normal development is good for cases in which prompt surgical evacuation of the hematoma is successful and there is no other parenchymal injury.

Manage intraparenchymal hemorrhage appropriately !

*Most require symptomatic and supportive care *Consult neurosurgeon with a large IPH with severe neurologic compromise *Diagnose and treat any coexisting pathology, such as infection/sinus venous thrombosis *Monitor head growth and neurologic status for days to weeks following IPH, to rule out hydrocephalus or remaining vascular malformation *Explain prognosis to the parents—small IPH has relatively few or no long-term neurologic consequences and a large IPH may result in a lifelong seizure disorder, hemiparesis or other type of cerebral palsy, feeding difficulties, and cognitive impairments.

Manage intracerebellar hemorrhage appropriately !

*Conservative management mostly *? role of craniotomy and evacuation of blood clot.

Manage subarachnoid hemorrhage appropriately!

*Symptomatic therapy only *Blood transfusions + vasopressors and neurosurgical intervention, if in rare cases, with a very large SAH presenting with a catastrophic syndrome (profound depression, seizures, and/or brainstem signs)

* *Ensure* ABCs, Pulse Oximetry, CR monitor, BP, urine output.

* ABG analysis and electrolytes, blood sugar,serum creatinine, co-agulation studies and echocardiogram if necessary.

* *DO PROVIDE SUPPORTIVE THERAPY WHERE APPROPRIATE !*

* *Support ABC's* Mechanically Ventilate for respiratory failure

Identify shock, hypoxia and metabolic acidosis and manage with Inotropes, fluid resuscitation and mechanical ventilation and control seizures aggressively with anticonvulsants

* *Avoid events* associated with wide swings in arterial and venous pressures.

1)Seizures. 2)Excess motor activity. 3) Apnea. 4) Crying 5) Pneumothorax

* *Monitor carefully the fluids, electrolytes and glucose levels with correction of* hypovolemia, hyponatremia, hypocalcemia and hypoglycemia and limitation of fluids if there is SIADH.

* *Restore* normal blood volume and hematocrit with packed cell transfusions.

* *Monitor DIC (Platelet counts, Hb, PCV, PT, PTT and fibrin split products)* and treat with FFP, platelet transfusions or whole fresh blood

* *Explain prognosis (shortandlong-term) to the parents! Educate and support the parents.*

* *Monitor for the development of post hemorrhagic hydrocephalus-* By *serial head circumference* measurements and by *USG head scan studies* and if is *symptomatic* (increasing HC, apnea, bradycardia, lethargy, a bulging AF, widely split sutures) and *progressive*, a Ventriculo Peritoneal shunt placement is necessary.

Serial LPs, ventricular taps, reservoirs, and externalized ventricular drains -*temporizing measures* but with increased risk of infection and "puncture porencephaly" due to injury to the surrounding parenchyma.

Acetazolamide and furosemide are carbonic anhydrase inhibitors that can be used to decrease CSF production. However, their combined use often produces electrolyte disturbances and nephrocalcinosis, and may be associated with a worse long term neurologic outcome. For these reasons, the use of acetazolamide and furosemide together has fallen out of favour.

---

*Pearl/Peril/Pitfall: Beware of Complications ICH-IVH! *Obstructive hydrocephalus*Nonobstructive hydrocephalus *Developmental impairment*Cerebral palsy*Seizures.*

TABLE 4   Risk factors involved in the ICH of term baby

A. Subdural hemorrhage

a. Large fetal head in comparison with size of birth canal and with rigid pelvic structures.

b. Vaginal breech delivery.

c. Malpresentation (breech, face, brow, foot).

d. Skull is unusually compliant and/or pelvic structures unusually rigid.

e. Labor is either very short (not enough time for dilation) or too long (head subjected to prolonged compression / molding)

f. Forceps, vacuum extraction, or rotational maneuvers required to effect delivery.

Pathophysiology: *Excessive vertical molding and frontal - occipital elongation, or oblique expansion of the head results in stretching of the falx and tentorium. *Venous sinuses are stretched, with possible rupture of the vein of Galen or cerebellar bridging veins. *Tear of dura, including the falx or tentorium may also occur.

B. Intraparenchymal hemorrhage

a. Coagulopathy b. Trauma c. Venous thrombosis d. Hypoxia-ischemia e. Extracorporeal membrane oxygenation therapy f. Arteriovenous malformation g. Aneurysm h. Tumor i. Secondary thrombosis: Protein C deficiency, Protein S deficiency, Factor V Leiden

C. Intracerebellar hemorrhage: a. Respiratory distress b. hypoxic events c. Prematurity d. Trauma

D. Subarachnoid hemorrhage

a. Primary hemorrhage may be precipitated by trauma (term baby) or hypoxia (preterm) b. Secondary to an extension of the above three types of ICH

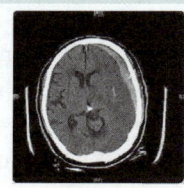

Subdural Hematoma

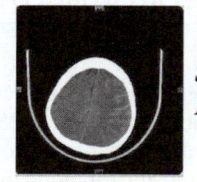

Subarachnoid Hemorrhage

TABLE 5   ICH of term baby—Clinical presentations

A) Subdural hemorrhage

(a) Decreased level of consciousness. (b) Seizure activity. (c) Asymmetry of motor function. (d) Determined by the extent of associated hypoxic-ischemic encephalopathy injury. (e) Often minimal to no clinical symptoms for first 24 hours due to slowly enlarging hematoma. (f) On day 2 or 3: *signs of increasing intracranial pressure* due to block in CSF flow in Posterior fossa: Full fontanel, irritability, lethargy. (g) *Signs of brainstem disturbance:* Dilated, poorly reactive pupil on same side as the hemorrhage, Respiratory abnormalities, facial paralysis, Doll's eye reflex: normal to abnormal. (h) Chronic subdural effusion: present within the first 6 months of life with enlarging OFC.

B) Intraparenchymal hemorrhage

(a) Acute onset of neurological signs at 1–5 days of age after a period of apparent normality (b) Seizures, hemiparesis or gaze preference, along with irritability/lethargy (c) In contrast, Clinically silent in a preterm baby, unless the hemorrhage is quite large.

C) Intracerebellar hemorrhage

(a) May have a history of hypoxic-ischemic insult. (b) Catastrophic deterioration with apnea, bradycardia, decreasing hematocrit values and blood CSF may occur. (c) Signs appear within the first 3 weeks, most commonly within the first 2 days of life. (d) Term infants may have a history of difficult breech delivery.

D) Subarachnoid hemorrhage

(a) Most commonly no symptoms develop. (b) Seizure activity may begin on day 2 of life, especially in the term infant. (c) Infant looks healthy between seizures: "well baby with seizures" (Volpe, 2001). (d) Recurrent apnea (more common in Preterm infants).

TABLE 6   ICH of term baby-diagnosis

A. Subdural hemorrhage

(a) History, clinical signs, CT head scan (b) MRI head scan proved to be quite sensitive to small hemorrhage and can establish timing of ICH and is superior for detecting contusion, thromboembolic infarction or hypoxic-ischemic injury that may occur in some infants with various risk factors associated (c) A CT head scan is much quicker and adequate in an unstable infant with increased ICP who may require neurosurgical intervention (d) When there is clinical suspicion of large SDH, a lumbar puncture (LP) should not be performed until after the CT scan is obtained, and the LP may be contraindicated if there is a large hemorrhage within the posterior fossa or supratentorial compartment. (e) With a smaller SDH, an LP should be performed to rule out infection in the Newborn with signs, such as seizures, depressed mental status, or other systemic signs of illness.

B) Intraparenchymal hemorrhage

(a) MRI is superior for demonstrating the extent and age of the hemorrhage and the presence of any other parenchymal abnormality (b) MR Angiography can be useful to demonstrate a vascular anomaly, lack of flow distal to an arterial embolus, or sinus venous thrombosis (c) LP should be performed to rule out infection, unless there is significant mass effect or herniation.

C) Intracerebellar hemorrhage

(a) CT head scan to define the hemorrhage (b) MRI only if CT scan is unable to provide definitive diagnostic information.

D) Subarachnoid hemorrhage

(a) Diagnosis of exclusion. Other forms of intracranial bleeding are eliminated by CT scan. (b) Lumbar puncture demonstrates uniformly blood -stained CSF.

Pearl/Peril/Pitfall: History of the patient can be entirely noncontributory in periventricular hemorrhage–intraventricular hemorrhage (PVH-IVH). Caregivers or parents might note nonspecific subtle signs. However, in some patients, events that result in loss of autoregulation of cerebral blood flow can be obtained.

TABLE 7   ICH in the newborn—do's and don'ts

Do's

* Do give IV Vitamin K before delivery to all women receiving Phenobarbital or Phenytoin during the pregnancy.

* Do minimize traumatic brain injury by judicious management of cephalopelvic disproportion and operative delivery (forceps, vacuum) .

* Do treat maternal ITP/alloimmune thrombocytopenia with steroids, IV immunoglobulin, or fetal platelet transfusion and cesarean section .

* Do give single course of antenatal steroids-betamethasone to pregnant women of 24–34 week gestation at risk for preterm delivery to reduce the risk of death, Grade III and IV IVH and PVL.

* Do try low-dose prophylactic Indomethacin (0.1mg/kg/day for 3days) to VLBW infants to reduce the incidence of severe IVH

* Do provide tenacious care of the LBW infants avoiding acidosis, hypocarbia, hypoxia, hypotension, wide fluctuations in Neonatal blood pressure, and pneumothorax.

* Do perform a routine USG head scan in all preterm <34 wk GA for detecting silent IVH, as clinical signs are nonspecific.

* Do perform a follow-up USG head scan at 34-40 wk post menstrual age to evaluate adequately for PVL changes

* Do perform a serial USG head scan q2-7 days to assess for posthemorrhagic hydrocephalus(PHH)

* Do organize a permanent VP shunt if PHH has persisted for >4wks despite conservative therapy

Don'ts

* Don't administer hyperosmolar IV solutions rapidly (sodium bicarbonate to correct acidosis, fluids to correct shock) to prevent wide fluctuations in blood pressure.

* Don't under/over ventilate to prevent hypercarbia and hypocarbia respectively so as to reduce ICH and PVL .

* Don't try acetazolamide and furosemide in posthemorrhagic hydrocephalus, because of electrolyte disturbances, nephrocalcinosis and worse long-term neurodevelopmental outcome.

* Don't perform an LP, until CT head scan is obtained, if there is a clinical suspicion of a large subdural hemorrhage.

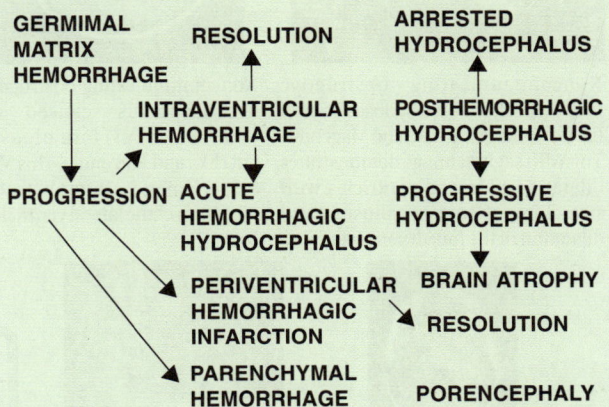

Progression of Germinal Matrix hemorrhage

KEY POINTS FOR CLINICAL PRACTICE

1. The diagnosis, management, and prognosis of ICH varies according to the ICH location and size, and the infant's GA. There is often a combination of two or more types of ICH, as an ICH in one location often extends into an adjacent compartment; for example, extension of a parenchymal hemorrhage into the subarachnoid space or ventricles.

2. The diagnosis depends on clinical features such as seizures, lethargy/irritability and focal neurodeficits and is confirmed with an appropriate neuroimaging study.

3. USG head scan is the preferred imaging technique for screening GMH-IVH in preterm infants because it is noninvasive, portable, reproducible and sensitive and specific for detection of IVH. MRI head scan is superior to CT head scan for Intraparenchymal hemorrhage for detecting the extent and age of hemorrhage and the presence of any other vascular anomaly or parenchymal abnormality.

4. With a large ICH, pressor support or volume replacement may be required because of significant blood loss. More commonly, management is focused on treating complications such as seizures or the development of posthemorrhagic hydrocephalus.

5. The presence and severity of parenchymal injury, whether due to hemorrhage, infarction, or other neuropathology, is usually the best predictor of outcome.

REFERENCES and FURTHER READING: 1)Volpe J. Intraventricular hemorrhage and brain injury in the premature infant: neuropathology and pathogenesis. Clinics in Perinatology 1989;16(2):361-386 2) Volpe J. Intraventricular hemorrhage and brain injury in the premature infant: diagnosis, prognosis and prevention. Clinics in perinatology 1989;16(2):387-411. 3)An Atlas of Neonatal Brain Sonography by Paul Govaert, Gent University Hospital and Linda S. de Vries, Wilhelmina Kinderziekenhuis. with contributions of Frank van Bel, Erik Beek, Dirk Voet, An Bael, Linde Goossens 4) Periventricular Hemorrhage-Intraventricular Hemorrhage in eMedicine, Author: David J Annibale, MD 5)Cohen HL, HallerJO. Advances in *pennatal* neurosonography. AJR 1994; 163:801-

Pearl/Peril/Pitfall: Although all infants who are born prematurely should be considered at risk for PVH-IVH, neonates delivered at less than 32 weeks' gestation are at significant risk. Beyond approximately 32 weeks' gestation, the germinal matrix has regressed to the point that hemorrhage is significantly less likely. Risk of developing PVH-IVH is inversely proportional to gestational age.

31

Hydrocephalus

@*Normal route of CSF from production to clearance is the following: From the choroid plexus, the CSF flows to the lateral ventricle, then to the interventricular foramen of Monro, the third ventricle, the cerebral aqueduct of Sylvius, the fourth ventricle, the 2 lateral foramina of Luschka and 1 medial foramen of Magendie, the subarachnoid space, the arachnoid granulations, the dural sinus, and finally into the venous drainage.*

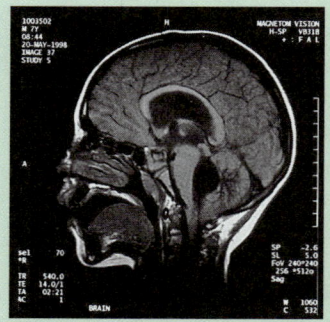
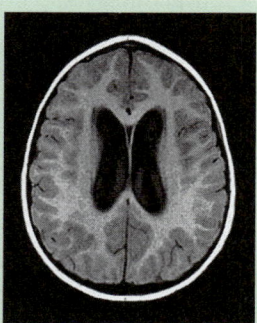
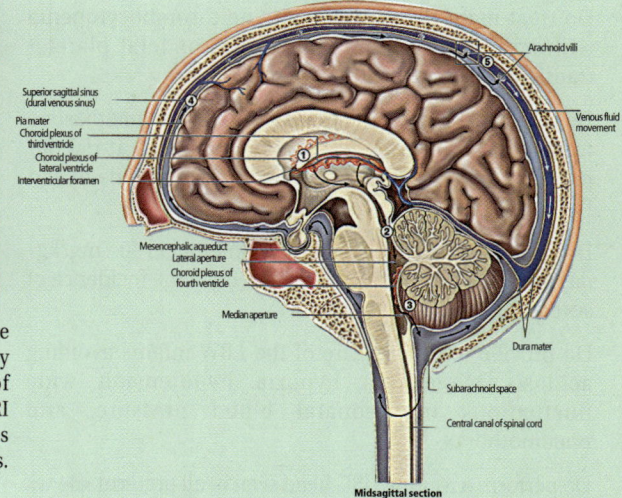

Noncommunicating obstructive hydrocephalus caused by obstruction of the foramina of Luschka and Magendie. This MRI sagittal image demonstrates dilatation of lateral ventricles with stretching of corpus callosum and dilatation of the fourth ventricle.

Noncommunicating obstructive hydrocephalus caused by obstruction of foramina of Luschka and Magendie. This MRI axial image demonstrates dilatation of the lateral ventricles.

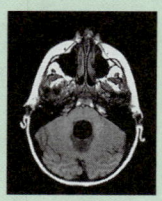
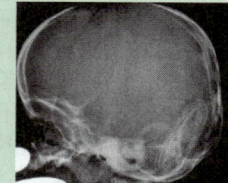
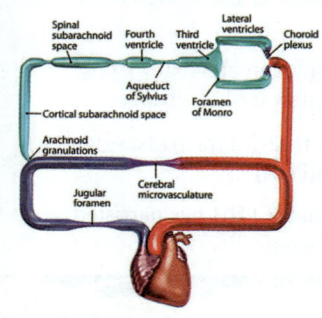
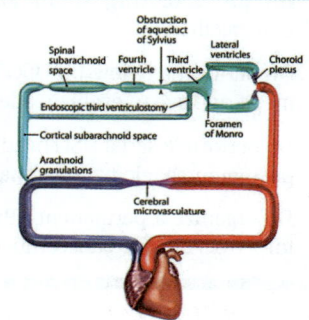

Non communicating obstructive hydrocephalus caused by obstruction of foramina of Luschka and Magendie. This MRI axial image demonstrates fourth ventricle dilatation.

Skull radiograph showing complete migration of a ventriculoperitoneal shunt into the subgaleal space in the occipital region.

REVIEW OF CLINICAL PROBLEMS

1. What are the signs and symptoms of increased intracranial pressure in infants ?
   Ans: Refer to Table 3 of the Chapter.

2. Mention CT/MRI criteria for acute hydrocephalus .
   Ans: Refer to the "No. 5" of the "BIRD`S EYE VIEW/OVERVIEW/SYNOPSIS" of the Chapter.

3. Discuss Three types of Shunt Malfunction .
   Ans: Refer to Table "4" of the Chapter.

4. Mention the Medicolegal pitfalls in the diagnosis and management of Hydrocephalus
   Ans: Refer to Table 5 of the Chapter.

5. How do you classify different causes of Hydrocephalus?
   Ans: Refer to Table "1" of the Chapter.

LEARNING OBJECTIVES

After completing this article, readers will be able to

1. Monitor Neonatal Head Circumference routinely and plot it on centile chart.

2. Recognize the developing Hydrocephalus in early stage before irreversible CNS insult supervenes.

3. Consult Pediatric Neurosurgeon for the preferred surgical intervention over medical therapies.

4. Diagnose Shunt malfunction/infection and liaise with Pediatric Neurosurgeon for Shunt revision.

5. Provide good parental support and communication regarding prognosis and prevent medicolegal pitfalls.

* ***Pearl/Peril/Pitfall :*** *Although hydrocephalus is a multifactorial disorder, the processes responsible for neurologic impairment can be classified into primary and secondary mechanisms. Primary mechanisms include mechanical compression and stretching of brain parenchyma, ischemia and anoxia, cerebral edema, and blood brain barrier dysfunction. These processes lead to secondary mechanisms, which include cytologic and cytoarchitectural alterations of neurons, reduced size and numbers of cerebral microvessels, axonal degeneration and demyelination, and so on. Shunting studies suggest that neuronal cell death may not play a major role until severe stages of hydrocephalus and that some impairments in connectivity can be reversed. Relatively early shunting may alleviate many of the pathologic features of hydrocephalus, but residual impairments in neurotransmitter levels and dependence on anaerobic respiration leave the treated hydrocephalic brain vulnerable to subsequent insults.*-McAllister JP 2nd, **Chovan P.-Department of Neurological Surgery, Wayne State University School of Medicine, Detroit, Michigan 48201, USA.**

BIRD'S EYE VIEW/OVERVIEW/SYNOPSIS

1. Hydrocephalus can be defined broadly as a disturbance of formation, flow, or absorption of cerebrospinal fluid (CSF) that leads to an increase in volume occupied by this fluid in the CNS. This condition also could be termed a hydrodynamic disorder of CSF. Acute hydrocephalus occurs over days, subacute hydrocephalus occurs over weeks, and chronic hydrocephalus occurs over months or years. Conditions such as cerebral atrophy and focal destructive lesions also lead to an abnormal increase of CSF in CNS. In these situations, loss of cerebral tissue leaves a vacant space that is filled passively with CSF. Such conditions are not the result of a hydrodynamic disorder and therefore are not classified as hydrocephalus. Benign external hydrocephalus is a self-limiting absorption deficiency of infancy and early childhood with raised intracranial pressure (ICP) and enlarged subarachnoid spaces. The ventricles usually are not enlarged significantly, and resolution within 1 year is the rule.

2. Communicating hydrocephalus occurs when full communication occurs between the ventricles and subarachnoid space. It is caused by overproduction of CSF (rarely), defective absorption of CSF (most often), or venous drainage insufficiency (occasionally). Noncommunicating hydrocephalus occurs when CSF flow is obstructed within the ventricular system or in its outlets to the arachnoid space, resulting in impairment of the CSF from the ventricular to the subarachnoid space.

3. Congenital hydrocephalus applies to the ventriculomegaly that develops in the fetal and infancy periods, often associated with macrocephaly. The most common causes of congenital hydrocephalus are obstruction of the cerebral aqueduct flow, Arnold-Chiari malformation or Dandy–Walker malformation; these patients may stabilize in later years due to compensatory mechanisms but may decompensate, especially following minor head injuries. During these decompensations, determining the extent to which any new neurological deficits may be due to the new acute event, compared with hydrocephalus that may have gone unnoticed for many years, is difficult.

4. Normal CSF production is 0.20-0.35 mL/min; most CSF is produced by the choroid plexus, which is located within the ventricular system, mainly the lateral and fourth ventricles. The capacity of the lateral and third ventricles in a healthy person is 20 mL. Total volume of CSF in an adult is 120 mL. ICP rises if production of CSF exceeds absorption. This occurs if CSF is overproduced, resistance to CSF flow is increased, or venous sinus pressure is increased. CSF production falls as ICP rises. Compensation may occur through transventricular absorption of CSF and also by absorption along nerve root sleeves. Temporal and frontal horns dilate first, often asymmetrically. This may result in elevation of the corpus callosum, stretching or perforation of the septum pellucidum, thinning of the cerebral mantle, or enlargement of the third ventricle downward into the pituitary fossa (which may cause pituitary dysfunction).

5. Table 1 enlists the most common causes of accelerating head growth in Neonates and children. Table 2 classifies the causes of a large head(Macrocephaly) following a normal growth curve. Table 3 shows the signs of Increased Intracranial pressure in Infants. Ultrasonography through the anterior fontanelle in infants is useful for evaluating subependymal and intraventricular hemorrhage and in following infants for possible development of progressive hydrocephalus. CT can assess the size of ventricles and other structures. MRI can evaluate for Chiari malformation or cerebellar or periaqueductal tumors. It affords better imaging of the posterior fossa than CT. CT/MRI criteria for acute hydrocephalus include the following: *Size of both temporal horns is greater than 2 mm, clearly visible. In the absence of hydrocephalus, the temporal horns should be barely visible. *Ratio of the largest width of the frontal horns to maximal biparietal diameter (i.e., Evans ratio) is greater than 30% in hydrocephalus. *Transependymal exudate is translated on images as periventricular hypoattenuation (CT) or hyperintensity (MRI T2-weighted and fluid-attenuated inversion recovery [FLAIR] sequences). *Ballooning of frontal horns of lateral ventricles and third ventricle (i.e., "Mickey mouse" ventricles) may indicate aqueductal obstruction. *Upward bowing of the corpus callosum on sagittal MRI suggests acute hydrocephalus.

6. It has long been believed that "hydrocephalus is mainly a white matter disease", and axonal degeneration has been commonly observed. Likewise, periventricular reactive gliosis has been well documented. Certainly there is no correlation between cognitive outcome and thickness of cerebral mantle (until the latter is less than 2 cm). However, cytoarchitectural studies have shown that, in untreated hydrocephalus, the neurones become hyperchromatic and pyknotic. Electron microscopic studies have shown that the dendrites are affected early in hydrocephalus and that there is a relatively short window of opportunity for this to be reversed by shunting. Positron emission tomography, and NMR spectroscopy revealed the consequences of hydrocephalus on cerebral metabolism. The degree of reversibility of these cellular changes depends on the duration of the hydrocephalus.

7. **Treatment options**-NON-SURGICAL-Diuretics are still often used in neonatal patients with post-haemorrhagic hydrocephalus (PHH) despite reports of side effects such as acidosis, CO_2 retention, electrolyte disturbance, etc. A recent multicentre randomised controlled trial actually showed a higher rate of shunt placement and increased neurological morbidity in the group receiving diuretics. Fortunately the incidence of PHH is decreasing with better general care, careful control of blood pressure, temperature, and blood gases, better ventilation, and the appropriate use of antenatal steroids and postnatal surfactant, but it remains a significant challenge. Repeated ventricular taps risk not only infection but also the development of "puncture porencephaly" and again are inadvisable.

8. *Surgical Management is the Preferred therapeutic option*- A ventriculoperitoneal (VP) shunt is used most commonly. The lateral ventricle is the usual proximal location. The advantage of this shunt is that the need to lengthen the catheter with growth may be obviated by using a long peritoneal catheter. The atrium was initially the preferred site for placement of the distal catheter, but atrial shunts have a unique set of complications including endocarditis and glomerulonephritis. They also migrate from the atrium with linear growth of the child, needing surgical revision of the distal catheter.

9. There are three ways in which shunts can malfunction: (*a*) they can become infected; (*b*) they can fail mechanically; (*c*) they can overdrain or underdrain (termed a "functional" failure). Refer the Table 4 for the summary of 3 Types of Shunt Malfuction.

10. *Patients with shunt-dependent hydrocephalus should be admitted for consideration of shunt revision if shunt malfunction or infection is suspected. *In children, shunt revisions are scheduled according to growth rate. Overall, about 50–55% of shunted hydrocephalic children will achieve an intelligence quotient (IQ) of greater than 80, with verbal cognitive skills being superior to nonverbal ones. Not surprisingly, epilepsy appears to be an important predictor of poor intellectual outcome in shunted hydrocephalic children, with an IQ > 90 being seen in 66% of children without epilepsy compared with 24% of children with epilepsy.

---

* *Pearl/Peril/Pitfall: Although CSF dynamics may seem of purely academic interest, from a clinical perspective, the distinction between communicating and obstructive hydrocephalus remains important as it effects treatment options.*

THE EVALUATION-DECISION-ACTION-PLAN/ALGORITHM FOR THE DIAGNOSIS AND MANAGEMENT OF *A NEONATE WITH HYDROCEPHALUS*.

SUBJECTIVE FINDINGS

Hx of- Symptoms -excessively enlarging OFC, a full or bulging fontanel (soft spot located on the top of the head) *increasing head circumference *seizures *bulging eyes and an inability of the baby to look upward with the head facing forward *very noticeable scalp veins *increased irritability *high-pitched cry *poor feeding *projectile vomiting *sleepiness or less alert than usual *developmental delays *Hx of-* etiological factors such as, infection prematurity, bleeding inside the head, birth injury, abnormal blood vessel formation inside of the head, trauma, tumour *Hx of-*abnormal fetal USG Scans-In many cases, hydrocephalus does not develop until the third trimester of the pregnancy and, therefore, may not be seen on ultrasounds performed earlier in pregnancy.

Determine whether it is Congenital/Acquired in origin- *Requires* Detailed A/N and Perinatal Hx.

OBJECTIVE FINDINGS

Assess ABCDs - vitals, BP, CRT, O_2 sats, sensorium-alert/lethargic?, seizures and focal neurological signs (cranial nerve signs)+abnormal posturing, ability to suck and swallow (phonation and feeding difficulties due to corticobulbar dysfunction) , apnea/choking,

Look for signs and symptoms of increased ICP-Refer to Table 3 , Unequal Pupils, Tone and Postural abnormalities (more so in lower limbs), abnormal movements, Hyper/Hypoventilation etc., Optic nerve atrophy due to compression of dilated 3rd ventricles.

Perform complete physical + neuroexamination and *examine parents and siblings , if X-linked Aqueductal stenosis is being considered.* Assess for Shunt malfunction, if aVP Shunt is *in situ.*

INVESTIGATIONS

*No specific blood tests are recommended in the workup for hydrocephalus.
*Genetic testing and counseling might be recommended when X-linked hydrocephalus is suspected.
*Evaluate cerebrospinal fluid (CSF) in posthemorrhagic and postmeningitic hydrocephalus for protein concentration and to exclude residual infection.
*CT/MRI Brain Scan
*After shunt insertion, confirm correct positioning of installed hardware with a plain radiograph. EEG if seizure occurs.

Neonate with suspected hydrocephalus

Check whether the large head (Macrocephaly) is due to Hydrocephalus/Megalencephaly/Thickening of the Skull/Hemorrhage into the subdural or epidural spaces! If Hydrocephalus is confirmed (by the History, Physical examination and Imaging), determine whether is it Obstructive or Communicating.

Hydrocephalus is the main cause of macrocephaly at birth in which intracranial pressure is increased. Children with anatomical megalencephaly are often macrocephalic at birth but have normal ICP. Children with metabolic megalencephaly are usually normocephalic at birth and develop megalencephaly from cerebral edema during the Neonatal period. Increased thickness of the skull bones does not cause macrocephaly at birth or in the Neonatal period but develops during infancy.

Management depends on the underlying cause of Hydrocephalus!

Congenital Aqueductal Stenosis: Three quarters of affected fetuses have other malformations, usually spina bifida. Voluntary termination of such pregnancies is common. Ventriculoperitoneal shunt is the procedure of choice for Neonates and small infants.

Congenital brain tumors: Complete resection of brain tumors is unusual, with the exception of Choroid plexus papilloma.

Dandy-Walker Malformation: Decompression of the cyst alone provides immediate relief of symptoms; however, hydrocephalus recurs, and VP Shunting is required in 2/3 rds of affected children.

Communicating Hydrocephalus: (usually due to meningitis/subarachnoid hemorrhage)- *Do perform a routine USG head scan in all preterm <34 wk GA for detecting silent IVH, as clinical signs are nonspecific. *Do perform a follow-up USG head scan at 34-40 wk post menstrual age to evaluate adequately for PVL changes *Do perform a serial USG head scan q2–7 days to assess for posthemorrhagic hydrocephalus(PHH) *Do organize a permanent VP shunt if PHH has persisted for >4wks despite conservative therapy.

Benign enlargement of Subarachnoid spaces: Most affected infants develop normally and do not require ventricular shunts. *Plot head circumference measurements monthly for 6 months after diagnosis to be certain that growth is paralleling the normal curve. Repeat CT is unnecessary, unless head growth deviates from the normal curve, neurological examination is abnormal, or development is delayed.*

Chiari Malformations: Refer to Section "Chiari malformations -Surgery" for the details of management.

Ensure ABCs, Monitor Vitals, BP, O_2 sats., Raised ICP, Seizures, Apneas-Bradys, Focal neurodeficits.

Notify Pediatric Neurosurgeon for further input and surgical intervention, where appropriate.

If raised ICP is clinically evident, Ensure to *maintain head midline *elevate head of bed 30^0 *maintain normothermia *avoid noxious stimuli *do not use hypotonic infusions *do not lower BP (associated with Cushing`s response).

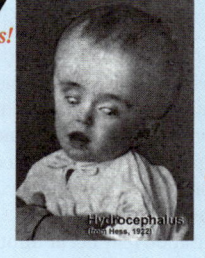

Hydrocephalus
(from Hess, 1922)

Check for the presence of VP Shunt/reservoir

NO
* Mannitol 0.5–1.0 g/kg IVB over 15–20 min. q 3–4 hours
* Insert bladder catheter
* Monitor labs q3–4 hours

*Intracranial hemorrhage-neurosurgical intervention
*Brain tumour/ abscess/cyst-IV Dexamethasone 1-2 mg/kg then 1–1.5 mg/kg/day in divided doses.
*Meningitis and Hyponatremia-Treat accordingly.

YES
Suspected shunt malfunction?
* May need to tap reservoir/ventricles
* Urgent Neurosurgical intervention

Suspected shunt infection?
* CSF complete analysis, C/S
* Do not delay Broad spectrum antibiotics if unstable

Transfer to NICU and Continue neuro resuscitation

---

* *Pearl/Peril/Pitfall: Patients with shunts should be reevaluated periodically, including assessment of distal shunt length in growing children. The first follow-up examination usually is scheduled 3 months after surgery, and CT scan or MRI of the head should be done at that time. Follow-up is performed every 6-12 months in the first 2 years of life. In children aged 2 years and older, follow-up is performed every 2 years*

TABLE 1   Differential diagnosis of accelerating head growth

Hydrocephalus

Noncommunicating

Aqueductal stenosis/gliosis (TORSCHH, Congenital, X- linked)

Malformations (Chiari II, Dandy-Walker-Cystic dilation of the 4th ventricle, the acqueduct, the 3rd and both lateral ventricles due to atretic foramen of Magendie and 1 or 2 foramina of Luschka.)and others), Neoplasm, Others (Arachnoid cyst, infection, etc.)

Communicating

Obstruction of arachnoid villi (posthemorrhagic (prematurity), inflammatory- Meningitis (especially bacterial), external hydrocephalus, hydranencephaly)

Arterial pressure in the venous system (AVM, Vein of Galen aneurysm)

Increased production of CSF(Choroid plexus papilloma)

Obstruction of CSF flow over the convexities (achondroplasia)

Increased brain mass

Edema (toxic-metabolic, AA, urea cycle, galactosemia, others)

Neoplasm

Extracerebral fluid

Subdural fluid collections (effusions, hematoma, empyema, others)

Extracranial fluid

Hematoma (subgaleal, subperiosteal [cephalhematoma], scalp[caput])

AA = aminoaciduria; AVM = arteriovenous malformation; CSF = cerebrospinal fluid; TORSCHH = Toxoplasmosis, Rubella, Syphilis, Cytomegalovirus, Herpes simplex, HIV, etc. Adapted from Current Management in Child Neurology, Bernard L.Maria 1999. B.C Decker Inc.

TABLE 2   Differential diagnosis of the large head without signs or symptoms of increased pressure

Megalencephaly with metabolic disease

Storage of metabolites (mucopolysaccharidoses, Alexander, Canavan, GM-2, others)

Anatomic megalencephaly

Unilateral

Isolated developmental anomaly of brain

With hamartomatous anomalies of brain and somatic structures

Bilateral

Familial magalencephaly

Asymptomatic

Symptomatic

With extracerebral fluid collections

Syndromes

Neurocutaneous syndromes

Other migrational defects (agenesis of CC, wide CSP, Riley-Smith, etc.)

With excessive somatic growth (Sotos, Weaver, Proteus, Beckwith, etc.)

With small stature (Russell-Silver, etc.)

Thickened extracerebral tissues

Subdural fluid collections (effusions)

Subgaleal, Subperiosteal, Scalp fluid/organizing hematomas

Skull thickening (osteodysplasias, rickets, anemia, others)

CC = corpus callosum; CSP = cavum septum pellucidum.
Adapted from Current Management in Child Neurology, Bernard L.Maria 1999. B.C Decker Inc.

TABLE 3   Signs and symptoms of increased intracranial pressure in infants

Behavioral signs	Physical signs
Decreased activity	Accelerating head growth
Poor feeding	Split/spread sutures (Macewen's sign)
Irritability	Tense anterior fontanelle
Lethargy	Dilated scalp veins
Vomiting	Setting-sun sign
(None)	Sixth nerve palsy
	Opisthotonus spasticity
	*Papilledema

*Rarely present in the Neonate, regardless of the degree of increased intracranial pressure.

TABLE 5   Medicolegal pitfalls

* Failure to recognize signs and symptoms of new onset hydrocephalus.

* Failure to recognize signs and symptoms of shunt malfunction or shunt infection, and failure to refer to a neurosurgeon immediately when these are suspected.

* Failure to inform patients with shunts and family members concerning the lifelong possibility of shunt complications.

TABLE 4   Essentials of shunt malfunction

A) Shunt infection: Most studies have reported rates of the order of 5–10% and significantly higher than this for Neonatal shunts.The role of antibiotic prophylaxis has been studied by metaanalysis, and antibiotic cover is recommended. Most shunt infections occur in the first six months after the operation and the most common organisms are staphylococci (Staphylococcus epidermidis, 40%; Staphylococcus aureus, 20%). Other species seen include coryneforms, streptococci, enterococci, aerobic Gram-negative rods, and yeasts. Most shunt infections result from contamination with the patient's own skin flora, which underlines the need for meticulous attention to surgical technique. Unfortunately, once a shunt is infected, it is almost always necessary to remove it and insert a temporary external ventricular drain.

B) Mechanical failure: The use of Kaplan-Meier curves to display shunt survival has led to a far greater understanding of shunt failure. Virtually all the studies to date have shown an exponential curve, with about 40% of shunts failing (including infection) in the first year and then about 5% a year. Over 50% of first shunt failures are due to obstruction, with the vast majority of these occurring at the ventricular catheter. This is almost certainly a consequence of the fact that all shunts overdrain, so that the ventricular catheter comes to lie against the ependyma and choroid plexus of the ventricle, and these tissues can then become incorporated into and block the holes at the end of the catheter. Although it is reassuring to see collapsed ventricles on a scan, this is probably not ideal for long term shunt functioning. Very occasionally, patients develop slit ventricle syndrome, which is transient symptoms of raised ICP in the setting of a scan that shows small or non-existent ventricles.

C) Functional failure: The cause of functional failure is usually overdrainage. The underlying problem is one of siphoning from the ventricle to the level of the distal tube (over a metre in an adult). This overdrainage can result in subdural hematoma, low pressure symptoms (postural headache and nausea), and craniosynostosis.

Pearl/Peril/Pitfall: In particular, it became clear that there are three ways in which shunts can malfunction: (a) they can become infected; (b) they can fail mechanically; (c) they can overdrain or underdrain (termed a "functional" failure).

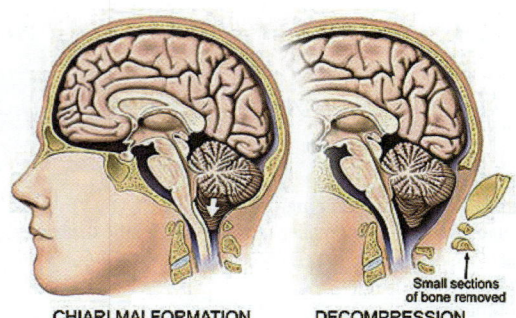

CHIARI MALFORMATION   DECOMPRESSION

Small sections of bone removed

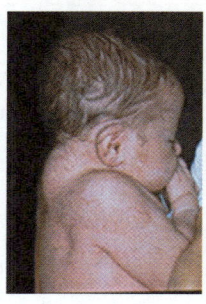 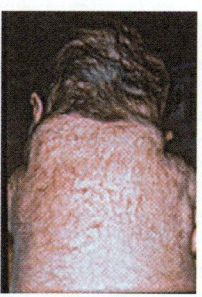

Type II Chiari Malformation: This malformation is characterized by downward displacement of the medulla, fourth ventricle, and cerebellum into the cervical spinal canal, as well as elongation of the pons and fourth ventricle. This type occurs almost exclusively in patients with myelomeningocele. Myelomeningocele is a congenital condition in which the spinal cord and column do not close properly during fetal development, resulting in an open spinal cord defect at birth. Other abnormalities associated with myelomeningocele include hydrocephalus (fluid in the brain), cardiovascular abnormalities (heart problems), imperforate anus (incomplete or no anus) as well as other gastrointestinal abnormalities. The symptoms associated with a Chiari II malformation can also be caused by problems related to myelomeningocele and hydrocephalus. These symptoms include: · Alteration in the pattern of breathing, including periods of apnea (brief periods of cessation of breathing) · Depressed gag reflex · Involuntary, rapid, downward eye movements · Loss of arm strength.

Type III Chiari Malformation: This malformation includes a form of dysraphism with a portion of the cerebellum and/or brainstem pushing out through a defect in the back of the head or neck. These malformations are very rare and are associated with a high early mortality rate, or severe neurological deficits in patients that survive. If treatment is undertaken, then early operative closure of the defect is necessitated. Hydrocephalus, which is commonly present, must also be treated through shunting. Additional severe birth defects are often present, which may require extensive treatment. Infants with Chiari III malformation may have life-threatening complications.

Syringomyelia / Hydromyelia: When CSF forms a cavity or cyst within the spinal cord, it is known as syringomyelia or hydromyelia. These are chronic disorders involving the spinal cord developing, expanding or extending over time. As the fluid cavity expands, it can displace or injure the nerve fibers inside the spinal cord. Syringomyelia/Hydromyelia Symptoms. A wide variety of symptoms can occur, depending upon the size and location of the syrinx. Loss of sensation in an area served by several nerve roots is one typical symptom, as is the development of scoliosis. Syringomyelia can arise from several causes. Chiari malformation is the leading cause of syringomyelia, although the direct link is not well understood. It is thought to be related to the interference of normal CSF pulsations caused by the cerebellar tissue obstructing flow at the foramen magnum. This condition can also occur as a complication of trauma, meningitis, tumor, arachnoiditis, or a tethered spinal cord. In these cases, the syrinx forms in the section of the spinal cord damaged by these conditions. As more people are surviving spinal cord injuries, increased cases of post-traumatic syringomyelia are being diagnosed. Hydromyelia is usually defined as an abnormal widening of the central canal of the spinal cord. The central canal, a very thin cavity in the middle of the spinal cord, is a remnant of normal development.

Treatment: Treatment of Chiari malformations and syringomyelia is very dependent on the exact type of malformation, as well as progression in anatomy changes or symptoms.

Chiari I malformations that are asymptomatic should be left alone. There is no indication for "prophylactic" surgery on these. If the malformation is defined as symptomatic, or is causing a syrinx, treatment is usually recommended. **Chiari** II malformations are treated if the patient is symptomatic, and physicians have determined that there are no complications from hydrocephalus. In some patients, consideration of a tethered cord is also explored. In many infants who become symptomatic from a Chiari II malformation, the symptom onset and progression are severe and rapid, and this requires an urgent or emergency approach.

Surgery: Surgical treatment of these malformations depends on the type of malformation. The goal of surgery is to relieve the symptoms, or stop the progression of the syrinx or symptoms. Chiari I malformations may be treated surgically with only local decompression of the overlying bones, decompression of the bones and release of the dura (a thick membrane covering the brain and spinal cord), or decompression of the bone and dura and some degree of cerebellar tissue resection. Decompression is performed under general anesthesia. It consists of removing the back of the foramen magnum and often the back of the first few vertebrae to the point where the cerebellar tonsils end. This provides more space for the brainstem, spinal cord, and descended cerebellar components.tissue graft is often spliced into this opening to provide even more room for the unimpeded passage of CSF. Occasionally, the cavity within the spinal cord resulting from hydromyelia can be drained with a diverting shunt tube. This tube can divert the fluid from inside the spinal cord to outside the cord, or be directed to either the chest or abdominal cavity. These procedures can be done together or separately. **Chiari II** decompression is treated similarly, but is usually restricted to decompressing the tissues in the spinal canal and leaving the back of the skull alone. **The goal of Chiari surgery** is Optimal decompression of nerve tissue· Reconstruction of normal CSF flow around and behind the cerebellum.

Outcome: The benefits of surgery should always be weighed carefully against its risks. Although some patients experience a reduction in their symptoms, there is no guarantee that surgery will help every individual. Nerve damage that has already occurred usually cannot be reversed. Some surgical patients need repeat surgeries, while others may not achieve symptom relief.

Endoscopic view of the Foramen of Monro. The arrow is on the fornix and pointing to the Foramen of Monro. The arrowhead points to the choroid plexus in the lateral ventricle entering the foramen.

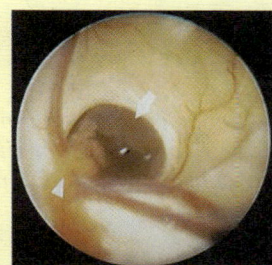 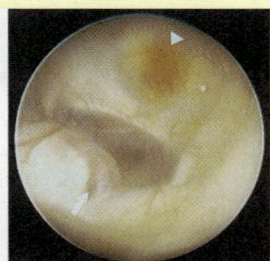

Endoscopic view of the floor of the third ventricle. The structures seen are the basilar artery bifurcation (arrow) immediately anterior to the mamillary bodies. The third ventriculostomy stoma is made anterior to the basilar artery. The arrowhead points to the infundibulum at the base of the pituitary stalk.

*Third ventriculostomy : Open third ventriculostomy (TV)—literally making a hole to connect the third ventricle with the subarachnoid space:TV has grown in popularity as an alternative to shunt placement for patients with triventricular (obstructive) hydrocephalus *Endoscopic TV entails entering the lateral ventricle, passage through the Foramen of Monro, identification of the mamillary bodies, and then perforation of the floor of the third ventricle just anterior to the bifurcation of the basilar artery. *However aesthetically appealing it is, there is no point in performing a TV if the absorptive capacity is abnormal. Unfortunately, there is no easy and reliable method of determining absorptive capacity. * A number of recent studies have described "success" rates of 49–100% with endoscopic TV; however, most of these studies have been descriptive and the outcome measures vague. *Failure to complete the procedure for technical reasons has been reported in up to 26% of patients and, not surprisingly, the main complication is hemorrhage secondary to vascular damage. Other reported complications include cardiac arrest, diabetes insipidus, inappropriate antidiuretic hormone, subdural hematoma, meningitis, and cerebral infarction. *The rate of shunt infection after failed TV is as yet unknown but needs to be quantified. As the potential operative risks with TV are greater than with shunting, careful patient selection is of paramount importance.
Courtesy: Hydrocephalus—what's new? P CHUMAS, A TYAGI, J LIVINGSTON Departments of Neurosurgery and Paediatric Neurology, Division of Paediatric Neurosciences, Leeds General Infirmary, Leeds LS1 3EX,UK Arch Dis Child Fetal Neonatal Ed 2001;85:F149–F154

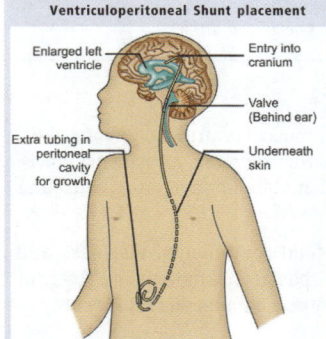

Ventriculoperitoneal Shunt placement

Enlarged left ventricle
Entry into cranium
Valve (Behind ear)
Extra tubing in peritoneal cavity for growth
Underneath skin

Surgery may be needed for some cases of hydrocephalus. Surgery usually involves placing a mechanical shunting device into the baby's head to help drain the extra CSF from the brain and redirect the extra fluid to another part of the body to be absorbed. A common type of shunt is the ventriculoperitoneal shunt. The shunt consists of three parts: *a tube that is placed inside of the ventricular space *a reservoir and valve to control the flow of CSF *tubing that is directed under the skin to the abdomen, or less commonly to the heart or lung area. Potential complications from the shunts or surgery can include the following: *infection *shunt malfunction that results in under-drainage or over-drainage of the CSF *bleeding. Other complications may include fever, vomiting, irritability, redness and swelling along the area of the tubing, or decreased alertness or lethargy.These complications require prompt medical evaluation.

KEY POINTS FOR CLINICAL PRACTICE

1. Congenital hydrocephalus applies to the ventriculomegaly that develops in the fetal and infancy periods, often associated with macrocephaly. The most common causes of congenital hydrocephalus are obstruction of the cerebral aqueduct flow, Arnold-Chiari malformation or Dandy–Walker malformation. These patients may stabilize in later years due to compensatory mechanisms but may decompensate, especially following minor head injuries.

2. Communicating hydrocephalus occurs when full communication occurs between the ventricles and subarachnoid space. It is caused by overproduction of CSF (rarely), defective absorption of CSF (most often), or venous drainage insufficiency (occasionally). Noncommunicating hydrocephalus occurs when CSF flow is obstructed within the ventricular system or in its outlets to the arachnoid space, resulting in impairment of the CSF from the ventricular to the subarachnoid space.

3. Ultrasonography through the anterior fontanelle in infants is useful for evaluating subependymal and intraventricular hemorrhage and in following infants for possible development of progressive hydrocephalus. CT can assess the size of ventricles and other structures. MRI can evaluate

for Chiari malformation or cerebellar or periaqueductal tumors. It affords better imaging of the posterior fossa than CT.

4. Treatment options-NON-SURGICAL-Diuretics are still often used in neonatal patients with post-hemorrhagic hydrocephalus (PHH) despite reports of side effects such as acidosis, CO2 retention, electrolyte disturbance, etc. A recent multicentre randomized controlled trial actually showed a higher rate of shunt placement and increased neurological morbidity in the group receiving diuretics.

5. Surgical Management is the Preferred therapeutic option- A ventriculoperitoneal (VP) shunt is used most commonly. There are three ways in which shunts can malfunction: (a) they can become infected; (b) they can fail mechanically; (c) they can overdrain or underdrain (termed a "functional" failure). *Patients with shunt-dependent hydrocephalus should be admitted for consideration of shunt revision if shunt malfunction or infection is suspected. *In children, shunt revisions are scheduled according to growth rate. Overall, about 50–55% of shunted hydrocephalic children will achieve an intelligence quotient (IQ) of greater than 80, with verbal cognitive skills being superior to non-verbal ones

REFERENCES AND FURTHER READING : 1) Rekate HL. A contemporary definition and classification of hydrocephalus. Semin Pediatr Neurol. Mar 2009;16(1):9-15. 2)Partington MD. Congenital hydrocephalus. Neurosurg Clin N Am. Oct 2001;12(4):737-42, ix. 3) du Plessis AJ. Posthemorrhagic hydrocephalus and brain injury in the preterm infant: dilemmas in diagnosis and management. Semin Pediatr Neurol. Sep 1998;5(3):161-79. 4)Frim DM, Scott RM, Madsen JR. Surgical management of neonatal hydrocephalus. Neurosurg Clin N Am. Jan 1998;9(1):105-10. 5)McAllister JP, Chovan P. Neonatal hydrocephalus. Mechanisms and consequences. Neurosurg Clin North Am 1998;9:73–93

32 Floppy Infant—Neonatal Hypotonia

@ *Neonatal Hypotonia- Although specific treatments are not always available, accurate diagnosis is critical to predict the clinical course, associated manifestations, complications, prognosis, and provide genetic counseling*

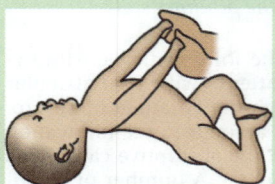 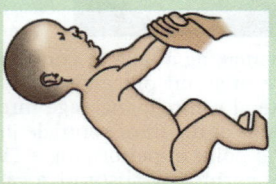 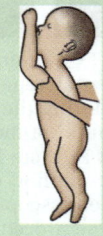 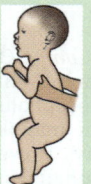

Vertical suspension response is elicited by holding the neonate with both hands under the axillas and lifting the neonate up. A hypotonic neonate shows poor shoulder support, the head drops, and the lower extremities remain extended and limp.

A normal neonate shows good shoulder and head support and flexion at the hips, knees, and ankles.

The arm traction response is obtained by slowly pulling the neonate by the hands to achieve a sitting position. A hypotonic neonate shows head lag, no arm pull is felt by the examiner, the arms remain extended as the body is pulled up, and the legs remain in contact with the bed.

A normal neonate shows minimal head lag, a backward pull is felt by the examiner as the neonate's arms are pulled, and there is flexion of the elbows, knees, and ankles.

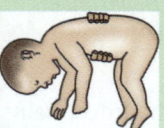 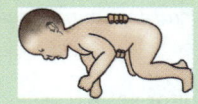

Horizontal suspension response is elicited by placing the neonate face down and lifting the neonate by the trunk. A hypotonic neonate bends ventrally and the head and limbs drop straight down like a rag doll. A normal neonate straightens the torso, briefly lifts the head up, and flexes the elbows, hips, knees, and ankles

Summary of types of Hypotonias

Central hypotonia

Site of lesion: Brain, brainstem, spinal cord (above the origin of the cranial nerve nuclei or anterior horn cells).

Causes: Brain malformations, chromosomal aberration: e.g. Down's syndrome, Prader-Willi syndrome, cerebellar hypoplasia.

Clues to diagnosis: History of brain insult, seizures, dysmorphic features, lack of interest in surroundings, abnormal head size, normal spontaneous movements, normal or increased reflexes, persistence of primitive reflexes, organomegaly.

Peripheral hypotonia

Site of lesion: Cranial nerve nuclei, anterior horn cell, nerve roots, peripheral nerves, neuromuscular junction or muscle.

Causes: Spinal cord injury, spinal muscular atrophy, poliomyelitis, peripheral neuropathy, Guillain-Barre syndrome, myasthenia gravis, infantile botulism, congenital or metabolic myopathy, muscular dystrophy.

Clues to diagnosis: Decreased fetal movements, alertness and responsiveness, weakness with little spontaneous movements, absent or decreased reflexes, fasciculations, muscle atrophy, and sensory loss.

Mixed hypotonia

Features of both central and peripheral hypotonia due to combined central and peripheral pathology (e.g. peroxisomal, lysosomal, and mitochondrial disorders, or any cause of peripheral hypotonia with an acquired hypoxic ischemic brain insult)

REVIEW OF CLINICAL PROBLEMS

1. How do you differentiate Neuromuscular Hypotonia from Central Hypotonia?
   Ans: Refer to the Evaluation-Decision-Action-plan/algorithm for the diagnosis and management of a Neonate with Hypotonia.

2. What are the differential diagnoses of Central Hypotonia in Neonatal period?
   Ans: Refer to the Table 1 of the Chapter.

3. What are the patterns of weakness in Neuromuscular Hypotonia?
   Ans: Refer to the Table 2 of the Chapter.

4. How do you diagnose and manage Transient Neonatal Myasthenia?
   Ans: Refer to the Synopsis of conditions causing Neuromuscular Hypotonia.

5. Mention the important aspects of history and physical examination in the evaluation of Neonatal Hypotonia.
   Ans: Refer to the Evaluation-Decision-Action-plan/algorithm for the diagnosis and management of a Neonate with Hypotonia..

LEARNING OBJECTIVES

After completing this article, readers will be able to

1. Recognize signs & symptoms of neuromuscular disorders
2. Diagnose causes of infantile weakness or hypotonia
3. Diagnose causes of acute or subacute weakness
4. Diagnose causes of progressive weakness
5. Refer patients with neuromuscular disorders to appropriate specialists for assistance in diagnosis
6. Coordinate care of patients with neuromuscular disorders (neurologist, physiatrist, pulmonologist, orthopedist, genetic counselling, cardiologist etc.)
7. Provide acute care & preventive care for patients with neuromuscular disorders (supportive care)
8. Help patient & family in end-of-life decisions & care

Pearl/Peril/Pitfall : EMG is a good initial diagnostic test for floppy children with neurogenic cause (SMA) having 80% sensitivity. Paradoxically, in most severe SMA type I, EMG was only 50% sensitive suggesting that diagnosis of SMA may be missed on EMG alone. Muscle biopsy is needed for precise characterization with immune and enzyme histochemistry and electron microscopy.

1. Neonatal hypotonia (Floppy infant) is a very significant symptom in a term baby and should never be ignored. *Preterm infants are normally hypotonic and muscle tone increases as the gestational maturity proceeds.* Generalized hypotonia may be due to abnormalities in a variety of anatomical sites: 1.*Brain* (asphyxia); 2.Spinal cord (trauma); 3. *Anterior horn cell* (spinal muscular atrophy); 4.*Nerve root* (brachial plexus injury). This causes hypotonia only of the affected limb; 5.*Peripheral nerve* (trauma); 6.*Neuromuscular junction* (myasthenia gravis); 7.*Muscle* (congenital dystrophy).

2. The presence of hypotonia is confirmed by the clinical findings such as **a)**frog-legged posturing when lying supine with lack of spontaneous movement **b)**Head lag when pulled to sitting posture from supine position **c)**Head falling forward and the arms hanging limply at the infant's side in the sitting posture **d)**slipping through fingers when vertically suspended by the arms under the infant's axillae **e)**_unable to_ lift the head & straighten the back & maintain flexion of the limbs (inverted "U" in prone suspension - Landau posture) **f)**Positive scarf sign.

3. Then, *Confirm* the presence of **weakness/paralysis** by the clinical finding - lack of movement against gravity (e.g. fails to kick the legs, hold up the arms, or attempt to stand when held) or in response to stimuli such as tickling or slight pain. This finding helps to differentiate *central hypotonia* from *neuromuscular hypotonia*—In central hypotonia, hypotonia occurs without weakness while in neuromuscular hypotonia the infant will be both hypotonic & weak. (See the *Evaluation-Decision-Action-Plan/Algorithm*).

4. *Beware of the fact* that an infant with a congenital neuromuscular disorder may suffer perinatal asphyxia or spinal cord injury during the course of a difficult delivery & consequently he/she may have several levels of the nervous system involved simultaneously.

5. *Central hypotonia* (Non paralytic) has various causes (refer to Table 1 of the Chapter) which should be differentiated by the use of laboratory, imaging, and neurophysiologic methods to evaluate the regions of nervous system such as cerebrum, brainstem, cerebellum, and spinal cord. The *Evaluation-Decision-Action-Plan/Algorithm* describes the essential aspects of diagnosis & management a Neonate with *Central Hypotonia.* Generalized hypotonia must be differentiated from decreased generalized movements due to pain. Neonates with generalized hypotonia and neonates with decreased movement due to pain have the same posture, yet during arm traction and during vertical and horizontal suspensions the typical hypotonic responses are not present in neonates with decreased generalized movement due to pain. Neonates with decreased generalized movement due to pain become stiff and cry during any of these maneuvers.

6. *Neuromuscular hypotonia* results from diseases that involve the motor neuron in the brainstem, anterior horn cell, peripheral nerves, neuromuscular junction, and the muscle itself—the *systematic evaluation* should include (history, general physical examination, neurologic examination and diagnostic studies such as serum Creatine Kinase [CK], Electro Myogram [EMG], Nerve Conduction Velocity [NCV], measurements and muscle biopsy and nerve biopsy. Specific genetic diagnosis by Polymerase Chain Reaction [PCR]).Table 3 of the Chapter classifies common and uncommon causes of Neonatal hypotonia; central hypotonia is more common than neuromuscular hypotonia obviously Refer to the Table 4 of the Chapter for the essentials of various investigations necessary for the differential diagnosis of neuromuscular hypotonia.

7. The *Evaluation-Decision-Action-Plan/Algorithm* also describes the essential aspects of diagnosis & management of a Neonate with *Neuromuscular hypotonia; a)History* should determine the duration of the problem, the distribution of the weakness (proximal, distal, or diffuse), associated symptoms such as pain, cramping, sensory loss, fatiguability, and urine changes, and family history of neuromuscular disorders, onset and vigour of intrauterine fetal movements, occurrence of poly/oligo hydramnios, presentation at birth (breech is more common in neuromuscular disorders), and the difficulty of the delivery, occurrence of neonatal respiratory distress, feeding difficulties, strength of the cry, presence of seizures or encephalopathy indicative of central hypotonia). *b)General physical examination* should identify the infant's alertness, respiratory distress, ptosis, weak cry, facial weakness, ocular muscle palsy, inability to suck, swallow, apnea/choking, arthrogryposis, exclusion of dysmorphic syndromes (Down, Prader-Willi, Marfan, Ehler-Danlos, Dysautonomia, Turner, LMB, etc.) systemic diseases such as malnutrition, chronic medical illness (CHD, BPD, Uremia, RTA), metabolic disease (hypercalcemia, Lowe disease, Pompe disease, Leigh disease etc.) and endocrinopathy (hypothyroidism). Look for congenital anomalies such as micrognathia,prominent forehead, high arched palate and undescended testes (congenital neuromuscular disorders due to weakened gubernaculum) *(c)Neurologic examination* should determine the degree of weakness, changes in or the presence or absence of deep tendon reflexes, and the presence or absence of sensory findings.

8. Table 5 of the Chapter gives the essential featur*es of diagnosis & management* of various causes of **Neonatal hypotonia**.General Management of neuromuscular hypotonia includes: Cardio-respiratory support pending definitive evaluation; Optimize nutrition(nasogastric tube feeding); Minimize Orthopedic deformities; Prepare family for chronic care needs.

9. An increasing number of recognized gene deletions may be detected by molecular genetics to enable the prenatal diagnosis. DNA may be extracted & stored for future genetic analysis.

10. The advent of investigative techniques, immunohistochemical/ultrastructural studies on muscle and nerve, and genetic studies have resulted in many benign essential hypotonia getting classified into specific disorders.

Difficulty of Feeding in the Alert Newborn

Congenital myotonic dystrophy, Familial dysautonomia, Genetic myasthenic syndromes, Hypoplasia of bulbar motor nuclei, Infantile neuronal degeneration, Myophosphorylase deficiency, Neurogenic arthrogryposis, Prader-Willi syndrome, Transitory neonatal myasthenia

Clues to Motor Unit Disorders

Absent or depressed tendon reflexes
Failure of movement on postural reflexes
Fasciculations
Muscle atrophy
No abnormalities of other organs

Clues to Cerebral Hypotonia

Abnormalities of other brain functions
Dysmorphic features
Fisting of the hands
Malformations of other organs
Movement through postural reflexes
Normal or brisk tendon reflexes
Scissoring on vertical suspension

---

* ***Pearl/Peril/Pitfall:*** *If the underlying cause is known, treatment is tailored to the specific disease, followed by symptomatic and supportive therapy for the hypotonia. In very severe cases, treatment may be primarily supportive, such as mechanical assistance with basic life functions like breathing and feeding, physical therapy to prevent muscle atrophy and maintain joint mobility, and measures to try to prevent opportunistic infections such as pneumonia.*

THE EVALUATION-DECISION-ACTION-PLAN/ALGORITHM FOR THE DIAGNOSIS AND MANAGEMENT OF *A NEONATE WITH HYPOTONIA (FLOPPY INFANT).*

SUBJECTIVE FINDINGS

Hx of Symptoms such as level of consciousness, and activity,spontaneous movements, limpy baby(hypotonic) on handling, poor suck, generalized *frog-leg* posturing / tonic posturing (often thought to be a seizures),muscular twitchings,strength of cry,frank seizures,breathing difficulties etc.,

Hx of polyhydramnios, reduced fetal movements, breech presentation, abnormal labor,birth asphyxia.

Hx of consanguinity,delayed milestones, and childhood deaths in the family. *Inquire from the mother & examine for signs of Myotonic dystrophy or Myasthenia gravis.*

OBJECTIVE FINDINGS

Assess ABCDs—vitals, BP, CRT, O₂ sats, sensorium-alert/lethargic? seizures and focal neurological signs (cranial nerve signs)+abnormal posturing, ability to suck & swallow,apnea/choking,

Look for reduced tone, power, and muscle bulk, ptosis, myotonia + fasciculations (may not be present), dysmorphic features, arthrogryposis, facial weakness, undescended testes, common congenital anomalies.

Perform complete physical + neuroexamination and *examine parents for Myotonia & Myasthenia!*

INVESTIGATIONS

Blood FBC, differential, platelets, hematocrit, blood cultures, ABG analysis, *Blood sugar,* BUN, creatinine, electrolytes, Ca⁺⁺, Mg⁺⁺,Phosphate, LTFs, drug screen, ammonia,bilirubin, TFTs, serum CK with isoenzymes MM,MB&BB aldolase, Tensilon/Neostigmine test. Acetylcholine receptor antibodies

Urine analysis
Imaging CXR, , USG /CT/MRI BRAIN SCAN

Perform COMPLETE SEPSIS SCREEN + LP if not C/I- FBC, CRP, blood & urine cultures, CXR etc.,

CONSIDER ECG,plasma amino acids,urine organic acids, serum lactate,pyruvate,DNA analysis- PCR,*EMG, NCV,Muscle &/or sural nerve biopsy,CSF ANALYSIS,when clinical course demands.*

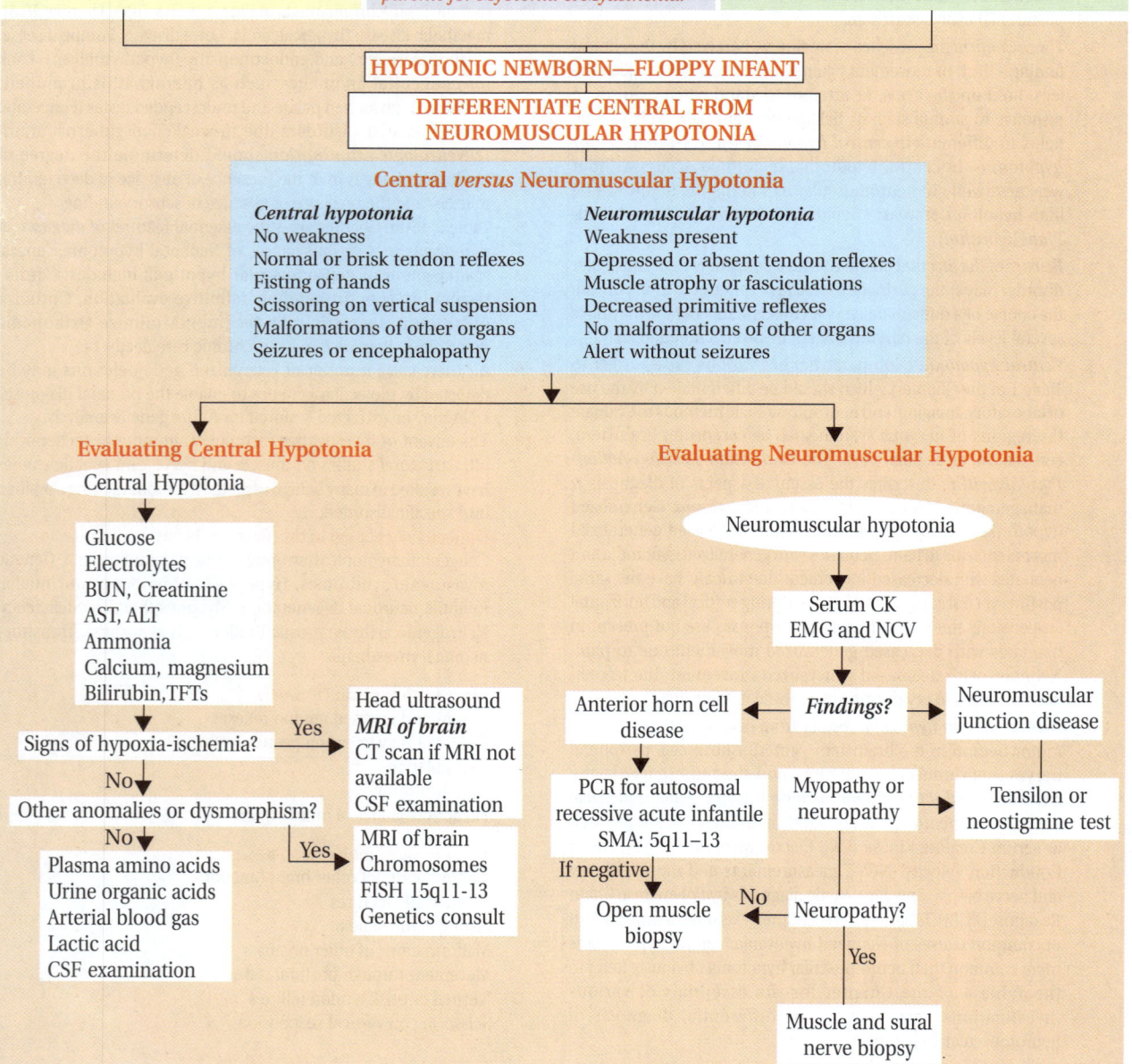

HYPOTONIC NEWBORN—FLOPPY INFANT

DIFFERENTIATE CENTRAL FROM NEUROMUSCULAR HYPOTONIA

Central *versus* Neuromuscular Hypotonia

Central hypotonia	*Neuromuscular hypotonia*
No weakness	Weakness present
Normal or brisk tendon reflexes	Depressed or absent tendon reflexes
Fisting of hands	Muscle atrophy or fasciculations
Scissoring on vertical suspension	Decreased primitive reflexes
Malformations of other organs	No malformations of other organs
Seizures or encephalopathy	Alert without seizures

Evaluating Central Hypotonia

Central Hypotonia

Glucose
Electrolytes
BUN, Creatinine
AST, ALT
Ammonia
Calcium, magnesium
Bilirubin,TFTs

Signs of hypoxia-ischemia? — **Yes** →

No ↓

Other anomalies or dysmorphism?

No ↓   **Yes** →

Plasma amino acids
Urine organic acids
Arterial blood gas
Lactic acid
CSF examination

Head ultrasound
MRI of brain
CT scan if MRI not available
CSF examination

MRI of brain
Chromosomes
FISH 15q11-13
Genetics consult

Evaluating Neuromuscular Hypotonia

Neuromuscular hypotonia

Serum CK
EMG and NCV

Anterior horn cell disease ← *Findings?* → Neuromuscular junction disease

PCR for autosomal recessive acute infantile SMA: 5q11–13

If negative ↓

Myopathy or neuropathy

Tensilon or neostigmine test

Open muscle biopsy ← **No** — Neuropathy?

Yes ↓

Muscle and sural nerve biopsy

Pearl/Peril/Pitfall: Muscle tone is the amount of tension or resistance to movement in a muscle. It is not the same as muscle weakness, which is a reduction in the strength of a muscle, but it can coexist with muscle weakness. Muscle tone indicates the ability of a muscle to respond to a stretch.

TABLE 1 Differential diagnosis of central hypotonia

Hypoxic-ischemic encephalopathy

Central nervous system malformations (neuronal migrational anomalies, cerebellar hypoplasias)

Intracranial hemorrhage (subdural, subarachnoid, intraventricular)

Intracranial infection (meningitis, encephalitis, congenital infections)

Sepsis (Group B streptococcal, Gram-negative)

Acute metabolic disorders (glucose, electrolytes, ammonia, calcium, magnesium, bilirubin)

Inborn metabolic disorders (amino acids, organic acids, urea cycle, peroxisomal)

Endocrine disorders (hypothyroid, CAH)

Chromosomal disorders (Down syndrome, Prader-Willi syndrome)

Intrapartum intoxications (narcotics, $MgSO_4$, local anesthetic in infant scalp)

Trauma (cerebral, spinal cord)

Cyanotic congenital heart disease (especially tetralogy of Fallot)

TABLE 2 Differential diagnosis of neuromuscular hypotonia

Motor Neuron	Spinal muscular atrophy	Generalized weakness, often spares the diaphragm, facial muscles, pelvis, and sphincters
Nerve	Peripheral neuropathies	Distal muscle groups involved
Neuromuscular junction	Myasthenia syndromes infantile botulism	Bulbar, oculomotor muscles exhibit greater degree of involvement
Muscle	Congenital myopathies, metabolic myopathies, congenital muscular dystrophy congenital myotonic dystrophy	weakness is prominent, proximal musculature, hypoactive reflexes, joint contractures

TABLE 3 Neonatal hypotonia-common & uncommon causes

Common causes :

Prematurity, Neonatal encephalopathy (Hypoxia, Hypoglycemia, Infection), Drugs administered to baby or mother

Uncommon/Rare causes :

Neuromuscular- (anterior horn cell, peripheral nerves, muscles), Spinal muscular atrophy, Congenital muscular dystrophy, Congenital myopathy, Congenital myotonic dystrophy, Neonatal myasthenia, *Metabolic-* IEM Renal tubular acidosis, Hypothyroidism, *Central CNS origin-*chromosomal disorders, Connective tissue disorders, Prader - Willi syndrome CNS malformations, Benign congenital hypotonia

TABLE 4 Neonatal hypotonia-essentials of diagnostic investigations

* *Preliminary diagnostic tests* include complete blood count, ESR, CK, liver function tests, CXR, ECG, & pulmonary function studies.

* *Serum Creatine Kinase (CK)-* mild elevation occurs in rapidly progressive neuropathic conditions, such as Werdnig - Hoffmann disease, but significant elevation (upto 50 times the upper normal) occurs in infants with several forms of congenital muscular dystrophy. CPK has 3 isozymes: MM for skeletal muscle, MB for cardiac muscle, & BB for brain. Many diseases of motor unit may not be associated with elevated enzymes.

* *EMG* - normal in central hypotonia, shows fasciculations & fibrillations - denervation pattern in anterior horn cell disease (W-H disease), fibrillations in peripheral nerve disease, decremental response in myasthenia, incremental response in botulism, short duration + small amplitude motor unit potentials + myopathic polyphasic potentials in myopathies.

* *Imaging of muscle* - MRI is quite useful in identifying inflammatory myopathies of immune (dermatomyositis) or infectious (viral, bacterial, parasitic) origin. MRI is the study of choice to image the spinal cord, nerve roots, or plexus (e.g.. brachial).

* *Nerve Conduction Velocity (NCV)* - because the NCV study measures only the fastest conducting fibres in a nerve, 80% of total nerve fibers must be involved before slowing in conduction is detected. Neuropathies of various types are detected by decreased conduction. The site of a traumatic nerve injury may also be localized. Peripheral neuropathies primarily affect either the axons or the myelin sheath. Demyelinating neuropathies cause greater slowing of conduction times where as axonal neuropathies demonstrate diminished action potential amplitudes.

* *Muscle biopsy* - single most definitive diagnostic procedure available for the evaluation of the infant with neuromuscular hypotonia. Accurate diagnosis of the structural myopathies requires an open biopsy rather than a needle biopsy. The specimen is subjected to histologic, histochemical, electron microscopic, & biochemical studies (mitochondrial cytopathies, acid maltase, carnitine palmityltransferase) to identify various myopathies. Muscle biopsy is normal in central hypotonia & in neuromuscular disorders. It shows denervation pattern in diseases affecting anterior horn cell & peripheral nerve. Interpretation is technically difficult in neonates.

* *Nerve biopsy-* sural nerve biopsy is helpful in many neuropathies whose clinical manifestations are predominantly motor. Sural nerve is a pure sensory nerve that supplies a small area of skin on the lateral surface of the foot. When sural nerve is severed behind the lateral malleolus of the ankle, regeneration of the nerve occurs in more than 90% of cases so that permanent sensory loss is not experienced. Electron microscopy is performed on most nerve biopsy specimen because many morphologic alterations cannot be appreciated at the resolution of a light microscope.

* *Molecular genetic markers by means of PCR technique* have fast replacing muscle biopsy as the mainstay of diagnosis especially in diseases such as W-H disease & congenital myotonic dystrophy. Prenatal diagnosis of some of these disorders may also be available.

Pearl/Peril/Pitfall: Parents of an hypotonic child must follow the treating physician's orders for treatment of the underlying cause. They must exercise special care when lifting and carrying the hypotonic infant to avoid causing an injury to the child. If lifted under the armpits, the hypotonic infant's arms will raise with no resistance and easily slip between the hands.

TABLE 5 Differential diagnosis of conditions causing neuromuscular hypotonia.

1. *MYOTONIC DYSTROPHY(MD):* *Severe neonatal form of MD appears in a minority of involved infants born to mothers with MD and is characterized by generalized hypotonia & weakness at birth along with prominent facial wasting *May require gavage feeding or prolonged ventilatory support for respiratory muscle weakness or apnea *Gaseous distention of stomach & small intestines occurs due to poor peristalsis from smooth muscle weakness *Polyhydramnios secondary to swallowing difficulties in utero, immobile face, triangular mouth (inverted v-shaped upper lip),thin cheeks,concave temporal fossae,cataracts are the important findings *Myotonia is not a feature until the about age 5 yr but mother is always affected(shake hands with her for demonstrating her inability to relax the grip) *Learning difficulties, Endocrine abnormalities,cardiac conduction problems rather than cardiomyopathy, unlike most other muscular dystrophies may occur later *Diagnosis is by clinical manifestations in typical cases and by muscle biopsy + DNA analysis of blood to demonstrate the abnomal expansion of CTG(Cytosine-Thymine-Guanine) repeat on chromosome 19 at 19q13 locus;prenatal diagnosis also feasible *Treatment is symptomatic and supportive only.

2. *WERDNIG-HOFFMAN DISEASE:* SMA type 1-acute spinal muscular atrophy*Progressive severe degeneration of anterior horn cells in spinal cord and cranial nerve motor nuclei due to deletion of 2 genes at 5q11.2-13.3 transmitted in a autosomal recessive pattern with prenatal and postnatal diagnosis possible *Diminished fetal movements, respiratory distress at birth, alertness despite hypotonia & weakness, impaired suck & swallow, fasciculations of the tongue, areflexia, frog-leg posturing commonly obvious *Lower limbs>upper limbs, Proximal muscles>Distal muscles involved *Paralysis of bulbar muscles, loss of cough reflex, and an inaudible cry occur as the disease advances *EMG shows spontaneous fasciculations and fibrillations.*CK is normal or moderately elevated(5 times upper limit of normal).*Rapid deterioration & respiratory death occur in the first 2 years of life.*Treatment is supportive only, given the poor prognosis.

3. *TRANSIENT NEONATAL MYASTHENIA:* *20% of infants born to mothers with acquired Myasthenia gravis develop this self-limiting but potentially life-threatening form and is due to transplacental transfer of maternal antibodies directed against the acetylcholine receptor (AchR) *Onset is within a few hours of birth and always within the first 3 days *Typical features include severe generalized hypotonia,poor suck and swallow, facial weakness, weak cry, dysphagia, fatigability during feeds, ptosis (50%), ophthalmoplegia and respiratory failure demanding mechanical ventilation *Once the first signs appear ,diagnosis can be confirmed by IM NEOSTIGMINE(single dose of 0.04- 0.15 mg/kg) which results in improvement in 15-30 minutes and lasts for 1-3 hours, allowing ample observation of the infant`s feeding, crying, antigravity limb movements and respiration. Perform this test on the NICU to meet potential cardiac arrhythmia or cholinergic crisis *Edrophonium (Tensilon) is not recommended because of too brief effect to assess and cardiac arrhythmias reported in neonates* High serum concentration of AchR antibodies in the mother and in the infant, are further evidence, but their absence does not rule out the diagnosis *EMG shows decremental response to repetitive nerve stimulation ; motor nerve conduction velocity remains normal *Treat with gavage feeding, mechanical ventilation, oral Pyridostigmine 5-10 mg,4 hourly/oral Neostigmine bromide 0.4 mg/kg every 4-6 hr for only a few days or occasionally for a few weeks, especially to allow feeding. Anticholinesterases are gradually weaned off when the infant is no longer symptomatic, between 1-4 months of age

4. *CONGENITAL MYASTHENIC SYNDROMES* *Congenital / Familial infantile myasthenia-Autosomal recessive & presynaptic form presents with hypotonia and bulbar+respiratory muscle paralysis which gradually improves*Sudden apnea & respiratory arrest in the course of intercurrent infection or fever in infancy is characteristic *May be asymptomatic in between these attacks *diagnosis is based on history, examination, EMG studies, Neostigmine test, response to acetylcholinesterase inhibitors, and by muscle biopsy *Long-term treatment with Neostigmine/ Pyridostigmine may be used *Congenital end plate acetylcholinesterase deficiency-autosomal recessive, synaptic or postsynaptic type does not show response or worsening on anticholinesterase administration.

5. *INFANTILE BOTULISM:* *Normal at birth but develop symptoms between the ages 10 days-6 months*Clinical features include marked hypotonia, weakness, areflexia, bulbar dysfunction, ophthalmoplegia, ptosis,mydriasis, preservation of DTR, constipation,apnea and respiratory insufficiency *Diagnosis is by culturing *Clostridium botulinum* from stools & by EMG showing incremental response to repetitive nerve stimulation*Treatment needs respiratory support & antitoxin therapy*symptoms last 2-6 weeks

6. *PERIPHERAL NERVE DISEASE:* *Hypotonia and generalized weakness,more pronounced distally with absent DTR, cranial nerve and respiratory muscle involvement,feeding difficulties, and joint contractures are common *A generalized peripheral neuropathy is very rare in neonates*Giant axonal neuropathy,inflammatory neuropathies,metabolic neuropathies (Leigh`s disease), and sensory neuropathies are some examples*Muscle biopsy shows denervation pattern & EMG shows fibrillations *Sensory deficits,elevated CSF protein,depressed nerve conduction velocity and abnormal nerve biopsy are other important findings.

7. *METABOLIC AND TOXIC JUNCTION DISORDERS* *Hypermagnesemia from therapy with Magnesium sulphate for maternal eclampsia may produce severe weakness, apnea, bulbar dysfunction, and autonomic dysfunction *Aminoglycosides may produce a very similar picture.

8. *ACUTE SPINAL CORD INJURY:* *Obstetric history is compatible with cervical trauma*Clinical features include flaccid paralysis,hyposthesia(sensory level) usually at cervical level,with varying respiratory insufficiency and neurogenic bladder,Horner syndrome; initially areflexic, later hyperreflexic *Evaluation is by MRI spinal cord (edema,hemorrhage); paraspinal EMG may confirm and localize diagnosis *Management includes avoiding further neck movement acutely, maintaining airway & ventilation, supporting BP* Early high-dose steroid administration has been suggested but not studied in the neonate.

AUTOIMMUNE MG: Neonatal and Juvenile Forms

CHILDHOOD MYASTHENIA GRAVIS: TYPES

	Neonatal	Congenital	Familial	Acquired Infantile	Recurrent Juvenile	Arthrogryposis
Maternal MG	+	–	–		–	+
Onset	0 to 3 days post natal	Birth to 1 year	Birth More in Orientals		> 1 year	Congenital
Weakness	Generalized	Ocular ± Generalized	Respiratory Generalized		Ocular ± Generalized	Generalized
Time course	Remission 1 to 6 weeks	Fixed weakness	Fatal early, or improvement > 2 years		Improvement over years	Static
Family history	± Other sibs Mother Untreated	Often	Usual		Rare	Other sibs Mother Untreated
Anti-AChR antibodies	Most	–	–		50% More in Orientals	+ vs Fetal AChR

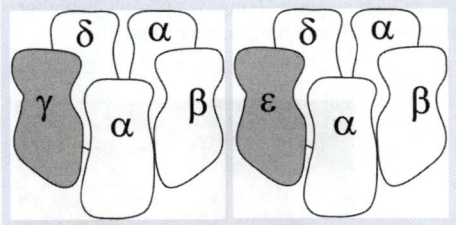

Fetal AChR   Adult AChR

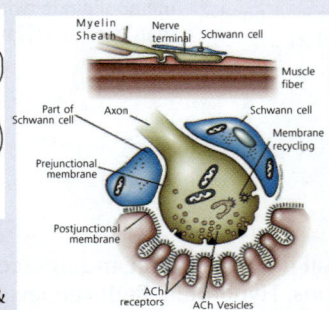

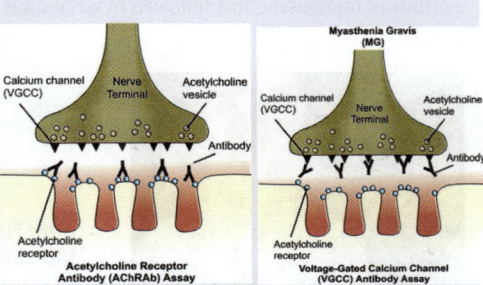

MYASTHENIA GRAVIS Acetylcholine Receptor & Acetylcholine Receptor Autoantibodies (AChRAb) Human muscle acetylcholine receptors (AChR) exist as two developmentally regulated subtypes; The fetal AChR is pentameric with stoichiometry of $2\alpha : \beta : \gamma : \delta$. In the adult subtype, expression of the ε subunit is induced and replaces the γ subunit within the AChR pentamer

Autoantibodies to the Acetylcholine receptor (AChRAb) can be detected in 80-90% of patients with myasthenia gravis. Myasthenia gravis (MG) is a neuromuscular disorder which results from a disruption of normal nerve-to-muscle signal transmission. The immunopathologic mechanisms by which normal signal transmission is disrupted are thought to be: blocking of the receptor as a result of the direct binding of the autoantibody, disruption of ACh binding to the receptor due to steric hindrance caused by autoantibody binding at sites adjacent to the ACh binding site, destruction of the muscle membrane as a result of complement activation by autoantibodies, increased receptor turnover due to autoantibody-receptor cross-linking.

KEY POINTS FOR CLINICAL PRACTICE

1. Neonatal Hypotonia has many causes and is classified *anatomically* in a centrifugal fashion, i.e. central in origin, or from the spinal cord, the peripheral nerves, the neuromuscular junction, or the muscles themselves.

2. Neonatal Hypotonia is more commonly due to *central causes* such as sepsis, hypoglycemia, hypoxic-ischemic encephalopathy and must be ruled out promptly and effectively.

3. Neuromuscular Hypotonia is often associated with a normal level of consciousness, decreased or normal DTR, poor limb recoil, and minor dysmorphic features or congenital anomalies, *whereas* Central Hypotonia is associated with decreased consciousness, seizures, cranial nerve signs, normal or brisk reflexes, strong limb recoil, a tendency for muscle to improve with time, and major congenital anomalies.

4. As the causes of Neonatal Hypotonia are legion, the approach to investigating hypotonia is determined to a large part by the *clinical impression* of the suspected underlying cause.

5. Management of Neuromuscular Hypotonia often involves cardiorespiratory support pending definitive evaluation; gavage feeds to optimize nutrition, orthopedic support to minimize deformities and preparing the family for chronic care needs.

REFERENCES AND FURTHER READING: 1) Neonatal Hypotonia, ALAN HILL, MD, PHD*Current Management in Child Neurology, Third Edition* Bernard L. Maria, 2)Dubowitz V.Muscle disorders in childhood. 2nd ed. Philadelphia PA):W.B. Saunders; 1995. 3) Volpe JJ. Neurology of the newborn. 4th ed. Philadelphia (PA): W.B. Saunders; 2001. 4)Royden-Jones H, Devivo D, Darras BT.Neuromuscular diseases of infancy, childhood and adolescence: a clinician's approach. Philadelphia (PA): Butterworth-Heinemann; 2003. 5)Fenichel GM. Neonatal Neurology 3rd edition. Churchill Livingston Inc. 1990

33 Respiratory Failure in a Neonate

@ *The differentiation between cardiac, respiratory, metabolic, neurologic, and other causes of hypoxia leading to the Respiratory Failure in a Newborn Infant is a common difficulty.*

Most of the Sick Neonates would not deteriorate suddenly; but many times we detect it suddenly-*Anonymous*

Signs of Respiratory Distress *Nasal Flaring and Head Bobbing *Signs of significantly increased respiratory effort—Tachypnea, Retractions, Grunting, Seesaw Chest Movements, Stridor/Wheeze

Signs of Respiratory Failure *Cyanosis *Decreased level of responsiveness *Poor skeletal muscle tone *Inadequate respiratory rate, effort, or chest expansion *Apnea

Disordered Control of Breathing *Hypoventilation which may be due to—Abnormal breathing pattern "breathing funny"— Inadequate respiratory rate or effort despite increased need— periods of increased effort followed by decreased effort

Signs of Respiratory Arrest: *Mottling; peripheral and central cyanosis *Unresponsive to voice and touch *Absent chest wall motion *Absent respirations *Weak to absent pulses *Bradycardia or asystole *Limp muscle tone

Summary of Differences in Infants *Infants are obligate nose breathers until 2-3 months old *Upper airway is relatively more sensitive to inhalation agents, more prone to collapse *Have less oxygen reserve, so hypoxemia occurs relatively more rapidly *Have metabolic rate twice as high as adult *Lung compliance is higher than in adults *Have less reserve in lung surface area.

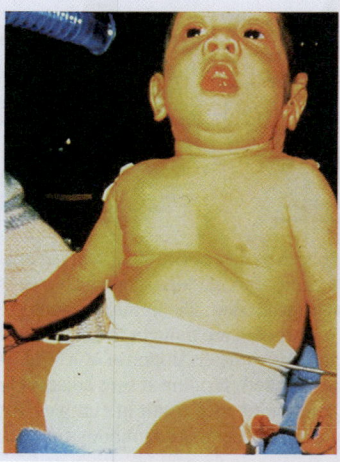

Note: Nasal flare, Subcostal and Intercostal Retractions, Hypotonia, Reduced level of Consciousness; This infant obviously has to be *intubated and Mechanically Ventilated* for an Impending Respiratory Failure/Arrest.

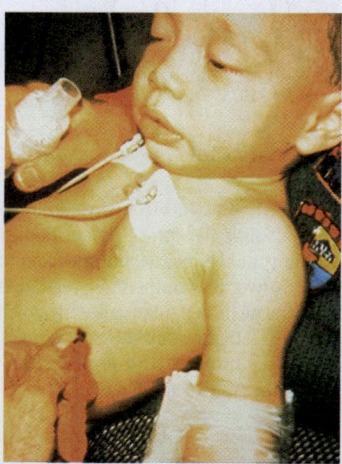

REVIEW OF CLINICAL PROBLEMS

1. Name the **exceptions to** 'Respiratory Failure which is usually' associated with hypoxemia and distress?
   Ans: Refer to the "No. 2" of the "BIRD'S EYE VIEW/OVERVIEW/ SYNOPSIS" of the Chapter.

2. What are the Indications for ET intubation and mechanical ventilation in a Neonate with Respiratory distress/depression?
   Ans: Refer to the Evaluation-Decision-Action Plan/Algorithm to diagnose and manage a Neonate with Respiratory Failure.

3. What are Clues to the likely etiology that can be picked up on examination of the Neonate with Respiratory Failure?
   Ans: Refer to the "Table 3 of the Chapter.

4. How do you differentiate between various causes of Neonatal Respiratory Failure?
   Ans: Refer to Table 8 of the Chapter.

5. How do you manage a Neonate with acute Respiratory Failure?
   Ans: Refer to the Evaluation-Decision-Action Plan/Algorithm to diagnose and manage a Neonate with Respiratory Failure.

LEARNING OBJECTIVES

After completing this article, readers will be able to

1. Recognize Neonates at risk for Respiratory Failure.

2. Institute immediate, effective, simple measures to stabilize Neonates with Respiratory Failure.

3. Delineate the common differential diagnosis of Respiratory Failure in the Newborn.

4. Become more aware of the treatment options for Hypoxic Respiratory Failure in preterm/term infants.

5. Refer Neonates with Respiratory Failure not responding to initial measures to appropriate tertiary care center for assistance with diagnosis and management.

Pearl/Peril/Pitfall: The clinical management of respiratory failure in the newborn often focuses on lung parenchymal stiffness due to immaturity, surfactant deficiency, infiltrates, and other causes. However, health care personnel should also consider the airway, which plays an important role in gas exchange and lung mechanics. The airway can be easily injured, and an injured airway can significantly alter both the acute and chronic course of lung disease in infants. Further, there are developmental changes that affect the susceptibility of the neonatal airway to injury. Recognizing and preventing causes of airway injury can help to ensure optimal outcomes for the critically ill neonate.

BIRD'S EYE VIEW/OVERVIEW/SYNOPSIS

1. *Respiratory failure is defined as the inability of the respiratory apparatus to maintain adequate oxygenation of the blood, with or without CO_2 retention to meet the metabolic demands of the body ; the resulting low PaO_2, high $PaCO_2$ and pH changes affecting the lungs, heart, kidneys and brain.* It arises from derangements in pulmonary gas exchange; a) Hypoventilation b) Diffusion impairment c) Intrapulmonary shunting and d) ventilation-perfusion (V/Q) mismatch. Acute respiratory failure is the most common problem seen in the preterm and term infants admitted to Neonatal intensive care units. *In preterm infants,* the most common cause of acute respiratory failure is respiratory distress syndrome caused by surfactant deficiency. Acute respiratory failure *in term and near term infants* is usually a result of meconium aspiration syndrome, sepsis, pulmonary hypoplasia, and primary pulmonary hypertension of the Newborn.

2. *Beware of the exceptions:* a) Hypoxemia is not always related to respiratory failure [E.g. right to left cardiac shunts, high altitude with low ambient O_2 concentration, Methemoglobinemia] b) Overt respiratory failure may occur without manifesting signs of respiratory distress [E.g. Neuromuscular disease-Myotonic dystrophy, Myasthenia-Transient Neonatal/Congenital], *while* a Neonate may display signs of severe respiratory distress with no pulmonary disease [E.g.: severe metabolic acidosis with Kussmaul respirations often resulting from Severe sepsis, Ductus-dependent Cardiac Malformations, Acute Renal Failure, NEC, Congenital Adrenal Hyperplasia, and Inborn Errors of Metabolism, especially Organic acidemias]. CNS pathology (Grade 2-3 HIE, IVH-ICH, Meningitis, CNS Malformations *may present as* other Neurologic features (respiratory depression, coma, areflexia, weakness) and a variety of respiratory patterns, including bradypnea, apnea, and Cheyne-Stokes breathing. *A precise assessment of the adequacy of Oxygenation and Ventilation must be based on both clinical and laboratory data.*

3. Respiratory failure can be classified into 2 types, *which usually co-exist in variable proportion.* The PaO_2 is low in both, where as the $paCO_2$ is high only in patients with type II respiratory failure. Refer to the Table 1 of the Chapter.

4. Primary pulmonary disease is the most common etiology for cyanosis and hypoxia in this population (American Academy of Pediatrics, 2002). The prudent clinician, however, will routinely consider alternatives, so as not to cause delayed diagnosis and its associated negative consequences for the infant with a less common disorder. Primary lung disease causes alveolar hypoventilation, decreased lung compliance, ventilation-perfusion inequality, intrapulmonary right-to-left shunts, and a resultant varying degree of hypoxia in the Newborn. Logically, as such, the entire spectrum of Neonatal respiratory disorders may present with cyanosis. *In general, hypoxia associated with pulmonary disease presents as tachypnea, grunting, flaring, chest retractions, arterial blood gas usually showing carbon dioxide retention, rise in PaO_2 when supplemental oxygen is used, and evidence of lung disease on chest radiograph.* There are numerous diagnoses included in the category of primary pulmonary disease, including: *Transient Tachypnea of the Newborn *Tracheoesophageal Fistula and Esophageal Atresia *Aspiration Syndromes *Respiratory Distress Syndrome *Pneumonia *Pulmonary Hemorrhage *Pulmonary Hypoplasia *Pulmonary Lymphangiectasia *Congenital Pulmonary Cysts *Pulmonary Lobar Emphysema. Refer to the Table 6 of the Chapter for* the Classification of Disorders: Primary Pulmonary Disease, Airway Obstruction, and Extrinsic Compression of the Lungs and Airway.(Refer to the Individual Chapters for the details of the diagnosis and management of common primary Respiratory diseases in Neonates.)

5. *Sepsis and hypotension:* Outside of primary pulmonary disease, perhaps the next most common abnormality presenting with hypoxia in the term Newborn is sepsis. The clinical signs of Neonatal sepsis are nonspecific and often camouflaged or associated with other Neonatal diseases such as respiratory distress syndrome, metabolic disorders, intracranial hemorrhage, and asphyxia. As such, infection is considered and empirically treated with nearly all unexpected events of hypoxia in the term Newborn.

6. *Central nervous system (CNS)* disorders and neuromuscular diseases can cause altered control of respiration and result in hypoxia in the term Neonate. This compromised neurologic control of respiration can be a result of a congenital neurologic disorder, due to seizures or CNS infection, or as a result of neurologic injury. Refer to the common Neurological conditions that can cause respiratory failure, hypoxia, and cyanosis enlisted in the Table 6 of the Chapter.

7. Other causes of Neonatal respiratory Failure are of Cardiac, Hematologic, Metabolic and Endocrinal in origin. A summary of these categories of disorders, along with characteristic history and typical physical, laboratory, and radiologic findings can be found in Table 8 of the Chapter. Methemoglobinemia is the rare but great impersonator in the evaluation of cyanosis of the Newborn. Methemoglobinemia causes reduced blood-oxygen carrying capacity due to abnormal hemoglobin or enzyme deficiency. Examination generally reveals a markedly cyanotic infant without respiratory distress, who has an arterial PaO_2 that is normal, although the infant will have low oxygen saturation values. Arterial blood obtained from such an infant is often described as "chocolate" in color. In the general population, methemoglobinemia is caused by ingestion of toxic agents such as nitrites, but in the term Newborn, methemoglobinemia instead is related to congenital absence of methemoglobin reductase.

8. *The Evaluation-Decision-Action Plan/algorithm* summarizes the essential aspects of history taking, physical examination, relevant investigations to diagnose and manage Respiratory Failure in Neonates.

9. Treatment of the hypoxic infant depends on accurate diagnosis. Initially, however, respiratory support with oxygen, CPAP (continuous positive airway pressure), or mechanical ventilation is indicated in most cases. In congenital heart disease, medication used to maintain the patency of the PDA (patent ductus arteriosus) may be necessary to maintain tissue perfusion until surgical correction can be achieved. In PPHN (persistent pulmonary hypertension), the goal of the therapy is to lower the pulmonary-to-systemic vascular resistance ratio and thus reduce shunting. ECMO (extracorporeal membrane oxygenation) has been used with success, while supportive measures are in place, and newer medical therapies such as inhaled nitric oxide are now improving upon those successes. Given the often vague signs of Neonatal infection, which includes hypoxia of various etiologies, evaluating for suspected sepsis while excluding other disease processes, is uniformly prudent for the clinician. Treatment with appropriate broadspectrum antibiotics is standard at the time of suspicion and prior to laboratory confirmation of infection. Where cyanosis is secondary to poor cardiovascular function in any form of shock, volume expanders and inotropic agents are important at maintaining adequate tissue oxygenation. Red blood cell transfusion to support oxygen-carrying capacity and metabolic and electrolyte management to optimize cardiac function are fundamental. For emergency conditions, such as pneumothorax, evacuation by the bedside clinician is often warranted, even before specialized Neonatal care. Obstructive lesions may also require urgent bedside palliation prior to definitive treatment (i.e., oral airway for choanal atresia or Pierre Robin Sequence, tracheal intubation, and gastrointestinal evacuation for diaphragmatic hernia). Where gastroesophageal reflux is identified, medical management with H2 blockers is often effective, as well as other pharmacologic remedies and formula thickening, for the management of events that cause hypoxia. Unusual conditions, such as methemoglobinemia, are treated more uniquely under the guidance of subspecialists, and after further targeted diagnostic tests are interpreted. Similarly, the treatment of hypoventilation as a function of metabolic or neuromuscular disorder, while initially supported by oxygen administration and ventilation, may require more specialized therapies.

10. Differentiating between the many etiologies for Newborn hypoxia and Respiratory Failure is undoubtedly an incredible challenge for the pediatric specialist in the Newborn nursery. While there are several common causes for Newborn cyanosis—primary pulmonary disease and sepsis—a myriad of disorders spanning all organ systems exist as possibilities.

Pearl/Peril/Pitfall: Despite implementation of alternative strategies such as Extra Corporeal Membrane Oxygenation. (ECMO), high frequency ventilation, inhalational nitric oxide, and liquid ventilation, conventional ventilation remains the mainstay of treatment of respiratory failure in newborns.

THE EVALUATION-DECISION-ACTION-PLAN/ALGORITHM FOR THE DIAGNOSIS AND MANAGEMENT OF *A NEONATE WITH ACUTE RESPIRATORY FAILURE*

SUBJECTIVE FINDINGS

Obtain Quick and Relevant History which should be *with a goal and purpose* to identify the etiology, whenever possible for the Neonatal Respiratory Failure.: Refer to the Table 4 of the Chapter.

OBJECTIVE FINDINGS

Assess ABCDs, vitals, BP, O_2 sats, work of breathing central cyanosis, CRT, pulses, Urine output *Look for clinical clues to suggest an underlying cause for the respiratory failure-Refer to the Table 3 for a review of possible underlying etiologies* *Perform* systemic examination to assess the complications of hypoxia/hypercarbia/hypotension associated with Respiratory Failure (MODS-acute renal failure, CHF, CNS dysfunction, DIC, NEC etc.,)

INVESTIGATIONS

Blood FBC, differential, platelets, **hematocrit,** reticulocyte count, Group and type and cross match, Smear, coagulation screen (PT, APTT, fibrinogen, thrombin time, bleeding time and clotting time), blood cultures, ABG analysis, **Blood sugar,** BUN, creatinine, electrolytes, Ca^{++} Mg^{++}, LTFs, drug screen

Urine analysis

Imaging- CXR, plain abdominal x-ray, USG scan/CT scan of head,

Perform- partial sepsis screen (**defer LP**)-(FBC, CRP, blood and urine cultures, CXR etc.,)

Consider - ECG, 2D ECHO, MRI brain scan, Metabolic screen, when clinical course demands.

Identify the Contraindications for CPAP 1)The need for ventilation because of ventilatory failure—inability to maintain oxygenation and the arterial PaCO2 <60 mm Hg and pH > 7.25. 2) Upper airway abnormalities (cleft palate, choanal atresia). 3)Tracheo-esophageal fistula.4) Diaphragmatic hernia. 5)Hypoventilation due to CNS Depression/Neuromuscular Weakness

Recognizing failure of CPAP administration

Decreasing pH (<7.25), Increasing $PaCo_2$ (>50 - 60 mm Hg)*, Increasing FIO_2 (>0.6 to 0.7), Decreasing PaO_2 (<60 to 80 mm Hg)†, Nasal CPAP > 12 cm H_2O, Frequent apnea with bradycardia.

* Higher ranges may apply with permissive hypercapnia, †Range should be consistent with clinical state and the presence of congenital heart anomalies.

Indications for et intubation and mechanical ventilation: Absolute: Major Apnea with failure to respond promptly to Bag and Mask Resuscitation *Relative:* *ELBW <28 wks GA in labor suite, *Recurrent minor apnea unresponsive to CPAP and Methylxanthines *Deteriorating Respiratory Status—PaO2<50 mm Hg in FiO_2 0.6(<32 wks GA)/ PaO2<50 mm Hg in FiO2 0.8(>32 wks GA), pH<7.25, PaCO2>50mm Hg(<32 wks GA)/ pH<7.20,PaCO2>60mm Hg(>32 wks GA) *Cerebral edema due to HIE

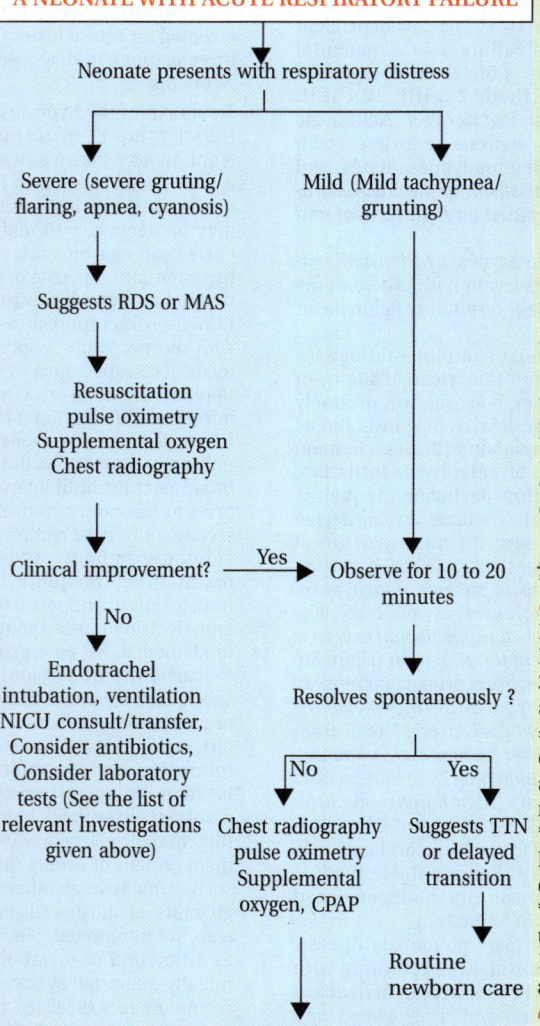

A NEONATE WITH ACUTE RESPIRATORY FAILURE

Neonate presents with respiratory distress

Severe (severe gruting/ flaring, apnea, cyanosis)

Mild (Mild tachypnea/ grunting)

Suggests RDS or MAS

Resuscitation pulse oximetry Supplemental oxygen Chest radiography

Clinical improvement? — Yes → Observe for 10 to 20 minutes

No

Endotrachel intubation, ventilation NICU consult/transfer, Consider antibiotics, Consider laboratory tests (See the list of relevant Investigations given above)

Resolves spontaneously ?

No → Chest radiography pulse oximetry Supplemental oxygen, CPAP

Yes → Suggests TTN or delayed transition → Routine newborn care

Apply "rule of two hours". NICU consult/transfer (and consider laboratory tests or antibiotics) if any of following is present: 1) Abnormality on chest radiograph 2) >40% oxygen needed to oxygenate 3) Condition deteriorates 4) Condition does not improve within two hours 5) Criteria for diagnosing Respiratory Failure -Table 2 of the Chapter.

Indications for high frequency oscillatory ventilation 1) Barotrauma—pulmonary airleaks— a) Pneumothorax b)Pulmonary Interstitial Emphysema (PIE) bronchopleural fistulas and pneumo-pericardium 2) Respiratory failure unresponsive to conventional ventilation, e.g. RDS, Pneumonia, 3) Persistent pulmonary hypertension of the newborn (PPHN), MAS, Hypoplastic lungs, diaphragmatic hernia 4) Pulmonary hemorrhage

Indications for INO therapy: Hypoxic respiratory failure can occur as a primary developmental defect or as a comorbidity from a secondary disorder (persistent pulmonary hypertension of the newborn [PPHN], meconium aspiration syndrome [MAS], sepsis, pneumonia, hyaline membrane disease, congenital diaphragmatic hernia [CDH], or pulmonary hypoplasia); *the best examples of INO's beneficial effects on oxygenation and on reducing the need for extracorporeal membrane oxygen (ECMO) with infants suffering hypoxic respiratory failure.*

Indications for extracorporeal membrane oxygenation ECMO criteria:·Oxygenation Index >30. OI = (Mean Airway Pressure × FiO_2)/ PaO_2 *Note: RA = 21, 100% = 100 *on 3 arterial blood gases at least 30 minutes apart *$AaDO_2$ > 600 for 8 hours Note: $AaDO_2$ = (760–46) – PaO_2 – $PaCO_2$) *Acute deterioration with PaO2 <35 mmHg *Shock and acidosis with pH <7.25 *Predicted mortality of at least 80% Exclusion Criteria: *Intracranial hemorrhage greater than Grade I *Lethal chromosomal anomaly *Major cardiac lesion *<34 weeks gestational age *<2,000gms *Coagulopathy that is ongoing uncorrectable *Mechanical ventilation for > 14 days *Severe neurologic insult or asphyxia *Patients who could potentially qualify for ECMO should have a cardiac Echo and cranial ultrasound performed in a timely manner so that, should they meet ECMO criteria, these results are known. Blood gases, ventilator settings, and FiO_2 should be followed closely so it is known when the critical OI or AaDO2 values are met.*

Pearl/Peril/Pitfall : Hypoxemia is caused by one of the following abnormalities:*Alveolar ventilation (V) and pulmonary perfusion (Q) mismatch *Intrapulmonary shunt *Hypoventilation *Abnormal diffusion of gases at the alveolar-capillary interface *Reduction in inspired oxygen concentration *Increased venous desaturation with cardiac dysfunction plus one or more of the above 5 factors.

TABLE 1 **Types of respiratory failure**

Findings	Causes	Examples
TYPE I Hypoxia with Normocapnia	Ventilation-Perfusion Mismatch (V/Q Mismatch	* Hyaline membrane disease(HMD) * Congenital pneumonia * Atelectasis *MAS *BPD
	Diffusion Impairment	* Pulmonary edema, *HMD * Pulmonary Interstitial Emphysema
	Shunt	* Congenital Cystic Adenomatoid Malformation * Pulmonary AV Malformation
TYPE II Hypoxia with Hypercapnia	Hypoventilation	* Neuromuscular Disease-Myotonic Dystrophy, Myasthenia * CNS depression due to respiratory depressants, severe HIE, IVH-ICH, Meningo-Encephalitis, CNS Malformations

Risk factors for neonatal hypoxia

* Maternal diabetes
* Preeclampsia
* Other significant maternal morbidities
* Multiple gestation
* Maternal drug addiction
* Other maternal drug use/administration
* Abnormal prenatal sonogram, especially for cardiac or pulmonary defect
* Abnormal serum alpha-fetoprotein or amniocentesis
* Oligohydramnios
* Polyhydramnios
* Large-for-dates infant
* Meconium-stained fluid
* Instrumented or cesarean delivery
* Prenatal infection
* Placental abruption or other maternal hemorrhage
* Suspected intrapartum infection
* Uterine rupture
* Shoulder dystocia
* Cord prolapse or other cord restriction
* Use of general anesthesia or systemic maternal sedatives/analgesia
* Nonreassuring fetal tracing
* Nonreassuring biophysical profile/non–stress testing

First impression of respiratory emergencies

Assessment	Respiratory distress	Respiratory failure	Respiratory arrest
Mental status	Alert, irritable, anxious, restless	Decreased level of responsiveness or responsive to pain	Unresponsive to voice or touch
Muscle tone	Able to maintain sitting position (children older than 4 mo)	Normal or decreased	Limp
Body position	May assume tripod position	May assume tripod position May need support to maintain sitting position as he/she tires	Unable to maintain sitting position (infant older than 7 to 9 mo)
Respiratory rate	Faster than normal for age	Tachypnea with periods of bradypnea; slowing to bradypnea/agonal breathing	Absent
Respiratory effort	Intercostal retractions Nasal flaring Neck flaring Neck muscle use Seesaw respirations	Inadequate respiratory effort or chest excursion	Absent
Audible airway sounds	Stridor, wheezing, grunting,	Stridor, wheezing, grunting, gasping	Absent
Skin color	Pink or pale; central cyanosis resolves with oxygen administration	Central cyanosis despite oxygen administration; mottling	Mottling; peripheral and central cyanosis

Pearl/Peril/Pitfall: The mnemonic MSOAPP can be used to remember the preparation essential for a safe tracheal intubation procedure. ·M = Monitors (heart rate, blood pressure, pulse oximetry, capnography for CO_2 detection) ·S = Suction and catheters ·O = Oxygenation with a bag-valve mask ·A = Apparatus (laryngoscope, endotracheal tubes appropriate for the patient's age and endotracheal tubes 0.5 size smaller and larger, stylets, oral airways) ·P = Pharmacy (medications for amnesia and paralysis) ·P = People (respiratory therapist, nurse, a skilled set of hands).

TABLE 2   Assessment of respiratory failure

Score	Upper Chest	Lower Chest Retrac	Xiphoid Retrac	Nasal Flare	Grunt
0	Sync	None	None	None	None
1	Lag on Insp	Just Visible	Just Visible	Minimal	Steth Only
2	See-Saw	Marked	Marked	Marked	Naked Ear

A score of 6 or more is indicative of impending respiratory failure

A) CLINICAL CRITERIA 1) FOR PRETERM BABIES
SILVERMAN-ANDERSON RETRACTION SCORE

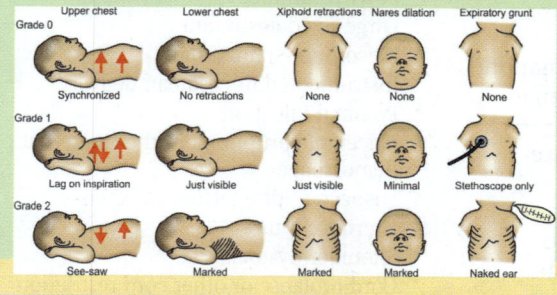

RESPIRATORY DISTRESS SCORING

2) FOR TERM BABIES DOWNE'S SCORE IN TERM BABIES

Score	Respiratory Rate/min	Cyanosis	Air entry	Retractions	Grunt
0	<60	None	Good	None	None
1	60–80	In air	Diminished	Mild	Audible with Stethoscope
2	> 80 or apneic	In 40% O_2	Barely audible	Moderate/severe	Audible with naked ear

A score of 6 or more is indicative of impending respiratory failure

B) LABORATORY CRITERIA pH-<7.1–7.2, PaO_2<50 mmHg (6.6kPa) In FiO_2> 0.6 $PaCO_2$>60mmHg (8kPa)

In infants weighing <1500g $PaCO_2$ should be modified to > 50mmHg-preventing the risk of intracerebral Hemorrhage (ICH) at high $PaCO_2$

ABG Score

Parameters	0	1	2	3
PaO_2mmHg	>60	50–60	<50	<50
PH	>7.3	7.20–7.29	7.1–7.19	<7.1
$PaCO_2$mmHg	<50	50–60	61–70	>70

A score of 3 or more on the ABG indicates the need for CPAP or mechanical ventilation. A pH of <7.2 with hypercarbia (pCO2>60mm) or a pO2<50mm Hg in FiO2 of 0.8 is suggestive of frank respiratory failure.

TABLE 4   Diagnostic approach to respiratory distress

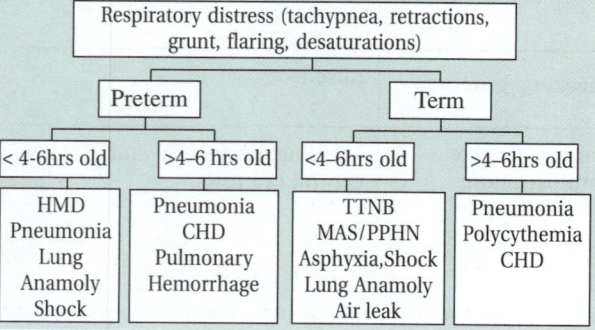

TABLE 3   Clinical Examination

Clues to the likely etiology can be picked up on examination of the Neonate

1. A preterm baby weighing <1500 gms with retractions and grunt is likely to have HMD.(*Note that an Infant of Diabetic Mom , usually a LGA can have RDS due to HMD.*)

2. A term baby born through meconium stained amniotic fluid with an increase in the AP diameter of the chest (barrel chest) is likely to be suffering from MAS.(*Note that a baby with MAS may have had Birth Asphyxia and developed PPHN as well*).

3. A depressed baby with poor circulation is likely to have neonatal sepsis with or without congenital pneumonia. (*Note that a septic looking baby may have several noninfectious underlying causes such as Congenital adrenal hyperplasia, Ductus-dependent CHD, Inborn Errors of Metabolism or non-bacterial causes such as Herpes meningoencephalitis, Fungal sepsis, Perinatal Tuberculosis, etc.*)

4. A near term baby with no risk factors and mild distress may have TTNB.(*Note Transient Tachypnea of the Newborn is a diagnosis by EXCLUSION of life-threatening underlying causes mentioned already*)

5. An asphyxiated baby may have PPHN.(Note that Birth Asphyxia is a Multisystem disorder with several clinical manifestations that can cause respiratory distress and/or depression leading to Respiratory Failure; CHF, Acute Renal Failure, Pulmonary Hemorrhage, Raised ICP, ICH-IVH, DIC, NEC, etc.)

6. A growth retarded baby with a plethoric look may have polycythemia.

7. A baby with respiratory distress should be checked for an air leak by placing a cold light source over the chest wall in a darkened room.

8. A baby presenting with tachypnea and a cardiac murmur may have a congenital heart disease.

9. Inability to pass a 5F catheter through the nostril of a term baby is suggestive of choanal atresia.

10. Insertion of a 10F nasogastric tube may show coiling in the mediastinum of patients who have concomitant esophageal atresia. This finding is diagnostic of TEFs associated with esophageal atresia.

TABLE 5   Review of antenatal and peripartum events

a) Were there any risk factors in the antepartum period or evidence of fetal distress prior to delivery? (Birth asphyxia or PPHN) **b)** Did the mother receive antenatal steroids if it was a preterm delivery? (Antenatal steroids decrease the incidence of HMD by 50%) **c)** Was there a history of premature rupture of membranes and fever? (congenital pneumonia or sepsis) **d)** Was there meconium stained amniotic fluid? (MAS is a possibility) e) A look at the antenatal ultrasonography (USG) for the amount of amniotic fluid would tell us the status of the fetal lung. (congenital anomalies of lung) **f)** Was resuscitation required at birth? (resuscitation trauma/PPHN/acidosis) **g)** Did the distress appear immediately or a few hours after birth? (HMD appears earlier than pneumonia) **h)** Was it related to feeding or frothing at the mouth? (tracheo-esophageal fistula or aspiration) **i)** Does the distress decrease with crying? (choanal atresia). For babies presenting later with distress we have to ask a few other questions :- a) Is the distress associated with feed refusal and lethargy? (sepsis, pneumonia) b) Did the distress appear slowly after starting feeds? (IEM). c) Is there a family history of early neonatal deaths? (CHD, IEM).

(**Courtesy:** Surg Cdr SS Mathai, Col U Raju, Col M Kanitkar AFMC, PUNE)

Pearl/Peril/Pitfall: Management of acute respiratory failure begins with a determination of the underlying etiology. While supporting the respiratory system and ensuring adequate oxygen delivery to the tissues, initiate an intervention specifically defined to correct the underlying condition.

TABLE 6 Etiological causes of neonatal respiratory failure

1. **PRIMARY PULMONARY DISEASE**

   Transient tachypnea of the newborn, Tracheoesphageal fistula, esophageal atresia, Aspiration syndromes, Respiratory distress syndrome, Pneumonia, Pulmonary hemorrhage, Pulmonary hypoplasia, Pulmonary lymphangiectasia, Congenital pulmonary cysts, Pulmonary lobar emphysema.

2. **AIRWAY OBSTRUCTION**

   Choanal atresia, choanal stenosis, Pierre-Robin sequence, Macroglossia, Right aortic arch, Thyroid goiter, Cystic hygroma, Laryngomalacia, Tracheomalacia, Tracheal stenosis, subglottic stenosis, Subglottic hemangioma/hematoma, Bronchomalacia, bronchial stenosis, laryngeal web, Vocal cord paralysis, Foreign body aspiration, Mucous plugging.

3. **EXTRINSIC COMPRESSION OF THE LUNGS AND AIRWAY**

   Pneumothorax, Pneumomediastinum, Pleural Effusion, Chylothorax, Congenital diaphragmatic hernia, Mediastinal masses, Thoracic dystrophies, thoracic dysplasias, Extralobar sequestration, Right/double aortic arch, Tracheal vascular ring, Pulmonary artery sling, Cricoid cartilage malformation.

4. **NEUROLOGIC CONDITIONS THAT CAN CAUSE RESPIRATORY FAILURE, HYPOXIA, AND CYANOSIS**

   a. **Reduction of tone—decreased respiratory effort:** Congenital hydrocephalus, Werdnig-Hoffman disease, Neurologic malformations, i.e. Chiari malformation, Spinal muscle atrophy, Dejerine-Sottas disease, Muscular dystrophy, Charcot-Marie-Tooth disease, Neurogenic arthrogryposis, Phrenic nerve paralysis, Congenital myasthenia, Congenital myopathies, Congenital neuropathies, CNS malignancies.

   b. **Epileptiform activity—apnea:** Seizures resulting from congenital neurologic disorder or genetic syndrome, Seizures resulting from CNS injury, Seizures resulting from infection, Seizures resulting from metabolic derangement.

   c. **Increased ICP, Impaired circulation and brain structures:** multifaceted effect on respiratory control, can cause seizures/apnea, Hypoxic-ischemic encephalopathy, Intraventricular hemorrhage, Subdural hemorrhage, Subarachnoid hemorrhage, Hemorrhagic infarction, Intracerebellar hemorrhage.

   d. **Can cause reduction in tone, seizures, increased ICP, apnea :** Bacterial infection: Group B streptococcus, Escherichia coli, Listeria monocytogenes, Viral infection: Syphilis, toxoplasmosis, Herpes simplex, Rubella, Cytomegalovirus

5. **CARDIOVASCULAR CONDITIONS THAT CAN CAUSE RESPIRATORY FAILURE, HYPOXIA, AND CYANOSIS:**

   Congenital Heart Disease: Ductus dependent cardiac malformations(Obstructive lesions-both Rt sided and Lt sided, Rt-to -Lt shunt lesions), Arrhythmias, Acquired Heart problems-Myocarditis,Cardiomyopathy, Congestive Heart Failure and Cardiogenic shock-due to cardiac and various noncardiac causes, PDA in a Preterm infant,Vascular rings,ALCAPA

6. **PERSISTENT PULMONARY HYPERTENSION (PPHN)**

7. **METABOLIC**

   Hypoglycemia, Hypo/Hyperthermia, Acidosis, Adrenal insufficiency/failure, Sepsis with MODS

8. **HEMATOLOGICAL**

   Anemia due to various causes, Polycythemia, Methemoglobinemia

9. **Thoracic dystrophies or dysplasias:** Now exceedingly uncommon, these problems result from shortened ribs, an elongated thoracic cage and a resultant respiratory compromise. Many are associated with other congenital defects or dwarfism. Jeune syndrome (or "asphyxiating thoracic dystrophy") is one such complex disorder, which often results in death during infancy.

TABLE 7 Comparing congenital heart disease with newborn pulmonary hypertension

Prenatal sonogram	Often suggests cardiac anomaly	Usually unremarkable
Perinatal events	Usually unremarkable	Often with events that put infant at risk for hypoxia
Pa O$_2$	With cyanotic lesions, unable to increase PaO$_2$ above 100 mm Hg despite Hg or supplemental oxygen	Infant may have a history of PaO$_2$ greater than 100 mm can obtain that level with therapy
Pa CO$_2$	Usually normal	Often elevated as lung disease a frequent component
Physical examination	Infant typically in no respiratory distress; heart murmur typical, but without hypotension	Respiratory distress common, as is hypotension; heart murmur less common
Echocardiogram	Demonstrates structural heart defect that produces shunting across pulmonary and systemic circulations	Suggests right-to-left shunting at the PFO and/or PDA without structural abnormality of the heart
Treatment	Usually surgical, sometimes in staged procedures; maintenance of PDA may need to be achieved with prostaglandins until surgery	Usually medical, most commonly requiring ventilation, supplemental oxygen, pressors and nitric oxide

Pearl/Peril/Pitfall: The physician must identify the affected area in the respiratory system that contributes to the respiratory failure. Identification can be achieved by dividing the respiratory system into 3 anatomic parts: (1) the extrathoracic airway, (2) the lungs responsible for gas exchange, and (3) the respiratory pump that ventilates the lung and that includes the nervous system, thorax, and respiratory muscles.

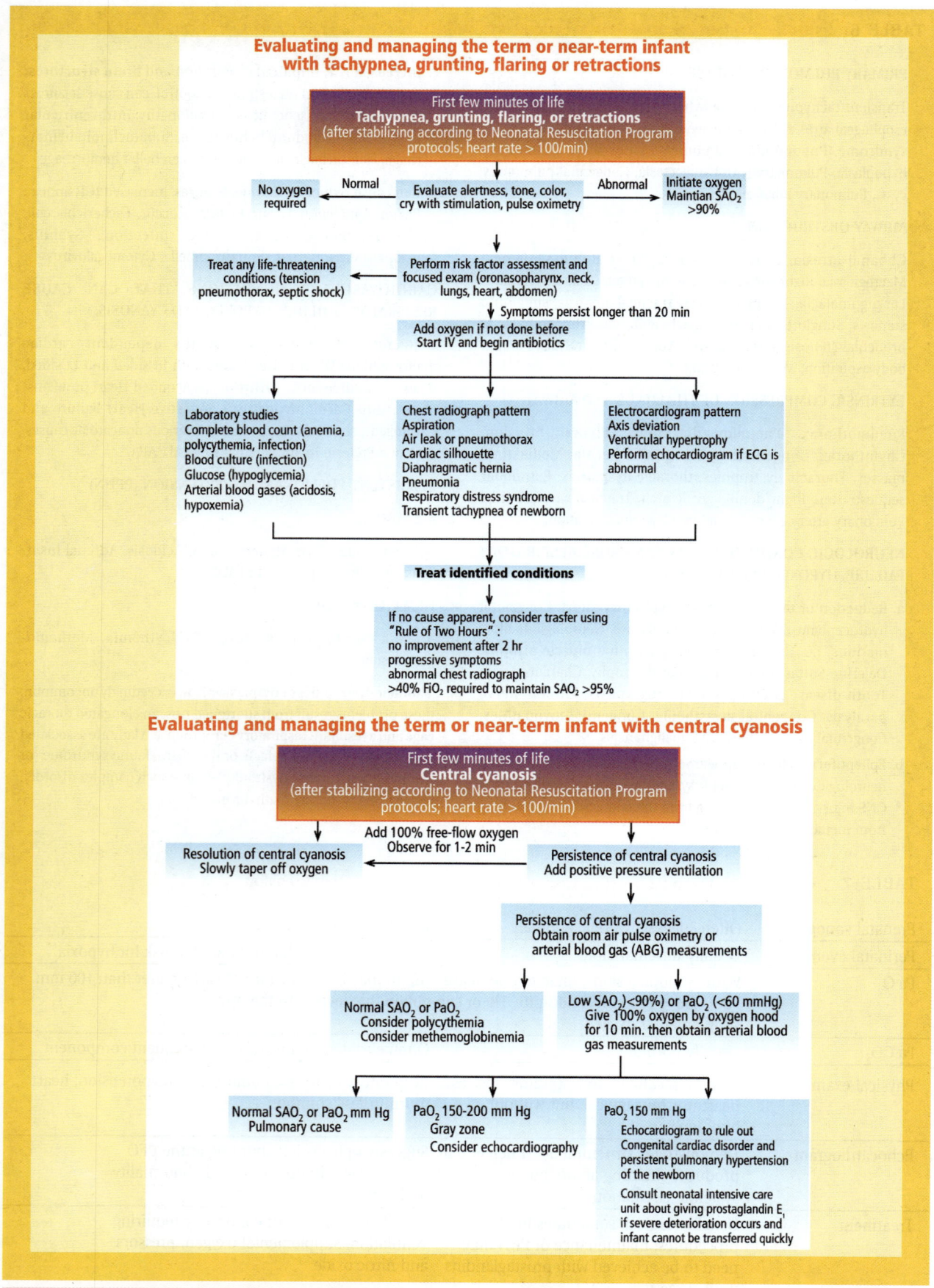

Evaluating and managing the term or near-term infant with tachypnea, grunting, flaring or retractions

First few minutes of life
Tachypnea, grunting, flaring, or retractions
(after stabilizing according to Neonatal Resuscitation Program protocols; heart rate > 100/min)

No oxygen required ← Normal — Evaluate alertness, tone, color, cry with stimulation, pulse oximetry — Abnormal → **Initiate oxygen Maintian SAO_2 >90%**

Treat any life-threatening conditions (tension pneumothorax, septic shock) ← Perform risk factor assessment and focused exam (oronasopharynx, neck, lungs, heart, abdomen)

Symptoms persist longer than 20 min

Add oxygen if not done before
Start IV and begin antibiotics

Laboratory studies
Complete blood count (anemia, polycythemia, infection)
Blood culture (infection)
Glucose (hypoglycemia)
Arterial blood gases (acidosis, hypoxemia)

Chest radiograph pattern
Aspiration
Air leak or pneumothorax
Cardiac silhouette
Diaphragmatic hernia
Pneumonia
Respiratory distress syndrome
Transient tachypnea of newborn

Electrocardiogram pattern
Axis deviation
Ventricular hypertrophy
Perform echocardiogram if ECG is abnormal

Treat identified conditions

If no cause apparent, consider trasfer using "Rule of Two Hours" :
no improvement after 2 hr
progressive symptoms
abnormal chest radiograph
>40% FiO_2 required to maintain SAO_2 >95%

Evaluating and managing the term or near-term infant with central cyanosis

First few minutes of life
Central cyanosis
(after stabilizing according to Neonatal Resuscitation Program protocols; heart rate > 100/min)

Add 100% free-flow oxygen
Observe for 1-2 min

Resolution of central cyanosis
Slowly taper off oxygen ← **Persistence of central cyanosis**
Add positive pressure ventilation

Persistence of central cyanosis
Obtain room air pulse oximetry or arterial blood gas (ABG) measurements

Normal SAO_2 or PaO_2
Consider polycythemia
Consider methemoglobinemia

Low SAO_2)<90%) or PaO_2 (<60 mmHg)
Give 100% oxygen by oxygen hood for 10 min. then obtain arterial blood gas measurements

Normal SAO_2 or PaO_2 mm Hg
Pulmonary cause

PaO_2 150-200 mm Hg
Gray zone
Consider echocardiography

PaO_2 150 mm Hg
Echocardiogram to rule out Congenital cardiac disorder and persistent pulmonary hypertension of the newborn

Consult neonatal intensive care unit about giving prostaglandin E_1 if severe deterioration occurs and infant cannot be transferred quickly

---

Pearl/Peril/Pitfall : Patients with acute respiratory acidosis require admission to the ICU for close monitoring and possible advanced airway management. Correct electrolyte abnormalities associated with muscle weakness, such as hypophosphatemia, hypokalemia, hypomagnesemia, and hypocalcemia. Narcotics, sedatives, or other respiratory depressants should be cautiously administered when the patient is breathing spontaneously and shows signs of increased respiratory work.

TABLE 8	Differentiating between the many etiologies for newborn hypoxia and respiratory failure :				
	Typical history and clinical findings				
Congenital cardiac defects and distress	May have abnormal fetal echocardiogram, maternal diabetes	Unremarkable	None or mild	Significant murmur	Low paO_2 despite high supplemental oxygen, abnormal cardiac silhouette on X-ray
Pulmonary hypertension (usually associated with a second category)	Often unremarkable	Often with evidence fetal stress/distress	Mild to severe respiratory distress	Variable, depending on associated category	Low paO_2 despite supplemental oxygen
Primary pulmonary disease	Often unremarkable, sometimes gestational diabetes	Often unremarkable, but may have evidence fetal stress/distress, history cesarean birth, or delivery at 36–37 weeks	Mild to severe respiratory distress	Often unremarkable	Abnormal bilateral lung fields on X-ray
Airway obstruc-tion	May have abnormal fetal sonogram	Unremarkable	Moderate to severe respiratory distress	Notable or palpable obstruction	Abnormal neck/chest X-ray or CT
Extrinsic compression of the lungs	May have abnormal fetal sonogram	Unremarkable	Moderate to severe respiratory distress	Chest asymmetry	Lesion on chest X-ray or CT
Central nervous system/neuromuscular diseases congenital disorder	May have abnormal fetal sonogram, may have evidence abnormal fetal movement	Malpresentation common	Apnea	Hypotonia, seizures,	Abnormal CT, EEG, or nerve/muscle studies
Central nervous system/neuromuscular diseases-injury	Often unremarkble, sometimes LGA	Often with evidence fetal stress/distress	Apnea	CNS depression or irritability, seizures, increased ICP, anemia	Abnormal head CT
Sepsis and hypotension	Often unremarkble, may have history UTI, poor prenatal care	Often with evidence fetal stress/distress	Apnea, mild to severe respiratory distress	Hypotension, poor perfusion, hypotonia	Abnormal CBC, elevated CRP
Hematologic disorders inherited and acquired (acquired disorders usually associated with a second category)	unremarkble, or may have family history	Often unremarkble if inherited disorder	None, or mild if developing hypovolemia	Petechiae, purpura, ecchymoses, hematomas, prolonged bleeding with heelstick	Abnormal clotting studies, anemia
Metabolic abnormalities	Often unremarkble, but may have family history of metabolic disorder, or may have history of drug use	unremarkble	Apnea (associated with seizures)	Hypotonia, tremors	Metabolic acidosis, electrolyte and Glucose abnor-malities, positive toxicology screen

*   *Pearl/Peril/Pitfall : Failure to respond to a child with impending or existing respiratory failure can lead to life-threatening hypoxemia with resultant end-organ perfusion abnormalities, especially hypoxic ischemic encephalopathy. Using sedative medications in a nonintubated patient can worsen respiratory acidosis, leading to unrecognized CO_2 narcosis.*

Beware of the factors that determine the development of respiratory failure in the presence of abnormalities in mechanical function of the respiratory system !

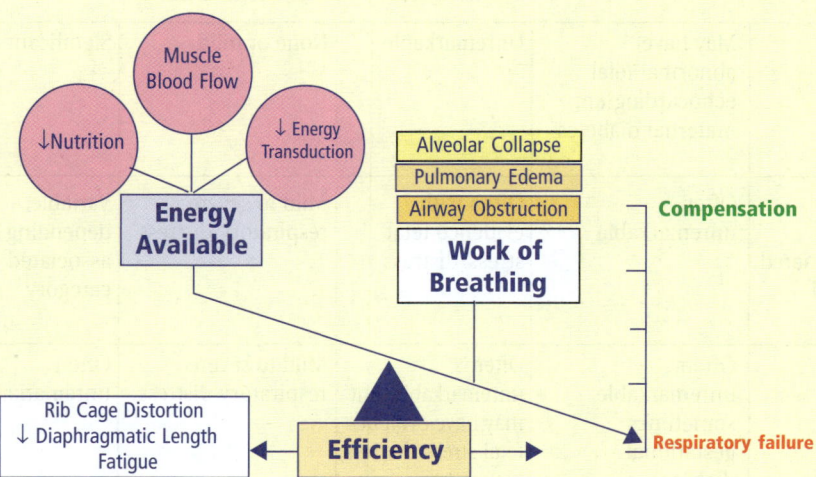

* If the demands exceed the capabilities of the respiratory muscles, respiratory failure develops.

* Under normal circumstances, energy availability greatly exceeds energy demands, and even substantial increases in the work of breathing can be compensated.

* However, when efficiency is reduced by rib cage distortion, overinflation of the lungs, or respiratory muscle fatigue, insufficient energy is transformed into work and the balance moves in the direction of respiratory failure.

* Alveolar collapse, pulmonary edema and airway obstruction increase the work of breathing; malnutrition, decreased muscle blood flow in shock states reduce the energy available.

* *There is a significant amount of interaction between the respiratory system and other organ systems. A certain degree of respiratory insufficiency can be tolerated by itself, but with additional stresses such as fluid overload, infections, myocardial dysfunction and metabolic abnormalities, decompensation readily occurs*

KEY POINTS FOR CLINICAL PRACTICE

1. **Respiratory failure** is defined as the inability of the respiratory apparatus to maintain adequate oxygenation of the blood, with or without CO_2 retention to meet the metabolic demands of the body ; the resulting low PaO_2, high $PaCO_2$ and pH changes affecting the lungs, heart, kidneys and brain.

2. **In preterm infants,** the most common cause of acute respiratory failure is respiratory distress syndrome caused by surfactant deficiency. Acute respiratory failure **in term and near term infants** is usually a result of meconium aspiration syndrome, sepsis, pulmonary hypoplasia, and primary pulmonary hypertension of the Newborn. Other causes of Neonatal respiratory Failure are of Cardiac, Hematologic, Metabolic and Endocrinal in origin.

3. In general, hypoxia associated with pulmonary disease presents as tachypnea, grunting, flaring, chest retractions, arterial blood gas usually showing carbon dioxide retention, rise in PaO_2 when supplemental oxygen is used, and evidence of lung disease on chest radiograph. **A precise** assessment of the adequacy of Oxygenation and Ventilation must be based on both clinical and laboratory data.

4. Central nervous system (CNS) disorders and neuromuscular diseases can cause altered control of respiration and result in hypoxia in the term Neonate. This compromised neurologic control of respiration can be a result of a congenital neurologic disorder, due to seizures or CNS infection, or as a result of neurologic injury.

5. *INDICATIONS FOR ET INTUBATION AND MECHANICAL VENTILATION:* **Absolute:** Major Apnea with failure to respond promptly to Bag and Mask Resuscitation **Relative :** *ELBW <28 wks GA in labour suite, *Recurrent minor apnea unresponsive to CPAP and Methylxanthines *Deteriorating Respiratory Status- PaO_2<50 mm Hg in FiO_2 0.6(<32 wks GA)/ PaO_2<50 mm Hg in FiO_2 0.8(>32 wks GA), pH<7.25, $PaCO_2$>50mm Hg (<32 wks GA)/pH<7.20,$PaCO_2$>60mm Hg (>32 wks GA) *Cerebral edema due to HIE.

REFERENCES AND FURTHER READING 1) Kopelman, A. E., and Mathew, O. P. (1995). Common respiratory disorders of the newborn. Pediatrics in Review, 16, 209-217. 2)Fanaroff, A. A., Miller, M. J., and Martin, R. J. (2002). The respiratory system: Other pulmonary problems. In: A. A. Fanaroff and R. J. Martin (Eds.). Neonatal-Perinatal Medicine (p. 840). St Louis: Mosby. 3)Verklan, M. T. (2006). Persistent pulmonary hypertension of the newborn: Not a honeymoon anymore. Journal of Neonatal and Perinatal Nursing, 20, 98-112. 4)Cifuentes, J., Segars, A. H., and Carlo, W. (2003). Respiratory system management and complications. In C. Kenner (Ed.), *Comprehensive neonatal nursing* (pp. 348-362). St. Louis, MO: WB Saunders. 5)Plessis, A. J. (2005). Perinatal asphyxia and hypoxic-ischemic brain injury. In A. Spitzer (Ed.), Intensive care of the fetus and neonate (pp. 775- 802). Philadelphia, PA: Mosby.

Pearl/Peril/Pitfall : Failure to aggressively manage acute respiratory failure with assisted ventilation can lead to an otherwise avoidable respiratory and/or cardiovascular arrest. Do not treat alveolar hypoventilation with supplemental oxygen; it must be treated with an augmentation of ventilation.

34 Neonatal Respiratory Distress Syndrome

@ *IT IS IMPORTANT TO BE AWARE - that two or more respiratory disorders may co-exist in the one infant: for e.g., RDS and Congenital Pneumonia in preterm infants after PROM or in the presence of chorioamnionitis, and meconium aspiration and congenital sepsis in term infants with respiratory distress*

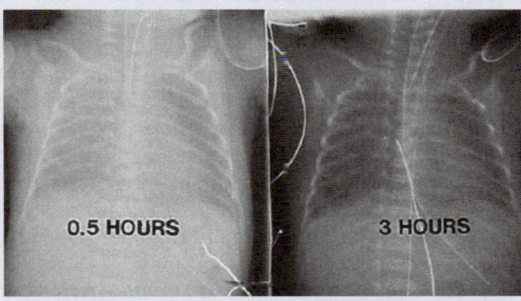

0.5 HOURS   3 HOURS

Chest radiographs in a premature infant with respiratory distress syndrome before and after surfactant treatment. Left: Initial radiograph shows poor lung expansion, air bronchogram, and reticular granular appearance. Right: Repeat chest radiograph obtained when the neonate is aged 3 hours and after surfactant therapy demonstrates marked improvement.

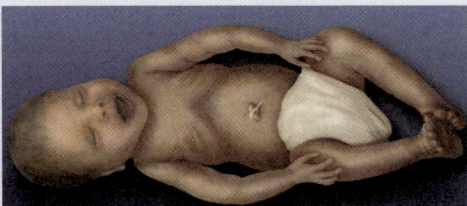

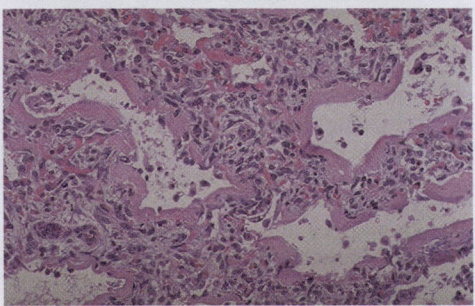

Microscopic appearance of lungs of an infant with respiratory distress syndrome. Hematoxylin and eosin stain shows hyaline membranes (pink areas).

PREMATURE BIRTH INTERRUPTS LUNG DEVELOPMENT

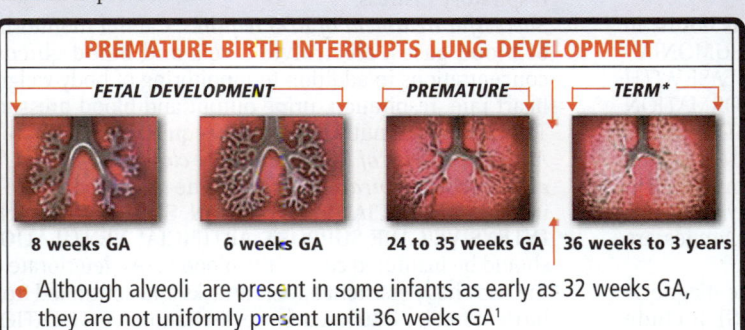

FETAL DEVELOPMENT		PREMATURE	TERM*
8 weeks GA	6 weeks GA	24 to 35 weeks GA	36 weeks to 3 years

- Although alveoli are present in some infants as early as 32 weeks GA, they are not uniformly present until 36 weeks GA[1]

* Pictures are artistic renditions of lung development and are designed to emphasize terminal acinus development and not the entire conducting airway system. Adapted from Moore 2003[2]
[1]Langston C. et at. am Rev Respir Dis. 1984; 129:607-613.
[2]Moore KL, Persaud TVN. In : The developing human : clinically oriented embryology. 7th ed., Philadelphia, PA: Saunders. 2003:241 253

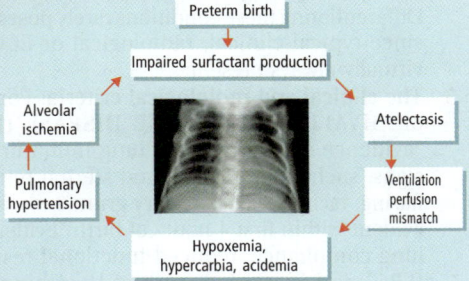

Preterm birth → Impaired surfactant production → Atelectasis → Ventilation perfusion mismatch → Hypoxemia, hypercarbia, acidemia → Pulmonary hypertension → Alveolar ischemia

REVIEW OF CLINICAL PROBLEMS

1. Name the clinical and radiological criteria for the diagnosis of Hyaline membrane disease?
   Ans: Refer to the "No. 5" of the "BIRD'S EYE VIEW/OVERVIEW/ SYNOPSIS" of the Chapter.

2. What are the 5 possibilities of respiratory illness starting *de novo* 4 hours after delivery of a Neonate ?
   Ans: Refer to the "No. 4" of the "BIRD'S EYE VIEW/OVERVIEW/ SYNOPSIS" of the Chapter.

3. What are the several co-existing diagnoses that can complicate RDS in a Neonate?
   Ans: Refer to the Evaluation-Decision-Action Plan/Algorithm to diagnose and manage a Neonatal RDS.

4. Mention the diagnostic and therapeutic priorities in evaluating a Neonate with Respiratory distress?
   Ans: Refer to Tables 5 and 6 of the Chapter.

5. What are usual causes of poor response to Surfactant therapy?
   Ans: Refer to the "No. 10" of the "BIRD'S EYE VIEW/OVERVIEW/ SYNOPSIS" of the Chapter.

LEARNING OBJECTIVES

After completing this article, readers will be able to

1. Anticipate respiratory problems in any High-Risk delivery and monitor for respiratory deterioration continuously.

2. Intervene early in the course of illness, before decompensation sets in, which may lead to Multiorgan Dysfunction and Exclude extrapulmonary causes of respiratory distress (cardiac, CNS, sepsis, hematologic, metabolic).

3. Differentiate surgical causes of Respiratory distress from medical causes promptly, to inform pediatric surgeon for further support and management.

4. Treat Hyaline Membrane Disease with Surfactant replacement, CPAP, Mechanical ventilation in addition to general supportive measures.

5. Refer Neonates with RDS & Respiratory Failure not responding to initial measures to appropriate tertiary care center for assistance with diagnosis and management.

Pearl/Peril/Pitfall: We need to suspect surgical conditions if there are any obvious malformations (cleft palate, micrognathia) or if there is a scaphoid abdomen (diaphragmatic hernia). Presence of frothing or history suggestive of aspiration may give a clue to the presence of a tracheo-esophageal fistula (TEF). Worsening of condition during resuscitation at birth by bag and mask ventilation -think of diaphragmatic hernia.

BIRD'S EYE VIEW/OVERVIEW/SYNOPSIS

1. **The new born with clinical signs of acute respiratory distress:** Central Cyanosis, Tachypnea (>60bpm), Tachycardia (>160 bpm), Retractions, Grunting, and Nasal flaring- **demands immediate attention.** A review of the maternal Hx, the age of onset of respiratory distress (within the first 4 hours of life or **DE NOVO** after 4 hours of life), a thorough physical examination and a Chest X-ray will greatly aid the clinician in assessing this problem further.

2. **Neonatal respiratory distress:** A major reason for morbidity and mortality in the Neonate, is an alarming symptom of pulmonary disorders in most cases. *The differential diagnosis of respiratory distress includes Pulmonary, Cardiac, Hematologic, Infectious, Anatomic, and Metabolic disorders that may directly or indirectly involve the lungs.*

3. **Echocardiography:** Easily differentiates isolated primary pulmonary hypertension (PPHN) from cyanotic congenital heart disease or ascertaining whether a baby who undoubtedly has surfactant - deficient RDS also has coexisting congenital heart disease (cyanotic or otherwise). HYPEROXIA TEST - can differentiate severe RDS and PPHN form cyanotic congenital heart disease.(Refer to Tables 7 & 8 of the Chapter)

4. **Respiratory illness starting de novo after four hours:** In essence there are *only five possibilities:* * PNEUMONIA - bacterial and viral * CONGENITAL HEART DISEASE WITH PULMONARY EDEMA * CONGENITAL MALFORMATION * THE DYSPNEA OF ACIDEMIA DUE TO UNDERLYING METABOLIC DISEASE * rare, late-onset lung disease of the VLBW baby (e.g. Wilson Mikity syndrome, CPIP). Differentiating these conditions rarely poses any problems, since typical clinical, radiological or ECG changes are virtually always present.

5. **The clinical and radiological criteria:** For the diagnosis of **HYALINE MEMBRANE DISEASE (RDS)** include *evidence of prematurity *lung immaturity *abnormal signs, such as intercostal and sternal retractions, nasal flaring, tachypnea, expiratory grunt and central cyanosis evident within first 4 hours of birth *evidence of reduced lung compliance, reduced functional residual capacity (FRC) and increased work of breathing *evidence of abnormal gas exchange (hypoxemia, hypercapnia, cyanosis) of sufficient severity to require oxygen and or continuous or intermittent positive pressure ventilatory support for >24hours (*Blood gases show respiratory and metabolic acidosis along with hypoxia. *Respiratory acidosis occurs because of alveolar atelectasis and/or overdistension of terminal airways. *Metabolic acidosis is primarily lactic acidosis, which results from poor tissue perfusion and anaerobic metabolism. *Hypoxia occurs from right-to-left shunting of blood through the pulmonary vessels, patent ductus arteriosus (PDA), and/or patent foramen ovale.)* *an abnormal chest radiogram with diffuse, parenchymal reticulogranular densities and air bronchograms (atelectasis) and underinflation during a good inspiratory effort at 6–24 hours of age (updated by Walther and Taeusch).*The prominent air bronchograms represent aerated bronchioles superimposed on a background of collapsed alveoli. *The cardiac silhouette may be normal or enlarged. Cardiomegaly may be the result of prenatal asphyxia, maternal diabetes, PDA, an associated congenital heart anomaly, or simply poor lung expansion. *These findings may be altered with either early surfactant therapy or a PDA or with mechanical ventilation. *The radiologic findings of respiratory distress syndrome cannot be reliably differentiated from those of pneumonia, which is most commonly caused by group B beta-hemolytic streptococci. If the radiograph shows streaky opacities, the diagnosis of *Ureaplasma* or *Mycoplasma* pneumonia should be considered and confirmed by means of tracheal aspirate cultures grown in the appropriate medium. *Echocardiographic evaluation is performed in selected infants to assist in diagnosing PDA and in determining the direction and degree of shunting on Doppler study. It is also useful in diagnosing pulmonary hypertension, assessing cardiac function, and excluding structural heart disease.* The classical signs of RDS are outdated because very immature infants may present with apnea at birth and intubation at birth for assisted ventilation and surfactant treatment modifies the course of RDS.

6. *It is important to be aware—that two or more respiratory disorders may coexist in the one infant:* For e.g. RDS and Congenital Pneumonia in preterm infants after **PROM** or in the presence of chorioamnionitis, and meconium aspiration and congenital sepsis in term infants with respiratory distress.

7. *Successful treatment of RDS requires:* Careful monitoring of blood gases, electrolyte levels and blood glucose concentrations in addition to monitoring of body weight, heart rate, respiration, urine output and blood pressure. Total parenteral nutrition may be required.

8. *All babies at risk of RDS—should be closely monitored for evidence of respiratory failure:* The treatment of RDS involves **ARTIFICIAL VENTILATION, SURFACTANT AND INTENSIVE CARE SUPPORT. ARTIFICIAL VENTILATION** should be instituted early if the blood gases deteriorate or the baby has persistent apneic attacks and continued from birth in babies intubated for resuscitation. VENTILATION should be adjusted to maintain; pH above 7.25, PaO_2, 6–10 kPa (45–75mmHg), $PaCO_2$ 5-7 kPa (37.5–52.5 mmHg).

9. **Surfactant treatment:** All babies < 28 weeks, if no antenatal steroids given, male sex, need for intubation in resuscitation, require prophylactic surfactant. For infants of 32 weeks gestation and greater, early rescue treatment is recommended, when endotracheal intubation becomes necessary to treat RDS. At gestational ages in between (from 28–31 weeks) early CPAP is recommended with surfactant given as soon as endotracheal intubation is needed. Although reduced, the incidence and severity of complications of respiratory distress syndrome can result in clinically significant morbidities. Sequelae of respiratory distress syndrome include septicemia, bronchopulmonary dysplasia (BPD), PDA, pulmonary hemorrhage, apnea/bradycardia, necrotizing enterocolitis (NEC), retinopathy of prematurity (ROP), hypertension, failure to thrive, intraventricular hemorrhage (IVH), and periventricular leukomalacia (PVL) with associated neurodevelopmental and audiovisual handicaps. *Direct attention to anticipating and minimizing these complications and to preventing premature delivery whenever possible are strategic goals.*

10. **Beware of the causes of a poor response to surfactant therapy—Wrong diagnosis**—lung hypoplasia, pneumonia, ARDS, congenital heart disease. **Wrong dose**-inadequate to overcome surfactant inactivation. **Wrong Place**—given in to 1 lung or into esophagus. **Wrong Condition**—correct hypothermia, acidosis, and hypotension before treatment.

Pearl/Peril/Pitfall: Pulse oximetry is used as a noninvasive tool to monitor oxygen saturation, which should be maintained at 90-95%. However, it is unreliable for determining hyperoxia because of the flat-top portion of the S -shaped oxygen-hemoglobin dissociation curve.

THE EVALUATION-DECISION-ACTION-PLAN/ALGORITHM FOR THE DIAGNOSIS AND MANAGEMENT OF *NEONATAL RESPIRATORY DISTRESS SYNDROME*

SUBJECTIVE FINDINGS

Hx of age of onset of respiratory distress - within first 4 hours of life or *de novo* after 4 hrs of life.

Hx of antenatal and natal factors like - prematurity, maternal diabetes, hydramnios/oligohydramnios, meconium stained liquor, post maturity, traumatic/ breech delivery, PROM and prolonged labor, fetal bradycardia/ tachycardia, cord prolapse, c/s, etc.

Hx of Apgar scores and details of resuscitation, associated symptoms like stridor, wheezing, frothy bleeding from the mouth etc.

OBJECTIVE FINDINGS

Assess ABCs, disability, O_2 sats, CRT, vitals, BP, Urine output

Look for "clues" which suggest most likely associated condition (refer to Table 2)

Perform thorough physical examination, focussing the "clinching" findings of specific conditions

Assess and Reassess the SILVERMAN ANDERSON and DOWNE'S SCORINGS depending on the gestational age

Beaware that two or more respiratory disorders may co-exist in one infant-*v.i.*

INVESTIGATIONS

Initial tests - at admission: 1)Hematocrit, blood counts 2)C-reactive Protein 3)Blood glucose 4)Chest X-ray including abdomen 5)Arterial blood gas Analysis

Follow-up investigations: 1)Echocardiogram 2)Biochemistry-calcium, electrolytes 3)Lumbar puncture and CSF analysis 4)Blood culture 5)Gastric aspirate analysis and culture 6)Cranial ultrasound

Special investigation—to be done if indicated: 1)CT scan—head 2)Muscle biopsy and EMG 3)Hemolytic workup including hemoglobin electrophoresis 4)Infantogram

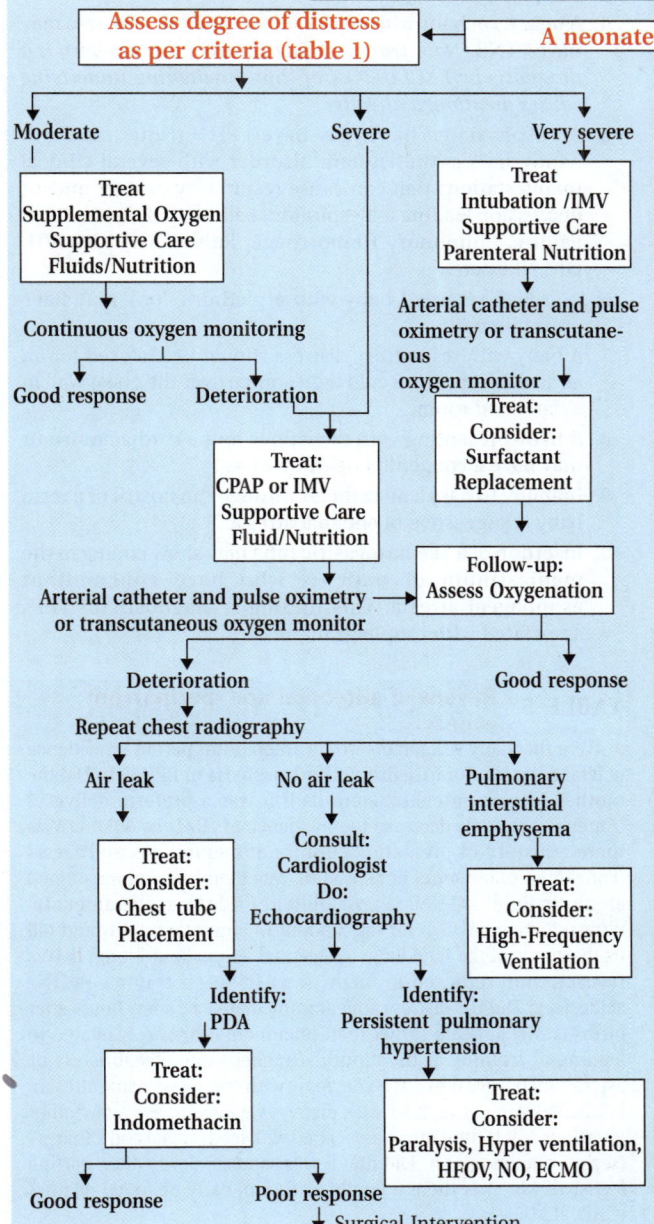

Assess degree of distress as per criteria (table 1) ← A neonate with respiratory distress

Etiology of respiratory distress

Preterm Infant	Preterm and Fullterm
Respiratory distress syndrome	Bacterial sepsis (GBS)
Erythroblastosis fetalis	Transient tachypnea (Term > preterm)
Nonimmune hydrops	Spontaneous pneumothorax
Pulmonary hemorrhage	Congenital anomalies (e.g. congenital lobar emphysema, cystic adenomatoid malformation, diaphragmatic hernia)
Full-Term Infant	
Meconium aspiration	Congenital heart disease
Pneumonia	Pulmonary hypoplasia
Polycythemia	Viral infection (e.g. herpes simplex, CMV)
Amniotic fluid aspiration	Inborn metabolic errors
Primary pulmonary hypertension of the Neonate	

CMV, Cytomegalovirus; GBS, group B streptococcus

Several diagnoses may coexist and complicate the course of respiratory distress syndrome, including the following:
*Pneumonia is usually secondary to group B beta-hemolytic streptococci (not common in India) and often coexists with respiratory distress syndrome. *Metabolic problems (e.g. hypothermia, hypoglycemia) may occur. *Hematologic problems (e.g. anemia, polycythemia, jaundice) may occur. *Transient tachypnea of the newborn usually occurs in term or near-term neonates, often after cesarean delivery. The chest radiograph of an infant with transient tachypnea shows good lung expansion and, often, fluid in the horizontal fissure. *Aspiration syndromes may result from aspiration of amniotic fluid, blood, or meconium. Aspiration syndrome is observed in more mature infants and is differentiated by obtaining a history and by viewing the chest radiographs. *Pulmonary air leaks, e.g. pneumothorax, interstitial emphysema, pneumomediastinum, pneumopericardium) may occur. In premature infants, these complications may be due to excessive positive-pressure ventilation. In rare cases, spontaneous pneumothorax may occur in large infants. *Congenital anomalies of the lungs, e.g. diaphragmatic hernia, chylothorax, congenital cystic adenomatoid malformation of the lung, lobar emphysema, bronchogenic cyst, pulmonary sequestration) and heart (e.g. cardiac anomalies) are uncommon in premature infants. These entities can be diagnosed on the basis of chest radiographic or echocardiographic findings. On rare occasions, they coexist with respiratory distress syndrome.*

Pearl/Peril/Pitfall: *The radiologic findings of respiratory distress syndrome cannot be reliably differentiated from those of pneumonia, which is most commonly caused by group B beta-hemolytic streptococci. If the radiograph shows streaky opacities, the diagnosis of Ureaplasma or Mycoplasma pneumonia should be considered and confirmed by means of tracheal aspirate cultures grown in the appropriate medium.*

TABLES 1 AND 2   Assessment of respiratory failure

Score	Upper Chest	Lower Chest Retrac	Xiphoid Retrac	Nasal Flare	Grunt
0	Sync	None	None	None	None
1	Lag on Insp	Just Visible	Just Visible	Minimal	Steth Only
2	See-Saw	Marked	Marked	Marked	Naked Ear

A score of 6 or more is indicative of impending respiratory failure

A)CLINICAL CRITERIA 1) FOR PRETERM BABIES
SILVERMAN-ANDERSON RETRACTION SCORE

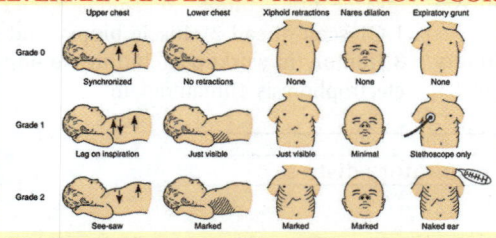

RESPIRATORY DISTRESS SCORING

2) FOR TERM BABIES
DOWNE'S SCORE IN TERM BABIES

Score	Respiratory Rate/min	Cyanosis	Air Entry	Retractions	Grunt
0	<60	None	Good	None	None
1	60-80	In air	Diminished	Mild	Audible with Stethoscope
2	> 80 or apneic	In 40% O$_2$	Barely audible	Moderate/severe	Audible with naked ear

A score of 6 or more is indicative of impending respiratory failure

B) LABORATORY CRITERIA pH-<7.1–7.2, PaO$_2$<50mmHg (6.6kPa) In FiO$_2$> 0.6 PaCO$_2$>60mmHg (8kPa)

In infants weighing <1500g PaCO$_2$ should be modified to > 50mmHg-preventing the risk of intracerebral Hemorrhage (ICH) at high PaCO$_2$

ABG Score

Parameters	0	1	2	3
PaO$_2$ mmHg	>60	50–60	<50	<50
PH	>7.3	7.20–7.29	7.1-7.19	<7.1
PaCO$_2$ mmHg	<50	50–60	61-70	>70

A score of 3 or more on the ABG indicates the need for CPAP or mechanical ventilation. A pH of <7.2 with hypercarbia (pCO2>60mm) or a pO2<50mm Hg in FiO2 of 0.8 is suggestive of frank respiratory failure.

TABLE 4   Diagnostic approach to respiratory distress

```
Respiratory distress (tachypnea, retractions,
grunt, flaring, desaturations)
           |
    ┌──────┴──────┐
  Preterm        Term
```

< 4-6hrs old	>4–6 hrs old	<4–6hrs old	>4–6hrs old
HMD Pneumonia Lung Anamoly Shock	Pneumonia CHD Pulmonary Hemorrhage	TTNB MAS/PPHN Asphyxia,Shock Lung Anamoly Air leak	Pneumonia Polycythemia CHD

TABLE 3   Clinical examination

Clues to the likely etiology can be picked up on examination of the Neonate

1. A preterm baby weighing <1500 gms with retractions and grunt is likely to have HMD. (*Note that an Infant of Diabetic Mom, usually a LGA can have RDS due to HMD.*)

2. A term baby born through meconium stained amniotic fluid with an increase in the AP diameter of the chest (barrel chest) is likely to be suffering from MAS.(*Note that a baby with MAS may have had Birth Asphyxia and developed PPHN as well*).

3. A depressed baby with poor circulation is likely to have neonatal sepsis with or without congenital pneumonia.(*Note that a septic looking baby may have several noninfectious underlying causes such as Congenital adrenal hyperplasia, Ductus-dependent CHD,Inborn Errors of Metabolism or non-bacterial causes such as Herpes meningoencephalitis, Fungal sepsis, Perinatal Tuberculosis etc.*)

4. A near term baby with no risk factors and mild distress may have TTNB.(*Note Transient Tachypnea of the Newborn is a diagnosis by EXCLUSION of life-threatening underlying causes mentioned already*)

5. An asphyxiated baby may have PPHN.(Note that Birth Asphyxia is a Multisystem disorder with several clinical manifestations that can cause respiratory distress and/or depression leading to Respiratory Failure;CHF, Acute Renal Failure, Pulmonary Hemorrhage, Raised ICP, ICH-IVH, DIC,NEC, etc.)

6. A growth retarded baby with a plethoric look may have polycythemia.

7. A baby with respiratory distress should be checked for an air leak by placing a cold light source over the chest wall in a darkened room.

8. A baby presenting with tachypnea and a cardiac murmur may have a congenital heart disease.

9. Inability to pass a 5F catheter through the nostril of a term baby is suggestive of choanal atresia.

10. Insertion of a 10F nasogastric tube may show coiling in the mediastinum of patients who have concomitant esophageal atresia. This finding is diagnostic of TEFs associated with esophageal atresia.

TABLE 5   Review of antenatal and peripartum events

a) Were there any risk factors in the antepartum period or evidence of fetal distress prior to delivery? (Birth asphyxia or PPHN) **b)** Did the mother receive antenatal steroids if it was a preterm delivery? (Antenatal steroids decrease the incidence of HMD by 50%) **c)** Was there a history of premature rupture of membranes and fever? (congenital pneumonia or sepsis) **d)** Was there meconium stained amniotic fluid? (MAS is a possibility) e) A look at the antenatal ultrasonography (USG) for the amount of amniotic fluid would tell us the status of the fetal lung. (congenital anomalies of lung) **f)** Was resuscitation required at birth? (resuscitation trauma/PPHN/acidosis) **g)** Did the distress appear immediately or a few hours after birth? (HMD appears earlier than pneumonia) **h)** Was it related to feeding or frothing at the mouth? (tracheo-esophageal fistula or aspiration) **i)** Does the distress decrease with crying? (choanal atresia). For babies presenting later with distress we have to ask a few other questions :- a) Is the distress associated with feed refusal and lethargy? (sepsis, pneumonia) b) Did the distress appear slowly after starting feeds? (IEM). c) Is there a family history of early neonatal deaths? (CHD, IEM).

(Courtesy: Surg Cdr SS Mathai, Col U Raju, Col M Kanitkar AFMC, PUNE)

Pearl/Peril/Pitfall: *Management of acute respiratory failure begins with a determination of the underlying etiology. While supporting the respiratory system and ensuring adequate oxygen delivery to the tissues, initiate an intervention specifically defined to correct the underlying condition.*

TABLE 6	Initial laboratory evaluation of respiratory distress
TEST	**RATIONALE**
Chest roentgenogram	To determine reticular granular pattern of RDS ; to determine presence of pneumothorax, cardiomegaly, life threatening congenital anomalies
Arterial blood gas	To determine severity of respiratory compromise, hypoxemia, hypercapnia, and type of acidosis. The severity determines treatment strategy.
Complete blood count	Hemoglobin/hematocrit to determine anemia and polycythemia, White blood count to determine neutropenia/sepsis. Platelet count and smear to determine DIC
Buffy coat smear Blood culture Blood glucose	For Gram stain of bacteria To recover potential pathogen To determine presence of hypoglycemia, which may produce or occur simultaneously with respiratory distress; and to determine stress hyperglycemia
Echocardiogram, electrocardiogram	In the presence of a murmur, cardiomegaly, refractory hypoxia; to determine structural heart disease or persistent fetal circulation (PFC)

TABLE 7	Priorities in initial evaluation of infant with respiratory distress
ASSESS	**RESPONSE**
Ventilation	Provide oxygen as indicated by cyanosis. Ventilate by mask and bag or through endotracheal tube if infant is unable to move sufficient air.
Circulation	Listen to heart, measure blood pressure, pulse, hematocrit. Provide blood or other volume expander if infant is in shock or anemic.
Temperature	Provide sufficient heat to bring axillary temperature to 37.5°C and to prevent peripheral vasoconstriction.
Causes of respiratory distress	Locate cardiac impulse. Transilluminate. Obtain chest radiograph.
Level of maturity	Estimate gestational age by appearance and responses. **Weigh infant.**
Possibility of infection	Obtain cultures of blood, amniotic fluid, blood count. Administer antibiotics.
Metabolic status	Measure pH, blood gases, blood glucose, electrolytes & treat according to findings.
History	Review with parents events of pregnancy and family history, and keep them informed realistically of the changing status of the infant.

Differential Diagnosis of Respiratory Distress in the Newborn: Most common causes*

Transient tachypnea of the Newborn
Respiratory distress syndrome Type-I (hyaline membrane disease)
Meconium aspiration syndrome
Less common but significant causes
Delayed transition
Infection (e.g. pneumonia, sepsis)

Nonpulmonary causes (e.g. anemia, congenital heart disease, congenital malformation, medications, neurologic or metabolic abnormalities, polycythemia, upper airway obstruction)
Persistent pulmonary hypertension of the Newborn
Pneumothorax
*—Listed in order of incidence

Medical

Respiratory distress syndrome (RDS)
Wet lung (transient tachypnea, RDS II)
Aspiration syndromes (meconium, blood)
Persistent pulmonary hypertension of the Newborn fistula
Pneumonia/sepsis
Polycythemia—hyperviscosity
Pulmonary edema
Hypoplastic lungs
Cardiac lesions
Hypoglycemia
Hypovolemia
Central nervous system

Surgical

Pneumothorax
Diaphragmatic hernia/eventration
Lobar emphysema
Esophageal atresia with or without TE

Pleural effusion
Cystic lesions
Mass lesions
Airway disorders (upper, laryngeal, lower)
Phrenic nerve paralysis

Pearl/Peril/Pitfall: Surgical causes of neonatal respiratory distress are due to airway obstruction, pulmonary collapse or displacement and parenchymal disease or insufficiency. Any two or all three mechanisms may occur simultaneously in the same baby.

| TABLE 8 | Hyperoxia test to differentiate neonatal cyanosis |

In cases of Neonatal cyanosis with breathing difficulties (either tachypnea or dyspnea)-

Do HYPEROXIA (Oxygen Challenge) TEST and Interpret according to the following table.

A) **Technique** - Used to evaluate etiology of cyanosis in Neonates. Obtain baseline arterial blood gases (ABG) or pulse oximetry saturation at $FiO_2=0.21$, then place infant in oxygen hood at $FiO_2=1$ (100%) for a minimum of 10 minutes, and repeat ABG or pulse oximetry. Pulse oximetry will not be useful for following the change in oxygenation once the saturations reach 100% (approximately $PO_2 \geq 90mmHg$)   (1 kPa = 7.5mmHg)

B) Interpretation	$FiO_2 = .21$ PaO_2 (% saturation)		$FiO_2 = 1.00$ PaO_2 (% saturation)	$PaCo_2$
Normal	70 (95)		> 200 (100)	35
Pulmonary disease	50 (85)		> 150 (100)	50
Neurologic disease	50 (85)		> 150 (100)	50
Methemoglobinemia	70 (95)		> 200 (100)	35
Cardiac disease				
Separate circulation*	<40 (<75)		<50 (<85)	35
Restricted PBF†	<40 (<75)		<50 (<85)	35
Complete mixing without restricted PBF‡	50 (85)		<150 (<100)	35
Persistent pulmonary hypertension	Preductal	Postductal		
PFO (no R to L shunt)	70 (95)	<40 (<75)	Variable	35-50
PFO (with R to L shunt)	<40 (<75)	<40 (<75)	Variable	35-50

PBF, Pulmonary blood flow *D-transposition of the great arteries (D-TGA) with intact ventricular septum. † Tricuspid atresia with pulmonary stenosis or atresia; pulmonary atresia or critical pulmonary stenosis with intact ventricular septum; or tetralogy of Fallot.

‡ Truncus, total anomalous pulmonary venous return, single ventricle, hypoplastic left heart, D-TGA with ventricular septal defect, tricuspid atresia without pulmonary stenosis or atresia.

From Less MH: *J pediatr* 77:484, 1970; Kitterman
J A: Pediatr Rev 4:13, 1982; Jones RWA et al: *Arch Dis Child* 51 : 667, 1976.

| TABLE 9 | Differentiating causes of respiratory distress in the newborn. *Courtesy* Dr. Meharban Singh |

	Respiratory	Cardiac	Hematological	Neurological
Antenatal history	Preterm labor Rupture of membranes	Antenatal US scan with cardiac or other anomalies	H/o blood group incompatibility Hydrops Placenta previa	IUGR Oligohydramnios Decreased fetal movements
Intranatal history	Foul smelling liquor Meconium staining Prolonged labor Unclean vaginal examination	Generally uneventful	Antepartum hemorrhage Pallor, limp at birth Milking of cord Unattended birth	Difficult or prolonged labor Difficult delivery Delayed or absent cry Prolonged resuscitation
Postnatal history	Onset soon after birth	Onset usually on day 3–7	Onset a few hours after birth	Onset at birth, seizures
Examination	Unequal air entry or poor air entry with lung signs	Poor or unequal pulses Abnormal 2nd heart sound Cardiac murmurs	Pallor Hepatosplenomegaly	Shrill cry Encephalopathy Abnormal tone and reflexes
Investigations	Abnormal chest X-ray	Abnormal echocardiogram	Low < 30% or high >60% hematocrit Abnormal Coomb's test Abnormal hemoglobin	Abnormal neurosonogram EEG, BAER
Course	Worsening over 3 days followed by improvement	Progressive worsening	Marked improvement if treated with exchange transfusion	Worsening over 1 week followed by gradual improvement

Pearl/Peril/Pitfall : Right-to-left shunts sometimes occur with noncardiac disease, however, giving a false-positive result on the hyperoxia challenge test. Examples include hypoglycemia, asphyxia, pneumonia, aspiration, diaphragmatic hernia, pulmonary hypoplasia, persistent pulmonary hypertension, and polycythemia. Even if a noncardiac source is suspected, echocardiography is recommended to exclude cardiac defects.

Supportive care for infants with respiratory distress syndrome

Treatment

1. a) Trained staff nurses (ratio of 1:2), respiratory therapists, and monitoring equipment.

    b) Available trained physicians, nurse practitioners.

2. Precise temperature control to maintain infant in neutral temperature

3. a) pH, PaO_2, $PaCO_2$, and HCO_3 measurements at least every 4 h. Maintain PaO_2 at 50–80 mm Hg. Continuous PaO_2 or SaO_2 is optimal.

    b) Monitor blood pressure.

    c) Attempt to keep pH > 7.25. If $PaCO_2$ >60 or PaO_2

    d) Lower environmental oxygen slowly when RDS infant is still ill.

    e) Limit $NaHCO_3$ to 8 mEq/kg/d.

4. Surfactant therapy (requires endotracheal tube).

5. IV glucose 60 mL/kg 1st day, 80–100 mL/kg 2nd day with body weight determination for small infants to calculate if larger amounts of H_2O required. May require 150 mL/kg or more

6. Controlled oxygen administration: warmed and humidified, using a hood.

7. Continually monitor respiration, heart rate, and temperature as well as blood pressure.

8. Frequent determinations of blood sugar and hematocrit (Na, K, and Cl every 12-24 h).

9. Transfuse if central hematocrit < 35 during acute phase of illness.

10. Record all observations (laboratory, nurse's notes, etc.) on single form.

11. Urinary output, blood urea nitrogen, creatinine, and when indicated urinary pH, electrolytes, and osmolality.

12. Minimize routing procedures such as suctioning, handling, and auscultation.

Logic

1. (a) and (b) Early management of complications and notification of change in course (e.g. apnea, bleeding from catheter).

2. Maintains minimal oxygen consumption and carbon dioxide production.

3. a) To determine requirements for oxygen and additional HCO_3. Permits continual assessment of infant's condition and limits toxic effects of oxygen.

    b) Recognize hypoperfusion, hypovolemia, patent ductus arteriosus.

    c) Same as (a)

    d) Prevents greater than expected decrease in PaO_2 when environmental oxygen is reduced (right-to-left shunt etiology?).

    e) Prevents hypernatremia with possible brain damage.

4. Therapeutic approach to underlying etiology of RDS.

5. Need to balance fluid and partial caloric requirements while minimizing the risk of fluid overload problems (e.g. patent ductus arteriosus).

6. Prevents large swings in environmental oxygen concentration and temperature and decreases water requirements.

7. prevents hypoxemia and acidemia with apneic episodes.

8. Necessary for calculating general metabolic requirements.

9. For adequate oxygen carrying capacity.

10. Permits immediate correlation of many variables.

11. Evaluation of renal function and blood flow to the kidney An increase in output occurs as the infant starts to improve.

12. Prevents iatrogenic decreases in PaO_2.

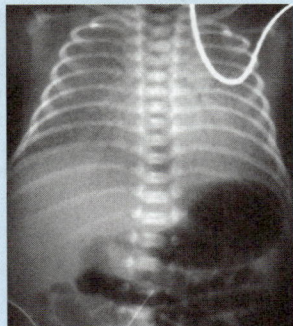

Respiratory Distress Syndrome (Surfactant deficient) Imaging findings
*Typically, diffuse "ground-glass" opacification of both lungs with air bronchograms and hypoaeration
*Hypoaeration from loss of lung volume (may be counteracted by respiratory therapy)
*Fine granular pattern
*Prominent air bronchograms
*Bilateral and symmetrical distribution

NB: Neonatal pneumonia can have a similar appearance. The classic findings may not be present because of the early intervention with surfactant and ventilatory support with intubation.

RDS complicated with Air leaks: Diffuse ground-glass appearance to both lungs with a left-sided tension pneumothorax and pneumomediastinum (oro gastric tube is in distal esophagus)

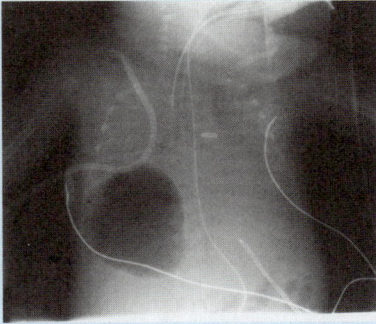

Large, right lower lobe pneumatocele is shown, compromising ventilation in a premature infant with RDS and superimposed RSV pneumonitis. Progression of pulmonary interstitial emphysema (PIE) to single or multiple pneumatoceles is uncommon, but may be seen in extremely premature infants with respiratory distress syndrome (RDS) on mechanical ventilation, after bacterial pneumonia and after suction catheter-induced airway trauma. While most premature infants with pneumatoceles are managed conservatively, mechanical decompression may be necessary.

Pearl/Peril/Pitfall : Although the precise mechanism of pulmonary hemorrhage following surfactant therapy remains unclear, it has been suggested that improved ventilation and decreased pulmonary vascular resistance following surfactant administration promotes left-to-right shunting through the ductus arteriosus, producing hemorrhagic pulmonary edema .

Guidelines on the use of Antenatal Corticosteroids to Prevent Respiratory Distress Syndrome (Royal College of Obstetricians and Gynecologist's Guidelines): Recommendations

*The benefits of antenatal administration of corticosteroids to fetuses at risk of preterm delivery vastly outweigh the potential risks. These benefits include not only a reduction in the risk of RDS but also substantial reduction in mortality and IVH. *All women between 24 and 36 weeks of pregnancy at risk of preterm delivery are candidates for antenatal corticosteroids therapy. *Fetal race, gender and availability of surfactant therapy should not influence the decision to use antenatal corticosteroid therapy. *Patients eligible for therapy with tocolytic agents should also be eligible for treatment with antenatal corticosteroids. *Treatment should consist of either 2 doses of 12 mg of betamethasone, IM, given 24 hours apart; or 4 doses of 6 mg of dexamethasone, IM, given 12 hours apart. The optimal benefit begins 24 hours after initiation of therapy and last 7 days. *Because treatment for less than 24 hours is still associated with a significant reduction in neonatal mortality, antenatal corticosteroids should be given unless immediate delivery is anticipated. *Antenatal corticosteroid use is recommended in women with preterm PROM less than 34 weeks gestation in the absence of clinical chorioamnionitis. *In women with complicated pregnancies for whom delivery prior to 34 weeks of gestation is likely, antenatal corticosteroid use is recommended unless there is evidence that corticosteroids will have an adverse effect on the mother or delivery is imminent. *There is evidence to show that repeated doses of corticosteroids may impose a risk to both mother and fetus hence there is a need to be cautious in its use and where possible, amniotic fluid phosphatidyl glycerol should be estimated. Caution should also be applied to antenatal corticosteroid use in poorly controlled diabetes in pregnancy.

Guidelines on the Use of Surfactant in the Treatment of Respiratory Distress Syndrome: Recommendations

*Surfactant should be given as early as possible to all preterm infants on mechanical ventilation for RDS. *However larger infants greater than 32 weeks may only require exogenous surfactant if the FiO_2 is > 0.5–0.6 *The use of surfactant does not obviate the need for antenatal steroids or strategies to reduce the incidence of preterm birth. *Until further evidence becomes available, it should be used only under neonatal intensive care conditions (*monitoring facilities for oxygen and cardiorespiratory status and close supervision of ventilation and fluid therapy*) *and administered by experienced, trained personnel. *Where an infant is born away from neonatal intensive care facilities exogenous surfactant may be administered by personnel trained in endotracheal intubation before transfer for intensive care.

Guidelines on the Use of Oxygen in the Newborn : Recommendations

*An understanding is required that Retinopathy of Prematurity (ROP) is currently not preventable in some neonates, even with optimal monitoring of oxygen therapy. Many factors other than hyperoxia may contribute to the pathogenesis in this condition.*Nevertheless, supplemental oxygen should only be used when there are specific indications such as respiratory distress, cyanosis or documented hypoxia.*In an emergency when oxygen is needed, it should be used without restriction, and concern for ROP should not override the need to save a life. Transient elevations of PaO_2 do not cause ROP.*The use of supplemental oxygen beyond the emergency period should be monitored by means of regular arterial PaO_2 measurements. Arterialized capillary sampling is an acceptable alternative if arterial sampling is not possible.*Term infants requiring oxygen therapy for periods longer than a few hours and all preterm infants requiring oxygen should be managed in a facility where monitoring of oxygen therapy is available. When this is not possible, the concentration of oxygen administered should be just enough to abolish cyanosis. It should be safe in the term neonate to administer oxygen for a few hours without monitoring arterial oxygen.*Transcutaneous oxygen measurement and/or pulse oximetry allow for continuous monitoring of oxygen therapy. The recommended levels of SaO2 are 89 to 95%. This should be supported by intermittent arterial blood gas analysis. A recommended range for most preterm neonates would be a PaO2 of 50-80 mmHg (6.7 –10.7 kPa).*In some neonates, efforts to keep the PaO2 within this range may result in unacceptable episodes of hypoxia. In such a situation, it might be necessary to accept PaO2 levels above this range. Such decisions should be documented clearly.*Institutions should have a written protocol for the documentation and monitoring of oxygen therapy. *Recognizing the benefits of early detection and treatment of ROP, eye examination at 4-6 weeks of age is recommended for: all babies less than 32 weeks gestation at birth or weight less than 1250gm. other babies above 32 weeks and 1250 gm depending on individual risk as assessed by the clinician. *Eye examination should be repeated at 2-4 weekly intervals until vascularisation reaches Zone 3 or there is no longer a risk of threshold disease. If threshold disease develops then ablative therapy should be considered for at least one eye within 72 hours of detection. (Every effort should be made to provide such a service for all these neonates)

Postnatal Corticosteroids for the Prevention and Treatment of Chronic Lung Disease in Preterm Infants: Recommendations (with Grading according to strength of evidence)

*The benefits and risks of postnatal corticosteroid use in oxygen dependant preterm infants should be weighed up in each individual case. (Grade A) *Postnatal corticosteroids should be reserved for situations where there is evidence of chronic lung disease such as failure of the X-ray to clear and continued high ventilator settings after 7 days and it is apparent that weaning may not be possible without steroids. (Grade A)*Postnatal corticosteroids for the purpose of preventing or treating CLD should not be given to infants below 7 days of age. (Grade A)*A suggested regime would be a starting dose of 0.5mg/kg/day tapering after 3 days, keeping the duration of treatment to a minimum (Grade A).*These recommendations should be revised when data becomes available from ongoing trials (DART Study, Doyle 2000) (Grade A)*Each Pediatric department should develop its own written policy on the indications of postnatal steroids.*Antenatal corticosteroids remain proven and beneficial in reducing RDS and their use should not be influenced by these new recommendations on the use of postnatal steroids (Grade A).

Courtesy: Perinatal Society of Malaysia

Pearl/Peril/Pitfall : The term hyaline membrane disease is now less commonly used in clinical practice to describe the constellation of pathologic, clinical, and radiologic findings produced by pulmonary surfactant insufficiency in infants. In general, hyaline membranes are not specific histologic evidence of surfactant deficiency, but they may form in the aftermath of a variety of primary bronchiolar insults. Thus, hyaline membranes are considered a byproduct, not the cause, of respiratory failure in neonates with immature lungs. Respiratory distress syndrome is currently used to denote surfactant deficiency and should not be used for other causes of respiratory distress. However, some authors consider the term nonspecific and imprecise, because it connotes a constellation of signs and symptoms that may accompany other causes of lung disease. In recognition of the underlying pathogenesis of the disease process, the alternative term surfactant deficiency disorder has been proposed.

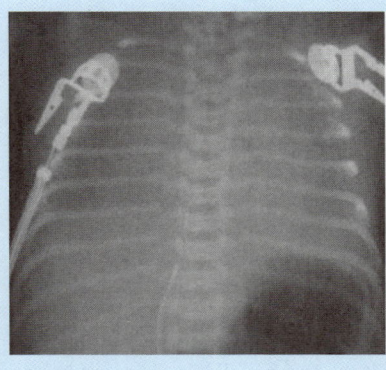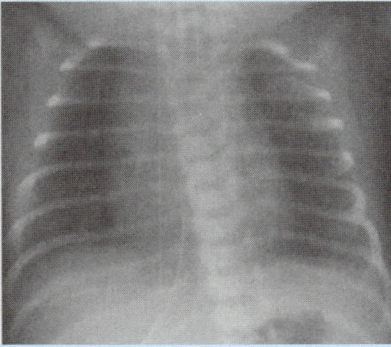

Symmetric surfactant effect in a 36 week-gestational-age infant of a diabetic mother. (a) Pretreatment radiograph shows diminished lung expansion, diffuse bilateral reticulogranular opacities, and air bronchograms, findings consistent with severe RDS. (b) Repeat radiograph, obtained 6 hours after endotracheal administration of one dose of surfactant, reveals marked improvement in lung aeration and vascular definition.

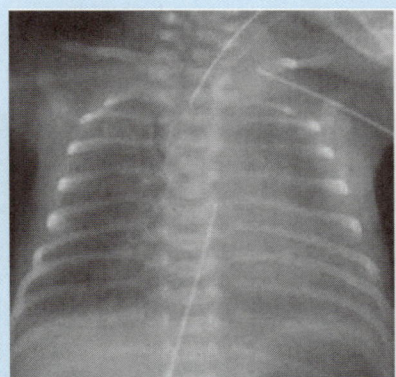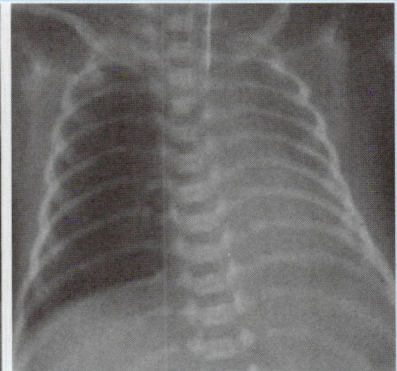

Asymmetric surfactant effect in a 2-day-old, 32-week-gestational age newborn with RDS. a)Frontal chest radiograph demonstrates multifocal residual consolidations that mimic pneumonia or meconium aspiration syndrome.b) Asymmetric distribution of endotracheal surfactant into the right mainstem bronchus in a 1-day-old preterm neonate with RDS. Frontal radiograph of the chest shows a clear hyperexpanded right lung, shift of mediastinal structures to the left, and persistence of diffuse left lung opacification.

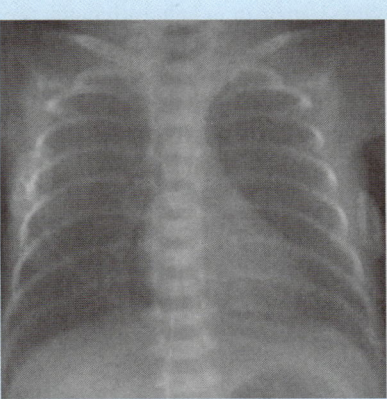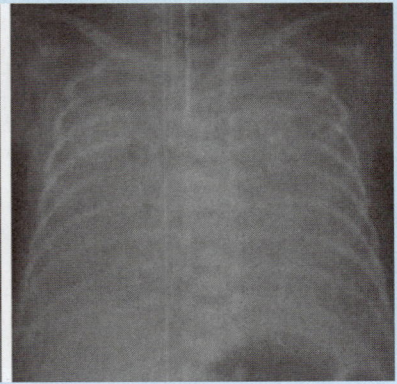

Pulmonary hemorrhage in a 26-week-gestational-age neonate following prophylactic surfactant therapy. (a) Frontal chest radiograph obtained after one dose of surfactant and during treatment with nasal CPAP shows hyperinflated lungs with faint symmetric residual opacities. (b) Repeat radiograph, obtained after 24 hours for evaluation of sudden respiratory decompensation and bloody endotracheal aspirates, shows dense bilateral airspace consolidation.

Factors stimulating surfactant release
- <u>Antenatal steroids</u>
- Thyroxine
- Prolactin
- Narcotic drugs
- Alcohol
- Tobacco smoking
- IUGR
- Labor and vaginal delivery

Factors inhibiting surfactant release
- Hypoxia, acidosis
- Hypothermia
- Sepsis
- Hyperinsulinemia
- Hyperglycemia
- Multiple pregnancy
- Male sex
- Delivery by C/section without labor

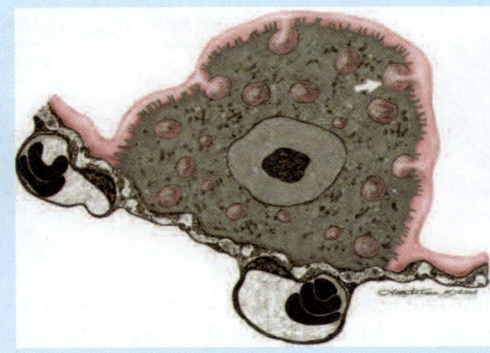

Endogenous surfactant delivery. Diagram of a type II pneumocyte demonstrates migration of lamellar bodies (arrow) from the nucleus to the apical cell surface, where surfactant (in pink) is released into the alveolus by exocytosis.

Pearl/Peril/Pitfall: Term infants of mothers with poorly controlled diabetes may also present with RDS, because fetal hyperinsulinism interferes with the glucocorticoid axis that governs surfactant biosynthesis.

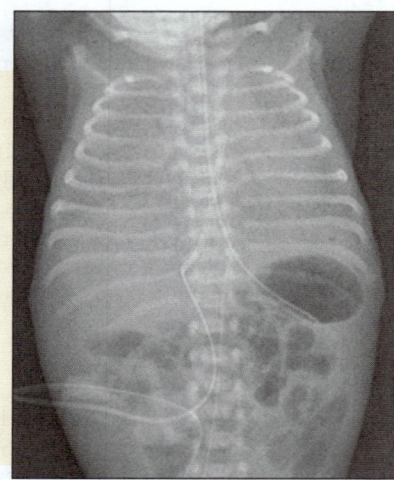

Respiratory Distress Syndrome (RDS) is a clinical diagnosis but one which is often interchanged with the terms Hyaline Membrane Disease (a pathological diagnosis) and Surfactant Deficiency (a term describing the typical appearances on radiographs of infants with RDS). The typical radiological features of Surfactant Deficiency are: *Small volume lungs *Homogenous "ground glass" opacity *Air bronchograms These classical radiological appearances have been altered by interventions such as CPAP (which tends to result in lungs which are of normal size) and surfactant administration (which is often given prior to the radiograph being taken, and can result in less homogenous appearances). The differential diagnosis includes: *Pneumonia (particularly Group B Streptococcus) *Retained Fetal Lung Fluid/TTN The image shows that the heart is all but obscured by the diffuse, homogenous lung fields. The baby has been intubated and there are umbilical catheters in situ.

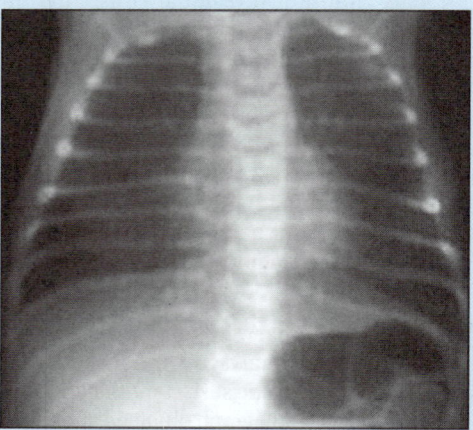

Transient Tachypnoea of the Newborn (TTN, also called Retained Fetal Lung Fluid or "Wet Lung") is a diagnosis of exclusion. Typical radiologic features are ill-defined but include: *Increased central vascular markings ("star-burst" appearance) *Hyperaeration *Evidence of interstitial and pleural fluid *Prominent interlobar fissures *Cardiomegaly Because the symptoms and radiological features are non-specific, infection should be considered in the differential diagnosis. Typically, respiratory symptoms resolve within the first 24-hours of life, but occasionally can persist longer.

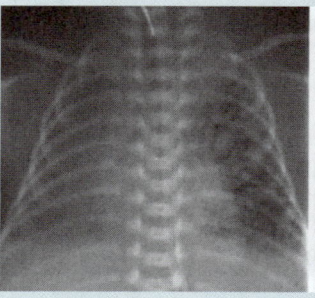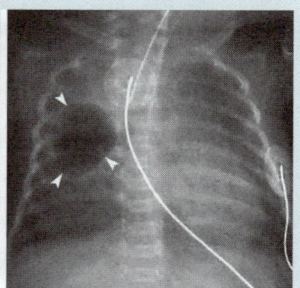

(Lt)Unilateral acute PIE in a premature infant who underwent positive-pressure ventilation for RDS. Frontal radiograph shows a profusion of irregular cystic lucencies within the left lung. Granular consolidation of the right lung is consistent with uncomplicated RDS. (Rt)"Pseudocyst" in a premature infant who underwent mechanical ventilation. Frontal chest radiograph shows a large, rounded, right juxtahilar gas collection with a smooth thin wall (arrowheads).

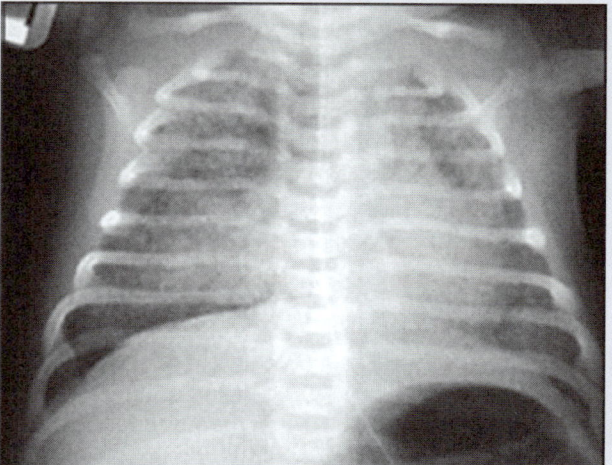

Meconium stained amniotic fluid (MSAF) occurs in about 12% of deliveries. Meconium aspiration is defined by meconium aspirated from below the vocal cords. However, **Meconium Aspiration Syndrome (MAS)** defines a wide array of respiratory symptoms associated with MSAF. MAS usually presents as respiratory distress and cyanosis. Pulmonary hypertension is common. The radiograph usually shows *Coarse infiltrates *Widespread consolidation *Hyperinflation *Pleural effusions are not uncommon *Pneumothorax and pneumomediastinum may be present Because the symptoms and radiological features are non specific, infection should be included on the differential diagnosis.

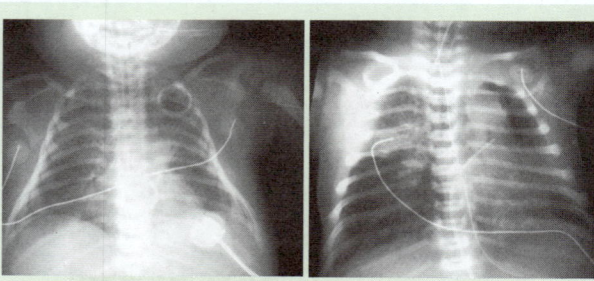

The chest radiograph appearances of **pneumonia** are not specific, and frank lobar consolidation as seen in adults and older children is rare. More commonly, there is coarse opacity of one or more regions of the lung parenchyma. However, these appearances can also be seen with retained fetal lung fluid, meconium aspiration, aspiration of gastric contents, and pulmonary hemorrhage. Pleural effusions are not uncommon in infection, but again may be seen with other conditions.

Pearl/Peril/Pitfall : Surfactant replacement therapy and mechanical ventilation are not universally effective in premature infants with RDS, possibly because of uneven surfactant distribution or concurrent sepsis, acidosis, or patent ductus arteriosus.

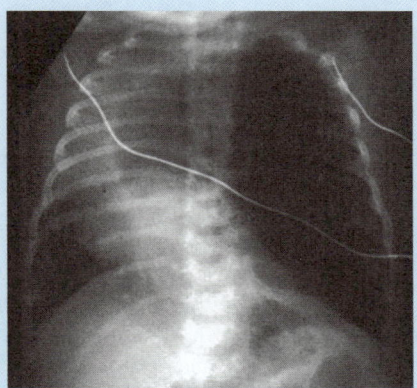

A frontal radiograph of the chest in a neonate shows marked overdistension of the left upper lobe with mediastinal shift to the right. **Congenital Lobar Emphysema:** In CLE, the involved lobe crossing the midline and the compressed normal lung can be seen. This appearance does not change during expiration or in the decubitus position. Vascularity of the involved site is attenuated. The intercostal spaces in the involved site appear widened, and the hemidiaphragm is flattened. Lucent, anteriorly herniated lung pushes the lung posteriorly, as seen on the lateral view. The lesion must be differentiated from contralateral lung hypoplasia and ipsilateral pneumothorax. Most commonly involves the left upper lobe, then right upper or middle lobes • believed to result from deficiency of bronchial cartilage causing collapse during expiration and air-trapping in the lobe • can rupture and result in true pneumothorax • symptoms can be triggered by viral infection or just progress over time after birth . Treatment:AIRWAY, BREATHING, CIRCULATION !! - congenital lobar emphysema needs a surgical consult —Avoid chest tube, if possible, for pure lobar emphysema

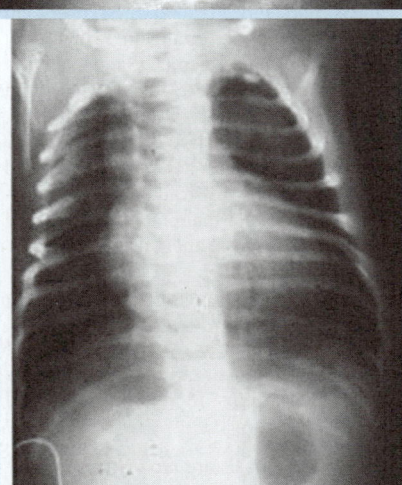

There is extraventilatory air in both the right and left chest. The left lung field demonstrates a collection of air (black) adjacent to the ribs. The left lung has partially deflated (collapsed) and can be seen pushed toward the center. There is also a right pneumothorax. The heart and its associated midline structures (mediastinum) is not shifted to either the right or the left, suggesting that there is not a lot of air pressure associated with either of these collections of air.

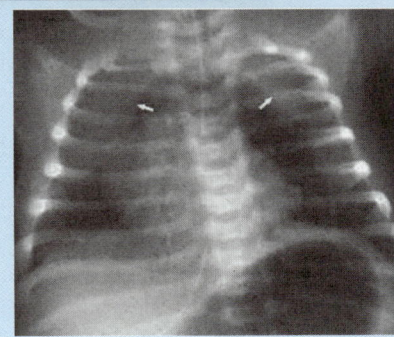

Pneumopericardium occurs when the extraventilatory air leakage dissects along the major blood vessels in the chest and forms a collection of air around the heart. In this radiograph, the dark black area surrounding the heart is the pneumopericardium. There are several tubes (which are appear as white lines) which have been placed, one of which is draining away air from the pneumopericardium as it collects.

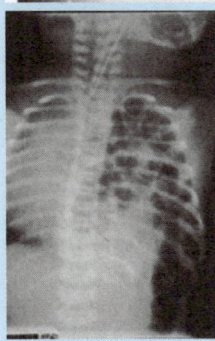

The air-filled loops of bowel can be seen in the left chest. The air-filled loops of intestine are have traversed from the abdomen to the left chest. This indicates that there must be a hole in the left diaphragm has not kept the intestines confined to the abdomen but has allowed them to enter the chest as well. The air-filled loops of intestine take up room and have pushed the heart and other midline structures into the right chest. **Lt CDH**

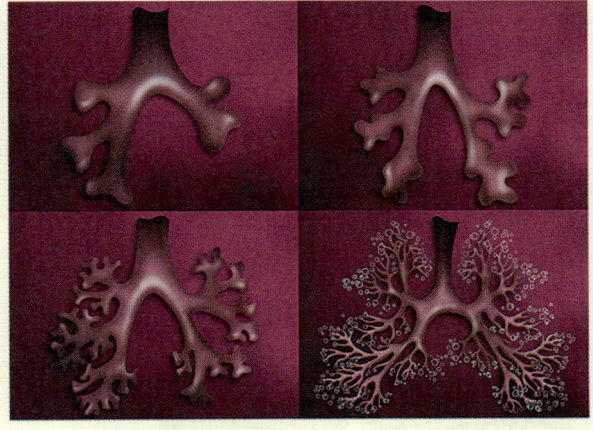

Pneumomediastinum. Frontal chest radiograph shows the lobes of the thymus (arrows), which are displaced superolaterally by a large central lucent area.

Normal lung development

The lung arises from the embryonic foregut, starting with the development of the main bronchi during the third week of gestation. The developing lung expands caudally into the surrounding mesenchyme and blood vessels, smooth muscle, cartilage and fibroblast components are derived from this tissue. The endodermally derived epithelium lining the airways gives rise to the conducting airways and alveoli. Beyond this early embryonic period, four stages of lung development are recognized. In all of these, airway and blood vessel development and differentiation proceed in parallel.

Pseudoglandular (5 to 17 weeks)
• Development of bronchial tree & acinar tubules
Canalicular (16 to 26 weeks)
• Capillary proliferation & thinning of mesenchyme
• Differentiation of Type II alveolar pneumocytes from around 20 weeks
Saccular (24 to 38 weeks)
• Development & expansion of peripheral air spaces
• Early alveolar septum formation
Alveolar (36 weeks to > 2 years post term)
• Thinning of alveolar septa & capillary remodelling

---

* *Pearl/Peril/Pitfall : Several explanations have been proposed for asymmetric radiographic improvement following surfactant therapy: (a) maldistribution of surfactant into the right mainstem bronchus, (b) insufficient surfactant requiring additional applications, and (c) regional differences in aeration before surfactant treatment.*

Congenital cystic adenomatoid malformation

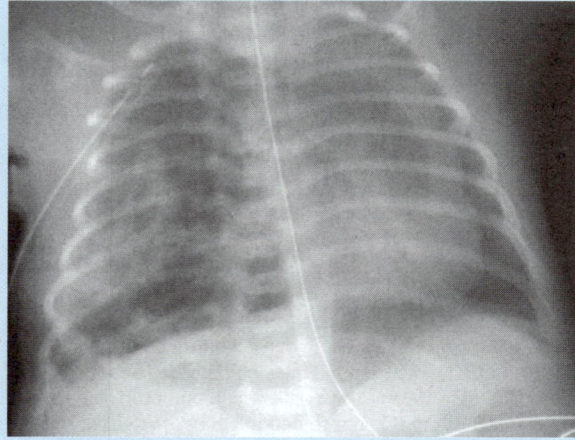

Chest X-ray reveals an inhomogeneous opacity of the lower part of the right lung

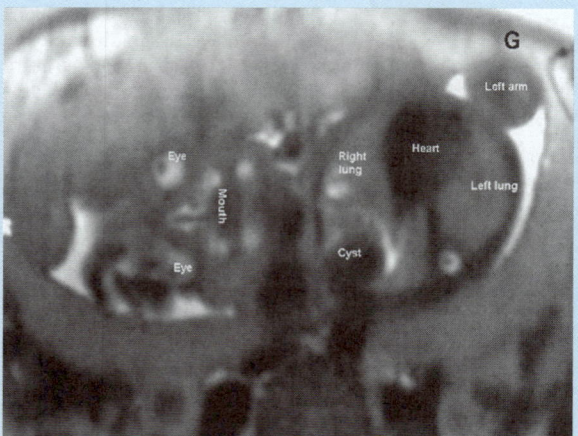

Fetal MRI suggests the diagnosis of a cystic adenomatoid malformation of the lung

CCAM was described for the first time by Ch'in and Tang in 1949. Since then, approximately 500 cases have been reported. The incidence is 1/25'000 to 1/35'000 gestation. It is the most frequent congenital anomaly of the lung and represents 25% of these conditions. Generally, only one pulmonary lobe is abnormal, and most frequently CCAM is located on the right side. However, diffuse CCAM of both lungs have been described.

CCAM results from an anomaly of lung development occurring in the 6th to 7th week of gestation. Several pathogenic hypotheses are plausible (impairment of the lung vascularization, infection, bronchial obstruction) but no single mechanism has been clearly identified. Several classifications of CCAM have been proposed, based on Stocker's work. In Stocker's classification, type I represents 60 to 70 % of all CCAMs and is characterized by large cysts over 2 cm in diameter and lined by a pseudo-stratified epithelium with mucus cells. In type II, cysts are smaller (< 1 cm in diameter) and lined by a cuboid epithelium. Type III represents only 10% of all CCAMs and looks macroscopically like a solid mass, with small microscopic cysts. Other congenital anomalies can be associated with CCAM, for example bilateral renal agenesis, sirenomelia, trisomy 18, congenital cardiopathies, anomalies of the digestive tract (labio-maxillo-palatine defects, esophageal cyst, intestinal malrotation, imperforate anus, Meckel's diverticulum), and vertebral anomalies.

The differential diagnosis includes diaphragmatic hernia, lung sequestration, congenital lobar emphysema, atresia of airways, bronchogenic cyst, mediastinal teratoma or pericardial cyst. The possible consequences of the development of CCAM in utero are pulmonary hypoplasia, polyhydramnios, fetal hydrops or fetal ascites.

In CCAM, risk factors for poor prognosis are type III, size of the lesion, involvement of both lungs, associated pulmonary hypoplasia, fetal hydrops, polyhydramnios or shift of the mediastinum. The natural history of CCAM depends on the size of the cysts, on their pathophysiological effects and on the size of the normal lung parenchyma. Overall, mortality in CCAM is reported to be 10 %. Respiratory distress or pneumothorax in the newborn or recurrent pulmonary infections in the older child can be the presenting signs. Some CCAMs are fortuitously diagnosed on chest X-rays later in life.

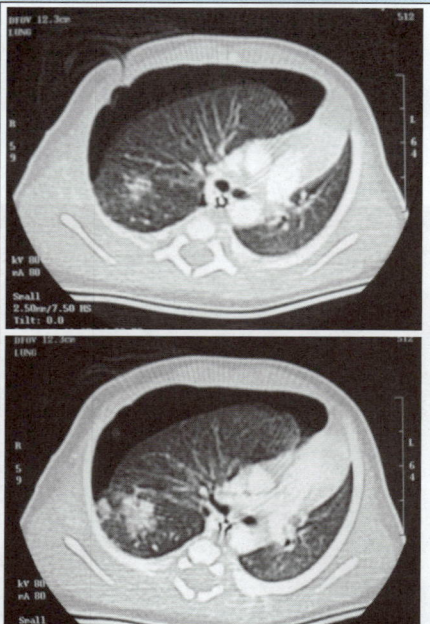

CT scan performed at 10 hours of life reveals a tension pneumothorax and an inhomogeneous mass with several cysts of varying sizes, located in the right pleural cavity

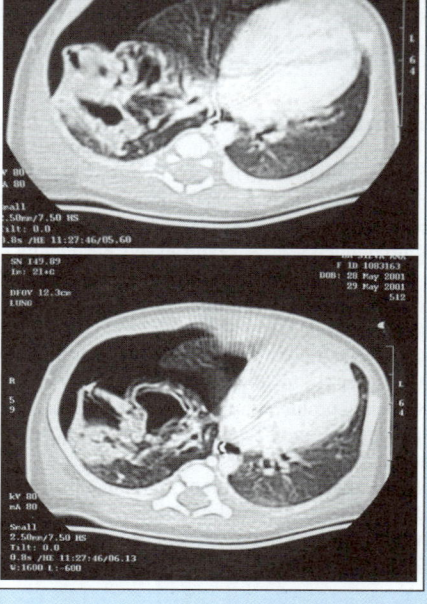

Pearl/Peril/Pitfall: Antenatal steroids and postnatal surfactant replacement independently and additively reduce mortality, the severity of respiratory distress syndrome, and air leaks in preterm infants.

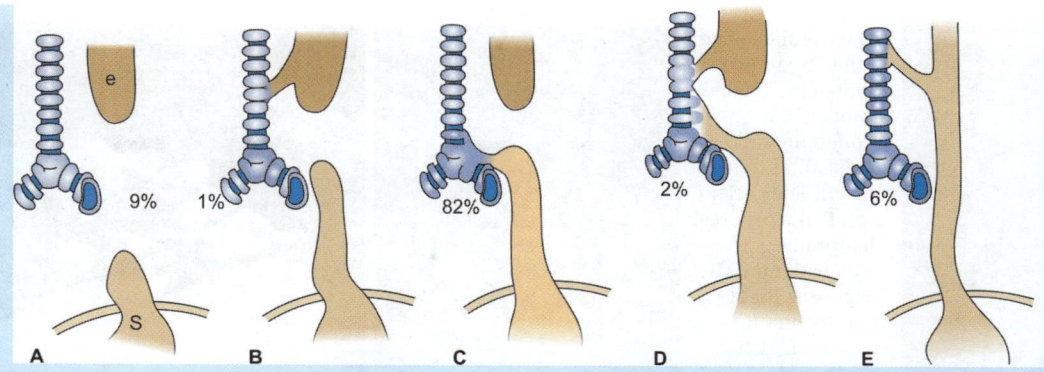

Drawings illustrate a classification scheme for esophageal atresia and tracheoesophageal fistula. *A* = atresia without fistula, *B* = atresia with upper fistula, *C* = atresia with lower fistula, *D* = atresia with both lower and upper fistulas, *E* = tracheoesophageal fistula with no atresia.(H-type) *e* = esophagus, *s* = stomach. Types A and B are similar radiographically, as are types C and D.

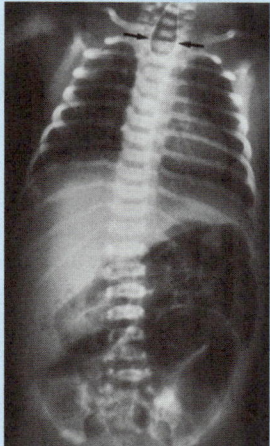

Esophageal atresia with lower fistula (type C). On a frontal radiograph, a catheter is seen coiled within the upper esophageal pouch (arrows). Air is also present in the gastrointestinal tract, indicating communication between the lower esophageal segment and the respiratory tree. The bowel dilatation is the result of an imperforate anus associated with esophageal atresia.

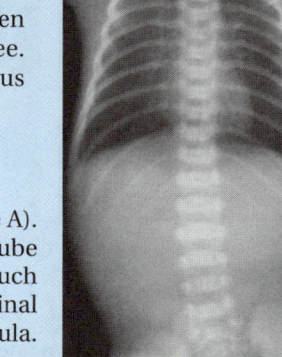

Esophageal atresia without fistula (type A). Frontal radiograph shows a radiopaque tube curling into the upper esophageal pouch (arrows). No air is present in the gastrointestinal tract; therefore, there is no distal fistula.

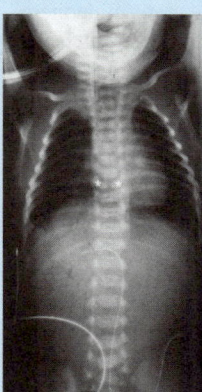

Vertebral, anorectal, cardiac, tracheal, esophageal, renal, and limb (VACTERL) association. Frontal radiograph in a patient with esophageal atresia (EA) without a tracheoesophageal fistula (TEF). Note the catheter in the proximal pouch and the butterfly vertebra (asterisks) at the level of T8 in this patient with associated VACTERL

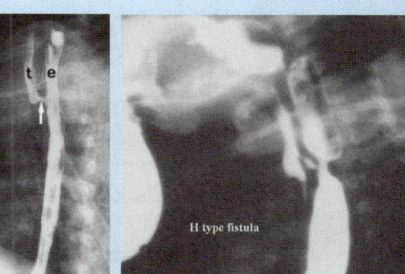

Tracheoesophageal fistula without atresia (type E). Esophagogram shows a fistula (arrow) arising from the anterior portion of the esophagus (*e*) and passing cephalad to the posterior portion of the trachea (*t*).

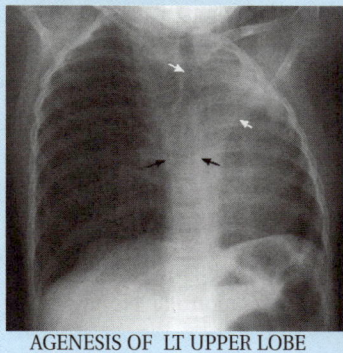
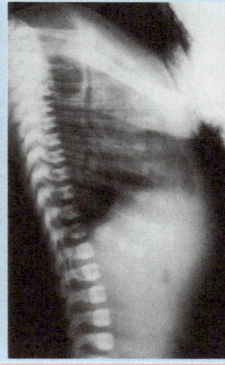
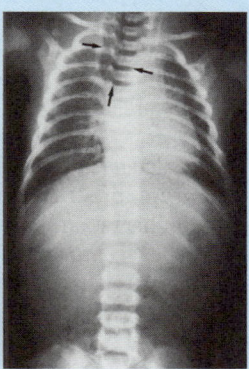

AGENESIS OF LT UPPER LOBE

Esophageal atresia with fistula (type D). **(a)** Frontal radiograph shows air within the distended upper esophageal pouch (arrows). The presence of gas in the bowel indicates fistulous communication between the lower esophageal segment and the trachea. **(b)** Lateral radiograph more clearly demonstrates the distended upper esophageal pouch with resulting pressure deformity of the trachea. An upper fistula was also found at surgery.

Pearl/Peril/Pitfall: Remember that not all newborns fit easily into a diagnostic category. A recent prospective study found that fewer than half of symptomatic newborns met textbook criteria for a specific diagnosis. Some infants were assessed early in the clinical course, and signs and symptoms resolved spontaneously before a disorder declared itself. Other infants had a more prolonged course but still were discharged with a nonspecific diagnosis.

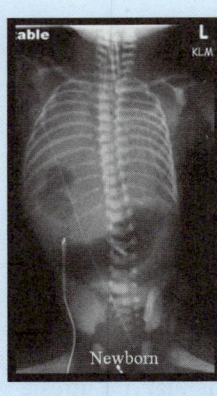

The NG tube coiled in the proximal esophagus. Dilated stomach and duodenum and mediastinal shift to the left. The patient is on Extracorporeal Membrane Oxygenation(ECMO). Diagnosis: Right Diaphragmatic Hernia, TE Fistula and Duodenal Atresia

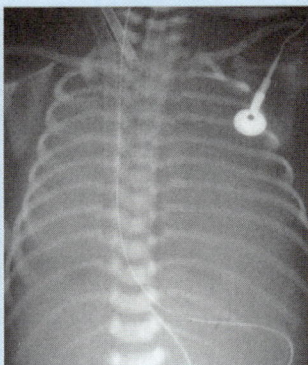

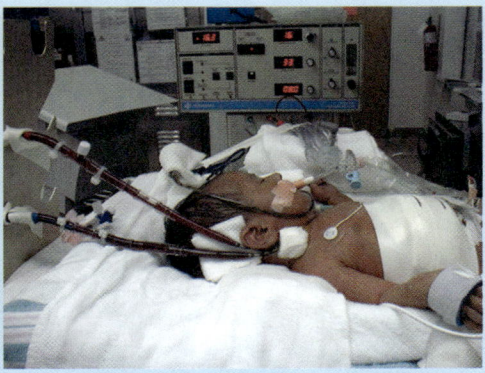

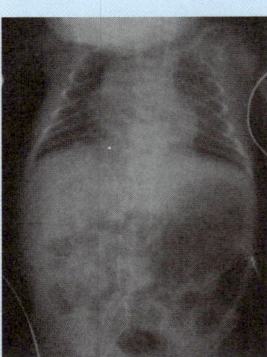

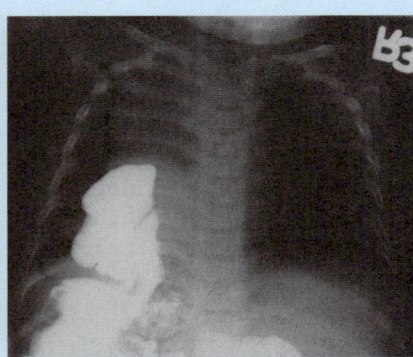

Diagnosis: Foramen of Morgagni Hernia -Usually, it appears as a right cardiophrenic angle mass, which if it contains bowel could be seen as lucent mass. If herniated omentum is present, thin linear densities may be seen which represents omental vessels. On lateral chest X-rays it appears as anterior cardiophrenic mass with the differential. It mostly appears as a right cardiophrenic mass, which could be (a) Homogenous right cardiophrenic mass Pericardial fat pad, Lipoma, Morgagni hernia containing omentum, Atelectasis, Pneumonia, Pericardial and Mediastinal cysts

(b) Heterogeneous right cardiophrenic mass Teratoma, Thymoma, Liposarcoma, Diaphragmatic or Pleural abscess.

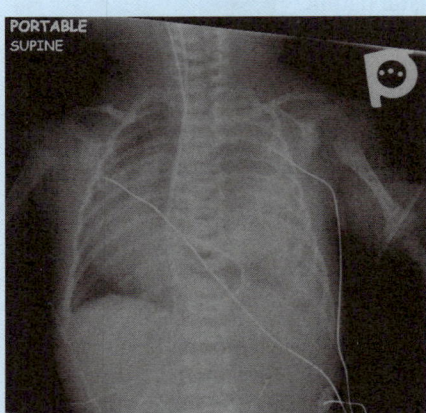

The radiograph demonstrates an endotracheal tube (indicative of respiratory distress) and a feeding tube looping up to terminate in the lower thorax (suggesting that the stomach is in the lower thorax.) Diagnosis: LT Congenital Diaphragmatic Hernia

Respiratory Distress Syndrome: Summary

Respiratory distress syndrome (RDS) is seen primarily in the preterm neonate and is due mostly to pulmonary surfactant deficiency. Lung atelectasis leads to ventilation-perfusion mismatching, hypoxia, and eventual respiratory failure in the untreated infant who has RDS. RDS is diagnosed by physical findings consistent with respiratory distress and characteristic radiographic findings. Treatment of RDS begins antenatally with the administration of maternal steroids to women at risk of preterm delivery between 24 and 34 weeks' gestation. The use of repeat doses of antenatal steroids is under investigation but is currently not recommended outside of randomized, controlled trials. SRT has been approved for use since 1990 and has been successful in decreasing rates of RDS. Natural surfactant is currently recommended for use, but synthetic surfactant that contains proteins to mimic surfactant proteins is being investigated. In general, prophylactic use of surfactant is recommended over rescue treatment in infants at high risk for developing RDS, but the determination of which infants are at high risk for developing RDS remains a clinical one. The push toward use of less invasive ventilation strategies in the treatment of RDS has led to several trials of nasal continuous positive airway pressure (nCPAP). Results of the SUPPORT trial are pending, but the COIN trial has concluded that nCPAP use in infants who have RDS is not detrimental. Inhaled nitric oxide for RDS still requires investigation on safety and efficacy. Several other treatments have been studied, but as of yet, only inositol administration shows promise in the treatment of RDS. Several complications of the recommended treatments for RDS have been identified, but the benefits far outweigh the risks. Finally, there remains a need for long-term follow-up studies on preterm infants treated for RDS to assess neurodevelopmental outcomes.

Pearl/Peril/Pitfall : Transient tachypnea of the newborn. Also known as wet lung, this condition is a retrospective diagnosis of exclusion and the most common cause of neonatal respiratory distress. Air bronchograms that suggest pneumonia and reticulonodular patterns typical of respiratory distress syndrome are usually absent.

Guidelines for good practice in the management of Neonatal respiratory distress syndrome
Report of the second working group of the British Association of Perinatal Medicine. *Executive Summary, January 1999*

All women between 23 and 34 completed weeks of gestation with threatened premature delivery are suitable for antenatal steroids, which reduce the risk of RDS.

* Preterm infants of less than 30 weeks gestation who require intubation for resuscitation should receive surfactant as soon as possible (prophylaxis). Other infants should be given surfactant if they require intubation for ventilation (see below) and the diagnosis of RDS is confirmed (rescue).

* Choice of surfactant preparation is largely a matter of individual preference. There is some evidence to support natural surfactant preparations but their rapid mode of action means that good monitoring is essential. Two doses are better than one, but more doses are not necessary.

* All infants at risk of RDS should be closely monitored for evidence of respiratory failure. Artificial ventilation should be instituted early if the blood gases deteriorate or the baby has persistent apnoeic attacks, and continued from birth in very preterm infants intubated for resuscitation (see above).

* Any ventilator designed for babies can be used, and the settings tailored to minimize asynchrony. On the whole, synchrony is achieved at ventilator rates of around 60 breaths per minute with inspiratory times of about 0.3 seconds. There is at present no evidence that any method of ventilation is better than conventional ventilation for the treatment of Neonatal RDS. There is evidence that faster rates are associated with fewer pneumothoraces.

* Randomized controlled trials comparing different levels of blood gas control in RDS have not been done. There is consensus that ventilation should be adjusted to maintain the following:
#pH above 7.25 #PaO_2 in the range 6–10 kPa (45–75 mmHg) #$PaCO_2$ in the range above 5kPa (above 37.5 mmHg). Upper limit depends on pH #Successful treatment of RDS requires careful monitoring of blood gases, electrolyte levels and blood glucose concentrations in addition to monitoring of heart rate, respiration and blood pressure. Total parenteral nutrition may be required. #Failure to respond to surfactant is rare, and advice from an experienced Neonatologist should be sought for an infant who remains in more than 60% oxygen requiring high ventilator pressures (more than 26/6 cm water) after two doses of surfactant. #Steroid therapy has been shown to reduce the duration of mechanical ventilation and should be considered in babies who are still artificially ventilated and requiring oxygen at two weeks of age. Early steroids before 2 weeks can cause neurodevelopmental sequelae. #Units which routinely ventilate babies for RDS should meet the standards set by the BAPM. These units should collect information about their results, including follow up information, in order to publish an annual report which meets the requirements of the BAPM minimum dataset.

KEY POINTS FOR CLINICAL PRACTICE

1. THE NEW BORN WITH CLINICAL SIGNS OF ACUTE RESPIRATORY DISTRESS—Central Cyanosis, Tachypnea (>60 bpm), Tachycardia (>160 bpm), Retractions, Grunting, and Nasal flaring- demands immediate attention. A review of the maternal Hx, the age of onset of respiratory distress (within the first 4 hours of life or DE NOVO after 4 hours of life), a thorough physical examination and a Chest X-ray will greatly aid the clinician in assessing this problem further.

2. The differential diagnosis of respiratory distress includes Pulmonary, Cardiac, Hematologic, Infectious, Anatomic, and Metabolic disorders that may directly or indirectly involve the lungs.

3. ECHOCARDIOGRAPHY Easily differentiates isolated primary pulmonary hypertension (PPHN) from cyanotic congenital heart disease or ascertaining whether a baby who undoubtedly has surfactant - deficient RDS also has coexisting congenital heart disease (cyanotic or otherwise). HYPEROXIA TEST—can differentiate severe RDS and PPHN from cyanotic congenital heart disease.

4. IT IS IMPORTANT TO BE AWARE that two or more respiratory disorders may coexist in the one infant, e.g. RDS and Congenital Pneumonia in preterm infants after PROM or in the presence of chorioamnionitis, and meconium aspiration and congenital sepsis in term infants with respiratory distress. ALL BABIES AT RISK OF RDS - should be closely monitored for evidence of respiratory failure. The treatment of RDS involves ARTIFICIAL VENTILATION, SURFACTANT AND INTENSIVE CARE SUPPORT. ARTIFICIAL VENTILATION should be instituted early if the blood gases deteriorate or the baby has persistent apneic attacks and continued from birth in babies intubated for resuscitation. VENTILATION should be adjusted to maintain ; pH above 7.25, PaO_2, 6–10 kPa (45–75 mmHg), $PaCO_2$ 5–7 kPa (37.5–52.5 mmHg).

5. Recent advances include (1) the use of antenatal steroids to enhance pulmonary maturity; (2) appropriate resuscitation facilitated by placental transfusion and immediate use of continuous positive airway pressure (CPAP) for alveolar recruitment; (3) early administration of surfactant; (4) the use of gentler modes of ventilation, including early use of "bubble" nasal CPAP to minimize damage to the immature lungs; and (5) supportive therapies, such as diagnosis and management of patent ductus arteriosus (PDA), fluid and electrolyte management, trophic feeding and nutrition, and use of prophylactic fluconazole.

REFERENCES AND FURTHER READING 1)Horbar JD, Carpenter JH, Buzas J, et al. Timing of initial surfactant treatment for infants 23 to 29 weeks' gestation: is routine practice evidence based?. *Pediatrics*. Jun 2004;113(6):1593–602. 2) McGettigan MC, Adolph VR, Ginsberg HG, Goldsmith JP. New ways to ventilate newborns in acute respiratory failure. *Pediatr Clin North Am*. Jun 1998;45(3):475-509. 3) Murray PG, Stewart MJ. Use of Nasal Continuous Positive Airway Pressure During Retrieval of Neonates With Acute Respiratory Distress. *Pediatrics*. March 2008;121:e754-e758. 4)Sinha SK, Gupta S, Donn SM. Immediate Respiratory Management of the Preterm Infant. *Seminars in Fetal and Neonatal Medicine*. February 2008;13:24-29. 5) Su PH, Chen JY. Inhaled Nitric Oxide in the Management of Preterm Infants with Severe Respiratory Failure. *Journal of Perinatology*. February 2008;28:112–116.

Pearl/Peril/Pitfall: Certain causes of respiratory distress have very specific treatments. Choanal atresia requires use of an oral airway. Robin syndrome is treated by placing the newborn in the prone position and may require insertion of a nasopharyngeal tube to bypass the retropositioned tongue. Pneumothorax is treated by aspiration with a 21- or 23-gauge needle at the fourth intercostal space in the anterior axillary line. Diaphragmatic hernia requires placement of an endotracheal tube and orogastric evacuation of stomach contents.

35 Meconium Aspiration Syndrome (MAS)

@ *Most infants born through meconium stained amniotic fluid require no interventions, but it is important to monitor these well appearing infants closely for signs of respiratory distress for 12-24 hr. One should always observe the infants for tachypnea, cyanosis, grunting, nasal flaring, and accessory muscle use (retractions).*

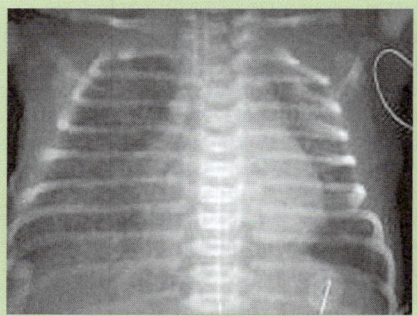
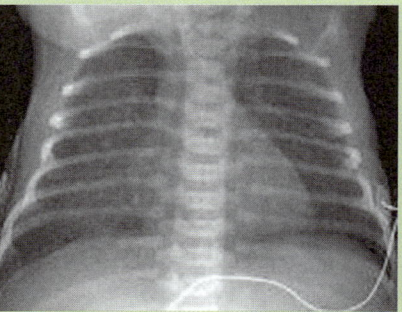
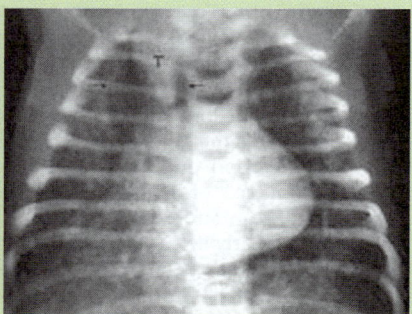

1.Meconium aspiration: Radiograph obtained shortly after birth shows ill-defined, predominantly perihilar opacities in the lungs ; these are more severe on the right than on the left. The lungs are hyperexpanded. The neonate's heart size is within normal limits.

2. Meconium aspiration: Radiograph obtained 2 days after Image 1 shows almost complete resolution of the pulmonary opacities

3.Meconium aspiration: Radiographic findings in a more severe case of meconium aspiration. This initial radiograph obtained shortly after birth shows patchy, coarse parenchymal opacities and severe hyperexpansion. In addition, pneumomediastinum is present on the right (arrows), outlining the right lobe of the thymus (T).

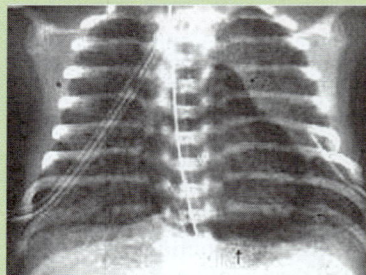

4.Meconium aspiration: *Follow-up radiograph in the patient in Image 3 obtained after placement of bilateral thoracostomy tubes for pneumothoraces shows pneumopericardium (arrows) and extensive imaging lucencies in the lungs. These findings indicate pulmonary interstitial emphysema*

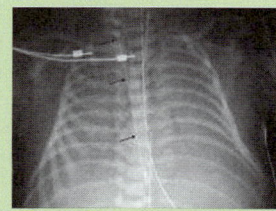

5.Meconium aspiration: Radiographic abnormalities in a patient with meconium aspiration who was treated with extracorporeal membrane oxygenation (ECMO). The lungs are airless because of pulmonary bypass. Cannula (arrows) enters from the right neck and extends to the right atrium, providing venous-venous ECMO. An endotracheal tube, a nasogastric tube, and an umbilical artery catheter are also in place

REVIEW OF CLINICAL PROBLEMS

1. Name Perinatal conditions associated with an increased risk of meconium stained amniotic fluid ? *Ans: Refer to the"No. 1" of the "BIRD'S EYE VIEW/OVERVIEW/ SYNOPSIS" of the Chapter.*

2. Mention the prophylactic management guidelines for MAS .
   Ans: Refer to Table 3 of the Chapter.

3. What are the indications for mechanical ventilation in an infant with MAS? *Ans: Refer to the"No. 9" of the "BIRD'S EYE VIEW/OVERVIEW/SYNOPSIS" of the Chapter.*

4. How do you manage a depressed baby born through thick meconium liquor ?
   Ans: Refer to Delivery room management of MAS.

5. Discuss the pathogenesis of MAS?
   Ans: Refer to the Figure 2 of the Chapter.

LEARNING OBJECTIVES

After completing this article, readers will be able to

1. Manage at delivery Neonates born with meconium stained amniotic fluid.

2. Recognize the signs of aspiration of meconium, blood, or gastric contents.

3. Recognize the common complications of aspiration, including pneumothorax, pulmonary hypertension, and chemical pneumonitis, HIE, Myocardial ischemia etc.,

4. Initiate urgent treatment of aspiration, including tracheal intubation, alkalinization, and evacuation of pneumothorax if necessary, pending referral or transfer to a Neonatal specialist.

5. Refer Neonates with MAS and Respiratory Failure not responding to initial measures to appropriate tertiary care center for assistance with diagnosis and management.

Pearl/Peril/Pitfall: *The term meconium is derived from ancient Greek word meconium-arion, or opium-like, from the Greek word mekoni meaning poppy juice. In the time of Aristotle, the term was used because it was believed that the substance induced fetal sleep.*

BIRD'S EYE VIEW/OVERVIEW/SYNOPSIS

1. *Meconium Aspiration syndrome (MAS)* is a serious pulmonary disorder of term or post term babies usually born through thick meconium (*rare in preterms and its presence may suggest Listeriosis*), potentially preventable and is associated with persistent pulmonary hypertension. In an infant born through meconium stained amniotic fluid, the risk and severity of MAS is influenced by a) the severity of concurrent asphyxia b) the degree of contamination of the amniotic fluid with meconium c) the presence of meconium in the airways(nasopharynx, trachea) at delivery. *Perinatal conditions associated with an increased risk of meconium stained amniotic fluid include*—*Maternal hypertension *Maternal diabetes mellitus *Maternal heavy cigarette smoking *Maternal chronic respiratory or cardiovascular disease *Postterm pregnancy *Pre-eclampsia/eclampsia *Oligohydramnios *Intrauterine growth retardation *Poor biophysical profile *Abnormal fetal heart rate patterns.

2. The incidence of meconium staining of the liquor is 10% of all labors at term (15–20% after 41 weeks); although 60% of the babies exposed to meconium staining of the liquor have meconium in the trachea, only 20% develop pulmonary disease. Before 37weeks of gestation, the risk of MSAF is <2%, whereas the risk after 42weeks of gestation is nearly 44%. *Meconium stained liquor is a poor marker of fetal asphyxia unless there are coexisting changes in the CTG or fetal pH (CTG = Cardiotocogram). (Refer to Figure 1* for the Mechanism of Respiratory Involvement following the delivery of a baby through Meconium stained amniotic fluid).

3. Consider the diagnosis of MAS in any infant born through meconium stained amniotic fluid who develops symptoms of respiratory distress, with onset soon after birth; CXR - in the MAS initially (within 1–2 hrs after birth) shows airtrapping with widespread patchy opacities (Atelectasis) with patchy areas of increased lucency (Emphysema). The chemical effects like pneumonitis, pleural effusion and pneumothorax + other air leaks are more prominent after 8–12 hrs. *Chest radiography is essential for the following:* *To confirm the diagnosis of meconium aspiration syndrome and determine the extent of intrathoracic pathology *To identify areas of atelectasis and air block syndromes *To assure appropriate positioning of the endotracheal tube and umbilical catheters.X-ray findings may not correlate with clinical condition (often worse) of the baby. In isolation, chest radiographs are neither sensitive nor specific for the diagnosis of meconium aspiration syndrome.

4. Meconium seems to be toxic to the lungs in many ways, and it may be difficult to determine which mechanisms predominate at a given point in time. (*Refer to Figure 2* for an outline of pathogenesis of MAS). They are a) mechanical obstruction of airways (partial - "ball - valve" or complete) b) chemical pneumonitis c) vasoconstriction of pulmonary vessels d) inactivation of surfactant.

5. Secondary bacterial infection of the lungs is another complication of MAS: also, infants who are infected *in utero* have a higher incidence of perinatal asphyxia and meconium aspiration, and therefore MAS may be superimposed on a congenital pneumonia. Because of the similarities in the clinical and radiographic manifestations of meconium aspiration and bacterial pneumonia, it is very difficult to diagnose a superimposed bacterial infection during the acute phase of MAS; therefore, one must have a high index of suspicion. Broad spectrum antibiotics (Ampicillin + Gentamicin + Ceftazidime) should be given after obtaining blood cultures.

6. *Figure 3* summarizes the delivery room management of infants born through meconium stained amniotic fluid. *Endotracheal intubation and Intratracheal suctioning should be done, in infants with low Apgar scores, respiratory distress, "thick/thin meconium staining, but depressed".* Avoid positive pressure ventilation, if possible, until tracheal suctioning is accomplished. The infant's general condition must not be ignored in persistent attempts to clear the trachea. Accomplish the suctioning procedure (with maximum pressure of 100 mmHg) rapidly, and initiate ventilation with 100% oxygen before significant bradycardia (< 60bpm) occurs. *Beware of* the other reported complications of intratracheal suctioning, such as bleeding, laryngospasm, air way trauma, stridor, apnea, and cyanosis.

7. Most infants born through meconium stained amniotic fluid require no interventions, but it is important to monitor these well appearing infants closely for signs of respiratory distress for 12–24 hr. One should always observe the infants for tachypnea, cyanosis, grunting, nasal flaring, and accessory muscle use (retractions). The chest may appear barrel shaped as a result of overinflation secondary to a ball-valve effect as the meconium plugs the lower airways. Rales and Rhonchi may be auscultated.

8. *The Evaluation-Decision-Action Plan/algorithm* summarizes the essential aspects of history taking, physical examination, relevant investigations to diagnose meconium aspiration syndrome and also the principles of timely management of MAS and its common complications.

9. *Mechanical ventilation* is indicated if the infant develops severe Meconium Aspiration Syndrome evidenced by a) impending respiratory failure b) PPHN c) hemodynamic compromise d) airleaks e) co-existing sepsis f) apneas and g) ABG analysis - pH <7.20, HCO_3 <14, PaO_2 <50 mmHg, $PaCO_2$ >60mmHg, oxygen saturations <90%, breathing in > 10lts/min of oxygen.(*Refer to the section for ventilation strategies for Meconium aspiration syndrome*). Recent advances in neonatal intensive care i.e. Surfactant, High Frequency Oscillatory Ventilation (HFOV), inhaled Nitric Oxide and ECMO (ExtraCorporeal Membrane Oxygenation) have substantially reduced the mortality and morbidity related to MAS in the developed nations. Replication of these results in the developing countries, however, is a difficult task due to limited resources and the high incidence of MAS.

10. Optimal care of an infant born through meconium stained amniotic fluid involves collaborations between obstetrician and pediatrician, each with separate but important roles. *As always, effective communication and advanced preparation and anticipation of potential problems form the cornerstone of this partnership.* Since meconium aspiration can occur prior to the time of delivery because of chronic asphyxia and infection, perhaps the most important preventive strategy is good prenatal care, including the detection and prevention of fetal hypoxemia and the avoidance of post-date deliveries.

Pearl/Peril/Pitfall: In an infant born through MSAF, the risk and severity of MAS is influenced by the severity of concurrent asphyxia* the degree of contamination of the amniotic fluid with meconium* the presence of meconium in the airways (nasopharynx, trachea) at delivery. Of these, asphyxia is the single most important risk factor for MAS, and is presumed to relate to the influx of MSAF into the lung during hypoxic fetal gasping. MAS can occur, however, in meconium-stained infants that are in good condition at birth.*

THE EVALUATION-DECISION-ACTION-PLAN/ALGORITHM FOR THE DIAGNOSIS AND MANAGEMENT OF *A NEONATE WITH MECONIUM ASPIRATION SYNDROME (MAS)*

SUBJECTIVE FINDINGS

Hx of meconium stained liquor, low Apgar scores at 5 mins, depressed neonate at birth, onset of respiratory distress in delivery room or in the first 6 hr of life

Hx of intrapartal risk factors for sepsis like - prolonged fever, febrile mother, foul liquor, multiple vaginal examinations, preterm labour (*consider listeriosis, if meconium stained*)

Hx of risk factors for meconium stained amniotic fluid- Refer to Table No 2 of the Chapter

OBJECTIVE FINDINGS

Assess ABCs, vitals, BP, O_2 sats, work of breathing (End-expiratory grunting, Alar flaring, Intercostal retractions, Tachypnea) central cyanosis, CRT, pulses, Urine output, signs suggestive of sepsis/birth asphyxia/CCF. *Look for* Barrel chest in the presence of air trapping, Auscultated rales and rhonchi (in some cases), Yellow-green staining of fingernails, umbilical cord, and skin *Assess* the respiratory status by Downe's score (Refer to the Chapter on "A Neonate with Respiratory Distress") periodically. *Perform* systemic examination to assess the complications of asphyxia.

INVESTIGATIONS

Blood FBC with hematocrit and platelets, glucose, blood culture, ABG analysis, electrolytes, Ca^{++}, Mg^{++}, creatinine, BUN, bleeding and clotting profile. *CXR* for patchy areas of atelectasis with hyperinflation, pneumonitis, pleural effusion, airleaks, cardiomegaly. *It is important to assess the positioning of tubes (endotracheal, nasogastric), lines (umbilical arterial/venous catheters, peripherally inserted central catheters), and other devices.* *CT/MRI Head scan* in case of HIE and seizures. *Echocardiogram* to assess pulmonary hypertension/congenital heart disease if any co-existing.

A NEONATE WITH MECONIUM ASPIRATION SYNDROME (MAS)

Secure IV access and *correct* hypoglycemia, hypocalcemia, acidosis and *maintain* normothermia and electrolytes. *Catheterize* the bladder to monitor urine output. *Ensure minimal handling.* *Give* broadspectrum IV antibiotics to cover for sepsis and pneumonitis

Ensure ABCs, give supplemental oxygen to maintain O_2 sats > 95%, monitor pulse oximetry, BP, CR monitor, CVP if necessary. *Treat* shock with 10ml/kg NS and then restrict fluids 2/3 rds of maintenance (SIADH may be a problem around 24 hours of age).

ASSESS DEGREE OF RESPIRATORY DISTRESS
(As per serial Clinical Assessment and ABG analysis)

MILD DISTRESS

* *Give oxygen* to maintain O_2 sats above 95%

* *Nurse the infant* in neutral thermal environment

* *Assess and Reassess* the severity of respiratory distress (Downe's score and ABG analysis) periodically.

* *Monitor, Correct and maintain* the disturbances in blood glucose, calcium, magnesium, electrolytes, hematocrit (maintain it > 40%).

* *Observe* these babies for 12-24 hr for sudden deterioration due to pulmonary hypertension or pneumothorax.

* *Maintain adequate systemic blood volume and pressure* (on higher side of the normal) with saline, plasma or blood and use IV Dobutamine infusion 5-10 mcg/kg/min early if myocardial ischemia complicates Meconium Aspiration Syndrome.

* Feeds may be comforting in mild cases of MAS but *withhold* feeds in severe cases until the respiratory distress improves.

* *Evaluate for co-existing problems* like CNS(HIE), renal (acute renal failure), thrombocytopenia, bleeding and clotting abnormalities and treat accordingly.

* *Chest physiotherapy* may exacerbate pulmonary hypertension during the acute stage; but during convalescence, it may be helpful in the management of collapse consolidation of lobes secondary to retention of secretions.

* *Anticipate the complications* a) PPHN b) Airleaks c) Infection d) Respiratory failure e) Birth asphyxia (co-morbidity) and manage them as discussed elsewhere.

* *Pneumothorax* requires 100% oxygen, sedation, analgesia if asymptomatic; if symptomatic/ on ventilator, institute intercostal drainage. Pneumomediastinum-conservative care. Pneumopericardium - pericardial drainage.

MODERATE TO SEVERE DISTRESS

* Worsening Downe's score(>7) * Apneas

* ABG - pH < 7.20 and HCO_3 < 14, PaO_2 < 50mm Hg, $PaCo_2$ >60mm Hg, SaO_2 <90% in 100 % oxygen* Circulatory insufficiency - tachycardia, prolonged CRT, Hypotension or shock, oliguria

* PPHN(labile oxygenation, refractory hypoxia, single S_2 ± normal CXR, right upper limb and left lower limb SaO_2 difference > 10% or ABG PaO_2 difference > 20 mmHg, 2d Echo - elevated pulmonary artery pressures with structurally normal heart, (A - a) O_2 gradient > 400)

Start conventional mechanical ventilation with PIP 30–35 cm H_2O, inspiratory time 0.4–0.5 seconds, rate 20-25 bpm (I : E = 1: 2), 0.8- 1 FiO_2, more rapid rates with prominent pneumonitis. Avoid Hyperventilation ($PaCO_2$<30 mmHg)

Start High Frequency Ventilation (jet/oscillatory), if the infant with severe MAS fails to improve with conventional ventilation and he/she develops air leak syndromes. The frequency varies from 250-350 bpm to > 1000 with 20-25% lower pressure (advantages - less barotrauma and increased mobilization of airway secretions)

Administer surfactant to those infants whose clinical status continues to deteriorate and who require escalating support.(If the oxygenation index >40 for 2hr)

Manage PPHN with High Frequency Ventilation + Nitric Oxide + Inotropes + Surfactant (Refer to the Chapter on a Neonate with PPHN). ECMO may be indicated in approximately 40% of infants with MAS treated with inhaled Nitric oxide: High survival rates (93-100%) reported.

Pearl/Peril/Pitfall : Intrapartum events initiating the meconium passage may cause the infant to have long-term neurologic deficits, including CNS damage, seizures, mental retardation, and cerebral palsy.

Fig. 1: Mechanism of respiratory involvement following MSAF

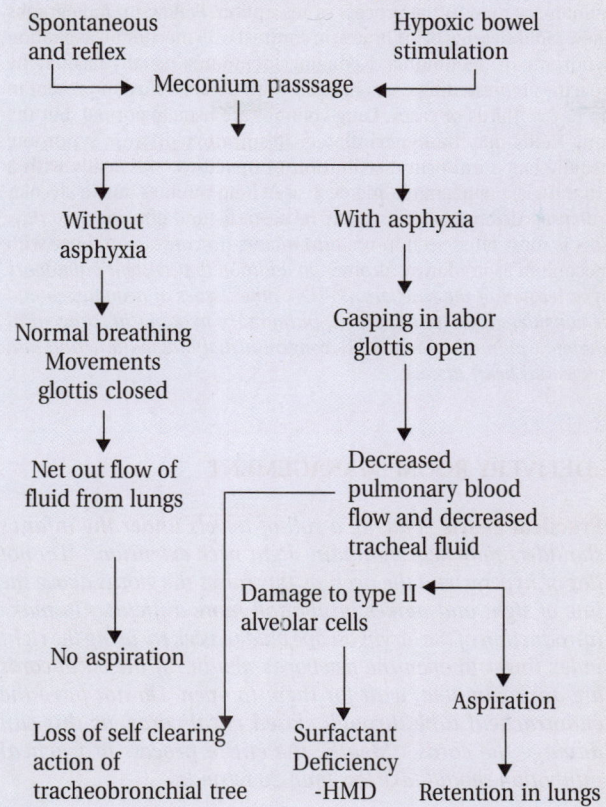

Spontaneous and reflex / Hypoxic bowel stimulation → Meconium passsage

Without asphyxia → Normal breathing Movements glottis closed → Net out flow of fluid from lungs → No aspiration → Loss of self clearing action of tracheobronchial tree

With asphyxia → Gasping in labor glottis open → Decreased pulmonary blood flow and decreased tracheal fluid → Damage to type II alveolar cells → Surfactant Deficiency -HMD / Aspiration → Retention in lungs

Fig. 2: Pathogenesis of MAS

Adapted with permission, from Wiswell TE, Bent RC. Pediatr Clin North Am 1977;24:467.

Meconium Stained Amniotic Fluid → Meconium Aspiration

Large plugs (upper airway obstruction) → Death / Acute hypoxia → Vasocon-striction-PPHN → Incomplete → Ball valve obstruction → Pneumomediastinum Pneumothorax Increased PaCO$_2$

Diffuse particle spread → Lower airway obstruction → Mechanical obstruction / Chemical Inflammation (cytokine activation) / Infection → Complete → Atelectasis → Right to left shunt, V-Q mismatch → Drop in PaO$_2$

→ Hypoxia
→ Hypercapnia
→ Acidosis → Metabolic / Respiratory

TABLE 1	Indications and contraindications for selective ET intubation and tracheal suctioning in a baby born through MSAF

The *indication* for selective intubation and tracheal suctioning of the *nonvigorous infant* includes any infant born through meconium-stained amniotic fluid (MSAF) who is nonvigorous. The NRP defines a nonvigorous infant as an infant who meets one or more of the following conditions: *Depressed respirations *Depressed muscle tone *Heart rate <100 bpm. <u>The consistency of the meconium in the amniotic fluid (thin versus thick) is no longer used to determine the need for tracheal suctioning.</u> Contraindications :A contraindication to selective intubation and tracheal suctioning of an infant born through meconium-stained amniotic fluid (MSAF) is *apparent vigor.* The NRP defines a vigorous infant as one with all of the following: *Strong respiratory effort *Good muscle tone *Heart rate >100 bpm.

TABLE 2	Factors that promote the passage of meconium in utero include the following

*Placental insufficiency *Maternal hypertension *Pre-eclampsia *Oligohydramnios *Maternal drug abuse, especially of tobacco and cocaine *Maternal infection-<u>chorioamnionitis</u> *Fetal gasping secondary to hypoxia *Inadequate removal of meconium from the airway prior to the first breath *Use of positive pressure ventilation (PPV) prior to clearing the airway of meconium.

TABLE 3	MAS—Prophylactic Management Guidelines

1. *Prevent intrauterine hypoxia*: Intrapartum O$_2$ administration to the mother, Saline amnio infusion to dilute the meconium and to counter the adverse effects of oligohydramnios and consequent compression of the umbilical cord *(Cochrane Review- needs additional trials to recommend/refute it)*

2. *Prevent intrauterine meconium aspiration:* There is no advantage in oral and pharyngeal suction as the head delivers and this is no longer indicated, regardless of the baby`s condition at birth. (Cochrane Conclusion)

3. *Prevent/Reduce postnatal aspiration:* a) In a depressed/distressed baby born through MSAF, *Inspect the airway* with a laryngoscope and continue aspiration under direct vision, pass ET tube if meconium is visible at the cords or below and apply suction directly. Don't give positive pressure ventilation if possible, until the meconium has been removed *(Commence normal resuscitation if the baby becomes profoundly bradycardic < 60 BPM).* b)Aspirate the gastric contents when resuscitation is completed to avoid vomiting and aspiration. Saline Bronchial lavage—is of unproven value. *Surfactant lavage of the airways—new and more effective method to remove meconium.*

Pearl/Peril/Pitfall: Oxygen- It cannot be overemphasized that administration of oxygen is critically important in infants with MAS, and in many infants is the only respiratory therapy needed. The pulmonary vasculature in the term infant is exquisitely sensitive to oxygen tension, and failure to overcome hypoxemia almost inevitably will lead to progressive pulmonary hypertension. Oxygen should be administered early and liberally in any baby suspected of having inhaled meconium. The suggested target range for oxygen saturation is 94-98%; target PaO$_2$ 60–90 mmHg. Oxygen toxicity is not an important consideration in the term infant.

Diagnosis: Meconium aspiration syndrome is a clinical diagnosis. Presence of meconium in amniotic fluid is required to cause meconium aspiration syndrome (MAS), but not all neonates with meconium-stained fluid develop meconium aspiration syndrome. The presence of thick particulate meconium in the amniotic fluid increases the likelihood of prenatal aspiration. Green urine may be observed in newborns with meconium aspiration syndrome less than 24 hours after birth. Meconium pigments can be absorbed by the lung and can be excreted in urine. It is suspected with meconium in the amniotic fluid at the time of birth and with respiratory distress in the Newborn. Classically, babies with this disease are post-term, they show signs of weight loss, and they have yellow-stained nails and umbilical cords. The inflammatory process of meconium aspiration may have various presentations on chest radiography, and it is initially indistinguishable from transient tachypnea of the newborn or neonatal pneumonia. Without visualization of meconium below the vocal cords during resuscitation, the diagnosis is made on the basis of the clinical course and the results of follow-up imaging studies.

Differential diagnosis and other problems to consider: <u>Transient tachypnea of the newborn:</u> usually has patchy opacities caused by pulmonary fluid in the process of resorption. Follow-up radiographs show rapid clearing of infiltrates, in contrast with meconium aspiration syndrome or pneumonia. <u>Neonatal pneumonia</u> usually has patchy opacities representing consolidation, with pleural effusion present in up to two thirds of cases. Lung volumes are usually normal, but the lung fields may be hyperinflated. <u>Respiratory distress syndrome</u> usually has a uniform distribution of opacities, classically with a ground-glass appearance and decreased lung volumes due to alveolar collapse. Air bronchograms may be seen. Pleural effusions are rare. This is most often seen in preterm infants (in contrast to those with meconium aspiration syndrome). *In addition to persistent pulmonary hypertension of the newborn (PPHN), other issues of neonates should be considered, including sepsis, pulmonary hypoplasia, congenital anatomic pulmonary anomalies, congenital diaphragmatic hernia, and congenital heart disease.*

MECONIUM ASPIRATION SYNDROME: DELIVERY ROOM MANAGEMENT

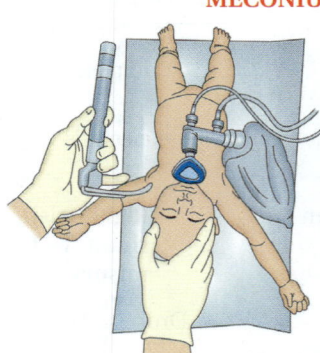

Positioning
For intubation and tracheal suctioning, place the infant on a flat surface, ideally under a radiant warmer. The head should be in midline position with neck slightly extended into the so-called "sniffing" position. Avoid flexion and hyperextension of the neck.

Practical Pearls *Placing a roll of towels under the infant's shoulders may help maintain slight neck extension. *Do not flex or hyperextend the neck, as this raises the glottis above the line of sight and makes intubation more difficult. *To make introduction of the laryngoscope blade easier, try using the right index finger to open the newborn's mouth. *If the vocal cords are approximated, wait for them to open. Do not force the endotracheal tube through closed vocal cords, as this can damage the cords. *Ideally, the entire process of tracheal intubation should take less than 20 seconds.*

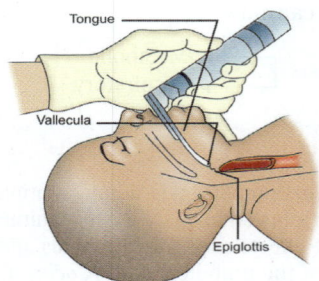

Intubation and tracheal suctioning
*Hold laryngoscope in the left hand. *Stabilize infant's head with the right hand. *Introduce the laryngoscope blade into the right side of mouth and sweep tongue to the left using the laryngoscope blade. *Advance the laryngoscope blade until tip is positioned on top of the epiglottis or immediately anterior to the epiglottis in the vallecula. *Gently lift the laryngoscope blade upward to elevate the epiglottis and tongue to reveal the vocal cords. Do not "rock back" with laryngoscope blade, as this may damage the alveolar ridge. *Identify the vocal cords and attempt to verify the presence of meconium below the level of the cords. If meconium is present, the posterior pharynx may need to be suctioned with a DeLee suction catheter to improve visualization of the cords.

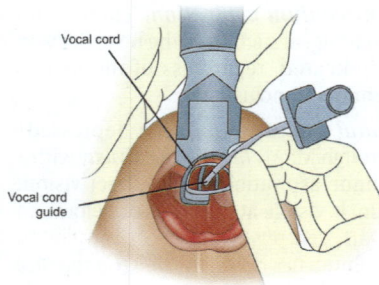

Stabilization: Stabilize the endotracheal tube in position by using an index finger to hold endotracheal tube against the hard palate. Remove the laryngoscope blade while holding the endotracheal tube in place. Attach a meconium aspirator, connected to a medical suction device with continuous pressure of –80 to –120 mmHg, to the endotracheal tube. Occlude the suction-control port on the meconium aspirator to apply suction.

Suctioning: While applying suction, withdraw the endotracheal tube over 3-5 seconds. If a substantial amount of meconium is returned by suction, the intubation and suction should be repeated until the aspirated material is cleared or the newborn's heart rate falls below 100 bpm

Visualization: While the clinician maintains direct visualization of the vocal cords, an assistant places the endotracheal tube into the clinician's right hand. Advance the endotracheal tube through open vocal cords until the vocal cord guide on the endotracheal tube is at the level of the cords.

Pearl/Peril/Pitfall: If the baby is apparently vigorous at birth (heart rate >100, spontaneous respiration, reasonable tone), intubation and tracheal suction is not indicated, unless the baby subsequently has poor respiratory effort or early respiratory distress.

Prevention of meconium aspiration syndrome (MAS)

*Prevention is paramount. *Obstetricians should monitor fetal status in an attempt to identify fetal stress. *When meconium is detected, administering amnioinfusion with warm, sterile saline is theoretically beneficial; it dilutes the meconium in the amniotic fluid, thereby minimizing the severity of the aspiration. However, routine amnioinfusion to prevent meconium aspiration syndrome is not well-supported by current evidence. *Current recommendations no longer advise routine intrapartum suctioning for infants born to mothers with meconium staining of the amniotic fluid. *When aspiration occurs, intubation and immediate suctioning of the airway can remove much of the aspirated meconium. *No clinical trials justify suctioning based on the consistency of meconium. Do not perform the following harmful techniques in an attempt to prevent aspiration of meconium-stained amniotic fluid: *Squeezing the chest of the baby *Inserting a finger into the mouth of the baby *The American Academy of Pediatrics Neonatal Resuscitation Program Steering Committee has promulgated guidelines for management of the baby exposed to meconium. The guidelines are under continuous review and are revised as new evidence-based research becomes available. **The current guidelines are as follows:** *If the baby is not vigorous (defined as minimal or absent respiratory effort, poor muscle tone, or heart rate <100 beats/min): Use direct laryngoscopy, intubate, and suction the trachea immediately after delivery. Suction for no longer than 5 seconds. If no meconium is retrieved, do not repeat intubation and suction. If meconium is retrieved and no bradycardia is present, reintubate and suction. If the heart rate is low, administer positive pressure ventilation and consider suctioning again later. *If the baby is vigorous (defined as good respiratory effort, crying, good muscle tone, and heart rate >100 beats/min): Do not electively intubate. Clear secretions and meconium from the mouth and nose with a bulb syringe or a large-bore suction catheter. *In either case: The remainder of the initial resuscitation steps should ensue and include drying, stimulating, repositioning, and administering oxygen as necessary.

NICU care for a baby with mas:

*Maintain an optimal thermal environment to minimize oxygen consumption. *Minimal handling is necessary because these infants are easily agitated, which causes right-to-left shunting, leading to hypoxia and acidosis. *Sedation is often necessary to decrease agitation. *Continue respiratory care. Oxygen therapy via hood or positive pressure is crucial in maintaining adequate arterial oxygenation. If mechanical ventilation is required, make concerted efforts to minimize the mean airway pressure and to use as short an inspiratory time as possible. Oxygen saturations should be maintained at 90–95%. *Surfactant therapy is now commonly used to replace displaced or inactivated surfactant and as a detergent to remove meconium. Although surfactant use does not appear to affect mortality rates, it appears to reduce the severity of disease and progression to extracorporeal membrane oxygenation (ECMO). Studies are ongoing to evaluate the potential role of pulmonary lavage with surfactant. *Although conventional ventilation commonly is initially used, high-frequency oscillation and jet ventilation are alternative effective therapies. Hyperventilation to induce hypocapnia and compensate for metabolic acidosis is no longer a primary therapy for pulmonary hypertension because hypocarbia may result in decreased cerebral perfusion ($PaCO_2$ <30 mm Hg). Prolonged alkalosis has been shown to cause neuronal injury in animals and humans, providing another reason to avoid alkalosis in these patients. *Ventilator therapy aimed at minimizing mean airway pressure and tidal volume should be used if pulmonary interstitial emphysema or a pneumothorax is present. *For treatment of persistent pulmonary hypertension of the newborn (PPHN), inhaled nitric oxide is the pulmonary vasodilator of choice. *Pay careful attention to systemic blood volume and blood pressure. Volume expansion, transfusion therapy, and systemic vasopressors are critical in maintaining systemic blood pressure greater than pulmonary blood pressure, thereby decreasing the right-to-left shunt through the patent ductus arteriosus. *ECMO is used if all other therapeutic options have been exhausted. Although effective in treating meconium aspiration syndrome, ECMO is associated with a high incidence of poor neurologic outcomes.

Medicolegal Pitfalls:

*Many infants who have experienced meconium aspiration syndrome (MAS) have had prenatal and postnatal periods of hypoxia and acidosis; therefore, these individuals are at increased risk of significant CNS damage. *Typically, medicolegal action is initiated by parents whose newborn develops long-term sequelae from significant perinatal hypoxia. Although the delivering physician is the primary focus of such a lawsuit, additional liability to other healthcare professionals may ensue from a poorly planned and executed resuscitation. *Commonly, the providers of the tertiary intensive care are included in these lawsuits, which are usually due to complications of necessary complex and aggressive care. Although other organ systems may be damaged by the initial insult and subsequent therapy, they are rarely the basis of legal action.

Prognosis:

*Most infants with meconium aspiration syndrome have complete recovery of pulmonary function. *Intrapartum events initiating the meconium passage may cause the infant to have long-term neurologic deficits, including CNS damage, seizures, mental retardation, and cerebral palsy.

Complications:

*Children with meconium aspiration syndrome may develop chronic lung disease as a result of intense pulmonary intervention. *Infants with meconium aspiration syndrome have a slightly increased incidence of infections in the first year of life because the lungs are still in recovery.

Transfer:

Although initial stabilization is necessary at community hospitals, infants with meconium aspiration syndrome frequently require high-frequency ventilation, inhaled nitric oxide (NO), or extracorporeal membrane oxygenation (ECMO). Therefore, in the event of significant aspiration, transferring these infants to a regional neonatal ICU (NICU) as soon as possible is important.

Pearl/Peril/Pitfall : Ventilatory strategies are set to prevent air-trapping by allowing enough expiratory time and/or apply high frequency ventilation. Animal studies suggest optimum oxygenation can be achieved by supplying enough PEEP for alveolar recruitment. Babies at risk of pulmonary hypertension need to remain at all times in optimal inspired oxygen to keep PaO2 100-120 mmHg or SaO2 > 98%. CO2 should be targeted at the normal range (35-40 mmHg) to provide an optimal pH. Sedation and paralysis should be started if the baby is not synchronized with the ventilator.

MECONIUM ASPIRATION SYNDROME-VENTILATION STRATEGIES:

Continuous positive airway pressure and conventional mechanical ventilation in the treatment of meconium aspiration syndrome : J P Goldsmith Abstract -Meconium aspiration syndrome (MAS) is a complex syndrome that ranges in severity from mild respiratory distress to severe respiratory failure, persistent pulmonary hypertension of the newborn and sometimes death. Understanding of the syndrome's complicated pathophysiology will help determine the appropriate treatment strategy, including the use of continuous positive airway pressure (CPAP), conventional mechanical ventilation (CMV) and other therapies. Approximately 30 to 50% of infants diagnosed with MAS will require CPAP or mechanical ventilation. The optimum modes of ventilation for MAS are not known. Very few studies have been conducted to determine ventilatory strategies. Despite the introduction, over the last two decades, of innovative ventilatory treatments for this disease (for example, surfactant, high-frequency ventilation, inhaled nitric oxide, extracorporeal membrane oxygenation), the majority of infants can be successfully managed with CPAP or mechanical ventilation alone. Journal of Perinatology (2008) 28, S49–S55; doi:10.1038/jp.2008.156.

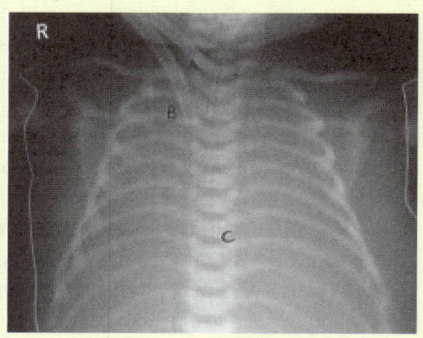

Figure 1 Chest radiograph of infant with severe meconium aspiration syndrome showing typical "white out" appearance 24 hours after institution of venoarterial extracorporeal membrane oxygenation support. The arterial cannula (A) has been inserted into the right common carotid artery, with its tip in the aortic arch; the venous cannula (B) has been inserted into the right internal jugular vein and its tip (C) lies in the right atrium.

Role of ECMO in Severe MAS

Infants with severe MAS are relatively "ideal" candidates for ECMO in that: *almost all are > 34 weeks gestation and weigh > 2 kg (cut off for ECMO) *they have a potentially reversible respiratory problem *associated pulmonary hypertension, although severe, is almost always reversible *these infants need the "lung rest" that ECMO provides *ECMO is an effective form of treatment for infants meeting the criteria *as a subgroup, patients with MAS have a very favourable outcome. ECMO support is usually required for between 100 and 120 hours18 in MAS, the shortest duration for any neonatal diagnosis. However, this duration will inevitably be significantly increased if high pressure/volume ventilation has led to air leaks before cannulation. While on ECMO, the infant receives "resting ventilation" with slow background ventilation with a moderate level of PEEP to maintain lung expansion (rate 10/min, pressures 20/10). Serial radiographs often show a complete "white out" during the first two to three days (fig 1), with subsequent reappearance of air bronchograms and resolution of the changes as the lungs recover.

Alternatives to ECMO in severe MAS: Other forms of treatment have been suggested for neonates with MAS, including surfactant, inhaled nitric oxide, and even liquid ventilation. However, despite some improvements in oxygenation even within these trials, there were still neonates who required ECMO support. Indeed these various forms of support and therapy are not necessarily mutually exclusive. For instance, surfactant has also been used in neonates supported with ECMO, resulting in improved pulmonary mechanics, reduced time on ECMO, and reduced disease complications.

Courtesy: P J DAVIS and L S SHEKERDEMIAN *Arch Dis Child Fetal Neonatal Ed* 2001; 84:F1–F3

KEY POINTS FOR CLINICAL PRACTICE

1. Meconium aspiration syndrome (MAS) occurs when meconium-stained amniotic fluid (MSAF) is aspirated into the lungs of an infant prior to, during, or immediately after birth. Intrauterine gasping resulting in aspiration of meconium has been shown in animal models exposed to hypoxia. MAS occurs in approximately 5% of infants born through MSAF. Even with modern neonatal intensive care, the mortality rate from MAS remains as high as 3–5%.

2. The *indication* for selective intubation and tracheal suctioning of the *nonvigorous infant* includes any infant born through meconium-stained amniotic fluid (MSAF) who is nonvigorous. The NRP defines a nonvigorous infant as an infant who meets one or more of the following conditions: *Depressed respirations *Depressed muscle tone *Heart rate <100 bpm. *The consistency of the meconium in the amniotic fluid (thin versus thick) is no longer used to determine the need for tracheal suctioning.*

3. Most infants born through meconium stained amniotic fluid require no interventions, but it is important to monitor these well appearing infants closely for signs of respiratory distress for 12–24 hr. One should always observe the infants for tachypnea, cyanosis, grunting, nasal flaring, and accessory muscle use (retractions).

4. *Mechanical ventilation* is indicated if the infant develops severe Meconium Aspiration Syndrome evidenced by **a)** impending respiratory failure **b)** PPHN **c)** hemodynamic compromise **d)** airleaks **e)** coexisting sepsis **f)** apneas and **g)** ABG analysis—pH <7.20, HCO_3 <14, PaO_2 <50 mmHg, $PaCO_2$ >60mmHg, oxygen saturations <90%, breathing in > 10lts/min of oxygen.

5. Recent advances in neonatal intensive care i.e. Surfactant, High Frequency Oscillatory Ventilation (HFOV), inhaled Nitric Oxide and ECMO (ExtraCorporeal Membrane Oxygenation) have substantially reduced the mortality and morbidity related to MAS in the developed nations. Replication of these results in the developing countries, however, is a difficult task due to limited resources and the high incidence of MAS.

REFERENCES AND FURTHER READING **1)**2005 American Heart Association (AHA) guidelines for cardiopulmonary resuscitation (CPR) and emergency cardiovascular care (ECC) of pediatric and neonatal patients: neonatal resuscitation guidelines. *Pediatrics.* May 2006;117(5):e1029-38. **2)** Dargaville PA, South M, McDougall PN. Surfactant and surfactant inhibitors in meconium aspiration syndrome. *J Pediatr.* Jan 2001;138(1):113-5. **3)** Glantz JC, Woods JR. Significance of amniotic fluid meconium. In: *Maternal-Fetal Medicine.* 1999:393-403. **4)**Ranzini AC, Chan L. Meconium and fetal-neonatal compromise. *In: Intensive Care of the Fetus and Neonate.* 1996: 297-303 **5)** Abman SH, Kinsella JP. Inhaled nitric oxide therapy for pulmonary disease in pediatrics. *Curr Opin Pediatr.* Jun 1998;10(3):236-42

Pearl/Peril/Pitfall : *One must remember that those babies may have an urgent need for oxygen, so an extended period of time spent intubating and aspirating meconium should be avoided. The babies born through meconium who present in between the aforementioned scenario's should be managed with a focus on normal resuscitation guidelines with attention to the airway (suction if necessary), breathing (proper bag and mask ventilation or intubation) and circulation.*

36 Apnea of Prematurity/Neonatal Apnea

@ Before a diagnosis of AOP is made, other causes of apnea in neonates must be excluded. Precise diagnosis of AOP requires multichannel recordings, which are most commonly measurements of nasal airflow, thoracic impedance, heart rate, and O_2 saturation. Expanded testing may include electroencephalography and/or use of an esophageal pH probe with a high thoracic Clark electrode.

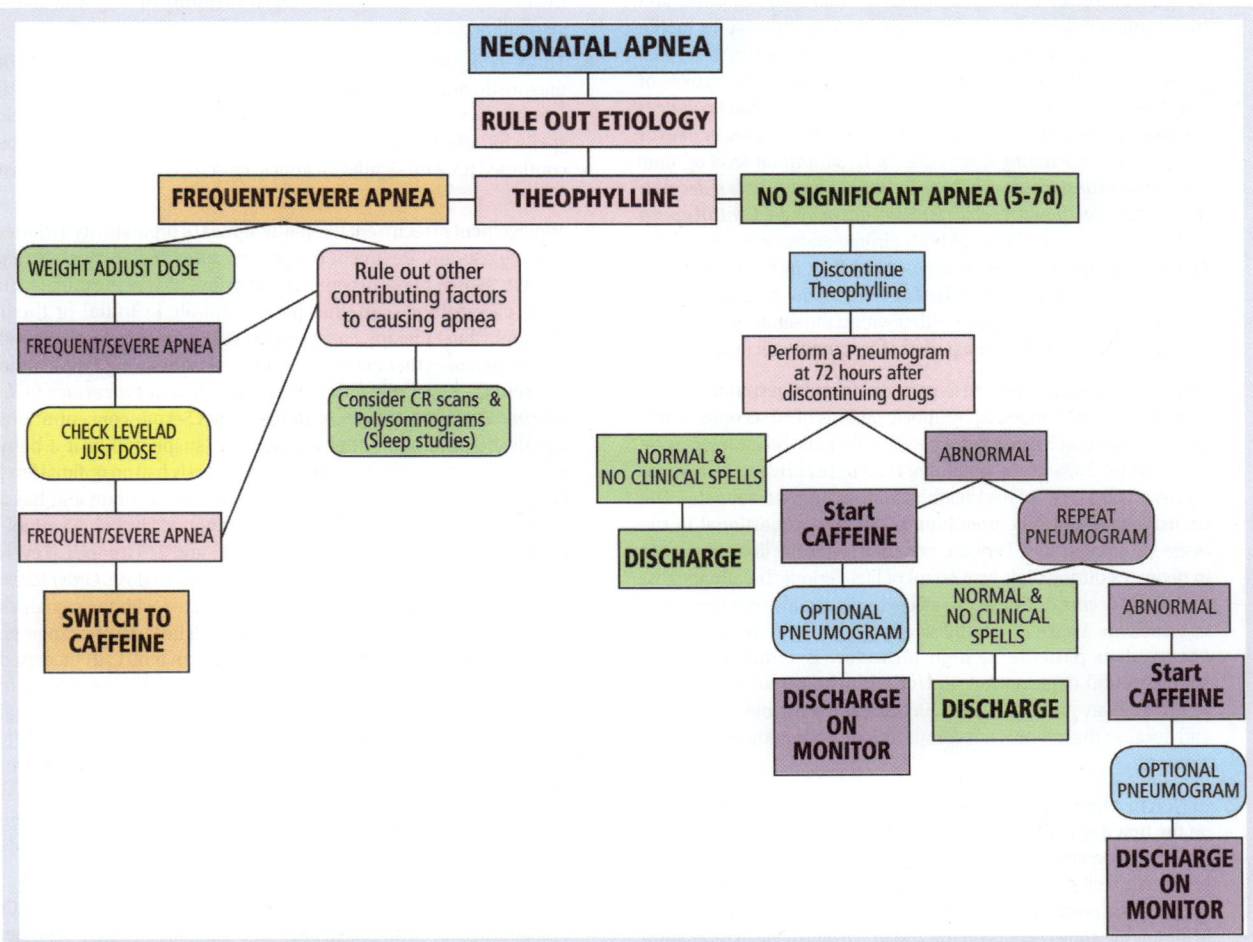

REVIEW OF CLINICAL PROBLEMS

1. Name the recommended procedures to manage an acute severe apneic episode.
   Ans: Refer to the "No.5" of the "BIRD'S EYE VIEW/OVER-VIEW/SYNOPSIS" of the Chapter.

2. Mention the differential diagnoses should you consider in a baby with significant apnea.
   Ans: Refer to Table 1 and Fig. 2 of the Chapter.

3. What are the investigations to be done to determine the treatable causes of apnea?
   Ans: Refer to the Evaluation-Decision-Action Plan/ Algorithm to diagnose and manage a Neonatal Apnea and Table 1.

4. How do you manage Neonatal Apnea generally and specifically? *Ans: Refer to Tables 2 and 3 of the Chapter.*

5. How do you assess the severity of Neonatal Apnea?
   Ans: Refer to Table 4 of the chapter.

LEARNING OBJECTIVES

After completing this article, readers will be able to

1. Treat apnea with acute resuscitation followed by diagnosis and treatment of specific causes.

2. Understand that apnea of prematurity is a *diagnosis of exclusion* and apnea on day 1 may not be due to idiopathic apnea of prematurity—consider sepsis or impending respiratory failure (esp. when there is underlying surfactant deficiency).

3. Recognize that a sudden increase in severity/frequency of apneic episodes suggests new pathology.

4. Initiate symptomatic control of recurrent apnea with medication or CPAP or ventilatory support.

5. Counsel parents that apnea of prematurity is not a risk factor for SIDS.

Pearl/Peril/Pitfall: When all causes of apnea other than prematurity are excluded during the diagnostic workup, AOP is the presumptive etiology. Caregivers must decide which intervention is appropriate given the severity of the patient's apnea, bradycardia, and O_2 desaturation.

BIRD'S EYE VIEW/OVERVIEW/SYNOPSIS

1. **APNEA OF PREMATURITY/NEONATAL APNEA** is defined as cessation of breathing for > 15 seconds in a term infant and > 20 seconds in a preterm infant with or without bradycardia (<100 BPM/mt) and/or color changes (cyanosis). Short apneic episodes (10 seconds) are rarely associated with bradycardia (**but can occur in ELBW {<1000gms} babies**), whereas longer ones (>20 seconds) have a higher incidence of bradycardia. After 30-45 seconds, pallor and hypotonia are seen and infants may be unresponsive to tactile stimulation. Bradycardia follows the apnea by 1–2 seconds in >95% of cases ; vagal responses and rarely heart block are causes of bradycardia without apnea. *Bradycardia in a premature neonate is considered clinically significant when the heart rate slows by at least 30 bpm from the resting heart rate. An O_2 saturation level of more than 85% is considered pathologic in this age group, as is a decrease in O_2 saturation should it persist for 5 seconds or longer.* **Central apnea** is defined as the cessation of both airflow and respiratory effort. *Obstructive apnea* is the cessation of airflow in the presence of continued respiratory effort. *Mixed apnea* contains elements of both central and obstructive apnea, either within the same apneic pause or at different times during a period of respiratory recording.

   Periodic breathing is defined as periods of regular respiration for as long as 20 seconds followed by apneic periods of 10 seconds or less that occur at least 3 times in succession . Periodic breathing may be observed for 2-6% of the breathing time in healthy term neonates and as much as 25% of the breathing time in preterm neonates. The occurrence of periodic breathing is directly proportional to the degree of prematurity. Periodic breathing typically does not occur in neonates during their first 2 days of life. Periodic breathing most frequently occurs during active sleep, but it can also happen when neonates are awake or quietly sleeping. This pattern, commonly observed in patients at high altitudes, is eliminated with supplemental oxygenation and/or with the use of continuous positive airway pressure (CPAP). Because the prognosis is excellent and because the infant is not compromised, no treatment is usually required.

2. **APNEA in a term infant on any day of life and in a premature baby on the first day of life is never physiologic;** it usually requires a full work-up to determine the underlying cause. The onset of apnea in a previously well premature neonate after the second week of life is also a critical event that warrants immediate investigation (the onset of idiopathic apnea occurs on the 2nd to 7th day of life in premature babies).

3. **Idiopathic apnea in premature infants is a diagnosis of exclusion** ; any baby who develops symptomatic apneic attacks must be carefully assessed to exclude the causes of secondary apnea, including **SEPSIS** . The most common pattern of idiopathic apnea in preterm neonates is a mixed etiology (50–75%), with obstructive apnea preceding (usually) or following central apnea. Short episodes of apnea are usually central, whereas prolonged ones are often mixed. Idiopathic apnea of prematurity occurs in infants that are usually < 34 weeks' gestation, weight < 1800gms.

4. The differential diagnosis in a baby with significant apnea should always include **infection, hypoglycemia, and seizures,** since these are potentially serious disorders for which early treatment is crucial. Routine history, physical examination, and lab. tests, will identify the causes of apnea such as maternal administration of CNS depressants, hypoxemia, hypothermia, anemia, hypocalcemia, and PDA, **but gastroesophageal reflux, intracranial hemorrhage, and upper airway obstruction are causes that can be missed unless they are considered and explored.**

5. **Recommended procedures to manage an acute apneic episode include** a) Stimulation of the infant. If the episodes are brief and not associated with systemic features, this may be all that is necessary b) Suction of the upper airways is indicated when obstruction is the likely cause c) Manual ventilation with a face mask and bag d) Intubation and intermittent positive-pressure ventilation will be necessary when the baby fails to respond to bag-and-mask ventilation, or when severe apneic attacks occur frequently.

6. The *E-D-A plan/algorithm* summarizes the essential aspects of diagnostic and therapeutic management of Neonatal apnea. All infants < 34 weeks of gestational age should be monitored for apneic spells for atleast the first week of life and monitoring should be continued until no significant apneic episode is detected for at least 5 days.

7. **Management of recurrent Idiopathic apnea of prematurity includes a)** Diagnosis and treatment of specific causes (e.g., hypoglycemia, anemia, sepsis) **b)** Nasal continuous positive airway pressure (4 cm H_2O) **c)** Xanthine (**caffeine {now available in India}** or theo/aminophylline) therapy, commencing with a loading dose followed by maintenance therapy, and serum level monitoring { difficult in our setting}, especially for aminophylline. *It is not necessary to do routine levels of Caffeine on stable babies.* Serum concentrations should be obtained either if toxicity is suspected or if a baby continues to have apnea and has not previously had an optimal level documented. Note that the assay is not very accurate and has a coefficient of variation of 15%, so that a reported level of 165 mmol/L has a 95% chance of being between 115 and 215 mmol/L. Levels should not be checked within 6 hours of previous dose. Order levels the day before assay is to be done (clearly dated with the next day's date). Levels to be done at 0830 hours. Therapeutic range is: 135–200 m mol/L, toxicity is unlikely at <400 m mol/L. **d)** Increased environmental oxygen only as necessary to maintain adequate baseline oxygen saturation (babies with apneic attacks have normal lungs and Retinopathy of Prematurity is a significant risk if O_2 is administered indiscriminately). Often associated with treatment of anemia. **e)** Assisted ventilation if all else fails. There are no fixed guidelines on the initiation of any of these treatments, as the assessment of apnea tends to be subjective, and each baby needs individual assessment.

8. Role of home apnea monitoring in preventing Sudden Infant Death Syndrome (SIDS)—though it reduces the parental anxiety at home, there is no evidence that it reduces the risk of a major life-threatening event occurring out of hospital, nor do they prevent death; babies have died despite being monitored. *It is essential that the parents are shown how to apply basic resuscitation skills to their infant prior to giving them an apnea monitor, in case the baby is found apneic or collapsed at home.*

9. The relationship between apnea, desaturation and bradycardia is not simple as summarized in Figure 1 of the Chapter.

10. Data still support the traditional belief that discharge from the NICU is appropriate after the infant has been free of symptomatic apnea for approximately 5–7 days (usually after 34 weeks of corrected gestational age). There is no evidence that the two-fold increased risk of Sudden Infant Death Syndrome (SIDS) is lessened by any treatment modality (including home monitoring), so parental reassurance is most appropriate in this situation. It is worth noting, however that premature infants who appear to have outgrown apnea of prematurity can have recurrence of apnea during severe respiratory tract infections or after general anesthesia as late as several months following discharge, so short-term monitoring may be indicated in these cases.

Pearl/Peril/Pitfall : Of the two methylxanthines in use, caffeine, which is just as effective, has potential therapeutic advantages over theophylline due to its higher therapeutic ratio and thus less side effects, more reliable enteral absorption and the longer half life allows once daily administration. The standard dosing with caffeine citrate is 20 mg/kg load (IVI or oral) and then 5 mg/kg/day (IVI or Oral). Blood levels do not need to be monitored routinely.

THE EVALUATION-DECISION-ACTION-PLAN/ALGORITHM FOR THE DIAGNOSIS AND MANAGEMENT OF *NEONATAL APNEA*

SUBJECTIVE FINDINGS

Do always resuscitate the "apneic" baby and stabilize fully before embarking on to more detailed evaluation.

Hx of apneic episode(s) - frequency and severity and Magnitude of the intervention required to alleviate the event (its/their resuscitation details)

Hx of feed intolerance, lethargy, temperature instability, volume and route of feeding, possibility of nasal obstruction due to vomitus, milk, mucus or meconium or choanal atresia

Hx of tachypnea, respiratory distress, cyanosis, jitteriness, CNS depression/ irritability, seizures, hypotonia.

OBJECTIVE FINDINGS

Assess ABCs and disability (altered sensorium, seizures, responsiveness and pupils), Vitals, O_2 sats, CRT, Pulses, BP, Hydration, Urine output. *Monitor the baby's cardiac, neurologic, and respiratory status. Observe the infant for any signs of breathing difficulty, desaturation, or bradycardia during feeding !*

Look for signs of Sepsis, CNS depression, Cardio respiratory involvement, abdominal distention and/ or bilious aspirates, severe pallor.

Perform head to toe examination to identify the multitude of causes of Neonatal apnea mentioned elsewhere in the Chapter (Figure 2).

Reassess the condition of the infant, periodically in case of any recurrence of apneas.

INVESTIGATIONS

Carry out lab investigations to determine treatable causes of apnea, depending on the prevailing clinical condition. **FBC,** bacterial cultures of blood, urine, cerebrospinal fluid (CSF), tracheal aspirate and other potential sites of infection; **chest X-ray; blood glucose;** serum electrolytes, including calcium, magnesium and sodium; **arterial blood gases** and **continuous monitoring of oxygen saturation, TcPO2 and perhaps PCO2;** ultrasound/CT examination of the head; if gastro-esophageal reflux is suspected, a number of further investigations may be undertaken, including an **intra-esophageal pH probe and/or contrast study;** **Echocardiogram** to exclude PDA, in special circumstances; further neurological investigation may be necessary, i.e. electroencephalogram (EEG), polygraphic sleep studies

SUGGESTED ALGORITHM FOLLOWING AN APNEA / BRADYCARDIA ALARM

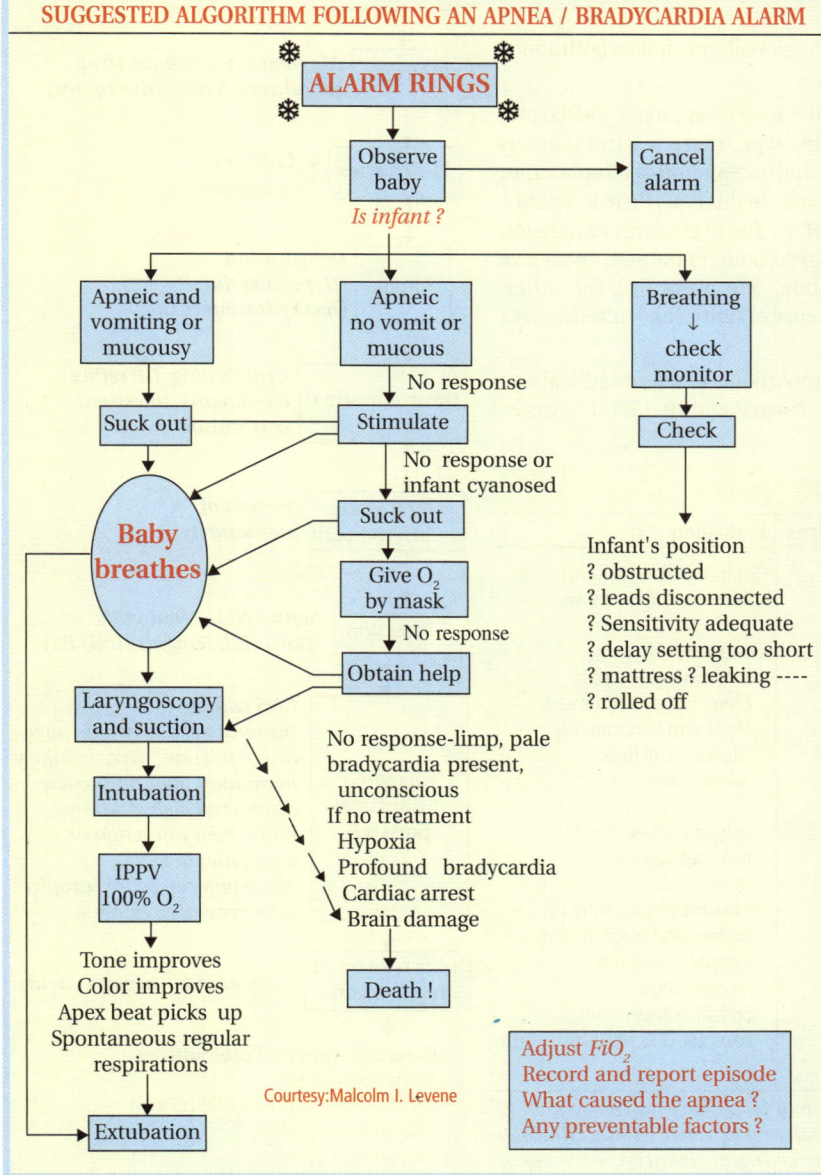

Courtesy:Malcolm I. Levene

Adjust FiO_2
Record and report episode
What caused the apnea ?
Any preventable factors ?

* When a monitor alarm sounds, <u>one should remember to respond to the infant, not the monitor,</u> checking for bradycardia, cyanosis and airway obstruction.

* Heart rate(ECG monitoring) should be monitored always, as none of the available apnea monitors will detect obstructive apnea, until the infant stops fighting for breath.

* <u>Pulse oximeter monitoring is the best method for detecting apnea in routine clinical setting, as it allows the detection of two harmful consequences of apnea(hypoxemia and bradycardia).</u>

* Periodic breathing consists of cycles of hyperventilation(15–20 seconds) alternating with periods hypoventilation and eventual apnea lasting about 3 seconds and is common in preterm babies.

* Clinically significant apnea can be defined as a cessation of respiration lasting for 20 seconds or more accompanied by bradycardia(<100 bpm) and/ or cyanosis. After 30–45 seconds, pallor and hypotonia are seen and infants may be unresponsive to tactile stimulation.

* All infants < 34 weeks of gestational age should be monitored for apneic spells for at least the first week of life and monitoring should be continued until no significant apneic episode is detected for at least 5 days.

* After the first apneic spell, the infant should be evaluated for a possible underlying cause. Be alert to the possibility of a precipitating cause in infants who are > 34 weeks of gestational age.

* Evaluation after an episode of significant apnea, irrespective of gestational age and postnatal age of the infant should include history, description and timing of apneas, and physical examination, especially cardiorespiratory system, neuro behavioral data, evidence of infection, capillary refill time and blood pressure.

Pearl/Peril/Pitfall : Discharge home occurs when staff and parents are satisfied with a period off the monitor (usually one week). In the absence of some unusual clinical indication predischarge pneumograms and use of apnoea monitors at home are discouraged, as there is no evidence of need and their use could impair the parental development of normal family relations by perpetuating an ICU attitude

Fig. 1

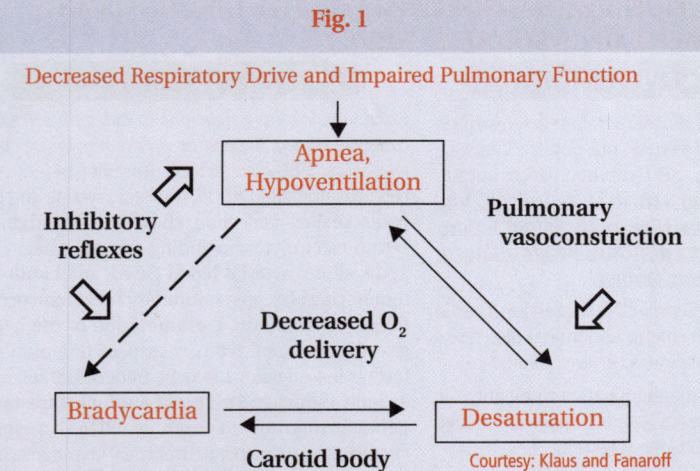

Decreased Respiratory Drive and Impaired Pulmonary Function

Apnea, Hypoventilation

Inhibitory reflexes

Pulmonary vasoconstriction

Decreased O₂ delivery

Bradycardia — Desaturation

Carotid body

Courtesy: Klaus and Fanaroff

* The relationship between apnea, desaturation and bradycardia is not simple as summarized in the adjacent figure. Decreased central respiratory drive is the usual initiating event, with reflex bradycardia presumably triggered by the resultant desaturation.

* Excitation of inhibitory reflexes may also occasionally precipitate both apnea and bradycardia.(Hering-Breuer reflex).

* Based on the polygraphic recording, neonatal apnea may be categorized into three major types: *Central apnea*: In this type, there is simultaneous cessation of respiratory effort and air flow due to cessation of motor output from the respiratory center. *Obstructive apnea*: In this type, there is absence of airflow despite presence of respiratory effort due to an obstructive lesion in the upper pharynx. *Mixed apnea*: In this type, both central and obstructive apneas develop during the same episode, one preceding the other. Experience shows that frequency of occurrence of central and mixed apneas in preterm neonates is more or less equal.

* Incidence of neonatal apnea is inversely proportional to the gestational age. 80% below 28–30 weeks, 50% between 30–32 weeks and 10–15% at 34 weeks of gestational age.

TABLE 1   Evaluation of an infant with apnea

Potential cause	Associated history of signs	Evaluation
Infection	Feeding intolerance, lethargy, temperature instability	Complete blood count, cultures if appropriate
Impaired oxygenation	Cyanosis, tachypnea, respiratory distress	Continuous oxygen monitoring, arterial blood gas measurement, chest x-ray examination
Metabolic disorders	Jitteriness, poor feeding, lethargy, CNS depression, irritability	Glucose, calcium, electrolytes
Drugs	CNS depression, hypotonia, maternal history	Magnesium, screen for toxic substances in urine
Temperature instability	Lethargy	Monitor temperature of patient and environment
Intracranial pathology	Abnormal neurologic examination, seizures	Cranial ultrasound examination
Gastroesophageal reflux	Difficulty with feeds	Specific observation, contrast UGI study/pH study

UGI = upper gastrointestinal. Analysis of the stool for different toxins related to botulism may reveal a cause in an infant with apnea, constipation, clinically significant hypotonia, difficulty swallowing or crying, or absent eye movements.

Fig.2: Potential causes of neonatal apnea and bradycardia

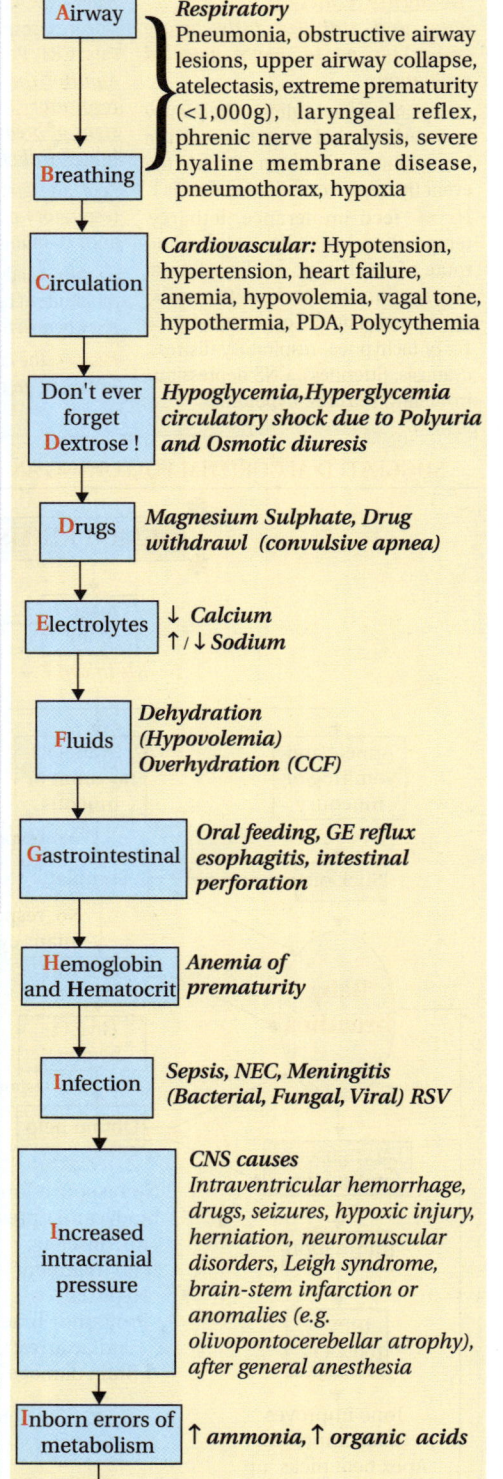

Airway
Breathing
Respiratory
Pneumonia, obstructive airway lesions, upper airway collapse, atelectasis, extreme prematurity (<1,000g), laryngeal reflex, phrenic nerve paralysis, severe hyaline membrane disease, pneumothorax, hypoxia

Circulation
Cardiovascular: Hypotension, hypertension, heart failure, anemia, hypovolemia, vagal tone, hypothermia, PDA, Polycythemia

Don't ever forget Dextrose !
Hypoglycemia, Hyperglycemia circulatory shock due to Polyuria and Osmotic diuresis

Drugs
Magnesium Sulphate, Drug withdrawl (convulsive apnea)

Electrolytes
↓ *Calcium*
↑ / ↓ *Sodium*

Fluids
Dehydration (Hypovolemia) Overhydration (CCF)

Gastrointestinal
Oral feeding, GE reflux esophagitis, intestinal perforation

Hemoglobin and Hematocrit
Anemia of prematurity

Infection
Sepsis, NEC, Meningitis (Bacterial, Fungal, Viral) RSV

Increased intracranial pressure
CNS causes
Intraventricular hemorrhage, drugs, seizures, hypoxic injury, herniation, neuromuscular disorders, Leigh syndrome, brain-stem infarction or anomalies (e.g. olivopontocerebellar atrophy), after general anesthesia

Inborn errors of metabolism
↑ *ammonia,* ↑ *organic acids*

Idiopathic Apnea of prematurity
Always should be
A DIAGNOSIS OF EXCLUSION
of above identifiable predisposing diseases !

Pearl/Peril/Pitfall: In cases of airway obstruction, stridor, or unexplained pathologic obstructive apnea, helpful upper airway evaluations include lateral neck radiography, head and neck 3-dimensional tomography, and otolaryngologic evaluation (e.g., fiberoptic assessment of the larynx through the nose during spontaneous breathing).

TABLE 2	Neonatal apnea-general management guidelines

1. *Airway and breathing*: *Avoid* vigorous suctioning of the oro-pharynx, and positions of extreme flexion or extention of the neck to reduce the likelihood of airway obstruction and withhold oral feeds for at least 24 hours. *Provide* supplemental humidified oxygen to maintain oxygen saturation above 90%, if intermittent hypoxemia is identified by pulse oximetry. *Handle* the low birth weight infants carefully and *pay attention* to feeding techniques, with avoidance of stomach distention and rapid feeding. *Nurse* the infant in the prone position and consider altering feeding regimen, i.e., a continuous milk infusion may be better tolerated than intermittent feeds or transpyloric feeding.

2. *Circulation*: *Transfuse* with packed RBC, if the haematocrit is < 25-30% and the infant has episodes of apnea and bradycardia that are frequent or severe while Aminophylline levels are therapeutic. *Avoid* swings in environmental temperature and decrease it to lower end of the thermoneutral range. *Treat* cardiac failure (diuretics and if indicated, Digoxin). *Manage* hemodynamically significant PDA if confirmed, after discussing with a Pediatric Cardiologist.

3. *Dextrose*: *Monitor for* hypoglycemia and correct it with an IV infusion containing 10% Dextrose, till the apneic attacks are controlled.

4. *Electrolytes, fluids and acid-base balance*: *Monitor and correct* the disturbances and maintain the milleu—interior within the normal limits.

5. *Gastrointestinal causes*: *Treat* Gastroesophageal reflux by **1.** Small frequent feeds **2.** Prone nursing position with head end elevation **3.** Antacid, e.g. Gaviscon or Ranitidine (H_2 antagonist) **4.** Cisapride (prokinetic) with ECG evaluation for prolonged QT interval **5.** Surgical fundoplication in very severe cases.

6. *Infection*: *Make sure to rule out* sepsis and Necrotizing Enterocolitis before treating other causes ; when in doubt *always start* broadspectrum antibiotics after performing full septic screen with CSF analysis. *Beware of* fungal / viral septicemia in a predisposing Newborn baby.

TABLE 3	Neonatal apnea-specific management guidelines

Step I **TACTILE STIMULATION** by regular stroking of the infant/by rocking or undulating the baby has been shown to reduce the number of apneic episodes, but is a not a feasible method for routine use. *Skin to skin contact by Kangaroo - mother - care (KMC) has been shown to control apneic episodes which are resistant to other conventional modes of management. If the apneic spells are severe and repeated, i.e. i) > 1 episode requiring bag and mask ventilation or oxygen supplementation within 24 hours, ii) > 2 episodes per hour requiring tactile stimulation - go to Step II, III and IV in the order of increasing invasiveness and risk.*

Step II: **DRUG THERAPY - THEOPHYLLINE/AMINOPHYLLINE Dosing:** no adjustment in dosing is necessary when switching between Theo and Amino in Neonates ·**Loading Dose: 6mg/kg** · **Maintenance Dose: 4mg/kg/d** divided Q8h (consider Q12h for infants <1,500gms).**Checking Levels:** *If patient continues to have persistent apnea and bradycardia spells *If patient is exhibiting signs/symptoms of toxicity (irritability, tachycardia, feeding intolerance, etc.) *Order as trough levels. *Therapeutic ranges: *Theophylline: 6–10mcg/ml · Caffeine: 8–20 mcg/ml **Adjusting Doses:** *if steady state level (Theo level 72h or Caffeine level 5 days after dose changes), calculate new dose (per pharmacy) *if non-steady state level, consider a partial loading dose and increase maintenance dose by 20% (notify pharmacy). It is generally discontinued after 34 weeks of gestational age, if no apneic spells occur for 5–7 days. It stimulates the CNS respiratory center, antagonizes adenosine (a neurotransmitter that can cause respiratory depression) and improves diaphragmatic efficiency. Tachycardia and diuresis are common side effects. *Oral Caffeine citrate* 20 mg of Caffeine base/kg/dose as loading dose followed by maintenance doses of 2.5–5mg/kg/daily in 1 dose

beginning 24 hours after the loading dose also can be used (now available in India) to decrease the frequency of apneic spells (serum levels are to be maintained at 5–20 micro grams/ml). Don't use *Doxapram*, because of its toxic manifestations. (seizures and hypertension). Drugs have no prophylactic role.

Step III: **NASAL CPAP**—at low levels (3–4 cm water) can reduce the number of mixed and obstructive apneic spells. It maintains the upper airway patency, increases the functional residual capacity and PaO_2 and stabilizes the chest wall. Always decompress the stomach by Oro-gastric tube to avoid overdistention of stomach due to CPAP administration. Nasal CPAP is ineffective in central apnea, but is quite an effective therapy for obstructive and mixed apnea.

Step IV: **MECHANICAL VENTILATION** - if all the previously mentioned interventions fail to control the apneic episodes, start mechanical ventilation to avoid major physiological changes associated with apneic episodes (only minimal pressures and rates are usually required). *(Always avoid hyperoxia, since this is a sure recipe for Retinopathy Of Prematurity {ROP}).* Measure Blood Gases and aim to keep PaO_2 in the range of 50-70mmHg (6.5-9.1KPa). The initial ventilator settings should be; 25% of O_2, rate 25/mt, inspiratory time 0.3 second, pressures 13/2 cms H_2O. Once the baby is intubated and attached to the ventilator at these settings , the blood gases can be checked, and it is then usually possible to drop back to IMV at 5-10 breaths/mt in most cases. It is often very difficult to wean a baby with recurrent apnea off IMV, and this may take 10-14 days in some cases. *Renew the search for underlying illness promptly !*

Treatment of Apnea with Methylxanthines (Theophylline, Caffeine) *Indications*: *To treat infants who are having frequent (5 or more episodes per day) or severe (requiring vigorous stimulation or CPR) apnea or bradycardia. Prior to prescribing theophylline or caffeine, treatable causes of apnea should be excluded, i.e., anemia, seizures, sepsis, hypoxemia, metabolic abnormalities, or gastroesophageal reflux. *To normalize an abnormal pneumogram prior to discharge. *To facilitate weaning from ventilatory support. *Scans while Patients are receiving Theophylline or Caffeine. If an infant has experienced no clinical apnea for 5–7 days while receiving theophylline or caffeine at therapeutic levels and discharge is anticipated within 2–3 weeks, theophylline and caffeine should be discontinued. A pneumogram can be obtained within 48–72 hours of discontinuing theophylline and within 72–96 hours of discontinuing

caffeine. <u>Apnea of prematurity or abnormal scans</u> :If the pneumogram is abnormal and the infant is otherwise ready for discharge, caffeine is started and the infant is referred to the Infant Apnea Program who does outpatient management of apnea of prematurity, home apnea monitors, and also gastroesophageal reflux. An infant discharged home on caffeine will also be placed on a home apnea monitor. Parents will be instructed by the Infant Apnea Program nurses in administration of caffeine, infant CPR, and use of a home monitor. Infants receiving theophylline should be changed to caffeine prior to discharge. Twenty mg/kg/day of caffeine citrate as a loading dose should be given, followed by 5 mg/kg/day maintenance dose. A caffeine serum level should be obtained prior to the second maintenance dose; if the infant is discharge before that time, at least one trough level (prior to a maintenance dose) needs to be obtained.

Pearl/Peril/Pitfall: Management includes correction of any aggravating factors and adequate monitoring of breathing movements (impedance apnoea alarm) and heart rate. If oxygenation is inadequate between apnoeas (PaO2<60) then a small increase in environmental oxygen, e.g. 23–25% may reduce the severity of apnoea. Care must be taken to avoid hyperoxia since the lungs are relatively normal and these immature infants are at risk of retinopathy.

TABLE 4 Assessment of severity of neonatal apnea

Apnea type	Type of intervention	Treatment indication
Spontaneous	No intervention required	Frequent episodes associated with desaturations (SaO_2 <80%) and/or bradycardia (HR <90); e.g. one or more per hour over a long period of time such as 12–24 hours
Mild	Light touch, stroke back Associated with desaturations <80% and bradycardia <90	Multiple episodes; more than 6 over a 12hour period or 12 over a 24hour period
Moderate	Move infant, i.e. roll over, reposition, etc. Oxygen administered	More than 2 episodes in a 24 hour period
Severe	Prolonged vigorous stimulation PPV with or without oxygen	More than 1 episode in a 24 hour period

Note: Apnea, bradycardia, and/or cyanotic spells associated with feeding, handling, suctioning, mucus plugging, etc. should not be counted when determining whether to initiate methylxanthine therapy.

Areas of Uncertainty in Clinical Practice

* **Minimizing apnea after extubation from PPV**

Both CPAP and theophylline will reduce post-extubation apnea.

* **The place of blood transfusion in treatment of apnea** Presence and severity of apnea correlate poorly with the presence of anemia. Theophylline has been shown superior to blood transfusion in improving symptoms of apnea in anemic infants (but in a very small study). The clinical benefits from transfusion appear greater the more severe the level of anemia (the effects are trivial when the haemoglobin is about 10g/dL).

* **Doxapram as medication for symptomatic control of apnea** Doxapram cannot be recommended for the treatment of apnea because of concerns about its safety.

* **Caffeine and Prematurity (CAP) Trial :** The CAP trial, which contained a number of infants managed in Melbourne, found that caffeine reduced the rates of death or disability, cerebral palsy and cognitive delay at 18-21 months corrected age when compared with placebo. Follow up to 5 years of age is ongoing.

* **Use of oxygen by nasal cannulae to control apnea**

High oxygen flows given by nasal cannulae may achieve significant positive distending pressures. Possible side effects include inadequate heating and humidification leading to temperature control problems and increased nasal irritation. Pressures generated are not able to be monitored with this system.

Adverse Effects of Methylxanthine Therapy

*Excessive diuresis *Increased cerebral metabolic rate (X2-3) *Decreased anoxic survival in animal studies *Increased cardiac output *Decreased cerebral blood flow *Increased blood sugar levels *Increased plasma glycerol *Increased lung glycogen metabolism *Decrease cholesterol synthesis in glial cells *Decreased cerebral cell growth and division *Decreased retinal blood flow

Principles of therapy for apnea of prematurity-A Summary!

Therapy for Apnea of Prematurity can be divided arbitrarily into four groupings based on proposed pathogenic mechanisms that might result in apnea. Institution of interventions should occur in the order of increasing invasiveness and risk. Debate regarding risk of interventions persists, some authors advocating use of methylxanthines prior to CPAP therapy.

Increase afferent input into the respiratory centers
* Cutaneous or vestibular stimulation
* Avoid hyperoxia

Treatment of primary depression of respiratory center
* Treat infection
* Correct metabolic disturbances
* Administer central nervous system stimulants (aminophylline, theophylline, caffeine, doxapram)

Treatment of hypoxemia
* Treat HMD, pneumonia, aspiration, etc.
* Increase inspired oxygen
* Apply continuous positive airway pressure (CPAP)
* Prone positioning
* Treat congestive heart failure
* Close patent ductus arteriosus
* Transfuse with packed red blood cells

Avoidance of triggering reflexes
* Beware of suction catheters
* Avoid nipple feedings (feed by tube or intravenously)
* Avoid hyperinflation and hyperventilation during bagging
* Avoid cold stimuli to the face Place infant in the prone position
* Avoid severe flexion of neck
* Treat gastroesophageal reflux

Courtesy: Dennis E. Mayock, M.D. Associate Professor, Pediatrics/ Neonatology University of Washington Seattle, Washington 98195.

Pearl/Peril/Pitfall : The breathing and heart rate of infants born at less than 34 weeks gestation (or more mature infants who are very ill) is usually monitored to detect apnea/bradycardia that may warrant clinical attention. The nursing staff grade events and keep a chart. Grade 1 = Apnoea > 15-20 seconds and/or bradycardia and/or cyanosis associated with cessation of effective breathing efforts, which respond quickly to stimulation. Grade 2 = As above or more prolonged, and responding slowly to stimulation or requiring bag and mask resuscitation.

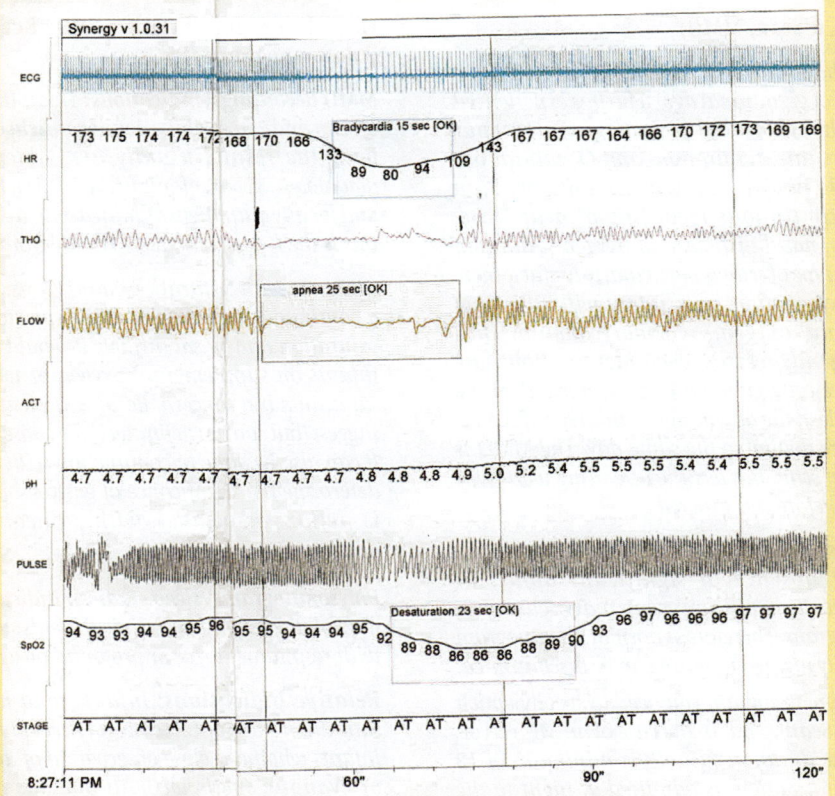

Central apnea is defined as the cessation of both airflow and respiratory effort. ECG = electrocardiogram; HR = heart rate; THO = thoracic impedance; FLOW = air flow; ACT = ; SpO2 = peripheral oxygen saturation; STAGE = sleep stage.

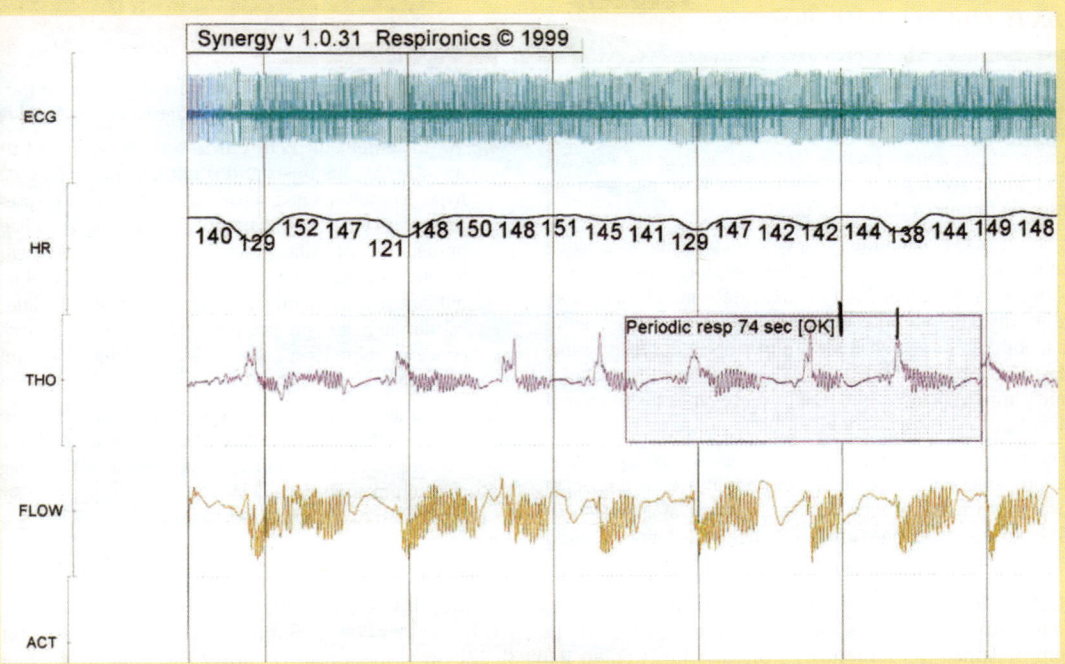

Polysomnogram. Periodic breathing is defined as periods of regular respiration for as long as 20 seconds followed by apneic periods no longer than 10 seconds that occur at least 3 times in succession. ECG = electrocardiogram; HR = heart rate (bpm); THO = thoracic movement; FLOW = flow the from nose and mouth; ACT = gross body movement.

Pneumograms (CR-scan, MMU)

All infants less than 34 weeks gestational age and any infant (regardless of gestational age) who has experienced clinical apnea should have a pneumogram (12-hour recording of heart rate, respiration, and O₂ saturation) performed prior to discharge. A Cardiorespiratory Scan (CR Scan) is a continuous recording of heart rate, breathing pattern, nasal airflow, and oxygen saturation (by pulse-ox); this type of scan is particularly useful if there is concern over oxygenation, as in infant with BPD and/or on supplemental oxygen. A Memory Monitor Unit (MMU) recording only records when monitor limits are violated (therefore only giving a brief "snapshot" of the monitored variables); the advantage to this type of scan is that the results are available the same day. The MMU is the routine type of scan, but ask the attending what type of scan is desired before it is ordered.

*A **pneumogram is not a test for SIDS**: It does document the presence or absence of significant apnea or bradycardia. Clinically significant events may occur before or after a pneumogram. Therefore, a normal pneumogram does not necessarily mean a monitor can be discontinued.*

When ordering a pneumogram you need to specify which type (MMU or CR Scan), and, in the case of an MMU, you need to specify the duration (usually a minimum of 12 hours, although if a patient is admitted at night to the Apnea Center, it may end up being less than 12 hours until morning.

Guidelines for Studies: CR Scans, MMUs and Polysomnograms (PSG)

***MMU Recordings** Indications: This is the most routine type of scan and can easily be done overnight or over several days, with the results usually available within hours of downloading. For infants in the NICU who have had "spells" and for any outpatient admitted with a diagnosis of "apnea", this is the type of scan that would be ordered.*

***CR Scans with Saturation** Indications: This type of scan is a continuous recording of HR, respiratory pattern, oxygen saturation and nasal airflow. It would be appropriate for infants on supplemental oxygen or with BPD where O2 saturation is a concern. Because it measures airflow, it can suggest (but can not definitively diagnose) obstructive apnea. It can also be done in conjunction with a pH probe to help determine the significance of gastroesophageal reflux (i.e., is reflux associated with apnea, bradycardia or desaturation).*

***Polysomnograms (sleep studies): Indications:** Infants with unexplained significant clinical events suggesting a problem with respiratory drive or profound airway obstruction.*

***Relative indications:** Infants who had an abnormal saturation study or CR scan and need additional evaluation. Infants who need close observation of apneic, bradycardic, or cyanotic spells without obvious etiology. Further evaluation of infants who have cyanotic or bradycardic episodes with feedings. Suspected Munchausen by proxy.*

KEY POINTS FOR CLINICAL PRACTICE

1. Apnea is the most common problem of ventilatory control in the premature infant frequently prolonging hospitalization and the need for cardiopulmonary monitoring. The standard definition of apnea is cessation of inspiratory gas flow for 20 seconds, or for a shorter period of time if accompanied by bradycardia (heart rate less than 100 beats per minute), cyanosis, or pallor.

2. Apnea has been classified into three types depending on whether inspiratory muscle activity is present. If inspiratory muscle activity fails following an exhalation, it is termed Central Apnea. If inspiratory muscle activity is present without airflow, this is termed Obstructive Apnea. If both central and obstructive apnea occur during the same episode, this is termed Mixed Apnea. It is important to characterize a patient's apnea episodes into one or more types for treatment consideration.

3. Apnea is only a symptom and frequently occurs secondary to other disease processes. However, 'Apnea of Prematurity' is a specific diagnosis and also one of exclusion. Other causes of apneic spells should be pursued if the apnea progresses in severity, fails to respond to appropriate therapy, severe episodes occur on the first day of life, or it appears at a gestational age where it should not occur.

4. Management of recurrent Idiopathic apnea of prematurity includes a) Diagnosis and treatment of specific causes (e.g., hypoglycemia, anemia, sepsis) b) Nasal continuous positive airway pressure (4 cm H_2O) c) Xanthine (caffeine {now available in India} or theo/aminophylline) therapy, commencing with a loading dose followed by maintenance therapy, and serum level monitoring { difficult in Indian setting}, especially for aminophylline. Doxapram cannot be recommended for the treatment of apnea because of concerns about its safety. d) Initiate mechanical ventilation, if all else fails.

5. Avoidance of Triggering Reflexes is important *Beware of suction catheters *Avoid nipple feedings (feed by tube or intravenously) *Avoid hyperinflation and hyperventilation during bagging *Avoid cold stimuli to the face *Place infant in the prone position *Avoid severe flexion of neck *Treat gastroesophageal reflux

REFERENCES AND FURTHER READING : **1)**A Primer on Apnea of Prematurity L.A. Stokowski Adv Neonatal Care 2005 5 155-170 **2)** Apnoea of Prematurity RJ Martin, JM Abu-Shaweesh, TM Baird Paediatr Respir Rev 2004 5 (Suppl A) S377-82 **3)**Current Options in the Management of Apnea of Prematurity J Bhatia Clin Paediatr 2000 39 327-36 **4)**Abendroth D, Moser DK, Dracup K, Doering LV. Do apnea monitors decrease emotional distress in parents of infants at high risk for cardiopulmonary arrest? *J Pediatr Health Care.* 1999;13:50–57 **5)** High-Flow Nasal Cannulae in the Management of Apnea of Prematurity: A comparison with conventional nasal continuous positive airway pressure C.Sreenan, R.P.Lemke, A. Hudson-Mason, H.Osiovich Pediatrics 2001 107(5) 1081-3

Pearl/Peril/Pitfall : *Major concern for the parents is whether their baby will have apnea at home and die from sudden infant death syndrome (SIDS). Epidemiological studies indicate that while preterm infants are at increased risk of SIDS this is not related to apnea of prematurity. However, an insult such as RSV infection or pertussis can cause a recurrence of apnea in the first few months after discharge. Polygraphic studies at discharge from neonatal units do not predict future SIDS*

37 Neonatal Pulmonary Hemorrhage

@ *The onset of Pulmonary Hemorrhage is characterized by oozing of bloody fluid from the nose and mouth or endotracheal tube with associated rapid worsening of the respiratory status, cyanosis and, in severe cases, shock. Bleeding may be noted from other sites. Radiographic findings range from patchy infiltrates to complete opacification of lung fields.*

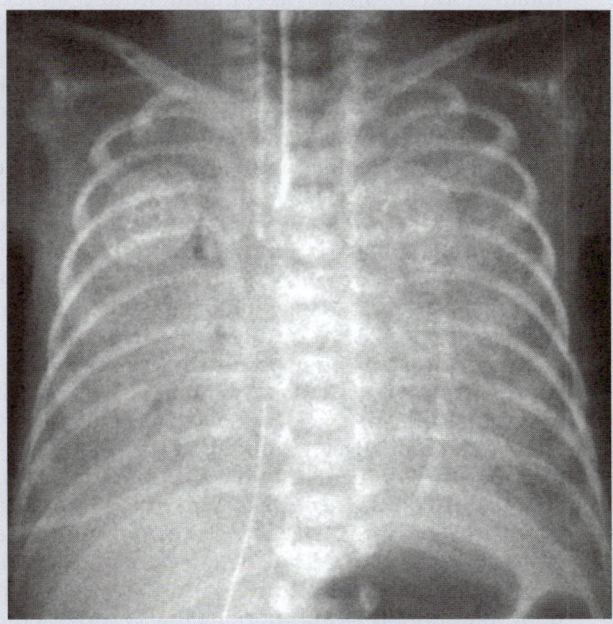

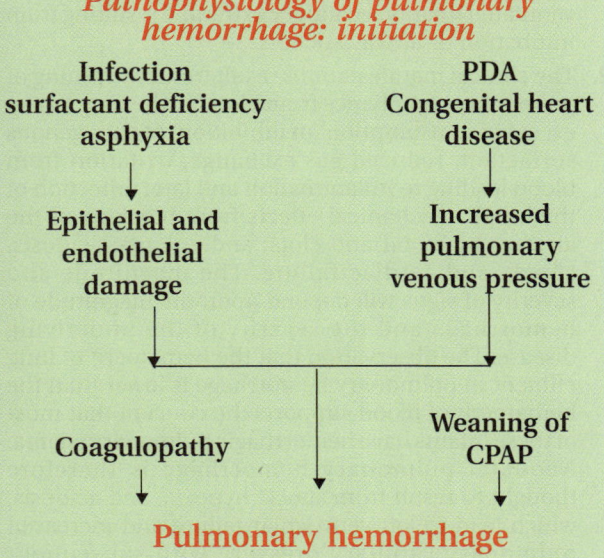

Pathophysiology of pulmonary hemorrhage: initiation

Infection surfactant deficiency asphyxia	PDA Congenital heart disease
↓	↓
Epithelial and endothelial damage	Increased pulmonary venous pressure

Coagulopathy · Weaning of CPAP

Pulmonary hemorrhage

Prematurity is the factor most commonly associated with P-Hem; other associated factors are those that predispose to perinatal asphyxia or bleeding disorders, including toxemia of pregnancy, maternal cocaine use, erythroblastosis fetalis, breech delivery, hypothermia, infection, Respiratory Distress Syndrome, administration of exogenous surfactant (in some studies) and ECMO. Although the pathogenesis is uncertain, it is probable that P-Hem is hemorrhagic pulmonary edema, as the hematocrit is lower than blood and the concentration of small proteins is higher than in plasma. It is postulated that the infant suffers an asphyxial insult with resultant myocardial failure; this increases pulmonary microvascular pressure resulting in pulmonary edema. Subsequently, there is frank bleeding into the pulmonary interstitial and alveolar spaces. Contributing factors include factors that favor increased filtration of fluid from pulmonary capillaries (*e.g.* low concentration of plasma proteins, high alveolar surface tension, lung damage, hypervolemia).

REVIEW OF CLINICAL PROBLEMS

1. Name the risk factors for Neonatal Pulmonary Hemorrhage
   Ans: Refer to Table No 1 of the Chapter.

2. Mention the *role of surfactant* in the etiology and treatment of Pulmonary Hemorrhage.
   Ans: Refer to the "No. 9" of the "BIRD'S EYE VIEW/OVERVIEW/ SYNOPSIS" of the Chapter.

3. What are the investigations to be done in the event of Pulmonary Hemorrhage?
   Ans: Refer to the Evaluation-Decision-Action Plan/Algorithm to diagnose and manage Neonatal Pulmonary Hemorrhage.

4. When should you suspect Pulmonary Hemorrhage Clinically?
   Ans: Refer to the "No. 6" of the "BIRD`S EYE VIEW/OVERVIEW/ SYNOPSIS" of the Chapter.

5. How do you manage Neonatal Pulmonary Hemorrhage generally and specifically?
   Ans: Refer to the Evaluation-Decision-Action Plan/Algorithm to diagnose and manage Neonatal Pulmonary Hemorrhage.

LEARNING OBJECTIVES

After completing this article, readers will be able to

1. Suspect pulmonary hemorrhage, if encountered with Sudden clinical deterioration in an otherwise stable Neonate.

2. Assess and stabilize ABCs, before investigating for the underlying cause of Pulmonary Hemorrhage.

3. Recognize the significant PDA in a Preterm baby with vigilant monitoring, who presents with Pulmonary Hemorrhage and manage it adequately

4. Counsel Parents about the prognosis after clinically significant Pulmonary Hemorrhage.

5. Follow preventive strategies like antenatal steroids, avoiding hypothermia, hypoxia, sepsis if possible.

Pearl/Peril/Pitfall: The onset of P-Hem is characterized by oozing of bloody fluid from the nose and mouth or endotracheal tube with associated rapid worsening of the respiratory status, cyanosis and, in severe cases, shock. Bleeding may be noted from other sites.

BIRD'S EYE VIEW/OVERVIEW/SYNOPSIS

1. Pulmonary hemorrhage is clinically defined as the presence of hemorrhagic fluid in the trachea and oronasopharynx that is accompanied by a respiratory decompensation requiring increased respiratory support or intubation within 60mts of the appearance of the fluid. It should be distinguished from the relatively common occurrence of minor blood staining of respiratory secretions, occurring in ventilated infants secondary to trauma resulting from intubation or airway suction.

2. The clinical manifestations result from: worsening of pulmonary compliance from blood in the lung tissue; excessive consumption (or inhibition) of endogenous surfactant; reduced gas exchange; irritation from blood leading to inflammation and later, infection of the lungs; mechanical effects from blocking of the airways by blood and clots; and anemia, acidosis, shock, and cardiac failure. The magnitude and severity of signs will depend upon the magnitude of hemorrhage and the severity of the underlying disease. The observation that the hematocrit of lung effluent in pulmonary hemorrhage is lower than the hematocrit of blood supports the concept that most of these infants have hemorrhagic pulmonary edema. Neonatal pulmonary hemorrhage is therefore thought to result from shock, hypoxia, and acidosis, which lead to left ventricular failure and increased pulmonary capillary pressure with subsequent hemorrhagic pulmonary edema.

3. Table 1 describes the risk factors i.e. conditions pre-disposing the infant to increased left ventricular filling pressure, increased pulmonary blood volume, compromised pulmonary venous drainage, or poor cardiac contractility. Increased pulmonary blood flow and compromised ventricular function accompanying a symptomatic patent ductus arteriosus in a preterm infant is a significant risk factor. Thrombocytopenia and vascular leak accompanying conditions such as sepsis appears to increase the risk. Coagulopathy is also associated with the occurrence of pulmonary hemorrhage, although it is unclear whether it is an inciting factor or a result of the hemorrhage.

4. Treatment with exogenous surfactant increases left to right ductal shunting and pulmonary blood flow, increasing the likelihood of hemorrhagic pulmonary edema by about 50%, mostly in the smallest prematurely born infants. It has been suggested that the risk of pulmonary hemorrhage following surfactant therapy can be reduced by judicious use of fluids and by closure of the ductus arteriosus.

5. Pulmonary haemorrhage has been reported following a host of insults including sepsis, asphyxia, congenital heart disease, left ventricular failure, intrauterine growth retardation and hypothermia. The heterogeneity of documented underlying disorders emphasizes that the pulmonary hemorrhage is a non-specific end result of these conditions.

6. One should suspect pulmonary hemorrhage, when an otherwise stable infant suddenly deteriorates (usually between the second and fourth day of life) with hypoxia, hypercapnia, and mixed acidosis with an increase in ventilator setting requirements associated with grossly bloody or blood-tinged tracheal and oropharyngeal effluent and shock. *Consider pulmonary hemorrhage, even in the absence of blood or blood-tinged orotracheal effluent, since the bleeding may be interstitial.* In cases of localized, small pulmonary hemorrhage with gradual evolution of signs, the diagnosis of pulmonary hemorrhage is established by exclusion of other causes. Cardiac murmur, and/ or other signs of PDA (full pulses, wide pulse pressure and an active precordium) may be found in 65% of preterm infants with pulmonary hemorrhage. Preterm infants often become inactive, whereas term infants may become agitated due to sudden hypoxia. A sudden deterioration of respiratory function often occurs with increased signs of respiratory distress, cyanosis, poor chest movement and fine crackles, indicative of pulmonary edema on chest auscultation.

7. The *E-D-A Plan/Algorithm* describes the essential aspects of rapid initial assessment, immediate attention with an ABC resuscitation sequence followed by vigorous airway suction, positive pressure ventilation, cautious fluid administration and inotropic support as appropriate. It also reviews the essential investigations (Hemoglobin, platelets and hematocrit, CXR, echocardiogram, ABG analysis, sepsis and coagulation screen, viral and fungal cultures as appropriate) and the supportive measures to be instituted. The mainstay of treatment is: *Maintenance of oxygenation *Control of cardiac failure with hemodynamic support *Correction of hematological abnormalities *Treatment of the underlying problem. After initial resuscitation, management should focus on maintaining stability.

8. IPPV(Intermitent Positive Pressure Ventilation) is required in all infants with massive pulmonary hemorrhage. The main aim is to improve oxygenation and preventing further bleeding. A high PEEP(6-8cm of H2O) and a long inspiration time(0.4-0.5) provides adequate oxygenation and redistributes lung fluid back into the interstitial space, improving gas exchange and ventilation perfusion mismatch. HFO's role is unproven in the management of pulmonary hemorrhage and may be potentially dangerous.

9. Although administration of exogenous surfactant is associated with onset of pulmonary hemorrhage, paradoxically further surfactant administration may be beneficial after the event to prevent secondary surfactant deficiency/inactivation due to contamination with Hb and RBC lipids.

10. Antenatal corticosteroids, vigilant monitoring for the signs of PDA in extremely small preterm infants with RDS requiring assisted ventilation are important to prevent pulmonary hemorrhage.

---

* ***Pearl/Peril/Pitfall :*** *Immediate treatment of P-Hem should include tracheal suction, oxygen and positive pressure ventilation. To assist in decreasing P-Hem, mean airway pressure should be increased, either by a relatively high PEEP (i.e., 6 to 10 cmH2O) or by high frequency ventilation.*

THE EVALUATION-DECISION-ACTION-PLAN/ALGORITHM FOR THE DIAGNOSIS AND MANAGEMENT OF *NEONATAL PULMONARY HEMORRHAGE*

SUBJECTIVE FINDINGS

Hx of Sudden clinical deterioration in an otherwise stable neonate, in association with grossly bloody/blood tinged tracheal or oropharyngeal effluent.

Hx of initial passage of small amounts of blood coming up the E.T. Tube/oropharynx-may be followed by massive hemorrhage leading to shock, apnea, dyspnea, pallor, restlessness, hypoxemia.

Hx of cardiac murmur and/ or other signs of PDA or other causes of Lt to Rt shunts.

Consider pulmonary hemorrhage in the presence of systemic shock and sudden deterioration, even in the absence of blood or blood tinged orotracheal effluent, since the bleeding may be interstitial.

OBJECTIVE FINDINGS

Assess ABCs, disability, O_2 sats, CRT, BP, Vitals, Urine output

Look for the presence of blood/blood tinged orotracheal effluent, presence of PDA murmur and other signs of PDA

Look for signs of cardiac failure-tachycardia, gallop rhythm, hepatomegaly etc.

Look for bleeding from multiple sites- skin, GIT, Urinary, CNS

Look for reduced chest air entry and for wide spread crepitations.

Look for signs of sepsis

INVESTIGATIONS

Blood FBC with hematocrit, platelets, differential count, coagulation screen, ABG analysis, blood sugar, electrolytes, albumin, creatinine, BUN, Ca^{++}, blood cultures, CRP

CXR

Urine analysis to rule out major bleeding in the kidney

Echocardiogram even in the absence of a typical PDA murmur

Cranial ultra sound examination to rule out intracranial hemorrhage

---

A NEONATE WITH PULMONARY HEMORRHAGE

Ensure airway and breathing by a)vigorous airway suction b)positive pressure ventilation at higher rate, PEEP of 6–8 cm H_2O and a higher mean airway pressure

Ensure frequent E.T.Tube suction to prevent airway obstruction and tube blockage and adequate humidification of ventilator gases to prevent clotting of bloody secretions. Don't apply chest physiotherapy immediately after pulmonary hemorrhage

Consider administering exogenous surfactant for continued treatment of RDS or to treat secondary surfactant deficiency resulting from inhibition by hemoglobin and plasma proteins after pulmonary hemorrhage.

High frequency ventilation controversial, not clinically proven and potentially dangerous

Explain prognosis to the parents :

Institute antishock measures—transfuse with blood, plasma or platelets as indicated and *support* systemic blood pressure with inotropic agents. *Correct* acidosis through restoration of adequate ventilation and blood pressure. *Correct* metabolic acidosis with bicarbonate therapy as indicated

Restrict fluids, if signs of fluid overload, CCF or PDA occur in infants with pulmonary hemorrhage. Echocardiography may be helpful to assess LV function, need for pressor support, and the possible contribution of a PDA.

Commence IV broadspectrum antibiotics after an infection screen performed, as bacterial sepsis is common in infants with pulmonary hemorrhage

Treat pre-existing coagulation abnormalities or secondary DIC, as a consequence of pulmonary hemorrhage with platelet transfusion and FFP, as appropriate

Manage hemodynamically significant PDA with indomethacin/ibuprofen if no contraindications exist(e.g. severe thrombocytopenia-<20,000/cumm and renal failure); consider surgical ligation if medical management fails or contraindications to medical treatment exist

*Pulmonary hemorrhage-outcome

Clinically significant PH (moderate–severe)
- Mortality 27%
- Majority from respiratory failure
* BPD
- 50% of survivors
- Greatly increased duration of MV and
* Oxygen
- 100% were on Oxygen at 28 days
- Survival without BPD 33%
* CNS morbidity increased
- IVH 53%
- Increased severity of IVH
- PVL 13%

Treatment of pulmonary hemorrhage
All anecdotal
* PEEP—Improves lung mechanics—Tamponades bleeding
* HFOV and HFJV—Tendency to use higher MAP
* Surfactant—Inactivation of Surfactant by blood component
* Steroids—Balance short term vs long term

Pearl/Peril/Pitfall: Prematurity is the factor most commonly associated with P-Hem; other associated factors are those that predispose to perinatal asphyxia or bleeding disorders, including toxemia of pregnancy, maternal cocaine use, erythroblastosis fetalis, breech delivery, hypothermia, infection, Respiratory Distress Syndrome, administration of exogenous surfactant (in some studies) and ECMO.

TABLE 1   Infants at risk for neonatal pulmonary hemorrhage

A. Host factors

1. <28 weeks gestation and/or <1,000 gm birth weight
2. Small for gestational age
3. Twin

B. Etiology and underlying clinical considerations

1. Respiratory distress syndrome (RDS), especially following treatment with either synthetic or natural exogenous surfactant
2. Patent ductus arteriosus (PDA)
3. Pulmonary interstitial emphysema (PIE) and/or pneumothorax
4. Systemic or pulmonary infections: bacterial, viral, or fungal (*Listeria* and *Hemophilus influenzae* are notorious)
5. Severe metabolic acidosis during the first week of life
6. Hypothermia, hypoglycemia, and shock during the first week of life
7. Extracorporeal membrane oxygenation (ECMO) - severe pulmonary hemorrhage might develop even after decannulation

8. Disseminated intravascular coagulation (DIC) from any cause
9. Trauma to the vocal cords, trachea, or other laryngeal and oropharyngeal structures (difficult and/or traumatic intubation
10. In experimental animals, inhaled Nitric Oxide (NO) at concentrations of 80ppm has been shown to cause pulmonary hemorrhage because of increased production of Nitrogen Dioxide (1ppm).

* Although most infants who develop pulmonary hemorrhage have the predisposing factors of extreme prematurity and underlying asphyxia and stress, there are a few case reports describing previously healthy, term infants with pulmonary hemorrhage associated with an inborn error of the urea cycle and elevated blood ammonia.

* Although disseminated intravascular coagulation may precede pulmonary hemorrhage, most infants with pulmonary hemorrhage do not have a coagulopathy. Pulmonary hemorrhage generally presents within the first week of life, and the mortality rate after pulmonary hemorrhage is estimated to be 75% to 90%.

KEY POINTS FOR CLINICAL PRACTICE

1. Pulmonary hemorrhage (P-Hem) is an acute, catastrophic event characterized by discharge of bloody fluid from the upper respiratory tract or the endotracheal tube. The incidence of P-Hem is 1 in 1,000 live births

2. Prematurity is the factor most commonly associated with P-Hem; other associated factors are those that predispose to perinatal asphyxia or bleeding disorders, including toxemia of pregnancy, maternal cocaine use, erythroblastosis fetalis, breech delivery, hypothermia, infection, respiratory distress syndrome, administration of exogenous surfactant (in some studies) and ECMO.

3. Radiographic findings range from patchy infiltrates to complete opacification of lung fields. Hematocrit of the P-Hem fluid is usually 15 to 20% less than blood.

4. Immediate treatment of P-Hem should include tracheal suction, oxygen and positive pressure ventilation. To assist in decreasing P-Hem, mean airway pressure should be increased, either by a relatively high PEEP (*i.e.* 6 to 10 cmH$_2$O) or by high frequency ventilation. Correct underlying abnormalities, especially disorders of coagulation. When blood loss is large, prompt blood transfusion may be needed to maintain an adequate circulating blood volume. The outcome is dependent on the cause of P-Hem. Mortality is 30 to 40%.

5. Antenatal corticosteroids, vigilant monitoring for the signs of PDA in extremely small preterm infants with RDS requiring assisted ventilation are important to prevent pulmonary hemorrhage.

REFERENCES AND FURTHER READING 1)Fanaroff aa, Martin rj. Neonatal-Perinatal Medicine: Diseases of the Fetus and Infant, 7th Edition, St Louis, MO:Mosby, 2001. 2) Raju TNK, Langenberg P. Pulmonary hemorrhage and exogenous surfactant therapy: a meta analysis. *JP* 1993 123:603-10. 3) Greenough A, Roberton NRC Acute respiratory disease in the newborn ;NRC Roberton's Textbook of Neonatology, 4th edition 4) Kluckow M, Evans N. Ductal shunting, high pulmonary blood flow, and pulmonary hemorrhage. *JP* 2000, 137-68-72.5) Manual of neonatal care John P Cloherty 6th edition Lippincot Williams and Wilkins.

Pearl/Peril/Pitfall : Although the pathogenesis is uncertain, it is probable that P-Hem is hemorrhagic pulmonary edema, as the hematocrit is lower than blood and the concentration of small proteins is higher than in plasma. It is postulated that the infant suffers an asphyxial insult with resultant myocardial failure; this increases pulmonary microvascular pressure resulting in pulmonary edema. Subsequently, there is frank bleeding into the pulmonary interstitial and alveolar spaces. Contributing factors include factors that favor increased filtration of fluid from pulmonary capillaries (e.g., low concentration of plasma proteins, high alveolar surface tension, lung damage, hypervolemia).

38 Neonatal Thoracic Airleak Syndrome

@ *Pneumothorax must be considered in mechanically ventilated infants who develop unexplained alterations in hemodynamics, pulmonary compliance, or oxygenation and ventilation. Clinical signs of pneumothorax range from insidious changes in vital signs to the complete cardiovascular collapse that frequently accompanies a tension pneumothorax.*

Ectopic air leaks can occur in Newborn infants. There are several types: *Pulmonary interstitial emphysema (PIE)—air in the interstitial lung spaces. *Pneumothorax—air in the pleural space. *Pneumomediastinum—air in the anterior mediastinum. *Pneumopericardium—air in the pericardial space. *Pneumoperitoneum—air in the peritoneal cavity. *Pneumoscrotum—air in the scrotum. *Air embolus—air descending into pulmonary veins and disseminating throughout the blood stream. *Surgical emphysema—air in the subcutaneous tissue.

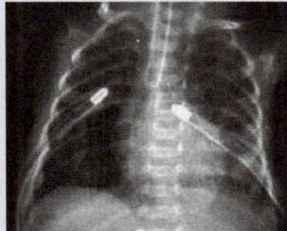

Bilateral Pneumothorax and PIE with ICD

The method of transillumination (TI) or diaphanoscopy in the field of pediatrics was first mentioned for the diagnostics of the hydrocephalus in the sixties of the last century. In the following decades, this method was applied for the quick identification of pneumothorax and pneumoperitoneum and for the diagnosing a hydrocele in the neonatal period.

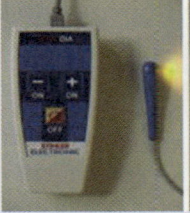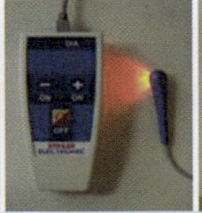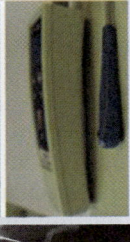

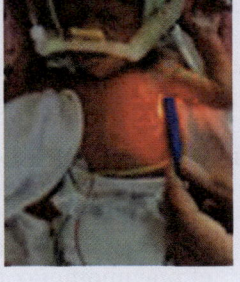

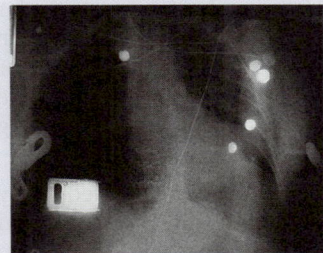

This picture shows a chest radiograph with 2 abnormalities: (1) tension pneumothorax and (2) potentially life-saving intervention delayed while waiting for X-ray results. *Tension pneumothorax* is a clinical diagnosis requiring emergent needle decompression, and therapy should never be delayed for X-ray confirmation.

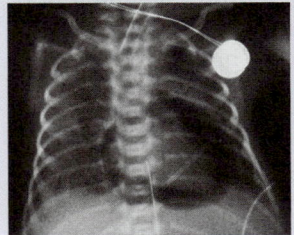

Pneumopericardium. There is an obvious pocket of air that completely surrounds the heart, and the pericardial space, normally not visible, is readily apparent. In most instances, this finding represents an acute, life-threatening emergency, marked by the physical changes seen in this infant: sudden deterioration in respiratory status, cyanosis, and decreased and distant heart sounds. Note Pulmonary Interstitial Emphysema as well.

REVIEW OF CLINICAL PROBLEMS

1. Name the diagnostic and therapeutic aspects of a Significant Pneumothorax in a Neonate.
   Ans: Refer to the "No.3" of the "BIRD'S EYE VIEW/OVERVIEW/SYNOPSIS" of the Chapter.

2. Mention the complications of a Significant Pneumothorax in a Neonate.
   Ans: Refer to the "No.4" of the "BIRD'S EYE VIEW/OVERVIEW/SYNOPSIS" of the Chapter.

3. What are the investigations to be done to determine the presence of Thoracic air leaks?
   Ans: Refer to the Evaluation-Decision-Action Plan/Algorithm to diagnose and manage Neonatal Thoracic Air leaks.

4. How do you manage Pneumopericardium?
   Ans: Refer to the Evaluation-Decision-Action Plan/Algorithm to diagnose and manage Neonatal Thoracic Air leaks.

5. Discuss the essentials of diagnosis and management of Pulmonary Interstitial Emphysema? *Ans: Refer to the "No.9" of the "BIRD'S EYE VIEW/OVERVIEW/SYNOPSIS" of the Chapter.*

LEARNING OBJECTIVES

After completing this article, readers will be able to

1. Consider Pneumothorax in any Neonate presented with an Acute Collapse.

2. Transilluminate the chest for possible Pneumothorax, when a mechanically ventilated Neonate develops unexplained sudden/gradual (over a brief period) deterioration in oxygenation and ventilation.

3. Institute chest tube drainage in all symptomatic Neonates and in Tension Pneumothoraces.

4. Anticipate and manage the complications of a Significant Pneumothorax.

5. Identify other air leaks such as Pneumopericardium, Pneumomediastinum, Pneumoperitoneum and Pulmonary Interstitial Emphysema and manage them appropriately.

Pearl/Peril/Pitfall: Treatment of tension pneumothorax requires immediate surgical drainage and placement of a chest tube. For treatment of pneumothorax that does not involve tension or cardiovascular compromise, inhalation of 100% oxygen, usually for 4 to 6 hours, can be used as a nitrogen washout method in term infants. Premature infants should not be treated with hyperoxia because they are at risk for ROP.

BIRD'S EYE VIEW/OVERVIEW/SYNOPSIS

1. Thoracic Air leak refers to a collection of gas outside the pulmonary space, which include a variety disorders like a)pneumothorax b)pneumomediastinum c) pneumo-pericardium d) pulmonary interstitial emphysema, e) pneumoperitonium and f)subcutaneous emphysema. Air leak syndromes arise by a common pathway that involves damage of the respiratory epithelium, usually by high transpulmonary pressures. Damaged epithelium allows air to enter the interstitium causing pulmonary interstitial emphysema. With continued high transpulmonary pressures, air dissects toward the visceral pleura and/or hilum via peribronchial or perivascular spaces.

2. The incidence, risk factors and a brief pathophysiology of air leak syndromes are summarized in Table 1.

3. Pneumothorax must be considered in mechanically ventilated infants who develop unexplained alterations in hemodynamics, pulmonary compliance, or oxygenation and ventilation. Clinical signs of pneumothorax range from insidious changes in vital signs to the complete cardiovascular collapse that frequently accompanies a tension pneumothorax. Spontaneous pneumothorax occurs in 1% of normal term infants around the time of birth; only about 10% of these are symptomatic. Diagnosis is made using the combination of clinical signs, physical examination, ABG analysis, transillumination, and radiography. Asymptomatic pneumothoraces need no treatment other than careful observation of the infant. A small, symptomatic pneumothorax may respond to increasing the inspired oxygen content concentration to 100%, as resorption of the extra-alveolar air occurs via Nitrogen washout (should not be used for preterm infants at risk of ROP). Needle aspiration is not recommended, other than as a diagnostic procedure when the infant is in extremis and there are no other diagnostic aids immediately available. Chest tube drainage must always be instituted in symptomatic preterm babies, in all babies who are receiving mechanical ventilation (unless the pneumothorax is very small and not associated with any deterioration in clinical conditions) and in all those with tension pneumothoraces.

4. The complications of significant pneumothorax include a) profound ventilatory and circulatory compromise and death b)IVH secondary to fluctuating cerebrovascular pressures, impaired venous return, hypercapnia, hypoxia and acidosis c)SIADH.

5. Pneumomediastinum, results from the dissection of pulmonary interstitial air into the mediastinum or when direct trauma occurs to the airways or the posterior pharynx: diagnosed by distant heart sounds, air collections on chest X-ray are central and elevate or surround the thymus *(spinnaker sail sign)*. Management includes a) observation for other airleaks b)reducing the mean airway pressure in mechanically ventilated infants, if possible, c)rarely, mediastinostomy may be necessary if the air is under tension and does not decompress into the pleural space, the retroperitoneum, or the soft tissues of the neck.

6. Pneumopericardium is the least common form of air leak in Newborns but the most common cause of cardiac tamponade; most cases occur in preterm infants with RDS treated with mechanical ventilation, preceded by PIE and pneumomediastinum and the mortality is around 80%. The diagnostic and therapeutic management of pneumopericardium has been summarized in the E-D-A Plan/Algorithm to manage airleaks in the Newborn.

7. Pneumoperitoneum is the intraperitoneal air which may result from extrapulmonary air that decompresses into the abdominal cavity and is of little clinical importance, *but must be differentiated from intraperitoneal air resulting from a perforated viscus.*

8. Subcutaneous emphysema can be detected by palpation of crepitus in the face, neck, or supraclavicular region; usually of no clinical significance, large collections of air in the neck can partially occlude or obstruct the compressible, cartilaginous trachea of the premature infant. Always exclude Co-existing Thoracic airleaks.

9. PIE (Pulmonary Interstitial Emphysema) frequently develops in the first 48 hrs of life, most often in mechanically ventilated, extremely preterm infants with RDS or sepsis. The interstitial air can be localized or can spread to involve significant portions of one or both lungs. It can dissect toward the hilum and the pleural surface via the adventitial connective tissue surrounding the lymphatics and pulmonary vessels, and can compromise lymphatic drainage and pulmonary blood flow. PIE decreases lung compliance, increases residual volume and dead space, and enhances ventilation/perfusion mismatch. The interstitial air may be ruptured into the pleural space and mediastinum and can result in pneumothorax and pneumomediastinum, respectively. The E-D-A Plan/ Algorithm summarizes the essential aspects of the diagnosis and management of PIE. (Refer to Chapter 39 for more details).

10. Systemic air embolism is a rare but fatal complication of pulmonary air leak and may be the result of disruption of the pulmonary venous system or by inadvertent injection through an intravascular catheter. The presence of air bubbles in blood withdrawn from an umbilical artery catheter can be diagnostic.

Pearl/Peril/Pitfall : Prompt recognition of air leak is essential for effective therapy. Unexpected changes in ventilatory requirements or status and abrupt fall in blood pressure, heart rate, respiratory rate, and PO_2 may indicate an air leak. Transillumination of the thorax can be useful in the diagnosis of pneumothorax and the response to therapy.

THE EVALUATION-DECISION-ACTION-PLAN/ALGORITHM FOR THE DIAGNOSIS AND MANAGEMENT OF *NEONATAL THORACIC AIR LEAK SYNDROME*

SUBJECTIVE FINDINGS

Hx of risk factors like sepsis, pneumonia, RDS and mechanical ventilation in preterms

Hx of MAS, pneumonia, congenital malformations and mechanical ventilation in term infants

Hx of respiratory distress, cyanosis, episodes of apnea and bradycardia, abdominal distention—either with sudden onset or gradual deterioration.

Hx of Spontaneous onset—in delivery room or post operatively.

OBJECTIVE FINDINGS

Assess ABCs, O_2 sats, Vitals, BP, CRT, disability and Urine output

Look for chest asymmetry with expansion of the affected side, shift in the point of maximum cardiac impulse, diminished or distant breath sounds on the affected side

Perform Transillumination test with a high intensity fibreoptic light source to demonstrate a pneumothorax (less sensitive in infants with chest wall edema or severe PIE)

CXR AP view confirms the clinical diagnosis - Needle aspiration may confirm the diagnosis and be therapeutic, in a rapidly deteriorating clinical situation.

INVESTIGATIONS

ABG Analysis demonstrates hypoxia and hypercarbia with respiratory and/or mixed acidosis because of circulatory compromise.

CXR findings in air leaks

a) Pneumothorax: hyperlucent hemithorax, separation of visceral from the parietal pleura, flattening of the diaphragm, and mediastinal shift.

b) PIE: Two patterns are seen; cyst like and linear

c) Pneumomediastinum: Central air collections and elevate the thymus.

d) Pneumopericardium: Air surrounds the heart and air under the inferior surface of the heart is diagnostic.

A NEONATE WITH AIR LEAKS

NEONATAL PNEUMOTHORAX

→ Dx clinical Fiberoptic light source CXR

Asymptomatic—Small ← → *Symptomatic*

↳ Observe

↳ Monitor—Vital signs blood gases

No assisted ventilation   Assisted ventilation

Spontaneous resolution

Clinically well tolerated ← *Clinically not well tolerated*   *Institute Pleural drainage*

↓   ↓

100% O_2 with N_2 wash out -Short duration - Monitor PO_2 carefully to avoid O_2 toxicity

-Clinical or Biochem deterioration ↓BP ↓CVP evidence of *tension*

Resolution   No Resolution → *INSTITUTE Pleural drainage*

* Drainage by aspiration using a syringe and butterfly is not recommended, other than as a diagnostic procedure when the infant is in extremis and there are no other diagnostic aids immediately available. Care must be taken not to remove too much air, otherwise the lung may be punctured by the needle and when the drain is subsequently inserted, it is likely to be inserted directly into the lung parenchyma.

* Although asymptomatic pneumothoraces need no treatment other than careful observation of the infant, a pneumothorax must always be drained in symptomatic preterm babies, in all babies who are receiving mechanical ventilation and in all those with tension pneumothoraces.

* Persistent pneumothorax refractory to routine measures may improve with High-Frequency Oscillation Ventilation (HFOV); some infants require ECMO.

* Sometimes one has to place catheters under ultrasound or fluoroscopic guidance to drain air collections that are inaccessible by standard techniques.

PIE (Pulmonary interstitial emphysema)

* *Diagnosed by* CXR showing either linear or cyst like radiolucencies in a preterm infant with RDS or sepsis, most often mechanically ventilated. May be accompanied by hypotension, bradycardia, hypercarbia, hypoxia and acidosis.

* *Managed by* decreasing mean airway pressure by lowering PIP, PEEP and inspiratory time. Minimize ET Suctioning and manual PPV. Position the infant with the affected lung dependent, if the PIE is unilateral. Initiate HFOV(High Frequency Oscillatory Ventilation) earlier to improve the chances of survival.

Pneumomediastinum

* *Diagnosed by* central air collection resulting in "wind - blown spinnaker sail" sign on CXR (a lobe or lobes of the thymus being elevated off the heart); best seen on lateral view.

* *Managed by* observation for any cardiorespiratory compromise, which occurs rarely and needs mediastino-stomy drainage. Otherwise it doesn't require any drainage procedure.

Pneumopericardium

* *Diagnosed by* air surrounding the heart including the inferior surface of the heart, shown on CXR AP view. ECG with decreased voltages is consistent with pneumo-pericardium.

* *Managed by* expectantly if asymptomatic and by needle aspiration if cardiac tamponade (Hypotension, Bradycardia, cyanosis, decreased pulse pressure) ensues.

Pneumoperitoneum

* *Diagnosed by* air under the diaphragm on plain abdominal X-ray. The presence of an intra abdominal air-fluid level, leakage of radiographic isotonic contrast agents, analysis of oxygen saturation levels or PO2 in intraperitoneal air can be used to distinguish whether the air leak is pulmonary or gastrointestinal in origin.

* *Managed* conservatively if evidence of pulmonary air leak precedes or simultaneously appears with pneum-operitoneum: laparotomy required in cases of bowel perforation.

Pearl/Peril/Pitfall: Pneumothorax during respiratory distress is associated with an increased risk of intraventricular hemorrhage, chronic lung disease, and death. Pneumothoraces occur in critically ill ventilated neonates despite treatment with antenatal corticosteroids, surfactant, and less aggressive ventilation in persistent pulmonary hypertension of the newborn.

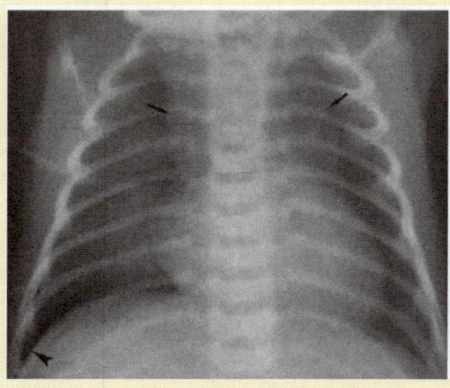
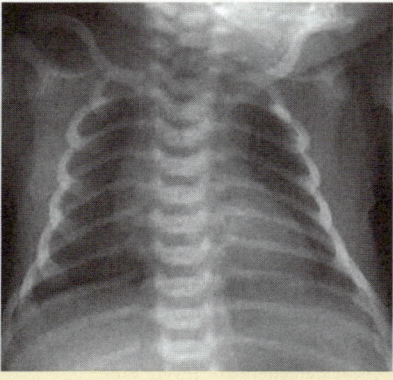
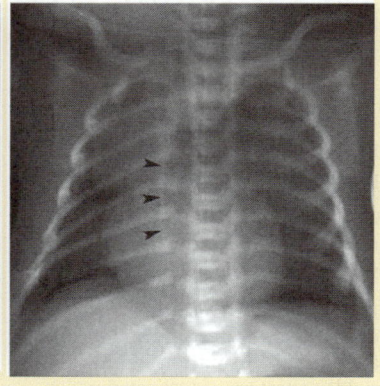

Bilateral pneumothoraces. **(a)** Anteroposterior chest radiograph shows juxtamediastinal lucencies and bisagittal compression of the lobes of the thymus (arrows), producing a "figure 8" configuration contour. A "deep sulcus sign" (arrowhead) is seen in the right lung. **(b)** On a radiograph obtained after spontaneous resolution of air leak, the mediastinal contour appears normal. **(c)** Frontal chest radiograph obtained with the infant rotated toward the right reveals the anterior junction line (arrowheads) outlined by pleural gas. Both diaphragm leaflets and the right aspect of the cardiothymic silhouette are abnormally well defined

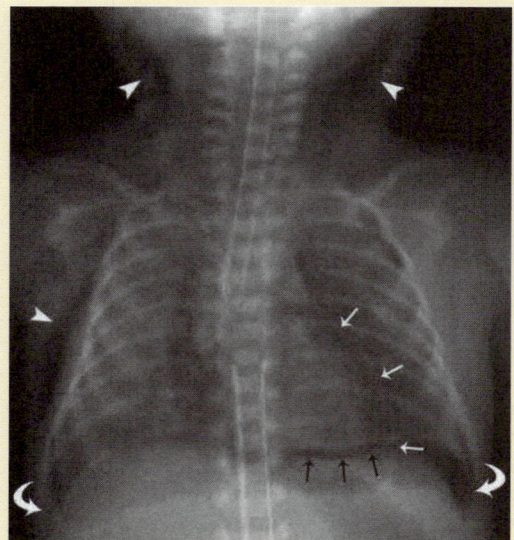

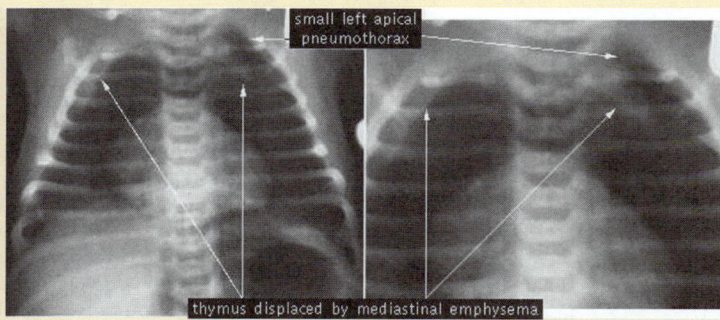

Pneumomediastinum. Frontal chest radiograph shows the lobes of the thymus (arrows), which are displaced superolaterally by a large central lucent area.
(Spinnaker sail sign)

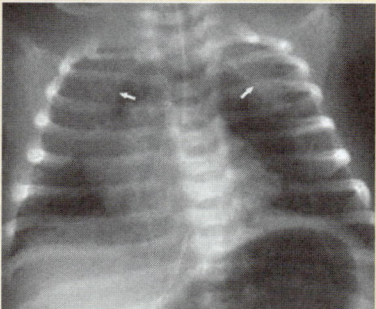

Extensive air leak in a premature neonate who received positive-pressure assisted ventilation for treatment of RDS. Frontal chest radiograph demonstrates a thin pericardial membrane (straight white arrows), which is defined medially by intrapericardial gas and laterally by pleural or mediastinal gas. Extrapleural gas outlines the medial aspect of the left diaphragm (black arrows). Bilateral pneumothoraces produce deep sulcus signs (curved arrows). Mediastinal gas tracks into the cervical soft tissues and right lateral chest wall (arrowheads). The tip of the endotracheal tube enters the right mainstem bronchus.

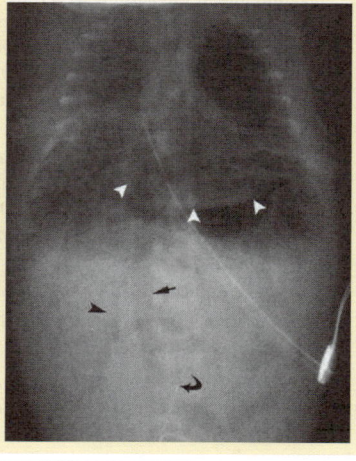

Systemic air embolism in the setting of diffuse bilateral PIE. Frontal radiograph of the chest and abdomen shows elevation and compression of the base of the heart (white arrowheads) by tension pneumopericardium. The cardiac chambers are filled with gas, and intraluminal gas is demonstrated in the inferior vena cava (straight arrow), hepatic veins (black arrowhead), and abdominal aorta surrounding the tip of the umbilical artery catheter (curved arrow). Both lungs are overexpanded by innumerable cystic lucencies representing PIE. (Courtesy of Gael J. Lonergan, MD, Austin Radiological Association, Austin, Tex.)

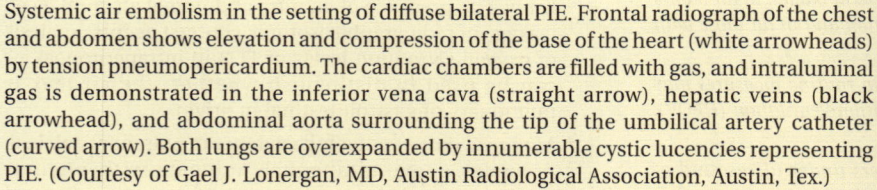

Pearl/Peril/Pitfall : *Unintentional overventilation was not associated with pneumothoraces. In the hours before diagnosis, there was increased clinical intervention, including reintubation; this was less so in those diagnosed by transillumination. The study did not elucidate whether such interventions caused the pneumothorax or were secondary to a failure to diagnose it. (Arch Dis Child Fetal Neonatal Ed 2001;85:F201–F203).*

Severe Air Leak Syndrome Management
by Alan R. Spitzer, MD
Case:

You have been caring for the following infant for the past week when he suddenly deteriorates. He is an 820 g infant born to Gravida 3 Para 0, now 1, mother at 26½ weeks gestation. Pregnancy was complicated by pre-term premature rupture of membranes at 21 weeks' gestation, requiring hospitalization since that time. The mother was given two courses of prenatal glucocorticoids, one course immediately after admission to the hospital and a second course 10 days prior to delivery. The mother received tocolytic therapy throughout the period of hospitalization with magnesium sulfate. Approximately 24 hours before delivery, the mother's temperature rose to 100.8o F and she began to contract. Because of the concern of infection, the mother was allowed to deliver. Apgar scores for this infant were 6 and 8 at one and five minutes respectively. Shortly after birth, however, the child was noted to be grunting and retracting, and he subsequently received two doses of surfactant. He required mechanical ventilation for severe RDS, and at the time of his event, he was in 78% oxygen, with pressures of 22/6 cm H2O at a rate of 40 breaths per minute. An arterial blood gas two hours before deterioration revealed a pH of 7.31, pCO2 of 48 torr, and a pO2 of 76 torr. Transillumination of the chest at the time of deterioration revealed bilateral air leaks and chest tube insertion was promptly initiated, since the pulse oximetry demonstrated of a saturation of only 58%. After bilateral chest tune insertion, the saturation increased, but only to 74%, and the following radiograph was obtained:

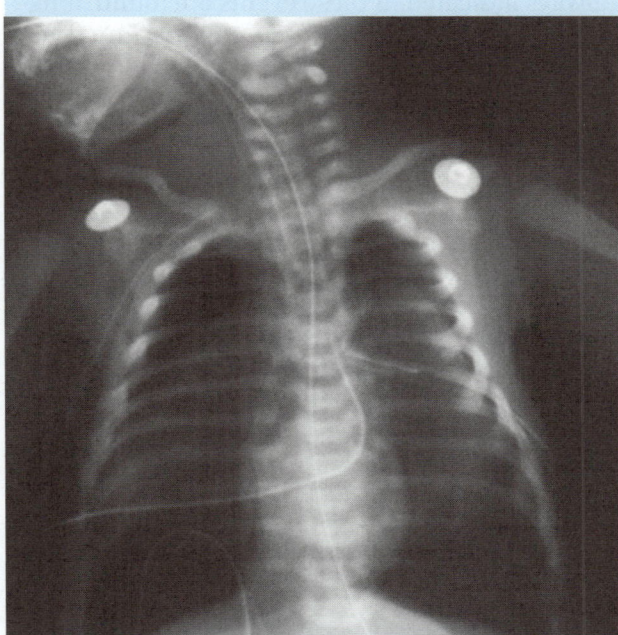

Image courtesy: Neil Ackerman, MD

Points for Discussion

1. What abnormalities still exist in this infant on the radiograph?
2. Why does the cardiac silhouette appear the way it does?
3. What should the chest tube management be at this time?
4. What are the likely sequelae from this series of events?

Discussion

This infant demonstrates the numerous hazards that one often encounters with air leak syndromes and the reasons why they are so feared. Air leaks can occur at any time in the premature infant who needs any form of respiratory assistance. Even oxygen administration itself is associated with a greater risk of air leak. That risk is compounded with the use of high flow nasal cannula, CPAP, or mechanical ventilation. In infants below 1500 grams birth weight, the risk of significant air leaks is about 10–15% with CPAP and about 30% with mechanical ventilation.

Once an air leak has occurred that requires intervention, it is not uncommon to have recurring problems for some period of time. Often, the recurrence of air leaks can leave the NICU staff stressed for days with an infant's care, since it seems that every time one moves away from the bedside for even a moment, the patient has developed a new tension pneumothorax. In the current radiograph, however, several problems exist that may explain why this child continues to manifest ongoing problems. First of all, there are still bilateral tension pneumothoraces. It is possible to recognize that the air leaks are under tension because the infant has both a highly compressed cardiac silhouette and deeply depressed diaphragms, residing at the T11–T12 level. While we often assume that a pneumothorax under pressure will shift the cardiac silhouette to the side opposite the air leak, when there are bilateral air leaks, the heart remains in the midline, but becomes severely constricted as the increased intrathoracic pressure inhibits cardiac filling. It should be noted that this type of cardiac silhouette can be seen in the absence of actual tension pneumothoraces, and may also occur with severe pulmonary interstitial emphysema. The interstitium of the lung fills with air in such situations, expanding the non-exchangeable gas volume to a severe degree that it acts to compress the heart, thereby impeding cardiac filling. In these cases, the creation of a pneumothorax by the insertion of chest tubes and lung perforation may be necessary and the only way to evacuate the air that is compressing the heart and the lung. While this approach sounds counterintuitive, it may be life-saving in some situations. In addition to the bilateral pneumothoraces, it is evident that the chest tube insertion is suboptimal. The chest tube on the right side has not entered the pleural space and is extrathoracic. On the left, the tube enters the chest through the 6th intercostal space and appears to be reasonably well placed, although one cannot tell from the AP view alone whether it lies anteriorly or posteriorly. Only a cross-table lateral radiograph will clarify this issue. One should remember that air leaks typically lie superior in a supine infant, so that a chest tube that is placed inferiorly may look as if it is in a good place on the AP view, but may be of little value to the infant and should be removed if it sits beneath the lung. From this X-ray, several steps should be immediately implemented. The right chest tube should be pulled and a new one placed in the 5th intercostal space in the mid to anterior axillary line. The most common error that is made in placing a chest tube is the failure to position the baby appropriately prior to the chest tube insertion.

Pearl/Peril/Pitfall: A pattern of increasing ventilation and an apparent need to reintubate or initiate resuscitative procedures in ventilated babies must be accompanied by a prompt search for a pneumothorax. This should include transillumination of the chest.

Pearl/Peril/Pitfall: During pneumopericardium tamponade of the heart occurs: ·cardiac output decreases ·heart rate increases ·perfusion becomes poor ·blood pressure and pulse pressure drop ·heart sounds become muffled.

Infants are often left supine for chest tube insertion, which is incorrect. When a chest tube is inserted with the child lying supine, the tube typically hits the lateral aspect of the lung and tracks inferiorly. The infant should be placed instead on his or her side, with the air leak that is being addressed in the superior position. This allows the air to rise and also forces the lung posteriorly so that a better track for an anterior chest tube can be achieved. One should also never neglect local anesthesia for chest tube placement. While an argument can be made that in many instances CO_2 narcosis accomplishes adequate anesthesia in and of itself, the extreme pain associated with a chest wall incision mandates that the child have appropriate measures for pain relief.

A cross-table lateral film should be taken immediately after the re-insertion of the right chest tube, as well as an AP view, to insure evacuation of air. Since the chest tube on the left has not completely drained the pleural space of free air, a second tube may be necessary. An anterior chest tube can be inserted in the second interspace in the mid-clavicular line if necessary. One must be careful to avoid the nipple area (often difficult to perceive in the smallest neonates) in both male and female infants, as the breast bud may be injured. Sometimes the second tube can be avoided by gently massaging the chest to break up loculations of air that may not be immediately evacuated even by a well-placed chest tube. Starting negative pressure for air evacuation should be about -10 to -15 cm H2O. It should be noted that the bubbling in the suction chamber of the chest tube evacuation device does not need to be loud and vigorous. Vigorous bubbling does not evacuate air any better and only serves to give the nurse at the bedside a serious headache over the course of the shift. Slow, gentle bubbling is sufficient.

If a tension pneumothorax cannot be successfully evacuated, one should take the following steps: 1) Be certain that the chest tube position is appropriate. A chest tube that sits inferiorly will not drain air that lies superiorly in the infant. 2) Be sure that the chest tube insertion has not created a bronchopleural fistula. Many chest tube insertions, because of the difficulty of the procedure (popping a chest tune into the pleural space is one of the most frightening feelings in neonatal medicine), will commonly perforate the lung. In most cases, air evacuation should still be adequate while one awaits closure of the air leak, though slightly higher negative pressures may be required. In rare cases, however, the airway itself is penetrated and this may need surgical intervention if the air leak continues to be profound. 3) Consider increasing the negative pressure to enhance air drainage from the pleural space.

A tension pneumothorax in the tiniest infants is one of the common precursors to bronchopulmonary dysplasia (BPD). While BPD is not inevitable after a severe air leak, the risk of BPD does increase significantly in the very low birth weight infant, and it may be helpful to counsel the family accordingly. There may be a long NICU ventilator course after a pneumothorax, and preparation of the family may make management easier in the long run. In addition, a severe tension pneumothorax virtually always affects the cerebral circulation, raising the potential for both intraventricular hemorrhage (IVH) and periventricular leukomalacia (PVL). Following a tension pneumothorax, a bedside ultrasound is always indicated. If these events are found, long-term neurological outcome may be impaired, though again, many infants will have multiple chest tube insertions and ultimately be entirely fine.

@The Editor is grateful to Dr *Alan R. Spitzer, MD for this great Instructive Case Study*.

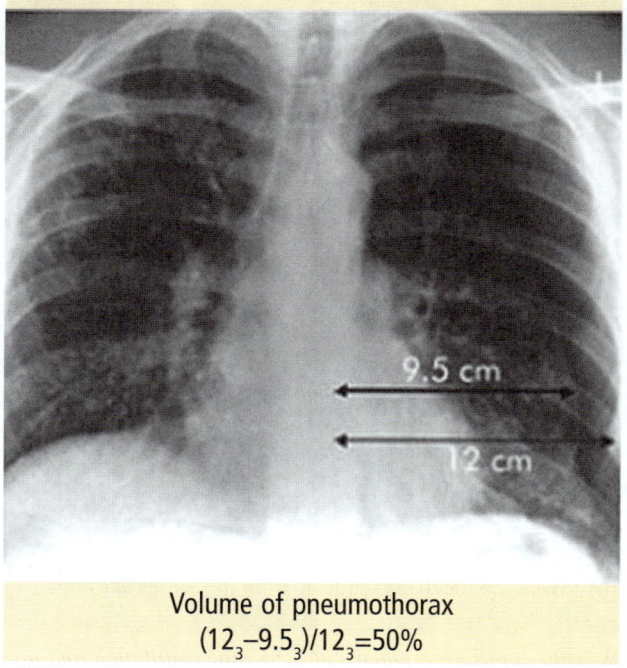

Volume of pneumothorax
$(12_3 - 9.5_3)/12_3 = 50\%$

Pearl/Peril/Pitfall: *Pneumomediastinum and pneumopericardium that does not unduly stress the infant can also be managed with 100% oxygen therapy. Tension pneumopericardium is life threatening, must be drained surgically, and is associated with a high incidence of morbidity and mortality.*

TABLE 1   Incidence and risk factors for thoracic airleaks in neonate

Estimates for the overall incidence of air leak in normal term infants range from 0.07–1%

A. The incidence of air leak varies depending on:
1. Degree of perinatal hypoxemia
2. Technique of resuscitation
3. Concomitant respiratory disease
4. Type and Style of assisted ventilation
5. Quality of radiographs and their interpretation
B. The likelihood of Pneumothorax being symptomatic without underlying lung disease is small and many go undetected.
C. Several disease states increase the risk of pulmonary air leaks
1. Respiratory distress syndrome (RDS), incidence 5–20%
2. Meconium aspiration syndrome (MAS), incidence 20–50%
3. Pulmonary hypoplasia
4. Pulmonary Interstitial Emphysema (PIE)

* *Pneumothorax results when the pleural surface is ruptured with air leaking into the pleural space.*
* *Pneumomediastinum results when air, following the path of least resistance enters the mediastinum.*
* *Pneumopericardium results as above when air dissects into the pericardium.*
* *Subcutaneous emphysema occurs when air from the mediastinum egresses into the fascial planes of the neck and skin.*
* *Pneumoperitoneum results from the dissection of retroperitoneal air, from pneumomediastinal decompression, into the peritoneum. (It can also occur from a ruptured abdominal viscus.)*

Needle aspiration: Needle aspiration is an emergency procedure only. Care must be taken to avoid laceration of the lung or puncturing blood vessels. Needle aspiration is not recommended, other than as a diagnostic procedure when the infant is in extremis and there are no other diagnostic aids immediately available. Chest tube drainage must always be instituted in symptomatic preterm babies, in all babies who are receiving mechanical ventilation(unless the pneumothorax is very small and not associated with any deterioration in clinical conditions) and in all those with tension pneumothoraces. **Equipment** *21gauge butterfly needle *3 way stopcock *10 ml syringe *70% Isopropyl alcohol swab *1 pair sterile gloves **Procedure** *Infant supine, prepare area with alcohol wipe *Insert needle into the pleural space (directly over the top of the rib in the 2nd or 3rd intercostal space in the mid-clavicular line) until air is aspirated into the syringe, then expel air through the 3-way stopcock. Ongoing Care Following needle aspiration insertion of an intercostal catheter is required for on-going management. It may be necessary to seek help with this procedure -consultation and assistance will be available with the receiving NICU. Refer to "Essential Neonatal Procedures" section.

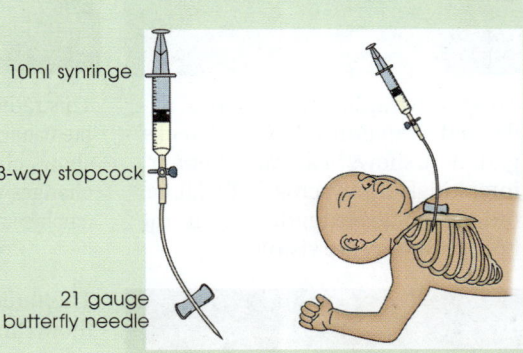

10ml synringe
3-way stopcock
21 gauge butterfly needle

KEY POINTS FOR CLINICAL PRACTICE

1. Pneumothorax must be considered in mechanically ventilated infants who develop unexplained alterations in hemodynamics, pulmonary compliance, or oxygenation and ventilation. Clinical signs of pneumothorax range from insidious changes in vital signs to the complete cardiovascular collapse that frequently accompanies a tension pneumothorax. Spontaneous pneumothorax occurs in 1% of normal term infants around the time of birth; only about 10% of these are symptomatic.

2. Diagnosis is made using the combination of clinical signs, physical examination, ABG analysis, transillumination, and radiography. Asymptomatic pneumothoraces need no treatment other than careful observation of the infant.

3. Pneumopericardium is the least common form of air leak in Newborns but the most common cause of cardiac tamponade; most cases occur in preterm infants with RDS treated with mechanical ventilation, preceded by PIE and pneumomediastinum and the mortality is around 80%.

4. *Chest tube drainage must always be instituted in symptomatic preterm babies, in all babies who are receiving mechanical ventilation(unless the pneumothorax is very small and not associated with any deterioration in clinical conditions) and in all those with tension pneumothoraces.*

5. The complications of significant pneumothorax include a)profound ventilatory and circulatory compromise and death b)IVH secondary to fluctuating cerebrovascular pressures, impaired venous return, hypercapnia, hypoxia and acidosis c) SIADH.

REFERENCES AND FURTHER READING 1)Kuhns LR, Bednarek FJ, Wyman ML. Diagnosis of pneumothorax or pneumomediastinum in the neonate by transillumination. Pediatrics. 1975;56:355. 2) Arda IS, Gurakan B, Aliefendioglu D, Tuzun M. Treatment of pneumothorax in newborns: use of venous catheter versus chest tube. Pediatr Int. 2002;44:78. 3) Banagle RC, Outerbridge EW, Aranda JV. Lung perforation: a complication of chest tube insertion in neonatal pneumothorax. J Pediatr. 1979;94:973. 4) Primhak RA. Factors associated with pulmonary air leak in premature infants receiving mechanical ventilation. J Pediatr. 1983;102:764. 5) Yeh TF, Pildes RS, Salem MR. Treatment of persistent tension pneumothorax in a neonate by selective bronchial intubation. Anesthesiology. 1978;49:37.

Pearl/Peril/Pitfall: Pneumothoraces fall into two major groups: spontaneous pneumothorax in otherwise healthy, fullterm infants, which most often occurs within minutes of birth, and pneumothorax in infants with significant pulmonary disease, which frequently occurs several days after birth, during therapy for pulmonary disease.

39 A Neonate with Pulmonary Interstitial Emphysema (PIE)

@ *Pulmonary interstitial emphysema occurs most frequently in smaller infants being treated by mechanical ventilation for primary lung disease. In this clinical setting, PIE is associated with a mortality rate of more than 50%. Unilateral PIE can be managed by placing the infant with the affected side down for 24 to 48 hours. Selective bronchial intubation and high-frequency or jet ventilation have been used to treat unilateral PIE. Careful attention to peak and mean inspiratory pressures may be beneficial in preventing and treating PIE. High frequency ventilation may be helpful. Bronchopulmonary dysplasia is a frequent sequel in infants surviving PIE.*

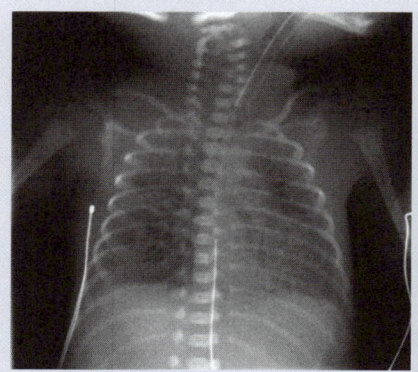 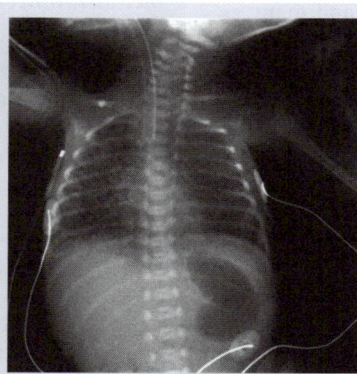

This radiograph, obtained from a 1-day-old premature infant at 24 weeks' gestation, shows bilateral pulmonary interstitial emphysema (PIE). Linear radiolucencies extending up to the lung periphery are visible.

This radiograph, obtained from a premature infant at 26 weeks' gestation, shows characteristic radiographic changes of pulmonary interstitial emphysema (PIE) of the right lung.

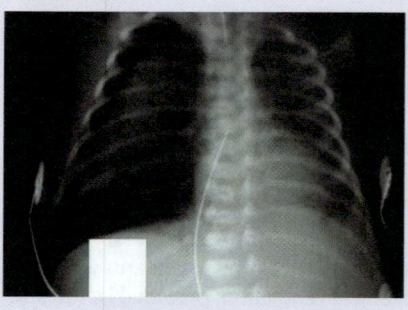

This radiograph shows pneumothorax and pulmonary interstitial emphysema (PIE) on the right side. Interstitial air prevents collapse of the underlying lung by a tension pneumothorax. In such cases, extreme caution is required during drainage of a pneumothorax to avoid perforation of the underlying lung

Pulmonary Interstitial Emphysema (PIE)

Collection of gases outside of normal air passage which is inside the connective tissue of the peribronchovascular sheaths, interlobular septa and visceral pleura results in compressing adjacent functional lung tissue, vascular structures and impedance of oxygenation, ventilation as well as blood pressure. Roentgenography: There are two basic radiographic appearance
1. Linear radiolucencies; coarse and non branching, 3–8 mm, and vary in width but rarely exceed 2 mm
2. Cyst like radiolucencies; 1–4 mm, though generally round, they may appear oval or slightly lobulated

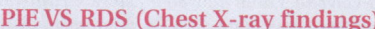

PIE VS RDS (Chest X-ray findings)

PIE: Coarse radiolucencies appear in the lung periphery or when the lucencies do not branch in a pattern consistent with the normal bronchial tree
RDS: Long smooth, branching, linear radiolucencies decrease in caliber from the hilum and frequently disappear at the lung periphery.

REVIEW OF CLINICAL PROBLEMS

1. Name the risk factors for the development of Pulmonary Interstitial Emphysema (PIE).
   Ans: Refer to the "No.1" of the BIRD'S EYE VIEW/ OVERVIEW/SYNOPSIS" of the Chapter.

2. Mention the different Treatment modalities being used in the management of PIE.
   Ans: Refer to Table 1 of the Chapter.

3. What are the Preventive aspects of PIE?
   Ans: Refer to Table 2 of the Chapter.

4. What is the role of surgery in treating PIE?
   Ans: Refer to the "No.8" of the "BIRD'S EYE VIEW/ OVERVIEW/SYNOPSIS" of the Chapter.

5. Mention the complications of PIE.
   Ans: Refer to the Evaluation-Decision-Action Plan/ Algorithm to diagnose and manage a Neonate with PIE.

LEARNING OBJECTIVES

After completing this article, readers will be able to

1. Anticipate the development of PIE in clinical situations associated with the known risk factors involved.

2. Manage PIE with different Ventilation Strategies appropriate to the clinical situation.

3. Beware of the complications of PIE-Pulmonary and CNS.

4. Explain the prognosis to parents

5. Consult Pediatric Pulmonologist and Pediatric Surgeon when indicated.

Pearl/Peril/Pitfall: *Pulmonary interstitial emphysema (PIE) is a radiographic and pathologic diagnosis. In most cases, the discovery of pulmonary interstitial emphysema may be preceded by a decline in the baby's clinical condition. Hypotension and difficulty in oxygenation and ventilation can suggest the development of pulmonary interstitial emphysema.*

BIRD'S EYE VIEW/OVERVIEW/SYNOPSIS

1. Pulmonary interstitial emphysema (PIE) is a collection of gases outside of the normal air passages and inside the connective tissue of the peribronchovascular sheaths, interlobular septa, and visceral pleura secondary to alveolar and terminal bronchiolar rupture. Pulmonary interstitial emphysema is more frequent in premature infants who require mechanical ventilation for severe lung disease. Once pulmonary interstitial emphysema is diagnosed, intensive respiratory management is required to reduce mortality and morbidity.Risk factors include the following: *Prematurity *Respiratory distress syndrome (RDS) *Meconium aspiration syndrome (MAS) *Amniotic fluid aspiration *Infection - Neonatal sepsis, pneumonia, or both *Low Apgar score or need for positive pressure ventilation (PPV) during resuscitation at birth *Use of high peak airway pressures on mechanical ventilation *Incorrect positioning of the endotracheal tube in one bronchus.Studies reflecting international frequency demonstrated that 2-3% of all infants in NICUs develop pulmonary interstitial emphysema. When limiting the population studied to premature infants, this frequency increases to 20–30%, with the highest frequencies occurring in infants weighing fewer than 1000 g.The mortality rate associated with pulmonary interstitial emphysema is reported to be as high as 53–67%.Development of pulmonary interstitial emphysema within the first 24–48 hours after birth is often associated with extreme prematurity, very low birth weight, perinatal asphyxia, and/or neonatal sepsis and frequently indicates a grave prognosis

2. Positive pressure ventilation (PPV) and reduced lung compliance are significant predisposing factors. However, in extremely premature infants, pulmonary interstitial emphysema can occur at low mean airway pressure and probably reflects increased sensitivity of the underdeveloped lung to stretch. Pulmonary interstitial emphysema has been rarely reported in the absence of mechanical ventilation or continuous positive airway pressure. The process of pulmonary interstitial emphysema is initiated when air ruptures from the alveolar airspace and small airways into the perivascular tissue of the lung. Infants with RDS have an initial increase in interstitial and perivascular fluid that rapidly declines over the first few days of life. This fluid may obstruct the movement of gas from ruptured alveoli or airways to the mediastinum, causing an increase of PIE. Another possible mechanism for entrapment of air in the interstitium is the increased amount of pulmonary connective tissue in the immature lung. The entrapment of air in the interstitium may result in a vicious cycle that causes compression atelectasis of the adjacent lung, which then necessitates a further increase in ventilatory pressure with still more escape of air into the interstitial tissues.

3. Plenat et al described two topographic varieties of air leak: intrapulmonary pneumatosis and intrapleural pneumatosis. In the intrapulmonary type, which is more common in premature infants, the air remains trapped inside the lung and frequently appears on the surface of the lung, bulging under the pleura in the area of interlobular septa. This phenomenon develops with high frequency on the costal surface and the anterior and inferior edges but can involve all of the pulmonary areas. In the intrapleural variety, which is more common in more mature infants with compliant lungs, the abnormal air pockets are confined to the visceral pleura, often affecting the mediastinal pleura. The air of pulmonary interstitial emphysema may be located inside the pulmonary lymphatic network.The extent of pulmonary interstitial emphysema can vary. It can present as an isolated interstitial bubble, several slits, lesions involving the entire portion of one lung, or diffuse involvement of both lungs. Pulmonary interstitial emphysema does not preferentially localize in any one of the 5 pulmonary lobes.

4. Pulmonary interstitial emphysema compresses adjacent functional lung tissue and vascular structures and hinders both ventilation and pulmonary blood flow, resulting in impedance of oxygenation, ventilation, and blood pressure. This further compromises the already critically ill infant with a significant increase in mortality and morbidity. Pulmonary interstitial emphysema can completely regress or decompress into adjacent spaces, causing pneumomediastinum, pneumothorax, pneumopericardium, pneumoperitoneum, or subcutaneous emphysema. Admission/transfer to a NICU is indicated for patients with pulmonary interstitial emphysema (PIE). A thoracentesis set should be readily available due to the possibility of air leak, including pneumothorax and pneumopericardium

5. **The Evaluation-Decision-Action Plan/algorithm** summarizes the essential aspects of history taking, physical examination, relevant investigations to diagnose Pulmonary Interstitial Emphysema(PIE) and also the principles of timely management of PIE and its common complications.

6. The roentgenologic appearance of pulmonary interstitial emphysema (PIE) can be confused with the following: *Air-bronchogram in respiratory distress syndrome (RDS) *Aspiration pneumonia *Pulmonary edema *Distended airways in patients on a ventilator. Other differential diagnosis of persistent pulmonary interstitial emphysema includes the following: *Congenital cystic adenomatoid malformation *Lymphangiectasia *Bronchogenic cysts *Congenital lobar emphysema *Cystic lymphangioma *Sequelae of prior infection *Diaphragmatic hernia

7. **Different treatment modalities have been used to manage pulmonary interstitial emphysema (PIE), with variable success.**These include a) lateral decubitus position with the affected lung in a dependent position b)selective intubation of the contralateral bronchus to decompress the overdistended lung tissue and to avoid exposing it to high positive inflationary pressures c) HFJV d) HFOV e) 3 day course of dexamethasone (0.5 mg/kg/d) f) chest physiotherapy with intermittent 100% oxygen in localized and persistent compressive pulmonary interstitial emphysema g) artificial pneumothorax, and multiple pleurotomies-Refer to the Table No. 1of the Chapter for the details.

8. Lobectomy is indicated in a small number of patients with localized pulmonary interstitial emphysema when spontaneous regression is not occurring and medical management has failed. Although clear guidelines for surgical intervention are difficult to establish, it should be reserved for infants in whom the risks of recurring complications outweigh those of surgery. It seems most helpful in infants who develop severe lobar emphysema.

9. Monitoring for physical and psychomotor development in a neonatal follow-up care program or equivalent program is important because most infants with pulmonary interstitial emphysema are premature and are at risk for developmental delay. In addition, pulmonary interstitial emphysema has been associated with increased risks of intraventricular hemorrhage (IVH) and periventricular leukomalacia (PVL), which also increase the risks of developmental delay in these infants. Patients with chronic lung disease may need pediatric pulmonology follow-up care.

10. **Prognosis and prevention** *Long-term follow-up data are scarce. *Gaylord et al demonstrated a high (54%) incidence of chronic lung disease in survivors of pulmonary interstitial emphysema compared with their nursery's overall incidence of 32%. In addition, 19% of the infants developed chronic lobar emphysema; 50% received surgical lobectomies.Although the primary risk factor for pulmonary interstitial emphysema, prematurity, is rarely preventable, attention should be given to the use of as little mechanical ventilatory support as is necessary for the patient's very fragile lungs. Because pneumothorax is a known complication, anticipatory guidance for this possibility should be provided for all those caring for the infant. Appropriate personnel should be readily available to address this complication.

Pearl/Peril/Pitfall: The chest radiographs of infants with PIE have been described as demonstrating a salt-and-pepper pattern in which the radiolucent interstitial air is juxtaposed to lung parenchyma. Radiolucent air is present in the pleural space in a pneumothorax.

THE EVALUATION-DECISION-ACTION-PLAN/ALGORITHM FOR THE DIAGNOSIS AND MANAGEMENT OF *NEONATAL PULMONARY INTERSTITIAL EMPHYSEMA*

SUBJECTIVE FINDINGS

Pulmonary interstitial emphysema (PIE) is a radiographic and pathologic diagnosis. In most cases, the discovery of pulmonary interstitial emphysema may be preceded by a **Hx of** decline in the baby's clinical condition. Hypotension and difficulty in oxygenation and ventilation or baby can present with pneumothorax/PIE apparent following reexpansion of a collapsed lung after drainage of a pneumothorax. **Hx of** *Prematurity *Respiratory distress syndrome (RDS)*Meconium aspiration syndrome (MAS) *Amniotic fluid aspiration*Infection - Neonatal sepsis, pneumonia, or both*Low Apgar score or need for positive pressure ventilation (PPV) during resuscitation at birth*Use of high peak airway pressures on mechanical ventilation*Incorrect positioning of the endotracheal tube in one bronchus.

OBJECTIVE FINDINGS

Assess ABCDs, vitals, BP, O_2 sats, work of breathing central cyanosis, CRT, pulses, Urine output *Look for* *No specific signs of pulmonary interstitial emphysema are reported.* Overinflation of the chest wall and crepitations on auscultation on the affected side may be present *Assess* for *ONGOING* development of "PIE associated morbidity" such as air leaks, IVH and BPD*Perform* systemic examination to assess the complications of hypoxia/hypotension associated with PIE.

INVESTIGATIONS

Blood FBC with hematocrit and platelets, glucose, blood culture, ABG analysis, electrolytes, Ca^{++}, Mg^{++}, creatinine, BUN, bleeding and clotting profile.

CXR for patchy areas of atelectasis with hyperinflation, pneumonitis, pleural effusion, air leaks, cardiomegaly. *It is important to assess the positioning of tubes (endotracheal, nasogastric), lines (umbilical arterial/venous catheters, peripherally inserted central catheters), and other devices.*CT/MRI Head scan in case of HIE and seizures* Echocardiogram to assess pulmonary hypertension/congenital heart disease if any co-existing.

A NEONATE WITH PULMONARY INTERSTITIAL EMPHYSEMA (PIE)

Ensure General Supportive Measures mandatory for any severely ill Neonate!

* **Ensure** ABCs, give supplemental oxygen to maintain O_2 sats > 95%, monitor pulse oximetry, Invasive BP, CR monitor, CVP if necessary. **Treat** shock and hypotension with 10ml/kg NS and IVI of Dopamine/Noradrenaline/Adrenaline and Dobutamine
* **Secure** IV access and **correct** hypoglycemia, hypocalcemia, acidosis and **maintain** normothermia and electrolytes. **Catheterize** the bladder to monitor urine output. **Ensure** minimal handling. **Give** broadspectrum IV antibiotics to cover for sepsis and pneumonitis.
* **Start** TPN, as it is very important to the overall nutritional management of these sick infants.
* **Ensure** that a thoracentesis set should be readily available due to the possibility of air leak, including pneumothorax and pneumopericardium.
* **Explain** prognosis to parents-Gaylord et al demonstrated a high (54%) incidence of chronic lung disease in survivors of pulmonary interstitial emphysema compared with their nursery's overall incidence of 32%. In addition, 19% of the infants developed chronic lobar emphysema; 50% received surgical lobectomies.
* **Consult** pediatric pulmonology and pediatric surgery specialists when appropriate !
* **Beware of** the complications of PIE:
  *Death   *Respiratory insufficiency
  *Other air leaks   *Pneumomediastinum
  *Pneumothorax   *Pneumopericardium
  *Pneumoperitoneum   *Massive air embolism

  *Subcutaneous emphysema (rare)
  *Chronic lung disease of prematurity
  *Intraventricular hemorrhage
  *Periventricular leukomalacia.

* **Try:** Lateral decubitus positioning for unilateral PIE—*place* the infant in the lateral decubitus position with the affected lung in a dependent position
* **Intubate** the mainstem bronchus of the contra-lateral side to decompress the overdistended lung tissue and to avoid exposing it to high positive inflationary pressures-in infants with severe localized pulmonary interstitial emphysema

PIE: VENTILATION STRATEGIES

* Best is to prevent-Refer to the Table 2 of the Chapter for preventive measures.
* Appropriate ventilation strategies
  – Avoidance of hyperventilation
  – Accept the blood gases: $PaCO_2$: 45–60 mmHg (? higher), PaO_2 45–52mm Hg, pH>7.25, Consider paralysis to minimize the risk of extension of air leaks
  – Avoidance of "hand bagging"
  – Avoidance of derecruitment of the lung
  – Don't loose PEEP (Low PEEP results in poor Compliance)
  – Low tidal volume ventilation <5 ml/kg
  – Early use of high frequency ventilation
  – HFJV/HFOV
?? 3-day course of dexamethasone (0.5 mg/kg/d)- Take informed consent from the parents after explaining about the possible long-term Neuro-developmental adverse effects due to postnatal steroids, chest physiotherapy with intermittent 100% oxygen in localized and persistent compressive pulmonary interstitial emphysema.
* artificial pneumothorax, and multiple pleurotomies.

Pearl/Peril/Pitfall: Unilateral PIE can be managed by placing the infant with the affected side down for 24 to 48 hours. Selective bronchial intubation and high-frequency or jet ventilation have been used to treat unilateral PIE.

| TABLE 1 | Different treatment modalities have been used to manage pulmonary interstitial emphysema (PIE), with variable success. |

Lateral decubitus positioning *This conservative approach has been used with success and is most effective in infants with unilateral pulmonary interstitial emphysema. The infant is placed in the lateral decubitus position with the affected lung in a dependent position. This therapy can result in plugging of dependent airways and improved oxygenation of the nondependent lung. The latter allows for overall decreased ventilatory settings. The combination of the above factors helps in resolution of pulmonary interstitial emphysema. *In different case studies of lateral decubitus position as a treatment of unilateral pulmonary interstitial emphysema in infants, pulmonary interstitial emphysema resolved in 48 hours to 6 days with minimal recurrence and a low failure rate. Lateral decubitus positioning should be considered as an early first-line therapy in the management of unilateral pulmonary interstitial emphysema. Lateral decubitus positioning has been used successfully for patients with bilateral pulmonary interstitial emphysema when one side is more significantly affected.

Selective main bronchial intubation and occlusion *Many case reports detail successful treatment of severe localized pulmonary interstitial emphysema in infants with selective intubation of the contralateral bronchus to decompress the overdistended lung tissue and to avoid exposing it to high positive inflationary pressures. Selective bronchial intubation of the right main bronchus is not a difficult procedure; the left side may be more difficult. The endotracheal tube of the same diameter as for a regular intubation is inserted 2–4 cm beyond its usual position. It is introduced with the bevel on the end of the tube positioned so that the long part of the tube is toward the bronchus to be intubated. This increases the chance of entering the correct bronchus as the tube is advanced into the airway. Turning the infant's head to the left or right moves the tip of the endotracheal tube to the contralateral side of the trachea and may help in selective tube placement. *Weintraub et al have described a method for left selective bronchus intubation using a regular Portex endotracheal tube in which an elliptical hole 1 cm in length has been cut through half the circumference 0.5 cm above the tip of the oblique distal end. With the side with the elliptical hole directed to the left lung, left selective bronchus intubation can be easily and repeatedly accomplished. Another method of selective intubation is the use of a small fiberoptic bronchoscope to direct the endotracheal tube tip into the desired bronchus. Selective intubation under fluoroscopy can also be considered. *Potential complications of the selective intubation/ ventilation include atelectasis in the affected lung, injury to bronchial mucosa with subsequent scarring and stenosis, acute hypoventilation or hypoxemia if ventilating one lung is inadequate, excessive secretions, hyper-inflation of the intubated or nonoccluded lung, upper lobe collapse when intubating the right lung, and brady-cardia. Despite potential risks, selective bronchial intubation is a desirable alternative to lobectomy in a persistent, severe, localized pulmonary interstitial emphysema causing mediastinal shift and compression atelectasis and not responding to conservative management. This procedure should be attempted before any surgical intervention.

High-frequency ventilation *Keszler et al studied use of high-frequency jet ventilation (HFJV) in 144 newborns with pulmonary interstitial emphysema. They concluded that HFJV was safe and more effective than rapid-rate conventional ventilation in the treatment of newborns with pulmonary interstitial emphysema. With HFJV, similar oxygenation and ventilation was obtained at lower peak and mean airway pressures, suggesting that, in infants with pulmonary interstitial emphysema, a reduction in the amount of air leaking into the interstitial spaces would occur. *Similar effects can be achieved by use of HFOV. *In a study by Clark et al, 27 low birth weight infants who developed PIE and respiratory failure while on conventional ventilation were treated with HFOV. Surviving patients showed continued improvement in oxygenation and ventilation at an increasingly lower fraction of inspired oxygen (FiO_2) and proximal airway pressure with resolution of pulmonary interstitial emphysema, whereas nonsurvivors progressively developed chronic respiratory insufficiency with continued pulmonary interstitial emphysema from which recovery was not possible. Overall survival in nonseptic patients was 80%. *They found HFOV to be effective in the treatment of pulmonary interstitial emphysema and hypothesized that interstitial air leak is decreased during HFOV because adequate ventilation is provided at lower peak distal airway pressures. Although this mode of ventilation has inherent risks, it can be a very effective tool in experienced hands for the treatment of severe diffuse pulmonary interstitial emphysema. Care must be taken in smaller infants who require a high amplitude to ventilate because the active exhalation during HFOV may cause small airway collapse and exacerbate gas trapping.

Other treatment modalities *Case reports and/or case series describe different approaches for the management of pulmonary interstitial emphysema, including 3-day course of dexamethasone (0.5 mg/kg/d), chest physiotherapy with intermittent 100% oxygen in localized and persistent compressive pulmonary interstitial emphysema, artificial pneumothorax, and multiple pleurotomies.

*Despite success claimed by the authors, the efficacy of these treatment modalities from these case reports seems questionable. With advancements in respiratory care, these treatment modalities rarely are used.

Surgical care: Lobectomy is indicated in a small number of patients with localized pulmonary interstitial emphysema when spontaneous regression is not occurring and medical management has failed. Although clear guidelines for surgical intervention are difficult to establish, it should be reserved for infants in whom the risks of recurring complications outweigh those of surgery. It seems most helpful in infants who develop severe lobar emphysema.

Consultations: All infants with pulmonary interstitial emphysema need to be under the care of a neonatologist. In some cases, pediatric pulmonology and pediatric surgery consultations are appropriate.

Diet: The overall importance of appropriate nutritional management of ill newborns cannot be overstressed. Most of these infants are treated with total parenteral nutrition and require diligent attention.

Pearl/Peril/Pitfall: Pulmonary interstitial emphysema occurs most frequently in smaller infants being treated by mechanical ventilation for primary lung disease. In this clinical setting, PIE is associated with a mortality rate of more than 50%.

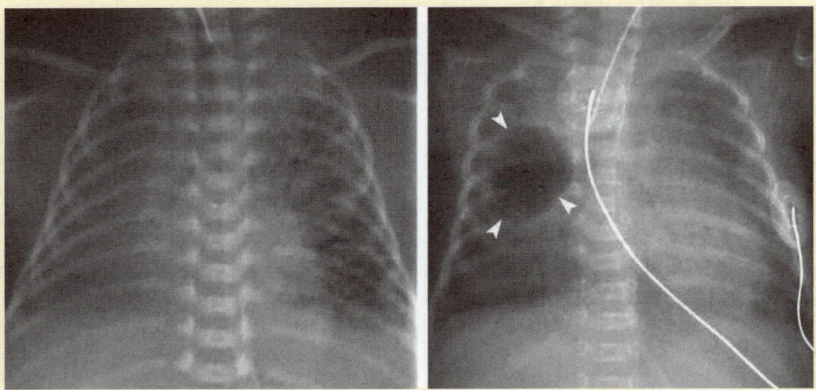

a) Unilateral acute PIE in a premature infant who underwent positive-pressure ventilation for RDS. Frontal radiograph shows a profusion of irregular cystic lucencies within the left lung. Granular consolidation of the right lung is consistent with uncomplicated RDS. **b)** "Pseudocyst" in a premature infant who underwent mechanical ventilation. Frontal chest radiograph shows a large, rounded, right juxtahilar gas collection with a smooth thin wall (arrowheads).

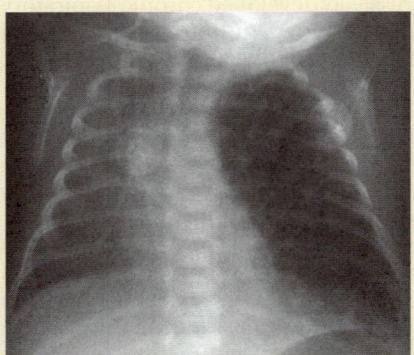
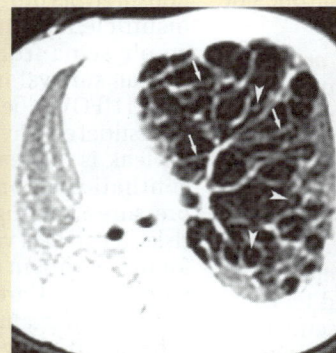
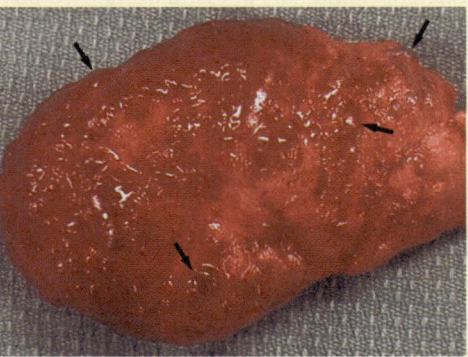

Diffuse persistent PIE in a 3-week-old girl with a history of positive-pressure mechanical ventilation. **(a)** Frontal chest radiograph shows overexpansion of most of the left lung by multiple cystic lucencies, producing contralateral mediastinal displacement and left retrocardiac compressive atelectasis. **(b)** Axial CT scan shows multiple collections of interstitial gas in the left upper lobe that surround lines (arrows) and dots (arrowheads) of soft-tissue attenuation. **(c)** Photograph of the resected left upper lobe shows the surface of the lung blistered by multiple subpleural cysts (arrows).

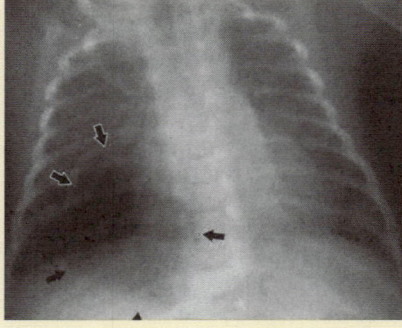
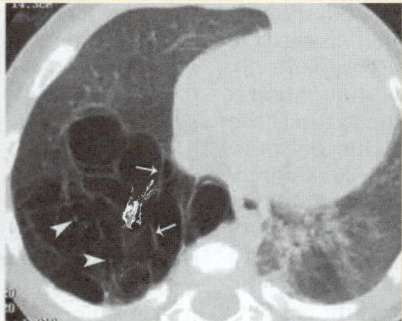
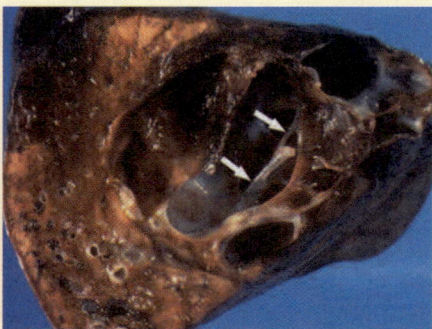

Localized persistent PIE in a 1-year-old boy delivered at 27 weeks gestational age. **(a)** Frontal chest radiograph shows a circumscribed lucent lesion at the medial right lung base with a smooth, lobulated, thin wall (arrows). **(b)** Axial CT scan shows an aggregate of thin-walled, gas-containing cysts in the right lower lobe that contains lines (arrows) and dots (arrowheads) of soft-tissue attenuation. **(c)** Photograph of the cut surface of the resected specimen shows a bronchovascular bundle (arrows) surrounded by gas within a multiloculated cystic mass.

Courtesy: Geoffrey A. Agrons, MD Sherry E. Courtney, MD J. Thomas Stocker, COL, MC, USA, Richard I. Markowitz, MD

Pearl/Peril/Pitfall : The temporal relationship between the acquisition of acute PIE and the subsequent development of persistent PIE in a neonate with a history of intubation and positive-pressure mechanical ventilation usually excludes other causes of a complex radiolucent chest mass, such as congenital lobar overinflation and cystic pulmonary airway malformation.

TABLE 2 — Prevention of PIE

Surfactant *Prophylactic surfactant administration to infants (<30–32 weeks' gestation) judged to be at risk of developing respiratory distress syndrome (RDS) compared with selective use of surfactant in infants with established RDS has been demonstrated to decrease the risk of pulmonary interstitial emphysema. *Metaanalysis of early surfactant replacement therapy with brief ventilation compared with later, selective surfactant replacement and continued mechanical ventilation suggests a trend towards a decreased incidence of air leak syndromes in premature infants in the early surfactant group. Early surfactant treatment, less invasive ventilatory support, or both could be responsible factors for the observed beneficial trend. *According to one report, in infants with respiratory distress, multiple doses of animal-derived surfactant extract resulted in greater improvements in oxygenation and ventilatory requirements, a decreased risk of pneumothorax, and a trend toward improved survival.

High-frequency ventilation *In a study comparing high-frequency positive pressure ventilation (HFPPV) to conventional ventilation, Pohlandt et al reported a reduction in the risk of pulmonary interstitial emphysema with HFPPV. Review of different trials of elective high-frequency oscillatory ventilation (HFOV) versus conventional ventilation for acute pulmonary dysfunction in preterm infants suggests an increase in the incidence of air leak syndromes including but not limited to pulmonary interstitial emphysema in the HFOV group. *A prospective randomized multicenter study of HFOV versus conventional ventilation in premature infants with RDS showed no difference in the incidence of pulmonary interstitial emphysema. Limited data regarding rescue HFOV for pulmonary dysfunction in the preterm infant also showed no difference in the rate of pulmonary interstitial emphysema. *Cochrane reviews of trials of elective high-frequency jet ventilation (HFJV) versus conventional ventilation for RDS demonstrated no significant difference in the incidence of air leak syndrome in the individual trials or in the overall analysis *In summary, current literature suggests that elective or rescue high-frequency ventilation does not prevent the development of pulmonary interstitial emphysema.

Other considerations *Different modes of conventional ventilation: No significant difference in the rate of pulmonary interstitial emphysema was found either in pooled analysis within subgroups or overall pooled analysis of trials comparing volume-targeted versus pressure-limited ventilation in the neonate. *Avoid use of high peak inspiratory pressure (PIP). *Be careful (watch manometer) during manual ventilation.

KEY POINTS FOR CLINICAL PRACTICE

1. Pulmonary interstitial emphysema often occurs in conjunction with respiratory distress syndrome (RDS), but other predisposing etiologic factors include meconium aspiration syndrome (MAS), amniotic fluid aspiration, and infection.

2. Positive pressure ventilation (PPV) and reduced lung compliance are significant predisposing factors. However, in extremely premature infants, pulmonary interstitial emphysema can occur at low mean airway pressure and probably reflects increased sensitivity of the underdeveloped lung to stretch. Pulmonary interstitial emphysema has been rarely reported in the absence of mechanical ventilation or continuous positive airway pressure.

3. Once pulmonary interstitial emphysema is diagnosed, intensive respiratory management is required to reduce mortality and morbidity

4. **Different treatment modalities have been used to manage pulmonary interstitial emphysema (PIE), with variable success.** These include a) lateral decubitus position with the affected lung in a dependent position b) selective intubation of the contralateral bronchus to decompress the overdistended lung tissue and to avoid exposing it to high positive inflationary pressures c) HFJV d) HFOV e) 3-day course of dexamethasone (0.5 mg/kg/d) f) chest physiotherapy with intermittent 100% oxygen in localized and persistent compressive pulmonary interstitial emphysema g) artificial pneumothorax, and multiple pleurotomies.

5. Although the primary risk factor for pulmonary interstitial emphysema, prematurity, is rarely preventable, attention should be given to the use of as little mechanical ventilatory support as is necessary for the patient's very fragile lungs. Because pneumothorax is a known complication, anticipatory guidance for this possibility should be provided for all those caring for the infant. Appropriate personnel should be readily available to address this complication

REFERENCES AND FURTHER READING: 1)Plenat F, Vert P, Didier F, Andre M. Pulmonary interstitial emphysema. *Clin Perinatol.* Sep 1978;5(2):351-75. 2) Cunningham K, Paes BA, Symington A. Pulmonary interstitial emphysema: a review. *Neonatal Netw.* Aug 1992;11(5):7-16, 29-31. 3) Greenough A, Dixon AK, Roberton NR. Pulmonary interstitial emphysema. *Arch Dis Child.* Nov 1984;59(11):1046-51. 4)Schwartz AN, Graham CB. Neonatal tension pulmonary interstitial emphysema in bronchopulmonary dysplasia: treatment with lateral decubitus positioning. *Radiology.* Nov 1986;161(2):351-4. 5)Chalak LF, Kaiser JR, Arrington RW. Resolution of pulmonary interstitial emphysema following selective left main stem intubation in a premature newborn: an old procedure revisited. *Paediatr Anaesth.* Feb 2007;17(2):183-6.

Pearl/Peril/Pitfall: Several examples of persistent PIE have been reported in neonates who received no assisted ventilation or only nasal CPAP . In ambiguous cases, the specific line-and-dot pattern seen at CT can be helpful in making the diagnosis of persistent PIE, and CT is superior to radiography in characterizing pulmonary lobar involvement in cases that will be managed surgically.

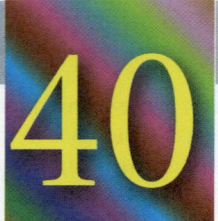

40 A Neonate with Congenital Pneumonia

@ *The 3 categories of congenital pneumonia are: (1) true congenital pneumonia, (2) intrapartum pneumonia, and (3) postnatal pneumonia. Not all pneumonia diagnosed in the first 24 hours of life is infectious; nonetheless, many cases are infectious and benefit from targeted antimicrobial therapy.*

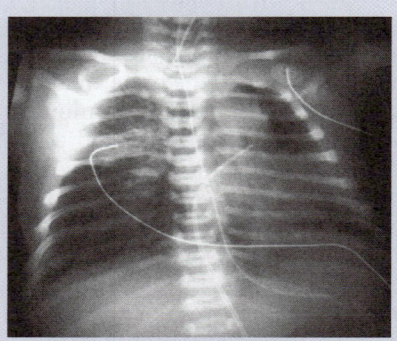

Anteroposterior chest radiograph in an infant born at 28 weeks' gestation was performed following apnea and profound birth depression. Subtle reticulogranularity and prominent distal air bronchograms were consistent with respiratory distress syndrome, prompting exogenous surfactant and antimicrobial therapy. Initial smear of endotracheal aspirate revealed few neutrophils but numerous, small, gram-negative coccobacilli. Culture of blood and tracheal aspirate yielded florid growth of nontypeable *Haemophilus influenzae*.

One of the most common forms of perinatal congenital infection arises from bacterial agents that ascend the birth canal and may be seen in association with premature rupture of membranes (PROM) and acute chorioamnionitis. Seen here is a congenital pneumonia with many *neutrophils* filling immature bronchioles.

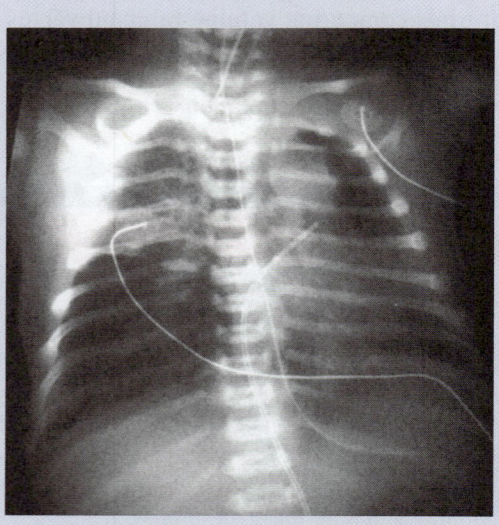

Patchy infiltrates most prominent along left cardiothymic margin in a full-term infant (note proximal humeral ossific nuclei) born to an afebrile woman 18 hours after membranes ruptured. The infant was initially vigorous but developed gradual onset of progressive respiratory distress beginning at 2 hours and prompting endotracheal intubation and transfer to a tertiary center at age 10 hours. Note blunting of the right costophrenic angle, a thin radiodense rim along the lateral right hemithorax, and a fluid line in the right major fissure, all consistent with pleural effusion. Gram staining of pleural fluid recovered at thoracentesis indicated occasional gram-negative bacilli. Tracheal aspirate, pleural fluid, and blood all yielded *Escherichia coli* upon culture. The dense right upper lobe may appear to suggest lobar infiltrate, but upward bowing of the fissure is more suggestive of volume loss, as in atelectasis, than the bulging picture expected with dense pneumonic change. This lobe appeared normal and appropriately inflated on a subsequent film 2 hours later, also suggestive of atelectasis. Umbilical venous catheter and endotracheal tube were positioned properly on the follow-up film.

REVIEW OF CLINICAL PROBLEMS

1. What are the risk factors for the development of Congenital Pneumonia?
   Ans: Refer to Table 1 of the Chapter.
2. Mention the complications of Neonatal Pneumonia
   Ans: Refer to the "No. 9" of the "BIRD'S EYE VIEW/OVERVIEW/ SYNOPSIS" of the Chapter.
3. What are the radiological features of congenital pneumonia?
   Ans: Refer to the section on Radiography—Congenital Pneumonia
4. How do you manage Neonatal Pneumonia generally and specifically?
   Ans: Refer to the Evaluation-Decision-Action Plan/Algorithm to diagnose and manage a Neonatal Pneumonia.
5. Mention the usual organisms that cause Neonatal Pneumonia.
   Ans: Refer to Table 2 of the Chapter.

LEARNING OBJECTIVES

After completing this article, readers will be able to

1. Identify Congenital Pneumonia promptly and Treat it effectively.
2. Expect the complications of Pneumonia and deal with them efficiently.
3. Understand that the therapy of Congenital Pneumonia is Multifaceted, not just IV Antibiotics alone.
4. Initiate respiratory support when the neonate with Congenital Pneumonia is complicated with Respiratory Failure.
5. Counsel parents about the prognosis of Congenital Pneumonia.

Pearl/Peril/Pitfall : Pneumonia acquired through the transplacental route is most commonly of viral origin. Rubella, varicella-zoster, cytomegalovirus (CMV), herpes simplex virus (HSV), and human immunodeficiency virus (HIV) are acquired by this route. Transplacentally acquired pneumonitis is also associated with adenoviral, enteroviral, and influenza viral infections.

BIRD'S EYE VIEW/OVERVIEW/SYNOPSIS

1. **Congenital pneumonia** frequently occurs in Newborn infants, although reported rates vary considerably depending on the diagnostic criteria used and the characteristics of the population under study. Most reports cite frequencies in the range of 5-50 per 1000 live births, with higher rates in the settings of maternal chorioamnionitis, prematurity, and meconium in the amniotic fluid. Among infants with congenital pneumonia associated with proven blood-borne infection, mortality is in the range of 5–10%, with rates as high as 30% in infants with very low birth weight. Pneumonia is a contributing factor in 10–25% of all deaths that occur in neonates younger than 30 days. Diagnosis in the clinical setting is usually based on a combination of historical, physical, radiographic, microbiologic, and laboratory findings.

2. Prenatal features that suggest an increased risk for congenital pneumonia include the following: *Unexplained preterm labor *Rupture of membranes before the onset of labor *Membrane rupture more than 18 hours before delivery *Maternal fever (>38°C/100.4°F) *Uterine tenderness *Foul-smelling amniotic fluid *Infection of the maternal genitourinary tract *Previous infant with neonatal infection *Nonreassuring fetal well-being test results *Fetal tachycardia *Meconium in the amniotic fluid *Recurrent maternal urinary tract infection *Gestational history of illness consistent with an organism known to have transplacental pathogenic potential. *Recognition, prevention, and treatment of these problems are major factors in the care of high-risk newborn infants.* Intrapartum antibiotic therapy reduces the risk of postpartum maternal infection and infection of the infant in the presence of some of these risk factors but does not eliminate the risk. The potential for selection of pathogens resistant to antibiotics used for intrapartum therapy remains controversial. Absence of these risk factors does not exclude pneumonia.

3. Pneumonia that becomes clinically evident within 24 hours of birth may originate at 3 different times. The 3 types often overlap, and assigning a particular pneumonic episode to one of these categories may be difficult. The 3 categories of congenital pneumonia are: (1) true congenital pneumonia, (2) intrapartum pneumonia, and (3) postnatal pneumonia. Not all pneumonia diagnosed in the first 24 hours of life is infectious; nonetheless, many cases are infectious and benefit from targeted antimicrobial therapy. Organisms responsible for infectious pneumonia typically mirror those responsible for early onset neonatal sepsis. This is not surprising in view of the role that maternal genitourinary and gastrointestinal tract flora play in both processes. Group B *Streptococcus* was the most common bacterial isolate in most locales from the late 1960s to the late 1990s, when the impact of intrapartum chemoprophylaxis in reducing neonatal and maternal infection by this organism became evident. *Escherichia coli* has become the most common bacterial isolate among very low birth weight infants (≤ 1500 g) since that time. Other prominent bacterial organisms include the following: *Nontypeable *Haemophilus influenzae* *Other gram-negative bacilli *Listeria monocytogenes* *Enterococci *Occasionally, *Staphylococcus aureus* (Table 2).

4. Among nonbacterial potential pathogens, *U urealyticum* has been recovered quite frequently from endotracheal aspirates shortly after birth in infants with very low birth weight and has been associated with various adverse pulmonary outcomes, including bronchopulmonary dysplasia. However, whether this organism is causal or simply a marker of increased risk is unclear. Agents of chronic congenital infection, such as cytomegalovirus, *Treponema pallidum, Toxoplasma gondii,* and others, may cause pneumonia in the first 24 hours of life. Clinical presentation usually involves other organ systems as well. *Chlamydia* organisms presumably are transmitted at birth during passage through an infected birth canal, although most infants are asymptomatic during the first 24 hours and develop pneumonia only after the first 2 weeks of life. Respiratory pathogens, such as respiratory syncytial virus, influenza, adenovirus, and others, may be transmitted by contact with infected family members or caregivers shortly after birth, but infection by these organisms rarely becomes apparent during the first 24 hours.

5. *The Evaluation-Decision-Action Plan/algorithm* summarizes the essential aspects of history taking, physical examination, relevant investigations to diagnose Congenital Pneumonia and its management.

6. **Therapy in infants with Neonatal pneumonia is multifaceted.** The goals of therapy are to eradicate infection and provide adequate support of gas exchange to ensure the survival and eventual well being of the infant. Options for targeted treatment of inflammation independent of antimicrobial therapy are severely limited. Considerable speculation suggests that current antimicrobial agents, directed at killing invasive organisms, may transiently worsen inflammatory cascades and associated host injury because dying organisms release proinflammatory structural and metabolic constituents into the surrounding microenvironment. This is not to imply that eradicating invasive microbes should not be a goal; however, other methods of eradication or methods of directly dealing with the pathologic inflammatory cascades await further definition. Even if the infection is eradicated, many hosts develop long-lasting or permanent pulmonary changes that affect lung function, the quality of life and susceptibility to later infections.

7. The duration of antimicrobial therapy for Neonatal pneumonia has not been rigorously assessed in comparative trials. **Most clinicians treat infants for 7-10 days if clinical signs resolve rapidly.** If positive results on culture were found at a normally sterile site, treatment for 7-10 days following sterilization is prudent. Longer periods of therapy may be warranted if a sequestered focus, such as empyema or abscess, is seen or if metastatic infection develops.

8. *Respiratory support :* *Adequate gas exchange depends not only on alveolar ventilation, but also on perfusion and gas transport capacity of the alveolar perfusate. Preservation of pulmonary and systemic perfusion is essential, using volume expanders, inotropes, afterload reduction, blood products, and other interventions (eg, inhaled nitric oxide) as needed. Excellent lung mechanics do little good if perfusion is not simultaneously adequate. *Criteria for institution and weaning of supplemental oxygen and mechanical support are similar to those for other Neonatal respiratory diseases. *Beware of remarkable heterogeneity of lung disease, with multiple subpopulations of normally inflated, hyperinflated, atelectatic, obstructed, fluid-filled, and variably perfused alveoli that may require multiple adjustments of ventilatory pressures, flows, rates, times, and modalities.

9. *Complications:* *Restrictive pleural effusion *Infected pleural effusion *Empyema *Systemic infection with metastatic foci *Pulmonary Hypertension, Persistent-Newborn *Air leak syndrome, including pneumothorax, pneumomediastinum, pneumopericardium, and pulmonary interstitial emphysema *Airway injury *Obstructive airway secretions *Hypoperfusion *Chronic lung disease *Hypoxic-ischemic and cytokine-mediated end-organ injury.

10. *Prognosis:* *Although quantitation of risk is difficult and strongly influenced by gestational age, congenital anomalies, and coexisting cardiovascular disease, there is a consensus that congenital pneumonia increases the following: *Chronic lung disease *Prolonged need for respiratory support *Childhood otitis media *Reactive airway disease *Complications attendant to these conditions *Continued growth and development of pulmonary and other tissues offers good prospects for long-term survival and progressive improvement in infants who survive.

Pearl/Peril/Pitfall: Most pneumonias result from an ascending vaginal infection associated with prolonged labor and premature rupture of the membranes, although the infection occasionally may be acquired hematogenously or during vaginal passage.

THE EVALUATION-DECISION-ACTION-PLAN-ALGORITHM FOR THE DIAGNOSIS AND MANAGEMENT OF *A NEONATE WITH CONGENITAL PNEUMONIA*

SUBJECTIVE FINDINGS

Hx of presentation Respiratory distress, increased O2 requirements,Sepsis picture-fever, jaundice,poor feeding, lethargy, hypothermia, seizures, apnea/desats./bradys etc., Review antenatal screening tests for infection, such as serologic tests for syphilis and birth canal tests for *Neisseria gonorrhoeae*, *Chlamydia* species, or group B *Streptococcus*, as well as any treatment courses and testing for cure. *Hx of* Prenatal features that suggest an increased risk for congenital pneumonia—Refer to the Table No 1 of the Chapter. Absence of these risk factors does not exclude pneumonia.

OBJECTIVE FINDINGS

Assess ABCDs, vitals, BP, O_2 sats, work of breathing central cyanosis, CRT, pulses, Urine output *Look for* Systemic findings - Similar to signs and symptoms seen in sepsis or other severe infections *Temperature instability *Skin rash *Jaundice at birth *Tachycardia *Glucose intolerance *Abdominal distention *Hypoperfusion *Oliguria *Localized findings *Conjunctivitis *Vesicles or other focal skin lesions *Unusual nasal secretions *Erythema, swelling, growth, unusual drainage, Hepatomegaly from infection, cardiac impairment, or increased intravascular volume. Apparent hepatomegaly may result if therapeutic airway pressures result in generous lung inflation and downward displacement of a normal liver.

INVESTIGATIONS

* *Blood* FBC with hematocrit and platelets, glucose, blood culture, ABG analysis, electrolytes, Ca^{++}, Mg^{++}, creatinine, BUN, bleeding and clotting profile. Culture of specimens from endotracheal aspiration and full sepsis screen (CRP, microESR, I:T ratio, Band cells, Urine c/s, Skin/conjunctival swabs C/S, CSF C/S, CXR) *CXR—Refer to the Table 3 for radiographic details in congenital pneumonia
* *Echocardiogram* to assess pulmonary hypertension/congenital heart disease if any co-existing.

A NEONATE WITH CONGENITAL PNEUMONIA

Secure IV access and *correct* hypoglycemia, hypocalcemia, acidosis and *maintain* normothermia and electrolytes. *Catheterize* the bladder to monitor urine output. *Ensure* minimal handling. *Give* broadspectrum IV antibiotics to cover for sepsis and pneumonitis-Ampicillin+Aminoglycoside+3rd 'G' Cephalosporin

Ensure ABCs, give supplemental oxygen to maintain O_2 sats > 95%, monitor pulse oximetry, BP, CR monitor, CVP if necessary. *Treat* shock with 10ml/kg NS and then restrict fluids 2/3 rds of maintenance (SIADH may be a problem around 24 hours of age)

ASSESS DEGREE OF RESPIRATORY DISTRESS
(As per serial Clinical Assessment and ABG analysis)

Mild distress

@ If appropriate respiratory, hemodynamic, or nutritional support cannot be safely and effectively administered at the hospital of birth, stabilize and transfer the neonate to a tertiary care NICU.

* *Give oxygen* to maintain O_2 sats above 95% * *Nurse the infant* in neutral thermal environment * *Assess and Reassess* the severity of respiratory distress (Downe's score and ABG analysis) periodically. * *Monitor, Correct and maintain* the disturbances in blood glucose, calcium, magnesium, electrolytes, hematocrit (maintain it > 40%).Nutritional support: Attempts at enteral feeding often are withheld in favor of parenteral nutritional support until respiratory and hemodynamic status is sufficiently stable. *Observe* these babies for 12-24 hr for sudden deterioration due to pulmonary hypertension or pneumothorax. *Maintain adequate systemic blood volume and pressure:* Preservation of pulmonary and systemic perfusion is essential, using volume expanders, inotropes, afterload reduction, blood products, and other interventions (e.g., inhaled nitric oxide) as needed.RBCs should be administered to ensure a hemoglobin concentration of 13-16 g/dL in the acutely ill infant to ensure optimal oxygen delivery to the tissues.

* *Evaluate for co-existing problems* like CNS(HIE), renal (acute renal failure), thrombocytopenia, bleeding and clotting abnormalities and treat accordingly. * *Chest physiotherapy* Gentle vibration and percussion is used in some centers to mobilize the secretions, although appropriately designed studies do not support its use. At least one report cautions that long-term routine percussion may be associated with brain injury in premature infants with a birth weight less than 1500 g. *Many clinicians elect to *administer surfactant* when mechanical ventilation is required with greater than 60% oxygen concentration. Time to clinical response and requirement for multiple doses are both reported to be greater than in infants with respiratory distress syndrome. *Anticipate the complications* a) PPHN b) Air leaks c) Infection d) Respiratory failure e) Birth asphyxia (co-morbidity) and manage them as discussed elsewhere.

Moderate to severe distress

* Worsening Downe's score(>7) * Apneas
* ABG - pH < 7.2 and HCO_3 < 14, PaO_2 < 50mm Hg, $PaCO_2$ >60mm Hg, SaO_2 <90% in 100 % oxygen* Circulatory insufficiency - tachycardia, prolonged CRT, Hypotension or shock, oliguria
* PPHN(labile oxygenation, refractory hypoxia, single $S_2 \pm$ normal CXR, right upper limb and left lower limb SaO_2 difference > 10% or ABG PaO_2 difference > 20mmHg, 2d echo—elevated pulmonary artery pressures with structurally normal heart, (A - a) O_2 gradient > 400).

→ *Start conventional mechanical ventilation* with PIP 30–35 cms H_2O, inspiratory time 0.4–0.5 seconds, rate 20–25 bpm (I : E = 1: 2), 0.8–1 FiO_2, more rapid rates with prominent pneumonitis. Avoid Hyperventilation (PaCO2<30mmHg).

→ *Start high frequency ventilation (jet/oscillatory)*, if the infant with severe Pneumonia fails to improve with conventional ventilation and he/she develops air leak syndromes. The frequency varies from 250–350 bpm to > 1000 with 20–25% lower pressure (advantages—less barotrauma and increased mobilization of airway secretions)

→ *Administer surfactant* to those infants whose clinical status continues to deteriorate and who require escalating support.(If the FiO_2 >0.6 ON VENTILATOR)

→ *Manage PPHN* with High Frequency Ventilation + Nitric Oxide + Inotropes + Surfactant (Refer to the Chapter on a Neonate with PPHN). ECMO may be indicated in approximately 40% of infants with MAS treated with inhaled nitric oxide: High survival rates (93–100%) reported.

---

* *Pearl/Peril/Pitfall :* Dense, bilateral air-space filling with air bronchograms is a common and rather characteristic radiographic finding in neonatal pneumonia. Less pronounced, diffuse, bilateral alveolar densities are also frequently present, occasionally tending to a patchy, unilateral, or central distribution.

TABLE 1 — Congenital pneumonia-prenatal risk factors

*Unexplained preterm labor *Rupture of membranes before the onset of labor *Membrane rupture more than 18 hours before delivery *Maternal fever (>38°C/100.4°F) *Uterine tenderness *Foul-smelling amniotic fluid *Infection of the maternal genitourinary tract *Previous infant with neonatal infection *Nonreassuring fetal well-being test results *Fetal tachycardia *Meconium in the amniotic fluid *Recurrent maternal urinary tract infection *Gestational history of illness consistent with an organism known to have transplacental pathogenic potential

TABLE 2 — Organisms that may cause pneumonia in the neonate

Bacterial	Viral	Other
Group B streptococcus	Cytomegalovirus	*Candida albicans* (and other fungi)
Escherichia coli	Adenovirus	Ureaplasma
Klebsiella	Rhinovirus	Chlamydia
Staphylococcus aureus	Respiratory syncytial virus	Syphilis
Listeria monocytogenes	Parainfluenza	*Pneumocystsis jiroveci* (carinii)
Enterobacter	Enterovirus	Tuberculosis
Haemophilus influenza	Rubella	
Pneumococcus		
Pseudomonas		
Bacteroides		
Citrobacter		
Streptococci viridans		
Acinetobacter		
Stenotrophomonas maltophilia		

Radiography—Congenital pneumonia

*Numerous radiographic patterns are consistent with neonatal pneumonia and a multitude of other pathologic processes. A synthesis of all available information and careful consideration of the differential diagnosis is essential to establishing the diagnosis, although empiric antimicrobial treatment usually cannot be deferred because of inability to prospectively exclude the diagnosis. *A well-centered, appropriately penetrated, anteroposterior chest radiography is essential, although other views may be warranted to clarify anatomic relationships and air-fluid levels. *Be aware that any image reflects conditions only at the instant when the study was performed. Because neonatal lung diseases, including pneumonia, are dynamic, initially suggestive images may require reassessment based on subsequent clinical course and findings in later studies. *When considering pneumonia, devote particular attention to the following: *Costophrenic angles *Pleural spaces and surfaces *Diaphragmatic margins *Cardiothymic silhouette *Pulmonary vasculature *Right major fissure *Air bronchograms overlying the cardiac shadow *Lung expansion *Patterns of aeration *Diffuse relatively homogeneous infiltrates that resemble the ground-glass pattern of respiratory distress syndrome are suggestive of a hematogenous process, although aspiration of infected fluid with subsequent seeding of the bloodstream cannot be excluded. *Patchy irregular densities that obscure normal margins are suggestive of antepartum or intrapartum aspiration, especially if such opacities are distant from the hilus. *Patchy irregular densities in dependent areas that are more prominent on the right side are more consistent with postnatal aspiration. *Generalized hyperinflation with patchy infiltrates suggests partial airway obstruction from particulate or inflammatory debris, although the contribution of positive airway pressure from respiratory support must be considered. Pneumatoceles (especially with air-fluid interfaces) and prominent pleural fluid collections also support the presence of infectious processes.

Limitations of cultures

*A number of factors may interfere with the ability to grow a likely pathogen from the sites noted, including (but not limited to) the following: (1) pretreatment with antibiotics that limit in vitro but not in vivo growth, (2) contaminants that overgrow the pathogen, (3) pathogens that do not replicate in currently available culture systems, and (4) patients in whom the process is inflammatory but not infectious, such as meconium aspiration. Techniques that may help overcome some of these limitations include antigen detection, nucleic acid probes, PCR-based assays, or serologic tests. Quantitative measurements of C-reactive protein, procalcitonin, cytokines (e.g., interleukin-6), and batteries of acute-phase reactants have been touted to be more specific but are plagued by concerns regarding limited positive predictive value. *Lag from infection to abnormalities *Use of serial measurements, especially high negative predictive value

Ultrasonography:
Ultrasonography may be helpful in selected circumstances. Ultrasonography is particularly useful for identifying and localizing fluid in the pleural and pericardial spaces. However, the presence of air within the lungs limits the use of ultrasonography.

CT scanning or MRI:
These imaging modalities may be helpful in selected circumstances. CT or MRI may be helpful for evaluating suspected tumors, aberrant vessels, sequestered lobes, or other primary pulmonary anomalies and for establishing the presence of infiltrate, atelectasis or other acquired processes.

Thoracentesis:
*If significant pleural fluid is detected radiographically or sonographically, consider thoracentesis for Gram stain, culture, and biochemical tests. This procedure may be therapeutic as well as diagnostic if the pleural fluid is impinging on lung or cardiac function.

Pearl/Peril/Pitfall: Radiographic changes of hyaline membrane disease may be distinguished from pneumonia occasionally by the presence of a pleural effusion. Finally, an unusually late development of the transient tachypnea pattern or persistence of changes beyond 1–2 days should suggest the presence of infection.

Radiographic findings in neonatal pneumonia

Phillip J. Haney1 Mark Bohlman2 Chen-Chih J. Suns
AJR:143, July 1984 : NO/% age
Alveolar densities—23/77
  Dense bilateral with air bronchograms—10/33
  Patchy bilateral—3/10
  Right greater than left—2/7
  Central, perihilar distribution—1/3
Air bronchograms—15/50
Pulmonary interstitial emphysema—7/23
Overinflation—5/17
Granular densities (hyaline membrane disease)—4/13
Dilated vessels—3/10
Pneumothorax—3/10
Pleural effusion—3/10
Normal—3/10
Thickened minor fissure—3/10
Pneumomediastinum—1/3
Bilateral reticular densities—1/3

Neonatal pneumonia in developing countries

T Duke:Arch Dis Child Fetal Neonatal Ed 2005;90:F211–F219. doi: 10.1136/adc.2003.048108
Common organisms Isolated- S pyogenes, Staph aureus, S pneumoniae ,Escherichia coli, Salmonella spp, Group B Streptococcus, Klebsiella pneumoniae,Enterobacter, H influenzae, Group G Streptococcus, Pseudomonas, Enterococcus spp, Acinetobacter

Definition of Neonatal pneumonia used in one Indian study

(Mathur NB, Garg K, Kumar S. Respiratory distress in neonates with special reference to pneumonia. Indian Pediatr 2002;39:529–37.)

A Neonate with respiratory distress (any of: rapid, noisy, or difficult breathing; respiratory rate >60/min; chest retractions; cough; grunting) who has: (a) a positive blood culture or (b) any two or more of the following:

(1) Predisposing factors
 – Maternal fever (>38°C)
 – Foul smelling liquor
 – Prolonged rupture of membranes (>24 hours)

(2) Clinical picture of sepsis
 – Poor feeding
 – Lethargy
 – Poor reflexes
 – Hypothermia or hyperthermia
 – Abdominal distention

(3) Radiograph suggestive of pneumonia (nodular or coarse patchy infiltrate, diffuse haziness or granularity, air bronchogram, lobar or segmental consolidation); radiological changes not resolved within 48 hours

(4) Positive sepsis screen (any of the following)
 – Bands >20% of leucocytes
 – Leucocyte count out of reference range
 – Raised C reactive protein
 – Raised erythrocyte sedimentation rate

Conclusions: The global burden of Neonatal pneumonia is huge. Efficient interventions must be targeted at all levels of the health services and communities. Unlike for pneumonia in older infants and children, where effective interventions against two bacteria (S pneumonia and H influenzae) will substantially reduce disease prevalence, the aetiology of neonatal pneumonia is more complex. Interventions that will reduce mortality from Neonatal pneumonia will be broad based and have a range of general positive effects: improved maternal health, better management of other common neonatal conditions, and reduced long term childhood and adult morbidity. Rising rates of resistance to affordable antibiotics may mean that case fatality rates from Neonatal pneumonia will increase in developing countries, emphasizing the need to explore widely applicable preventive and treatment measures.

KEY POINTS FOR CLINICAL PRACTICE

1. Although pneumonia is an important cause of morbidity and mortality among newborn infants, it remains a difficult disease to prospectively identify and treat. Clinical manifestations are often nonspecific, sharing respiratory and hemodynamic signs with a host of noninflammatory processes. Radiographic and laboratory findings also have limited predictive value.

2. Diagnosis in the clinical setting is usually based on a combination of historical, physical, radiographic, microbiologic, and laboratory findings. Physical findings may be pulmonary, systemic, or localized. Many extrapulmonary findings are nonspecific and may be seen in many other common neonatal conditions. Some signs of respiratory distress cannot be manifested if the infant is affected by other processes that result in apnea, such as poor tolerance of labor, exposure to transplacental respiratory depressants, or CNS anomaly or injury.

3. Therapy in infants with Neonatal pneumonia is multifaceted. The goals of therapy are to eradicate infection and provide adequate support of gas exchange to ensure the survival and eventual well being of the infant. At most institutions, initial empiric therapy consists of ampicillin and either gentamicin or cefotaxime. Dosage regimens vary according to gestational and postnatal age, as well as renal function.

4. Adequate gas exchange depends not only on alveolar ventilation, but also on perfusion and gas transport capacity of the alveolar perfusate. Preservation of pulmonary and systemic perfusion is essential, using volume expanders, inotropes, afterload reduction, blood products, and other interventions (e.g. inhaled nitric oxide) as needed. Excellent lung mechanics do little good if perfusion is not simultaneously adequate. Criteria for institution and weaning of supplemental oxygen and mechanical support are similar to those for other neonatal respiratory diseases.

5. Many clinicians elect to administer surfactant when mechanical ventilation is required with greater than 60% oxygen concentration. Time to clinical response and requirement for multiple doses are both reported to be greater than in infants with respiratory distress syndrome.

REFERENCES AND FURTHER READING 1)Haney PJ, Bohlman M, Sun CC. Radiographic findings in neonatal pneumonia. *AJR Am J Roentgenol.* Jul 1984;143(1):23-6. 2) Gauvin F, Dassa C, Chaibou M, et al. Ventilator-associated pneumonia in intubated children: comparison of different diagnostic methods. *Pediatr Crit Care Med.* Oct 2003;4(4):437-43. 3) Bone RC, Grodzin CJ, Balk RA. Sepsis: a new hypothesis for pathogenesis of the disease process. *Chest.* Jul 1997;112(1):235-43. 4)Duke T. Neonatal pneumonia in developing countries. *Arch Dis Child Fetal Neonatal Ed.* May 2005;90(3):F211-9. 5) Barnett ED, Klein JO. Bacterial infections of the respiratory tract. In: Remington JS, Klein JO, eds. *Infectious Diseases of the Fetus and Newborn Infant.* 6th ed. Philadelphia, Pa: Elsevier Saunders Co; 2006:297-317.

Pearl/Peril/Pitfall : Premature infants are affected more often than full-term infants. Symptoms vary; the infant may be stillborn or manifest immediate severe respiratory distress in some cases, whereas in others the only indication of disease may be hypothermia. Early diagnosis requires identification of pathogenic organisms in the amnion, gastric aspirate, or tracheal aspirate.Direct Lung Aspiration is advocated by some authors to isolate the Causative organism.

41 Congenital Diaphragmatic Hernia (CDH)

@ *Prompt intubation, avoidance of bag-mask ventilation, placement of a nasogastric tube to provide intestinal decompression, and ongoing care in an intensive care nursery by individuals experienced in the management of the Newborn who has CDH now is the norm.*

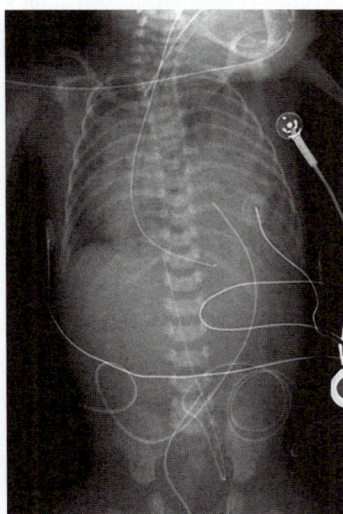

Prenatal Diagnosis Both prenatal ultrasonography and measurement of maternal serum alpha-fetoprotein (MS-AFP) have been found to be useful in identifying infants who have CDH. MS-AFP levels are obtained routinely during the 18th week of pregnancy, and low levels have been associated with CDH as well as trisomy 18 and 21. Thus, a low MS-AFP concentration should prompt additional diagnostic testing. Ultrasonography now is considered the gold standard for diagnosing CDH antenatally. Suggestive findings include polyhydramnios, an absent or intrathoracic stomach bubble, and mediastinal and cardiac shift away from the side of the hernia. The differential diagnosis includes congenital cystic adenomatoid malformation, cystic teratoma, extrapulmonary sequestration, bronchogenic cysts, and neurogenic tumors.

Radiograph of a 1-day-old infant with a moderate-sized congenital diaphragmatic hernia (CDH). Note the air- and fluid-filled bowel loops in the left chest, the moderate shift of the mediastinum into the right chest, and the position of the orogastric tube

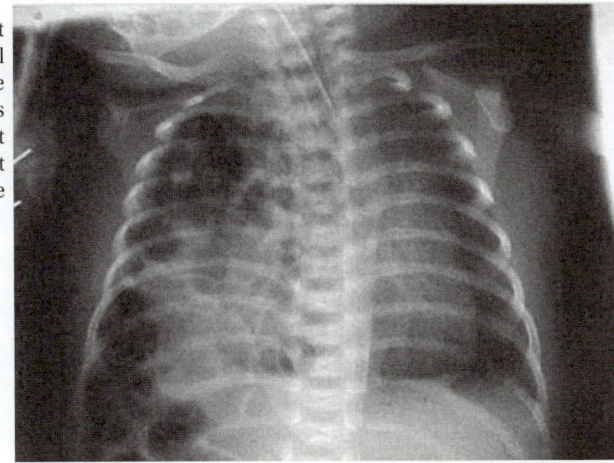

RIGHT CONGENITAL DIAPHRAGMATIC HERNIA

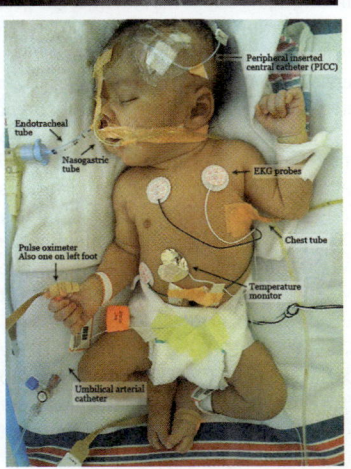

*All infants with a CDH will need to be cared for in the Neonatal Intensive Care Unit (NICU). Specific treatment will be determined by the baby's physician based on the following: * baby's overall health and medical history * the severity of the problem and the degree of breathing difficulty * baby's tolerance for specific medications, procedures, or therapies * parental opinion or preference*

REVIEW OF CLINICAL PROBLEMS

1. What are the principles of Prenatal Counseling and Evaluation, once C D H has been diagnosed in utero ?
   Ans: Refer to the "No.2" of the "BIRD'S EYE VIEW/OVERVIEW/ SYNOPSIS" of the Chapter.
2. Mention the essentials of resuscitation of an infant born with C D H.
   Ans: Refer to the Evaluation-Decision-Action Plan/Algorithm to diagnose & manage a Neonate with C D H.
3. Discuss Ventilation Strategies for C D H.
   Ans: Refer to the Section on Ventilation Strategies-CDH
4. Name the differential diagnoses to consider in an infant born with C D H.
   Ans: Refer to Table 3 of the Chapter.
5. Mention the key determinants of mortality for C D H.
   Ans: Refer to Table 2 of the Chapter.

LEARNING OBJECTIVES

After completing this article, readers will be able to:

1. Delineate the studies used for prenatal diagnosis of Congenital Diaphragmatic Hernia (CDH).
2. Describe prenatal therapies currently being investigated for the treatment of CDH.
3. Provide Proper Resuscitation and Stabilization of a Neonate with CDH before organizing Transfer to a Tertiary center.
4. Delineate the options available for ventilation of the Neonate who has CDH.
5. Describe the potential complications that can be experienced by surviving infants who have CDH.

Pearl/Peril/Pitfall: Cardiac ultrasonography: The incidence of associated cardiac anomalies is high (~25%); therefore, cardiac ultrasonography is needed shortly after birth. Cardiac defects may be relatively minor (atrial septal defect) or life-threatening (transposition of great vessels, hypoplastic left heart). In addition, echocardiography is helpful in assessing myocardial function and determining whether the left ventricular mass is significantly decreased.

BIRD'S EYE VIEW/OVERVIEW/SYNOPSIS

1. Congenital diaphragmatic hernia (CDH) is a congenital anomaly that presents with a broad spectrum of severity dependent upon components of pulmonary hypoplasia and pulmonary hypertension. While advances in neonatal care have improved the overall survival of CDH in experienced centers, mortality and morbidity remain high in a subset of CDH infants with severe CDH. Most diaphragmatic hernias are posterolateral defects of the Bochdalek type, although Morgagni and pars sternalis hernias do occur. The incidence of CDH ranges from 0.08 to 0.45 per 1,000 births. The explanation for this variation in incidence most likely is underdiagnosis related to early deaths among neonates who are severely affected. Eighty-five percent of defects are left-sided, 13% are right-sided, and 2% are bilateral. Most studies have found an equal representation of genders, although a 1.25 male-to-female ratio was reported in one large population-based study.

2. **Prenatal Counseling and Evaluation:** Once CDH has been diagnosed antenatally by ultrasonography, it is important to determine if the defect is isolated or associated with other anomalies known to affect outcome. Level 2 ultrasonography to screen for other anatomic abnormalities should be performed, and amniocentesis should be considered to identify chromosomal abnormalities. After this evaluation, the medical team must present the various management options to the parents, which generally include pregnancy termination or delivery at a tertiary level center that has multimodality support available. The option of pregnancy termination depends on the gestational age at the time of diagnosis. Fetal surgery now is available to selected infants diagnosed prenatally as an experimental procedure at a few research centers.

3. **Prenatal therapies:** Refer to the section "Prenatal therapies" for CDH. The future of fetal surgery for CDH is yet to be determined. Its success will depend both on accurate identification of the fetus who has a poor prognosis and the demonstration of an increased survival with in utero surgery over conventional postnatal therapy for this subgroup of fetuses.

4. **Delivery Room and Immediate Intensive Care :** Antenatal diagnosis of CDH has allowed optimal immediate care of affected infants. Parents can be educated about the diagnosis and potential treatment modalities, and the delivery of medical and surgical care can be coordinated by perinatology, neonatology, and pediatric surgical services. Birth at a tertiary care center that has pediatric surgery and neonatology services as well as advanced therapies is desirable. Prompt intubation, avoidance of bag-mask ventilation, placement of a nasogastric tube to provide intestinal decompression, and ongoing care in an intensive care nursery by individuals experienced in the management of the newborn who has CDH now is the norm.

5. *The Evaluation-Decision-Action Plan/algorithm* summarizes the essential aspects of history taking, physical examination, relevant investigations to diagnose Congenital Diaphragmatic Hernia. Chest radiography *Obtain a chest radiograph if congenital diaphragmatic hernia is suspected. Placement of an orogastric tube prior to the study helps decompress the stomach and helps determine whether the tube is positioned above or below the diaphragm. *Typical findings in a left-sided posterolateral congenital diaphragmatic hernia include air-filled or fluid-filled loops of the bowel in the left hemithorax and shift of the cardiac silhouette to the right. Examine the chest radiograph for evidence of pneumothorax. Emergency surgery was the standard approach to CDH during the 1980s because it was believed that reduction of the hernia would lead to improvement in the respiratory status by allowing the lung to re-expand. With the discovery that the lung was hypoplastic, not atelectatic, and that abnormal arteriolar muscularization and resulting pulmonary hypertension were important in the pathophysiology of CDH, delayed surgical repair was introduced. Currently, most infants who have CDH are stabilized before operative intervention. The mean age at the time of surgery for infants not treated with extracorporeal membrane oxygenation (ECMO) is 73 hours (range, 0 to 443 h). Several recent articles report on the success of a multimodality approach using a combination of therapies, including delayed surgery, HFOV, inhaled nitric oxide (iNO), low ventilator pressures, permissive hypercapnea, surfactant replacement, and ECMO. These single centers cite survival rates of 80% to 90% with a multimodal approach. Multicenter studies are needed to confirm the efficacy and safety of this approach.

6. **CONVENTIONAL MECHANICAL VENTILATION** Attempts should be made to prevent conditions known to raise pulmonary vascular resistance (hypoxemia, acidosis, hypotension, and hypercarbia). Ventilation with low peak inspiratory pressures is desirable because contralateral pneumothorax can result in added cardiorespiratory instability and decompensation. Sedation and paralysis often are employed if hypoxia persists despite other medical treatments. **GENTLE VENTILATION :** Wung et al first described the use of gentle ventilation in infants who had persistent pulmonary hypertension of the newborn. This therapeutic approach also has been applied in the management of infants who have CDH. It is based on the concept that overdistention of the lungs will cause pulmonary hypertension and result in lung injury due to barotrauma. The goal is to maintain preductal saturation at greater than 90% with minimal, but adequate ventilatory support that does not involve the use of paralysis, hyperventilation, or alkalosis. $PaCO_2$ levels up to 60 mm Hg are tolerated. If hypoxemia persists, tolazoline or dobutamine is added. ECMO is reserved for infants who fail this management strategy. In one comparison of survival for infants who had CDH during several time periods and employing various therapeutic strategies, the use of gentle ventilation, delayed surgery (mean age at surgery, 100 h), and no chest tube resulted in the highest survival (94%) and a low requirement for ECMO. Despite the lack of conclusive evidence that ECMO improves survival, it remains a mainstay of therapy for the infant who has CDH.

7. **HIGH-FREQUENCY OSCILLATORY VENTILATION (HFOV)** HFOV has been shown to reduce the need for ECMO in term infants who have respiratory failure. CDH has been associated with failure of HFOV and the need for ECMO more often than other causes of neonatal respiratory failure.

8. **Surfactant replacement** in affected infants after birth has been associated with poor results unless the surfactant is administered prior to the first breath (prophylactically) instead of as a rescue.

9. Lack of improvement in oxygenation with iNO use prior to ECMO or CDH repair has been documented. However, significant improvement in oxygenation may occur when iNO follows ECMO and CDH repair.

10. CDH survivors have a number of significant medical issues after hospital discharge, including chronic lung disease, gastroesophageal reflux, growth failure, reherniation, volvulus, scoliosis, sensorineural hearing loss, and developmental delay. (Refer to the Section of the Chapter for various medical issues in CDH survivors). Despite several decades of investigation and a vast array of new therapeutic approaches, the optimal therapeutic strategy for the newborn who has CDH remains undetermined. Ongoing data collection and the development of multicenter clinical trials should clarify which therapies are most likely to be of benefit.

Pearl/Peril/Pitfall : Cranial ultrasonography: CNS defects (neural tube defects, hydrocephalus) may be associated with congenital diaphragmatic hernia. However, bedside cranial sonography is generally performed when an infant is considered for extracorporeal support. In that circumstance, the goal is to evaluate for intraventricular bleeding and hypoxic-ischemic changes, as well as to rule out intracranial anomalies.

THE EVALUATION-DECISION-ACTION-PLAN/ALGORITHM FOR THE DIAGNOSIS AND MANAGEMENT OF *A NEONATE WITH CONGENITAL DIAPHRAGMATIC HERNIA*

SUBJECTIVE FINDINGS

History * congenital diaphragmatic hernia (CDH) is diagnosed based on prenatal ultrasonography findings in approximately one half of affected infants. Infants may have a prenatal history of *polyhydramnios.

*Infants most commonly present with respiratory distress and cyanosis in the first minutes or hours of life, although a later presentation is possible. The respiratory distress can be severe, requiring aggressive resuscitative measures.

OBJECTIVE FINDINGS

Assess ABCDs, vitals, BP, O_2 sats, work of breathing central cyanosis, CRT, pulses, Urine output *Look for* specific signs of CDH such as*Infants frequently exhibit a scaphoid abdomen, barrel-shaped chest, and signs of respiratory distress (retractions, cyanosis, grunting respirations).*In left-sided posterolateral hernia, auscultation of the lungs reveals poor air entry on the left, with a shift of cardiac sounds over the right chest. In patients with severe defects, pneumothorax signs (poor air entry, poor perfusion) may also be found.*Perform* systemic examination to assess the complications of hypoxia/hypotension associated with CDH.

INVESTIGATIONS

Blood FBC with hematocrit & platelets, glucose, blood culture, ABG analysis, electrolytes, Ca^{++}, Mg^{++}, creatinine, BUN, bleeding & clotting profile. *Chromosome studies* include appropriate deletion analysis (on chromosomes 1q, 8p, and 15q) *CXR* Place an orogastric tube prior to the study to decompress the stomach and to determine whether the tube is positioned above or below the diaphragm.*CT/MRI Head scan* (the goal is to evaluate for intraventricular bleeding and hypoxic-ischemic changes, as well as to rule out intracranial anomalies) *Renal ultrasonography* to exclude genitourinary anomalies *Echocardiogram* to assess pulmonary hypertension/ congenital heart disease if any co-existing.

A NEONATE WITH CONGENITAL DIAPHRAGMATIC HERNIA (CDH)

Resuscitation : Resuscitation will be individualized according to the condition of the baby and the response to initial steps in resuscitation. Ventilation using a bag and mask should be minimized. If endotracheal intubation is required make sure the tube is not inserted too far. Positive pressure ventilation should be accompanied by inspiratory pressure or volume monitoring, when available. IPPV, if required, should be provided by a mechanical ventilator at the earliest opportunity. A large bore nasogastric tube (Ryles tube 10F) should be passed once the baby has been stabilized in the delivery room. Physical contact with the parents should be facilitated before transfer. Preductal saturation monitoring should be undertaken during any transfers. Saturations in the 70's and 80's are satisfactory provided sufficient ventilatory support is provided to ensure adequate tidal volume. This is the most difficult situation to get right and in the absence of portable volume monitors a highly experienced clinician must be supervising this period.

Ongoing Stabilization *establish venous access - if the baby's condition is poor and the circulation compromised rapidly place a UV catheter *measure blood pressure and assess the circulation to determine the need for volume support *obtain a chest X Ray *if the baby's condition remains poor obtain a blood gas by the most expedient route (arterial stab) and adjust support accordingly *arterial access *if urgent - cannulate the UA *if non urgent then either the procedure can be deferred until the baby has been transferred, or a right radial (i.e. preductal) line sited *do not waste time (and arteries) if the first attempt is unsuccessful *sedate and muscle relax the baby who remains in poor condition despite attempts at optimizing ventilation. In particular muscle relaxants should be considered if the baby requires high pressure IPPV (e.g. a mean airway pressure of > 14) *surfactant administration (survanta, one ampoule) is optional. Some babies with CDH tolerate this procedure very poorly The baby with a best preductal pO2 <70 mmHg, or a persistent respiratory or metabolic acidosis despite 3-6 hours of attempting to optimize ventilatory and circulatory support has a very poor prognosis.

Stabilization —immediate priorities

* achieve acceptable gas exchange *saturations > 75%
* pCO_2 at a level that allows the pH to be > 7.20 while minimizing the chances of inducing lung injury or air leak. *monitor preductal saturations *apply a transcutaneous pCO2 monitor
* Consult level 3 centre Units reporting very high survival concentrate on minimizing lung injury especially in the initial hours after birth and rarely exceed PIP of 25. If available use a synchronized mode of ventilation

Continuing Management *requires a team of neonatologists, pediatric surgeons and pediatric intensivists *continuous monitoring of transcutaneous pCO_2, tidal and minute volumes *the lowest FiO_2 that results in a preductal saturation > 85% is maintained, especially in the initial hours of care. Permissive hypercarbia is strongly advocated *preductal arterial access is desirable if the infant's condition is marginal *assessment for dysmorphism - including echocardiography, renal and cranial sonography, a karyotype should be considered *an ongoing metabolic acidosis requiring repeated large doses of base suggests myocardial ischemia, sepsis or strangulated bowel *the principles of management and escalation of therapy include *use of muscle relaxants and sedatives *synchronized ventilation (SIMV or A/C) with tidal/minute volume monitoring *HFOV +/- Inhaled nitric oxide if the baby has unsatisfactory gas exchange after a reasonable trial of conventional ventilation, or there is an ongoing need for high ventilatory pressures or FiO_2 *jet ventilation if there is overt gas trapping or air leak *ECMO - less than 10% of babies need this *surgery - after ventilatory and circulatory support weaned to satisfactory levels (e.g. FiO_2 < 0.4 and mean airway pressure < 14) *discharge to a level II unit considered after *full enteral nutrition established for at least one week *respiratory status indicates significant reserve *audiology - arranged prior to discharge if possible *long term follow up required.

Pearl/Peril/Pitfall: The size of the diaphragmatic defect correlates with mortality and morbidity in live born infants with congenital diaphragmatic hernia, and this factor may have a much larger impact than other known risk factors: the defect size is likely to be a marker for the degree of pulmonary hypoplasia.

TABLE 1	Genetic Counseling—CDH

*CDH can occur as an isolated finding, as part of a genetic syndrome or chromosome abnormality, or as part of a complex but nonsyndromic set of findings.

*Kindreds representing both syndromic and nonsyndromic CDH consistent with autosomal dominant, autosomal recessive, and X-linked patterns of inheritance have been reported and some pedigrees suggest incomplete penetrance.

*The recurrence risk in subsequent pregnancies depends on whether the CDH is isolated, complex but nonsyndromic, or caused by a genetic syndrome or chromosome abnormality. Sibling recurrence for isolated Bochdalek hernia, the most common type of defect, is generally low (~1–2%); however, pedigrees consistent with monogenic inheritance have been reported, albeit rarely.

*Prenatal diagnosis is possible by ultrasound examination, but a diaphragmatic defect may be missed. MRI is especially useful for the prenatal diagnosis of thoracic lesions that are atypical or complicated by multiple abnormalities and for assessing lung volumes.

TABLE 2	CDH: Key Determinants of Mortality

* Whether the CDH is isolated or complex. Higher mortality occurs with complex CDH associated with a chromosome abnormality, a single gene disorder, and/or the coexistence of major malformations. The presence of a cardiovascular malformation also indicates a worse prognosis [Cohen et al 2002].
* The size of the diaphragm defect [Congenital Diaphragmatic Hernia Study Group 2007]
* The degree of pulmonary hypoplasia
* Whether the liver is up in the chest or remains down below the diaphragm [Albanese et al 1998]. Individuals with a large amount of "liver up" CDH have higher mortality than those whose liver remains down below the diaphragm.
* The severity of pulmonary hypertension in the perinatal period. Pulmonary hypertension, which may progress to a late or chronic phase, is often not responsive to medical therapy [Kinsella et al 2005].
* Whether the hernia is right-sided, left-sided, or bilateral. Some, but not all, studies show that a right-sided hernia is associated with greater mortality than a left-sided hernia [Skari et al 2000]. Bilateral CDH always confers a high mortality.

TABLE 3	CDH: Differential Diagnosis

Bronchogenic (foregut duplication) cysts result from abnormal budding of the ventral foregut [Knudtson & Grewal 2004]. They contain several components of the bronchi, including respiratory epithelia, mucous glands, and cartilage and may occur anywhere along the length of the trachea or esophagus. Most are diagnosed incidentally, although cysts can become infected or if large enough, can compress the esophagus and/or trachea.

Congenital cystic adenomatoid malformation (CCAM) is a developmental abnormality of the lung resulting from abnormal cell proliferation and decreased programmed cell death of lung tissue. Abnormally formed bronchi connect to the CCAM. Type I CCAM is most common and is distinguished by relatively large cysts and mucin production. Symptoms can result when CCAMs grow in size and compress structures in the mediastinum.

Cystic teratomas are benign tumors most often found in the anterior mediastinum [Jaggers & Balsara 2004]. They consist of several differentiated cell types derived from endoderm, ectoderm, and/or mesoderm. Cystic teratomas of the mediastinum are uncommon, comprising fewer than 10% of all tumors in that region.

Neurogenic tumors are the most common lesion found in the posterior mediastinum. They are likely to be of neural crest origin; the majority are benign. Examples include: neurilemoma, neurofibroma, ganglioneuroma, pheochromocytoma, and neuroblastoma. CT and MRI are helpful in establishing the diagnosis.

Paraesophageal hernia occurs when a portion of the stomach and sometimes part of the peritoneal sac containing the spleen or colon move into the chest cavity through the (normally occurring but) generally enlarged or dilated esophageal hiatus. More accurately, paraesophageal hernias are a type of hiatal hernia, in which the stomach gets "stuck" in the chest, rather than sliding back and forth between the thorax and abdomen. Approximately 5–10% of (acquired) hernias are paraesophageal. They are rare in infancy and most commonly present in older adults.

Pulmonary agenesis refers to partial or complete absence of lung tissue that is caused by failure of lung bud development. It is often associated with additional congenital malformations.

Pulmonary sequestration results from primitive lung tissue that is not connected to the tracheobronchial tree. Sequestration may be intrapulmonary, occurring within the pleura of the normal lung, or extrapulmonary, occurring outside the normal lung within its own pleural sac. Extrapulmonary sequestration seems to arise from an accessory lung bud and often has associated anomalies, such as CDH. The most common presenting symptom is respiratory, such as recurrent chest infections. MRI can accurately distinguish between pulmonary sequestration and CCAM [Quinn et al 1998].

Although all of the above lesions can remain undetected, respiratory symptoms usually develop at some point. Bronchogenic cysts, CCAM, and pulmonary sequestration should be surgically resected within the first few months of life to maximize growth of the surrounding normal lung tissue [Laberge et al 2005].

Pearl/Peril/Pitfall: Chromosome deletions on chromosomes 1q, 8p, and 15q have been reported in association with congenital diaphragmatic hernia. Deletions of chromosomes 8p and 15q appear to be associated with heart malformations. Chromosome abnormalities have been reported in as many as 30% of infants with congenital diaphragmatic hernia, which has been described as part of trisomy 13, trisomy 18, trisomy 21, and Turner syndrome (monosomy X) & Pallister-Killian syndrome (tetrasomy 12p mosaicism).

Ventilation Strategies-CDH

Conventional Mechanical Ventilation

Prevent conditions known to raise pulmonary vascular resistance (hypoxemia, acidosis, hypotension, and hypercarbia). *Institute* ventilation with low peak inspiratory pressures to avoid contralateral pneumothorax which can result in added cardiorespiratory instability and decompensation. *Employ* sedation and paralysis if hypoxia persists despite other medical treatments.

High-Frequency Oscillatory Ventilation (HFOV)

HFOV has been shown to reduce the need for ECMO in term infants who have respiratory failure. CDH has been associated with failure of HFOV and the need for ECMO more often than other causes of neonatal respiratory failure .Several recent articles report on the success of a multimodality approach using a combination of therapies, including delayed surgery, HFOV, inhaled nitric oxide (iNO), low ventilator pressures, permissive hypercapnea, surfactant replacement, and ECMO. Multicenter studies are needed to confirm the efficacy and safety of this approach.

Gentle Ventilation

The goal is to maintain preductal saturation at greater than 90% with minimal, but adequate ventilatory support that does not involve the use of paralysis, hyperventilation, or alkalosis. $PaCO_2$ levels up to 60 mm Hg are tolerated. If hypoxemia persists, tolazoline or dobutamine is added. ECMO is reserved for infants who fail this management strategy.

Intratracheal Pulmonary Ventilation (ITPV)

ITPV has been shown to maintain low airway pressures while decreasing ventilated anatomic dead space and increasing carbon dioxide removal in animal models of severe pulmonary hypoplasia. There is one report of ITPV use in two infants who had CDH on ECMO. Additional clinical experience will be needed before the usefulness of this technique in infants who have CDH is determined.

ECMO

Despite the lack of conclusive evidence that ECMO improves survival, it remains a mainstay of therapy for the infant who has CDH. Criteria for the selection of infants most likely to benefit from ECMO remain imprecise. It has been suggested that it is possible to avoid ECMO in those who have CDH and overwhelming pulmonary hypoplasia by requiring a preductal PaO_2 of greater than 100 torr and a $PaCO_2$ of less than 50 torr.

Currently, ECMO is used both in the preoperative patient who fails to stabilize scores and a higher incidence of hypotonia when compared with other ECMO survivors. Infants who have CDH have been shown in numerous studies to have longer periods of hospitalization and higher rates of chronic lung disease, both of which affect development. Longer term follow-up of larger with medical management and in the postoperative patient who deteriorates after repair. It is clear that infants who

have CDH and require ECMO preoperatively have more severe pulmonary hypoplasia and pulmonary hypertension and, thus, lower survival rates. The timing of the repair on or following ECMO remains controversial. The CDH Study Group reported that 33% of infants receiving ECMO were repaired on bypass. The risks of operating on ECMO (bleeding) must be weighed against the risks of operative repair after ECMO decannulation (recurrence of pulmonary hypertension). Two studies have concluded that mortality and morbidity are lower if the repair is undertaken after decannulation from ECMO.

Surfactant Replacement

Surfactant replacement in affected infants after birth has been associated with poor results unless the surfactant is administered prior to the first breath (prophylactically) instead of as a rescue. Several authors reporting increased survival rates include surfactant treatment as part of their management strategy.

Inhaled Nitric Oxide (iNO)

iNO has been shown in several large randomized clinical trials of infants who have hypoxic respiratory failure to improve oxygenation significantly and decrease the need for ECMO. However, the response to iNO has been suggested to be disease-specific; infants who have CDH experience little improvement with iNO therapy. Lack of improvement in oxygenation with iNO use prior to ECMO or CDH repair has been documented. However, significant improvement in oxygenation may occur when iNO follows ECMO and CDH repair. Both surfactant and partial liquid ventilation as well as administration of iNO following CDH repair and ECMO may allow iNO to be delivered to terminal lung units, thereby improving ventilation perfusion matching.

Partial Liquid Ventilation (PLV)

PLV may have an important role in the management of infants who have CDH. Perfluorocarbon is instilled into the trachea to a physiologic functional residual capacity, and gas ventilation techniques are continued. PLV has been shown to be effective in recruiting and stabilizing noncompliant alveoli, resulting in a significantly increased PaO_2 and pulmonary compliance in infants who have CDH and are receiving ECMO. iNO has been used in conjunction with PLV in an animal model of CDH, and a significant increase in oxygenation and reduction in pulmonary hypertension over PLV alone was observed. Clearly, PLV alone or in combination with other therapies offers promise for improved survival among infants who have CDH, and clinical trials are underway.

Lung Transplantation

To date there has been a single case report of successful lung transplantation in a newborn who had CDH following ECMO. At the age of 5 years, the transplanted lung was removed after the side effects of immunosuppression (growth failure, infection, hirsutism, and hypertension) became increasingly problematic. Balloon occlusion of the pulmonary artery to the transplanted lung during cardiac catheterization demonstrated that pneumonectomy.

Pearl/Peril/Pitfall : Infants with congenital diaphragmatic hernia are critically ill and require meticulous attention to detail for subsequent medical care, including continuous monitoring of oxygenation, blood pressure, and perfusion. A minimal stimulation approach that reduces handling and invasive procedures, such as suctioning, is suggested.

would be tolerated. Patient selection, donor lung size, availability, and the long-term risks of immuno-suppression remain barriers to the wider use of lung transplantation in the patient who has CDH.

Prognosis-outcome Survival

Mortality from CDH continues to be high, ranging from 20% to 60%. Data from neonatal or referral centers operating on relatively selected cases, primarily those with isolated left-sided Bochdalek hernia, report 80%-90% survival [Downard et al 2003]. However, population-based studies of outcome for all prenatally diagnosed CDH cases report mortality of at least 50%, if pregnancy terminations are included [Colvin et al 2005]. In a meta-analysis, Stege et al [2003] observed that approximately one-quarter of all prenatally diagnosed cases were electively terminated, 3% spontaneously miscarried, and 3% were stillborn; 31% of the liveborns died, the majority within the first 24 hours of life. When all resources, including ECMO, are provided, reported survival rates range from 40-90%. The ELSO registry reports the ECMO survival rate at 52%. *CDH survivors have a number of significant medical issues after hospital discharge, including chronic lung disease, gastroesophageal reflux, growth failure, reherniation, volvulus, scoliosis, sensorineural hearing loss, and developmental delay.*

Lung Function and Chronic Lung Disease

Almost all individuals with CDH have some degree of pulmonary hypoplasia. Many infants require oxygen supplementation and diuretics following surgical correction of CDH. Given the remarkable growth and recuperative capacity of the lung, these treatments can usually be discontinued within the first two years of life. By early childhood, few children have respiratory symptoms at rest; however, formal testing even in older children shows small airway obstruction and diminished blood flow on ventilation-perfusion (V-Q) scan, especially to the lung ipsilateral to the hernia. Limited exercise tolerance can be a lifelong problem. Intermittent wheezing requiring bronchodilator use is common in persons with CDH, and they are at risk for respiratory decompensation with intercurrent illness. It is not clear whether the severity of long term pulmonary morbidity can be predicted based on the severity of the perinatal respiratory disease. The long-term clinical significance of abnormal pulmonary function testing in these children will be better defined as a greater number of severely affected children survive. More recent studies of infants treated with ECMO have shown that only 22% were using oxygen at discharge.

Gastroesophageal Reflux: The incidence of significant gastroesophageal reflux is very high in patients who survive congenital diaphragmatic hernia, and studies document an incidence of 45-85%. The need for a diaphragmatic patch may be a significant predictor of gastroesophageal reflux. Severe reflux may result in chronic aspiration and is, therefore, aggressively treated. Although most infants can be medically treated with H2-blockers or proton pump inhibitors in combination with a motility agent such as metoclopramide, surgical intervention is sometimes required.

Failure to Thrive: Failure to thrive is common, and, in some studies, more than 50% of patients are below the 25th percentile for height and weight during the first year of life. In one study, one third of infants required gastrostomy tube placement to improve caloric intake. The need for supplemental oxygen at the time of discharge is a significant predictor for subsequent growth failure. Possible causes include increased caloric requirements due to chronic lung disease, oral aversion after prolonged intubation, poor oral feeding due to neurologic delays, and gastroesophageal reflux.

Reherniation: The incidence of reherniation is increased with the use of synthetic patch repairs and ranges from 5% to 80%. The timing of the reherniation appears to vary. Symptoms occurring with reherniation are usually respiratory, such as coughing and wheezing, or feeding difficulties.

Volvulus: Patients who have CDH have malrotation, and a small number will have obstruction of the small bowel due to midgut volvulus or adhesions. If unrecognized, this complication can be life-threatening.

Scoliosis: Chest wall and spinal deformities are found in children and adults who have CDH. A study of 60 adult CDH survivors (mean age, 29 y) documented chest asymmetry in 48%, pectus excavatum in 18%, and significant scoliosis with a Cobb angle of at least 10 degrees in 27%. The incidence of these abnormalities was greatest among those who had a large diaphragmatic defect and those who had undergone thoracotomy versus laparotomy. It is likely that repair of a large defect causes tension, which may interfere with normal development of the thoracic cage and promote asymmetry. Other authors have noted lower incidences of chest wall and spinal deformities, but these reports have had shorter periods of follow-up. Clearly, CDH survivors should be monitored for these abnormalities.

Hearing loss: Risk factors for hearing impairment in the newborn population include low birthweight, use of ototoxic medications such as aminoglycosides and furosemide, hyperbilirubinemia, congenital infections, meningitis, and hyperventilation. Hyperventilation with the induction of a respiratory alkalosis has been associated with the development of a progressive high-frequency sensorineural hearing loss. One study documented hearing loss in 52.5% of infants who had persistent pulmonary hypertension that was associated with exposure to high pH levels and long periods of ventilation. The reported incidence of hearing loss in ECMO survivors has ranged from 4% to 28%. A recent study of hearing in CDH survivors treated with and without ECMO found almost 60% to have sensorineural hearing loss. This hearing loss is progressive, and normal results on a hearing screen at discharge do not preclude the development of later hearing loss. Regular hearing screening is a necessity for CDH survivors.

Developmental outcome: In early reports of long-term survivors, neurologic abnormalities and mild-to-moderate developmental delay were common, especially among those receiving ECMO (extracorporeal membrane oxygenation) treatment. Information about developmental outcomes using more current practice standards is limited by lack of prospective studies testing with standard developmental assessment tools. However, emerging data indicate that most children who are not diagnosed with a chromosome abnormality or syndrome have full-scale IQ scores in the low-average or average range, with virtually none having intellectual disability (i.e. IQ score <70) [Bouman et al 2000; S Freedman, personal communication]. However, these children with normal IQs remain vulnerable to learning disabilities, attention problems, and behavior problems [Friedman et al 2008, Peetsold et al 2009].

CDH: Practice points

* The most important prenatal negative predictor in leftsided CDH is the presence of liver in the chest.

* The postnatal care are of CDH has evolved from previous aggressive ventilation and emergent operation to current permissive hypercapnea, physiologic stabilization, and elective surgical repair.

* When available, ECMO is considered for almost all infants with CDH who fail conventional therapy as a means of stabilizing pulmonary hypertension and lung protection

CDH: Research directions

* More accurate prenatal parameters need development to allow standardization of results between centers and appropriate design of clinical trials in CDH.

* The efficacy, timing, duration, and patient selection of tracheal occlusion for severe CDH need careful study.

* As survival improves and in the assessment of treatment efficacy, morbidity and quality of life measures need more attention.

Pearl/Peril/Pitfall: The medical problems of pulmonary hypoplasia and PPHN are largely responsible for the outcome of congenital diaphragmatic hernia and that the severity of these pathophysiologies is largely predetermined in utero. Herniated viscera in the chest does not appear to exacerbate the pathophysiology as long as bowel decompression with a nasogastric tube is continuous.

CDH: Principles of Prenatal Care

* referral for tertiary level obstetric ultrasound
* if the diagnosis is confirmed referral to a multidisciplinary fetal diagnostic/management team

Objectives

* establish an accurate description of the abnormalities present
* specify ultrasound features relevant to CDH using a standard form
* degree of mediastinal shift * liver/stomach position
* lung:head ratio * liquor volume
* fetal echocardiogram performed by a Paediatric cardiologist, if associated congenital heart disease suspected
* establish a fetal karyotype, if informed parental consent given
* provide informed and supportive counselling for the family including a written summary of any discussion with the parents. This summary should include a description of the abnormalities and most likely diagnoses, management options available, and possible outcomes

Ongoing Management

* referral to a Pediatric Thoracic Surgeon if not previously arranged
* regular general obstetric surveillance
* repeat ultrasounds at 24, 30 and 34 weeks to assess fetal growth and features of the CDH as defined above

Intervention

* prenatal steroid therapy - recommended according to usual indications. Clinical trials are under consideration for use at mature gestations
* fetal operative intervention (tracheal ligation) is an unproven therapy : not recommended outside of clinical trials (currently in progress overseas)

KEY POINTS FOR CLINICAL PRACTICE:

1. Ultrasonography now is considered the gold standard for diagnosing CDH antenatally. Suggestive findings include polyhydramnios, an absent or intrathoracic stomach bubble, and mediastinal and cardiac shift away from the side of the hernia. The differential diagnosis includes congenital cystic adenomatoid malformation, cystic teratoma, extrapulmonary sequestration, bronchogenic cysts, and neurogenic tumors

2. Once CDH has been diagnosed antenatally by ultrasonography, it is important to determine if the defect is isolated or associated with other anomalies known to affect outcome. Prompt intubation, avoidance of bag-mask ventilation, placement of a nasogastric tube to provide intestinal decompression, and ongoing care in an intensive care nursery by individuals experienced in the management of the newborn who has CDH now is the norm.

3. Currently, most infants who have CDH are stabilized before operative intervention. The mean age at the time of surgery for infants not treated with extracorporeal membrane oxygenation (ECMO) is 73 hours (range, 0 to 443 h). Currently, ECMO is used both in the preoperative patient who fails to stabilize with medical management and in the postoperative patient who deteriorates after repair. It is clear that infants who have CDH and require ECMO preoperatively have more severe pulmonary hypoplasia and pulmonary hypertension and, thus, lower survival rates. The timing of the repair on or following ECMO remains controversial.

4. Both surfactant and partial liquid ventilation as well as administration of iNO following CDH repair and ECMO may allow iNO to be delivered to terminal lung units, thereby improving ventilation perfusion matching.

5. Despite several decades of investigation and a vast array of new therapeutic approaches, the optimal therapeutic strategy for the newborn who has CDH remains undetermined. Ongoing data collection and the development of multicenter clinical trials should clarify which therapies are most likely to be of benefit.

REFERENCES AND FURTHER READING : 1) The Neonatal Inhaled Nitric Oxide Study Group (NINOS). Inhaled nitric oxide and hypoxic respiratory failure in infants with congenital diaphragmatic hernia. *Pediatrics*. 1997;97:83-845 2) Van Meurs KP, Robbins ST, Reed VL, et al. Congenital diaphragmatic hernia: long-term outcome in neonates treated with extracorporeal membrane oxygenation. *J Pediatr*. 1993;122:893-899 3) Wung JT, Sahni R, Moffitt ST, Lipsitz E, Stolar CJH. Congenital diaphragmatic hernia: survival with very delayed surgery, spontaneous respiration and no chest tube. *J Pediatr Surg*. 1995;30:406-409 4) Schnitzer JJ, Thompson JE, Hedrick HL. A new ventilator improves CO_2 removal in newborn lambs with congenital diaphragmatic hernia. *Crit Care Med*. 1999;27:109-112 5) Reyes C, Chang LK, Waffarn F, Mir H, Warden MJ, Sills J. Delayed repair of congenital diaphragmatic hernia with early high-frequency oscillatory ventilation during preoperative stabilization. *J Pediatr Surg*. 1998;33:1010-1016

---

* *Pearl/Peril/Pitfall : Long-term morbidity: As noted, survivors are at risk for significant long-term morbidity, including chronic lung disease, growth failure, gastroesophageal reflux, hearing loss, and neurodevelopmental delay. The risk appears to be highest in infants with severe lung disease (need for supplemental oxygen), need for patch closure of the diaphragm, and need for gastrostomy tube feeding.*

42 Neonatal Persistent Pulmonary Hypertension (PPHN)

@ *Oxygenation is often assessed by using the oxygenation index (OI), which accounts for the postductal PaO_2 and the ventilator settings. The OI is calculated as the mean airway pressure multiplied by the fraction of inspired oxygen (FiO_2) and the 100, and the product is divided by the postductal PaO_2. An OI of 40 typically prompts consideration of ECMO support.*

Persistent pulmonary hypertension of the newborn (PPHN) is the result of elevated pulmonary vascular resistance to the point that venous blood is diverted to some degree through fetal channels (i.e. the ductus arteriosus and foramen ovale) into the systemic circulation and bypassing the lungs, resulting in systemic arterial hypoxemia. This disorder can be classified into *three forms* dependent on the likely etiology of the pulmonary hypertension:

A. **PPHN associated with pulmonary parenchymal disease**, such as hyaline membrane disease, meconium aspiration, or transient tachypnea of the newborn as the cause of alveolar hypoxia *known as secondary PPHN or appropriate PPHN *alveolar oxygen tension appears to be the major determinant of pulmonary artery vasoconstriction.

B. **PPHN with radiographically normal lungs** and no evidence of parenchymal disease *frequently called Persistent Fetal Circulation (PFC), or primary or inappropriate PPHN

C. **PPHN associated with hypoplasia of the lungs** *most often in the form of diaphragmatic hernia *associated with an anatomic reduction in capillary number.

This syndrome is usually noted in term or post-term infants. The baby presents clinically with cyanosis and respiratory distress, with tachypnea, but with minimal retractions during the first day of life. The infants chest radiograph may be normal (as noted in infants with primary PPHN, i.e. PFC) or demonstrate various abnormalities compatible with aspiration, pneumonia, diaphragmatic hernia, or hyaline membrane disease.

Supplemental oxygen is needed in an attempt to correct arterial hypoxemia. With a large right-to-left shunt through a patent ductus arteriosus, an oxygen tension gradient may be noted between the preductal arterial circulation (i.e. right upper extremity) and the postductal arterial circulation (i.e. lower extremities). However, this gradient may not be present if substantial shunting is present at the level of the foramen ovale. Systemic hypotension is a late finding usually resulting from both heart failure and persistent hypoxemia. Chest radiography *Chest radiography is useful in determining whether underlying parenchymal lung disease (e.g. meconium aspiration syndrome, pneumonia, surfactant deficiency) is present. Chest radiography also assists in excluding underlying disorders, such as congenital diaphragmatic hernia. *In newborns with idiopathic persistent pulmonary hypertension of the newborn, the lung fields appear clear, with decreased vascular markings. *Heart size is typically normal or slightly.

The diagnosis is confirmed echocardiographically. The most appropriate treatment of Persistent Pulmonary Hypertension of the Newborn remains unclear . Substantial variation in clinical practice exists between institutions. However, basic treatment goals do exist . *In order of increasing aggressiveness and invasiveness:* *Improve alveolar oxygenation *Minimize pulmonary vasoconstriction *Maintain systemic blood pressure and perfusion *Consider induction of an alkalotic state *Consider a trial of vasodilatation (Inhaled nitric oxide) *Consider extracorporeal membrane oxygenation support .

REVIEW OF CLINICAL PROBLEMS

1. When should you suspect PPHN clinically ?
   Ans: Refer to the "No.1" of the "BIRD'S EYE VIEW/OVERVIEW/ SYNOPSIS" of the Chapter.

2. How do you interpret Differential Pulse Oximeter readings in assisting the diagnosis of PPHN ?
   Ans: Refer to the "No.2 a" of the "BIRD'S EYE VIEW/OVERVIEW/ SYNOPSIS" of the Chapter.

3. What are the investigations to be done to determine the Etiology and Degree of Pulmonary Hypertension ?
   Ans: Refer to the Evaluation-Decision-Action Plan/Algorithm to diagnose and manage Neonatal PPHN.

4. How do you manage Neonatal PPHN?
   Ans: Refer to the Evaluation-Decision-Action Plan/Algorithm to diagnose and manage Neonatal PPHN.

5. Name the Clinical signs that favor cyanotic congenital heart disease over PPHN.
   Ans: Refer to the "No.3" of the "BIRD'S EYE VIEW/OVERVIEW/ SYNOPSIS" of the Chapter.

LEARNING OBJECTIVES

After completing this article, readers will be able to

1. Recognize fetal blood flow patterns and postnatal changes in pulmonary vascular resistance after lung inflation and oxygenation.

2. Recognize factors that aggravate Persistent Pulmonary Hypertension of the Newborn and Institute Preventive measures Pre and Post natally.

3. Diagnose and initiate treatment for Persistent Pulmonary Hypertension of the Newborn, and refer as needed for assistance in diagnosis or management.

4. Exclude Cyanotic CHD, and Secondary causes of Pulmonary Hypertension.

5. Counsel parents about treatment and prognosis of PPHN.

Pearl/Peril/Pitfall: Sedation and analgesia with opioids is often necessary to achieve adequate mechanical ventilation in patients with persistent pulmonary hypertension of the newborn (PPHN). Muscle paralysis may be used for the same purpose; however, this method is controversial because adverse circulatory effects and alveolar collapse in dependent regions of the lung may develop. The administration of a surfactant may be helpful if parenchymal disease is present.

BIRD'S EYE VIEW/OVERVIEW/SYNOPSIS

1. **PPHN of the newborn** is a condition that results from a failure of the normal postbirth decrease in pulmonary vascular resistance, leading to a variable degree of right-to-left shunting through to persistent fetal channels, the foramen ovale and ductus arteriosus, and severe hypoxemia. *Suspect PPHN clinically* if there is *history of perinatal asphyxia/ meconium aspiration syndrome/sepsis or pneumonia/polycythemia/pulmonary hypoplasia/ congenital diaphragmatic hernia / congenital heart disease (Refer to Table 1). *Hypoxemia in a Newborn out of proportion to the degree of parenchymal lung disease *Intermittent cyanosis, especially to painful stimuli *Loud single S2 *Tricuspid regurgitant murmur *A prominent RV impulse.

2. **PPHN is essentially a diagnosis of exclusion**: it should routinely be considered in evaluating the cyanotic newborn. Among cases of suspected PPHN, the most common alternative diagnoses are uncomplicated severe pulmonary parenchymal disease, sepsis and congenital heart disease.

   a) *Differential pulse oximeter readings* - A difference > 5% between preductal (right radial artery) and postductal (left radial, umbilical, or tibial arteries) oxygen saturations is considered indicative of a right - to- left ductal shunt.A difference of > 10–15mmHg between preductal and postductal PaO_2 is also considered suggestive of a right - to - left ductal shunt. No difference can be found if the right - to-left shunting (may be predominantly at the atrial level and the ductus may not be patent at all). Oximeter probes can be placed on preductal (right hand) and postductal (right or left foot) sites to assess for right-to-left shunt at the level of the ductus arteriosus. Remember that sites on the left hand should be avoided because it may be preductal or postductal. b) *Hyperoxia test* PPHN should be considered if marked improvement in oxygenation (>30mmHg increase in PaO_2) is noted on hyperventilating the infant (lowering the $PaCO_2$ to 25-30mmHg and increasing pH to 7.5–7.7). Little or no response is expected in infants with cyanotic congenital heart disease (Refer to Table 5).

   c) *Radiography*: Nonspecific, may suggest or exclude associated conditions. Clear lung fields or only minor disease in the face of severe hypoxemia is strongly suggestive of PPHN, if cyanotic congenital heart disease has been ruled out by Echocardiogram.

   d) *Echocardiography/Doppler study:* Indicated to rule out cyanotic congenital heart disease and to identify patients with myocardial dysfunction.

   e) *Cardiac catheterization:* May be important to rule out TAPVR, which can not be ruled out by 2D Echo.

3. *Clinical signs that favour cyanotic congenital heart disease over PPHN include* cardiomegaly, weak pulses, active precordium, pulse differential between upper and lower extremities, pulmonary edema, Grade-III+ murmur, and persistent pre- and postductal arterial oxygen tension (PaO_2) at or < 40mmHg.

4. *The severity of the PPHN can be assessed by measuring* **OXYGENATION INDEX (OI)**

$$OI = \frac{FiO_2 \times mean\ airway\ pressure \times 100}{PaO_2\ (post\ ductal)}$$

$OI > 15$ = severe respiratory failure

$OI > 30\text{–}35$ = failure to respond to existing mode of ventilatory support : try HFOV + NO

$OI > 40$ = ECMO support is mandatory

5. The preventive measures to deal with PPHN are *listed in Table 2. The management goals include:* 1) establish the diagnosis 2) reduce the pulmonary artery pressure either pharmacologically and / or by mechanical ventilation 3) correct myocardial dysfunction 4) stabilize the patient and treat associated conditions (Refer to E-D-A-Algorithm).

6. *General stabilization measures include :* a) careful and intensive monitoring b) fluid management c) correction of acidosis, hypovolemia, hypoglycemia, hypocalcemia, hypomagnesemia, and hypothermia d) minimal handling e) maintain hemoglobin above 15g/dL to maintain adequate oxygen carrying capacity f) assure adequate systemic blood pressure—Dopamine along with Dobutamine IVI help to optimize cardiac output, enhance systemic blood pressure, and reduce pulmonary vascular resistance g) treat sepsis with antibiotics h) correct mechanical problems (eg : pneumothorax, pleural effusions, ascites).

7. *Measures to reduce pulmonary artery pressure include:* a) hyperventilation b) metabolic alkalinization c) vasodilator therapy d) analgesia, sedation and /or muscle paralysis e) high frequency oscillatory ventilation (HFOV) together with nitric oxide (NO) therapy f) ECMO (Refer Tables 3 and 4).

8. *Inhaled NITRIC OXIDE is a promising therapy for PPHN* it relaxes the pulmonary vasculature (at 6-20 ppm -parts per million-upto 80ppm can be tried) like natural endothelium derived NO. Potential toxicities include methemoglobinemia (at above 40 ppm) and lung injury from metabolites (nitrates and nitrites). Inhaled Nitric Oxide is most effective when administered after adequate alveolar recruitment, which can be accomplished among infants PPHN with diffuse pulmonary disease by the concomitant use of HFOV and/or Surfactant treatment.

9. ECMO is often lifesaving therapy for infants with PPHN who fail conventional mangement and/or iNO treatment. The overall survival rate is around 80% with ECMO and is dependent upon underlying disease: lower rates for congenital diaphragmatic hernia and lung hypoplasia.

10. Long term sequelae in survivors is about 20% : include psychomotor delay and sensorineural deafness from alkalinization and hyperventilation. The outcome of PPHN is good if it is acute or secondary to a reversible lung disease, such as MAS. The outlook is less optimistic, if PPHN is secondary to chronic in utero hypoxia and ischemia or to pulmonary hypoplasia, such as congenital diaphragmatic hernia or congenital renal dysplasia.

Pearl/Peril/Pitfall : Neurologic sequelae ·Although most surviving newborns with persistent pulmonary hypertension of the newborn have normal neurodevelopmental outcomes, as many as 25% have significant neurodevelopmental sequelae. ·Prolonged hyperventilation is associated with an increased prevalence of neurodevelopmental sequelae, especially sensorineural hearing loss.

THE EVALUATION-DECISION-ACTION-PLAN/ALGORITHM FOR THE DIAGNOSIS AND MANAGEMENT OF *PERSISTENT PULMONARY HYPERTENSION OF THE NEWBORN (PPHN)*

SUBJECTIVE FINDINGS

Hx of cyanosis and tachypnea without apnea and retractions/grunting in a term /postterm baby, beginning 6–12 hours after birth.

Hx of meconium staining/birth asphyxia.

Hx of maternal ingestion of NSAIDs in the third trimester.

Hx of antenatal scan findings like chronic intrauterine asphyxia, congenital diaphragmatic hernia, oligohydramnios, etc.

Hx of perinatal sepsis (PROM > 24 hours, maternal fever > 38.5°C, etc.)

OBJECTIVE FINDINGS

Assess ABCs, BP, O_2 Sats (Preductal and postductal), vitals, CRT, Urine output.

Look for dysmorphic features -Potter's facies

Assess CVS Prominent RV impulse, single and loud S2, soft regurgitant systolic murmur of TR, gallop rhythm of myocardial dysfunction occasionally

Assess RS Abnormal breath sounds.

Observe any significant decreases in pulse oximetry reading with routine nursing care or minor stress

Observe for other variable findings associated with secondary causes of PPHN

INVESTIGATIONS

a. Differential pulse oximeter readings (preductal and postductal)
b. Hyperoxia test
c. CXR
d. 2D Echocardiography
e. Blood - Full blood count, (haemoglobin and haematocrit) with platelets (thrombocytopenia in 60% of the babies with PPHN), ABG analysis, electrolytes with calcium, magnesium, blood glucose, blood cultures.
f. ECG (ST segment depression suggestive of ischemia)
g. Rarely Cardiac catheterization

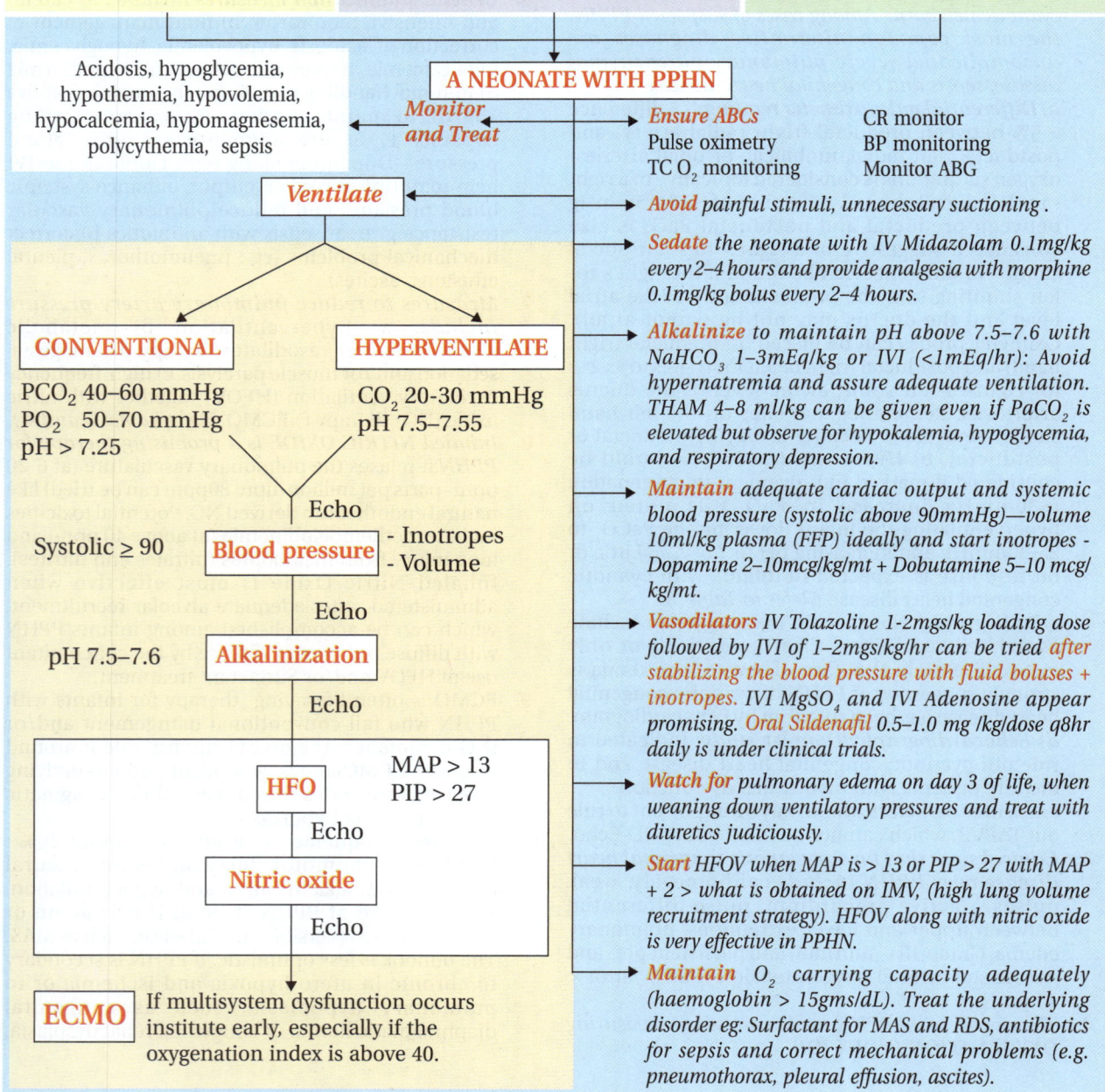

A NEONATE WITH PPHN

Acidosis, hypoglycemia, hypothermia, hypovolemia, hypocalcemia, hypomagnesemia, polycythemia, sepsis

Monitor and Treat

Ensure ABCs   CR monitor
Pulse oximetry   BP monitoring
TC O_2 monitoring   Monitor ABG

Ventilate

Avoid painful stimuli, unnecessary suctioning .

Sedate the neonate with IV Midazolam 0.1mg/kg every 2–4 hours and provide analgesia with morphine 0.1mg/kg bolus every 2–4 hours.

CONVENTIONAL
PCO₂ 40–60 mmHg
PO₂ 50–70 mmHg
pH > 7.25

HYPERVENTILATE
CO₂ 20-30 mmHg
pH 7.5–7.55

Alkalinize to maintain pH above 7.5–7.6 with $NaHCO_3$ 1–3mEq/kg or IVI (<1mEq/hr): Avoid hypernatremia and assure adequate ventilation. THAM 4–8 ml/kg can be given even if $PaCO_2$ is elevated but observe for hypokalemia, hypoglycemia, and respiratory depression.

Echo

Systolic ≥ 90   **Blood pressure**   - Inotropes - Volume

Maintain adequate cardiac output and systemic blood pressure (systolic above 90mmHg)—volume 10ml/kg plasma (FFP) ideally and start inotropes - Dopamine 2–10mcg/kg/mt + Dobutamine 5–10 mcg/kg/mt.

Echo

pH 7.5–7.6   **Alkalinization**

Vasodilators IV Tolazoline 1-2mgs/kg loading dose followed by IVI of 1–2mgs/kg/hr can be tried *after stabilizing the blood pressure with fluid boluses + inotropes.* IVI $MgSO_4$ and IVI Adenosine appear promising. *Oral Sildenafil 0.5–1.0 mg /kg/dose q8hr daily is under clinical trials.*

Echo

HFO   MAP > 13   PIP > 27

Watch for pulmonary edema on day 3 of life, when weaning down ventilatory pressures and treat with diuretics judiciously.

Echo

Nitric oxide

Start HFOV when MAP is > 13 or PIP > 27 with MAP + 2 > what is obtained on IMV, (high lung volume recruitment strategy). HFOV along with nitric oxide is very effective in PPHN.

Echo

ECMO   If multisystem dysfunction occurs institute early, especially if the oxygenation index is above 40.

Maintain O_2 carrying capacity adequately (haemoglobin > 15gms/dL). Treat the underlying disorder eg: Surfactant for MAS and RDS, antibiotics for sepsis and correct mechanical problems (e.g. pneumothorax, pleural effusion, ascites).

Pearl/Peril/Pitfall: The use of paralytic agents is highly controversial and typically reserved for newborns who cannot be treated with sedatives alone. Be aware that paralysis, in particular with pancuronium, may promote atelectasis of dependent lung regions and promote ventilation-perfusion mismatch.

TABLE 1	Neonatal PPHN—etiopathogenic factors

A. Normal pulmonary vascular morphology/myocardial dysfunction or increased vascular reactivity from vasoconstrictive stimuli.

1. Associated with asphyxia
   a. Vasoconstrictive effects of hypoxia, hypercarbia, acidosis
   b. Myocardial dysfunction (especially left ventricle) leading to pulmonary venous hypertension and subsequent PPHN with right-to-left shunting through the ductus arteriosus

2. Associated with meconium aspiration syndrome (MAS)
   a. Alveolar hypoxia results in vasoconstriction
   b. Gas trapping and lung overdistention contribute to increased pulmonary vascular resistance.
   c. Concomitant effects of severe parenchymal lung disease
   d. Some infants will also have morphological changes in pulmonary vasculature (see B)

3. Sepsis / pneumonia
   a. Infection initiates an inflammatory response
   b. Release of cytokines and other vascular mediators increases pulmonary vascular resistance
   c. Severe parenchymal lung disease aggravates hypoxemia

4. Thrombus or microthrombus formation with release of vasoactive mediators

5. Hyperviscosity syndrome

B. Morphologically abnormal pulmonary vasculature

1. Abnormal extension of vascular smooth muscle, with thickening and increased resistance deeper into the pulmonary vascular tree. May be related to chronic intrauterine hypoxia.
   a. Some cases of MAS
   b. *In utero* closure of the ductus arteriosus
   c. Idiopathic PPHN

2. Abnormally small lungs with decreased cross-sectional area of the pulmonary vascular bed and muscular thickening and distal extension
   a. Pulmonary hypoplasia (either primary or secondary)
   b. Congenital diaphragmatic hernia
   c. Cystic adenomatoid malformation

C. Structurally abnormal heart disease

1. Left ventricular outflow tract obstruction

2. Anomalous pulmonary venous return

3. Ebstein's anomaly

4. Left ventricular cardiomyopathy

5. Any structural abnormality which results in a obligatory right-to-left shunt

TABLE 2	Neonatal PPHN preventive measures

A. Prenatal

1. Pregnancies found to be complicated by conditions associated with PPHN (e.g. congenital diaphragmatic hernia, prolonged oligohydramnios) should be referred to a high-risk center capable of caring for the infant following delivery.

2. Identification and appropriate obstetrical management of other at-risk pregnancies (e.g. meconium-staining, chorioamnionitis, post dates)

B. Postnatal

1. Adequate resuscitation

2. Avoidance of hypothermia, hypovolemia, hypoglycemia

3. Avoidance of acidosis, hypoxia, and hypercarbia

4. Prompt treatment of suspected sepsis, hypotension, or other problems

PULMONARY ARTERIAL HYPERTENSION CYCLE

Pearl/Peril/Pitfall : In newborns with severe airspace disease who require high peak inspiratory pressures (i.e., >30 cm H_2O) or mean airway pressures (>15 cm H_2O), consider high-frequency ventilation (HFV) to reduce barotraumas and associated air leak syndrome. When HFV is used, the goal should still be to optimize lung expansion and FRC and to avoid overdistension.

TABLE 3   **Ventilation strategy to manage a child with severe PPHN**

1. *Conventional ventilation*: This uses the least amount of support possible to achieve gas exchange and pH which is marginally acceptable, to avoid barotrauma. A pH $\geq$ 7.25, a $PaCO_2$ 55–60 mmHg, and PaO_2 50–70 mmHg are the targets for conventional ventilation. The lowest possible mean airway pressure (MAP) and PEEP, and an FiO_2 of 1 (100% oxygen) initially are utilized to achieve the targets. Weaning should be gradual and in small steps *(attempt several small ventilator / FiO_2 changes than one large one)*. The use of sedatives and skeletal muscle relaxants is discouraged. A transitional phase of PPHN occurs at 3–5 days of age. Vascular reactivity diminishes and support can be decreased at a faster rate. Once the baby reaches an FiO_2 of < 0.3 to 0.4, PIP 18, and PEEP 4 cm H_2O, extubation has to be considered.

2. *Hyperventilation*: This attempts to take advantage of the vasodilatory effects of alkalosis and hypocarbia on the pulmonary vasculature. Decrease the $PaCO_2$ to the critical value (20–30mmHg), below which there is a sharp rise in PaO_2. Respiratory alkalosis so produce can be augmented by infusion of sodium bicarbonate, to keep the pH > 7.5. A PaO_2 between 80-100mmHg and the target pH > 7.3 are to be achieved with a rate of 80-100/mt, PIP > 35 cm H_2O, PIP around 4-5 cm H_2O, I:E ratio 1:1, inspiratory time 0.2-0.3 seconds. Ventilatory changes and decrease in adjunctive support is done very slowly. Once a PaO_2 100-150mmHg is achieved, a gradual and steady weaning down of FiO_2 is done till it reaches 0.7. Then the CO_2 is not so critical and pulmonary vasculature is not labile. *Low psychomotor development and sensorineural hearing loss are more common in babies who had PCO_2 < 15mmHg.*

3. Many clinicians prefer a *"middle of the road"* approach, where physiologically normal blood gases and pH are targeted by using ventilator support that is somewhere in between those approaches described above.

4. *Consider high frequency oscillatory ventilation (HFOV)*, if the MAP is above 13 and PIP > 27 cm and the oxygenation index is > 30.

TABLE 4   **Management goals in aggressive hyperventilation approach and a more conservative ventilation approach in persistent pulmonary hypertension of the newborn**

	Hyperventilation	*Conservative ventilation*
Target pH	$\geq$ 7.3	$\geq$ 7.25
Target $PaCO_2$ (mmHg)	20-25	40-60
Target PaO_2 (mmHg)	80-100	50-70
Rates (breaths per min)	Upto 100	Matched to patient's rate
Peak inspiratory pressure (cm H_2O)	high (may be >35) cm H_2O)	Minimum needed to produce chest expansion
Inspiratory time (s)	short (0.2-0.3 sec)	Long (-0.6 sec)

TABLE 5   **Hyperoxia test**

In cases of Neonatal cyanosis with breathing diffculties (either tachypnea or dyspnea) *Do HYPEROXIA (Oxygen Challenge) TEST and Interpret according to the following table.* A) Technique Used to evaluate etiology of cyanosis in neonates. Obtain *baseline arterial blood gases (ABG)* or pulse oximetry saturation at FiO_2=0.21, then place infant in oxygen hood at FiO_2 =1 (100%) for a minimum of 10 minutes, and *repeat ABG* or pulse oximetry. Pulse oximetry will not be useful for following the change in oxygenation once the saturations reach 100% (approximately $pO_2 \geq$ 90mm Hg) (1 kPa = 7.5mmHg)

B) Interpretation	FiO_2 = .21		FiO_2 = 1.00	
	PaO_2 (% saturation)		PaO_2 (% saturation)	$PaCO_2$
Normal	70 (95)		> 200 (100)	35
Pulmonary disease	50 (85)		> 150 (100)	50
Neurologic disease	50 (85)		> 150 (100)	50
Methemoglobinemia	70 (95)		> 200 (100)	35
Cardiac disease				
Separate circulation*	<40 (<75)		< 50 (<85)	35
Restricted PBF †	<40 (<75)		< 50 (<85)	35
Complete mixing without restricted PBF	‡ 50 (85)		<150 (<100)	35
Persistent pulmonary hypertension	Preductal	Postductal		
PFO (no R to L shunt)	70 (95)	<40 (<75)	Variable	35–50
PFO (with R to L shunt)	<40 (<75)	<40 (<75)	Variable	35–50

PBF, Pulmonary blood flow *D-Transposition of the great arteries (D-TGA) with intact ventricular septum. †Tricuspid atresia with pulmonary stenosis or atresia ; pulmonary atresia or critical pulmonary stenosis with intact ventricular septum ; or tetralogy of Fallot. ‡ Truncus, total anomalous pulmonary venous return, single ventricle, hypoplastic left heart, D-TGA with ventricular septal defect, tricuspid atresia without pulmonary stenosis or atresia. From Less MH : *J Pediatr* 77:484, 1970 ; Kitterman JA : *Pediatr Rev* 4:13, 1982 ; Jones RWA et al : *Arch Dis Child* 51 : 667, 1976.

PPHN—General considerations

*The care of newborns with persistent pulmonary hypertension of the newborn (PPHN) requires meticulous attention to detail. Continuous monitoring of oxygenation, blood pressure, and perfusion is critical.

*When one cares for newborns, use a minimal stimulation protocol to minimize the need to handle the patient and to perform invasive procedures, such as suctioning.

*Management of fluid and electrolyte levels, particularly calcium, is important. An adequate circulating blood volume is necessary to maintain right ventricular filling and cardiac output; however, repeated bolus administration of crystalloid and colloid solutions does not provide additional benefit.

*Inotropic support with dopamine, dobutamine, and/or milrinone alone or in combination, is frequently helpful in maintaining adequate cardiac output and systemic blood pressure while avoiding excessive volume administration. Although dopamine is frequently used as a first-line agent, other agents, such as dobutamine and milrinone, are helpful when myocardial contractility is poor.

PPHN—Medicolegal pitfalls

*The main pitfall in the treatment of persistent pulmonary hypertension of the newborn is in recognizing its existence and severity. Although inhaled nitric oxide (iNO) is an effective pulmonary vasodilator, extracorporeal membrane oxygenation (ECMO) remains the only therapy that has been proven to be life-saving for persistent pulmonary hypertension of the newborn. Timely transfer to an ECMO center is life saving for newborns with severe persistent pulmonary hypertension of the newborn. *Identifying and maintaining communication with clinicians at an ECMO center is especially important given the widespread availability of iNO therapy. Continuous delivery of NO is required during transport. The referring center is responsible for determining what transport capabilities are available in order to administer a successful therapeutic iNO program.

KEY POINTS FOR CLINICAL PRACTICE

1. Persistent pulmonary hypertension of the Newborn is defined as the failure of the normal circulatory transition that occurs after birth. It is a syndrome characterized by marked pulmonary hypertension that causes hypoxemia and right-to-left extrapulmonary shunting of blood. Because a patent foramen ovale and patent ductus arteriosus are normally present early in life, elevated pulmonary vascular resistance in the Newborn produces extrapulmonary shunting of blood, leading to severe and potentially unresponsive hypoxemia. With inadequate pulmonary perfusion, Neonates are at risk for developing refractory hypoxemia, respiratory distress, and acidosis.

2. This syndrome is usually noted in term or post-term infants. The baby presents clinically with cyanosis and respiratory distress, with tachypnea, but with minimal retractions during the first day of life. The infants chest radiograph may be normal (as noted in infants with primary PPHN, i.e. PFC) or demonstrate various abnormalities compatible with aspiration, pneumonia, diaphragmatic hernia, or hyaline membrane disease. Supplemental oxygen is needed in an attempt to correct arterial hypoxemia. With a large right-to-left shunt through a patent ductus arteriosus, an oxygen tension gradient may be noted between the preductal arterial circulation (i.e. right upper extremity) and the postductal arterial circulation (i.e. lower extremities). However, this gradient may not be present if substantial shunting is present at the level of the foramen ovale.

3. In Newborns with idiopathic persistent pulmonary hypertension of the newborn, the lung fields appear clear, with decreased vascular markings. *Heart size is typically normal or slightly The diagnosis is confirmed echocardiographically. *Measures to reduce pulmonary artery pressure include*: a) hyperventilation b) metabolic alkalinization c) vasodilator therapy d) analgesia, sedation and /or muscle paralysis e) high frequency oscillatory ventilation (HFOV) together with nitric oxide (NO) therapy f) ECMO.

4. Oxygenation is often assessed by using the oxygenation index (OI), which accounts for the postductal PaO_2 and the ventilator settings. The OI is calculated as the mean airway pressure multiplied by the fraction of inspired oxygen (FiO_2) and the 100, and the product is divided by the postductal PaO_2. An OI of 40 typically prompts consideration of ECMO support. Baseline criteria for Newborns considered for ECMO are generally as follows: *Gestation of more than 34 weeks *Weight more than 2000 g *No major intracranial hemorrhage on cranial sonograms (i.e., larger than a grade II hemorrhage) *Reversible lung disease or mechanical ventilation for 7-14 days *No evidence of lethal congenital anomalies or inoperable cardiac disease.

5. Overall, the survival rate for Newborns with persistent pulmonary hypertension of the Newborn is greater than 90% when all resources, including ECMO, are provided. Pulmonary recovery is typically complete, and survivors do not have residual pulmonary disease. Although most surviving Newborns with persistent pulmonary hypertension of the Newborn have normal neurodevelopmental outcomes, as many as 25% have significant neurodevelopmental sequelae. Prolonged hyperventilation is associated with an increased prevalence of neurodevelopmental sequelae, especially sensorineural hearing loss.

REFERENCES AND FURTHER READING : 1)Walsh-Sukys MC, Tyson JE, Wright LL, et al. Persistent pulmonary hypertension of the newborn in the era before nitric oxide: practice variation and outcomes. *Pediatrics*. Jan 2000;105(1 Pt 1):14-20. [Medline]. 2) Abman SH. Neonatal pulmonary hypertension: a physiologic approach to treatment. *Pediatr Pulmonol Suppl*. 2004;26:127-8. [Medline]. 3) Steinhorn RH. Nitric oxide and beyond: new insights and therapies for pulmonary hypertension. *J Perinatol*. Dec 2008;28 Suppl 3:S67-71. 4)Ziegler JW, Ivy DD, Kinsella JP, Abman SH. The role of nitric oxide, endothelin, and prostaglandins in the transition of the pulmonary circulation. *Clin Perinatol*. Jun 1995;22(2):387-403. 5) Alano MA, Ngougmna E, Ostrea EM Jr, Konduri GG. Analysis of nonsteroidal antiinflammatory drugs in meconium and its relation to persistent pulmonary hypertension of the newborn. *Pediatrics*. Mar 2001;107(3):519-23. [Medline].

Pearl/Peril/Pitfall: Metabolic acidosis and respiratory acidosis require correction. Sodium bicarbonate is typically used to correct metabolic acidosis. However, if carbon dioxide clearance is a problem, administering bicarbonate may produce a respiratory acidosis. In these situations, tromethamine (THAM) 1-2 mmol/kg may be a useful alternative, although THAM should never be administered to patients with anuria or uremia

43 Bronchopulmonary Dysplasia (BPD) and Chronic Lung Disease (CLD)

@ *Babies with BPD have a degree of pulmonary hypertension, and are therefore likely to benefit from a more generous oxygen administration regimen rather than from a restrictive policy, however the corrected gestational age and the state of vascularization of the retina needs to be taken into consideration before saturation targets are liberalized. Whilst there is some logic to this approach, there is indirect evidence from randomized controlled trials conducted for other reasons suggesting that a more liberal oxygen policy in these babies can actually increase the pulmonary morbidity. RCT's are in progress to address this question.*

* *CONCEPTUAL EQUATION 1:* **IMMATURE LUNG + MECHANICAL VENTILATION + SUPPLEMENTAL OXYGEN= LUNG DAMAGE AND LUNG INFLAMMATION.**

* *CONCEPTUAL EQUATION 2:* **LUNG DAMAGE+LUNG INFLAMMATION+TIME= BPD WITH OR WITHOUT EVENTUAL CLD.**

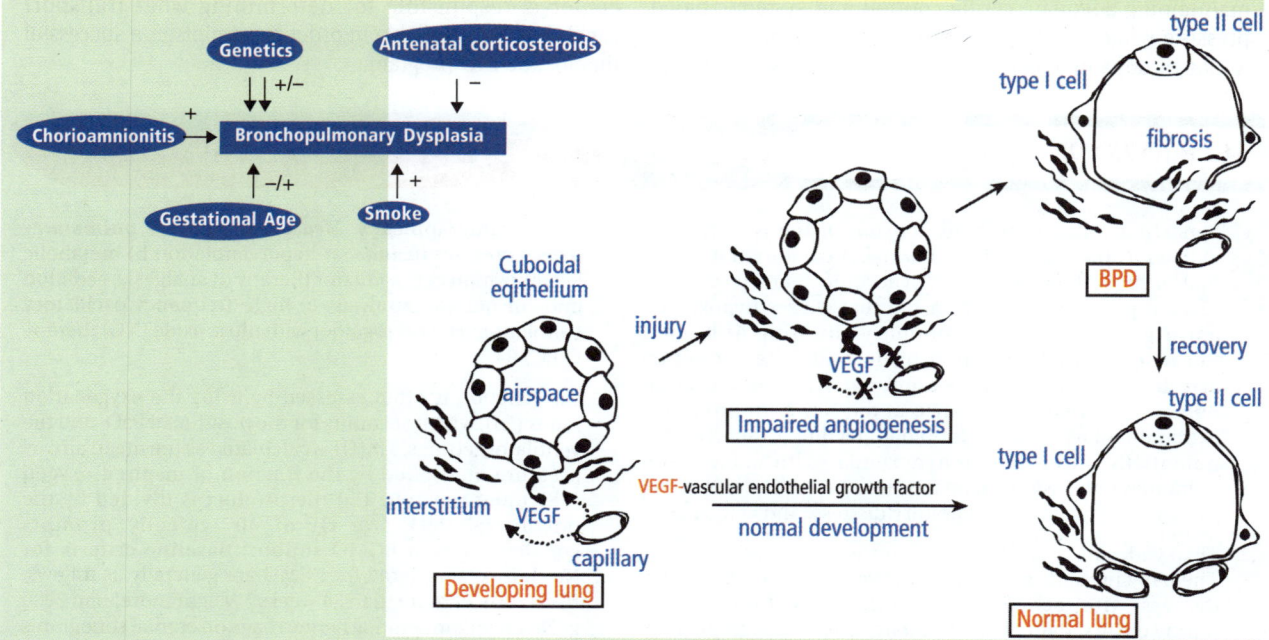

REVIEW OF CLINICAL PROBLEMS

1. Discuss the Current Preventive Strategies for BPD/CLD.
   Ans: Refer to Table 3 of the Chapter.

2. How do you manage Evolving/Established BPD ?
   Ans: Refer to Table 4 of the Chapter.

3. What are the Essentials of Ventilatory management for BPD/CLD?
   Ans: Refer to the Evaluation-Decision-Action Plan/ Algorithm to diagnose and manage a Neonate with BPD/ CLD.

4. Discuss the Role of Postnatal Steroids in the management of BPD/CLD.
   Ans: Refer to SECTION on BPD: Postnatal Steroids.

5. How do you explain to Parents about the Prognosis for BPD/CLD?
   Ans: Refer to SECTION on BPD:Prognosis.

LEARNING OBJECTIVES

After completing this article, readers will be able to

1. Understand the clinical presentation of BPD/CLD.

2. Recognize promptly the CLD infants with signs of growth failure, intercurrent viral illnesses, Pulmonary hypertension and right heart failure, respiratory failure due to various complications.

3. Manage CLD and its complications promptly and appropriately.

4. Ensure proper follow-ups for infants with CLD, especially for monitoring the ongoing problems, such as cor pulmonale, systemic hypertension, neurodevelopmental delays, etc.

5. Provide good parental support and communication regarding prognosis and preventative measures.

Pearl/Peril/Pitfall: *Over the past decade the clinical definition of BPD has evolved from oxygen dependency at 28 days of age to oxygen dependency at 36 weeks corrected gestational age. The National Institute for Health in the USA has further divided this definition into mild (in supplemental oxygen at 28 days of age, but in air by 36 weeks corrected age), moderate (requiring <30% supplemental oxygen at 36 weeks corrected age and severe (in >30% supplemental oxygen and/or requiring positive pressure support, CPAP or ventilation, at 36 weeks corrected age). BPD is the single most important factor determining length of stay in babies born at less than 29 weeks. The most severely affected babies are the most premature, particularly 23 - 26 week gestation babies.*

BIRD'S EYE VIEW/OVERVIEW/SYNOPSIS

1. *BPD AND CLD* are both the result of incompletely resolved/abnormally repaired lung disease which occurred in the Neonatal period. **BPD** can be diagnosed on the 28th day of life in infants who continue to require supplemental oxygen, have an abnormal physical examination with tachypnea, crackles or wheezes and retractions and have an abnormal CXR (*Bancalari's definition of BPD, 1979*). An infant is said to have **Chronic Lung Disease** if, at 36 weeks postconceptional age, there is a continued requirement for supplemental oxygen, an abnormal PE and CXR as described for BPD, regardless of the cause or need for mechanical ventilation (*Shennan, 1988*). Many infants who meet the criteria for BPD on the 28th day of life will be sufficiently recovered by 36 weeks postconceptional age that they do not meet criteria for the diagnosis of CLD. This is due to the survival of ELBW infants making BPD a less specific diagnosis. The diagnosis of CLD is a better predictor of clinical respiratory difficulty during infancy. For VLBW infants who require ventilation support, 60% are oxygen dependent at 28 days of age, and 30% remain oxygen dependent at 36 weeks of postconceptional age.

2. Most Neonates with BPD are born preterm, usually at <32 weeks gestational age, and have had surfactant deficiency RDS treated with supplemental oxygen, mechanical ventilation and surfactant replacement therapy. Occasionally, Neonates born at more advanced ages and ventilated for conditions other than RDS will develop BPD. The primary etiological factors in the development of BPD and CLD are: *a)* an immature lung *b)* direct injury to the lung by oxygen and mechanical ventilation (barotrauma and volutrauma) and *c)* injury to the lung which occurs when lung inflammation is initiated by supplemental oxygen and mechanical ventilation.

3. *Classic BPD* was originally described by Northway in 1966, and its diagnosis was based on progressive radiographic changes in preterm infants who had prolonged ventilator and oxygen dependence as a consequence of their treatment for RDS. Northway described 4 distinct radiographic stages of BPD: *a)* RDS *b)* diffusely hazy *c)* diffusely bubbly, interstitial pattern, and *d)* hyperaeration, focal hyperlucency, and alternating strands of opacification. As many infants do not have the classic radiologic changes, the term Chronic Lung disease is now preferred. In 1996, Cherukupalli and colleagues analyzed morphologic and biochemical lung features of infants with BPD. *Four distinct pathologic stages* were identified: acute lung injury, exudative bronchiolitis, proliferative bronchiolitis, and obliterative fibroproliferative bronchiolitis. At present, pathologic examination of extremely low-birth-weight infants dying from BPD reveal greatly reduced total numbers of alveoli and septa. This condition is commonly referred to as the *new BPD*. Infants with BPD today may have worsening airway obstruction after they are discharged from the NICU. Additional research is needed to improve our understanding of the complex interactions of prematurity and environmental influences on pulmonary development and the effects of postnatal treatments on improving Neonatal morbidity and mortality.

4. Surfactant deficient preterm lung, under the influence of deficient anti-oxidant defences, protease inhibitors, barotrauma + volutrauma from prolonged mechanical ventilation, and free oxygen radicle damage from supplemental oxygen gets injured initially. This injury initiates an influx of neutrophils into the lung with consequent lung inflammation and protease/antiprotease imbalance, which is thought to play an important role in the lung injury/ abnormal repair that leads to BPD/CLD.

5. *Why do some Neonates develop BPD/CLD, while others show complete resolution of RDS ?* Risk factors include; strong family history of asthma, HLA-A2 haplotype, male sex, poor nutritional status of VLBW and ELBW infants, deficiency of selenium, copper, zinc, iron, essential fatty acids, vitamins A and E, colonization of VLBW infants with Ureaplasma urealyticum etc.,

6. *The E-D-A Plan/Algorithm* summarizes the essential aspects of history taking, physical examination, relevant investigations to diagnose BPD/CLD and also the principles of current management of BPD/CLD and its common complications. *Chest radiography is helpful in determining the severity of BPD and in differentiating BPD from atelectasis, pneumonia, and air leak syndrome.* Chest radiographs may demonstrate decreased lung volumes, areas of atelectasis and hyperinflation, pulmonary edema (PE), and pulmonary interstitial emphysema (PIE). Hyperinflation or interstitial abnormalities on chest radiograph appears to be correlated with the development of airway obstruction later in life. Most recently, CT and MRI studies of infants with BPD have provided detailed images of the lung. High-resolution CT may detect radiographic abnormalities not readily identified with routine chest radiography.

7. Inadequate oxygenation and periodic arterial desaturation can lead to pulmonary vascular disease and Cor pulmonale. Pulse oximetry is ideal for assessing the adequacy of oxygenation. Oxygen saturation should be monitored in all behavioral states as desaturation may occur during sleep or associated with feedings.

8. Providing optimal nutritional management is important in resolving CLD. Infants should be closely monitored for growth failure and a thorough evaluation should be pursued if growth failure occurs.

9. RSV and other illnesses can lead to severe respiratory failure in infants with CLD. Preventative measures should be emphasized to the family and the infant should be closely monitored for early signs of infection.

10. Future management of BPD will involve strategies that emphasize prevention. Because few accepted therapies currently prevent BPD, many therapeutic modalities (e.g., mechanical ventilation, oxygen therapy, nutritional support, medication) are used to treat BPD. Practising Neonatologists have observed reduced severities of BPD in the postsurfactant era. Maintaining PPV and oxygen therapy for longer than 4 months and discharging patients to facilities for prolonged mechanical ventilation is now unusual.

Pearl/Peril/Pitfall : Infants developing BPD require 20 to 40% more calories than their age-matched healthy controls. Their caloric requirement varies from 120 to 150 Kcal/kg/day. This can be achieved by fortifying breast milk with human milk fortifier (HMF) or infant formula.

THE EVALUATION-DECISION-ACTION-PLAN/ALGORITHM FOR THE DIAGNOSIS AND MANAGEMENT OF *A NEONATE WITH BPD/CLD*

SUBJECTIVE FINDINGS

Hx of Premature baby usually<32 wks' GA, who is still oxygen dependent, tachypneic, wheezy with retractions on the 28th day of life(BPD), or at 36 weeks postconceptional age(CLD)

Hx of intrapartal risk factors, such as RDS, supplemental O2, Mechanical ventilation, VLBW/ELBW infants deficient in caloric reserves and micronutrients, chorioamnionitis, and strong family history of asthma etc.,

Hx of ongoing problems-growth failure, pulmonary hypertension, right heart failure,intercurrent viral illnesses, RAD, recurrent Chest infections, GERD and Aspiration, feeding difficulties

OBJECTIVE FINDINGS

Assess ABCs, vitals, BP, O_2 sats, work of breathing, central cyanosis, CRT, pulses, Urine output *Look for* Systemic hypertension, LVH, Pulmonary hypertension/edema, RVH, failure to thrive/increased work of breathing/frank respiratory failure *Assess for* signs suggestive of sepsis/chest infection/RAD/Cor pulmonale, *Perform* systemic examination to assess the complications of CLD-Postnatal infection and/or sepsis, PVL, severe intraventricular hemorrhage, ventriculomegaly, hearing impairment, and severe retinopathy of prematurity

INVESTIGATIONS

Blood FBC with hematocrit and platelets, glucose, blood culture, ABG analysis, electrolytes, Ca^{++}, Mg^{++}, creatinine, BUN, bleeding and clotting profile.

CXR decreased lung volumes, areas of atelectasis and hyperinflation, pulmonary edema (PE), and pulmonary interstitial emphysema (PIE). Hyperinflation or interstitial abnormalities

High-resolution CT may detect radiographic abnormalities not readily identified with routine chest radiography.

Echocardiogram to assess pulmonary hypertension/right heart failure if any co-existing.

A NEONATE WITH BPD/CLD

Ensure: Nutritional requirements of a Neonate/Infant with BPD/CLD-*Caloric requirements up to 150kcal/kg/day - 20-40% >age-matched controls without respiratory distress. *Avoid prolonged periods of TPN,due to adverse effects of intralipid on the lungs. *Prefer the nutrient-enriched (higher intake of protein, calcium,phosphorus, and zinc) Enteral feeds @120ml/kg /day, using either a concentrated feed up to 30kcal/oz *or* calorie supplementation.

Avoid: Excess fluid intake; if their weight gain is >20gm/kg/day on a daily 150ml/kg/day fluid regimen, suspect incipient heart failure and consider diuretics to be continued. *Monitor ABG, Electrolytes- sodium, potassium, chloride, and calcium and give appropriate supplements if these become abnormal *Perform serial renal USG Scans to check for the development of nephrocalcinosis secondary to chronic furosemide therapy.

Treat: Chest infections promptly- with physiotherapy, antibiotics, or antiviral therapy, as appropriate. *Culture the ET/NP secretions, if their respiratory status/radiological findings deteriorate. *Send NP secretions for immuno-fluorescence screening for RSV,adeno and influenza and consider ribavirin therapy, if such infections are identified and other causes of respiratory deterioration (PDA) have been excluded.

Give: Immunoprophylaxis with Palivizumab against RSV for babies discharged home on supplemental oxygen, and for other CLD babies, if they are <6 mo of age at the start of the RSV season.*Immunize them with routine vaccines , but a killed polio , once CLD babies reach 2 mo of age, even though they remain on the NICU.*Consider immunization against influenza, especially for CLD babies receiving home oxygen therapy.

Monitor: For *systemic hypertension* frequently transient and responds to antihypertensive medication; identify the underlying causes such as corticosteroids *or* renal damage due to prolonged UAC usage/nephrocalcinosis from chronic diuretic therapy.

Monitor: For *pulmonary hypertension* clinically and echocardiographically and maintain O_2sats. >95%, if it is detected.

Ensure: ABCs, give supplemental oxygen to maintain O_2 sats >92%, monitor pulse oximetry, BP, CR monitor; If pulmonary hypertension is detected- by single S2 and TR murmur + Echocardiography (25% of patients), aim for O_2 SATs >95%.

Ventilator management
*Keep the PIPs and FiO_2 at the minimum compatible with achieving a PaO_2 of 50–70mmHg and O_2 sats of at least 92%. *Consider a PEEP level of 6cmH_2O, after the 1st week to improve oxygenation without adversely affecting CO_2 elimination. (this strategy may not be successful in babies with severe cystic BPD.) *Allow Permissive Hypercapnia, provided that there is no evidence of a respiratory acidosis (pH<7.25) *Keep the sedation to the minimum to promote the infant`s respiratory efforts to come out of the ventilator dependency.
PTV may not generate sufficient flow or pressure to exceed the critical trigger level. HFOV can improve oxygenation who deteriorate acutely, but may cause overexpansion in those who have cystic BPD. *Consider a Tracheostomy in babies who remain fully ventilated after 3 mo of age.*Weaning—Try to wean the baby from the ventilator frequently, ignoring a rise in $PaCO_2$ unless the pH falls below 7.25. Methylxanthines may be useful to hasten weaning, in babies <1 mo of age. Avoid corticosteroids because of possible long-term adverse effects on neurodevelopmental outcome. Nasal CPAP is useful for those who have acquired tracheobronchomalacia, but may be poorly tolerated. Avoid reintubation and ventilation, unless the baby suffers from frequent/troublesome apnea, a severe metabolic acidosis indicating respiratory fatigue or a marked deterioration in blood gases. Consider chest physiotherapy and more FiO_2 as the 1st line of treatment for worsening blood gases, which usually be due to atelectasis associated with secretions.

Transfuse (PRBC 15ml/kg) babies with O_2 requirements >30%, if their Hematocrit falls below 40%.Check the Hemogram on a weekly basis, once they do not require respiratory support and transfuse only those babies who have symptomatic anemia with a poor reticulocyte response.

Pearl/Peril/Pitfall: Infants with 'BPD spells' (sudden episodes of deterioration due to marked expiratory airflow limitation) may require sedation and muscle relaxation to reduce agitation.

TABLE 1 Pharmacologic treatment of BPD/CLD

Drug	Dose	Comments
INHALED BRONCHODILATORS		
Salbutamol	supplied as 0.5% solution, 5 mg/kg. Admin. 0.02–0.04 ml/kg, diluted to 1.5–2.0 ml with normal or 1/2 normal saline every 4–6 h or as needed (0.1–0.2 mg/kg)	Bronchodilator of choice for acute bronchoconstriction. Do not administer if heart rate 180 beats/min, MDI with spacer may be superior to nebulizer.
Ipratropium bromide	Supplied as 0.02% solution. Dose is 0.13–0.4 ml/kg, 0.025–0.08 mg/kg up to 0.18 mg in 2–2.5 ml normal saline. Given every 6 h by nebulization	Experience in infants is limited. Do not exceed 0.9 ml of ipratropium solution. May be mixed with albuterol if used within 1 h. Protect from exposure to light
Cromolyn sodium	Given by nebulization. Dose is 20 mg every 6 h	Contraindicated during acute respiratory difficulty. Often requires 2–4 weeks to elicit effect
DIURETICS		
Furosemide	1–2 mg/kg/day orally, May be divided every 12 h	Most efficacious diuretic, highest frequency of adverse effects. Best diuretic for acute volume overload. Alternate day use may minimize complications but be effective.
Hydrochlorthiazide	1–2 mg/kg/dose every 12 h	Usually provides adequate diuresis for continuing management. Effect on lung function may require several days. Lower frequency and magnitude of adverse effects compared to furosemide.
Spironolactone	1–3 mg/kg/dose orally every 12 h	Generally used with another diuretic to minimize urinary potassium loss and hypokalemia. If used alone, not a very effective diuretic.
METHYLXANTHINES		
Theophylline	Oral loading dose is 5 mg/kg maintenance is 2 mg/kg every 8–12 h	Maintenance requirements vary widely, serum levels should be monitored and kept between 80–110 mmol/L peak and 55 mmol/L Trough
Caffeine base	10 mg/kg loading dose, 2.5 mg/kg once daily	Convenient dosing schedule for outpatients. Level should be 5–25 mg/ml
Caffeine citrate	20 mg/kg loading dose, 5 mg/kg once daily	Same as for base form of drug.

TABLE 2 Definition of BPD

	Gestational age	
	< 32 weeks	> 32 weeks
Time point of assessment	36 weeks PMA or discharge*	> 28 days but < 56 days postnatal age or discharge*
Treatment with oxygen	**> 21% for atleast 28 days**	**> 21% for at least 28 days**
BPD		
Mild	Breathing room air at 36 weeks PMA or discharge*	Breathing room air at 56 days postnatal age or discharge*
Moderate	Need* for <30% oxygen at 36 weeks PMA or discharge*	Need* for <30% oxygen at 56 days postnatal age or discharge*
Severe	Need for ≥ 30% oxygen and/or positive pressure (IMV/CPAP) at 36 weeks PMA or discharge*	Need for ≥ 30% oxygen and/or positive pressure (IMV/CPAP) at 56 days postnatal age or discharge*

*- Whichever comes first From Jobe AH, Bancalari E: BPD. Am J Respir Crit Care Med 2001; 163: 1723-29.
(PMA, Postmenstrual age; BPD, bronchopulmonary dysplasia; IMV, intermittent mandatory ventilation; CPAP, continuous positive airway pressure)

Pearl/Peril/Pitfall : Most neonates with BPD ultimately survive. As infants, patients are at increased risk for repeated and serious pulmonary infections (eg, RSV), asthma, cardiac dysfunction, and neurologic impairments. Infants with severe BPD remain at high risk for pulmonary morbidity and mortality during the first 2 years of life.

TABLE 3	Preventive strategies and their current status			
Strategies	Proven benefit	Promising (needs more studies)	Probably beneficial (effects ±)	No benefit
Ventilatory	–	NIPPV Volume targeted ventilation Permissive hypercapnia Permissive hypoxemia	Early CPAP Patient triggered modes	High frequency ventilation
Fluids and nutrition		Aggressive early enteral and parenteral nutrition	Fluid restriction	
Pharmacological	Vitamin A Postnatal steroids (but harmful as well)	Superoxide dismutase	Antenatal steroids Exogenous surfactant Methylxanthines iNo therapy Diuretics	Antenatal TRH prophylactic indomethacin / ibuprofen Inhaled steroids Bronchodilators Mast cell stabilizers

(NIPPV, Nasal intermittent positive pressure ventilation; CPAP continuous positive airway pressure; iNO, inhaled nitric oxide; TRH, Thyrotropin releasing hormone)

Courtesy: M. Jeeva Sankar, Ramesh Agarwal, Ashok K Deorari, Vinod K Paul

Division of Neonatology, Department of Pediatrics, All India Institute of Medical Sciences Ansari Nagar, New Delhi–110029

TABLE 4	Management of Evolving or Established BPD*	
	Evolving BPD (2–4 weeks age)	Established BPO (> 4 weeks age)

Ventilatory strategies	* Minimizing ventilatory support (e.g. using nCPAP whenever possible)
	 * Tolerating slightly higher $PaCO_2$ (45–55 mm Hg provided pH > 7.25)
	 * Target SPO_2: 88–93%
	 * if on IMV:
	 * Use PTV if possible
	   * Slow rates (25/40/min)
	   * Moderate PEEP (4–5 cm H_2O)
	   * Moderate Ti (0.35–0.45 sec)
	   * Low tidal volume (3–6 mLkg)
	   * Early extubation to CPAP
		* Minimizing ventilatory support
		
		 * Tolerating higher $PaCo_2$ (55–60 mm Hg provided pH >7.25)
		 * Target SPO_2: 89–94%
		 * if on IMV:
		 * Use PTV if possible
		   * Slow rates (20/40/min)
		   * Moderate PEEP (4–8 cm H_2O)
		   * Longer Ti (0.4–0.7 sec)
		   * Larger tidal volume (5–8 mL/kg)

Pharmacological strategies	* Methylxanthines to facilitate extubation * Steroids:@ consider in ELBW infants on ventilator support even after 10–14 days of age * Specific management: * Diuretics for features of pulmonary edema * Bronchodilators for bronchospasm	* Steroids:@ individualize based on the clinical condition * Specific management: * Bronchodilators for bronchspasm * Sedation and muscle relaxation for 'BPD spells'
Others	* Nutrition: * Increase daily calorie intake to 120 to 150 Kcal/kg/d * Give expressed breast milk fortified with HMF * Use fat supplementation (e.g. MCT oil) for providing additional calories * Give multivitamin supplements to meet RDA	*Same as for evolving BPD

@ Could result in potentially harmful effects including adverse neurodevelopmental outcomes; counsel parents before initiation of therapy. (n CPAP, nasal continuous positive airway pressure ; IMV, intermittent mandatory ventilation; PTV, patient triggered ventialtion; PEEP, positive end expiratory pressure; Ti, inspiratory time; HMF, human milk fortifier; MCT, medium chain triglycerides; RDA, recommended dietary allowance)

Pearl/Peril/Pitfall: During feeding and certain parts of sleep are the times where a baby's oxygen demand is higher. Therefore if one is looking to see if a baby will manage in less oxygen saturations should be monitored over several feed periods or for several hours during sleep For babies in headbox/tent oxygen do not wean oxygen by more than 1% in a 24 hour period even if the saturations are 100%.

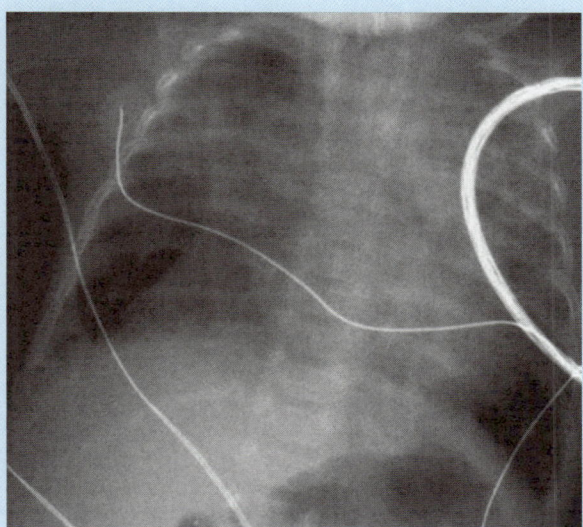
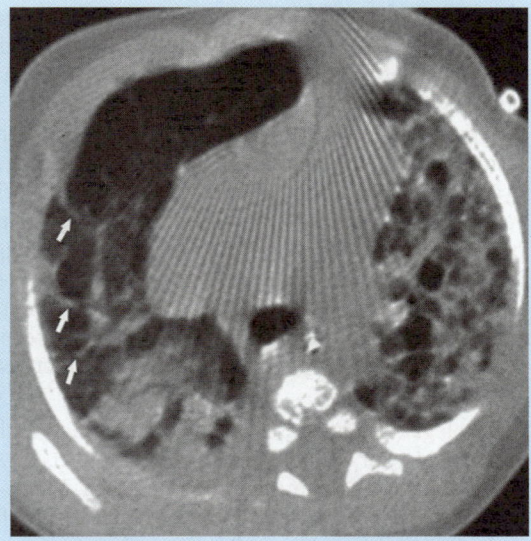

"Classic" severe BPD in a 3-month-old premature infant. (a) Frontal radiograph shows heterogeneous aeration, coarse strandlike areas of opacity, and intervening cystic lucencies. (b) Axial CT scan demonstrates right upper lobe regional air trapping anteriorly, architectural distortion with fibrotic subpleural parenchymal bands (arrows) and subsegmental atelectasis posteriorly, and diffuse coarse reticular opacities in the left lung.

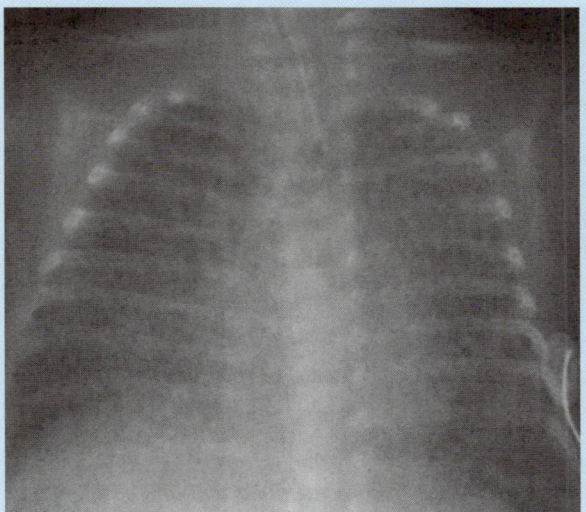
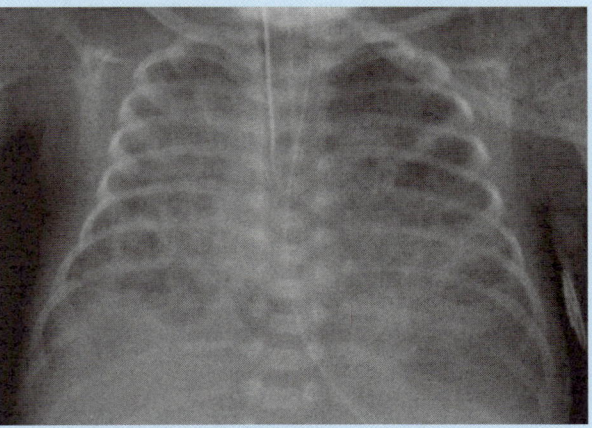

BPD in a 33-day-old preterm infant. Frontal chest radiograph demonstrates uniform distribution of reticular opacities and small cystic lucencies

Stage 4 BPD. **Differential diagnosis**
- Pulmonary interstitial emphysema (PIE) may look identical
- Smaller air-containing spaces in PIE (bubbly appearance)
- Left-to-right shunt such as a patent ductus arteriosus
- Infection, especially with non group A beta streptococci
- Congestive heart failure and pulmonary edema

This is usually a sequel of significant lung disease in the immediate newborn period. Classically, four stages were described by Northway in 1967. *Stage 1 was the homogenous appearance of RDS

* Stage 2 was a generalized opacity, frequently seen towards the end of the first week of life

* Stage 3 marked the onset of chronic changes, with a bubbly appearance

* Stage 4 consisted of a inhomogenous appearance with hyperinflation, bleb formation, irregular fibrous streaks, and cardiomegaly (from cor pulmonale). Other scoring systems have followed. These have largely been used in research rather than in clinical practice. The lung fields are generally "bubbly" and "streaky" with localized areas of hyperaeration in the right lower lobe and left lower lobe. The strongest risk factor for neonatal CLD is now gestation. Ventilation and oxygen may play a role in the pathogenesis, as may infection with organisms such as *Ureaplasma*.

Pearl/Peril/Pitfall: BPD/CLD Complications—Postnatal infection and/or sepsis, PVL, severe intraventricular hemorrhage, ventriculomegaly, hearing impairment, and severe retinopathy of prematurity are all important confounding variables that can greatly affect an infant's outcome.

BPD/CLD Prognosis: *Most neonates with BPD ultimately survive. *As infants, patients are at increased risk for repeated and serious pulmonary infections (e.g. RSV), asthma, cardiac dysfunction, and neurologic impairments. *Infants with severe BPD remain at high risk for pulmonary morbidity and mortality during the first 2 years of life. *Rehospitalization for impaired pulmonary function is most common during the first 2 years of life. *Hakulinen and associates (1990) found a gradual decrease in symptom frequency among children aged 6-9 years compared with infants aged 0-2 years. *In children and adults with a history of BPD, high-resolution chest CT reveals lung abnormalities that are directly correlated with the degree of pulmonary dysfunction. *The infant with severe BPD is at high risk for long-term pulmonary and neurologic sequelae. *Persistent right ventricular hypertrophy or fixed pulmonary hypertension unresponsive to oxygen supplementation is associated with a poor prognosis. *Northway (1992) followed up pediatric patients with BPD to adulthood and reported that patients had airway hyperreactivity, abnormal pulmonary function, and hyperinflation, as noted on chest radiography. *Bader et al (1987) and Blayney et al (1991) found persistence of respiratory symptoms and abnormal pulmonary function in children aged 7 and 10 years. Postnatal infection and/or sepsis, PVL, severe intraventricular hemorrhage, ventriculomegaly, hearing impairment, and severe retinopathy of prematurity are all important confounding variables that can greatly affect an infant's outcome

Medicolegal Pitfalls: *Associated confounding problems in infants with BPD can be severe, and delayed diagnosis can be catastrophic. For example, if an infant with BPD and superimposed sepsis is treated with systemic corticosteroids, the infant may have serious complications or death. When steroids (hydrocortisone, dexamethasone) are administered with indomethacin, the risk of spontaneous intestinal perforation is significantly increased. *Careful discussions between parents and caregivers should be undertaken before corticosteroids are given to high-risk infants.

Home oxygen: *Criteria for Home Oxygen—General*·Appropriate social/home environment including reasonable accessibility to medical care ·Baby is on 4 hourly or demand oral feeding regimen ·Baby is normothermic in an open cot ·Satisfactory growth ·All babies discharged from tertiary units on home oxygen have specific Paediatric Thoracic specialist follow up. **Criteria for Home Oxygen—Respiratory**·Baby must pass an "air test". The oxygen is turned off, the nasal prongs removed and the baby monitored over 30 minutes ·If saturations are maintained >86% for 30 minutes the test should be repeated in 48 hours. If a second test is satisfactory the baby is eligible for discharge on home oxygen on respiratory grounds. In other words the baby has demonstrated a reasonable level of respiratory reserve.

Prevention: *The multifactorial etiology of BPD compounds its prevention. *Prenatal steroid therapy and postnatal surfactant has improved survival and mitigated the severity of BPD. Prevention of preterm birth and chorioamnionitis should reduce the incidence of BPD. *Meticulous attention to optimal oxygenation, ventilation (early extubation, increased use of CPAP), and fluid management may decrease the incidence and severity of BPD. New therapies, such as iNO and/or recombinant human antioxidants, may also improve short and long-term outcomes. *Maximizing nutritional support, careful monitoring of fluid intake, and judicious use of diuretics promote lung healing. *Evidence regarding the use of high-frequency ventilation to prevent BPD is inconclusive.

BPD : Postnatal steroids

Postnatal steroids may produce a short-term improvement in lung mechanics that can facilitate extubation or a reduction in ventilatory requirements in ventilator-dependant infants with evolving / established chronic lung disease. However, they have not been shown to have any effect on the duration of oxygen requirement or longer term evolution of chronic lung disease. There are significant adverse effects associated with the use of postnatal steroids, including an increased risk of long term neurodevelopmental abnormalities. For this reason, the use of postnatal steroids is *contentious and limited to infants* with either steadily increasing ventilation requirements or those infants who cannot be weaned from ventilation after all other treatments and interventions have been exhausted.

The use of Postnatal steroids has been reviewed according to timing of administration in three recent meta-analyses.

* **Early (<96 hours)** Infants treated with early steroids were extubated earlier and showed a reduced incidence of chronic lung disease (either at 28 days postnatal or 36 weeks postmenstrual age). However, there was no benefit over control infants in mortality or other short-term neonatal morbidity. There were reports relating an increased risk of cerebral palsy and developmental delay among steroid-treated survivors.

* **Moderately early (7–14 days)** Infants treated with steroids at between 7 to 14 days had reduced neonatal mortality, earlier extubation (within 7 days) and a reduced incidence of chronic lung disease (either at 28 days postnatal or 36 weeks postmenstrual age). There were no effects on other short-term morbidity. There is little available long-term follow up data for this group of infants.

* **Late (>3 weeks)** Infants treated with steroids after 3 weeks of age were more likely to be extubated and showed a reduced incidence of chronic lung disease (either at 28 days postnatal or 36 weeks postmenstrual age). There was no effect on overall mortality.

Pearl/Peril/Pitfall : Babies with BPD have a degree of pulmonary hypertension, and are therefore likely to benefit from a more generous oxygen administration regimen rather than from a restrictive policy, however the corrected gestational age and the state of vascularization of the retina needs to be taken into consideration before saturation targets are liberalized . Whilst there is some logic to this approach, there is indirect evidence from randomized controlled trials conducted for other reasons suggesting that a more liberal oxygen policy in these babies can actually increase the pulmonary morbidity. RCT's are in progress to address this question.

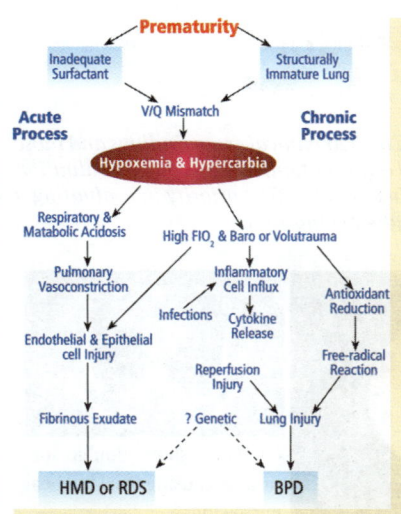

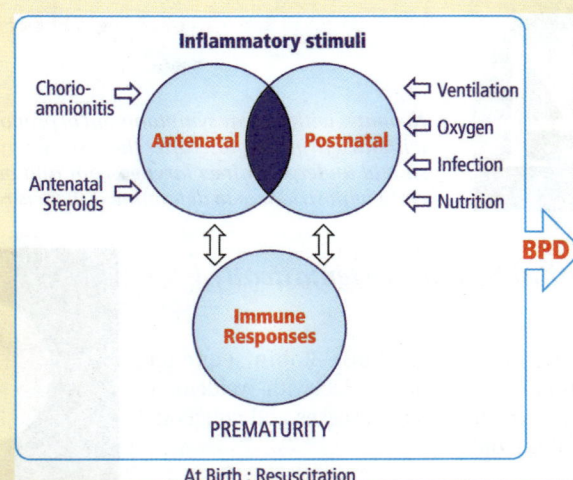

Schematic of interactions between inflammation and immune responses in the pathogenesis of BPD/CLD

BPD—Pathophysiology

KEY POINTS FOR CLINICAL PRACTICE

1. BPD is the single most important factor determining length of stay in babies born at less than 29 weeks. The most severely affected babies are the most premature, particularly 23–26 week Tertiary unit babies with BPD (actual or evolving) fall into three broad groups *babies dependant on endotracheal mechanical ventilation (MV) *babies dependant of Nasal CPAP *babies who are oxygen dependant, usually by nasal prongs gestation babies.

2. Endotracheal ventilation is increasingly being replaced by NCPAP, for even the tiniest babies many are being managed with NCPAP from birth. Results from a recent randomised controlled trial have shown that 50% of babies 25–28 weeks gestation are able to manage without ever requiring intubation and ventilation, and that infants of this age who commence NCPAP from birth have no increased risk of death or BPD, and in fact are less likely to be in oxygen at 28 days of age.

3. For those who do require intubation and ventilation there is an intense focus on minimizing ventilator associated lung injury from the moment a baby is placed on a ventilator. Synchronised modes of MV with close monitoring of tidal volumes are key features of current practice. In addition there is a more liberal approach to carbon dioxide control, allowing CO_2 to rise into the 50's and 60's providing the pH remains better than 7.25. Babies who require endotracheal ventilation are aggressively weaned and extubated to NCPAP often within 1–2 days of birth. Oxygen damages delicate lung tissue as well as the immature retina. Pulse oximetry targets are typically set between 85 to 94% in the first weeks after birth

4. Dexamethasone is effective in achieving short-term improvement in the status of ventilator dependant babies as well as longer term reductions in BPD, however, there is now level evidence showing that dexamethasone in the first week of life is associated with an increased risk of cerebral palsy in survivors. safety of corticosteroids used later in the course of evolving BPD between 14–28 days is unresolved and the Cochrane review of current evidence suggests reserving the use of late corticosteroids to infants who cannot be weaned from mechanical ventilation, and minimising the dose and duration of treatment. In light of this evidence frequency of the use of steroids for BPD in NICUs has dramatically declined in the past 5 years and a "low" dose regimen (e.g. 0.15–0.25mg/kg/day) weaned and ceased over a 7–10 day period is recommended. There is no evidence for efficacy in non ventilated babies therefore diuretic therapy should be weaned and ceased once babies are stable off mechanical ventilation

5. Providing optimal nutritional management is important in resolving CLD. Infants should be closely monitored for growth failure and a thorough evaluation should be pursued if growth failure occurs. Vitamin A supplementation reduces death and oxygen requirements at 36 weeks corrected gestational age. These babies require term follow up throughout childhood There is an increased pulmonary morbidity in the first 2 years of life. Parents should be counselled about this morbidity and ways to minimise it. Influenza vaccine is recommended for infants with ongoing cardiac, respiratory or neurological illnesses at 6 months of age. Recommendations are 2 doses, 4 weeks apart Influenza vaccine is not officially recommended for these babies RSV prophylaxis is not routinely recommended, the American Academy of Pediatrics recommends use of RSV prophlaxis for infants <2yrs, with BPD requiring treatment within the last 6 months, who are discharged home prior to the RSV season. The Department of Health in the UK recommends its use in children <2yrs with BPD on home oxygen or who have had prolonged use of oxygen.

REFERENCES AND FURTHER READING : 1)Jobe A, Bancalari E. Bronchopulmonary Dysplasia, NICHD/NHLBI/ORD Workshop Summary. Am J Respir Crit Care Med. 163 1723-1729, 2001 2) Halliday HL and Ehrenkranz RA. Early postnatal corticosteroids for the prevention of chronic lung disease in preterm babies. Cochrane Neonatal group, Cochrane database of systematic reviews, Issue 3, 2001. 3) Darlow BA, Graham PJ. Vitamin A supplementation to prevent mortality and short and long-term morbidity in very low birthweight infants. Cochrane Database Syst Rev. 2007 Oct 17;(4):CD000501. Review. 4) CLD in the Newborns M. Jeeva Sankar, Ramesh Agarwal, Ashok K Deorari, Vinod K Paul *Division of Neonatology, Department of Pediatrics All India Institute of Medical Sciences Ansari Nagar, New Delhi –110029* 5) Barrington KJ and Finer NN. Treatment of Bronchopulmonary Dysplasia - A Review. Clinics in Perinatology 25 1 March 1998 177-202

Pearl/Peril/Pitfall: Vitamin A is essential for maintaining the integrity of respiratory tract epithelial cells. Very preterm infants are relatively deficient in vitamin A which has been shown to be associated with CLD. A large RCT of 807 infants with a birth weight of less than 1000 g has shown that a large dose of intramuscular vitamin A (5000 units three times a week for 4 weeks from birth) decreases the risk of CLD (OR 0.89; 95%CI 0.8–0.99).

Congenital Stridor

@ *Neonates with airway symptoms out of proportion to their clinical exam findings and those without a firm diagnosis after the history, physical examination, and radiologic evaluation should undergo a direct laryngoscopy and bronchoscopy. The first priority in evaluating a child with stridor is to determine if there is respiratory compromise.*

Approach Congenital Stridor Systematically !

1. **Supraglottic-*inspiratory stridor***
   Choanal atresia, Micrognathia (e.g. Pierre-Robin sequence, Treacher-Collins syndrome), Macroglossia Beckwith-Weidemann and down syndromes, glycogen storage diseases and congenital hypothyroidism, lingual thyroid

2. **Glottic (laryngeal) and subglottic-*biphasic stridor***
   Laryngomalacia(*usually inspiratory but can present with biphasic stridor in severe cases*),Vocal cord paralysis, Subglottic (or tracheal) stenosis, laryngeal web, cystic hygroma, Subglottic hemangiomata, laryngotracheo-esophageal cleft.

3. **Intrathoracic-*expiratory stridor***
   tracheomalacia, Vascular rings, Mediastinal masses (e.g. cyst, teratoma , lymphoma, lymphadenopathy).

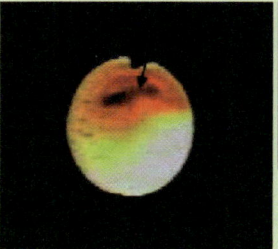

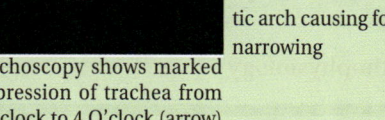

Bronchoscopy shows marked compression of trachea from 10 O'clock to 4 O'clock (arrow) by an extra-mural pulsating mass.

CT thorax shows double aortic arch causing focal tracheal narrowing

Courtesy: YT CHAN, DKK NG, ASF CHONG, JCS HO. HK J Paediatr (new series) 2003;8:126-129

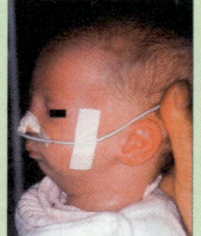

A newborn infant with Pierre-Robin syndrome. Note the micrognathia.

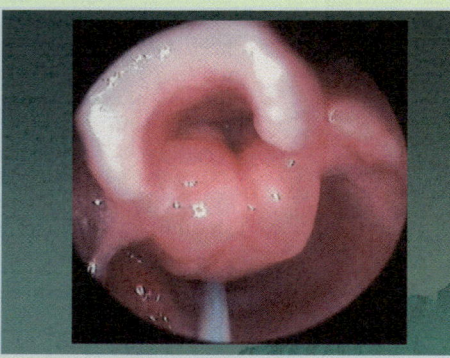

Laryngomalacia "Floppy Larynx"

* Omega shaped epiglottis
* Short (A-P) and Tall tethered Aryepiglottic folds
* Associated Reflux in 75%
* Soft Cartilage?
* Redundancy of Mucosa?
* Associated Neuromuscular immaturity, Muscular Hypotonia?

REVIEW OF CLINICAL PROBLEMS

1. Describe the essential points to be clarified in obtaining the history and physical examination of a Neonate presented with Stridor.
   Ans: Refer to the *Evaluation-Decision-Action Plan/Algorithm* to diagnose and manage *a Neonate with Congenital Stridor.*
2. Mention the Pitfalls in the diagnosis of Congenital Stridor.
   Ans: Refer to the"No. 8" of the *"BIRD'S EYE VIEW/OVERVIEW/ SYNOPSIS" of the Chapter.*
3. What are the indications for surgical intervention in a Neonate with Congenital Stridor ?
   Ans: Refer to the"No. 10" of the *"BIRD'S EYE VIEW/OVERVIEW/ SYNOPSIS" of the Chapter.*
4. Name the Imaging modalities that are useful in evaluating a Neonate with Congenital Stridor .
   Ans: Refer to the Evaluation-Decision-Action Plan/Algorithm to diagnose and manage a Neonate with Congenital Stridor.
5. Describe the essential features of *Laryngomalacia, the most common cause of Congenital Stridor.*
   Ans: Refer to the Table 1 of the Chapter.

LEARNING OBJECTIVES

After completing this article, readers will be able to

1. **Approach the evaluation of Congenital Stridor systematically and to recognize the different causes of airway obstruction in a Neonate-Infant.**

2. **Assess the urgency for either medical or surgical intervention.**

3. **Recognize the role of endoscopy in the evaluation of Congenital Stridor.**

4. **Distinguish between laryngomalacia and tracheo-malacia.**

5. **Tailor the management to each condition and its degree of severity.**

Pearl/Peril/Pitfall: Vocal cord paralysis accounts for 10% of all congenital laryngeal lesions and is, after laryngomalacia, the second most frequent cause of neonatal stridor. Unilateral vocal cord paralysis occurs more often on the left side because of the longer course of the recurrent laryngeal nerve, which makes it more vulnerable to injury. Unilateral dysfunction may result from birth trauma, trauma during thoracic surgery or compression by mediastinal masses of cardiac, pulmonary, esophageal, thyroid or lymphoid origin. Bilateral vocal cord paralysis is more commonly associated with central nervous system problems including perinatal asphyxia, cerebral hemorrhage, hydrocephalus, bulbar injury and Arnold-Chiari malformation.

BIRD'S EYE VIEW/OVERVIEW/SYNOPSIS

1. Congenital Stridor presents at birth or within the first few weeks (4–6) of life.Stridor is a clinical sign characterized by monophonic, audible breath sounds (noisy breathing) that usually originates from the extrathoracic airways. The presence of stridor indicates a partial obstruction of the upper airways, glottis, or trachea. The pitch of the stridor is determined by the degree of airway obstruction and the velocity of the airflow; the loudness and tone of the sound also varies by the specific cause.Stridor results from partial obstruction of an airway with turbulent flow characteristics. Such respiratory tract areas are the upper airway, glottis, and trachea. The obstruction can be fixed or variable. Variable extrathoracic obstructions are primarily associated with inspiratory stridor. This is because, during inspiration, extrathoracic intraluminal airway pressure is negative relative to atmospheric pressure, leading to collapse of supraglottic structures. During expiration, intrathoracic pressure is positive and tends to collapse the airway. Thus, stridor caused by intrathoracic obstructions tends to be more prominent upon expiration. Stridor heard during both phases of respiration is usually due to either a fixed airway obstruction or to 2 areas of obstruction (i.e. intrathoracic and extrathoracic).

2. Congenital Stridor is rarely life-threatening. Immediately life-threatening obstruction from congenital lesions such as severe micrognathia are apparent at birth, and are treated with emergent tracheotomy. Bilateral vocal cord paralysis and subglottic hemangioma may present as causes of congenital stridor that are life-threatening. Significant airway obstruction can lead to respiratory distress and failure to thrive, secondary to the increased work of breathing.

3. **Laryngomalacia** is the most common cause of Congenital Stridor. Patients typically have high-pitched inspiratory stridor that increases with crying and when supine. It rarely interferes with feeding. Symptoms are usually present at birth or within the first 4-6 weeks of life. Laryngomalacia usually resolves of its own accord within 18-24 months.Vocal cord paralysis may cause a patient to have a weak cry. Patients may also be worse with feeding. Ruling out underlying conditions that may result in vocal cord paralysis, in particular neurologic conditions such as Arnold-Chiari malformation, is important. Bilateral paralysis is more commonly associated with neurologic problems and is a life-threatening emergency.**Subglottic stenosis** can be congenital or acquired. Stridor of subglottic stenosis is typically biphasic. Acquired forms usually arise from endotracheal (ET) intubation.

4. Papillomas (human papilloma virus types-6 and11) are found most frequently on the vocal cords, affecting the voice and the airway causing hoarseness and stridor. They frequently enlarge and can spread to adjacent areas of the larynx or airway, including the nose and palate. They are thought to be transmitted vertically during birth by passage through the vaginal canal. The treatment of recurrent laryngeal papillomatosis is multiple endoscopic excisions. Several adjuvent medical therapies are being tried, but none are universally effective. In most children, recurrent respiratory papillomatosis eventually becomes quiescent for unknown reasons and may leave a scarred, although functional, larynx. Airway hemangioma may or may not be found with cutaneous hemangioma. Cutaneous hemangioma in the region of the mandible and neck should raise suspicions in a stridulous infant. Girls are affected 3 times more commonly than boys and are seen more commonly in premature infant. The most common site of airway involvement is the subglottis. The stridor usually develops by 2 months of age and the hemangiomas encroach on the airway, causing progressive obstruction when they proliferate during the first year. Medical therapy involves high-dose prednisone (5mg/kg/day, with the monitoring side effects). If steroid therapy fails to produce enduring improvement in the airway, surgical removal of the obstructing hemangioma may be necessary. Although interferon has been used successfully to treat life-threatening hemangiomas, its use is limited because spastic diplegia has occurred in some infants.

5. *Vascular ring* the double aortic arch is the most common complete vascular ring, encircling both the trachea and esophagus compressing both. With rare exception, these patients are symptomatic by 3 months of age. Respiratory symptoms predominate (stridor, coarse wheezing, and croupy cough), but dysphagia + vomiting may be present. Respiratory compromise can be severe and may lead to apnea, respiratory arrest and even death. Barium swallow, which shows a posterior indentation of the esophagus by the ring, is the mainstay of diagnosis. Chest X-ray and echocardiogram may miss abnormalities. CT scan with contrast or MRI angiography or bronchoscopy can define the information needed for the surgeon. Right aortic arch with left ligamentum arteriosum or PDA, pulmonary artery sling, anomalous innominate or left carotid artery, and aberrant right subclavian artery all but the latter can present with tracheal compression. Any condition (CHDs) that produces significant pulmonary hypertension increases the size of the pulmonary arteries, which, in turn, causes compression of the left main bronchus. Correction of underlying pathology to relieve pulmonary hypertension relieves the airway compression. Patients with significant symptoms require surgical correction, especially those with double aortic arch. Patients usually improve following correction but may have persistent but milder symptoms of airway obstruction due to associated tracheomalacia.

6. The *E-D-A plan/algorithm* summarizes the essential aspects of an infant who presents with Congenital stridor. Fiberoptic laryngoscopy and bronchoscopy, are valuable diagnostic tools for the evaluation of Congenital Stridor, offer several important advantages over radiographic imaging, including the following:*Lesions can be directly visualized. Evidence of inflammation or bleeding can be observed. Characteristics of the lesion, such as vascularity, can be determined.*Biopsies and bronchoalveolar lavage samples can be taken if necessary. *The examination is conducted while the patient is actively breathing, allowing assessment of dynamic events.In cases of suspected gastroesophageal reflux (GER), 24-hour mid esophageal pH monitoring may be helpful in establishing the diagnosis.

7. The prognosis for Congenital Stridor depends on the specific cause. In general, it is very good. For conditions such as laryngomalacia, the condition is self-limited and resolves on its own. For other conditions, such as subglottic stenosis, surgical correction is curative.

8. *The major medical pitfall in evaluation of Congenital Stridor is failure to make the diagnosis.* *Infants are frequently diagnosed with congestion or asthma. *True viral upper respiratory infections in infants younger than 1 month are rare. *Persistently abnormal noisy breathing is unlikely to be associated with a viral illness and warrants further investigation.

9. Medical care is primarily supportive because many causes of Congenital Stridor resolve spontaneously over time. For those that do not, such as vascular rings, surgical treatment is usually definitive. However, in some patients, tracheomalacia persists for some time after such a repair. In severe cases of Congenital Stridor, nonsurgical therapy may have a role prior to definitive surgical correction.

10. Surgical management depends on the specific lesion that causes stridor. Management is tailored to each condition and its degree of severity.*In general, indications for surgical correction include the following: *Inability to maintain a patent airway *Feeding difficulties or failure to thrive *Inability to maintain adequate oxygenation. Some of the surgical procedures used to treat congenital stridor include the following: *Epiglottoplasty for laryngomalacia *Tracheostomy for severe subglottic stenosis or tracheomalacia *Division of a vascular ring *Tracheoplasty for complete tracheal rings.

Pearl/Peril/Pitfall : *Unilateral choanal atresia does not usually cause any clinical problem unless the contralateral side is obstructed, for example, as a result of an upper respiratory tract infection. Bilateral choanal atresia is a life-threatening condition and a well-recognized cause of airway obstruction and respiratory distress in the newborn.*

THE EVALUATION-DECISION-ACTION-PLAN/ALGORITHM FOR THE DIAGNOSIS AND MANAGEMENT OF *A NEONATE WITH CONGENITAL STRIDOR*

SUBJECTIVE FINDINGS

Hx of **Stridor:** Time of onset: gradual, progressive, Persistent versus intermittent, or sudden, characteristics of cry, Relationship of stridor to feeding, Aspiration or reflux, Cyanosis, *Previous prolonged/repeated intubations,* Careful repeated questioning for aspirated foreign body, Presence of other congenital abnormalities.

Hx of pregnancy (fetal movements, distress), delivery (trauma, HIE), feeding problems.

OBJECTIVE FINDINGS

Assess ABCs, vitals, BP, O_2 sats, work of breathing, central cyanosis, CRT, pulses, Urine output, signs suggestive of sepsis/birth asphyxia/CCF., , ability to feed.

Assess for Stridor, pitch, duration, and timing of the stridorous sound, Careful inspection of the patient in the parent's arms, choanal patency, jaw and tongue size, Respiratory rate and degree of distress, Tachypnea and onset of fatigue, Flaring of nasal alae and other signs of respiratory effort, Auscultation of stridor, Skin lesions (e.g. hemangiomas), Neurologic status.

INVESTIGATIONS

Blood FBC with hematocrit and platelets, glucose, blood culture, ABG analysis, electrolytes, Ca^{++}, Mg^{++}, creatinine, BUN, bleeding and clotting profile. (depending on the presentation)

Imaging *X-ray – AP and lateral neck/chest: look for soft tissue masses and delineate the airway *Barium swallow: extrinsic compressors of the trachea will probably also compress the esophagus. *Echocardiography/CT with contrast/MRI: to exclude vascular rings or slings.* *Flexible fibre-optic nasopharyngoscopy and laryngoscopy: performed by ENT surgeon with patient awake - can visualize supraglottic and laryngeal lesions, observe laryngomalacia and vocal cord movement *Operative laryngoscopy/bronchoscopy: performed under GA – see better views of subglottic area and can biopsy lesions or drain cysts.

Although important, pre-endoscopy assessment including history, physical examination and radiological examination, is only a guide to the type and degree of pathology found during endoscopy.

Identify choanal atresia, micrognathia, macroglossia, *Lingual Thyroid or Thyroglossal Cyst, Hypothyroidism,* Down syndrome

A NEONATE WITH CONGENITAL STRIDOR

Assess severity — Airway emergency

Stable airway → Stabilize airway / Endotracheal intubation / Tracheostomy

Clinical Assessment / Detailed history / Physical examination

Acute Stridor or Acute on Chronic — Chronic Stridor

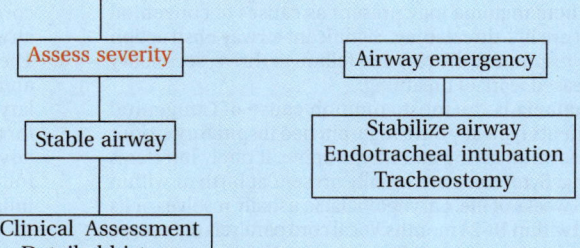

Laryngeal
Vocal cord paralysis
Subglottic stenosis
Subglottic hemangioma
Foreign body

Tracheal
Vascular ring
Bronchogenic cysts
Tracheal stenosis
Tracheitis
Cystic hygroma

Non anatomic
GERD
Hypocalcemic tetany

Chronic Stridor → Plain X-ray / Fiberoptic endoscopy

Mild symptoms Laryngomalacia suspected → Consider reflux management → Observe → Improves

Mod/severe symptoms Laryngomalacia suspected or diagnosis uncertain → Microlaryngoscopy and bronchoscopy

No improvement → Microlaryngoscopy and bronchoscopy

---

*Direct examination of the airway is often necessary to confirm the diagnosis and is essential in children with persistent stridor. Flexible fiberoptic bronchoscopy is widely used in the evaluation of airways in children. However, rigid bronchoscopy performed under general anesthesia gives a better view of the airway, especially the part below the level of the vocal cords. Rigid bronchoscopy also allows tissue biopsy and removal of foreign bodies using forceps. *A barium swallow is a useful method if vascular compression or gastroesophageal reflux is suspected. Gastrografin should be used as the contrast medium if tracheoesophageal fistula is suspected. *Videofluoroscopy is useful in the diagnosis of tracheomalacia, foreign body aspiration and vocal cord dysfunction. *Computed tomographic (CT) scan and magnetic resonance imaging (MRI) may be obtained to visualize the airway and the surrounding soft tissue structures, including any evidence of vascular compression. *Treatment of stridor should be directed at the underlying cause.

*The airway should be established immediately in children with severe respiratory distress or actual airway obstruction. This can be done by endotracheal intubation. After adequate ventilation is achieved by intubation, tracheostomy can be performed if deemed necessary. *Supportive measures may include oxygen, humidified air, intravenous fluids, suction and aerosol treatments with steroids and beta-adrenergic drugs.

Pearl/Peril/Pitfall: Subglottic Hemangioma. A subglottic hemangioma occurs more commonly in girls, with a female-to-male ratio of 2:1. The lesion is usually submucosal. No color change or, at most, a slight bluish discoloration is evident. It is frequently associated with hemangiomas elsewhere on the body. The stridor is biphasic and exaggerated by crying or straining as the lesion tends to become engorged.

TABLE 1   Congenital stridor-causes and differential diagnosis

Differential diagnosis of stridor can be divided into supralaryngeal, laryngeal, tracheal, and nonanatomic categories.

Supralaryngeal causes of stridor: Supralaryngeal causes include choanal atresia, vallecular cysts, thyroglossal cysts, and tongue dermoid or teratoma. *Choanal Atresia.* Choanal atresia, although rare, is the most common congenital anomaly of the nose. Choanal atresia results from a persistence of the bucconasal membrane in the posterior nares at the posterior margin of the hard palate. Unilateral choanal atresia does not usually cause any clinical problem unless the contralateral side is obstructed, for example, as a result of an upper respiratory tract infection. Bilateral choanal atresia is a life-threatening condition and a well-recognized cause of airway obstruction and respiratory distress in the newborn. A lingual thyroid is due to a failure of descent of the thyroid gland. A thyroglossal cyst arises from remnants of the thyroglossal duct. Clinically, a thyroglossal cyst presents as a smooth, discrete mass in the midline of the neck anywhere from just above the hyoid bone to the thyroid gland. Typically, the mass moves upward when the tongue is protruded. A lingual thyroid or thyroglossal cyst, if large enough, may cause airway obstruction and stridor.

Laryngeal causes of stridor:

a. *Laryngomalacia:* The most common cause of persistent stridor in infants, usually is seen the first 2–6 weeks of life (may be present at birth).It has a male-to-female ratio of approximately 2:1. It is worse in the supine position, with increased activity, with upper respiratory infections, and during feeding. Usually a benign congenital disorder in which the cartilaginous support for the supraglottic structures is under developed. At the child grows, the cartilages become more rigid and support the larynx, so the stridor resolves. Symptoms increase in severity upto 6 months, although gradual improvement can begin at any time. Diagnosis is established by direct flexible laryngoscopy, which shows inspiratory collapse of an omega shaped epiglottis (with or without long, redundant arytenoids). The aryepiglottic folds and false vocal cords are drawn into the laryngeal lumen, which results in a substantial narrowing of the lumen on inspiration. Because 15–60% of infants with laryngomalacia have synchronous airway anomalies, complete bronchoscopy is undertaken for patients with moderate to severe obstruction. With associated dysphagia, a contrast swallow study and esophagogram may be indicated. When the work of breathing is moderate to severe, airway films and chest radiographs are indicated. Most children will outgrow the condition by 12–18 months. More severe cases may fail to thrive secondary to airway obstruction and poor feeding or night time obstructive symptoms and desaturations or associated GERD (Gastro Esophageal Reflux Disease). These children require supraglottoplasty i.e. surgical trimming of the supraglottis. Laryngopharyngeal reflux is managed aggressively.

b. *Tracheomalacia:* It may be confused with laryngomalacia and the two differ in etiology, natural history, and treatment.

	Laryngomalacia	Tracheomalacia
Stridor	Inspiratory only	Biphasic or expiratory
Etiology	Weak cartilage of the larynx or inadequate neuromuscular tone of the larynx	Widened tracheal rings (primary) Extrinsic compression (secondary)
Symptoms in severe cases	Failure to thrive, cyanosis, or apnea	Reflux apnea ("dying spell")
Associated findings	Gastroesophageal reflux common	Chronic cough (may be "barking") Cardiovascular abnormalities Gastroesophageal reflux
Endoscopic findings	Collapse of epiglottis, arytenoids, or both on inspiration Normal trachea	Normal larynx Posterior tracheal wall "fish mouth" to anterior wall May be short or long segment Bronchomalacia
Treatment	Expectant management Supraglottoplasty in severe cases	Aortopexy if innominate artery compression Tracheostomy in severe cases
Natural history	Spontaneous resolution by 18months old	Recurrent "croup" episodes Narrow segment less critical with growth

c. *Congenital subglottic stenosis* - third most common cause of stridor, which is biphasic or primarily inspiratory and is recurrent or persistent typically. First symptoms often occur with a respiratory tract infections as edema and thickened secretions of a common cold narrow an already compromised airway. Narrowing of the subglottic airway can occur because the first tracheal ring is trapped within the cricoid cartilage, a deformity of the cricoid cartilage, or excess soft tissue within the cricoid cartilage. The diagnosis is made by rigid endoscopy under general anesthesia. The glottis of the neonate measures approximately 7mm in the sagittal plane and 4mm in the coronal plane. The vocal cords are 6-8mm long, with the posterior aspect composed of the cartilaginous process of the arytenoid. The subglottic diameter measures approximately 4.5 by 7 mm . A diameter of less than 3.5 mm is suggestive of a subglottic stenosis. Tracheostomy is often required when airway compromise is severe. Surgical intervention (laryngotracheal reconstruction using a cartilage graft from rib to expand the airway) is ultimately required to correct the stenosis.

Pearl/Peril/Pitfall: Intubation. Intubation may result in vocal cord paralysis, laryngotracheal stenosis, subglottic edema and laryngospasm. Any of the above, alone or in combination, may lead to airway obstruction and stridor

Acquired subglottic stenosis due to prolonged intubation may be complicated by associated GERD, which should be controlled because gastric refluxate may contribute to the laryngeal inflammation. Heliox (Oxygen-21% + Helium-79%) has been recommended as a temporary measure to promote laminar flow in patients who have upper airway obstruction. Heliox doesn't treat the airway lesion directly, but decreases the work of breathing and allows time for a reversible lesion, such as post extubation laryngeal edema, to resolve. Nebulized epinephrine also commonly is used to treat post extubation stridor. IV steroids has been shown efficacious in treating post extubation stridor.

d. *Vocal cord paralysis* may cause a patient to have a weak cry. Patients may also be worse with feeding. Unilateral vocal cord paralysis occurs more often on the left side because of the longer course of the recurrent laryngeal nerve, which makes it more vulnerable to injury. Unilateral dysfunction may result from birth trauma, trauma during thoracic surgery or compression by mediastinal masses of cardiac, pulmonary, esophageal, thyroid or lymphoid origin. Bilateral vocal cord paralysis is more commonly associated with central nervous system problems including perinatal asphyxia, cerebral hemorrhage, hydrocephalus, bulbar injury and Arnold-Chiari malformation. The vocal cords may also be injured by direct trauma from endotracheal intubation attempts or during deep airway suction. In vocal cord paralysis, the stridor is typically biphasic. In unilateral vocal cord paralysis, the infant's cry is weak and feeble; however, there is usually no respiratory distress. In bilateral vocal cord paralysis, the voice is usually of good quality, but there is marked respiratory distress.

Other laryngeal abnormalities leading to stridor include webs, cysts, hemangiomas, papillomata, and laryngo-tracheoesophageal clefts. A laryngeal web results from a failure of the embryonic airway to recanalize. Most laryngeal webs occur at the level of the vocal cords and are anterior in location. A laryngeal cyst typically occurs in the aryepiglottic fold or in the epiglottis. A laryngeal cyst usually contains mucus from minor salivary glands. A laryngocele arises as a dilatation of the saccule of the laryngeal ventricle. A laryngeal web, cyst or laryngocele may present with stridor, usually at birth or soon after.

* Tracheal causes of stridor:

* Extrinsic compression of the trachea by vascular abnormalities is a common cause of stridor. Anomalies that may lead to stridor include double aortic arch, innominate artery compression, aberrant right sub-clavian vein, and *pulmonary artery sling. * Bronchogenic cysts* can also cause extrinsic compression of the trachea. *Tracheomalacia* may be observed in association with laryngomalacia or as an isolated lesion. (*v.s*) *Tracheal stenosis can be a complication of long-term ET intubation (Intubation may result in vocal cord paralysis, laryngo-tracheal stenosis, subglottic edema and laryngospasm. Any of the above, alone or in combination, may lead to airway obstruction and stridor.)* or a congenital lesion. ·Complete tracheal rings are a subset of tracheal stenosis with severe biphasic airway sounds.

*Nonanatomic causes of stridor: Cardio-vocal syndrome occurs when cardiac abnormalities lead to compression of the recurrent laryngeal nerve. Foreign body may be present. *Gastroesophageal reflux (GER)* has been associated with stridor, although no controlled studies have been performed to demonstrate that GER is actually responsible for the stridor.

Vocal cord paralysis accounts for 10% of all congenital laryngeal lesions and is, after laryngomalacia, the second most frequent cause of neonatal stridor. An overview of etiologies of vocal cord paralysis in all pediatric age groups is given in the Table below:

Etiology	Unilateral VCP	Bilateral VCP
CNS (most brainstem)	Infrequent	Common
PNS	Infrequent	Common (myasthenia gravis)
Trauma	Common (thoracic surgery, ETT)	Infrequent
Neoplasm	Common (skull base tumor)	Infrequent
Inflammatory	Infrequent	Infrequent
Cardiovascular anomaly	Common (VSD)	Infrequent
Metabolic	Infrequent (chemotherapy)	Infrequent
Genetic	Infrequent	Infrequent
Idiopathic	Common	
Common		

CNS: central nervous system (Arnold-Chiari malformation, leukodystrophy, encephalocele, myelomeningocele, hydrocephalus, cerebral or nuclear dysgenesis); PNS: peripheral nervous system; ETT: endotracheal tube; VCP: vocal cord paralysis; VSD: ventricular septal defect

Pearl/Peril/Pitfall : Tracheomalacia. Tracheomalacia is characterized by abnormal tracheal collapse secondary to inadequate cartilaginous and myoelastic elements supporting the trachea. Tracheal narrowing occurs with expiration and causes stridor.[11] The stridor may not be present at birth but appears insidiously after the first weeks of life. The stridor is usually aggravated by respiratory tract infections and agitation. The word "stridor" is derived from the Latin word "stridulus," which means creaking, whistling or grating. Stridor is a harsh, vibratory sound of variable pitch caused by partial obstruction of the respiratory passages that results in turbulent airflow through the airway. Although stridor may be the result of a relatively benign process, it may also be the first sign of a serious and even life-threatening disorder. Stridor is a distressing symptom to its victims and their parents, and presents a diagnostic challenge to physicians.

THE CHILD WITH RECURRING DESATURATION BY ALAN R. SPITZER, MD

Case

A former 680 gram 25 week gestation infant has been treated with mechanical ventilation since shortly after birth. Attempts to wean this infant have not been successful, and he is now 42 days old on a conventional ventilator with the following settings: FiO$_2$ 0.44, PIP 21 cm H$_2$O, PEEP 5 cm H$_2$O. With each reduction in peak pressure or end expiratory pressure, the nursing staff notes that he has increased oxygen desaturation, frequently needing hand ventilation with a bag and mask with these episodes. During periods of crying or agitation, he is particularly prone to these events. A trial of bronchodilators is initiated, but the infant's condition does not change, and increasing the frequency of dosing only seems to make him even worse. In frustration, you refer him for bronchoscopy, which reveals the following image:

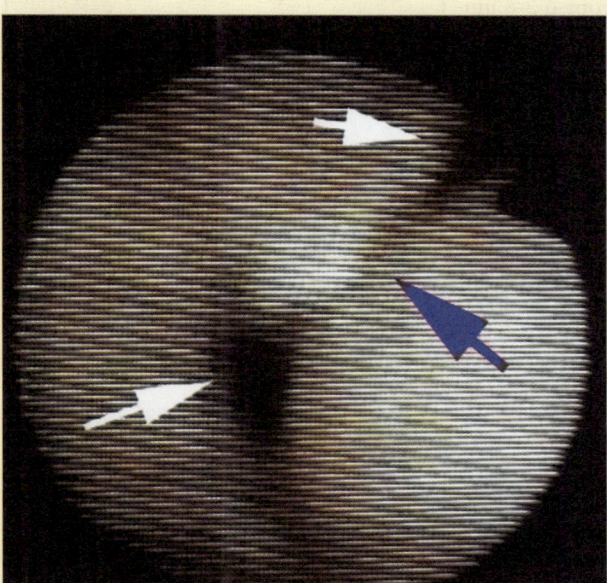

Discussion Points

1. What is the diagnosis?
2. What is happening at the blue and the white arrows?
3. What other tests might be helpful at this point?
4. Should bronchodilators be continued?
5. What treatment(s) would be most helpful?

Discussion: This child has **tracheobronchomalacia**. The image reveals a buckling of the trachea at the site of the blue arrow, in which it folds upon itself during expiration, while the white arrows point out the mainstem bronchi, which are simultaneously severely narrowed. Tracheobronchomalacia is actually quite common in many extremely low birth weight (ELBW) premature infants who are ventilated for longer than two weeks. Approximately 30% of infants with BPD will have this problem. The continued force of positive pressure within the airway causes progressive distension of the airway. Because of the lack of adequate cartilaginous support, the airway becomes increasingly soft and compliant. During expiration, the airway collapses and airflow is reduced to a very low level, which can be revealed on either pulmonary function tests, or careful inspection of pulmonary graphics now supplied with many neonatal ventilators.

While inspiration may also be affected to some degree, the expansion of the chest wall and lowering of the diaphragm during inspiration usually maintains airway patency. In expiration, however, the airway narrows, as seen in this infant, and exhalation of carbon dioxide becomes increasingly difficult. When agitated, the expiratory pressure that even a small pre-term infant can generate significantly exceeds the end distending pressure that is being provided. Because the airway also has a liquid lining layer (often increased from the inflammatory response to oxygen and mechanical ventilation), the surface tension of the liquid lining is difficult for the infant to overcome when the airway walls adhere, and the airway cannot be readily reopened. Agitation from hypoxia increases and progressively worsens the situation. An infant does not need to be agitated to have this happen, however. Often, during periods of sleep, the relaxation of airway muscle tone will simply cause the airway to narrow and the same sequence of events may occur as described above.

Because bronchodilators tend to decrease airway tone, they are detrimental in tracheobronchomalacia. Since these infants are often mistaken for having bronchospasm, the tendency is to increase the frequency of treatments, which only produces further deterioration in the child's clinical status. In general, unless bronchospasm can be documented by pulmonary function testing, bronchodilators should be avoided in the chronically ventilated patient. While some infants do have demonstrable bronchospasm that is responsive to bronchodilator therapy on PFTs, the majority of patients will not respond to these drugs and they tend to be used excessively and unnecessarily in many patients.

The correct approach to tracheobronchomalacia is twofold: Increased end expiratory pressure will help stabilize the airway and prevent some, though not all, of the airway collapse. A PEEP as high as 10–12 cm H$_2$O may be needed in some infants, though such cases are not common and many infants will do well at a PEEP of 7-8 cm H$_2$O, especially if bronchodilators are discontinued. During bronchoscopy, one can often visualize the airway open dramatically at a critical PEEP level, and a PEEP "grid" can be performed either during bronchoscopy or with PFT testing, by slowly increasing PEEP to see where airway mechanics are most satisfactory.

In addition, concentration on nutritional support of the infant is critical. Because these infants are so difficult to feed when they are desaturating, feeds are often repeatedly held. Once the airway is stabilized, feeding can be continued more satisfactorily and growth can be achieved at a steadier pace. As the infant grows, the airway enlarges, ultimately reaching a size in which the collapse is less problematic and weaning can proceed. The addition of cartilage also aids in recovery.

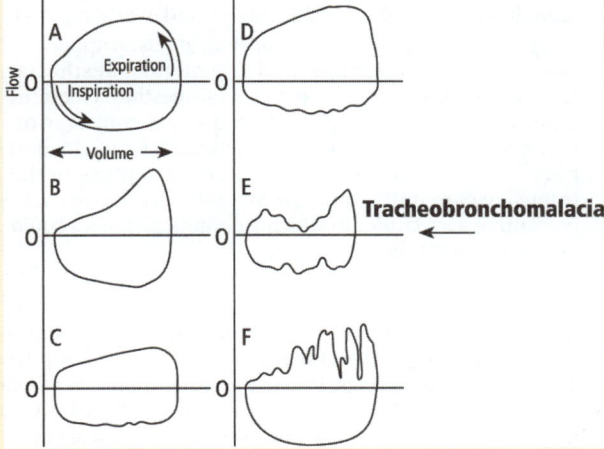

Pearl/Peril/Pitfall: *The vocal cords may also be injured by direct trauma from endotracheal intubation attempts or during deep airway suction. In vocal cord paralysis, the stridor is typically biphasic. In unilateral vocal cord paralysis, the infant's cry is weak and feeble; however, there is usually no respiratory distress. In bilateral vocal cord paralysis, the voice is usually of good quality, but there is marked respiratory distress.*

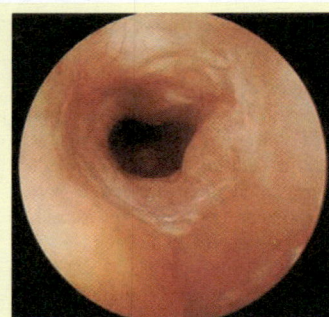

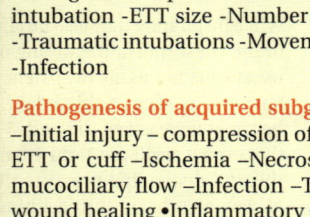

Acquired SGS: ¨95% of cases of SGS ¨90% due to long-term or prior intubation -Duration of intubation -ETT size -Number of intubations -Traumatic intubations -Movement of the ETT -Infection

Pathogenesis of acquired subglottic stenosis –Initial injury – compression of mucosa by an ETT or cuff –Ischemia –Necrosis –Decreased mucociliary flow –Infection –Three stages of wound healing •Inflammatory •Proliferative – granulation tissue •Scar formation – contraction and remodeling.

Management of SGS:¨Observation–Reasonable in mild cases, esp. congenital SGS (Cotton-Myer grade I and mild grade II) •If no retractions, feeding difficulties, or episodes of croup requiring hospitalization •Follow growth curves •Repeat endoscopy q 3-6 mo ¨Tracheostomy –Often the initial step in treatment of pediatric acquired SGS –May be avoided in patients with congenital SGS – Allows time for the infant to mature •Lungs – BPD •Wt. – 10 kg (Cotton) –2%-5% mortality in children •Accidental decannulation and plugging.

Surgery for SGS ¨I. Endoscopic –Dilation – Laser ¨II. Open procedure–Expansion procedure (with trach and stent or SS-LTR) •Laryngotracheoplasty •Laryngotracheal reconstruction.

Courtesy: Subglottic Stenosis (SGS)- Christopher D. Muller, M.D. Anna M. Pou, M.D. University of Texas Medical Branch Galveston, TX Department of Otolaryngology – Head and Neck Surgery.

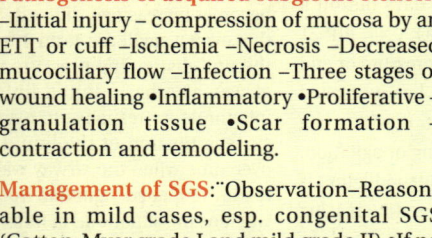

Classification	From	To
Grade I	No Obstruction	50% Obstruction
Grade II	51% Obstruction	70% Obstruction
Grade III	71% Obstruction	99% Obstruction
Grade IV	No Detectable Lumen	

Cotton-Myer grading system for subglottic stenosis

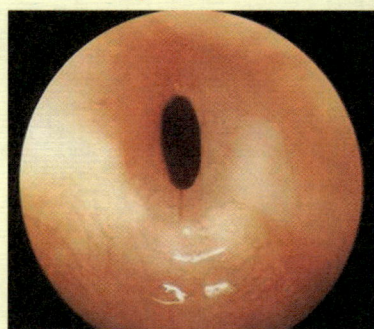

Congenital SGS

KEY POINTS FOR CLINICAL PRACTICE

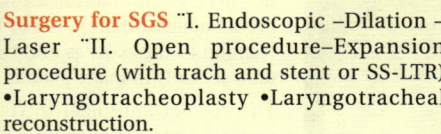

1. Stridor is the sound caused by abnormal air passage into the lungs and can exist in different degrees and be caused by obstruction located anywhere in the extra-thoracic (nose, pharynx, larynx, trachea) or intra-thoracic airway (tracheobronchial tree). Stridor may be congenital or acquired, acute, intermittent or chronic. Laryngotracheomalacia is the most common cause of congenital, chronic stridor. Stridor is a clinical sign and not a diagnosis.

2. The golden standard in the workup of stridor is an upper and lower airway endoscopy under general anesthesia. Endoscopic examination under general anesthesia requires a multidisciplinary approach and close cooperation between anesthesiologist, pediatrician, ENT surgeon and nursing staff. Following this procedure, a place in the intensive care unit should be available for those cases presenting with stridor in which a definite diagnosis could not yet be established.

3. Laryngomalacia is the most common congenital laryngeal anomaly. Inspiratory stridor often does not present until two weeks after birth and resolves by 18 months of age. Most cases are managed with watchful waiting. Severe cases require a surgical intervention.

4. Bilateral vocal cord paralysis is usually idiopathic. In certain cases, paralysis may occur secondary to central nervous system abnormality including Arnold-Chiari malformation, cerebral palsy, hydrocephalus, myelomeningocele, spina bifida, or hypoxia. Severe cases may necessitate endotracheal intubation and tracheostomy.

5. Congenital subglottic stenosis is the third most common laryngeal anomaly. It is defined as a diameter of less than 4mm of the cricoid region in a full-term infant, and less than 3mm in a premature infant. This condition is the most common laryngeal anomaly that requires tracheotomy in newborns. Laryngotracheoplasty may be required to achieve decanulation.

REFERENCES and FURTHER READING 1)Belmont JR, Grundfast K. Congenital laryngeal stridor (laryngomalacia): etiologic factors and associated disorders. *Ann Otol Rhinol Laryngol.* Sep-Oct 1984;93(5 Pt 1):430-7. 2) Berdon WE, Baker DH. Vascular anomalies and the infant lung: rings, slings, and other things. *Semin Roentgenol.* Jan 1972;7(1):39–64. 3) Cotton RT. Pediatric laryngotracheal stenosis. *J Pediatr Surg.* Dec 1984;19(6):699–704 4)Cotton RT. Pediatric laryngotracheal stenosis. *J Pediatr Surg.* Dec 1984;19(6):699–704 5) Parnell FW, Brandenburg JH. Vocal cord paralysis. A review of 100 cases. *Laryngoscope.* Jul 1970;80(7):1036-45.

Pearl/Peril/Pitfall: External Compression. Tracheal compression may result from vascular anomalies such as double aortic arch, right aortic arch with left ligamentum arteriosum, anomalous innominate artery, anomalous left common carotid artery, anomalous left pulmonary artery or aberrant subclavian artery. The child may prefer to keep the neck hyperextended. The stridor resulting from tracheal compression is often aggravated by feeding.

45 A Newborn Baby with Suspected Cardiac Problem

@ *"It is helpful to consider not only the type of presentation but also the usual timing of presentation, when making a diagnosis of cardiac disease in the Newborn." Essentially, heart disease in the Newborn presents in one of the 7 main ways: a) asymptomatic b)cyanosis, with/ without respiratory distress c)respiratory distress (CHF) with/without cyanosis d) collapse/ shock e) an associated lesion/syndrome/dysmorphology f) premature baby with significant PDA g) birth asphyxia with transient myocardial ischemia and pulmonary edema.*

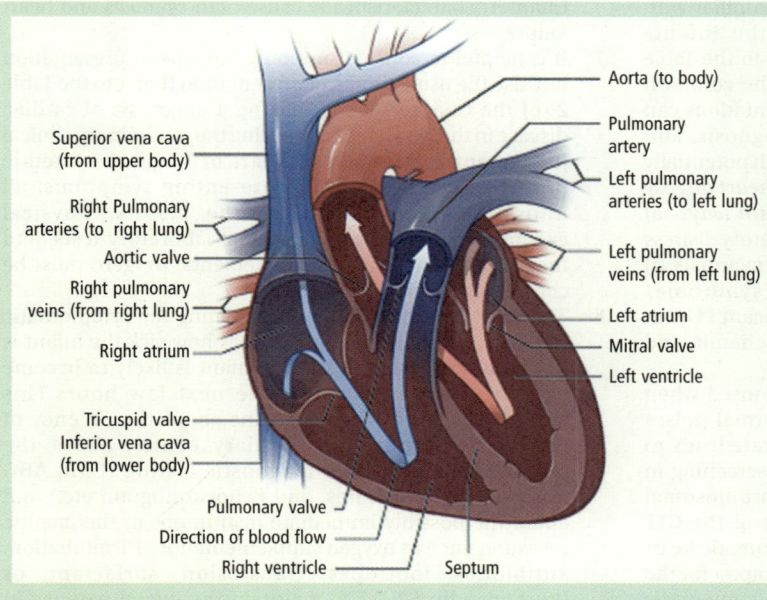

Aorta (to body)
Pulmonary artery
Left pulmonary arteries (to left lung)
Superior vena cava (from upper body)
Left pulmonary veins (from left lung)
Right Pulmonary arteries (to right lung)
Aortic valve
Right pulmonary veins (from right lung)
Left atrium
Right atrium
Mitral valve
Left ventricle
Tricuspid valve
Inferior vena cava (from lower body)
Pulmonary valve
Direction of blood flow
Right ventricle
Septum

We can classify congenital heart defects into several categories in order to better understand the problems the baby will experience. They include:

* Problems that cause **too much** blood to pass through the lungs (*Increased Pulmonary Blood Flow*); These defects allow oxygen-rich blood that should be traveling to the body to re-circulate through the lungs, causing increased pressure and stress in the lungs. (*Respiratory Distress due to CHF*), e.g. large PDA in a Preterm, large VSD, AV Canal defect

* Problems that cause **too little** blood to pass through the lungs (*Decreased Pulmonary Blood Flow*); These defects allow blood that has not been to the lungs to pick up oxygen (and, therefore, is oxygen-poor) to travel to the body. The body does not receive enough oxygen with these heart problems, and the baby will be *cyanotic,* or have a blue coloring, e.g. Tricuspid Atresia, Pulmonary Atresia.

* Problems that cause too little blood to travel to the body(*decreased Systemic Blood Flow/Cardiac Output*) : These defects are a result of underdeveloped chambers of the heart or blockages in blood vessels that prevent the proper amount of blood from traveling to the body to meet its needs, e.g. Critical AS, Coarctation of Aorta. *Again, in some cases there will be a **combination** of several heart defects, making for a more complex problem that can fall into several of these categories, e.g. Hypoplastic Left Heart Syndrome, TAPVR.

REVIEW OF CLINICAL PROBLEMS

1. Name the 7 types of presentations a Neonate with a suspected Heart problem do present clinically
   Ans: Refer to the"No. 2"of the "BIRD'S EYE VIEW/OVERVIEW/ SYNOPSIS"of the Chapter, and to the Table 1 of the Chapter.

2. Mention the Typical timing and mode of CHD Presentation in Neonates-Infants.
   Ans: Refer to the Table 2 of the Chapter.

3. What are the **Indications for Referral of Newborns and Infants to a Pediatric Cardiologist**?
   Ans: Refer to the Table 6 of the Chapter.

4. How do you manage a Neonate with an Asymptomatic Heart murmur ?
   Ans: Refer to the Evaluation-Decision-Action Plan/Algorithm to diagnose and manage a Neonate with an Asymptomatic Heart murmur.

5. Discuss common surgical procedures for CHD.
   Ans: Refer to the Table 3 of the Chapter.

LEARNING OBJECTIVES

After completing this article, readers will be able to

1. Recognize the "7" different clinical presentations of heart disease in Neonates.

2. Stabilize the ABCDs of a sick Neonate adequately before seeking for the cardiologist`s help.

3. Consult a local cardiologist with pediatric expertise, for confirming the most likely clinical diagnosis.

4. Start IVI PROSTAGLANDIN E2, to maintain the ductal patency in a Neonate with/likely with a ductus-dependent CHD.

5. Establish lines of referral, consultation, and communication about the transport of these high-risk infants to a tertiary referral center-(Neonatal/ Cardiac).

Pearl/Peril/Pitfall: It is useful to classify congenital heart disease according to the pathophysiology of the major heart lesion, in particular, whether the lesion is associated with cyanosis ('blue') or is acyanotic ('pink'), also whether the lesion is associated with abnormal flow between the cardiac chambers (abnormal 'shunt'), obstruction to flow, abnormal connections of the major vessels or abnormal mixing.

BIRD'S EYE VIEW/OVERVIEW/SYNOPSIS

1. Accurate and timely diagnosis of a *symptomatic Newborn* due to Congenital heart disease is extremely important (whether premature or term baby) to minimize the morbidity and mortality. Many serious pulmonary and cardiac disorders that affect Newborns become obvious or are exacerbated as the normal postnatal cardiopulmonary adaptations unfold leading to dramatic changes in gas exchange and circulation at the moment of birth.

2. Every Pediatrician/Neonatologist should be familiar with the common clinical presentations of the infants demanding cardiovascular evaluation (Refer to the Table No 1 of the Chapter).This familiarity with the common cardiovascular causes of these different presentations can provide earlier insight into the correct diagnosis, and management for better than 90% of infants with potentially serious cardiovascular problems. *Essentially, heart disease in the Newborn presents in one of the 7 main ways-* a) asymptomatic b)cyanosis, with/without respiratory distress c)respiratory distress (CHF) with/without cyanosis d) collapse/shock e) an associated lesion/syndrome/ dysmorphology f) premature baby with significant PDA g) birth asphyxia with transient myocardial ischemia and pulmonary edema.

3. **Asymptomatic heart disease** is usually diagnosed when incidental finding of a heart murmur, abnormal pulses (absent femorals), abnormal heart rhythm/rate leads to detailed cardiac evaluation. Routine cardiac screening in cases of various dysmorphic syndromes, chromosomal abnormalities, or congenital abnormalities of the GIT system also enables early diagnosis of asymptomatic heart disease.(Refer to the Table 8,9 and 10 of the Chapter for the pathological features of an infant with an asymptomatic heart murmur which suggest the possibility of a serious (duct-dependent) heart lesion.) Innocent heart murmurs are diagnosed by the absence of any other features of cardiac disease as well as the presence of certain positive murmur characteristics. (Refer to E-D-A plan/ algorithm "Neonate with an asymptomatic murmur".)

4. **Central cyanosis** (bluish discoloration of tongue, mucous membranes, and the peripheral skin, and is usually apparent clinically at O_2 sats. of 85% or below) is one of the most significant signs of serious cardiac abnormality; hence, prompt recognition and diagnostic evaluation are mandatory. *Clinical features of cardiac cyanosis include;* a)differential cyanosis (lower limbs more cyanosed than upper limbs) -seen in neonates with right-to-left ductal shunting associated with PPHN or an aortic arch obstruction. b) worsening of cyanosis with crying/agitation c) central cyanosis with minimal respiratory distress d) ABG Analysis:low $PaO2$ with normal $PaCO_2$ d) no response to challenge with 100% inspired oxygen (Hyperoxia Test) e) abnormalities on CVS examination: precordial hyper-activity, heart murmur, and unequal peripheral pulses f) CXR- abnormal cardiac size/shape and abnormal pulmonary vascularity g) abnormal ECG (normal ECG does not exclude serious cardiac abnormality in neonates). Refer to Tables 10 and 11.

5. **Collapse/Shock** in a neonate can be caused by cardiac, respiratory, metabolic, and CNS conditions. Cardiac conditions which may present with collapse are listed in the Table No. 2 of the Chapter. Left heart obstructive lesions are the most common causes. In addition to duct-dependent cardiac lesions, SVT should be considered if the heart rate is >250bpm. Myocardial disease such as cardiomyopathy, either dilated or hypertrophic as seen in infants of diabetic mothers, myocardial ischemia following perinatal distress or anomalous origin of the left coronary artery are rare causes. Pericardial effusion with tamponade occasionally occurs.

6. **Cardiac conditions presenting with respiratory distress** usually do so through congestive heart failure (Refer to the Table No.1 of the Chapter) , some of these conditions may present with collapse and in retrospect a period of respiratory distress may have been present prior to collapse. Some cardiac conditions (listed in the Table 1 of the Chapter) characteristically cause both cyanosis and heart failure.

7. It is helpful to consider not only the type of presentation but also the usual timing of presentation (Refer to the Table 2 of the Chapter) when making a diagnosis of cardiac disease in the Newborn.In reaching the preliminary clinical judgement as to whether heart or lungs or systemic problems are causing the presenting symptoms, all information available from the history, physical examinations(serial examinations) laboratory tests, and therapeutic trials(such as supplemental oxygen) must be considered quickly but carefully.

8. The most important issue in evaluating the symptomatic Newborn due to cardiac problem is how sick the infant is now and how much sicker the infant is likely to become without intervention over the next few hours.This determines and drives decisions about the urgency of possible transport to a tertiary center, about the performance of further diagnostic testing (CXR, ABG Analysis, blood cultures, and Echocardiogram etc.) and about the possibly immediate institutions of therapeutic measures such as oxygen supplementation, ET intubation, antibiotics, inotropes, transfusion, surfactant, or Prostaglandin E2 IVI to maintain the ductal patency in ductus-dependent cardiac malformations.

9. Although in >90% of times a single diagnosis account for all symptoms in a given newborn, it is obviously important not to overlook a second diagnosis when 2 diseases co-exist, e.g. failure to recognize TGV in term baby with obvious meconium aspiration pneumonia can be calamitous.

10. *The Evaluation-Decision-Action-Plan/Algorithm* describes the essential aspects of diagnosis and management of a Neonate with a suspected cardiac problem.When a Neonate/infant presents with respiratory failure/CHF or shock, the initial approach to stabilization is determined by the symptoms at the presentation. If a duct-dependent cardiac lesion is suspected, reopening of the ductus with an IVI of Prostaglandin E2 should be a priority, particularly when immediate cardiac evaluation is not available. Failure to reopen the ductus in infants who are critically ill with ductal-dependent CHD is often fatal. Giving PGE2 to an infant who later proves to have sepsis or inborn error of metabolism seldom causes harm. Reopening of the ductus stabilizes infants with ductal-dependent CHD until a definitive evaluation or palliative or corrective surgery can be accomplished. In small infants and at higher doses, there is a significant incidence of apnea with PGE2 infusion, requiring mechanical ventilation in up to 10% of infants receiving it. It is important to establish lines of referral, consultation, and communication about the transport of these high risk infants to the tertiary referral center for preop/postoperative care. Serial assessments and adjustments in management are usually required throughout transport in infants with symptomatic CHD. The preterm infant with significant PDA and cardiac failure secondary to left-to-right shunting may require surgical ligation of the ductus if indomethacin/ibuprofen therapy fails. The care of these infants preoperatively is focused on the management.

Pearl/Peril/Pitfall: Recognizable chromosomal abnormalities are present in 25% of children with CHD. The diagnosis of a chromosomal abnormality should lead to active assessment for CHD.

THE EVALUATION-DECISION-ACTION- PLAN/ALGORITHM FOR THE DIAGNOSIS AND MANAGEMENT OF *A SICK NEWBORN BABY WITH SUSPECTED CARDIAC PROBLEM*

SUBJECTIVE FINDINGS

Postnatal Hx of symptom free interval, central and/or peripheral cyanosis, respiratory distress, feeding difficulties, prematurity, acute collapse-shock-CCF in a previously well baby, asymptomatic but significant heart murmur, obvious multiple congenital anomalies (eg., VACTERAL association)

Natal Hx of birth wt, APGAR scores, resuscitation details, mode of delivery, PROM/meconium stained labor, asphyxia

Antenatal Hx of maternal infections, medications, diabetes, SLE, drug abuse (including smoking, alcohol), amniocentesis and fetal USG SCAN results, fetal dysrhythmias/congenital heart block/SVT.

OBJECTIVE FINDINGS

Assess ABCDs and monitor CRT, O_2 sats (differential pulse oximetry), *4-limb BP,* core-peripheral temperature difference, RR, HR, central and peripheral pulses, urine output.

Determine whether the baby is in preterminal (*"pre arrest"*) conditions such as apnea, gasping or RR <20 bpm, shock, extremely lethargic or unresponsive limpy baby, bleeding, etc. and *intervene with appropriate resuscitation of ABCDs promptly.*

Note the other alarming signs such as: convulsions, irritability, pallor, central cyanosis, hypothermia, abdominal distention, bilious vomiting, petechiae and ecchymoses, vesicles, etc. (*signs suggestive of sepsis, asphyxia, CCF, NEC due to PDA*)

Note dysmorphic features (facies), obvious congenital malformations/stigmata of congenital infections

Perform CVS examination cardiac impulse, heart sounds, gallop, murmurs, breath sounds, rales, cardiomegaly, hepatomegaly.

INVESTIGATIONS

Blood FBC, TC, DC, **Hct**, Platelets, CRP, Blood cultures, **ABG analysis, electrolytes,** calcium and magnesium, **blood sugar,** creatinine, BUN, coagulation profile.

CXR for cardiomegaly/plethoric *or* oligemic lung fields, respiratory infections/air leaks , etc.

Consider carboxyhemoglobin or methemoglobin levels.

Urine analysis and culture

Laboratory studies for cardiac diagnosis Hyperoxia test, 15-lead ECG, 2D ECHO AND COLOR DOPPLER, Cardiac catheterization (before surgery)

MRI cardiac scanning in difficult cases

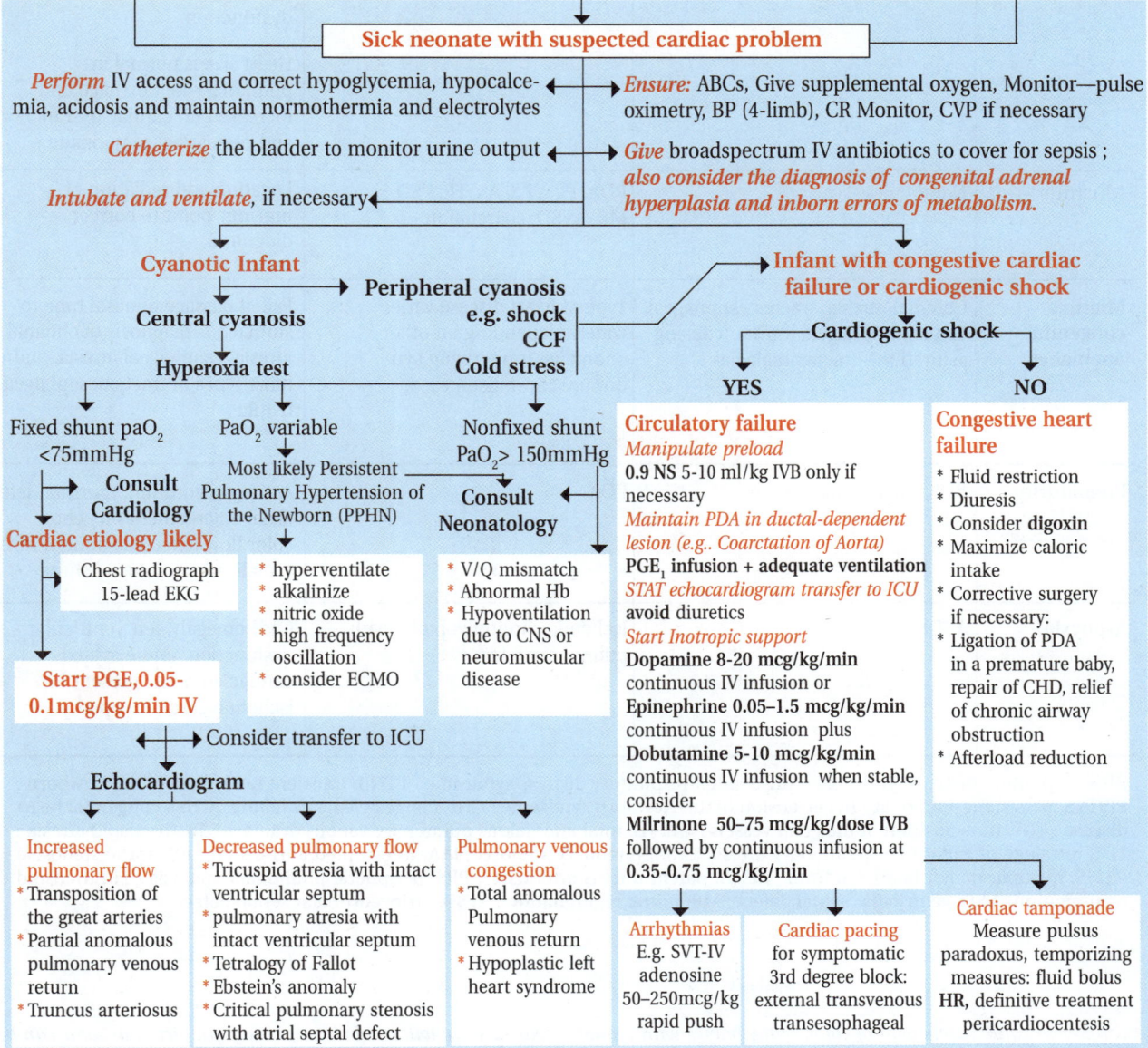

Sick neonate with suspected cardiac problem

Perform IV access and correct hypoglycemia, hypocalcemia, acidosis and maintain normothermia and electrolytes

Ensure: ABCs, Give supplemental oxygen, Monitor—pulse oximetry, BP (4-limb), CR Monitor, CVP if necessary

Catheterize the bladder to monitor urine output

Give broadspectrum IV antibiotics to cover for sepsis ; *also consider the diagnosis of congenital adrenal hyperplasia and inborn errors of metabolism.*

Intubate and ventilate, if necessary

Cyanotic Infant

Central cyanosis

Peripheral cyanosis e.g. shock CCF Cold stress

Hyperoxia test

Infant with congestive cardiac failure or cardiogenic shock

Cardiogenic shock

YES   NO

Fixed shunt paO_2 <75mmHg

Consult Cardiology

Cardiac etiology likely

Chest radiograph 15-lead EKG

Start PGE,0.05-0.1mcg/kg/min IV

PaO_2 variable

Most likely Persistent Pulmonary Hypertension of the Newborn (PPHN)

* hyperventilate
* alkalinize
* nitric oxide
* high frequency oscillation
* consider ECMO

Nonfixed shunt PaO_2> 150mmHg

Consult Neonatology

* V/Q mismatch
* Abnormal Hb
* Hypoventilation due to CNS or neuromuscular disease

Circulatory failure
Manipulate preload
0.9 NS 5-10 ml/kg IVB only if necessary
Maintain PDA in ductal-dependent lesion (e.g.. Coarctation of Aorta)
PGE₁ infusion + adequate ventilation
STAT echocardiogram transfer to ICU
avoid diuretics
Start Inotropic support
Dopamine 8-20 mcg/kg/min continuous IV infusion or
Epinephrine 0.05–1.5 mcg/kg/min continuous IV infusion plus
Dobutamine 5-10 mcg/kg/min continuous IV infusion when stable, consider
Milrinone 50–75 mcg/kg/dose IVB followed by continuous infusion at 0.35-0.75 mcg/kg/min

Congestive heart failure
* Fluid restriction
* Diuresis
* Consider **digoxin**
* Maximize caloric intake
* Corrective surgery if necessary:
* Ligation of PDA in a premature baby, repair of CHD, relief of chronic airway obstruction
* Afterload reduction

Consider transfer to ICU

Echocardiogram

Increased pulmonary flow
* Transposition of the great arteries
* Partial anomalous pulmonary venous return
* Truncus arteriosus

Decreased pulmonary flow
* Tricuspid atresia with intact ventricular septum
* pulmonary atresia with intact ventricular septum
* Tetralogy of Fallot
* Ebstein's anomaly
* Critical pulmonary stenosis with atrial septal defect

Pulmonary venous congestion
* Total anomalous Pulmonary venous return
* Hypoplastic left heart syndrome

Arrhythmias
E.g. SVT-IV adenosine 50–250mcg/kg rapid push

Cardiac pacing
for symptomatic 3rd degree block: external transvenous transesophageal

Cardiac tamponade
Measure pulsus paradoxus, temporizing measures: fluid bolus **HR,** definitive treatment pericardiocentesis

Pearl/Peril/Pitfall : Routine newborn examination of the cardiovascular system is not just auscultation and should include: ·Assessment of color. ·Assessment of peripheral pulses including femorals. ·Assessment of the precordial impulses. ·Auscultation for normal heart sounds and murmurs.

TABLE 1   Seven commonly occurring presentations of infants needing cardiovascular evaluation

Presentation	Lung diseases	Heart/systemic diseases	Differentiating points
Respiratory distress	RDS, pneumonia, ARDS, meconium aspiration, TTNB, diaphragmatic hernia, PPHNS (Pulmonary causes), congenital lobar emphysema	CHF (any cause), absent pulmonary valve, PPHNS (cardiac causes)	Cardiomegaly is not present in pulmonary causes but is common in cardiac causes
Cyanosis	Idiopathic PPHNS	Cyanotic CHD, with either increased (TGV, truncus, TAPVD, TA) or decreased (TOF, PA, critical PS, Ebstein anomaly) pulmonary blood flow	Idiopathic PPHNS ; normal cardiac contour, clear lungs/ decreased pulmonary vessels. Cyanotic CHD : either increased pulmonary vessels or abnormal cardiac contour
	Determine the time of onset of cyanosis, presence of differential cyanosis (PDA with COA, PPHN, HLHS), presence of reverse differential cyanosis (upper limb O_2 sats. < those of lower limb) [as in TGA with COA + PDA], presence of acidosis and circulatory shock and perform hyperoxia test		
Shock	pulmonary hemorrhage, tension pneumothorax	IAA, coarctation, AS, HLHS, cardiomyopathy, pneumopericardium, pericardial tamponade, sepsis	Hematocrit of secretions from endotracheal tube : > 30% in pulmonary hemorrhage, <10% in pulmonary edema from cardiac dysfunction. Heart size is normal in pulmonary hemorrhage and increased in cardiac dysfunction and pericardial tamponade
Murmur	None	PDA, PPS, PS, AS, TR, VSD, MR, AVSD, coarctation	Location and radiation of murmur point to correct diagnosis
Multiple congenital anomalies	Choanal atresia, tracheoesophageal fistula, esophageal atresia (causing aspiration), tracheomalacia	Type of heart disease varies widely, depending on other anomalies/underlying syndrome, chromosomes	Failed passage of nasal tube to stomach is diagnosis of choanal atresia, esophageal atresia, and most types of tracheoesophageal fistula
Prematurity	RDS, pneumonia	PDA	Active precordium, murmur, left atrial enlargement on echo, color flow detected shunt in PDA visualization of ductal shunt
Asphyxia	ARDS	Ischemic cardiomyopathy with pulmonary edema	Cardiomegaly, left ventricular dysfunction, and elevated cardiac enzymes present in ischemic cardiomyopathy

RDS, respiratory distress syndrome ; ARDS, adult respiratory distress syndrome ; TTNB, transient tachypnea of the Newborn ; PPHNS, persistent pulmonary hypertension of the Newborn syndrome ; CHF, congestive heart failure ; CHD, congenital heart disease ; TGV, transposition of the great vessels ; TAPVD, total anomalous pulmonary venous drainage ; TA, Tricuspid atresia ; TOF, tetralogy of Fallot ; PA, pulmonary atresia ; PS, pulmonary stenosis ; IAA, interrupted aortic arch ; AS, aortic stenosis ; HLHS, hypoplastic left heart syndrome ; PDA, patent ductus arteriosus ; PPS, peripheral pulmonary stenosis ; TR, tricuspid regurgitation ; VSD, ventricular septal defect ; MR, mitral regurgitation ; AVSD, atrioventricular septal defect

Pearl/Peril/Pitfall: Assessment of color. Many babies with cyanotic heart disease will be obviously blue from birth but some can be quite subtle, particularly with common mixing situations or ductal dependent pulmonary circulations before ductal constriction. This is further confused by babies often having blue lips and extremities in the first day or two after birth. Looking at the tongue can be helpful in babies with blue lips but, if in doubt, put an oxygen saturation monitor on the baby's foot.

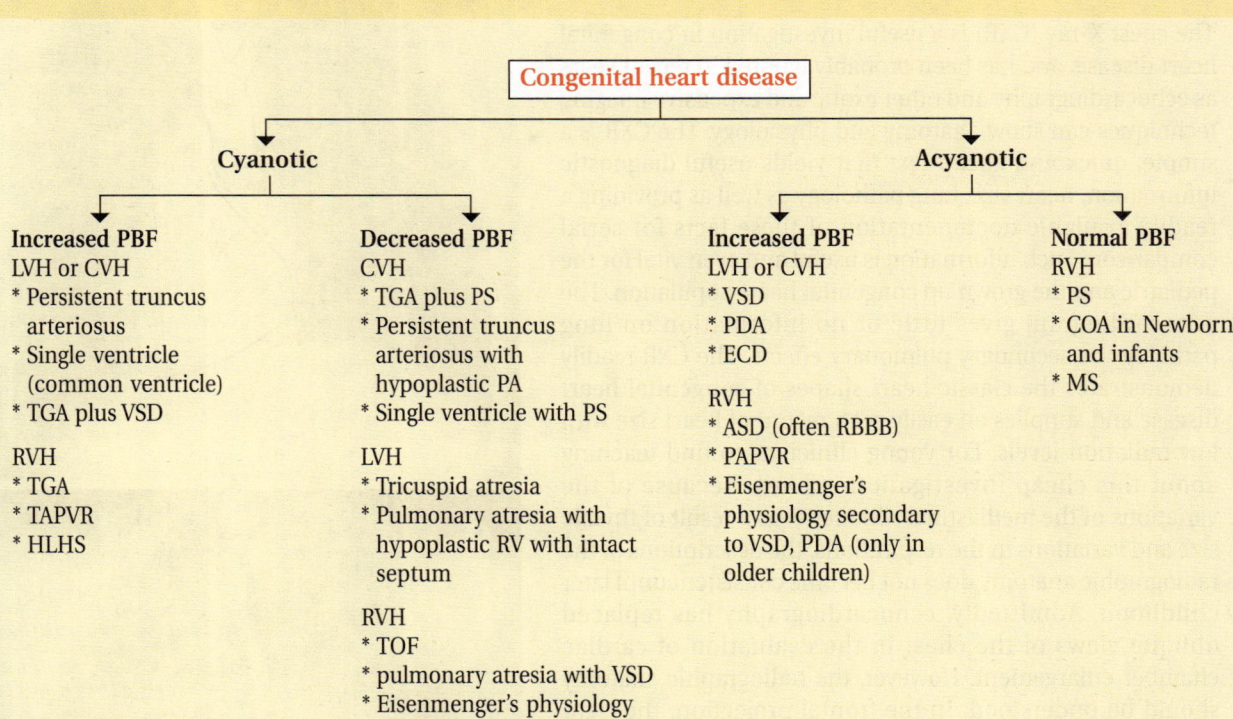

Fig. 1: Algorithm to arrive at a diagnosis of congenital heart disease

Congenital heart disease

Cyanotic

Increased PBF
LVH or CVH
* Persistent truncus arteriosus
* Single ventricle (common ventricle)
* TGA plus VSD

RVH
* TGA
* TAPVR
* HLHS

Decreased PBF
CVH
* TGA plus PS
* Persistent truncus arteriosus with hypoplastic PA
* Single ventricle with PS

LVH
* Tricuspid atresia
* Pulmonary atresia with hypoplastic RV with intact septum

RVH
* TOF
* pulmonary atresia with VSD
* Eisenmenger's physiology secondary to ASD, VSD, PDA (only in older children)

Acyanotic

Increased PBF
LVH or CVH
* VSD
* PDA
* ECD

RVH
* ASD (often RBBB)
* PAPVR
* Eisenmenger's physiology secondary to VSD, PDA (only in older children)

Normal PBF
RVH
* PS
* COA in Newborn and infants
* MS

* The above algorithm is based on the presence of absence of central cyanosis (documented by hyperoxia test to exclude pulmonary / CNS causes of cyanosis), and on the status of pulmonary blood flow (PBF) on chest X-ray whether normal, increased, or decreased. The presence of right ventricular hypertrophy (RVH) or left ventricular hypertrophy (LVH) or both further narrows the possibilities.

* It should be remembered that normal ECG and normal pulmonary vascular markings on chest x-ray films do not rule out congenital heart disease. In fact, many mild acyanotic heart defects don't show abnormalities on the ECG or chest X-ray films; diagnosis of these defects rests primarily on findings from the physical examination, particularly on auscultation.

* ECG findings are helpful in making the diagnosis (in addition to ventricular hypertrophy) occasionally E.g.. a) a superiorly oriented QRS axis [i.e. left anterior hemiblock] in an acyanotic infant suggests endocardial cushion defect [ECD], where as in a cyanotic infant it suggests tricuspid atresia b) supraventricular tachycardia or congenital heart block.

* ECG Criteria for right ventricular hypertrophy in the Newborn - 1) S waves in lead 1, ≥ 12mm 2) R waves in aVR, ≥ 8mm 3)Important abnormalities in VI such as : a) Pure R waves (without S) in VI, ≥10mm b) R waves VI, ≥ 25mm c) qR pattern in VI (also seen in 10% of normal newborns) d) Upright T waves in VI in newborns more than 3 days of age (with upright T in V6) 4) QRS axis greater than + 180 degrees

* ECG criteria for left ventricular hypertrophy - 1) LAD for the patient's age 2) QRS voltage in favor of the LV (in the presence of normal QRS duration) a) R in I, II, III, aVL, aVF, V5, or V6 greater than the upper limits of the normal for age b) S in VI or V2 greater than upper limits of normal age 3) Abnormal R/S ratio in favor of the LV : R/S ratio in VI and V2 less than the lower limits of normal for the patient age 4) Q in V5 and V6, 5mm or more, as well as tall symmetric T waves in the same leads ("LV diastolic overload") 5) In the presence of LVH, a wide QRS-T angle with the T axis outside the normal range indicates "strain" pattern ; this is manifested by inverted T waves in lead I or aVF.

CHD, congenital heart defect; *PBF,* pulmonary blood flow; LVH, left ventricular hypertrophy ; CVH, combined ventricular hypertrophy ; VSD, ventricular septal defect ; PDA, patent ductus arteriosus ; ECD, endocardial cushion defect ; RVH right ventricular hypertrophy ; ASD, atrial septal defect ; RBBB, right bundle branch block ; PAPVR, partial anomalous pulmonary venous return ; AS, aortic stenosis ; AR, aortic regurgitation ; COA, coarctation of the aorta ; MR, mitral regurgitation ; PS, Pulmonary stenosis ; MS, mitral stenosis ; TGA, transposition of the great arteries ; TAPVR, total anomalous pulmonary venous return ; HLHS, hypoplastic left heart syndrome ; PA, Pulmonary artery ; RV, right ventricle ; TOF, tetralogy of fallot.

Pearl/Peril/Pitfall: Assessment of peripheral pulses. In post-ductal coarctation or preductal coarctation with a constricting duct, weak femoral pulses may be the only clinical pointer. Unfortunately in the latter condition, while the duct is still patent, the femorals may be easily palpable. Feeling the femorals can be difficult in a vigorous baby. One useful technique is to hold the leg in your hand and run your thumb up the medial border of the quadriceps muscle, your thumb will usually fall on the femoral pulse while your hand can limit the leg movement.

The Normal Chest Radiograph

The chest X-ray (CXR) is a useful investigation in congenital heart disease, and has been probably ignored in recent years as echocardiography and other exotic and expensive imaging techniques can show anatomy and physiology. The CXR is a simple, quick and cheap test that yields useful diagnostic information, heart size, lung pathology as well as providing a readily available documentation of these facts for serial comparison. Such information is useful and even vital for the pediatric and the grown up congenital heart population. The echocardiogram gives little or no information on lung pathology or secondary pulmonary effects. The CXR readily demonstrates the classic heart shapes of congenital heart disease and supplies an easily seen record of heart size with low radiation levels. For young clinicians to find teaching about this cheap investigation is hard. Because of the variations of the mediastinal silhouette, as a result of thymic size and variations in the respirations, the descriptions of the radiographic anatomy does not become consistent until later childhood. Admittedly, echocardiography has replaced oblique views of the chest in the evaluation of cardiac chamber enlargement. However, the radiographic anatomy should be understood. In the frontal projection, the right cardiac border is the right atrium and the left cardiac border is normally the outflow tract of the left ventricle. Above the left ventricular convexity, there is a normal prominence of the undivided portion of the pulmonary artery. The convexity above this is the aortic arch which displaces the trachea slightly to the right. In spite of anatomic textbooks, the left atrial appendage rarely contributes to the left heart silhouette. In the right anterior oblique view, the anterior chamber is the right ventricle, and the convexity above it is the pulmonary artery; posteriorly, the inferior shadow is the right atrium, and above it lies the left atrium. Enlargement of the left atrium will displace the esophagus (outlined with contrast material) to the right and posteriorly. Also, a normal left aortic arch will produce indentation of the anterior border of the esophagus. The main advantage of this view is demonstration of left atrial enlargement. In the left anterior oblique view, the anterior chamber is the right ventricle, and the posterior chamber is the inflow tract of the left ventricle. Increased convexity of the anterior cardiac chamber suggests right ventricular dilation. If the esophagus contains contrast media, a right aortic arch indenting the esophagus can be identified. The main advantage of this view is to evaluate right and left ventricular dilation. In the lateral view, the right ventricle constitutes the lower half to two-thirds of the anterior cardiac border, and lies behind the sternum. The upper third constitutes the right ventricular outflow tract and the main pulmonary artery. The upper half of the posterior cardiac border consists of the left atrium and the lower half is the left ventricle.

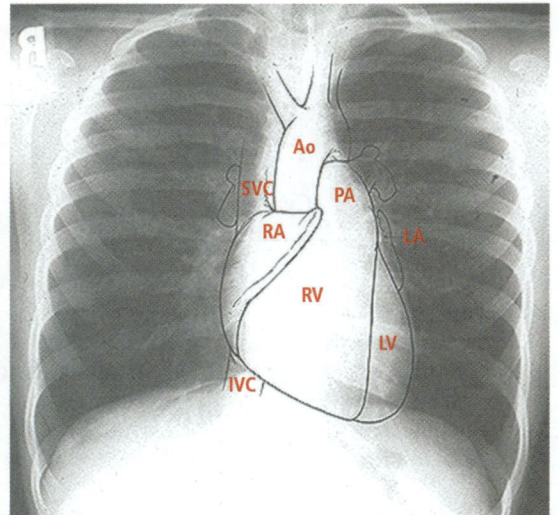

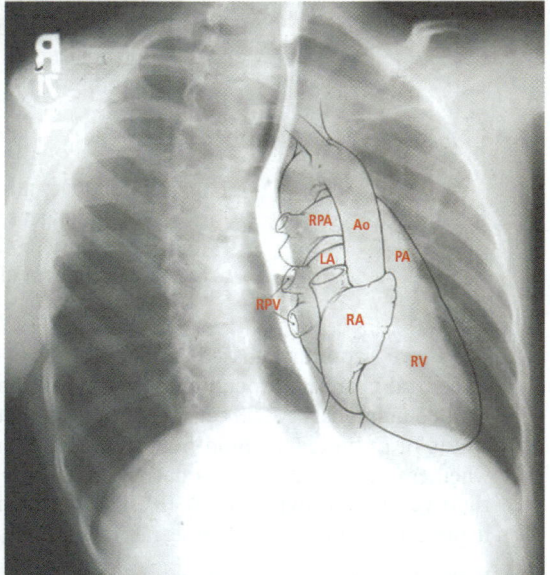

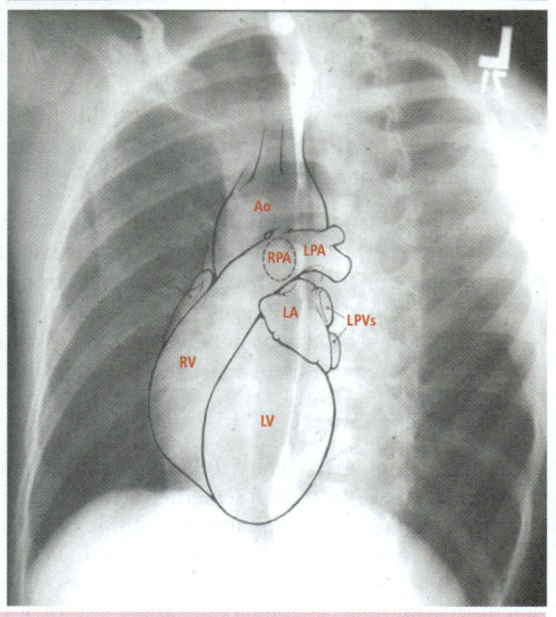

Pearl/Peril/Pitfall: Shock /cardiovascular collapse. This is the classic presentation of the ductal dependent obstructive left ventricle conditions (hypoplastic left heart, critical aortic stenosis and coarctation). In these conditions, the only way blood can reach the systemic circulation is via the ductus. They are often asymptomatic while the duct is patent and then collapse any time during the first week when it closes. They present pale and shocked with respiratory distress and weak pulses. The liver is invariably very large. They can be mistaken for a septic picture. Diagnosis is with echocardiography. Treatment depends on re-opening the duct with prostaglandin E2.

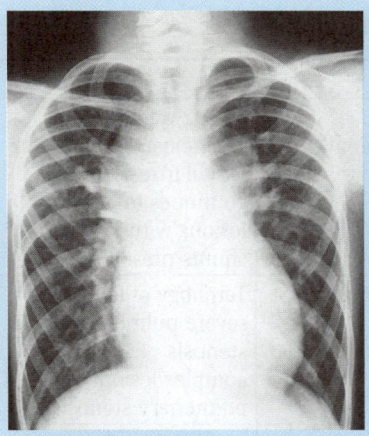

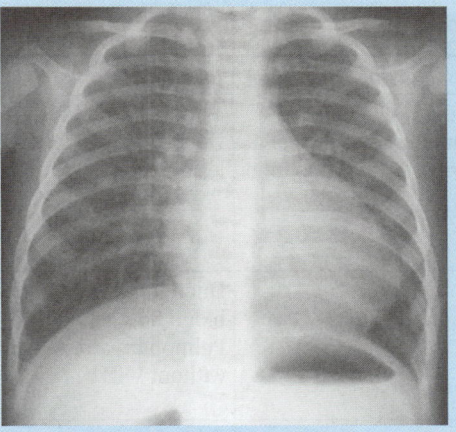

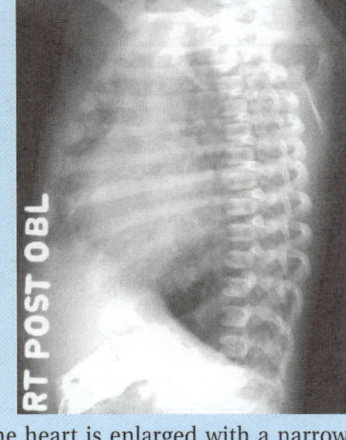

A classic picture of the 'snowman' or 'cottage loaf' heart shape due to **total anomalous pulmonary venous drainage into a left superior vena cava (SVC).** The confluence of pulmonary veins joins behind the heart and enters the ascending limb of the left SVC which appears as a dilated vessel on the right of the upper mediastinal edge. This large venous flow enters the transverse crossing vein or innominate vein making the convex roof of the cottage loaf, and joins the right SVC causing dilatation of the left side of mediastinum. As one looks at this film, there is, beneath these venous shadows, the lower part of the cottage loaf made up of dilated right atrium and ventricular mass which is the right ventricle. There is considerable increase in the size of pulmonary vessel arteries and veins (pulmonary plethora). This is due to increased pulmonary blood flow shown throughout the lungs.

Transposition of the Great Arteries (D-TGA) The heart is enlarged with a narrow "pedicle" giving the so called "egg on a string" appearance. The superior mediastinum appears narrow due to the antero-posterior relationship of the transposed great vessels and "radiologic-absence of the thymus". The stress of hypoxia in the newborn period is believed responsible for thymic regression. Right posterior oblique view demonstrates widening of structures in the superior mediastinum due to the anteroposterior relationship of the aorta and pulmonary artery.

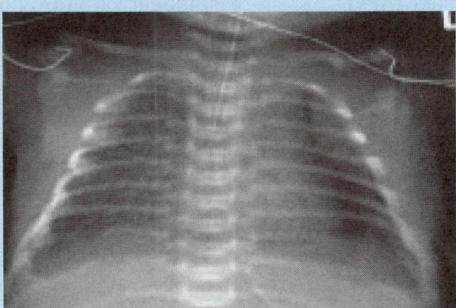

Chest radiograph of a hypoxic infant referred on the first day of life for extracorporeal membrane oxygenation support with a presumed diagnosis of persistent pulmonary hypertension secondary to meconium aspiration. Cardiac echocardiography showed an obstructed **infradiaphragmatic total anomalous pulmonary venous connection**

Hypoplastic left heart syndrome. There is marked cardiomegaly with passive venous congestion. The endotracheal tube, nasogastric tube and umbilical arterial line are in appropriate position.

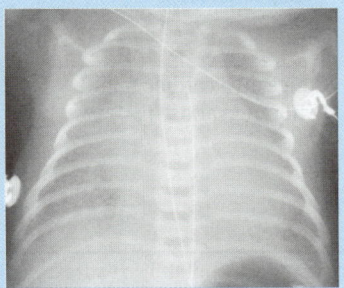

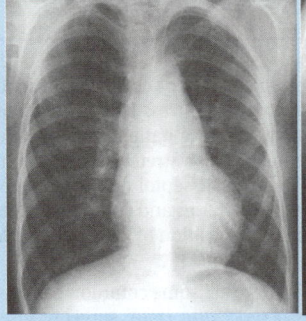 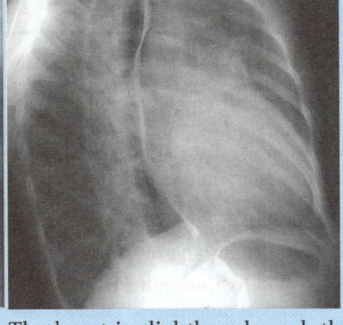

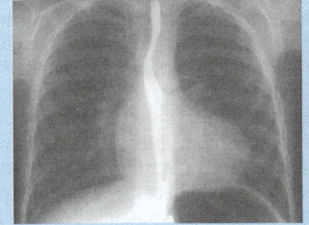 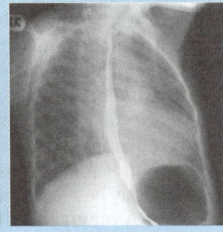

Patent ductus arteriosus: A. The heart is slightly enlarged, the main pulmonary artery convex, and the aortic arch prominent above the MPA. There are increased pulmonary vascular markings. B. Right anterior oblique view demonstrates the esophagus to be indented by a large left aortic arch in addition to posterior displacement by the dilated left atrium.

Tetralogy of fallot A. PA chest radiograph shows normal heart size which is "boot-shaped" (from coeur-en-sabot, literally translated *boot shaped*). There are diminished pulmonary vascular markings and a prominent left sided aortic arch (indentation in left of trachea). B. Right anterior oblique views shows upturned apex and decreased pulmonary vascular markings

Pearl/Peril/Pitfall : Echocardiography. This is the definitive test and in situations where there is early access to these skills, most of the other investigations become superfluous. Early echocardiography to exclude CHD should be arranged in the following situations. Any baby with signs suggestive of CHD . Any baby with a persisting murmur on newborn examination. Any baby with severe hypoxic respiratory failure. Any baby with Down syndrome. Any baby with malformations that might be associated with CHD.

TABLE 2 — Typical timing and mode of presentation of congenital heart disease in the neonate

	Early	Intermediate	Late
	0–24 hours High pulmonary vascular resistance, arterial duct open	4 hours - 2weeks Duct closing - 'duct dependent' lesions present	After 2 weeks Duct closed.pulmonary vascular resistance continues to fall and lesions with left-to-right shunts present
Cyanosis (without congestive failure or respiratory distress)	TGA	Duct dependent for pulmonary blood flow, e.g. Pulmonary atresia with or without VSD	Tetralogy of fallot with severe pulmonary stenosis complex lesions with pulmonary stenosis
		Critical pulmonary stenosis (with right-to-left interatrial flow), Tricuspid atresia with small VSD, Complex lesions with severe pulmonary stenosis Duct dependent for mixing, TGA (simple and complex)	
Cyanosis with congestive failure or respiratory distress	Obstructed TAPVD (usually infradiaphragmatic) Severe Ebstein's anomaly	Pulmonary arteriovenous fistula (rare) partially obstructed TAPVD	Mixed circulations with unobstructed pulmonary blood flow, e.g. Unobstructed TAPVD (cardiac or supracardiac), common atrerial trunk, Tricuspid atresia with a large VSD. Some complex lesions with high pulmonary blood flow.*
Collapse/shock		Left heart obstuction, e.g., Aortic coarctation or interruption, HLHS, Aortic stenosis	
Congestive cardiac failure (without cyanosis)		Left heart obstruction with a left-to-right shunt, e.g. Aortic coarctation ± VSD Systemic arteriovenous fistulae, e.g. cerebral	Left-to-right shunts, e.g. Large VSD, complete AV septal defect, PDA, aortopulmonary window Complex lesions

Types of congenital heart surgery : The repair of congenital heart disease has three major goals. Most ideal is total *correction* of the given disorder. This results in the heart being anatomically normal in the sequence of blood flow. Obviously, it is not possible to reestablish such a normal sequence of chambers and valves for many forms of complex congenital heart disease, and *partial correction* may be the only achievable goal. The third major intent of surgery is *palliation*. Palliative surgery does not correct the problem, but rather minimizes the problems that result from any given disorder. In some instances, palliation may be elected until the child becomes a candidate for total correction. A variety of different shunts are possible between the aorta and the pulmonary arteries to supply ample blood to the lungs for oxygenation. Although there is a strong tendency in many institutions to totally correct this problem in infancy, there are some situations where early total correction is not possible and palliative procedures must be performed.

Reparative Congenital Heart Surgery: Pediatric Cardiothoracic Surgeons perform many types of reparative heart surgery. Some of the more common procedures include : · Repairing or closing ventricular or atrial septal defects and atrioventricular valves. This is done with stitches or a patch (artificial or made from the patient's own tissue). More about atrial and ventricular septal defects · Stretching or widening the pulmonic valve and closing a ventricular septal defect to correct Tetralogy of the Fallot · Moving the great arteries and coronary arteries back to their normal position to cure transposition of the great arteries · Widening a narrow aorta to treat coarctation

Palliative Congenital Heart Surgery : Here are some common palliative surgical procedures: · Blalock-Taussig procedure. Here, surgeons insert a tube to connect the aorta to the pulmonary artery to increase the flow of blood to the lungs. · Fontan procedure. This procedure helps patients with a single ventricle by allowing deoxygenated blood flow into the lungs and avoiding the heart. The one heart ventricle then pumps oxygenated blood. · Pulmonary artery band. A band is placed around the pulmonary artery in order to restrict the flow of blood to the lungs.

*Pearl/Peril/Pitfall: At a practical level, differentiating between an innocent and significant murmur can be difficult and the Various data would suggest all newborn babies with murmurs should be investigated. However the following clinical pointers suggest that a murmur may be significant:·Other abnormal cardiac signs as detailed above. *Loudness and radiation. If a murmur is easy to hear and particularly if it radiates to other areas, then it will often be significant. If you're struggling to hear it in one area then it's more likely to be a transitional innocent murmur. *Persistence. Transitional murmurs are just that and often go away, even within the space of a day. If a murmur persists, it should be investigated however soft it is. *Abnormal heart sounds. Likewise if the heart sounds aren't normal, a murmur should always be investigated. The commonest abnormal heart sound in CHD is a loud S2.*

TABLE 3   **Common surgical procedures in surgery for congenital heart disease**

Procedure	Description	Intent	Result
Blalock-Hanlen*	Surgical removal of the atrial septum	PAL	Increases mixing of blood
Blalock-Taussig	Subclavian artery to PA anastamosis	PAL	Increase PULM flow
Brock's*	Closed PVotomy and infundibulectomy	PAL	Increase PULM flow
Central Shunt	Conduit or anastamosis	PAL	Increase PULM flow
Damus-Kaye -Stansel	PA end to side anastamosis to AO, valved conduit between RV-MPA	COR	Increase flow to AO and PA when there is AO stenosis and two VENT. Reestablishes RV to PA continuity
Fontan	Anastamosis or conduit between RA and PA	PC	Increase PULM flow in cases of univentricular morphology or TA
Glenn's	SVC to PA anastamosis	PAL	Increase PULM flow
Great Arterial Switch	AO and PA moved to proper ventricles, coronaries reimplanted	COR	Creates normal relationship between the VENT and GA
Konno	Replacement of AV with AV annular	COR	Alleviates sub-AO obstruction and replaces abnormal AV
Mustard's	Atrial switch using intra-atrial baffle made of pericardium	COR	Reestablishes proper flow sequence to PA and AO in TGA
Norwood	PA anastamosis to AO, conduit from AO to MPA	PAL	Increase flow to AO for sub AO obstruction and only one VENT
Park	Atrial septostomy with catheter blade	PAL to TGA	Increases mixing of blood
Patch	Closes an opening or surgical incision	COR	Closes a shunt
PDA Ligation	Ties off PDA	COR	Closes a shunt
Potts-Smith-Gibson*	Descend AO to PA shunt	PAL	Increases PULM flow
PA Band	Constrictive band around MPA	PAL	Decreases PULM flow
Rashkind	Atrial septostomy with catheter balloon	PAL	Increases mixing of blood for TGA or TA
Rastelli's	Valved conduit from RV to PA, VSD closure	COR	Increase PULM flow, may reestablish proper sequence of flow to AO and PA
Senning	Atrial switch using intra-atrial babble made of atrial wall flaps	COR	Reestablishes proper flow sequence to PA and AO in TGA
Valvectomy	PV excision	PAL	Relieve PV obstruction
Valvotomy	Surgical opening of obstructed valve	COR	Open obstructed valve
Valve replacement	Replaces any valve	COR	Relieve obstruction or regurgitation
Valvuloplasty	Repair of any valve	COR	Relieve regurgitation
Waterston*	Ascending AO to RPA	PAL	Increase PULM flow

Pearl/Peril/Pitfall: CHD is only one of several conditions that can present with cyanosis. The differential should include: *Respiratory problems. *Apnea *Seizures *Methemoglobinemia (very rare but always remembered) While babies with cyanotic heart disease may present blue at birth, in many it is less obvious. The oxygen saturation has to be below 80% before cyanosis becomes clinically obvious. In some cyanotic conditions, the resting saturations will be in the 80's and so will not be obvious. Conditions that do this include anything where there is common mixing (transposition with VSD, unobstructed TAPVD, single ventricles) or ductal dependent conditions while the duct is patent (tricuspid or pulmonary atresia). Ductal dependent lesions eventually present with rapidly progressive cyanosis as the duct closes but the mixing situations may take some time to present. If there is any doubt about a baby, put a saturation monitor on the foot. If it is persistently less than 90%, further investigations should be initiated.

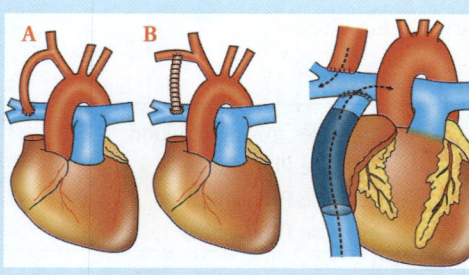

Blalock-Taussig operation **Fontan operation**

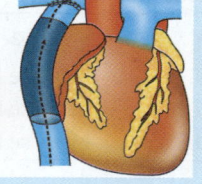

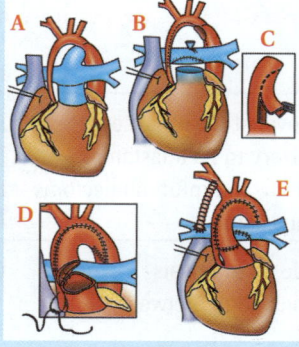

Norwood operation

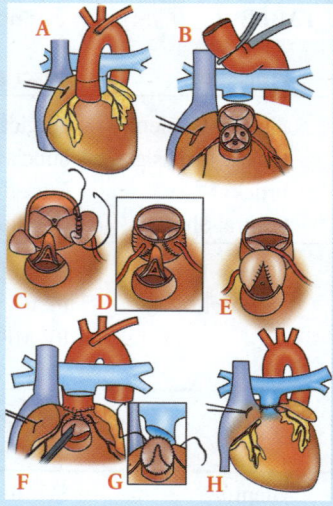

Jatene operation for TGA

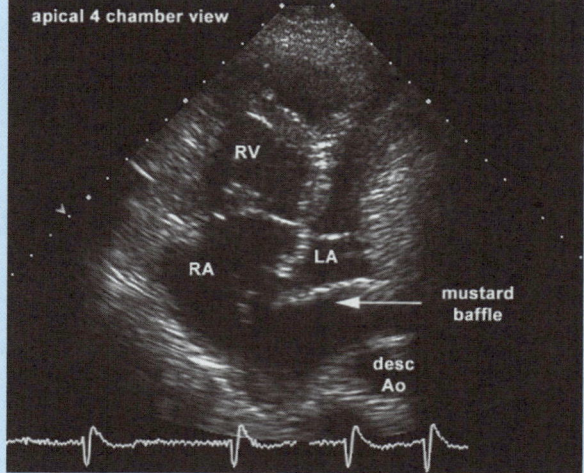

The Mustard procedure as applied to patients with d-transposition of the great arteries employs a baffle to direct oxygenated pulmonary venous return into the right atrium and thence into the right ventricle which is the pumping ventricle for the aorta and the systemic circulation.

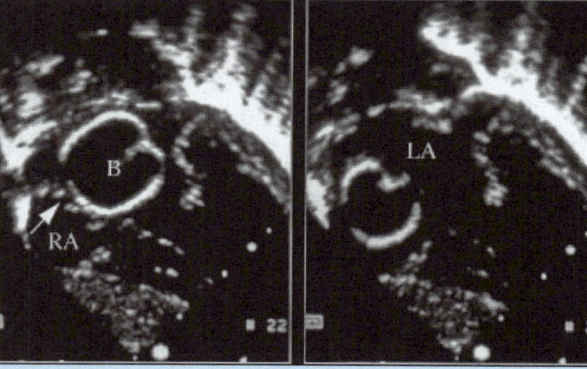

Balloon atrial septostomy in a neonate with transposition of the great arteries. The septostomy catheter has been inserted into the umbilical vein, and has been passed from the right atrium (RA) across the foramen ovale (arrow). After inflation of the balloon (B) in the left atrium (LA), the catheter is pulled back across the atrial septum, thus enlarging the interatrial communication.

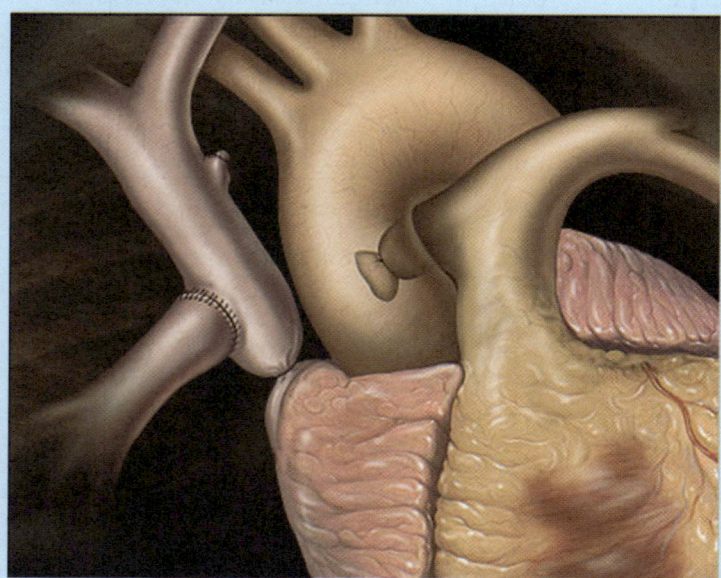

Since the late 1950's the **Glenn shunt**, as the SVC-to-right pulmonary artery anastomosis is called, has been performed on patients with diverse cyanotic congenital heart disease to improve pulmonary blood flow.

The Glenn shunt does not create volume overload of the ventricle or increased work for the ventricle, as is the case in systemic-pulmonary artery shunts. It provides venous flow to the lung fields for oxygenation, rather than an arteriovenous mixture. The venous return is under relatively low pressure, unlike systemic-pulmonary artery shunts, and the risk for pulmonary artery distortion and late pulmonary vascular obstructive disease is substantially less.

The Glenn shunt is palliative—not corrective. Depending on the diagnosis and the surgical era, the Glenn shunt may be the only palliation for the cyanotic patient, one of several palliative surgeries, or a step prior to corrective surgery or the Fontan form of total right heart bypass.

TABLE 4 — Causes and clinical findings of central cyanosis

Central nervous system depression

Causes
- perinatal asphyxia
- Heavy maternal sedation
- Intrauterine fetal distress

Findings
- Shallow irregular respiration
- poor muscle tone
- Cyanosis that disappears when stimulated or oxygen is given to the patient

Pulmonary disease

Causes
- Parenchymal lung disease (e.g., hyaline membrane disease, atelectasis)
- Pneumothorax or pleural effusion
- Diaphragmatic hernia
- PPHN (or persistent fetal circulation syndrome)

Findings
- Tachypnea and respiratory distress with retraction and expiratory grunting
- Rales and/or decreased breath sounds on auscultation
- Chest x-ray film that may reveal causes (as listed previously)
- Oxygen administration that improves or abolishes cyanosis

Cardiac disease

Causes
- Cyanotic CHD with right-to-left- shunt

Findings
- Tachypnea but usually without retraction
- Lack of rales or abnormal breath sounds unless CHF supervenes
- Heart murmur that may be absent in serious forms of cyanotic CHD
- A continuous murmur (of PDA) that may indicate restricted PBF through the ductus, Chest X-ray films that may show cardiomegaly, abnormal cardiac silhouette, increased or decreased PVMs
- Little or no increase in PO_2 with oxygen administration

TABLE 5 — Causes of heart failure in the newborn

Congestive heart failure is a syndrome that results from the inability of the heart to provide adequate support for the metabolic requirements of the body. Symptoms are related to the failing heart and venous congestion. These include tachycardia, hepatomegaly, JVD. However, extracardiac symptoms may sometimes be the primary manifestation of CHF, and these include tachypnea, wheezing, poor feeding, and failure to thrive.

oxygen delivery (DO_2) = cardiac output (CO) x arterial O_2 content (CaO_2)

cardiac output = stroke volume × heart rate

components of stroke volume = preload, cardiac contractility and afterload

In early CHF, cardiac contractility and other compensatory mechanisms maintain adequate cardiac output. When these compensatory mechanisms are exhausted, cardiogenic shock becomes manifest.

Structural heart Failure in the Newborn

At birth
- HLHS
- Severe TR or PR
- Large systemic AV fistula

First week
- TGA
- Premature infants with large PDA (Now earlier with surfactant therapy)
- TAPVR below diaphragm

1 to 4 weeks
- Critical AS or PS
- COA

Noncardiac causes
- Birth asphyxia resulting in transient myocardial ischemia
- Metabolic : hypoglycemia, hypocalcemia
- Severe anemia (as seen in hydrops fetalis)
- Overtransfusion or overhydration
- Neonatal sepsis, congenital adrenal hyperplasia

Primary myocardial disease
- Myocarditis
- Transient myocardial ischemia (with or without birth asphyxia)
- Cardiomyopathy (seen in infant of diabetic mother)

Disturbances in heart rate
- SVT
- Atrial flutter/fibrillation
- Congenital heart block (when associated with CHD)

TABLE 6 — Indications for referral of newborns and infants to a pediatric cardiologist

1. **Cyanosis**
   a. >2 hours after birth (assumes normal temperature and BP)
   b. O_2 sat. consistently <90% in 100% FiO_2

2. **Congestive heart failure**
   a. Heart rate >160bpm at rest
   b. Respiratory rate >60bpm at rest
   c. +/- murmur
   d. +/- cardiomegaly on CXR

3. **Shock**
   a. Hypotension
   b. delayed CRT
   c. +/- acidosis (sepsis has been ruled out)

4. **Symptomatic arrhythmias**
   a. Heart rate persistently >200bpm
   b. Heart rate persistently-<80bpm in a newborn and<60bpm in an infant

5. **Syndrome/Dysmorphism**
   a. Down syndrome
   b. VACTERAL anomalod
   c. Infant of a diabetic mother
   d. CATCH 22

Pearl/Peril/Pitfall: Major CHD can manifest as severe respiratory distress with high oxygen requirements and can closely mimic primary respiratory disease and or PPHN. Skinner reported a series of 34 such babies referred for assessment of PPHN of whom one had CHD. Obstructed total anomalous pulmonary venous drainage is the classic condition that does this. In this condition, the pulmonary veins drain to systemic veins or the right atrium. If this drainage is obstructed, pulmonary venous congestion and oedema results in a respiratory clinical presentation. This condition is also one of the easiest to miss on echocardiography because the intracardiac anatomy is often normal. Transposition of the great arteries and coarctation of the aorta are the other conditions that can present this way.

THE EVALUATION-DECISION-ACTION- PLAN/ALGORITHM FOR THE DIAGNOSIS AND MANAGEMENT OF *A NEONATE WITH AN ASYMPTOMATIC HEART MURMUR*

*Heart murmurs in the Newborn may be *a)*Innocent (functional, physiologic, benign) or *b)*Pathologic. * >50% of term infants and 2/3rds of preterms were found to have an Innocent heart murmur at some time during 1st week of life. *It is important to note that Innocent heart murmurs have positive characteristics as well as being associated with no other clinical evidence of cardiovascular disease. *4 common Innocent murmurs in the Newborn period are: 1) Pulmonary flow murmur of the Newborn; 2) Transient systolic murmur of PDA; 3) Transient systolic murmur of Tricuspid regurgitation (without structural heart disease); 4) Vibratory innocent murmur (counterpart of Still`s murmur in older children). * Many serious cardiac conditions have unimpressive or even no murmurs(e.g., severe cyanotic heart defect, such as TGA or Pulmonary atresia with a closing PDA). Infants who are in severe CHF may not have a loud murmur until the myocardial function is improved through anticongestive measures. Therefore, other auscultatory and general cardiovascular signs are very important in assessing the significance of a heart murmur. *Most pathological heart murmurs should be audible during 1st month of life, with the exception of an ASD; heart murmurs of stenotic/obstructive lesions (e.g., AS, PS, COA) are audible immediately after birth and persist, because these murmurs are not affected by the level of pulmonary vascular resistance. Lesions associated with left-to right shunts frequently cause no murmur in the immediate newborn period(due to high PVR in the1st week of life) and may not be detected until a 6–8 week routine check, when the PVR falls significantly. For example, a heart murmur of a small VSD becomes audible shortly after birth, whereas that of a large VSD may not become audible until the PVR falls significantly. The continuous murmur of a large PDA may not appear for 2–3 weeks. Instead, it is a crescendo systolic murmur with slight or no diastolic component;best audible at the left infraclavicular area. A Newborn with a large ASD may not have a heart murmur;it appears late in infancy with insidious onset and becomes loud after a year or two, when the distensibility of the RV becomes maximal. *If a structural abnormality is suspected as the cause of an asymptomatic heart murmur(because of certain clinical features given below), an ECG and CXR should be performed. These investigations may have diagnostic features and are of some help in deciding the severity of the lesion and therefore timescale in which cardiology review and Echocardiography are indicated.

Determine the innocent nature of the heart murmur!

1.Pulmonary flow murmur of the Newborn *the most common heart murmur in the Newborn infant and more common in premature and small for dates than in fullterm infants. *heard best at the ULSB and transmits well to both sides of the chest, axillae, and the back. *it is soft, usually not louder than a grade 2/6 in intensity. *ECG and CXR are normal *it is not transient, usually lasting for weeks or up to 6 months.

2.Transient systolic murmur of PDA *audible at the ULSB and in the left infraclavicular area on the 1st day *usually disappears shortly thereafter. *it is usually only systolic and crescendic up to the S2 and with a grade 2/6 in intensity.* it is believed to originate from a closing ductus arteriosus, but no definite evidence that it can be heard whilst closing normally.

3.Transient systolic murmur of Tricuspid Regurgitation *sounds like a VSD murmur and maximally heard at the LLSB *it disappears in a day or two as the PVR falls *more common in infants who had perinatal stress or Neonatal asphyxia, because they tend to maintain high PVR for a longer period.

4.Vibratory innocent murmur *a counterpart of Still`s murmur in older children, best audible at the LLSB or near the apex and has a low frequency, vibratory quality *ejection systolic in timing unlike a regurgitant VSD murmur *rarely heard in Newborn period and lasts for years.

Determine the pathologic nature of the heart murmur!

Look for clinical features suggestive of a Pathologic murmur

*no weight loss after birth/excessive weight gain, especially if feeding poorly (may suggest incipient heart failure) *any suggestion of symptoms- if dusky, a transcutaneous hyperoxia test may help *any doubt about quality of femoral pulses suggests Coarctation Of Aorta *right arm systolic BP> 20 mm Hg above leg pressure (4 limb BP measurement) suggests Coarctation Of Aorta *murmur loudest between scapulae suggests COA, innocent pulmonary murmur well heard front and sides as well. *louder in intensity (grade 3/6 or more), longer in duration, a diastolic component and less variable with time and heart rate*cardiomegaly on CXR and ventricular hypertrophy on ECG * a neonate with cardiac symptoms and associated dysmorphic features or congenital anomalies of other organ systems.

Management of neonate with an asymptomatic heart murmur

*If no symptoms or other signs of cardiac disease are present(normal ECG and CXR) and the murmur has features compatible with an innocent one, discharge from hospital, but the family should be warned about important signs and follow-up arranged for 4-6 weeks time .*A baby with an asymptomatic heart murmur should not be allowed home until it is clear that no form of duct-dependent CHD is present; this is usually apparent on clinical grounds. If there is any doubt, either a further period of observation in hospital is indicated or, preferably, echocardiography should be arranged.*If symptoms or other signs of cardiac disease exist or if no signs/symptoms are present but the murmur has features suggesting a structural lesion, an ECG and CXR should be performed and cardiology referral made for a detailed Echocardiography. The echocardiogram is essential for anatomical diagnosis and also to plan subsequent therapy and follow-up.

TABLE 7	Common congenital heart lesions
Cyanotic	**Acyanotic**
Decreased pulmonary blood flow	Atrial septal defect
Pulmonary atresia	Ventricular septal defect
Tricuspid atresia	Patent ductus arteriosus
Tetralogy of Fallot	Left-sided obstructive lesions
Transposition of the great vessels	Coarctation of the aorta
	Aortic stenosis (atresia)
Increased pulmonary blood flow	Mitral stenosis (atresia)
	Hypoplastic left heart syndrome (HLHS)
Total anomalous pulmonary venous return	

TABLE 8	Differential diagnosis of sick newborn infants : Pulmonary vascularity	
Normal vascularity	**Decreased vascularity**	**Increased vascularity**
Lung diseases	Idiopathic PPHNS	Cyanotic CHD (ITAPVD, truncus arteriosus, tricuspid atresia)
Systemic diseases	Tetralogy of Fallot	CHF (HLHS, critical aortic stenosis, critical coarctation interrupted aortic arch
Incidental CHD	Pulmonary atresia	Shunts (PDA, VSD, AVSD, AVM)

PPHNS, persistent pulmonary hypertension of the newborn syndrome ; CHD, congenital heart disease ; ITAPVD, infradiaphragmatic total anomalous pulmonary venous drainage ; CHF, congestive heart failure ; HLHS, hypoplastic left heart syndrome ; PDA, patent ductus arteriosus ; VSD, ventricular septal defect ; AVSD, atrioventricular septal defect ; AVM, arteriovenous malformation

TABLE 9	Work of breathing and congenital heart disease
Normal work of Breathing	**Increased work of Breathing**
Cyanotic CHD with decreased pulmonary blood flow : pulmonary atresia, PS, Tricuspid atresia (+small VSD/or PS) Cyanotic CHD with inadequate mixing : TGV	Cyanotic CHD with increased pulmonary blood flow : TAPVD, truncus arteriosus, tricuspid atresia (+large VSD, no PS) Shunts : PDA, VSD, AVSD, AVM, pulmonary venous congestion : HLHS, asphyxia, hypoglycemia, EFE, cardiomyopathy

CHD, congenital heart disease ; VSD, ventricular septal defect; PS, pulmonary stenosis ; TGV, transposition of the great vessels; TAPVD, total anomalous pulmonary venous drainage ; PDA patent ductus arteriosus ; AVSD, atrioventricular septal defect; HLHS, hypoplastic left heart syndrome ; EFE, endocardial fibroelastosis ; AVM, arteriovenous malformation.

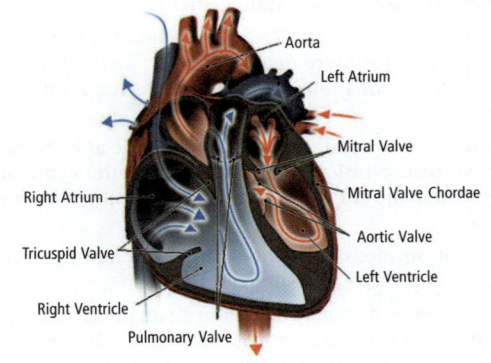

Aorta
Left Atrium
Mitral Valve
Mitral Valve Chordae
Right Atrium
Aortic Valve
Tricuspid Valve
Left Ventricle
Right Ventricle
Pulmonary Valve

Heart and Valves

TABLE 10	Differential diagnosis from heart position, size, and shape in symptomatic newborn infants			
Position	**Size**	**Contour/shape**	**Pulmonary artery**	**Diagnosis**
Normal	Normal	Normal	Normal	Lung/systemic disease
Normal	Normal	Snowman/Figure of 8	Normal	Supracardiac TAPVD
Normal	Normal	Egg on side	Not seen	TGV
Normal	Normal	Boot-shaped	Not seen	Pulmonary atresia, TOF, tricuspid atresia
Normal	Increased	Right atrial enlargement	Normal	Critical pulmonary stenosis/Ebstein anomaly, ASD, AVSD
Normal	Decreased	Normal	Normal	ITAPVD
Right chest	Any	Any	Any	Complex CHD

TAPVD, total anomalous pulmonary venous drainage ; TGV, transposition of the great vessels ; TOF, tetralogy of Fallot ; IAA, interrupted aortic arch ; EFE, endocardial fibroelastosis ; VSD, ventricular septal defect ; PDA, patent ductus arteriosus ; ITAPVD infradiaphragmatic total anomalous pulmonary venous drainage, CHD, congenital heart disease ; ASD, atrial septal defect ; AVSD atrioventricular septal defect.

Pearl/Peril/Pitfall: Temmerman et al found that a CXR helped in the diagnosis of heart disease in only 7% of cases. In babies with Downs syndrome, CXR had a sensitivity of 44% but specificity of 98% for CHD while ECG had a sensitivity of 41% and specificity of 100%. So if either of these tests are abnormal, they help, but if they're normal it doesn't exclude heart disease.

Antenatally diagnosed major congenital heart disease management at delivery and in NICU

The major cardiac lesions diagnosed antenatally can be generally divided into three groups:

* Duct-dependent for systemic blood flow (e.g. Hypoplastic Left Heart Syndrome, critical aortic stenosis, interrupted aortic arch).

* Duct-dependent cyanotic lesions (e.g. pulmonary atresia, transposition of the great arteries)

* Rhythm disturbances (e.g. congenital heart block, fetal supraventricular tachycardia

Management in Labor

* A copy of the fetal echocardiography report(s), and Fetal Medicine Panel report if applicable, should be obtained so accurate information is available.

* The obstetric service should notify the Level 3 neonatal registrar that delivery is anticipated. The registrar should inform the neonatal unit clinical charge nurse and the neonatal specialist on duty or on call.

* The paediatric cardiologist on call should be informed during normal working hours if the mother is in labor or is going to be induced or electively delivered by caesarean section.

* The paediatric cardiologist has usually already met with the parents to explain what is planned post-delivery.

Immediate Delivery Room Management

* Most infants with major congenital heart disease will not require additional resuscitation at birth and will be asymptomatic of their cardiac disease for hours or days postnatally.

* **An infant who is cyanosed and bradycardic at birth requires effective resuscitation, and the cause of the cyanosis and bradycardia should be assumed to be respiratory and not cardiac.**

* Resuscitation measures may include the administration of oxygen and positive pressure ventilation.

* Cardiac lesions that are responsible for an infant being in poor condition at birth are rare (e.g. severe Ebstein's anomaly, or other cardiac conditions such as arrhythmia, particularly if accompanied by *fetal hydrops.

* Following resuscitation and assessment, the infant should be transferred to NICU as soon as practical. The parents should be given the opportunity to hold their baby if the baby's condition allows this.

Initial Management in NICU

Initial management will depend on the underlying cardiac lesion and the anticipated neonatal problems.

* Infants should be admitted to Level 3 NICU.

* Cardiorespiratory and oxygen saturation monitoring should be commenced as soon as possible.

* If the infant is unwell or requiring significant support, take blood cultures and commence antibiotics.

*Intravenous access

* If the infant requires significant ventilatory support, arterial and venous access should be obtained.

* Infants with lesions*dependent on the duct for systemic blood flow, a double lumen umbilical venous catheter should be inserted.

* For infants with other lesions it is not necessary to insert umbilical catheters if the baby is otherwise well.

* Ongoing Care in NICU

Duct-dependent for Systemic Blood Flow
With severe left-sided obstructive lesions systemic blood flow is dependent on right-to-left flow through a patent ductus arteriosus, so these babies are duct-dependent. Examples: Hypoplastic Left Heart Syndrome, critical.

*Insert a double lumen umbilical venous catheter *Commence a*prostaglandin infusion at an initial dose of 10 nanograms/kg/min. *Do not over-oxygenate the infant (over-oxygenation will result in increased pulmonary blood flow and reduced systemic blood flow). *Accept oxygen saturations of 75% or above. Reduce inspired oxygen if saturations >85%.

Contact the paediatric cardiologist on call *The baby is to remain nil by mouth. *If the infant requires assisted ventilation, ensure that the baby is not over-ventilated. The aim should be to initially ventilate to keep a low-normal arterial pH. Sedation, muscle relaxation, and controlled hypoventilation to further reduce arterial pH may be necessary if there is excessive pulmonary blood flow and reduced systemic blood flow (oxygen saturations >85%, low MAP, tachycardia, cool peripheries).

Duct-dependent Cyanotic Lesions

These lesions are duct-dependent either to ensure adequate pulmonary blood flow (e.g. pulmonary atresia, critical pulmonary stenosis) or to ensure adequate mixing between the systemic and pulmonary circulations (transposition of the great arteries). *Commence a *prostaglandin infusion at an initial dose of 10 nanograms/kg/min. *Ensure that at least one extra IV leur is available in the event that the PGE1 infusion tissues. *If the systemic oxygen saturation is below 75%, call the paediatric cardiologist on call. *If the infant develops apnoea or the systemic oxygen saturation is below 75% despite prostaglandin, they should be ventilated. *If the infant develops apnoea but has a systemic oxygen saturation of 75% or above, the dose of prostaglandin can be reduced (but not below 5 nanograms/kg/min). If apnoea continues, the infant should be ventilated. *If the infant is delivered after midnight but is stable, the paediatric cardiologist should be contacted in the morning by 0700 hours. If unstable, contact the paediatric cardiologist on call.

Rhythm Disturbances

Many infants are asymptomatic despite rhythm disturbances which have been detected antenatally or postnatally. Some infants may require significant resuscitation, particularly if they are hydropic. Hydropic infants require the attendance of a neonatal specialist. Severely hydropic infants may require emergency insertion of intercostal and/or abdominal drains at delivery.

Congenital Heart Block

*In the case of complete heart block with fetal hydrops, delivery should be planned in consultation with the paediatric cardiologist and/or paediatric cardiac surgeon on call as urgent pacing may be necessary. *Transfer to NICU as quickly as possible. *Intravenous access should be obtained. *It is preferable but not essential to obtain a 12-lead ECG soon after admission to NICU. *If the heart rate is above 55bpm and the infant is stable, contact the paediatric cardiologist non-urgently. *If the heart rate is below 55bpm, contact the paediatric cardiologist on call. *Do not commence chronotropic agents (e.g.. isoprenaline) without first discussing management with the paediatric cardiologist.

Tachyarrhythmias
*Be aware that some pregnant mothers are treated with one or more anti-arrhythmic medications when the fetus has SVT, in order to treat the fetus, thus the baby may have anti-arrhythmic medication(s) on board at delivery. *If the tachycardia is still present after delivery, transfer to NICU as quickly as possible *Intravenous access should be obtained. *Obtain a 12-lead ECG soon after admission to NICU. *Contact the paediatric cardiologist on call to discuss further management. *If the tachycardia has resolved by delivery and the infant is stable, the baby can be admitted to the postnatal ward under paediatric care. The baby should have Q4H observations initially. Arrange review by the neonatal specialist on call the following morning with a 12 lead ECG available.

Neonatal Echocardiography

Over recent years echocardiography has changed from a purely research tool to an essential part of adequate management of the critically ill newborn. In the hypotensive or shocked infant, there is no better way to find a treatable underlying cause of their circulatory failure such as myocardial dysfunction, a large ductal shunt, pericardial effusion, or hypertrophic cardiomyopathy in infants of mothers with diabetes. A large ductal shunt sufficient to cause severe reduction in effective cardiac output and even cardiorespiratory collapse after extubation can be clinically silent and may only be revealed by echocardiography. Similarly, septic vegetations or thrombi on valves or central lines can only be seen this way, and it is feasible to assess pulmonary arterial pressure non-invasively in most ill newborns. Echocardiographic evaluation of ductal shunting is necessary before treatment, relatively easy to learn, and aortic coarctation can be excluded in this group before giving indomethacin by confirming that pure left to right ductal shunting is present using Doppler in association with good foot pulses. Each unit should have one consultant with special skills in echocardiography. Some trainees in neonatology may usefully elect to spend a year or more within a paediatric cardiac centre to train in echocardiography and CHD. Each trainee should attend a course in basic echocardiography and paediatric echocardiography, currently available from the British Society of Echocardiography, and/or a specialist course in echocardiography for the neonatologist. The neonatologist echocardiographer should have ongoing, regular, and documented contact with a local paediatric cardiac unit allowing continued exposure to echocardiography in CHD and allowing for specialist audit. Some form of certification of competence needs to be organized through a body as yet unspecified.

Which infants should be referred to the Pediatric cardiologist?

*Those with clinically suspected congenital heart disease *Those ventilated for severe persistent hypoxemia, particularly if extracorporeal membrane oxygenation is being considered *Those in whom an adequate echocardiogram is not obtained by the neonatologist or where echocardiography reveals previously unsuspected CHD.

Which infants can reasonably be assessed by a trained neonatologist echocardiographer?

*The hypotensive or shocked newborn in the first few hours of life without clinical evidence of congenital heart disease *Those requiring assessment of ductal and/or interatrial shunting *Those with a central line to assess its position or to exclude vegetation or thrombus *Those in whom pulmonary arterial pressure or cardiac output needs to be assessed (once CHD has been excluded by a paediatric cardiologist in infants with persistent hypoxemia).

Echocardiography is an essential part of modern neonatal intensive care. Its use should not be limited to cardiologists in the diagnosis and assessment of CHD but should be extended to the routine care of critically ill neonates. As with any investigative tool, echocardiography should be used in combination with clinical acumen and not as a replacement. Paediatric cardiologists should not be worried about neonatologists learning echocardiography, rather they should encourage, support and supervise them—live video links may even help to avoid unnecessary transfer to cardiac centres of cyanotic infants without CHD. Being involved in establishing guidelines for the safe practice of neonatal echocardiography is surely better than ignoring it.

Courtesy: J R SKINNER *Department of Cardiology, Bristol Children's Hospital, St Michael's Hill, Bristol BS2 8BJ, UK.*

Telemedicine in Pediatric Cardiology

Telemedicine can broadly be defined as the application of modern telecommunication systems for clinical purposes. The essential feature is that there is remote consultation: the doctor and patient are in different places often separated by large distances. Such remote consultation usually requires the transfer of images from the referral centre to a centre of expertise. Telemedicine lends itself particularly to those specialties where images are crucial to diagnosis. Thus there have been many applications in radiology with remote reporting of radiographs, computed tomography, and magnetic resonance images. In pathology remote reporting on frozen sections and other histological specimens has been successfully performed. Recently, remote consultation on fetal ultrasound images has been reported.5 In cardiology the simplest applications are in the transmission of electrocardiograms. **Application to paediatric cardiology:** The major application in paediatric cardiology is in the transmission of echocardiographic images to provide remote diagnosis. This is particularly relevant to the diagnosis of congenital heart disease (CHD) in the neonate, where early diagnosis and institution of appropriate management may be crucial to the outcome for the patient. Many such babies are born in district general hospitals where there is not immediate access to a paediatric cardiologist, thus transfer to a paediatric cardiology centre is usually necessary. The main benefit of a telemedicine link is to be able to provide a remote diagnosis from transmitted echocardiographic images before deciding whether patient transfer is indicated. There is a double benefit in that those with serious CHD are diagnosed and transferred early and those in whom CHD is excluded are not subjected to an unnecessary and potentially hazardous journey. A consultant paediatric cardiologist usually interprets transmitted images. Live transmission is preferable to transmission of prerecorded studies as it allows the paediatric cardiologist to guide the person performing the scan so that all the views necessary to reach a diagnosis are obtained. **Common diagnostic difficulties for the neonatologist:** In terms of life or death of the patient, the defects that must be diagnosed are those causing cyanotic heart disease, major obstructive lesions of the left or right heart, and total anomalous pulmonary venous drainage (TAPVD). Cyanotic lesions such as transposition of the great arteries, pulmonary or tricuspid atresia, and other complex lesions with univentricular hearts do not usually present diagnostic difficulty if standard views can be obtained during the transmitted echocardiography. The diagnosis of TAPVD is the one likely to provide the most difficulty and is obviously a crucial one to make, particularly in babies where the differential diagnosis is persistent pulmonary hypertension. The correct diagnosis of supracardiac TAPVD can be made with the transmitted scan, on which the pulmonary venous confluence and the ascending vein could be seen. The exclusion of a diagnosis of TAPVD requires a combination of imaging the pulmonary veins entering the left atrium and the demonstration of normal Doppler flow from them into left atrium. For those with limited experience in echocardiography, obtaining good aortic arch views is one of the areas that causes most difficulty. The diagnosis of coarctation of aorta is essentially a clinical one, and if the femoral pulses are weak or absent in association with an arm–leg blood pressure gradient, the patient will require transfer to the regional centre for a definitive diagnosis. The other common diagnostic dilemma for the neonatologist is in deciding whether the premature infant has a PDA, and, if there is one, how much is it contributing to the clinical condition of the patient? It is not practical to use a telemedicine link to confirm or exclude a PDA in all premature infants with this clinical problem. There is a case, however, for transmitting scans on ventilator dependent babies with chronic lung disease to determine whether a significant shunt through a PDA is exacerbating the problem. It is very useful in this situation to be able to answer the question by remote echocardiography and avoid transferring the ventilated patient.

Courtesy : Consultant Paediatric Cardiologist, Royal Belfast Hospital For Sick Children, 180 Falls Road, Belfast BT12 6BE, UK

Pearl/Peril/Pitfall: Residents: What to do?·Examine all babies' cardiovascular system thoroughly. Don't just focus on murmurs. ·If you find anything abnormal, get the baby reviewed by a more senior member of the team. ·If in doubt arrange an echocardiogram.

Table 11 — Differential diagnosis of neonatal cyanotic heart diseases

| Sign/Symptom | Decreased Pulmonary Blood Flow* ECG (QRS) Axis | | | | Increased Pulmonary Blood Flow* ECG Ventricular Forces | | |
	<0°† Tricuspid Atresia	0–90° Critical PS PA/IVS	90–150° TOF	>150° Complex CHD with PS or PA	Normal d-TGA	Abnormal TAPVC	HLHS
Systolic murmur	0 or long	0 or long	Short	0 or long	0	0	0 or long
Pulses	N or ↓	N or ↓	N or ↑	N	N	0 – +	0 – +
S2	Single	Single	Single	Single	Single	±split†	Single
Hepatomegaly	+	+	0	0	0	+++↑	+++↑
CXR findings	CM (↑RA)	CM (↑RA)	"Boot"† Right arch	CM	"Egg shape"	No CM Edema†	CM Edema†
Other ECG	LVH, RAE,↓RV	RAE,↑RV	RVH	RVH	N (RVH)†	RAE, RVH	RVH, LV
PO₂ (mmHg)	30–60	30–60	30–60	30–60	<30	<30	30–90†

*Chest radiograph
†Important differential feature.
+ present; 0=absent; ↓decreased: ↑increased.
CHD, congenital heart disease; CM, cardiomegaly; CXR, chest radiograph; d-TGA, d-transposition of great arteries; ECG, electrocardiogram;
HLHS, hypoplastic left heart syndrome; VS, intact ventricular septum; LVH, left ventricular hypertrophy; N, normal; PA, pulmonary atresia;
Po2, arterial oxygen tension; PS, pulmonary stenosis; RAE, right atrial enlargement; RV, right ventricle shadow; RHV, right ventricular hypertrophy;
TAPVC, total anomalous pulmonary venous connection (obstructed); TOF, tetralogy of Fallot.

KEY POINTS FOR CLINICAL PRACTICE

1. Critical congenital heart disease (CHD) is that presenting in early infancy with life threatening congestive heart failure or ductal-dependence (dependence on the ductus arteriosus to provide either blood flow to the lungs or to the systemic circulation). Patients with critical congenital heart disease can be divided into 4 general categories: those with *inadequate pulmonary blood flow*, such as Pulmonary Atresia; those with *inadequate systemic blood flow*, such as coarctation of the aorta; those with *inadequate mixing*, such as transposition of the great arteries; and those with *inadequate gas exchange*, such as total anomalous pulmonary venous connection.

2. Accurate and timely diagnosis of a *symptomatic Newborn* due to Congenital heart disease is extremely important (whether premature or term baby) to minimize the morbidity and mortality. Newborn presents in one of the 7 main ways- a) asymptomatic b)cyanosis, with/without respiratory distress c)respiratory distress (CHF) with/without cyanosis d) collapse/shock e) an associated lesion/syndrome/dysmorphology f) premature baby with significant PDA g) birth asphyxia with transient myocardial ischemia and pulmonary edema.

3. The most important issue in evaluating the symptomatic Newborn due to cardiac problem is how sick the infant is now and how much sicker the infant is likely to become without intervention over the next few hours.This determines and drives decisions about the urgency of possible transport to a tertiary center, about the performance of further diagnostic testing (CXR, ABG Analysis, blood cultures, and Echocardiogram etc.,) and about the possibly immediate institutions of therapeutic measures such as oxygen supplementation, ET intubation, antibiotics, inotropes, transfusion, surfactant, or Prostaglandin E2 IVI to maintain the ductal patency in ductus-dependent cardiac malformations.

4. It is important to establish lines of referral, consultation, and communication about the transport of these high risk infants to the tertiary referral center for preop/postoperative care. Serial assessments and adjustments in management are usually required throughout transport in infants with symptomatic CHD.

5. The preterm infant with significant PDA and cardiac failure secondary to left-to-right shunting may require surgical ligation of the ductus if indomethacin/ibuprofen therapy fails. The care of these infants preoperatively is focused on the management of the pulmonary disease and prematurity.

REFERENCES and FURTHER READING : 1)Wren C, Richmond S, Donaldson L. Presentation of congenital heart disease in infancy: implications for routine examination. *Arch Dis Child Fetal Neonatal Ed* 1999;**80**:F49–53 . 2) Kuehl KS, Loffredo CA, Ferencz C. Failure to diagnose congenital heart disease in infancy. *Pediatrics* 1999;**103**:743–7.3)Critical Congenital Heart Disease Dr. Gina Baffa, MD NICUniversity.org 4)Skinner JR. Echocardiography on the neonatal unit: a job for the neonatologist or the cardiologist? *Arch Dis Child* 1998;**78**:401–7. 5)Randolph GR, Hagler DJ, Khandheria BK, *et al*. Remote telemedicine interpretation of neonatal echocardiograms: impact on clinical management in a primary care setting. *J Am Coll Cardiol* 1999;**34**:241–5.

Pearl/Peril/Pitfall: Hyperoxia test (alias Nitrogen Washout). This is used for differentiating cardiac from non cardiac causes of cyanosis. Most babies with cyanotic heart conditions will not increase pO₂ significantly if placed in 100% oxygen. Babies are placed in 100% oxygen for 10 minutes, a preductal (either arm) arterial pO2 is measured. A pO2 over 150 mmHg makes cyanotic CHD unlikely. A pO₂ under 150 mmHg is most likely to be CHD but severe respiratory problems and/or PPHN are not completely excluded.

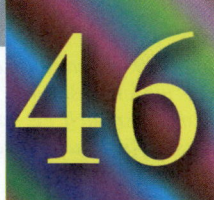

Neonatal Cyanosis

@ Hypoxia denotes inadequate oxygenation at the cellular level and is most commonly characterized by cyanosis. In general, hypoxia is discovered on clinical exam by the presence of cyanosis—the blue discoloration of the skin, tongue, and mucous membranes.

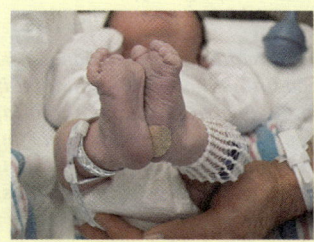

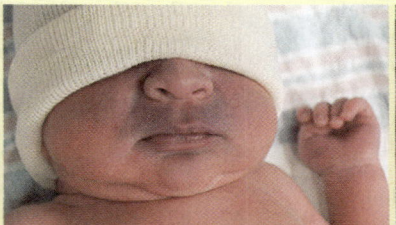

Perioral cyanosis: Another newborn with perioral cyanosis clearly demonstrates that although the philtrum and upper chin have a dark tint, the lips and tongue are bright pink.

Acrocyanosis: The cyanosis of the feet is apparent in comparison to the parent's hand and the baby's chin in the background.

Perioral cyanosis: A blue color around the lips and philtrum is a relatively common finding shortly after birth. This is part of acrocyanosis. The skin in this infant is visibly well perfused, and the tongue and mucous membranes in the mouth were pink, a finding that assures the examiner that central cyanosis is not present. This finding resolved spontaneously over the next 48 hours.

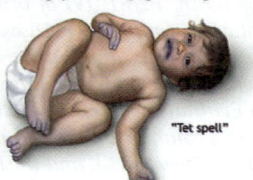

Children with Tetralogy of Fallot exhibit bluish skin during episodes of crying or feeding.

"Tet spell"

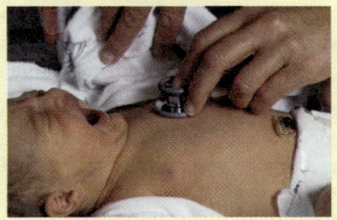

Lack of cyanosis does not always ensure a healthy baby, however, because newborns can tolerate a large decrease in PaO_2 without detectable cyanosis. Infants with oxygen saturation in the mid-80% range can often appear pink and only later be discovered to be hypoxic after vital signs become unstable.

Cyanotic spell (hypoxic spell, Tet spell) is characterized by a rapid and deep respiration, irritability, prolonged crying, increasing cyanosis, and decreasing intensity of the heart murmur in an infant with a known cyanotic congenital heart disease (**Eg:** Tetralogy of Fallot and Tricuspid Atresia).

Effect of hemoglobin concentration on the recognition of cyanosis

Hgb (g)	Reduced Hgb (g)	SaO$_2$	Total Hgb-Reduced Hgb/Total Hgb
20	3	85	(20-3)/20
8	3	62	(8-3)/20

These data show the expected levels of saturation for two hypothetical babies: one with a normal hemoglobin (20 g/dL) vs. one with a low hemoglobin (8 g/dL). Both babies have a fixed reduced hemoglobin level of 3 grams. The infant with the hemoglobin of 20 will have a saturation of 85%, and may appear cyanotic. However, the severely anemic infant may not appear cyanotic until the saturation is critically low. (*Beware of an APGAR Score of 10, in an anemic & underperfused Newlyborn baby!*)

Clin Pediatr Emerg Med. 2008 September; 9(3): 169–175. doi: 10.1016/j.cpem.2008.06.006

REVIEW OF CLINICAL PROBLEMS

1. Name the life-threatening causes of central cyanosis.
   Ans: Refer to Table 1 of the Chapter.

2. Mention the suggested steps in the management of a cyanotic newborn.
   Ans: Refer to Table 3 of the Chapter.

3. Discuss the essential management of ductus-dependent CHD. *Ans: Refer to Table 6 of the Chapter.*

4. What is the easiest way to remember the groups of causes of Central Cyanosis?
   Ans: Refer to the "No.4" of the "BIRD'S EYE VIEW/ OVERVIEW/SYNOPSIS" of the Chapter.

5. Mention the important subjective & objective findings you should ask/look for in a Cyanotic Newborn/Infant.
   Ans: Refer to the Evaluation-Decision-Action Plan/ Algorithm to diagnose & manage Neonatal Cyanosis.

LEARNING OBJECTIVES

After completing this article, readers will be able to:

1. Differentiate Central versus Peripheral Cyanosis.

2. Recognize promptly the ductus-dependent CHD and start IVI Prostin as soon as possible.

3. Start IV Antibiotics to cover for Sepsis, in any Cyanotic and/ or shocked Infant.

4. Evaluate further to confirm/exclude Cyanotic CHD, PPHN after liaising with Pediatric Cardiologist.

5. Stabilize the Hypoxic infants and organize the Transfer to Higher center for advanced management.

Pearl/Peril/Pitfall : DON'T ASSUME THAT ACROCYANOSIS IS NORMAL IN A LETHARGIC NEONATE !!! *-It may indicate the presence of CHF and/or Shock, Cold Injury, Polycythemia etc.,*

BIRD'S EYE VIEW/OVERVIEW/SYNOPSIS

1. **"CYANOSIS"** refers to a dusky purple-blue color caused by an absolute amount of reduced hemoglobin(>5g of reduced hemoglobin/dL) and is most readily apparent in superficial capillary-rich sites such as the lips,tongue,mucous membranes, and nail beds. It was shown in Neonates that cyanosis was evident when 3 to 4 g/100 mL of deoxygenated Hb was present. Most physicians recognize definite cyanosis when arterial oxygen saturation is under 85%, but under optimal conditions of normal vision, good ambient light, light skin pigmentation, and normal hemoglobin concentration, minor degrees of cyanosis at arterial oxygen saturation levels of 90–92% can be detected in Newborn because of high level of haemoglobin. Infants with mild desaturation can have a "ruddy" complexion with reddish discoloration of cheeks. Cyanosis is less apparent clinically when there is severe anemia because the concentration of reduced hemoglobin is limited by the anemia. Conversely, cyanosis may occur with normal arterial oxygen saturation when the hematocrit is greatly increased(polycythemia).

2. It is essential to distinguish peripheral from central cyanosis. *Peripheral cyanosis* occurs with normal arterial oxygen saturation and is caused by slowed peripheral circulation with excessive oxygen extraction by the tissues, and thus an increased concentration of reduced hemoglobin at the venous end of the capillaries. This occurs in a cold environment, polycythemia, heart failure, Shock, Vaso-spasm, arterial or venous obstruction, or even in normal newborn infants (acrocyanosis); the extremities are cold and blue, but the tongue is pink. Peripheral cyanosis may resolve with gentle warming of extremities. *Central cyanosis*, on the other hand, is caused by arterial desaturation and is best seen in the tongue and oral mucous membranes, which are always warm and have a high blood flow. *Central cyanosis is always a sign of severe pathology and has respiratory, cardiac, CNS, hematologic and metabolic causes (Refer to the Table 1 of the Chapter)*. Central cyanosis if caused by pulmonary conditions, is accompanied by rapid respirations + retractions + grunt. If it is caused by CNS depression the respirations tend to be irregular and weak and often slow. Cyanosis unaccompanied by obvious signs of respiratory difficulty suggests cyanotic congenital heart disease or methemoglobinemia. Episodes of cyanosis may also be the initial sign of hypoglycemia, shock, sepsis, or pulmonary hypertension *(Refer to the Table 2 of the Chapter)*.

3. *Differential central cyanosis* (cyanosis of toes but not the fingers) occasionally is seen because of right-to-left ductal shunting of desaturated blood with pulmonary hypertension or aortic arch obstruction. *Reverse differential cyanosis* (fingers but not the toes are blue) occurs, when there is transposition of great arteries with right-to-left shunting of saturated blood through the ductus. Clubbing of the fingers and toes occurs in cyanotic CHD, but seldom under 1 year.

4. *The easiest way to remember the groups of causes of central cyanosis is to consider the path that oxygen takes from the nose to the peripheral tissues: a) Oxygen supply Eg: seizures, IVH, apnea, respiratory depressants can cause hypo-ventilation and decreased oxygen supply and cyanosis b) Conducting airway Eg: Airway obstruction due to choanal atresia, laryngomalacia, TE fistula, diaphragmatic hernia, congenital lobar emphysema, pneumothorax c) Diffusion Eg:* pneumonia, HMD, pulmonary edema cause a diffusion. gradient and cyanosis which responds to oxygen d) Ventilation and perfusion mismatch Eg: Intrapulmonary shunting due to serious diffuse lung disease, cyanotic congenital heart disease e) Oxygen carriage Eg: Methemoglobinemia and anemia (tissue hypoxia, but not usually cyanosed) f) Oxygen delivery Eg:- Hypovolemia and shock, hypoglycemia, acidosis, cold stress, polycythemia.

5. *Most cases of central cyanosis require urgent action:(100% oxygen supplements by hood, intubation and ventilation if hypoventilating, correcting hypoglycemia, hypothermia, hypocalcemia, and IV antibiotics for possible Sepsis) leaving little time for a detailed history and physical examination. Any infant who is acidotic, febrile, or in respiratory distress, with or without cyanosis should be assumed to be septic : following a full septic work-up the child should be treated with IV antibiotics.*

6. Investigations to manage an infant with central cyanosis should include; chest X-ray, ECG, Echocardiogram, ABG analysis in room air and in 100% of oxygen (hyperoxia test) (Refer to the Tables 3 of the Chapter and to the Chapter 42 "Neonatal PPHN for hyperoxia test details.)

7. *Start an infusion of Prostaglandin E2/E1 (IVI of prostin 0.05–0.1 mcg/kg/mt), if Cyanotic Congenital Heart Disease is suspected and appears to be ductus-dependent (Eg: pulmonary atresia with or without VSD, tricuspid atresia, HLHS, severe COA) (Refer to Evaluation-Decision-Action-Plan/Algorithm). Beware of the 3 common side effects of IV prostin infusion are apnea (12%) fever (14%), and flushing (10%); less common side effects include tachycardia/ bradycardia, hypotension, and cardiac arrest. If clinical condition deteriorates, consider TAPVR and discontinue infusion.*

8. Only the most severe of Tetralogy of Fallot present as a cyanotic neonate. The less severe forms present with cyanotic spells, or with a loud murmur on routine check. *Cyanotic spell* (hypoxic spell, Tet spell) is characterized by a rapid and deep respiration, irritability, prolonged crying, increasing cyanosis, and decreasing intensity of the heart murmur in an infant with a known cyanotic congenital heart disease (Eg: Tetralogy of Fallot and Tricuspid Atresia). The spells occur usually in the morning after crying, feeding, or defecation with peak incidence between 2–4 months of age. A severe spell may lead to limpness, convulsion, cerebrovascular accident or even death. Therefore a cyanotic spell requires immediate recognition and appropriate treatment (Refer to the Table 4 of the Chapter).

9. If the methemoglobinemia is suspected (chocolate colored arterial blood, normal PaO_2), order a test of the methemoglobin level and treat with methylene blue 0.1–0.2ml/kg IV over 5–10 minutes as a 1% solution mixed with normal saline.

10. PPHN (Persistent Pulmonary Hypertension of the Newborn) requires hyperventilation, alkalinization, inotropes, inhaled nitric oxide + high frequency oscillation, and ECMO in severe cases and correction of acidosis, hypocalcemia and hypoglycemia.

Pearl/Peril/Pitfall : Cardiac Neonate may appear quite comfortable with only mild tachypnea and cyanosis and no respiratory distress - infant is often described as "happily tachypneic" - cyanosis due to pulmonary pathology will usually present with retractions, nasal flaring, and grunting • cardiac cyanosis will worsen with crying, improve with rest—pulmonary cyanosis will improve with crying due to increased ventilation

THE EVALUATION-DECISION-ACTION-PLAN/ALGORITHM FOR THE DIAGNOSIS AND MANAGEMENT OF *CENTRALLY CYANOTIC INFANT*

SUBJECTIVE FINDINGS

Postnatal Hx of symptom free interval, central and/or peripheral cyanosis-Hx of onset (did it occur in the nursery, shortly after coming home) severity, permanent or paroxysmal nature of cyanosis and whether the cyanosis becomes worse after feeding, respiratory distress, feeding difficulties, prematurity, acute collapse-shock-CCF in a previously well baby, asymptomatic but significant heart murmur, obvious multiple congenital anomalies(eg.,VACTERAL association)

Hx of hypoxic spells (Cyanotic Spells) (infants were breathing fast and deep during the spell or were holding their breath)

Natal Hx of birth wt, APGAR scores, resuscitation details, mode of delivery, PROM/meconium stained labor, asphyxia

Antenatal Hx of maternal infections, medications, diabetes,SLE,drug abuse(including smoking,alcohol), amniocentesis & fetal USG SCAN results, fetal dysrhythmias/congenital heart block/SVT

OBJECTIVE FINDINGS

Assess ABCDs and monitor CRT, O_2 sats (pre & postductal), BP, core-peripheral temperature difference, RR, HR, central & peripheral pulses, urine output.

Determine whether the baby is in preterminal ("pre arrest") conditions such as apnea, gasping or RR <20 bpm, shock, extremely lethargic or unresponsive limpy baby, bleeding etc.. and *intervene with appropriate resuscitation of ABCDs promptly.*

Look for cyanosis of tongue, mucous membranes, respiratory distress,lethargy/ irritability, convulsions. *Note- dysmorphic features (facies),* obvious congenital mal-formations

Examine-CVS- Tachycardia,precardial activity, murmur, thrill, gallop,unequal pulses. RS Tachypnea, retractions, wheeze, crackles. P/A Hepatomegaly.

INVESTIGATIONS

Blood FBC, TC, DC, **Hct**, Platelets, CRP, Blood cultures, **ABG analysis, electrolytes,** calcium and magnesium, **blood sugar**, creatinine, BUN, coagulation profile.

CXR for cardiomegaly/plethoric *or* oligemic lung fields, respiratory infections/air leaks etc.,

Consider carboxyhemoglobin or methemoglobin levels.

Urine analysis & culture

Laboratory studies for cardiac diagnosis Hyperoxia test, 15-lead ECG, 2D ECHO AND COLOR DOPPLER, Cardiac catheterization (before surgery)

MRI cardiac scanning in difficult cases

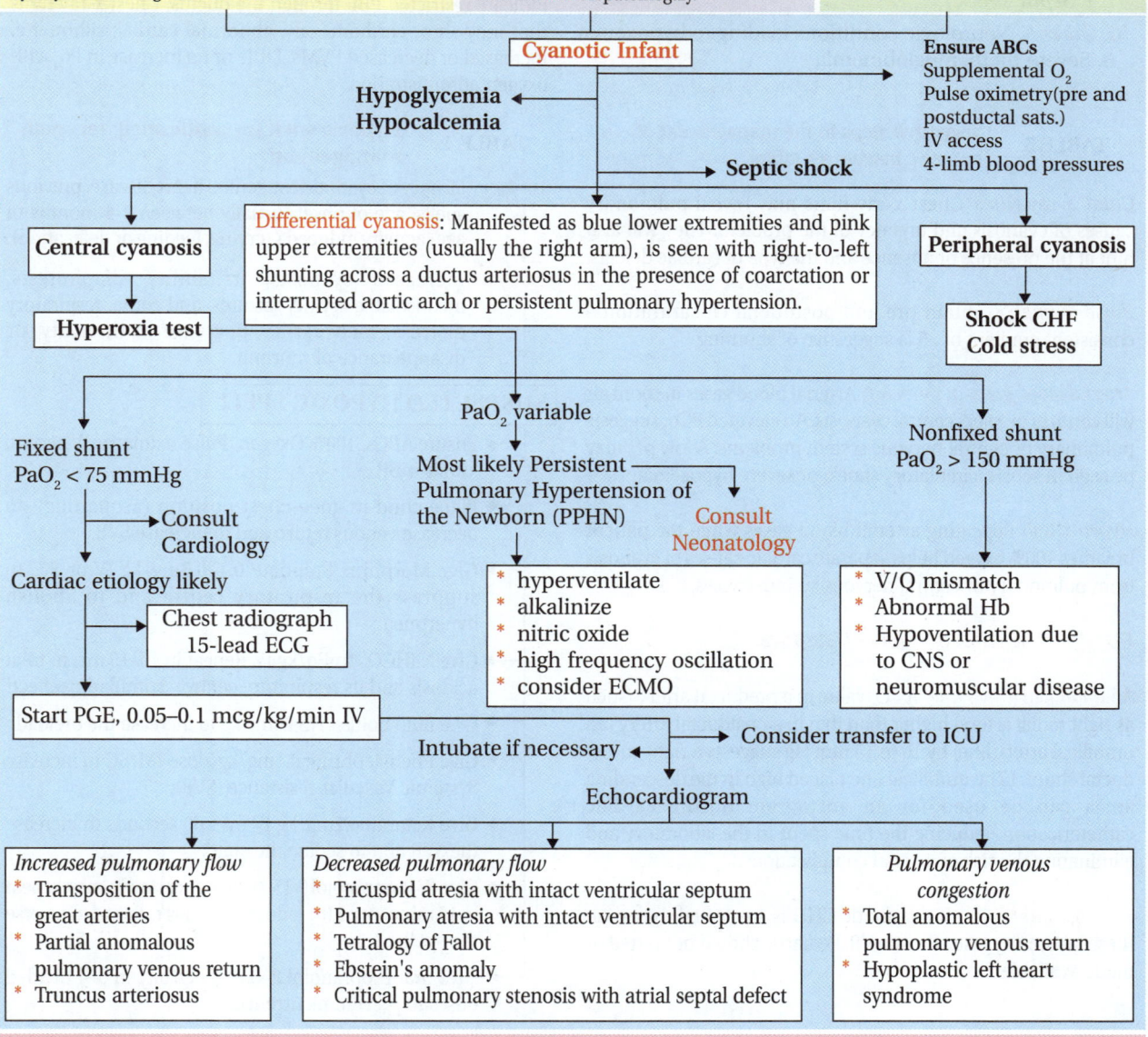

Cyanotic Infant

Hypoglycemia
Hypocalcemia

Septic shock

Ensure ABCs
Supplemental O_2
Pulse oximetry(pre and postductal sats.)
IV access
4-limb blood pressures

Central cyanosis

Differential cyanosis: Manifested as blue lower extremities and pink upper extremities (usually the right arm), is seen with right-to-left shunting across a ductus arteriosus in the presence of coarctation or interrupted aortic arch or persistent pulmonary hypertension.

Peripheral cyanosis

Hyperoxia test

Shock CHF
Cold stress

PaO_2 variable

Fixed shunt
PaO_2 < 75 mmHg

Most likely Persistent Pulmonary Hypertension of the Newborn (PPHN)

Consult Neonatology

Nonfixed shunt
PaO_2 > 150 mmHg

→ Consult Cardiology

Cardiac etiology likely

Chest radiograph 15-lead ECG

* hyperventilate
* alkalinize
* nitric oxide
* high frequency oscillation
* consider ECMO

* V/Q mismatch
* Abnormal Hb
* Hypoventilation due to CNS or neuromuscular disease

Start PGE, 0.05–0.1 mcg/kg/min IV

Intubate if necessary ← Consider transfer to ICU

Echocardiogram

Increased pulmonary flow
* Transposition of the great arteries
* Partial anomalous pulmonary venous return
* Truncus arteriosus

Decreased pulmonary flow
* Tricuspid atresia with intact ventricular septum
* Pulmonary atresia with intact ventricular septum
* Tetralogy of Fallot
* Ebstein's anomaly
* Critical pulmonary stenosis with atrial septal defect

Pulmonary venous congestion
* Total anomalous pulmonary venous return
* Hypoplastic left heart syndrome

Pearl/Peril/Pitfall: CONGENITAL HEART DISEASE causing CYANOSIS - Tetralogy of Fallot (TOF) - may be overlooked in nursery Tricuspid atresia, Transposition of the Great Arteries (TGA), Total Anomalous Pulmonary Venous Return (TAPVR), Truncus Arteriosus - may be overlooked in the nursery, Pulmonary atresia or stenosis other less common lesions .

TABLE 1	Life-threatening causes of cyanosis

1. Respiratory
A. Decreased inspired O_2 concentration
B. Upper airway obstruction/disruption
C. Chest wall immobility
D. Tension pneumothorax
E. Massive hemothorax
F. Lung disease leading to hypoxemia

II. Vascular

A. Cardiac
1. Cyanotic congenital defects
2. Congestive heart failure
3. Cardiogenic shock

B. Pulmonary
1. Pulmonary edema
2. Primary pulmonary hypertension of the Newborn
3. Pulmonary embolism
4. Pulmonary hemorrhage

C. Peripheral
1. Septic shock

III. Other A. Neurologic conditions leading to hypoxemia
B. Severe methemoglobinemia

TABLE 2	Causes and clinical findings of central cyanosis

Central Nervous System Depression—*Causes*: Perinatal asphyxia, Heavy maternal sedation, Intrauterine fetal distress. *Findings* : Shallow irregular respiration, Poor muscle tone, Cyanosis that disappears when stimulated or oxygen is given to the patient.

Pulmonary Disease—*Causes*: Parenchymal lung disease (e.g., hyaline membrane disease, atelectasis), Pneumothorax or pleural effusion, Diaphragmatic hernia, PPHN (or persistent fetal circulation syndrome). *Findings*: Tachypnea and respiratory distress with retraction and expiratory grunting, Rales and/or decreased breath sounds on auscultation, Chest x-ray film that may reveal causes (as listed previously), Oxygen administration that improves or abolishes cyanosis.

Cardiac Disease—*Causes*: Cyanotic CHD with right-to-left shunt. *Findings* : Tachypnea but usually without retraction, Lack of rales or abnormal breath sounds unless CHF supervenes, Heart murmur that may be absent in serious forms of cyanotic CHD, A continuous murmur (of PDA) that may indicate restricted PBF through the ductus, Chest x-ray films that may show cardiomegaly, abnormal cardiac silhouette, increased or decreased PVMs, Little or no increase in Po_2 with oxygen administration.

TABLE 3	Suggested steps in the management of cyanotic newborn / infant

Chest X-ray films Chest x-ray films may reveal pulmonary causes of cyanosis and urgency of the problem. They will also hint at the presence or absence and the type of cardiac defects.

Pulse oximetry obtain pre and postductal O_2 saturations-consistent gradient of >5 is suggestive of shunting.

Arterial blood gases in room air Arterial blood gases in room air will confirm or reject central cyanosis. An elevated PCo_2 suggests pulmonary or central nervous system problems. A low pH may be seen in sepsis, circulatory shock, or severe hypoxemia.

Hyperoxitest Repeating arterial blood gases while the patient breathes 100% oxygen helps separate cardiac causes of cyanosis from pulmonary or central nervous system causes.

ECG if cardiac origin of cyanosis is suspected.

An umbilical artery line A PO_2 value in a preductal artery (such as right radial artery) higher than that in a postductal artery (an umbilical artery line) by 10 to 15 mm Hg suggests a right-to-left ductal shunt. (The umbilical line placed high in the descending aorta can be used for an aortogram during cardiac catheterization, reducing the time spent in the laboratory and eliminating the risk of arterial complications.)

Prostaglandin E_1, E_2 If a cyanotic CHD is suspected based on these laboratory tests, Prostin VR Pediatric should be started or made available.

TABLE 4	Hypoxic spell (cyanotic spell, tet spell) management

Ask for : History of cyanotic congenital heart disease, previous spells, age of onset (usually between 2-4 months of age) activity induced ? (crying, feeding or defecation).

Look for: Increased cyanosis, irritability, diaphoresis, inconsolable crying, seizures, and coma, respiratory distress, tachycardia, decrease in intensity, or disappearance of murmur.

SUSPECTED HYPOXIC SPELL

- Ensure ABCs, 100% Oxygen, Pulse oximetry, IV access, Monitor BP.
- Place child in knee-chest position (=squatting), to decrease venous return and to increase SVR.
- Give Morphine Sulphate 0.1–0.3mg/kg IV or SC, to suppress the respiratory centre and to abolish hyperpnea.
- Give $NaHCO_3$ 1mEq/kg IV. Repeat in 10–15 mts to treat acidosis and its respiratory centre - stimulating effect.
- Give fluid bolus - NS 20ml/kg to increase the preload
- Give Phenylephrine 0.1mg/kg/dose IM/SC to increase Systemic Vascular resistance (SVR).
- Give Ketamine 2mg/kg IV over 60 seconds to increase the SVR and to sedate the child.
- Give IV Propranolol 0.15–0.25 mg/kg slowly, may repeat in 15 minutes x 1 (to reduce the heart rate and to reverse the spell).
- Give oral Propranolol 2–6 mgs/kg/day in 3–4 divided doses to prevent recurrence.

Pearl/Peril/Pitfall: Differentiating between the many etiologies for newborn hypoxia is undoubtedly an incredible challenge for the pediatric specialist in the newborn nursery. While there are several common causes for newborn cyanosis—primary pulmonary disease and sepsis—a myriad of disorders spanning all organ systems exist as possibilities.

ASSESSMENT OF NEONATAL TACHYPNEA AND CENTRAL CYANOSIS

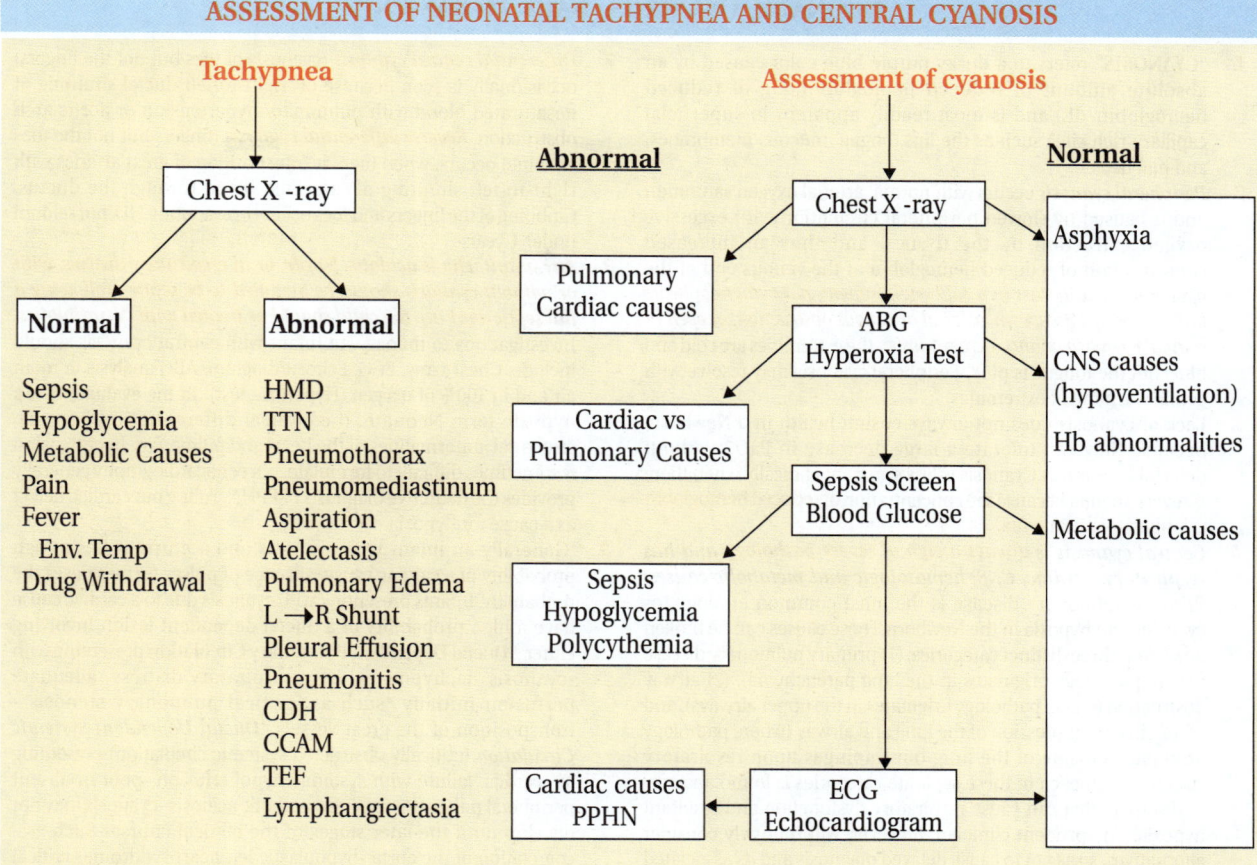

Tachypnea

Chest X -ray

Normal

Sepsis
Hypoglycemia
Metabolic Causes
Pain
Fever
  Env. Temp
Drug Withdrawal

Abnormal

HMD
TTN
Pneumothorax
Pneumomediastinum
Aspiration
Atelectasis
Pulmonary Edema
L →R Shunt
Pleural Effusion
Pneumonitis
CDH
CCAM
TEF
Lymphangiectasia

Assessment of cyanosis

Abnormal

Chest X -ray

Pulmonary
Cardiac causes

ABG
Hyperoxia Test

Cardiac vs
Pulmonary Causes

Sepsis Screen
Blood Glucose

Sepsis
Hypoglycemia
Polycythemia

Cardiac causes
PPHN

ECG
Echocardiogram

Normal

Asphyxia

CNS causes
(hypoventilation)

Hb abnormalities

Metabolic causes

Courtesy: P. Sasidharan/PCNA 51(2004) 999-1021

Essential beginning assessments in a Cyanotic Neonate include:

* Distinguishing between acrocyanosis (the normal peripheral cyanosis of hands and feet) and central cyanosis (of mucous membranes and tongue)

* Assessing the difference between cyanosis and bruising

* Assessing vital signs, including blood pressures in both upper and lower extremities

* Obtaining O2 saturation levels at both preductal (right hand) and postductal (left arm and lower extremities) sites

* Diagnosing tachycardia or bradycardia

* Diagnosing cyanosis with concomitant respiratory distress

* Observing tachypnea, grunting, flaring, or retractions

* Listening to breath sounds auscultated over all lung fields

* Evaluating for heart murmur

* Finding pulses in all extremities

* Assessing vigor, responsiveness, and cry *Determining gestational age, size for that age, and presence of features that might suggest a genetic disorder (e.g., low-set ears, spacing of eyes/toes/nipples, microcephaly or macrocephaly, atypical eye slant, nasal bridge flattening) *Clearing airway obstruction

* Evaluating what the infant was doing before the hypoxia. How long were the symptoms present before the clinician's evaluation? Feeding is a culprit for gastroesophageal reflux, and bathing is a culprit for hypoglycemia and hypothermia. Any of these conditions can result in hypoxia and cyanosis.

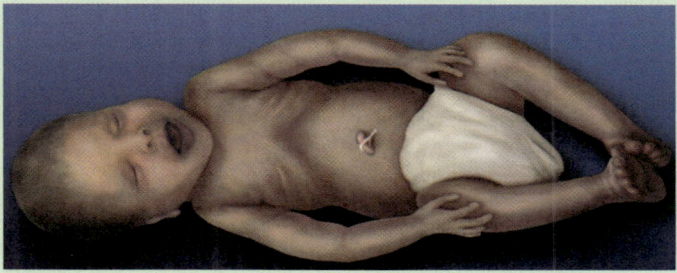

Clinical features of neonatal respiratory distress.
Drawing depicts a representative preterm newborn with RDS exhibiting substernal and intercostal retractions, nasal flaring, and circumoral cyanosis. (Illustration by Aletta Ann Frazier, MD, Department of Radiologic Pathology, Armed Forces Institute of Pathology.) **Primary pulmonary disease is the most common etiology for cyanosis and hypoxia in the Newborn.**

NEONATAL CYANOSIS : BACK TO BASICS

1. "CYANOSIS" refers to a dusky purple-blue color caused by an absolute amount of reduced hemoglobin(>5g of reduced hemoglobin/dL) and is most readily apparent in superficial capillary-rich sites such as the lips,tongue ,mucous membranes, and nail beds.

2. *Peripheral cyanosis* occurs with normal arterial oxygen saturation and is caused by slowed peripheral circulation with excessive oxygen extraction by the tissues, and thus an increased concentration of reduced hemoglobin at the venous end of the capillaries. *This occurs in a cold environment, polycythemia, heart failure, Shock, Vasospasm, arterial or venous obstruction, or even in normal newborn infants (acrocyanosis);* the extremities are cold and blue, but the tongue is pink. Peripheral cyanosis may resolve with gentle warming of extremities.

3. Lack of cyanosis does not always ensure health in a Newborn, because they can tolerate a large decrease in PaO2 without detectable cyanosis.Cyanosis is less apparent clinically when there is severe anemia because the concentration of reduced hemoglobin is limited by the anemia.

4. *Central cyanosis is always a sign of severe pathology and has respiratory, cardiac, CNS, hematologic and metabolic causes;* Primary pulmonary disease is the most common etiology for cyanosis and hypoxia in the Newborn.These causes can be broken down into **three distinct** categories: (1) primary pulmonary disease (where pathology originates in the lung parenchyma), (2) airway obstruction (where pathology originates in the upper airways), and (3) extrinsic compression of the lung and airway (where pathology originates outside of the lung but impinges upon respiratory structures). In each of these separate categories is found an array of disorders that can cause respiratory dysfunction and resultant hypoxia. The prudent clinician, however, will routinely consider alternatives, so as not to cause delayed diagnosis and its associated negative consequences for the infant with a less common disorder.

5. Methemoglobinemia is the rare but great impersonator in the evaluation of cyanosis of the Newborn. Methemoglobinemia causes reduced blood-oxygen carrying capacity due to abnormal hemoglobin or enzyme deficiency. Examination generally reveals a markedly cyanotic infant without respiratory distress, who has an arterial PaO2 that is normal, although the infant will have low oxygen saturation values. Arterial blood obtained from such an infant is often described as "chocolate" in color.

6. Central cyanosis if caused by pulmonary conditions, is accompanied by rapid respirations + retractions + grunt. If it is caused by CNS depression the respirations tend to be irregular and weak and often slow. Cyanosis unaccompanied by obvious signs of respiratory difficulty suggests cyanotic congenital heart disease or methemoglobinemia. *Episodes of cyanosis may also be the initial sign of hypoglycemia, shock, sepsis, or pulmonary hypertension.*

7. *Differential central cyanosis* (cyanosis of toes but not the fingers) occasionally is seen because of right-to-left ductal shunting of desaturated blood with pulmonary hypertension or aortic arch obstruction. *Reverse differential cyanosis* (fingers but not the toes are blue) occurs, when there is transposition of great arteries with right-to-left shunting of saturated blood through the ductus. Clubbing of the fingers and toes occurs in cyanotic CHD, but seldom under 1 year.

8. *Any infant who is acidotic, febrile, or in respiratory distress, with or without cyanosis should be assumed to be septic : following a full septic work-up the child should be treated with IV antibiotics.* Investigations to manage an infant with central cyanosis should include; Chest x-ray, ECG, Echocardiogram, ABG analysis in room air and in 100% of oxygen (Hyperoxia test). In the evaluation of a hypoxic term Neonate, the clinical differentiation between structural abnormalities of the heart and pulmonary hypertension is sometimes difficult to formulate, but echocardiography generally provides the definitive diagnosis of PPHN, ruling out cardiac defect as a cause for hypoxia.

9. Generally an infant with cyanosis and a murmur has a high probability of a cardiac cause, absence of pulses further raises the probability. Infants presenting with cyanosis due to a cardiac cause have a high probability of a ductal dependent lesion involving either: *Ductal Dependent Pulmonary Circulation presenting with -cyanosis -tachypnea without respiratory distress -adequate perfusion initially *such as -critical pulmonary stenosis -transposition of the great vessels *Ductal Dependent Systemic Circulation* (critically obstructed systemic circulation) presenting as -cardiac failure with systemic hypoperfusion -poor or absent peripheral pulses -increasing metabolic acidosis -cyanosis may not develop until the later stages of the clinical course -Such as -coarctation of the aorta -hypoplastic left heart syndrome -critical aortic stenosis * **Management:** Aim to maintain adequate tissue perfusion and ductal patency rather than correcting the cyanosis. *minimise pulmonary blood flow *moderate PEEP (4-6 cm H_2O) *ventilate in air if possible *aim for a CO_2 of 37 - 45 mmHg *SaO_2 75-85% *maximise tissue perfusion *fluid resuscitation (saline 10ml/kg boluses) *low dose inotropes (dopamine/dobutamine) - management of *shock *sodium bicarbonate if BE > -10 (dose (mmol) = BE *wt/4) *consider paralysis if infant distressed *achieve ductal patency with Prostaglandin E1.

10. *"How often have I said to you that when you have eliminated the impossible, whatever remains, however improbable, must be the truth?* Sherlock Holmes (Sir Arthur Conan Doyle) - Beware of the less common causes of extrinsic compression of the airway and lungs in the newborn include: *Right/Double Aortic Arch *Tracheal Vascular Ring *Pulmonary Artery Sling *Cricoid Cartilage Malformation.*

Reverse Differential Cyanosis in the Newborn

Differential cyanosis: PPHN may be associated with a variety of perinatal diseases. There may be intracardiac shunting of deoxygenated blood from the right atrium to the left atrium across a PFO and from the pulmonary artery to the descending aorta across a PDA. If the intracardiac shunting occurs primarily or exclusively at the level of the PDA, there may be differential cyanosis, with a preductal PaO2 that is at least 20 mm Hg greater (or O2 sat that is at least 5% greater) than the postductal PaO2 (or O2 sat). Reverse *differential cyanosis*, with a preductal PaO2 less than the postductal PaO2, is a much rarer clinical presentation.A rare, formerly fatal condition, usually seen with dextrotransposition of the great arteries (with persistent pulmonary hypertension or aortic interruption/ coarctation), it can be treated successfully with oxygen, prostaglandin E1, atrial septotomy, nitric oxide, bosentan, or extracorporeal membrane oxygenation, followed by the arterial switch operation.

Courtesy: Reverse Differential Cyanosis: A Treatable Newborn Cardiac Emergency, Thomas C. Martin, MD *NeoReviews* 2011;12;e270-e273

Diagnostic and therapeutic approach to reverse differential cyanosis in the newborn

1. Perform resuscitation and provide support, fluids, cultures, and antibiotics, as indicated.
2. Administer oxygen as treatment and for diagnosis (hyperoxia test).
3. If infant is cyanotic, perform echocardiography immediately.
4. Start PGE1, before echocardiography if necessary, or immediately after.
5. If dTGA is present, perform BAS as soon as possible.
6. If O_2 sat fails to improve, begin nitric oxide.
7. If O_2 sat fails to improve, consider @bosentan (or sildenafil).
8. If O_2 sat fails to improve, consider restricting PDA flow (stop PGE1).
9. If O_2 sat fails to improve, consider ECMO.
10. Perform arterial switch when stable for 3 to 7 days.

BAS balloon atrial septostomy, dTGA dextrotransposition of the great arteries, ECMO extracorporeal membrane oxygenation,O_2 sat oxygen saturation, PDA patent ductus arteriosus, PGE1 prostaglandin E1 @Bosentan, an oral endothelin-1 receptor antagonist, was used successfully in two patients who haddTGA and PPHN at a dose of 1.0 mg/kg every 12 hours.

TABLE 5	Presentations of ductal dependent congenital heart disease	
Cyanosis	**Shock with congestive Heart Failure**	**Shock without congestive Heart Failure**
Pulmonary atresia	Aortic atresia	Coarctation
Critical pulmonary stenosis	Mitral atresia	Interrupted arch
Tetralogy of Fallot	HLHS	
Tricuspid atresia		
Transposition of the great vessels		

Congenital heart defects that result in ↓↓ blood flow to the lungs or systemic blood flow are dependent on the pulmonary-systemic shunt from the patent ductus arteriosus to maintain pulmonary and systemic blood flow. Closure of the ductus arteriosus causes marked worsening of obstruction to pulmonary blood flow with right to left shunt and cyanosis in right-sided congenital lesions and decreased systemic blood flow with shock in left sided obstructive lesions. *Obstructive right heart lesions-**Pulmonary atresia *Pulmonary stenosis *Tricuspid atresia *Tetralogy of Fallot *Obstructive left heart lesions-**Aortic stenosis *Severe coarctation of the aorta *hypoplastic left heart syndrome *Mixed lesion -* D - TGV without VSD or ASD.

TABLE 6	Essential management of a ductal -dependent CHD

* If a duct-dependent cardiac malformation is confirmed by an ECHOCARDIOGRAM, start *IVI PROSTAGLANDIN E2 @0.005-0.05 micrograms/kg/min* to maintain the ductal patency until some palliative surgery is done as soon as possible; at a low dose initially and increase at 15-30 minute intervals if no response.(dilute 500 micrograms in 500 ml of 5% dextrose, that is 1 microgram/ml. Starting dose-0.3ml/kg/hr=0.005 *micrograms/kg/min. Double the dose in 20 minutes if SaO2 is unchanged.)*

* If cardiology consultation is not readily available, empirical treatment of an infant with suspected heart disease is appropriate.Giving PGE2 to an infant who later proves to have sepsis or inborn error of metabolism seldom causes harm.

* *IVI PROSTAGLANDIN E2* can be administered in a peripheral IV line, but a central line is preferred. If an UVC cannot be obtained, two peripheral lines are recommended. One should observe for central apnea, fever, and hypotension. Prostaglandin is contraindicated in the presence of TAPVR with Obstruction.

* Always Ensure ABCs- Provide ventilatory support (avoid high PEEP, which can increase pulmonary vascular resistance) in the presence of apnea, pulmonary edema or persistent acidosis, IVI inotropic(IVI Dobutamine @ 5-10 mcg/kg/min) support after volume expansion with NS 5-10 ml/kg if hypovolemic, IVI Dopamine @3-5 mcg/kg/min to improve renal perfusion, half-correct the metabolic acidosis guided by the base deficit and give Furosemide 1mg/kg/dose IV in cardiac failure to reduce the increased extravascular fluid volume.

* Oxygen for cyanotic infants is not contraindicated. Oxygen is a potent pulmonary vasodilator and may increase pulmonary blood flow;this may be beneficial for infants with decreased pulmonary blood flow. *The goal of oxygen therapy is to correct hypoxemia, not cyanosis.* The oxygen saturation need not increase to normal range. High saturation may indicate excessive pulmonary blood flow that is unnecessary and possibly deleterious.

TABLE 7	Structural lesions presenting with respiratory distress or collapse in the early Newborn period. All may have Cyanosis if PPHN or shocked; all have cardiomegaly with congested lung fields on chest X-ray

Condition	Pulses	Cyanosis	Precordium	Auscultation	ECG	Extracardiac associations
Hypoplastic left heart	Weak, femoral stronger if DA open	Mild	Active	Gallop	Small LV voltages	Uncommon
Aortic arch interruption	Strong Proximal to lesion	None	Active	Gallop, LVOT, systolic murmur	LV/RV+ T↓V$_{5-6}$	Common (DiGeorge)
Coarctation	Weak femoral	None	Active	Gallop, EC, LVOT, systolic murmur, Murmur between scapulae	RA+ RV+ T↓V$_{5-6}$	Uncommon (Turner)
Critical aortic stenosis	Weak	None	Active	Gallop, EC, LVOT, systolic murmur	LV+ ST↓ , T↓V$_{5-6}$	Uncommon

Central Cyanosis—Differential Diagnosis:

*Because central cyanosis is an indicator of significant hypoxia, it is always a cause of concern in the term infant; differentiation is needed among **cardiac, respiratory, and other causes of hypoxia**. For systematic ease, causes of hypoxia and central cyanosis can be divided into broad categories.*

Causes of Hypoxia and Central Cyanosis in the Newborn

● Structural abnormality of the heart and great vessels
● Pulmonary hypertension ● Primary pulmonary disease
● Airway obstruction ● Extrinsic compression of the lungs Central nervous system/neuromuscular diseases ● Hematologic disorders
● Sepsis and hypotension ● Metabolic abnormalities

Pearl/Peril/Pitfall : *Although primary pulmonary disease is the most common etiology for cyanosis and hypoxia in the newborn population, the prudent clinician needs to consider alternatives, in order to ensure a timely diagnosis and avoid negative consequences for the infant with a less common disorder.*

TABLE 8	Differential diagnosis of a cyanosed infant				
	Breathing pattern	Right and left SaO$_2$ difference	pCO$_2$	Severe metabolic acidosis	Response to 100% O$_2$
Primary Pulmonary Disease	Tachypnoea, grunting and recession	No difference	↑	no	↑PaO$_2$ and SaO$_2$
Cardiac	Tachypnoea, slow/deep breathing	+/-(usually 5–10%)	Normal or ↓	Present	No significant change
PPHN	Tachypnoea, recession and grunting may be present	>10–15%	Normal or ↑	+/–	+/-
Sepsis	Respiratory distress may be present	No difference	Normal or↑	+/–	Moderate↑ PaO$_2$ or SaO$_2$

(PPHN = Persistent Pulmonary Hypertension of the Newborn)

*History and presentation may allow the cause to be easily identified but often differentiating cause is difficult without echocardiography, especially in infants with relatively little respiratory distress. Transporting infants with severe cyanosis is difficult whatever the aetiology and stabilization prior to transport is particularly important. Fortunately with adequate stabilization, the overall transport-related mortality in infants with suspected cardiac disease is 0.7%. Echocardiography is the gold standard for the assessment of congenital heart disease in infancy.

KEY POINTS FOR CLINICAL PRACTICE

1. Confirm central cyanosis with arterial blood gas (ABG) in room air, if possible, a sample from the right arm is the best site. Assess the history and examination for cause, including four limb BP *an upper to lower limb systolic difference of > 10mmHg is significant and suggestive of Coarctation of the Aorta *hypotension in a cyanotic infant is a serious finding. Correct metabolic acidosis and systemic hypoperfusion if present with fluid boluses and bicarbonate.

2. Hyperoxia Test (HT): HT is not as reliable as an echocardiogram and is not as important as resuscitation and attendance to cardiorespiratory support, especially if acidosis or respiratory distress is present. HT has many limitations especially when only saturations are measured and not arterial PaO2 and should only be used in conjunction with a thorough clinical assessment.

3. Echocardiography is the gold standard for the assessment of congenital heart disease in infancy. *All infants with central cyanosis should be commenced on parental antibiotics (Differentiating the infant in severe septic shock from other causes of cyanosis is very difficult and no safe clinical measures exist) early until further investigation is possible. *Differentiating PPHN from ductal dependent pulmonary cardiac lesions can be very difficult; if uncertainty exists a PG infusion is generally the safest option for transport.

4. Generally an infant with cyanosis and a murmur has a high probability of a cardiac cause, absence of pulses further raises the probability. Infants presenting with cyanosis due to a cardiac cause have a high probability of a ductal dependent lesion involving either: **Ductal dependent Pulmonary circulation** presenting with *cyanosis *tachypnea without respiratory distress *adequate perfusion initially *such as -critical pulmonary stenosis -transposition of the great vessels OR **Ductal dependent systemic circulation** (critically obstructed systemic circulation) presenting as *cardiac failure with systemic hypoperfusion *poor or absent peripheral pulses *increasing metabolic acidosis *cyanosis may not develop until the latter stages of the clinical course *Such as -coarctation of the aorta -hypoplastic left heart syndrome -critical aortic stenosis.

5. **Management of cardiac causes of cyanosis:** Aim to maintain adequate tissue perfusion and ductal patency rather than correcting the cyanosis. *minimise pulmonary blood flow ·moderate PEEP (4-6 cm H$_2$0) *ventilate in air if possible *aim for a CO$_2$ of 37–45 mmHg ·SaO$_2$ 75–85%·maximize tissue perfusion *fluid resuscitation (saline 10ml/kg boluses) *low dose inotropes (dopamine/ dobutamine) *shock *sodium bicarbonate if BE > -10 (dose (mmol) = BE *wt/4)*consider paralysis if infant distressed *achieve ductal patency with Prostaglandin E1.

REFERENCES & FURTHER READING : 1) Penny DJ, Shekerdemian LS. Management of the neonate with symptomatic congenital heart disease. Arch Dis Child Fetal Neonatal Ed 2001; 84: F141 - F145 2) Hellstr?m-Westas L et al. Long-distance transports of newborn infants with congenital heart disease. Pediatr Cardiol 2001; 22: 380-384 3) Pickert CB, Moss MM, Fiser DH. Differentiation of systemic infection and congenital obstructive left heart disease in the very young infant. *Pediatr Emerg Care* 1998;**14**:263–7. 4) Hsu, D., & Gersony, W. (2005). Medical management of congenital heart disease. In A. Spitzer (Ed.), *Intensive care of the fetus and neonate* (pp. 929-938). Philadelphia: Mosby. 5) Nouri, S. (1997). Congenital heart defects: Cyanotic and acyanotic. *Pediatric Annals, 26,* 95-98.

Pearl/Peril/Pitfall: Cyanosis is based on amount of deoxygenated blood and not the percentage, • normally deoxygenated Hgb = 2 g/dl in the venules; need another 3 g/dl to appear cyanotic pO2 • polycythemic infants (neonates) may be cyanotic but still delivering O$_2$ to the tissues. ex: hgb 20 g/dl→if deoxy 3 g/dl →oxygenated hgb 17/20 = 85% oxygenated • anemic infants may not appear cyanotic yet still hypoxic, and not delivering O2 to the tissues ex: hgb 6 g/dl →deoxy 3 →oxygenated hgb 3/6 = 50% oxygenated • may not appear cyanotic until the 02 sats drop to 50% .

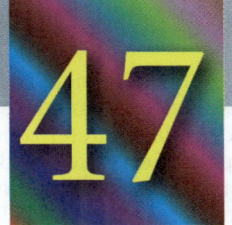

47

Congestive Heart Failure in a Neonate—CHF

@ *"In early CHF, increased cardiac contractility and other compensatory mechanisms maintain adequate cardiac output. When these compensatory mechanisms are exhausted, cardiogenic shock and collapse becomes manifest resulting in inadequate perfusion of vital organs."*

The Frank-Starling relationship. Ventricular output corresponds to ventricular filling volume or pressure. A decrease in contractility at any filling volume is associated with a decrease in cardiac output. A cardiac output insufficient to meet metabolic needs at any filling pressure (*lower curve/left*) is associated with fatigue at rest or "exercise." As contraction deteriorates, increased ventricular residual volumes lead to congestive symptoms (Congestive Heart Failure).

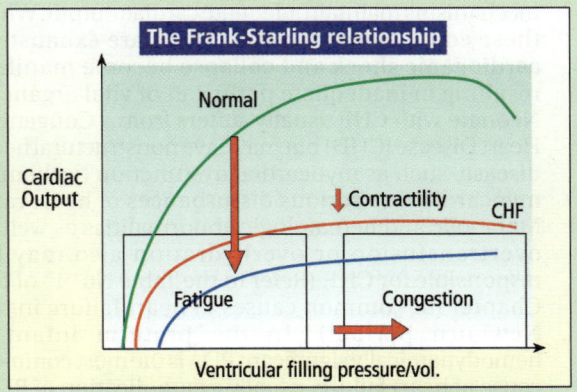

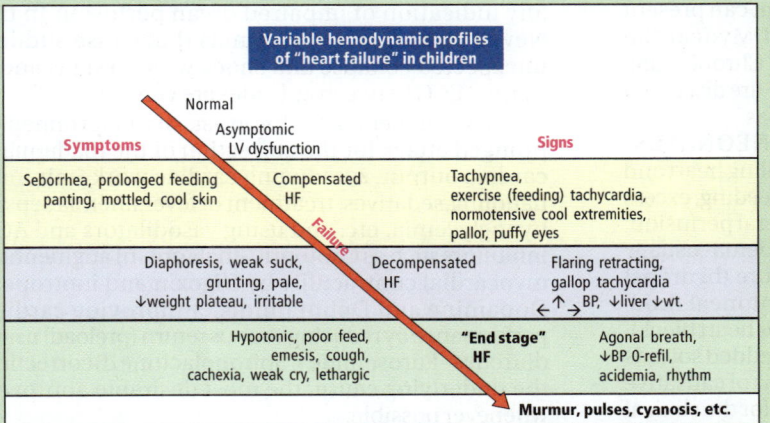

Symptoms and signs of heart failure (HF) in children vary with condition, age, and stage (early or late). This illustration of evolving signs and symptoms of HF in Newborns, infants, and children indicates how these are associated with advancing clinical HF.

BP, blood pressure; LV, left ventricular

REVIEW OF CLINICAL PROBLEMS

1. How do you recognize heart failure in a Neonate clinically? *Ans : Refer to the "No. 2" of the "BIRD'S EYE VIEW/OVERVIEW/ SYNOPSIS" of the Chapter, and to the "Table 2" of the Chapter.*

2.. Mention the essential investigations to evaluate CHF in a Neonate. *Ans: Refer to the "No. 4" of the 'BIRD'S EYE VIEW/ OVERVIEW/SYNOPSIS" of the Chapter..*

3. What is the most important issue to be determined in the acute management of CHF in Neonates ? *Ans: Refer to the "No. 5" of the 'BIRD'S EYE VIEW/OVERVIEW SYNOPSIS" of the Chapter.*

4. How do you manage a Neonate with CHF *without shock? Ans : Refer to the Evaluation-Decision-Action Plan/ Algorithm to diagnose and manage a Neonate with Congestive Heart Failure.*

5. How do you diagnose and manage heart failure in an Infant of Diabetic Mother? *Ans : Refer to the CHF IN NEONATES-SPECIAL SITUATIONS.*

LEARNING OBJECTIVES

After completing this article, readers will be able to:

1. Recognize the signs and symptoms of Heart failure in Neonates, early in the clinical course.

2. Recognize and diagnose the major causes of Neonatal Heart failure.

3. Interpret physical findings and laboratory studies associated with Heart failure in Neonates.

4. Institute initial medical therapy of Heart failure promptly and adequately.

5. Refer to Pediatric Cardiology team for assistance in diagnosis, treatment, and follow-up.

* *Pearl/Peril/Pitfall : CHF signs are due to pulmonary overcirculation and sympathetic stimulation, or due to left ventricular failure ! • poor feeding, diaphoresis (especially while eating), tachypnea, tachycardia, hepatomegaly, cardiomegaly and finally, pallor, mottling, hypotension, and oliguria • difficulty feeding is a fairly constant feature, with the neonate tiring and diaphoretic • heart rates above 180–200 when the neonate is at rest suggest increased autonomic activity to compensate for a failing myocardium • respiratory rates above 50 - 60/ minute, usually without increased depth, is an early sign.*

BIRD'S EYE VIEW/OVERVIEW/SYNOPSIS

1. *Congestive Heart Failure (CHF) is a clinical syndrome in which the heart is unable to pump enough blood to the body to meet its metabolic needs, to dispose of venous return adequately, or a combination of the two, despite various compensatory hemodynamic and neurohumoral mechanisms.* In early CHF, increased cardiac contractility and other compensatory mechanisms maintain adequate cardiac output. When these compensatory mechanisms are exhausted, cardiogenic shock and collapse become manifest resulting in inadequate perfusion of vital organs. A Neonate with CHF usually suffers from a Congenital Heart Disease (CHD) but may have nonstructural heart disease, such as myocardial dysfunction (ischemia, myocarditis) or serious disturbances of heart rate. Metabolic and hematologic abnormalities as well as overtransfusion or overhydration also may be responsible for CHF. (Refer to the Table No "1" of the Chapter for common causes of heart failure in the Newborn period.). In the preterm infant a hemodynamically significant PDA is the most common cause of heart failure, usually a complication of RDS. Three nonstructural heart situations that can present with CHF in a Neonate are Transient Myocardial Ischemia, Infant of a diabetic mother, and Chronic Lung Disease. Arrhythmias that can cause CHF are discussed in the Chapter- 48 " Neonatal Arrhythmias".

2. **CLINICAL FEATURES OF CHF IN NEONATES-** Symptoms and signs are related to the failing heart and venous congestion. *These include;* poor feeding, excess or unexpected weight gain, poor peripheral perfusion, clammy mottled skin, cold sweatiness, edema- usually late but characteristic of fetal heart failure (hydrops) often with pericardial, pleural and peritoneal fluid, tachycardia(unless cause of heart failure is heart block), hepatomegaly, respiratory distress with added sounds in chest, gallop rhythm, and specific signs of causative lesion. (Refer to Table No 2 of the Chapter for the clinical features of Neonatal heart failure classified according to the underlying hemodynamics.)

3. The clinical picture of CHF in the Newborn period may simulate other conditions, such as sepsis, meningitis, pneumonia or bronchiolitis. Moreover, the features of Neonatal heart failure can be masked or caused by respiratory disease and by circulatory collapse from any cause. Cardiac disease will also cause respiratory distress if there is marked pulmonary venous engorgement or metabolic acidosis has developed. Most causes of heart failure will be associated with other cardiovascular signs and with cardiomegaly on CXR, which together usually allow the distinction to be made with confidence.

4. The Essential investigations to evaluate CHF in a Neonate should include; *CXR*—absence of cardiomegaly almost rules out the diagnosis of CHF and its presence *per se* does not mean CHF is present, because some infants with large left-to-right shunt lesions have cardiomegaly without heart failure *ECG*- helps to determine the type of defect (arrhythmias, cardiac ischemia, chamber hypertrophy) but not helpful in deciding whether CHF is present. *ECHOCARDIO-GRAPHY- 2D WITH COLOR DOPPLER-* confirms the anatomical diagnosis and the hemodynamics of cardiac diseases and has resulted in a dramatic reduction in the need for diagnostic cardiac catheterization and can be used to guide interventions such as Balloon Atrial Septostomy. Echo may be able to determine the cause of CHF and is also useful in serial evaluation of the efficacy of therapy. *MRI HEART IMAGING-* provides excellent images of heart, but in the Newborn, echocardiography usually yields more than adequate information. ABG ANALYSIS, ELECTROLYTES, FBC, BLOOD GLUCOSE, CALCIUM ETC., are useful in the management of CHF.

5. *The Evaluation-Decision-Action-Plan/Algorithm* describes the essential aspects of diagnosis and management of a *Neonate with CHF. It is crucial to determine the presence of shock and collapse in a Neonate with CHF, which indicates the presence of a ductus-dependent LV outflow tract obstructive lesion, such as HLHS, COA, Critical AS, Interrupted Aortic arch or aortic atresia.* Along with timely and effective CPR, an IVI of Prostaglandin E2/E1 should be started when the diagnosis is established or if there is any indication of impaired organ perfusion. In the Newborn period, arrhythmias that cause sudden unexpected collapse and shock with no signs and a normal ECG between episodes are very rare.

6. The management of CHF consists of a determined 4-pronged attack for the correction of the inadequate cardiac output. *a)* reducing cardiac work (minimal handling, sedatives, treatment of fever, anemia sepsis, hypoglycemia, etc. and using vasodilators and ACE inhibitors such as Captopril/Enalapril, b) augmenting myocardial contractility by Digoxin and inotropes-Dopamine and Dobutamine, c) improving cardiac performance by reducing venous return (preload) using diuretics -Furosemide + Spironolactone d) correcting the underlying cause, the most desirable approach whenever possible.

7. Admit Neonates with CHF, if severely ill with shock, marked respiratory distress, or altered mental status into a NICU and monitor continuously arterial BP, CVP, and urine output. Administer Oxygen, and monitor ABGs frequently. Intubate and Ventilate, if the neonate is severely agitated with borderline oxygenation or evidence of impending respiratory failure. Consider Morphine sulfate for agitation only if the patient is intubated and well monitored.

8. If the cause is a congenital cardiac anomaly amenable to surgery, medical treatment is indicated to prepare the patient for surgery and in the immediate postoperative period while the heart is recovering from the effects of cardiopulmonary bypass.

9. In contrast, if the cause of heart failure is reversible, such as myocarditis/transient myocardial ischemia, medical management provides temporary relief from symptoms and may allow the patient to recover.

10. If the lesion is not reversible, heart failure management usually allows the infant to return to normal activities for some period and delay, sometimes for years, a consideration for heart transplantation.

Pearl/Peril/Pitfall: Neonates and infants younger than 2 months are the most likely group to present with congestive heart failure related to structural heart disease. The systemic or pulmonary circulation may depend on the <u>patency of the ductus arteriosus</u>, *especially in patients presenting in the first few days of life. In these patients, prompt cardiac evaluation is mandatory. Myocardial disease due to primary myopathic abnormalities or inborn errors of metabolism must be investigated. Respiratory illnesses, anemia, and known or suspected infection must be considered and appropriately managed.*

THE EVALUATION-DECISION-ACTION- PLAN/ALGORITHM FOR THE DIAGNOSIS AND MANAGEMENT OF *A NEONATE WITH CONGESTIVE HEART FAILURE (CHF)*

SUBJECTIVE FINDINGS

Postnatal Hx of symptom free interval, central and/or peripheral cyanosis, respiratory distress, feeding difficulties, prematurity, acute collapse-shock-CCF in a previously well baby, asymptomatic but significant heart murmur, obvious multiple congenital anomalies (eg. VACTERAL association).

Natal Hx of birth wt, APGAR scores, resuscitation details, mode of delivery, PROM/meconium stained labor, asphyxia.

Antenatal Hx of maternal infections, medications, diabetes, SLE, drug abuse (including smoking, alcohol), amniocentesis and fetal USG SCAN results, fetal dysrhythmias/congenital heart block/SVT.

OBJECTIVE FINDINGS

Assess ABCDs and monitor CRT, O_2 sats (differential pulse oximetry), *4-limb BP,* core-peripheral temperature difference, RR, HR, central and peripheral pulses, urine output.

Determine whether the baby is in preterminal (*pre arrest*) conditions such as apnea, gasping or RR <20 bpm, shock, extremely lethargic or unresponsive limpy baby, bleeding, etc. and *intervene with appropriate resuscitation of ABCDs promptly.*

Note the other alarming signs such as convulsions, irritability, pallor, central cyanosis, hypothermia, abdominal distention, bilious vomiting, petechiae and ecchymoses, vesicles, etc.(*signs suggestive of sepsis, asphyxia, CCF, NEC due to PDA*).

Note- dysmorphic features (*facies*), obvious congenital malformations/stigmata of congenital infections.

Perform CVS and systemic examination cardiac impulse, heart sounds, gallop, murmurs, breath sounds, rales, cardiomegaly, hepatomegaly.

INVESTIGATIONS

Blood FBC, TC, DC, **Hct**, Platelets, CRP, Blood cultures, **ABG analysis, electrolytes,** calcium and magnesium, **blood sugar**, creatinine, BUN, coagulation profile.

CXR for cardiomegaly/plethoric *or* oligemic lung fields, respiratory infections/air leaks etc.

Consider carboxyhemoglobin or methemoglobin levels.

Urine analysis and culture.

Laboratory studies for cardiac diagnosis Hyperoxia test, 15-lead ECG, 2D ECHO AND COLOR DOPPLER, Cardiac catheterization (before surgery).

MRI cardiac scanning in difficult cases.

A NEONATE WITH CONGESTIVE HEART FAILURE (CHF)

Intubate and ventilate, if necessary-*SHOCK and HYPOTENSION *APNEA *COLLAPSE -Avoid high PEEP (increased PEEP may decrease preload)

→ *Ensure* ABCs, Give supplemental oxygen, Monitor—pulse oximetry, BP (4-limb), CR Monitor, CVP if necessary, continuous BP monitoring

→ *Perform* IV access and correct (and maintain the normal range) hypoglycemia, hypocalcemia, anemia, polycythemia, acidosis and maintain normothermia and electrolytes

Catheterize the bladder to monitor urine output ←

WITH SHOCK ←   → *WITHOUT SHOCK*

Circulatory Failure

Manipulate preload

0.9 NS 5–10 ml/kg IVB only if necessary

PGE_1 or PGE_2 infusion + adequate ventilation

STAT echocardiogram and transfer to ICU

avoid diuretics

Start Inotropic support

Dopamine 8–20 mcg/kg/min continuous IV infusion

or

epinephrine 0.05-1.5 mcg/kg/min continuous IV infusion plus

---

dobutamine 5–10 mcg/kg/min continuous IV infusion when stable, consider

milrinone 50–75 mcg/kg/dose IVB followed by continuous infusion at 0.35–0.75 mcg/kg/min

Control rhythm disturbances-pacing, drugs-Refer to the Chapter "NEONATAL ARRHYTHMIAS"

Transfer to specialist cardiac unit for urgent Echocardiogram and surgical intervention

---

Congestive heart failure

* Rest (occasional sedation-Morphine sulfate 0.1–0.2mg/kg/dose, s/c, every 4hrs or phenobarbital 2–3 mg/kg/dose by mouth/IM every 8 hrs)-semi-Fowler position, temperature and humidity control + oxygen

* Fluid restriction *Diuresis

* Consider **digoxin-*refer to the Table 4***

* Maximize caloric intake-150 cal/kg/day @24–28 cal/oz concentration while limiting fluid intake

* Afterload reduction, only after stabilization to avoid hypotension

* ECHO for anatomical diagnosis

* Corrective surgery if necessary

* Ligation of PDA in a premature baby

* Truncus arteriosus/TAPVR-early surgical repair

* VSD/PDA/AVSD-optimal medical therapy to control CHF and early surgery if medical therapy fails:

* failure to thrive

* persistent heart failure

* development of pulmonary hypertension

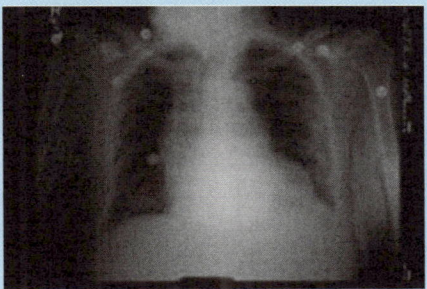

Chest radiograph shows signs of congestive heart failure (CHF)

Pearl/Peril/Pitfall: *The evaluation of serum electrolyte levels in the patient with congestive heart failure may demonstrate hyponatremia secondary to water retention. Elevated potassium levels may represent renal compromise or even tissue destruction due to low cardiac output. Significant tissue hypoxia increases serum lactate concentration and depletes the serum bicarbonate level.*

TABLE 1 Causes of heart failure in the newborn

A. Structural heart defects

At birth
a. Hypoplastic left heart syndrome (HLHS)
b. Volume overload lesions:
   Severe tricuspid or pulmonary insufficiency
   Large systemic AV fistula

First week
a. Transposition of the great arteries (TGA)
b. PDA in small premature infants
c. HLHS (with more favorable anatomy)
d. TAPVR, particularly those with pulmonary venous obstruction
e. Others:
   Systemic AV fistula
   Critical As or PS

First to four week
a. Coarctation of the aorta (preductal, with associated anomalies)
b. Critical aortic stenosis
c. Large left-to-right shunt lesions (VSD, PDA) in premature infants
d. All other lesions listed above

Four to six week
Some left-to-right shunt lesions such as endocar dial cushion defect

Six week to four months
a. Large VSD
b. Large PDA
c. Others such as anomalous left coronary artery from the pulmonary artery. (ALCAPA)

B. Noncardiac causes
a. Birth asphyxia (resulting in transient myocardial ischemia
b. Metabolic:hypoglycemia, hypocalcemia
c. Severe anemia (as seen in hydrops fetalis)
d. Neonatal sepsis.

C. Primary myocardial disease
a. Myocarditis
b. Transient myocardial ischemia (w/wo birth asphyxia)
c. Cardiomyopathy (seen in infant of diabetic mother)

D. Disturbances in heart rate
a. Supraventricular tachycardia (SVT, or PAT)
b. Atrial flutter/fibrillation
c. Congenital heart block (when associated with CHD)

Adapted from Pediatric Cardiology for Practioners—by Myung K. Park

TABLE 2 Signs and symptoms of heart failure in the newborns

History

Feeding difficulty: *Slowness to feed (>30 min) *pallor and sweating with feeding *Breathlessness and irritability during feeding *failure to gain weight

Physical examination

Signs of impaired myocardial function and compromised tissue perfusion—*Tachycardia (heart rate of >150/min), gallop rhythm, and thready pulse *Cardiomegaly (clinical and radiographic) *Reduced urine output (<1ml/kg per h) *Metabolic acidosis *Vascular collapse/ shock: pale, mottled skin, cold extremities, prolonged capillary refill time (>3s), increased toe-core temperature difference (>2° C), and impalpable pulses.

Signs of pulmonary venous congestion: *Tachypnea (respiratory rate of >60/min) *Subcostal or intercostal recession *Wet lung fields on chest radiograph *Frank pulmonary edema *Wheezing or basal rales *Cyanosis

Signs of systemic venous congestion: Hepatomegaly (>3 cm or progressive) *Excess weight gain (>30 gm/ 24h) despite feeding difficulties.

TABLE 3 Suggested preparation of prostaglandin E_1

Add 1 ampule (500 µg/1 mL) to:	Concentration (µg/mL)	ml/hr X weight (kg), needed to infuse 0.1µg/ kg/min
200 mL	2.5	2.4
100 mL*	5	1.2
50 mL	10	0.6

* Usually the most convenient dilution, provides one-fourth of maintenance fluid requirement. Usually mix in dextrose-containing solution for Newborns.

TABLE 4 Oral digoxin dosage for CHF

Age	TDD* (µg/kg)	Maintenance*+ (µg/kg/day)
Prematures	20	5
Newborns	30	8
Under 2 yr	40–50	10–12
Over 2 yr	30–40	8–10

TDD, total digitalizing dose.

*IV dose is 75% of the oral dose. +Maintenance dose is 25% of the TDD in two divided doses, 12 hours apart

Pearl/Peril/Pitfall: Congestive heart failure in the fetus, or hydrops, can be detected by performing fetal echocardiography. In this case, congestive heart failure may represent underlying anemia (e.g., Rh sensitization, fetal-maternal transfusion), arrhythmias (usually supraventricular tachycardia), or myocardial dysfunction (myocarditis or cardiomyopathy). Curiously, structural heart disease is rarely a cause of congestive heart failure in the fetus, although it does occur.

TABLE 5 — Diuretic agents and dosages

Preparation	Route	Dosage
Thiazide Diuretics		
Chlorothiazide (Diuril)	Oral	20-40 mg/kg/day in 2-3 divided doses
Hydrochlorothiazide	Oral	2-4 mg/kg/day in 2-3 divided doses
Loop diuretics		
Furosemide (Lasix)	IV	1 mg/kg/dose
	Oral	2–3 mg/kg/day in 2–3 divided doses
Ethacrynic acid	IV	1 mg/kg/dose
Aldosterone antagonist		
Spironolactone	Oral	2–3 mg/kg/day in 2–3 divided doses

DIURETICS—IMPORTANT PRACTICAL ASPECTS

*In a patient with cardiogenic shock, diuretics can precipitously decrease preload and lead to further decrease in cardiac output, and should therefore be avoided. * In a patient with *CHF without shock*, IV Furosemide 1–2mg/kg /initial dose usually results in a brisk diuresis within an hour of administration, and if no response, a 2nd dose (2–4mg/kg/dose) may be tried. *When changing from an effective parenteral to oral dose of Furosemide, the dose should be increased by 50-80%. * Potassium chloride supplementation (3-4mEq/kg/day) is usually required unless the potassium-sparing diuretic Spironolactone is given concomitantly. When Furosemide is administered every other day, dietary potassium supplementation may be adequate to maintain normal serum potassium levels.*Hydrochlorthiazide in combination with spironolactone is a convenient option for chronic use in CHF, to avoid nephrocalcinosis associated with Furosemide *Furosemide may increase the nephro- and ototoxicity of concurrently used aminoglycoside antibiotics.* Hypochloremic metabolic alkalosis due to Furosemide therapy predisposes to digitalis toxicity. * Diuretic induced hyponatremia may become difficult to manage in patients with severe heart failure.

TABLE 6 — Dosages of vasodilators

Drug	Route and dosage	Comments
Hydralazine	(IV) 1.5 mcg/kg/min, or 0.1–0 2 mg/kg/dose, evert 4–6 hours (maximum 2 mg/kg every hours) (O) 0.75–3.0 mg/kg/day, in two to four doses (maximum 200 mg/day)	It may cause tachycardia, and it may be used with propranolol. It may cause gastrointestinal symptoms, neutropenia, and lupus like syndrome.
Nitroglycerin	(IV) 0.5-2.0 mcg/kg/min (maximum 6.0 mcg/kg/min)	Start with a small dose and titrate based on its effects.
Captopril	(O) Newborn: 0.1–0.4 mg/kg/dose, 1to 4 times a day infants : 0.5-6.0 mg/kg/day, 1 to 4 times a day Child: 12.5 mg/dose, 1 to 2 times a day	It may cause hypotension, dizziness, neutropenia and proteinuria, hyperkalemia The dose should be reduced in patients with impaired renal function.
Enalapril	(O) 0.1 mg/kg, once or twice daily dizziness, or syncope.	The patient may develop hypotension,
Nitroprusside	(IV) 0.5-8 mcg/kg/min (e.g. fatigue, nausea, disorientation), hepatic dysfunction, or light sensitivity.	It may cause thiocyanate or cyanide toxicity
Prazosine	(O) First dose: 5 mcg/kg; increase to 25–150 mcg/kg/day, in four doses	It has fewer side effects than hydralazine; orthostatic hypotension or tachyphylaxis may develop

IV, Intravenous; O, oral.

VASODILATORS-IMPORTANT PRACTICAL ASPECTS

*ACE Inhibitors (Captopril, Enalapril) reduce the afterload by producing arterial dilatation and also reduce the preload by venodilatation and can cause hypotension and should therefore be avoided during resuscitation phase of neonate with cardiogenic shock. * Afterload reducers (*v.s*) are especially useful in improving low cardiac output principally by decreasing impedance to ventricular ejection;these effects are especially helpful after cardiac surgery in children. * All IV Vasodilators must be used cautiously in patients with moderate to severe lung disease;their use has been associated with increased intrapulmonary shunting and acute reductions of PaO_2. *Milrinone, a phosphodiesterase inhibitor, given by IVI @0.25–1mcg/kg/min, after an initial loading dose of 50–75 mcg/kg/dose IVB is useful in treating patients with low cardiac output who are refractory to standard therapy and has been shown to be highly effective in managing low-output state in children after open heart surgery. Hypotension is the main side effect and can generally be managed by volume expansion and IVI of inotropes. Amrinone is a similar drug , but can cause reversible thrombocytopenia.

* *Pearl/Peril/Pitfall :* The goals of medical therapy for congestive heart failure include reducing the preload, enhancing cardiac contractility, reducing the afterload, improving oxygen delivery, and enhancing nutrition.

CHF IN NEONATES-SPECIAL SITUATIONS

1. *Transient myocardial ischemia:* *Characterized by ischemic myocardial dysfunction and presents with cyanosis or with CHF and a low output state *A preceding history of perinatal hypoxia and or hypoglycemia is common. *The patient (usually a term infant born with low APGARs) usually has a systolic murmur of TR/MR (due to papillary muscle infarction indicated by elevated serum levels of Creatine kinase MB fraction). CHF with Gallop rhythm develops in 1/3rd of patients. Rarely, hypotension and vascular collapse occurs. *ECG shows generalized flat T waves and minor ST-segment depression due to subendocardial ischemia and sometimes abnormal Q waves due to anterior/inferior infarction.*CXR shows varying degrees of cardiomegaly with wet lungs in severely affected neonates *ECHO reveals varying degrees of myocardial dysfunction, including an enlarged LA and/or LV, decreased contractility of the LV, especially of the posterior wall, and mitral regurgitation.All of these abnormalities tend to improve over 1-2 weeks *These neonates usually have evidence of pulmonary hypertension, bidirectional shunts at the atrial and/or ductal levels, and TR. *ABG Analysis shows mildly reduced PaO_2 and pH but usually without CO_2 retention. *Mild cases require only supportive measures- oxygen ,correction of acidosis, hypothermia, hypoglycemia, fluid restriction, diuretics etc., *More severely affected infants need ventilatory assistance and Inotropic support with IVI of Dopamine and Dobutamine *They usually recover within a few days unless the ischemia is associated with severe acidosis, CNS damage, or advanced Sepsis.

2. *Myocarditis:* *Usually the result of a viral infection (coxsackie, rubella, and varicella), but can be due to bacterial, fungal, or autoimmune etiology. *May occur as an isolated or as a component of a generalized illness with associated hepatitis and/or encephalitis. *The infant presents with signs and symptoms of CHF and/or arrhythmia *The course is frequently fulminant and fatal *However, full recovery of ventricular function may occur if the infant can be supported and survive the acute illness. *Supportive care includes- oxygen supplements, diuretics, inotropic agents, afterload reduction, and mechanical ventilation *ECMO and Ventricular Assist devices can be considered in severe cases *Digoxin can potentiate the arrhythmia or complete heart block.

3. *Infant of diabetic mother:* *CHF should be suspected ,if a plethoric/mildly cyanotic IDM develops progressive distress from birth, tachypnea, tachycardia (>160bpm), ejection systolic murmur/pansystolic murmur and gallop rhythm * The differential diagnosis of CHF in an IDM include; a) a CHD, with VSD, TGA and COA b) Hypertrophic cardiomyopathy with or without LV outflow tract obstruction *IDMs also are at increased risk of PPHN. They are often affected by conditions that promote the persistence of pulmonary hypertension, such as hypoglycemia, perinatal asphyxia, respiratory distress syndrome, and polycythemia. *ECHO shows hypertrophic cardiomyopathy+/- LV outflow tract obstruction in 10-20% of these infants, asymmetrical septal hypertrophy or an associated CHD. *Treatment is symptomatic and supportive; Digoxin and other inotropes are contraindicated because they may worsen the obstruction. In most cases, hypertrophy spontaneously resolves within the first 6-12 months of life.Beta- adrenergic blockers, such as propranolol, may help the LV outflow tract obstruction, but treatment usually is not necessary.

4. *Chronic lung disease:* *Suspect Chronic Right heart failure-Cor Pulmonale (chronic pulmonary hypertension), if a premature baby(in 50% of premature infants with birth weights of 500-750g and about 10% of premature infants weighing <1500g who are machanically ventilated) develops respiratory distress, pulmonary rales, soft murmur of TR/nonspecific ejection systolic murmur and hepatomegaly *ECHO shows dilated RV and thickened LV posterior wall in >80% of infants; this may account for pulmonary edema and systemic hypertension in these patients *Treatment is supportive only- consists of a) nutritional b) hydrochlorothiazide 2mg/kg dose every 12hr with spironolactone 1.5 mg/kg every 12 hr c) oxygen therapy d) digoxin may be tried, with uncertain beneficial effects. *At least 15% of severely affected infants die in the 1st year. Most surviving infants are asymptomatic by 2 years, and signs or symptoms are rare after 5 years.

5. *Supraventricular tachycardia:* *Newborns with sustained SVT become restless and tachypneic with feeding difficulties and eventually develop signs of CHF and shock within 24-48 hours(in 20% of patients after 36 hours and in 50% of them after 48 hours) after onset. * Although rare, SVT diagnosed in utero may present with severe CHF at birth and has a high mortality rate, requiring prenatal digitalization of mother. Therapy is usually is instituted in the mother by IV loading of Digoxin (8–12 mcg/kg) over 24 hours, followed by a relatively large oral maintenance dose of 0.5-0.75 mg/day. Fetal digoxin levels usually similar to maternal levels, although the ratio of fetal to maternal digoxin ranges from 0.6-1. * If the neonate with SVT is in CHF, Cardioversion may be performed, followed by digitalization and diuretics.

KEY POINTS FOR CLINICAL PRACTICE:

1. *Congestive Heart Failure (CHF) is a clinical syndrome in which the heart is unable to pump enough blood to the body to meet its metabolic needs, to dispose of venous return adequately, or a combination of the two, despite various compensatory hemodynamic and neurohumoral mechanisms.*

2. A Neonate with CHF usually suffers from a Congenital Heart Disease (CHD) but may have nonstructural heart disease, such as myocardial dysfunction (ischemia, myocarditis) or serious disturbances of heart rate. Metabolic and hematologic abnormalities as well as overtransfusion or overhydration also may be responsible for CHF. Three nonstructural heart situations that can present with CHF in a Neonate are Transient Myocardial Ischemia, Infant of a diabetic mother, and Chronic Lung Disease.

3. The clinical picture of CHF in the Newborn period may simulate other conditions, such as sepsis, meningitis, pneumonia or bronchiolitis. Moreover, the features of Neonatal heart failure can be masked or caused by respiratory disease and by circulatory collapse from any cause. *ECHOCARDIOGRAPHY- 2D WITH COLOR DOPPLER- confirms the anatomical diagnosis and the hemodynamics of cardiac diseases and* has resulted in a dramatic reduction in the need for diagnostic cardiac catheterization and can be used to guide interventions such as balloon atrial septostomy.Echo may be able to determine the cause of CHF and is also useful in serial evaluation of the efficacy of therapy

4. Admit Neonates with CHF, if severely ill with shock, marked respiratory distress, or altered mental status into a NICU and monitor continuously arterial BP, CVP, and urine output.Administer Oxygen, and monitor ABGs frequently. Intubate and Ventilate, if the Neonate is severely agitated with borderline oxygenation or evidence of impending respiratory failure.

5. The management of CHF consists of a determined **4-pronged attack** for the correction of the inadequate cardiac output. *a)* reducing cardiac work (minimal handling,sedatives, treatment of fever,anemia sepsis,hypoglycemia, etc. and using vasodilators and ACE inhibitors such as Captopril/Enalapril *b)*augmenting myocardial contractility by Digoxin and inotropes-Dopamine and Dobutamine.*c)* improving cardiac performance by reducing venous return (preload) using diuretics -Furosemide+Spironolactone *d)* correcting the underlying cause, *the most desirable approach whenever possible.*

REFERENCES and FURTHER READING 1) Kay JD,Colan SD, Graham TP Jr:CHF in Pediatric patients. Am Heart J 2001;142:923-8. 2) Clark BJ 3rd: Treatment of heart failure in infants and children. Heart Dis 2000;2:354-61 3) Nohria A et al: Medical management of advanced heart failure. JAMA 2002;287:628-40 4) Shaddy RE : Optimizing treatment for chronic CHF in children, Crit Care Med 2001;29 (suppl):237-40 5) Wren C, Richmond S, Donaldson L. Presentation of congenital heart disease in infancy: implications for routine examination. *Arch Dis Child Fetal Neonatal Ed* 1999;**80**:F49–53.

Pearl/Peril/Pitfall: ED TREATMENT OfCHF:• AIRWAY, BREATHING, CIRCULATION !! • Oxygen and ventilatory support as needed • Lasix 1mg/kg IV • Dopamine or Dobutamine for systemic hypotension • Echocardiogram • Any neonate this ill deserves a septic workup and antibiotics until sure of diagnosis !! • Admit child to a Neonatal or Pediatric ICU CONSULT A PEDIATRIC CARDIOLOGIST OR THE NEONATAL ICU IN THE AREA !!

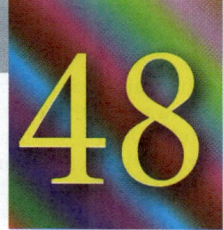

Neonatal Arrhythmias

48

@ *"Infants with an arrhythmia may be asymptomatic or present with heart failure or very rarely with collapse due to shock and/or hypotension."*

CARDIAC RHYTHM DISTURBANCES IN NEONATES

Heart condition	Supraventricular arrhythmias	Ventricular arrhythmias
Structurally normal heart	Atrial flutter Atrial ectopic tachycardia Reentrant SVT (AVNRT, PJRT, AVRT) Wolff-Parkinson-White syndrome	PVCs* AIVR* LQTS (torsade de pointes Idiopathic VT/VF
Congenital heart disease	Reentrant tachycardia Intra-atrial reentry tachycardia Micro-reentry tachycardia Atrial flutter Atrial ectopic tachycardia Occasional reentrant SVT	Incisional reentrant VT Poly/monomorphic VT
Cardiomyopathy	Atrial ectopic tachycardia	Poly/monomorphic VT

*Benign arrhythmia not requiring treatment.

AIVR, automatic ideoventricular rhythm, AVNRT, atrioventricular nodal reentry tachycardia; LQTS, long QT syndrome; PJRT, permanent junctional reciprocating tachycardia; PVCs, premature ventricular contractions; SVT, supraventricular tachycardia; VF, ventricular fibrillation; VT, ventricular tachycardia.

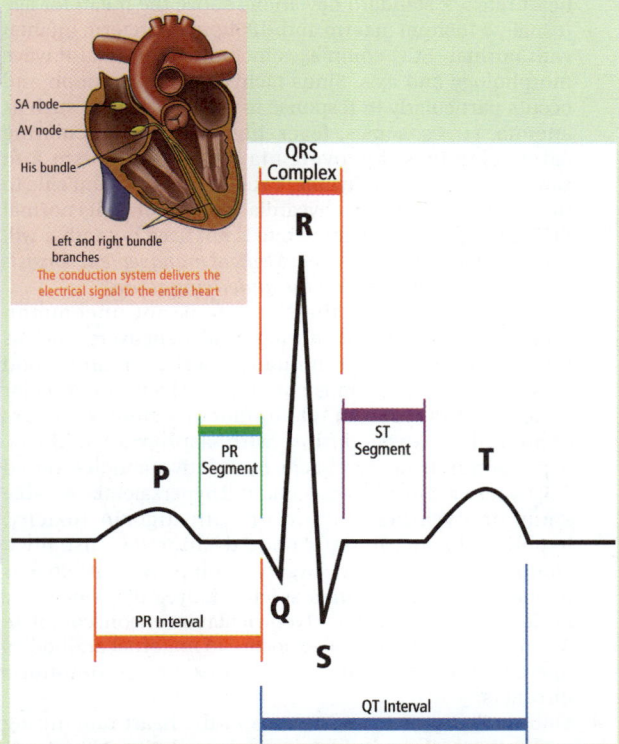

Pearl/Peril/Pitfall:Although premature ventricular depolarizations are usually benign, their identification should prompt evaluation for possible structural or functional heart disease, electrolyte abnormalities (e.g., hypokalemia, hyperkalemia, and hypocalcemia), hypoglycemia, hypoxia, or the congenital long-QT syndrome. Premature ventricular complexes may also be related to administration of drugs (e.g., dopamine, dobutamine, epinephrine, caffeine, aminophylline, theophylline, digoxin, or other antiarrhythmic medications).

REVIEW OF CLINICAL PROBLEMS

1. How do you differentiate Sinus tachycardia from a SVT ? *Ans: Refer to the"No. 2" and "No. 6" of the "BIRD'S EYE VIEW/OVERVIEW/SYNOPSIS"of the Chapter.*

2. How do you manage an unstable Neonate with a sustained SVT for >48 hours? *Ans: Refer to the"No.7 b)" of the "BIRD'S EYE VIEW/OVERVIEW/SYNOPSIS"of the Chapter.*

3. How do you diagnose and manage a Neonate with Wolff-Parkinson-White Syndrome? *Ans : Refer to the"No. 6" of the "BIRD'S EYE VIEW/OVERVIEW/ SYNOPSIS"of the Chapter.*

4. What are the essential aspects of history taking and physical examination, when a Neonate is found to have a significant arrhythmia? *Ans : Refer to the Evaluation-Decision-Action Plan/Algorithm to diagnose and manage Arrhythmias in Neonate.*

5. How do you manage a Neonate with VT/VF? *Ans : Refer to the"No.8" of the "BIRD'S EYE VIEW/OVERVIEW/ SYNOPSIS"of the Chapter.*

LEARNING OBJECTIVES

After completing this article, readers will be able to

1. Evaluate a Neonate with an arrhythmia while simultaneously assessing the electrophysiology and hemodynamic status.

2. Resuscitate the Neonate with an arrhythmia with shock and hypotension effectively and timely by *supporting, stabilizing and maintaining ABCDs, before definitive diagnosis is made.*

3. Identify various ECG patterns of Neonatal arrhythmias.

4. Understand the indications and contraindications of antiarrhythmic drugs in Neonates.

5. Consult a Pediatric Cardiologist, about combination drug therapy and cardiac pacing in severe arrhythmias.

* *Pearl/Peril/Pitfall : Identification and treatment of arrhythmias in newborns is challenging and differs from older children, and the natural history of arrhythmias presenting in the neonatal period is often dramatically different.Diagnostic methods: •15 lead electrocardiogram (standard 12 lead plus V3R, V4R, V7) •Heart rate determination (ECG strip, count number of QRS complexes in 6 sec x 10) •Blood pressure (intra-arterial or indirect).*

BIRD'S EYE VIEW/OVERVIEW/SYNOPSIS

1. The heart rate of a healthy Neonate shows considerable variations depending on the state of sleep or activity. The normal resting heart rate of the Neonate varies between 110bpm-150bpm with a mean heart rate of 120bpm. During quiet sleep some term infants have a resting heart rate as low as 90–100bpm.

2. Sinus tachycardia in the Neonate is defined as persistent heart rate > 2 standard deviations above the mean for age (usually >160bpm in term and>180bpm in preterm infants) with normal ECG complexes including a normal P wave morphology and axis. Sinus tachycardia is common and occurs particularly in response to systemic events such as anemia, stress, sepsis, fever, high levels of circulating catecholamines, hypovolemia, hyperthyroidism and xanthine (e.g. aminophylline) toxicity. An important clue to the existence of sinus tachycardia, in addition to its normal ECG morphology, is that the rate is not fixed but rather will vary by 10% to 20% over time. *Medical management consists of identifying and treating the underlying cause.*

3. Sinus bradycardia in the Neonate is not uncommon especially during sleep or during vagal maneuvers , such as bowel movements. If the infant's perfusion and blood pressure are normal, transient bradycardia is not of major concern. Bradycardia <80bpm consistently occurs commonly in association with asphyxia, acidosis, hypothermia, hypothyroidism, obstructive jaundice, raised ICP, hypertension, hypocalcemia and hyperkalemia. A stable sinus bradycardia may occur with digoxin toxicity, hypothyroidism, or sinus node dysfunction (usually a complication of cardiac surgery). Complete heartblock is frequently detected *in utero* as fetal bradycardia, which may be due to anatomic defects (ventricular inversion, complete AVcanal defect) or to fetal exposure to maternal antibodies like anti Ro and SS Ro of SLE and other autoimmune disorders.

4. Sinus arrhythmia is an increase in the heart rate during inspiration and results in a regular irregularity of heart rate in time with the respiratory cycle. Sinus arrest or pauses result in an occasional abnormally long pause(>1.6 sec) between P waves, producing an irregular irregularity of the heart rate. Neither is common in the newborn infant. These two variations of normal are of no significance of themselves. If they are very pronounced, they can be a marker of sinoatrial dysfunction which may be associated with symptomatic bradycardia or tachycardia.

5. Benign supraventricular and ventricular ectopic beats are also common, and most subside spontaneously in the absence of structural heart defects. Very frequent ventricular ectopics, the presence of a family history suggesting a long QT syndrome, cardiac physical signs or ECG abnormalities-particularly a long QT or evidence for heart disease- are an indication for echocardiography and 24-hour ECG monitoring (looking for VT). Isolated ventricular ectopics with a normal heart rate require no treatment and will resolve within 2 months; if they do not, echocardiography and 24-hour ECG monitoring should be performed and repeated.

6. *Supraventricular Tachycardia- SVT* is the most common symptomatic arrhythmia in all children including Neonates. SVTs usually have a heart rate - >230bpm, "fixed" frequently with no beat-to-beat variation in rate, rapid onset and termination in 'reentrant' types,variable in duration and narrow QRS complexes on the ECG. The infant is asymptomatic initially, but later becomes irritable, fussy, and refuse feedings. CHF usually does not develop before 24 hours of continuous SVT. However, heart failure is seen in 20% of patients after 36 hours and in 50% after 48 hours.

SVT in the neonate is almost always "reentrant", involving either an accessory AV pathway and the AV node, or due to atrial flutter. Approximately 40–50% of these patients will manifest short PR interval and preexcitation (delta wave) on QRS upstroke on the ECG when not in tachycardia (WOLFF-PARKINSON-WHITE Syndrome.) The QRS complexes are narrow when SVT occurs unless aberrant conduction occurs, which is very unusual in the Newborn. P waves may be visible between QRS complexes, but if they are, they have an abnormal axis. Any form of structural heart disease, myocardial tumours, myocarditis, electrolyte disturbances or indwelling right atrial lines should be considered as causes, but the heart is usually normal. Myocardial dysfunction and mitral regurgitation develop secondary to the arrhythmia and can be expected to resolve once control is achieved.

7. Treatment of SVT consists of **a)** when the Neonate is stable hemodynamically—vagal maneuver like facial immersion in cold water for a maximum of 10 seconds can be successful; if this fails IV Adenosine should be used. It has 85% success rate in restoring sinus rhythm and it may unmask atrial flutter if present. **b)** if these measures fail and the baby is collapsed, synchronized DC shock should be given. Digoxin should be given if heart failure is marked;Propranolol may be used instead if heart failure is not present. If the rhythm is well tolerated, it is acceptable to give Digoxin at least 6-12 hours to work, even if the loading doses have been used. If Digoxin successfully maintains the patient in sinus rhythm, it is typically continued for 6-12 months.W-P-W Syndrome is managed with Propranolol, as digoxin potentiates antegrade conduction across the accessory pathway. Amiodarone or procainamide can be added if necessary, but only after consultation with a pediatric cardiologist. *In utero* SVT is confirmed by fetal echocardiography, and a search for CHD and fetal hydrops may be made. Maternal treatment with digoxin, flecainide etc., is successful; if not, in the presence of fetal hydrops ,fetal SVT is an indication for cesarean section, as the fetal heart rate will not be a reliable indicator of fetal distress.

8. Wide complex tachycardias like Ventricular tachycardia-VT and Ventricular fibrillation(very rare and preterminal)-VF are rare in Neonates relatively, and are associated with severe systemic illnesses such as hypoxemia, shock, electrolyte disturbances, digoxin toxicity, and catecholamine toxicity. VT consists of wide and frequently bizarre QRS complexes with a rapid rate of 150-250bpm and the rhythm may be paroxysmal/sustained;if paroxysmal, fusion beats may be seen. This ECG pattern is simulated by SVT with aberration seen in patients with W-P-W Syndrome. VT is potentially a unstable rhythm commonly with hemodynamic consequences. If unstable/VF occurs, full CPR, and DC cardioversion/defibrillation(1-2J/kg to start with) should be instituted, to be followed by IVB Lidocaine 1-2 mg/kg, then to be followed by an IVI of Lidocaine 20-50 mcg/kg/min.Once the infant has been resuscitated, the underlying problems should be evaluated and treated.

9. *The Evaluation-Decision-Action- Plan/Algorithm* describes the essential aspects of diagnosis and management of various Neonatal arrhythmias, including heart block. Tables Nos 1,2,3 describe the essential features of their diagnosis and management. Table No 4 enlists the useful anti-arrhythmic drugs' doses, common adverse effects and therapeutic levels.

10. Transesophageal overdrive pacing is a very effective maneuver for terminating tachyarrhythmias. A placement of permanent epicardial pacemaker leads is the best option for complete heart block with symptoms.

---

* *Pearl/Peril/Pitfall :* Pathologic supraventricular tachyarrhythmias can be differentiated from sinus tachycardia by usually faster rates>230 BPM, abnormal P wave axis or PR interval, and (when present) by an abrupt onset and termination or wide QRS complexes.

THE EVALUATION-DECISION-ACTION- PLAN/ALGORITHM FOR THE DIAGNOSIS AND MANAGEMENT OF *ARRHYTHMIAS IN NEONATE*

SUBJECTIVE FINDINGS

Postnatal Hx **Determine** the onset, duration,severity,and frequency of recurrence of the rapid heart rate *Note* symptoms related to CHF -poor feeding, rapid breathing

Note any predisposing condition/precipitating factor—CHD, infection, (myocarditis), fever, anemia, hypovolemia xanthine (aminophylline) toxicity, hypoxia, shock, digoxin toxicity, electrolyte disturbances, high circulating catecholamines, thyroid problems, cardiac surgery etc.

Natal Hx of birth wt, APGAR scores, resuscitation details, mode of delivery, PROM/meconium stained labor, asphyxia

Antenatal Hx of maternal infections, medications,diabetes, SLE, drug abuse (including smoking, alcohol), amniocentesis and fetal USG SCAN results, fetal dysrhythmias/congenital heart block/SVT

OBJECTIVE FINDINGS

Assess ABCDs and monitor CRT, O_2 sats, BP, core-peripheral temperature difference, RR, HR (brady/tachy), central and peripheral pulses, urine output.

Determine whether the baby is in preterminal ("pre arrest") conditions such as apnea, gasping or RR <20 bpm, shock, extremely lethargic or unresponsive limpy baby, bleeding etc. and *intervene with appropriate resuscitation of ABCDs promptly.*

Note the other alarming signs such as signs of CHF,irritability,somnelence,cyanosis,hypo/hyperthyroidism,seizures,

Note dysmorphic features (facies), obvious congenital malformations/structural CHD/stigmata of congenital infections

Perform CVS and systemic examination quickly to identify the problems which require *emergent life saving procedures* such as DC cardioversion, CPR, IV Adenosine, IV Lidocaine/Amiodarone etc.,

INVESTIGATIONS

Perform ECG and Echocardiogram

Blood FBC, TC, DC, **Hct**, Platelets, CRP, Blood cultures, **ABG analysis, electrolytes,** calcium and magnesium, **blood sugar,** creatinine, BUN, coagulation profile,cardiac enzymes

CXR for respiratory infections/cardiomegaly/air leaks

Urine analysis and culture

Observe **nursing charts** for episodes of apnea, bradys, desaturations, tachys, hypoglycemia, and interventions to maintain the baby's temperature (a record of both environmental and core temperature, along with observation for other signs of sepsis)

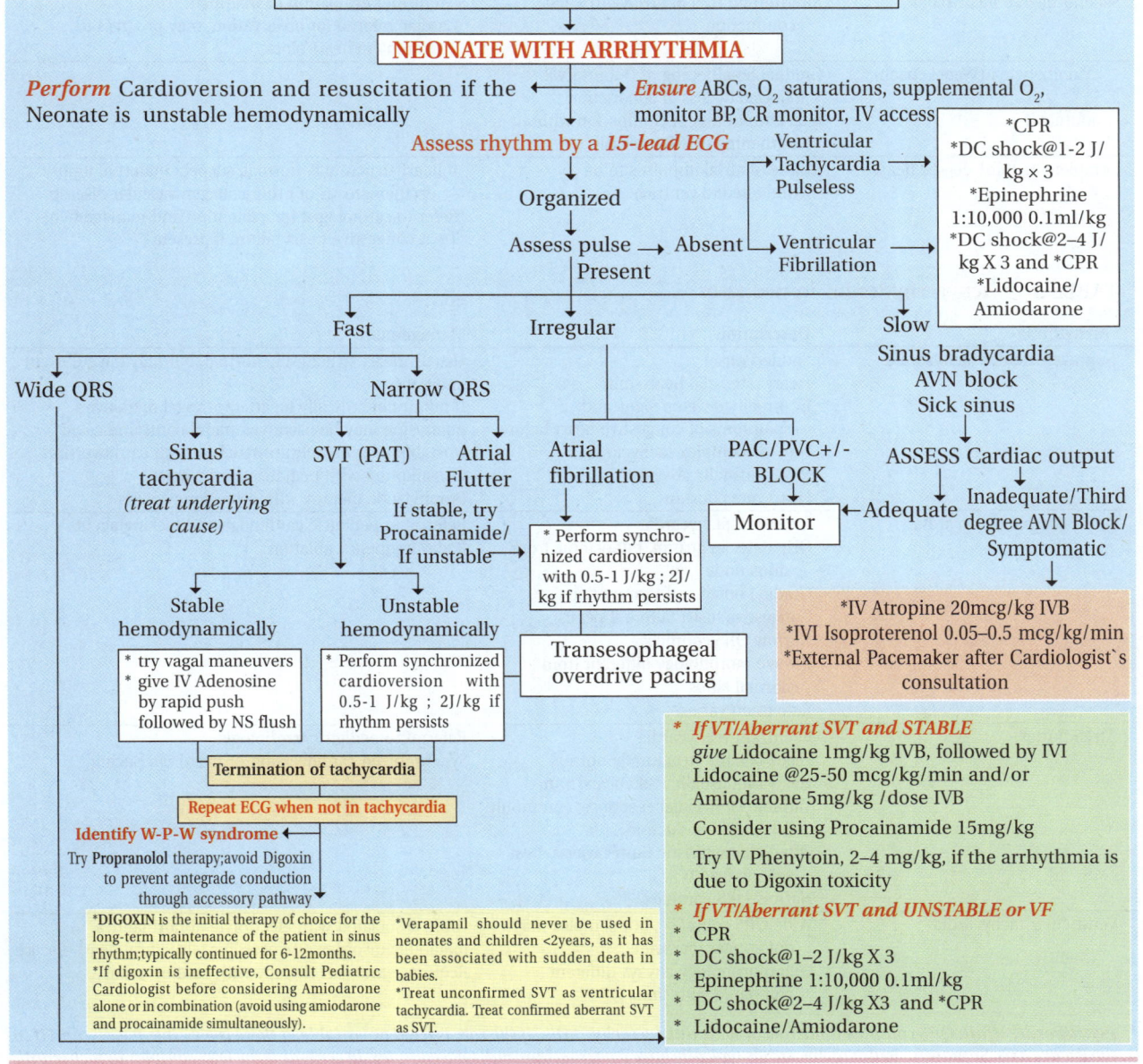

* **Pearl/Peril/Pitfall:** *In neonates with central venous catheters, frequent atrial premature depolarizations may be as a result of contact of the catheter with an atrial wall, and constitute an indication to withdraw the catheter from the atrium.*

TABLE 1 — Benign arrhythmias in the neonate

Arrhythmia	Description	Management
Sinus arrhythmia	Benign arrhythmia Phasic variation in heart rate	If P wave axis normal, no further evaluation necessary
Premature atrial contractions	Benign arrhythmia P wave morphology different from normal beat QRS complex same as normal beat	Rarely associated with electrolyte abnormalities, myocarditis, or structural heart disease If no risk factors present, no further evaluation necessary If central line in place, consider movement. Evaluate for atrial thrombus
Premature ventricular contractions	No P wave Abnormal QRS complex	Evaluate for metabolic abnormalities, prolonged Q-T syndrome, myocarditis, structural heart disease Review medications and classes If isolated premature ventricular contractions have uniform morphology of QRS complex, no further evaluation necessary

TABLE 2 — Bradyarrhythmias in neonates

Arrhythmia	Description	Management
Second-degree heart block	Intermittent loss of atrioventricular conduction	No further evaluation or treatment Cardiac referral for observation; may progress to complete heart block
Mobitz type I (Wenckebach)	Gradual lengthening of P-R interval followed by loss of conduction	
Mobitz II	Intermittent loss of conduction without lengthening of P-R interval	
Complete or third-degree heart block	Failure of atrial impulses to be conducted to ventricle	If heart structurally normal, suspect maternal lupus erythematosus or other collagen vascular disease Refer to cardiologist for evaluation and management Treat congestive heart failure if present

TABLE 3 — Tachyarrhythmias in neonates

Arrhythmia	Description	Management
Supraventricular tachycardia	Sudden onset Heart rate >250 beats/min Eventually develop signs and symptoms of congestive heart failure Narrow-complex tachycardia P wave usually absent Heart rate constant	Usually heart structurally normal, but may have Ebstein anomaly If infant not critically ill, attempt vagal maneuvers Adenosine may be used; verapamil contraindicated Unstable patients require synchronized cardioversion Consultation with pediatric cardiologist Prophylactic therapy with β-blocking agents
Atrial ectopic tachycardia	Incessant tachycardia Originates in atrium, but ectopic from sinus node Gradual onset and termination Congestive heart failure if persists Narrow QRS complex P wave morphology different from normal sinus Rate often varies	Referral to pediatric cardiologist β-blocking agents Radio frequency ablation
Atrial flutter	Reentrant tachycardia Heart usually structurally normal Heart rate usually >300 beats/min Variable ventricular response, commonly 2:1 or 3:1 conduction Often characteristic flutter waves, best seen in lead II Narrow QRS complex	Referral to pediatric cardiologist Synchronized cardioversion or overdrive pacing
Ventricular tachycardia	Wide QRS complex , but complex may not appear that wide QRS morphology always different compared with sinus QRS	Often associated with electrolyte abnormalities, metabolic disorders, myocarditis, structural heart disease Requires emergent therapy with cardioversion

* *Pearl/Peril/Pitfall: QRS complex is narrow or wide during tachycardia, if the rate is fixed or variable, if there is a visible P wave and if so, the P wave axis. Supraventricular tachycardias typically have a narrow (normal) QRS complex. In general, if the QRS complex in tachycardia remains wide, the rhythm should be considered ventricular tachycardia. However, it is not uncommon for the first few beats of SVT to be wide because of aberrant conduction (right or left bundle branch block) before changing to a narrow QRS complex.*

A. Tachyarrhythmias with narrow QRS

1. Reentry tachycardias

Diagnosis	Findings on ECG	Treatment
Atrial flutter 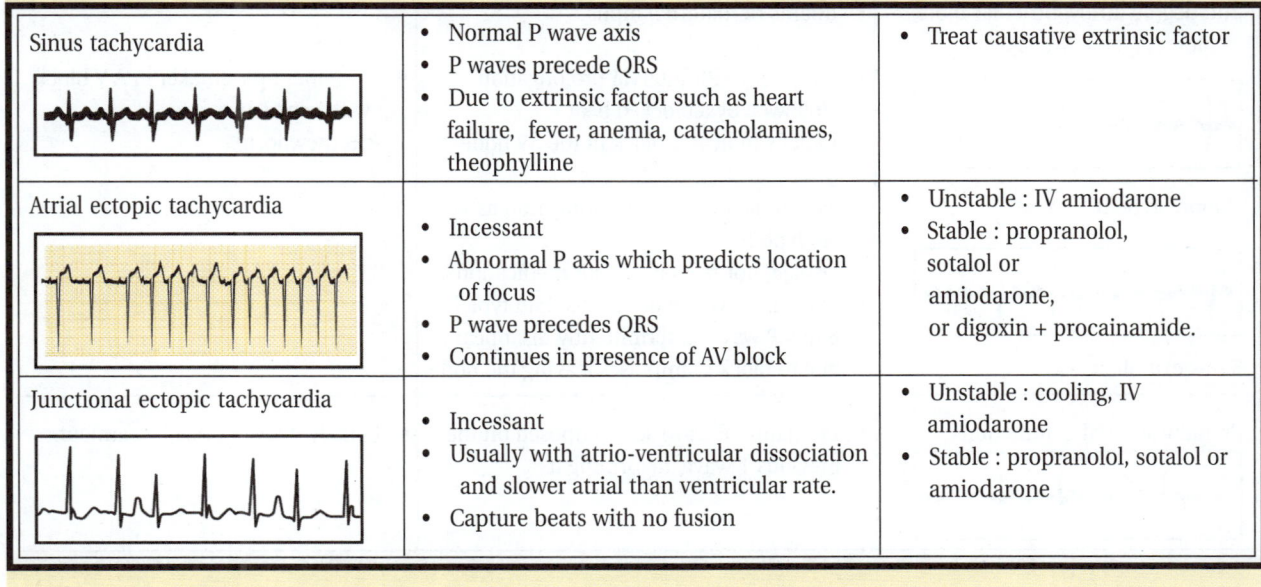	• 'Sawtooth" flutter waves • AV block does not terminate atrial rhythm • Atrial rate up to 500 in Newborns • Variable AV conduction common	• Unstable : esophageal pacing or electrical cardioversion • Stable : digoxin, propranolol, or digoxin + procainamide
Accessory pathway mediated tachycardia (WPW)	• P follows QRS, typically on upstroke of T -Superior or rightward P wave axis • AV block always with P wave • After termination, WPW have pre-excitation	• Stable : Vagal maneuvers. adenosine propranolol or digoxin
Permanent form of junctional reciprocating tachycardia (PJRT)	• Incessant P wave precedes QRS • Inverted P waves in II, III, AVF • AV block always terminates tachycardia • May terminate with QRS or P wave • No pre-excitation after termination	• No response : Procainamide or flecainide
Atrioventricular node reentry	• P usually not visible, superimposed on QRS • AV block usually terminates tachycardia.	
Atrial and sinoatrial reentry	• P present, precedes next QRS • Terminates with QRS rather than P • AV block does not terminate atrial rhythm • P axis may be superior or inferior	• Unstable : electrical cardioversion • Stable : propranolol, procaina-mide or amiodarone
Atrial fibrillation	• "Irregularly irregular" • No two RR intervals exactly the same • P waves difficult to see, bizarre and chaotic	• Unstable : electrical cardioversion • Stable : digoxin + procainamide

II. Increased automaticity

Sinus tachycardia	• Normal P wave axis • P waves precede QRS • Due to extrinsic factor such as heart failure, fever, anemia, catecholamines, theophylline	• Treat causative extrinsic factor
Atrial ectopic tachycardia	• Incessant • Abnormal P axis which predicts location of focus • P wave precedes QRS • Continues in presence of AV block	• Unstable : IV amiodarone • Stable : propranolol, sotalol or amiodarone, or digoxin + procainamide.
Junctional ectopic tachycardia	• Incessant • Usually with atrio-ventricular dissociation and slower atrial than ventricular rate. • Capture beats with no fusion	• Unstable : cooling, IV amiodarone • Stable : propranolol, sotalol or amiodarone

B. Tachyarrhythmias with wide QRS

Diagnosis	Findings on ECG	Treatment
Ventricular tachycardia (VT)	• Often with AV dissociation • Capture beats with narrower QRS than other beats; fusion beats	• Unstable : electrical cardioversion • Stable ; lidocaine, procainamide
Ventricular FIBRILLATION	• Complete chaotic rhythm • Rapid and irregular rhythm	(1) asynchronous cardioversion 2j/kg (2) asynchronous cardioversion 2j/kg (3) asynchronous cardioversion 4j/kg (4) lidocaine + asynch. cardioversion
SVT with pre-existing bundle branch block	• QRS morphology similar to that in sinus rhythm • QRS morphology is that of right or left bundle branch block	• Unstable : esophageal pacing or electrical cardioversion • Stable : vagal maneuvers, adenosine, propranolol or digoxin
Antidromic SVT in WPW	• QRS morphology similar to pre-excited sinus rhythm, but wider • Never with AV dissociation	• No response : procainamide or flecainide

C. Bradyarrhythmias

Diagnosis	Findings on ECG	Treatment
Sinus bradycardia	• Slow atrial rate with normal P waves • 1:1 conduction • Due to underlying causes such as hypoxia, acidosis, increased intracranial pressure, abdominal distention, hypoglycemia,hypothermia, digoxin, propranolol	• Vigorous resuscitation and supportive care • A B C • O_2 • Treat underlying causes
Atrioventricular block	• Atrioventricular dissociation • Regular R-R intervals • Regular P-P intervals • Atrial rate > ventricular rate • P which occur after T have no effect on R-R interval	• Unstable : A B C O_2 Atropine, isoproterenol infusion Temporary transvenous pacing • Stable : Treat underlying causes
2nd degree atrioventricular block - Mobitz type I (Wenckebach)	• Infants of maternal lupus • Progressive PR interval prolongation followed by a blocked beat • Usually indicates block in the AV node	• Permanent pacemaker in A V block with ventricular rate <55 (newborn)
-Mobitz type II Sinus exit block	• No characteristic PR prolongation as seen in type 1. • Usually not reversible with medications. • Type II has worse prognosis than type I. • Sinus P waves intermittently disappear due to block of impulses leaving the node.	
Premature atrial contractions	• Premature P wave superimposed on the previous T wave, deforming it	• Usually does not need treatment.

TABLE 4   Treatment options for SVT

Vagal stimulation

The diving reflex stimulates the vagal reflex which may cause conversion to sinus rhythm.

1. Initially try facial cooling:
   - Fill a polythene bag with cold water and ice cubes.
   - Place this over the baby's forehead, eyes, nose, mouth and cheeks for 15 s.
2. If this fails, try immersion:
   - Wrap the baby in a towel and immerse the head and face completely in a basin full of water and ice for 5 s.
   - Ensure the nose and mouth are immersed and do not worry about aspiration as the baby will be rendered temporarily apneic as a reflex reaction to the cold water.
   - There may be short period of nodal bradycardia before a return to sinus rhythm.
3. If vagal stimulation fails, try adenosine.

Adenosine

- Impairs conduction of electrical impulses through the atrioventricular node and is very effective in the treatment of SVT.
- Short half-life (15 s), so there is no cumulative effect and there is no depressant action on the myocardium.
- Give adenosine by a rapid bolus IV.
- Flush the line with saline immediately afterwards.
- Start with 50 micrograms/kg. IV.
- Increase in increments of 50 micrograms/kg. IV at 2-min intervals until sinus rhythm is restored.
- The maximum dose is 300 micrograms/kg.
- Adenosine is antagonized by theophylline.
- Adenosine has such a short half-life that SVT may recur unless a further regular antiarrhythmic agent is started.

Possible side-effects are sinus bradycardia, AV block and flushing, but these are rare and resolve within 40 s.

Following a return to sinus rhythm

- ECG for evidence of WPWS (slow upstroke of delta wave preceding QRS).
- Echocardiogram.
- There may be non-specific ischemic changes on the ECG for 24 h afterwards and it may take 24 h for the CXR to return to normal.
- Color and peripheral circulation should improve more dramatically followed by diuresis, with hepatomegaly and the gallop rhythm regressing over 24 h.
- Seek specialist advice.
- Regular antiarrhythmic: Digoxin 5 mcg/kg twice a day orally. In the presence of WPWS or pre-existing heart disease. digoxin alone may be unsuccessful but other drug such as propranolol, flecainide or amiodarone require specialist advice. Fetal SVT can be retreated by giving the mother digoxin or flecainide but again this requires specialist advice.

Synchronized DC cardioversion

- Always successful in converting SVT to sinus rhythm.
- Repeated use causes myocardial damage.
- SVT may recur unless regular antiarrhythmic therapy is started.
- Establish IV access and have facilities available for intubation and positive pressure ventilation.
- Sedate with IV midazolam.
- Give oxygen by face mask.
- Use Neonatal defibrillator paddles.
- Disconnect the ECG monitor from the infant.
- Apply one paddle to the apex of the heart and the other to the right sternal border and ensure there is no electrode gel bridging the gap between the 2 two paddles.
- Give an initial shock of 0.5–1 J/kg ensuring that the shock is synchronized.

Because it is almost always successful, DC cardioversion should be first line treatment in the very ill infant.

TABLE 5   Distinguishing tachyarrhythmias in Neonates and Infants

	Sinus tachycardia	SVT	Atrial flutter	VT
History	Sepsis, fever, hypovolemia etc.	Usually otherwise normal	Most have a normal heart	Many with abnormal heart
Rate	Almost always < 230 b/min	Most often 260-300 b/min	Atrial 300-500 b/min. Vent. 1:1 to 4:1 conduction	200-500 b/min
R-R interval variation	Over several seconds may get faster and slower	After first 10-20 beats. extremely regular	May have variable block (1:1, 2:1, 3:1) giving different ventricular rates	Slight variation over several beats
P wave axis	Same as sinus almost always visible P waves	60% visible P waves, P waves do not look like sinus P waves	Flutter waves (best seen in LII, LIII, aVF, V₁)	May have sinus P waves continuing unrelated to VT (AV dissociation), retrograde P waves, or no visible P waves
QRS	Almost always same as slower sinus rhythm	After first 10-20 beats; almost always same as sinus	Usually same as sinus, may have occasional beats different from sinus	Different from sinus (not necessarily 'wide')

SVT = Supraventricular tachycardia
VT = Ventricular tachycardia

Adapted from *European Heart Journal* (2002) **23,** 1329–1344 Guidelines for the interpretation of the Neonatal ECG, A Task Force of the European Society of Cardiology, P. J. Schwartz et al.

TABLE 6	Drugs used in the treatment of neonatal arrhythmias		
Medication (class)	**Oral dose**	**IV dose**	**Common adverse effects**
Adenosine		50 mcg/kg; may increase to 250 mcg/kg if no effect (IV push)	Hypotension, flushing, chest pain, heart block, Afib
Digoxin	*Load*: Preterm: 20mcg/kg in 3 doses; full-term: 30 mcg/kg in 3 doses *Maintenance*:Preterm: 5-7.5 mcg/kg div q12h; full-term: 6-10 mcg/kg div q12h	75%-80% oral dose *Load*: Preterm: 15mcg/kg in 3 doses; full term: 20 mcg/kg in 3 doses *Maintenance*:Preterm: 3-4 mcg/kg div q12h; full-term: 6-8 mcg/kg div q12h	AV, SA block, bradycardia, nausea/ vomiting, toxicity with hypocalcemia or K abnormality
Procainamide (IA)	15-50 mg/kg/day in 4-8 div doses	*Load*: 3-6 mg/kg/dose over 5 minutes; repeat dose over 10 minutes up to a maximum of 15 mg/kg. *Maintenance*: 20-80 mg/kg/min	Hypotension, AV block, nausea/ vomiting, lupus-like syndrome
Lidocaine (IB)		1 mg/kg/dose (bolus); 20-50 mcg/kg/min (infusion); decrease with hepatic or renal dysfunction	Hypotension, heart block, CNS effects, respiratory depression
Propranolol (II)	0.25 mg/kg/dose q6-8h, usual dosage range 2-4 mg/kg/day divided q6-q8h	0.01 mg/kg/over 10 min; repeat q6-8h, may increase slowly to 0.15 mg/kg/dose q6-8h	Hypotension, bradycardia, conduction block, hypoglycemia, bronchospasm, weakness
Amiodarone (III)	5 mg/kg q12h for 7 days, then 2-5 mg/kg/day; decreased with liver dysfunction	5 mg/kg/dose over 30 min; may repeat up to 15 mg/kg on day 1 *Maintenance*: 3-10 mg/kg/min	Thyroid/hepatic dysfunction, AV block, hypotension, corneal deposits, proarrhythmia

TABLE 7	Approach to ECG interpretation of an arrhythmia

QRS complexes	Rate	Slow/norm/fast	P waves	Seen/not seen	
	Rhythm	Regular/irregular		Rate	Slow/normal/fast
		If irregular: premature/ delayed		Rhythm	Regular/irregular
	Configuration	Normal/abnormal			If irregular:
					Premature/delayed
				Axis	Normal/abnormal
				Relationship to	None/constant/variable
				QRS complexes	If consult:
					before/within/after
					If before, PR interval:
					Normal/long
					Fixed/changing

KEY POINTS FOR CLINICAL PRACTICE

1. *Sinus tachycardia* (a heart rate >160bpm in term and>180bpm in preterm infants) is always secondary, usually to non-cardiac causes, such as fever, pain, respiratory failure, anemia, fluid overload, septicemia, and drugs(methyl xanthines and inotropes).Medical management consists of identifying and treating the underlying cause.

2. *Supraventricular tachycardia* SVT is the most common symptomatic arrhythmia in all children including Neonates. SVTs usually have a heart rate - >230bpm, "fixed" frequently with no beat-to-beat variation in rate, rapid onset and termination in 'reentrant' types,variable in duration and narrow QRS complexes on the ECG. If IV Adenosine fails to convert it to a sinus rhythm and the baby is collapsed, synchronized DC shock should be given. Digoxin should be given if heart failure is marked;Propranolol may be used instead, if heart failure is not present.

3. *In utero SVT* is confirmed by fetal echocardiography, and a search for CHD and fetal hydrops may be made. Maternal treatment with digoxin, flecainide etc., is successful; if not, in the presence of fetal hydrops, fetal SVT is an indication for cesarean section, as the fetal heart rate will not be a reliable indicator of fetal distress.

4. *Wide complex tachycardias like Ventricular tachycardia-VT and Ventricular fibrillation(very rare and preterminal)-VF* are rare in Neonates relatively, and are associated with severe systemic illnesses such as hypoxemia, shock, electrolyte disturbances, digoxin toxicity, and catecholamine toxicity. Once the infant has been resuscitated, the underlying problems should be evaluated and treated.

5. VT is potentially a unstable rhythm commonly with hemodynamic consequences. If unstable/VF occurs, full CPR, and DC cardioversion/ defibrillation(1–2J/kg to start with) should be instituted, to be followed by IVB Lidocaine 1-2 mg/kg, then to be followed by an IVI of Lidocaine 20-50 mcg/kg/min.Once the infant has been resuscitated, the underlying problems should be evaluated and treated.

REFERENCES AND FURTHER READING 1)Roberton's Text Book of Neonatology,4th Edition 2) Deal BJ, Keane JF, Gillette PC, *et al.* Wolff-Parkinson-White syndrome and supraventricular tachycardia during infancy:management and follow-up. *J Am Coll Cardiol* 1985;5:130–5. 3) Eronen M, Siren M, Ekblad H, *et al.* Short- and long-term outcome of children with congenital complete heart block diagnosed in utero or as a newborn. *Pediatrics* 2000;**106**:86–91.4) Van Hare GF: Indications for radiofrequency ablation in the Pediatric population. J Cardiovasc Electrophysiology 1997;8:952 5)Esberger SP:Junctional Tachycardia Br Med J 2002; 324:662–65.

Pearl/Peril/Pitfall: In approximately 50% of infants with congenital heart block, there is an associated cardiovascular malformation (e.g., l-transposition of the great arteries, heterotaxy syndrome, endocardial cushion defect). In the absence of structural heart disease, the heart block is usually related to maternal autoantibodies (anti- Ro and/or anti-La) that cross the placenta and interact with the developing conduction system . These antibodies are associated with maternal connective tissue disease, particularly lupus erythematosis and Sjögren syndrome. In newborns with heart block and no structural cardiac abnormalities, testing of their mothers for these antibodies is indicated because they may have no signs or symptoms of connective tissue disease.

Patent Ductus Arteriosus in a Preterm Infant

@ *"Ductus-dependent complex cardiac lesions should be ruled out before instituting duct closure therapy, for which PGE$_2$ IVI is necessary to maintain the ductus patent".*

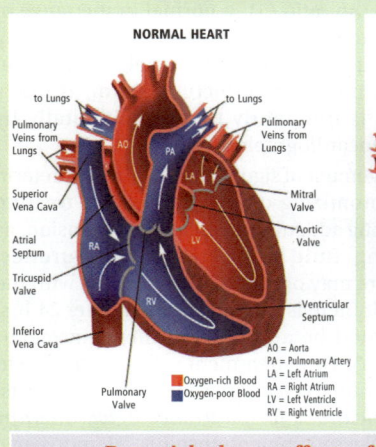

NORMAL HEART

to Lungs | to Lungs
Pulmonary Veins from Lungs | Pulmonary Veins from Lungs
Superior Vena Cava | Mitral Valve
| Aortic Valve
Atrial Septum |
Tricuspid Valve | Ventricular Septum
Inferior Vena Cava |
Pulmonary Valve

AO = Aorta
PA = Pulmonary Artery
LA = Left Atrium
RA = Right Atrium
LV = Left Ventricle
RV = Right Ventricle

■ Oxygen-rich Blood
■ Oxygen-poor Blood

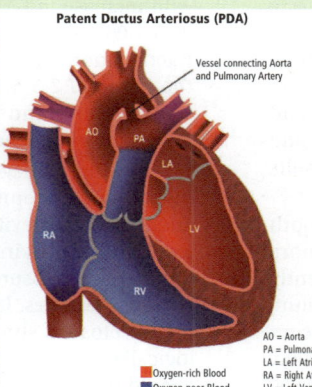

Patent Ductus Arteriosus (PDA)

Vessel connecting Aorta and Pulmonary Artery

AO = Aorta
PA = Pulmonary Artery
LA = Left Atrium
RA = Right Atrium
LV = Left Ventricle
RV = Right Ventricle

■ Oxygen-rich Blood
■ Oxygen-poor Blood
■ Mixed Blood

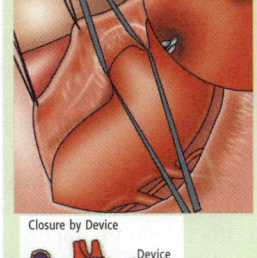

Closure by Device

Device

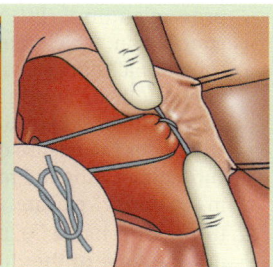

PDA Closure by Ligation/Occlusion by a Device.

Potential adverse effects of therapies for closing patent ductus arteriosus

Surgical Ligation
Atelectasis, Pulmonary Edema
LV Dysfunction, Hypotension
Intraventricular Hemorrhage
Pneumothorax
   Vocal cord/Diaphragm Palsy
Surgical site infection
   /Dehiscence
Chylothorax, Pleural effusion
Bleeding, Pulmonary
artery/Bronchus ligation,
Rib deformity, Scoliosis,
Increased risk of BPD and
Neurosensory impairment

Medical Closure
Oliguria, Fluid retention
Hyponatremia, Hyperkalemia
Hypoglycemia
Platelet Dysfunction,
Bleeding
Renal failure
Intestinal Perforation
Altered CBF Autoregulation
Sepsis?,
Respiratory
deterioration?
Increased risk
of BPD and
Neurosensory
impairment

PDA—SUMMARY—CONCLUSIONS

- Ligation, indomethacin, and ibuprofen are effective measures to achieve ductal closure (reducing rates of symptomatic PDA and ductal ligations)
- Prophylactic indomethacin reduces the incidence of severe IVH, but does not improve neurodevelopmental outcomes
- Interventions to close the ductus - prophylactically or for asymptomatic or symptomatic PDA - do not reduce the incidence of death, BPD, NEC or other morbidities
- Short-term benefits may be illusory or overestimated, so those who advocate treatment based on biological plausibility are wrong twice (false predicate, potentially dangerous conclusion)

REVIEW OF CLINICAL PROBLEMS

1. How do you recognize that a PDA is significant clinically and confirm it hemodynamically ?
   Ans: Refer to the "No. 3" and "No. 4" of the "BIRD'S EYE VIEW/ OVERVIEW/SYNOPSIS"of the Chapter.

2. Mention the duct-dependent complex cardiac malformations, where ductus should be treated with *PGE$_1$ IVI* to maintain its patency, until some palliative procedure will be planned.
   Ans: Refer to the " Table 1" of the Chapter.

3. What are the contraindications to start/discontinue Indomethacin therapy in treating sig.PDA ?
   Ans: Refer to the Evaluation-Decision-Action Plan/Algorithm to diagnose and manage a Neonate with PDA.

4. What are the indications for surgical closure of PDA?
   Ans: Refer to the"No. 9" of the "BIRD'S EYE VIEW/ OVERVIEW/SYNOPSIS"of the Chapter.

5. Describe the supportive measures that may help in the spontaneous closure of sig. PDA.
   Ans: Refer to the Evaluation-Decision-Action Plan/Algorithm to diagnose and manage a Neonate with PDA.

LEARNING OBJECTIVES

After completing this article, readers will be able to

1. Suspect PDA in preterm infants, especially those weighing <1,000 g or <28 wks' GA.

2. Diagnose clinically by the typical symptoms and signs of a clinically significant PDA.

3. Confirm the diagnosis of a PDA by the 2-D ECHO and COLOR DOPPLER study, preferably done by a Pediatric Cardiologist.

4. Refer those infants with significant PDA to a higher center, where facilities for pharmacotherapy and/or surgical closure are readily available.

5. Counsel the parents about the complications, and the cost factor involved, in case the surgical closure of a significant PDA is to be attempted after the failure of pharmacotherapy.

***Pearl/Peril/Pitfall** : Echocardiography is indicated in any child with unexplained congestive heart failure to assess cardiac function and identify potential cardiovascular causes, particularly anatomic lesions. On the other hand, congestive heart failure itself is not an echocardiographic diagnosis; therefore, the underlying etiology is best identified by means of detailed history taking and physical examination, and often chest radiography.*

BIRD`S EYE VIEW/OVERVIEW/SYNOPSIS

1. Patent Ductus Arteriosus (PDA) is a vital conduit in the fetal circulation and it diverts pulmonary blood flow toward the placenta when the lungs are nonfunctioning and pulmonary vascular resistance is high. Shortly after birth in full-term infants, an increase in arterial oxygen tension, drop in ductal blood pressure, and decrease in serum prostaglandin $E_2(PGE_2)$ produce ductal smooth muscle contraction, which limits ductal blood flow and produces "functional" duct closure. Because the ductal wall media is dependent on luminal oxygen delivery, local hypoxia develops. Local hypoxia causes smooth muscle death and stimulates the release of transforming growth factor b and subsequent intimal Proliferation, which ultimately results in "anatomic" closure.

2. In preterm babies <28 weeks' GA, the intrinsic smooth muscle tone of the ductus is decreased, and it is more sensitive to PGE_2. Thus, the immature ductus frequently fails to close functionally, which in turn may result in failure of anatomic closure. The incidence of clinically significant PDA in preterm infants varies from 7% (birth weight >1500g, or ≥ 33 weeks'GA) to 50% (birth weight <1000g, or 28 weeks' GA). The incidence of PDA also varies with the severity of RDS and is influenced by acute perinatal stress, hypoxia, acidosis, fluid therapy, surfactant therapy, and prenatal medication. During the acute stage of RDS, PGE levels are elevated, and this may influence ductal patency. With resolution of RDS, there is a reduction in pulmonary vascular resistance, a rise in pulmonary blood flow, and a congestive circulatory state. This may increase ventilatory requirements and increase the risk of developing CLD, NEC, and pulmonary hemorrhage. The current use of exogenous surfactant has caused the symptomatic PDA to present earlier than it did during the presurfactant era. Steroids decrease the sensitivity of the ductus to PGE; hence, prenatal administration of steroids decreases the incidence of PDA.

3. The PDA in preterm infants may be subclinical (no murmur) or clinical (murmur present), while clinical PDA may be nonsignificant (no cardiopulmonary dysfunction) or significant (with cardiopulmonary dysfunction). In the absence of a ductus murmur, a PDA can be diagnosed noninvasively only by Doppler echocardiography. A nonsignificant clinical PDA presents with only a heart murmur (at the left sternal border, second intercostal space), which is largely systolic, although it may continue into the diastolic phase. **Significant clinical PDA** *Precordial murmur (commonly purely systolic) in the pulmonary area *Hyperactive precordium *Bounding pulses *Widened pulse pressure (>25mm Hg) *Resting tachycardia *Frequent apnea *Carbon dioxide retention *Cardiomegaly on chest radiograph *Failure to wean off the ventilator at the expected time or unexplained deterioration of respiratory status. *Pulmonary plethora or congestion with cardiomegaly on chest radiograph.

4. **2-D ECHO and Color Doppler** is more sensitive and specific than clinical signs. The initial echocardiogram should be "complete"; that is, it should look for other cardiovascular anomalies that might influence management of the ductus. Examples of important coexisting anomalies include aortic coarctation, pulmonary hypertension, or complex "ductal dependent" cardiac lesions (Refer to Table 1 of the Chapter) *Ductus-dependent complex cardiac lesions should be ruled out before instituting duct closure therapy for which PGE_1*

IVI is necessary to maintain the ductus patent. Additional findings should be evaluated by a Pediatric cardiologist. More limited echocardiograms can be performed serially to assess for spontaneous closure or the results of pharmacologic treatment. Hemodynamically significant PDA shows chamber enlargement (left atrial enlargement with increase in LA/Ao ratio (>1.3; normal in the range of 0.66-1.06), high LV function index shown by LV shortening fraction; normal value 34 ±3% and the ductal size will be in the range of 2.5-5mm. A small ductus (<2mm) is rarely symptomatic and is frequently found incidentally by auscultation or echocardiography.

5. The first-line management of significant PDA in the preterm infant involves epitomizing oxygen delivery by treating anemia and achieving adequate arterial oxygen tension, as well as employing fluid restriction and diuretics. Spontaneous closure may occur in 25% of infants with the 1st line measures. If there is no improvement after 24 hrs, ductal closure should be attempted either pharmacologically or by surgery. Drug treatment with Indomethacin should be tried first unless a contraindication to it exists; *Relative contraindications for pharmacological therapy include-* * Shock *Necrotizing enterocolitis *Hemorrhagic disease *Thrombocytopenia (platelets <50,000/mm³) *Recent (<48 h) intraventricular hemorrhage *Renal impairment (blood urea >30 mg/dL creatinine >1.8mg/dL or persistent oliguria of <1ml/kg per h).

6. **Indomethacin** may be given as an IVI for 30-60 minutes either in conventional doses(0.2 mg/kg/dose at 0, 12, and 36 hours);this regimen may be repeated once *or* as a prolonged course administered as 0.1 mg/kg/dose once a day for 5 or 6 days.A 5-day course of Indomethacin has been shown to reduce relapse rate, and a 6-day lower dose course is associated with lower relapse rates and less biochemical disturbance.The success rates of Indomethacin varies with birth weight; the closure rate was 69% for infants with a weight of 470–1000 g and 83% for those with a weight of 1000–1500 g.In the smaller weight range, 27% of patients required 2 courses of therapy, whereas 13% required 2 courses in the greater weight range.

7. **Ibuprofen** in 3 doses of 10 mg/kg; 5 mg/kg and 5 mg/kg at an interval of 24 hrs each (IV preferably if available or Oral) has been shown to be as effective in closing a PDA as Indomethacin but with a better safety profile(more normal urine output, less elevation of BUN and creatinine,less decrease in mesenteric blood flow, and improved autoregulation of cerebral blood flow).

8. **The Evaluation-Decision-Action Plan/Algorithm** describes the essential aspects of the diagnosis and management of PDA in a Neonate.

9. **Surgical closure** is the best option for those symptomatic infants who do not respond to a 2nd treatment with Indomethacin or cannot tolerate it due to side effects. Surgical complications include;pneumothorax, pleural effusion-chylothorax, Horner syndrome, phrenic and recurrent laryngeal nerve injuries and inadvertent ligation of left pulmonary artery or transverse aortic arch.

10. **Full term infants and children with a PDA** are very unlikely to respond to pharmacologic methods of closure.Standard surgical occlusion with a ligature, clips, or both is achieved either with left lateral thoracotomy or with a Video-Assisted Thoracoscopy.

Pearl/Peril/Pitfall: Just prior to the 3rd indomethacin dose, obtain an echocardiogram. If there is echocardiographic evidence of patency of the ductus (even if there are no clinical signs), give 4th, 5th, and 6th doses of indomethacin (0.1 mg/kg at 24 h intervals). Repeat the echocardiogram after the 6th dose.

THE EVALUATION-DECISION-ACTION-PLAN / ALGORITHM FOR THE DIAGNOSIS AND MANAGEMENT OF *A NEONATE WITH PATENT DUCTUS ARTERIOSUS.*

SUBJECTIVE FINDINGS

Hx of apnea for unexpected reasons in a preterm baby recovering from RDS, increasing oxygen requirement/dependency, failure to wean off the ventilator.

Hx of incidental finding of a "murmur" in an asymptomatic preterm/term infant

Hx of associated factors such as hypoxia, acidosis, systemic hypotension, excessive fluid administration, sepsis, anemia, hypoalbuminemia, phototherapy

Hx of symptoms suggestive of NEC, Renal dysfunction, sepsis, IVH etc.,

OBJECTIVE FINDINGS

Assess ABCDs and monitor CRT, O_2 sats, BP, core-peripheral temperature difference, RR, HR, central and peripheral pulses, urine output.

Assess for bounding peripheral pulses, widened pulse pressure(>25 mm Hg), hyperdynamic precordium, a continuous or systolic murmur with or without extension into diastole or an apical diastolic murmur, multiple clicks resembling the shaking of dice.

Assess for signs of CHF such as cardiomegaly, hepatomegaly and pulmonary edema on CXR.

INVESTIGATIONS

Blood FBC, differential, *platelets*, *hematocrit,* Group and type and cross match, Smear, coagulation screen (PT, APTT, fibrinogen, thrombin time, bleeding time and clotting time), blood cultures, ABG analysis, *Blood sugar,* BUN, *creatinine,* electrolytes, Ca^{++} Mg^{++}, LTFs(including albumin). *Urine analysis and Intake-Output chart.*
Imaging CXR, plain abdominal x-ray, USG scan/CT scan of head, if IVH is suspected.
2-D ECHO and COLOR DOPPLER is mandatory to confirm and treat PDA and to exclude Duct-dependent complex cardiac malformations.

PRETERM INFANT WITH PATENT DUCTUS ARTERIOSUS

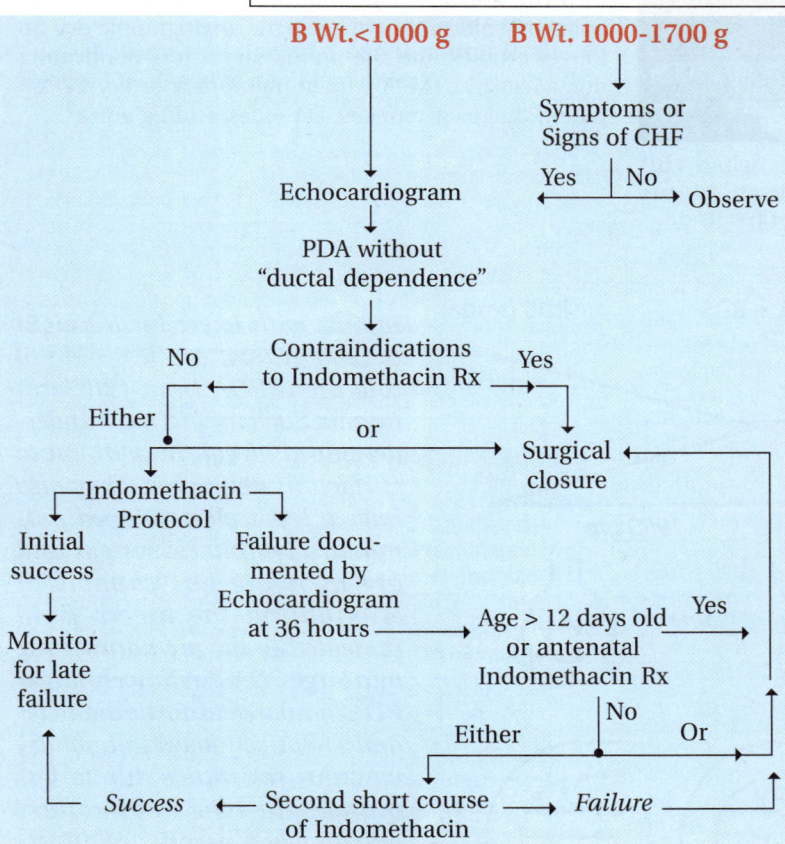

* *Monitor for* platelets, BUN, creatinine, electrolytes daily before initiating and during therapy with Indomethacin.

* *Monitor for* urine output- if at any time during therapy with Indomethacin the urine output drops to <0.5 ml/kg/hr, don`t administer the next dose and consider surgical closure of PDA.

* IV Indomethacin is administered in doses mentioned in the Table No 2 at 0, 12 and 36 hrs.

* *CONTRAINDICATIONS TO* Indomethacin Thrombocytopenia(<50,000/cu mm), bleeding disorders, oliguria(<1 ml/kg/hr), NEC, Isolated intestinal perforation and an elevated plasma creatinine(>1.8 mg/dL).

* *INDICATIONS FOR SURGICAL CLOSURE OF PDA:* Failure of/Contraindications to pharmacologic therapy.

* *ROLE OF FUROSEMIDE* Furosemide can prevent renal side effects of Indomethacin without reducing its efficacy. Monitor for electrolyte disturbances. Note that Furosemide also promotes ductal patency by stimulating renal PGE_2 production. It is the diuretic of choice during CHF state but use chlorthiazide 20 mg/kg/dose once or twice daily with amiloride 0.2 mg/kg, as Furosemide causes electrolyte disturbances and nephrocalcinosis.

* *ROLE OF DOPAMINE* Though it improves urine output, it does not affect or prevent a rise in plasma creatinine levels or the incidence of oliguria.

* Ibuprofen in 3 doses of 10 mg/kg; 5 mg/kg and 5 mg/kg at an interval of 24 hrs each (IV preferably if available or Oral) has been shown to be as effective in closing a PDA as Indomethacin without reducing cerebral, mesenteric, or renal blood flow velocity. Compared to Indomethacin, Ibuprofen reduces the risk of oliguria, but may increase the risk for CLD and pulmonary hypertension.

PDA : SUPPORTIVE MEASURES

A) *Intubate and ventilate,* for apnea and cardiorespiratory failure and pulmonary hemorrhage to maintain oxygenation and manage co_2 retention. B)*Restrict* fluids to about 80- 100 ml/kg/day and give Furosemide 1–2 mg/kg/dose once a day if there is evidence of fluid overload. Digitalis is not very useful because myocardial contractility is increased rather than reduced in infants with PDA. C)*Maintain* Hematocrit >40% in a ventilated baby and >35% in a non-ventilated baby. D)*Treat* sepsis with IV broadspectrum antibiotics. E)*Correct* thrombocytopenia, electrolyte imbalance and hypoalbuminemia. F) *Cover* the chest of the preterm infant <1000g during phototherapy, as light exposure relaxes the ductus and prevents PDA from closing.

---

* *Pearl/Peril/Pitfall :* Echocardiography Usually done at 3 days in infants <28 weeks' gestation or <1000g. ·Other babies are investigated on clinical suspicion. Rules out (most) congenital heart disease. ·It is important to rule out duct dependent lesions, especially coarctation. ·Pulmonary stenosis may be masked by a large PDA.

Echocardiography of the PDA : The ductus can be well visualized from the left parasternal area (A) with low velocity flow back into the pulmonary artery from the aorta (B). After therapy with indomethacin the PDA significantly decreases in size (C) with color Doppler flow in a smaller jet (D), and a high velocity, restrictive spectral Doppler pattern (E). (MPA = main pulmonary artery, RPA = right pulmonary artery, Ao = aorta, PDA = patent ductus arteriosus, DA = descending aorta, LPA = left pulmonary artery).

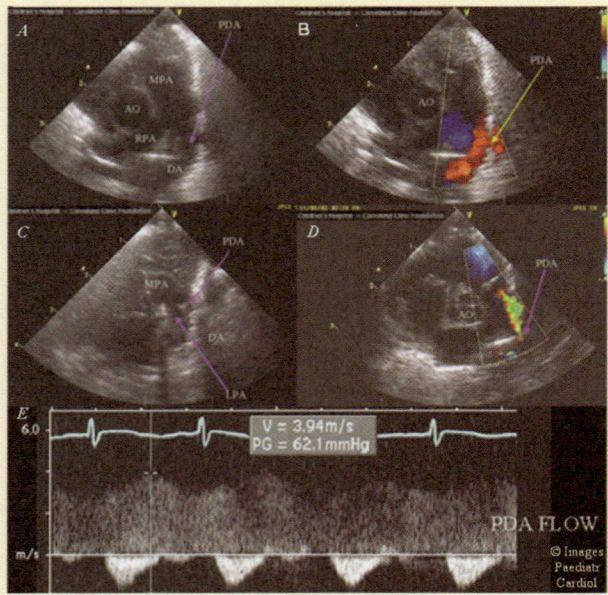

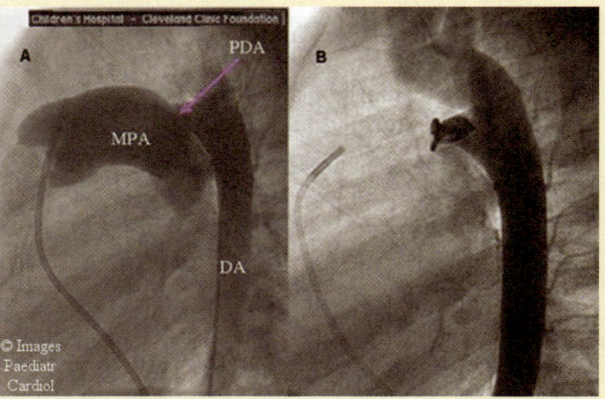

Closure of a PDA by coil catheterization (A) Injection into the aorta reveals a large PDA at baseline. (B) Following placement of a coil the angiographic dye no longer crosses into the pulmonary artery confirming ductal closure. (MPA = main pulmonary artery, PDA = patent ductus arteriosus, DA = descending aorta)

Courtesy: Mehta SK, Younoszai A, Pietz J, Achanti BP. Pharmacological closure of the patent ductus arteriosus. Images Paediatr Cardiol 2003;14:1-15

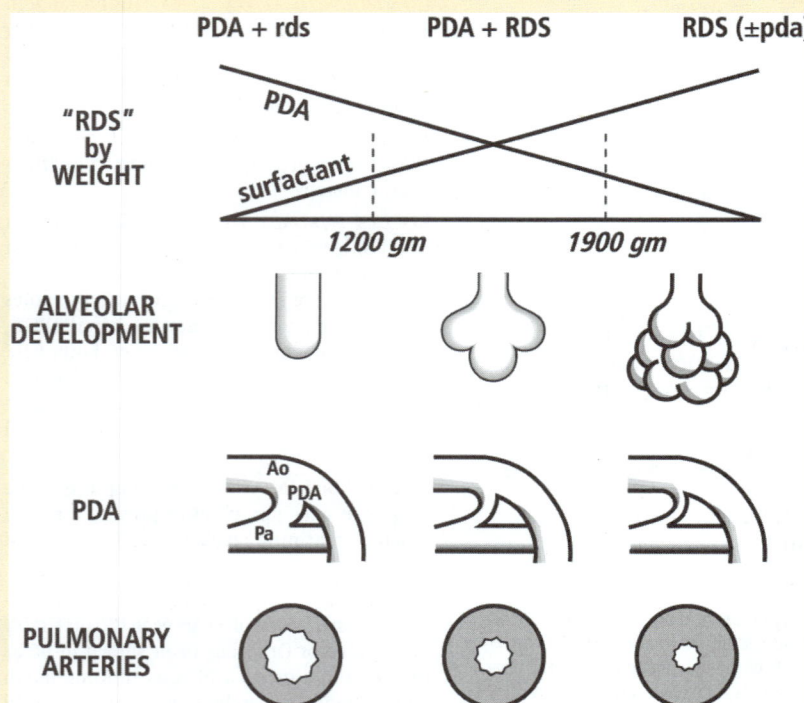

Infants with lower birth weight (<1200 grams) are less able to tolerate a PDA than full term infants. Such infants have underdeveloped alveoli in addition to surfactant deficiency. They also have a less well developed pulmonary lymphatic system and are therefore less capable of eliminating the excess fluid presented to the premature lung by a large PDA. A relatively larger PDA compared to aortic diameter and a relatively lower pulmonary vascular resistance due to less muscle in the pulmonary vascular bed permits relatively larger pulmonary blood flow. This also steals significant blood flow from vessels distal to the duct such as the gut.

Pearl/Peril/Pitfall: Management During Indomethacin Treatment: Because indomethacin decreases gastrointestinal blood flow, infants should be kept NPO until at least 48 h after the indomethacin therapy has been completed. Because indomethacin may cause a transient decrease of urine output (similar to excessive ADH action), IV fluids should be adjusted every 8–24 h, taking into consideration not only fluid intake in mL/kg, but more importantly, the relationship between urine output and fluid intake. An acceptable output to intake ratio in these circumstances is between 0.3 and 0.7, taking the infant's anticipated weight change into consideration. A decrease in serum Na+ should prompt additional fluid restriction because of retention of free water with indomethacin administration.

TABLE 1   Presentations of ductal dependent congenital heart disease

Cyanosis	Shock with congestive Heart Failure	Shock without congestive Heart Failure
Pulmonary atresia	Aortic atresia	Coarctation
Critical pulmonary stenosis	Mitral atresia	Interrupted arch
Tetralogy of Fallot	HLHS	
Tricuspid atresia		
Transposition of the great vessels		

Congenital heart defects that result in ↓↓blood flow to the lungs or systemic blood flow are dependent on the pulmonary-systemic shunt from the patent ductus arteriosus to maintain pulmonary and systemic blood flow. Closure of the ductus arteriosus causes marked worsening of obstruction to pulmonary blood flow with right to left shunt and cyanosis in right-sided congenital lesions and decreased systemic blood flow with shock in left sided obstructive lesions. Obstructive right heart lesions-*Pulmonary atresia *Pulmonary stenosis *Tricuspid atresia *Tetralogy of Fallot Obstructive left heart lesions-*Aortic stenosis *Severe coarctation of the aorta *hypoplastic left heart syndrome *Mixed lesion - D - TGV without VSD or ASD.

TABLE 2   Indomethacin therapy for patent ductus arteriosus

AGE AT FIRST DOSE	Dose (mg/kg IV)		
	Ist	2nd	3rd
< 48 hr	0.2	0.1	0.1
2-7 days	0.2	0.2	0.2
>7days	0.2	0.25	0.25

TABLE 3   PDA—Preventive measures

1. Antenatal Steroids reduces the incidence and severity of clinically significant PDA.
2. In view of the current concerns about postnatal dexamethasone therapy and adverse neurodevelopmental outcome, it cannot be recommended.
3. Fluid restriction (<140 ml/kg/day) during the first week of life reduces the incidence of clinically significant PDA.
4. Inappropriate use of plasma expanders for hypotension may predispose to the development of a clinically significant PDA.
5. Prophylactic Indomethacin therapy decreases the incidence of clinically significant PDA without convincingly improving morbidity and mortality, and is therefore *not generally* recommended. 6)Prophylactic ductal ligation in infants <1,000 g does not reduce mortality or morbidity(apart from decreasing the incidence of NEC) would result in surgery being performed in many infants who do not require it.

KEY POINTS FOR CLINICAL PRACTICE

1. The frequency that a premature infant will develop a hemodynamically significant left-to-right shunt through a PDA is inversely proportional to advancing age and birth weight.

2. The clinical consequences of PDA are related to the degree of left-to-right shunting with its associated increase in blood flow to the lungs (CHF, and pulmonary hemorrhage) and decrease in blood flow to the kidneys(oliguria) and intestines(NEC).

3. 2-D ECHO and Color Doppler should be performed by a pediatric cardiologist preferably, to confirm the presence and severity of PDA as well as to exclude the duct-dependent complex cardiac malformations, before initiating PDA closure with pharmacologic therapy.

4. Prophylactic Indomethacin therapy is recommended in babies <1,000 g, when their PDA first becomes apparent, regardless of the presence of symptoms or signs of a significant left-to-right shunt. For infants weighing >1000g, Indomethacin is to be tried only after cardio-respiratory symptoms and signs of a hemodynamically significant PDA develops.

5. Surgical closure is *indicated for* a)those infants who fail to respond to Indomethacin /Ibuprofen therapy (i.e. after 2 successive courses of 3–4 days apart in infants >1,000 g, 3–4 days apart, or after one course in infants of birth weight <1,000g), b)infants showing strong contra-indications or side effects to Indomethacin/Ibuprofen, c) infants <1,000g with a large, clinically significant PDA,without attempting any pharmacologic therapy.

REFERENCES and FURTHER READING 1)Treatment of Patent Ductus Arteriosus in the Preterm Infant: What is the Evidence? William E. Benitz, M.D. Division of Neonatal and Developmental Medicine Stanford University School of Medicine Lucile Packard Children's Hospital 2)Gellis and Kagan`s Current Pediatric Therapy, 17th edition. 3)Nelson Text Book of Pediatrics, 18th edition 4)Manual of Neonatal Care, John P. Cloherty, 6th edition. 5)Knight DB Treatment of PDA in Preterm infants Seminars in Neonatology 2001 6;63–73.

*Pearl/Peril/Pitfall: Fluid restriction *While on indomethacin, reduce by 20-40ml/kg/day. *There is no evidence that fluid restriction per se results in closure of the duct but there are studies suggesting that early, liberal fluid intakes are associated with a higher incidence of PDA.*

50 Neonatal Systemic Hypertension

@ *Hypertension in newborn infants primarily is of renal origin, although cardiac, endocrine, and pulmonary causes have been described as well. Therefore, the pathophysiology depends on the organ system involved. For example, hypertension related to renal emboli primarily is a high renin form of hypertension, whereas the hypertension associated with bronchopulmonary dysplasia (BPD) is likely related to hypoxia. Such differences in pathophysiology are very important because they can guide the clinician with respect to evaluation and treatment.*

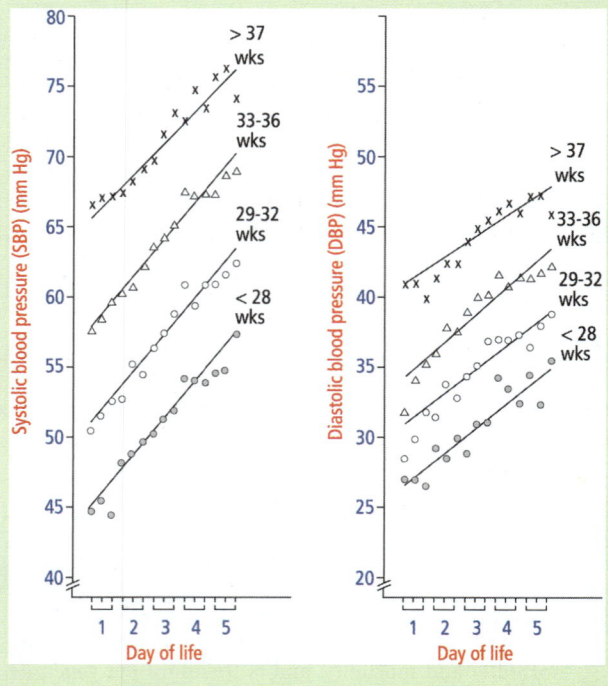

How BP to be measured ?

- Upper extremity preferred.
- First apply cuff, then wait 5 min before taking BP measurements.
- If "elevated", i.e SBP > 95% for PCA, repeat Q1H × 3. Use same extremity as the initial measurement.
- **Infant must be in resting state, in between feeds, prone position preferred**—Cuff must fit **2/3 of the length** of the ARM, and the inflating portion of the cuff must encircle at least 75% of the width of the arm.

Measurements

- 3 consecutive measures at least an hour apart.
- If **2/3** of measurements are >95% for age, then consider as hypertension, and proceed with initiation of diagnostic work-up, NOT necessarily treatment.
- **Source**: Is this an arterial BP or oscillatory BP measurement? Are the 2 sources concordant if available?

Hypertensive crisis

- Defined as a "sustained" systolic blood pressure > 25-30mm Hg above the 95% for Post conceptional age.
- Repeat blood pressure within 15 minutes from the initial measurement. If values are consistent, then **must** initiate diagnostic workup **and** treatment.
- NEED confirmation and monitoring via arterial access or Doppler.

While receiving treatment:

Labs: Creatinine, electrolytes every 2 weeks, **Imaging:** Echocardiogram (baseline ventricular size and function). **Other studies:** Ophthalmologic evaluation for hypertensive retinopathy. **Consults:** Cardiology, renal and ophthalmology. Urology if needed.

REVIEW OF CLINICAL PROBLEMS

1. Name the categories of Neonates, that require direct Invasive Arterial pressure monitoring.
   Ans: Refer to the"No.3" of the ''BIRD`S EYE VIEW/ OVERVIEW/SYNOPSIS" of the Chapter.
2. Mention the common symptoms and signs of Neonatal Hypertension.
   Ans: Refer to the"No.5" of the ''BIRD'S EYE VIEW/ OVERVIEW/ SYNOPSIS" of the Chapter.
3. What are the investigations to be done to determine the treatable causes of Neonatal Hypertension?
   Ans: Refer to the Evaluation-Decision-Action Plan/ Algorithm to diagnose and manage Neonatal Hypertension.
4. How do you evaluate Neonatal Hypertension?
   Ans: Refer to the Evaluation-Decision-Action Plan/ Algorithm to diagnose and manage Neonatal Hypertension.
5. Discuss the prognosis of Neonatal Hypertension.
   Ans: Refer to the Section "Neonatal hypertension: prognosis".

LEARNING OBJECTIVES

After completing this article, readers will be able to

1. Monitor High-Risk Sick Neonates for the presence of Hypertension.
2. Recognize the underlying causes of Neonatal Hypertension,(especially Renal/Endocrine/ Cardiac).
3. Treat the treatable causes of neonatal Hypertension, such as drugs (dexamethasone and aminophylline, high doses of adrenergic agents, prolonged use of pancuronium, or administration of phenylephrine ophthalmic drops, Thrombosed UAC, etc.)
4. Explain prognosis to the parents.
5. Organize The Outpatient Follow-up care for long-term sequelae of Neonatal Hypertension.

Pearl/Peril/Pitfall: *BP in newborns depends on various factors, including gestational age, postnatal age, and birth weight. Hypertension can be observed in various situations in the modern NICU and is especially common in infants who have undergone umbilical arterial catheterization. A careful diagnostic evaluation should lead to determination of the underlying cause of hypertension in most infants. Tailor treatment decisions, which may include intravenous therapy, oral therapy, or both, to the severity of the hypertension. Hypertension resolves in most infants over time, although a small number of infants may have persistent BP elevation throughout childhood.*

BIRD'S EYE VIEW/OVERVIEW/SYNOPSIS

1. Neonatal Hypertension remains arbitrarily defined as systolic blood pressure more than 90 mm Hg and diastolic blood pressure more than 60 mm Hg in the full-term Newborn and systolic blood pressure more than 80 mm Hg and diastolic blood pressure more than 50 mm Hg in the preterm infant. In the ELBW infant (birth weight < 1,000 gm), however, even the arbitrary limits of hypertension are not agreed on. Mean blood pressure increases with postnatal age by 1-2 mm Hg/day during the first week and by approximately 1 mm Hg per week during the first 6 weeks of life. Systolic blood pressure in Newborn infants usually stabilizes at a mean of 92 mm Hg (95% confidence interval 72-112) at a postconceptional age of 44-48 weeks, irrespective of gestation at birth. *As a very rough guide, mean BP should be at least equal to the baby's, gestation in weeks. The lower limit of normal systolic BP in mm Hg on the first day = (7.5 X birth weight in kg) + 30. The lower limit of normal diastolic BP in mm Hg on the first day = (5 X birth weight in kg) + 10.*

2. Hypertension is quite unusual in healthy term infants. The most common causes of hypertension seen in Neonatal intensive care units are thrombosis of renal artery due to umbilical arterial catheterization, chronic lung disease, ECMO, and Coarctation of aorta. The actual incidence of hypertension in Neonates ranges from 0.7%–3.2%. Automatic oscillometry is the most commonly used noninvasive technique that provides an accurate, reproducible, and convenient estimate of blood pressure (including the mean blood pressure) in most Newborns, provided that the approximate size cuff is used with a cuff width - to - arm circumference ratio of 0.44 to 0.55. In VLBW Newborns as well as in cases of extreme hypotension, some inaccuracy is possible. To minimize errors it is better to follow the suggested guidelines: **a)** Obtain an average of 3 measurements **b)** Obtain BP measurements during quite or sleep state **c)** Use of mean BP to monitor BP changes .

3. Direct arterial BP monitoring (invasive) is the 'gold standard' but can only be justified in ill infants. It should be used in all children who have an indwelling arterial catheter already in situ for measurement of ABGs. It should be considered in the following categories: * infants in the acute phase of RDS and requiring ventilation * an infant in whom indirect methods of BP measurements suggest significant hypo- or hypertension *any infant on inotropic drugs to support the circulation.

4. BP is usually recorded in the right arm. *However, if any discrepancy exists between the arm pulses or between arm and leg pulses, BP should be recorded in all four limbs.* The doppler ultrasound method is reliable for measurement of systolic values, but it can not accurately detect the diastolic blood pressure. The traditional methods using auscultation, palpation, or the flush technique are insensitive, especially when the stroke volume is low.

5. Approximately 1/3rd of patients with Neonatal hypertension remain asymptomatic. In those who develop clinical signs, the findings are rather nonspecific, and the presence or severity of the signs and symptoms is not related to the magnitude of the blood pressure elevation. They may present with signs of CVS dysfunction (congestive cardiac failure, decreased or unequal pulses, cardiomegaly, hepatomegaly, vasomotor instability), respiratory system (tachypnea, cyanosis), CNS dysfunction (tremors, seizures, lethargy, coma, apnea, abnormal muscle tone, opisthotonus, asymmetrical reflexes, facial palsy, hypertensive retinopathy, cerebral edema, and hemorrhage), and the kidneys (dehydration, sodium wasting, oliguria/anuria, renal enlargement). Abdominal distention, edema, fever, and failure to thrive may occur. Approximately 50% of the Newborns with hypertension exhibit signs of hypertensive retinopathy, including a decreased ratio of the arterial to venous caliber, vascular tortuosity, and exudate formation.

6. *The E-D-A Plan/Algorithm* summarizes the essential aspects of history taking, physical examination, relevant investigations to diagnose the Neonatal hypertension. If the clinical or laboratory findings indicate, further studies may be warranted to rule out other, less frequent conditions associated with Neonatal hypertension, including endocrine disorders and pheochromocytoma.

7. In asymptomatic Newborns, with only mild to moderate elevation of blood pressure and without an identified cause, close observation, with no aggressive anti-hypertensive treatment, is recommended, unless clinical or echocardiographic evidence of hypertension develops.

8. The definitive therapy of Neonatal hypertension is to treat the primary cause whenever possible (e.g., removal of the umbilical catheter, discontinuation of an offending medication). In asymptomatic Newborns with severe hypertension and in all symptomatic Newborns even with only mild to moderate blood pressure elevation, treatment of the hypertension with antihypertensive agents is the presently accepted clinical practice *Refer to the Table 3.*

9. Mild hypertension may respond to diuretic therapy using furosemide or thiazide diuretic with or without spironolactone. In the long-term diuretic treatment of Neonatal hypertension, thiazide diuretics are preferred over furosemide because of long-term furosemide treatment is associated with potentially detrimental side effects, including severe electrolyte imbalance resulting in failure to thrive, calciuria, nephrocalcinosis, and osteopenia. For moderate to severe hypertension Hydralazine alone are in combination with a b-blocker (propranolol) can be tried. Captopril should not be used in the Newborn except with expert advice as there may be rapid deterioration in renal function.

10. Significant (BP consistently > 97th centile) symptomatic hypertension in the Newborn may be treated initially with IV agents and direct IA BP monitoring. These infants usually present with either cardiac failure or seizures. Asymptomatic hypertension can be treated orally. Aim to reduce systolic and diastolic BP to less than the 95th centile for weight and postnatal age. Aim for one third of the desired BP reduction in not less than the first 6 h; remaining two thirds over the next 24 h. All the drugs in Table 3 may cause relative or absolute hypotension, which is as dangerous as hypertension. Patients discharged on anti-hypertensives: Renal outpatient follow-up. Consider cardiology outpatient follow-up if patient has BPD, is being discharged home on oxygen AND being treated for HTN. Consider ophthalmologic follow-up.

Pearl/Peril/Pitfall : *For infants with extremely severe blood pressure (BP) elevation, angiography may be necessary. Although some investigators have used aortography via the umbilical artery catheter, formal renal arteriography using the traditional femoral vascular approach is much more accurate for diagnosing renal arterial stenosis, primarily because of the high incidence of intrarenal branch vessel abnormalities observed in children with fibromuscular dysplasia (FMD). Depending on the expertise available, this may need to be deferred until the infant is larger.*

THE EVALUATION-DECISION-ACTION-PLAN/ALGORITHM FOR THE DIAGNOSIS AND MANAGEMENT OF *HYPERTENSION IN THE NEWBORN*

SUBJECTIVE FINDINGS

Hx of non specific symptoms such as feeding difficulties, irritability or lethargy, asymptomatic and detected on routine monitoring of vital signs. *Hx of* symptoms suggestive of congestive cardiac failure or cardiogenic shock. *Hx of* CNS symptoms such as seizures, apnea or coma. Is **drug withdrawal** (illicit AND/OR iatrogenic drugs) a possibility? Were recent **boluses** of fluid, blood products administered? *Hx of* exposure to medications (steroids), inadvertent overdose of Dopamine/ Dobutamine, UA catheterization with thrombosis, excessive administration of salt or water. *Hx of* any symptoms suggestive of other systemic causes of hypertension in the Neonate (*Refer to Table 2*). Review medical diagnoses: SGA infant, BPD, IVH, ROP, history of renal dysfunction, history of/or current umbilical artery line, history of pneumothorax, PDA.

OBJECTIVE FINDINGS

Assess ABCs, O_2 sats, Vitals, BP, CRT, disability, AF, and Urine output.

Assess BP (by automatic oscillometry-dinamap) in all 4 limbs to rule out coarctation of aorta and look for ambiguous genitalia (CAH with hypertension), source of pain/ discomfort

Perform careful cardiac and abdominal examination for heart murmur, flank mass, epigastric bruit etc.

Remember that approximately 1/3rd of Neonates with hypertension remain asymptomatic.

Perform fundus examination as 50% of Newborns with hypertension exhibit signs of hypertensive retinopathy.

INVESTIGATIONS

Blood FBC with hematocrit, platelets, differential count, ABG analysis, blood sugar, electrolytes, albumin, creatinine, BUN, Ca^{++}, Phosphorus. Consider 17-OH progesterone, aldosterone, cortisol, $plasma renin activity, TFTs, in selected cases.

Urine Urine analysis for blood, protein, microscopy for cells and casts, culture and consider VMA: Creatinine and HVA: Creatinine ratios (send spot sample followed by 6-24hr timed collection). Save frozen urine for steroid profile.Urine toxicology screen if soon after birth.

IMAGING: CXR, ECG, Echocardiogram and Renal Ultrasound Consider doppler flow studies of aortic, renal artery and renal vein blood flow, arteriography if renal vascular disease is suspected.

Consider Investigations such as MCUG, DTPA, MAG-3 and DMSA if a renal cause is suspected.

Evaluate for the possibility of a tumour, if there is a palpable renal mass.

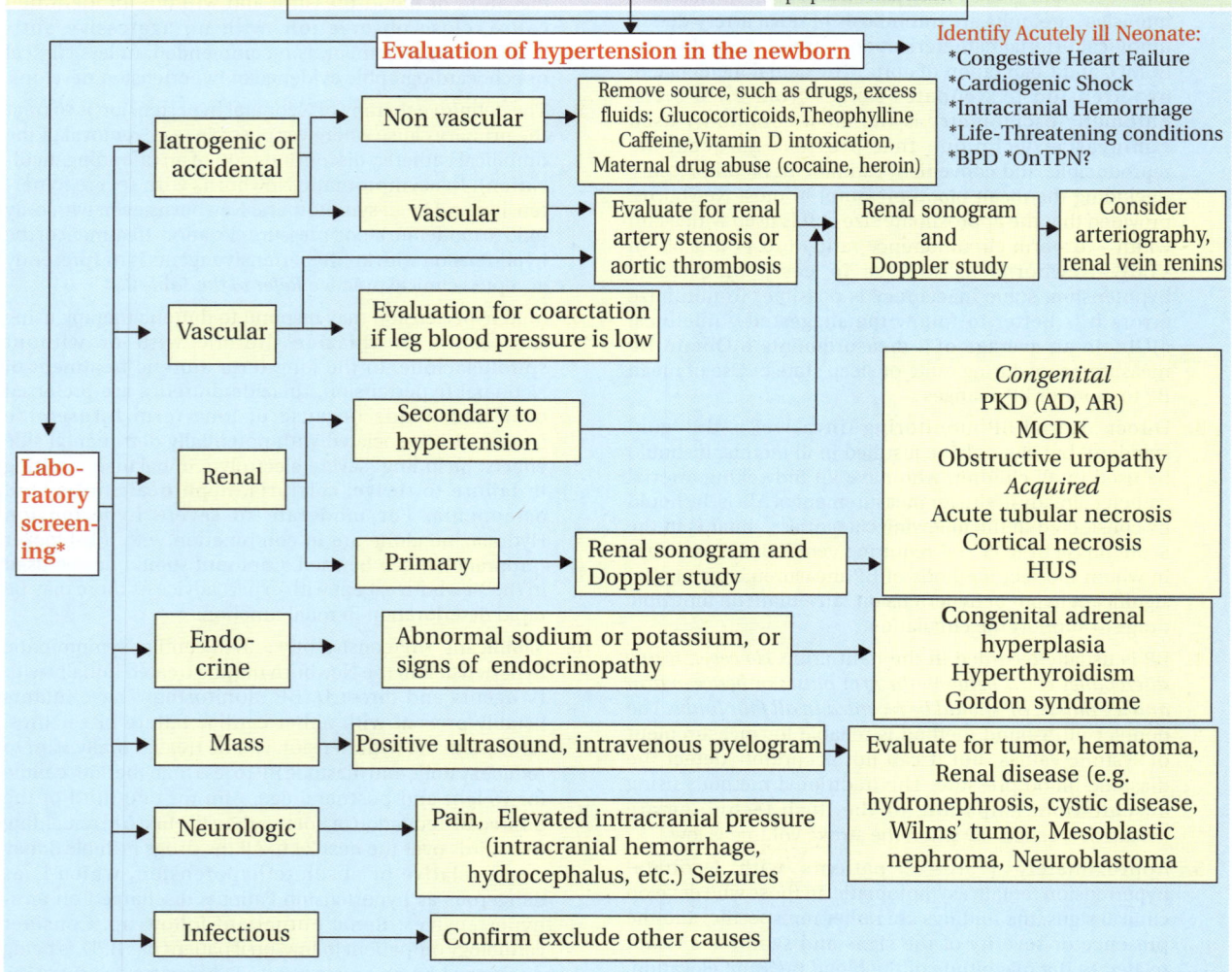

Evaluation of hypertension in the newborn

Identify Acutely ill Neonate:
*Congestive Heart Failure
*Cardiogenic Shock
*Intracranial Hemorrhage
*Life-Threatening conditions
*BPD *OnTPN?

Iatrogenic or accidental
- **Non vascular** → Remove source, such as drugs, excess fluids: Glucocorticoids,Theophylline Caffeine,Vitamin D intoxication, Maternal drug abuse (cocaine, heroin)
- **Vascular** → Evaluate for renal artery stenosis or aortic thrombosis → Renal sonogram and Doppler study → Consider arteriography, renal vein renins

Vascular → Evaluation for coarctation if leg blood pressure is low

Laboratory screening*

Renal
- **Secondary to hypertension** → *Congenital* PKD (AD, AR) MCDK Obstructive uropathy *Acquired* Acute tubular necrosis Cortical necrosis HUS
- **Primary** → Renal sonogram and Doppler study

Endocrine → Abnormal sodium or potassium, or signs of endocrinopathy → Congenital adrenal hyperplasia Hyperthyroidism Gordon syndrome

Mass → Positive ultrasound, intravenous pyelogram → Evaluate for tumor, hematoma, Renal disease (e.g. hydronephrosis, cystic disease, Wilms' tumor, Mesoblastic nephroma, Neuroblastoma

Neurologic → Pain, Elevated intracranial pressure (intracranial hemorrhage, hydrocephalus, etc.) Seizures

Infectious → Confirm exclude other causes

* Urinalysis, urine culture, blood urea nitrogen, creatinine, electrolytes, carbon dioxide, plasma renin activity
$ Proposed renin ranges in non-hypertensive children 0–12 month: 15 or less (ng/ml/hr)

Pearl/Peril/Pitfall: Measurement of plasma renin activity (PRA) is usually recommended as part of the laboratory assessment in newborns with hypertension, although elevated peripheral renin levels may not signify the presence of underlying pathology because renin values are typically high in infancy. In addition, plasma renin levels may be falsely elevated by medications that are commonly used in the neonatal ICU (NICU), such as aminophylline. Furthermore, many laboratories have switched from measurement of PRA to the direct renin assay, which is easier to perform. However, normative values for the direct renin assay in neonates are not widely available. Keep these factors in mind when interpreting renin values.

Neonatal Hypertension-Prognosis *The long-term prognosis for most infants with hypertension is quite good. For infants with hypertension related to an umbilical arterial catheter, the hypertension usually resolves over time. These infants may require increases in their antihypertensive medications in the first several months following discharge from the nursery as they undergo rapid growth. Following this, weaning the patient off antihypertensive therapy is usually possible by making no further dose increases as the infant continues to grow. Home BP monitoring by the parents is a crucially important component of this process. Provide proper equipment, either a Doppler or oscillometric device, for all infants discharged from the NICU on long-term antihypertensive medications. Such infants may benefit from referral to a comprehensive pediatric hypertension clinic if their primary care provider is inexperienced in managing hypertension. *Other forms of Neonatal hypertension may persist beyond infancy. In particular, polycystic kidney disease (PKD) and other forms of renal parenchymal disease may continue to cause hypertension throughout childhood. Infants with renal venous thrombosis (RVT) may also remain hypertensive, and some of these children ultimately benefit from nephrectomy. Persistent or recurrent hypertension may also be observed in children who have undergone repair of renal arterial stenosis or coarctation of the aorta. Reappearance of hypertension in these situations should prompt a search for restenosis using the appropriate imaging studies. *BP in newborns depends on various factors, including gestational age, postnatal age, and birth weight. Hypertension can be observed in various situations in the modern NICU and is especially common in infants who have undergone umbilical arterial catheterization. A careful diagnostic evaluation should lead to determination of the underlying cause of hypertension in most infants. Tailor treatment decisions, which may include intravenous therapy, oral therapy, or both, to the severity of the hypertension. Hypertension resolves in most infants over time, although a small number of infants may have persistent BP elevation throughout childhood. The received wisdom is that an asymptomatic neonate with a systolic pressure consistently between the 95th and 99th centiles and with no end organ involvement should be observed but not treated, in the expectation that the hypertension will settle.

Surgical care: Surgery is rarely indicated for treatment of Neonatal hypertension, except for specific diagnoses, such as ureteral obstruction, aortic coarctation, or certain tumors. Unilateral renal venous thrombosis (RVT) is commonly treated with nephrectomy to avoid the need for long-term drug therapy. For infants with renal arterial stenosis, managing the infant medically may be necessary until growth is sufficient to undergo definitive repair of the vascular abnormalities. Infants with malignant hypertension secondary to polycystic kidney disease (PKD) may require bilateral nephrectomy. Fortunately, such severely affected infants are quite rare.

TABLE 1	Systolic blood pressure in preterm infants with birth weight <1500 g during the first week of life		
Age	**n**	**Systolic Blood Pressure (mmHg)**	**+ 2 SD* (mmHg)**
1	44	39.2 ± 7.6	54.4
2	37	45.3 ± 7.8	60.9
3	33	45.2 ± 7.8	60.8
4	27	46.0 ± 8.9	63.8
5	23	46.0 ± 8.7	63.4
6	22	47.5 ± 9.9	67.3
7	19	51.1 ± 9.9	70.9

Educate the parents of infants who develop hypertension requiring drug therapy about the expected effects and side effects of their infant's antihypertensive medications. In addition, arrange home BP monitoring equipment and educate the parents in its use prior to the infant's discharge from the NICU. Parents must monitor the BP of all infants discharged on antihypertensive medications on a regular basis (i.e. usually daily); parents should call the prescribing clinician if the infant's BP exceeds or falls below the target range.

TABLE 2   Causes of neonatal hypertension

Vascular
Renal artery thrombosis
Aortic thrombosis
Coarctation of the aorta
Hypoplastic aorta
Renal vein thrombosis
Thrombosis of the ductus arteriosus
Renal artery stenosis/intimal hyperplasia
Idiopathic arterial calcification

Renoparenchymal
Acute renal failure
Polycystic kidney disease
Renal cortical and medullary necrosis
Hypoplastic, dysplastic kidney
Acute renal infection
Pyelonephritis with scarring
Obstructive uropathy
Constrictive perirenal hematoma or urinoma
Congenital mesoblastic nephroma
Nephrolithiasis
Following pyeloplasty of a hydronephrotic kidney
Multicystic kidney

Endocrine
Pheochromocytoma
Neuroblastoma
Adrenal disorders (hyperplasia, hyperaldosteronism, carcinoma, hematoma)
Hyperthyroidism

Other
Drugs (corticosteroids, theophylline, pancuronium, intrauterine cocaine exposure, phenylephrine eye drops)
Extracorporeal membrane oxygenation (ECMO)
TPN
Bronchopulmonary dysplasia (BPD)
Increased intracranial pressure/ seizures
Fluid and electrolyte overload
Following closure of an abdominal wall defect

Diet A low-sodium diet may assist in treatment of infants with persistent hypertension; however, because most infant formula is relatively low in sodium content, no special dietary modifications are usually necessary in the neonatal period. Currently available **drugs** for continuous infusion include sodium nitroprusside, labetalol, esmolol, fenoldopam and nicardipine. Nicardipine,(1-5 mcg/kg/min IV constant infusion) which is a dihydropyridine calcium channel blocker, has been reported to be effective most often in neonates and appears to have some advantages compared with older drugs that may make it the drug of choice in this population. Regardless of the drug chosen, continuously monitor BP via an indwelling arterial catheter or by frequently repeated (every 10–15 min) cuff readings so that the rate of infusion can be titrated to achieve the desired degree of BP control.

Pearl/Peril/Pitfall : Assess the clinical status of the infant and correct any easily correctable iatrogenic causes of hypertension (eg, infusions of inotropic agents, volume overload, pain) prior to instituting drug therapy. Next, choose an antihypertensive agent that is most appropriate for the specific clinical situation.

TABLE 3   Antihypertensive agents used in the treatment of hypertension in newborn

Medication Diuretics	Route	Dose	Comments
Furosemide	IV, oral (q8h, q12h, q24h)	1–2mg/kg/dose	Hyponatremia, hypokalemia, hypochloremia, hypercalciuria, nephrocalcinosis, osteopenia, ototoxicity, growth retardation
Chlorothiazide	IV, oral	5–50 mg/kg/day (q12h)	Hyponatremia, hypokalemia, hypochloremia, calcium sparing
Spironolactone	Oral	1–3 mg/kg/day	Weak diuretic, hyperkalemia
Adrenergic blockers			
Beta-adrenergic blockers			
Propranolol	Oral	0.5–2 mg/kg/day	Precipitation of heart failure, bronchospasm, hypoglycemia, decreased renin release, recommended in combination with hydralazine
Alpha1/beta-adrenergic blockers			
Labetalol	IV	0.25–1 mg/kg/hr	Limited experience in neonatal hypertensive emergencies
Vasodilators			
Hydralazine[A]	IV	0.1-2 mg/kg/dose (q6–12h)	Reflex tachycardia, paroxysmal atrial tachycardia, emesis, diarrhea, positive ANA assay (SLE-like syndrome)
	Oral	0.25–1 mg/kg/dose (q6–12h)	
Diazoxide[A]	IV	1–3 mg/kg/dose	Hypotension, hyperglycemia, sodium and water retention
Nitroprusside[A]	IV	0.2–10 mcg/kg/min	Thiocyanate and cyanide toxicity, methemoglobinemia; drug must be protected from light due to increased photochemical degradation
Angiotensin—Converting Enzyme Inhibitors			
Captopril	Oral	10–50 mcg/kg/dose (q8-24h) May titrate to 0.5 mg/kg/dose	Oliguria, renal failure, hyperkalemia, apnea, seizures, cough
Enalapril	IV	5–15 mcg/kg/dose (q8-24h)	Oliguria, renal failure, hyperkalemia, cough

[A] Recommended in neonatal hypertensive emergencies. ANA. antinuclear antibody; SLE, systemic lupus erythematosus.

Ca-Channel Blockers-Nicardipine -IV Infusion: Initially 0.5mcg/kg/min- **Maintenance**: 0.5–2mcg/kg/min-Used only as a drip for **severe HTN-May cause reflex tachycardia.**

KEY POINTS FOR CLINICAL PRACTICE

1. In most Newborns, hypertension is discovered on routine monitoring of vital signs. Other presentations of Neonatal hypertension to be aware of in acutely ill infants include congestive heart failure (CHF) and cardiogenic shock, which are potentially life threatening. Fortunately, these consequences of hypertension gradually resolve with appropriate BP reduction.

2. Proper identification of hypertension in the Newborn requires accurate BP measurement. Fortunately, in most acutely ill infants, BP is usually monitored directly via an indwelling arterial catheter, either in the radial or umbilical artery. This method provides the most accurate BP readings and is clearly preferable to other methods. In infants who do not have indwelling umbilical lines, automated oscillometric devices are an acceptable alternative method of BP measurement.

3. The physical examination should begin with 4-extremity BP measurements in order to rule out aortic coarctation. Assess the general appearance of the infant and pay particular attention to the presence of dysmorphic features that may indicate an underlying genetic syndrome. Perform careful cardiac and abdominal examinations to rule out CHF or renal anomalies. Examine the genitalia to rule out congenital adrenal hyperplasia (CAH).

4. Usually only a limited set of laboratory data are needed in the evaluation of Neonatal hypertension. Obtain serum electrolyte, creatinine, and BUN levels as well as urinalysis in order to look for renal parenchymal disease. Obtain endocrinologic studies, such as cortisol, aldosterone, or thyroxine, when pertinent history is noted. Perform renal ultrasonography with Doppler of the renal vessels in all hypertensive infants. Accurate renal ultrasonography may help uncover potentially correctable causes of hypertension (e.g. renal venous thrombosis [RVT]); it may detect aortic thrombi, renal arterial thrombi, or both; and it can reveal anatomic renal abnormalities or other congenital renal parenchymal disease.

5. The definitive therapy of Neonatal hypertension is to treat the primary cause whenever possible (e.g., removal of the umbilical catheter, discontinuation of an offending medication).

REFERENCES and FURTHER READING :1) Seliem WA, Falk MC, Shadbolt B, Kent AL. Antenatal and postnatal risk factors for neonatal hypertension and infant follow-up. *Pediatr Nephrol.* Dec 2007;22(12):2081-7. **2**)Zubrow AB, Hulman S, Kushner H, Falkner B. Determinants of blood pressure in infants admitted to neonatal intensive care units: a prospective multicenter study. Philadelphia Neonatal Blood Pressure Study Group. *J Perinatol.* Nov-Dec 1995;15(6):470-9. **3**)Flynn JT. Neonatal hypertension: diagnosis and management. *Pediatr Nephrol.* Apr 2000;14(4):332-41. **4**)Roth CG, Spottswood SE, Chan JC, Roth KS. Evaluation of the hypertensive infant: a rational approach to diagnosis. *Radiol Clin North Am.* Sep 2003;41(5):931-44. **5**) Adelman RD. Long-term follow-up of neonatal renovascular hypertension. *Pediatr Nephrol.* Jan 1987;1(1):35-41.

*   *Pearl/Peril/Pitfall : Monitor blood pressure (BP) regularly in neonates with hypertension until the infant is ready for discharge from the neonatal ICU (NICU). Infants treated with ACE inhibitors or diuretics should have electrolyte levels and renal function monitored periodically until discharge.*

Neonatal Vomiting

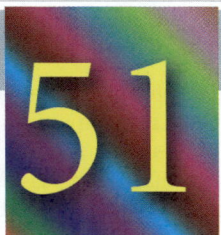

51

@ *Before 1912, early successful operative treatments of pyloric stenosis included gastroenterostomy, pyloroplasty, and forcible dilatation via gastrostomy (Loreta operation). In 1912, Rammstedt observed an uneventful recovery in a patient following pyloroplasty, in which sutures that were used in reapproximating the seromuscular layer had been disrupted. Following this observation, Rammstedt left the split muscle layer unsutured in all subsequent repairs. The Rammstedt pyloromyotomy, whether performed through a right-upper-quadrant incision, an umbilical incision, or via laparoscopy, remains the standard operation for pyloric stenosis today.*

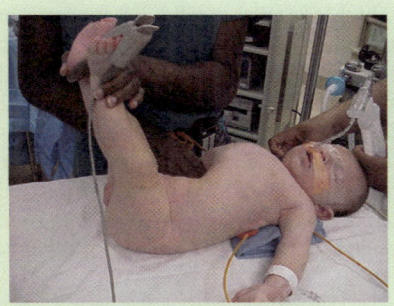

Technique used for examining an infant with pyloric stenosis. The infant is best examined from the right, with mild pressure applied using the first 3 fingers of the right hand in a cephalad direction. Careful examination reveals an oblong, smooth, hard mass that is 1-2 cm in length. This mass is the hypertrophied pylorus and is commonly referred to as an olive.

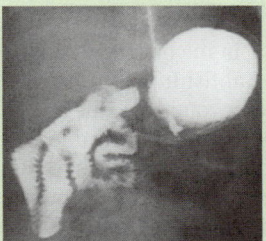

Upper GI shows *malrotation without midgut volvulus:* The duodenojejunal junction is low and to the right of the spine on the frontal view

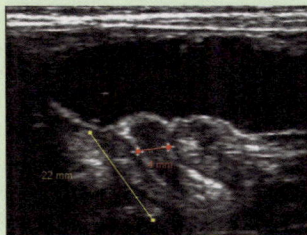

Longitudinal ultrasonogram of pyloric stenosis. Pyloric stenosis is diagnosed by the demonstration of an elongated sausage-shaped mass with a pyloric diameter greater than 14 mm, a muscular thickness greater than 4 mm, and a length of more than 16 mm.

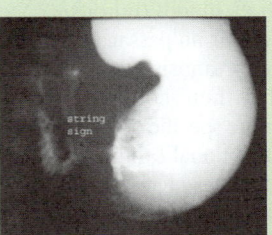

Malrotation with midgut volvulus: Most pediatric surgeons will prefer the upper gastrointestinal study because it confirms the position of the ligament of Treitz and demonstrates small bowel loops hanging completely into the right side of the abdomen. The duodenal loop will be dilated and obstructed (corkscrew appearance), it will lack the classic "C" shape, and it won't cross the spine back into its normal left-sided location.

@*The commonest cause for vomiting in the first two days of life is undoubtedly a neonatal gastritis due to irritation from swallowed liquor & debris from the birth canal. One or two stomach washouts with normal saline suffice to identify the debris & the altered maternal blood & to cure the problem. The baby remains well throughout. If the baby is sick, other signs such as bloody/bilious vomiting, abdominal distension, delayed or no passage of meconium, respiratory distress/apnea/cyanosis etc. are present or the vomiting persists, then complete investigation is necessary to exclude more specific organic causes.*

REVIEW OF CLINICAL PROBLEMS

1. What are the sinister clinical features of Neonatal Vomiting?
   Ans: Refer to the Evaluation-Decision-Action Plan/Algorithm to diagnose & manage Neonatal Vomiting.

2. *What causes should you consider in a Sick Neonate with vomitings with normal Abdominal X-ray ?*
   Ans: Refer to the Table "1" of the chapter.

3. What are the essential aspects of History and Physical Examination in evaluating Neonatal Vomiting?.
   Ans: Refer to the Evaluation-Decision-Action Plan/Algorithm to diagnose & manage Neonatal Vomiting.

4. When should you intubate & ventilate a Neonate with Vomitings?
   Ans: Refer to the Evaluation-Decision-Action Plan/Algorithm to diagnose & manage Neonatal Vomiting.

5. Mention the complications of Persistent Neonatal Vomiting.
   Ans: Refer to the "No.10" of the "BIRD'S EYE VIEW/ OVERVIEW/ SYNOPSIS" of the Chapter.

LEARNING OBJECTIVES

After completing this article, readers will be able to

1. Differentiate Pathologic Vomiting from Physiological /Self-limiting types of regurgitation/posseting.

2. Investigate Bloody/Bilious Vomitings promptly, as it is sinister always, unless proved otherwise.

3. Understand the significance of *Red Flags* in Neonatal Vomiting, suggestive of Organic causes.

4. Evaluate neonatal vomiting with relevant History and Physical examination and appropriate investigations.

5. Consult pediatric surgeon for further diagnosis and management of ? surgical causes of Neonatal Vomiting.

* *Pearl/Peril/Pitfall : Infection (Sepsis/Meningitis/UTI/NEC) should be at the top of the list of differential diagnoses of Neonatal Persistent Vomiting because of its prevalence and disastrous consequences if untreated in the neonatal period. Fever is not always seen in association with neonatal infections.*

BIRD'S EYE VIEW/OVERVIEW/SYNOPSIS

1. *Posseting* (the regurgitation of small amounts of milk after feeds) is common in the Neonatal period and is easily distinguished from *pathological vomiting* by experienced mothers and midwives. *Regurgitation & vomiting* both indicate underlying disorders (vomiting is a more serious problem). *Rumination* is a rare disorder, where the baby regurgitates small amounts of food into the mouth which is then chewed with apparent self-gratification. It usually presents after the Neonatal period.

2. Neonatal vomiting in the first week of life may be due to difficulties in establishing appropriate feeding. The commonest cause for vomiting in the first two days of life is undoubtedly a Neonatal gastritis due to irritation from swallowed liquor & debris from the birth canal. One or two stomach washouts with normal saline suffice to identify the debris & the altered maternal blood & to cure the problem. The baby remains well throughout.

3. If the baby is sick, other signs such as bloody/bilious vomiting, abdominal distention, delayed or no passage of meconium, respiratory distress/apnea/cyanosis etc. are present or the vomiting persists, then complete investigation is necessary to exclude more specific organic causes. *Refer to Table 1* for possible functional & organic causes of vomiting presenting in the first week of life. *Refer to Table 2* for appropriate investigations for the underlying etiology of early Neonatal vomiting.

4. *Persisting of vomiting/vomiting after the first week of life:* Babies presenting after the first week of life tend to have acquired problems although lower intestinal obstructions, malrotation & NEC in the VLBW baby may present later. Consideration of the baby's clinical state allows a fairly rapid differentiation.

   * **Baby well:**
     abdomen normal
       posseting
       feeding disorder
       gastroesophageal reflux
       gastrointestinal food allergy
       pyloric stenosis
       urinary tract infection

   * **Baby unwell:**
     abdomen distended
       late obstruction
       peritonitis/appendicitis
       intussusception
       NEC

   Persisting of vomiting/vomiting after the first week of life:

   Persistent vomiting even in a relatively well baby, especially if accompanied by poor growth, may indicate a more serious underlying disorder. *If investigations are normal, a feeding disorder is excluded & the vomiting still persists then the differential diagnosis usually rests between a dietary food intolerance & gastroesophageal reflux.*

5. Vomiting may occur with many disturbances that don't obstruct the digestive tract, such as milk allergy, sepsis, UTI, meningitis, increased intracranial pressure, metabolic disorders like galactosemia, organic acidemias, hyper ammonemias, and salt-losing variety of congenital adrenal hyperplasia. Appropriate investigation is necessary to confirm the underlying diagnosis *(Refer to Table 2)*.

6. *Neonatal gastrointestinal obstruction* may be heralded by a number of significant signs including a)maternal polyhydramnios b)persistent bilious vomitings c)abdominal distension d)failure to pass meconium. Bile stained vomiting suggests intestinal obstruction beyond the duodenum, but may also be idiopathic and also occurs in NEC. Bile-stained vomit, which is green, should be distinguished from vomit which contains yellow colostrum or from vomit which contains swallowed meconium. Abdominal X-rays (kidney-ureter-bladder (KUB) and cross-table lateral views) should be performed in Neonates with persistent emesis and in all infants with bile-stained emesis to detect air-fluid levels, distended bowel loops, characteristic patterns of obstruction (double bubble: duodenal atresia), and pneumoperitoneum (intestinal perforation). *A contrast swallow roentgenogram with small bowel follow-through is indicated in the presence of bilious emesis.*

7. Vomiting associated with congenital hypertrophic pyloric stenosis may begin any time after birth, & it is non-bilious but doesn't assume its projectile pattern before the second or third week. Vomiting with obstipation is common early sign of Hirschsprung disease. Vomiting from esophageal obstruction occurs with the first feeding & the diagnosis should be made before the infant has trouble with oral feedings and develops aspiration pneumonia. *(Refer to Table 2 for appropriate investigations to diagnose these).*

8. *The Evaluation-Decision-Action-Plan / Algorithm* describes the essential aspects of history taking, examination & relevant investigations to diagnose & manage the various causes of vomiting in the Neonatal period. *Refer to the Chapter 52* for detailed investigation & management of gastrointestinal obstruction in the Neonatal period.

9. Infantile achalasia (cardiospasm), a rare cause of vomiting in Newborn infants, is demonstrable roentgenographically by obstruction at the cardiac end of the esophagus without organic stenosis. Regurgitation of feedings because of continuous relaxation of the esophageal-gastric sphincter, or chalasia, is a cause of vomiting. Keeping the infant in a semi-upright position, thickening the feeding, or administering prokinetic drugs can control it.

10. Significant & persistent vomiting due to any cause in the Newborn period can cause severe dehydration, electrolyte losses, prerenal failure, if prolonged intrinsic renal failure. Correction of fluid & electrolyte disturbances is paramount, while performing the investigations to identify the underlying causes. ABG analysis & electrolytes should be monitored serially to correct the losses as appropriate. Surgical disorders when identified will require prompt transfer to a pediatric surgical unit with appropriate measures such as nil oral, reliable & continuous NG decompression, IV fluid therapy, IV antibiotics to cover for sepsis, maintaining normothermia & correction of fluid & electrolyte losses etc. Bloody vomiting in the Neonate is well discussed in the *Chapter 57   GIT Bleeding in the Neonate.*

---

* *Pearl/Peril/Pitfall: A negative laboratory profile (i.e., normal peripheral leukocyte count and differential, normal CSF findings, normal glucose levels) in a neonate who is symptomatic is not as reassuring as it would be in an older child. Neonate's history of lethargy, poor feeding, and persistent vomiting raises concern about sepsis, despite his/her normal physical examination and laboratory findings.*

THE EVALUATION-DECISION-ACTION-PLAN/ALGORITHM FOR THE DIAGNOSIS AND MANAGEMENT OF *NEONATAL VOMITING*

SUBJECTIVE FINDINGS

Hx of type, amount and constitution of feed.

Hx of frothy/bloody/bilious/milk only type of vomiting.

Hx of posseting/rumination/maternal postnatal depression/anxiety, poor feeding techniques.

Hx of abdominal distention, jaundice, delayed or no meconium passage, bleeding per rectum, symptoms of sepsis such as poor feeding, diarrhea, fever, hypothermia, lethargy etc. in a Sick Neonate.

Hx of perinatal asphyxia (raised ICT), birth trauma & family history suggestive of inborn errors of metabolism.

OBJECTIVE FINDINGS

Assess ABCDs, hydration status, O_2 sats, Vitals CRT, BP, urine output, AF, petechiae and purpura & pass NG tube to verify the gastric aspirates & to exclude esophageal atresia.

Determine whether the baby sick or well.

Check anorectal region for patency & position of the anus and for passage of meconium.

Verify the hernial orifices, presence of abdominal distention, visible gastric/intestinal peristalsis, abdominal tenderness, masses, and perform *testfeed* to identify palpable pyloric tumor.

Perform complete systemic examination for signs of sepsis, meningitis, obstructive uropathy (urine stream) trauma, cardiac, metabolic & endocrine disorders (CAH salt losing type).

INVESTIGATIONS

Blood FBC with hematocrit & platelets, ABG analysis with electrolytes, blood glucose, calcium $^{++}$, Mg^{++}, BUN & creatinine, LFTs, urine analysis & culture, blood culture, CRP $\pm$ LP, coagulation studies (PT, APTT, D-dimer & FDP) if clinically indicated. Stool cultures for proctocolitis.

Imaging CXR/AXR with large NG tube to exclude esophageal atresia & TE fistula, AXR for intestinal obstruction, NEC, renal USG scan for obstructive uropathy, barium swallow/pH study for hiatus hernia & gastroesophageal reflux, Color Doppler Testes as dictated by clinical impression.

NEONATAL VOMITING

Perform IV access & correct fluid & electrolyte disturbances in a Neonate with significant vomiting associated with dehydration, possible surgical causes.

Refer to the chapter 57 "GIT bleeding in the Neonate" for bloody vomitings in the Neonate.

Beware of that If evaluated early in the clinical course, pyloric stenosis may present without the "classic" findings of projectile Non-bilious vomiting, "olive" on abdominal examination, weight loss, and hypochloremic, hypokalemic metabolic alkalosis.

Intubate & ventilate if Neonatal vomiting is likely to be due to a) raised ICT, secondary to hypoxic-ischemic encephalopathy & meningitis, b) diaphragmatic hernia, c) complicated by aspiration pneumonia/ARDS

Exclude common problems like a) mucous gastritis b) feeding problems (winding or burping) c) posseting.

Ensure ABCs, Pulse oximetry, O2 supplements, in any sick infant with vomiting.

Give IV broadspectrum antibiotics to cover for sepsis in a sick Neonate with vomiting; *consider* the diagnosis of salt-losing Congenital Adrenal Hyperplasia and Inborn Errors of Metabolism in cases of Neonatal vomiting associated with family history of consanguinity & unexplained Neonatal deaths.

BILIOUS VOMITING

Consider the following causes in the differential diagnosis of bilious emesis

Pathophysiology	Proximal Intestinal	Distal Intestinal Obstruction
Differential Diagnosis	Duodenal atresia Annular pancreas Malrotation with or without volvulus Jejunal obstruction, atresia	Ileal atresia Meconium ileus Colonic atresia Meconium plug-hypoplastic left colon syndrome Hirschsprung disease
Physical examination	Abdominal distention not prominent	Abdominal distention
Diagnosis	Abdominal X-ray: "double bubble" Upper GI Sweat test Mucosal rectal biopsy	Abdominal x-ray; dilated loops of bowel Contrast enema

Always suspect

INT. OBSTRUCTION

Check Ano-Rectal Region passage of Meconium ?
Plain X-ray (erect)

Watch & Repeat X-Ray SOS

ABNORMAL   NORMAL

E.g. INT.ATRESIA MECONIUM ILEUS

Clinical Condition LowBirth Wt?

INFECTION
Culture-Urine Blood

F & E Homeostasis

Surgery

LP

Observe carefully

Antibiotics?

Red flags in Neonatal vomiting, suggestive of an organic disease

* Presence of a bulging AF- suggesting cerebral edema or an intracranial hemorrhage * Drowsiness * Failure to suck well, failure to demand feeds * Bile-stained vomiting- suggests GIT obstruction below the ampulla of Vater, but may occur when there is a serious infection or birth injury. * Abdominal distention (may be absent in the presence of high intestinal obstructions) * Presence of a palpable abdominal mass (meconium ileus, enlarged kidneys, reduplication of the intestine or a palpable bladder * Visible peristalsis * dehydration * fever * failure to pass meconium in the first 24hrs * failure to gain weight, or loss of weight after the first 2 or 3 days * maternal polyhydramnios with frothy oral secretions $\pm$ choking spells with vomit after the first feed (TEF + EA) * stridor (vascular ring) * bloody vomitus * family history of consanguinity & unexplained Neonatal deaths (inborn errors of metabolism & Congenital salt-losing form of adrenal hyperplasia.)

---

* **Pearl/Peril/Pitfall :** *Vomiting outside of the immediate neonatal period should prompt a work-up for gastrointestinal anatomic anomalies that cause obstruction (e.g. malrotation, volvulus, intestinal atresia or stenosis, incarcerated hernia) and those that do not cause obstruction (e.g., gastric antral web, gastric duplication, hiatal hernia, hypertrophic pyloric stenosis, pylorospasm, and gastroesophageal reflux disease [GERD]).*

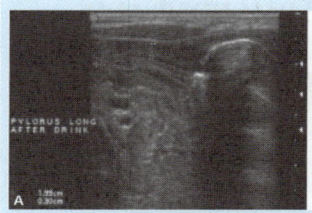
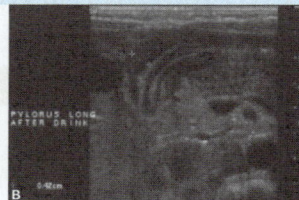

Figure 1. Ultrasound of a Neonate with suspected CHPS. (A) Pyloric length of 19 mm is visible. (B) Pyloric width (i.e., muscle thickness) of 4 mm is visible. Both images are consistent with the ultrasound diagnostic criteria for pyloric stenosis.
Courtesy: *Marina Catallozzi, MD, and Angelo P. Giardino, MD, PhD.*

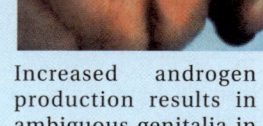

Increased androgen production results in ambiguous genitalia in Newborn girls

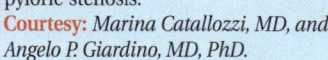

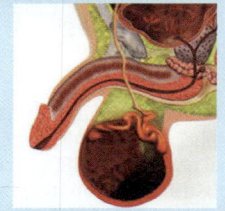

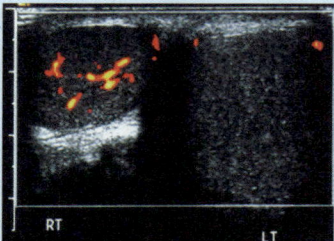

When encountered with a Neonate who presents with "Persistent-Significant" bilious/non-bilious Vomitings associated with lethargy and/or irritability, Pediatrician/Neonatologist should examine Hernial orifices (Incarcerated Inguinal Hernia in a premature baby commonly), Genitalia (Testicular Torsion, Clitoromegaly in a girl Neonate with suspected Congenital Adrenal Hyperplasia). High index of suspicion is necessary to exclude an UTI/Meningitis (LP, SPA, Blood C/S) and/or Sepsis. GIT problems are to be excluded anyway, irrespective of other Clinical findings.

Testicular torsion: Transverse power Doppler image of both testes illustrates an enlarged, avascular left testicle.

Inguinal Hernia

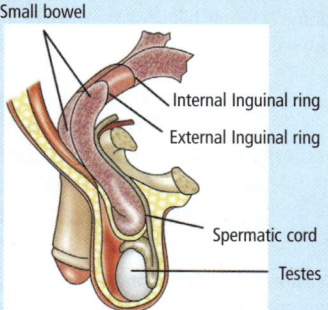

Small bowel

Internal Inguinal ring

External Inguinal ring

Spermatic cord

Testes

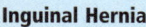

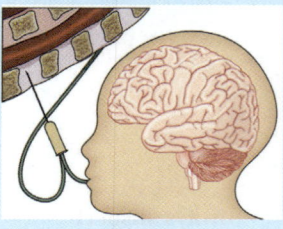
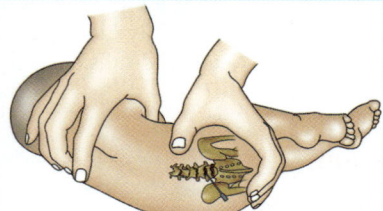
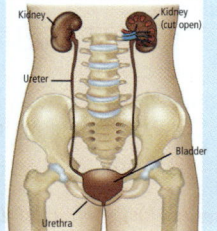
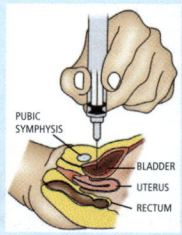

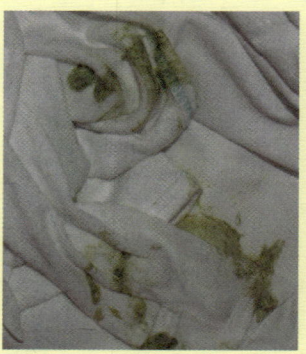

This is an example of bilious emesis. The green color of bile is clearly present here. This newborn was thought to be well and was tolerating feedings for several days before the sudden onset of this abnormal emesis. Malrotation with volvulus was diagnosed and the infant underwent emergent surgical correction. Emesis like this is never normal.

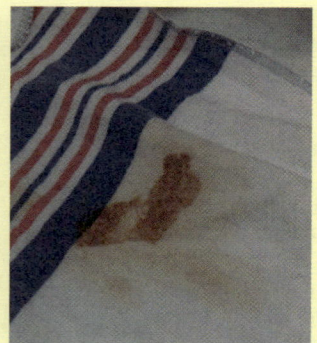

During the process of delivery, a newborn will occasionally swallow small amounts of maternal blood. When this is spit back up after delivery (usually during the first 24 hours), it typically causes some anxiety for caregivers. The appearance above, where the blood appears to be partially digested, is common, but bright red blood can also be of maternal origin. In an otherwise well newborn, close observation is the only necessary intervention. If doubt exists about the origin of the blood, an Apt test can be performed on the sample.

APT Test - now used to differentiate between maternal or fetal blood in the stool or vomitus—fetal Hgb (infant) is alkaline-resistant - adult Hgb (mom) will change to alkaline hematin upon the addition of alkali.

1. Rinse the bloody diaper or stool with water to obtain a pink supernatant hemoglobin solution—fresh red blood must be used; melena or coffee-ground blood will falsely appear as "adult" Hgb.

2. Centrifuge the mixture or strain through filter paper. (Supernate should be pink due to presence of blood).

3. To 5 parts supernate, add 1 part of 1% sodium hydroxide

4. Within 2 min, a yellow-brown color indicates the Hgb is swallowed maternal blood (Hgb A) ; persistent pink color indicates the Hgb is fetal (F) * (A control test with known infant or mom's blood is advisable).

Modified APT Test 1. apply 10–20% NaOH solution directly to the stain in the diaper until a margin of solution was absorbed into the diaper past the stain 2. Read color change off the diaper Mcrury's study showed if blood was > 30 minutes old, test was unreliable ; blood was oxidized by the air and changed color from red to brown - could be mistaken for maternal blood.

TABLE 1 — Neonatal vomiting in the first week of life

1. Vomitus
* Frothy
  - tracheoesophageal fistula
* Blood
  - maternal - swallowed
  - hemorrhagic disease
  - gastric erosions/stress ulcers
* Bile
  - intestinal obstruction
  - intestinal perforation/peritonitis
  - intestinal pseudo-obstruction
* Milk only
  - feeding disorder
  - gastroesophageal reflux
  - food allergy

2. Baby well: abdomen normal
* AXR - fluid level
  - duodenal/intestinal atresia

  - meconium ileus
  - large bowel obstruction/Hirschsprung's disease
* AXR - no fluid levels
  - gastroesophageal reflux
  - milk allergy

3. Baby sick
* Abdomen normal: AXR - no or occasional fluid levels + watery diarrhea
  - sepsis/urinary tract infection
  - increased intracranial pressure/meningitis
  - renal tract disorders
  - metabolic disorders
* Abdomen distended/tender: AXR - fluid levels (watery diarrhea or bloody diarrhea)
  - NEC
  - obstruction/perforation
  - volvulus
  - intussusception

TABLE 2 — Neonatal vomiting—etiology and investigations

Etiology	Investigations	Etiology	Investigations
Feeding disorders		Acquired	
Overfeeding	Feeding history and	Pseudo-obstruction/sepsis	Full blood count,
Air swallowing	observation		sepsis screen
Maternal stress	Family history	NEC	AXR-free or intramural gas
Esophageal disorders		Proctocolitis	Stool cultures
Tracheoesophageal	CXR/AXR with large	Food allergy	Dietary manipulation
fistula/frothy vomit day 1	nasogastric tube	Incarceration/strangulation	Inspection
Hiatus hernia	Barium swallow/pH study	Inguinal herniae	AXR
Gastric disorders		*Extraintestinal disorders*	
(Gastritis)		Intracranial lesions	
Maternal debris	Stomach washout	Asphyxia, meningitis	
Blood-hemorrhagic disease	Clotting screen	Intracranial hemorrhage	CT/MRI head scan
of the Newborn		Hydrocephalus/SOL	
Maternal stress illness	History	Renal disorders	
Pyloric stenosis	Test feed	Urinary tract infection	MSU/bag urine
	Ultrasound/barium meal	Obstructive uropathy	Renal ultrasound
		Metabolic disorders	
Small intestinal disorders		Galactosemia	Urine sugar
Congenital		Hyperammonemias	Urine amino acids
Duodenal atresia	AXR	Phenylketonuria	Urine amino acids
Extrinsic duodenal obstruction	AXR	Organic acidemias	pH urine
Malformation	AXR	Congenital adrenal	Electrolytes (Na/K)
Volvulus	AXR	hyperplasia	
Meconium ileus	AXR (calcification)	Drugs	Theophylline
Intestinal duplication	AXR		

AXR, abdominal X-ray; CXR, chest X-ray; MSU, mid stream urine; NEC, necrotizing enterocolitis; SOL, space occupying lesion.

KEY POINTS FOR CLINICAL PRACTICE

1. In many Neonates, it is simply regurgitation from overfeeding/failure to burp the infant adequately. When only small amounts come up after feeds & the child is well, taking the feeds normally & gaining weight, disease is unlikely.

2. Always look for the sinister clinical features of Neonatal vomiting, suggestive of the presence organic disease (Refer to Red flags given in the *E-D-A Algorithm*) & evaluate further.

3. Bilious vomiting often indicates intestinal obstruction at or beyond the second portion of the duodenum & *represents a potential surgical emergency; sepsis & NEC and visceral neuro/*

myopathies can cause non obstructive bilious vomiting.

4. Assessment should always include the overall clinical condition of the Neonate & other symptoms & signs, as well as the volume, frequency & contents of the vomitus. *If the baby is sick, other signs are present or the vomiting persists, complete investigation is required.*

5. It is important to correct fluid & electrolyte and acid base disturbances due to severe, persistent Neonatal vomiting, irrespective of the underlying etiology, while investigating further.

REFERENCES & FURTHER READING 1) Godbole P, Stringer MD: Bilious Vomiting in the Newborn: How often is it pathologic? J Pediatric Surgery-2002, 2) Primary Care of the Newborn—4th edition by Henry M. Seidel 3) Symptoms of Disease in Childhood by T.J. David. 4) Manual of Neonatal Care by Cloherty - 6 th edition 5) Nelson Text Book of Pediatrics - 18th edition

* *Pearl/Peril/Pitfall : CHPS–Conservative medical management (i.e., small frequent feeds and administration of atropine) has been previously attempted. However, it has resulted in slower improvement and a higher mortality rate. Surgical treatment(the Ramstedt pyloromyotomy remains the surgical procedure of choice. after medical stabilization (with a focus on rehydration and correction of electrolyte abnormalities) is curative.*

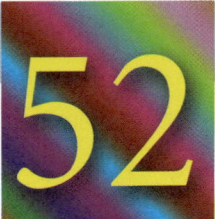

Neonatal Gastrointestinal Obstruction (GIT)

@ *Imaging is a mainstay to diagnosis of intra-abdominal pathology and should be readily performed in an infant with suspected intestinal obstruction. Noninvasive techniques, such as plain radiography and ultrasonography, can be performed at the bedside and can yield valuable information. Fluoroscopy (Gastrografin enema) may be both diagnostic and therapeutic but should be performed with caution in an infant at risk for intestinal perforation. If possible, consult with surgical colleagues prior to performing any invasive or contrast procedure because the order in which various tests are performed could impact the value of subsequent diagnostic pursuits.*

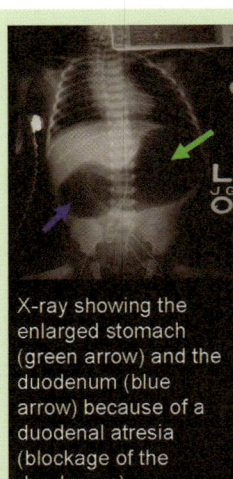

X-ray showing the enlarged stomach (green arrow) and the duodenum (blue arrow) because of a duodenal atresia (blockage of the duodenum).

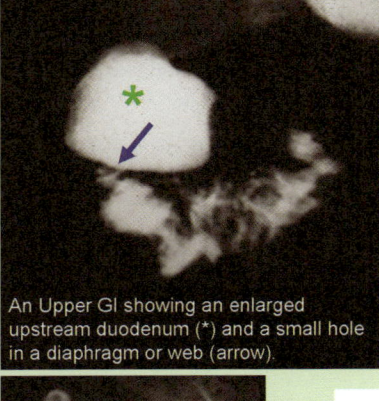

An Upper GI showing an enlarged upstream duodenum (*) and a small hole in a diaphragm or web (arrow).

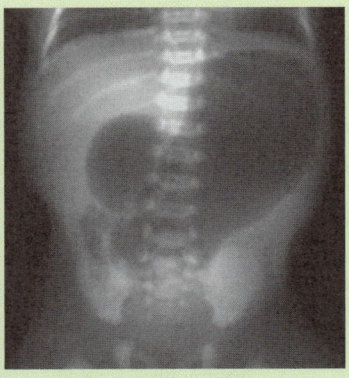

Supine radiograph shows a "double bubble" with some distal small bowel gas.
Diagnosis: Annular pancreas. The differential diagnosis includes duodenal atresia with a "Y" connection of the biliary tree and midgut volvulus.

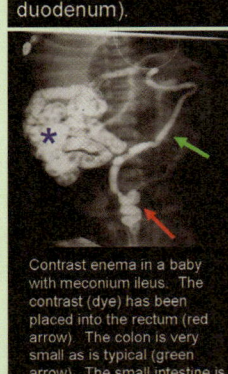

Contrast enema in a baby with meconium ileus. The contrast (dye) has been placed into the rectum (red arrow). The colon is very small as is typical (green arrow). The small intestine is filled with "pebbles" of meconium (stool, *).

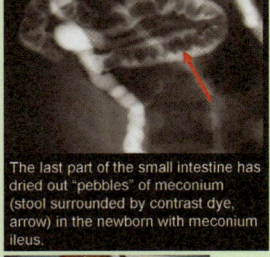

The last part of the small intestine has dried out "pebbles" of meconium (stool surrounded by contrast dye, arrow) in the newborn with meconium ileus.

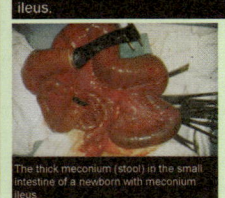

The thick meconium (stool) in the small intestine of a newborn with meconium ileus.

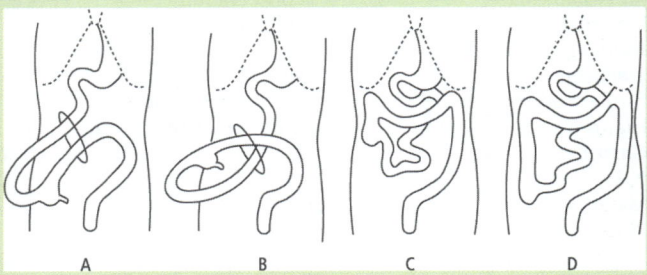

Drawings illustrate the stages of intestinal rotation. In *A*, the duodenum has rotated 90° counterclockwise to lie to the right of the superior mesenteric artery. The distal large bowel also rotates 90° counterclockwise. In *B*, the duodenum has rotated another 90° counterclockwise. In *C*, the duodenum has rotated its final 90° counterclockwise with the duodenojejunal flexure lying to the left of the midline. The cecum continues to rotate. In *D*, the normally rotated bowel is depicted.

REVIEW OF CLINICAL PROBLEMS

1. When should you suspect GIT Obstruction in a Neonate?
   Ans: Refer to the "No. 1" of the "BIRD`S EYE VIEW/OVERVIEW/ SYNOPSIS" of the Chapter.

2. Name the Common exceptions *one should be aware of* when dealing with Neonatal GIT obstruction.
   Ans: Refer to the "No. 2" of the "BIRD'S EYE VIEW/OVERVIEW/ SYNOPSIS" of the Chapter.

3. How do you manage GIT Obstruction preoperatively?
   Ans: Refer to the "No. 6" of the "BIRD`S EYE VIEW/OVERVIEW/ SYNOPSIS" of the Chapter.

4. What are the Differential diagnoses of Failure to pass Meconium?
   Ans: Refer to the Section "Failure to pass Meconium" of the Chapter.

5. How do you evaluate and manage Neonatal GIT Obstruction?
   Ans: Refer to the Evaluation-Decision-Action Plan/Algorithm to diagnose & manage Neonatal GIT Obstruction.

LEARNING OBJECTIVES

After completing this article, readers will be able to:

1. Be aware of GIT surgical emergencies in an ill appearing Neonate.

2. Consider Bilious vomitings pathological until proven otherwise, *whether associated with abdominal distention or not.*

3. Examine the genitalia(imperative) especially in boys, to exclude the possibility of an incarcerated hernia or testicular torsion.

4. Consult Pediatric Surgeon early in the course of illness, ensuring conservative management meanwhile.

5. Be able to search for associated Congenital anomalies- VACTERL Association if any, & Counsel the parents about the prognosis.

* **Pearl/Peril/Pitfall:** *Volvulus can present in one of three ways: (1) sudden onset of bilious vomiting and abdominal pain in a neonate, (2) history of feeding problems with bilious vomiting that appears like a bowel obstruction, and, less commonly, (3) failure to thrive with severe feeding intolerance. Bilious vomiting in a neonate is always worrisome and is a surgical emergency until proven otherwise.*

BIRD'S EYE VIEW/OVERVIEW/SYNOPSIS

1. *Neonatal gastrointestinal obstruction* occurs in about 1/1000 Newborn babies, may be associated with maternal polyhydramnios and should be suspected when the infant presents with some or all of the following features *a)* If the NG tube aspirate is > 20ml immediately after birth *b)* Frequent, Persistent, Copious, Vomitings with or without bile-staining *c)* Abdominal distention *(the higher the obstruction in the intestine, the earlier, the infant will present with vomiting and less prominent the distention will be ; the opposite is true for lower intestinal obstructions E.g., :- Jejunoileal atresia, meconium ileus, meconium plug syndrome, Hirschsprung's disease) d)* Visible deep peristalsis *e)* Delayed or no passage of meconium *(>90% of full term Newborn infants pass meconium within the first 24 hours, and most of the remainder do so within 36 hours. About 20% of VLBW infants do not pass meconium within the first 24 hours) f)* If a changing stool is never seen *g)* Dehydration and collapse due to excessive vomitings.

2. *Beware of the exceptions 1)* Meconium stools may be passed initially if the obstruction is in the upper part of the small intestine or if the obstruction developed late in intrauterine life *2)* Bile - stained vomit, which is green should be distinguished from vomit which contains yellow colostrum or from vomit which contains swallowed meconium *3)* There is little or no abdominal distention if the obstruction is high in the intestinal tract involving the duodenum or proximal jejunum *4)* Meconium plug syndrome and Hirschsprung's disease may present with distention and delayed stooling (>24 hours) without any vomitings *5)* Vomiting may occur with many other disturbances that do not obstruct the digestive tract, such as milk allergy, adrenal hyperplasia of the salt-losing variety, galactosemia, hyperammonemias, organic acidemias, increased intracranial pressure, septicemia, meningitis, and urinary tract infections. *6)* Palpable abdominal mass may be due to meconium ileus, enlarged kidneys, duplication of intestine or a palpable bladder.

3. *Neonatal intestinal obstruction* may be *PARTIAL/ COMPLETE, CONGENITAL (Intrinsic / Extrinsic)/ ACQUIRED, ANATOMICAL/FUNCTIONAL, SIMPLE/ STRANGULATING, HIGH (Proximal) / LOW (Distal) or any combination of these variables.*

4. *History and physical examination almost always suggest bowel obstruction and imaging is used to confirm the diagnosis and localize the area of obstruction:* (Plain abdominal X-rays with CXR {supine, erect and decubitus views), USG Scan of abdomen, upper GI water soluble contrast studies, water soluble contrast enemas).

5. No laboratory studies are diagnostic of obstruction or differentiate simple obstruction from obstruction associated with bowel infarction. Obstruction high in the gastrointestinal tract is often associated with hypochloremic metabolic alkalosis. Marked leukocytosis with or without thrombocytopenia, metabolic acidosis, and hematochezia suggests bowel infarction /infection/ Sepsis. Urinalysis may be helpful in diagnosis of Sepsis and imperforate anus.

6. All babies with presumed intestinal obstruction should be transported to a pediatric surgical centre with *a)* Nil oral and NG decompression [FG 10 catheter] with continuous aspiration of gastric contents to prevent gastric rupture, pulmonary aspiration or respiratory compromise secondary to diaphragmatic compression *b)* Correction of shock, dehydration, and fluid and electrolyte disturbances with appropriate fluids and electrolytes *c)* Broadspectrum antibiotic coverage [Ampicillin + Amikacin + Ceftazidime + Metronidazole] if there is any suspicion of volvulus or any question of bowel integrity. *d)* With stabilization of the Newborn ABC 's, blood sugar, calcium and body temperature *e)* Well - functioning IV line.

7. *The definitive treatment for most of these conditions [with the exception of meconium plug syndrome, small left colon syndrome, and some cases of meconium ileus] is SURGERY. Patients with strangulation must have immediate surgical relief before the bowel infarcts, resulting in gangrene and intestinal perforation. Extensive intestinal necrosis results in short - gut syndrome. Postoperatively the Newborn fluid requirement is two-thirds the standard maintenance level for the 1st 24-48 hours + continuing losses which must be replaced.*

8. It is important to think of *malrotation of the intestine* in any infant with unexplained attacks of vomiting, & exclude the condition with upper GI contrast series. The vomiting & obstruction may be intermittent, leading one to conclude incorrectly that there is no organic cause. The danger of malrotation is the constant danger of volvulus, with strangulation & fatal infarction of the intestine. Recently, in specialized centers the use of an abdominal ultrasound examination has been shown to be a useful though not entirely reliable method to detect malrotation. It is a life-threatening surgical emergency if not recognized & treated promptly.

9. Nonoperative conservative management is usually limited to children with suspected adhesions or inflammatory strictures that may resolve with nasogastric decompression or anti-inflammatory medications. If clinical signs of improvement are not evident within 12-24 hr, then operative intervention is usually indicated.

10. *The Evaluation-Decision-Action-Plan/Algorithm* describes essential aspects of assessment and management of GIT Obstruction in Neonates.

---

* *Pearl/Peril/Pitfall : Congenital adrenal hyperplasia (CAH) can cause bilious vomiting without anatomical obstruction, and it can present in the first few weeks of life. CAH results in adrenal insufficiency with decreased cortisol levels and salt wasting. Infants will present with hypotension and electrolyte imbalance (low Na+, high K+). It is more likely that CAH will be seen in male infants in the ED. Female newborns who have this condition are less commonly missed in the newborn nursery because the accumulation of androgenic compounds affects the external genitalia to a greater extent.*

THE EVALUATION-DECISION-ACTION-PLAN/ALGORITHM FOR THE DIAGNOSIS AND MANAGEMENT OF *SUSPECTED NEONATAL GASTROINTESTINAL OBSTRUCTION*

SUBJECTIVE FINDINGS

History Maternal polyhydramnios, persistent and frequent vomitings, bile-stained vomitus, abdominal distention, delayed or no passage of meconium, increased salivation with choking at the first feed, intermittent vomitings {think of malrotation with constant danger of volvulus, with strangulation and fatal infarction of the intestine}

OBJECTIVE FINDINGS

General Fussy, lethargic, irritable, inconsolable. Dysmorphic features
Skin Turgor, Rash, Petechiae.
HEENT Sunken eyes, Sunken Fontanel.
CVS Tachycardia, shock & Heart Murmurs?
RS Tachypnoea, retractions.
GIT Distended abdomen, tenderness or palpable mass.
GU Groin bulge, anal stenosis, imperforate anus.

INVESTIGATIONS

Blood Hb, TC, DC, Hematocrit, Platelets, Cultures, Glucose, Electrolytes, ABG, Urea, Creatinine, Group and Type, Cross match, Bleeding time, Clotting Time.
Urine Analysis and Culture.
Imaging CXR, 3-view AXR {Supine, erect and prone cross table lateral view}, USG SCAN, Contrast Studies {Upper GI & Enema}

Malrotation of the bowel -

* May be unsuspected in a healthy neonate for days or weeks, and then cause acute bilious vomiting and abdominal distention
* Per se it is not dangerous, but the bowel is poorly fixed to a narrow vascular pedicle permitting it to twist {VOLVULUS}, occluding the superior mesenteric artery and producing extensive bowel necrosis.
* VOLVULUS is a true surgical emergency; bloody stools are ominous.
* Contrast {water soluble} study is usually necessary for confirmation.
* Repair consists of mobilization and repositioning of the bowel; remove frankly necrotic intestine and perform an ostomy of the proximal viable intestine.
End - to- end anastomosis may be possible in some cases.

SUSPECTED GI OBSTRUCTION

Shock ←

→ **Notify Pediatric Surgeon !**

→ **Hypoglycemia**

Ensure ABCs, Supplemental O$_2$ IV access, Monitor BP, CR monitor, Pulse oximetry

Fluid Resuscitation
0.9 NS or LR 20mL/kg IVB follow with Maintenance IVF
Correct metabolic acidosis

Insert **OG/NG tube** to assess patency/ allow decompression *reliably & Continuously!*

Difficulty in passing tube

NON BILIOUS

NG Aspirate

Tube passes easily

BILIOUS

Begin antibiotics

Radiographic signs of malrotation include absence of the splenic and hepatic flexures and a cecum positioned in the right upper quadrant; in volvulus, colonic obstruction is observed.

Chest radiograph
Tube coiled in chest TEF

DISTENDED   NONDISTENDED

Abdominal radiograph
may show early obstruction

Non-projectile emesis
GERD=Gastro Esophageal Reflux Disease

Projectile emesis with palpable olive-pyloric stenosis, obtain US to confirm

NONDISTENDED
Imaging
UGI - abnormal
    duodenal atresia
    malrotation
    jejunal atresia
    ileal atresia (may be distended)
    adhesion/band (may be distended)
UGI - normal
    non-surgical ileus
    CNS-related
    sepsis
Abdominal Radiograph—NEC (pneumatosis)

Contrast enema
Intussusception, Hirschsprung's, meconium ileus, small left colon, meconium plug, colonic atresia, NEC stricture

DISTENDED ←

Imperforate anus, hernia

BE AWARE OF THE BASICS! *1. Normally air can be demonstrated radiologically in the jejunum by 15-60 minutes, in the ileum by 2-3 hours and in the colon by 3 hr of birth. 2. Absence of rectal gas at 24 hours is abnormal; the absence of rectal gas is not specific for Hirschsprung's disease, being more commonly seen in infants with sepsis and necrotizing enterocolitis. 3. The vomiting associated with pyloric stenosis may begin any time after birth but does not assume its characteristic pattern before the 2nd-3rd week. 4. It is difficult to accurately differentiate small from large bowel obstruction in children < 2yrs. 5. Ultrasonography is helpful in identifying pyloric stenosis, malrotation and volvulus or intussusception and in differentiating pyloric stenosis from other cause of proximal obstruction. 6. Contrast studies of the bowel are indicated when plain films or sonograms fail to identify the source of obstruction. 7. Water soluble contrast studies avoid the risk of barium contamination of the peritoneum when there is significant chance of perforation not detected by the presence of pneumoperitoneum on plain films. 8. Water soluble contrast enemas are useful in diagnosing malrotation, meconium ileus, meconium plug and intussusception. 9. Calcification within the peritoneal cavity usually indicates meconium peritonitis. Rarely obstruction with intraluminal calcification may be associated with rectourinary fistula, colonic aganglionosis or intestinal atresia. 10.*
Pearl/Peril/Pitfall: If the small bowel obstruction is caused by mechanical compression, high-pitched bowel sounds with "rushes" can be heard. When intraluminal pressure becomes higher than the venous and arterial pressures, ischemia develops in the bowel and hematochezia might be seen. As with most abdominal emergencies in children, hematochezia is a late finding.

GASTROINTESTINAL OBSTRUCTION IN NEONATES & YOUNG INFANTS-DIFFERENTIAL DIAGNOSIS

Lesion	Clinical presentation	Association	Diagnosis	Management	Cautions
Esophageal atresia, T-E fistula	Excessive salivation coughing, gagging, cyanosis, pneumonia	VACTERL {25%} Cardiac {35%} GI {24%} - duodenal, atresia, imperforate anus	Pass NG tube with CXR + AXR . {tube coils back} without TEF → gasless abdomen {10%}	Drain proximal pouch Surgery - divide fistula, esophagoesophagostomy	Keep head of the the baby elevated 45º to minimize aspiration.
Pyloric stenosis	Projectile nonbilious emesis, palpable olive	Family history, certain ABO groups	History/physical exam,UGI/ US, electrolytes (⁻Cl⁻, ⁻K⁺ metabolic alkalosis}	NPO, correct electrolytes surgery, pyloromyotomy	Pre- operative resuscitation
Duodenal atresia	Bilious emesis usual {85% distal to ampulla} maternal polyhydramnios	Annular pancreas, malrotation, Down syndrome {30%}, prematurity {25-50%}	Abdominal radiograph- *"double bubble" sign*	NPO, NG, IV fluids, antibiotics, surgery, duodenoduodenostomy	Rule out malrotation and volvulus
Malrotation	Bilious emesis	Diaphragmatic hernia, abdominal wall defects, CHD, heterotaxia, duodenal atresia	UGI or BE, abdominal radiograph-double bubble sign	NPO, NG, IV fluids, antibiotics, surgery, Ladd procedure and appendectomy	Risk for midgut volvulus, treat immediately
Jejunal atresia	Bilious emesis, mild distention, jaundice	Multiple atresia {6–20%}, malrotation {10%} Hirschsprung's disease (15%)	UGI or BE	NPO, NG, IV fluids, antibiotics, surgery, bowel resection and anastomosis	Apple peel or Christmas tree variant-familial, premature {50%}, malrotation {50%}
Ileal atresia	Bilious emesis, distention, jaundice		Abdominal radiograph ; air fluid levels, calcium=meconium peritonitis {10%}, BE		Higher mortality with multiple atresias, meconium ileus and peritonitis due to antenatal perforation
Post-op adhesions	Pain, anorexia, nausea, vomiting, distention	Previous intra-abdominal surgery or infection	Abdominal radiograph, UGI, consider CT scan	NPO, NG, IV fluids, antibiotics, surgery, adhesiolysis	Beware of internal hernias and closed loop obstruction
Hernia	Palpable mass in the groin, pain, emesis	Mainly in boys {6:1}, usually right sided {60%}	Physical examination	Sedation and reduction, surgery: herniorrhaphy	High risk of incarceration in premies < 1yr, may contain ovaries {risk of torsion} in females
Intussusception	Well nourished, sudden intermittent pain {81%}, emesis, bloody stools {58%}, RUQ mass {57%}	HSP, hemophilia, lymphoma, CF	Physical examination, abdominal radiograph, contrast enema	NPO, NG, IV fluids, contrast enema (air reduction 95% successful), surgery, reduction and resection	Be aware of pathologic lead points in 2-8%, and post-op intussusception
Hirschsprung's disease	Bilious emesis, distention, failure to pass meconium, alternating obstipation and diarrhea	Familial, Down syndrome {10%}	BE, suction rectal biopsy	NPO, NG, IV fluids, antibiotics, surgery: resection and pullthrough	Prone to enterocolitis {50%}, suction biopsy must be done above, dentate line
Meconium ileus	Bilious emesis, distention, failure to pass meconium	CF {20%}, volvulus/ atresia/perforation {25%}	Abdominal radiograph: ground glass/soap bubble, calcium indicates antenatal perforation, contrast enema	Uncomplicated : N-acetylcysteine or hyperosmolar enema or operate, irrigate and close complicated :operate, irrigate and close or stomas in select cases	Genetic studies and sweat test to check for CF
Colonic atresia	Bilious emesis, distention	Skeletal anomalies, small bowel atresia, ocular defects, Hirschsprung, diaphragmatic hernia	Abdominal radiograph, BE	NPO, NG, IV fluids, antibiotics surgery: resection and stoma or anastomosis	Prone to perforate at transverse colon
Meconium plug syndrome	Bilious emesis, distention, failure to pass meconium	Hirschsprung {10%}	Contrast enema	Contrast enema	Consider sweat test, suction rectal biopsy to rule out Hirschsprung
Small left colon	Bilious emesis, distention, failure to pass meconium	Diabetic mothers, use of magnesium during labor	Contrast enema	Contrast enema and time	
NEC stricture	Emesis, distention, prematurity, feeding intolerance, NEC	Umbilical lines, hyperosmolar formula, prematurity, use of indomethacin	Abdominal radiograph, BE	NPO, NG, IV fluids, antibiotics, surgery: resection and anastomosis	Should fully evaluate the colon before surgery
Imperforate anus	Usually boys, improperly placed anus, absent anus	VACTERL, CHD, GI-duodenal atresia, TEF	Physical examination, abdominal radiograph (include prone and cross table lateral views), US, urinalysis	Dilate anal stenosis, surgery {for imperforate anus}:colostomy and staged pull-through	Need to determine if high or low lesion

ROLE OF IMAGING IN THE DIAGNOSIS OF CONGENITAL ANOMALIES OF THE GASTROINTESTINAL TRACT

* Plain radiograph is a useful, simple and most inexpensive tool in the evaluation of the Neonate with gastrointestinal (GI) obstruction. Unlike adults and older children, in Neonates the small and large bowel usually cannot be distinguished. The gas is distributed throughout the small and large bowel where a little fluid is present resulting in sharp bowel-air interfaces which appear as multiple closely apposed rounded or polyhedral structures on plain radiograph. The precise level of obstruction may be evident in high GI obstruction but is difficult to determine in a low gut obstruction. **High GI obstruction** occurs most commonly at the level of duodenum and proximal jejunum and plain radiography alone is often diagnostic. Bilious vomiting indicates obstruction distal to the ampulla of Vater. Although there is little role of contrast examintion in high gut obstruction, GI contrast examination should be performed in obstructions presenting beyond first few days of life to rule out malrotation and midgut volvulus. The stomach is emptied through a nasogastric tube before upper GI contrast study is undertaken. The causes of high obstruction include pyloric atresia, duodenal atresia, malrotation with midgut volvulus or Ladd's bands and proximal jejunal atresia. Partial obstruction results from jejunal stenosis, peritoneal bands, duplication cyst, malrotation and Meckel's diverticulum. **Low Intestinal Obstruction:** Failure to pass meconium in the first 24-48 hours of life may be due to structural or functional reasons. The causes include ileal or colon atresia, Anorectal malformations, Hirschsprung's disease, meconium plug syndrome, and neonatal small left colon syndrome.

* Barium suspension is not used in cases of suspected perforation or if there is a risk of barium inspissations. Aspiration into lungs should be avoided while using contrast agents because commonly used high osmolality ionic contrast may produce severe pulmonary edema. Hypertonic water-soluble ionic contrast media may be useful in relieving obstruction in meconium ileus by drawing water into the bowel lumen. However, this may cause fluid and electrolyte imbalance. Therefore, infant should be hydrated and serum electrolytes monitored before the procedure. Non-ionic low osmolality contrast media are preferred in most circumstances. Barium is preferred in cases of suspected Hirschsprung's disease or other conditions where delayed films have diagnostic value.

* Ultrasonography (US) is often the first modality to be used in investigation of child with abdominal lump or suspected hypertrophic pyloric stenosis. US is highly accurate in the diagnosis of hypertrophic pyloric stenosis and extremely useful in the investigation of mass lesions such as enteric duplication cysts and mesenteric or omental cysts. US is the modality of choice for prenatal screening, but occasionally additional imaging information is needed.

* MRI is being increasingly used for prenatal imaging of congenital anomalies. The use of fast sequences like single shot fast spin echo and echoplanar imaging has enabled successful prenatal MR imaging. Esophageal, duodenal, or small bowel atresia can be diagnosed on antenatal MRI. On MRI, the signal intensity differences of the dilated bowel may provide additional information complementary to the US in identifying the site of obstruction. The proximal small bowel (fluid content) appears hyperintense on single-shot fast spin echo (SSFSE) and hypointense on T1-weighted fast spin echo (FSE) imaging. In contrast, the distal small bowel and colon appear hypointense on SSFSE and hyperintense on T1- weighted FSE imaging due to presence of meconium. CT and MRI has assumed a greater importance as these provide excellent anatomic details which may be necessary for correct diagnosis as well as treatment planning. This is particularly true in evaluation of congenital anomalies such as esoph ageal/enteric duplications, vascular rings and anorectal anomalies. Magnetic resonance imaging has proven to be the single stop modality to answer all the crucial questions such as level and type of anorectal malformation, type of fistula, developmental state of the sphincter muscle complex, and the presence of associated anomalies. Spinal radiographs must be examined carefully for abnormalities, because spinal pathology has profound effect on the outcome. Normal radiographic and sonographic appearance of spinal anatomy in children with anorectal malformation makes MRI superfluous, but if radiographs or ultrasound are uninformative/abnormal, MRI should be used to accurately depict possible intraspinal pathology. Sonography of the urinary tract for associated renal anomalies is essential in all patients with anorectal malformation. It is important to be familiar with the role nad usefulness of the various imaging modalities so that these can be used judiciously to avoid unnecessary radiation exposure while minimizing the patient discomfort.

DEVELOPMENTAL LESIONS OF THE NEONATAL GASTROINTESTINAL TRACT CAN BE GROUPED AS FOLLOWS:

Structural

Attributed to embryologic maldevelopment
- Esophageal atresia with or without fistula
- Antro-pyloric atresia
- Antral diaphragm
- Duodenal atresia
- Duodenal stenosis

Intrinsic: windsock duodenum
Extrinsic: annular pancreas
- Midgut malrotation with peritoneal bands
- Duplication or mesenteric cyst
- Anorectal atresia

Attributed to in utero vascular (ischemic) complication
- Jejuno-ileal atresia
- Colonic atresia or stenosis
- Complicated meconium ileus

Functional
- Meconium plug syndrome and its variants
- Megacystis-microcolon-intestinal hypoperistalsis

Structural and Functional Combined
- Hypertrophic pyloric stenosis
- Midgut volvulus (complicating midgut malrotation)
- Uncomplicated meconium ileus
- Colonic aganglionosis

Courtesy: Arun Kumar Gupta and Bhuvnesh Guglani *Department of Radiodiagnosis, All India Institute of Medical Sciences, New Delhi, India.* Indian Journal of Pediatrics, Volume 72—May, 2005

* *Pearl/Peril/Pitfall : Patients with uncomplicated meconium ileus may be successfully treated with a diatrizoate maglumine (Gastrografin) enema performed while adequate intravenous fluid is being administered. The hypertonicity of the radiopaque agent (1,900 mOsm per L) draws fluid into the bowel to facilitate passage and expulsion of the tenacious meconium.[21] This treatment is successful in 16 to 50 percent of patients.*

The first stool is passed within 24 hours of birth in 99 percent of healthy full-term infants and within 48 hours in all healthy full-term infants. Failure of a full-term newborn to pass meconium within the first 24 hours should raise a suspicion of intestinal obstruction. Among premature infants, however, one study revealed that only 37 percent of 844 preterm infants passed their first stool in the first 24 hours; 32 percent had delayed passage of the first stool beyond 48 hours. In 99 percent of the preterm infants, the first stool was passed by the ninth day after birth.

Failure to pass meconium combined with progressive abdominal distention, refusal to feed and vomiting of bilious intestinal contents are the classic clinical signs of intestinal obstruction in neonates. Abdominal examination often reveals distended loops of bowel, which may be visible or palpable. Anal inspection is essential to exclude the presence of anal atresia, perineal fistula with anal atresia, the membranous form of anal atresia and anal stenosis.

Plain radiographs of the abdomen do not allow differentiation of small bowel obstruction from large bowel obstruction. The differential diagnosis for small bowel obstruction in neonates includes duodenal atresia, malrotation and volvulus, jejunoileal atresia, meconium ileus and meconium peritonitis. Bilious vomiting, with or without abdominal distention, is usually the first sign of small bowel obstruction.

In many cases of suspected neonatal intestinal obstruction, the clinical history and physical examination combined with plain abdominal radiographs, contrast enema radiographic examination, anorectal manometry and rectal biopsy eventually yield the diagnosis. The most difficult management decision is to decide between conservative management and emergency surgery. Ideally, all newborns suspected of having bowel obstruction should receive treatment at a center where a pediatric surgeon is available.

Hirschsprung's Disease

Hirschsprung's disease, or congenital aganglionic megacolon, has an overall incidence of one in 4,000 live births. It accounts for 20 to 25 percent of the cases of neonatal bowel obstruction. The disease affects four times as many boys as girls, and 8 percent of patients with Hirschsprung's disease also have Down syndrome. The abnormal bowel innervation affects the internal anal sphincter. Most often, the rectosigmoid is involved, but a variable length of gut can be involved. A 30-year retrospective study revealed that the mean age at diagnosis has decreased to 2.6 months because of vigilance on the part of physicians, the use of anorectal manometry for assessment of the anal sphincter and early rectal biopsy to confirm the clinical diagnosis.

A common presentation of Hirschsprung's disease in the newborn is failure to pass meconium during the first few days of life, with subsequent passage of a meconium plug followed by sparse bowel movements. Gastrointestinal bleeding and diarrhea are danger signs for Hirschsprung's disease-associated enterocolitis. Enterocolitis can be fatal and is thought to be due to proliferation of bacteria as a result of stasis. Physical examination often reveals the anus and rectum to be narrow and empty of stool. Plain abdominal radiographs show gas and stool in the colon and often the distention with stool or gas does not reach distally to the pelvic rim (*Figure 1a*). Barium enema radiographic examination, performed with the colon unprepared, may reveal a transition zone that separates the small- to normal-diameter aganglionic bowel from the dilated bowel above (*Figure 1c*). A transition zone may not be recognizable in up to 25 percent of Neonates with classic Hirschsprung's disease (*Figure 1b*). Similarly, a transition zone may not be discernible in patients with ultrashort-segment Hirschsprung's disease, in patients with total colonic aganglionosis in whom the transition zone is above the colon and in patients who had an emergency colostomy. The presence of barium in the 24-hour delayed film is also suggestive of Hirschsprung's disease. Diagnosis depends on the anorectal manometry and rectal biopsy. **Treatment**-Surgery to remove or bypass the diseased bowel is required in all children with Hirschsprung's disease. In most neonates, a colostomy is initially placed into the normal bowel for decompression, followed by corrective surgery in three to six months. Occasionally, a primary pull-through procedure is performed.

Meconium plug syndrome is the mildest and most common form of functional distal obstruction in the newborn. It is a transient form of distal colonic or rectal obstruction caused by inspissated, immobile meconium. The incidence of meconium plug syndrome is estimated to range from one case in 500 to one case in 1,000 neonates. The etiology of this disorder is unclear. The plain abdominal radiograph often reveals generalized gaseous distention of intestinal loops of small and large bowel filling the entire abdomen, but with no fluid levels. Contrast enema is diagnostic, showing the outline of the meconium plug (*Figure 2*), and also therapeutic if the plug is passed afterward. In some newborns, rectal stimulation with a thermometer, digital rectal examination or a saline enema induces passage of the plug. After the plug is passed, bowel movements are normal, and all symptoms resolve. However, even neonates with organic disease, such as Hirschsprung's disease, may pass a meconium plug and do well for a period of time. Therefore, continued observation is required in infants who pass a meconium plug and, if symptoms persist, further work-up is required.

Meconium Ileus-Another cause of neonatal bowel obstruction by thick tenacious meconium is meconium ileus. Meconium ileus accounts for about 30 percent of cases of intestinal obstruction in newborns. In approximately 50 percent of the newborns with meconium ileus, the gut is undamaged and continuity is not disrupted; the obstruction is merely due to intraluminal meconium. In the other infants, meconium ileus is associated with volvulus, atresia or perforation. Cystic fibrosis is the underlying disorder in most infants with meconium ileus. Meconium ileus occurs in 15 percent of patients with cystic fibrosis. Typically, abdominal distention is present at birth. Within hours, as air is swallowed, the distention increases, and the infant vomits bile-stained material. Thickened bowel loops are often palpable and visible through the abdominal wall. Massive distention, abdominal tenderness or abdominal erythema indicates the presence of complications. Rectal examination is often difficult because of the small caliber of the rectum. Abdominal radiographs may reveal a distended bowel, few air-fluid levels and, in the right lower abdomen, meconium mixed with air, which has a ground-glass appearance on plain film. The presence of calcifications, free air or very large air-fluid levels suggests complications. The difference between meconium ileus and meconium plug syndrome is in the site and severity of the obstruction. Contrast enema radiographic examination demonstrates a microcolon, often with no bowel contents. Reflux of contrast into the small bowel reveals the plugs. The small bowel is of narrow caliber below the plug and dilated above the plug. Simple meconium ileus may be successfully treated by administration of a diatrizoate meglumine (Gastrografin) enema and plenty of intravenous fluids; the

* ***Pearl/Peril/Pitfall:*** *Bilious vomiting in a neonate is considered to be a surgical emergency until proven otherwise; however, in early presentations of volvulus, vomitus can be nonbilious, and a misdiagnosis of acute gastroenteritis might result.*

success rate is 16 percent to 50 percent. If the Gastrografin enema is unsuccessful, operative evacuation of the obstructing meconium by irrigation will be necessary. Complications such as atresia, perforation and meconium peritonitis always require immediate surgery, including resection, intestinal anastomosis and ileostomy.

Small Left Colon Syndrome

A rare cause of neonatal intestinal obstruction is small left colon syndrome, a functional distal bowel obstruction secondary to transient dysmotility in the descending colon. With this disorder, abdominal distention often develops after the newborn has passed meconium. More than 50 percent of newborns with small left colon syndrome are infants of mothers who have diabetes or an abnormal glucose tolerance test. Other infants are hypoglycemic or septic and, in others, an association with hypothyroidism, hypermagnesemia and maternal use of psychotropic drugs has been reported.

Plain radiograph shows dilated intestinal loops (*Figure 3a*) and, often, air-fluid levels. Contrast studies show the colon to be shortened and to lack the usual tortuosity from the anus to the splenic flexure. A sharp transition zone is seen at the splenic flexure (*Figure 3b*).

Rectal biopsy in patients with small left colon syndrome shows ganglion cells, contrary to the absence of ganglion cells in patients with Hirschsprung's disease. The ganglion cells can be normal, immature or hyperganglionic. The clinical course in newborns with small left colon syndrome varies in severity from mild symptoms, which may be relieved by the contrast enema, to severe bowel obstruction requiring a temporary transverse colostomy. Newborns with small left colon syndrome eventually have normal intestinal motility.

Anorectal Malformations

One in 4,000 to one in 8,000 newborns is born with an anorectal malformation. A spectrum of anomalies of the lower intestinal tract and the genitourinary structures occurs from a failure of the completion of the complex embryologic developmental sequences in which the growth of the urorectal septum, lateral mesoderm structures and ectodermal structures form the normal rectum and lower urinary tract.

Anal Stenosis Anal stenosis accounts for approximately 20 percent of anorectal malformations. The anus is very small, and a central black dot of meconium is present. Intense efforts are required to pass a ribbon-like stool. The diagnosis of anal stenosis is established by demonstration of a small, tight anus. Occasionally, an anal web may be the cause of the small anus. Anal dilatation is the usual treatment for anal stenosis and may need to be continued for several months. **Anal Atresia**- Anal atresia affects males and females with equal frequency. Perineal inspection reveals the absent anus (*Figure 4*). Broadly classified, anal atresia is characterized as "high" or "low," depending on whether the rectum ends above the levator muscle or partially descends through this muscle. Often, the rectum ends in a fistula. In the high type of anal atresia, the fistula often ends in the prostatic urethra in males and in the vagina in females (*Figure 5*).

Patients with a low type of anal atresia usually have a well-formed sacrum, a prominent midline groove and a prominent anal dimple. The low lesions are associated with a cutaneous fistula to the perineum. The orifice is small, located in the perineum anterior to the center of the external anal sphincter, close to the scrotum in the male and the vulva in the female. The abnormal anterior position anorectal malformation. About 50 percent have urologic problems. *The mnemonic VACTERL is used to describe the association of a combination of vertebral defects, anal atresia, cardiac defects, tracheoesophageal fistula with esophageal atresia, renal defects and radial upper limb hypoplasia.*

Anal atresia requires surgical correction. The goal is to preserve bowel, urinary and sexual function. A colostomy is initially performed in neonates with high anal atresia. If a fistula is present on the perineum or in the vagina, it can be gently dilated to allow the gas and meconium to pass. Low lesions, including those with perineal fistulas, can be corrected electively when the infant's condition is stable.

Other Causes of Failure to Pass Meconium

Various maternal medical conditions can cause a delay in meconium passage. In addition, maternal drug use, such as illicit drugs, magnesium sulfate and ganglionic blocking agents, can affect the infant and interfere with the passage of meconium. Neonatal medical conditions that can be associated with a failure to pass meconium include hypothyroidism, hypercalcemia, hypokalemia, sepsis and congestive heart failure.

Hypoganglionosis and neuronal intestinal dysplasia type A can produce symptoms and radiographic findings similar to those of Hirschsprung's disease. Both of these diseases are rare. They can affect part of or all of the gastrointestinal tract and sometimes occur in combination with Hirschsprung's disease. Histologically, hypoganglionosis is characterized by a reduced number of ganglion cells. In neuronal intestinal dysplasia type A, histologic features include hypoplasia or aplasia of the sympathetic innervation of the myenteric plexus and mucosa, along with mucosal inflammation.

Neuronal intestinal dysplasia type B may be manifested in the newborn period as meconium plug syndrome, small left colon syndrome or megacystis-microcolon-intestinal hypoperistalsis syndrome. The biopsy shows a dysplastic submucosal plexus and numerous giant ganglia, with many giant and small ganglion cells.

Various medications, partial or total parenteral nutrition, or surgery to remove or bypass segments of bowel may be necessary in patients with hypoganglionosis and neuronal intestinal dysplasia.

Another rare cause of neonatal intestinal obstruction is the megacystis-microcolon-intestinal hypoperistalsis syndrome. In this disorder, the small bowel is dilated and shortened, and the colon is a microcolon (*Figure 6*). There is an abundance of ganglion cells in the entire gastrointestinal tract. All patients with this syndrome have megacystis and megaureters, and most eventually die of complications from the disorder.

---

* *Pearl/Peril/Pitfall: Duodenal atresia occurs in 1 per 5,000 to 10,000 live births, involving male infants more commonly than female infants. Down syndrome occurs in about one-quarter of these patients; congenital heart disease occurs in about 20 percent of them. Abdominal plain film shows a characteristic "double-bubble" sign, demonstrating the bubbles in the stomach and the dilated proximal duodenum; this confirms the diagnosis. The prognosis is excellent unless the patient has associated serious congenital anomalies.*

FAILURE TO PASS MECONIUM: DIAGNOSING NEONATAL INTESTINAL OBSTRUCTION

Differential Diagnosis of Conditions That May Be Associated with Failure to Pass Meconium in the Newborn

Diagnosis	Frequency	Abnormal findings	Therapy
Hirschsprung's disease	1/4,000	Tight anus, empty rectum, transition zone	Surgery
Meconium plug syndrome	1/500 to 1/1,000	Meconium plugs	Rectal stimulation, enema
Meconium ileus	1/2,800	Abdominal distention at birth, Cystic fibrosis	Enema with intravenous fluids, surgery
Anorectal malformation	1/4,000 to 1/8,000	Absent anus, tight anus or fistula	Dilatation, surgery
Small left colon syndrome	Rare	Transition zone* at splenic flexure	Enema, rarely, colostomy
Hypoganglionosis	Rare surgery	Transition zone*	Medical, TPN,
Neuronal intestinal dysplasia type A	Rare	Transition zone,* mucosal inflammation	Medical, surgery
Neuronal intestinal dysplasia type B	Rare	Megacolon	Medical, rarely, surgery
Megacystis-microcolon -intestinal hypoperistalsis syndrome	Very rare megacystis	Microcolon,	TPN

TPN = total parenteral nutrition.

*—Transition zone (from small- to large-diameter bowel) refers to radiographic visualization on contrast study.

Anorectal Manometry When possible, anorectal manometry should be performed in all newborns with symptoms of lower bowel obstruction. With anorectal manometry, changes in anal pressure are recorded during and after rectal distention. When ganglion cells are present, rectal distention with a balloon inhibits the internal anal sphincter, resulting in a fall in anal pressure, called the rectosphincteric reflex (*See Figure given below-upper half*). In patients with Hirschsprung's disease, the rectosphincteric reflex is absent (*See Figure given below-lower half*). Anorectal manometry is most helpful in excluding the diagnosis of Hirschsprung's disease in a newborn. If the rectosphincteric reflex is absent, the diagnosis of Hirschsprung's disease needs to be confirmed by rectal suction biopsy, which shows no ganglion cells and markedly increased acetylcholinesterase staining of increased coarse neural fibers within the muscularis mucosae and the lamina propria.

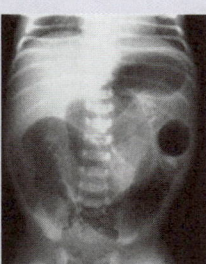

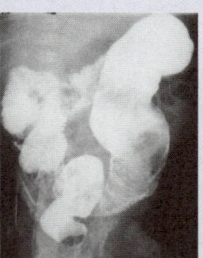

Figure1a Plain abdominal radiograph demonstrating numerous loops of dilated bowel. Small bowel obstruction cannot be differentiated from large bowel obstruction. No gas is visible in the rectum.

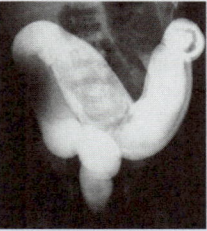

Figure 1b Barium enema radiograph showing an incompletely filled, dilated colon. This examination confirms that most of the dilated bowel on the plain film is the colon. No transition zone is visible

Figure 1c Barium enema radiograph performed when the infant was six weeks of age, revealing a transition zone in the distal portion of the sigmoid colon, with marked dilatation of the descending colon and the left side of the transverse colon. These findings are consistent with Hirschsprung's disease.

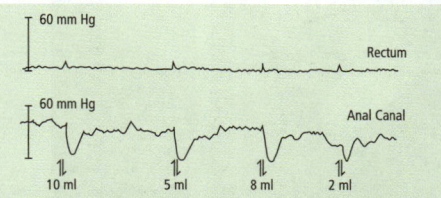

Anorectal manometric recording of a newborn with delayed passage of stool, showing a normal rectosphincteric reflex as demonstrated by the drop in anal pressure in response to rectal distention. The volume indicated is the volume used for rapid rectal distention. Rectal distention inhibits the internal anal sphincter, resulting in a fall in anal canal pressure.

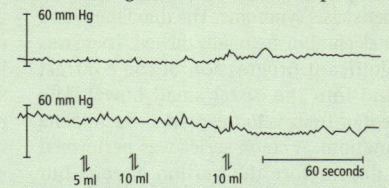

Anorectal manometric recording of a newborn with Hirschsprung's disease. The rectosphincteric reflex is absent, manifested by no change in the anal canal pressure in response to rectal distention.

* *Pearl/Peril/Pitfall : Before touching the abdomen, the examiner should look for any obvious abnormalities such as distension, masses, or peristaltic waves. If a child is crying, it should be remembered that the abdomen is relatively soft during the child's inhalation, which might be the best time to detect masses. To elicit areas of tenderness or peritoneal signs, a quieter, calm child is helpful.*

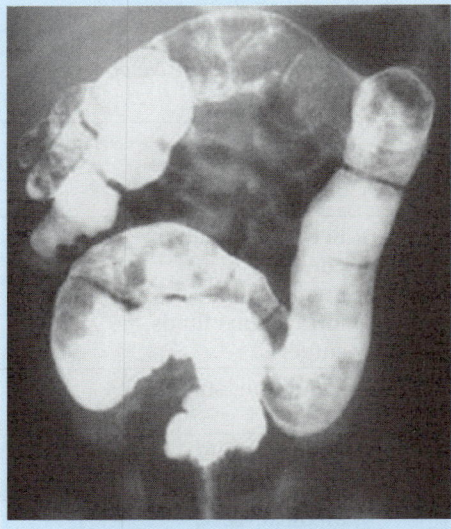

Figure 2 Barium radiograph of a newborn with meconium plug syndrome. Barium outlines multiple plugs of meconium. This infant passed the multiple plugs after the barium enema and then continued to pass normal meconium.

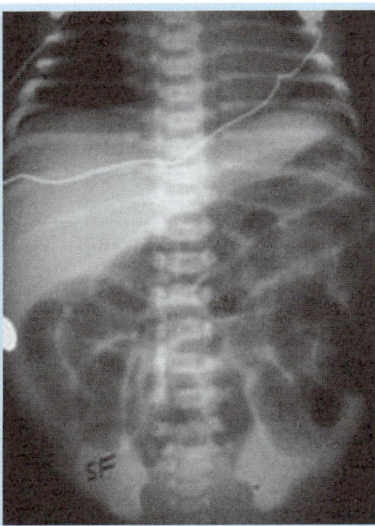

Figure 3a Plain radiograph of an infant with small left colon syndrome. Dilated intestinal loops are visualized.

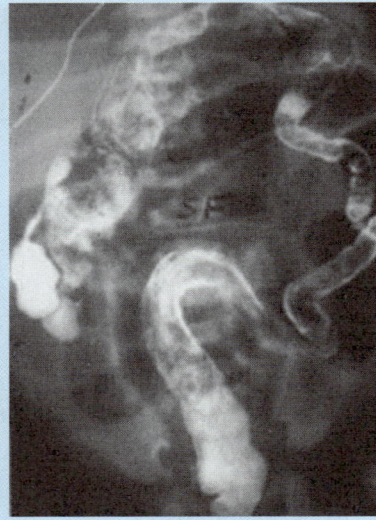

Figure 3b Barium enema radiograph of the infant in Figure 3a, showing a sharp transition zone at the splenic flexure

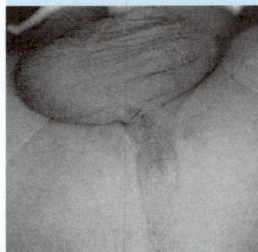

Figure 4 Imperforate anus in a male infant.

Figure 5 Barium enema radiograph showing evidence of imperforate anus and a vaginal fistula. Barium is present in the vagina (arrow). "PC" marks the pubococcygeal line.

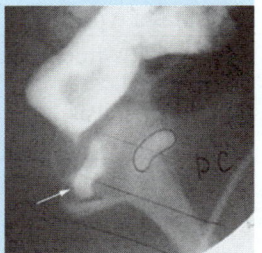

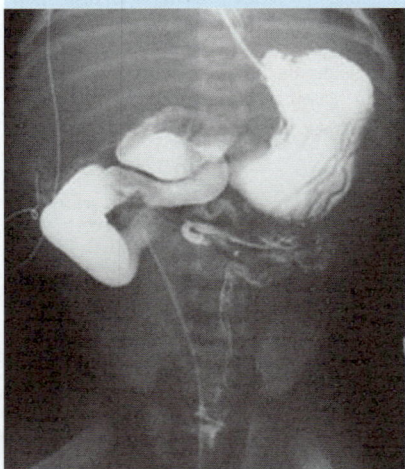

Figure 6 Barium enema radiograph in an infant with megacystis - microcolon - intestinal hypoperistalsis syndrome. The duodenum and proximal jejunum are mildly dilated. There was no significant progression of the contrast medium into the distal small bowel. The ligament of Treitz is to the right of the midline (malrotation). A colon series was performed three days before the barium enema, but contrast is still visible in the tortuous and abnormally positioned small colon. In addition, the urinary bladder is large and thickened, and reflux is present in the right dilated system.

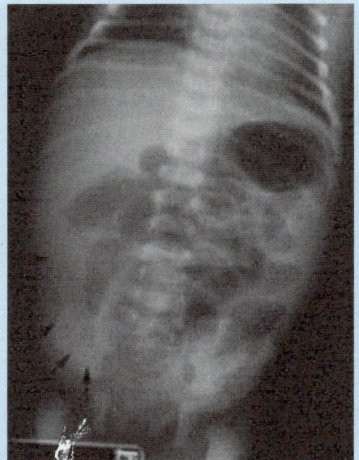

With meconium ileus, three cardinal signs of intestinal obstruction are generally evident including generalized abdominal distention, bilious vomiting, and failure to pass meconium within 48 hours. Plain radiographs of the abdomen may be extremely helpful. In patients with simple obturation obstruction, the characteristic radiologic features include varying-sized loops of distended intestine, a relative absence of air-fluid levels, and a "soap bubble" appearance of portions of the abdomen (Neuhauser's sign), particularly the right lower quadrant . Other disorders that may share some of these radiologic findings include Hirschsprung's disease, ileal atresia, and meconium plug syndrome.

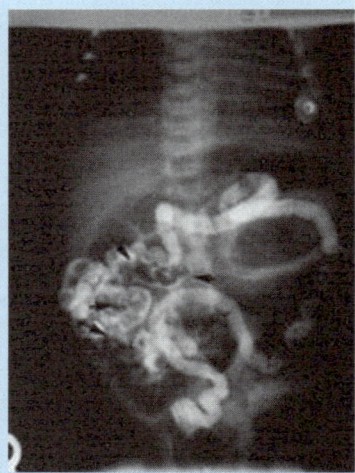

When simple meconium ileus is suspected, a contrast enema study should be performed. The classic finding is a microcolon along with pellet-like meconium when contrast is refluxed into the terminal ileum

---

* Pearl/Peril/Pitfall: *Meconium peritonitis is an aseptic peritonitis caused by spillage of meconium into the abdominal cavity during the development of jejunoileal atresia. Extravasation of meconium causes an intense chemical and foreign body reaction with characteristic calcifications, vascular fibrous proliferation and cyst formation.*

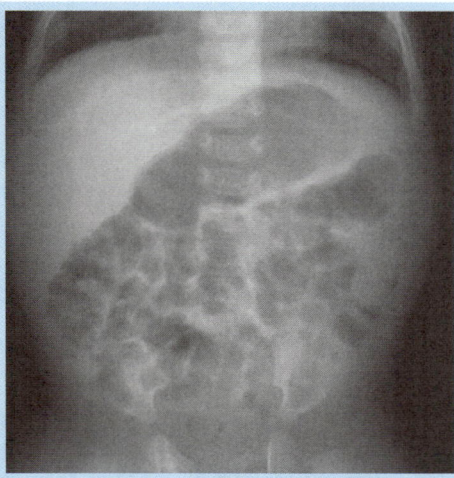

Frontal view of the abdomen shows multiple calcifications scattered in the pelvis and inguinal region. Diagnosis : Meconium peritonitis. Meconium ileus was not the etiology in this case.

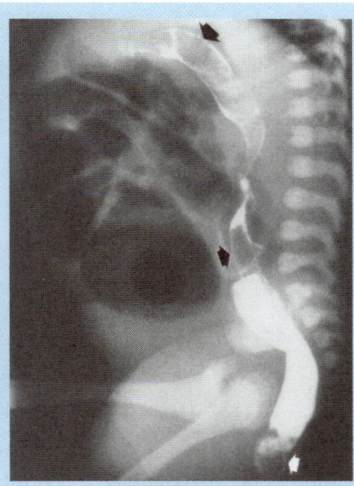

Meconium plug syndrome: Image from a barium enema study shows a normal-sized rectum and colon with inspissated meconium filling defects (arrows).

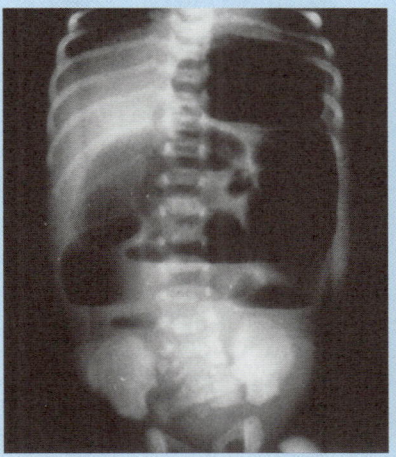

Ileal atresia (a) Upright radiograph shows multiple air-fluid levels occupying the entire abdominal cavity. (b) Image from a barium enema study shows numerous dilated, air-filled loops of bowel and a small, unused colon (functional microcolon).

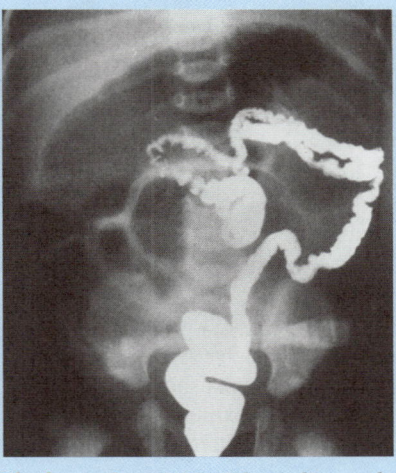

Ileal atresia: (a) Upright radiograph shows multiple air-fluid levels occupying the entire abdominal cavity. (b) Image from a barium enema study shows numerous dilated, air-filled loops of bowel and a small, unused colon (functional microcolon).

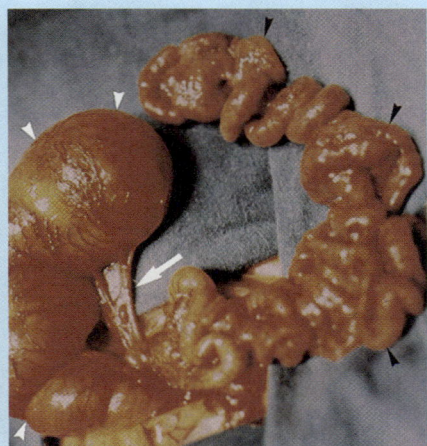

Gross specimen demonstrates apple peel small bowel. Note the distention of the proximal small bowel (white arrowheads), the shortening of the dorsal mesentery (arrow), and the distal spiraled segment of the small bowel (black arrowheads).

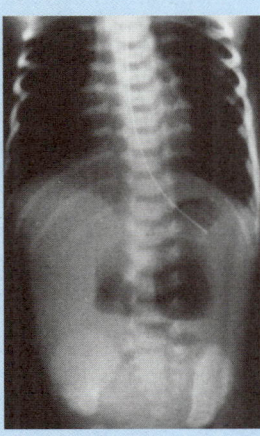

Jejunal atresia. (a) Supine radiograph in a neonate with associated esophageal atresia shows three dilated loops of bowel. *st* = stomach. (b) Upright radiograph obtained in a different patient shows air-fluid levels in the stomach and the first part of the small bowel. No distal gas is seen.

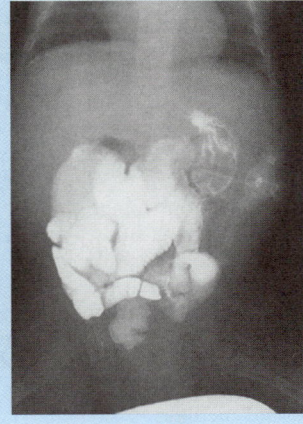

Frontal view of the abdomen from an enema shows extensive bowel resection and barium opacifying the remaining bowel. Note the dilated small bowel in the right upper quadrant; this occurs after surgery to increase absorptive capacity but can also result in decreased motility. Short bowel syndrome due to multiple intestinal atresias.

---

* *Pearl/Peril/Pitfall: Meconium peritonitis is an aseptic peritonitis caused by spillage of meconium into the abdominal cavity during the development of jejunoileal atresia. Extravasation of meconium causes an intense chemical and foreign body reaction with characteristic calcifications, vascular fibrous proliferation and cyst formation.*

IMAGING IN NEONATAL GIT OBSTRUCTION

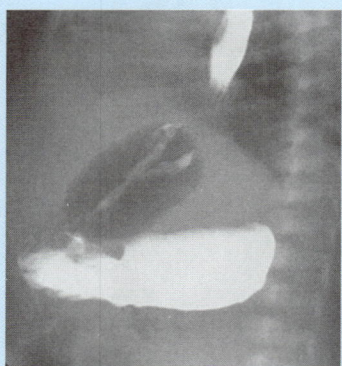

Lateral image from an Upper GI shows obstruction to the passage of barium at the 2nd portion of the duodenum and there is gas in decompressed loops distal to this level. **Diagnosis:** Duodenal atresia and "Y" connection.

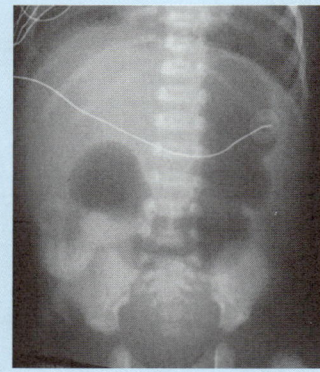

Supine abdominal radiograph shows a "double bubble" and exaggerated gastric incisura. **Diagnosis:** Associated duodenal atresia and imperforate anus.

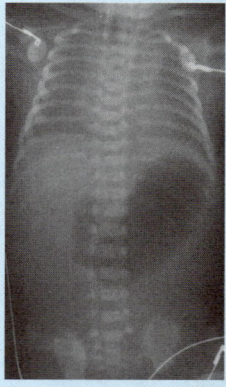

Supine chest and abdominal radiograph shows the catheter cannot be advanced beyond the proximal esophagus and there is a "double bubble". Esophageal atresia, duodenal atresia, and distal fistula.

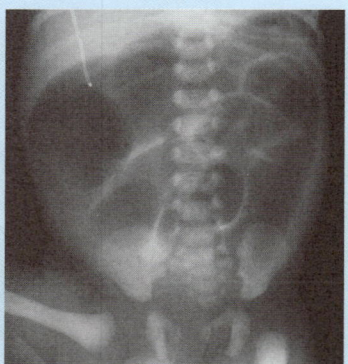

Supine radiograph of the abdomen shows diffusely dilated loops of bowel throughout the abdomen (small and large bowel are difficult to differentiate in the infant). **Diagnosis:** Ileal Atresia.

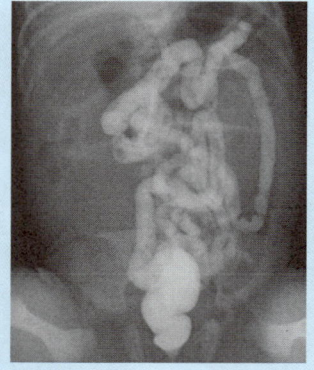

Water soluble enema shows microcolon and dilated proximal bowel loops. **Diagnosis:** Jejunal atresia.

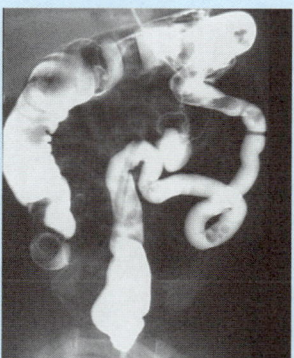

Contrast enema shows small caliber of the left colon with apparent "transition" at level of splenic flexure. Note normal recto-sigmoid index ("R" and "S" lines). **Diagnosis:** Neonatal small left colon.

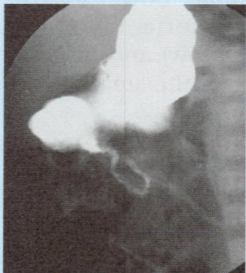

Upper GI: the "corkscrew" sign **Diagnosis:** Malrotation with midgut volvulus.

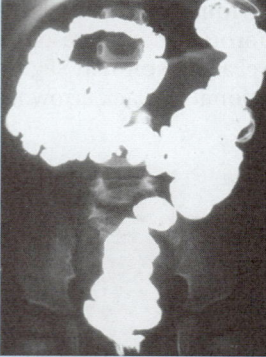

Malrotation. On an image from a barium enema study, the intestine occupies an intermediate position between that of nonrotation and the normal postnatal position. The cecum and the terminal ileum are displaced upward and medially.

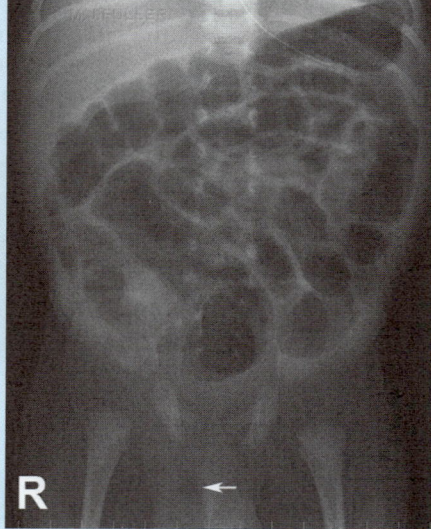

The arrowed structure is air in bowel which has herniated into the scrotum. Clearly, if this anatomy had not been included on the image, the diagnosis would have been missed. If the request form suggests that there is a possibility of **inguinal hernia,** the scrotum should be included in the abdominal image (unnatural as that may be). If the request form lists "obstruction" as a differential diagnosis, ask the referring doctor if he/she wants the scrotum included.

***** *Pearl/Peril/Pitfall : Most patients with midgut malrotation develop volvulus within the first week of life. Bilious vomiting is the initial symptom, but abdominal distention is not remarkable. The bowel can be involved in strangulation at any time and at any age. Once midgut ischemia occurs, unstable hemodynamics, intractable metabolic acidosis and necrosis with perforation develop, putting the patient at critical risk.*

TYMPANITIC ABDOMEN IN NEWBORNS AND NEONATES

* Tympanitic abdominal distention may occur in healthy infants, in infants who have systemic conditions, and in Newborns who have congenital causes of intestinal obstruction.

Some healthy infants experience mild distention because of air swallowing with crying or feeding. This distention is variable, greatest after feeding or fussing, and absent at other times. Vomiting is absent, and the stooling pattern and physical examination are normal. This transient generalized distention responds to changes in feeding technique and burping and in consoling techniques for the crying infant.

* In the ill Newborn, many systemic conditions cause a paralytic intestinal ileus characterized by quiet, nontender abdominal distention: sepsis, birth asphyxia, hypothyroidism, and electrolyte imbalance. Newborns who have pneumonia or respiratory distress may also develop distention from aerophagia.

* The most common cause of acquired abdominal distention in premature infants is necrotizing enterocolitis (NEC). Definitive radiographic evidence of NEC includes findings of (1) pneumatosis intestinalis and (2) gas visible in the portal venous system of the liver.

* Congenital causes of proximal gastrointestinal obstruction causing distention in the Newborn include intestinal atresias, annular pancreas, abnormalities of intestinal rotation, and fixation . The most common proximal gastrointestinal obstruction is duodenal atresia, characterized by polyhydramnios in 50% of patients and the onset of bilious vomiting in the 1st hours of life in conjunction with focal epigastric distention. Upright plain-film radiographs are diagnostic of duodenal obstruction when they demonstrate the double-bubble sign. Occasionally, evacuating the stomach of bile and amniotic fluid and instilling air are necessary to appreciate duodenal obstruction. Intestinal atresias are medical emergencies in so far as urgent decompression via nasogastric suction is indicated to diminish the risk of aspiration and gastrointestinal perforation. Malrotation is seen in up to 19% of patients who have intrinsic duodenal obstruction; a barium enema should establish normal intestinal rotation in infants whose surgery is deferred.

* Upper abdominal distention is a common, though not universal, finding in Newborns and infants who have symptomatic intestinal malrotation, the majority of whom will have bilious vomiting in the first 4 weeks of life. Approximately 25% of infants who have malrotation may have nonbilious vomiting; a high index of suspicion is warranted, given the severe morbidity of a delay in diagnosis. Plain-film radiographs may demonstrate a distended stomach or duodenal distention that has a paucity of gas distally. Most significantly, plain-film radiographs may appear normal. Therefore a stable infant thought to have malrotation should undergo an upper gastrointestinal series, which is diagnostic when the duodenal-jejunal junction is seen on the right side of the midline or when a beak or corkscrew obstruction is noted in the 2nd or 3rd part of the duodenum. Symptomatic malrotation is an operative emergency whether or not signs of intestinal ischemia (hematochezia, acidosis, shock, a blue-gray tinge to the abdomen, or peritonitis) have developed.

* Congenital causes of lower intestinal obstruction include distal intestinal atresias, meconium ileus, Hirschsprung disease, small left colon syndrome, and anorectal malformations. Newborns who have lower intestinal obstruction typically develop generalized tympanitic distention over the course of 24 to 48 hours, with bilious vomiting and failure to pass meconium. Although an imperforate anus or an incarcerated hernia will be apparent on physical examination, differentiation of the remaining causes of lower intestinal obstruction involves radiographic evaluation.

* Marked tympanitic abdominal distention can be a manifestation of pneumoperitoneum, which is demonstrated by upright and cross-table lateral abdominal radiographs revealing free air within the peritoneum. When pneumoperitoneum is associated with peritonitis, intestinal perforation is likely, and the causes include NEC, volvulus, an intestinal obstruction causing perforation, appendicitis, and spontaneous perforations. In infants on a respirator, pneumoperitoneum may occur without peritonitis as a complication of pneumomediastinum when air tracks down through diaphragmatic fenestrations into the peritoneal cavity.

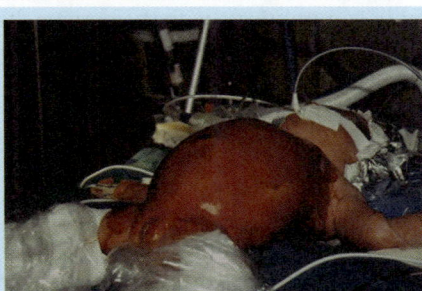
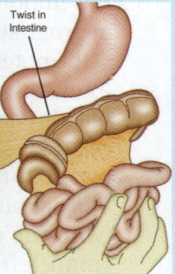
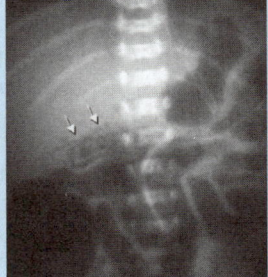
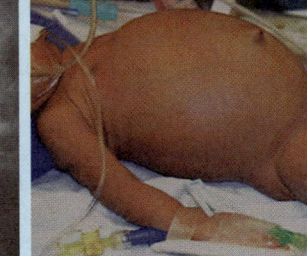

Typical distended abdomen noted in a baby with meconium at birth

Midgut volvulus. The colon is tightly coiled around the base of the small bowel mesentery. The bowel must be rotated in a counterclockwise manner to reduce the volvulus.

Anteroposterior image shows necrotizing enterocolitis with pneumatosis intestinalis

* *Pearl/Peril/Pitfall : When dilated bowel loops and air-fluid levels are demonstrated, the diagnosis of a surgical abdomen is suggested, and urgent consultation with a pediatric surgeon is indicated, preferably in a pediatric surgical center. Gastric decompression, hydration and secured airway must be completed before initiating transport of the patient.*

DIFFERENTIAL DIAGNOSIS BASED ON LEVEL OF GI OBSTRUCTION

Level	Nonbilious, Nondistended	Bilious, Nondistended	Bilious, Distended	Nonbilious, Distended
Esophageal	▓ ↕			
TEF	▓			
Gastric	▓			
GERD	▓			
Pyloric stenosis	▓ ↕			
Small bowel		▓ ↕		
Duodenal atresia		▓		
Malrotation		▓		
Jejunal atresia		▓ ↕		
Ileal atresia			▓	▓ ↕
Adhesive band			▓	▓
Hernia			▓	▓
Intussusception			▓	▓
Neoplasm			▓	▓
Colon			▓	▓
Hirschsprung			▓	▓
Meconium ileus			▓	▓
Small left colon			▓	▓
Meconium plug			▓	▓
Colonic atresia			▓	▓
NEC stricture			▓	▓
Neoplasm			▓	▓
Rectal			▓	▓
Imperforate anus			▓ ↕	▓ ↕

Bilious vomiting in the newborn: Rapid diagnosis of intestinal obstruction : Summary of evaluation and management: When a Neonate develops bilious vomiting, one should suspect a surgical condition. After a focused physical examination, a nasogastric or orogastric catheter should be placed for gastric decompression to prevent further vomiting and aspiration. This should be done before any diagnostic or therapeutic maneuvers are performed. Establishment of an intravenous line should follow for administration of fluid, electrolytes and nutrition. When the patient is hemodynamically stabilized, appropriate imaging studies of the abdomen should be performed. These would include plain abdominal films and/or contrast studies. When dilated bowel loops and air-fluid levels are demonstrated, the diagnosis of a surgical abdomen is suggested, and urgent consultation with a pediatric surgeon is indicated, preferably in a pediatric surgical center. Gastric decompression, hydration and secured airway must be completed before initiating transport of the patient. Intestinal obstruction with bilious vomiting in Neonates can be caused by duodenal atresia, malrotation and volvulus, jejunoileal atresia, meconium ileus, and necrotizing enterocolitis.

KEY POINTS FOR CLINICAL PRACTICE:

1. GIT obstruction in the Neonate should be suspected, when the following symptoms present: feeding intolerance, abdominal distention, recurrent & persistent vomitings, bilious emesis, increased gastric residual (>25-30ml), maternal history of polyhydramnios, excessive oral secretions & trisomy 21.

2. Always stabilize the Neonate with IV access, fluids, electrolytes, acid base balance, radiant warmer and perform a full examination & investigate further after discussing with an experienced pediatric surgeon.

3. It is important to communicate with the parents the appropriate level of concern, the need for consultation, & the potential need for surgery.

4. Intestinal malrotation & midgut volvulus is a potentially life-threatening condition, which needs upper GI contrast studies to confirm/exclude it, to prevent mortality & morbidity.

5. The definitive treatment for most of these conditions [with the exception of meconium plug syndrome, small left colon syndrome, and some cases of meconium ileus] is SURGERY.

REFERENCES & FURTHER READING : 1)Nerwich N, Shi E. Neonatal duodenal obstruction: a review of 30 consecutive cases. Pediatr Surg Int 1994;9:47-50. 2) Rescorla FJ, Shedd FJ, Grosfeld JL, Vane DW, West KW. Anomalies of intestinal rotation in childhood: analysis of 447 cases. Surgery 1990;108:710-5. 3)Donnellan WL, Kimura K. Malrotation, internal hernias, congenital band. In: Donnellan WL, ed. Abdominal surgery of infancy and childhood. Austria-United States: Harwood Academic, 1996:1-27. 4) Rescorla FJ, Grosfeld JL. Intestinal atresia and stenosis: analysis of survival in 120 cases. Surgery 1985;98:668-76. 5)O'Neill JA Jr, Grosfeld JL, Boles ET Jr, Clatworthy HW Jr. Surgical treatment of meconium ileus. Am J Surg 1970;119:99-105.

* *Pearl/Peril/Pitfall: The malrotated bowel itself does not cause any significant problem. However, because of the narrow axis, the midgut can at any time twist around the axis, perhaps triggered by peristaltic action. The tighter the twist, the more the midgut suffers from obstruction of the lumen, obstruction of venous and lymphatic return from the midgut, and obstruction of arterial inflow, thus threatening midgut viability. Unless it is treated in a timely manner, bowel strangulation results in an ischemic loss of extensive bowel, causing the short-gut syndrome.*

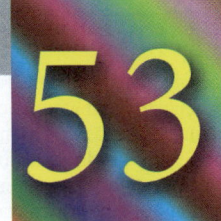

53 Neonatal Jaundice and Hyperbilirubinemia

@ *UNCONJUGATED VS CONJUGATED* •*consider unconjugated hyperbili when direct (conjugated) < 15% of total - unconjugated form is neurotoxic at certain concentrations—kernicterus—CNS changes due to deposits of unconj bilirubin in nuclei of the brain—depending upon gestational age, neonates at risk with bilirubin > 10–20 mg/dl (now being re-investigated) —usually due to hemolytic hyperbilirubinemia; extremely rare for physiologic •consider conjugated hyperbili when direct (conjugated) > 25–30% of total —conjugated form is not toxic, but indicates a potentially serious pathological disorder.*

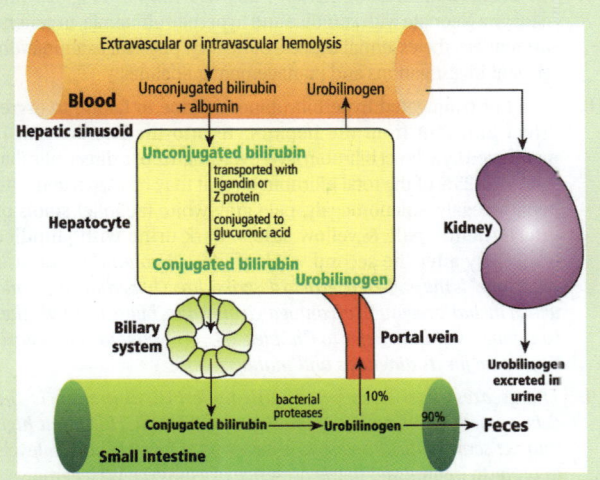

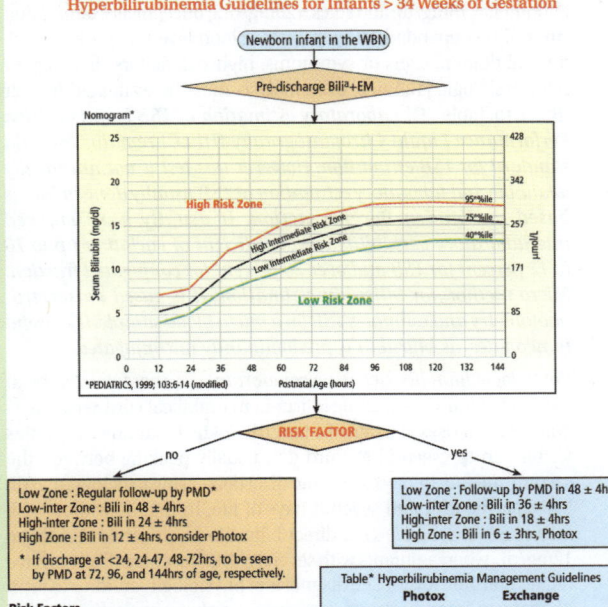

Hyperbilirubinemia Guidelines for Infants > 34 Weeks of Gestation

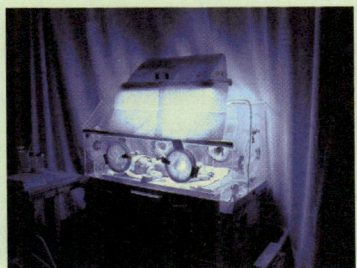

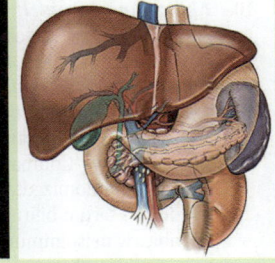

Low Zone : Regular follow-up by PMD*
Low-inter Zone : Bili in 48 ± 4hrs
High-inter Zone : Bili in 24 ± 4hrs
High Zone : Bili in 12 ± 4hrs, consider Photox

* If discharge at <24, 24-47, 48-72hrs, to be seen by PMD at 72, 96, and 144hrs of age, respectively.

Low Zone : Follow-up by PMD in 48 ± 4hrs
Low-inter Zone : Bili in 36 ± 4hrs
High-inter Zone : Bili in 18 ± 4hrs
High Zone : Bili in 6 ± 3hrs, Photox

Risk Factors
1. Family history of jaundice or hemolysis
2. Near term infants (34-38wks) Late preterms
3. Polycythemia
4. Internal or external bleeding
5. Postnatal hemolysis
6. Increase Bili rise (>0.5mg/dl/hr)
7. Increased Bili production (high ETCOc)
8. Hypoxemia, acidosis, sepsis, hypoalbuminemia

Abbreviations
Bili = Total bilirubin
EM = Educational material
ETCOc = End tidal volume corrected CO
Photox = Phototherapy
PMD = Attending pediatrician
WBN = Well Baby Nursery

Table* Hyperbilirubinemia Management Guidelines

	Photox	Exchange
<24hrs	10-12 (7-10)	20 (18)
25-48hrs	12-15 (10-12)	20-25 (20)
49-72hrs	15-18 (12-15)	25-30 (>20)
>72hrs	18-20 (12-15)	25-30 (>20)

Bilirubin levels expressed in mg/dl
In brackets are Bili levels for infants with risk factors
*PEDIATRICS, 1994; 94:558-565 (modified)

a) Bilirubin can be obtained either by blood sample or by transcutaneous measurement

This algorithm is a suggested practice guidelines and do not intend to replace clinical judgement.

REVIEW OF CLINICAL PROBLEMS

1. Name the Risk factors for Jaundice & Hyperbilirubinemia.
   Ans: Refer to the Table 1 of the Chapter.

2. Mention the Categories of Neonatal Jaundice that need prompt investigation to determine the cause of Jaundice.
   Ans: Refer to the Evaluation-Decision-Action Plan/ Algorithm to diagnose & manage Neonatal Jaundice & Hyperbilirubinemia

3. *What are the Diagnostic features of various types of Neonatal Jaundice ?*
   Ans: Refer to the Table 2 of the Chapter.

4. How do you classify the various causes of Indirect Hyperbilirubinemia in a Neonate?
   Ans: Refer to the Table 4 of the Chapter.

5. Describe the Non-Invasive assessment of Neonatal Jaundice.
   Ans: Refer to the Section "Noninvasive Assessment of Neonatal Jaundice".

LEARNING OBJECTIVES

After completing this article, readers will be able to

1. Differentiate pathological jaundice from physiological Jaundice in a Neonate.

2. Monitor for Indirect Hyperbilirubinemia and manage it appropriately to avoid advanced bilirubin toxicity.

3. Identify the risk factors for Jaundice in a term infant and manage them adequately.

4. Identify the potentially preventable causes of Kernicterus.

5. Ensure neurodevelopmental & hearing follow-up of neonates discharged having been treated for severe indirect hyperbilirubinemia.

---

* Pearl/Peril/Pitfall: *Currently, clinicians should not solely rely on cephalocaudal jaundice progression to estimate bilirubin levels during the birth hospitalization or to predict subsequent severe Neonatal hyperbilirubinemia. However, the complete absence of jaundice (when reliably recognized) may predict that these infants will not develop significant hyperbilirubinemia.*

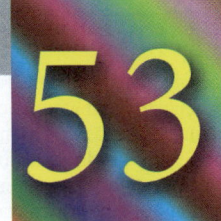

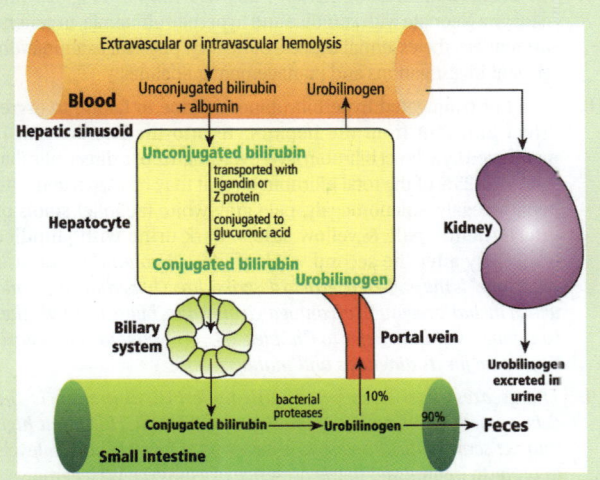

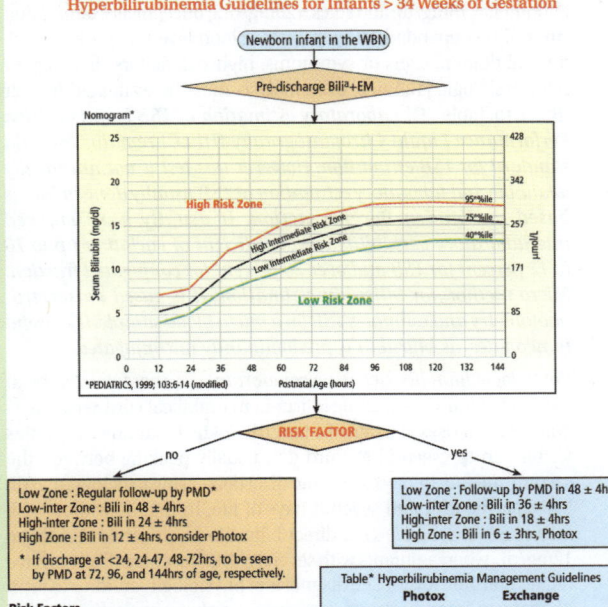

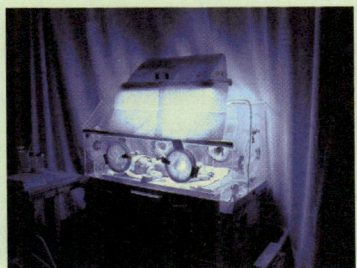

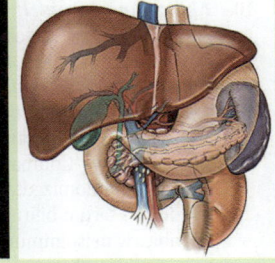

BIRD'S EYE VIEW/OVERVIEW/SYNOPSIS

1. Jaundice & hyperbilirubinemia in Neonates is mostly a benign problem (observed in 60% of term infants and 80% of preterm infants during the first week of life), _but if untreated severe indirect hyperbilirubinemia is potentially neurotoxic, and conjugated direct hyperbilirubinemia often signifies a serious hepatic or systemic illness_.

2. Jaundice usually begins on the face and, as serum levels increase, progresses to the abdomen and then the feet. Dermal pressure may reveal the anatomic progression of jaundice (face = 5mg/dL; mid-abdomen = 15mg/dL and soles = 20mg/dL), but clinical examination can not be depended on to estimate blood levels. Jaundice to the mid- abdomen, signs or symptoms, high-risk factors that suggest nonphysiologic jaundice, or hemolysis must be evaluated further (Refer to Table 1). *Laboratory estimation of TSB based on High Performance Liquid Chromatography (HPLC) remains the gold standard for TSB estimation. However this test is not universally available and laboratory estimation of TSB usually done in labs is based on Vanden Bergh reaction. It usually have marked interlaboratory variability with coefficient of variation up to 10 to 12 percent for TSB and over 20 percent for conjugated fraction. Micro method for bilirubin estimation: It is based on spectrophotometry and estimates TSB on a micro blood sample. It is useful in neonates, as bilirubin is predominantly unconjugated.*

3. *Physiologic Jaundice (Icterus Neonatorum)* - is characterized by a) the level of indirect-reacting bilirubin in umbilical cord serum is 1-3mg/dL, and rises at a rate of < 5mg/dL/24 hr b) jaundice becomes visible on the second to third day, usually peaking between the second and fourth days at 5-6mg/dL c) decreasing to below 2mg/dL between the fifth and seventh days of life. In infants without risk factors *(Refer to Table 1)*, indirect bilirubin levels rarely rise above 12mg/dL, whereas infants with several risk factors more likely to have higher bilirubin levels. The diagnosis of physiologic jaundice in term or preterm infants can be established *only by excluding known causes of jaundice* on the basis of the history, clinical and laboratory findings *(Refer to Table 2)*.

4. One should make a search to determine the cause of jaundice if 1) it appears in the 1st 24-36 hr of life, 2) serum bilirubin is rising at a rate faster than 5mg/dL/24 hr, 3) serum bilirubin is greater than 12 mg/dL in full-term (especially in the absence of risk factors) or 10-14 mg/dL in preterm infants, 4) jaundice persists after 10-14 days of life, or 5) direct-reacting bilirubin is greater than 2 mg/dL at any time. Among other factors suggesting a nonphysiologic cause of jaundice are a family history of hemolytic disease, pallor, hepatomegaly, splenomegaly, failure of phototherapy to lower bilirubin, vomiting, lethargy, poor feeding, excessive weight loss, apnea, bradycardia, abnormal vital signs (including hypothermia), light-colored stools, dark urine positive for bilirubin, and signs of kernicterus.

5. *Persistent or prolonged physiologic jaundice beyond 8 days in term infants and 14 days in preterm infants,* suggests hemolysis, hereditary glucuronyl transferase deficiency, breast milk jaundice, hypothyroidism, or intestinal obstruction, UTI, hepatitis / TORSCH infections etc.

6. *Unconjugated hyperbilirubinemia may be caused or increased by any factor that 1)* increases the load of bilirubin to be metabolized by the liver (hemolytic anemias, polycythemia, shortened red cell life as a result of immaturity or transfused cells, increased red cell life as a result of immaturity or transfused cells, increased

enterohepatic circulation, infection), 2) damages or reduces the activity of the transferase enzyme (genetic deficiency, hypoxia, infection, possibly hypothermia and thyroid deficiency), 3) competes for, and blocks the transferase enzyme (drugs and other substances requiring glucuronic acid conjugation for excretion), or 4) leads to an absence or decreased amounts of the enzyme or to reduction of bilirubin uptake by liver cells (genetic defect, prematurity) *(Refer to Table 4)*.

7. *The Evaluation-Decision-Action-Plan/Algorithm* to diagnose and manage a Neonate with jaundice and hyperbilirubinemia, in general summarizes the essential aspects of history, physical examination, relevant investigations and management guidelines.

8. Direct or conjugated hyperbilirubinemia (due to failure to excret direct bilirubin from the hepatocyte into the Duodenum) is manifested by a direct bilirubin level over 2mg/dL or a direct bilirubin level > 20-25% of the total bilirubin level. It may be associated with hepatomegaly, splenomegaly, pale gray-white (acholic) stools or intermittently pale & yellow stools, dark urine with jaundice (especially after the second week of life). _"Neonatal cholestasis syndrome" is the preferred term to describe direct hyperbilirubinemia which includes retention of conjugated bilirubin, bile acids, and other components of bile (Refer to Chapter 54, on Neonatal Cholestasis Syndrome for its diagnosis and management)._

9. *The greatest risk associated with hyperbilirubinemia is the development of bilirubin encephalopathy (KERNICTERUS) at high indirect serum bilirubin levels.* It develops at lower bilirubin levels in preterm infants and in the presence of asphyxia, IVH, hemolysis or drugs that displace bilirubin from albumin *(Refer to The E-D-A-Plan / Algorithm to diagnose and manage KERNICTERUS)*. KERNICTERUS does occur in patients with breast milk jaundice that is very uncommon. The exact serum bilirubin level that is harmful for VLBW (< 1500gms) infants is unclear.

10. *Management guidelines of indirect hyperbilirubinemia* (e.g. supportive measures to ensure adequate fluid and caloric intake and bowel function, phototherapy, exchange transfusion) should be modified in any sick infant with acidosis, hypercapnia, hypoxemia, asphyxia, sepsis, hypoalbuminemia (< 2.5g/dL), or signs of KERNICTERUS. **Intravenous immunoglobulin combined with phototherapy**—Compared with phototherapy alone, this has been shown in randomized, controlled trials to significantly reduce the maximum serum bilirubin and the need for exchange transfusion in babies with isoimmune hemolytic jaundice. Other outcomes that were significantly reduced were duration of phototherapy and length of hospitalization. However, such was the problem with small numbers and weak design, that the authors of this Cochrane Review did not recommend the routine use of this treatment, and suggested that the results of further RTCs of higher quality be awaited. They suggested that in circumstances where there was a strong need to avoid transfusion, that it may be justified.

The indications for phototherapy and exchange transfusion are summarized in Tables 3 & 5. Refer to the section "Essential Neonatal Guidelines & Practical Procedures" respectively, for the details of phototherapy & exchange transfusion. The American Academy of Pediatrics subcommittee on hyperbilirubinemia provided an updated guidelines providing a framework for the prevention and management of hyperbilirubinemia in newborn infants of 35 or more weeks' gestation (Refer to Table 3 & 5)

---

* *Pearl/Peril/Pitfall : APPEARANCE OF JAUNDICE • within first 24 hours of birth (ALWAYS PATHOLOGIC): Rh disease, concealed hemorrhage, sepsis, rubella, or congenital toxoplasmosis • first appearing on the 2nd or 3rd day: "physiologic", Crigler-Najjar • first appearing after 3rd day and within 1st week: breast feeding jaundice, sepsis, syphilis, TORCH, infections • first appearing after day 7: breast milk jaundice, sepsis, congenital biliary atresia, hepatitis, syphilis, TORCH infections, galactosemia, congenital hemolytic anemias (ex spherocytosis or G6PD deficiency) • first appearing after day 14: NOT PHYSIOLOGIC OR BREAST MILK RELATED !! PATHOLOGICAL UNTIL PROVEN OTHERWISE !!*

* *Pearl/Peril/Pitfall: BREAST-MILK JAUNDICE "LATE" (different than breast-feeding jaundice!) • A diagnosis by Exclusion; occurs in 1–2% of breast-milk fed babies; usually family history of same • breast milk may contain a glucuronidase that may inhibit glucuronyl transferase activity • bilirubin increases between 4th–7th day of life, (classically appears during 2nd week of life) peaks during the 3rd week of life; gradually decreases then plateaus to persist for 3–10 weeks—infant usually will be resolving his physiological jaundice then suddenly start to turn yellow again • levels = 10–30mg/dL • If breast feeding is stopped for 2–4 days, then levels rapidly decline and breast feeding can be resumed without a return of bilirubin to its previously high levels.*

THE EVALUATION-DECISION-ACTION-PLAN/ALGORITHM FOR THE DIAGNOSIS AND MANAGEMENT OF *NEONATAL JAUNDICE & HYPERBILIRUBINEMIA*

SUBJECTIVE FINDINGS

Hx of onset of jaundice (< 24 hrs), term or preterm baby, sick or well baby, associated with pallor, poor feeding, tempetature instability, distress, excessive weight loss/dehydration, pale stools, dark urine, fever.

Hx of obstetric trauma, oxytocin use, maternal diabetes / Rh sensitization, medications during pregnancy (G-6-PD-def.,) delayed cord clamping.

Hx of jaundice, anemia, splenectomy or liver disease in the family and siblings.

Hx of breast feeding / delayed or infrequent stooling/poor caloric intake.

OBJECTIVE FINDINGS

Assess signs of systemic illness—fever, hypothermia, pallor, seizures, abdominal distention, hepatosplenomegaly, omphalitis, evidence of hypothyroidism, extravascular blood (bruising, cephalhematoma etc.,).

Assess whether the baby is premature / IUGR / term AGA !

Look for stigmata of intrauterine infections (TORSCH) like microcephaly, petechiae, hepatosplenomegaly or chorioretinitis.

Assess for the clinical features of KERNICTERUS *(refer to E-D-A-Algorithm to diagnose & manage the most dreaded complication of severe indirect hyperbilirubinemia).*

INVESTIGATIONS

Blood Total serum bilirubin with direct & indirect fractions, FBC, differential platelets, reticulocyte count, smear, hematocrit & RBC indices, blood group, type & direct Coombs test of the infant, blood group, type & indirect Coombs test of the mother, G-6-PD screen, LFTs, TORSCH screen, blood cultures, electrolytes, ABG analysis.

If direct hyperbilirubinemia is evident— Refer to the Chapter 54, on Neonatal Cholestasis Syndrome.

Urine analysis, & Culture sensitivity, reducing substances.

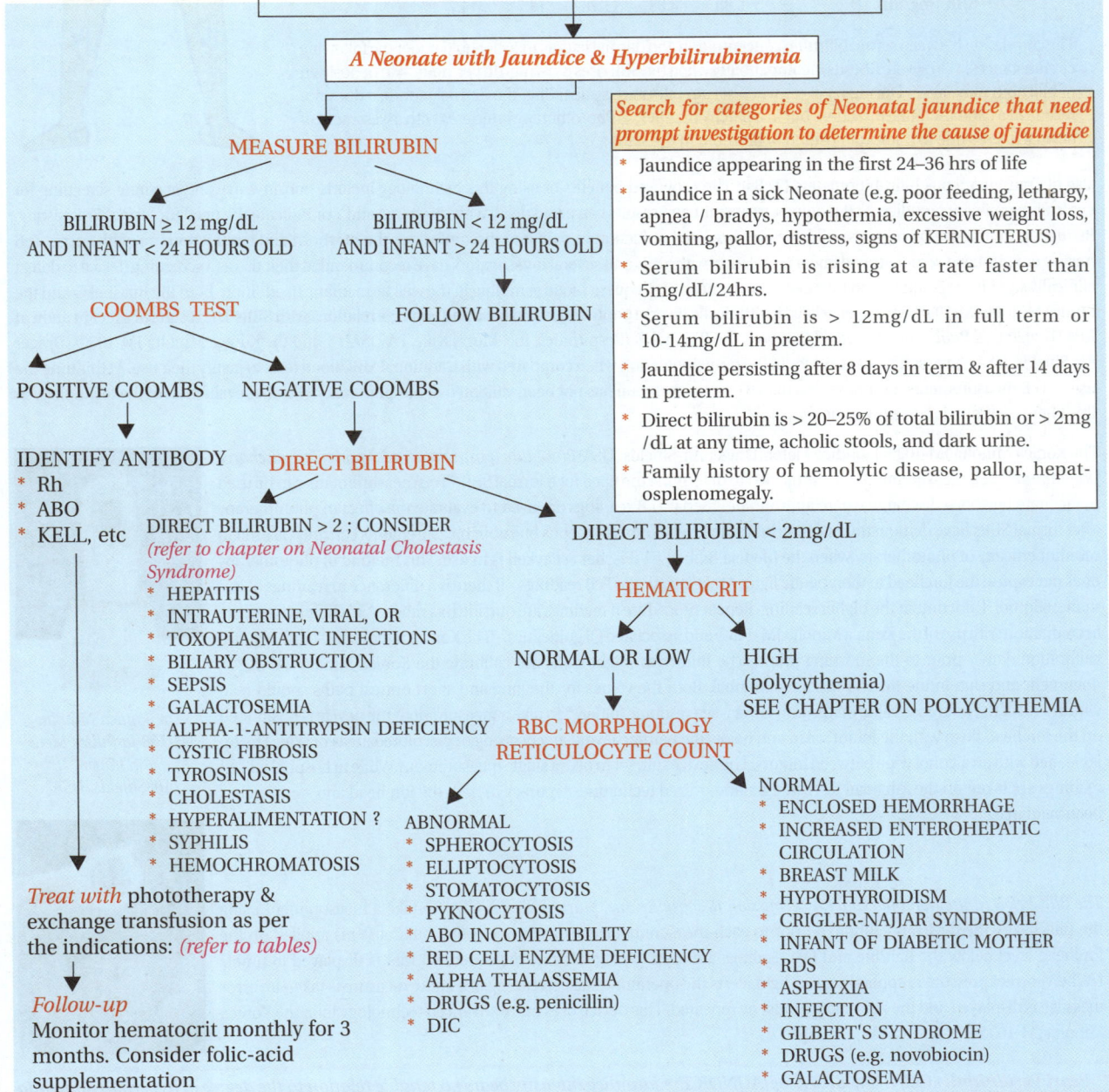

A Neonate with Jaundice & Hyperbilirubinemia

MEASURE BILIRUBIN

BILIRUBIN ≥ 12 mg/dL AND INFANT < 24 HOURS OLD

BILIRUBIN < 12 mg/dL AND INFANT > 24 HOURS OLD

COOMBS TEST

FOLLOW BILIRUBIN

POSITIVE COOMBS

NEGATIVE COOMBS

IDENTIFY ANTIBODY
* Rh
* ABO
* KELL, etc

DIRECT BILIRUBIN

Search for categories of Neonatal jaundice that need prompt investigation to determine the cause of jaundice

* Jaundice appearing in the first 24–36 hrs of life
* Jaundice in a sick Neonate (e.g. poor feeding, lethargy, apnea / bradys, hypothermia, excessive weight loss, vomiting, pallor, distress, signs of KERNICTERUS)
* Serum bilirubin is rising at a rate faster than 5mg/dL/24hrs.
* Serum bilirubin is > 12mg/dL in full term or 10-14mg/dL in preterm.
* Jaundice persisting after 8 days in term & after 14 days in preterm.
* Direct bilirubin is > 20–25% of total bilirubin or > 2mg /dL at any time, acholic stools, and dark urine.
* Family history of hemolytic disease, pallor, hepatosplenomegaly.

DIRECT BILIRUBIN > 2 ; CONSIDER
(refer to chapter on Neonatal Cholestasis Syndrome)
* HEPATITIS
* INTRAUTERINE, VIRAL, OR TOXOPLASMATIC INFECTIONS
* BILIARY OBSTRUCTION
* SEPSIS
* GALACTOSEMIA
* ALPHA-1-ANTITRYPSIN DEFICIENCY
* CYSTIC FIBROSIS
* TYROSINOSIS
* CHOLESTASIS
* HYPERALIMENTATION ?
* SYPHILIS
* HEMOCHROMATOSIS

DIRECT BILIRUBIN < 2mg/dL

HEMATOCRIT

NORMAL OR LOW

HIGH (polycythemia) SEE CHAPTER ON POLYCYTHEMIA

RBC MORPHOLOGY RETICULOCYTE COUNT

ABNORMAL
* SPHEROCYTOSIS
* ELLIPTOCYTOSIS
* STOMATOCYTOSIS
* PYKNOCYTOSIS
* ABO INCOMPATIBILITY
* RED CELL ENZYME DEFICIENCY
* ALPHA THALASSEMIA
* DRUGS (e.g. penicillin)
* DIC

NORMAL
* ENCLOSED HEMORRHAGE
* INCREASED ENTEROHEPATIC CIRCULATION
* BREAST MILK
* HYPOTHYROIDISM
* CRIGLER-NAJJAR SYNDROME
* INFANT OF DIABETIC MOTHER
* RDS
* ASPHYXIA
* INFECTION
* GILBERT'S SYNDROME
* DRUGS (e.g. novobiocin)
* GALACTOSEMIA

Treat with phototherapy & exchange transfusion as per the indications: *(refer to tables)*

Follow-up
Monitor hematocrit monthly for 3 months. Consider folic-acid supplementation

* *Pearl/Peril/Pitfall :* 10 DAY OLD INFANT WITH ONE DAY OF JAUNDICE • breast milk related ???, pathologic ??? • history and physical exam directed at signs of sepsis, hemolysis • check birth history for mom's blood type, thyroid screen • labs - CBC, reticulocyte, total and direct bili, peripheral smear.

NONINVASIVE ASSESSMENT OF NEONATAL JAUNDICE

The incidence of clinical jaundice in newborn infants is reported to be as high as 60 to 80 per cent during the first days following birth. Jaundice is safe for most term infants but high levels of unconjugated bilirubin can cause brain damage in susceptible newborns. Preventative, screening and management strategies therefore remain a significant practice issue during the early postnatal period.

This high incidence of jaundice combined with a relatively low incidence of adverse outcomes and the shortening of postnatal stay means that peak serum bilirubin levels (SBRs) often occur after discharge. Thus effective screening and surveillance are essential to ensure that infants with severe hyperbilirubinemia are not missed. Importantly it is still not known at what level bilirubin can cause a significant risk of brain damage. However SBRs over 450 micromol/L have been associated with kernicterus in the term infant with co morbidities such as sepsis or hemolysis.

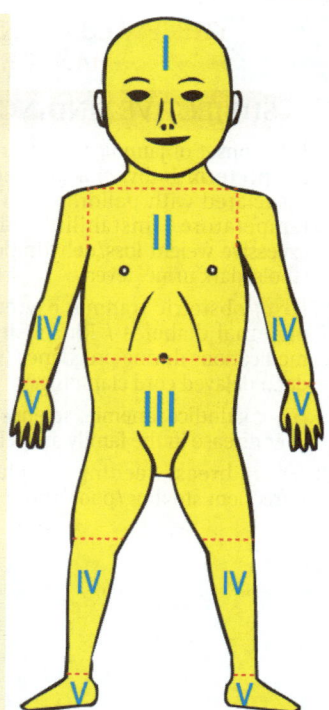

Rather than estimating the level of jaundice by simply observing the baby's skin color, one can utilize the cephalocaudal progression of jaundice. Kramer drew attention to the observation that jaundice starts on the head, and extends towards the feet as the level rises. This is useful in deciding whether or not a baby needs to have the SBR measured. Kramer divided the infant into 5 zones; the SBR range associated with progression to the zones is as follows:(1mg/dL=17.1umol/L or 5mg/dL=85.4umol/L)

Zone	1	2	3	4	5
SBR (umol/L)	100	150	200	250	>250
SBR (mg/dL)	5.88	8.88	11.76	14.7	>14.7

The correlation between serum bilirubin concentration and dermal icterus may not hold under the following circumstances: 1) In severe Rhesus incompatibility when the SBR rises by >1mg/dL per hour, skin deposition of bilirubin may lag. 2) During recovery when serum bilirubin is subsiding, the dermal jaundice does not recede in a caudal-cranial direction, but in a patchy manner. 3) Phototherapy interferes with assessment of dermal icterus due to photo-deposition of bilirubin in the skin.

Use of Transcutaneous Bilirubinometers (TcBs): The proposed benefits of using this technology include non-invasive and accurate screening for clinically significant jaundice. TcB readings are instant and results can avoid delay with discharge and / or indicate the need for formal SBR testing. Reduction in invasive blood tests will have an associated reduction in pain and discomfort for the newborn and a reduction in health costs. TcB measurements have demonstrated linear correlation with SBRs and several investigators have recommended their use as a screening device to detect clinically significant jaundice and thus decrease the need for frequent blood sampling in the well term infant. In addition, both the BiliChek® and the Konica Minolta JM-103® have been trialed in ethnically diverse populations and have had good correlations with SBRs.The results of a recent audit at *RPA Women and Babies* demonstrated that both the BiliChek® (Respironics, Inc. Murrysville, PA USA) – and the Konica Minolta JM-103® (Dräger Air-Shields, USA) have sufficient accuracy in the term population when compared with traditional SBR blood tests to justify their use. At this time the use of TcB measurements for infants less than 37 weeks gestation has not been validated in our population. Further evaluation of the technology in this high-risk group is currently underway.

The Konica Minolta JM-103® Jaundice Meter (Dräger Air-Shields, USA)*Procedure (postnatal wards / midwifery discharge programme)* *TcB measurements are performed to determine the need for a formal SBR *TcB measurements can be used to facilitate newborn discharge where appropriate *Serial TcB readings are used to evaluate the effect of phototherapy after formal SBRs have demonstrated falling bilirubin levels. Transcutaneous bilirubin measurements can only be used to monitor efficacy of phototherapy when the Medela Bilibed ™ (Fischer & Paykel) is in use. This method of phototherapy does not expose the forehead to therapeutic light. *Take two single TcB readings – if there is a difference in readings of less than ± 60µmol/L document the higher reading. Repeat procedure if readings are outside this range. *All clinicians require accreditation with use of the Konica Minolta JM-103® and associated QI guidelines. *The Konica Minolta JM-103® requires calibration daily - prior to the morning round. The midwives (night shift) will calibrate the Konica Minolta JM-103®, document and sign in the JM-103 Resource Manual. Both the values for the long and short optical paths should read within ±1.0 of the reference value on the unit cover – see resource folder. *To take a measurement the device is positioned on the forehead flush with the infant's skin and below the hairline. Avoid any bruising or discolored areas of skin. The tip is cleaned with an alcohol wipe between infants. The devices are set to take a single measurement.While in hospital all TcB readings are taken on the forehead to ensure a standardized technique. Accuracy of both the forehead and sternum has been validated.

*The Konica Minolta
JM-103 Jaundice Meter
(Dräger
Air-Shields, USA)*

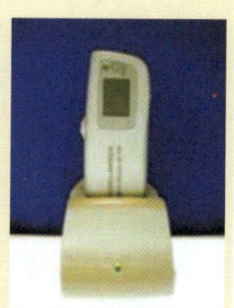

The BiliChek® in use (reproduced with permission Respironics, Inc. Murrysville, PA USA):To take a measurement using the BiliChek®, the device is calibrated prior to each measurement; the disposable probe (BiliCal ™) is applied on the forehead level below the hairline and five readings are used to generate one measurement that is displayed in µmol/L.When correct pressure is applied a green light alerts the operator to take a reading, if a faulty measure is taken an error message is displayed and the last reading must be repeated. This device uses more advanced technology than the Konica Minolta JM-103®.

---

* **Pearl/Peril/Pitfall :** *CLINICAL SIGNS of JAUNDICE • jaundice intensity bears no reliable relation to the degree of hyperbilirubinemia, however, typically starts at the head/neck area and spreads to chest and extremities • more difficult to diagnose jaundice in a neonate than in the adult (bilirubin level 4 - 6mg/dl before clinically visible) - if unsure, press a clean glass slide onto skin to view yellow color • unconjugated form tends to be bright yellow or orange • conjugated/direct form tends to be greenish or muddy yellow.*

SCREENING FOR HYPERBILIRUBINEMIA IN TERM INFANTS: SUMMARY

Signs of jaundice < 24 hours of age	**Do SBR** – *see jaundice policy* for additional investigations
Signs of jaundice > 24 hours of age +Risk factors (maternal antibodies; history of G6PD)	**Do SBR** – *see jaundice policy* for additional investigations
Signs of jaundice 24–48 hours of age Well infant / no risk factors	**Do SBR** If TcB measurement > 140μmol/L (>8mg/dL)
Signs of jaundice 48–72 hours of age Well infant / no risk factors	**Do SBR** If TcB measurement > 200μmol/L (>12mg/dL)
Signs of jaundice >72 hours of age Well infant / no risk factors	**Do SBR** If TcB measurement > 260μmol/L (>15mg/dL)
Phototherapy using the Medela Bilibed ™ Well infant / no other risk factors	**Do SBR** – if level falling, Monitor jaundice using TcB

Indications for SBR blood tests: *preterm infants with clinically significant jaundice *all infants less than 24 hours of age who present with jaundice*all infants with hemolysis or other significant risk factors for jaundice*term infants 24 – 48hours of age where the TcB reading is greater than 8mg/dL*term infants 48 – 72 hours of age where the TcB reading is greater than 12mg/dL*term infants greater than 72 hours of age where the TcB reading is greater than 15mg/dL *first jaundice level after initiation of phototherapy on the postnatal ward or in the home*all infants receiving overhead phototherapy.

*The potential harms associated with using invasive blood tests to measure SBRs and over diagnosing jaundice include:*infant pain and discomfort*infection*maternal distress*interruption to breast feeding and *maternal infant separation.

*The potential harms associated with underdiagnosis of moderate to severe jaundice include:*sensorineural hearing loss*bilirubin encephalopathy (hypertonia, arching, opisthotonos, high pitched cry)*kernicterus.

Risk factors for jaundice in the term infant: Several factors increase the risk for jaundice in the otherwise well term infant. These include a history of hyperbilirubinemia in a previous sibling, infants less than 38 weeks gestation, Asian ethnicity and infants who are breast feeding, Asian race and a gestational age less than 38 weeks are strong predictors for maximum SBRs over 25mg/dL. Maisels et al (1988) also reported a strong relationship between breast feeding (p < .0001) and greater than seven per cent weight loss (p = .0001) and hyperbilirubinemia. The list of complex factors that advance bilirubin toxicity in the at risk newborn include *high levels of unconjugated bilirubin* (excessive bruising, increased entero hepatic bilirubin production, or hemolysis - Rh or ABO incompatibility and glucose-6-phosphate dehydrogenase deficiency), low serum albumin levels (prematurity) and / or *impaired binding of bilirubin to albumin* (acidosis, sepsis, hypothermia, hypoglycemia) and *decreased bilirubin solubility / increased bilirubin deposition* (acidosis, anaemia, sepsis, poor perfusion or respiratory distress).

Breast milk jaundice: This occurs infrequently, peaks in the 2nd or 3rd week, and may persist at moderately high levels for 3-4 weeks before declining slowly. *It is a diagnosis of exclusion.* In an otherwise well infant, it is considered a benign condition. If feeding with breast milk is stopped, the serum bilirubin usually falls, however this would very rarely be indicated. The potential harms of stopping breast feeding would outweigh any risks of a mild or moderate hyperbilirubinemia. The etiology is unknown, but there is some support for both a hormonal factor in the milk acting on the infant's hepatic metabolism, and an enzyme (lipase) facilitating intestinal absorption of bilirubin.

Pathological jaundice

1) "Too Early" (< 24–36 hours of age): *always pathological *usually due to hemolysis, with excessive production of bilirubin *babies can be born jaundiced with -very severe hemolysis— hepatitis (unusual)—causes of hemolysis (decreasing order of probability) *ABO incompatibility *Rh immunization *sepsis *rarer causes—other blood group incompatibilities—red cell enzyme defects, e.g. G6PD deficiency—red cell membrane defects, e.g. hereditary spherocytosis

2) "Too High" (24 hours - 10 days of age): If the serum bilirubin concentration exceeds 12–15mg/dL, over this time, various causes include *mild dehydration/insufficient milk supply (breast-feeding jaundice) *hemolysis - continuing causes as discussed under "too early" *breakdown of extravasated blood (e.g. cephalhematoma, bruising, CNS hemorrhage, swallowed blood) *polycythemia (increased RBC mass) *infection - a more likely cause during this time *increased enterohepatic circulation (e.g. gut obstruction)

3) "Too Long" (> 10 days of age, especially > 2 weeks): The major clue to diagnosis is whether the elevated bilirubin is mostly unconjugated (>85%) or whether the conjugated fraction is substantially increased (>15% of the total). Causes of persistent unconjugated hyperbilirubinemia *breast milk jaundice (diagnosis of exclusion, cessation not necessary)*continued poor milk intake *hemolysis *infection (especially urinary tract infection) *hypothyroidism

* *Pearl/Peril/Pitfall :* GUIDELINES FOR TREATMENT OF PHYSIOLOGICAL JAUNDICE (AAP: Practice parameter: management of hyperbilirubinemia in the healthy term newborn 1994) **full term infant with negative history and exam for pathology: • unconjugated level < 12 mg/dl, just follow - increase frequency of feedings - take infant out into sun - cover eyes — avoid added glucose water, suppositories • unconjugated level > 15 - 17 mg/dl, ?? consider stopping breast feeding temporarily - CAUTION: many mom's will never go back to breast feeding when told to stop temporarily !

TABLE 1 — Jaundice risk factors for neonatal hyperbilirubinemia

J aundice visible on the 1st day of life

A sibling with Neonatal jaundice or anemia

U nrecognized hemolysis (ABO, Rh, other blood group, incompatibility) ;

U DP- glucuronyl transferase deficiency (Crigler-Najjar, Gilbert disease)

N onoptimal feeding (formula or breast-feeding)

D eficiency of Glucose-6-phosphate dehydrogenase

I nfection (viral, bacterial).

I nfant of diabetic mother.

I mmaturity (prematurity)

C ephalhematoma or bruising.

C entral hematocrit > 65% (polycythemia)

E ast Asian, Mediterranean, Native American heritage

TABLE 2 — Diagnostic features of the various types of neonatal jaundice

Diagnosis	Nature of Van den Bergh Reaction	Jaundice Appears	Jaundice Disappears	Peak Bilirubin concentration mg/dL	Peak Bilirubin concentration Age in days	Bilirubin rate of accumulation (mg/dL/day)	Remarks
"Physiologic jaundice":							Usually relates to degree of maturity
Full-term	Indirect	2–3 days	4–5 days	10–12	2–3	<5	
Premature	Indirect	2–3 days	7–9 days	15	6–8	<5	
Hyperbilirubine-mia due to metabolic factors							Metabolic factors: hypoxia, respiratory distress, lack of carbohydrate
Full-term	Indirect	2–3 days	Variable	>12	1st wk	<5	Hormonal influences : cretinism, hormones, Gilbert syndrome
Premature	Indirect	3–4 days	Variable	>15	1st wk	<5	Genetic factors : Crigler Najjar syndrome, Gilbert syndrome Drugs : vitamin K, novobiocin
Hemolytic	Indirect states and hematoma	May appear in 1st 24 hr	Variable	Unlimited	Variable >5	Usually ABO, Kell	Erythroblastosis : Rh, Congenital hemolytic states : spherocytic, nonspherocytic Infantile pyknocytosis Drugs : vitamin K Enclosed hemorrhage-hematoma
Mixed hemo-lytic and hepatotoxic factors	Indirect and direct	May appear in 1st 24 hr	Variable	Unlimited	Variable	Usually >5	Infection : bacterial sepsis, pyelonephritis, hepatitis, toxoplasmosis, cytomegalic inclusion disease, rubella, syphilis Drugs : vitamin K
Hepato-cellular damage	Indirect and direct	Usually 2-3 days, may appear by 2nd wk	Variable	Unlimited	Variable	Variable, can be > 5	Biliary atresia ; paucity of bile ducts, familial cholestasis, galactose-mia ; hepatitis and infection

From Brown AK ; PCNA -1962: 9;589

TABLE 3 — Suggested maximal indirect serum bilirubin concentration (mg/dl) in preterm infants

Birth weight (g)	Uncomplicated	Complicated*
< 1,000	12–13	10–12
1,000–1,250	12–14	10–12
1,251–1,499	14–16	12–14
1,500–1,999	16–20	15–17
2,000–2,500	20–22	18–20

Phototherapy is usually started at 50–70% of the maximal indirect level. If values greatly exceed this level, if phototherapy is unsuccessful in reducing the maximal bilirubin level, or if signs of kernicterus are evident, exchange transfusion is indicated.

*Complications include perinatal asphyxia, acidosis, hypoxia, hypothermia, hypoalbuminemia, meningitis, intraventricular hemorrhage, hemolysis, hypoglycemia, or signs of kernicterus.

*   Pearl/Peril/Pitfall : *A Cochrane review of fibreoptic phototherapy for Neonatal jaundice showed that fibreoptic devices were less effective in decreasing the bilirubin level than conventional phototherapy except in preterm infants. Combining a fibreoptic device with conventional phototherapy was more effective than conventional phototherapy alone.*

Hemolytic disease of newborn (Erythroblastosis Fetalis):

Erythroblastosis fetalis is caused by the transplacental passage of maternal antibody active against RBC antigens of the infant and is characterized by an increased rate of RBC destruction. It continues to be an important cause of anemia and jaundice in newborn infants despite the development of a method of preventing maternal isoimmunization by Rh antigens. **Common causes of HDN:** Rh system antibodies, ABO system antibodies **Uncommon causes—**Kell system antibodies **Rare causes—**Duffy system antibodies, MNS and s system antibodies, **No occurrence in HDN:** Lewis system antibodies, P system antibodies. Although the Rh antibody was and still is the most common cause of severe HDN, other alloimmune antibodies belonging to Kell (K and k), Duffy (Fya), Kidd (Jka and Jkb), and MNSs (M, N, S, and s) systems do cause severe HDN. Blood group incompatibilities other than Rh or ABO (c, E, K, and so on) account for less than 5% of hemolytic disease of the newborn. The direct Coombs test is invariably positive, and exchange transfusion may be indicated for hyperbilirubinemia and anemia. Hemolytic disease, anemia, and hydrops fetalis as a result of anti-Kell antibodies are not predictable from the previous obstetric history, amniotic fluid OD_{450} bilirubin determinants, or the maternal antibody titer. Erythroid suppression may contribute to the anemia; PUBS is beneficial in actually measuring the fetal Hct.

Hemolytic disease of newborn caused by ABO incompatibility:

Hemolysis associated with ABO incompatibility exclusively occurs in type-O mothers with fetuses who have type A or type B blood, although it has rarely been documented in type-A mothers with type-B infants with a high titer of anti-B IgG. In mothers with type A or type B, naturally occurring antibodies are of the IgM class and do not cross the placenta, whereas 1% of type-O mothers have a high titer of the antibodies of IgG class against both A and B. They cross the placenta and cause hemolysis in fetus. Hemolysis due to anti-A is more common than hemolysis due to anti-B, and affected neonates usually have positive direct Coombs test results. However, hemolysis due to anti-B IgG can be severe and can lead to exchange transfusion. Because A and B antigens are widely expressed in various tissues besides RBCs, only a small portion of antibodies crossing the placenta are available to bind to fetal RBCs. In addition, fetal RBCs appear to have less surface expression of A or B antigen, resulting in few reactive sites; hence the low incidence of significant hemolysis in affected neonates. This results in hyperbilirubinemia as a predominant manifestation of incompatibility (rather than anemia), and peripheral blood film frequently reveals a large number of spherocytes and few erythroblasts, unlike what is seen in Rh incompatibility (erythroblastosis fetalis), in which blood film reveals a large number of nucleated RBCs and few spherocytes. Most cases are mild, with jaundice being the only clinical manifestation. The infant is not generally affected at birth; pallor is not present, and hydrops fetalis is extremely rare. The liver and spleen are not greatly enlarged, if at all. Jaundice usually appears during the 1st 24 hr. Rarely, it may become severe, and symptoms and signs of kernicterus develop rapidly. The hemoglobin level is usually normal but may be as low as 10-12 g/dL (100-120 g/L). Reticulocytes may be increased to 10-15%, with extensive polychromasia and increased numbers of nucleated RBCs. In 10-20% of affected infants, the unconjugated serum bilirubin level may reach 20 mg/dL or more unless phototherapy is administered. Phototherapy may be effective in lowering serum bilirubin levels. In rare severe cases, treatment is directed at correcting dangerous degrees of anemia or hyperbilirubinemia by exchange transfusions with type O blood of the same Rh type as the infant. Indications for this procedure are similar to those previously described for hemolytic disease caused by Rh incompatibility. Some infants with ABO hemolytic disease may require transfusion of packed RBCs at several weeks of age because of slowly progressive anemia. Post-discharge monitoring of hemoglobin/Hct is essential in newborns with ABO hemolytic disease.

Hemolytic disease of newborn caused by Rh incompatibility:

The Rh antigenic determinants are genetically transmitted from each parent and determine the Rh type and direct the production of a number of blood group factors (C, c, D, d, E, and e). Each factor can elicit a specific antibody response under suitable conditions; 90% are due to D antigen and the remainder to C or E. When Rh-positive blood is infused into an Rh-negative woman through error or when small quantities (usually more than 1 mL) of Rh-positive fetal blood containing D antigen inherited from an Rh-positive father enter the maternal circulation during pregnancy, with spontaneous or induced abortion, or at delivery, antibody formation against D antigen may be induced in the unsensitized Rh-negative recipient mother. Once sensitization has taken place, considerably smaller doses of antigen can stimulate an increase in antibody titer. Initially, a rise in IgM antibody occurs, which is later replaced by IgG antibody; the latter readily crosses the placenta and causes hemolytic manifestations.

Hemolytic disease rarely occurs during a first pregnancy because transfusions of Rh-positive fetal blood into an Rh-negative mother tend to occur near the time of delivery, too late for the mother to become sensitized and transmit antibody to her infant before delivery. The fact that 55% of Rh-positive fathers are heterozygous (D/d) and may have Rh-negative offspring and that fetal-to-maternal transfusion occurs in only 50% of pregnancies reduces the chance of sensitization, as does small family size, in which the opportunities for its occurrence are reduced. Finally, the capacity of Rh-negative women to form antibodies is variable, some producing low titers even after adequate antigenic challenge. Thus, the overall incidence of isoimmunization of Rh-negative mothers at risk is low, with antibody to D detected in less than 10% of those studied, even after five or more pregnancies; only about 5% ever have babies with hemolytic disease. When the mother and fetus are also incompatible with respect to group A or B, the mother is partially protected against sensitization by the rapid removal of Rh-positive cells from her circulation by her pre-existing anti-A or anti-B, which are IgM antibodies and do not cross the placenta. The risk of Rh immunization after the delivery of the first child to a nulliparous Rh-negative mother is 16% if the Rh-positive fetus is ABO compatible with its mother, 2% if the fetus is ABO incompatible, and 2-5% after an abortion. The ABO-incompatible RBCs are rapidly destroyed in the maternal circulation, reducing the likelihood of exposure to the immune system. The degree of Rh sensitization of the mother is directly related to the amount of fetomaternal hemorrhage (i.e., 3% with <0.1 mL compared with 22% with >0.1 mL). Once a mother has been sensitized, her infant is likely to have hemolytic disease. The severity of Rh illness tends to worsen with successive pregnancies. The possibility that the first affected infant after sensitization may represent the end of the mother's childbearing potential for Rh-positive infants argues urgently for the prevention of sensitization when possible. Such prevention consists of the injection of anti-D gamma globulin (RhoGAM) into the mother immediately after the delivery of each Rh-positive infant. Before the establishment of modern therapy, 1% of all pregnant women developed Rh alloimmunization. Since the advent of routine prophylaxis of at-risk women, incidence of Rh sensitization has declined from 45 cases per 10,000 births to 10.2 cases per 10,000 births, with less than 10% requiring intrauterine transfusion. Alloimmunization due to Kell antigen accounts for 10% of severely affected fetuses. Currently, anti-D is still one of the most common antibodies found in pregnant women, followed by anti-K, anti-c and anti-E. Of those fetuses who require intrauterine transfusions, 85%, 10%, and 3.5% were due to anti-D, anti-K, and anti-c, respectively. ABO incompatibility frequently occurs during the first pregnancy and is present in approximately 12% of pregnancies, with evidence of fetal sensitization in 3% of live births. Less than 1% of births are associated with significant hemolysis.

Hemolytic disease of the Newborn (HDN) is characterized by one or more of the following **clinical presentations:** *Rapidly progressive severe hyperbilirubinemia or prolonged hyperbilirubinemia *Positive maternal antenatal antibody findings and/or diagnosis of anemia or fetal hydrops *Positive neonatal direct Coombs test (direct antiglobulin test) *Hemolysis on blood film findings. The infant born to an alloimmunized mother shows clinical signs based on the severity of the disease. The typical diagnostic findings are jaundice, pallor, hepatosplenomegaly, and fetal hydrops in severe cases (**Erythroblastosis fetalis**). The jaundice typically manifests at birth or in the first 24 hours after birth with rapidly rising unconjugated bilirubin level. Occasionally, conjugated hyperbilirubinemia is present because of placental or hepatic dysfunction in those infants with severe hemolytic disease. Anemia is most often due to destruction of antibody-coated RBCs by the reticuloendothelial system, and, in some infants, anemia is due to intravascular destruction. The suppression of erythropoiesis by IVT of adult Hb to an anemic fetus can also cause anemia. Extramedullary hematopoiesis can lead to hepatosplenomegaly, portal hypertension, and ascites. Anemia is not the only cause of hydrops. Excessive hepatic extramedullary hematopoiesis causes portal and umbilical venous obstruction and diminished placental perfusion because of edema. Increased placental weight and edema of chorionic villi interfere with placental transport. Fetal hydrops results from fetal hypoxia, anemia, congestive cardiac failure, and hypoproteinemia secondary to hepatic dysfunction. Commonly, hydrops is not observed until Hb drops below approximately 4 g/dL (Hct <15%). Clinically significant jaundice occurs in as many as 20% of ABO-incompatible infants.

Before treatment, the direct Coombs test is usually positive, and anemia is generally present. The cord blood hemoglobin content varies and is usually proportional to the severity of the disease; with hydrops fetalis it may be as low as 3-4 g/dL. Alternatively, despite hemolysis, it may be within the normal range because of compensatory bone marrow and extramedullary hematopoiesis. The blood smear typically shows polychromasia and a marked increase in nucleated RBCs. The reticulocyte count is increased. The white blood cell count is usually normal but may be elevated; thrombocytopenia may develop in severe cases. Cord bilirubin is generally between 3 and 5 mg/dL; direct-reacting (conjugated) bilirubin may be substantially elevated. Indirect-reacting bilirubin rises rapidly to high levels in the 1st 6 hr of life. After intrauterine transfusions, cord blood may show a normal hemoglobin concentration, negative direct Coombs test, predominantly type O Rh-negative adult RBCs, and a relatively normal smear. Marked elevation of both indirect- and direct-reacting bilirubin levels has been reported in these infants.

In the absence of a positive direct Coombs test result, other causes of pathologic jaundice should be considered, including intrauterine congenital infections; erythrocyte membrane defects (e.g., hereditary spherocytosis, hereditary elliptocytosis, hereditary pyropoikilocytosis); RBC enzyme deficiencies (e.g., glucose-6-phosphate dehydrogenase [G6PD] deficiency, pyruvate kinase deficiency, triosephosphate isomerase deficiency); and nonhemolytic causes (e.g., enclosed hemorrhages, hypothyroidism, gastrointestinal obstruction, and metabolic diseases). Similarly, hydrops can occur from nonimmune hematologic disorders that cause anemia, such as hemoglobinopathies (e.g., ± -thalassemia major), cardiac failure due to dysrhythmia, congenital heart defects, and infections (e.g. syphilis, cytomegalovirus [CMV], parvovirus).

Treatment of a Severely affected Liveborn Infant: Severe hemolytic disease accounts for the remaining 25% of the alloimmunized newborns who are either stillborn or hydropic at birth. The fetal hydrops is predominantly caused by a capillary leak syndrome due to tissue hypoxia, hypoalbuminemia secondary to hepatic dysfunction, and high-output cardiac failure from anemia. About half of these fetuses become hydropic before 34 weeks' gestation and need intensive monitoring and management of alloimmunized gestation as described earlier. Mild hydrops involving ascites reverses with IVTs in only 88% of cases with improved survival but severe hydrops causing scalp edema and severe ascites and pleural effusions reverse in 39% of cases and are associated with poor survival. Ensure *the following care of the neonate promptly!* * Skillful Neonatal Resuscitation * Availability of Fresh, low-titer, group O, irradiated Rh-negative blood cross-matched against maternal serum *Supportive therapy-ABCs, temperature stabilization, Correction of anemia with a small transfusion of compatible PRBC, Volume expansion for hypotension, Assisted ventilation for respiratory failure and monitoring before proceeding with Exchange Transfusion.

Mild hemolytic disease accounts for 50% of newborns with positive direct antibody test results. Most of these newborns are not anemic (cord Hb >14 g/dL) and have minimal hemolysis (cord bilirubin <4 mg/dL). Apart from early phototherapy, they require no transfusions. However, these newborns are at risk of developing severe late anemia by 3–6 weeks of life. Therefore, monitoring their Hb levels after hospital discharge is important. Moderate hemolytic disease accounts for approximately 25% of affected neonates.

Moderate HDN is characterized by moderate anemia and increased cord bilirubin levels. These infants are not clinically jaundiced at birth but rapidly develop unconjugated hyperbilirubinemia in the first 24 hours of life. Peripheral smear shows numerous nucleated RBCs, decreased platelets, and, occasionally, a large number of immature granulocytes. These newborns often have hepatosplenomegaly and are at risk of developing bilirubin encephalopathy without adequate treatment. Early exchange transfusion with type-O Rh-negative fresh RBCs with intensive phototherapy is usually required. Use of IVIG in doses of 0.5–1 gm/kg in a single or multiple dose regimen have been able to effectively reduce need for exchange transfusion. These newborns are also at risk of developing late hyporegenerative anemia of infancy at 4–6 weeks of life. *Antenatal Diagnosis and Management: Women at risk for alloimmunization should undergo an indirect Coombs test and antibody titers at their first prenatal visit. If positive, obtain a paternal blood type and genotype with serologic testing for other Rh antigens (C, c, E, e). The presence of measurable antibody titer at the beginning of pregnancy, a rapid rise in titer, or a titer of 1:64 or greater suggests significant hemolytic disease, although the exact titer correlates poorly with the severity of disease. If a mother is found to have antibody against D antigen at a titer of 1:16 or greater at any time during a subsequent pregnancy, the severity of fetal disease should be monitored by amniocentesis, Percutaneous Umbilical Blood Sampling (PUBS), and ultrasonography.

Indicators for severe hemolytic disease of the newborn (HDN) include mothers who have had previous children with hemolytic disease, rising maternal antibody titers, rising amniotic fluid bilirubin concentration, and ultrasonographic evidence of fetal hydrops (e.g. ascites, edema, pleural and pericardial effusions, worsening biophysical profile, decreasing Hb levels). The major advance in predicting the severity of hemolytic disease was the delta-OD 450 reported by Liley in 1961.[1] The serial values of deviation from baseline at 450 nm, the wavelength at which bilirubin absorbs light, are plotted on a Liley curve against the gestational weeks. The values above 65% on zone 2 indicate direct fetal monitoring by cordocentesis. Hct levels below 30% or a single value in zone 3 are indications for intrauterine transfusion. The modified Liley curve developed by Queenan (see Media file 2) is used to correct for gestations of less than 24 weeks because bilirubin levels normally peak at 23-25 weeks' gestation in unaffected fetuses. In a recent prospective evaluation, the Queenan curve predicted moderate anemia with a sensitivity of 83% and a specificity of 94%, whereas the sensitivity and specificity for severe anemia were 100% and 79%, respectively. The delta-OD 450 value that plots out in the intrauterine transfusion zone of Queenan curve indicates the need for FBS.

*Treatment of An Unborn Infant: With ultrasonographic guidance, a needle is introduced into an umbilical vein at the cord insertion into the placenta or into its intrahepatic portion, and a fetal blood sample is obtained. The blood sample is confirmed to be of fetal origin by rapid alkaline denaturation test. All the relevant fetal tests (eg, blood type, direct antibody test, reticulocyte count, platelet count, Hb level, Hct level, serum albumin level, erythropoietin level) are performed. If the Hb level is less than 11 g/dL or if the Hct level is less than 30%, an IVT is started. Packed RBC are given by slow -push infusion after cross matching with the mother's serum. The cells should be obtained from a CMV-negative donor and irradiated to kill lymphocytes to avoid Graft vs host disease. The position of the needle is confirmed by noting the turbulence in the fetal vessel on injection of saline. The fetus is frequently paralyzed with pancuronium in order to prevent the displacement of the needle by fetal movements. The transfusion is performed in 10-mL aliquots to a volume of approximately 50 mL/kg estimated body weight using ultrasonography or until an Hct level of 40% is reached. The procedure is promptly discontinued if cardiac decompensation is noted on ultrasonography findings. Severely anemic fetuses do not tolerate acute correction of their Hct to normal values, and the initial Hct should not be increased by more than 4-fold at the time of first IVT. They should then be monitored every 2-7 days. The IVT is repeated when it reaches a value that reflects critical anemia in the fetus. A loss of 1% of transfused cells per day can be anticipated. Transfusions should achieve a post-transfusion Hct of 45–55% and can be repeated every 3–5 wk. Indications for delivery include Pulmonary maturity, fetal distress, complications of PUBS, or 35–37 wk of gestation.

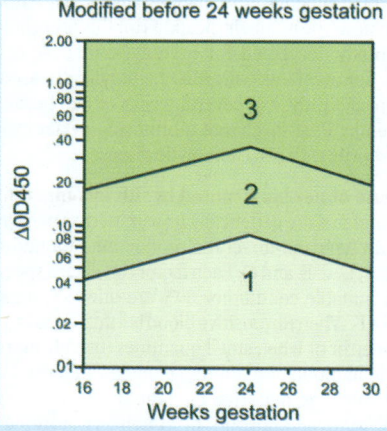

Modified Liley curve for gestation of less than 24 weeks showing that bilirubin levels in amniotic fluid peak at 23-24 weeks' gestation.

Managing patients with a previously affected fetus

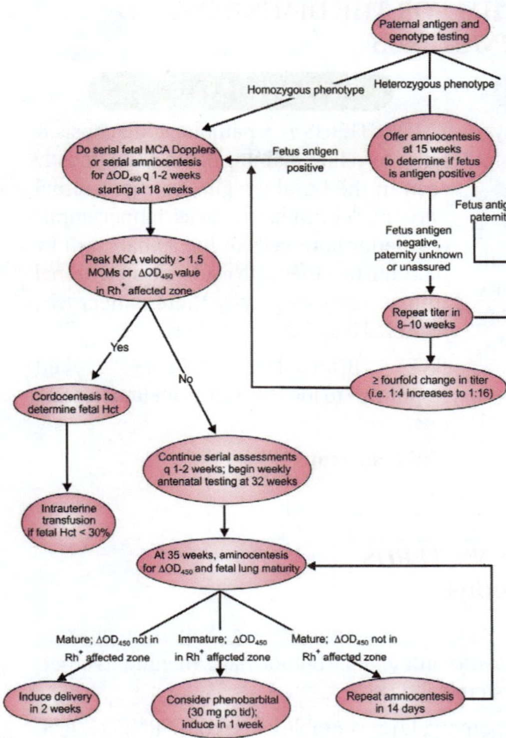

Paternal antigen and genotype testing

- Homozygous phenotype → Do serial fetal MCA Dopplers or serial amniocentesis for ΔOD$_{450}$ q 1-2 weeks starting at 18 weeks → Peak MCA velocity > 1.5 MOMs or ΔOD$_{450}$ value in Rh$^+$ affected zone → Yes → Cordocentesis to determine fetal Hct → Intrauterine transfusion if fetal Hct < 30%
- No → Continue serial assessments q 1-2 weeks; begin weekly antenatal testing at 32 weeks → At 35 weeks, amniocentesis for ΔOD$_{450}$ and fetal lung maturity
- Heterozygous phenotype → Offer amniocentesis at 15 weeks to determine if fetus is antigen positive
  - Fetus antigen positive →
  - Fetus antigen negative, paternity assured → Deliver at term
  - Fetus antigen negative, paternity unknown or unassured → Repeat titer in 8–10 weeks → < fourfold change in titer / ≥ fourfold change in titer (i.e. 1:4 increases to 1:16)
- Antigen negative paternity assured → Deliver at term

At 35 weeks, amniocentesis for ΔOD$_{450}$ and fetal lung maturity →
- Mature; ΔOD$_{450}$ not in Rh$^+$ affected zone → Induce delivery in 2 weeks
- Immature; ΔOD$_{450}$ in Rh$^+$ affected zone → Consider phenobarbital (30 mg po tid); induce in 1 week
- Mature; ΔOD$_{450}$ not in Rh$^+$ affected zone → Repeat amniocentesis in 14 days

Managing a first sensitized pregnancy

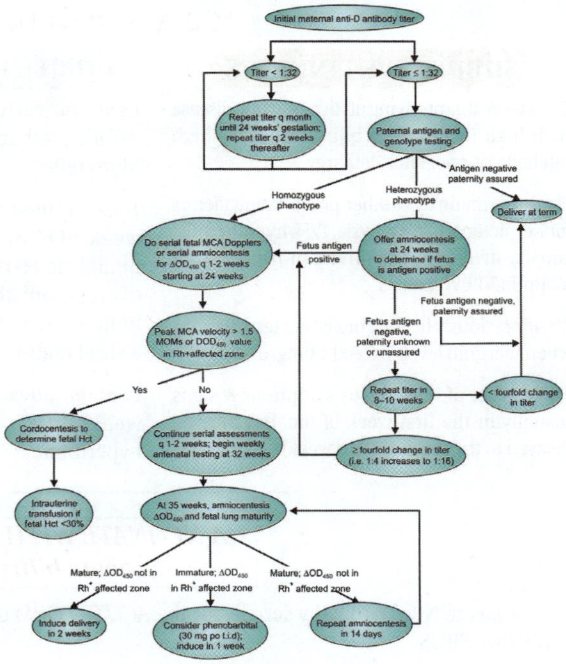

Initial maternal anti-D antibody titer
- Titer < 1:32 → Repeat titer q month until 24 weeks' gestation; repeat titer q 2 weeks thereafter
- Titer ≤ 1:32 → Paternal antigen and genotype testing
  - Homozygous phenotype → Do serial fetal MCA Dopplers or serial amniocentesis for ΔOD$_{450}$ q 1-2 weeks starting at 24 weeks → Peak MCA velocity > 1.5 MOMs or ΔOD$_{450}$ value in Rh+ affected zone → Yes → Cordocentesis to determine fetal Hct → Intrauterine transfusion if fetal Hct <30%
    - No → Continue serial assessments q 1-2 weeks; begin weekly antenatal testing at 32 weeks → At 35 weeks, amniocentesis ΔOD$_{450}$ and fetal lung maturity
  - Heterozygous phenotype → Offer amniocentesis at 24 weeks to determine if fetus is antigen positive
    - Fetus antigen positive →
    - Fetus antigen negative, paternity assured →
    - Fetus antigen negative, paternity unknown or unassured → Repeat titer in 8–10 weeks → < fourfold change in titer / ≥ fourfold change in titer (i.e. 1:4 increases to 1:16)
  - Antigen negative paternity assured → Deliver at term

At 35 weeks, amniocentesis ΔOD$_{450}$ and fetal lung maturity →
- Mature; ΔOD$_{450}$ not in Rh$^+$ affected zone → Induce delivery in 2 weeks
- Immature; ΔOD$_{450}$ in Rh$^+$ affected zone → Consider phenobarbital (30 mg po t.i.d); induce in 1 week
- Mature; ΔOD$_{450}$ not in Rh$^+$ affected zone → Repeat amniocentesis in 14 days

Queenan curve for ΔOD$_{450}$ values

Graph: ΔOD_{450} nm (y-axis 0.00–0.20) vs Weeks' gestation (x-axis 14–40).
- Intrauterine death risk
- Rh positive (affected)
- Indeterminate
- Rh negative (unaffected)

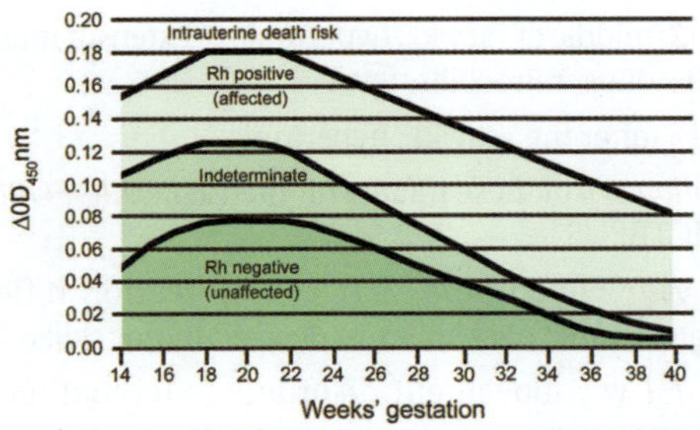

Queenan Curve: Modified Liley curve that shows delta-OD 450 values at 14-40 weeks' gestation.

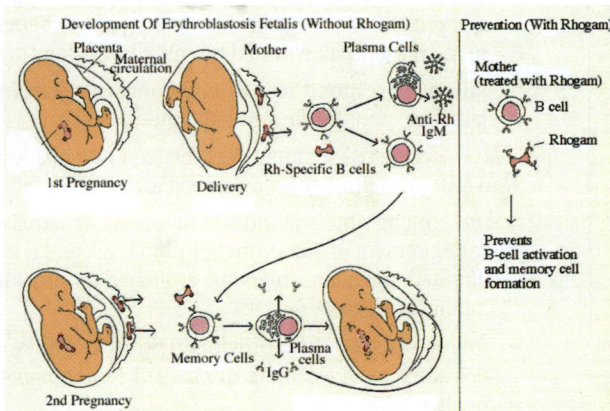

Development Of Erythroblastosis Fetalis (Without Rhogam) — Prevention (With Rhogam)

1st Pregnancy; Placenta; Maternal circulation; Mother; Rh-Specific B cells; Plasma Cells; Anti-Rh IgM; Delivery
2nd Pregnancy; Memory Cells; Plasma cells; IgG
Mother (treated with Rhogam); B cell; Rhogam → Prevents B-cell activation and memory cell formation

Rh Incompatability

Hemolytic disease of the newborn (HDN) often occurs as a result of rhesus incompatibility. It occurs when an Rh-negative mother carries an Rh-positive fetus. The fetal red blood cells are separated from the mother's circulation by the layer of cells in the placenta called the trophoblast. However, during late pregnancy, and especially during the process of childbirth, the fetal red blood cells may escape into the mother's circulation. Once these cells reach the mother's circulation, they are perceived as foreign and therefore provoke an antibody response. Antibodies to fetal red blood cells are not usually made before first childbirth. Repeated pregnancies provoke high antibody levels in the mother. Maternal IgG antibodies provoked in this way can cross the placenta and reach the fetal circulation, where they react with the fetal red blood cells and cause their destruction and eventually death.

Prevention of RH Sensitization: IM inj. of RhoGAM (Human anti-D globulin 1ml=300mcg) within 72 hrs of delivery of an Rh-positive infant, ectopic pregnancy, abdominal trauma in pregnancy, amniocentesis, chorionic villus biopsy, or abortion reduces the risk of initial sensitization of Rh-negative mothers from 20% to <1%. RhoGAM, if given at 28-32 wk and again at birth (40 wk) is more effective than a single dose.

Refer to Page 754, Essential Neonatal Clinical Guidelines: for the differentiation of Clinical and Laboratory Features of Immune Hemolysis Due to Rh Disease and ABO Incompatibility
Refer to Page 1026, Essential Neonatal Procedures: for the practical aspects of Exchange Transfusion

THE EVALUATION-DECISION-ACTION-PLAN/ALGORITHM FOR THE DIAGNOSIS AND MANAGEMENT OF *NEONATAL KERNICTERUS*

SUBJECTIVE FINDINGS

Hx of term-infants dying of Rh hemolytic disease with high (>20mg/dL) bilirubin levels, high pitched cry, poor suck, lethargy.

Hx of prematurity & other potentiating factors for Kernicterus like asphyxia, IVH, hypothermia, sepsis, drugs that displace bilirubin from albumin, VLBW babies.

Hx of previously healthy breast fed term infants, when bilirubin levels exceed 30mg/dL.

Hx of onset of Kernicterus symptoms & signs (usually in the first week of life, but may be delayed to the second -third week).

OBJECTIVE FINDINGS

Look for early signs (first 1–2 days) (subtle); lethargy, poor feeding, loss of Moro reflex.

Look for subsequent signs (middle of 1st week) like prostration, gravely ill, diminished tendon reflexes, respiratory distress, opisthotonos with a bulging fontanel, twitching of the face or limbs, a shrill high-pitched cry.

Look for advanced signs (after the 1st week) like convulsions, spasm & hypertonia.

INVESTIGATIONS

KERNICTERUS is a pathologic diagnosis & refers to yellow staining of the brain (mostly seen in the basal ganglia, various cranial nerve nuclei, cerebellar nuclei, hippocampus & anterior horn cells of the spinal cord) by bilirubin together with evidence of neuronal injury. Microscopically there is necrosis, neuronal loss & reactive gliosis.

BAER (Brain-stem auditory evoked responses) to identify sensorineural hearing loss.

MRI brain scan & EEG.

A NEONATE WITH SUSPECTED KERNICTERUS (acute bilirubin encephalopathy)

Examine the Newborn baby serially for the *ACUTE FORM* of KERNICTERUS

* *Phase 1* (1st 1–2 days): poor sucking, stupor, hypotonia, seizures

* *Phase 2* (middle of 1st wk) : hypertonia of extensor muscles, opisthotonos, retrocollis, fever

* *Phase 3* (after the 1st wk) ; hypertonia

Ensure Follow-up of these infants for the *CHRONIC FORM* of KERNICTERUS

* *First year :* hypotonia, active deep tendon reflexes, obligatory tonic neck reflexes, delayed motor skills

* *After 1st yr :* movement disorders (choreoathetosis, ballismus, tremor), upward gaze, sensorineural hearing loss

* *Look for* mild form like mild to moderate neuromuscular incoordination, partial deafness, or "minimal brain dysfunction", occurring singly or in combination : these problems may be inapparent until the child enters school.

Exclude mimicking diagnoses, e.g. Sepsis, asphyxia, hypoglycemia, intracranial hemorrhage, meningitis other acute systemic illnesses.

Identify potentially preventable causes of KERNICTERUS

* early discharge (<48hr) with no early follow-up (within 48 hr of discharge); this problem is particularly important in near-term infants (35–37 wk gestation).

* failure to check the bilirubin level in an infant noted to be jaundiced in the 1st 24 hr

* failure to recognize the presence of risk factors for hyperbilirubinemia

* underestimating the severity of jaundice by clinical (i.e. visual) assessment

* lack of concern regarding the presence of jaundice

* delay in measuring the serum bilirubin level despite marked jaundice or delay in initiating phototherapy in the presence of elevated bilirubin levels ; and

* failure to respond to parental concern regarding jaundice, poor feeding, or lethargy.

Follow-up high risk infants as per the recommendations from AAP (American Academy of Pediatrics)

* any infant who is jaundiced before 24 hr requires measurement of the serum bilirubin level, and if it is elevated, the infant should be evaluated for possible hemolytic disease, and

* follow-up should be provided within 2-3 days of discharge to all Neonates discharged earlier than 48 hr after birth.

Effects of Bilirubin Toxicity in Newborns

Early	Late	Chronic
Lethargy	Irritability	Athetoid cerebral palsy
Poor feeding	Opisthotonos	High-frequency hearing loss
High-pitched cry	Seizures	Paralysis of upward gaze
Hypotonia	Apnea	Dental dysplasia
	Oculogyric crisis	Mild mental retardation
	Hypertonia	
	Fever	

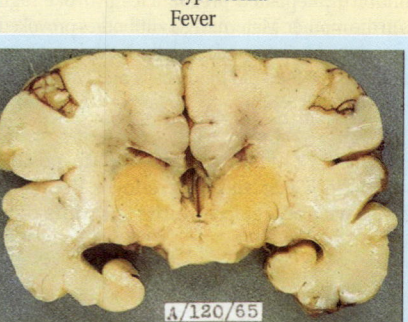

The yellow staining in the brain of a Neonate is known as kernicterus. There is a coronal section of medulla on the left and cerebral hemisphere on the right demonstrating kernicterus in deep grey matter of hemisphere and brain stem. Increased unconjugated bilirubin, which accounts for the kernicterus, is toxic to the brain tissue. Kernicterus is more likely to occur with prematurity, low birth weight, and increased bilirubin levels.

* *Pearl/Peril/Pitfall :* Eye care ·Eye pads are required for the infants comfort if overhead white or blue fluorescent lights are used : ·Size N720 (micro) if < 1500g ·Size N721 (small) if 1500 - 2500g ·Size N722 (large) if > 2500g ·Eye pads should be removed 4 hourly and eye cares attended with normal saline. ·There have never been human studies showing that retinal damage occurs from with phototherapy.

TABLE 4	Causes of unconjugated hyperbilirubinemia in the neonates

Excessive production of bilirubin (hemolysis)
- Blood group heterospecificity (incompatibility)
  - Rh
  - ABO
  - Minor blood group
- Red blood cell enzyme abnormalities
  - Glucose-6-phosphate dehydrogenase
  - Pyruvate kinase
- Sepsis
- Red blood cell membrane defects
  - Hereditary spherocytosis, elliptocytosis, poikilocytosis
- Extravascular blood

Polycythemia
Impaired conjugation or excretion
- Hormonal deficiency
  - Hypothyroidism
  - Hypopituitarism
- Disorders of bilirubin metabolism
  - Crigler-Najjar syndrome : Type I
  - Crigler-Najjar syndrome : Type II (Arias disease)
  - Gilbert disease
  - Lucey-Driscoll syndrome
Enhanced enterohepatic circulation
- Intestinal obstruction, pyloric stenosis
- Ileus, meconium plugs, cystic fibrosis

TABLE 5	Approach to indirect hyperbilirubinemia in healthy term infants without hemolysis*

Treatment Strategies		Intensive Phototherapy & Preparation for Exchange	Exchange Transfusion if Phototherapy Fails‡
Age (hr)	Phototherapy	Transfusion†	
<24	§	§	§
24-48	≥15-18	≥25	≥20
49-72	≥18-20	≥30	≥25
>72	≥20	≥30	≥25
>2 wk	¶	¶	¶

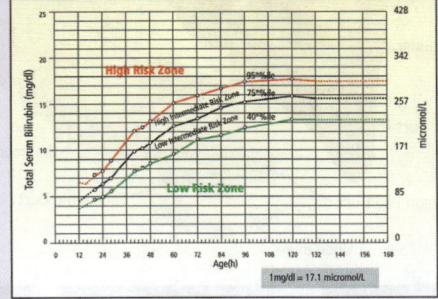

1mg/dl = 17.1 micromol/L

*With hemolysis, exchange transfusion is initiated with an indirect bilirubin level of 20 or higher at any age. The precise level of unconjugated bilirubin in healthy breast-fed term infants that requires therapy is unknown. Treatment options include continued breast-feeding and initiation of phototherapy or interrupted breast-feeding (use formula as a substitute), with or without phototherapy. If any signs of kernicterus are noted during evaluation or treatment as suggested anywhere in the table or any level of bilirubin, emergency exchange transfusion must be performed. †If the initial bilirubin value is high, intense phototherapy should be initiated and preparation made for exchange transfusion. If phototherapy fails to reduce the bilirubin level to the levels noted on the column to the right, initiate exchange transfusion. ‡Intensive phototherapy should be initiated for bilirubin levels in this column and usually reduces serum bilirubin levels 1-2mg/dL in 4-6 hr. Such treatment is often associated with administration of intravenous fluids at 1-1.5 times maintenance ; oral alimentation should also continue. § Jaundice in the 1st 24 hr of life is not seen in "healthy" infants. Hyperbilirubinemia of this degree within 48 hr of birth is unusual and should suggest hemolysis, concealed hemorrhage, or causes of conjugated (direct) hyperbilirubinemia. ¶ Jaundice suddenly appearing in the 2nd wk of life or continuing beyond the 2nd wk of life with significant hyperbilirubinemia levels to warrant therapy should be investigated in detail because it most probably is due to a serious underlying cause such as biliary atresia, galactosemia, hypothyroidism, or neonatal hepatitis.

KEY POINTS FOR CLINICAL PRACTICE

1. The diagnosis of physiologic jaundice in term or preterm infants can be established *only by excluding known causes of jaundice* on the basis of the history, clinical and laboratory findings.

2. One should make a search to determine the cause of jaundice if 1) it appears in the 1st 24–36 hr of life, 2) serum bilirubin is rising at a rate faster than 5mg/dL/24 hr, 3) serum bilirubin is greater than 12 mg/dL in full-term (especially in the absence of risk factors) or 10–14 mg/dL in preterm infants, 4) jaundice persists after 10-14 days of life, or 5) direct-reacting bilirubin is greater than 2 mg/dL at any time. *Persistent or prolonged physiologic jaundice beyond 8 days in term infants and 14 days in preterm infants*, suggests hemolysis, hereditary glucuronyl transferase deficiency, breast milk jaundice, hypothyroidism, or intestinal obstruction, UTI, hepatitis / TORSCH infections etc.

3. The aim of phototherapy is to decrease the level of unconjugated bilirubin in order to prevent acute bilirubin encephalopathy, hearing loss and kernicterus. Lamps emitting light between the wavelengths of 400 - 500 nanometres (peak at 460nm) are specifically used for administering phototherapy as bilirubin absorbs this wavelength of light. The light is visible blue light and contains no ultraviolet light. The decision to start phototherapy is based on the level and rate of rise of serum bilirubin, the gestational and postnatal age of infant and the underlying cause of the hyperbilirubinemia. Factors that influence the efficacy of phototherapy include: the light wavelength and irradiance, bilirubin level, birthweight, gestational age, postnatal age, surface area exposed, skin thickness and pigmentation and the etiology of the jaundice.

4. The incidence of Rhesus iso-immunization has dramatically declined since the implementation of prophylaxis (treatment of Rh-negative mothers with anti-D antibody following birth of an Rh-positive baby, or in association with miscarriages, termination, ectopic pregnancies and other invasive procedures). Factors which increase the risk of kernicterus for a given SBR level include: *prematurity *acidosis *hypoalbuminemia *rapidly rising SBR. **Kernicterus** (bilirubin encephalopathy) *Early: This clinical syndrome includes hypertonia progressing to opthistotonia, seizures, and often death. At autopsy, such babies display evidence of bilirubin staining of the basal ganglia. *Late: Survivors may go on to develop sensorineural hearing impairment and cerebral palsy, often with ataxia and chorioathetosis.

5. The American Academy of Pediatrics subcommittee on hyperbilirubinemia provided an updated guidelines providing a framework for the prevention and management of hyperbilirubinemia in newborn infants of 35 or more weeks' gestation.

REFERENCES & FURTHER READING : 1) AAP Subcommittee on Hyperbilirubinemia; Pediatrics 114; 297, 2004 2) Centers for Disease Control & Prevention: Kernicterus in full term infants- US, 1994-1998 3) Dennery PA et all: Neonatal Hyperbilirubinemia, N Engl J Med 2001; 344;581 4) Primary Care of the Newborn by Henry M. Saidel -4th edition 5) Nelson Textbook of Pediatrics - 18th edition.

54 Neonatal Cholestasis Syndrome

@ *Percutaneous liver biopsy is widely regarded as the most valuable study for evaluating Neonatal cholestasis. Morbidity is low in patients without coagulopathy. When examined by an experienced pathologist, an adequate biopsy specimen can differentiate between obstructive and hepatocellular causes of cholestasis, with 90% sensitivity and specificity for biliary atresia.*

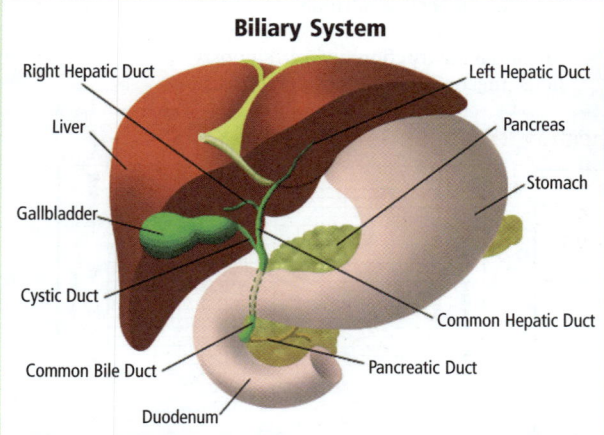

Biliary System

Right Hepatic Duct

Liver

Gallbladder

Cystic Duct

Common Bile Duct

Duodenum

Left Hepatic Duct

Pancreas

Stomach

Common Hepatic Duct

Pancreatic Duct

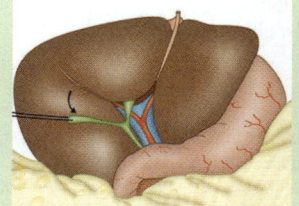

Operative view of complete extra-hepatic biliary atresia

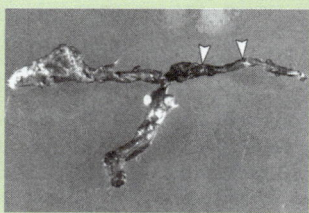

Hepatobiliary ultrasonographic-triangular cord (TC) sign the sensitivity and specificity of these findings, even in the most experienced centers, probably do not exceed 80%.

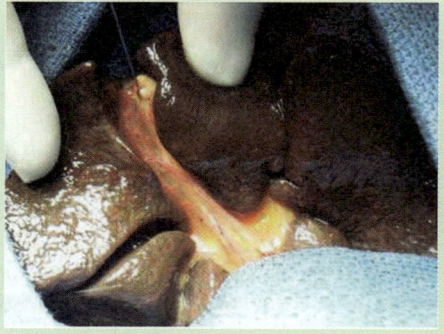

Intraoperative cholangiogram:
Biliary atresia

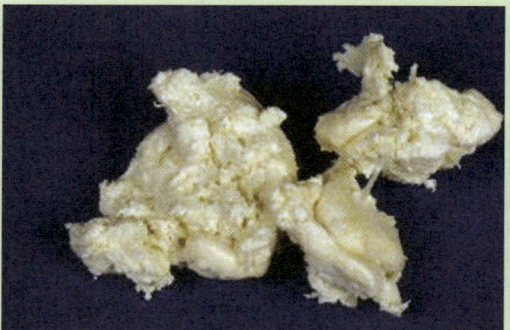

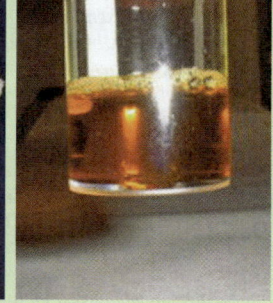

Acholic stools & dark urine which stains the diaper are typical of Neonatal Cholestasis Syndrome.

REVIEW OF CLINICAL PROBLEMS

1. Mention consequences of prolonged Neonatal Cholestasis.
   Ans: Refer to the "Figure 2" of the Chapter.

2. How do you classify Direct Hyperbilirubinemia clinically?
   Ans: Refer to the Table "2" of the Chapter.

3. Discuss the role of important investigations in the diagnosis of Neonatal Cholestasis?.
   Ans: Refer to the Table "5 & 6" of the Chapter.

4. How do you investigate Neonatal Cholestasis Syndrome?
   Ans: Refer to the Evaluation-Decision-Action Plan/ Algorithm to diagnose and manage Neonatal Cholestasis Syndrome.

5. Describe the essential aspects of Kasai Procedure.
   Ans: Refer to the Section KASAI PROCEDURE.

LEARNING OBJECTIVES

After completing this article, readers will be able to:

1. Identify the Cardinal signs of Cholestasis-Acholic stools & Dark Urine staining the nappy.

2. Evaluate Neonatal Cholestasis in a Step-wise manner, initially excluding Potentially life-threatening conditions, such as Sepsis, Galactosemia and Endocrinopathies.

3. Understand the role of Investigations in the diagnostic evaluation of Neonatal Cholestasis.

4. Liaise with Pediatric Surgeon to manage EHBA before 60 days of life for an improved outcome.

5. Counsel the parents about the prognosis and the clinical course and complications after Kasai procedure.

* *Pearl/Peril/Pitfall : Neonatal cholestasis should be ruled out in infants presenting with jaundice that persists after 2 weeks of life. It is important to check fractionated serum bilirubin levels in these patients and immediately refer the patients with conjugated hyperbilirubinemia to a pediatric gastroenterologist for further evaluation.*

BIRD'S EYE VIEW/OVERVIEW/SYNOPSIS

1. *Neonatal Cholestasis is defined as prolonged elevation of serum levels of direct (conjugated) bilirubin, i.e. > 2mg/dL (34 micromols/lt) or a direct bilirubin level > 20% of total bilirubin level beyond the first 14 days of life.* Jaundice that appears after 2 week of age, progresses after this time, or doesn't resolve at this time should be evaluated and a direct bilirubin level determined. It may be associated with hepatomegaly, splenomegaly, pale stools, and dark urine.

2. *Cholestasis in a Neonate may be due to infectious, genetic, metabolic, or undefined abnormalities giving rise either to mechanical obstruction of bile flow or to functional impairment of hepatic excretory function and bile secretion (Refer to Table 1).*

3. *Idiopathic Neonatal hepatitis* is the most common cause of Neonatal Cholestasis (60%), but this diagnosis is to be made after all other *known causes have been excluded*. Biliary atresia is the second most common cause (30%). *In the Newborn intensive care unit,* the most common causes of elevated conjugated bilirubin, in decreasing order of frequency, are hyperalimentation (TPN), idiopathic hepatitis, biliary atresia, alpha-1- antitrypsin deficiency, intrauterine infections (TORSCH), choledochal cyst, galactosemia, and increased bilirubin load from hemolytic disease *(inspissated bile syndrome).* Neonatal cholestasis may be divided into extrahepatic and intrahepatic disease *(Refer to Figure 1).*

4. The clinical features of any form of **Cholestasis** are similar. In an affected Neonate, the diagnosis of certain entities, such as Sepsis, hypothyroidism and galactosemia, is relatively simple.In most cases, however, the cause of Cholestasis is more obscure. *Differentiation among biliary atresia, idiopathic Neonatal Hepatitis, and intrahepatic Cholestasis is particularly difficult (Refer to Table 2 & 3).* Conjugated bilirubin is found in the urine ; urobilinogen is not. The term **cholestasis** includes retention of conjugated bilirubin, bile acids, and other components of bile.

5. The evaluation of the Neonate/infant with Cholestatic jaundice should follow a logical, cost—effective sequence as described in the Evaluation-Decision-Action-Plan / Algorithm. In contrast to unconjugated hyperbilirubinemia, which may be physiologic, *Cholestasis in the Neonate is always pathologic and prompt differentiation is imperative (Refer to Table 5, 6 & 7).*

   Step 1: differentiate direct from indirect hyperbilirubinemia

   Step II: recognize Cholestatic conditions for which specific therapy is available e.g., sepsis, endocrinopathy (hypothyroidism or panhypopituitarism), galactosemia or tyrosinemia, cystic fibrosis, alpha 1 antitrypsin deficiency, congenital syphilis, herpes, CMV, etc. The hepatitis A,B,C viruses rarely cause Neonatal Cholestasis.

   Step III: Differentiate extrahepatic biliary atresia from Neonatal hepatitis *(Refer to Table 3).*

6. *The affected Neonates with Cholestasis (with any form) are at increased risk for chronic complications,* which reflect various degrees of residual hepatic functional capacity and are due directly or indirectly to diminished bile flow *(Refer to Figure 2).*

7. *Extra Hepatic Biliary Atresia (EHBA)* (Syn-Progressive Obliterative Cholangiopathy): the incidence is 1/10,000–15,000 live births, and it constitutes 30% of the Neonatal Cholestasis syndrome characterized by passing persistently acholic stools, dark urine, jaundice with dark green hue, hepatomegaly, well-appearing infant at the time of initial presentation, hepatobiliary ultrasonographic-triangular cord (TC) sign, hepatobiliary scintigraphy with technetium—labeled iminodiacetic acid (HIDA) derivatives showing normal uptake and absent excretion into the intestine & Percutaneous liver biopsy showing bile ductular proliferation, the presence of bile plugs, and portal or perilobular edema and fibrosis, with the basic hepatic lobular architecture intact. When EHBA is suspected, Intraoperative Cholangiogram and Hepatic Porto-enterostomy (Kasai procedure) should be performed in the first 8-10 weeks of life because the bile flow can be established in 80-90% of cases if done early; whereas if the surgery is delayed for > 3 months of age, the bile flow can be established in 10-20% cases only. Good prognostic factors for EHBA surgery are surgery done under 60 days of life, minimal or no fibrosis on histology, good bile flow after surgery and absence of cholangitis in immediate postoperative period or first year of life and availability of surgical expertise.

8. *Liver transplantation,* with 10 year survival rate of 85-90% is the choice of therapy for EHBA if 1) failed Kasai procedure 2) progressive liver disease in spite of successful Kasai procedure 3) late presentation of EHBA (unoperated) are encountered.

9. *The suggested medical management of persistent Cholestasis* has been summarized in the *Table 4.*

10. *Prognosis and Outcome:* Prognosis of Neonatal Hepatitis is very good, if diagnosed early and appropriate treatment is instituted depending upon the etiology. In idiopathic Neonatal hepatitis 70-80 percent recover; 10-20 percent may have progressive liver disease and very small percentage of 1-2 percent may develop cirrhosis. Death occurs due to sepsis, bleeding or acute liver failure. In EHBA even after successful portoenterostomy 1/3 die during first year of operation, 1/3 die by 10 years of age whereas 1/3 survive after 10 with some compromised liver functions. With liver transplantation survival of EHBA has improved to 90 percent in best centres.

---

* *Pearl/Peril/Pitfall : Conjugated hyperbilirubinemia, pale stools and dark urine are the cardinal features of neonatal cholestasis. Early recognition and a stepwise diagnostic evaluation of the infant with cholestasis are essential in successfully treating or managing the complications of the metabolic and infectious liver diseases of the infant as well as surgically relieving obstruction in patients who have biliary atresia.*

THE EVALUATION-DECISION-ACTION-PLAN/ALGORITHM FOR THE DIAGNOSIS AND MANAGEMENT OF *NEONATAL CHOLESTASIS SYNDROME*

SUBJECTIVE FINDINGS

Hx of risk factors such as : premature, sick Neonates, prolonged TPN in LBW babies, sepsis, TORSCH infections, inspissated bile from hemolytic disease, Parental Consanguinity (genetic & metabolic causes)

Hx of Neonatal infection—UTI, sepsis and viral infection.

Hx of jaundice, dark urine staining the nappy, light or acholic stools, bleeding tendency, malabsorption, irritability/pruritus, progressive liver disease (ascites, variceal bleeding, hypersplenism) end-stage liver disease.

Hx of endocrinopathy suggestive of hypo-thyroidism / panhypopituitarism.

Hx of Neonatal Cholestasis in the siblings & family.

OBJECTIVE FINDINGS

Look for jaundice, hepatomegaly, spleno-megaly, petechiae, chorioretinitis + cataracts, & microcephaly (TORSCH).

Assess growth parameters, vitals, nutritional status, neurologic signs.

Examine the nappies for pale acholic stools & staining of dark urine.

Check carefully for signs of sepsis, snuffles, ascites, pneumonia, & CCF.

Look for dysmorphic features suggestive of various syndromes causing Neonatal Cholestasis *(Refer to Table 7).*

Assess for features suggestive of progressive liver disease & end- stage liver disease .

INVESTIGATIONS

(Refer to Table 5) + *perform the following investigations.*

Blood FBC, differential, platelets, Reticulocyte count, Coombs test, blood cultures,TORSCH screen, hepatitis B markers.

Exploratory laparotomy & Operative Cholangiography.

Urine cultures.

Stop TPN with aminoacids, & if this is the cause, the liver dysfunction will usually resolve.

A Neonate with Cholestasis (direct bilirubin > 2mg/dL or > 20% of total bilirubin

Ultrasound *Absent gallbladder, *"triangular cord" sign* *Low sensitivity; operator dependent *Evaluates for other anatomic abnormalities

ALT, AST
g-Glutamyltranspeptidase
Alkaline phosphatase
Consider :
Bacterial and viral cultures

Identify :
Bacterial/viral infections

Do :
Ultrasonography

INFECTIONS

Bacterial

Infection found Infection likely

Treat with antibiotics

Chole-stasis resolves Cholestasis continues

Consider change of antibiotics

Cholestasis resolves Cholestasis continues

Viral
* CMV
* Rubella
* Herpes
* Hepatitis B
* AIDS

Positive if any Negative

Observe/ treat accordingly

Protozoal
* Toxoplasmosis
* Malaria
Listeriosis

Positive Negative

Treat accordingly

Chole-stasis resolves Cholestasis continues

Congenital sypilis

Treat with penicillin

Chole-stasis resolves Chole-stasis conti-nues

Consider metabolic work up

Abnormal

Identify :
Choledochal cyst
Duplication
Cholelithiasis
Abscess
Tumor
Liver/pancreatic cysts

Biliary atresia

Intrahepatic Extrahepatic
Consult :
Surgeon,
Gastroent-erologist

Treat :
Surgery

Normal (or absent gallbladder)

Identify :
Prolonged (TPN) hyperalimentation

Do :
Radionuclide scan
P/C liver biopsy
I/O cholangiography

Treat :
Consider :
Increase Enteral Feedings
Discontinue TPN

Idiopathic Neonatal Hepatitis

The "3 - Step" process to differentiate neonatal cholestasis syndrome

Step - 1 : differentiate direct from indirect hyperbilirubinemia

Step- II : recognize Cholestatic conditions for which specific therapy is available e.g., sepsis, endocrinopathy (hypothyroidism or panhypopituitarism), galactosemia or tyrosinemia, cystic fibrosis, alpha 1 antitrypsin deficiency , congenital syphilis, herpes, CMV etc. The hepatitis A,B,C viruses rarely cause Neonatal Cholestasis.

Step - III : differentiate extrahepatic biliary atresia from Neonatal hepatitis *(Refer to Table 3)*

TABLE 1 — Differential diagnosis of neonatal and infantile cholestasis

INFECTIOUS
Generalized bacterial sepsis
Viral hepatitis
    Hepatitis A,B,C (rare)
    Cytomegalovirus
    Rubella virus
    Herpes virus HSV, HHV 6 and 7
    Varicella virus
    Coxsackievirus
    Echovirus
    Reovirus type 3
    Parvovirus B19
    HIV
Others
    Toxoplasmosis
    Syphilis
    Tuberculosis
    Listeriosis

TOXIC
Parenteral nutrition related
Sepsis (e.g., urinary tract) with endotoxemia
Drug related

METABOLIC
Disorders of amino acid metabolism
    Tyrosinemia
Disorders of lipid metabolism
    Wolman disease
    Niemann-Pick disease (type C)
    Gaucher disease
Disorders of carbohydrate metabolism
    Galactosemia
    Fructosemia
    Glycogenosis IV
Disorders of bile acid biosynthesis
Other metabolic defects
    a_1-Antitrypsin deficiency
    Cystic fibrosis
    Idiopathic hypopituitarism

Hypothyroidism
Zellweger (cerebrohepatorenal) syndrome
Neonatal iron storage disease
Indian childhood cirrhosis/infantile copper overload
Hemophagocytic lymphohistiocytosis (HLH)
Congenital disorders of glycosylation
Mitochondrial hepatopathies

GENETIC/CHROMOSOMAL
Trisomy E
Down syndrome
Donahue syndrome (leprechaunism)

INTRAHEPATIC DISEASES
Intrahepatic cholestasis-persistent
    "Idiopathic" neonatal hepatitis
    Alagille syndrome (arteriohepatic dysplasia)
    Intrahepatic biliary hypoplasia or paucity of
        intrahepatic bile ducts (nonsyndromic)
    Progressive familial intrahepatic cholestasis (PFIC)
Intrahepatic cholestasis - recurrent
    Familial benign recurrent cholestasis associated with
        lymphedema (Aagenaes)
Congenital hepatic fibrosis
Caroli disease (cystic dilatation of intrahepatic ducts)

EXTRAHEPATIC DISEASES
Biliary atresia
Sclerosing cholangitis
Bile duct stenosis
Choledochal-pancreaticoductal junction anomaly
Spontaneous perforation of the bile duct
Choledochal cyst
Mass (neoplasia, stone)
Bile/mucous plug ("Inspissated bile")

MISCELLANEOUS
Langerhans cell histiocytosis
Shock and hypoperfusion
Associated with enteritis
Associated with intestinal obstruction
Neonatal lupus erythematosis
Myeloproliferative disease (21-trisomy)

TABLE 2 — Causes of direct hyperbilirubinemia in the infant

Well-appearing infant	Ill-appearing infant
Biliary atresia	Sepsis
Choledochal cyst	Urinary tract infection
a_1-Antitrypsin deficiency	Intrauterine infection
Hepatitis B	Neonatal hemochromatosis
Alagille syndrome	Metabolic disease
Urinary tract infection	Tyrosinemia
Idiopathic neonatal hepatitis	Galactosemia
Dubin-Johnson syndrome	Fructose intolerance
Total parenteral nutrition	Fatty acid oxidation disorders
Progressive familial intrahepatic cholestasis	Mitochondrial enzyme defects
type 3 (not types 1 and 2)	Carbohydrate deficient glycoprotein syndrome
Bile acid synthesis and metabolism disorders	Hypopituitarism
Bile plug syndrome	Idiopathic neonatal hepatitis
Cystic fibrosis	

* **Pearl/Peril/Pitfall** : *Percutaneous liver biopsy is the single most definitive investigation in the evaluation of neonatal cholestasis. The characteristic findings in biliary atresia include bile duct proliferation, bile plugs and portal tract edema and fibrosis. These findings should be differentiated from those seen in idiopathic neonatal hepatitis that include diffuse cell swelling, giant cell transformation and focal hepatocellular necrosis. Liver biopsy can also demonstrate viral inclusion bodies suggesting cytomegalovirus or herpes simplex infection.*

Figure 1

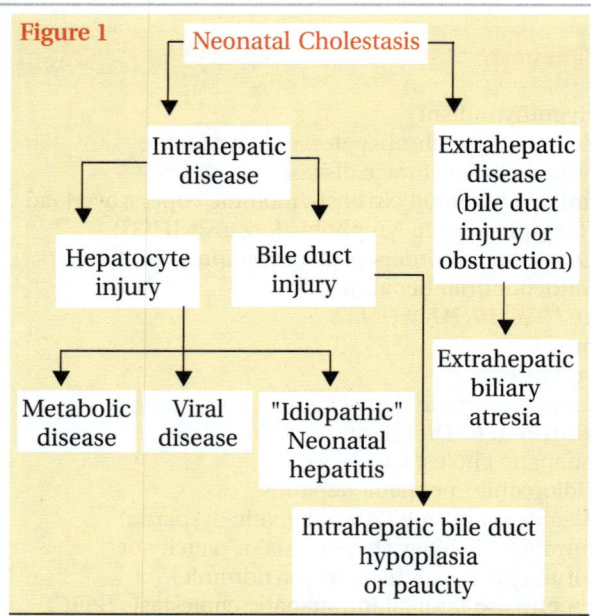

Neonatal cholestasis. Conceptual approach to the group of diseases presenting as cholestasis in the Neonate. There are areas of overlap-patients with extrahepatic biliary atresia may have some degree of intrahepatic injury. Patients with "idiopathic" Neonatal hepatitis may in the future be determined to have a primary metabolic or viral disease.

Figure 2   *Consequences of Prolonged Cholestasis*

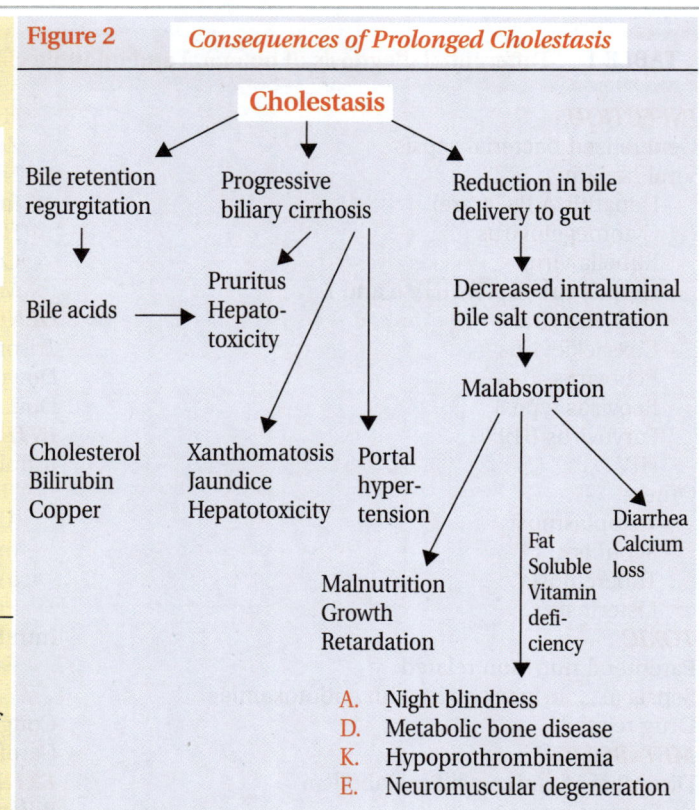

A.	Night blindness
D.	Metabolic bone disease
K.	Hypoprothrombinemia
E.	Neuromuscular degeneration

TABLE 3   DIFFERENCES BETWEEN NEONATAL HEPATITIS AND EXTRA HEPATIC BILIARY ATRESIA (EHBA)

	Features	Neonatal Hepatitis	EHBA
1.	Onset	Anytime in Neonatal period	End of first week
2.	Gestation	Preterm or Small for Date	Term baby
3.	Appearance	May be sick looking	Well looking
4.	Jaundice	Mild-moderate	Moderate-severe
5.	Stools	Incompletely Acholic	Totally Acholic(Clay-colored)
6.	Activity and feeding	Normal or slow	Normal
7.	Hepatosplenomegaly	Early presentation	Late presentation
8.	Liver	Mild to Moderate,Soft	Moderate to Large,Firm to Hard
9.	Multisystem Involvement	Often present	Rare,Polysplenia may be present
10.	Urinary urobilin	+	-
11.	Stercobilin in stools	+	-
12.	Serum alkaline phosphatase*	+++	
13.	S.G.O.T. and S.G.P.T.*	Severe derangement	Mild to moderate derangement
14.	Serum alpha-fetoproteins	May be raised	Absent
15.	Alpha 1-antitrypsin	May be deficient	Generally normal
16.	Australia antigen	±	-
17.	Tc 99 m-para isopropyl IDA (iminodiacetic acid hepato biliary scintigraphy)	Radioactivity seen in the intestine	No radioactivity seen in the intestine
18.	Liver biopsy*	Giant cells predominate	Hypoplasia and dilatation of bile canaliculi predominate
19.	Operative cholangiogram	Normal	Block may be visualized

*These parameters do not show any distinctive differences after the age of 2 to 3 months.

Adapted from **Care Of the Newborn** *by Dr Meharban Singh, 6th Edition & IAP Textbook of Pediatrics -Dr VS Sankaranarayanan*

TABLE 4	Treatment of complications of chronic cholestatic liver disease		
Indication	**Treatment**	**Dose**	**Toxicity**
Intrahepatic cholestasis	Phenobarbital	3–10 mg/kg/d	Drowsiness, irritability, interference with vitamin D metabolism
	Cholestyramine/colestipol hydro-chloride	250–500 mg/kg/d	Constipation, acidosis, binding of drugs, increased steatorrhea
	Ursodeoxycholic acid	15–20 mg/kg/d	Transient increase in pruritus
Pruritus	Phenobarbital or cholestyramine/colestipol (or both)	Same as above	
	Antihistamines :		Drowsiness
	diphenhydramine hydrochloride	5–10 mg/kg/d	
	hydroxyzine	2–5 mg/kg/d	
	Ultraviolet light B	Exposure as needed	Skin burn
	Carbamazepine	20-40 mg/kg/d	Hepatotoxicity, marrow suppression, fluid retention
	Rifampin	10 mg/kg/d	Hepatotoxicity, marrow suppression
	Ursodeoxycholic acid	15–20 mg/kg/d	Transient increase in pruritus
Steatorrhea	Formula containing medium-chain triglycerides (e.g., Pregestimil)	120–150 calories/kg/d	Expensive for infants
	Oil supplement containing medium-chain triglycerides	1–2 mL/kg/d	Diarrhea, aspiration
Malabsorption of fat-soluble vitamins	Vitamin A	10,000–25,000 units/d	Hepatitis, pseudotumor cerebri, bone lesions
	Vitamin D	800–5000 units/d	Hypercalcemia, hypercalciuria
	25-Hydroxycholecalciferol	3–5 mg/kg/d (vitamin D)	Hypercalcemia, hypercalciuria
	1, 25-Dihydroxycholecalciferol	0.05–0.2mg/kg/d (vitamin D)	Hypercalcemia, hypercalciuria
	Vitamin E (oral)	25–200 IU/kg/d	Potentiation of vitamin K deficiency TPGS,[1] 15–25 IU/kg/d
	Vitamin E (intramuscular)	1–2 mg/kg/d	Muscle calcifications
	Vitamin K (oral)	2.5 mg twice per week to 5 mg/d	
	Vitamin K (intramuscular)	2–5 mg each 4 wk	
Malabsorption of other nutrients	Multiple vitamin	1–2 times the standard dose	
	Calcium	25–100 mg/kg/d	Hypercalcemia, hypercalciuria
	Phosphorus	25–50 mg/kg/d	Gastrointestinal intolerance
	Zinc	1mg/kg/d	Interference with copper and iron absorption

[1]*D-alpha tocopheryl polyethylene glycol-1000 succinate (water-soluble vitamin E)*

TABLE 5	Value of specific tests in the evaluation of patients with suspected neonatal cholestasis
Serum bilirubin fractionation	Documents cholestasis
Assessment of stool color	Indicates bile flow into intestine
Urine/serum bile acids measurement	Confirms cholestasis; may indicate inborn error of bile acid biosynthesis
Hepatic synthetic function (albumin,coagulation profile)	Indicates severity of hepatic dysfunction
α_1-antitrypsin phenotype	Suggests (or excludes) PiZZ
Thyroxine and TSH	Suggests (or excludes) endocrinopathy
Sweat chloride/mutation analysis	Suggests (or excludes) cystic fibrosis
Urine/serum amino acids and urine reducing substances	Suggests (or excludes) metabolic liver disease
Ultrasonography	Suggests (or excludes) choledochal cyst; may detect the triangular cord
(TC) sign suggesting biliary	atresia
Hepatobiliary scintigraphy	Documents bile duct patency or obstruction
Liver biopsy	Distinguishes biliary atresia from neonatal hepatitis; Suggests alternative diagnosis

Pearl/Peril/Pitfall : Conditions like sepsis, metabolic disorders like galactosemia, glycogen storage disorders and other endocrinopathies that are potentially life threatening and need immediate intervention should be ruled out first. Once they have been excluded, the next step is to rule out biliary atresia.

TABLE 6	Important investigations to diagnose neonatal cholestasis syndrome

1. *Ultrasound hepatobiliary scan* *accurately identifies a) choledochal cyst b) choledocholithiasis c) bile plug syndrome & d) Caroli's disease (cystic dilation of intrahepatic ducts) *ultrasonographic TC (Triangular Cord sign), which represents a cone-shaped fibrotic mass cranial to the bifurcation of the portal vein, may be seen in patients with biliary atresia. This is very specific for EHBA in expert hands *the gall bladder is either not visualized or a micro-gall bladder is seen in patients with biliary atresia : children with intrahepatic cholestasis caused by idiopathic Neonatal hepatitis, cystic fibrosis, or TPN may have similar ultrasonographic findings *in patients with EHBA, ultrasound may detect associated anomalies such as abdominal polysplenia and vascular malformations

2. *Hepatobiliary scintigraphy* *a sensitive but not specific test for EHBA and it fails to identify other structural abnormalities of the biliary tree or vascular anomalies *the administration of phenobarbital (5mg/kg/day) for 5 days before the scan is recommended because it may enhance biliary excretion of isotope (technetium - labelled iminodiacetic acid derivatives - HIDA) *the hepatic uptake of the agent is normal in patients with EHBA but excretion into the intestine is absent *although the uptake may be impaired in Neonatal hepatitis, excretion into the bowel will eventually occur : obtaining a follow-up scan after 24 hrs is of value to determine the patency of the biliary tree *the lack of the specificity of the test and the need to wait for 5 days makes this procedure less practical and of limited usefulness in the evaluation of children suspected to have biliary atresia.

3. *Percutaneous liver biopsy* *a valuable procedure in the evaluation of Neonatal hepatobiliary diseases and provides the most reliable discriminatory evidence *in Neonatal hepatitis, there is severe, diffuse hepatocellular disease, with distortion to lobular architecture, marked infiltration with inflammatory cells, and focal hepatocellular necrosis ; the bile ductules show little alteration *biliary atresia is characterized by bile ductular proliferation, the presence of bile plugs, and portal or perilobular edema and fibrosis, with the basic hepatic lobular architecture intact *giant cell transformation is found in infants with either condition and has no diagnostic specificity *the histologic changes seen in patients with idiopathic Neonatal hepatitis may also occur in various diseases, including alpha-1-antitrypsin deficiency, galactosemia, and, various forms of intrahepatic cholestasis *in best hands histopathology can differentiate Neonatal hepatitis and EHBA upto 95% ; in 5% cases there can be overlap problems to label.

4. *Intraoperative cholangiography* *the gold standard to confirm the diagnosis of EHBA, when above given investigations don't suggest EHBA *the presence of gall bladder along with the dye showing in duodenum and after clamping the common bile duct showing dye in intrahepatic radicles rules out EHBA *if dye is not going to duodenum or there is no extrahepatic biliary tree this confirms EHBA *there is advantage of taking wedge biopsy of liver and Kasai's porto-enterostomy can be done simultaneously in EHBA. *MR cholangiography may replace diagnostic laparotomy and surgical cholangiography in jaundiced neonates in whom no bowel excretion is seen on cholescintigrams. (see next page)*

TABLE 7	Important syndromes of neonatal cholestasis

1. *Alagille syndrome (arteriohepatic dysplasia)* *the most common syndrome incorporating intrahepatic bile duct paucity *clinical features are varied and nonspecific *clinical features include abnormal facies (broad forehead, deep-set, widely spaced eyes, long—straight nose, underdeveloped mandible), ocular abnormalities (posterior embryotoxon), CVS abnormalities (peripheral pulmonary stenosis and TOF), vertebral arch defects and failure of anterior vertebral arch fusion (butterfly vertebra) and tubulointerstitial nephropathy. Growth retardation and defective spermatogenesis may reflect nutritional deficiency *prognosis for prolonged survival is good but patients are likely to have pruritus, xanthomas with markedly elevated serum cholesterol levels, and neurologic complications of vitamin E deficiency if untreated *mutations in human jagged 1 gene (JAG 1), which encodes a ligand for the notch receptor, are linked to Alagille syndrome.

2. *Zellweger syndrome* (cerebrohepatorenal syndrome)- *a rare autosomal recessive genetic disorder marked by progressive degeneration of liver and kidneys and is fatal within 6-12 months *the incidence is 1/1,00,000 and the affected infants have severe, generalized hypotonia and markedly impaired neurologic function with psychomotor retardation *patients have an abnormal head shape and unusual facies, hepatomegaly, renal cortical cysts, stippled calcifications of the patellas and greater trochanter, and ocular abnormalities *hepatic cells on ultrastructural examination show an absence of peroxisomes. *Unusual problems in prenatal development, an enlarged liver, high levels of iron and copper in the blood, and vision disturbances are among the major manifestations of Zellweger syndrome.*The PXR1 gene has been mapped to chromosome 12; mutations in this gene cause Zellweger syndrome. The PXR1 gene product is a receptor found on the surface of peroxisomes - microbodies found in animal cells, especially liver, kidney and brain cells. The function of peroxisomes is not fully understood, although the enzymes they contain carry out a number of metabolically important reactions. The PXR1 receptor is vital for the import of these enzymes into the peroxisomes: without it functioning properly, the peroxisomes can not use the enzymes to carry out their important functions, such as cellular lipid metabolism and metabolic oxidations.

3. *Byler disease* (Progressive Intrahepatic Cholestasis): *characterized by unique structural abnormalities in the bile canalicular membrane and the affected patients present with failure to thrive, steatorrhea, pruritus, rickets, and low gamma GT levels and cirrhosis *the major clinical differentiation from Alagille syndrome is the absence of bile duct paucity and extrahepatic features.

4. *Dubin-Johnson syndrome* *autosomal recessive disorder involving hepatocyte secretion of bilirubin glucuronide and also involves several organic anions normally excreted from the liver cell into bile *bile acid secretion is normal, and serum bile acid levels are normal *urinary coproporphyrin excretion is normal in quantity ; however due to a defect in porphyrin excretion, coproporphyrin I constitutes 80% of the total (coproporphyrin III is normally > 75% of the total) *cholangiography fails to visualize the biliary tract and radiology of the gall bladder is also abnormal *conjugated hyperbilirubinemia + hepatic lysosomal pigment + normal life span.

5. *Aagenaes syndrome* (idiopathic familial intrahepatic cholestasis associated with lymphedema of the lower extremities) *affected patients usually present with episodic cholestasis with elevation of serum aminotransferases, alkaline phosphatase, & bile acids *asymptomatic between the episodes and the biochemical indices improve.

---

* *Pearl/Peril/Pitfall :* Idiopathic neonatal hepatitis, also known as giant cell hepatitis, accounts for approximately 30% to 60% of the cases of neonatal cholestasis. It is a diagnosis of exclusion and diagnosed by the presence of the classic pathological findings.

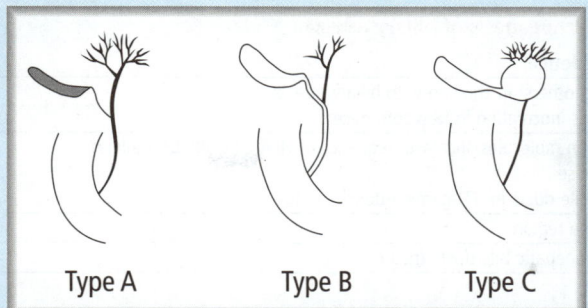

Type A   Type B   Type C

Drawing shows the three types of biliary atresia. Type A has complete fibrous obliteration of the entire extrahepatic bile duct. Type B shows a patent but extremely hypoplastic common bile duct with atretic hepatic ducts. Type C has a cystic dilatation of the common hepatic duct with an atretic common bile duct.

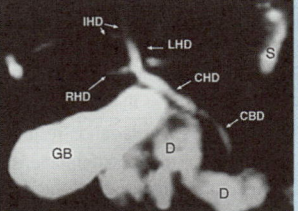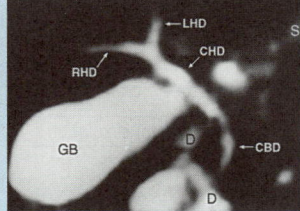

MR cholangiography can be used to depict the major biliary structures of Neonates and small infants and to exclude biliary atresia as the cause of Neonatal cholestasis by allowing visualization of the biliary tract.

MR cholangiograms in a 3-month-old nonjaundiced male infant. S = stomach, D = duodenum. (a) T2-weighted turbo SE image (3,000/700 [effective]) with 2D acquisition by using an MIP algorithm clearly depicts the gallbladder (GB), common bile duct (CBD), common hepatic duct (CHD), right and left hepatic ducts (RHD, LHD), and the second-order intrahepatic ducts (IHD). (b) T2-weighted IR turbo SE image (7,000/1,000 [effective]/50) with 3D acquisition by using an MIP algorithm shows the biliary structures up to the right and left hepatic ducts (RHD, LHD). The second-order intrahepatic duct is not visible. CBD = common bile duct, CHD = common hepatic duct, GB = gallbladder.

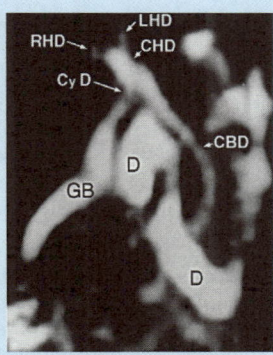

MR cholangiogram in a 3-day-old nonjaundiced male neonate. T2-weighted turbo SE image (3,000/700 [effective]) in steep oblique projection shows the gallbladder (GB), cystic duct (CyD), common bile duct (CBD), common hepatic duct (CHD), and right and left hepatic ducts (RHD, LHD), but the second-order intrahepatic ducts are not shown. D = duodenum.

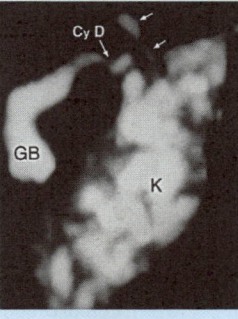

MR cholangiogram in a 32-day-old female infant with paucity of intrahepatic ducts and infantile polycystic kidney disease. T2-weighted turbo SE image (3,000/700 [effective]) obtained with steep oblique coronal projection depicts the gallbladder (GB), cystic duct (Cy D), and extrahepatic bile duct (arrows). Also seen is the enlarged right kidney (K) with small hyperintense cystic lesions

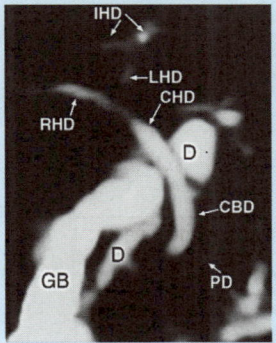

MR cholangiogram in a 46-day-old female infant with neonatal hepatitis. T2-weighted turbo SE image (3,000/700 [effective]) obtained from frontal projection shows clearly visible gallbladder (GB), common bile duct (CBD), common hepatic duct (CHD), and right and left hepatic ducts (RHD, LHD) and faintly visible second-order intrahepatic ducts (IHD). The pancreatic duct (PD) is also seen. D = duodenum.

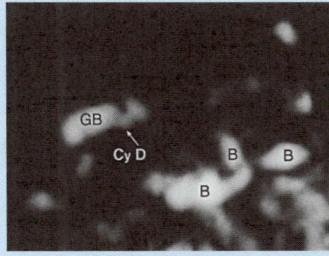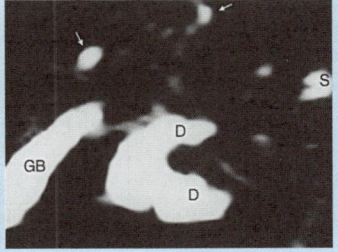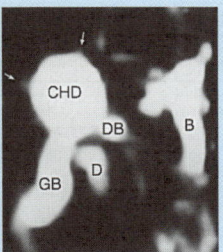

MR cholangiograms in patients with biliary atresia. (a) Biliary atresia in a 32-day-old male infant (patient 1). T2-weighted turbo SE image (3,000/700 [effective]) obtained with coronal oblique projection shows an atrophic gallbladder (GB) and cystic duct (Cy D). The common bile duct, common hepatic duct, and intrahepatic ducts are not visible. B = bowel. (b) Biliary atresia in a 57-day-old female infant (patient 3). T2-weighted turbo SE image (3,000/700 [effective]) in coronal oblique projection demonstrates a normal gallbladder (GB) without visualization of the common bile duct or common hepatic duct. Only incomplete intrahepatic ducts (arrows) are visible. D = duodenum, S = stomach. (c) Biliary atresia in a 23-day-old male neonate (patient 6). T2-weighted turbo SE image (3,000/700 [effective]) in slightly oblique coronal projection shows cystic dilatation of the common hepatic duct (CHD), a small gallbladder (GB), and partially visible hepatic ducts (arrows). The common bile duct is not visible. B = bowel, D = duodenum, DB = duodenal bulb. COURTESY:Twei-Shiun Jaw, MD, Yu-Ting Kuo, MD, Gin-Chung Liu, MD, Shaou-Hsium Chen, MD and Chien-Kuo Wang, MD July 1999 Radiology, 212, 249-256

* **Pearl/Peril/Pitfall:** Cholestasis is a complication of parenteral nutrition (PN) in preterm infants. Though a clear etiology has not been identified, it is felt that the immaturity of the enterohepatic circulation plays a role in the pathogenesis. Risk factors for the development of parenteral nutrition associated liver disease include prematurity, sepsis, early initiation and prolonged parenteral nutrition, lack of enteral feeds and preexisting liver disease.

Mechanisms implicated in the pathogenesis of biliary atresia	
Mechanisms	**Evidence**
Viral infections	Detection of viruses (CMV, rotavirus, among others) in children with biliary atresia. Animal model of atresia induced by rotavirus inoculation in Newborn mice.
Immune dysregulation	Increased expression of intercellular adhesion molecules. Increase frequency of HLA-B12, B8, DR3 alleles. Hepatic profile with predominant T_H1 response. Prevention of inflammatory obstruction of bile ducts in IFN-gamma-deficient mice.
Toxins	Associated cases at the same time and in the region.
Defect in prenatal circulation	Intrauterine devasculaization results in extrahepatic bile duct strictures.
Morphogenetic effects	Coexistence of other malformations. Defects in the remodeling of the ductal plate. Mutations in laterality genes 9CFC1, ZIC3) in patients with atresia and laterality defects. Epigenetic factors : increased expression of regulatory genes in children with embryonic atresia. *inv* mouse : model or bile duct obstruction and *situs inversus*.

Classification of EHBA according to the site of extrahepatic biliary obstruction

Type	Prevalence	Characteristics
Type 1	~ 5%	Obliteration of the common bile duct, while proximal ducts are patent. the gallbladder usually contains bile.
Type 2	~ 3%	Atresia of hepatic ducts, the gallbladder does not contain bile and the transsection of proximal remnants shows two distinct bile duct lumens.
Type 3	> 90 %	Atresia involving the right and left hepatic ducts. Obstruction to the level of the Porta hepatis. Absence of proximal lumens at the Porta hepatis.

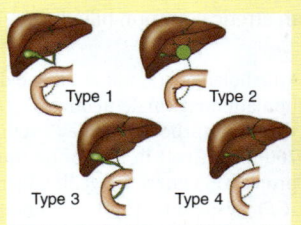
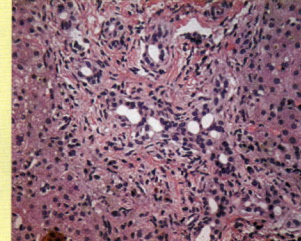

Bile ductular proliferation in liver biopsy specimen (hematoxylin and eosin stain) from patient with biliary atresia. Also note hepatocellular bile staining as a consequence of cholestasis.

In short, if the biopsy suggests obstruction, laparotomy with operative cholangiography is indicated, since only this procedure can confirm or rule out the possibility of atresia. In fact, the establishment of diagnosis is still a challenge, and the combined analysis of all information allows for higher accuracy.

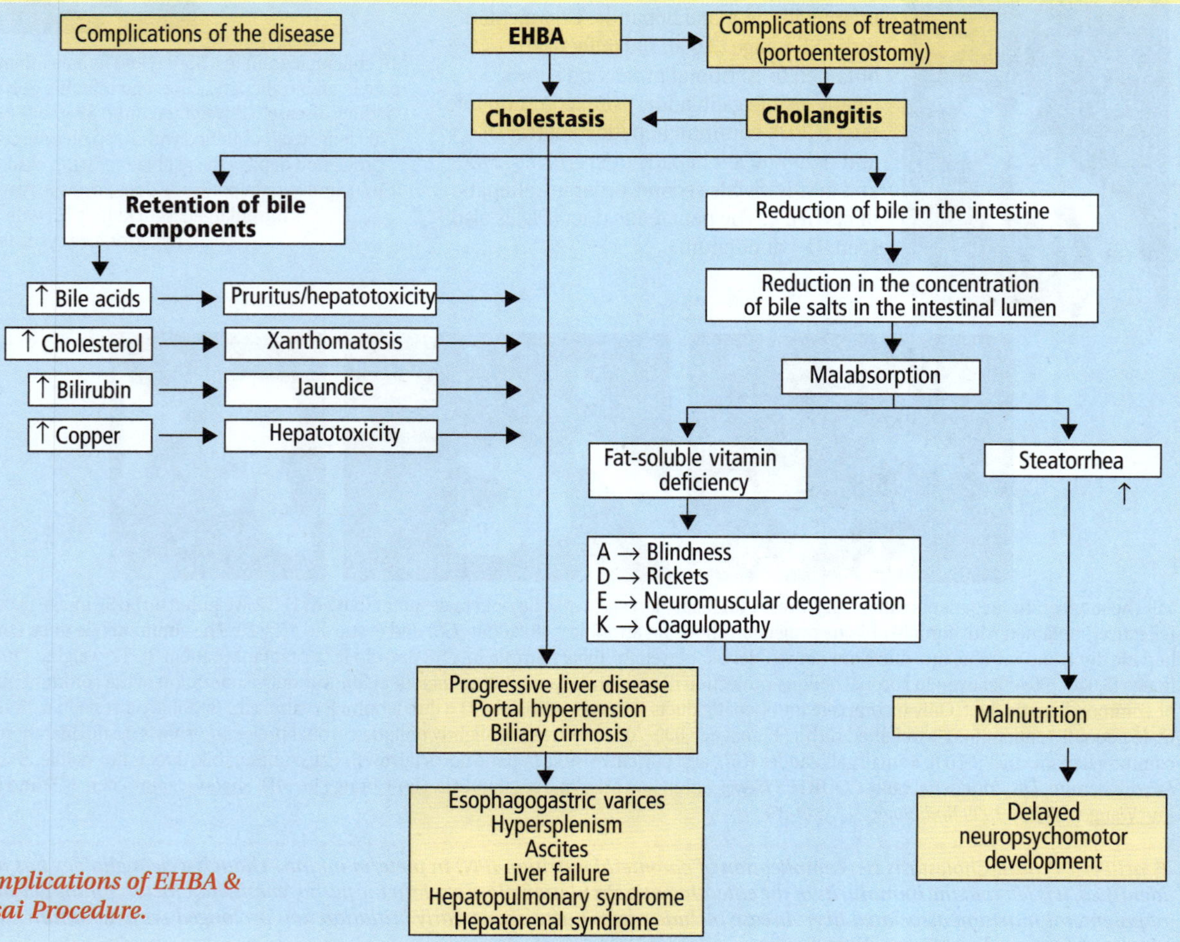

Courtesy: Elisa de Carvalho,Cláudia Alexandra Pontes Ivantes Jorge A. Bezerra, J. Pediatr. (Rio J.) vol.83 no.2 Porto Alegre Mar./Apr. 2007.

Complications of the disease → **EHBA** → Complications of treatment (portoenterostomy)

Cholestasis ← **Cholangitis**

Retention of bile components

↑ Bile acids → Pruritus/hepatotoxicity
↑ Cholesterol → Xanthomatosis
↑ Bilirubin → Jaundice
↑ Copper → Hepatotoxicity

Reduction of bile in the intestine

Reduction in the concentration of bile salts in the intestinal lumen

Malabsorption

Fat-soluble vitamin deficiency

Steatorrhea

A → Blindness
D → Rickets
E → Neuromuscular degeneration
K → Coagulopathy

Progressive liver disease
Portal hypertension
Biliary cirrhosis

Malnutrition

Esophagogastric varices
Hypersplenism
Ascites
Liver failure
Hepatopulmonary syndrome
Hepatorenal syndrome

Delayed neuropsychomotor development

Complications of EHBA & Kasai Procedure.

@Kasai Procedure: resection of the obliterated bile duct w/ creation of a Roux-n-Y hepatoportoenterostomy *Timing of procedure* predicts the prognosis *<60 days-bile flow returned in 80-90% cases *Only 30% with complete drainage *>90 days-bile flow returned in ~20% cases *Usually require a liver transplant within one year *The **experience of the center** performing the Kasai is one of the most important factors determining surgical outcome.

@Post-operative Management *Prophylactic Abx to prevent cholangitis *Ursodiol: enhance bile flow *No special diet needed unless concern with poor bile drainage*MCTformula ie…Alimentum, Pregestimil) *Fat-soluble vitamins: A, D, E, K *+/-short term, high dose steroid therapy.

@If Kasai Fails? *+/-support for revision of Kasai procedure if fails *Despite clinical improvement after a Kasai, 70–80% pts will eventually require liver transplantation *Indications for Liver Transplant: *operation not successful in restoring bile flow initially (~20%) *late referrals (generally >120 days) *develop end-stage liver disease despite bile drainage (ie portal hypertension, recurrent cholangitis, ascites, growth failure) *Liver Transplant results: *one-yr survival rates >90% b/c reduced size allografts and living-related donors.

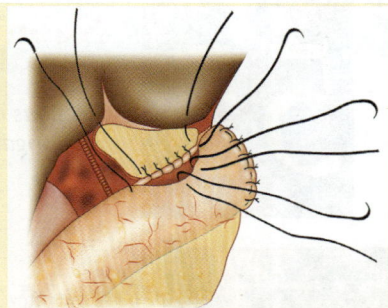

Hepatoporto-enterostomy (Kasai procedure)

Many technical variants are possible, according to the anatomical pattern of the biliary remnant:

- in type 1 BA: cholecysto-enterostomy, or hepatico enterostomy.

- in type 2 BA: cysto-enterostomy. This operation can be performed only if the hilar cyst communicates with the dystrophic intra-hepatic bile ducts (cholangiography).

- in type 3 BA: hepatoporto-cholecystostomy. The patent galbladder, cystic duct and common bile duct are preserved. The gallbladder is mobilised with preservation of its pedicle. An anastomosis is performed between the gallbladder and the transsected tissue in the porta hepatis. Since there is no direct contact between the porta hepatis and the intestine, this operation is expected to reduce the risk of post operative cholangitis. Its specific complications are: bile leaks and post-operative biliary ascites, kinking and obstruction of cystic duct and common bile duct.

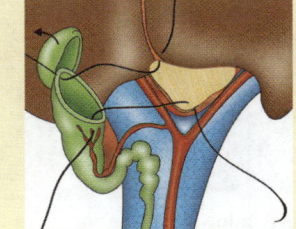

Hepatoporto-cholecystostomy

Ascending cholangitis is the most common postoperative complication seen with the Kasai procedure. Patients present with fever, abnormal liver function tests, worsening jaundice and an elevated ESR. Blood cultures are not always positive. The common pathogens are usually gram-negative rods, though gram-positive rods like Hemophilus influenza have also been identified. These patients are treated with broadspectrum intravenous antibiotics. In patients with refractory cholangitis, prophylactic oral antibiotics like oral neomycin or trimethoprim-sulfamethoxazole have shown some success in decreasing the rates of cholangitis.

KEY POINTS FOR CLINICAL PRACTICE:

1. Cases with suspected extrahepatic biliary atresia (EHBA) should be referred to Pediatric Surgeon without loss of time. Even if liver biopsy is suggestive of Neonatal hepatitis but the baby continues to have persistently pale stools, the patient should be referred to a Pediatric Surgeon.

2. In a sick baby with cholestatic jaundice possibilities of galactosemia, toxoplasmosis, herpes, tyrosinemia, sepsis, malaria, etc. should be considered. In babies apparently looking healthy and passing pale stools, serious consideration should be given to search for obstructive causes like EHBA or choledochal cyst on priority.

3. NCS cases who are passing pigmented stools and do not look sick may be having neonatal hepatitis, ductal paucity, rarely metabolic/storage disorders or hypothyroidism; this group of children (passing pigmented stools) are unlikely to have biliary atresia. Work up of these cases should be based on a rational approach and all unnecessary investigations should be avoided. In all cases of Neonatal Cholestasis, administer diet rich in calories and medium chain triglycerides and adequate proteins. Fat and water soluble vitamin supplementation is mandatory.

4. Liver biopsies of babies with suspected EHBA are an emergency and should be reported on priority basis. A uniform diagnostic criteria need to be followed at all the centers. In case of any doubt about the histopathological diagnosis, the slides should be sent for second opinion to other centers with more experience without losing time.

5. Liver transplantation may remain the only option for infants with EHBA with decompensated liver disease (ascites and/or encephalopathy) or failed portoenterostomy.

REFERENCES & FURTHER READING : 1)*Guibaud L, Lachaud A, Touraine R, et al. MR cholangiography in neonates and infants: feasibility and preliminary applications. AJR 1998; 170:27-31.*2)*Kasai M. Treatment of biliary atresia with special reference to hepatic portoenterostomy and its modifications. Prog Pediatr Surg 1974; 6:5 52.*3)*Laurent G, Bret PM, Reinhold C, Atri M, Barkun AN. Bile duct obstruction and choledocholithiasis: diagnosis with MR cholangiography. Radiology 1995; 197:109-115.*4)*Yachha SK, Mohindra S. Neonatal cholestasis syndrome: Indian scene. Indian J Pediatr 1999; 66 (SS1): S94-S96. 5)*Haber BA, Russo P: Biliary atresia. Gastroenterol Clin North Am 2003; 32:891-911.

---

* *Pearl/Peril/Pitfall: EHBA-If all the initial diagnostic tests are inconclusive, operative exploration and intraoperative cholangiography should be performed. a1-Antitrypsin deficiency has similar presentation and should be ruled out before laparotomy.*

55 Neonatal Necrotizing Enterocolitis (NEC)

@ *"Bilious or feculent vomiting and bleeding per rectum in babies must always be investigated, but not all causes are serious."*

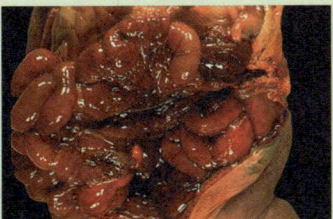 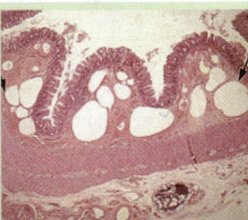 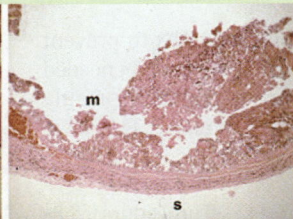 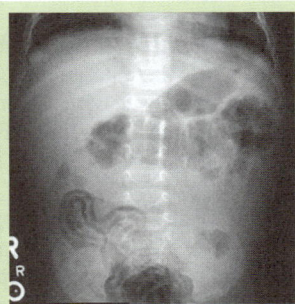

A complication of prematurity and low birth weight is neonatal necrotizing enterocolitis (NEC) in which ischemia results in focal to confluent areas of bowel necrosis, most often in the terminal ileum. Seen at autopsy here is a dark red appearance to the small intestine of a premature neonate.

Pathologic findings in NEC. (**a**) Histologic section of small bowel (original magnification, 100; hematoxylin- eosin stain). Intramural gas is seen as rounded bubbles in the submucosa (arrows). There is hyperemia of the serosa. (**b**) Histologic section of small bowel (original magnification, 100; hematoxylin-eosin stain). The bowel is affected much more severely than in **a**. There is necrosis of the mucosa, submucosa, and muscularis with intraluminal necrotic debris on the mucosal side of the bowel wall *(m)*. Only the serosa appears intact. *s* serosal surface of bowel wall.

Pneumatosis intestinalis

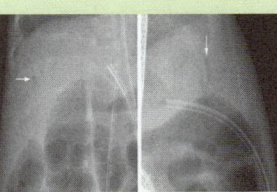

Portal Venous Pneumatosis

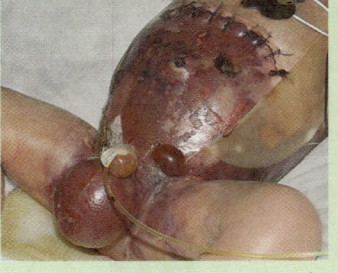 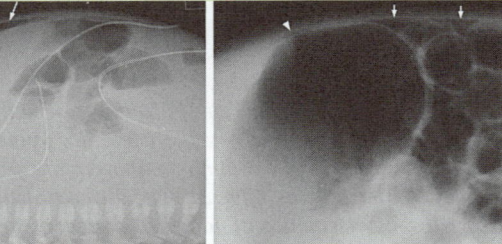 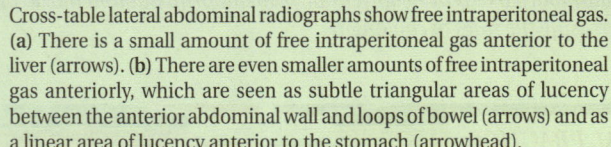 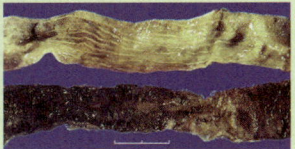

This child's disease appears to be necrotizing enterocolitis (NEC) totalis. Only a profound disseminated coagulopathy could have caused such devastation

Cross-table lateral abdominal radiographs show free intraperitoneal gas. (**a**) There is a small amount of free intraperitoneal gas anterior to the liver (arrows). (**b**) There are even smaller amounts of free intraperitoneal gas anteriorly, which are seen as subtle triangular areas of lucency between the anterior abdominal wall and loops of bowel (arrows) and as a linear area of lucency anterior to the stomach (arrowhead).

Normal (top) versus necrotic section of bowel in NEC

REVIEW OF CLINICAL PROBLEMS

1. What are the risk factors involved in NEC and the preventive strategies to reduce its incidence?
   Ans: Refer to the "No. 1"&"No. 2"of the "BIRD`S EYE VIEW/ OVERVIEW/SYNOPSIS" of the Chapter and also to the Figure No "1" of the Chapter.
2. How do you make a therapeutic decision in managing NEC? *Ans: Refer to the "No. 6" of the "BIRD'S EYE VIEW/ OVERVIEW/SYNOPSIS" of the Chapter.*
3. What are the mimicking conditions, which must be considered in the differential diagnosis of NEC ?
   Ans: Refer to the Evaluation-Decision-Action Plan/ Algorithm to diagnose & manage a Neonate with NEC.
4. How do you approach the Neonatal Pneumoperitoneum? *Ans: Refer to the Figure "2" of the Chapter.*
5. Discuss the role of surgery in managing NEC?
   Ans: Refer to the "No. 9" of the "BIRD'S EYE VIEW/ OVERVIEW/SYNOPSIS" of the Chapter and also to the Table "5" of the Chapter.

LEARNING OBJECTIVES

After completing this article, readers will be able to

1. Be exceedingly vigilant in assessing very preterm infants for NEC, for a protracted postnatal period(10-12 weeks)

2. Diagnose NEC, with a high index of suspicion because of its highly variable signs and symptoms, their onset (acute/insidious) and the time of illness (within the 1st week/thereafter).

3. Assess the severity of NEC, by following Modified Bell`s Staging serially.

4. Manage NEC, by paying attention to acute care as well as long term care.

5. Counsel the parents about the complications and prognosis of NEC- for both short-term & long-term.

* Pearl/Peril/Pitfall : Blood culture: Obtaining a blood culture is recommended before beginning antibiotics in any patient presenting with any signs or symptoms of sepsis or necrotizing enterocolitis. Although blood cultures do not grow any organisms in most cases of necrotizing enterocolitis, sepsis is one of the major conditions that mimics necrotizing enterocolitis and should be considered in the differential diagnosis. Therefore, identification of a specific organism can aid and guide further therapy.

BIRD`S EYE VIEW/OVERVIEW/SYNOPSIS

1. **NEC (Necrotizing Enterocolitis)** - A condition seen primarily in Premature Neonates, characterized by partial or full-thickness intestinal ischemia and necrosis (usually involves the terminal ileum) of unknown etiology and of speculative pathophysiology (Refer to Figure "1" of the Chapter). *NEC is essentially due to an ischemic vascular insult of an immature bowel, which initiates mucosal injury followed by reperfusion injury leading to bowel necrosis aggravated/compounded by bacteria and luminal substrate (feeds).* Prematurity is the single greatest risk factor for NEC. Maternal cocaine ingestion, umbilical arterial catheters, PDA and Indomethacin, Aminophylline and Caffeine, high dose dopamine and adrenaline, hypothermia, polycythemia can compromise mesenteric blood flow significantly & predispose the infant to develop NEC. It is the most common serious surgical disorder among NICU babies, causing significant Neonatal morbidity and mortality (20–40% with NEC complicated by perforation).

2. Preventing NEC is the ultimate goal, which is possible only by preventing premature birth. *If prematurity cannot be avoided, follow certain preventive strategies such as* a)prenatal steroid therapy to induce GI maturation b)oral immunoglobulins (IgA & IgG supplements of feeds) c)breast feeds (incidence is lower & alone it cannot prevent NEC) d)very slow introduction of feedings along with polyunsaturated fatty acids e)oral trials of PAF (Platelet Aggregation Factor) antagonistis f)oral probiotics

3. *As early diagnosis of NEC is the most important factor in determining the outcome.* Suspect the NEC with a high- index in the high risk Neonates (Refer to Table 1 of the Chapter). The onset of NEC can be sudden or insidious : abrupt clinical deterioration may be indistinguishable from the sepsis syndrome (Refer to Table "3" of the Chapter).

4. NEC usually presents in the first week of life or 3–7 days after the onset of initial enteral feeds : abdominal distention is the most frequent early sign associated with increased volume of gastric aspirate and/or bilious aspirate, ileus, apnea and other signs of sepsis, blood per rectum, frank signs of shock and peritonitis and perforation.

5. Confirm the clinically suspected NEC by diagnostic serial abdominal radiographs (AP and cross-table lateral or left lateral decubitus views), surgery, or autopsy. No laboratory tests are specific for NEC : however some tests are valuable in confirming diagnostic impressions (Refer to *the Evaluation-Decision-Action-Plan / Algorithm*). Abdominal X-ray if shows pneumatosis intestinalis (presence of gas within the bowel wall) is pathognomonic for NEC : other findings include abnormal bowel gas pattern, ileus, free peritoneal air, and/ or intrahepatic portal venous air. Radiological findings can often be subtle and confusing : for Eg: perforation of an abdominal viscus will not always cause pneumoperitoneum and conversely, pneumoperitoneum doesn't necessarily indicate abdominal perforation from NEC. Therefore seek careful serial review (KUB film- AP & lateral views q6-8hr x 48-72hr) of the X-rays with a pediatric surgeon/radiologist to assist in interpretation and to plan for further appropriate studies.

6. Follow the well known BELL staging of NEC modified by Walsh and Kliegman, as it provides a basis for therapeutic decision-making based on clinical stage of disease (Refer to Table "1" of the Chapter.).

   1. *Stage* I (suspect) clinical signs and symptoms, nondiagnostic radiographs.

   2. *Stage* II (definite) clinical signs and symptoms, pneumatosis intestinalis on radiograph.

   b)Moderately ill with systemic toxicity

   3. *Stage III* (advanced) clinical signs and symptoms, pneumatosis intestinalis on radiograph, and critically ill.
      a)Impending IP (Intestinal Perforation)
      b)Proven IP (Intestinal Perforation)
   NEC is the most common cause of pneumoperitoneum in a premature infant, but it must be distinguished from pneumoperitoneum secondary to gas that dissects from the thorax to the abdominal cavity after pulmonary interstitial emphysema, pneumothorax or pneumomediastinum. If there is uncertainty, paracentesis, an upper GIT contrast study, or both should be performed to exclude the possibility of an intestinal perforation. (Refer to Figure "2" of the Chapter.)

7. The incidence of NEC is 8–12% in infants < 1.5Kgs. 60-80% of the cases occur in high-risk premature infants and 10-25% occur in low-risk full term infants. NEC represents 2-5% of NICU admissions. An estimated 0.3-2.4 cases occur in every 1000 live births. The mean gestational age of infants with NEC is 30–32 weeks. The mean age of onset is 12 days, and the mode is 3 days. More than 90% of infants have been fed prior to the onset of this disease.

8. *The differential diagnosis of NEC includes* a) pneumonia and sepsis b) surgical causes including malrotation with obstruction (complete or intermittent), malrotation with midgut volvulus, gastric perforation, mesenteric vessel thrombosis c) infectious enterocolitis (campylobacter bloody diarrhea) d) severe forms of inherited metabolic disease (Eg: galactosemia with Esch.coli sepsis) e) feeding intolerance.

9. *The medical management of NEC includes* (Refer to Table "2" of the Chapter for the medical interventions and goals of therapy). a) stabilize ABCs b) allow gastrointestinal rest by nothing by mouth, NG tube decompression, monitoring for abdominal girth and vital signs and GIT bleeding, removing the unbilical catheters c) IV antibiotics (Ampicillin, Gentamicin + Metronidazole or Clindamycin) to cover for aerobes and anaerobes for about 14 days (after blood, urine, stool and CSF cultures) d) Injection Vitamin K, Platelet transfusions to correct severe thrombocytopenia and packed RBC to maintain the hematocrit above 35% and whole blood exchange transfusion for severe neutropenia e) strict monitoring of fluid intake and output to maintain urine output of 1–3 ml/kg/hr and serial monitoring of ABG, Electrolytes, Urea, Creatinine to check for impending renal failure from ATN, coagulative necrosis f) anticipating the neurological complications (seizures) and treating promptly g) Total Parenteral Nutrition (TPN) h) family support. *The Evaluation-Decision-Action Plan/Algorithm describes the essential aspects of diagnosis & management of NEC.*

10. *The surgical management is necessary* for a) intestinal perforation (20-30%) b) evidence of a persistent, fixed sentinel loop over 24 hours c) right lower quadrant mass d) abdominal wall erythema (peritonitis) e) spontaneous intestinal perforation in VLBW infants, a different clinical entity from NEC (Refer to Table "5" of the Chapter.).

11. Explain - prognosis of NEC to the parents (Refer to Table No "4" of the Chapter.). In uncomplicated cases of NEC, the long-term prognosis may be comparable with that of LBW infants, but those with stage IIB & stage III NEC have a higher incidence of growth delay. NEC requiring surgical intervention may have more serious sequelae including increased morbidity & mortality secondary to infection, respiratory failure & TPN associated hepatic disease, rickets & significant developmental delay.

Pearl/Peril/Pitfall: NEC-Metabolic acidosis: Low serum bicarbonate (<20) in a baby with a previously normal acid-base status is also concerning. It is seen in conjunction with poor tissue perfusion, sepsis, and bowel necrosis.

THE EVALUATION-DECISION-ACTION-PLAN/ALGORITHM FOR THE DIAGNOSIS AND MANAGEMENT OF *NECROTIZING ENTEROCOLITIS IN NEWBORN (NEC)*

SUBJECTIVE FINDINGS

Hx of prematurity

Hx of Increasing gastric residuals and bilious vomitings

Hx of change in stool pattern

Hx of factors related to NEC - birth asphyxia, respiratory distress, PDA, polycythemia, umbilical catheterizations, congenital heart disease, exchange transfusion.

Hx of hyperosmolar feedings

Since early features are often nonspecific, a high index of suspicion is the most reliable approach to early diagnosis

OBJECTIVE FINDINGS

Observe for

a) *systemic signs*: Respiratory distress, apnea and/or bradycardia, lethargy, temperature instability, irritability, poor feeding, shock, prolonged capillary refill time, acidosis, oliguria, bleeding diathesis,

b) *Abdominal signs*: Distension, tenderness, gastric aspirates, vomiting of bile, blood, or both, ileus, wall erythema or induration, persistent localized abdominal mass, ascites and bloody stools.

INVESTIGATIONS

Abdominal X-rays: AP and left lateral decubitus views, *Serial films (every 6-8 hrs)* to check the NEC progression are mandatory. Recognize that free air is sometimes missed on the AP views : *left lateral decubitus films may be more sensitive to identify silent perforations.*

Blood: CBC, Platelets, CRP, Cultures, ABG analysis, Electrolytes, Clotting studies, Urea, Creatinine, LFT.

Stool : Occult blood and clinitest

Urine: Microscopy and cultures

CSF: Cultures if necessary

*Nil oral with IV fluids
*NG tube drainage
*FBC & Electrolytes
*KUB film q6-8hr x 48hr
*Blood culture
*IV ampicillin & gentamicin x 48hr
*Stool Heme test & Clinitest

NEWBORN WITH NECROTIZING ENTEROCOLITIS

Suspect NEC Stage I —— **ASSESS DEGREE OF ILLNESS**

Severe (Stage II definite)

Discontinue feeding

Treat:
Nasogastric Tube
IV Antibiotics

Repeat abdominal radiography q6-12h
Reassess clinical signs

Good response

Poor response

Maintain NPO 7-10 days after normal abdominal film

Treat :
Consider :
Surgery

NEC-DIFFERENTIAL DIAGNOSIS

A. *Pneumonia and Sepsis* - Adbominal tenderness and distention will be absent.

B. *Malrotation with obstruction / midgut volvulus, gastric perforation* -Explorative laparotomy is often necessary to differentiate.

C. *Campylobacter enterocolitis* - Bloody diarrhea present but not associated with any other enteric or systemic signs of NEC.

D. *Galactosemia with Esch.coli Sepsis* - Overlaps with some signs of NEC.

E. *Feeding intolerance in premature babies* - With hold enteral feeds and give IV fluids and antibiotics for 72 hrs, until this benign disorder can be distinguished from NEC.

F. *Diarrhea is uncommon presence of NEC in the absence of bloody stools* : this sign should point away from NEC.

Very severe (Stage III advanced)

Discontinue feeding

Stabilize Circulation
Initiate Ventilation for
Respiratory Failure

Request surgical consultation

Treat :
Nasogastric Tube
IV Antibiotics
(including
anaerobic coverage -
MTZ)

Treat :
Consider :
Fresh Frozen Plasma
Platelet Infusion
Packed Cells

Maintain NPO
10-14 days

Treat :
Central or Peripheral Hyperalimentation (TPN)
Continue IV Antibiotics 7-14 days

Treat :
Introduce Enteral Feedings
with Elemental Formula

Follow-up:
Barium Enema in 6-8 wk
to Diagnose Stricture

Treat : Consider : Surgery Indications :

1) Failure to respond to medical management
2) Perforation
3) Fixed sentinel loop over 24 hrs
4) Right lower quadrant mass
5) Abdominal wall erythema
6) Stricture development in 6-8 wks after recovery

Pearl/Peril/Pitfall : NEC-The pertinent physical findings in patients who develop necrotizing enterocolitis can be primarily GI, primarily systemic, indolent, fulminant, or any combination of these. A high index of clinical suspicion is essential to minimize potentially significant morbidity or mortality.

Figure 1: Etiological factors in nec. Major factors are enclosed in boxes

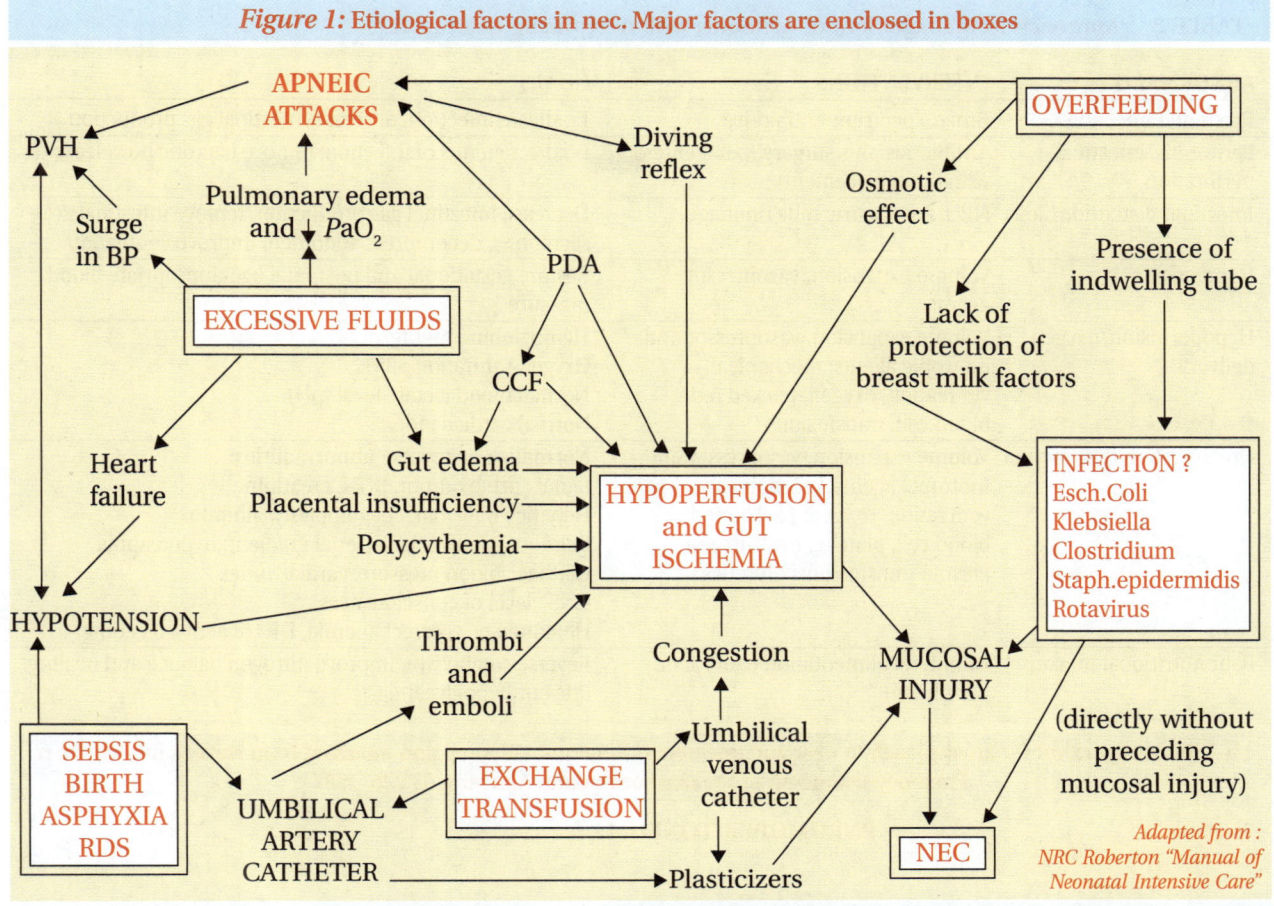

TABLE 1	Modified bell's staging criteria for necrotizing enterocolitis			
Stage	Systemic signs	Intestinal signs	Radiologic signs	Treatment
1. Suspected A	Temperature instability, apnea, bradycardia	Elevated pregavage residuals, mild abdominal distention, occult blood in stool	Normal or mild ileus	NPO, antibiotics x 3 days
B	Same as IA	Same as IA, plus gross blood in stool	Same as IA	Same as IA
II. Definite A: *Mildly ill*	Same as IA	Same as, I plus absent bowel sounds, abdominal tenderness	Ileus, intestinal pneumatosis	NPO, antibiotics × 7–10 days
B: *Moderately ill*	Same as I, Plus mild metabolic acidosis, mild thrombocytopenia	Same as I, plus absent bowel sounds, definite abdominal tenderness, abdominal cellulitis, right lower quadrant mass	Same as IIA, plus portal vein gas, with or without ascites	NPO, antibiotics × 14 days
III. Advanced A: *Severely ill, bowel infarct*	Same as IIB, plus hypotension, bradycardia, respiratory acidosis, metabolic acidosis, disseminated intravascular coagulation, neutropenia	Same as I and II, plus signs of generalized peritonitis, marked tenderness, and distention of abdomen	Same as IIB, plus definite ascites	NPO, antibiotics × 14 days, fluid resuscitation, inotropic support, ventilator therapy, paracentesis
B: *Severely ill : bowel perforated*	Same as IIIA	Same as IIIA	Same as IIB, plus pneumoperitoneum	Same as IIA, plus surgery

Pearl/Peril/Pitfall : NEC-Presenting symptoms may include subtle signs of feeding intolerance that progresses over several hours to a day, subtle systemic signs that may be reported enigmatically by the nursing staff as "acting different," and, in advanced disease, a fulminant systemic collapse and consumption coagulopathy.

TABLE 2 Approach to management of neonates with necrotizing enterocolitis

ABNORMALITY	INTERVENTIONS	GOALS
Presumed infection	Broad-spectrum antibiotics	Eradicate infection, decrease intestinal gas production
Peritonitis/intestinal perforation	Antibiotics plus surgery (paracentesis) with drain placement)	Eradicate nidus of infection; remove necrotic bowel, ascites
Intestinal distention/ileus	NPO, nasogastric tube drainage	Decrease intestinal gas production, remove intestinal secretions, decompress abdomen, improve ventilation
Hypotension	Volume expansion, vasopressor agents	Restore gestational and postnatal age-appropriate blood pressure
Hypoperfusion/oxygen delivery	Volume expansion, vasopressor and inotropic agents; mechanical ventilation, oxygen, packed red blood cell, transfusions	Hemoglobin, 12–14g/dl Oxygen saturation >95% Normal blood lactate level (pH) Normal cardiac index
Organ system dysfunction	Volume expansion, vasopressor and Inotropic agents; mechanical ventilation, oxygen; packed red blood cell, platelet, fresh-frozen Plasma transfusions; diuretics	**Normalize or reverse abnormalities:** Renal : urine output, BUN, creatinine Hepatic : bilirubin, coagulopathy, albumin Pulmonary : alveolar-arterial gradient, hypercapnia Cardiac : blood pressure, cardiac index CNS : level of consciousness Hematologic : correct anemia, DIC (if active bleeding)
Poor nutritional intake	Parenteral alimentation (central or peripheral)	Reverse catabolism, improve nitrogen balance and healing, Prevent hypoglycemia

FIGURE 2: Algorithm for an approach to neonatal pneumoperitoneum. (Adapted and modified from stevens m, richetts rr: Pneumoperitoneum in the newborn infant. Ann surg 53:226, 1987

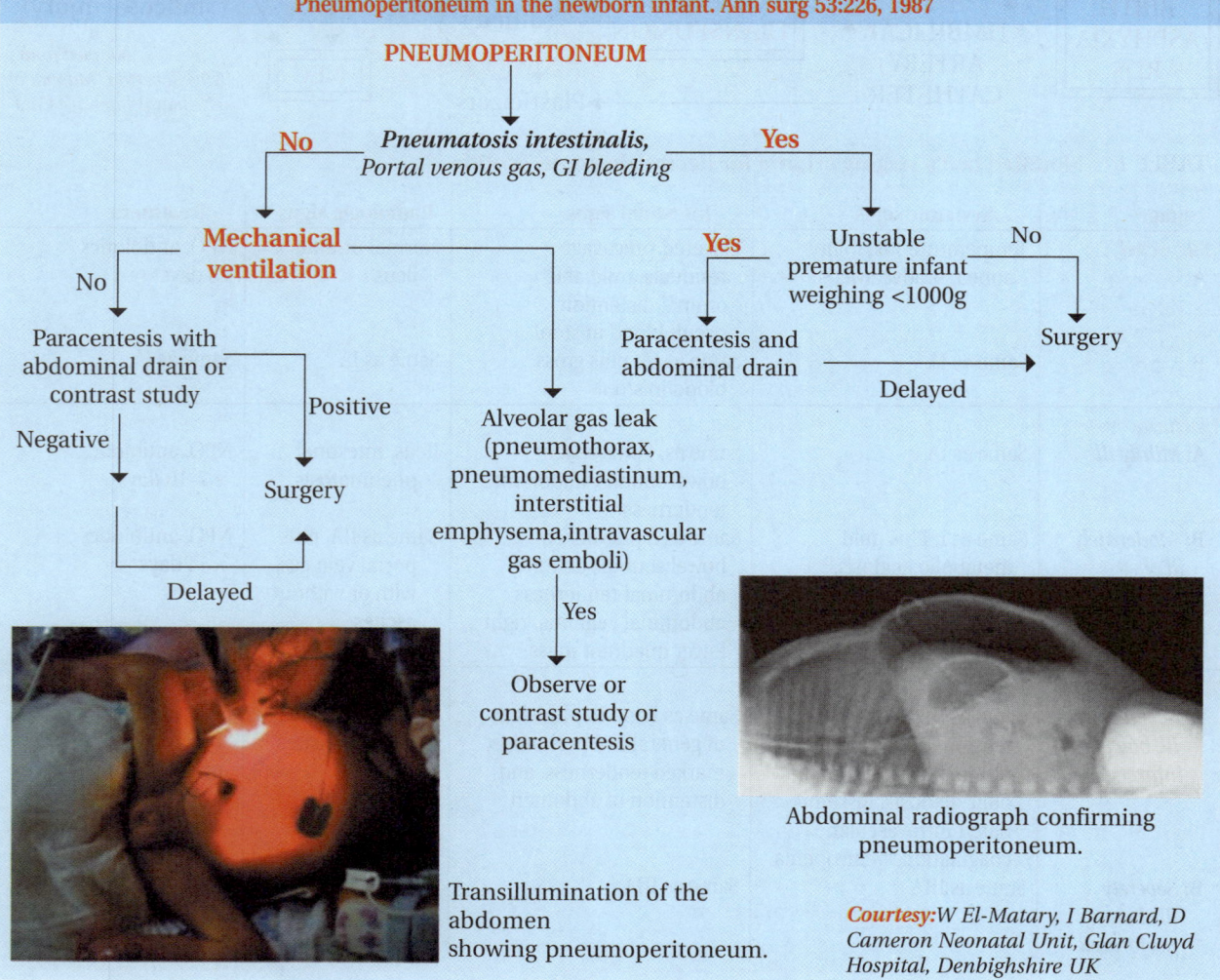

Transillumination of the abdomen showing pneumoperitoneum.

Abdominal radiograph confirming pneumoperitoneum.

Courtesy: W El-Matary, I Barnard, D Cameron Neonatal Unit, Glan Clwyd Hospital, Denbighshire UK

Pearl/Peril/Pitfall : NEC-Presentation•Abdominal distention - 83%•Explosive foul-smelling diarrhea - 69%•Bilious vomiting - 51%•Fever - 34%•Lethargy - 27%•Colonic perforation / shock - 2.5%.

NEONATAL GASTROINTESTINAL PERFORATION

Neonatal gastrointestinal perforation most commonly occurs as a complication of necrotizing enterocolitis (42% of cases), where it is associated with a high mortality of 62%.2 3 Spontaneous or idiopathic perforation, usually involving the terminal ileum, is the next most common presentation in 22%,2 and is associated with a lower mortality of 14%. Evidence of free air on abdominal radiograph often tips the balance between conservative management and operative treatment. _**Clinical suspicion is supported by radiological signs, which may be subtle and must be sought specifically.**_ A review of 105 cases of perforated necrotizing enterocolitis found that abdominal radiographs show evidence of free intraperitoneal gas in only 63% of cases, with 21% showing ascites but not free air, and 16% showing neither feature.4 A confounding factor is that a pneumoperitoneum could also be due to air tracking from the chest in ventilated patients. Radiographs may need to be repeated frequently in order to pick up tell tale signs as early as possible.Several signs are pathognomonic of pneumoperitoneum, regardless of the age group. A common sign is a collection of gas in the right upper quadrant adjacent to the liver, lying mainly in the subhepatic space and the hepatorenal fossa,which is visible as an oval or triangular gas shadow not obviously in continuity with the rest of the bowel. Clear visualization of the outer as well as the inner wall of a bowel loop— Rigler's sign—is a valuable indication of a pneumoperitoneum. *Sign of · pneumoperitoneum *Gas outside the bowel wall causes both sides (the mucosal and the serosal surfaces) of the bowel wall to be depicted *Usually indicates a large amount of *pneumoperitoneum

Small triangular collections of gas between loops of bowel may sometimes be identified. Reflections of the peritoneum normally present on the inner surface of the anterior abdominal wall are not usually identified, but may be visualized by free gas when it lies on either side. Thus the falciform ligament in particular, and occasionally the umbilical ligaments and urachus, may sometimes be identified in the presence of free air. The falciform ligament appears as a white streak, and when surrounded by the oval lucency of a pneumoperitoneum, supposedly resembles the seam of an American football. Hence the "football sign", visible on supine view. Relatively large amounts of gas may accumulate and show up beneath the diaphragm (cupola sign), or on the upper part of the abdomen in a decubitus or "shoot through" lateral film. A gasless abdomen may also represent perforation. Ultrasonography may be help to assess the presence and the character of ascites, and is particularly helpful in the context of a gasless abdomen. The presence of particulate matter most likely indicates perforation. Early diagnosis of intestinal perforation is imperative to allow prompt surgical intervention. In the absence of expert radiological opinion, a low threshold for performing decubitus films with the right side up is advised, as free gas is most easily perceived separate from other bowel, lateral to the liver. A systematic review of all radiographs is advisable so that signs are not missed, especially when films are taken to assess positions of tubes and lines. An awareness of the clinical presentation and main radiological signs will enable the diagnosis to be made more promptly even in centres without paediatric surgical expertise.

Reference: Courtesy-M K Farrugia, A S Morgan, K McHugh, E M Kiely Great Ormond St Hospital for Sick Children, London, UK; Arch Dis Child Fetal Neonatal Ed 2003;88:F75.

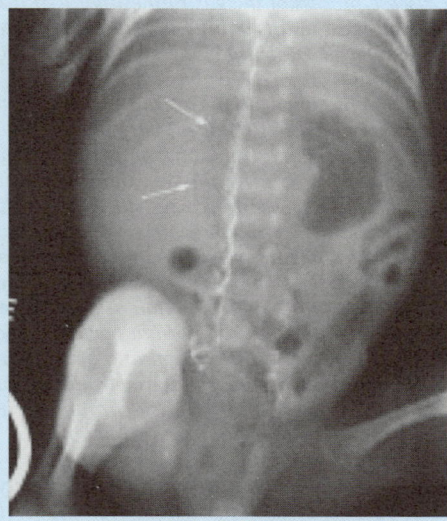

Intraperitoneal air visible as a central oval lucency: the football sign.

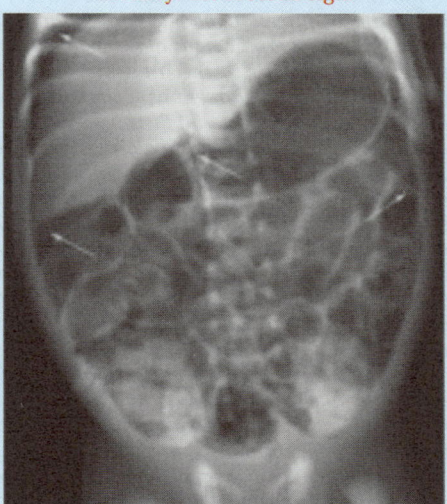

Abdominal radiograph showing free subdiaphragmatic and subhepatic air, falciform ligament outlined by intraperitoneal air; Rigler's Sign in upper left quadrant (arrowed).

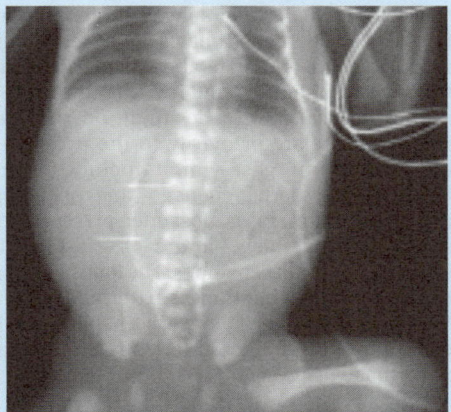

Free air outlining falciform ligament (arrowed).

---

*   _**Pearl/Peril/Pitfall:**_ _NEC-Once the diagnosis is made, gastric decompression and intravenous administration of fluid and antibiotics should be started. Complete blood cell count, arterial pH and blood gas determination, and electrolyte assays are mandatory. Surgery is indicated when free peritoneal gas or clinical deterioration develop. Intractable metabolic acidosis and thrombocytopenia are also critical signs of bowel ischemia, indicating surgical treatment._

@NEC-SUMMARY- *Necrotizing enterocolitis (NEC) is primarily a disease process of the gastrointestinal (GI) tract of premature Neonates that results in inflammation and bacterial invasion of the bowel wall. Despite advances in the care of premature infants, NEC remains one of the leading causes of morbidity and mortality in this population. It occurs in 1-5% of all Neonatal intensive care admissions and 5-10% of all very low birthweight (<1500 g) infants. Although research has presented an interesting array of potential contributing factors, the precise aetiology of this multifactorial disease process remains elusive. Historically, it was believed that NEC arose predominantly from ischemic injury to the immature GI tract, yet alternate plausible hypotheses indicate that many factors are likely to be involved. These may include issues related to the introduction and advancement of enteric feeding, alterations in the normal bacterial colonization of the GI tract, bacterial translocation and activation of the cytokine cascade, decreased epidermal growth factor, increased platelet activating factor, and mucosal damage from free radical production. Clinical manifestations of NEC may be vague, including increased episodes of apnea, desaturations, bradycardia, lethargy and temperature instability. There may also be GI-specific symptoms such as feeding intolerance, emesis, bloody stools, abdominal distention and tenderness, and abdominal wall discoloration. Laboratory values may be indicative of infection, coagulation abnormalities and fluid retention. Radiographic signs may include ileus, dilated or fixed intestinal loops, air in the intestinal wall or free air in the abdomen. Medical treatment typically consists of bowel rest and decompression, antibacterial therapy, and management of other hematological or electrolyte imbalances. Increased respiratory and cardiovascular support is sometimes needed. In Neonates who do not respond adequately to medical management, or if pneumoperitoneum is present, surgical intervention may occur with either use of a peritoneal drain or laparotomy. Advances in antenatal and neonatal care have resulted in increased survival of extremely preterm Neonates. As this at-risk population continues to increase, an effective preventative strategy for NEC is needed. One preventative strategy is the use of antenatal corticosteroids to enhance maturation of the fetus if preterm delivery is likely. Recommendation of use of breast milk, early initiation of trophic feeds and judicious advancement of enteric feeds are current postnatal strategies. Other preventative strategies that have been investigated include the use of oral antibacterials, antioxidants, supplementation of arginine and epidermal growth factor, none of which have changed clinical practice. Recent promising data indicate that prophylactic use of probiotics may play a role in preventing the onset of NEC. However, more large-scale, definitive studies are needed.*

Imaging Findings for Necrotizing enterocolitis - Plain film

*Plain abdominal radiography is the current modality of choice for the evaluation of Neonates suspected of having NEC. *The timing of follow-up plain abdominal radiographs depends on the severity of the NEC and may vary from 6 to 24 hourly. *The main observations to be made on the plain abdominal radiograph relate primarily to the presence, amount, and distribution of gas, which includes intraluminal gas, *pneumatosis, *portal venous gas, and *pneumoperitoneum. *In normal Neonates, gas is most often present through most of the small and large bowel and each gas-filled loop causes an impression on adjacent loops. The loops develop a multifaceted configuration, giving the gas pattern a "mosaic" appearance. *Dilatation with loss of the mosaic pattern and the development of rounded or elongated loops is more suggestive that an abnormality is present.

Bowel Gas Pattern

*In NEC, bowel dilatation is a nonspecific finding best appreciated on the plain abdominal radiograph and may be the only sign present in many patients with either mild or severe forms of the disease. The dilatation is usually due to an ileus and may be generalized or focal, depending on the extent of bowel involvement. It is the commonest sign, being present in over 90% of patients, with the remaining 10% showing only minor or nonspecific disturbances of bowel gas pattern. *Dilatation of bowel is an early sign and may even precede the clinical features of NEC by several hours. *The degree of dilatation usually correlates well with the clinical severity of the disease and the distribution of the dilated loops in serial examinations is related to clinical progression. *Worrisome if the dilated loops maintain the same appearance as fixed loops on follow-up plain abdominal radiographs. This suggests the development of full-thickness necrosis and may precede clinical deterioration including signs of peritonitis.

Pneumatosis

*Pneumatosis is also an early sign that may precede clinical signs. *Although intramural gas may be present in other neonatal conditions, it is most commonly seen in NEC and thus has been considered a virtually pathognomonic sign of NEC. *Pneumatosis is more commonly present in the distal small bowel and large bowel and is therefore most commonly seen in the right lower quadrant. *On plain abdominal radiographs, intramural gas may be diffuse or localized and appears as linear or rounded radiolucencies. *The linear lucencies often appear curvilinear; they represent intramural gas in the subserosa and appear as black lines on the radiograph, which can occasionally be confused with overlapping bowel loops filled with gas. *A clue to differentiating intramural gas from overlapping loops are the white lines that often accompany the black lines of intramural gas. The white lines represent the mucosa and submucosa, which are lifted off the serosa and are contrasted by the subserosal intramural gas and the intraluminal gas.

Portal venous gas

*In NEC, portal venous gas is an extension of intramural gas that enters the veins of the bowel wall and passes into the portal venous system. *Portal venous gas has been reported on plain abdominal radiographs in up to 30% of neonates with NEC, and these are usually, but not always, the more severely affected cases. Portal venous gas is not always associated with a fatal outcome. *On a supine plain abdominal radiograph, portal venous gas appears as branching, linear, radiolucent vessels that may extend from the region of the main portal vein toward the periphery of both hepatic lobes, and the extent depends on the amount of portal venous gas present.

Pneumoperitoneum

*Free gas in the peritoneal cavity results from bowel perforation, which most commonly occurs in the distal ileum and proximal colon. *It is the only universally accepted radiologic indication for surgical intervention. *On the cross-table lateral view, free gas may appear as triangular lucencies between loops of bowel anteriorly just beneath the abdominal wall or as small bubbles or linear gas collections anterior to the liver. *On the left lateral decubitus view, small amounts of gas may be seen between the right lobe of the liver and the right lateral abdominal wall. *On the supine view, large amounts of gas may give rise to the *football sign, where the gas outlines the whole of the peritoneal cavity, the undersurface of the diaphragm, and the falciform ligament (the lacing of the football). *Smaller amounts of free gas may give rise to lucency below the diaphragm without giving rise to the full-blown football sign. *Even on the supine view, smaller amounts of free gas may be detected when both sides of the bowel wall are outlined (*Rigler sign).

REFERENCE: Monica Epelman, Alan Daneman, Oscar M. Navarro, Iris Morag, Aideen M. Moore, Jae Hong Kim, Ricardo Faingold, Glenn Taylor, and J. Ted Gerstle. Necrotizing Enterocolitis: Review of State-of-the-Art Imaging Findings with Pathologic Correlation. RadioGraphics 2007 27: 285-305.

Pearl/Peril/Pitfall : NEC-Abdominal plain films taken at an interval of six to eight hours initially and daily in the following seven to 10 days are helpful in diagnosis and evaluation of the clinical progress. Distended loops with thickened bowel wall, pneumatosis cystoides intestinalis, air in the portal vein and/or free air are the radiographic findings. Daily change in bowel gas pattern is a good prognostic sign because it excludes ileus and bowel necrosis.

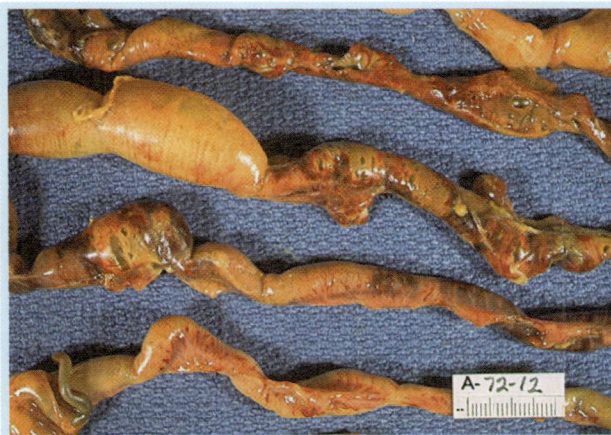

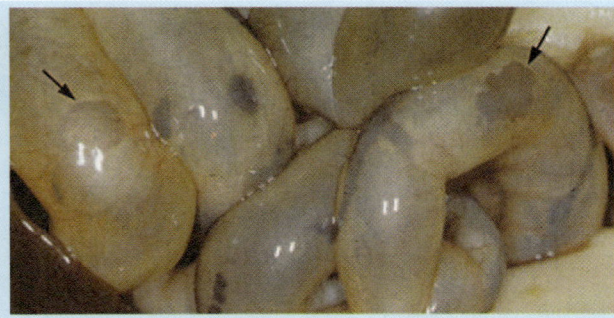

Segments of intestine affected by necrotizing enterocolitis (NEC). The classic findings of diffuse NEC are seen in this image. Patchy areas of necrosis are seen with questionable intestinal viability.

Neonatal necrotizing enterocolitis, gross pathology
Courtesy: Centers for disease control and prevention

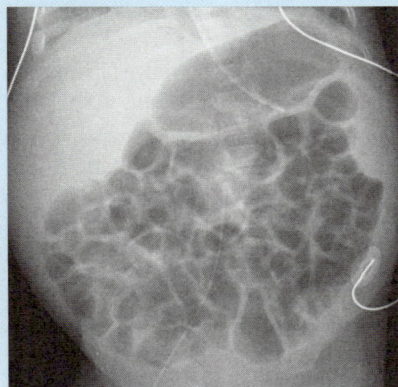

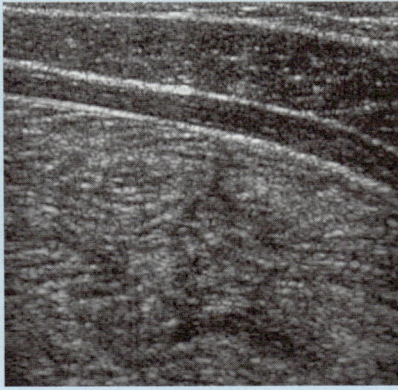

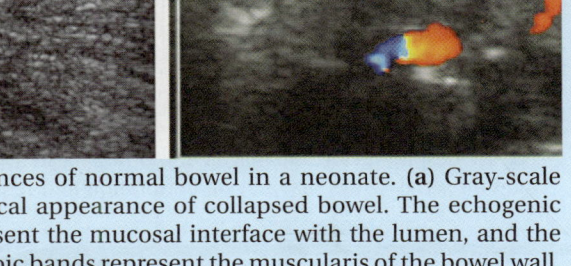

Supine radiograph of the abdomen of a normal neonate shows a normal bowel gas pattern. Gas is distributed throughout the small and large bowel, and it is difficult to differentiate the small bowel from the large bowel. Each loop causes impressions on adjacent loops, giving each loop a multifaceted appearance; the overall pattern resembles that of a mosaic. The loops are generally not rounded or elongated.

Sonographic appearances of normal bowel in a neonate. (a) Gray-scale image shows the typical appearance of collapsed bowel. The echogenic linear markings represent the mucosal interface with the lumen, and the surrounding hypoechoic bands represent the muscularis of the bowel wall. (b) Color Doppler image of normal collapsed bowel shows color dots of flow in the arteries of the bowel wall.

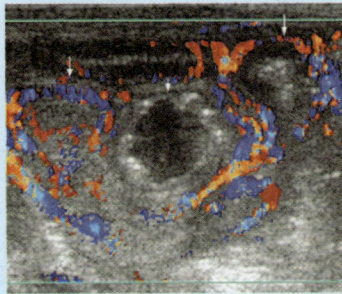

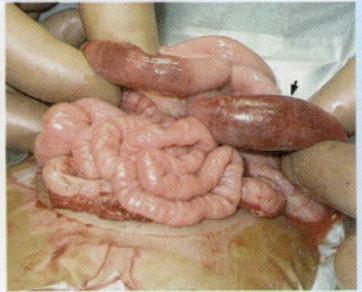

Courtesy: Necrotizing Enterocolitis:

Review of State-of the- Art Imaging Findings with Pathologic Correlation

Monica Epelman, MD, Alan Daneman, MD , Oscar M. Navarro, MD Iris Morag, MD, Aideen M. Moore, MD Jae Hong Kim, MD Ricardo Faingold, MD, Glenn Taylor, MD ,J. Ted Gerstle, MD, **Radio Graphics 2007;** 27:285–305.

NEC and bowel necrosis in a neonate. (a) Color Doppler sonogram shows three bowel loops (arrows). The two outer loops (long arrows) are markedly hyperemic, with flow around the entire circumference of each loop and some prominent mesenteric vessels. The central loop has an irregular wall with focal thinning at one site (short arrow) and small hyperechoic foci suggestive of intramural gas. There is no flow in the wall, a finding highly suggestive of necrosis. (b) Intraoperative photograph of the bowel shows the necrotic bowel loop (arrow).

---

* ***Pearl/Peril/Pitfall:*** *NEC-The usual onset is 10 to 12 days of age, with presenting symptoms of gastric retention, bilious vomiting, ileus, abdominal distention and bloody stools. Bradycardia, hypothermia, apneic spells and hypotension are later signs of progressive deterioration. Abnormal hemorrhage, hyperbilirubinemia and oliguria are late findings.*

TABLE 3	Sudden compared with insidious presentation of Necrotizing enterocolitis
Sudden onset	**Insidious onset**
Full-term or preterm infants	Usually preterm
Acute catastrophic deterioration	Evolves during 1 to 2 days
Respiratory decompensation	Feeding intolerance
Shock/acidosis	Change in stool pattern
Marked abdominal distention	Intermittent abdominal distention
Positive result of blood culture	Occult blood in stools

TABLE 4 NEC—Prognosis

A. NEC with perforation is associated with a mortality of 20-40%.

B. Recurrent NEC is a rare complication.

C. Subacute or intermittent symptoms of bowel obstruction due to stenosis or strictures of the colon and, less frequently, of the small bowel are seen in ~ 10-20% of cases. A barium enema is usually confirmatory.

D. Infants undergoing extensive surgical resection require long-term parenteral nutrition, enterostomy care, and management of short gut syndrome. Chronic electrolyte imbalance and failure to thrive are common.

E. In the absence of short gut syndrome, growth, nutrition, and gastrointestinal function appear to catch up and are normal by the end of the first year.

TABLE 5 Role of surgery in NEC

* Always consult a pediatric surgeon early in the course of treatment, to make him familiar with the case and to provide additional evaluation.

* Ideally surgery should be performed after intestinal necrosis develops, but before perforation and peritonitis occur, noninvasive diagnosis of intestinal necrosis with abdominal MRI is being studied. Brown paracentesis fluid with organisms on gram stain suggests perforation.

* An infant with increasing abdominal distention, abdominal wall erythema, an abdominal mass, a worsening clinical picture despite medical management, or a persistent fixed loop on serial X-rays may have a perforation and requires operative intervention consisting of explorative laparotomy, resection of necrotic bowel, and external ostomy diversion.

* Peritoneal drainage may be helpful in patients in extremis with peritonitis who are too unstable to withstand surgery.

* Strictures occur in 25–35% of patients with or without surgery and are most common in the large bowel, which need surgical repair around 6-8 wks after the recovery from NEC. A barium enema is necessary to establish the presence of a stricture.

* NEC requiring surgical intervention may have a more serious sequelae, including increased morbidity and mortality secondary to infection, respiratory failure, TPN associated hepatic disease, rickets, and significant developmental delay.

KEY POINTS FOR CLINICAL PRACTICE

1. Necrotizing EnteroColitis (NEC) is the most common serious surgical disorder among NICU infants & is a significant cause of Neonatal morbidity & mortality. *Prematurity is the single greatest risk factor;* approximately 10% of infants with NEC are full-term. More than 90% of infants have been fed before the onset of NEC.

2. NEC is a heterogeneous disease resulting from complex interactions between mucosal injury secondary to a variety of factors such as *ischemia, luminal substrate, & infection and poor host protective mechanisms in response to injury.*

3. Early diagnosis of NEC is the most important factor in determining outcome, which is accomplished by careful clinical observation of non-specific signs (systemic as well as abdominal), with *a high index of suspicion in infants at risk.*

4. Consider various differential diagnoses such as a)pneumonia & sepsis b)surgical abdominal catastrophes such as malrotation with obstruction, midgut volvulus, intus- susception, gastric perforation & mesenteric vessel thrombosis c)isolated intestinal perforation in ELBW infants d)galactosemia with E.coli sepsis e)severe allergic colitis f) feeding intolerance.

5. Assess the severity of NEC by modified Bell staging & manage accordingly. *Promptly consult pediatric surgeon & consider surgery in an infant with increasing abdominal distention, an abdominal mass, a worsening clinical picture despite medical management, or a persistent fixed loop on serial radiographs suggestive of perforation.*

6. Prognosis of NEC depends on the staging of the disease; in uncomplicated cases the long-term prognosis may be comparable with that of other LBW infants. Those with stage IIB or stage III NEC have a higher incidence of growth delay. Surgically intervened cases of NEC have more serious sequelae including increased morbidity & mortality.

REFERENCES & FURTHER READING 1) Henry MC, Moss RL. Current issues in the management of necrotizing enterocolitis. Semin Perinatol 2004; 28: 221–233. 2) Hsueh W, Caplan MS, Qu XW, Tan XD, De Plaen IG, Gonzalez-Crussi F. Neonatal necrotizing enterocolitis: clinical considerations and pathogenetic concepts. Pediatr Dev Pathol 2003; 6: 6–23 3) Recognition and medical management of NEC by Kanto WP et al : Clin. Perinatol 1994 : 21 : 335 4) Lessin MS, Luks FI, Wesselhoeft CW, Gilchrist BF, Iannitti D, DeLuca FG. Peritoneal drainage as definitive treatment for intestinal perforation in infants with extremely low birth weight (<750 g). J Pediatr Surg 1998; 33: 370–372. 5)Tam AL, Camberos A, Applebaum H. Surgical decision making in necrotizing enterocolitis and focal intestinal perforation: predictive value of radiologic findings. J Pediatr Surg 2002; 37: 1688–1691.

* *Pearl/Peril/Pitfall : NEC-Physical findings include erythema and edema of the abdominal wall, absence of bowel sounds, abdominal distention, visible and/or palpable loops of the bowel, guarding and lethargy. It should be kept in mind that physical findings do not always or accurately reflect an intestinal catastrophe, especially in a weak premature infant.*

56 Neonatal Abdominal Mass

@ *The neonate, infant, or child with an abdominal mass needs rapid clinical evaluation. Age, history, and physical examination provide initial guideposts to diagnosis. Imaging studies, particularly sonography, may provide a specific diagnosis.*

Hydronephrosis secondary to ureteropelvic junction obstruction and multicystic kidney disease are the two most common causes of abdominal masses of urologic origin. **Many are diagnosed on antenatal sonogram, which remains the diagnostic procedure of choice for cystic & solid masses that are palpable at birth. Early consultation among the pediatrician, pediatric radiologist, pediatric surgeon, and, in the case of prenatal diagnosis, the obstetrician can expedite this process. Diagnosis should be achieved in an orderly, timely, accurate and cost-effective manner.**

Differential diagnosis of abdominal masses in newborns

Renal masses: hydronephrosis (ureteropelvic junction obstruction, posterior urethral valves, vesicoureteric reflux), cystic disease of the kidneys (multicystic dysplastic kidneys, polycystic kidneys), renal vein thrombosis, tumors (Wilms' tumor, mesoblastic nephroma).

Gastrointestinal masses: duplication cyst, complicated meconium ileus (intraperitoneal meconium cyst), mesenteric or omental cyst, hypertrophic pyloric stenosis.

Nonrenal retroperitoneal masses: adrenal hemorrhage, tumors (neuroblastoma, teratoma, rhabdomyosarcoma, sacrococcygeal teratoma).

Genital masses: hydrometrocolpos, ovarian mass (simple cyst, torsion, teratoma).

Hepatobiliary masses: infections (viruses, bacteria), lysosomal storage diseases (glycogen storage diseases), congestive heart failure, tumors (hepatoblastoma), choledochal cyst, hemolytic anemias.

Splenomegaly: infections (viruses, spirochetes), congenital hemolytic anemias (hereditary spherocytosis, thalassemia, hemoglobinopathies), storage disorders (Gaucher's disease, Niemann-Pick disease), mucopolysaccharide disorders (Hurler's syndrome).

REVIEW OF CLINICAL PROBLEMS

1. Name the Imaging studies useful in evaluating an Abdominal mass in a Neonate.
   Ans : Refer to the "No. 3" of the "BIRD'S EYE VIEW/ OVERVIEW /SYNOPSIS" of the Chapter.

2. Mention the Essential aspects of History & Physical examination of a Neonate with an abdominal Mass.
   Ans : Refer to the Evaluation-Decision-Action Plan/ Algorithm to diagnose & manage a Neonate with an abdominal Mass.

3. How do you classify the Neonatal abdominal masses?
   Ans : Refer to the Table "1" of the Chapter.

4. How do you plan initial investigations when evaluating an Abdominal mass in a Neonate?
   Ans : Refer to the Table "2" of the Chapter.

5. Describe the Differential diagnosis for Adrenal masses in Neonates.
   Ans : Refer to the "No. 8" of the "BIRD'S EYE VIEW/ OVERVIEW/ SYNOPSIS" of the Chapter.

LEARNING OBJECTIVES

After completing this article, readers will be able to

1. Take proper history, including prenatal scan results and carefully perform postnatal evaluation of Neonatal abdominal mass.

2. Consult Pediatric radiologist, Pediatric surgeon/ Urologist and, in the case of prenatal diagnosis, the obstetrician to expedite the diagnostic process.

3. Understand the role of a wide array of sophisticated imaging techniques which have become available to aid in the diagnosis of an abdominal mass, in addition to fetal ultrasonography.

4. Treat nonsurgical variety (i.e. organomegaly or bladder distention conservatively.

5. Counsel the parents about the prognosis and the clinical course of abdominal mass, depending on the cause.

---

* *Pearl/Peril/Pitfall : Although history and physical examination, plain radiographs and ultrasonography will confirm most diagnoses, severe unilateral hydronephrosis, hemorrhagic neuroblastoma, and intraperitoneal cysts may provide diagnostic difficulties. Masses identified by prenatal ultrasound need careful evaluation as they may represent normal structures, nonsignificant variants, or physiologically significant anomalies.*

BIRD'S EYE VIEW/OVERVIEW/SYNOPSIS

1. The presence of an abdominal mass in the Neonatal period is common, occurring in approximately 1 infant in 1000 live births. Despite this relatively high incidence, the finding of an abdominal mass in a Neonate can be alarming for both parents and physicians. Most of the abdominal masses in Neonates are *benign* and over half of them arise from the urinary tract. *Hydronephrosis secondary to ureteropelvic junction obstruction and multicystic kidney disease are the two most common causes of abdominal masses of urologic origin.* Many are diagnosed on antenatal sonogram, which remains the diagnostic procedure of choice for cystic & solid masses that are palpable at birth. Early consultation among the pediatrician, pediatric radiologist, pediatric surgeon, and, in the case of prenatal diagnosis, the obstetrician can expedite this process. Diagnosis should be achieved in an orderly, timely, accurate and cost-effective manner.

2. Table 1 lists the differential diagnosis of neonatal abdominal masses by location. Renal & adrenal masses are retroperitoneal in location. Because the ovary is not a pelvic organ in a Newborn, ovarian cysts/teratoma can float freely throughout the abdomen. Physical examination may significantly narrow the diagnostic possibilities, even if it doesn't provide any absolute answer; large masses may fill the entire abdomen, making it impossible to determine the site of origin on examination. Hard, nodular masses are usually malignant tumors. A highly mobile mass is usually a mesenteric cyst, a duplication, or an ovarian cyst.

3. The imaging studies that are most useful in evaluating a Newborn with an abdominal mass include a) A plain abdominal radiograph might reveal a mass effect or bowel obstruction, can help localize the mass, and can sometimes provide useful information about the mass itself, such as the presence of calcifications or stool. b) An abdominal ultrasound is extremely useful in the majority of cases because if can show whether the mass is cystic or solid, can reveal the effect on adjacent anatomic structures, and often can identify the exact anatomic location of the mass. c) Further information can be provided with abdominal computed tomography, magnetic resonance imaging or urologic imaging.

4. Multicystic kidneys, hydronephrosis, hydroureter, and bladder outlet obstruction, due to posterior urethral valves in male infants are imaged by ultrasound. These conditions require immediate pediatric urologic consultation to repair or drain. Hydronephrosis results from obstruction at the ureteropelvic junction, ureterovesicular junction, or the bladder outlet and can be unilateral or bilateral. With hydronephrosis, sonography shows a dilated renal pelvis surrounded by and communicating with several cystic structures (calyces). Renal scintigraphy can demonstrate the level of obstruction and assess renal function. The management of children with hydronephrosis may be supportive as many cases resolve spontaneously. Decompression may be required when there is risk of significant renal compromise or ongoing infection. Resection of nonfunctioning kidneys is indicated for complications such as infections and severe hypertension. Renal vein thrombosis is a rare but important cause of a smooth flank mass and hematuria, which develop concurrently in an ill Newborn after an episode of asphyxia, sepsis, or dehydration or in an infant whose mother has diabetes. Unilateral multicystic kidneys and other nonobstructive renal anomalies are followed closely for signs of infection or impaired renal function. Nephromegaly may the result of cystic dysplasia, renal vein thrombosis, or nephroblastoma. Discrete renal masses are most likely mesoblastic nephromas, which are benign. Wilms tumor is rare in Newborns, distinguished from nephroma at surgery or by evidence of metastasis.

5. Nonrenal cystic masses in female infants are usually ovarian in origin & include simple follicular cysts, hemorrhagic cysts, and teratomas. Most of the ovarian cysts arise in response to antenatal hormonal stimulation & may subsequently resolve after birth. Potential complications such as torsion, hemorrhage into the cyst, and the rupture are somewhat related to the size of the cyst; the risk of malignancy depends on whether the cyst is simple (homogeneous) or complex. Most authorities recommend carefully following up on asymptomatic cysts with serial ultrasonograpy for several months if they are echo free & <5cm in diameter. If the cyst causes compressive symptoms, has any solid components, or is >5cm in diameter, it should be excised, possibly laparoscopically.

6. The differential diagnosis of nonrenal and nonovarian intra-abdominal cysts includes mesenteric and omental cysts, meconium cysts from cystic fibrosis, enteric duplication cysts, and choledochal cysts. Choledochal cysts typically are associated with proximal biliary ductular dilation, but also may be seen with distal biliary atresia. Indications for surgical intervention in female Newborns with an abdominal cyst include size greater than 4-5 cm, intracystic septa or debris, or any sign of biliary or bowel obstruction. Any male with an intra-abdominal cyst of nongenitourinary origin should undergo surgical exploration.

7. Primary hepatic masses are extremely rare in the Neonate & include hemangioma, hemangioendothelioma & malignant hepato-blastoma, which can be differentiated by CT/MRI findings. Serum alpha-fetoprotein is usually elevated in hepatoblastoma. Small to moderate hemangiomas can be observed or treated medically with corticosteroids or alpha-interferon. Most large or symptomatic hemangiomas (causing pain, heart failure, thrombocytopenia) and all hemangioendotheliomas and hepatoblastoma require hepatic resection.

8. The differential diagnosis of adrenal masses includes adrenal hemorrhage, neuroblastoma, and teratoma. When a neonate has a palpable flank mass after a traumatic or breech delivery, the possibility of an adrenal hemorrhage should be considered, as should hepatic and splenic hematomas. Neuroblastoma is the most common malignancy in the Newborn period, with generally an excellent prognosis. For this reason, adrenal lesions may be followed for several months, anticipating resolutions of an adrenal hemorrhage & even of a neuroblastoma.

9. Pelvic masses in female Neonates are typically of ovarian origin, including benign teratomas and, rarely, germ cell tumors. Sacrococcygeal teratomas usually have a significant external component in Newborns, are often benign, and generally can be excised completely at surgery. Rhabdomyosarcomas are rare in neonates. They typically arise from the genitourinary tract and are biopsied, pretreated with chemotherapy, and then surgically excised or irradiated.

10. *The Evaluation- Decision -Action Plan/Algorithm* describes the essential aspects of the diagnosis & management of Neonatal abdominal masses. Distended bladder should be considered in the differential diagnosis of abdominal masses; 90% of Newborns void during the first 24hrs of life & essentially all void by 48hrs of life unless there is a problem such as a) posterior urethral valves b) neurogenic bladder c) pelvic/vaginal rhabdomyosarcoma (rare) d) ureterocele obstructing the bladder outlet. Hydrometrocolpos is rare. Many abdominal masses are of the nonsurgical variety (i.e., organomegaly or bladder distention). Most masses requiring surgical intervention are benign (87%), and the prognosis for Neonates with an abdominal mass is good. Female Newborns may have a lower abdominal or pelvic mass from hydrometrocolpos, which develops as a result of an upper or lower vaginal obstruction in combination with a secretory response to a high level of maternal estrogens in utero. An imperforate hymen will be evident on the genital examination as a bulging round membrane within the introitus. Rectal examination can be diagnostic for the presence of a dilated vagina in higher obstructions. Maternal estrogens may also induce the development of a large functional or follicular ovarian cyst in Newborns.

---

* *Pearl/Peril/Pitfall : A scaphoid abdomen suggests the presence of a diaphragmatic hernia. In newborns with abdominal distension, it is important to determine whether the condition is secondary to excess air inside or outside the bowel, fluid in the peritoneal cavity, an enlarged viscus, or a tumor in the abdomen.*

THE EVALUATION-DECISION-ACTION-PLAN / ALGORITHM FOR THE DIAGNOSIS AND MANAGEMENT OF *NEONATAL ABDOMINAL MASS*

SUBJECTIVE FINDINGS

Hx of relevant Antenatal and Postnatal factors- *Was there a prenatal ultrasound performed with *any unusual findings*? *Are there any GI symptoms such as vomiting and poor feeding? *How much amniotic fluid was present? (oligos/polyhydramnios) *Any family history of masses or renal disease (generally noncontributory)?

Hx of *Any prenatal interventions, such as amniocentesis or pigtail catheter placement?

OBJECTIVE FINDINGS

Assess ABCDs, hydration status, O$_2$ sats, CRT, BP, urine output.

Determine *the location of the mass- flank, mid abdomen, or suprapubic *Is the mass solid, cystic, smooth, or tender? *Note the size, shape, texture, mobility of the mass *Is there hepatosplenomegaly? Other physical findings unrelated to the mass- facies, rectal, lung exam, other anomalies

Assess for Potter sequence(lung hypoplasia, urinary obstruction and oligos), bulging hymen, a sign of hydrometrocolpos, skin metastases (neuroblastoma).

INVESTIGATIONS

Suggested initial evaluation of abdominal mass *Radiologic imaging *Plain abdominal radiograph *Sonogram *Computed tomography scan or magnetic resonance imaging@

Laboratory studies Complete blood count with differential Electrolytes (including calcium, phosphorus) blood urea nitrogen, creatinine, Uric acid and lactate dehydrogenase, Urinalysis

Urine homovanillic acid and vanillylmandelic acid *Serum chorionic gonadotropin and alpha-fetoprotein

@If clinically indicated.

Neonate with an abdominal mass

Physical examination to possibly identify origin of mass

Abdominal radiograph

Radiographic findings suggestive of intestinal obstruction

Gastrointestinal study using contrast medium; consultation with Pediatric radiologist or surgeon

Radiographic study not diagnostic

Other potentially helpful diagnostic tests: complete blood count, serum electrolyte levels, urinalysis, abdominal US, CT scaning with or without contrast medium, MRI, voiding cystourethrography (to identify lower urinary tract abnormalities), catecholamine levels (to diagnose neuroblastoma)

Hepatomegaly

With hyperbilirubinemia

Elevated indirect or mixed bilirubin level

Differential diagnosis hemolytic anemia, congestive heart failure, drugs, or toxins

Elevated direct bilirubin level

With splenomegaly

Differential diagnosis Viral (TORSCH) infection, bacterial infection, metabolic disorder

Without splenomegaly

Abdominal US with or without biliary scanning or liver biopsy

Differential diagnosis: choledochal cysts, biliary atresia, neonatal hepatitis, prolonged parenteral nutrition, drugs, or toxins

Without hyperbilirubinemia

With splenomegaly

Abdominal US with or without Doppler flow studies

Differential diagnosis: vascular malformation or obstruction, liver tumor, metabolic disease

Without splenomegaly

Abdominal US

Differential diagnosis: tumor, malnutrition, maternal diabetes

---

* **Pearl/Peril/Pitfall :** *Abdominal radiograph- will show gas pattern, displacement of organs may identify location of the mass. May also show calcifications associated with neuroblastoma, meconium peritonitis, and hepatoblastoma.*

TABLE 1 — Differential diagnosis of abdominal mass in children

Neonates	Wilms' tumor
Renal	Lymphoma
Hydronephrosis*	Liver
Multidysplastic kidney*	Hepatoblastoma*
Mesoblastic nephroma*	Embryonal sarcoma†
Renal vein thrombosis†	**Gastrointestinal**
Polycystic kidney disease†	Duplication
Wilms' tumor†	Meckel's diverticulum
Rhabdoid tumor†	Fecal mass
Pelvic	**Pelvic**
Ovarian cyst	Ovarian cysts
Hydrocolpos	Teratomas
Hydrometrocolpos	**Other**
Gastrointestinal duplication	Omental or mesenteric cyst
Infants and children	*Common.
Retroperitoneal	†Rare.
Neuroblastoma	

TABLE 2 — Suggested initial evaluation of abdominal mass

Radiologic imaging
Plain abdominal radiograph
Sonogram
Computed Tomography scan or Magnetic Resonance Imaging*
Laboratory studies
Complete blood count with differential
Electrolytes (including calcium, phosphorus) blood urea nitrogen, creatinine
Uric acid and lactate dehydrogenase
Urinalysis
Urine homovanillic acid and vanillylmandelic acid*
Serum chorionic gonadotropin and alpha-fetoprotein*

If clinically indicated.

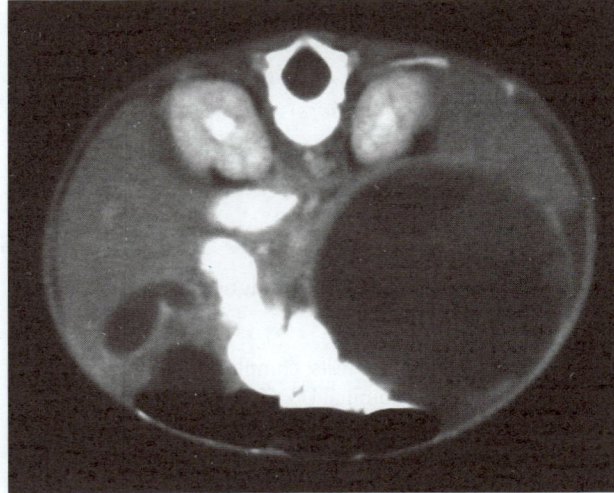

Abdominal computed tomography scan revealing a well-circumscribed cystic mass compressing the stomach and pancreas.

ABDOMINAL MASS IN NEONATE

Abdominal radiograph → Ultrasound
Normal → Stop
Obstruction
Mass
MUC → Renal cystic / Renal solid
Upper GI-series or Barium enema
Ultrasound → Other
Nuclear medicine
CT/MRI

KEY POINTS FOR CLINICAL PRACTICE

1. Abdominal masses in Neonates are most often benign and of genitourinary origin. Malignant abdominal masses are more likely to be encountered beyond the Neonatal age and mainly include neuroblastomas, Wilms' tumors, and lymphomas.

2. Hydronephrosis secondary to ureteroplevic (UPJ) junction obstruction & multicystic kidney disease are the two most common causes of abdominal masses of urologic origin in Neonates.

3. Plain abdominal radiographs should be the first imaging studies to evaluate an abdominal mass, while sonography is an inexpensive, radiation-free adjunct imaging modality that can determine the origin and extent of an abdominal mass. Ultrasound examination, both antenatally & postnatally remains the diagnostic procedure of choice for cystic & solid masses that are palpable at birth; CT/MRI studies are helpful to provide further information of the masses.

4. Surgical excision is indicated for ovarian cysts >5cm in size, causing compressive symptoms & has solid components, & choledochal cyst. Bladder outlet obstruction generally is secondary to posterior urethral valves in male infants & requires immediate urologic consultation to repair or drain.

5. Abdominal masses in Neonates reflect a wide spectrum of diseases, from lesions that can cause significant morbidity and mortality, to conditions readily corrected surgically, to entities which may be safely observed. Diagnosis should be achieved in an orderly, timely, accurate and cost-effective manner.

* *Pearl/Peril/Pitfall : The majority of masses are of benign origin and greater than 50% are of renal origin. The majority will be diagnosed with a good history, physical examination, and ultrasound evaluation.*

REFERENCES & FURTHER READING : 1) Chandler JC, Gauderer MW. The neonate with an abdominal mass. Pediatr Clin North Am 2004;51: 979–97, ix. 2) Pinto E, Guignard JP. Renal masses in the neonate. Biol Neonate 1995;68:175–84. 3) Strickland JL. Ovarian cysts in neonates, children and adolescents. Curr Opin Obstet Gynecol 2002;14:459–65. 4) Rizk D, Chapman AB. Cystic and inherited kidney diseases. Am J Kidney Dis 2003;42:1305–17. 5) Glick RD, Hicks MJ, Nuchtern JG, et al. Renal tumors in infants less than 6 months of age. J Pediatr Surg 2004; 39:522–5.)

* *Pearl/Peril/Pitfall : Initial light palpation of all 4 quadrants and the flank areas is essential. A second circuit of palpation can allow deeper examination. Percussion helps detect organ or mass size and assists in differentiating the underlying components.*

57 Neonatal GIT Bleeding

@ *A prothrombin time (PT), activated partial thromboplastin time (aPTT), fibrinogen levels, and a platelet count should be included in the initial workup for vitamin K deficiency bleeding (VKDB) in a newborn. A thrombin clotting time (TCT) is optional.*

Evaluation and Decision Process in GI bleeding

* *Assess the hemodynamic status of patient and stabilize the patient*

* *Establish the level of bleeding*

* *Establish a differential diagnosis based on broad diagnostic categories.*

Assessment of the Severity of the Acute Presentation

* *Appearance of the patient*
* *Hemodynamic status of the patient*
* *Clinical presentation*
* *Character of the bleeding*
  – *Coffee ground emesis or melena suggests a lower rate of bleeding. *Fresh blood quickly changes to brown in an acid environment • Intestinal bacteria oxidize hemoglobin to hematin giving blood a tarry appearance*
  – *Bright red blood may indicate either a low or very high rate of bleeding*
* *Estimated volume of blood lost* and * *Hematocrit*

Immediate Laboratory Studies

* *Type and Cross*
* *CBC with platelet count*
* *Hematocrit is an unreliable initial index of acute blood loss*
* *MCV is a good screen for acute vs. chronic GI blood loss*
* *PT/PTT*
* *Comprehensive metabolic panel*

Intravenous therapy for active GI Bleeding

* *Restoration of intravascular volume*
* *Crystalloid, colloid, or blood*
* *Because both intravascular and extravascular volumes are reduced in acute GI bleeding, crystalloid (normal saline, Ringer's lactate) is the solution of choice for initial resuscitation*
* *Colloid solutions or blood are used only when blood loss is massive because in this situation respiratory insufficiency or shock lung may develop with fall in plasma oncotic pressure*
* *Restoration of oxygen carrying capacity-Blood*

REVIEW OF CLINICAL PROBLEMS

1. How do you classify the common causes of Neonatal GIT Hemorrhage?
   Ans : Refer to the Table 1 of the Chapter.

2. How do you approach a Bleeding Neonate?
   Ans : Refer to Figure "1" of the Chapter.

3. Discuss the differences between various forms of Vitamin K deficiency bleeding (VKDB) in Neonates.
   Ans : Refer to the Table 2 of the Chapter.

4. What are the essentials of management of moderate-severe Neonatal GIT Bleeding?
   Ans : Refer to the "No. 5" of the "BIRD'S EYE VIEW/OVERVIEW/SYNOPSIS" of the Chapter.

5. Describe the essential aspects of History & Physical examination, when evaluating a Neonate with GIT Bleeding.
   Ans : Refer to the Evaluation-Decision-Action Plan/Algorithm to diagnose & manage a Neonate with GIT Bleeding.

LEARNING OBJECTIVES

After completing this article, readers will be able to:

1. Prevent Vitamin K deficiency bleeding (VKDB) in Neonates by giving IM Vitamin K Prophylaxis without exception.

2. Promptly treat VKDB with IV Vitamin K, FFP, Packed RBCs or Fresh whole Blood Transfusion.

3. Evaluate for other causes of GIT Bleeding: a) trauma (e.g. broken rectal thermometer); b) Meckel's diverticulum ; c) malrotation ; d) peptic ulceration; e) rectal polyps/ hemangiomas; f) colitis; g) intussusception; h) gut reduplication.

4. Liaise with Pediatric Surgeon for managing severe, intractable, recurrent GIT Bleeding.

5. Check for Bleeding from other sites—Pulmonary, Renal, CNS-which may indicate MODS+DIC.

* *Pearl/Peril/Pitfall: A newborn's hospital chart should have a specific place for documentation of dose and administration. Failure to provide vitamin K at birth and subsequent bleeding presents a legal liability for physicians and hospitals. If parents refuse prophylaxis, document the discussion of the risks and benefits along with the parents' refusal in the medical record of the infant.*

BIRD'S EYE VIEW/OVERVIEW/SYNOPSIS

1. GIT bleeding in the Newborn (which can present in 4 ways - Hematemesis, Hematochezia, Melena or occult bleeding) mostly results from swallowed maternal blood (30%) at delivery / from a cracked nipple / local trauma from nasogastric tube, laryngoscopy, overvigorous laryngeal suction and fissure-in-ano. But it may be a potentially serious problem and may result from the presence of a stress - induced peptic ulcer, esophagitis, bleeding disorder or congenital anomalies of the GIT (Refer to Table 1).

2. The initial assessment should rapidly address the need for resuscitation, and whether the bleeding is ongoing. Recognition of shock should not rely on hypotension, a late and ominous finding in infancy. The evaluation of this problem involves a systematic approach by historical data, a detailed examination and followed by an investigational work-up to establish the diagnosis (Refer to the Evaluation-Decision-Action-Plan / Algorithm to manage a Neonate with GIT bleeding).

3. Differentiation of upper from lower GIT bleeding will guide the order of investigations and the therapy. Hematemesis is clear guide of upper bleeding (proximal to the ligament of Treitz), melena suggests a source far from the rectum (from the esophagus, stomach, or duodenum), and hematochezia can occur with small intestinal or colonic or rectal bleeding (from a source distal to the ligament of Treitz). As little as 3ml of ingested blood may result in the passage of 1 or more blood containing stools in the first 24 hours. If larger volumes are ingested, melena may persist for 2-3 days. While bleeding sufficient to produce hematemesis usually results in melena, less than half patients with melena have hematemesis.

4. Minor degrees of GIT bleeding are very common and the causes (v.s.) should be excluded before embarking on complex studies of clotting system or diagnosing serious intra-abdominal disease. Perform Apt test to exclude swallowed maternal blood (Refer to E-D-A-Plan / Algorithm). If bleeding persists, *consider the serious differential diagnoses for hematemesis or blood in the stools as follows*: 1. Necrotizing enterocolitis; 2. hemorrhage diatheses of various types, including hemorrhagic disease of the Newborn, and DIC. 3. Steroids ; 4. rare causes : a) trauma (e.g. broken rectal thermometer); b) Meckel's diverticulum; c) malrotation; d) peptic ulceration; e) rectal polyps/ hemangiomas; f) colitis; g) intussusception; h) gut reduplication.

5. Treatment of all moderate and severe cases of Neonatal GIT bleeding includes assessment, resuscitation, appropriate venous access, consultation with a Pediatric surgeon, then identification and treatment of the cause.

6. Management involves principles of emergency treatment in a Neonate comprising of ensuring ABCs, correcting hypothermia, hypoglycemia, hypocalcemia, electrolyte disturbances, and specific interventions including use of injection Vitamin K (IV only to prevent large hematoma from IM injection), fresh frozen plasma, packed RBC, platelets, coagulation factors, and whole blood as per need.

7. *Hemorrhagic disease of the newborn:* Classically it occurs at 2–7 days old generally in breast-fed term healthy infants and can be prevented by Vitamin K supplementation at birth. Early form presents within the first 24–48 hours and is associated with severe Vitamin K deficiency in utero. The usual cause is maternal medication that interferes with Vitamin K. e.g., Phenobarbitone, Phenytoin, INH, Rifampicin, Warfarin. It can not be prevented by Vitamin K supplementation at birth. Late form presents from 2 weeks–6 months of age and usually associated with disorders that reduce Vitamin K absorption. e.g. alpha-1 antitrypsin deficiency, biliary atresia, liver disease and malabsorptive states. Breast-fed babies are also at risk. It is prevented by repeated doses of oral Vitamin K at birth and in the first weeks of life (Refer to Table 2).

8. Bleeding from other sites (along with GIT bleeding) suggests DIC or another coagulopathy including hemorrhagic disease of the Newborn and Congenital Coagulopathies. The initial screening tests should include a) prothrombin time (PT - measures activity of factors II, V, VII, & X) b) APTT - measures factors II, V, VIII, IX, X, XI & XII c) Thrombin time (TT) prolonged by quantitative and qualitative disorders of fibrinogen, the presence of inhibitory factors such as fibrin / FDPs & the presence of Heparin d) Fibrinogen level e) Platelet count (Refer to Figure 1 for a diagnostic Algorithm for bleeding in Neonates.)

9. NEC usually causes lower GI bleeding and it is a rare cause of upper GI bleeding and indicates extensive disease (Refer to Chapter 55 on NEC for its diagnosis and management).

10. Failure of conservative therapy warrants early endoscopic and/or surgical management. The outcome of GIT bleeding in the Neonate is generally good with early prompt diagnosis and effective intervention. It is not associated with significant mortality except in those with a severe primary illness. > 50% of cases of GI bleeding in the Neonates have no clear diagnosis (Idiopathic), which resolve within several days usually.

---

* *Pearl/Peril/Pitfall : Breast milk is a poor source of vitamin K (breast milk levels are 1-4 ¼ g/L). The recommended dietary intake of vitamin K is 1 ¼ g/ kg/d. Exclusively breastfed infants have intestinal colonization with lactobacilli that do not synthesize vitamin K; thus, reduced production of menaquinones increases the neonatal risk of developing a hemorrhagic disorder if not supplemented with vitamin K. Formula-fed infants have higher fecal concentrations of vitamin K_i because of dietary intake and significant quantities of fecal menaquinones, reflecting the gut's microflora.*

THE EVALUATION-DECISION-ACTION-PLAN/ALGORITHM FOR THE DIAGNOSIS AND MANAGEMENT OF *A NEONATE WITH GI TRACT BLEEDING*

SUBJECTIVE FINDINGS

Hx of bloody vomitus / aspirate / stools.

Hx of bleeding from other sites (e.g. hematuria, pulmonary hemorrhage, CNS hemorrhage, venepuncture sites).

Hx of premature birth, birth weight, APGAR scores, PROM, resuscitation details, maternal & Neonatal medications like steroids, indomethacin, anticonvulsants, ATDs, Theophylline etc.

Hx of Vitamin K administration at birth ?

Is the baby breast - fed ?

Is the baby sick or stable hemodynamically?

Hx of bloody diarrhea only after starting cow's milk feeds (allergic colitis) ?

OBJECTIVE FINDINGS

Assess ABCDs and monitor CRT, O_2 sats, BP, core-peripheral temperature difference, RR, HR, central & peripheral pulses, urine output.

Assess severity of bleeding, bleeding from other sites (pulmonary, CNS, cutaneous & renal) and obvious cause of bleeding if any ?

Carefully examine the abdomen for distention, tenderness, lump, perforation, peritonitis.

Exclude the causes of ingested blood or blood from trauma, e.g. swallowed maternal blood at birth and from cracked nipples (Apt test), NG tube/laryngoscopic trauma.

INVESTIGATIONS

Blood FBC, differential, platelets, hematocrit, reticulocyte count, MCHC, Smear, coagulation screen (PT, APTT, fibrinogen, thrombin time, bleeding time & clotting time) FDPs & D-dimer test, blood cultures, ABG analysis, BUN, Creatinine, Blood sugar, electrolytes. LTFs, *Urine analysis.*
Radiological CXR, Plain abdominal X-ray, barium contrast radiography, ultrasonography.
Endoscopy Upper GI & lower GI
Technetium scan (for Meckel's diverticulum)
CT scan (for duplication cyst & hemangioma)
MRI (for bowel inflammation or hematoma)
Stool & vomitus for Naked eye examination & occult blood, Stool microscopy & cultures.

A Neonate with GI tract bleeding

Apt - Downey Test : *Mix* one part vomitus/stool with 5 parts water. *Centrifuse* at 2000 RPM x 2 mts, & mix the 5 parts supernatant to 1 part 0.1 N NaOH. Fetal hemoglobin, which is more resistant to alkali denaturation than adult hemoglobin, remains pink whereas maternal hemoglobin turns brown.

Ensure ABCs, pulse oximetry, IV access, monitor BP & CRT. *Pass* NG tube to confirm the presence of bleeding and to document ongoing blood loss. *Perform* Apt- Downey test to exclude swallowed maternal blood. *Consider* ET intubation and *assist* ventilation in Neonates with respiratory insufficiency, altered mental status, ongoing hematemesis. *Treat* shock with 20ml/kg NS IV bolus, repeat PRN & consider packed RBC 15ml/kg *(maintain hematocrit above 40%)* IV (may require FFP & platelets in massive bleed). *Correct* hypoglycemia, hypothermia, acid-base, & electrolytes disturbances. *Start* IV broadspectrum antibiotics to cover for sepsis related DIC. *Search* for CNS / pulmonary / renal bleeding.

Determine the following :
* Is it really blood ?
* Is the Neonate hemodynamically stable ?
* Is the bleeding from the upper or lower GI tract ?
* What is the site & severity of bleeding ?
* Is the bleeding acute, chronic or ongoing ?

A Neonate with Upper GI tract bleeding

Stop bleeding with epinephrine lavage (1:10,000). 0.1ml + 10ml of sterile water can be used if tepid water lavages don't stop the bleeding. Don't use ice water, as the Neonate may become hypothermic.

Give Inj. Vitamin K 2mgs IV along with FFP 10ml/kg every 12-24 hours. Monitor PT, PTT, platelet count & fibrinogen levels.

Give Inj. Ranitidine 1mg/kg IV every 12 hours. Maintain record of abdominal girth and watch for abdominal distention and tenderness. *Withhold* all the drugs known to cause upper GI bleeding. *Treat* reflux esophagitis with prone positioning + head end elevation + thickening of the feeds + Cisapride + Sucralfate etc.

If DIC is present , *treat* the underlying condition and support blood pressure with multiple transfusions of colloid with platelets as needed.

Bleeding stops
* Keep Nil oral x 3 days
* Start breast feeding
* Close observation for feed intolerance
  → No intolerance
  → Full feeds → Start hematinics early

Bleeding continues
Investigate cause
Medical & Surgical treatment
→ Bleeding stopped

A Neonate with Lower GI tract bleeding

Exclude anal fissure by simple anal examination & by the presence of bright red blood that streaks the stool. If present, treat with local demulcent cream, stool softeners & avoid PR examinations.

Watch for abdominal signs of acute abdomen (distention, tenderness, mass, bilious vomitings / aspirates, absent bowel sounds, increasing abdominal girth etc.)

If negative : *Nil oral *IV fluids + Dopamine & / or Dobutamine IVI+ IV antibiotics*Maintain ventilation / oxygenation / metabolic homeostasis / normal coagulation by FFP, platelets, vitamin K, & packed RBC.

If positive: *Nil oral & NG decompression continuously & reliably *IV fluids + Inotropes + IV antibiotics * *Consult Pediatric surgeon* *Investigate* with upper GI & lower GI contrast studies, USG scan & / or endoscopy *Exclude* volvulus of mid gut *(abdominal distention may be absent)* always *If NEC is suspected, isolate the baby, repeat AXR 12-24 hourly, watch for signs of perforation, start TPN & *liaise with* Pediatric Surgeon *(refer to chapter on NEC).*

Low grade bleed
Investigate (endoscopy & Isotope scan)

Bleeding Stopped
Start feeds Hematinics

Meckel's diverticulum → Surgery

Gastric peptic ulcer disease → H$_2$ blocker, Sucralfate

Proctocolitis Exclude cow's milk protein from the baby's & mother's diet

---

* **Pearl/Peril/Pitfall :** *Hemorrhagic Disease of Newborn -Infants with vitamin K deficiency bleeding typically have a prolonged PT with platelet counts and fibrinogen levels within the normal range for Newborns. Thrombocytopenia or a prolonged aPTT should prompt workup for other causes of bleeding during the Neonatal period.*

TABLE 1	Causes of GIT hemorrhage in a neonate

Common	Less common
Upper Gastrointestinal Hemorrhage	
Hemorrhagic disease	
Swallowed maternal blood	Vascular malformation
Gastritis	Esophageal/gastric duplications
Reflux esophagitis	Structural anomalies
Mallory-Weiss syndrome	Gastric polyp
Peptic ulcer disease	Gastric teratoma
Primary coagulopathy	Leiomyoma
Iatrogenic trauma-gavage tube	
Perinatal asphyxia	
Idiopathic	
Lower Gastrointestinal Hemorrhage	
Anal fissure	Iatrogenic trauma
Upper GI tract bleeding	Primary coagulopathy
Necrotizing enterocolitis	Vascular malformation
Milk allergy	Enterocolitis of Hirschsprung's disease
Malrotation with volvulus	Small bowel/colon duplications

TABLE 2	Forms of Vitamin K deficiency bleeding (VKDB) in infancy

Early form	Classic form	Late form
	Age	
< 24 hr	Days 2–7	0.5–6 mo
Causes and Risk Factors		
Medications during pregnancy		Marginal VK content in breast milk due to low VK intake and absorption
Anticonvulsants	Breast-feeding	Cystic fibrosis
Oral anticoagulants	Inadequate VK intake	Diarrhea
(rifampin, isoniazid)		α_1 AT deficiency
Antibiotics		Hepatitis
(rarely idiopathic or hereditary)		Celiac disease
Localization in Order of Frequency		
ICH	ICH	ICH (> 50%)
GI	GI	GI
Umbilicus	Umbilicus	Skin
Intraabdominal	ENT region	ENT region
Cephalhematoma	Injection sites	Injection sites
	Circumcision	Urogenital tract
		Intrathoracic
Frequency Without VK Prophylaxis		
Very rare	1.5%-1/10,000 births	4-10/10,000 births *
Prophylaxis		
	Adequate VK supply	Adequate VK supply
Discontinue or replace of offending medications	Early and adequate breast-feeding	Adequate breast-feeding
Maternal VK prophylaxis	Formula	Formula
	VK prophylaxis	VK prophylaxis†

More common in southeast Asia. †Single intramuscular injection is better than single oral ; repeated small doses are closer to physiologic conditions. Warning signs : Neonatal icterus, poor feeding, failure to thrive, any form of bleeding. ICH, intracranial bleed ; GI, gastrointestinal bleed ; ENT region, ear, nose, and throat region.

* **Pearl/Peril/Pitfall** : Hemorrhagic Disease of Newborn -*In the absence of intracranial hemorrhage, the prognosis for vitamin K deficiency bleeding in an otherwise healthy infant is excellent. *Prognosis after intracranial hemorrhage depends on the extent and location of the hemorrhage. *Long-term sequelae of intracranial hemorrhage may include motor and intellectual deficits.*

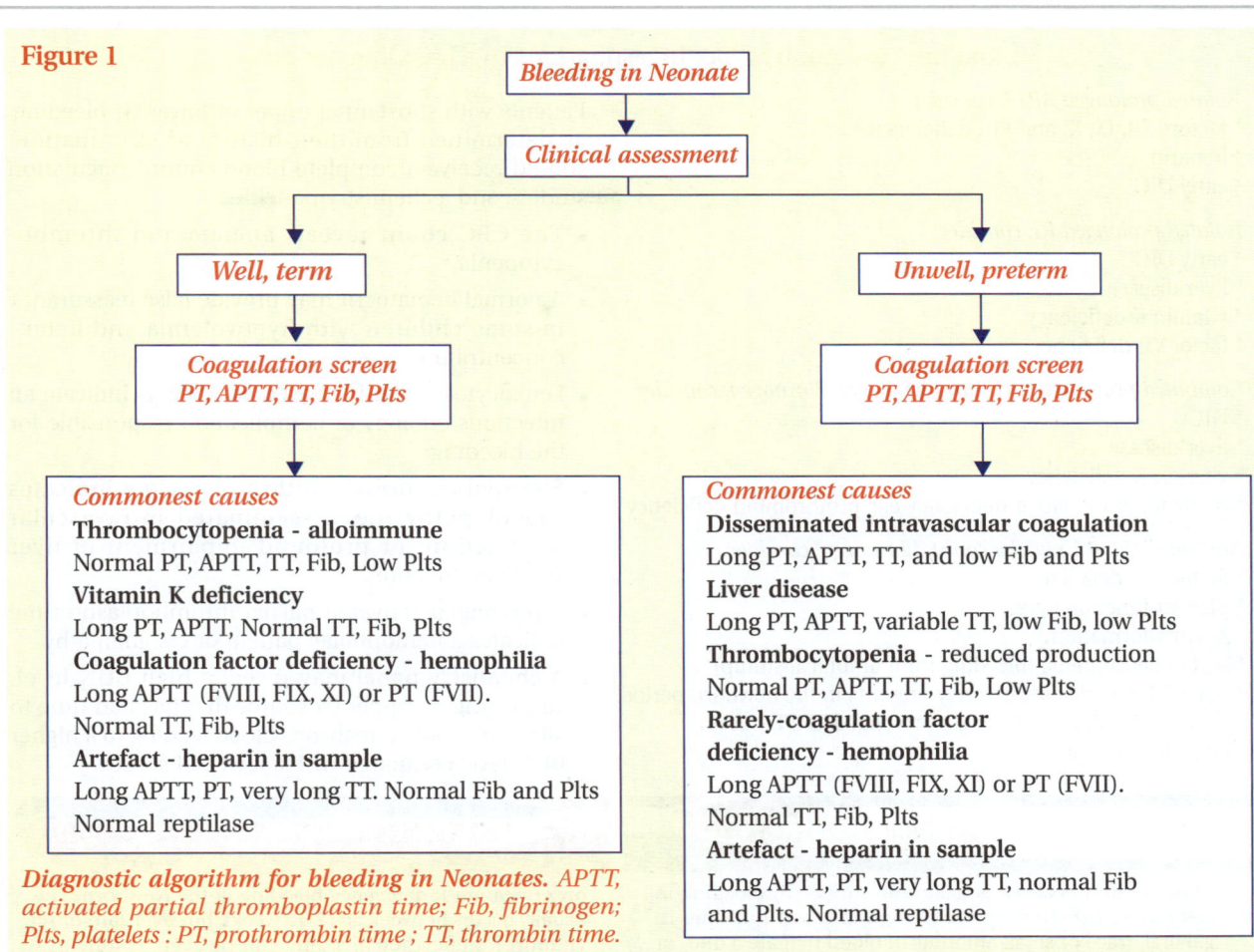

Figure 1

Diagnostic algorithm for bleeding in Neonates. *APTT, activated partial thromboplastin time; Fib, fibrinogen; Plts, platelets : PT, prothrombin time ; TT, thrombin time.*

TABLE 3	Normal values for laboratory screening tests in the neonate		
Laboratory test	Premature infant having received vitamin K	Term infant having received vitamin K	Child over 1 to 2 months of age
Platelet count /ml Platelets on peripheral blood smear	150,000–400,000 10–20/Platelets/oil immersion field, including 1 or 2 small clumps	1,50,000–4,00,000 Same as premature infant	1,50,000–4,00,000 Same as premature infant
PT (sec.)*	14–22	13–20	12–14
PTT (sec.)*	35–55	30–45	25–35
Fibrinogen (mg/dl)	150–300	150–300	150–300

Key : PT = prothrombin time ; PTT = partial thromboplastin time.

*Normal values may vary from laboratory to laboratory, depending on the particular reagent employed. In full-term infants who have received vitamin K, the PT and PTT values generally fall within the normal "adult" range by several days (PT) to several weeks (PTT) of age. Small premature infants (under 1500 gm) tend to have longer PT and PTT than larger babies. In infants with hematocrit levels greater than 60%, the ratio of blood to anticoagulant (sodium citrate 3.8%) in tubes should be 19:1 rather than the usual ratio of 9:1 ; otherwise, spurious results will be obtained, since the amount of anticoagulant solution is calculated for a specific volume of plasma. Blood drawn from heparinized catheters should not be used. The best results are obtained when blood from a clean venipuncture is allowed to drip directly into the tube from the needle or scalp vein set. Factor levels II, VII, IX, and X are decreased. Three-day-old full-term baby not receiving vitamin K has levels similar to a premature baby. Factor XI and XII levels are lower in preterm infants than in term infants and account for prolonged PTT. Fibrinogen, factor V, and factor VII are normal is premature and term infants. Factor XIII is variable.

* *Pearl/Peril/Pitfall : Hemorrhagic Disease of Newborn *Intracranial bleeding is rare and usually associated with other causes of bleeding, particularly thrombocytopenia; however, intracranial hemorrhage has been reported in vitamin K deficiency bleeding and can be fatal. *Investigate any neurologic symptoms with imaging. MRI exposes the neonate to no radiation and is becoming the preferred way to study the brain because tissue damage can be better defined.*

Rapid interpretation of lab. Investigations in a bleeding neonate

- *Isolated prolonged APTT, consider*
  * factors XII, IX, XI and VIII deficiencies
  * heparin
  * early DIC

- *Isolated prolonged PT, consider*
  * early DIC
  * liver disease
  * vitamin K deficiency
  * factor VII deficiency

- *Combined prolonged APTT and PT+/- low fibrinogen, consider*
  * DIC
  * liver disease
  * vitamin K deficiency
  * rarely inherited factor deficiency e.g. prothrombin deficiency

- *Normal APTT, PT, platelet count, fibrinogen, consider*
  * factor XIII deficiency
  * platelet function defect
  * A-V malformation
  * severe neutropenia (bleeding from umbilical stump)
  * Von Willebrand Disease rarely presents in the newborn period. Factor XII deficiency causes a prolonged APTT, but no clinical bleeding.

Patients with substantial upper or lower GI bleeding, as determined from their history or examination, should receive a complete blood count, coagulation studies, and a chemistry panel.

- The CBC count reveals anemia and thrombocytopenia.

- A normal hematocrit may provide false reassurance in some children with hypovolemia and hemoconcentration.

- Leukocytosis with increased bands may indicate an infectious etiology or complication responsible for the bleeding.

- Elevated abnormal prothrombin time indicates coagulopathy (i.e. disseminated intravascular coagulation) or profound impairment of liver synthetic function.

- A prolonged activated partial thromboplastin time indicates a hemophiliac patient or coagulopathy.

- A chemistry panel may reveal a high BUN level, suggesting an upper GI source that has had time to allow the body to reabsorb blood leading to a higher BUN level compared with a lower GI source.

KEY POINTS FOR CLINICAL PRACTICE

1. Most common causes of gastrointestinal (GI) bleeding in Neonates and children are benign and self-limiting. In general, trace or small amounts of blood that are a one- or first-time occurrence are not of emergent concern. If a Neonate is actively spitting up or vomiting blood, or if it is significant enough to require placement of a nasogastric tube, one can use the Apt-Downey test to differentiate between maternal and fetal blood.

2. Patients with substantial upper or lower GI bleeding, as determined from their history or examination, should receive a complete blood count, coagulation studies, and a chemistry panel. Imaging for emergency Neonatal GI bleeding may begin with barium contrast studies (barium swallows, upper GI series, small bowel follow-throughs, or barium enemas-For Neonates with malrotation with midgut volvulus, it may reveal a corkscrew of small bowel or a bird's beak if complete obstruction is present.A Meckel scan uses technetium-99m pertechnate to highlight the ectopic gastric mucosa.

3. Classic vitamin K deficiency bleeding usually occurs after 24 hours and as late as the first week of life. Classic vitamin K deficiency bleeding is observed in infants who have not received prophylactic vitamin K at birth. Infants who have classic vitamin K deficiency bleeding are often ill, have delayed feeding, or both. Bleeding commonly occurs in the umbilicus, GI tract (i.e., melena), skin, nose, surgical sites (i.e., circumcision), and, uncommonly, in the brain. Late-onset vitamin K deficiency bleeding in the Newborn. This usually occurs between age 2-12 weeks; however, late-onset vitamin K deficiency bleeding can be seen as long as 6 months after birth. This disease is most common in breastfed infants who did not receive vitamin K prophylaxis at birth.

4. Endoscopy reveals the source in 90% of patients with upper GI bleeding, and endoscopy is beneficial in predicting the likelihood of continued bleeding. Patients with severe upper GI bleeding should receive endoscopy within the first 12 hours of the hemorrhagic episode if they are sufficiently stable because early endoscopy improves the diagnostic index. The site of upper GI bleeding can be identified in 90% of cases when endoscopy is performed within 24 hours. For lower GI bleeds, colonoscopy can reveal the source of bleeding more effectively than barium enema, and it has 80% sensitivity. NEC usually causes lower GI bleeding and it is a rare cause of upper GI bleeding and indicates extensive disease.

5. Failure of conservative therapy warrants early endoscopic and / or surgical management. The outcome of GIT bleeding in the Neonate is generally good with early prompt diagnosis and effective intervention. It is not associated with significant mortality except in those with a severe primary illness. > 50% of cases of GI bleeding in the Neonates have no clear diagnosis (Idiopathic), which resolve within several days usually.

REFERENCES & FURTHER READING : 1) *Gastrointestinal hemorrhage in Neonates : Criticare Pediatrics volume 14, Page 389* 2) *Nelson text book of Pediatrics - 18th edition* 3)Goyal A, Treem WR, Hyams JS. Severe upper gastrointestinal bleeding in healthy full-term neonates. *Am J Gastroenterol.* Apr 1994;89(4):613-6. 4) Loh DL, Munro FD. The role of laparoscopy in the management of lower gastro-intestinal bleeding. *Pediatr Surg Int.* Jun 2003;19(4):266-267. 5)Arain Z, Rossi TM. Gastrointestinal bleeding in children: an overview of conditions requiring nonoperative management. *Semin Pediatr Surg.* Nov 1999;8(4):172-80.

* *Pearl/Peril/Pitfall: Currently, the following 3 forms of vitamin K are known: *K_1: Phylloquinone is predominantly found in green leafy vegetables, vegetable oils, and dairy products. Vitamin K given to neonates as a prophylactic agent is an aqueous, colloidal solution of vitamin K_1. *K_2: Menaquinone is synthesized by gut flora. *K_3: Menadione is a synthetic, water soluble form that is no longer used medically because of its ability to produce hemolytic anemia.*

58 Neonatal Ascites

@ *Prenatal diagnosis of urinary ascites has been made with fetal ultrasonography. Signs and symptoms of urinary ascites includes abdominal distention, acidosis, elevated BUN and creatinine levels, and electrolyte abnormalities. Respiratory distress may be present, and, in advanced cases, Potter syndrome may be present. Most patients are male and are younger than 1 month.*

USG Imaging can detect as little as 50–100 ml of free fluid in the abdominal cavity and may also be used to safely direct needle insertion during the performance of diagnostic or therapeutic paracentesis.

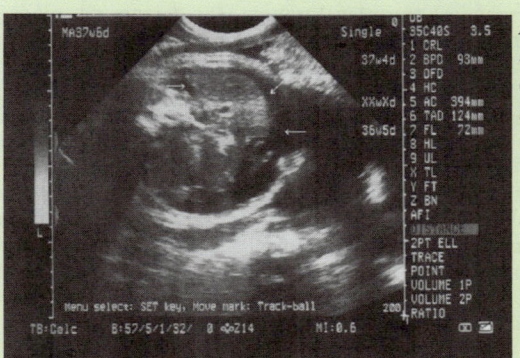

Ascites in the abdominal cavity during the antenatal period (white arrows)

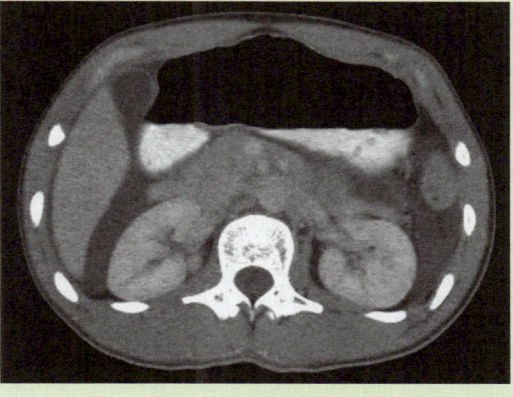

CT demonstrates free intraperitoneal fluid due to urinary ascites.

Neonatal management of congenital Chylothorax
Conservative approach

* Management of underlying disease
* Repeated thoracocenteses
* Continuous drainage
* Dietary modifications (medium chain triacylglycerol diet or total parenteral nutrition)
* Chest tube pleurodesis
* Chemical(intrapleural injection of povidone iodine) or mechanical pleurodesis
* High positive end expiratory pressure during mechanical ventilation

Surgical approach
* Thoracoscopic pleurodesis
* Pleuroperitoneal pump
* Surgical abrasion
* Ligation of the thoracic duct (by thoracoscopy or thoracotomy)
* Thoracic duct to azygous vein anastomosis and lung transplantation (lymphangioleiomyomatosis)

REVIEW OF CLINICAL PROBLEMS

1. Mention the common causes of Neonatal Ascites. *Ans : Refer to the Table 1 of the Chapter.*

2. Name the Components of Routine analysis of Ascitic Fluid. *Ans : Refer to the Table "2" of the Chapter.*

3. Mention the Essential aspects of History & Physical examination of a Neonate with Ascites. *Ans: Refer to the Evaluation-Decision-Action Plan/Algorithm to diagnose & manage a Neonate with Ascites.*

4. How do you manage Chylous Ascites in a Neonate? *Ans : Refer to the Evaluation-Decision-Action Plan/Algorithm to diagnose & manage a Neonate with Ascites.*

5. Discuss Urinary Ascites in Neonates. *Ans: Refer to the "No. 5" of the "BIRD`S EYE VIEW/OVERVIEW/SYNOPSIS" of the Chapter & to the Evaluation-Decision-Action Plan/Algorithm to diagnose & manage a Neonate with Ascites.*

LEARNING OBJECTIVES

After completing this article, readers will be able to:

1. Provide General management of Ascites, whilst awaiting the LAB. results or surgical correction of underlying conditions.

2. Evaluate for the common differential diagnoses of Neonatal Ascites.

3. Discuss with Pediatric Radiologist for the appropriate Imaging modalities to confirm/exclude the causes of Neonatal Ascites.

4. Search for & manage the Iatrogenic Causes of Neonatal Ascites.

5. Liaise with Pediatric Surgeon, if surgical causes of Neonatal Ascites are to be dealt with.

* *Pearl/Peril/Pitfall : The term ascites is of Greek origin, from the word askos, which means "bag" or "bladder." The condition has been recognized since antiquity. Ascites may consist of transudates (thin, low protein count, and low specific gravity) or exudates (high protein count and specific gravity). The etiology of ascites may differ among neonates and older children.*

BIRD'S EYE VIEW/OVERVIEW/SYNOPSIS

1. **Ascites in newborns and neonates:** The Newborn with ascites has a distended, nontympanitic abdomen with bulging and dullness in the flanks, findings that may be mimicked by a massively dilated bladder, a severely hydronephrotic kidney, or a large ovarian cyst. *In the Newborn, ascites results most often from a perforation within an obstructed urinary tract; in boys, posterior urethral valves are a common precipitant.* Ascites also occurs as a complication of congestive heart failure or of liver disease caused by congenital infections, galactosemia, or a lysosomal storage disease, and *it has been reported in association with intestinal malrotation.* Chylous ascites is a rare condition that occurs when lymphatic fluid leaks directly into the peritoneum because of a malformation or perforation of the intestinal lymphatics occurring in utero. Idiopathic or benign ascites is a diagnosis of exclusion and resolves without treatment. Beyond the Neonatal period, ascites occurs most commonly as a consequence of chronic liver disease with cirrhosis and portal hypertension. Refer to the Table 1of the Chapter for a list of common causes of Neonatal Ascites.

2. Ascites may occur as an isolated phenomenon or in conjunction with other causes of generalized edema such as immune/nonimmune hydrops. The differential diagnosis, management and prognosis may be significantly different in an isolated collection of peritoneal fluid from that of the more generalized edema characteristic of hydrops.

3. USG Imaging can detect as little as 50–100 ml of free fluid in the abdominal cavity and may also be used to safely direct needle insertion during the performance of diagnostic or therapeutic paracentesis. CT/MRI Imaging are less helpful and not always immediately available/applicable in a sick Neonate.

4. **Ascitic Fluid analysis:** Laboratory analysis of the paracentesis fluid will establish the diagnosis in most cases. The fluid should be removed under sterile conditions and 10–20 ml of Peritoneal fluid is sufficient for diagnostic purposes and should include the **routine analysis** *as outlined in the Table 2 of the Chapter.* A WBC count of >500cells/ cumm with a DC showing predominantly neutrophils suggests infection.Lower cell counts with a DC of predominantly (>75%) lymphocytes suggests a chylous etiology, particularly if the Triglyceride level is elevated. If the infant has been fed, total fat levels in ascitic fluid can rise significantly, and Triglyceride levels may exceed 1500 mg/dL. An ascites -serum creatinine ratio of >1 is suggestive, if not diagnostic, of an intraperitoneal urinary leak. Patients with Portal hypertension have serum-to-ascites albumin gradients >1.1 g/dL, whereas etiologies unrelated to portal hypertension have levels <this value.

5. **Urinary Ascites:** The most common cause of isolated ascites in a Newborn is Neonatal urinary ascites secondary to urinary obstruction and extravasation of urine into the abdominal cavity. The presence of Oliguria, elevated BUN and Serum Creatinine, Renal USG Scan, Paracentesis as mentioned before, a VCUG, and a MAG3 Isotope Scan would establish a diagnosis. In infants with Posterior Urethral Valves, it is possible to insert ureterostomy/nephrostomy drains under fluoroscopic guidance to divert the urine flow until the infant stabilizes and operative ablation can be undertaken. Although good renal function is preserved in many cases with urological and with good NICU support, follow-up with a nephrologist is recommended. Initial treatment is usually directed at relieving the associated obstruction to urinary outflow. Urinary tract decompression, rehydration, correction of electrolyte abnormalities, and antibiotics are the initial treatment. Catheter bladder drainage followed by cystoscopic ablation of the valves is indicated for posterior urethral valves. Drainage of the upper tract may be necessary in rare circumstances. Direct repair of the perforation site is usually unnecessary.

The Evaluation-Decision-Action-Plan/Algorithm describes the essential aspects of diagnosis & management of the common causes of Neonatal Ascites.

6. Chylous ascites occurs as a result of damage or obstruction of the thoracic duct and related lymph channels and is relatively uncommon in the Newborn period. It may be a manifestation of inflammation or an underlying congenital malformation and can be secondary to surgical trauma. The diagnosis is made by paracentesis, when the characteristic milky-appearing ascitic fluid is found to have a high level of triglycerides with a lymphocytic predominance. Significant nutritional deficiencies may result from losses and an inability to ingest appropriate calories. Conservative and medical management with TPN, Enteral nutrition with Medium Chain Triglycerides and EFA supplements is optimal in most of the cases. Surgical intervention carries high mortality and is indicated only when a surgically correctable lesion is apparent, when failure of medical treatment is persistent, or when ascites recurs after a normal diet is reintroduced. Successful use of a modified peritoneovenous shunt has been reported in infants with persistent/ recurrent ascites.

7. Hepatobiliary causes are suggested by jaundice, hepatosplenomegaly and investigations like abdominal USG scan, Paracentesis, Fibroblast cultures in conjunction with genetic and metabolic studies (Urinary oligosaccharides) help in elucidating the precise diagnosis.Biliary atresia needs a Kasai portoenterostomy initially and a Liver transplantation ultimately. Management of patients with hepatobiliary ascites is directed at controlling the amount of ascites with diuretics, salt restriction, and paracentesis as needed while the exact etiology of the disorder is being determined. Infectious causes may either resolve spontaneously over time (hepatitis) or require specific therapies(syphilis, toxoplasmosis). Metabolic disorders such as tyrosinemia and Galactosemia may show resolution of hepatic dysfunction after the institution of specific therapeutic modalities. Other inherited metabolic diseases caused by a primary hepatic enzyme deficiency may be an indication for liver transplantation in early infancy.

8. Meconium peritonitis (Fetal ascites as early as 18 wks GA, Pseudo-cyst formation, or calcification) is managed by decompression, fluid replacement, antibiotic therapy, and surgical excision of affected bowel with enterostomy.

9. Bacterial peritonitis after perforation associated with NEC demands Mechanical ventilation, vigorous IV fluid resuscitation, pressor support, NG decompression, TPN, IV Antibiotics for both aerobic and anaerobic organisms, and surgical exploration after medical stabilization- with removal of affected necrotic bowel and enterostomy placement as needed. Premature infants with an ELBW (<1,000gm) may undergo placement of a peritoneal drain in lieu of immediate surgery.Infection may lead to excess peritoneal fluid;tuberculous fluid collections and Salmonella organisms are observed in patients in the developing world. Treatment is directed at the underlying condition.

10. General management of Neonatal ascites include Correction of fluid and electrolyte, nutritional, hemodynamic, renal and hematologic disturbances, IV antibiotic coverage while awaiting negative culture results that exclude an infectious etiology or until surgical correction of the underlying lesion has been performed.

---

* Pearl/Peril/Pitfall : Chylous ascites is rare. Most cases occur in infancy, with a male predominance, and are of congenital origin. Signs and symptoms of chylous ascites are nonspecific and include abdominal distention and poor feedingUltrasonography or CT scanning may reveal the fluid and may help rule out underlying causes (e.g., mesenteric cyst, tumor). The diagnosis is confirmed with paracentesis; the fluid has a markedly elevated triglyceride content (>1500 mg/dL) and a predominance of lymphocytes (>75%).

THE EVALUATION-DECISION-ACTION-PLAN/ALGORITHM FOR THE DIAGNOSIS AND MANAGEMENT OF *NEONATAL ASCITES*

SUBJECTIVE FINDINGS

Hx of - symptoms suggestive of ascites- abdominal distention, respiratory distress, non-specific symptoms of poor feeding, poor weight gain, oliguria. poor urinary stream, bilious vomitings(malrotation)

Hx of mild jaundice (direct hyperbili- rubinemia), feeding intolerance, and a distended nontender abdomen.

Hx of Fetal ascites (may be identified during prenatal ultrasonography)

OBJECTIVE FINDINGS

Assess - airway, breathing, circulation & disability by observing the vitals, BP, O_2 sats, color, CRT, pulses, sensorium, *In the infant or child, the signs of ascites include shifting dullness to percussion, a fluid wave, and abdominal distention. *An increased respiratory rate or frank respiratory distress may be the result of diaphragmatic elevation. *The liver, spleen, or both may be ballottable. Signs of peritoneal irritation are usually absent, depending on the underlying etiology.* Look for jaundice, Potter`s facies, Acidosis, CHF and Hepatosplenomegaly.

INVESTIGATIONS

Blood - FBC with hematocrit & platelets, ABG analysis with electrolytes, calcium ++, Mg++, BUN & creatinine, urine analysis & culture, blood culture if infection is suspected, Blood glucose.

Ascitic Fluid Analysis (Refer to the Table No2 of the Chapter)

IMAGING- Plain Abdominal X-Ray, USG Scan, CT/MRI, ECHOCARDIOGRAM as indicated.

Chromosomal and Blood studies as indicated

Identify the Iatrogenic causes ← **NEONATAL ASCITES** → *Ensure* ABCs, Supplemental O_2 IV access, Monitor BP, CR monitor, Pulse oximetry

---

* *Ascites may occur (particularly while the patient is in the Neonatal Intensive Care Unit [NICU]) as a result of iatrogenic gastric perforation from gastric catheters and/or tubes and with intraperi- toneal feedings. Similarly, umbilical catheter perfora- tion may result in the leakage of parenteral nutritional fluid into the peritoneal cavity. Treatment usually requires exploration and repair of the injury site.*

* Determine whether Ascites is an isolated event or associated with Pleural effusion/pericardial effusion-Hydrops
* Determine the Nature of Ascitic Fluid- Urinary/Chylous/Biliary/ Infectious-Inflammatory
* Identify the underlying cause of the Ascites
* Direct the treatment at the underlying condition

Chylous ascites	Nonchylous ascites
Intestinal malrotation	Obstruction in GU system
Trauma	Fetal hydrops (immune & nonimmune)
Lymphatic causes	Congenital heart disease
Trauma	Intrauterine supraventricular tachycardia
Lymphatic obstruction	Lysosomal storage diseases
Lymphatic rupture	Sialodosis
Lymphangiectasia	GM1 gangliosidosis
	Intrauterine infections (CMV & toxoplasmosis)
	Pancreatic ascites
	Intraperitoneal malignancy
	Neural tube defects
	Alpha-1-antitrypsin deficiency
	Congenital Budd-Chiari syndrome
	Obstruction/perforation of the biliary ducts
	Duplication of the small bowel
	Eosinophilic hernia
	Cutis marmorata telangiectasia
	Meconium peritonitis
	Intestinal malrotation
	Cystic adenomatoid malformation of the lung

GU, genitourinary; CMV, cytomegalovirus

Treat Chylous Ascites: After surgical causes (e.g.,malrotation, obstruction, neoplasia) have been ruled out with appropriate imaging studies, more than one half of patients respond to nonoperative treatment with parenteral nutrition and bowel rest for 2-4 weeks. Some authors advocate the initial use of diets rich in medium-chain triglycerides (eg, Portagen) rather than complete bowel rest. Aspiration of the fluid may be necessary if it compromises respiration.If the chylous ascites is refractory to nonsurgical treatment (i.e., if it fails to resolve after 6 wk of nothing by mouth [NPO], total parenteral nutrition [TPN], or both) or if a surgically correctable underlying cause is identified, exploratory laparotomy or laparoscopy is necessary. Administration of a high-fat diet or whole milk with Sudan dye immediately before surgery may help in identifying the site of leakage. Although the site may be anywhere in the retroperitoneum or mesentery, the most common location is the base of the superior mesenteric vessels. Ligation of the leak site with the use of fibrin glue is performed. If direct repair fails, a peritoneovenous shunt may be needed.If the chylous ascites is refractory to nonsurgical treatment (i.e., if it fails to resolve after 6 wk of nothing by mouth [NPO], total parenteral nutrition [TPN], or both) or if a surgically correctable underlying cause is identified, exploratory laparotomy or laparoscopy is necessary. Administration of a high-fat diet or whole milk with Sudan dye immediately before surgery may help in identifying the site of leakage. Although the site may be anywhere in the retroperitoneum or mesentery, the most common location is the base of the superior mesenteric vessels. Ligation of the leak site with the use of fibrin glue is performed. If direct repair fails, a peritoneovenous shunt may be needed. These must often be individually customized for infants. These must often be individually customized for infants.

Treat Urinary Ascites : Initial treatment is usually directed at relieving the associated obstruction to urinary outflow. Urinary tract decompression, rehydration, correction of electrolyte abnormalities, and antibiotics are the initial treatment. Catheter bladder drainage followed by cystoscopic ablation of the valves is indicated for posterior urethral valves. Drainage of the upper tract may be necessary in rare circumstances. Direct repair of the perforation site is usually unnecessary.

Biliary Ascites: Biliary ascites in Neonates is rare. The usual clinical presentation is that of ascites with mild jaundice (direct hyperbilirubinemia), feeding intolerance, and a distended nontender abdomen. A small percentage of infants are more acutely ill, but most have a gradual progression of symptoms. It almost always occurs in infants younger than 3 months. Hepatobiliary scanning with iminodiacetic acid (IDA) demonstrates extraductal radionuclide in the peritoneal cavity. Ultrasonography is usually necessary to rule out congenital anomalies and obstructing lesions. Paracentesis reveals elevated bilirubin levels in the fluid.The treatment of biliary ascites due to spontaneous perforation is drainage, either open or laparoscopic. Intraoperative cholangiography is performed through the gallbladder, and simple external drainage is used at the site of perforation. The perforation usually seals in a few weeks. The cholecystostomy tube can be left in place to verify ductal continuity and the absence of obstruction before the drain is removed. No attempt should be made to repair or reconstruct the duct.

---

* *Pearl/Peril/Pitfall :* Hepatocellular disease (eg, storage disease, neonatal or viral hepatitis, alpha1-antitrypsin deficiency) may result in ascites. Evaluation and treatment of the underlying disease is essential. Paracentesis reveals the presence of fluid with a high serum- to-ascites albumin gradient (>1.1 g/dL). Spontaneous bacterial peritonitis may complicate the course of the disease. Treatment of the ascites consists of sodium and fluid restriction and diuretics (usually spironolactone).

TABLE 1	Causes of neonatal ascites

Genitourinary Tract	Infection
Bladder outlet obstruction	Cytomegalovirus
Congenital nephrotic syndrome	Parvovirus
	Toxoplasmosis
Ovarian cyst with torsion	Syphilis
Ureteropelvic junction obstruction	Chlamydia
Cloacal anomalies	

Gastrointestinal	Cardiac
Meconium peritonitis	Arrythmias
Congenital diaphragmatic Hernia	Congenital heart disease
	Artetiovenous malformations
Midgut volvulus	

Hepatobiliary	Chromosomal
Hepatitis	Trisomy 21
Hepatic necrosis	Turner's syndrome
Tumors	Lysosomal Storage Disease
Biliary atresia	Wolman's disease
Hepatic fibrosis	GM gangliosidosis

Lymphatic	Salla's disease
Thoracic duct obstruction	Gaucher's disease
	Sialidosis

TABLE 2	Routine analysis of ascitic fluid

Macroscopic appearance – straw colored, turbid, bloody, chylous, cell count and differential

Chemistry profile – protein, albumin, amylase, triglyceride

Cytology

Gram stain and bacterial culture

pH, lactate dehydrogenase

ETIOLOGY: Neonatal ascites is usually biliary, urinary, or chylous. In older children, trauma, infection, hepatocellular disease, pancreatic ascites, gynecologic or GI abnormalities, neoplasia, and other miscellaneous causes predominate.

*Biliary ascites in Newborns is the result of spontaneous perforation of the bile duct, usually at the junction of the common bile duct and the cystic duct. The cause of these perforations is unknown; elevated intraductal pressure from a long common channel, congenital weakness of the wall of the duct, vascular insufficiency at the level of the ductal wall, and pancreatic reflux have all been proposed. Perforation of a choledochal cyst can be causative. Bile ascites in older children may occur as a result of trauma or after cholecystectomy.

*Urinary ascites in Neonates is usually due to intraperitoneal bladder or ureteric or upper tract perforation as a result of distal obstruction. Posterior urethral valves are the most common cause; for this reason, males are affected much more often than females. Complex urinary anomalies (eg, persistent cloaca) may allow reflux of urine through the genital tract into the peritoneal cavity, without the presence of a perforation. Useful information may be gained from an analysis of the ascitic fluid because only in urinary ascites can the urea and creatinine concentrations of the ascitic fluid exceed those of plasma (although, because of the back diffusion across the peritoneum, these concentrations will be midway between those for urine and plasma). An additional point of differentiation is that with ascitic fluid of other origin the protein concentration is usually much higher. The diagnosis of a ruptured bladder can, if necessary, be confirmed with a micturating cystogram.

*Chylous ascites may occur in Neonates, with a slight male predominance. Neonatal chylous ascites is almost always idiopathic, but a congenital lymphatic abnormality is thought to be the usual underlying cause. Trauma (particularly nonaccidental trauma) with disruption of lymphatic ducts is well described in infants and older children. External compression of the lymphatics due to malrotation, hernia, intussusception, and neoplasia is another cause. Malignancy is an uncommon cause of ascites in children.

Other causes vary in incidence by age and geography. After the newborn period, infections such as tuberculosis are more frequent in underdeveloped areas, whereas hepatobiliary disease and neoplasia are more common in developed countries.

KEY POINTS FOR CLINICAL PRACTICE

1. Fetal ascites may be identified during prenatal ultrasonography. In the infant or child, the signs of ascites include shifting dullness to percussion, a fluid wave, and abdominal distention. An increased respiratory rate or frank respiratory distress may be the result of diaphragmatic elevation. The liver, spleen, or both may be ballottable. Signs of peritoneal irritation are usually absent, depending on the underlying etiology.

2. Plain radiography may demonstrate a diffuse glassy-hazy opacification, with separation of bowel loops. Ultrasonographic findings confirm ascites. Paracentesis and analysis of the fluid are often necessary for a specific diagnosis.

3. The most common cause of isolated ascites in a Newborn is Neonatal urinary ascites secondary to urinary obstruction and extravasation of urine into the abdominal cavity.

4. Neonatal chylous ascites is almost always idiopathic, but a congenital lymphatic abnormality is thought to be the usual underlying cause.

5. The differential diagnosis, management and prognosis may be significantly different in an isolated collection of peritoneal fluid from that of the more generalized edema characteristic of hydrops.

REFERENCES & FURTHER READING : 1)Haller JO, Condon VR, Berdon WE, et al. Spontaneous perforation of the common bile duct in children. *Radiology.* Sep 1989;172(3):621-4. 2)Scott TW. Urinary ascites secondary to posterior urethral valves. *J Urol.* Jul 1976;116(1):87-91. 3)Adams MC, Ludlow J, Brock JW III, Rink RC. Prenatal urinary ascites and persistent cloaca: risk factors for poor drainage of urine or meconium. *J Urol.* Dec 1998;160(6 Pt 1):2179-81. 4)Chye JK, Lim CT, Van der Heuvel M. Neonatal chylous ascites— report of three cases and review of the literature. *Pediatr Surg Int.* Apr 1997;12(4):296-8. 5)Sooriakumaran P, McAndrew HF, Kiely EM, et al. Peritoneovenous shunting is an effective treatment for intractable ascites. *Postgrad Med J.* Apr 2005;81(954):259-61.

* *Pearl/Peril/Pitfall : Cardiac abnormalities (e.g., congestive failure, physiologic right-sided heart obstruction, severe valvular regurgitation) may result in ascites. Management is directed at the underlying lesion.*

59 Neonatal Diarrhea

@ *The causes of Diarrhea are either infectious or non infectious: The infectious causes are either inflammatory (usually bacterial) or non inflammatory (usually viruses, parasites). The non infectious causes are many & include a)Feeding difficulty b)Anatomic defects c)Malabsorption d)Endocrinopathies e)Food poisoning f)Neoplasms g)Miscellaneous.*

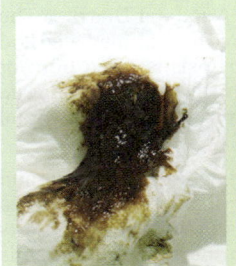
Meconium Stools

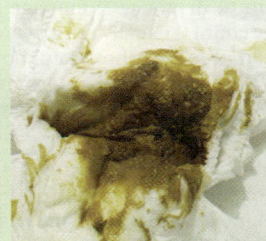
Transitional Stools

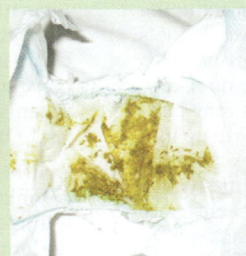
Breastfed Stools

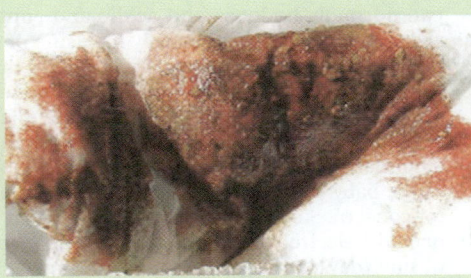
Bloody Stools

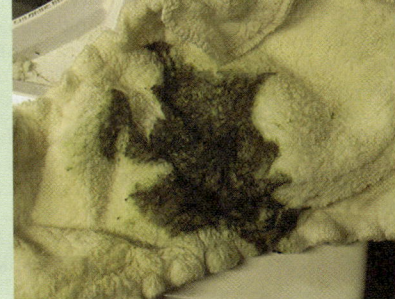

Green stools in a healthy baby may indicate a sensitivity/allergy to a medication or a food or a Viral infection or simply a foremilk-hindmilk imbalance.

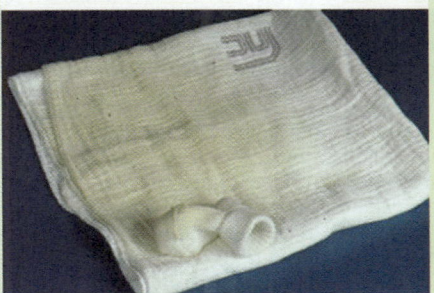

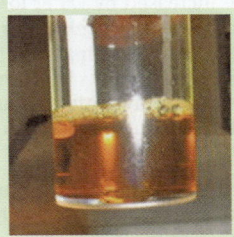

Acholic Stools (**Chalky white poop**) associated with Dark Urine-Neonatal Cholestasis Syndrome(EHBA)

Often mistaken for blood in the urine, **urate crystals** are a frequent intermittent finding in the first week. The characteristic appearance of pink-orange material is sufficient to make the diagnosis. No laboratory analysis is needed.

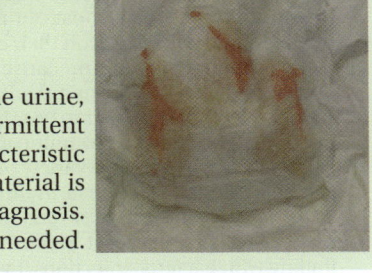

REVIEW OF CLINICAL PROBLEMS

1. What are the usual causes of Diarrhea in a Neonate?
   Ans: Refer to the Table "1" of the Chapter.

2. Discuss the mechanisms of Diarrhea.
   Ans: Refer to the Table "2" of the Chapter.

3. How do you investigate Neonatal diarrhea?.
   Ans: Refer to the Evaluation-Decision-Action Plan/ Algorithm to diagnose and manage Neonatal Diarrhea.

4. When should you notify a Pediatric surgeon , if a Neonate presents with diarrhea?
   Ans: Refer to the Evaluation-Decision-Action Plan/ Algorithm to diagnose & manage Neonatal Diarrhea.

5. How do you differentiate Secretory from Osmotic Diarrhea ?
   Ans: Refer to the Table 3 of the Chapter.

LEARNING OBJECTIVES

After completing this article, readers will be able to:

1. Understand the differences between Diarrhea and normal Breastfed stools and other physiological variations in healthy Neonate's bowel movements.

2. Admit those Neonates with alarming symptoms associated with diarrhea, i.e. fever, toxic appearance, bloody diarrhea, moderate-severe dehydration, acidosis, suspected surgical abdomen, renal failure, malabsorption-malnutrition etc.

3. Correct Fluid, Electrolyte, Acid-Base, Glucose, Hematocrit, disturbances secondary to Diarrhea & Dehydration.

4. Investigate SPUR-severe/persistent/unresponsive/ recurring cases of Neonatal Diarrhea by organizing referral to/consultation with a Pediatric Gastroenterologist.

5. Treat the underlying causes of Diarrhea, rather than the symptom of diarrhea alone.

* *Pearl/Peril/Pitfall : Disorders that interfere with absorption in the small bowel tend to produce voluminous diarrhea, whereas disorders compromising colonic absorption produce lower volume diarrhea. Dysentery i.e., small volume, frequent bloody stools with mucus, tenesmus, & urgency) is the predominant symptom of colitis.*

BIRD'S EYE VIEW/OVERVIEW/SYNOPSIS

1. Diarrhea indicates an increase in water content in stools, which results in looser, watery, mucusy, green, or runnier than usual consistency, increased frequency of bowel movements, or both; newborns often stool 8 – 12 times a day, sometimes passing small, watery stools mixed with yellow, seedy pieces. They also may have several stools each day that are runnier and more mucusy than usual. These are all normal variations and are not a cause for concern. Stools of Breastfed infants can normally be loose and acidic and contain reducing sugars. Infants may occasionally have one or several stools that are much more loose and foul smelling than usual. This is probably due to a variation in diet or may be for no reason at all. It is not a cause for concern. Some infants may have persistent loose, runny stools that never seem to firm up into a normal stool. This can go on for one or two weeks. As long as the baby is thriving, not acting sick, there is little reason for concern. Stool output of > 10g/kg/day(an excessive loss of fluid & electrolyte in the stool ;young infant passes 5gm/kg of stool/day normally: adult limit 200gms /24hrs) suggests higher than normal stool output that is not necessarily a practical definition. **Greenish or Yellow/Brown, grainy or seedy:** This is the transition between meconium and a regular breastfed stool and begins as mom's milk is coming in on the second, third or fourth day of life. There may be three stools each day, ten, or even twenty(often mistaken for diarrhea). Occasionally, even a baby in the first week of life will skip a day and have no bowel movements at all.

2. Neonatal diarrhea can be due to Infectious and Non-Infectious causes (enlisted in the Table 1 of the Chapter).

3. The pathogenesis of most episodes of diarrhea can be explained by secretory, osmotic, or motility abnormalities or a combination of these (Refer to Table 2 of the Chapter). Intestinal infections – most of these are not serious, not treatable, and will resolve on their own with time: *Rotavirus – one of the most common causes of diarrhea, especially during late fall and winter months. It causes very foul smelling, watery, green or brown diarrhea that can persist for weeks. Fever and vomiting are common at the onset of the illness. Other viruses – there are a variety of these, none of which are serious. *Bacteria – these include E. Coli, Salmonella, *Campylobacter fetus* and several others. Vomiting and fever may be present at the onset. Blood in the diarrhea is a common finding with bacterial infections. Even these infections rarely require antibiotic treatment. *Parasites – there are a variety of these. They are usually caught from contaminated water (e.g. Giardia) or during travel to foreign countries. The telltale sign of a parasite is very watery diarrhea that lasts beyond two weeks. *CONTAGIOUS – these are all generally contagious as long as the diarrhea continues. The identified risk factors are gestational age less than 37 weeks, birth weight of less than 2500 gms, formula feeding and hospital stay of more than 10 days. Prophylactic usage of antibiotics have proven to be non-beneficial in reducing the acquisition of diarrhoea. Anticipation of the problem in those that are at risk and persistent surveillance to detect cases would be of paramount importance in reducing the overall morbidity.

4. *Diarrhea* may be a symptom of overfeeding (especially high–caloric density formula), acute gastroenteritis, or malabsorption, or it may be a nonspecific symptom of infection. Diarrhea may occur in conditions accompanied by compromised circulation of part of the intestinal or genital tract, such as mesenteric thrombosis, necrotizing enterocolitis, strangulated hernia, intussusception, and torsion of the ovary or testis.

5. *Several clinical signs that warrant admission and further evaluation and management include:* *Bloody diarrhea. This can be a sign of a bacterial illness or an allergy(Cow`s milk protein intolerance). *Moderate to severe dehydration *Child is acting lethargic (limp, and less responsive to touch or words, won't focus on mother). *Increased abdominal pain. *Continued weight loss of more than 5% of body weight. Refer to the Evaluation-Decision-Action Plan/Algorithm to diagnose & manage Neonatal Diarrhea. The leukocyte count is usually not elevated in viral-mediated and toxin-mediated diarrhea. Leukocytosis is often but not constantly observed with enteroinvasive bacteria. *Shigella* organisms cause a marked bandemia with a variable total white blood cell count.

6. Diarrheal episodes are classically distinguished into acute and chronic (or persistent) based on their duration. Acute diarrhea is thus defined as an episode that has an acute onset and lasts no longer than 14 days; chronic or persistent diarrhea is defined as an episode that lasts longer than 14 days. The distinction, supported by the World Health Organization (WHO), has implications not only for classification and epidemiological studies but also from a practical standpoint because protracted diarrhea often has a different set of causes, poses different problems of management, and has a different prognosis.

7. *Rapid dehydration:* The physiological characteristics of the Newborn baby result in more rapid dehydration during diarrhoea than occurs with older infants. The more premature the infant, the greater the risk of severe dehydration. Reduced fluid intake may result if the Neonate is unable to take breastmilk from its mother due to poor sucking ability or lethargy due to illness. The fluid loss from the body caused by diarrhoea and vomiting may be increased by water loss through the skin due to fever and from the upper respiratory tract by rapid breathing, especially in hot, dry climates. It is essential to: *recognize diarrhoea immediately *prevent dehydration occurring or undertake early rehydration *treat any other illness in the infant *restore adequate food intake as soon as possible.

8. *Drug therapy:* Antibiotics and other drugs do more harm than good in newborn infants and should never be given. The only possible exception is where the cause of the diarrhoea has been clearly identified as shigella, campylobacter or, giardia.

9. *Early feeding:* The Newborn infant should be breastfed as soon as possible after birth. Feeding both during and after the diarrhoea is essential. Newborns have very limited nutritional reserves to combat starvation and quickly become hypoglycemic. After an episode of diarrhea, an infant needs extra food intake to rebuild reserves and prevent the cycle of diarrhoea and malnutrition. Breastfeeding should always be encouraged. Bottle-feeding carries a high risk of infection and good hygienic standards must be observed to prevent recurrence of diarrhea. In some cultures, inappropriate semi-solid and solid foods are sometimes given to the very young infant with disastrous consequences.

10. Management of diarrhoeal disease in the Newborn requires accurate diagnosis and quick responses from health personnel and mothers, with emphasis on preventing dehydration by increasing fluid intake and on ensuring adequate calorie intake through suitable feeding. Neonates with diarrhoea should be closely monitored to ascertain those who need early referral to a hospital or other health facility.

---

* *Pearl/Peril/Pitfall : Well designed RCTs with adequate sample size and independent of any competitive interest, studying the efficacy and safety of racecadotril (Racecadotril, an enkephalinase inhibitor, reinforces the physiological activity of endogenous enkephalins. The antisecretory mechanism involves activation of d opiate receptor leading to reduction in secretion of intracellular CAMP.) in acute childhood diarrhea, are needed before we reach any conclusion regarding the role of the drug in the management of acute diarrhea.*

THE EVALUATION-DECISION-ACTION-PLAN/ALGORITHM FOR THE DIAGNOSIS AND MANAGEMENT OF *NEONATAL DIARRHEA*

SUBJECTIVE FINDINGS

Hx of onset, duration, frequency, pattern, & severity of the diarrhea, Blood/Mucus in the stools? Document type & amount of feed (Breast &/or Bottle), Formula dilution, sterilization, frequency of urination. Note Associated symptoms such as vomiting(Bilious?), excessive crying due to crampy abdominal pain, poor appetite, fever, cough, coryza, rash, weight loss, mental status, & decreased activity level.

Hx of Precipitating factors like IV Antibiotics, Home made remedies, Phototherapy, Maternal drugs etc.,
Hx of diarrhea in the Family, recent travel, epidemiological outbreaks of diarrhea in the community.

OBJECTIVE FINDINGS

Assess ABCDs, hydration status, O_2 sats, CRT, BP, urine output. *Determine* the mental status, noting any irritability, lethargy, seizures, abnormal movements or focal neurologic signs.

Assess the Neonate's ability to suck and swallow the milk normally/eagerly/poorly(not able to drink).

Note systemic signs such as Skin rashes, Hepatosplenomegaly, Lymphadenopathy, respiratory distress, Bleeding-GIT, Skin, urine, Failure to thrive etc.,

Perform complete systemic examination

INVESTIGATIONS

Blood FBC with hematocrit & platelets, ABG analysis with electrolytes, blood glucose, calcium ++, Mg++, BUN & creatinine, blood culture, CRP ± LP, coagulation studies (PT, APTT, D-dimer & FDP) if clinically indicated.

Stool smear for Leukocytes and cultures if persistent, intractable, containing blood.

Urine urine analysis & culture to exclude UTI causing Parenteral diarrhea.

CSF Analysis if Meningitis is being suspected to cause Parenteral diarrhea.

Imaging CXR to exclude pneumonia, aspiration.

NEONATAL DIARRHEA

Assess for Dehydration & Manage it according to the Flow chart given on the Next page.

Ensure ABCs, BP, Pulse oximetry, O2 supplements, in any sick infant with Diarrhea

---

Assess for the presence of risk factors for admission (Potentially Serious) and further Evaluation and Management, such as

1. Fever greater than 38.5°C (101.3°F)-usually associated with intestinal inflammation due to invasive bacteria (e.g.*Shigella*, *Salmonella*, or *Campylobacter* species), enteric viruses, or toxin-induced damage due to *Clostridium difficile.*
2. Blood in the stools,
3. Toxic appearance, crampy abdominal pain, seizures, altered sensorium, poor intake, persistent vomiting etc
4. Moderate-Severe dehydration with Weight loss >5% of body weight.
5. Suspecting Parenteral Diarrhea- Sepsis, UTI, Pneumonia, Meningitis etc.,
6. ?Neonatal Drug Withdrawal Syndrome/ Maternal Grave`s disease with /?Neonatal Hyperthyroidism
7. Immuno suppression/deficiency/Allergy- preterms on antibiotics, steroids, fungal infections, Indwelling vascular catheters, maternal HIV Positive status, Cow`s milk Protein Intolerance

Hospitalize & Perform IV access & correct fluid & electrolyte disturbances in a neonate with significant Diarrhea associated with dehydration, possible systemic causes *Treat with IV Antibiotics after taking Stool, Blood, Urine for Microscopy & Cultures. and modify the antibiotics according to Culture Sensitivity Results:

E.coli- IV Gentamicin

Clostridium difficile- Discontinue Antibiotics, Consider Vancomycin/Metronidazole

Salmonella-IV Ceftriaxone

Shigella- IV Ceftriaxone/Cefaperazone

Yersinia- IV Gentamicin

Giardiasis-Metronidazole

*Treat the underlying conditions appropriately!

Notify pediatric surgeon if considering/suspecting the following clinical conditions causing Neonatal Diarrhea.

1. Is it due to NEC?
2. Is it due to Intestinal Obstruction?
3. Is it due to Postoperative diarrhea secondary to Short Bowel syndrome/Blindloop syndrome?
4. Is it due to Cholestasis?
5. Is it due to Hirschsprung disease (enterocolitis) ?
6. Is it due to Strangulated Hernia, Intussusception, Torsion Testis / Ovary?

Acute, self-limited process likely
1. Mild diarrhea & dehydration
2. Well looking infant with good oral intake, normal urine output, without any risk/predisposing factors for serious systemic infection/Surgical causes.

* Continue Breast feeding.
* Start Oral Rehydration Therapy with New ORS-Refer to Table No- 5.
* Zinc supplementation 10mg/day -May not be helpful in infants<3 mo; need more studies to decide the issue.
* Avoid irrational antibiotics, antimotility agents, & harmless but unnecessary drugs.

Refer Neonates with SPUR Symptoms, i.e., Severe / Persistent /Unresponsive / Recurring types of Diarrhea to a Pediatric Gastroenterologist for further Evaluation & Management.
e.g. Malabsorption-Malnutrition
Metabolic problems - Galactosemia, Tyrosinemia, Enterkinase deficiency

Ensure to perform Complete Stools Examination in Neonatal Diarrhea with Alarming / SPUR SYMPTOMS !

stool examination for occult blood, stool examination for fecal leucocytes
stool culture , serum electrolytes, laboratory evaluation for ova and parasites
stool assay for C. difficile toxin, endoscopy.

@No investigations are routinely required in acute diarrhea. Majority of the cases need no investigations. In a small proportion the following situations may require investigations. *Stool culture should be done in cases of bloody diarrhea and cholera only. *When diarrhea is prolonged beyond 5 days than stool examination for giardiasis and amebiasis is justified. Confirmation is with a fresh stool sample showing trophozoites *To confirm a case of secondary lactose intolerance stool pH and reducing sugar can be done. *Diarrhea associated with clinical signs of electrolyte imbalance or metabolic acidosis may need serum sodium, serum potassium or blood gas analysis *Complete blood count, peripheral blood smear, chest radiography, urine culture should be done wherever needed in case of sepsis or if extra-intestinal infection is clinically evident.

---

* *Pearl/Peril/Pitfall :* A meta-analysis 84 published in 2006 concluded that there is insufficient evidence about the prophylactic or therapeutic role of probiotics (The competitive blockage of receptors thereby preventing the adhesion & invasion of the virus, enhanced immune response, down regulation of the host's secretory & motility defenses and /or inactivation of the virus particles by substances produced by the lactobacilli could be the possible mechanisms.) in acute childhood diarrhea in the developing world where the main burden of the disease lies.

PROBLEM : A 3 week old infant with a recent Pre illness weight of 3 kg was brought with 3 days Hx of gastroenteritis with 10% dehydration (current illness weight 2.7kgs). His serum sodium on admission was 137mEq/L. How do you assess, evaluate and manage his fluid and electrolyte problems ?

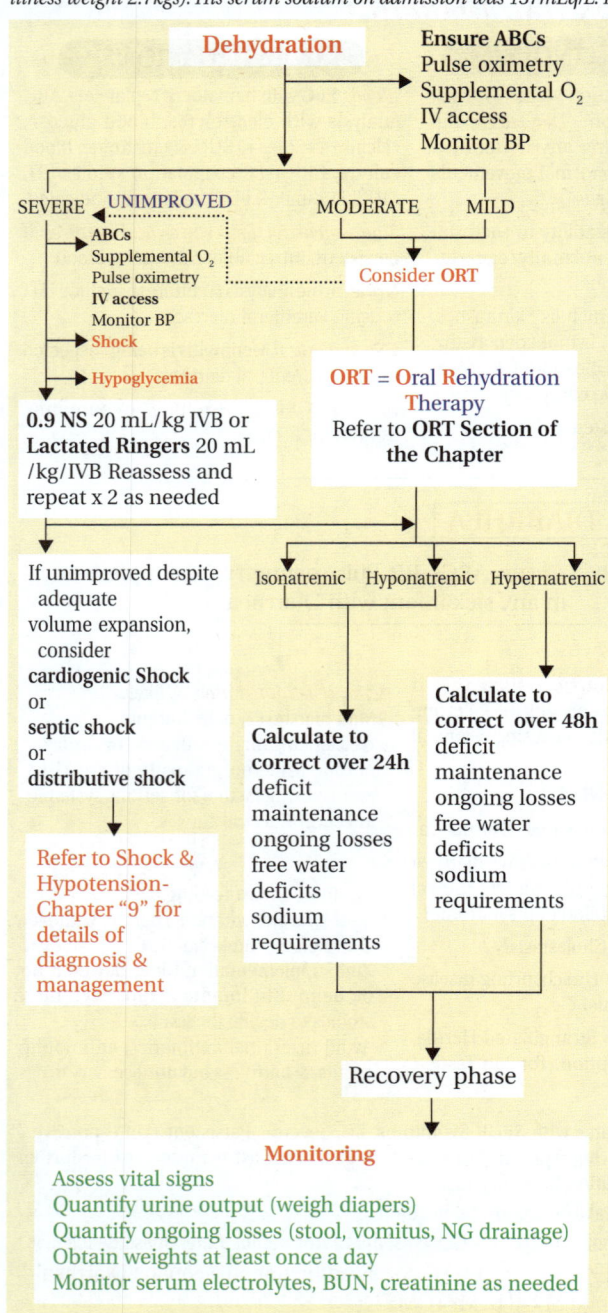

Dehydration

Ensure ABCs
Pulse oximetry
Supplemental O_2
IV access
Monitor BP

SEVERE UNIMPROVED — MODERATE MILD

ABCs
Supplemental O_2
Pulse oximetry
IV access
Monitor BP
Shock

Hypoglycemia

0.9 NS 20 mL/kg IVB or Lactated Ringers 20 mL/kg/IVB Reassess and repeat x 2 as needed

Consider **ORT**

ORT = Oral Rehydration Therapy
Refer to **ORT Section of the Chapter**

If unimproved despite adequate volume expansion, consider **cardiogenic Shock** or **septic shock** or **distributive shock**

Isonatremic Hyponatremic Hypernatremic

Refer to Shock & Hypotension-Chapter "9" for details of diagnosis & management

Calculate to correct over 24h deficit maintenance ongoing losses free water deficits sodium requirements

Calculate to correct over 48h deficit maintenance ongoing losses free water deficits sodium requirements

Recovery phase

Monitoring
Assess vital signs
Quantify urine output (weigh diapers)
Quantify ongoing losses (stool, vomitus, NG drainage)
Obtain weights at least once a day
Monitor serum electrolytes, BUN, creatinine as needed

If weight loss is unknown, estimate severity of dehydration from signs and symptoms of extracellular fluid loss (ECF)
CLINICAL OBSERVATION IN DEHYDRATION*

	Older child: 3% (30mL/kg)	6% (60mL/kg)	9% (90mL/kg)
Examination	Infant:5% (50mL/kg)	10% (100mL/kg)	15% (150mL/kg)
Dehydration	Mild	Moderate	Severe
Skin turgor	Normal	Tenting	None
Skin (touch)	Normal	Dry	Clammy
Buccal mucosa/lips	Moist	Dry	Parched/cracked
Eyes	Normal	Deep set	Sunken
Tears	Present	Reduced	None
Fontanelle	Flat	Soft	Sunken
CNS	Consolable	Irritable	Lethargic/obtunded
Pulse rate	Normal	Slightly increased	Increased
Pulse quality	Normal	Weak	Feeble/impalpable
Capillary refill	Normal	=2 sec	> 3 sec
Urine output	Normal	Decreased	Anuric

* For the same degree of dehydration, clinical symptoms are generally worse for hyponatremic dehydration than for hypernatremic dehydration. May not be reliable in Neonates.

B. Isonatremic dehydration calculations for the index case
ISONATREMIC DEHYDRATION CALCULATIONS *
Example : 3-kg infant with 10% dehydration ($\geq$3 days). Serum Na^+ = 137. Illness weight = 2.7kg.

	H_2O (mL)	Na^+ (mEq)	K^+(mEq)
Maintenance 3x100	300	9	6
DEFICIT	300		
0.6 x 0.3 L x 145 =		26	--
0.4 x 0.3 L x 150 =		--	18
24-**HOUR TOTAL**	600	35	24
FLUID SCHEDULE			
First 8 hr 1/3 maintenance	100	3	2
+ 1/2 deficit	150	13	9
FIRST 8 - HR TOTAL	250	16	11

Exact calculations : 250mL/8 hr = 31 mL/hr ; 16mEq Na^+ /0.250 L = 64 mEq/L ; 11 mEq K^+ /0.250 L = 44 mEq/L)

Next 16 hr 2/3 maintenance	200	6	4
+ 1/2 deficit	150	13	9
NEXT 16-HR TOTAL	350	19	13

Exact calculations : 350 mL/16 hr = 22 mL/hr ; 19 mEq Na^+ / 0.350 L = 54 mEq/L ; 13 mEq K^+/0.350 L = 37 mEq/L)
A convenient fluid for this patient would be D_5 1/2 NS + 40 mEq/L KCl
* In the absence of hypokalemia, 20 to 30 mEq/L of potassium is commonly used and is usually adequate ; monitor carefully for hyperkalemia and adequate urine output if high concentrations of potassium are used.Potassium infusion rates should not exceed 1.0 mEq/kg/hr, if rate exceeds 0.5mEq/kg/hr, the patient should be placed on a cardiorespiratory monitor.

USEFUL FORMULAE
1. Na^+ deficit (mEq) = fluid deficit (L) x proportion from ECF x Na^+ concentration (mEq / L) in ECF, for Eg: in the above case 0.3 L x 0.6 x 145 = 26mEq.
2. K^+ deficit (mEq) = fluid deficit (L) x proportion from ICF × K^+ concentration (mEq / L) in ICF, for Eg: in the above case 0.3 L x 0.4 x 150 = 18 mEq.
3. Formula for electrolyte deficits (in excess of ECF / ICF electrolyte losses) mEq required = desired concentration (mEq/L) - present concentration (mEq/L) x distribution factor x baseline weight before illness, for Eg: if the above case shows serum Na^+ 115mEq/L the excess Na^+ deficit will be :

   (135 - 115) x 0.6 x 3= 36 mEq

   to this you have to add expected Na^+ deficit if it were just isonatremic dehydration i.e., 26 mEq as calculated above.

4. HCO_3^- deficit (mEq) = desired HCO_3^- - measured HCO_3^- x 0.6 x baseline weight before illness, for Eg: if the HCO_3^- is 10 mEq /L then HCO_3^- deficit = (23-10) × 0.6 × 3 = 23.4 mEq. Metabolic acidosis is a biochemical derangement that results from an underlying disease process, therefore treatment should be aimed at correction of the disease. It needs correction only when the pH is < 7.2 and HCO_3^- - 10mEq/L. Give only 50% of calculated deficit slowly over 6-12 hours. Consider rapid correction (over 30mts) if the pH is < 7. If ABG available the HCO_3^- deficit will be; base deficit x body weight (kg) x 0.6. Beware of the untoward side effects of HCO_3^- therapy; 1. Hypokalemic cardiac toxicity 2. Hypocalcemic tetany in the renal failure 3. CCF due to Na^+ excess 4.Hypernatremia with IVH in premature babies 5.Hypercarbia in a child with respiratory depression ($NaHCO_3 \rightarrow Na^+ + H_2O + CO_2$).
5. Anion gap = (serum Na^+ + K^+)-(serum Cl + HCO_3^-) normal range = 12 mEq/L + 4 mEq/L .

TABLE 1 — Etiology of diarrhea in newborn

1. GI infections in order of frequency: viral, entero-pathogenic Escherichia coli (EPEC), Salmonella, Pseudomonas, Klebsiella, Enterobacter, Proteus, Staphylococcus aureus, Campylobacter fetus, and Shigella, Viral infections in infants younger than 2 months of age are usually asymptomatic. After 3 months of age, rotavirus becomes the most common infectious cause of diarrhea in infants.

2. Sepsis

3. Overfeeding

4. Antibiotics

5. Milk/formula protein allergy

6. NEC

7. *Malabsorption syndromes:* These can be post-infectious, or can be caused by cystic fibrosis, human immunodeficiency virus (HIV), or other congenital malabsorptive conditions (rare: Shwachman syndrome, congenital lactase deficiency, microvillus inclusion disease, glucose galactose malabsorption, congenital sucrase-isomaltase deficiency).

8. Cholestasis (biliary atresia, Alagille syndrome).

9. Familial chloridiarrhea.

10. Phototherapy-The colon plays a part in the pathogenesis of secretory diarrhea and that both hyperbilirubinemia and phototherapy are necessary for such an effect to develop.

11. Bowel resection (short bowel syndrome, blind loop syndrome).

12. Hirschsprung disease (enterocolitis).

13. Intestinal obstruction (diarrhea may be an initial symptom).

14. Metabolic : galactosemia, tyrosinemia, enterkinase deficiency.

15. Maternal drugs during breast-feeding (antibiotics, sulfasalazine, ergotamine).

TABLE 2 — Mechanisms of diarrhea

Primary Mechanism	Defect	Stool Examination	Examples	Comment
Secretory	Decreased absorption, increased Secretion: electrolyte transport	Watery, normal osmolality; osmols = 2 × (Na$^+$ + K$^+$) neuroblastoma, congenital	Cholera, toxigenic Escherichia coli;carcinoid, VIP chloride diarrhea, Clostridium difficile, cryptosporidiosis (AIDS) Phototherapy	Persists during fasting, bile salt malabsorption also may increase intestinal water secretion; no stool leukocytes
Osmotic	Maldigestion, transport defects, ingestion of unabsorbable solute	watery,acidic, + reducing substances; increased osmolality; osmosis >2 x (Na$^+$ + K$^+$)	Lactase deficiency, glucose-galactose malabsorption, lactulose, laxative abuse	Stops with fasting, increased breath hydrogen with carbohydrate malabsorption, no stool leukocytes
Motility — Increased motility	Decreased transit time	Loose to normal-appearing stool, stimulated by gastrocolic reflex	Irritable bowel syndrome, thyrotoxicosis, postvagotomy dumping syndrome	Infection also may contribute to increased motility
Decreased motility	Defect in neuromuscular unit(s) Stasis (bacterial overgrowth)	Loose to normal-appearing stool	Pseudo-obstruction, blind loop	Possible bacterial overgrowth
Mucosal inflammation	Inflammation, decreased mucosal surface area and/or colonic reabsorption, increased motility	Blood and increased WBCs in stool	Celiac disease, Salmonella, Shigella, amebiasis, Yersinia, Campylobacter, rotavirus enteritis	Dysentery = blood, mucus, and WBCs

VIP = vasoactive intestinal peptide; WBC = white blood cell   *Adapted from Nelson Essentials of Pediatrics ,3rd edition Philadelphia, WB Saunders,1998.*

TABLE 3 — Differential diagnosis of osmotic versus secretory diarrhea

	Osmotic diarrhea	Secretory diarrhea
Volume of stool	<200mL/24hr	>200mL/24hr
Response to fasting	Diarrhea stops	Diarrhea continues
Stool Na+	<70 mEq/L	>70 mEq/L
Reducing substances*	Positive	Negative
Stool pH	<5	>6

Sucrose is not reducing agent. Add 5 drops of 0.1 N HCI to a stool sample before adding reducing agent (clinitest tablet)

* *Pearl/Peril/Pitfall : Diarrhea and Failure to thrive and malnutrition *Reduced muscle and fat mass or peripheral edema may be clues to the presence of carbohydrate, fat, and/or protein malabsorption. *Giardia organisms can cause intermittent diarrhea and fat malabsorption.*

TABLE 4	Composition of new ORS				
New ORS	**Grams/litre**	**%**	**New ORS**		**mmol/litre**
Sodium chloride	2.6	12.683	Sodium		75
Glucose, anhydrous	13.5	65.854	Chloride		65
Potassium chloride	1.5	7.317	Glucose, anhydrous		75
Trisodium citrate, dihydrate	2.9	14.146	Potassium		20
			Citrate	10	
Total	**20.5**	**100.00**	**Total osmolarity**		**245**

TABLE 5	ORT in the management of diarrhea

No dehydration Replace stool loses with ORS* Continue age appropriate feeding.

Mild dehydration (3–5% volume loss) Repletion phase—Hydration should be restored by administering ORT at a volume of 50 mL/kg over four hours. Additional ORS is given to replace ongoing loss of stool*. Reassessment of the patient's hydration status and replacement of ongoing losses should occur at least every two hours. Maintenance phase - Once repletion is completed, feeding and fluids should be started. ORT is continued for ongoing diarrheal losses.

Moderate dehydration (6-9% volume loss) Repletion phase - Hydration should be restored by administering ORT at a volume of 100 mL/kg over four hours. Additional ORS is given to replace ongoing loss of stool*. At the end of each hour, the patient's hydration status and continuing stool and emesis losses should be calculated, with the total hourly loss added to the amount to be given over the next hour. Maintenance phase - Once repletion is completed, feeding and fluids should be started. ORT is continued for ongoing diarrheal losses.

Severe dehydration (10 % or greater volume loss.)

Repletion phase - Emergent intravenous therapy with rapid infusion of 20 mL/kg of isotonic saline should be given. As the patient's clinical condition stabilizes and his/her level of consciousness returns to normal, therapy can be changed to ORT. A nasogastric tube can be used in patients who have a normal mental status but may be too weak to adequately drink the necessary volume of fluid. The intravenous line should remain in place until it is certain there is successful transition to ORT. ORT therapy is started at a volume of 100 mL/kg over four hours. Additional ORS is given to replace ongoing loss of stool*. At the end of each hour, the patient's hydration status and continuing stool and emesis losses should be calculated, with the total hourly loss added to the amount to be given over the next hour. Maintenance phase - Once repletion is completed, feeding and fluids should be started. ORT is continued for ongoing diarrheal losses.

* 1 mL of ORS should be administered for each gram of diarrheal stool or, 10 mL/kg of body weight of ORS should be administered for each watery or loose stool, and 2 mL/kg of body weight for each episode of emesis.

Limitations of ORT use

*Altered mental status with concern for aspiration *Abdominal ileus *Underlying disorder that limits intestinal absorption of ORT (eg, short gut, carbohydrate malabsorption) * Severe dehydration *If stool output continues to be excessive, and ORT is unable to adequately rehydrate the child. *If there is severe and persistent vomiting, and inadequate intake of ORS, intravenous therapy is recommended.

Indications for shift from Low Lactose to Lactose Free Diet

1. Purge rate of more than 15 loose stools per day after 48 hours.
2. Persistence of dehydration after 48 hours of admission.
3. Loss of weight or no gain of weight despite adequate calories for two consecutive days.

KEY POINTS FOR CLINICAL PRACTICE

1. Acute diarrhea is defined as the abrupt onset of abnormally high fluid content in the stool (more than the normal value of approximately 10 mL/kg/d). This situation typically implies an increased frequency of bowel movements, which can range from 4-5 to more than 20 times per day.
2. **Several clinical signs associated with neonatal diarrhea that warrant admission and further evaluation and management include:***Bloody diarrhea. This can be a sign of a bacterial illness or an allergy (Cow's milk protein intolerance). *Moderate to severe dehydration *Child is acting lethargic (limp, and less responsive to touch or words, won't focus on mother). *Increased abdominal pain. *Continued weight loss of more than 5% of body weight.
3. It is essential to: * recognise diarrhea immediately *prevent dehydration occurring or undertake early rehydration * treat any other illness in the infant * restore adequate food intake as soon as possible and * avoid harmful and unnecessary drugs.
4. One should notify a Pediatric Surgeon , if Surgical causes of Neonatal Diarrhea are being suspected and refer those Neonates with SPUR, i.e. Severe-Persistent-Unresponsive-Recurrent types of Diarrhea to a Pediatric Gastro-enterologist.
5. Management of diarrheal disease in the Newborn requires accurate diagnosis and quick responses from health personnel and mothers, with emphasis on preventing dehydration by increasing fluid intake and on ensuring adequate calorie intake through suitable feeding. Neonates with diarrhoea should be closely monitored to ascertain those who need early referral to a hospital or other health facility.

REFERENCES & FURTHER READING : 1) King CK, Glass R, Bresee JS, Duggan C. Managing acute gastroenteritis among children: oral rehydration, maintenance, and nutritional therapy. *MMWR Recomm Rep.* Nov 21 2003;52:1-16.2)Guandalini S. Treatment of acute diarrhea in the new millennium. *J Pediatr Gastroenterol Nutr.* May 2000;30(5):486-9. 3)Coffin SE, Elser J, Marchant C, et al. Impact of acute rotavirus gastroenteritis on pediatric outpatient practices in the United States. *Pediatr Infect Dis J.* Jul 2006;25(7):584-9. 4)Sullivan PB. Nutritional management of acute diarrhea. *Nutrition.* Oct 1998;14(10):758-62. 5)Bellemare S, Hartling L, Wiebe N, et al. Oral rehydration versus intravenous therapy for treating dehydration due to gastroenteritis in children: a meta-analysis of randomised controlled trials. *BMC Med.* Apr 15 2004;2:11.

Inborn Errors of Metabolism (IEM)

@ *"Even if the disorder is not treatable, establishing the diagnosis in the index case is crucial for prenatal diagnosis in subsequent pregnancies*

* Most IEMs with acute life-threatening presentation can be categorized based on findings of initial laboratory evaluations with the presence of at least 1 of the following : * Metabolic acidosis: Metabolic acidosis usually with elevated anion gap occurs with many IEMs and is a hallmark of organic acidemias. Manifestations include tachypnea, vomiting, lethargy. *Hypoglycemia: *Hyperammonemia: Early manifestations include anorexia, abdominal pain, headache, irritability, fatigue, late-tachypnea, vomiting, lethargy, seizures, coma, and death. Ammonia level greater than 100 mcg/dL in the neonate and greater than 80 mcg/dL beyond the neonatal period is considered elevated. Ammonia is highest in the urea cycle defects often exceeding 1000 mcg/dL and causing primary respiratory alkalosis sometimes with compensatory metabolic acidosis. Ammonia in organic acidemias, if elevated, rarely exceeds 500 mcg/dL, and in fatty acid oxidation defects is usually less than 250 mcg/dL. *Major exceptions include nonketotic hyperglycinemia (lethargy, coma, seizures, hypotonia, spasticity, hiccups, apnea), and pyridoxine deficiency (encephalopathy, intractable seizures). * If a child has died, attempting to diagnose a metabolic disease is still important because of the possibility that presently asymptomatic siblings are affected or that future children will be affected. *Plasma, serum, urine, and possibly CSF, skin, and selected organ specimens should be collected and frozen. If permission for autopsy is not granted, as appropriate, discuss with the family the possibility/importance of obtaining vitreous humor, skin biopsy, and/or organ needle biopsy for evaluation. *Pictures and/or radiographs may be useful in the child with dysmorphism.

Distinguishing findings of inborn errors of metabolism with hyperammonemia

Findings	UCD	OA	FAO	MSUD
Metabolic acidosis	–	++	±	±
Respiratory alkalosis	+	–	–	–
Hypoglycemia	–	±	+	±
Ketones	Appropriate	High	Appropriate/Low	Appropriate/High
Lactic acidosis	–	±	±	±
Hyperammonemia	++	+	±	±

*UCD-urea cycle disorders; OA-organic acidemias; FAO-fatty acid oxidation disorders; MSUD-maple syrup urine disease

Adapted from Weiner, DL. Metabolic Emergencies. In: Textbook of Pediatric Emergency Medicine, 5th ed, Fleisher, GR, Ludwig, S, Henretig, FM (Eds) 2006.

In summary: The laboratory studies for any infant suspected of having an inborn error of metabolism would include: CBC with differential, urinalysis, blood gases, serum electrolytes, blood glucose, plasma ammonia, urine reducing substances, urine ketones if acidosis or hypoglycemia is present, plasma and urine amino acids (quantitative), urine organic acids, and plasma lactate. Remember to measure an ammonia level in every sick infant. When evaluating the patient with an elevated ammonia level, it helps to know if the patient is acidotic or not; normoglycemic or hypoglycemic; and ketotic or not. Hyperammonemia is a true medical emergency. TIME works against you! It is important to recognize hyperammonemia early since the neurologic insult can be devastating.

REVIEW OF CLINICAL PROBLEMS

1. Discuss the General principles of management of Inborn Errors of Metabolism .
   Ans : Refer to the Table "1" of the Chapter.

2. Mention Stage 1 level of investigations for diagnosing IEMs.
   Ans :Refer to the Table "3" of the Chapter.

3. What are the Investigations to be done for suspected inborn errors, if a child dies without a diagnosis ?
   Ans : Refer to the Table "6" of the Chapter.

4. How do you institute acute management of Hyperammonemia?
   Ans : Refer to the Table "9" of the Chapter.

5. How do you evaluate a Neonate with suspected IEM?
   Ans: Refer to the Evaluation-Decision-Action Plan/ Algorithm to diagnose & manage a Neonate with IEM.

LEARNING OBJECTIVES

After completing this article, readers will be able to:

1. Consider Inborn Errors of Metabolism *in the differential diagnosis of a severely ill Neonate/infant & undertake special studies if the index of suspicion is high.*

2. Institute acute management of IEM, while organizing transfer to a tertiary center for further evaluation and management.

3. Collect specimens for necessary investigations, *if an infant is dying or has died of what may be a metabolic disease.*

4. Prevent next sibling from being affected by Genetic counseling and Prenatal diagnosis and Neonatal Screening, where appropriate.

5. Counsel the parents about the prognosis and the clinical course and long-term management of disorder under consideration.

Pearl/Peril/Pitfall: Neonates with Inborn Errors of Metabolism are misdiagnosed to have Sepsis or other disorders;moreover Sepsis often accompanies IEM and may confound diagnosis further. While the diseases individually are rare, they collectively account for a significant proportion of neonatal and childhood morbidity and mortality. Diagnosis is important not only for treatment and prognostication but also for genetic counseling and antenatal diagnosis in subsequent pregnancies.

BIRD'S EYE VIEW/OVERVIEW/SYNOPSIS

1. Inborn Errors of Metabolism (IEM), a significant cause of mortality & morbidity in Neonates & children need early recognition & appropriate treatment. Even if the disorder is not treatable, establishing the diagnosis in the index case is crucial for prenatal diagnosis in subsequent pregnancies. Pediatricians, therefore, need to know when to suspect IEM, how to investigate it & the basis of initial management. About 100 different IEM may present clinically in the Neonatal period. Their overall incidence is as high as 1 in 2,000, although IEM are individually rare.

2. Most IEM are transmitted as autosomal recessive genetic traits. A history of parental consanguinity, unexplained neonatal deaths, or severe illness in the immediate family should alert the clinician to the possibility of an IEM. Some IEM, such as the urea cycle disorder ornithine trans-carbamylase (OTC) deficiency, are X-linked. As in any X-linked disorder, the severely affected family member could have been a maternal uncle, or a brother, or perhaps a mildly affected mother, sister, or maternal aunt.

3. *Consider an Inborn Error of Metabolism in the differential diagnosis of a severely ill Neonatal infant & undertake special studies if the index of suspicion is high.* IEM causing clinical manifestations in the Neonatal period are usually severe and are often lethal if proper therapy is not initiated promptly. Clinical findings are usually nonspecific & similar to those seen in infants with sepsis. Most Neonates with IEM are born at term and appear normal at birth. Because the infant undergoes marked endogenous fat & protein catabolism leading to a rapid accumulation of toxic metabolites, clinical illness usually becomes apparent within the first 48-72hrs of life (although some disorders may not occur until later).

4. A progressive encephalopathy is by far the most common form of presentation, although the onset of symptoms may initially be subtle with poor feeding, vomiting & lethargy. This is then followed by more severe problems such as apnea, seizures & coma. With a few exceptions, it is incorrect to believe that feeding needs to be established before an IEM becomes manifest. *Other types of presentations include* a) metabolic acidosis with tachypnea and respiratory alkalosis with hyperammonemia b)hypoglycemia (ketotic & nonketotic) c)liver dysfunction d)dysmorphism e) cardiomyopathy & arrhythmias. Refer to Table 2 for IEM disorders with an acute presentation in the Newborn period.

5. Metabolic investigations for Neonates with an acute illness are divided into 3 stages. Stage I investigations are those that would normally be undertaken in any sick child, but the results of which may point towards the diagnosis of an IEM. Stage II investigations should be undertaken if an IEM is suspected but needs to be considered early in the course of the disease. Stage III investigations are more specialized tests that may be indicated in certain situations. Refer to Tables 3,4, & 5. For children with a more slowly progressive illness, investigations will depend upon the history and clinical findings. In both cases it is extremely important to discuss the timing and method of collection of samples with the laboratory or with a specialist pediatrician.

6. Most IEMs that present in the Newborn period have late onset variants, usually because certain mutation allow for the production of enzyme with a little residual activity. Some disorders, however, even with a complete loss of enzyme function, characteristically present in late infancy or early childhood. These become manifest after an episode of metabolic stress, for example, an intercurrent infections or prolonged fasting. e.g. fatty acid oxidation defects like medium chain acyl CoA dehydrogenase deficiency. Although an acute illness is the usual manifestation of this group of inborn errors some disorders may have a more chronic & insidious onset with developmental delay and failure to thrive.

7. *The Evaluation-Decision-Action-Plan/Algorithm* provides guidelines to diagnose & manage an IEM in the Neonate. Measurements of serum ammonia, ABG analysis & blood sugar are often very helpful in differentiating major causes of IEM in the Neonate. Elevation of blood ammonia usually caused by defects of urea cycle enzymes, which have normal serum pH & bicarbonate values. Serum ammonia is also elevated but along with acidotic pH with increased anion gap in infants with certain organic acidemias. When both ammonia, pH, and bicarbonate values are normal, consider amino-acidopathies or galactosemia; galactosemic infants may also manifest cataracts, hepatomegaly, ascites, & jaundice.

8. The general principles of an acute illness due to an Inborn Error of Metabolism or listed in Table 1 which include a) Supportive care b) Reduction of load on the affected metabolic pathway c) Removal of toxic metabolites and d) Stimulation of residual enzyme activity.

9. *If an infant is dying or has died of what may be a metabolic disease, it is very important to make a specific diagnosis in order to help the parents with genetic counseling for future reproductive planning.* Table 6 lists samples that should be collected in this situation. Urine is usually the best biological material for analysis & a suprapubic bladder aspiration should be undertaken if no sample has been taken prior to death. Photographs should be taken and a full skeletal radiologic screening done of any infant with dysmorphism. A full autopsy should be done if permitted.

10. Inborn Errors of Metabolism can be prevented by prenatal diagnosis (by amniocentesis, chorionic villous biopsy and fetal liver biopsy) done by analysis of fetal DNA or gene tracking by RFLPs (Restriction Fragment Length Polymorphisms) which is possible only in a few highly specialized laboratories. Newborn screening may identify some disorders like PKU, Maple syrup urine disease, galactosemia, biotinidase deficiency & congenital adrenal hyperplasia.

Pearl/Peril/Pitfall : Clinical pointers towards an underlying IEM include · Deterioration after a period of apparent normalcy · Parental consanguinity · Family history of neonatal deaths · Rapidly progressive encephalopathy and seizures of unexplained cause · Severe metabolic acidosis · Persistent vomiting · Peculiar odor.

THE EVALUATION-DECISION-ACTION-PLAN/ALGORITHM FOR THE DIAGNOSIS AND MANAGEMENT OF *A NEONATE WITH INBORN ERROR OF METABOLISM (IEM)*

SUBJECTIVE FINDINGS

Hx of

* Unexplained sibling death, esp, male infant.

* Consanguinity of parents.

* Symptoms associated with feeding, fasting, infection, surgery.

* Improvement when milk feeds are stopped with relapse on reintroduction.

* More than one feature of an IEM present.

* Infant well in first few hours/days. Symptoms develop with the onset of intense catabolism & the introduction of feeds containing proteins.

OBJECTIVE FINDINGS

Assess ABCDs, O2 sats, BP, CRT, Urine output.

Look for facial dysmorphism, cataracts, acidotic breathing (Kussmaul's), central hyperventilation, hypotonia, seizures, lethargy, coma and failure to thrive.

Examine the skin for dermatitis & alopecia.

Note abnormal body/urine odors.

Look for jaundice, hepatomegaly in a Neonate presented with seizures & hypoglycemia.

Assess CVS for cardiomyopathy & arrhythmias in an infant with hypotonia & failure to thrive.

INVESTIGATIONS

Refer to Tables 3,4 & 5 for Stage I, Stage II & Stage III investigations for diagnosing IEM in a stepwise manner. *Smell the neonate for Key urine odors ,which may suggest a diagnosis of an inborn errors of metabolism* *Cabbage: Tyrosinemia, type I *Cat urine: 3-methylcrotonyl-CoA carboxylase deficiency *Fish: Trimethylaminuria *Hops: Oasthouse urine disease *Maple syrup: Maple syrup urine disease *"Mousy" or musty: Phenylketonuria *Sweaty feet or cheesy: Isovaleric acidemia; glutaric aciduria, type II

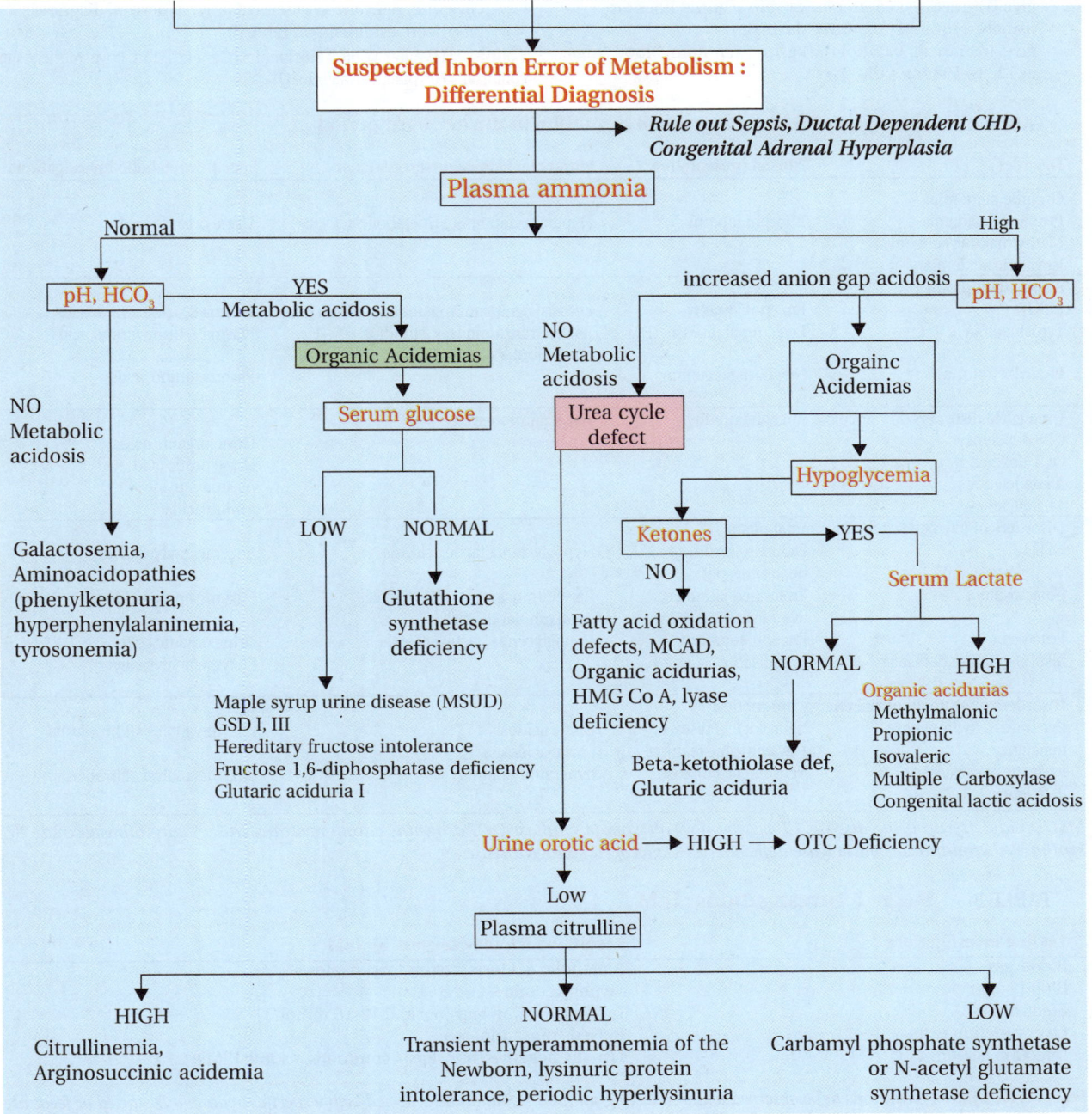

Suspected Inborn Error of Metabolism : Differential Diagnosis

→ *Rule out Sepsis, Ductal Dependent CHD, Congenital Adrenal Hyperplasia*

Plasma ammonia

Normal — High

pH, HCO₃ — YES Metabolic acidosis — increased anion gap acidosis — **pH, HCO₃**

Organic Acidemias

NO Metabolic acidosis

Orgainc Acidemias

NO Metabolic acidosis

Serum glucose

Urea cycle defect

Hypoglycemia

Galactosemia, Aminoacidopathies (phenylketonuria, hyperphenylalaninemia, tyrosonemia)

LOW — NORMAL

Ketones — YES

NO

Serum Lactate

Glutathione synthetase deficiency

Maple syrup urine disease (MSUD) GSD I, III Hereditary fructose intolerance Fructose 1,6-diphosphatase deficiency Glutaric aciduria I

Fatty acid oxidation defects, MCAD, Organic acidurias, HMG Co A, lyase deficiency

NORMAL — HIGH

Organic acidurias Methylmalonic Propionic Isovaleric Multiple Carboxylase Congenital lactic acidosis

Beta-ketothiolase def, Glutaric aciduria

Urine orotic acid → HIGH → OTC Deficiency

Low

Plasma citrulline

HIGH

Citrullinemia, Arginosuccinic acidemia

NORMAL

Transient hyperammonemia of the Newborn, lysinuric protein intolerance, periodic hyperlysinuria

LOW

Carbamyl phosphate synthetase or N-acetyl glutamate synthetase deficiency

---

* **Pearl/Peril/Pitfall :** *Abnormal Urine/Body odor is characteristic of some IEMs. MSUD- Maple syrup or Burnt sugar, Isovaleric acidemia and Glutaric aciduria type II-Sweaty feet smell, PKU-mousy/mushy, beta methyl crotonyl aciduria-tom cat urine, Methionine malabsorption-cabbage, Trimethyl aminuria-rotten fish, Tyrosenemia-rancid/fishy odor.*

TABLE 1 — General principles of management of acute illness due to an inborn error of metabolism

1. Supportive care

- intensive care is often necessary
- establish arterial and central venous access
- maintain adequate respiratory support(assisted ventilation should be considered early)
- correct hypothermia, hypoglycemia and dehydration
- treat cerebral oedema if present
- correct significant metabolic acidosis with intravenous sodium bicarbonate (0.5-2 mmol/h)
- monitor electrolytes and blood gases
- treat with antibiotics as septicemia is commonly associated with metabolic decompensation.

2. Reduce load on the affected metabolic pathway

- stop all exogenous protein
- give IV glucose at 5-10 mg/kg/min (central lines are usually required for >10% dextrose)
- give insulin at 0.05-0.1 U/kg/hr (maintain blood sugar at 126 to 198 mg / dL)

3. Removal of toxic metabolites

- give IV 1-carnitine at 100-200 mg/kg/day (but may be contraindicated in certain fat oxidation defects)
- maintain adequate urine output if possible)
- dialysis may be required if poor urine output, hypernatremia, metabolic acidosis. or in order to remove specific toxic substrates or metabolites (for example ammonia in urea cycle disorders or organic acidemias. leucine in maple syrup urine disease. propionate in propionic acidemia). Hemodialysis is usually the most effective method.

4. Stimulation of residual enzyme activity

- Give the relevant co-factor(if any) where a diagnosis has been established (Table 6)

Courtesy: J H Walter. Willink Biochemical Genetics Unit, Royal Manchester Children's Hospital, Pendlebury,UK

TABLE 2 — Examples of IEM with acute presentation in the newborn period

Disorder	Clinical presentation	Initial biochemical investigations	Specific metabolic investigations
Organic acidemias			
Propionic acidemia	Encephalopathy	Hyperammonemia ± metabolic acidosis	Urine organic acids
Methylmalonic acidemia			
Isovaleric acidemia			
Aminoacidopathies			
MSUD	Encephalopathy	Ketosis(significant metabolic acidosis rare)	Plasma & urine aminoacids
Tyrosinaemia	Liver/renal disease	Raised transaminases, jaundice, renal tubular disease	Plasma & urine amino acids
Phenylketonuria	Newborn screening		Plasma amino acids
Urea cycle disorders	Encephalopathy	Hyperammonemia	
CPS deficiency			Urine organic acids
OCT deficiency			Urine orotic acid
AS deficiency			plasma & urine
AL deficiency			Amino acids
Disorders of glucose & galactose metabolism			
GSD I	Failure to thrive, hepatomegaly	Hypoglycemia,lactic acidosis	Enzyme analysis(liver)
Galactosemia	Prolonged jaundice, liver disease, sepsis	Raised transaminases, jaundice, renal tubular disease	Enzyme analysis(blood)
Fructose 1,6-bisphosphatase deficiency	Encephalopathy, liver disease	Hypoglycemia, lactic acidosis	Urine organic acids Enzyme analysis(liver)
Disorders of mitochondrial energy production			
Pyruvate dehydrogenase deficiency	Neurological disease, ± dysmorphic features	Lactic acidosis	Enzyme analysis(fibroblasts)
Pyruvate carboxylase deficiency	Neurological disease	Lactic acidosis, hyperammonemia	Enzyme analysis(fibroblasts)

MSUD:maple syrup urine disease; CPS:carbamoyl phosphate synthase;OCT:ornithine carbamoyltransferase:AS:argininosuccinate synthase;AL:argininosuccinate lyase deficiency;GSD:glycogen storage disease.

TABLE 3 — Stage 1 Investigations : IEM

1st line investigations	Results which may suggest an IEM
Blood gas	Metabolic acidosis/respiratory alkalosis
Blood sugar	Hypoglycemia
Electrolytes	Increased anion gap (normal 12-16 mmol/1)
Liver function tests	Raised transaminases
Infection screen	Usually negative (but sepsis common in some IEMs)

Pearl/Peril/Pitfall : Precautions to be observed while collecting samples 1. Should be collected before specific treatment is started or feeds are stopped, as may be falsely normal if the child is off feeds. 2. Samples for blood ammonia and lactate should be transported in ice and immediately tested. Lactate sample should be arterial and should be collected after 2 hrs fasting in a preheparinized syringe. Ammonia sample is to be collected approximately after 2 hours of fasting in EDTA vacutainer. Avoid air mixing. Sample should be free flowing. 3. Detailed history including drug details should be provided to the lab. (sodium valproate therapy may increase ammonia levels).

| TABLE 4 | Stage 2 Investigations : IEM | Courtesy: J H Walter. Willink Biochemical Genetics Unit, Royal Manchester Children's Hospital, Pendlebury,UK |

2nd line investigations	Indications	Comments
Blood ammonia	Encephalopathy	Normal <80mmol/1(usually > 200 in organic acidemia,>500 in urea cycle disorder)
Blood lactate	Encephalopathy,acidosis, unexplained multi-system disorder	Normal <2.5 mmol/1(exclude poor tissue perfusion and cardiac disease)
Insulin,c-peptide,growth hormone, cortisol	Hypoglycemia	Endogenous hyperinsulinism, surreptitious insulin injection and other endocrine causes of hypoglycemia
Urine reducing substances	Liver/renal disease	Unreliable for diagnosis of galactosemia
Urine ketones	Encephalopathy, hypoglycemia, metabolic acidosis	Ketosis unusual in newborn, suggests IEM. Hypoketosis in older infants with hypoglycemia suggests disorder of fatty acid oxidation or hyperinsulinism
Urine/plasma amino acids	Encephalopathy, hyperammonemia, hypoglycemia, metabolic acidosis	Aminoacidoathies, characterization of urea cycle disorders
Urine organic acids	Encephalopathy, hyperammonemia, hypoglycemia, metabolic acidosis	Fat oxidation defects (only reliable during acute metabolic decompensation) and organic acidemias
Urine orotic acid	Hyperammonemia	OCT deficiency
Beutler test	Liver disease	Screening test for galactosemia, unreliable if blood transfusion within 3 months
Urine succinylacetone	Liver disease	Specific test for tyrosinemia
Alpha$_1$ antitrypsin	Liver disease	
Plasma carnitine	Encephalopathy, hyperammonemia, hypoglycemia, metabolic acidosis, cardiomyopathy, liver disease	Primary and secondary carnitine deficiencies
CSF lactate	Encephalopathy, fits	Unexplained neurological disease.>2.5 mmol/1 suggests disorder of mitochondrial energy metabolism
Very long chain fatty acids, DHAP-AT	Unexplained neurological disease, particularly if associated with dysmorphic features	Peroxisomal disorders
Transferrin iso-electric focusing	Unexplained multi-system disorder	Carbohydrate deficient glycoprotein syndrome
Urine mucopolysaccharides and oligosaccharides	Chronic progressive neurological disease, organomegaly, certain dysmorphic features	Screening test for some lysosomal disorders

| TABLE 5 | Stage 3 Investigations : IEM |

3rd line investigations	Comments
DNA analysis	For specific mutation analysis(if available). Consult specialist laboratory.
Enzyme assays	For specific disorders. Tissue required dependent upon suspected disorder. Consult specialist laboratory

| TABLE 6 | Investigations for suspected inborn errors, if child dies without a diagnosis |

3rd line investigations	Comments
5 ml red cells at +4° C 5 ml plasma at-20° C 10-20 ml urine at-20° C Skin biopsy for fibroblast culture (collect into skin biopsy medium) Muscle & liver biopsy Post-mortem	Consult specialist laboratory to discuss analysis of samples. skin should be taken after cleaning to prevent bacterial contamination. Muscle and liver samples should be collected for histology (consult pathology laboratory), and put into liquid nitrogen for enzyme analyses. Samples taken prior to or immediately after death are most suitable.

| TABLE 7 | Examples of disorders for which co-factor responsive variants have been described |

Disorder	Co-factor	Therapeutic dose	Frequency of responsive variants
Methylmalonic acidemia	Vitamin B$_{12}$	1 mg IM weekly	Some (usually partial response)
Biotinidase deficiency	Biotin	5–10 mg/d	All cases
Multiple carboxylase deficiency	Biotin	10–40 mg/d	Most
Glutaric aciduria type II	Riboflavin	20–40 mg/d	Rare
Homocystinuria	Pyridoxine	50–500 mg/d	Approximately 50%
Carnitine transporter defect	Carnitine	100 mg/kg/d	All
MSUD	Thiamine	10–50 mg/d	Rare
Respiratory chain disorders	Ubiquinone	100–300 mg/d	Anecdotal evidence

Pearl/Peril/Pitfall: Genetic counseling and prenatal diagnosis: Most of the IEM are single gene defects, inherited in an autosomal recessive manner, with a 25% recurrence risk. Therefore when the diagnosis is known and confirmed in the index case, prenatal diagnosis can be offered, wherever available for the subsequent pregnancies.

TABLE 8	Acute management of hypoglycemia

1. Insert IV cannula (central venous access is required for persistent hypoglycemia)
2. Collect 5 ml blood for investigations(1 ml fluoride, 2 ml heparin, 2 ml clotted.
3. If symptomatic give bolus dose of 10% dextrose of 2 ml/kg(200 mg/kg) over 5 min.
4. Start infusion of 10% dextrose at 4 ml/kg/hr(~7mg/kg/min).
5. Re-check glucose after 15 min. Increase infusion rate to 8 ml/kg/hr of 10% dextrose(~13 mg/kg/min of glucose) if still hypoglycemic.(higher rates will be required for hyperinsulinism).
6. Collect the next available urine specimen for organic acid analysis.

TABLE 9	Acute management of hyperammonemia (NH_4^+ >120m mol/1)

1. Stop all exogenous protein

2. Inhibit endogenous catabolism
   - correct metabolic acidosis if present
   - give maintenance fluids as 10%-15% glucose (aim for blood sugars of 126 - 180 mg/dL)
   Combine with continuous insulin infusion at 0.05-0.1 U/kg/hr

3. Intravenous medication. Start if ammonia>180 mmol/1

	Sodium benzoate mg/kg	Sodium phenylbutyrate mg/kg	Arginine 10% mg/kg(ml/kg)	L-Carnitine mg/kg
Priming infusion (Make up in 30 ml/kg of 10% glucose and give over 90 min)	250	250	200(2)	
Maintenance (Make up in 30 ml/kg of 10% glucose and give as continuous infusion over 24 h) Monitor NH_4^+ , sodium,potassium and blood gases ever 4-8 h	250	250	200(2)	100-200

4. Dialysis. For ammonia levels> 400mmol/1, or if <400 mmol/1 but with no decrease after 4 h of intravenous medication. Hemodialysis is preferable (better clearance of NH_4^+) but if not available peritoneal dialysis or hemofiltration should be used. Dialysis will also remove toxic metabolites that accumulate in organic acidemias.

5. Patients with urea cycle disorders will need to continue on oral medication following recovery.Supportive care: treatment of sepsis, seizures, ventilation. Avoid sodium valproate. Courtesy: J H Walter. Willink Biochemical Genetics Unit, Royal Manchester Children's Hospital, Pendlebury,UK

KEY POINTS FOR CLINICAL PRACTICE:

1. Inborn Errors of Metabolism (IEM) are a significant cause of mortality & morbidity in Neonates & infants, but with early recognition & appropriate treatment the outcome for many disorders can be good.

2. Specific diagnosis, even in an infant in whom death seems inevitable, is of great importance for genetic counseling (including prenatal diagnosis) of the family; every effort should be made to determine the diagnosis while the infant is alive, because postmortem examination is not always helpful.

3. A specific diagnosis may be established by measurement of abnormal metabolites in body fluids, by assay of the specific enzyme activity, or by identification of the mutant gene.

4. Since most disorders of IEM are autosomal recessive in inheritance, a family history is usually absent but parental consanguinity & a similar clinical illness in other family members increases the likelihood of an inherited disorder being present.

5. Inborn Errors of Metabolism present with nonspecific symptoms & signs often in the Neonatal period, & mimic more common acquired conditions such as infections (sepsis & meningitis), heart diseases, asphyxia & hyperinsulinemia. The key to the early diagnosis & management of IEM is to have a high index of suspicion.

REFERENCES & FURTHER READING : 1) Investigation and initial management of suspected metabolic disease by JH. Walter (1997 Current Pediatrics U.K). 2) Nelson Text Book of Pediatrics -18th edition. 3) Pediatric Acute Care- 2nd edition- Lippincott. 4) Inherited Metabolic Diseases, Holton.J (ed). Edinburgh, Churchill Livingstone. 1994. 5) Physician's Guide to the Lab Diagnosis of Metabolic Diseases- Blau.N, Duran.M, London: Clapman & Hall medical, 1996.

Pearl/Peril/Pitfall : Most of the IEMs are Autosomal Recessive in inheritance except OTC Deficiency, Fabry`s disease,Menkes and Hunter`s diseases which are X-linked Recessive in nature.

Pearl/Peril/Pitfall : IEM should be considered in the differential diagnosis of any sick neonate along with common acquired causes such as sepsis, hypoxic-ischemic encephalopathy, duct-dependant cardiac lesions, congenital adrenal hyperplasia and congenital infections.

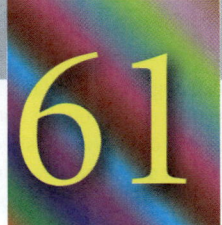

Congenital Hypothyroidism

@ Congenital Hypothyroidism—Presentation *The usual mode of presentation is by the presence of an elevated TSH detected on the 48-72 hour screen (except in secondary or tertiary disease) *Neonates are often subclinically affected and only detected on routine screening *clinical features include: ·dry skin ·hoarse cry ·puffy face ·prominent tongue ·listless ·umbilical hernia ·hypothermia ·bradycardia ·failure to thrive *Neonates may also present with jaundice due to an unconjugated hyperbilirubinemia (glucuronyl transferase deficiency).*

Hypothalamo-pituitary-thyroid axis

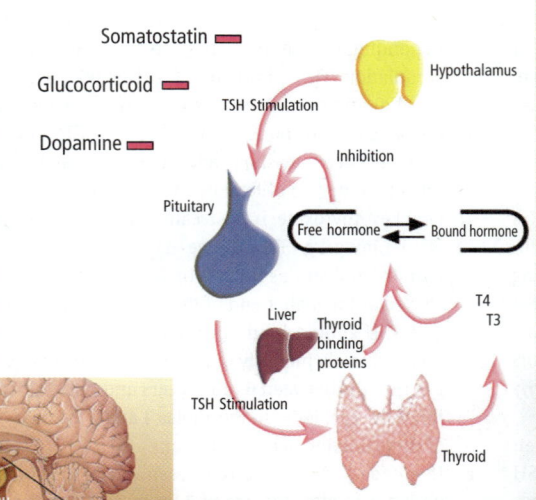

THYROID REGULATION

Somatostatin —
Glucocorticoid —
Dopamine —

TSH Stimulation
Inhibition
Hypothalamus
Pituitary
Free hormone ⇌ Bound hormone
Liver
Thyroid binding proteins
T4
T3
TSH Stimulation
Thyroid

"5–8% of affected infants can escape detection by screening because of errors in sample collection or laboratory routine, and _an awareness of early symptoms and signs must be maintained_."

TRH
Hypothalamus
Pituitary Gland
TSH
Thyroid Gland
T₃ & T₄

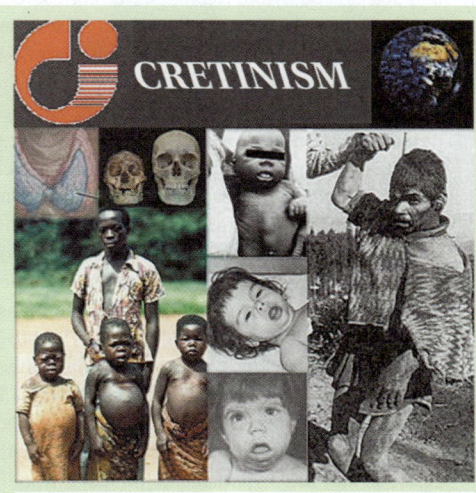

CRETINISM

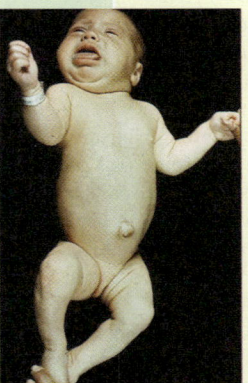

Congenital hypothyroidism

- Incidence 1 in 3,000
- One of the most common *treatable* causes of mental retardation
- Because newborns are asymptomatic at birth, screening programs developed worldwide

REVIEW OF CLINICAL PROBLEMS

1. How do you diagnose Congenital Hypothyroidism?
   Ans: Refer to the "No. 1" of the "BIRD'S EYE VIEW/OVER VIEW/ SYNOPSIS" of the Chapter.

2. What are the "early symptoms and signs" should you assess for a suspected Congenital Hypothyroidism?
   Ans: Refer to the the Table 2 of the Chapter.

3. What are the "objective findings" should you search for in an infant with suspected Congenital Hypothyroidism?
   Ans: Refer to the Evaluation-Decision-Action Plan/Algorithm to diagnose & manage Congenital Hypothyroidism.

4. Mention the "essential investigations" to evaluate Congenital Hypothyroidism?
   Ans: Refer to the Table 3 of the Chapter.

5. How do you manage Congenital Hypothyroidism?
   Ans: Refer to the Nos. 7, 8, 9 and 10 of the "BIRD'S EYE VIEW/ OVERVIEW/SYNOPSIS" of the Chapter. Also refer to the Tables No 4 and 5 of the Chapter.

LEARNING OBJECTIVES

After completing this article, readers will be able to:

1. Ensure appropriate neonatal screening for congenital hypothyroidism.

2. Recognize abnormal screening tests, and perform laboratory evaluation on all infants with possible congenital hypothyroidism.

3. Recognize signs and symptoms of congenital hypothyroidism.

4. Ensure *timely and appropriate* treatment of infants with congenital hypothyroidism, with the assistance of or a referral to a Pediatric endocrinologist.

5. Ensure *adequate follow-up* of infants with Congenital Hypothyroidism.

* **Pearl/Peril/Pitfall :** Congenital Hypothyroidism: The incidence is 1 in 3000-3500 with some geographic variation. ·75% due to dysgenesis -agenesis -ectopia ·10% due to dyshormonogenesis-often autosomal recessive -Pendred's syndrome = peroxidase deficiency associated with sensorineural deafness ·5% due to hypothalamic-pituitary (H-P) deficiency -secondary hypothyroidism -tertiary hypothyroidism ·10% due to intrauterine causes -iodine exposure -maternal antithyroid antibodies.

BIRD'S EYE VIEW/OVERVIEW/SYNOPSIS

1. Most Newborn infants with Congenital Hypothyroidism are asymptomatic at birth, even if there is complete agenesis of the Thyroid gland, possibly because of transplacental passage of moderate amounts of maternal T4, which provides fetal levels(approximately 33% of normal at birth);these low serum T4 and concomitantly elevated levels of TSH make it possible to screen and detect hypothyroid Neonates. Newborn Screening is done on the filter paper blood spots collected at 2-5 days of age, as the serum TSH levels normally elevated during the first 24-48 hours of life due to Neonatal TSH surge. It was introduced in the early 1970s in the developed world and was remarkably successful in the early detection of infants with the classic types of Congenital Hypothyroidism, allowing treatment in a timely fashion and preventing mental retardation. A serum T4 of <7micro gm/dL or 90 nmol/L, with a serumTSH in excess of 20 micro IU/mL or 20 m IU/L, at 3-5 days of life suggests Congenital Hypothyroidism. All infants with suspicious screening tests must be confirmed by measurement of serum T4 and TSH concentrations.After 7 days of age,a serum T4 of <6micro gm/dL, with a TSH of >50micro IU/mL or 50 m IU/L indicates primary Congenital Hypothyroidism. A serum T4 in the range of 6-11micro gm/dL with a TSH level of 20-50micro IU/mL or 20- 50 m IU/L is suggestive, and repeat testing is necessary. This approach misses infants with delayed TSH elevation and with hypothalamic/pituitary hypothyroidism. *5-8% of affected infants can escape detection by screening because of errors in sample collection or laboratory routine, and an awareness of early symptoms and signs must be maintained.*

2. Transient conditions of Neonatal hypothyroidism are seen frequently in sick or preterm infants. These include maternal TSH Receptor blocking antibodies, maternal exposure to iodine-containing compounds, Down syndrome and prematurity. Premature infants <28 wk of gestation may have problems resulting from a combination of immaturity of the hypothalamic-pituitary-thyroid axis and loss of maternal contribution of thyroid hormone and so may be candidates for temporary thyroid hormone replacement;further studies are needed.

3. Most cases of Congenital Hypothyroidism are not hereditary and result from thyroid dysgenesis (75-85% of cases). 10% of cases may be familial, usually caused by an inborn error of thyroxine hormone synthesis. 5% of cases are the result of transplacental passage of maternal TRB(blocking)Ab also known as (TBII(Thyroid Binding Inhibitory Immunoglobulin).

4. In about 1/3rd of cases of Thyroid dysgenesis, even sensitive radionuclide scans can find no remnants of thyroid tissue(aplasia) and other 2/3rds of them, rudiments of thyroid tissue are found in an ectopic location, anywhere from the base of the tongue (lingual thyroid) to the normal position in the neck (hypoplasia). The exact cause of thyroid dysgenesis is unknown in most cases;occurs sporadically, but may be familial with genetic component.

5. The early and late clinical features of Congenital Hypothyroidism are given in the Table 2 of the Chapter; infants with low thyroxine levels are more likely to have clinical signs such as lethargy, feeding difficulties, prolonged jaundice, umbilical hernia, and macro-glossia. Such infants are more likely to have an aplastic rather than hypoplastic or ectopic gland. A gestation over 40 weeks,, induction of labor,and a birth weight > 3,500g are all more common.

6. *The Evaluation-Decision-Action- Plan/Algorithm* describes the essential aspects of the diagnosis and management of Congenital Hypothyroidism. 123 I-sodium iodide isotope scintigraphy can help to pinpoint the underlying cause in infants with Congenital Hypothyroidism,but treatment should not be unduly delayed for this study. Isotope uptake into a normally sited gland usually indicates the presence of one of the recessively-inherited thyroxine biosynthetic defects, while absent uptake in the normal site usually indicates thyroid agenesis/hypoplasia and sublingual uptake indicates ectopic thyroid tissue. Transient hypothyroidism due to maternal antibodies is also associated with absent uptake of isotope. Ultrasound of thyroid gland is useful to confirm the presence of normally sited thyroid tissue, but is less helpful in identifying sublingual thyroid tissue or confirming agenesis or hypoplasia of the gland. Thyroglobulin levels will be low in agenesis or thyroxine synthetic defects and elevated in thyroid dysgenesis, depending on the quantity of thyroid tissue and degree of TSH stimulation. TRH stimulation test;TSH release measured at 30, 60 and 120 minutes will show a subnormal response in Pituitary CH and a delayed response in hypothalamic CH. Bone age evaluation by X-ray knee may show delay in epiphyseal maturation and may reflect the degree of fetal hypothyroidism.

7. Oral Levothyroxine, is the treatment of choice;initial starting dose is 10-15mcg/kg (37.5-50mcg/day). Newborns with more severe hypothyroidism, as judged by a serum T4<3mcg/dL, should be started at the higher end of the dosage range. Levels of T4/free T4 and TSH should be monitored at recommended intervals, i.e. approximately monthly in the 1st 6 months of life, and then every 2–3 months between 6 mo-2 years and maintained in the normal range for age. Refer to the Tables 4 and 5 for dose and monitoring of thyroxine replacement therapy.

8. If needed, definitive reassessment of thyroid status can be undertaken after the age of 2 years, to rule out the possibility of transient hypothyroidism,when brief cessation of therapy will have no adverse effect. Discontinuation of therapy for 4 weeks results in a marked increase in TSH levels in children with permanent hypothyroidism. This reassessment of thyroid status is unnecessary in infants with proven thyroid ectopia or in those who manifest elevated levels of TSH after 6-12 mo of therapy because of poor compliance or an inadequate dose of T4.

9. Prompt, early thyroxine replacement, close monitoring, and maintenance of T4 levels in the upper half of reference range has significantly improved neurodevelopment, even in the most severe cases of CH. Subtle neurocognitive deficits may persist, including poor visuospatial abilities, attention, and memory skills,despite early therapy.

10. A formal hearing assessment is recommended in the hypothyroid infant because of the 10 fold increase in the hearing loss in these babies.

Summary of Management of Congenital Hypothyroidism (CH)

Initial work-up: Detailed history and physical examination. Referral to pediatric endocrinologist. Recheck serum TSH and FT4, Thyroid ultrasonography and/or thyroid scan

Medications: L-T4: 10–15 micro gram/kg by mouth once daily

Monitoring: Recheck T4, TSH, 2–4 wk after initial treatment is begun, Every 1–2 mo in the first 6 mo. Every 3–4 mo between 6 mo and 3 y of age. Every 6–12 mo from 3 y of age to end of growth

Goal of therapy: Normalize TSH and maintain T4 and FT4 in upper half of reference range, Assess permanence of CH

If initial thyroid scan shows ectopic/absent gland, CH is permanent. If initial TSH is <50 mU/L and there is no increase in TSH after newborn period, then trial off therapy at 3 y of age. If TSH increases off therapy, consider permanent CH

Pearl/Peril/Pitfall: Gene mutations have been implicated in all forms of congenital hypothyroidism and in some cases result in an expanded phenotype including respiratory distress, choanal atresia, renal malformation and mental delay (independent of degree of hypothyroidism).

THE EVALUATION-DECISION-ACTION-PLAN/ALGORITHM FOR THE DIAGNOSIS AND MANAGEMENT OF *CONGENITAL HYPOTHYROIDISM*

SUBJECTIVE FINDINGS

Newborn screening for T4 & TSH at days 3–5 should be done for all Newborn infants, as infants with Congenital Hypothyroidism are born with little or no clinical evidence of thyroid hormone deficiency. Laboratory errors occur, however, and awareness of early symptoms and signs must be maintained, with a high index of suspicion mandatory due to non-specific presentation.

History of-early symptoms suggestive of Neonatal hypothyroidism-sleepy, placid baby with poor feeding and choking spells during nursing,apneic episodes,noisy respirations, nasal obstruction, typical RDS picture as well, cry little(parental impression:"good baby"), constipation. abdominal distention,umbilical hernia, prolonged jaundice, transient hypothermia *Maternal history of* Graves disease with hyperthyroidism and may have been treated with PTU, methimazole, ^{131}I, iodides, or surgery, History of Hashimoto disease

History of Previous cases of Neonatal hypothyroidism in the family

OBJECTIVE FINDINGS

Assess ABCDs and monitor CRT, O_2 sats, BP, core-peripheral temperature difference, RR, HR, central & peripheral pulses, urine output

Look for goitre(Most neonatal goitres result from maternal ingestion of goitrogens/iodine deficiency), large, Anterior, and, Posterior, fontanelle (>5mm), pallor, perioral cyanosis, jaundice, subnormal temperature<35⁰C, cold mottled skin, respiratory distress, hoarse cry, noisy respirations and/or apneas

Late signs (After 6 weeks) Typical cretin facies; depressed nasal bridge,narrow forehead, puffy eyelids, large tongue, large patent fontanelle, thick dry coarse skin, coarse hair, hyporeflexia, bradycardia, anemia, growth failure, delayed development (Table 2)

Assess for the associated congenital anomalies; cardiac, neurologic, ophthalmic-occur in 10% of infants with Congenital Hypothyroidism.

Look for micropenis,refractory hypoglycemia, cleft lip/palate, hypospadias or nystagmus, if secondary/tertiary hypothyroidism is suspected.

INVESTIGATIONS

Blood FBC, TC, DC, **Hct**, Platelets, CRP, Blood cultures, **LFTs, ABG analysis, electrolytes,** calcium & magnesium, **blood sugar**, creatinine, BUN, coagulation profile. (for general management of any sick neonate)

Refer to Table 3 for **LABORATORY EVALUATION OF CONGENITAL HYPOTHYROIDISM**

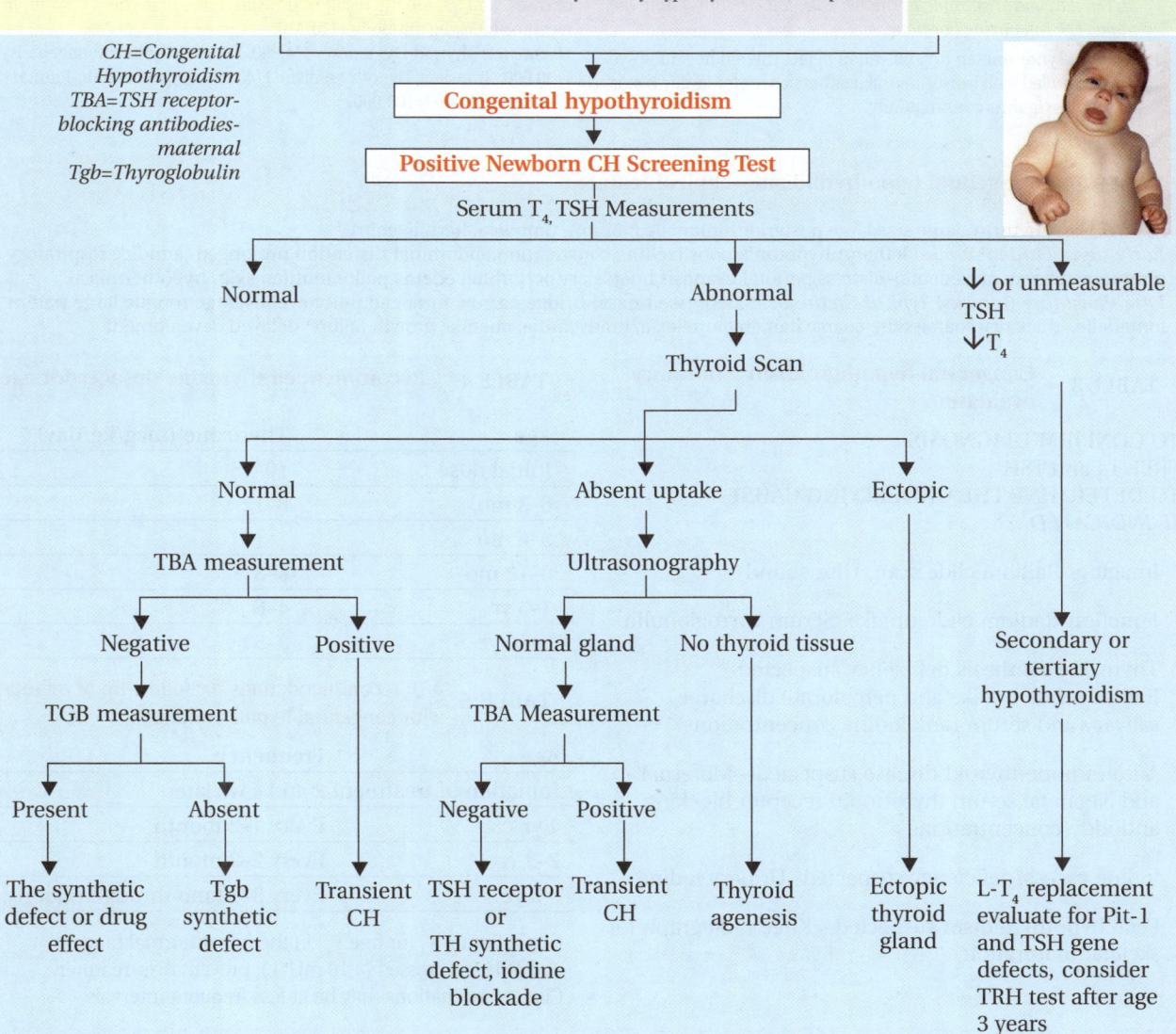

CH=Congenital Hypothyroidism
TBA=TSH receptor-blocking antibodies-maternal
Tgb=Thyroglobulin

Congenital hypothyroidism

Positive Newborn CH Screening Test

Serum T_4, TSH Measurements

- Normal
- Abnormal → Thyroid Scan
- ↓ or unmeasurable TSH ↓T_4

Thyroid Scan:
- Normal → TBA measurement
- Absent uptake → Ultrasonography
- Ectopic

TBA measurement:
- Negative → TGB measurement
- Positive → Transient CH

TGB measurement:
- Present → The synthetic defect or drug effect
- Absent → Tgb synthetic defect

Ultrasonography:
- Normal gland → TBA Measurement
- No thyroid tissue → Thyroid agenesis

TBA Measurement:
- Negative → TSH receptor or TH synthetic defect, iodine blockade
- Positive → Transient CH

Ectopic → Ectopic thyroid gland

↓ or unmeasurable TSH → Secondary or tertiary hypothyroidism → L-T_4 replacement evaluate for Pit-1 and TSH gene defects, consider TRH test after age 3 years

---

* *Pearl/Peril/Pitfall:* Congenital Hypothyroidism-Confirmatory investigations include·T4 and TSH levels ·thyroid scan (showing absent, lingual or increased uptake of radioisotope) ·X-ray distal femoral epiphysis (absence implying prolonged/prenatal hypothyroidism) ·assessment and imaging of pituitary gland, if indicated.

| TABLE 1 | Etiologic classification of congenital hypothyroidism |

Primary hypothyroidism
  Defect of fetal thyroid development
    Aplasia, hypoplasia, ectopia (dysgenesis)
  Defect in thyroid hormone synthesis (AR inheritance)
  (e.g. goitrous hypothyroidism)
    Iodide transport defect
    Thyroid peroxidase defect
        Thyroid oxidase mutations:homozygotic-permanent;heterozygotic-transient
    Thyroglobulin synthesis defect
    Deiodination defect
  Defect in thyroid hormone transport
  Iodine deficiency (endemic goiter)
    Neurologic type
    Myxedematous type
  Maternal antibodies
    Thyrotropin receptor-blocking antibody (TRBAb, also termed thyrotropin-binding inhibitor immunoglobulin)
  Maternal Medications
    Radioiodine, iodides
    Propylthiouracil, methimazole
    Amiodarone
ACTH, adrenocorticotropic hormone; FSH, follicle-stimulating hormone; LH, luteinizing hormone.

Pendred syndrome-an organification defect thyroid hormone synthesis coupled with sensorineural deafness;check for family history of deafness/goitre/consanguinity.

Central (hypopituitary) hypothyroidism
PIT-1 mutations
Deficiency of thyrotropin (TSH), growth hormone, and prolactin
PROP-1 mutations
Deficiency of TSH, growth hormone, prolactin, LH, FSH, ± ACTH
Thyrotropin-releasing hormone (TRH) deficiency
        Isolated?
        Multiple hypothalamic deficiencies (e.g., septo-optic dysplasia)
TRH unresponsiveness
        Mutations in TRH receptor
TSH deficiency
        Mutations in b - chain
Multiple pituitary deficiencies (e.g. craniopharyngioma)
TSH unresponsiveness
        G_s a mutation (e.g., type 1A pseudohypoparathyroidism)
        Mutation in TSH receptor
*Thyroid Dysgenesis- aplasia,hypoplasia(1/3rd), ectopic gland (2/3rds) is the most common cause of Congenital Hypothyroidism,accounting for 85% of cases. The exact cause of it is unknown in most cases. It occurs sporadically, but familial cases have been reported occasionally. *Defect in thyroid hormone synthesis, an inborn error is responsible for it in 10% of cases, and 5% are the result of transplacental maternal Thyrotropin receptor-blocking antibody (TRBAb).*
Incidence: Thyroid Dysgenesis-1/4,000, Thyroid Dyshormonogenesis-1/30,000, Transient Hypothyroidism-1/40,000, Hypothalamic-Pituitary Hypothyroidism-1/100,000.

| TABLE 2 | Congenital hypothyroidism—clinical features |

At birth: Postmaturity, large size,large posterior fontanelle (>5mm), umbilical hernia, goitre
Early signs(within 6 weeks) lethargy,hypotonia,poor feeding,constipation,abdominal distention,prolonged jaundice,respiratory symptoms(airway myxedema)-distress,perioral cyanosis,hoarse cry,periorbital edema,pallor,mottled skin, hypothermia
Late signs(after 6 weeks) Typical Cretin facies;depressed nasal bridge,narrow forehead,puffy eyelids,large tongue,large patent fontanelle, thick dry coarse skin, coarse hair, hyporeflexia, bradycardia, anemia, growth failure, delayed development

| TABLE 3 | Congenital hypothyroidism laboratory evaluation |

TO CONFIRM DIAGNOSIS
FREE T4 and TSH
TO DETERMINE THE UNDERLYING CAUSE-
IF INDICATED

* Imaging- Radionuclide scan, Ultrasound

* Function-Radionuclide uptake, Serum thyroglobulin

* Thyroxine synthesis deficiency suspected-Radionuclide uptake and perchlorate discharge, salivary and serum radioiodine concentrations

* Autoimmune thyroid disease suspected—Maternal and Neonatal serum thyrotropin receptor blocking antibody concentrations

* Iodine excess/deficiency suspected- Urinary iodine

* Fetal hypothyroidism suspected—Knee radiograph for skeletal maturation

| TABLE 4 | Recommended thyroxine dosages for age |

Age	Thyroxine (mcg/kg/day)
Initial dose	10–15
0–3 mo	8–12
3–6 mo	7–10
6–12 mo	6–8
1–3 yr	4–6
3–10 yr	3–5

| TABLE 5 | AAP recommendations for follow-up of infants with congenital hypothyroidism |

Age	Frequency
Initiation of treatment 2 and 4 wk later	
1 yr	Every 1–2 month
2–3 yr	Every 2–3 month
> 3 yr	Every 3–12 mo through puberty

Goals: Serum T_4 (or free T_4) in the upper normal range and TSH suppressed (< 10 mU/L), prevent overtreatment, Clinical evaluations may be at less frequent intervals

* **Pearl/Peril/Pitfall:** *Congenital Hypothyroidism—Management Thyroxine replacement therapy should be commenced as soon as possible at a dose of 8–10 microgram/kg/day in a single daily dose. Tablets should be ground up between two teaspoons and mixed with a few drops of milk. This solution should be transferred to a small, plastic feeding spoon and deposited on the back of the tongue immediately prior to feeds.*

Transient Neonatal Hypothyroidism: This group of conditions can be subdivided into 4 main categories. Cause and biochemical profiles are as follows.

Transient Hypothyroxinemia
Immaturity of H-P axis (<30 wks gest'n)
- low serum T4 levels seen in approx. 50% of infants delivered before 30 weeks gestation
- normal or low TSH levels
- corrects spontaneously over 4-8 weeks
- no treatment required

Transient primary hypothyroidism -Maternal anti- hypothyroidism thyroid therapy, iodine deficiency, maternal Ab's, idiopathic
- low serum T4 levels and high TSH levels
- seen in approx. 20% of premature infants (incidence increases as gestation decreases)

- usually develops within 1-2 weeks ex-utero and often superimposed upon transient hypothyroxinemia
- repeated screening cards should be sent on all infants <30 wks (test at 48 hrs and then again at 28 days)
- hypothyroidism may persist for 2-3 months treatment recommended

Transient hyperthyrotropinemia -Erroneous assay, iodine deficiency or excess, idiopathic
- rare (1 in 16-19,000 births)
- elevated TSH for 3-9 months before reducing spontaneously
- no treatment required but need careful follow-up to exclude partial dyshormonogenesis or ectopia

Low T3/T4 syndrome ("sick euthyroid") -Prematurity, (In preterm infants) surgical stress, sepsis, malnutrition-no treatment required

Courtesy: http://www.rch.org.au/nets/ handbook/index.cfm?doc_id=819

	T3	T4	TSH
Low T3 syndrome	decreased	Normal	Normal
Low T4 syndrome	decreased	decreased	Normal

Preterm baby & Thyroid Function: When a baby is born preterm, the level of T4 is lower than that of term babies and correlates with gestational age and birth weight. Levels of TSH and T3 are normal to low, free T4 concentrations are also low, and thyroglobulin levels are high (reflecting increased thyroid gland production of poorly iodinated thyroid hormone precursor). Responses of TSH and T3 to TRH are normal, reflecting that the site of *immaturity is the hypothalamus.* In addition, hypothyroxinemia is in part secondary to reduced levels of thyroid binding globulin. These data would suggest that the hypothyroxinemia of prematurity is physiological. The more preterm the baby the more pronounced is this hypothyroxinemia. Although there is an increase in the incidence of transient primary hypothyroidism in these babies (when the TSH level is also raised), in the majority, the hypothyroxinemia is associated with a normal TSH level. The severity of the neonatal illness is also reflected in the T4 levels, with infants who require ventilatory assistance for respiratory distress syndrome having the lower T4 levels, possibly suggesting non-thyroidal illness (sick euthyroid syndrome), which may be an adaptive response to illness resulting in a depressed metabolic rate. The reason for this

hypothyroxinemia is multifactorial, including the loss of the maternal T4 contribution, immaturity of the hypothalamic-pituitary axis, the responsiveness of the thyroid gland to TSH, and immaturity of peripheral tissue deiodination. Iodine balance is negative in the first few weeks after birth in these very low birthweight babies, suggesting an inability to augment thyroidal iodine uptake and increase T4 secretion. These changes are further compounded by iodine deficiency in areas of the world with low environmental iodine, and by the use of iodine-containing antiseptics, drugs, and contrast agents. Thus, although severe hypothyroxinemia is associated with neonatal morbidity and developmental disability, it is unclear whether in those with normal thyrotropin levels (and no abnormalities of the hypothalamic-pituitary axis) this is an association (usually in the sickest infants) or the cause. The data to date do not support supplementation with thyroid hormones in these babies, and indeed it may be detrimental to long term neurological outcome. The possible advantage to those babies born at 25 and 26 weeks gestation requires further clarification before recommendation of thyroid hormone supplementation.

KEY POINTS FOR CLINICAL PRACTICE:

1. Most cases of Congenital Hypothyroidism are not hereditary and result from thyroid dysgenesis (85% of cases). 10% of cases may be familial, usually caused by an inborn error of thyroxine hormone synthesis. 5% of cases are the result of transplacental passage of maternal TRB(blocking)Ab also known as (TBII(Thyroid Binding Inhibitory Immunoglobulin).

2. *Newborn Screening for T4 & TSH at days 3-5 should be done for all Newborn infants, as infants with congenital hypothyroidism are born with little or no clinical evidence of thyroid hormone deficiency. Laboratory errors occur, however, and awareness of early symptoms and signs must be maintained, with a high index of suspicion mandatory due to non-specific presentation.* A serum T4 of <7micro gm/dL or 90 nmol/L, with a serumTSH in excess of 20 micro IU/mL or 20 m IU/L, at 3-5 days of life suggests Congenital Hypothyroidism. All infants with suspicious screening tests must be confirmed by measurement of serum T4 and TSH concentrations.

3. Oral Levothyroxine, is the treatment of choice;initial starting dose is 10-15mcg/kg(37.5-50mcg/day). Newborns with more severe hypothyroidism, as judged by a serum T4<3mcg/dL, should be started at the higher end of the dosage range. Levels of T4/free T4 and TSH should be monitored at recommended intervals, i.e., approximately monthly in the 1st 6 months of life, and then every 2-3 months between 6 mo-2 years and maintained in the normal range for age.

4. Prompt, early thyroxine replacement, close monitoring, and maintenance of T4 levels in the upper half of reference range has significantly improved neurodevelopment, even in the most severe cases of CH. Subtle neurocognitive deficits may persist, including poor visuospatial abilities, attention, and memory skills,despite early therapy.

5. A formal hearing assessment is recommended in the hypothyroid infant because of the 10 fold increase in the hearing loss in these babies.

REFERENCES & FURTHER READING : 1)Gruters A, Krude H. Update on the management of congenital hypothyroidism. *Horm Res.* 2007;68 Suppl 5:107-11. **2)**LaFranchi S. Congenital hypothyroidism: etiologies, diagnosis, and management. *Thyroid.* Jul 1999;9(7):735-40. **3)**Rovet JF. Congenital hypothyroidism: long-term outcome. *Thyroid.* Jul 1999;9(7):741-8. *4)*Postellon DC. Diagnosis and treatment of congenital hypothyroidism. *Compr Ther.* Feb 1983;9(2):41-4. **5)**LaFranchi SH, Austin J. How should we be treating children with congenital hypothyroidism?. *J Pediatr Endocrinol Metab.* May 2007;20(5):559-78.**6)**Pediatric Endocrinology Sperling MA, WB Saunders 1996, Philadelphia.

Pearl/Peril/Pitfall: Congenital Hypothyroidism-Prognosis The prognosis is usually one of normal intellectual and physical development if treatment is commenced promptly and monitored closely. Overtreatment may result in craniosynostosis and has been implicated in causing attention deficit hyperactivity disorder.

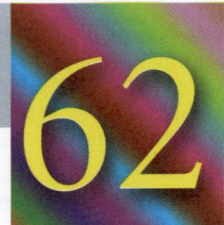

Neonatal Hyperthyroidism (Thyrotoxicosis)

@ *Most infants have a goitre. Central nervous system signs include irritability, jitteriness, and restlessness. Eye signs such as periorbital edema, lid retraction, and exophthalmos may be present even in the absence of maternal eye signs. Exophthalmos can occur even in thyrotoxicosis secondary to causes other than maternal Graves' disease. Cardiovascular signs include tachycardia and arrhythmias, but may progress to cardiac failure. Systemic and pulmonary hypertension may be present.*

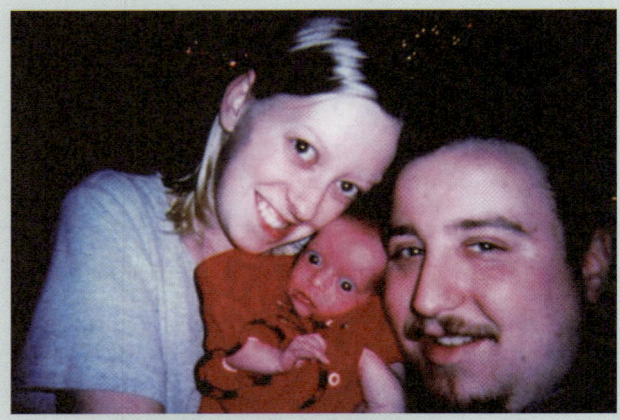

A baby with neonatal hyperthyroidism secondary to maternal Grave's disease. Note the prominent eyes in the baby and mother in whom Grave's disease developed after radioiodine therapy for Hodgkin's disease. In contrast, the father was unaffected.
Courtesy:Rosalind S. Brown, M.D.Boston, MA 02115 University of Massachusetts Medical Center Department of Pediatricshttp://www.thyroidmanager.org/chapter/disorders-of-the-thyroid-gland-in-

Neonatal Thyrotoxicosis

• Only occur with 5% of thyrotoxic mothers.

• Severity consistent in future pregnancies.

• 20% mortality if untreated.

• Evolves rapidly, evident by day 7 of life, unless TRAB blocking antibody is present.

• Associate with cranial synostosis and learning difficulties, if not treated.

• Fetal thyrotoxicosis in rats leads to abnormal CNS myelination.

• Parents should be aware of potential learning problems (early school years should be monitored).

• Symptomatic neonatal hyperthyroidism should be considered a medical emergency. Prompt and adequate institution of treatment may prevent severe damage in the newborn. Graves disease during pregnancy needs to be monitored closely to avoid complications due to the free passage of antibodies through the placenta and the development of clinical manifestations.

"The symptoms and signs of Neonatal Hyperthyroidism are non-specific and mimic those of narcotic withdrawal in infants of addicted mothers or Neonatal sepsis. A high index of suspicion is required in a symptomatic Neonate when an antenatal history of thyroid dysfunction is lacking."

REVIEW OF CLINICAL PROBLEMS

1. How do you diagnose and manage Fetal Hyperthyroidism?
   Ans: Refer to the"No. 2" of the "BIRD`S EYE VIEW/OVERVIEW/ SYNOPSIS" of the Chapter.

2. What are the "important aspects of history" you should elicit in evaluating Neonatal Hyperthyroidism?
   Ans: Refer to the Evaluation-Decision-Action Plan/ Algorithm to diagnose & manage Neonatal Hyperthyroidism.

3. What are the "objective findings" you should search for in an infant with suspected Neonatal Hyperthyroidism?
   Ans: Refer to the Evaluation-Decision-Action Plan/Algorithm to diagnose & manage Neonatal Hyperthyroidism.

4. Mention the "essential investigations" to evaluate Neonatal Hyperthyroidism.
   Ans: Refer to the Evaluation-Decision-Action Plan/Algorithm to diagnose & manage Neonatal Hyperthyroidism.

5. How do you manage Neonatal Hyperthyroidism?
   Ans: Refer to the Nos. 6, 7, 8, 9 and 10 of the "BIRD'S EYE VIEW/OVERVIEW/SYNOPSIS" of the Chapter & to the Table 2 of the Chapter.

LEARNING OBJECTIVES

After completing this article, readers will be able to:

1. Recognize and treat Neonatal Hyperthyroidism early to ensure the best outcome.

2. Have a high index of suspicion in a symptomatic infant when an antenatal history of thyroid dysfunction is lacking.

3. Maintain close observation until treatment has been successfully stopped and the infant is well, because fatal acute recurrent thyrotoxicosis has occurred at this stage.

4. Follow-up affected infants for at least 6 months-1 year with regular monitoring of TFTs.

5. Address complications like craniosynostosis and psychomotor retardation.

Pearl/Peril/Pitfall : Neonatal Hyperthyroidism—In the neonate, symptoms and signs of thyrotoxicosis may be apparent at birth or may be delayed for several days, because of either the effect of maternal antithyroid drugs or the effect of coexistent blocking antibodies, but are usually apparent by 10 days of life. However, overt thyrotoxicosis has been reported to occur as late as 45 days after birth.

1. Neonatal Hyperthyroidism is a rare disorder with an incidence of 1:25,000-1:40,000 live births, and a mortality rate of 15-20% in the 1970s, which can be lowered with the benefits of modern NICU care for the most severely affected infants. It is caused by the transplacental passage of *IgG TSH Receptor- stimulating antibodies -TRS Ab* from a mother with active/inactive/treated Grave's disease or with other autoimmune thyroid disease, but the clinical onset, severity and course may be modified by the concurrent passage of *TRB Ab(TBII(Thyroid Binding Inhibitory Immunoglobulin)*-Blocking Antibodies and by the transplacental passage of antithyroid drugs taken by the mother.The disease is usually transient, resolving within the timespan of the circulating antibodies.The antibodies have a half-life of approximately 12 days, hence the condition is transient with a duration of 3-12 weeks.Early recognition and treatment are essential to ensure the best outcome. A rare , Autosomal dominant, nonimmune cause of Neonatal Hyperthyroidism is characterized by an activating mutation of the TSH receptor;this condition results in permanent hyperthyroidism and may require thyroid gland ablation.

2. Acquisition of *IgG TSH Receptor- stimulating antibodies* increases dramatically between 22-28 weeks' GA at around a time when fetal thyroid becomes fully responsive to stimulation. There is an increased rate of miscarriage, stillbirth,IUGR, Premature birth, advanced bone age, and craniosynostosis, and later intellectual impairment in those babies significantly affected in utero. *Fetal tachycardia-160bpm,the presence of a goitre and growth retardation detected by ultrasound during the 3rd trimester can all be used as an indirect measure of fetal hyperthyroidism-treatment is warranted to avoid further complications* The mother should be given low doses of antithyroid drugs which readily cross the placenta to depress the fetal thyroid. Their efficacy can be monitored by the fetal heart rate. This in utero treatment will influence the Neonatal picture. Hence, an infant who is initially hyperthyroid can subsequently become hypothyroid(requiring thyroxine replacement) and an initially hypothyroid infant can become hyperthyroid.

3. Only 1–5% of mothers with Grave's disease give birth to Neonates who will go on to develop hyperthyroidism. Onset of symptoms is usually within 24–48 hours of birth, but may be delayed by 5-10 days to allow degradation of the maternal derived antithyroid drug, in those infants of mothers treated antenatally with antithyroid drugs.

4. Measurements of maternal *TSI(TRSAb) and TBII(Thyroid Binding Inhibitory Immunoglobulin)* levels may be predictive for the likelihood of but not widely used because of their low sensitivity and specificity.

5. *The symptoms and signs of Neonatal Hyperthyroidism are non-specific and mimic those of narcotic withdrawal in infants of addicted mothers or Neonatal sepsis.* A high index of suspicion is required in a symptomatic Neonate when an antenatal history of thyroid dysfunction is lacking. *Refer to the Table 1 of the Chapter for the common signs and symptoms of Neonatal Hyperthyroidism.* The infant is extremely restless, irritable, and hyperactive, and appears anxious and unusually alert. The eyes are opened widely and appear exophthalmic. There may be extreme tachycardia, tachypnea, hyperthermia, jaundice, loss of weight despite voracious appetite, and hepatosplenomegaly.The most severely affected infants who have the highest mortality present in high output CHF compounded by atrial tachyarrhythmias which can be difficult to control. The infant may die if therapy is not instituted promptly. The serum level of T4 is markedly elevated, and the TSH is suppressed.

6. *The Evaluation-Decision-Action- Plan/Algorithm* describes the essential aspects of the diagnosis and management of Neonatal Hyperthyroidism. The majority of infants are asymptomatic at birth and remain so. Those who develop symptoms are likely to do so within the 1st 48 hr and observation on the postnatal wards, initially is justified. However, due to the variable time of onset(especially when antenatal antithyroid drugs have been used) asymptomatic infants should be assessed at frequent intervals after birth for at least the 1st 2 weeks and TFTs performed at the 1st sign of clinical symptoms. The parents should be taught the important clinical symptoms and given instructions to seek pediatric advice immediately if any are present. In symptomatic infants when the diagnosis is strongly suspected, particularly when there is an antenatal history of Grave's disease, treatment should be commenced without awaiting results of TFTs as delay may result in progressive deterioration.

7. General supportive measures such as adequate oxygenation, hydration,calorie intake, and temperature control are essential. The infant should be nursed with the minimum of external stimuli. Thyroid enlargement may compromise the airway and head position with slight elevation and mild extension is usually sufficient. Rarely , intubation and ventilation are required; often in the most severely affected infants with cardiac failure.

8. *The most important initial therapy for the Neonatal Hyperthyroidism regardless of etiology is beta-adrenergic blockade using Propranolol to control the features of sympathetic nervous system overactivity, and Lugol's iodine to inhibit the hormone synthesis as well as release.* Sedatives for irritable and restless infant, Digoxin for tachyarrhythmias, diuretics for heart failure, hydrocortisone to inhibit the peripheral conversion of free T4 to free T3, Double volume Exchange blood Transfusion to reduce free T4 and free T3 levels are used when necessary.

9. Antithyroid drugs- Propylthiouracil or Carbimazole are the mainstay of treatment, after a euthyroid state is achieved. Refer to the Table 2 of the Chapter for dose ,duration(4-8 weeks usually), and tapering method of these drugs.

10. *Affected infants should be followed up for at least 6 months and possibly up to 1 year of age with bimonthly monitoring of TFTs.* Late onset hypothyroidism may occur due to the persistence of blocking antibodies, or delay in pituitary-thyroid axis responsiveness. Complications such as craniosynostosis may need to be dealt with in their own right. Intellectual development is normal in most treated infants with Neonatal Hyperthyroidism, though some may show injury from in utero Hyperthyroidism.

Pearl/Peril/Pitfall : Neonatal Hyperthyroidism-β-Blockers are effective in controlling symptoms caused by adrenergic stimulation. In addition, they inhibit deiodination of T4 to T3. Propranolol may be used in a dose of 0.27–0.75 mg/kg 8 hourly. However, it can cause serious hypoglycemia, bradycardia, and hypotension, so babies require close monitoring. Specific treatment for cardiac failure may be required, for example with digoxin and diuretics.

THE EVALUATION-DECISION-ACTION-PLAN/ALGORITHM FOR THE DIAGNOSIS AND MANAGEMENT OF *NEONATAL HYPERTHYROIDISM*

SUBJECTIVE FINDINGS

History of symptoms suggestive of Neonatal Thyrotoxicosis, such as agitation, diarrhea, vomiting, fever, flushing, failure to thrive despite high caloric intake, LBW/ PREMATURITY with wasting etc.,

Presenting symptoms may mimic those of narcotic withdrawal in an addicted mother/neonatal sepsis

History of Previous cases of Neonatal Thyrotoxicosis in a family.

Maternal history of Graves disease with hyperthyroidism and may have been treated with PTU, methimazole, ^{131}I, iodides, or surgery, History of Hashimoto disease.

A High Index of suspicion is required in a symptomatic Neonate when an antenatal history of Thyroid dysfunction is lacking.

OBJECTIVE FINDINGS

Assess ABCDs and monitor CRT, O_2 sats, BP, core-peripheral temperature difference, RR, HR, central & peripheral pulses, urine output.

Look for Irritable wasted LBW/PREMATURE infant, tachycardia, hypertension, thyroid enlargement, Eye signs-lid retraction, periorbital edema, exophthalmos, jaundice, purpura, polycythemia, hepatosplenomegaly, signs of CHF, Tachyarrhythmias-SVT, Atrial Flutter and Atrial Fibrillation with rapid ventricular rate, rarely DIC.

Assess for **Microcephaly** and Craniosynostosis. Perform Neurologic examination.

Determine gestational age by dates, ultrasonography during pregnancy, or Dubowitz examination.

INVESTIGATIONS

Blood FBC, TC, DC, **Hct**, Platelets, CRP, Blood cultures, **ABG analysis**, **electrolytes**, calcium & magnesium, **blood sugar**, LFTs, creatinine, BUN, coagulation profile.(for general management of any sick neonate).

Urine for toxicologic screen for illicit substances.

TFTs Free T3, T4, TSH, TSH Receptor antibodies

X-Ray Knee for advanced bone age.

For selected cases: ECG and ECHO, auditory and visual evoked potentials, motor conduction, velocity tests, skull radiographs.

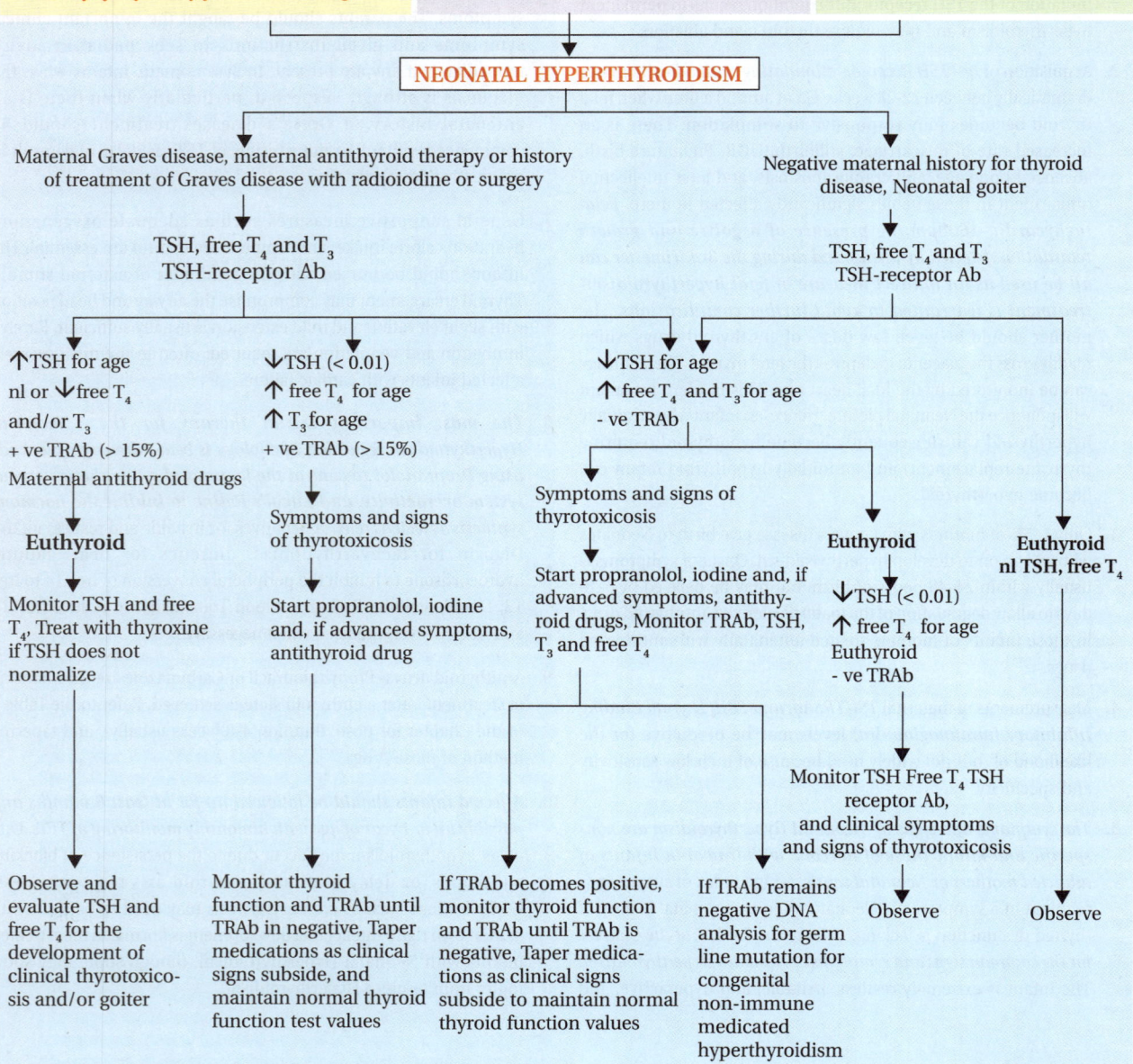

NEONATAL HYPERTHYROIDISM

Maternal Graves disease, maternal antithyroid therapy or history of treatment of Graves disease with radioiodine or surgery

TSH, free T_4 and T_3 TSH-receptor Ab

↑TSH for age nl or ↓free T_4 and/or T_3 + ve TRAb (> 15%) Maternal antithyroid drugs

Euthyroid

Monitor TSH and free T_4, Treat with thyroxine if TSH does not normalize

Observe and evaluate TSH and free T_4 for the development of clinical thyrotoxicosis and/or goiter

↓TSH (< 0.01) ↑ free T_4 for age ↑ T_3 for age + ve TRAb (> 15%)

Symptoms and signs of thyrotoxicosis

Start propranolol, iodine and, if advanced symptoms, antithyroid drug

Monitor thyroid function and TRAb until TRAb in negative, Taper medications as clinical signs subside, and maintain normal thyroid function test values

Negative maternal history for thyroid disease, Neonatal goiter

TSH, free T_4 and T_3 TSH-receptor Ab

↓TSH for age ↑ free T_4 and T_3 for age - ve TRAb

Symptoms and signs of thyrotoxicosis

Start propranolol, iodine and, if advanced symptoms, antithyroid drugs, Monitor TRAb, TSH, T_3 and free T_4

If TRAb becomes positive, monitor thyroid function and TRAb until TRAb is negative, Taper medications as clinical signs subside to maintain normal thyroid function values

If TRAb remains negative DNA analysis for germ line mutation for congenital non-immune medicated hyperthyroidism

Euthyroid

↓TSH (< 0.01) ↑ free T_4 for age Euthyroid - ve TRAb

Monitor TSH Free T_4 TSH receptor Ab, and clinical symptoms and signs of thyrotoxicosis

Observe

Euthyroid nl TSH, free T_4

Observe

*** Pearl/Peril/Pitfall:** Babies at high risk of neonatal thyrotoxicosis : Mother: Raised thyroid binding immunoglobulin levels in pregnancy, Thyroid binding immunoglobulin level not assessed, Clinical thyrotoxicosis in third trimester, Thionamide required in third trimester, Family history of TSH receptor mutation Baby: Evidence of fetal thyrotoxicosis.*

TABLE 1	Signs and symptoms in neonatal hyperthyroidism

Mild to Moderately Severe

Tachycardia > 160/min	Hypertension
Irritability	Diarrhea
Flushing	Jaundice
Poor weight gain despite high caloric intake	Thyroid enlargement
Eye signs - Lid retraction	Hepatosplenomegaly
- Periorbital edema	Purpura (due to thrombocytopenia)
- Exophthalmos	Polycythemia

Severe

Tachycardia > 200/min
Arrhythmias - Atrial flutter
  - Supraventricular tachycardia
  - Atrial fibrillation with rapid
Ventricular rate
Cardiac failure

TABLE 2	Drugs to treat neonatal hyperthyroidism

Sedatives*, e.g. Chloral Hydrate 25 mg/kg/dose 8 hourly.
Beta blocker*, e.g. Propranolol 1–2 mg/kg/day (3 divided doses).
Antithyroid drugs*
  Propylthiouracil(PTU) 5–10 mg/kg/day (3 divided doses)
  Carbimazole 0.5–1.0 mg/kg/day (3 divided doses)
  Lugol's iodine (5% iodine and 10% Potassium iodide solution = 126 mg iodine/ml-1 drop every 8 hours
Corticosteroids,   e.g. Hydrocortisone 2–4mg/kg/dose IV 6–8 hourly, 1–2 days

Given orally or via nasogastric tube.
Current recommendations state that breastfeeding should continue, and both ATDs are considered safe. Both appear in human milk (methimazole more than propylthiouracil) but in low concentrations. Clinical studies of breastfed infants have shown that they have normal thyroid function.

PRACTICAL ASPECTS OF THE MANAGEMENT OF NEONATAL HYPERTHYROIDISM

*Propranolol is the initial drug to be used to control sympathetic overactivity, but should be used with caution or avoided if cardiac failure is present *Lugol`s iodine is used early in all except the most mildly symptomatic infants and has the most rapid onset of action, inhibiting hormone synthesis as well as release. *Radiographic iodine-containing agents such as sodium ipodate(0.5 mg every 3 days) have also been used in the treatment of Neonatal Hypothyroidism, partly because of the relatively rapid response.*All infants should be rendered euthyroid/minimally hyperthyroid clinically by 72h of treatment. Once control is established, iodide can be stopped after 7-10 days, with a reduction in the dose of Propranolol. *Antithyroid drug-Propylthiouracil has a faster onset of action than Carbimazole and inhibits peripheral conversion of freeT4 to the more biologically active T3, in addition to its main action of inhibiting thyroid hormone synthesis. * Antithyroid drugs and Propranolol can be gradually tapered down over the next 4-8 weeks with careful monitoring of clinical state and TFTs.

*Antithyroid drugs can be reduced when the free T4 falls below normal range or when the TSH starts to rise.An alternative approach is to maintain the infant on a dose of antithyroid drugs for 6-8 weeks and then stop;close monitoring is required as the infant may become clinically hypothyroid during treatment. *Duration of treatment is usually 4-8 weeks and rarely exceeds 3 months. Sometimes prolonged treatment is necessary in some cases due to the presence of other antibodies which enhance TSI(TRSAb) action. *Sedatives for irritable and restless infant, Digoxin for tachyarrhythmias , diuretics for heart failure, hydrocortisone to inhibit the peripheral conversion of free T4 to free T3, Double volume Exchange blood Transfusion to reduce free T4 and free T3 levels are used when necessary. *Affected infants should be followed up for at least 6 months and possibly up to 1 year of age with bimonthly monitoring of TFTs. Late onset hypothyroidism may occur due to the persistence of blocking antibodies, or delay in pituitary-thyroid axis responsiveness.

KEY POINTS FOR CLINICAL PRACTICE:

1. Neonatal Hyperthyroidism is a rare, *transient, but potentially fatal disorder* if not recognized early on its clinical course, which is highly variable, due to the concurrent presence of TRB(Blocking)Ab and by the transplacental passage of antithyroid drugs taken by the mother.

2. The symptoms and signs of Neonatal Hyperthyroidism are *non-specific and mimic* those of narcotic withdrawal in infants of addicted mothers or Neonatal sepsis. A high index of suspicion is required in a symptomatic Neonate when an antenatal history of thyroid dysfunction is lacking.

3. The majority of infants are asymptomatic at birth and remain so. Those who develop symptoms are likely to do so within the 1st 48 hr and observation on the postnatal wards, initially is justified. However, due to the variable time of onset(especially when antenatal antithyroid drugs have been used) asymptomatic infants should be assessed at frequent intervals after birth for at least the 1st 2 weeks and TFTs performed at the 1st sign of clinical symptoms.Complications from hyperthyroidism include the following: * Congestive heart failure (CHF) * Craniosynostosis (neonates) * Developmental delay (neonates) * Hypothyroidism *Hypercalcemia

4. The *Key to successful management* of Neonatal Hyperthyroidism is, first anticipation and prevention, then control of thyroid status(with Propranolol, Lugol`s iodine, Propylthiouracil,sedatives and supportive measures) until the disease runs its self limited course for a period of 4-8 weeks , rarely 3 months.

5. Affected infants should be followed up for at least 6 months and possibly up to 1 year of age with bimonthly monitoring of TFTs. Late onset hypothyroidism may occur due to the persistence of blocking antibodies, or delay in pituitary-thyroid axis responsiveness.

REFERENCES & FURTHER READING : 1)Skuza KA, Sills IN, Stene M, et al. Prediction of neonatal hyperthyroidism in infants born to mothers with Graves' disease. J Pediatr 1996;128:264–7. 2)Transue D, Chan J, Kaplan M. Management of neonatal Graves' disease with iopanoic acid. J Pediatr 1992;121:472–4. 3) Watson WJ, Fiegen MM. Fetal thyrotoxicosis associated withnonimmune hydrops. Am J Obstet Gynecol 1995;172:1039–40. 4) Ramsay I. Fetal and neonatal hyperthyroidism. Contemp Rev Obstet Gynaecol 1991;3:74–8. 5)Tamaki H, Amino N, Aoza M, et al. Universal predictive criteria for neonatal overt thyrotoxicosis requiring treatment. Am J Perinatol 1988;5:152–8.

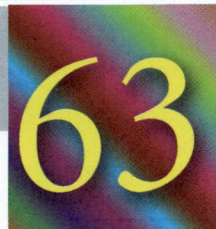

Neonatal Adrenocortical Insufficiency/Crisis

@ *Male infants with CAH appear normal at birth. Thus the diagnosis may not be made in boys until signs of adrenal insufficiency develop. Because patients with this condition can deteriorate quickly, infant boys are more likely to die than infant girls.*

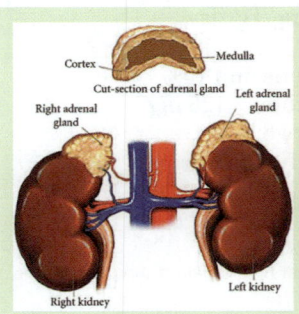

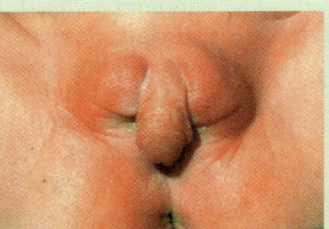

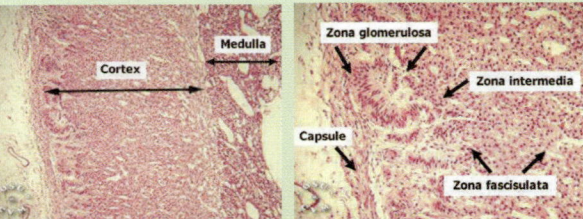

Congenital adrenal hyperplasia in a female infant

Function of the adrenal cortex *Zona glomerulosa cells secrete mineralocorticoids (principal one is aldosterone). These steroid hormones act on the kidney to: *Increase Na^+ reabsorption *Increase K^+ secretion

*Zona fasciculata and reticularis cells secrete glucocorticoids (e.g., cortisol, cortisone, corticosterone) which control glucose metabolism.

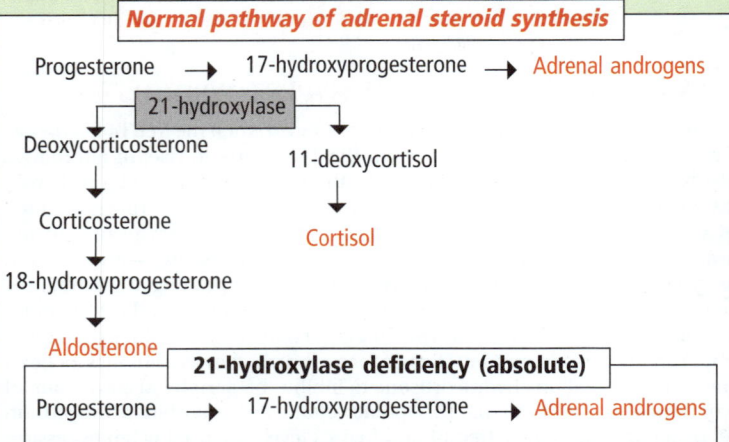

Normal pathway of adrenal steroid synthesis

Progesterone → 17-hydroxyprogesterone → Adrenal androgens

21-hydroxylase

Deoxycorticosterone → 11-deoxycortisol

Corticosterone → Cortisol

18-hydroxyprogesterone

Aldosterone

21-hydroxylase deficiency (absolute)

Progesterone → 17-hydroxyprogesterone → Adrenal androgens

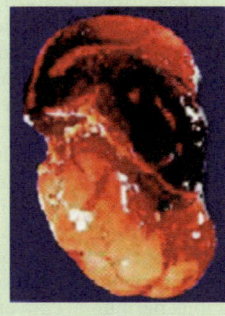

Adrenal hemorrhage in the neonate may lead to severe anemia and shock due to acute adrenal insufficiency

REVIEW OF CLINICAL PROBLEMS

1. How do you diagnose & manage Adrenal hemorrhage/necrosis in a Neonate?
   Ans: Refer to the "No. 2" of the "BIRD'S EYE VIEW/ OVERVIEW/SYNOPSIS" of the Chapter.

2. Discuss the essential aspects of diagnosis and management of Acute Adrenal Insufficiency in a Neonate.
   Ans: Refer to the Evaluation-Decision-Action Plan/ Algorithm to diagnose & manage a Neonate with Neonatal Adrenocortical insufficiency / Crisis.

3. *What are the Clinical Indicators of CAH due to Classic or severe 21-Hydroxylase Deficiency ?.*
   Ans: Refer to the Table "2" of the Chapter.

4. Discuss the Principles of Management of Classic CAH?
   Ans: Refer to the Table "3" of the Chapter.

5. How do you differentiate the various forms of CAH?
   Ans: Refer to the Table "4" of the Chapter.

LEARNING OBJECTIVES

After completing this article, readers will be able to:

1. Consider adrenal insufficiency in the differential diagnosis of any unexplained Neonatal collapse, shock, acidosis, hyponatremia with hyperkalemia.

2. Institute acute management of adrenal insufficiency promptly to prevent morbidity and mortality.

3. Ensure regular follow-up of children with CAH for growth, development, hypertension, serum electrolytes, bone age etc.

4. Prevent next sibling from being affected by Genetic counseling and prenatal diagnosis and Neonatal Screening.

5. Educate parents and affected children (when grown up) to understand the pathophysiology of their disease and the importance of glucocorticoid and mineralocorticoid replacement during crisis.

* *Pearl/Peril/Pitfall: The diagnosis of congenital adrenal hyperplasia depends on the demonstration of inadequate production of cortisol, aldosterone, or both in the presence of accumulation of excess concentrations of precursor hormones. For example, the distinguishing characteristic of 21-hydroxylase deficiency is a high serum concentration of 17-hydroxyprogesterone (usually >1000 ng/dL) and urinary pregnanetriol (metabolite of 17-hydroxyprogesterone) in the presence of clinical features suggestive of the disease (e.g., salt wasting, clitoromegaly or ambiguous genitalia [in a female patient], precocious pubic hair, excessive growth, premature phallic enlargement in the absence of testicular enlargement, hirsutism, oligomenorrhea, female infertility).*

BIRD'S EYE VIEW/OVERVIEW/SYNOPSIS

1. Adrenocortical insufficiency in a Neonate results from a number of causes in addition to the well known Congenital Adrenal Hyperplasia (CAH); Refer to the Table 1 of the Chapter. Hypocortisolemia may be relative/absolute, depending on the level of endogenous glucocorticoid secretion by the adrenal gland. It may result from loss of adrenal function(primary) or from lack of pituitary ACTH stimulation to the adrenal gland(secondary). It also includes deficiency of mineralocorticoid secretion.

2. Adrenal hemorrhage/necrosis mostly results from birth trauma, with an increased incidence in preterm infants and after septic shock,prolonged or complicated labour. Bilateral adrenal hemorrhage has been described in neonatal tuberculosis or syphilis. The bleeding may be sufficient to form a palpable mass, especially if unilateral, or may rupture into the peritoneum and cause intestinal obstruction or a scrotal hematoma. There may also be signs of acute blood loss or at a later stage, anemia and jaundice. If both adrenal glands are infarcted, the baby can present acutely with hypoglycemia, shock, and Addisonian features. Ultrasound is useful to confirm suspected hemorrhage.Adrenal calcification has been observed as early as the 5th day, but usually occurs much later. The presentation of adrenocortical insufficiency may be delayed but the regenerative capacity of the adrenal is great, and most adrenal hemorrhage is not associated with significantly impaired function. *Waterhouse-Friderchson syndrome* -acute adrenal insufficiency from adrenal hemorrhage and infarction complicating septicemic illness with DIC is a rare event in the Newborn, but can cause circulatory collapse and death.

3. *Adrenal crisis* may supervene in all forms of adrenal insufficiency pre- or post diagnosis. It may develop insidiously or be precipitated by acute illness or surgery. Hypoglycemia can occur independently of salt and water loss. Clinical features include poor feeding, poor weight gain, and then vomiting, diarrhea, vascular collapse, prostration and coma. Metabolic acidosis, hyponatremia, and hyperkalemia all may be present indicating mineralocorticoid deficiency. Treatment of acute adrenal crisis must be *immediate and vigorous*.

4. *Congenital adrenal hyperplasia* (CAH) is a group of autosomal recessive disorders with a deficiency of one of the enzymes necessary for cortisol synthesis by the adrenal cortex. CAH differs from other causes of primary adrenal insufficiency in that precursor steroids accumulate proximal to the blocked enzymatic conversion. Because cortisol is not synthesized efficiently, ACTH levels are high, leading to hyperplasia of the adrenal cortex and levels of precursor steroids that may be hundreds of times normal. Although several enzymes are necessary for steroid synthesis, 90% are caused by deficiency of 21-hydroxylase enzymatic activity. Complete deficiency of 21-hydroxylase activity causes the "classic", or severe form of the disorder that presents (1 in 15,000-20,000 births) infancy with simple virilizing (25%) or salt-losing (75%) forms. Partial deficiency of 21-hydroxylase activity, the "nonclassic" form, is milder, without ambiguous genitalia, and presents later in childhood or young adulthood. Refer to the Table No 4 of the Chapter for the essential diagnostic features of various types of CAH. For common clinical Indicators of "Classic" or Severe 21-Hydroxylase Deficiency-Refer to the Table 2 of the Chapter.

5. In fact, CAH should be considered in the differential diagnosis of "*any sick Newborn*"with various clinical presentations such as *a)* female infant with ambiguous genitalia *b)* acute collapse due to shock *c)* vomiting, diarrhea, dehydration, lethargy and failure to thrive *d)* electrolyte disturbances with "hyponatremia+ hyperkalemia" and metabolic acidosis *e)* hypoglycemia *f)* family history of sibling deaths.

6. *The Evaluation-Decision-Action- Plan/Algorithm* describes the essential aspects of the diagnosis and management of Neonatal Adrenocortical insufficiency/crisis. Patients with salt-losing disease have typical laboratory findings associated with cortisol and aldosterone deficiency, including hyponatremia, hyperkalemia, metabolic acidosis, and often hypoglycemia, but these abnormalities can take 1-2 week or longer to develop after birth. Blood levels of 17-hydroxyprogesterone are markedly elevated, However , levels of this hormone are high during the first 2-3 days of life, even in unaffected infants and especially if they are sick or premature. Diagnosis of 21-hydroxylase deficiency is most reliably established by measuring 17-hydroxyprogesterone before and 30 or 60 minutes after an IV Bolus of 0.125–0.25 mg of ACTH 1-24.

7. Male infants with CAH appear normal at birth. Thus the diagnosis may not be made in boys until signs of adrenal insufficiency develop. Because patients with this condition can deteriorate quickly, infant boys are more likely to die than infant girls. Newborn Screening based on the 17-hydroxyprogesterone levels of dried blood spots is effective in preventing many cases of adrenal crisis in affected males.

8. The *goals of therapy* for Classic CAH are a)to achieve normal growth b)to achieve normal pubertal development c)to achieve normal sexual function d)to discuss establishment of a satisfactory gender identity and e)to discuss fertility issues.Refer to the Table 3 of the Chapter for the most comprehensive management of Classic CAH.

9. *Congenital adrenal hypoplasia or atrophy of the glands* (1 in 12,500 births) is a well recognized cause of an adrenal crisis in the Neonatal period and later childhood. The clinical and biochemical picture in the neonatal period is very similar to CAH but 17-hydroxyprogesterone levels are not raised in Congenital Adrenal *Hypoplasia.* In addition to X-linked recessive and autosomal recessive forms it has been described in association with IUGR,metaphyseal dysplasia and genital anomalies (IMAGE).

10. Once a child is diagnosed with CAH, future pregnancies in the family can be monitored. Prenatal diagnosis of 21-hydroxylase is possible in the 1st trimester by analysis of DNA obtained by chorionic villus sampling or during the 2nd trimester by amniocentesis. This facilitates the prenatal treatment of affected female infants through the maternal therapy with dexamethasone from 6 weeks`gestation.

---

* *Pearl/Peril/Pitfall : Patients with salt-wasting forms of adrenal hyperplasia do not need potassium supplementation because they are usually hyperkalemic. However, patients with 11-hydroxylase and 17-alpha-hydroxylase deficiency may be hypokalemic and may require potassium. After appropriate diagnostic studies are performed or after the results are known, glucocorticoid therapy, mineralocorticoid therapy, or both may be started.*

THE EVALUATION-DECISION-ACTION-PLAN/ALGORITHM FOR THE DIAGNOSIS AND MANAGEMENT OF *NEONATAL ADRENOCORTICAL INSUFFICIENCY/CRISIS*

SUBJECTIVE FINDINGS

History of poor feeding,vomiting,poor weight gain,diarrhea, seizures,apneas,and shock with acute collapse, with a median age at presentation of around 12 days(in a typical case of salt-losing CAH due to 21alpha-hydroxylase deficiency).

History of virilized female infants,often mistakenly presumed to be males with hypospadias and cryptorchidism;males appear normal,therefore diagnosis is delayed until signs of adrenal insufficiency develop.

Natal Hx of birth wt, APGAR scores, resuscitation details, mode of delivery, PROM/meconium stained labor, asphyxia (*?pointing towards the common causes of adrenal hemorrhage—History of-* prematurity, birth trauma,prolonged / complicated labor, bleeding tendency, perineal/scrotal bruising, suspected sepsis)

Family Hx of unexplained Neonatal deaths and consanguinity *Antenatal Hx of* maternal Cushing syndrome/large doses of steroid therapy.

OBJECTIVE FINDINGS

Assess ABCDs and monitor CRT, O_2 sats, BP, core-peripheral temperature difference, RR, HR, central & peripheral pulses, urine output.Donot ever forget Dextrose-search for hypoglycemia and correct immediately after stabilizing ABCs.

Determine whether the baby is in preterminal ("pre arrest") conditions such as apnea, gasping or RR <20 bpm, shock, extremely lethargic or unresponsive limpy baby, bleeding etc.. and intervene with appropriate resuscitation of ABCDs promptly.

Note the other alarming signs such as convulsions, irritability, pallor, central cyanosis, hypothermia, abdominal distention,palpable abdominal mass, bilious vomiting, petechieae and ecchymoses, scrotal/perineal bruising, etc. *Note: dysmorphic features (facies),* obvious congenital malformations, *virilization of female infants,* evidence for birth trauma stigmata of congenital infections (tuberculosis,syphilis).

Perform systemic examination quickly to exclude the problems which may require emergent life saving measures such as pneumothorax, upper airway obstruction, bowel obstruction, PDA etc..

INVESTIGATIONS

Blood FBC, TC, DC, **Hct**, Platelets, CRP, Blood cultures, **ABG analysis, electrolytes,** calcium & magnesium, **blood sugar**, LFTs, creatinine, BUN, coagulation profile.(for general management of any sick neonate) *Adrenocortical hormone tests-* ↓cortisol,↑ACTH, ↑↑baseline & ACTH stimulated 17- Hydroxy progesterone (reliable after 24 hours of age), serum androgens (androstenedione), plasma renin

Imaging Pelvic ultrasound to exclude renal malformations and to identify enlarged echogenic adrenals, and adrenal hemorrhage, *CXR, CT Brain scan and Echo* to exclude pulmonary, CNS and cardiac ductal-dependent causes of acute collapse in a Neonate, if clinically indicated.

Karyotyping- a top priority, when the genitalia are ambiguous *Genotyping if available*-for CYP21/6p21.3 mutations, if CAH due to 21-hydroxylase deficiency is suspected.

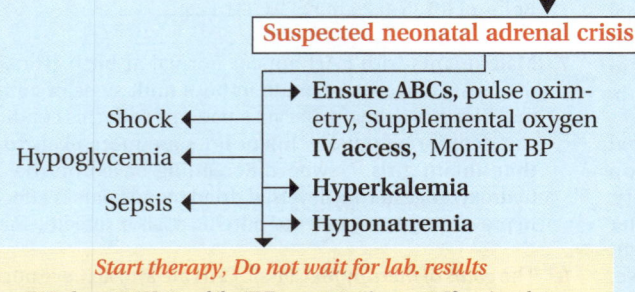

Suspected neonatal adrenal crisis

Shock ← → **Ensure ABCs,** pulse oximetry, Supplemental oxygen **IV access,** Monitor BP

Hypoglycemia ←

Sepsis ← → **Hyperkalemia**

→ **Hyponatremia**

Start therapy, Do not wait for lab. results

IV Bolus-0.9 NS 20 ml/kg/IVB over 10 minutes & If patient has hypoglycemia, give 10% Dextrose 5-10 ml/kg IVB,then continue rehydration fluid using **D₅ 0.9 NS**

Hydrocortisone -10 mg IV STATIM, then 100-200mg/Sq meter/day as 4-hourly bolus therapy or ,ideally by continuous IVI

cortisone acetate 1–5 mg/kg/d IM div q 12-24 h

OR, IF VENOUS ACCESS IS DIFFICULT, HYDROCORTISONE IM CAN BE GIVEN.

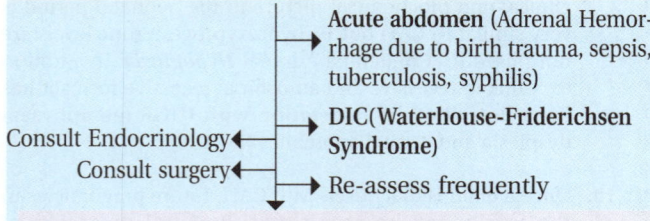

→ **Acute abdomen** (Adrenal Hemorrhage due to birth trauma, sepsis, tuberculosis, syphilis)

Consult Endocrinology ← **DIC(Waterhouse-Friederichsen Syndrome)**

Consult surgery ← → Re-assess frequently

Once patient is stable

1. Begin fludrocortisone 0.05–0.3mg QD when patient begins PO intake, and if hydrocortisone dose has been decreased to <100 mg/d.

2. Taper IV **hydrocortisone** by decreasing the dose by 1/3 QD until at maintenance dose(20 mg/m2/day)

3. In patients with salt-losing states, begin deoxycorticosterone acetate 1-3 mg until tolerating oral intake. check all doses with Endocrinology.

CAH-LONG-TERM THERAPY

Glucocorticoid replacement therapy is necessary for all cases of CAH, after managing the adrenal crisis, to suppress ACTH, and hence androgen levels-*Oral Hydrocortisone @15-20 mg/m2/24 hr in 3 divided doses regimen* is appropriate in most infants. Affected infants usually require dosing at the high end of this range. Double the dose with moderate stress, like URTI,ASOM, Mild Acute GE and triple the dose with severe stress like pneumonia, Acute GE with dehydration.*IM/IV Hydrocortisone@50-75mg/m2/day in 4 divided doses is necessary with severe stress associated with, vomiting, ileus, surgery* *Therapy is modified to maintain linear growth along percentile lines & to keep the 17-hydroxyprogesterone levels in the high-normal range or several times normal; low normal levels can usually be achieved only with excessive glucocorticoid doses. Overtreatment results in relative obesity and growth retardation;undertreatment results in progressive virilization and bone age advancement.* Glucocorticoid therapy must be individualized; continued indefinitely in all patients with classical 21-hydroxylase deficiency but may not be necessary in patients with nonclassical disease unless signs of androgen excess are present.

Mineralocorticoid replacement therapy Only those with the salt-losing form of CAH require *9-alpha-Fludrocortisone@0.05-0.3 mg/day in 2 divided doses and also often require sodium chloride,1-3 g/day supplementation*.Older infants and children are usually maintained with 0.05-0.1mg daily of Fludrocortisone. Therapy is evaluated by monitoring of vital signs; tachycardia and hypertension are signs of overtreatment with mineralcorticoids. Measure serum Electrolytes and Plasma Renin Activity in early infancy as therapy is adjusted.

Surgical treatment Virilized female infants with ambiguity of the external genitalia require reduction Clitoroplasty(not a clitorectomy), and vaginoplasty with correction of the urogenital sinus.

Prenatal diagnosis(DNA analysis after chorionic villus sampling) and Genetic Counseling to facilitate treatment of affected females - with dexamethasone@20mcg/kg prepregnancy weight daily in 2–3 divided doses,if started by 6 wk gestation ameliorates virilization of the external genitalia.

---

* **Pearl/Peril/Pitfall:** *Salt-wasting forms of adrenal hyperplasia are accompanied by low serum aldosterone concentrations, hyponatremia, hyperkalemia, and elevated plasma renin activity (PRA), indicating hypovolemia. In contrast, hypertensive forms of adrenal hyperplasia (i.e., 11-beta-hydroxylase deficiency and 17-alpha-hydroxylase deficiency) are associated with suppressed PRA and, often, hypokalemia.*

TABLE 1 — Neonatal causes of adrenocortial insufficiency

Primary

Congenital adrenal hyperplasia
Deficiency of glucocorticoid and mineralocorticoid
• 21a-hydroxylase deficiency, salt-losing
• 11b-hydroxylase deficiency, (in early life)
• 3b-hydroxylase dehydrogenase deficiency
• Lipoid CAH (steroidogenic acute regulatory protein and side-chain cleavage defects)
• 21a-hydroxylase deficiency, non-salt-losing
• 11b-hydroxylase deficiency
• 17a-hydroxylase deficiency
  Deficiency of glucocorticoid
• Corticosterone methyl oxidase deficiency I
• Corticosterone methyl oxidase deficiency II
Early abnormalities of steroidogenesis
Smith-Lemli-Opitz (7-dehydrocholesterol reductase deficiency)
Lysosomal acid lipase deficiency (Wolman's syndrome)

Congenital adrenal hypoplasia
  X-linked (abnormalities of DAX-1/NROB1)
  Autosomal recessive
  IMAGE association
Adrenal hypoplasia in association with SF-1 mutations
Adrenoleukodystrophy
Adrenal necrosis or hemorrhage
Acute infection (Waterhouse-Friderichsen syndrome)
Isolated glucocorticoid deficiency
  Familial glucocorticoid therapy
  Triple-A syndrome
Iatrogenic, post glucocorticoid therapy

Secondary

Hypopituitarism
Withdrawal from glucocorticoid therapy
Maternal Cushing's

TABLE 2 — Indicators of "classic" or severe 21-hydroxylase deficiency

Females
Ambiguous genitalia
Clitoromegaly
Partial posterior fusion labioscrotal folds
Single urogenital sinus
Signs of salt-losing (see below) if present

Males
Dehydration and/or shock
Failure to thrive
Vomiting, spitting up or formula changes without relief of symptoms
Hyponatremia (Na < 130 mg/dL) with Hyperkalemia (K > 6 mg/dL)

Salt - Losing type
Vomiting
Lethargy
Shock
Severe Hyponatremia (Na < 130 mg/dL)
Hyperkalemia (K > 6 mg/dL)
Acidosis

TABLE 3 — Management of classic congenital adrenal hyperplasia

Category & Specific Managements

Coordination of care
♦ Newborn : initial referral for assistance in diagnosis
♦ Referral to pediatric endocrinologist and tertiary care center for long term management of condition.
♦ Assist pediatric endocrinologist with referral and follow-up- for patients who require surgical intervention
♦ Communicate regularly with specialists

Parent education
♦ Instruct parents as follows:
  Whom to call when child is sick, What to do in an emergency, Importance of regular health maintenance visits, Importance of regular follow-up with specialist, Adherence.

Acute illness
♦ Adequately treat stress Treat underlying illness appropriately
♦ Consult pediatric endocrinologist regularly for any questions regarding treatment of acute illness
♦ Refer patients who are not responding adequately to treatment

Health maintenance
♦ Ensure immunization, including pneumococcal and annual influenza
♦ Regularly monitor growth and provide growth data to pediatric endocrinologist
♦ Monitor adherence with long-term treatment
♦ Carefully follow development

Adapted from Practical Pediatric Endocrinology By Anurag Bajpai, Jyoti Sharma, PSN Menon

TABLE 4 — Comparison of different forms of CAH

Deficiency	Mineralocorticoid	Glucocorticoid	Androgen	BP	Ambiguity	Diagnosis	Treatment
21-Hydroxylase							
CSW	Low	Low	Elevated	Low	Female	17-OHP	HC and Flu
CV	Normal	Normal	Elevated	Normal	Female	17-OHP	HC and Flu
NC	Normal	Normal	Elevated	Normal	None	ACTH stimulation	HC
3bHSD	Low	Low	Low	Low	Male	17-OH pregnenolone	HC and Flu
					Female	↓ Delta 5:Delta 4	
11-Hydroxylase	Elevated	Low	Elevated	Elevated	Female	DOC	HC
17-Hydroxylase	Elevated	Low	Low	Elevated	Male	18-hydroxyl DOC	HC
Star	Low	Low	Low	Low	Male	Low steroid precursors	HC and Flu

BP - Blood Pressure, HC - Hydrocortisone, Flu - Fludrocortisone, CSW - Classical salt wasting,
CV - Classical virilizing, NC - Non-classical

* Pearl/Peril/Pitfall : Imaging studies of the adrenal gland are generally not useful in the evaluation of patients with suspected adrenal hyperplasia. However, CT scanning of the adrenal gland can be useful in excluding bilateral adrenal hemorrhage in patients with signs of acute adrenal failure without ambiguous genitalia or other clues of adrenal hyperplasia. Pelvic ultrasonography may be performed in an infant with ambiguous genitalia to demonstrate a uterus or associated renal anomalies, which are sometimes found in other conditions that may result in ambiguous genitalia (e.g. mixed gonadal dysgenesis, Denys-Drash syndrome).

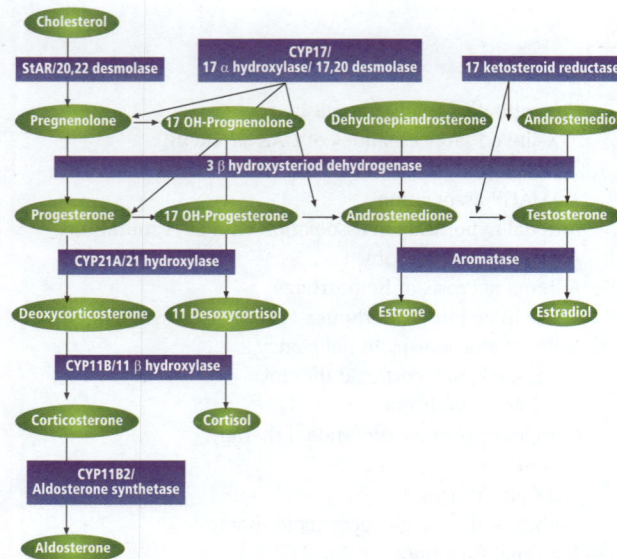

Steroidogenic pathway for cortisol, aldosterone, and sex steroid synthesis. A mutation or deletion of any of the genes that code for enzymes involved in cortisol or aldosterone synthesis results in congenital adrenal hyperplasia. The particular phenotype that results depends on the sex of the individual, the location of the block in synthesis, and the severity of the genetic deletion or mutation

Diagnostic Criteria for Late-onset Circulatory Collapse in VLBW Infants (LCC)

* *One week or longer since birth*
* *No inotropic agent administered*
* *Mean blood pressure ≤80% of that in the previous stable state or systolic blood pressure lower than 40 mm Hg*
* *Urine volume of ≤ 0.5mL/kg per hour over the past 8 hours or ≤1.0 mL/kg per hour over the past 24 hours*
* *Increased body weight*

* No other apparent cause of hypotension (It is important to exclude other disorders such as sepsis, PDA, and necrotizing enterocolitis, in which circulatory failure may occur, but the specific treatment for those diseases may be helpful.) LCC is associated with hypotension involving relative adrenal insufficiency that occurs after the respiratory and circulatory dynamics have stabilized. There seems to be little doubt that the prematurity of adrenal function (i.e., relative adrenal insufficiency) is involved in LCC. The severity of the condition varies, from mild disease that requires a single dose of steroid to severe disease that requires repeated steroid administration. Although LCC is a form of circulatory failure, no highdose steroid administration is necessary, unlike for septic shock. Hydrocortisone administered at 0.5 to 2 mg/kg per dose is effective for most cases. The blood pressure rises within several hours after steroid administration, and the urine volume is restored. When the initial treatment is not effective, the steroid dose can be increased to a several times higher dose. However, a thorough examination for the presence of other diseases should be performed. When hypotension persists, it may aggravate CLD and cause PVL, serving as a poor neurologic prognostic factor. Thus, detailed elucidation of the pathogenesis to facilitate early diagnosis and treatment is essential through cooperative studies.

Courtesy: Masayuki Miwa, MD,* Satoshi Kusuda, MD,† Kazushige Ikeda, MD* *NeoReviews* 2009;10;e381-e386

KEY POINTS FOR CLINICAL PRACTICE:

1. Adrenocortical insufficiency in a Neonate results from a number of causes in addition to the well known Congenital Adrenal Hyperplasia (CAH). Hypocortisolemia may be relative/absolute, depending on the level of endogenous glucocorticoid secretion by the adrenal gland. It may result from loss of adrenal function(primary) or from lack of pituitary ACTH stimulation to the adrenal gland (secondary). It also includes deficiency of mineralocorticoid secretion.

2. Adrenal hemorrhage/necrosis mostly results from birth trauma, with an increased incidence in preterm infants and after septic shock, prolonged or complicated labor. Bilateral adrenal hemorrhage has been described in neonatal tuberculosis or syphilis. The bleeding may be sufficient to form a palpable mass, especially if unilateral, or may rupture into the peritoneum and cause intestinal obstruction or a scrotal hematoma.

3. *Adrenal Crisis* may supervene in all forms of adrenal insufficiency pre- or post diagnosis. It may develop insidiously or be precipitated by acute illness or surgery. Hypoglycemia can occur independently of salt and water loss. Clinical features include poor feeding, poor weight gain, and then vomiting, diarrhea, vascular collapse, prostration and coma. Metabolic acidosis, hyponatremia, and hyperkalemia all may be present indicating mineralcorticoid deficiency.

4. Patients with salt-losing CAH have typical laboratory findings associated with cortisol and aldosterone deficiency, including hyponatremia, hyperkalemia, metabolic acidosis, and often hypoglycemia, but these abnormalities can take 1-2 week or longer to develop after birth. Blood levels of 17-hydroxyprogesterone are markedly elevated, However, levels of this hormone are high during the first 2-3 days of life, even in unaffected infants and especially if they are sick or premature. 21-hydroxylase deficiency in males is generally not identified in the Neonatal period because the genitalia are normal.

5. The *goals of therapy* for Classic CAH are a)to achieve normal growth b)to achieve normal pubertal development c)to achieve normal sexual function d) to discuss establishment of a satisfactory gender identity and e)to discuss fertility issues.

REFERENCES & FURTHER READING : 1)Carlson AD, Obeid JS, Kanellopoulou N, et al. Congenital adrenal hyperplasia: update on prenatal diagnosis and treatment. *J Steroid Biochem Mol Biol.* Apr-Jun 1999;69(1-6):19-29. 2)White PC. Neonatal screening for congenital adrenal hyperplasia. *Nat Rev Endocrinol.* Sep 2009;5(9):490-8 3)Merke DP, Cutler GB Jr. New approaches to the treatment of congenital adrenal hyperplasia [clinical conference]. *JAMA.* Apr 2 1997;277(13):1073-6. 4)Speiser PW, White PC. Congenital adrenal hyperplasia due to steroid 21-hydroxylase deficiency. *Clin Endocrinol (Oxf).* Oct 1998;49(4):411-7. 5)Pang S. Congenital adrenal hyperplasia. *Endocrinol Metab Clin North Am.* Dec 1997;26(4):853-91.

Pearl/Peril/Pitfall : As with all forms of adrenal insufficiency, the need for coverage with stress doses of glucocorticoids must be emphasized and reemphasized periodically because caretakers are often reluctant to provide stress doses when needed and are particularly reluctant to administer injectable glucocorticoids when the patient is unable to take oral medication or when he or she is severely lethargic. Disastrous consequences can result.

Ambiguous Genitalia

64

@ *Male phenotypic development can be viewed as a 2-step process: 1) testis formation from the primitive gonad (sexual determination) and 2) internal and external genitalia differentiation by action of factors secreted by the fetal testis (sexual differentiation). The first step is very complex and involves interplay of several transcription factors and signaling cells. Dosage imbalances in genes involved in DSD-Disorders of sexual development (deletions or duplication) have been identified as a not rare cause of these disorders. The dosage effect on gonadal development is sex limited, deletions or duplications of such genes can therefore manifest only in 46,XY or 46,XX subjects.*

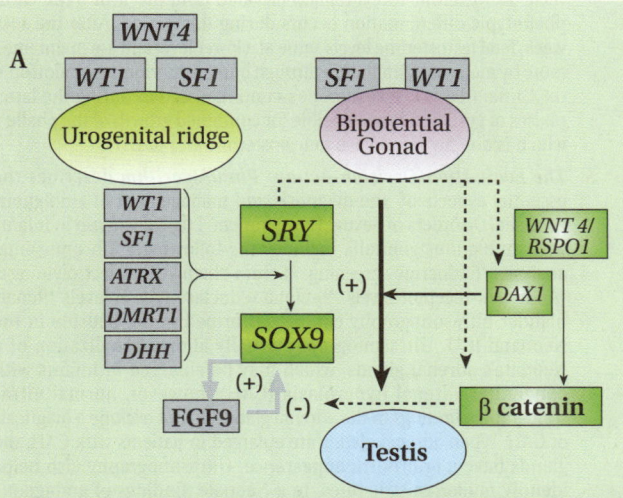

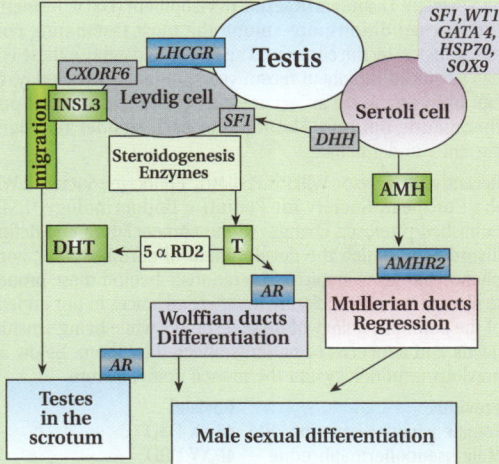

Summary of the molecular events in sex determination indicating the genes in which molecular defects can cause gonadal disorders in animal models. Some of these disorders were confirmed in humans. Sf1, Wnt4 and Wt1 are expressed in the urogenital ridge whose development results in formation of the gonads, kidneys and adrenal cortex. Several genes, Wt1, Sf1, Lhx9, Lim1, Gata4, Dmrt1, Emx2, Dhh, Wnt4 and Fgf9, are expressed in bipotential gonad. Sf1 and Wt1 up-regulate Sry expression in pre-Sertoli cells and initiates the male gonad development. Sry strongly up-regulates Sox9 in Sertoli cells. Sox9 up-regulates Fgf9 and Fgf9 maintains Sox9 expression, forming a positive feed-forward loop in XY gonads. The balance between Fgf9 and Wnt4/Rspo1 signals is shifted in favor of Fgf9, establishing the male pathway. If Wnt4/Rspo1 is over expressed activating the b-catenin pathway this system blocks Fgf9 and disrupt the feed-forward loop between Sox9 and Fgf9. Sry inhibits beta-catenin-mediated Wnt signaling. Overexpression in either DAX1 (locus DSS) or WNT4/RSPO1 antagonizes testis formation. On the other hand, Dax1 regulates the development of peritubular myoid cells and the formation of testicular cords. Dmrt1, Atrx and Dhh are also involved in testes determination.

The second step, male sex differentiation, is a more straightforward process. Anti Müllerian hormone (AMH) secreted by the testicular Sertoli cells acts on its receptor in the Müllerian ducts to cause their regression. Testosterone secreted by the testicular Leydig cells acts on the androgen receptor in the Wolffian ducts to induce the formation of epidydimis, deferent ducts and seminal vesicles. Summary of the molecular events in sex differentiation indicating the genes in which molecular defects cause 46,XY DSD in humans. After testis determination, hormones produced by the male gonad induce the differentiation of internal and external genitalia acting on their specific receptor. The regulation of AMH gene requires cooperative interaction between SOX9 and SF1, WT1, GATA4 and HSP70 at the AMH promoter. Combinatorial expression of DHH and SF1 is required for Leydig cell development. SF1 regulates gonadal steroidogenesis. The Leydig cells also produce the INSL3, which causes the testes to descend to the scrotum. Testosterone is further reduced to dihydrotestosterone (DHT), which acts on the androgen receptor of the prostate and external genitalia to cause its masculinization.

REVIEW OF CLINICAL PROBLEMS

1. Mention the Revised Nomenclature for Ambiguous genitalia.
   Ans: Refer to the"No. 2" of the "BIRD'S EYE VIEW/OVERVIEW/SYNOPSIS" of the Chapter.

2. Discuss the logical work-up for a Neonate born with Ambiguous genitalia.
   Ans: Refer to the Nos. "5,6 & 7" of the "BIRD'S EYE VIEW/OVERVIEW/SYNOPSIS" of the Chapter.

3. What are the management options for a Neonate born with Ambiguous Genitalia?
   Ans: Refer to the Nos "8,9 & 10" of the "BIRD'S EYE VIEW/OVERVIEW/SYNOPSIS" of the Chapter.

4. How do you plan relevant investigations depending on the clinical findings in an infant with Ambiguous Genitalia?
   Ans: Refer to the Table "2"of the Chapter.

5. Discuss the interpretation of Clinical findings in an infant with Ambiguous Genitalia.
   Ans: Refer to the Table "3"of the Chapter.

LEARNING OBJECTIVES

After completing this article, readers will be able to:

1. Be very careful in her/his choice of words during the diagnostic period and do not sign the birth certificate until a definite decision as to the sex of rearing has been reached.

2. Be aware of associated metabolic problems.

3. Appreciate that palpable gonads imply the presence of testicular tissue.

4. Understand that decisions as to sex of rearing may have no relationship to karyotypic, gonadal or genital status in isolation.

5. Counsel the parents that there is some ongoing controversy as to when is the appropriate time to make decisions as to sex of rearing and who should be party to those decisions.

BIRD'S EYE VIEW/OVERVIEW/SYNOPSIS

1. *Infants born with ambiguous genitalia represent a true medical and social emergency.* Salt-wasting nephropathy occurs in 75% of infants born with CAH, *the most common cause of ambiguous genitalia.* If unrecognized, the resulting hypotension can cause vascular collapse and death. Male infants with this syndrome may be phenotypically normal, and the diagnosis may be missed. Modern treatment of infants with ambiguous genitalia involves a *team-oriented approach.* This gender-assignment team usually involves neonatologists, geneticists, endocrinologists, surgeons, counselors, and ethicists. The goal is to provide appropriate medical support and counseling regarding care and therapy. Disorders of sexual development (DSD), formerly termed intersex conditions, are among the most fascinating conditions encountered by the clinician. The ability to diagnose these conditions has advanced rapidly in recent years. In most cases today, clinicians can promptly make an accurate diagnosis and counsel parents on therapeutic options. The topic of early gender reassignment is currently under debate.

2. Recently, the Lawson Wilkins Pediatric Endocrine Society (LWPES) and the European Society for Pediatric Endocrinology (ESPE) have published proposed changes to the nomenclature and definitions of disorders in which the development of chromosomal, gonadal, or phenotypic sex is atypical. The rationale behind these proposals was to change the nomenclature to reflect advances in our understanding of the pathophysiology of these disorders while being sensitive to the needs and concerns of patients affected by them. Below are listed previous terminology and the revised nomenclature.

Previous	Revised
Female pseudohermaphrodite	46,XX DSD
Male pseudohermaphrodite	46,XY DSD
True hermaphrodite	Ovotesticular DSD
XX male	46,XX testicular DSD
XY sex reversal	46,XY complete gonadal dysgenesis

3. **Gonadal differentiation:** During the second month of fetal life, the indifferent gonad is guided to develop into a testis by genetic information present on the short arm of the Y chromosome. Testis-determining factor (TDF) is a 35–kilobase pair (kbp) sequence on the 11.3 subband of the Y chromosome, an area termed the sex-determining region of the Y chromosome (SRY). When this region is absent or altered, the indifferent gonad develops into an ovary. The existence of patients with 46,XX testicular DSD, who have testicular tissue in the absence of an obvious Y chromosome or SRY genetic material, clearly requires other genetic explanations. Other genes important to testicular development include *DAX1* on the X chromosome, *SF1* on band 9q33, *WT1* on band 11p13, *SOX9* on bands 17q24-q25, and *AMH* on band 19q13.3. Fetal ovaries develop when the *TDF* gene (or genes) is absent. When testicular tissue is absent, the fetus morphologically begins and completes the internal sex duct development and external phenotypic development of a female. When testicular tissue is present, two produced substances appear to be critical for development of male internal sex ducts and an external male phenotype, namely, testosterone and müllerian-inhibiting substance (MIS) or AMH.

4. Testosterone is produced by testicular Leydig cells and induces the primordial wolffian (mesonephric) duct to develop into the epididymis, vas deferens, and seminal vesicle. MIS is produced by the Sertoli cells of the testis and is critical to normal male internal duct development. MIS represses müllerian duct development, while testosterone stimulates wolffian duct development. The external genitalia of both sexes are identical during the first 7 weeks of gestation. Without the hormonal action of the androgens testosterone and dihydrotestosterone (DHT), external genitalia appear phenotypically female. In the gonadal male, differentiation toward the male phenotype actively occurs over the next 8 weeks. This differentiation is moderated by testosterone, which is converted to 5-DHT by the action of an enzyme, 5-alpha reductase, present within the cytoplasm of cells of the external genitalia and the urogenital sinus. DHT is bound to cytosol androgen receptors within the cytoplasm and is subsequently transported to the nucleus, where it leads to translation and transcription of genetic material. In turn, these actions lead to normal male external genital development from primordial parts, forming the scrotum from the genital swellings, forming the shaft of the penis from the folds, and forming the glans penis from the tubercle. The prostate develops from the urogenital sinus Incomplete masculinization occurs when testosterone fails to convert to DHT or when DHT fails to act within the cytoplasm or nucleus of the cells of the external genitalia and urogenital sinus. The timing of this testosterone-related developmental change begins at approximately 6 weeks of gestation with a testosterone rise in response to a surge of luteinizing hormone (LH). Testosterone levels remain elevated until the 14th week. Most phenotypic differentiation occurs during this period. After the 14th week, fetal testosterone levels settle at a lower level and are maintained more by maternal stimulation through human chorionic gonadotropin (hCG) than by LH. Testosterone's continued action during the latter phases of gestation is responsible for continued growth of the phallus, which is directly responsive to testosterone and to DHT.

5. *The Evaluation-Decision-Action-Plan/Algorithm* describes the essential aspects of the diagnosis and management of ambiguous genitalia/Disorders of Sexual Development. Logical workup in infants with ambiguous genitalia includes the following: *Chromosomal analysis *Endocrine screening *Serum chemistries/electrolyte tests *Androgen-receptor levels *5-alpha reductase type II levels *Renal/bladder ultrasonography can be performed at the bedside in the Neonatal ICU. Ultrasonography usually allows visualization of a Neonate's adrenal glands, which may be enlarged in infants with congenital adrenal hyperplasia (CAH); however, normal ultrasonographic findings in the adrenal glands do not exclude a diagnosis of CAH. When adrenal glands are enlarged in patients with CAH, the glands have a cribriform appearance. Ultrasonography also helps identify müllerian structures. In a Neonate, findings of ambiguous genitalia, enlarged adrenal glands, and evidence of a uterus are virtually pathognomonic for CAH.

6. *Genitography helps determine ductal anatomy. In a Neonate with ambiguous genitalia, a catheter can be inserted into the distal urogenital sinus (urethra). Contrast is injected to outline the internal ductal anatomy. Findings may indicate normal urethral anatomy, an enlarged utricle, a müllerian remnant in a male, a common urogenital sinus, or an area of vaginal and urethral confluence in female neonates. *CT scanning and MRI are usually not indicated but may help identify internal anatomy.

7. Exploratory laparotomy/gonadal biopsy: Open exploration may help identify internal duct anatomy and allow gonadal tissue to be obtained for histologic characterization; however, many authors advocate laparoscopy for this purpose. Diagnostic laparoscopy/gonadal biopsy: A laparoscope may be inserted just inferior to the umbilicus under general anesthesia, allowing rapid identification and delineation of the internal duct anatomy without the morbidity associated with open exploration. Biopsy of gonads may be performed laparoscopically by placing additional trocars. Histologic analysis of gonadal biopsy specimens may identify ovarian tissue, testicular tissue, ovotestes, or streak gonads.

8. Medical therapy for intersex conditions depends on the underlying cause and is indicated for the conditions associated with ambiguous genitalia, including congenital adrenal hyperplasia (CAH). Supplemental hormone therapy may be implemented if gonadal function is compromised.

9. Surgical Care*In a virilized female, the surgical procedure is termed feminizing genitoplasty and includes vaginoplasty and clitoroplasty. *Undervirilized males typically have hypospadias requiring surgical reconstruction. Gender reassignment may be considered in patients with male pseudohermaphrodism and genital inadequacy.

10. Treatment for intersex states is controversial. No one debates the need to address and treat underlying physiologic problems such as those associated with congenital adrenal hyperplasia (CAH). The controversy revolves around issues of gender reassignment. Gender assignment by the physician and family may not correlate with gender preference by the patient in adulthood. Remember that the most important sex organ is the brain, which may undergo hormonal imprinting in utero.

*** *Pearl/Peril/Pitfall :* •Be very careful in your use of terms when discussing the baby with ambiguous genitalia. Appropriate, non-gender orientated terms are listed as follows. Suggested phenomenology when dealing with babies with ambiguous genitalia.*FEMALE-She,Clitoris,Labia,Ovaries,Vagina, urethra *AMBIGUOUS-Your baby,Phallus,Folds,Gonads,Urogenital sinus*MALE-He,Penis,Scrotum,Testes,Urethra. •The situation should be treated as a medical emergency, with pediatric endocrine advice being sought immediately .Never refer to the baby in question as "it".*

THE EVALUATION-DECISION-ACTION-PLAN/ALGORITHM FOR THE DIAGNOSIS AND MANAGEMENT OF *NEONATAL AMBIGUOUS GENITALIA*

SUBJECTIVE FINDINGS

History of

- Drug ingestion during pregnancy?
- Any recent androgenic changes in the mother suggesting androgen excess?
- Are there few (or no) male offspring in families on mother's side?
- Any siblings dying in the newborn period?
- Any siblings with over-virilization or precocious puberty?
- Any history of infection or exposure to teratogens?

OBJECTIVE FINDINGS

Genital ambiguity can be quantified according to the Prader scale (Figure 1). Other relevant clinical details include •gonads palpable in the labioscrotal or inguinal regions •size of the phallus •pigmentation of the genitalia ·syndromic features •metabolic condition of the baby (paying particular attention to glucose, sodium and potassium) The baby's mother should also be examined for signs of hyperandrogenism. Care should be taken in the interpretation of examination findings in growth retarded or premature female neonates. These children may exhibit atrophic labia and clitoral oedema giving them an appearance of "pseudo-ambiguity". It is a moot point where the boundary lies between severe perineal hypospadias and genital ambiguity. Inability to palpate the gonads in this situation may be indicative of a diagnosis other than isolated hypospadias.

INVESTIGATIONS

Blood should be sent for •electrolytes •gonadotropins (LH, FSH) •testosterone •urgent karyotype •serum 17-hydroxyprogesterone (17OHP) levels (after day 3 of life) *Pelvic ultrasound* (carried out by an experienced sonographer) should be undertaken as soon as possible.*Other investigations* which may or may not be subsequently relevant include·genitogram ·human chorionic gonadotropin stimulation test *Androgen-receptor levels, 5-alpha reductase type II levels (to assess testosterone and dihydrotestosterone synthesis capability).

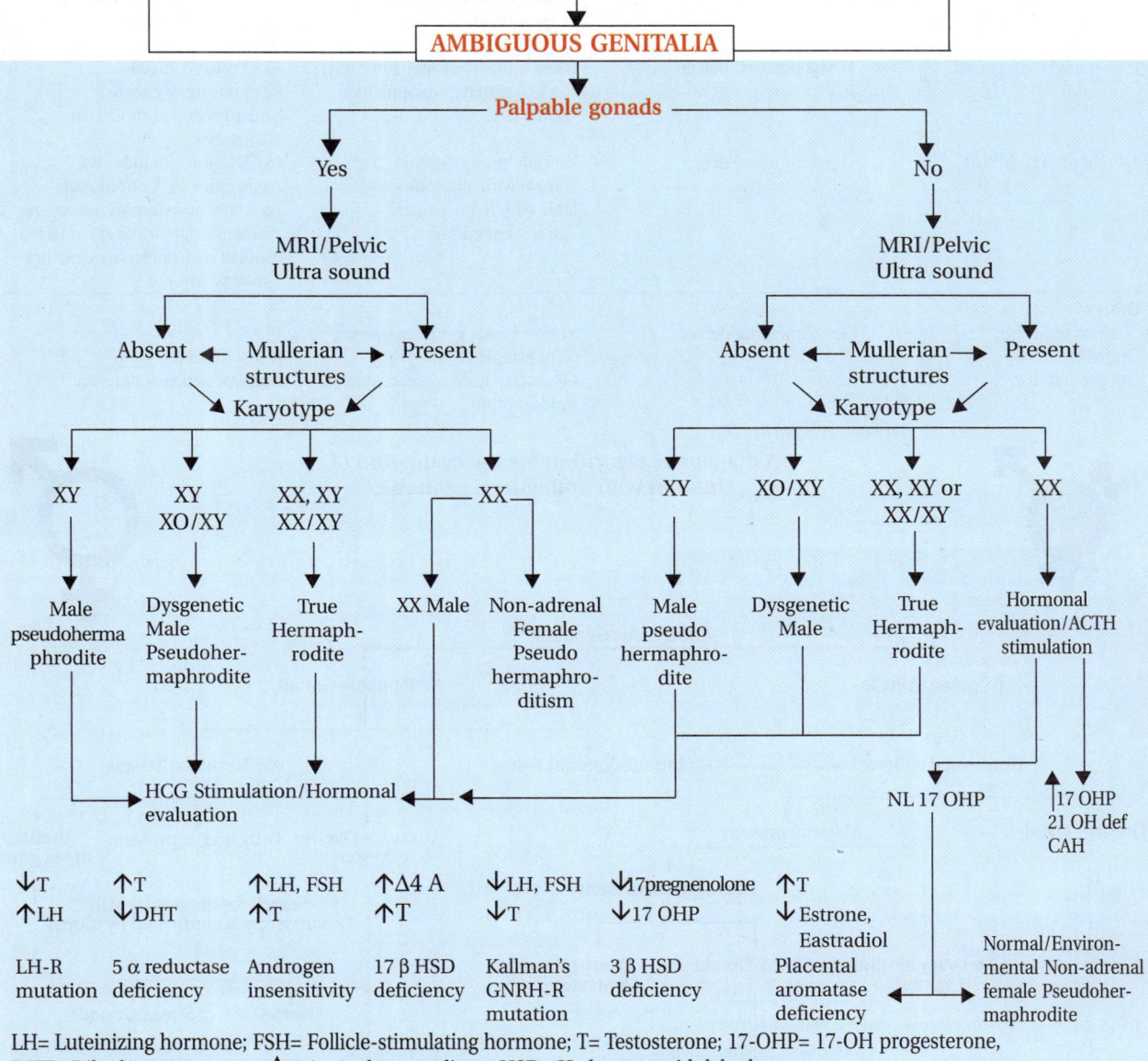

LH= Luteinizing hormone; FSH= Follicle-stimulating hormone; T= Testosterone; 17-OHP= 17-OH progesterone, DHT= Dihydrotestosterone; Δ 4 A= Androstenedione; HSD= Hydroxysteroid dehydrogenase

---

* **Pearl/Peril/Pitfall :** *Parents may seek advice regarding the naming of their infant. The usual advice is to select non-ambiguous names (i.e. using gender specific names) since it is thought that by encouraging the use of ambiguous (non-gender specific) names, one is implying an ongoing sense of "ambiguity".*

TABLE 1	Categories and characteristics of disorders with ambiguous genitalia		
Diagnosis	**Defect**	**External appearance**	**Karyotype, internal status**
Female Pseudohermaphroditism	Fetal exposure to virilizing	Virilization depends on extent	46, XX
Congenital adrenal hyperplasia	substances	of androgen exposure in	Ovarian tissue only
Progestin induced	Congenital fetal metabolic	utero; mild clitoromegaly	Mullerian structures present
Maternal androgen induced	defect	to fully male-appearing phallus	
Indeterminate	Coming from the mother	No palpable gonads	
Male Pseudohermaphroditism	Several possible defects	Variable presentations	46,XY
Androgen insensitivity	Defective androgen synthesis	Near-normal male	Testicular tissue only
Androgen receptor defect	Target tissue insensitivity	Inguinal hernias	Wolffian structures present
(5a-reductase)	to androgen	Cryptorchidism	Mullerian structures may be
	Failure of mullerian regression		present
	Other uncertain causes		
Vanishing testis syndrome		Small phallus	
Persistent mullerian duct syndrome		Hypospadias	
Indeterminate		Intermediate genitalia	
		Near-normal or normal female	
Mixed gonadal dysgenesis	Developmental defect	Usually incompletely virilized	Most 46, XY/45,XO
		male	Testis, streak gonad present
		Small phallus	Mullerian structures may be
		Cryptorchidism	present on the side of the streak
		Hypospadias	gonad
Pure gonadal dysgenesis	Developmental defect	Often initially normal; infertility,	46,XX; 46,XY; 45,XO
		lack of sexual development	Bilateral streak gonads
		noted later	Underdeveloped mullerian
			structures
True hermaphroditism	Developmental defect	Variable presentations	46,XX (approximately 70%);
		Female with clitoromegaly	remainder 46, XY or mosaic
		Male with hypospadias,	Testicular and ovarian tissues are
		undescended testes	present (separate or as ovotestis)
			Wolffian and mullerian structures
			may be present
Others			
Cloacal exstrophy	Developmental defect	External male genitalia severely	46,XY
Aphallia		compromised	Testes present
Microphallus		Cloacal exstrophy - bifid phallus	Wolffian structures present
		and scrotum	

A diagnostic algorithm for the evaluation of children with ambiguous genitalia.

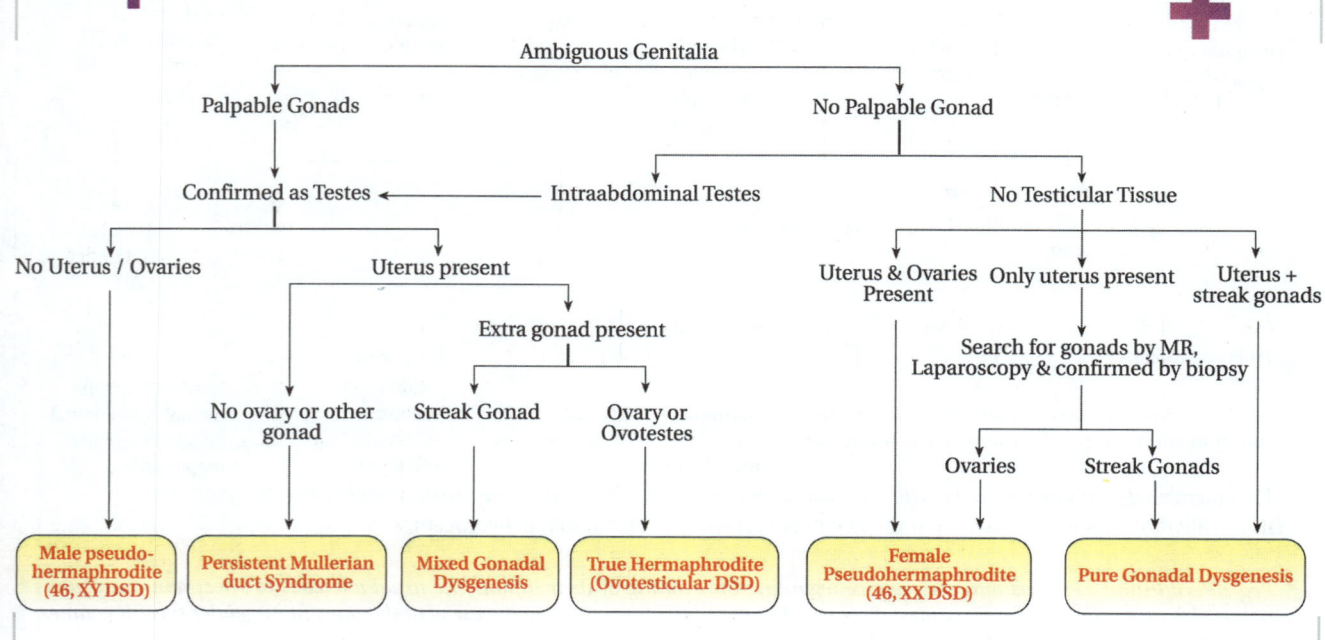

Development of male internal and external genitalia in human embryo.

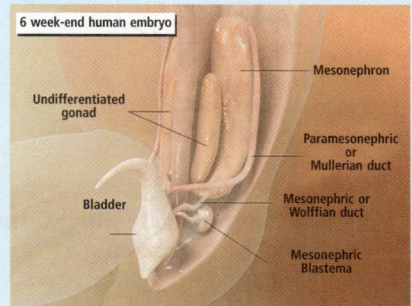

The development of male internal genitalia in human embryo-The 6-wk-end embryo is equipped with both male and female genital ducts derived from mesonephrons.

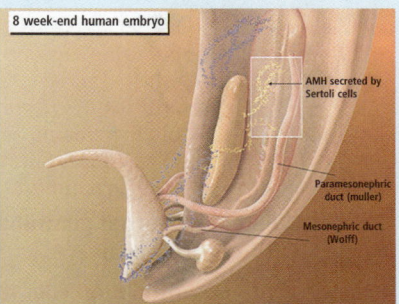

The development of male internal genitalia in human embryo- The regression of the Müllerian ducts is mediated by the action of AMH secreted by the fetal Sertoli cells.

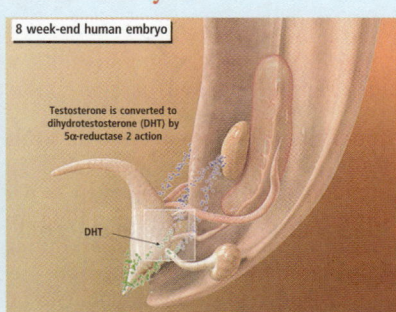

The development of male internal genitalia in human embryo—The stabilization and differentiation of the Wolffian ducts are mediated by testosterone synthesized by the fetal Leydig cells. The enzyme 5a-reductase 2 converts testosterone to dihydro-testosterone (DHT). The Wolffian ducts differentiate into epididymis, vas deferens and seminal vesicles. DHT contributes to prostate differentiation.

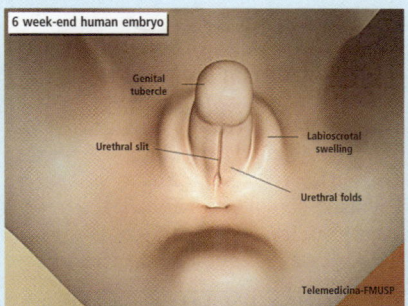

The development of male external genitalia in human embryo- At the 8-wk-end embryo the external genitalia of both sexes are identical and have the capacity to differentiate in both direction: male or female. The DHT stimulates growth of the genital tubercle and induces fusion of urethral folds and labioscrotal swellings. It also inhibits growth of vesicovaginal septum preventing the development of the vagina.

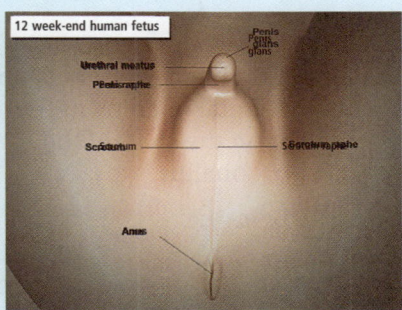

At the 12-week-end embryo the male external genitalia is entirely formed.

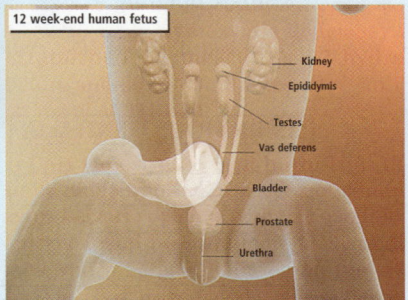

Development of male internal and external genitalia in human embryo. At the 12-week-end embryo both internal and external genitalia are completely formed

Courtesy: *Berenice Bilharinho Mendonca, MD Professor of Medicine, Head of the Division of Endocrinology, Hospital das Clinicas of the University of São Paulo School of Medicine, São Paulo, Brazil,* **Sorahia Domenice, MD** *Assistant Professor of Endocrinology, Division of Endocrinology, Hospital das Clinicas of the University of São Paulo School of Medicine, São Paulo,* **Brazil Ivo J P Arnhold, MD** *Associate Professor of Endocrinology, Division of Endocrinology, Hospital das Clinicas of the University of São Paulo School of Medicine, São Paulo, Brazil,* **Elaine M F Costa, MD** *Assistant Professor of Endocrinology, Division of Endocrinology, Hospital das Clinicas of the University of São Paulo School of Medicine, São Paulo, Brazil*

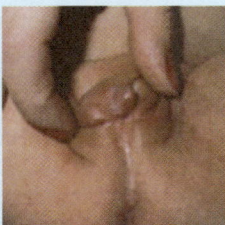

A female patient with the 46,XX karyotype with mild virilization due to congenital virilizing adrenal hyperplasia secondary to 21-hydroxylase deficiency. Despite the mild clitoromegaly, this patient has fusion of the labial-scrotal folds and salt wasting.

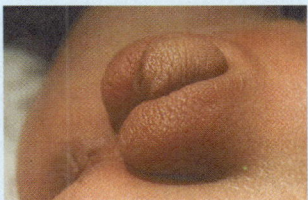

Severe virilization in a female patient with the 46,XX karyotype with congenital adrenal hyperplasia secondary to 21-hydroxylase deficiency. This patient also has salt wasting.

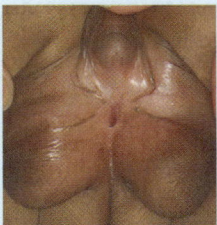

Patient with 46,XY disorder of sexual development. Note the masculinized appearance of the genitalia with an enlarged phallus and scrotal appearance of the labia

* *Pearl/Peril/Pitfall : Ambiguous Genitalia-Physical Examination: Although physical examination is useful, a diagnosis should not be made solely on examination findings. However, the following information is useful in determining what investigations are required.·Are gonads palpable? -25% of infants with undescended testes and hypospadias have an intersex disorder -Gonads palpable in the perineum almost always indicate a male karyotype·Is the penile length normal? -Measure stretched length with a spatula from the symphysis pubis to the stretched tip (not foreskin) of the penis -Normal stretched length >3cm at term -<2.5cm at term indicates a microphallus -Is there reasonable penile girth on palpation? -Is the phallus straight or is there chordee present?·Where is the urethral opening? ·How fused are the labioscrotal folds? ·Is the scrotum hypoplastic? ·Is the anus normally sited? ·Are there any other physical abnormalities?*

Figure 1: Prader staging system for the degree of virilisation of the external genitalia.

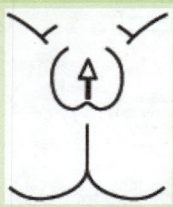
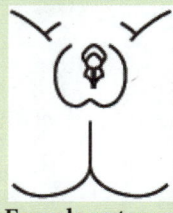
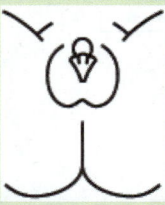

Prader 0: Normal female external genitalia.

Prader 1: Female external genitalia with clitoromegaly.

Prader 2: Clitoromegaly with partial labial fusion forming a funnel-shaped urogenital sinus.

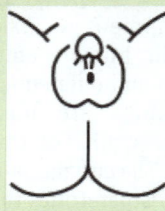
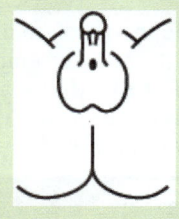
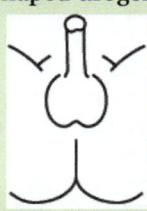

Prader 3: Increased phallic enlargement. Complete labioscrotal fusion forming a urogenital sinus with a single opening.

Prader 4: Complete scrotal fusion with urogenital opening at the base or on the shaft of the phallus.

Prader 5: Normal male external genitalia.

Courtesy: *(Prader Von, A. (1954). Helv. Pediatr. Acta. 9: 231-248.)*

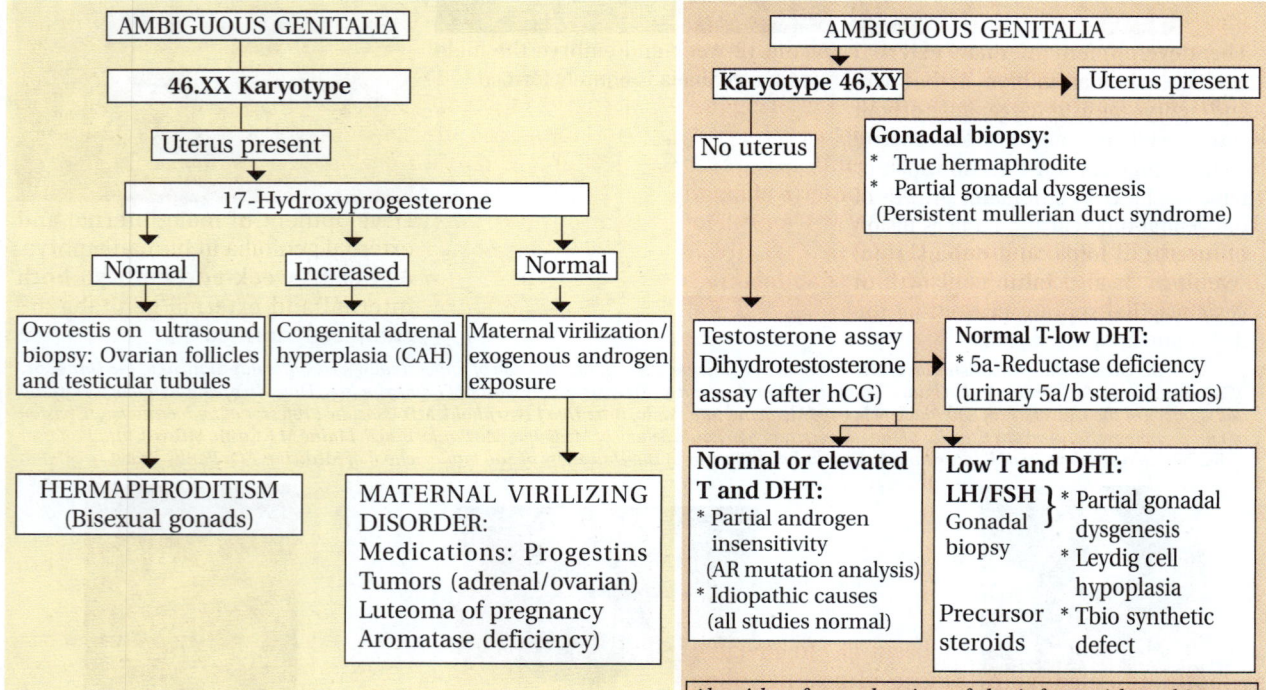

Algorithm for evaluation of the 46,XX infant with ambiguous genitalia. The presence of a uterus would be determined radiographically by ultrasound examination, genitourethrogram, or magnetic resonance imaging.

Algorithm for evaluation of the infant with ambiguous genitalia and 46, XY karyotype. The presence or absence of a uterus would be determined by radiographic imaging including ultrasound examination, genitourethrogram, or magnetic resonance imaging, as appropriate. Testosterone (T) and dihydrotestosterone (DHT) levels ideally should be obtained after human chorionic gonadotropin (hCG) stimulation. AR, androgen receptor; FSH, follicle-stimulating hormone; LH, luteinizing hormone.

* **Pearl/Peril/Pitfall :** •*Differential diagnoses* •*Gonads palpable, 46XY -gonadal dysgenesis -partial androgen insensitivity -biosynthetic defect in either testosterone or dihydrotestosterone production* •*Gonads impalpable, 46XX -Congenital adrenal hyperplasia -gonadal dysgenesis -exogenous androgen exposure* •*Mosaic karyotype -gonadal dysgenesis.*

TABLE 2	Investigations for ambiguous genitalia	
Features identified	**Differential diagnosis**	**Most appropriate tests**
No gonads palpable; uterus present (digital examination or ultra sonography); hyperpigmentation	CAH (21-hydroxylase deficiency or 11 β - hydroxylase deficiency)	Serum 17- OHP, Electrolytes, glucose, Chromosomes, Urogenital sinugram.
Gonad (s) palpable; no uterus; affected sibling, uncle or aunt	Either partial AIS or defect in testosterone biosynthesis	Chromosomes, hCG stimulation test, pelvic Ultrasound, Urogenital sinugram, Gonadal biopsy.
Asymmetric labioscrotal folds; gonad(s) palpable; uterus present; Tuner syndrome features*	Mixed gonadal dysgenesis or true hermaphroditism	Gonadal biopsy, Chromosomes, Urogenital sinugram, pelvic and abdominal ultrasonogram, test urine for albumin, urea, and electrolytes

AIS, androgen insensitivity syndrome; CAH, congenital adrenal hyperplasia. * Peripheral edema, small upturned nails, fish-shaped mouth, high-arched palate, cardiac murmur, webbed neck. *From Warne GL: Disorders of sexual differentiation. Endocrinal Metab Clin North Am 1998; 27:954*

TABLE 3	Diagnostic interpretation of clinical findings in an infant with ambiguous genitalia			
Clinical Findings	**Congenital adrenal Hyperplasia (CYP21)**	**Partial androgen Insensitivity Syndrome**	**XY Gonadal Dysgenesis**	**Testosterone Biosynthetic Defect**
Genitalia symmetric	+	+	-	+/-
Hyperpigmentation	+	-	-	+/-
Gonad (s) palpable	-	+	+	+
Uterus present	+	-	+/-	-
Dysmorphic facies	-	-	+/-	-
Systemic illness	+/-	-	-	+/-
Positive family history	Siblings	Sibling, uncle, or aunt	Sibling	Sibling

+, present; -, absent; +/-, present or absent.
From warne GL: Disorders of sexual differentiation. Endocrinol Metab Clin North Am 1998;27:954

KEY POINTS FOR CLINICAL PRACTICE

1. Approximately 1 in 4,500 births are complicated by ambiguous genitalia. This situation is rarely anticipated and can be a source of great distress for parents, delivery room and nursery staff. Often there can be pressure on medical staff to "make it better" and assign a gender to the child arbitrarily in the first few hours after birth. **This must be avoided at all costs.**

2. Evaluation of a Newborn with ambiguous genitalia requires a team effort. The most common disorder of sexual development (DSD), congenital adrenal hyperplasia (CAH), results in virilization of a 46,XX female and thus is classified under the heading of 46,XX DSD. The clinician's challenge is to distinguish CAH from other less common causes of ambiguous genitalia.

3. Genital ambiguity can be quantified according to the Prader scale. Other relevant clinical details include gonads palpable in the labioscrotal or inguinal regions -size of the phallus, pigmentation of the genitalia, syndromic features , metabolic condition of the baby (paying particular attention to glucose, sodium and potassium). The baby's mother should also be examined for signs of hyperandrogenism. Blood should be sent for electrolytes, gonadotropins (LH, FSH), testosterone, urgent karyotype, serum 17-hydroxyprogesterone (17OHP) levels (after day 3 of life). Pelvic ultrasound (carried out by an experienced sonographer) should be undertaken as soon as possible. Other investigations which may or may not be subsequently relevant include·genitogram ·human chorionic gonadotropin stimulation test (to assess testosterone and dihydrotestosterone synthesis capability) Androgen-receptor levels, 5-alpha reductase type II levels.

4. Exploratory laparotomy/gonadal biopsy: Open exploration may help identify internal duct anatomy and allow gonadal tissue to be obtained for histologic characterization; however, many authors advocate laparoscopy for this purpose. Diagnostic laparoscopy/gonadal biopsy: A laparoscope may be inserted just inferior to the umbilicus under general anesthesia, allowing rapid identification and delineation of the internal duct anatomy without the morbidity associated with open exploration. Biopsy of gonads may be performed laparoscopically by placing additional trocars.

5. From a medicolegal standpoint, the best approach to managing these cases is to provide parents with as much information as possible so that they can make informed decisions. Adequate counseling and support for parents is vital. The ideal management method is a team approach including neonatologists, geneticists, endocrinologists, surgeons, counselors, and ethicists.

REFERENCES & FURTHER READING : *1)*Allen TD. Disorders of sexual differentiation. *Urology.* Apr 1976;7(4 Suppl):1-32.*2)* de Grouchy J. Cytogenetics in intersex states. In: Josso N, ed. *The Intersex Child, Pediatric and Adolescent Endocrinology.* S Karger AG; 1981:21-8.*3)*Faure C, Garel L. Radiology in intersex states. In: Josso N, ed. *The Intersex Child, Pediatric and Adolescent Endocrinology.* S Karger AG; 1981:40-50.*4)*Forest MG. Inborn errors of testosterone biosynthesis. In: Josso N, ed. *The Intersex Child, Pediatric and Adolescent Endocrinology.* 1981. S Karger AG; 133-55.*5)* Hughes IA, Houk C, Ahmed SF, Lee PA. Consensus statement on management of intersex disorders. *Arch Dis Child.* Apr 19 2006.

* *Pearl/Peril/Pitfall : Ongoing Management Decision as to sex of rearing is made after opinions have been sought from the endocrine and surgical teams. It should be undertaken with the baby's parents after all the relevant investigation results have been discussed. The decision that will be influenced by an amalgam of ·the baby's karyotype ·gonadal status ·internal and external genital duct status ·potential for fertility and adequate sexual function · cultural influences Do not complete the baby's birth certificate until the sex of rearing has been decide.*

65

Neonatal Anemia

@ *"Asphyxia pallida presents at birth with pallor and cyanosis(which improves with supplemental oxygen), respiratory failure, bradycardia, & normal central venous pressure. This disorder must be distinguished clinically from acute hemorrhage because specific immediate therapy is needed for each disorder."*

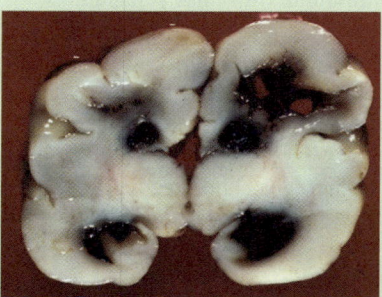

Intracranial Hemorrhage can result in severe anemia in the Newborn.

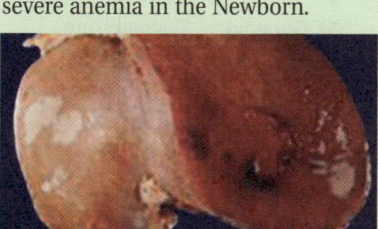

Subcapsular hematoma of liver may cause severe Neonatal anemia and even shock.

Reticulocytes with polyribosomal remnants (RNA) staining dark in their cytoplasm. They are slightly larger than the completely mature erythrocytes and are often found in the peripheral bloodstream at times when blood cells are being formed unusually rapidly (as during or after certain blood diseases).

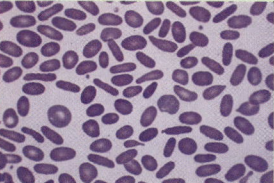

Elliptocytosis is a hereditary disorder of the red blood cells (RBCs). In this condition, the RBCs assume an elliptical shape, rather than the typical round shape.

Spherocytosis is a hereditary disorder of the red blood cells (RBCs), which may be associated with a mild anemia. Typically, the affected RBCs are small, spherically shaped, and lack the light centers seen in normal, round RBCs

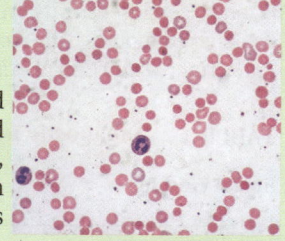

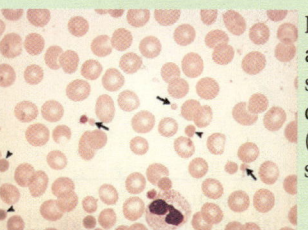

Microspherocytes: hemolytic anemia, Rh deficiency syndrome, ABO · hemolytic disease of the newborn (HDN), hereditary spherocytosis .

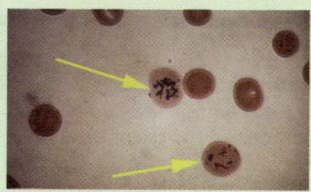

REVIEW OF CLINICAL PROBLEMS

1. How do you differentiate Asphyxia pallida from pallor due to Acute blood loss?
   Ans: Refer to the"No. 3" of the "BIRD'S EYE VIEW/ OVERVIEW/SYNOPSIS" of the Chapter, to the Table 5 & to the Table 10.

2. Discuss the essential aspects of diagnosis and management of Neonatal Anemia.
   Ans: Refer to the Evaluation-Decision-Action Plan/ Algorithm to diagnose & manage Neonatal Anemia.

3. What are the risks of Blood Transfusion to Preterm Infants?
   Ans: Refer to the Table 11 of the Chapter.

4. How do you differentiate Rh Immune Hemolysis from ABO Incompatibility?
   Ans: Refer to the Table 7 of the Chapter.

5. How do you approach to differentiate Neonatal Anemia?
   Ans: Refer to the Table 2 of the Chapter.

LEARNING OBJECTIVES

After completing this article, readers will be able to:

1. Describe the best methods of evaluating Neonatal Anemia.

2. Understand the Differential approach to Neonatal Anemia.

3. List the mechanisms of Anemia Of Prematurity.

4. Follow the safe Transfusion Guidelines to reduce the risks of Blood Transfusions, especially to the Preterms.

5. Know the Indications for Recombinant Human Erythropoietin.

* *Pearl/Peril/Pitfall: The decision of whether a particular hemoglobin (Hb) value is sufficiently low to meet the criteria for neonatal anemia must be based on the infant's birthweight, postnatal age, and the site of blood sampling. Failure to consider these factors adequately can lead to errors in diagnosis and unnecessary laboratory tests. At birth and for the first 2 to 3 months of life, healthy preterm infants have lower Hb levels than term infants. Normative data for postnatal Hb levels are readily available in standard neonatology and pediatric textbooks. Values below two standard deviations of the mean are diagnostic of anemia. It is also important to appreciate that Hb determinations performed on capillary blood samples, especially in the first days of life, are higher than those obtained from venous or arterial samples because of red blood cell (RBC) sludging in low-flow capillaries with resultant transudation of plasma.*

BIRD'S EYE VIEW/OVERVIEW/SYNOPSIS

1. *Neonatal anemia* is defined as hemoglobin less than the normal range of hemoglobin for birth weight and postnatal age (central venous hemoglobin < 13g/dL and capillary hemoglobin < 14.5g/dL) (Refer to Table 3 of the Chapter). A "physiologic" decrease in hemoglobin content is noticed at 8-12 week in term infants (Hb 11g/dL) and at about 6 week in premature infants (7–10g/dL). This exaggerated physiologic anemia of prematurity is related to a combination of decreased RBC mass at birth, increased iatrogenic losses from laboratory blood sampling, shorter RBC life span, inadequate erythropoietin production, and rapid body growth. In the absence of clinical complications associated with prematurity, infants will remain asymptomatic during this process.

2. *Anemia in the Newborn infant results from one of three processes* : **1)** loss of RBCs, (hemorrhagic anemia) the most common cause **2)** increased destruction of RBCs, or hemolytic anemia ; or **3)** underproduction of RBCs, or hypoplastic anemia (Refer to Table 4, 6, 7 & 8 of the Chapter).

3. *Hemorrhagic anemia,* if due to acute blood loss usually results in severe distress at birth, initially with a normal hemoglobin level, no hepatosplenomegaly, and early onset of shock. In contrast, if it is due to chronic blood loss **in utero**, produces marked pallor, less distress, a low hemoglobin level with microcytic indices with compensatory reticulocytosis, and if severe heart failure, often without cyanosis (because of <5g/dL of deoxyhemoglobin).The liver is often enlarged because of compensatory extramedullary erythropoiesis. Both forms have significant rates of perinatal morbidity & mortality if they remain unrecognized. Neither form has significant elevation of bilirubin levels. *Asphyxia pallida* presents at birth with pallor and cyanosis, which improves with supplemental oxygen, respiratory failure, bradycardia, & normal central venous pressure (Refer to Table 5 & 10 of the Chapter). This disorder must be distinguished clinically from acute hemorrhage because specific immediate therapy is needed for each disorder.

4. Anemia appearing in the first few days after birth is also most frequently a result of hemolytic disease of the Newborn. Other causes are hemorrhagic disease of the Newborn, bleeding from an improperly tied / clamped umbilical cord, large cephalhematoma, intracranial hemorrhage, or subcapsular bleeding from rupture of the liver, spleen, adrenals, or kidneys. Rapid decreases in hemoglobin or hematocrit values during the first few days of life may be the initial clue to these conditions. *Jaundice with unconjugated hyperbilirubinemia of >10–12 mg/dL, pallor, tachypnea, hepatosplenomegaly with or without hydrops fetalis, signify the hemolytic anemia*. Compensatory reticulocytosis is invariably present. There may be evidence of drug ingestion late in the 3rd trimester ; IUGR; a family member with splenectomy, anemia, jaundice, or cholelithiasis; maternal autoimmune disease; Mediterranean or Asian ethnic background.

5. *Hypoplastic anemia* is rare and is characterized by presentation after 48hr of age, absence of jaundice, and reticulocytopenia. The normal reticulocyte values are 3%-7% during the first day of life and 1–3% during the second & third days. The congenital causes are a) Diamond - Blackfan Syndrome b) Atransferrinemia c) Congenital leukemia d) Sideroblastic anemia. The acquired causes are rubella and syphilis, aplastic crisis and aplastic anemia. The presence of neutropenia and/or thrombocytopenia suggests the possibility of infection/leukemia.

6. *Fetomaternal hemorrhage* occurs in 30–50% of pregnancies and the risk is increased with PET, instrumentation, and with Cesarean Section. In 8% of pregnancies, the volume of hemorrhage is > 10ml. *The Kleihauer-Betke test* demonstrates significant amounts of fetal hemoglobin (an acid elution technique, when stained with eosin, fetal RBCs stain darkly whereas adult RBCs don't stain and appear as "ghost cells") and RBCs in maternal blood. New and more accurate *Flow Cytometry* detects fetal cells in maternal blood.

7. **Twin-Twin transfusion syndrome (TTTS)** occurs in 13-33% of twin pregnancies only in monozygotic multiple births, in the presence of a monochorial placenta. The difference in Hb concentration between twins is > 5g/dL. The anemic donor may develop CCF, whereas the recipient plethoric twin may manifest signs of the hyperviscosity syndrome.*Refer to the Chapter 19 "Twins and Multiple births" for details.*

8. *The Evaluation-Decision-Action-Plan/Algorithm* to diagnose and manage a Neonate with anemia summarizes the essential aspects of history, physical examination, relevant investigations & decision making about the general and specific aspects of management (Refer to Table 2 of the Chapter for the differential diagnosis of Neonatal anemia).

9. *Treatment of neonatal anemia* by blood transfusion depends on the severity of symptoms, the hemoglobin level, and the presence of co-morbid diseases (e.g. BPD, cyanotic CHD, HMD that interfere with oxygen delivery). The need for treatment with blood should be balanced against the risks of transfusion, including hemolytic transfusion reactions, exposure to blood product preservatives, volume overload, possible increased risk of ROP and NEC, graft versus host reaction, transfusion acquired infection (CMV, HIV, Hepatitis B & C) *(Refer to Table 1 for transfusion guidelines in Neonates).*

10. *Recombinant human erythropoietin (r-HuEPO)* IV / SC has been used to prevent / treat chronic anemia associated with prematurity, BPD, and hyporegenerative anemia of erythroblastosis fetalis. It must be supplemented with oral iron and vitamin E. Treatment with erythropoietin & iron doesn't have a major impact on transfusion requirements & routine use of erythropoietin in VLBW infants is not recommended. (Refer to Table 9 & 11.)

---

* *Pearl/Peril/Pitfall: Evaluating the etiology of neonatal anemia can be a daunting task. The numerous and diverse causes of this condition can be grouped into three broad pathogenetic categories: 1) decreased erythrocyte production, 2) increased erythrocyte destruction, and 3) blood loss. The importance of obtaining a complete and accurate history and performing a physical examination for diagnosing anemia cannot be overemphasized. In particular, the infant's family history and the mother's obstetric history often are of critical importance in narrowing down the etiologic possibilities.*

THE EVALUATION-DECISION-ACTION-PLAN/ALGORITHM FOR THE DIAGNOSIS AND MANAGEMENT OF *NEONATAL ANEMIA*

SUBJECTIVE FINDINGS

Hx of pallor, shock, CCF, jaundice < 24 hrs especially, respiratory distress, obvious blood loss / concealed hemorrhage (e.g. IVH with altered sensorium, seizures, and bulging fontanelle)

Hx of 3rd trimester vaginal bleeding *(abruptio or placenta previa)* or amniocentesis, twins, maternal chills or fever postpartum, C/S, obstetric trauma, unattended / precipitous delivery, perinatal fetal distress or a low APGAR score.

Hx of IUGR & Rh negative mothers.

Hx of drug ingestion late 3rd trimester (G6 PD deficiency), a family member with splenectomy, anemia, jaundice, or cholelithiasis, maternal autoimmune disease, Asian ethnic background.

Hx of prematurity.

OBJECTIVE FINDINGS

Assess ABCDs, CRT, BP, vitals, respiratory distress, urine output

Look for jaundice greater than expected degree in the Newborn, hepatosplenomegaly, stigmata of congenital infections, signs of congestive cardiac failure.

Differentiate pallor due to acute blood loss from pallor due to Neonatal asphyxia (asphyxia pallida - *Refer to Table 5).*

Suspect hepatic hemorrhage, when a previously healthy infant goes into shock with an increasing right upper quadrant mass, shifting dullness & free fluid on AXR.

INVESTIGATIONS

Blood FBC (RBC indices), hematocrit, reticulocytes, peripheral blood smear *(spherocytes of ABO hemolysis & hereditary spherocytosis, elliptocytes, pyknocytes of G6PD deficiency, helmet cells of DIC)* Coomb's test (positive in isoimmune / auto-immune hemolysis) both direct & indirect.

Other selected lab studies Blood group & type of mother and Neonate, Kleihauer - Betke test, TORSCH screen, coagulation profile + FDPs, placental examination & cranial + abdominal ultrasonography for occult hemorrhage, RBC enzyme studies, analysis of globin chain ratio, RBC membrane studies.

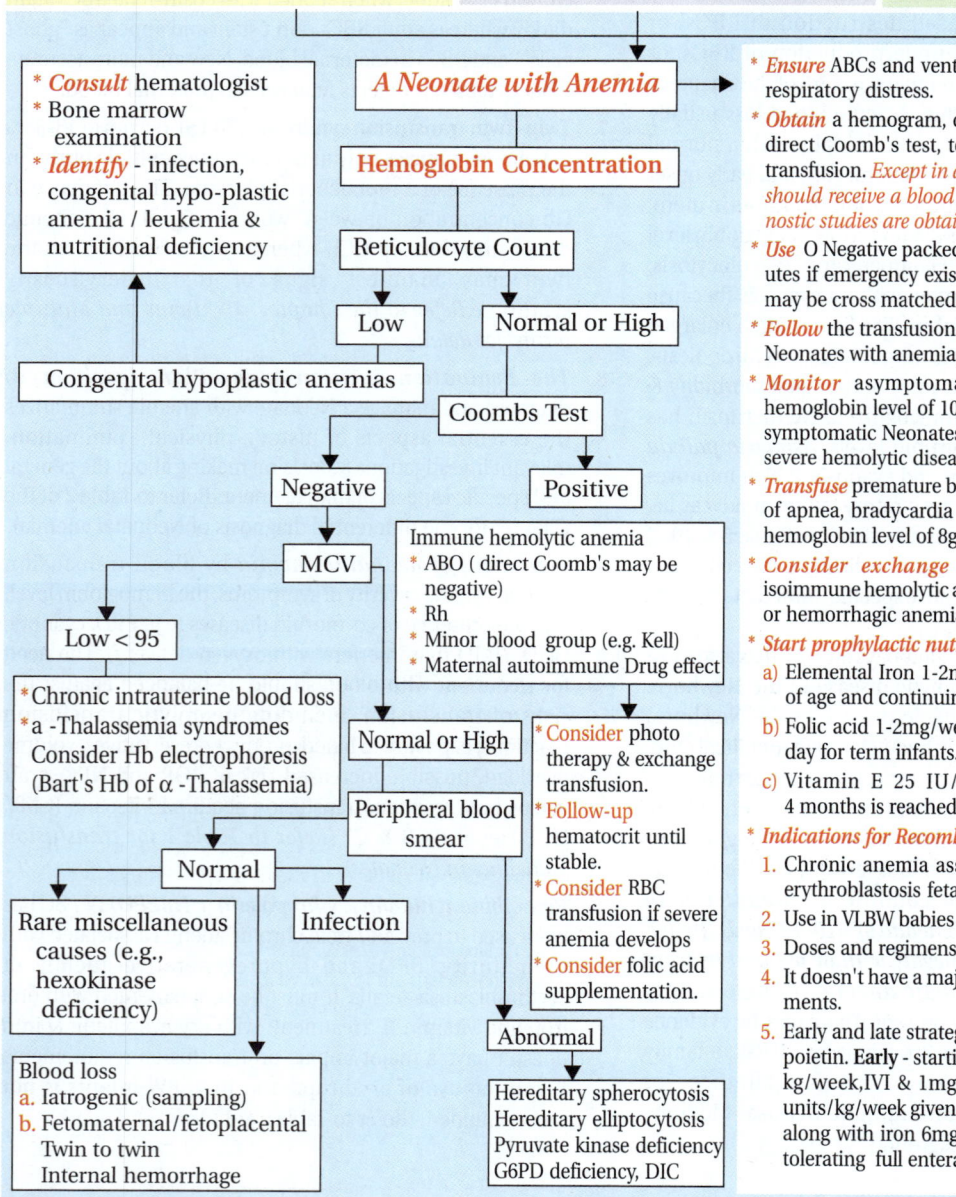

* *Consult* hematologist
* Bone marrow examination
* *Identify* - infection, congenital hypo-plastic anemia / leukemia & nutritional deficiency

A Neonate with Anemia

Hemoglobin Concentration

Reticulocyte Count → Low / Normal or High

Congenital hypoplastic anemias

Coombs Test → Negative / Positive

MCV

Low < 95

*Chronic intrauterine blood loss
*a -Thalassemia syndromes
Consider Hb electrophoresis (Bart's Hb of α -Thalassemia)

Immune hemolytic anemia
* ABO (direct Coomb's may be negative)
* Rh
* Minor blood group (e.g. Kell)
* Maternal autoimmune Drug effect

Normal or High

Peripheral blood smear → Normal / Infection

Rare miscellaneous causes (e.g., hexokinase deficiency)

Blood loss
a. Iatrogenic (sampling)
b. Fetomaternal/fetoplacental Twin to twin Internal hemorrhage

* *Consider* photo therapy & exchange transfusion.
* *Follow-up* hematocrit until stable.
* *Consider* RBC transfusion if severe anemia develops
* *Consider* folic acid supplementation.

Abnormal

Hereditary spherocytosis
Hereditary elliptocytosis
Pyruvate kinase deficiency
G6PD deficiency, DIC

* *Ensure* ABCs and ventilate the Neonate if in shock & in respiratory distress.

* *Obtain* a hemogram, differential, blood type & Rh type, direct Coomb's test, total bilirubin before giving blood transfusion. *Except in an emergency, no anemic Newborn should receive a blood transfusion before adequate diagnostic studies are obtained.*

* *Use* O Negative packed RBC 10-15ml/kg over 10-15 minutes if emergency exists at birth (if time permits blood may be cross matched to the mother's blood).

* *Follow* the transfusion protocol *(Refer to Table 1)* for the Neonates with anemia, but not in emergency crisis.

* *Monitor* asymptomatic full-term infants with a hemoglobin level of 10g/dL *while transfuse immediately* symptomatic Neonates after abruptio - placenta or with severe hemolytic disease of the Newborn.

* *Transfuse* premature babies who have repeated episodes of apnea, bradycardia despite theophylline therapy & a hemoglobin level of 8g/dL or lower.

* *Consider exchange transfusion* for DIC, severe isoimmune hemolytic anemia, chronic hemolytic anemia or hemorrhagic anemia with increased CVP.

* *Start prophylactic nutritional supplementation*
a) Elemental Iron 1-2mg/kg/day, beginning at 2 month of age and continuing through 1 year of age.
b) Folic acid 1-2mg/week for preterm infants ; 50mcg / day for term infants.
c) Vitamin E 25 IU/day until a corrected age of 4 months is reached.

* *Indications for Recombinant Human Erythropoietin*
1. Chronic anemia associated with prematurity, BPD, erythroblastosis fetalis.
2. Use in VLBW babies is *controversial*.
3. Doses and regimens vary.
4. It doesn't have a major impact on transfusion requirements.
5. Early and late strategies have been used for erythropoietin. **Early** - starting on day 1 or 2, 1200-1400 units/kg/week,IVI & 1mg/kg/day of iron. **Late** - 500-700 units/kg/week given 3-5 times a week subcutaneously along with iron 6mgs/kg/day as soon as the infant is tolerating full enteral feeds.

* *Pearl/Peril/Pitfall:* The more immature the infant, the more likely the development of AOP. AOP is not typically a significant issue for infants born beyond 32 weeks' gestation. The nadir of the hemoglobin level is typically observed when the tiniest infants are aged 4-10 weeks, with concentrations of 8-10 g/dL if birthweight was 1200-1400 grams, or 6-9 g/dL if birthweight was less than 1200 grams. AOP spontaneously resolves by the time most patients are aged 3-6 months.

TABLE 1 — Transfusion guidelines for neonatal anemia

Hct/Hgb	Respiratory Support and / or Symptoms	Transfusion Volume
Hct $\leq$ 35/Hgb $\leq$ 11	Infants requiring moderate to significant mechanical ventilation (MAP > 8 cm H_2O and FiO_2 > 0.4)	15mL/kg PRBC * over period 2-4 hr
Hct $\leq$ 30/Hgb $\leq$ 10	Infants requiring minimal respiratory support (any mechanical ventilation or endotracheal / nasal CPAP > 6 cm H_2O and FiO_2 $\leq$ 0.4)	15mL/kg PRBCs over period of 2-4 hr
Hct $\leq$ 25/Hgb $\leq$ 8	Infants not requiring mechanical ventilation but who are receiving supplemental O_2 or CPAP with an FiO_2 $\leq$ 0.4 and in whom 1 or more of the following is present : * $\leq$ 24 hr of tachycardia (HR > 180) or tachypnea (RR > 80) * An increased oxygen requirement from the previous 48 hr, defined as a $\geq$ 4-fold increase in nasal canula flow (i.e., 0.25 to 1 L/min) or an increase in nasal CPAP $\geq$ 20% from the previous 48 hr (i.e., 5 to 6 cm H_2O) * Weight gain < 10 g/kg/day over the previous 4 days while receiving $\geq$ 100 kcal/kg/day * An increase in episodes of apnea and bradycardia (>9 episodes in a 24-hr period or $\geq$ 2 episodes in 24 hr requiring bag and mask ventilation) while receiving therapeutic doses of methylxanthines * Undergoing surgery	20 mL/kg PRBCs over period of 2-4 hr (divided into 2-10 mL/kg volumes if fluid sensitive)
Hct $\leq$ 20/Hgb $\leq$ 7	Asymptomatic and an absolute reticulocyte count < 100 000 cells/ mL	20 mL/kg PRBCs over period of 2-4 hr (2–10 mL/kg volumes)

Packed RBCs. The volume of transfusion may be calculated as follows:

$$\text{Weight in Kilogram} \times \text{blood volume per kilogram} \times \frac{(\text{Hct desired} - \text{Hct observed})}{\text{Hct of blood to be given}} = \text{volume of transfusion}$$

The average newborn blood volume is 80mL/kg; the Hct of packed RBCs is 60% to 80% and should be checked before transfusion. Generally transfuse 15 to 20 mL/kg; larger volumes may need to be divided.

Hct = hematocrit ; Hgb = hemoglobin ; MAP = mean airway pressure ; FiO_2 = fractional inspired oxygen ; PRBC = packed red blood cells ; CPAP = continuous positive airway pressure ; HR = heart rate ; RR = respiratory rate. *RBC should be irradiated prior to transfusion.

A hemoglobin of 14g/dL corresponds to a RBC mass of 31 mL/kg. This implies that a transfusion of 2mL RBC/kg increases the hemoglobin concentration by approximately 1 g/dL. Packed RBCs (hematocrit approximately 67%) contain 2 mL of RBC/3 mL packed RBC. Whole blood (hematocrit approximately 33%) contains 2mL RBC/6 mL whole blood. Thus, the transfusion of 3 mL packed RBC/kg or 6mL whole blood/kg increases hemoglobin concentration by approximately 1g/dL.

TABLE 2 — Differential approach to anemia in newborn period

Hemoglobin	Reticulocytes	Bilirubin	Coombs Test	Clinical Considerations
Decreased	Normal/decreased	Normal	Negative	Physiologic anemia of infancy and prematurity Hypoplastic anemia
Decreased	Normal/increased	Normal	Negative	Hemorrhagic anemia
Decreased	Normal/increased	Increased	Positive	Immune-mediated hemolysis
Decreased	Normal/increased	Increased	Negative	Acquired or hereditary RBC defects Enclosed hemorrhage with resorption of blood Coombs-negative ABO incompatibility

TABLE 3 — RBC Values in term and premature infants during the 1st week of life

	Hgb (g/100 mL)	Hct (%)	Reticulocytes (%)	Nucleated RBCs (cells/1000 RBCs)
Term				
Cord blood	17.0 (14–20)	53.0 (45–61)	< 7	< 1.00
Day 1	18.4	58.0	< 7	<0.40
Day 3	17.8	55.0	< 3	<0.01
Day 7	17.0	54.0	<1	0
Premature *(weighing less than 1500 g)*				
Cord blood	16.0 (13.0–18.5)	49	< 10	<3.00
Day 7	14.8	45	< 3	<0.01

* **Pearl/Peril/Pitfall :** *Patient Education in Anemia Of Prematurity-*Explain the normal course of anemia. *Explain criteria for and risks of transfusions. *Explain advantages and disadvantages of erythropoietin (EPO) administration.*

TABLE 4	Causes of hemorrhagic anemia in newborns

Fetal hemorrhage
- Spontaneous fetomaternal hemorrhage
- Hemorrhage following amniocentesis
- Twin-twin transfusion
- Nuchal cord

Placental hemorrhage
- Placenta previa
- Abruptio placentae
- Multilobed placenta (vasa previa)
- Velamentous insertion of cord
- Placental incision during cesarean section

Umbilical cord bleeding
- Rupture of umbilical cord with precipitous delivery
- Rupture of short or entangled cord

Postpartum hemorrhage
- Bleeding from umbilicus
- Cephalhematomas, scalp hemorrhages
- Hepatic rupture, splenic rupture
- Retroperitoneal hemorrhages

TABLE 6	Causes of hemolytic anemia during the newborn period

Immune

Isoimmune : Rh and ABO incompatibility

Maternal immune disease : Autoimmune hemolytic anemia, systemic lupus erythematosus

Drug induced : Penicillin

Acquired red blood cell (RBC) disorders

Infection : Cytomegalovirus, toxoplasmosis, syphilis, bacterial sepsis

Disseminated and localized intravascular coagulation, respiratory distress syndrome

Hereditary RBC disorders

Membrane defects : Hereditary spherocytosis, hereditary elliptocytosis

Enzyme abnormalities : Glucose-6-phosphate dehydrogenase pyruvate kinase

Hemoglobinopathies : Alpha- thalassemia syndromes, gamma/ beta-thalassemia

TABLE 5	Comparative clinical findings in neonatal asphyxia and acute hemorrhage

	Neonatal asphyxia	Acute blood loss
Heart rate	Decreased	Increased
Respiratory rate	Decreased	Increased
Intercostal retractions	Present	Absent
Skin color	Pallor with cyanosis	Pallor without cyanosis
Response to oxygen and assisted ventilation	Marked Improvement	No significant change

TABLE 7	Clinical and laboratory features of immune hemolysis due to rh disease and ABO incompatibility

	Rh disease	ABO incompatibility
Clinical Features		
Frequency	Unusual	Common
Pallor	Marked	Minimal
Jaundice	Marked	Minimal to moderate
Hydrops	Common	Rare
Hepatosplenomegaly	Marked	Minimal
Laboratory Features		
Blood type		
Mother	Rh (-)	O
Infant	Rh (+)	A or B
Anemia	Marked	Minimal
Direct Coomb's test	Positive	Frequently negative
Indirect Coomb's test	Positive	Usually positive
Hyperbilirubinemia	Marked	Variable
RBC morphology	Nucleated RBCs	Spherocytes

TABLE 8	Etiology of neonatal anemia

	Blood loss	Decreased production	Hemolysis
Common	Fetal-maternal bleed Placenta previa Abruptio placentae Twin-twin transfusion	Perinatal-congenital infections	Rh ABO Minor groups
Rare	Vasa previa Rupture of umbilical cord Hepatic hematoma Splenic hematoma Nuchal cord	Parvovirus Diamond-Blackfan syndrome Osteopetrosis Congenital leukemia Congenital neuroblastoma Sideroblastic anemia	RBC enzyme deficiency Hemoglobinopathy RBC membrane disorders Disseminated intravascular coagulopathy

***** ***Pearl/Peril/Pitfall:*** *Neonatal Anemia—Physical examination: Tachycardia and hypotension suggest acute, significant blood loss. Jaundice suggests hemolysis, either systemic (from ABO incompatibility or G6PD deficiency) or localized (from breakdown of sequestered blood in cephalhematomas). Hepatosplenomegaly suggests either hemolysis or heart failure. Hematomas, ecchymoses, or petechiae suggest bleeding diathesis; congenital anomalies may suggest a bone marrow failure syndrome.*

TABLE 9 — Transfusion guidelines for premature infant

1. Asymptomatic infants with Hct <21% and reticulocytes <100, 000/μL)

2. Infants with Hct <31% and hood O2 <36% or mean airway pressure <6 cm H_2O by CPAP or IMV or >9 apneic and bradycardic episodes per 12h or 2/24 h requiring bag and mask ventilation while on adequate methylxanthine therapy or HR > 180/min or RR >80/min sustained for 24h or weight gain or <10 g/d for 4 d on 100Kcal/kg/d or having surgery.

3. Infants with Hct <36% and requiring >35% O2 or mean airway pressure 6-8 cm H_2O by CPAP or IMV

   CPAP = continuous positive airway pressure by nasal or endotracheal route; HR = heart rate; Hct = hematocrit; IMV = intermittent mandatory ventilation; RR = respiratory rate.

From the multicenter trial of recombinant human erythropoietin for preterm infants.

Source: Data from Straus RG. Erythropoietin and neonatal anemia (Editorial). N Engl J Med 1994;330:1227.

TABLE 10 — Pale newborn: Anemia *versus* asphyxia

Organ system	Hemorrhagic	Anemia hemolytic	Anemia asphyxia
Neurologic	Normal or hyperalert/hyperirritable ("catecholamine response")	Normal	Abnormal transition period, hypotonic, decreased arousal state, seizures in first 12–48 hr of life.
Respiratory	Tachypnea, no oxygen requirement	Normal	Respiratory distress, oxygen requirement
Cardiovascular	Tachycardia, hypotension	May vary from normal to hydrops, depending on degree of anemia	Bradycardia or normal heart rate; variable congestive heart failure and blood pressure
Hematologic	Drop in hematocrit/hemoglobin	Anemic from birth, hepatosplenomegaly, jaundice, positive Coombs test	Hematocrit/hemoglobin remains stable over time; may develop thrombocytopenia and DIC from hypoxic injury to marrow

TABLE 11 — Premature infants- mechanisms of anemia and risks of blood transfusion

Etiology of anemia of prematurity	Risks of blood transfusion in preterm infants	Measures to reduce the risk of infection associated with transfusion
• Frequent blood sampling • Low reticulocyte levels • Low levels of endogenous erythropoietin • Poor response to endogenous erythropoietin • Shortened life span of neonatal erythrocytes	• Fluid overload • Transfusion associated infection: Hepatitis B and C viruses Human immunodeficiency virus Cytomegalovirus • Hemolytic transfusion reactions • Immune mediated transfusion reactions • Extravasation injury • Graft versus host disease (rare)	• Screen donors for transmissible viruses • Limit exposure to multiple donors—multiple pediatric packs from single adult donor • Use cytomegalovirus antibody negative blood • Irradiate transfusion packs • Use leucocyte depletion filters (removes cytomegalovirus)

KEY POINTS FOR CLINICAL PRACTICE

1. Anemia in Neonates may be physiologic, or it may be caused by blood loss, decreased RBC production, or increased RBC destruction (hemolysis). Physiologic anemia: Normal physiologic processes often cause normocytic-normochromic anemia in term and preterm infants. Physiologic anemias do not generally require extensive evaluation or treatment.

2. Symptoms and signs are similar regardless of the cause but vary with severity and rate of onset of the anemia. Neonates are generally pale and, if anemia is severe, have tachypnea, tachycardia, and sometimes a flow murmur; hypotension is present with acute blood loss. Jaundice may be present with hemolysis.

3) Evaluation of Neonatal Anemia involves thorough Perinatal history, comprehensive physical examination and relevant investigations to differentiate 3 major underlying causes of pathological Neonatal Anemia.

4. Need for treatment varies with degree of anemia and associated medical conditions; otherwise healthy term and preterm infants with mild anemia generally do not require treatment. Treatment is directed at the underlying diagnosis. Some patients require transfusion or exchange transfusion of packed RBCs. Transfusion: Transfusion is indicated to treat severe anemia. Guidelines for when to transfuse vary, but one accepted set is:· Hb ≤" 12 g/dL (Hct ≤" 36%) in the 1st 24 h of life ·≥ 10% decrease in Hb in 1 wk ·≥ 10% acute blood loss ·Hb ≤12 g/dL in a Neonate requiring intensive care ·Hb ≤11 g/dL in a Neonate with chronic O_2 dependency ·Hb ≤ 7 g/dL in a stable infant with late (i.e., 4 to 6 wk) anemia.

5. At this time, no agreement regarding the safety, timing, dosing, route, or duration of therapy has been established. In short, the cost-benefit ratio for Recombinant human erythropoietin has yet to be clearly established, and this medication is not universally accepted as a standard therapy for an infant with AOP.

REFERENCES & FURTHER READING : 1)Schwarz KB, Dear PR, Gill AB, et al. Effects of transfusion in anemia of prematurity. *Pediatr Hematol Oncol.* Oct-Nov 2005;22(7):551-9. *2) Nelson text book of Pediatrics - 18th edition 3)*Strauss RG. Practical issues in neonatal transfusion practice. *Am J Clin Pathol.* Apr 1997;107(4 Suppl):S57-63.*4)*Carbonell-Estrany X, Figueras-Aloy J, Alvarez E. Erythropoietin and prematurity—where do we stand?. *J Perinat Med.* 2005;33(4):277-86. *5)*Salsbury DC. Anemia of prematurity. *Neonatal Netw.* Aug 2001;20(5):13-20.

* *Pearl/Peril/Pitfall : Before the 1st transfusion, if not already done, maternal and fetal blood should be screened for ABO and Rh types and the presence of atypical RBC antibodies, and a DAT should be performed on the infant's RBCs. Blood for transfusion should be the same as or compatible with the neonate's ABO and Rh group and with any ABO or RBC antibody present in maternal or neonatal serum. Neonates produce RBC antibodies only rarely, so in cases where the need for transfusion persists, repeat antibody screening is usually not necessary until 4 mo of age.*

66

Neonatal Polycythemia

@ *American Academy of Pediatrics states, "The accepted treatment of polycythemia is partial exchange transfusion (PET). However there is no evidence that exchange transfusion affects the long term outcome."*

DEFINITIONS

* *Polycythemia* is increased total RBC mass Central venous hematocrit > 65%.

* Above 65%, blood viscosity rises exponentially.

* *Polycythemic hyperviscosity* is increased viscosity of the blood resulting from increased numbers of RBCs.

* Not all polycythemic infants have symptoms of hyperviscosity.

CLINICAL PRESENTATION

* Symptoms are non-specific!
* CNS: lethargy, hyperirritability, proximal muscle hypotonia, vasomotor instability, vomiting, seizures, cerebral infarction (rare).
* Cardiopulmonary: respiratory distress, tachycardia, CHF, pulmonary hypertension.
* GI: feeding intolerance, sometimes NEC.
* GU: oliguria, ARF, renal vein thrombosis, priapism.
* Metabolic: hypo-glycemia/-calcemia/-magnesemia.
* Heme: hyperbili, thrombocytopenia.
* Skin: ruddiness.

MANAGEMENT

Asymptomatic infants

* Expectant observation unless central venous hematocrit >75% (consider partial exchange transfusion).
* Can do a trial of rehydration over 6-8 hr if dehydrated.
* Usually at > 48 hours of age and weight loss > 8-10%
* Give 130-150 ml/kg/d.
* Check central hematocrit q6 hours.
* Normal peak is at 2-4 hours of age for acute polycythemia.

MANAGEMENT

Symptomatic infants with central HCT > 65%

* Partial exchange transfusion is advisable but debatable.

* For exchange can use normal saline, Plasmanate, 5% albumin, or FFP

* Volume exchanged = (Weight (kg) x blood volume) x (hct - desired hct) / hct.

Blood volume is 80 ml/kg.

Exchange can be done via UVC that is not in the liver, low UAC, or PIV.

REVIEW OF CLINICAL PROBLEMS

1. Which of the Neonates should be screened for Poly-cythemia?
   Ans: Refer to the Table 2 of the Chapter.

2. Discuss the clinical signs associated with Neonatal Polycythemia-Hyperviscosity Syndrome.
   Ans: Refer to the Table 3 of the Chapter.

3. How do you calculate the volume of blood to be ex-changed in performing Partial ET for symptomatic Neonatal Polycythemia-Hyperviscosity Syndrome?
   Ans: Refer to the Evaluation-Decision-Action Plan/ Algorithm to diagnose & manage Neonatal Polycythemia-Hyperviscosity Syndrome.

4. Discuss the etiology of Neonatal Polycythemia-Hypervis-cosity Syndrome.
   Ans: Refer to the Table 1 of the Chapter.

5. What is the long-term prognosis of Neonatal Poly-cythemia-Hyperviscosity Syndrome?
   Ans: Refer to the"No. 9" of the "BIRD`S EYE VIEW/OVER-VIEW/SYNOPSIS" of the Chapter.

LEARNING OBJECTIVES

After completing this article, readers will be able to:

1. Screen High-Risk Neonates for Polycythemia-Hyperviscosity Syndrome.

2. Determine the underlying cause & Evaluate for complications of Neonatal Polycythemia-Hyperviscosity Syndrome.

3. Institute correction of dehydration & Perform Partial ET in symptomatic Polycythemia-Hyperviscosity Syndrome.

4. Manage Complications of Neonatal Poly-cythemia—Hyperviscosity Syndrome.

5. Counsel the parents about the long-term prognosis of Polycythemia-Hyperviscosity Syndrome.

* **Pearl/Peril/Pitfall :** *The terms polycythemia and hyperviscosity are often used interchangeably but are not equivalent. Polycythemia is significant only because it increases risk for hyperviscosity syndrome. Hyperviscosity syndrome is symptoms and signs caused by sludging of blood within vessels. Sludging occurs because increased RBC mass causes a relative decrease in plasma volume and a relative increase in proteins and platelets.*

BIRD'S EYE VIEW/OVERVIEW/SYNOPSIS

1. *Neonatal polycythemia (a free flowing central venous hematocrit > 65% & / or a hemoglobin > 22g/dL, during the first week of life) is usually caused by one of two conditions: increased intrauterine erythropoiesis or fetal hypertransfusion (Refer to Table 1).* Other causes seen in older children such as arterial hypoxemia (cyanotic heart disease, pulmonary disease), abnormal hemoglobins, or hypersecretion of erythropoietin by tumors are rare, and primary polycythemia or polycythemia vera are virtually nonexistent.

2. *In normal term infants, delayed clamping of the cord leading to an increased transfer of placental blood to the infant is the most common cause of polycythemia.* Placental insufficiency and chronic intrauterine hypoxia, as seen typically in *small for gestational age infants,* most commonly underlie increased intrauterine erythropoiesis. The American Academy of Pediatrics recommends that the high risk Neonates like SGA, LGA, infants of diabetic mothers and twins should have at least one screening of hematocrit done at 8hrs after birth using venous blood.

3. *As the hematocrit increases, blood viscosity increases, especially above hematocrit of 65%.* Hyperviscosity is the cause of clinical symptoms in infants presumed to be symptomatic from polycythemia. Many polycythemic infants are also hyperviscous, but this is not invariably the case. *The terms polycythemia and hyperviscosity are not interchangeable.*

4. *Most polycythemic infants have no symptoms, particularly if the polycythemia becomes apparent only upon routine Neonatal screening.* Symptoms, when present, are usually attributable to hyperviscosity and poor tissue perfusion or to associated metabolic abnormalities such as hypoglycemia and hypocalcemia *(Refer to Table No-2 for the symptoms of hyperviscosity, which may occur independently of polycythemia / hyperviscosity and must be considered in the differential diagnosis.)*

5. *Following diagnosis, an attempt should be made to determine the cause of polycythemia (Refer to Table No-1).* The condition is particularly common in infants of diabetic mothers or those with Down syndrome and may also occur in the setting of maternal hypertension. However, no apparent cause is found in most cases. Studies to determine the effects of polycythemia are dictated by the clinical findings but should usually *include* serum bilirubin, glucose, calcium, BUN, and creatinine levels.

6. *Severe complications of polycythemia—hyperviscosity include* seizures, pulmonary hypertension, severe respiratory distress with or without CCF, peripheral gangrene, NEC, & renal failure from renal vein thrombosis & priapism.

7. *The Evaluation-Decision-Action-Plan/Algorithm to diagnose and manage a Neonate with polycythemia / hyperviscosity* summarizes the current management. Asymptomatic infants although have an increased risk of late, mild neuropsychologic handicaps, prospective studies have failed to demonstrate major benefit from partial exchange transfusion. *Because co-existing hypoglycemia is an important determinant of adverse neurologic outcome, careful monitoring and maintenance of adequate glucose levels and hydration are important.* Most advocate partial exchange transfusion if the hematocrit is > 75%, even if the baby is asymptomatic. Before a diagnosis of polycythemia is considered, it is mandatory to exclude dehydration. If the birth weight is known, re-weighing the baby and looking for excessive weight loss would help in the diagnosis of dehydration. If this is present, it should be corrected by increasing fluid intake. The hematocrit should be measured once again after correction of dehydration. Once a diagnosis of polycythemia is made, associated metabolic problems including hypoglycemia should be excluded. Two modes of therapy have been described for polycythemia.

8. *Symptomatic infants need partial exchange transfusion with normal saline or with 5% albuminated saline, to lower the hematocrit and viscosity and to improve acute symptoms .* Unlike FFP, these products don't carry a risk of transmitting viral infections. Calculation of the total volume of blood to be exchanged for diluent uses the following formula.

Exchange volume :

observed hematocrit - desired hematocrit × blood volume

   (mL/kg) × weight (kg)/ observed hematocrit

Blood volume varies between 75ml/kg for baby with birth weight of 4 kg &, 110ml/kg for baby weighing 1000gm & thus has an inverse relationship - smaller the baby more the blood volume. 85-90ml/kg is considered for most of the neonates with normal birth weight. For e.g. a 3 kg dyspneic infant with an 80% hematocrit requires a partial exchange transfusion.

Blood volume = 3 kg × 90mL/kg = 270 mL

$$\frac{Observed\ Hct - desired\ Hct = \quad 80-55}{Observed\ Hct = \quad\quad\quad 80}$$

Therefore, volume of exchange =270mL × 0.31= 83.7ml. As a rough guide, the volume of blood to be exchanged is usually 25–30 ml/kg.

9. *The long-term prognosis of polycythemic infants is unclear.* Reported adverse outcomes include speech deficits, abnormal fine motor control, reduced IQ, school problems, and other neurologic abnormalities. It is thought that the underlying etiology (e.g. chronic intrauterine hypoxia) and hyperviscosity contribute to adverse outcomes. The outlook of asymptomatic polycythemia is less certain & remains to be explored.

10. *Partial exchange transfusion may reduce but not eliminate the risk of neurologic sequelae. Only low birth weight & small for gestational age are the risk factors for poor developmental outcome.* A causal relationship exists between partial exchange transfusion and an increase in gastrointestinal tract disorders and necrotizing enterocolitis.

---

* *Pearl/Peril/Pitfall : Asymptomatic infants should be treated with IV hydration. Symptomatic infants should undergo an isovolumic partial exchange transfusion to reduce the Hct to 55% and thereby decrease blood viscosity; blood is removed in 5 mL/kg (about 10 to 12 mL) aliquots and replaced with an equal volume of 0.9% saline. Asymptomatic infants whose Hct remains persistently > 70% despite hydration may also benefit from this procedure.*

THE EVALUATION-DECISION-ACTION-PLAN/ALGORITHM FOR THE DIAGNOSIS AND MANAGEMENT OF *NEONATAL POLYCYTHEMIA - HYPERVISCOSITY SYNDROME*

SUBJECTIVE FINDINGS

Review the perinatal history to identify the various causes of polycythemia-hyperviscosity in Neonates.

(Refer to Table 1,2 & 3 for etiology and symptoms)

OBJECTIVE FINDINGS

Look for the following nonspecific symptoms & signs of polycythemia - hyperviscosity

Lethargy	Apnea
Irritability	Hypotonia
Tremors, abnormal cry	Seizures
Hypoglycemia	Poor feeding
Vomiting	Cyanosis
Hepatomegaly	Acidosis
Thrombocytopenia	Jaundice
Cardiac failure	Respiratory distress
NEC	Persistent pulmonary
Oliguria	Hypertension
Hematuria	Peripheral gangrene
Renal vein	Plethora/prolonged
thrombosis	CRT

INVESTIGATIONS

Blood FBC, platelets,Group/Type & Crossmatch, venous & capillary hematocrit, blood sugar, serum calcium and bilirubin, BUN, creatinine.

CXR , ECG, ECHO if cardiorespiratory symptoms present.

CT/MRI Brain scan & EEG if seizures, hypotonia, irritability & lethargy present.

Ultrasound kidneys if renal failure due to renal venous thrombosis is suspected.

Blood cultures & ABG analysis if sepsis & respiratory distress are present.

A Neonate with Polycythemia—Hyperviscosity syndrome

BASICS

The relationship between viscosity and hematocrit is linear below a hematocrit of 60–65%, but increases exponentially above this. Viscosity is much greater in small vessels than in large ones.

The interrelationship between polycythemia and hyperviscosity and their contribution towards clinical signs is described below :

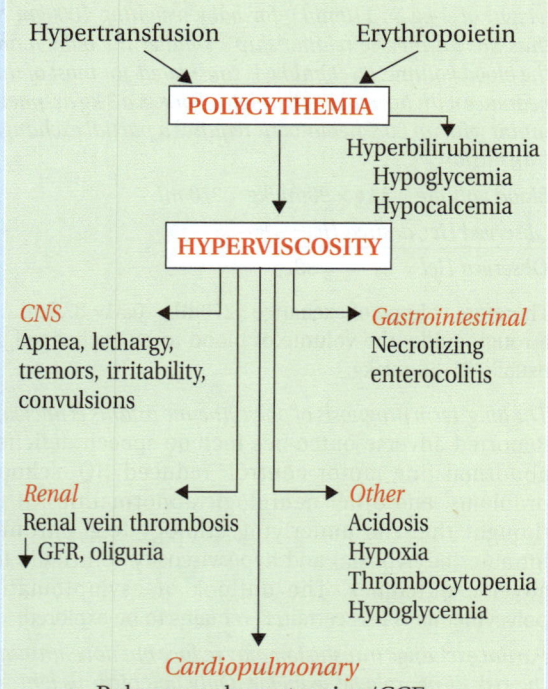

Hypertransfusion   Erythropoietin

POLYCYTHEMIA

Hyperbilirubinemia
Hypoglycemia
Hypocalcemia

HYPERVISCOSITY

CNS
Apnea, lethargy, tremors, irritability, convulsions

Gastrointestinal
Necrotizing enterocolitis

Renal
Renal vein thrombosis
↓GFR, oliguria

Other
Acidosis
Hypoxia
Thrombocytopenia
Hypoglycemia

Cardiopulmonary
Pulmonary hypertension/CCF
Symptomatic pulmonary plethora

---

* *Ensure* ABCs *& ventilate* if the Neonate is in respiratory distress with or without pulmonary hypertension and in congestive cardiac failure & having CNS symptoms like altered sensorium, seizures etc.

* *Monitor* urine output and treat for renal failure as per the protocol for any renal failure *(refer to Chapter 72 on Neonatal Acute Renal Failure)*.

* *Suspect* NEC in case of any co-existing abdominal distention, bilious aspirates, absent bowel sounds and feed intolerance. *Manage* NEC as per the protocol *(refer to Chapter 55 on Neonatal NEC)*.

* *Monitor, correct and maintain within normal range* hypoglycemia, hypocalcemia, acidosis, hypothermia, hyperbilirubinemia, thrombocytopenia, hypomagnesemia, thrombosis, bleeding tendency.

* *Consider* IV broadspectrum antibiotics to cover for sepsis.

* *Monitor* asymptomatic infants - *Repeat* venous hematocrit 6-12 hrs until it is below 65%. *Ensure* adequate fluid intake (monitor urine specific gravity). *Give* partial exchange transfusion 30ml/kg saline / 5% albuminated saline over 30 minutes, if venous hematocrit is above 75% (avoid FFP).

* *If symptomatic* (e.g. cardiorespiratory or neurological signs and symptoms) : give partial exchange transfusion and aim at reducing the hematocrit to about 55% by the following formula.

Exchange volume :

$$\frac{observed\ hematocrit - desired\ hematocrit\ \times\ blood\ volume\ (mL/kg) \times weight\ (kg)}{observed\ hematocrit}$$

Where blood volume is usually 90mL/kg but in infants of diabetic mothers it may be lower (80-85mL/kg).

For e.g. a 3 kg dyspneic infant with an 80% hematocrit requires a partial exchange transfusion.

Blood volume = 3 kg × 90mL/kg = 270mL

$$\frac{Observed\ Hct-desired\ Hct}{Observed\ Hct} = \frac{80-55}{80} = 0.31$$

Therefore, volume of exchange = 270mL × 0.31 = 83.7mL.

* *Partial exchange transfusion* : *Perform* through an umbilical arterial / venous catheter. *Ensure* that the tip of the umbilical arterial catheter below the 3rd lumbar vertebra (i.e., below the origins of the renal & inferior mesenteric arteries) and the tip of umbilical venous catheter should be in the right atrium or inferior vena cava and not in the portal circulation. If the catheter tip can not be advanced through the ductus venosus and remains in the portal system - *only withdraw* the blood *but infuse* exchange fluid into a peripheral vein to avoid NEC.

TABLE 1 — Etiology of neonatal polycythemia

Active (Increased intrauterine erythropoiesis)

Intrauterine hypoxia
  Placental insufficiency
    Small-for-gestational-age infants
  Postmaturity
  Toxemia of pregnancy
  Drugs (propranolol)
Severe maternal heart disease
Maternal smoking
Maternal diabetes

Neonatal hyperthyroidism or hypothyroidism
Congenital adrenal hyperplasia
Chromosome abnormalities
  Trisomy 13
  Trisomy 18
  Trisomy 21 (Down syndrome)
Hyperplastic visceromegaly (Beckwith syndrome)
Decreased fetal erythrocyte deformability

Passive (Secondary to Erythrocyte Transfusions)

From Oski FA, Naiman JL : Hematologic Problems in the Newborn.

TABLE 2 — Screening for polycythemia

Screening is recommended for the following:

a. Small for gestational age (SGA) infants

b. Infants of diabetic mothers (IDM)

c. Large for gestational age (LGA) infants

d. Monochorionic twins especially the larger twin

e. Morphological features of growth retardation.

Courtesy-AIIMS Protocol-Deorari AK, Paul VK et al

TABLE 3 — Clinical signs associated with neonatal polycythemia—hyperviscosity syndrome

A. *Central nervous system:* There may be an altered state of consciousness, including lethargy and decreased activity, hyperirritability, proximal muscle hypotonia, vasomotor instability, and vomiting. Seizures, thromboses, and cerebral infarction are extraordinarily rare.

B. *Cardiopulmonary system:* Respiratory distress and tachycardia may be present. Congestive heart failure with cardiomegaly may be seen but is rarely clinically prominent. Pulmonary hypertension may occur but is not usually severe unless other predisposing factors are present.

C. *Gastrointestinal tract:* Feeding intolerance occurs occasionally. Necrotizing enterocolitis has been reported but rarely without other factors (e.g., IUGR), which casts doubt on the primary cause.

D. *Genitourinary tract:* Oliguria, acute renal failure, renal vein thrombosis.

F. *Hematologic disorders:* There may be hyperbilirubinemia, thrombocytopenia, or reticulocytosis (with enhanced erythropoiesis only).

TABLE 4 — Practical aspects of diagnosis and management of neonatal polycythemia—hyperviscosity syndrome

* *Hematocrit* should be measured at age 2–4 hours in all infants at risk for polycythemia e.g. infants of diabetic mothers, infants of hypertensive mothers, IUGR / large for dates, trisomy 21.

* *Simple phlebotomy* is contraindicated because it decreases arterial blood pressure as well as blood volume. The decrease in systemic arterial blood pressure will decrease blood flow and thus increase viscosity and its effects.

* *Acidosis* decreases deformability of RBCs and thereby increases blood viscosity. Therefore correct acidosis and maintain the pH above 7.25.

* Because of the association of *NEC* with polycythemia, infants with polycythemia who are *thrombocytopenic* should not be given enteral feedings until the platelet count increases to normal. Thrombocytopenia is thought to result from consumption of platelets in microthrombi and is indicative of obstruction in microcirculation.

* Some polycythemic infants present with *persistent pulmonary hypertension* and findings that mimic cyanotic congenital heart disease. Echocardiogram should be obtained to differentiate between the two conditions. *(v.i.)*

* In screening apparently healthy Newborns for polycythemia, account must be taken of a number of physiologic variables that influence the hematocrit during the first 12 hrs of life :

1) time of cord clamping - immediate clamping (within 30 seconds) minimizes placental transfusion 2) Age at sampling - values increase from birth to a peak at 2 hrs, gradually decreasing to cord levels around 12–18 hrs 3) Site of sampling - values from blood extracted by the heelstick method exceed those from venous blood (that difference can be minimized by prewarming the heel) 4) Method of hematocrit determination - spun values are higher than those obtained by electronic cell counter and show better correlation with blood viscosity.

* *One way to standardize and simplify screening for polycythemia is as follows :* At birth, clamp the cord at about 30 to 45 seconds; at 4 to 6 hours of age obtain a blood sample from a warmed heelstick and perform a spun hematocrit. If the result is greater than 70%, repeat the test on a venous sample. A venous hematocrit of 65% or more indicates polycythemia. By this approach, 1% to 5% of Newborns are polycythemic ; the range largely reflects differences in altitude at which the study population resides. Because the hematocrit is lower with increasing prematurity, polycythemia is less frequently seen in preterm infants than in term babies.

* *Polycythemia—hyperviscosity in the Newborn* period mimics *cyanotic congenital heart disease* as it can produce cyanosis, enlarged heart, increased pulmonary vascular markings and palpable liver. However cyanotic congenital heart disease doesn't produce polycythemia in the Newborn period (while in older children it can produce physiologic polycythemia that allows adequate oxygen transport to occur in the presence of arterial hypoxemia). *Rapid disappearance of the cardiac abnormalities following recognition and treatment of polycythemia (by partial exchange transfusion) differentiates it from the cyanotic congenital heart disease.*

* *Partial exchange transfusion with FFP* has been associated with the appearance of the *NEC*, whereas purified plasma protein derivatives such as albumin haven't.

* *Pearl/Peril/Pitfall : Diagnosis of polycythemia is by Hct; diagnosis of hyperviscosity syndrome is clinical. Capillary samples often overestimate Hct so a venous Hct, preferably spun, should be obtained before the diagnosis is made; most published studies of polycythemia use spun Hcts, which are generally higher than those obtained on automated counters. Laboratory measure of viscosity is not readily available.*

NEONATAL POLYCYTHEMIA & HYPERVISCOSITY : SUMMARY OF TREATMENT

Treatment for asymptomatic patients

- Hct 65–75%: Perform cardiorespiratory monitoring and monitoring of Hct and glucose levels every 6 hours and observe the patient for symptoms.

- Hct more than 75% on repeated measurements: Consider partial exchange transfusion.

Treatment for symptomatic patients

- Hct 60–65%: Consider alternative explanations for the symptoms. Although polycythemia and hyperviscosity may be the etiology of the symptoms, other causes for the symptoms must be excluded.

- Hct more than 65% with symptoms attributable to polycythemia and hyperviscosity: Perform partial exchange transfusion.

Partial exchange transfusion

- Perform a partial exchange transfusion by using an umbilical venous catheter to reduce the central Hct to 50–55%.

- The total blood volume to be exchanged is determined as follows: [blood volume(patient's Hct – desired Hct)]/(patient's Hct), where blood volume = the patient's weight in kilograms multiplied by 90 mL/kg.

- Normal saline is the replacement fluid of choice for exchange transfusions because it is effective and inexpensive. As alternatives, Plasmanate, 5% albumin, or fresh frozen plasma can be used. However, none of these is more effective than normal saline. In addition, both 5% albumin and fresh frozen plasma are blood products, and certain religious beliefs prohibit their use. Lastly, these colloid products have been associated with complications such as NEC.

- Sterile technique is required.

- An exchange transfusion can be performed in 3 ways, depending on the type of vascular access that is available. Regardless of the method used, aliquots should not exceed approximately 5 mL/kg delivered or removed over 2–3 minutes.

- If only a single umbilical venous catheter is in place, use a push-pull technique. With this technique, the withdrawal of blood is alternated with the administration of replacement fluid through the single catheter. Do not remove more than 5 mL/kg in any single withdrawal.

- If both umbilical venous and arterial catheters are in place, withdraw blood from the arterial catheter while administering the replacement fluid through the venous catheter.

- If a venous or arterial umbilical catheter and a peripheral venous catheter are in place, the former can be used for blood withdrawal, while the latter is used to simultaneously and continuously infuse the replacement fluid.

Screening guidelines for high risk infants with suspected polycythemia/hyperviscosity

Age	Screening technique
Birth	Dextrostix for all high-risk infants (eg, IUGR, infants of diabetic mothers, Down's syndrome, Congenital Adrenal Hyperplasia, Hypo-and Hyperthyroidism, Beckwith-Wiedemann syndrome, etc)
6–8 hours	Peripheral Hct determination in symptomatic infants > 34 weeks' gestation. Venous hematocrit determination when peripheral Hct is significantly elevated (> 70%).
Any time	When available, evaluate viscosity for symptomatic infants with moderately elevated Hct (>55-64%). In the absence of viscosity measurements, estimate viscosity by assessing total protein and red cell smear for abnormalities in RBC shape.

KEY POINTS FOR CLINICAL PRACTICE

1. Polycythemia is defined as a central venous hematocrit of over 65%, whereas hyperviscosity is defined as viscosity >14.6 cP at a shear rate of 11.5/s as measured by a viscometer. The relationship between hematocrit & viscosity is linear below a hematocrit of 60%, but viscosity increases exponentially at a hematocrit of 70% or greater. Besides hematocrit, viscosity is altered by other factors, such as fibrinogen & local blood flow. *Dehydration as a cause of increased hematocrit should always be ruled out before diagnosing and intervening for polycythemia.*

2. SGA, LGA, infants of diabetic mothers and twins should be screened for polycythemia at 8hrs of age and monitor for symptoms and signs of Polycythemia and Hyperviscosity.

3. Asymptomatic infants with a hematocrit between 60–70% can usually be managed by increasing fluid intake and repeating the hematocrit in 4–6hrs. Most Neonatologists perform a partial exchange transfusion when the venous hematocrit is >70% in the absence of symptoms (controversial)

4. All infants with symptomatic polycythemia should receive a partial exchange transfusion, although the efficacy of it improving neurological outcomes is uncertain.

5. The prognosis of infants with the polycythemia depends largely on the primary cause of polycythemia.

REFERENCES & FURTHER READING : 1) Swetnam SM et all. Hemodynamic consequences of Neonatal Polycythemia. J Pediatrics-1987 2) OhW. Neonatal Polycythemia & Hyperviscocity. PCNA-1986 3) Text Book of Neonatology by Rennie JM, Roberton NRC (Eds)-1999-3rd editon 4)Dempsey EM, Barrington K. Short and long term outcomes following partial exchange transfusion in the polycythaemic newborn: a systematic review. Arch Dis Child Fetal Neonatal Ed. 2006;91:F2-6. 5)Deorari AK, Paul VK, Shreshta L, Singh M. Symptomatic neonatal polycythemia: Comparison of partial exchange transfusion with saline versus plasma. Indian Pediatr 1995;32:1167–71

* Pearl/Peril/Pitfall : Normal saline is the replacement fluid of choice for exchange transfusions because it is effective and inexpensive. As alternatives, Plasmanate, 5% albumin, or fresh frozen plasma can be used. However, none of these is more effective than normal saline. In addition, both 5% albumin and fresh frozen plasma are blood products, and certain religious beliefs prohibit their use. Lastly, these colloid products have been associated with complications such as NEC.

Neonatal Bleeding and Bruising

@ Neonatal hemostatic abnormalities can present diagnostic and therapeutic challenges to the physician. Developmental deficiencies and/or increases of certain coagulation proteins, coupled with acquired or genetic risk factors, can result in a hemorrhagic or thromboembolic emergency. The timely diagnosis of a congenital hemorrhagic or thrombotic disorder can avoid significant long-term sequelae. However, due to the lack of randomized clinical trials addressing the management of neonatal coagulation disorders, treatment strategies are usually empiric and not evidence-based.

Signs and symptoms of neonatal bleeding disorders.

- Umbilical stump oozing
- Post-venipuncture/heel stick bleeding
- Significant caput succedaneum and /or cephalohematomas without significant birth trauma
- Prolonged post-circumcision bleeding
- Intracranial hemorrhage in a term or late preterm infant

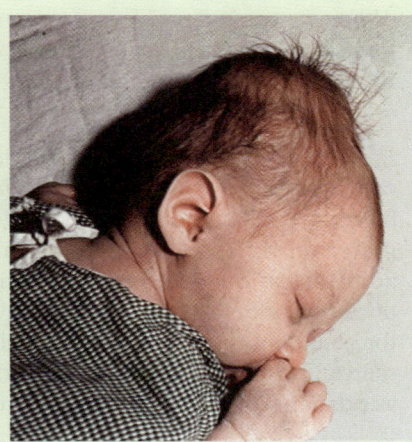

Immune thrombocytopenia. An infant born with a cephalohematoma.

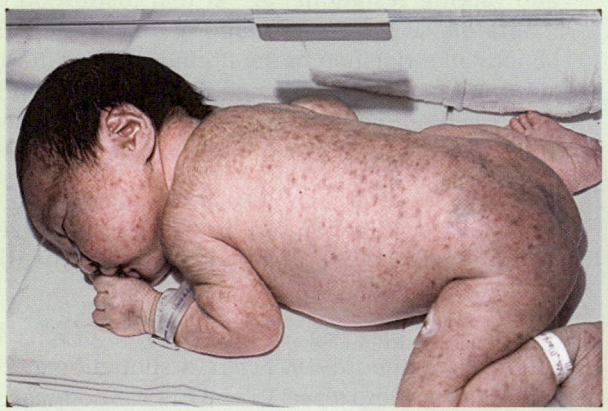

Immune Thrombocytopenia. An infant born with neonatal lupus syndrome and severe thrombocytopenia. Note extensive bruising and petechiae.

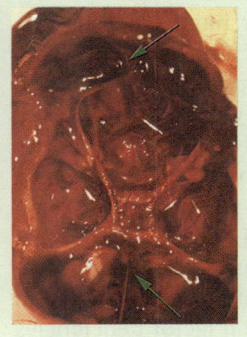

Immune Thrombocytopenia. Neonatal brain at autopsy showing extensive subdural hemorrhage.

REVIEW OF CLINICAL PROBLEMS

1. How do you classify Fetal & Neonatal Thrombocytopenia?
   Ans: Refer to the Table 1 of the Chapter.

2. Discuss the differences between Early onset Thrombocytopenia and Late onset Thrombocytopenia.
   Ans: Refer to the Table 2 of the Chapter.

3. How do you differentiate Alloimmune Thrombocytopenia from Autoimmune Thrombocytopenia ?
   Ans: Refer to the Table 6 of the Chapter.

4. What are the common causes of Bleeding in "well" and "sick" infants?
   Ans: Refer to the Table 7 of the Chapter.

5. Discuss the Guidelines for Neonatal Platelet Transfusions.
   Ans: Refer to the Table "4" of the Chapter.

LEARNING OBJECTIVES

After completing this article, readers will be able to:

1. Recognize Neonatal Bleeding disorders early and Investigate them promptly to prevent mortality and morbidity.

2. Appreciate the differences-clinical/lab, of Neonatal bleeding between Well babies and Sick babies.

3. Interpret the Laboratory tests for coagulation so as to come to the most likely cause of Neonatal Bleeding.

4. Institute the appropriate management of the bleeding disorder, mostly empirically due to lack of evidence-based Guidelines.

5. Counsel the parents about the prognosis and the clinical course and long-term management of disorder under consideration.

*   ***Pearl/Peril/Pitfall :*** *Neonates are susceptible to bleeding for various reasons ·immaturity of the hemostatic system because of quantitative and qualitative deficiency of coagulation factors ·maternal disease and drugs ·birth trauma ·other conditions eg sepsis and asphyxia.*

BIRD`S EYE VIEW/OVERVIEW/SYNOPSIS

1. *The diagnosis and management* of acquired and congenital hemostatic disorders in Newborns differ from those of older patients owing to a unique hemostatic system at birth and age - related pathologic conditions. Physiologic levels of many coagulation proteins are low, making the diagnosis of some inherited and acquired hemostatic problems difficult. *Although acquired problems are more frequent, severe forms of congenital factor deficiencies often first present in early infancy and should seriously be considered in otherwise healthy infants.*

2. *Evaluation* of any infant with hemorrhagic complications includes *a careful history* of family bleeding problems, outcome of previous pregnancies, maternal illnesses (especially infections), drug administration (maternal and neonatal), and documentation that Vitamin K was given at birth. Note the gestational history, method of delivery, and APGAR scores. Consider risk factors for bacterial infection such as prematurity, PROM, fetal distress during labor.

3. *In the physical examination* note the extent (localized versus diffuse) and type of bleeding (petechiae, purpura, ecchymoses, mucosal bleeding, umbilical cord bleeding or GI hemorrhage.) Assess the cardiovascular status for signs of intravascular volume depletion (rapid blood loss or sepsis). Severe jaundice, hepatosplenomegaly, respiratory distress, or signs of sepsis suggest a generalized acquired bleeding disorder (DIC). Congenital hemostatic defects present most typically in an otherwise well-appearing child with unexplained bleeding. Look carefully for a cavernous hemangioma and consider the possibility of intracranial hemorrhage. Hemarthrosis, a common presentation of severe congenital factor deficiencies in older children, rarely occurs in Newborns. In otherwise healthy infants, the most common causes of bleeding are thrombocytopenia secondary to transplacental passage of a maternal antiplatelet antibody, Vitamin K deficiency and less commonly, a congenital coagulation factor deficiency. Although sick infants may have an underlying congenital deficit, acquired disorders such as DIC and liver failure are more common.

4. *The initial laboratory evaluation* of infants with bleeding complications should include a PT, APTT, TCT, fibrinogen level, platelet count, and on rare occasion, a bleeding time. Abnormalities in these tests usually guide the selection of additional tests such as specific factor assays and paracoagulation tests. For a male child in whom hemophilia A or B is suspected, specific factor assays should be performed regardless of the APTT value. Deficiencies of FXIII and α_2AP do not prolong the screening tests and must be measured directly if they are suspected. Differentiation of congenital and acquired deficiencies from physiologic values can be difficult for some coagulation proteins, a problem unique to newborns.

5. The commonly encountered diagnosis along with the laboratory abnormalities and differential diagnosis in 'SICK' & 'WELL' infants are shown *in Table 7.*

6. In most Neonates the diagnoses of bleeding is clarified with 3 screening tests ; platelet count, prothrombin time (PT), and activated partial thromboplastin time (APTT) *(refer to figure 4, describing the algorithm of coagulation tests and their interpretation).* A PT > 17 seconds in a Neonate at any gestational age and a PTT > 45–50 seconds in term infant should be considered abnormal. In preterm infant, the PTT is useful only if one has normal values for the Neonate and varying gestational age at that institution or laboratory. If the PT, PTT and platelets are truly abnormal, estimation of the fibrinogen level, fibrin split products are performed. If the fibrinogen is decreased, along with the presence of FDP and D-dimer, a diagnosis of DIC is made.

7. *The E-D-A-Plan/Algorithm* to diagnose and manage a Neonate with bleeding the bruising summarizes salient features of diagnostic and therapeutic interventions.

8. Treat serious bleeding with fresh frozen plasma. If Vitamin K has not been given, it should be given immediately, with a repeat PT and PTT 4–6 hours later; a marked improvement strongly suggests Vitamin K deficiency.

9. An isolated prolongation of the PTT suggests a congenital defect in hemostasis or heparin effect. Order clotting assays for factors VIII, IX and XI. Treat serious bleeding with FFP (or cryoprecipitate or factor concentrate for confirmed factor VIII or IX deficiency) and consider a hematology consultation.

10. An isolated prolonged PT suggests factor VII deficiency, Vitamin K deficiency, or early liver disease. Besides controlling the bleeding in a sick neonate, therapy should be primarily focused on the underlying disease state such as septicemia, herpes simplex, necrotizing enterocolitis, shock, hypovolemia, hypoxia, acidosis, and ITP. Blood products should be administered judiciously. If the Neonate has isolated thrombo-cytopenia, a platelet count should be performed in the mother. She may have thrombocytopenia associated with pre-eclampsia or idiopathic thrombocytopenic purpura.

---

* *Pearl/Peril/Pitfall : Vitamin K deficiency bleeding (VKDB) refers to bleeding that occurs as a consequence of vitamin K deficiency during the first six months of life. Previously known as hemorrhagic disease of the newborn, it was renamed to emphasize that bleeding problems during the neonatal period are not confined to those arising from vitamin K deficiency and that bleeding secondary to vitamin K deficiency may occur beyond the first month of life.*

THE EVALUATION-DECISION-ACTION-PLAN /ALGORITHM FOR THE DIAGNOSIS AND MANAGEMENT OF *NEONATAL BLEEDING AND BRUISING*

SUBJECTIVE FINDINGS

Hx of localized versus diffuse bleeding from multiple sites.

Hx of bleeding from the umbilicus / from mucous membranes / following circumcision / from venepuncture sites / into the scalp (large cephalhematoma) / into the skin (large ecchymoses) / into the joints (hemarthrosis) / ICH / GI tract / pulmonary hemorrhage etc.

Hx of hemorrhagic diatheses in the family members, maternal SLE, ITP, drugs like anticonvulsants & ATDs, infections, birth trauma.

Hx of vitamin K administration at delivery.

OBJECTIVE FINDINGS

Asses ABCs and disability (convulsions, coma, pupils, fundi, doll's eyes, movements), CRT, BP, urine output.

Determine whether the pattern of bleeding : localized or diffuse from multiple sites & the type of bleeding (petechiae, purpura / ecchymoses / frank blood) .

Check whether is it swallowed maternal blood or is it due to nasogastric tube trauma !

Check whether the stool is normal in colour, but with streaks of blood (anal fissure / rectal trauma). Look for congenital malformations, syndromes & for hepatosplenomegaly.

Determine whether the baby is healthy or sick in appearance !

INVESTIGATIONS

Blood Hb, Hematocrit, TC, DC, Platelets, Smear, Bleeding Time, Clotting Time, PT, APTT, Thrombin Clotting Time (TCT), fibrinogen level, specific factor assays. (factor VIII, IX, XIII, α_2AP etc.), Group, Type, Cross match, Blood cultures, TORSCH titers, Bone marrow studies, Coomb's test.

Maternal blood studies platelets, rapid HPA-1a (PL A1) phenotyping & anti-HPA-1a (PLA1) alloantibodies.

LFTs, FDPs, d-dimer test.

Ultrasound scanning of kidneys (renal vein thrombosis), CT brain scan (IVH or ICH)

In the sick Newborn consider blood cultures, ABG analysis, CXR, AXR & urine analysis.

A NEONATE WITH BLEEDING AND BRUISING

Perform *Apt test to exclude swallowed maternal blood syndrome *(refer to box on right side of this Algorithm)*

Identify "sick infant" and correct hypoglycemia, hypothermia, electrolyte & acid-base disturbances. *Give* IV broadspectrum antibiotics to cover for sepsis *(after full septic screen with LP only after stabilization)*. Ventilate if necessary (eg. circulatory failure, raised ICT, severe RDS).

Ensure ABCs, *treat* shock with 20ml/kg NS or O Negative whole fresh blood transfusion + IV Dobutamine infusion if necessary 10mcg/kg / mt IVI). *Give* Vitamin K 2mgs IV after obtaining PT & PTT on cord blood. *Give* fresh frozen plasma 10ml/kg, if the PT is greatly prolonged and fails to improve with Vitamin K.

Verify the coagulation screen (PT, PTT, platelet count)

Normal coagulation screen

Consider : Bleeding time
Consult : Hematologist

Identify :
Mild von Willebrand disease
Platelet function defect
Drugs (aspirin)
Factor XIII deficiency
α_2-Antiplasmin deficiency
Plasminogen activator inhibitor deficiency
Trauma, Vascular abnormality

Isolated thrombocytopenia
(refer to next page for its evaluation)

Apt devised the following test for this differentiation : (1) Rinse a blood-stained diaper or some grossly bloody (red) stool with a suitable amount of water to obtain a distinctly pink supernatant hemoglobin solution. (2) Centrifuge the mixture and decant the supernatant solution. (3) To five parts of the supernatant fluid add one part of 0.25 N (1%) sodium hydroxide. Within 1-2 min a color reaction takes place : a yellow-brown color indicates that the blood is maternal in origin ; a persistent pink indicates that it is from the infant. A control test with known adult or infant blood, or both, is advisable.

Abnormal coagulation screen

Increased PT, increased PTT, decreased platelets	Increased PT, increased PTT, normal platelets	Normal PT, increased PTT, normal platelets	Increased PT, normal PTT, normal platelets
Do : Fibrinogen, FDP, D-dimer	**Do :** Fibrinogen, FDP, D-dimer	**Do :** Factor assays (VIII, IX, XI) Von Willebrand assays	**Do :** Factor VII assay Liver function tests
Consider : Liver function tests Viral cultures	**Consider :** Liver function tests		
Identify : Consumptive coagulopathy (sepsis, NEC, asphyxia, acidosis, respiratory distress, cavernous hemangioma) Liver disease	**Identify :** Vitamin K deficiency Liver disease DIC (severe asphyxia) Congenital deficiencies (factors I, II, V, X) Heparin effect	**Identify :** Congenital deficiencies (factors VIII, IX, XI) Severe von Willebrand disease Heparin effect	**Identify :** Factor VII deficiency Liver disease Mild vitamin K deficiency
Treat : Consider : Fresh Frozen Plasma, Platelet Transfusion, Vitamin K	**Treat : Consider :** Fresh Frozen Plasma, Vitamin K, Protamine Sulfate	**Treat : Consider :** Factor Concentrate (VIII, IX, von Willebrand) Fresh Frozen Plasma (XI)	**Treat : Consider :** Vitamin K Fresh Frozen Plasma

* *Pearl/Peril/Pitfall : Owing to the physiological increase in vWF concentrations at birth, type I disease does not usually manifest until later in life, and, even where there is a family history, it is not usually possible to make a diagnosis of this condition during the newborn period.*

THE EVALUATION-DECISION-ACTION-PLAN/ALGORITHM FOR THE DIAGNOSIS AND MANAGEMENT OF *NEONATAL ISOLATED THROMBOCYTOPENIA*

SUBJECTIVE FINDINGS

Hx of maternal drug ingestion (aspirin, indomethacin, quinine, hydralazine, thiazide, heparin), maternal infections (TORSCH, Bacterial or viral), DIC, HELLP syndrome (hemolysis, elevated liver enzymes, low platelets), maternal ITP, SLE.

Hx of thrombocytopenia in the family or hx of intracranial hemorrhage in a sibling and previous episodes of bleeding).

Hx of birth asphyxia, NEC, bacterial or candida sepsis, congenital leukemia, trisomies 13, 18 or 21, Fanconi's anemia, TAR syndrome (thrombocytopenia - absent radius syndrome).

OBJECTIVE FINDINGS

Assess ABCDs as usual & check whether the Neonate is well or sick & resuscitate the sick Neonate promptly before investigating further.

Look for petechiae (< 60,000/cumm), mucosal bleeding (<20,000/cumm, ICH (severe thrombocytopenia) physical malformations suggestive of TAR syndrome, Rubella syndrome, Giant hemangioma (Kasabach-Merritt syndrome), hepatosplenomegaly (e.g. TORSCH, congenital leukemia).

Large ecchymoses and muscle hemorrhages are more likely to be due to coagulation disturbances than to platelet disturbances.

INVESTIGATIONS

Maternal studies Maternal low platelet count suggests autoimmune thrombocytopenia or inherited thrombocytopenia (X - linked recessive/ autosomal dominant), maternal serum and whole blood sample for rapid HPA - 1a (PLA1) phenotyping + screen for anti HPA- 1a alloantibodies.

Neonatal studies Platelet count, full blood count, group and type, Coomb's test, coagulation studies and other studies if indicated (eg. TORSCH titers, bacterial cultures, bone marrow studies if decreased platelet production is present).

(refer to Table 9 *for differentiating decreased platelet production versus increased platelet destruction*).

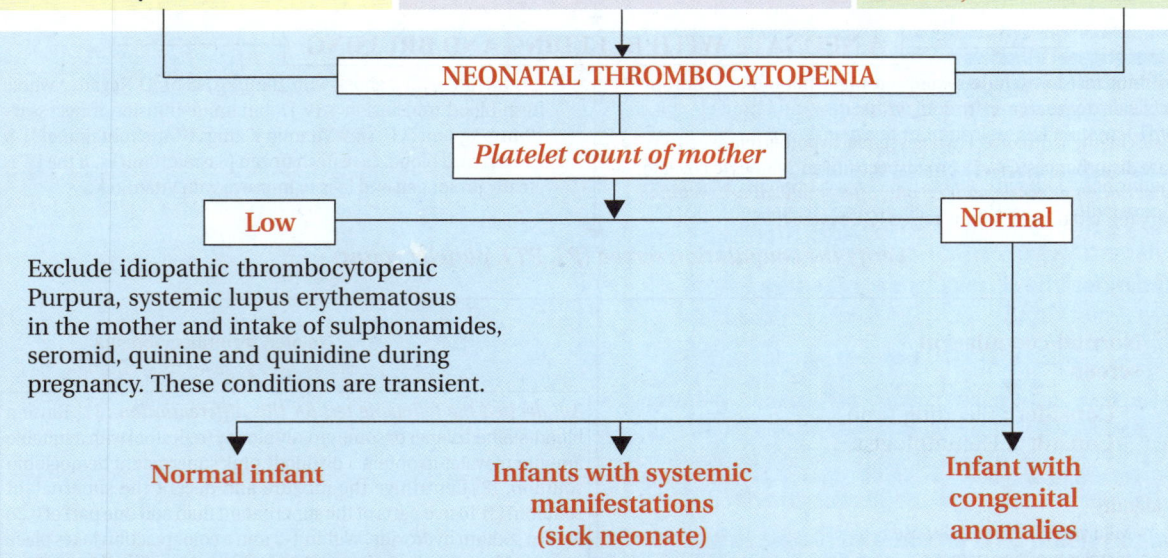

NEONATAL THROMBOCYTOPENIA

Platelet count of mother

Low — **Normal**

Exclude idiopathic thrombocytopenic Purpura, systemic lupus erythematosus in the mother and intake of sulphonamides, seromid, quinine and quinidine during pregnancy. These conditions are transient.

Normal infant	**Infants with systemic manifestations (sick neonate)**	**Infant with congenital anomalies**
1. Thiazides during pregnancy. Depression of megakaryocytes in the bone marrow.	1. Intrauterine infections.	1. Giant hemangioma.
2. Platelet iso-immunization. Estimate platelet antibodies in the maternal blood.	2. DIC.	2. Hypoplasia or aplasia of megakaryocytes in the bone marrow. Exclude rubella syndrome and Fanconi's anemia with absent radii.
3. Pancytopenia without congenital anomalies.	3. Renal vein thrombosis.	
	4. Cyanotic heart disease.	
	5. Congenital leukemia.	

Neonatal Thrombocytopenia - Management (1) *Treat* the underlying cause (eg. Sepsis) & stop the drugs known to cause thrombocytopenia 2) *Give* platelet concentrate 10-15 ml/kg (to increase the platelet count by 1 lakh /cumm), if the platelet count is < 25-30,000/cumm or if the neonate is unwell with platelet count below 50,000/cumm 3) *The* plasma in platelets should be ABO and Rh compatible with the infants RBC's & repeat the platelet count 1 hour post transfusion. 4) *For alloimmune thrombocytopenia* (with platelets < 20,000/cumm) - give HPA - 10 & HPA - 5b negative ABO & Rh D compatible platelets until the platelet count stabilize. Consider exchange transfusion and washed maternal platelets, if this is not available. Give high dose immunoglobulin (0.5g/kg) for 2 days but will not work immediately. Monitor without any intervention, if the platelet counts are 20-50,000/cumm. Prednisone 2mgs/kg/day may be beneficial in immune thrombocytopenia. 5) *For autoimmune thrombocytopenia* - (eg. maternal ITP, SLE, etc.) prevent ICH during vaginal delivery (C/S may be indicated). Maternal IV immunoglobulin and corticosteroids 2 weeks prior to delivery may be beneficial. Give short course of steroids to the infant. Newer treatments include recombinant thrombopoietin, interleukin - II.

* **Pearl/Peril/Pitfall :** *Although neonatal platelet numbers are normal, studies of platelet function suggest that neonatal platelets are hyporeactive compared with adult platelets. Despite this, the bleeding time, which can be viewed as an in vivo assessment of the platelet vessel wall interaction, is shortened in normal healthy neonates. This probably reflects multiple factors including increased concentrations of von Willebrand factor (vWF), the presence of large vWF multimers, and the high neonatal packed cell volume.*

TABLE 1	Classification of fetal and neonatal thrombocytopenias

Fetal : Alloimmune, Congenital infection (e.g. CMV, toxoplasma, rubella, HIV), Aneuploidy (e.g. trisomies 18, 13, 21, or triploidy) Autoimmune (e.g. ITP, SLE), Severe Rh hemolytic disease, Congenital/inherited (e.g. Wiskott-Aldrich syndrome)

Early onset Neonatal (<72 hours)

Placental insufficiency (e.g. PET, IUGR, diabetes) Perinatal asphyxia, Perinatal infection (e.g. E coli, GBS, Haemophilus influenzae), DIC, Allo-immune, Autoimmune (e.g. ITP, SLE) Congenital infection (e.g. CMV, toxoplasma, rubella, HIV), Thrombosis (e.g. aortic, renal vein), Bone marrow replacement (e.g. congenital leukaemia), Kasabach-Merritt syndrome, Metabolic disease (e.g. propionic and methylmalonic acidemia), Congenital/inherited (e.g. TAR, CAMT)

Late onset Neonatal (>72 hours)

Late onset sepsis, NEC, Congenital infection (e.g. CMV, toxoplasma, rubella, HIV), Autoimmune, Kasabach-Merritt syndrome, Metabolic disease (e.g. propionic and methylmalonic acidemia) Congenital/inherited (e.g. TAR, CAMT)

The most common conditions are highlighted. CMV, Cytomegalovirus; ITP, idiopathic thrombocytopenic purpura; SLE, systemic lupus erythematosus; PET, pre-eclampsia; IUGR, intrauterine growth restriction; E coli Escherichia coli; GBS, group B streptococcus; DIC, disseminated intravascular coagulation; TAR, thrombocytopenia with absent radii; CAMT.

TABLE 2	Comparison of natural history of early and late onset thrombocytopenia in neonates

Early	Late
Mild to moderate (platelet nadir rarely <50 x10⁹/l)	Severe (platelet nadir frequently <50 × 10⁹/l)
Evolves slowly over several days	Rapid onset and progression over 24–48 hours
Associated with	*Associated with*
Complicated pregnancies (PET, IUGR, maternal diabetes)	Sepsis and NEC
Rarely requires specific treatment	Multiple platelet transfusions often required
Mechanism	*Mechanism*
Impaired platelet production	Combined platelet consumption and impaired production

PET, Pre-eclampsia; IUGR, intrauterine growth restriction; NEC, necrotizing enterocolitis.

TABLE 3	Congenital and inherited thrombocytopenias that may present in the fetus or neonate

Thrombocytopenia (with abnormal platelet function)	Thrombocytopenia (without marked thrombocytopathy)
Bernard-Soulier syndrome	Fanconi's anemia
Wiskott-Aldrich syndrome	TAR syndrome
X-linked thrombocytopenia	Amegakaryocytic thrombocytopenia
Chediak-Higashi syndrome	Giant platelet syndromes (e.g.
Quebec platelet disorder	May-Hegglin anomaly, Sebastian
Some giant platelet syndromes	syndrome, Fechtner syndrome)
(e.g. Montreal syndrome)	Autosomal dominant thrombocytopenia

TABLE 4	Guidelines for platelet transfusion in the newborn

Platelet count (x10⁹/l)	Non-bleeding neonate	Bleeding neonate	NAITP (proven or suspected)
<30	Consider transfusion in all patients	Transfuse	Transfuse (with HPA compatible platelets)
30–49	Do not transfuse if clinically stable Consider transfusion if: • <1000 g and <1 week of age • clinically unstable (e.g. fluctuating blood pressure or perfusion) • previous major bleeding (e.g. grade 3–4 IVH or pulmonary hemorrhage) • current minor bleeding (e.g. petechiae, puncture site oozing or blood stained ET secretions) • concurrent coagulopathy • requires surgery or exchange transfusion	Transfuse	Transfuse (with HPA compatible platelets if any bleeding)
50–99	Do not transfuse	Transfuse	Transfuse (with HPA compatible platelets if major bleeding present)
>99	Do not transfuse	Do not transfuse	Do not transfuse

NAITP, Neonatal alloimmune thrombocytopenia; HPA, human platelet antigen; IVH, intraventricular hemorrhage; ET, endotracheal.

* *Pearl/Peril/Pitfall : It is important that infants presenting with abnormal bleeding are appropriately investigated for hemophilia and other inherited bleeding disorders. In particular, physiological prolongation of the APTT must be interpreted with care, and it should also be noted that a mildly reduced FVIII concentration is not incompatible with a normal APTT. Factor assays should therefore always be performed if bleeding appears excessive.*

Certain Neonatal conditions are associated with severe and prolonged thrombocytopenia . The mechanisms of thrombocytopenia associated with these conditions, along with platelet production indices, can be used to predict the patient's probable response to platelet transfusion

TABLE 5	Severe and prolonged thrombocytopenia		
Cause	**MPV**	**RP%**	**Mechanism**
Alloimmune	High	High	Immune reticulo-endothelial destruction
NEC/necrotic bowel	High	High	Platelet adhesion to damaged epithelium
Fungal sepsis	High	High	Platelet adhesion to damaged epithelium
Marrow failure	Normal	Low	Impaired production
Liver disease	Normal	Low	Impaired Tpo production

MPV = mean platelet volume; RP = reticulated platelets; NEC = necrotizing enterocolitis

TABLE 6	Alloimmune and autoimmune thrombocytopenia	
	Alloimmune thrombocytopenia	**Autoimmune thrombocytopenia**
Platelet antigens	Antigens on fetal platelets not found on maternal platelets–most commonly HPA - 5b	Antigens common to both maternal and fetal platelets–most commonly GPIIB/IIIA and GPIb/IX complexes
Platelet count	Generally severe birth thrombocytopenia with counts often < 20,000/ul	Generally mild thrombocytopenia with birth counts often > 50,000/ul
Time of presentation	Platelet count usually very low at birth	Platelet count can even be normal at birth and fall over several days
Maternal history	Normal maternal platelet count. No history of ITP, SLE, or hypothyroidism	Low maternal platelet count (unless splenectomy). Possible history of ITP, SLE, hypothyroidism
Intracranial hemorrhage	10 – 20%	< 1 – 2%
Treatment	Antigen negative or maternal platelets and IVIG and/or methylprednisone	IVIG and/or methylprednisolone
Resolution of thrombocytopenia	Usually within 1 – 2 weeks	Slower resolution, usually 3 – 4 weeks after birth as nadir may occur at 3 – 4 days.

Case Studies: Will These Infants Benefit From Platelet Transfusion?

The following case studies illustrate the considerations used to determine whether an infant with thrombocytopenia will benefit from platelet transfusion. Questions to ask about each case study are: (1) What is the kinetic mechanism causing the infant's thrombocytopenia; and (2) What do you predict will be the infant's response to a platelet transfusion?

Case 1. 27 weeks' gestation AGA (appropriate for gestational age) Neonate who had normal platelet count at birth. Now 25 days old, recovering from NEC, still taking nothing by mouth and on antibiotics. Platelet count has been 30-40,000/mcL for 1 week. Mean platelet volume is 12 fL; reticulated platelets 10%.

> *Answer:* The underlying cause of the thrombocytopenia in this situation is accelerated platelet usage or destruction. Platelets transfused into this infant are likely to have a short survival.

Case 2. 37 weeks' gestation nondysmorphic Neonate whose platelet count has been < 50,000/mcL since birth. At 5 days of age, stools are hematest-positive and platelet count is 18,000/mcL. MPV is 7.3 fL; reticulated platelets 1%.

> *Answer* : In this case, the underlying cause of low platelets is reduced platelet production. Transfused platelets will have a normal survival.

Neonatal thrombocytopenia is a clinical problem that can be either benign or serious, depending upon factors such as the underlying cause and the health of the Neonate. By evaluating not only platelet counts but also indices of platelet production, the practitioner can gain a better understanding of the significance of the infant's thrombocytopenia and the appropriate therapy.

---

* *Pearl/Peril/Pitfall : Much of the management of DIC thus continues to centre around the use of supportive treatment with fresh frozen plasma, cryoprecipitate, and platelets to try to maintain adequate hemostasis. Although the use of blood products and the thresholds set for transfusion are largely empirical, it would appear reasonable to institute replacement therapy, particularly where there is an increased risk of bleeding. Guidelines for the transfusion of platelets suggest that the platelet count should be maintained above 50 x10⁹/l by the transfusion of platelet concentrates (10–15 ml/kg). Fresh frozen plasma (10–15 ml/kg) can be used to replace hemostatic proteins, although cryoprecipitate (5–10 ml/kg) is a better source of fibrinogen, which should be kept above 1 g/l.24.*

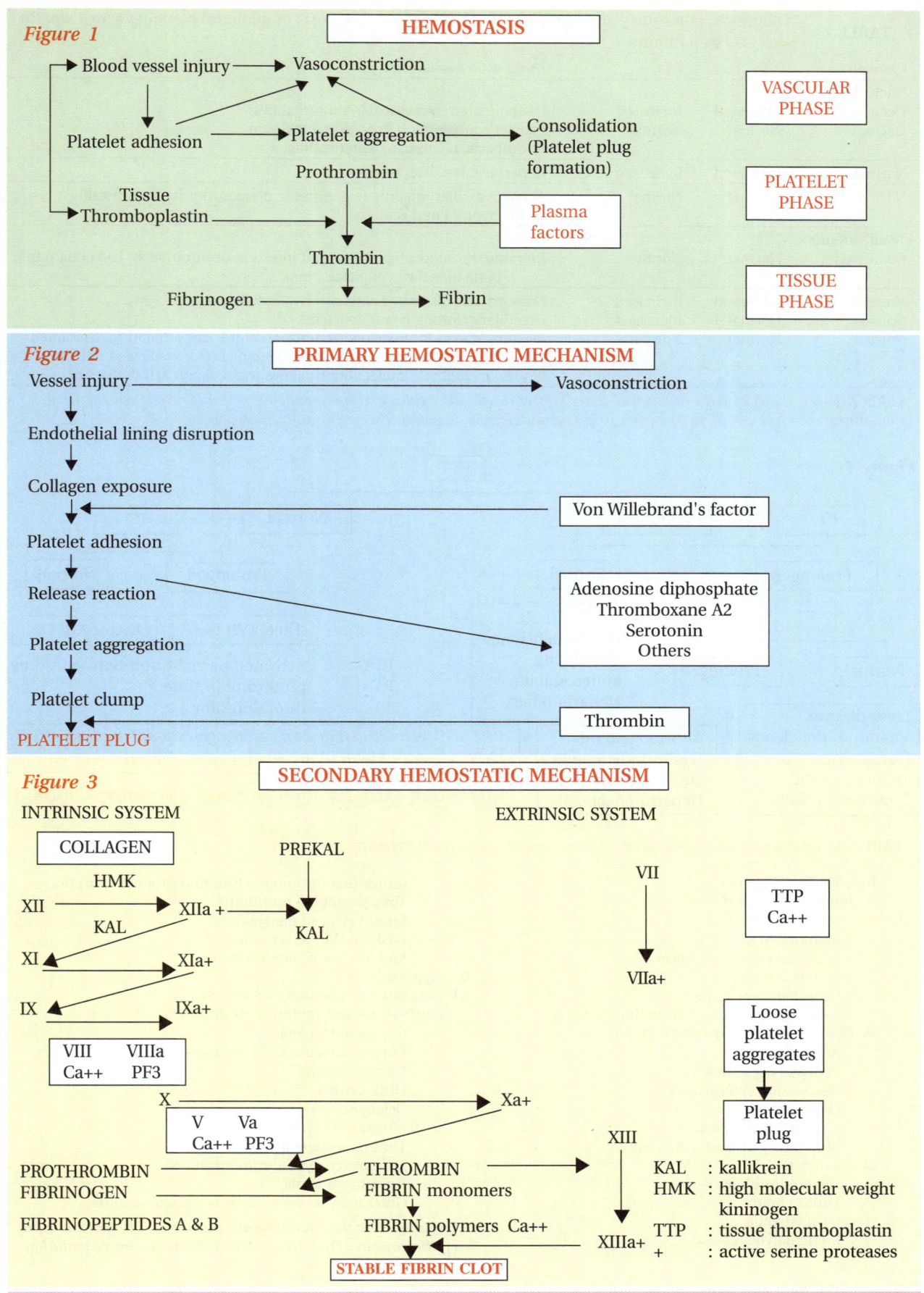

Figure 1

HEMOSTASIS

Blood vessel injury → Vasoconstriction

Platelet adhesion → Platelet aggregation → Consolidation (Platelet plug formation)

Tissue Thromboplastin

Prothrombin

Plasma factors

Thrombin

Fibrinogen → Fibrin

VASCULAR PHASE

PLATELET PHASE

TISSUE PHASE

Figure 2

PRIMARY HEMOSTATIC MECHANISM

Vessel injury → Vasoconstriction

Endothelial lining disruption

Collagen exposure

Von Willebrand's factor

Platelet adhesion

Release reaction

Adenosine diphosphate
Thromboxane A2
Serotonin
Others

Platelet aggregation

Platelet clump

Thrombin

PLATELET PLUG

Figure 3

SECONDARY HEMOSTATIC MECHANISM

INTRINSIC SYSTEM   EXTRINSIC SYSTEM

COLLAGEN   PREKAL   VII   TTP Ca++

HMK
XII → XIIa + → KAL
KAL

XI → XIa+

IX → IXa+

VIII   VIIIa
Ca++   PF3

X → Xa+

V   Va
Ca++ PF3

PROTHROMBIN → THROMBIN

FIBRINOGEN → FIBRIN monomers

FIBRINOPEPTIDES A & B

FIBRIN polymers Ca++

VIIa+

Loose platelet aggregates

Platelet plug

XIII

XIIIa+

KAL : kallikrein
HMK : high molecular weight kininogen
TTP : tissue thromboplastin
 +   : active serine proteases

STABLE FIBRIN CLOT

* *Pearl/Peril/Pitfall* : The presence of a family history of a bleeding disorder or of a previously affected infant can also be an important diagnostic pointer. Obstetric complications and problems at delivery can also affect the hemostatic system resulting in coagulation activation and DIC. Finally both maternal and neonatal drugs, particularly with regard to vitamin K metabolism, may be highly relevant at this time.

TABLE 7	Diagnosis, laboratory abnormalities and differential diagnosis of neonatal bleeding & bruising in sick and well infants			
Platelets	*PT*	*PTT*	*Diagnostic possibilities*	
"Sick" infant				
Decreased	Increased	Increased	Disseminated intravascular abnormalities	
Decreased	Normal	Normal	Platelet consumption (infection, renal vein thrombosis, necrotizing enterocolitis)	
Normal	Increased	Increased	Heparinisation, liver disease	
Normal	Normal	Normal	Altered vascular integrity (e.g. extreme prematurity, hyperosmolality, severe hypoxia and acidosis)	
"Well" infants				
Decreased	Normal	Normal	Immune thrombocytopenia, occult infection or thrombosis, leukemia (rare), bone marrow hypoplasia (rare).	
Normal	Increased	Increased	Hemorrhagic disease of newborn (vit. K deficiency)	
Normal	Normal	Increased	Hereditary clotting factor deficiency	
Normal	Normal	Normal	Bleeding due to local factors (trauma, anatomic abnormalities), Disrupted vessel from anatomical lesion (ulcer, hemangioma), swallowed mother's blood. Qualitative platelet abnormalities (rare), factor XIII deficiency.	

A SICK INFANT is one with the presence of severe asphyxia, acidosis, hypoxia, hypothermia, hypovolemia, hypoglycemia, seizures, prematurity with severe RDS, hypotension, or perinatal infection, hepatosplenomegaly, congenital anomalies,

Figure 4

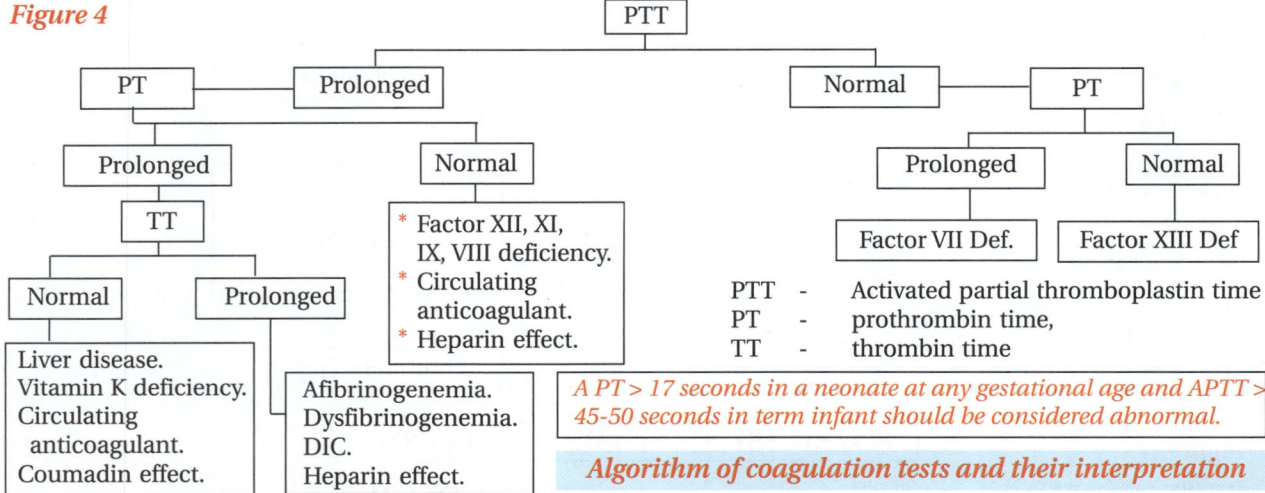

PTT - Activated partial thromboplastin time
PT - prothrombin time,
TT - thrombin time

A PT > 17 seconds in a neonate at any gestational age and APTT > 45-50 seconds in term infant should be considered abnormal.

Algorithm of coagulation tests and their interpretation

TABLE 8	Disease states associated with neonatal thrombocytopenia

I.   **Increased destruction**
     A. *Immune mediated*
          Maternal ITP
          Maternal SLE
          Maternal hyperthyroidism
          Maternal drugs
          Maternal preeclampsia
          Neonatal alloimmune thrombocytopenia
     B. *Nonimmune—likely related to DIC*
          Asphyxia
          Perinatal aspiration
          Necrotizing enterocolitis
          Hemangiomas
          Neonatal thrombosis
          Respiratory distress syndrome
     C. *Unknown*
          Hyperbilirubinemia
          Phototherapy
          Polycythemia
          Rh hemolytic disease

Congenital thrombotic thrombocytopenic purpura
Total parenteral nutrition
Inborn error of metabolism
Wiskott-Aldrich syndrome
Multiple congenital anomalies
II. **Hypersplenism**
III. **Decreased production of platelets**
     A. *Bone marrow replacement disorders*
          Congenital leukemia
          Congenital leukemoid reactions
          Neuroblastoma
          Histiocytosis
          Osteopetrosis
     B. *Bone marrow aplasia*
          Thrombocytopenia absent radii
          Amegakaryocytic thrombocytopenia
          Fanconi's anemia
          Other marrow hypoplastic or aplastic disorders

ITP, idiopathic thrombocytopenic purpura ; SLE, systemic lupus erythematosus ; DIC, disseminated intravascular coagulation

* **Pearl/Peril/Pitfall :** *Although acquired disorders most often present in sick term or preterm infants, many inherited disorders manifest in otherwise healthy infants. Recognition of the clinical setting in which bleeding occurs is therefore an important clue to the underlying diagnosis. Investigation requires careful observation of age dependent features, which are especially important during the early weeks of life.*

TABLE 9 Investigations for classifying thrombocytopenia by mechanism

Laboratory Parameter	Increased Platelet Destruction	Decreased Platelet Production
Platelet size	Increased	Normal
Platelet survival	Decreased	Normal
Platelet associated IgG	Often very increased	Usually normal or slightly increased
Bleeding time	Usually prolonged	Prolonged
Other cell lines	Usually normal	Often abnormal
Megakaryocytes	Normal or increased	Decreased
Other bone marrow Cell lines	Normal	Often decreased or abnormal

TABLE 10 Forms of Vitamin K deficiency bleeding (VKDB) in infancy

Early Form	Classic form	Late form
	Age	
< 24 hr	Days 2–7	0.5–6 mo
Medications during pregnancy	**Causes and risk factors**	Marginal VK content in breast milk due to low VK intake and absorption
Anticonvulsants	Breast-feeding	Cystic fibrosis
Oral anticoagulants (rifampin, isoniazid)	Inadequate VK intake	Diarrhea
Antibiotics (rarely idiopathic or hereditary)		α_1 AT deficiency
		Hepatitis
		Celiac disease
	Localization in order of frequency	
ICH	ICH	ICH (> 50%)
GI	GI	GI
Umbilicus	Umbilicus	Skin
Intraabdominal	ENT region	ENT region
Cephalhematoma	Injection sites	Injection sites
	Circumcision	Urogenital tract
		Intrathoracic
	Frequency without VK prophylaxis	
Very rare	1.5%-1/10,000 births	4-10/10,000 births *
	Prophylaxis	
	Adequate VK supply	Adequate VK supply
Discontinue or replace of offending medications		
Maternal VK prophylaxis	Early and adequate breast-feeding	Adequate breast-feeding
	Formula	Formula
	VK prophylaxis	VK prophylaxis†

*More common in southeast Asia. †Single intramuscular injection is better than single oral ; repeated small doses are closer to physiologic conditions. Warning signs : neonatal icterus, poor feeding, failure to thrive, any form of bleeding. ICH, intracranial bleed ; GI, gastrointestinal bleed ; ENT region, ear, nose, and throat region.

TABLE 11 Normal values for hemostasis screening tests in the newborn*

Test	30-36 weeks gestation		Term infant	
	Day1	Day 30	Day 1	Day 30
Prothrombin Time (sec)	Mean : 13.0 Range : 10.6-16.2	Mean : 11.8 Range : 10.0-13.6	13.0 + 1.43	11.8 ± 1.25
Activated partial thromboplastin Time (sec)	Mean : 53.6 Range : 27.5-79.4	Mean : 44.7 Range : 26.9-62.5	42.9 + 5.8	40.4 ± 7.42
Thrombin clotting time (sec)	Mean : 24.8 Range : 19.2-30.4	Mean 24.4 Range 18.8-29.9	23.5 ± 2.38	24.3 ± 2.44
Fibrinogen (g/L)	Mean : 2.43 Range : 1.50-3.73	Mean : 2.54 Range : 1.50-4.14	2.83 ± 0.58	2.70 ± 0.54
Platelet count (x 10⁹ /L)	Range 150-400	Range : 150-400	Range : 150-400	Range : 150-400

*Data from Andrew M et al. All infants received vitamin K at birth

* *Pearl/Peril/Pitfall : At birth, concentrations of the vitamin K dependent (FII, FVII, FIX, FX) and contact factors (FXI, FXII) are reduced to about 50% of normal adult values and are further reduced in preterm infants. Similarly, concentrations of the naturally occurring anticoagulants, antithrombin, protein C, and protein S, are low at birth, and, as a consequence, both thrombin generation and thrombin inhibition are reduced in the newborn period. Plasminogen is the major protein involved in fibrinolysis, and again this is reduced during the neonatal period, resulting in a relatively hypofibrinolytic state.*

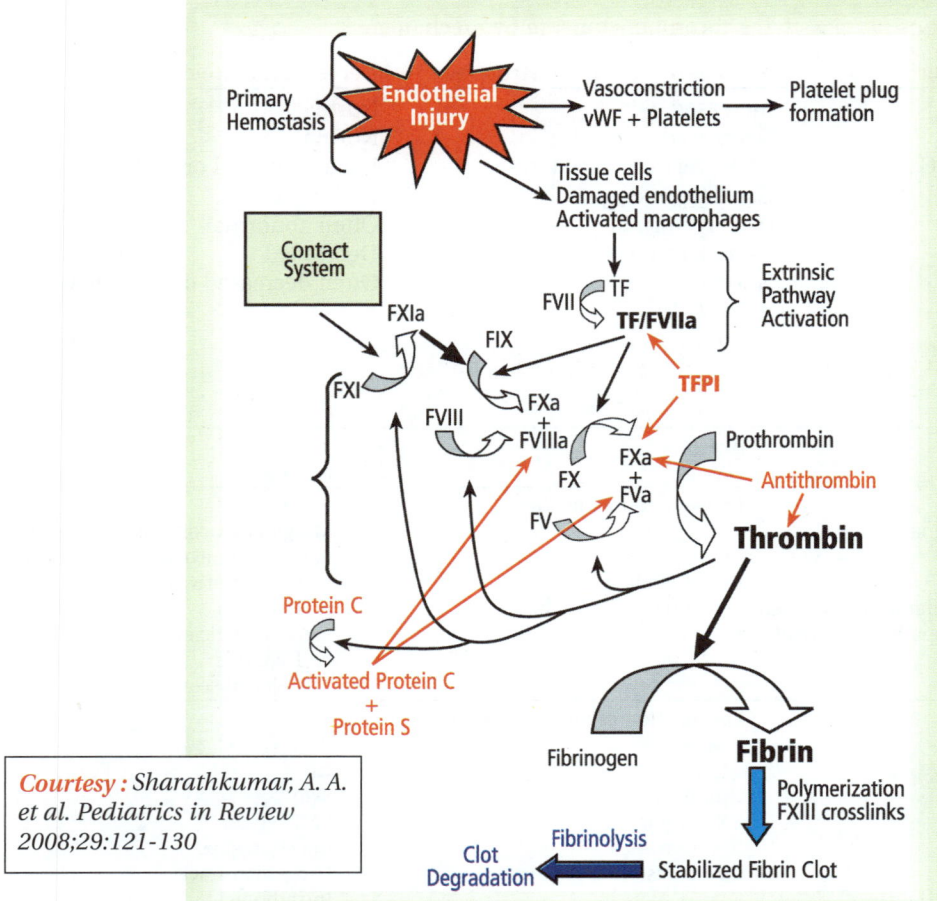

Courtesy : Sharathkumar, A. A.
et al. Pediatrics in Review
2008;29:121-130

KEY POINTS FOR CLINICAL PRACTICE

1. A number of different coagulation disorders may manifest with bleeding problems during the neonatal period. Early recognition of abnormal bleeding together with careful use of appropriate diagnostic investigations and recognition of those features unique to the neonatal haemostatic system should facilitate prompt diagnosis and appropriate management for these infants. Bleeding in an otherwise well neonate is much more suggestive of an inherited coagulation or an immune mediated thrombocytopenia, whereas a sick preterm neonate is more likely to have a consumptive coagulopathy with disseminated intravascular coagulation (DIC).

2. The diagnosis of vitamin K deficiency may be suspected from the results of coagulation screening where initially there is isolated prolongation of the prothrombin time, followed by prolongation of the APTT, in association with a normal fibrinogen concentration and a normal platelet count. Confirmation of the diagnosis requires measurement of the specific vitamin K dependent factors (II, VII, IX, X) which are corrected by the administration of vitamin K.

3. DIC always occurs as a secondary event, and a number of perinatal and neonatal problems are associated with this complication: birth asphyxia, acidosis, respiratory distress syndrome, infection, necrotizing enterocolitis, meconium aspiration, aspiration of amniotic fluid, brain injury, hypothermia, giant hemangioma, homozygous protein C/S deficiency, thrombosis, malignancy. As in older children and adults, once established, DIC is often associated with increased mortality.

4. Thrombocytopenia presenting in the first 72 hours of life is usually secondary to placental insufficiency and caused by reduced platelet production; fortunately most episodes are mild or moderate and resolve spontaneously. Thrombocytopenia presenting after 72 hours of age is usually secondary to sepsis or necrotizing enterocolitis and is usually more severe and prolonged. Platelet transfusion remains the only treatment. Finally, ensuring accurate diagnosis and determining effective fetal and neonatal treatment for NAITP, the thrombocytopenia currently identifiable as directly causing most mortality and morbidity, should remain a goal for all fetal medicine specialists, hematologists, and Neonatal pediatricians.

5. Although acquired problems are more frequent, severe forms of congenital factor deficiencies often first present in early infancy and should seriously be considered in otherwise healthy infants.

REFERENCES & FURTHER READING : 1)Guidelines for the use of platelet transfusions. Br J Haematol 2003;122: 10.2)Andrew M, Paes B, Milner R, et al. Development of the coagulation system in the full-term infant. Blood 1987;70:165–72 3)Blanchette VS, Rand ML. Platelet disorders in newborn infants: diagnosis and management. Semin Perinatol 1997;21:53–62. 4)Sutor AH, von Kries R, Cornelissen EAM, et al. Vitamin K deficiency bleeding in infancy. Thromb Haemost 1999;81:456–61. 5)Roberts I, Murray NA. Neonatal thrombocytopenia: causes and management. Arch Dis Child Fetal Neonatal Ed 2003;88:F359–64.

* *Pearl/Peril/Pitfall: Neonatal hemostatic abnormalities can present diagnostic and therapeutic challenges to the physician. Developmental deficiencies and/or increases of certain coagulation proteins, coupled with acquired or genetic risk factors, can result in a hemorrhagic or thromboembolic emergency. The timely diagnosis of a congenital hemorrhagic or thrombotic disorder can avoid significant long-term sequelae. However, due to the lack of randomized clinical trials addressing the management of neonatal coagulation disorders, treatment strategies are usually empiric and not evidence-based.*

Neonatal Neutropenia

68

@ *"The classical signs of acute bacterial infection are the presence of an increased percentage of band neutrophils and toxic granulation of immature and mature neutrophils followed after 1-2 days by a mature neutrophilia and after 3-5 days by eosinophilia. During the 1st 2 weeks of life, a band-segmented neutrophil ratio of >0.3 has been considered to be abnormal. By contrast, there is no increase in band cells or toxic granulation in viral infections; instead atypical viral lymphocytes are seen, particularly in congenital CMV infection,where they may persist for several months."*

A number of disease processes can present during the neonatal period with neutropenia, but three distinct immune-mediated conditions share a common pathophysiologic origin in antibody-mediated destruction of neutrophils: alloimmune neonatal neutropenia (ANN), neonatal autoimmune neutropenia, and autoimmune neutropenia of infancy (AINI) (a relatively less well-defined category).

Basic causes of neonatal Neutropenia

Decreased Neutrophil Production
Bone marrow failure syndromes
–Kostmann syndrome
–Reticular dysgenesis
–Shwachman-Diamond syndrome
–Cartilage-hair hypoplasia
–Cyclic neutropenia
Maternal conditions leading to placental insufficiency
–Pregnancy-induced hypertension
–Diabetes mellitus
Increased Neutrophil Destruction
Immune-mediated neutropenias
–Alloimmune neonatal neutropenia
–Neonatal autoimmune neutropenia
–Autoimmune neutropenia of infancy
 Sepsis
Necrotizing enterocolitis
Decreased Production and Increased Destruction of Neutrophils
 Congenital or acquired infections
Drug-induced neutropenia
Idiopathic neutropenia of prematurity
 Pseudoneutropenia

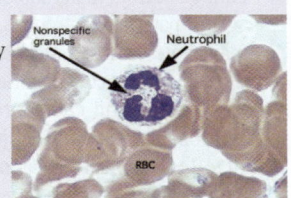

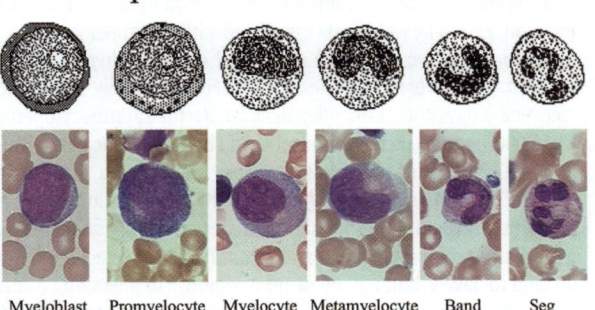

Manroe *et al.* 1979 106 neonates

Neutrophil Maturation in the Marrow

| Myeloblast | Promyelocyte | Myelocyte | Metamyelocyte | Band | Seg |

--PROLIFERATIVE POOL-- ----STORAGE POOL----

COURTESY: Robert D. Christensen, MD

REVIEW OF CLINICAL PROBLEMS

1. What are the important aspects of History & Physical examination to evaluate a Neonate with Neutropenia?
   Ans : Refer to the Evaluation-Decision-Action Plan/Algorithm to diagnose & manage Neonatal Neutropenia.

2. Discuss the essential investigations to evaluate a Neonate with Neutropenia.
   Ans : Refer to the Evaluation-Decision-Action Plan/Algorithm to diagnose & manage Neonatal Neutropenia.

3. What are the Clinical Indications of Severity in a Neonate with Neutropenia?
   Ans : Refer to the Evaluation-Decision-Action Plan/ Algorithm to diagnose & manage Neonatal Neutropenia.

4. Discuss the Therapeutic options for severe & persistent Neonatal Neutropenia.
   Ans : Refer to the Table "2" of the Chapter.

5. How do you classify the causes of Neonatal Neutropenia?
   Ans : Refer to the Table "1" of the Chapter.

LEARNING OBJECTIVES

After completing this article, readers will be able to:

1. Search for clinical clues to explain Neonatal Neutropenia.

2. Differentiate Transient & self-limited Neonatal Neutropenia from the prolonged & severe category.

3. Monitor the full blood counts twice weekly for 6 weeks and treat the intercurrent problems, such as infections, failure to thrive, systemic complications.

4. Refer the Neonates with severe persistent unresponsive and recurrent neutropenia to a pediatric hematologist for further evaluation.

5. Counsel the parents about the prognosis and the clinical course of neutropenia, if known.

---

* *Pearl/Peril/Pitfall :* Neonatal Neutropenia Evaluation-Differential count, Evaluation of blood smear, CBC on mother, Neutrophil antigen typing - Mother, Antineutrophil antibodies - Mother,Antineutrophil antibodies Baby, Marrow aspirate or biopsy.

BIRD'S EYE VIEW/OVERVIEW/SYNOPSIS

1. The normal values for neutrophil counts vary both with gestational age and with postnatal age, particularly over the 1st few days of life. *Neonatal Neutropenia requiring worth monitoring and/or further investigation* is pragmatically and flexibly defined as a neutrophil count<2,000cells/cumm at birth and up to 24–48 hours, and <1,000 cells/cumm thereafter and during 1st month of life.

2. Neutropenia is fairly common and transient in preterm infants but is uncommon in term infants. In preterms the commonest cause is IUGR and/or maternal hypertension/toxemia. The second most frequent cause in preterm infants, and the most common cause in term infants, is neutropenia secondary to bacterial or viral infection.Refer to the Table 1 of the Chapter for the principal causes of Neonatal Neutropenia.

3. *Neutropenia and Infection:* A short-lived (<6–12hours) neutropenia is a normal response in any bacterial infection, but neutropenia lasting >12 hours in the setting of acute bacterial infection is a poor prognostic sign. The classical signs of acute bacterial infection are the presence of an increased percentage of band neutrophils and toxic granulation of immature and mature neutrophils followed after 1-2 days by a mature neutrophilia and after 3–5 days by eosinophilia. During the 1st 2 weeks of life, a band-segmented neutrophil ratio (I:T Ratio) of >0.3 has been considered to be abnormal. By contrast, there is no increase in band cells or toxic granulation in viral infections; instead atypical viral lymphocytes are seen, particularly in congenital CMV infection,where they may persist for several months. Maternal diabetes, hypoglycemia, meconium aspiration, and APGAR score <6 at 5 minutes can all result in an increased I:T Ratio but generally will not be associated with neutropenia.

4. *Neutropenia associated with IUGR and maternal hypertension, toxemia, and diabetes-* resolves spontaneously, usually starting to recover 2-3 days after birth; *often associated with* thrombocytopenia <1,50,000/cumm, increased number of circulating nucleated RBC (>20/100 WBC) and there will be severe neutropenia (<300 cell/cumm). The *main clinical significance* of this form of neutropenia is *firstly* that recognition of its natural history prevents unnecessary treatment and investigations, and *secondly* that affected Neonates do tend to have a 'blunted' neutrophil response to infection,i.e., the neutrophil response is both delayed and sometimes inadequate, which may lead to an increased frequency and duration of bacterial infections.

5. *Congenital and Inherited Neutropenias* All of these are rare, but should be considered where the neutropenia is prolonged, if there is a relevant family history/consanguinity, or if the baby has typical dysmorphic features (e.g. thumb/radial abnormalities in Fanconi`s anemia). Kostmann`s syndrome (autosomal recessive/autosomal dominant) is severe congenital neutropenia, in which neutrophil production is reduced due to an 'arrest' of differentiation at the myelocyte/promyelocyte stage. The affected infants usually present with severe infections within a few weeks of birth associated with marked neutropenia (<200/cumm), a marked compensatory monocytosis and absent antineutrophil antibodies. Before the use of rhG-CSF, 2/3rds of these patients died of fatal infections before reaching adolescence.

6. *Alloimmune Neonatal Neutropenia:* Occurs after transplacental transfer of maternal alloantibodies directed against antigens on the infant`s neutrophils, analogous to Rh hemolytic disease. Prenatal sensitization induces maternal IgG antibodies to neutrophil antigens on fetal cells. The antibodies are usually complement activating and are frequently directed to neutrophil-specific antigens. The pathogenesis of alloimmune neonatal neutropenia usually involves phagocytosis of antibody-coated neutrophils by splenic macrophages. The tests used most commonly to diagnose immunemediated neutropenia include the granulocyte agglutination test (GAT), granulocyte immunofluorescence test (GIFT), and the monoclonal antibody immobilization of granulocyte antigens (MAIGA) assay. Symptomatic infants may present with delayed separation of the umbilical cord, mild skin infections (*Staphylococcus aureus*), fever, and pneumonia within the 1st 2 wk of life; these resolve with antibiotic therapy. The neutropenia is often severe and associated with fever and infections due to the usual microbes that cause neonatal disease. By 7 wk of age, the neutrophil count usually returns to normal, reflecting the duration of maternal antibodies in the infant`s circulation.Treatment consists of supportive care and appropriate antibiotics for clinical infections. In severe cases, where there is clinical deterioration despite antibiotics, plasma exchange and/or rhG-CSF (10 mcg/kg/day) may be helpful.

7. *Neonatal Autoimmune Neutropenia* Mothers with autoimmune disease may give birth to infants who develop transient neutropenia. The duration of the neutropenia depends on the time required for the infant to clear the maternally transferred IgG antibody. It persists in most cases for a few weeks to months. Neonates almost always remain asymptomatic. Administration of IVIG can transiently increase the neutrophil counts in these infants.

8. *The Evaluation-Decision-Action-Plan/Algorithm* describes the essential aspects of the diagnosis and management of Neonatal Neutropenia. Until it is clear from cultures and the infant`s clinical course that sepsis is not the etiology, IV broadspectrum antibiotics should be initiated and continued. Persistent neutropenia should have FBC with differential cell counts twice weekly for 5-6 weeks in order to evaluate the periodicity of neutrophil counts suggestive of a *cyclic process*. Cyclic neutropenia is autosomal dominant when familial; not usually diagnosed in the Neonate. In healthy infants with no apparent cause for neutropenia, Neonatal isoimmune/alloimmune neutropenia should be considered. Antineutrophil antibodies from maternal serum in such cases are typically reactive against paternal neutrophils. In some cases a bone marrow aspirate may be necessary to exclude the possibility of an intrinsic marrow disorder such as congenital leukemia. A bone marrow biopsy should be given careful consideration in neonates who have severe neutropenia (0.5×10^3/mcL [0.5×10^9/L]) that persists for more than 10 to 14 days (most causes of transient neutropenia should resolve in this period) or if it is unresponsive to 3 to 5 days of therapy with recombinant human granulocyte-colony-stimulating factor (rhG-CSF). Bone marrow evaluation may be helpful in excluding a diagnosis of severe congenital neutropenia (SCN) (Kostmann syndrome). Unlike patients who have SCN and have a promyelocyte/myelocyte arrest with few maturing forms, infants who have immune-mediated neutropenia frequently have relatively normaltohypercellular marrow, with several bands and mature neutrophils.

9. *Schwachman-Diamond syndrome* is a rare multiorgan disease caused by inactivating mutations of the SBDS gene located on chromosome 7 and is characterized by metaphyseal chondrodysplasia, dwarfism, pancreatic exocrine deficiency, and severe neutropenia (< 200-400/cumm). Clinical manifestations begin in neonatal age with diarrhea, weight loss, failure to thrive, eczema, otitis media, and pneumonia. The neutropenia responds to rhG-CSF. The illness may progress to bone marrow hypoplasia leading to moderate thrombocytopenia and aplastic anemia or leukemia.

10. The prognosis varies greatly with the cause and severity of the neutropenia obviously. In severe and persistent cases, it is poor in spite of antibiotic therapy.

Pearl/Peril/Pitfall : Neonatal Neutropenia Evaluation-Marrow aspirate or biopsy- It seldom if ever reveals the precise diagnosis. However, it can help categorize the condition as being the result of diminished production or accelerated destruction.

THE EVALUATION-DECISION-ACTION-PLAN/ALGORITHM FOR THE DIAGNOSIS AND MANAGEMENT OF *NEONATAL NEUTROPENIA*

SUBJECTIVE FINDINGS

History of fever, hypothermia, diarrhea, recurrent skin and respiratory-urinary-GIT infections, failure to thrive.

History of IUGR, preterm baby, infant of diabetic mother, multiple births with TTTS, Birth asphyxia, *drugs* -penicillins, barbiturates, antithyroids, and antipyretics.

History of Previous cases of Neonatal neutropenia in a family- congenital & inherited causes of neutropenia.

Maternal history of CMV infection, maternal hypertension/toxemia, maternal autoimmune disorders, perinatal bacterial infections, drugs like thiazides, antithyroids, gold salts.

Review the serial laboratory investigations already done and observe the trends in neutrophils, and other cells, to determine whether the neutropenia is an isolated one or there is pancytopenia.

OBJECTIVE FINDINGS

Assess ABCDs and monitor CRT, O₂ sats, BP, core-peripheral temperature difference, RR, HR, central & peripheral pulses, urine output.

Identify skin abscesses, cellulitis, perirectal abscesses, Pneumonia, fungal infections, UTI, NEC, SEPSIS, MENINGITIS etc.,

Look for physical stigmata of Fanconi's anemia(thumb & radial), features of IUGR, Down syndrome.

Assess for Failure to thrive, pallor, petechiae, jaundice, hepatosplenomegaly.

Determine the *degree of illness*-asymptomatic/mild/moderate to severe and *duration of illness*.

*depending on the **SPUR** signs and symptoms, i.e. *S*evere/*S*ystemic-*P*ersistent/*P*rogressive-*U*nresponsive/*U*nusual-*R*ecurrent/*R*ecalcitrant.

INVESTIGATIONS

Blood FBC, TC, DC, **Hct**, Platelets, Group/Type & Crossmatch, CRP, *Blood cultures & full septic screen*, **ABG analysis, electrolytes,** calcium & magnesium, **blood sugar,** creatinine, BUN, coagulation profile.(for general management of any sick neonate).Blood - *Repeat* FBC,TC, I:T Ratio, DC, Hct, Platelets, detailed peripheral blood film, antineutrophil antibodies, immunoglobulins, CD8 T cell and NK cell numbers.

Urine analysis, culture/sensitivity.

Radiographic bone survey of bone abnormalities.

For selected cases: Bone marrow Aspiration and Biopsy, cytogenetics, HIV-1/2 PCR, serologic tests for TORSCH and Hepatitis A,B,C.

NEONATAL NEUTROPENIA

Assess degree of illness

Mild → Repeat CBC with differential and platelet count in 6-8 wk → Neutropenia resolves / Chronic neutropenia

Moderate or severe

Indications of severity of illness
* Failure to thrive
* Persistent/Recurrent Neutropenia
* Immature WBC & Pancytopenia
* Unexplained Hepatosplenomegaly/Lymphadenopathy
* Family H/O genetic/metabolic problems

When to Worry? ANC <500/µL for 2 days or more or ANC 500-1000/µL for a week or more

Chronic neutropenia → Reassess degree of illness → **Mild** / **Moderate or severe**

Mild: *Consult:* Pediatric Hematologist → Follow-up : Biweekly CBC with Differential and platelets for 6 wk → Identify : Chronic idiopathic neutropenia, Cyclic neutropenia

Moderate or severe: *Consult:* Pediatric Hematologist

Neutropenia: specific therapy
geared to the particular diagnosis.
meticulous attention to good hygiene- hand washing, gloves.
granulocyte-colony stimulating factor (G-CSF) often can stimulate transient neutrophil production in many disorders.
granulocyte transfusions only during life-threatening sepsis.
prophylactic antibiotic schedules when infection is not discovered- to be considered individually, based on severity.

Consider: Bone marrow aspiration/biopsy, Immunological evaluation-Immunoglobulins, Lymphocyte subsets & function, Neutrophil antibody, ANA,HIV tests, maternal and family member neutrophil counts, in vitro granulocyte colony cultures to classify mechanism of neutropenia

Identify: Autoimmune/Alloimmune Neutropenia, Infection (HIV, CMV,HepatitisB/C), Malignancy, Metabolic disease, Schwachman-Diamond syndrome, Fanconi's anemia, Severe Congenital Neutropenia.

---

* *Pearl/Peril/Pitfall : Neonatal Neutropenia Evaluation- Metamyelocytes and bands are less pliable than are segmented neutrophils. On that basis, immature neutrophils might be slightly less capable of vascular exit and tissue migration (chemotaxis).*

TABLE 1	Causes of neonatal neutropenia

1. Placental insufficiency
  a) Maternal hypertension
  b) Intrauterine growth restriction
  c) Maternal diabetes
2. Infection
  a) Acute, perinatal bacterial infection, e.g. group B streptococcus
  b) Congenital infections, e.g. Rubella, CMV
  c) Postnatal bacterial & fungal infections
  d) Postnatal viral infections, e.g. CMV
3. Necrotizing enterocolitis
4. Idiopathic Neutropenia of Prematurity
5. Drug Induced Neutropenia
6. Transient Neutropenia-Donor of a Twin -Twin Transfusion syndrome & severe Rh hemolytic disease
	6. Immune
	Alloimmune neonatal neutropenia -ANN
	Neonatal autoimmune neutropenia -NAN
	Autoimmune neutropenia of infancy
	7 . Genetic
	  a) Trisomies : 21, 13 and 18
	  b) Kostmann's syndrome
	  c) Schwachman's syndrome
	  d) Pearson's syndrome
	  e) Reticular dysgenesis
	  f) Metabolic disorders, e.g. hyperglycinemia, isovaleric, Propionic and methylmalonic acidemia
	  g) Cartilage-hair hypoplasia
	8 . Marrow replacement
	  a) Congenital leukemia

TABLE 2 — Neonatal persistent and severe neutropenia -therapeutic options

Role of IVIG in the Treatment of Severe and Prolonged Neonatal Neutropenia :Intravenous immunoglobulin (IVIG) has been used at doses of 0.3 to 1 g/kg for 3 to 5 days with moderate success in both ANN(alloimmune neonatal neutropenia) and NAN(neonatal autoimmune neutropenia , offering response rates of approximately 50%. The primary mechanism of action of IVIG is through the blockade of the Fc receptors of the reticuloendothelial system, which allows antibodycoated neutrophils to escape phagocytosis by the macrophages. However, in most cases, the effects are transient, necessitating repeat dosing.

rhG-CSF:(recombinant myeloid growth factors such as G-CSF)- Neupogen is *not* recommended for varieties of neonatal neutropenia likely to be transient (or mild): Sepsis, PIH/SGA, Twin-Twin, Rh hemolytic, idiopathic Neonates who have ANN usually respond very well to rhG-CSF treatment at doses of 5 to 10 mcg/kg per day administered intravenously or subcutaneously. In most patients, a "response" (two- to threefold increase in neutrophil counts,

concentrations 1.010^3/mcL [1.010^3/L]) is evident within 24 to 48 hours, and no more than 2 to 3 weeks of treatment is required.rhG-CSF has been used successfully in AINI at dose similar to those used for ANN. In these patients, a rise in the neutrophil count usually is seen within 4 days, and remission lasts until the cessation of therapy.

Corticosteroids constitute the third major treatment strategy for the management of immune-mediated neutropenia, although effects in infants have been inconsistent. A greater benefit may be seen for infants who have AINI as opposed to ANN, but most studies have only included small numbers of patients. Exchange transfusions have not been effective in treatingimmune-mediated neutropenia.

Granulocyte Transfusions: Multiple experiments in septic, neutropenic neonatal animals indicate that leukocyte transfusions can be life saving. Used infrequently because of practical problems with rapid procurement and administration. No capacity for storage. "Comeback" rG- Comeback in adult oncology, with rG CSF priming of donors. Cells should be irradiated to prevent GVHD.

KEY POINTS FOR CLINICAL PRACTICE:

1. **Neonatal Neutropenia requiring worth monitoring and/or further investigation** is pragmatically and flexibly defined as a neutrophil count<2,000cells/ cumm at birth and up to 24–48 hours, and <1,000 cells/cumm thereafter and during 1st month of life.

2. Neutropenia is fairly common and transient in preterm infants but is uncommon in term infants. In preterms the commonest cause is IUGR and/or maternal hypertension/toxemia. The second most frequent cause in preterm infants, and the most common cause in term infants, is neutropenia secondary to bacterial or viral infection.

3. A short-lived (<6-12hours) neutropenia is a normal response in any bacterial infection, but neutropenia lasting >12 hours in the setting of acute bacterial infection is a poor prognostic sign. **Neutropenia associated with IUGR and maternal hypertension,** **toxemia, and diabetes-** resolves spontaneously, usually starting to recover 2-3 days after birth.

4. **Alloimmune Neonatal Neutropenia:** Occurs after transplacental transfer of maternal alloantibodies directed against antigens on the infant's neutrophils, analogous to Rh hemolytic disease. By 7 wk of age, the neutrophil count usually returns to normal, reflecting the duration of maternal antibodies in the infant`s circulation. **Congenital and Inherited Neutropenias-** All of these are rare, but should be considered where the neutropenia is prolonged, if there is a relevant family history/consanguinity, or if the baby has typical dysmorphic features (e.g. thumb/ radial abnormalities in Fanconi`s anemia).

5. The **prognosis** varies greatly with the cause and severity of the Neutropenia obviously. In severe and persistent cases, it is poor in spite of antibiotic therapy.

REFERENCES & FURTHER READING : 1)James RM, Kinsey SE : The investigation of chronic neutropenia in children.Arch Dis Child 2006; 852-858 2) Boxer l et all :Neutropenia; causes and consequences. Semin Hematol 2002;39:75-81 3)Nelson Text Book of Pediatrics, 18th edition 4)Neutropenia in NICU-Akhil Maheshwari, MD,Robert D. Christensen,NeoReviews Vol.5 No.10 October 2004 e431

* **Pearl/Peril/Pitfall :** *Neonatal Neutropenia-*<u>Alloimmune: neutrophils. Mother has a normal ANC. Mother has IgG antibody against an antigen on the fetal (and paternal) neutrophils</u> *Maternal Autoimmune: Mother has a low ANC. Mother has IgG antibody against her own neutrophil antigens. Neonatal Autoimmune: Mother has a normal ANC. Baby has autoantibodies against antigens on his/ her own neutrophils.*

69 Blood Component Therapy in Neonates

@ *As blood products convey a risk of transmitting potentially serious infections and are increasingly costly, it is clearly important to define evidence-based and/or standardized protocols for blood product use in Neonatal medicine.*

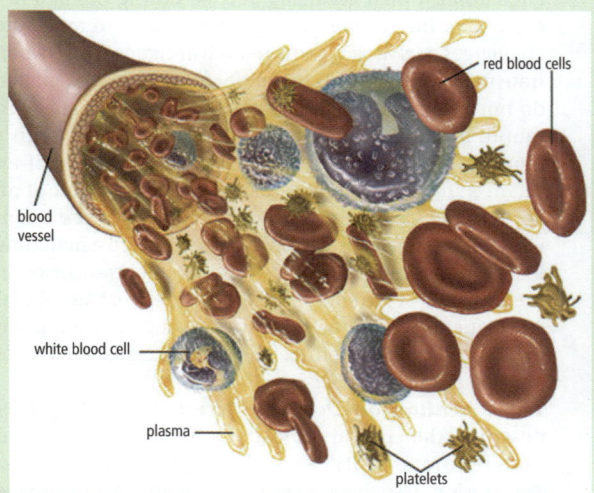

red blood cells

blood vessel

white blood cell

plasma

platelets

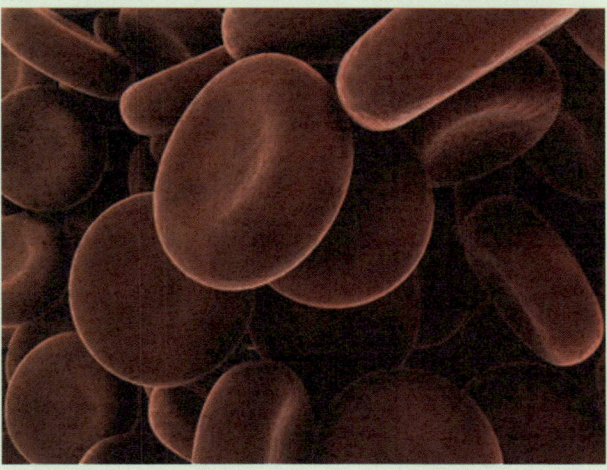

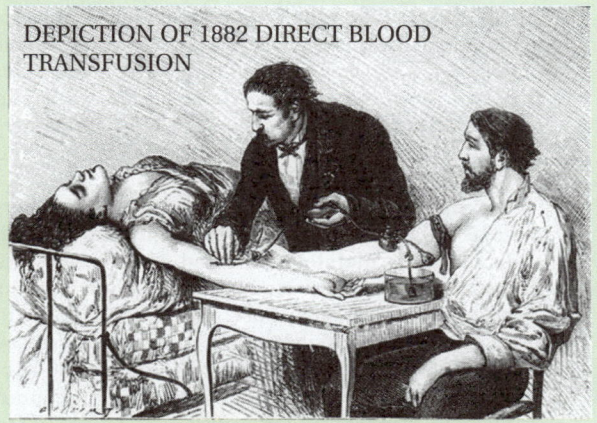

DEPICTION OF 1882 DIRECT BLOOD TRANSFUSION

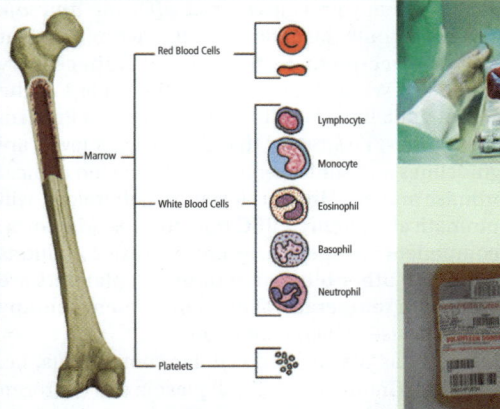

Red Blood Cells

Marrow

White Blood Cells

Lymphocyte

Monocyte

Eosinophil

Basophil

Neutrophil

Platelets

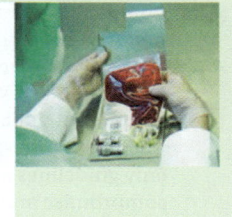

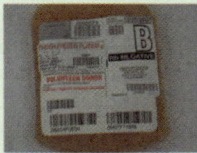

REVIEW OF CLINICAL PROBLEMS

1. Mention "3" Clinical Indications in a sick Neonate, where Whole blood is the First Choice of Transfusion ?
   Ans: Refer to the"No. 3" of the "BIRD'S EYE VIEW/OVERVIEW/ SYNOPSIS" of the Chapter.
2. What are the *"Requirements"* that a Neonatal Blood Trans fusion should meet? *Ans: Refer to the"No. 5" of the "BIRD'S EYE VIEW/OVERVIEW/SYNOPSIS" of the Chapter.*
3. What are the clinical indications for using "Leukocyte -reduced blood products" & "Irradiated components" in Neonates?
   Ans: Refer to the Evaluation-Decision-Action Plan/Algorithm to diagnose & manage Neonatal Blood Component Therapy.
4. How do you recognize and manage "Risks" associated with Neonatal blood transfusions?
   Ans: Refer to the Evaluation-Decision-Action Plan/ Algorithm to diagnose & manage a Neonate with Transfusion Associated Risks.
5. Mention Compatible blood group of the donor, when a Neonate with "O" BLOOD GROUP needs FFP transfusion and Why ?
   Ans: Refer to the Table 5 of the of the Chapter.

LEARNING OBJECTIVES

After completing this article, readers will be able to:

1. Restrict the use of blood components only on the basis of strict clinical and laboratory criteria, when no other alternative therapy is available and the benefits clearly outweigh the risks.
2. Understand the indications, dosage, and effects of blood components used for Neonatal transfusions.
3. Recognize and prevent hemolytic reactions and transmission of infectious agents when blood products have to be given to the Neonates.
4. Define evidence-based and/or standardized protocols for blood component use in Neonatal medicine.
5. Audit regularly and review the protocols/guidelines for the administration of all blood products to sick Neonates.

* *Pearl/Peril/Pitfall: The need for exchange transfusion has been reduced due to improved bilirubin surveillance, phototherapy, immunoprophylaxis with anti-Rh immunoglobulin, and intrauterine transfusions of nonmaternal red blood cells. Exchange transfusions are necessary in infants where other methods to reduce bilirubin have failed or the rate of rise in bilirubin demands immediate exchange.*

BIRD'S EYE VIEW/OVERVIEW/SYNOPSIS

1. Nearly 85% of ELBW infants require transfusions during their hospital stay, *without any "set guidelines"* for transfusion of blood component therapy. Neonatal transfusion remains *opinion—based rather than evidence-based,* and there is a wide diversity of opinion and practice between different clinicians and institutions. As blood products convey a risk of transmitting potentially serious infections and are increasingly costly, it is clearly important to define evidence-based and/or standardized protocols for blood product use in Neonatal medicine.

2. The *usual indications* for an *early transfusion* in Neonates are: *Exchange Transfusion *Significant Anemia at birth *Significant acute hemorrhage *Iatrogenic blood losses (cumulative sampling losses for diagnostic purposes) *Prenatal hematological disorders such as rhesus isoimmunization. Neonates may require *late transfusion* for *severe NEC *severe sepsis *surgery with significant blood loss *symptomatic anemia of any cause (producing tachycardia, apnea, feeding difficulties, and poor weight gain.*)

3. **Whole blood *versus* Component therapy:** Apart from a few indications, such as *Acute blood loss>20% blood volume &/or shock *Exchange transfusion *Cardiac surgery & ECMO, Whole blood transfusion has limited utility in contemporary Neonatal blood transfusion practice. Blood Component therapy provides *correct, effective and safe replacement* of only the deficient cells/factors, without exposing the recipient to the evils of unnecessary components of Whole blood. Refer to the Table 1 of the Chapter for guidelines for PRBC transfusions in Preterm Neonates. It must be stressed that these trigger levels are only guidelines and some Neonates will have no clinical compromise at these Hb/Hcrt levels and, therefore, will not automatically require PRBC transfusions. Moreover, each component has specific optimal storage conditions (In contrast to other blood components, platelets are stored at room temperature) and component therapy maximizes the use of blood donations.

4. Whole blood has plasma and cellular components, i.e. RBC, Platelets, Granulocytes. Fresh plasma can be frozen at -30° C and used as FFP in future or pooled to be converted into components like cryoprecipitate, albumin, gamma globulin, anti-D globulin and plasma proteins. One can modify and manipulate these components, and get neocyte packs, frozen RBC, washed RBC or Platelets, UV light/Gamma- irradiated RBC or Platelets. One can select a specific donor and get CMV-negative blood components, HLA-matched blood components or blood products from specific minor blood group compatible donor. Lastly one can get stem cells from the umbilical cord blood of a Newborn for stem cell transplant.

5. *Neonatal blood transfusion should meet the following requirements:* *The blood used should have been screened for infection with CMV, HIV, HBV, and HCV. *Blood and its components should also be free from bacterial/parasital infection. *Use of small subunits derived from one pack (octopus or satellite units) is encouraged to reduce donor exposure, especially for premature infants who are expected to require multiple simple transfusions for anemia of prematurity. *For massive transfusions (such as exchange transfusion/

ECMO), fresh whole blood <48-72 hours old or reconstituted whole blood (washed packed red cells and FFP) is required. *In the immediate newborn period, samples from both the Neonate and mother should be grouped to determine the ABO and Rhesus group and screened for atypical red cell alloantibodies. Newborn infants have IgG antibodies derived from the maternal circulation, which gradually decline during the first 3-4 months of life. They have a poor response to antigenic challenges such as allogenic red cell antigens. Thus, when transfused with red cells that differ from their own, infants do not respond by making alloantibodies until after 3rd month of life. Any antibodies detected in a Newborn`s blood sample are maternal in origin. Therefore, if an infant`s initial antibody screen is negative, blood of an appropriate group and type can be issued to the infant without the need for further typing and crossmatching for the first 3 months of life. *Components transfused in the first year of life should be CMV-negative. *All cellular components should be leukocyte- reduced at the point of manufacture to reduce the risk of transmission of infectious agents.

6. *The Evaluation-Decision-Action-Plan/Algorithm* describes the clinical indications for Whole blood and blood components and their practical aspects. Transfusion Associated risks in a Neonate are classifiable into *a) Infectious b) Noninfectious*-acute (immunologic/nonimmunologic)/delayed. *Refer to the Tables 8 & 9 of the Chapter for an organized classification. The Evaluation-Decision-Action- Plan/Algorithm* to diagnose and manage **"Transfusion Associated risks in a Neonate"** explains the details of their prevention, diagnosis, and management.

7. **Leukoreduced blood components:** Leukoreduction filters remove ~99.9% of WBC from RBC and platelets. In addition, most platelets collected by apharesis are leukoreduced even without additional filtration. Benefits of leukoreduction include a) decreased immunization to antigens on leukocytes such as HLA antigens b) decreased rate of Nonhemolytic febrile transfusion reactions c) minimization of a possible but controversial immuno-modulatory effect of blood transfusions and d) decreased rate of CMV transmission.

8. *Irradiation of blood components:* Unless blood is emergently needed, all PRBCs, platelets, and granulocytes are irradiated to prevent TAGVHD, especially among those at risk, such as Premature <1,500g, Immune compromised newborns especially those with cellular immuno-deficiency, who require Intrauterine transfusions, and who receive transfusion from a relative donor (mother/father/siblings).

9. In order to maintain best practice, Neonatal units must construct, adhere closely to, and regularly audit and review guidelines for the administration of all blood products to sick Neonates.

10. Neonatologists should continue to recognize that very little is actually known about the significant short- and long-term effects of blood product use in Neonates. This should continue to stimulate the design and conduct of high-quality, randomized, controlled trials of blood component use in Neonates in order to define and refine the best evidence-based practice.

---

* *Pearl/Peril/Pitfall : A Cochrane review on preterm infants found no overall significant clinical benefit to using albumin compared with saline. These conclusions regarding the use of albumin as well as the increased cost, potential for pulmonary edema, anticoagulant properties, and minor risk of infection must seriously be taken into consideration before making the decision to give albumin over a crystalloid solution.*

THE EVALUATION-DECISION-ACTION- PLAN/ALGORITHM FOR THE DIAGNOSIS AND MANAGEMENT OF NEONATAL BLOOD COMPONENT THERAPY

Evaluate the neonate for the clinical indications!	Decide what is appropriate? Blood/Component	ESSENTIAL PRACTICAL ASPECTS & REMARKS

* Acute blood loss>20% blood volume &/or shock

* Exchange transfusion *Cardiac surgery & ECMO

Whole blood *10ml/kg of Whole blood will raise the Hb by 1–1.5g/dL.*Stored at 1–4°C with a shelf life of 21–42 days, but it has 100% of all the components only in the first 4–6 hours of collection. *Platelets and labile clotting factors V &VIII fall to<1% by 4-48 hours of storage. Do not use stored blood of >2–3days old, when used just after cardiopulmonary bypass and that of >5–7 days old when used in other situations. *Do not misuse Whole blood to provide platelets,clotting factors and to replace blood loss without shock. *Avoid it unless strictly indicated, because of its disadvantages, such as hyperkalemia, metabolic acidosis, hypocalcemia, volume overload,especially in a sick preterm, plasma-borne infections, urticaria,allergic reactions,CMV transmission and GVHD due to its lymphocyte content.

* Anemia due to blood loss in antenatal/natal/postnatal periods, obvious/occult third space loss

* Iatrogenic blood loss to the "laboratory" >10% of blood volume

* Anemia of prematurity with poor weight gain,apneic spells, acidosis, poor feeding unexplained by other causes.

* Late anemia following Exchange transfusion

* Major surgery and acute blood loss without shock

Packed RBC *Refer to the Table No "1" and No "2" of the Chapter for the specific indications for PRBC.*Volume and Rate of PRBC transfusion : a) Volume of PRBC = Blood volume (ml/kg) x (desired minus actual hematocrit) divided by the hematocrit of the transfused PRBC b) Rate of transfusion should be <10ml/kg/hr in the absence of CHF, and it should not be >2ml/kg/hr in the presence of CHF. * A full term Neonate has 70–80ml/kg and a preterm 100ml/kg of blood volume *Transfusions of >25ml/kg are rarely required except in acute hemorrhage. *PRBC is made by centrifugation of Whole blood and it contains 22–50% of original plasma, nearly 100% of neutrophils, and lymphocytes as at the time of collection but has <10% platelets and clotting factors. Ideal Hematocrit for PRBC is 70–75%. For Newborns, while doing exchange transfusion, Hcrt can be adjusted to 50–55% using additional FFP/Albumin. *PRBC shelf life is only 24 hours, once packed. *Each 9ml/kg PRBC transfusion will increase Hb level by 3 g/dL. *Ensure meticulous monitoring of input, output, and vital signs during blood transfusion. *NAT - Nucleic Acid amplification Testing identifies viral antigens in the window period before antibodies develop and is available for HIV, HCV, and West Nile Virus.

* Thrombocytopenia as per the guidelines given in the Table 3 of the Chapter.

* Platelet Dysfunction-Primary/ Secondary

Platelets *Indications for Platelet transfusion in nonimmune thrombocytopenia depend on the level of sickness in the Newborn as highlighted in the Table 3 of the Chapter. *In alloimmune thrombocytopenia use Human Platelet Antigen (HPA) compatible platelets, which generally are *Maternal platelets* meticulously washed and irradiated with an aim to maintain the platelet count >30 x 10^9/L;if no such HPA compatible platelets are available, an alternative approach is the use of IVIG @1g/kg/day on 2 consecutive days or 0.5g/kg/day for 4 days, alone or in combination with random donor platelet transfusion. *In autoimmune thrombocytopenia, the goal is to keep the platelet count >30 x 10^9/L;IVIG@1g/kg/day for 2 days is given if the counts are less than acceptable minimum. *The usual recommended dose of platelets is 1 unit/10 kg body weight, which amounts to 5ml/kg. The predicted rise in platelet count from a 5ml/kg dose would be 20–60 × 10^9/L; doses up to 10–20ml/kg may be used in case of severe thrombocytopenia. *Platelets are stored at 20–22°C on a constant agitator and should be transported quickly and infused rapidly over 20–30 minutes to prevent loss due to aggregation. One should use ABO/Rh identical/compatible donor. *Single donor platelets (SDP) also called platelet concentrate, obtained by apheresis from a single donor over a 4-6 hr period are more effective than Random Donor Platelet/platelet pack (RDP) and exposes the patient to a single donor.

* Newborn <2weeks of age with sepsis and has Absolute Neutrophil Count (ANC) < 300/cumm and in a septic Newborn who has ANC <500/cumm and does not respond to adequate antibiotics and antifungals and in septic newborns who have known neutrophil functional disorder.

Granulocytes-GTX: The dose of Granulocytes recommended is 1–2 × 10^9/kg body weight in 10–15 ml/kg of volume. It can be repeated 12-24 hourly for 5 days. As the GTX pack has plenty of lymphocytes, it is advisable to irradiate it before use in Newborns, especially prematures, to prevent Transfusion associated GVHD. *The donor should be ABO, Rh compatible and preferably CMV -NEGATIVE. *GTX should be stored at room temperature and they have shelf life of only 24 hours. *In the Neonate, many Neonatologists prefer to use alternative therapies such as IV Immunoglobulin and G-CSF/GM-CSF (Granulocyte-Macrophage Colony Stimulating Factor).

THE EVALUATION-DECISION-ACTION- PLAN/ALGORITHM FOR THE DIAGNOSIS AND MANAGEMENT OF *NEONATAL BLOOD COMPONENT THERAPY*

Evaluate the Neonate for the Clinical indications!	*Decide what is appropriate? Blood/Component*	ESSENTIAL PRACTICAL ASPECTS & REMARKS

* Neonatal indications

*a.*hemorrhage secondary to vitamin K deficiency

*b.*DIC with bleeding

*c.*bleeding in congenital coagulation factor deficiency when more specific treatment is either unavailable or inappropriate.

d. reconstitution of RBC concentrates to simulate whole blood for use in massive transfusion (e.g. exchange transfusion or cardiovascular surgery)

Fresh frozen plasma (FFP) & cryoprecipitate *Prophylactic use of FFP transfusion to prevent IVH in premature infants is *not* recommended.*FFP is *unnecessary* in partial exchange transfusion for the treatment of Neonatal hyperviscosity syndrome because safer crystalloid/colloid solutions are available. *TRALI-* Transfusion Associated Acute Lung Injury is more likely since more plasma containing antibodies that react with the patient`s HLA Antigens causing lung injury.*FFP is *not* indicated for correction of hypovolemia or as immunoglobulin replacement therapy, asymptomatic stable neonates with "physiologically" prolonged indices of coagulation and in non-bleeding thrombocytopenic Neonates, unless there is good laboratory evidence of concurrent DIC. *FFP should be group AB (since this contains neither anti-A nor anti-B) or compatible with recipient`s ABO RBC antigens*Usual dose of FFP- *10-15 ml/kg with the larger dose given if possible in order to limit donor exposure where repeated dosing is likely;* repeat doses as needed q8 hour. *Cryoprecipitate is prepared from FFP by thawing at 2-4ºC and is stored at -20ºC ,given at a dose of 5ml/kg; it contains about 80-100 U of factor VIII in 10-25 ml of plasma, 300mg of fibrinogen and varying amounts of factor XIII.It is useful in treating DIC associated with hypofibrinogenemia, inherited afibrinogenemia or hypofibrinogenemia and factor VIII deficiency if factor VIII concentrate is not immediately available.

* Preterm<1,500g
* Intrauterine transfusion
*Transfusion from a relative donor, especially mother, father, or siblings
* Immune compromised newborns especially those with cellular immunodeficiency

Irradiated blood components *All the blood products, such as whole blood, packed RBC, platelets, and granulocyte concentrates can lead to Transfusion Associated Graft Versus Host Disease (TAGVHD) and hence need to be irradiated with Gamma irradiation @2,500–3,500 cGy;once irradiated the shelf life is only for 28 days. *Frozen "acellular" products, such as FFP and cryoprecipitate, do not require irradiation.

* Patients requiring recurrent blood transfusions *but to avoid* NHFTR- Non Hemolytic Febrile Reactions, HLA alloimmunization, Trans-mission of leukotropic Viruses (CMV, EBV, HTLV-1,HIV), Transfusion Associated GVHD, and TRALI (Transfusion Associated Acute Lung Injury)

Leukocyte reduced blood components and frozen RBC *Leukocyte depletion/ reduction defined as achieving a concentration of $< 5 \times 10^6$ leukocytes per unit of RBC. * Methods of Leukocyte depletion/reduction include: a)centrifugation and removal of buffy coat (pre-storage) b) use of leukocyte filters (pre and post storage) c)washing of RBC with saline d)freezing and thawing of RBC. *Transfusion-associated CMV* can be nearly eliminated by transfusing leukocyte-reduced cellular blood products or by selecting CMV-Negative blood donors.

* *Pearl/Peril/Pitfall: Washed RBCs, leukocyte-poor RBCs, and irradiated RBCs are three methods used to reduce white blood cells (WBCs) from RBCs. Washed RBCs refers to the process of washing RBCs with 0.9% sodium chloride to remove >95% of the nonviable RBCs and 85 to 90% of the WBCs as well as extracellular potassium. This technique is very effective at reducing the risk of graft versus host disease (GVHD) but is limited by having a 24-hour shelf life.*

* *Pearl/Peril/Pitfall : One donor red cell unit can be stored in satellite bags using a sterile docking device to transfer the blood without altering the expiration date. Stored RBCs generally have a shelf life of 35 to 42 days. Lee found a 64% reduction in multiple donor exposure by using dedicated eight-packs of unwashed packed RBCs up to the date of expiration. Thus, the risk of infection theoretically decreases as the number of different donors decreases.*

TABLE 1   Guidelines for red cell transfusion for preterm neonates

Assisted ventilation		CPAP			Breathing spontaneously	
< 28 days	≥ 28 days	< 28 days	≥ 28 days	FiO$_2$>0.21	Well in air	
FiO$_2$≥0.3	FiO$_2$<0.3					
Hb<12g/dl or	Hb<11g/dl or	Hb<10g/dl or	Hb<10g/dl or	Hb<8g/dl or	Hb<8g/dl or	Hb<7g/dl or
PCV<0.40	PCV<0.35	PCV<0.30	PCV<0.30	PCV<0.25	PCV<0.25	PCV<0.20

RBC transfusion may be considered at higher thresholds than the above for Neonates with:
- Hypovolemia (unresponsive to crystalloid infusion)
- Septic shock
- Necrotizing enterocolitis
- Undergoing/recovering from major surgery.

TABLE 2   Guidelines for neonatal & pediatric red blood cell transfusions*

Infants within the first 4 month of life
Hemoglobin of < 13.0 g/dL and *severe pulmonary disease*
Hemoglobin of < 10.0 g/dL and *moderate pulmonary disease*
Hemoglobin of < 13.0 g/dL and *severe cardiac disease*
Hemoglobin of < 10.0 g/dL and *major surgery*
Hemoglobin of < 8.0 g/dL and *symptomatic anemia*

Children and adolescents
Acute loss of > 25% of circulating blood volume
Hemoglobin of < 8.0 g/dL in the perioperative period
Hemoglobin of < 13.0 g/dL and *severe cardiopulmonary disease*
Hemoglobin of < 8.0 g/dL and *symptomatic chronic anemia*
Hemoglobin of < 8.0 g/dL and *marrow failure*

* words in *italics* must be defined for local transfusion guidelines.Hemotocrit estimated by Hb g/dL x 3

TABLE 4   Requirements for neonatal blood transfusion

* The blood used should have been screened for infection with CMV, HIV, HBV, and HCV.

* Blood and its components should also be free from bacterial infection.

* Use of small subunits derived from one pack(octopus or satellite units) is encouraged to reduce donor exposure.

* For massive transfusions (such as exchange transfusion/ ECMO), fresh whole blood <48hours old or reconstituted whole blood (washed packed red cells and FFP) is required.

* In the immediate newborn period, maternal blood is required to ensure compatibility.

TABLE 5   Donor—recipient blood group compatibility

Infant's blood group & antibodies	Compatible donor red cells	Compatible donor plasma
O with Anti-A & Anti-B	O	AB, O, A, B,
A with Anti-B	O, A,	AB, A
B with Anti-A	O, B	AB, B
AB with None	O, A, B, AB	AB

TABLE 3   Guidelines for neonatal & pediatric platelet transfusions

INFANTS WITHIN THE FIRST 4 MO OF LIFE

PLTs < 100 × 10^9/L and only *when actively bleeding*

PLTs < 50 × 10^9/L and sick and bleeding *or invasive procedure-Surgery/Exchange Transfusion or ELBW Infant Or <1 week old or previous* major bleeding tendency (grade 3/4 IVH)

PLTs < 30 × 10^9/L even *asymptomatic* and *clinically stable*

PLTs < 100 × 10^9/L and *clinically unstable*

PLTs at any count, but with PLT dysfunction plus bleeding or an invasive procedure

CHILDREN AND ADOLESCENTS

PLTs < 50 × 10^9/L and bleeding

PLTs < 50 × 10^9/L and an invasive procedure

PLTs < 20 × 10^9/L and *marrow failure with hemorrhagic risk factors*

PLTs < 10 × 10^9/L and *marrow failure without hemorrhagic risk factors*

PLTs at any count, but with PLT dysfunction plus bleeding or an invasive procedure

* words in *italics* must be defined for local transfusion guidelines. (PLTs, platelets.)

TABLE 6   Traditional indications for fresh frozen plasma (FFP) use in neonates

* These are poorly defined clinical indications traditionally misused

* Now there is accumulating evidence from a number of studies in Neonates to show that the use of FFP is not appropriate in these clinical situations (with the exception of treatment of DIC). *As a result, FFP administration to Neonates has now dramatically reduced and this probably represents the greatest evidence-based improvement in Neonatal Transfusion Medicine.

* Treatment of proven or suspected DIC.

* Prevention of intraventricular hemorrhage in preterms.

* Blood volume replacement.

* Adjuvant therapy during sepsis (addition of opsonizing factors).

* During episodes of thrombocytopenia.

* To correct prolonged indices of coagulation, not accompanied by clinical signs of bleeding or other laboratory findings consistent with DIC e.g. thrombocytopenia or red cell fragmentation.

* *Pearl/Peril/Pitfall : Leukocyte-poor RBCs refers to RBC concentrates after approximately 70% of WBCs are removed using one of the following techniques: inverted spin, manual removal or an automated processor, sedimentation, neutralization, centrifuging, washing, freezing, or filtration. These processes are time consuming, expensive, and result in a significant loss of RBC mass.*

THE EVALUATION-DECISION-ACTION- PLAN/ALGORITHM FOR THE DIAGNOSIS AND MANAGEMENT OF *A NEONATE WITH TRANSFUSION ASSOCIATED RISKS*

SUBJECTIVE FINDINGS

History of febrile reaction occurring within 30-60 minutes after the transfusion has started, *rash, urticaria* typically beginning minutes after the infusion started, *increasing pallor, oliguria, jaundice, hematuria, shock, bleeding, tachypnea, distress,* soon after an ABO - incompatible blood/component infusion, due to human error. *Past Hx of similar events?*

History of large volume transfusion@rapid rate (volume overload & CHF), *large volume transfusion stored blood >5-7 days after collection*(Hyperkalemia,Metabolic acidosis, Hypernatremia, Hypocalcemia)

History of a premature infant having received recurrent blood transfusions/transfusion from a related donor/in utero transfusion without irradiated blood products(TAGHVD).

OBJECTIVE FINDINGS

Assess ABCDs and monitor CRT, O_2 sats(differential pulse oximetry), *BP,* core-peripheral temperature difference, RR, HR, central & peripheral pulses, urine output. *Note fever,tachycardia,mental status changes, oozing/bleeding from IV sites, oliguria, changes in urine color.*

Determine whether the baby is in preterminal (*"pre arrest"*) conditions such as apnea, gasping or RR <20 bpm, shock, extremely lethargic or unresponsive limpy baby, bleeding etc.. and *intervene with appropriate resuscitation of ABCDs promptly.*

Note the other alarming signs suggestive of MODS acute renal failure, respiratory failure, DIC, Hemoglobinuria, Hyperbilirubinemia, & CNS dysfunction.

Perform CVS and systemic examination cardiac impulse, heart sounds, gallop, murmurs, breath sounds, rales, cardiomegaly, hepatomegaly.

INVESTIGATIONS

Blood FBC, TC, DC, **Hct**, Platelets, CRP, Blood cultures, **ABG analysis, electrolytes,** calcium & magnesium, **blood sugar,** LFTs creatinine, BUN, coagulation profile - PT, APTT, DIC PANEL

REPEAT GROUP and TYPE and CROSS-MATCH, DIRECT AND INDIRECT COOMBS, DONOR & RECIPIENT GRAM STAIN/CULTURE.

CXR for cardiomegaly/pulmonary edema.

Urine analysis(hemo/myo globin) & culture.

Inform Blood Transfusion Service & Start Work-up!

A NEONATE WITH TRANSFUSION ASSOCIATED RISKS

Ensure the Safety of Blood and Blood components: a) Screen donors b) Test donated blood for HIV,HBV, HCV, and Syphilis c) Screen the donors for viruses each time they donate d) give leukodepleted blood products to all neonates ideally obtained from a CMV-Negative donors e)restrict transfusions and avoid them unless essential (the only way to prevent transfusion associated variant Creutzfeldt-Jacob disease(PRIONS).

Beware of the possibilities: a) Hepatitis B/C may not be detected because of low viremia and mutant strain undetectable by routine ELISA *b)* preterms have 10-30% seroconversion rate for CMV, if they are transfused with CMV-Positive blood *c)* Bacterial infections can be transmitted because of asymptomatic bacteremia in the donor and due to inadequate skin sterilization in collecting the blood *d)* Malaria is still transmissible, as the screening tests for Plasmodium spe. are insensitive

Ensure ABCs, Give supplemental oxygen, Monitor - pulse oximetry, BP (4-limb), CR Monitor, CVP if necessary,continuous BP monitoring.

Perform IV access and correct (& maintain the normal range)hypoglycemia,hypocalcemia,anemia, Hyperbilirubinemia, acidosis & maintain normo-thermia & electrolytes.

Catheterize the bladder to monitor urine output.

Enforce strict guidelines for patient identification and issue of blood and minimize the human error to prevent immune mediated hemolysis. *Newborns must be screened for maternal RBC antibodies, including ABO antibodies if NON-O RBCs are to be given as first transfusion; if the initial results are negative, no further testing is needed for the first 3months of life.

Allergic reactions

* Rash &Urticaria may occur.

* Rare in Neonates, &generally mild; respond to antihistamines-diphendramine 1mg/kg IV/IM

* Use IgA deficient products or washed RBCs for future transfusions

* Anaphylaxis is very rare indeed and may require IV epinephrine 1:10,000 0.1 ml/kg, IV hydrocortisone 1 mg/kg and diphendramine 1mg/kg IV/IM

Hemolytic reactions

*Acute hemolytic reaction secondary to infusion of ABO-incompatible plasma present in PRBC or Platelet concentrates occurs most commonly, because of clerical error involving misidentification of the patient or blood sample *Newborns tolerate <5ml/kg of ABO-incompatible plasma generally well and they do not manifest the usual symptoms of hemolysis that are observed in older patients, such as fever, hypotension, chills,back pain, palpitations, vomiting etc.,*It may present as increased pallor, presence of plasma free hemoglobin, hyperbilirubinemia, hemoglobinuria, hyperkalemia, and metabolic acidosis *Sometimes Acute Renal Failure, DIC, Acute Respiratory Failure and/or shock may complicate the issue, if the transfusion is not stopped immediately.

Discontinue the Transfusion *Give 0.9% NS@20ml/kg IVB with forced diuresis by IV Furosemide 1–2 mg/kg *Send Labs and *start work-up* as instructed in the Table 7 of the Chapter. *Manage* SHOCK/ARF/DIC/RESPIRATORY FAILURE as per the guidelines/protocols of the Institution.

Consider IV Broadspectrum antibiotics, if an infectious cause is suspected. *Intubate & ventilate,* if necessary-*SHOCK &HYPOTENSION *APNEA *COLLAPSE *ARF & PULMONARY EDEMA-CHF *DIC.

Nonhemolytic febrile reactions (NHFTR)

>2°C rise in body Temperature/with hypotension

* Suspect bacterial contamination
* Perform Gram`s stain and culture on the remaining blood product
* Provide IV antibiotic coverage for Gram-negative bacteria, Staph.aureus, Staph.epidermidis

<2°C rise in body Temperature

* Usually mild & due to host antibody response to donor leukocyte antigens
* Pause the transfusion and provide thermoneutral environment ?paracetamol ?hydrocortisone *Use leukocyte reduced blood products in future.

---

* **Pearl/Peril/Pitfall :** *A third method utilized to remove WBCs from RBCs is irradiation. Irradiating RBCs with 1,500 to 5,000 Gy of radiation prohibits T lymphocyte proliferation. The combination of irradiation and washing RBCs can remove up to 95% of the T lymphocytes.*

TABLE 7 — Workup of acute transfusion reactions

Transfusionist

Stop transfusion; treat patient symptomatically; document symptoms on report form; draw posttransfusion specimens; send specimens, unit, and report form to transfusion service

Transfusion service

A. All reactions verify that the unit was intended for recipient

B. Febrile reactions to RBC

Recheck recipient and unit ABO/Rh type
Perform direct antiglobulin test (DAT) on recipient RBC
Visually inspect recipient's plasma for the hemoglobin
If DAT positive or free hemoglobin present, repeat serologic crossmatch on unit
If serologic incompatibility or hemolysis is found, perform testing to identify specificity of antibody
If hemolytic workup is negative, consider WBC-mediated reaction.
If patient shows signs of sepsis that were not present before transfusion Grain stain and culture unit and patient

C) Febrile reactions to platelets

Perform posttransfusion platelet count
If poor rise in platelet count, consider testing patient for anti HLA antibodies
If good increment, consider other WBC-related or cytokine reactions
If patient shows signs of sepsis that were not present before transfusion Grain stain and culture unit and patient

D) Allergic reactions

Mild symptoms; no testing indicated
Severe (eg, hypotension, angioedema): test patient and / or donor for IgA deficiency and anti-IgA antibodies

E) Pulmonary edema

Consider fluid overload
Consider testing patient or donor for anti-WBC antibodies- TRALI-(transfusion-related acute lung injury)

TABLE 8 — Noninfectious complications of transfusion

Hemolysis Recipient antibodies to transfused RBC : alloimmunization to red blood cell and leukocyte antigens (uncommon in infants),Osmotic, thermal, or mechanical lysis of cells before infusion, hemolytic transfusion reaction due to mismatched blood transfusion (medical error).

Nonhemolytic Febrile Transfusion Reactions-NHFTR : Recipient antibodies to WBC in blood product, Cytokines in blood product, Bacteria in blood product

Allergic Recipient sensitivity to plasma in blood product, Anti-IgA (in IgA-deficient recipient)

Pulmonary edema Volume overload,CHF from rapid or large volume transfusions, Anti-WBC antibodies in blood product or recipient **Electrolyte & Acid-base disturbances**-hyperkalemia from stored blood,hypernatremia from blood stored in CPD, hypocalcemia and hypomagnesemia due to citrate binding in CPD UNIT, metabolic acidosis from large transfusions with stored blood, Hypoglycemia due to a rebound to high glucose content of stored blood, Hypothermia when given via central line.

GVHD with in utero and massive transfusions.

TABLE 9 — Infectious agents transmissible by blood

Viruses

Hepatitis B,C
Retroviruses: HIV-1 and HIV-2, human T-cell leukemia viruses, types I and II (HTLV-I/II)
Cytomegalovirus (CMV), parvovirus B19, and Epstein-Barr virus (EBV) (mainly in immunosuppressed recipients), variant Creutzfeldt-Jacob disease(PRIONS)

Bacteria

Associated with asymptomatic bacteremia in blood donors (Yersinia enterocolitica, Salmonella, and other gram-negative organisms)
caused by contamination during collection (skin flora) or processing of blood)

Syphilis

Parasites

Malaria, babesiosis, trypanosoma cruzi, leishmaniasis

KEY POINTS FOR CLINICAL PRACTICE

1. As blood products convey a risk of transmitting potentially serious infections and are increasingly costly, it is clearly important to define evidence-based and/or standardized protocols for blood product use in Neonatal medicine. In order to maintain best practice, Neonatal units must construct, adhere closely to, and regularly audit and review guidelines for the administration of all blood products to sick Neonates.

2. Blood Component therapy provides **correct, effective and safe replacement** of only the deficient cells/factors, without exposing the recipient to the evils of unnecessary components of Whole blood. Moreover, each component has specific optimal storage conditions (In contrast to other blood components, platelets are stored at room temperature) and component therapy maximizes the use of blood donations.

3. Components transfused in the first year of life should be CMV-negative. All cellular components should be leukocyte- reduced at the point of manufacture to reduce the risk of transmission of infectious agents.

4. Unless blood is emergently needed, all PRBCs, platelets, and granulocytes are to be irradiated to prevent TAGVHD, especially among those at risk, such as Premature <1,500g, Immune compromised Newborns especially those with cellular immunodeficiency, who require Intrauterine transfusions, and who receive transfusion from a relative donor, especially mother, father, or siblings.

5. Acute hemolytic reaction secondary to infusion of ABO-incompatible plasma present in PRBC or Platelet concentrates occurs most commonly, because of clerical error involving misidentification of the patient or blood sample.

REFERENCES & FURTHER READING : 1) Busch MP et all. Current and emerging infectious risks of blood transfusions. JAMA 2003;289:959-962. 2) Maier RF et all. Changing practices of red cell transfusions in infants with birth weights <1,000 g. J.Pediatr 2000;136: 220-224 3) British Committee for Standards in Hematology Transfusion service<www.bcshguidelines.com> 4) AIIMS Neonatal Division Guidelines for Neonatal blood transfusion. 5) Textbook of Neonatal Hematology-Oncology 2003 ed.MR Lokeswar and Nitin Shah.

* **Pearl/Peril/Pitfall** : Many neonatology groups prefer to use fresh blood (<5 to 7 days) because of concerns regarding storage and hyperkalemia, shortened RBC life, hyperglycemia, hypernatremia, acidosis, renal toxicity (adenine, mannitol), and increased oxyhemoglobin affinity (decreased 2,3-DPG levels).

70

Neonatal Disseminated Intravascular Coagulation (DIC)

@ *"The cornerstone of DIC management remains the successful treatment of the underlying problem. In the absence of clinical manifestations, Newborns probably do not require therapy for the hemostatic disorder itself. In the presence of clinically significant bleeding, therapeutic intervention with plasma products is indicated and often improves hemostasis. For infants between these two ends of spectrum , treatment is dictated by the severity of hemostatic impairment and the underlying problem."*

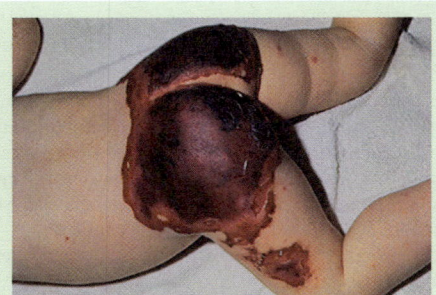

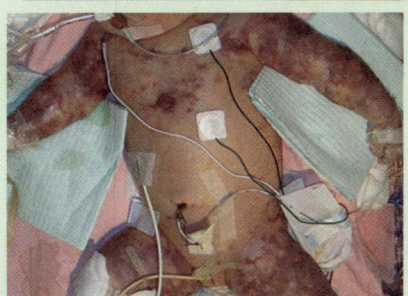

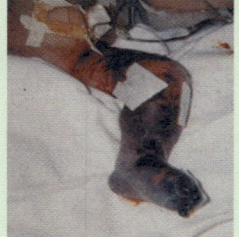

DIC: Purpura fulminans

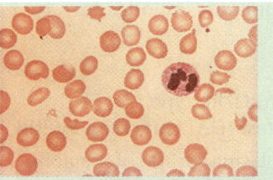

DIC-PBS: showing Schistocytes & Thrombocytopenia

The International Society on Thrombosis and Hemostasis (ISTH) scoring system for overt DIC

1. Risk assessment : does the patient have an underlying disorder known to be associated with overt DIC?
   If yes : Proceed   If no : Do not use this algorithm
2. Order global coagulation tests (platelet count, prothrombin time, fibrinogen, fibrin-related marker)
3. Score global coagulation test results-Apply newborn normal range of laboratory values.
 Platelet count (>100=0; <100=1; <50=2)
Elevated fibrin related marker (e.g. D-dimers; fibrin degradation products)
  Prolonged prothrombin time (<3s=0; >3 but <6s=1; >6s=2)
Fibrinogen level (>1.0gL⁻¹=0; <1.0gL⁻¹=1)
  4. Calculate score
  If >5:compatible with overt DIC : repeat score daily
  If <5: suggestive (not affirmative) for non-overt DIC: repeat next 1-2 days
The sensitivity and specificity of this scoring system are more than 90%. However, the algorithm should only be applied in the presence of an underlying disorder known to be associated with DIC. Recent observations have suggested that scoring for rates of change in the PT, platelet count, and D-dimer levels can help identify non-overt DIC in the early stages.

REVIEW OF CLINICAL PROBLEMS

1. Mention the common Neonatal conditions, which can be complicated by DIC.
Ans: Refer to the Table "1" of the Chapter.

2. What are the usual presenting symptoms and signs of DIC in a Neonate ?
Ans: Refer to the"No. 5" of the "BIRD`S EYE VIEW/OVER-VIEW/SYNOPSIS" of the Chapter.

3. Discuss the essentials of diagnosis of Neonatal DIC.
Ans: Refer to the"No. 7" of the "BIRD`S EYE VIEW/OVER-VIEW/SYNOPSIS" of the Chapter.

4. How do you differentiate Neonatal DIC from Coagulopathy of liver disease?
Ans: Refer to the Table 2 of the Chapter.

5. How do you manage Neonatal DIC?
Ans: Refer to the Evaluation-Decision-Action Plan/ Algorithm to diagnose & manage Neonatal DIC.

LEARNING OBJECTIVES

After completing this article, readers will be able to:

1. Anticipate DIC in the common Neonatal problems, which can predispose the baby to be hypoxic, acidotic, and hypotensive and to have tissue necrosis and/or endothelial damage.

2. Diagnose DIC in Neonates by a combination of clinical manifestations and the usual laboratory abnormalities.

3. Differentiate DIC from coagulopathy of liver disease and to monitor for the end-organ damage due to major vessel thromboses and/or bleeding in severe DIC.

4. Treat the underlying triggering conditions promptly and effectively to ward off DIC in its early stages.

5. Counsel the parents about the prognosis and the clinical course of DIC; primarily dependent on the outcome of the treatment of the primary disease and prevention of end-organ damage.

* *Pearl/Peril/Pitfall : Neonatal DIC: Fibrinolysis-Unregulated generation of thrombin and deposition of fibrin provide a strong stimulus to the fibrinolytic system. Whether fibrinolysis is a primary or secondary event is uncertain, but most believe that the fibrinolytic system is activated in response to the initiation of coagulation. In response to thrombin generation and endothelial injury, tPA is released from the endothelium. The continued activity of the fibrinolytic system contributes to the consumption of coagulation factors and to development of the hemorrhagic diathesis.*

BIRD'S EYE VIEW/OVERVIEW/SYNOPSIS

1. Disseminated Intravascular Coagulation (DIC)/Consumption Coagulopathy is not a primary diagnosis, but a secondary process to a variety of primary associated / triggering disease states enlisted in the Table 1 of the Chapter. It is an acquired pathologic process characterized by tissue factor-mediated diffuse coagulation activation in the host. DIC involves dysregulated, excessive thrombin generation, with consequent intravascular fibrin deposition and consumption of platelets and procoagulant factors. *Microthrombi, composed of fibrin and platelets, may produce hemolytic anemia (microangiopathic), tissue hypoxia—ischemia, end-organ damage, multiorgan dysfunction, and death.* The fibrinolytic system is frequently activated in DIC, leading to plasmin-mediated destruction of fibrin and fibrinogen; this results in fibrin-fibrinogen degradation products (FDPs) which exhibit anticoagulant and platelet-inhibitory functions.

2. Any life-threatening pathologic process associated with hypoxia, acidosis, tissue necrosis, shock, and/or endothelial damage may trigger DIC. The excess production of thrombin is central to the process of DIC. In addition to the conversion of fibrinogen to fibrin, thrombin has numerous other effects relative to the coagulation cascade. Although the clinical symptoms are primarily hemorrhagic, the initiating event is usually excessive activation of clotting that consumes both the physiologic anticoagulants, (protein C, protein S, antithrombin III) and procoagulants resulting in a deficiency of factor V, factor VIII, Prothrombin, Fibrinogen, and Platelets. Anticoagulant proteins C and S and antithrombin III also play a role in DIC. Congenital homozygous deficiencies of proteins C and S may result in Neonatal DIC. Low levels of antithrombin III are noted during DIC, and infusion of antithrombin III concentrate may aid in the recovery from DIC. Commonly, the clinical result of this sequence of events is hemorrhage. The hemostatic dysregulation may also result in thromboses in the skin, kidneys, and other organs.

3. The sick newborn is particularly more prone to DIC because of decreased synthesis of coagulation proteins, an underdeveloped reticuloendothelial system, and the tendency to develop hypoxia, acidosis, and shock. Physiologic anticoagulants, (protein C, protein S, antithrombin III) also decrease during 1st week of life. At birth plasminogen levels are decreased to 50% of adult values whereas tissue plasminogen activator (tPA) concentrations are increased. Overall, there is activation of fibrinolytic activity at birth and this is evidenced by shortened euglobulin lysis time and increased concentrations of D-dimer.

4. DIC occurs in sick Neonates, most commonly premature infants, unlike bleeding due to vitamin K deficiency or Inherited factor deficiencies. DIC process may occur rapidly or slowly and with varying degrees of severity. Intensity and duration of activation of the hemostatic system, degree of impaired blood flow, and liver function all influence the clinical severity of DIC. Some infants with laboratory evidence of DIC may show little or no clinical signs, whereas those clinically affected usually present with multiorgan failure and/or bleeding from multiple sites.

5. Signs of DIC may include a) diffuse bleeding tendency-ecchymoses, petechiae, purpura (*failure to look for purpura in a febrile/hypothermic infant, and to recognize it as a possible sign of disseminated intravascular coagulation (DIC), could lead to an adverse outcome.*), persistent oozing from venepuncture/surgical/gingival sites, hematuria, GIT bleeding or pulmonar/CNS hemorrhage. b) signs of shock, often including end-organ dysfunction such as acute renal failure, respiratory failure, ARDS, increased intracranial pressure due to CNS ischemia and/or hemorrhage c)evidence of thrombotic lesions-major vessel thrombosis, purpura fulminans. The clinical appearance of each patient heavily depends on the underlying cause. In many instances, determining if clinical manifestations are a result of DIC or an underlying disorder is difficult.

6. *The Evaluation-Decision-Action-Plan/Algorithm* describes the essential aspects of the clinical and laboratory diagnosis and the management of Neonatal DIC. Refer to Table 2 of the Chapter for a differential diagnosis of common haemostatic conditions, especially from coagulopathy of liver disease.

7. The diagnosis of DIC is based on compatible clinical features in conjunction with abnormalities of specific coagulation tests. Laboratory findings in severe DIC are characterized by prolonged PT, APTT, depletion of fibrinogen, factor V, factor VIII, increased fibrin degradation products, thrombocytopenia, and a microangiopathic hemolytic anemia with fragmented, burr, and helmet shaped schistocytes. Clinical judgment in conjunction with these tests provide a means of working towards a diagnosis of DIC, although no single test results alone are confirmatory. Yet diagnosis of DIC in the Newborn is difficult, and no clear-cut diagnostic criteria are available. The diagnostic difficulties are due to an overlap of physiologic and pathologic values for several procoagulant and anticoagulant factors, physiologically elevated markers of thrombin formation and fibrinolysis, and the limited blood volume available for diagnostic work-up. D-dimers are increased but measurement is not necessary for diagnostic purposes and is often not done in Neonates because of the need for an extra blood sample; results should also be interpreted with caution as D-dimers are not specific and can be found in healthy Neonates with no evidence of coagulopathy. Organ involvement and concurrent illness dictate the need for additional laboratory studies.

8. The cornerstone of DIC management remains the successful treatment of the underlying problem. In the absence of clinical manifestations, Newborns probably do not require therapy for the hemostatic disorder itself. In the presence of clinically significant bleeding, therapeutic intervention with *plasma products (Refer to the Evaluation-Decision-Action- Plan/Algorithm)* is indicated and often improves hemostasis. For infants between these two ends of spectrum, treatment is dictated by the severity of hemostatic impairment and the underlying problem. In general, the more pronounced the laboratory abnormalities, the greater the risk of bleeding or thrombotic complications.

9. Replacement Therapy for DIC is guided by the laboratory assessment and the *reasonable goals in the treatment of DIC are to maintain platelet counts >50,000/cumm, fibrinogen levels >1g/L, and PT values at normal levels for postnatal and gestational ages.*

10. Since many of the Neonatal disorders causing DIC are of brief in duration, optimum patient management is rewarding and complete recovery is more likely, provided there is no significant end-organ damage. Follow-up care with subspecialists may be required depending on the patient's underlying disorder and clinical course.

---

* *Pearl/Peril/Pitfall : Neonatal DIC: Failure to look for purpura in a febrile child, and to recognize it as a possible sign of disseminated intravascular coagulation (DIC), could lead to an adverse outcome. Recognizing and treating the underlying cause is critical.*

THE EVALUATION-DECISION-ACTION-PLAN/ALGORITHM FOR THE DIAGNOSIS AND MANAGEMENT OF *NEONATAL DISSEMINATED INTRAVASCULAR COAGULATION (DIC)*

SUBJECTIVE FINDINGS

History of a sick baby commonly a *preterm* with persistent oozing from venepuncture sites or bleeding from GIT, ecchymosis, petechiae and purpura, hematuria, pulmonary hemorrhage, and ICH in some.(*in contrast,* bleeding due to vit. K deficiency or inherited factor deficiencies occur in a well baby).

History of associated conditions causing severe hypoxia and/or acidosis peripartum hemorrhage, severe birth asphyxia, sepsis, RDS, Meconium aspiration syndrome, hypothermia, apneic episodes, polycythemia, NEC, Hemolytic disease of the Newborn.

Note that some infants with laboratory evidence of DIC may show little or no clinical signs, whereas those clinically affected usually present with multiorgan failure and/or bleeding from multiple sites.

OBJECTIVE FINDINGS

Assess ABCDs and monitor CRT, O_2 sats, BP, core-peripheral temperature difference, RR, HR, central & peripheral pulses, urine output

Identify petechiae, ecchymoses, epistaxis, oozing of blood from venepuncture sites/ surgical/gingival sites, *Purpura fulminans,* hematuria, hemoptysis, GIT bleeds, necrotic digits, acrocyanosis, poor perfusion, tone, hypotension etc., *Look for* renal, hepatic, pulmonary, or CNS manifestations which often accompany DIC. Most patients are critically ill.*Determine* the *degree of illness-* asymptomatic / mild/moderate to severe and *duration of illness. Verify the Laboratory profile of the patient for DIC and exclude other hematologic conditions-Refer to the Table 1 of the Chapter.*

INVESTIGATIONS

Blood FBC, TC, DC, **Hct**, Platelets, peripheral blood smear, Group/Type & Crossmatch, CRP, *Blood cultures & full septic screen,* **ABG analysis, electrolytes,** calcium & magnesium, **blood sugar,** LFT, creatinine, BUN, **coagulation profile.**(for general management of any sick neonate). Blood - Repeat FBC,TC, I:T Ratio, DC, Hct, Platelets, detailed peripheral blood film (fragmented, burr or helmet-shaped schistocytes due to microangiopathic hemolytic anemia), PT, APTT, TT, Fibrinogen, Fibrin split/degradation products, D-dimer(-nonspecific and can be found in healthy Neonates with no evidence of coagulopathy)
Urine analysis, culture/sensitivity CXR/CT or MRI Brain scan for ICH

NEONATAL DIC

Identify and Treat the underlying disease process.Because DIC is not the primary disease but a manifestation of underlying illness, diagnosing the initiating disorder is crucial.

Note that bleeding quickly ceases, and there is improvement of the abnormal laboratory findings, if the underlying problem can be controlled.

Ensure ABCs, Give supplemental oxygen, Monitor - pulse oximetry, BP (4-limb), CR Monitor, CVP if necessary,continuous BP monitoring.

Restore normal homeostasis by correcting the shock,acidosis, and hypoxia, that usually complicate DIC.

*If no bleeding/asymptomatic-*Monitor vital signs and for evidence of bleeding; Urine dipstick & Stool guaiac

If symptomatic with bleeding

Rationale for use of HEPARIN

* To date, no evidence is available to support the use of Heparin for infants with DIC.
* Heparin reduces the generation of excess thrombin in the early stages of DIC, and has to be initiated prior to micro-thrombus formation to provide at least theoretical benefit.
* Efficacy of Heparin treatment also depends on the AT-Prothrombin ratio, which may be low in Neonatal sepsis, resulting in a reduced Heparin sensitivity.
* Unfractionated Heparin @a loading dose of 75 units/kg IV over 10 minutes then 28units/kg/hr IVI can be tried, if DIC is associated with thromboembolic complication or evidence of extensive fibrin deposition.
* During Heparin therapy, pay careful attention to replacement therapy to maintain an adequate platelet count and thus limit bleeding complications.

The Argument that Replacement therapy may *"fuel the fire"* is theoretical , and this association has not been proved.

* *Administer* FFP 10–15 ml/kg IV over 1–2 hours for significant bleeding associated with elevated PT (4 seconds more than the normal value for an age-matched control).*Monitor* PT, APTT q6 hr and may repeat dose as needed.
* *Give* Cryoprecipitate,if hypofibrinogenemia is documented.
* *Give* Platelets, if the platelet count is <50,000/ cumm.
* *Exchange Transfusions* can be useful for fulminant DIC, especially associated with liver disease, but their effects are transient unless the underlying problem resolves.

Purpura fulminans is severe, extensive hemorrhage into the skin associated with fever and hypotension. It may be caused by infections, such as meningococcemia and varicella, or by protein C deficiency. Cutaneous purpuric or hemorrhagic lesions rapidly develop and spread and may progress to frank gangrene.

APC-Activated Protein C concentrate and AT- shown to be not useful in Neonatal DIC. Further well-designed controlled trials are required to determine their safety and efficacy.

In the absence of definitive clinical trials, reasonable goals in the treatment of DIC are to maintain platelet counts >50,000/cumm, fibrinogen levels >1g/L, and PT values at normal levels for postnatal and gestational ages.

---

* *Pearl/Peril/Pitfall : Neonatal DIC: Fibrin or fibrinogen degradation products and D-dimers are usually elevated due to the rapid generation of fibrin and breakdown of cross-linked fibrin polymers. Although sensitive, these tests are not specific. Fibrinogen levels are often decreased, as is antithrombin III. The PT and the aPTT are usually prolonged on screening tests but may be normal in an individual in the early phase of DIC ("non overt DIC").Thrombocytopenia is an almost universal finding, and the CBC count with smear review may reveal findings suggestive of DIC, such as increased platelet size, schistocytes, and helmet cells.*

TABLE 1 Disorders associated (*triggering events*) with DIC in the newborn

♦ Septicemia ♦ NEC ♦Birth asphyxia ♦Hyaline membrane disease ♦Meconium aspiration syndrome ♦Apneic episodes ♦Hypothermia ♦Polycythemia ♦Abruptio placentae ♦Hemolytic disease of Newborn ♦ Brain injury ♦ Purpura fulminans ♦ Dead twin fetus

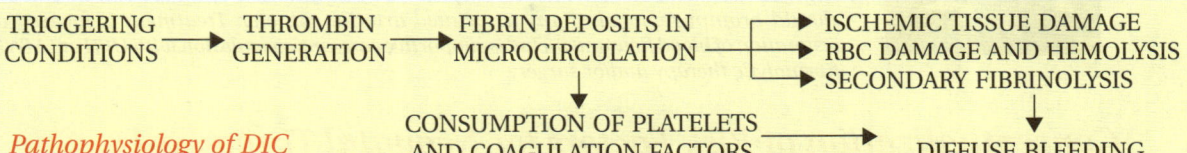

TRIGGERING CONDITIONS → THROMBIN GENERATION → FIBRIN DEPOSITS IN MICROCIRCULATION → ISCHEMIC TISSUE DAMAGE / RBC DAMAGE AND HEMOLYSIS / SECONDARY FIBRINOLYSIS

Pathophysiology of DIC → CONSUMPTION OF PLATELETS AND COAGULATION FACTORS → DIFFUSE BLEEDING

TABLE 2 Laboratory profile for DIC and other hematologic conditions

	DIC	Liver disease	Vitamin K deficiency/ Warfarin use	Heparin use	Massive blood transfusion
PT	↑	↑	↑	↑	↑
PTT	↑	↑	↑	↑	↑
TT	↑	↑	N	↑	N/↑
Platelet count	↓	N/↓	N	N/↓	↓
Fibrinogen	↓	↓	N	N	↓
D-dimer	⊕	Negative/ weakly positive	Negative	Negative	Negative
Schistocytes	Yes	Yes	No	No	No
FDP	↑	N/↑	N	N	N
Anti-thrombin III	↓	↓	N	N	↓
Factor VIII	↓	N/↑	N	N	↓
Factor V	↓	↓	N	N	↓
Factor II	↓	↓	↓	N	↓
Protein C,S	↓	↓↓	↓↓	N	↓

N = normal *NB*- In practice, no single laboratory test can be used to confirm or exclude DIC in a Neonate. Normal tests do not rule out activation of the coagulation and fibrinolytic systems.

KEY POINTS FOR CLINICAL PRACTICE

1. DIC is not a primary diagnosis, but a secondary pathological process triggered by hypoxia, acidosis, tissue necrosis, shock, and/or endothelial damage, and is associated with asphyxia, sepsis, NEC, meconium aspiration syndrome, RDS, apneic episodes, hypothermia, and hemolytic disease of newborn.

2. Although the clinical symptoms are primarily hemorrhagic, the initiating event is usually excessive activation of clotting that consumes both the physiologic anticoagulants, (protein C, protein S, antithrombin III) and procoagulants resulting in a deficiency of factor V, factor VIII, Prothrombin, Fibrinogen, and Platelets. Commonly, the clinical result of this sequence of events is hemorrhage. The hemostatic dysregulation may also result in thromboses in the skin, kidneys, and other organs.

3. Signs of DIC may include a) diffuse bleeding tendency-ecchymoses, petechiae, purpura, persistent oozing from venepuncture/surgical/gingival sites, hematuria, GIT bleeding or pulmonary/CNS hemorrhage. b) signs of shock, often including end-organ dysfunction such as acute renal failure, respiratory failure, ARDS, increased intracranial pressure due to CNS ischemia and/or hemorrhage c)evidence of thrombotic lesions- major vessel thrombosis, purpura fulminans.

4. The diagnosis of DIC is based on compatible clinical features in conjunction with abnormalities of specific coagulation tests. Laboratory findings in severe DIC are characterized by prolonged PT, APTT, depletion of fibrinogen, factor V, factor VIII, increased fibrin degradation products, thrombocytopenia, and a microangiopathic hemolytic anemia with fragmented, burr, and helmet shaped schistocytes.

5. The cornerstone of DIC management remains the successful treatment of the underlying problem. In the absence of clinical manifestations, Newborns probably do not require therapy for the hemostatic disorder itself. In the presence of clinically significant bleeding, therapeutic intervention with **plasma products** is indicated and often improves hemostasis.

REFERENCES & FURTHER READING : 1)Smith OP, Hann IM. Essential Pediatric Hematology. London: Martin Dunitz, 2002 2) Nathan and Oski`s Hematology of infancy and childhood, 6th ed. WB Saunders, 2003 3) Toh CH et al; DIC:Old disease, new hope. BMJ 2003;327:974-977.4)Levi M et al: DIC :N Engl J Med 1999;341: 586-592. 5) Franchini M et al : Update on the treatment of DIC. Hematology 2004;9: 81-85.

* *Pearl/Peril/Pitfall : Neonatal DIC: The most important prognostic factor is the ability to correct the underlying cause and arrest the ongoing derangement of the coagulation system.*

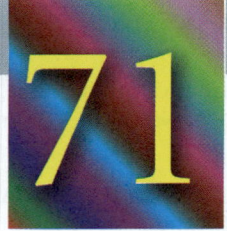

Thromboembolism in Neonates

@ Complications of UACs include mesenteric ischemia, hypertension, renal dysfunction/ failure, limb loss and congestive heart failure. High UAC positioning has been associated with fewer clinical complications. Suspicion or confirmation of an arterial thrombosis should prompt removal of any associated arterial catheter. Treatment is focused on restoration of blood flow and includes supportive care, anticoagulation with UFH or LMWH, fibrinolytic therapy and/or surgery.

Conceptualization of Risk Factors for Neonatal Thrombosis.

Maternal Factors
Infertility
Oligohydramnios
Thrombotic states
PET
Autoimmunity
Diabetes
Chorioamnionitis

Neonatal Thrombo-sis

Fetal/Neonatal Factors
Catheters
CHD
Infection
RDS
Dehydration
Birth Asphyxia
Polycythemia
Inherited Thrombophilias

Courtesy: Matthew A Saxonhouse, MD,FAAP NICU University of Florida

REVIEW OF CLINICAL PROBLEMS

1. What risk factors should you consider when taking History in evaluating Neonatal Thromboembolism?
Ans: Refer to the Table "1" of the Chapter.

2. Discuss the essential features of Neonatal Thromboembolism.
Ans: Refer to the Tables 2 & 6 of the Chapter.

3. What Imaging & Laboratory Investigations are useful in evaluating Neonatal Thromboembolism?
Ans: Refer to the Table "7" of the Chapter.

4. Discuss the recommended therapy and dosing of Neonatal antithrombic agents.
Ans: Refer to the Table "3" of the Chapter & to the Section "Medical management" of Neonatal Thromboembolism.

5. How do you prevent Iatrogenic Neonatal Thromboembolism?
Ans: Refer to the Section "Prevention" of Catheter related Neonatal Thromboembolism.

LEARNING OBJECTIVES

After completing this article, readers will be able to:

1. Delineate potential causes of vascular thromboembolic disease in Neonates.

2. Describe methods of diagnosing Neonatal vascular thromboembolism.

3. Delineate the anticoagulation/thrombolytic therapies used in Neonates.

4. Review potential complications of Neonatal thrombolytic therapies.

5. Individualize the Treatment strategies for each Neonate, taking into consideration age and clinical status.

* Pearl/Peril/Pitfall : Catheter related venous thrombosis (non-cardiac): umbilical venous catheters and peripherally inserted venous catheters- Due to the high complication rates from umbilical venous catheters (UVCs), the US Centers for Disease Control and Prevention (CDC) have recommended that the use of UVCs be limited to 14 days . Long term complications of venous TE include chronic venous obstruction with cutaneous collateral circulation, chylothorax, portal hypertension and post-thrombotic syndrome. Suspicion or confirmation of a venous thrombus warrants either prompt catheter removal, or 3-5 days of anticoagulant therapy followed by catheter removal (to reduce the risk for emboli at the time the catheter is pulled out) . While the latter is an approach favored by many physicians, there are no studies to support this practice, so it remains at the physician's discretion.

BIRD'S EYE VIEW/OVERVIEW/SYNOPSIS

1. The group of critically ill Newborns presents the largest patient population in childhood suffering from (TE) thromboembolism. Making decisions regarding therapeutic strategies is a challenge for the intensive care physician as the clinical significance of Neonatal thrombosis varies from asymptomatic incidents to life- or limb-threatening events; moreover, appropriate evidence-based treatment algorithms are lacking. 15% of all babies admitted to Neonatal intensive care unit (NICU) and 50% of all preterm Neonates with a birth weight of <1000 g are instrumented with an umbilical venous catheter . Unfortunately, together with asphyxia, sepsis, and prematurity, catheterization is among the most important risk factors for thrombosis in the Neonatal period.

2. Whereas arterial TEs other than Neonatal stroke or renal artery thrombosis are usually found at the site of insertion of an arterial catheter or arterial vascular access, venous thromboses are predominantly located in the renal vein, portal vein, and the inferior and superior vena cava . Other frequently affected locations include the femoral and axillary veins and the right atrium.Neonatal arterial ischemic stroke is most frequently caused by large vessel infarcts involving the carotid circulation in more than 2/3 of cases. In many of these infants, either perinatal complications or cardiac disease can be identified .

3. Although the hemostatic system of the term and preterm Neonate is significantly different from that of children and adults, most authors refer to the hemostatic potential of the "healthy" Neonate as being balanced, neither promoting hemorrhage nor thrombosis. On the pro-coagulant side, especially the vitamin K-dependent coagulation factors (II, VII, IX, and X) and the components of the contact system (FXI, FXII, prekallikreine and high molecular weight kininogen) show significantly reduced plasma activities in Neonates compared to children and adults. Although interpretation of values requires caution as corrected gestational age plays a major role, plasma activities of these components can be as low as 30% in the Neonate versus 80% to 120% in adults. Adult plasma concentrations are not achieved before the sixth month of life. However, the vitamin K-dependent inhibitors of coagulation, protein C and protein S, are also reduced in the Neonatal period, counterbalancing the reduced clotting potential of Neonatal plasma. In fact, both antithrombin and protein C concentrations are decreased to approximately 30% of adult values in term and even lower in preterm Newborns. Neonatal platelets have been reported to be hypo-reactive; however, this deficiency seems to be balanced by increased von Willebrand factor activity, resulting in overall normal platelet function. The activity of the fibrinolytic system in the Newborn is reduced compared to adults and older children due to both decreased plasma activity of plasminogen and increased plasma levels of plasminogen activator inhibitor (PAI). The latter fact may explain the high rate of TE associated with intravascular devices in Newborns; however, to date there is no evidence that the Neonatal hemostatic system either protects from or promotes thrombus formation. Of course, additional risk factors, e.g., critical illness or congenital thrombophilia, have to be considered separately from the immaturity of Neonatal hemostasis. Given the significant differences between the plasma factor concentrations in different age groups, a detailed knowledge on the development of hemostasis is critical for the intensivist in order to adapt pharmacological approaches and interpret results from laboratory tests in the Neonate with TE.

4. Critical illness is a well-recognized risk factor for TE in all age groups. Immobilization, rapid changes in intravascular volume and extensive intravascular instrumentation contribute to the enhanced risk of venous and arterial thrombosis in patients in intensive care units. In Neonates, this risk is further increased by the fact that indwelling catheters are large compared to the diameter of the vessel, in most cases obstructing approximately 50% of the lumen. Hence, it is not surprising that almost 90% of thromboembolic events in Neonates are caused by intravascular devices. Additional risk factors include, but are not limited to, asphyxia, maternal diabetes, poor cardiac output and dehydration. Neonates are born with a high hematocrit and tend to contract their intravascular volume within the first days of life, making them even more prone to thromboembolic events.

5. Neonates with sepsis develop an acquired pro-thrombotic state due to increased consumption of already limited supplies of coagulation inhibitors. Furthermore, plasma activity of PAI-1 is increased in sepsis and levels of protein C are reduced. The latter fact has been reported to correlate with poor outcomes in adults and Neonates. Ongoing consumption of coagulation factors and platelets resulting in microcirculatory thrombosis likely contributes to sepsis-induced multi-organ failure and death. Macro-circulatory thrombotic events are rare in this setting but can occur, especially in babies who have UACs or UVCs in situ.

6. *Congenital thrombophilia: Neonates with TE should undergo an extensive screening, including resistance to activated protein C (APC-R), protein C, protein S, and antithrombin activity, concentration of clot-table fibrinogen, plasminogen activity, activities of coagulation factors VIIIC and XII, Lp(a), histidine-rich glycoprotein, heparin cofactor II, antiphospholipid antibodies, lupus anticoagulants, as well as fasting homocysteine concentrations. In addition, DNA-based assays (i.e. factor V G1691A mutation, factor II G20210A variant and MTHFR C677T genotype) should be performed.* Whereas DNA-based mutation analysis can be performed at any time point, protein-based assays should not be carried out in the first 6–8 months after the event and oral anticoagulation is recommended to be discontinued at least 14–30 days before plasma samples for thrombophilia diagnosis are drawn. An obvious clinical picture is associated with either homozygous or double heterozygous congenital protein C deficiency. These infants develop the life-threatening complication of purpura fulminans within the first days of life. Notably, patients with prothrombotic mutations and polymorphisms are most likely to develop thrombosis when triggering elements, such as placement of catheters, prolonged immobilization, or surgery, are also present.Cyanotic congenital heart diseases (CHD) with secondary polycythemia and a hyperviscous state are associated with a reduction in blood flow and subsequent thrombosis. In CHD, the incidence of venous TE in infants <6 months of age is about 50% and even higher in arterial TE (70%). The increasing number of surgical procedures carried out in the Neonatal period potentiates the risk for TE events. Trans-catheter interventions in Newborns, which are mostly performed using venous access from the femoral or umbilical vein, incur the risk for transient or permanent occlusion of the lower body veins.

7. *Refer to Tables 1, 2, 3 ,4, 5, & 6 of the Chapter for the risk factors, clinical features, investigations/imaging modalities for the evaluation of Neonatal Thromboembolism, recommended therapy & dosing of Neonatal antithrombic agents & the contraindications to thrombolytic therapy.*

8. Registry data and case studies have demonstrated that the majority of symptomatic Neonatal Thromboses, particularly spontaneous events (i.e. not catheter-related), are associated with either multiple prothrombotic defects or the combination of prothrombotic defects and other acquired risk factors. Therefore, it is currently recommended that Neonates with thrombosis (regardless of risk factors) undergo testing for a full panel of genetic prothrombotic traits .

9. **Management of neonatal thrombosis:** If anticoagulation or thrombolysis are deemed necessary, the current dosing guidelines listed in Table 3 should be used. Before initiating antithrombotic therapy, however, the clinician must decide that the benefits of therapy outweigh its risks, especially in the premature infant. In regard to anticoagulation treatment, the choice is either UFH or LMWH.

10. The lack of randomized clinical trials addressing the management of Neonatal hemorrhagic and TE emergencies forces Neonato-logists to base their medical decisions on limited evidence from case reports and expert opinions. *The ultimate goal is to treat effectively without causing additional harm.* This can be difficult when treatments for both hemorrhage and thrombosis have significant risks, which need to be balanced against the benefits of treatment. Randomized clinical trials investigating treatment options for Neonatal hemorrhage and thrombosis are critically needed.

TABLE 1 — Risk factors for pathologic neonatal thromboses

Maternal Risk factors	Delivery Risk Factors	Neonatal Risk Factors	
Infertility and its treatment	Emergent cesarean section	Central Catheters	Polycythemia
Oligohydramnios	Severe bradycardia	Congenital heart disease	Pulmonary hypertension
Thrombotic states during pregnancy	Instrumentation	Sepsis	Prothrombotic disorders
Preeclampsia		Birth asphyxia	
Diabetes		Respiratory distress syndrome	Surgery
Chorioamnionitis		Dehydration	Extracorporeal membrane
Prolonged rupture of membranes		Congenital nephritic/nephrotic syndrome	oxygenation (ECMO)
Autoimmune disorders		Necrotizing enterocolitis	Medications (steroids, heparin)

TABLE 2 — Pathologic neonatal thromboses

Type of Blood Vessel	Type/Location	Presenting Symptoms	Imaging Modality
Arterial	Ischemic perinatal Stroke	Seizures, lethargy, apnea, poor feeding	MRI
	Iatrogenic/Spontaneous* (aorta, or large arterial vessel)	Line dysfunction, extremity blanching and /or cyanosis, pulseless extremity, thrombocytopenia, acute renal failure	Contrast angiography Ultrasound
	Catheter related	Persistent infection, persistent thrombocytopenia, line dysfunction.	Ultrasound/echocardiography CT or MRI
	Intracardiac (right atrium)	Infection, right heart failure	Echocardiography
Venous	Renal vein thrombosis	Macroscopic hematuria, palpable abdominal mass, thrombocytopenia, hypertension	Ultrasound
	Cerebral sinovenous thrombosis	Seizures, fever, lethargy	MRI
	Portal venous thrombosis	Thrombocytopenia, liver failure	Ultrasound

*Mainly related to umbilical arterial and peripheral arterial catheters

Courtesy: M A Saxonhouse and M C Sola-Visner

TABLE 3 — Recommended therapy and dosing of neonatal antithrombotic agents.

Clinical Indication	Medication	Traditional Dosing	Current Recommended Dosing	Complications
Asymptomatic or symptomatic thrombus but non-limb or organ threatening	UFH	75 units/kg IV over 10 minutes, then 28 units/kg/hour	< 28-weeks gestation: 25 units/kg IV over 10 minutes, then 15 units/kg/hour 28-37-weeks gestation : 50 units/kg over 10 minutes, then 15 units/kg/hour > 37-weeks gestation: 100 units/kg over 10 minutes, then 28 units/kg/hour	Bleeding Heparin induced Thrombocytopenia
Asymptomatic or symptomatic thrombus but non-limb threatening	LMWH	1.5 mg/kg SQ q 12 hours	Term Neonates 1.7 mg/kg SQ q 12 hours Preterm Neonates 2.0 mg/kg SQ q 12 hours	Bleeding
Limb/life threatening thrombus	rTPA	N/A	0.06 mg/kg/hour + UFH at 10 units/kg/hour	Bleeding

UFH = Unfractionated heparin; LMWH = Low molecular weight heparin; rTPA = Recombinant Tissue Plasminogen Activator

TABLE 4 — Contraindications to thrombolytic therapy. Rules should also be applied to anticoagulation therapy but clinical judgment recommended.

Absolute contraindications

1. Central nervous system surgery or ischemia (including birth asphyxia within ten days)
2. Active bleeding
3. Invasive procedure within three days
4. Seizures within 48 hours

Relative contraindications

1. Platelet count < 50, 000 /µl
2. Platelet count < 100,000/µl in neonate on mechanical ventilation, presence of chest tubes, other risks for potential hemorrhage
3. Fibrinogen concentration < 100 mg/dl
4. INR > 2
5. Severe coagulation deficiency
6. Hypertension

TABLE 5   Diagnosis of thromboembolism in neonates

Diagnosis: The clinical picture of vascular incidents in neonates is extremely variable and largely dependent on the location and the size of the thrombus or embolus. Presentation may vary from discrete symptoms or asymptomatic events to life or limb threatening acute events. Although in the following sections TE will be categorized as arterial, venous, and CNS events, one needs to keep in mind that several right-to-left (i.e., venoarterial) shunts remain patent for a considerable time even in the term Neonate. Thus, a paradoxical embolus cannot be ruled out even in the absence of congenital heart disease. **Arterial :** Arterial vascular events, accounting for about half of all TE in the Neonatal population, are almost always directly related to arterial vascular catheterization of central or peripheral arteries. This underscores the need for meticulous clinical observation in children with arterial access in place. Obvious signs include ischemia of limbs or trunk, pale or cold extremities distal to the catheterization site, weak or absent palpability of the pulse (pulse oximeters will also show this) and decreased or immeasurable blood pressure. Signs of necrotizing enterocolitis such as feed intolerance, bilious gastric aspirates, blood-stained stools, and bowel wall pneumatosis in an infant with UAC should raise the suspicion of mesenteric infarction. Diagnostic work-up for renal failure in children with UAC should include a Doppler flow study of the renal arteries to avoid missing out on the diagnosis of renal artery thrombosis. Elevated blood pressure might also hint at decreased renal perfusion. There are some reports of aortic thrombosis in the Neonate mimicking coarctation of the aorta with significant blood pressure differences in upper and lower body blood pressure readings; thus, the simple investigation of upper and lower body blood pressure measurements should be performed in any infant with hypertension diagnosed by measurements obtained from the upper body. **Venous:** Limb swelling, pain, and cyanotic or hyperemic color should raise the suspicion of venous thrombosis. Renal vein thrombosis may present with an abdominal mass and hematuria or proteinuria; hence, these symptoms should ring a bell especially in Neonates with risk factors such as prematurity, asphyxia, critical illness, femoral CVL, and male sex Signs of impaired liver function, hepatomegaly and splenomegaly should raise the suspicion of PVT; however, only about 10% of children with PVT develop acute clinical symptoms. Thrombosis of the inferior vena cava can present with signs resembling obstruction of the renal vein (hematuria, retroperitoneal mass); however, these will occur bilaterally when the inferior vena cava is affected. In addition, the lower limbs may be edematous and, if blood flow is substantially impaired, the child may be in respiratory distress and may have high blood pressure. **Pulmonary embolism:** Pulmonary embolism (PE) is a rare event in the Neonatal period. Clinical signs of massive ventilation/perfusion mismatch, difficult oxygenation, and signs of right heart failure should raise the suspicion of PE, especially in babies with congenital heart disease. In the few cases reported in the literature, diagnosis of PE was confirmed by lung perfusion scans or angiography. **Central nervous system:** In contrast to the clinical picture in adults, Neonatal stroke does not usually present with hemiplegia. The leading clinical symptoms in central nervous system TE in Neonates are seizures and lethargy. The diagnosis of ischemic stroke as well as of sinus vein thrombosis can initially be confirmed by cerebral ultrasound through the open fontanel followed by cranial magnetic resonance imaging (MRI). **Post-thrombotic syndrome:** TEs that remain clinically asymptomatic in the Neonatal period can become evident later in life when children or adolescents present with venous collaterals, post-thrombotic syndrome (featuring edema, purpura, eczematous dermatitis, pruritus, ulceration, and/or cellulitis), reduced limb growth or other late complications such as portal hypertension. Any of these symptoms can be the result of a vascular accident in the Neonatal period.

TABLE 6   Clinical signs and symptoms of thromboembolism in critically ill neonates

Early	Extremities	Intestine	Kidney	Aorta	CNS	Lung
Arterial	Extremities Pale and/or cold Pulse weak or absent Blood Pressure reduced	Feed Intolerance Gastric aspirates bilious Stools bloody Bowel wall pneumatosis	Blood pressure elevated	Blood Pressure higher in arms than in legs	Lethargy seizures (No hemiplegia)	Right heart failure Oxygen saturation low Ventilation/perfusion mismatch
Venous	Swelling Pain Cyanosis Hyperemia	Portal vein Liver function impaired Splenomegaly	Hematuria Proteinuria Abdominal mass	Inferior Vena cava Hematuria Lower limb edema Both Kidneys palpable Respiratory distress	Lethargy, seizures	
Late	Venous collaterals Limb growth reduced Post-thrombotic syndrome	Portal vein Portal hypertension GI hemorrhage Hepatic atrophy Splenomegaly	blood pressure abnormalities	Inferior vena cava Leg and abdominal pain Varicose veins post-thrombotic syndrome	Neurodevelopmental delay cognitive impairment Cerebral palsy	Right heart hypertrophy

TABLE 7 — *Imaging and Laboratory*

Ultrasound

Imaging by using either echocardiography or abdominal ultrasound is the most commonly applied diagnostic method to confirm clinical suspicion of TE or to screen babies for clinically silent disease. However, despite its advantages as point of care testing (minimal invasiveness and no use of radiation), the overall performance of ultrasound to detect thrombi is poor. One study comparing echocardiographic investigations to venograms reported a sensitivity of 21%–43% and specificities ranging from 76% to 94% . This study concluded that venography is required to accurately diagnose UVC related TE in Neonates. Since in this study 4% of all infants investigated were incorrectly diagnosed as having central venous thrombosis, the confirmation with contrast venography might avoid exposing an infant unnecessarily to potentially hazardous treatment.

Contrast venogram

Still regarded as the gold standard in the diagnosis of Neonatal catheter-induced TE, a contrast venogram exposes the infant to radiation and contrast agent. A recent study, using 1.5 to 2 ml of iohexol™ administered by hand injection over 1 to 2 sec and fluoroscopy times of 5–15 sec, reported a 100% agreement between two blinded radiologists about presence or absence of thrombi. In one of 14 babies with thrombosis a disagreement between the two examiners was reported in regards to the extension of the thrombus. A portable image intensifier allows contrast venography to be performed on the NICU as long as radiation exposure guidelines are taken into consideration.

MRI angiography

MRI angiography is recommended for the diagnosis of ischemic neonatal stroke and is an option in Neonatal pulmonary embolism. The need for transport limits the practicability in the most critically ill and very preterm Neonatal patients.

Laboratory

Initial laboratory work-up in a neonate in whom thrombosis is suspected should include a full blood count as well as a coagulation screening with determination of prothrombin time, thrombin time and activated partial thromboplastin time.

D-dimers

D-dimers, which are elevated as an acute phase reaction in all patients with infection or systemic inflammatory response syndrome (SIRS), are a positive finding in almost all critically ill Neonates. Conversely, negative D-dimers are relatively accurate in ruling out thrombosis in most patients, including Neonates.

Platelets

In almost all Neonates, platelet numbers decrease after birth. However, a sudden and severe drop in platelet counts should alert the intensivist. Although the differential diagnosis for thrombocytopenia in the Neonate is broad, including auto- and allo-antibodies as well as effects of medications and consumption, thrombocytopenia remains one of the most sensitive indicators for micro- (in the setting of sepsis) or macro-circulatory thrombosis.

Prevention

Obviously, strategies to prevent thrombus formation are of utmost importance in critically ill Neonates. Since the majority of TE in Neonates is catheter-related, optimal management and careful consideration of the necessity of these devices might give the intensivist a unique chance to improve outcome. Since even small thrombi might act as a nidus for infection, prevention of clot formation is of double benefit for the patient.

Umbilical catheters

Data suggest that UAC-related thrombosis can be minimized by high umbilical positioning, end-hole and single-lumen construction. Low-dose heparin infusion is recommended for UACs with some studies suggesting that even low doses 0.25 IU/ml are effective. The incidence of heparin-induced thrombocytopenia (HIT II) in preterm Newborns seems to be extremely low, thus promoting the use of unfractionated heparin (UFH) to ensure line patency. Time in situ should be minimized and many Neonatologists would see no indications for a UAC in a baby with stable hemodynamics and low to moderate ventilation parameters. Although some reports indicate that indwelling UACs in sick infants may not carry an increased risk of thrombosis during the first 5 days of use , a study published by Boo and colleagues showed that the only significant risk factor associated with the development of abdominal aortic thrombosis following insertion of UAC was longer duration of UAC in situ (for every additional day of UAC in situ, adjusted OR of developing thrombosis was 1.2, 95% CI: 1.1, 1.3; p = 0.002). When the use of UVC was audited by the study group for complications in perinatal care, it become apparent that UVC were inserted in approximately 50% of infants with a birth weight of 1000 g or less . Heparin was used in the infusate in the majority of the participating centers. As in UACs, the duration of use seems to be of importance in avoiding thrombus formation. In the report of the study group, the UVC was removed after a median of 4.4 days, the Center for Disease Control recommends removal after 14 days at the latest. However, one study recently compared long- and short-term use of UACs in premature Neonates and did not find an increased risk of thrombosis in the long-term group in which UACs were in situ for up to 28 days. Nevertheless, 9 of the 45 small for gestational age babies in the study developed a thrombus which was detected by echocardiography.

Other central venous catheters

Whereas percutanously placed peripheral silastic catheters in general have a lower incidence of thrombosis compared to centrally placed catheters, the highest incidence in CVCs is seen in femoral lines. Internal jugular access shows a lower rate of thrombosis compared to subclavian. Heparin infusion is utilized in most centers for CVCs in Neonates, especially for those placed in the femoral vein. The effectiveness of heparin infusion in percutanously placed peripheral silastic catheters has been controversial: A 2005 Cochrane review did not recommend the routine use of heparin for silastic catheters, whereas a recently published prospective study documented lower catheter occlusion rates but similar incidences of thrombosis in the heparin vs the placebo group. These findings lead to the publication of an update of the 2005 Cochrane review in 2008, in which the use of heparin at a dose of 0.5 IU/kg/h is recommended to maintain line patency, although this regimen does not reduce the risk of catheter-related thrombosis. Heparin-coated catheters might become an interesting option in the future to prevent both catheter occlusion as well as catheter-related thrombosis. However, a recent Cochrane review could not yet confirm a clear advantage of heparin-coated catheters in children and studies in Neonates have not yet been undertaken.

Management

Acute: When to treat TE in critically ill Neonates is a challenging question for everybody involved in the care of these infants. Since withholding anticoagulation is an equally active decision as commencing treatment, the individual risk/benefit ratio has to be carefully considered.

Potential benefits of antithrombotic therapy include complete or partial re-canalization of the obstructed vessel with consequently decreased tissue hypoperfusion in the affected area; limb saving in the scenario of acute arterial occlusion; avoidance of detrimental long term morbidity from conditions such as portal hypertension, hepatic post thrombotic syndrome, renal hypertension, impaired renal function, renal shrinkage, discrepancies in limb growth, claudication, and paraplegia.

The major potential risk of antithrombotic therapy, especially in Neonates, is a hemorrhagic event that is potentially massive and life threatening, in particular intracranial hemorrhage. Since low molecular weight heparins show a particularly favorable risk/benefit ratio, the decision *not* to treat TE will most likely be restricted to those infants with an exceptionally high risk of hemorrhage, e.g., very immature preterm Neonates within the first days of life or established intraventricular hemorrhage (IVH). Other relative contraindications for anticoagulant therapy include thrombocytopenia with platelet counts of less than 50,000/μl and history of high grade IVH. In most other patients, heparin therapy might be considered appropriate for clinically symptomatic TE.

The appropriateness of thrombolytic therapy will always depend on the individual patient. However, since the risk of hemorrhage, especially in systemic allied thrombolytic therapy remains unclear, most would restrict this therapeutic approach to life or limb threatening vessel obstructions.

Guidelines on treatment of clinically asymptomatic clots (detected for example during routine imaging in critically ill neonates) are not published and individual decision-making remains necessary. A majority of clinicians might decide to treat clots which obstruct more than 50% of the lumen of a major vessel (including the portal venous system) with low molecular weight heparin (LMWH) in the absence of contraindications. This approach takes both the potential long-term consequences of even asymptomatic TE in major vessels as well as the potential danger that the thrombus size may increase into account.

Medical

Unfractionated heparin

Unfractionated heparin has been the standard medication for prophylaxis and treatment of TE for many years. Due to unfavorable pharmacokinetics and pharmacodynamics and the imminent danger of HIT, UFH was almost completely replaced by low molecular weight heparins in adult medicine with the exception of anticoagulation during extracorporeal circulation. In neonatal medicine, however, UFH are still widely used to prevent and treat TE. Despite the lack of studies on LMWH in the neonatal population, the low incidence of HIT II , and the availability of protamine for potential reversal of UFH action, support its use in preterm and term neonates. Dosages of >25 IU/kg/h are usually required to achieve a targeted prolongation of the aPTT to 70 sec and above.

Low molecular weight heparin

Low molecular weight heparin has widely replaced UFH in prophylaxis and treatment of acute TE in adult patients due to superior efficacy, safety and pharmacokinetics. In Neonatal patients, the data available are still limited. However, LMWH is increasingly used in NICU in the post-acute treatment of venous and arterial TE as well as in prevention of thrombosis in high-risk patients. Subcutaneous enoxaparin seems to be the most frequently used substance in term and preterm neonates. Data published on the use of enoxaparin in 12 preterm and 4 term infants found no serious adverse events and a resolution of TE in 71% of the patients. Anti-Xa level is usually targeted at 0.4–0.6 IU/ml in prophylaxis and at 0.6–0.8 IU/ml in treatment scenarios. Preterm infants require longer to achieve an anti-Xa level within target range compared to term infants (6 vs 2 days) and were found to require higher doses of enoxaparin (2.1 mg/kg/12 h vs 1.7 mg/kg/12 h).

Recent evidence also suggests a starting dose of 1.7 mg/kg/12 h in term and 2 mg/kg/12 h in preterm neonates. Efficacy was reported to be 59%–100%. Cessation of anticoagulation can be achieved by terminating the medication 12–24 h prior to planned surgical procedures. In contrast to common belief, protamine is able to antagonize anti-Xa activity of LMWH in part and anti-IIa activity of LMWH completely. In a recent case report, an overdose of 40 mg of enoxaparin in a Neonate was successfully antagonized with 35 mg of protamine given in the preceding 4.5–7.5 h.

Streptokinase: Streptokinase is infrequently administered in the Neonatal period due to decreased fibrin specificity and high antigenicity compared to rtPA. In the few patients described in the literature, doses of 1000–2000 IU/kg/h have been used.

rtPA (recombinant tissue plasminogen activator): If thrombolytic therapy is utilized, rtPA is mostly favored due to high fibrin specificity with poor activation of free plasmin, lack of antigenicity and short half life (4 min in plasma, 45 min for thrombolytic effects). Dosing varies between different reports, ranging from 0.3 to 9 mg/kg/24 h. Plasminogen levels are low in neonates compared to adults, pointing towards a possible requirement for higher doses of rtPA. Administration of fresh frozen plasma (FFP) prior to utilization of thrombolytics may increase success rates by providing sufficient plasminogen levels. Frequent monitoring of fibrinogen levels and FFP administration if fibrinogen levels fall below 100 mg/dl are required.
Urokinase As with streptokinase, the decreased fibrin specificity and the antigenicity of urokinase compared to rtPA limit its use in Neonates. In the small number of Neonatal patients which are described in the literature, doses of 1000 up to 10,000 IU/kg/h have been reported, although the majority of patients received 2000 IU/kg/h or less .

Some studies, which include small numbers of term neonates, investigated urokinase as treatment or prevention of catheter occlusion and/or catheter infection with some success in older children and adults. However, this treatment is not sufficiently evaluated in the Neonatal population to be recommended.

Duration of treatment: The administration of fibrinolytics such as rtPA, streptokinase, and urokinase is usually rather short in duration. These agents are stopped either after a few days or when revascularization has been achieved (as determined clinically or via imaging). In contrast, LMWH is increasingly used in therapeutic concentrations for prolonged therapies of 6 weeks or even up to 3 months, since late revascularization occurs in adults and in children and Neonates, as the few studies performed in these patient groups have shown.

Interventional Catheter-directed thrombolysis: Catheter-directed thrombolysis (CDT) has been reported in 13 patients in the Neonatal period. In these reports, rtPA (dosage 0.01–0.1–0.5 mg/kg/h [min–median–max]) was used in 8 patients, while 4 patients received streptokinase and one was treated with urokinase. In contrast to systemic thrombolytic therapy, efficacy of CDT seems to be superior (82% vs 62% of complete clot lysis, 16% vs 8% partial clot lysis, 8% vs 21% failure). The safety profile also favors CDT with a rate of one intraventricular hemorrhage (IVH) in 13 patients with CDT compared to 2 IVH, one intra abdominal bleed, one kidney rupture, one mucosal bleed and one puncture site bleed in 38 neonates with systemic thrombolysis. *Surgical* Surgical clot removal and vessel reconstruction may become necessary in the rare event of life or limb threatening arterial thromboembolism and in the even rarer event of massive venous thrombosis.

Conclusion: Critically ill Neonates are at major risk of venous and arterial thromboembolic events. Since indwelling catheters are the main contributing factor, a significant proportion of these events might be preventable by critically re-evaluating especially the indication for umbilical artery and venous catheter on a daily basis and using heparin prophylaxis in those babies where catheterization of the umbilical vessels cannot be discontinued. While therapy of established thrombus formation with unfractionated or low molecular weight heparin needs to be weighed carefully against the "lost chance" of not applying therapy, thrombolysis or mechanical clot removal should be restricted to the rare scenarios of acute life threatening vessel occlusion. All Neonates with a history of thromboembolic events warrant a follow-up with an emphasis on the development of post-thrombotic syndrome, portal hypertension and an investigation for congenital thrombophilic risk factors. A detailed knowledge of developmental hemostasis is necessary to guide therapy and monitoring in Neonates with thrombotic events.

Thrombosis in the critically Ill Neonate—Therapeutic options and Mechanisms of action.

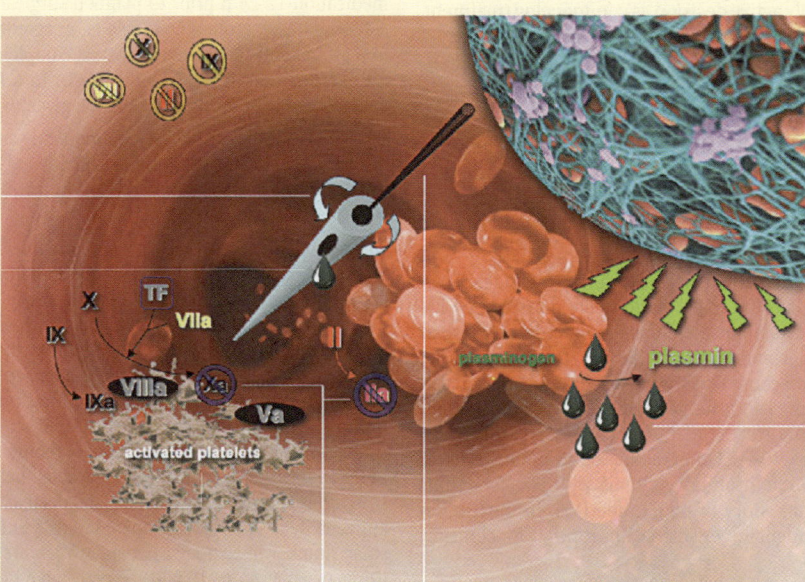

Vitamin K antagonists eg. warfarin

Mechanical clot lysis
Catheter interventions
Local application of rtPA

Platelet antagonists eg., ASA or clopidogrel

Heparin
Unfractionated

Prophylaxis
Avoid femoral lines

Systemic Thrombolysis rtPA, urokinase, streptokinase

Courtesy: Alex Veldman, Marcel F Nold, Ina Michel-Behnke.

KEY POINTS FOR CLINICAL PRACTICE:

1. Among children, Newborn infants are most vulnerable to development of thrombosis and serious thromboembolic complications. Amongst Newborns, those neonates who are critically ill, both term and preterm, are at greatest risk for developing symptomatic thromboembolic disease.

2. The most important risk factors are inflammation, DIC, impaired liver function, fluctuations in cardiac output, and congenital heart disease, as well as exogenous risk factors such as central venous or arterial catheters.

3. In most clinically symptomatic infants, diagnosis is made by ultrasound, venography, or CT or MRI angiograms. However, clinically asymptomatic vessel thrombosis is sometimes picked up by screening investigations or during routine imaging for other indications.

4. Acute management of thrombosis and thromboembolism comprises a variety of approaches, including simple observation, treatment with unfractionated or low molecular weight heparin, as well as more aggressive interventions such as thrombolytic therapy or catheter-directed revascularization. Long-term follow-up is dependent on the underlying diagnosis. In the majority of infants, stabilization of the patients' general condition and hemodynamics, which allows removal of indwelling catheters, renders long-term anticoagulation superfluous.

5. Nevertheless, in certain types of congenital heart disease or inherited thrombophilia, long-term prophylaxis may be warranted.

REFERENCES & FURTHER READING : 1) Andrew M, Paes B, Johnston M, et al. 1990. Development of the hemostatic system in the neonate and young infant. *Am J Pediatr Hematol Oncol,* 12:95–104. 2)Barrington KJ. 2000. Umbilical artery catheters in the newborn: effects of position of the catheter tip. *Cochrane Database Syst Rev,* 2: CD000505. 3)Andrew ME, Monagle P, deVeber G, et al. 2001. Thromboembolic disease and antithrombotic therapy in newborns. *Hematology Am Soc Hematol Educ Program,* 358–74. 4)Malowany JI, Knoppert DC, Chan AK, et al. 2007. Enoxaparin use in the neonatal intensive care unit: experience over 8 years. *Pharmacotherapy,* 27:1263–71. 5)Nowak-Gottl U, Bidlingmaier C, Krumpel A, et al. 2008. Pharmacokinetics, effi cacy, and safety of LMWHs in venous thrombosis and stroke in neonates, infants and children. *Br J Pharmacol,* 153:1120

* *Pearl/Peril/Pitfall: Acute complications of RVT include adrenal hemorrhage, extension of the clot into the IVC, renal failure, hypertension and death. Genetic prothrombotic conditions have been found in 43-67% of patients with RVT. In the absence of uraemia or extension into the IVC in patients with unilateral RVT, current recommendations are to provide either supportive care with monitoring for extension or anticoagulation with UFH or LMWH for up to three months. In cases of unilateral RVT with extension into the IVC, anticoagulation with UFH or LMWH should be instituted for three months. Thrombolytic therapy plus anticoagulation with UFH, followed by anticoagulation with UFH or LMWH, should be reserved for patients with bilateral RVT and renal failure.*

72 Acute Renal Failure in Neonates

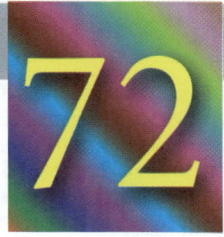

@ *Neonatal Renal Failure is most commonly caused by Sepsis, Birth Asphyxia, Respiratory distress, CHD with CHF, NEC, Nephrotoxins and Obstructive Uropathy.*

@ *A careful assessment of clinical indicators of volume status, including heart rate, blood pressure, skin turgor, capillary refill, oral mucosa integrity, and fullness of the anterior fontanelle, is essential. Other pertinent data that must be monitored include body weight, fluid intake, urine and stool output, serum electrolytes, and urine osmolarity or specific gravity.*

Causes of acute renal failure

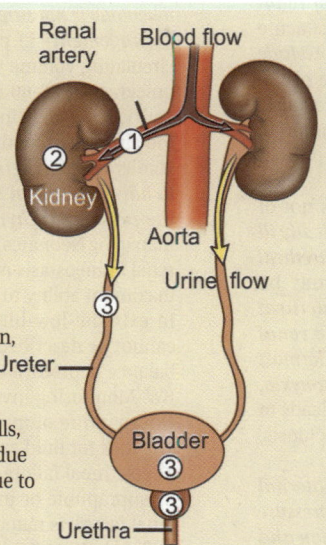

1. **Prerenal**
   Sudden and severe drop in blood pressure (shock) or interruption of blood flow to the kidneys from severe injury or illness.

2. **Intrarenal**
   Direct damage to the kidneys by inflammation, toxins, drugs, infection, or reduced blood supply.

3. **Postrenal**
   Posterior Urethral valves, Fungus balls, Renal Calculi, Extrinsic obstruction due to SC Teratoma, Hematocolpos or due to Neurogenic bladder.

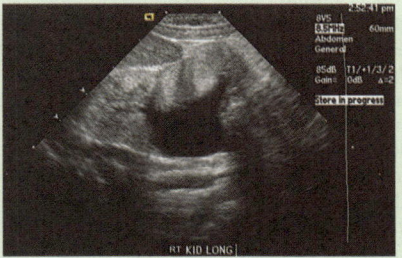

Sonogram of the right kidney in a patient with grade V vesicoureteral reflux. Hydronephrosis and increased echogenicity indicating renal dysplasia secondary to reflux nephropathy. *US is an integral part of the evaluation of renal insufficiency and failure in Neonates. High-resolution US allows improved characterization of the renal parenchyma and more precise description of renal architecture. Recognition of the US appearance and characteristics of different pathogeneses aids in the establishment of a differential diagnosis. Prompt diagnosis permits earlier intervention and may prevent progression of renal insufficiency to renal failure in some patients.*

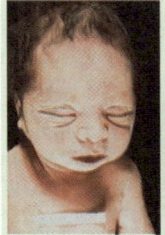

Potter's syndrome is incompatible with life outside the uterus and is found in 0.2% to 0.4% of the autopsies performed on stillborn infants or those who die soon after birth. The characteristic facial features include hypertelorism, redundant skin, Mongolian palpebral fissure, epicanthal fold, specific suborbital crease, depressed nasal bridge, parrot-beak nose, posteriorly rotated low-set ears, receding small chin, a crease below lower lip, bow legs, clubfoot, hip dislocation, wide and broad hands, and a short neck (Figures 1 and 2).

During nephrogenesis, the essential interaction between the ureteric bud and metanephric mesenchyme is controlled by genes, transcription factors, and growth factors. The genetic disorder often occurs prior to day 31 of fetal development. The ureteric bud which forms the kidneys fails to develop and the absence of the kidneys causes a deficiency of amniotic fluid after the weeks 12 to 16. Renal agenesis when accompanied by these characteristic features is called "Potter's disease". Kidneys normally produce the amniotic fluid (as urine) which is necessary for normal lung development. Oligohydramnios causing a continuous pressure of uterine wall on the fetal chest wall and the pressure of fetal intraabdominal organs on the diaphragm are the main causes of lung hypoplasia and insufficiency in Potter's syndrome. The degree of hypoplasia depends on the degree and duration of oligohydramnios as well as the stage of lung development at which oligohydramnios occurs.

REVIEW OF CLINICAL PROBLEMS

1. How do you differentiate Prerenal from Intrinsic Renal Failure in Neonates ?
   Ans: Refer to the Table 1 and 6 of the Chapter.

2. Discuss the essential aspects of Management of Hyperkalemia in Neonatal ARF.
   Ans: Refer to the Table "3" of the Chapter.

3. Mention the Clinical Indications for instituting Peritoneal Dialysis in Neonatal ARF.
   Ans: Refer to the Evaluation-Decision-Action Plan/ Algorithm to diagnose & manage a Neonate with ARF.

4. Discuss the Essential aspects of History taking and Physical examination in evaluating Neonatal ARF.
   Ans: Refer to the Evaluation-Decision-Action Plan/ Algorithm to diagnose & manage a Neonate with ARF.

5. Mention the usual causes of Seizures in Neonatal ARF.
   Ans: Refer to the Evaluation-Decision-Action Plan/ Algorithm to diagnose & manage a Neonate with ARF.

LEARNING OBJECTIVES

After completing this article, readers will be able to:

1. Define the types and delineate the causes of acute renal failure (ARF) in Neonates.

2. Describe the laboratory tests and imaging studies used to diagnose ARF.

3. Explain the roles of fluid balance, diuretics, dopamine, and nutrition in the management of Neonatal ARF.

4. Describe the approaches to treating hyponatremia, hyperkalemia, calcium-phosphorus perturbations, acidosis, and hypertension in ARF.

5. Review the outcome and prognosis for ARF in Neonates.

Pearl/Peril/Pitfall : Neonatal ARF: Physical examination: Look for abdominal masses. These are often renal or related to genito urinary system. Look for other congenital anomalies which are often associated with renal abnormalities. They are low set ears, ambiguous genitalia, anal atresia, abdominal wall defect, vertebral anomalies, meningomyelocele, pneumothorax, hemihypertrophy, persistent urachus, hypospadiasis, and cryptorchidism.

BIRD'S EYE VIEW/OVERVIEW/SYNOPSIS

1. *Acute renal failure* in the Neonate is diagnosed when the urine output is < 0.5ml/kg/hr in the first day and <1ml/kg/hr thereafter *with a serum creatinine level >1.5mg/dL and if it rises at a rate of 0.3mgs/dL/day).* (normal serum creatinine - 0.8-1.0mgs/dL at day 1, 0-7-0.8mgs/dL at 3 days and < 0.6mgs/dL by 7 days of life). *Higher values suggest renal disease except in LBW infants, in whom a creatinine level of < 1.6mgs/dL is considered normal. Rule of thumb ; if the creatinine doubles , then 50% of renal function has been lost.* Oliguria is usually the first sign of acute renal failure, *although a normal urine output doesn't exclude the diagnosis,* (nonoliguric renal failure) and because of the practical difficulties in measuring a baby's urine output, oliguria may escape observation. Hypercatabolism, which is common in sick infants, leads to uremia and hyperkalemia due to protein breakdown despite a normal GFR.

2. Although delayed micturition in a healthy Neonate is not of concern until 24 hours after birth, *urine output in a critically ill Neonate should be assessed by 8-12 hours of life, using urethral catheterization if indicated.* Acute Renal Failure may be secondary to *circulatory insufficiency without structural damage (pre-renal), parenchymal damage (intrinsic renal failure) or due to urinary tract obstruction (post-renal). The most common causes of Neonatal acute renal failure are asphyxia, sepsis and severe respiratory illness.* Acute renal failure leads to problems with fluid volume overload, hyperkalemia, acidosis, hypocalcemia, and hyperphosphatemia.

3. *Most of the conditions can be established by taking the maternal and infant history, examining the baby (including blood pressure and catheterization of the bladder), screening for infection and performing a renal and bladder ultrasound scan, to exclude / confirm urinary tract obstruction.*

4. *Differentiation between pre-renal and intrinsic renal failure is often more difficult, and may be further complicated by the fact that the former may lead to the latter.* Renal failure indices are often less helpful in the Neonate because a low protein diet and a high urinary Na$^+$ excretion affect both osmolality and those indices which rely on urinary Na$^+$. Among urinary indices utilized to differentiate oliguric Neonatal ARF from prerenal oliguria, a fractional excretion of sodium greater than 3% or a renal failure index (RFI) greater than 3 are helpful in confirming ARF. Such indices must be viewed with caution in very premature infants who may have a physiologically high sodium excretion rate and in Neonates with the nonoliguric form of ARF. All indices are less reliable in preterm infants, and a high fractional excretion of Na$^+$ (FeNa) in particular doesn't necessarily indicate renal failure. If doubt exists about the prerenal component, an IV Isotonic fluid challenge (15ml/kg of Normal saline) with a simultaneous bolus of 2mg/kg of frusemide, can be useful *but is clearly ill advised in a hypotensive, edematous, ventilated 1kg baby who is already requiring inotropic support because of risk of fluid overload.*

5. The *Evaluation-Decision-Management Plan/Algorithm* describes the essential aspects of History, Physical Examination, and Investigations and the management issues of a Neonate with Acute Renal Failure. **Urine microscopic analysis:** The presence of granular casts hyaline casts, RBC, proteins and tubular cells suggests an intrinsic cause. **Ultrasonography and doppler:** useful in ruling out congenital anomalies like polycystic kidneys, dysplasia of kidneys and obstructive causes of renal failure like posterior urethral valves. Renal doppler studies are helpful in diagnosing vascular thrombosis. **Voiding cysto-urethrography** can identify lesions of the lower urinary tract that cause obstruction, such as posterior urethral valves. **Differentiate acute from chronic renal failure:** Clinical setting as shown by prenatal, natal and post natal events generally would tell about the reversibility of the renal failure. Pointers to underlying irreversible renal problem: Family history of congenital/hereditary renal disease, Prenatal USG showing oligohydraminos and significant renal anomalies, Maternal intake of drugs like NSAIDs, Post natal USG showing bilateral renal anomalies, Presence of known external markers and other congenital organ anomalies. *Unless proved otherwise it is better to treat one as reversible renal failure when one is not sure.*

6. *Management-* 1) pre-renal failure is managed by restoring circulating volume with blood or isotonic saline 10-20ml/kg IV quickly over 30-60 minutes, maintaining a urine output above 1ml/kg/hr and giving frusemide 2-4mg/kg. With hypotension, in the absence of fluid depletion, give an infusion of Dopamine 5-10micro grams /kg/mt. *Overall low dose dopamine does not seem to have any role in the prevention or treatment of ARF except in the presence of hypotension or CHF (Cochrane study).* While managing Neonates one has to keep in mind the fact that, at birth, renal homeostasis is limited in healthy preterm infants (e.g., the maximum ability to concentrate urine is 700 to 800 mOsm/L).

7. In extreme-low-birth-weight (ELBW) infants, renal function cannot be described as "homeostatic," and fluid and electrolyte balance is precarious. Problems are greatest in infants <1250 g BW. Monitoring involves: Weighing the Neonate every 8 hours. Hourly urine output measurement. Measure abdominal girth and look for fluid excess. Rewriting fluid advice at least 8 hours. 2) post renal failure due to obstruction is relieved by surgery or by suprapubic or urethral catheter as appropriate 3) intrinsic renal failure is managed by conservative treatment with control of fluid balance and hyperkalemia, in most cases as the oliguria is usually short-lived.

8. *peritoneal dialysis* is seldom required but should be instituted urgently if there is : 1) severe fluid overload +/ - pulmonary edema 2) severe metabolic acidosis (pH < 7.2 with PaCO$_2$ < 40mmHg) 3) hyperkalemia (K$^+$ > 8mmol/lt) not responding to medical measures 4) intractable hypoglycemia. *5) Consider dialysis if CNS prognosis considered good in a baby with HIE .* Raising creatinine alone is not an indication for dialysis. Before embarking on dialysis ethical factors must be considered. *Consider the following issues:* 1. Is the renal defect reversible? 2. How long is dialysis likely to be required? 3. Other medical problems and their reversibility. 4. Parental views. Generally one need not hesitate to undertake dialysis in a Neonate weighing > 1.5 kg who is likely to survive without severe neurological deficits and whose renal disease is reversible.

9. *Continuous renal replacement therapy (CRRT)* using arterio venous hemofiltration through an extracorporeal circuit is becoming a more frequently employed modality for renal replacement therapy in the hemodynamically unstable Neonate. (with high risk for intracranial bleeding due to heparinization)

10. *Neonates with acute renal failure have variable prognosis* ; Prerenal failure if treated promptly carries an excellent prognosis. Post renal ARF has a variable outcome that is dependent on degree of associated renal dysplasia. *Infants with intrinsic ARF have the poorest prognosis with mortality rates as high as 50%.* The mortality of oliguric Neonatal renal failure may be as high as 60% in medical ARF and even higher in Neonates with congenital heart disease, or with anomalies of the genitourinary system. In contrast, nonoliguric renal failure in Neonates has an excellent prognosis. Long-term abnormalities in glomerular filtration rate and in renal tubular function are common in survivors of Neonatal ARF: *Long- term sequelae seen in survivors of Neonatal ARF include hypertension, impaired urinary concentrating ability, renal tubular acidosis and impaired renal growth.*

Pearl/Peril/Pitfall: Acute renal failure (ARF) is a very common problem in the Neonatal intensive care unit. The Newborn kidney has a very low glomerular filtration rate (GFR) that is maintained by a delicate balance between vasoconstrictor and vasodilatory forces. (1) Although sufficient for growth and development under normal conditions, the low GFR of the Newborn kidney limits postnatal renal functional adaptation to endogenous and exogenous stresses. (2) This limited response predisposes the newborn to the development of ARF and is even more pronounced in the low birthweight infant (i.e., <2,500g due to preterm birth or intrauterine growth restriction). (3) Given this predisposition, early identification of ARF in the Neonate is essential to preserving renal function.

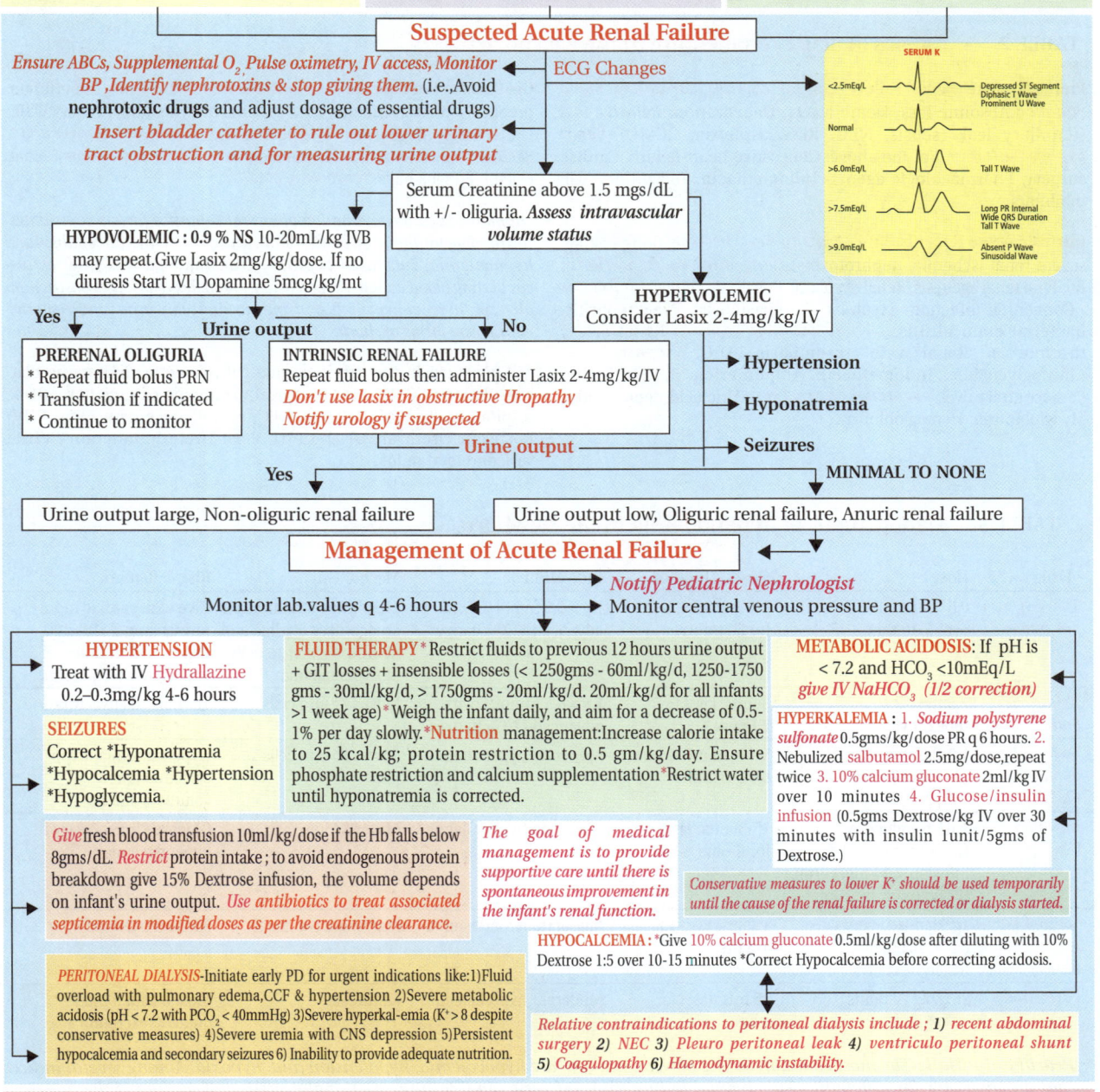

THE EVALUATION-DECISION-ACTION-PLAN/ALGORITHM FOR THE DIAGNOSIS AND MANAGEMENT OF *NEONATAL ACUTE RENAL FAILURE*

SUBJECTIVE FINDINGS

Hx of Hypovolemia Blood loss, plasma loss, insensible loss (phototherapy in VLBW infants), GI losses (D&V), polyuria, inadequate intake (fluid restriction after birth asphyxia).

Hx of Hypoxic - Ischemic Encephalopathy and Hx of risk factors for Septicemia or severe respiratory illness, NEC.

Hx of Maternal Diabetes-Renal vein thrombosis. Hx of oligohydramnios - Potter's syndrome. Hx of Nephrotoxic drugs (aminoglycosides, indomethacin, frusemide). Hx of congestive heart failure. Hx of force of the infant's urinary stream (posterior urethral valves.

OBJECTIVE FINDINGS

Look for Symptoms and signs of renal failure
* *Symptoms of renal failure*, e.g. poor feeding, vomiting, seizures, bleeding, cardiac arrhythmias.
* *Signs*, e.g. fluid overload (hypertension, edema, excess weight gain, hepatomegaly, tachypnoea), fluid depletion (poor peripheral perfusion, hypotension), renal abnormality (palpable kidney, bladder).

Look for the presence of any congenital anomalies associated with renal abnormalities (e.g. Potter's syndrome, VACTERL, Epispadias).

INVESTIGATIONS

Weight, BP, Infection Screen, Renal Ultra Sound.
Urine Multistix, Microscopy, Urea, Electrolytes, Creatinine, Osmolality.
Blood Electrolytes, Urea, Creatinine, ABG analysis, Osmolality, Calcium, Mg++, Glucose, Albumin, Full blood count, Clotting studies, LFTs. ECG and CXR
Renal Ultrasound is helpful in the identification of congenital renal disease and urinary tract obstruction.

Micturating cystourethrogram should be performed in neonates with suspected posterior urethral valves, vesicoureteral reflux, or bladder abnormality.

Suspected Acute Renal Failure

Ensure ABCs, Supplemental O₂, Pulse oximetry, IV access, Monitor BP ,Identify nephrotoxins & stop giving them. (i.e.,Avoid **nephrotoxic drugs** *and adjust dosage of essential drugs)*

ECG Changes

Insert bladder catheter to rule out lower urinary tract obstruction and for measuring urine output

SERUM K

<2.5mEq/L	Depressed ST Segment / Diphasic T Wave / Prominent U Wave
Normal	
>6.0mEq/L	Tall T Wave
>7.5mEq/L	Long PR Internal / Wide QRS Duration / Tall T Wave
>9.0mEq/L	Absent P Wave / Sinusoidal Wave

Serum Creatinine above 1.5 mgs/dL with +/- oliguria. *Assess intravascular volume status*

HYPOVOLEMIC : 0.9 % NS 10-20mL/kg IVB may repeat.Give Lasix 2mg/kg/dose. If no diuresis Start IVI Dopamine 5mcg/kg/mt

HYPERVOLEMIC Consider Lasix 2-4mg/kg/IV

Yes — Urine output — **No**

PRERENAL OLIGURIA
* Repeat fluid bolus PRN
* Transfusion if indicated
* Continue to monitor

INTRINSIC RENAL FAILURE
Repeat fluid bolus then administer Lasix 2-4mg/kg/IV
Don't use lasix in obstructive Uropathy
Notify urology if suspected

→ Hypertension
→ Hyponatremia
→ Seizures

Urine output

Yes — **MINIMAL TO NONE**

Urine output large, Non-oliguric renal failure

Urine output low, Oliguric renal failure, Anuric renal failure

---

Management of Acute Renal Failure

Monitor lab.values q 4-6 hours
Notify Pediatric Nephrologist
Monitor central venous pressure and BP

HYPERTENSION
Treat with IV Hydrallazine 0.2–0.3mg/kg 4-6 hours

SEIZURES
Correct *Hyponatremia *Hypocalcemia *Hypertension *Hypoglycemia.

FLUID THERAPY * Restrict fluids to previous 12 hours urine output + GIT losses + insensible losses (< 1250gms - 60ml/kg/d, 1250-1750 gms - 30ml/kg/d, > 1750gms - 20ml/kg/d for all infants >1 week age)* Weigh the infant daily, and aim for a decrease of 0.5-1% per day slowly.*Nutrition management:Increase calorie intake to 25 kcal/kg; protein restriction to 0.5 gm/kg/day. Ensure phosphate restriction and calcium supplementation*Restrict water until hyponatremia is corrected.

METABOLIC ACIDOSIS: If pH is < 7.2 and HCO₃ <10mEq/L *give IV NaHCO₃ (1/2 correction)*

HYPERKALEMIA : 1. *Sodium polystyrene sulfonate* 0.5gms/kg/dose PR q 6 hours. 2. Nebulized *salbutamol* 2.5mg/dose,repeat twice 3. 10% calcium gluconate 2ml/kg IV over 10 minutes 4. Glucose/insulin infusion (0.5gms Dextrose/kg IV over 30 minutes with insulin 1unit/5gms of Dextrose.)

Give fresh blood transfusion 10ml/kg/dose if the Hb falls below 8gms/dL. *Restrict* protein intake ; to avoid endogenous protein breakdown give 15% Dextrose infusion, the volume depends on infant's urine output. *Use antibiotics to treat associated septicemia in modified doses as per the creatinine clearance.*

The goal of medical management is to provide supportive care until there is spontaneous improvement in the infant's renal function.

Conservative measures to lower K⁺ should be used temporarily until the cause of the renal failure is corrected or dialysis started.

HYPOCALCEMIA : *Give 10% calcium gluconate 0.5ml/kg/dose after diluting with 10% Dextrose 1:5 over 10-15 minutes *Correct Hypocalcemia before correcting acidosis.*

PERITONEAL DIALYSIS-Initiate early PD for urgent indications like:1)Fluid overload with pulmonary edema,CCF & hypertension 2)Severe metabolic acidosis (pH < 7.2 with PCO₂ < 40mmHg) 3)Severe hyperkal-emia (K⁺ > 8 despite conservative measures) 4)Severe uremia with CNS depression 5)Persistent hypocalcemia and secondary seizures 6) Inability to provide adequate nutrition.

Relative contraindications to peritoneal dialysis include ; 1) recent abdominal surgery 2) NEC 3) Pleuro peritoneal leak 4) ventriculo peritoneal shunt 5) Coagulopathy 6) Haemodynamic instability.

---

* *Pearl/Peril/Pitfall : Babies with ARF have to be monitored for several metabolic derangements like hyponatremia, hyperkalemia, hypocalcemia, and acidosis and have to be managed accordingly. Fluid balance should be precise in order to avoid fluid overload. It is difficult to provide adequate calories due to fluid restriction. Dialysis has to be instituted to preempt complications. Peritoneal dialysis is the easiest and safest modality. These babies need long term follow up as they are prone for long term complications.*

TABLE 1   Diagnostic indices suggestive of prerenal or intrinsic renal failure in the Newborn

	Prerenal Acute Renal Failure	Intrinsic Acute Renal Failure
Urine flow rate (mL/kg/h)	Variable	Variable
Urine osmolality (mOsm/L)	>400	$\leq$ 400
Urine/plasma osmolar ratio	>1.3	$\leq$ 1.0
Urine/plasma creatinine ratio	29.2 $\pm$ 1.6‡	9.7 $\pm$ 3.6‡
Urine [Na+] (mEq/L)	10-50	30-90
FENa° (%)	<0.3 (0.9 $\pm$ 0.6)‡	>3.0 (4.3 $\pm$ 2.2)‡
RFI†	<3.0 (1.3 $\pm$ 0.8)‡	>3.0 (11.6 $\pm$ 9.6)‡
Response to fluid challenge ($\pm$ furosemide)	Increased urine output	No effect on urine output

° Fractional excretion of sodium (FENa) = (Urine [Na+] / Serum [Na+]) / (Urine [Cr] / Serum [Cr]) × 100.
† Renal failure index (RFI) = Urine [Na+] / (Urine [Cr] / Serum [Cr]) ‡ Mean $\pm$ SD.

TABLE 2   Causes of acute renal failure in the Newborn*

Prerenal Acute Renal Failure *Loss of effective circulating blood volume ;* Absolute loss, Hemorrhage, Dehydration, **Relative loss** -Capillary leak (sepsis, NEC, RDS, asphyxia, ECMO) *Renal hypoperfusion ;* All of the above, Congestive heart failure, Cardiac surgery, Pharmacologic agents- Indomethacin, Tolazoline, ACE inhibitors.

Intrinsic Acute Renal Failure *Acute tubular necrosis* (long-lasting, severe renal ischemia, nephrotoxins) *Congenital malformations ;* Bilateral renal agenesis, Renal dysplasia, Polycystic kidneys, *Infections ;* Congenital infections (syphilis, Toxoplasmosis), Pyelonephritis, Bacterial endocarditis, *Renal vascular causes ;* Renal artery thrombosis, Renal vein thrombosis, DIC, *Nephrotoxins;* Aminoglycosides, Indomethacin, Amphotericin B, Methicillin, Radiocontrast dyes *Intrarenal obstruction ;* Uric acid nephropathy, Myoglobinuria, Hemoglobinuria.

Obstructive Renal Failure *Congenital malformations ;* Imperforate prepuce, Urethral stricture, PUV, Urethral diverticulum, Primary VUR, Ureterocele, Megaureter, PUJ obstruction, *Extrinsic compression ;* Sacrococcygeal teratoma, Hemotocolpos *Intrinsic obstruction ;* Renal calculi, Fungus balls *Neurogenic bladder*.

In many cases, a combination of several causative factors contributes to the development of acute renal failure. For instance, absolute hypovolemia, increased capillary leak-induced loss in effective circulating blood volume, hypotension, and reflex renal vasoconstriction all result in renal hypoperfusion and ensuing renal injury in Newborns with severe forms of shock.

ACE, angiotensin-converting enzyme; DIC, disseminated intravascular coagulation ; ECMO, extracorporeal membrane oxygenation ; RDS, respiratory distress syndrome. NEC, necrotizing enterocolitis. PUV, Posterior Urethral Valves ; PUJ, Pelvi Ureteric Junction ; VUR, vesicoureteral reflux.

TABLE 3   Management of hyperkalemia in the Newborn

Drug	Dose	Onset, Duration	Indication	Mechanism	Risk & Remark
10% Calcium gluconate	0.5-1ml/kg IV over 5-10 min.	1-2 minutes, lasts for 30 minutes	K+ > 6.5 mmol/L with advanced ECG changes	Membrane stabilization antagonizes cardiac and neuromuscular toxicity of hyperkalemia	Give with cardiac monitoring. Stop if HR <100 Repeat in 5 minutes, if abnormal ECG persists.
Nebulized Salbutamol	2.5mgs/dose repeat twice	30mts, lasts for 2 hours	K+ > 6.5 mmol/L with advanced ECG changes	Moves K+ into cells	Tremors, tachycardia
Sodium bicarbonate (3.75%)	1.0-2.0mEq/kg (IV over 10 min)	5-10 minutes, lasts for 2-6 hours	Moderate hyperkalemia	Moves K+ into cells	Hypernatremia, hypocalcemic tetany, volume overload
Insulin & Glucose	1 IU/5 g glucose (IV bolus or infusion $\leq$ 14 mg/kg/min (IV bolus or infusion)	15-30mts, lasts for 4-6hrs	Moderate hyperkalemia	Moves K+ into cells	Glucose Unnecessary if hyperglycemia +
Sodium polystryrene sulfonate	1g/kg dose every 6 h as needed (orally/rectally)	1-2 hrs, lasts for 4-6 hrs	Moderate hyperkalemia	Exchanges Na+ for K+	Sodium overload
Furosemide	2mg/kg IV bolus	15 mts, lasts for 4 hrs	Moderate hyperkalemia	Kaliuresis	Most useful if inadequate K+ excretion +.

* **Pearl/Peril/Pitfall :** *The most common causes of Neonatal ARF are hypovolemia, hypotension and, hypoxia. Among several indices that are available for differentiating prerenal failure from intrinsic renal failure, fractional excretion of sodium is the preferred index. Diagnostic fluid challenge with or without frusemide is a bed side method for differentiating prerenal failure from intrinsic renal failure. (Cautious fluid challenge, if no signs of fluid overload or heart failure are present. Normal saline 10–20 ml/kg is infused over 1-2 h. If urine is produced, it is probable prerenal renal failure. If no urine or little urine is produced in 1 h post infusion, IV furosemide 1 mg/kg is given. If still no or only little urine is produced, it is probable parenchymal renal failure.)*

TABLE 4   Urine collection itself needs extra attention

a. Suprapubic aspiration is the most reliable method, esp, for detecting infection.

b. Diaper urine specimens are enough for pH and qualitative determinations of presence of glucose, protein, and blood.

c. - Bag collections are adequate for specific gravity, pH, electrolytes, protein, glucose and sediments.

d. - For quantification of the urine volume you need either bag collections or bladder catheterization. Catheterization is used if an infant has failed to pass urine by 36 – 48 hrs and is not hypovolemic.

Rising plasma creatinine:

Serum creatinine values on first two days reflect maternal values. Normally creatinine level falls quickly from 0.8 mg/dl at birth to 0.5 mg/dl at 5–7 days and reach a stable level of 0.3 to 0.4 by 9 days. (Refer Table 5). The rate of fall in creatinine is slower in premature infants as they start with a lower GFR. Anything outside this is considered abnormal.

One has to be careful in interpreting creatinine (when estimated by Jaffe's method) in the presence of high bilirubin (which is not uncommon in the neonate). Creatinine level is spuriously low in the presence of high bilirubin. One can get around this problem by doing something called rate blanking. This compensates for the bilirubin up to about 30 mg/dl. Creatinine by immuno nephelometric method is not interfered by bilirubin or ketones. Estimation of Cystatin C, which is evolving as a better marker for estimation of renal function, would even be better.

TABLE 5   Normal serum creatinine values in term and preterm infants

Age (days)	<28 wk	29–32 wk	33–36 wk	>37 wk
7	0.95 (1.31)	0.94 (1.40)	0.77 (1.25)	0.56 (0.96)
14	0.81 (1.17)	0.78 (1.14)	0.62 (1.02)	0.43 (0.65)
28	0.66 (0.94)	0.59 (0.97)	0.40 (0.68)	0.34 (0.54)

TABLE 6   Differentiate retention from renal failure

Palpate bladder / Attempt to express bladder

Urine found in bladder or urine expressed		No urine or minimal urine in bladder
Good stream	Poor stream	Confirm absence of urine by Ultrasonogram
	Obstructive uropathy : • Urethral valves • Bilateral ureteroceles	If none Presumed prerenal or Parenchymal renal failure
Action : Repeated bladder expression, or Catheter, till spontaneous resolution	Action : Consider catheter Assess anatomy of urinary tract by sonography Assess renal function Exclude UTI	

Courtesy: J. Balasubramaniam, Kidney Care centre. Tirunelveli, Tamil Nadu. India

* **Pearl/Peril/Pitfall :** *Birth asphyxia and neonatal sepsis are still common; more so in developing countries where obstetric and newborn resuscitation facilities are not universally available yet. Combination of dehydration, sepsis, shock, and nephrotoxic drugs is not an uncommon situation in neonatal ICU. These lead to high incidences of neonatal renal failure. The inciting insults can sometimes be so subtle and occult that the cause of renal failure may seem unobvious. They are often reversible if identified and managed in time.*

PERITONEAL DIALYSIS IN THE NEW BORN-PRACTICAL ASPECTS - Peritoneal dialysis is preferred over hemodialysis in the Newborn because it is similarly effective, safer and technically less demanding and it should be started when the Newborn is still hemodynamically stable so that this treatment modality can affect morbidity and mortality from acute renal failure.

Procedure - 1) *Ventilate* the baby as the Neonate in **ARF** doesn't tolerate the diaphragmatic splinting which occurs when peritoneum is full of dialysate, so the dialysate has to be run in and out sequentially with no ""resting" phase.

2) *Empty* the bladder by inserting a urinary catheter.

3) *Insert* a 19G IV cannula through the right iliac fossa into the peritoneal cavity and instil warmed dialysis fluid to fill the cavity, which allows the PD catheter to be more safely introduced, with a lower risk of damaging the bowel.

4) *Insert* the PD cannula at a point midway between the umbilicus and the left anterior superior iliac crest and secure with a purse string suture.

5) *Use* an Isotonic dialysis solution (1.36% glucose) for biochemical and metabolic indications. *Use* a hypertonic solution (3.86% glucose) for fluid overload but hyperglycemia is a risk.

6) *Undertake* the dialysis in the following sequence: a) allow the fluid to drain from the peritoneal cavity; b) for each cycle, run in 20-30 mL/kg of prewarmed and heparinized (1 unit/ml) dialysis fluid over 10 min; c) allow this to remain in the cavity for 20-30 min, so that dialysis occurs; d) let fluid drain out under gravity for 20 min. Each cycle therefore lasts about 1 h; e) accurately record the volumes in and out ; and f) perform microscopy of the dialysate every 24h to detect infection.

7) *ADD* potassium 4 mmol/L to the dialysate once the baby's level is below this.

8) *Hourly exchanges* usually result in obligate ultrafiltration even when 1.5% Dextrose concentration is used, so that parenteral or central fluid intake is needed to avoid volume depletion and prolongation of acute renal failure.

9) *Continue* the dialysis until the fluid balance is satisfactory and/or the potassium concentration is below 6mmol/Lt; once this has been achieved, with the conservative management of renal failure, the baby probably only need peritoneal dialysis for about 8 hrs a day until renal function returns, although this may take up to 3 weeks.

Suggested water, sodium and potassium intakes (these may need considerable modification from day to day depending on clinical course) for various weight† babies in kilograms.

Day	Water				Sodium				Potassium
	<1	<1.5	<2.5	>2.5	<1	<1.5	<2.5	>2.5	All weights
1	100	80	60	60	0	0	0	0	0
2	120	100	90	90	5	4	3	1	0-2
3	150	130	120	110	5*	4	3	1	2-3
4	180	150	150	130	5*	4	3	1	2-3
5	200	180	170	150	5*	4	3	2	2-3
6	200	180	170	150	5*	4	3	2	2-3
7	200	180	170	150	5*	4	3	2	2-3
8-13	200	180	170	150	5*	4	3	2	2-3
14-20	180	160	150	150	4	3	2	1	2-3
21-27	160	160	150	150	3	2	2	1	2-3
>28	160	150	150	150	2	2	2	1	2-3

These figures are for infants nursed in incubators or cots. Infants under radiant warmers may require much higher volumes of water.

* Commonly higher requirements. Check blood sodium daily.

†Use birthweight or most recent weight, whichever is greater.

Increases IWL	Decreases IWL
1. Severe prematurity, 100-300%	1. Humidification in incubator, 50-100%
2. Open warmer bed, 50-100%	2. Plastic head shield in incubator, 30-50%
3. Forced convection, 30-50%	
4. Phototherapy, 30-50%	3. Plastic blanket under radiant warmer, 30-50%
5. Hyperthermia, 30-50%	
6. Tachypnea, 20-30%	4. Tracheal intubation with humidification, 20-30%

*SENSIBLE WATER LOSSES - Urine : Smaller preterm infants without systemic hypotension and prerenal renal failure usually lose 30-40ml/kg/day water in the urine during the first day of life and around 120ml/kg/day on the 3rd day after birth. In stable more mature preterm infants born after 28th week of gestation, it will be 90-150ml/kg/day. **Stool :** Term baby loses 10ml/kg/day and the preterm loses 7ml/kg/day during the first week of life. Water losses in the stool increase thereafter and are influenced by the type of feeding and the frequency of stooling. **Excessive fluid intake (> 150-160ml/kg/day) may predispose the premature baby to develop significant PDA.*

The Relationship Between Metabolism and Maintenance

ROUTE	LOSS/GAIN	ML REPLACEMENT/ 100 KCAL METABOLIZED ENERGY
Insensible:		
Skin	Loss	25
Respiration	Loss	15
Urine	Loss	60
Stool	Loss	10
Water of oxidation	Gain	10
Total for Maintenance		100

Insensible Water Loss (IWL) in preterm infants

Birth Weight (g)	Average IWL (ml/kg/day)
>750–1000	64
1001–1250	56
1251–1500	38
1501–1750	23
1751–2000	20
2001–3250	20

* Pearl/Peril/Pitfall : *Neonatal ARF:When interpreting FENa, one has to keep in mind that the Na reabsorption capacity of premature kidney is limited, resulting in high FENa (> 3%) even in prerenal states unlike in adults where it is < 1%. In premature neonates with oliguria, if FENa is <3%, we may assume that the renal failure is incipient and that there is enough residual renal function to retain salt. The usefulness of FENa is uncertain if a diuretic has been already given.*

FLUID AND ELECTROLYTE PROBLEMS
ASSOCIATED WITH SPECIFIC CLINICAL CONDITIONS

Extreme Prematurity: Preterm neonates have more water (at 23 weeks' gestation, 90% water composed of 60% ECF and 30% ICF), and they may lose 10-15% of their weight in the first week of life. Small for gestational age (SGA) preterm infants may have a higher proportional body water content (90% for SGA infants vs 84% for appropriate for gestational age [AGA] infants at 25-30 weeks' gestation). Insensible water loss (IWL) is water loss that is not readily measured, and consists mostly of water lost via evaporation through the skin (two thirds) or respiratory tract (one third). Sensible water loss: Other measurable sources of fluid include urine, stool (e.g., diarrhea and ostomy), nasogastric (NG) or orogastric (OG) drainage, and cerebrospinal fluid (CSF) (eg, ventricular drainage). Ventilated infants receive humidified gas. Therefore, IWL from the lungs is eliminated in these infants The average water requirement for an infant with birth weight between 500 and 750 grams in the first week of life is estimated to be about 170 mL/kg/day if the infant is in an incubator with low ambient humidity and without phototherapy and perhaps 150 mL/kg/day if moderate humidity is added to the incubator. The requirement would be 210 to 220 mL/kg/day if a radiant warmer or overhead phototherapy is used and 250 to 270 mL/kg/day if both radiant warmer and photo therapy are used. Infants born at gestational ages younger than 26 weeks present special problems in fluid and electrolyte management. These infants have large IWL , in some cases more than 200 mL/kg/day if the infant is nursed under a radiant warmer. The large IWL of extremely premature infants results from their meager skin barrier to evaporation and their large ratio of surface area to body weight. In the first week of life, the water requirement may be even higher in infants born after only 22 or 23 weeks of gestation. In these extremely premature infants, the cutaneous IWL and consequently the total water requirement decrease toward the end of the first week of life, as the stratum corneum matures and becomes less permeable to water. Extremely premature infants, unless hyponatremic from maternal hypotonicity , should initially be started on electrolyte-free solutions of glucose (5 g/dL) in water or solutions that provide sodium in a dose of 2 to 3 mEq/kg/day as sodium acetate or sodium bicarbonate. The latter bases compensate for respiratory acidosis while allowing hypercapnia with the goal of minimizing lung trauma. Administering some or all of the maintenance sodium as sodium acetate or sodium bicarbonate also serves to mitigate the metabolic acidosis present in many extremely premature infants as a result of renal immaturity and transient renal tubular acidosis. If sodium is not begun initially, it should be added by the second day, provided the serum sodium concentration is below 145 mEq/L. Some of the smallest preterm infants have sodium requirements of as much as 6-8 mEq/kg/d because of the decreased capacity of the kidneys to retain sodium. Hyperkalemia is a very common problem in extremely premature infants during the first week of life. This potentially dangerous condition results from potassium release from catabolized cells in the presence of immature distal renal tubular function . Hyperkalemia is exacerbated if dehydration and oliguria occur as a result of inadequate water intake. No potassium should be given to extremely premature infants until the serum potassium concentration falls below 4 mEq/L. If the serum potassium concentration exceeds 7 mEq/L, rectal administration of a potassium binding resin should be considered.

Perinatal Asphyxia: After birth asphyxia, it is advisable to restrict water intake in anticipation of possible increased AVP secretion (also known as inappropriate antidiuretic hormone secretion) or acute renal failure. In a term infant, insensible water losses are approximately 20 to 25 mL/kg per day, and stool loss is minimal. Fluid requirements during the first day of life in an anuric term infant are approximately 30 mL/kg per day. Insensible losses for an anuric premature infant may be as high as 80 mL/

kg per day, depending on gestational age. During the first 24 hours of life, the water intake for asphyxiated infants should be limited to IWL plus urine output minus about 20 mL/kg/day to allow for some physiologic contraction of the extracellular water volume. If urine production is normal by the third postnatal day, water intake can be restored to a normal level. During the oliguric phase of acute renal failure, potassium should not be administered unless the serum potassium concentration is less than 3.5 mEq/L. With acute renal failure resulting from hypoxia or ischemia, the initial period of oliguria may be followed by a diuretic phase with polyuria. If urine output increases and body weight falls below the expected level (i.e., the weight before fluid retention began), the intake of water must be increased to prevent dehydration. This diuretic phase may be accompanied by large losses of sodium and other electrolytes, which must be replaced. Replacement of the urinary sodium losses is facilitated by measuring the volume and sodium concentration in an aliquot of urine from a timed collection.

Respiratory Distress Syndrome and Bronchopulmonary Dysplasia: The renal function in preterm babies may be further compromised in the presence of hypoxia and acidosis due to RDS. Positive pressure ventilation may lead to increased secretion of aldosterone and ADH, leading to water retention. Symptomatic patent ductus arteriosus (PDA) is more likely to occur in the presence of RDS. Results from various studies have shown that restricted water intake has a beneficial effect on the incidence of PDA, CLD, NEC and death. Hence fluid therapy in sick preterm infants should be monitored strictly using the above mentioned clinical and laboratory criteria.

Symptomatic Patent Ductus Arteriosus: The management of fluid regimens in preterm infants who have or are at risk of a HSDA (hemodynamically significant patent ductus arteriosus) remains a challenge. In the first few days after birth, careful fluid restriction to meet physiologic requirements while avoiding dehydration may reduce the risk of a PDA. Routine fluid restriction in ELBW infants who have proven HSDAs and during pharmacologic treatment with indomethacin cannot be advocated because this may cause end-organ hypoperfusion and caloric restriction, with subsequent long-term complications. Clinicians should strive to achieve a delicate balance between pulmonary overcirculation and systemic hypoperfusion with fluid administration. Concurrent diuretic therapy is only indicated if there are signs of pulmonary edema or left ventricular failure. Postligation cardiac syndrome due to left ventricular dysfunction is not an uncommon complication of PDA surgical ligation and requires careful monitoring postoperatively. Clinical management entails early fluid restriction with or without diuretic therapy and inotropic drugs, especially in the presence of pulmonary edema. Fluids should be scrutinized carefully and regimentally delivered to optimize pulmonary and systemic perfusion (Qp/Qs).

Infants of diabetic mothers: These infants receive i.v. glucose because of increased danger of hypoglycemia; however, they frequently do not receive sodium and have been found to develop rather substantial hyponatremia at 24 h if this is not added at or before this time. This danger is greater the greater rate of glucose needed to maintain blood glucose. Addition of sodium should be considered at 16-18 h.

Sepsis and Necrotizing Enterocolitis : Systematic reviews of randomized clinical trials of varying fluid intake in premature infants have identified overhydration as a risk factor in the pathogenesis of NEC . Infants with septicemia who also have meningitis may develop inappropriate ADH secretion, reducing their water requirement. Infants with septicemia or

---

* Pearl/Peril/Pitfall : *Neonatal ARF:Clinical setting as shown by prenatal, natal and post natal events generally would tell about the reversibility of the renal failure. Pointers to underlying irreversible renal problem:Family history of congenital/hereditary renal disease, Prenatal USG showing oligohydraminos and significant renal anomalies, Maternal intake of drugs like NSAIDs, Post natal USG showing bilateral renal anomalies, Presence of known external markers and other congenital organ anomalies.Unless proved otherwise it is better to treat one as reversible renal failure when one is not sure.*

NEC may also develop shock from endotoxin production or from hypovolemia due to loss of intravascular water and protein to the interstitial and peritoneal spaces or to the intestinal lumen, or from frank hemorrhage resulting from thrombocytopenia, disseminated intravascular coagulopathy, or intestinal injury. In infants with shock, it is essential to replace lost water and solutes in the form of blood products or other solute-containing fluids. Even if properly treated, septic shock may cause renal injury, which then further complicates fluid and electrolyte management.

Pyloric Stenosis: Infants with pyloric stenosis are likely to be dehydrated and may have hypochloremic metabolic alkalosis and hypokalemia. The alkalosis may cause lethargy, hypoventilation, and, in severe cases, tetany. Parenteral fluid therapy consists of replacing the deficits of water, potassium, and chloride. The chloride should initially be given as sodium chloride. Potassium chloride should be added after adequate urination has been established. In most cases, control of vomiting, correction of dehydration, and replacement of chloride and potassium deficits will restore the blood acid-base status to normal.

Abdominal Wall Defects: Infants born with abdominal wall defects (gastroschisis or omphalocele) have increased IWL from the exposed viscera and require extra water prior to surgical repair. This is especially true of infants with gastroschisis because there is no membrane covering the extruding organs. Once the abdominal wall has been closed, evaporative water loss is no longer increased, although there may still be abnormal loss of water into the peritoneal cavity or interstitial fluid compartment.

Diarrhea: Because of their limited renal concentrating ability, Newborn infants are quicker to develop severe dehydration, hypovolemia, and cardiovascular collapse. Therefore, rapid establishment of intravenous access for vascular expansion is of the utmost importance in Newborn infants with moderate to severe dehydration from diarrhea. After stabilization, fluid and electrolyte deficits should be estimated as described in the Chapter No. 59 "Neonatal Diarrhea". Water and electrolytes should be given to correct established deficits, meet maintenance requirements, and counteract ongoing losses. Metabolic acidosis is a frequent finding in diarrheal dehydration. During initial volume reexpansion, preexisting acidosis may worsen as the body bicarbonate is further diluted with bicarbonate-free replacement fluids. Prerenal azotemia is common with diarrheal dehydration. It usually corrects spontaneously within several days as the infant is rehydrated. Oral fluids and feeding should be withheld during recovery from diarrheal dehydration. *Oral rehydration has been used successfully in older children with diarrhea, but there has been less experience with this technique in newborn infants . For this reason, oral rehydration is not recommended for newborn infants in areas where adequate personnel and supplies are available to maintain parenteral infusions. However, oral rehydration provides an important alternate therapy when intravenous therapy is not feasible for economic or technical reasons.* The appropriate period of fasting for diarrhea depends on the severity and duration of the diarrheal episode. As a rule, a more severe, protracted bout requires a longer period of fasting. How long diarrheal stools persist following the onset of fasting also helps to determine the duration of fasting. Reintroduction of oral fluids should be carried out with extreme care. Aggressive refeeding may precipitate a recurrence of diarrhea or even protracted chronic diarrhea and malabsorption with consequent growth failure.

Fluid and Electrolyte Management of Neonatal Surgical Patients: If a condition that requires surgery (e.g., pyloric stenosis) results in dehydration and electrolyte or acid-base disturbance, the infant should be restored as close as possible to normal fluid, electrolyte, and acid-base status before surgery. Otherwise, the risks of anesthesia and surgery might be increased by dehydration, acidosis, alkalosis, or abnormal serum potassium concentration. During surgery, the prescribed fluid and electrolyte therapy should be continued with the same fluid composition and rate of infusion unless additional intraoperative losses require replacement. The anesthesiologist and surgeons should be apprised of the plan for parenteral fluid therapy to avoid errors resulting from lack of communication. The operative losses of fluid and blood should be recorded and replaced either during surgery or shortly thereafter. During the initial postoperative period, some infants have reduced urine output as a result of fluid loss from the vascular compartment or increased secretion of AVP. Therefore, the fluid provided for maintenance may need to be reduced during the immediate postoperative period. However, this reduction may be offset by the extra fluid required to replace abnormal operative and postoperative losses. Fluid requirements may be twice or three times that noted above. The more extensive the procedure the greater the needs! These infants may require 125-150 ml/kg/day immediately postoperative with subsequent increases as determined by blood pressure measurements and urine output. Isotonic saline also may be required because of third spacing of fluid into tissues and other spaces, e.g., the bowel lumen. Strict I&O is mandated. Gastric drainage is replaced q8-12h, depending on volume, with isotonic saline. Colloid also may be needed because of rapid fluid shifts, decreases in arterial pressure, and increases in capillary filling time (i.e., > 3 sec.). A system of careful monitoring of fluid and electrolyte balance is essential in the surgical patient, as in other ill Newborn infants.

Recommendations

1. Initiate fluid therapy at 60-80 ml/kg/d with D10W, (80–150 ml/kg/d for infants ? 26 weeks).

2. Infants <1500 g should be covered with a saran blanket and strict I&O should be followed. For infants < 26 weeks the saran blanket should be applied directly upon the infant to minimize IWL.

3. Infants <1000 g should have electrolytes and weights recorded every 6-8 hours; every 12 hours for infants 1000-1500 grams.

4. For serum Na+ >145 mEq/L, increase infusate by ~10 mL/kg/d without Na+ in the infusate.

5. Increase fluids for urine output <0.5 mL/kg/hr by ~10 mL/kg or, in infant ? 26 weeks, calculate IWL and change fluids accordingly.

6. Infuse Na+ free fluids (including flushes) until serum Na+ <145 and good urine output is established (post diuretic phase). Then add 3-5 mEq/kg/d Na+.

7. Add KCl (2-3 mEq/kg/d) to IV fluids after urine output is well established and K+ <5 mEq/L (usually 48-72 hours).

8. Increase fluid administration gradually over the first week of life to 120-130 cc/kg/d by day 7, allowing for expected physiologic weight loss.

9. In VLBW infants, avoid the infusion of parenteral solutions containing <200 mOsmol/L (i.e., D3W), to minimize local osmotic hemolysis and thereby reduce renal K load.

10. **During** the first few days of life, appropriate fluid and electrolyte balance is reflected by a urine output of approximately 1 to 3 mL/kg per hour, a urine specific gravity of approximately 1.008 to 1.012, and an approximate weight loss of 5% in term infants and 15% in premature infants with very low birthweight. *The goal of early management is to allow initial ECF loss over the first 5 to 6 days as reflected by weight loss, while maintaining normal tonicity and intravascular volume as reflected by blood pressure, heart rate, urine output, serum electrolyte levels, and pH. Subsequent fluid management should maintain water and electrolyte balance, including requirements for body growth.*

*Pearl/Peril/Pitfall : Neonatal ARF: fluid and electrolyte balance requires precise control. To individualize fluid and electrolyte therapy, frequent monitoring is needed. Monitoring involves:*Weighing the neonate every 8 hours. *Hourly urine output measurement. *Measure abdominal girth and look for fluid excess. *Rewriting fluid advice at least every 8 hours.*

OUTLINE OF FLUID THERAPY IN THE NEWBORN

Intravenous solution	Concentration for use in maintenance fluids	Variation
Basic fluid for i.v. therapy	10% dextrose (1mmol=18mg)	Decrease to 5% if hypergly-cemia (>160mgs/dL) +/- glycosuria Increase if blood glucose <27mgs/dL
Sodium	30-50 mmol/l (1/5-1/3 normal saline)	Omit (a) in infants < 1.2kg on days 1-2 (b) if plasma Na>140mmol/l Increase to 77 mmol/l (1/2 N.saline) if i.v. being used to supplement oral feeding and Na < 125 mmol/l, or in any infant with Na < 120 mmol/l
Potassium	20mmol/l	Omit (a) on day 1 (b) if K⁺ > 5.5 mmol/l Increase to 40 mmol/l if (a) K⁻ < 3.0 mmol/l (b) if K⁺ is 3.0-4.0mmol/l but total fluid intake (i.v. + oral) < 60 ml/kg/24 hours Increase to 80 mmol/l (a) if K⁺ < 2.0 mmol/l (b) if K⁺ 2.0-2.5 mmol/l but total fluid intake (i.v. + oral) <60 ml/kg/24 hours

Intravenous solution	Concentration for use in maintenance fluids	Variation
Calcium	Nil for maintenance	Give 5ml 10% calcium gluconate/ kg/ 24 hours if Ca < 1.75 mmol Give 10 ml/kg/day if Ca < 1.5 mmol/l
Infusion rate	Infusion rate 60ml/ kg on days 1–2	Remember (a) bolus infusions (b) fluid used to sustain or clear intravenous catheter. *May* need to be inc-reased by 50–75 ml/ kg 24 hours if nursed under radiant heater and infant looks dry. Increase towards 100-150 ml/ kg by day 5, if infant is : (a) not edematous (b) passing urine satisfactorily Increase much faster if clinically shocked or if dehydrated Decrease rate (and sodium) (a) if inappropriate ADH secretion (b) + + edema

The most important principle of fluid and electrolyte management of the sick preterm and term infant is to find means to prevent or at least to decrease the likelihood of significant pulmonary and extra pulmonary edema formation. Restrict fluids and electrolytes, use blood transfusions rather than colloid or crystalloid for volume support if appropriate and provide sufficient nutrition to achieve the goal.

Weight Document daily or twice daily and aim for a weight loss of 1-2% per day for 5 days. Adjust volumes of maintenance fluid accordingly. Urine Output Monitor continuously using nappy weights, or urine collection system. Review results 8 hourly. Aim for a urine output of at least 0.5ml/kg/ hour on the first day, and 2-7ml/kg/hour thereafter. Adjust maintenance fluid, blood pressure support (Inotropes) to achieve this. Urine output below 1ml/kg/hour for > 8 hours requires renal failure management.

Na⁺ Measure daily or twice daily. Omit added Na⁺ until urine output is established. Increase input if low Na⁺ (<125mEq/lt) considered to be due to Na⁺ depletion ; otherwise restrict fluid.

Glucose Monitor glucose 6 hourly, during intensive care.

K⁺ Monitor daily or twice daily. Omit on day 1 and if renal failure developing. Calcium Monitor daily

KEY POINTS FOR CLINICAL PRACTICE:

1. Acute renal failure (ARF) is a frequent clinical condition in Neonatal intensive care units. Plasma creatinine concentrations should be used with some caution for ARF diagnosis in the first days of life. An intravenous fluid challenge allows differentiation of prerenal failure and intrinsic renal failure. Based on the site of origin of insult it can be of 3 types: a) Pre renal (75–80%) b) Intrinsic renal (10-15%) c) Post renal (5%).

2. ARF is traditionally suspected if Plasma creatinine is more than 1.5 mg/dL for at least 24 to 48 hrs if mother's renal function is normal and Serum creatinine is rising more than 0.3 mg/dL/day. Serum creatinine fails to fall below maternal plasma creatinine within 5-7 days The above definitions can be used with a reasonable degree of accuracy in term Neonates. In preterm Neonates, the physiological decline in plasma creatinine can extend over 2–3 weeks. In fact the plasma creatinine can rise transiently and then decline. The plasma creatinine remains elevated due to reabsorption of creatinine across permeable tubules.

3. All clinical conditions associated with hypovolemia, hypoxemia, and hypotension in the newborn infant may lead to renal insufficiency, the leading causes being perinatal anoxia-ischemia and sepsis.

4. The initial treatment mainly relies on correction of hypotension, acidosis, and hypoxemia, in order to reduce renal vasoconstriction and improve renal perfusion.

5. If necessary, the main renal replacement therapy is usually peritoneal dialysis even if skilled medical and nursing personnel are available in some neonatal intensive care units to perform hemofiltration and hemodiafiltration safely.

REFERENCES & FURTHER READING : 1)Gouyon J B, Guignard J P, Management of acute renal failure in newborns. PediatrNephrol 2000,14:1037-1044. 2)Philippe SF Jacquelyyn RE, Tivadar T, Seri I. In Acute and chronic renal failure, Avery's diseases of newborn, editors William Taeusch, Roberta Ballard, and Christine A. Gleason, 2005, 8 edition, Saunders. 1298-1306 3)Mathew O.P. et al. Neonatal renal failure: Usefulness of diagnostic indices. Pediatrics 65:57,1980. (Modified) 4) Andreoli SP. Acute renal failure. Curr Opin Pediatr. Apr 2002;14(2):183-8. 5) Pietrement C, Malot L, et al. Neonatal Acute Renal Failure Secondary to Maternal Exposure to Telmisartan, Angiotensin II Receptor Antagonist. J Perinatol. 2003 May;23(3):254-5. 6)Neonatal Renal Failure J. Balasubramaniam Kidney Care centre. Tirunelveli, Tamilnadu. India balas@vsnl.com.

Pearl/Peril/Pitfall : Neonatal ARF: Before embarking on dialysis ethical factors must be considered. Consider the following issues: 1. Is the renal defect reversible? 2. How long is dialysis likely to be required? 3. Other medical problems and their reversibility. 4. Parental views. Generally one need not hesitate to undertake dialysis in a neonate weighing > 1.5 kg who is likely to survive without severe neurological deficits and whose renal disease is reversible.

Neonatal Hyponatremia

73

@ *"It is vitally important to understand that low serum sodium can reflect either a low body sodium or can result from dilution, because the management of the two situations is quite different ".*

Steps in the Evaluation of Hyponatremia

♦ Calculate plasma osmolality
♦ Measure plasma osmolality
  • When low; defines true hypo-osmolal state or clinical hyponatremia
  • Consider plasma glucose, protein and lipids
♦ Evaluate volume status of patient
  • Volume depletion
  • Volume expansion
  • Euvolemia
♦ Measure urine sodium

Syndrome of Inappropriate ADH Release (Bartter's Criteria)

Hyponatremia and true hypoosmolality by definition
Euvolemia clinical
Urine less than maximally dilute (urinary osmolality usually > 200 mOsm/kg of H_2O)
Normal renal, cardiac, hepatic, adrenal, pituitary, and thyroid function
No history of antidiuretic drugs
No emotional or physical stress
Urinary sodium > 20 mEq/liter[α]

[α]Urinary sodium may be < 20 mEq/liter if the patient is volume deleted or on low sodium intake.

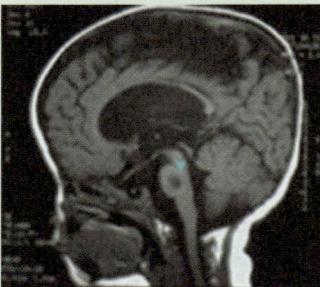

Central pontine myelinolysis may occur due to rapid correction of hyponatremia. Central pontine myelinolysis should be suspected in a Neonate with hyponatremia that in the course of correction of the hyponatremia develops cranial nerve dysfunction and quadriparesis. Magnetic resonance imaging is the study of choice . Central pontine myelinolysis. [A] MRI of the brain (T1-weighted image) demonstrating a round lesion in the central pontine area. [B] MRI of the brain (T2-weighted image) demonstrating an oval lesion in the central pontine area.

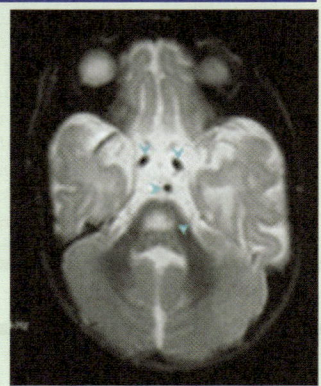

REVIEW OF CLINICAL PROBLEMS

1. What are the clinical features of Hyponatremia in Neonates?
   Ans: Refer to the Evaluation-Decision-Action Plan/ Algorithm to diagnose & manage a Neonate with Hyponatremia.
2. How do you diagnose and manage SIADH ?
   Ans: Refer to the "No. 8" of the "BIRD`S EYE VIEW/ OVERVIEW/SYNOPSIS" of the Chapter.
3. What are the causes of Hypotonic Hyponatremia due to ECF volume depletion ?.
   Ans: Refer to the "No.5" of the "BIRD`S EYE VIEW/OVER-VIEW/SYNOPSIS" of the Chapter.
4. How do you investigate Hyponatremia in the Neonatal period and manage it?
   Ans: Refer to the Evaluation-Decision-Action Plan/ Algorithm to diagnose & manage a Neonate with Hyponatremia.
5. When do you seek for Hypertonic hyponatremia (serum osmolality >295mOsm/L)?
   Ans: Refer to the "No.4" of the "BIRD`S EYE VIEW/OVER-VIEW/SYNOPSIS" of the Chapter.

LEARNING OBJECTIVES

After completing this article, readers will be able to:

1. Understand that Hyponatremia in Neonates can be due *either to water overload or to sodium depletion*.

2. Differentiate the 3 different clinical presentations of *Hypotonic hyponatremia*.

3. Diagnose SIADH presentation and its underlying conditions for managing effectively.

4. Treat the Neuroemergency secondary to *rapid & severe Hyponatremia* promptly.

5. Be careful about the preterm infants, as they can develop *late Hyponatremia*.

* *Pearl/Peril/Pitfall: Hyponatremia (less than 130 mmol/ L) is more frequently seen because of the high FENa during the diuretic phase. It may also be noted during the first day of life if the mother has received large amounts of hypotonic intravenous fluids. Hyponatremia is also seen following therapy with indomethacin without prior proper reduction of fluid intake, and later on when diuretics are used for the treatment of CLD.*

BIRD'S EYE VIEW/OVERVIEW/SYNOPSIS

1. Hyponatremia (serum sodium <130mEq/L) represents a deficit of sodium in relation to body water content and may be due to either total body sodium deficit or free water excess. When hyponatremia is caused by total body sodium deficit, free water may be decreased (hyponatremia with ECF volume contraction or dehydration), normal (hyponatremia with neither dehydration nor edema) or increased (hyponatremia with volume expansion or edema).

2. Depending on the osmolality of the serum, hyponatremia may be hypotonic, isotonic, or hypertonic. The most common manifestation of hyponatremia in the Neonate is hypotonic hyponatremia due to excessive administration or retention of free water.

3. Isotonic pseudohyponatremia (serum osmolality 285-295mOsm/L) or factitious hyponatremia occurs with hyperlipidemia and hyperproteinemia, where the total body sodium, total body water content, and sodium concentration in the aqueous phase are all within normal limits, but sodium concentration measured in the total plasma compartment is reduced. Under physiologic conditions, 93% of total plasma volume is an aqueous phase that contains the electrolytes and the remaining 7% is a solid phase composed primarily of lipids and proteins. In hyperlipidemia or hyperproteinemia, the solid phase increases at the expense of aqueous phase, and serum sodium concentration measured in the total plasma compartment decreases.

4. Hypertonic hyponatremia (serum osmolality >295mOsm/L) occurs because of the presence of an osmotically active substance in the plasma, such as glucose or mannitol. Hypertonicity, in turn causes water to shift from the intracellular space into the interstitium and the intravascular compartment, leading to a decrease in the plasma sodium concentration. With a serum glucose concentration in excess of 100mg/dL, every 100-mg/dL rise in plasma glucose results in a 1.6-mEq/L decrease in the serum sodium concentration. One should suspect this diagnosis, if hyponatremia is detected along with a serum osmolality is >295mOsm/L or if the measured serum osmolality is 20mOsm/L higher than the calculated serum osmolality.

5. Hypotonic hyponatremia due to ECF volume depletion occurs with predisposing factors such as diuretic use, osmotic diuresis (glycosuria), VLBW with renal water and Na wasting, adrenal or renal tubular salt-losing disorders, gastrointestinal losses (vomiting, diarrhea), and third-space losses of ECF (skin sloughing, early necrotizing enterocolitis [NEC]). It also occurs in cerebral salt wasting and during recovery from an acute renal insult (asphyxia, shock). Although cerebral salt wasting is uncommon in Neonates, this condition must be differentiated from SIADH. In contrast to patients with SIADH, patients with cerebral salt wasting have decreases in plasma volume as well as plasma aldosterone and vasopressin levels and a normal plasma uric acid concentration. The diagnosis of hyponatremia due to ECF volume depletion is by observing decreased weight, poor skin turgor, tachycardia, rising BUN and metabolic acidosis. If renal function is mature, the Newborn may develop decreased urine output, increased urine specific gravity, and low FE-Na. Treatment consists of replacement of both the free water and the sodium deficit + ongoing losses.

7. Hypotonic hyponatremia due to ECF volume excess occurs with predisposing factors such as sepsis with decreased cardiac output, late NEC, heart failure, abnormal lymphatic drainage, medications (muscle paralysing agents, indomethacin therapy), liver failure, acute renal failure and hypoproteinemia (congenital nephrotic syndrome). The diagnosis is based on clinical signs of edema and weight gain, decreasing urine output, increasing BUN and urine specific gravity, and a low FE-Na in infants with mature renal function. Therapy is directed towards treating the underlying disorder and restricting the water to alleviate hypotonicity. Sodium restriction and improving cardiac output may be beneficial.

8. Hypotonic hyponatremia with normal ECF volume occurs with excess fluid administration and the SIADH. Weight gain usually occurs without edema. Excessive fluid administration without SIADH results in low urine specific gravity and high urine output. In contrast, SIADH leads to decreased urine output and increased urine osmolality. *Urine sodium excretion in infants with SIADH varies widely and reflects sodium intake.* The diagnosis of SIADH presumes no volume-related stimulus to ADH release, such as reduced cardiac output or abnormal renal, adrenal, or thyroid function. Therapy includes essentially water restriction and treating the underlying cause of SIADH. In severe cases, serum sodium <120mEq/L ± seizures and altered sensorium, give Furosemide 1mg/kg IV q6hr and replace urinary sodium excretion with 3% sodium chloride 3–4 ml/kg initial dose depending on the severity, until the serum sodium reaches 120mEq/L. Then complete correction of hyponatremia should be performed more slowly over 24–48hrs to prevent pontine and extrapontine myelinolysis.

9. *The Evaluation-Decision-Action-Plan/Algorithm* describes the essential aspects of the diagnosis & management of Neonatal hyponatremia. Hyponatremia is relatively rare in the first 48–72hrs of life.

10. It is vitally important to understand that low serum sodium can reflect either a low body sodium or can result from dilution, because the management of the two situations is quite different as discussed above.

---

* *Pearl/Peril/Pitfall: Hyponatremia with weight loss suggests sodium depletion and would merit sodium replacement. When associated with weight gain Hyponatremia points toward water excess and requires fluid restriction.*

* *Pearl/Peril/Pitfall : The normal maintenance fluid required on the 1st day ranges from 2.5-3.5ml/kg/hr in Newborns. This volume would increase to 5-6ml/kg/hr by the end of the first week and 7-8ml/kg/hr thereafter.*

THE EVALUATION-DECISION-ACTION-PLAN/ALGORITHM FOR THE DIAGNOSIS AND MANAGEMENT OF *NEONATAL HYPONATREMIA*

SUBJECTIVE FINDINGS

Hx of predisposing factors for hyponatremia due to hypovolemia diarrhea and vomiting, third-space losses (NEC, skin sloughing), diuretic use, osmotic diuresis (hyperglycemia), VLBW with renal water & sodium wasting, adrenal/renal tubular salt-losing disorders.

Hx of predisposing factors for hyponatremia due to hypervolemia sepsis with decreased cardiac output, late NEC, CCF, neuromuscular paralysis, indomethacin therapy, hypo-proteinemia, liver failure and acute renal failure.

Hx of predisposing factors for hyponatremia due to Isovolemia SIADH, asphyxia, meningitis, pneumothorax, positive-pressure ventilation, IVH, pain, opiate administration and excess fluid administration.

OBJECTIVE FINDINGS

Assess Airway, Breathing, Circulation and Disability by observing the vitals, BP, O_2 sats, color, CRT, pulses, urine output, sensorium, focal neurologic deficits, seizures, abnormal movements, tone and reflexes, etc.

Assess body weight (increased/decreased), skin turgor, edema or dehydration, oliguria/anuria/polyuria, hypotension/hypertension.

Perform complete physical examination to identify systemic causes of hyponatremia such as CCF, renal failure, SIADH, adrenal insufficiency, NEC, liver disease.

INVESTIGATIONS

Blood FBC with TC,DC, Platelets, ABG electrolytes, BUN, creatinine, osmolality, glucose, LFTs.

Urine Specific gravity, creatinine, urea, electrolytes, osmolality, accurate intake and output, daily twice weights.

Serum osmolality-normal range 280–295mOsm/L

$$= 2 \times Na^+ + \frac{glucose\ (mg/dL)}{18} + \frac{blood\ urea/6\ or}{BUN/2.818}$$

Imaging studies may be indicated depending on the underlying etiology of the hyponatremia (e.g. *chest radiograph* in a patient with congestive heart failure). Usually, a *head CT scan* is indicated in the patient with altered mental status to ensure that no other underlying cause for the mental status is present.

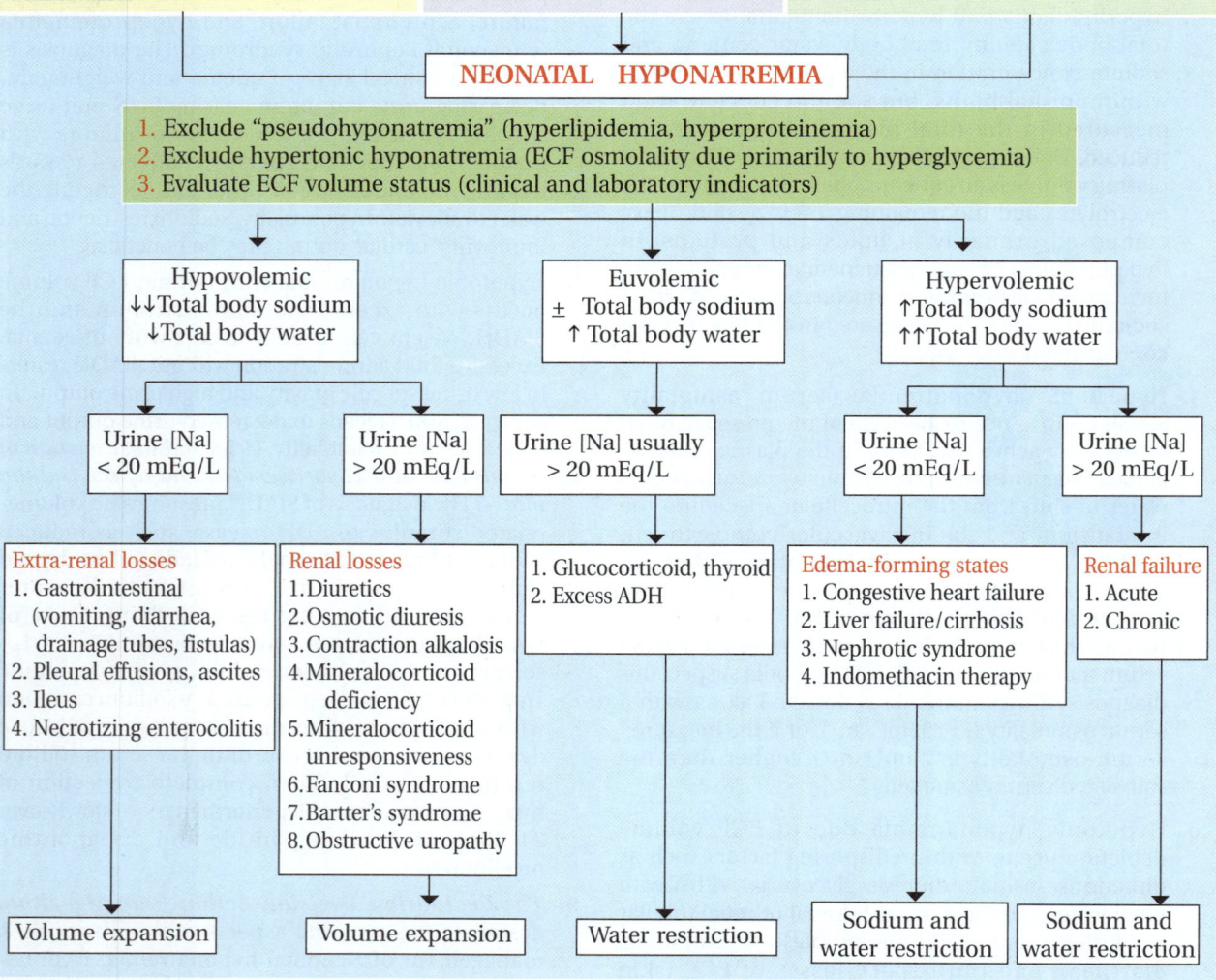

NEONATAL HYPONATREMIA

1. Exclude "pseudohyponatremia" (hyperlipidemia, hyperproteinemia)
2. Exclude hypertonic hyponatremia (ECF osmolality due primarily to hyperglycemia)
3. Evaluate ECF volume status (clinical and laboratory indicators)

Hypovolemic
↓↓Total body sodium
↓Total body water

Euvolemic
± Total body sodium
↑ Total body water

Hypervolemic
↑Total body sodium
↑↑Total body water

Urine [Na] < 20 mEq/L

Urine [Na] > 20 mEq/L

Urine [Na] usually > 20 mEq/L

Urine [Na] < 20 mEq/L

Urine [Na] > 20 mEq/L

Extra-renal losses
1. Gastrointestinal (vomiting, diarrhea, drainage tubes, fistulas)
2. Pleural effusions, ascites
3. Ileus
4. Necrotizing enterocolitis

Renal losses
1. Diuretics
2. Osmotic diuresis
3. Contraction alkalosis
4. Mineralocorticoid deficiency
5. Mineralocorticoid unresponsiveness
6. Fanconi syndrome
7. Bartter's syndrome
8. Obstructive uropathy

1. Glucocorticoid, thyroid
2. Excess ADH

Edema-forming states
1. Congestive heart failure
2. Liver failure/cirrhosis
3. Nephrotic syndrome
4. Indomethacin therapy

Renal failure
1. Acute
2. Chronic

Volume expansion

Volume expansion

Water restriction

Sodium and water restriction

Sodium and water restriction

---

* **Pearl/Peril/Pitfall :** *Renal Impairment* *Restrict intake to insensible water loss + urine output. *Monitor fluid balance, serum electrolytes and weight carefully. *In early Acute Tubular Necrosis, consider a pre-renal cause. *Fractional excretion of sodium may help sort this out. ·FE Na⁺ >2.5% in term infants suggests renal failure. ·FE Na⁺<2.5% in term infants suggests pre-renal failure. ·FE Na⁺ is high in preterm infants because of tubular immaturity.
*FE Na⁺ =Urine [Na] x Serum Creatinine /Serum [Na⁺] x Urine Creatinine

* **Pearl/Peril/Pitfall:** *Hyponatremia is defined as a serum sodium level less than 130 mEq/L. Usually, this is not a cause for concern until the serum sodium has dropped to less than 125 mEq/L. Remember that hyponatremia usually results from excessive free water intake relative to insensible and sensible water loss. However, especially in the extremely premature infant or infants with increased sodium losses, inadequate sodium intake can contribute to the development of hyponatremia. Gastrointestinal Losses-If there are significant gastric aspirates, replace these ml for ml with 0.9% NaCl plus 10mmolKCl per 500ml.Restricting sodium intake in preterm infants in the first few days may also reduce the incidence of chronic lung disease.*

Causes of hyponatremia in Neonates

Primary water excess

- Excess intake
    - To mother: large intrapartum infusion of sodium free fluid
    - To baby: excessive intravenous intake

- Impaired excretion
    - Intrinsic renal failure
    - Indomethacin
    - Appropriate or inappropriate ADH secretion
    - Adrenocortical failure

Mixed

- Water excess and sodium depletion
    - Sodium and water depletion treated with continued infusion of sodium-free fluid
    - Chronic lung disease treated with long-term diuretic therapy

- Water excess disproportionate to whole body sodium excess
    - Congestive cardiac failure
    - Liver failure
    - Nephrotic syndrome

Primary sodium depletion

- Insufficient intake
    - Maternal laxative or diuretic abuse
    - Use of non-sodium-supplemented donor breast milk for preterm babies

- Excessive loss
    - Renal
    - Diuretics including xanthines
    - Tubular dysfunction
    - Pyelonephritis
    - Nephrotoxic agents
    - Obstructive uropathies

- Endocrine
    - Salt-losing forms of congenital adrenal hyperplasia
    - Hypoaldosteronism

- Gastrointestinal
    - External
    - Vomiting
    - Ileostomy/colostomy loss

- Sequestered
    - Ileus
    - Obstruction
    - Necrotizing enterocolitis

- Central nervous system
    - Following repeated drainage of CSF in posthemorrhagic hydrocephalus
    - Cerebral salt wasting

KEY POINTS FOR CLINICAL PRACTICE:

1. **Hyponatremia** (Serum Sodium< 130 mEq/L) in Neonates is mainly due to water overload during the 1st week of life but thereafter Sodium depletion becomes more important. It is critical that a definitive diagnosis is made as the appropriate treatment may be either fluid restriction or Sodium supplementation.

2. In *Premature infants,* a high incidence of "late" hyponatremia is well recognized and, in contrast to the first postnatal week, this is due to total body Sodium depletion and there is poor weight gain or even weight loss. Term infants require as little as 1mEq/kg/24 h of Sodium, after the 1st week of life whereas immature infants may require 8–12 mEq/kg/24h if "late" hyponatremia is to be avoided.

3. An *acute fall in Serum Sodium* usually reflects impaired water excretion/retention but may occur following a single dose of furosemide or with sudden GIT losses, as in NEC.

4. The Serum Sodium concentration at birth reflects *the maternal value;* often, a low serum Sodium at birth suggests that the mother has received a large volume of salt-poor IV fluid during labor, resulting in an excess of water to the baby. Newborn hyponatremia has also been described following *maternal diuretic and laxative abuse.*

5. In severe cases, with serum sodium <120mEq/L $\pm$ seizures and altered sensorium, give *Furosemide 1mg/ kg IV q6hr* and replace urinary Sodium excretion with *3% Sodium chloride 3–4 ml/kg initial dose* depending on the severity, until the Serum Sodium reaches 120mEq/L. Then complete correction of hyponatremia should be performed more slowly over 24-48hrs to prevent pontine and extrapontine myelinolysis.

REFERENCES & FURTHER READING : 1) *Avner ED: Clinical disorders of water metabolism: Hyponatremia and hypernatremia. Pediatr Ann 24:23-30, 1995.* 2) Nelson Text Book of Pediatrics, 18th edition 3) Manual of Neonatal Care, John P. Cloherty, 6th edition. 4) Avery's diseases of the Newborn, 8th edition 5) Roberton`s Text Book of Neonatology,4th Edition.

* *Pearl/Peril/Pitfall:* Preterm neonates have more water (at 23 weeks' gestation, 90% water composed of 60% ECF and 30% ICF), and they may lose 10-15% of their weight in the first week of life. Small for gestational age (SGA) preterm infants may have a higher proportional body water content (90% for SGA infants vs 84% for appropriate for gestational age [AGA] infants at 25-30 weeks' gestation).

74

Neonatal Hypernatremia

@ *"Hypernatremia does not indicate total body sodium content, which can be high, low, normal depending on the cause of hypernatremia and total body water content. Patients with hypernatremia can have Hypovolemia or Euvolemia or Hypervolemia."*

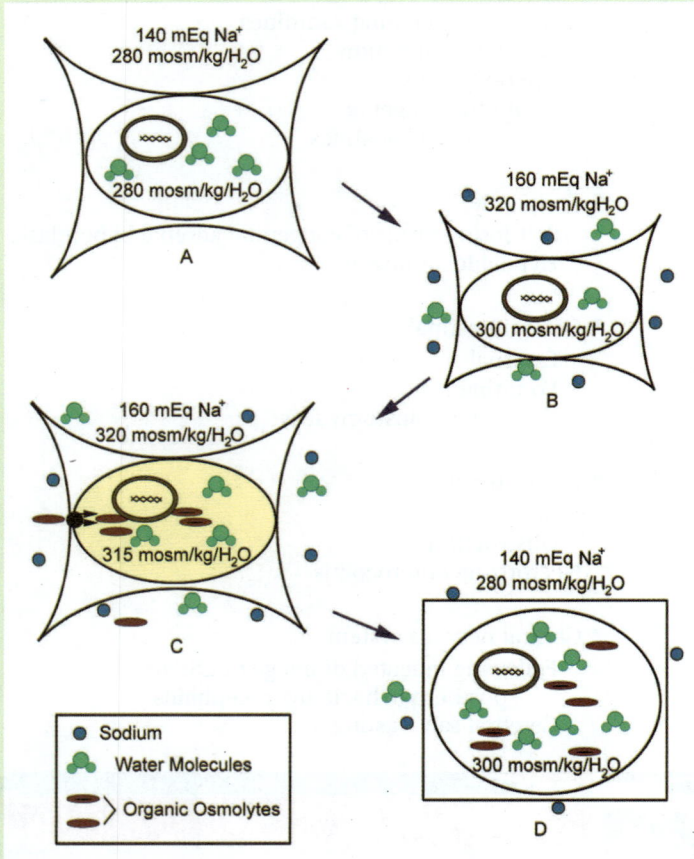

Sodium
Water Molecules
Organic Osmolytes

Figure A: Normal cell.

Figure B: Cell initially responds to extracellular hypertonicity through passive osmosis of water extracellularly, resulting in cell shrinkage.

Figure C: Cell actively responds to extracellular hypertonicity and cell shrinkage in order to limit water loss through transport of organic osmolytes across the cell membrane, as well as through intracellular production of these osmolytes.

Figure D: Rapid correction of extracellular hypertonicity results in passive movement of water molecules into the relatively hypertonic intracellular space, causing cellular swelling, damage, and ultimately death.

REVIEW OF CLINICAL PROBLEMS

1. What are the 3 different types of Hypernatremia in Neonates?
   Ans: Refer to the "No. 1" of the "BIRD`S EYE VIEW/ OVERVIEW/SYNOPSIS" of the Chapter.

2. Why do Neonates & infants are worst affected with Hypernatremic dehydration ?
   Ans: Refer to the "No. 3" of the "BIRD`S EYE VIEW/ OVERVIEW/SYNOPSIS" of the Chapter.

3. How do you correct Hypernatremia to prevent CNS injury?
   Ans: Refer to the "No.6" of the "BIRD`S EYE VIEW/ OVERVIEW/SYNOPSIS" of the Chapter.

4. What are the major goals of therapy in the treatment of severe and chronic hypernatremic dehydration ?
   Ans: Refer to the Evaluation-Decision-Action Plan/ Algorithm to diagnose & manage a Neonate with Hypernatremia.

5. How do you monitor the treatment of Hypernatremia?
   Ans: Refer to the Table 4 of the of the Chapter.

LEARNING OBJECTIVES

After completing this article, readers will be able to

1. Understand that Hypernatremia in Neonates can be due *either to water depletion or to sodium overload.*

2. Differentiate the 3 different types of Hypernatremia in Neonates.

3. Manage Hypernatremia in Neonates and its underlying conditions effectively.

4. Treat the Neuroemergency secondary to *rapid and severe hypernatremia* promptly.

5. Be careful about the complications during therapy of Hypernatremia in Neonates.

---

* Pearl/Peril/Pitfall: *Hypernatremia is defined as a serum sodium level greater than 150 mEq/L. Usually, this is not a cause for concern until the serum sodium level has risen to greater than 150-155 mEq/L. Hypernatremia is commonly seen in the first few days of life in ELBW preterm infants and is most often the result of inadequate free water intake to compensate for very high IWLs.*

BIRD'S EYE VIEW/OVERVIEW/SYNOPSIS

1. *Hypernatremia (serum sodium >150mEq/L)* reflects a deficiency of water relative to total body sodium content and **usually/most often** a disorder of water balance rather than that of sodium balance. Hypernatremia does not indicate total body sodium content, which can be high, low, normal depending on the cause of hypernatremia and total body water content. Patients with hypernatremia can have Hypovolemia or Euvolemia or Hypervolemia. *Hypovolemic hypernatremia* occurs in Neonates with diarrhea, VLBW infants with excessive sweating and radiant warmers, inadequate breast feeding, maternal breast milk with high sodium content, hyperventilation, osmotic diuresis due to diabetes mellitus, mannitol or glycerol and renal dysplasia. *Euvolemic hypernatremia* occurs with diabetes insipidus with intact thirst mechanism and with medications such as amphotericin, phenytoin and aminoglycosides. *Hypervolemic hypernatremia* occurs with improperly mixed formula/ORS, iatrogenic IV $NaHCO_3$ administration to correct the acidosis without correcting the underlying cause, IV hypertonic saline and rarely primary hyperaldosteronism. (Refer to Table 1 of the Chapter).

2. Neonates with hypernatremic dehydration tend to have better preservation of intravascular volume because of the shift of water from the intracellular space to the extracellular space, resulting in intracellular dehydration. *This maintains BP and urine output, and allows hypernatremic infants to be less symptomatic initially and potentially become more dehydrated (>10% loss in body weight) late in the course of the condition.* Neonates are irritable, restless, weak, and lethargic; some infants have a high-pitched cry and hyperpnea. Periods of lethargy may be interspersed with periods of irritability. Hypernatremia, even without dehydration, causes CNS symptoms that tend to parallel the degree of sodium elevation and the acuity of the increase. CNS cellular dehydration results in decrease in brain volume resulting in tearing of intracerebral veins and bridging blood vessels as the brain moves away from the skull and the meninges. Patients can have subarachnoid, subdural, and parenchymal hemorrhages. Seizures and coma are possible sequelae of the hemorrhage, even though seizures are more common during treatment. Fever can both be a contributing cause and a result of hypernatremic dehydration.

3. Hypernatremia is associated with *Hyperglycemia and mild Hypocalcemia; the mechanisms are unknown.* Thrombotic complications occur in severe Hypernatremic dehydration and include stroke, dural sinus thrombosis, peripheral thrombosis and renal vein thrombosis possibly due to Hypercoagulability associated with Hypernatremia. Mortality in an acute case with Na+ >160mEq/L is 50% and the worst outcome is in babies < 6 months. *Infants are worst affected with hypernatremic dehydration because of a) immaturity of the kidney to excrete an excess Na+ load b) limited ability to express thirst and c) reliance on others to provide appropriate fluids.*

4. In the critically ill infant, the etiology of hypernatremia may be multifactorial, and the treatment is less straight forward. However thorough analysis of the medical history and the changes in clinical signs, laboratory findings, and body weight usually aid in determining the major etiologic factor and thus the treatment of the more complex cases of serum sodium abnormalities.

5. With combined sodium and water deficits, analysis of the urine differentiates renal and nonrenal etiologies. When the losses are extrarenal, the kidney responds to volume depletion with low urine volume, a concentrated urine, and sodium retention (urine sodium less than 20 mEq/L). With renal causes, the urine volume is not appropriately low, the urine is not maximally concentrated, and the urine sodium may be inappropriately elevated (>20mEq/L).

6. *The Evaluation-Decision-Action-Plan/Algorithm* describes the essential aspects of the diagnosis & management of hypernatremia in the Neonates. *Table 2* outlines the plan of treatment of hypernatremic dehydration. *Hypernatremia should not be corrected rapidly, because of that dangers of overly rapid correction, such as cerebral edema and seizures. The goal is to decrease the serum sodium by 12mEq/L/day, @ 0.5mEq/L/hour in chronic severe hyponatremia, whereas in acute hypernatremia reducing the serum concentration by 1mEq/L/hr (24mEq/L/day) is appropriate.*

7. The most important component of correcting moderate or severe hypernatremia is frequent monitoring of the serum sodium so that fluid therapy can be adjusted to provide adequate correction, neither too slow nor too fast as mentioned above. The first priority is to restore intravascular volume with normal saline. Administer IVI of 3% sodium chloride 4ml/kg to treat seizures because of an overly rapid decrease of the serum sodium during correction of hypernatremic dehydration to reverse cerebral edema. Do not allow hypotonic oral feeds, which may contribute to a rapid decrease in serum sodium. *Always address the underlying cause of hypernatremia.*

8. When hypernatremia is due to sodium intoxication and the hypernatremia severe (> 180mEq/L), it may not be possible to administer enough water to rapidly correct the hypernatremia without worsening volume overload. In this situation Peritoneal Dialysis allows for safe and gradual removal of the excess sodium. In less severe cases the addition of a loop diuretic (frusemide 2mg/kg/dose q6hrs) increases removal of excess sodium and water, decreasing the risk of volume overload. With sodium overload, hypernatremia is corrected with sodium - free IV fluid (5% dextrose in water).

9. Hyperglycemia from hypernatremia is not usually treated with insulin because the acute decrease in glucose, by lowering plasma osmolality, may precipitate cerebral edema (reduce IV fluid glucose concentration from D5 to D2.5). Treat secondary hypocalcemia as needed. Potassium concentration of the IV fluids is dictated by the serum potassium concentration and the level of renal function.

10. Although MRI brain imaging before discharge provides information on potential insults associated with the hypernatremia and its treatment, *long-term neuro-developmental follow-up* should be arranged for every neonate who had experienced severe hypernatremic dehydration.

---

* *Pearl/Peril/Pitfall : Very rarely, hypernatremia is the result of excessive administration of sodium in either the diet or IVFs. A common cause of excessive administration of sodium is associated with the administration of sodium bicarbonate to infants with pulmonary hypertension or metabolic acidosis in an effort to increase blood pH levels.*

THE EVALUATION-DECISION-ACTION-PLAN/ALGORITHM FOR THE DIAGNOSIS AND MANAGEMENT OF *NEONATAL HYPERNATREMIA*

SUBJECTIVE FINDINGS

Hx of Diarrhea, VLBW infants with increased renal & insensible water loss, radiant warmer, osmotic diuresis, Improper formula mixing, Hypertonic rehydration solutions, Hx of polyuria & Polydipsia (DI & DM), Burns and heat stroke, Breast milk high sodium, inadequate breast milk intake, medications with renal insult—Amphotericin, aminoglycosides, phenytoin.

OBJECTIVE FINDINGS

Assess airway, breathing, circulation & disability by observing the vitals, BP, O_2 sats, color, CRT, pulses, urine output, sensorium, focal neurologic deficits, seizures, abnormal movements, tone & reflexes, etc.

Look for weight loss or weight gain, dry and parched mucous membranes, Sunken fontanel, Doughy skin, Tachycardia, Hypotension etc.

Determine whether the Neonate is hypovolemic/hypervolemic/Euvolemic.

INVESTIGATIONS

Blood FBC, TC, DC, Platelets, blood glucose, Serum sodium, potassium, calcium, bicarbonate, ABG analysis, serum osmolality, BUN, creatinine.

Urine Analysis, SpGr, C/S, osmolality, urine electrolytes

Intake and output chart

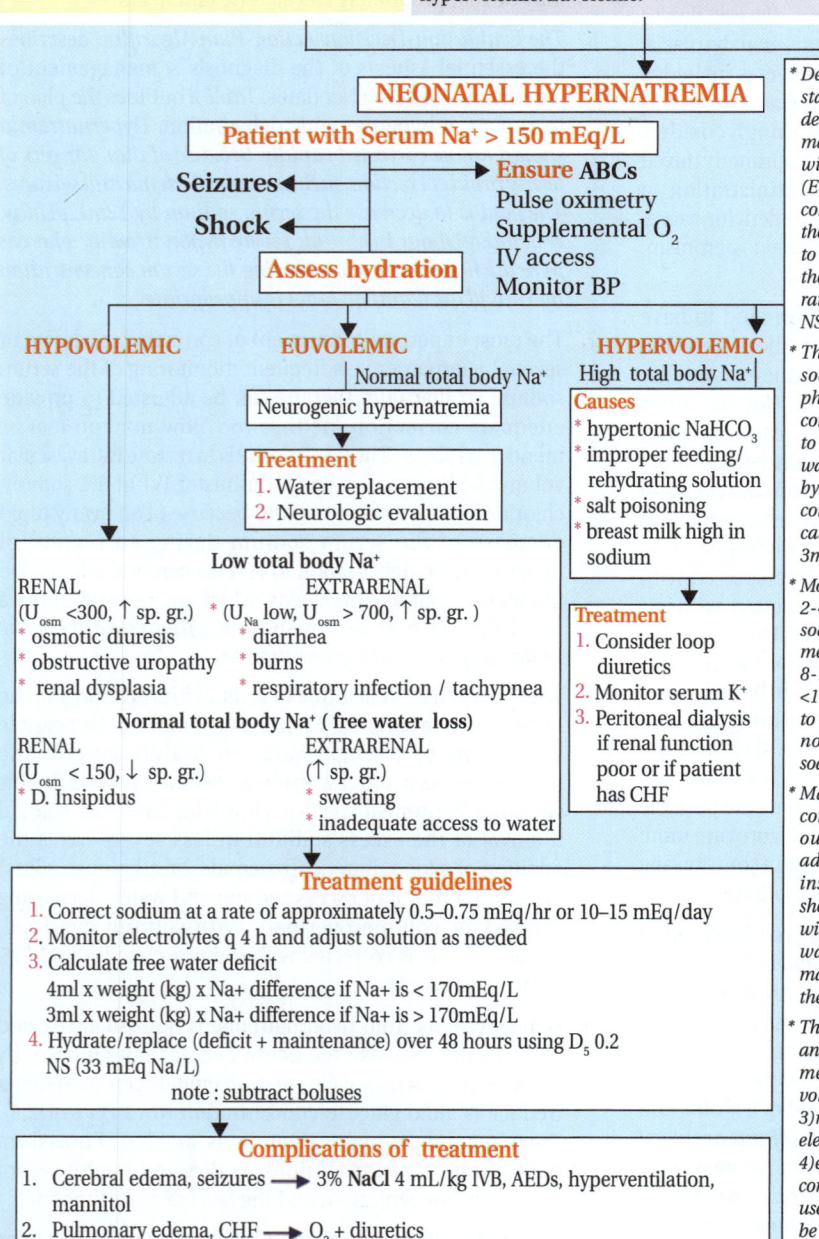

NEONATAL HYPERNATREMIA

Patient with Serum Na⁺ > 150 mEq/L

Seizures ◄

Shock ◄

► **Ensure ABCs**
Pulse oximetry
Supplemental O_2
IV access
Monitor BP

Assess hydration

HYPOVOLEMIC

EUVOLEMIC
Normal total body Na⁺
Neurogenic hypernatremia

Treatment
1. Water replacement
2. Neurologic evaluation

HYPERVOLEMIC
High total body Na⁺

Causes
* hypertonic $NaHCO_3$
* improper feeding/rehydrating solution
* salt poisoning
* breast milk high in sodium

Treatment
1. Consider loop diuretics
2. Monitor serum K⁺
3. Peritoneal dialysis if renal function poor or if patient has CHF

Low total body Na⁺

RENAL
(U_{osm} <300, ↑ sp. gr.)
* osmotic diuresis
* obstructive uropathy
* renal dysplasia

EXTRARENAL
* (U_{Na} low, U_{osm} > 700, ↑ sp. gr.)
* diarrhea
* burns
* respiratory infection / tachypnea

Normal total body Na⁺ (free water loss)

RENAL
(U_{osm} < 150, ↓ sp. gr.)
* D. Insipidus

EXTRARENAL
(↑ sp. gr.)
* sweating
* inadequate access to water

Treatment guidelines
1. Correct sodium at a rate of approximately 0.5–0.75 mEq/hr or 10–15 mEq/day
2. Monitor electrolytes q 4 h and adjust solution as needed
3. Calculate free water deficit
   4ml x weight (kg) x Na+ difference if Na+ is < 170mEq/L
   3ml x weight (kg) x Na+ difference if Na+ is > 170mEq/L
4. Hydrate/replace (deficit + maintenance) over 48 hours using D_5 0.2 NS (33 mEq Na/L)

note : subtract boluses

Complications of treatment
1. Cerebral edema, seizures ⟶ 3% **NaCl** 4 mL/kg IVB, AEDs, hyperventilation, mannitol
2. Pulmonary edema, CHF ⟶ O_2 + diuretics
3. Hypocalcemia ⟶ add **calcium gluconate** 10% 10 mL to 500 mL of IV fluids
4. Renal tubular injury and azotemia ⟶ PERITONEAL DIALYSIS

* *Dextrose 5% with 1/4 normal saline is an appropriate starting IV solution for a neonate with hypernatremic dehydration, whereas dextrose 5% with 1/2 normal saline may be a better choice in a 3 yr old. For difficult patients with severe hypernatremia, having two IV solutions (E.g.: D5 1/4 NS and D5 1/2 NS, both with the same concentration of potassium) at the bed side can facilitate the adjustment in the sodium concentration of the IV fluids to modify the rate of decrease in serum concentration. If the serum sodium concentration decreases too rapidly, the rate of D5 1/2 NS can be increased and the rate of D5 1/4 NS can be decreased.*

* *The amount of free water required to decrease serum sodium concentration by 1mEq/L is 4ml/kg under physiologic circumstances. However when the sodium concentration is >170 mEq, ≤ 3ml/kg of free water is needed to achieve the same effect. Therefore the amount of free water required to decrease serum sodium concentration by 12mEq/L (ideal rate of decrease in serum sodium concentration within 24hrs to prevent cerebral edema) is calculated as : free water required = current weight(kg) x 3ml/kg x 12mEq/L = 36ml/kg/day x current weight(kg)*

* *Monitor serum electrolytes, BUN, serum creatinine every 2-4hrs until an appropriate rate of decline in serum sodium concentration has been established. Then lab measurements can be relaxed to every 4-6hrs (and later to 8-12hrs), until the serum sodium concentration is <145mEq/L. This approach provides a reasonable chance to gradually decrease serum sodium concentration to the normal range over 5-7days depending on the initial sodium values.*

* *Maintenance fluid calculations must take into consideration the usually significantly decreased urine output. Therefore, free water maintenance fluid administration should be based only on calculated insensible losses (30-40ml/kg/day), and urine output should initially be replaced volume for volume every 4-6hrs with a solution tailored to the urinary sodium and free water losses. To calculate the replacement and maintenance free water requirements, one must also know the free water content of the intravenous fluids used.*

* *The major goals of fluid therapy in the treatment of severe and chronic hypernatremic dehydration are 1) establishment and maintenance of appropriate intravascular volume, 2)replacement of water and electrolyte deficits, 3)replacement of ongoing urine and stool water and electrolyte losses as well as insensible water losses, and 4)establishment of a rate of decline in serum sodium concentration that does not exceed 12mEq/L/day. Boluses used for stabilization of the intravascular volume should be given through the use of intravenous fluids with a sodium concentration either equal to the serum sodium concentration or at most 10mEq/L less than that concentration.*

Pearl/Peril/Pitfall : *When hypernatremia (of any etiology) occurs, cells become dehydrated. Either the osmotic load of the increased sodium acts to extract water from the cells or a portion of the burden of the body's free water deficit is borne by the cell. (Sodium, primarily an extracellular ion, is actively pumped out of most cells and is the primary determinant of serum osmolarity.) Dehydrated cells shrink from water extraction. The effects of cellular dehydration are seen principally in the CNS, where stretching of shrunken neurons and alteration of membrane potentials from electrolyte flux lead to ineffective functioning. If shrinkage is severe enough, stretching and rupture of bridging veins may cause intracranial hemorrhage.*

TABLE 1 — Conditions causing neonatal hypernatremia

Hypovolemic hypernatremia:

Inadequate breast milk intake	Excessive sweating
Diarrhea	Renal dysplasia
Radiant warmers	Osmotic diuresis

Euvolemic hypernatremia: *(most cases of diabetes insipidus present with hypovolemia, as the Neonates and young infants do not usually have control over their fluid intake)*

Decreased production of antidiuretic hormone:

Central diabetes insipidus, head trauma, central nervous system tumors (craniopharyngioma), meningitis, or encephalitis

Decrease or absence of renal responsiveness:

Nephrogenic diabetes insipidus, extreme immaturity, renal insult and medications such as amphotericin, phenytoin, aminoglycosides

Hypervolemic hypernatremia:

- Improperly mixed formula
- $NaHCO_3$ administration
- NaCl administration
- Primary hyperaldosteronism

TABLE 2 — Typical patterns of physical signs in moderate - severe dehydration

Sign	Isonatremic	Hyponatremic	Hypernatremic
Skin			
Color	Gray	Gray	Gray
Temperature	Cold	Cold	Cold
Turgor	Poor	Very poor	Fair
Feel	Dry	Clammy	Thick, doughy
Mucous membrane	Dry	Dry	Parched
Eyeball	Sunken and soft	Sunken and soft	Sunken
Fontanel	Sunken	Sunken	Sunken
State of consciousness	Lethargic	Very lethargic	Hyperirritable
Pulse	Rapid	Rapid	Moderately rapid
Blood pressure	Low	Very low	Moderately

TABLE 3 — Treatment of hypernatremic dehydration

Restore intravascular volume

Normal saline : 20 mL/kg over 20 min (Repeat until intravascular volume restored)

Determine the time for correction based on the initial sodium concentration

[Na]: 145-157 mEq/L : 24 hr, [Na]: 158–170 mEq/L : 48 hr, [Na]: 171-183 mEq/L : 72 hr, [Na]: 184-196 mEq/L : 84 hr

Administer fluid at a constant rate over the time for correction

Typical fluids : D5 1/4 NS or D5 1/2 NS (both with 20 mEq/L KCl unless contraindicated)

Typical rate : 1.25-1.5 times maintenance

Follow serum sodium concentration

Adjust fluid based on clinical status and serum sodium concentration

Signs of volume depletion : administer NS (20mL/kg)

Sodium decreases too rapidly

Increase sodium concentration of intravenous fluid, or

Decrease rate of intravenous fluid

Sodium decreases too slowly

Decrease sodium concentration of intravenous fluid, or

Increase rate of intravenous fluid

Replace ongoing losses as they occur.

TABLE 4 — Monitoring therapy

Monitoring therapy: Fluid and electrolyte replacement is based on estimations of deficits and ongoing maintenance requirements. Assess the child and monitor biochemistry frequently.

Monitor : 1. pulse and BP, 2. serum - Na^+, K^+, Urea, creatinine and osmolality (Ca^{2+}, and glucose if required), 3. urine - Na^+, K^+, urea and osmolality, 4. total input and output of fluids (and electrolytes if necessary) preferably by flow sheet, 5. accurate monitoring of weight change with therapy can be very helpful.

Indicators of decreased vascular volume (and ECF) may include:

1. tachycardia, decreased BP, decreased CVP, increased respiratory rate 2. decreased peripheral perfusion 3. metabolic acidosis 4. increased hematocrit, increased serum osmolality 5. increased blood urea and creatinine 6. decreased urine output, increased urine osmolality.

These variables are seen to revert towards normal with appropriate rehydration and management.

KEY POINTS FOR CLINICAL PRACTICE

1. *Hypernatremia (serum sodium >150mEq/L) reflects a deficiency of water relative to total body Sodium content and usually/most often a disorder of water balance rather than that of Sodium balance. Hypervolemic hypernatremia occurs with improperly mixed formula/ORS, iatrogenic IV $NaHCO_3$ administration to correct the acidosis without correcting the underlying cause, IV hypertonic saline and rarely primary hyperaldosteronism.*

2. Neonates with hypernatremic dehydration tend to have better preservation of intravascular volume because of the shift of water from the intracellular space to the extracellular space, resulting in intracellular dehydration. *This maintains BP and urine output, and allows hypernatremic infants to be less symptomatic initially and potentially become more dehydrated (>10% loss in body weight) late in the course of the condition.*

3. *Hypernatremia should not be corrected rapidly, because of that dangers of overenthusiastic correction, such as cerebral edema and seizures. The goal is to decrease the Serum Sodium by 12mEq/L/day, @ 0.5mEq/L/hour in chronic severe hyponatremia, whereas in acute hypernatremia reducing the serum concentration by 1mEq/L/hr (24mEq/L/day) is appropriate.*

4. *Always address the underlying cause of hypernatremia.*

5. *Long-term neurodevelopmental follow-up should be arranged for every Neonate who had experienced severe hypernatremic dehydration.*

REFERENCES & FURTHER READING : 1) Avner ED: Clinical disorders of water metabolism: Hyponatremia and hypernatremia. Pediatr Ann 24:23-30, 1995. 2) Nelson Text Book of Pediatrics, 18th edition 3) Manual of Neonatal Care, John P. Cloherty, 6th edition. 4) Avery's diseases of the Newborn, 8th edition 5) Roberton`s Text Book of Neonatology ,4th Edition

* *Pearl/Peril/Pitfall : Hypernatremia with weight loss suggests dehydration and would require fluid correction over 48 hours. Hypernatremia with weight gain suggests salt and water overload and is an indication for sodium and fluid restriction.*

75

Neonatal Hypokalemia

@ *The causes for hypokalemia can be grouped into four main categories: Spurious hypokalemia, redistribution hypokalemia, extrarenal potassium loss, and renal potassium loss.*

HYPOKALEMIA

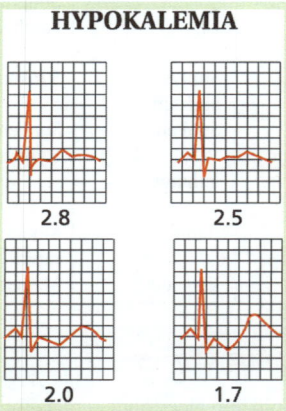

2.8   2.5

2.0   1.7

ECG changes in hypokalemia: Prominent U waves after T waves in hypokalemia. (Increased prominence of U waves (small positive deflection after T wave, best seen in V2 and V3) and Flattening or inversion of T waves Depression of ST segment Ventricular ectopia.

HYPERKALEMIA

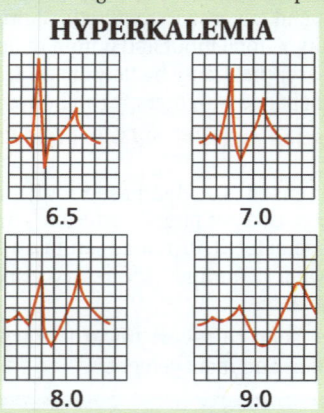

6.5   7.0

8.0   9.0

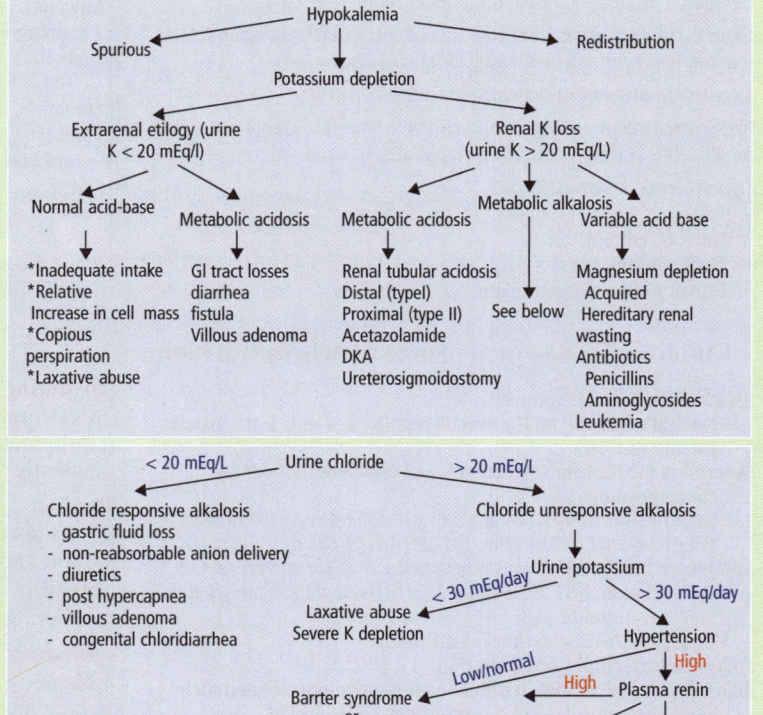

REVIEW OF CLINICAL PROBLEMS

1. Mention the renal causes of Neonatal Hypokalemia.
   Ans: Refer to the Table 1 of the Chapter.

2. What are the essential clinical manifestations of Neonatal Hypokalemia? *Ans: Refer to No 7 of the Bird's eye view/Overview/Synopsis of the Chapter.*

3. How do you evaluate Neonatal Hypokalemia?
   Ans: Refer to the Evaluation-Decision-Action Plan/Algorithm to diagnose and manage Neonatal Hypokalemia.

4. How do you manage life-threatening Neonatal Hypokalemia? *Ans: Refer to the Evaluation-Decision-Action Plan/Algorithm to diagnose and manage Neonatal Hypokalemia.*

5. How do you prevent the commonest cause of Neonatal Hypokalemia?
   Ans: Refer to No 9 of the Bird's eye view/Overview/Synopsis of the Chapter.

LEARNING OBJECTIVES

After completing this article, readers will be able to:

1. Identify the common causes of Neonatal Hypokalemia.

2. Diagnose the acute and gradual presenting symptoms of Neonatal Hypokalemia.

3. Differentiate the underlying causes of acid-base disorder often co-existing with Hypokalemia.

4. Treat Neonatal Hypokalemia depending on the severity and underlying disorder.

5. Prevent/reduce Neonatal Hypokalemia by using potassium-sparing diuretics and by adequate dietary potassium supplements.

* *Pearl/Peril/Pitfall: Hypokalemia is defined as a serum potassium level of less than 3.5 mEq/L. Unless the patient is receiving digoxin therapy, hypokalemia is rarely cause for concern until the serum potassium level is less than 3.0 mEq/L. Hypokalemia often results from chronic diuretic use and unreplaced electrolyte loss from NG drainage.*

BIRD'S EYE VIEW/OVERVIEW/SYNOPSIS

1. *Neonatal hypokalemia* (Serum Potassium <3.5 mEq/L) is a common problem in the NICU; and is due to causes secondary to 4 basic mechanisms (a) Spurious (b) Transcellular shifts (c) Decreased intake d) Losses which can be due to Extrarenal or Renal. *Refer to the Table 1 of the Chapter for a practical classification of Neonatal Hypokalemia.* Blood levels of less than 2.5–3.0 mEq/L are considered moderate hypokalemia. Levels less than 2.5 mEq/L are considered severe hypokalemia. Spurious/ Pseudohypokalemia may be seen with sampling errors, particularly if a blood sample is taken upstream of an infusion of saline, dextrose, or other fluids that contain little or no potassium. Clues to sampling errors include other serum level abnormalities that reflect sampling of a mixture of blood and the fluid that is infused.

2. *Iatrogenic Medication-related Hypokalemia is the most common cause in the Newborn;* Diuretics, Theophylline, Insulin, Amphotericin B, Aminoglycosides, Penicillins and Corticosteroids cause hypokalemia in Neonates through various mechanisms as enlisted in the Table 1 of the Chapter.

3. Redistribution hypokalemia is caused by the entry of potassium into cells. Only a small amount of total body potassium is located in the extracellular compartment. As a result, a small shift of potassium from the extracellular space to the intracellular space can cause a change in plasma potassium concentration. During this shift, alkalosis may occur. A rough guide to the degree of shift is that the serum potassium concentration falls by about 0.3 mEq/L for each 0.1 increase in pH. Alkalosis often results from disorders that deplete total body potassium. As a result, true depletion of total body stores is usually present as well as a redistribution hypokalemia when metabolic alkalosis is present. Increased beta2-adrenergic activity is an important one for therapists to keep in mind. A potassium shift into the cells may also result from another common respiratory drug, theophylline. This generally occurs only during theophylline toxicity (>20 mg%). The mechanism for this is unknown; however, this hypokalemia may aggravate serious arrhythmias that sometimes occur in severe theophylline toxicity.

4. Severe diarrhea results in loss of potassium with HCO_3- resulting in hypokalemia and metabolic acidosis. Sweat has a potassium concentration of roughly 9 mEq/L; increased transepidermal losses due radiant warmers can result in Hypokalemia in premature infants.

5. Renal potassium depletion conditions also tend to be associated with acid-base disorders. It is useful to classify the various causes of renal potassium loss according to whether they typically occur together with metabolic acidosis, metabolic alkalosis, or have no specific acid-base disorder. *Refer to the Table 1 of the Chapter for a practical classification of Neonatal Hypokalemia.* Metabolic alkalosis is usually associated with hypokalemia since conditions that cause metabolic alkalosis also lead to potassium depletion. In many types of metabolic alkalosis, the excess HCO_3- acts as a poorly reabsorbable anion and "carries" more sodium to the collecting tubule, leading to increased sodium-potassium exchange and urinary potassium loss.

6. Recovery from acute renal failure, postobstructive diuresis, and osmotic diuresis can all lead to renal potassium loss. Magnesium depletion is a very important cause of renal potassium loss. *It is difficult to correct the potassium loss until the magnesium deficit is corrected first. If magnesium depletion is not corrected, urinary potassium loss will continue despite large replacement doses of potassium.*

7. *The Evaluation-Decision-Action-Plan/Algorithm* describes the essential aspects of the diagnosis and management of hypokalemia in Neonates. Physical examination findings may frequently be within the reference range. Occasionally, muscle weakness is evident. Cardiac arrhythmias and acute respiratory failure from muscle paralysis are life-threatening complications that require immediate diagnosis. Cardiovascular examination findings may also be within normal limits. Occasionally, tachycardia with irregular beats may be heard. Severe hypokalemia may manifest as bradycardia with cardiovascular collapse. Hypoactive bowel sounds may suggest hypokalemic gastric hypomotility or ileus. Although ECG changes may be helpful if present, their absence should not be taken as reassurance of normal cardiac conduction. The ECG in hypokalemia may appear normal or may have only subtle findings immediately before clinically significant dysrhythmias. ECG findings may include the following: *Ventricular dysrhythmia *Prolongation of QT interval *ST-segment depression *T-wave flattening *Appearance of U waves *During therapy, monitor for changes associated with overcorrection and hyperkalemia, including a prolonged QRS, peaked T waves, brady-arrhythmia, sinus node dysfunction, and asystole. Medical therapy is aimed at potassium supplementation by the enteral (i.e. oral or through feeding tubes) or parenteral route. Transient, asymptomatic, or mild hypokalemia may resolve spontaneously, or it may be treated using enteral potassium supplements.

8. Intravenous administration of potassium is used for profound, life-threatening hypokalemia and in infants who are unable to tolerate oral administration. Potassium is very irritating veins and must be given slowly over time. There is also an increased risk of acute hyperkalemia with the intravenous route and the patient must be closely monitored. Usual dose for potassium replacement: 0.5-1 mEq/kg IV; not to exceed 30–40 mEq/dose. Infusion rate not to exceed 0.3–0.5 mEq/kg/h for noncritical hypokalemia; however, this rate may be inadequate in life-threatening hypokalemia. Infusion rates: $\geq$0.5 mEq/kg/h can be delivered but requires ECG monitoring to detect potentially fatal arrhythmia, especially ventricular dysrhythmia, because it can rapidly lead to cardiac arrest. PO supplementation is based on body weight, ranging from 2–4 mEq/kg/d PO in divided doses to avoid gastric distress. Potassium chloride is the preferred salt for patients with preexisting alkalosis. Avoid treating a patient on the basis of a low serum potassium value that is false because of a sampling or laboratory error (or failing to treat a patient with symptoms of actual hypokalemia because of an elevated serum potassium value.)

9. Because many medications (particularly loop diuretics, mineralocorticoids, catecholamines, methylxanthines, alkalinizing agents) may be responsible for hypokalemia, eliminating or reducing the doses of these medications may be helpful in preventing or minimizing hypokalemia If current medications are responsible for hypokalemia, substitution of potassium-sparing alternatives may help reduce degree of hypokalemia and may help minimize requirements for potassium supplementation.

10. With adequate control of potassium levels and resolution of any predisposing condition, prognosis is excellent. Ongoing communication is essential for reducing the risks and in therapy, especially in patients with chronic conditions associated with hypokalemia (Bartter, Gitelman. RTA, etc.)

---

* *Pearl/Peril/Pitfall : Severe hypokalemia can produce cardiac arrhythmias, ileus, and lethargy. When significant, this condition is treated by slowly replacing potassium either intravenously or orally. Rapid administration of KCl is not recommended because it is associated with life-threatening cardiac dysfunction.*

THE EVALUATION-DECISION-ACTION-PLAN/ALGORITHM FOR THE DIAGNOSIS AND MANAGEMENT OF *NEONATAL HYPOKALEMIA*

SUBJECTIVE FINDINGS

Hx of persistent vomiting, nasogastric suction, secretory diarrhea, diuretic therapy, chloride deficient formula.

Hx of renal losses-polyuria, failure to thrive, vomitings.

Hx of low/nil potassium in IV fluid therapy, a premature baby with chronic lung disease on diuretic therapy.

Hx of drugs/toxins such as Theophylline, diuretics, Salbutamol Nebs., steroids, Amphotericin B, Aminoglycosides

Hx of muscle weakness, abdominal distention, breathing irregularities, shock in acute presentation

OBJECTIVE FINDINGS

Assess ABCs, disability (altered sensorium, seizures, focal neurodeficits), vitals, BP, Urine output & capillary refil time.

Look for dehydration *or* hypertension, hypokalemia related symptoms, such as ileus, apathy, weakness of limbs, apneas, respiratory paralysis, arrhythmias, hypoventilation and its effects (hypoxia and hypercarbia).

Note signs consistent with pyloric stenosis, chronic lung disease, sepsis, congenital heart disease & Bartter syndrome.

INVESTIGATIONS

Blood ABG analysis, electrolytes, BUN, creatinine, osmolality, ketones, glucose, culture, calcium, magnesium, FBC with differential & platelets, drug screen.

Urine analysis, pH, electrolytes, drug screen, culture, 17ketosteroids *Others* consider imaging, ECG, Echocardiogram depending on the suspected underlying disease.

Determine, if Metabolic alkalosis is evident on ABG Analysis a)whether the urinary chlorides below 15mEq/L or above 20mEq/L b)whether the urinary potassium is below 30mEq/day or above 30mEq/day. *Serum* renin and aldosterone concentrations differentiate children with a metabolic alkalosis, a high urinary chloride level, and elevated blood pressure.

SUSPECTED HYPOKALEMA < 3.5 mEq/L

Ensure ABCs, Supplemental O_2, BP monitoring, IV access, Treat shock, pulse oximetry, correct hypoglycemia & hypocalcemia, Treat Sepsis, start reliable NG decompression and IV fluid rehydration

Hx of vomiting, diarrhea or GI tubes or fistulas — YES →

GI LOSSES
Vomiting
Diarrhea
Gastric suctioning
Intestinal fistulas
Laxative abuse
Ureterosigmoidostomy
Villous adenoma

NO

Check Urine K⁺

Urine K⁺ < 20 mEq/l

Transcellular shifts
Alkalosis (metabolic or
    respiratory)
Insulin or glucose therapy
Catecholamine (stress
    beta agonist therapy
    for asthma)
Treatment of anemia
    (megaloblastic)
Blood transfusion
    (washed RBCs)
Hypothermia
Periodic paralysis
    hypokalemic

Nutritional deficiency
prolonged, excessive sweating

Urine K⁺ > 20 mEq/l

Renal tubular damage
    (nephritis, toxins,
    hypercalcemia)
Diuretics
Excess mineralocorticoid
    effect : primary
    hyperaldosteronism
    Licorice
    Cushing's syndrome
Volume depletion (vomiting)
Nonreabsorbable anions
    (penicillins, bicarbonate,
    ketones)
Renal tubular disorders (RTA,
    Fanconi's, Bartter's,
    Gitelman's or Liddle's
    syndromes)
Hypomagnesemia

MANAGEMENT
a. In urgent situations with impending cardiorespiratory arrest - give IV potassium chloride 15%, 0.25–0.5 ml/kg/dose over 1 hour (0.5–1 m Eq/kg/dose) cautiously preventing hyperkalemia.
(Monitor Serum K⁺ closely !)
b. In less urgent situations, start IV fluids with KCl, maximum of 10ml/500ml (20mEq), monitoring serum potassium 6-8 hourly until correction and maintenance by oral supplements done.
c. Oral Potassium is safer in elective situations (potclor contains 20mEq in 15ml) 1–2mEq/kg/day in 3–4 doses.

*Patients with acidosis and hypokalemia can receive potassium citrate/acetate. *If hypophosphatemia is present, then some of the potassium deficit can be replaced with potassium phosphate. *For patients with excessive urinary losses, potassium sparing diuretics are effective, but use them cautiously in patients with renal insufficiency. *If hypokalemia, metabolic alkalosis and volume depletions are present (e.g. with gastric losses), then restoration of intravascular volume with adequate chloride will decrease urinary potassium losses. *Disease - specific therapy is effective in many of the genetic tubular disorders. *Hypokalemic patients treated with Digoxin should be given potassium supplements.

---

* Pearl/Peril/Pitfall: *Patients with hypokalemia often have no symptoms, especially if the hypokalemia is mild (serum potassium 3.0–3.5 mEq/L). Neuromuscular (most prominent manifestations): *Skeletal muscle weakness (proximal > distal muscles, lower limbs > upper) may range from mild weakness to total paralysis, including respiratory muscles; may lead to rhabdomyolysis and/ or respiratory arrest in severe cases*Smooth-muscle involvement may lead to GI hypomotility, producing ileus and constipation *Cardiovascular: -Ventricular arrhythmias; higher risk if underlying CHF, LVF, cardiac ischemia -Hypotension -Cardiac arrest.*

TABLE 1	Causes of hypokalemia in neonates

SPURIOUS
* High WBC count*Sampling errors

MASKED
* Hemolysed blood sample

TRANSCELLULAR SHIFTS
* Alkalemia *Insulin *β-adrenergic agonists : Salbutamol Nebs.
* Theophylline

DECREASED INTAKE
* Inadequate maintenance of IV Potassium

EXTRARENAL LOSSES (Skin and GIT)
* Diarrhea
* Vomiting (CHPS)/NG Tube losses
* Increased sweating

RENAL LOSSES

A. *With metabolic acidosis*
 *Renal Tubular Acidosis-Distal & Proximal
 *Ureterosigmoidostomy

B. *With metabolic alkalosis*
 1. *Low urinary chloride:* vomiting/NGT suction, Chloride-osing diarrhea, Cystic Fibrosis, Low Chloride Formula, Posthypercapnia, Previous diuretic use
 2. *High urinary chloride and normal blood pressure-* Bartter Syndrome, Gitelman Syndrome, Diuretics - Current usage, AD Hypoparathyroidism
 3. *High urinary chloride and high blood pressure:* Renal artery stenosis, Congenital Adrenal Hyperplasia due to 17α and 11β- Hydroxylase deficiency

C. *Without specific Acid-Base disturbance:* Tubular Toxins-Amphoterecin, Aminoglycosides, Interstitial nephritis, Diuretic phase of Acute Tubular Necrosis, Postobstructive diuretic phase, Hypomagnesemia, High urinary anions- Penicillins.

KEY POINTS FOR CLINICAL PRACTICE:

1. *Neonatal Hypokalemia* (Serum Potassium <3.5mEq/L) is a common problem in the NICU; and is due to causes secondary to **4** basic mechanisms **a)** Spurious **b)** Transcellular shifts **c)** Decreased Intake **d)** Losses which can be due to Extrarenal or Renal.

2. *Iatrogenic Medication-related Hypokalemia is the most common cause in the Newborn;* Diuretics,Theophylline, Insulin, Amphotericin B, Aminoglycosides, Penicillins and Corticosteroids cause Hypokalemia in Neonates

3. Renal potassium depletion conditions also tend to be associated with acid-base disorders. It is useful to classify the various causes of renal potassium loss according to whether they typically occur together with metabolic acidosis, metabolic alkalosis, or have no specific acid-base disorder.

4. There are a number of potentially serious problems associated with Hypokalemia such as: Neuromuscular manifestations such as fatigue, paralysis, weakness, respiratory muscle dysfunction, and rhabdomyolysis. Gastrointestinal problems include constipation and ileus. There are a number of cardiac arrhythmias and ECG changes that can occur such as prominent U waves, T wave flattening, and ST segment changes. Transient, asymptomatic, or mild Hypokalemia may resolve spontaneously, or it may be treated using enteral potassium supplements.

5. Intravenous administration of potassium is used for profound, life-threatening hypokalemia and in infants who are unable to tolerate oral administration. Potassium is very irritating veins and must be given slowly over time. There is also an increased risk of acute hyperkalemia with the intravenous route and the patient must be closely monitored. With adequate control of potassium levels and resolution of any predisposing condition, prognosis is excellent.

REFERENCES & FURTHER READING : **1)** Rose BD. Introduction to disorders of potassium balance. In: *Clinical Physiology of Acid-Base and Electrolyte Disorders.* 1989:715-56. **2)** Jospe N, Forbes G. Fluids and electrolytes—clinical aspects. *Pediatr Rev.* Nov 1996;17(11):395-403; quiz 404. **3)** Rodriguez-Soriano J. Bartter and related syndromes: the puzzle is almost solved. *Pediatr Nephrol.* May 1998;12(4):315-27. **4)** Landau D. Potassium handling in health and disease: lessons from inherited tubulopathies. *Pediatr Endocrinol Rev.* Dec 2004;2(2):203-8. **5)** Wood EG, Lynch RE. *Fluid and Electrolyte Balance.* 1998:703-22.

* *Pearl/Peril/Pitfall :* *Neonatal Hypokalemia-Workup for cause:* ·*Excessive renal potassium loss: Urinary potassium is >20 mEq/d in presence of hypokalemia ·In patient with excessive renal potassium loss and hypertension, plasma renin and aldosterone levels should be determined to differentiate adrenal from nonadrenal causes of hyperaldosteronism. ·If hypertension is absent and patient is acidotic, renal tubular acidosis should be considered. ·If hypertension is absent and serum pH is normal to alkalotic, high urine chloride (>10 mEq/d [>10 mmol/d]) suggests hypokalemia secondary to diuretics or Bartter syndrome; low urine chloride (<10 mEq/d [<10 mmol/d]) suggests vomiting as probable cause.*

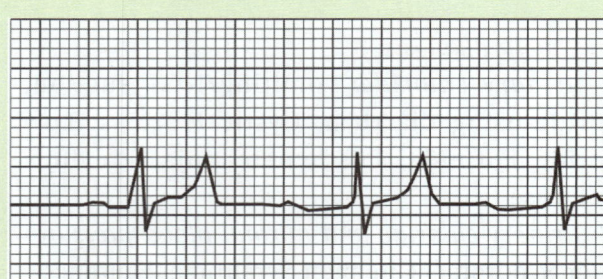

Neonatal Hyperkalemia

@ *True hyperkalemia is caused by one of 3 basic mechanisms, although the root cause for any individual patient is often multifactorial; *Increased K⁺ intake *Transcellular K⁺ shifts *Decreased K⁺ excretion.*

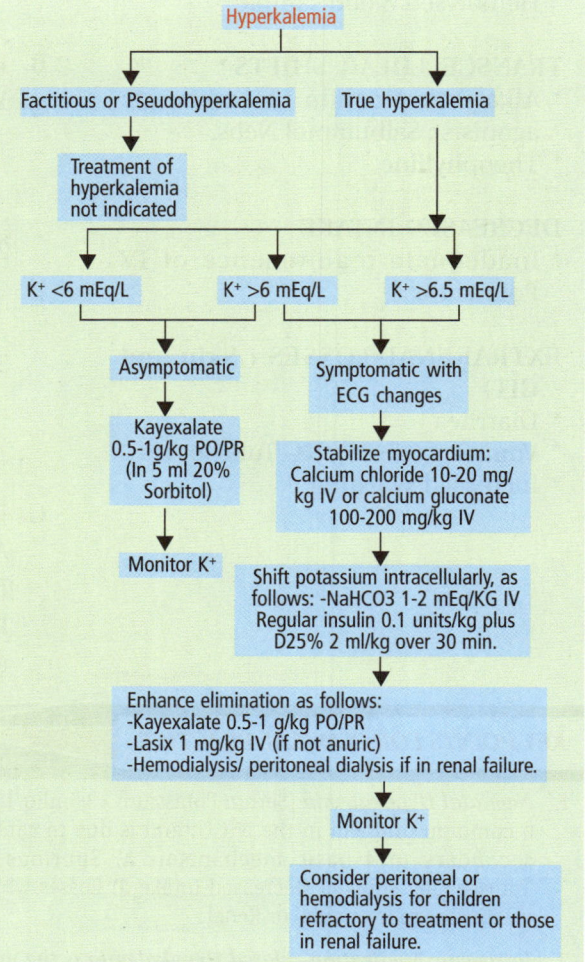

Hyperkalemia and ECG : The ECG findings progress with increasing serum K from peaked T waves (increased rate of repolarization), flattened P waves and increasing PR interval (suppression of atrial conductivity), to QRS widening and slurring) and finally supraventricular/ ventricular tachycardia, bradycardia, or ventricular fibrillation.

Pseudohyperkalemia

Pseudohyperkalemia occurs when laboratory reports of potassium do not reflect actual values. The most common cause is lysis of red cells in a phlebotomy specimen. Potassium released from platelets can lead to spuriously high levels of potassium in a blood sample allowed to clot to collect serum. Pseudo-hyperkalemia can be excluded by repeating the sample collection as atraumatically as possible and obtaining serum and plasma potassium levels. In patients with pseudohyperkalemia, the plasma potassium will be normal in the face of an elevated serum potassium.

REVIEW OF CLINICAL PROBLEMS

1. Describe "Spurious" Neonatal Hyperkalemia.
   Ans: Refer to No 4 of the Bird`s eye view/Overview Synopsis of the Chapter.

2. What are the indications for Dialysis in Neonatal Hyperkalemia?
   Ans: Refer to No 8 of the Bird`s eye view/Overview/ Synopsis of the Chapter.

3. How do you evaluate Neonatal Hyperkalemia?
   Ans: Refer to the Evaluation-Decision-Action Plan/ Algorithm to diagnose and manage Neonatal Hyperkalemia.

4. How do you manage life-threatening Neonatal Hyperkalemia?
   Ans: Refer to the Evaluation-Decision-Action Plan/ Algorithm to diagnose and manage Neonatal Hyperkalemia.

5. Mention the medications that can cause Neonatal Hyperkalemia.
   Ans: Refer to Table 1 of the Chapter.

LEARNING OBJECTIVES

After completing this article, readers will be able to:

1. Identify the common causes of Neonatal Hyperkalemia;determine the inciting cause and to prevent recurrence.

2. Diagnose the ECG changes of Neonatal Hyperkalemia.

3. Treat Neonatal Hyperkalemia with 3 primary goals of immediate management: (1) immediate stabilization of the myocardial cell membrane, (2) rapidly shifting potassium intracellularly, and (3) enhancing total body potassium elimination.

4. Coordinate and Communicate with Various specialists depending on the underlying cause of Neonatal Hyperkalemia.

5. Stop all exogenous sources of potassium and discontinue drugs associated with Hyperkalemia.

* *Pearl/Peril/Pitfall: The most common causes of Neonatal ARF are hypovolemia, hypotension and, hypoxia. Among several indices that are available for differentiating prerenal failure from intrinsic renal failure, fractional excretion of sodium is the preferred index. Diagnostic fluid challenge with or without frusemide is a bed side method for differentiating prerenal failure from intrinsic renal failure.*

BIRD'S EYE VIEW/OVERVIEW/SYNOPSIS

1. *Hyperkalemia* (normal serum K level in a nonhemolyzed blood specimen at normal pH is 3.5–5.5 mEq/L), is seen in ill VLBW infants who have been hypotensive and are in renal failure. *Neonates tolerate levels of 3–6 mEq/L extremely well, but outside this range treatment is required.* Upto 50% of VLBW infants born before 25 weeks of gestation manifest serum K levels > 6 mEq/L in the first 48hrs of life. The most common cause of sudden unexpected Hyperkalemia in the NICU is medication error.

2. Hyperkalemia is essentially caused by 3 basic mechanisms *a) Increased intake*—IV or oral, blood transfusions *b)Transcellular shifts*—acidosis, digitalis intoxication, tissue necrosis, hemolysis, hematomas, GIT bleeding, hypothermia, asphyxia/ischemia, IVH, trauma *c)Decreased excretion*—renal failure, oliguria, hyponatremia, congenital adrenal hyperplasia, medications such as ACE inhibitors, potassium sparing diuretics. *Hyperkalemia should be anticipated and screened in the above clinical scenarios* (Table 1).

3. The most important effects of Hyperkalemia are due to the role of potassium in membrane polarization affecting the cardiac conduction system with the potential for lethal arrhythmia. The ECG findings progress with increasing serum K from peaked T waves (increased rate of repolarization), flattened P waves and increasing PR interval (suppression of atrial conductivity), to QRS widening and slurring (conduction delay in ventricular conduction tissue as well as in the myocardium itself), and finally supraventricular/ventricular tachycardia, bradycardia, or ventricular fibrillation. The ECG findings may be the first indication of Hyperkalemia. Asystole may occur.

4. *Spurious Hyperkalemia* occurs with *a)* tissue ischemia during difficult blood drawing *b)* hemolysis *c)* thrombocytosis *d)* leukocytosis. For every 100,000/cumm increase in the platelet count, the serum potassium level increases by approximately 0.15 mEq/L. Elevated WBC counts, typically >200,000/cumm, can cause a dramatic elevation in the serum K concentration. Analysis of a plasma sample usually provides an accurate results. It is important to analyze the sample promptly to avoid K release from cells. This occurs if the sample is stored in the cold, whereas storage at room temperature can lead to cellular uptake of K and spurious hypokalemia.

5. Initial laboratory evaluation of suspected Hyperkalemia should include creatinine, BUN, ABG analysis. Many causes of Hyperkalemia produce a metabolic acidosis; a metabolic acidosis worsens Hyperkalemia by the transcellular shift of K out of cells. Renal insufficiency is a common cause of the combination of metabolic acidosis and Hyperkalemia. This association is also seen in congenital adrenal hyperplasia with aldosterone insufficiency. *In contrast to a Neonate in renal failure, the infant with salt losing form of congenital adrenal hyperplasia is volume depleted.* Hyponatremia occurs in both the conditions (**dilutional** in renal failure and **hypovolemic** in congenital adrenal hyperplasia).

6. *The Evaluation-Decision-Action-Plan / Algorithm* describes the essential aspects of history taking, clinical examination and laboratory evaluation and the management of Neonatal Hyperkalemia. Once Hyperkalemia is diagnosed, remove all sources of exogenous K (IV and Oral), rehydrate the patient if necessary, and eliminate arrhythmia promoting factors. *The clinical condition, ECG, and actual serum K level all affect the choice of therapy for hyperkalemia. Refer to Table 2* for pharmacologic treatment of Neonatal Hyperkalemia.

7. The treatment of Hyperkalemia has *three basic goals:* 1) to stabilize the heart to prevent life-threatening arrhythmias 2) to dilute and shift K into the cell and 3) to remove K from the body. *Calcium* stabilizes the cell membrane of heart cells, preventing arrhythmias. Calcium gluconate 10% 1-2 ml/kg IV over 5-10 minutes under cardiac monitoring is the most useful in the NICU. Calcium should be given over 30 minutes in a patient receiving digitalis because it may cause arrhythmias. *Bicarbonate* causes potassium to move intracellularly, lowering the plasma K level. Insulin causes potassium to move intracellularly, but it must be given with glucose to avoid hypoglycemia. The combination of insulin and glucose works within 30 minutes. Nebulized salbutamol/albuterol, by stimulation of b_1 - receptors, leads to rapid intracellular movement of potassium. To excrete potassium from the body, sodium polystyrene sulfonate (Kayexalate), an exchange resin given rectally or orally and furosemide are the useful drugs. The former is not recommended in preterm babies because they are prone to hypomotility and are at risk for NEC.

8. *Peritoneal dialysis is seldom required but should be instituted urgently if there is : 1)* severe fluid overload +/- pulmonary edema *2)* severe metabolic acidosis (pH < 7.2 with $PaCO_2$ < 40mmHg) *3)* Hyperkalemia (K+ > 8mEq/lt) not responding to medical measures *4)* intractable hypoglycemia. *5)* Consider dialysis if CNS prognosis considered good in a baby with HIE. *Continuous Renal Replacement Therapy (CRRT) using arterio-venous haemofiltration through an extracorporeal circuit is becoming a more frequently employed modality for renal replacement therapy in the hemodynamically unstable Neonate. (high risk for intracranial bleeding due to heparinization).*

9. Chronic management of Hyperkalemia includes reducing intake through dietary changes and eliminating or reducing medications that cause Hyperkalemia. Some patients require medications to increase potassium excretion. These include sodium polysterene sulfonate and loop/thiazide diuretics.

10. Some infants with chronic renal failure may need to start dialysis to allow adequate caloric intake without Hyperkalemia. It is unusual for an older child to require dialysis principally to control chronic Hyperkalemia. The disorders that are due to a deficiency in aldosterone respond to replacement therapy with fludrocortisone.

---

* *Pearl/Peril/Pitfall : (* Spurious/Pseudohyperkalemia - first exclude hemolysis by inspecting a centrifuged blood specimen's supernatant fluid => pseudohyperkalemia is present when the plasma potassium [heparinized tube] is more than 0.3mEq/L greater than the serum potassium).*

THE EVALUATION-DECISION-ACTION-PLAN/ALGORITHM FOR THE DIAGNOSIS AND MANAGEMENT OF *HYPERKALEMIA IN NEONATES*

SUBJECTIVE FINDINGS

HISTORY SUGGESTIVE OF ACUTE RENAL FAILURE?

Hx of Hypovolemia Blood loss, plasma loss, insensible loss (phototherapy in VLBW infants), GI losses (D&V), polyuria, inadequate intake (fluid restriction after birth asphyxia). *Hx of Hypoxic - Ischemic Encephalopathy and Hx of risk factors for Septicemia or severe respiratory illness, NEC.*

Hx of Maternal Diabetes Renal vein thrombosis. Hx of oligohydramnios - Potter's syndrome. Hx of Nephrotoxic drugs (aminoglycosides, indomethacin, frusemide). Hx of congestive heart failure. Hx of force of the infant's urinary stream (posterior urethral valves.)

History suggestive of SPURIOUS HYPER-KALEMIA AND TRANSCELLULAR SHIFTS and MEDICATIONS CAUSING HYPERKALEMIA- Refer to the Table 1 of the Chapter.

OBJECTIVE FINDINGS

Look for Symptoms and signs of renal failure

* **Symptoms of renal failure**, e.g. poor feeding, vomiting, seizures, bleeding, cardiac arrhythmias.

* **Signs**, e.g. fluid overload (hypertension, edema, excess weight gain, hepatomegaly, tachypnea), fluid depletion (poor peripheral perfusion, hypotension), renal abnormality (palpable kidney, bladder).

Look for the presence of any congenital anomalies associated with renal abnormalities (e.g. Potter's syndrome, VACTERL, Epispadias).

INVESTIGATIONS

Weight, BP, Infection Screen, Renal Ultra Sound.

Urine Multistix, Microscopy, Urea, Electrolytes, Creatinine, Osmolality.

Blood Electrolytes, Urea, Creatinine, ABG analysis, Osmolality, Calcium, Mg++, Glucose, Albumin, Full blood count, Clotting studies, LFTs.

ECG and CXR

Renal Ultrasound is helpful in the identification of congenital renal disease and urinary tract obstruction.

Micturating cystourethrogram should be performed in Neonates with suspected posterior urethral valves, vesicoureteral reflux, or bladder abnormality.

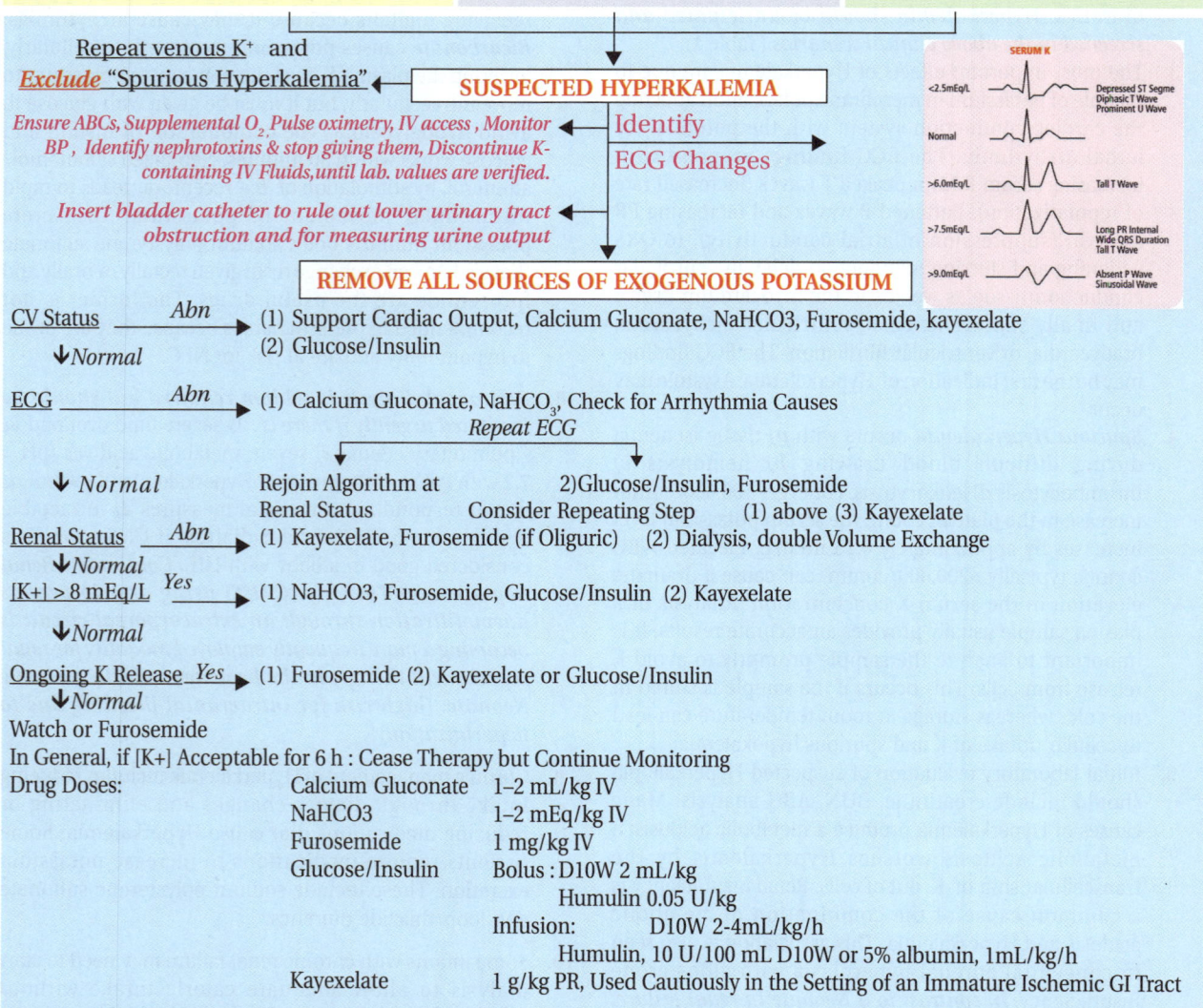

Repeat venous K⁺ and
Exclude "Spurious Hyperkalemia" ← **SUSPECTED HYPERKALEMIA**

Ensure ABCs, Supplemental O₂, Pulse oximetry, IV access , Monitor BP , Identify nephrotoxins & stop giving them, Discontinue K-containing IV Fluids,until lab. values are verified.

Identify ECG Changes

Insert bladder catheter to rule out lower urinary tract obstruction and for measuring urine output

REMOVE ALL SOURCES OF EXOGENOUS POTASSIUM

CV Status — *Abn* → (1) Support Cardiac Output, Calcium Gluconate, NaHCO3, Furosemide, kayexelate
↓*Normal*   (2) Glucose/Insulin

ECG — *Abn* → (1) Calcium Gluconate, NaHCO₃, Check for Arrhythmia Causes
                    Repeat ECG

↓ *Normal*   Rejoin Algorithm at   2)Glucose/Insulin, Furosemide
               Renal Status   Consider Repeating Step   (1) above (3) Kayexelate

Renal Status — *Abn* → (1) Kayexelate, Furosemide (if Oliguric)   (2) Dialysis, double Volume Exchange
↓*Normal*
[K+] > 8 mEq/L — *Yes* → (1) NaHCO3, Furosemide, Glucose/Insulin (2) Kayexelate

↓*Normal*

Ongoing K Release — *Yes* → (1) Furosemide (2) Kayexelate or Glucose/Insulin
↓*Normal*
Watch or Furosemide
In General, if [K+] Acceptable for 6 h : Cease Therapy but Continue Monitoring

Drug Doses:
	Calcium Gluconate	1–2 mL/kg IV
	NaHCO3	1–2 mEq/kg IV
	Furosemide	1 mg/kg IV
	Glucose/Insulin	Bolus : D10W 2 mL/kg
		Humulin 0.05 U/kg
		Infusion: D10W 2-4mL/kg/h
		Humulin, 10 U/100 mL D10W or 5% albumin, 1mL/kg/h
	Kayexelate	1 g/kg PR, Used Cautiously in the Setting of an Immature Ischemic GI Tract

Treatment of hyperkalemia (CV = cardiovascular; Nl = normal; Abn = abnormal; ECG = electrocardiogram; GI = gastrointestinal). For a given algorithm outcome proceed by administering the entire set of treatments labeled (1). If unsuccessful in lowering [K+] or improving clinical condition, proceed to the next set of treatments, for example, (2) and then (3).

* ***Pearl/Peril/Pitfall :*** ECG *There is no definite correlation between any ECG changes and the serum potassium - the relationship depends on individual patient sensitivity and the rapidity of development of the hyperkalemia (* ECG signs may be absent if the onset of hyperkalemia is slow - as seen in chronic renal failure - even though the serum potassium is in the range of 7 - 7.5meq/L; by contrast, acute hyperkalemia can produce ECG signs at much lower serum potassium levels).*

TABLE 1   Causes of hyperkalemia in the Newborn

SPURIOUS (PSEUDOHYPERKALEMIA)
LABORATORY VALUE
Hemolysis
Tissue ischemia during blood drawing
Thrombocytosis
Leukocytosis
INCREASED INTAKE
Intravenous or oral
Blood transfusions
TRANSCELLULAR SHIFTS
Acidosis
Rhabdomyolysis
Tumor lysis syndrome
Tissue necrosis
Hemolysis/hematomas/gastrointestinal bleeding
Succinylcholine
Digitalis intoxication
Fluoride intoxication
β -Adrenergic blockers
Exercise
Hyperosmolality
Insulin deficiency
Malignant hyperthermia (MIM 145600)
Hyperkalemic periodic paralysis (MIM 170500)

DECREASED EXCRETION
Renal failure
Primary adrenal disease
    Acquired Addison disease
    21-hydroxylase deficiency (MIM 201910)
    3 β -hydroxysteroid dehydrogenase deficiency (MIM 201810)
    Lipoid congenital adrenal hyperplasia (MIM 201710)
    Adrenal hypoplasia congenital (MIM 300200)
    Aldesterone synthase deficiency (MIM 203400)
    Adrenoleukodystrophy (MIM 300100)
Hyporeninemic hypoaldosteronism
    Urinary tract obstruction
    Sickle cell disease (MIM 603903)
    Kidney transplant
    Lupus nephritis
Renal tubular disease
    Pseudohypoaldosteronism type I (MIM 264350 and 177735)
    Pseudohypoaldosteronism type II (MIM 745260)
    Urinary tract obstruction
    Sickle cell disease
    Kidney transplant
Medications
    Angiotensin-converting enzyme inhibitors
    Angiotensin II blockers
    Potassium-sparing diuretics
    Calcineurin inhibitors
    Nonsteroidal anti-inflammatory drugs
    Trimethoprim
    Heparin
    Drug-induced potassium channel syndrome
MIM, database number from the Mendelian Inheritance in Man

TABLE 2   Management of hyperkalemia in the Newborn

Drug	Dose	Onset, Duration	Indication	Mechanism	Risk & Remark
* 10% Calcium gluconate	0.5–1ml/kg IV over 5–10 min.	1–2 minutes, lasts for 30 minutes	K+ > 6.5 mmol/L with advanced ECG changes	Membrane stabilization antagonizes cardiac and neuromuscular toxicity of hyperkalemia	Give with cardiac monitoring. Stop if HR <100 Repeat in 5 minutes, if abnormal ECG persists.
* Nebulized Salbutamol	2.5mgs/dose repeat twice	30mts, lasts for 2 hours	K+ > 6.5 mmol/L with advanced ECG changes	Moves K+ into cells	Tremors, tachycardia
* Sodium bicarbonate (3.75%)	1.0-2.0mEq/kg (IV over 10 min)	5–10 minutes, lasts for 2–6 hours	Moderate hyperkalemia	Moves K+ into cells	Hypernatremia, hypocalcemic tetany, volume overload
* Insulin & Glucose	1 IU/5 g glucose (IV bolus or infusion ≤ 14 mg/kg/min (IV bolus or infusion)	15–30mts, lasts for 4–6hrs	Moderate hyperkalemia	Moves K+ into cells	Glucose unnecessary if hyperglycemia +
* Sodium polystryrene sulfonate	1g/kg dose every 6 h as needed (orally/rectally)	1–2 hrs, lasts for 4–6 hrs	Moderate hyperkalemia	Exchanges Na+ for K+	Sodium overload
* Furosemide	2mg/kg IV bolus	15 mts, lasts for 4 hrs	Moderate hyperkalemia	Kaliuresis	Most useful if inadequate K+ excretion +.

* *Pearl/Peril/Pitfall* : *Calcium gluconate* special warnings: *calcium should be given slowly over 20 - 30 minutes in a digitalized patient by diluting the calcium in 25 ml of normal saline and giving the calcium by an infusion pump - high risk of increased myocardial toxicity in the digitalized patient *calcium is contraindicated in digoxin-toxic patients and hypercalcemic states *don't give calcium in solutions containing bicarbonate. *An alternative is to consider using magnesium instead of calcium to stabilize the myocardium.*

* *Pearl/Peril/Pitfall:* *Intravenous administration of insulin (together with glucose) effectively manages hyperkalaemia in neonates (Ditzenberger, 1999), but the response is unpredictable, and carries the risk of hypoglycemia, hyperosmolarity, and volume overload (Helfrich, 2001). No good, randomized trials for its use in neonates have been identified. Intravenous salbutamol is rapidly effective and side effects, including elevated heart rate, mild vasomotor flushing and mild tremor are all short-lasting (Helfrich, 2001; Kemper, 1996; Murdoch, 1991).*

* *Pearl/Peril/Pitfall :* *Do some VLBW infants without renal failure suffer from hyperkalaemia? Extremely premature babies may develop hyperkalaemia without significant renal impairment due to release of potassium from catabolized cells, as well as shift of intracellular potassium to the extracellular spaces. This may be exacerbated by dehydration.*

POTASSIUM-Normal values
<1,000 gm: 6.4 mEq/l
1,001 – 1,500 gm: 6.0
1,501 – 2,000 gm: 5.4
2,001 – 2,500 gm: 5.6

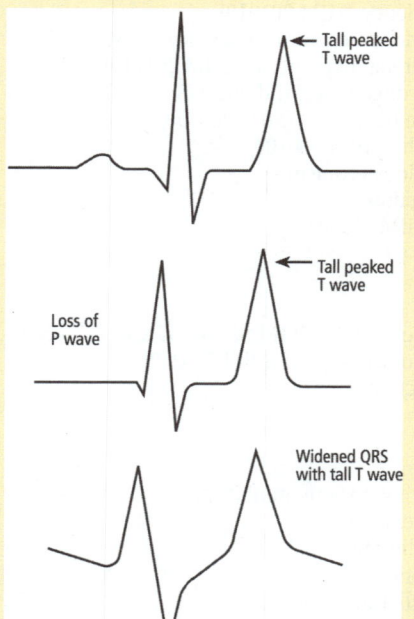

Typical electrocardiograph changes seen in patients with hyperkalemia.

* When the etiology of hyperkalemia remains unclear, calculation of the transtubular potassium gradient (TTKG) using the following formula may be useful:

TTKG = (K$^+$ urine X Osm plasma)/(K$^+$ plasma X Osm urine)

* The normal TTKG varies from 5-15. In the setting of hyperkalemia with normal renal excretion of potassium, the TTKG should be greater than 10. A TTKG of less than 8 in the setting of hyperkalemia implies inadequate potassium excretion, which is usually secondary to aldosterone deficiency or unresponsiveness. Checking a serum aldosterone level may be helpful.

An ECG is essential in all children in whom hyperkalemia is suspected. ECG reveals the sequence of changes as follows: *Serum K$^+$ 5.5-6.5 mEq/L - Tall, peaked T waves with narrow base, best seen in precordial leads *Serum K$^+$ 6.5-8.0 mEq/L - Peaked T waves, prolonged PR interval, decreased or disappearing P wave, widening of QRS, amplified R wave *Serum K$^+$ greater than 8.0 mEq/L - Absence of P wave; progressive QRS widening, intraventricular/fascicular/bundle branch blocks; progressive widening of QRS, eventually merging with the T wave just before cardiac arrest, forming the sine wave pattern.

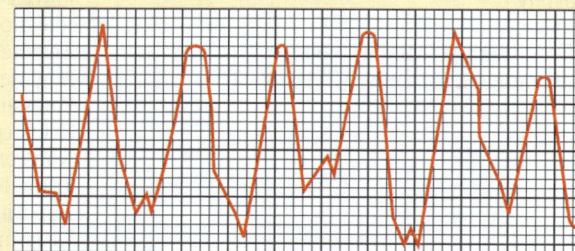

KEY POINTS FOR CLINICAL PRACTICE

1. Hyperkalemia is defined as a serum potassium level greater than 6 mEq/L measured in a nonhemolyzed specimen. Hyperkalemia is of far more concern than hypokalemia, especially when serum potassium levels exceed 6.5 mEq/L or if ECG changes have developed.

2. ECG manifestations of hyperkalemia are a progression from peaked T waves, as the earliest sign, to a widened QRS configuration, bradycardia, tachycardia, supraventricular tachycardia (SVT), ventricular tachycardia, and ventricular fibrillation.

3. Causes of hyperkalemia include potassium release from damaged neuronal cells and breakdown of RBCs following intraventricular hemorrhage (IVH), trauma and intravenous hemolysis. In addition, severe acidosis and decreased urinary potassium excretion contribute to elevations in serum potassium. Finally, hyperkalemia may be one of the earliest manifestations of congenital adrenal hyperplasia.

4. The treatment of Hyperkalemia has *three basic goals:* 1) to stabilize the heart to prevent life-threatening arrhythmias 2) to dilute and shift K into the cell and 3) to remove K from the body. Intravenous calcium is effective in reversing electrocardiographic changes and reducing the risk of arrhythmias but does not lower serum potassium. Serum potassium levels can be lowered acutely by using intravenous insulin and glucose, nebulized beta2 agonists, or both. (Refer to Table 2 of the Chapter.)* Remember: - to change to a solution without K - hold gentamicin pending evaluation of renal status - high potassium without EKG changes (although unlikely) still needs treatment - check for factitious causes first - hyperkalemia is worsened by hypocalcemia, hypomagnesemia.

5. Medications are administered to enhance potassium excretion, including intravenous furosemide 1 mg/kg or rectally administered sodium polystyrene sulfonate (Kayexalate) 1 g/kg (do not use sorbitol-containing products and do not administer orally). Several hours must pass before any effect is observed with either of these medications. Dialysis or exchange transfusion may be used to assist in more rapidly removing potassium from the body.

REFERENCES & FURTHER READING : 1) Mildenberger E. Versmold HT. Pathogenesis and therapy of non-oliguric hyperkalaemia of the premature infant. Eur J Pediatr, 2002; 161:415-22 2) Nelson Text Book of Pediatrics, 18th edition 3) Manual of Neonatal Care, John P. Cloherty, 6th edition. 4) Avery GB, Fletcher MA, MacDonald MG (eds). Neonatology: pathophysiology and management of the Newborn. JB Saunders 2005, 8th edition 5) The Northern Neonatal Network. Neonatal Formulary (3rd Ed), BMJ Publishing 2000.

* *Pearl/Peril/Pitfall : What level of hyperkalaemia should prompt treatment? The criteria on which to treat hyperkalaemia have ranged from 6.8 to 7.5 mmol/L, but 6.5 mmol/L may be a better level at which to begin treatment, as rhythm disturbances are to be expected above 7.0 mmol/L (Grammatikopoulos, 2003). If treatment is not initiated until symptoms appear (or the serum level exceeds 7.0 mmol/L), the potential for success is reduced (Ditzenberger, 1999). Mortality rates may be as high as 80% once arrhythmias have appeared (Singh, 2002).*

77

Neonatal Hypocalcemia

@ *Early-onset Neonatal hypocalcemia* typically occurs during the first few days of life, with the lowest concentrations of serum calcium being reached at 24-48 hrs of age, whereas late-onset Neonatal hypocalcemia occurs towards the end of the first week of life.

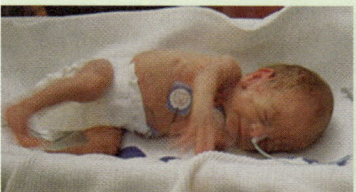 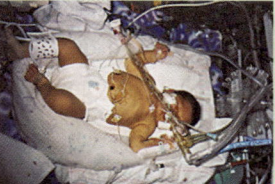 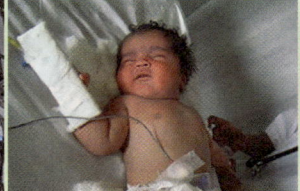 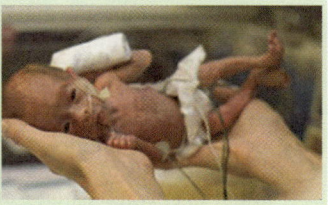

Premature/ELBW baby   **Asphyxiated baby**   **Infant of diabetic mum**   **IUGR Baby**

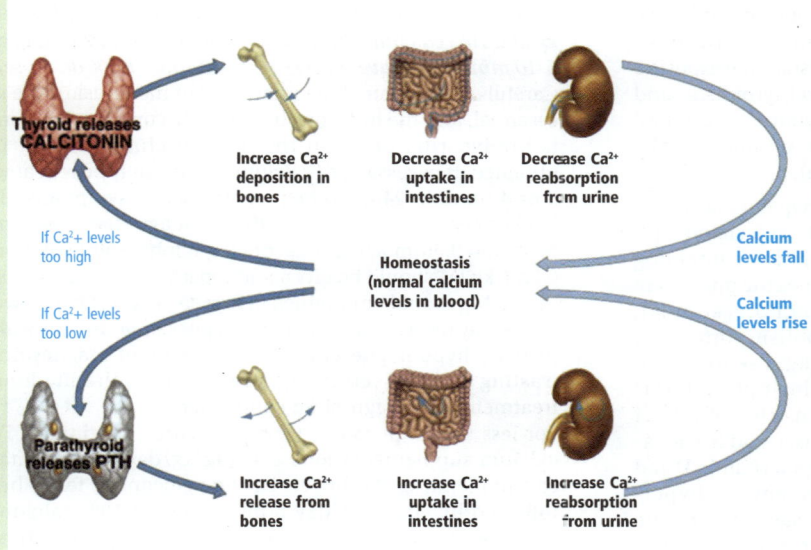

@Early Neonatal Hypocalcemia (within 48-72 h of birth)

*Prematurity: Possible mechanisms include poor intake, decreased responsiveness to vitamin D, increased calcitonin, and hypoalbuminemia leading to decreased total but normal ionized calcium. *Birth asphyxia: Delayed introduction of feeds, increased calcitonin production, increased endogenous phosphate load, and alkali therapy all may contribute to hypocalcemia. *Diabetes mellitus in the mother: Magnesium depletion in mothers with diabetes mellitus causes hypomagnesemic state in the fetus. This hypomagnesemia induces functional hypoparathyroidism and hypocalcemia in the infant. A high incidence of birth asphyxia and prematurity in infants of diabetic mothers are also contributing factors. *Intrauterine growth retardation (IUGR): Infants with IUGR may have hypocalcemia if they are also preterm or have had perinatal asphyxia;per se IUGR is not a factor in causing Neonatal Hypocalcemia.

REVIEW OF CLINICAL PROBLEMS

1. How do you evaluate Neonatal Hypocalcemia?
   Ans: Refer to the Evaluation-Decision-Action Plan/Algorithm to diagnose and manage Neonatal Hypocalcemia.
2. Discuss the essential aspects of Calcium Therapy for Neonatal Hypocalcemia.
   Ans: Refer to the Evaluation-Decision-Action Plan/Algorithm to diagnose and manage Neonatal Hypocalcemia.
3. How do you prevent Early and Late onset types of Neonatal Hypocalcemia?
   Ans:Refer to 9 and 10 of Bird's eye view/Overview/Synopsis of the Chapter.
4. Mention the Medicolegal Pitfalls in Neonatal Hypocalcemia.
   Ans:Refer to Table 3 of the Chapter
5. What are the important differential diagnoses of Neonatal Hypocalcemia?
   Ans: Refer to Table 4 of the Chapter

LEARNING OBJECTIVES

After completing this article, readers will be able to:

1. Anticipate early onset hypocalcemia in the high-risk neonates and monitor serum ionized calcium levels regularly.
2. Treat acute symptomatic hypocalcemia promptly by stabilizing the ABCDs, if seizures occur.
3. Differentiate other causes of neonatal seizures (seizures usually do not respond to the usual antiseizure medications until calcium is intravenously administered.)
4. Prevent late onset hypocalcemia by avoiding phosphate rich Cow's milk and by ensuring adequate vitamin D stores during pregnancy.
5. Counsel the parents about the prognosis of different types of neonatal hypocalcemia depending on the underlying etiology.

* *Pearl/Peril/Pitfall : Late neonatal hypocalcemia (3–7 d after birth, though occasionally as late as age 6 wk) *Exogenous phosphate load: This is most commonly seen in developing countries. Hypocalcemia is caused by feeding with phosphate-rich formula or cow's milk. Whole cow's milk has 7 times the phosphate load of breast milk (956 vs 140 mg/L in breast milk). *Magnesium deficiency *Transient hypoparathyroidism of newborn *Hypoparathyroidism due to other causes *Gentamicin use: Data have suggested association with gentamicin use, especially with the newer every-24-hour dosing schedule*

BIRD'S EYE VIEW/OVERVIEW/SYNOPSIS

1. *Neonatal hypocalcemia* is defined as a total serum calcium concentration of < 7mg/dL (< 1.75 mmol/L) in preterm infants, and below 8mg/dL (< 2 mmol/L) in term infants *or an ionized calcium concentration of <4mg/dL (< 1 mmol/L).* In VLBW infants, ionized calcium values of 0.8-1 mmol/L are common, without any associated clinical symptoms usually. But in larger infants and in infants of >32 weeks gestation, symptoms may readily occur with an ionized calcium concentration of < 1 mmol/L.

2. Based on onset, Neonatal hypocalcemia has been classified as either early or late, although the distinction may not be clear-cut. **Early-onset Neonatal hypocalcemia** typically occurs during the first few days of life, with the lowest concentrations of serum calcium being reached at 24–48 hrs of age, whereas late-onset Neonatal hypocalcemia occurs towards the end of the first week of life. Early-onset Neonatal hypocalcemia represents an exaggeration of the physiologic decrease in serum calcium during the first few days of life, and is most commonly associated with prematurity, birth asphyxia, obstetric trauma, fetal distress, maternal insulin-dependent diabetes, gestational exposure to anticonvulsants, maternal hyperparathyroidism, and Neonatal illness- respiratory distress syndrome, cerebral injury, hypoglycemia, and sepsis. (**Refer to Table 1 for the list of causes of Neonatal hypocalcemia**).

3. **Late-onset hypocalcemia**, which is less frequent than early-onset hypocalcemia, is most commonly associated with administration of relatively high phosphate-containing formula feeds(Whole cow's milk has 7 times the phosphate load of breast milk (956 vs 140 mg/L in breast milk), disturbed maternal vitamin D metabolism, intestinal malabsorption of calcium, hypomagnesemia, and hypoparathyroidism. Formula with a high phosphorus content and a low calcium-to-phosphorus ratio of 1.3–1.4 (breast milk contains 150 mg phosphorus/L and has a Ca-to-P ratio of 2.3), immaturity of parathyroid, vitamin D and renal function causing phosphorus retention, hyper-phosphotemia, and inability to support calcium levels are the important factors in the pathogenesis of late-onset hypocalcemia.

4. Early-onset hypocalcemia in preterm Newborns is often asymptomatic but may show apnea, seizures, or abnormalities of cardiac function. In the Neonatal period the main clinical signs are jitteriness, tremors, and generalized or focal seizures; infants may also be lethargic, feed poorly, vomit, and have abdominal distention. Frank convulsions are seen more commonly with late-onset Neonatal hypocalcemia. The degree of irritability of the infants does not appear to correlate with serum calcium levels. The classic signs of peripheral hyperexcitability of motor nerves, such as carpopedal spasm and laryngospasm are uncommon in Newborn infants.

5. The diagnosis of hypocalcemia is based on the determination of ionized or total calcium. In addition to a history and physical examination, certain data are useful when there is not a clear cause for hypocalcemia: serum total calcium, ionized calcium, P, Mg, Glucose and ABG analysis. ECG determination of prolonged QTc (>0.40 second) suggests hypocalcemia. *Although the QTc cannot precisely predict the ionized calcium concentration, may be useful to monitor the response to calcium therapy.*

6. When the infant is refractory to therapy or there are unusual findings in the initial evaluation, additional data may be of value to diagnose the less common causes of Neonatal hypocalcemia (e.g. primary hypoparathyroidism, malabsorption, and disorders of vitamin D metabolism). Based on the factors that can contribute to hypocalcemia, the etiology can be determined from the laboratory findings. Elevated serum P concentration (>8mg/dL) suggests P loading (a clue to high dietary P intake), renal insufficiency, or hypoparathyroidism. Absence of thymic shadows on chest x-ray may suggest DiGeorge sequence (Karyotyping to assess for 22q11 and 10p13 deletion). Hypercalciuria associated with hypocalcemia supports a deficiency of PTH. Low serum 25-hydroxyvitamin D concentration (<11ng/mL) indicates vitamin D deficiency.

7. *The Evaluation-Decision-Action-Plan/Algorithm* describes the essential aspects of the diagnosis and management of hypocalcemia in Neonates. *For emergency treatment of hypocalcemic crisis with seizures, tetany, or apnea, 1–2 ml/kg of a 10% calcium gluconate should be administered over 5-10 minutes intravenously (in 1:1 dilution in 5% dextrose).* Careful observation of the infant and of the infusion site is essential, and the infusion should be discontinued if there is bradycardia or when the desired clinical result is obtained. If necessary, IV calcium therapy may be repeated 3 or 4 times in 24hrs to help control acute symptoms. If hypocalcemia is associated with hypomagnesemia (serum Mg below 0.6mmol/L [1.5mg/dL] Mg sulphate 50% solution 0.2ml/kg IM should be given and repeated after 12–24 hrs. Serum Mg should be obtained before each dose. One or two doses may resolve transient hypomagnesemia. Infants with primary hypomagnesemia have permanent magnesium wasting and low serum Mg levels and require life long treatment with magnesium supplements.

8. For less urgent purposes (asymptomatic), continuous IV calcium supplementations @ 80mg/kg/day of elemental calcium (8ml/kg/day of 10% calcium gluconate) for 48 hrs followed by 40mg/kg/day (4ml/kg/day of 10% calcium gluconate) for 24 hrs is generally sufficient to restore normocalcemia. After normocalcemia is achieved, a step wise reduction of IV calcium may help to prevent rebound hypocalcemia and then discontinue. Vitamin D metabolites are not recommended for clinical management of early hypocalcemia because of their variable response and potential side effects.

9. Because late-onset hypocalcemia is usually symptomatic, the goals of therapy are to reduce the P load and to increase calcium absorption by using feedings with a Ca/P ratio ≥ 4:1, which can be accomplished by the use of low-P feedings, such as human milk or low-P formula, in conjunction with an oral calcium supplement. Hypoparathyroidism requires therapy with 1, 25-(OH)$_2$D and life long calcium supplementation.

10. The essential measures to prevent early-onset Neonatal hypocalcemia in ill neonates, include **a)** IV or oral calcium supplementation (80mg/kg/day) **b)** early feeding and provision of Ca to the gut **c)** judicious use of bicarbonate administration **d)** avoidance of respiratory alkalosis. Regular follow-up monitoring of serum calcium is necessary in those infants who continue to have hypocalcemia (some of these infants may have permanent hypoparathyroidism or transient but prolonged hypoparathyroidism).

---

* *Pearl/Peril/Pitfall :* *Late-Onset Neonatal Hypocalcemia, if refractory to treatment requires further investigations-*A CT scan may be done to look for Basal ganglion calcifications *An ophthalmic (for cataract) and the hearing evaluation is also important *An ECHO may be done in case a De George syndrome is suspected. If the hypocalcemia is present with hyperphosphatemia and a normal renal function than hypoparathyroidism should be strongly suspected.*

THE EVALUATION-DECISION-ACTION-PLAN/ALGORITHM FOR THE DIAGNOSIS AND MANAGEMENT OF *NEONATAL HYPOCALCEMIA*

SUBJECTIVE FINDINGS

Hx of - predisposing conditions for early-onset hypocalcemia, such as prematurity, infant of diabetic mother, RDS, sepsis, birth asphyxia, alkalosis and bicarbonate therapy, phototherapy, exchange transfusion with citrate-buffered blood etc.,

Hx of - predisposing conditions for late-onset hypocalcemia, such as high phosphate load in the diet (cow's milk derived formula), congenital hypoparathyroidism (DiGeorge sequence or as part of Kenny-Caffey syndrome) or vitamin D deficiency due to various causes.

Hx of - non specific symptoms such as jitteriness, tremors, seizures, tetany, apnea, poor feeding and lethargy.

OBJECTIVE FINDINGS

Assess ABCs, disability (altered sensorium, seizures, focal neurodeficits), vitals, BP, Urine output & capillary refil time.

Determine whether the symptoms are of early-onset (first 24-48 hrs of life) or of late-onset (at the end of the first week of life).

Note that laryngospasm and carpopedal spasm signs are uncommon in the Newborn.

Most infants are asymptomatic and therefore monitor serum calcium as per the schedule

- preterms (1-1.5kg) : 24, 48hrs of life

- preterms (<1kg): 12, 24, 48 hrs of life

- sick or stressed infants : 12, 24, 48 hrs of life

INVESTIGATIONS

Blood - Serum calcium - total and ionized fractions, PO_4, Mg, ABG analysis, alkaline phosphatase, glucose.
Urine Drug Screen
ECG - for prolonged QTc interval (> 0.4 second).
CXR - for absence of thymic shadow, aortic arch position (DiGeorge sequence).
In selected cases - PTH levels, Urine calcium/creatinine ratio, maternal calcium, phosphate and alkaline phosphatase levels, 25(OH) D., CT Scan for basal ganglia calcifications, Hearing and Eye(cataract) evaluations and ECHO for Di George sequence.
Others (e.g. malabsorption workup, lymphocyte count, T-cell numbers and function, maternal and family screening)

HYPOCALCEMIA IN NEONATES

Ensure ABCs, pulse oximetry, Supplemental O₂, IV access & Monitor BP

Low ionized serum Ca++ (<0.75-1.1mmol/L or <3-4.4 mg/dL)

SYMPTOMATIC

YES
seizures, tetany, hypotension, or arrhythmias

NO

Calcium gluconate 10% IV

Give 1-2 ml/kg (9-18mg elemental calcium/kg) in 1:1 dilution in 5% dextrose over 10 minutes. Repeat in 10 minutes if no response.

Then start maintenance IV calcium gluconate 10% infusion @ 8ml/kg/day for 48 hrs. Then give 4ml/kg/day of 10% IV gluconate for 24 hrs more. Commonly as little as 2-3 days of treatment is needed, *because most causes of hypocalcemia in the neonate are transient.*

Other causes

Transient Early onset neonatal

Calcium supplements PO

Observation

Refractory hypocalcemia

check Mg⁺⁺ & serum albumin
Hypomagnesemia
Hypoalbuminemia
albumin 0.5-1.0 g/kg. IV
repeat as necessary

If Mg⁺⁺ & albumin normal, determine other etiology

PTH↓

PTH N/↑

<10 d age transient physiologic

>10 d age with normal Mg++ Hypoparathyroidism

serum phosphorus

phosphorus↑

normal phosphorus

vitamin D level

↓phosphorus intake **phosphate binders**

BUN, creatinine abnormal

Renal insufficiency

ESSENTIAL ASPECTS OF CALCIUM THERAPY FOR HYPOCALCEMIA

*Calcium concentration reported as mgs/dL can be converted to molar units by dividing by 4 **(e.g., 8mg/dL converts to 2.0 mmol/L)** *At birth, the umbilical serum calcium level is elevated (10-11 mg/dL). In healthy term babies, calcium concentrations decline for the first 24-48 hrs; the nadir is usually 7.5-8.5 mg/dL. Thereafter, calcium concentrations progressively rise to the mean values observed in older children. *Rapid IV infusion of calcium can cause a sudden elevation of serum calcium, leading to bradycardia or other dysrhythmias. Therefore it should be done with careful cardiovascular monitoring. Extravasation of calcium solutions into subcutaneous tissues can cause severe necrosis and subcutaneous calcifications. Never give Calcium through an UAC; it may be given through an UVC if the tip of the UVC is definitely placed in the inferior vena cava. *IV calcium solutions are incompatible with sodium bicarbonate, hence calcium carbonate will precipitate. Infusion by means of the umbilical vein may result in hepatic necrosis if the catheter is lodged in a branch of portal vein. *If the ionized calcium level drops to 1mmol/L or less (>1,500gm) or 0.8 mmol/L or less (< 1,500gm), a continuous IV calcium infusion may be commenced. (either through the TPN or IV fluids) - a dose of 40-50mg/kg/day of elemental calcium is typical. (4 to 5 ml/kg/day 10% Calcium Gluconate)

*To prevent the onset of hypocalcemia for newborns complicated by cardiovascular compromise (e.g., severe respiratory distress syndrome, asphyxia, septic shock, PPHN), it is essential to start a continuous calcium infusion, by means of a central catheter, to maintain an ionized calcium 1-1.4 mmol/L (<1,500 gm) or 1.2 - 1.5 mmol/L (>1,500gm).
* Emergency calcium therapy for active seizures or profound cardiac failure thought to be associated with severe hypocalcemia consists of 100-200 mg/kg (or 1-2 ml/kg) of 10% calcium gluconate (9-18 mg of elemental calcium/kg) by IV infusion over 10-15 minutes. *After normocalcemia is achieved, a step wise reduction of IV calcium may help to prevent rebound hypocalcemia: 8ml of 10% calcium gluconate/kg/day for the first day, 4ml/kg/day next day and half again and then discontinue. Alternatively, if infants can tolerate oral fluids, calcium gluconate can be given orally at the same doses (divided into 4-6 doses) after initial correction. (may not be practical in sick infants because oral calcium can stimulate bowel movements).*If hypocalcemia is associated with **hypomagnesemia** (serum Mg below 0.6mmol/L or <1.5mg/dL), Mg sulphate 50% solution (500mg or 4mEq/mL) 0.2ml/kg IV or IM (may cause local tissue necrosis) should be given and repeated after 12-24 hrs. Serum Mg should be obtained before each dose. *Commonly calcium therapy is required for 2-3 days, because most causes of hypocalcemia in the neonate are transient.

---

*   *Pearl/Peril/Pitfall : Prophylactic Measure for Late-Onset Neonatal Hypocalcemia: Preterm < 32 wks, Sick IDM, Severe asphyxia 40 mg/kg/day for 3 days(4ml/kg/day of 10% Calcium gluconate)IV or oral if can tolerate per oral• Treatment is for 72 hours• Continuous infusion is better than bolus • Symptomatic babies: treatment is 48 hrs continuous infusion In case the hypocalcemia does not correct by the above by, 72 hours, then investigate for causes of late hypocalcemia*

TABLE 1 — Causes of neonatal hypocalcemia

Early-onset Hypocalcemia (< 48 hr of age)
Prematurity
Perinatal distress/asphyxia
Infants of diabetic mothers
Intrauterine growth restriction

Late-onset Hypocalcemia (> 3–7 days of age)
- **Increased phosphate load**
  Cow's milk, advanced renal insufficiency
- **Hypomagnesemia**
- **Vitamin D deficiency**
  Maternal vitamin D deficiency
  Malabsorption
  Renal insufficiency
  Hepatobiliary disease
- **PTH resistance**
  Transient neonatal pseudohypoparathyroidism
- **Hypoparathyroidism**
  Primary
  Hypoplasia, aplasia of parathyroid glands. - (Di George's syndrome), CATCH 22 syndrome (Cardiac anomaly, Abnormal facies, Thymic aplasia, Cleft palate, Hypocalcemia with deletion on chromosome 22)
  Activating mutations of the calcium sensing receptor (CSR)
  <u>Secondary</u>
  Maternal hyperparathyroidism
- **Metabolic syndromes**
  Kenny-caffey syndrome.
  Long-chain fatty acyl CoA dehydrogenase deficiency
  Kearns-Sayre syndrome

- **Iatrogenic**
  Citrated blood products
  Lipid infusions
  Bicarbonate therapy
  Diuretics (loop diuretics)
  Glucocorticosteroids
  Phosphate therapy
  Alkalosis
  Phototherapy

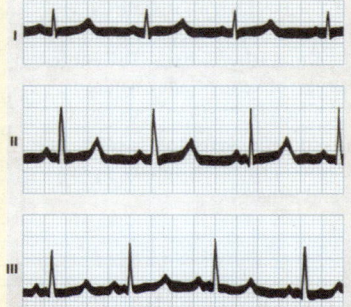

Long QT interval with normal T waves Prolongation of the ST segment with little shift from the baseline

For Neonatal Hypomagnesemia and Neonatal Hypermagnesemia-
Refer to Appendix-I: Neonatal Pearls of Wisdom to Remember!!!
Page 1121

TABLE 2 — Etiology of hypocalcemia related to pth

* Transient/ physiologic (neonatal)	* Pseudohypoparathyroidism
	* Renal failure
* Hypopara-thyroidism	* Liver disease/malabsorption
	* Vitamin D deficiency
* Hypomagnesemia	* Drugs: furosemide, aminoglycoside, cimetidine
* Pancreatitis	* Heparin, theophylline
	* Alkalosis
	* Cardiopulmonary bypass
	* Fat embolism
	* Sepsis
	* Blood transfusion

Etiology of hypocalcemia in the neonatal period

Prenatal (maternal factors)	Perinatal	Postnatal
* Vitamin D deficiency	* Perinatal stress	* Postnatal stress
* Hyperpara-thyroidism	* Hypoxia/ anoxia	* RDS
* Physiologic ↑ PTH (diabetes)	* Prematurity. IUGR	* Sepsis/Shock
		* NAHCO3 infusion
		* Post transfusion

Transient or late onset Neonatal (3-10 d age)

* physiologically underactive PTH glands are unable to respond to high phosphate diet

* high phosphate decreases serum calcium through calcium phosphate deposits

Etiology of hypocalcemia related to other factors

Hypomag-nesemia	Hyperphos-phatemia	Vitamin D deficiency
* Decreased intake	* Increased intake	
* Increased intracellular uptake	* Cell lysis	
* Renal and / or GI loss	* Renal failure and/or ↓PTH	

TABLE 3 — Medicolegal pitfalls : Neonatal hypocalcemia

*Intravenous infusion with calcium-containing solutions can cause severe tissue necrosis. This can cause contractures and may require skin grafting. Integrity of the intravenous site should be ascertained before administering calcium through a peripheral vein. *Necrosis of liver can occur after calcium infusion through an umbilical vein catheter placed in a branch of the portal vein. The position of all umbilical vein catheters must be confirmed radiologically before infusing calcium-containing solutions. *Rapid infusion of calcium-containing solutions through arterial lines can cause arterial spasm and, if administered via an umbilical artery catheter, intestinal necrosis.

TABLE 4 — Differential diagnosis : Neonatal hypocalcemia

Hypernatremia, Hyponatremia, Hypoglycemia, Aseptic Meningitis, Hypomagnesemia, Bacterial Meningitis, Neonatal Sepsis Hypoparathyroidism, Intracranial bleeding, Narcotic withdrawal, Pseudohypoparathyroidism, Malabsorption Syndromes, Rickets, osteomalacia, or rachitis (i.e., vitamin D deficiency), Hyperphosphatemia, Hypoalbuminemia , Renal failure, Anoxia, Metabolic disease affecting vitamin D, seizures.

* *Pearl/Peril/Pitfall :* <u>*Fast Facts about Calcium:*</u> *1) Plasma Calcium concentration falls by 0.8 mg/dL or 0.2 mmol/L for every 1g/dL fall in the Plasma Albumin concentration. 2) PTH levels: PTH is decreased in hypoparathyroidism. *Urine calcium/creatinine ratio: Ratio > 0.2 is suggestive of hypoparathyroidism.*

Mechanisms for the development of neonatal hypocalcemia

Agent	Problem	Clinical association
Ca (Calcium)	Decreased intake or absorption	Prematurity; malabsorption syndrome
Ca2+ (Ionized Calcium)	Increased Ca complex	Chelating agent (e.g. citrated blood for exchange transfusion, long-chain free fatty acid)
Mg (Magnesium)	Decreased tissue store or absorption	Maternal hypomagnesemia; specific Mg malabsorption
PO4 (Phosphate)	Increased	Endogenous and exogenous (e.g. dietary, enema) phosphate loading
pH	Increased	Respiratory or metabolic alkalosis (i.e. shifts Ca from ionized to protein-bound fraction)
Parathyroid Hormone	Decreased production	Maternal hyperparathyroidism; hypoparathyroidism; DiGeorge syndrome; Hypomagnesemia
Calcitonin	Increased	Infant of diabetic mother, birth asphyxia, prematurity
1,25-dihydroxy vitamin D	Decreased end-organ responsiveness	Prematurity

Adapted from Koo WWK, Tsang RC. Calcium and magnesium homeostasis. In: Avery GB, Fletcher MA, MacDonald MGJB, eds. Neonatology: Pathophysiotherapy and Management of the Newborn. 4th ed. Philadelphia: J.B. Lippincott Company, 1994:592.

Although total serum calcium levels are often measured and reported, ionized calcium is the active and physiologically important component. Total calcium level includes both the ionized fraction and the bound fraction. The ionized calcium level is affected by the albumin level, blood pH, serum phosphate, serum magnesium, and serum bicarbonate and may be reduced by exogenous factors that may bind calcium, such as citrate from transfused blood or free fatty acids from total parenteral nutrition (TPN). At a physiologic pH of 7.4, 40% of total calcium is bound to albumin; 10% is complexed with bicarbonate, phosphate, or citrate; and the remaining 50% is free ionized calcium. The normal range for ionized calcium is 1-1.25 mmol/L (4-5 mg/dL).

The concentration of calcium in the serum is critical to many important biologic functions, including the following:*Calcium messenger system by which extracellular messengers regulate cell function *Activation of several cellular enzyme cascades *Smooth muscle and myocardial contraction *Nerve impulse conduction *Secretory activity of exocrine glands

Hypocalcemia manifests as CNS irritability and poor muscular contractility. Low calcium levels decrease the threshold of excitation of neurons, causing them to have repetitive responses to a single stimulus. Because neuronal excitability occurs in both sensory and motor nerves, hypocalcemia produces a wide range of peripheral and CNS effects, including paresthesias, tetany (i.e., contraction of hands, arms, feet, larynx, bronchioles), seizures, and even psychiatric changes in children. Tetany is not caused by increased excitability of the muscles. Muscle excitability is depressed because hypocalcemia impedes acetylcholine release at neuromuscular junctions and, therefore, inhibits muscle contraction. However, the increase in neuronal excitability overrides the inhibition of muscle contraction. Cardiac function may also be impaired because of poor muscle contractility.

KEY POINTS FOR CLINICAL PRACTICE:

1. Hypocalcemia is defined as a total serum calcium concentration of less than 2.1 mmol/L (8.5 mg/dL) in children, less than 2 mmol/L (8 mg/dL) in term neonates, and less than 1.75 mmol/L (7 mg/dL) in preterm neonates.

2. Based on onset, Neonatal hypocalcemia has been classified as either early or late, although the distinction may not be clear-cut. **Early-onset Neonatal hypocalcemia** typically occurs during the first few days of life, with the lowest concentrations of serum calcium being reached at 24–48 hrs of age, whereas late-onset Neonatal hypocalcemia occurs towards the end of the first week of life.The diagnosis of hypocalcemia is based on the determination of ionized or total calcium. In addition to a history and physical examination, certain data are useful when there is not a clear cause for hypocalcemia: serum total calcium, ionized calcium, P, Mg, Glucose and ABG analysis. ECG determination of prolonged QTc (>0.40 second) suggests hypocalcemia. *Although the QTc cannot precisely predict the ionized calcium concentration, may be useful to monitor the response to calcium therapy.*

3. Early-onset Neonatal hypocalcemia represents an exaggeration of the physiologic decrease in serum calcium during the first few days of life, and is most commonly associated with prematurity, birth asphyxia, obstetric trauma, fetal distress, maternal insulin-dependent diabetes, gestational exposure to anticonvulsants, maternal hyperparathyroidism, and Neonatal illness-respiratory distress syndrome, cerebral injury, hypoglycemia, and sepsis.

4. **Late-onset hypocalcemia**, which is less frequent than early-onset hypocalcemia, is most commonly associated with administration of relatively high phosphate-containing formula feeds(Whole cow's milk has 7 times the phosphate load of breast milk (956 vs 140 mg/L in breast milk), disturbed maternal vitamin D metabolism, intestinal malabsorption of calcium, hypomagnesemia, and hypoparathyroidism. Formula with a high phosphorus content and a low calcium-to-phosphorus ratio of 1.3-1.4 (breast milk contains 150mg phosphorus/L and has a Ca-to-P ratio of 2.3), immaturity of parathyroid, vitamin D and renal function causing phosphorus retention, hyperphosphotemia, and inability to support calcium levels are the important factors in the pathogenesis of late-onset hypocalcemia.Refractory Hypocalcemia demands further investigations to pinpoint the rare underlying etiology.

5. *For emergency treatment of hypocalcemic crisis with seizures, tetany, or apnea, 1–2 ml/kg of a 10% calcium gluconate should be administered over 5–10 minutes intravenously (in 1:1 dilution in 5% dextrose).* Careful observation of the infant and of the infusion site is essential, and the infusion should be discontinued if there is bradycardia or when the desired clinical result is obtained. If necessary, IV calcium therapy may be repeated 3 or 4 times in 24hrs to help control acute symptoms. If hypocalcemia is associated with hypomagnesemia (serum Mg below 0.6mmol/L [1.5mg/dL] Mg sulphate 50% solution 0.2ml/kg IM should be given and repeated after 12–24 hrs.

REFERENCES & FURTHER READING : 1) Newfield RS. Recombinant PTH for initial management of neonatal hypocalcemia. *N Engl J Med.* Apr 19 2007;356(16):1687-8. **2)** Gertner JM. Disorders of calcium and phosphorus homeostasis. *Pediatr Clin North Am.* Dec 1990;37(6):1441-65.**3)** Singh J, Moghal N, Pearce SH, Cheetham T. The investigation of hypocalcaemia and rickets. *Arch Dis Child.* May 2003;88(5):403-7.**4)** Mimouni F, Tsang RC. Neonatal hypocalcemia: to treat or not to treat? (A review). *J Am Coll Nutr.* Oct 1994;13(5):408-15. **5)** Guise TA, Mundy GR. Clinical review 69: Evaluation of hypocalcemia in children and adults. *J Clin Endocrinol Metab.* May 1995;80(5):1473-8.

78 Neonatal Hypercalcemia

@ *Symptomatic (or serum calcium >14mg/dL) hypercalcemia requires emergency medical treatment with volume expansion using normal saline (10-20ml/kg over 15-30 minutes), followed by furosemide 1mg/ kg/dose IV q6-8 hr to induce calciuria.*

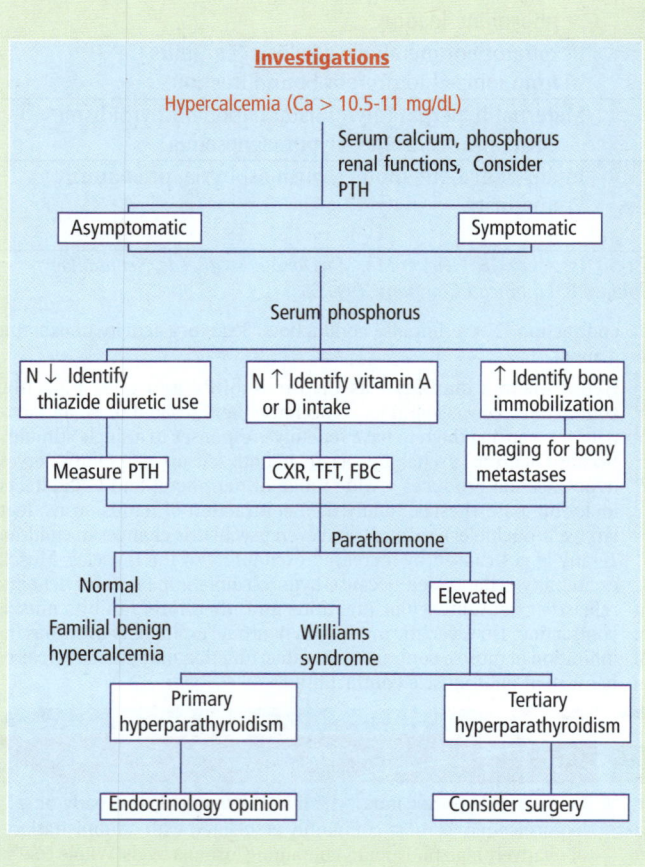

Investigations

Hypercalcemia (Ca > 10.5-11 mg/dL)

Serum calcium, phosphorus renal functions, Consider PTH

Asymptomatic — Symptomatic

Serum phosphorus

- N ↓ Identify thiazide diuretic use
- N ↑ Identify vitamin A or D intake
- ↑ Identify bone immobilization

Measure PTH — CXR, TFT, FBC — Imaging for bony metastases

Parathormone

Normal — Elevated

Familial benign hypercalcemia — Williams syndrome

Primary hyperparathyroidism — Tertiary hyperparathyroidism

Endocrinology opinion — Consider surgery

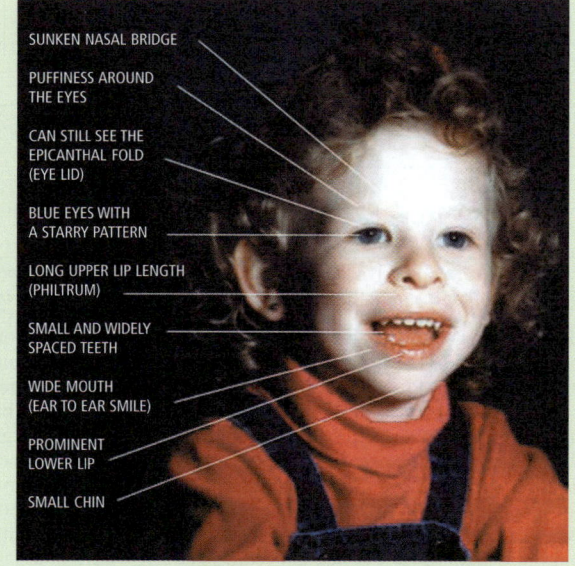

SUNKEN NASAL BRIDGE
PUFFINESS AROUND THE EYES
CAN STILL SEE THE EPICANTHAL FOLD (EYE LID)
BLUE EYES WITH A STARRY PATTERN
LONG UPPER LIP LENGTH (PHILTRUM)
SMALL AND WIDELY SPACED TEETH
WIDE MOUTH (EAR TO EAR SMILE)
PROMINENT LOWER LIP
SMALL CHIN

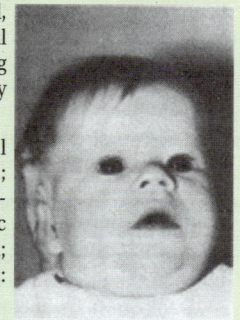

Williams syndrome: broad forehead, short palpebral fissures, low nasal bridge, anteverted nostrils, long filtrum, full cheeks, and relatively large and often downturned mouth

* Gene map locus 7q11.23 Clinical features: mental retardation; peculiar cognitive profile; dysmorphic facies; supravalvular aortic stenosis; infantile hypercalcemia; growth deficiency] [Inheritance: most cases are sporadic]

REVIEW OF CLINICAL PROBLEMS

1. What are the important aspects of History in evaluating Neonatal Hypercalcemia?
   Ans: Refer to the Evaluation-Decision-Action Plan/Algorithm to diagnose and manage Neonatal Hypercalcemia.

2. What Imaging modalities are useful in evaluating Neonatal Hypercalcemia?
   Ans: Refer to the Section "Imaging -Hypercalcemia' of the Chapter.

3. How do you manage Symptomatic Neonatal Hypercalcemia ?
   Ans : Refer to the Evaluation-Decision-Action Plan/Algorithm to diagnose and manage Neonatal Hypercalcemia.

4. Mention the Important associations of Hyperparathyroidism in Neonates.
   Ans : Refer to the "No.5" of the "BIRD`S EYE VIEW/OVERVIEW/ SYNOPSIS"of the Chapter.

5. What are the well recognized complications of Neonatal Hypercalcemia?
   Ans : Refer to the "No.6" of the "BIRD`S EYE VIEW/OVERVIEW/ SYNOPSIS"of the Chapter.

LEARNING OBJECTIVES

After completing this article, readers will be able to:

1. Anticipate Hypercalcemia in the High-Risk Neonates and monitor Serum Calcium levels regularly.

2. Treat acute symptomatic Hypercalemia promptly by stabilizing the ABCDs, if Hypertension/seizures occur.

3. Differentiate various causes of Neonatal Hypercalcemia.

4. Monitor for Complications of Neonatal Hypercalcemia.

5. Counsel the parents about the prognosis of different types of Neonatal Hypercalcemia depending on the underlying etiology.

* *Pearl/Peril/Pitfall : The use of Ca and P supplementation alone is inappropriate for the treatment or prevention of osteopenia with or without fractures or rickets, since bone growth requires protein and multiple other nutrients for matrix formation and mineralization.*

BIRD'S EYE VIEW/OVERVIEW/SYNOPSIS

1. Neonatal hypercalcemia (total serum calcium level >11mg/dL and serum ionized calcium level >1.5mmol/L) occurs in association with several clinical entities listed in Table 1. It may be asymptomatic and discovered incidentally during routine screening or may manifest dramatically, especially if serum calcium is >14mg/dL and be life threatening, requiring immediate medical intervention.

2. Normally, the parathyroid-renal axis prevents hypercalcemia via inhibition of parathyroid hormone secretion (PTH) and 1, 25 $(OH)_2$ D synthesis, which reduces calcium absorption from the intestine, mobilization from bone, and reabsorption from the kidney. An elevated serum calcium, therefore, indicates that there is inappropriate calcium influx to the ECF from one or more of these pools. Because the kidney is the principal organ for calcium balance, hypercalcemia usually means the renal capacity to excrete calcium has been exceeded. In fact, abnormalities in distal tubular resorption are involved in the pathogenesis of many hypercalcemic conditions (e.g., hyperparathyroidism) and renal impairment frequently accompanies many hypercalcemic syndromes.

3. Idiopathic Neonatal/infantile hypercalcemia occurs in the constellation of Williams Syndrome (hypercalcemia, supravalvular aortic stenosis or other cardiac anomalies, "elfin" facies, psychomotor retardation) and in a familial pattern without the Williams phenotype. Increased calcium absorption has been demonstrated, but enhanced vitamin D sensitivity and impaired calcitonin secretion are proposed as possible mechanisms. A low-calcium diet usually controls hypercalcemia. The hypercalcemia rarely persists beyond several months and resolves spontaneously, but hypercalciuria may persist. In children with idiopathic infantile hypercalcemia without Williams phenotype, serum calcium levels remain elevated for a prolonged period which may be an exaggerated increase in serum 1, 25 $(OH)_2$ D in response to exogenous PTH administration. Therefore, in addition to dietary calcium restriction and avoidance of vitamin D, glucocorticoid therapy to reduce GIT calcium absorption is sometimes warranted.

4. Hypercalcemia should be sought in all infants with subcutaneous fat necrosis (*v.i*) which is frequently associated with a history of difficult delivery, trauma, hypothermia, or asphyxia. Laboratory evaluation shows high blood 1, 25 $(OH)_2$ D levels and usually normal phosphorus and alkaline phosphatase. Granulomatous (macrophage) inflammation of the necrotic lesions causes unregulated 1, 25 $(OH)_2$ D synthesis and induces hypercalcemia. It may persist for days to weeks and treatment consists of glucocorticoids, intravascular volume expansion, furosemide diuresis, and a low-calcium, low-vitamin D diet.

5. Hyperparathyroidism is an important cause of hypercalcemia in the Neonates, associated with a) maternal hypoparathyroidism b) multiple endocrine adenomatosis c) renal tubular acidosis with secondary hyperparathyroidism d) familial (benign) hypercalcemic hypocalciuria e) homozygous severe familial primary hyperparathyroidism.

6. Hypercalcemia may present dramatically with poor feeding, vomiting, constipation, polyuria, hypertension, tachypnea, dyspnea, hypotonia, lethargy, and seizures. Extraskeletal calcifications in the kidney, skin, subcutaneous tissue, falx cerebri, arteries, myocardium, lung, or gastric mucosa. Nephrocalcinosis, nephrolithiasis, diffuse bone undermineralization and osteitis fibrosa are well-recognized hypercalcemic complications.

7. *The Evaluation-Decision-Action-Plan/Algorithm* describes the essential aspects of the diagnosis and management of hypercalcemia in Neonates. The clinical history, serum and urine mineral levels of phosphorus, and the urinary calcium: creatinine ratio ($[U_{Ca}/U_{Cr}]$) should suggest a likely diagnosis. **a)** **Very** elevated serum calcium level (> 15 mg/dL) usually indicates primary hyperparathyroidism or, in VLBW infants, phosphate depletion. **b)** **Low** serum phosphorus level indicates phosphate depletion, hyperparathyroidism, or familial hypocalciuric hypercalcemia. **c)** **Very** low U_{Ca}/U_{Cr} suggests familial hypocalciuric hypercalcemia. Specific serum hormone levels (PTH, 25(OH)D, 1,25(OH)$_2$D) will confirm the diagnostic impression in cases where obvious manipulations of diet/TPN are not apparent. A level very low serum alkaline phosphatase activity suggests hypophosphatasia (confirmed by increased urinary phosphoethanolamine level). Radiography of hand/wrist may suggest hyperparathyroidism (demineralization, subperiosteal resorption) or hypervitaminosis D (submetaphyseal rarefaction). ECG sign of Hypercalcemia - Shortened QT interval may not be obvious even in patients who have deranged plasma concentrations that are clinically significant.

8. Symptomatic (or serum calcium >14mg/dL) hypercalcemia requires emergency medical treatment with volume expansion using normal saline (10–20 ml/kg over 15–30 minutes), followed by furosemide 1mg/kg/dose IV q6–8 hr to induce calciuria. When severe hypercalcemia is associated with hypophosphatemia, 30–50 mg/kg/day oral or IV phosphorus as a phosphate salt may be given. The goal of phosphate therapy is to maintain serum phosphorus levels around 3–5mg/dL. The oral route is preferable because of the potential for serious complications with IV phosphate treatment. In more severe and resistant cases, prednisone 2 mg/kg/day may be added, to suppress intestinal calcium absorption and increase renal excretion; glucocorticoids are ineffective in hyperparathyroidism.

9. Low-calcium, low-vitamin D diets are an effective adjunctive therapy for hypervitaminosis A or B, subcutaneous fat necrosis, and Williams Syndrome. Calcitonin or biphosphonates use as antihypercalcemic agents is of limited experience in Newborns.

10. Parathyroidectomy with autologous reimplantation may be indicated for severe persistent Neonatal hyperparathyroidism.

Subcutaneous fat necrosis (SCFN): A rare disorder that occurs in term or post-term neonates. Typical lesions include smooth, erythematous, subcutaneous nodules or plaques located on the cheeks, shoulders, back, buttocks, or thighs. Lesions usually develop within the first weeks of life and regress over the following weeks without treatment. Although the etiology of SCFN is unclear, subcutaneous stress e.g. hypoxemia, leading to adipocyte necrosis may be a critical step in the pathogenesis. Maternal predisposing risk factors include gestational diabetes mellitus, preeclampsia, cocaine use, smoking, calcium channel blocker use during pregnancy, and thrombosis. Hypothermia, hypoxemia, infections and cutaneous trauma during delivery, as well as newborn anemia and tendency for thrombosis are also implicated. Generally benign, complications like hypercalcemia. thrombocytopenia, hypoglycemia, hypertriglyceridemia, lactic acidosis, anemia, and hyperferritinemia associated with it may cause long-term sequelae and even mortality. The most serious metabolic complication, hypercalcemia, may take up to 6 months to develop after the onset of skin lesions. Common clinical presentation ranges from no symptoms, to lethargy, hypotonia, vomiting, polyuria, dehydration, and failure to thrive. In severe cases, metastatic calcification occurs in kidneys, myocardium, major vessels, liver, and brain, compromising these organs' function and even causing organ failure. Management includes i.v. normal saline, loop diuretics, steroids, and low calcium and vitamin D formula. Cases resistant to these measures can be treated with corticosteroids, bisphosphonate, and calcitonin. Serum calcium level needs to be monitored at least biweekly for up to 6 months or until resolution of fat necrosis. Included in the differential diagnosis for SCFN is sclerema neonatum (SN), a panniculitis affecting ill preterm neonates in the first week of life. Unlike SCFN, which is local and self limiting, SN rapidly generalizes and carries a grave prognosis with 75 percent mortality. On histology, the two entities differ in their level of inflammation. Sclerema neonatum typically shows minimal inflammation on biopsy, with normal epidermis and dermis and needle-shaped crystals arranged radially in adipocytes. Subcutaneous fat necrosis characteristically has needle-like clefts in histiocytes, although they may be seen less commonly in adipocytes as well. The crystals are formed from triglycerides of stearic and palmitic acids, which make up the panniculus of the neonate.

Pearl/Peril/Pitfall: Subcutaneous fat necrosis, which manifests in neonate as violaceous plaques or nodules overlying fatty areas, can lead to life-threatening hypercalcemia at age 1-6 months. It is likely mediated by prostaglandin E (PGE) or due to macrophage production of 1,25-dihydroxyvitamin D. Treatment includes corticosteroids and symptomatic support of patient

THE EVALUATION-DECISION-ACTION-ALGORITHM FOR THE DIAGNOSIS AND MANAGEMENT OF *HYPERCALCEMIA IN NEONATES*

SUBJECTIVE FINDINGS

Hx of maternal/familial hypercalcemia or hypocalcemia, parathyroid disorders, nephrocalcinosis or familial hypocalciuric hypercalcemia, High maternal or neonatal supplies of vitamin D and/or A Drugs during pregnancy (thiazide, lithium), Traumatic birth
Hx of TPN adjustment by removing the phosphorus due to concern about excess sodium/potassium intake, in VLBW infants.
Hx of feeding difficulties or poor linear growth.
Hx of evidence for hyperparathyroidism - hypotonia, encephalopathy, constipation, poor feeding, vomiting, polyuria, anemia, hepato-splenomegaly and extraskeletal calcifications, including nephrocalcinosis.

OBJECTIVE FINDINGS

Assess ABCs, disability (altered sensorium, seizures, focal neurodeficits), vitals, BP, Urine output & capillary refil time.
Look for hypertension, subcutaneous fat necrosis, dehydration, growth restriction hypotonia, encephalopathy and seizures.
Search for features suggestive of Williams Syndrome - "elfin" facies, supravalvular aortic stenosis and psychomotor retardation.
Identify the features, such as craniotabes, fractures (hyperparathyroidism), bone dysplasia (hypophosphatasia) and evidence of hyperthyroidism. Take Eye specialist opinion

INVESTIGATIONS

Blood Calcium, ionized calcium, phosphorus, alkaline phosphatase, specific hormone levels - PTH, 25(OH)D, 1,25(OH)$_2$D, FBC with differential and platelets, serum creatinine, ABG analysis and electrolytes.
Urine Urinary calcium : creatinine ratio, creatinine, cyclic adenosine monophosphate
Radiography of hand/wrist. *Imaging* Refer to the section on Imaging & Hypercalcemia
Echocardiogram if Williams Syndrome is suspected, to identify cardiac lesions. ECG-QT interval
FISH for the detection of elastin locus deletions (7q 11.23) for Williams Syndrome

---

HYPERCALCEMIA IN NEONATES

Asymptomatic or Mild
(Serum Calcium <14mg/dL)

* Restrict dietary calcium, eliminate vitamin D supplements and limit the exposure to sunlight.

Symptomatic or Severe
(Serum Calcium >14mg/dL)

* Volume expansion with NS 10-20ml/kg over 15-30 minutes, followed by IV furosemide 1-2 mg/kg/dose q6-8hr to excrete calcium. For neonates, specifically, Oski recommends 5% dextrose (D5) in one-half isotonic sodium chloride solution with 30 mEq/L potassium chloride at 2 times the maintenance dose along with 2-3 mg/kg/d furosemide and adequate phosphate supplementation to maintain normal levels. Strongly consider surgical correction of primary hyperparathyroidism
* Give phosphorus supplements @ 30-50mg/kg/day of oral phosphorus, when severe hypercalcemia is associated with hypophosphatemia, to maintain serum phosphorus levels in a range of 3-5mg/dL
* Add prednisone, 2mg/kg/day, in more severe and resistant cases, to suppress intestinal calcium absorption and to increase renal excretion. (Glucocorticoids are effective in hypervitaminosis A and D and subcutaneous fat necrosis, but are ineffective in hyperparathyroidism).
* Parathyroidectomy with autologous reimplantation - indicated for severe persistent neonatal hyperparathyroidism.
* Peritoneal or hemodialysis with a low-Ca dialysate may be considered in severely symptomatic patients refractory to medical therapy.

TABLE 1   Causes of neonatal hypercalcemia

Iatrogenic (calcium salts)
Parathyroid hyperfunction
  Neonatal severe primary hyperparathyroidism (NSPHP)
    Ca^{2+}-sensing receptor mutation homozygosity
  Familial (benign) hypercalcemic hypocalciuria (FBHH)
    Ca^{2+}-sensing receptor mutation heterozygosity
  Neonatal hyperparathyroidism associated with multiple endocrine adenomatosis
  Renal tubular acidosis with secondary hyper-parathyroidism
  Neonatal hyperparathyroidism secondary to maternal hypoparathyroidism
Williams syndrome (elastin gene locus deletions)
Idiopathic infantile hypercalcemia ("Lightwood-type")
Phosphate depletion
Hypervitaminosis D
  Vitamin D intoxication
  Subcutaneous fat necrosis
Blue diaper syndrome
Hypercalcemia associated with skeletal dysplasias
  Infantile hypophosphatasia
  Jansen metaphyseal chondrodysplasia (activating mutations of the PTH/PTHrP receptor)
Other causes
  Tumor-associated hypercalcemia, Congenital lactase deficiency, Acute adrenal insufficiency, Hypervitaminosis A, Thyrotoxicosis, Prolonged ECMO

ECMO, extracorporeal membrane oxygenation; PTH, parathyroid hormone; PTHrp, parathyroid hormone-related protein. **Blue diaper syndrome** is a selective defect in the intestinal transport of tryptophan. The diagnosis is confirmed by analyzing urine indoles.

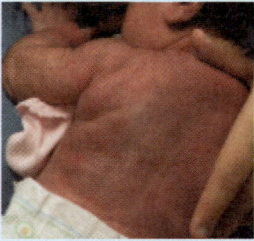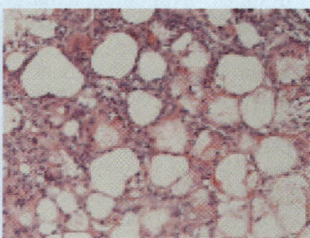

Subcutaneous fat necrosis on the back and shoulders of the newborn: showing small, firm, erythematous plaque. **Biopsy** shows a lobular panniculitis with an infiltrate of mixed inflammatory cells. Needle shaped clefts, in radial array, are seen in adipocytes and giant cells. *c/f* Sclerema neonatum typically shows minimal inflammation on biopsy, with normal epidermis and dermis and needle-shaped crystals arranged radially in adipocytes. **Courtesy:** Wenhong Zhou et al, Dermatology Online Journal

---

* ***Pearl/Peril/Pitfall :*** *Hypercalcemia: Patients in whom the diagnosis should not be missed are those with a dangerous underlying etiology, neonates, and children with ECG changes, altered mental status, dehydration, or renal failure.*

IMAGING STUDIES & HYPERCALCEMIA

* Plain radiography may reveal demineralization, pathologic fractures, bone cysts, and bony metastases.

* Renal imaging, ultrasonography, CT urography, or intravenous pyelography (IVP) may reveal evidence of calcifications or stones.

* Perform ultrasonography of the parathyroid glands if hyperplasia or adenoma is a primary diagnosis. A sestamibi nuclear scan may be helpful in locating a parathyroid adenoma.

* Other imaging tests may be necessary to exclude alternative diagnoses (e.g., gallstone vs hypercalcemic pancreatitis) or to find a primary or associated malignancy if the laboratory tests or history produce suspicious findings.

TABLE 2 Normal laboratory values

All laboratories have different reference-range values, examples of which are listed in the table below.

Laboratory Test	Reference Range	Normal Response to Increased Calcium
Serum calcium	8.5-10.2 mg/dL	NA
Ionized calcium	1-1.3 mmol/L*	NA
PTH (intact)	10-55 pg/mL	Decrease
Serum phosphate	Age-dependent	Increase
1,25-dihydroxyvitamin D	36-108 pmol/L	Decrease
Alkaline phosphatase	68-217 U/L	Normal
Urine calcium	4 mg/kg/d	Increase
Urine Ca/Cr ratio	See note†	Increase
Urine cAMP‡	<5 mol	Decrease

Note that 1 mmol/L equals 4 mg/dL. †In infants younger than 7 months, the reference range is less than 0.86; in infants aged 7-18 months, the reference range is less than 0.6. By age 6-7 years, the adult reference range of less than 0.21 is reached. ‡The urine cAMP level generally parallels the PTH level.

KEY POINTS FOR CLINICAL PRACTICE:

1. Neonates with Hypercalcemia may be asymptomatic or may have vomiting, hypotonia, hypertension, or seizures. Neonatal primary hyperparathyroidism can begin as soon as the parathyroid glands, functional in the first trimester of pregnancy, become hyperplastic. Infants have malaise, constipation, and vomiting; serum calcium and parathyroid hormone (PTH) concentrations are elevated, and serum phosphate concentration is decreased. Aminoaciduria occurs. Rarefaction of bones leads to easier fracturing. Rehydration with isotonic sodium chloride solution and forced diuresis with furosemide are urgently required, as well as administration of subcutaneous calcitonin. Definitive treatment is performed by means of surgical resection, often with reimplantation of a small amount of tissue into a more accessible ectopic site (e.g., forearm).

2. Secondary hyperparathyroidism is a Neonatal response to maternal hypocalcemia with similar symptoms to primary hyperparathyroidism, except that the child undergoes a progression from hypocalcemia to normocalcemia to hypercalcemia quickly after birth. PTH is generally elevated. During the first few months, the parathyroid glands and skeletal lesions normalize; therefore, only symptomatic nonsurgical treatment is required.

3. Subcutaneous fat necrosis, which manifests in Neonate as violaceous plaques or nodules overlying fatty areas, can lead to life-threatening hypercalcemia at age 1-6 months. It is likely mediated by prostaglandin E (PGE) or due to macrophage production of 1,25-dihydroxyvitamin D. Treatment includes corticosteroids and symptomatic support of patient. Idiopathic infantile hypercalcemia is a poorly understood disorder possibly related to non–malignancy-associated PTH-related protein (PTHrP), which spontaneously resolves by age 12 months.

4. Williams syndrome, which is associated with a deletion of elastin genes on chromosome 7, occurs as transient Neonatal hypercalcemia, perhaps secondary to increased sensitivity to vitamin D. The syndrome is associated with characteristic elfin facies, mental retardation, and supravalvar aortic stenosis. Generally, hypercalcemia is symptomatic, with poor feeding and constipation, and spontaneously remits by age 9-18 months. Treatment is a dietary restriction of calcium to 100 mg/d and limited vitamin D intake. Hydrocortisone at 10-25 mg/kg/d or calcitonin is sometimes helpful.

5. In more severe and resistant cases, prednisone 2mg/kg/day may be added, to suppress intestinal calcium absorption and increase renal excretion; glucocorticoids are ineffective in hyperparathyroidism.

REFERENCES & FURTHER READING : 1) Hsu YH, Chen HI. Acute respiratory distress syndrome associated with hypercalcemia without parathyroid disorders. *Chin J Physiol.* Dec 2008;51(6):414-8. 2) Nelson Text Book of Pediatrics, 18th edition 3) Cheung M. Drugs used in paediatric bone and calcium disorders. *Endocr Dev.* 2009;16:218-232 4) Mundy GR. *Calcium Homeostasis: Hypercalcemia and Hypocalcemia.* 1989 5) Rodd C, Goodyer P. Hypercalcemia of the newborn: etiology, evaluation, and management. *Pediatr Nephrol.* Aug 1999;13(6):542-7.

* *Pearl/Peril/Pitfall : When testing for hypervitaminosis D, assess the serum levels of 25-hydroxyvitamin D because they reflect the intake of vitamin D better than levels of 1,25-dihydroxyvitamin D. The exception to this is when 1,25-dihydroxyvitamin D is overingested or overproduced.*

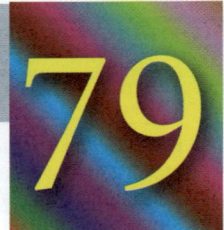

79 Osteopenia (Metabolic Bone Disease) of Prematurity

@ *Metabolic Bone disease (MBD)usually occurs in premature neonates but may also occur in full term neonates. The clinical manifestations of MBD are: hypotonia, enlarged fontanel, widened cranial sutures, frontal bossing and rachitic rosary. Radiological findings include prominent costochondral junctions and epiphyseal flaring and widening. The triad of rachitic rosary, low 25-hydroxyvitamin D and high alkaline phosphatase is diagnostic of neonatal rickets.*

The transition from fetal to Neonatal calcium metabolism. Ca, calcium; CT, calcitonin; 1,25(OH)$_2$D, 1,25-dihydroxycholecalciferol; PTH, parathyroid hormone.

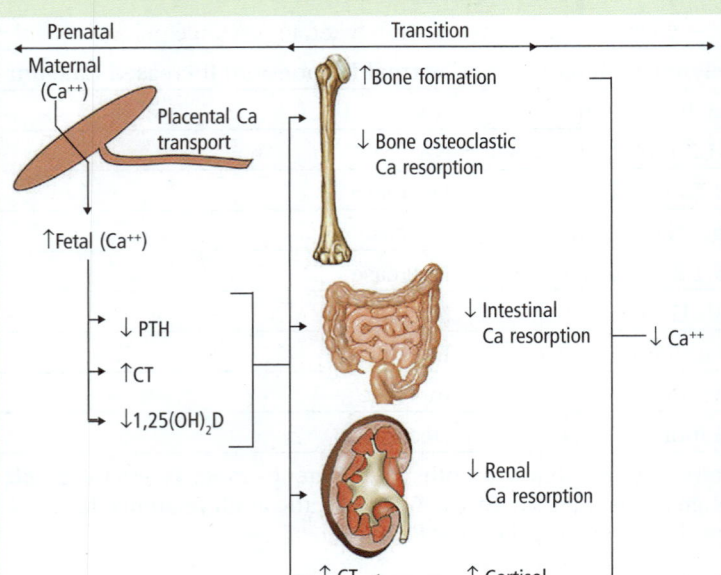

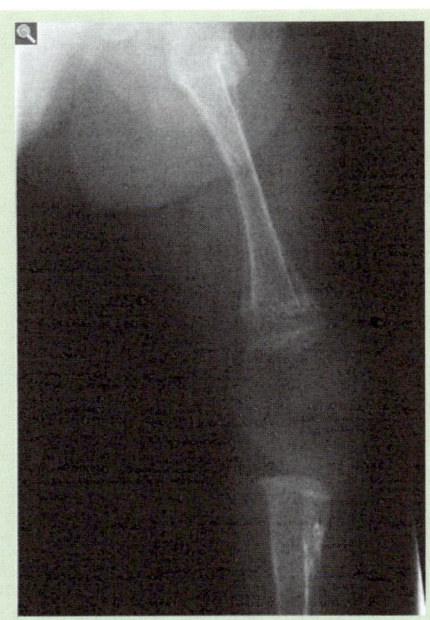

Severe osteoporosis associated with prematurity and bronchopulmonary dysplasia

*Diagnosis of metabolic bone disease: *biochemical tests of osteopenia of prematurity are not definitive *serum Phosphate: suspicious if <1.5, likely if < 1.1 mmol/L *the alkaline phosphatase (ALP) is more elevated than usual for preterm babies. Levels above 600 or 800 IU/L are quoted. However, the ALP only rises high if there is bone turnover. If the condition is very severe the ALP may not be very high *the calcium level may be normal, elevated or even low *a bone x-ray will show very poor mineralization and as the infants grow can show changes of rickets or fractures *an abnormal Ca^{++} : PO$_4$ ratio in the urine. In normal infants it is less than 1.0 (both measured in mmol/L)) .Risk Factors: *<30 weeks gestation.*<1000g birthweight. *Delayed establishment of full enteral feeds/prolonged parenteral nutrition. *Enteral feeds with low mineral content or bioavailability (unfortified EBM, standard term formula). *Chronic use of medications that increase mineral excretion (diuretics, dexamethasone, sodium bicarbonate). *Cholestatic jaundice.*

REVIEW OF CLINICAL PROBLEMS

1. What is the usual pathogenesis of Osteopenia of Prematurity ?
   Ans: Refer to the "No.2" of the "BIRD`S EYE VIEW/ OVERVIEW/SYNOPSIS' of the Chapter.

2. Mention the risk factors involved in causing Osteopenia of Prematurity.
   Ans: Refer to the Table 1 of the Chapter.

3. Describe the radiological signs of Osteopenia of Prematurity.
   Ans: Refer to the "No.6" of the "BIRD`S EYE VIEW/ OVERVIEW/SYNOPSIS" of the Chapter.

4. How do you interpret the Lab. data in different types of rickets?
   Ans: Refer to the Table 2 of the Chapter.

5. Discuss the management guidelines for Osteopenia of Prematurity.
   Ans: Refer to the Evaluation-Decision-Action Plan/Algorithm to diagnose and manage a Neonate with Osteopenia of Prematurity.

LEARNING OBJECTIVES

After completing this article, readers will be able to:

1. Anticipate and Search for Osteopenia of Prematurity (Metabolic Bone Disease) in Premature babies associated with High-Risk Factors.

2. Interpret biochemical and Radiological features of Osteopenia of Prematurity.

3. Consider other Nutritional deficiencies, such as Zinc and treat them appropriately.

4. Manage Osteopenia of Prematurity adequately and Ensure proper follow-up of the affected infants for ongoing bone disease, until biochemical & Radiological normalcy achieved.

5. Provide good parental support and communication regarding prognosis and preventative measures.

Pearl/Peril/Pitfall : Hypercalcemia can cause symptoms at levels as low as 12 mg/dL and consistently causes symptoms at 14 mg/ dL.Neonates may be asymptomatic or may have vomiting, hypotonia, hypertension, or seizures.If hypercalcemia is symptomatic, the differential diagnosis rests heavily on the predominating symptom.

BIRD'S EYE VIEW/OVERVIEW/SYNOPSIS

1. Osteopenia (postnatal bone mineralization that is inadequate to fully mineralize bones) commonly occurs in VLBW infants. It develops during the first postnatal weeks. Signs of rickets, such as epiphyseal dysplasia and skeletal deformities usually become evident after 6 weeks postnatal age or by term-corrected gestational age. The risk of bone disease is greatest for the sickest, most premature infants. It occurs in >30% of infants weighing <1,500gm., and in >50% of those weighing <1,000gm. The incidence and severity of this disorder is inversely related to gestational age, birth weight, and directly related to postnatal morbidity. Eg., BPD, NEC, or TPN and delay in achieving full enteral feeds.

2. The pathogenesis of osteopenia of prematurity differs from nutritional rickets seen in older children in two aspects: **a)** Vitamin D deficiency is typically not the primary cause in most cases, and **b)** There is no hyperparathyroidism. The most frequent cause is inadequate availability of phosphorus and calcium which may occur in sick preterm infants on prolonged parenteral fluids, unsupplemented human milk, formulas not designed for use in preterm infants, long-term steroid use, furosemide therapy and with renal phosphorus wasting secondary to renal tubular acidosis, Fanconi Syndrome, or X-linked hypophosphatemic rickets. Demands for rapid growth in the third trimester are met by intrauterine mineral accretion rates of approximately 120mg of calcium and 60mg of phosphorus/kg/day. Poor mineral intake and absorption after birth result in undermineralized new and remodeled bone.

3. Vitamin D deficiency as a primary cause of osteopenia of prematurity is far less frequent than mineral deficiency. Maternal vitamin D deficiency can cause congenital rickets. Inadequate vitamin D intake or absorption produces nutritional rickets but this is not the primary cause of osteopenia in preterm infants. Hepatobiliary rickets results largely from vitamin D malabsorption. Chronic renal failure, chronic use of phenytoin and phenobarbitone (which increase 25(OH)D metabolism) and hereditary pseudo-vitamin D deficiency: type I (abnormality or absence of 1-a-hydroxylase activity) or type II (tissue resistance to 1, 25-$(OH)_2$ D). **Refer to Table 1** for various risk factors involved in the development of osteopenia of prematurity.

4. The disorder is clinically silent during early stages of bone demineralization. Later clinical signs include respiratory insufficiency or failure to wean from a ventilator, hypotonia, pain on handling due to pathologic fractures, decreased linear growth with sustained head growth, frontal bossing, enlarged anterior fontanel and widened cranial sutures, craniotabes (posterior flattening of the skull), "rachitic rosary" (swelling of costochondral junctions), Harrison grooves (indentation of the ribs at the diaphragmatic insertions), and enlargement of wrists, knees, and ankles. Some infants may manifest with crying on handling, and decreased movement of the affected limb (pseudo-paralysis).

5. There are no diagnostic biochemical tests. Serum calcium values may remain normal until late in the course. Low serum phosphate concentrations (3 mg/dL) have low sensitivity but high specificity. Low concentrations of inorganic phosphate (1.8 mmol/L [5.5 mg%], with elevated alkaline phosphatase (900 international units/L) may be more sensitive (100%) and specific (70%) for diagnosing inadequate intake and low bone mineral density. Concentrations of 1, 25 (OH)2 vitamin Dare elevated, but routine vitamin D and PTH measurements are not required for diagnosis. Serum alkaline phosphatase (ALP) is the sum of three isoforms (liver, intestine, and bone), of which the bone isoform contributes about 90%. Elevated values are seen with normal growth, healing rickets, fractures, or copper deficiency; low concentrations are seen with zinc deficiency, malnutrition, and congenital hypophosphatasia. ALP is correlated negatively with phosphate concentrations; high values (1,200 units/L) have been associated with short stature in childhood. Isolated elevations in ALP without calcium and phosphorus abnormalities may occur with transient hyperphosphatasia of infancy. C-terminal procollagen peptide or propeptide of type I collagen correlates with collagen turnover and bone formation in preterm infants. Osteocalcin may be elevated but is of limited utility in preterm infants.

6. Diagnosis has been based on criteria that include clinical signs, radiologic findings, biochemical markers, measurement of BMC, and postmortem analysis of bone structure and mineral composition. No screening tests are sensitive and specific. Radiographic signs include widening of epiphyseal growth plates, cupping, fraying, and rarefaction of the metaphyses and subperiosteal new-bone formation, osteopenia of skull, spine, scapula and ribs. A loss of upto 40% of bone mineralization can occur without radiographic changes. Chest films may show osteopenia and sometimes rachitic changes. Wrist or knee films can be useful. Measurement of bone mineral content (BMC) by Dual-Energy X-ray Absorptiometry (DEXA) or ultrasonography remains investigational. Quantitative ultrasonography, using broadband ultrasonographic measurement, speed of sound (SOS), or bone transmission time, has been employed to assess bone density. Ultrasonography offers several advantages. It measures both qualitative and quantitative bone properties, such as bone mineralization and cortical thickness, elasticity, and microarchitecture.

7. *The Evaluation-Decision-Action-Plan/Algorithm* describes the essential aspects of the diagnosis and management of the osteopenia of prematurity. The AAP recommends 140-160mg of calcium/100 cal., 95-108mg of phosphorus/100cal., and 400IU/day of vitamin D regarding mineral intake enterally in preterm infants. This can be done by a) fortification of human milk b) preterm formula (calcium 120-140mg/dL and phosphorus 60-70mg/dL).

8. The adequacy of mineral intake is indicated by 1) increase in serum P to normal levels (>1.8 mmol/L, or >5.5mg/dL) 2) decrease in serum alkaline phosphatase activity 3) increase in P concentration to >1.2mg/dL in a spot urine sample. Absence of phosphate in urine suggests inadequate mineral intake 4) resolution of hypercalciuria (calcium/creatinine ratio < 2 in a spot urine sample).

9. When the ELBW infants are on TPN, it is recommended that intakes for preterm infants should be-50–60 mg of calcium/dL, 40-45mg of P/dL and 160 IU of vitamin D/dL upto a maximum of 400 IU/day. It may not be possible to deliver calcium and phosphorus in amounts necessary to match intrauterine accretion.

10. Human milk fortification or the use of premature infant formula can usually be discontinued after the infant weighs approximately 2,000 to 2,200 g and tolerating enteral feeds well. It may be continued longer for infants who are fluid restricted or have a markedly elevated alkaline phosphatase activity or radiologic evidence of osteopenia.

Stimulation: In preterm infants, mechanical stimulation by passive exercises to improve bone mineralization has yielded conflicting outcomes. Improved BMC, bone length, and bone area have been reported in individual studies. Current evidence does not justify the standard use of physical activity programs in preterm infants.

Minimizing Furosemide and Corticosteroid Use: Changing to the use of thiazide diuretics, although of theoretical advantage, has not been shown to prevent osteopenia.

Malabsorption: Infants at risk of cholestasis and malabsorption may benefit from additional supplementation with fat-soluble vitamins and use of specialized formula to facilitate fat absorption.

Pearl/Peril/Pitfall : With the current practice of early discharge of preterm infants from neonatal units, it is possible that some nutritional rickets could be diagnosed after hospital discharge; if there are associated fractures, it may be misdiagnosed as child abuse, as is the case with fractures from other medical illnesses.

THE EVALUATION-DECISION-ACTION-PLAN/ALGORITHM FOR THE DIAGNOSIS AND MANAGEMENT OF OSTEOPENIA (METABOLIC BONE DISEASE) OF PREMATURITY

SUBJECTIVE FINDINGS

Hx of VLBW/ELBW infants and the use of fluid restriction, prolonged TPN, long-term steroid use.

Hx of a fracture noticed by the parents or incidentally on x-rays taken for other purposes.

Hx of rapid increase in alkaline phosphatase.

Hx of symptoms such as hypotonia, crying on handling, and decreased movement of the affected limb (pseudoparalysis).*Clinically, MBD manifests between 6 and 12 weeks of age and may remain asymptomatic for weeks until overt rickets or fractures develop.*

OBJECTIVE FINDINGS

Look for respiratory insufficiency with late onset, failure to wean from the ventilator, enlarged AF, craniotabes (posterior flattening of the skull with "ping-pong ball" sign), frontal bossing, decreased linear growth with disproportionate large head, costochondral beading (rachitic rosary), Harrison Grooves (indentation of the ribs at the diaphragmatic insertions), and enlargement of wrists, knees, and ankles.

Assess for hypotonia and pain on handling due to pathologic fractures.

INVESTIGATIONS

Blood serum calcium, phosphorus, alkaline phosphatase, serum $25(OH)D_3$ if liver disease is suspected.
Reserve measurement of serum $1, 25$-$(OH)_2 D$ or parathyroid hormone for complicated / refractory cases. *Imaging* X-rays of wrists, knees, skull, scapula, ribs. Quantitative ultrasonography, using broadband ultrasonographic measurement, speed of sound (SOS), or bone transmission time
Dual-Energy X-ray Absorptiometry (DEXA) for assessing bone mineralization (accurate, reproducible and have low radiation exposure).

OSTEOPENIA (METABOLIC BONE DISEASE) OF PREMATURITY

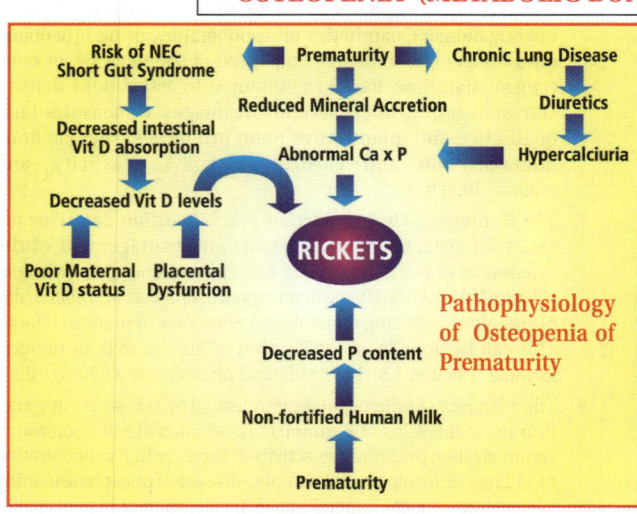

Pathophysiology of Osteopenia of Prematurity

Conversion factors (One of the problems with this area is that the USA, and many books, work in mg, while Australia and Europe use mmol/L)
Ca^{++} 1 mmol = 40 mg, PO_4^- 1 mmol = 31 mg
Mg^{++} 1 mmol = 24 mg

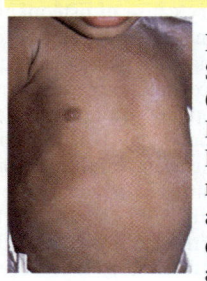
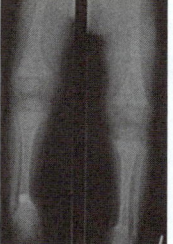

Later Clinical Signs of Osteopeniaof Prematurity [A] Rachitic rosary noted few days after birth; [B] epiphyseal flaring and widening

Guidelines for the treatment of osteopenia of prematurity

1. Initiate early enteral feeding in VLBW infants, to enhance the establishment of full-volume enteral intake, leading to increased calcium accumulation and decreased osteopenia.
2. Prefer mineral-fortified human milk or "premature" formulas for preterm infants weighing <1,800 to 2,000 g and for Small for gestational infants weighing <1,800 to 2,000 ; their use at 120 kcal/kg/day can prevent and treat metabolic bone disease of prematurity.
3. Avoid elemental mineral supplementation of human milk (less desirable than the use of prepackaged fortifiers containing calcium and phosphorus) because of concern over medication error and potential hyperosmolarity. Also avoid addition of both calcium and phosphorus supplements directly to milk or formula as it may lead to the formation of a precipitate.
4. Discourage the long-term use of specialized formulas in VLBW infants, including soy and elemental formulas , as it may increase the risk for osteopenia.
5. Provide smaller amounts of calcium (usually up to 40 mg of elemental calcium/kg/day) and/or sodium or potassium phosphate (usually up to 20 mg of elemental phosphorus) in babies with radiologic evidence or rickets not responding to fortified human milk or premature formula. (in babies whose birth weights were <800 g or who had a prolonged hospital course including long-term Total parenteral nutrition (TPN), fluid restrictions, or bronchopulmonary dysplasia.)
6. Ensure adequate vitamin D stores by an intake of 150 to 400 IU/day (Max. 800 IU/day). Try dihydrotachysterol (DHT) or calcitriol for the rare defects in vitamin D metabolism
7. Prefer thiazide diuretic to Furosemide to prevent latter induced renal calcium wasting. Minimize steroid use.
8. Avoid nonessential handling and vigorous chest physiotherapy in preterm infants with severely undermineralized bones. Institute daily passive physical activity (range of motion, 5-10 minutes) to enhance both growth and bone mineralization.
9. Monitor serum calcium, phosphorus, and alkaline phosphate levels periodically, in infants receiving human milk with added fortifier or premature formula.
10. Discontinue Human milk fortification or the use of premature infant formula after the infant weighs approximately 2,000 to 2,200 g and tolerating enteral feeds well. (may be continued longer for infants who are fluid restricted or have a markedly elevated alkaline phosphatase activity or radiologic evidence of osteopenia.)
11. Use a transitional formula at hospital discharge, in infants with birth weight <1,500 g that has calcium and phosphorus contents midrange between that of preterm formulas and formulas designed for fullterm infants.
12. Provide vitamin D supplementation based an American Academy of Pediatrics (AAP) guidelines for fullterm infants (200 IU/day) or higher (many would recommend 400 IU/day for this population) for LBW infants discharged from hospital and who are on unsupplemented mother's milk are at risk for persistent osteopenia. Arrange a follow-up measurement of serum phosphorus and alkaline phosphatase activity at 4 to 8 weeks postdischarge.

Pearl/Peril/Pitfall: The primary underlying cause in preterm infants appears to be mineral deficiency, particularly Ca and P, which was demonstrated more than 2 decades ago and confirmed by many investigators; vitamin D deficiency is of secondary importance.

TABLE 1   Etiological factors osteopenia of prematurity

Deficiency of Calcium and Phosphorus is the principal cause
a. Diets low in mineral content predispose preterm newborns to metabolic bone disease.
b. Unsupplemented human milk.
c. Long-term use of parenteral nutrition.
d. Formulas not designed for use in preterm infants (e.g. full-term, elemental, soy-based).
e. Furosemide therapy causes renal calcium wasting. It is not likely the principal contributor to osteopenia however for most preterm infants.
f. Long-term steroid use.
g. Renal phosphorus wasting.

Vitamin D deficiency-Far less frequent cause of OPP
a. Maternal vitamin D deficiency can cause Congenital rickets.
b. Inadequate vitamin D intake or absorption produces nutritional rickets but this is not the primary cause of osteopenia in preterm infants.
c. Hepatobiliary rickets results largely from vitamin D malabsorption.
d. Chronic renal failure (renal osteodystrophy).
e. Chronic use of phenytoin or phenobarbital increases 25 (OH) D metabolism.
f. Hereditary Pseudo-vitamin D deficiency: type I (abnormality or absence of 1-a-hydroxylase activity) or type II (tissue resistance to 1, 25-$(OH)_2$ D_3).

TABLE 2   Laboratory data in different types of rickets

	Phosphate Deficiency (Rickets of Prematurity)	Calcium Deficiency	Vitamin D Deficiency
Calcium	N,↑	↓↓	↓↓
Phosphorus	↓↓	↓	↓
Alkaline Phosphatase	↑↑	↑↑	↑↑
Calcidiol 25 (OH) D	N	N	↓↓
Calcitriol 1,25 $(OH)_2$ D	↑	↑	N↑
Parathormone	N,↓	↑	↑

KEY POINTS FOR CLINICAL PRACTICE:

1. Most postnatal cases of MBD and osteopenia are diagnosed incidentally during the radiographic investigation of skeletal complications such as fractures, or nonskeletal problems such as respiratory illness. Radiographic features such as generalized bone demineralization and widening, cupping, and fraying of the distal metaphyses confirm the presence of osteopenia and rickets.

2. Serial biochemical changes commonly include persistently low serum inorganic phosphate, elevated serum alkaline phosphatase activity more than five times the normal adult upper limit, and elevation of other bone turnover markers in serum and urine. Serum Ca is usually normal except in late severe nutritional vitamin D deficiency rickets.

3. The **Risk Factors for Osteopenia of Prematurity include:** *<30 weeks gestation. *<1000g birthweight. *Delayed establishment of full enteral feeds/prolonged parenteral nutrition. *Enteral feeds with low mineral content or bioavailability (unfortified EBM, standard term formula). *Chronic use of medications that increase mineral excretion (diuretics, dexamethasone, sodium bicarbonate). *Cholestatic jaundice.

4. In preterm infants receiving infant formulae with lower Ca and P content (compared to the preterm infant formulae currently available), normal vitamin D status as indicated by serum 25-OHD concentrations has been reported in infants who received daily supplements of 400 to 2,000 IU vitamin D. However, for enterally fed preterm infants given adequate volumes of high Ca-, high P-, and vitamin D-fortified preterm infant formula, or human milk fortified with commercial human milk fortifiers, a daily total intake of 400 IU vitamin D should be adequate; additional vitamin D supplementation may be excessive. **Extra phosphate supplementation.** If a baby needs supplementation then a solution of phosphate 0.8 mmol/ml is made by dissolving one tablet of Sandoz phosphate in 20 ml water. Begin supplementation with 3 mmol/kg/day in 3 divided doses (i.e. 1 mmol/kg/dose tds). The dose should then be titrated against the blood phosphate level over the following weeks. Stop phosphate supplements if the serum phosphate is >1.8 mmol/L.

5. Biochemical monitoring of nutritional rickets includes measurement of serum Ca, P, and alkaline phosphatase and avoiding hypercalciuria (less than 0.15 mmol [6 mg/kg/day], especially in human-milk-fed preterm infants) at 1- to 2-week intervals until stable and then at 1- to 2-month intervals. Bone turnover markers, IPTH, vitamin D metabolites, and any other abnormal biochemical parameters should be monitored at 1- to 2-month intervals. All biochemical monitoring should be continued until standard radiographs show completion of healing and remodelling of skeletal defects. Radiographs of the wrists and fracture site(s) should be taken at 2- to 4-month intervals.

REFERENCES & FURTHER READING : **1)** 1 Groh-Wargo S, Thompson M, Hovasi Cox J, Hartline J. Nutritional Care for High-Risk Newborns, 3rd Edition, Illinois, Precept Press, 2000 **2)** Koo WWK, Steichen JJ. Osteopenia and rickets of prematurity. In: Polin R, Fox W, eds. *Fetal and neonatal physiology*, 2nd ed. Philadelphia: WB Saunders, 1998:2335-2349.**3)** Koo WWK. Laboratory assessment of nutritional metabolic bone disease in infants. *Clin Biochem* 1996;29:429-438.**4)** Koo WWK, Sherman R, Succop P, et al. Fractures and rickets in very low birth weight infants: conservative management and outcome. *J Pediatr Orthop* 1989;9:326- **5)** Lyon AJ, McIntosh N, Wheeler K, et al. Radiological rickets in extremely low birthweight infants. *Pediatr Radiol* 1987;17:56-58. 330.

*** Pearl/Peril/Pitfall :** *Skeletal manifestations of disturbed mineral metabolism in infants usually present as osteopenia or rachitic changes on standard radiographs. True fetal or congenital rickets is rare.*

Metabolic Acidosis in Neonates

80

@ *"The presence of metabolic acidosis in the Newborn should be suspected from the clinical presentation and the history of predisposing conditions, including perinatal depression, respiratory distress, blood or volume loss, sepsis, and congenital heart disease associated with poor systemic perfusion or cyanosis."*

METABOLIC ACIDOSIS CAN BE IDENTIFIED IN *6 STEPS* USING INFORMATION FROM THE ABG ANALYSIS AND SERUM ELECTROLYTE CONCENTRATIONS!

Step - I

Determine whether the patient is alkalemic or acidemic on the basis of arterial pH (normal, 7.35-7.45). Blood with pH less than 7.35 is acidemic.

Step - II

Determine whether the primary disorder causing acidemia is metabolic or respiratory. The normal serum level of HCO_3-is 18 to 22 mEq/L. A serum HCO_3-level of less than 18 mEq/L indicates a primary metabolic acidosis.

Step - III

Determine whether gap or nongap acidosis is present. The anion gap is calculated as Na^+- $(HCO_3^- + Cl^-)$, and the normal anion gap is **8-16.** (Average 12±4)

Step - IV

Determine whether the respiratory system is appropriately compensating by excreting and lowering CO_2 (normal PCO_2, 36-44 mm Hg). **Winter formula,** $(HCO_3^- \times 1.5) + 8 \pm 2 = pCO_2$, is an accurate way to calculate the expected pCO_2. The last 2 digits of the pH should roughly equal the pCO_2. (the "quick look" method).

Step - V

Determine whether another metabolic disorder is present in patients with a high anion gap acidosis. Calculate the delta anion gap acidosis. Calculate the delta anion gap as follows: delta gap = (anion gap - 10) / (24 - HCO_3^-). The normal value is between 1 and 1.6. A low delta gap suggests the presence of a concomitant nongap acidosis, whereas a delta gap greater than 1.6 suggests the presence of a concomitant metabolic alkalosis.

Step - VI

Calculate the Urinary Anion gap (urine Na^+ + urine K^+ - urine Cl^-), an indirect measure of ammonium secretion; helpful to differentiate GIT loss from renal pathologies as a cause of normal plasma anion gap acidosis. A negative urinary anion gap (<0) suggests appropriate renal excretion of ammonium and points to GIT loss as the cause of the acidosis. Conversely, a zero/positive anion gap suggests impaired ammonia production and a renal etiology for the acidosis.

REVIEW OF CLINICAL PROBLEMS

1. What are the common causes of Metabolic acidosis with increased anion gap in Neonates?
   Ans: Refer to the "No.5" of the "BIRD`S EYE VIEW/OVERVIEW/ SYNOPSIS"of the Chapter.

2. How does Metabolic acidosis manifest clinically?
   Ans: Refer to the "No.6" of the "BIRD`S EYE VIEW/OVERVIEW/ SYNOPSIS"of the Chapter.

3. How do you assess and evaluate a sick Neonate for suspected Metabolic acidosis?.
   Ans: Refer to the Evaluation-Decision-Action Plan/Algorithm to diagnose & manage a Neonate with Metabolic acidosis.

4. How do you manage a sick Neonate with severe Metabolic acidosis?
   Ans: Refer to the Evaluation-Decision-Action Plan/Algorithm to diagnose & manage a Neonate with Metabolic acidosis.

5. Mention the specific therapies to address the underlying cause of Metabolic acidosis?
   Ans: Refer to the Evaluation-Decision-Action Plan/Algorithm to diagnose & manage a Neonate with Metabolic acidosis.

LEARNING OBJECTIVES

After completing this article, readers will be able to:

1. Suspect Metabolic acidosis in any sick Neonate and to discern the cause from the history and physical examination.

2. Confirm Metabolic acidosis by ABG Analysis and to calculate the Anion gap to differentiate the 2 groups of metabolic acidosis.

3. Perform specific laboratory evaluation of electrolytes, renal function, lactate, serum and urine amino acids, depending on the diagnosis that is suspected clinically.

4. Assess the severity of Metabolic acidosis and responsiveness of the underlying pathologic process to clinical management.

5. Use temporizing buffer therapy judiciously aimed at increasing the arterial pH to 7.25-7.30 in cases of severe acidosis.

* ***Pearl/Peril/Pitfall :*** **Syndrome of late metabolic acidosis of prematurity:** First described in the 1960s, otherwise healthy premature infants at several weeks of age demonstrated mild to moderate increased anion gap acidosis and decreased growth. All the infants were receiving high-protein cow's milk formula, and they demonstrated higher net acid excretion compared with controls. Because of the use of special premature infant formulas and changes in regular formulas with decreased casein-to-whey ratios and lower fixed acid loads, Late metabolic acidosis is being rarely seen.

BIRD'S EYE VIEW/OVERVIEW/SYNOPSIS

1. Metabolic acidosis is a common problem, particularly in the critically ill Newborn, and it occurs when the drop in pH is caused by the accumulation of acid other than H_2CO_3 by the ECF, resulting in loss of available HCO_3^-, or by the direct loss of HCO_3^- from body fluids. Metabolic acidosis is most commonly caused by inadequate tissue perfusion (shock) caused by hypovolemia, decreased cardiac output, or sepsis. Hypoxemia caused by lung or heart disease often contributes to the tissue hypoxia and resulting lactic acidosis seen with hypoperfusion states. Sepsis in the Newborn, as in older individuals, may cause metabolic acidosis by decreasing perfusion ("cold shock") and by interfering with cellular aerobic metabolism ("warm shock"). To compensate for metabolic acidosis, term Neonates and infants will attempt to lower PCO_2 by hyperventilating; however, compensation is usually not complete, that is, not to a pH of 7.4. A suggested guideline for the desired PCO_2 is as follows: The last two digits of the pH should equal the expected PCO_2. If the actual PCO_2 is much higher than expected, there may also be a respiratory acidosis. Premature infants are often not able to compensate for a metabolic acidosis by hyperventilation and respiratory alkalosis. After treating the primary underlying problem causing the metabolic acidosis, slow infusions of sodium bicarbonate are often given *Essentially, Metabolic Acidosis is a decrease in the buffering capacity (Sodium Bicarbonate) of the blood, which results from three basic mechanisms;* a)loss of bicarbonate from the body (GI tract - diarrhea or Kidneys - proximal RTA) b)impaired ability to excrete acid by the kidney (distal RTA) c)addition of acid to the body (*exogenous* - poisoning by salicylate/ ethylene glycol *endogenous* - inborn errors of metabolism/lactic acidosis/ketoacidosis.

2. **Metabolic Acidosis - Pathophysiology**
   HCO_3^- loss or $\downarrow H^+$ load $\rightarrow \downarrow HCO_3 \rightarrow$ metabolic acidosis compensation decreases the magnitude of the pH change but does not completely normalize the pH. Lungs - elimination of CO_2, full effect achieved by 12–24 h, Kidneys - production and secretion of NH_3 and excretion of titratable acids; full effect achieved by 5-7 days In a patient with an isolated metabolic acidosis, there is a predictable decrease in the blood CO_2 concentration; $PCO_2 = 1.5 \times (HCO_3^-) + 8 \pm 2$. A mixed acid - base disturbance is present if the respiratory compensation is not appropriate. If the PCO_2 is > predicted, then the child has a concurrent respiratory acidosis. A lower PCO_2 than predicted indicates a concurrent respiratory alkalosis or, less commonly , an isolated respiratory alkalosis. Because the appropriate respiratory compensation for a metabolic acidosis never normalizes the patient's pH, the presence of a normal pH & a low bicarbonate concentration only occurs if some degree of respiratory alkalosis is present. (*then differentiation is possible only by clinical history & physical examination*).

3. **Plasma anion gap** is the difference between the measured serum cations & the measured anions. It is also the difference between the unmeasured cations (e.g. K^+, Mg^{++}, Ca^{++}) and the unmeasured anions (eg. Albumin, Phosphate, Urate, Sulfate) **Sodium - (Chloride + Bicarbonate) = 8-16.** The plasma anion gap divides patients with metabolic acidosis into two diagnostic groups: normal anion gap or increased anion gap (**Refer to Table 1**). In clinical practice, although a serum anion gap value >16mEq/L is highly predictive of lactic acidosis and a value <8mEq/L is highly predictive of the absence of lactic acidosis, an anion gap value between 8 and 16mEq/L cannot be used to differentiate between lactic and nonlactic acidosis in the critically ill newborn. Therefore, the measurement of serum lactate is indicated when one suspects lactic acidosis and the anion gap is in the normal range.

4. A **normal anion gap metabolic acidosis** most commonly occurs in the Newborn as a result of bicarbonate loss from the ECF space through the kidneys/ the GIT. Hyperchloremia develops with the HCO_3^- loss because a proportionate rise in serum chloride concentration must occur to maintain the ionic balance or to correct the volume depletion in the ECF compartment. The most common cause of normal anion gap metabolic acidosis in the preterm newborn is a mild, developmentally regulated, proximal renal tubular acidosis with renal

HCO_3^- wasting. In infants with this disorder, the serum HCO_3^- usually stabilizes at 14–18 mEq/L in the early postnatal period. In proximal RTA there is low threshold for the reabsorption of bicarbonate; patients can acidify the urine only when plasma bicarbonate falls below the lowered renal threshold (15mEq/ L). In distal RTA, the kidney is unable to excrete an acid urine at any plasma bicarbonate concentration. Impaired distal tubular hydrogen ion excretion results in excessive urinary loss of both Potassium & Phosphorus, leading to hypokalemic acidosis.

5. An **increased anion gap metabolic acidosis** (**Refer to Table 1 and Figure 1**) in the Newborn is most commonly due to lactic acidosis secondary to tissue hypoxia, as seen in asphyxia, hypothermia, severe respiratory distress, sepsis, other severe neonatal illnesses. An increased anion gap metabolic acidosis occurs when there is an increase in unmeasured anions. For example lactate anions in lactic acidosis, ketoacids in diabetic ketoacidosis, phosphate, urate, and sulfate in renal failure, formate in methanol intoxication, glycolate in ethylene glycol intoxication, lactate & ketoacids in salicylate intoxication. In inborn errors of metabolism, the unmeasured anions depend on the specific etiology & may include ketoacids, lactate, and/ or other organic anions. In a few inborn errors of metabolism, the acidosis occurs without generation of unmeasured anions &, thus , the anion gap is normal (**Refer to Figure 1**).

6. **The clinical manifestations of the metabolic acidosis** are related to the degree of acidemia; children with appropriate respiratory compensation & less severe acidemia have fewer manifestations than those with a concomitant respiratory acidosis. *At a serum pH < 7.20, the cardiac contractility is impaired with an increased risk of cardiac arrhythmias, especially if predisposed by the presence of congenital heart disease or electrolyte disorders.* Severe acidemia also causes a)lethargy & coma b)worsening of pulmonary hypertension c)insulin resistance, increased protein degradation & reduced ATP synthesis d) increased serum potassium concentration by moving it from the ICF to ECF. e)Failure to thrive if the metabolic acidosis is chronic.

7. *The E-D-A Plan/Algorithm to diagnose & manage a Neonate with metabolic acidosis* summarizes the essential aspects of clinical & laboratory evaluation and management. The presence of metabolic acidosis in the Newborn should be suspected from the clinical presentation and the history of predisposing conditions, including perinatal depression, respiratory distress, blood or volume loss, sepsis, and congenital heart disease associated with poor systemic perfusion or cyanosis. Metabolic acidosis is confirmed by ABG analysis; specific laboratory evaluation of electrolytes, renal function, lactate, and serum and urine aminoacids may be undertaken, depending on the diagnosis that is suspected clinically.

8. *Repairing of the underlying disorder is the most effective therapeutic approach for children with a metabolic acidosis.* (e.g., insulin therapy in diabetic ketoacidosis, restoration of adequate perfusion in lactic acidosis). In children with RTA or chronic renal failure, long term base therapy is necessary. In children with acute renal failure & metabolic acidosis base therapy is necessary until their kidney's ability to excrete hydrogen normalizes.

9. *Sodium bicarbonate* is the most widely used buffer in the treatment of metabolic acidosis in the Neonatal period. The indications and contraindications and the potential disadvantages of sodium bicarbonate administration in acute metabolic acidosis are summarized in **Table 2**. *THAM (Tromethamine)* has more rapid intracellular buffering capability, direct lowering ability of PCO_2 levels, and it does not cause an increase in sodium load. It is the recommended buffer therapy in life-threatening situations of combined metabolic and respiratory acidosis.

10. *Peritoneal dialysis* is helpful in correcting metabolic acidosis due to renal insufficiency but it may not correct metabolic acidosis in patients with concomitant renal failure & lactic acidosis. **Hemodialysis** is helpful for correcting the metabolic acidosis due to methanol/ethylene glycol intoxication. **Carbicarb** corrects metabolic acidosis with less generation of CO_2, an advantage in patients with respiratory insufficiency.

Pearl/Peril/Pitfall : The adverse hemodynamic effects of a deteriorating metabolic acidosis are profound and, if untreated, can be life threatening. An increase in acidity causes pulmonary vasoconstriction and an increase in pulmonary hypertension. These developments can lead to Right ventricular failure. At an arterial pH <7.2, generalized myocardial depression eventually occurs. In arteriolar smooth muscle, a decrease in pH leads to systemic vasodilation, which can cause hypotension & circulatory failure. In patients with underlying lung disease, the burden imposed by the compensatory increase in minute ventilation will progress to respiratory muscle fatigue and failure.

THE EVALUATION-DECISION-ACTION-PLAN/ALGORITHM FOR THE DIAGNOSIS AND MANAGEMENT OF *METABOLIC ACIDOSIS IN NEONATES*

SUBJECTIVE FINDINGS

Hx of vomiting, diarrhea, failure to thrive, polyuria, fever, seizures.

Hx of predisposing factors such as perinatal depression, respiratory distress, blood or volume loss, sepsis, congenital heart disease with poor systemic perfusion/cyanosis, renal disease, diarrhea and vomiting, hypothermia, known hypoglycemic syndrome & inborn errors of metabolism, Neonatal Diabetes mellitus, toxin ingestion.

Hx of unexplained Neonatal deaths & metabolic disorders in the family.

OBJECTIVE FINDINGS

Assess ABCs, disability (altered sensorium, seizures, focal neurodeficits), vitals, BP, Urine output & capillary refil time.

Look for hyperventilation & Kussmaul breathing (deep rapid respirations) & smell for unusual body odors which may suggest inborn errors of metabolism.

Note signs consistent with respiratory distress, sepsis, congenital heart disease and CNS disorder (hypoxic-ischemic encephalopathy).

INVESTIGATIONS

Blood ABG analysis, electrolytes, chloride, BUN, creatinine, osmolality, ketones, glucose, culture, calcium, magnesium, FBC with differential & platelets, drug screen, LFTs.

Urine analysis, pH, ketones, reducing substances, electrolytes, drug screen, culture *others*-consider imaging, *Metabolic* plasma lactate, ammonia, serum amino acids, urine amino acids & organic acids ECG, Echocardiogram depending on the suspected underlying disease.

Calculate anion gap = $Na^+ - (HCO_3^- + Cl^-)$ *normal anion gap is 12mEq/l (range 8-16).*

Calculate serum osmolality = $2 \times (serum\ Na^+ + K^+) + (BUN / 2.8)$ or Urea/6 + (Blood glucose-mg/dL/18).

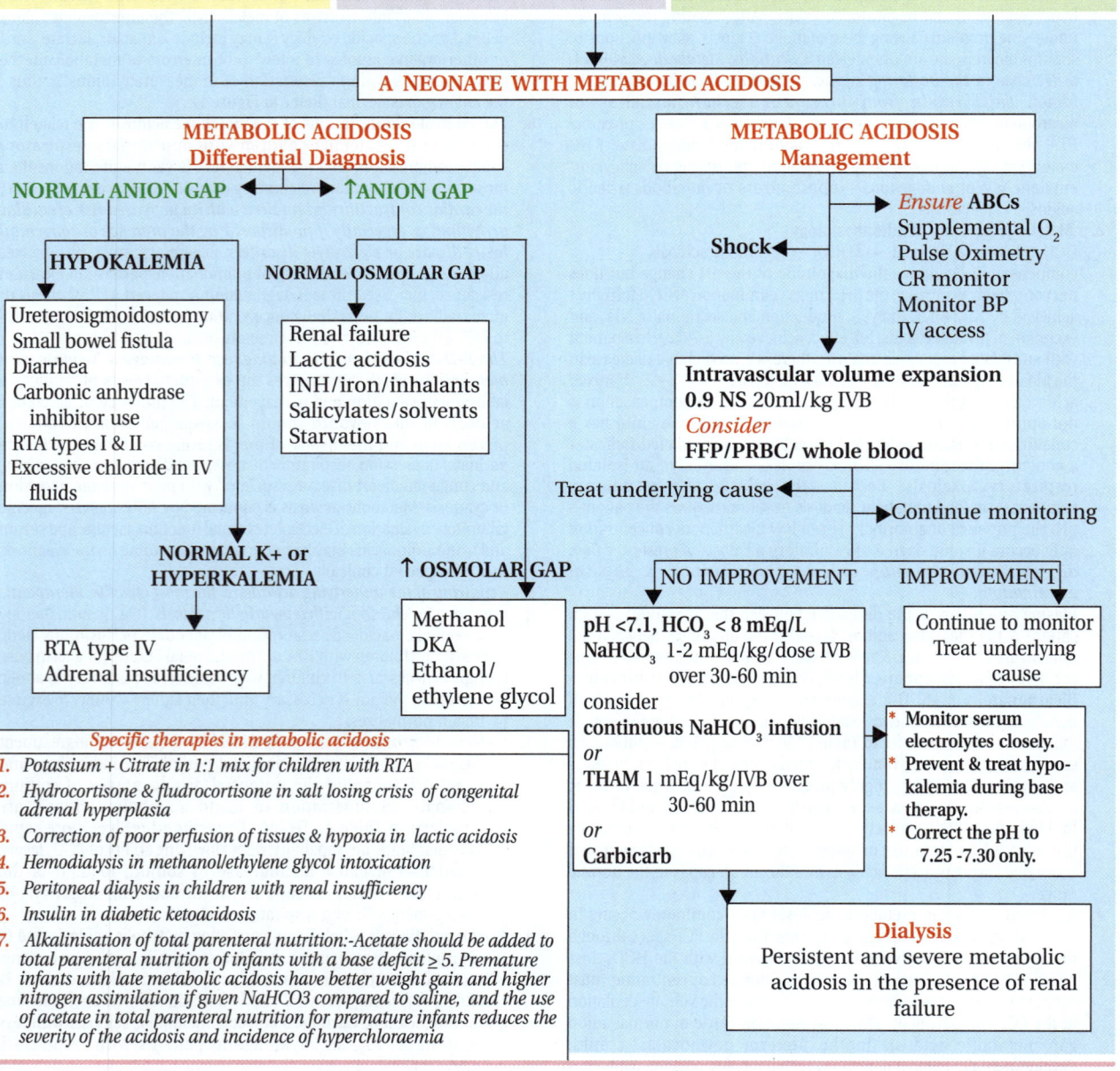

A NEONATE WITH METABOLIC ACIDOSIS

METABOLIC ACIDOSIS
Differential Diagnosis

NORMAL ANION GAP ⟷ ↑ANION GAP

HYPOKALEMIA

NORMAL OSMOLAR GAP

Ureterosigmoidostomy
Small bowel fistula
Diarrhea
Carbonic anhydrase inhibitor use
RTA types I & II
Excessive chloride in IV fluids

Renal failure
Lactic acidosis
INH/iron/inhalants
Salicylates/solvents
Starvation

NORMAL K+ or HYPERKALEMIA

↑ OSMOLAR GAP

RTA type IV
Adrenal insufficiency

Methanol
DKA
Ethanol/ ethylene glycol

METABOLIC ACIDOSIS
Management

Shock ←

Ensure ABCs
Supplemental O_2
Pulse Oximetry
CR monitor
Monitor BP
IV access

Intravascular volume expansion
0.9 NS 20ml/kg IVB
Consider
FFP/PRBC/ whole blood

Treat underlying cause ← → Continue monitoring

NO IMPROVEMENT   IMPROVEMENT

pH <7.1, HCO$_3$ < 8 mEq/L
NaHCO$_3$ 1-2 mEq/kg/dose IVB over 30-60 min
consider
continuous NaHCO$_3$ infusion
or
THAM 1 mEq/kg/IVB over 30-60 min
or
Carbicarb

Continue to monitor
Treat underlying cause

* **Monitor serum electrolytes closely.**
* **Prevent & treat hypokalemia during base therapy.**
* **Correct the pH to 7.25 -7.30 only.**

Dialysis
Persistent and severe metabolic acidosis in the presence of renal failure

Specific therapies in metabolic acidosis

1. *Potassium + Citrate in 1:1 mix for children with RTA*
2. *Hydrocortisone & fludrocortisone in salt losing crisis of congenital adrenal hyperplasia*
3. *Correction of poor perfusion of tissues & hypoxia in lactic acidosis*
4. *Hemodialysis in methanol/ethylene glycol intoxication*
5. *Peritoneal dialysis in children with renal insufficiency*
6. *Insulin in diabetic ketoacidosis*
7. *Alkalinisation of total parenteral nutrition:-Acetate should be added to total parenteral nutrition of infants with a base deficit ≥ 5. Premature infants with late metabolic acidosis have better weight gain and higher nitrogen assimilation if given NaHCO3 compared to saline, and the use of acetate in total parenteral nutrition for premature infants reduces the severity of the acidosis and incidence of hyperchloraemia*

* ***Pearl/Peril/Pitfall :*** *Given that plasma lactate is now frequently measured in sick neonates, it is important to have a logical approach to high lactate levels. It is firstly necessary to consider whether the sample is adequate - capillary or venous lactate levels may be very high in the face of normal arterial lactate. If arterial lactate is persistently high (> 3 mmol/L), the differential diagnosis is as follows-*Severe organ dysfunction leading to decrease tissue perfusion/oxygen delivery, or increased metabolic demand *perinatal asphyxia *congenital heart disease (duct-dependent lesions) *sepsis *untreated seizures. · Primary lactic acidoses -*disorders of pyruvate metabolism *mitochondrial disorders. · Secondary lactic acidoses other metabolic diseases may be associated with lactic acidosis, for example. *fatty acid oxidation defects *organic acidoses *urea cycle defects *sulphite oxidase deficiency*

Renal Tubular Acidosis in Neonates

The hyperchloremic metabolic acidosis with normal anion gap, in a neonate can have the following causes, to be differentiated, to institute the appropriate therapy.

Distal renal tubular acidosis
Congenital subclinical hypothyroidism
Obstructive uropathy
Early uremic acidosis
Bicarbonate loss
—Proximal renal tubular acidosis
—Diarrhea
—Intestinal fistula
—Ureterosigmoidostomy
—Medications: cholestyramine, magnesium sulfate, calcium chloride
Acid loading
—Ammonium chloride
—Arginine hydrochloride

* When a metabolic acidosis is identified, it is necessary to evaluate for other pathologic causes of the acidosis. For a preterm newborn, prophylactic antibiotic administration during an evaluation for infection or necrotizing enterocolitis is appropriate, as is ruling out anemia or intracranial hemorrhage as a cause of acidosis.

* Ultrasonography of the kidneys is appropriate to rule out hydronephrosis and hydroureters of obstructive uropathy.

* The history excludes bicarbonate losses from diarrhea; intestinal fistula; ureterosigmoidostomy; or ingestion of calcium chloride, magnesium sulfate, or cholestyramine, Acid loading.

* Normal BUN, serum Creatinine excludes early uremic acidosis.

* Rapid stabilization in clinical status with adequate alkali therapy (4.5 mEq/kg per day of bicarbonate is consistent with RTA, classically defined as a normal anion gap hyperchloremic acidosis without impaired glomerular filtration. It effectively rules out the likelihood of underlying infection, tissue ischemia, or a disorder causing decreased cardiac output.

* RTA is caused by either impaired renal reabsorption of bicarbonate ion (HCO3), or impaired urinary acidification/impaired acid hydrogen (H) excretion. Three types of RTA occur, named for the site of the abnormality within the renal tubule or the most noteworthy feature: type I (distal), type II (proximal), and type IV (hyperkalemic). Type 3 RTA-Infants who have mild, distal renal tubular acidification defect combined with mild proximal bicarbonate reabsorption defect were classified previously as having type 3 RTA. This has been reclassified as a subtype of type 1 RTA that occurs primarily in preterm infants.

* Type I (distal) RTA is caused by diminished acid secretion in the distal tubule. Characteristically, this type of RTA presents with hypokalemia as potassium is lost in the urine as a cation replacement for hydrogen. Hypocitraturia develops as citrate reabsorption is upregulated to create new bicarbonate, and the concentration of calcium in the urine also increases. The cause of hypercalcuria is not completely clear, but most likely results from increased calcium release from bone as a buffer, downregulation of calcium transport proteins in the kidney, and high distal sodium delivery contributing to more calcium excretion. As a result of the increased urine pH and the elevated calcium concentrations, nephrocalcinosis and nephrolithiasis are seen commonly. The diagnosis of type I RTA is confirmed by a high urine pH (6.5) in the setting of a normal anion gap hyperchloremic metabolic acidosis associated with lethargy, vomiting, and dehydration. In some cases, the systemic pH is normal or nearly normal, making diagnosis unclear. In this instance, an oral acid challenge (with either ammonium or furosemide/fludrocortisone) should be administered, and if the urine pH remains above 5.5, the diagnosis can be made.

* Type II (proximal) RTA is caused by a reduction in the threshold for bicarbonate resorption in the proximal tubule to 15 mEq/L (15 mmol/L). In this group of disorders, there is no resorption above that threshold, and because bicarbonate normally is almost all filtered and subsequently recovered, the defect results in pronounced urinary losses. The diagnosis can be made by measuring urine pH, which in type II RTA is inappropriately

high (often 7.6 or greater, and rarely below 7.0) in the face of a metabolic acidosis. If the serum bicarbonate value drops below 14 to 15 mEq/L (14 to 15 mmol/L), the resorption threshold is met and the kidney can produce acid urine. As a result, proximal RTA usually is milder than the distal (type I) form. More often, proximal RTA occurs as a part of Fanconi syndrome, characterized by renal wasting of sodium, potassium, glucose,

Diagnostic evaluation for RTA: Studies and Interpretation

1. Fresh, spot urine pH Type 1 RTA, urine pH consistently >5.5. Type 2 RTA, urine pH <5.5.
2. Serum electrolytes Metabolic acidosis with serum total CO_2 <17.5 mEq/L (17.5 mmol/L) for all types of RTA, usually associated with hyperchloremia and normal anion gap.
   Normal serum urea nitrogen, creatinine, and creatinine clearance.
3. 24-h urine for calcium, citrate, potassium, and oxalate: Hypercalciuria, hypocitraturia, and potassium wasting are associated with type 1 RTA. Rule out hyperoxaluria.
4. Ultrasonography of the kidneys: Nephrocalcinosis in undiagnosed, untreated, or inadequately treated RTA.
5. Urine minus blood PCO_2 Normal values, >20 mm Hg: Proximal, type 2 RTA, >20 mm Hg Distal, type 1 RTA, <20 mm Hg
6. Tubular reabsorption of bicarbonate (TRB): Bicarbonate wasting or TRB >15% in type 2 RTA and <5% in type 1 RTA at normalized serum total CO_2.
7. Tubular reabsorption of phosphate (TRP): TRP <60% filtered load of phosphate in Fanconi syndrome and other proximal tubular defects in reabsorption of phosphate. If Fanconi syndrome is suspected, 24-h urine collection is needed to confirm the aminoaciduria and potassium wasting.
8. Renal acidification studies If metabolic acidosis is clearly present, with total CO_2 <17.5 mEq/L (17.5 mmol/L), there is no need for further acidification. If the metabolic acidosis is unclear, the renal ability to acidify can be tested maximally after ammonium chloride or arginine hydrochloride acid loading. The net acid excretion of <70 mcEq/min per $1.73m^2$ confirms a distal tubular acidification defect.

phosphorous, and amino acids. This presentation is part of several inborn errors of metabolism, including cystinosis, tyrosinemia, galactosemia, Wilson disease, and hereditary fructose intolerance.

*Type I RTA is easier to treat because of the lower alkali requirement (Bicitra 3 to 4 mEq/kg per day) to maintain acid-base equilibrium. The large bicarbonate wasting of type II RTA may require up to 14 mEq/kg per day. The larger dose and frequency of dosing makes compliance a problem. Additional therapy or dietary manipulation is determined by the presence of any associated metabolic disease. Vitamin D and phosphate are appropriate treatments for patients with rickets and hypophosphatemia and may improve the acidification defect. Patients with fructose intolerance should avoid fructose.

* Type IV RTA is due to either aldosterone deficiency or aldosterone resistance that results in an inability to excrete hydrogen and potassium ions. Retention of these ions gives rise to systemic metabolic acidosis and hyperkalemia. The latter features distinguish type IV RTA from the hypokalemia, which commonly characterizes the first two types of RTA. Aldosterone deficiency may result from congenital adrenogenital syndrome, and aldosterone resistance may follow relief of posterior urethral valve obstruction or prostatic hypertrophy.

* Follow-up of RTA : Studies & Interpretation

Serum total CO2: Adequate base therapy to maintain serum total CO_2 >22 mEq/L (22 mmol/L). Spot urine calcium/ creatinine ratio: Adequate base therapy to maintain urine calcium/ creatinine ratio to <0.20 mg/mg. Ultrasonography of the kidneys: Monitor nephrocalcinosis

* Prognosis is dependent to a large part on the nature of any underlying disease, if present. Patients with treated isolated proximal or distal RTA will generally demonstrate improvement in growth, provided serum bicarbonate levels can be maintained in the normal range. Patients with systemic illness and Fanconi syndrome may have ongoing difficulties with growth failure, rickets, and signs and symptoms related to their underlying disease.

* The underlying causes of Type I RTA & Type II RTA are classified as Genetic & Acquired. Type II RTA can occur as a transient developmental problem in the neonate and young infant. Commonly, term infants have a normal mild RTA, with serum bicarbonate concentrations of 20 to 24 mEq/L (20 to 24 mmol/L), and preterm infants may have values as low as 15 mEq/L (15 mmol/L). Such transient failure of bicarbonate resorption usually improves progressively during infancy, although in some reported cases, maturation was delayed as long as 6 years.

TABLE 1	Common causes of metabolic acidosis in neonates
Increased Anion Gap :	Lactic acidosis due to tissue hypoxia, Asphyxia, hypothermia, shock, Sepsis, respiratory distress syndrome, Inborn errors of metabolism, Congenital lactic acidosis, Organic acidosis, Late metabolic acidosis, Toxins (e.g., benzyl alcohol)
Normal Anion Gap :	Renal / GIT bicarbonate loss, Bicarbonate wasting due to immaturity, Renal tubular acidosis, Gastrointestinal bicarbonate loss, Small bowel drainage: ileostomy, fistula, Diarrhea, Excessive chloride in IV fluids, Aldosterone deficiency

TABLE 2 Base therapy in metabolic acidosis

* Dose of sodium bicarbonate (mEq) = base deficit (mEq/L) × body weight (kg) x 0.3. Most clinicians would use half of the calculated total correction dose for initial therapy to avoid overcorrection of metabolic acidosis. Subsequent doses of sodium bicarbonate are then based on the results of further blood gas measurements

* Metabolic acidosis is a biochemical derangement that results from an underlying disease process, therefore, treatment should be aimed at correction of the disease.

* Severe metabolic acidosis with pH < 7.1 and/or HCO_3^- < 6-8 mEq/L can have deleterious effects on the myocardium and other organ systems. Correction of acidosis and low HCO_3^- is therefore recommended.

* Bicarbonate should not be given if ventilation is inadequate, because its administration results in an increase in PCO2 with no improvement in pH and an increase in intracellular/CNS acidosis.

* Disadvantages of $NaHCO_3$ administration:

  1. - sodium load - hypernatremia/hyperosmolality can cause intracranial bleed in premature infants

  2. Hypercarbia: $NaHCO_3 \ll Na^+ + H_2O + CO_2$

  3. May aggravate pre-existing hypocalcemia and hypokalemia by inducing cellular shifts

* Other therapeutic options for correction of metabolic acidosis:

THAM (Tromethamine) lowers PCO2 by covalently binding H+ and thus shifting the equilibrium of the reaction

$H^+ + HCO_3^- \leftrightarrow H_2CO_3 \leftrightarrow H_2O + CO_2$ to the left resulting in a decrease in CO_2 and an increase in HCO_3. The initial dose is 1-2 mEq/kg or 3.5ml - 6ml/kg given IV using the 0.3M solution, with the rate of administration not exceeding 1ml/kg/minute. Once a blood gas measurement has been obtained, the dose of THAM required to raise the pH can be estimated using the formula *dose of tromethamine in mL = base deficit (mEq/L) x body weight (kg).*

Side effects:1.Acute respiratory depression, most likely secondary to an abrupt decrease in $PaCO_2$ levels as well as from rapid intracellular correction of acidosis in the cells of the respiratory center 2.White matter damage in preterms due to decreased cerebral blood flow secondarily to hypocapnea 3.Hyponatremia 4. Hypoglycemia 5.Hyperkalemia, 6.an increase in hemoglobin oxygen affinity, and diuresis followed by oliguria

* **Carbicarb** an equimolar solution of $NaHCO_3 + Na_2CO_3$

  $Na_2CO_3 + CO_2 + H_2O ® 2H_2CO_3 + 2Na^+$

* **DCA** (dichloroacetate) activates pyruvate dehydrogenase kinase and decreases lactate production. Still in experimental stage in the newborn and cannot be recommended at this time. Regardless of the buffer used, care should be taken to avoid overtreatment, to minimize adverse effects of the buffer itself and of rapid swings in pH, and to direct therapy toward the underlying problem.

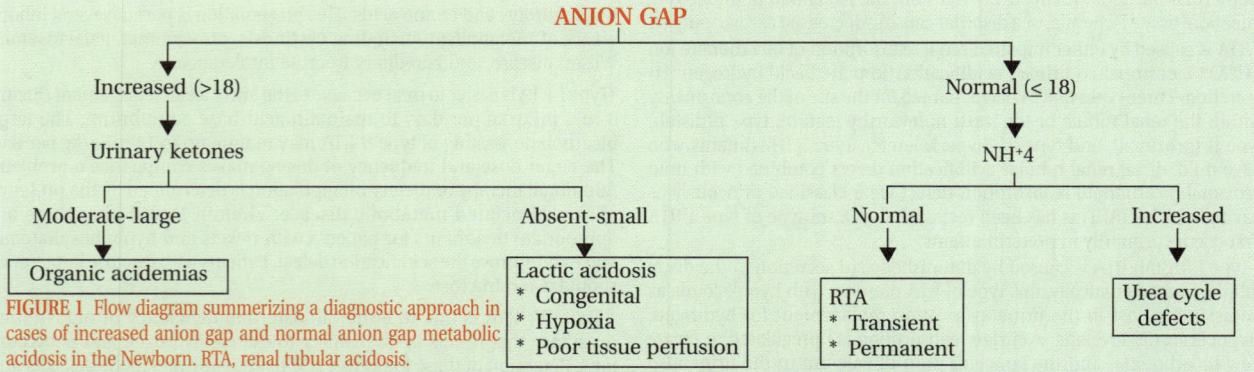

FIGURE 1 Flow diagram summerizing a diagnostic approach in cases of increased anion gap and normal anion gap metabolic acidosis in the Newborn. RTA, renal tubular acidosis.

KEY POINTS FOR CLINICAL PRACTICE:

1. A *Systematic approach to Metabolic acidosis* is required in order to identify correctly its etiology and therefore the appropriate management.

2. The commonest cause of metabolic acidosis in NICU is tissue hypoxia, which causes lactic acidosis as seen in *asphyxia,anemia, hypothermia, severe respiratory distress,shock,sepsis, NEC,* and other severe Neonatal illnesses.

3. Consider an Inborn error of metabolism especially in term infants, particularly where there is a family history of *unexplained neonatal illnesses and/or deaths and consanguinity.* "Screening tests" for **metabolic disease***odor of baby and urine (but most babies with malodorous urine do not have metabolic disease) *blood glucose *serum ammonia *acid-base status *anion gap ($[Na^+ + K^+] - [Cl^- + HCO3^-]$, normal < 12 mmol) *lactate - arterial sample *liver function tests *urinary reducing substances (Clinitest). Remember that glucose is a reducing substance, so if the Clinitest is positive, check the urine specifically for glucose using a glucose oxidase strip *urinary ketones

*urine metabolic screen. A sample of 5-10 mL of freshly-collected urine is needed for this test; the sample can be frozen prior to analysis if necessary. As much clinical information as possible should be included on the request card to assist in the interpretation of the results In only a few cases will the results of the above "screening" tests pinpoint the exact metabolic defect. They will, however, identify infants with a high likelihood of having a metabolic disease, in whom further tests would be performed as appropriate.

4. At a serum pH < 7.20, the cardiac contractility is impaired with an increased risk of cardiac arrhythmias, especially if predisposed by the presence of congenital heart disease or electrolyte disorders.

5. In most conditions, correcting the pH to 7.25 to 7.30 is adequate. In addition, the recommendations for buffer treatment in metabolic acidosis, although widely practiced, are largely empiric without the backing of substantial evidence-based experimental evidence.Repairing of the *underlying disorder* is the most effective therapeutic approach for children with a metabolic acidosis.

REFERENCES & FURTHER READING : 1) Driscoll P et al A simple guide to Blood Gas Analysis. 1997 BMJ:London 2) Nelson Text Book of Pediatrics, 18th edition 3)Fall PJ. A stepwise approach to acid-base disorders. Practical patient evaluation for metabolic acidosis and other conditions. *Postgrad Med*. Mar 2000;107(3):249-50, 253-4, 257-8 passim. 4) Levraut J, Grimaud D. Treatment of metabolic acidosis. *Curr Opin Crit Care*. Aug 2003;9(4):260-5. 5)Szaflarski N, Hanson CW 3rd. Metabolic acidosis. *AACN Clin Issues*. Aug 1997;8(3):481-96.

Metabolic Alkalosis in Neonates

81

@ *"The symptoms in patients with a metabolic alkalosis are often related to the underlying diseases and associated electrolytes disturbances. Neonates with chloride(saline)-responsive causes of metabolic alkalosis often have symptoms related to volume depletion, such as thirst and lethargy. In contrast, Neonates with chloride(saline)-unresponsive causes may have symptoms related to hypertension."*

Metabolic Alkalosis
(e.g. $HCO_3 > 28$ mmol/L or B.E. > plus 4.0 mEq/L, pH > 7.45)

This occurs where the plasma HCO_3 or base excess is abnormally high. Causes include hypochloremia (the level of bicarbonate and chloride in plasma are reciprocally related), which may be due to diuretic therapy or upper gastrointestinal obstruction (e.g. pyloric stenosis). The baby may also be trying to compensate for a respiratory acidosis, although the pH will never become alkalotic (as the baby will never over-compensate). The treatment of a metabolic alkalosis is to treat the underlying cause (e.g. chloride replacement) or the underlying cause of the respiratory acidosis.

What are the abnormal 'maintenance factors' of Metabolic Alkalosis?

The four factors that cause maintenance of the alkalosis (by increasing bicarbonate reabsorption in the tubules or decreasing bicarbonate filtration at the glomerulus) are:
* Chloride depletion
* Reduced glomerular filtration rate (GFR)
* Potassium depletion
* ECF volume depletion

Chloride depletion is the most common factor

Volume depletion and potassium depletion may coexist in some disorders (e.g. vomiting). Severe potassium depletion alone can cause a metabolic alkalosis but this is typically only of mild to moderate degree. The mechanism seems to be related to an intracellular shift of H^+ ('intracellular acidosis') in exchange for K^+. The alkalosis is generated predominantly due to non-renal mechanisms. Renal mechanisms are frequently involved in causing the potassium depletion (e.g. in syndromes of mineralocorticoid excess).

Volume depletion has long been implicated in maintenance of an alkalosis. The idea is that hypovolemia is associated with increased fluid and sodium reabsorption in the proximal tubule and bicarbonate is reabsorbed in preference to chloride; the alkalosis thus being maintained. The role of volume depletion has probably been overemphasized: the coexisting chloride depletion is the most important factor responsible for persistence of the alkalosis. *Correction of the volume deficit without correction of the chloride deficit will not result in correction of the alkalosis. These deficits are often corrected together with a saline infusion.*

Diuretics can cause excess renal loss of fixed acid anions and result in alkalosis. Their use can also cause depletion of chloride, water (hypovolemia) and potassium. These factors together maintain the alkalosis. For an alkalosis to develop in patients on diuretic therapy, there generally has to some decrease in chloride intake as well (e.g. if the patient is on a 'salt restricted' diet). A continued normal oral chloride intake (usually as NaCl) prevents patients on diuretics from getting an alkalosis.

REVIEW OF CLINICAL PROBLEMS

1. What are the clinical features of Metabolic Alkalosis in Neonates?
   Ans: Refer to the "No. 8" of the "BIRD'S EYE VIEW/OVERVIEW/ SYNOPSIS" of the Chapter.

2. How do you differentiate the 2 types of Metabolic Alkalosis in Neonates?
   Ans: Refer to the "No. 2" of the "BIRD'S EYE VIEW/OVERVIEW/ SYNOPSIS" of the Chapter.

3. How do you assess a Neonate with suspected Metabolic Alkalosis clinically and investigate further?
   Ans: Refer to the Evaluation-Decision-Action Plan/Algorithm to diagnose & manage a Neonate with Metabolic Alkalosis.

4. How do you manage Metabolic Alkalosis in Neonates?
   Ans: Refer to the Evaluation-Decision-Action Plan/Algorithm to diagnose & manage a Neonate with Metabolic Alkalosis.

5. How do you manage a preterm infant with mixed Metabolic alkalosis and Respiratory acidosis?
   Ans: Refer to the "No.7" of the "BIRD`S EYE VIEW/OVERVIEW/ SYNOPSIS" of the Chapter.

LEARNING OBJECTIVES

After completing this article, readers will be able to:

1. Identify the underlying diseases causing Metabolic Alkalosis in Neonates.

2. Differentiate the *chloride(saline)-responsive causes of metabolic alkalosis* from *chloride(saline)-unresponsive causes.*

3. Anticipate and search for a mixed metabolic alkalosis and respiratory acidosis in a preterm infant with chronic lung disease.

4. Treat metabolic alkalosis depending on the severity of the alkalosis and the underlying etiology.

5. Address the management of underlying etiological conditions causing and/or perpetuating Metabolic Alkalosis in Neonates.

* *Pearl/Peril/Pitfall : The effects of the alkalosis are often difficult to distinguish from the effects of associated problems such as hypovolemia, potassium and chloride depletion. This makes it more difficult to characterize the effects of the alkalosis itself. Adverse Effects of Alkalosis—decreased myocardial contractility -arrhythmias -decreased cerebral blood flow-confusion-mental obtundation -neuromuscular excitability—impaired peripheral oxygen unloading (due shift of oxygen dissociation curve to left). The disorder is associated with significantly increased morbidity and mortality especially in critically ill patients. The compensatory rise in arterial pCO_2 will tend to counteract some of these effects (e.g. the effect on cerebral blood flow).*

BIRD'S EYE VIEW/OVERVIEW/SYNOPSIS

1. Metabolic alkalosis is characterized by a primary increase in the extracellular HCO_3^- concentration sufficient to raise the arterial pH >7.45. *In the Newborn, metabolic alkalosis occurs when there is a loss of H^+, a gain of HCO_3^-, or a depletion of the ECF volume with the loss of more chloride than HCO_3^-.* It is important to understand that metabolic alkalosis generated by any of these mechanisms can be maintained only when factors limiting the renal excretion of HCO_3^- are also present (e.g. renal insufficiency or concurrent volume depletion).

2. Table 1 of the Chapter classifies the various causes of metabolic alkalosis into two categories, i.e. *chloride responsive and chloride resistant.* In **chloride responsive type of metabolic alkalosis,** the patient is volume depleted due to extrarenal losses of fluid and the urinary chloride level is below 15mEq/L. The volume depletion in these patients is due to losses of sodium and potassium, but the loss of chloride is usually > that of sodium and potassium combined. Because chloride losses are the dominant cause of the volume depletion, the patients require chloride to correct their volume depletion and metabolic alkalosis. In contrast, the patients with an elevated urinary chloride level (>20mEq/L), do not respond to volume repletion and hence they are called **chloride resistant.**

3. The serum bicarbonate concentration is increased with a metabolic alkalosis, although a respiratory acidosis also leads to a compensatory elevation of the serum HCO_3^- concentration. With a simple metabolic alkalosis, however, the pH is elevated; alkalemia is present. Patients with respiratory acidosis are acidemic. A metabolic alkalosis, by decreasing ventilation, causes appropriate respiratory compensation. PCO_2 increases by 7mmHg for each 10-mEq/L increase in the serum bicarbonate concentration. Appropriate respiratory compensation never exceeds a PCO_2 of 55-60mmHg. *The patient has a concurrent respiratory alkalosis if the PCO_2 is lower than the expected compensation. A greater than expected PCO_2 occurs with a concurrent respiratory acidosis.*

4. Metabolic alkalosis resulting from a loss of H^+ from the body (either GIT or renal loss) *most commonly caused by* continuous nasogastric aspiration, persistent vomiting, and diuretic treatment in the Newborn period. Less common causes of H^+ losses are congenital chloride-wasting diarrhea, certain forms of congenital adrenal hyperplasia, hyper-aldosteronism, posthypercapnia, and Bartter syndrome.

5. Metabolic alkalosis resulting from a gain of HCO_3^-, occurs during the administration of buffer solutions to the Newborn. It is usually due to chronic excessive administration of HCO_3^-, lactate, citrate, or acetate in IV fluids and blood products, with rapid resolution commonly. However, if the alkalosis is severe and urine output is limited, inhibition of the carbonic anhydrase enzyme by the administration of acetazolamide may enhance elimination of bicarbonate.

6. Metabolic alkalosis resulting from a loss of ECF containing disproportionally more chloride than HCO_3^-, so-called **contraction alkalosis** occurs with loss of gastric fluid (emesis, nasogastric suction) and with diuretics. Contraction alkalosis responds to administration of saline to replete the intravascular volume and potassium supplementation.

7. In a *preterm infant with chronic lung disease* on long term diuretic treatment, a mixed acid-base disorder occurs. Such a Newborn initially has a chronic respiratory acidosis that is partially compensated by renal HCO_3^- retention. Prolonged or aggressive use of diuretics can lead to total-body potassium depletion and contraction of the ECF volume, thus exacerbating the metabolic alkalosis. The routine use of potassium chloride supplements, and close monitoring of serum sodium, chloride, and potassium levels are recommended during long-term diuretic therapy to prevent the common iatrogenic problems like hypokalemia, hyponatremia and hypochloremia.

8. *The Evaluation-Decision-Action-Plan/Algorithm* describes the essential aspects of the diagnosis and management of metabolic alkalosis in Neonates. The symptoms in patients with a metabolic alkalosis are often related to the underlying diseases and associated electrolytes disturbances. Neonates with chloride-responsive causes of metabolic alkalosis often have symptoms related to volume depletion, such as thirst and lethargy. In contrast, Neonates with chloride-unresponsive causes may have symptoms related to hypertension. *Alkalemia leads to hypokalemia (through redistribution and renal losses), hypocalcemic tetany (through decreased ionic calcium as a result of increased binding of calcium to albumin), arrhythmias, increased risk of digoxin toxicity, decreased cardiac output, decreased ventilation (through a compensatory increase in the PCO_2) and hypoxia (through the decrease in ventilatory drive) in patients with underlying lung disease.*

9. Patients with a metabolic alkalosis and a high urinary chloride level or saline/chloride unresponsive are separated based on blood pressure. *Neonates with normal blood pressure* may have Bartter syndrome or Gitelman syndrome. *Excess base administration is another diagnostic possibility, but this is usually apparent from the history.* Other causes with high blood pressure, such as primary hyperaldosteronism, Cushing syndrome, renovascular hypertension, congenital adrenal hyperplasia due to 17α-hydroxylase, and 11β-hydroxysteroid dehydrogenase deficiency are uncommon in the Neonatal period.

10. *The approach to treatment of metabolic alkalosis depends on the severity of the alkalosis and the underlying etiology.* Intervention is often unnecessary in children with a mild metabolic alkalosis ($HCO_3^- < 32$), due to diuretic therapy for congenital heart disease; in contrast, intervention may be appropriate in a child with a worsening mild metabolic alkalosis due to nasogastric suction (pyloric stenosis). Treatment may be indicated in a patient with combined respiratory alkalosis and metabolic alkalosis, because of risk for severe alkalemia. In contrast in a patient with a concurrent respiratory acidosis, the severity of pH elevation is more important than the compensatory increase in bicarbonate concentration.

---

* *Pearl/Peril/Pitfall : The main principles are : *Correct the primary cause of the disorder. *Correct those factors which maintain the disorder (esp, chloride administration in the common Cl⁻ deficient cases). Repletion of chloride, potassium and ECF volume will promote renal bicarbonate excretion and return plasma bicarbonate to normal.*

THE EVALUATION-DECISION-ACTION-PLAN/ALGORITHM FOR THE DIAGNOSIS AND MANAGEMENT OF *METABOLIC ALKALOSIS IN NEONATES*

SUBJECTIVE FINDINGS

Hx of persistent vomiting, nasogastric suction, secretory diarrhea, diuretic therapy, chloride deficient formula.

Hx of symptoms suggestive of co-existing problems like hypokalemia, hypocalcemia, hypertension, dehydration, hypoxia and hypercarbia.

Hx of a premature baby with chronic lung disease on diuretic therapy.

Hx of chronic excessive alkali administration, lactate, citrate, acetate in IV fluids and blood products.

OBJECTIVE FINDINGS

Assess ABCs, disability (altered sensorium, seizures, focal neuro-deficits), vitals, BP, Urine output & capillary refill time.

Look for dehydration *or* hypertension, hypocalcemic tetany, hypokalemia related symptoms, arrhythmias, hypoventilation and its effects (hypoxia and hypercarbia).

Note signs consistent with pyloric stenosis, chronic lung disease, sepsis, congenital heart disease & Bartter syndrome.

INVESTIGATIONS

Blood ABG analysis, electrolytes, BUN, creatinine, osmolality, ketones, glucose, culture, calcium, magnesium, FBC with differential & platelets, drug screen.

Urine analysis, pH, electrolytes, drug screen, culture
Others consider imaging, ECG, Echocardiogram depending on the suspected underlying disease.

Determine a) whether the urinary chlorides below 15mEq/L or above 20mEq/L b) whether the urinary potassium is below 30mEq/day or above 30mEq/day.

Serum renin and aldosterone concentrations differentiates children with a metabolic alkalosis, a high urinary chloride level, and elevated blood pressure.

NEONATE WITH METABOLIC ALKALOSIS

URINE CHLORIDES

<15 mEq/L
Saline responsive
Metabolic alkalosis

>20mEq/L
Saline unresponsive
Metabolic alkalosis

Pyloric stenosis, Vomiting, Upper GI suction, Congenital chloride diarrhea, Laxative abuse, Diuretic abuse, Cystic fibrosis, Chloride-deficient formula in infants, Poorly reabsorbable anion administration, Abrupt relief of chronic hypercapnia, Post-treatment of organic acidemias.

Primary hyperaldosteronism (extremely rare in pediatrics)

Hyperreninemic hypertension, Renal artery stenosis, Cushing's syndrome, congenital adrenal insufficiency due to 17alpha-OH deficiency, 11beta-OH deficiency, Licorice, Liddle's -syndrome, *Bartter syndrome*, Severe potassium deficiency. Massive blood product transfusion.

---

* *BARTTER SYNDROME* is a rare form of renal potassium wasting, characterized by hypokalemia, normal blood pressure, vascular insensitivity to pressor agents, and elevated plasma concentrations of renin and aldosterone.

* *PATHOGENESIS* - Primary defect in chloride reabsorption in the ascending limb of the loop of Henle → leads to extra sodium chloride presentation to the distal tubule → sodium is reabsorbed in exchange for potassium → urinary potassium wasting → Hypokalemia induced → stimulates prostaglandins synthesis → leads to the activation of renin - angiotensin - aldosterone system by increasing renin release and by stimulating aldosterone synthesis → exacerbates renal potassium wasting.

* Some patients may also have hypercalciuria, hyperuricemia, hypomagnesemia and urinary sodium wasting.

* Gitelman syndrome is similar but presents in older children and young adults with muscle weakness, carpopedal spasms /tetany.

URINE POTASSIUM

> 30mmol/day
Laxative abuse
Severe K⁺/Mg Depletion

<30mmol/day
Blood pressure

Low/normal → **BARTTER**

High

Plasma Renin

High unilateral renal vein renin ← High ← Low

Yes | No

Renovascular HTN JGA tumor

Malignant or Accelerated HTN

Plasma aldosterone

Cushing syndrome, Liddle syndrome, licorice ingestion, 17alpha-hydroxylase deficiency, 11beta-hydroxylase deficiency, and 11beta-hydroxysteroid dehydrogenase deficiency — Low

High

Primary Aldosteronism Glucocorticosteroid remediable hypertension

---

* *Metabolic alkalosis—Principles of management* **a) Address the underlying etiology** decrease or discontinue nasogastric suction, and add a gastric proton pump inhibitor to reduce gastric secretions and losses of HCL, eliminate or reduce the dose of diuretics, adequate potassium chloride supplementation or the addition of a potassium sparing diuretic, correction of the volume deficit with sufficient NaCl and KCl etc. **b) In children with Bartter syndrome and Gitelman syndrome** - therapy includes oral potassium supplementation and potassium sparing diuretics. Children with Gitelman syndrome often require magnesium supplementation, whereas children with severe Bartter syndrome often benefit from indomethacin. **c) In children with the chloride-resistant causes of a metabolic alkalosis** - that are associated with hypertension, volume repletion is contraindicated because it exacerbates the hypertension and does not repair the metabolic alkalosis. Ideally, treatment focuses on eliminating the excess aldosterone effect (e.g. resection of adrenal adenomas, repair the renovascular disease, glucocorticoid administration for congenital adrenal hyperplasia due to 17*alpha* - hydroxylase, and 11*beta*- hydroxysteroid dehydrogenase deficiency).

TABLE 1 Common causes of metabolic alkalosis in neonates

a) Chloride responsive (Urinary chloride < 15mEq/L):

Gastric losses (vomiting/nasogastric suction)
Diuretics (loop or thiazide)
Posthypercapnia (chloride loss during metabolic acidosis)

Pyloric stenosis
Chloride-losing diarrhea

b) Chloride resistant (Urinary chloride > 20 mEq/L):

High blood pressure
17α - hydroxylase deficiency
11β - hydroxylase deficiency
11β - hydroxysteroid dehydrogenase deficiency
Renin - secreting tumour
Renovascular disease
Adrenal adenoma/hyperplasia
Glucocorticoid -remediable-aldosteronism
Cushing syndrome

Normal blood pressure
Base administration
Massive blood product transfusion
Bartter syndrome
Gitelman syndrome

METABOLIC ALKALOSIS is usually iatrogenic in premature infants related to diuretic use or GI losses and occurs in combination with contracted intravascular and ECF volumes.

Cause of metabolic alkalosis	Treatment
Compensation for respiratory acidosis	Correct ventilation
Diuretic Rx (especially furosemide) (contraction alkalosis)	Decrease diuretic dose, add spironolactone, replace K+ and Cl- deficit
Loss of gastric fluid from vomiting or diarrhea with Cl-loss	Replace deficit and give fluids and electrolytes to keep pace with continuing losses.
Increased alkali load from feedings (alkalosis of prematurity)	-Cl- administration as KCl or Arginine Cl
Excessive administration of alkali (Excess acetate in parenteral nutrition)	-Cl- as KCl or Arginine Cl
Bartter syndrome (rare)	Replace electrolyte losses

KEY POINTS FOR CLINICAL PRACTICE

1. *In the Newborn, metabolic alkalosis occur when there is a loss of H^+, a gain of HCO_3^-, or a depletion of the ECF volume with the loss of more chloride than HCO_3^-. A metabolic alkalosis requires BOTH an **initiating process** and a **maintaining process**. Without an abnormal process maintaining it, the alkalosis will rapidly correct as the kidney pours out HCO3 in the urine. The initiating cause in most cases is loss of gastric acid (e.g. **vomiting** or **diuretic** use. Chloride depletion is the abnormality that impairs renal bicarbonate excretion.*

2. *In CHLORIDE/SALINE responsive type of metabolic alkalosis, the patient is volume depleted due to extrarenal losses of fluid and the urinary chloride level is below 15mEq/L.In contrast, the patients with an elevated urinary chloride level (>20mEq/L), do not respond to volume repletion and hence they are called CHLORIDE resistant.*

3. *In a preterm infant with chronic lung disease on long term diuretic treatment, a mixed acid-base disorder occurs. Such a Newborn initially has a chronic respiratory acidosis that is partially compensated by renal HCO_3^- retention. Prolonged or aggressive use of diuretics can lead to total-body potassium depletion and contraction of the ECF volume, thus exacerbating the metabolic alkalosis.*

4. *Alkalemia leads to hypokalemia (through redistribution and renal losses* Hypokalemia is the most common associated electrolyte abnormality and can be life-threatening itself *), hypocalcemic tetany (through decreased ionic calcium as a result of increased binding of calcium to albumin), arrhythmias, increased risk of digoxin toxicity, decreased cardiac output, decreased ventilation (through a compensatory increase in the PCO_2) and hypoxia (through the decrease in ventilatory drive) in patients with underlying lung disease.*

5. Hypoxemia may occur and oxygen delivery to the tissues may be reduced. Factors involved in impaired arterial oxygen content are:
   - Hypoventilation (due respiratory response to metabolic alkalosis)
   - Pulmonary microatelectasis (consequent to hypoventilation)
   - Increased ventilation-perfusion mismatch (as alkalosis inhibits hypoxic pulmonary vasoconstriction)
   Peripheral oxygen unloading may be impaired because of the alkalotic shift of the hemoglobin oxygen dissociation curve to the left. The body's major compensatory response to impaired tissue oxygen delivery is to increase cardiac output but this ability is impaired if hypovolemia and decreased myocardial contractility are present.

REFERENCES & FURTHER READING : 1) Vantyghem MC, Douillard C, Binaut R, and Provot F. *[Bartter's syndromes].* Ann Endocrinol (Paris) 1999 Dec; 60(6) 465–72. 2) Nelson Text Book of Pediatrics, 18th edition 3) Naka T, Bellomo R. Bench-to-bedside review : treating acid-base abnormalities in the intensive care unit—the role of renal replacement therapy. *Crit Care.* Apr 2004;8(2):108-14. 4) Avery's diseases of the Newborn, 8th edition 5) Fall PJ. A stepwise approach to acid-base disorders. Practical patient evaluation for metabolic acidosis and other conditions. *Postgrad Med.* Mar 2000;107(3):249-50, 253-4, 257-8 passim.

* *Pearl/Peril/Pitfall : Metabolic alkalosis There are 2 aspects of prevention for a metabolic alkalosis : *Prevention of the primary or initiating process, and/or *Prevention of the factors that are involved in maintaining the alkalosis. Patients with nasogastric drainage and pyloric obstruction should receive adequate fluid replacement using a chloride containing fluid. Patients receiving thiazide diuretics likewise need to have adequate chloride intake.*

Respiratory Acidosis in Neonates

82

@ *Patients with a respiratory acidosis are often tachypneic/dyspneic in an effort to correct the inadequate ventilation. CNS depression and neuromuscular diseases cause respiratory acidosis and failure without producing obvious respiratory distress.*

*Potentially preventable patient deaths have occurred because of ventilation-related problems. Changes in circulatory and respiratory status can be detected sooner with capnography than with pulse oximetry. It is also essential to monitor the partial pressure of arterial carbon dioxide ($PaCO_2$) levels in the blood, because both low and high $PaCO_2$ levels may give rise to complications in Neonates. Life-threatening airway malfunctions can be averted with the use of continuous capnometry monitoring. End-tidal carbon dioxide ($EtCO_2$) measurement is a continuous and noninvasive measurement of blood carbon dioxide tensions with fast response time to changes in blood CO_2 levels and internal calibrating ability. It will also reduce the blood loss associated with repeated arterial blood gas sampling. The correlation between mainstream $EtCO_2$ and $PaCO_2$ is good. *Neonates with pulmonary disease will have a lower correlation. Surfactant therapy improves the correlation. EtCO2 monitoring is helpful in trending or screening for abnormal PaCO$_2$ values.*

*One common problem in the management of infants with BPD is distinguishing a primary, chronic, respiratory acidosis with metabolic compensation from a diuretic-induced metabolic alkalosis with respiratory compensation. In infants with BPD, lung mechanics, ventilation/perfusion relations, and work of breathing are abnormal. This results in a chronically high PCO_2—a primary respiratory acidosis. Renal compensation causes bicarbonate retention, bringing the pH back towards normal, but compensation is usually not complete, that is, pH remains <7.40. Diuretics are used to improve lung mechanics, to decrease lung water, and to improve gas exchange. Thiazide and especially loop diuretics result in a loss of chloride, potassium, and sodium, and in retention of bicarbonate. When high doses of diuretics are used without salt replacement, metabolic alkalosis can result, with pH values >7.40. Under these circumstances, respiratory drive can be depressed, worsening the hypoventilation. Lowering the dose of diuretics, changing from a loop to a thiazide diuretic, replacement of salt, or use of acetazolamide to lower plasma bicarbonate are strategies that can be used to minimize this problem.

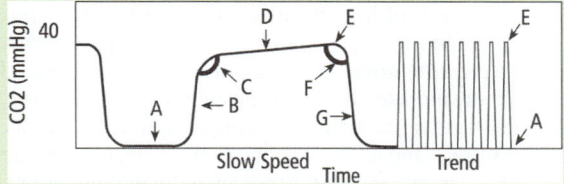

Fig.1. Normal features of a capnogram.

A: Baseline, represents the beginning of expiration and should start at zero.

B: The transitional part of the curve represents mixing of dead space and alveolar gas.

C: The alpha angle represents the change to alveolar gas.

D: The alveolar part of the curve represents the plateau average alveolar gas concentration.

E: The end-tidal carbon dioxide value.

F: The beta angle represents the change to the inspiratory part of the cycle. G: The inspiration part of the curve shows a rapid decrease in carbon dioxide concentration.

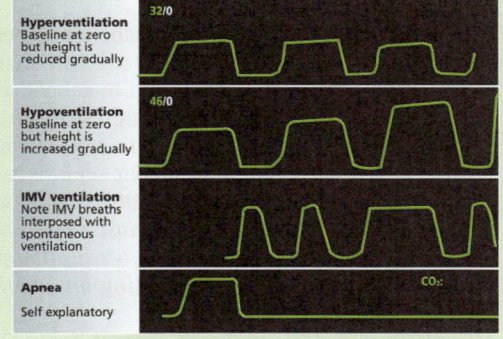

Hyperventilation
Baseline at zero but height is reduced gradually

Hypoventilation
Baseline at zero but height is increased gradually

IMV ventilation
Note IMV breaths interposed with spontaneous ventilation

Apnea
Self explanatory

REVIEW OF CLINICAL PROBLEMS

1. What are the common causes of Respiratory Acidosis in Neonates?
   Ans: Refer to the Table 1 of the Chapter.

2. Discuss the clinical features of various disorders causing Respiratory Acidosis in Neonates.
   Ans: Refer to the Table 2 of the Chapter.

3. How do you assess the severity of respiratory acidosis & failure?
   Ans: Refer to the Table 3 of the Chapter.

4. How do you Evaluate & manage respiratory Acidosis in Neonates?
   Ans: Refer to the Evaluation-Decision-Action Plan/Algorithm to diagnose & manage a Neonate with Respiratory Acidosis.

5. Mention the Criteria for Intubation & Mechanical ventilation in a Neonate with Respiratory Acidosis.
   Ans: Refer to the Evaluation-Decision-Action Plan/Algorithm to diagnose & manage a Neonate with Respiratory Acidosis.

LEARNING OBJECTIVES

After completing this article, readers will be able to:

1. Search for the presence of respiratory acidosis in a Neonate with breathing difficulties- either distress or depression of respiratory system (Central to Peripheral).

2. Monitor for respiratory acidosis by Et CO_2, Tc CO_2, ABG analysis and Identify the indications for Instituting ET intubation and Mechanical ventilation.

3. Understand the systemic effects of acute respiratory acidosis.

4. Assess the severity of Respiratory acidosis and responsiveness of the underlying pathologic process to clinical management.

5. Differentiate acute from chronic respiratory acidosis & manage each appropriately.

* **Pearl/Peril/Pitfall:** *The tendency to develop neurologic abnormalities in acute respiratory acidosis is due to the rapid reduction in CSF pH. CO_2 is lipid soluble and rapidly crosses the blood brain border, leading to a decline in CSF pH. In contrast, HCO_3^- is a polar compound that does not readily cross the blood border and thus is not available to counteract the actions of CO_2. Thus acute respiratory acidosis promotes a greater fall in CSF pH than acute metabolic acidosis, which may explain why neurologic abnormalities are seen less often in the latter. In chronic respiratory acidosis, the CO_2 accumulates at a much slower rate, allowing renal compensation to return the arterial pH and ultimately CSF pH toward normal. Therefore neurologic abnormalities are also seldom seen in chronic respiratory acidosis.*

BIRD'S EYE VIEW/OVERVIEW/SYNOPSIS

1. *Respiratory acidosis* is an inappropriate increase in blood Carbon dioxide (PCO_2), usually due to a decrease in the effectiveness of Carbon dioxide removal by the lungs, causing a decrease in the arterial blood pH < 7.35. The causes of respiratory acidosis in a Neonate are either pulmonary or nonpulmonary. (*Refer to Table 1* for various causes of respiratory acidosis in the Newborn). *Mild to moderate lung disease* often causes a respiratory alkalosis as a result of hyperventilation secondary to hypoxia or stimulation of lung *mechano/chemo receptors. Only more severe lung disease* causes a respiratory acidosis. Upper airway diseases, by impairing air entry into the lungs, may decrease ventilation, producing a respiratory acidosis. CNS disorders and narcotic depression can decrease the activity of the central respiratory center, reducing ventilatory drive causing a respiratory acidosis. Respiratory muscle failure due to various causes can prevent adequate ventilation and causes a respiratory acidosis.

2. Respiratory acidosis is acutely compensated (<12-24hr) by the non-HCO_3^- intracellular buffers without noticeable renal compensation: plasma HCO_3^- increases by 1mEq/L for each 10-mmHg increase in the Pco_2. With a chronic respiratory acidosis, there is more significant renal compensation, which occurs over 3–4 days and causes a predictable increase in the serum bicarbonate concentration: plasma HCO_3^- increases by 4 mEq/L for each 10-mmHg increase in the Pco_2.

3. A mixed disorder is present if the metabolic compensation is inappropriate. A higher than expected bicarbonate value occurs in the setting of a concurrent metabolic alkalosis (e.g., premature baby with chronic lung disease on diuretic therapy). A lower than expected bicarbonate value occurs in the setting of a concurrent metabolic acidosis (e.g., RDS patient with sepsis). *Evaluating whether conpensation is appropriate during a respiratory acidosis requires clinical knowledge of the acuity of the process, because the expected compensation is different depending on whether the process is acute or chronic.*

4. A respiratory acidosis is always present if a patient has acidemia/ decrease in pH and elevated Pco_2. However, an elevated Pco_2 also occurs as appropriate respiratory compensation for a simple metabolic alkalosis, but the patient has alkalemia/increase in pH. During a mixed disturbance, a patient can have respiratory acidosis and a normal or even a low Pco_2. This may occur in a patient with a metabolic acidosis; a respiratory acidosis is present if the patient does not have appropriate respiratory compensation (the Pco_2 is higher than expected, based on the severity of the metabolic acidosis).

5. Patients with a respiratory acidosis are often tachypneic/ dyspneic in an effort to correct the inadequate ventilation. *CNS depression and neuromuscular diseases cause respiratory acidosis and failure without producing obvious respiratory distress.* An arterial pH < 7.20 impairs cardiac contractility and the normal response to catecholamines, in both the heart and the peripheral vasculature. *Hypercapnia causes vasodilation in the cerebral vasculature but produces vasoconstriction of the pulmonary circulation.* Respiratory acidosis increases the risk of cardiac arrhythmias, especially in a child with underlying cardiac disease. Acute respiratory acidosis is usually more symptomatic than chronic respiratory acidosis. Symptoms are also increased by concurrent hypoxia/metabolic acidosis.

6. Cerebral blood flow increases by about 10% for each rise of 7.5 mmHg in pCO_2. Because of the role of increased cerebral blood flow in the etiology of Germinal matrix hemorrhage-IVH it is prudent to keep the Pco_2 below 52.5-56mmHg in very preterm babies at risk from this complication.

7. *The Evaluation-Decision-Action-Plan/Algorithm* describes the essential aspects of the diagnosis and the management of respiratory acidosis in Neonates. The Pco_2 measurements in RDS are *valuable* in the following situations: **1)A steadily rising PCO_2 at any stage in the disease is an indication that ventilatory assistance is likely to be needed. 2)A sudden rise in PCO_2 may be an indication of acute changes in the baby's condition, e.g. pneumothorax, collapsed lobes, misplaced endotracheal tube. 3) A swift rise in PCO_2 (often accompanied by hypoxaemia) during an attempt to wean a baby off IPPV or CPAP indicates that the time was not appropriate for that change in therapy. 4) A gradual rise in Pco_2 at the end of the first week in a low birth weight baby on a ventilator who has previously been stable, may herald the development of a PDA or chronic lung disease.**

8. *Beware of the fact,* that in many Neonates respiratory acidosis may be multifactorial: an infant with chronic lung disease, an intrinsic lung disease, may worsen due to respiratory muscle dysfunction from severe hypokalemia as a result of diuretic therapy. Conversely, a child with spinal muscular atrophy may worsen because of aspiration pneumonia.

9. Respiratory acidosis is best managed by treating the underlying etiology. *Mechanical ventilation is necessary for hypoxia that responds poorly to oxygen, a slowly responsive underlying lung/CNS disease, if the sick neonate appears to be tiring and respiratory arrest seems likely and if there is concomitant metabolic acidosis.* In patients with a chronic respiratory acidosis, it is best to avoid mechanical ventilation because extubation is often difficult. However, an acute illness may necessitate mechanical ventilation in an infant with a chronic respiratory acidosis. When intubation is necessary, the PCO_2 should be lowered only to the patients normal base line, and this should be done gradually. A rapid lowering of the PCO_2 can cause a severe metabolic alkalosis, potentially leading to complications such as cardiac arrhythmias, decreased cardiac output, and decreased cerebral blood flow.

10. In patients with a chronic respiratory acidosis, the respiratory drive is often less responsive to hypercarbia and more responsive to hypoxia. Hence, with chronic respiratory acidosis, excessive use of oxygen can blunt the respiratory drive and therefore increase the PCO_2. In these patients, oxygen must be used cautiously.

* *Pearl/Peril/Pitfall : Key Fact: A rise in arterial pCO_2 is a potent stimulus to ventilation so a respiratory acidosis will rapidly correct unless some abnormal factor is maintaining the hypoventilation. This feedback mechanism is responsible for the normal tight control of arterial pCO_2. The factor causing the disorder is also the factor maintaining it. The prevailing arterial pCO_2 represents the balance between the effects of the primary cause and the respiratory stimulation due to the increased pCO_2. Other than by ventilatory assistance, the pCO_2 will return to normal only by correction of the cause of the decreased alveolar ventilation. An extremely high arterial pCO_2 has direct anesthetic effects and this will lead to a worsening of the situation either by central depression of ventilation or as a result of loss of airway patency or protection.*

THE EVALUATION-DECISION-ACTION-PLAN/ALGORITHM FOR THE DIAGNOSIS AND MANAGEMENT OF *RESPIRATORY ACIDOSIS IN A NEONATE*

SUBJECTIVE FINDINGS

Hx of predisposing conditions causing acute respiratory distress, such as neonatal RDS in a premature baby, Meconium Aspiration Syndrome in a term baby, congenital pneumonia, pulmonary edema secondary to PDA, pulmonary hemorrhage and aspiration.

Hx of predisposing conditions causing acute respiratory depression, such as hypoxic-ischemic encephalopathy, increased ICP, head trauma, medications-narcotics, barbiturates, benzodiazepines, anesthesia, vecuronium, aminoglycosides etc.

Hx of respiratory muscle paralysis secondary to myasthenia, myotonic dystrophy, diaphragmatic paralysis or botulism.

OBJECTIVE FINDINGS

Assess ABCs, disability (altered sensorium, seizures, focal neurodeficits), vitals, BP, Urine output & capillary refill time,

Determine whether the Neonate has acute or chronic and has mild/moderate/severe respiratory acidosis depending on the clinical history and ABG analysis.

Determine whether the respiratory acidosis is an isolated or is a mixed disorder depending on the appropriate respiratory compensation, if metabolic alkalosis or metabolic acidosis is co-existing.

Determine the response to naloxone in a Neonate depressed at birth possibly due to maternal opiate administration within 4hrs before delivery. (never give naloxone to a Neonate born to a drug addicted mother, as it precipitates acute withdrawal symptoms).

INVESTIGATIONS

Blood **ABG analysis**, electrolytes, BUN, creatinine, glucose, culture, calcium, magnesium, FBC with differential & platelets, drug screen.

CXR to diagnose pulmonary disease

CT/MRI brain scan and a lumbar puncture potentially to evaluate the CNS causes.

ECG & Echocardiogram to identify cardiac arrhythmias and reduced cardiac output.

Alveolar oxygen arterial oxygen (A-a gradient) gradient is useful for distinguishing poor respiratory effort and intrinsic lung disease: it is increased if the hypoxemia is due to intrinsic lung disease.

RESPIRATORY ACIDOSIS IN A NEONATE

Look for signs of inadequate ventilation - tachypnea or apnea or inadequate respiratory rate for clinical condition, nasal flaring, retractions, agitation/anxiety, altered mental status.

Recognize respiratory failure by the clinical indicators - marked tachypnea (early), bradypnea/apnea (late), tachycardia (early), bradycardia (late), increased/decreased/no respiratory effort, cyanosis, poor to absent distal air movement, stupor or coma.

Beware of the fact that respiratory failure may occur without typical signs of respiratory distress, in Neonates with central depression or neuromuscular weakness. Clinical signs of disordered control of breathing include **a)** variable/irregular respiratory rate (tachypnea alternating with bradypnea), **b)** **variable** respiratory effort **c)** **shallow** breathing (frequently resulting in hypoxemia and hypercarbia) and **d)** central apnea (i.e. apnea without any respiratory effort).

The PCO_2 measurements in RDS are valuable in the following situations: 1)A steadily rising $PaCO_2$ at any stage in the disease is an indication that ventilatory assistance is likely to be needed. 2)A sudden rise in $PaCO_2$ may be an indication of acute changes in the baby's condition, e.g. pneumothorax, collapsed lobes, misplaced endotracheal tube. 3) A swift rise in $PaCO_2$ (often accompanied by hypoxaemia) during an attempt to wean a baby off IPPV or CPAP indicates that the time was not appropriate for that change in therapy. 4) A gradual rise in $PaCo_2$ at the end of the first week in a low birth weight baby on a ventilator who has previously been stable, may herald the development of a PDA or chronic lung disease.

In patients with a chronic respiratory acidosis (e.g. premature baby with chronic lung disease), it is best to avoid mechanical ventilation because extubation is often difficult. However, an acute illness may necessitate mechanical ventilation in an infant with a chronic respiratory acidosis. When intubation is necessary, the PCO_2 should be lowered only to the patient's normal base line, and this should be done gradually. A rapid lowering of the PCO_2 can cause a severe metabolic alkalosis, potentially leading to complications such as cardiac arrhythmias, decreased cardiac output, and decreased cerebral blood flow.

Ensure ABCs, Pulse oximetry, Capnography(Et CO_2), Tc CO_2, Administer oxygen, Cardiac monitor, protect airway and apnea monitor, BP, ideally from the arterial catheter.

Monitor ABG 3-4 hrly for PCO_2, arterial pH and base deficit (*hypercarbia secondary to impaired ventilation, even if the pulse oximeter indicates adequate oxyhemoglobin saturations*).

Determine—Where is the lesion? Upper airway obstruction/lower airway obstruction/lung parenchymal disease/CNS or neuromuscular disordered control of breathing (**Refer to the Table 2**). **Note** *that respiratory problems do not always occur in isolation.* A neonate may demonstrate one or more types of respiratory distress or failure. For e.g. a neonate may have disordered control of breathing due to hypoxic-ischemic encephalopathy and then develop pneumonia or meconium aspiration syndrome.

Assess for the severity of respiratory distress or failure (**Refer to the Chapter 34 "Neonatal RDS"** for Downe's score in term babies and for Silverman-Anderson retraction score for preterm babies).

Intubate & ventilate if there is a slowly responsive underlying disease, hypoxia that responds poorly to oxygen and CPAP, concomitant metabolic acidosis, or if the neonate appears to be tiring and respiratory arrest seems likely.

Criteria for intubation and positive pressure ventilation
Absolute
* Major apnea with failure to respond promptly to bag and mask resuscitation

Relative
* ELBW infants <28 weeks gestational age in the labor suite
* Recurrent minor apnea unresponsive to CPAP and methylaxanthines
* Deteriorating respiratory status

  $PaO_2 \leq 50$ mmHg in FiO_2 $0.6 \leq 32$ weeks gestation
  $PaO_2 \leq 50$ mmHg in FiO_2 $0.8 > 32$ weeks gestation
  pH <7.25, $PaCO_2 > 50$ mmHg ≤ 32 weeks gestation
  pH <7.20, $PaCO_2 > 60$ mmHg > 32 weeks gestation
* Cerebral edema due to hypoxic-ischemic encephalopathy

---

* *Pearl/Peril/Pitfall :* The effects on the cardiovascular system are a balance between the direct and indirect effects. Typically, the patient is warm, flushed, sweaty, tachycardic and has a bouncing pulse. The clinical picture may be modified by effects of hypoxemia, other illnesses and the patient's medication. Arrhythmias may be present particularly if significant hypoxemia is present or sympathomimetics have been used. Acutely the acidosis will cause a right shift of the oxygen dissociation curve. If the acidosis persists, a decrease in red cell 2,3 DPG occurs which shifts the curve back to the left.

TABLE 1 — Causes of respiratory acidosis in neonates

a. **Pulmonary disease**

Pneumonia, Pneumothorax, Pulmonary edema, Pulmonary hemorrhage, Respiratory distress syndrome, Bronchopulmonary dysplasia, Hypoplastic lungs, Meconium Aspiration Syndrome, Bronchiolitis.

b. **Upper airway disease**

Aspiration, obstructive apnea, vocal cord paralysis, hemangioma (extrinsic/intrinsic)

c. **Neuromuscular disorders**

Myotonic dystrophy, Myasthenia gravis, diaphragmatic paralysis, medications such as muscle paralysing agents, aminoglycosides etc. Botulism, spinal muscular atrophies.

d. **CNS depression**

Hypoxic-Ischemic Encephalopathy, Increased intracranial pressure, medications such as narcotics, barbiturates, benzodiazepines, anesthesia etc., birth trauma with head injury.

e. **Miscellaneous** asphyxiating thoracic dystrophy, kyphoscoliosis etc.,

TABLE 2 — Clinical features of disorders causing respiratory acidosis in neonates

a. **Upper airway obstruction (i.e. the airways outside the thorax):** typical signs are observed predominantly during inspiration and may include *tachypnea *increased inspiratory respiratory effort (retractions and nasal flaring) *change in voice (e.g. hoarseness), cry *stridor (usually inspiratory but may be biphasic) *poor chest rise *poor air entry on auscultation. Other signs, such as cyanosis, drooling, cough, or seesaw breathing may be present. Respiratory rate is often mildly elevated because rapid rates create turbulent flow and further increase the resistance to airflow.

b. **Lower airway obstruction (i.e. the airways within the thorax) :** typical signs occur during expiration and include *tachypnea *wheezing (expiratory most common) *increased respiratory effort (retractions,

nasal flaring, and prolonged expiration) *prolonged expiratory phase associated with increased expiratory effort (i.e. expiration is an active rather than a passive process) *cough.

c. **Lung parenchymal disease :** typical signs include *tachypnea (often marked) *tachycardia *increased respiratory effort *grunting *hypoxemia (may be refractory to supplementary oxygen) *crackles (rales) *diminished breath sounds.

d. **Disordered control of breathing :** typical clinical signs are *variable/irregular respiratory rate (tachypnea alternating with bradypnea) *variable respiratory effort *shallow breathing (frequently resulting in hypoxemia and hypercarbia) *central apnea (i.e. apnea without any respiratory effort).

TABLE 3 — ABG analysis to assess the severity of respiratory acidosis and failure

LABORATORY CRITERIA pH-<7.1–7.2, PaO_2<50mmHg (6.6kPa) In FiO_2> 0.6 $PaCo_2$>60mmHg (8kPa). In infants weighing < 1500 g $PaCO_2$ should be modified to 50mmHg preventing the risk of intracerebral Hemorrhage (ICH) at high $PaCO_2$

Parameters	ABG Score			
	0	1	2	3
PaO_2 mmHg	>60	50-60	<50	<50
PH	>7.3	7.20-7.29	7.1-7.19 <7.1	
$PaCO_2$ mmHg	<50	50-60	61-70	>70

A score of 3 or more indicates the need for CPAP mechanical ventilation

KEY POINTS FOR CLINICAL PRACTICE

1. *Respiratory acidosis* is an inappropriate increase in blood Carbon dioxide (PCO_2), usually due to a decrease in the effectiveness of Carbon dioxide removal by the lungs, causing a decrease in the arterial blood pH < 7.35.

2. *CNS depression and neuromuscular diseases cause respiratory acidosis and failure without producing obvious respiratory distress, in contrast to Airways and lung parenchymal diseases.*

3. *Beware of the fact,* that in many Neonates respiratory acidosis may be multifactorial: an infant with chronic lung disease, an intrinsic lung disease, may worsen due to respiratory muscle dysfunction from severe hypokalemia as a result of diuretic therapy. Conversely, a child with spinal muscular atrophy may worsen because of aspiration pneumonia.

4. Respiratory acidosis is best managed by treating the underlying etiology. *Mechanical ventilation is necessary for a)hypoxia that responds poorly to oxygen, b)a slowly responsive underlying lung/CNS disease, if the sick Neonate appears to be tiring and respiratory arrest seems likely and c) if there is concomitant metabolic acidosis.*

5. *In patients with a chronic respiratory acidosis (e.g. premature baby with chronic lung disease), it is best to avoid mechanical ventilation because extubation is often difficult. However, an acute illness may necessitate mechanical ventilation in an infant with a chronic respiratory acidosis.*

REFERENCES & FURTHER READING : 1) Narins RG, Gardner LB. Simple acid-based disturbances. Med Clin North Am 1984;65:321. 2) Shapiro BA, Peruzzi WT, Templin R. Clinical application of blood gases, 5th edition 1994 Mosby-Year Book St. Louis. . 3) Kirpalani H, Kechagias S, Lerman J. Technical and clinical aspects of capnography in neonates. J Med Eng Technol 1991;15:154-161. 4) Avery`s diseases of the Newborn, 8th edition 5) Siggaard-Andersen O. Acid- Base Balance. Encyclopedia of respiratory medicine, 2004; 1-5.

* *Pearl/Peril/Pitfall: Important effects of Hypercapnia *Stimulation of ventilation via both central and peripheral chemoreceptors *Cerebral vasodilation increasing cerebral blood flow and intracranial pressure *Stimulation of the sympathetic nervous system resulting in tachycardia, peripheral vasoconstriction and sweating *Peripheral vasodilation by direct effect on vessels *Central depression at very high levels of pCO_2.*

Respiratory Alkalosis in Neonates

83

@ *Although neonates with primary lung disease may initially have a respiratory alkalosis, worsening of the disease, combined with respiratory muscle fatigue, often causes respiratory failure and the development of a respiratory acidosis.*

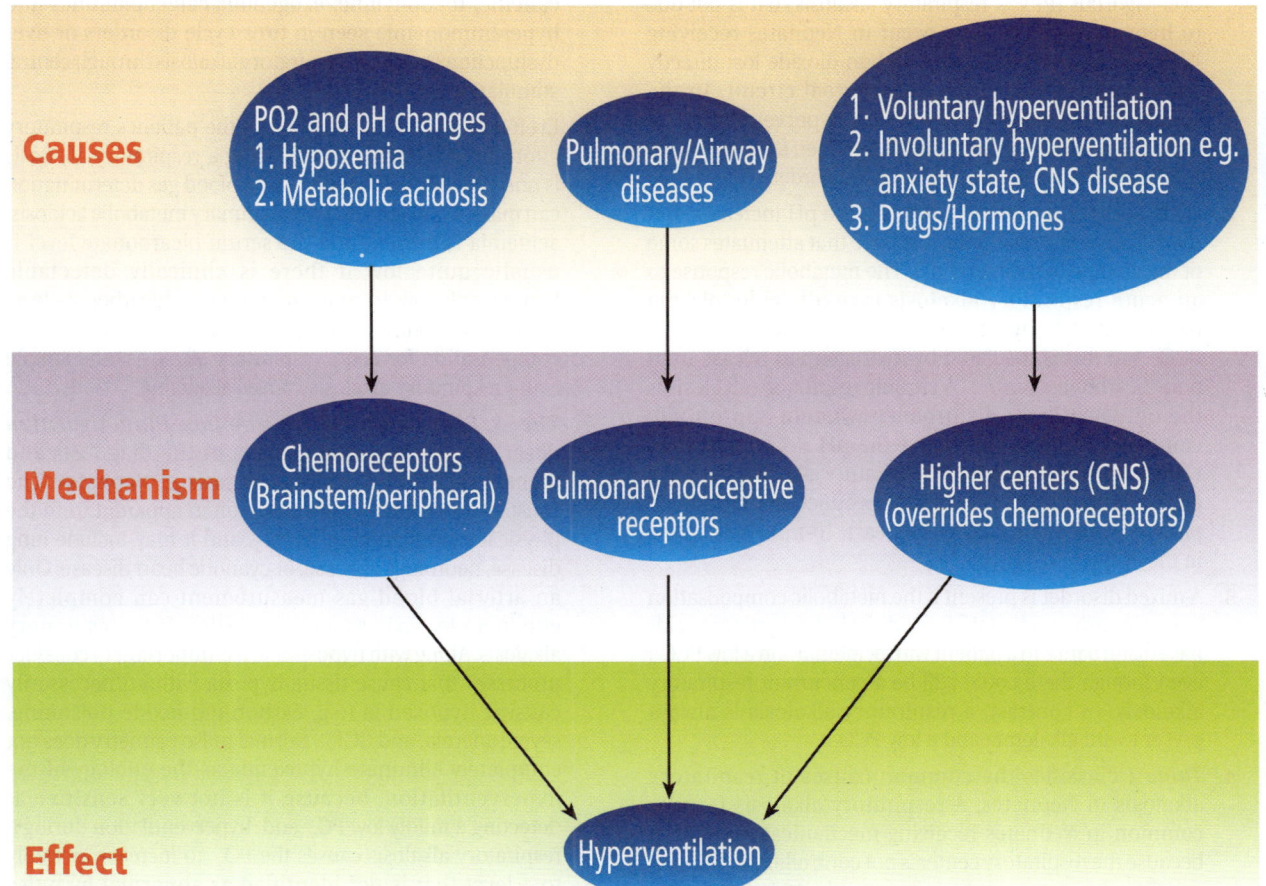

Causes

PO2 and pH changes
1. Hypoxemia
2. Metabolic acidosis

Pulmonary/Airway diseases

1. Voluntary hyperventilation
2. Involuntary hyperventilation e.g. anxiety state, CNS disease
3. Drugs/Hormones

Mechanism

Chemoreceptors (Brainstem/peripheral)

Pulmonary nociceptive receptors

Higher centers (CNS) (overrides chemoreceptors)

Effect

Hyperventilation

REVIEW OF CLINICAL PROBLEMS

1. Mention the common causes of Respiratory Alkalosis.
   Ans: Refer to the Table No 1 of the Chapter.

2. How do you evaluate Respiratory Alkalosis?
   Ans: Refer to the Evaluation-Decision-Action Plan/Algorithm to diagnose and manage Respiratory Alkalosis in Neonates.

3. Mention the cause of Respiratory Alkalosis in a Neonate not due to Hyperventilation.
   Ans: Refer to No 1 of the Bird`s eye view/Overview/Synopsis of the Chapter.

4. How do you manage Respiratory Alkalosis?
   Ans: Refer to the Evaluation-Decision-Action Plan/Algorithm to diagnose and manage Respiratory Alkalosis in Neonates.

5. What CNS & Lung INSULT, can happen due to severe Respiratory Alkalosis in Neonates?
   Ans: Refer to No 8 of the Bird`s eye view/Overview/Synopsis of the Chapter.

LEARNING OBJECTIVES

After completing this article, readers will be able to:

1. Search for the common causes of Respiratory Alkalosis in Neonates.

2. Confirm Respiratory Alkalosis in Neonates by ABG Analysis, as hyperventilation is not clinically detectable.

3. Manage Respiratory Alkalosis in Neonates by instituting specific treatment of underlying cause.

4. Avoid Iatrogenic Hyperventilation by adjusting ventilator settings.

5. Be careful about the preterm infants, as they can develop *PVL & CLD* secondary to severe Respiratory Alkalosis.

---

* **Pearl/Peril/Pitfall** : *Respiratory alkalosis- Hypoxemia is an important cause of respiratory stimulation and consequent respiratory alkalosis. The decrease in arterial pCO_2 inhibits the rise in ventilation. The hypocapnic inhibition of ventilation (acting via the central chemoreceptors) may leave the patient with an impaired state of tissue oxygen delivery. Adaptation occurs over a few days and the central chemoreceptor inhibition is lessened and ventilation increases. The number one priority is correction of any co-existing hypoxemia- Correction of hypoxemia is the most urgent concern and is many times more important than correction of the respiratory alkalosis. Administration of oxygen in sufficient concentrations and sufficient amounts is essential. Attention to other aspects necessary to improve oxygen delivery and minimize tissue oxygen consumption is important.*

BIRD'S EYE VIEW/OVERVIEW/SYNOPSIS

1. Respiratory alkalosis is an inappropriate reduction in the blood carbon dioxide concentration i.e. a PCO_2 below 32 mmHg and pH>7.40, is usually secondary to *hyperventilation* which is stimulated by a variety of stimuli such as hypoxia, cerebral irritation, metabolic acidosis or brain damage. However, it is commonly iatrogenic, due to over-vigorous IPPV. A respiratory alkalosis that is not due to hyperventilation may occur in Neonates receiving ECMO or hemodialysis, with carbon dioxide lost directly from the blood in the extracorporeal circuit. In the spontaneously breathing Newborn hyperventilation is most often caused by fever, sepsis, retained fetal lung fluid, mild aspiration pneumonia, or CNS disorders.

2. With a simple respiratory alkalosis, the pH increases, but there is a normal metabolic response that attenuates some of the change in the blood pH. The metabolic response to an acute respiratory alkalosis is predictable: plasma bicarbonate falls by 2 for each 10-mmHg decrease in the PCO_2 and this is mediated by hydrogen ion release from non-bicarbonate buffers. A chronic respiratory alkalosis is the only acid-base disturbance wherein appropriate compensation may normalize the pH > 7.4. Metabolic compensation for a chronic respiratory alkalosis develops gradually and takes 2-3 days to produce the full effect: plasma bicarbonate falls by 4 for each 10-mmHg decrease in the PCO_2.

3. A mixed disorder is present if the metabolic compensation is inappropriate. A metabolic acidosis is the dominant acid-base disturbance in a patient with acidemia and a low PCO_2, even though there could still be a concurrent respiratory alkalosis. In contrast, a respiratory alkalosis is always present with alkalemia and a low PCO_2.

4. *Table 1* classifies the common causes of respiratory alkalosis in Neonates. A respiratory alkalosis is quite common in Neonates receiving mechanical ventilation because the respiratory center is not controlling ventilation and these Neonates may have decreased metabolic rate and less carbon dioxide production because of sedation and paralytic medications. The physiologic response to decreased carbon dioxide production is to decrease ventilation, which does not occur in a Neonate who cannot reduce his ventilatory effort.

5. A variety of stimuli can increase the ventilatory drive and cause a respiratory alkalosis, such as arterial hypoxemia or tissue hypoxia secondary to primary lung disease, severe anemia, carbon monoxide poisoning, aspiration, hypotension, CCF, cyanotic heart disease, pneumothorax, and RDS. *Although Neonates with primary lung disease may initially have a respiratory alkalosis, worsening of the disease, combined with respiratory muscle fatigue, often causes respiratory failure and the development of a respiratory acidosis.* Hyperventilation in the absence of lung disease occurs with direct stimulation of the central respiratory center, which occurs with CNS diseases, such as meningitis, hemorrhage, and trauma. Sepsis can cause respiratory alkalosis due to cytokine release that stimulates the central respiratory center as well as a compensatory mechanism to the underlying metabolic acidosis. Although the exact mechanisms are not clear, liver disease causes a respiratory alkalosis that is usually proportional to the degree of liver failure. Certain medications, such as caffeine, theophylline, exogenous catecholamines and hyperammonemia seen in urea cycle disorders or liver dysfunction can cause respiratory alkalosis through central stimulation.

6. Even with careful observation of the patient's respiratory effort, hyperventilation producing a respiratory alkalosis is not clinically detectable. Only a blood gas determination can make the diagnosis. With a primary metabolic acidosis, acidemia is present and the serum bicarbonate level is usually quite low if there is clinically detectable hyperventilation. In contrast, the serum bicarbonate level never goes below 17mEq/L as part of the metabolic compensation for acute respiratory alkalosis, and simple acute respiratory alkalosis causes alkalemia.

7. *The Evaluation-Decision-Action-Plan/Algorithm* describes the essential aspects of the diagnosis and management of respiratory alkalosis in Neonates. The cause of a respiratory alkalosis is often apparent from the physical examination or history, and it may include lung disease, neurologic disease, or cyanotic heart disease. Only an arterial blood gas measurement can completely eliminate hypoxia as an explanation for a respiratory alkalosis. Along with hypoxemia, it is important to consider processes that cause tissue hypoxia without necessarily causing hypoxemia (e.g. carbon monoxide poisoning, severe anemia, and CCF). Normal pulse oximetry does not completely eliminate hypoxemia as the etiology of the hyperventilation, because it is not very sensitive at detecting a mildly low PO_2 and hyperventilation during a respiratory alkalosis causes the PO_2 to increase, possibly to a level that is not identified as abnormal by pulse oximetry.

8. *It is very important to avoid hyperventilation during resuscitation and mechanical ventilation in the management of the sick preterm newborn, because findings suggest an association between hypocarbia (PCO_2 < 20 mmHg) and the development of periventricular leukomalacia (PVL) and chronic lung disease.*

9. The treatment of Neonatal respiratory alkalosis consists of the specific management of the underlying process causing hyperventilation. Mechanical ventilator settings are adjusted to correct iatrogenic respiratory alkalosis, unless the hyperventilation has a therapeutic purpose (e.g., treatment of increased intracranial pressure).

10. Because alkalemia causes more calcium bind to albumin, it is important to correct hypocalcemia related tetany and seizures secondary to severe respiratory alkalosis. A respiratory alkalosis also causes a mild reduction in the serum potassium level due to redistribution.

---

* **Pearl/Peril/Pitfall:** *Only one respiratory acid-base disorder can be present at one time. A patient cannot have both a respiratory alkalosis and a respiratory acidosis. Essentially this is because a person cannot be both hyperventilating and hypoventilating at the same time. More than one metabolic acid-base disorder can be present at the one time. A patient can have a lactic acidosis and then develop a metabolic alkalosis (e.g. due to vomiting) and end up with a HCO_3 level & pH which are normal. This is possible if the acidosis and the alkalosis exactly balance each other. This patient is then said to have both a metabolic acidosis AND a metabolic alkalosis. It is therapeutically useful to know this rather then to say there is no acid-base disorder present.*

THE EVALUATION-DECISION-ACTION-PLAN / ALGORITHM FOR THE DIAGNOSIS AND MANAGEMENT OF *RESPIRATORY ALKALOSIS IN NEONATES*

SUBJECTIVE FINDINGS

Hx of predisposing conditions which can increase the ventilatory drive - hypoxia secondary to pneumonia, sepsis, pulmonary edema, severe anemia, aspiration, cyanotic heart disease, high altitude, pneumothorax and RDS.

Hx of predisposing conditions which stimulate the central respiratory center directly - meningitis, CNS hemorrhage and trauma, fever, pain, medications (caffeine, theophylline, catacholamines etc.,) hyperammonemia, mechanical ventilation and ECMO.

OBJECTIVE FINDINGS

Assess ABCs, disability (altered sensorium, seizures, focal neurodeficits), vitals, BP, Urine output & capillary refill time.

Look for hypocalcemic tetany/seizures, hypokalemia related symptoms.

Perform complete physical examination to identify the underlying causes of respiratory alkalosis (Refer to Table 1), which may include lung disease, neurologic disease, or cyanotic heart disease.

Note whether the neonate is spontaneously breathing/mechanically ventilated.

INVESTIGATIONS

Blood ABG analysis, electrolytes, BUN, creatinine, osmolality, ketones, glucose, culture, calcium, magnesium, FBC with differential & platelets, drug screen, LFTs.

CXR to identify lung pathology.

Echocardiogram if cyanotic heart disease is suspected.

Serum ammonia if an inborn error of metabolism/liver dysfunction is suspected.

CT/MRI brain scanning if CNS pathology is to be excluded.

RESPIRATORY ALKALOSIS IN NEONATES

Identify Hypocalcemia and Hypokalemia and manage them appropriately. *Control* fever, pain or anxiety due to an underlying disease.

Adjust Mechanical ventilator settings to correct iatrogenic respiratory alkalosis and to prevent PVL changes in a preterm baby (never allow PCO_2 to fall below 20mmHg).

Administer IV broadspectrum antibiotics after full septic screen, if sepsis is suspected to be the underlying cause of respiratory alkalosis.

Ensure ABCs, Pulse oximetry, Administer oxygen, Cardiac monitor, protect airway and apnea monitor, BP, ideally from the arterial catheter.

Monitor ABG 3-4 hrly for PCO_2, arterial pH and base deficit (pulse oximetry is not very sensitive at detecting a mildly low PO_2 and severe anemia, CCF, and carbon monoxide poisoning cause tissue hypoxia without necessarily causing hypoxemia).

Focus the management on the underlying disease, as there is seldom a need for specific treatment of respiratory alkalosis.

TABLE 1   Causes of respiratory alkalosis in neonates

a. Hypoxemia/tissue hypoxia Pneumonia, pulmonary edema, cyanotic heart disease, congestive cardiac failure, severe anemia, aspiration, hypotension, carbon monoxide poisoning, pulmonary embolism.

b. Lung receptor stimulation Pneumonia, pulmonary edema, pneumothorax, RDS

c. Central stimulation Fever, pain, liver failure, sepsis, medications such as caffeine, theophylline, catecholamines, etc. mechanical ventilation, hyperammonemia, ECMO and CNS disease (meningitis, trauma, hemorrhage etc.)

KEY POINTS FOR CLINICAL PRACTICE

1. Respiratory alkalosis is an inappropriate reduction in the blood carbon dioxide concentration i.e. a PCO_2 below 32 mmHg and pH>7.40, is usually secondary to *hyperventilation* which is stimulated by a variety of stimuli such as hypoxia, cerebral irritation, metabolic acidosis or brain damage. However, it is commonly iatrogenic, due to overvigorous IPPV.

2. In the spontaneously breathing Newborn hyperventilation is most often caused by fever, sepsis, retained fetal lung fluid, mild aspiration pneumonia, or CNS disorders.

3. The metabolic response to an acute respiratory alkalosis is predictable: plasma bicarbonate falls by 2 for each 10-mmHg decrease in the PCO_2 and this is mediated by hydrogen ion release from non-bicarbonate buffers. A chronic respiratory alkalosis is the only acid-base disturbance wherein appropriate compensation may normalize the pH > 7.4.

4. Hyperventilation in the absence of lung disease occurs with direct stimulation of the central respiratory center, which occurs with CNS diseases, such as meningitis, hemorrhage, and trauma. Sepsis can cause respiratory alkalosis due to cytokine release that stimulates the central respiratory center as well as a compensatory mechanism to the underlying metabolic acidosis.

5. The treatment of Neonatal respiratory alkalosis consists of the specific management of the underlying process causing hyperventilation. Mechanical ventilator settings are adjusted to correct iatrogenic respiratory alkalosis, unless the hyperventilation has a therapeutic purpose (e.g., treatment of increased intracranial pressure).

REFERENCES & FURTHER READING : 1) Paulev PE, Siggaard-Andersen O. Clinical application of the pO2-pCO2 diagram. *Acta Anaesthesiol Scand* 2004; 48: 1105-1114. 2) Taeusch HW, Ballard RA (Eds). Avery's Diseases of the Newborn 8th Ed. W.B. Saunders Company, Philadelphia. 2005.

* *Pearl/Peril/Pitfall : Respiratory alkalosis: Key points regarding compensation in respiratory alkalosis: *Role of Kidney : The effector organ for compensation is the kidney. *Slow Response: The renal response has a slow onset and the maximal response takes 2 to 3 days to be achieved. *Outcome: The drop in bicarbonate results in the extracellular pH returning only partially towards its normal value.*

84

Prenatal Hydronephrosis

@ *The main considerations in evaluating a fetus with antenatal hydronephrosis are gestational age, laterality of the lesion, the presence of unfavorable prognostic factors, volume of amniotic fluid, and overall fetal well-being.*

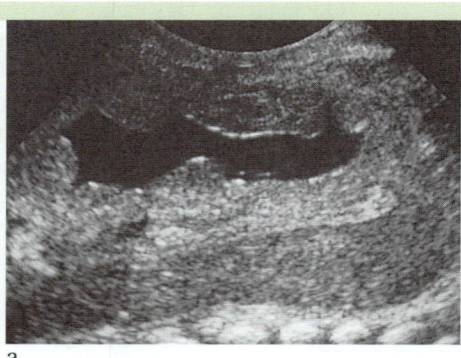 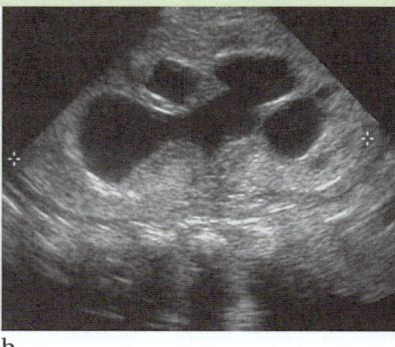 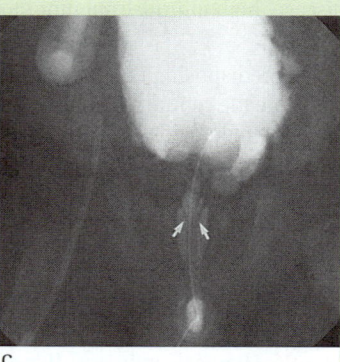

a.   b.   c.

Posterior urethral valves in a 1-day-old boy. **(a)** US scan shows a markedly thickened bladder wall. **(b)** US scan shows a hydronephrotic kidney with associated dysplastic parenchymal changes of increased echogenicity and loss of corticomedullary differentiation. **(c)** Voiding cystourethrogram shows the posterior urethral valves (arrows) at both sides of an indwelling catheter. The bladder is heavily trabeculated.

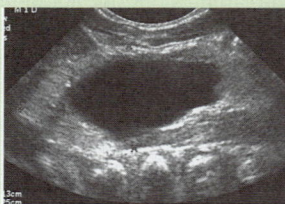 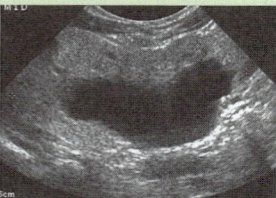

a.   b.

Bilateral obstruction of the ureteropelvic junction in a 1-day-old boy. **(a, b)** US scans of the right **(a)** and left **(b)** kidneys show marked dilatation of the collecting system and diffuse renal dysplasia with increased parenchymal echogenicity and thinning.

Hydronephrosis in the Fetus and Neonate

Criteria for Surgery or Observation

Consider Surgery:
* Anteroposterior diameter >30 mm
* Anteroposterior diameter >20 mm with calyceal dilation
* Renal function <30%
* Worsening renal function
* Worsening hydronephrosis
* Symptoms

Continued Observation:
* Prophylactic antibiotics
* Renal ultrasonography every 2 to 12 months, as indicated
* Repeat renography if ultrasonography documents worsening or symptoms develop
* Discharge if improved, surgery if indicated

REVIEW OF CLINICAL PROBLEMS

1. Mention the usual causes of Prenatal Hydronephrosis.
   Ans: Refer to the Table 1 of the Chapter.

2. How do you grade Prenatal Hydronephrosis?
   Ans: Refer to the Table 2 of the Chapter.

3. What sort of inquiries should be done on finding Fetal Hydronephrosis?
   Ans: Refer to No 4 of the Bird's eye view/Overview/Synopsis of the Chapter.

4. How do you evaluate Prenatal Hydronephrosis postnatally?
   Ans: Refer to the Evaluation-Decision-Action Plan/Algorithm to diagnose and manage Prenatal Hydronephrosis.

5. What differential diagnoses should you consider while evaluating Prenatal Hydronephrosis?
   Ans: Refer to the Evaluation-Decision-Action Plan/Algorithm to diagnose and manage Prenatal Hydronephrosis.

LEARNING OBJECTIVES

After completing this article, readers will be able to:

1. Identify significant renal & urinary tract abnormalities causing Prenatal Hydronephrosis.

2. Avoid unnecessary testing in physiologic/insignificant Prenatal Hydronephrosis.

3. Consider the common Differential diagnoses of Prenatal Hydronephrosis, during evaluation.

4. Liaise early with Pediatric Urologist when significant obstructive uropathy is the working diagnosis.

5. Communicate with parents about the course, investigations, prophylaxis for VUR/UTI, & Prognosis for the underlying diagnosis, where appropriate.

Pearl/Peril/Pitfall : Evaluation and management of the neonate or infant in the outpatient setting is directed by the underlying cause of antenatal and postnatal hydronephrosis. Arranging appropriate follow-up with other subspecialties may also be necessary if the prenatal and postnatal evaluation warrants this type of management.

BIRD'S EYE VIEW/OVERVIEW/SYNOPSIS

1. Hydronephrosis is the most common pathologic finding in the urinary tract on prenatal screening by ultrasonography, accounting for 50% of all abnormal findings; a significant fetal anomaly in 1% of pregnancies, of which 20-30% of cases are genitourinary in origin. If not for prenatal ultrasonographic detection, many of these urologic anomalies would manifest, as they did in the past, later in life as pyelonephritis, symptomatic flank or abdominal pain, renal calculi, hypertension, or even end-stage renal disease. Antenatal hydronephrosis has received significant attention since prenatal ultrasonography became a mainstream screening tool; however, the management and treatment remains controversial in terms of patient outcome.

2. Most anomalies of the urinary tract discovered in the prenatal period are characterized by hydronephrosis or dilatation of the upper urinary tract. Intuitively, these lesions may be considered obstructive in nature; however, antenatal hydronephrosis can be the result of nonobstructive processes, such as vesicoureteral reflux, nonrefluxing nonobstructed megaureter, and prune belly syndrome. Obstructive lesions, particularly bilateral lesions, are more harmful to the developing kidneys, and the urine produced is a major component of amniotic fluid necessary for normal lung development and prevention of compression deformities. Therefore, differentiation of obstructive lesions and nonobstructive lesions is extremely important in determining the eventual outcome of the fetus. However, this may not be possible until the child is born.

3. Obstructive lesions and lesions that affect both kidneys are uniformly more threatening than nonobstructive and unilateral lesions. The survival rate with unilateral renal obstruction approaches 100%, with only 15-25% of patients requiring surgery at 4 years' follow-up. In the presence of a bilateral obstructive process, oligohydramnios is the best predictor of an adverse outcome. Obstructive lesions and lesions that affect both kidneys are uniformly more threatening than nonobstructive and unilateral lesions. The survival rate with unilateral renal obstruction approaches 100%, with only 15-25% of patients requiring surgery at 4 years' follow-up. In the presence of a bilateral obstructive process, oligohydramnios is the best predictor of an adverse outcome. Fetal urine is a significant component of the amniotic fluid volume, and maintenance of adequate volumes is essential for normal lung development. If oligohydramnios is present, pulmonary hypoplasia and compression deformities of the skeletal system can result and significantly influence quality of life and survival (Potter syndrome).

4. The finding of antenatal hydronephrosis should prompt a series of inquires regarding onset, fetal sex, oligohydramnios, laterality, severity of hydronephrosis, bladder cycling, other anomalies, prior pregnancy complications, and family history of urologic disease. Ultrasonographic evaluation can provide important information, such as sex of the fetus, unilateral or bilateral disease, renal anterior-posterior (AP) pelvic diameter, bladder distension, bladder sagittal length, volume of amniotic fluid, and associated pathologic conditions. For example, Reuss et al found that 16 of 31 (55%) fetuses with bilateral hydronephrosis and oligohydramnios had an associated structural or chromosomal abnormality. Other aspects of the history that can be helpful in identifying the cause of hydronephrosis include family and maternal history.

5. Numerous pathologic entities can cause antenatal hydronephrosis. Antenatal hydronephrosis without associated urinary tract anomaly is the etiology in the vast majority of infants with hydronephrosis (79-84%) and has been termed isolated antenatal hydronephrosis (IAHN). IAHN is believed to be caused by a physiologic dilatation of the developing ureter. *The goal of evaluation is to differentiate benign physiologic dilation from significant obstructive disease or reflux.*

6. *The Evaluation-Decision-Action-Plan/Algorithm* describes the essential aspects of history taking, clinical examination and laboratory evaluation and the management of Prenatally diagnosed Hydronephrosis. Renal AP pelvic diameter is used to evaluate the significance of dilation. In one series, 94% of fetuses with a renal AP diameter of greater than 2 cm, 50% with an AP diameter of 1-1.5 cm, and only 3% with an AP diameter of less than 1 cm required surgery or at least long-term monitoring for a significant urinary tract lesion. More recently, a renal AP pelvic diameter of at least 4 mm before 33 weeks' gestation and at least 7 mm after 33 weeks' gestation is considered significant. Caliectasis correlates best with the presence of a significant dilation or an obstructive process. The presence of a distended bladder without functional emptying is important in developing a differential diagnosis. A filled bladder should be visualized, with functional emptying observed every 30-60 minutes. A system that does not function in this manner suggests the presence of posterior urethral valves, prune belly syndrome, or the often-fatal urethral atresia. In these cases, the bladder and (sometimes) the upper urinary tract are massively dilated. The measurement of fetal sagittal bladder length (FSBL) in combination with the presence of pelviectasis has been suggested as a tool to determine the outcome of antenatal hydronephrosis. The presence of megacystis, determined as FSBL of greater than gestational age (GA) plus 12, in association with pyelectasis, suggests the presence of posterior urethral valve or vesicoureteral reflux. Renal architecture, renal size, and echogenicity of the renal parenchyma are important in developing a differential and determining the potential function of the kidney. Increased echogenicity may be associated with renal dysplasia.

7. The final consideration for the imaging team is a global assessment of the fetus. Finding abnormalities in other systems is not uncommon when a urologic abnormality is detected. One series showed that 55% of fetuses with bilateral hydronephrosis and oligohydramnios had an associated structural or chromosomal abnormality. These anomalies are commonly of cardiovascular, neurologic, and orthopedic origin, but they can be found elsewhere and should be sought during the imaging evaluation.

8. **Surgical Care:** Intervention for a fetus with antenatal hydronephrosis is controversial for various reasons. First, obtaining an accurate diagnosis with current technology is difficult. Second, the natural history of each disease process causing antenatal hydronephrosis is variable and has not been fully elucidated. Finally, the lack of data regarding the success and complications of intervention has impeded progress in defining specific indications for treatment.

9. A management strategy has been developed based on initial and serial prenatal ultrasonographic findings. Significant unilateral hydronephrosis does not require prenatal intervention; however, it should be evaluated in the postnatal period with follow-up renal ultrasonography (if needed), voiding cystourethrography, and diuretic renography. Bilateral hydronephrosis without bladder distension is more significant and should be monitored prenatally with serial ultrasonographic examinations to monitor for bladder distension and development of oligohydramnios. Postnatal evaluation should be performed as above. A fetus that presents with bilateral hydronephrosis and a distended bladder should raise serious concern for an obstructive process, such as urethral atresia or urethral valves.

10. The most common inpatient and/or outpatient medication prescribed in the setting of antenatally detected hydronephrosis persisting in the postnatal period is a prophylactic antibiotic against urinary tract infection. This medication is required to prevent urinary tract infections and possible renal damage that may result from pyelonephritis. This medication is not prescribed to all patients with hydronephrosis and is administered to patients based on the underlying cause of their hydronephrosis. Generally, a penicillin-based antibiotic is appropriate in this age group. Most neonates with antenatal hydronephrosis have an excellent prognosis. Prognosis is largely dependent on the underlying etiology of the dilated collecting system. Severe bilateral hydronephrosis that is associated with obstruction and oligohydramnios detected early in gestation is the best predictor of an adverse outcome.

Pearl/Peril/Pitfall : Although renal pelvic dilatation is a transient, physiologic state in most cases, urinary tract obstruction and vesicoureteral reflux (VUR) are also causal. These conditions can prevent normal renal development and/or cause renal injury. However, the majority of cases of antenatal hydronephrosis are not clinically significant and can lead to unnecessary testing of the newborn baby and anxiety for patients and healthcare providers.

THE EVALUATION-DECISION-ACTION-ALGORITHM FOR THE DIAGNOSIS AND MANAGEMENT OF *PRENATAL HYDRONEPHROSIS*

SUBJECTIVE FINDINGS

Hx of onset, fetal sex, oligo-hydramnios, laterality, severity of hydronephrosis, bladder cycling, other anomalies, prior pregnancy complications, and family history of urologic disease.

Hx of family and maternal history.

OBJECTIVE FINDINGS

* Failure to void within the first 48 hours of life favors the diagnosis of obstructive uropathy(PU Valves or Urethral Atresia); remember that the observation of spontaneous voiding with normal urinary stream within first 24 hours of life does not rule out an obstructive process

Assess for palpable kidneys, bladder, hypertension, Potter facies and other dysmorphic features

Determine renal anterior-posterior (AP) pelvic diameter(Refer to the Table 2 of the Chapter),bladder distension, bladder sagittal length, volume of amniotic fluid, and associated pathologic conditions, unilateral or bilateral disease,

INVESTIGATIONS

Imaging Postnatal follow-up renal ultrasonography (if needed), voiding cystourethrography, and diuretic renography.

RENAL FUNCTION TESTS AND URINANALYSIS ANS C/S AS INDICATED *clinically.*

Differential diagnoses

Posterior Urethral Valves

Radiographic Evaluation of the Pediatric Urinary Tract

Ureteropelvic Junction Obstruction

Vesicoureteral Reflux

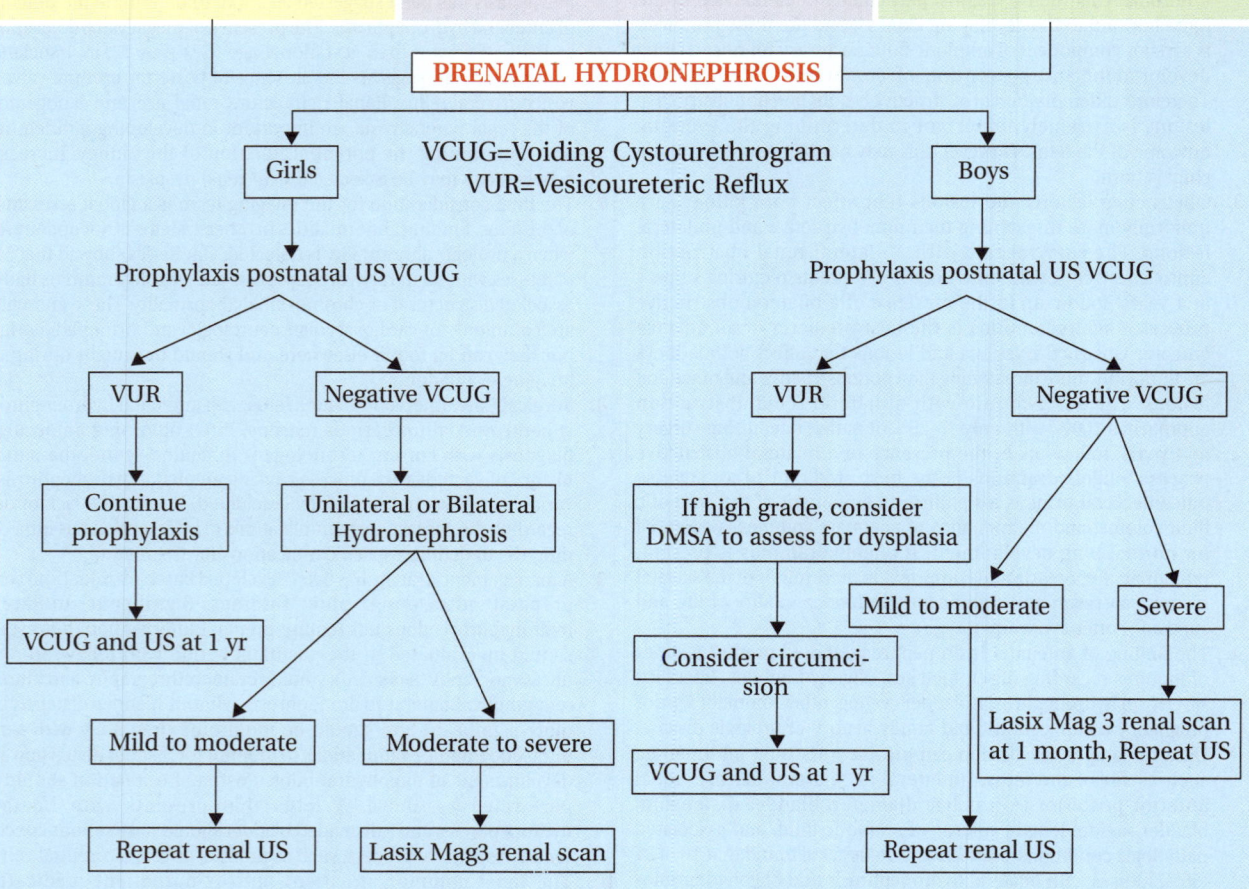

The clinical spectrum of posterior urethral valves (PUVs) includes the stillborn fetus with Potter's syndrome, the Newborn baby with significant pulmonary hypoplasia and renal failure that leads to early Neonatal death, the prenatally detected or clinically presenting case that responds to early aggressive management of obstruction, infection and bladder dysfunction, and patients where the effects of obstruction are more subtle and diagnosis is delayed possibly into adult life. Although resecting the obstructing valve leaflets is relatively straightforward nowadays using state-of-the-art equipment, patients with PUVs have a constellation of associated problems that pose a continued threat to renal function through childhood. Clinicians looking after boys with PUVs need to be aware of the complex pathophysiology of the condition, the need for ongoing appropriate specialist investigation and follow-up throughout life, and the frequent occurrence of chronic renal failure despite the provision of expert multidisciplinary care.***Surgical Treatment, most commonly a Pyeloplasty of a Pelviureteric Junction anomaly is advocated by most urologists when the following conditions exist;** *a symptomatic PUJ Anomaly *declining function in the dilated kidney *moderate pelvic dilation with dilatation of the calyses *an increasing pelvic dilatation *bilateral moderate-to-severe dilatation of the pelvis.*

* ***Pearl/Peril/Pitfall :*** *The goal of postnatal management of infants with antenatal hydronephrosis is to identify patients with significant renal and urinary tract abnormalities while avoiding unnecessary testing in patients with physiologic or clinically insignificant hydronephrosis. Evaluation includes physical examination and the use of radiologic studies to detect renal and urinary tract abnormalities including obstructive uropathy or vesicoureteral reflux (VUR).*

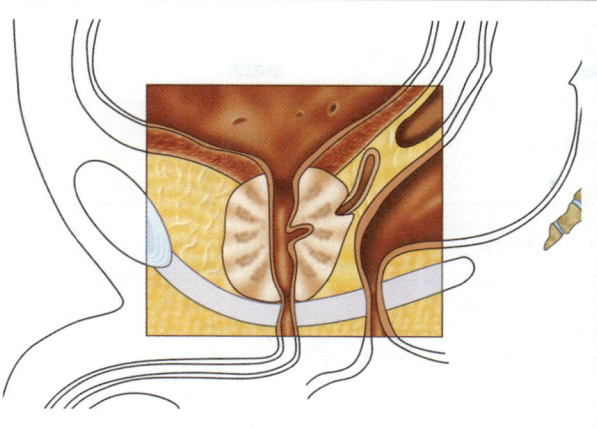

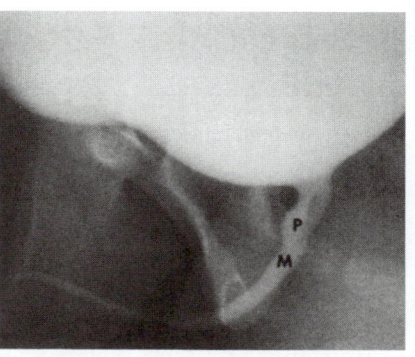

The male urethra The male urethra is divided into five anatomic divisions. The glandular portion, the cavernous or penile portion, and the bulbous portion form the "anterior urethra." The prostatic portion, P, that part within the prostate gland, and the membranous portion, M, the short part traversing the pelvic floor, are the "posterior urethra." It is with the posterior urethra that we are mainly concerned here.

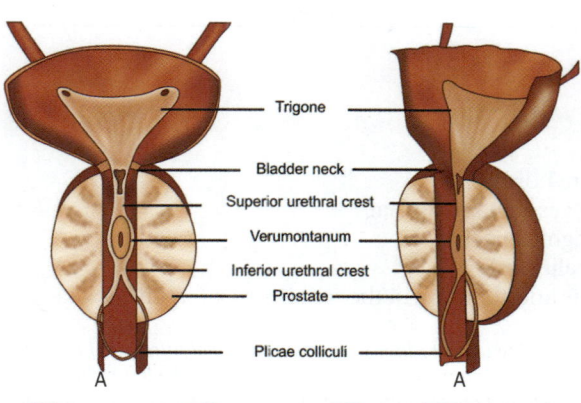

The posterior urethra: The important anatomic structures concerned in the morphology of posterior urethral valves are shown in these frontal (A) and oblique (B) diagrams of the bladder base and posterior urethra. The inferior urethral crest, the midline extension of the verumontanum, terminates in two to four plicae colliculi (or fins). These pass downward while encircling the urethra, ending anteriorly close to the midline at a more caudal level.

Courtesy: *Posterior urethral valves*
Roderick I. Macpherson, M.D.* Richard E. Leithiser, M.D.* L. Gordon, M.D.* W.R. Turner, M.D.t. Volume 6, Number 5 1 September, 1986 Radiographics

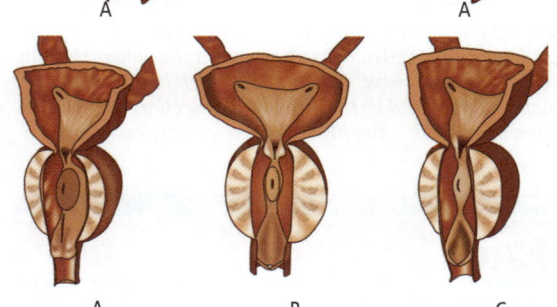

Types of posterior urethral valves The original classification of the types of posterior urethral valves proposed by Young *(27)* in 1919 is still in use today. (A) Type I posterior urethral valves (arrow) are mucosal folds extending anteroinferiorly from the caudal aspect of the verumontanum, often fusing anteriorly at a lower level. They are derived from the plicae colliculi and constitute the vast majority of valves. (B) Type 2 posterior urethral valves (arrow) are mucosal folds extending anterosuperiorly from the verumontanum toward the bladder neck. A rare occurrence, they are probably an effect rather than a cause of bladder obstruction. (C) Type 3 posterior urethral valves (arrow) are disc-like membranes located below the verumontanum and unrelated to it. They constitute a small percentage of posterior urethral valves.

The pathophysiology and subsequent pathologic effects of posterior urethral valves must be understood in order for one to appreciate their clinical and radiologic features as well as the problems in their management.

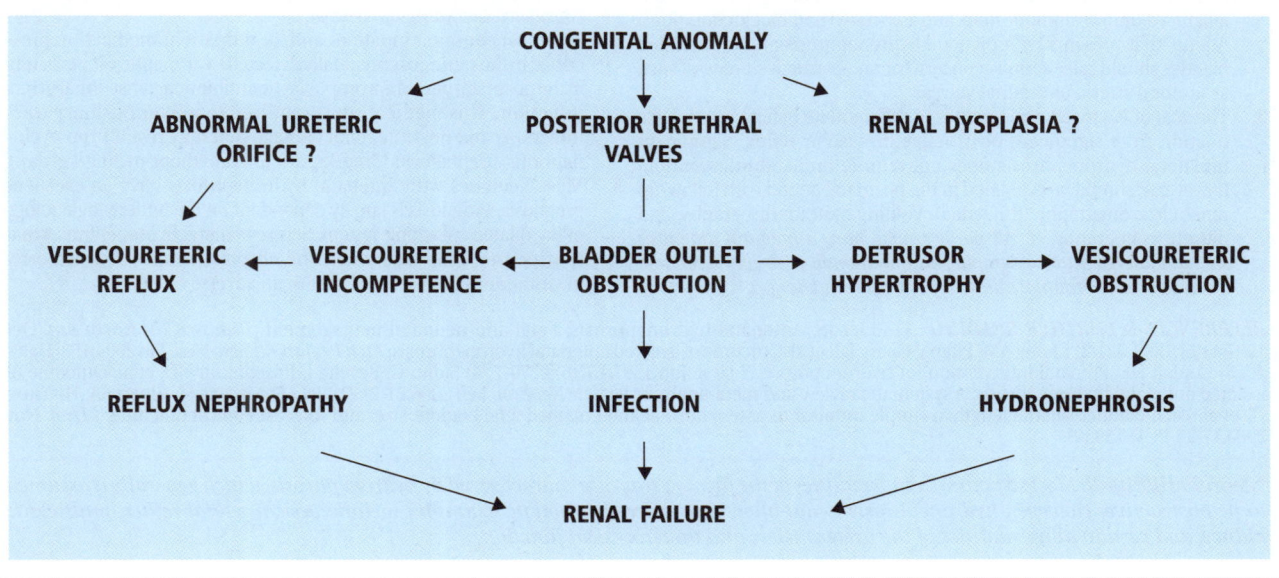

TABLE 1 Causes of prenatal hydronephrosis and ultrasound characteristics

	Ipsilateral ureter	Bladder
UPJO	Normal	Normal
Vesicoureteral reflux	Dilated or normal	Dilated or normal
Ureterocele	Dilated	Dilated or normal (cystic mass-ureterocele)
Ectopic ureter	Often dilated	Normal
Posterior urethral valves	Often dilated (bilateral)	Thick wall, increased postvoid residual
Multicystic kidney	Normal	Normal
Primary obstructive or nonrefluxing nonobstructing mega-ureter	Dilated	Normal
Urethral ureter	Dilated (bilateral)	Thick wall, not emptying (oligohydramnios)
Retrocaval ureter	Dilated proximal and normal distal	Normal
Prune belly syndrome	Dilated	Dilated

UPJO=Ureteropelvic Junction Obstruction

TABLE 2 Fetal hydronephrosis grading scale

Grade I   : Pelvic APD is 1 cm and the calyces are normal
Grade II   : Pelvic APD is 1 to 1.5 cm but the calyces remain normal
Grade III : Pelvic APD is >1.5 cm and there is slight caliectasis
Grade IV   : Pelvic APD >1.5 cm with moderate caliectasis
Grade V   : APD is >1.5 cm with severe caliectasis and thinning of the renal cortex (<2 mm thick)

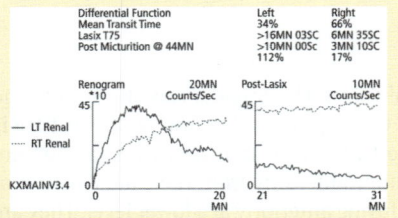

MAG3 Diuretic Renogram showing a left kidney with ipsilateral Pelviureteric junction obstruction anomaly. The dotted line represents the radioactivity in the left kidney; the plain line represents the radioactivity in the right kidney. The right kidney takes up the radioactive marker promptly and then within 20 minutes, as shown by the down-sloping line, has excreted the marker. This is normal curve. In contrast, the left kidney has poor uptake, indicating reduced function, confirmed by the differential function of 34%, and by 30 minutes the radioactivity remains high, showing impaired urinary excretion.

KEY POINTS FOR CLINICAL PRACTICE:

1. Hydronephrosis is the most common pathologic finding in the urinary tract on prenatal screening by ultrasonography, accounting for 50% of all abnormal findings. The finding of antenatal hydronephrosis should prompt a series of inquires regarding onset, fetal sex, oligohydramnios, laterality, severity of hydronephrosis, bladder cycling, other anomalies, prior pregnancy complications, and family history of urologic disease.

2. Ultrasonographic evaluation can provide important information, such as sex of the fetus, unilateral or bilateral disease, renal anterior-posterior (AP) pelvic diameter, bladder distention, bladder sagittal length, volume of amniotic fluid, and associated pathologic conditions. A fetus that presents with bilateral hydronephrosis and a distended bladder should raise serious concern for an obstructive process, such as urethral atresia or urethral valves.

3. The goal of Postnatal evaluation is to differentiate benign physiologic dilation *from* significant obstructive disease or reflux. Significant unilateral hydronephrosis does not require prenatal intervention; however, it should be evaluated in the postnatal period with follow-up renal ultrasonography (if needed), voiding cystourethrography, and diuretic renography. *1. All patients who have a prenatal diagnosis should undergo ultrasonographic examination in postnatal week 1. a. Those who have minimal dilation (15 mm) are discharged. b. Those who have bilateral disease should undergo VCUG and renography. Severe cases should be considered for surgical intervention according to the criteria Refer to table given above; milder disease is followed with observation. c. Those who have unilateral disease are considered for surgery if the dilation is severe; the others are followed with repeat ultrasonography after 8 to 12 weeks of observation. 2. If follow-up ultrasonography documents improvement, the patient can be discharged. If there is persistent hydronephrosis of Grade 2 or higher, renography is performed and surgery or continued observation is considered according to the criteria.*

4. The most common inpatient and/or outpatient medication prescribed in the setting of antenatally detected hydronephrosis persisting in the postnatal period is a prophylactic antibiotic against urinary tract infection. This medication is required to prevent urinary tract infections and possible renal damage that may result from pyelonephritis. (Cephalexin 15mg/kg/day or Trimethoprim 2mg/kg/day.)

5. Most Neonates with antenatal hydronephrosis have an excellent prognosis. Prognosis is largely dependent on the underlying etiology of the dilated collecting system. Severe bilateral hydronephrosis that is associated with obstruction and oligohydramnios detected early in gestation is the best predictor of an adverse outcome.

REFERENCES & FURTHER READING : 1) Elder JS. Antenatal hydronephrosis. Fetal and neonatal management. *Pediatr Clin North Am.* Oct 1997;44(5):1299-321. 2) Cheng AM, Phan V, Geary DF, et al. Outcome of isolated antenatal hydronephrosis. *Arch Pediatr Adolesc Med.* Jan 2004;158(1):38-40. 3) Coplen DE. Prenatal intervention for hydronephrosis. *J Urol.* Jun 1997;157(6):2270-7. 4) Sidhu G, Beyene J, Rosenblum ND, et al. Outcome of isolated antenatal hydronephrosis: a systematic review and meta-analysis. *Pediatr Nephrol.* Feb 2006;21(2):218-24. 5) Maizels M, Alpert SA, Houston JT, et al. Fetal bladder sagittal length: a simple monitor to assess normal and enlarged fetal bladder size, and forecast clinical outcome. *J Urol.* Nov 2004;172(5 Pt 1):1995-9.

Pearl/Peril/Pitfall: Most structural abnormalities of the urinary tract are characterized by hydronephrosis, which generally is assumed to be obstructive. However, hydronephrosis is not often caused by obstruction; examples include vesicoureteral reflux, multicystic kidney, and certain abnormalities of the ureteropelvic and ureterovesical junction.

85 Neonatal Urinary Tract Infection and Vesicoureteric Reflux

@ *Clinical presentation of UTI in children may be nonspecific, and the appropriateness of certain diagnostic tests remains controversial. The diagnostic work-up should be tailored to uncover functional and structural abnormalities such as dysfunctional voiding, vesicoureteral reflux and obstructive uropathy. A more aggressive work-up, including renal cortical scintigraphy, ultrasound and voiding cystourethrography, is recommended for patients at greater risk for pyelonephritis and renal scarring, including infants less than one year of age and all children who have systemic signs of infection concomitant with a UTI.*

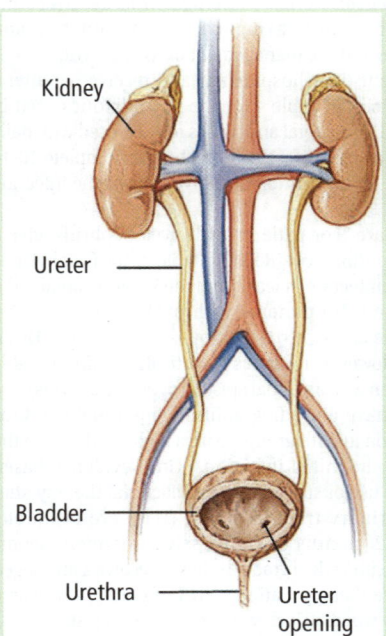

Urinary tract infection (UTI) in childhood affects many children but it can be difficult to diagnose, especially in infancy where it is believed that most renal damage occurs. UTI can point the way to underlying congenital abnormalities of the urinary tract which are uncommon, as are the long-term sequelae of renal scarring, hypertension and chronic renal failure. It is now appreciated that many infants have reflux associated damage before birth with associated renal dysplasia. Investigations in children with a UTI remain controversial with ultrasonography being sufficient in experienced hands and only selected patients undergoing cystography and radionuclide imaging. Gross vesicoureteric reflux (VUR) is rare and most mild to moderate VUR resolves spontaneously. Although there is no randomized controlled trial to date low dose prophylactic antibiotics are used in the majority of children in whom VUR is detected with surgery being reserved for those with problematical infections or anatomical abnormalities. Familial reflux is increasingly recognized.

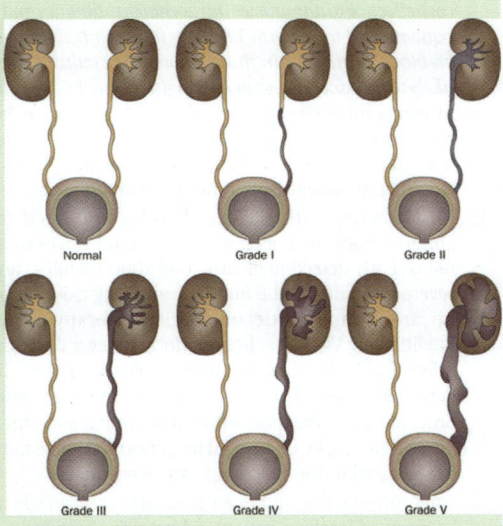

The severity of VUR has been most commonly reported using the classification of the International Reflux Study. This classification defines grade I as reflux into the ureter only, and grade II as reflux into a non-dilated pyelocalyceal system. Grade III VUR demonstrates dilatation of the collecting system. Grade IV involves more-extensive dilation with blunting of the calyces and tortuosity of the ureter, and grade V VUR is associated with massive dilation of the collecting system and severe tortuosity of the ureter. Grading of Vesicoureteric Reflux: International System of Radiographic Reflux Study Group 1985

REVIEW OF CLINICAL PROBLEMS

1. Discuss the pros and cons of the diagnostic imaging modalities for evaluating UTI.
   Ans: Refer to the Table 3 of the Chapter.

2. How do you grade the Vesicoureteric Reflux ?
   Ans: Refer to Figure given above.

3. How do you evaluate UTI & for VUR?
   Ans: Refer to the Evaluation-Decision-Action Plan/ Algorithm to diagnose and manage Neonatal UTI & VUR.

4. How do you manage UTI in a Neonate?
   Ans: Refer to No 6, 7 & 8 of the Bird's eye view/Overview/ Synopsis of the Chapter.

5. How do you manage VUR in a Neonate?
   Ans: Refer to No 9 & 10 of the Bird`s eye view/Overview/ Synopsis of the Chapter.

LEARNING OBJECTIVES

After completing this article, readers will be able to:

1. Identify/Confirm UTI in a Neonate Promptly, with a high index of suspicion.

2. Treat Neonatal UTI with Parenteral Antibiotics adequately & check for urine sterilization.

3. Plan further investigations to identify Vesicoureteral Reflux and Congenital urinary tract abnormalities.

4. Prevent further UTI with Prophylactic medications, until imaging shows no evidence for VUR.

5. Continue Preventive therapy if VUR is present and discuss with Pediatric Urologist whether any surgical intervention is necessary or not.

Pearl/Peril/Pitfall : The most accurate evaluation of renal scarring and renal function is performed with intravenously injected[99m] Tc DMSA or GH. DMSA accumulates in the distal tubular cells and provides excellent visualization of the renal cortex, correlating with histopathologic findings in 95% of experimental animals.

BIRD'S EYE VIEW/OVERVIEW/SYNOPSIS

1. The organisms associated with neonatal urinary tract infection mirror those that cause neonatal sepsis. For communityacquired neonatal disease, infection with *E. coli* is most common. Although GBS can be isolated from the urine of infants with GBS sepsis, primary urinary tract infection is rare. The frequency of health care–associated urinary tract infection has increased with the survival of infants with VLBW. Pathogens causing health care–associated infections include *E. coli*, other gram-negative enteric bacilli, *Enterococcus, Candida,* and CONS. Urinary tract infection (UTI) in the Neonatal period is considered a serious bacterial illness requiring the completion of a full workup for sepsis including an LP, followed by 7 to 14 days of parenteral antibiotics. These recommendations are predicated on the belief that UTI in Neonates is frequently secondary to bacteremia rather than to an ascending infection, as is seen in older children. Their young age is believed to place Neonates at an increased risk for dissemination of infection to the CNS, and when such dissemination occurs, there is often a lack of typical clinical signs suggestive of meningitis; and there is no correlation between the presence of bacteremia and the peripheral WBC count or the intensity of fever. Hence, these parameters could not be used to predict spread of infection beyond the urinary tract. It appears that in the nontoxic- appearing Neonate with the only high-risk criterion being a positive urinalysis (more than 10 leukocytes per HPF in unspun urine), the risk for serious complications, such as meningitis, is low. *Based on the apparent low risk of meningitis in Neonates with UTI, it would appear to be safe, less invasive, and more cost-effective to administer intravenous antibiotics and monitor these patients and to perform LPs only in patients with positive findings on blood cultures or in those whose urine cultures yield a pathogen likely to be associated with meningitis (namely, group B streptococci).* At this point, CSF culture results may be negative, but changes in cytochemical and immunologic measures of CNS infection may be used in conjunction with the patient's clinical status to determine length of treatment with intravenous antibiotics.

2. All Neonates with UTI need to be evaluated for structural abnormalities, such as posterior urethral valves or vesicoureteral reflux. Early detection of structural abnormalities can help prevent severe morbidity in the future by ensuring close outpatient follow-up and prophylactic or surgical therapy when indicated. Traditionally, VCUG has been performed several weeks after an acute infection. However, recent studies have shown some benefit and no detriment when VCUG was done early in the treatment course. In order to ensure that patients with abnormal anatomy and/or reflux are not missed, VCUG should be performed while the patient is still hospitalized unless follow-up can be ensured.

3. Large, prospective studies are needed to confirm whether LP should be reserved for those patients whose urine cultures grow organisms likely to cause CNS infection (group B streptococci) or whose blood cultures become positive. Once therapy has been started and the patient shows clinical improvement, follow-up urine cultures are redundant. Repeated catheterization is invasive and provides no new information. In most cases, a short course of parenteral antibiotics (3 to 5 days) can be followed by oral antibiotic therapy. Once afebrile and clinically improved, patients can be discharged on a regimen of oral antibiotics, to finish 14 days of treatment, if compliance and follow-up are ensured. *Suprapubic aspiration is the method of choice for obtaining urine for culture and sensitivity. A culture of a urinary specimen from a sterile bag attached to the perineal area that shows no or scant growth (<10,000 colony-forming units [CFUs]/mL) is strong evidence of absent urinary tract infection (UTI).* Refer to Table 2. However, the false-positive rate is so high that this method of urine collection is not suitable for diagnosing a UTI. Urinalysis does not substitute for urine culture to document the presence of a UTI. However, it can help in identifying febrile children who should receive antibacterial treatment while culture results from a properly collected urine specimen are pending.

4. Morbidity associated with pyelonephritis is characterized by hypertension, low-birth-weight neonates.systemic symptoms, such as fever, abdominal pain, vomiting, and dehydration. Bacteremia and clinical sepsis may occur. Neonates with pyelonephritis also may have cystitis. Long-term complications of pyelonephritis are hypertension, impaired kidney function, end-stage renal disease (ESRD), and complications of pregnancy (e.g. UTI, pregnancy-related.

5. *The Evaluation-Decision-Action-Plan/Algorithm* describes the essential aspects of history taking, clinical examination and laboratory evaluation and the management of UTI & VUR.

6. Infants with UTI are usually hospitalized and receive parenteral antibiotic therapy. Refer to Table 4 for the IV Antibiotics used in Neonates to treat UTI. Parenteral antibiotics may be used with daily follow-up until the patient is afebrile for 24 hours. Complete 10-14 days of therapy with an oral antibiotic active against the infecting bacteria.

7. **Further Inpatient Care** *For patients with pyelonephritis, give a suppressive dose of antibiotics -(Refer to Table 5 for Prophylactic agents) to prevent reinfection at least until the VCUG is obtained if one is to be obtained. *In patients with pyelonephritis, some clinicians discontinue antibacterial therapy 1-2 days after VCUG, if no VUR is present. *However, in studies of cortical scanning, roughly one half of the children with an initial episode of pyelonephritis have VUR, and one half have no radiographically identifiable reflux. Reinfection is common in both groups, with a high incidence in the first 6 months after the initial infection. *Until evidence-based guidelines about the use of suppressive antibacterial therapy after an initial febrile urinary tract infection (UTI) are available, recommending 6-12 months of suppressive treatment seems reasonable. Patients with VUR of grade III should receive a prolonged course of suppressive therapy. Patients VUR of grade IV or worse should be referred to a pediatric nephrologist or urologist.

8. **Further Outpatient Care** *For children with uncomplicated acute pyelonephritis *Although children with a febrile UTI may qualify for outpatient care, they still are at risk for kidney damage. Initial use of a parenteral antibiotic may increase the likelihood of promptly ceasing the bacterial proliferation in the renal tissue. *If the patient is not allergic to a cephalosporin, initial treatment may consist of a single dose of ceftriaxone 75 mg/kg IV/IM q12-24h (try cefotaxime in Neonates) *If the patient is allergic to cephalosporin, initial treatment may be gentamicin 2.5 mg/kg IV/IM as a single dose. *Start treatment with an oral antibacterial agent at therapeutic doses within the next 12-18 hours if the patient's response is satisfactory. *Arrange for follow-up, usually telephone follow-up, at 24 hours to monitor the response to treatment and at 48 hours to modify treatment the results of antibacterial sensitivity studies indicate a need to change. *Arrange for a follow-up visit after 7–10 days to check the patient's clinical course.

9. Intervention for VUR remains a controversial topic. Guidelines for medical and surgical management are constantly being reassessed. For many years, the emphasis on the investigation of the child with UTI has centered on diagnosis of VUR. More recently, some authors have suggested that the focus should be whether the child has renal scarring or is at risk for renal scarring. The natural tendency for VUR to resolve spontaneously during childhood warrants initial medical management of most patients with low-grade reflux.

10. The primary goals in the management of VUR are the prevention of pyelonephritis and renal scarring. Antibiotic prophylaxis should be instituted from the first day of life in all infants in whom VUR figures in the differential diagnosis. In children with VUR, prophylaxis is usually continued until the reflux spontaneously resolves or is surgically corrected. The requirement for early postnatal surgical intervention is virtually confined to relieving outflow obstruction (usually boys with posterior urethral valves) and relieving gross hydronephrosis.

Pearl/Peril/Pitfall : Direct radionuclide cystography with a^{99m} Tc-labeled agent (sulfur colloid, diethylenetriamine penta-acetate [DTPA], or pertechnetate) is a well-accepted alternative to fluoroscopic VCUG for screening asymptomatic siblings or offspring, for follow-up examination of children with VUR, for postoperative evaluation after ureteral reimplantation, and for excluding VUR when it is not seriously considered (especially in girls).

THE EVALUATION-DECISION-ACTION-PLAN/ALGORITHM FOR THE DIAGNOSIS AND MANAGEMENT OF *NEONATAL UTI AND VUR*

SUBJECTIVE FINDINGS

Hx of **High index of suspicion is warranted** because of non-specific symptoms such as jaundice, poor feeding, irritability, & weight loss **Suggestive of pyelonephritis;** fever, nausea, vomiting, diarrhea, abdominal/ flank pain may be present. Cystitis doesn't cause fever, but may be manifested as dysuria, suprapubic pain, frequency, & malodorous urine.

Hx of risk factors for UTI- Prematurity, instrumentation, boys>girls up to 1st year, anatomic abnormalities on prenatal USG Scan(obstructive uropathy), formula-fed>breast-fed, wiping from back to front.

OBJECTIVE FINDINGS

Assess for palpable Kidneys, Bladder, Hypertension, Potter facies and other dysmorphic features *Failure to void within the first 48 hours of life favors the diagnosis of obstructive uropathy (PU Valves or Urethral Atresia); remember that the observation of spontaneous voiding with normal urinary stream within first 24 hours of life does not rule out an obstructive process.*

Determine systemic involvement of invasive bacteria of UTI- Pneumonia, Septic Arthritis, Meningitis,Osteomyelitis, etc. All Neonates with UTI need to be evaluated for structural abnormalities, such as posterior urethral valves or vesicoureteral reflux.

INVESTIGATIONS

Blood FBC with differential & platelets, Blood cultures, ABG analysis, electrolytes, BUN, creatinine, osmolality, ketones, glucose, calcium, magnesium.

Urinanalysis (SPA has been considered the "gold standard" for obtaining urine for detecting bacteria in bladder) urine accurately. ANS C/S AS INDICATED *clinically. CSF Analysis and C/S, IF clinically indicated as part of full sepsis screen.*

Imaging Postnatal follow-up renal ultrasonography (if needed), voiding cystourethrography, and diuretic renography.

Differential diagnosis

Posterior urethral valves, radiographic evaluation of the pediatric urinary tract, ureteropelvic junction obstruction, vesicoureteral reflux.

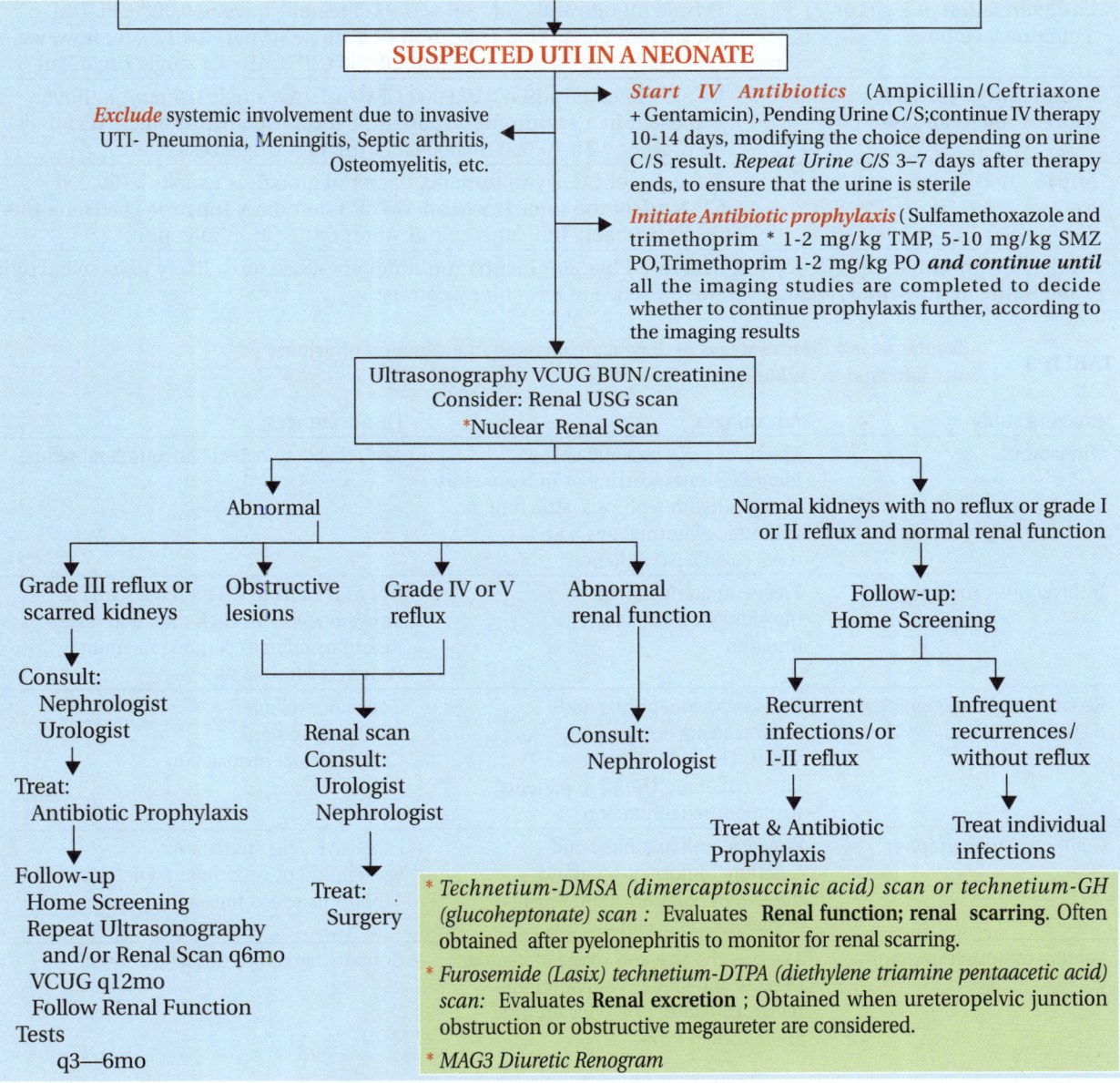

SUSPECTED UTI IN A NEONATE

Exclude systemic involvement due to invasive UTI- Pneumonia, Meningitis, Septic arthritis, Osteomyelitis, etc.

Start IV Antibiotics (Ampicillin/Ceftriaxone + Gentamicin), Pending Urine C/S;continue IV therapy 10-14 days, modifying the choice depending on urine C/S result. *Repeat Urine C/S 3–7 days after therapy ends, to ensure that the urine is sterile*

Initiate Antibiotic prophylaxis (Sulfamethoxazole and trimethoprim * 1-2 mg/kg TMP, 5-10 mg/kg SMZ PO,Trimethoprim 1-2 mg/kg PO *and continue until* all the imaging studies are completed to decide whether to continue prophylaxis further, according to the imaging results

Ultrasonography VCUG BUN/creatinine
Consider: Renal USG scan
*Nuclear Renal Scan

Abnormal

Normal kidneys with no reflux or grade I or II reflux and normal renal function

Grade III reflux or scarred kidneys

Obstructive lesions

Grade IV or V reflux

Abnormal renal function

Follow-up: Home Screening

Consult:
Nephrologist
Urologist

Renal scan
Consult:
Urologist
Nephrologist

Consult:
Nephrologist

Recurrent infections/or I-II reflux

Infrequent recurrences/ without reflux

Treat:
Antibiotic Prophylaxis

Treat & Antibiotic Prophylaxis

Treat individual infections

Follow-up
Home Screening
Repeat Ultrasonography and/or Renal Scan q6mo
VCUG q12mo
Follow Renal Function
Tests
q3—6mo

Treat:
Surgery

* *Technetium-DMSA (dimercaptosuccinic acid) scan or technetium-GH (glucoheptonate) scan :* Evaluates **Renal function; renal scarring**. Often obtained after pyelonephritis to monitor for renal scarring.

* *Furosemide (Lasix) technetium-DTPA (diethylene triamine pentaacetic acid) scan:* Evaluates **Renal excretion** ; Obtained when ureteropelvic junction obstruction or obstructive megaureter are considered.

* *MAG3 Diuretic Renogram*

* **Pearl/Peril/Pitfall** : The goal of postnatal management of infants with antenatal hydronephrosis is to identify patients with significant renal and urinary tract abnormalities while avoiding unnecessary testing in patients with physiologic or clinically insignificant hydronephrosis. Evaluation includes physical examination and the use of radiologic studies to detect renal and urinary tract abnormalities including obstructive uropathy or vesicoureteral reflux (VUR).

TABLE 1   Urinalysis for Presumptive Diagnosis of Uti*

Method	Findings
Bright-field or phase-contrast microscopy of centrifuged urinary sediment	Bacteria
Gram stain of uncentrifuged or centrifuged urinary sediment	Bacteria
Nitrite and leukocyte esterase test	Positive = UTI likely
Nitrite test	Positive = UTI probable
Leukocyte esterase test	Positive = Nonspecific

*Negative microscopic findings for bacteria do not rule out a UTI, nor do negative results of dipstick testing for nitrite and leukocyte esterase.

TABLE 2   Quantitative urine culture for the diagnosis of UTI*

Method	Finding
Suprapubic aspiration	If a UTI is present, bacteria are likely to be proliferating in bladder urine with growth of any organism except 2000-3000 CFU/mL coagulase-negative staphylococci.
Catheterization in a girl or a circumcised boy	Febrile infants and children with UTI usually have >50,000 CFU/mL of midstream clean-void collection in a single urinary pathogen; however, UTI may be present with 10,000-50,000 CFU/mL of a single organism.*
Midstream clean-void collection in a girl or uncircumcised boy	UTI is indicated when >100,000 CFU/mL of a single urinary pathogen is present in a symptomatic patient. Pyuria usually present. A UTI may be present with 10,000-50,000 CFU/mL of a single bacterium.*
Any method in a girl or boy	If the patient is asymptomatic, bacterial growth is usually >100,000 CFU/mL of the same organism on different days. If pyuria is absent, this result probably indicates colonization rather than infection.

*Patients with urinary frequency (i.e. decreased bladder incubation time) are those most likely to have bacteria proliferating in the urinary bladder in the presence of low colony counts.

TABLE 3   Advantages and disadvantages of diagnostic imaging in evaluation of urinary Tract infection in children

Imaging study	Advantages	Disadvantages
Ultrasound	Measures renal size and shape. Identifies renal scarring or inflammatory changes hydronephrosis, structural or anatomic abnormalities and renal calculi. No radiation	Not reliable to detect vesicoureteral reflux,
Intravenous urography	Precise anatomic image of the kidneys. Estimates renal function	Not as reliable to detect renal scarring or pyelonephritis. High radiation dose Risk of reaction to contrast medium Poor detail in infants
Renal cortical scintigraphy (DMSA, DTPA)	Detects pyelonephritis and renal scarring even in early stages. Useful in neonates. Little radiation. Useful in patients with poor renal function.	Does not evaluate collecting system. Cannot detect obstruction
Computed tomography	Provides both anatomic and functional information about the kidney. Possibly more sensitive in diagnosing pyelonephritis.	Expensive. High radiation Few clinical or experimental data to support its use at present
Voiding cystourethrography	Assesses the size and shape of bladder. Detects and grades vesicoureteral reflux. Evaluates posterior urethral anomalies in boys	Gonadal radiation. Catheterization

*Pearl/Peril/Pitfall: The most accurate evaluation of renal scarring and renal function is performed with intravenously injected[99m] Tc DMSA or GH. DMSA accumulates in the distal tubular cells and provides excellent visualization of the renal cortex, correlating with histopathologic findings in 95% of experimental animals.

VUR is graded according to the International Reflux Classification outlined by the International Reflux Study Group in 1985. This classification scheme is widely accepted and no new schemes have been introduced. *Grade I - Reflux into the ureter only *Grade II - Reflux into the collecting system, without dilatation. *Grade III - Reflux into the collecting system with mild dilatation, slight ureteral tortuosity, and no or slight blunting of the fornices *Grade IV - Moderate dilatation and/or tortuosity of the ureter and moderate dilatation of the renal pelvis and calyces, with complete obliteration of the sharp angle of the fornices but maintenance of the papillary impressions in the majority of calyces *Grade V - Gross dilatation and tortuosity of the ureter, with gross dilatation of the renal pelvis and calyces and nonmaintained papillary impressions

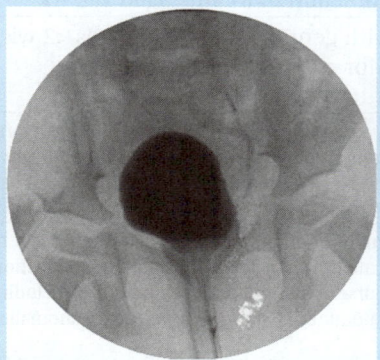

Voiding cystourethrogram (VCUG) shows grade I left VUR. Incidentally noted is vaginal reflux

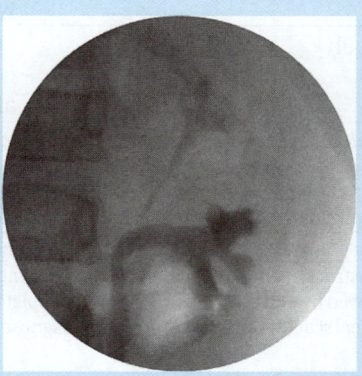

Voiding cystourethrogram (VCUG) demonstrates grade II VUR into the upper-pole moiety of a duplex collecting system and grade III VUR to the lower-pole moiety.

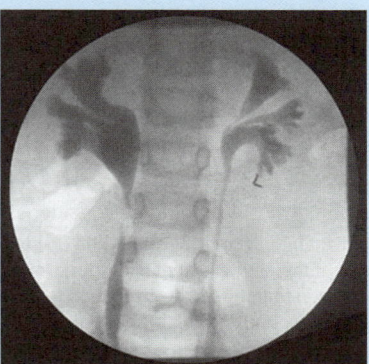

Voiding cystourethrogram (VCUG) demonstrates bilateral grade III reflux. The renal pelvis is mildly dilated on the right. There is some mild blunting of the calyceal fornices and loss of papillary impressions in the upper poles bilaterally.

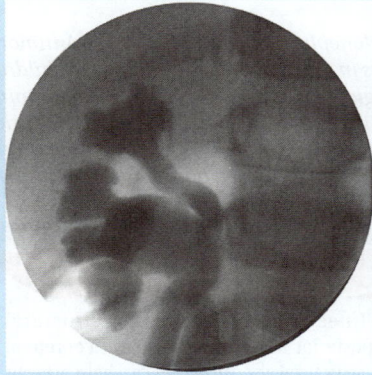

Voiding cystourethrogram (VCUG) demonstrates high-grade IV vesicoureteral reflux in a patient.

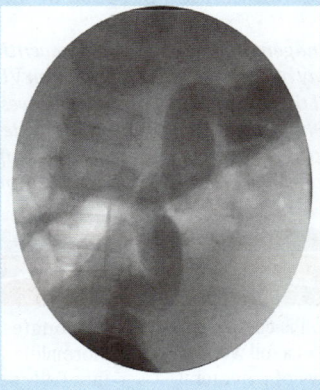

Voiding cystourethrogram (VCUG) demonstrates a tortuous, dilated ureter in a patient with grade V.

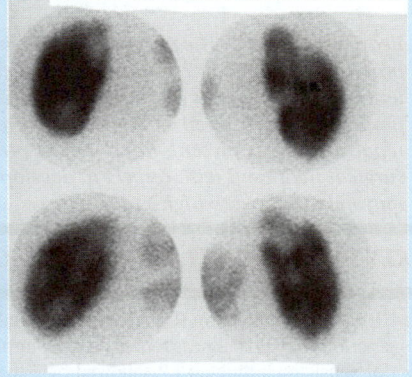

Dimercaptosuccinic acid (DMSA) scans demonstrate photopenia at the right superior pole consistent with scarring in this patient with vesicoureteral reflux.

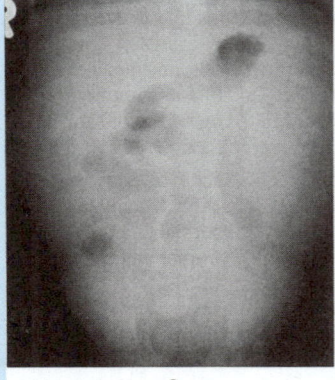

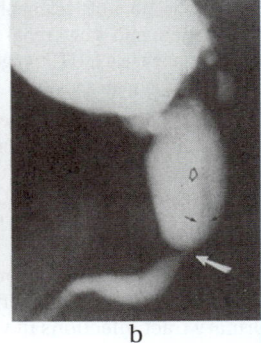

a   b

Urine ascites associated with posterior urethral valves This infant had abdominal distention at birth. (A) The abdominal radiograph shows the typical features of ascites; increased abdominal girth and bowel loops floating centrally. The diagnosis of ascites was confirmed by sonography. (B) Voiding cystourethrography shows typical posterior urethral valves (arrow). Note the visibility of the verumontanum (open arrow) and the valve cusps (small arrows) within the dilated posterior urethra.

Pearl/Peril/Pitfall: Intrarenal reflux appears as contrast medium extending from the calyces into the polar renal collecting tubules in the form of striations. This can be identified most often in neonates and infants with moderate or severe reflux (5-15%). The presence of intrarenal reflux does not change the grade or treatment of VUR.

TABLE 4	Antibiotic agents for parenteral treatment of UTI	
Drug	**Dosage and route**	**Comment**
Ceftriaxone	50–75 mg/kg/d IV as a single dose or divided q12h	Do not use in infants <6 wk of age; parenteral antibiotic with long half-life; may displace bilirubin from albumin
Cefotaxime	150 mg/kg/d IV divided q6-8h	Safe to use in infants <6 wk of age; used with ampicillin in infants aged 2–8 wk
Ampicillin	100 mg/kg/d IV divided q8h	Used with gentamicin in Neonates <2 wk of age; for enterococci and patients allergic to cephalosporins

Gentamicin : *Term neonates <7 d: 3.5-5 mg/kg/dose IV q24h. Infants and children <5 y: 2.5 mg/kg/dose IV q8h or single daily dosing with normal renal function or 5-7.5 mg/kg/dose IV q24h, Children ≥5 y: 2-2.5 mg/kg/dose IV q8h or single daily dosing with normal renal function of 5-7.5 mg/kg/dose IV q24h. Monitor blood levels and kidney function if therapy extends >48 h.Vancomycin and an aminoglycoside should be considered for empirical therapy of health care–associated urinary tract infections.*

Sterilization of the urine should be documented by repeat culture after 48 hours of therapy. Treatment duration is usually 10 days, but can be longer if there is persistent bacteriuria, anatomic obstruction, or a perinephric abscess.In uncomplicated cases of primary urinary tract infection, parenteral therapy can be given for 5 to 7 days, followed by oral antibiotic therapy to complete the course of treatment. Imaging studies, including renal ultrasound and voiding cystourethrogram or renal scan, should be performed to diagnose any anatomic or physiologic urinary tract anomalies.

TABLE 5	Antibiotic agents to prevent reinfection
Agent	**Single daily dose**
* Cephalexin	10–15mg/kg/day
Sulfamethoxazole and trimethoprim*	1–2 mg/kg TMP, 5–10 mg/kg SMZ PO
Trimethoprim	1–2 mg/kg PO

* Do not use nitrofurantoin or sulfa drugs in infants younger than 6 weeks. Reduced doses of an oral first-generation cephalosporin, such as cephalexin at 10 mg/kg, may be used until the child reaches the age of 6 weeks. Ampicillin or amoxicillin are not recommended because of the high incidence of resistant *E coli*.

* Pearl/Peril/Pitfall : *The primary goals in the management of VUR are the prevention of pyelonephritis and renal scarring. Antibiotic prophylaxis should be instituted from the first day of life in all infants in whom VUR figures in the differential diagnosis. In children with VUR, prophylaxis is usually continued until the reflux spontaneously resolves or is surgically corrected. Some advocate stopping prophylaxis in children older than 7 or 8 years who have mild or moderate (grade I-III) VUR, particularly when no evidence of prior renal scarring is present. Randomized prospective studies have shown no significant difference between medical treatment and surgical treatment with respect to development of new scars or progression of preexisting scars. However, only surgical treatment may help those with high-grade reflux.*

KEY POINTS FOR CLINICAL PRACTICE:

1. Urinary tract infection (UTI) in the Neonatal period is considered a serious bacterial illness requiring the completion of a full workup for sepsis including an LP, followed by 7 to 14 days of parenteral antibiotics. These recommendations are predicated on the belief that UTI in Neonates is frequently secondary to bacteremia rather than to an ascending infection, as is seen in older children.

2. It appears that in the nontoxic- appearing Neonate with the only high-risk criterion being a positive urinalysis (more than 10 leukocytes per HPF in unspun urine), the risk for serious complications, such as meningitis, is low. *Based on the apparent low risk of meningitis in Neonates with UTI, it would appear to be safe, less invasive, and more cost-effective to administer intravenous antibiotics and monitor these patients and to perform LPs only in patients with positive findings on blood cultures or in those whose urine cultures yield a pathogen likely to be associated with meningitis (namely, group B streptococci).*

3. All Neonates with UTI need to be evaluated for structural abnormalities, such as posterior urethral valves or vesicoureteral reflux. Early detection of structural abnormalities can help prevent severe morbidity in the future by ensuring close outpatient follow-up and prophylactic or surgical therapy when indicated.

4. Morbidity associated with pyelonephritis is characterized by systemic symptoms, such as fever, abdominal pain, vomiting, and dehydration. Bacteremia and clinical sepsis may occur. Neonates with pyelonephritis also may have cystitis. Long-term complications of pyelonephritis are hypertension, impaired kidney function, end-stage renal disease (ESRD), and complications of pregnancy (e.g.., UTI, pregnancy-related hypertension, low-birth-weight Neonates.)

5. Finally, postponing completion of a VCUG until several weeks after discharge results in noncompliance in nearly half of the patients. In order to ensure that patients with abnormal anatomy and/or reflux are not missed, VCUG should be performed while the patient is still hospitalized unless follow-up can be ensured.

REFERENCES & FURTHER READING : 1) Dick PT, Feldman W: Routine diagnostic imaging for childhood urinary tract infections: A systematic overview. J Pediatr 128:12, 1996. **2)** Crain EF, Gershel JC: Urinary tract infections in febrile infants younger than 8 weeks of age. Pediatr 86:363, 1990. **3)** Ginsberg CM, McCracken GH jr.: Urinary tract infections in young infants. Pediatr 69:409, 1982. **4)** Drew JH, Acton CM: Radiologic findings in newborn infants with urinary infection. Arch Dis Child 51:628, 1976. **5)** Lerner GR, Fleischmann LE, Perlmutter AD: Reflux nephropathy. Pediatr Clin N Am 34:747, 1987.

* Pearl/Peril/Pitfall : *Urinalysis does not substitute for urine culture to document the presence of a UTI. However, it can help in identifying febrile children who should receive antibacterial treatment while culture results from a properly collected urine specimen are pending.*

Perinatal Tuberculosis

86

@ *Timely diagnosis of Perinatal Tuberculosis require a high index of suspicion, as there are no typical clinical signs or radiographic findings-the affected infant is commonly born prematurely, but clinical signs typically don't appear until the baby is 2-4 wks of age.*

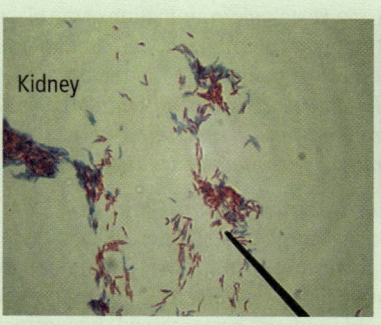

Kidney

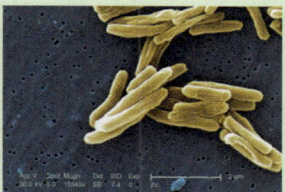

Electron Microscopic Picture of *Mycobacterium tuberculosis* (MTB)

This is an acid fast stain of *Mycobacterium tuberculosis* (MTB). Note the red rods—hence the terminology for MTB in histologic sections or smears: acid fast bacilli.

Revised diagnostic criteria for congenital tuberculosis. The infant must have proven tuberculous lesions and at least one of the following: (1) lesions in the first week of life; (2) a primary hepatic complex or caseating hepatic granulomas; (3) tuberculous infection of the placenta or the maternal genital tract; or (4) exclusion of the possibility of postnatal transmission by a thorough investigation of contacts, including the infant's hospital attendants, and by adherence to existing recommendations for treating infants exposed to tuberculosis. *Different patterns of restriction-fragment-length polymorphism in the M. tuberculosis isolates from the mother and the infant would exclude congenital transmission, although identical patterns could result from either congenital or postnatal transmission.*

—*Michael F. Cantwell.*

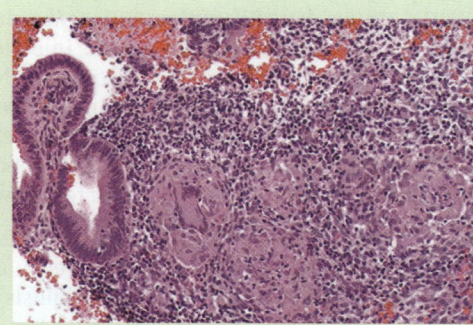

Granulomas are not always well-formed, but there should at least be epithelioid cells. Giant cells are often present. Other inflammatory cell components include lymphocytes, plasma cells, and occasional neutrophils. Collagenization usually indicates a healing response. As granulomas heal, they can become calcified

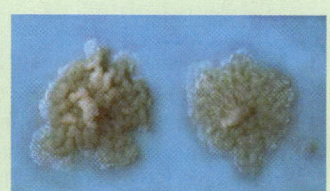

MTB Colonies

REVIEW OF CLINICAL PROBLEMS

1. Mention the "Diagnostic Criteria" of Perinatal Tuberculosis.
   Ans: Refer to the No "1" BIRD'S EYE VIEW/OVERVIEW SYNOPSIS of the Chapter.

2. What are the "essential features" of History and Physical Examination of a Neonate with suspected Perinatal Tuberculosis?
   Ans: Refer to the Evaluation-Decision-Action Plan/Algorithm to diagnose & manage Perinatal Tuberculosis.

3. Mention the essential investigations for diagnosing Perinatal Tuberculosis.
   Ans: Refer to the Evaluation-Decision-Action Plan/Algorithm to diagnose & manage Perinatal Tuberculosis.

4. Mention the common clinical signs of Perinatal Tuberculosis.
   Ans: Refer to the Table 1 of the Chapter.

5. How do you manage an asymptomatic infant born to a mother with suspected Perinatal Tuberculosis?
   Ans: Refer to the Evaluation-Decision-Action Plan/Algorithm to diagnose & manage Perinatal Tuberculosis.

LEARNING OBJECTIVES

After completing this article, readers will be able to:

1. Understand that clinical manifestations of Perinatal Tuberculosis are non specific and resemble those of bacterial sepsis and other congenital infections.

2. Maintain a high index of suspicion for the timely diagnosis and management of Perinatal Tuberculosis.

3. Recognize that successful management of Perinatal Tuberculosis depends on early recognition and treatment of the disease.

4. Investigate the mother and household contacts for active tuberculosis and manage them appropriately.

5. Monitor the Neonate for adverse effects of ATD Therapy and Prevent the Perinatal Tuberculosis by control of the disease among women of child bearing age.

---

* *Pearl/Peril/Pitfall : Infants may acquire tuberculosis (TB) by transplacental spread through the umbilical vein to the fetal liver, by aspiration or ingestion of infected amniotic fluid, or via airborne inoculation from close contacts (family members or nursery personnel). All neonates with suspected congenital TB should have chest x-ray and culture of tracheal aspirates, gastric washings, urine, and CSF for acid-fast bacilli. Skin testing is not extremely sensitive but should be performed; biopsy of the liver, lymph nodes, lung, or pleura may be needed to confirm diagnosis.*

BIRD'S EYE VIEW/OVERVIEW/SYNOPSIS

1. Perinatal Tuberculosis is comparatively rare (hardly 300 cases of true perinatal tuberculosis were reported so far), because of a) infertility, a common sequel of genital tuberculosis b) perinatal morbidity due to Prematurity, IUGR, LBW rather than due to perinatal tuberculosis itself c) under reporting of cases from developing countries. *The diagnostic criteria for Perinatal Tuberculosis (Cantwell et al, 1994) are* **a)** the Neonate must have proven Tuberculous lesions **b)** lesions in the infant in the first week of life **c)** a primary hepatic complex or caseating hepatic granulomas in the infant (percutaneous liver biopsy) **d)** tuberculous infection of the placenta or maternal genital tract, and **e)** exclusion of postnatal transmission by thorough investigation of contacts.

2. Perinatal Tuberculosis is acquired by **a)** hematogenous spread of the tuberculous bacilli from the placenta via the umbilical vein **b)** aspiration in utero of infected amniotic fluid from either placental or endometrial infection **c)** ingestion of infected amniotic fluid or secretions during delivery **d)** postnatal infection from contact with a contagious mother or caregiver or ingestion of infected breast milk from a mother with tuberculous breast abscess. It is difficult to differentiate between the truely congenital & postnatally acquired infection. This differentiation is of epidemiological importance primarily, as management & prognosis do not differ significantly between the two modes of transmission.

3. The clinical manifestations of Perinatal Tuberculosis are non specific and resemble those of bacterial sepsis and other congenital infections. The affected infant is commonly born prematurely, but clinical signs typically do not appear until he or she is 2–4 wks of age. The clinical features vary as per the site & size of caseous lesions. *The only lesion in the Neonate that is unquestionably associated with Congenital infection is a primary complex in the liver; all others may be acquired congenitally or postnatally.* **Refer to Table 1** for the most common symptoms and signs of Perinatal Tuberculosis. *It is important to maintain a high index of suspicion for the timely diagnosis & management of Perinatal Tuberculosis, as there are no typical clinical signs or radiographic findings .*

4. The diagnosis should be suspected in an infant with signs & symptoms of bacterial or congenital infection whose response to antibiotic and supportive therapy is poor & evaluation for other infections is unrevealing. *The most important clue for rapid diagnosis of perinatal tuberculosis is a maternal or family history of Tuberculosis.* Frequently, the mother's disease is discovered only after the Neonate's diagnosis is suspected.

5. The infant's tuberculin skin test is negative initially but may become positive in 1-3 month. A positive acid-fast stain of an early morning gastric aspirates of a Newborn usually indicates tuberculosis. Direct acid-fast stains on middle ear discharge, bone marrow, tracheal aspirates, or liver biopsy can be useful. The CSF should be examined & cultured, although the yield for M.*tuberculosis* is low. PCR assays are available for testing of specimens such as gastric aspirates, respiratory secretions, & CSF, but they are not recommended for routine use because their sensitivity is similar to that of culture, and both false-positive & false-negative results occur.

6. Examination of the mother should include a tuberculin skin test, and chest X-ray. Histologic examination of the placenta, if available is strongly recommended, and an endometrial biopsy may also help in confirming the maternal disease. *The mother with tuberculosis should also undergo serologic testing for HIV antibody, and, if she is seropositive, the infant should be evaluated for perinatally acquired HIV infection.*

7. *The Evaluation-Decision-Action-Plan/Algorithm* to diagnose and manage the Perinatal Tuberculosis outlines the essential aspects of history taking, physical examination and appropriate investigations as well as management of the affected infant and mother. The successful management of Perinatal Tuberculosis depends on early recognition and treatment of the disease. Empiric therapy is provided often to Neonates and should not be delayed while awaiting culture results, epidemiologic investigation, and follow-up tuberculin skin testing. The regime recommended by IAP working group consists of **a)** a "two month course" with 3 drugs (INH-5mg/kg/day, Rifampicin-10 mg/kg/day, Pyrazinamide -25mg/kg/day) along with injection Streptomycin-20mg/kg/day, IM, in view of high primary INH resistance **b)** a "seven month course" with 2 drugs (INH and Rifampicin). In multidrug resistant tuberculosis, the general regime is 12–18 month course of 4 drugs (INH + Rifampicin + Pyrazinamide + Ethambutol, but the specific regime will depend on the results of the drug sensitivity tests.

8. Steroids (Prednisolone 1–2 mg/kg/day for 4–8 weeks) are indicated for **a)** Meningitis **b)** Miliary tuberculosis **c)** Peritonitis and pleural or pericardial effusions **d)** Endobronchial Tuberculosis/segmental lesions **e)** Genitourinary tuberculosis/sinus formation. *Breastfed infants & Neonates must receive Pyridoxine supplements.*

9. Monitoring the infant for clinical signs of hepatotoxicity with the INH and Rifampicin, optic neuritis with Ethambutol, auditory and vestibular toxicities with Streptomycin should be considered when these agents are used to treat the infant, *(LFTs, hearing and vision should be periodically monitored).* Separation of the baby from the mother and discontinuing breast feeding is desirable when **a)** mother is so sick to need admission **b)** MDR tuberculosis is suspected **c)** a sputum positive mother who hasn't been put on antituberculous drug therapy **d)** there is proven or expected default.

10. The mortality rate of Perinatal Tuberculosis is very high because of delayed diagnosis; many children will have complete recovery with prompt diagnosis and adequate chemotherapy. Prevention requires the control of the disease among women of child bearing age.

---

* *Pearl/Peril/Pitfall : Well-appearing neonates whose mothers had a positive skin test but a negative chest x-ray and no evidence of active disease should have a skin test q 3 mo for 1 yr. If the test is positive, chest x-ray and cultures for acid-fast bacilli are obtained as above.*

THE EVALUATION-DECISION-ACTION-PLAN/ALGORITHM FOR THE DIAGNOSIS AND MANAGEMENT OF *PERINATAL TUBERCULOSIS*

SUBJECTIVE FINDINGS

Hx of Neonatal symptoms suggestive of bacterial sepsis - (Refer to Table 1), with poor response to antibacterial & supportive therapy.

The onset of Neonatal symptoms can be sudden & overwhelming, or insiduous & prolonged. The mean age of onset is 2-3wks of life (may present at birth).

Maternal history suggestive of active Tuberculosis - prematurity, sterility, IUGR. Genital Tuberculosis is often asymptomatic. Hx of medical diagnosis & treatment for maternal tuberculosis & other household contacts (*may not be present*).

OBJECTIVE FINDINGS

Look for respiratory distress, fever, hepatosplenomegaly, lethargy and/or irritability, failure to thrive, lymph-adenopathy, nasal/ear discharge, skin lesions, jaundice, seizures

Timely diagnosis of Perinatal Tuberculosis require a high index of suspicion, as there are no typical clinical signs or radiographic findings the affected infant is commonly born prematurely, but clinical signs typically don't appear until the baby is 2-4 wks of age.

50% of mothers of infants with Perinatal Tuberculosis were not diagnosed with Tuberculosis at the time their infants demonstrated clinical signs.

INVESTIGATIONS

Blood FBC with hematocrit and platelets, ABG analysis with electrolytes, Blood glucose, Ca^{++}, Mg^{++}, BUN and creatinine, urine analysis and culture, blood cultures to exclude bacterial sepsis, Liver function tests.

CXR to identify lung infiltrates, hilar/mediastinal lymph-adenopathy, miliary pattern (50%), pleural effusion, etc.

Mantoux test negative initially; may become positive in 6–12 wk time, almost 4 wks after clinical presentation.

Acid fast staining and culture of early morning gastric aspirate, tracheal aspirate, middle ear discharge, CSF, Urine, bone marrow biopsy, liver biopsy, lymphnode biopsy, skin biopsy

HIV status of the baby and the mother

> *Investigate mother & household contacts for an evidence for tuberculosis !*

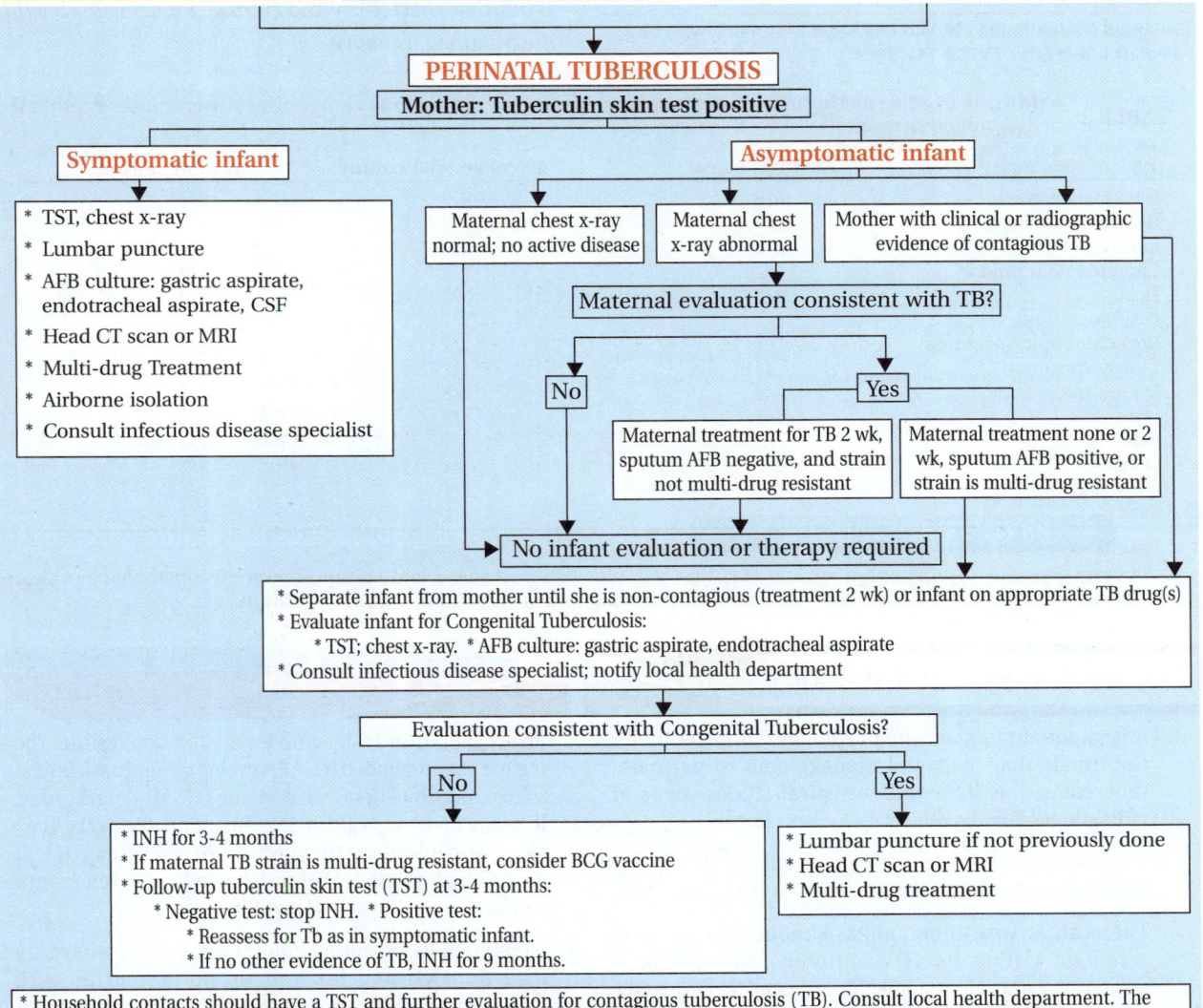

PERINATAL TUBERCULOSIS

Mother: Tuberculin skin test positive

Symptomatic infant

* TST, chest x-ray
* Lumbar puncture
* AFB culture: gastric aspirate, endotracheal aspirate, CSF
* Head CT scan or MRI
* Multi-drug Treatment
* Airborne isolation
* Consult infectious disease specialist

Asymptomatic infant

Maternal chest x-ray normal; no active disease | Maternal chest x-ray abnormal | Mother with clinical or radiographic evidence of contagious TB

Maternal evaluation consistent with TB?

No → Yes

Maternal treatment for TB 2 wk, sputum AFB negative, and strain not multi-drug resistant | Maternal treatment none or 2 wk, sputum AFB positive, or strain is multi-drug resistant

No infant evaluation or therapy required

* Separate infant from mother until she is non-contagious (treatment 2 wk) or infant on appropriate TB drug(s)
* Evaluate infant for Congenital Tuberculosis:
    * TST; chest x-ray. * AFB culture: gastric aspirate, endotracheal aspirate
* Consult infectious disease specialist; notify local health department

Evaluation consistent with Congenital Tuberculosis?

No

* INH for 3-4 months
* If maternal TB strain is multi-drug resistant, consider BCG vaccine
* Follow-up tuberculin skin test (TST) at 3-4 months:
    * Negative test: stop INH. * Positive test:
        * Reassess for Tb as in symptomatic infant.
        * If no other evidence of TB, INH for 9 months.

Yes

* Lumbar puncture if not previously done
* Head CT scan or MRI
* Multi-drug treatment

* Household contacts should have a TST and further evaluation for contagious tuberculosis (TB). Consult local health department. The mother should receive treatment for latent tuberculosis infection. All persons with tuberculosis should be tested for Human immunode-ficiency virus (HIV) infection.
…Acid-fast bacillus (AFB) culture of amniotic fluid and placenta, if available; placenta for histopathologic examination.
Includes mother with chest radiographic findings consistent with old, healed tuberculosis.
BCG, bacille Calmette-Guerin; CSF, cerebrospinal fluid; CT, computed tomography; INH, isoniazid; MRI, magnetic resonance imaging.

---

* *Pearl/Peril/Pitfall : Neonates with active TB: The American Academy of Pediatrics recommends treatment once/day with INH (10 to 15 mg/kg po), rifampin (10 to 20 mg/kg po), pyrazinamide (20 to 40 mg/kg po), and streptomycin (20 to 40 mg/kg IM) for 2 mo, with INH and rifampin continued for another 10 mo.*

TABLE 1	Clinical signs of congenital tuberculosis in 58 infants	
Sign	No. of patients	% of patients
Respiratory distress	44	76
Hepatosplenomegaly with/without splenomegaly	38	65
Fever	33	57
Lymphadenopathy	19	33
Poor feeding	18	31
Lethargy/irritability	16	30
Abdominal distention	15	26
Failure to thrive	9	15
Ear discharge	9	15
Rash	5	9
Abdominal fundo-scopic findings	4	7
Jaundice	4	7
Seizures	3	5
Bloody diarrhea	3	5
Ascites	3	5

Adapted from Abughali N, Van Der Kuyp F, Annable W, et al: Pediatr Infect Dis J 13:738-741, 1994.

@ The clinical presentation of Neonatal TB is nonspecific but is usually marked by multiple organ involvement. The Neonate may look acutely or chronically ill. Fever, lethargy, respiratory distress, hepatosplenomegaly, or failure to thrive may indicate TB in a Neonate with a history of exposure.

@ All Neonates with suspected congenital TB should have chest X-ray and culture of tracheal aspirates, gastric washings, urine, and CSF for acid-fast bacilli. Skin testing is not extremely sensitive but should be performed; biopsy of the liver, lymph nodes, lung, or pleura may be needed to confirm diagnosis. Well-appearing neonates whose mothers had a positive skin test but a negative chest X-ray and no evidence of active disease should have a skin test q 3 mo for 1 yr. If the test is positive, chest X-ray and cultures for acid-fast bacilli are obtained as above.

TABLE 2	Results of diagnostic procedures performed on 29 infants with Congenital tuberculosis reported from 1980 to 1994*		
Type of specimen	Acid-fast smear	Mycobacterial culture	Smear or culture
Gastric aspirate	8/9	8/9	9/11
Endotracheal aspirate	7/7	7/7	7/7
Ear discharge	2/2	1/1	2/2
Cerebrospinal fluid	1/2	1/2	1/2
Urine	0/2	0/2	0/2
Peritoneal fluid	1/1	1/1	1/1
Bronchoscopic specimen	1/1	1/1	1/1
Biopsy specimen	14/19	11/12	16/21
Lymph node	7/8	6/6	7/8…
Liver	4/6	1/2	4/6…
Skin	1/3	1/1	1/3
Lung	1/1	1/1	2/2
Bone marrow	---	1/1	1/1
Ear	1/1	1/1	1/1

* Results expressed as no. positive results/no. patients tested.
…All biopsy specimens of lymph node and liver that tested negative on smear and culture showed histopathologic changes consistent with tuberculosis (i.e., gaint cell transformation of granulomas, with or without caseation).

KEY POINTS FOR CLINICAL PRACTICE:

1. It is important to maintain a high index of suspicion for the timely diagnosis and management of perinatal tuberculosis, as there are no typical clinical signs or radiographic findings.

2. The most important clue for rapid diagnosis of perinatal tuberculosis is a maternal or family history of Tuberculosis.

3. The mother with tuberculosis should also undergo serologic testing for HIV antibody, and, if she is seropositive, the infant should be evaluated for perinatally acquired HIV infection.

4. Empiric therapy is provided often to Neonates and should not be delayed while awaiting culture results, epidemiologic investigation, and follow-up tuberculin skin testing. The regime recommended by IAP working group consists of a) a "two month course" with 3 drugs (INH-5 mg/kg/day, Rifampicin-10 mg/kg/day, Pyrazinamide -25 mg/kg/day) along with injection Streptomycin-20 mg/kg/day, IM, in view of high primary INH resistance b) a "seven month course" with 2 drugs (INH and Rifampicin).

5. Monitoring the infant for clinical signs of hepatotoxicity with the INH and Rifampicin, optic neuritis with Ethambutol, auditory and vestibular toxicities with Streptomycin should be considered when these agents are used to treat the infant, (LFTs, hearing & vision should be periodically monitored).

REFERENCES & FURTHER READING : 1) Cantwell MF, Shehab ZM, Costello AM. Congenital Tuberculosis. NEJ of Med1994;330 (15):1051 2) Mallory MD. Jacobs RF, Congenital Tuberculosis. Semin Pediatr Infect Dis 1999;10(3):177 3) Jacobs RF et al. Management of TB in pregnancy and newborn. Clin Perinatol 1988;15(2):305 4)CDCP. The role of BCG vaccine in the prevention and control of TB in the US Morb Mortal WKLY rEP 1996;45 (RR-4):1-18 5) World Health Organisation; Research for Action : understanding and controlling tuberculosis in India;2000,12

Congenital Malaria

87

@ *A classic presentation of malaria may not occur in the newborn, since these parasites can only use reticulocytes for replication and these cells are scarce in newborns due to depressed erythropoiesis after birth*

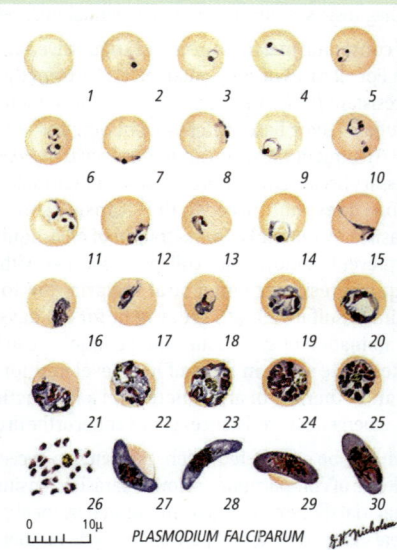

A: The stages of *P. falciparum*. **1:** Normal red cell; **Figs. 2-18:** Trophozoites (among these, **Figs. 2-10** correspond to ring-stage trophozoites); **Figs. 19-26:** Schizonts (**Fig. 26** is a ruptured schizont); **Figs. 27, 28:** Mature macrogametocytes (female); **Figs. 29, 30:** Mature microgametocytes (male). **Illustrations from:** Coatney GR, Collins WE, Warren M, Contacos PG. The Primate Malarias. Bethesda: U.S. Department of Health, Education and Welfare; 1971.

Ring-form trophozoites (rings) of *Plasmodium falciparum* are often thin and delicate, measuring on average 1/5 the diameter of the red blood cell. Rings may possess one or two chromatin dots. They may be found on the periphery of the RBC (accolé, appliqué) and multiply-infected RBCs are not uncommon. Ring forms may become compact or pleomorphic depending on the quality of the blood or if there is a delay

Trophozoites of *P. falciparum* in thin blood smears

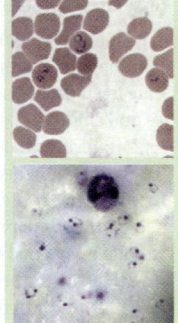

Rings of *P. falciparum* in a thick blood smear.

Malaria is transmitted by mosquitoes in the genus *Anopheles*. These mosquitoes are not only vectors of malaria, but also serve as the definitive host for *Plasmodium* spp., as the sexual stages of the parasite take place in the mosquito. Different species and species complexes of *Anopheles* transmit malaria in different parts of the world. However, of the over 200 species of *Anopheles* in the world, less than half are vectors of human malaria. Anopheline mosquitoes can be separated by other genera by possessing palps that extend the same length as the proboscis. Also, many anopheline mosquitoes assume a "head-stand" position when taking a blood meal from the mammalian host.

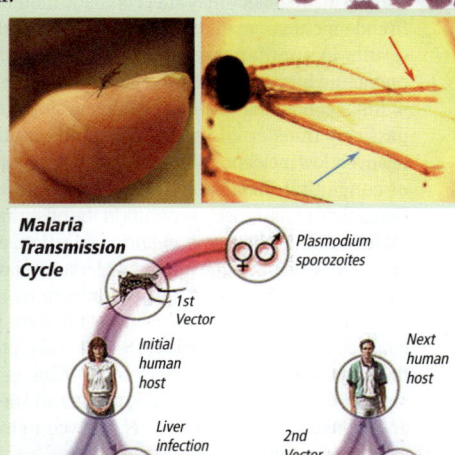

Malaria Transmission Cycle
Plasmodium sporozoites
1st Vector
Initial human host
Next human host
Liver infection
Blood infection
2nd Vector
In utero transmission

REVIEW OF CLINICAL PROBLEMS

1. Discuss the adverse effects of Malaria during pregnancy.
   Ans: Refer to No 2 of the Bird`s eye view/Overview/Synopsis of the Chapter.

2. How do you evaluate a Neonate with suspected Congenital Malaria?
   Ans: Refer to the Evaluation-Decision-Action Plan/Algorithm to diagnose and manage Neonatal/Congenital Malaria.

3. How do you manage Congenital Malaria?
   Ans: Refer to No 7 of the Bird`s eye view/Overview/Synopsis of the Chapter.

4. Mention the Objective findings you should look for in a Neonate with Congenital Malaria?
   Ans: Refer to the Evaluation-Decision-Action Plan/Algorithm to diagnose and manage Neonatal/Congenital Malaria.

5. Discuss the Rapid Diagnostic Tests to detect Plasmodium spe.
   Ans: Refer to Section "An overview of the Laboratory Diagnosis of Malaria-CDC Recommendations."

LEARNING OBJECTIVES

After completing this article, readers will be able to:

1. Suspect Congenital Malaria in a Neonate with fever, sepsis like picture, pallor, hepatosplenomegaly, jaundice etc.,

2. Institute rapid diagnostic methods to screen and confirm by finding parasites by thick and thin smear examination.

3. Manage Neonates with proven Congenital Malaria with appropriate antimalarials and supportive therapy.

4. Prevent Congenital Malaria based on avoidance of exposure and use of chemoprophylaxis.

5. Treat resistant *P. falciparum* spe. with Artemesinin derivatives when necessary.

* *Pearl/Peril/Pitfall : Unless the parasitemia is severe, malarial infection is unlikely in neonates because of the protection offered by the placenta, presence of maternal antibodies and preponderance of fetal red blood cells. The symptoms and signs closely mimic sepsis and hence a high index of suspicion is needed to diagnose this condition.*

BIRD`S EYE VIEW/OVERVIEW/SYNOPSIS

1. Congenital malaria is a rare disease. So far, 300 cases are reported in literature. There are some arguments about the definition of congenital malaria. Normally, symptoms occur 10 to 30 days postpartum. However, the disease can be seen in a day-old baby or be delayed for weeks or months. *Congenital Malaria* is defined as malaria acquired by the fetus or newborn directly from the mother, either in utero or during delivery. In endemic areas it is difficult to differentiate between congenitally acquired malaria from postnatal infection acquired through mosquito bite or blood transfusion. It appears that placenta acts as a barrier to the malarial parasite & its transplacental transmission is further blocked if mother is immune. More likely, vertical transmission occurs by transfusion of parasitized maternal RBCs through a breach in the placental barrier that may occur either prematurely during pregnancy or during labor. Parasites in umbilical cord blood or fetal blood then may be cleared spontaneously, resulting in no disease manifestations, or may proliferate, with development of clinical signs of disease. Transmission of malaria by breast-feeding does not occur.

2. Malaria in pregnancy may affect both the mother & fetus adversely. In endemic areas, maternal peripheral/placental parasitemia often results in spontaneous abortions, miscarriages, stillbirths, premature births, IUGR & Neonatal deaths. The relative resistance of RBCs containing fetal hemoglobin against malarial parasites & passively transferred IgG from immune mothers may explain relatively low incidence of congenital malaria. (only about 300 cases of congenital malaria are reported in the world literature). Congenital malaria usually occurs in the offspring of a nonimmune mother with *P. vivax* or *P. malariae* infection, although it can be observed with any of the human malaria species. Host factors that can decrease the risk of malarial infections include abnormal hemoglobin and malaria-speciûc antibodies. Erythrocytes with fetal hemoglobin or hemoglobin S are less likely to become infected than erythrocytes with hemoglobin A. Women living in endemic areas are continuously exposed to malaria and develop antimalarial antibodies. Maternal antibody is believed to exhibit a protective effect for the fetus.

3. The diagnosis of congenital malaria is often delayed because of its nonspecific features & the lack of clinical suspicion. The clinical features often resemble those due to sepsis or other congenital infections & include fever, irritability, anorexia, vomiting, diarrhea, jaundice, hepatosplenomegaly, hemolytic anemia & thrombocytopenia. The disease manifests around 2-8 wks of age; the prolonged interval between birth & onset of clinical manifestations may be explained by transmission late in pregnancy or at delivery, so that multiple erythrocytic life cycles are required to produce clinically evident disease, or by the presence & amount of transplacentally acquired maternal antimalarial antibodies. Preterm infants, who do not benefit from passive immunity, may manifest clinical signs of malaria earlier than full-term infants.Congenital malaria often is complicated by bacterial illnesses in developing countries. In rare cases, malaria can be complicated by hypoglycemia; central nervous system infection; splenic rupture; renal failure; and, in *P. falciparum* infections, blackwater fever (severe hemolysis, hemoglobinuria, and renal failure). Untreated *P. falciparum* infection is associated with a high case-fatality rate.

4. The diagnosis of congenital malaria is based on microscopic demonstration of parasites on thick & thin blood smears. For detection of organisms, a **thick blood film** is preferred because it concentrates the RBCs. Identification of the *Plasmodium* species, however requires a **thin blood film**. Specimens for smears should be obtained from both the infant & the mother, and quantification of the parasitemia is helpful to assess the response to therapy.

5. Maternal history of fever with rigors & positive smear for malarial parasites during late pregnancy is often available. The condition should be differentiated from other intrauterine infections.

6. *The Evaluation-Decision-Action-Plan/Algorithm* describes the essential aspects of diagnosis & management of congenital malaria.

7. The management of congenital malaria consists of supportive care & antimalarial therapy. For all cases of congenital malaria, except those due to chloroquine-resistant *P. falciparum*, the recommended therapy is oral chloroquine sulfate (10mg base/kg followed by 5mg base/kg at 6, 24, and 48 hrs later). Treatment with primaquine for *P.vivax or P.ovale* infections is not necessary because, as in transfusion-acquired malaria, congenital infection does not involve the transmission of exoerythrocytic parasites. Parenteral administration of chloroquine should be avoided to prevent cardiovascular collapse associated with it. In cases of chloroquine-resistant congenital malaria due to *P. falciparum*, oral quinine sulfate 25mg/kg/day q8hr for 3-5 days is recommended. A combination of artesunate and mefloquine can be used rather than artesunate alone in areas of high level multidrug resistance. Combination therapy of artesunate with a long acting antimalarial prevents emergence of resistance against either of the drug.

8. Exchange transfusion may be considered when parasitemia exceeds 10% or if there is evidence of complications at lower parasite densities. The efficacy of antimalarial therapy should be monitored by means of sequential blood smears for percentage of parasitemia. The mother of an infant with congenital malaria should be screened for malaria. Even if the smear is negative, by definition she is harboring a *plasmodium* infection and should be treated accordingly. Mothers may breast-feed while receiving antimalarial drugs. Only very small concentrations of antimalarial drugs are detected in breast milk; the amount is neither harmful to the infant nor protective against malaria.

9. Most cases of congenital malaria respond rapidly to therapy & the short-term outcome generally has been favorable. Because delay in diagnosis & treatment can result in significant morbidity & mortality, the differential diagnosis of fever, in infants born to mothers who have lived or traveled in areas where malaria is endemic must include congenital malaria.For women with history of travel to or immigration from an area in which malaria is endemic or with a history of malaria before delivery, clinicians should remain alert to the diagnosis of malaria in the Neonate or infant. Malaria blood films should be obtained from such Neonates and infants should they become ill. For women with a confirmed diagnosis of malaria during the peripartum or postnatal periods, the need for presumptive treatment of the Neonate or infant with an antimalarial appropriate for the mother's infecting species and region of acquisition should be considered. In certain cases, educating the mother about the risk for congenital malaria in her infant and instructing her to seek medical care for her infant if the infant had symptoms of malaria might be sufficient. In other cases, presumptive treatment of the Newborn might be warranted.

10. The prevention of congenital malaria is based on avoidance of exposure & use of chemoprophylaxis. Chloroquine prophylaxis for pregnant women during third trimester is recommended by WHO. Currently Mefloquine is the prophylactic drug of choice, including during the first trimester, for pregnant women who may be exposed to chloroquine-resistant *P.falciparum*. Doxycycline & atovaquone-proguanil should not be used during pregnancy to prevent malaria. In practice, implementation of antenatal malaria prevention is limited by lack of access to medical care, poor compliance with therapy, and widespread presence of chloroquine-resistant organisms.

---

* *Pearl/Peril/Pitfall: Neonatal Malaria or Congenital Malaria—The febrile newborn should be evaluated for malaria especially if there is a history of prolonged labor or in the presence of maternal malaria infection.*

THE EVALUATION-DECISION-ACTION-PLAN/ALGORITHM FOR THE DIAGNOSIS AND MANAGEMENT OF *NEONATAL CONGENITAL MALARIA*

SUBJECTIVE FINDINGS

Hx of fever, severe anemia in pregnant women living in endemic areas.

Hx of associations with abortion, still births, prematurity, fetal growth retardation (known problems with congenital malaria).

Hx of nonspecific Neonatal symptoms such as fever, diarrhea, vomiting, jaundice, anorexia.

OBJECTIVE FINDINGS

Look for anemia, fever, jaundice, irritable Neonate with poor feeding, apnea, resp.distress, jaundice

Examine the abdomen for hepatosplenomegaly

Remember, that the clinical features of congenital malaria are nonspecific & often resemble those due to sepsis or other congenital infections.

Fever is almost uniformly present, but without the characteristic paroxysmal pattern.

Beware of the fact that the diagnosis of congenital malaria is often delayed because of its nonspecific features & the lack of clinical suspicion.

INVESTIGATIONS

Blood FBC with hematocrit & platelets, reticulocyte count, ABG analysis with electrolytes, Blood glucose, calcium++, Mg++, BUN & creatinine, urine analysis and culture, blood cultures to exclude bacterial sepsis, Liver function tests.

Peripheral blood thick smears for detection of organisms and thin smears for identification of *plasmodium* species <u>Microscopic examination remains the "gold standard" for laboratory confirmation of malaria.</u>

*Rapid Diagnostic Tests to detect Plasmodium spe.
*PCR for Molecular Diagnosis-Refer to Overview of the current diagnostic methods in Malaria

---

NEONATAL CONGENITAL MALARIA

Screen mother of an infant with congenital malaria for malarial infection & treat her accordingly.

Monitor for hypoglycemia & treat it energetically, as it is associated with increased mortality & neurologic sequelae.

Ensure ABCs, pulse oximetry, BP, CR monitor

Correct shock, DIC, thrombocytopenia, renal failure, ARDS, hemolytic anemia, CNS complications with appropriate NICU management

Consider exchange transfusion, when parasitemia is >10%

* Treat the infant with Chloroquine sulfate - 10mg base/kg followed by 5mg base/kg at 6, 24, & 48hrs later.

* For Chloroquine-resistant *P.falciparum* - give oral quinine sulfate, 25mg/kg/day, in 3 divided doses for 5 days or Trimethoprim - sulfamethoxazole (8mg/kg/day of Trimethoprim in 2 divided doses for 5 days). *Artemisinin derivatives are safe and highly effective in the treatment of resistant falciparum malaria.*

* Parenteral administration of chloroquine has been associated with cardiovascular collapse & should be reserved for severe cases if oral administration is not possible.

* Treatment with Primaquine is not necessary because, as in transfusion-acquired malaria, congenital infection doesn't involve the transmission of exoerythrocytic parasites of *P.vivax* & *P.ovale*.

KEY POINTS FOR CLINICAL PRACTICE:

1. Congenital malaria is acquired from the mother prenatally or perinatally & is a serious problem in tropical areas & it can cause abortions, stillbirths, IUGR & Neonatal deaths.

2. The clinical features of congenital malaria are nonspecific & often resemble those due to sepsis or other congenital infections, which must be differentiated. The first sign or symptom most commonly occurs between 10 & 30 days of age (range 14hr to several months of age).The most common clinical features in 80% of cases are fever, anemia, and splenomegaly. Other signs and symptoms include hepatomegaly, jaundice, regurgitation, loose stools, and poor feeding.

3. Fever is almost uniformly present, but without the characteristic paroxysmal pattern.

4. The recommended therapy for congenital malaria consists of a) supportive therapy b) oral chloroquine sulfate c) oral quinine sulfate for chloroquine-resistant P. falciparum.

5. The efficacy of antimalarial therapy should be monitored by means of sequential blood smears for percentage of parasitemia. The mother of an infant with congenital malaria should be screened & treated for malaria, even if the smear is negative.

REFERENCES & FURTHER READING : 1) Hindi RD, Azimi PH: Congenital malaria due to *Plasmodium falciparum*. Pediatr 66:977, 1980. 2) Hulbert TV: Congenital malaria in the United States: Report of a case and review. Clin Infect Dis 14:922, 1992. 3) Larkin GL, Thuma PE: Congenital malaria in a hyperendemic area. Am J Trop Med Hyg 45:587, 1991. 4) 8. Ibhanesebhor SE. Clinical characteristics of neonatal malaria. J Trop Pediatr 1995; 41: 330-333. 5) Ibhanesebhor SE, Okolo AA. Malaria parasitemia in neonates with predisposing risk factors for neonatal sepsis: Report of six cases. Ann Trop Pediatr 1992; 12: 297-302.

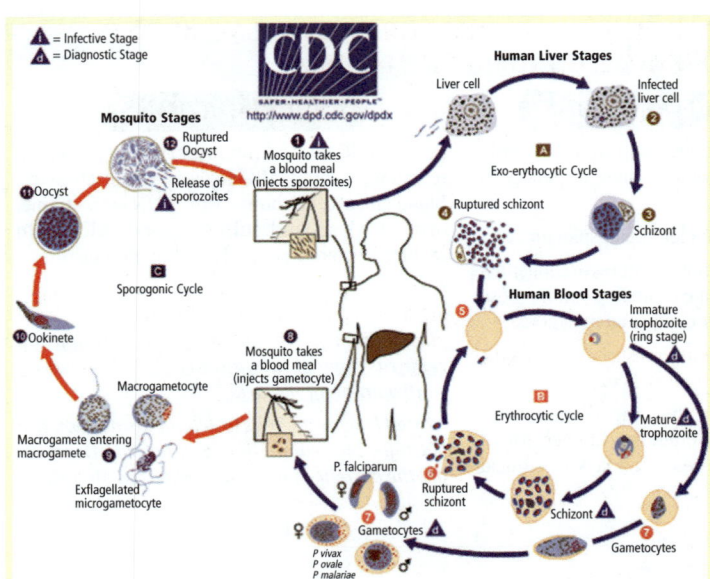

⚠ = Infective Stage
⚠ = Diagnostic Stage

CDC
SAFER·HEALTHIER·PEOPLE*
http://www.dpd.cdc.gov/dpdx

The malaria parasite life cycle involves two hosts. During a blood meal, a malaria-infected female *Anopheles* mosquito inoculates sporozoites into the human host 1. Sporozoites infect liver cells. 2. and mature into schizonts. 3. which rupture and release merozoites. 4. (Of note, in *P. vivax* and *P. ovale* a dormant stage [hypnozoites] can persist in the liver and cause relapses by invading the bloodstream weeks, or even years later.) After this initial replication in the liver (exo-erythrocytic schizogony A), the parasites undergo asexual multiplication in the erythrocytes (erythrocytic schizogony B). Merozoites infect red blood cells. 5. The ring stage trophozoites mature into schizonts, which rupture releasing merozoites. 6. Some parasites differentiate into sexual erythrocytic stages (gametocytes). 7. Blood stage parasites are responsible for the clinical manifestations of the disease.

The gametocytes, male (microgametocytes) and female (macrogametocytes), are ingested by an *Anopheles* mosquito during a blood meal. 8. The parasites' multiplication in the mosquito is known as the sporogonic cycle C. While in the mosquito's mid-gut, the microgametes penetrate the macrogametes generating zygotes. 9. The zygotes in turn become motile and elongated (ookinetes). 10. which invade the midgut wall of the mosquito where they develop into oocysts. 11. The oocysts grow, rupture, and release sporozoites. 12. which make their way to the mosquito's salivary glands. Inoculation of the sporozoites into a new human host perpetuates the malaria life cycle 1.

@Presumptive Treatment: In highly endemic areas (particularly in Africa), the great prevalence of asymptomatic infections and lack of resources (such as microscopes and trained microscopists) have led peripheral health facilities to use "presumptive treatment". Patients who suffer from a fever that does not have any obvious cause are presumed to have malaria and are treated for that disease, based only on clinical suspicion, and without the benefit of laboratory confirmation. This practice is dictated by practical considerations and allows the treatment of a potentially fatal disease. But it also leads frequently to incorrect diagnoses and unnecessary use of antimalarial drugs. This results in additional expenses and increases the risk of selecting for drug-resistant parasites.

KEY MORPHOLOGICAL DIFFERENCES BETWEEN HUMAN PLASMODIUM SPECIES IN BLOOD

Key Morphological Differences Between Human Plasmodium Species in Blood Smears

	vivax	ovale	malariae	falciparum
Ring Stage				
Trophozoite				
Schizont				
Segmenter				sequestered
Gametocytes				

The ring forms of all four species are very similar and difficult to distinguish. *P. falciparum* rings tend to be a little smaller and more numerous than the other species. The presence of a large number of rings in the absence of more mature stages, as well as multiply-infected erythrocytes, is highly suggestive of *P. falciparum*. Erythrocytes infected with *P. vivax* and *P. ovale* are enlarged and exhibit Schüffner's dots as the rings mature into trophozoites. The trophozoites of *P. vivax* are often ameboid, whereas *P. ovale* tends to be more compact. The *P. malariae* trophozoite is very compact and the host erythrocyte is not enlarged. Mature asexual forms of *P. falciparum* are rarely found in the peripheral circulation. The typical number of merozoites produced per schizont is: *P. vivax* 14-20 (up to 24), *P. ovale* 6-12 (up to 18), *P. malariae* 8-10 (up to 12), and *P. falciparum* 16-24 (up to 36). *P. falciparum* exhibits crescent-shaped gametocytes whereas the other species are all round to oval. *P. vivax* and *P. ovale* gametocytes are in enlarged erythrocytes with Schüffner's dots and are difficult to distinguish from each other. *P. malariae* gametocytes do not modify the host erythrocyte. Gametocytes can be distinguished from trophozoites by their large size (nearly filling the erythrocyte) and a single nucleus. Mature microgametocytes tend to stain lighter than macrogametocytes and have a more diffuse nucleus.

* **Pearl/Peril/Pitfall:** *Neonatal Malaria or Congenital Malaria - It may present with progressive pallor and hepatosplenomegaly without fever. Congenital infection manifests within 2-3 weeks after birth whereas acquired infection presents at 4-6 weeks.*

An overview of the Laboratory Diagnosis of Malaria-CDC Recommendations

Microscopic Diagnosis: Blood smear stained with Giemsa, showing a white blood cell (on right side) and several red blood cells are infected with *Plasmodium falciparum* (on left side). Malaria parasites can be identified by examining under the microscope a drop of the patient's blood, spread out as a "blood smear" on a microscope slide. Prior to examination, the specimen is stained (most often with the Giemsa stain) to give to the parasites a distinctive appearance. ***This technique remains the gold standard for laboratory confirmation of malaria.*** However, it depends on the quality of the reagents, of the microscope, and on the experience of the laboratorian. Disadvantages- In many developing countries, microscopy is not reliable because the microscopists are insufficiently trained and supervised and are overworked, the microscopes and reagents are of poor quality, and often the supply of electricity is unreliable. Conversely in non-endemic countries, laboratory technicians are often unfamiliar with malaria and may miss the parasites.

Antigen Detection: A Rapid Diagnostic Test (RDT) is an alternate way of quickly establishing the diagnosis of malaria infection by detecting specific malaria antigens in a person's blood. Various test kits are available to detect antigens derived from malaria parasites. Such immunologic ("immuno-chromatographic") tests most often use a dipstick or cassette format, and provide results in 2-15 minutes. These "Rapid Diagnostic Tests" (RDTs) offer a useful alternative to microscopy in situations where reliable microscopic diagnosis is not available. Malaria RDTs are currently used in some clinical settings and programs. However, before malaria RDTs can be widely adopted, several issues remain to be addressed, including improving their accuracy; lowering their cost; and ensuring their adequate performance under adverse field conditions. *Technique*-A blood specimen collected from the patient is applied to the sample pad on the test card along with certain reagents. After 15 minutes, the presence of specific bands in the test card window indicate whether the patient is infected with *Plasmodium falciparum* or one of the other 3 species of human malaria. It is recommended that the laboratory maintain a supply of blood containing *P. falciparum* for use as a positive control. **Disadvantages**-The use of the RDT does not eliminate the need for malaria microscopy. The RDT may not be able to detect some infections with lower numbers of malaria parasites circulating in the patient's bloodstream. Also, there is insufficient data available to determine the ability of this test to detect the 2 less common species of malaria, *P. ovale* and *P. malariae*. Therefore all negative RDT's must be followed by microscopy to confirm the result. In addition, all positive RDTs should also followed by microscopy. The currently approved RDT detects 2 different malaria antigens; one is specific for *P. falciparum* and the other is found in all 4 human species of malaria. Thus, microscopy is needed to determine the species of malaria that was detected by the RDT. In addition, microscopy is needed to quantify the proportion of red blood cells that are infected, which is an important prognostic indicator.

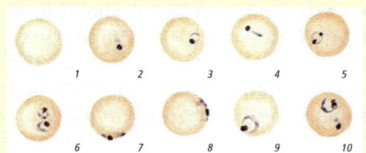

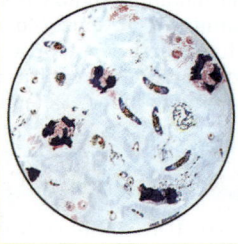

Normal red blood cell and ring-form trophozoites (rings) of *P. falciparum:* **Fig. 1:** Normal red cell; **Figs. 2-10:** Increasingly mature ring-form parasites

Serology: Indirect Fluorescent Antibody Test Malaria antibody detection is performed using the indirect fluorescent antibody (IFA) test. The IFA procedure can be used to determine if a patient has been infected with *Plasmodium*. Because of the time required for development of antibody and also the persistence of antibodies, serologic testing is not practical for routine diagnosis of acute malaria. However, antibody detection may be useful for:*Screening blood donors involved in cases of transfusion-induced malaria when the donor's parasitemia may be below the detectable level of blood film examination *Testing a patient with a febrile illness who is suspected of having malaria and from whom repeated blood smears are negative *Testing a patient who has been recently treated for malaria but in whom the diagnosis is questioned. Species-specific testing is available for the four human species: *P. falciparum*, *P. vivax*, *P. malariae*, and *P. ovale*. Cross reactions often occur between *Plasmodium* species and *Babesia* species. Blood stage *Plasmodium* species schizonts (meronts) are used as antigen. The patient's serum is exposed to the organisms; homologous antibody, if present, attaches to the antigen, forming an antigen-antibody (Ag-Ab) complex. Fluorescein-labeled anti-human antibody is then added, which attaches to the patient's malaria-specific antibodies. When examined with a fluorescence microscope, a positive reaction is when the parasites fluoresce an apple green color. Enzyme immunoassays have also been employed as a tool to screen blood donors, but have limited sensitivity due to use of only *Plasmodium falciparum* antigen instead of antigens of all four human species. *Molecular diagnosis:* Morphologic characteristics of malaria parasites can determine parasite species, however, microscopists may occasionally fail to differentiate between species in cases where morphologic characteristics overlap (especially *Plasmodium vivax* and *P. ovale*), as well as in cases where parasite morphology has been altered by drug treatment or improper storage of the sample. In such cases, the *Plasmodium* species can be determined by using confirmatory molecular diagnostic tests. In addition, molecular tests such as PCR can detect parasites in specimens where the parasitemia may be below the detectable level of

*A: Agarose gel (2%) analysis of a PCR diagnostic test for species-specific detection of Plasmodium DNA. PCR was performed using nested primers of Snounou et al.*Lane S: Molecular base pair standard (50-bp ladder). Black arrows show the size of standard bands. *Lane 1: The red arrow shows the diagnostic band for P. vivax (size: 120 bp). *Lane 2: The red arrow shows the diagnostic band for P. malariae (size: 144 bp). *Lane 3: The red arrow shows the diagnostic band for P. falciparum (size: 205 bp). *Lane 4: The red arrow shows the diagnostic band for P. ovale (size: 800 bp). REFERENCE-Centers for Disease Control and Prevention,1600 Clifton Rd, Atlanta, GA 30333, U.S.A*

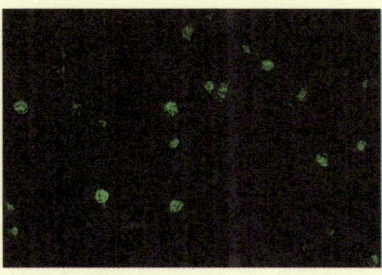

Indirect fluorescent antibody (IFA) test. The fluorescence indicates that the patient serum being tested contains antibodies that are reacting with the antigen preparation (here, Plasmodium falciparum parasites).

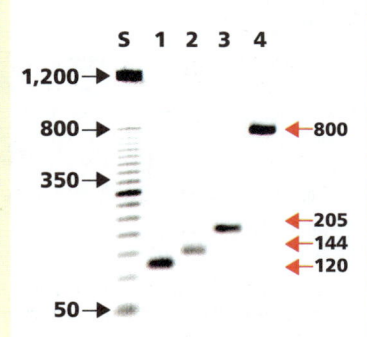

blood film examination. The method currently used at CDC is described below. *Species-specific PCR diagnosis of malaria* Plasmodium genomic DNA is extracted from 200 µl whole blood using the QIAamp Blood Kit (Cat. No. 29106; Qiagen Inc., Chatsworth, CA.) or a similar product that can yield the comparable concentration of genomic DNA from the same volume of blood. Detection and speciation of *Plasmodium* is done with a two step nested PCR using the primers of Snounou et al. In the first step (PCR1), 1 µl of extracted DNA is amplified using genus specific primers; in the second step (PCR2), 1 µl of PCR1 amplification product is further amplified using species specific primers. Ten µl of each PCR2 amplified DNA product is separated by 2% agarose gel electrophoresis, stained for 15 min with ethidium bromide and visualized by UV illumination.

CONGENITAL MALARIA

Vertical transmission of malaria, diagnosed by finding parasites in the Neonate within 7 days of birth is rare. Congenital malaria has caused death in the camps.

Physical examination: Asymptomatic, fever, irritability, feeding problems, hepatosplenomegaly, anemia, jaundice.

Differential Diagnosis

Neonatal sepsis, CMV, herpes simplex, rubella, toxoplasmosis, syphilis

Investigations

Neonates born to mothers with malaria (PF or PV) in the last 7 days before delivery need a malaria smear irrespective of the clinical picture. This should be done 1) at birth and 2) at 7 days of age OR 3) if the clinical condition of the Neonate is worrying.

Treatment
*A Neonate with malaria can deteriorate VERY quickly. The first dose should be parenteral. IV (or IM) Artesunate: or, if unavailable, IM Artemether: Then artesunate 2 mg/kg/day for 7 days. IV or IM Quinine: If using quinine check blood glucose 2-4 hourly. In the event of difficulty gaining IV access in small babies, IM quinine may be used. Nasogastric tube can be used to administer glucose. Frequent breast-feeding is essential. If the Neonate is stable otherwise, a combination course of oral artesunate (total dose of 12 mg/kg can be given as 2 mg/kg/day for 5 days and 1 mg/kg/day for 2 days) and oral mefloquine on day 2 in split dose of 15 mg/kg and 10 mg/kg 12 hours apart. Remark: Quinine, chloroquine and mefloquine are excreted in the breast milk, but the suckling Neonate would receive only a few mg/day. Maternal hypoglycemia, a common complication of malaria or its treatment with quinine, may cause marked fetal bradycardia and other signs of fetal distress.

INTRAVENOUS (IV) ARTESUNATE TREATMENT SCHEDULE
H0, H12, H24 Artesunate 2.4 mg/kg.
Then every 24 hours: Artesunate 2.4 mg/kg daily until the patient can tolerate oral medication.
Artesunate can be given intramuscularly in the same dose as IV.

OR

INTRAMUSCULAR (IM) ARTEMETHER TREATMENT SCHEDULE
If injectable artesunate is unavailable, IM artemether may be used.
H0 Artemether 3.2mg/kg
H24 Artemether 1.6mg/kg every 24 hours until oral medication is tolerated.

OR

INTRA VENOUS (IV) QUININE TREATMENT SCHEDULE
H0 to H4 20 mg/kg given over four hours (preferably in a burette)
H8 10 mg/kg given over 2 hours and this is repeated every 8 hours (H16, H24 etc... total **daily** dose 30 mg/kg).

OR

INTRAMUSCULAR (IM) QUININE TREATMENT SCHEDULE
H0 20 mg/kg is given in 2 simultaneous injections in the 2 antero-lateral thighs after 50 % dilution of the quinine in sterile water.
H8 10 mg/kg is given in one IM injection every 8 hours using the same dilution.
Oral treatment will replace parenteral therapy as soon as the patient can eat and drink.

COMA - MANAGEMENT STEPS: A TO K

A, B C, D, E, F, G, H, I, J, K

    A IRWAY

    B REATHING

    C IRCULATION

    D ON'T FORGET: HYPOGLYCEMIA AND MALARIA

    E VALUATE FOR MENINGITIS

    F ITTING?

    G CS AND GENERAL OBSERVATIONS

    H YDRATION

    I NCREASING PARASITEMIA?

    J UST CONFIRM HEMOGLOBIN OR HEMATOCRIT

    K EEP CARING - good nursing care (position, eyes, clean, NG, food?)

Pearl/Peril/Pitfall : Malaria prevention measures in pregnant women such as insecticide-treated nets and intermittent presumptive treatment should be a priority for malaria control programmes to prevent low birth weight, anaemia, intrauterine growth retardation, premature delivery and neonatal malaria.

Congenital Syphilis

88

@ *All pregnant women should be screened for syphilis with the VDRL test at the first prenatal visit, and in high-risk populations should be repeated at 28-32 weeks gestation and at delivery. All positive VDRL pregnant women should be confirmed with a treponemal test (FTA-ABS).*

Early Congenital Syphilis

Early manifestations are varied, with multi-system Involvement

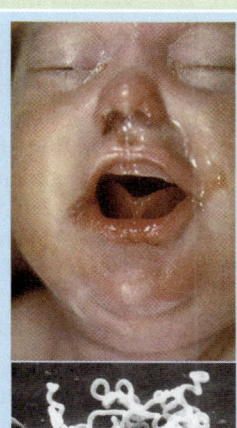
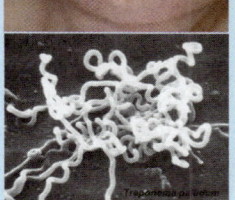

- Jaundice – due to hepatitis
- Generalized lymphadenopathy –epitrochlear nodes
- Coombs – hemolytic anemia, thromobocytopenia, leukopenia, leukocytosis
- Hydrops fetalis
- Mucocutaneous: rhinitis (highly infectious), "snuffles", mucous patches
- Hepatosplenomegaly- diffuse inflammation, scarring
- Maculopapular rash
- Desquamation
- Pemphigus syphiliticus (vesicular bullous eruptions of palms and soles)
- Petechial lesions
- Bony lesions, osteochondritis, periostitis, pseudoparalysis
- Syphilitc leptomeningitis
- Chorioretinitis,salt and pepper fundus, glaucoma
- Pancreatitis

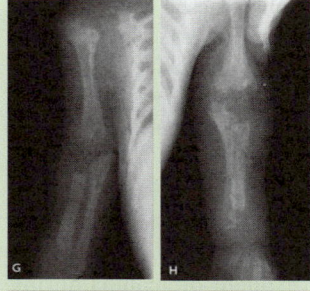

Congenital Syphilis: A much more chronic, untreated infection. The destructive metaphysitis is advanced, with complete disruption of the proximal end of the right humerus, the distal end of the left humerus, and the proximal left radius and ulna. There is a florid periosteal reaction, with new bone and cortical thickening, giving a "bone within a bone" appearance, particularly in all the bones of the left arm and in the right radius.

Definitive diagnosis can be made by dark-field microscopy on specimen from skin lesions, placenta, umbilicus

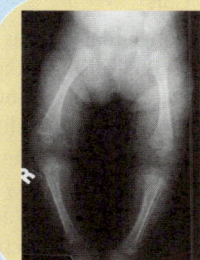

Radiographic findings of bony involvement include metaphyseal lucent bands, which may be a nonspecific response to systemic illness or may be due to syphilitic granulation tissue in the metaphyses. A more specific finding is localized bony destruction of the medial portion of the proximal tibial metaphysis (Wimberger's sign). Other findings include metaphyseal serration ("sawtooth metaphyses"), and diaphyseal involvement with periosteal reaction. Other entities that can mimic Wimberger's sign include neonatal hyperparathyroidism and osteomyelitis. Bony destruction in congenital syphilis may lead to pathologic fractures, and may mimic battered child syndrome.

REVIEW OF CLINICAL PROBLEMS

1. What clinical clues would suggest a diagnosis of Congenital Syphilis ?
   Ans: Refer to the Table 1 of the Chapter.

2. How do you investigate a Neonate with suspected Congenital Syphilis?
   Ans: Refer to the Evaluation-Decision-Action Plan/ Algorithm to diagnose and manage Congenital Syphilis.

3. Discuss the Follow-Up management after Treatment or Prophylaxis for Congenital Syphilis.
   Ans: Refer to the Table 3 of the Chapter.

4. How do you manage Congenital Syphilis ?
   Ans: Refer to the Evaluation-Decision-Action Plan/ Algorithm to diagnose and manage Congenital Syphilis.

5. Discuss the recommended treatment for pregnant women with Syphilis.
   Ans: Refer to the Table 2 of the Chapter.

LEARNING OBJECTIVES

After completing this article, readers will be able to:

1. Screen all pregnant women for VDRL and treat all positive cases adequately after confirmatory tests.

2. Screen both symptomatic and asymptomatic infants born to mothers with maternal nontreponemal and treponemal serology positive and Monitor for Clues suggestive of Congenital Syphilis

3. Treat all infants with presumptive diagnosis of Congenital syphilis with regimens effective for *neurosyphilis* because this cannot be reliably excluded.

4. Evaluate infants and their mothers at risk for syphilis or are infected for other sexually transmitted diseases such as hepatitis B, gonorrhea, chlamydia and HIV.

5. Observe Universal sterile precautions when handling infants with congenital syphilis until therapy has been administered for at least 24 hrs.

---

* ***Pearl/Peril/Pitfall :*** *Late congenital syphilis usually does not manifest until after 2 yr of life and causes gummatous ulcers that tend to involve the nose, septum, and hard palate and periosteal lesions that result in saber shins and bossing of the frontal and parietal bones. Neurosyphilis is usually asymptomatic, but juvenile paresis and tabes may develop. Optic atrophy, sometimes leading to blindness, may occur. Interstitial keratitis, the most common eye lesion, frequently recurs, often resulting in corneal scarring. Sensorineural deafness, which is often progressive, may appear at any age. Hutchinson's incisors, mulberry molars, and maldevelopment of the maxilla resulting in "bulldog" facies are characteristic, if infrequent, sequelae.*

BIRD'S EYE VIEW/OVERVIEW/SYNOPSIS

1. Congenital Syphilis results from transplacental passage of *Treponema pallidum, at any stage of pregnancy but ordinarily occurs during the second half of pregnancy.* Fetuses infected early may die in utero or are at high-risk for significant neurodevelopmental morbidity. The usual outcome of a 3rd trimester infection is the birth of an apparently normal infant who becomes ill within the first few weeks of life. Whereas virtually all infants born to women with primary or secondary syphilis have congenital infection, only 50% are clinically symptomatic. Early latent infection results in a 40% infant infection rate, & late latent infection results in a 6–14% infant infection rate.

2. The risk factors most commonly associated with congenital syphilis are lack of prenatal care and cocaine drug abuse, and trading of sex for drugs, in addition to inadequate prenatal care and poor treatment of syphilis during pregnancy.

3. All pregnant women should be screened for syphilis with the VDRL test at the first prenatal visit, &, in high-risk populations should be repeated at 28-32 weeks gestation & at delivery. All positive VDRL pregnant women should be confirmed with a treponemal test (FTA-ABS). When a woman presents in labor with no history of prenatal care of if results of previous testing are unknown, an STS should be performed at delivery and the infant should not be discharged from the hospital until the test results are known. In women at very high risk, consideration should be given to a repeat STS 1 month postpartum to capture the rare patient who was infected just before delivery but had not yet seroconverted.

4. Untreated syphilis during pregnancy as a transmission rate of 100% & fetal and perinatal death occurs in 40% of affected infants. Approximately 66% of infected & surviving infants are asymptomatic at the time of birth and are identified only by routine prenatal screening of mothers; if they are untreated, symptoms develop within weeks or months. *Refer to Table 1* for clinical clues that suggest a diagnosis of early congenital syphilis. If untreated, late manifestations appear after 2 years of age & may include neurosyphilis, bony changes (frontal bossing, short maxilla, high patalal arch, saddle nose, Hutchinson teeth) interstitial keratitis, 8th nerve deafness etc.

5. Symptomatic infants should be thoroughly evaluated and treated. (*Refer to the E-D-A-Plan/Algorithm* for the diagnosis and management of congenital syphilis).

6. Asymptomatic infants considered at risk for congenital syphilis because the maternal nontreponemal and treponemal serology is positive should be evaluated if (1) maternal treatment was inadequate, unknown, or undocumented; (2) maternal treatment was ≤30 days before delivery; (3) the mother was treated with erythromycin or another nonpenicillin regimen; or (4) the maternal nontreponemal titers did not decrease sufficiently to demonstrate a cure (4-fold or greater). If the maternal treatment was adequate and ≥1 mo before delivery, the infant's positive nontreponemal test result represents passively acquired antibody and the infant does not need treatment at delivery, but follow-up serology should be obtained. If the maternal evaluation is incomplete, these infants are assumed infected and treated.

7. *The Evaluation-Decision-Action-Plan/Algorithm* describes the essential aspects of diagnosis & management of congenital syphilis. For infants with proven/highly probable disease or abnormal physical findings, complete evaluation including serologic tests (VDRL/RPR), complete blood count with differential and platelet count, long bone radiographs, ophthalmology examination, auditory brain stem response, and other tests as indicated should be performed. For infants with a positive VDRL/RPR test result & normal physical examination, whose mothers were inadequately treated, further evaluation is not necessary if 10 days of parenteral therapy is administered.

8. It is now accepted that all infants with a presumptive diagnosis of congenital syphilis should be treated with regimens effective for *neurosyphilis* because this cannot be reliably excluded. A positive CSF VDRL test result in a newborn warrants treatment for neurosyphilis, even though it might reflect passive transfer of antibodies from serum to CSF.

9. Congenital syphilis is treated with crystalline penicillin G (1-1.5 lakhs units/kg/day divided every 12hr IV for the first week of life, and every 8hr thereafter given for 10 days). Treated infants should be followed up serologically to confirm decreasing nontreponemal antibody titers. (*Refer to Table 3*). In a very low risk neonate (asymptomatic, whose mother was treated appropriately, without evidence of relapse or reinfection, a low and stable VDRL titer), no evaluation is necessary. Such an infant can be treated with a single dose of benzathine penicillin G 50,000 units/kg IM. *All seroreactive infants should have a physical examination and nontreponemal titer every 2–3 months until the test becomes nonreactive/the titer decreases 4-fold. If the titer is found to increase/remain reactive at 6–12 months, the infant should undergo reevaluation for signs of active syphilis and retreatment should be seriously considered. If the CSF VDRL test result remains positive at any 6-month interval, retreatment is recommended. If it is negative, but the CSF cell count &/or protein concentration are not declining or remain abnormal at 2 years, retreatment is recommended.*

10. Infants and their mothers at risk for syphilis or are infected with syphilis should be evaluated for other sexually transmitted diseases such as hepatitis B, gonorrhea, chlamydia and HIV. Nasal secretions (snuffles) and open syphilitic lesions are highly infectious. Universal sterile precautions should be observed when handling infants with congenital syphilis until therapy has been administered for at least 24 hrs. Those who have had close contact with an infected infant or mother before precautions were taken should be examined & tested for infection and treatment should be considered.

---

* *Pearl/Peril/Pitfall: Maternal infection is usually detected by antenatal screening using a non-treponemal test (e.g. VDRL) but note there is a risk of false-positive results (due to concomitant infection or autoimmune disease) and confirmation with a specific treponemal test (e.g. FTA-ABS) is required.*

THE EVALUATION-DECISION-ACTION-PLAN/ALGORITHM FOR THE DIAGNOSIS AND MANAGEMENT OF *CONGENITAL SYPHILIS*

SUBJECTIVE FINDINGS

Hx of risk factors for Congenital Syphilis -lack of prenatal health care, illicit drug use (Cocaine use especially), no serologic test for syphilis done during pregnancy, a negative serologic test in the first trimester, without repeat test later in pregnancy, delay in/failure of treatment of a pregnant woman identified as having syphilis.

Hx of Neonatal symptoms suggestive of early congenital syphilis-most affected infants are asymptomatic at birth; symptoms usually develop within the first 3 months of life (Refer to Table No-1)

OBJECTIVE FINDINGS

Look for the most common signs of early congenital syphilis - snuffles, jaundice, pneumonia, anemia, skin & mucocutaneous lesions, hepatomegaly, splenomegaly, osteochondritis, periostitis, pseudoparalysis

In syphilis, pseudoparalysis appears within the first 3 mo of life; in scurvy, it seldom manifests before 5 mo of life.

Signs of CNS involvement seldom appear in the Newborn, even though 1/3rd to 1/2 of those infected suffer such involvement.

Additional diagnoses associated with Congenital Syphilis include - nonimmune hydrops, nephrosis, & myocarditis.

INVESTIGATIONS

Blood - FBC with TC, DC, platelets

Nontreponemal tests - Rapid Plasma Reagin (RPR) test, VDRL test, & Automated Reagin Test (ART).

Treponemal tests - FTA-ABS test & TP-Particle Agglutination Test.

CSF-cell count, proteins, CSF VDRL tests, FTA-ABS of CSF.

New tests under investigation-1)FTA-ABS 19S immunoglobulin M test 2)Polymerase Chain Reaction (PCR).

Dark-field visualization of *Treponema* in scrapings from any lesion/any body fluid.

Radiographs of long bones for osteochondritis & periostitis.

Other tests as clinically indicated - LFTs, ophthalmologic examination, auditory brainstem responses, CXR & cranial ultrasonography.

CONGENITAL SYPHILIS

Recommended Treatment of Pregnant Patients with Syphilis (Refer to Table 2) ←→ **Follow-Up After Treatment or Prophylaxis for Congenital Syphilis (Refer to Table 3)**

Recommended Treatment of Neonates (≤4 wk of age) With Proven or Possible Congenital Syphilis

CLINICAL STATUS	EVALUATION	ANTIMICROBIAL THERAPY*
Proven or highly probable disease†	CSF analysis for VDRL, cell count, and protein CBC and platelet count Other tests as clinically indicated (e.g., long bone radiography, liver function tests, ophthalmologic examination	Aqueous crystalline penicillin G, 100,000-150,000 U/kg/day, administered as 50,000 U/kg/dose IV every 12 hr during the 1st 7 days of life and every 8hr thereafter for a total of 10 days **OR** Penicillin G procaine, 50,000 U/kg/day IM in a single dose for 10 days
Normal physical examination and serum quantitative nontreponemal titer the same of <4-fold the maternal titer:		Aqueous crystalline penicillin G IV for 10 days‡ **OR** Penicillin G procaine, 50,000 U/kg/day IM in a single dose for 10 days §
(a) 1. Mother was not treated or inadequately treated or has not documented treatment; 2. mother was treated with erythromycin or other nonpenicillin regimen; 3. mother received treatment <4 wk before delivery	CSF analysis for VDRL, cell count, and protein CBC and platelet count Long bone radiography	
(b) 1. Adequate maternal therapy given >4 wk before delivery; 2. mother has no evidence of reinfection or relapse	None	**OR** Penicillin G benzathine, 50,000 U/kg IM in a single dose Clinical, serologic follow-up, and penicillin G benzathine, 50,000 U/kg IM in a single dose ~
(c) Adequate therapy before pregnancy and mother's nontreponemal serologic titer remained low and stable during pregnancy and at delivery	None	None ¶

* If >1 day of therapy is missed, the entire course should be treated

† Abnormal physical examination, serum quantitative nontreponemal titer that is 4-fold greater than the mother's titer, or positive result of dark-field or fluorescent antibody test of body fluid(s).

‡ Penicillin G benzathine and penicillin G procaine are approved for IM administration only.

§ A complete evaluation (CSF analysis, bone radiography, CBC) is not necessary if 10 days of parenteral therapy is administered but may be useful to support a diagnosis of congenital syphilis. If a single dose of penicillin G benzathine is used, then the infant must be evaluated fully, the full evaluation must be normal, and follow-up must be certain. If any part of the infant's evaluation is abnormal or not performed or if the CSF analysis is uninterpretable, the 10 day course of penicillin is required.

~ Some experts would not treat the infant but would provide close serologic follow-up.

¶ Some experts would treat with penicillin G benzathine, 50,000 U/kg, as a single IM injection if follow-up is uncertain.

CBC, complete blood count, CSF, cerebrospinal fluid, VDRL, Venereal Disease Research Laboratory (test).

* **Pearl/Peril/Pitfall :** *Early congenital syphilis* The infant may fail to thrive and have a characteristic "old man" look, with fissured lesions around the mouth (rhagades) and a mucopurulent or blood-stained nasal discharge causing snuffles. A few infants develop meningitis, choroiditis, hydrocephalus, or seizures, and others may be mentally retarded. Within the 1st 3 mo of life, osteochondritis (chondroepiphysitis), especially of the long bones and ribs, may cause pseudoparalysis of the limbs with characteristic radiologic changes in the bones.

TABLE 1	Clues that suggest a diagnosis of congenital syphilis*
Epidemiologic background	**Clinical findings**
Untreated early syphilis in the mother	Osteochondritis, periostitis
Untreated latent syphilis in the mother	Snuffles, hemorrhagic rhinitis
An untreated mother who has contact with a known syphilitic during pregnancy	Condylomata lata Bullous lesions, palmar/plantar rash
Mother treated for syphilis during pregnancy with a drug other than penicillin	Mucous patches Hepatomegaly, splenomegaly
Mother treated for syphilis during pregnancy without follow-up to delivery	Jaundice Non immune hydrops fetalis Generalized lymphadenopathy Central nervous system signs; elevated cell count or protein in cerebrospinal fluid Hemolytic anemia, diffuse intravascular coagulation, thrombocytopenia Pneumonitis Nephrotic syndrome Placental villitis or vasculitis (unexplained enlarged placenta) Intrauterine growth restriction

* Arranged in decreasing order of confidence of diagnosis

From Remington JS, Klein JO, Wilson CB, Baker CJ (editors): *Infectious Diseases of the Fetus and Newborn Infant*, 6th ed. Philadelphia, Elsevier/Saunders, 2006, p 556

TABLE 2	Recommended treatment of pregnant patients with syphilis		
Stages of syphilis	**Drug (Penicillin G)**	**Route**	**Dose (units)**
Early (<1 yr duration) Primary, secondary, or early latent	Recommended		
HIV antibody-negative	Benzathine	IM	2.4 million single dose; possibly repeat in 1 wk
HIV antibody -positive*	Benzathine *Alternative* Penicillin desensitization†	IM	2.4 million single dose; possibly repeat weekly x 2
Latent (>1 yr duration)‡	*Recommended* Benzathine *Alternative* Penicillin desensitization	IM	2.4 million weekly x 3 wk
Neurosyphilis	*Recommended* Aqueous *Alternative* Procaine	IV IM	3-4 million every 4 hr x 10-14 days 2.4 million daily x 10-14 days

* With normal cerebrospinal fluid findings, if performed.

† For details, see MMWR Morb Mortal Wkly Rep 47:28, 1998.

‡ Lumbar puncture to exclude neurosyphilis is recommended for HIV-antibody positive patients.

§ Probenecid, 500 mg orally QID X 10-14 days, should also be prescribed.

HIV = human immunodeficiency virus; IM=intramuscular; IV=intravenous

From Remington Js, Klein Jo (eds): Infectious Diseases of the Fetus and Newborn Infant. 5th ed. Philadelphia,

---

* *Pearl/Peril/Pitfall:* Early congenital syphilis (birth through 1st few months of life) causes characteristic bullous eruptions or a macular, copper-colored rash on the palms and soles and papular lesions around the nose and mouth and in the diaper area. Generalized lymphadenopathy and hepatosplenomegaly often occur.

Patient category	Follow-up procedures
Patients receiving diagnosis of congenital syphilis	1. Reagin testing every 2–3 months for the first 15 months, then every 6 months until result is negative or stable at low titer. 2. Treponemal antibody test after 15 months of age. 3. Repeat cerebrospinal fluid evaluation 6 months after treatment if patient received treatment for or shown any signs of central nervous system disease. 4. Careful developmental evaluation, vision testing, and hearing testing before 3 years of age or at time of diagnosis.
Patients receiving treatment in utero or at birth because of maternal syphilis	1. Reagin testing at birth and then every 3 months until test is negative. 2. Treponemal antibody test after 15 months of age.
Women receiving treatment for syphilis during pregnancy	1. Reagin testing monthly until delivery, then every 6 months until test result is negative. 2. Retreatment any time there is a four fold increase in reagin titer.

TABLE 3   Follow-up after treatment or prophylaxis for congenital syphilis

KEY POINTS FOR CLINICAL PRACTICE:

1. Congenital syphilis is a multisystem infection caused by Treponema pallidum and transmitted to the fetus via the placenta. Transplacental transmission occurs in 90% of untreated women, with highest risk early in the disease. Early signs are characteristic skin lesions, lymphadenopathy, hepatosplenomegaly, failure to thrive, blood-stained nasal discharge, perioral fissures, meningitis, choroiditis, hydrocephalus, seizures, mental retardation, osteochondritis, and pseudoparalysis.

2. Early congenital syphilis: Diagnosis is usually suspected based on maternal serologic testing, which is routinely performed early in pregnancy, and often in the 3rd trimester and at delivery. Neonates of mothers with positive tests should have a thorough examination, darkfield microscopy of any skin or mucosal lesions, and a quantitative nontreponemal serum test (e.g., rapid plasma reagin [RPR], venereal disease research laboratory [VDRL]); cord blood is not used for serum testing because results are less sensitive and specific. The placenta or umbilical cord should be analyzed using darkfield microscopy or fluorescent antibody staining. Infants with clinical signs of illness or suggestive serologic test results also should have lumbar puncture with CSF analysis for cell count, VDRL, and protein; CBC; liver function tests; and long-bone x-rays.

3. Diagnosis is confirmed by microscopic visualization of spirochetes in samples from the neonate or the placenta. Diagnosis based on neonatal serologic testing is complicated by the transplacental transfer of maternal IgG antibodies, which can cause a positive test in the absence of infection; however, a neonatal titer > 4 times the maternal titer would not generally result from passive transfer, and diagnosis is considered confirmed or highly probable. Maternal disease acquired late in pregnancy may be transmitted before development of antibodies. Thus, in neonates with lower titers but typical clinical manifestations, syphilis is also considered highly probable.

4. Early congenital syphilis: In confirmed or highly probable cases, 2002 CDC guidelines recommend aqueous penicillin G 50,000 units/kg IV q 12 h for the 1st 7 days of life, and q 8 h thereafter for a total of 10 days, or procaine penicillin G 50,000 units/kg IM once/day for 10 days. This regimen also is used for infants considered to have possible syphilis if the mother was untreated or her treatment status is unknown, she was treated < 4 wk before delivery, or she was inadequately treated (a nonpenicillin regimen, or maternal titers did not decrease 4-fold). Infants with possible syphilis whose mothers were adequately treated and who are clinically well can be given a single dose of benzathine penicillin 50,000 units/kg IM. If close follow up is assured, some clinicians instead obtain nontreponemal serology monthly for 3 mo, and at 6 mo, and treat with a full antibiotic course if titers rise or are positive at 6 mo.

5. Follow up: All seropositive infants and those whose mothers were seropositive should have VDRL or RPR titers q 2 to 3 mo until the test is nonreactive or the titer has decreased 4-fold. In uninfected and successfully treated infants, nontreponemal antibody titers are usually nonreactive by 6 mo. Passively acquired treponemal antibodies may be present for longer, perhaps 15 mo. If VDRL or RPR remain reactive past 6 to 12 mo or titers increase, the infant should be reevaluated (including lumbar puncture for CSF analysis, and CBC with platelet count, long bone x-rays, and other tests as clinically indicated). Retreatment of the mother in subsequent pregnancies is necessary only if serologic titers remain positive. Women who remain seropositive after adequate treatment may have been reinfected and should be retreated.

REFERENCES & FURTHER READING : 1) [Guideline] Screening for syphilis infection in pregnancy: U.S. Preventive Services Task Force reaffirmation recommendation statement. Ann Intern Med. May 19 2009;150(10):705-9. 2) American Academy of Pediatrics. Syphillis. In: Red Book: Report of the Committee on Infectious Diseases. 26th ed. 2003:595-607. 3) Chakraborty R, Luck S. Managing congenital syphilis again? The more things change ... Curr Opin Infect Dis. Jun 2007;20(3):247-52. 4) Chau J, Atashband S, Chang E, Westerberg BD, Kozak FK. A systematic review of pediatric sensorineural hearing loss in congenital syphilis. Int J Pediatr Otorhinolaryngol. March 2009; 5)Brion LP, Manuli M, Rai B. Long-bone radiographic abnormalities as a sign of active congenital syphilis in asymptomatic newborns. Pediatrics. Nov 1991;88(5):1037-40.

* *Pearl/Peril/Pitfall : Pregnant women should be routinely tested for syphilis and retested if they acquire other sexually transmitted diseases during pregnancy. In 99% of cases, adequate treatment during pregnancy cures both mother and fetus. However, in some cases, treatment late in pregnancy eliminates the infection but not some signs of syphilis that appear at birth.*

89 Congenital Toxoplasmosis and Rubella

@ *All Neonates suspected to have Congenital Toxoplasmosis based on symptoms, maternal acute Toxoplasma infection during pregnancy, or maternal HIV with a history of chronic Toxoplasma infection should be evaluated.*

Congenital toxoplasmosis is produced by the obligate intracellular protozoan parasite Toxoplasma gondii. This protozoan parasite is more likely to cross the placenta in the last trimester of pregnancy; nevertheless, central nervous system and ocular manifestations are more frequent in fetuses infected during the first trimester. Microcephaly may occur in neonates with central nervous system toxoplasmosis infection but macrocephaly due to hydrocephalus as a result of aqueductal stenosis may also occur. Seizures often occur. Toxoplasmosis produces parenchymatous and periventricular calcifications. Porencephaly and hydranencephaly may also occur. Cerebrospinal fluid pleocytosis is often present. Hepatomegaly, hyperbilirubinemia, and anemia are systemic manifestations of congenital toxoplasmosis.

Chorioretinitis is present in most neonates with central nervous system involvement .Chorioretinitis is usually bilateral and involves the macular region.

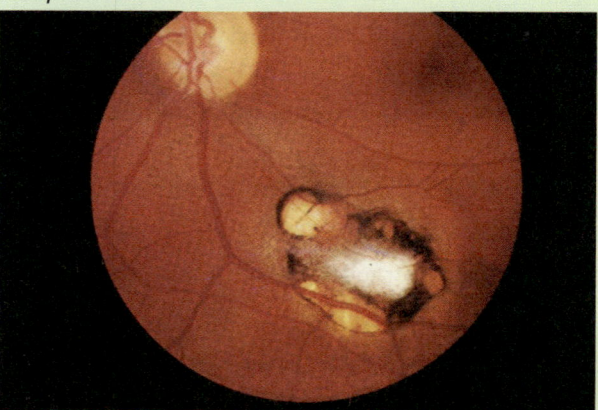

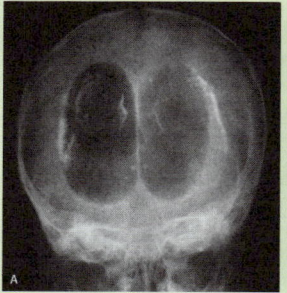
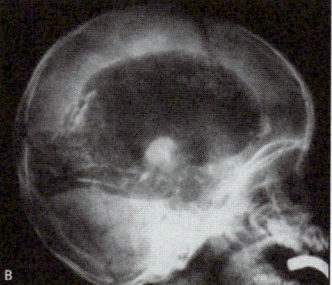

Congenital toxoplasmosis with intracranial hyrocephalus. The grossly dilated lateral ventricles are outlined with air on (A) AP and (B) lateral radiographs after pneumoencephalography. There is spreading of the cranial sutures due to increased intracranial pressure. There is extensive calcification lining the walls of the dilated lateral ventricles, mimicking exactly the intracranial calcifications seen in cytomegaloviral infections.

REVIEW OF CLINICAL PROBLEMS

1. Mention the "common symptoms and signs" of Congenital Toxoplasmosis.
   Ans: Refer to the Table 2 of the Chapter.

2. How do you evaluate a Neonate with suspected Congenital Toxoplasmosis?
   Ans: Refer to the Evaluation-Decision-Action Plan/ Algorithm to diagnose and manage Congenital Toxoplasmosis.

3. Mention the Treatment Guidelines for Congenital Toxoplasmosis.
   Ans: Refer to the Table 5 of the Chapter.

4. Mention the multidisciplinary team useful in managing a Neonate with Congenital Toxoplasmosis.
   Ans: Refer to the "No. 8" of the ''BIRD`S EYE VIEW/ OVERVIEW/SYNOPSIS" of the Chapter.

5) How do you prevent Antenatal transmission of Congenital Toxoplasmosis ?
   Ans: Refer to the Table 3 of the Chapter.

LEARNING OBJECTIVES

After completing this article, readers will be able to:

1. Understand that clinical manifestations of *Congenital Toxoplasmosis* are non specific & resemble those of bacterial sepsis and other congenital infections.

2. Screen all high-risk Neonates for the timely diagnosis and management of *Congenital Toxoplasmosis.*

3. Institute an early recognition and treatment of *Congenital Toxoplasmosis.*

4. Prevent Antenatal transmission of *Toxoplasmosis.*

5. Monitor the Neonate for the sequelae of *Congenital Toxoplasmosis.*

---

* *Pearl/Peril/Pitfall: In suspected congenital toxoplasmosis, serologic tests, MRI or CT imaging of the brain, CSF analysis, and a thorough eye examination by an ophthalmologist should be performed. CSF abnormalities include xanthochromia, pleocytosis, and increased protein concentration. The placenta is inspected for characteristic signs of T. gondii infection. Nonspecific laboratory findings include thrombocytopenia, lymphocytosis, monocytosis, eosinophilia, and elevated transaminases.*

1. Congenital toxoplasmosis is asymptomatic in 80% of infected Newborns, although thorough evaluation may demonstrate eye and CNS abnormalities in about 20% of cases. Clinically apparent disease is present in about 10–25% of infected infants. CNS involvement is the hallmark of Congenital Toxoplasmosis infection; the "Classic triad" of the disease consists of Chorioretinitis, Intracranial Calcifications, and Hydrocephalus. Their presence should alert the clinician to the diagnosis. Chorioretinitis (focal necrotizing retinitis) is often bilateral with macular involvement and even the optic nerve and can lead to complications such as blindness, iridocyclitis, and cataracts. Intracranial Calcifications (visualized best by CT Scan) may be single/multiple but typically generalized and located in the caudate nucleus, choroid plexus, meninges, and subependyma; may also occur periventricularly as in Cytomegalovirus infection. In contrast to Hydrocephalus (resulting from the extensive periaqueductal and periventricular vasculitis with necrosis that causes obstruction of the ventricular system), Microcephaly can also occur indicating severe brain damage.

2. Table 2 of the Chapter enlists common clinical findings among infants with Congenital Toxoplasmosis. Apart from the CNS manifestations discussed above, the multisystem involvement is evident by the presence of fever, jaundice, hepatosplenomegaly, generalized lymphadenopathy, skin rash, anemia, pneumonitis, thrombocytopenia, eosinophilia, hypo/hyperthermia, CSF Lymphocytic pleocytosis and elevated protein, microphthalmia, glaucoma, and metaphyseal bony lucencies.

3. Infection of the fetus occurs as a consequence of maternal primary infection during pregnancy or rarely, just before conception. Reactivation of latent Toxoplasma infection during pregnancy does not lead to fetal infection except among immunocompromised women such as those infected with HIV. Acute maternal infection which is usually acquired early in pregnancy may lead to fulminant fetal infection resulting in stillbirth, nonimmune fetal hydrops, preterm birth, and perinatal death. Placental infection is an important intermediary step, and up to 16 weeks may elapse between placental infection and subsequent fetal infection. 15% of infants are infected, when maternal infection occurs in the first trimester (30% in 2nd trimester and 60% in 3rd trimester and usually 90% of which are subclinical); however the severity of clinical manifestations is greatest when maternal infection is acquired early in pregnancy.

4. The differential diagnosis includes; CMV, Rubella, Syphilis, HSV, Hepatitis B, Sepsis, Immune Thrombocytopenia, Histiocytosis, Metabolic disorders, Hemolytic diseases, Congenital leukemia, Congenital lymphocytic choriomeningitis. Diagnosis may be made by serology, Polymerase Chain Reaction (PCR), Histology, or isolation of the parasite.

5. *The Evaluation-Decision-Action-Plan/Algorithm* to diagnose & manage Congenital Toxoplasmosis outlines the essential aspects of history taking, physical examination & appropriate investigations as well as management of the affected infant & mother.

6. Table 5 of the Chapter gives an outline of guidelines for the treatment of Congenital Toxoplasmosis. Therapy is recommended, regardless of symptoms, to prevent the high incidence of sequelae, resolve acute symptoms, and improve outcomes. As current medications do not eradicate T.gondii and primarily act against the tachyzoite form not tissue cysts, especially from neural tissue and the eye, extended therapy until 1 year of age is recommended.

7. Refer to the Table 3 of the Chapter for Antenatal screening: this allows early diagnosis of acute maternal, fetal, and neonatal infection, and improves outcomes. Positive Sabin-Feldman dye tests should be confirmed by Ig M double-sandwich ELISA. Ig G avidity can help establish the timing of infection. It is strongly recommended that a Toxoplasma reference laboratory confirm all serology suggesting infection before treatment, fetal testing, or abortion.

8. Multidisciplinary consultation with ophthalmologist, Audiologist, neurosurgeon, neurodevelopmental pediatrics, and infectious disease specialists is usually helpful for patient management.

9. Primary prevention strategies seek to prevent cases of congenital infection by preventing cases of maternal infection, involving pre- or early pregnancy counseling on how to avoid exposure.To reduce mother-to-child transmission and morbidity from congenital toxoplasmosis, some high-incidence countries such as Austria and France have chosen a secondary prevention strategy and implemented nationwide programmes to detect and treat acute Toxoplasma infections during pregnancy. In women with evidence of acute infection spiramycin is usually prescribed and amniocentesis performed. In the event of fetal infection, pyrimethamine and sulfonamides is the treatment of choice and termination is discussed if fetal abnormalities are detected on ultrasound.

10. Finally, tertiary prevention attempts to lessen the severity of disease sequelae through early detection and treatment of congenital disease. Proponents of this idea recognize that most congenital disease is subclinical at birth, but that sequelae often develop over time. Tertiary prevention also involves considering termination of pregnancy for severely affected fetuses.

---

* *Pearl/Peril/Pitfall : Congenital toxoplasmosis is caused by transplacental acquisition of Toxoplasma gondii. Signs, if present, are prematurity, intrauterine growth restriction, jaundice, hepatosplenomegaly, myocarditis, pneumonitis, rash, chorioretinitis, hydrocephalus, intracranial calcifications, microcephaly, and seizures. Diagnosis is by serology.*

THE EVALUATION-DECISION-ACTION-PLAN/ALGORITHM FOR THE DIAGNOSIS AND MANAGEMENT OF *CONGENITAL TOXOPLASMOSIS*

SUBJECTIVE FINDINGS

Hx of Neonatal symptoms suggestive of Congenital Toxoplasmosis-Refer to the Table 2 of the Chapter.

Hx of maternal infection acute/chronic with sporadic abortion, past Hx of still birth, prematurity, fetal hydrops, perinatal death

Asymptomatic subclinical infections can only be diagnosed by universal screening of all neonates in high risk populations.

OBJECTIVE FINDINGS

Assess airway, breathing, circulation & disability by observing the vitals, BP, O_2 sats, color, CRT, pulses, sensorium, focal neurologic deficits, seizures, abnormal movements, tone & reflexes etc.

Look for - signs of multisystem involvement- Refer to the Table 2 of the Chapter.

INVESTIGATIONS

Refer to the Table 1 of the Chapter given below for the relevant investigations to diagnose and follow-up of Congenital Toxoplasmosis.

TABLE 1   Postnatal: Suggested evaluation & treatment program for infants with congenital toxoplasma infection

Initial evaluation

Complete physical examination
Cranial CT scan
CSF protein, glucose, cell count, PCR, SEROLOGY, ISOLATION OF PARASITES
Complete eye examination by a pediatric ophthalmologist
Complete blood count, liver function tests (especially ALT, bilirubin)
Serum glucose-6-phosphate dehydrogenase screen (prior to initiating sulfadiazine)
Urine culture for cytomegalovirus
Pediatric neurology assessment if apparent symptomatic CNS disease

Follow-up evaluation

Complete blood counts to monitor for drug toxicity:*
    1–2 times/week while on daily pyrimethamine
    1–2 times/month while on every other day pyrimethamine
Complete pediatric examination, including neurodevelopmental assessment every month
Pediatric ophthalmology examination every 3 months until 18 months of life, then yearly thereafter.†
Pediatric neurology examination every 3-6 months until 1 year of age ‡
Serum IgG and IgM determinations every 3 months until 18 months of age

Treatment regimen

Pyrimethamine 1 mg/kg daily for 2–6 months, then 1 mg/kg every other day to complete 1 year of therapy
Sulfadiazine 100 mg/kg in 2 divided doses each day for 1 year
Folinic acid (leukovorin) 10 mg 3 times/week with dose increased as needed for pyrimethamine toxicity

---

* Counts should be done at the more frequent interval if there is an intercurrent illness or any occurrence of neutropenia. Folinic acid (leucovorin) dose should be increased if the absolute neutrophil count (ANC) falls below 1000, and pyrimethamine should be temporarily withheld if the ANC falls below 500. Persistent neutropenia despite withholding of pyrimethamine may be caused by sulfadiazine. Measurement of serum ALT and creatinine, and obtaining a urinalysis every 3 months may be useful in monitoring for side effects of sulfadiazine.

† Frequency of examinations adjusted as needed if retinal disease present.

‡ Frequency and duration of pediatric neurology follow-up determined by the presence of neurologic abnormalities.

Source: Guerina, N.G. Congenital infection with *Toxoplasma gondii*. Pediatr. Ann. 23:138, 1994.

TABLE 2	Signs and symptoms in 210 infants with proved congenital toxoplasma infection*	
Finding	**No. examined**	**No. positive (%)**
Prematurity	210	
Birthweight <2,500 g		8(3.8)
Birthweight 2,500-3,000 g		5 (7.1)
Intrauterine growth restriction		13 (6.2)
Icterus	201	20 (10)
Hepatosplenomegaly	210	9 (4.2)
Thrombocytopenic purpura	210	3 (1.4)
Abnormal blood count (anemia, eosinophilia)	102	9 (4.4)
Microcephaly	210	11 (5.2)
Hydrocephaly	210	8 (3.8)
Hypotonia	210	12 (5.7)
Convulsions	210	8 (3.8)
Psychomotor retardation	210	11 (5.2)
Intracranial calcification x-ray	210	24 (11.4)
Ultrasound	49	5 (10)
Computed tomography	13	11 (84)
Abnormal electroencephalogram	191	16 (8.3)
Abnormal cerebrospinal fluid	163	56 (34.2)
Microphthalmia	210	6 (2.8)
Strabismus	210	111 (5.2)
Chorioretinitis	210	
Unilateral		34 (16.1)
Bilateral		12 (5.7)

*infants were identified by prospective study of infants born to women who acquired *Toxoplasma gondii* infection during pregnancy. Data adapted from Couvreur J, Desmonts G, Tournier G, et al: A homogeneous series of 210 cases of congenital toxoplasmosis in 0-11 mo old infants detected prospectively. Ann Pediatr (Paris) 1984;31:815-819

TABLE 3	Antenatal prevention of congenital toxoplasmosis

- Routine one time screening of pregnant women for TORCH infections - not recommended.
- Prevent INFECTION or Reduce Manifestations in the fetus

a. Prevent infection of mother
    Prevent infection with OOCYSTS excreted by CATS
       wash fruits & vegetables thoroughly before consumption
       wear gloves while gardening.
       Prevent access of flies, cockroaches, etc. to food
    Prevent infection from meat, eggs & milk
       Cook meat to 'welldone'
       Wash hands thoroughly after handling meat
       Cook eggs, don't drink unpasteurized milk
    Prevent infection via blood transfusion or organ transplantation.
       Don't use blood products and organs from seropositive donors for seronegative recipients

b. Treat acutely infected mother during pregnancy to reduce transmission (60%) - SPIRAMYCIN 1 gram every 8 hrs for 3 weeks, followed by 2 wk break and continued till delivery.

c. Identify Infected fetus by USG, Amniocentesis & fetal blood sampling (PUBS) for culture, PCR, specific IgM, total IgM & Blood chemistries

d. When fetal infection is confirmed OPTIONAL Termination of pregnancy in the 1st & 2nd trimester. If termination is not an option - treat mother intensively with PYRIMETHAMINE 100 mg Bd on day 1 then 500 mg/d thereafter + FOLINIC Acid 10–20 mg/d + sulfadiazine 1.5 gm bd from 24 wks of gestation. Alternate this regimen with SPIRAMYCIN every 3 weeks. Follow-up with serial ultrasounds.

* *Pearl/Peril/Pitfall: The rate of transmission to the fetus is higher in women infected later during pregnancy. However, those infected earlier in gestation generally have more severe disease. Overall, 30 to 40% of women infected during pregnancy will have a congenitally infected child.*

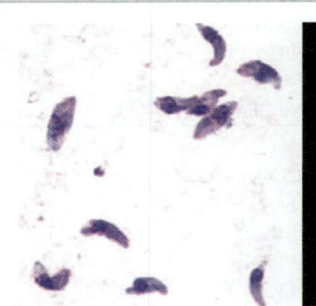
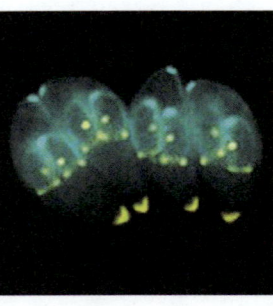

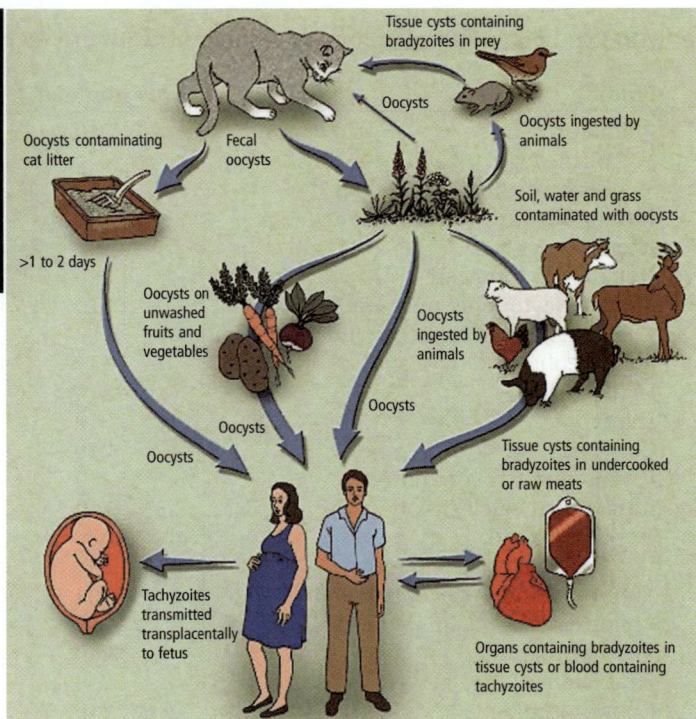

"*Toxoplasma gondii* tachyzoites, stained with Giemsa, from a smear of peritoneal fluid obtained from a mouse inoculated with *T. gondii*. Tachyzoites are typically crescent shaped with a prominent, centrally placed nucleus."

Pathways for Toxoplasma gondii infection. The feline intestinal tract is the only source for the production of *T. gondii* oocysts. Transmission to humans usually occurs through the ingestion of oocysts from contaminated sources (e.g., soil, cat litter, garden vegetables, water) or the ingestion of tissue cysts in undercooked meat from infected animals. Although fetal infection most often occurs after acute *T. gondii* infection in a pregnant woman, it also can occur after the reactivation of latent infection in an immunocompromised pregnant woman. Redrawn with permission from Lynfield R, Guerina NG. Toxoplasmosis. Pediatr Rev 1997;18(3):75–83.

| TABLE 4 | Frequency of clinical findings in infants with congenital infections |

Clinical Findings	Rubella	Toxoplasma	CMV	Syphilis	HSV
Intrauterine growth restriction	+++	±	++	++	±
Reticuloendothelial system					
Jaundice	+	++	+++	+++	+
Hepatitis	±	+	+++	+++	+
Hepatosplenomegaly	+++	++	+++	+++	+
Anemia	+	+++	++	+++	–
Thrombocytopenia	++	±	+++	++	+
Disseminated intravascular coagulation	–	–	±	–	++
Adenopathy	++	++	–	++	–
Dermal erythropoiesis	+	–	+	–	–
Skin rash	–	+	–	++	+++
Bone abnormalities	++	–	±	++	–
Eye					
Cataracts	++	±	±	±	–
Retinopathy	++	+++	+	±	+++
Microphthalmia	+	±	±	–	±
Central nervous system					
Microcephaly	+	+	++	–	±
Meningoencephalitis	++	+++	+++	++	+++
Brain calcification	±	++	++	–	+
Hydrocephalus	–	++	±	±	++
Hearing defect	+++	+	+++	+	–
Pneumonitis	++	+	±	+	±
Cardiovascular					
Myocarditis	+	±	±	±	–
Congenital defect	+++	–	–	–	–

±, rare; +, 5% to 20%; ++, 20% to 50%; +++, more than 50%; CMV, cytomegalovirus; HSV, herpes simplex virus.

CONGENITAL RUBELLA SYNDROME

Congenital rubella is a viral infection acquired from the mother during pregnancy. Signs are multiple congenital anomalies that can result in fetal death. Diagnosis is by serology and viral culture. There is no specific treatment. Prevention is by routine vaccination. Congenital rubella typically results from a primary maternal infection. Despite widespread vaccination, 10 to 20% of postpubertal people lack antibody. Rubella is believed to invade the upper respiratory tract, with subsequent viremia and dissemination of virus to different sites, including the placenta. The fetus is at highest risk for developmental abnormalities when infected during the 1st 16 wk of gestation, particularly the 1st 8 to 10 wk. Early in gestation, the virus is thought to establish a chronic intrauterine infection. Its effects include endothelial damage to blood vessels, direct cytolysis of cells, and disruption of cellular mitosis.

Symptoms and Signs Rubella in a pregnant woman may be asymptomatic or characterized by upper respiratory tract symptoms, fever, lymphadenopathy (especially in the suboccipital and posterior auricular areas), and a maculopapular rash. This illness may be followed by joint symptoms. In the fetus there may be no effects, multiple anomalies, or death in utero. The most frequent abnormalities include intrauterine growth restriction, meningoencephalitis, cataracts, retinopathy, hearing loss, cardiac defects (patent ductus arteriosus and pulmonary artery stenosis), hepatosplenomegaly, and bone radiolucencies. Others are thrombocytopenia with purpura, dermal erythropoiesis resulting in bluish red skin lesions, adenopathy, and interstitial pneumonia. Close observation is needed to detect subsequent hearing loss, mental retardation, abnormal behavior, endocrinopathies, or a rare progressive encephalitis.

Diagnosis Pregnant women routinely have a serum rubella titer measured early in pregnancy. Titer is repeated in seronegative women who develop symptoms or signs of rubella; diagnosis is made by seroconversion or a e" 4-fold rise between acute and convalescent titers. Virus may be cultured from nasopharyngeal swabs. Infants suspected of having congenital rubella should have antibody titers and viral cultures. Persistence of rubella-specific IgG in the infant after 6 to 12 mo suggests congenital infection. Increased rubella-specific IgM antibodies also indicate rubella. Specimens from the nasopharynx, urine, CSF, buffy coat, and conjunctiva may grow virus; the laboratory should be notified that rubella virus is suspected. In a few centers, diagnoses can be made prenatally by isolating the virus from amniotic fluid, detecting rubella-specific IgM in fetal blood, or applying reverse transcriptase–PCR (RT-PCR) techniques to fetal blood or chorionic villus biopsy specimens. Other tests include a CBC with differential, CSF analysis, and radiologic examination of the bones to detect characteristic radiolucencies. Thorough ophthalmologic and cardiac evaluation is also useful.

Treatment No specific therapy is available for maternal or congenital rubella infection. Women exposed to rubella early in pregnancy should be informed of the potential risks to the fetus. Some experts recommend administering immune globulin (0.55 mL/kg IM) for exposure early in pregnancy but this use does not guarantee prevention, and routine use is not recommended by the American Academy of Pediatrics.

Prevention Rubella can easily be prevented by vaccination. Infants should receive vaccination for rubella together with measles and mumps vaccinations at 12 to 15 mo of age and again at entry to grade school or junior high school Postpubertal females who are not known to be immune to rubella should be vaccinated. (Caution: *Rubella vaccination is contraindicated in immunodeficient or pregnant women.*) After vaccination, women should be advised not to become pregnant for 28 days. Efforts should also be made to screen and vaccinate high-risk groups, such as hospital and child care workers, military recruits, and college students.

REFERENCES & FURTHER READING: 1)CDC. Rubella and congenital rubella syndrome - United States, 1994-1997. MMWR 1997;46:350-4. 2) Greaves WL, Orenstein WA, Stetler HC, et al. Prevention of rubella transmission in medical facilities. JAMA 1982;248:861-4.

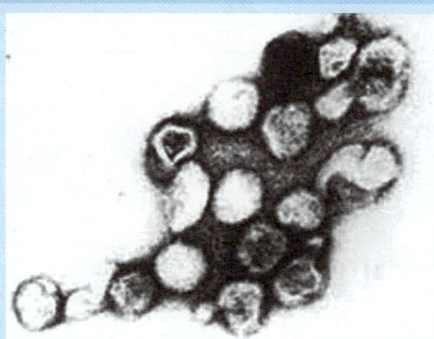

Rubella Virus, transmission electron micrograph (Image: CDC USA):Rubella virus (Latin, *rubella* = little red), also known as "German Measles" (due to early citation in German medical literature), infection during pregnancy can cause congenital rubella syndrome (CRS) with serious malformations of the developing fetus. The type and degree of abnormality relates to the time of maternal infection.

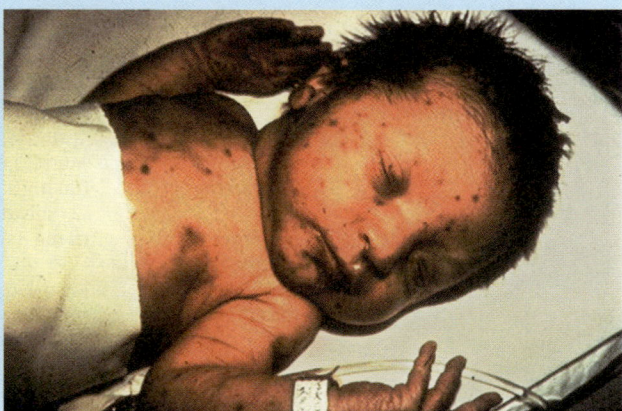

Congenital Rubella (Image: CDC USA)

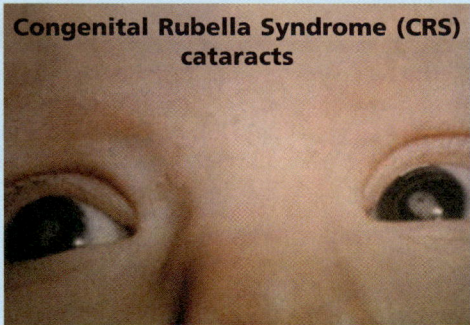

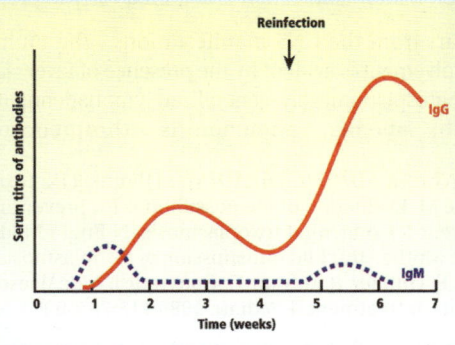

Typical serological events following acute rubella infection. Note that in reinfection, rubella-specific IgM is usually absent or present at a low level transiently

TABLE 5 Treatment guidelines for congenital toxoplasmosis

	Therapy	Dosage (Oral unless specified)	Duration
In Pregnant women with acute toxoplasmosis: For first 21 weeks of gestation or until term if fetus not infected	Spiramycin	1 g q 8hr without food	Until fetal infection documented or excluded at 21 wks; if fetal infection documented, replaced with pyrimethamine, leucovorin, and sulfadiazine (see below)
If fetal infection confirmed after 18th week of gestation or if infection acquired in last few weeks of gestation	Pyrimethamine and	Loading dose: 100 mg/day in 2 divided doses for 2 days followed by 50 mg/day	Until delivery
	Sulfadiazine and	Loading dose: 75 mg/kg/day in 2 divided doses (maximum, 4 g/d) for 2 days; then 100 mg/kg/day in 2 divided doses (maximum, 4 g/day)	Until delivery
	Leucovorin†	10-20 mg qd	Until delivery
Congenital Toxoplasma infection in infant	Pyrimethamine and	Loading dose: 2 mg/kg/day for 2 days; then 1 mg/kg/day for 2 or 6 months; then 1 mg/kg/day on Mon, Wed, and Fri each week	≥ 1 yr
	Sulfadiazine and	100 mg/kg/day in 2 daily divided doses	≥ 1 yr
	Leucovorin (folinic acid)†	10 mg 3 times weekly	≥ 1 yr
	Corticosteroids (prednisone)‡	1 mg/kg/daily in 2 daily divided doses	Until resolution of elevated (≥ 1 g/dL) CSF protein or active chorioretinitis that threatens vision

†Monitor blood and platelet counts weekly; adjust dosage for megaloblastic anemia, granulocytopenia, or thrombocytopenia.
‡When signs of inflammation or active chorioretinitis have subsided, dosage can be tapered and drug discontinued; use only in conjunction with pyrimethamine, sulfadiazine, and leucovorin.

KEY POINTS FOR CLINICAL PRACTICE:

1. CNS involvement is the hallmark of Congenital Toxoplasmosis infection; the "Classic triad" of the disease consists of Chorioretinitis, Intracranial calcifications, and Hydrocephalus. Their presence should alert the clinician to the diagnosis.

2. 15% of infants are infected, when maternal infection occurs in the first trimester (30% in 2nd trimester and 60% in 3rd trimester and usually 90% of which are subclinical); however the severity of clinical manifestations is greatest when maternal infection is acquired early in pregnancy.

3. Apart from the CNS manifestations , the multisystem involvement is evident by the presence of fever, jaundice, hepatosplenomegaly, generalized lymphadenopathy, skin rash, anemia, pneumonitis, thrombocytopenia,

eosinophilia, hypo/hyperthermia, CSF Lymphocytic pleocytosis and elevated protein, microphthalmia, glaucoma, and metaphyseal bony lucencies.

4. Multidisciplinary consultation with ophthalmologist, Audiologist, neurosurgeon, neurodevelopmental pediatrics, and infectious disease specialists is usually helpful for patient management.

5. Therapy is recommended, regardless of symptoms, to prevent the high incidence of sequelae, resolve acute symptoms, and improve outcomes. As current medications do not eradicate T.gondii and primarily act against the tachyzoite form not tissue cysts, especially from neural tissue and the eye, extended therapy until 1 year of age is recommended.

REFERENCES & FURTHER READING : 1)Frenkel JK. Toxoplasmosis. Pediatr Clin North Am. 1985;32: 917–932. 2) Foulon W, Naessens A, Derede M. Evaluation of the possibilities for preventing congenital toxoplasmosis. Am J Perinatol. 1994;11(1):57–62. 3) Desmonts G, Couvreur J. Congenital toxoplasmosis. N Engl J Med. 1974;290:1110–6. 4)Dunn D, Wallon M, Peyron F, Petersen E, Peckham C, Gilbert R. Mother-to-child transmission of toxoplasmosis: Risk estimates for clinical counseling. Lancet. 1999;353:1829–33. 5)Hohlfeld P, Daffos F, Thulliez P, Aufrant C, Couvreur J, MacAleese J, et al. Foetal toxoplasmosis: outcome of pregnancy and infant follow-up after in utero treatment. J Pediatr. 1989;115:765–9.)

* Pearl/Peril/Pitfall : Serology is important in diagnosing maternal and congenital infection; there are numerous tests, some of which are performed only in reference laboratories. The most reliable are the Sabin-Feldman dye test, the indirect fluorescent antibody (IFA) test, and the direct agglutination assay. Acute maternal infection is suggested by seroconversion or a e" 4-fold rise between acute and convalescent IgG titers. However, maternal IgG antibodies may be detectable in the infant through the 1st year. PCR analysis of fetal blood and amniotic fluid may prove a better method. Tests to isolate the organism include inoculation into mice and tissue culture.

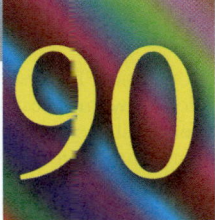

Perinatal Herpes

@ An infant with skin lesions at birth should be investigated for herpes infection by PCR testing of the vesicles. The diagnosis of herpetic skin lesions in a newborn should lead to careful examination of CNS, eyes and abdominal organs.

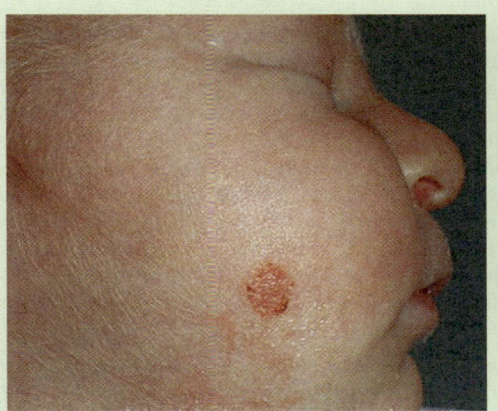

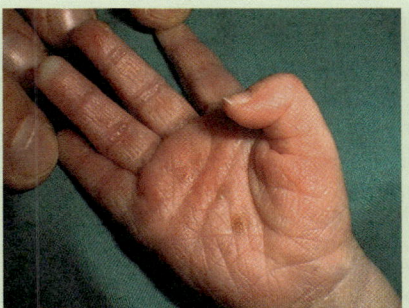

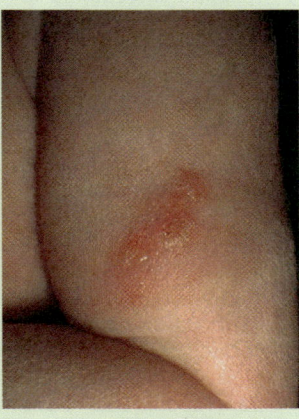

Multiple grouped Herpetic vesicles on an erythematous base on the upper limbs and face

Cerebral ultrasound on day of life 6 showed extensive bilateral periventricular calcifications and encephaloclastic areas in the left parietal and in both temporal lobes. These findings were later confirmed by MRI

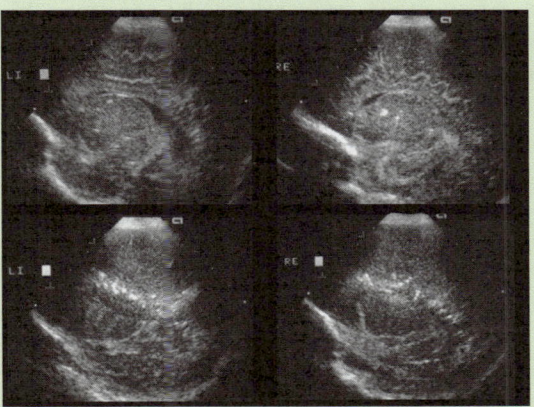

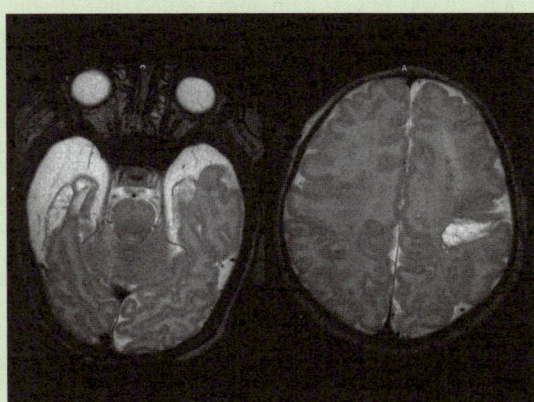

REVIEW OF CLINICAL PROBLEMS

1. Mention the "3 Categories" of Perinatal HSV infection.
   Ans: Refer to "No. 3" of the "BIRD'S EYE VIEW/OVERVIEW/ SYNOPSIS" of the Chapter.

2. Describe the management of an infant born to a woman with active genital HSV infection.
   Ans: Refer to the Table 1 of the Chapter.

3. What are the risk factors for HSV acquisition by the Neonate ?
   Ans: Refer to "No. 2" of the "BIRD'S EYE VIEW/OVERVIEW/ SYNOPSIS" of the Chapter.

4. How do you manage a Neonate with disseminated Herpes?
   Ans: Refer to the Evaluation-Decision-Action Plan/Algorithm to diagnose & manage Neonatal Herpes.

5. What should you look for, when performing a physical examination of a Neonate with suspected Perinatal Herpes?
   Ans: Refer to the Evaluation-Decision-Action Plan/Algorithm to diagnose & manage Neonatal Herpes.

LEARNING OBJECTIVES

After completing this article, readers will be able to:

1. Suspect Neonatal Herpes in any Neonate with antibiotic unresponsive sepsis and disseminated multiorgan dysfunction.

2. Diagnose Neonatal Herpes promptly, and treat effectively.

3. Anticipate the need for the provision of Intensive Care, if CNS is involved manifesting as apneas, seizures, and lethargy.

4. Follow-up of Neonatal survivors of Perinatal Herpes for long-term neurological sequelae such as psychomotor retardation and seizures.

5. Prevent Nursery cross-infections by observing the Universal Sterile Precautions.

** **Pearl/Peril/Pitfall** : Neonatal herpes simplex virus infection is usually transmitted during parturition. Signs are typically a vesicular eruption and subsequent disseminated disease. Diagnosis is by viral culture, histology, serology, or molecular biology. Treatment is with high-dose parenteral acyclovir and supportive care.*

BIRD`S EYE VIEW/OVERVIEW/SYNOPSIS

1. Neonatal Herpes is an uncommon but potentially fatal infection of the fetus or more likely the Newborn. Herpes simplex virus type 2 (HSV-2) is the predominant cause of Neonatal disease (75–80%), also the predominant cause of recurrent genital disease of mothers. Most HSV infections during pregnancy represent recurrent disease. Risk of Neonatal infection is about 50% for those with primary maternal HSV genital infection, as against only 5% for those with recurrent infection. *The amount and duration of maternal virus shedding is likely to be greatest with primary infections and less passive immunity to the HSV also increases the risk of transmission in primary infections.*

2. Most of the Neonatal infections (>95%) occur as a result of intrapartum transmission; the risk factors for HSV acquisition by the Neonate during passage through birth canal include **a)** Cervical HSV infection **b)** Multiple genital lesions **c)** Prematurity **d)** Rupture of membranes more than 4hrs **e)** Scalp electrode or other internal monitoring **f)** Chorioamnionitis **g)** Vaginal delivery **h)** Absent or low titers of transplacentally acquired neutralizing HSV antibodies. Postnatal infection may result from transmission of virus from the cold sore of a mother or medical attendant to the baby. Antenatal transmission has been documented but is uncommon, which may result in spontaneous abortion before 20 wks of gestation and a wide range of clinical manifestations in survivors such as localized skin/eye/disseminated multiorgan involvement and congenital malformations.

3. Most infants with perinatal/postnatal HSV infection are normal at birth, illness developing after 3 days of age. *It is critical to recognize that most mothers of infants with Neonatal HSV do not have a history of HSV. Overt Herpetic disease in the maternal genital tract is evident in only about 1/3 rd of patients.* The morbidity and mortality of Neonatal HSV best correlates with 3 categories of disease. 1)Localized skin, eye, and mouth (SEM) disease 30–40% 2) Encephalitis/CNS disease-20% 3)Disseminated multiorgan herpes - 50%. Less than half of infants with any form of HSV infections have fever, only 30-40% of patients have the classic vesicular skin lesions at presentation, and only 2/3rds of patients have skin lesions at any time during infection.

4. Disseminated herpes usually begins toward the end of the first week of life. Skin vesicles may be the first or a later sign, but they do not appear at all in almost half of patients. Systemic symptoms, although insiduous in onset, progress rapidly. Poor feeding, lethargy, and fever may be accompanied by irritability or convulsions if the CNS is involved. These symptoms are followed rapidly by jaundice, respiratory distress/apnea, hypotension, DIC and shock. This form of disease is indistinguishable at its onset from both neonatal enterovirus infection and bacterial sepsis. Mortality without treatment is >80% and with treatment it is still 50% and 50% of the survivors have severe neurologic impairments.

5. Infants with encephalitis typically presents at 8-17days of life with clinical findings suggestive of bacterial meningitis, including irritability, lethargy, poor feeding, poor tone, and seizures. Fever is relatively uncommon, and only about 60% have skin vesicles. If untreated, 50% will die and most survivors have severe neurologic sequelae. Infants with SEM disease (skin, eye, mouth) generally present at 5–11 days of life and typically develop a few small vesicles, particularly on the presenting part or at sites of trauma such as with scalp electrode placement. If untreated, infants with SEM disease may progress to develop encephalitis or disseminated disease involving the brain, lungs, liver, heart, and adrenals.

6. *The Evaluation-Decision-Management-Plan/Algorithm* describes the essential aspects of the diagnosis and management of the 3 different categories of Neonatal Herpes. Evaluation of the Neonate with suspected HSV infection should include cultures of suspicious lesions as well as eye and mouth swabs, and PCR of CSF. Culture or antigen detection should be used in evaluating lesions associated with suspected acute genital herpes. Because most HSV diagnostic tests take at least a few days to complete, treatment should not be withheld but rather initiated promptly in order to ensure the maximum therapeutic benefit.

7. *Encephalitis in the Neonatal period tends to be more global, that is, not limited to the temporal lobe (EEG and MRI Brain).* In HSV meningo-encephalitis there can be an increase in lymphocytes and protein, the glucose may be normal/reduced, and RBC may be present. Disseminated infections may cause elevated liver enzymes, thrombocytopenia, and abnormal coagulation.

8. *Refer to Table No-1* for the management of the infant born to a woman with active genital HSV infection. Cesarean Section should be performed on women with signs and symptoms suggesting genital HSV infection at the onset of labor, *preferably within 4hrs of ruptured membranes*. It is not known whether cesarean delivery can reduce the risk of Neonatal herpes when the membranes have been ruptured for > 4-6hrs. If no maternal genital lesions are identified, vaginal delivery is appropriate, but a cervical swab should be obtained for culture. If the culture is positive or if the Neonate develops signs and symptoms of Neonatal HSV, IV Acyclovir therapy should be started.

9. After the appropriate specimens are collected and sent for viral culture and PCR analysis, the Neonate should receive Acyclovir, 60mg/kg/day IV divided into 3 doses given every 8 hr, for 14 days in SEM disease and 21 days in disseminated/CNS disease. Herpetic keratoconjunctivitis should receive topical ophthalmic antiviral therapy along with parenteral treatment.

10. Prevention of Neonatal HSV infection is important and includes various measures such as **a)** contact isolation of infants and mothers **b)** careful handwashing and wearing gloves **c)** avoiding breast feeding if there are breast lesions **d)** wearing face mask, if active oral HSV present etc.The mother, the father, visitors and medical staff on the rooming-in ward must be informed and take the necessary precautionary measures (sealed cover of the lesions to prevent direct contact with the skin or mucosa of the Neonate). Medical staff with oral herpes simplex who observe these precautions need not be suspended from caring for Neonates Finally, ultimate elimination of Neonatal HSV likely will require development of an effective HSV vaccine that protects against genital HSV-2 and HSV-1 infection and/or disease.

---

* *Pearl/Peril/Pitfall : Transplacental transmission of virus and hospital-acquired spread from one neonate to another by hospital personnel or family may account for about 15% of cases. Mothers of neonates with HSV infection tend to have no history or symptoms of genital infection at the time of delivery.*

THE EVALUATION-DECISION-ACTION-ALGORITHM FOR THE DIAGNOSIS AND MANAGEMENT OF *PERINATAL HERPES*

SUBJECTIVE FINDINGS

Hx of risk factors for HSV acquisition by the Neonate during passage through the birth canal; *prematurity, PROM >6hrs, multiple genital lesions, cervical HSV infection, fetal scalp pH monitoring, vaginal delivery, chorioamnionitis etc.*

Hx of Neonatal symptoms suggestive of bacterial sepsis, especially if the mother has primary HSV lesions of the genital tract.

It is critical to recognize that most mothers of infants with Neonatal HSV do not have a history of HSV

Consider HSV infection in the differential diagnosis of any Neonatal illness, manifested as fever, jaundice, apnea, shock & hypotension, DIC, pneumonia, seizures & altered sensorium.

OBJECTIVE FINDINGS

Assess airway, breathing, circulation & disability by observing the vitals, BP, O₂ sats, color, CRT, pulses, sensorium, focal neurologic deficits, seizures, abnormal movements, tone & reflexes etc.

Identify skin, mucocutaneous vesicles, keratoconjunctivitis.

Search for disseminated multiorgan involvement - pneumonitis, DIC, seizures & shock, liver & adrenal manifestations.

Suspect CNS infection alone, in the absence of SEM disease if the Neonate becomes symptomatic at 10–14 days of life with lethargy, seizures, hypotonia and temperature instability.

INVESTIGATIONS

Blood FBC with hematocrit & platelets, ABG analysis with electrolytes, calcium ++, Mg++, BUN & creatinine, urine analysis & culture, blood culture if infection is suspected, Blood glucose.

Virus culture & direct fluorescent antibody technique From the herpetic vesicle, oropharynx, nasopharynx, conjunctivae, stool, & urine.

CSF analysis for elevated protein level & pleocytosis & viral culture and PCR serial CSF examinations are more important, as initial values may be within normal limits.

EEG & CT/MRI Brain for HSV encephalitis, LFTs, coagulation profile, neutropenia & thrombocytopenia & CXR for diffuse interstitial pneumonitis.

PERINATAL HERPES

Treat infants with IV Acyclovir 60mg/kg/day, divided into 3 doses given every 8hrs for 14 days in SEM disease & 21 days in disseminated/CNS disease.

Start topical ophthalmic antiviral therapy along with parenteral treatment for Herpetic keratoconjunctivitis (after consultation with an ophthalmologist).

Suspect Neonatal herpes a)in any Neonate with suggestive signs born to a mom with a history of genital herpes b)in any Newborn with antibiotic unresponsive sepsis, especially with low platelets, elevated LFTs, DIC, early pneumonitis & unexplained lymphocytic meningitis.

Intubate & ventilate, if the Neonate develops apnea, respiratory distress, seizures, altered sensorium, hypotension & shock & DIC

Correct shock & hypotension with fluid bolus + IVI of inotropes & manage DIC as per protocol (Refer to Chapter No. 70 on DIC in Neonates)

Consider Herpes in any Newborn with vesicular eruption; take dermatologist's opinion if in doubt, as the differential diagnosis of vesicular eruptions in the Newborns is extensive.

At the end of treatment repeat CSF analysis, HSV PCR, viral & bacterial culture and monitor CBC & LFTs weekly, creatinine twice weekly, repeat MRI, ophthalmic examination during first week & at 6 months, brain stem auditory evoked response & neurodevelopmental follow-up at 6 & 12 months of age.

TABLE 1 **Management of the child born to a woman with active genital herpes simplex virus (HSV) infection**

Maternal primary or first-episode infection:
* Consider offering an elective cesarean section, regardless of lesion status at delivery, or if membranes ruptured >4 h
* Swab infant's conjunctivae and nasopharynx, and possibly collect urine for DFA and culture to determine exposure to HSV
* Treat with acyclovir if DFA or culture positive or signs of Neonatal HSV.

If cesarean section performed after 24h of ruptured membranes or if vaginal delivery unavoidable:
* Swab infant's conjunctivae and nasopharynx, and collect urine for DFA and culture to determine exposure to HSV.

Recurrent infection, active at delivery:
* Cesarean section after 4 h of ruptured membranes or unavoidable vaginal delivery.
* Swab infant's conjunctivae and nasopharynx, and possibly collect urine for DFA and culture to determine exposure to HSV
* Treat with acyclovir if culture positive or signs of HSV infection.

DFA = direct fluorescent antibody.

@ The *five factors* known to influence transmission of HSV from mother to Neonate are: 1. Type of maternal infection (primary versus. recurrent) 2. Maternal antibody status; 3. Duration of rupture of membranes; 4. Integrity of mucocutaneous barriers (e.g., use of fetal scalp electrodes);and 5. Mode of delivery (cesarean versus vaginal delivery).Patients with disseminated or SEM disease generally present to medical attention at 10 to 12 days of life, whereas patients with CNS disease on average present somewhat later at 16 to 19 days of life.

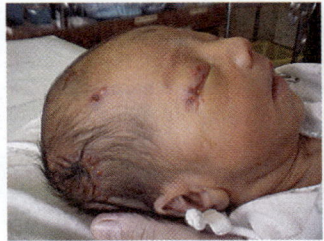 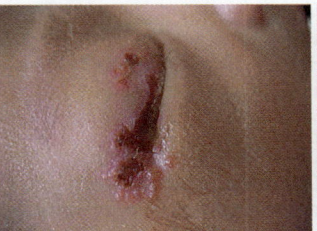 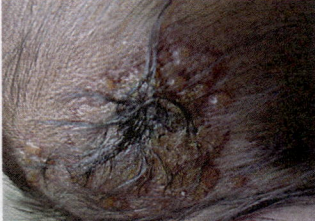 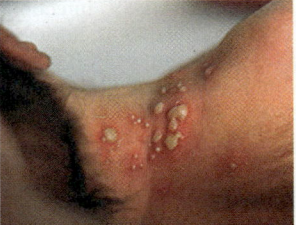

Neonatal Herpes Infection Courtesy:Virat Sirisanthana, M.D.Department of Pediatrics, Chiang Mai University

DIAGNOSIS OF NEONATAL HERPES

CLINICAL: The possibility of Neonatal herpes infection must be especially considered in case of: – characteristic skin or mucosal lesions – conjunctivitis, particularly if there is injection of the conjunctiva, bulbi, or keratitis – seizures and/or lethargy without any other explanation – fever or other systemic symptoms without any other explanation. In suspected cases of neonatal HSV infection the following examinations must be performed : – cultures of vesicular, conjunctival, oropharyngeal, stool/rectal swabs, urine and blood – lumbar puncture with HSV-PCR (CSF cultures are less sensitive) – routine laboratory tests including transaminases and coagulation tests – cerebral imaging and/ or ophthalmological examination if indicated.

SEROLOGIC METHODS: serologic studies play no role in establishing the diagnosis of neonatal HSV disease

VIRAL CULTURE: Isolation of HSV by culture remains the definitive diagnostic method of establishing Neonatal HSV disease. If skin lesions are present, a scraping of the vesicles should be transferred in appropriate viral transport media on ice to a diagnostic virology laboratory. Such specimens are inoculated into cell culture systems, which then are monitored for cytopathic effects characteristic of HSV replication. Typing of an HSV isolate then may be done by one of several techniques. Other sites from which virus may be isolated include the cerebrospinal fluid (CSF), urine, blood, stool or rectum, oropharynx, and conjunctivae. Specimens for viral culture from multiple body sites (with the exception of CSF) may be combined before plating in cell culture to decrease costs since, with the exception of CNS involvement, the important information gathered from such cultures is the presence or absence of replicating virus, rather than its precise location. Of the sites routinely cultured for HSV, skin or eye/conjunctival cultures consistently provided the greatest yields regardless of disease classification, with 90 percent or more of cultures being positive. In a recent study, 58 (94%) of 62 patients had a positive skin or eye culture; 33 (48%) of 69 patients had a positive mouth/oropharyngeal culture; and 17 (40%) of 42 patients with CNS involvement (CNS disease or disseminated disease with CNS involvement) had a positive CSF or brain biopsy culture.

Polymerase Chain Reaction (PCR): The diagnosis of Neonatal HSV infections has been revolutionized by the application of PCR to clinical specimens, including CSF and blood. Because of the very power of the technology, however, the variability in performance of PCR among laboratories warrants brief consideration. Interlaboratory standards that assure that identical specimens processed in two different laboratories will yield identical results are lacking. Furthermore, the performance of PCR is highly dependent on the manner in which the specimen was collected and maintained before reaching the laboratory for PCR analysis. Given these caveats, interpretation of PCR results, either positive or negative, must be correlated with the patient's clinical presentation and disease course in determining their ultimate clinical or diagnostic significance. A negative PCR result does not in and of itself rule out neonatal HSV disease.

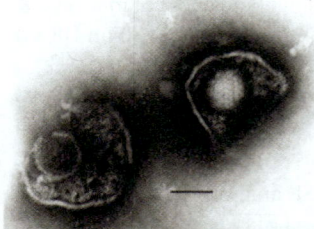

Herpesviruses have an envelope surrounding an icosahedral capsid, approximately 100nm in diameter, which contains the dsDNA genome. When the envelope breaks and collapses away from the capsid, negatively stained virions have a typical "fried-egg" appearance.

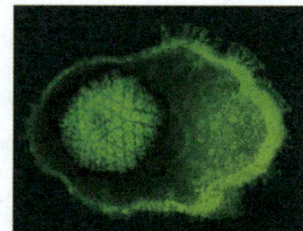

KEY POINTS FOR CLINICAL PRACTICE:

1. Neonatal herpes simplex virus (HSV) infection usually is acquired during the birth process, as the Neonate comes in contact with the virus during passage through an infected birth canal. After an incubation period which can last as long as 2 to 4 weeks, Neonatal HSV disease then manifests in 1 of 3 ways: (1) disseminated disease, with visceral organ involvement (including infection of the brain in two-thirds to three-quarters of patients); (2) central nervous system disease (with no other visceral organ involvement, but with skin lesions in two-thirds of patients); or (3) disease limited to the skin, eyes, and/or mouth (i.e. SEM disease).

2. Diagnostic advances in recent years have focused primarily on applying polymerase chain reaction technology to babies suspected of having Neonatal HSV disease.

3. Treatment of Neonatal HSV disease with intravenous acyclovir has improved the likelihood of survival substantially, although neurologic morbidity remains a common sequelae, especially among survivors of central nervous system disease.

4. Despite these advances, the duration of time from onset of symptoms and initiation of antiviral therapy has remained unchanged for the past 20 years. The surest way to improve outcomes rapidly at this point is to raise awareness of Neonatal HSV disease, resulting in the establishment of earlier diagnoses and more rapid institution of antiviral therapy.

5. In the longer term, development of a bedside nucleic acid detection kit for real-time detection of HSV DNA in the maternal genital tract at the time of delivery could identify which babies are at risk of developing Neonatal HSV disease.

REFERENCES & FURTHER READING : 1) **Arvin AM, Prober CG.** 1993. Analysis of the epidemiology and pathogenesis of herpes simplex virus (HSV) infections in pregnant women and infants using the HSV-2 glycoprotein G antibody assay. Infect Agents Dis. 1993 Dec;2(6):375-82. Review. 2) Kohl S.. Neonatal herpes simplex virus infection. Clin Perinatol 1997;24:129-50 3) **Gonzalez-Villasenor LI.** 1999. A duplex PCR assay for detection and genotyping of Herpes simplex virus in cerebrospinal fluid. Mol Cell Probes. 1999 Aug;13(4):309-14. PMID: 10441204. 4) Grose, C. (1994). "Congenital infections caused by varicella zoster virus and herpes simplex virus." Sem in Pediatr Neurol 1994;1:43-9. 5) **Raguin G, Malkin JE.** 1997. Genital herpes: epidemiology and pathophysiology. Update and new perspectives. Ann Med Interne (Paris). 1997;148(8):530-3. Review.

* *Pearl/Peril/Pitfall : Acyclovir decreases the mortality rate by 50% and increases the percentage of children who develop normally from 10 to 50%; dose is 20 mg/kg IV q 8 h for 14 to 21 days. Vigorous supportive therapy is required, including appropriate IV fluids, alimentation, respiratory support, correction of clotting abnormalities, and control of seizure disorders. Herpetic keratoconjunctivitis requires concomitant systemic acyclovir and topical therapy with a drug such as trifluridine.*

Congenital/Neonatal Varicella

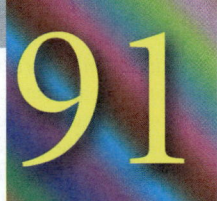

91

@ *With neonatal disease, the presence of a typical vesicular rash and a maternal history of peripartum varicella or postpartum exposure are all that is required to make the diagnosis.*

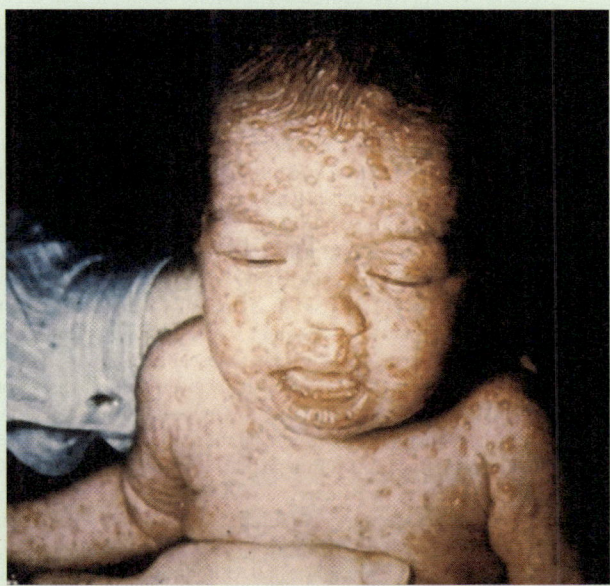

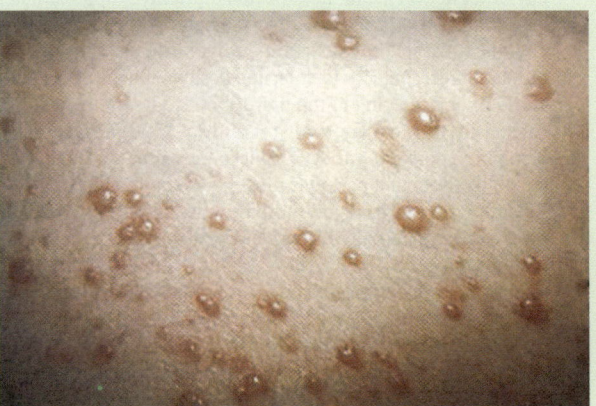

NEONATAL VARICELLA: The pleomorphic rash characteristic of varicella. Papules, vesicles, and pustules are concurrently present.

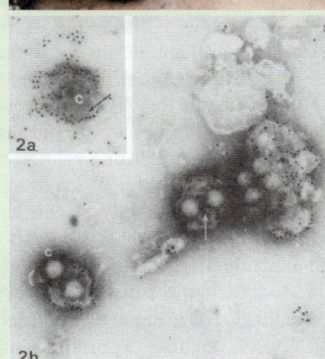

VZV meningitis: Neonates with VZV infection may present with a vesicular rash, typically 9-15 days after their mothers develop a rash. However, Mustonen (1998) and Pignotti (2004) reported 5 neonates who had no cutaneous symptoms despite having culture-proven VZV meningitis. Complications include pneumonitis, hepatic dysfunction, and DIC.

Immunofluorescence on endotracheal aspirate can demonstrate varicella zoster virus (VZV), and VZV DNA can be demonstrated by polymerase chain reaction of endotracheal aspirate, cerebrospinal and vesicle fluids.

REVIEW OF CLINICAL PROBLEMS

1. Mention the *"Potential consequences"* of VZV infections during pregnancy?
   Ans: Refer to the Table 1 of the Chapter.

2. What are the *"essential features"* of Congenital Varicella Syndrome?
   Ans: Refer to the Table 2 of the Chapter.

3. Discuss the *essentials of diagnosis* of Neonatal Varicella.
   Ans: Refer to the "No. 6" of the "BIRD'S EYE VIEW/OVERVIEW/ SYNOPSIS" of the Chapter.

4. How do you prevent further cases of Neonatal Varicella?
   Ans: Refer to the "No. 8" of the "BIRD'S EYE VIEW/OVERVIEW/ SYNOPSIS" of the Chapter.

5. How do you *manage* Neonatal Varicella?
   Ans: Refer to the Evaluation-Decision-Action Plan/Algorithm to diagnose & manage Neonatal Varicella.

LEARNING OBJECTIVES

After completing this article, readers will be able to:

1. Differentiate Neonatal Varicella from Congenital Varicella Syndrome.

2. Prevent/Modify Neonatal Varicella by screening and passively immunizing susceptible pregnant women.

3. Diagnose Neonatal Varicella and differentiate from Herpes/entero/coxsakie viral infections and other vesiculobullous skin lesions in a Neonate

4. Treat Neonatal Varicella and its complications promptly and effectively.

5. Prevent Nursery outbreaks by observing the Universal Sterile Precautions and by giving VZIG to all the exposed Neonates.

* *Pearl/Peril/Pitfall : The use of VZIG can modify the clinical course, usually preventing more severe infection. However, although decreased, the risk of death is not eliminated. Therefore, VZIG does not always prevent severe or fatal varicella in this high risk group. Expectant treatment with close observation, followed by prompt initiation of antiviral treatment on suspicion of neonatal varicella, is recommended.*

BIRD'S EYE VIEW/OVERVIEW/SYNOPSIS

1. Neonatal varicella (chickenpox) affects approximately 25% of Newborns whose mothers developed varicella within the peripartum period. The onset of disease usually occurs 13 to 15 days after the onset of maternal rash. The greatest risk for severe disease is seen when maternal varicella occurs in the 5 days before or 2 days after delivery. Neonatal symptoms generally begin 5-10 days after delivery, and the expected mortality is approximately 30%. Maternal varicella can infect the baby by (1) transplacental viremia, (2) ascending infection during birth, or (3) respiratory droplet /direct contact with infectious lesions after birth. Neonatal chickenpox occurring in the first 10 to 12 days of life has to be caused by intrauterine transmission of VZV because of the incubation period of varicella. Chickenpox after the 10th to 12th day of the Neonatal period is most likely acquired by postnatal VZV infection and has a low morbidity rate as most Neonates are protected by maternally derived antibodies. However, premature infants younger than 28 weeks' gestation or below 1000 g birth weight are at an increased risk for severe varicella during the first 6 weeks after birth.

2. When the Neonatal varicella rash develops within 10 days of life, it is presumed to result from *in utero* transmission. When in utero transmission of Varicella-Zoster virus occurs before the peripartum period, there is no obvious clinical impact in most fetuses; however, congenital varicella syndrome can occur.

3. If the mother develops varicella > 5 days prior to delivery, she still may pass virus to the soon-to-be-born child, but infection is attenuated due to transmission of maternal antibody across the placenta. *This moderating effect of maternal antibody occurs if delivery occurs after 30wk of gestation, when maternal IgG is able to cross the placenta.*

4. *Congenital varicella syndrome* most commonly occurs with maternal V-ZV infection in weeks between 6-20 of gestation. The characteristic findings include cicatricial skin lesions, ocular defects, CNS abnormalities, IUGR, and early death (*Refer to Table 2*)

5. Postnatal varicella acquired in the Newborn period as a result of postnatal exposure is a mild disease generally. Rarely, severe disseminated disease occurs in newborns exposed shortly after birth. It appears that the primary mode of transmission of V-ZV is through respiratory droplets from patients with chickenpox. Spread through contact with vesicular lesions also can occur. Typically, individuals with chickenpox are contagious from 1-2 days before and 5 days after the onset of rash. Conventionally, a patient is no longer considered contagious when all vesicular lesions have dried and crusted over. The incubation period for primary disease extends from 10–21 days, with most infections occurring between 13–17 days.

6. With Neonatal disease, the presence of a typical vesicular rash and a maternal history of peripartum varicella or postpartum exposure are all that is required to make the diagnosis. Laboratory confirmation can be made by a)culture of vesicular fluid b) 4-fold rise in V-ZV antibody titer by the fluorescent antibody to membrane antigen (FAMA) assay or by ELISA. Immunofluorescent antibody test from cells at the base of a vesicle can detect antigen, which is sensitive, specific, and rapid and should be the preferred method of diagnosis when vesicles are present. The *most sensitive and specific* method for the detection of VZV in clinical specimens is the amplification of conserved sequences of viral DNA by polymerase chain reaction.This technique is clearly the method of choice for the investigation of skin swabs or biopsies, liquor specimens, tissue samples, and amniotic fluid for the prenatal diagnosis of fetal infections. The isolation of VZV in cell culture is not useful for a rapid and sensitive diagnosis of Neonatal chickenpox as VZV is extremely labile and cell-associated.

7. *The Evaluation-Decision-Action-Plan / Algorithm* describes the essential aspects of diagnosis and management of congenital and perinatal varicella (chickenpox). Infants with perinatal varicella acquired from maternal infection near the time of delivery are at risk for severe disease. In this setting IV Acyclovir therapy, 60mg/kg/day in 3 divided doses, q8hr for 7 days should be given, along with IM VZIG (Varicella-Zoster Immune Globulin) 125 units, within 72 hrs of delivery/exposure to attenuate V-ZV infection. Infants with congenital infection, resulting from in utero transmission before the peripartum period, are unlikely to have active viral disease, so antiviral therapy is not indicated.

8. *Prevention of further cases of varicella is very important 1) Exposure in early and mid-pregnancy* - Pregnant women exposed to varicella will usually be VZV-immune and there is almost always an opportunity to test for anti-VZV antibodies before having to give VZIG. The risk of varicella syndrome seems highest in the second trimester (2–3% risk) and lower in the first trimester (around 0.4% risk). It is unclear whether VZIG given following exposure will protect the fetus against varicella syndrome; however, if the woman is susceptible and in the first 20 weeks of pregnancy VZIG is usually given and is likely to be successful in at least modifying the maternal disease. Herpes zoster in pregnancy seems to confer little risk to the fetus and does not justify intervention. Although there is less evidence that VZIG is needed later in pregnancy, it may also be given to women between 21 and 36 weeks gestation. The recommended dose is 125 U/10 kg of body weight, up to a maximum of 625 U administered intramuscularly or 0.5 ml /kg intramuscularly and 1 ml /kg intravenously, respectively. Although passive immunization of pregnant women may theoretically reduce the risk of fetal infection, there is no evidence that this prevents Neonatal varicella. Thus, the primary reason for VZIG is to prevent severe chickenpox and complications in the mother. *1) Exposure in late pregnancy* - If the woman is susceptible and near term (within 4 weeks), then VZIG should be given. Although it may not prevent infection, it will usually ameliorate the severity of infection when given up to 10 days after contact. *3)Exposed Neonates* - Varicella-zoster immunoglobulin should be given to the Newborn if the mother has developed varicella or herpes zoster in the 7 days before or after birth. VZIG should also be given to any exposed premature Neonate (prior to 28 weeks or under 1 kg birth weight) even if the mother is immune, because maternal antibody is poorly transferred to the preterm fetus. Intravenous acyclovir is sometimes used prophylactically in the mother and in her baby where maternal infection occurs just before delivery. Maternal zoster during the perinatal period does not cause problems for newborn infants as the infants possess specific maternal IgG class antibodies and there is no viremic spread of VZV.

9. Vaccination of women who are not immune to varicella should decrease the incidence of congenital and perinatal varicella. Women should not receive the vaccine if they are pregnant or in the 3 months before pregnancy. Additionally, Acyclovir should also be considered for seronegative women exposed to varicella during pregnancy beginning 7-9 days postexposure and continuing 7 days.

10. Nursery outbreaks by nosocomial spread of virus can occur and steps should be taken to minimize the risk. Universal sterile precautions should be observed. VZIG can be given to all other exposed neonates, but this can be withheld from full-term infant whose mothers have a history of varicella. Neonates at < 28 week GA should be given VZIG postexposure regardless of maternal status.

---

* *Pearl/Peril/Pitfall : As administration of VZIG can prolong the incubation period, this period of vigilance should extend to 30 days. VZIG may also modify disease and may lead to atypical rashes, such as occurred in the infants reported here.*

THE EVALUATION-DECISION-ACTION-PLAN/ALGORITHM FOR THE DIAGNOSIS AND MANAGEMENT OF *CONGENITAL / NEONATAL VARICELLA (CHICKEN POX)*

SUBJECTIVE FINDINGS

Hx of susceptible pregnant woman exposed to varicella/acquiring primary varicella during pregnancy beginning 7–9 days post exposure and continuing 7 days.

Hx of maternal varicella occurring 5 days before or 2 days after delivery (greatest risk for severe neonatal disease).

Hx of Neonatal skin rash developing within 10 days of life (indicates in utero transmission) or between 13-15 days after the onset of maternal rash (indicates peripartal transmission).

Hx of prematurity (<28wks of GA & <1,000gm)

Hx of postnatal contact with nursery/community personnel with active varicella.

OBJECTIVE FINDINGS

Examine the infant for Congenital varicella syndrome (*vide infra*). *Post natal varicella is generally a mild disease. Rarely severe disseminated disease occurs in newborns exposed shortly after birth*-encephalitis, pneumonitis, purpura, hemorrhagic vesicles, hematuria, GIT bleeding, secondary bacterial sepsis with group A streptococci & S. aureus etc. The **differential diagnosis** includes herpes simplex virus (HSV) and enterovirus infections. A vesicular rash or bullae present at birth or within a few days have been noted in most infants with congenital HSV infections. Intrauterine transmission of coxsackie virus during the late pregnancy may also lead to varicella - like congenital skin lesions.

INVESTIGATIONS

Blood look for initial leukopenia during the first 72hrs followed by a relative & absolute lymphocytosis, mild thrombocytopenia, mildly elevated LFTs.

Direct fluorescent antibody test for VZV, from cutaneous lesions & by PCR amplification

VZV IgG antibodies with 4-fold rise confirmatory of acute infection. VZV IgM antibodies are not useful for clinical diagnosis.

Viral culture of vesicular fluid not reliable because the virus is quite labile.

CXR for pneumonia, *CSF* analysis for CNS complications.

NEONATAL VARICELLA (CHICKEN POX)

A. Exposed susceptible women	Protected by VZIG + IV Acyclovir
B. Maternal varicella 5 days before - 2 days after delivery	1. Administer VZIG (Varicella-Zoster Immune Globulin) 125 UNITS, IM, within 72hrs of exposure (50% may still develop mild disease) 2. Monitor for development of skin lesions & Treat with IV Acyclovir 60 mg/kg/day in 3 divided doses - q8hr if any progression 3. Premature infants (<28wk of gestation & <1,000gm) should be given VZIG post exposure regardless of maternal status 4. Defer breast feeding, until the mother is likely to be viremic &/or infectious (when all vesicular lesions have dried and crusted over)
C. Infants with community acquired Chickenpox with pneumonia, Hepatitis, encephalitis	IV Acyclovir 60 mg/kg/day in 3 divided doses - q8hr Rx for 7/7 days or until *no new lesions* have appeared for 48 hrs

*Following prophylactic treatment with VZIG, asymptomatic Newborns should be under surveillance in the hospital for 2 weeks, that is, to the end of incubation period. When a Neonate who has received VZIG is discharged home, it should be made clear to the parents that prompt hospital review should be undertaken if the baby becomes unwell or develops rash. Passive immunization of the Newborn may modify the clinical course of Neonatal varicella but it does not prevent the disease and, although decreased, the risk of death is not eliminated. *Therefore, acyclovir therapy should be administered promptly at a dosage of 10 to 15 mg/kg every 8 hours intravenously for 5 to 7 days on suspicion of Neonatal chickenpox. Prophylactic intravenous acyclovir can prevent Neonatal varicella or reduce the severity of the disease markedly. *To reduce the mortality from Neonatal chickenpox, the date of delivery may also be postponed allowing maternal antibodies to pass the placental barrier. No therapy is indicated for Neonatal chickenpox if the maternal rash onset is more than 7 days before delivery. Mothers and Newborns suffering from or being at risk of varicella have to be isolated on maternity wards. *Active immunization with a live -attenuated varicella vaccine (VZV Oka strain) should be offered to nonpregnant women of child - bearing age without a history of varicella to provide them protective VZV-specific immunity. The available vaccines proved to be safe and lead to complete protection from severe chickenpox. Pregnancy should be avoided for at least 4 weeks following vaccination. Varicella vaccine, as all live -attenuated vaccines, is contraindicated in pregnant women. Several industrialized countries consider universal immunization of all susceptible children.

TABLE 1	VZV infections and their potential consequences during pregnancy

Maternal varicella / zoster timing	*Consequences for mother/fetus/term neonate*
Varicella at any stage	Intrauterine death, neonatal or infantile zoster
Varicella in first 20 weeks	Congenital varicella syndrome (risk: 2%, mortality: 30%)
Varicella in third trimester	Maternal pneumonia (risk: 10–20%, mortality: 10–45%)
Varicella near term 5 to 6 days before delivery	Neonatal varicella at ages up to 10–12 days (risk: 20–50%, mortality: 0%)
Varicella 4 to 5 days before to 2 days after delivery:	Neonatal varicella 0–4 days after birth (risk: 20–50%, mortality: 0–3%) Neonatal varicella between 5 and 10 to 12 days after birth (risk: 20–50%, mortality: 30%)
Normal zoster at any stage	No risk for severe maternal, fetal or neonatal infections

* *Pearl/Peril/Pitfall: When a neonate who has received VZIG is discharged home, it should be made clear to the parents and all health workers involved that if the baby becomes unwell in any way and/or develops any sort of rash, prompt hospital review, with the possibility of intravenous acyclovir, should be undertaken.*

TABLE 2	Congenital varicella syndrome

Infectivity rate	
* 25% of fetuses	VZV embryopathy; Rate up to 2% (in the first 20 wk of pregnancy)
* Fetal Infection at 6–12 wks of GA	Maximal Interruption with limb development (Shortened/malformed)
* Fetal infection at 16–20 wks GA	Eyes (cataracts, Optic Atrophy, Microphthalmia, Chorioretinitis) Brain (Microcephaly, Hydrocephaly, Aplasia, Calcifications) Damage to cervical or lumbosacral cord—hypoplasia of an extremity, motor and sensory deficits, anisocoria, Horner syndrome, absent deep tendon reflexes, anal/urinary sphincter dysfunction.
* *Diagnosis based on Hx of Gestational chickenpox + Stigmata seen in the fetus*	
* Chorionic villous sampling and fetal blood collection for viral DNA (PCR) - not useful to distinguish between infection and disease. If negative Reassuring.	
* VZIG, IV Acyclovir—No Proven efficacy, but can be tried. Acyclovir should only be considered when the benefit to the mother outweighs the potential risk to the fetus.	
* POSTNATALLY	– VZV embryopathy nonprogressive – No persistent viral replication – No Treatment is indicated

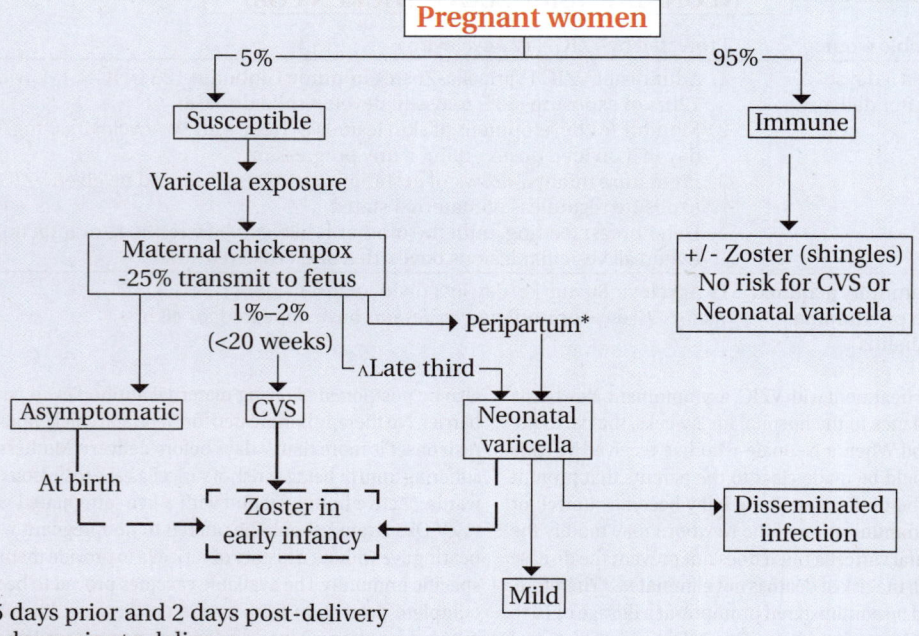

*Between 5 days prior and 2 days post-delivery
∧2 weeks-5 days prior to delivery

Fig. 1: Overview of varicella infection during pregnancy. *Peripartum* is defined as between 5 days before and 2 days after delivery; *Late third trimester* is defined as between 2 weeks and 5 days before delivery. *Dotted lines* denote potential outcome. CVS = Congenital Varicella Syndrome

KEY POINTS FOR CLINICAL PRACTICE:

1. Neonatal varicella is mostly caused by maternal chickenpox acquired during the last 3 weeks of pregnancy. Transplacentally transmitted infections occur in the first 10 to 12 days of life, whereas chickenpox after that time is most likely acquired by postnatal infection.

2. If the mother develops rash between days 4 and 5 antepartum to day 2 postpartum, generalized neonatal varicella leading to death occurs in up to 20% of affected cases. Neonatal chickenpox within the first 4 days after birth has usually been found to be mild. A fatal outcome has been reported in 23% of cases if Neonatal chickenpox occurs between 5 and 10 to 12 days of age.

3. Serological methods have been widely used to confirm clinical diagnosis. For rapid virological diagnostics, amplification of viral DNA in skin swabs by polymerase chain reaction is the method of choice.

4. To prevent severe Neonatal chickenpox, passive immunization varicella-zoster immune globulin (VZIG) is indicated. If varicella occurs, acyclovir treatment has to be administered promptly.

5. Clear instructions to parents and health professionals may prevent avoidable morbidity and mortality in this group of patients.

REFERENCES & FURTHER READING : 1)Sauerbrei A, Wutzler P. The congenital varicella syndrome. J Perinatol 2000;20:548–54. 2) Huang YC et al. Prophylaxis of intravenous immunoglobulin and acyclovir in perinatal varicella. Eur J Pediatr 2001;160:91-94 3) Pollard AJ et al. Potentially lethal bacterial infection associated with varicella zoster virus. BMJ 1996; 313: 283-285 4) Royal College of Paediatrics and Child Health: Manual of childhood infections (2nd edition). 5)Holland P, Isaacs D, Moxon ER. Fatal neonatal varicella infection. Lancet 1986;2:1156.

92 Congenital and Perinatal Cytomegalovirus (CMV) Infection

@ *Symptomatic Neonates have a mortality rate of up to 30%, and 70 to 90% of survivors have some neurologic impairment, including hearing loss, mental retardation, and visual disturbances. In addition, 10% of asymptomatic Neonates eventually develop neurologic sequelae. Because hearing defects are a concern, close monitoring after the Neonatal period is needed. No specific therapy is available. Ganciclovir decreases viral shedding in Neonates with congenital CMV and prevents hearing deterioration at 6 mo. When therapy stops, the virus is again shed; therefore, its role in treatment remains controversial.*

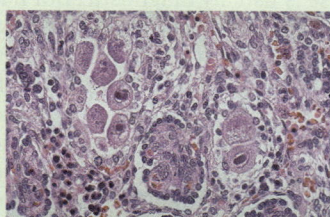

Cytomegalovirus, Congenital Kidney: Microscopic

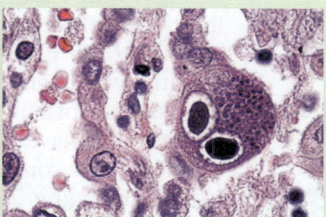

Histologically, the detection of the distinct "owl's eye" inclusion bodies on tissue sample can be a highly specific method for determining organ involvement of CMV.

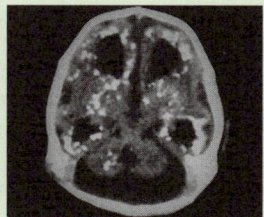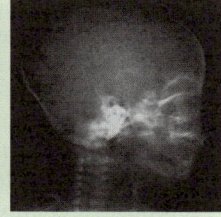

Congenital CMV infection-Microcephaly and Intracranial Calcifications (Periventricular).

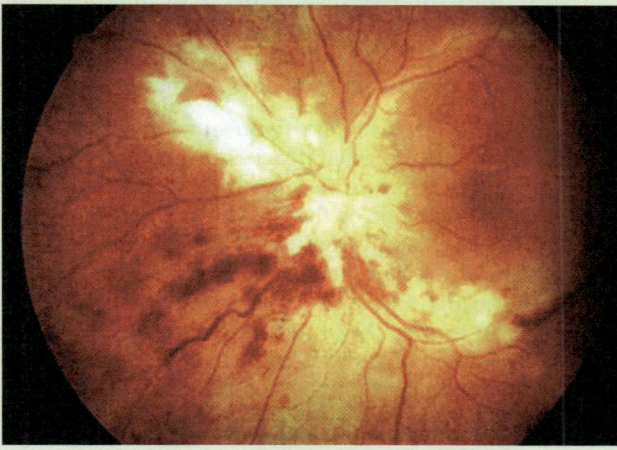

Pizza pie" Retinopathy of CMV

You are looking at a mixture of cotton wool spots, infiltrates, and hemorrhages. This combination spells death for the retina. The virus gets into the vascular endothelium, closes off blood vessels, and spreads through tissue like wildfire. The entire retina can be destroyed within weeks.

This is a moderately advanced stage. The earliest sign may be a cotton wool spot. This presents a diagnostic problem, because cotton wool spots are also a non-infectious sign of microvascular occlusion in early HIV disease. Still, any severely immunocompromised patient who develops a cotton wool spot must be presumed to have early CMV retinitis and watched carefully. CMV retinitis may also start in the retinal periphery with infiltrates and vitreous floaters. CMV retinitis is most often seen in immunocompromised patients (HIV, organ transplant) and in neonates whose mothers are infected. In adults, it is associated with very low suppressor T-cell counts. It may be the presenting sign of systemic or central nervous system CMV infection. Treatment with systemic ganciclovir or foscarnet can arrest this process. These medications can also be delivered through a reservoir sewn onto the sclera.

REVIEW OF CLINICAL PROBLEMS

1. Describe the features of Congenital CMV Infection.
   Ans: Refer to the Table 1 of the Chapter.

2. How do you prevent primary CMV infection of pregnant women ?
   Ans: Refer to the Evaluation-Decision-Action Plan/Algorithm to diagnose and manage Congenital and Perinatal CMV Infection.

3. What investigations are needed to diagnose Congenital CMV infection ?
   Ans: Refer to the Evaluation-Decision-Action Plan/Algorithm to diagnose and manage Congenital & Perinatal CMV Infection.

4. Discuss the treatment aspects of Congenital CMV infection.
   Ans: Refer to the Evaluation-Decision-Action Plan/Algorithm to diagnose and manage Congenital & Perinatal CMV Infection.

5. How does the CMV differ from Herpes/Varicella viruses?
   Ans: Refer to No 8 of the Bird`s eye view/Overview/Synopsis of the Chapter.

LEARNING OBJECTIVES

After completing this article, readers will be able to:

1. Describe the common means of CMV transmission.
2. Describe the major manifestations of CMV infection.
3. Describe how to diagnose, treat and prevent CMV infection.
4. Educate Nonimmune pregnant women that they attempt to limit exposure to the virus- should always wash their hands thoroughly after exposure to urine and respiratory secretions from children.
5. Ensure Neurodevelopmental follow-up of infants with Congenital CMV infection.

* *Pearl/Peril/Pitfall : Congenital CMV is diagnosed if the virus is isolated from urine or other body fluids obtained within the 1st 2 wk of life. After 2 wk, positive cultures may indicate perinatal or congenital infection. Infants may shed CMV for several years after either type of infection. A CBC and differential and liver function tests may be helpful. A cranial ultrasound or CT examination and an ophthalmologic evaluation should also be performed.*

BIRD'S EYE VIEW/OVERVIEW/SYNOPSIS

1. CMV (Human Cytomegalovirus, the largest of the herpes viruses with double-stranded DNA viral genome) is the most common cause of Congenital infection, which occasionally causes the syndrome of Cytomegalic inclusion disease (hepatosplenomegaly, jaundice, petechiae, purpura, microcephaly, afebrile pneumonitis, chorioretinitis, sensorineural deafness, CNS manifestations) in Neonates. The incidence of Congenital CMV infection ranges from 0.2 to 2.4% of all live births, with the higher rates among low socioeconomic populations. The risk for fetal infection is greatest with maternal primary CMV infection (30%) and much less likely with recurrent infection (<1%). Perinatal transmission is common, accounting for an incidence of 10-60% through the first 6 months of life. *The most important perinatal sources of virus are genital tract secretions at delivery and breast milk.* Among CMV-seropositive mothers, virus is detectable in breast milk in 96%, with postnatal transmission occurring in approximately 38% of infants, resulting in symptomatic infection in nearly 50% of VLBW infants. Infected infants excrete virus for years in saliva and urine.

2. Only 5% of all congenitally infected infants have severe disease, another 5% have mild involvement, and 90% are born with subclinical, but still chronic, CMV infection. Asymptomatic congenital CMV infection is likely the leading cause of sensorineural hearing loss, which occurs in approximately 7% of all infants with congenital CMV infection, whether symptomatic at birth or not. **In symptomatic infants, the characteristic signs and symptoms include:** *IUGR, prematurity, hepato-splenomegaly, jaundice, blueberry muffin-like rash, thrombocytopenia and purpura, and microcephaly and intracranial calcifications.* Other neurologic problems include chorioretinitis, sensorineural hearing loss, and mild increases in CSF protein.

3. Perinatally acquired CMV infection may occur from a) intrapartum exposure to virus within the maternal genital tract b) postnatal exposure to infected breast milk c) exposure to infected blood/blood products d) nosocomially through urine or saliva. All perinatally infected term infants are asymptomatic. But preterms are mostly symptomatic with higher frequency for long term developmental and neurological abnormalities. Occasionally perinatally acquired CMV infection is associated with pneumonitis and sepsis-like syndrome. Premature and ill full term infants may have neurologic sequelae and psychomotor retardation.

4. CMV infection is more common among HIV-1 infected infants, and coinfected infants may have rapid progression of HIV-1 disease. Therefore screening for CMV in HIV-exposed infants is important.

5. Congenital CMV infection should be suspected in any infant having a) typical symptoms of infection b) if there is a maternal history of seroconversion c) if there is a mononucleosis-like illness in pregnancy. The diagnosis is made if CMV is identified in urine, saliva, blood, or respiratory secretions and defined as *congenital* infection if found within the first 2 wks of life and as *perinatal* infection if after 4 wks of life.

6. The definitive method for diagnosis of congenital CMV infection is virus isolation/PCR, which should be performed at or shortly after birth. Urine and saliva are the best specimens for culture. Serology for CMV IgG and IgM with 4-fold rise is usually diagnostic, but has limitations (Refer to Table 2 for interpretation). IgM anti-CMV (by ELISA) has 95% specificity and 70% sensitivity in diagnosis of congenital CMV infection. If the diagnosis of congenital CMV infection is made, the infant should have a thorough physical and neurologic examination, a computed tomography (CT) scan of the brain (or magnetic resonance imaging [MRI]), an ophthalmologic examination, and a hearing test. Laboratory tests include a complete blood count, liver function tests, and cerebrospinal fluid (CSF) examination (if the CSF PCR is positive for CMV, the infant should be classified as having CNS disease).

7. *The Evaluation-Decision-Action-Plan / Algorithm* describes the essential aspects of diagnosis and management of congenital/perinatal CMV infection and the CDCP recommendations for screening of pregnant women at risk of developing CMV infection.

8. The CMV virus differs from herpes simplex and varicella viruses in that it lacks the enzyme thymidine kinase. This feature renders it resistant to antiviral agents that depend on the enzyme for their action, such as Acyclovir. Ganciclovir and more recently valganciclovir have been effective in the treatment of and prophylaxis against dissemination of CMV. Hyperimmune CMV immunoglobulin may benefit infants with congenital CMV, especially those with a fulminant presentation.

9. Prenatal diagnosis of congenital CMV infection can be established by isolation of the virus from amniotic fluid obtained by amniocentesis or from fetal blood (by quantitative PCR). Pregnant women with primary CMV who receive CMV hyperimmune globulin may have a reduced risk for delivering congenitally infected infant. No recommendations for therapeutic abortion have been made so far, even if primary maternal infection is documented. Two live attenuated CMV vaccines have been developed, but their efficacy has not been clearly established.

10. The most important means of prevention of CMV infection are basic hygiene and handwashing for pregnant women, especially after contact with urine, diapers, oral secretions, and other body fluids. Currently, there is no evidence to support the antiviral therapy for CMV infection during pregnancy.

---

* *Pearl/Peril/Pitfall : Transfusion-associated perinatal CMV disease can be avoided by giving preterm neonates blood products from CMV-seronegative donors or products that have been treated to make them noninfectious. Development of a vaccine against CMV is under investigation.*

THE EVALUATION-DECISION-ACTION-PLAN/ALGORITHM FOR THE DIAGNOSIS AND MANAGEMENT OF *CONGENITAL/ PERINATAL CYTOMEGALOVIRUS (CMV) INFECTION*

SUBJECTIVE FINDINGS

Suspect congenital CMV infection in any infant having typical symptoms of infection (Refer to Table 1) or if there is a maternal history of seroconversion or a mononucleosis—like illness in pregnancy.

OBJECTIVE FINDINGS

Look for early manifestations of symptomatic CMV infection : petechiae /purpura (79%), hepatosplenomegaly (74%), jaundice (63%), prematurity & "blue berry muffin" spots, pneumonitis.

Assess for sequelae on follow-up disproportionate microcephaly (48%) with periventricular intracranial calcifications, ventricular dilatation, cortical atrophy, low IQ scores below 50, sensorineural deafness, motor spasticity, visual problems, dental defects, etc.

INVESTIGATIONS

Blood Identify hemolytic anemia, thrombocytopenia & atypical lymphocytosis, direct hyperbilirubinemia & elevated hepatic transaminases.

CXR for hyperinflation, diffuse increased pulmonary markings, thickened bronchial walls, & focal atelectasis (CMV pneumonitis).

CT/MRI head scan 90% of CMV- infected infants with abnormal scan will have CNS sequelae.

Virus isolation (spin - enhanced culture or "shell vial") from urine, saliva, breast milk, buffy coat, bronchoalveolar washings, cervical secretions confirms active CMV infection.

CMV PCR or CMV antigen tests - costly & mostly unavailable.

Serology for CMV IgG/IgM 4-fold rise is usually diagnostic but have several limitations (Refer to Table 2).

CONGENITAL & PERINATAL CYTOMEGALOVIRUS (CMV) INFECTION

* Diagnose the congenital infection by PCR/culture of URINE & SALIVA shortly after birth.
* If congenital CMV infection diagnosed—do a through physical, Neurological exam, a CT of brain & ophthalmic exam, hearing test, a CBC, LFT & CSF exam.
* Look for the most characteristic signs & symptoms a) IUGR, PREMATURITY b) Hepatosplenomegaly & jaundice c) Thrombocytopenia & purpura d) Microcephaly & intracranial calcifications, chorioretinitis, sensorineural hearing loss, mild in CSF protein.
* Allow breast feeding because of rare symptomatic infection in TERM infants & protective maternal IgG for preterms against CMV. (Freezing Milk at 20°C will reduce the titer of CMV but will not eliminate active virus).

* Use CMV free blood products in all instances of Neonatal transfusions esp. for premature Newborn.
* No highly effective therapy currently available - GANCICLOVIR 6 mg/kg/dose every 12hr IV for the first 6 wk of life along with CMV IVIG (400mg/kg on days 1, 2, & 7, and 200mg/kg/ on day 14) found to be effective in CMV chorioretinitis & GIT disease, but like viral excretion, often recur on cessation.
* GANCICLOVIR toxicity (neutropenia, thrombocytopenia, liver dysfunction, reduction in spermatogenesis, GIT & renal abnormalities) is frequent & often severe. FOSCARNET is an alternative antiviral agent.

Prevent primary CMV infection of pregnant women as for Centers for Disease Control & Prevention recommendations

1. Pregnant women practise hand-washing with soap and water after contact with diapers or oral secretions.
2. Pregnant women who develop a mononucleosis-like illness during pregnancy should be evaluated for CMV infection and counseled about risks to the unborn child.
3. Antibody testing can confirm prior CMV infection.
4. Recovery of CMV from the cervix or urine of women near delivery does not warrant a cesarean section.
5. The benefits of breastfeeding outweigh the minimal risk of acquiring CMV.
6. There is no need to screen for CMV or exclude CMV-excreting children from schools or institutions.

Figure 1: **Consequences of human CMV in pregnancy**

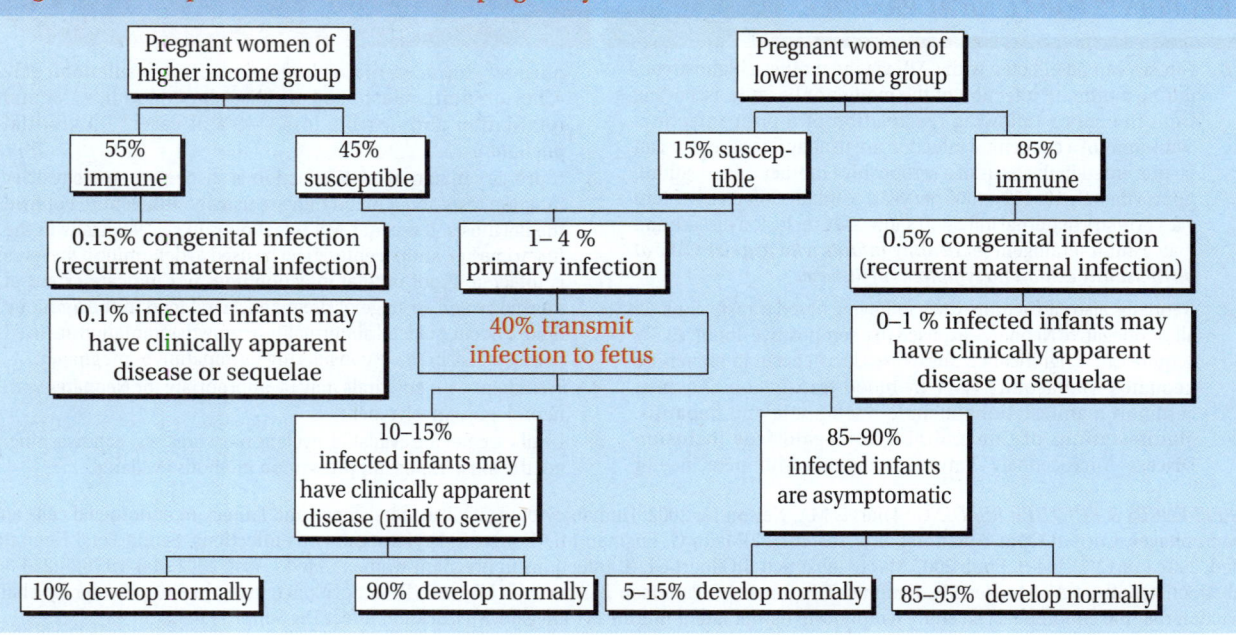

TABLE 1	Characteristics of the 285 Infants Enrolled in the National Congenital Cytomegalovirus Disease Registry (January 1, 1990, through December 31, 1993)		
Characteristic		**No. of Infants affected**	**% of Infants affected**
Non-neurologic abnormalities:			
Petechiae or purpura		154	54
Small for gestational age		114	40
Hepatosplenomegaly		135	47
Jaundice at birth		108	38
Pneumonia		24	8
Neurologic abnormalities:			
One or more of the following abnormality		194	68
Intracranial calcifications		106	37
Microcephaly		104	36
Unexplained abnormality		78	27
Hearing impairment		70	25
Chorioretinitis		30	11
Seizures		25	9
Neonatal death*			
Laboratory findings:			
Platelet count $\leq 75,000/mm^3$		136	48
Direct bilirubin level ≥ 3 mg/dL		102	36
Alanine aminotransferase level > 100 U/L		66	23
Hemolytic anemia		32	11
*Data not systematically collected.			

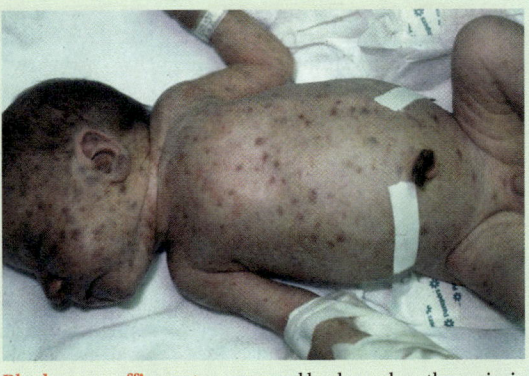

Blueberry muffin spots are caused by dermal erythropoiesis in profound intrauterine anemia. They have been described in Rh disease, twin-to-twin transfusions and intrauterine infections (i.e. parvovirus B19, CMV, HSV, toxoplasmosis and lues) . It is not clear if circulating hematopoietic cells settle down in the skin or if dermal mesenchymal cells have the potency to differentiate in situ to blood producing cells. Lack of circulating erythroblasts seem to favor the latter mechanism.

Data from Istas AS, Demmler GH, Dobbins JG, Stewart JA: Surveillance for congenital cytomegalovirus disease: A report from the National Congenital Cytomegalovirus Disease Registry. Clin Infect Dis 20:665-670, 1995.

TABLE 2	Laboratory diagnosis of CMV using maternal and neonatal serology		
Time	**Mother** IgG mother	**Baby** IgG baby	**Suspected CMV Infection IgG Status of Baby Interpretation**
Birth	Negative	Negative	Excludes CMV Infection (<40% of instances)
Birth	Positive	Positive	Possibly Transplacental Transfer, repeat IgG at 1 month
1 mth	Positive	Negative or decreased titre	No infection in the baby
1 mth	Positive	Positive	Possible infection in the baby
>3 mth	Positive	Positive or increased titre	Infected baby

KEY POINTS FOR CLINICAL PRACTICE:

1. Fetuses can be infected with CMV via the mother's bloodstream during a primary infection of the mother or by virus ascending from the cervix following reactivation of a prior infection. Symptoms of a congenital infection are usually less severe or can be prevented in the fetus of a seropositive mother (reactivation). Approximately 10–15% (4000 per year) of infants infected in utero via a primary maternal infection show CMV inclusion disease and may exhibit teratogenesis. *Healthy infants who acquire CMV at birth usually exhibit no symptoms of disease.*

2. Neonates also can acquire CMV following blood transfusions. Of all seronegative Neonates exposed to a seropositive donor, 13.5% acquire CMV. Significant clinical disease can occur in premature neonates who acquire CMV by blood transfusion. The most common manifestations include pneumonia and hepatitis. **Manifestations of Congenital Cytomegalovirus Inclusion Disease** ·Microcephaly ·Thrombocytopenia with ·petechiae or purpura ·Intracerebral calcification ·Hepatosplenomegaly ·Chorioretinitis ·Rash ·Seizure disorders ·Jaundice ·Mental retardation and hearing loss (1–3% of cases) ·Interstitial pneumonia.

3. If primary maternal CMV infection is suspected, serology, liver function tests and a blood film are usually sufficient to confirm the diagnosis. If recent CMV infection is likely, especially in the first trimester, amniocentesis can be used to determine if the fetus is infected. Proof of fetal infection does not indicate extent of morbidity and so stage of pregnancy, viral load in the amniotic fluid, evidence of fetal abnormality or growth retardation are used to assess risk in those considering termination of pregnancy.

4. Treatment with antivirals may be appropriate for Neonates with neurological involvement.

5. Until vaccines are available, hygiene measures, e.g. handwashing, are the most important prevention methods available.

REFERENCES & FURTHER READING : 1)Jarvis MA, Nelson JA. 2002. Human cytomegalovirus persistence and latency in endothelial cells and macrophages. Current Opin. Microbiol. 5(4):403-407. 2)Malm G, Engman ML; Congenital cytomegalovirus infections. Semin Fetal Neonatal Med. 2007 Jun;12(3):154-9. Epub 2007 Mar 6. [abstract] 3)Gilbert GL; 1: Infections in pregnant women.; Med J Aust. 2002 Mar 4;176(5):229-36. [abstract] 4)Koffron AJ, Mueller KH, Kaufman DB, Stuart FP, Patterson B, Abecassis MI.1995. Direct evidence using in situ polymerase chain reaction that the endothelial cell and T-lymphocyte harbor latent murine cytomegalovirus. Scand J Infect Dis Suppl 99:61-2.

93 Perinatal Hepatitis B and Hepatitis C

@ *An infant weighing less than 2 kg whose mother is HBsAg positive should receive the first dose of hepatitis B vaccine and HBIG within 12 hours of birth. Do not count the hepatitis B vaccine dose as the first dose in the vaccine series. Reinitiate the full hepatitis B vaccine series at age 1–2 months.*

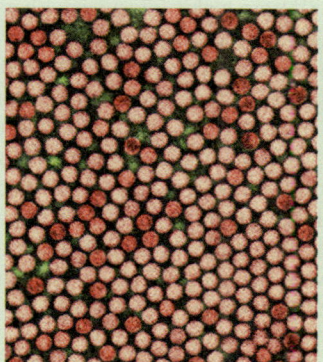

Hepatitis B virus-HBV is a 42-nm DNA virus classified in the *Hepadnaviridae* family. Hepatitis B virus (HBV) infection in a pregnant woman poses a serious risk to her infant at birth. Perinatal HBV transmission can be prevented by identifying HBV-infected (i.e. Hepatitis B surface antigen [HBsAg]-positive) pregnant women and providing Hepatitis B immune globulin and Hepatitis B vaccine to their infants within 12 hours of birth.

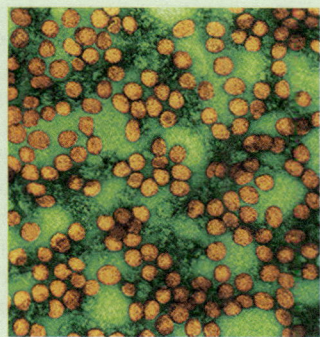

Hepatitis C Virus-It belongs to the Flavivirus family and is an enveloped RNA virus that buds (single stranded; yellow fever is prototype). Hepatitis C virus is associated with chronic liver disease and also with primary liver cancer in some countries. It is most commonly spread by blood contact, through blood transfusions or shared infected needles. There is currently no vaccine for hepatitis C.

Summary of hepatitis B vaccination recommendations

for infants, children, and adolescents CDC-MMWR December 23, 2005

Maternal hepatitis B surface antigen (HBsAg) testing

- All pregnant women should be tested routinely for HBsAg.

Vaccination of infants *At birth*

- Infants born to mothers who are HBsAg positive should receive hepatitis B vaccine and hepatitis B immune globulin (HBIG) <12 hours of birth.
- Infants born to mothers whose HBs Ag status is unknown should receive hepatitis B vaccine <12 hours of birth. The mother should have blood drawn as soon as possible to determine her HBsAg status; if she is HBsAg positive, the infant should receive HBIG as soon as possible (no later than age 1 week).
- Full-term infants who are medically stable and weigh >2,000 g born to HBsAg-negative mothers should receive single-antigen hepatitis B vaccine before hospital discharge.
- Preterm infants weighing <2,000 g born to HBs Ag negative mothers should receive the first dose of vaccine 1 month after birth or at hospital discharge.

After the birth dose

- All infants should complete the hepatitis B vaccine series with either single-antigen vaccine or combination vaccine, according to a recommended vaccination schedule
- Infants born to HBsAg-positive mothers should be tested for HBsAg and antibody to HBsAg after completion of the hepatitis B vaccine series at age 9–18 months.

Vaccination of children and adolescents

- All unvaccinated children and adolescents aged <19 years should receive the hepatitis B vaccine series.

REVIEW OF CLINICAL PROBLEMS

1. How do you manage Preterms <2 kg, depending on the maternal hepatitis B surface antigen (HBsAg) status ?
   Ans: Refer to the Table 2 of the Chapter.

2. How do you modify Hepatitis B Vaccination schedule, in relation to Maternal Hepatitis B surface antigen (HBsAg) status ?
   Ans: Refer to the Table 1 of the Chapter.

3. How do you interpret the POST VACCINATION TEST FOR HBs Ag & ANTI HBs AT 9–15 MONTHS OF AGE ?
   Ans: Refer to the Evaluation-Decision-Action Plan/Algorithm to diagnose and manage Perinatal Hepatitis B & C.

4. What Historical information should you elicit, while evaluating Perinatal Hepatitis B & C ?
   Ans: Refer to the Evaluation-Decision-Action Plan/Algorithm to diagnose and manage Perinatal Hepatitis B & C.

5. Discuss the clinical course and prognosis of Neonatal Hep.B infection.
   Ans: Refer to No 8 of the Bird's eye view/Overview/Synopsis of the Chapter.

LEARNING OBJECTIVES

After completing this article, readers will be able to:

1. Prevent Neonatal Hepatitis B transmission from Hep.B positive Mom by giving vaccination & Hepaglob simultaneously within 12 h of birth & by completing the vaccine series.

2. Understand that there is currently no vaccine for Hepatitis-C, although research is underway.

3. Perform Postvaccination testing for HBs Ag and anti-HBs at 9–15 months of age.

4. Ensure that Universal precautions should be in effect in all Newborn nurseries, so the risk of exposure to blood and body secretions should be minimized.

5. Discuss the issue of breast feeding with the mother on individual basis, though CDC states that maternal Hep B/C is not a contraindication to breastfeed.

---

* *Pearl/Peril/Pitfall: Maternal-infant HBV transmission results primarily from maternal-fetal microtransfusions during labor or contact with infectious secretions in the birth canal. Transplacental transmission is unusual. Postpartum transmission occurs rarely through exposure to infectious maternal blood, saliva, stool, urine, or breast milk.*

BIRD'S EYE VIEW/OVERVIEW/SYNOPSIS

1. Hepatitis B (DNA virus) and Hepatitis C (RNA virus) viruses are of major importance in the Newborn period. Both are transmitted vertically from the infected mothers and can cause chronic carrier stage, acute and chronic hepatitis, cirrhosis and hepatocellular carcinoma.

2. Hepatitis B is transmitted from infected mothers to their Newborns primarily resulting from exposure to maternal blood at the time of delivery. Acute maternal HBV infection during late pregnancy/near the time of delivery may result in 50–75% transmission rate. When acute maternal HBV infection occurs during the first and second trimesters of pregnancy, there is generally little risk to the Newborns, because antigenemia is usually cleared by term and anti-HBs is present. Transplacental transfer (occurs in Taiwan) has not been found in other parts of the world.

3. *The risk of transmission of Hepatitis B to the Neonate is greatest, if the mother also is HBe antigen positive (this makes them, 80-90% chance of becoming carriers of HBsAg).* But any patient positive for HBsAg is potentially infectious. Acute infection in the mother or baby can be diagnosed by the presence of clinical symptoms & a positive HBsAg or anti-HBc IgM. The chronic carrier state is defined as the presence of HBsAg on to occasions, 6 months apart, or the presence of HBsAg without anti-HBc IgM. (*Refer to Table 1* for diagnostic serologic tests for Hepatitis B infection & their interpretation).

4. Pregnant women with higher HBV viral loads are potentially also more likely to transmit HBV to their infants. Therapy with Lamivudine, Tenofovir or Adefovir, or Etanercept may reduce the possibility of transmission. It is recommended that all pregnant women be screened for HBsAg early in gestation. When there is any concern about a possible infectious contact, development of acute hepatitis, or high-risk behavior in a nonimmunized woman, testing should be repeated.

5. All infants born to mothers confirmed to be positive for HBsAg should receive hepatitis B immuno globulin 200 units IM within the first 12 hrs of life at a different site along with recombinant Hepatitis B vaccine. The vaccine is repeated at 6 wks, 10 wks and 12 months. Breast feeding of unimmunized infants by infected mothers doesn't appear to confer a greater risk of Hepatitis on offspring than does formula feeding, despite the possibility that cracked nipples may result in ingestion of contaminated maternal blood by a nursing infant. Routine immunoprophylaxis of infants born to HBs Ag - positive mothers with HB vaccine and HBIG may eliminate theoretical risks.

6. Postvaccination testing for HBs Ag and anti-HBs should be at 9-15 months of age. If the result is positive for anti-HBs, the child is immune to HBV. If the result is positive for HBs Ag only, the parent should be counseled and the child evaluated by a Pediatric Hepatologist. If the result is negative for both HBs Ag and anti-HBs, a second complete Hepatitis B vaccine series should be administered, followed by testing for anti-HBs to determine if subsequent doses are needed. Routine postvaccination testing of immunized infants born to HBs Ag negative woman or with anti-Hbs is not recommended. The 3 dose series (at 0–2 months, 1–4 months and 6–18 months of age) can be completed even if the interval between doses is longer than recommended.

7. In one study in Taiwan, cesarean delivery in conjunction with maternal immunization dramatically reduced the incidence of perinatally acquired HBV from highly infective mothers. These results are promising & may offer a potential adjunctive therapy for very high-risk situations for e.g., HBsAg/HBe positive women. Currently, no specific recommendations can be made regarding mode of delivery. Universal precautions should be in effect in all newborn nurseries, so the risk of exposure to blood and body secretions should be minimized. Immunization of health care workers is also strongly recommended. Post exposure prophylaxis of non immunized persons should be done with Hepatitis B immune globulin after sending the blood samples for Hepatitis serology.

8. *The Evaluation-Decision-Action-Plan/Algorithm* describes the essential aspects of diagnosis and management of perinatally acquired Hepatitis B and Hepatitis C infections. Infants with Hepatitis B infection do not show clinical or chemical signs of disease at birth. Without immuno-prophylaxis, the usual pattern is the development of chronic antigenemia with mild and often persistent enzyme elevations, beginning at 2–6 months of age. Less commonly, the infection becomes clinically manifest, with jaundice, fever, hepatomegaly, and anorexia, followed by either recovery or chronic active hepatitis. Rarely, fulminant hepatitis is seen and can be fatal. Approximately 5%–10% of infants born to HBeAg positive mothers become chronic HBV carriers despite combined active and passive immuno-prophylaxis with HBIG and HBV vaccine. Infants who become infected with HBV perinatally have a 90% risk of chronic infection, and 15–25% of those with chronic infection die of HBV-related liver disease (primarily hepatocellular carcinoma) as adults.

9. There is no therapy for acute Hepatitis B infection. Interferon (IFN-ALPHA) and lamivudine have been approved for treatment of chronic hepatitis B in children, but success is widely variable. Adefovir for HBV treatment in pediatrics is being investigated.

10. Hepatitis C, the main cause of non-A, non-B, parenterally transmitted hepatitis can be transmitted to 5% of infants born to hepatitis C infected women vertically. HCV is transmitted at a higher frequency if the mother is also HIV infected. It can be transmitted via hematogenous in utero mode or/ via passage through the birth canal, but the exact mode of transmission is unknown. The CDCP currently states that maternal HCV infection is not a contraindication to breast feeding. The decision to breast-feed should be discussed with the mother on an individual basis. Refer to the E-D-A algorithm for the essential features of Hepatitis C infection in the Neonates.

---

* *Pearl/Peril/Pitfall : Separating a neonate from its HBsAg-positive mother is not recommended, and breastfeeding does not appear to increase the risk of postpartum HBV transmission, particularly if HBIG and hepatitis B virus vaccine have been given. However, if a mother has cracked nipples, abscesses, or other breast pathology, breastfeeding could potentially transmit HBV.*

THE EVALUATION-DECISION-ACTION-PLAN/ALGORITHM FOR THE DIAGNOSIS AND MANAGEMENT OF *PERINATAL HEPATITIS - B & HEPATITIS C*

SUBJECTIVE FINDINGS

Hx of high risk groups for Hepatitis B infection: mothers born in endemic areas, persons with high-risk behaviour (IV drug abuse, multiple sex partners), close contacts with HBV-infected persons, & those receiving multiple blood/blood products transfusions, health care providers.

Hx of screening status for HBsAg in pregnant woman (should be a routine procedure) & for HBe positive woman (high viral replication & high infectivity).

Hx of Hepatitis during late pregnancy or/near the time of delivery (50–75% transmission rate).

Hx of risk factors for Hepatitis-C infection- IV drug abusers, transfusion recepients, dialysis patients & sexual partners of HCV-infected persons.

OBJECTIVE FINDINGS

Assess mother for symptoms and signs of Hepatitis such as jaundice, abdominal pain, anorexia, nausea & vomiting and malaise.

Look for maternal chronic liver disease (25% of Hepatitis-B infected patients develop chronic active Hepatitis & 60% of Hepatitis-C infected patients develop chronic disease.

Newborn babies are usually asymptomatic even when infected with Hepatitis-B or C, because of long incubation periods (45–160 days for HBV infection & 40–90 days for HCV infection).

INVESTIGATIONS

Hepatitis B make the diagnosis by specific serology & by the detection of viral antigens (*Refer to Table 1* for interpretation). Infectivity correlates best with HBeAg positivity, but any patient positive for HBsAg is potentially infectious.

Hepatitis-C maternal ELISA for detection of antibodies to 3 proteins (c100-3, c22-3, & c33c) & maternal RIA for antibodies to these 3 proteins & to another antigen, 5-5-1.

HCV RNA PCR to detect viral genome must be performed on infants born to HCV infected mothers (to exclude the passively acquired maternal HCV antibodies).

PERINATAL HEPATITIS - B

HBs Ag Positive PREGNANCY
(Screen all women during Pregnancy)
Whether High Risk +

Mode of Transmission

Vaginal Passage (>90%)
Transplacental
Breast Milk (Some Risk)

Treat Supportively LSCS not recommended Currently

Out Come

Infant Born to HBs AG Positive Woman

Neonatal Hepatitis Chronic HbS Ag Carrier — 90% If not Treated

Give

a) Hepatitis 'B' Vaccine

Engerix-10mcgms=0.5ml IM at Birth, 6 weeks and 14 weeks

+ HBIG 200 IU (esp, for whose mothers positive for HBe Antigen Deep IM *Within 12 hrs of Birth at a different site*

NB-IAP recommends four doses schedule of Hepatitis B Vaccine at birth, 6 weeks, 10 weeks and 12 months for optimal protection (if HBIG is not available)

b) Breast Milk-not contraindicated
(May need 'Formula' in case of cracked nipples, Mastitis & in mothers with HBe antigen Positive)

DO

A POST VACCINATION TEST FOR HBs Ag & ANTI HBs AT 9–15 MONTHS OF AGE

ANTI-HBs Positive	HBs Ag Negative Anti HBs Negative	HBs Ag Positive only Anti HBs Negative
IMMUNE CHILD	Treat with 2nd Complete Hepatitis 'B' Vaccine Series	
REASSURE PARENTS	TEST FOR Anti HBs For Subsequent doses	*Counseling *Evaluation by Pediatric Hepatologist

PERINATAL HEPATITIS- C

* Most Neonates perinatally infected with HCV do not show clinical symptoms or at most have hepatomegaly. They may have elevated liver ALT either briefly/intermittently (most commonly between 3 and 6 months of age). HCV-RNAPCR results may be negative initially at birth but typically become positive by 1–2 wks of age & remain so until at least 5 years of age.

* Confirmatory serologic anti-HCV IgG antibody tests should be delayed until exposed infants are atleast 18 months old, when at least 90% will have cleared maternal antibody.

* Liver ultrasonograpy is usually normal or may consist of a mild increase in Echogenicity. Liver biopsies, when performed, typically demonstrate mild-moderate chronic persistent hepatitis.

* Infants & children with persistent elevations in liver transaminases should be referred to a pediatric gastroenterologist for evaluation & management.

* Interferon & Ribavirin combination therapy may help in achieving remission in symptomatic persons with chronic HCV infection. Side effects of this therapy include fever, and myalgias, and the risk/benefit ratio must be taken into account.

* Most children remain viremic until at least 5-6 years of age, & most develop chronic, persistent Hepatitis. Cirrhosis may develop in as many as 20% of chronic disease cases, but may be less likely in pediatric patients.

* *Prevention* - a) screen blood products for antibody to HCV & discard the product if antibody positive. b) *no benefit* to immune globulin given to the exposed infant or to the needle-stick recipient, as products containing antibody are excluded from the lot. c) currently no vaccine for Hepatitis-C, although research is underway. d) infants with HCV should receive routine Hepatitis-B immunization and also Hepatitis A vaccination at 2 years of age. e) parents should be advised to avoid unnecessary administration of hepatotoxic drugs.

---

* **Pearl/Peril/Pitfall :** *Infrequently, infected neonates develop acute hepatitis B, which is usually mild and self-limited. They develop jaundice, lethargy, failure to thrive, abdominal distention, and clay-colored stools. Occasionally, severe infection with hepatomegaly, ascites, and hyperbilirubinemia (primarily conjugated bilirubin) occurs. Rarely the disease is fulminant and even fatal. Fulminant disease occurs more often in neonates whose mothers are chronic carriers of hepatitis B.*

TABLE 1 Hepatitis B vaccine schedules for Newborn infants, by Maternal Hepatitis B surface antigen (HBsAg) status*

Maternal HBsAg status	Single-antigen vaccine		Single antigen + combination vaccine	
	Dose	Age	Dose	Age
Positive	1†	Birth (<12 hrs)	1†	Birth (<12 hrs)
	HBIG§	Birth (<12 hrs)	HBIG	Birth (<12 hrs)
	2	1–2 mos	2	2 mos
	3¶	6 mos	3	4 mos
			4¶	6 mos (Pediarix) or 12–15 mos (Comvax)
Unknown**	1†	Birth (<12 hrs)	1†	Birth (<12 hrs)
	2	1–2 mos	2	2 mos
	3¶	6 mos	3	4 mos
			4¶	6 mos (Pediarix) or 12–15 mos (Comvax)
Negative	1†,††	Birth (before discharge)	1†,††	Birth (before discharge)
	2	1–2 mos	2	2 mos
	3¶	6–18 mos	3	4 mos
			4¶	6 mos (Pediarix) or 12–15 mos (Comvax)

* See Table 2 for vaccine schedules for preterm infants weighing <2,000 g.

† Recombivax HB or Engerix-B should be used for the birth dose. Comvax and Pediarix cannot be administered at birth or before age 6 weeks.

§ Hepatitis B immune globulin (0.5 mL) administered intramuscularly in a separate site from vaccine.

¶ The final dose in the vaccine series should not be administered before age 24 weeks (164 days).

** Mothers should have blood drawn and tested for HBsAg as soon as possible after admission for delivery; if the mother is found to be HBsAg positive, the infant should receive HBIG as soon as possible but no later than age 7 days.

†† On a case-by-case basis and only in rare circumstances, the first dose may be delayed until after hospital discharge for an infant who weighs >2,000 g and whose mother is HBsAg negative, but only if a physician's order to withhold the birth dose and a copy of the mother's original HBsAg-negative laboratory report are documented in the infant's medical record.

TABLE 2 Hepatitis B immunization management of preterm infants weighing <2,000 g, by maternal hepatitis B surface antigen (HBSAG) status

Maternal HBsAg status	Recommendation
Positive	• HBIG* + hepatitis B vaccine (<12 hrs of birth)
	• Continue vaccine series beginning at age 1–2 mos according to recommended schedule for infants born to HBsAg-positive mothers (see Table1)
	• Do not count birth dose as part of the vaccine series.
	• Test for HBsAg and antibody to HBsAg after completion of the vaccine series at age 9–18 mos (i.e., next well-child visit).
Unknown	• HBIG + hepatitis B vaccine (<12 hrs of birth)
	• Test mother for HBsAg.
	• Continue vaccine series beginning at age 1–2 mos according to recommended schedule based on the mother's HBsAg result (see Table1).
	• Do not count birth dose as part of the vaccine series.
Negative	• Delay first dose of hepatitis B vaccine until age 1 mo or hospital discharge.
	• Complete the vaccine series (see Table 1).

* *Hepatitis B immune globulin*

* *Pearl/Peril/Pitfall : Of the recognized forms of primary viral hepatitis, only hepatitis B virus (HBV) is an important cause of neonatal hepatitis. Other viral infections (e.g, cytomegalovirus, herpes simplex virus) may cause liver inflammation along with their other manifestations.*

Typical interpretation of serologic test results for Hepatitis B virus infection

HBsAg*	Total anti-HBc†	IgM§ anti HBc	Anti HBs¶	Interpretation
–**	–	–	–	Never infected
+††§§	–	–	–	Early acute infection; transient (up to 18 days) after vaccination
+	+	+	–	Acute infection
–	+	+	–	Acute resolving infection
–	+	–	+	Recovered from past infection and immune
+	+	–	–	Chronic infection
–	+	–	–	False positive (i.e., susceptible); past infection; "low-level" chronic infection;¶¶ passive transfer to infant born to HBsAg-positive mother
–	–	–	+	Immune if concentration is >10 mIU/mL,*** passive transfer after hepatitis B immune globulin administration

Serologic marker

* Hepatitis B surface antigen. † Antibody to hepatitis B core antigen. § Immunoglobulin M. ¶ Antibody to HBsAg. ** Negative test result. †† Positive test result. §§ To ensure that an HBsAg-positive test result is not a false positive, samples with repeatedly reactive HBsAg results should be tested with a licensed (and, if appropriate, neutralizing confirmatory) test. ¶¶ Persons positive for only anti-HBc are unlikely to be infectious except under circumstances in which they are the source for direct percutaneous exposure of susceptible recipients to large quantities of virus (e.g., blood transfusion or organ transplant). *** Milli-International Units per milliliter.

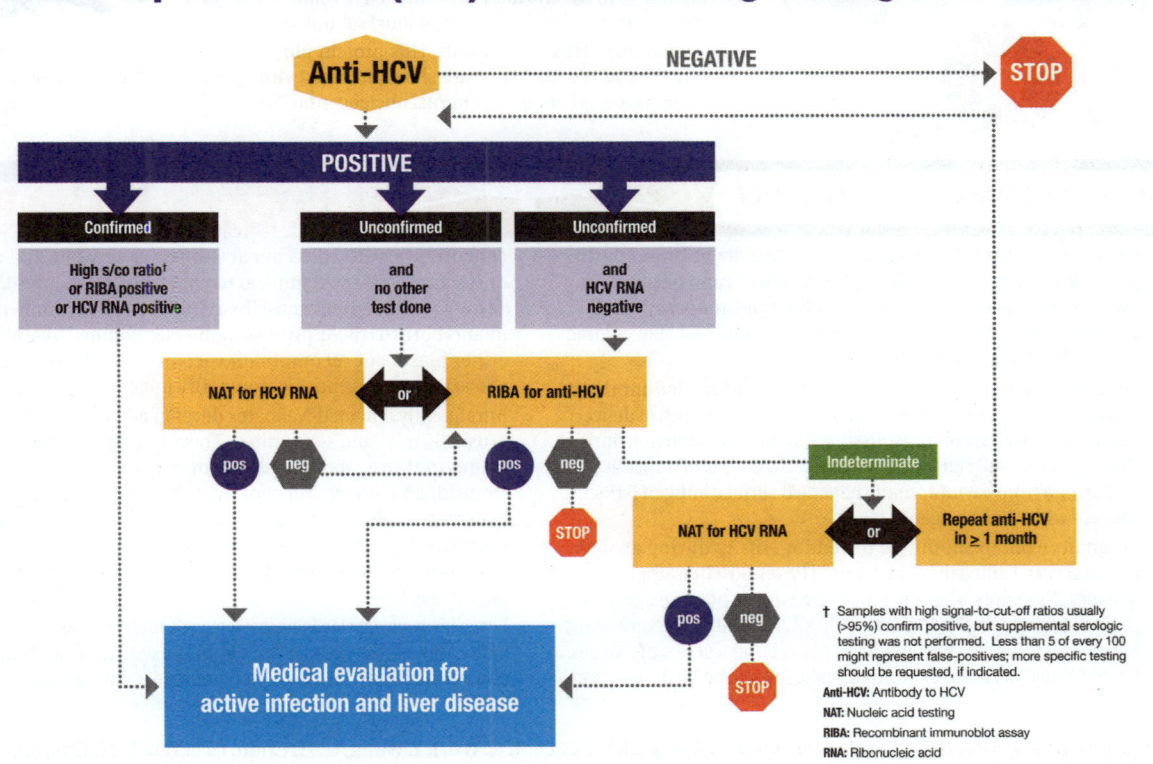

Hepatitis C Virus (HCV) Infection Testing for Diagnosis

† Samples with high signal-to-cut-off ratios usually (>95%) confirm positive, but supplemental serologic testing was not performed. Less than 5 of every 100 might represent false-positives; more specific testing should be requested, if indicated.

Anti-HCV: Antibody to HCV
NAT: Nucleic acid testing
RIBA: Recombinant immunoblot assay
RNA: Ribonucleic acid

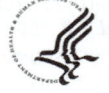

DEPARTMENT OF HEALTH & HUMAN SERVICES
Centers for Disease Control and Prevention
Division of Viral Hepatitis

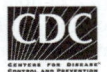

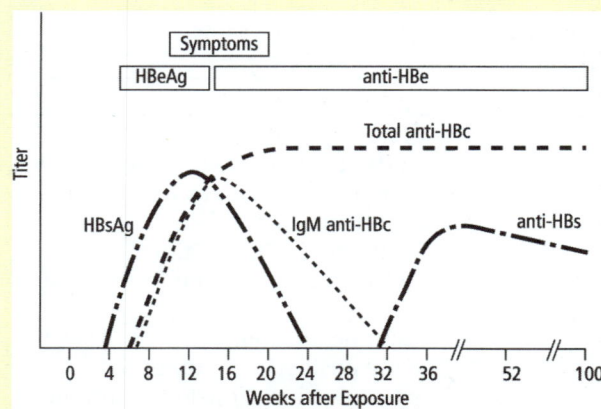

Because the clinical symptoms of HBV infection are indistinguishable from other forms of viral hepatitis, definitive diagnosis is dependent on serologic testing for HBV infection. A variety of tests are available to make the diagnosis of HBV infection. Acute HBV infection is characterized by the presence of HBsAg in serum and the development of IgM class antibody (IgM anti-HBc). Detection of HBsAg has evolved from immunodiffusion methods to reversed passive hemagglutination assays and to the more sensitive enzyme immunoassays and radioimmunoassays, which can detect HBsAg at concentrations of ≥0.1 ng/ml. HBeAg is also detectable during acute infection. During convalescence, HBsAg and HBeAg are cleared, and anti-HBs, anti-HBc, and anti-HBe develop. Anti-HBs is a protective antibody that neutralizes the virus. The presence of anti-HBs following acute infection indicates recovery and immunity from reinfection. Anti-HBs is also detected among persons who have received hepatitis B vaccine. Immunoassays for the detection of total anti-HBc involve both IgM and IgG class antibody to the core protein and indicate current or past exposure to virus and viral replication. IgG anti-HBc appears shortly after HBsAg among persons with acute disease and generally persists for life; therefore, total anti-HBc is not a good marker for persons with acute disease. The detection of IgM anti-HBc is diagnostic of acute HBV infection.

Structure and organization of the HBV genome HBV is the smallest DNA virus known: it has only 3,200 bp in its genome, which is uniquely organized in a partly double-stranded, circular pattern The minus strand of the DNA is almost a complete circle and contains overlapping genes that encode both structural proteins (pre-S, surface, and core) and replicative proteins (polymerase and X protein). The plus strand of the DNA is shorter and variable in length.

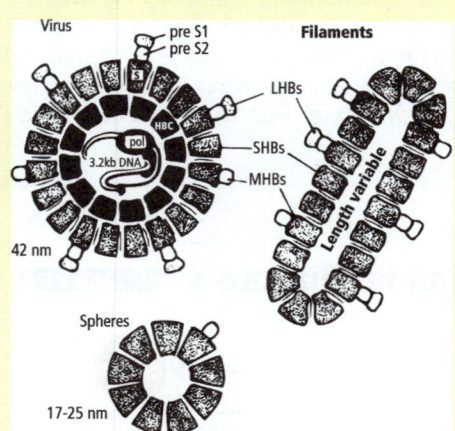

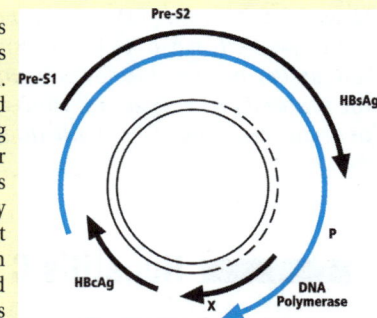

HBV is a double-stranded, enveloped DNA virus of the *Hepadnaviridae* family, which replicates in the liver and causes hepatic dysfunction. HBsAg is found on the surface of the virus and is also produced in excess amounts, circulating in the blood as 22-nm spherical and tubular particles. The inner core of the virus contains HBcAg, HBeAg, a single molecule of partially double-stranded DNA, and a DNA-dependent DNA polymerase. HBsAg can be identified in serum 30 to 60 days after exposure to HBV and persists for variable periods. Individual subunits containing SHBs protein only, HBs protein plus pre-S2 (MHBs), and HBs protein plus pre-S1 and pre-S2 (LHBs) are shown in intact virus, among filaments and spheres. The virus particles contain an internal nucleocapsid (HBc) and viral genome. pol, polymerase.

KEY POINTS FOR CLINICAL PRACTICE

1. Neonatal hepatitis B virus infection is usually acquired during parturition. It is usually asymptomatic but can cause chronic subclinical disease. Symptomatic infection produces jaundice, lethargy, failure to thrive, abdominal distention, and clay-colored stools. Diagnosis is by serology.

2. HBV infection occurs during delivery from infected mothers. Maternal acute hepatitis B occurring within 2 to 3 month of delivery has about a 70% risk of transmission, but disease occurring during the 1st or 2nd trimester has only about 5% risk. Risk of transmission is also high from asymptomatic hepatis B surface antigen (HBsAg) carriers with the e antigen.

3. Pregnant women should be tested for HBsAg during an early prenatal visit. Failing that, they should be tested when admitted for delivery. Neonates whose mothers are HBsAg-positive should be given 1 dose of HBIG 0.5 mL IM within 12 h of birth. Recombinant hepatitis B virus vaccine should be given IM in a series of 3 doses. (Note: Doses vary among proprietary vaccines.) The 1st dose is given concurrently with HBIG but at a different site. The 2nd and 3rd doses are given 1 to 2 mo and 6 mo, respectively, after the first. Testing for HBsAg and anti-HBs at 9 to 15 mo is recommended. In infants born to HBeAg positive mothers, combined treatment with either plasma or recombinant vaccines and HBIG is 79 to 98% efficacious in preventing chronic HBV infection.

4. Infrequently, infected Neonates develop acute hepatitis B, which is usually mild and self-limited. They develop jaundice, lethargy, failure to thrive, abdominal distention, and clay-colored stools. Occasionally, severe infection with hepatomegaly, ascites, and hyperbilirubinemia (primarily conjugated bilirubin) occurs. Rarely the disease is fulminant and even fatal. Fulminant disease occurs more often in Neonates whose mothers are chronic carriers of hepatitis B.

5. Long-term prognosis is unknown, although HBsAg carriage early in life appears to increase the risk of subsequent liver disease (e.g. chronic hepatitis, cirrhosis, hepatocellular carcinoma).

REFERENCES & FURTHER READING : 1) Lo, K. J., Y. T. Tsai, S. D. Lee, T. C. Wu, J. Y. Wang, G. H. Chen, C. L. Yeh, B. N. Chiang, S. H. Yeh, and A. Goudeau. 1985. Immunoprophylaxis of infection with hepatitis B virus in infants born to hepatitis B surface antigen-positive carrier mothers. J. Infect. Dis. **152**:817–822 2) Rosner, G, Lurie, Y, Blendis, L, Halpern, Z, Oren, R (2006). Acute hepatitis B in the era of immunisation: pitfalls in the identification of high risk patients.. *Postgrad. Med. J.* 82: 207–210 3) Chien, Y.-C., Jan, C.-F., Kuo, H.-S., Chen, C.-J. (2006). Nationwide Hepatitis B Vaccination Program in Taiwan: Effectiveness in the 20 Years After It Was Launched. *Epidemiol Rev* 28: 126-135 4) Summers, J., P. M. Smith, and A. L. Horwich. 1990. Hepadnavirus envelope proteins regulate covalently closed circular DNA amplification. J. Virol. **64**:2819-2824 5) Jenkins, C. N. H., McPhee, S. J., Wong, C., Nguyen, T., Euler, G.L. (2000). Hepatitis B Immunization Coverage Among Vietnamese-American Children 3 to 18 Years Old. *Pediatrics* 106: 78e–78

Congenital and Perinatal HIV Infection

@ *Proviral DNA PCR: This test is usually performed only in Newborns because conventional serologic testing is useless in these patients (maternal antibodies may persist for 9–18 months). Two or more negative results separated by at least one month is considered a negative result.*

HIV contains the 3 species-defining retroviral genes— *gag* (group-specific antigen; the inner structural proteins), *pol* (polymerase; also contains integrase and protease—the viral enzymes—and is produced as a C-terminal extension of the Gag protein), and *env* (envelope; the outer structural proteins responsible for cell-type specificity). HIV-1 has 6 additional accessory genes— *tat, rev, nef, vif, vpu,* and *vpr*. HIV-2 does not have *vpu* but instead has the unique gene *vpx*. The only other virus known to contain the *vpu* gene is simian immunodeficiency virus in chimpanzees (SIV$_{cpz}$), which is the simian equivalent of HIV. Interestingly, chimpanzees with active HIV-1 infection are resistant to disease. The accessory proteins of HIV-1 and HIV-2 are involved in viral replication and may play a role in the disease process. The outer part of the genome consists of long terminal repeats (LTRs) that contain sequences necessary for gene transcription and splicing, viral packaging of genomic RNA, and dimerization sequences to ensure that 2 RNA genomes are packaged. The dimerization, packaging, and gene-transcription processes are intimately linked; disruption in one process often subsequently affects another. The LTRs exist only in the proviral DNA genome; the viral RNA genome contains only part of each LTR, and the complete LTRs are re-created during the reverse-transcription process prior to integration into the host DNA.

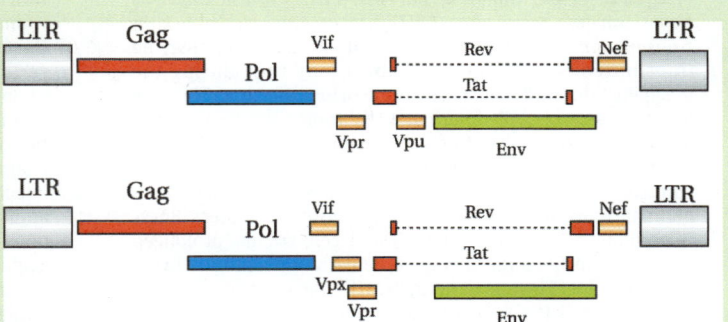

Genome layouts of HIV-1 (upper) and HIV-2 (lower)

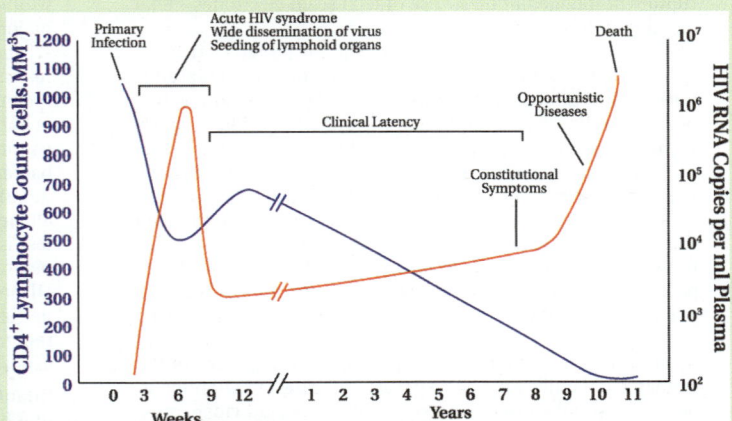

Timeline of CD4 T-cell and viral-load changes over time in untreated human immunodeficiency virus (HIV) infection.

REVIEW OF CLINICAL PROBLEMS

1. Mention the Recommended schedule of Tests for evaluating HIV-exposed Neonate-Infant.
   Ans: Refer to the Table 1 of the Chapter.

2. Discuss the indications & interventions for providing Prophylaxis against infections associated with HIV infection in infants.
   Ans: Refer to the Table 5 of the Chapter.

3. What Anti Pneumocystis pneumonia Regimens are available?
   Ans: Refer to the Table 3 of the Chapter.

4. How do you interpret HIV infection and usual pattern of test results in Newborns of women with HIV infection ?
   Ans: Refer to the Table 6 of the Chapter.

5. Discuss Obstetric/Perinatal aspects of management which may reduce vertical transmission.
   Ans: Refer to the Evaluation-Decision-Action Plan/Algorithm to diagnose and manage Neonatal HIV Exposure/Infection.

LEARNING OBJECTIVES

After completing this article, readers will be able to:

1. Prevent/Reduce the Vertical Transmission rates of HIV from HIV + ve mother to Neonates/Infants.

2. Exclude/Confirm Neonate's HIV status as per current CDC recommendations.

3. Understand the importance of interpretation of various Tests for HIV Infection and their timing to perform.

4. Provide prophylaxis against HIV and Its related opportunistic infections in HIV confirmed Neonates/Infants.

5. Search for co-infections, such as HBV, Hep C, CMV, Syphilis, Toxoplasmosis, TB, etc. in the Neonate, mother, father/living partner, siblings irrespective of their age.

---

* *Pearl/Peril/Pitfall: The HIV DNA PCR test is the recommended initial screening tool in infants born to HIV-positive mothers. The test has a sensitivity of 93.2 percent and a specificity of 94.9 percent; however, it is less accurate in neonates. In infants with a low risk of transmission, the positive predictive value of the HIV DNA PCR test is 55.8 percent during the first month after birth and 83.2 percent after the first month.*

BIRD'S EYE VIEW/OVERVIEW/SYNOPSIS

1. *HIV is a blood-borne, sexually transmissible virus. The virus is typically transmitted via sexual intercourse, shared intravenous drug paraphernalia, and mother-to-child transmission (MTCT), which can occur during the birth process or during breastfeeding. The most common route of infection varies from country to country and even among cities, reflecting the population in whom HIV was introduced initially and local practices. Co-infection with other viruses that share similar routes of transmission, such as hepatitis B, hepatitis C, and human herpes virus 8 (HHV 8; also known as Kaposi sarcoma herpes virus [KSHV]), is common. Mother to baby transmission :* HIV (Human Immunodeficiency Virus) may be transmitted from mother to baby at any time during the pregnancy, during labour, or as a result of breastfeeding. This type of transmission is called perinatal HIV transmission or vertical transmission or mother-to-child transmission of HIV. Without interventions the rate of mother to baby transmission is approximately 25–30%. Factors associated with increased risk of perinatal transmission include *acute stage of the mother's illness *high maternal viral load *low CD4 (T cell) count *prolonged rupture of the membranes *vaginal delivery *premature delivery *breastfeeding. The rate of perinatal HIV transmission can be as low as 1-2% if the following strategies are used *perinatal prophylactic antiretroviral therapy (to mother and newborn) *elective Cesarean section *formula feeding. Other strategies that are thought to be beneficial include the avoidance of *artificial rupture of the membranes *use of fetal scalp electrodes *fetal blood sampling.

2. All HIV positive antenatal patients should be referred to an Infectious Diseases consultant for continuation of maternal anti-retroviral treatment during pregnancy. Women who are HIV positive and pregnant require an integrated multidisciplinary approach to care. Experienced HIV physicians, obstetricians, midwives and social workers should work closely during the pregnancy, preferably as early as possible. This is important to *establish an early rapport with the parents *offer counseling on the current strategies to minimize the risk of perinatal HIV transmission *prepare them for when the baby is born *offer postnatal antiretroviral prophylaxis *offer pneumocystis carinii pneumonia prophylaxis *complete the testing process involved in establishing a diagnosis in the baby *provide education to staff involved in the management of the woman. The privacy of the woman and family must be respected and care and attention to her needs should also be observed. Health care providers must not assume that partners, parents, relatives, friends or even other health care workers are informed of the woman's HIV status. Neither can they assume that the woman is prepared for any or all of these contacts to know. Health care professionals need to be guided by the woman's wishes in this regard.

3. **Antenatal maternal management:** Data from the AIDS Clinical Trials Group study demonstrated a significant decrease in perinatal HIV transmission (~ 70% reduction from 25% to 8%) when pregnant women and their babies received a 3 part AZT (zidovudine) regimen *AZT during pregnancy (after the 14th week of gestation) *intrapartum intravenous AZT *6 weeks of AZT to babies. If the mother is not already receiving treatment, this should be started as soon as HIV status is confirmed positive. Ideally treatment should commence during the second trimester and no later than the beginning of the third trimester and continue throughout pregnancy. Prescribing of anti-retrovirals to pregnant women is complex and should be referred to an Infectious Diseases consultant.

4. **Perinatal management:** AZT (Zidovudine) is the anti-retroviral agent of choice for use during delivery to decrease perinatal transmission. For other anti-retroviral agents that may also be used during delivery to decrease perinatal transmission, consult an Infectious Diseases consultant for further advice. Zidovudine is an anti-retroviral agent. It is used for the treatment of HIV infection and provides protection for the baby during delivery, and decreases perinatal transmission when taken by the baby for 6 weeks after birth. Elective Cesarean Section: A loading dose is usually required followed by a continuous infusion starting 4 hours prior to a planned caesarean. Once the umbilical cord is clamped, intravenous treatment can be ceased. **Breastfeeding** is **NOT** recommended in women with HIV due to the risk of viral transmission through breast milk. Formula feeds are preferred.

However, skin-to-skin contact between mother and baby should still be encouraged.

5. *The Evaluation-Decision-Action-Plan/Algorithm* to diagnose & manage Congenital/Perinatal HIV Infection outlines the essential aspects of history taking, physical examination and appropriate investigations as well as management of the affected infant & mother. There are no known contraindications to the use of short-term steroids to promote fetal lung maturity in women with HIV. There are no known contraindications to an HIV positive woman having either a general or epidural anesthetic.

6. **Obstetric/Perinatal aspects of management** which may reduce vertical transmission are summarized in the Table 2 of the Chapter.

7. **Neonatal management: Neonatal management should always be in consultation with an Infectious Disease Consultant Diagnosis of HIV in Neonates :** Whilst the diagnosis of HIV infection in adults is readily established by the detection of HIV antibodies, the situation is more complex in babies born to HIV positive women. During the pregnancy, the fetus passively acquires maternal HIV antibodies across the placenta. This does not mean the fetus is infected but rather has "acquired" the antibodies from the mother. The babies will always test "HIV antibody positive" as the test will detect antibodies derived from the mother. Therefore, the HIV antibody test alone cannot be relied on in these babies, since all babies born to HIV positive women will test positive to HIV antibodies (and in the vast majority of cases are unlikely to be infected). It can take up to 12-18 months for a baby to clear these maternal antibodies. For this reason, a sensitive nucleic acid based technique called the "PCR" (polymerase chain reaction) is used to detect the presence of HIV in babies. Multiple negative tests to age 6 months are required to confirm an "uninfected" status in exposed infants. In uninfected babies, it is recommended that the child have a "final" test at 18 months (the HIV antibody test) to show that the baby has cleared all the passively acquired HIV antibodies. If a PCR is positive, the test is always repeated as soon as possible (on a new sample) before it is confirmed that the baby is infected. All babies born to HIV positive women should be followed into adulthood by a Pediatrician. Refer to the Table 1 of the Chapter for the recommended schedule of tests for the diagnosis of HIV-1 exposed infants.

8. **Infant AZT dosages** After clamping of umbilical cord or within 6 to 8 hours of delivery, start oral zidovudine and continue for 6 weeks *2mg/kg/dose every 6 hours or *4mg/kg/dose twice a day. If infant vomits more than 15 minutes after dose, give next dose at next scheduled time. If infant vomits within 15 minutes of a dose, give another dose if possible. Ensure that the entire bottle of zidovudine syrup is sent home with the infant (it is sufficient to complete the six weeks of therapy). Each 5mL of zidovudine syrup contains 50mg zidovudine. If infant unable to tolerate oral feeds, start zidovudine infusion. Infant IV infusion - 1.5mg/kg/dose over 30 minutes every 6 hours, dilute to 4mg/ml, compatible with 5% Dextrose or N Saline.

9. **Pneumocystis (PCP) prophylaxis:** PCP prophylaxis is recommended for all babies born to HIV infected women. It is commenced at 6 weeks and continues until testing at 3 months confirms the absence of HIV infection in formula fed infants. This is discussed with the parents to assist them in making informed decision. Treatment is with Co-Trimoxazole. There are several regimens. One suggested regimen is 0.5 ml/kg/day for 6 weeks (dose based on the trimethroprim component). Refer to Table 3.

10. **Immunizations :** Routine childhood immunizations (DTPa -hep B, Hib, poliovirus vaccine, MMR, meningococcal and pneumococcal disease) should be given to all babies according to the schedule. Inactivated injectable polio vaccine given subcutaneously is administered instead of the oral polio vaccine to all babies born to HIV infected mothers to minimise the risk of OPV strains being transmitted to immunocompromized members of the family. MMR is safe for contacts and for all patients except those with severely compromised immune function. It is preferable to give MMR rather than expose a child to the risk of infection with wild type measles. Varicella vaccine is recommended for children aged 12 months or more with normal immune function.

THE EVALUATION-DECISION-ACTION-PLAN/ALGORITHM FOR THE DIAGNOSIS AND MANAGEMENT OF *NEONATAL HIV EXPOSURE/INFECTION*

SUBJECTIVE FINDINGS

Hx of Maternal HIV infection (for newborns, infants, and children): Steps taken to reduce the risk of transmission at birth include cesarean delivery and prenatal antiretroviral therapy in the mother and antiretroviral therapy in the Newborn immediately after birth.

Hx of Family and Social dynamics-Poverty, substance abuse, promiscuity, nil/irregular antenatal care etc.,

OBJECTIVE FINDINGS

Assess the following! *Eliminating mother-to-child transmission of HIV requires early engagement in prenatal care, skilled counseling and HIV testing (and sometimes repeat testing), carefully chosen and intensely monitored antiretroviral prophylaxis, testing and close follow up of the exposed infant, and – throughout – sensitive and supportive care.*

INVESTIGATIONS

In addition to HIV tests described below the HIV-exposed Newborn should be tested for syphilis, hepatitis B, and hepatitis C if the mother has not been screened. If the mother is hepatitis B surface antigen–positive, the infant should receive hepatitis B immunoglobulin and hepatitis B vaccine at birth, and hepatitis vaccine again at one to two months of age and six months of age.

CONGENITAL/PERINATAL HIV INFECTION

Time of ZDV	Regimen Administration
Antepartum	Oral administration (to the pregnant woman) of 100 mg ZDV 5 times daily, initiated at 14-34 weeks gestation and continued throughout the pregnancy.
Intrapartum	During labor Intravenous administration (to the pregnant women) of ZDV in a 1 hour-initial dose of 2 mg/kg body weight, followed by a continuous infusion of 1 mg/kg body weight/hour until delivery.
Postpartum	Oral administration of ZDV to the Newborn infant (ZDV syrup at 2 mg/kg body weight/dose every 6 hours) for the first six weeks of life, beginning at 8-12 hours after birth.

TABLE 1 Laboratory monitoring and treatment of infants born to women with HIV infection

Age	Category of intervention	Test or treatment indicated
Newborn	Evaluation	ELISA for antibody to HIV (and Westron blot if ELISA positive). A well documented history of HIV infection in mother can replace ELISA testing in the Newborn. HIV DNA PCR (polymerase chain reaction)[a] -complete blood count with differential
	Treatment	ZDV (AZT) for prophylaxis against vertical transmission. Advise against breast feeding if safe alternatives are available
4 weeks	Evaluation	HIV DNA PCR[a], Hematocrit (to check for anemia from ZDV)
	Treatment	Continue ZDV
6 weeks	Treatment	Stop ZDV
		Begin treatment with trimethoprim/sulfamethoxazole for prophylaxis against Pneumocystis carinii pneumonia
4 months	Evaluation	HIV DNA PCR[a] (if prior testing negative)
	Treatmemt	Stop treatment with trimethoprim/sulfamethoxazole when the 4 month HIV DNA PCR returns and is negative. Continue if HIV DNA PCR testing is positive.
18 months	Evaluation	ELISA for antibody to HIV (Western blot confirmation if ELISA positive). IF negative, in the presence of prior negative HIV DNA PCR testing and absence of symptoms of HIV infection, patient is a "sero-reverter," and HIV infection is definitively excluded at the present time. If positive, repeat.

[a] Any positive HIV DNA PCR is repeated as soon as possible to confirm the diagnosis. Infants diagnosed with HIV infection are treated as outlined in Federal Guidelines for care. Patients should have HIV DNA PCR testing in the nursery. Cord blood should not be used for HIV DNA PCR testing, as false positives can occur. If mother is suspected of having non-B subtype HIV, she should be tested using HIV DNA PCR during pregnancy. If the mother is positive by HIV DNA PCR, then the HIV DNA PCR test can be used to test for HIV infection in the infant. If the mother is negative by HIV DNA PCR testing, the infant should be tested using HIV RNA tests optimized for identification of non-B subtype HIV, e.g., the Bayer HIV-1 Versant Assay version 3.0 or higher. Consult with a specialist with experience in care of persons with HIV. Follow-up to show absence of antibody to HIV at 12 to 18 months of age is imperative.

| TABLE 2 | Reduction of perinatal HIV transmission: Clinical scenarios and management recommendations |

Clinical scenario—Management recommendations

Antiretroviral therapy

Scenario 1: HIV-infected pregnant woman not previously exposed to antiretroviral drugs: Antiretroviral drug therapy is selected based on the same parameters used in nonpregnant HIV-infected women. The regimen should include orally administered zidovudine (Retrovir) during pregnancy and intravenously administered zidovudine during labor.

Scenario 2: HIV-infected woman receiving antiretroviral drugs during current pregnancy: Continuation of antiretroviral drug therapy should be considered. Zidovudine should be incorporated into the regimen and should be given intravenously during labor.

Scenario 3: HIV-infected woman in labor with no previous antiretroviral drug therapy: Consider one of four regimens: 1. Single dose of orally administered nevirapine given to the mother at the onset of labor, and single dose given to the Newborn by 48 hours after birth 2. Orally administered lamivudine-zidovudine given to the mother during labor and to the Newborn for 1 week after birth 3. Intravenously administered zidovudine given to the mother during labor, and orally administered zidovudine given to the Newborn for 6 weeks after birth 4. Two doses of orally administered nevirapine and intravenously administered zidovudine given to the mother during labor, and orally administered zidovudine given to the Newborn for 6 weeks after birth

Scenario 4: Infant of an HIV-infected mother who did not receive antiretroviral drugs during pregnancy or labor Give orally administered zidovudine to the Newborn for 6 weeks after birth. Consider use of additional antiretroviral drugs.

Mode of delivery

Scenario A: HIV-infected woman presenting late in pregnancy, not receiving antiretroviral drug therapy and unlikely to have laboratory evaluations before delivery.-Begin antiretroviral drug therapy. Consider elective cesarean section at 38 weeks of gestation.

Scenario B: HIV-infected woman initiating prenatal care in third trimester, receiving highly active antiretroviral drug therapy but with a viral load of >1,000 copies per mL-Continue antiretroviral drug therapy as long as the viral load is dropping appropriately. Consider elective cesarean section at 38 weeks of gestation.

Scenario C: HIV-infected woman on highly active antiretroviral drug therapy with an undetectable viral load-Whether elective cesarean section has any additional benefit is unclear. The risk of vertical transmission of HIV is less than 2 percent with vaginal delivery.

Scenario D: HIV-infected woman who has elected cesarean section for delivery but presents in labor-Begin intravenous administration of zidovudine. If delivery is imminent, vaginal delivery may be used, with oxytocin (Pitocin) augmentation considered. If a long labor is anticipated, consider proceeding with cesarean section. The risk of vertical transmission of HIV is increased with rupture of membranes for longer than 4 hours. HIV = human immunodeficiency virus. *Adapted from* Public Health Service Task Force recommendations for the use of antiretroviral drugs in pregnant HIV-1 infected women for maternal health and interventions to reduce perinatal HIV-1 transmission in the United States. Living document: January 24, 2001. Retrieved February 2001, from http://www.hivatis.org/trtgdlns.html#Perinatal.

Prevention of Pneumocystis pneumonia

Pneumocystis pneumonia (PCP) is the most common serious opportunistic infection in HIV-1-infected children. This condition is caused by Pneumocystis jiroveci (formerly Pneumocystis carinii). It is recommended that PCP prophylaxis be started at or near the completion of ZDV prophylaxis (four to six weeks of age) but discontinued when HIV-1 infection is reasonably excluded. PCP prophylaxis would, therefore, be discontinued when results of two virological assays performed on two separate samples, one after one month of age and the other after two to four months of age, are known to be negative. Drugs and dosing regimens for PCP prophylaxis in the infant are listed in the following Table. . Infants who are HIV-1-infected should remain on PCP prophylaxis until 12 months of age, at which time they should receive PCP prophylaxis according to guidelines.

| TABLE 3 | Regimens for pneumocystis pneumonia prophylaxis in infants |

Drug	Dose	Route	Schedule
Trimethoprim sulfamethoxazole	Trimethoprim, 150 mg/m²/day, with sulfamethoxazole, 750 mg/m²/day	PO	Twice daily for 3 days/week
Dapsone	2 mg/kg	PO	Once daily
	4 mg/kg	PO	Once weekly
Pentamidine	4 mg/kg	IV	Every 2 to 4 weeks
Atovaquone	Infants 1–3 months of age: 30mg/kg	PO	Once daily
	Infants 4–24 months of age: 45 mg/kg	PO	Once daily
IV Intravenous; PO Oral			

Screening for Tuberculosis: The reemergence of tuberculosis has coincided with the spread of HIV. Infants infected with HIV and all children living with an HIV-positive person are at increased risk for tuberculosis. HIV-infected pregnant women should be screened for tuberculosis before delivery. Infants should be kept away from any person with active pulmonary disease until that person is no longer considered to be contagious. Infants and young children exposed to a person with active tuberculosis should have a purified protein derivative (PPD) skin test and a chest radiograph. A positive PPD test in HIV-exposed or HIV-infected children is 5 mm of induration. Even if the PPD test is negative, infants who have been exposed to tuberculosis should be given isoniazid (INH) for three months. Then, the PPD test should be repeated. If the test is negative, isoniazid may be discontinued. If the test is positive, prophylaxis is continued. All HIV-infected children should have a screening PPD test annually, starting at 12 months of age. Immunizations and TB screening should be provided for HIV-1-exposed infants in accordance with national guidelines.

TABLE 4 Clinical categories of children with human immunodeficiency virus (HIV) infection

Category N: Not symptomatic
No signs or symptoms or only one of the conditions listed in category A

Category A: Mildly symptomatic
Having two or more of the following conditions:
Lymphadenopathy
Hepatomegaly
Splenomegaly
Dermatitis
Parotitis
Recurrent or persistent upper respiratory infection, sinusitis, or otitis media

Category B: Moderately symptomatic
Having symptoms attributed to HIV infection other than those in category A or C

Examples : Anemia, neutropenia, thrombocytopenia,Bacterial meningitis, pneumonia, sepsis (single episode), Candidiasis, oropharyngeal, persisting more than 1mo, Cardiomyopathy, Cytomegalovirus infection with onset < age 1mo, Diarrhea, recurrent or chronic, Hepatitis, Herpes simplex virus recurrent stomatitis, bronchitis, pneumonitis, esophagitis at < 1 month of age, Herpes zoster- two or more episodes or more than one dermatome, Leiomyosarcoma, Lymphoid interstitial pneumonia, Nephropathy, Nocardiosis, persistent fever, Toxoplasmosis with onset < age 1 mo, Varicella, complicated.

Category C: Severely symptomatic
Serious bacterial infections, multiple or recurrent
Candidiasis, esophageal or pulmonary
Coccidioidomycosis, disseminated
Cryptosporidiosis or isosporiasis with diarrhea > 1 mo
Cytomegalovirus infection with onset > age 1 mo
Encephalopathy
Herpes simplex virus: Persistent oral lesions, or bronchitis, pneumonitis, esophagitis at > age 1mo
Histoplasmosis
kaposi sarcoma
Lymphoma
Mycobacterium tuberculosis, extrapulmonary
Mycobacterium infection, other species, disseminated
Pneumocystis jiroveci pneumonia
Progressive multifocal leukoencephalopathy
Salmonella septicemia, recurrent
Toxoplasmosis of the brain with onset > age 1 mo
Wasting syndrome

Maternal health information should be reviewed to determine if the HIV-1-exposed infant may have been exposed to maternal coinfections including TB, syphilis, toxoplasmosis, hepatitis B or C, cytomegalovirus and herpes simplex virus. Diagnostic testing and treatment of the infant are based on maternal findings. Pediatricians should provide counseling to parents and caregivers of HIV-1-exposed infants about HIV-1 infection, including anticipatory guidance on the course of illness, infection control measures, care of the infant, diagnostic tests, and potential drug toxicity.

TABLE 5 Prophylaxis of infections associated with HIV

Infection	Intervention	Indication
Hepatitis B virus (HBV)	HBV vaccination	Hepatitis B negative
Hepatitis A virus (HAV)	HAV vaccination virus, or high-risk exposures	Coinfected with HBV or hepatitis C
Streptococcus pneumoniae	Pneumococcal vaccination (23-valent polysaccharide) cell count less than 200 cells per mm³	CD4+ cell count greater than 200 cells per mm³(200 × 10⁹ per L) CD$_4^+$ [CIII]
Influenza	Inactivated vaccine	Annually
Pneumocystis jiroveci pneumonia	Trimethoprim/sulfamethoxazole SMX; Bactrim, Septran)	CD4+ cell count less than 200 cells per mm³ or CD4+ cell count less than 14 percent or history of AIDS diagnosis or history of oral thrush
Toxoplasmosis	TMP-SMX (100 × 10⁹ per L) and toxoplasma IgG+	CD4+ cell count less than 100 cells per mm³
Mycobacterium avium intracellulare complex	Azithromycin or (50 × 10⁹ per L) clarithromycin	CD4+ cell count less than 50 cells per mm³
Tuberculosis	Isoniazid (INH)	

* *Pearl/Peril/Pitfall : Testing family members-The infant's father and all siblings should be offered testing for HIV-1 infection. Testing should be strongly recommended. The age of the sibling should not be a deterrent to testing because it is possible that perinatally infected children may remain asymptomatic for many years, even into adolescence. *Pearl/Peril/Pitfall: Zidovudine (Retrovir) prophylaxis is recommended for most infants exposed to HIV in utero to decrease the risk of vertical transmission. Beginning eight hours after birth, these neonates should receive zidovudine in a dosage of 2 mg per kg every six hours for at least six weeks. Mild anemia is the primary side effect of zidovudine prophylaxis in infants. The anemia is maximal at six weeks of life and resolves spontaneously by 12 weeks without treatment.*

TABLE 6	HIV infection and usual Pattern of Test results in Newborns of women with HIV infection

HIV infection Category	Test	Infant's age when testing performed and usual result of testing				
		Day of birth	1 month	4 months	> 6 months	18 months
Not infected Seroreverter[a]	ELISA/WB	+	+	+	+/−	−
	HIV DNA PCR	−	−	−	−	−
Infected in utero	ELISA/WB	+	+	+	+	+
	HIV DNA PCR	+	+	+	+	+
Peri-partum	ELISA/WB	+	+	+	+	+
	HIV DNA PCR	−	+/−	+	+	+
via breast milk	ELISA/WB	+	+	+	+	+
	HIV DNA PCR	−	−/+	+/−	+	+

[a] Non-transmitted maternal infection.

Obstetric/Perinatal aspects of management which may reduce vertical transmission:

*avoid early artificial rupture of membranes (ARM) *if artificial rupture of membrane (ARM) is undertaken, careful use of the amnihook is necessary so that scalp integrity is maintained *assess fetal wellbeing using non-invasive methods - avoid the use of fetal scalp electrodes and fetal blood sampling. An open wound may allow direct entry of HIV from mother to infant *the use of forceps or Ventouse extraction may cause a loss of skin integrity increasing the risk of transmission, however this does not preclude their use as required *on delivery of the head, gently wipe the baby's eyes free of secretions *suction is not generally required, but if it is, be gentle to avoid damage to mucous membranes *clamp the cord as soon as possible, milking between the clamps in a direction away from the baby *place a sponge over the cord before cutting to prevent spurting of blood *once born, towel dry the baby. Cleanse the baby as soon as possible *prior to any procedures on the Neonate that will disrupt skin or mucous membrane integrity, ensure the area is thoroughly cleaned. An example is the administration of IMI Vitamin K *ensure that standard precautions are utilised when handling/cleaning up blood/body fluid spillage.

KEY POINTS FOR CLINICAL PRACTICE:

1. The management of infants whose mothers are infected with the human immunodeficiency virus (HIV) involves minimizing the risk of vertical transmission of HIV, recognizing Neonatal HIV infection early, preventing opportunistic infections, and addressing psychosocial issues.

2. Maternal antiretroviral drug therapy during pregnancy and labor, followed by six weeks of Neonatal zidovudine therapy, can significantly decrease the risk of vertical transmission. Additional antiretroviral drugs may be needed in some high-risk Newborns. Elective cesarean section also may prevent vertical transmission of HIV.

3. Virologic tests allow early diagnosis of HIV infection, facilitating the timely initiation of aggressive treatment and the prevention of opportunistic infections. Even when tests are negative, infants must be closely monitored until age 18 months to completely rule out HIV infection.

4. Prophylaxis for Pneumocystis carinii pneumonia should be initiated when HIV-exposed infants are six weeks old and should be continued for at least four months, regardless of negative virologic tests, because P. carinii pneumonia is often the initial presentation of HIV infection in infants.

5. Laboratory monitoring, screening for perinatal infections, appropriate social support, and other modifications of standard infant care are also necessary.

REFERENCES & FURTHER READING : 1) The mode of delivery and the risk of vertical transmission of human immunodeficiency virus type 1—a meta-analysis of 15 prospective cohort studies. The International Perinatal HIV Group. N Engl J Med 1999; 340:977-987. 2) Breastfeeding and the use of human milk: Policy Statement. American Academy of Pediatrics. Pediatrics, February 2005; 115 (2): 496-506. 3) Connor EM, Sperling RS. Reduction of maternal-infant transmission of human immunodeficiency virus type 1 with zidovudine (AZT) treatment. N Engl J Med 1994; 331:1173-1180. 4) HIV infection in pregnancy and neonatal diagnosis: A guide to management. Sydney Children's Hospital, Royal Hospital for Women and Albion Street Centre. 5) Simonds RJ, Oxtoby MJ, Caldwell MB, Gwinn ML, Rogers MF. Pneumocystis carinii pneumonia among US children with perinatally acquired HIV infection. *JAMA.* 1993;270:470–3.

95 Neonatal Tetanus

@ *"Neonatal Tetanus is an entirely vaccine preventable Neonatal infection but when manifested it needs to be treated with expensive modern technology."*

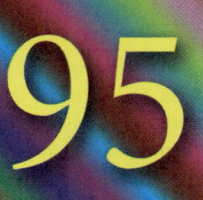

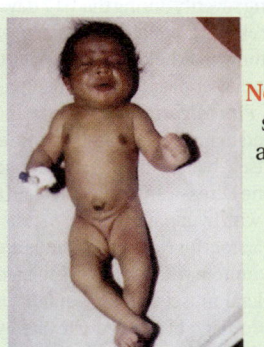

Neonatal tetanus. Newborn showing risus sardonicus and generalized spasticity.

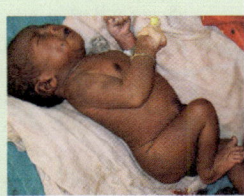

Neonatal tetanus. A, This newborn demonstrates the trismus (locked jaw) and fixed smile of risus sardonicus that are typical of tetanus. Note as well the clenched fists and fanned toes. B, Viewed from the side, his opisthotonic posturing is more evident. (Courtesy Jonathan Spector, MD, Boston.)

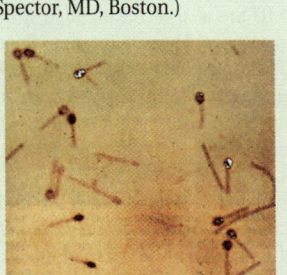

Clostridium tetani Gram stain: Round terminal spores give cells a "Drumstick" or "Tennis racket" appearance

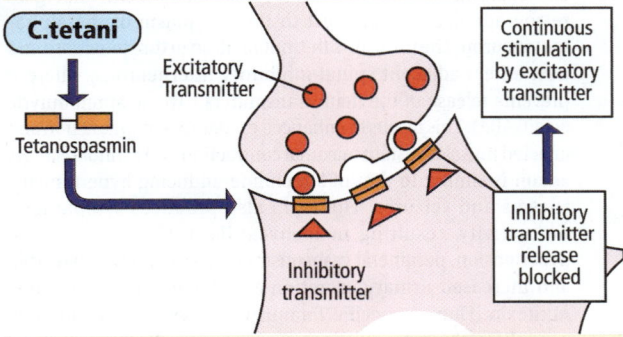

Neonatal tetanus. Tonic contractions of lumbar and abdominal musculature occur next, and result in opisthotonus in extension.

Mechanism of action of Tetanus Toxin

C.tetani

Tetanospasmin

Excitatory Transmitter

Inhibitory transmitter

Continuous stimulation by excitatory transmitter

Inhibitory transmitter release blocked

REVIEW OF CLINICAL PROBLEMS

1. Describe the *essential features* of Neonatal Tetanus.
   Ans: Refer to the "No. 4" of the "BIRD'S EYE VIEW/OVERVIEW/ SYNOPSIS" of the Chapter.

2. What are the *poor prognostic factors* of Neonatal Tetanus?
   Ans: Refer to the Evaluation-Decision-Action Plan/Algorithm to diagnose & manage Neonatal Tetanus.

3. Mention the *complications* of Neonatal Tetanus.
   Ans: Refer to the "No. 4" of the "BIRD'S EYE VIEW/OVERVIEW/ SYNOPSIS" of the Chapter.

4. How do you *manage* Neonatal Tetanus?
   Ans: Refer to the Evaluation-Decision-Action Plan/Algorithm to diagnose & manage Neonatal Tetanus.

5. Describe the pathogenesis of Neonatal Tetanus.
   Ans: Refer to the "No. 3" of the "BIRD'S EYE VIEW/OVERVIEW/ SYNOPSIS" of the Chapter.

LEARNING OBJECTIVES

After completing this article, readers will be able to:

1. Prevent Neonatal Tetanus from occurring by actively immunizing pregnant women, passively immunizing the Newborn of unimmunized mothers, aseptic management of umbilical cord at birth.

2. Diagnose Neonatal Tetanus promptly and institute appropriate general management.

3. Provide muscle relaxation along with assisted ventilation to improve the survival from Neonatal Tetanus.

4. Search for complications of Neonatal Tetanus and treat them promptly and effectively.

5. Ensure active immunization of survivors from Neonatal Tetanus.

Pearl/Peril/Pitfall: A significant level of immunity in mothers (and in infants after 6 weeks of age) can be achieved from vaccination with two doses of adsorbed tetanus toxoid given at least four weeks apart. The primary series of two doses should be reinforced by a third dose given 6 to 12 months later. The duration of immunity after three doses of tetanus toxoid is thought to be at least five years, with a total of five doses providing lifelong immunity.

BIRD`S EYE VIEW/OVERVIEW/SYNOPSIS

1. Neonatal(or Umbilical) Tetanus *(Tetanus Neonatorum),* though entirely preventable through active immunization of pregnant women with tetanus toxoid and by aseptic management of the umbilical cord at birth, still kills approximately 5 lachs of infants each year, with about 80% of deaths in just 12 tropical Asian and African countries. It occurs even in developed countries, among migrant workers, immigrants from developing world, and other patients with limited access to health care and nil/inadequate immunization against tetanus.

2. In rural India, the walls of the village houses are made of a mixture of earth and cowdung, and the ash of cowdung fires is used to dress the umbilical stump. Infection of the umbilical stump caused by septic management of the cord and harmful cultural practices are the main reasons for the high frequency of Neonatal Tetanus in rural communities in the tropics. Neonatal Tetanus is known as the "8-day disease" in the Punjab, because so many babies die of tetanus on the 8th day of life.

3. *Clostridium tetani*- a motile Gram-positive, spore-forming obligate anaerobe whose natural habitat worldwide is soil, dust, animal feces, though usually absent from human feces. Spores of *Cl.tetani* are highly resistant to heat, chemicals, and antibiotics, but can be destroyed if autoclaved. They can survive many years in dry dust or earth. During germination and growth in anaerobic conditions, the organism produces 2 toxins-tetanospasmin and tetanolysin. Unlike many clostridia, *Cl.tetani* is not a tissue-invasive organism and instead causes illness through its toxin the *tetanospasmin,* a potent exotoxin with high affinity for nervous tissue. *It is the 2nd most poisonous substance known, surpassed in potency only by Botulinum toxin.* Tetanus toxin binds at the neuromuscular junction and enters the motor nerve by endocytosis, after which it undergoes retrograde axonal transport to the cytoplasm of the alpha-motoneuron. The toxin exits the motoneuron in the spinal cord and next enters adjacent spinal inhibitory interneurons, where it prevents release of the neurotransmitters Glycine aminobutyric acid(GABA). This results in enhanced excitatory synaptic action and affected muscles sustain maximal contraction and cannot relax. Its action is similar to that of strychnine, inducing hypertonicity, spasms and seizures. The toxin also produces sympathetic overactivity, resulting in tachycardia, arrhythmias, labile hypertension, peripheral vasoconstriction, sweating, hypercarbia and increased urinary excretion of catecholamines. Tetanus Antitoxin (Human specific Tetanus immunoglobulin) can only neutralize unbound circulating toxin and has no effect on toxin fixed in nerve cells, but should be given as soon as possible in order to neutralize toxin that diffuses from the contaminated umbilicus into the circulation before the toxin can bind at distant muscle groups.

4. Most Neonatal Tetanus cases occur between 3 -10days after birth, though the incubation period is 3 days-3 weeks, the severity of the disease being greater with a shorter incubation period. The infant usually presents with difficulty in sucking (due to upper lip spasm), excessive irritability, restlessness and Trismus (the presenting sign in >50% of cases), caused by spasm of the masseter muscles. This is followed by stiffness of the neck muscles and difficulty in swallowing. Spasm of the facial muscles produces risus sardonicus. Tonic contractions of lumbar and abdominal musculature occur next, and result in opisthotonus in extension. This is accompanied by flexion and adduction of the arms and clenching of the fists. Spasms which initially last a few seconds become more prolonged, and may persist for minutes as the disease progresses. The Neonate is conscious and crying because of intense pain from muscle spasms that become more powerful. These spasms are easily precipitated by any tactile, visual or auditory stimulus. Fever is a feature, probably because of both rigidity and spasms of

muscles. Laryngeal and respiratory muscle spasms may lead to airway obstruction, asphyxia, and cyanosis. Tetanus is often fatal in the Neonate, with mortality as high as 50-90%. Broncho-pneumonia, aspiration pneumonia and atelectasis are common complications.When assisted ventilation and intensive care are available, the death rate can be substantially reduced. The natural history of tetanus is one of increasing severity during the 1st 7 days, followed by a plateau in the 2nd week and gradual abatement over the next 2–6 weeks. The umbilical stump may hold remnants of dirt, dung, clotted blood, or serum, or it may appear relatively benign.

5. *The Evaluation-Decision-Action- Plan/Algorithm* describes the essential aspects of the diagnosis and management, and prognosis of Neonatal Tetanus. Diagnosis is easy but meningitis, metabolic disorders such as Maple Syrup Urine Disease, infantile Gaucher`s disease and Di George`s syndrome with hypoparathyroidism must be considered, when predisposing factors for Neonatal Tetanus are absent and trismus is an isolated symptom without any associated stimulus provoked spasms of skeletal muscles. Management of Neonatal Tetanus is based on the provision of an adequate airway and ventilation, neutralization and elimination of toxins,prevention of spasms and convulsions and maintaining hydration and nutrition. The aim of treatment is to sustain the patient until the effects of toxins resolve.

6. General management includes skillful nursing care to prevent aspiration pneumonia and atelectasis, to minimize stimuli causing spasms, to control fever, and correction of fluid, electrolyte, and acid-base disturbances.

7. Human Tetanus Specific Immunoglobulin in a single dose of 250 IU/kg IV is sufficient to neutralize systemic tetanus toxin, but total doses as high as 3,000–6,000 IU are also recommended without proven benefit. The use of Intrathecal Human Tetanus Specific Immunoglobulin 250IU STAT appears to confer additional therapeutic benefit by bathing and travelling along with nerve roots to inactivate the toxin.There is no convincing evidence that periumbilical infiltration of antitoxin has a significant effect on the outcome of Neonatal Tetanus.

8. IV Penicillin G 1lakh units/kg/day in 4 divided doses for 10 days remains the antibiotic of choice to eliminate *Cl. tetani.* Concomitant infections should be treated with appropriate broad-spectrum antibiotics.

9. The mortality from Neonatal Tetanus has been strikingly reduced by the use of sedatives, muscle relaxants and Assisted Ventilation, and this approach should be used wherever the facilities to apply it available.

10. Neonatal Tetanus does not produce prolonged immunity and survivors require standard tetanus immunizations. Active immunization of pregnant women with 2 doses of Tetanus Toxoid, 0.5ml each, separated by 2 months affords excellent immunity.

Risk factors for tetanus *neonatorum*

1) Low anti-tetanus vaccination coverage in potential childbearing women; 2) Home birth assisted by a traditional midwife or other non-capacitated provider without appropriate tools and personnel; 3) Inappropriate prenatal care (and/or poorly qualified caregivers) in remote areas; 4) Early hospital discharge and insufficient infant and mother postpartum follow-up; 5) Insufficient hygienic care of the umbilical cord stump and the newborn;6) Low maternal education level; 7) Low family social and economic levels; 8) No access to health education

Measures that are considered essential for tetanus *neonatorum* prophylaxis and control

Health education and communication actions, Prenatal care, Vaccination, Birth care, Postpartum care

---

* *Pearl/Peril/Pitfall : Infants born to immune mothers acquire temporary immunity for about five months. However, if an infant is born less than 15 days after the mother's second or subsequent dose of tetanus toxoid, the infant will not be protected because the vaccine will not have had time to stimulate the production of antibodies.*

THE EVALUATION-DECISION-ACTION-PLAN/ALGORITHM FOR THE DIAGNOSIS AND MANAGEMENT OF *NEONATAL TETANUS*

SUBJECTIVE FINDINGS

Determine the incubation period, time of onset(appearance of symptoms to first generalized spasm), and the maternal immunization history.

Note the feeding difficulties, irritability, restless crying, spasms and seizures, apneic and blue episodes.

History of previously affected child-(as many as a third of Neonatal Tetanus cases occur in infants born to mothers of another affected child).

OBJECTIVE FINDINGS

Assess ABCDs and monitor CRT, O_2 sats, BP, core-peripheral temperature difference, RR, HR, central & peripheral pulses, urine output

Look for Trismus, Risus Sardonicus, flexion and adduction of the arms and clenching of fists +extension of legs in an Opisthotonic posture, Abdominal rigidity, hypo/hyperthermia, poor sucking & swallowing reflexes, conscious and irritable infant, hypo/hypertension, apneic episodes and central cyanosis, tendency of general spasms to get triggered by tactile, visual, or auditory stimuli.

Assess for complications, such as aspiration pneumonia, bronchopneumonia, asphyxia, atelectasis.

Examine the umbilicus for signs of omphalitis or fascitis and seek other possible entrance sites.

INVESTIGATIONS

Blood FBC, TC, DC, **Hct**, Platelets, CRP, Blood cultures, **ABG analysis, electrolytes,** calcium & magnesium, **blood sugar,** creatinine, BUN, coagulation profile.(for management purposes)

The Neonatal Tetanus is a clinical diagnosis, because of its most dramatic presentation; the typical setting is a Newborn baby born to an unimmunized mother who was injured(through septic umbilical cord management) within preceding 2 weeks, who presents with Trismus, other rigid muscles, and clear sensorium

---

NEONATAL TETANUS

Identify: Inborn error of Metabolism ◄

Note the worsening prognosis!

While no other disease clinically resembles full-blown Neonatal tetanus, there are a number of medical conditions that can display one or more similar clinical characteristics. The differential diagnosis should take into account causes of Neonatal convulsions. In general, there are three etiologic categories of Neonatal convulsions: • Congenital (cerebral anomalies); • Perinatal (complicated delivery, perinatal trauma and anoxia, or intracranial hemorrhage); and • Postnatal (infections and metabolic disorders). None of these conditions produce trismus as tetanus does.

POOR PROGNOSTIC FACTORS
* Onset of symptoms within 1st week of life *Interval between Trismus and onset of spasms of <48 hours *Presence and intensity of fever *Tachycardia *High frequency and greater severity and duration of muscular spasms of larynx *the number and duration of apneic episodes

Treat:
Assure Adequate Airway
Administer Sedation/Muscle Relaxant
Insert Nasogastric Tube
Minimize Stimulation
Administer HTIG
Administer Antibiotics Pending Culture Results

Consider:
Surgical consultation for debridement

Assess response

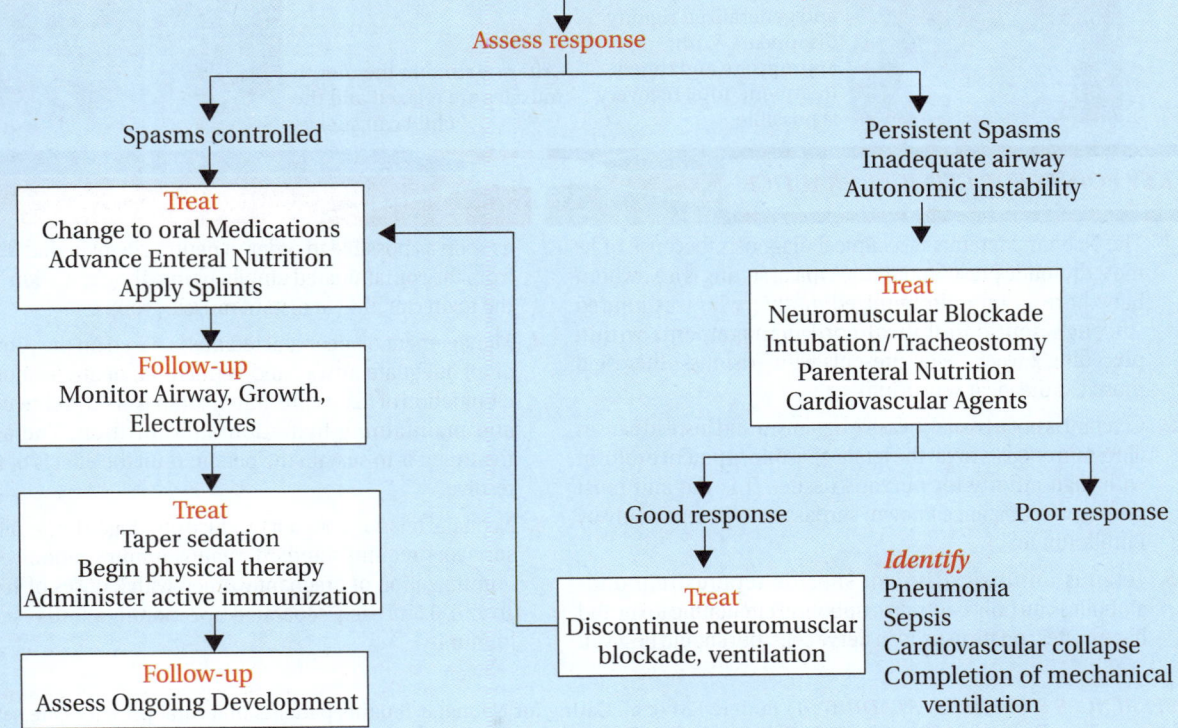

Spasms controlled

Treat
Change to oral Medications
Advance Enteral Nutrition
Apply Splints

Follow-up
Monitor Airway, Growth, Electrolytes

Treat
Taper sedation
Begin physical therapy
Administer active immunization

Follow-up
Assess Ongoing Development

Persistent Spasms
Inadequate airway
Autonomic instability

Treat
Neuromuscular Blockade
Intubation/Tracheostomy
Parenteral Nutrition
Cardiovascular Agents

Good response

Poor response

Treat
Discontinue neuromusclar blockade, ventilation

Identify
Pneumonia
Sepsis
Cardiovascular collapse
Completion of mechanical ventilation

---

*Pearl/Peril/Pitfall: *Trismus (a spasm of the masticatory muscles) apparently disturbs the proper movement of the lips that helps control sucking. The newborn becomes irritable and cries constantly. The mother may still manage to squeeze milk into the mouth or spoon-feed the infant, but the jaw's rigidity impedes swallowing.*

TABLE 1 Drugs used in treatment of neonatal tetanus

Passive immunization

- HTIG 500–6000 U IM (optimum therapeutic dose has not been established).

  IV immunoglobulin (dose not establish for this indication) Equine ATS 3000 IU IM in 2 divided doses.

Active immunization

- Diphtheria-tetanus-pertussis vaccine 0.5 ml IM (to age 5yr) Diphtheria-tetanus vaccine 0.5 ml IM (age 5 yr-adult).

Antibiotics

- Penicillin G 100,000 U/kg/24 hr IV in 4-6 divided doses for 10–14 days.

  Procaine penicillin 50,000 U/kg/day IM q24h to complete 10–14 days.

  Ampicillin 100 mg/kg/24 hr IM or IV in 4 divided doses.

  Gentamicin 7.5 mg/kg/24 hr IM or IV in 3 divided doses .

  Metronidazole 30 mg/kg/24 hr IM or IV in 3–4 divided doses.

Sedatives, Muscle relaxants

- Diazepam 0.2–0.8 mg/kg/24 hr PO in 3 or 4 divided doses up to 2.5-5 mg PO t.i.d.-q.i.d. for maintenance muscle relaxation. 0.25 mg/kg/dose IV q15 min for 2–3 doses for emergent control of spasms.
  Midazolam 0.1-0.2 mg/kg IV loading dose followed by continuous infusion of 2 µg/kg/min (titrate 0.4-6 µg/kg/min to achieve desired effect) for conscious sedation during mechanical ventilation.
  Phenobarbital 6-10 mg/kg/24 hr PO in 3-4 divided doses
  Vecuronium 0.1 mg/kg/ IV for intubation.
  Pancuronium 0.03-0.1 mg/kg IV q30-60min p.r.n. movement during mechanical ventilation.

Cardiovascular agents

  Dopamine 5–20 µg/kg/min continuous IV infusion.
  Esmolol 500 µg/kg/min loading dose IV over 1 min, followed by continuous infusion of 50–200 µg/kg/min.
  Labetalol 50-100 µg/kg/hr continuous IV infusion (not approved for infants).

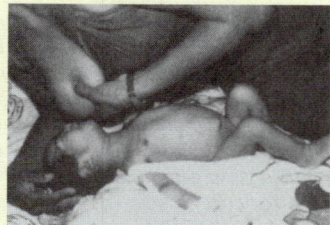

Difficulty sucking due to spasms of the oral (masticating) muscles is often the first sign of Neonatal tetanus

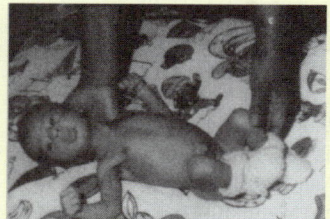

The child shows the first symptoms of widespread rigidity and trismus. Lips are pursed and the eyebrows are arched.

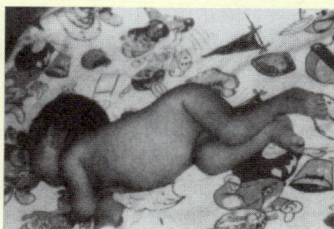

Opisthotonos (arched back) caused by spasms of the spinal muscles. Spasms become more frequent as the disease advances.

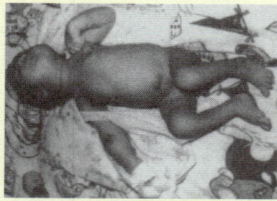

Spasms gradually cease and generalized rigidity disappears. With appropriate and timely treatment, total recovery is possible.

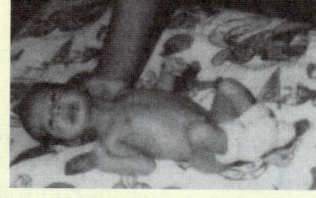

After treatment, the mouth muscles are relaxed and the child can suckle.

KEY POINTS FOR CLINICAL PRACTICE

1. The Neonatal tetanus is a clinical diagnosis, because of its most dramatic presentation;the typical setting is a Newborn baby born to an unimmunized mother who was injured (through septic umbilical cord management) within preceding 2 weeks, who presents with Trismus, other rigid muscles, and clear sensorium.

2. Cl.tetani is not a tissue-invasive organism and instead causes illness through its toxin the tetanospasmin, a potent exotoxin with high affinity for nervous tissue.. It is the 2nd most poisonous substance known, surpassed in potency only by Botulinum toxin.

3. Tetanus antitoxin (Human specific tetanus immuno-globulin) can only neutralize unbound circulating toxin and has no effect on toxin fixed in nerve cells, but should be given as soon as possible in order to neutralize toxin that diffuses from the contaminated umbilicus into the circulation before the toxin can bind at distant muscle groups.

4. Management of neonatal tetanus is based on the provision of an adequate airway and ventilation, neutralization and elimination of toxins,prevention of spasms and convulsions and maintaining hydration and nutrition. The aim of treatment is to sustain the patient until the effects of toxins resolve.

5. Neonatal tetanus does not produce prolonged immunity and survivors require standard tetanus immunizations. Active immunization of pregnant women with 2 doses of Tetanus Toxoid, 0.5ml each, separated by 2 months affords excellent immunity.

REFERENCES & FURTHER READING : 1) Einterz EM et al. Caring for Neonatal Tetanus patients in a rural primary care setting in Nigeria. J Trop Pediatrics 1991;37:179 2) Roberton`s Text Book of Neonatology ,4th Edition 3) Nelson Text Book of Pediatrics, 18th edition 4) Neonatal Tetanus Elimination Field Guide 2nd Edition 2005.

* *Pearl/Peril/Pitfall : Neonatal Tetanus- The child can die of apnea or serious anoxia during the spasms, or two to four days later due to acute gastroenteritis or complications from difficulty in swallowing that lead to pneumonia.*

96 Neonatal Conjunctivitis

@ *"Infants with a potentially sexually transmitted disease, such as gonorrhea or chlamydia, should undergo evaluation for other sexually transmitted diseases, such as syphilis and HIV, as should the mother and her sexual partner(s).*

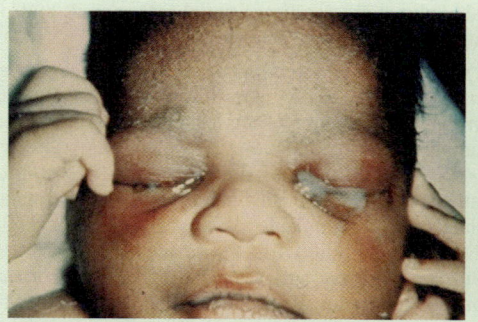

Severe purulent discharge and eyelid edema in a Newborn with gonococcal conjunctivitis (confirmed with Gram stain and culture)

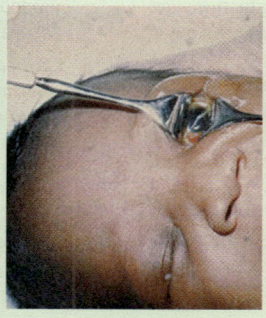

Cloudy cornea without ulcer in neonatal gonococcal conjunctivitis.

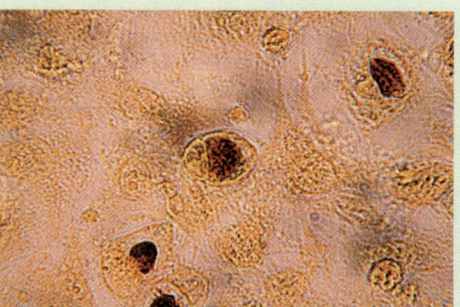

Chlamydia

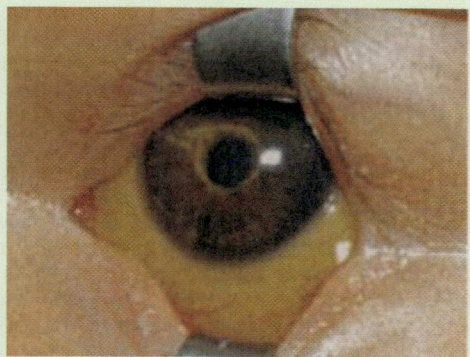

Pseudomonas aeruginosa endophthalmitis in a Neonate, showing a whitish ring around the pupil consistent with hypopyon material lying on the iris in the supine patient.

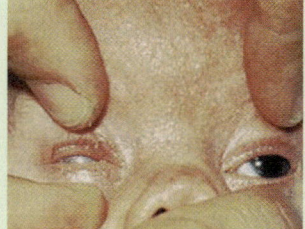

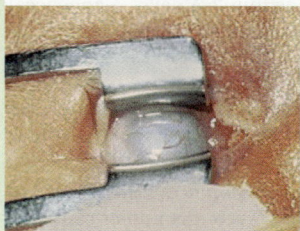

Pseudomonas aeruginosa endophthalmitis may be a devastating disease if not recognized and treated appropriately, especially in premature infants:

Appearance of both eyes at age 3 months showing small phthisical right eye with opaque vascularized scarred cornea.
-**Courtesy:H Gaili, G H A Woodruff**

REVIEW OF CLINICAL PROBLEMS

1. Describe the clinical presentation of Gonococcal Neonatal conjunctivitis.
   Ans: Refer to the "No. 4" of the "BIRD`S EYE VIEW/OVERVIEW/ SYNOPSIS" of the Chapter.
2. How do you diagnose and manage Chlamydial Neonatal conjunctivitis?
   Ans: Refer to the Evaluation-Decision-Action Plan/Algorithm to diagnose & manage Neonatal Conjunctivitis.
3. What are Medicolegal pitfalls in dealing with Neonatal Conjunctivitis?
   Ans: Refer to the "No. 8" of the "BIRD`S EYE VIEW/OVERVIEW/ SYNOPSIS" of the Chapter.
4. Name the Systemic complications of Neonatal Conjunctivitis.
   Ans: Refer to the Evaluation-Decision-Action Plan/Algorithm to diagnose & manage a Neonatal Conjunctivitis.
5. When should you consult an ophthalmic surgeon, while managing Neonatal Conjunctivitis ?
   Ans: Refer to the Evaluation-Decision-Action Plan/Algorithm to diagnose & manage a Neonatal Conjunctivitis.

LEARNING OBJECTIVES

After completing this article, readers will be able to:

1. Provide adequate and prompt prophylaxis against Neonatal Conjunctivitis.

2. Diagnose Neonatal Conjunctivitis by clinical presentation and to confirm with Gram stain, Giemsa stain and cultures of conjunctiva, where indicated.

3. Identify *life/sight threatening* complications/mimicking conditions and refer to an eye specialist, promptly.

4. Treat Neonatal Conjunctivitis timely and effectively.

5. Search for other STD in the mother and her sexual partner (s), and treat them promptly.

---

* *Pearl/Peril/Pitfall : Gonorrheal ophthalmia produces an acute purulent conjunctivitis that appears 2 to 5 days after birth or earlier with premature rupture of membranes. The neonate has severe eyelid edema followed by chemosis and a profuse purulent exudate that may be under pressure. If untreated, corneal ulcerations and blindness may occur. Conjunctivitis caused by other bacteria has a variable onset, ranging from 4 days to several weeks. Herpetic keratoconjunctivitis can occur as an isolated infection or with disseminated or CNS infection. It can be mistaken for bacterial or chemical conjunctivitis, but the presence of dendritic keratitis is pathognomonic.*

BIRD'S EYE VIEW/OVERVIEW/SYNOPSIS

1. By definition, Neonatal conjunctivitis presents during the first month of life and may be aseptic or septic. Aseptic Neonatal conjunctivitis most often is a chemical conjunctivitis that is induced by silver nitrate solution, which is used for prophylaxis of infectious conjunctivitis. Chemical conjunctivitis is not as common any more because of the use of erythromycin ointment in place of silver nitrate solution for the prophylaxis of infectious conjunctivitis. Bacterial, chlamydial, and viral infections are major causes of septic Neonatal conjunctivitis, *Chlamydia* being the most common infectious agent. Infants may acquire these infective agents as they pass through the birth canal during the birth process. The pathology of Neonatal conjunctivitis is influenced by the anatomy of the conjunctival tissues in the Newborn. The inflammation of conjunctiva may cause blood vessel dilation, chemosis, and excessive secretion. This reaction tends to be more serious due to the following: lack of immunity, absence of lymphoid tissue in the conjunctiva, and absence of tears at birth.

2. The epidemiology of Neonatal conjunctivitis has changed since silver nitrate solution was introduced to prevent gonococcal ophthalmia. *Chlamydia* has been reported as the most common infectious agent that causes ophthalmia neonatorum. In contrast, the incidence of gonococcal ophthalmia neonatorum has been reduced dramatically, from 100 per 1000 live births to 3 per 1000 live births. Antibiotics have significantly altered the prognosis of Neonatal conjunctivitis, especially with *Neisseria gonorrhoeae* infection.

3. Although clinical presentations vary with etiology, it is difficult to determine the exact cause of neonatal conjunctivitis on clinical grounds alone. Significant overlap in clinic presentations may be present. Chemical conjunctivitis secondary to silver nitrate solution application usually occurs in the first day of life, disappearing spontaneously within 2–4 days. Gonococcal conjunctivitis tends to occur 3–5 days after birth but can present later. Chlamydial conjunctivitis usually has a later onset than gonococcal conjunctivitis; the incubation period is 5–14 days. The incubation period for other nongonococcal, nonchlamydial conjunctivitis is longer, according to a previous report. Herpetic conjunctivitis usually occurs within the first 2 weeks after birth.

4. *Clinical presentation of Gonococcal conjunctivitis :* Gonococcal conjunctivitis tends to be more severe than other causes of ophthalmia neonatorum; there is a classic presentation of purulent conjunctivitis, which usually is bilateral. Corneal involvement has been reported, including diffuse epithelial edema and ulceration that may progress to perforation of the cornea and endophthalmitis. Patients also may have systemic manifestations (e.g., rhinitis, stomatitis, arthritis, meningitis, anorectal infection, septicemia). This type of conjunctivitis is the most serious, usually occurring 24-48 hours following birth. Typically, patients develop a hyperacute conjunctivitis, associated with marked lid edema, chemosis, and purulent discharge. A conjunctival membrane may be present. Corneal ulcer may occur and rapidly progress to perforation, if treatment is delayed. *Gonorrheal conjunctivitis must be absolutely excluded in every case of Neonatal conjunctivitis to avoid serious consequences.*

5. *Chlamydial conjunctivitis :* The presentation of chlamydial conjunctivitis may range from mild hyperemia with scant mucoid discharge to eyelid swelling, chemosis, and pseudomembrane formation. Blindness, although rare and much slower to develop than in gonococcal conjunctivitis, is not due to corneal involvement as in gonococcal conjunctivitis; eyelid scarring and pannus (as in trachoma) cause it. A follicular reaction does not occur because newborns have no requisite lymphoid tissue present in the conjunctiva. Like gonococcal conjunctivitis, chlamydial conjunctivitis also may be associated with extraocular involvement, including pneumonitis, otitis, and pharyngeal and rectal colonization. Patients typically present with unilateral or bilateral watery discharge, which may become more copious and purulent later. Although most cases are mild and self-limited, it occasionally may be severe. Pseudomembranes, thickened palpebral conjunctiva, significant peripheral pannus, and/or corneal opacification may be present.

6. *Clinical presentation of Neonatal conjunctivitis due to other bacterial agents :* usually is milder. *Herpes simplex keratoconjunctivitis* usually presents in infants with generalized herpes simplex with corneal epithelial involvement or vesicles on the skin (which surround the eye). Serious systemic complications, such as encephalitis, may occur in these Neonates due to their poor immunologic response. Although it rarely causes Neonatal conjunctivitis, *Pseudomonas* can lead to devastating consequences, such as rapid progression to corneal ulceration and perforation; if left untreated, it even can lead to endophthalmitis and subsequent death. *Herpetic conjunctivitis* This type typically occurs within the first 2 weeks after birth. Ocular involvement may follow systemic herpes infection or vesicular lesions on the skin or lid margins. Patients may present with nonspecific lid edema, moderate conjunctival injection, and nonpurulent and often serosanguinous discharge, which may be unilateral or bilateral. Microdendrites or geographic ulcers, rather than typical dendrites as seen in adults, are the most typical signs of herpetic keratitis in Newborns. Conjunctival membrane may be present.

7. *The Evaluation-Decision-Action- Plan/Algorithm* describes the essential aspects of the diagnosis and management of Neonatal Conjunctivitis. Laboratory studies for Neonatal conjunctivitis should include the following: Conjunctival scraping Gram stain and either Giemsa or calcofluor white stains, Culture on chocolate agar and/or Thayer-Martin for *N gonorrhoeae* Culture on blood agar for other bacteria. Rule out chlamydial infection with a conjunctival scraping Giemsa stain for intracytoplasmic inclusion bodies or, preferably, a direct immunofluorescent antibody assay. A culture for HSV is indicated if a corneal epithelial defect is present or if vesicles are present on the eyelids or other parts of the body, and if the diagnosis cannot be made on ocular examination.

8. *Medicolegal pitfalls:* include; *Failure to recognize or treat gonococcal conjunctivitis *Failure to provide preventive measures in Newborns *Failure to exclude other potential causes of acute red eye (e.g. preseptal cellulitis, orbital cellulitis).

9. *Special concerns:* *Consider the risk of transmission of chlamydia, gonococcus, herpes, and streptococcus to the fetus during the birth process. Obtain cervical cultures (if indicated), and manage appropriately. *Newborns with conjunctivitis are at risk for secondary infections, such as pneumonia, meningitis, and septicemia, which can lead to sepsis and death. *Infants with a potentially sexually transmitted disease, such as gonorrhea or chlamydia, should undergo evaluation for other sexually transmitted diseases, such as syphilis and HIV, as should the mother and her sexual partner(s).

10. *If untreated, corneal ulceration may occur in *N gonorrhoeae* infection and rapidly progress to corneal perforation. *When unrecognized and not immediately treated, *Pseudomonas* infection may lead to endophthalmitis and subsequent death. *Pneumonia has been reported in 10-20% of infants with chlamydial conjunctivitis. Neonatal conjunctivitis usually responds to appropriate treatment, and the prognosis generally is good.

---

* *Pearl/Peril/Pitfall : Chemical conjunctivitis secondary to silver nitrate usually appears within 6 to 8 h after instillation and disappears spontaneously within 48 to 96 h. Chlamydial ophthalmia usually occurs 5 to 14 days after birth. It may range from mild conjunctivitis with minimal mucopurulent discharge to severe eyelid edema with copious drainage and pseudomembrane formation. Follicles are not present in the conjunctiva, as they are in older children and adults.*

THE EVALUATION-DECISION-ACTION-PLAN/ALGORITHM FOR THE DIAGNOSIS AND MANAGEMENT OF *NEONATAL CONJUNCTIVITIS*.

SUBJECTIVE FINDINGS

History of **onset, duration severity of** symptoms such as mild, transient tearing and conjunctival injection,unilateral or bilateral watery discharge, which may become more copious and purulent later, systemic symptoms suggestive of sepsis, pneumonia and meningitis.

History of STD in the family? **Maternal history:** sexually transmitted diseases or exposure, results of high vaginal, cervical and urethral swabs in pregnancy, length of labor and duration of membrane rupture.

Newborns with conjunctivitis are at risk for secondary infections, such as pneumonia, meningitis, and septicemia, which can lead to sepsis and death.

OBJECTIVE FINDINGS

Assess Conjunctival erythema, Purulent discharge, Lid edema,chemosis,conjunctival membrane, Corneal ulcer,nonpurulent and often serosanguinous discharge, which may be unilateral or bilateral. *Look for* involvement of any other system, e.g. herpes vesicles, infected scalp pH site.

Identify the common differentiating features of Neonatal conjunctivitis/ eye discharge-*v.i*

Look for renal, hepatic, pulmonary, or CNS manifestations which may accompany conjunctivitis. *Determine* the *degree of illness-*asymptomatic/mild/moderate to severe and *duration of illness.* Suspect *congenital glaucoma ,if corneal clouding or proptosis, is associated with portwine stains in the ophthalmic region.*

INVESTIGATIONS

Laboratory studies for Neonatal conjunctivitis should include the following: Conjunctival scraping Gram stain and either Giemsa or calcofluor white stains Culture on chocolate agar and/or Thayer-Martin for *N gonorrhoeae* Culture on blood agar for other bacteria.

Rule out chlamydial infection with a conjunctival scraping Giemsa stain for intracytoplasmic inclusion bodies or, preferably, a direct immunofluorescent antibody assay. A culture for HSV is indicated if a corneal epithelial defect is present or if vesicles are present on the eyelids or other parts of the body, and if the diagnosis cannot be made on ocular examination.

Consider the risk of transmission of chlamydia, gonococcus, herpes, and streptococcus to the fetus during the birth process. Obtain cervical cultures (if indicated), and manage appropriately.

Neonatal Conjunctivitis

Identify **Sticky eyes**(clear /white discharge small in amount without inflammatory signs, innocuous), **nasolacrimal duct obstruction**(unilateral clear discharge without signs of inflammation), and **Chemical conjunctivitis** (usually occurs in the first day of life,mild, (transient tearing and conjunctival injection) disappearing spontaneously within 2-4 days.)- sterile on Gram stain and culture.

Differentiate from other serious causes of red eye-preseptal cellulitis/orbital cellulitis; *d/w* an ophthalmic surgeon, if suspected.

Beware of Pseudomonal Conjunctivitis, though rare- which can lead to devastating consequences, such as rapid progression to corneal ulceration and perforation; if left untreated, it even can lead to endophthalmitis and subsequent death; *if Gram stain finds Gram -ve bacilli, seriously consider Pseudomonas and consider sepsis screen and parenteral anti-Pseudomonal antibiotics.*

Identify Chlamydial pneumonia, systemic complications of bacterial/viral conjunctivitis-such as sepsis, meningoencephalitis, pneumonia,arthritis etc., and Consult an ophthalmologist if a congenital glaucoma is suspected .

History + PE+ Conjunctival Gram Stain + Culture + Giemsa stain for intracytoplasmic inclusion bodies of Chlamydiae + preferably, a rapid direct immunofluorescent antibody

---

Gonococcal conjunctivitis : the most serious, usually occurring 24-48 hours following birth. Typically, patients develop a hyperacute conjunctivitis, associated with marked lid edema, chemosis, and purulent discharge. A conjunctival membrane may be present. Corneal ulcer may occur and rapidly progress to perforation, if treatment is delayed *gram-negative diplococcus neutrophils on Gram stain*

* *Give a single dose of IV Ceftriaxone 25-50mg/kg, not to exceed 125mg and Clean eyes using sterile saline irrigation*
* *Admit and evaluate for Gonococcal invasive complications such as sepsis, meningitis, arthritis, etc.,*
* *Screen the infant and the mother and her sexual partner for Chlamydial and other STD ; Treat accordingly!*

Chlamydial conjunctivitis : Patients typically present with unilateral or bi-lateral watery /yellow discharge, which may become more copious and puru-lent later, eye lid swelling 5-14 days af-ter birth.
Although most cases are mild and self limited, it occasionally may be severe. Pseudomembranes, thickened palpe-bral conjunctiva, significant peripheral pannus, and or corneal opacification may be present. *Chlamydial conjunc-tivitis—Neutrophils, lymphocytes, plasma cells on Gram stain; basophilic intracytoplasmic inclusions in epithe-lial cells on Giemsa stain*
10–20% will develop pneumonia

* *Treat with Oral Erythromycin 50 mg/ kg/d PO divided qid for 14 d 0.5% ophthalmic ointment: Apply 0.5-1 cm to each conjunctival sac tid/qid for 3 wk;topical treatment is not adequate and unnecessary, when systemic therapy is given.*
* *Screen the mother and her partner for STD and treat appropriately.*

Herpetic conjunctivitis : This type typically occurs within the first 2 weeks after birth. Ocular involvement may follow systemic herpes infection or vesicular lesions on the skin or lid margins. Patients may present with nonspecific lid edema, moderate conjunctival injection, and nonpurulent and often serosanguinous discharge, which may be unilateral or bilateral. Microdendrites or geographic ulcers, rather than typical dendrites as seen in adults, are the most typical signs of her-petic keratitis in Newborns. Conjunctival membrane may be present. *Herpetic conjunctivitis—Lymphocytes, plasma cells, multinucleate giant cells on Gram stain; eosinophilic intranuclear inclusions in epi-thelial cells on Papanicolaou smear*

*Therapy of viral infections begins with me-chanical debridement of the involved rim along with a rim of normal epithelium. This is followed by the topical instillation of anti-viral medications such as vidarabine, trifluridine, and acyclovir *Oral Acyclovir 30mg/kg/day in 3divided doses for 10-14 days provides faster resolution and may prevent recurrent outbreaks.*

Other bacterial conjunctivi-tis: Various organisms (e.g. gram-positive and gram-negative bacteria) have been identified.
Classic clinical pictures are lid edema, conjunctival in-jection, chemosis, and dis-charge, which are variable and often indistinguishable from signs of other etiologies. The most commonly identi-fied gram-positive organisms include *Staphylococcus au-reus, Streptococcus pneumo-niae, Streptococcus viridans,* and *Staphylococcus epider-midis.* Gram-negative organ-isms, such as *Escherichia coli, Klebsiella pneumoniae, Ser-ratia marcescens,* and *Pro-teus, Enterobacter* have been implicated.

*Treat with topical erythro-mycin/soframycin/gentami-cin

---

* ***Pearl/Peril/Pitfall:*** *A neonate with gonorrheal ophthalmia is hospitalized to observe for possible systemic gonococcal infection and given a single dose of ceftriaxone 25 to 50 mg/kg IM to a maximum dose of 125 mg (some clinicians use 100 mg/kg). Frequent saline irrigation of the eye prevents secretions from adhering. Topical antimicrobial ointments alone are ineffective.*

OPHTHALMIC *PSEUDOMONAS* INFECTION IN INFANCY

Endogenous endophthalmitis results from hematogenous spread to the eye secondary to septicemia. In exogenous endophthalmitis, the infection develops initially in the eye as a result of corneal infection, perforating injury, or intraocular surgery. Diagnosis is confirmed by microscopy and culture of aspirated vitreous fluid. Culture of the purulent discharge is useful but less reliable in identifying the causative organism, being found in only two of our four cases. Nevertheless, growth of *P aeruginosa* from discharge from an eye in a sick child should alert the clinician to the risk of a sight threatening and life threatening illness. The most appropriate treatment for endophthalmitis is a combination of intravenous cephalosporin and aminoglycoside, for example, ceftazidime 50 mg/kg every 12 hours and gentamicin 4 mg/kg every 24 hours. As intraocular accumulation of intravenous antibiotics is poor, the use of intravitreal antibiotics is essential—for example, ceftazidime 2.25 mg in 0.1 ml. Topical treatment may be used, but not as sole treatment. Morbidity and mortality in pseudomonal endophthalmitis are high despite early diagnosis. For survivors, the usual result is blindness of the affected eye, with enucleation sometimes being necessary. **Key messages:** * Loss of red reflex, a change in the appearance of the iris, or purulent eye discharge can be clues to a life threatening ocular and systemic infection * Bilateral endophthalmitis can complicate neonatal pseudomonal septicemia, and is a grave prognostic sign for survival *Treatment of neonatal endophthalmitis should include intravitreal and intravenous antibiotics.

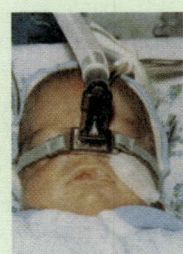 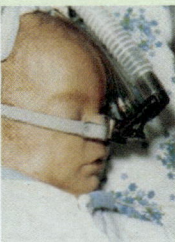

Serious eye infection due to *Ps aeruginosa* is usually a complication of injury to the corneal epithelium. This injury may be due to trauma, exposure, or any process that may damage the corneal epithelium, which is normally resistant to bacterial invasion. Neonates are unable to complain of eye pain or decreasing vision, making early diagnosis and treatment more difficult. It is important to avoid injuring the cornea when using nasal CPAP and that it is essential to ensure correct positioning of the fixation straps to avoid such injury. When *Pseudomonas* is isolated within a neonatal unit, prompt diagnosis of any sticky eye is indicated. Gram staining of the discharge should be performed urgently and swabs obtained for culture. As *Pseudomonas* spreads easily, both patient isolation and strict handwashing are indicated.

Demonstration (in another child) of possible mechanism for cornea injury by inappropriate placement of fixing straps of Infant Flow Driver nasal continuous positive airway pressure.

Courtesy: Exogenous Pseudomonas endophthalmitis: a cause of lens enucleation H Gaili, G H A Woodruff Arch Dis Child Fetal Neonatal Ed 2002;86:F204–F206

NEONATAL CONJUNCTIVITIS

Onset after Birth	Etiology	Pearl
< 24 hours	Chemical (e.g. silver nitrate prophylaxis)	Disappears within 2 to 4 days
2–4 days	Neisseria gonorrhoeae	Medical emergency due to corneal involvement and threat to vision
4–7 days	Staphylococcus aureus, Group B streptococcus, Streptococcus pneumoniae, Pseudomonas aeruginosa	
4–10 days	Chlamydia trachomatis	Treat with oral erythromycin
5–10 days	Haemophilus influenzae	Frequently hemorrhagic
6–14 days	Herpes simplex virus	Usually unilateral

KEY POINTS FOR CLINICAL PRACTICE:

1. Gonorrheal conjunctivitis must be absolutely excluded in every case of Neonatal conjunctivitis to avoid serious consequences. Corneal ulcer may occur and rapidly progress to perforation, if treatment is delayed.

2. Identify Chlamydial pneumonia, systemic complications of bacterial/viral conjunctivitis-such as sepsis, meningoencephalitis, pneumonia, arthritis, etc. and *Consult an ophthalmologist if a congenital glaucoma is suspected* .

3. Consider the risk of transmission of chlamydia, gonococcus, herpes, and streptococcus to the fetus during the birth process. Obtain cervical cultures (if indicated), and manage appropriately.

4. Infants with a potentially sexually transmitted disease, such as gonorrhea or chlamydia, should undergo evaluation for other sexually transmitted diseases, such as syphilis and HIV, as should the mother and her sexual partner(s).

5. ***Differentiate*** from other serious causes of red eye-preseptal cellulitis/orbital cellulitis; *d/w* an ophthalmic surgeon, if suspected.

REFERENCES & FURTHER READING : 1) de Toledo AR, Chandler JW. Conjunctivitis of the newborn. *Infect Dis Clin North Am*. Dec 1992;6(4):807-13.. 2) Fransen L, Klauss V. Neonatal ophthalmia in the developing world. Epidemiology, etiology, management and control. *Int Ophthalmol*. Jan 1988;11(3):189-96. 3) Rapoza PA, Chandler JW. *Neonatal conjunctivitis: diagnosis and treatment. American Academy of Ophthalmology: Focal Points*. Vol 1. 1988:1-11. 4) O'Hara MA. Ophthalmia neonatorum. *Pediatr Clin North Am*. Aug 1993;40(4):715-25. 5)Hammerschlag MR. Neonatal conjunctivitis. *Pediatr Ann*. Jun 1993;22(6):346-51.

* ***Pearl/Peril/Pitfall :*** *Conjunctival material is Gram stained, cultured for gonorrhea (e.g., on modified Thayer-Martin medium), and tested for chlamydia (e.g., by direct immunofluorescence, enzyme-linked immunosorbent assay, nucleic acid amplification techniques—samples must contain cells). Conjunctival scrapings can also be examined with Giemsa stain; if blue intracytoplasmic inclusions are identified, chlamydial ophthalmia is confirmed. Viral culture is obtained only if viral infection is suspected by skin lesions or maternal infection.*

97 Staphylococcal Scalded Skin Syndrome (SSSS)

@ *Staphylococcal scalded skin syndrome (SSSS) is the clinical term used for a spectrum of blistering skin diseases induced by the exfoliative (epidermolytic) toxins (ET) of Staphylococcus aureus. Current synonyms include Ritter's disease, bullous impetigo, pemphigus neonatorum, and staphylococcal scarlatiniform rash. It seems that the location of lesions depends on age. In neonates, the lesions are mostly found on the perineum or periumbilically, or both, while the extremities are more commonly affected in older children.*

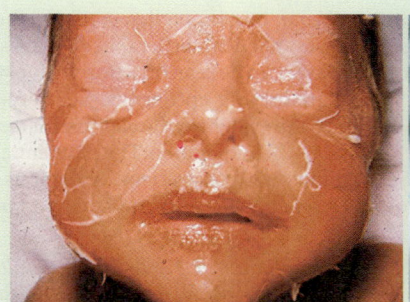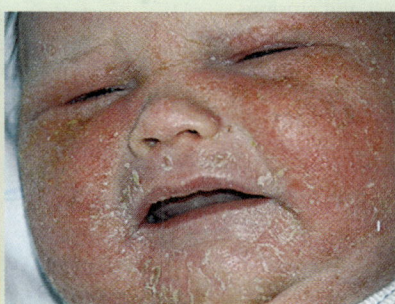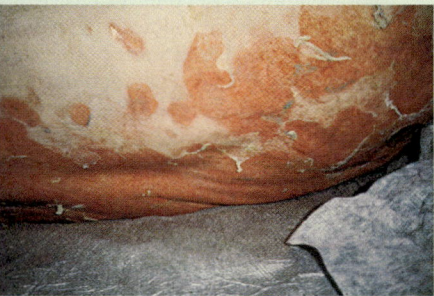

STAPHYLOCOCCAL SCALDED SKIN SYNDROME

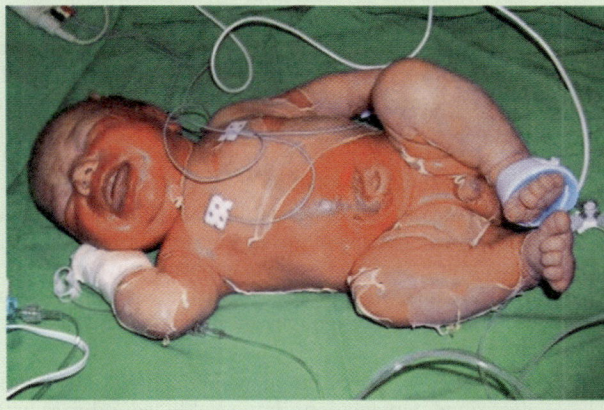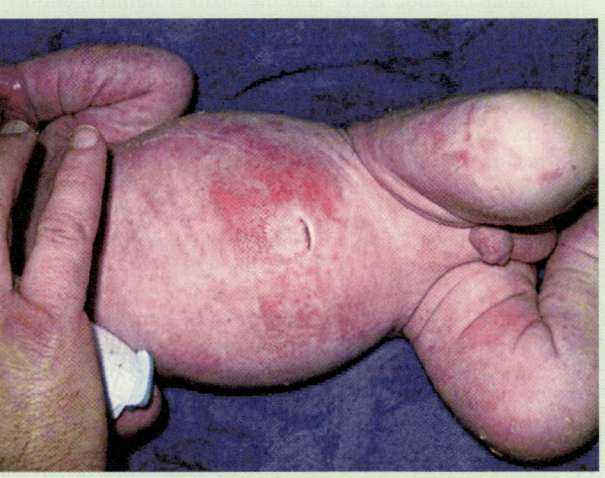

SSSS though looks ghastly during acute stage (Picture on Lt side) usually heals completely, without leaving scar (Picture on Rt side)

REVIEW OF CLINICAL PROBLEMS

1. Describe the clinical presentation of Staphylococcal Scalded Skin Syndrome ?
   Ans: Refer to the "No. 1" of the "BIRD'S EYE VIEW/OVERVIEW/ SYNOPSIS" of the Chapter.

2. How do you differentiate SSSS from Toxic Epidermal Necrolysis ?
   Ans: Refer to the "No. 4" of the "BIRD`S EYE VIEW/OVERVIEW/ SYNOPSIS" of the Chapter.

3. How do you manage SSSS ?
   Ans: Refer to the Evaluation-Decision-Action Plan/Algorithm to diagnose & manage a Neonate with SSSS.

4. Name the Systemic complications of Neonatal SSSS.
   Ans: Refer to the "No. 7" of the "BIRD`S EYE VIEW/OVERVIEW/ SYNOPSIS" of the Chapter.

5. What preventive measures should you take to control the Nursery/Hospital outbreaks of SSSS?
   Ans: Refer to the "No. 10 " of the "BIRD'S EYE VIEW/OVERVIEW/ SYNOPSIS" of the Chapter.

LEARNING OBJECTIVES

After completing this article, readers will be able to:

1. Diagnose Staphylococcal Scalded Skin Syndrome promptly by its typical clinical features.

2. Differentiate SSSS from the closely mimicking conditions like Toxic Epidermal Necrolysis, bullous impetigo, epidermolysis bullosa, pemphigus, drug eruption, erythema multiforme.

3. Identify complications of SSSS, such as dehydration, sepsis, pneumonia, hypothermia, and shock and manage them effectively.

4. Treat SSSS with a penicillinase-resistant synthetic penicillin (e.g. nafcillin)/Vancomycin, if MRSA is suspected.

5. Identify and treat asymptomatic carriers .

* *Pearl/Peril/Pitfall: The form and severity of SSSS will vary with the route of delivery of the toxin to the skin, ranging from the legalized bullous impetigo to generalized SSSS involving the entire skin surface. In the latter, patients are susceptible to poor temperature control, extensive fluid losses, and secondary infections. They may also develop sepsis and present with hypotension, neutropenia, and respiratory distress.*

BIRD'S EYE VIEW/OVERVIEW/SYNOPSIS

1. **Staphylococcal Scalded Skin Syndrome (SSSS)** also known as Ritter von Ritterschein disease (in Newborns), Ritter disease, and staphylococcal epidermal necrolysis, occurs in Neonates, infants and children < 5 year of age, caused by exfoliative toxin-producing strains of *S. aureus* (Phage group II, types 71 & 55) and *present with* abrupt onset of fever, irritability, and tender erythema of the skin, most marked in flexural areas and around the mouth and nose. Within 12–24 hours, extensive blisters and erosions form and may be followed by widespread superficial peeling of the skin in sheets, especially in Neonates and infants. Superficial separation of the skin after rubbing (Nikolsky sign) is present. Subsequent denudation of the skin with a moist, glistening, red surface at sites of prior blistering may lead to significant cutaneous fluid losses and secondary infection with resulting sepsis. The mucosal surfaces are spared. Older children may present with more mild forms of SSSS, with more localization of lesions and less toxicity.

2. Patients with SSSS usually have a primary infection at sites other than the skin, such as the nasopharynx, conjunctiva, throat, or middle ear, and the toxin is hematogenously disseminated . The clinical features of SSSS are related to cleavage of the epidermis in a superficial location, beneath stratum corneum or stratum granulosum. The increased susceptibility of infants may be related to immature mechanisms of renal clearance of the toxin. *Predisposing factors in older children and adults, in whom SSSS is rare, include renal failure, immunosuppression, and HIV I infection.* Staphylococcal scalded skin syndrome differs from bullous impetigo. Both are blistering skin diseases caused by staphylococcal exfoliative toxin. However, in bullous impetigo, the exfoliative toxins are restricted to the area of infection, and bacteria can be cultured from the blister contents. In staphylococcal scalded skin syndrome, the exfoliative toxins are spread hematogenously from a localized source potentially causing epidermal damage at distant sites

3. The desquamative phase begins after 2–5 days of cutaneous erythema ; healing occurs without scarring in 10-14 days. Patients may have pharyngitis, conjunctivitis, and superficial erosions of the lips, but intraoral mucosal surfaces are spared. Although some patients appear ill, many are reasonably comfortable except for the marked skin tenderness.

4. *SSSS must be distinguished from Toxic Epidermal Necrolysis (TEN).* TEN can often be distinguished by a history of drugs ingestion, the presence of Nikolsky sign only at sites of erythema, absence of perioral crusting , full-thickness epidermal necrosis, and blister cleavage plane in the lower most epidermis(at the level of basement membrane). SSSS should also be distinguished from other exanthems like Streptococcal Scarlet fever, Kawasaki disease, toxic shock syndrome, Measles, Roseola, erythema infectiosum, and a number of other blistering and exfoliating disorders including bullous impetigo, epidermolysis bullosa, pemphigus, drug eruption, erythema multiforme. In most cases the history, clinical presentation and physical examination aid in the differentiation of SSSS from these entities. (Refer to Table No. 1) Skin biopsy reveals a split in the superficial epidermis in SSSS, versus, full-thickness epidermal necrosis, and subepidermal blister formation in TEN. An inflammatory cell infiltrate is typically not present. Immunofluorescence and the presence of antibodies that are common in pemphigus foliaceous are not present in staphylococcal scalded skin syndrome (SSSS).

5. Although cultures of skin and blister fluid are characteristically negative, recovery of S. aureus from the blood nasopharynx, throat, or conjunctiva confirms the diagnosis of SSSS.In cases that demand a rapid diagnosis, the exfoliated corneal layer can be seen on a frozen biopsy specimen of the desquamating epidermis. Scattered acantholytic cells, which are evident in the cleftlike bullae, can also be seen in a TZANCK preparation. The differential diagnosis of SSSS include various exanthems (infectious/ toxic/unknown) which are overviewed in the Table No.1 of the Chapter.

6. *SSSS affected Neonates and infants < 1 year of age should be admitted to the hospital and started on IV penicillinase - resistant penicillin (cloxacillin or Cefazolin) after blood cultures are obtained.* In addition, any older child who is toxic or who has severe skin involvement with significant denudation should be admitted. IV Clindamycin may be added to inhibit bacterial protein (toxin) synthesis. Topical antibiotics are unnecessary but the skin should be gently moistened and cleansed with Burow solution/Dakin solution/Isotonic saline. Application of an emollient provides lubrication and decreases discomfort, once the skin dries and desquamation commences.

7. Most of the time, SSSS is a self-limited disorder with rapid recovery without any sequelae. But complications such as dehydration, shock, electrolyte imbalance, hypothermia / hyperthermia, pneumonia, septicemia, and cellulitis can occur and may cause increased morbidity and mortality (around 3%).

8. Aggressive supportive management include IV fluids, electrolyte management, impeccable wound care with minimal handling, and pain control.

9. *The Evaluation-Decision-Action-Plan/Algorithm* summarizes the essential aspects of history taking, physical examination and investigations along with the principles of the management of SSSS.*Cultures of bullae are negative in the absence of contamination.*Blood culture: Usually negative in Neonates (but positive in bullous impetigo) A Gram stain and/or culture from the remote infection site may confirm staphylococcal infection.A chest radiograph should be considered to rule out pneumonia as the original focus of infection.

10. *Prevention of SSSS includes:* *Avoidance of the primary staphylococcal infection that may lead to the toxic syndrome *Timely treatment of established staphylococcal infections *Identification and treatment of asymptomatic carriers (*In outbreaks of staphylococcal infections and staphylococcal scalded skin syndrome (SSSS), identifying and treating asymptomatic carriers is imperative. Universal precautions should be used at all times.*).Maternal antibodies transferred to infants in breast milk are thought to be partially protective, but neonatal disease can still occur possibly as a result of inadequate immunity or immature renal clearance of exotoxin.

---

* *Pearl/Peril/Pitfall: The two known toxins (ETA and ETB) act specifically in the zona granulosa of the epidermis, and even intraperitoneal inoculation will result in exfoliation. Immunocytochemical studies have shown that the toxin binds to the filaggrin group of proteins in keratohyalin granules, and because filaggrins act as intracellular anchors of desmosomes, many investigators have speculated that epidermal splitting is a result of rupture of these desmosomes, probably from proteolytic activity of the toxins.*

THE EVALUATION-DECISION-ACTION-PLAN/ALGORITHM FOR THE DIAGNOSIS AND MANAGEMENT OF *A NEONATE/INFANT WITH STAPHYLOCOCCAL SCALDED SKIN SYNDROME (SSSS)*

SUBJECTIVE FINDINGS

Hx of fever, irritability, tender erythema of the skin, most marked in flexural areas and around the mouth & nose in infants and children younger than 5 years.

Hx of conjunctivitis (may be purulent), pharyngitis, and superficial erosions of the lips, but intraoral mucosal surfaces are spared.

Hx of rapid progression of skin lesion - within 12–24 hours, extensive blisters and erosions form & may be followed by wide spread superficial peeling of the skin in sheets, especially in infants.

OBJECTIVE FINDINGS

Assess ABCDs, O$_2$ sats, BP, CRT, hydration status, urine output

Look for Fever (although patients may be afebrile), *Tenderness* to palpation, Warmth to palpation, *Diffuse erythematous rash*(Often begins centrally, Sandpaperlike, progressing into a wrinkled appearance, Accentuated in flexor creases), *Bullae* secondary cutaneous infection, sepsis, fluid & electrolyte disturbances. Exfoliation of skin, which may be patchy or sheetlike in nature, Facial edema, Perioral crusting, Most patients do not appear severely ill.

Note Nikolsky sign (superficial separation of the skin after rubbing) and sparing of the mucosal surfaces.

Differentiate from Toxic Epidermal Necrolysis (TEN) by a history of drugs ingestion, the presence of Nikolsky sign only at sites of erythema, absence of perioral crusting, full-thickness epidermal necrosis, and a blister cleavage plane in the lowermost epidermis in the TEN.In TEN, the mucous membranes are almost always affected (mouth, conjunctiva, trachea, esophagus, anus, vagina)Note the absence of strawberry tongue and palatal petechiae which are present in Streptococcal Scarlet fever.

INVESTIGATIONS

Blood FBC, CRP, gram staining & culture from skin swab, blood culture, electrolytes, BUN, creatinine, cultures from suspected sites of localized infection like impetigo, sites of skin trauma, or the nares, urinanalysis.

A more rapid diagnostic examination can be accomplished with Wright's or Giemsa staining of a "snip excision" of a blister roof or peeled epidermal fragment, which will demonstrate a superficial versus deep blister plane and enable a distinction between SSSS & TEN.

Although cultures of skin and blister fluid are characteristically negative, recovery of S.aureus from the blood, nasopharynx, throat, or conjunctiva confirms the diagnosis of SSSS.

A Neonate /Infant with Staphylococcal Scalded Skin Syndrome

Ensure impeccable wound care with minimal handling and pain control (gently moisten the skin and cleanse with Burow solution, Dakin solution, or isotonic saline and apply an emollient to provide lubrication and to decrease discomfort). *Topical antibiotics are unnecessary.*

Differentiate SSSS from the mimicking conditions Refer to Table No. 1 given below

Ensure ABCs, *Treat* shock, *correct* fluid and electrolyte disturbances

Search for complications like faulty temperature regulation (hypothermia / hyperthermia), pneumonia, septicemia & cellulitis and *manage them energetically* to decrease the morbidity and mortality.

Hospitalize affected Newborn and any child with severe disease for IV antibiotic therapy and aggressive supportive management . *Start* IV Cloxacillin 150mg/kg/day in 4 divided doses or IV Cefuroxime 150mgs/kg/day in 3 divided doses + IV Aminoglycoside - Netilmicin 6mgs/kg/day in 2 divided doses, to finish a 10 day course. *Consider adding IV Clindamycin 50mgs/kg/day in 4 divided doses to inhibit bacterial protein (toxin) synthesis. *Consider* IV Vancomycin 50mgs/kg/day in 3 divided doses, if MRSA (Methicillin Resistant Staph. aureus) is suspected. (Reports implicating MRSA and community-acquired methicillin Staphylococcus aureus (CA-MRSA) as a cause of staphylococcal scalded skin syndrome are increasing). Manage older children with localized involvement and no toxicity, as outpatients with oral antibiotics (Cloxacillin 100mgs/kg/day in 4 divided doses or Cephalexin 100mg/kg/day in 4 divided doses).

TABLE 1	Summary of selected bacterial exanthems

Disease (cause)	Exanthem	Associated findings	Diagnosis	Management (comment)
1.SSSS	tender erythema, blisters, peeling in sheets, early on, mostly in flexures & around nose & mouth	Fever, irritability, rhinitis	Skin biopsy, snip excision with frozen section, culture of S. aureus	Anti - Staphylococcal antibiotics, analgesia, fluid & electrolyte management in severe cases
2.Toxic shock Syndrome	Diffuse erythema/erythroderma desquamation later	Fever, hypotension, shock abnormalities in > 3 other organ systems	Clinical, diagnostic criteria, isolation of S. aureus or GABHS	Fluid management, pressor support, IV antibiotics
3.Scarlet Fever	Red papules superimposed on diffuse erythema (sunburn with goose pimples)	Palatal petechiae, strawberry tongue, exudative pharyngitis, fever, abdominal pain, headache, Pastia's lines - linear red streaks in folds	Throat culture	Penicillin
4.Kawasaki Disease	Polymorphous ; papular, morbilliform, erythema with desquamation	Conjunctivitis, cheilitis, fever, glossitis, lymphadenopathy, peripheral edema, hydrops of gall bladder	Clinical	IVIG & aspirin
5.Meningococcemia	Papules, petechiae, purpura on trunk, palms, soles	Fever, meningismus, circulatory collapse	Clinical ; blood & CSF cultures	IV Penicillin & treat shock contact prophylaxis

---

* Pearl/Peril/Pitfall : *The use of antiseptic neonatal umbilical cord care delays the time of cord separation. However, several studies have shown that nil antiseptic cord care practice has led to a significant increase in staphylococcal umbilical colonization, which in turn may lead to an increase in neonatal infections, including SSSS and methicillin resistant S aureus outbreaks.*

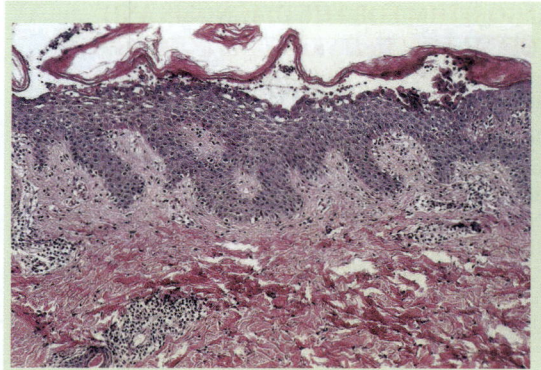

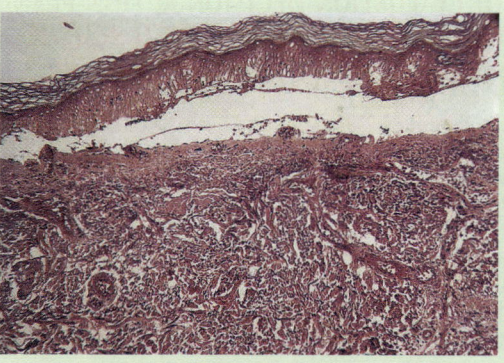

Drugs incriminated in etiology of TEN;
Ranitidine
Phenytoin
Vancomycin
Ceftazidime
Ethambutol
Nevirapine
Chloroquine
Clobazam
Ciprofloxacin
Penicillin
Sulfa drugs
Barbiturates

The staphylococcal scalded skin syndrome with subcorneal splitting. (H&E) may contain: *a few acantholytic cells *sparse neutrophils. Underlying dermis: *sparse, mixed inflammatory cell infiltrate: *in contrast to heavier dermal infiltrate in generalized bullous impetigo and pemphigus foliaceus

Toxic epidermal necrolysis (TEN): There is a subepidermal cell-poor blister with epidermal necrosis in the roof. (H&E). Sparse perivascular infiltrate of lymphocytes. Dermal infiltrate more prominent in cases that overlap with erythema multiforme.

* SSSS must be distinguished from Toxic Epidermal Necrolysis (TEN). TEN can often be distinguished by a history of drugs ingestion, the presence of Nikolsky sign only at sites of erythema, absence of perioral crusting, full - thickness epidermal necrosis, and blister cleavage plane in the lower most epidermis (at the level of the basement membrane). In SSSS, the mucous membranes are spared. In TEN, the mucous membranes are almost always affected (mouth, conjunctiva, trachea, esophagus, anus, vagina).

KEY POINTS FOR CLINICAL PRACTICE:

1. **Staphylococcal scalded skin syndrome (SSSS)** also known as Ritter von Ritterschein disease (in Newborns), Ritter disease, and staphylococcal epidermal necrolysis, occurs in Neonates, infants and children < 5 year of age, caused by exfoliative toxin-producing strains of *S. aureus* (Phage group II, types 71 & 55) and *present with* abrupt onset of fever, irritability, and tender erythema of the skin, most marked in flexural areas and around the mouth and nose. Within 12–24 hours, extensive blisters and erosions form and may be followed by widespread superficial peeling of the skin in sheets, especially in Neonates and infants. Superficial separation of the skin after rubbing (**Nikolsky sign**) is present. Subsequent denudation of the skin with a moist, glistening, red surface at sites of prior blistering may lead to significant cutaneous fluid losses/dehydration and secondary infection with resulting sepsis. The mucosal surfaces are spared.

2. In addition to symptomatic and supportive care, *Consideration* must be given for the sharply increasing rates of community-acquired *S aureus* infection (CA-MRSA). Prompt treatment with parenteral anti-staphylococcal antibiotics is essential. Most staphylococcal infections implicated in staphylococcal scalded skin syndrome have penicillinases and are resistant to penicillin. Nafcillin, oxacillin, or vancomycin is indicated. *Steroids are not indicated and may worsen immune function. Nonsteroidal anti-inflammatory agents and other agents that potentially reduce renal function should be avoided.*

3. Differentiating between staphylococcal scalded skin syndrome (SSSS) and more dangerous dermatologic conditions, such as toxic epidermal necrolysis (TEN) and pemphigus in the early stages of disease, can be difficult. Care should be taken to establish the correct diagnosis and as well to have a low threshold for speciality consultation as well as ICU and/or burn unit care.

4. Prognosis of staphylococcal scalded skin syndrome (SSSS) in children is excellent, with complete healing typically occurring in 10 days without significant scarring.

5. In outbreaks of staphylococcal infections and staphylococcal scalded skin syndrome (SSSS), identifying and treating asymptomatic carriers is imperative. Universal precautions should be used at all times.

REFERENCES & FURTHER READING : 1) Patel GK, Finlay AY. Staphylococcal scalded skin syndrome: diagnosis and management. *Am J Clin Dermatol.* 2003;4(3):165–75 2) Moss C, Gupta E. The Nikolsky sign in staphylococcal scalded skin syndrome. *Arch Dis Child.* Sep 1998;79(3):290. 3) Baartmans MG, Maas MH, Dokter J. Neonate with staphylococcal scalded skin syndrome. *Arch Dis Child Fetal Neonatal Ed.* Jan 2006;91(1):F25. 4) El Helali N, Carbonne A, Naas T, et al. Nosocomial outbreak of staphylococcal scalded skin syndrome in neonates: epidemiological investigation and control. *J Hosp Infect.* Oct 2005;61(2):130-8. 5) Ladhani S, Evans RW. Staphylococcal scalded skin syndrome. *Arch Dis Child.* Jan 1998;78(1):85–8.

** **Pearl/Peril/Pitfall:** Outbreaks of SSSS involving a large number of babies in neonatal wards are not uncommon and may persist for a long time if carriers of toxin producing S aureus are not rapidly identified and treated. While individual cases can easily be treated by the primary health care team, delays in recognizing an outbreak mean that carriers still working in the hospital will continue to infect more patients until identified, isolated, and treated. Staff should therefore ensure rigorous aseptic technique with hospital patients, particularly with neonates, and clinicians should beware of a possible outbreak, even if patients present with infection after hospital discharge.*

98 The Irritable and Crying Infant

@ *Irritability Definition *Irritability is excessive response to a stimulus. *Not a quantifiable symptom *Includes episodes of crying or fussiness despite attempts to comfort.*

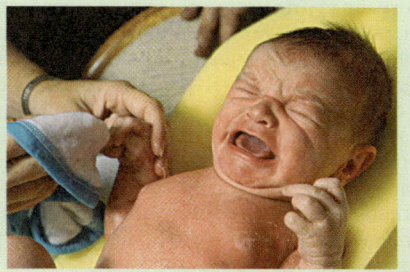

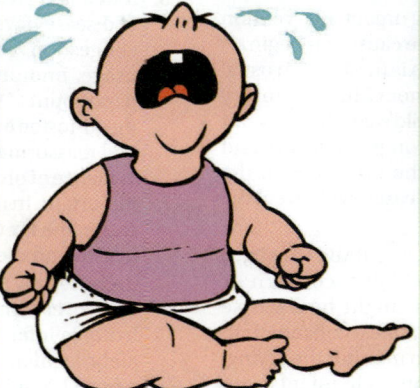

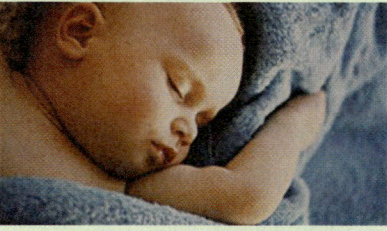

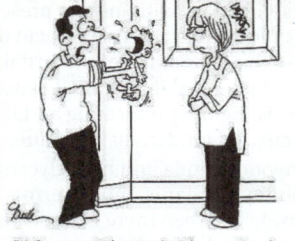

"Of course I know what he wants when he cries. He wants you."

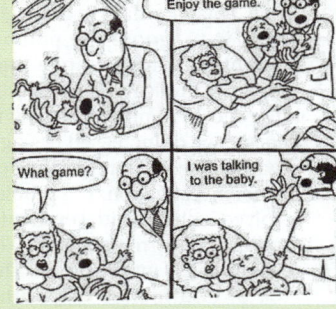

Enjoy the game.

What game?

I was talking to the baby.

Irritability—Physical exam *A thorough head-to-toe examination, including special attention to the eyes, ears, digits, and genitalia, is essential to establish a diagnosis. *Irritability and nonspecific crying episodes may be related to: *Foreign body in the ear or nose *Corneal abrasion *Hair wrapped around a digit or penis *Diaper rash *Nonspecific vaginitis *Balanitis *Insect and spider bites or stings *Vaccination pain. *A systematic search for injuries should be performed on any child with a history of trauma. *Inflicted injuries are more difficult to diagnose. *Signs may be subtle, and the history often is misleading. *Causes may be easily apparent, such as *fractures or dislocations.

Irritability—Diagnostic Procedures *Corneal abrasion:* Diagnosis is made by Wood lamp examination after instillation of fluorescein into the eye. *Acute myocarditis* should be considered in an irritable child with tachycardia, especially if accompanied by poor perfusion. :Electrocardiography may reveal sinus tachycardia with low-voltage QRS complexes, arrhythmias, and ST changes. *Anomalous left coronary artery originating from pulmonary artery* :Myocardial ischemia on electrocardiographic examination is almost universal. *Nonconvulsive status epilepticus* :Electroencephalography can be diagnostic.

REVIEW OF CLINICAL PROBLEMS

1. What organic causes of Infant Crying/Irritability you should be aware of ?
   Ans: Refer to the Table 1 of the Chapter.

2. Discuss the components of physical examination useful in reaching a diagnosis in a Crying infant.
   Ans: Refer to the Table 2 of the Chapter.

3. Describe various therapeutic management strategies you can follow in a Crying &/or Irritable infant.
   Ans: Refer to the Table 8 of the Chapter.

4. What is the most important procedure to be done, if all the evaluation of a Crying infant is negative ?
   Ans: Refer to No 8 of the Bird`s eye view/Overview/Synopsis of the Chapter.

5. Discuss the preliminary evaluative work-up to rule out serious conditions when dealing with a Crying &/or Irritable infant.
   Ans: Refer to the Evaluation-Decision-Action Plan/Algorithm to diagnose and manage a Neonate/Infant with excessive crying & Irritability.

LEARNING OBJECTIVES

After completing this article, readers will be able to:

1. Identify important signs and symptoms in the crying, afebrile infant.

2. Develop a differential diagnosis based on the clinical presentation of the crying infant.

3. Propose a diagnostic strategy for the workup of the crying infant.

4. Distinguish cases of minor illness from life- or limb threatening illnesses or injury.

5. Educate-Counsel-Comfort the parents and caregivers, if an infant is found to be crying due to psychological/social reasons.

* **Pearl/Peril/Pitfall :** *Unexplained irritability or lethargy, or a scalp hematoma in an irritable child, protracted vomiting, or neurologic deficits, all warrant computed tomography of the head. Plain films, ultrasonography, magnetic resonance imaging, and bone scanning can be helpful in the evaluation of: •Suspected bone abnormalities •Fractures •Osteomyelitis •Infarction in sickle cell disease •Joint processes •Septic arthritis, particularly of the hip •Trauma .*

BIRD'S EYE VIEW/OVERVIEW/SYNOPSIS

1. Excessive infant crying {SYN ; cross baby [fussy baby], colic, paroxysmal fussing, irritable infant} is the response to a variety of illness and physiologic disturbances, producing much parental anxiety even though an underlying cause is rarely found. *A cause for excessive crying is likely to be found if the infant is over 3 months of age, the crying is of recent onset, the child cannot be consoled, or there is an accompanying symptom.* Acute irritability may be associated with life-threatening illnesses requiring urgent intervention and stabilization before a search for the cause can begin. A parent who seeks care for an infant who is fussier than usual may arrive with a child who is in shock, in respiratory distress, or having a seizure. If the child's condition is not immediately life-threatening, then a complete history and thorough physical examination are the first steps in the evaluation of irritability, and, in many cases, will reveal the cause of the symptom.

2. Avoid 3 major pitfalls in managing a COLIC BABY ; **a)** Major pitfall is to ignore the parent's complaint, concern or downplay its importance. Indeed it might be a worse prognostic indicator if parents don't manifest concern than is they do. **b)** Another Pitfall - is to fail to monitor the crying. Persistence of increased crying is common in infants with organic diseases and an important clue to the need for further investigation. The problem of increased crying is not resolved with the initial evaluation but only when the crying (and the concern it generates) is resolved. **c)** PITFALL '3' is to focus solely on the infant. The physician should prevent lack of confidence in parenting skills or depressive symptoms in the parents which constitutes therapeutic success.

3. It is useful to know the normal crying times of the babies, to avoid overdiagnosis of Infantile Colic. In a 1962 study of 80 middle -class infants, Brazelton found the normal crying times, usually concentrated in the evening, to be as follows: 2 hr/day at 2 weeks of age ; 3 hr/day at 6 weeks of age ; 1 hr/day at 3 months of age. The clinical pattern of infant colic is well described. **a)** Attacks occur suddenly, usually in the evening **b)** They are characterized by a loud, almost continuous cry. **c)** They last several hours. **d)** the face of the infant is flushed, with occasional circumoral pallor **e)** The abdomen is distended and tense **f)** Legs are drawn up on the abdomen and the feet often cold. Legs may extend periodically during forceful cries. **g)** The fingers are clenched **h)** Relief is often noted from passage of flatus or feces **i)** The attack is not quelled for long by feeding, even though the infant may appear hungry and eats normally. **j)** The attack usually terminates from apparent exhaustion. No consistent etiology has been identified. It is also useful to know that an infant can be considered to have COLIC, if it cries for more than 3 hours a day for more than 3 days in a week for more than 3 weeks{wessel et all} {COLIC = KOLIKOS [Greek] = "pertaining to the colon"}.Infant colic is always a diagnosis of EXCLUSION !

4. Always try to identify infants with organic disease ; Gormally & Barr suggest atleast four clinical clues that increase the possibility that organic causes might be implicated. **a)** HIGH PITCHED cry with regular arching their backs during crying bouts and without manifesting a diurnal pattern {afternoon-evening clustering} **b)** Excessive crying alone was rare presentation of organic disease. Other symptoms by HISTORY {increased regurgitations, diarrhea, vomiting, respiratory distress} or by EXAMINATION {bruises, retinal Hemorrhages, etc} were almost always reported **c)** A late onset of increased crying in the 3rd month of following a switch from breast to formula may implicate cow's milk protein intolerance. **d)** It was common for the unusual or excessive crying of infants with organic disease to persist beyond 4 months. This justifies the importance of regular monitoring of the complaint until the crying resolves.

5. A detailed History {of crying itself + associated symptoms of disease {fever, poor weight gain, vomiting diarrhea, nasal congestion, cough, wheeze, + recent trauma, medication usage, immunizations {DPT esp.} + parental concerns is paramount . A deliberate, thorough physical examination {head-to-toe evaluation} is efficient in managing the patients and reassuring to the parents. An investigative search for an evidence of organicity depending on the clinical clues is also important. In irritable infants presenting without an obvious cause, the Hx will reveal the diagnosis in about 20%, the PE in 41% and the investigations in 20%.

6. Because only 50% of infants with meningitis initially present with fever : this diagnosis is very important to rule out in the irritable infant and because the differential of the irritable afebrile infant includes nonmeningial intracranial causes, a head CT should be obtained before performing an LP in these infants to rule out increased intracranial pressure.

7. Acidosis, hypernatremia, hypocalcemia and hypoglycemia are serious causes of irritability in infants. Inborn errors of metabolism should be considered when there is associated vomiting, neurologic symptoms, failure to thrive or a positive family history, including unexplained Neonatal deaths.

8. If all the evaluation is negative, then the most important evaluative procedure is monitoring the infant until the expected resolution of the crying occurs {not beyond the first 4 months} i) Direct the specific therapy at the pathophysiology of the organic condition. ii) For the remainder therapy can be directed a) at reducing the crying in the infant b) at reducing the psychological stressors.

9. The *Evaluation-Decision-Action Plan/Algorithm* outlines the essential diagnostic and management aspects of an Irritable and excessively crying Neonate-Infant.

10. Excessive crying by infants and children is very disturbing to parents. Irritability(excessive sensitivity to any stimulus or irritant) is often accompanied by inconsolable crying. 2 studies (Hunziker and Barr, 1986;St. James-Roberts and Halil, 1991) report that mean crying time in normal 1- to 3-mo-old infants was about 2 hrs/day. More crying occurred in the evening compared with other times of the day. As infants grew older, they were observed to cry less (Hunzikerand Barr, 1986). Whenever excessive crying or irritability occurs, it is important to determine its cause. Parents need an explanation, so they can understand and cope with this problem. Excessive crying or irritability must be taken seriously, especially when comforting and consoling fail to remedy the situation. Age of child and presence of illness narrow diagnostic possibilities. Complete history, including psychosocial and developmental history, and physical exam are often diagnostic. Infant can have normal physical exam with occult trauma (skull or extremity fracture), so that radiographs sometimes are necessary. Placement of fluorescein drops in eye may be diagnostic of corneal abrasion or foreign body. If physical exam is normal and crying does not persist after assessment, serious illness is unlikely.If crying persists, other investigations may be necessary, and these are guided by history and physical exam.

---

* *Pearl/Peril/Pitfall : Inguinal hernia • 60% of incarcerated inguinal hernias occur during the first year of life, with symptoms of irritability, • vomiting, and pain in the groin and abdomen. • Testicular examination is imperative in all boys with irritability or abdominal pain. • On examination, a nonfluctuant tender mass is present in the inguinal region and may extend down into the scrotum. • With the onset of ischemia of the involved bowel, pain becomes more intense and localized to the scrotum, and the infant may have bilious vomiting with the presence of bloody stools.*

THE EVALUATION-DECISION-ACTION-PLAN/ALGORITHM FOR THE DIAGNOSIS AND MANAGEMENT OF *A NEONATE/INFANT WITH IRRITABILITY AND EXCESSIVE CRYING*

SUBJECTIVE FINDINGS

*Complete history, including psychosocial and developmental history;*Be sure to ask the mother about any changes in the infant's behavior during the past 24 hours: Has he been vomiting? Has he seemed restless or unlike himself? Has his sucking reflex diminished? Does he cry when moved? Suspect child abuse if the infant's history is inconsistent with physical findings. (Refer to Table 5).

OBJECTIVE FINDINGS

Refer to the Tables 1, 2 and 6 for focussed examination depending on the presenting symptom and co-existing symptoms and signs *If the infant has High-pitched Cry-* Perform a neurologic examination. Remember that neurologic responses in Neonates and young infants are primarily reflex responses. Determine the infant's level of consciousness (LOC). Is he awake, irritable, or lethargic? Does he reach for an attractive object or turn toward the sound of a rattle? Observe his posture. Is he in the normal flexed position or in extension or opisthotonos? Examine muscle tone and observe the infant for signs of a seizure, such as a tremor and twitching..... Cont.. to the adjacent Box....,

INVESTIGATIONS

* Refer to the Main algorithm given below for appropriate investigations. Cont....Examine the size and shape of the infant's head. Is the anterior fontanel bulging? Measure the infant's head circumference, and check pupillary size and response to light. Unilateral or bilateral dilation and a sluggish response to light may accompany increased ICP. Finally, test the infant's reflexes; expect Moro's reflex to be diminished.

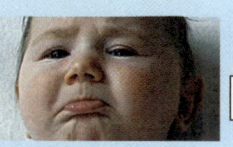

A NEONATE/INFANT WITH IRRITABILITY & EXCESSIVE CRYING

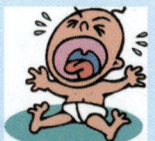

IRRITABLE NEONATE/INFANT

Take detailed History and perform complete physical examination {include fluorescein exam for corneal abrasions}

Abnormal physical examination

→ No →

Consolable during time of observation — No →

Yes ↓

Symptoms Compatible with teething in older infant

Yes → **Teething**

No ↓ → **First Episode** — No →

Yes ↓

Preliminary evaluation to rule out serious conditions:
CBC, ESR, CRP, ABG Analysis
Urine Analysis (and culture)
Stool guaiac (occult blood)
Lumbar puncture (consider CT prior to LP)
Consider additional work-up (if diagnosis not evident)
Skeletal survey or bone scan
Head CT (if not already done)
Electrolytes, calcium and glucose levels
Ophthalmology consult
Urine toxicology screen
ECG
UGI or endoscopy
± In patient observation

Tourniquet syndrome ; Foreign body (eye) Corneal abrasion ; Congestive heart failure Intussusception ; Other causes of acute abdomen Testicular torsion ; Tachyarrhythmias Hand-foot syndrome (sickle cell disease) "Shaken baby syndrome" (retinal hemorrhages) Septic arthritis/osteomyelitis (hip) ; Anal fissure (constipation) ; Encephalitis/meningitis ; Pseudotumor cerebri ; Incarcerated inguinal hernia.

UTI/pyelonephritis ; Intussusception ;Meningitis Encephalitis ; Intracranial hemorrhage (child abuse) Brain tumor ; Enteritis (allergic, infectious) Pseudotumor cerebri ; Sickle cell disease (**Based on additional work-up**) ; Unsuspected fractures (child abuse) ; Osteomyelitis/diskitis; Septic arthritis; Metabolic disorders (hyponatremia, hypoglycemia, hypocalcemia); Gastroesophageal reflux/esophagitis; Drugs/toxins; Supraventricular tachycardia; Anomalous coronary artery.

Normal growth and development Hx of similar episodes — No → go to next flow - chart below :

Yes → COLIC, NORMAL INFANT , CONSTIPATION

Abnormal results - Eg : - UTI, Intussusception, constipation / fissures, Sickle cell disease {pain crisis}

Obtain CBC with DC, Urine Analysis Stool guaiac

→ **Normal results (first episode)** → **Observe and follow-up in 24 hours** → **Irritability resolved**

Yes → Normal infant, vaccine reaction (DPT), teething, constipation, overstimulation, viral ilness.

No → Return to the above flow - chart and reevaluate !

→ **Normal results (Recurrent episodes)** → **Mild GI symptoms Present**

Yes → Trial of ISOMIL feeds - cow's milk protein hypersensitivity, if symptoms resolved

No → Skeletal survey, bone scan, UGI/endoscopy, Eyes evaluation → Child abuse, esophagitis, peptic ulcer disease, if the results are abnormal

* *Pearl/Peril/Pitfall :* Hypoxic or ischemic events & Irritable/crying infant • Carbon monoxide (CO) poisoning and methemoglobinemia cause irritability in response to hypoxia. -A history of smoke inhalation and exposure to an indoor gas stove or to automobile exhaust fumes is indicative. -Early findings with CO poisoning are influenza-like: -headache, irritability, and •-dizziness. -Prolonged exposure may result in altered mental status. •Methemoglobinemia—Characteristic blue-gray cyanosis that is not improved with oxygen, despite normal arterial oxygen tension, and chocolate brown appearance of arterial blood are the hallmarks of methemoglobinemia. -In infancy it may be hereditary; the hereditary form usually is mild. -May be acquired, related to: -Hypoxic events -Medication use (sulfonamides, topical anesthetics, metoclopramide) -Ingestion of products containing nitrites and nitrates (contaminated well water or foods with naturally occurring nitrates, such as spinach, green beans, carrots, and squash) • Diarrhea, probably caused by the nitrite-forming bacteria in the gut • Sickle cell anemia -Ischemia may cause a painful vasooclusive crisis. -Initial presentation in infants and younger children usually is irritability and dactylitis, and painful swelling of the hands and feet as a result of vascular stasis and ischemia.

Clinical pathway: Life-threatening or urgent causes of excessive crying in the neonate

Evidence of compensated shock ? — **YES** →
* Apply cardiac and pulse ox monitors
* Obtain IV access and administer a fluid bolus of 20 ml/kg normal saline
* Check bedside glucose and administer 10 ml/kg D$_{10}$ w if hypoglycemic
* Admit or transfer to NICU / PICUsetting

NO ↓

Temperature abnormality (fever or hypothermia)? — **YES** →
* Septic workup including lumbar puncture
* Administer antibiotics :
  Ampicillin 100 mg/kg IV
  Cefotaxime 50 mg/kg IV
* Admit or transfer to appropriate pediatric bed

NO ↓

Hypoxia without increased work of breathing and clear lungs? — **YES** →
Suspect a neuromuscular disease
* Administer supplemental oxygen
* Intubate if hypoxia persists despite oxygen administration
* Obtain a head CT and perform lumbar puncture if head CT is normal
* Admit or transfer to appropriate pediatric bed where a pediatric neurology consult can be obtained

NO ↓

Hypoxia with increased work of breathing with wheezes and/or crackles ? — **YES** →
Suspect cardiac or pulmonary disease
* Administer supplemental oxygen
* Intubate if hypoxia persists despite oxygen administration
* Obtain a chest X-ray

X-ray Results

If focal infiltrate (s):
* Administer antibiotics
* Admit to a pediatric bed

If a viral pattern is present :
* Perform viral testing for RSV
* Test for pertussis

If cardiomegaly or evidence of congestive heart failure:
* ECG
* Echocardiogram
* Troponin level
* Furosemide 1mg/kg IV
* Admit to a monitored pediatric bed

If chest X-ray is normal, consider viral testing (or alternative diagnoses).

NO ↓

Sustained heart rate greater than 200-220 beats per minute ? — **YES** →
Suspect supraventricular tachycardia
* Obtain 12-lead ECG
* Administer adenosine 0.1 mg/kg IV
  Repeat dose 0.2 mg/kg IV needed
* Synchronized cardioversion 0.5 J/kg
* Admit or transfer to pediatric bed with pediatric cardiology consult available

NO ↓

Bilious emesis ? — **YES** →
Suspect malrotation with midgut volvulus
* Prompt pediatric surgery consultation is required arrange transfer
* Upper GI study (if hemodynamically stable)

NO ↓

Paradoxical irritability, vomiting, full fontanel, with or without temperature instability ? — **YES** →
Suspect intracranial infection or nonaccidental Trauma
* Perform a lumbar puncture
  May consider CT scan prior to LP for children with a focal neurologic examination
* Administer empiric antibiotics
  Ampicillin 100 mg/kg IV,   Cefotaxime 50 mg/kg IV
* Admit or transfer to a pediatric bed with social work/ Child protective service consult

NO ↓

Vesicular rash or history of maternal genital herpes — **YES** →
Suspect herpes encephalitis
* Acyclovir 20 mg/kg I V

NO ↓

Irritability tremor, poor feeding, vomiting, diarrhea, tachycardia, hypertension ? — **YES** →
Suspect Neonatal withdrawal syndrome, congenital hyperthyroidism, or Neonatal hypoparathyroidism
* Obtain serum calcium, magnesium, and phosphorus levels (replace if low)
* Admit or transfer to an appropriate pediatric bed for social services consultation and/or endocrinologic workup

NO ↓

Consider more benign causes of excessive crying (including corneal abrasions and hair tourniquets). If etiology remains unclear, admission or transfer to a pediatric bed for observation and further evaluation is prudent

TABLE 1 — **Beware of the organic causes of crying that have physical findings** (Always examine 9 orifices + the umbilicus)

Common causes	Uncommon causes
Otitis media	General—failure to thrive
Nasal congestion/irritation	Eyes—glaucoma, corneal abrasion, foreign body
Constipation, gastroenteritis	Ears, nose, and throat - pharyngitis
And fissure	Cardiovascular—CHF, SVT, any cause of coronary insufficiency
Umbilical inflammation/infection	Gastrointestinal—intussusception, inguinal hernia, GE reflux, volvulus, acute abdominal conditions, pin worm infestation.
Mouth ulcers, thrush	Genitourinary—Urinary tract obstruction, meatal ulcer, torsion of the testis or ovary.
Skin - any pruritic or painful rash	Skeletal—fracture, subperiosteal hematoma, osteomyelitis
	Hair or thread twisted around digit/Penis/even the Uvula {Tourniquet Syndrome }
	Neurologic—Increased ICT

TABLE 2 — **The components of the physical examination useful in reaching a diagnosis**

Diagnostic Study whom proved	No. of patients for the Component Useful (n = 30)
Otoscopy	10
Rectal exam	4
Fluorescein staining of cornea	3
Inspection underneath clothing	2
Palpation of bones	2
Oral exam	2
Auscultation of heart (tachyarrhythmia)	2
Laryngoscopic exam of hypopharynx	1
Eversion of eyelid	1
Palpation of anterior fontanelle	1
Retinal exam	1
Neurologic exam	1

Always examine the hernial orifices for a strangulated hernia and look for the *TORSION OF THE TESTIS* and acute onset of screaming attacks should suggest the possibility of *INTUSSUSCEPTION*.

TABLE 3 — **The components of the investigations that identified the diagnosis**

Diagnostic Study	No. of patients (n = 30)
Skeletal roentgenography	2
Lumbar puncture/ Cerebrospinal fluid analysis	2*
Electrocardiography	2
CT scan of the head	2*
Barium enema	1
Esophagogram	1
Amino and organic acid studies	1
Urinalysis	1

* One patient, with Pseudotumor cerebri, required lumbar puncture and CT scan of the head to make the diagnosis.

TABLE 4 — **Types of cry**

Can we recognize the child's illness by hearing the type of the cry ? **Well, of course! it depends on our knowledge data base, past clinical experience, present keen and continuous observation mixed with common sense, art and wisdom.**

Types of Cry

Shrill, high-pitched cry
   cerebral irritability
   raised intracranial pressure

Whimper or lack of cry
   Seriously ill child

Hoarse cry
   Laryngitis
   congenital heart disease (rare)
   Faber disease (rare)

Grunting cry
   respiratory distress syndrome
   Pneumonia
   acute abdomen (rare)

Weak cry
   spinal muscular atrophy (rare)
   myasthenia gravis (rare)
   Prader-Willi syndrome (rare)

Hoarse gruff cry
   congenital hypothyroidism (rare)

High-pitched mewling cry
   cry-du-chat syndrome (rare)

Low-pitched growling weak cry
   de Lange syndrome (rare)

* A shrill, high pitched cry is a common feature of cerebral irritability (causes include hypoglycemia, hypoxic-ischemic encephalopathy, Neonatal drug withdrawal) and raised intracranial pressure (e.g., caused by meningitis, hydrocephalus or subdural hematoma).

* A whimpering cry, or the lack of any cry, are features of a seriously ill child.

* Grunting is a sound made during expiration when infants or small children breathe out against a partially closed glottis. Grunting respirations are a feature of the respiratory distress syndrome, pneumonia and children who have an acute abdomen (Eg: Intussusception and volvulus)

* Pearl/Peril/Pitfall : Metabolic system • Hypoglycemia, hypo- or hypernatremia, hypo- or hypercalcemia, hypomagnesemia, and inborn errors of metabolism can all cause irritability.· Hypoglycemia is defined as a glucose level d"40 mg/dL. • Can be a primary process • Can be caused by sepsis, ingestion, or cardiac or respiratory failure. Inborn errors of metabolism that cause irritability are those in which a toxic intermediate accumulates. • Organic and aminoacidemias and urea cycle disorders result in metabolic acidosis or hyperammonemia. • Symptomatic in the first few weeks of life, with • vomiting, poor feeding, irritability, and lethargy • When a milder degree of enzyme dysfunction is present, clinical disease may be triggered by a bacterial or viral illness.

TABLE 5 — Acute unexplained excessive crying in neonates and infants : Essential aspects of history

History of present illness
Onset and duration
Frequency: First episode or recurrent?
If recurrent: Frequency, time of occurrence, duration, prior evaluations
Interventions: What makes it better?
Associated activities: Feeding, sleep disturbance
Review of systems
Fever
Vomiting: Bilious, partially-digested food, bloody
Diarrhea: Frequency, consistency, bloody
Rhinorrhea, cough, respiratory distress
Rash
Abnormal behavior, movements, spells
Recent trauma
Exposures: Household, daycare
Feeding: breast, formula, solids, recent changes, amount, frequency
Formula: Type, changes
Breast: Maternal meds, drugs, nicotine, breast disease
Stooling: Frequency, consistency, blood, recent changes
Urination: Frequency, color, odor, time of last urination
Sleeping: More, less

Birth history
Prenatal: Maternal illness, meds (Rx, OTC), illicit drugs
Perinatal: Maternal GBS status, gestational age, complications, birth weight, Newborn screening
Past medical history
Illnesses, hospitalizations, weight gain, developmental milestones
Medications: Rx, OTC
Immunizations: What and when
Medication allergy
Family history
Inherited disease: i.e., SCD, hemophilia, asthma, mental illness
Medications in household
Social history
Number living in household
Siblings (ages)
Living arrangement: House, apartment, shelter
Daycare
Smoking exposure
Illicit drugs or alcohol in household

TABLE 6 — Acute unexplained excessive crying in neonates and infants: Differential diagnosis by system

HEENT
Trauma
Rash
Foreign body: eye, ear, nose, pharynx
Corneal abrasion
Glaucoma
Nasal congestion (< 6 months)
Thrush, stomatitis, pharyngitis

Neck
Torticollis
Adenitis
Mass
Retropharyngeal cellulitis/abscess
Chest
Hypoxia, hypercarbia
Mastitis (neonate)
Bronchiolitis
Pneumonia
Trauma

Cardiac
Congestive heart failure
Supraventricular tachycardia
Myocarditis
Coronary ischemia

Gastrointestinal (nonobstructive)
GERD
Allergic esophagitis
Congenital webs
Gastroenteritis
Constipation
Anal fissure
Appendicitis
Peritonitis
Protein milk allergy
Malabsorption

Gastrointestinal (obstructive)
Congenital small bowel stenoses
Pyloric stenosis
Malrotation/midgut volvulus
Intussusception
Hirschsprung's disease

Genitourinary
Testicular torsion
Inguinal hernia
Hydrocele
Urinary tract infection
Meatal stenosis
Balanoposthitis
Genital tourniquet

Musculoskeletal
Septic arthritis
Toxic synovitis
Osteomyelitis
Discitis
Developmental hip dysplasia
Rickets
Congenital syphilis
Digital tourniquet
Trauma (fracture, dislocation)

Dermatologic
Eczema
Diaper dermatitis
Insect bites
Black widow & brown recluse spider bites
Cellulitis

Hematologic
Sickle cell disease
Iron deficiency anemia

Neurologic
Meningoencephalitis
Intracranial hemorrhage, cerebral edema
Hydrocephalus
Pseudotumor cerebri
Migraine

Toxic-Metabolic
Prenatal drug use
Breast milk drug transmission
Immunizations
Toxic ingestion
Electrolyte abnormalities
Inborn errors of metabolism
Hypoglycemia
Hyperthyroidism

DIFFERENTIAL DIAGNOSIS OF LIFE— THREATENING CONDITIONS

Meningoencephalitis	Appendicitis (infant)
Sepsis	Intracranial hemorrhage
Pneumonia	Hydrocephalus
Bronchiolitis	Malrotation/midgut volvulus
Myocarditis	Intussusception
	Supraventricular tachycardia
	Coronary anomalies and aneurysms

TABLE 7   **The irritable and crying infant—fact is stranger than fiction**

1. Babies commonly cry when left alone and are quiet when picked up. Particular attention should be paid to whether the baby's crying worsens when pickedup {Paradoxical Irritability} - implying a pathologic process aggravated by movement.

2. Most babies from the age of 6 weeks or so, are not content to be left lying down with nothing to see. They are quiet when propped up so that they can see what is going on.

3. Symptoms { e.g. high fever, rash, loose stools, convulsions} are often wrongly attributed to TEETHING, but TEETHING can cause irritability, crying and a marked increase in salivation.

4. Excessive infant crying may provoke child abuse or be its result , therefore search for signs of physical abuse {observe carefully for an abnormal *parent-infant interaction* and note inconsistencies in the history.

5. Nasal congestion can cause excessive crying, as most infants are obligate nasal breathers and are bothered by nasal blockage.

6. BABIES CRY WHEN THEY ARE HUNGRY AND FOR OTHER REASONS , SUCH AS THIRST, DISCOMFORT {WIND, COLD, HEAT, ITCHING, WET NAPKIN, LOUD NOISES, TIREDNESS}, AND AS THEY GET OLDER THEY CRY WHEN THEY ARE CROSS /FRUSTRATED.

7. Not many parents can stand their babies crying intermittently throughout the night and the temptation is to feed them, not so much for nutrition, as to keep them quiet. They may react to this by vomiting.

8. Despite appropriate management, some babies cry excessively, and one can only ascribe it to the personality. Some babies seem to sense their mother's anxiety and tenseness and cry as a result. However, much crying by infants occurs without a discoverable cause.

9. Intolerance to cow's milk protein is a possible but uncommon cause of excessive crying. It is more likely as a cause if there are other symptoms attributable to cow's milk protein intolerance, such as loose stools, perioral erythema, eczema, wheezing and persistent rhinitis. The diagnosis can only be established by a therapeutic trial of cow's milk protein avoidance, followed by reintroduction of cow's milk to see if symptoms recur, followed by a further period of avoidance until tolerance to cow's milk protein has developed.

10. Most infants cry and fret while falling asleep. An intelligent and perceptive mother can readily differentiate between the cry due to hunger and cry as a signal of discomfort.

11. In infants and young children who cannot speak, the cry is the only signal to express their needs and draw attention to their discomfort, hunger, and painful or unpleasant conditions. Certain amount of crying is physiological and desirable and is believed to be akin to "exercise period", and "letting off the steam" to give vent to their anger, frustration and to seek attention.

12. Chronic constipation and crying while defecating are suggestive of ANAL FISSURE, while most healthy infants may cry before passing urine due to unpleasant sensation of full bladder ; however they become quiet, relaxed and dazed while passing urine.

13. Beware of drug induced excessive crying—a} Atropine derivatives, pseudoephedrine, antispasmodics, xanthine derivatives can cause excessive irritability and restlessness b} Excessive crying due to pseudotumor cerebri is a recognized side effect of excessive or prolonged intake of nalidixic acid, tetracyclines, corticosteroids, vitamin A etc., c}Prolonged and excessive local application of lignocaine over perianal area in an infant with anal fissure may lead to excessive irritability, restlessness and even seizures. d} Excessive and inconsolable crying is a recognized complication due to whole cell Pertussis component of DPT vaccination.

14. Abnormal and excessive crying at night should alert to the possibilities of exposure to cold or insect bites due to mosquitoes and bed bugs. Sudden episodes of crying at night may occur in female infants when pinworms wriggle through the vaginal orifice.

15. Infants with acute gastroenteritis often cry due to thirst but it is often misinterpreted as colic. When an infant with acute GE develops sudden constipation with passage of red currant jelly stools [not always] and episodes of inconsolable crying due to abdominal colic, it is highly suggestive of acute intussusception.

16. Crying or fussiness while feeding should alert to the possibility of nose block, thrush, aphthous ulcers and herpangina.

17. Note any gestures the infant makes during crying—flexion of thighs over abdomen with passage of flatus [intestinal colic], head banging [headache], poking fingers or pulling at ears [earache], touching or rubbing genitals [UTI], inability to move a limb [Pseudoparalysis due to scurvy, osteomyelitis , congenital syphilis, fracture and dislocation etc.], blinking, rubbing and watering of an eye [foreign body].

18. Hypoxia due to cardio respiratory disorders [bronchospasm and shock] is an important cause of restless and crying but the clinical picture is dominated by underlying condition and infant looks critically sick.

19. Unexplained episodes of severe abdominal pain and bone pains may occur due to vasoocclusive crises of sickle cell disease and in children with acute leukemia.

20. History of sudden choking, stridor and unilateral wheezing are diagnostic of a foreign body in the air passages [older sibling may have been playing with the infant by putting beads, toys with loose components causing inhalation / ingestion of foreign body].

Pearl/Peril/Pitfall : *Prescribed or over-the-counter medications may cause irritability, even when used as directed and certainly when overused. • β-Agonists • Antiepileptics • Decongestants • Antihistamines • Antitussives • Various cold medicines. Certain drugs of abuse are known to cause irritability. • Cocaine • Alcohol • Phencyclidine hydrochloride • Inhalants. Exposure in infants and children may occur: • By passive means • Transplacentally • By ingestion of human milk • By inhalation • By accidental ingestion. A positive history may be difficult to elicit, and toxicologic screen may not always be helpful; thus, a strong index of suspicion is needed.*

Educate Parents for mild fussiness-Home Care

1. Breastfeeding mothers should:
  *Avoid caffeine *Avoid antihistamines *Avoid exposure to secondary smoke

2. For infants under 3 months old:
  *Place the infant in a quiet, dark room to sleep.*Provide adequate time for your baby to sleep.
  *Continue breastfeeding every 2–4 hours.
  *Infants who are hungry after breastfeeding may require formula feedings.
  *Cuddle and rock your baby.*Learn how to feed your baby properly with burping
  *Do not place the infant face down to sleep
  *Remove cow's milk from the diet. *Provide soy formula, if indicated.

3. Treat causes of fussiness: *Anal fissure treatment *Constipation treatment *Diaper rash treatment
  *Remove an eyelash in the eye. *Remove hair wrapped around the finger or penis.

Crying: What should I do?

Why does my baby cry?

- Since your baby can't talk yet, crying is one way to tell you what they need. Your baby may be telling you that he is hungry, wet, tired, or wants to be held. Sometimes your baby cries at the same time everyday. Your babies crying may be caused because of "colic." Or crying just may be the way your baby deals with feeling tense.

- No matter why your baby cries, it is hard to listen to crying for a long time. If you try to stop the crying but it just doesn't work, it can be very frustrating.

- If you or your child's caregivers are sad, upset or tense your baby can sense this and may cry more.

What do I do when my baby cries all the time?

- If you think your baby needs food, feed them slowly. Burp your baby often.

- Offer your baby a pacifier. If you think your baby is teething, chill the pacifier.

- Check your baby's diaper. If it is wet or messy, change the diaper.

- Check to see if your baby is too hot or too cold. Check to see if clothes are loose and comfortable.

- Hold your baby against your chest, walk or gently rock them.

- Comfort your baby with hugs and kisses.

- Take your baby for a ride in a stroller or the car. Be sure your baby is safely strapped in the stroller or in an approved car seat in the car.

- Sing to your baby.

- Play soft music for your baby.

- Talk to your baby's doctor if crying is a problem.

Be patient. Your baby does not hate you or want to ruin your life. Your baby will outgrow the constant crying. It just takes time.

What can I do if I feel like it's too much to deal with?

When you feel that you just can't listen to the crying anymore:

- Wrap your baby in a soft blanket. Put your baby in a safe place, like a crib, with the side rails up. The room should be quiet, dark and a comfortable temperature. Close the door and take a break! If possible, see if someone else can take care of your baby for a half-hour or so.

- **Never pick up or hold your baby if you feel angry.**

- No matter how much the crying bothers you, **never shake your baby!** Hard shaking may cause brain damage, blindness, hearing loss, learning problems, seizures or even death. Letting your baby "cry it out" is much safer for your baby.

ALERT: Call your child's doctor, nurse, or clinic if you have any questions or concerns or if your child has special health care needs that were not covered by this information.

This teaching sheet is meant to provide you with additional information about your child's care. Diagnosis, treatment, and follow-up should be provided by your health care professional.

---

* **Pearl/Peril/Pitfall :** *Infants may be irritable after vaccination, with local erythema, swelling, and tenderness at the injection site. •Persistent, inconsolable crying lasting > 3 hours within 48 hours of receiving whole-cell pertussis DTP vaccine has been reported but not with the newer acellular pertussis DTaP vaccine. In some instances, the source of a child's irritability will be found only on thorough examination of the genitalia, which may reveal evidence of vaginitis, balanitis, or anal fissure. Diaper dermatitis, common after a diarrheal illness, with Candida infection or as an allergic reaction to the diaper material Insect and spider bites or stings.*

TABLE 8   The irritable and crying infant—therapeutic management strategies

1. **Infant colic:** Reassurance and parental education and advise prone positioning, gentle vibration and appropriate carrying, less stimulation and more soothing behavior. Elimination of cow's milk protein can be tried in colic infants with Diarrhea and Vomiting {Isomil feeds}. Prevent the possibility of extreme parental fatigue and possible child abuse. Hospitalize the baby for a short period to break the cycle of parental—infant fatigue and frustration. Medications like Colicaid or Neopeptin drops or Chloral hydrate 5–10 mgs/kg/dose can be tried empirically [don't use dicyclomine, phenobarbital, because of problematic side effects].

2. **Nasal congestion:** Saline nose drops - 2 drops 10 minutes before feeds and PRN to each nostril followed by gentle suction with a nasal aspirator and a cool mist Vaporizer can be tried.

3. **Otitis media:** Oral analgesics [Paracetamol, Ibuprofen, Codeine] and antibiotics {Cefixime or Co-amoxyclav}, nasal decongestants or antihistamine]

4. **Otitis externa:** Cleaning of debris with cotton pledgets, oral analgesics, sofracort - topical application or candibiotic ear drops q2–3 hours while the infant is awake.

5. **Anal fissure and constipation:** Sitz lukewarm baths, stool softeners [lactulose],Bacitracin/Soframycin, Hydro-cortisone, topical anesthetic cream sparingly.

6. **Mouth ulcers:** Adequate fluid intake, 1:1 mixture of lidocaine viscous 2% and diphenhydramine [Benadryl] elixir to be applied on the painful lesions with soft cotton bud [don't allow the infant to drink the solution, because toxicity with seizures may result].

7. **Oral thrush:** Clotrimozole paint [10 drops tds] to be smeared over the lesions until 2–3 days after visible evidence of infection has resolved.

8. **UTI :** Antibiotics and investigate for the underlying cause as per the protocol and prevent further infections.

9. **Hair tourniquet of Penis:** Use cool compresses to decrease penile swelling, then gently wash with warm water. Cut the hair carefully if the hair doesn't become free. Observe the infant until the swelling has resolved. Surgical intervention is frequently needed, especially for cases of penile strangulation.

10. **Obvious watering of the eye** [glaucoma, corneal abrasion, foreign body]: Have an ophthalmologist opinion and treat accordingly.

11. **Osteomyelitis and/or fracture:** Consult an Orthopedician and treat accordingly.

12. **Raised ICT:** CT scanning of the head, careful LP, intensive care according to the cause of raised ICT and stop offending drugs causing Pseudotumor cerebri.

13. **Inguinal hernia, intussusception, volvulus, acute abdominal conditions:** Consult Pediatric surgeon urgently and treat accordingly.

14. **Skin** [pruritic or painful rash]: Soothening agents, antibiotics [topical and oral], antiscabetic agents etc.

15. **CVS [CCF and SVT]** Obtain CXR, ECG and ECHO ; discuss with Paediatric cardiologist and treat accordingly.

KEY POINTS FOR CLINICAL PRACTICE:

1. Excessive infant crying {SYN ; cross baby [fussy baby], colic, paroxysmal fussing, irritable infant} is the response to a variety of illness and physiologic disturbances, producing much parental anxiety even though an underlying cause is rarely found.

2. When to Admit ? *Infants < 1 month of age who are irritable, for evaluation and observation *Children in whom child abuse and neglect are suspected *Children with a life-threatening condition, such as *meningitis or *brain tumor, that causes irritability.

3. Four clinical clues that increase the possibility that organic causes might be implicated. **a)** HIGH PITCHED cry with regular arching their backs during crying bouts and without manifesting a diurnal pattern (afternoon-evening clustering, etc.) were almost always reported. **b)** Excessive crying alone was rare presentation of organic disease. Other symptoms by HISTORY {increased regurgitations, diarrhea, vomiting, respiratory distress} or by EXAMINATION {bruises, retinal Hemorrhages, **c)** A late onset of increased crying in the 3rd month of following a switch from breast to formula may implicate cow's milk protein intolerance. **d)** It was common for the unusual or excessive crying of infants with organic disease to persist beyond 4 months. This justifies the importance of regular monitoring of the complaint until the crying resolves.

4. A detailed History {of crying itself + associated symptoms of disease {fever, poor weight gain, vomiting diarrhea, nasal congestion, cough, wheeze, + recent trauma, medication usage, immunizations {DPT esp.} + parental concerns is Paramount.

5. If all the evaluation is negative, then the most important evaluative procedure is monitoring the infant until the expected resolution of the crying occurs {not beyond the first 4 months} i) Direct the specific therapy at the pathophysiology of the organic condition. ii) For the remainder therapy can be directed a) at reducing the crying in the infant b) at reducing the psychological stressors.

REFERENCES & FURTHER READING : 1)Pawel BB, Henretig FM. Crying and colic in early infancy.In: Fleisher GR, Ludwig S, eds. Textbook of pediatric emergencymedicine, 4th ed. Philadelphia: Lippincott Williams & Wilkins, 2000:193–195. **2)** Barr RG, Gunnar M. The "transientresponsivity" hypothesis. In: Barr RG, et al., eds. Cryingas a sign, a symptom, & a signal. London: Mac Keith Press,2000:41–66. **3)** Schmitt BD. Colic: excessive crying in newborns. ClinPerinatol 1985;12:441–451. **4)** Carey WB. The effectiveness of parent counseling inmanaging colic. Pediatrics 1994;94:333–334. **5)** Berkowitz D, et al. "Infantile colic" asthe sole manifestation of gastroesophageal reflux. J Pediatr GastroenterolNutr 1997;24:231–233.

---

* *Pearl/Peril/Pitfall : Malrotation with midgut volvulus peaks during the first month of life but can occur anytime in childhood.*
  • *The neonate will be irritable initially.* • *As bowel becomes obstructed and necrotic, bilious vomiting and* • *shock may result from perforation.*

99 Apparent Life Threatening Event (ALTE)/ Near Miss SIDS

@ *"an episode that is frightening to the observer and is characterized by some combination of apnea (central or occasionally obstructive), color change (usually cyanotic or pallid but occasionally erythematous or plethoric), marked change in muscle tone (usually marked limpness), choking, or gagging."*

ALTE-History: Key questions related to the history of the episode include the following: *Who observed the event? Recognize that second-hand accounts may vary from the history provided by direct observers who were present at the time. *What was the description of the event? A caregiver's description of the infants' color, respiration, and muscle tone is key. Care must be taken to distinguish central cyanosis (lips and oral mucous membranes) from acrocyanosis (hands and feet). Infants who are coughing, choking, or gagging may exhibit a ruddy or plethoric facial color that may be interpreted as "turning blue." Determine whether apnea was present, and, if so, whether it appeared to be central (lack of respiratory effort) or obstructive (respiratory effort with inadequate airflow). Distinguish apnea that lasted more than 15–20 seconds from periodic breathing, in which respiratory rate and tidal volumes fluctuate and are accompanied by brief pauses in breathing that typically last less than 5-10 seconds. *Was the infant limp, or was muscle tone increased during or after the event? *Were any seizure like movements observed? *Was any resuscitation required, or did the event spontaneously resolve? Recall that caregivers may provide mouth-to-mouth resuscitation to spontaneously breathing infants with intact perfusion, fearing that the infant's life is threatened. *Was the infant born at term, or was the infant premature? *Were any pregnancy or labor and delivery complications reported? *Are any factors that predispose to Neonatal sepsis noted? *Has the infant previously exhibited symptoms of gastroesophageal reflux or aspiration of thin liquids? These symptoms may include coughing, choking, or gagging during or after feeding; frequent or excessive spitting-up; persistent nasal stuffiness; or frequent hiccups. Acid reflux disease is suggested by excessive irritability, arching, and straining behaviors displayed during or following a feeding. *Are the Newborn metabolic screening findings normal? *Does the family have a history of seizures, metabolic disorders, previous sudden infant death syndrome (SIDS), or unexplained death in infancy or childhood?

ALTE-Physical examination: A complete physical examination begins by obtaining a full set of vital signs, including pulse oximetry. *A full head-to-toe examination of the skin should be performed to look for skin lesions or signs of trauma. *The head and neck examination should note the characteristics of the anterior fontanelle (i.e., normal, bulging, or sunken). Nondilated funduscopic examination should be performed. If retinal hemorrhages are suspected, a formal dilated indirect examination may be necessary for further characterization. The nose and mouth should be examined for the presence of blood or formula. *The respiratory examination should include the respiratory rate, pattern of breathing, and adequacy of air exchange. The presence of stridor, wheezes, or crackles should be noted. *The cardiovascular examination should reveal whether murmurs are present and the adequacy and symmetry of pulses. In young infants, suspicion for ductal-dependent cardiovascular lesions may be heralded by a differential in blood pressure findings, oximetry findings, or both in the right upper extremity compared with measurements obtained from the lower extremities. *Abdominal distention or tenderness may indicate acute intestinal obstruction. Inguinoscrotal examination should evaluate for incarcerated inguinal hernia or testicular torsion. *Neurologic assessment begins with assessment of the infants' responsiveness. Determine whether lethargy is persistent or resolved and whether the muscle tone and reflexes are appropriate for age. Also, determine if any focal or lateralizing findings are present.

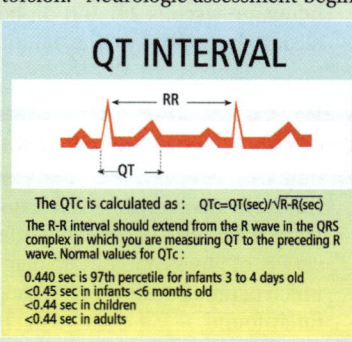

QT INTERVAL

The QTc is calculated as : $QTc=QT(sec)/\sqrt{R-R(sec)}$

The R-R interval should extend from the R wave in the QRS complex in which you are measuring QT to the preceding R wave. Normal values for QTc :

0.440 sec is 97th percentile for infants 3 to 4 days old
<0.45 sec in infants <6 months old
<0.44 sec in children
<0.44 sec in adults

REVIEW OF CLINICAL PROBLEMS

1. What is the differential diagnosis of an Apnea/ALTE in a Neonate/an Infant ?
   Ans: Refer to the Table 1 of the Chapter.

2. What 2 key questions you should always address while dealing with an ALTE?
   Ans: Refer to No 4 of the Bird's eye view/Overview/Synopsis of the Chapter.

3. Mention the essential features of History to elicit when an ALTE is being evaluated.
   Ans: Refer to the Table 2 of the Chapter.

4. What investigations you may include in evaluating an ALTE?
   Ans: Refer to the Table 4 of the Chapter.

5. Discuss how you can counsel parents about home monitoring after an ALTE.
   Ans: Refer to No 8 of the Bird`s eye view/Overview/Synopsis of the Chapter.

LEARNING OBJECTIVES

After completing this article, readers will be able to:

1. Evaluate an ALTE, while performing resuscitation of the infant where appropriate.

2. Formulate the diagnostic work-up, depending on the focussed History & Thorough physical examination.

3. Discuss with the Parents about pros & cons of Home Monitoring.

4. Understand that about 50% of ALTEs are idiopathic-no cause can be identifiable even after investigations.

5. Discuss the issue of lack of causal relationship between ALTE & SIDS with the parents to reassure them .

---

* ***Pearl/Peril/Pitfall :*** *Remember "The apnea monitoring business has become a religion. More people are living off of SIDS than dying from it." Jerold F. Lucey, ed. Pediatrics.*

* ***Pearl/Peril/Pitfall :*** *Standard and specific evaluation procedures are listed to help identify a cause for the ALTE. The most frequent problems associated with an ALTE are digestive (about 50%), neurological (30%), respiratory (20%), cardiovascular (5%), metabolic and endocrine (under 5%), or diverse other problems, including child abuse. Up to 50% of ALTEs remain unexplained. The finding of medical or surgical anomalies leads to specific treatments.*

1. An apparent life-threatening event (ALTE), is not a specific diagnosis, but a description of an acute, unexpected change in an infant's breathing behavior that was frightening to the caretaker and that included some combination of the following features : *Apnea — usually no respiratory effort (central) or sometimes effort with difficulty (obstructive) *Color change — usually cyanotic or pallid, but occasionally erythematous or plethoric *Marked change in muscle tone (usually limpness or rarely rigidity) *Choking or gagging In some cases, the observer fears that the infant has died. Recovery occurs only after stimulation or resuscitation. However, episodes are often mislabelled as "ALTEs" even when a parent reports that the child resumed normal breathing after simply being picked up and patted. Apnea is defined as the cessation of breathing for > 15 seconds, or less, if accompanied by Pallor, Cyanosis, and/or Bradycardia. The two sub-types are central and obstructive apnea. Apnea must be distinguished from periodic breathing, which is a normal breathing pattern seen in infants, consisting of > 2 second respiratory pauses with regular respirations, and it is not accompanied by color change or bradycardia.

2. Don't ever forget the first priority of the emergency pediatrician, after immediate resuscitation of the patient (refer to Figures 1 & 2), is to identify a Life-Threatening Condition—persistent/recurrent apnea, hypoxia, septic shock, and hypoglycemia. Note the general appearance, mental status, vital signs including a rectal temperature and blood pressure.

3. *Do follow the 3 essential pillars of the diagnosis* - namely quick and focused history (refer to table 2), thorough physical examination (an apnea is always potentially life-threatening, even in the absence of abnormal physical findings) and appropriate diagnostic studies to evaluate the child for several common etiologies (Refer to Table No. 4). The common causes include: *33–50%: GI (gastro-esophageal reflux). Has the infant previously exhibited symptoms of gastroesophageal reflux or aspiration of thin liquids? These symptoms may include coughing, choking, or gagging during or after feeding; frequent or excessive spitting-up; persistent nasal stuffiness; or frequent hiccups. Acid reflux disease is suggested by excessive irritability, arching, and straining behaviors displayed during or following a feeding. *15–30%: Neurologic (seizures) *11–20%: Respiratory (lower respiratory tract infections) *4%: ENT *1–5%: Cardiac *In approximately 25–50% of cases no cause can be identified.*

4. Always address the two key questions : 1) Is this episode of clinical significance ? and 2) What is the risk of recurrence ? Factors to consider include signs of another acute illness, the age of child, and other possible risk factors for clinically significant or recurrent apnea.

5. Remember only a small percentage of patients with ALTE are at risk for SIDS (sudden infant death syndrome) : In addition only a small percentage of infants succumbing to SIDS have prior episodes of apnea. ALTEs occur in the same age group as infants who die of sudden death.

6. Hospitalize the most patients for observation in order to reduce stress on the family and allow prompt completion of the evaluation (**Refer to the Evaluation-Decision-Action -Plan /Algorithm**). From retrospective studies, apparent life-threatening events have been associated with *gastroesophageal reflux disease;* viral lower respiratory tract infection; *pertussis; sepsis* and/or meningitis; seizures; metabolic disorders; cardiac dysrhythmia (e.g. long QT syndrome, supraventricular tachycardia); anemia; nonaccidental trauma; or structural CNS, cardiac (ductal-dependent lesion), or airway anomaly. If historical events are inconsistent with physical findings, suspect child abuse and ensure proper documentation. Drug overdose, either accidental or intentional, may also present with apnea. Several series document that apneic episodes may be falsely reported by parents seeking attention (i.e. Munchausen - by - proxy syndrome). Look for pinch marks on the nares, as parents may physically interfere with a child's respiratory efforts.

7. Since there is "lack of consensus in approach" (*reflux testing (pH probe study or upper GI) *sleep study *EEG *ECG *head CT *chest x-ray *lumbar puncture *medications for presumed infection or GER) direct the therapy at the underlying cause if one is found after the evaluation (for e.g.: IV antibiotics for possible sepsis/meningitis, anticonvulsants for seizures, anti-reflux therapy for GE reflux, cardiologist opinion for any congenital heart disease or arrhythmias). *If no definable cause is found, the parents of infants who have had ALTEs should be instructed in basic cardiopulmonary resuscitation prior to discharge (refer to Figures 1, 2 & Table 3).*

8. Tell the parents the fact, that with over 20 years of home monitoring, the sudden infant death rate did not change due to home monitoring. They should be aware of the possibility of frequent false alarms and many parents can not handle the stress associated with having a apnea monitor in the home. Infants with severe initial episodes or repeated severe episodes are now thought to be at significant increased risk and should probably be monitored in the home, for the sake of parental reassurance. No objective guidelines exist for instituting or terminating the monitoring; Empirically agree that it's use will be terminated by either of; 2 mos. with no events, or 6 mos. of age.

9. Oxygen therapy by reducing periodic breathing of infancy, by increasing the baseline saturation, by reducing the severity of desaturation with short apneas can be useful as therapy for recurrent ALTEs. Respiratory stimulants such as Caffeine or Aminophylline can be used in specific cases of central apnea or periodic breathing.

10. Do follow the good medical practice, which dictates that the parents should always be given the specific instructions regarding indications for another emergency room visit and a follow-up visit to a primary care provider. Well-appearing infants older than 30 days who have experienced a single apparent life-threatening event and who have normal initial screening findings may be safely discharged from the hospital with proper outpatient follow-up.

---

* *Pearl/Peril/Pitfall : Surveillance programmes with the use of home monitoring devices may be undertaken, preferably with cardiorespiratory monitors, and when possible, with event monitors, although no currently available home monitoring device is free of false alarms or offers complete protection.*

THE EVALUATION-DECISION-ACTION-PLAN/ALGORITHM FOR THE DIAGNOSIS AND MANAGEMENT OF *APNEA AND APPARENT LIFE-THREATENING EVENT (ALTE) IN CHILDREN*

SUBJECTIVE FINDINGS

Hx of ALTE's full description from the witnesses. Was the baby asleep (central apnea) or awake and struggling to breathe (obstructive apnea)?

Hx of resuscitation done?

Hx of relation with feeding, position, or gagging or breath holding.

Hx of perinatal events, respiratory symptoms, medications, prematurity, family history of SIDS, Are the Newborn metabolic screening findings normal?

OBJECTIVE FINDINGS

GEN Pallor, cyanosis, fever/hypothermia/ full head-to-toe examination of the skin *CVS* tachycardia, bradycardia, cardiac arrest, heart murmur *RESP* may be associated with stridor, wheezing, rhinorrhea, cough, respiratory arrest *CNS* macrocephaly, signs ↑ of ICP, hypotonia, seizures, lethargy, fundus examination for retinal hemorrhages (child abuse), *Abdominal* distention or tenderness may indicate acute intestinal obstruction. Inguinoscrotal examination should be evaluated for incarcerated inguinal hernia or testicular torsion

INVESTIGATIONS

Blood ABG/CBG, CBC, differential, electrolytes, serum lactate, BUN, creatinine, glucose, Ca++, Mg++, Drug screen, LFTs.

Urine urinalysis, drug screen.

Imaging chest radiograph, head CT scan, lateral neck radiograph.

Others sepsis work-up to include lumbar puncture, RSV nasal wash.

Consider EEG, ECG, esophagogram, sleep pneumogram, metabolic screen, esophageal PH monitoring.

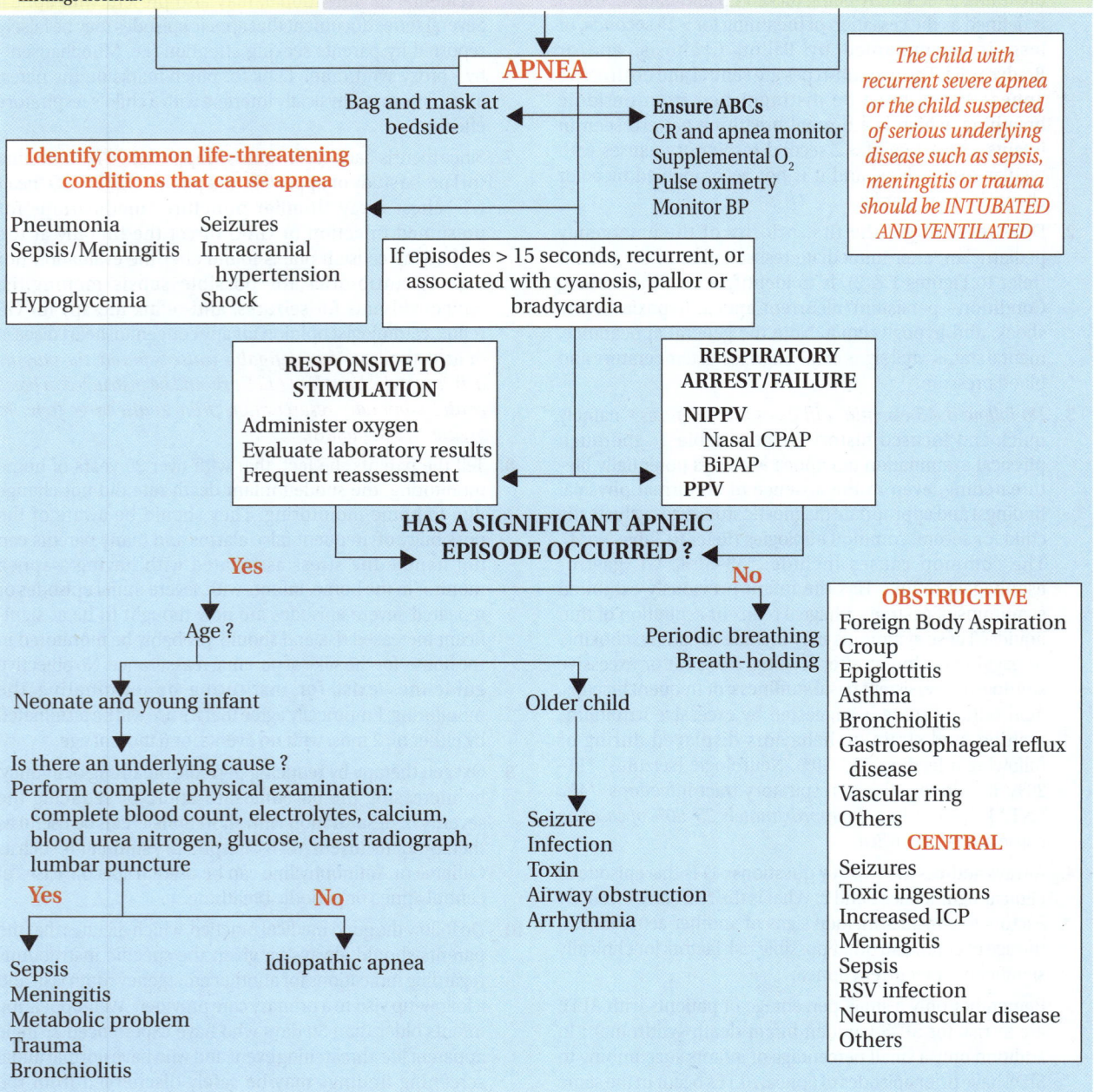

APNEA

Bag and mask at bedside

Ensure ABCs
CR and apnea monitor
Supplemental O₂
Pulse oximetry
Monitor BP

The child with recurrent severe apnea or the child suspected of serious underlying disease such as sepsis, meningitis or trauma should be INTUBATED AND VENTILATED

Identify common life-threatening conditions that cause apnea

Pneumonia	Seizures
Sepsis/Meningitis	Intracranial hypertension
Hypoglycemia	Shock

If episodes > 15 seconds, recurrent, or associated with cyanosis, pallor or bradycardia

RESPONSIVE TO STIMULATION

Administer oxygen
Evaluate laboratory results
Frequent reassessment

RESPIRATORY ARREST/FAILURE

NIPPV
　Nasal CPAP
　BiPAP
PPV

HAS A SIGNIFICANT APNEIC EPISODE OCCURRED?

Yes

Age?

No

Periodic breathing
Breath-holding

Neonate and young infant

Older child

Is there an underlying cause?
Perform complete physical examination:
　complete blood count, electrolytes, calcium,
　blood urea nitrogen, glucose, chest radiograph,
　lumbar puncture

Yes

No

Seizure
Infection
Toxin
Airway obstruction
Arrhythmia

Sepsis
Meningitis
Metabolic problem
Trauma
Bronchiolitis

Idiopathic apnea

OBSTRUCTIVE
Foreign Body Aspiration
Croup
Epiglottitis
Asthma
Bronchiolitis
Gastroesophageal reflux
　disease
Vascular ring
Others
CENTRAL
Seizures
Toxic ingestions
Increased ICP
Meningitis
Sepsis
RSV infection
Neuromuscular disease
Others

*　*Pearl/Peril/Pitfall: Infants with an ALTE present to medical attention because of an acute and unexpected change in behavior that alarmed the care giver. The initial episodes can occur during sleep, awake, or feeding. They are most commonly described as some combination of apnoea, color change (cyanotic or pallid, occasionally plethora), marked change in muscle tone (limpness, rarely rigidity), choking or gagging [41]. In most cases the observers reported that the episode appeared potentially life-threatening or they thought the infant had died, and that a prompt intervention was associated with normalization of the child's CRY, COLOR, AND ACTIVITY.*

TABLE 1 — Differential diagnosis of apnea

	Neonate, infant	Older child
Central nervous system	Infection (meningitis, encephalitis	Infection
	Seizure	Toxin
	Prematurity	Tumor
	Intraventricular hemorrhage	Seizure
	Increased intracranial pressure (ICP)	Increased ICP (trauma, hydrocephalus)
	Congenital anomaly (e.g., Arnold-chiari)	
	Breath-holding spell	Idiopathic hypoventilation ("Ondine's curse")
Upper airway	Laryngospasm (e.g., gastroesophageal reflux)	Obstructive sleep apnea
	Infection (e.g., croup)	Infection (epiglottitis, croup)
	Congenital anomaly (e.g., Down syndrome)	Foreign body
Lower airway	Infection (pneumonia, bronchiolitis)	Infection
	Congenital anomaly	Asthma
Other	Infant botulism	Guillain-Barre syndrome
	Hypocalcemia, hypoglycemia	Spinal cord injury
	Anemia	Flail chest
	Sepsis	Arrhythmia
	Arrhythmia	
	Sudden infant death syndrome (SIDS)	

TABLE 2 — Historical features of apnea

History	Significant apnea
Duration of event	Greater than 10 sec
Was child asleep or awake?	Either, but apnea during sleep is more worrisome
Color change	Pallor or cyanosis
Associated movements, posture, or change in tone	Seizure activity Hypotonia "He looked dead"
Resuscitative efforts and response	Color change or hypotonia requiring cardiopulmonary resuscitation to improve
Interval since last feeding	If shortly after feeding, consider gastroeso phageal reflux
Where event occurred	Association with sleep, trauma

Figure 2

THE SAFE APPROACH

Shout for help
Approach with care
Free from danger
Evaluate ABC

Figure 1

The overall sequence of basic life support in cardiopulmonary arrest
(CPR = Cardiopulmonary Resuscitation)

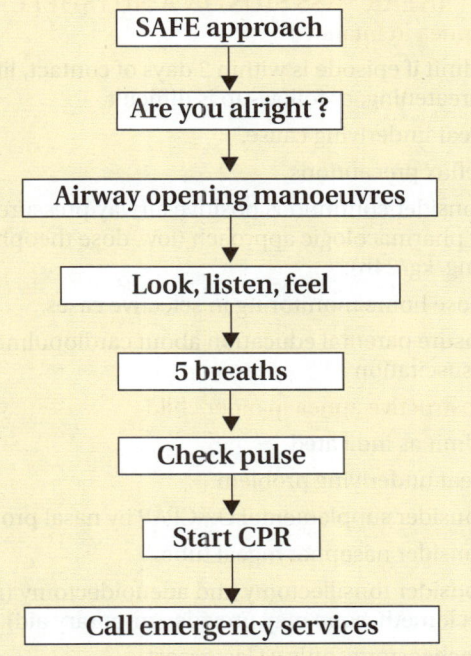

SAFE approach
↓
Are you alright ?
↓
Airway opening manoeuvres
↓
Look, listen, feel
↓
5 breaths
↓
Check pulse
↓
Start CPR
↓
Call emergency services

TABLE 3 — Summary of basic life support techniques in infants and children

	Infant	Small child	Larger child
Airway Head-tilt position	Neutral	Sniffing	Sniffing
Breathing Initial slow breaths	5	5	5
Circulation Pulse check	Brachial or femoral	Carotid	Carotid
Landmark	One finger-breadth below nipple line	One finger-breadth above xiphisternum	Two finger-breadths above xiphisternum
Technique	Two fingers or encircling	One hand	Two hands
Cardiopulmonary resuscitation Ratio	5:1	5:1	5:1 (15:2)
Cycles per minute	20	20	20 (4)

* ***Pearl/Peril/Pitfall** : ALTE:INVESTIGATIONS-These will be dictated by the clinical presentation, but will often include: • Full blood count and differential count, C-reactive protein. • Capillary blood gas • Urea & electrolytes, Ca++, fasting (pre-feed) blood glucose, liver function tests • Chest x-ray • ECG (measure QT interval) • Overnight oximetry with printout. If febrile, blood and urine cultures (consider lumbar puncture). In selected cases, the following investigations may be appropriate: • Metabolic: Lactate / pyruvate, ammonia, urine amino & organic acids, carnitine profile. • Barium swallow, pH monitoring. • ENT consultation (with PA and lateral neck x-ray). • EEG. • CT head (history or signs of head trauma, altered level of consciousness).*

KEY PRACTICAL PROCEDURE (s) TO DEAL WITH *APPARENT LIFE-THREATENING EVENT*

BAG AND MASK VENTILATION

Indication

(1) Apnea/gasping (2) Heart rate < 100/minute

Equipment: (1) Resuscitation bag (self-inflating, capacity 240-260ml) (2) Oxygen (90–100%) (3) Masks, (4) Oxygen equipment (source, flowmeter, tubing, etc.)

Procedure : The baby's neck should be slightly extended to ensure an open airway while he lies on his back. The appropriate sized self-inflating bag and mask are selected. The mask is placed in position so that it covers the mouth and the nose but not the eyes. Then, bagging is started at a rate of 40–60/minute for 15-30 seconds, using enough pressure to cause good chest movements. In case the chest fails to move adequately, change the position of the infant, suction the throat and then apply bag and mask carefully.

Evaluation : If heart rate > 100/minute and infant having spontaneous breathing, stop bagging (ventilation). If the infant is yet not having spontaneous breathing or is gasping, continue ventilation. If heart rate 60–100/minute and showing still an increase, continue ventilation and check for adequacy of ventilation from chest evaluation. If heart rate is 60–100/minute and is not increasing, continue ventilation. If heart rate < 80/minute, start chest compressions. If heart rate < 60/minute, continue to ventilate and begin chest compressions ; consider endotracheal intubation.

Signs of Improvement: (1) Rising heart rate (2) Spontaneous breathing, (3) Improving color.

Risks: Abdominal distention because of gastric distention from entry of air into stomach during ventilation.

Trouble shooting (If chest does not rise)

Action	Condition Corrected
1. Reapply mask	Inadequate seal
2. Reposition infant's head	Blocked airway
3. Check for secretions, suction if present	Blocked airway
4. Ventilate with mouth slightly open	Blocked airway
5. Increase pressure slightly	Inadequate pressures
If chest *still* does not rise, get a new bag, check it, and try again.	

CHEST COMPRESSION

Indications : If after 30 seconds of PPV with 100 percent oxygen, heart rate remains < 60/minute. The earlier recommendation of starting chest compression at heart rate of 60–80 and not rising stands withdrawn increasingly.

Site: Lower third of the sternum below the imaginary line drawn between two nipples.

Procedure: In the preferred thumb technique, thumbs are employed to compress the sternum while the fingers support the back and the hands encircle the torso. In the two-finger technique, the fingertips (middle finger with index finger or ring) are employed to compress the sternum. The other hand supports the Neonate's back. The rate of chest compression should be 90 compressions and 30 PPVs in one minute, making a total of 120 events. The depth of compression should be 1–2 cm. During the procedure, fingers of thumb must never be taken off the sternum, during both compression and release.

Evaluation : Thirty seconds of chest compression should be followed by rechecking of the heart rate. If heart rate < 80 / minute, the procedure should continue along with bad and mask ventilation with 100 percent oxygen. plus medication. If heart rate is > 80/minute, stop chest compression but continue ventilation until heart rate crosses 100/minute and the Neonate is breathing spontaneously.

Risks: Trauma to the chest in the form of fractures, pneumothorax and laceration of liver.

MANAGEMENT OF ALTE (NEAR MISS SIDS) IN A NUTSHELL

a. Apnea in infancy

Admit if episode is within 2 days of contact, life threatening, or follow-up is difficult.

Treat underlying cause.

Reflux precautions.

Consider continuous positive airway pressure (CPAP) or pharmacologic approach (low-dose theophylline-5mg/kg/24h).

Close home monitoring in selective cases.

Ensure parental education about cardiopulmonary resuscitation .

b. Obstructive apnea in older child

Admit as indicated.

Treat underlying problem.

Consider supplemental O_2, CPAP by nasal prongs.

Consider nasopharyngeal tube.

Consider tonsillectomy and adenoidectomy (nasal beclomethasone may provide temporary aid).

Tracheostomy only as last resort.

---

* *Pearl/Peril/Pitfall: ALTE:Possible Treatable Causes • Infection : bacterial : meningitis, septicaemia , viral : URTI, pertussis, RSV, etc. • Airway obstruction: congenital abnormalities, infection, hypotonia. • Gastro-oesophageal reflux • Metabolic problems : hypoglycemia, hypocalcaemia, etc. • Cardiac disease: congenital heart disease, arrhythmias, vascular ring. • Toxin / Drugs : accidental or non-accidental. • Neurological causes : head injury, seizures, infections etc. • Rarely apnoea may be a manifestation of child abuse (shaken baby, drug overdose, Münchhausen by proxy syndrome).*

Lack of causal relationship between ALTE and SIDS: An association between SIDS and ALTE had been suggested because of prior ALTE events in 5 percent of SIDS victims and early anecdotal reports of SIDS in infants with recurrent apnea . However, the vast majority of SIDS victims do not experience apnea prior to death. Furthermore, studies over the past two decades have failed to confirm a causal relationship between preexisting apnea and SIDS. Several other factors argue against a relationship between SIDS and ALTE: *ALTE refers to a heterogeneous group of problems ranging from benign to near-fatal, whereas SIDS denotes a fatal problem. *The case definition in ALTE depends upon parental observations, which have been shown to be unreliable in several studies *Over 80 percent of SIDS deaths occur between midnight and 6 AM , whereas 82 percent of ALTE episodes occur between 8 AM and 8 PM . *Interventions to prevent SIDS (e.g., supine sleeping) have not resulted in a decreased incidence of ALTE *The risk factors for SIDS and ALTE differ . In one prospective population-based study, prone sleeping, lack of breast feeding, and maternal smoking were risks for SIDS, whereas behavioral characteristics such as repeated apnea, pallor, history of cyanosis, and feeding difficulties were risk factors for ALTE.

TABLE 4	**ALTE-diagnostic evaluation**

ALTE-Diagnostic evaluation may include the following:

* A CBC count to screen for the presence of systemic viral or bacterial infection or anemia.

* Serum chemistry levels to assess for -hypoglycemia, -hyponatremia,-hyperkalemia, acidemia, -hypocalcemia, or elevation of serum lactate

* ABG to assess for acidosis or retention of carbon dioxide

* Serum or urine toxicology studies for suspected ingestions

* Specific bacterial or viral cultures to assess for -respiratory syncytial virus (RSV), pertussis, -bacteremia, or urinary tract infection

* ECG to assess for long QT syndrome and preexcitation that suggests supraventricular tachycardia or other dysrhythmia

* EEG to assess for epileptiform activity

* Upper GI contrast studies to assess for swallowing dysfunction, thin liquid aspiration, or upper-intestinal anatomic malformations

* Impedance pH monitoring to assess for gastroesophageal reflux disease

* Neuroimaging to assess for hemorrhage or structural CNS abnormality

* Polysomnography to assess for sleep-based disturbances in cardiorespiratory control.

KEY POINTS FOR CLINICAL PRACTICE:

1. An apparent life-threatening event (ALTE) is defined as an episode that is frightening to the observer and is characterized by some combination of apnea (central or obstructive), color change (cyanotic, pallid, erythematous or plethoric), change in muscle tone (usually diminished), and choking or gagging. In some cases, the observer fears that the infant has died.The cause of apparent life-threatening events (ALTEs) in infants reflects a differential diagnosis that includes an array of congenital or acquired disorders. As many as 50% of apparent life-threatening events may remain unexplained following a thorough evaluation. The apparent life-threatening events were associated with the following: *Gastroesophageal reflux disease - 26% *Pertussis - 9% *Lower respiratory tract infection - 9% *Seizure - 9% *Urinary tract infection - 8% *Factitious illness - 3% *Miscellaneous - 11%.

2. ALTE replaced the terms: *Aborted crib death *Near-miss sudden infant death syndrome *Change corrects erroneous implication of an association between ALTE and*sudden infant death syndrome (SIDS).

3. The evaluation and disposition of an infant following an apparent life-threatening event (ALTE) is directed by a thorough history of the event and a careful physical examination. In most cases, the infant is free of symptoms by the time medical evaluation occurs, allowing for a systematic approach to history-taking and physical examination.

4. In-hospital observation has been suggested for most infants following an apparent life-threatening event (ALTE). The initial evaluation of some infants reveals active ongoing symptoms and clearly suggests the need for hospitalization for further evaluation and treatment (e.g., sepsis). However, apparent life-threatening events that are the result of self-resolving episodes of choking or gagging associated with feedings in well-appearing infants may be observed in an outpatient setting.

5. Documenting cardiorespiratory monitors may be considered for preterm infants who are at high risk for recurrent apnea or bradycardia and for infants who depend on technology due to specific disorders of cardiorespiratory control.

REFERENCES & FURTHER READING: 1)McGovern, MC, Smith, MB. Causes of apparent life threatening events in infants: a systematic review. Arch Dis Child 2004; 89:1043. 2)Genizi, J, Pillar, G, Ravid, S, Shahar, E. Apparent life-threatening events: neurological correlates and the mandatory work-up. J Child Neurol 2008; 23:1305 3) Kahn, A. Recommended clinical evaluation of infants with an apparent life-threatening event. Consensus document of the European Society for the Study and Prevention of Infant Death, 2003. Eur J Pediatr 2004; 163:108. 4) Farrell, PA, Weiner, GM, Lemons, JA. SIDS, ALTE, apnea, and the use of home monitors. Pediatr Rev 2002; 23:3. 5) Apnea, sudden infant death syndrome, and home monitoring. Pediatrics 2003; 111:914.

---

* *Pearl/Peril/Pitfall :* ALTE: What was the description of the event? A caregiver's description of the infants' color, respiration, and muscle tone is key. Care must be taken to distinguish central cyanosis (lips and oral mucous membranes) from acrocyanosis (hands and feet). Infants who are coughing, choking, or gagging may exhibit a ruddy or plethoric facial color that may be interpreted as "turning blue." Determine whether apnea was present, and, if so, whether it appeared to be central (lack of respiratory effort) or obstructive (respiratory effort with inadequate airflow). Distinguish apnea that lasted more than 15-20 seconds from periodic breathing, in which respiratory rate and tidal volumes fluctuate and are accompanied by brief pauses in breathing that typically last less than 5-10 seconds.

Bronchiolitis

100

@ Prognosis of Bronchiolitis is excellent. Most children recover in 3 to 5 days without sequelae, although wheezing and cough may continue for 2 to 4 wk. Mortality is < 1% when medical care is adequate. An increased incidence of asthma is suspected in children who have had bronchiolitis in early childhood, but the association is controversial and the incidence seems to decrease as children age.

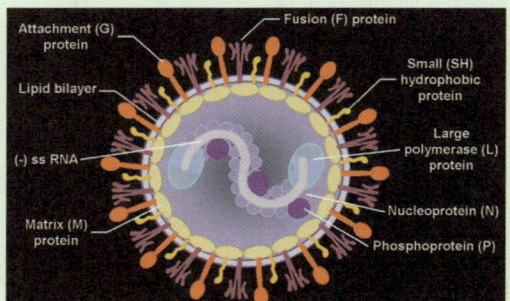

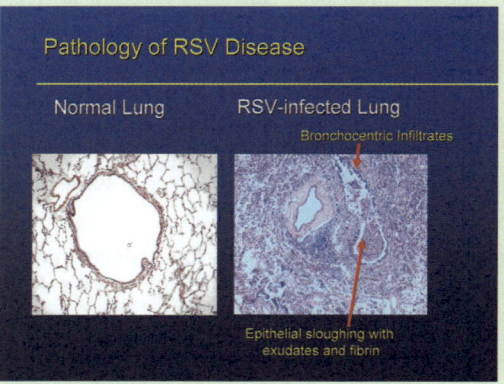

Pathology of RSV Disease

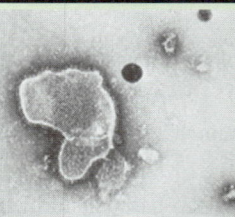

An electron micrograph of respiratory syncytial virus (RSV). RSV is the most common cause of bronchiolitis and pneumonia in children younger than 1 year. Image courtesy of CDC.

Courtesy: Mark Polak, MD
Professor of Pediatrics West Virginia University
SoMWVU Children's Hospital

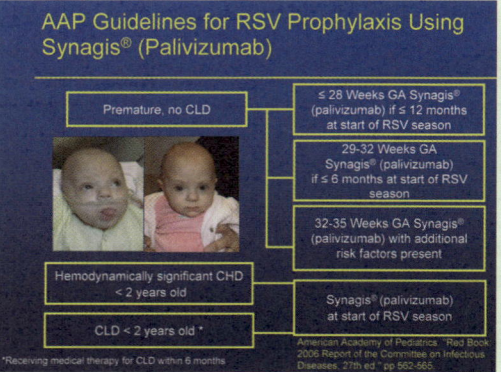

AAP Guidelines for RSV Prophylaxis Using Synagis® (Palivizumab)

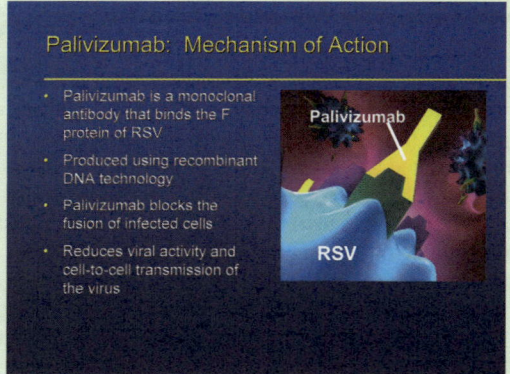

Palivizumab: Mechanism of Action

- Palivizumab is a monoclonal antibody that binds the F protein of RSV
- Produced using recombinant DNA technology
- Palivizumab blocks the fusion of infected cells
- Reduces viral activity and cell-to-cell transmission of the virus

REVIEW OF CLINICAL PROBLEMS

1. Discuss the clinical guidelines for Palivizumab (Synagis) prophylaxis (AAP).
   Ans: Refer to No 10 of the Bird's eye view/Overview/Synopsis of the Chapter.

2. What are the Evidence -Based Recommendations for the diagnosis & management of Bronchiolitis?
   Ans: Refer to the Table 1 of the Chapter.

3. Mention the important History to be elicited, when a Neonate/Infant is admitted with suspected Bronchiolitis.
   Ans: Refer to the Evaluation-Decision-Action Plan/Algorithm to diagnose and manage Bronchiolitis.

4. How do you monitor for the degree of illness in a child with Bronchiolitis?
   Ans: Refer to the Evaluation-Decision-Action Plan/Algorithm to diagnose and manage Bronchiolitis.

5. Discuss the management of Moderate-Severe Bronchiolitis.
   Ans: Refer to the Evaluation-Decision-Action Plan/Algorithm to diagnose and manage Bronchiolitis.

LEARNING OBJECTIVES

After completing this article, readers will be able to:

1. Diagnose Bronchiolitis clinically and assess the severity of illness for triaging the patients.

2. Provide the supportive therapy and hospitalize severe cases for monitoring and intervention if deterioration occurs.

3. Identify the High-risk groups for developing severe Bronchiolitis and protect them with palivizumab (Synagis) prophylaxis.

4. Prevent nosocomial spread of RSV by thorough hand washing and isolate the patients as a group in a bay

5. Follow-up Bronchiolitis patients for recurrent wheezing and Reactive Airway disease.

---

* **Pearl/Peril/Pitfall :** Bronchiolitis:In hospitalized children, 30 to 40% O_2 delivered by tent or face mask is usually sufficient to maintain O_2 saturation > 90%. Endotracheal intubation is indicated for severe recurrent apnea, hypoxemia unresponsive to O_2 therapy, or CO_2 retention or if the child cannot clear bronchial secretions.

BIRD'S EYE VIEW/OVERVIEW/SYNOPSIS

1. Bronchiolitis is a disorder most commonly caused in infants by viral lower respiratory tract infection (LRTI). It is the most common lower respiratory infection in this age group. It is characterized by acute inflammation, edema and necrosis of epithelial cells lining small airways, increased mucus production, and bronchospasm. Signs and symptoms are typically rhinitis, tachypnea, wheezing, cough, crackles, use of accessory muscles, and/or nasal flaring. Many viruses cause the same constellation of symptoms and signs. The most common etiology is the respiratory syncytial virus (RSV), with the highest incidence of RSV infection occurring between December and March. Ninety percent of children are infected with RSV in the first 2 years of life, and up to 40% of them will have lower respiratory infection.

2. Infection with RSV does not grant permanent or longterm immunity. Reinfections are common and may be experienced throughout life. Other viruses identified as causing bronchiolitis are human metapneumovirus, influenza, adenovirus, and parainfluenza. In the community setting, a number of factors have been associated with increased risk of acquiring RSV disease, including the following: Childcare attendance, Older siblings in preschool or school , Crowding, lower socioeconomic status, Exposure to environmental pollutants (e.g., cigarette smoke), Multiple birth sets (especially triplets or greater) , Minimal breastfeeding.

3. The illness may begin with URT symptoms and progress rapidly over 1-2 days to the development of diffuse small airway disease characterized by cough, coryza, wheezing and rales, low-grade fever (<101°F), and decreased oral intake. A family history of asthma and/or atopy is frequently obtained.In more advanced disease, retractions and cyanosis may be noted, and as many as 20% of patients may develop higher temperatures. The incidence of concomitant or secondary serious bacterial infection in association with RSV infection appears to be quite low (<1%), except for otitis media, which may occur in as many as 40% of cases. In very young infants, apnea out of proportion to respiratory signs and symptoms may be present, and, in infants younger than 6 weeks, a more nonspecific sepsislike picture has been described.

4. In addition to morbidity and mortality during the acute illness, infants hospitalized with bronchiolitis are more likely to have respiratory problems as older children, especially recurrent wheezing, compared with those who did not have severe disease. Severe disease is characterized by persistently increased respiratory effort, apnea, or the need for intravenous hydration, supplemental oxygen, or mechanical ventilation. It is unclear whether severe viral illness early in life predisposes children to develop recurrent wheezing or if infants who experience severe bronchiolitis have an underlying predisposition to recurrent wheezing.

5. Laboratory studies frequently are not indicated in the infant with bronchiolitis who is comfortable in room air, well hydrated, and feeding adequately. Nonspecific laboratory studies may include CBC count, serum electrolytes, urinalysis, and oxygen saturation measurement. The CBC count may reveal a normal or mildly elevated WBC count and an elevated percentage of band forms. Blood cultures, although obtained frequently, are rarely positive for pathogenic bacteria. An arterial blood gas may be indicated if carbon dioxide retention is a concern.

6. Specific diagnostic tests for confirmation of respiratory syncytial virus (RSV) infection are readily available. These tests can be performed on samples of secretions obtained by washing, suctioning, or swabbing the nasopharynx. Secretions can be analyzed for virus in the laboratory by culture and/or antigen revealing techniques. Newer molecular probes for revealing RSV in clinical specimens are being developed and may be more sensitive than the above assays, although they are not routinely available at this time. The antigen detection methods offer the potential for diagnosis within hours and may be obtained reliably in the absence of a sophisticated virology laboratory. However, monitoring of test performance is critical in maintaining appropriate sensitivity and specificity. Specific tests for RSV may be indicated for making decisions regarding therapy (e.g., withdrawal of unnecessary antibiotics), isolation of patients, and in educating parents and staff about the nature of RSV disease. Chest radiography is frequently obtained in children with severe RSV infection. Chest radiography typically reveals hyperinflated lung fields with a diffuse increase in interstitial markings. In 20-25% of cases, focal areas of atelectasis and/or pulmonary infiltrate are also noted. Generally, these findings are neither specific to RSV infection nor predictive of the course or outcome, except for the observation that infants who have the additional findings of atelectasis and/or pneumonia may have a more severe course with their illness.

7. In assessing an infant with RSV infection, several factors have been correlated with more severe disease and the need for hospitalization. Although infants in these groups (outlined below) are at increased risk for severe RSV disease compared to normal full-term infants based on percentage, many more children in the normal full-term group are admitted; thus, most admissions for RSV disease occur in otherwise normal infants. Family history of asthma and genetic factors also correlate with more severe RSV disease, although the exact relationship and mechanisms have not been elucidated. *Prematurity, especially birth at less than 35 weeks' gestation *Age younger than 3 months at time of infection *Chronic lung disease *Congenital heart disease *Congenital immunodeficiency (e.g., *severe combined immunodeficiency [SCID]) *Severe neuromuscular disease *Toxic appearance at time of presentation *Respiratory rate more than 70 per minute in room air *Atelectasis and/or pneumonitis on chest radiography *Oxygen less than 95% on room air.

8. Bronchiolitis is a clinical diagnosis that does not require diagnostic testing. Many of the commonly used management modalities have not been shown to be effective in improving the clinical course of the illness. This includes the routine use of bronchodilators, corticosteroids, ribavirin, antibiotics, chest radiography, chest physiotherapy, and complementary and alternative therapies.

9. Supportive care is the mainstay of therapy for respiratory syncytial virus (RSV) infection. If the child can take in fluids by mouth and tolerate room air, outpatient management, with close physician contact as needed, is reasonable, especially in the absence of significant underlying risk factors. For children who require hospitalization for RSV infection, supportive therapy is still the mainstay of care. Supportive care may include administration of supplemental oxygen (guided by respiratory rates, work of breathing, oxygen saturation, and arterial blood gases, as indicated), mechanical ventilation, and fluid replacement, as necessary. Refer to the Table No 1 of the Chapter for the Evidence-Based Recommendations to manage Bronchiolitis Cases. Antiviral therapy (Ribavirin) for severe RSV disease is indicated in high-risk patients. Treatment must be promptly initiated at the onset of the infection to effectively inhibit the replicating virus.

10. Attempts to develop a vaccine against RSV (as opposed to the passive protection discussed above) have been unsuccessful to date. Respiratory syncytial virus (RSV) transmission appears to occur via contact with infected secretions through hand-to-hand spread and/or fomites and respiratory droplets with an incubation period of 3-5 days. Aerosolized secretions appear to be less important in RSV transmission; thus, attention to handwashing and cleaning of environmental surfaces are important to prevent RSV transmission. In the hospital setting, isolation of patients infected with RSV as a group and wearing of mask and gown during close contact with infected children are important in controlling nosocomial spread. Transmission of RSV on pediatric units has been shown to be a significant problem.The AAP Committee on Infectious Diseases guidelines for candidates for palivizumab (Synagis) prophylaxis are as follows. *Infants younger than 24 months who have hemodynamically significant congenital heart disease (cyanotic or acyanotic lesions) or chronic lung disease and are off oxygen and/or pulmonary medications for less than 6 months at the start of RSV season *Premature infants born at less than 28 weeks' gestational age who are younger than 1 year chronological age at the start of RSV season *Premature infants born at 29-32 weeks' gestational age who are younger than 6 months chronological age at the start of RSV season *Infants born at 33-35 weeks' gestational age who are younger than 6 months chronological age and have at least 2 additional risk factors at the start of RSV season. A second-generation monoclonal antibody, motavizumab, has increased affinity for RSV compared with palivizumab and is currently under investigation.

* *Pearl/Peril/Pitfall : Bronchiolitis:Hydration may be maintained with frequent small feedings of clear liquids. For sicker children, fluids should be given IV initially, and the level of hydration should be monitored by urine output and specific gravity and by serum electrolyte determinations.*

THE EVALUATION-DECISION-ACTION-PLAN/ALGORITHM FOR THE DIAGNOSIS AND MANAGEMENT OF *BRONCHIOLITIS (RSV)*

SUBJECTIVE FINDINGS

Hx Fever (typically low-grade), Cough, Tachypnea, Cyanosis, Retractions, Wheezing, Rales, Sepsislike presentation or apneic episodes (in very young infants) *Identify* the **High-risk groups** for severe RSV infection include the following: *Premature infants in their first year of life (the younger the child is [gestational and chronological age] at the start of RSV season, the greater the risk) *Infants with chronic lung disease (e.g., bronchopulmonary dysplasia, *cystic fibrosis) during their first 2 years of life *Children with hemodynamically significant congenital heart disease, especially with increased pulmonary blood flow *Immunodeficient states *Children with metabolic and neuromuscular disorders *Children of multiple births (triplets or greater)

OBJECTIVE FINDINGS

Assess airway, breathing, circulation & disability by observing the vitals, BP, O2 sats, color, CRT, pulses, sensorium, focal neurologic deficits, Apnea, seizures, abnormal movements, tone & reflexes etc.

Identify the impending respiratory failure especially, in high-risk groups

Perform complete physical examination from head to toe including detailed neurological examination.

INVESTIGATIONS

Blood ABG/CBG, CBC, differential, electrolytes, serum lactate, BUN, creatinine, glucose, Ca^{++}, Mg^{++}, Drug screen

Imaging chest radiograph in high-risk groups to identify/rule out atelectasis, pneumonia, pneumothorax

Others RSV-ELISA nasal wash (If clinically indicated, Sepsis work-up to include lumbar puncture)

SUSPECTED BRONCHIOLITIS

Monitor for the degree of Illness;

Mild Respiratory Rate <60 bpm, good air entry, minimal or no retractions, no signs of dehydration

Moderate Resp.Rate>60bpm, moderate retractions, prolonged expiratory phase with decreased air exchange

Severe High-risk groups mentioned above, marked increase in work of breathing, O_2 sats <94% at sea level/ <90% at 5000 ft, signs of dehydration/systemic toxicity

Very severe Apnea/Arrest, Shock, Cyanosis on O_2 supplements, ABG Analysis-PaO_2<50 mmHg and $PaCO_2$>60mm Hg

Follow AAP Evidence-Based Recommendations/Options, if any doubt exists about the diagnostics/therapeutics.

Ensure ABCs -CR and apnea monitor Supplemental O_2, Pulse oximetry, Monitor BP

Mild-Moderate Illness

Ensure proper hydration*Consider a trial of Salbutamol/Albuterol(1.5–2.5mg in 3ml NS) Nebs. and Racemic/Regular epinephrine Nebs. 0.25–0.5 ml in 3 ml NS (Anticholinergic agents such as ipratropium have not been shown to alter the course of viral bronchiolitis.) *Parameters to measure its effectiveness include improvements in wheezing, respiratory rate, respiratory effort, and oxygen saturation. *Home care, if good response with feeding, breathing, sleeping, interacting, and smiling *Educate parents to return if their child develops fast breathing, chest indrawing, blue color, fever, or becomes too weak to eat *Assess in 24–48 hours *Revisit in 1-2 week

Severe illness
Provide Supportive care—fluids, O_2 supplements, Nebulized Bronchodilators, @ Ribavirin in High-Risk groups, IV antibiotics if bacterial illness is co-existing/cannot be differentiated
Continue Ongoing Monitoring-Serum potassium, glucose, ABG Analysis, ABCDs as needed

Poor Response

Good Response

Discharge home *Follow-up in 24-48 hours

@ Ribavirin - Analog of the nucleic acid guanosine. Ribavirin inhibits viral replication by an unknown mechanism. Reconstitute 6 g in 300 mL of distilled water to a concentration of 20 mg/mL . Administer as aerosol for 12–20 h/d for 3–7 d based on clinical response. Alternatively, 6 g in 100 mL of distilled water aerosol in 2-h pulses tid has been suggested as equally effective in small studies.

Very severe illness
Ensure ABCDs * Intubate and ventilate if apneic, shocked, and respiratory failure supervenes*Consider all the measures such as fluids, O_2 supplements, Nebulized Bronchodilators, Ribavirin in High-Risk groups, IV antibiotics if bacterial illness is co-existing/cannot be differentiated.
Consider Palivizumab (Synagis):A humanized monoclonal antibody directed against the F (fusion) protein of RSV. Administered monthly through the RSV season, it has been demonstrated to decrease the chances of RSV hospitalization in premature babies who are at increased risk for severe RSV-related illness. 15 mg/kg/dose IM every mo through RSV season (typically November through April in the northern hemisphere).

---

* **Pearl/Peril/Pitfall :** *3% saline, when combined with a Nebulized bronchodilator, does seem to shorten length of hospital stay in children who are admitted with diagnoses of bronchiolitis. — Howard Bauchner, MD Published in Journal Watch Pediatrics and Adolescent Medicine May 13, 2009.*

Life Threatening Bilateral Tension Pneumothorax Complicating Artificial Ventilation in an Infant with Severe RSV Bronchiolitis

A Case Report by YW *Hui,* WH *Choy,* KY *Chan* HK J Paediatr (new series) 2007;12:58-60

A 2-month-old girl, who was well all along, presented with a 3-day history of fever and coryzal symptoms. She was treated by private doctors with dexchlorpheniramine, ephedrine nasal drops and cefaclor. Her condition was getting worse and developed shortness of breath with noisy breathing and became drowsy and cyanotic. In the Accident & Emergency Department (AED), she was found to be in severe respiratory distress with marked chest recession, and cyanosis. The initial vital signs were heart rate 134/min, respiratory rate 40 breaths/min and SaO2 76%. Chest examination revealed poor air entry with occasional expiratory rhonchi. The liver edge was 2 cm below the right costal margin. Respiratory failure developed rapidly, prompting emergent intubation. An endotracheal tube of size 3.5 mm was inserted at a level of 11 cm at the lip. There was no foreign body found at the throat during intubation. She was supported with hand ventilation using Laerdal ambu bag. She improved and turned pink, but about 5 minutes later, she became cyanotic again despite continuous hand ventilation. The lung became very stiff to bagging and the heart rate dropped to 40/min, but the pulse was not palpated. The liver edge was 10 cm below the right costal margin. Cardiopulmonary resuscitation was initiated, and 3 doses of epinephrine were administered by intraosseous route. Tension pneumothorax was suspected and needle thoracostomy was performed and yielded 30 ml and 50 ml of air from left and right chest respectively. Her condition improved after the procedure. Chest X-radiograph (CXR) showed bilateral tension pneumothorax (Figure 1). Two chest tubes were immediately inserted (one on each side of chest) and she was transferred to the pediatric intensive care unit (PICU) for further care. In the PICU, she was sedated and paralysed with midazolam and atracurium infusions, and supported by mechanical ventilation. Chest examination revealed satisfactory air entry with prolonged expiratory phase, diffuse crepitation and rhonchi. The liver edge was 2 cm below the right costal margin The CXR revealed re-expansion of both lungs with diffuse haziness in the right middle zone (Figure 2). The first blood gas showed significant metabolic acidosis: pH 7.17, PaO2 67.7 mmHg, PaCO2 28.8 mmHg, bicarbonate 10.5 mmol/l and base excess -16.9. The complete blood picture was normal: white blood cell count 7.5 x 109/l (neutrophil/lymphocyte 3.7/3.1 x 10^9/l), hemoglobin 11.7 g/dl, platelet count 404 x 109/l. Nasopharyngeal aspirate (NPA) was positive for RSV, and negative for adenovirus, influenza A & B, parainfluenza and Chlamydia trachomatis. Per-nasal swab for Bordetella pertussis was negative. Endotracheal tube aspirate and blood for bacterial culture were also negative. The liver and renal function tests were normal. She was treated with intravenous cefotaxime. In view of the problem of air-trapping in severe acute bronchiolitis, the ventilation strategy of permissive hypercapnia was adopted in order to minimize further barotraumas to the lungs. She was being ventilated with pressure control mode using Infant Star ventilator. On day 1, the inspiratory/expiratory ratio was 1 to 4 and respiratory rate 25/min; the highest positive inspiratory pressure (PIP) and positive end-expiratory pressure (PEEP) were 27 cmH2O and 5 cmH2O respectively. Nebulised salbutamol was given through the ventilator circuit to relieve the small airway obstruction. She showed satisfactory response and her progress in the PICU was good. The highest PaCO2 was 70.1 mmHg (9.2 kPa) at 10 hours and the blood gas finally normalized at 36 hours of PICU care.

She was extubated on day 3. The left side chest tube was removed on day 5 and the right side chest tube on day 6. There was no recurrence of pneumothorax. She left the PICU on day 7 and was discharged from the hospital on day 11. She was last seen at the age of 1½ years old and was found to have normal development and the examination of the respiratory system was normal.

Discussion : Acute bronchiolitis is a common cause for childhood hospitalization. In US, Shay et al found that the annual bronchiolitis hospitalization rate was 31 per 1000 infants per year in 1996, and RSV was the most important cause of bronchiolitis. Most of the patients with acute bronchiolitis recover uneventfully. Spontaneous pneumothorax caused by RSV bronchiolitis is rare. A case of spontaneous bilateral pneumothorax was reported in 1987 by Pollack et al. Because of the small-sized pneumothoraces, the patient was successfully treated with simple aspiration. Pneumothoraces are divided into post-traumatic, iatrogenic and spontaneous which is further classified as primary spontaneous pneumothorax and secondary spontaneous pneumothorax. For post-traumatic pneumothorax, it can be penetrating or non-penetrating thoracic injury. Thoracocentesis, lung biopsy and artificial ventilation are examples causing iatrogenic pneumothorax. Primary spontaneous pneumothorax occurs in patients with no pre-existing lung disease whereas secondary spontaneous pneumothorax occurs in patients with predisposing lung disease or pulmonary anatomical abnormality such as hyaline membrane disease and congenital pulmonary hypoplasia in newborns, cystic fibrosis, bronchiolitis and asthma. In paediatric group of patients, primary spontaneous pneumothorax is the commonest and mainly occurs in teenagers with tall and slim stature. The other group of patients vulnerable to pneumothorax are those receiving ventilator therapy for their primary severe respiratory diseases including acute respiratory distress syndrome, pneumonia, asthma, bronchiolitis, pulmonary congenital diseases and foreign body aspiration. We report a case of life threatening bilateral tension pneumothorax complicating artificial ventilation in a patient suffering from RSV bronchiolitis. The patient was hypoxic and lapsed into respiratory failure which warranted emergent intubation and artificial ventilation. She showed good response in the beginning. During resuscitation, hand ventilation is usually performed too energetically i.e. using too high a pressure and rate. This is very risky in patient with air trapping conditions like asthma or bronchiolitis. The uncontrolled manual ventilation can result in more severe air trapping, and ultimately, the alveoli ruptured resulting in bilateral tension pneumothorax. Mechanical ventilation for patients with bronchiolitis is not an easy issue. The small airway obstruction and inflamed edematous alveoli makes the lungs very prone to exaggerated air trapping and barotraumas which will further cause air leaks in the lung such as pneumothorax and pneumomediastinum. Briassoulis et al found that there was strong positive correlation between the incidence of air leaks and high ventilatory pressure or large tidal volume which induced barotraumas to the lungs. In order to minimize excessive intrapulmonary pressure and further lung injury, we adopted the ventilation strategy of permissive hypercapnia. A slow respiratory rate and prolonged expiratory time was used to allow adequate time for expiration, so as to avoid further air trapping. PEEP was kept at a minimum level because high auto-PEEP.

---

* *Pearl/Peril/Pitfall :* Indications for hospitalization include accelerating respiratory distress, ill appearance (eg, cyanosis, lethargy, fatigue), apnea by history, hypoxemia, and inadequate oral intake. Children with underlying disorders such as cardiac disease, immunodeficiency, or bronchopulmonary dysplasia, which put them at high risk of severe or complicated disease, also should be considered candidates for hospitalization.

is a characteristic of bronchiolitis. PIP and FiO_2 were kept at optimal levels to prevent hypoxia. This strategy of permissive hypercapnia without hypoxia appears to have little serious adverse effect. The safe limits for pH and a main bronchus, obstruction of the tracheal tube, pneumothorax or equipment failure. Among these causes, tension pneumothorax is high in the list in patients with small airway obstruction; hence one has to look for clinical features of tension pneumothorax, which include hyperinflated chest, hyper-resonant percussion note, pushing down liver edge and poor lung compliance with limited air entry. Needle thoracostomy is a rapid and reliable bedside test as well as an emergency treatment for tension pneumothorax. CXR is the definite method of diagnosing pneumothorax, but it should not delay the resuscitation procedure in the critical condition. In summary, bronchiolitis is commonly an uneventful illness, but life-threatening complications like respiratory failure will occur. For those patients requiring artificial ventilation, precaution has to pay to minimize the risk of barotraumas and the subsequent tension pneumothorax. We advocate the strategy of permissive hypercapnia for both hand and mechanical ventilation in patients with respiratory failure complicating bronchiolitis. Tension pneumothorax is an uncommon but fatal complication of artificial ventilation on patients with air trapping lung disease such as bronchiolitis and asthma, so rapid diagnosis and prompt treatment is of upmost importance. PaCO2 are not known, but it has been suggested to keep the pH above 7.15 and PaCO2 below 80 mmHg. Similar ventilation strategy should apply to hand ventilation on this patient in the AED. One should bag gently and slowly to allow adequate time for expiration so as to minimize barotraumas. One can ensure complete expiration by listening to the expiratory breath sounds with auscultation. In case of sudden deterioration in an intubated patient, one should try to identify the causes with the use of the DOPE mnemonic suggested in pediatric advanced life support (PALS) provider course, which means displacement of the tracheal tube out of the airway or into a main bronchus, obstruction of the tracheal tube, pneumothorax or equipment failure. Among these causes, tension pneumothorax is high in the list in patients with small airway obstruction; hence one has to look for clinical features of tension pneumothorax, which include hyperinflated chest, hyper-resonant percussion note, pushing down liver edge and poor lung compliance with limited air entry. Needle thoracostomy is a rapid and reliable bedside test as well as an emergency treatment for tension pneumothorax. *CXR is the definite method of diagnosing pneumothorax, but it should not delay the resuscitation procedure in the critical condition.*

In summary, bronchiolitis is commonly an uneventful illness, but life-threatening complications like respiratory failure will occur. For those patients requiring artificial ventilation, precaution has to pay to minimize the risk of barotraumas and the subsequent tension pneumothorax. We advocate the strategy of permissive hypercapnia for both hand and mechanical ventilation in patients with respiratory failure complicating bronchiolitis. Tension pneumothorax is an uncommon but fatal complication of artificial ventilation on patients with air trapping lung disease such as bronchiolitis and asthma, so rapid diagnosis and prompt treatment is of upmost importance.

The Editor is grateful to YW *HUI*, WH *CHOY*, KY *CHAN* for this Instructive Case Study

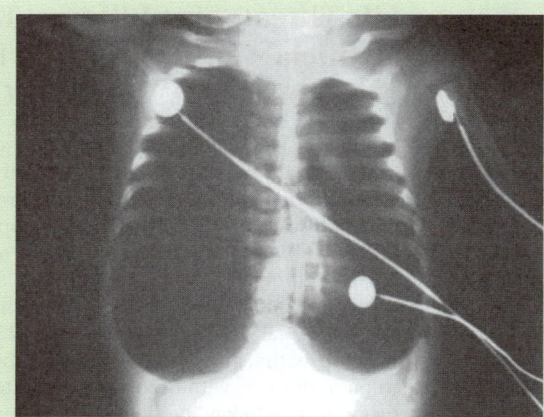

Fig. 1 : Chest radiograph showing bilateral pneumothorax

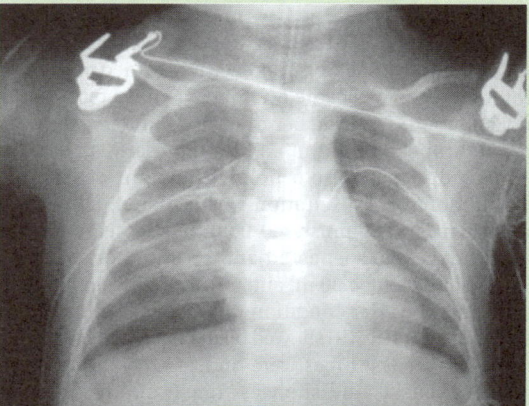

Fig. 2 : Chest radiograph showing re-expansion of bilateral lung fields with 2 chest tubes inserted.

References

1. Shay DK, Holman RC, Newman RD, Liu LL, Stout JW, Anderson LJ. Bronchiolitis-associated hospitalizations among US children, 1980-1996. JAMA 1999;282:1440-6.

2. Pollack J. Spontaneous bilateral pneumothorax in an infant with bronchiolitis. Pediatr Emerg Care 1987;3:33-5.

3. Gibson GJ, Geddes DM, Costabel U, et al. Respiratory Medicine. 3rd edition. London: W.B. Saunders; 2003.

4. Davis AM, Wensley DF, Phelan PD. Spontaneous pneumothorax in paediatric patients. Respir Med 1993;87:531-4.

5. Hui YW, Chan KW, Ko S, et al. Adolescent primary spontaneous pneumothorax: A hospital's experience. HK J Paediatr (new series) 2006;11:128-32.

6. Briassoulis GC, Venkataraman ST, Vasilopoulos AG, Sianidou LC, Papadatos JH. Air leaks from the respiratory tract in mechanically ventilated children with severe respiratory disease. Pediatr Pulmonol 2000;29:127-34.

7. Marini JJ. New options for the ventilatory management of acute lung injury. New Horiz 1993;1:489-503.

8. Bidani A, Tzouanakis AE, Cardenas VJ Jr, Zwischenberger JB. Permissive hypercapnia in acute respiratory failure. JAMA 1994; 272:957-62.

9. Feihl F, Perret C. Permissive hypercapnia. How permissive should we be? Am J Respir Crit Care Med 1994;150(6 Pt 1):1722-37.

10. Martin LD. New approaches to ventilation in infants and children. Curr Opin Pediatr 1995;7:250-61.

11. American Academy of Pediatrics, American Heart Association. PALS Provider Manual 2002.

* *Pearl/Peril/Pitfall : Many clinicians are concerned that patients with more severe disease may have "bacterial superinfections." This may result in the addition of antibiotics to a patient's treatment. Such concerns are typically based on illness severity, chest x-ray appearance, and an elevated white blood count. No data were found to support these assumptions.*

TABLE 1	AAP conclusions (evidence-based recommendations) for the diagnosis and management of bronchiolitis:

1a. Clinicians should diagnose bronchiolitis and assess disease severity on the basis of history and physical examination. Clinicians should not routinely order laboratory and radiologic studies for diagnosis (recommendation). **1b.** Clinicians should assess risk factors for severe disease such as age less than 12 weeks, a history of prematurity, underlying cardiopulmonary disease, or immunodeficiency when making decisions about evaluation and management of children with bronchiolitis (recommendation).

2a. Bronchodilators should not be used routinely in the management of bronchiolitis (recommendation). **2b.** A carefully monitored trial of -adrenergic or -adrenergic medication is an option. Inhaled bronchodilators should be continued only if there is a documented positive clinical response to the trial using an objective means of evaluation (option).

3. Corticosteroid medications should not be used routinely in the management of bronchiolitis (recommendation).

4. Ribavirin should not be used routinely in children with bronchiolitis (recommendation).

5. Antibacterial medications should only be used in children with bronchiolitis who have specific indications of the coexistence of a bacterial infection. When present, bacterial infection should be treated in the same manner as in the absence of bronchiolitis (recommendation).

6a. Clinicians should assess hydration and ability to take fluids orally (strong recommendation). **6b.** Chest physiotherapy should not be used routinely in the management of bronchiolitis (recommendation).

7a. Supplemental oxygen is indicated if SpO2 falls persistently below 90% in previously healthy infants. If the SpO2 does persistently fall below 90%, adequate supplemental oxygen should be used to maintain an SpO2 at or above 90%. Oxygen may be discontinued if SpO2 is at or above 90% and the infant is feeding well and has minimal respiratory distress (option). **7b.** As the child's clinical course improves, continuous measurement of SpO2 is not routinely needed (option). **7c.** Infants with a known history of hemodynamically significant heart or lung disease and premature infants require close monitoring as oxygen is being weaned (strong recommendation).

8a. Clinicians may administer palivizumab prophylaxis for selected infants and children with CLD or a history of prematurity (less than 35 weeks' gestation) or with congenital heart disease (recommendation). **8b.** When given, prophylaxis with palivizumab should be given in 5 monthly doses, usually beginning in November or December, at a dose of 15 mg/kg per dose administered intramuscularly (recommendation).

9a. Hand decontamination is the most important step in preventing nosocomial spread of RSV. Hands should be decontaminated before and after direct contact with patients, after contact with inanimate objects in the direct vicinity of the patient, and after removing gloves (strong recommendation). **9b.** Alcohol-based rubs are preferred for hand decontamination. An alternative is hand-washing with antimicrobial soap (recommendation). **9c.** Clinicians should educate personnel and family members on hand sanitation (recommendation).

10a. Infants should not be exposed to passive smoking (strong recommendation). **10b.** Breastfeeding is recommended to decrease a child's risk of having LRTD (recommendation).

KEY POINTS FOR CLINICAL PRACTICE:

1. Respiratory syncytial virus (RSV) transmission appears to occur via contact with infected secretions through hand-to-hand spread and/or fomites and respiratory droplets with an incubation period of 3-5 days. Aerosolized secretions appear to be less important in RSV transmission; thus, attention to handwashing and cleaning of environmental surfaces are important to prevent RSV transmission.

2. Bronchiolitis is a clinical diagnosis that does not require diagnostic testing. CXR, FBC, ABG Analysis are necessary, if the illness becomes severe in its clinical course.

3. Supportive care is the mainstay of therapy for respiratory syncytial virus (RSV) infection.

4. Antiviral therapy (Ribavirin) for severe RSV disease is indicated in high-risk patients. Treatment must be promptly initiated at the onset of the infection to effectively inhibit the replicating virus.

5. The AAP Committee on Infectious Diseases guidelines for candidates for palivizumab (Synagis) prophylaxis are as follows: *Infants younger than 24 months who have hemodynamically significant congenital heart disease (cyanotic or acyanotic lesions) or chronic lung disease and are off oxygen and/or pulmonary medications for less than 6 months at the start of RSV season *Premature infants born at less than 28 weeks' gestational age who are younger than 1 year chronological age at the start of RSV season *Premature infants born at 29-32 weeks' gestational age who are younger than 6 months chronological age at the start of RSV season *Infants born at 33-35 weeks' gestational age who are younger than 6 months chronological age and have at least 2 additional risk factors at the start of RSV season.

REFERENCES & FURTHER READING : 1)Diagnosis and Management of Bronchiolitis Subcommittee on Diagnosis and Management of Bronchiolitis PEDIATRICS Volume 118, Number 4, October 2006 1775 2)King VJ, Viswanathan M, Bordley WC, et al. Pharmacologic treatment of bronchiolitis in infants and children. *Arch Pediatr Adolesc Med.* 2004;158:127–137 3) Hartling L, Wiebe N, Russell K, Patel H, Klassen TP. Epinephrine for bronchiolitis. *Cochrane Database Syst Rev.* 2004;(1): CD003123 4) Edell D, Khoshoo V, Ross G, Salter K. Early ribavirin treatment of bronchiolitis. *Chest.* 2002;122:935–939 5) LaVia W, Marks MI, Stutman HR. Respiratory syncytial virus puzzle: clinical features, pathophysiology, treatment, and prevention. *J Pediatr.* 1992;121:503–510

*** Pearl/Peril/Pitfall :** Bronchiolitis: Young infants may present with recurrent apneic spells followed by more typical symptoms and signs over 24 to 48 h. Signs of distress may include circumoral cyanosis, deepening retractions, and audible wheezing. Fever is usually but not always present. Infants initially appear nontoxic and in no distress, despite tachypnea and retractions, but may become increasingly lethargic as the infection progresses.*

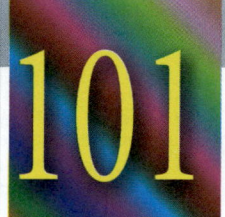

Sudden Infant Death Syndrome (SIDS)

@ **Sudden infant death syndrome (SIDS)** or **crib death** is a syndrome marked by the sudden death of an infant that is unexpected by history and remains unexplained after a thorough forensic autopsy and a detailed death scene investigation. The term **cot death** is often used in the United Kingdom, Ireland, Australia, India, South Africa and New Zealand

RISK FACTORS ASSOCIATED WITH SIDS

Maternal risk Factors	Neonatal risk Factors	Postnatal risk Factors
Maternal smoking during pregnancy	Exposure to passive smoking	Prone sleeping
Maternal age < 20 at first pregnancy	Intrauterine growth restriction	Soft sleep surfaces
Lack of prenatal care	Multiple births	Loose bedding
Illicit drug use	Preterm birth	Overheating
Low socioeconomic status	Low birth weight	Bed sharing
		Poor postnatal weight gain

Current Recommendations on Sleep Position and the Infant Sleep Environment

* Place the infant on its back for sleep on a firm tight fitting mattress in a crib that meets current federal safety standards

* Remove pillows, quilts, comforters, sheep skins, stuffed toys and other soft items from the crib

* Do not place the infant on a waterbed, sofa mattress, pillow or other soft surface to sleep

* Consider using a sleeper or sleepsack as an alternative to blankets or other covers

* Make sure that the infant's head remains uncovered during sleep

* Place the infant so that its feet are positioned at the foot of the crib

* If a thin blanket is used, tuck it around the crib mattress positioned up only as far as the infant's chest

SOURCES: American Academy of Pediatrics, National Institutes of Child Health and Human Development, Association of SIDS and Infant Mortality Programs, Consumer Product Safety Commission.

American Academy of Pediatrics "Back to Sleep" Recommendations Pediatr 2005; 116: 1245-1255

1. Infants should be placed exclusively on their back (supine) for every sleep. The side sleep position is not as safe as supine and is not recommended.

2. Use a firm safety-approved crib mattress with a tight fitting sheet. Pillows, quilts, comforters or sheepskins should not be placed under the infant.

3. Keep soft objects and loose bedding out of the crib. If blankets are used, they should be tucked in under the mattress so that infant's head is less likely to become covered by bedding.

4. Do not smoke during pregnancy. Avoid second-hand smoke exposure for the infant.

5. A room-sharing sleep arrangement is recommended. Bed-sharing is associated with a higher risk for SIDS.

6. Offer a pacifier when placing the infant down for sleep. Delay use of a pacifier until after one month of age for breast-fed infants.

7. Avoid overheating and overbundling.

8. Avoid commercial devices marketed to reduce the risk for SIDS.

9. Do not use home monitors as a strategy to reduce the risk for SIDS.

10. Avoid development of positional plagiocephaly. Positional flattening of the head can be reduced by alternating head position during placement for sleep and use of "tummy-time" when awake.

11. Continue "Back to Sleep" public awareness campaigns.

REVIEW OF CLINICAL PROBLEMS

1. Mention the Triple Risk Model to explain the basic cause of SIDS.
   Ans: Refer to the "No. 5" of the "BIRD`S EYE VIEW/OVERVIEW/ SYNOPSIS" of the Chapter.

2. What are the "Essentials of History Taking" When a SIDS occurs?
   Ans: Refer to the "No. 3" of the "BIRD`S EYE VIEW/OVERVIEW/ SYNOPSIS" of the Chapter.

3. What are the "essentials of Physical Examination" of the SIDS ?
   Ans: Refer to the "No. 4" of the "BIRD`S EYE VIEW/OVERVIEW/ SYNOPSIS" of the Chapter.

4. How do you organize the Parental support and counseling of SIDS victims?
   Ans: Refer to the Evaluation-Decision-Action Plan/Algorithm to diagnose and manage SIDS.

5. Mention the essentials of Parental Education to prevent/reduce SIDS.
   Ans: Refer to the "Educate the parents" section of the Chapter.

LEARNING OBJECTIVES

After completing this article, readers will be able to:

1. Identify the known risk factors associated with Sudden Infant Death Syndrome (SIDS).

2. Appreciate that ALTE has no causal relationship with SIDS and SIDS is a diagnosis to be made only after excluding all recognizable causes of Death.

3. Meet with the family to discuss the results of the autopsy and answer their questions.

4. Specify current recommendations on sleep position and the infant sleep environment as interventions to lower the risk of SIDS.

5. Discuss grief response to the loss and Provide Parental Support, Counseling and Education to reduce the incidence of SIDS.

---

* **Pearl/Peril/Pitfall :** *SIDS: Four major avenues of investigation aid in the determination of a SIDS death: postmortem lab tests, autopsy, death-scene investigation, and the review of victim and family case history.*

BIRD'S EYE VIEW/OVERVIEW/SYNOPSIS

1. Sudden infant death syndrome (SIDS) is defined as the sudden death of an infant younger than 1 year that remains unexplained after a thorough case investigation, including the performance of a complete autopsy, examination of the scene of death, and review of the clinical history.SIDS is one of the single most common causes of death in the postneonatal period (i.e. in infants aged 1 mo to 1 y). The occurrence of SIDS is rare during the first month of life, increases to a peak between 2 and 3 months of age, and then decreases. In conjunction with a more than 50% reduction in SIDS deaths since 1992, there has been a small shift in the age of death. A slightly higher proportion of deaths in the neonatal period and after 6 months of age were reported in 2001 than in 1992.

2. The following have been consistently identified across studies as *independent risk factors for SIDS*: prone sleep position, sleeping on a soft surface, maternal smoking during pregnancy, overheating, late or no prenatal care, young maternal age, preterm birth and/or low birth weight, and male gender.Despite intensive study and advances in the understanding of associated factors, the specific cause or causes of SIDS remain unknown.

3. **History** *Infants whose deaths are attributed to sudden infant death syndrome (SIDS) are typically found pulseless and apneic associated with a period of sleep. *A typical history is that of an infant who had been recently fed and then placed for sleep. When next checked, the infant is discovered without pulse or respiration. *Infants with SIDS are typically born full term without a history of significant pregnancy-related complications. *Approximately 12–20% of infants with SIDS are born prematurely (<37 weeks' gestation) or at low birth weight (<2500 g). *Before death, infants with SIDS are thought to be feeding well and gaining weight normally. *Generally, no outward signs of significant health-related concerns are observed. *Approximately 70% of infants with SIDS have a history of minor viral upper respiratory tract or GI illness in the week preceding the death; however, these illnesses are generally not marked by high fever, respiratory distress, or signs of dehydration.

4. **Physical** *Infants with SIDS often display a frothy blood-tinged discharge from the nose or mouth at the time of discovery. *Signs of livor mortis or rigor mortis are often present. *Care should be taken at the scene of death to examine for signs of obstruction of the external airways, accidental entrapment of the head, or other environmental factors (e.g. ambient temperature, source of heating for carbon monoxide exposures) that may have contributed to the death. *At autopsy, the infant usually exhibits signs of normal hydration and nutrition, which is evidence of proper care. *No signs of obvious or occult trauma should be present. *Gross examination of the organs generally reveals no evidence of a congenital abnormality or acquired disease process consistent with a recognizable cause of death. *Krous et al noted that intrathoracic petechiae are typically present on the surfaces of the thymus, pleura, and epicardium.*The frequency and severity of petechiae have been noted to be similar regardless of whether infants have been discovered facedown on the sleep surface or with face up or face to the side. This finding suggests that centrally mediated airway failure, such as that seen with apnea or ailed gasping rather than external airway obstruction, is likely in SIDS. *Microscopic examination may reveal minor inflammatory changes within the tracheobronchial tree or signs of passive congestion of the organs. Very mild myocardial lymphocyte and macrophage infiltration with scattered necrotic cardiomyocytes may be seen in SIDS and are not considered to be pathologic. *Histologically, the thymus and adrenal glands are normal.

5. *Triple risk model* *The cause or causes of SIDS are likely to be multifactorial. The triple risk model, proposed by Filiano and Kinney, suggests that SIDS represents an intersection of factors, including a vulnerable infant possessing intrinsic abnormalities in cardiorespiratory control, a critical period of development of homeostatic control mechanisms, and exogenous stressors. *Death occurs when vulnerable infants are subjected to stressors at times when normal defence mechanisms may be structurally, functionally, and/or developmentally deficient. *This model allows for the possibility of multiple potential stressors and for heterogeneity in underlying vulnerabilities that manifest as sudden unexplained infant death (SUID).

6. Establish a diagnosis of sudden infant death syndrome (SIDS) by excluding recognizable causes of sudden unexplained infant death (SUID). The necessary data set includes information obtained from the scene of death, infant and family medical and social history, and autopsy examination. Guidelines for the autopsy examination, including gross and microscopic dissections, and the role of toxicologic, microbiologic, radiographic, and other special procedures, are detailed by Krous and others. **Imaging Studies** *Obtain whole-body radiographs to evaluate for evidence of skeletal trauma. Special coned-down radiographic views may be necessary to further delineate subtle metaphyseal corner fractures of the long bones seen with nonaccidental forms of trauma. In many jurisdictions, toxicologic screening of serum and vitreous electrolyte analysis are routinely performed as part of the postmortem evaluation. If not routinely performed, obtain appropriate specimens and retain them for potential analysis.

7. Some conditions that may be undiagnosed and thus could be alternative diagnoses to SIDS include: *medium-chain acyl-coenzyme A dehydrogenase deficiency (MCAD deficiency), *infant botulism *long QT syndrome *infections with the bacterium *Helicobacter pylori* *shaken baby syndrome and other forms of*child abuse For example, an infant with MCAD deficiency could have died by 'classical SIDS' if found swaddled and prone with head covered in an overheated room where parents were smoking. Genes of susceptibility to MCAD and Long QT syndrome do not protect an infant from dying of classical SIDS. Therefore presence of a susceptibility gene, such as for MCAD, means the infant may have died either from SIDS or from MCAD deficiency. It is impossible for the pathologist to distinguish between them.

8. Though SIDS cannot be prevented, parents of infants are encouraged to take several precautions in order to reduce the likelihood of SIDS. AAP RECOMMENDATIONS to reduce the incidence of SIDS based on current evidence, are enlisted at the beginning of the Chapter.

9. Case reports or case series of infant homicide highlight the need for a thorough and competent death investigation that must include an evaluation of the infant and family medical history and review of the scene of death to accurately distinguish natural from nonnatural infant deaths.

10. After interpreting data from the Collaborative Infant Home Monitoring Study Group, the AAP has recommended that infant home monitoring not be used as a strategy to prevent SIDS but may be useful in some infants who have had an ALTE.

---

* *Pearl/Peril/Pitfall: SIDS: An autopsy provides clues as to the cause of death. In 15%-25% of sudden, unexpected infant deaths, specific abnormalities of the brain or central nervous system, the heart or lungs, or infection may be identified as the cause of death. The autopsy findings in SIDS victims are typically subtle and yield only supportive, rather than conclusive, findings to explain SIDS.*

THE EVALUATION-DECISION-ACTION-PLAN/ALGORITHM FOR THE DIAGNOSIS AND MANAGEMENT OF *SUDDEN INFANT DEATH SYNDROME-SIDS*

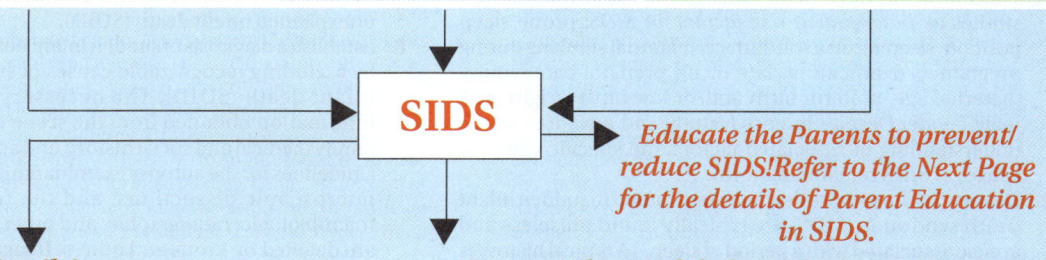

SUBJECTIVE FINDINGS	OBJECTIVE FINDINGS	INVESTIGATIONS
Hx THE EVENT`S details from the mum/caretakers, any identifiable Risk factors associated with SIDS,	*Refer to the Information given under "6" of the Bird's eye view/ overview/ synopsis of the Chapter.*	Establish a diagnosis of sudden infant death syndrome (SIDS) by excluding recognizable causes of sudden unexplained infant death (SUID). The necessary data set includes information obtained from the scene of death, infant and family medical and social history, and autopsy examination. *Guidelines for the autopsy examination, including gross and microscopic dissections, and the role of toxicologic, microbiologic, radiographic, and other special procedures are to be followed.*

Hx of resuscitation done ?

Hx of relation with feeding, position, or gagging or breath holding

Hx of perinatal events, respiratory symptoms, medications, prematurity, family history of SIDS, Are the newborn metabolic screening findings normal?

SIDS

Educate the Parents to prevent/ reduce SIDS!Refer to the Next Page for the details of Parent Education in SIDS.

Support the Family!

Ensure to be careful about the Special Concerns!

* Experts in the field of grief support describe the following strategies for supporting the family under these difficult circumstances:*At the time of death: Express condolences to the family. Encourage the parents and family to see and hold the infant if they feel that they are able to do so. Explain the local procedure that is followed after the death, including autopsy and death investigation by local authorities. If sudden infant death syndrome (SIDS) is suggested, reassure the family that they could not have done anything to prevent the death. Reassure the family that intense feelings of grief are normal and that resources are available for support. Autopsy findings. *Reviewing the autopsy findings: Meet with the family to discuss the results of the autopsy and answer their questions. Discuss grief response to the loss. *Long-term family support: Be available to families as needed.

*In addition to notifying the medical examiner or coroner, several other key individuals should be contacted immediately after the death. *The infant's primary health care providers should be notified of the death so that they may provide consolation and immediate guidance to the family. They can also provide the infant's relevant medical history. *If subspecialty health care providers cared for the infant, they should also be contacted for the same reasons. *Immediate and extended family members should be contacted to assist the family with grief support. *The family's religious institution and chaplain staff may also be contacted to offer consolation and guidance to the family. *In special cultural settings, family or tribal elders may need to be notified to assist the family following the death.

Lack of causal relationship between ALTE and SIDS — An association between SIDS and ALTE had been suggested because of prior ALTE events in 5 percent of SIDS victims and early anecdotal reports of SIDS in infants with recurrent apnea. However, the vast majority of SIDS victims do not experience apnea prior to death. Furthermore, studies over the past two decades have failed to confirm a causal relationship between preexisting apnea and SIDS. Several other factors argue against a relationship between SIDS and ALTE: *ALTE refers to a heterogeneous group of problems ranging from benign to near-fatal, whereas SIDS denotes a fatal problem. *The case definition in ALTE depends upon parental observations, which have been shown to be unreliable in several studies *Over 80 percent of SIDS deaths occur between midnight and 6 AM, whereas 82 percent of ALTE episodes occur between 8 AM and 8 PM. *Interventions to prevent SIDS (e.g., supine sleeping) have not resulted in a decreased incidence of ALTE *The risk factors for SIDS and ALTE differ. In one prospective population-based study, prone sleeping, lack of breast feeding, and maternal smoking were risks for SIDS, whereas behavioral characteristics such as repeated apnea, pallor, history of cyanosis, and feeding difficulties were risk factors for ALTE.

* *Pearl/Peril/Pitfall : SIDS: Rebreathing asphyxia: When a baby is facedown, air movement around the mouth may be impaired. This can cause the baby to re-breathe carbon dioxide that the baby has just exhaled. Soft bedding and gas-trapping objects, such as blankets, comforters, water beds, and soft mattresses, are other types of sleep surfaces that may impair normal air movement around the baby's mouth and nose when positioned facedown.*

The good news is that cradle boards may help reduce SIDS deaths because the baby is placed on his or her back. But cradle boards should not be used when the baby is a passenger in a motor vehicle. When transporting your baby, use an infant car seat that will protect him or her in case of a motor vehicle crash. The baby has been placed on his back. His clothing is loose fitting. The sheets on the mattress are tight fitting. The mattress provides the baby with a firm, flat surface. The crib does not have any stuffed animals, blankets, bumper pads, or pillows. By following these simple baby care practices, you can lower your baby's chance of dying of SIDS. The proper care of an infant is important for everyone who looks after a baby, not just parents, but also other members of the family including grandparents and other caregivers, such as foster parents, childcare providers and babysitters.

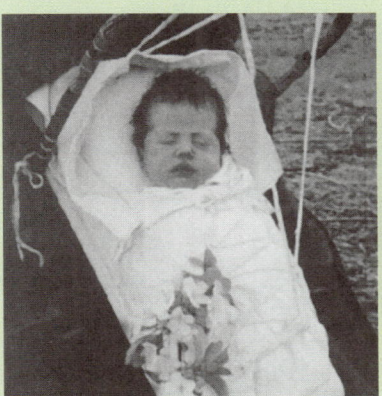
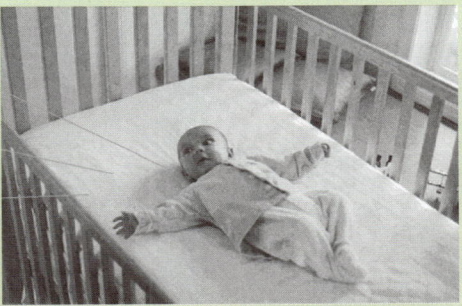
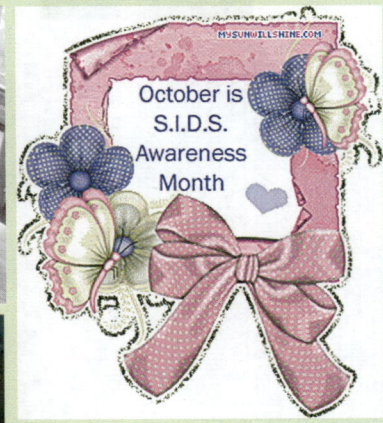
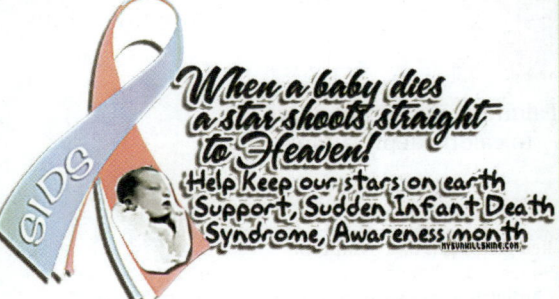

A separate but proximate sleeping environment is recommended: The risk of SIDS has been shown to be reduced when the infant sleeps in the same room as the mother. Infants may be brought into bed for nursing or comforting but should be returned to their own crib or bassinet when the parent is ready to return to sleep. The infant should not be brought into bed when the parent is excessively tired or using medications or substances that could impair his or her alertness.

KEY POINTS FOR CLINICAL PRACTICE

1. Although there is ongoing discussion about changing the definition, the current generally accepted definition of SIDS remains as follows: The sudden death of an infant under 1 year of age, which remains unexplained after a thorough case investigation, including performance of a complete autopsy, examination of the death scene, and review of the clinical history. A diagnosis of sudden infant death syndrome (SIDS) is established by excluding recognizable causes of sudden unexplained infant death (SUID).

2. The following have been consistently identified across studies as *independent risk factors for SIDS*: prone sleep position, sleeping on a soft surface, maternal smoking during pregnancy, overheating, late or no prenatal care, young maternal age, preterm birth and/or low birth weight, and male gender.

3. The necessary data set for the evaluation of SIDS includes information obtained from the scene of death, infant and family medical and social history, and autopsy examination.

4. Parental support, counseling and education about SIDS prevention/reduction are extremely important.

5. In most deaths attributed to SIDS, no history of child abuse, neglect, or parental psychiatric illness manifesting as Münchausen syndrome by proxy is present; however, case reports or case series of infant homicide highlight the need for a thorough and competent death investigation that must include an evaluation of the infant and family medical history and review of the scene of death to accurately distinguish natural from nonnatural infant deaths.

REFERENCES & FURTHER READING : 1)Mitchell EA, Hutchison L, Stewart AW (July 2007). "The continuing decline in SIDS mortality". *Arch Dis Child.* **92** (7): 625–6. doi:10.1136/adc.2007.116194. PMID 17405855. 2) The Changing Concept of Sudden Infant Death Syndrome: Diagnostic Coding Shifts, Controversies Regarding the Sleeping Environment, and **New Variables to Consider in Reducing Risk** PEDIATRICS Vol. 116 No. 5 November 2005 **1245** 3) Hauck FR, Herman SM, Donovan M, Iyasu S, Merrick Moore C, Donoghue E, Kirschner RH, Willinger M (2003). "Sleep environment and the risk of sudden infant death syndrome in an urban population: the Chicago Infant Mortality Study". *Pediatrics* **111**: 1207–14. doi:10.1542/peds.111.5.S1.1207 (inactive 2008-06-25). PMID 12728140. http://pediatrics.aappublications.org/cgi/content/abstract/111/5/S1/1207. 4) Pollack HA, Frohna JG. Infant sleep placement after the Back to Sleep campaign. *Pediatrics.* 2002;109:608–614 5) Apnea, sudden infant death syndrome, and home monitoring. Pediatrics 2003; 111:914.

* *Pearl/Peril/Pitfall : SIDS: Sudden infant death syndrome remains an unpredictable, unpreventable, and largely inexplicable tragedy. The baby is seemingly healthy without any sign of distress or significant illness prior to the incident. Death occurs rapidly while the infant is sleeping. Typically, it is a silent event. The baby does not cry. Minor upper respiratory or gastrointestinal symptoms are not uncommon in the last two weeks preceding SIDS.*

102

Failure to Thrive

@ *The key to diagnosing FTT is finding the time in busy clinical practice to accurately measure and plot a child's weight, height, and head circumference, and then assess the trend.*

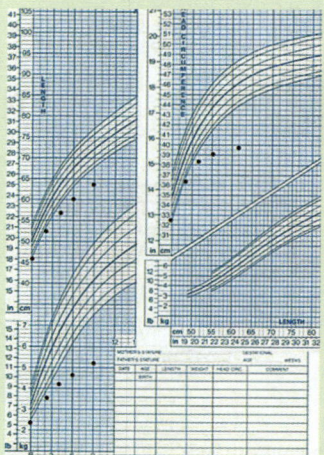

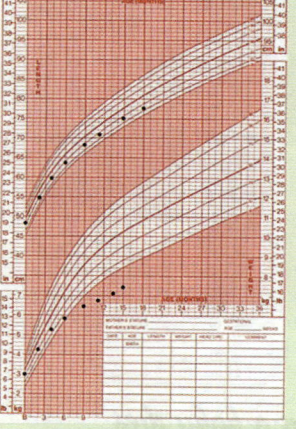

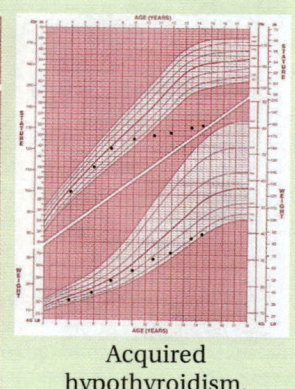

Acquired hypothyroidism.

Failure of growth in weight, length, and head circumference starting at birth, suggesting an organic etiology that occurred in utero.

Growth failure in length and weight with a normal head circumference in an infant with growth hormone deficiency.

Failure to thrive secondary to caloric deprivation.

* *Failure to thrive remains one of the greatest challenges for the practicing pediatrician. The process of the attempt at identification of the causes can be exhausting and expensive. The list of organic and nonorganic causes of this entity is extensive, and combinations of the 2 types of causes are common in specific children. Failure to thrive can have its roots in prenatal origins or can develop postnatally. Information from a careful extensive history and from a detailed physical examination may give important clues to the underlying diagnoses. Hospitalization and the involvement of a multispecialty team may be helpful in diagnosis.*

Red Flag Signs and Symptoms
Suggesting Medical Causes of Failure to Thrive
Cardiac findings suggesting congenital heart disease or heart failure (e.g., murmur, edema, jugular venous distention)
Developmental delay
Dysmorphic features
Failure to gain weight despite adequate caloric intake
Organomegaly or lymphadenopathy
Recurrent or severe respiratory, mucocutaneous, or urinary infection
Recurrent vomiting, diarrhea, or dehydration

REVIEW OF CLINICAL PROBLEMS

1. What screening investigations are useful in evaluating an infant with Failure to Thrive ?
   Ans: Refer to the Table 2 of the Chapter.

2. Classify the various causes of Failure to Thrive.
   Ans: Refer to the Table 1 of the Chapter.

3. What are the 4 main goals of performing Physical examination of an infant with FTT?
   Ans: Refer to No 4 of the Bird`s eye view/Overview/Synopsis of the Chapter.

4. Describe the benefits of Hospitalization in an infant with FTT.
   Ans: Refer to No 8 & 9 of the Bird`s eye view/Overview/Synopsis of the Chapter.

5. Discuss the clinical approach to FTT based on the presenting signs & symptoms.
   Ans: Refer to the Evaluation-Decision-Action Plan/Algorithm to diagnose and manage Failure To Thrive.

LEARNING OBJECTIVES

After completing this article, readers will be able to:

1. Define the Failure To Thrive, Identify by History, Physical examination, and if necessary screening investigations to exclude organic causes.

2. Measure Growth parameters & Plot them on Centile charts serially to find out the various patterns of Growth failure.

3. Hospitalize selected cases of FTT for diagnostic & therapeutic purposes.

4. Ensure that Interdisciplinary Team approach is to be followed to manage FTT.

5. Educate the parents to give 150 percent of the recommended daily caloric intake for their expected, not actual, weight for age.

Pearl/Peril/Pitfall: FTT:Early childhood is a critical period for growth and development, and early intervention for any child with FTT will maximize the potential for better outcomes. Given the evidence of long-term problems, all children who have been diagnosed with FTT need to be followed carefully for possible later sequelae.

BIRD'S EYE VIEW/OVERVIEW/SYNOPSIS

1. FTT is best defined as inadequate physical growth diagnosed by observation of growth over time using a standard growth chart (The National Center for Health Statistics (NCHS). Most practitioners diagnose FTT when a child's weight for age falls below the fifth percentile of the standard NCHS growth chart or if it crosses two major percentile lines. Recent research has validated that the weight-for-age approach is the simplest and most reasonable marker for FTT. Other growth parameters that can assist in making the diagnosis of FTT are weight for height and height for age. FTT is diagnosed if a child falls below the 10th percentile for either of these measurements.Body mass index (BMI) charts, which are available for individuals aged 2-20 years, have replaced the weight-for-stature charts. BMI is calculated by dividing weight in kilograms by height in meters squared. Accurate measurements are essential to the interpretation of growth charts. Scales need to be calibrated regularly; length should be measured carefully, and head circumference should be measured using standardized techniques. Alternate growth charts are available for children with Down syndrome, Turner syndrome, meningomyelocele, low birth weight, and very low birth weight. No matter which growth chart is used, the most valuable information is obtained by careful measuring and plotting on the same chart over time. Infants and children remain within 1-2 percentile curves over time.

2. Historically, FTT has been classified as organic or nonorganic.Usually, this distinction may not useful because most children have mixed etiologies. For example, a child may have a medical disorder that causes feeding problems and family stress. The stress can compound the feeding problem and aggravate FTT. A more useful classification system is based on pathophysiology—inadequate caloric intake, inadequate absorption, excess metabolic demand, or defective utilization. This classification leads to a logical organization of the many conditions that cause or contribute to FTT. Refer to the Table 1 of the Chapter for a list of basic causes of FTT.

3. RECOGNIZING FTT:The key to diagnosing FTT is finding the time in busy clinical practice to accurately measure and plot a child's weight, height, and head circumference, and then assess the trend. After determining that FTT is a concern, the evaluation should focus on a careful history, including an assessment of diet and feeding or eating behaviors, and past and current medical, social, and family history. Table 2 details items that should be covered in each category. It is important to ascertain the child's developmental status at the time of diagnosis because children with FTT have a higher incidence of developmental delays than the general population. Physicians should still be concerned about a child without developmental delays who is failing to thrive. FTT is primarily a growth disorder, not a developmental problem.

4. Physical examination: A complete physical examination is essential, with four main goals: (1) identification of dysmorphic features suggestive of a genetic disorder impeding growth; (2) detection of underlying disease that may impair growth;(3) assessment for signs of possible child abuse; and (4) assessment of the severity and possible effects of malnutrition. The severity of a child's undernutrition can be determined most easily by using the Gomez criteria. By comparing the child's current weight for age with the expected weight (50th percentile) at that age, the degree of malnutrition can be assessed. If the weight is less than 60 percent of expected, the FTT is considered severe, 61 to 75 percent denotes moderate FTT, and 76 to 90 percent is mild.

5. Parent-child interaction:Observing the interaction between a parent and child, especially during a feeding session in the office, may provide valuable information about the etiology of FTT.Parents can be asked to feed an infant or bring in a snack for a toddler. The assessment should be done at a time when the child is hungry. It is important to pay attention to a caregiver's ability to recognize the child's cues, the child's responsiveness, and the parental warmth and appropriate behavior toward the child.It is similarly important to observe the nature of the child's cues (clear or not), the child's temperament, and responses toward the parent. Developing a portrait of the relationship is key to guiding intervention.

6. Laboratory evaluation: Laboratory evaluation should be guided by history and physical examination findings only.If a diagnosis can be made and a cause for failure to thrive (FTT) can be identified, the history and physical examination usually supply the answer. Laboratory assessment has a limited value in determining the etiology of failure to thrive. Occasionally, laboratory test results are unexpectedly abnormal. For instance, blood dyscrasias, chronic urinary tract infections, chronic acidosis, and renal failure all can be diagnosed using these screening tests. However, only about 1% of the tests ordered produce abnormal results and help identify the etiology of failure to thrive.Children diagnosed with failure to thrive usually undergo certain screening tests, including the following: *CBC count *Urinalysis *Urine culture *Electrolytes, including creatinine and BUN *Liver function tests, including total protein and albumin. Prealbumin may be used as a nutritional marker. More specific tests may be indicated (depending on findings from the history and physical examination), including the following: *Human immunodeficiency virus (HIV) testing *Sweat chloride test *Thyroid function tests *Stool studies for parasites or malabsorption *Immunoglobulins *Purified protein derivative (PPD) skin test *Radiological studies. If concern surrounds possible growth hormone deficiency, the following may be obtained: *Serum insulinlike growth factor I (IGF-I) *Insulinlike growth factor binding protein (IGF-BP3)Serum immunoglobulin A tissue transglutaminase antibody (TTG-IgA), IgA-endomysial antibody (IgA-EMA), and immunoglobulin G antigliadin antibodies (AGA-IgG) may be used to screen for celiac disease when clinically indicated.Imaging Studies *A bone age may be helpful to distinguish genetic short stature from constitutional delay of growth.

7. Most children with failure to thrive (FTT) can be treated as outpatients; home visits and close clinical follow-ups often help determine the underlying reason for the failure to thrive. However, hospitalization sometimes is necessary for diagnostic and therapeutic reasons. Diagnostic benefits of admission may include observation of feeding, parental-child interaction, and dietary habits, as well as the ability to perform specific tests and consult subspecialists

8. Therapeutic benefits may result from hospitalization. Acute needs, such as dehydration, infection, anemia, or electrolyte imbalance, can be addressed and managed within the hospital. For instance, intravenous fluids, systemic antibiotic therapy, transfusion, and, possibly, parenteral nutrition often are in-hospital procedures. Of course, if an organic etiology is found for the failure to thrive in a particular child, specific therapy can be initiated during the hospitalization.

9. Another benefit of hospitalization may be the observation of parent-child interaction. In addition to observation of the feeding techniques of the parents, other interactions can be observed more easily in the hospital. For instance, the degrees to which parents bond, speak, and even interact with their children all can be observed during the hospital stay. If children gain weight easily during a hospitalization, the cause of the failure to thrive is most likely nonorganic.

10. When treating children with failure to thrive, an interdisciplinary team approach combining pediatric, nutritional, mental health, and social work expertise often is helpful. An interdisciplinary approach ensures that programs such as women, infants, and children (WIC); food stamps; and Medicaid can be accessed. Using an interdisciplinary approach is also helpful if appropriate home-based intervention needs to be arranged. Other advantages of using an interdisciplinary team include the fact that the family's psychosocial situation can be addressed and intervention can be provided. For example, an older child with a chronic illness and failure to thrive may benefit from referral to a psychologist. If neglect is suspected, child protective services can become involved as a result of this multidisciplinary approach. Subspecialists should be involved for the treatment of organic illness when identified.Infants may be given concentrated formulas, assuming renal function is normal. If this option is chosen, renal function must be normal because the osmolar load of the resultant formula is high. In cases in which this is a problem because of renal insufficiency, increasing the fat content of the formula may be useful as a way of delivering additional calories.

---

* *Pearl/Peril/Pitfall : SIDS: An autopsy provides clues as to the cause of death. In 15–25% of sudden, unexpected infant deaths, specific abnormalities of the brain or central nervous system, the heart or lungs, or infection may be identified as the cause of death. The autopsy findings in SIDS victims are typically subtle and yield only supportive, rather than conclusive, findings to explain SIDS.*

THE EVALUATION-DECISION-ACTION-PLAN/ALGORITHM FOR THE DIAGNOSIS AND MANAGEMENT OF *FAILURE TO THRIVE*

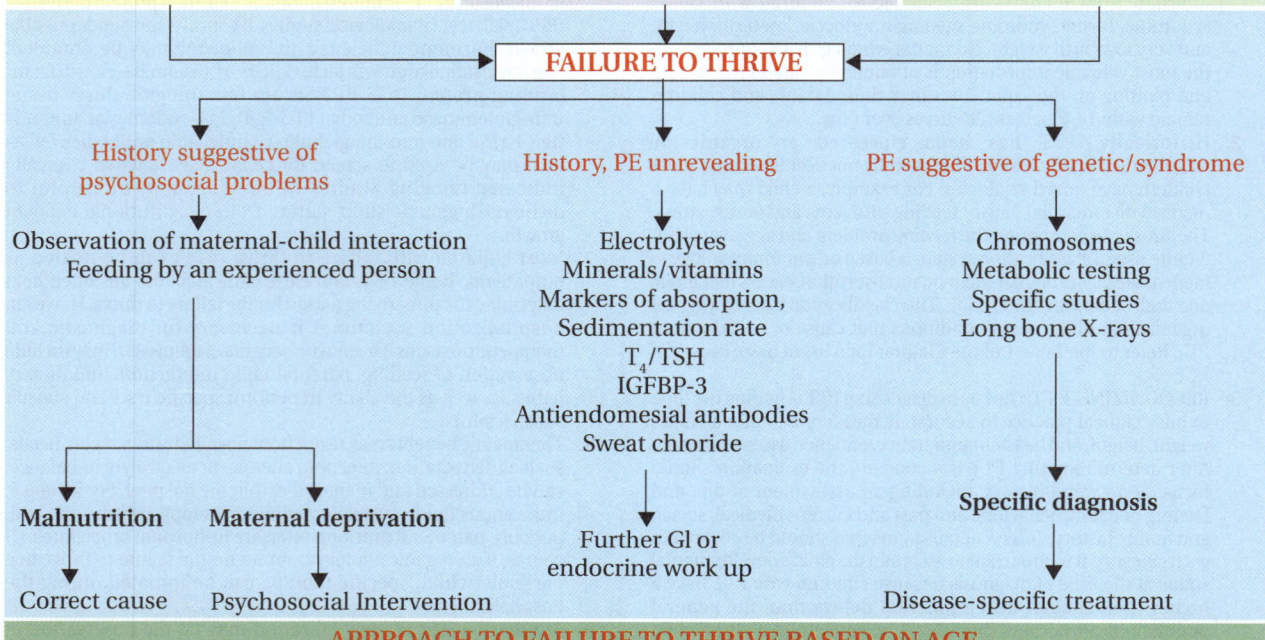

SUBJECTIVE FINDINGS

Hx of any problems in the nursery (meningitis, any history of signs of chronic conditions, such as cerebral palsy (CP), spasticity, seizures, and delayed development), dietary details- breast/formula, the frequency of feeds, number of wet diapers and stools each day, and a history of sequential weights, bowel habits of a child Family and social history should include other siblings, living conditions, stressors, and data on parents' growth history

Hx of prenatal events-*Smoking *Alcohol consumption *Use of medications *Any illness during the pregnancy.

OBJECTIVE FINDINGS

Plot the head circumference, height, and weight on a growth chart. Insisting on careful measurements during each examination is important; detect trends in growth rather than to rely on measurements at one particular visit. Evaluate for the pattern of failure to thrive. *Document* *Blood pressure *Respiration *Pulse rate *Oxygen saturation in certain clinical situations *Note·* *Edema *Wasting *Hepatomegaly *Rash or skin changes *Hair color and texture changes *Mental status changes *Signs of vitamin deficiency *Dysmorphism & *Perform* complete systemic examination.

INVESTIGATIONS

Laboratory assessment has a limited value in determining the etiology of failure to thrive. Occasionally, laboratory test results are unexpectedly abnormal. For instance, blood dyscrasias, chronic urinary tract infections, chronic acidosis, and renal failure all can be diagnosed using these screening tests. However, only about 1% of the tests ordered produce abnormal results and help identify the etiology of failure to thrive- Refer to the Table 2 of the Chapter.

FAILURE TO THRIVE

History suggestive of psychosocial problems → Observation of maternal-child interaction / Feeding by an experienced person → **Malnutrition** → Correct cause / **Maternal deprivation** → Psychosocial Intervention

History, PE unrevealing → Electrolytes / Minerals/vitamins / Markers of absorption, / Sedimentation rate / T_4/TSH / IGFBP-3 / Antiendomesial antibodies / Sweat chloride → Further GI or endocrine work up

PE suggestive of genetic/syndrome → Chromosomes / Metabolic testing / Specific studies / Long bone X-rays → **Specific diagnosis** → Disease-specific treatment

APPROACH TO FAILURE TO THRIVE BASED ON AGE

Age of Onset	Major Diagnostic Consideration
Birth to 3 mo	Psychosocial failure to thrive, perinatal infections, gastroesophageal reflux, inborn errors of metabolism, cystic fibrosis
3-6 mo	Psychosocial failure to thrive, human immunodeficiency virus infection, gastroesophageal reflux, inborn errors of metabolism, milk protein intolerance, cystic fibrosis, renal tubular acidosis
7-12 mo	Psychosocial failure to thrive (autonomy struggles), delayed introduction of solids, gastroesophageal reflux, intestinal parasites, renal tubular acidosis
12+mo	Psychosocial failure to thrive (coercive feeding, new psychologic stressor), gastroesophageal reflux

APPROACH TO FAILURE TO THRIVE BASED ON SIGNS AND SYMPTOMS

History/Physical Examination	Diagnostic consideration
Spitting, vomiting, food refusal	Gastroesophageal reflux, chronic tonsillitis, food allergies
Diarrhea, fatty stools	Malabsorption, intestinal parasites, milk protein intolerance
Snoring, mouth breathing, enlarged tonsils	Adenoid hypertrophy, obstructive sleep apnea
Recurrent wheezing, pulmonary infections	Asthma, aspiration
Recurrent infections	Human immunodeficiency virus disease
Travel to/from developing countries	Parasitic or bacterial infections of the gastrointestinal tract

Combined organic and nonorganic failure to thrive *Failure to thrive in a patient can result from the combination of both organic and nonorganic reasons. In one study, half of the cases with organic etiology had a psychosocial factor contributing to the failure to thrive. This is caused by a number of reasons. It is clear that illnesses in children, particularly chronic illnesses, can take their toll on families. Stresses from coping with chronic illnesses may lead to parental dysfunction, such as depression, alcohol or drug abuse, divorce, or chaotic home environments. Parental dysfunction and the resultant negative atmosphere in which children are reared affect their food intake. In addition, children may undergo personality changes when they have chronic diseases. Medications (e.g., steroids) are well known to cause behavioral changes, but the mere presence of a chronic illness also can result in resistance or noncompliance in many aspects of a child's life, including consumption of proper energy intake. *Many examples of children having both organic and nonorganic causes of failure to thrive exist. For example, children with CF, asthma, heart disease, and CP all have organic reasons for failure to thrive. In addition, the social pressures that children with these conditions experience can cause behavioral changes that result in decreased energy intake and, therefore, failure to thrive.

TABLE 1 — Selective differential diagnosis of failure to thrive

Inadequate caloric intake
- Incorrect preparation of formula (too diluted, too concentrated)
- Unsuitable feeding habits (food fads, excessive juice)
- Behavior problems affecting eating
- Poverty and food shortages
- Neglect
- Disturbed parent-child relationship
- Mechanical feeding difficulties (oromotor dysfunction, congenital anomalies,
- central nervous system damage, severe reflux)

Inadequate absorption
- Celiac disease
- Cystic fibrosis
- Cow's milk protein allergy
- Vitamin or mineral deficiencies (acrodermatitis enteropathica, scurvy)
- Biliary atresia or liver disease
- Necrotizing enterocolitis or short-gut syndrome

Increased metabolism
- Hyperthyroidism
- Chronic infection (human immunodeficiency virus or other immunodeficiency, malignancy, renal disease)
- Hypoxemia (congenital heart defects, chronic lung disease)

Defective utilization
- Genetic abnormalities (trisomies 21, 18, and 13)
- Congenital infections
- Metabolic disorders (storage diseases, amino acid disorders)

Nonorganic failure to thrive
- *Poor feeding or feeding-skills disorder
- *Dysfunctional family interactions
- *Difficult parent-child interactions
- *Lack of support (e.g., no friends, no extended family)
- *Lack of preparation for parenting
- *Family dysfunction (e.g., divorce, spouse abuse, chaotic family style)
- *Difficult child
- *Child neglect
- *Emotional deprivation syndrome
- *Feeding disorders (e.g., anorexia, bulimia)

TABLE 2 — Screening investigations for FTT

Blood-ABG/CBG, CBC, differential, electrolytes, BUN, creatinine, Liver function tests, including total protein and albumin, Prealbumin.

* If clinically indicated-*Human immunodeficiency virus (HIV) testing *Sweat chloride test *Thyroid function tests *Stool studies for parasites or malabsorption *Immunoglobulins *Purified protein derivative (PPD) skin test *Radiological studies.

Urine-urinalysis, urine C/S Imaging-Bone age Others-Serum immunoglobulin A tissue transglutaminase antibody (TTG-IgA), IgA-endomysial antibody (IgA-EMA), and immunoglobulin G antigliadin antibodies (AGA-IgG) may be used to screen for celiac disease when clinically indicated.

Consider-If concern surrounds possible growth hormone deficiency, the following may be obtained: *Serum insulinlike growth factor I (IGF-I) *Insulin like growth factor binding protein (IGF-BP3).

Summary of Organic Causes of Failure to Thrive:

Prenatal causes

Prematurity with complications, Maternal malnutrition, Toxic exposure in utero, Alcohol, smoking, medications, infections, IUGR, Chromosomal abnormalities.

Postnatal causes

Inadequate intake

Lack of appetite (e.g., iron deficiency anemia, CNS pathology, chronic infection), Inability to suck or swallow: CNS or muscular, Vomiting (e.g., CNS, metabolic, obstruction, renal) Gastroesophageal reflux and esophagitis.

Poor absorption and/or use of nutrients : GI disorder (e.g., CF, celiac disease, Shwachman-Diamond syndrome, chronic diarrhea) Renal - Renal failure, renal tubular acidosis Endocrine - Hypothyroidism, diabetes mellitus, growth hormone deficiency· Inborn error of metabolism Chronic infection (e.g., HIV, tuberculosis, parasites).

Increased metabolic demand

Hyperthyroidism
Chronic disease (e.g., heart failure, BPD)
Chronic inflammatory conditions (e.g., inflammatory bowel disease, systemic lupus erythematosus), Renal failure
Malignancy

KEY POINTS FOR CLINICAL PRACTICE:

1. Failure to thrive is a condition commonly seen by primary care physicians. Prompt diagnosis and intervention are important for preventing malnutrition and developmental sequelae. Medical and social factors often contribute to failure to thrive. Either extreme of parental attention (neglect or hypervigilance) can lead to failure to thrive.

2. About 25 percent of normal infants will shift to a lower growth percentile in the first two years of life and then follow that percentile; this should not be diagnosed as failure to thrive. Infants with Down syndrome, intrauterine growth retardation, or premature birth follow different growth patterns than normal infants.

3. Many infants with failure to thrive are not identified unless careful attention is paid to plotting growth parameters at routine checkups. A thorough history is the best guide to establishing the etiology of the failure to thrive and directing further evaluation and management.

4. All children with failure to thrive need additional calories for catch-up growth (typically 150 percent of the caloric requirement for their expected, not actual, weight). Few need laboratory evaluation. Hospitalization is rarely required and is indicated only for severe failure to thrive and for those whose safety is a concern.

5. A multidisciplinary approach is recommended when failure to thrive persists despite intervention or when it is severe.

REFERENCES & FURTHER READING : 1) Gahagan S, Holmes R. A stepwise approach to evaluation of undernutrition and failure to thrive. Pediatr Clin North Am 1998;45:169-87. 2) Wright CM. Identification and management of failure to thrive: a community perspective. Arch Dis Child 2000;82:5-9. 3) Powell GF. Nonorganic failure to thrive in infancy: an update on nutrition, behavior, and growth. J Am Coll Nutr 1988;7:345-53. 4) Failure to Thrive SCOTT D. KRUGMAN, M.D., Franklin Square Hospital Center, Baltimore, Maryland HOWARD DUBOWITZ, M.D., M.S., University of Maryland School of Medicine, Baltimore, Maryland SEPTEMBER 1, 2003 / VOLUME 68, NUMBER 5 www.aafp.org/afp AMERICAN FAMILY PHYSICIAN 5) Batchelor JA. Has recognition of failure to thrive changed? Child Care Health Dev 1996;22:235-40.

103 Gastroesophageal Reflux Disease (GERD)

@ *Diagnosis of GOR *usually clinical *barium swallow and ultrasound nonspecific (only useful to rule out structural abnormalities) *24-hour pH probe gold standard, although gastric contents must be **acid** *demonstration of acid in oral secretions by using litmus paper (wont diagnose reflux into lower oesophagus) *white oral secretions may be differentiated from milk if milk is tinged with methylene blue (few drops only) *endoscopy little data available for preterm infants *radio-nucleotide studies not standardized in preterm infants *esophageal manometry catheter size limits usefulness in VLBW .*

Algorithm for evaluation and "step-up" management of Gastroesophageal Reflux (GER).

Suspect GER

↓

History / Physical Exam R/O Other Diagnoses

↓

Complicated GER ? — Yes → * Acid suppression * Consider further evaluation

No ↓

Warning Signals ?

No ↓

Reassurance
Lifestyle changes
- Consider hypoallergenic formula (infants)
- Thickened feeds (infants)
- Re-evaluate

↓

* Symptoms improved ?
* Infants - Resolution by 18 mo ?

↓ Yes

Routine F/U

Pediatric GI consultation → No

↓

* Re-evaluate therapy
- "Step-up"
- "Step-down"
- Consider;
- UGI
- EGD/biopsy
- pH Monitoring

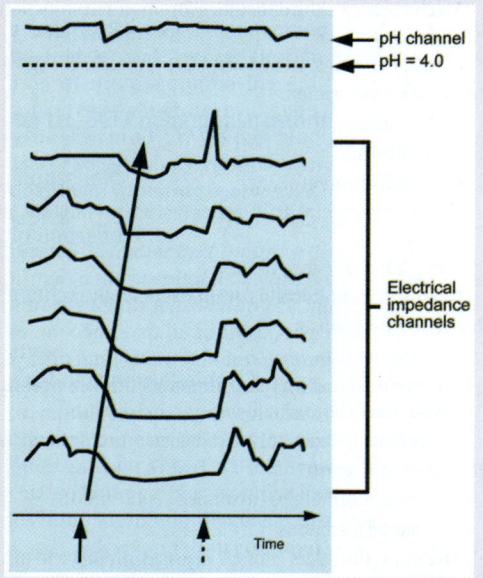

The image is a representation of concomitant intraesophageal pH and esophageal electrical impedance measurements. The vertical solid arrow indicates commencement of a nonacid gastroesophageal reflux (GER) episode (diagonal arrow). The vertical dashed arrow indicates the onset of a normal swallow. *Esophageal pH monitoring is not indicated in cases of obvious gastroesophageal reflux but is useful in demonstrating an association between reflux and symptoms in atypical presentations and in grading the risk of esophagitis.*

REVIEW OF CLINICAL PROBLEMS

1. What are the warning signs of disorders other than GERD in infants with Vomiting ?
   Ans: Refer to the Table 2 of the Chapter.

2. What diagnostic tests are useful in identifying Gastroesophageal Reflux?
   Ans: Refer to the Table 3 of the Chapter.

3. Discuss the conservative therapy/lifestyle changes in managing GERD.
   Ans: Refer to the Table 4 of the Chapter.

4. What Surgical options are available for severe GERD ?
   Ans: Refer to the Table 9 of the Chapter.

5. Discuss the essential aspects of history in evaluating a child with GERD.
   Ans: Refer to the Evaluation-Decision-Action Plan/ Algorithm to diagnose and manage a child with GERD.

LEARNING OBJECTIVES

After completing this article, readers will be able to:

1. Understand the differences between GER & GERD.

2. Search for the warning signs that would suggest other disorders than GERD.

3. Perform Diagnostic work-up for severe GERD, after d/w a Pediatric Gastroenterologist.

4. Institute Conservative therapy initially to manage GERD.

5. Liaise with Pediatric Gastroenterologist &/or Surgeon for surgical intervention in selected GERD cases.

---

* ***Pearl/Peril/Pitfall:*** *In the infant with suspected GER or GERD, the health care provider should observe the caretaker feeding the infant. This allows the provider to assess feeding technique, swallow function, as well as infant-caregiver interaction or bonding. The infant's height, weight, and head circumference should be documented at each visit*

BIRD'S EYE VIEW/OVERVIEW/SYNOPSIS

1. *Gastroesophageal Reflux (GER)*, defined as a passage of gastric contents into the esophagus, is a normal physiological process that occurs throughout the day in healthy infants and children. When refluxed material passes into the pharynx and out the mouth, then "spitting up" or vomiting occurs. 50% of all infants between 0-3 months of age and 2/3rds of 4–6 months old infants vomit atleast once per day. Postprandial regurgitation is the most common sign of GER in infants and may range from effortless spitting to forceful vomiting (Sondheimer, 2003). The prevalence of reflux decreases dramatically after 8 months of age : 50% of these infants outgrow the problem by the age 1 year, and virtually all do so by 18–24 months of age, and no evaluation or treatment is necessary, if not accompanied by color change or bradycardia.

2. In a small number of infants, GER may cause disease (GERD) characterized by chronic symptoms such as : a) Malnutrition from inadequate caloric intake as a result of discomfort or calorie loss from vomiting b) Esophageal symptoms of pain, inflammation, and bleeding , c) Airways symptoms of hoarseness and laryngitis, cough, apnea, exacerbation of reactive airways disease, or pneumonia (refer to Table No 1 of the Chapter) and d) changes in neurodevelopmental patterns.

3. The decision to perform tests or prescribe pharmacologic treatment should take into account that most neurologically normal infants have GER that is self-limited. There is no clear point at which "regurgitation" or "spitting up" becomes a disease to be evaluated and treated. To parents, the problem is defined by the volume and frequency of regurgitation, crying or apparent discomfort, or arching and posturing. To physicians, the disease is defined by complications, such as acid esophagitis, failure to thrive, or compromise of the respiratory tract (apnea or aspiration). Acid esophagitis may manifest as pain, with discomfort and posturing (Sandifer syndrome), or by ongoing inflammation with failure to thrive, or both. In approximately 25-50% of cases no cause can be identified. Three mechanisms have been identified that allow reflux of the gastric contents across the esophagogastric junction and into the esophagus: transient lower esophageal sphincter relaxations (TLESRs), hypotensive or incompetent lower esophageal sphincter (LES), and anatomic disruption of the esophagogastric junction (e.g., hiatal hernia). TLESRs are mediated primarily through vagal pathways and account for virtually all reflux episodes in healthy individuals and the majority of reflux episodes (50-88%) in those with GERD. TLESRs are primarily triggered by gastric distention after a meal (Orlando, 2001). Pharyngeal stimulation, cholecystokinin, and gastric acid secretion may contribute to an increased rate of TLESRs (Sherman, 2001). Reflux with normal LES pressure may occur with increased abdominal pressure, such as after meals, crying, defecating, and coughing. Infants are more predisposed to "spitting up or vomiting" than are adolescents and adults because of the small reservoir of their esophagus (Herbst, 2000).

4. The Pediatrician should consider other causes of vomiting rather than GER , in an infant with "WARNING SIGNS' (refer to Table 2 of the Chapter).

5. A thorough history and physical examination are generally sufficient to arrive at an uncomplicated GER, which obviates the need for any diagnostic testing. If none of the WARNING SIGNS or the potential complications are present, reassurance of the parents including education regarding the range of normal frequency for vomiting and the potential complications of GER is usually sufficient for management.

6. In case of GERD, the diagnostic approaches vary depending on the presenting symptoms, and in all cases, other treatable causes of the disorder must be considered during the diagnostic evaluation. No test serves as the "gold standard" for making a diagnosis of GERD : a series of tests is usually required to determine if a particular disorder is being caused by GER (Refer to Table 3 of the Chapter).

7. The *Evaluation-Decision-Action-Plan/Algorithm* describes the clinical approach to diagnose and manage GERD in children.

8. Management of GERD : Conservative therapy can be used in virtually anyone with symptoms that suggest gastroesophageal reflux. Pharmacologic therapy is used for children who are shown to have reflux disease, or in some specific instances, it may be used empirically for a limited time. Surgery may be indicated if reflux causes persistent vomiting with failure to thrive, chronic esophagitis, esophageal strictures, or chronic pulmonary disease that does not respond to 2 to 3 months of pharmacological therapy (Sondheimer, 2003). Surgical management involves the Nissen fundoplication procedure, in which the upper stomach (fundus) is wrapped around the bottom of the esophagus, creating a collar, to augment sphincter pressure (Sherman, 2001; Borowitz, 2002). The surgical success rate based on symptomatic relief in infants and children ranges from 57% to 97% (Farivar, 2001). The mortality rate due to surgery may range from 0 to 4.5%, and complications may occur in up to 45% of cases. The most common complications are breakdown of the fundoplication, small bowel obstruction, infection, atelectasis, perforation, persistent esophageal strictures, and esophageal obstruction (Farivar, 2001).

9. The emergency Pediatrician should identify ALTEs (Apparent Life-Threatening Events) associated with GERD,, which are frightening to the observer and are characterized by a combination of apnea, change in color (cyanosis, pallor, rubra), limpness / stiffness, and chocking / gagging. The first event usually occurs by 1-2 months of age. These are typically obstructive in nature and occur while the patient is awake, supine, and within 1 hour of a feeding. Diagnosis is generally best made from typical history. Episodes occur infrequently, so even carefully performed 24-hour esophageal pH monitoring combined with measurements of airflow and chest wall impedance may be unable to document episodes.Therapy includes thickened feedings, prokinetic and acid suppressant therapy, position therapy with prone positioning (SIDS may be increased). Antireflux surgery (laparoscopic fundoplication and P/C gastrojejunostomy) is effective, but because the episodes are self -resolving and decreased in frequency after age 6 months in most infants, surgery is very rarely indicated.

10. Cisapride has been shown to be an effective therapy for GERD, but been withdrawn in July 2000, because of the cardiac rhythm complications (QT interval prolongation). But it can be used in selected cases, with careful ECG monitoring to guide the therapy. Avoid drug interactions of Cisapride with macrolides and imidazoles. The pediatric health care provider should offer an ongoing, comprehensive clinical approach to the family based on considerations of growth and development, and the quality of interactions between the caregivers and child.

---

* *Pearl/Peril/Pitfall : According to the GER Guidelines of the North American Society for Pediatric Gastroenterology and Nutrition (Rudolph et al., 2001), a thorough history and physical examination with attention to warning signals is generally sufficient to allow the clinician to establish a diagnosis of GER, recognize complications, and initiate management.*

THE EVALUATION-DECISION-ACTION-ALGORITHM FOR THE DIAGNOSIS AND MANAGEMENT OF *A CHILD WITH GASTROESOPHAGEAL REFLUX DISEASE (GERD)*

SUBJECTIVE FINDINGS

Hx of onset, frequency, severity (quantity, degree of forcefullness, presence of bile or blood) of the vomiting.

Determine the type of formula, method of preparation, quantity ingested, and feeding position and technique.

Establish the time of vomiting in relation to the feeding.

Note associated symptoms such as - fever, cough, cold, respiratory distress, diarrhea, altered mental status, seizures and failure to thrive.

Inquire about perinatal deaths in the family (e.g.. inborn errors of metabolism & CAH).

OBJECTIVE FINDINGS

Assess hydration and circulatory status

Plot the infant's length, weight, and head circumference on a growth chart (to identify failure to thrive or rapid head growth)

Assess mental status: irritability, lethargy, seizures, or focal neurologic signs.

Search for any ASOM, aspiration pneumonia, RAD.

Observe a feeding and note the peristaltic waves.

Palpate abdomen for pyloric olive (CHPS)

INVESTIGATIONS

Blood FBC with differential, electrolytes, CRP, cultures, BUN, creatinine, ABG analysis, LFTs.

Urine Urinalysis, cultures

Imaging Upper endoscopy with biopsy to exclude Crohn disease and eosinophilic / infectious esophagitis.

Nuclear scintigraphy To detect aspiration in to the lungs

Esophageal pH monitoring (24 hrs) - Combined with a pneumogram.

Others CXR, CT scan, laryngoscopy/ bronchoscopy with lavage.

Degree of illness in Gastroesophageal Reflux

Mild
No signs of growth failure during infancy
and
No limitation of normal activities
and
No complications of reflux

Moderate
Symptoms of esophagitis (pain)
or
Signs of aspiration pneumonia /reactive airway disease
or
Growth failure
or
Anemia, asymptomatic upper GI bleeding

Severe
A life-threatening event, near miss sudden infant death
or
Active upper GI bleeding
or
Severe pain that limits normal activities
or
Severe dehydration
or
Malnutrition
or
Electrolyte/serum pH abnormality

Very Severe
Signs of shock
or
Altered mental status with coma or seizures

A CHILD WITH GASTROESOPHAGEAL REFLUX

Assess degree of illness

Mild | Moderate | Severe | Very severe

Severe → Hospitalize

Very severe → **Stabilize**
Respiratory Support
Circulatory Support
Hospitalize in ICU

Mild → **Treat**
Diet Modification
Prone Positioning
→ **Follow-up**
Assess in 2–4 wk
→ Improved / Not improved

Obtain : Upper GI series
Consider:
Radionuclide scan
Endoscopy
Esophageal pH monitoring

Reflux identified | Reflux not identified

Treat
Diet Modification
Thicken Feeds
Increase Frequency and Decrease Amounts
Avoid Caffeine, Soda, Gum, and Smoke in Older Patients
Prone positioning for Infants
Elevation of Head During Sleep for Older Patients
Consider :
Antacids
→ Improved / Not improved

Identify
Esophageal stricture or foreign body
Duodenal web
Diaphragmatic hernia
Hiatal hernia
Gastric outlet obstruction
Intestinal malrotation/ obstruction
Tracheoesophageal fistula
Vascular compression

Treat
Consider in infants :
Metoclopramide
Bethanechol , Cisapride
Consider for Esophagitis :
Lansaprazole

Not improved | Improved

Treat
Consider :
Nasoduodenal or Nasogastric
Tube Feedings
or Surgical Fundoplication

---

* ***Pearl/Peril/Pitfall:*** *The health care provider should educate parents regarding feeding and positioning interventions and reassure parents of their child's health. Growth charts should be shared with parents at each visit to document the infant's continued growth within standard percentiles. Helping the caregiver to understand symptoms and potential complications will enable the caregiver to seek appropriate treatment.*

TABLE 1	Complications of gastroesophageal reflux

Vomiting
- Parental frustration
- Iatrogenic weight loss from limitations on feeding to prevent vomiting
- Weight loss or inadequate weight gain from excessive vomiting

Esophagitis
- Dysphagia (may limit feedings, causing weight loss)
- Chest pain, heartburn
- Irritability and inconsolable crying in infants
- Hematemesis, anemia, melena
- Sandifer syndrome
- Globus sensation
- Barret esophagus
- Esophageal stricture

Respiratory disorders
- Cough, hoarseness, stridor
- Bronchospasm or wheezing
- Apnea (especially obstructive)
- Recurrent aspiration pneumonia or pulmonary fibrosis

TABLE 2	Warning signs of disorders other than Gastroesophageal reflux in the infant with vomiting

- Forceful or bilious vomiting
- Diarrhea
- Constipation
- GI bleeding
- Abdominal tenderness or distention
- Fever or lethargy
- Hepatosplenomegaly
- Bulging fontanelle, macro/microcephaly, seizures
- Onset of vomiting after 6 months of life

TABLE 3	Diagnostic tests to identify GE reflux

24 hr Esophageal pH monitoring This records the number and duration of acid reflux episodes into the lower and / or upper esophagus. Prolonged esophageal mucosal exposure (i.e. > 11% of a 24 hr period in an infant and > 6% in an older child) increased the risk for esophagitis, and therefore this test is helpful to determine the risk of esophagitis. 24 hr esophageal pH monitoring should be combined with a pneumogram that measures O_2 sats. and chest wall and air flow movements if one is attempting to establish a clearer cause - and - effect relationship between apnea episodes and GER ; however, these time - consuming and technically challenging tests often fail to clarify if apnea is caused by GER. A normal study doesn't exclude GER as a potential factor causing airway symptoms.

Upper gastrointestinal radiography (UGI) It is useful to diagnose anatomic abnormalities that present with non bilious vomiting as with GER, such as esophageal stricture, pyloric stenosis, antral webs, or disorders of esophageal motility such as achalasia. The UGI is not useful for diagnosis of GER because reflux of ingested radiographic contrast often occurs in normal individuals.

Upper endoscopy with biopsy Useful to evaluate if there is esophagitis or other sequelae of chronic esophageal acid exposure such as stricture or Barrett esophagus. In addition, it allows diagnosis of Crohn disease and eosinophilic / infectious esophagitis.

Nuclear scintigraphy Evaluates the distribution of isotope - labeled formula / food following normal feeding. Because GER may occur in normal individuals, documentation of these episodes is of little pathophysiological use unless aspiration in to the lungs is detected. If this occurs, it is a clear indication that airway protective mechanisms are deficient.

Other tests -Broncho alveolar lavage of lipid laden macrophages is a test for aspiration. It becomes positive as early as 6 hours and remains positive upto 3 days after an aspiration episodes. It cannot differentiate the source of aspirate (gastric acid versus oral feedings).

TABLE 4	Treatment of gastroesophageal reflux disease : Conservative therapy/"lifestyle changes"

Positional changes
- **Infant** : supine position with head elevated (unless high risk from GER, and then consider prone)
- **Older child** : head of bed elevation

Nutritional therapy
- **Infant**
  - Trial of hypoallergenic formula for 1 to 2 weeks
  - Thicken feedings
    - 1 to 2 tbsp rice cereal / oz formula
    - Commercial formulas with thickening agents
  - Increase caloric density of formula with concentration
  - Small frequent feeds (2.5 hours between feeds)
- **Child**
  - Avoid caffeinated beverages, peppermint, and chocolate
  - Weight loss if obese

- Rarely, nasogastric or nasojejunal feeding may be required

Pharmacologic therapy
- Antacids (only for relief of occasional symptoms in older children)
- Antisecretory agents
  - Histamine-2 receptor blockers (cimetidine, ranitidine, famotidine)
  - Proton pump inhibitors (omeprazole, lansoprazole, rabeprazole, pontoprazole)
- Prokinetic agents (cisapride where available)

Surgical therapy
- Nissen fundoplication
- Thal fundoplication
- Esophagogastric disconnection

---

* *Pearl/Peril/Pitfall :* Differential Diagnosis (of vomiting) • drugs e.g. theophylline and caffeine •inborn errors of metabolism •pyloric stenosis (GOR usually not projectile) •bowel obstruction (usually bile-stained vomiting) •sepsis (especially UTI) •necrotizing enterocolitis.

TABLE 5   Indications for PH monitoring recommendations by *NASPGHAN

Recommended only if it leads to clinically important alteration in diagnosis, treatment or prognosis.

1. Chronic laryngeal symptoms
2. Unexplained recurrent pneumonia
3. GER suspected as the cause of apnea : as part of multi-channel pneumocardiography test
4. Intractable reactive airway disease
5. Atypical chest pain
6. Barrett's esophagus : to determine whether the dosage of medication is optimal
7. Prior to surgery (fundoplication)
8. To evaluate the effectiveness of fundoplication

* NASPGHAN = North American Society for Pediatric Gastroenterology, Hepatology and Nutrition

TABLE 6   Typical dosage range of the generally used H₂ blocker and proton pump inhibitors

Drugs used for GERD therapy ≥ 8 weeks

Drug	Dose	Frequency
Cimetidine	20–40 mg/kg/day	(t.i.d, or q.i.d)
Ranitidine	5–10 mg/kg/day	(t.i.d, or q.i.d)
Omeprazole	0.8–3 mg/kg/day	(q.d. or b.i.d.)
Lansaprazole	0.8–3 mg/kg/day	(q.d. or b.i.d.)
Sucral fate	40–80 mg/kg/day	(max. q.i.d.)
Cisapride	0.8 mg/kg/day	(t.i.d. or q.i.d.)
Reglan	0.4–0.8 mg/kg/day	(t.i.d. or q.i.d.)

TABLE 7   Pharmacological agents affecting lower esophageal sphincter pressure

Agents	Lower esophageal sphincter pressure Increases	Decreases
Hormones & peptides	Angiotensin	Cholecystokinin
	Bombesin	Gastric inhibitory peptide
	Gastrin	Glucagon
	Motilin	Neurotensin
	Substance	Progesterone
	Vasopressin	Secretin
	Pancreatic polypeptide	Vasoactive intestinal peptide
Neurotrans-mitters	α-adrenergic agonists	α-adrenergic antagonists
	Anticholinesterase	Anticholinergics
	β-adrenergic antagonists	β-adrenergic agonists
	Cholinergic agonists	Dopamine
Other	Cisapride	Calcium channel blockers
	Domperidone	Cyclic adenosine monophosphate
	Histamine (H₁)	Histamine (H₂)
	Indomethacin	Lidocaine
	Metoclopramide	Morphine
	Prostaglandin F₂-α	Prostaglandins E₁ and E₂
	Serotonin (neural receptor)	Serotonin (muscle receptor)
		Theophylline

TABLE 8   Treatment for children with gastroesophageal reflux

Clinical condition	Treatment
Very mild reflux	Mother reassured Simple feeding advice
Mild reflux	Thickened feeds
Moderate reflux	Prokinetic drugs (consider risk benefit)
Reflux with esophagitis	Add histamine 2 blockers Proton pump inhibitor
Severe reflux	Consider continuous nasogastric tube feeding in children less than 1 year as an alternative to fundoplication
Failure of medical treatment	Fundoplication
Esophagitis with stricture	Fundoplication with dilatation

TABLE 9   Surgery for GERD

* *Fundoplication* Nissen (tight wrap, 360°) or Thal (loose wrap < 360° with or without a gastric drainage procedure (E.g.. Pyloroplasty) to improve gastric emptying ; an effective method for children with GERD refractory to aggressive pharmacotherapy, those with aspiration, chronic lung disease, or neurological devastation, esophageal stricture or Barrett's esophageal metaplasia.

* Preoperative accuracy of diagnosis of GERD and the skill of the surgeon are two of the most important predictors of successful outcome.

* Complications of fundoplication include ; herniation of the wrap through the hiatus, bowel obstruction due to adhesions, gas bloat, gastric dysmotility, & inability to belch or vomit when necessary.

* Laparoscopic fundoplication or alternatively the placement of a percutaneous gastrojejunostomy tube under endoscopic guidance reduce the morbidity in children with GERD, who require surgical intervention.

---

* *Pearl/Peril/Pitfall: The barium contrast UGI series is important, particularly in infants, to identify anatomic causes of recurrent regurgitation or vomiting, such as pyloric stenosis, malrotation, hiatal hernia, esophageal stricture, gastric outlet obstruction, or other anatomic abnormalities. The presence of reflux and delayed gastric emptying time may also be identified. However, the UGI series is not sufficiently sensitive or specific to provide a definitive diagnosis of GER (Rudolph et al., 2001).*

The goal of surgery for gastroesophageal reflux disease (GERD) is to reestablish the antireflux barrier, without creating obstruction to the food bolus. In general, the Nissen fundoplication, which is a complete 360° wrap, best controls the symptoms of gastroesophageal reflux; however, it may lead to more episodes of dysphagia (difficulty and discomfort with swallowing) and gas bloat than a partial wrap. Before operative intervention, patients should be evaluated with a thorough history and physical examination, and results of medical treatment (nonoperative therapy) should be well documented. In infants and young children, performing upper GI series (upper GI contrast study) prior to performance of fundoplication is advisable in order to rule out other possible pathologies that may be causing emesis. Surgical treatment of gastroesophageal reflux should be considered for the following patients:

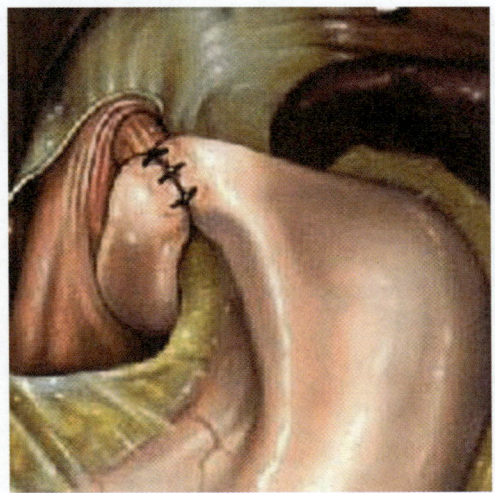

Diagram illustrating the Nissen fundoplication. Note how the stomach is wrapped around the esophagus (360º wrap).

* Infants and children who have failed "step-up" therapy for gastroesophageal reflux (typically over 12 wk) and those who cannot be weaned off of acid-reducing medications should be considered for surgical treatment.

* Those with an atypical presentation, especially respiratory, whose symptoms are clearly associated with gastroesophageal reflux (e.g. obstructive apnea temporally associated with reflux during pH monitoring) should be considered for surgical treatment. However, a period of medical therapy (including acid blockade) under close monitoring conditions should be attempted in many cases prior to recommending a surgical approach.

* Patients with complications of gastroesophageal reflux, such as aspiration, stricture of the esophagus, or Barrett esophagus should be considered for surgical treatment. Patients with neurologic impairment that requires feeding gastrostomy who are found to have pathologic reflux and remain medication dependent should also be considered for surgery.

* Patients with chronic reflux and recurrence of anastomotic stricture after repair of esophageal atresia should be considered for surgical treatment.

KEY POINTS FOR CLINICAL PRACTICE:

1. During an infant's first year of life, GER is a common occurrence and concern of families. The infant with uncomplicated GER may be managed conservatively with feeding schedule modifications, thickened feeds, changes in positioning, or a trial of formula change. Gastroesophageal reflux disease (GERD) is a pathological process in infants manifested by poor weight gain, signs of esophagitis, persistent respiratory symptoms or complications, and changes in neurobehavior. GERD may be a significant factor for the development of ALTE in infants.

2. The diagnosis of GERD needs to be assessed via the results of both clinical and radiological examinations as well as the 24 hour pH monitoring. The "gold standard" for the diagnosis of GERD is the 24 hour pH probe. The test is performed by transnasally placing a microelectrode into the lower esophagus, which measure and records intraesophageal pH usually every 4 to 8 seconds (Rudolph et al. 2001). Esophageal pH monitoring via a 24 hour probe provides information about the rate of gastric clearance and frequency of reflux. The pH probe quantifies esophageal acid exposure to determine if an association exists between atypical symptoms (chronic cough, stridor, wheezing, apnea, irritability, or opisthotonic posturing) and acid reflux. One episode of acid reflux is defined by a pH of < 4 for at least 15 to 30 seconds (Sandritter, 2003). The reflux index is the percentage of time during the pH probe study that the pH is < 4. The upper limit of normal for the reflux index in the first year of life is 12% and only 6% in children greater than 1 year of age.

3. Despite lack of randomized, controlled studies of non-pharmacological management of GER, life-style changes are generally recognized as the appropriate initial management of uncomplicated GER. Life style changes include the following modifications: (a) feeding schedule; (b) thickening of feedings; (c) positioning, and (d) formula changes.

4. Persistent problems and complications of GER, despite non-pharmacologic interventions, may warrant pharmacological (H2 blockers, e.g. Ranitidine Proton pump inhibitors, e.g. Omeprazole) intervention. If an UGI series has ruled out anatomic causes of recurrent regurgitation, pharmacologic management with the use of an acid suppressant is generally the first line of therapy.

5. Surgery may be indicated if reflux causes persistent vomiting with failure to thrive, chronic esophagitis, esophageal strictures, or chronic pulmonary disease that does not respond to 2 to 3 months of pharmacological therapy (Sondheimer, 2003). Surgical management involves the Nissen fundoplication procedure, in which the upper stomach (fundus) is wrapped around the bottom of the esophagus, creating a collar, to augment sphincter pressure.

REFERENCES & FURTHER READING : 1)Jung AD. Gastroesophageal reflux in infants and children. Am Fam Physician 2001;64:1853-60. 2)Wong WM, Wong BCY. Definition and diagnosis of gastroesophageal reflux disease. J Gastroenterol Hepatol 2004;19:S26-S32. 3) Mahajan L, Wylie R, Oliva L et al. Reproducibility of 24-hour intraesophageal pH monitoring in pediatric patients. Pediatrics 1998; 101:260-3. 4) Sarani B, Gleiber M, Evans SRT. Esophageal pH monitoring, indications and methods. J Clin Gastroenterol 2002;34:200-6. 5) Arad-Cohen N, Cohen A, Tirosh E. The relationship between gastroesophageal reflux and apnea in infants. J Pediatr 2000; 137: 321-6.

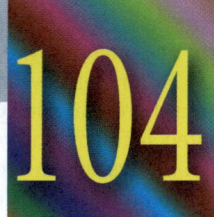

Febrile Neonate/Young Infant without a Focus

@ *Febrile neonates younger than 4 weeks old should have a full evaluation for sepsis. A full evaluation for sepsis consists of a complete blood cell count (CBC) with differential, blood culture, enhanced urinalysis (UA), urine culture, and a lumbar puncture (LP) to collect cerebrospinal fluid (CSF). CSF should be analyzed for cell counts, protein, glucose, and culture. CSF should be assayed for herpes simplex virus (HSV) using polymerase chain reaction (PCR) in all neonates in the first 28 days of life who appear ill, who have mucocutaneous lesions, or who have had a seizure.*

Fever is defined as a rectal temperature that exceeds 38°C (100.4°F). Direct the initial evaluation of these patients toward identifying occult bacteremia or other serious bacterial infections. Address the following questions:

- What laboratory studies are indicated for various age ranges?
- Which patients need in-depth evaluation and treatment?
- Which patients need treatment with antibiotics?
- Which patients should be hospitalized?
- Which patients can be sent home safely and what follow-up is appropriate for them?
- Are the diagnosis and treatment modalities for each patient cost-effective?
- What is the potential morbidity associated with testing and treatment?
- What are the parental (and patient) preferences for testing and treatment?

Diagnostic Goals and Challenges for Evaluating a febrile Neonate/Infant

1. Differentiate child with serious disease from child with minor acute illness.

2. Identify etiologic agent for fever early in the course of illness.

3. Identify children at risk for occult bacteremia.

4. Avoid unnecessary and expensive workups.

5. Recognize children with a possible immunodeficiency syndrome.

Management Goals for a Febrile Neonate/Infant

1. Treat potentially serious infection early.

2. Maximize comfort of patient during fever.

3. Hospitalize patient only when necessary.

4. Prevent complication of febrile seizure.

5. Alleviate parental anxiety.

6. Avoid unnecessary antibiotic use.

7. Use specialists when necessary.

REVIEW OF CLINICAL PROBLEMS

1. How do you evaluate an infant <90 days old with fever and nonlocalizing signs/symptoms?
   Ans: Refer to the Evaluation-Decision-Action Plan/Algorithm to diagnose & manage Febrile Neonate/Infant without localization of signs/symptoms.

2. Whom do you consider to have serious bacterial infections among febrile children, independent of their age?
   Ans: Refer to the Table 6 of the Chapter.

3. What are the Clinical factors which demand a low threshold for urgent investigation of a Febrile Neonate/Infant?
   Ans: Refer to the Table 2 of the Chapter.

4. Mention the components of Full septic Screen.
   Ans: Refer to the Table 4 of the Chapter.

5. Mention the important diagnostic clues in a febrile Neonate/Infant. *Ans: Refer to the Table 1 of the Chapter.*

LEARNING OBJECTIVES

After completing this article, readers will be able to:

1. Document temperature accurately, and understand the pathophysiology of fever.

2. Recognize the significance of fever in various age categories and have a logical approach to its evaluation.

3. Use signs, symptoms, and selected laboratory tests to identify the underlying cause of fever.

4. Have a treatment plan for fever and for the etiology of fever.

5. Recognize the need for specialist referral for treatment of infections or immunologic causes of fever

---

* **Pearl/Peril/Pitfall:** *Obtain blood culture before administering antibiotics. Neonates aged 0–30 days should be treated with combination of IV ampicillin and a third-generation cephalosporin or gentamicin. For infants aged 31–60 days, a third-generation IV cephalosporin alone is recommended as first-line therapy. IV ampicillin is recommended in addition to a third-generation cephalosporin for severely ill infants aged 31-60 days or for infants in this age group with UTI. In addition to the antibiotics discussed above, vancomycin should be considered in settings where MRSA is prevalent or suspected.*

BIRD'S EYE VIEW/OVERVIEW/SYNOPSIS

1. Consider a child is febrile, when his/her rectal temperature is 38°C (100.4°F) or higher. Oral temperatures > 37.6°C (99.7°F) and axillary temperatures > 37.3°C are considered to be elevated. Some diurnal variation exists in children > 2 yrs of age, with elevations of 1°C (1.8°F) occurring in the late afternoon or early evening. The tympanic membrane has been used with great accuracy and reproducibility but is not considered reliable in children younger than 6 months of age, and rectal temperatures should be measured in this age group. Oral and axillary temperatures usually are about 0.6° C (1° F) and 1.1° C (2° F) less than rectal temperatures, respectively.

2. *Admit infants younger than 1 month of age and do a full sepsis assessment before starting on broad-spectrum IV antibiotics, because they show limited signs of infection, often making it difficult to distinguish clinically between serious bacterial infections and self-limited viral illnesses.* No laboratory or historical factors should be used to exclude underlying bacterial infection, since there are no clear factors that are sensitive or specific enough to direct decision making. Pediatricians have historically considered that febrile infants younger than 2-3 months of age require a more detailed and invasive diagnostic evaluation than older children. The reasons for this are several, including the relative immaturity of infantile host defences and the potential for perinatally acquired infections, both of which result in an increased risk of bacteremia, sepsis, and significant bacterial focal infections. In addition, in this age group, the clinical assessment of "toxicity", or septic appearance, is difficult, as such judgment relies on observation of the child's responsiveness and behavior, which in babies is so developmentally limited.

3. Febrile children between 1–3 months of age, who appear ill and toxic require prompt hospitalization and immediate IV antibiotic therapy after cultures of blood, urine, and CSF. Infants younger than 3 months of age with fever who appear generally well ; who have been previously healthy ; who have no evidence of skin, soft tissue, bone, joint, or ear infection ; and who have a total WBC count of 5,000–15,000 cells / cumm, an absolute band count of < 1,500 /cumm, normal urine analysis (< 5 WBC/HPF), normal stools (< 5 WBC / HPF) ; who have good social situation are unlikely to have a serious bacterial infection—should have close follow-up as an outpatient/or admit for close observation, if the follow-up is difficult.

4. Infants between 3–36 months of age, who have a temperature < 39°C and who do not appear toxic can be observed as outpatients without performing diagnostic tests or administering antimicrobial agents. For non toxic-appearing infants with a rectal temperature of 39°C or greater, two options were suggested : (1) obtain a blood culture and give empirical antimicrobial therapy (ceftriaxone, a single dose of 50 mg/kg, not to exceed 1 g) or (2) if the WBC count is 15,000 / cumm or greater, obtain a blood culture and give empirical antimicrobial therapy. A third option, not offered in these guidelines, for selected infants is to obtain a blood culture and observe as outpatients without empirical antimicrobial therapy with return for re-evaluation within 24 hr. Lumbar punctures should be considered for febrile infants and children who are younger than 8 weeks old; have a full anterior fontanelle; are persistently irritable, inconsolable, or lethargic; or have a petechial rash. Chest radiographs should not be routinely performed for fever alone, in the absence of lower respiratory tract findings or hypoxemia.

Chest radiographs are most useful for those with high fever, focal pulmonary examination findings, rales, grunting, flaring, retractions, or hypoxia, or for the subset of patients with leukocytosis (if obtained) in the absence of an alternative source of fever. Regardless of the management option, the family should be instructed to return immediately if the child's condition deteriorates or new symptoms,such as rash,develop.

5. *Febrile children, independent of age, if develop petechiae with or without localizing signs are at high risk for life-threatening bacterial infections such as bacteremia, sepsis, and meningitis.* Since 8-20% of patients with fever and petechiae have a serious bacterial infection, and 7-10% have meningococcal sepsis or meningitis, management of these children includes prompt hospitalization, culture of blood and CSF, and administration of appropriate IV antibiotics.

6. Although temperatures above 40°C increase the risk of meningitis, hyperpyrexia (> 41°C) is not associated with higher rates of serious bacterial infections than temperatures of 40°C. As they result from CNS involvement or heat stroke, infants and children with hyperpyrexia should be carefully evaluated as for all children with fever.

7. *Immunocompromised children require an aggressive and anticipatory approach to potential infections, regardless of age and the height of fever* (refer to Table No 6 of the Chapter)

8. Occult bacteremia (6% of febrile children without a defined focus have positive blood cultures) is a significant problem and the high-risk group includes: age < 24 months, fever > 39.4°C (102.9°F), WBC > 15,000/cumm and ESR > 30 mm/hr . Evaluate them carefully to be certain that there is no underlying disease such as pneumonia or meningitis.All neonates aged 0-30 days and toxic-appearing children should be hospitalized for antibiotic treatments. Antibiotic treatment should not be discontinued until all culture results show no bacterial growth after 48 hours.

9. General management of fever includes a) Extra fluids b) Acetaminophen 15mgs/kg/dose q4hr c) Ibuprofen 5mgs/kg/dose q6hr d) Sponging with lukewarm water-only for children with febrile delirium, a febrile seizure, or any fever over 41.1°C.Give Acetaminophen always 30 minutes prior to sponging to prevent shivering which may ultimately raise the temperature. By contrast, heat stroke requires immediate cold water sponging (antipyretics are not beneficial).

10. **Patient Education:** Provide education to parents regarding the signs or symptoms of a serious bacterial infection, the importance of following the recommended immunization schedule and seeking immediate medical attention if a child should present any signs or symptoms of a serious bacterial infection.**Complications** *Serious bacterial infection *Septic shock *Organ damage from hypoperfusion or untreated infections *Long-term adverse effects later in life *Death *A child's immunizations should be kept up to date. *The importance of fever, especially during the first 3 months of an infant's life, should be emphasized. *The importance of close follow-up should be communicated. *Caretakers might ask their health care providers for educational materials or resources, and providers should be prepared to respond. The prognosis depends on the patient's age, the severity of the disease, the duration of the disease, the time from when the patient seeks medical care to treatment, the patient's medical history, and other factors.

---

* *Pearl/Peril/Pitfall : Evaluating febrile neonates for herpes simplex infection should be considered when the following risk factors are present: age younger than 3 weeks, vesicles, seizure, toxic or ill-appearing, CSF pleocytosis or red blood cells, or maternal history of herpes. Laboratory studies to screen for herpes infection may include vesicle fluid for culture and direct fluorescent antibody, swabbing nasopharynx, conjunctiva, and rectum for culture, or CSF for polymerase chain reaction testing and culture.*

THE EVALUATION-DECISION-ACTION-PLAN/ALGORITHM
FOR THE DIAGNOSIS AND MANAGEMENT *OF A FEBRILE CHILD*

Figure 1
**Algorithm for the management of a previously healthy infant
<90 days of age with a fever without localizing signs.**

| < 28 days old, rectal temperature ≥ 38°C | | Nontoxic-appearing, 28–90 days old, and "low-risk" infant, rectal temperature ≥ 38°C |

Low-risk criteria for febrile infants

Clinical criteria
Previously healthy
  Nontoxic clinical appearance
  No focal bacterial infection on
    examination (except
    otitis media)

Laboratory criteria
WBC count 5–15 × 10³/mm³ (<1500 bands/mm³)
Normal urinalysis (< 5 WBCs/HPF)
  on Gram-stained smear
When diarrhea present : < 5 WBCs/HPF in stool
When respiratory symptoms present :
  normal chest radiograph

No →

Admit to hospital
 Blood culture
 Urine culture
 Lumbar puncture
 Parenteral antibiotics

Yes

Outpatient management

Option 1
Blood culture, Urine culture,
Lumbar puncture, Ceftriaxone 50 mg/kg IM (to 1 g),
Return for reevaluation within 24 hr

Option 2
Urine culture
Blood culture
Careful observation

Follow-up of low-risk infants

All cultures negative
Afebrile
Well appearing
Careful observation

Blood cultures negative
Well appearing
Febrile
Careful observation
May consider second dose
of ceftriaxone

Blood culture positive
Admit for sepsis evaluation
and parenteral antibiotic
therapy pending results

Urine culture positive
If persistent fever, admit for sepsis
evaluation and parenteral antibiotic
therapy pending results
Outpatient antibiotics if afebrile & well

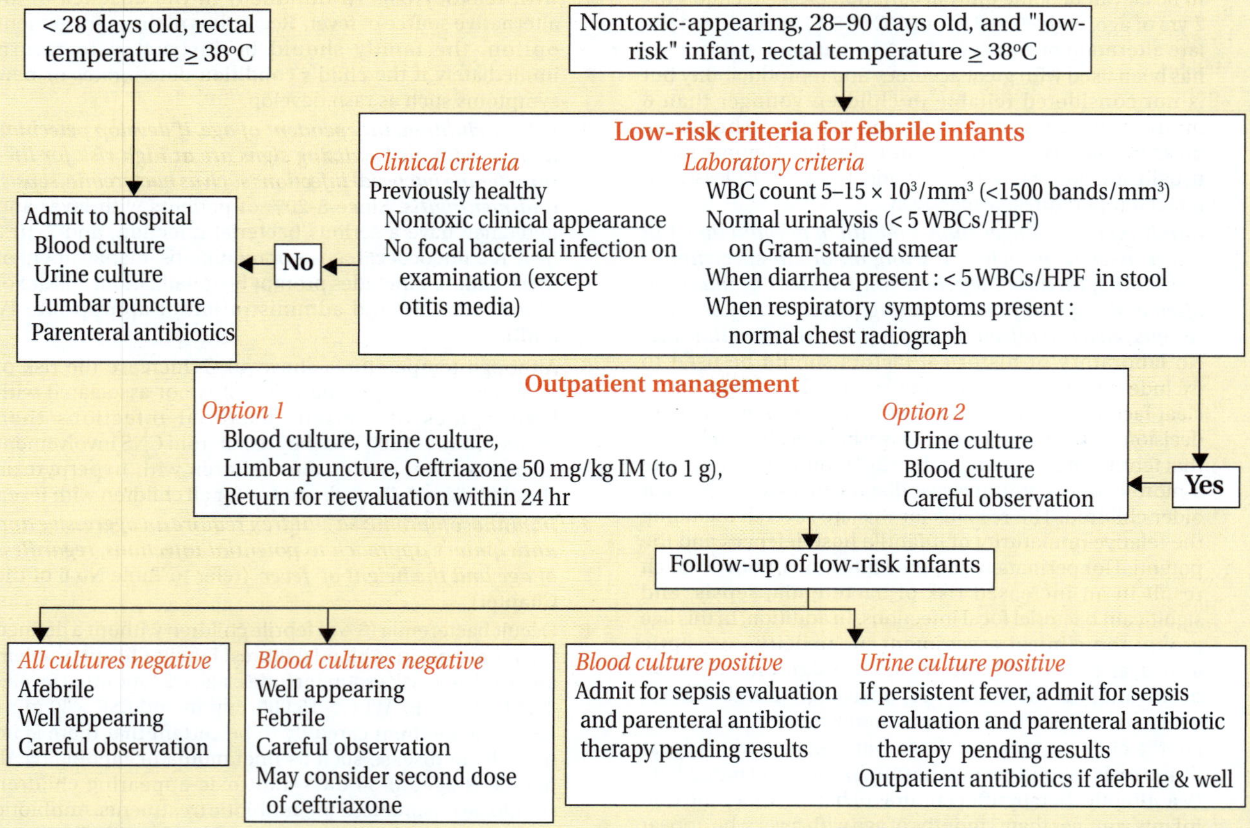

Figure 2
**Algorithm for the management of a previously healthy
child 91 days to 36 months of age with a fever without
localizing signs**

| 91-days-36 months, FWLS |

Child appears toxic

Yes / **No**

Admit to hospital , Sepsis workup, Parenteral antibiotics

Temperature ≥ 39.0°C

Yes / **No**

Urine culture : Males < 6 mo of age, Females <2 yr of age
Stool culture : Blood and mucus in stool or ≥ 5 WBCs/HPF in stool
Chest radiograph : Dyspnea, tachypnea, rales, or decreased breath sounds
Blood Culture : Option 1 : All children with temperature ≥ 39.0°C
Option 2 : Temperature ≥ 39.0°C and WBC count ≥ 15,000/mm³
Empiric antibiotic therapy after cultures obtained:
Option 1: All children with temperature ≥ 39.0°C
Option 2 : Temperature ≥ 39.0°C and WBC count ≥ 15,000/mm³
Consider antipyretic such as acetaminophen for symptomatic relief

No diagnostic tests or antibiotics
Consider antipyretic such as acetaminophen
 for symptomatic relief
Return if fever persists > 48hr or clinical
 condition deteriorates

Follow-up in 24-48 hr

Urine culture positive:
All organisms : Admit if febrile
or ill appearing. Outpatient
antibiotics if afebrile and well

Blood culture positive :Streptococcus pneumoniae
with persistent fever OR all other pathogens :
Admit for sepsis evaluation (including LP) and IV
antibiotics pending results

Blood culture negative:
Careful clinical observation
and follow-up : If clinical
deterioration, consider full
sepsis evaluation and IV
antibiotics pending results

Blood culture positive:
Streptococcus pneumoniae
when patient is afebrile
(without antipyretics) and
well appearing : Consider
repeat blood culture: May
consider lumbar puncture
if clinical suspicion present:
Complete 10 days of
antibiotics

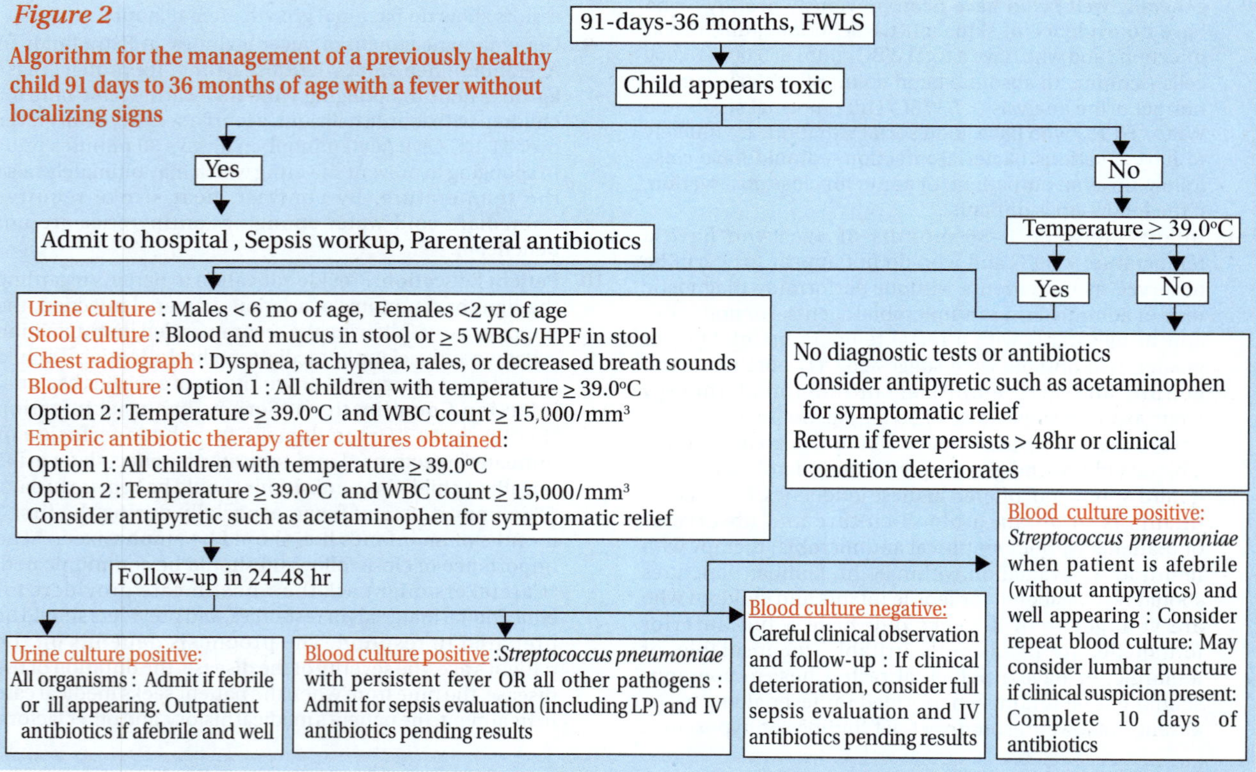

* *Pearl/Peril/Pitfall : Febrile Infants aged 5-8 weeks old:The threshold for performing an LP in these infants should be low, but an LP may be omitted in
well-appearing infants who have blood and urine studies obtained and when the following apply: *Reliable follow-up is possible in 12-24 hours.
*Clinicians are confident that parents or caretakers can comply with appropriate observation and follow-up. *No antibiotics have been started.*

TABLE 1 — Some diagnostic clues to evaluating the febrile infant/child

Prolonged fever
Bacterial infection, e.g. UTI, bacterial endocarditis
Other infections - viral, fungal, protozoal, tuberculosis
Kawasaki's disease
Drug reaction
Malignant disease
Connective tissue disorder (e.g. Still's disease)

Septicemia
Can be difficult to recognise in absence of rash before
  shock develops
Need to start antibiotics on clinical suspicion without
  waiting for culture results

Meningitis/encephalitis
Lethargy, loss of interest in surroundings,
  drowsiness/unconscious/seizures ?
Neck stiffness, arching of the back, bulging fontanelle,
  positive Kernig's sign (pain leg straightening) ?
Only non-specific symptoms and signs may be present
  in young children (< 18 months)

Upper respiratory tract infection
Very common, may be coincidental with another more
  serious illness

Otitis media
Always examine tympanic membranes in febrile
children

Diarrhea
Gastroenteritis ?
Fever with blood and mucus in the stool :
Shigella, salmonella, or *Campylobacter* ?

Tonsillitis
Erythema or exudate on the tonsils

Stridor
Epiglottitis ?
Viral croup ?
Bacterial tracheitis ?

Pneumonia
In infants, only raised respiratory rate and increased
respiratory effort may be present, with no abnormality on
auscultation - diagnosis may require chest X-ray

Urinary tract infection
Urine sample needed for any seriously ill young child or any
febrile illness that does not settle

Osteomyelitis or septic arthritis
Suspect if painful bone or joint or reluctance to move limb

Periorbital cellulitis
Redness and swelling of the eyelids.
May spread to orbit of the eye

Rash
Viral exanthem ?
Purpura from meningococcal infection

Abdominal pain
Appendicitis ?
Pyelonephritis ?
Hepatitis ?

Seizures
Febrile convulsions ? (> 6 Mo)
Meningitis ?
Encephalitis ?

TABLE 2 — Evaluation of the need for urgent investigation and treatment in the febrile child

Threshold for urgent investigation (septic screen) and intravenous antibiotics
Factors indicative of illness severity

LOW	HIGH
Young age (treat if < 2 months old)	Older child
Systemically ill	Not systemically ill
High or prolonged fever	Low grade fever
Features of potentially serious illness	No features of potentially
e.g. osteomyelitis, septic arthritis,	serious illness
septicemia, meningitis/encephalitis	Localised, minor illness,
No localising features	e.g. URTI, otitis media
Predisposition to infection e.g. immunodeficiency	Normal child

TABLE 3 — Life-theatening acute febrile illness

Infection
  Central nervous system
    Acute bacterial meningitis
    Encephalitis
    Cerebral Malaria
  Upper airway
    Acute epiglottitis
    Retropharyngeal abscess
    Laryngeal diphtheria (rare)
    Croup (severe)
  Pulmonary
    Pneumonia (severe)
    Tuberculosis, miliary

Cardiac
    Myocarditis
    Bacterial endocarditis
    Suppurative pericarditis
  Gastrointestinal
    Acute gastroenteritis (fluid/
      electrolyte losses)
    Appendicitis
    Peritonitis (other causes)
  Musculoskeletal
    Necrotizing myositis (gas
      gangrene)/fasciitis)

Systemic
    Meningococcemia
    Other bacterial sepsis
    Typhoid fever and its
      systemic complications
    Toxic shock syndrome
  Collagen-vascular
    Acute rheumatic fever
    Kawasaki disease
    Stevens-Johnson syndrome
  Miscellaneous
    Thyrotoxicosis
    Heat stroke
    Acute poisoning :atropine,
      aspirin, amphetamine, cocaine
    Malignancy

TABLE 4 — Septic screen

Full blood count including differential
white cell count

Blood culture

Acute-phase reactant, e.g. C-reactive
protein

Urine for microscopy, culture and
sensitivity

CSF (unless contraindicated) for
microscopy, culture and sensitivity

Chest X-ray

TABLE 5 — Clinical features of septicemia

History	Examination
Fever	Fever
Poor feeding	Purpuric rash
Miserable	(meningococcal
Lethargy	septicemia
History of focal infec-tion, e.g. meningitis, osteomyelitis, gastro-enteritis, cellulitis	Irritability
	Shock
	Multi-organ
	failure
Predisposing condi-tions, e.g. sickle cell disease, immunodefi-ciency	

Figure 3

Practical approach to the evaluation of the febrile child with or without a focus

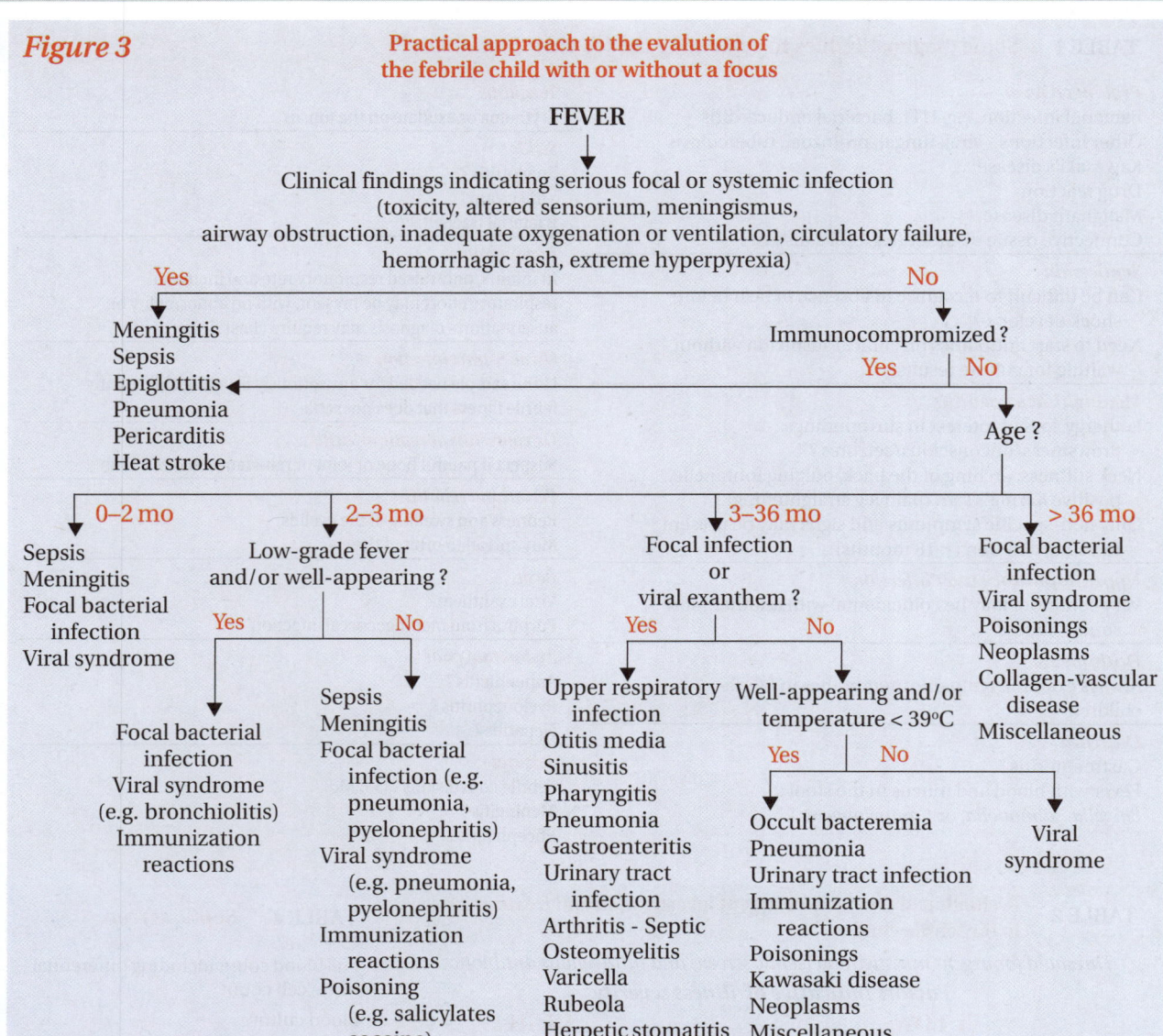

TABLE 6	Febrile patients at increased risk for serious bacterial infections

Risk Group	Diagnostic considerations
Immunocompetent Patients	
Neonates (<28 days)	Sepsis and meningitis caused by group B *streptococcus*, *Escherichia coli*, *Listeria monocytogenes*, and herpes simplex virus
Infants < 3 mo	Serious bacterial disease in 10–15%, including bacteremia in 5%, of febrile infants < 3 mo
Infants and children 3–36 mo	Occult bacteremia in 1.5%; increased risk with temperature > 39°C and white blood cell count >15,000/m L
Hyperpyrexia (> 40°C)	Meningitis, bacteremia, pneumonia, heatstroke, hemorrhagic shock-encephalopathy syndrome
Fever with petechiae	Bacteremia and meningitis caused by *Neisseria meningitidis*, *Haemophilus influenzae* type b, and *streptococcus pneumoniae*
Immunocompromised Patients	
Sickle cell disease	Sepsis, pneumonia, and meningitis caused by *S. pneumoniae*, osteomyelitis caused by *Salmonella* (as well as *staphylococcus*)
Asplenia	Bacteremia and meningitis caused by *N. meningitits*, *H.influenzae* type b, and *S. pneumoniae*
Complement/properdin deficiency	Sepsis caused by *N. meningitidis*
Agammaglobulinemia	Bacteremia, sinopulmonary infection
AIDS	*S. pneumoniae*, *H. influenzae* type b, and *Salmonella* infections
Congenital heart disease	Infective endocarditis ; brain abscess with right-to-left shunting
Central venous line	*Staphylococcus aureus*, coagulase-negative staphylococci, *Candida*
Malignancy	Bacteremia with gram-negative enteric bacteria, *S. aureus*, and coagulase-negative staphylococci ; fungemia with *Candida* and *Aspergillus*

Fever—Pathophysiology: Fever is a complex phenomenon, involving the highly coordinated interplay of autonomic, neuroendocrine, and behavioral responses to a variety of infectious and noninfectious inflammatory challenges. The febrile reaction is quite stereotyped and independent of precise causation. Various exogenous pyrogens (e.g. toxins, infectious agents, antigen–antibody complexes) produce fever in humans by inducing the production of proteins, collectively termed endogenous pyrogens, by phagocytic leukocytes. These enter the circulation and interact with specialized receptor neurons in the preoptic, anterior hypothalamus. Signaling there leads to the production of prostaglandins, particularly PGE2, which is believed to be the critical mediator of the febrile response, and impacts on hypothalamic neurons that reset the thermostatic set point and result in several responses.

The major effect is on the vasomotor center and results in peripheral vasoconstriction of cutaneous beds with redirection of blood flow to deeper tissues, thus minimizing skin heat loss. Additionally, sweating is decreased; vasopressin secretion falls, resulting in lowered extracellular fluid volume that requires heating; and behavioral modifications such as shivering and seeking a warmer environment are stimulated. These effects combine to elevate body temperature. Very rarely, fever is the result of central nervous system dysfunction (e.g. hypothalamic tumor, infarction) that alters the thermostatic set point directly, rather than via pyrogen induction. There is evidence that increased body temperature impairs replication of many microbes and may aid phagocytic bactericidal activity. The febrile response includes additional adaptive neuroendocrine effects. Glucose metabolism is lessened in favor of that based on lipolysis and proteolysis, thereby depriving bacteria of their preferred substrate. Fever induced anorexia also diminishes glucose availability to microbes. Hepatic synthesis of acute phase reactant proteins may result in binding divalent cations, which serve as growth factors for microorganisms. These effects combine to further enhance the host's response to microbial invasion.

KEY POINTS FOR CLINICAL PRACTICE:

1. Age is an important factor in bacteremia and sepsis for at least the following 4 reasons. First, the immune system is not fully developed in young children. Second, the important pathogens vary with age. Third, infants are not scheduled to receive the first PCV immunization until they reach at least 6 weeks old. Fourth, young infants do not have the ability to demonstrate signs of an illness.

2. Children can be septic without having hyperpyrexia; therefore, history taking, physical examination, and clinical judgment are still the most important factors in caring for sick children. History taking is an important part of clinical decision making.

3. Febrile neonates younger than 4 weeks old should have a full evaluation for sepsis. A full evaluation for sepsis consists of a complete blood cell count (CBC) with differential, blood culture, enhanced urinalysis (UA), urine culture, and a lumbar puncture (LP) to collect cerebrospinal fluid (CSF). CSF should be analyzed for cell counts, protein, glucose, and culture. Evaluating febrile neonates for herpes simplex infection should be considered when the following risk factors are present: age younger than 3 weeks, vesicles, seizure, toxic or ill-appearing, CSF pleocytosis or red blood cells, or maternal history of herpes. Laboratory studies to screen for herpes infection may include vesicle fluid for culture and direct fluorescent antibody, swabbing nasopharynx, conjunctiva, and rectum for culture, or CSF for polymerase chain reaction testing and culture.

4. Most febrile infants aged 5-8 weeks presenting to the ED warrant a full evaluation for SBI because they are difficult to judge clinically and because ED physicians can not ensure adequate follow-up. The threshold for performing an LP in these infants should be low, but an LP may be omitted in well-appearing infants who have blood and urine studies obtained and when the following apply: *Reliable follow-up is possible in 12–24 hours. *Clinicians are confident that parents or caretakers can comply with appropriate observation and follow-up. *No antibiotics have been started.

5. Provide education to parents regarding the signs or symptoms of a serious bacterial infection, the importance of following the recommended immunization schedule and seeking immediate medical attention if a child should present any signs or symptoms of a serious bacterial infection.

REFERENCES AND FURTHER READING: 1)Alpern ER, Henretig FM. Fever. In: Fleisher GR, Ludwg S, Henretig FM, eds. *Textbook of Pediatric Emergency Medicine.* 5th ed. Philadelphia, PA: Lippincott Williams & Wilkins; 2006:295-306. 2)Stanley R, Pagon Z, Bachur R. Hyperpyrexia among infants younger than 3 months. *Pediatr Emerg Care.* May 2005;21(5):291-4. 3) ACEP Clinical Policies Committee and Clinical Policies Subcommittee on Pediatric Fever. Clinical policy for children younger than three years presenting to the emergency department with fever. *Ann Emerg Med.* Oct 2003;42(4):530-45 4) Ishimine P. Fever without source in children 0 to 36 months of age. *Pediatr Clin North Am.* Apr 2006;53(2):167-94. 5) Avner JR, Baker MD. Management of fever in infants and children. *Emerg Med Clin North Am.* Feb 2002;20(1):49-67.

*** Pearl/Peril/Pitfall :** Infants/children older than 28 days old may be discharged home if they are well-appearing and meet all of the low-risk criteria, otherwise, admission is warranted. Low-risk criteria • Did not receive antibiotics within the past 48 hours • No dehydration, lethargy, irritability, or wheezing • No focal source of infection on physical examination (except otitis media) • Laboratory tests- CSF <8 WBC/hpf • WBC between 5 and 15,000 and band:poly <0.2 • UA <10 WBC/hpf • Chest radiograph without infiltrate (if obtained) • Caretaker is available by phone for follow-up and can bring the patient back to ED in 24 hours as needed.*

105

The Shaken Baby Syndrome

@ *Birth of a premature infant is associated with higher levels of parental anxiety, hostility, depression, and psychosocial adjustment. These levels are most likely related to the disruption of attachment secondary to medical complications and hospitalization. Differences in a preterm infant's behavior and a mismatch with parental expectations may further contribute to the infant's vulnerability. The most serious consequence of a caregiver's inability to cope with inconsolable crying is the development of frustration, anger, and intolerance, which can lead to physical abuse.*

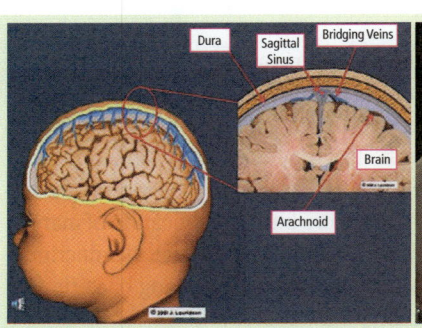
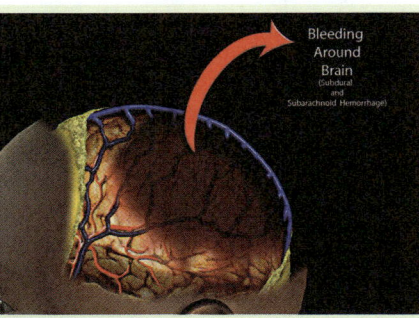
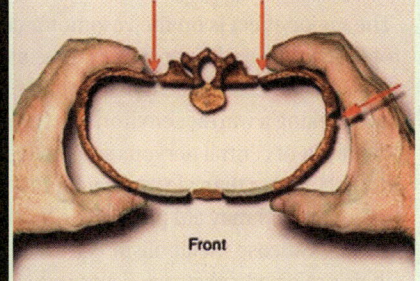

Note the location of the sagittal sinus and the bridging veins where subdural and subarachnoid hemorrhages occur in a shaking event.

Illustrates the narrow chest wall, and risk for rib fractures, when the chest is squeezed tightly during a shaking event.

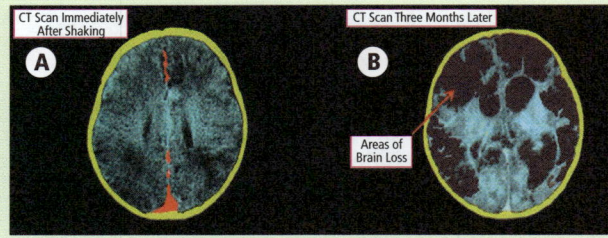
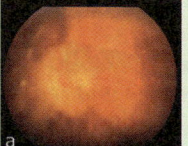
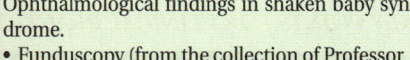
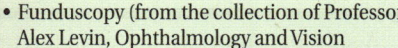
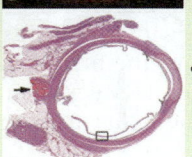
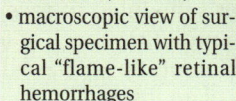
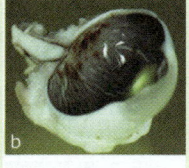
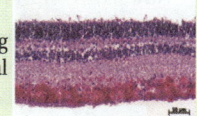

(A) This computerized tomography (CT) scan of the brain, obtained immediately following a shaking event, shows significant cerebral edema. Due to brain swelling, the gray and white matter of the brain are unable to be differentiated. The reddened areas signify fresh blood between the brain hemispheres. (B) shows the same brain, scanned 3 months after the shaking event. The dark area shows areas of brain loss. The child did not survive. *Courtesy:* Lauridson J, Levin A, Parrish R, Wicks A. 2002.

Ophthalmological findings in shaken baby syndrome.
• Funduscopy (from the collection of Professor Alex Levin, Ophthalmology and Vision Sciences, Hospital for Sick Children, University of Toronto, Canada) and
• macroscopic view of surgical specimen with typical "flame-like" retinal hemorrhages
• Histological ocular specimen showing bleeding in the optic nerve sheath (arrow) and retinal hemorrhages.
• Enlargement of the area marked in c)

REVIEW OF CLINICAL PROBLEMS

1. What special clinical features would suggest the occurrence of Shaken Baby Injury?
   Ans: Refer to the Table 2 of the Chapter.

2. Describe the role of Ophthalmoscopy in the evaluation of the Shaken Baby Syndrome.
   Ans: Refer to the Section "Retinal examination of the Shaken Baby Syndrome".

3. How do you stabilize a seriously injured Shaken Baby?
   Ans: Refer to No 8 of the Bird's eye view/Overview/Synopsis of the Chapter.

4. What Historical information & physical examination should you obtain while evaluating a Shaken Baby?
   Ans: Refer to the Evaluation-Decision-Action Plan/Algorithm to diagnose and manage the Shaken Baby Syndrome.

5. Discuss the preventive measures to be taken to reduce the incidence of the Shaken Baby Syndrome.
   Ans: Refer to the Section "Primary/Secondary/Tertiary preventive measures for the Shaken Baby Syndrome.

LEARNING OBJECTIVES

After completing this article, readers will be able to:

1. Consider the Shaken Baby Syndrome in the differential diagnosis of unexplained crying, irritability, poor feeding, neurological symptoms etc.,

2. Perform thorough evaluation of the Shaken infant, including detailed CNS, Retinal, Hematological, Skeletal survey, etc.

3. Stabilize acutely ill child & Arrange the follow-up of survivors for Neurodevelopmental, visual, hearing sequelae.

4. Ensure that parents/perpetrators are counseled to help with grief.

5. Prevent by warning the New Parents against the dangers of Shaking the babies.

* ***Pearl/Peril/Pitfall :*** *Obtain blood culture before administering antibiotics. Neonates aged 0–30 days should be treated with combination of IV ampicillin and a third-generation cephalosporin or gentamicin. For infants aged 31–60 days, a third-generation IV cephalosporin alone is recommended as first-line therapy. IV ampicillin is recommended in addition to a third-generation cephalosporin for severely ill infants aged 31-60 days or for infants in this age group with UTI. In addition to the antibiotics discussed above, vancomycin should be considered in settings where MRSA is prevalent or suspected.*

BIRD'S EYE VIEW/OVERVIEW/SYNOPSIS

1. Parent-infant stress syndrome or battered baby syndrome was first described in 1946, based on findings of retinal hemorrhage and intracranial hemorrhages associated with an episode of repetitive and violent shaking. *Shaken baby syndrome* is a medical term defined by pediatric radiologist John Caffey. It describes the violent shaking and resultant injuries sustained. The hallmark findings of SBS are lack of external injuries in the presence of intracranial and intraocular hemorrhages. If a history of accidental injury is provided, it is either inconsistent or inappropriate for the infant's developmental stage.

2. Shaken baby syndrome does not result from use of an infant swing, bouncing an infant or small child on the knee, or routine playing. It reflects the severe forces that accompany the perpetrator's rage, anger, and loss of control during the shaking episode. There is considerable debate as to whether shaking alone or shaking followed by forceful impact onto a surface leads to the constellation of findings. Based on this debate, the term *inflicted childhood neurotrauma* is a more accurate description of the injury, and the use of this term is supported by the National Institutes of Health. This term is not yet widely used

3. Cases of SBS have occurred as early as 8 days and as late as 4 years of age; most involve infants <6 months of age. The shaking can occur as an isolated event, as a pattern of repetitive shaking over several days to months, or in conjunction with other forms of abuse and neglect. The precise incidence of SBS is unknown. Prematurity, a prolonged stay in the newborn intensive care unit (NICU), and the presence of residual medical complications place preterm infants at a higher risk of abuse than their full-term counterparts. After hospital discharge, preterm infants may display atypical behavior; difficult temperaments, erratic sleep patterns, difficulty in consoling themselves, and feeding difficulties are common. Their parents, who have already been challenged by the unanticipated premature birth, must acquire the skills needed to care for their infant, often while managing their own residual disappointment, frustration, and anger. An increased awareness of the escalated risk factors for SBS and knowledge about preventative strategies that can be initiated in the hospital are essential for healthcare providers in the NICU.

4. Of infants who are shaken approximately one third will die, one third will suffer permanent brain injuries, and one third will survive with minimal long-term effects. Morbidity may include profound mental impairment or more subtle learning deficits and cognitive processing problems. Other reported problems include neuromotor impairment, such as paralysis, seizures, or cerebral palsy; visual impairments ranging from mild deficits to cortical blindness; and hearing impairments ranging from minor losses to complete deafness.

5. The presenting signs of infants with SBS are variable and depend on the degree of cerebral edema, increased ICP, and the extent of axonal injury present. The initial symptoms may be clouded by delays in seeking medical treatment. Parents do not voluntarily give a history of shaking. Presenting symptoms may be nonspecific, such as lethargy, irritability, poor feeding, or vomiting, and they are easily attributable to a viral etiology; however, there is typically no fever, diarrhea, or rhinorrhea. Bruising may or may not be present, and estimating the age of bruises is difficult and imprecise. Systemic disease, drugs that interfere with normal coagulation, dermatologic conditions, and cultural remedies, such as coining or cupping, may result in bruises that mimic those of inflicted trauma.

6. **Systematic Evaluation for Suspected SBS:** The clinical evaluation of the infant includes a complete history and physical examination, in addition to laboratory and diagnostic studies to rule out other conditions. A high index of suspicion, coupled with prompt and accurate investigation, is essential; the consequences of missing abuse as the diagnosis may result in further injury or even death at a later date. CT Scan Head is the initial diagnostic tool of choice for the evaluation of intracranial injury, primarily because of its availability, ability to quickly study unstable patients to determine the need for urgent neurosurgical intervention, comparatively lower cost, and strength in evaluating both soft tissue and bony structures. It can identify epidural, subdural, subarachnoid, and intracerebral hemorrhages. In the absence of a motor vehicle accident and related trauma, meningitis, or a bleeding diathesis, subdural fluid collections are suspicious for inflicted injuries. Complementary to CT imaging. MRI is generally obtained 1 to 2 days after the initial CT study. It is helpful in identifying more subtle injuries and detecting changes in the composition and age of intracranial blood. As hemoglobin ages, it oxidizes and breaks down, creating a predictable pattern on MRI. Old and new injuries can be accurately dated within days. During the first week after a bleed, the blood consists primarily of deoxyhemoglobin. Within 2 to 4 weeks the deoxyhemoglobin breaks down into methemoglobin. It is further degraded to the final byproduct, hemosiderin. **Skeletal Survey:** Obtain a skeletal survey of the hands, feet, long bones, skull, spine, and ribs to detect occult skeletal injuries. Suspicious findings suggesting other forms of abuse include skull fractures that are multiple, bilateral, or cross the suture lines; single or multiple fractures of the midshaft or metaphysis of long bones; or rib fractures in the absence of osteopenia. Repeat the skeletal survey 2 weeks after the initial study, because new fractures may not be apparent until they have begun to heal.

7. Retinal hemorrhages are best evaluated by a dilated fundoscopic examination, performed by a pediatric ophthalmologist. Retinal hemorrhages, in the absence of high-velocity witnessed trauma in children <4 years of age, are highly suggestive of SBS until proven otherwise. Retinal hemorrhages are found in 65% to 95% of shaken infants. Those associated with shaking are often too numerous to count, occur bilaterally in all layers of the eye, and can extend into the ora serrata. During a shaking episode, the rapid movement of the vitreous body disrupts the richly vascular layers of the retina. Subretinal, retinal, and preretinal hemorrhages develop from the stretching and shearing of the retinal layers and from the sudden increased intraocular pressure as a result of ICP.

8. The *Evaluation-Decision-Action Plan/Algorithm* outlines the essential diagnostic and management aspects of a Neonate/Infant with Shaken Baby syndrome. Management of the infant or child with subdural hemorrhages includes normalizing ICP, optimizing cerebral perfusion pressure and cerebral blood flow, preventing secondary injury, and avoiding complications associated with treatment. Interventions may include elevating the head of bed to 30°, intubation and optimization of gas exchange, sedation and pain control management, maintaining euvolemia, and administering osmotic agents. Hyperventilation is no longer recommended due to concerns of vasoconstriction contributing to poor cerebral blood flow and potential ischemia. Previously, mannitol (American Pharmaceutical Partners Inc, Schaumberg, Ill) was the gold standard for treating increased ICP. Recent studies advocate the use of small-volume hypertonic 3% saline to promote osmotic diuresis and decrease cerebral metabolic demands. Regardless of the osmotic agent used, maintain an euvolemic state with hyperosmolarity; perform strict intake and output measurements, serial serum electrolyte and osmolarity, and daily weights to monitor fluid balance. Serial hematocrit levels are used to identify progressive anemia. With increased ICP, subtle or acute changes in vital signs and level of consciousness can occur. Note any changes in vital signs or neurological checks. Monitor the infant or child for feeding intolerance, an early sign of increased ICP. Neurologic changes due to subdural bleeding may take as long as 24 to 48 hours to appear due to the venous origin of the bleed. If medical management is ineffective in decreasing ICP, surgical interventions, such as serial taps or insertion of drains, may be needed

9. After the acute stabilization, occupational and physical therapy is an essential element of the treatment regime. Inpatient evaluation and interventions set the stage for outpatient follow-up. Therapists can help the infant or child relearn lost skills and regain proper developmental sequences. In cases of permanent impairments, the therapist can assist in optimizing function and preventing further adverse sequelae.

10. The infant or child's emotional wellbeing is an important consideration in the hospital and at the time of discharge. Older children may need counseling as they cope with the abusive assault, especially if there are residual deficits. The nonperpetrating caregivers may need counseling to help with grief, which may be magnified if the infant or child suffers long-term permanent impairments. This grief can recur as different anticipated milestones are unmet.

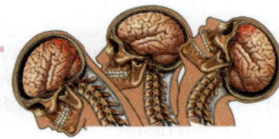
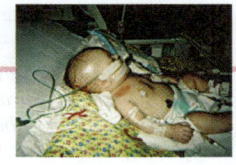

Shaken Baby Syndrome:
1/3 rd of all Shaken babies die in spite of the provision of maximal Intensive Care!

THE EVALUATION-DECISION-ACTION-PLAN/ALGORITHM FOR THE DIAGNOSIS AND MANAGEMENT OF *THE SHAKEN BABY SYNDROME*

SUBJECTIVE FINDINGS

Symptoms range from mild irritability, poor feeding, vomiting and lethargy to breathing difficulties, seizures, coma and death. SBS can be misdiagnosed with accidental trauma due to lack of information. More than 60% of the victims of Shaken Baby Syndrome are male. * Almost 80% of the perpetrators of Shaken Baby Syndrome are male. "SBS" victims range in age from a few days to a few months old; the average is six months. Infants who are premature and have congenital defects, developmental delays, or difficult temperament are at greater risk for child abuse, possibly due to poor parental bonding.

OBJECTIVE FINDINGS

Assess ABCDs - vitals, BP, CRT, O$_2$ sats, sensorium-alert/lethargic?, seizures & focal neurological signs (cranial nerve signs) + abnormal posturing, ability to suck & swallow, apnea/choking. *Look for* * Head turned to one side. * Unable to lift or turn head. * Pinpointed, dilated, or unequal size pupils. * Blood pooling in the eyes. * Pupils unresponsive to light. *Bulging or spongy forehead. * No smiling or vocalization, *Poor sucking or swallowing, *Rigidity, *Semi-consciousness, lethargy, or decreased muscle tone, * Difficulty breathing, * Seizures or spasms, *Swollen head, which may appear later.

INVESTIGATIONS

Blood - FBC, differential, platelets, *hematocrit,* reticulocyte count, Group & type & cross match, Smear, coagulation screen (PT, APTT, fibrinogen, thrombin time, bleeding time & clotting time), blood cultures, ABG analysis, *Blood sugar,* BUN, creatinine, electrolytes, Ca^{++} Mg^{++}, LTFs, drug screen

Urine analysis, Imaging- CXR, plain abdominal x-ray, USG scan/CT/MRI scan of head, Skeletal survey for fractures

Consult an Ophthalmologist to get detailed eye & Fundus examination done.

SUSPECTED SHAKEN BABY SYNDROME

Institute Supportive care, the mainstay of treatment in child abuse. • Blood pressure and vital signs should be supported and maintained. • Provide mechanical ventilation as needed. •Treat increased intracranial pressure, if present. • Organize surgical evacuation of subdural hematoma.

Identify Skin conditions which should be differentiated from the SBS-Bleeding diatheses, Mongolian blue spots, bullous impetigo, purpura etc.,

Identify Systemic Mimics of SBS, such as—Congenital Syphilis, Osteogenesis imperfecta, Metaphyseal chondrodysplasia, Sepsis-Meningitis,

Organize referral to the state or county protective (abuse) center to identify siblings who may be at risk of abuse.

Assess the Pattern of Injury

* Bruising/Soft tissue trauma-Do: Bleeding screen-Platelets, Bleeding times, PT, APTT *Identify Bruises, Bleeding disorder

* Skeletal trauma/Limitation of Movement-Do: Radiography, Skeletal Survey * Identify Fractures

* Abdominal Trauma- Do: Amylase, BUN,Creatinine, LFTs, Urinalysis and Consider CT/USG Scans *Identify Liver/Spleen/Kidney Hematoma/Laceration, Pancreatitis

* CNS Trauma/Neurological Signs-Do: CT/MRI

* Identify Cerebral edema, Skull Fracture(usually in the occipital or parietal bones), Subdural/Epidural Hematoma(subarachnoid hemorrhage, and even intraparenchymal hemorrhage can also occur)

* The key to diagnosis is the presence of retinal hemorrhages, which are seen in 80% of patients. *Retinal hemorrhage is considered the hallmark of shaken baby syndrome. *Retinal hemorrhages can be seen as early as 48 hours before any intracranial lesions can be detected on brain CT or MRI. •After vaginal delivery, retinal hemorrhages are occasionally seen without intracranial lesions.

Assess Cause of Injury

Accidental — Suspicious — Inflicted

Suspicious →
Consult:
Child Protection Team/
Senior Consultant Pediatrician

Accidental Injury — Suspicious for Intentional injury

Accidental → Assess for neglect

Not suspected — Suspected → Report to Local Child Protective Services

Inflicted → Report to Local Child Protective Services

Follow-up assessment in 2–4 wk

Ensure Follow-up: Further Inpatient Care *inpatient rehabilitation therapy may be indicated to manage the acute intracranial pathology, depending on the severity of injury *If long-term inpatient care is required, the patient should be transferred to a pediatric rehabilitation unit for maximal multidisciplinary care. Further Outpatient Care *The patient may require continued physical and occupational therapy after discharge. *Continued follow-up with a neurologist is recommended. *Closely watch the patient for spasticity, and control this with medication as needed. *Organize physical/occupational/speech therapy. *Arrange for a long-bone skeletal survey to check for new or healing fractures. Complications of Shaken Baby Syndrome-The main complications after shaken baby syndrome affect the neurologic and visual systems. *After retinal hemorrhages resolved, the following visual complications may occur: macular thinning, retinal pigment epithelial atrophy, and visual loss. *Wilkinson et al showed that the degree of retinal hemorrhage reflects the degree of neurologic injury. *Patients with bilateral retinal hemorrhages tend to have acute, severe neurologic injury. *Large subhyaloid hemorrhage, vitreous hemorrhage, or diffuse involvement of the fundus is likely to be associated with severe neurologic injury. *Neurologic complications include varying degrees of learning disabilities, spasticity and weakness, hydrocephalus, developmental delay, acquired microcephaly, seizures, hearing loss, and cortical blindness. *Antiepileptic medication may be indicated if evidence of seizures is noted. *Prognosis depends on the severity of the neurologic injury and the involvement of other organ systems.

* *Pearl/Peril/Pitfall :* Medical professionals strongly suspect shaking as the cause of injuries when a baby or small child presents with retinal hemorrhage, fractures, soft tissue injuries or subdural hematoma, that cannot be explained by accidental trauma or other medical conditions. About three quarters of cases involve retinal hemorrhaging. Additional effects of SBS are diffuse axonal injury, oxygen deprivation and swelling of the brain, which can raise intracranial pressure and damage delicate brain tissue.

Typical SBS-associated subdural hemorrhages are crescent-shaped, conforming to the calvarium and underlying cortex; they are most prominent in the posterior interhemispheric fissure and minimal over the convexities of the hemisphere. Hemorrhages occur due to the severe acceleration-deceleration and rotational injury to the infant's head during violent shaking; the cortical veins that drain the cortex and superficial venous sinuses are torn, causing subdural bleeding. Cerebral injury causes increased cerebral blood volume, leading to increased blood under pressure and symptoms of increased ICP (increased fullness of the fontanel, irritability, and vomiting). Subdural bleeds are not constrained by a tight dura allowing for clot expansion. They usually present more insidiously than epidural bleeds because of their venous origin. Treatment requires intensive medical and possibly surgical treatment. Multiple areas of hemorrhage at different stages of evolution are suggestive of repeated shaking events. An MRI is superior to CT scan when differentiating extra-axial collections, a common late sequelae of SBS. It is also helpful in evaluating white-matter-shearing injuries indicative of poor long-term neurodevelopmental outcome. The disadvantages of MRI include its high cost, lack of universal availability, safety and complexity for infants on life support, and the need for sedation in an already compromised infant. The infant's eyes must be dilated in order for peripheral bleeds to be detectable.

Retinal hemorrhages are often present in newborns due to birth trauma; these hemorrhages usually reabsorb within the first month. After the first month of life, they can occur with infections (viral, rickettsial, bacterial sepsis, subacute bacterial endocarditis), severe coagulopathies, severe accidental and nonaccidental trauma, and, on rare occasions, after prolonged cardiopulmonary resuscitation.

Prevention of SBS Healthcare providers in the NICU can play an important role in preventing SBS. Parents of preterm infants grieve the loss of their "normal" baby as they witness progress and setbacks during hospitalization and face uncertain futures.

Primary prevention Infants who require intensive care are often separated from their parents. Policies and practices that eliminate or reduce this separation are essential. Examples include encouraging parents to hold or touch their infant before transfer, promoting unrestricted visiting hours, and encouraging parents to have an active voice in developing the plan of care. The parents' presence at the bedside is an important opportunity for them to learn about their infant's individual behavior patterns; nurses should provide positive reinforcement as parents learn to care for their infant. Teach parents about normal and preterm development to help them develop realistic expectations of their infant. Encourage parents to verbalize their feelings of inadequacy and helplessness. Provide anticipatory guidance about normal emotions and frustrations and tell parents that it is common for these feelings to escalate after discharge. The universal theme in shaking events is that the infant or child was crying and the caregiver just wanted him or her to be quiet. Teach parents that it is normal for infants to cry for regular periods each day, and this behavior does not reflect negatively on their parenting abilities. Discuss concrete strategies for coping with an infant who is irritable and hard to console. Help the parents devise an emergency plan for situations when they can no longer tolerate the crying, so that they can take appropriate action before anger and frustration get out of control. A complete social history provides important background and context. Determine who lives in the household and identify their roles, relationships, stressors, and support systems. Every infant caregiver, including maternal boyfriends, grandparents, and other babysitters, need to know that shaking an infant can cause severe, permanent injuries or even death. Healthcare providers can disseminate this information to individual families and to the community through babysitter programs, Teach-In America programs at public schools, and other community programs. Identify community resources to support families after discharge. Anticipate ongoing financial challenges. Hospitalization costs, travels, meals, childcare expenses, and loss of income may cause undue and ongoing financial stress, particularly if a parent must stop working to take care of a special-needs infant.

Secondary and Tertiary Prevention

Secondary prevention is aimed at early identification of and intervention with families at risk of abuse. Risk factors might be noted during the infant's hospitalization or during follow-up appointments, when the parents may display unrealistic expectations of the infant and a lack of insight into normal preterm behaviors and development.

Tertiary prevention is aimed at preventing further abuse once it has occurred. Abusive parents need to be made aware of the help available to them, aid in problem solving, and assistance recognizing situations where abuse may be more likely to occur, so they can seek help in time to avoid the abuse.

Five controversies have been identified in the field of nonaccidental trauma to children. They pertain to the 5 major assumptions reflected in the sworn testimony of state medical experts.

- The first assumption is that shaking alone of a healthy child causes retinal hemorrhages and subdural hematomas. Biomechanical research and human case data suggest that shaking alone cannot cause these symptoms, but experts can state that short falls cannot.

- The second assumption is that falls over a short distance do not kill infants or children. However, findings from medical research and case studies do suggest that infants and children can and do die from such falls.

- The third controversy states that chronic subdural hematomas do not spontaneously rebleed. The literature about adult patients suggests that rebleeding can also occur in children with a subdural hematoma, with or without abuse.

- The fourth controversy is that a lucid interval is not a feature of pediatric head injury. However, the medical literature suggests the occurrence of a lucid interval in head injuries affecting children, as well as adults.

- The fifth controversy is that retinal hemorrhage occurs only in shaken baby syndrome. However, this hemorrhage is found in different situations, such as injuries related to childbirth, coagulation disorders, and CPR.

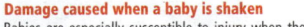

Damage caused when a baby is shaken
Babies are especially susceptible to injury when they are shaken because their connecting tissues and bones structure have not sufficiently developed to offer any protection

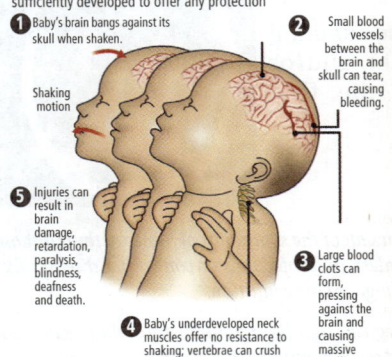

1. Baby's brain bangs against its skull when shaken.

Shaking motion

2. Small blood vessels between the brain and skull can tear, causing bleeding.

5. Injuries can result in brain damage, retardation, paralysis, blindness, deafness and death.

3. Large blood clots can form, pressing against the brain and causing massive swelling.

4. Baby's underdeveloped neck muscles offer no resistance to shaking; vertebrae can crush the spinal cord.

Common clinical symptoms associated with SBS *Poor feeding *Failure to thrive *Vomiting *Respiratory problems *Apnea *Weakness *Decreased tone *Lethargy *Altered level of consciousness *Irritability *Posturing *Seizures *Fixed and dilated pupils *Hypothermia *Bradycardia *Full or bulging fontanelles.

In 1998, Jayawant identified 9 characteristics of supposed and proven nonaccidental injury in children with subdural hematoma. These characteristics suggest a set of criteria that may be used to increase the precision of diagnosis.

- Boys account for two thirds of the children studied.
- Four fifths of the perpetrators are men.
- In about one eighth of all cases, the child and/or his or her siblings were previously abused by the same perpetrator.
- More than half of the caregivers change their stories several times.
- About half of all perpetrators eventually admit to shaking the child.
- About half of all patients have a hemoglobin level of less than 10 g/L at presentation.
- The skeletal survey is positive in 60% of cases involving nonaccidental injury.
- About 60% of patients have evidence of present or past trauma.
- Retinal hemorrhages are present in 80% of patients.

Selected differential diagnoses of SBS

Constellation-Remarks

* Accidental craniocerebral trauma: Serious accidents rare in infancy, often with SDH and fractures, very seldom with RH

* Perinatal: SDH found in 8%, RH in 34% of newborns; generally resorbed by four weeks with no ill effects

* Aneurysm/AVM: Rare as cause of bleeding in infancy; exclusion by imaging

* Arachnoid cyst/external hydrocephalus in BESS: SDH possible following trivial trauma, exceptionally associated with RH; diagnosis by imaging, possibly only after observation for some time.

* Meningoencephalitis: Postinfectious hygroma possible, exceptionally associated with RH; diagnosis by imaging, CSF, laboratory tests.

* Coagulopathies: SDH and RH possible; diagnosis by laboratory tests

* Terson syndrome: Very rare in infancy, in contrast to adulthood .

* Glutaraciduria type I: Exceptionally associated with SDH and RH; disease course generally features characteristic crises; usually already known (part of neonatal screening)

* Galactosemia: Intraocular bleeding described in exceptional cases; generally characteristic clinical picture featuring hepatosplenomegaly, jaundice, sepsis, cataract; usually already known.

* Osteogenesis imperfecta type I/type IV: Atypical fractures possible; generally characteristic clinical picture with positive family history, blue sclera, wormian bones; molecular genetic diagnosis in exceptional cases.

* Menkes syndrome: SDH described in isolated cases;characteristic clinical picture featuring microcephaly and typical trichopathy (kinky hair disease); diagnosis by laboratory tests

* Increased intrathoracic/ intravasal pressure: RH very exceptionally after resuscitation, fits; not after vomiting or coughing. SBS, shaken baby syndrome; SDH, subdural hemorrhage; RH, retinal hemorrhage; AVM, arteriovenous malformation; BESS, benign enlargement of the subarachnoid space

Subdural hematomas are localized between the periosteum and the arachnoid. Subdural hematomas are usually produced by trauma but the possibility of a clotting disorder should be considered. Subdural hematomas may be asymptomatic. Small subdural hematomas of the falx cerebri and the tentorium cerebri are frequently present after vaginal delivery in asymptomatic neonates. Most neonates with small subdural hematomas have normal neurological development. Large subdural hematomas may produce paroxysmal clinical events, decreased limb movements (monoparesis, hemiparesis, paraparesis, upper extremity diplegia, and quadriparesis), facial weakness, or coma. The study of choice to diagnose subdural hematoma in the cranial vault is CT of the brain. The study of choice to diagnose subdural hematoma in the spinal canal is MRI of the spine. The blood in subdural hematomas crosses the bone sutures (concave inner surface is convex) but does not enter into the fissures and sulci . The collection of blood is concave because it is not restricted by the individual periosteum of each bone. The treatment of subdural hematomas is dictated by the clinical manifestations. Drainage of the blood collection is necessary if symptoms are progressive or there are signs of impending herniation. Treatment of anemia and hyperbilirubinemia may be necessary.

Extra-axial hemorrhages and hematomas Extra-axial hematomas may be localized to the epidural, subdural, and arachnoid/subarachnoid spaces * The distinction between epidural and subdural hematomas is not always anatomically possible because both compartments may be simultaneously involved. Extra-axial hematomas are often related to trauma.

Epidural hematomas Epidural hematomas are located between the bone and the internal periosteum. They may occur in the anterior, medial, and posterior fossi, and in the spinal canal. Epidural hematomas are usually produced by trauma but the possibility of a clotting disorder should be considered. Epidural hematomas tend to produce paroxysmal clinical events, decreased limb movements (monoparesis, hemiparesis, paraparesis, upper extremity diplegia, and quadriparesis), facial weakness, or coma. The study of choice to diagnose epidural hematoma in the cranial vault is CT of the brain. The study of choice to diagnose epidural hematoma in the spinal canal is MRI of the spine. The blood in epidural hematomas does not cross the bone sutures, the inner surface the hematoma is convex, and the blood does not enter in the fissures. The convexity of the inner surface occurs because the blood pools in the center area of each bone since the periosteum is limited to each bone and is tightly attached to the bone edges. The treatment of epidural hematomas is dictated by their clinical manifestations. Drainage of the blood collection is necessary if symptoms are progressive or there are signs of impending herniation.

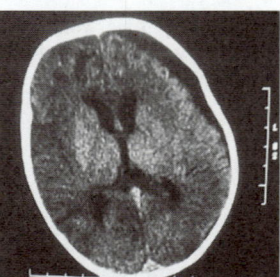

The key to diagnosing shaken baby syndrome is neuroimaging.

* CT scanning of the brain is sufficient to diagnose subdural hemorrhage (Lt side), cerebral edema (Rt side), and/or subarachnoid hemorrhage. CT is usually the first neuroimaging study obtained in the ED.

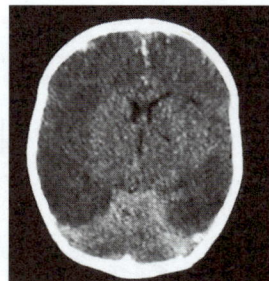

* *Pearl/Peril/Pitfall : Shaken Baby Syndrome : Shaken Baby Syndrome: No alternative condition mimics all of the symptoms of SBS exactly, but those that must be ruled out include hydrocephalus, sudden infant death syndrome (SIDS), seizure disorders, and infectious or congenital diseases like meningitis and metabolic disorders.[15] CT scanning and magnetic resonance imaging are used to diagnose the condition.*

* *Pearl/Peril/Pitfall : Shaken Baby Syndrome : SBS may be misdiagnosed and underdiagnosed, and caregivers may lie or be unaware of the mechanism of injury. Commonly, there are no externally visible signs of the condition, and there is no established set of symptoms that indicate it. Examination by an experienced ophthalmologist is often critical in diagnosing shaken baby syndrome, as particular forms of ocular bleeding are quite characteristic.*

Retinal hemorrhages are a cardinal manifestation of Shaken Baby Syndrome (SBS): Examination by ophthalmologists familiar with ocular findings in SBS, is an essential part of evaluating suspected child victims and in situations of unexplained life-threatening events or sudden death. Examination should be carried out with pupil dilation, either using eye drops, or through the naturally dilated pupils of the severely ill child. Ophthalmologists use the indirect ophthalmoscope to view the entire retina. Examination by non-ophthalmologists using only a direct ophthalmoscope is insufficient. After death, eyeball removal along with all orbital contents, is important to help to establish cause. Post mortem protocols have been published. In considering causation of retinal hemorrhage, it is important to detail types of retinal hemorrhage (preretinal, intraretinal, subretinal), number of hemorrhages, distribution of hemorrhages (confined to back [posterior pole] of the retina or spreading to edges [ora] of retina) and pattern of hemorrhages. Two-thirds of SBS victims have too numerous to count, multi-layered retinal hemorrhages extending to the ora. 15% have no retinal hemorrhages. Absence of retinal hemorrhage does not rule out child abuse. Traumatic retinoschisis is a particularly diagnostic lesion caused by traction applied to the retina by the vitreous jelly (which fills the eye and is attached firmly to the retina) as the child is submitted to repetitive acceleration-deceleration forces. The retina splits, creating a blood filled cystic cavity, not reported in otherwise well children except SBS victims and perhaps severe head crush injury which would otherwise be obvious by history. Multiple other causes of retinal hemorrhage are usually easy to diagnose by history, other medical findings, and laboratory/radiologic evaluations.

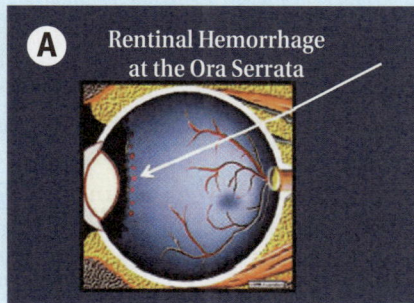
A Rentinal Hemorrhage at the Ora Serrata

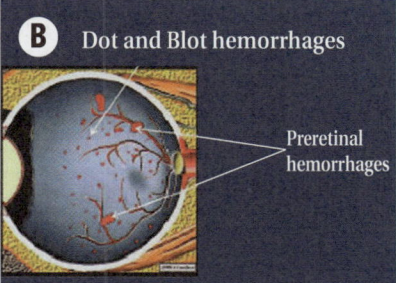
B Dot and Blot hemorrhages
Preretinal hemorrhages

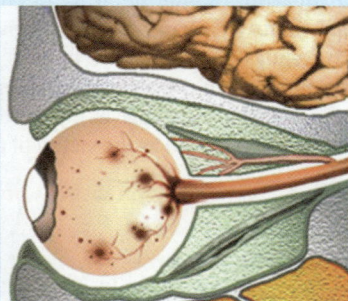

Courtesy: Alex V. Levin, M.D. MHSc, FAAP, FAAO, FRCSC

(A) Retinal hemorrhages in the Ora Serrata are generally caused by infant shaking and not by accidental trauma or other disease processes. (B) Circular hemorrhages in the deep layers of the retina are called dot and blot hemorrhages. Dot hemorrhages are smaller than blot hemorrhages. Reprinted with permission from Lauridson J, Levin A, Parrish R, Wicks A. 2002. Shaken Baby Syndrome: A Visual Overview. (Version 2.0) [Animated CD ROM], Ogden, Utah: The National Center on Shaken Baby Syndrome.

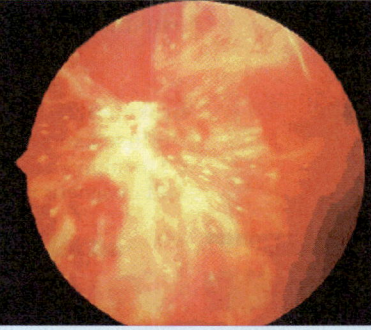
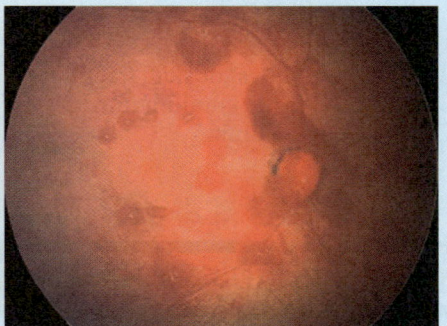

Retinal hemorrhages: These can be very extensive. They are most predominant at the posterior pole. They may be intraretinal, preretinal, subhyaloid or vitreal. They may obscure the retinal structures. Papilledema may or may not be present.

What can cause these Hemorrhages and Retinal changes in an infant?

1.Shaking Injuries 2.Birth Trauma 3.Subarachnoid or Subdural Hemorrhages 4.Blood Dyscrasias or bleeding disorders

Retinal hemorrhages are found in up to 80% of patients with suspected shake injury (Duhaime et al). There is some discussion whether shaking alone will cause these injuries or whether the injury is a combination of shaking and impact injury - Shaken and Slamming Injury. The picture of Retinal Hemorrhages with no history of very severe trauma should be treated as strong evidence of a SHAKEN BABY. The associated presence of retinal folds are seen only in cases of non-accidental trauma.

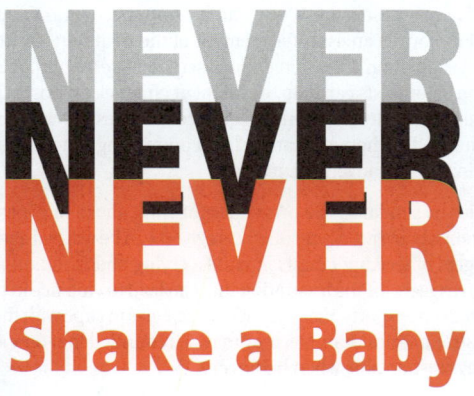
NEVER NEVER NEVER Shake a Baby

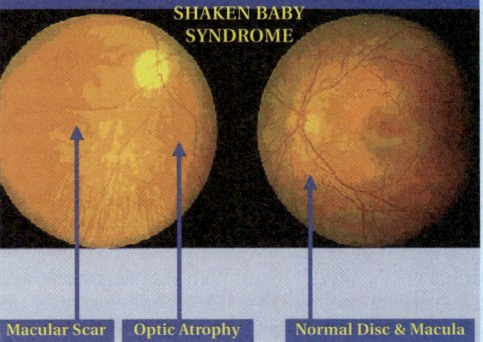
SHAKEN BABY SYNDROME
Macular Scar | Optic Atrophy | Normal Disc & Macula
Optic Atrophy & Macular DAMAGE FOLLOWING SHAKING.

Parental Advice: Hard shaking causes a baby's head to whip back and forth, slamming the brain repeatedly against the skull. When this happens, blood vessels to the brain are broken, causing the brain to swell and bleed. This can result in: * Brain damage * Spinal cord injury * Paralysis * Mental retardation * Blindness * Even DEATH. * Never shake a child for any reason. * Always provide support for a baby's head when holding, playing with or transporting him. * Learn what to do if a baby won't stop crying. Remember, all babies cry. * Make sure that everyone who cares for your baby knows the dangers of shaking a baby. * Always play gently with a baby. Never throw or toss a baby in the air.

Parent care: The nurse serves as a role model for the parents, demonstrating positive and constructive interactions with the infant or child. Discuss nonviolent methods of discipline and other ways to vent frustration so that anger toward the infant or child can be dissipated. This discussion is especially important when the infant or child is being returned to the home. Although the primary role of the healthcare providers is to serve as the infant's or child's advocates, they must also support parents and other family members, who may be experiencing overwhelming guilt, anger, and helplessness about the shaking event. Parents may need further explanation of tests that were performed, clarification of the meaning of the test results, and an opportunity to ask questions. Caregivers must examine their own feelings toward abusive parents so that they can form a relationship with the parents based on genuine concern, One approach is for the caregiver to view the abusive parent as the patient and the child as the victim of abuse. It is essential that healthcare providers document parent-infant interactions. Nurses and/or medical records may be subpoenaed to appear in court, making objective, accurate, factual documentation imperative.

Differential diagnosis: The differential diagnosis for irritability and bilateral subdural hemorrhages after a minor fall included:

*Bacterial or viral infection *Bleeding disorders *Cerebral aneurysm *Osteogenesis imperfecta *Metabolic disorders *Accidental injury *Nonaccidental head injury (SBS).

"It didn't take elaborate experiments to deduce that an infant would die from want of food. But it took centuries to figure out that infants can and do perish from want of love."
—Louise J. Kaplan, in "No Voice Is Ever Wholly Lost," 1995

TABLE 1	**Clinical features of head injury in young children**

Less specific features
Altered consciousness like drowsiness or coma
Vomiting
Convulsions or seizures

More characteristic features
Broken skull bone(s) or skull fracture(s)
Bleeding inside the cranium (intracranial bleeding)
Contusion of the brain

TABLE 2	**Specific features that suggest the occurrence of shaking**

The clinical feature	Documentation
Bleeding in the retina (retinal hemorrhage)	Ophthalmoscopy
Bleeding in the subdural space (subdural hematoma)	CT scan MRI Operation Autopsy
Broken nerve fibres (diffuse axonal injury)	Autopsy MRI

CT=computed tomography;
MRI=magnetic resonance imaging

KEY POINTS FOR CLINICAL PRACTICE

1. Shaken baby syndrome (SBS) or Battered Baby Syndrome is a form of child abuse that occurs when an abuser violently shakes an infant or small child, creating a whiplash-type motion that causes acceleration-deceleration injuries. SBS is often fatal and can cause severe brain damage, resulting in lifelong disability. Estimated death rates (mortality) among infants with SBS range from 15 to 38%; the median is 20–25%. Up to half of deaths related to child abuse are reportedly due to shaken baby syndrome. Nonfatal consequences of SBS include varying degrees of visual impairment (including blindness), motor impairment (e.g. cerebral palsy) and cognitive impairments.

2. Symptoms range from mild irritability, poor feeding, vomiting and lethargy to breathing difficulties, seizures, coma and death. In general, 1/3 die, 1/3 have major neurologic damage, and 1/3 survive in good condition. The severity of injury depends on the length of time the baby is shaken and severity of the shaking Injuries caused by shaking.

3. The clinical evaluation of the infant includes a complete history and physical examination, in addition to laboratory and diagnostic studies to rule out other conditions. A high index of suspicion, coupled with prompt and accurate investigation, is essential; the consequences of missing abuse as the diagnosis may result in further injury or even death at a later date. CT Scan Head is the initial diagnostic tool of choice for the evaluation of intracranial injury, primarily because of its availability, ability to quickly study unstable patients to determine the need for urgent neurosurgical intervention. Retinal hemorrhages are best evaluated by a dilated fundoscopic examination, performed by a pediatric ophthalmologist. Retinal hemorrhages, in the absence of high-velocity witnessed trauma in children <4 years of age, are highly suggestive of SBS until proven otherwise.

4. Acutely ill Shaken babies often demand Neurointensive care & supportive care. After the acute stabilization, occupational and physical therapy is an essential element of the treatment regime. Inpatient evaluation and interventions set the stage for outpatient follow-up. Therapists can help the infant or child relearn lost skills and regain proper developmental sequences. In cases of permanent impairments, the therapist can assist in optimizing function and preventing further adverse sequelae.

5. Prevention is similar to the prevention of child abuse in general. New parents, babysitters, and other caregivers can be warned about the dangers of shaking infants. A child's crying and irritation are common triggers for the frustration that can lead to violence in the caregiver. Some experts offer caregivers strategies to cope with their own frustrations; for example, they may be reminded that they are not always responsible when babies cry.

REFERENCES & FURTHER READING : 1)Carbaugh SF. Understanding shaken baby syndrome. Adv Neonatal Care . 2004; 4(2):105-114.2)Blumenthal I. Shaken baby syndrome. Postgrad Med J . 2002;78:732-735.3) Brain Injury Association of America http://www.biausa.org/ 4) American Academy of Pediatrics http://www.aap.org/5) Caring for Kids http://www.caringforkids.cps.ca/

* *Pearl/Peril/Pitfall : Shaken Baby Syndrome : Shaken Baby Syndrome: An estimated 1,200 to 1,400 cases of Shaken Baby Syndrome (SBS) occur each year in the United States. Only 1 out of 4 babies dies of Shaken Baby Syndrome. HOWEVER, the other three babies will need ongoing medical attention for the rest of their short lifespans. What about the Indian Statistics ?- Possibly Underdiagnosed/ Underestimated than the exact Incidence of SBS, which is unknown.*

The Septic—Appearing Infant

106

@ Treating the critically ill infant with empiric antibiotics after culturing the blood and urine is appropriate in most cases, as is identifying and treating hypoglycemia. An organized approach maximizes clear thinking and gives dying babies their best hope of making it out of the ED alive.

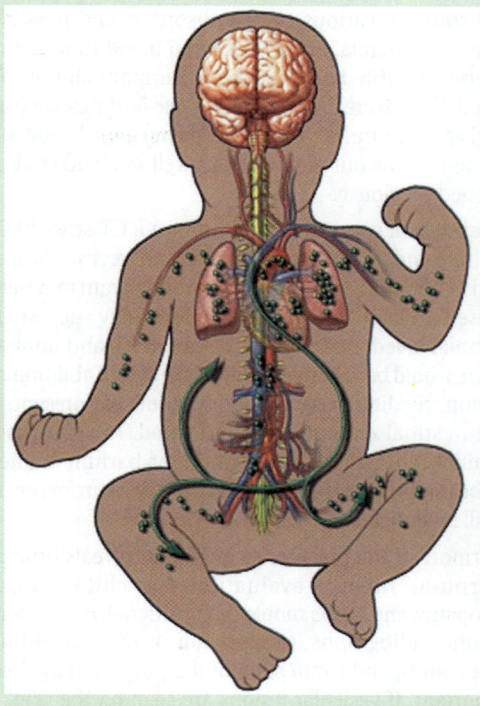

Sepsis, if complicated by Multiorgan Dysfunction Syndrome has to be differentiated from the Primary underlying organ/systemic diseases or *vice versa*.

Some Clinical Features of the Critically Ill/Septic—Appearing Infants.

- Depressed or altered mentation (i.e. "lethargy")
- Inappropriate cooperation (e.g. a full term Neonate who doesn't move for a blood draw; i.e. "apathy")
- Grunting respirations
- Head bobbing with breathing
- Increased work of breathing with or without retractions
- Progression from tachypnea to bradypnea (inappropriately slow respirations) to apnea
- Inability to feed or disinterest in feeding
- Sweating with feeds (suggestive of congestive heart failure)
- Decreased or floppy muscle tone, poor suck
- Skin changes including mottling, pallor, gray discoloration, cyanosis, petechiae
- Large, firm liver on exam (suggestive of congestive heart failure)
- Decreased peripheral pulses

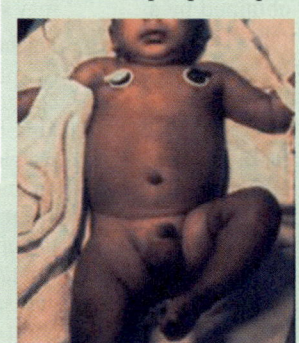

An infant with septic arthritis of the left hip. The child holds his hip rigidly in the classic position of flexion, abduction, and external rotation, a position that maximizes capsular volume. The patient is relatively comfortable as long as the hip joint remains immobile in this position.

REVIEW OF CLINICAL PROBLEMS

1. What are the common differential diagnoses in a Septic Appearing Neonate/Infant?
   Ans: Refer to the Table 1 of the Chapter.

2. How do you approach a Septic-Appearing Neonate/Infant with the characteristic physical findings?
   Ans: Refer to the Table 2 of the Chapter.

3. What relevant History & Physical examination should you obtain when a Septic-Appearing Neonate/Infant is being evaluated?
   Ans: Refer to the Evaluation-Decision-Action Plan/Algorithm to diagnose and manage a Septic-Appearing Neonate/Infant.

4. Mention the common causes of Metabolic acidosis other than Sepsis.
   Ans: Refer to the Evaluation-Decision-Action Plan/Algorithm to diagnose and manage a Septic-Appearing Neonate/Infant.

5. Discuss the Initial Resuscitation protocol to follow in a Septic-Appearing Neonate/Infant.
   Ans: Refer to the Evaluation-Decision-Action Plan/Algorithm to diagnose and manage a Septic-Appearing Neonate/Infant.

LEARNING OBJECTIVES

After completing this article, readers will be able to

1. Follow an organized approach to the critically ill or Septic-appearing infant to minimize chaos in the ED.

2. Presume that critically ill or Septic-appearing infant is septic and give empiric IV antibiotics, Unless another etiology is obvious.

3. Assess ABCDs & Stabilize them with top priority, before embarking to detailed history taking and investigations-Often the situation demands simultaneous intervention.

4. Go after multiple diagnoses while simultaneously treating life-threatening findings such as hypoglycemia and hypoxia.(The most effective strategy.)

5. Avoid the most costly mistake, i.e. to get a huge lawsuit for missing the big diagnosis, not preventing the preventable, or performing inadequate resuscitation.

---

* Pearl/Peril/Pitfall : 1. A critically ill or comatose infant is hypoglycemic until proven otherwise. 2. It is better to have a septic child undergo a barium enema than to miss intussusception. 3. Non-accidental trauma is always in the differential diagnosis. 4. The clock always ticks faster during these cases. If there is difficulty in getting IV access, immediately place an intraosseous needle. 5. A baby with green vomit has malrotation with midgut volvulus and needs emergent surgery until proven otherwise. 6. A critically ill or comatose infant has bacterial sepsis until proven otherwise, regardless of the temperature (high, low, or normal).

BIRD'S EYE VIEW/OVERVIEW/SYNOPSIS

1. The septic-appearing young infant/late Neonate (>7–14 days of life, discharged home without known risk factors), when brought to the ED, because he or she "just doesn't look right" to the parents the pediatrician immediately considers sepsis and manages reflexly with IV antibiotics. _Although this approach may be correct in most cases, one should remember that several other conditions may cause an infant to appear septic._ Table 1 of the Chapter classifies the various causes of septic - appearing infant. The most common disorders that mimic sepsis are 1) UTI 2) Viremia 3) CHF 4) Gastroenteritis with Dehydration. The remaining disorders, although uncommon, demand diagnostic consideration because they are potentially life threatening and yet treatable.

2. A complete history should be obtained. It is important to learn of any previous medical problems such as known heart disease or failure to thrive. The time of onset of symptoms, exposure to infection, medications given at home, and specific symptoms noted by the parents must be determined. Next, careful physical examination must be performed because specific findings may lead to a diagnosis other than sepsis.

3. After the physical examination, a complete laboratory evaluation should be performed. All sick infants should have a blood culture and urine culture obtained by a urethral catheter or suprapubic bladder tap. A lumbar puncture also should be performed unless the physical findings point strongly to a diagnosis other than sepsis or the infant is too ill to tolerate the procedure.

4. A chest radiograph is also essential to look for pulmonary infection and to evaluate the heart size. A FBC should be obtained; leukocytosis will add support to a suspicion of sepsis but also may be found in various other disorders, including viral infections, myocarditis, pericarditis, intracranial bleeds, NEC, appendicitis, intussusception, and methemoglobinemia.

5. Because metabolic problems (disturbances in acid-base balance, electrolytes, blood sugar) can result from sepsis or be the primary problem that mimics sepsis, all sick infants should have chemistries to evaluate serum sodium, potassium, chloride, glucose, and bicarbonate. If hyponatremia is found, water intoxication, aspiration toxicity, cystic fibrosis, and CAH should be considered. If there is also a marked hyperkalemia, CAH is most likely. If there is hypochloremic alkalosis or alkalosis alone, then pyloric stenosis, aspirin toxicity, or gastroenteritis should be considered. If there is hypoglycemia, it should be considered secondary to poor glucose reserves in an ill infant or related to drug (aspirin) toxicity, inborn errors of metabolism, CAH, or methemoglobinemia. If the serum bicarbonate is low, this should be confirmed with an arterial blood gas. If acidosis is present, poor perfusion caused by shock should be considered, as well as dehydration, drug toxicity, methemoglobinemia, appendicitis, CAH, and inborn errors of metabolism, as primary problems. Finally if laboratory tests are not revealing for a specific disorder or the patient does not improve quickly as an inpatient receiving antibiotics, stool and CSF isolates for viruses should be considered.

6. If the physical examination suggests a specific problem, it may be necessary to obtain additional laboratory tests. For instance, if the examination reveals pallor, cyanosis, or cardiac abnormality (muffled heart sounds, murmur, unexplained tachycardia, or arrhythmia) the physician should consider various cardiac disorders and possibly methemoglobinemia. An ECG, arterial blood to measure Pao_2, and possibly and an echocardiogram should be obtained. If there are unusual neurologic findings, such as a bulging fontanelle, a lumbar puncture should be performed to rule out meningitis as well as blood studies mentioned previously.

7. The presence of seizures should prompt a CT scan, EEG, and culture and treatment for herpes simplex virus, Also, if marked hypotonia is present, an electromyogram may help diagnose botulism. Retinal hemorrhages may suggest an intracranial bleed, and thus a CT scan, MRI, and lumbar puncture would be valuable studies. Likewise, if abdominal distention, rigidity, mass, or bloody stools are present, a gastrointestinal emergency is indicated. In such case, abdominal radiographs, ultrasound, or barium studies would be important diagnostic aids, but a workup for sepsis may still be indicated.

8. Furthermore, if the physical examination reveals bruises or purpura, further evaluation for child abuse, coagulopathy, and sepsis should be considered, In addition, long bone radiographs, coagulation profile (including platelet count), and Gram stain of the purpura may then be important. If vesicular lesions are seen on the skin, a Tzanck smear and culture for herpes should be obtained. If ambiguous genitalia are noted, blood should be drawn for 17-hydroxyprogesterone, renin, aldosterone, and cortisol to rule out CAH. Last, if wheezing is detected on chest examination, a nasopharyngeal swab should be sent for rapid slide detection of RSV or for culture of RSV.

9. The Evaluation-Decision-Action Plan/Algorithm describes the essential aspects of the History, Physical examination and relevant investigations when encountered with a septic and/or shocked Neonate/Young Infant.

10. Nightmare neonate • term infant, with usually normal Apgars, who suddenly deteriorates in the first 1–2 weeks of life after a well interval at home ——> presents to the ED in extremis !! COMMON CAUSES OF A CRASHING NEONATE S – Sepsis Viral (Herpes, Enterovirus) Bacterial (E.coli, Strep, Listeria), S—Seizures, I—Inborn Errors of Metabolism or other metabolic derangements, C—Congenital cardiac disease Ductus-dependent left-outflow obstruction lesions, Large left-to-right shunts Cardiomyopathies Dysrhythmias, e.g. SVT C—Congenital Adrenal Hyperplasia (CAH) C—CNS hemorrhages, AV malformation, Child abuse, Vitamin K deficiency (Hemorrhagic Disease of the Newborn) F - Formulas mix-ups, I—Intestinal disasters Volvulus Necrotizing enterocolitis, Incarcerated hernias, T—Toxins and other home remedies .

* _Pearl/Peril/Pitfall : The evaluation and appropriate management of the critically ill neonate requires knowledge of the physiologic changes and life-threatening pathologies that may present during this time period. A broad systematic approach to evaluating the neonate is necessary to provide a comprehensive yet specific differential diagnosis for a presenting complaint or symptom. Do not assume that every ill-looking Neonate/Infant is Septic, unless & until you can exclude other mimicking diagnoses._

THE EVALUATION-DECISION-ACTION-PLAN/ALGORITHM FOR THE DIAGNOSIS AND MANAGEMENT OF *THE SEPTIC-APPEARING INFANT (<2 MONTHS)*

SUBJECTIVE FINDINGS

Hx of presenting symptoms (lethargy, irritability, difficulty in feeding and breathing, diarrhea, bilious/blood vomiting, anorexia, skin rash or fever), and *determine onset, duration, progression, and severity,* Feeding details etc.,

Hx of previous medical problems such as known heart disease, failure to thrive, ongoing perinatal problems

Hx of unexplained neonatal deaths, CHD, in the family, exposure to infection, medications given at home

OBJECTIVE FINDINGS

Assess ABCDs and monitor CRT, O_2 sats, BP, core-peripheral temperature difference, RR, HR, central & peripheral pulses, urine output.

Note the other alarming signs such as - convulsions, irritability, pallor, central cyanosis, hypothermia, abdominal distention, bilious vomiting, petechiae and ecchymoses, vesicles, etc.. *Determine -* whether the baby is in preterminal ("pre arrest") conditions such as apnea, gasping or RR <20 bpm, shock, extremely lethargic or unresponsive limpy baby, bleeding etc.. and intervene with appropriate resuscitation of ABCDs promptly. *Note* abnormal body/urine odors *dysmorphic features (facies) Perform -* systemic examination quickly to identify the problems which require emergent life saving procedures

INVESTIGATIONS

Blood FBC, differential, platelets, *hematocrit,* reticulocyte count, Group & type & cross match, Smear, coagulation screen (PT, APTT, fibrinogen, thrombin time, bleeding time & clotting time), blood cultures, ABG analysis, *Blood sugar,* BUN, creatinine, electrolytes, Ca^{++} Mg^{++}, LTFs, drug screen *Urine analysis*

Imaging CXR, plain abdominal x-ray, USG scan/ CT scan of kidneys & bladder and head, *Perform-* Full sepsis screen with LP(*If the infant is stable ABCD wise)-*FBC, CRP, blood & urine cultures, CXR etc., *Consider -* ECG, 2D ECHO, MRI brain scan metabolic screen, Methemoglobin levels when clinical course demands. *Refer to Table No 2 for the relevant investigations*.

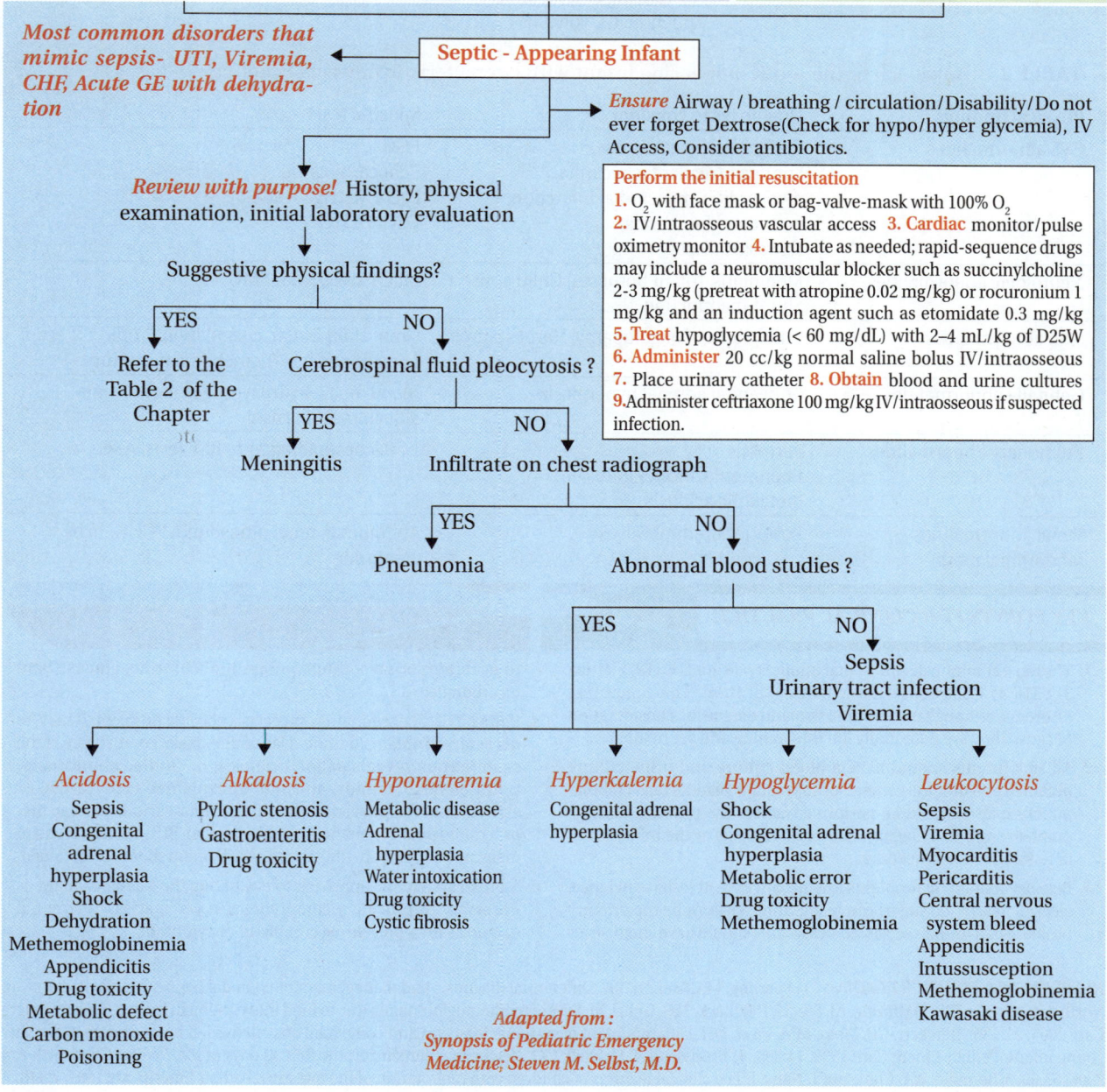

Most common disorders that mimic sepsis- UTI, Viremia, CHF, Acute GE with dehydration

Septic - Appearing Infant

Ensure Airway / breathing / circulation/Disability/Do not ever forget Dextrose(Check for hypo/hyper glycemia), IV Access, Consider antibiotics.

Review with purpose! History, physical examination, initial laboratory evaluation

Suggestive physical findings?

YES → Refer to the Table 2 of the Chapter

NO → Cerebrospinal fluid pleocytosis ?
- YES → Meningitis
- NO → Infiltrate on chest radiograph
  - YES → Pneumonia
  - NO → Abnormal blood studies ?
    - YES
    - NO → Sepsis / Urinary tract infection / Viremia

Perform the initial resuscitation
1. O_2 with face mask or bag-valve-mask with 100% O_2
2. IV/intraosseous vascular access 3. **Cardiac** monitor/pulse oximetry monitor 4. Intubate as needed; rapid-sequence drugs may include a neuromuscular blocker such as succinylcholine 2-3 mg/kg (pretreat with atropine 0.02 mg/kg) or rocuronium 1 mg/kg and an induction agent such as etomidate 0.3 mg/kg
5. **Treat** hypoglycemia (< 60 mg/dL) with 2–4 mL/kg of D25W
6. **Administer** 20 cc/kg normal saline bolus IV/intraosseous
7. Place urinary catheter 8. **Obtain** blood and urine cultures
9. Administer ceftriaxone 100 mg/kg IV/intraosseous if suspected infection.

Acidosis
Sepsis
Congenital adrenal hyperplasia
Shock
Dehydration
Methemoglobinemia
Appendicitis
Drug toxicity
Metabolic defect
Carbon monoxide
Poisoning

Alkalosis
Pyloric stenosis
Gastroenteritis
Drug toxicity

Hyponatremia
Metabolic disease
Adrenal hyperplasia
Water intoxication
Drug toxicity
Cystic fibrosis

Hyperkalemia
Congenital adrenal hyperplasia

Hypoglycemia
Shock
Congenital adrenal hyperplasia
Metabolic error
Drug toxicity
Methemoglobinemia

Leukocytosis
Sepsis
Viremia
Myocarditis
Pericarditis
Central nervous system bleed
Appendicitis
Intussusception
Methemoglobinemia
Kawasaki disease

Adapted from :
Synopsis of Pediatric Emergency Medicine; Steven M. Selbst, M.D.

* *Pearl/Peril/Pitfall :* "Sometimes I wonder whether today we take sufficient care to make a thorough physical examination before our patient starts off on the round of the laboratories, which have become so necessary that oftentimes we do not fully appreciate the value of our five senses in estimating the condition of the patient."—William Mayo,

TABLE 1	Differential diagnosis of the septic-appearing infant

Infectious diseases
- Bacterial sepsis
- Meningitis
- Urinary tract infection
- Viral infections–Enterovirus, respiratory
- Syncytial virus, herpes simplex
- Pertussis
- Congenital syphilis

Cardiac disease
- Congenital heart disease
- Supraventricular tachycardia
- Myocardial infarction
- pericarditis
- Myocarditis
- Kawasaki disease

Metabolic disorders
- Hyponatremia, hypernatremia
- Cystic fibrosis
- Inborn errors of metabolism
- Hypoglycemia
- Drugs/toxins–aspirins, carbon monoxide

Renal disorders
- Posterior urethral valves

Hematologic disorders
- Severe anemia
- Methemoglobinemia

Gastrointestinal disorders
- Gastroenteritis with dehydration
- Pyloric stenosis
- Intussusception
- Necrotizing enterocolitis
- Appendicitis, volvulus

Neurologic disease
- Infant botulism
- Shunt obstruction, infection
- Child abuse-intracranial hemorrhage

TABLE 2	Approach to the septic-appearing infant with characteristic physical findings

Physical findings	Diagnoses to consider	Specific tests
CVS abnormalities	Congenital heart disease, Supraventricular tachycardia, myocarditis, myocardial infarction, methemoglobinemia, Kawasaki disease	EGG Echocardiogram PaO_2, MetHgb level ECG, ECHO
Neurologic abnormalities	Meningitis, Infant botulism, Child abuse Shunt malfunction	LP, CT scan, MRI, EMG
Skin abnormalities	Child abuse, Coagulopathy, Herpes simplex	Gram stain lesion, coagulation profile, CT scan, Long bone films, Tzanck smear, culture
Genitalia abnormalities	Congenital adrenal hyperplasia	Blood for 17-hydroxyprogesterone, renin, aldosterone, cortisol
Pulmonary abnormalities	Pertussis Pneumonia, bronchiolitis, metabolic acidosis	PCR, chest radiograph, RSV tests, ABG
Renal abnormalities (abdominal mass)	Posterior urethral valves	Abdominal, renal ultrasound, VCUG, BUN, creatinine

KEY POINTS FOR CLINICAL PRACTICE

1. The most common disorders that mimic sepsis are 1) UTI 2) Viremia 3) CHF 4) Gastroenteritis with Dehydration. The remaining disorders, although uncommon, demand diagnostic consideration because they are potentially life threatening and yet treatable.

2. All sick infants should have a blood culture and urine culture obtained by a urethral catheter or suprapubic bladder tap. A lumbar puncture also should be performed unless the physical findings point strongly to a diagnosis other than sepsis or the infant is too ill to tolerate the procedure.

3. Because metabolic problems (disturbances in acid-base balance, electrolytes, blood sugar) can result from sepsis or be the primary problem that mimics sepsis, all sick infants should have chemistries to evaluate serum sodium, potassium, chloride, glucose, and bicarbonate.

4. If the physical examination suggests a specific problem, it may be necessary to obtain additional laboratory tests. For instance, if the examination reveals pallor, cyanosis, or cardiac abnormality (muffled heart sounds, murmur, unexplained tachycardia, or arrhythmia) the physician should consider various cardiac disorders and possibly methemoglobinemia. An ECG, arterial blood to measure Pao_2, and possibly an echocardiogram should be obtained.

5. A broad systematic approach to evaluating the Neonate/infant is necessary to provide a comprehensive yet specific differential diagnosis for a presenting complaint or symptom.

REFERENCES & FURTHER READING : 1) Sperling, MA, Menon, RK. Differential diagnosis and management of neonatal hypoglycemia. Pediatr Clin North Am 2004; 51:703. 2) Murone, AJ, Stucki, P, Roback, MG, Gehri, M. Severe methemoglobinemia due to food intoxication in infants. Pediatr Emerg Care 2005; 21:536. 3) Pickert, CB, Moss, MM, Fiser, DH. Differentiation of systemic infection and congenital obstructive left heart disease in the very young infant. Pediatr Emerg Care 1998; 14:263. 4) Brousseau, T, Sharieff, GQ. Newborn emergencies: the first 30 days of life. Pediatr Clin North Am 2006; 53:69. 5) Bonadio, WA, Clarkson, T, Naus, J. The clinical features of children with malrotation of the intestine. Pediatr Emerg Care 1991; 7:348.

* *Pearl/Peril/Pitfall : An infant with a history of sweating with feeds has congestive heart failure until proven otherwise. If after two or three fluid boluses the patient has no significant resolution of their tachycardia and/or has increasing respiratory distress, that child has myocarditis until proven otherwise.*

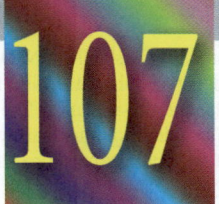

Surgical Neonate/Infant

@ *The collaboration between pediatrician and pediatric surgeon is very important in the case of a newborn particularly preterm and term low birth weight babies, where temperature regulation, fluid balance, assessment of metabolic disturbances, respiratory function, management of nutrition etc are vital for a successful outcome. Not only is a joint evaluation valuable for assessing the neonate prior to surgery, but also in the management of the neonate afterwards.*

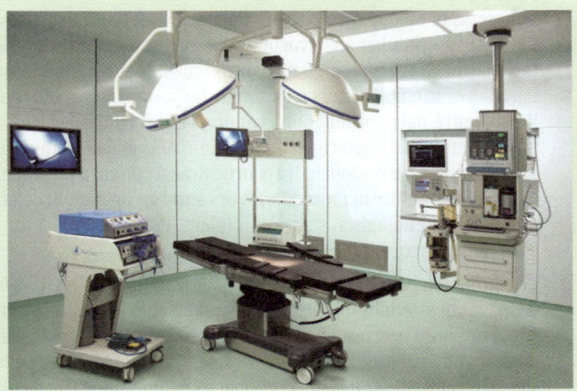

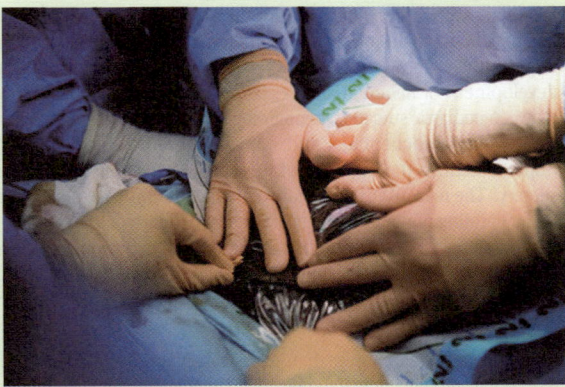

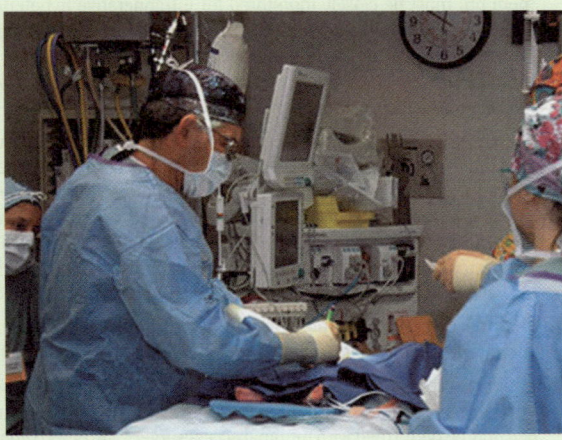

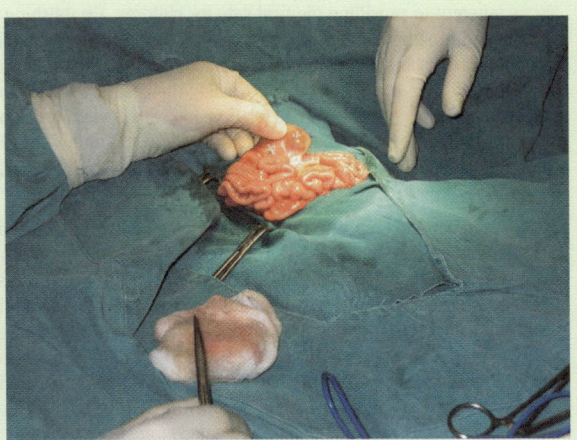

REVIEW OF CLINICAL PROBLEMS

1. How do you organize the transfer of the Surgical Neonate to a Tertiary center?
   Ans: Refer to the Table 2 of the Chapter.

2. Discuss the essentials of Pediatric surgeon's communication with the parents of the Surgical Neonate.
   Ans: Refer to the Table 4 of the Chapter.

3. How do you ensure good preoperative care of the Surgical Neonate?
   Ans: Refer to No 6 of the Bird's eye view/Overview/Synopsis of the Chapter and to the Table 5 of the Chapter.

4. What are the essentials of postoperative care of the Surgical Neonate ?
   Ans: Refer to the Table 6 of the Chapter.

5. Discuss the Neonatal Applications of Minimal Access Surgery.
   Ans: Refer to the Section "Minimal Access Surgery in a Neonate.

LEARNING OBJECTIVES

After completing this article, readers will be able to:

1. Understand the importance of Collaboration, Co-ordination and Communication between Pediatric surgeon, Neonatologist, Anesthetist, Radiologist, & the NICU Staff in delivering the best of Neonatal Surgical care.

2. Organize the Transfer of Surgical Neonate to a Tertiary Neonatal center.

3. Institute the Preoperative and Postoperative care of the Surgical Neonate.

4. Establish good and trusted communication with the anxious parents of the Surgical Neonate.

5. Know the Neonatal applications, advantages, disadvantages, and complications of Minimal Access Surgery (MAS).

* **Pearl/Peril/Pitfall:** *Not all congenital lesions need to be addressed to immediately. While some constitute dire emergencies others are dealt with after initial stabilization, still others have their specific unique optimal time zones for ideal management. Recognition of these will help both the referring neonatologist/pediatricians and the surgeon and ultimately translate into better overall management of the patient.*

BIRD'S EYE VIEW/OVERVIEW/SYNOPSIS

1. Paediatric surgery is the only surgical speciality which is defined by the patient's age rather than by a specific condition; a subspecialty of surgery involving the surgery of fetuses, Newborn, infants, children, adolescents, and young adults. **Neonatal surgery** refers to operations on children in the first month of life, almost always on an emergency or urgent basis. Many of these conditions are interesting and myriad, ranging from common in-born anomalies (cardio-vascular and gastro-intestinal) to fortunately rarer lethal conditions. The surgical treatment of neonates has enjoyed rapid development during the last 50 years. Neonatal surgery has now become an independent branch of general surgery, which requires the expertise of dedicated paediatric surgeons. Much of the development of neonatal surgery is due to the close collaboration between pediatric surgeons, neonatologists, anesthetists, pathologists, radiologists, biochemists, and nurses. There has been a steady improvement in the outcome of most neonatal diseases requiring surgery. The reasons for this improvement can be ascribed to a better understanding of the physiology of surgical neonates, to the advances in fluid management, nutrition, mechanical ventilation, and not least to refinements in surgical techniques. There is still considerable work to be done to improve the survival of neonates with severe conditions such as necrotizing enterocolitis (NEC).

2. Comprehensive care of the pediatric surgical patient is multifaceted and requires a thorough understanding of the surgical diseases encountered, the physiology of the pediatric population, and an awareness of unique issues inherent to providing medical care for children. Establishing a healthy and trusting relationship with child's parents or guardian, is essential. Parents and guardians are often anxious about the treatment of their child, and the responsibility to allay their fears lies with the pediatric surgeon. Fostering a good relationship with the family can be accomplished with skilled communication. Refer to Table 4 of the Chapter for the details of Parental Communication with the Pediatric Surgeon.

3. Advances in neonatal intensive care dictate that effective and efficient treatment of the sickest neonates can only be available by concentrating resources such as equipment and skilled staff in a few specialist paediatric centres that have responsibilities to a particular region. It is well established that the outcome of critically ill neonates is better if they are cared for in specialised tertiary centres. In addition, it has been shown that the prognosis for ill neonates is better if postnatal care is given in the same hospital in which they were born. However, not every critically ill neonate can and must be antenatally transferred. Neonates with congenital malformations will therefore have to be transported safely to the specialised centres, sometimes over considerable distances. Refer to Table 2 of the Chapter for the basics of Transfer of Surgical Neonate to a Tertiary center. The presence of a functioning nasogastric tube of adequate size reduces the risk of vomiting and aspiration during transportation.

4. The surgeon must obtain a complete and detailed history from the parents. The history, in concert with a well-performed physical examination, is the basis for a diagnosis and treatment plan. In an academic setting, the attending surgeon often sees the patient after a resident or medical student performs the initial evaluation. At this time, the surgeon must verify important points in the reported history and findings. This initial encounter with the surgeon also provides him or her with an opportunity to get to know the child and family.

5. Patients who have an isolated surgical problem and who are otherwise healthy do not require routine laboratory tests before surgery. In patients with other medical problems and those undergoing major operations, order a complete blood cell count, electrolyte tests, and coagulation studies. If clinically significant blood loss is anticipated, the patient's blood should be typed and screened or cross-matched so that blood can be immediately available if needed in the operating room.

6. **Establishing NPO status**: Anesthesia carries an inherent risk of the patient's vomiting and aspirating the stomach contents. NPO status should be discussed with the anesthesia team and assigned according to the guidelines and policies of the individual institution. General guidelines are as follows: · Solids or formula: Newborns and infants younger than 6 months should be assigned NPO status for 4 hours before surgery. Patients older than 6 months should be NPO for 6 hours before surgery. · Clear liquids: All patients should be NPO for 3 hours before surgery. Always consult the anesthesia team before complicated and unusual operations. These include procedures that involve repositioning the patient during the operation or manipulation of the great vessels or lungs. Notify the anesthesia team if the patient has a history of complications with previous anesthetics, malignant hyperthermia, or a coagulation disorder. Also, alert the anesthesia team if the patient has symptoms of an upper respiratory tract illness because this increases the risk of postintubation laryngotracheal edema. Preoperatively notify the anesthesia team about patients who might benefit from a caudal injection or an epidural catheter insertion for postoperative pain control. Preoperative pain consultation is appropriate if clinically significant postoperative pain is anticipated. The pain-management team can then proactively discuss postoperative pain treatment options with the family. In deciding whether to proceed with or cancel an operation, deferring to the anesthesiologists is always prudent. Refer to Table 5 for the essentials of Preoperative preparation of Neonates.

7. **Condition the patient's current medications:** Patients who have been taking corticosteroids long-term may not be able to mount a natural stress response because of chronic suppression of the hypothalamic-pituitary-adrenal axis. During the perioperative period, these patients should receive stress dosing of corticosteroids proportional to the stress of surgery. Patients who are taking antihypertensives should continue them but must be closely monitored for intraoperative hypotension. Other drugs that should be continued in the perioperative period include antiepileptics, drugs for asthma, and immunosuppressants. *Drugs that should be discontinued before surgery include anticoagulants, aspirin, nonsteroidal anti-inflammatory drugs (NSAIDs), and diuretics.*

8. **Obtaining consent from a parent or guardian,** for a procedure requires the clinician to discuss the indication for the procedure, describe the procedure, explain alternatives to the procedure, and declare the potential risks and complications. Bleeding and infection must always be mentioned, along with any other risks inherent to the surgery being performed. (Refer to the EDA Plan/Algorithm for the general principles of Diagnosis and Management of the Surgical Neonate.

9. Postoperative Management issues of the Surgical Neonate are summarized in the Table 6 of the Chapter.

10. Minimal access surgery-MAS has grown remarkably over the last twenty years and is continuing to expand. A lot of surgical operations in neonates can now be performed with minimal access surgery with good reported results. However few studies to date have been subjected to critical analysis and results must be interpreted with caution. With further advances and refinement in technology and technique, minimal access surgery should continue to expand and will be seen as a major changing trend in neonatal surgery. Historically, pediatric surgeons were slow to adapt to minimal access surgery (MAS) techniques compared with the adult surgical community. However, MAS now is widely established in infants and children. Differences in size and physiology have necessitated a number of surgical and technological modifications to apply MAS techniques to this population. The physiologic response to pneumoperitoneum in children is more pronounced than in adults. Peritoneal insufflation with carbon dioxide has been shown to cause hypercarbia, acidemia, and decreased oxygenation in the pediatric piglet model. In infants, however, there is no detrimental effect on blood pressure, heart ratwe, or oxygen saturation during short periods of pneumoperitoneum, and elevations in end-tidal CO_2 can be counteracted readily by increasing the minute ventilation. Hypercarbia-induced pneumoperitoneum in infants is associated with changes in cerebral blood flow and cardiac output. Nevertheless, laparoscopic procedures have been performed safely with proper anesthetic management in children who have even severe congenital cardiac abnormalities such as hypoplastic left heart syndrome. Hypothermia also can be a concern due to rapid insufflation of unwarmed CO_2 gas, mandating the moderation of flow rates. The benefits of MAS are evident with less adhesion, less postoperative pain, better cosmetic result and less length of hospital stay. It seems that the limit of MAS for neonates is not the technical feasibility but rather the right selection of those who would benefit.

THE EVALUATION-DECISION-ACTION-PLAN/ALGORITHM FOR THE DIAGNOSIS AND MANAGEMENT OF *SURGICAL NEONATE / INFANT*

SUBJECTIVE FINDINGS

Hx of presenting symptoms *Determine the onset, duration, frequency, severity, progression, recurrence with asymptomatic periods intervening,* such as persistent and frequent vomitings, bile-stained vomitus, abdominal distention, delayed or no passage of meconium, increased salivation with choking at the first feed, intermittent vomitings {think of malrotation with constant danger of volvulus, with strangulation and fatal infarction of the intestine}. Document pertinent negative findings. Aggravating or relieving factors. *Detailed antenatal/natal/postnatal Hx if relevant to various congenital malformations, which often present with surgical disposition.* Document the family history and the social history

OBJECTIVE FINDINGS

Assess ABCDs and monitor CRT, O_2 sats, BP, core-peripheral temperature difference, RR, HR, central & peripheral pulses, urine output. *General* Fussy, lethargic, irritable, inconsolable. Pallor, Jaundice, Dysmorphic features/Obvious malformations/syndromes *Skin* Turgor, Rash, Petechiae. *HEENT* Sunken eyes, and Fontanel. *CVS* Tachycardia, shock & Heart Murmurs ? *RS* Tachypnea, retractions. *GIT* Distended abdomen, tenderness or palpable mass. *GU* Groin bulge, anal stenosis, imperforate anus.

INVESTIGATIONS

Blood Hb, TC, DC, Hematocrit, Platelets, Cultures, Glucose, Electrolytes, ABG, Urea, Creatinine, Group & Type, Cross match, Bleeding time, Clotting Time, Chromosomal studies if indicated, LFTs.

Urine Analysis & Culture.

Imaging CXR, 3-view AXR {Supine, erect and prone cross table lateral view}, USG SCAN, Contrast Studies {Upper GI & Enema}, ECHOCARDIOGRAM, CT/MRI Brain, spine, abdomen, chest when clinically indicated.

Obtain Informed Consent from the parents-(the indication for the procedure, describe the procedure, explain alternatives to the procedure, and declare the potential risks and complications.)

Notify Pediatric Surgeon !

Monitor for & Correct as per protocol- Hypoxia, Hypoglycemia, Hypothermia, Dehydration, Acidosis, Sepsis &/or Peritonitis, Anemia, Bleeding, Jaundice, Oliguria-Anuria, Electrolyte disturbances, Seizures, Hypo/Hypertension & Hypocalcemia.

SUSPECTED SURGICAL NEONATE/INFANT

Shock

Ensure ABCs, Supplemental O_2, IV access, Monitor BP, CR monitor, Pulse oximetry, Institute Preoperative/Postoperative care.

Identify Obvious Congenital Anomalies, by their common clinical manifestations-Refer to Table 1

Identify CHD-Central cyanosis, Heart murmur, poor Peripheral pulses, RDS, Feeding problems, Hyperoxia test, CXR-cardiomegaly, ECG, ECHO confirmation-? Ductal-dependency—Start IVI Prostin & Organize transfer to Tertiary Cardiac center for further evaluation & management.

Fluid resuscitation
0.9 NS or RL 20mL/kg IVB follow with Maintenance IVF Correct metabolic acidosis

Insert **OG/NG tube** to assess patency/ allow decompression *reliably & Continuously!*

Difficulty in passing tube

NG Aspirate

Tube passes easily

Chest radiograph Tube coiled in chest TEF

NON BILIOUS

BILIOUS

Begin antibiotics

DISTENDED NONDISTENDED

Abdominal radiograph may show early obstruction

Projectile emesis with palpable olive-pyloric stenosis, obtain <u>US</u> to confirm

NONDISTENDED

Imaging
UGI abnormal
duodenal atresia, malrotation
jejunal atresia, ileal atresia (may be distended)
adhesion/band (may be distended)
UGI normal
non-surgical ileus
CNS-related sepsis
Abdominal radiograph
NEC (pneumatosis)

Non-projectile emesis GERD=Gastro Esophageal Reflux Disease

Contrast Enema
Intussusception, Hirschsprung's, meconium ileus, small left colon, meconium plug, colonic atresia, NEC stricture

DISTENDED

Imperforate anus, hernia

---

*Surgical evaluation and treatment of the Neonate with acute illness (Patients with intra-abdominal catastrophes) is one of the most challenging aspects of pediatric surgery. *The child's airway must be secured and maintained, breathing must provide adequate ventilation, and oxygenation, and circulation must adequately perfuse the end organs. *Children with signs of hypovolemic shock are most commonly those with ongoing hemorrhage, peritonitis, intestinal obstruction, Sepsis, vomiting, or diarrhea. *A patient in hypovolemic shock should be resuscitated with a 20-mL/kg bolus of warm lactated Ringer solution administered by means of peripheral or central venous line. If the child's condition responds inadequately and if further resuscitation is necessary, the choice of fluid (eg, crystalloid, colloid, blood) depends on the type of fluid that the child has lost. *In general, fluid lost because of peritonitis, and bowel obstruction may be replaced by lactated Ringer solution, which has an electrolyte composition similar to that of the fluid lost from the intravascular space. *Acid-base imbalances and electrolyte disturbances must be corrected before surgery. *Electrolytes and arterial blood gases must be monitored serially until corrected and stabilized. *Adequate volume resuscitation is crucial because anesthetic agents cause vasodilation. Therefore, patients with hypovolemia can have sudden hypotension with possible end-organ damage if they undergo anesthesia before receiving sufficient resuscitation. *The endpoint for volume resuscitation includes improvement in skin color and capillary refill and adequate urine output (1 mL/kg/h measured by using a urinary catheter).*

CONGENITAL ANOMALIES: A major cause of still births & neonatal deaths, but they are perhaps even more important as causes of acute illness & long-term morbidity. Early recognition of anomalies is important for planning care; with some, such as TE fistula, diaphragmatic hernia, choanal atresia, & intestinal obstruction, **immediate medical and surgical therapy** is essential for survival. Parents are likely to feel anxious & guilty on learning of the existence of congenital anomaly and require sensitive counseling.

TABLE 1	Common life-threatening congenital anomalies

Name	Manifestations
Choanal atresia	Respiratory distress in delivery room, apnea, unable to pass nasogastric tube through nares, Suspect CHARGE syndrome
Pierre Robin syndrome/sequence	Micrognathia, cleft palate, airway obstruction
Diaphragmatic hernia	Scaphoid abdomen, bowel sounds present in chest, respiratory distress
Tracheoesophageal fistula	Polyhydramnios, aspiration pneumonia, excessive salivation, unable to place nasogastric tube in stomach. Suspect VATER syndrome
Intestinal obstruction Volvulus, duodenal atresia, ileal atresia	Polyhydramnios, bile-stained emesis, abdominal distention. Suspect trisomy 21, Cystic fibrosis, cocaine
Gastroschisis, omphalocele	Polyhydramnios, intestinal obstruction
Renal agenesis, Potter syndrome	Oligohydramnios, anuria, pulmonary hypoplasia, pneumothorax
Neutral tube defects : anencephalus, meningomyelocele	Polyhydramnios, elevated α-fetoprotein, decreased fetal activity
Ductal-dependent congenital heart disease	Cyanosis, hypotension, murmur

CHARGE, coloboma of the eye, heart anomaly, choanal atresia, retardation, and genital and ear anomalies; VATER, vertebral defects, imperforate anus, tracheoesophageal fistula, and radial and renal dysplasia.

TABLE 2	Transfer of a Surgical Neonate

Referrals. Outside referrals are often transported by a team from the referring hospital. The surgical service should be consulted before patients with surgical problems are transported. The following set of instructions are to be followed .by the referral team:

1. The patient's specific problem(s) should be defined, if possible. The infant should be transferred in a transport incubator to prevent hypothermia. Under ideal circumstances facilities should be available for monitoring of the infant's temperature, heart rate, and inspired oxygen concentration. Mechanical ventilation is required for the critically ill infant and particularly for infants with diaphragmatic hernia and respiratory distress syndrome.

2. Nasogastric decompression is essential for all infants with intestinal obstruction but is also recommended for all surgical neonates to prevent vomiting and aspiration. A size 8 FG calibre tube is suitable for term infants but size 6 FG is more appropriate for preterm babies. The tube should be aspirated at frequent intervals to ensure that the stomach is evacuated of all its contents and should remain patent and on free drainage. A tube that is spigotted may promote reflux and is therefore more dangerous than no tube at all.

3. Copies of all relevant medical and nursing notes including details of the pregnancy and delivery should be sent to the regional centre.

4. Radiographs and results ot all relevant serological and bacteriological investigations should accompany the infant.

5. A valid consent for surgery should be immediately available. Ideally, the father should accompany the infant in order to discuss the planned procedure, but this may be impractical as he may be needed to care for the rest of the family at home.

6. A 10 ml specimen of clotted maternal blood will reduce the amount of infant's blood necessary for cross matching purposes. All neonates undergoing surgery require blood to be available for transfusion should the need arise.

7. Anticipated time of hospital arrival should be estimated. The chief surgical resident should be informed by the senior pediatric resident as soon as possible. The intensive care unit should be informed of the patient's expected problems and needs.

8. All other physicians who will be contributing to the patient's care (eg, neonatologist, radiologist, anesthesiologist) should be informed of the patient's problems and the anticipated arrival time.

9. If the patient is likely to require urgent operative intervention, the operating room staff should be informed.

10. Special instructions:

(a) *Esophageal atresia:* The blind upper oesophageal pouch should be kept empty, ideally by means of a double lumen Replogle tube maintained on continuous suction. This may be difficult to achieve during the ambulance journey and a wide calibre naso-esophageal tube, aspirated at regular intervals (5 to 10 minutes) will achieve the same effect. The infant should be kept in the prone position, which has been shown to reduce gastroesophageal reflux into the distal esophagus most effectively.

(b) *Diaphragmatic hernia:* A large calibre nasogastric tube should be passed immediately on diagnosis. This will restrict the amount of air entering the gastrointestinal tract, thereby minimizing compression on the pulmonary tissues. For infants with continuing respiratory distress and particularly for those less than 12 hours of age, endotracheal intubation and gentle mechanical ventilation are essential. Sudden deterioration of the infant's condition is frequently caused by a tension pneumothorax. Needle aspiration of the pleural cavity may be a life saving manoeuvre in these cases.

(c) *Gastroschisis and exomphalos:* The exposed intestine is a source of major heat and fluid loss. Both these losses may be restricted by wrapping the infant's torso in several layers of plastic wrap ('cling film'). An intravenous infusion of plasma (20 ml/kg/hour) and broad spectrum antibiotics (penicillin and gentamicin) should be given. Resuscitation of the shocked infant should be begun at the referring hospital and should continue ideally until the infant's condition has stabilized. There are, however, certain circumstances in which prolonged resuscitation may be counterproductive and where the delay in surgical treatment may jeopardize the infant's chances of survival (midgut volvulus, intestinal perforations, hemorrhage from a ruptured liver), and in these conditions close collaboration with the regional centre will determine the most propitious time for transfer. The mother should always be given the opportunity of seeing and handling her newly born infant before the transfer is effected. A digital photograph of the infant is of invaluable comfort to her during the difficult and uncertain period of the separation.

CRITICAL PERIODS IN HUMAN DEVELOPMENT*

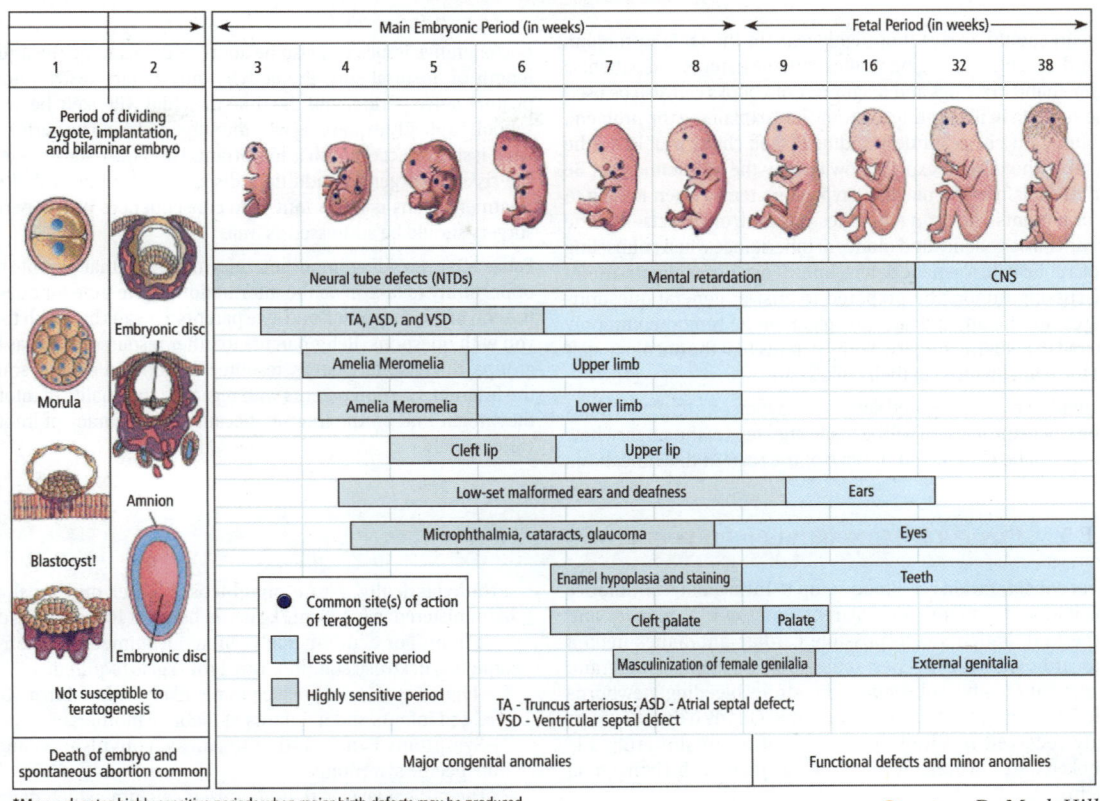

		Main Embryonic Period (in weeks)						Fetal Period (in weeks)			
1	2	3	4	5	6	7	8	9	16	32	38

Period of dividing Zygote, implantation, and bilarninar embryo

Morula — Embryonic disc — Amnion — Blastocyst! — Embryonic disc

Not susceptible to teratogenesis

- Neural tube defects (NTDs) / Mental retardation / CNS
- TA, ASD, and VSD
- Amelia Meromelia / Upper limb
- Amelia Meromelia / Lower limb
- Cleft lip / Upper lip
- Low-set malformed ears and deafness / Ears
- Microphthalmia, cataracts, glaucoma / Eyes
- Enamel hypoplasia and staining / Teeth
- Cleft palate / Palate
- Masculinization of female genitalia / External genitalia

● Common site(s) of action of teratogens
▢ Less sensitive period
▢ Highly sensitive period

TA - Truncus arteriosus; ASD - Atrial septal defect; VSD - Ventricular septal defect

Death of embryo and spontaneous abortion common | Major congenital anomalies | Functional defects and minor anomalies

*Mauve denotes highly sensitive periods when major birth defects may be produced.

Courtesy: Dr Mark Hill

TABLE 3 Optimal timing for pediatric surgical problems

Immediate surgery Trauma, intestinal obstruction, peritonitis, esophageal atresia with or without tracheo-esophageal fistula, congenital diaphragmatic hernia, foreign bodies, torsion testis, ruptured omphalocele and gastroschisis, low anorectal malformations and colostomy for high anorectal anomalies.

Surgery at diagnosis Hydrocephalus, spina bifida, craniosynostosis, cystic hygroma, branchial sinus and cyst, eventration of diaphragm, congenital lobar emphysema, duplication cyst, neoplasms, patent vitellointestinal duct, pyloric stenosis, extrahepatic biliary atresia, choledochal cyst, colostomy for Hirschsprung's disease, turn-in for exstrophy bladder, ureteropelvic junction obstruction, inguinal hernia, ectopic testis and undescended testis seen after 1 year or associated with hernia at any age.

Conditions requiring Staged Procedures Anorectal malformations, Hirschsprung's disease, exstrophy of bladder, large omphalocele.

Conditions requiring Observation Hydrocele, sternomastoid tumor, capillary hemangioma, preputial adhesions, umbilical hernia.

Inguinal Hernia Optimal time recommended for elective repair of indirect inguinal hernia in otherwise healthy children is within seven days of diagnosis to prevent complications. Avoid surgery for Congenital hydrocele till the age of two years. Inguinal hernia does not resolve on its own and merit surgical correction at the earliest after diagnosis. It is recommended that Undescended testis persisting beyond the age of one year should be surgically mobilized, brought down into scrotum and fixed there. It is done at an earlier age if associated with clinically diagnosed hernia. For perineal ectopic testis, it is advisable to perform orchidopexy at the time of diagnosis, as these do not reach the scrotum even if one waits. A retractile testis should be differentiated from undescended testis, it does not merit surgical correction and counselling is advisable. Hypospadias is being repaired as single stage procedure at 6-12 months of age. Many surgeons still prefer to wait till the age of 18-24 months of age for performing urethroplasty so that larger tissue is available. Most

Umbilical hernia need closure only if the umbilical ring size is larger than 1-2 centimeter at 4-5 years of age. It is important not to apply any pressure causing object like coin or dressing on the hernia during the period of observation as this causes skin maceration and complications. Repair of Cleft lip is guided by the 'Millard' rule of 10' *i.e.* cleft lip should be repaired when the child is 10 weeks of age, weighs at least 10 pounds and has a minimum hemoglobin of 10 g/dl. Surgery is also feasible at birth. This may achieve better heeling with less scar and avoids psychological trauma to the parents leading to parental detachment. The objective of the treatment of Cleft palate repair is to achieve normal speech, maxillo-facial growth, and hearing. To prevent deterioration in these functions of child, cleft palate repair is increasingly being done at a younger age (9–12 months) in contrast to earlier recommendations of 18 months. It is recommended to perform anterior palate repair at the time of lip repair when both are associated. Some surgeons prefer to close soft palate defects at 3-6 months. Residual hard palate is repaired at 15–18 months of age. Experience and personal preference of the surgeon and availability of necessary instruments is a prerequisite for performing early surgery. Tongue-tie- Pediatric surgeons and majority of pediatricians tend to believe that the condition is harmless, does not interfere with feeding and speech, and operative treatment is essentially carried out for cosmetic reasons and is not free of complications.Most pediatric surgeons tend to defer the division of frenulum till the age of two years or more and perform it only if deemed necessary at that age. Sternomastoid tumor- The condition usually resolves over a period of 6-12 months and does not require any surgical intervention. Indications of surgery include presentation after 1 year of age, development of strabismus or hemihypoplasia or no improvement by the age of one and a half years. Neural tube defects should be assessed and investigated adequately for associated anomalies and prognosis explicity explained to the parents. Intact lesions in the newborn should undergo surgery within 48 hours.

Courtesy: **Anup Mohta** *From the Department of Surgery, Guru Teg Bahadur Hospital and University College of Medical Sciences, Delhi 110 095, India.* Indian Pediatrics 2002; 39:648-653.

TABLE 4 — Parental communication with the pediatric surgeon

The surgeon should always thoroughly explain the child's problem. Reviewing the results of imaging studies with the parents and patient is helpful. Freehand drawings and diagrams from books can also be used to aid the surgeon in illustrating anatomy and explaining the problem. Parents often gain a better understanding of their child's problem if the surgeon takes the time to explain how or why the problem arose. Be prepared to explain embryology in layperson's terms when talking to parents of patients with congenital lesions and/or defects. Also be familiar with basic genetics and modes of inheritance when counseling parents of a child with a genetic defect. Knowledge in oncology is useful when discussing tumors; be prepared to answer general questions regarding chemotherapy and radiation regimens for tumors commonly encountered in pediatric surgery. Notify parents that the oncology staff is part of the team involved in their child's care.

The explanation of the proposed surgery in layperson's terms includes describing where the incision will be made, the steps of the surgery, how the incision will be closed, and the size of the scar. At this time, basic postoperative issues can also be addressed, including the anticipated length of hospital stay, the activity and dietary restrictions in the postoperative period, and the time the child will likely be away from school. Explicitly explaining why the surgery should be performed and what it should accomplish is important. This is also the time to discuss the risks of surgery. In addition, discussing options and alternative treatment plans is important. The consequences of not performing surgery should be addressed as well.

Pause after providing important information so that parents have the opportunity to take in all the information. Leave time for questions at the end of the encounter, and give parents a means by which to contact you with questions. Refer parents to other resources, such as support groups, the hospital's family resource center, and reliable sources on the Internet. Caution parents with regard to the quality of information they might find on the Internet because the accuracy of information varies widely.

TABLE 5 — Preoperative preparation for neonates

1. **General considerations** a. Blood setup b. Intravenous antibiotics (ampicillin and gentamicin) c. Parental consent for surgery and anesthesia d. Patients with possible cardiac anomalies need a electrocardiogram (ECG), chest radiograph, and echocardiogram. e. To prevent possible subsequent disastrous bleeding, newborns should be given 1 mg of vitamin K intramuscularly if they have not already received it. Vitamin K administration sometimes is overlooked during a difficult delivery of an infant with a congenital problem.
2. **Newborns with metabolic complications**
a. **Hypoglycemia.** Hypoglycemia is a particular risk in infants of diabetic mothers or infants who are small for their gestational age.
1) Symptoms can include jitteriness, seizures, apathy, hypotonia, apnea, and hypothermia, but these infants can be asymptomatic.
2) Glucose levels should be kept above 40 mg/100 mL.

Prophylactically, 4 to 8 mg glucose/kg per minute should be administered (e.g, 100 mL/kg per 24 hours of 10% aqueous dextrose solution). For acute hypoglycemia, an immediate push of 25% aqueous dextrose solution, 1 to 2 mL/kg, is required.
b. **Hypocalcemia.** Hypocalcemia is likely in low-birth-weight or stressed infants and in infants of diabetic mothers.
1) Symptoms can include jitteriness, convulsions, and other nonspecific symptoms.
2) The critical level is that of ionized calcium, which depends on serum total protein. Infants with acute symptomatic hypocalcemia should be started on 10% calcium chloride at 20 mg/kg per dose (0.2 mL/kg per dose) intravenously, slowly. Stop administration when clinical response is obtained. Monitor ECG continuously. Follow with calcium infusion up to 50 to 60 mg/kg per 24 hours.

TABLE 6 — Postoperative management of surgical neonate

Pain: Pain is a common issue in the evaluation of the postoperative patient, and one must attempt to differentiate the issues of anxiety and pain. Pain in patients who have undergone minor procedures (eg, hernia repair) is generally controllable with oral analgesics such as acetaminophen, ibuprofen, or oxycodone/acetaminophen. Pain control after major surgery (eg, laparotomy, thoracotomy) is more complex. Consider the use of intravenous patient-controlled analgesia (PCA) or parent- or nurse-controlled analgesia (PNCA). In select patients, epidural analgesia can be used and is sometimes preferred. The transition to oral pain medication should be made when the patient is tolerating a diet.

Postoperative nausea and vomiting: Postoperative nausea and vomiting (PONV) is a common problem encountered in the postoperative period. While the physiologic pathways and triggers surrounding PONV are complex, 4 drug classes can be used to manage this problem—anticholinergics, antihistamines, D_2 antagonists, and $5HT_3$ antagonists. Gastric distension can also cause nausea, and the index of suspicion should be high for this, especially if the patient was bagged without gastric decompression. Patients who have undergone abdominal surgery can also have a distended stomach due to gastrointestinal ileus. In many cases, gastric decompression can improve nausea if this is the cause.

Hydration status: Hemodynamic status and urine output are useful indicators of how well a child is resuscitated. A normotensive child who is not tachycardic is likely well-resuscitated; a child with tachycardia and/or hypotension may be hypovolemic. It is also important to try to account for the influence of anxiety and pain, which can raise the heart rate and blood pressure. Patients who third-space fluid may do so over a period of days and will require particularly careful monitoring of their fluid status during this time. Urine output is an objective measure of volume status. Urine output of 2 mL/kg/h is acceptable in neonates and infants, while 1 mL/kg/h is acceptable in older children. A hypovolemic patient should be resuscitated with 10 mL/kg boluses of isotonic fluid such as normal saline or lactated Ringer solution. Once the patient is intravascularly euvolemic, he or she should be placed on maintenance intravenous fluid. If repeated attempts at resuscitation fail, other reasons for hypotension should be considered, including ongoing bleeding and sepsis.

Laboratory studies: Most patients do not need laboratory studies in the postoperative period. A complete blood cell count, platelet count, and coagulation panel should be checked if ongoing blood loss is a concern. Electrolytes should be checked when there are significant fluid shifts or losses. Concern for infection should prompt an evaluation for leukocytosis, as well as culture studies.

MINIMAL ACCESS SURGERY (MAS) IN THE NEONATE

Minimal access surgery (MAS) is a milestone development in the history of surgery. Several small puncture wounds are used to perform surgical procedures that would otherwise require a large incision. The benefits of MAS have been well documented in adults. With advances in miniaturized instruments, video technology, new surgical techniques and anesthesia, MAS is increasingly performed in infants and neonates. Currently, it has been used in both neonatal chest and abdominal conditions. However, further clinical studies are required to document the benefit of MAS in neonates in the long term.

Advantages of minimal access surgery

· Laparoscopy often offers better visualization than open surgery, particularly better visualization of the hiatus and deep structures in the pelvis. · Minimal access surgery (MAS) offers dramatic advantages in terms of the quality of life after the operation. · Postoperative pain is reduced, which decreases postoperative narcotic use and its complications. This also aids in lower pulmonary complications. · Smaller wounds are associated with fewer wound complications, less scarring, and better cosmesis. · MAS results in reduction of postoperative adhesions. · Patients stay in the hospital for a shorter period and recover faster. · Patients are able to return to their normal activities faster (eg, feeding, school, work). · A child's quick recovery allows parents to return to work faster. · Video imaging allows surgical assistants, anesthesiologists, and nurses to view what the surgeon is doing and to actively participate in the procedure in their respective roles. · Laparoscopy can be performed in infants weighing less than 1.5 kg without significant mortality or morbidity.

Disadvantages of minimal access surgery

• Initial capital cost is associated with laparoscopy because new equipment and training are necessary.
• Operating time is longer and the complication rate is higher during the learning curve of the procedure.
• Loss of tactile sensation occurs, which is perhaps the major disadvantage of minimal access surgery (MAS). Intraoperative ultrasonography is helping to overcome this deficiency.
• With current technology, the video camera can provide only a 2-dimensional image, although 3-dimensional views are becoming available.
• Controlling bleeding laparoscopically is difficult.
• The number of instruments and angles in which they can be applied are limited. Robotic applications using wrist technology is improving this problem.

Complications of minimal access surgery

Technique-related complications

• Complications can be related to placement of the initial trocar or initial creation of pneumoperitoneum. Underlying vessels or viscera can be injured. These injuries can be minimized by the use of open technique for the first trocar placement.
• Complications can also arise from dissection during the procedure. These include direct injuries to hollow and solid organs, as well as thermal injury. These can also be minimized by careful and precise technique.

Carbon dioxide–related complications

• Carbon dioxide can be easily absorbed through the peritoneal surface, leading to hypercapnia. Elevation in carbon dioxide can lead to acidosis, which can have further metabolic and hemodynamic consequences.
• Insufflation of carbon dioxide can also cause cardiovascular compromise because of the previously mentioned venous tourniquet effect.
• Another serious, but fortunately rare, side complication is gas embolism; this is minimized by carbon dioxide use as opposed to use of other gases.
• Hypothermia can also ensue because of cold carbon dioxide insufflation, especially in small infants.
• These complications can be minimized by low pressure and warm humidified gas insufflation, slight hyperventilation, proper fluid resuscitation, and careful monitoring in the operating room.

Minimal Access Surgery and Neonatal Applications: A number of abdominal operations using laparoscopic approach have been performed in neonates. In some conditions, laparoscopy has virtually replaced open surgery as the operation of choice while in others it may be a good alternative.

1. *CHPS—Ramstedt's pyloromyotomy* has been regarded as the gold standard for the management of hypertrophic pyloric stenosis. Laparoscopic pyloromyotomy gives equally good result with excellent cosmetic effect and is becoming an increasingly popular alternative.

2. *Fundoplication with or without feeding gastrostomy* is a common procedure performed in neonates. Indications include gross oesophageal reflux, recurrent aspiration, and profound neurological impairment with failure to thrive. Laparoscopic approach has virtually replaced open surgery.

3. *Pull-through for Hirschsprung's Disease* The management of Hirschsprung's disease has gone through revolutionary changes from the traditional open two to three stage procedure to the open one stage procedure, and more recently to the laparoscopic-assisted or trans-anal one stage pull-through. All the traditional techniques of Swenson, Duhamel and Soave can be applied laparoscopically but the Soave (endorectal) technique is most commonly performed. The procedure involves laparoscopic localization with histological confirmation of the transitional zone, mobilization of the colon, trans-anal submucosal dissection, pull-through of the colon and anastomosis of the colon proximal to the transition zone to the anal region. Early result of the procedure has been satisfactory. Although further studies are necessary to determine the long-term outcome, it is likely that laparoscopic-assisted pull-through procedure is going to stay and will become increasingly popular.

4. *Pull-through for Imperforate Anus:* High type of imperforate anus has been traditionally managed with an initial defunctioning colostomy followed later by pull-through procedure using an abdominal perineal approach or posterior sagittal anorectoplasty. Laparoscopic-assisted pull-through for a high anomaly has been described. The fistula is first dissected and ligated using laparoscopic approach. The site of the sphincteric muscle complex is identified by muscle stimulation on the perineum. A tract is then made through the muscle complex into the pelvic cavity as guided by the laparoscope. This tract is then dilated and the large bowel is pulled through to the perineum and a neo-anus reconstructed. Short-term result has been promising though the long-term outcome of continence needs further study.

5. *The repair of intestinal atresia* is possible using laparoscopic approach. Laparoscopic repair for duodenal atresia has been reported. although cases with associated severe cardiac anomaly may limit its use. The proximal and distal segments are mobilized and then joined together using intracorporeal sutures. For more distal intestinal atresia, the dilated bowel loops may render laparoscopic approach more difficult and technically demanding.

6. *Malrotation and volvulus:* Malrotation with or without volvulus has been repaired using laparoscopic approach. The volvulus is untwisted and a Ladd's procedure performed. For cases with equivocal findings, laparoscopy can provide a diagnostic tool. In those cases with significant bowel ischaemia and dilatation, laparoscopic approach may be difficult and an open approach is preferable.

7. *Inguinal Hernia:* Laparoscopic herniotomy has been reported. Advantages include the detection of contralateral hernia allowing repair in the same setting, and the avoidance of potential injury to the vas deferens and cord vessels that might be associated with the conventional open repair while the hernia sac is being stripped off the vas and vessels.

8. *Intussusception* is a common cause of intestinal obstruction in infants but less so in neonates. Non-operative treatment using pneumatic or hydrostatic reduction usually suffices for 80–90% of cases. Laparoscopy may have a role in those cases with equivocal complete reduction or unsuccessful non-operative treatment.

9. *Laparoscopy has been used in operative cholangiogram* and liver biopsy in cases of prolonged jaundice. Sporadic cases of laparoscopic-assisted repair of biliary atresia and choledochal cysts have been reported. However the longterm results of these cases are not available and laparoscopic repair should only be used in selected cases.

10. *Ovarian and Pelvic Disorders* Laparoscopy has been used in the treatment of ovarian cysts in neonates and in the dissection of the pelvic portion of sacrococcygeal teratoma

11. *Necrotizing enterocolitis (NEC)* is the most common gastrointestinal emergency in neonates affecting mainly premature infants. Lack of specific indications for surgical intervention is occasionally encountered in critically ill babies with suspected NEC. Laparoscopy has been used in these cases either confirming the diagnosis or reviewing the extent of the disease, which can guide the subsequent management.

12. *Thoracoscopy* is not as commonly used as laparoscopy in neonates. It can be used for diagnostic purpose such as biopsy of lung lesions. Resections of thoracic lesions like cystadenomatoid malformations, sequestrations, mediastinal masses can be performed via thoracoscopy.

13. The *management of esophageal atresia* has gone through revolutionary changes. One of the recent advancement is the use of thoracoscopy to clip and divide the tracheoesophageal fistula and to join the proximal and distal oesophageal segments. Apart from the minimal wound pain and the excellent cosmetic effect, there is the avoidance of the potential musculoskeletal weakness that may result from the conventional open thoracotomy. However, thoracoscopy may not be applicable in babies who are premature or small for dates and with associated severe cardiac and pulmonary anomalies.

14. *Thoracoscopic or laparoscopic approach* has been used in the repair of **diaphragmatic hernia** in stable infants. Symptomatic eventration of the diaphragm can be plicated using a thoracoscopic technique.

15. *A patent ductus arteriosus* can be clipped using thoracoscopic means preserving the recurrent laryngeal nerve.

Courtesy: KKW LIU, MWY LEUNG, Current Trends in Minimal Access Surgery for Neonates, HK J Pediatrics 2007;12:125-129

KEY POINTS FOR CLINICAL PRACTICE:

1. Much of the development of Neonatal surgery is due to the close collaboration between pediatric surgeons, neonatologists, anesthetists, pathologists, radiologists, biochemists, and nurses. The reasons for this improvement can be ascribed to a better understanding of the physiology of surgical neonates, to the advances in fluid management, nutrition, mechanical ventilation, and not least to refinements in surgical techniques.

2. The surgeon must obtain a complete and detailed history from the parents. The history, in concert with a well-performed physical examination, is the basis for a diagnosis and treatment plan. *The goal of the physical examination is to identify the current surgical issues and to ensure that the organ systems other than the one being treated are healthy.*

3. Complete care of the pediatric surgical patient includes establishing a good rapport with the child's parents or guardian. The surgeon should always thoroughly explain the child's problem. Reviewing the results of imaging studies with the parents and patient is helpful. Freehand drawings and diagrams from books can also be used to aid the surgeon in illustrating anatomy and explaining the

problem. Parents often gain a better understanding of their child's problem if the surgeon takes the time to explain how or why the problem arose. Pause after providing important information so that parents have the opportunity to take in all the information. Leave time for questions at the end of the encounter, and give parents a means by which to contact you with questions.

4. Advances in Neonatal intensive care dictate that effective and efficient treatment of the sickest neonates can only be available by concentrating resources such as equipment and skilled staff in a few specialist pediatric centres that have responsibilities to a particular region. It is well established that the outcome of critically ill Neonates is better if they are cared for in specialised tertiary centres.

5. Minimal access surgery (MAS) has grown remarkably over the last twenty years and is continuing to expand. A lot of surgical operations in Neonates can now be performed with minimal access surgery with good reported results. With further advances and refinement in technology and technique, Minimal access surgery should continue to expand and will be seen as a major changing trend in Neonatal surgery.

REFERENCES & FURTHER READING : 1) **Thomas** DFM. Transfer of neonates for surgery. Hospital update 1982;8:955-63. 2) **Rice** HE, Caty MG, Glick PL. Fluid therapy for the pediatric surgical patient. *Pediatr Clin North Am*. Aug 1998;45(4):719-27. 3) Klein MD. Congenital Abdominal Wall Defects. In: Ashcraft KW, Holcomb III GW, Murphy JP. *Pediatric Surgery*. 4th ed. Philadelphia, PA: Elsevier Saunders; 2005:659-69. 4) Leape LL: *Patient Care in Pediatric Surgery.* Boston: Little, Brown, 1987. 5)Frequently Encountered Problems in Pediatric Surgery I: Neonatal Problems Hospital Physician,Richard K. Spence, MD, FACS Richard B. Wait, MD, FACS

Pearl/Peril/Pitfall : Special needs of preterm babies' fluid therapy are: conservative approach, consider body weight changes, sodium balance and ECF tonicity. They are susceptible to both sodium loss and sodium and volume overloading. High intravenous therapy can lead to patent PDA, bronchopulmonary dysplasia, enterocolitis and intraventricular hemorrhage. Impaired ability to excrete a sodium load can be amplified with surgical stress (progressive renal retention of sodium). Estimations of daily fluid requirements should take into consideration: (1) urinary water losses, (2) gastrointestinal losses, (3) insensible water losses, and (4) surgical losses (drains).

Common Neonatal Surgical Problems

108

CHPS-CONGENITAL HYPERTROPHIC PYLORIC STENOSIS

CHPS-Congenital Hypertrophic Pyloric Stenosis :
*Progressive narrowing of the pyloric canal by muscular hyperplasia and hypertrophy and mucosal edema. *Usually occurs in the first 3 to 6 weeks of life. It is extremely rare during the first week of life.*Epidemiology : 2-4 cases every 1,000 newborns; male-to-female ratio 4:1; *Clinical Presentation: Nonbilious vomiting (becoming projectile), cannot hold down water, leading to severe dehydration (metabolic alkalosis, decreased potassium and chloride ions). Serum pH is increased.Hypochloremic- Hypokalemic Saline responsive Metabolic alkalosis on ABG analysis in a severe case with Fluid & Electrolyte disturbances.
*Diagnosis: 1. Palpation of the pyloric olive. Contrary to the textbook description of its location in the right upper quadrant, the pyloric olive is more commonly found in the midline. If the pyloric olive can be felt, no further diagnostic tests are necessary. a. In an infant with a history that strongly suggests pyloric stenosis, emptying the stomach with a nasogastric tube to make the olive easier to feel is recommended. b. Palpating the olive is impossible if the infant is crying. 1) Crying can be suppressed by giving the infant a pacifier or a small amount of an oral electrolyte maintenance solution. 2) Patience on the part of the physician is important in this circumstance. c. When the infant is not crying, the physician should stand at the infant's left side and hold up the baby's feet with his or her left hand to relax the infant's belly. The physician should then gently palpate the epigastrium with the extended middle finger of the right hand, being careful not to dig into the baby's abdomen. 2. Barium study. Typical findings on barium study indicating pyloric stenosis are the "string" sign and the "double tract" sign. 3. Ultrasonography is the gold standard for diagnosis of pyloric stenosis. a. If the history is strongly suggestive of pyloric stenosis but a mass is not palpable, an ultrasound is a good diagnostic test in experienced hands. b. If pyloric stenosis is not the cause of vomiting, gastroesophageal reflux may also be diagnosed by ultrasound.

Treatment is surgical 1. Preoperative management. A clinical assessment of the patient's hydration should be made, and serum electrolyte levels should be checked immediately on admission to rule out a serious hypokalemic hypochloremic metabolic alkalosis. This should be corrected with appropriate potassium- and chloride containing intravenous fluids before elective pyloromyotomy.Children with severe dehydration have accelerated renal K+ and H+ losses due to an attempt to retain fluid and Na+ ions. The urine pH of severely dehydrated children may demonstrate a paradoxical aciduria because the renal mechanisms for acid resorption are lost in an attempt to retain Na+ and K+ ions. As the kidneys attempt to retain Na+, an initial compensatory excretion of K+ occurs. Then, as K+ deficit develops, the kidney attempts to retain both Na+ and K+; thus, it excretes H+ instead of K+, and paradoxical aciduria then occurs. This cycle can be broken only by

adequately replacing fluids and electrolytes. In cases of clinical dehydration, children with pyloric stenosis require rehydration with IV fluid therapy before surgery. Administer D5W with 0.45% NaCl IV at 1.5 times the maintenance rate. Severely dehydrated children should receive initial deficit fluid therapy with 0.9% NaCl. When urine output is demonstrated, KCl 10-20 mEq/L can be added to the fluids. Defer surgery for pyloric stenosis until the child is adequately rehydrated. The severity of dehydration can be estimated by physical examination and by measuring serum Cl- and HCO_3^+ levels. The degree of dehydration and the clinical response to fluid replacement therapy guide the duration of preoperative preparation in a child with pyloric stenosis. Optimal resuscitation is determined by normal skin turgor, moist mucous membranes, urine output of more than 1 mL/kg/h, serum HCO_3^- level less than 28 mEq/dL, and Cl- level of more than 100 mEq/dL. Enteral feeds can usually be started soon after uncomplicated pyloromyotomy, and full feeds can be given within 24-48 hours. Postoperative electrolyte abnormalities are rare.
2. Pyloromyotomy-The Ramstedt-Fredet pyloromyotomy, performed with the infant under general anesthesia, is universally acceptable as the preferred operation. The stomach should be emptied again just before induction of anesthesia to minimize the risk of aspiration. A transverse skin incision followed by vertical splitting the right rectus muscle and fascia is used most frequently. The right upper abdominal transverse muscle splitting gridiron incision (Robertson) is used by many as well. Because it provides a better cosmetic appearance, a supraumbilical, curvilinear incision has been used by some surgeons.
3. Postoperative management a. Feeding regimen-1) The patient should be given nothing orally for 6 hours after surgery. 2) Feeding can usually be initiated 6 to 8 hours postoperatively. Sugar water is generally given first, followed by formula or breast milk, using the following guidelines. This regimen can be advanced more rapidly or slowly depending on how the baby does. a) Sugar water, 30 mL every 2 hours, two times b) Formula or breast milk i) If sugar water is tolerated, the baby may be given halfstrength formula, 30 mL every 2 hours, two times. This is followed by fullstrength formula every 4 hours at liberty. ii) Breast milk may be substituted for formula but must be measured and fed by bottle. 3) If the infant vomits, feedings should cease for 2 hours. 4) All routine procedures (eg, taking vital signs, diaper changing, sponge bathing) should be completed before each feeding begins. b. Hospital discharge. Most infants may be discharged 24 hours after surgery. c. Surgical complications. Gastric and gastroesophageal reflux are the most common causes of persistent postoperative vomiting. Incomplete pyloromyotomy may be considered if vomiting continuous for more than 7 - 10 days postoperatively, if it is forceful, and if it follows every feeding. If the duodenum is inadvertently entered during the pyloromyotomy, and was noticed during the surgery, the perforated mucosa can be repaired or all layers should be closed and pyloromyotomy performed on other site, then the infant should remain on both nasogastric suction and intravenous antibiotics postoperatively for a minimum of 2 days.

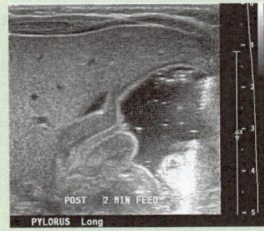

CHPS-Ultrasound findings include: "target sign" (hypertrophied hypoechoic muscle surrounding echogenic mucosa); elongated pylorus with thickened muscle; "cervix sign"; "antral nipple sign"; exaggerated peristalsis; and failure of the pylorus to open.

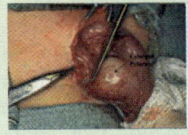 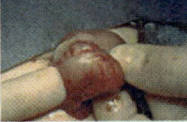

Intraoperative picture of the pylorus before and after the muscle has been divided. Note that the inside lining of the pylorus is left intact after the muscle is divided

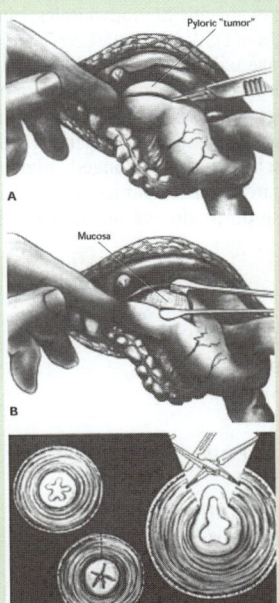

Fredet-Ramstedt pyloromyotomy. (A) Pylorus delivered into wound and seromuscular layer incised. (B) Seromuscular layer separated down to submucosal base to permit herniation of mucosa through pyloric incision. (C) Cross section demonstrating hypertrophied pylorus,depth of incision,and spreading of muscle to permit mucosa to herniate through incision.

REFERENCES: 1) Benson CO: Infantile Hypertrophic Pyloric Stenosis. In *Pediatric Surgery,* 4th ed. Welch KJ, et al, eds. Chicago: Year Book, 1986 2) O'Neill JA Jr. Grosfeld JL. Fonkalsrud EW. Coran AG., Caldamone AA. Hypertropic pyloric stenosis. Principles

GASTROSCHISIS AND OMPHALOCELE

GASTROSCHISIS (Greek for "belly cleft") Is a defect of the anterior abdominal wall just lateral to the umbilicus. The defect is almost always to the right of an intact umbilical cord and some cases are separated from the cord by an intact skin bridge. In contrast to omphalocele there is no peritoneal sac so that antenatal evisceration of the bowel occurs through a relatively small defect during intra uterine life. The irritating effect of the amniotic fluid (pH 7.0), which contains fetal urine and various growth factors, on the exposed bowel wall results in a chemical form of peritonitis characterized by a thick edematous membrane that is occasionally exudative. Omphalocele is a covered defect of the umbilical ring into which abdominal contents have herniated. The defect is thought to occur in the third week of intrauterine life when the midgut elongates and resides in the yoke sac outside of the embryonic celom. **Associated anomalies:** Associated anomalies should be ruled out, particularly in neonates with an omphalocele. The VACTERL constellation is often found in patients with omphalocele.
Management: Treatment begins immediately following delivery.
1. Medical treatment: a) Hypothermia is usually the immediate life-threatening problem. **b)** Systemic intravenous antibiotics (ampicillin/gentamicin) are given to protect contaminated amnion and viscera. Infection can be devastating if a mesh closure is necessary. **c)** Intravenous hydration with balanced salt solution and colloid is essential. Fluid requirements in a neonate with gastroschisis can range up to 2.5 times that of a healthy newborn in the first 24 hours of life. As a general rule, the more matted and inflamed the exposed viscera appear, the greater the fluid requirements of the infant. Initial resuscitation of an infant with gastroschisis is generally begun with a 10-mL to 20-mL/kg bolus of 0.9% NaCl or RL solution in addition to maintenance fluids. Additional isotonic fluid is administered until urine output is established. The infant's ongoing fluid needs are tailored to his or her specific hemodynamics, but volumes are generally 120–175 mL/kg/d of D5W with 0.45% NaCl with added potassium.The patient's acid-base balance should be closely monitored because metabolic acidosis is common as a result of poor perfusion related to hypovolemia. An orogastric tube is placed in the stomach to prevent the patient from swallowing air and aspirating intestinal contents because an infant with gastroschisis has a prolonged, adynamic ileus. The infant should be given parenteral antibiotics and kept in a thermoneutral environment. Because omphalocele occurs early in gestation, other associated anomalies of midline structures are frequently present, most commonly in the heart. Pulmonary hypoplasia is also a serious associated problem and is related to the compression of the developing lungs. Because the defect is covered, fluid resuscitation is typically not as vigorous as it is in patients with gastroschisis.Patients with ruptured omphalocele had a larger fluid requirement than those with gastroschisis or an intact omphalocele sac.

2.Surgical management for gastroscisis
The abdominal wall defect is enlarged 1 to 2 cm cephalad and caudad to improve the mechanical advantage for reducing the exposed viscera. Primary abdominal repair may not be possible in 40 - 50 % of cases. Too tight a closure may result in cardiorespiratory compromise from diaphragmatic elevation and ventilatory restriction, vena caval compression that reduces venous return, and diminished bowel perfusion leading to intestinal ischemia and necrosis. Some infants require a staged closure using a Dacron reinforced Silastic Silo as a temporary extra - abdominal housing. As a result of prolonged adynamic ileus and exposure of the bowel to the amniotic fluid, it takes long for the bowel to commence normal peristalsis, necessitating, in almost all infants, TPN for adequate caloric support.

Surgical Treatment for Omphalocele a) The sac or exposed intestines should be covered by a barrier-type dressing. A large circumferential dressing is applied last. **b)** With gastroschisis in particular, it is essential that the bowel be supported, usually with the patient on his or her side and the bowel supported by towels, to prevent strangulation of the bowel and consequent bowel ischemia. **c)** Gastrointestinal decompression by nasogastric tube is imperative to minimize further gastrointestinal distention and prevent aspiration of gastric contents. **d)** Small defects (2 cm) can be managed by direct primary closure of the abdominal wall. Medium-sized defects are managed by careful removal of the sac at its base with suture ligation of the umbilical vein, the two umbilical arteries and the urachus. The liver and then the bowel are reduced into the abdomen. If the abdominal wall fascia cannot be approximated, skin closure with creation of a small ventral hernia may be used in some patients. Some may use prosthetic material to bridge the gap or staged-closure using a Dacron-reinforced silastic silo as a temporary locale for the bowel. Non-operative management using topical application of an escharotic (0.25% merbromin and 0.5% silver nitrate) agent is an alternative choice of treatment.

CLINICAL FINDINGS IN INFANTS WITH ABDOMINAL WALL DEFECTS

	Omphalocele	Gastroschisis
Location	Umbilical ring	Lateral to umbilical cord
Defect size	Large (2–10 cm)	Small (2–4 cm)
Cord	Inserts in sac	Normal insertion (left of defect)
Sac	Present	None
Contents	Liver, bowel	Bowel, gonads
Bowel	Normal	Matted, inflamed
Malrotation	Present	Present
Small abdomen	Present	Present
Intestinal function	Normal	Poor function initially
Other anomalies	Common (30–70%)	Unusual except for bowel atresia

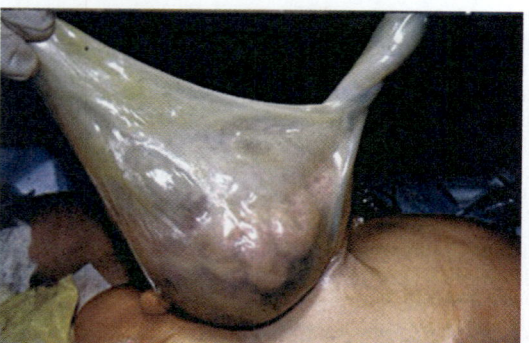

OMPHALOCELE

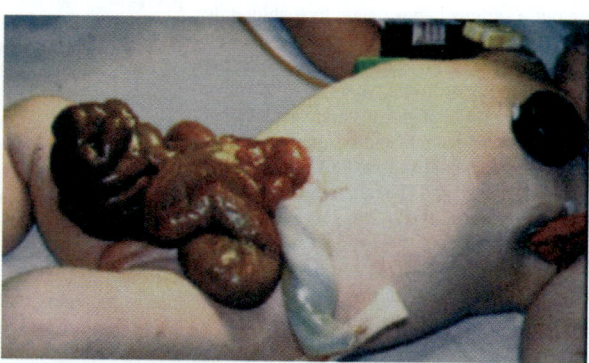

GASTROSCHISIS

ESOPHAGEAL ATRESIA AND TRACHEOESOPHAGEAL FISTULA

Esophageal Atresia

1. **Definition:** Esophageal atresia (EA) with distal tracheo-esophageal fistula (TEF) is the most common congenital anomaly of the esophagus, followed by EA without TEF also known as pure esophageal atresia and pure TEF. Incidence is 1 in every 2500 live births.

2. **Embryology:** The trachea and esophagus initially begin as a ventral diverticulum of the foregut during the third intrauterine week of life. A proliferation of endodermal cells appears on the lateral aspect of this growing diverticulum. These cell masses will divide the foregut into trachea and esophageal tubes. Whether interruption of this normal event leads to tracheo-esophageal anomalies, or whether during tracheal growth, atresia of the esophagus results because of the fistulous fixation of the esophagus to the trachea remains to be proven. Thirty percent of infants with this syndrome are premature.

3. **Clinical presentation:** Respiratory distress due to: 1) Clinical signs include: **a)** Excessive salivation **b)** Choking during feeding **2)** Patients with esophageal atresia may also present with: **a)** Recurrent aspiration/reflux pneumonia **b)** Right upper lobe pneumonia and atelectasis. Contrast studies are rarely needed and of potential disaster (aspiration). Correct dehydration, acid-base disturbances, respiratory distress and decompress proximal esophageal pouch (Reploge tube).

4. **Associated anomalies:** Evaluate for associated conditions which occurs in 30 % of patients. Such as **VACTERL** association (3 or more): - Vertebral anomalies (i.e. hemivertebrae, spina bifida) - **A**nal malformations (i.e. imperforate anus)—**C**ardiac malformations (i.e. VSD, ASD, Tetralogy Fallot)—**T**racheo-**E**sophageal fistula (must be one of the associated conditions) - **R**enal Deformities (i.e. absent kidney, hypospadia, etc.) - **L**imb dysplasia

5. **Diagnosis :** 1) Diagnosis confirmed by observing a coiling nasogastric tube in a proximal pouch on radiograph. 2) Barium/water soluble gastrgraphin preferably / (0.5 ml) may be *carefully* instilled in the proximal pouch, only if there is diagnostic dilemma. During this procedure, the child is to be accompanied by the doctor to the x-ray room. 3) Radiographs should include the neck and abdomen **a)** If air is seen in the intestine, the diagnosis is esophageal atresia with distal tracheoesophageal fistula is the most likely diagnosis.

6. **Treatment : 1) Peri-operative Management a)** If present, right upper lobe pneumonia and atelectasis should be corrected with antibiotics before surgery. **b)** The baby should be kept in a reverse Trendelenburg's position. **2) Operative Management** A gastrostomy should be performed as soon as possible **a)** Vigorous chest physical therapy and suctioning should be performed. **1.** The gastrostomy tube should be placed to gravity. **2.** Saliva should be suctioned from the blind proximal pouch either by continuous sump tube (Replogle) or by oral suctioning every 15 minutes. **b)** An extrapleural division and closure of the tracheoesophageal fistula with end-to-end anastomosis without undue tension should be performed. In certain types of tracheoesophageal fistula with esophageal atresia or in premature infants, a delayed anastomosis may be considered.

7. **Outcome:** Most important predictors of outcome if the patient presents immediately are: birth weight, severity of pulmonary dysfunction, and presence of major congenital cardiac disease. **Complication after surgery:** anastomotic leak, stricture, gastroesophageal reflux, tracheomalacia and recurrent TEF. **Increased survival:** Is associated with improvements in perioperative care, meticulous surgical technique and aggressive treatment of associated anomalies.

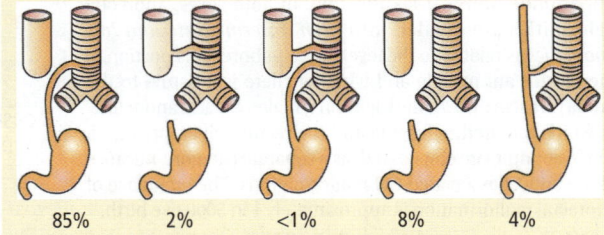

85%   2%   <1%   8%   4%

Anatomical variations of esophageal atresia and tracheoesophageal fistula, indicating relative frequency

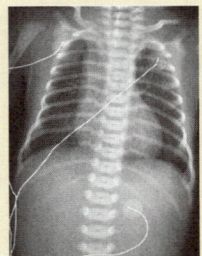

Isolated esophageal atresia (EA). Frontal view of the chest and abdomen demonstrates a catheter in the proximal pouch in this patient with EA. Note the absence of bowel gas in this patient with EA, but it is not associated with a tracheoesophageal fistula (TEF).

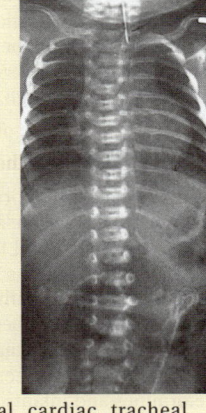

Esophageal atresia (EA) with distal tracheoesophageal fistula (TEF). Frontal view of the chest and abdomen of a neonate demonstrates a tube in the proximal pouch in this patient with EA. The presence of bowel gas implies the presence of a distal TEF, making this the most common type of EA/TEF.

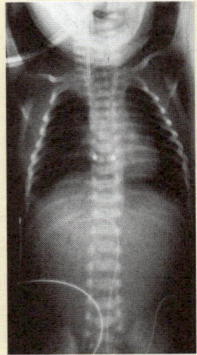

Vertebral, anorectal, cardiac, tracheal, esophageal, renal, and limb (VACTERL) association. Frontal radiograph in a patient with esophageal atresia (EA) without a tracheoesophageal fistula (TEF). Note the catheter in the proximal pouch and the butterfly vertebra (asterisks) at the level of T8 in this patient with associated VACTERL.

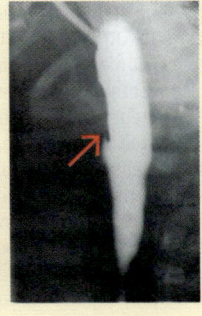

H-type tracheoesophageal fistula (TEF). Oblique barium esophagogram demonstrates a fistula (arrow) arising from the anterior esophagus and extending anterosuperiorly to the trachea.

Which babies develop tracheoesophageal fistula or esophageal atresia? These two problems are not thought to be inherited. However, they are often seen when a baby has other birth defects, such as: trisomy 13, 18, or 21 *other digestive tract problems (such as diaphragmatic hernia, duodenal atresia, or imperforate anus) *heart problems (such as ventricular septal defect, tetralogy of Fallot, or patent ductus arteriosus) *kidney and urinary tract problems (such as horseshoe or polycystic kidney, absent kidney, or hypospadias) *muscular or skeletal problems *VACTERL syndrome (which involves Vertebral, Anal, Cardiac, TE fistula, Renal, and Limb abnormalities). Up to one-half of all babies with TE fistula or esophageal atresia have another birth defect.

ANORECTAL MALFORMATIONS

Imperforate Anus —Classification: In both sexes, anorectal deformities are divided into *high, intermediate and low anomalies* as related to the level of the puborectalis portion of the levator ani muscle and whether there is a fistula to the urinary tract in male or the vagina in females. Cloacal anomalies, in which the urethra, vagina and the rectum all empty into a single conduit, are considered, as a separate category, because of the critical associated GU malformations. The incidence of anorectal malformation is approximately 1 in 5000 live birth.

Initial management of the newborn with imperforate anus :
The first decision in the assessment of the newborn with an anorectal anomaly is whether a colostomy is required. Although it is always better to err on the side performing a colostomy, there are many anomalies in which one is unnecessary. The examination of the perineum is paramount because it may provide evidence of a low lying fistula or meconium beneath the membranous covering typical of a low lesion. In contrast , a flat or "rocker–bottom" perineum may be observed, which indicates poor sphincter or levator muscle development typical of a high anomaly (Anatomically, it ends above the level of puborectalis portion of the levator ani muscle.) It is best to wait 24 hrs to allow progression of gas or meconium down close to or onto the perineum before finalizing the assessment. Of the female malformations, 95% are of the low variety, whereas most male anomalies are high.

Surgical management of imperforate anus :

1. Initial treatment in the neonate:

Male and female newborn who have low anomalies in the form of an anocutaneous fistula, ano vestibular fistula or anal stenosis usually can be treated initially with dilatation. In the past, anocutaneous fistulas regularly were dilated and repair performed several months later, but in more recent years, more pediatric centers have been performing anoplasty shortly after birth unless contraindicated by some other condition. Male and female infants suspected of intermediate or high-lying deformities and infants whose internal anatomy cannot be determined with certainty should have a colostomy performed. The most satisfactory approach is to perform colostomy at the junction between the descending colon and the sigmoid colon, leaving sufficient length to permit a subsequent pull-through procedure without having a take down the colostomy. Many surgeons believe that loop colostomy to be sufficient.

2.Definitive operation is done when the surgeon determines the infant can best tolerate the procedure, when the infant is a minimum of three months of age. **Posterior Sagittal Anorectal plasty (PSARP)-** *Pena de Vries posterior sagittal anorectoplasty* The incision is made from the exposed rectal opening (fistula) to the rectum. The true rectal sphincter, containing the rectal nerves and muscles is identified and the fistula is brought down and sutured to the rectum. This creates anal opening where the infant's rectal muscles and nerves are located, in order to maximize the infant's ability to control bowel movements in the future. The colostomy is not closed during this operation. The infant will continue to stool through the colostomy to allow the new operative site to heal. About eight weeks later an operation will be done to close the colostomy. The anastomosis created at the PSARP operation must be completely healed. The child must be monitored closely for regular bowel movements and minimal straining. Stool softeners may be prescribed. Initially the infant may stool with each diaper change. It is common for the child to develop a diaper rash. Children with imperforate anus must be followed by for most of their lives. Greater than 95% of those who have had a simple anoplasty for a low-lying lesion are continent, but constipation is a frequent problem and must be managed. In children who have had a PSARP performed, the results in terms of continence are directly related to the anomaly. 65% to 75% of children with intermediate and high anomalies report satisfactory continence, which usually includes the need for a bowel management program.

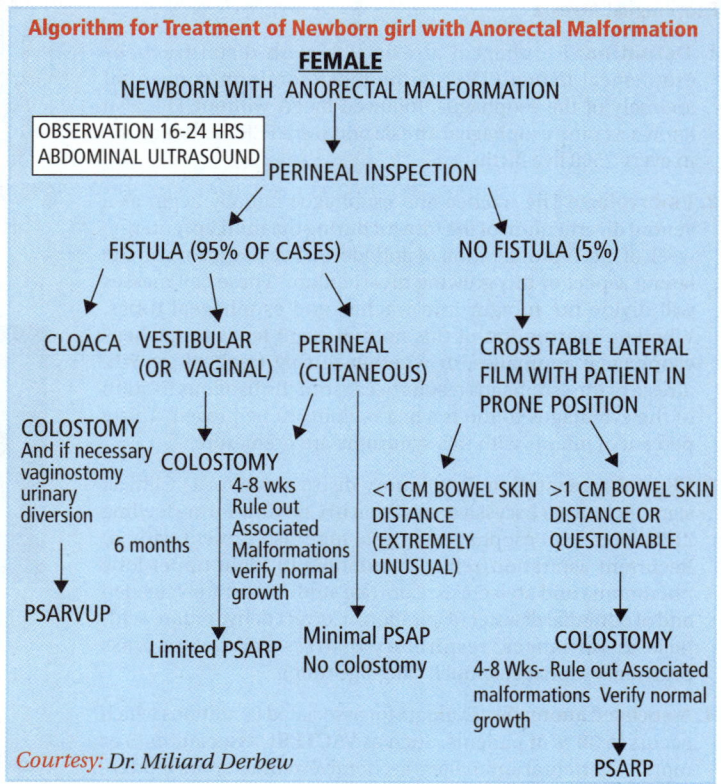

Algorithm for Treatment of Newborn girl with Anorectal Malformation

FEMALE
NEWBORN WITH ANORECTAL MALFORMATION

OBSERVATION 16-24 HRS ABDOMINAL ULTRASOUND → PERINEAL INSPECTION

FISTULA (95% OF CASES) — NO FISTULA (5%)

CLOACA / VESTIBULAR (OR VAGINAL) / PERINEAL (CUTANEOUS) / CROSS TABLE LATERAL FILM WITH PATIENT IN PRONE POSITION

COLOSTOMY And if necessary vaginostomy urinary diversion — 6 months → PSARVUP

COLOSTOMY 4-8 wks Rule out Associated Malformations verify normal growth → Limited PSARP

Minimal PSAP No colostomy

<1 CM BOWEL SKIN DISTANCE (EXTREMELY UNUSUAL)

>1 CM BOWEL SKIN DISTANCE OR QUESTIONABLE → COLOSTOMY 4-8 Wks- Rule out Associated malformations Verify normal growth → PSARP

Courtesy: Dr. Miliard Derbew

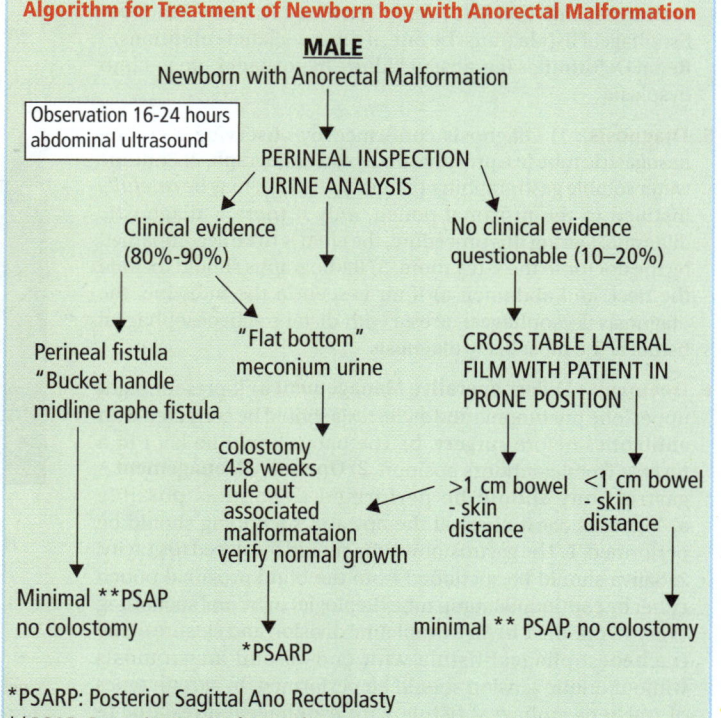

Algorithm for Treatment of Newborn boy with Anorectal Malformation

MALE
Newborn with Anorectal Malformation

Observation 16-24 hours abdominal ultrasound → PERINEAL INSPECTION URINE ANALYSIS

Clinical evidence (80%-90%) — No clinical evidence questionable (10–20%)

Perineal fistula "Bucket handle midline raphe fistula → Minimal **PSAP no colostomy

"Flat bottom" meconium urine → colostomy 4-8 weeks rule out associated malformataion verify normal growth → *PSARP

CROSS TABLE LATERAL FILM WITH PATIENT IN PRONE POSITION

>1 cm bowel - skin distance

<1 cm bowel - skin distance → minimal ** PSAP, no colostomy

*PSARP: Posterior Sagittal Ano Rectoplasty
**PSAP: Posterior Sagittal Ano plasty

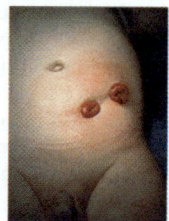

Recommended colostomy with divided stomas, the proximal stoma in the descending colon.

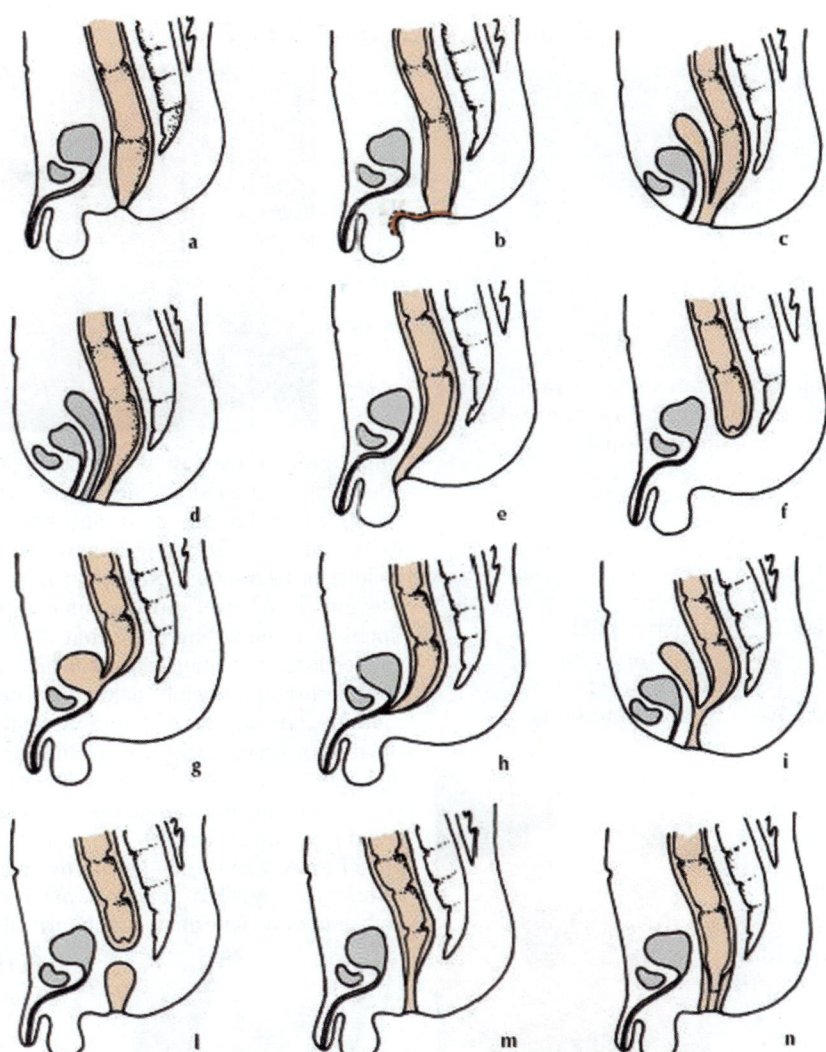

Classification according to the level of the atretic rectal cul-de-sac with respect to the pubococcygeal line (the radiological landmark for the upper border or the levator ani muscle assessed with MRI, no longer with Wangensteen-Rice invertogram 12–24 hours after birth, when swallowed air has reached rectum and can act as a natural contrast agent; puborectal muscular flonde) and the sex : ·

High ARM : cul-de-sac above the level of the pubococcygeal line ·**anorectal atresia with rectovesical or rectourethral (high rectovaginal or rectocloacal in female) fistula** ·**anorectal atresia without fistula** ·**rectal atresia** Epidemiology : male-to-female ratio 3:1.

Intermediate ARM : cul-de-sac at the level of the pubococcygeal line ·**anorectal atresia with bulbar rectourethral (rectovestibular or low rectovaginal) fistula** ·**anorectal atresia without fistula**.

Low ARM : cul-de-sac below the level of the pubococcygeal line ·**incomplete covered anus (with anocutaneous perineal or scrotal/anovestibular fistula) and anal stenosis (ectopic anus)** ·**complete covered anus (without fistula) or membranous anus** Epidemiology : male-to-female ratio 1:3 +/- associated fistula.

 Denis Browne classification (simpler than 1984 Wingspread conference classification) : ·**stenotic anus (fig. a)** Symptoms and signs : constipation, abdominal distention, tooth-paste stools => fecal retention => fecalomas => abdominal occlusion

Therapy: progressive anal dilatation ·**aproctia** : congenital absence or imperforation of the anus. ·**imperforate, membranous or Denis Browne microscopic anus / anal atresia / atresia ani / proctatresia** : persistence of the anal membrane, so that the anus is closed. The defect is not always complete; sometimes a narrow opening permits the passage of the bowel contents. When the anus is completely imperforate, there is simply a dimple in the skin of the perineum; this condition is often associated with atresia of the lower rectum Therapy: perforation of the membrane and progressive anal dilatation. ·**covered anus (fig. b)** : lack of anal pit and orifice accompanied by a blackish line along the raphe in the male, small vaginal opening in the female ·**ectopic anus** · **anus vesicalis** : anomalous opening of the rectum into the bladder, the anus being imperforate · **anus vestibularis** : anomalous opening of the rectum on the vulva, the anus being imperforate

*in the female : · **low vaginal (subhymenal) or vulvar anus** (forquette anus) (fig. c) (more common) · **ectopic anus with barrel gun perineum (fig. d)** (anal orifice is separated by vaginal opening by a tract of skin) (less common)

*in the male - **perineal anus (fig. e)** (more common), **scrotal anus** (less common), **anorectal atresia** (the most severe ARM)

f : **anorectal atresia without fistulas** **g** : anorectal atresia with rectovesical fistula **h** : anorectal atresia with rectourethral fistula **i** : anorectal atresia with high suprahymenal vaginal fistula.

ANORECTAL MALFORMATIONS

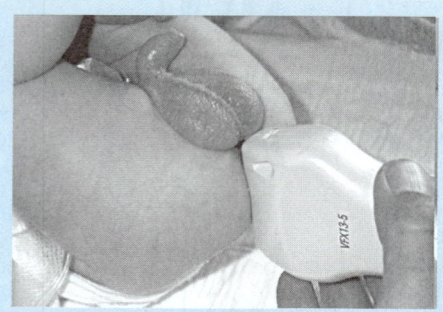

1-day-old boy with imperforate anus. Photograph shows placement of linear transducer for **transperineal sonographic examination.**

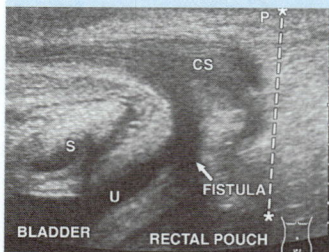

Transperineal Sonography for determining type of Imperforate Anus

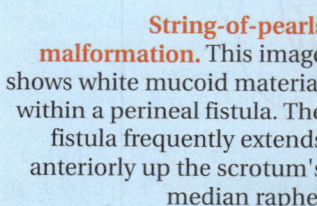

String-of-pearls malformation. This image shows white mucoid material within a perineal fistula. The fistula frequently extends anteriorly up the scrotum's median raphe.

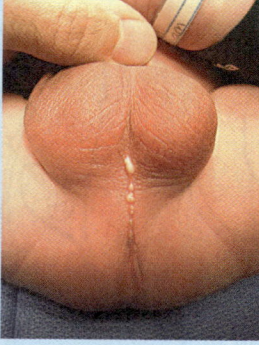

Bucket-handle malformation. The appearance of a band of skin overlying the sphincteric muscle complex is a common sign in a child born with imperforate anus and perineal fistula.

Cloaca. This is the classic appearance of a girl with a cloacal malformation with a single perineal orifice. The genitals appear quite short, which is a finding consistent with cloaca.

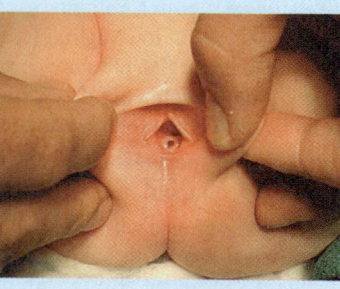

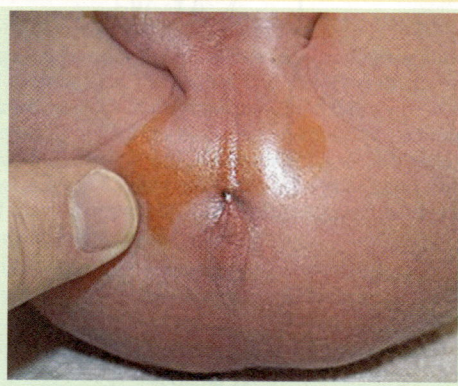

Imperforate anus may include a single abnormality or a combination of abnormalities of the rectum (the end of the intestine near the anus) and anus (the opening of the rectum to the skin). There are many forms of this birth defect that may include the following: 1. The absence of an anal opening, which prevents any bowel movements completely. 2. The anal opening in the wrong place that is often too small. 3. A connection, or opening called a fistula, between the rectum and the urethra, bladder or vagina. This may cause bowel movements to pass out of these abnormal openings. 4. In girls, the rectum, urethra, vagina can join together to form a single opening. This is called a cloaca and it is very rare. There is no known cause for imperforate anus and most cases are isolated and do not run in families. The birth defect occurs in about one of every 4,000–5,000 newborns and is somewhat more common in boys than girls. Males are twice as likely to have a high or intermediate anorectal abnormality.

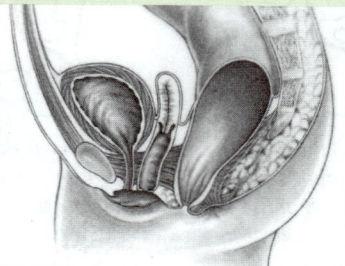

Perineal Fistula

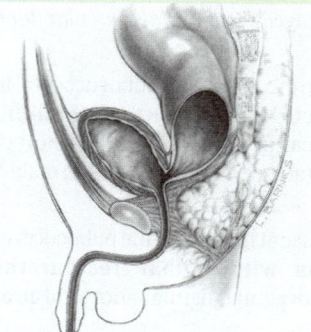

Rectovesicle Fistula

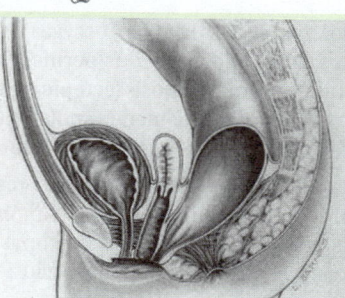

Rectovestibular Fistula

INGUINAL HERNIA AND HYDROCELE

Inguinal hernia Swelling in inguinal region (can extend to scrotum in males, or to labia in females) secondary to persistence of a wide processus vaginalis, with herniation of bowel (or, in females, the ovary) Incidence: term newborns, 0.5% to 1%; premature newborns, 5% to 10%; location on right side (~60%), left side (40%), or both sides (10%), with bilateral hernias more common in premature newborns (~62% of affected infants).

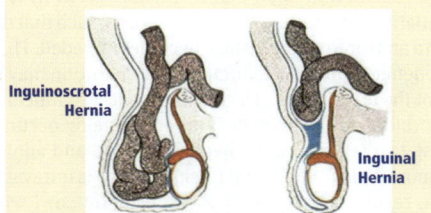

Clinical features: soft, nontender,Difficult to define the upper margin of the swelling (unlike hydroceles) reducible bulge in the inguinal canal, off the midline, especially at times of increased intra-abdominal pressure, with possible extension into scrotum/labia; when incarcerated, tenderness and tenseness of hernia, with discoloration of overlying skin,May transilluminate.

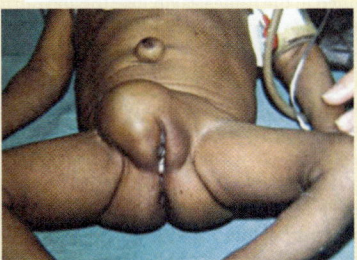

Complications: incarceration and strangulation

Treatment: If reducible and infant in NICU – non-urgent surgical referral for surgical repair prior to discharge. If *reducible* and infant at home—discuss with surgical registrar (will usually be repaired within 1-2 weeks). If incarcerated, **urgent** surgical referral (elective surgical repair as soon as possible after diagnosis.)

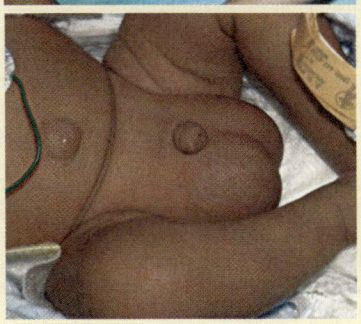

Incarcerated inguinal hernia 1. **Definition.** Incarcerated inguinal hernia in a child is a patent processus vaginalis with an intra-abdominal organ within it. This condition is age related, occurring most often in infants during the first year of life. **a.** Incarcerated inguinal hernia in boys often contains bowel. **b.** Incarcerated inguinal hernia in girls often contains ovary and tube. 2. **Etiology** is not known. 3. **Clinical presentation.** Both boys and girls invariably are noted to have a lump in the groin. 4. **Differential diagnosis** a. **In boys,** differentiating an incarcerated hernia from a hydrocele of the cord is imperative. 1) **External examination** a) A hydrocele of the cord is often tense. b) The end of the hydrocele can be distinguished from the testis itself. c) The proximal end of the cord can be detected. 2) **Rectal examination** can also distinguish the two conditions. a) The inside of the abdominal wall at the level of the internal ring should be palpated. b) If the vas and the ring are easily palpable, an incarceration cannot be present. c) If the physician is still unsure of the diagnosis, palpation on the other side can be compared. b. **In girls,** differential diagnosis is hydrocele of the canal of Nuck. 5. **Treatment** a. **Treatment of boys** 1) **Manual reduction.** Most incarcerated inguinal hernias can be reduced manually, obviating emergency surgery. Some hernias reduce easily;others require several attempts. a) If necessary, the patient should be sedated with an appropriate barbiturate (e.g, pentobarbital sodium 2 to 3 mg/kg body weight, morphine 0.1 mg/kg). b) Occasionally, simply holding the patient in a very steep Trendelenburg's position reduces the hernia because of the pull of the mesentery. c) If the hernia does not spontaneously reduce with the patient in Trendelenburg's position, an assistant should hold the infant above the knees in a frog-leg position to relax the abdominal wall. d) The physician should use the fingers of one hand to attempt to fix the hernia while gradually pressing the incarcerated mass with the other hand. i) The physician should try to milk the bowel contents out of the incarcerated bowel until it "pops" back within the abdomen. ii) A considerable length (i.e., 5 minutes) of steady pressure may be required to produce the desired reduction, so the physician should be in a comfortable position.

This is a typical appearance of bilateral inguinal hernias. In contrast to hydrocele, inguinal hernias are associated with a fullness in both the inguinal area and the scrotum and can usually be reduced with digital pressure. At times bowel sounds may even be appreciated over the area of the mass. This infant is preterm, a risk factor for the presence of hernias. While the scrotum may transilluminate with either hydrocele or hernia, other clinical features will usually differentiate the two conditions.

2) Postreduction management

a) If manual reduction of the hernia is successful, the patient is always admitted to the hospital, and the repair is performed electively within 24 to 48 hours after the inguinal edema has resolved. b) High ligation of the sac is the operation performed in both boys and girls.

3) **Surgical management.** Emergency surgical intervention is required if the hernia cannot be manually reduced or if there is postreduction evidence of persistent intestinal obstruction or nonviable bowel.

b. **Treatment of girls.** Because the blood supply to the ovary is usually not impaired, these hernias can generally be repaired on a semielective basis. As with boys, treatment consists of manual reduction followed by high ligation of the sac.

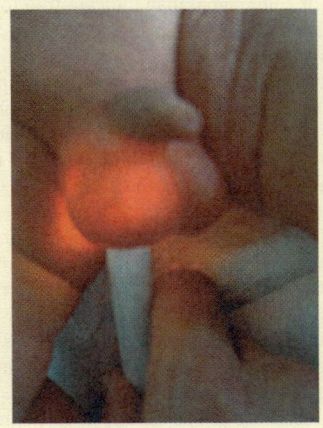

6. **Complications.** Hemorrhagic infarction of the testicle is an unfortunate complication of an incarcerated hernia. Reduction will usually reinstitute blood flow to the testis. Incarceration of an ovary in a girl generally has no sequelae.

7. **Incarcerated inguinal hernia in a premature infant** a. An inpatient premature infant with multiple problems can have a hernia repaired just before discharge home.b. An infant with a history of prematurity (gestational age less than 36 weeks at birth) should be admitted overnight after hernia repair for apnea monitoring. This pertains until the child reaches a postconceptional age of at least 50 weeks.

Hydrocele: Persistence of the processus vaginalis results in peritoneal fluid in the scrotum around the testis or spermatic cord *Clinical features:* painless, tense, fluctuant scrotal mass that transilluminates; upper border usually movable away from inguinal canal; possibly, testis not palpable. Treatment: Except <u>Reassurance</u> none usually needed, because hydroceles generally decrease in size and resolve over the first year of life; if not resolved by the age of 1 to 2 years, consideration of elective surgical repair; for communicating hydrocele (i.e., one that fluctuates in size), same treatment as for inguinal hernia.

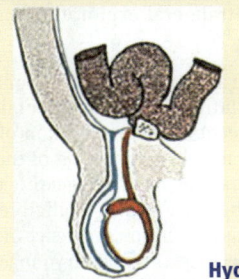

Hydrocoele

TORSION TESTIS

Testicular torsion is an acute vascular event in which the spermatic cord becomes twisted on its axis, such that the blood flow to and/or from the testicle becomes impeded. This results in ischemic injury and infarction. The condition may result in loss of the testis. Testicular torsion can be a significant source of morbidity in the neonate. This abnormality occurs in boys during two age peaks, the neonatal period and adolescence. The more typical adolescent torsion usually is intravaginal and is the result of twisting of the spermatic cord while it is suspended in the tunica vaginalis. Torsion during the neonatal period usually is extravaginal, with the spermatic cord and its adjacent tunica twisting as a unit. Neonatal testicular torsion is divided into two groups: (l) prenatal testicular torsion presenting at birth (torsion in utero) and (2) postnatal testicular torsion (torsion within the first 30 days of life). In a literature review, it was found that 72.4% of neonatal torsions were prenatal and 27.5% occurred during the postnatal period. Only 0.5% of cases had difficulty in establishing the onset of presentation. Numerous studies have found that spermatic cord torsion was extravaginal and supravaginal accounting for 92% of cases. In a solo case this was found to be intravaginal. The differential diagnosis includes inguinal hernia with or without incarceration, torsion of testis appendix, hydrocele, hematocele, epididymoorchitis, idiopathic infarction of the testis, ectopic splenic or adrenal rests, and benign and malignant tumors of the testis and epididymis. In contrast to postnatal torsion, the prenatal or in utero torsion in the newborn mostly is insidious and asymptomatic. The patient has an edematous hemiscrotum at birth, with a scrotal swelling that does not transmit tight. In most cases, there are no associated symptoms such as pain or pyrexia. Perinatal torsion of the spermatic cord does not appear to be related to prematurity, low-birthweight mode of delivery, or perinatal trauma and both sides are affected equally. Doppler sonography can also provide information helpful in diagnosing other conditions that mimic acute testicular torsion clinically. This is particularly true for epididymitis. The absence of color flow signal is diagnostic of acute testicular torsion. Infectious causes of acute testicular pain usually lead to hyperemia and increased vascular flow. Antenatal and neonatal testicular torsion can be a more difficult diagnosis to make. Normal testicular blood flow during the antenatal period is low. The absence of color signal may indicate true torsion or may be technical in nature, reflecting the difficulty in detecting normal but slow blood flow by Doppler imaging. Power Doppler sonography (also known as color Doppler energy, amplitude Doppler sonography, color amplitude imaging, color intensity Doppler sonography, and sonographic angiography) is very sensitive to low flow rates and can help diagnose acute testicular torsion in a newborn infant. It depends on the integrated power of the Doppler sonographic signal, as opposed to conventional color Doppler sonography, which relies on the mean Doppler frequency shift. The goals of surgical exploration include (1) confirmation of the diagnosis of torsion, (2) detorsion of the involved testis, (3) assessment of the viability of the involved testis, (4) removal (if nonviable) or fixation (if viable) of the involved testis, and (5) fixation of the contralateral testis, when appropriate. Because of the concern regarding the possibility of asynchronous testicular torsion, contralateral exploration and fixation is widely performed.

Neonate with acute scrotum at birth or a few days after birth: Recommendations are controversial. Although most authorities recommend exploration of the ipsilateral side-orchiectomy mostly and fixation of the contralateral testis-orchiopexy, some have suggested that observation is acceptable because of the negligible salvage rate of the ischemic testis and the low incidence of contralateral torsion. The risk of anesthesia in children younger than 1 year may also factor into decision-making process.

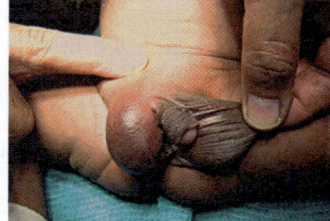
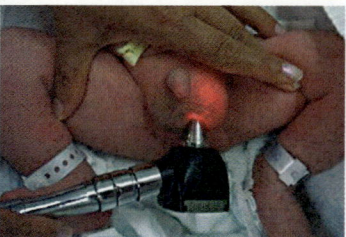

Rt Testicular Torsion: Because of the pathology that is occuring in the right testicle, the right scrotum does not transilluminate equally with the left.

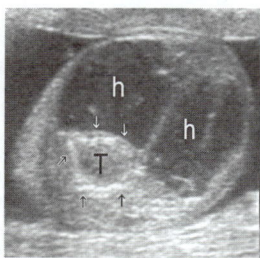

Testicular torsion in a newborn with discoloration of the right testicle at birth. Longitudinal US scan shows the testis (T) surrounded by a highly echogenic tunica (arrows), which is probably calcified. A complex hydrocele (h) with several septa occupies the scrotal sac.

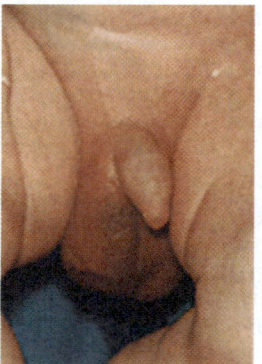

Scrotal bruising due to idiopathic haemorrhage in a 3 day old infant. A similar appearance can follow a difficult breech delivery, although the swelling usually affects both sides and cutaneous bruising may be more prominent. Most cases resolve spontaneously, but progress should be monitored. Spontaneous idiopathic scrotal haemorrhage has been reported in normally delivered infants, though they are usually large for their gestational age. Although the clinical features are similar to those of a torsion, one sign to distinguish idiopathic haemorrhage is a small but separate bruise over the superficial inguinal ring.

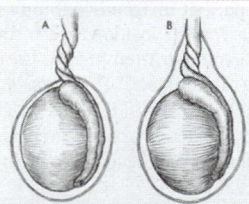

Testicular torsion: (A) extravaginal; (B) intravaginal.

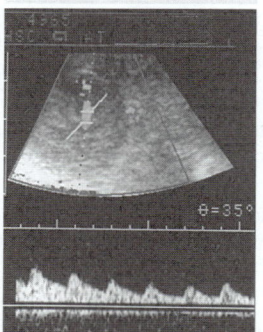

Power Doppler sonogram of right testicle, transverse plane. Power Doppler sonographic signal (*arrow*) was obtained in the central portion of the testicle, although none had been obtained using routine color Doppler sonography. **B,** Power Doppler sonogram with spectral tracing of right testicle, transverse plane. An arterial waveform was obtained from the insonated central testicular vessel.

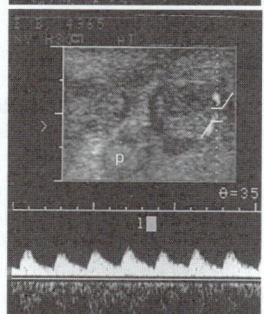

Power Doppler sonogram with spectral tracing of left testicle, transverse plane. No central flow was seen in the left testicle; only peripheral flow was observed. The spectral pattern proves this flow to be arterial. p, Penis.

MYELOMENINGOCELE

Myelomeningocele remains the most complex congenital malformation of the central nervous system that is compatible with life. This lesion results when the neural tube fails to fold normally during postovulatory Days 21 to 27. **Myelomeningocele** is a condition in which the spinal cord and nerve roots herniate into a sac comprising the meninges. This sac protrudes through the bone and musculocutaneous defect. The spinal cord often ends in this sac, in which it is splayed open, exposing the central canal. The splayed-open neural structure is called the neural placode. Certain neurologic anomalies, such as hydrocephalus and Chiari II malformation, accompany myelomeningocele. In addition, myelomeningoceles have a higher incidence of associated intestinal, cardiac, and esophageal malformations, as well as renal and urogenital anomalies. Most neonates with myelomeningocele have orthopedic anomalies of their lower extremities and urogenital anomalies due to involvement of the sacral nerve roots. A **Meningocele** is simply herniation of the meninges through the bony defect (spina bifida). The spinal cord and nerve roots do not herniate into this dorsal dural sac. These lesions are important to differentiate from myelomeningocele because their treatment and prognosis are so different from myelomeningocele. Neonates with a meningocele usually have normal findings upon physical examination and a covered (closed) dural sac. Neonates with meningocele do not have associated neurologic malformations such as hydrocephalus or Chiari II. A subtype of spina bifida is called **lipomeningocele, or lipomyelomeningocele,** which is a common form of neural tube defect treated by pediatric neurosurgeons. These lesions have a lipomatous mass that herniates through the bony defect and attaches to the spinal cord, tethering the cord and often the associated nerve roots. The lipomyelomeningocele can envelop both dorsal and ventral nerve roots, only the dorsal nerve roots, or simply the filum terminale and conus medullaris. These lesions do not have associated hydrocephalus but have a more guarded prognosis than simple meningoceles. The surgical correction of these lesions is more complex, and the retethering rate, in which an additional surgery is required, is as high as 20% in some series. In a third, rare type of **Spina bifida cystica called myelocystocele,** the spinal cord has a large terminal cystic dilatation resulting from hydromyelia. The posterior wall of the spinal cord is often attached to the skin (ectoderm) and is undifferentiated, thus giving rise to a large terminal skin-covered sac. The vast majority of the lesions are dorsal, although a small minority (approximately 0.5%) are ventral in location. The most common ventral variant is an anterior sacral meningocele, which is most often discovered in females as a pelvic mass. **Spina bifida occulta** In this group of neural tube defects, the meninges do not herniate through the bony defect. This lesion is covered by skin (i.e., closed), therefore rendering the underlying neurologic involvement occult or hidden. These patients do not have associated hydrocephalus or Chiari II malformations. Often, a skin lesion such as a hairy patch, dermal sinus tract, dimple, hemangioma, or lipoma points to the underlying spina bifida and neurologic abnormality present in the thoracic, lumbar, or sacral region. Presence of these cutaneous stigmata above the gluteal fold signifies the presence of an occult spinal lesion. Dimples below the gluteal fold signify a benign, nonneurologic finding such as a pilonidal sinus. This is an important point for differentiating the lesions that have neurologic involvement from those that do not. An experienced pediatrician or surgeon should examine any neonate with cutaneous stigmata on the back around the gluteus. *A good rule of thumb is that a lesion (eg, pit, tract) below the gluteal crease is often a pilonidal sinus and needs no further evaluation. Those tracts, pits, or lesions above the gluteal fold should be evaluated further.* Lesions that are questionable can be scanned with ultrasonography in a neonate or with MRI in an older child. Ultrasonography or MRI delineates the presence or absence of a tethered cord or other spinal anomaly. Plain radiology can reveal a panoply of anomalies, such as fused vertebrae, midline defects, bony spurs, or abnormal laminae. An MRI is often useful in evaluating for a split cord malformation (i.e., diastematomyelia), in which a bony spur splits the spinal cord, or a duplication of the spinal cord and nerve roots (diplomyelia). More commonly, the neurosurgeon is searching for tethering of the spinal cord by a sinus tract or thickened filum that can cause traction on the spinal cord with subsequent neurologic deficits as the child grows. A growing body of evidence indicates that the surgical repair of these lesions is more effective when performed prophylactically. Once the patient experiences a significant neurologic deficit, such as a neurogenic bladder or leg weakness, from these occult spinal lesions, the surgical remedy may not return the patient to the baseline neurologic status.

Detailed clinical examination is required to assess · site and level of lesion · motor and sensory level · presence of clinical hydrocephalus · presence of hindbrain herniation e.g. stridor, apnoea, swallowing difficulty · presence of musculoskeletal deformity or anomalies of other organ systems . **Management:** Infants need referral and transport to a neonatal centre for assessment by a co ordinated team of specialists experienced in dealing with these lesions so that a treatment policy can be discussed with the parents. Before and during transport · the lesion, especially if ruptured, should be covered with a sterile non-adherent dressing · the infant should be nursed in the prone position and the defect protected e.g. by foam rubber cut into a doughnut. IV access is required to provide antibiotics e.g. Penicillin and Gentamicin (preferably after blood is taken for culture). IV fluids are required if an excessive delay before oral feeds can commence is anticipated, respiratory difficulty or hypoglycemia is present. *Fetal surgery to close the defect and thus possibly reduce the incidence of hydrocephalus and long term neurological complications remains experimental.* Cesarean section before the onset of labor is usually the desired mode of delivery since this has been associated with improved neurological outcomes. *The multidisciplinary team is critical to the ultimate success and long-term management of these patients. The initial closure is just the beginning of the medical care that these children will require. An integrated team of neurosurgeons, orthopedists, urologists, physiatrists, therapists, and nurses is important to long-term care. Children born with myelomeningocele have the opportunity to live normal, healthy, and productive lives in the majority of cases.* Consistent and frequent long-term medical follow up is essential to achieving this goal.

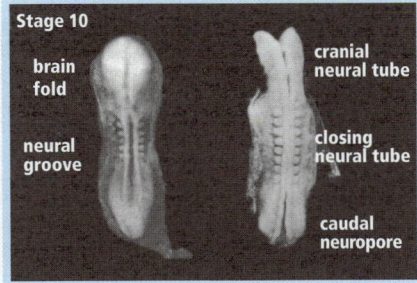

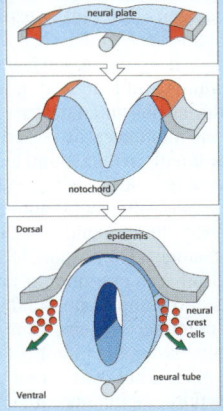

Research over the last 20 years has suggested a relationship between maternal diet and the birth of an affected infant, and recent evidence has confirmed that folic acid, a water soluble vitamin, found in many fruits (particularly oranges, berries and bananas), leafy green vegetables, cereals and legumes, may prevent the majority of neural tube defects.

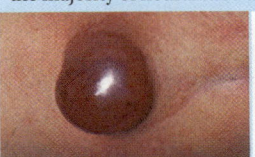 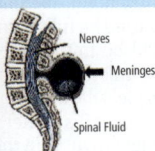

Meningocele: In this condition we have a defect in the posterior vertebra arches with protrusion of the neural covering to the surface of the skin. The lesion appears as a cystic lesion covered with a thin membrane. The lesion contains cerebrospinal fluid but no neural elements. Occasionally the lesion is covered with normal skin. Clinical examination reveals no neurological deficits and x-ray of the spine shows a defect in the posterior arches of the vertebral column. These cases are managed by excision of the sac and watertight closure of the neural covering. This is followed by closure of the overlying muscles and skin.

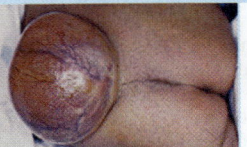 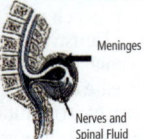

The lumbar region of a newborn baby with **Myelomeningocele.** In these cases there is herniation of neural elements to skin surface. The lesion appears as a mass covered by thin and occasionally transparent membrane, which is false dura, and within the sac there is cerebrospinal fluid and either part of the spinal cord or spinal nerve roots.

CLEFT LIP AND CLEFT PALATE

Cleft lip and cleft palate (CL/CP) are the most commonly occurring craniofacial birth defects. Although some CL/CPs are detected on prenatal ultrasound, the majority are immediately recognized in the delivery room. Parents will be anxious about what the future may hold for their child. The way the news is delivered will influence how the family understands, responds, and ultimately copes with the challenge of parenting an infant with CL/CP. An understanding of the etiology of CL/CP is important and will assist the clinician in performing a focused history and risk analysis. Review the infant's family history carefully, identifying any other family members who have an isolated CL, isolated CP, or CL with CP. Note the infant's relationship to affected family members. A history of 2 or more affected family members may suggest a syndromic cleft. Explore the severity and nature of the anomaly and the racial and ethnic background of the family. Identify antenatal exposures to potential teratogens. Specifically, explore the use of prescribed medications, recreational substances, tobacco, and alcohol, noting the timing, duration, and dose of each exposure. Review the use of protective agents, such as prenatal vitamins and folic acid, prior to conception and throughout the pregnancy. Review the antenatal care including the timing of ultrasounds, if performed, the anomalies visualized (if any), and the growth status of the fetus. Improvements in ultrasound technology have led to detection of CL as early as 13 weeks gestation, using level II high-resolution vaginal ultrasound. Three-dimensional ultrasound allows even better examination of the fetal face and displays abnormalities accurately and clearly. Perform a Focused Physical Assessment- The purpose of a systematic physical assessment in the newborn period is to examine for any anomalies, establish a baseline for observations and comparisons, and initiate referrals for continued care of identified or potential problems. Complete a systematic head-to-toe physical examination to assess the infant for other malformations. Other minor or major anomalies, when associated with an isolated CP, may indicate an underlying syndrome. Infants with CL/CP have a 10% chance of having an associated syndrome. With a CL, it is imperative that this systematic examination be completed before a feeding, due to the potential presence of a CP. Observe the infant's face, looking for symmetry of the eyes, nose, and mouth when the infant is both quiet and crying. Note atypical features and evaluate for asymmetry of features or movement. Assess the spacing of the eyes and the width of the nasal bridge. When evaluating the mouth, note the length of the philtrum and size of the mouth, tongue, and jaw. The mouth should be in the midline of the face and appear symmetrical in shape and movement. It should be in proportion with the tongue and chin. The lips should be fully formed, continuous, and without scars or irregularities. A CL will be immediately apparent; clefts can range from a small niche to a complete separation that extends upward into the floor of the nose. Visually inspect the infant's palate; use a light and maneuvers that encourage the infant to open his or her mouth. Palpate the hard and soft palates with a gloved finger to rule out the presence of a hard or soft palate cleft. Assess the infant's suck; note the pattern, coordination, and strength of propulsion. The strength of the suck depends on the infant's gestational age and environmental state. Assess for the presence or absence of a gag reflex. If the infant has been fed, obtain a complete feeding history, focusing on feeding interest, vigor, and coordination of suck and swallow. Note reports of choking episodes that may suggest a CP. Observing the infant during a feeding provides excellent insight into feeding tolerance and effectiveness. The treatment for CL is surgical closure and reconstruction. If both CL and CP are present, the CL is typically closed at 3 months of age, as long as the child is free of infection and no other complications are present. The goals for surgery of the CL are: · Continuity of the muscle · Symmetry of the floor and sil of the nostril · Natural appearance of the Cupid's bow · Minimal scarring. The 2 most common surgical techniques for CL repair are the Tennison-Randall triangular flap and the Millard rotational advanced technique. Most surgeons agree that operative repair of the palate should occur before the child reaches 18 months of age and speech patterns have been established. The goals of palatal surgery are to: · Construct a symmetrical nose with open, functional nostrils; · Create alveolar integrity of the cleft area; · Minimize growth retardation of the maxilla; · Create an intact palate that will support normal speech development. The birth of an infant with CL/CP is an emotional time for parents who must face the loss of the perfect child. Parents deserve immediate, accurate, and complete information regarding the etiology, treatment options, and the long-term prognosis of their infant. Sucking for children with a cleft palate is difficult because of the poorly formed roof of the mouth The infant should be held in an upright position to help keep the food from coming out of the nose Small, frequent feedings are recommended. Water should be used to end feeding as it will facilitate cleaning of the cleft (Semmler & Hunter, 1990). Efficient and safe feeding should be the goal when selecting feeding methods for infants with cleft lip and palate.

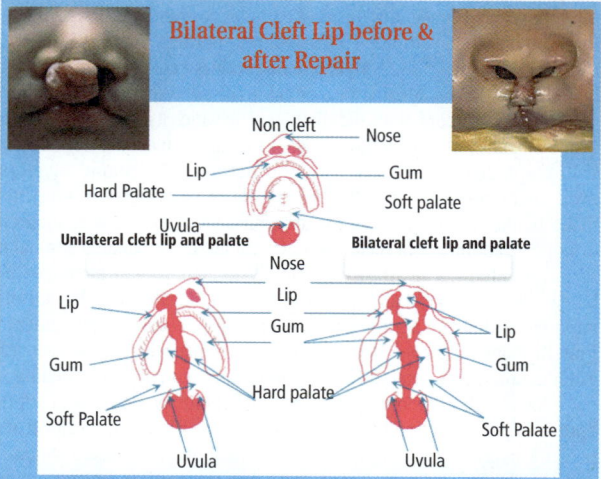

Bilateral Cleft Lip before & after Repair

Supplemental feedings should be considered if feeding is not completed in 20 to 30 minutes as this may lead to loss of calories and energy (Glass & Wolf, 1999). Haberman Feeder® This is a specially designed bottle system with a valve to help control the air the baby drinks and to prevent milk from going back into the bottle. Syringes: These may be used in hospitals following cleft surgery and may also be used at home. Typically, a soft, rubber tube is attached on the end of the syringe, which is then placed in the infant's mouth.

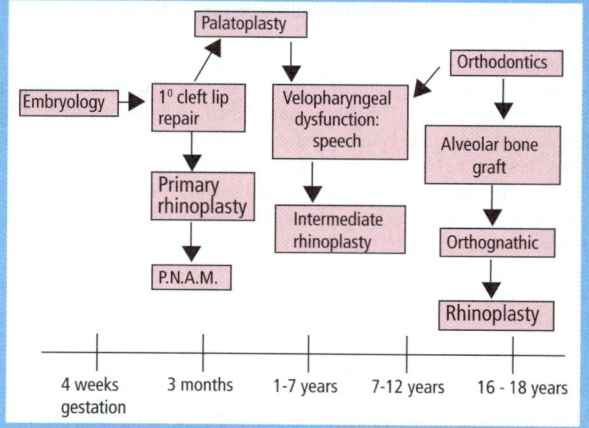

Type	Definition	Examples
Unilateral Cleft	Cleft occurs on 1 side of the face. It is important to document which side is involved	
Bilateral Cleft	Cleft occurs on both sides of the face	
Incomplete	Only the lip and anterior part of maxilla are involved.	
Complete Cleft Lip and Palate	Cleft involves the lip, the hard and soft palate, and thea anterior part of the maxilla.	

INTUSSUSCEPTION

Intussusception, a common gastrointestinal (GI) emergency in children, develops when a proximal segment of the gastrointestinal tract (intussusceptum) telescopes into a distal portion (intussuscipiens), most commonly located near the ileocecal valve. Its incidence is highest between 5 and 9 months of age with a male predominance of 3:2. , being uncommon in neonates. The majority of pediatric cases involve the ileocolic (or ileocecal) portion of the intestine. The most common location of idiopathic intussusception is at the hepatic flexure. When the intussusceptum invaginates and pulls along the mesentery, there is compromise of venous return. This is followed by engorgement of the intussusceptum, edema and bleeding from the mucosa which lead to currant jelly stools. Finally the arterial blood supply of the intestine gets compromised leading to necrosis, perforation and/or shock. Children less than 3 months and greater than 2 years old are most likely to have a "lead point" or specific identified cause, such as (in decreasing order of incidence): meckel diverticulum, duplications, polyposis and lymphomas. Hyperplasia of the intestinal Peyer's patches have been identified as the leading point in infant cases. Most cases are reported during summer and spring which favor a not fully understood infectious mechanism. Peyer's patches hyperplasia can occur secondary to viruses such as adenovirus, enterovirus, echovirus and human herpes virus 6. The most common surgical complication of patients with Henoch Schönlein Purpura is intussusception. Its incidence is also increased in the postoperative period probably due to edema or adhesions. *The typical triad of severe intermittent abdominal pain, currant jelly stools and vomiting is seen in less than 20% of cases.* Bouts of abdominal pain may be evidenced by pulling of knees against the abdomen with an interim asymptomatic healthy child. In ileocolic intussusception palpation of the abdomen may reveal a sausage-shaped mass which is located in the RUQ. A wide spectrum of symptoms may range from painless intussusception to constipation, dehydration, diarrhea, intestinal prolapse, rectal bleeding, sepsis, shock, syncope, vomiting and altered mental status (lethargy and irritability). Lethargy is seen most frequent in infants and young children with or without history of gastrointestinal symptoms. Altered mental status has been hypothesized to be secondary to a combination of factors such as dehydration, electrolyte imbalance, and endorphins or toxic metabolic products released from the ischemic bowel which can affect the brain. Recurrent intussusception is present in only 5-8% of children and is most common after hydrostatic versus surgical reduction. Fifty percent of recurrent intussusception cases occur within 48 hours of a prior episode (but have been reported up to 18 months later). Most postoperative intussusception cases are located in the small bowel. **Plain abdominal films** (supine frontal and left lateral decubitus) are the first imaging studies used in the ED. However, they lack sensitivity (45%) and may give many false negatives. Classic intussusception radiological signs are: Absence of air in the ascending colon (RUQ and RLQ). Soft tissue density in the upper abdomen (up to 60% of patients). Small bowel obstruction signs: small bowel dilation, air fluid levels. *Target sign:* 2 concentric lines seen in RUQ which corresponds with mesenteric fat of intussusceptum. *Crescent Sign:* Semilunar lucency seen within course of colon and corresponds to air trapping between 2 intestinal surfaces. **Ultrasound** is a fast, non-invasive and simple reproducible test. It's sensitivity (98-100%) and specificity (88–100%) is high, but is clearly operator dependant. At some centers it has displaced radiographs as the initial imaging test of choice. Other indications for its use are: suspected cases of intussusception where abdominal x-rays are non-conclusive, evaluation for reducibility, presence of a lead point mass, potential incomplete reduction after enema and intussusception limited to small bowel. Classic findings include: the *target lesion or doughnut sign* on transverse imaging and the *pseudokidney sign* on longitudinal imaging. **Computed tomography (CT) scan** is usually not indicated in children, since the diagnosis is generally confirmed by ultrasound or enema. The CT scan involves high costs, radiation exposure and sedation risk which is overall less convenient for this population group. Contrast enemas (barium, water-soluble and air) are diagnostic and therapeutic techniques, with reduction rates of 70 to 90%. **Barium enema** is no longer considered the gold standard for non-surgical treatment, though its use is still extensive. Risks with barium enema such as shock and bowel perforation (secondary peritonitis, infection and adhesions) should never be overlooked. This test should be considered only after stabilizing the child, adequate hydration, and consultation with a pediatric surgeon. The only current absolute contraindication for barium enema is full bowel necrosis. Air enema's use has increased due to its lower perforation risk, less radiation exposure, faster and better reduction rate. One study compared air vs. contrast enema reporting success rates of 76% and 63% respectively. Intussusception recurrence rates for air versus liquid enema are reported to be similar, approximately 10%. **Air enema** is now considered the gold standard treatment of intussusception in children. Surgical intervention is needed only in unstable patients with non-operative reduction contraindications or in prior unsuccessful reduction attempts. Barium enemas should be avoided in children with evidence of peritonitis, severe shock, sepsis, perforation or extreme ages. Enema reduction should be attempted 3 times at the most before considering it unsuccessful and submitting the patient to surgery. Poor enema reduction rate is determined by (in descending order): symptoms longer than 24 hours, age less than 3 months, dehydration and intussusception of the rectum. Repeat enema is both safe and effective in recurrent intussusception. Spontaneous reduction occurs in approximately 10–17% of patients, being most common in the small bowel. Clinical suspicion is the key factor in making a diagnosis of intussusception and should be considered by the ED physician even in absence of typical signs and symptoms.

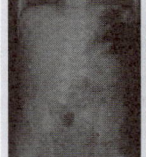 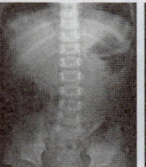 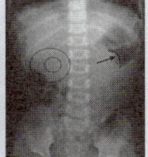

Absence of air in the ascending colon Target sign and crescent sign

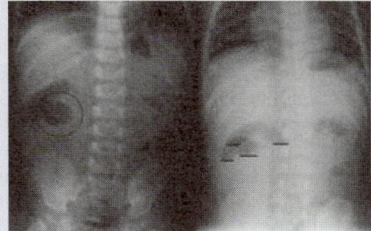

Small bowel obstruction signs: left: small bowel dilation (smooth bowel walls) and right: few air fluid levels.

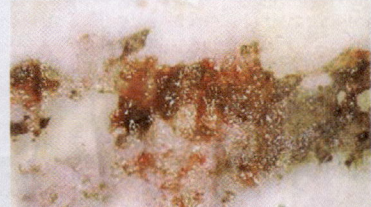

Bloody mucoid stool(the currant jelly stool in 60%)

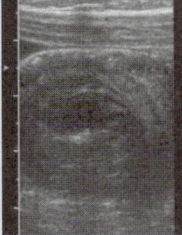

Ultrasound image of target sign

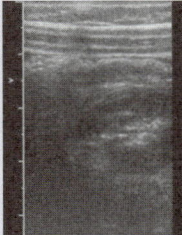

Ultrasound image of pseudo-kidney sign

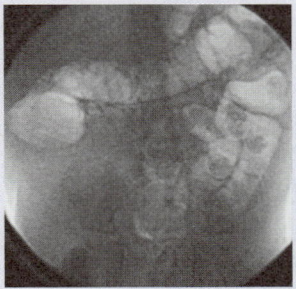

Air enema with intussusception near the hepatic flexure. Coiled spring appearance which corresponds with barium in lumen of intussusceptum.

Courtesy: Carol Pineda MD & Madhu Hardasmalani MD Division of Pediatric Emergency Department St Joseph's Children's Hospital Paterson, NJ The Internet Journal of Pediatrics and Neonatology™ ISSN: 1528-8374

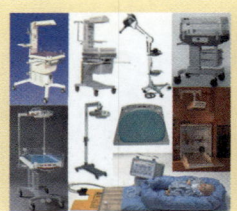 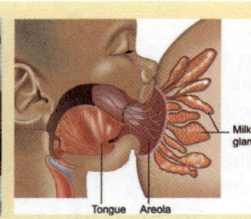 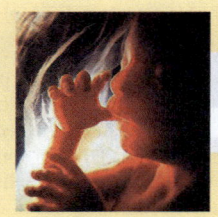

Section II

ESSENTIAL NEONATAL CLINICAL GUIDELINES

A **medical guideline** (also called a **clinical guideline**, **clinical protocol** or **clinical practice guideline**) is a document with the aim of guiding decisions and criteria regarding diagnosis, management, and treatment in specific areas of healthcare. In contrast to previous approaches, which were often based on tradition or authority, modern medical guidelines are based on an examination of current evidence within the paradigm of evidence-based medicine. They usually include summarized consensus statements, but unlike the latter, they also address practical issues. Modern clinical guidelines briefly identify, summarize and evaluate the best evidence and most current data about prevention, diagnosis, prognosis, therapy including dosage of medications, risk/benefit and cost-effectiveness. Additional objectives of clinical guidelines are to standardize medical care, to raise quality of care, to reduce several kinds of risk (to the patient, to the healthcare provider, to medical insurers and health plans) and to achieve the best balance between cost and medical parameters such as effectiveness, specificity, sensitivity, resoluteness, etc. It has been demonstrated repeatedly that the use of guidelines by healthcare providers such as hospitals is an effective way of achieving the objectives listed above, although they are not the only ones. The Essential Clinical Guidelines are intended to cover common situations and are not meant to be encyclopedic. Providers need to consider their *personal level of comfort and expertise as well as their NICU practice setting* when evaluating and managing difficult and more complex case scenarios. If significant components of the process cannot be accomplished in the primary/secondary care setting, referral should be made to a Tertiary Sub-Specialist/Higher Referral Center. It is not the intention in promulgating these guidelines to interfere with the provider/patient relationship, nor are these guidelines intended to represent the standard of care in any given circumstance. These guidelines are recommendations to be used at the sole discretion of the provider and are not meant to dictate the manner or style of clinical practice employed in rendering services to a particular patient.

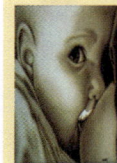 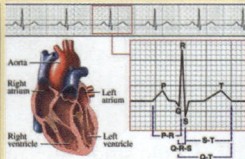 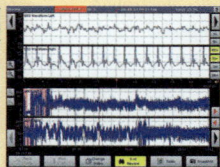 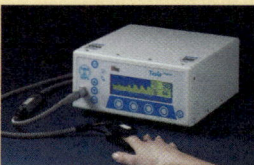 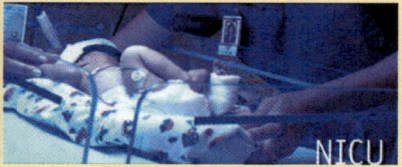

CONTENTS

CONTENTS

SELF ASSESSMENT REVIEW OF ESSENTIAL NEONATAL CLINICAL GUIDELINES

1. Which of the following is *not to be followed* , if you want to reduce/avoid pitfalls during Neonatal Resuscitation?

   a)Strictly follow the guidelines of the NRP. **b)** Mock codes with manikins should be used to maintain resuscitation skills. c)Avoid hypoglycemia during the postresuscitation stabilization period. **d)**Capnography and colorimetric CO_2 monitors should be used to document that the endotracheal tube is in the trachea. e)Unlimited number of individuals who serve as the team leader of Newborn resuscitations.

2. All of the following are the Contraindications to Breast Feeding, *except..,* **a)**Chemotherapy with cytotoxic drugs, such as cyclophosphamide,methotrexate, or doxorubicin **b)** Galactosemia in the infant c)Herpes simplex active breast lesions d) Maternal HIV infection in a poor illiterate mother from a developing country e)**Active** untreated Tuberculosis in mother.

3. All of the following statements about Fetal-Neonatal Circulation are correct, *except..,*

   a)Deoxygenated fetal blood is conducted to the placenta via the two umbilical arteries. **b)** Oxygenated blood from the placenta passes through the single umbilical vein and enters the inferior vena cava (IVC). c)Fetal Blood flowing through the foramen ovale and into left atrium passes into the left ventricle where it is ejected into the ascending aorta. This relatively oxygen rich blood passes predominantly to the head and upper extremities.d)Postnatal (Neonatal)circulation is Parallel, and the Fetal circulation is Series in nature e)Postnatally,The ductus arteriosus constricts due to the high partial pressure of oxygen. The process is usually complete within 2 days after birth.

4. All of the following factors will shift the Oxyhemoglobin dissociation curve to left, causing increasing affinity of Hb toward oxygen with consequently poor tissue release of oxygen *except..,*

   a)Low Carbon Monoxide (pCO) **b)**Hypothermia **c)**Hypocarbia d)Alkalosis e) Fetal Hemoglobin.

5. The Factors needed in the palliative care of extremely preterm infants should include all *except..,*
   a)Warmth b)Dignity c)Nil Privacy d)Pain relief e)Human contact

6. All of the following statements about a Newlyborn infant are correct *except..,*
   a)Approximately 70% of normal Newborn infants excrete meconium during the 1st 24hrs, & 95% of infants pass atleast one stool within 24hrs.b)Approximately 2/3rds of Newborn infants urinate within 12hrs of birth, & virtually all Newborn infants have voided atleast once within 24hrs. c)Jaundice after 1st 24hr may be "physiologic" or may be due to septicemia, hemolytic anemia, galactosemia, hepatitis, congenital biliary atresia, inspissated bile syndrome after E.fetalis, syphilis, herpes simplex, or other congenital infections. d)Mottling, an example of general circulatory instability, may be associated with serious illness or related to a transient fluctuation in skin temperature. e) PERSISTENT TACHYPNEA, FLARING OF ALAE NASI, GRUNTING, RETRACTIONS & RALES - are *not accepted* as normal events during the 1st period of reactivity.

7. All of the following Congenital Anomalies are associated with Maternal Polyhydramnios, except..,
   a)Omphalocele b)Potter syndrome c)Tracheoesophageal fistula d)Anencephalus e)Duodenal atresia

8. All of the following Suggestions for "Breaking Bad News" in the NICU, With Skill and Empathy are essential *except..,*

   a)Use trained translators as needed b)Start telling a lone parent without his or her spouse and/or a preferred support person present c)Enable the parents to touch the deceased child before or during the interview d)Hold or touch the child with obvious care e)Recognize that parents are primarily responsible for their child.

9. All of the following indicate the good adaptive Parental responses to the Stress of their baby`s NICU Admission, except..,
   a)Frequent visits and calls **b)** Development of comfortable interaction with infant during hospitalization c) Confidence in assuming total responsibility for infant d) Debilitating preoccupation with infant's condition e)Realistic view of infant and potential needs at time of discharge

10. All of the following issues are essential in maintaining "Good Practice in Handover" when a shift changes take place except..,

    a)Each NICU needs to identify the relevant staff who need to attend. The ideal model includes all grades of staff from each specialty or ward. The senior nurse and/or ANNPs should be present. **b)** The room should be free from distraction and not used by others at that time. Access to results, x-rays and telephones should be available. c) Attendance at handover should take priority over all other work *except emergencies.* d)Handover will not be needed at each change of shift. e)Daily involvement of senior clinicians is essential, to ensure that appropriate level management decisions are made and also to convey the seriousness with which the organization takes the process.

11. Absolute Contraindications to early Newborn discharge include all except:
    a)Jaundice at < 24 hours **b)**Mother treated with antibiotics in labor for GBS prophylaxis/UTI c)Known or suspected narcotic addiction or withdrawal d)Birth weight < 2500 g e)Oral defects (clefts, micrognathia).

12. All of the following statements are correct about the limitations of APGAR Scores, except..,
    a)It is appropriate to use an Apgar score alone to establish the diagnosis of asphyxia. **b)** The incidence of low Apgar scores is inversely related to birth weight, and a low score is limited in predicting morbidity or mortality. c)Elements of the score such as tone, color, and reflex irritability partially depend on the physiologic maturity of the infant.d)The healthy preterm infant with no evidence of asphyxia may receive a low score only because of immaturity. e)A number of factors may influence an Apgar score, including but not limited to drugs, trauma, congenital anomalies, infections, hypoxia, hypovolemia, and preterm birth.

13. Whilst Communicating with Parents following Perinatal death, you should say to grief-stricken parents/relatives all of the following things except..,
    a)"Cry when you feel like crying". **b)**"Do you have any questions?" c)"You can have more children" d) "We can talk again later" e) "I feel sad" or "I am sad for you"

14. Regarding Postnatal Weight loss/gain of a Neonate all of the following statements are correct, except..,

    a)Typical Postnatal Weight loss in a Term infant is 5-10% of Birth weight and in a Preterm infant it will be 15% of birth weight. **b)**The Clinician's goal is to limit the degree and duration of initial weight loss in preterms and to facilitate regain of birth weight within 21-28 days of life. c)The nadir in Weight loss usually occurs by 4-6 days of life, with birth weight regained by 14-21 days of life.d) After achieving birth weight, the goals of: 10-20 g/kg/day weight gain (15–20 g/kg/day for infants <1,500 g), approximately 1 cm/week in length, and 0.5-1 cm/week in head circumference) Excess Weight gain (> 50 g/day) indicates either Catch-up growth in a healthy baby or excess fluid retention in a sick baby secondary to cardiac (PDA) & renal failure, SIADH, Chronic lung disease etc.

15. All of the following are well recognized *Advantages* of Gastro-intestinal Priming with Minimal Enteral Nutrition except..,

    a)Shortens time to regain birth weight b) Enhances enzyme maturation c)Improves feeding tolerance d)Improves gastrointestinal motility e)Has no effect on mineral absorption, mineralization.

16. All of the following clinical factors increase the Insensible water loss in a critically ill Neonate, except..,

a) Increased skin permeability at birth b) Increased BSA to weight ratio c) Phototherapy d) Radiant warmer bed e) Humidified Incubators.

17. All of the following are acute consequences of Untreated Pain in Neonates, except..,

a) Periventricular Intraventricular hemorrhage b) Increased chemical and hormone release c) Breakdown of fat and carbohydrate stores d) Prolonged hypoglycemia e) Higher morbidity for NICU patients.

18. All of the following risk factors are important in the etiology of Developmental Dysplasia of Hips, except..,

a) Breech birth b) Polyhydramnios c) Cesar for breech d) Infants with phenylketonuria e) Postmaturity.

19. All of the following Pitfalls about Pulse Oximetry are described correctly, except..,

a) Pulse Oximetry doesn't detect CO_2 levels, so has limitation in the assessment of the patient with respiratory failure due to CO_2 retention {type II respiratory failure} b) It gives erroneous information if patient is poorly perfused E.g.: - hypothermia, shock, cardiac failure and some cardiac arrhythmias and in severe anemia {Hb < 5 gms/dL}. c) It gives falsely low reading, if carboxyhemo-globin or methemoglobin are present in the blood in elevated levels d) Excessive patient movement and shivering can give false readings {since the sensor must identify every pulse beat to calculate the SaO_2, movement can interfere with sensing} e) IV dyes such as methylene blue, indigocarmine and indocyanine also give false readings ; however the readings are not affected by jaundice, and anemia {except if hemoglobin < 5gms/dL as mentioned above}.

20. Surfactant Production is increased by all of the following factors except..,

a) Cold stress (<35°C) b) Maternal PIH c) Maternal Opiate addiction) d) A/N Corticosteroids e) PROM

21. The Different Ways to increase MAP of a conventional Mechanical ventilator include all except..,

a) Increase inspiratory flow rate, producing a square-wave inspiratory pattern; b) Increase PIP c) Reverse the inspiratory-expiratory (I/E) ratio or prolong the inspiratory time without changing the rate; d) Decrease the PEEP e) Increase ventilatory rate by reducing expiratory time without changing the inspiratory time.

22. Explicit consent recommended : (Whenever explicit consent is obtained, whether verbal or signed, this should be recorded in the notes.) in all of the following Neonatal investigations, interventions and treatments except..,

a) Clinical photographs and video-recordings b) ROP screening c) Genetic testing (incl. karyotype) d) MRI / CT with or without contrast e) Treatment for ROP.

SELF ASSESSMENT REVIEW OF ESSENTIAL NEONATAL CLINICAL GUIDELINES : ANSWERS

1. e) To avoid pitfalls during Neonatal Resuscitation, One should *limit the number of individuals* who serve as the team leader of Newborn resuscitations. Hospital should consider using Neonatologists, hospitalists, nurse practitioners, respiratory therapists, or nurses to serve as the skilled team leader. Refer to Essential Clinical Guidelines 10.2. for details.(PITFALLS IN COMMON NEONATAL PROBLEMS).

2. d) Refer to Essential Clinical Guidelines 13 for details.(Essentials of breast feeding).

3. d) Fetal Circulation is *Parallel*, in contrast to Postnatal *Series* Circulation. Refer to Essential Clinical Guidelines 21.14 for details.(It Pays To Know the Essential Differences Between....,).

4. a) Refer to Essential Clinical Guidelines 21.16 for details.(It Pays To Know the Essential Differences Between....,).

5. c) The parents can spend time with their baby, and should be aware that their baby may show signs of life, such as occasional gasps, after birth. Privacy and sensitive support for parents and family with subsequent follow up are essential. Refer to Essential Clinical Guidelines 7 for details.(PERINATAL MANAGEMENT AT THE THRESHOLD OF VIABILITY).

6. e) Refer to Essential Clinical Guidelines 12 for details.(ALERTING AND/OR ALARMING NEONATAL SYMPTOMS).

7. b) Refer to Essential Clinical Guidelines 12 for details.(ALERTING AND/OR ALARMING NEONATAL SYMPTOMS).

8. b) Refer to Essential Clinical Guidelines 8 for details.(How to Break Bad News in the NICU ?).

9. d) Refer to Essential Clinical Guidelines 5 for details.(How to Support the Stressful Parents of a Neonate admitted in the NICU?).

10. d) Refer to Essential Clinical Guidelines 23 for details.(Good Practice in Handover).

11. d) Refer to Essential Clinical Guidelines 30 for details. (DISCHARGE AND FOLLOW-UP OF NICU PATIENTS).

12. a) Refer to Essential Clinical Guidelines 32 for details.(APGAR SCORING SYSTEM).

13. c) Refer to Essential Clinical Guidelines 34 for details.(DEATH OF A NEONATE IN THE NICU OR AT HOME).

14. b) Refer to Essential Clinical Guidelines 50 for details. (MONITORING

15. e) Refer to Essential Clinical Guidelines No. 55 for details.(GUT PRIMING/TROPHIC FEEDING/MINIMAL ENTERAL NUTRITION).

16. e) Refer to Essential Clinical Guidelines No. 56 for details.(TOTAL PARENTERAL NUTRITION-TPN).

17. d) Refer to Essential Clinical Guidelines No. 57 for details.(RECOGNITION AND MANAGEMENT OF PAIN IN NEONATES).

18. d) Refer to Essential Clinical Guidelines No. 70 for details. (Developmental Dysplasia of the Hip (DDH)).

19. c) Refer to Essential Clinical Guidelines No. 76 for details. (PULSE OXIMETRY (5th VITAL SIGN)).

20. a) Refer to Essential Clinical Guidelines No. 83 for details. (SURFACTANT- REPLACEMENT THERAPY FOR RESPIRATORY DISTRESS IN THE PRETERM AND TERM NEONATE).

21. d) Refer to Essential Clinical Guidelines No. 84 for details. (The ABC`s of Conventional Mechanical Ventilation).

22. b) Refer to Essential Clinical Guidelines No. 99 for details. (CONSENT FOR COMMON NEONATAL INVESTIGATIONS, INTERVENTIONS AND TREATMENTS).

NICU SURVIVAL TIPS FOR A RESIDENT DOCTOR

 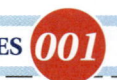
1. While you are the doctor, in general the nurses know more about nursing, the nutritionists know more about nutrition, and the respiratory therapists know more about ventilators than we do. *Please listen to them and use their expertise to learn.* Do not be afraid to ask them for help if you are at a loss for what to do. You can learn a lot of tricks and practical stuff. They know more than you can read desperately searching thick neonatology books for different problems.

2. Take ownership of your patients, think about them critically and come up with your own plan. The attendings will listen to what you have to say and help you fine tune it. *The more you think about your patients, the more you will learn.*

3. Be confident. You have graduated from medical school and are bright. *Nurses respect a confident but not cocky resident.* They are sometimes reluctant to listen to a resident that is weak and timid in their decision making. Learning to strike a balance between these two will be one of the most important lessons you will learn initially.

4. You are now a physician in the Neonatalogy / Pediatrics department, and you have an important role to fill. *You are no longer a student that should be worried about what you could be pimped about, what your grade will be or when you will be able to study for the shelf exam.* You are not getting graded but you are constantly being evaluated, both formally and informally. You will receive feedback on your performance rather than a grade for your work.

5. So now that you are here, relax and approach residency with a team attitude. *Take care of your patients, but reach out and help your fellow interns.* Help each other with admits, orders, lab followups, and phone calls, because in the end we all like to get home at a reasonable time. Also, be able to rely on each other to take care of your patients when you sign out. You will need to work hard when you're here, but be able to leave the hospital when it's time.

6. You are now part of a team that cares for patients. You have many resources at your hands including nursing, social work, dietetics, PT, OT, wound care, child life, subspecialists, and many others. *Don't be afraid to use these services as they will help tailor an individual plan for each of your patients.*

7. You have heard many times from many people to be nice to nurses. They are an integral part of the medical team and your relationships with them can greatly impact your experience as a resident. Now that you are a physician, you will interact with them differently than when you were a medical student. Ideally, it is a relationship based on mutual respect. You will rely on each other to ensure proper medical care for your patients. *Particularly in the ICUs, the nursing staff knows a great deal about patient management.* Always remember that first impressions are important and to treat others as you would like to be treated.

8. Remember that even though you are a physician, some of them have been in nursing longer than you have been alive. Don't be surprised if during your first code in the ICU, the nurses are running the show. However, remember that your patient is your responsibility. Nurses will often have protocols while you have to worry about the specifics of your patient's case. They may have suggestions for you and the team. At the same time, they appreciate when you explain why you are doing a new treatment or changing a plan. *It will make it easier if everyone is on the same page and understands the plan.*

9. *Remember to stay calm.* Some staff members will panic during seizures, codes, and other unexpected situations. If you are calm, they will be calm and more confident of your abilities. Efficiency-One of the hardest and most important aspects of internship is learning how to become an efficient resident. The key to efficiency is organization, especially during rounds. *Make a to-do list for each patient* as you develop the plan during rounds. This can be written in the cross cover section for each patient on the patient list, on a back page of the list or on a separate page all together, you decide what works for you. After the rounds, discuss what tasks you

want your medical student to take care of and then complete your list in a time sensitive manner. For example, discharge patients first (you can write an order to discharge home once seen by attending if this is approved during rounds), write time sensitive orders, then call remaining consults that your medical student is not. Finally arrange any other studies needed and write remaining orders (next-day labs). If possible, bring order sheets/charts on rounds and write orders for fellow interns as they present their plan. *Plan ahead.* Try to discuss discharge plans when applicable the day before, including follow up appointments and reviewing discharge medications. Find out what prescriptions are needed and try to write them the day before. Instruct the family to have them filled prior to discharge; this will identify any insurance issues that may arise. It is much easier to have it taken care of by social work/discharge planner while the patient is still in the hospital!

10. *Be sure to spend time talking to families.* You will know them best and there is often more to the story than what is initially apparent. They value you as their doctor and will remember your name and what you say. • Communication and unified plans are important. Speaking with all specialists involved in a patient's care is very necessary so that you and the families are on the same page and not frustrated.

More Essential NICU Survival Tips :

1. **Infection control:** Start your day at the unit with the **three minute mandatory scrub-in procedure** every morning. Wash hands or use hand sanitizer between babies to prevent spread of infection. Wear gloves when examining patients. Use stethoscopes provided at bedsides of babies (not your own)

2. **Communication:** Please speak to your specific attending regarding their preference for problem based or systems based notes. If you are called to see a baby for a problem, write a note indicating the problem you were called for, your assessment, and what evaluation and/or therapy was done. Fill out the order sheet first. Let the nurse know about your orders. Do not forget that you have to visit the mother and inform her about the actions taken to stabilize her baby, and then every 1-2 days for updates. Document communication (or attempts) in chart. Primary care providers should be updated prior to discharge for continuity of care.

3. **Procedure note:** Write a procedure note in the chart after completion of any procedure: include procedure, indication, consent obtained, sedation, patient preparation, and complications.

4. **Prevent medication errors:** Observe the 6 rights for administering medications:*Right patient *Right drug *Right dose *Right route*Right time *Right documentation.*Always get the calculation counter-checked by another person and initial it.*

5. **Early PICC (peripherally inserted central catheter):** For any babies you anticipate will need TPN for > 1 week, or who will be working up slowly on feeds, consider a PICC line early (within first 3 days of life). This will increase the chance of success, and save the baby needle sticks.

6. **Be time efficient:** To realize the value of ONE YEAR, ask a student who failed a grade. ..To realize the value of ONE MONTH, ask a mother who gave birth to a premature baby....To realize the value of ONE WEEK, ask the editor of a weekly newspaper....To realize the value of ONE HOUR, ask the lovers who are waiting to meet....To realize the value of ONE MINUTE, ask a person who missed the train...To realize the value of ONE SECOND, ask a person who just avoided an: accident...To realize the value of ONE MILLISECOND, ask the person who won a silver medal in the Olympics. Treasure every moment that you have...during your NICU posting.

References:

1. NICU Survival Guide.pub medicine.mercer.edu/.../files/.../ NICU_Survival_GuideSavannah   2.NICU Survival Guide www.peds.ufl.edu/residency/resources/nicu-survival-guide

NEONATAL MEDICINE GOALS AND OBJECTIVES FOR RESIDENT TRAINING

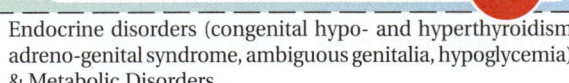

General objectives

@ Obtain a broad understanding of the medical problems afflicting infants during the first month of life.

@ Acquire an understanding of, and appreciation for, prenatal care of high risk patients

@ Learn generally applicable principles in the NICU setting: physiology, ethics, reading, critiquing and applying the medical literature the use of the National Library of Medicine database to access medical literature

Specific objectives: Be adept in neonatal resuscitation procedures and obtain NALS /AAP/AHA certification in neonatal resuscitation (NRP) by the end of the R-1 year. Get materials from attending during your first UW rotation (Newborn or NICU).

@ Accurately obtain a history of pregnancy and perinatal events relevant to the newborn and understand the unique aspects of the physical examination of the premature and newly born full term infant, including gestational age determination and assessment and management of LGA and SGA infants.

@ Understand the broad medical, social, and economic consequences of **prematurity**, including factors related to, or influencing, its incidence and the incidence of disorders unique to premature infants (e.g. lungs, eyes,).

@ Understand the broad medical, social, and economic consequences of **congenital defects** including factors related to, or influencing, its incidence.

@Be familiar with birth weight and gestational age-related neonatal morbidity and mortality statistics and comparisons of perinatal, neonatal and infant mortality rates, regionally, nationally and internationally.

@ Be competent in the assessment and management of the infant in the delivery room with a background knowledge of transitional physiology (cardiopulmonary, metabolic and temperature changes).

@ Recognize the clinical presentation and provide appropriate management of emergencies presenting the first month of life including respiratory distress with/without cyanosis, shock, bleeding, or life threatening neurologic abnormalities.

@ Understand the physiology, pathophysiology, diagnosis, and treatment of acute and chronic respiratory disorders in the premature and full term infant, including hyaline membrane disease, apnea, meconium aspiration, persistent pulmonary hypertension, transient tachypnea, pneumonia, pneumothorax, pulmonary interstitial emphysema, diaphragmatic hernia, pleural effusions, congenital pulmonary disorders, and bronchopulmonary dysplasia.

@ Demonstrate knowledge of the clinical and laboratory diagnosis, pathophysiology, and treatment of the following disorders of premature and full term infants.

 *Infection: Neonatal sepsis (bacterial, viral, fungal), Congenitally acquired infections (HIV, CMV, toxoplasmosis, syphillis, rubella), Localized infections (omphalitis, skin, osteomyelitis, arthritis, urinary tract).Understand the peculiarities of host defense mechanisms in the newborn.

* Hyperbilirubinemia (physiologic, hemolytic, obstructive).

* Metabolic disorders (hypoglycemia, infant of diabetic mother, hypo- and hypercalcemia, inborn errors of protein, organic acid and amino acid metabolism).

* Gastrointestinal disorders (necrotizing enterocolitis, bowel obstruction, gastrointestinal bleeding, abdominal wall defects).

* Cardiovascular disorders (presentation of congenital heart disease in the neonatal period, patent ductus arteriosus, congenital cardiomyopathies, hypertension).

* Hematologic disorders (neonatal coagulopathy, polycythemia, anemia).

* Renal disorders (acute renal failure, congenital malformation of the urogenital tract including agenesis, dysgenesis, cystic disease, obstructive uropathies, exstrophy of bladder).

* Endocrine disorders (congenital hypo- and hyperthyroidism, adreno-genital syndrome, ambiguous genitalia, hypoglycemia), & Metabolic Disorders .

* Thermoregulation

* Neurologic disorders (seizures, hydrocephalus, hypoxic-ischemic injury, neonatal asphyxia, intraventricular hemorrhage and outcome).

NICU CAREER —A Summary

1. For many junior doctors the experience of working in a neonatal unit (as part of a pediatric attachment) provides lasting memories of endless rounds of blood gases, cannulations, baby checks, all-powerful midwives, and attending deliveries of newborn babies because of meconium stained liquor. If, however, you can see past this stage, you will discover that neonatology is an exciting and advancing specialty that is rapidly progressing in training, research, and technology.

2. Neonatologists work closely with the obstetricians, and the delivery unit is usually where the action starts. But care starts before the baby is born. Perinatal liaison meetings are held regularly with obstetricians, specialists in fetal medicine, and clinical geneticists. Other relevant specialists, such as cardiologists, surgeons, and urologists are often involved if they can contribute to the management of babies in whom specific problems have been diagnosed before delivery. The outcome for anticipated problems is better than for problems discovered at birth. Arrangements can be made to deliver these babies electively, in the presence of appropriate personnel and equipment.

3. Many babies in the neonatal unit receive respiratory support and are monitored with regular measurements of blood gases and serum electrolytes. Premature babies and ill term babies need their cardiovascular status monitored and maintained. Babies are supported with parenteral nutrition until they are able to tolerate breast milk and often require arterial and central venous catheters. In addition, premature infants need monitoring of their glucose concentrations and regular ultrasound examinations of their developing brains. Therefore, trainees will soon acquire basic practical skills such as managing the neonatal airway, emergencies in the delivery room, assisted ventilation, securing arterial and central venous access, and ultrasound examination of the head. At registrar level, neonatology combines fine practical skills with ongoing clinical management, and opportunities exist for trainees interested in echocardiography and perinatal counselling.

4. Trainees learn good communication skills: they often have to relay news to parents and are involved in helping parents through the bereavement process. Personal qualities such as empathy, kindness, and humility come into play here.

5. Over the past two decades there has been a decreasing trend in mortality and morbidity in premature infants. Many challenges remain, however, such as preventing the consequences of prematurity, minimizing neurological damage resulting from hypoxia and ischaemia in term infants and improving subsequent developmental outcome. The research goes on.

The pros and cons of a career in Neonatology

Advantages : *Immensely rewarding *Dedicated staff and colleagues *One of the larger subspecialities in paediatrics *Predicted likely expansion in consultant numbers *Can be practised in academic or research orientated setting as well as in a predominantly clinical setting in district hospitals *Great scope for innovative research *Opportunities to cultivate special interests such as perinatal counselling *Work with the whole family

Disadvantages: *Physically, mentally and emotionally demanding *Highly intensive workload *"Out of hours" work at consultant level *Junior consultants may be expected to be resident on call in the future (but with fewer hours in total per week).

Courtesy: Peter Tarczy-Hornoch, M.D. & David Woodrum, M.D. University of Washington Academic Medical Center |

CHANGING TRENDS IN NEONATOLOGY & PEDIATRICS A CHALLENGE TO THE "ALREADY TRAINED"

Objective Learning Points-

1. Change is inevitable & only thing constant in life is a change. Changing trends are so diverse that while we have to keep pace with scientific advances that are mostly beneficial, we may have to keep away from irrational & unethical practices that are so widely prevalent, which is a great challenge to the "already trained".

2. For practicing pediatrician, aim should be to achieve work satisfaction, peer acceptance, community respect, healthy life & happy family. It is futile to be after "vitamin M" without achieving other goals (after all, we know that storable vitamins are toxic).

3. Discourage managing quantity at the cost of quality. It is pity that patient often spends a lots of money & in return gets little time, short description & long prescription. The only rational solution is developing group practice to share responsibility & maintain quality.

4. Use appropriate communication skills (father-child pattern = authoritative, sibling pattern = gently suggestive, departmental store pattern = options are given to parents after pros & cons are explained) with patience, politeness, transparency & with peer respect.

5. Use CPA (Consumer Protection Act) as a boon for self imposed improvement by proper documentation, timely referral & detailed explanation to allay anxiety of parents & seek full cooperation from parents.

6. Realize that learning is an investment for better management and bright future; learning has to be need based & priority given to practical applications.

7. A super specialist (actually a sub specialist) is one who knows everything about "a thing" but nothing about anything else, while a generalist is one who knows something about everything but not everything about anything. Super specialist must be an excellent generalist & a generalist must go through the standard guidelines brought out by sub speciality chapters.

8. Literature search & discussion with peers after proper documentation of clinical material contribute significantly to practical application in the community (documentation + storing + analysis + interpretation)

9. HIT (History, interpretation, Investigation and then Treatment) should replace MISS pattern (Manage first without diagnosis, if not improved, they Investigate next & if no diagnosis is reached, they enquire about Symptoms & Signs) of practice.

10. Change yourself to meet the challenges given below, or hang your stethoscope & proclaim yourself as illiterate pediatrician of 21st century, who cannot learn, unlearn & relearn.

    a. *Variable clinical presentation of infectious diseases* due to age of the child, nutritional status, previous exposure to infection, large infective load, intercurrent viral infection or immunosuppressive drugs, drug resistance, partially treated cases, changing epidemiology of natural infection & vaccinations.

    b. *Increasingly diagnosed conditions*: Dengue, Leptospirosis, Resurgence of Diphtheria & Plague, increased incidence of Asthma, Sinusitis, GE reflux, Autism, Kawasaki disease, Cystic fibrosis, Sarcoidosis etc. need to be considered in the present scenario of clinical practice.

    c. *Sophisticated investigative modalities with confusing interpretations* - men behind the machines must develop experience & expertise for proper interpretation.

    d. *New management (preventive + therapeutic) strategies* - neonatal screening, antenatal diagnosis, growth & development monitoring, routine monitoring of blood pressure, eye refraction & dental hygiene, chemo-prophylaxis against UTI & maternal transmission of Hepatitis B or HIV, inhalation therapy for persistent asthma, IVIG for kawasaki, blood component therapy, early surgical correction of congenital malformations such as obstructive uropathy & biliary atresia. Pediatricians have a challenge to face as early diagnosis is just not enough & close monitoring is necessary, as prognosis remains guarded. Interventional cardiology, minimal invasive surgery & finally robotic surgery are some of the advances that are already on the anvil & need to be known for their future utility.

    e. *Educated parents with easy access to information about the disease* - evidence based medicine with consideration of ground reality is the need of modern scientific practice, to meet this challenge.

Strategies to avoid professional malpractice litigation

*Stay current by reading journals and textbooks, and by attending continuing medical education conferences

*Maintain professional ties with a large medical center

*When facing a difficult situation, consider consulting with a colleague *Maintain open communication with parents and families

*Practice timely documentation of procedures, communication, complications, and persons present

*Document telephone advice

*Be aware of state laws that affect your practice reality is the need of modern scientific practice, to meet this challenge.

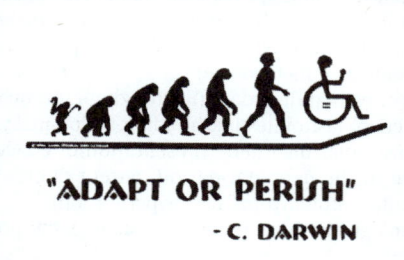

"ADAPT OR PERISH"
- C. DARWIN

Courtesy: **DR. Y.K. Amdekar, Mumbai**

The experience of parenting a premature infant in the NICU is often overwhelming. Although the health of our baby(s) is our greatest concern, in the day to day life in the NICU, it is the little things that medical professionals do that make a difference. Preemie parents from all over the world came together (via www.preemie-l.org) to create a list for nurses and doctors that will help them understand the intricate needs and desires of parents and families. Please feel free to print this list and give it to anyone who may benefit from it.

Please Do... ***Do:** Ask me what I like to be called. I may or may not want to be called "mom." I would like to be called by my first name. ***Do:** Send me a Polaroid/Digital photo of my baby when I can't get out of bed because I have had a C-section. ***Do:** When referring to my baby, please don't call him "your baby" (as if he is your baby) or "the baby." He is your patient, but he is my baby. The best possible way to refer to my baby is by calling him by his first name. ***Do:** Give me a tour of the nursery soon after I arrive so I know where the pumping room is, where to store breast milk, the lounge, bathroom, etc. (Remember if I am groggy or having a difficult time coping, I might need a second tour later.) ***Do:** Make a cute nametag for my baby's bed. ***Do:** If you are the nurse caring for my baby, acknowledge me when I come in the room so I know who you are. ***Do:** Tell us when I can speak with the doctor. ***Do:** Promote attachment between parents and their babies. Show me that you are confident I will not cause my child any harm. ***Do:** Tell me how to read stress cues so I know the best time to touch my baby and when to stop. ***Do:** Show me how to do things that I can do to help care for my baby. ***Do:** Realize that once I am able to do some kind of activity for my baby, it is really stressful to have a staff member decline my doing it because they are unable to help. ***Do:** Acknowledge when we do things correctly, praise us, thank us! ***Do:** Tell me how to touch my baby in a developmental and soothing way. ***Do:** Allow me to hold my baby as early as possible-it is the best part of being a parent. ***Do:** Help me to do Kangaroo Care as early as possible. Please check on me during this time to make sure I am okay. ***Do:** Encourage us to make a tape to leave in the isolette; singing, talking, or telling stories for my baby. Tell me what I can do to decorate my baby's bed. ***Do:** Create an environment for my baby that seems healing and supportive (i.e.. No harsh lights or minimal noise, but cluster care when possible). ***Do:** Put up a big sign that says, "SHHHH...BABIES ARE SLEEPING!!!!" ***Do:** Quietly set things down on the isolette—remember the sound inside is much louder! ***Do:** Take pictures (with a Digital camera I have left for you) of our babies when we're not there, or when we're cuddling or spending time with our babies. We may not think to get our cameras out at those special moments, and we may be missing some big ones when we can't be there. ***Do:** Talk to my child and explain that you are about to touch them. ***Do:** If you find it necessary to shave my baby's head for an IV, please save a lock of hair from the "haircut." ***Do:** Provide support without judging. ***Do:** Realize that every parent is different and responds differently. Find out how we want to deal with things. ***Do:** Understand that parents, like our children, will have "crisis days" and they may not coincide with the status of my baby. ***Do:** Work to build genuine connections with parents. Even when there is nothing concrete or specific that you can do, your presence, attention, and compassion bring strength and comfort. ***Do:** Help parent of preemies build a community by removing obstacles preventing families from finding comfort in the experiences of others. ***Do** what you can to create an environment in which parents can talk and support one another. ***Do:** Provide honest information and clear explanations. Please allow us to ask questions. ***Do:** Let us know when tests are being done on our babies (even if it means a quick call to home) and explain what they're for-in parent's terms. (Also let us know if any scheduled tests/procedures have been cancelled and why.) ***Do:** Let us know that we are allowed to read our baby's chart. ***Do:** Give us access to as much information as possible. Have a parent library with current books, videos, and a list of websites available. We would love to be able to buy books right there in the hospital-please encourage your gift shop to stock a supply of books and resources that we may purchase to help us through this process. ***Do:** Give us complete information that is significant to future possible outcomes (concerning all drugs, procedures and alternatives that we can choose from). ***Do:** Realize that the truth is always easier for us to deal with in the long run. If a bleak prognosis can be expected, that prognosis won't be any easier if it comes as a complete and total shock later on. ***Do:** Respect parents enough to allow them to feel all their jumbled emotions without running away or minimizing what they feel. ***Do:** Talk with us about other things than our baby to help us pass the time and get our minds off things (maybe even ask us about the birth or things unrelated to our baby). It's nice to be treated as a friend. ***Do:** Support us if we are unable to breast-feed/express milk and must use formula for whatever reason. ***Do:** Refer me to a lactation specialist if I am having trouble lactating or feeling uncomfortable with pumping milk or breast-feeding. ***Do:** Please respect my efforts in pumping my breast milk and breast feeding my baby. Thaw only what breast milk is necessary for each feeding-it is a precious commodity! Please say only encouraging remarks about my breast-feeding efforts. ***Do:** Do ask me if I would like to have a screen put up when I am trying to nurse my baby, as it is a very exposing experience with these tiny babies. Please check in with me often when I'm behind the screen, especially when the alarms are going off. ***Do:** Make sure to let me know when my supply of breast milk is running low so I can make sure to bring some in. ***Do:** Dress my baby in her own clothes whenever possible. ***Do:** Find out our schedules so we can be there for feedings, baths, and maybe even a quick holding during weights and isolette changes. ***Do:** Encourage me to write notes to be left on my child's bed that share my special knowledge of my child with the staff. ***Do:** Give credence to a parent's intuition about their child. If I tell you, "Something is wrong", act on that information as if it were true. ***Do:** Congratulate us on our baby's milestones! (Diapers finally taped on, larger diapers, changing to a new type of bed, going to a lower oxygen setting, getting off the vent/CPAP, wearing clothes, learning to suck/swallow, being held, etc.) ***Do:** If you have not cared for my baby before, please read the chart carefully and note what times I usually come by. ***Do:** Put graduate pictures of former patients in the waiting room. ***Do:** Laugh with us. ***Do:** Cry with us. ***Do:** Treat us like real parents.

Please Don't...

Don't: Call me "Mom." Please ask me what I would prefer to be called. **Don't:** Move the baby without telling me ahead of time, or at least meeting me at the door. **Don't:** Tell me how I should be feeling or that I "need to be patient." **Don't:** Dismiss or diminish my concerns. I am not used to seeing my baby have bradycardias or color changes. **Don't:** Assume that I don't care for or love my baby if I don't touch him. I may be very scared or overwhelmed. **Don't:** Tell me my baby had a bradycardia because I was touching him, feeding him, or doing something wrong. **Don't:** Please never treat me as if I am stupid. All of the medical terms and information are very difficult to understand and comprehend at times, especially since I am probably feeling a tremendous amount of stress. **Don't:** Write harsh judgements about me in the nurse's notes, unless the information you are recording is known to you without question from both observation and communication. **Don't:** Assume anything about me or my family if we are unable to visit regularly. My family may be very loving and supportive, but cannot come to the NICU for other reasons. **Don't:** Sound annoyed or make insensitive comments when I call to check on my baby. The phone is sometimes my only connection to my precious baby. **Don't:** Do the tasks that I have already been doing (bath, diapers, feedings, etc.) if you know I am on the way to the nursery. It takes away what little parenting I can do. **Don't:** Act as if breast-feeding is not crucial for my baby. There is enough scientific evidence of its importance to preemies that it should be encouraged to breastfeed. However, if I am unable to produce milk, please do not make me feel inadequate by comparing me to all the other mothers who have no problem with lactating. **Don't:** Talk loudly or keep the lights on unnecessarily. **Don't:** Please be careful to not share information about a baby with the wrong person. Please check and double check that you have the correct information with the correct parent. **Don't:** Talk about a baby in a negative way when the parents are gone. It is morally wrong, very unprofessional, and may also hurt other parent's feelings (wondering what they say about my baby when I am not here). **Don't:** Try to instill your personal views (philosophies, religion, or ethics) on us. Allow us the same freedom to choose and have our views, as you were allowed to choose and have yours. (This includes miracles happening in the NICU.) **Don't:** Be afraid of my emotions, or of your own. **Don't:** Let me travel this difficult journey alone.

Edited by: Dianne Maroney Andrea O'Brien Sheri DeBari

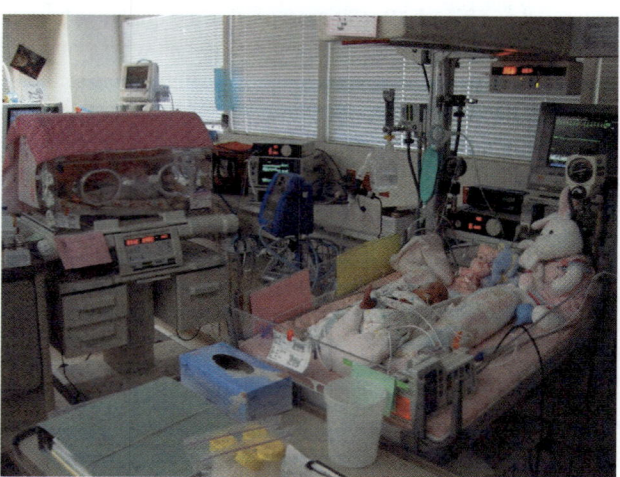

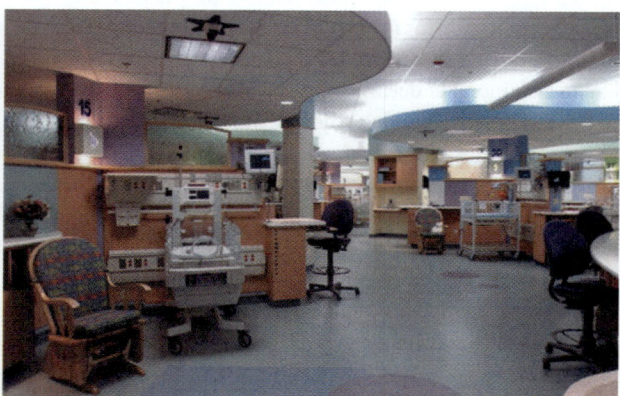

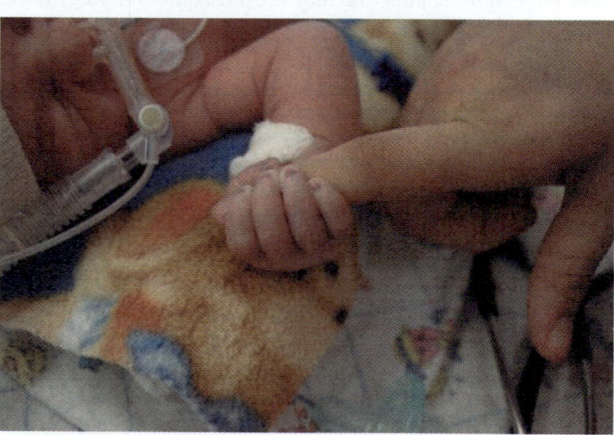

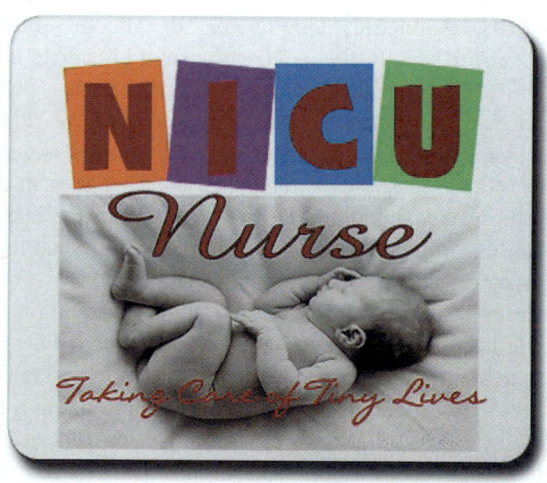

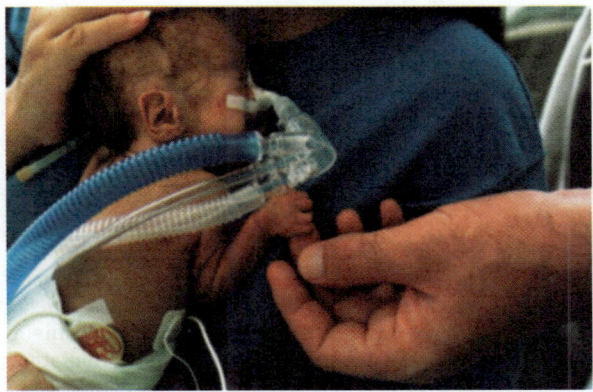
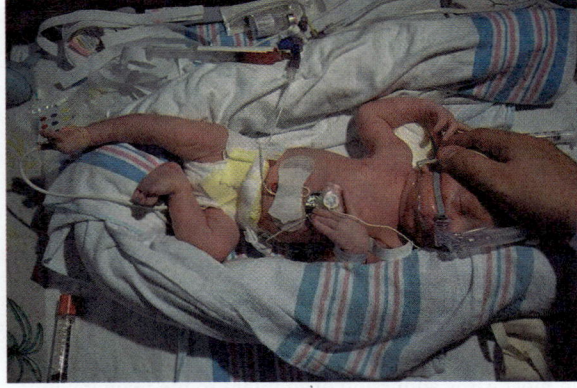

Seeing their baby receive intensive care can be terrifying for parents; allowing parents to touch/cuddle their baby whenever possible, if they comply with the infection control measures can be helpful in controlling their stress.

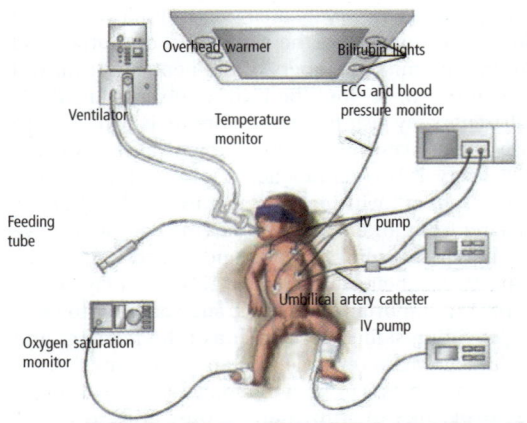
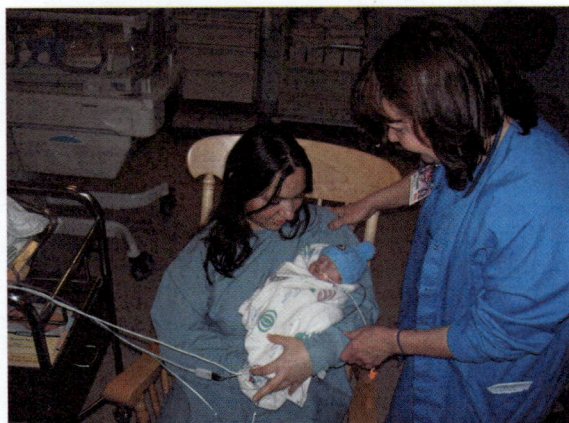

The environment of the Neonatal Intensive Care Unit, which can be hot, noisy and "high tech," is usually alien to parents

Guidelines for Respectful Communication with Parents

* Provide open, truthful communication at all times
* Use easily understandable language
* Identify areas of medical uncertainty
* Create an environment for communication that encourages parents' participation and their becoming as fully informed as possible
* Identify and remove barriers that limit parents' role in communication (e.g. language, physical distance)
* Communicate with parents: at the time of admission, at any crisis point in their child's NICU course, via periodic reviews of longer stay patients, and other unstructured opportunities
* Encourage parents to seek clarification of information at any point by requesting an appointment with the child's responsible physician
* Provide information as accurately as possible and with as much certainty of diagnosis and prognosis as is possible in each clinical situation
* Assess family communication preferences, and attempt to communicate within those parameters
* Be preemptive in communication (i.e., foresee what problems or issues may arise in the child's course)
* Be proactive in communication in any clinical situation in which a poor outcome is predicted
* Convene meetings with both parents when important decisions need to be made
*Keep parents informed of any special investigations/tests that are planned in the course of management of their child
* Recognize the need for time for processing and absorption of information
* Ensure consistency and continuity of communication in the face of medical staff changes
* Practice open, honest, and timely disclosure regarding medical error

A Holistic Approach to the NICU Care!

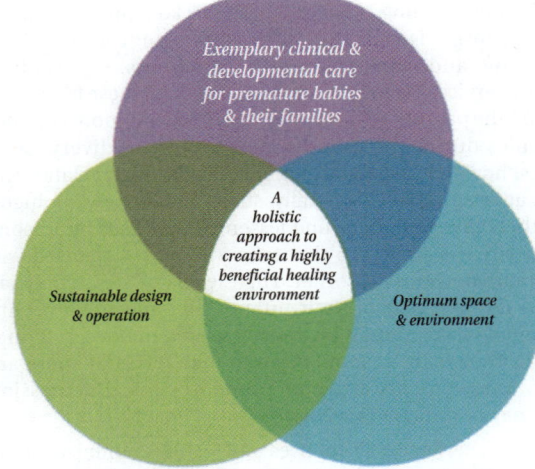

Exemplary clinical & developmental care for premature babies & their families

A holistic approach to creating a highly beneficial healing environment

Sustainable design & operation

Optimum space & environment

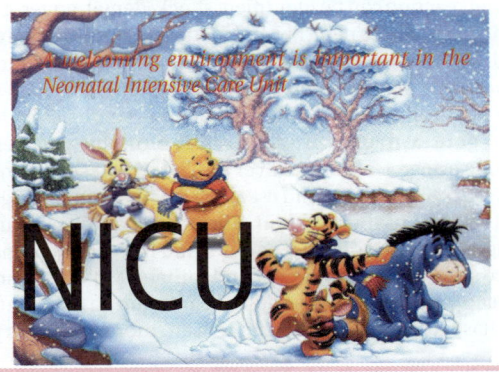

A welcoming environment is important in the Neonatal Intensive Care Unit

NICU

HOW TO SUPPORT THE STRESSFUL PARENTS OF A NEONATE ADMITTED IN THE NICU?

Supporting parents in the Neonatal unit: Parents find it very stressful when their baby is admitted to the neonatal unit for any reason. Different sources of stress have been identified, and certain occasions (such as discharge from hospital or bereavement) are particularly difficult. These experiences impact on families in positive and negative ways, and people adopt a range of coping mechanisms. Staff should adopt a holistic approach to care that acknowledges the uniqueness of each family and supports them appropriately. During pregnancy, most women and their partners do not give serious consideration to the possibility of preterm delivery or illness in their newborn baby. In most cases admission of an infant to the neonatal unit is unexpected and is stressful for the parents. If a problem is diagnosed antenatally, parents can be forewarned. For most admissions to the neonatal unit, however, there is little or no time to prepare the family. Parents are unfamiliar with the potentially complex problems their infant is facing and they are unsure of the future. Incomprehension and uncertainty are major sources of stress. In addition, maternal health is often compromised at this time.

Sources of stress experienced by parents: • Maternal ill health • Separation from their baby • Strange, "hostile" environment • Unfamiliar staff • Appearance and condition of the baby • Complex medical problems to understand • Sudden changes • Uncertainty • Lack of information • Physical demands • Financial hardship. A degree of separation exists between the mother and baby when the infant is admitted to the neonatal unit, and this may extend over many months. Although in some places a visit to the neonatal unit is a routine part of antenatal care, the neonatal unit is an alien environment to most parents. Units are often noisy, bright, and hot. They can be overcrowded and parts of every unit will be "high tech." Parents rarely know the neonatal unit staff before their baby is admitted, and the language and behaviors they encounter can contribute to an overwhelming feeling of isolation. The sickest preterm infants may be in hospital for many months, and visiting can be difficult, exhausting, and a financial drain for parents, especially as neonatal services become more centralized. All these factors put strain on the parents' relationship: breakdown is more common in couples during the months after preterm delivery. Some couples, however, feel the experience makes their relationship closer, at least initially. Generally, stress and anxiety are higher in mothers than in fathers, and lessen as time goes by. In some parents stress is similar to that seen in adults diagnosed with post-traumatic stress disorder. High levels of stress may last beyond the first year of their infant's life, and the level and duration of stress may not be directly related to how preterm or how sick their baby is. In addition to high levels of stress and anxiety, these parents are more prone to clinical depression, which may be difficult to recognize.

Coping mechanisms : Responses and feelings reminiscent of a classic grief reaction can be identified: shock, denial, anger, guilt, acceptance, and adjustment. Several models explore how parents cope with having their baby in the neonatal unit. A great variety of mechanisms are seen, however, and a single model will probably not fit all parents. Some of the coping strategies include trying to gain a deeper understanding of the problems, establishing a degree of control over the situation, seeking social support from other people, and escaping from or minimizing the apparent severity of the situation. These mechanisms are used to varying degrees in individual parents, and there is a systematic difference seen between mothers and fathers. Mothers tend to look for support from others and to search for an explanation for what has happened, whereas fathers are more likely to try to minimize the situation, often by concentrating on supporting their partner.

Limiting parental stress : A better understanding of the sources of stress and how parents might try to cope allows appropriate care of the family. When designing neonatal units, great emphasis is placed on effective layout, lighting, and noise reduction. Facilities for families to stay close to their baby are usually provided, and parent rooms allow mothers and fathers to relax and meet other parents. Play areas for siblings can be incorporated into some units. This more "family-orientated" approach to care is helped by less restricted visiting policies in neonatal units. Most units will allow parents and siblings open access to their baby if they comply with local infection control measures. Having transitional care areas as an integral part of the neonatal unit or as a separate area (for example, as part of the postnatal ward) minimizes the separation of mother and baby. When time permits, members of the neonatal team will often meet with parents before the birth to discuss any likely admission. Parents may visit the unit before their baby is born to familiarizes themselves with the environment and some of the staff. After delivery, it is good practice to discuss medical and nursing issues in detail with parents and to involve them in decision making from an early stage. Parents will often have immediate access to recordings, results, and clinical notes. They can also help care for their preterm baby. This care may extend beyond simple but important measures, such as "skin to skin" contact, to providing skilled care such as tube feeding, oral toileting, and intensive "developmental care" programs. Parents of other preterm babies can give personal support through "buddying" programs or informally. Counseling through organizations, such as the Premature Baby Charity (BLISS) in the United Kingdom, or formal support can be helpful even for families whose babies are not critically ill. Written information about the neonatal unit and, where appropriate, describing specific conditions or procedures may be useful. Routine contact between the neonatal unit and social services may allow financial support to be provided for the parents.

Death and decision making: Babies, particularly extremely preterm infants, may die despite continuing intensive treatment and full medical support. In addition, a decision to limit active treatment may be made because of the inevitability of death or a prognosis that indicates a very poor quality of life. Death, however it comes about, is a desperate time for the families who are affected. Parents want to be involved in decision making at these times. They need full and frank information, given in a compassionate manner by experienced staff who know the family and their baby. In most cases, the decision to stop or limit treatment is made with senior medical and nursing staff. Family, friends, and external bodies (such as religious leaders and support groups) do not often have a substantial role in the decision to withdraw treatment but they do contribute to family support afterwards. Bereaved parents often need factual information that may help explain why their baby has died. Without autopsy, important information can be missed, and in most neonatal units, postmortem examination will always be considered and offered to the parents if appropriate. High profile cases of procedural inadequacies and anxieties about organ retention have contributed to a fall in the number of autopsies carried out. This drop is increased by a parent's natural reluctance to authorize further "suffering" for their infant and a lack of awareness of the questions that remain unanswered.

Discharge home: Discharge home, although an exciting time for families, can also be a time of extreme anxiety, and so a formal

699

How to Support the Stressful Parents of a Neonate Admitted in the NICU?

Parental tasks

| Realistically perceive infant's medical condition and needs | Adapt to infant's hospital environment | Assume primary caretaking role | Assume total responsibility for infant upon discharge | Cope with death of infant |

Maladaptive responses
Failure to visit infant or call
Emotional withdrawal from infant
Difficulty interacting comfortably with infant during hospitalization
Resistance to providing minimal caretaking during hospitalization
Failure to achieve sense of parental competence
Failure to achieve sense of attachment to infant
Distortion of medical information received
Debilitating preoccupation with infant's condition
Ascribing blame for infant's condition
Fear of taking infant home
Distorted view of infant and potential needs at time of discharge
Failure to verbalize needs and concerns to staff and family
Hostility towards and distrust of staff

Adaptive responses
Frequent visits and calls
Emotional involvement with infant
Development of comfortable interaction with infant during hospitalization
Interest in assuming maximum amount of caretaking during hospitalization
Growing sense of parental competence
Objective interpretation of medical information received
Acceptance of and constructive adaptation to infant's condition
Objective understanding of the causes of infant's condition
Confidence in assuming total responsibility for infant
Realistic view of infant and potential needs at time of discharge
Free verbalization of needs and concerns to staff and family
Realistic view of expectations of staff

Unhealthy outcome
Disturbed parent-child relationship
Failure to thrive
Vulnerable child syndrome
Deterioration of marital and family equilibrium

Healthy outcome
Positive parent-child relationship
Maintenance of marital and family equilibrium

Maladaptive and adaptive parental responses during crisis period, showing unhealthy and healthy outcomes.

LEARNING OBJECTIVES　　**CONCEPTS**

Describe the interventions to facilitate parental attachment with the at-risk Newborn.

1. Assess the parent's level of understanding of the infant's problem
2. Prepare and facilitate the parents' viewing of the infant
3. Promote touching and facilitate parental participation in care of the infant.
4. Facilitate parental adjustment to the infant's special needs.

Identify the special initial and long-term needs of parents of at-risk Infants.

1. Initially, the parents need to understand the infant's problem, including expected treatments.
2. Need to understand routine well-baby care.
3. Need to understand how to perform any special procedures needed to care for the infant.
4. Need referral for normal infant screening procedures.
5. Need to understand normal growth and development of infants.
6. Need to have medical follow-up arranged.
7. Need referral for any special equipment required at home.

approach to "discharge planning" is often adopted. Mothers "room in" with their baby to promote bonding, establish feeding, and learn practical skills that might be needed. Support for the family in the community once the infant is discharged can also be arranged, including specialist neonatal nurses, primary care health staff (for example, health visitors, general practitioners), social workers, and national or local family support groups.. Although managing the immediate stress of discharge home is important, it needs to be recognized that although practical issues may become easier to manage as time passes, for some families considerable levels of stress and anxiety remain long after the discharge itself. Psychological support should be an integral part of neonatal follow up programs.

Summary points • Having a preterm baby is stressful • Parents manage stress and anxiety in many ways that are not necessarily consistent across different families, religions, and cultures • Men and women differ in how they cope with stress and bereavement • Appropriate support for parents should be an integral part of neonatal care. Family-centered care is a philosophy of care that embraces a partnership between staff and families. Families, patients, and staff benefit in a family-centered care environment and the design of the newborn intensive care unit (NICU) must not interfere with its successful implementation. Unrestricted parental presence in the NICU, parental involvement in infant caregiving, and open communication with parents are basic tenets of family-centered care. By virtue of their continual presence and role in the NICU, nurses are in a unique position to support family-centered care.

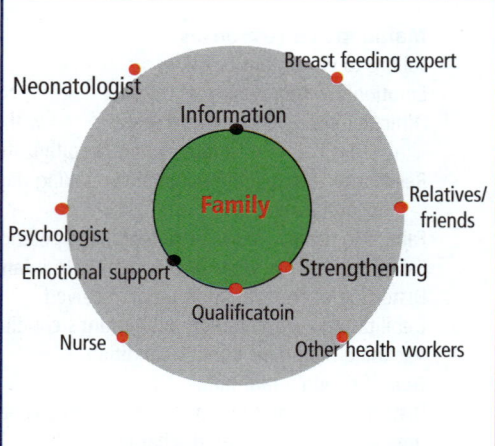

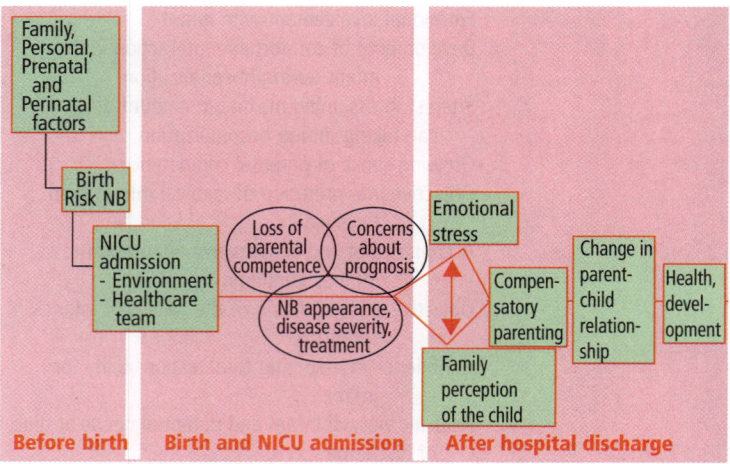

Figure shows the effects of birth and NICU admission of newborns and possible triggers of stress to parents and family members. Emphasis is placed on the importance of knowing the family, personal, prenatal and perinatal history of parents in order to better understand what families carry with them in terms of life experience, enabling them to come to terms with the birth and hospitalization of their children.

Family is the focus of attention which, in turn, provides help by developing strategies for emotional, strengthening and information support, enhancing the healthy perception about the birth and NICU admission of a risk newborn, in addition to restoring parental competence. The support group should use formal support, provided by an interdisciplinary team, and informal support, provided by family members, throughout the process. Intergenerational support also plays a crucial role and so does parent-to-parent support.

FAMILY CENTERED CARE- MAJOR COMPONENTS
- Acknowledging the family as the constant in a child's life
- Developing collaborative work between parents and the NICU staff
- Sharing complete and reliable information about the Newborn with the family
- Respecting the individuality, strength, and coping ability of the family
- Respecting racial, ethnic, cultural and socioeconomic diversities of the families
- Encouraging parent-to-parent support during the NICU stay
- Enabling parent's participation and skills in caring for the Newborn in the NICU
- Planning flexible, accessible programs that meet the needs of the family
- Ensuring emotional and financial support to the families

Parents' closeness and involvement with their baby can be supported through encouraging:
- positive reassuring touch
- comfort or containment holding
- skin-to-skin or 'kangaroo' care
- nappy changing and providing other care
- expressing breast milk
- giving milk feeds.

Family-centred policies are needed on:
- introduction and orientation to the unit for parents and families;
- supporting parental contact, including engagement with fathers and partners and skin-to-skin or 'kangaroo', care;
- supporting breast-feeding, provision of breastpumps and access to donor breastmilk;
- exchanging information with parents, good practice includes parent folders, parent update meetings, baby-logs and diaries;
- preparation and planning for transfers between levels of care and discharge home;
- contact with and use of staff in specialist roles;
- access to social and psychological support, including counselling and local parent support groups.

Key points
Role and identity as a parent intrinsically involves:
protecting + nurturing the newborn,
BUT Admission to neonatal care is associated with
*Separation
*Marginalisation
*Lack of responsibility
*Loss of nurturing and protective role
Neonatal care with a family focus aims to minimise adverse effects with:
*A family-centred care philosophy
*Family-friendly facilities
*Development of specialist roles
*Family oriented staff training and support

Courtesy: Peter W Fowlie, Hazel McHaffie

Ophthalmic disorders manifesting in the newborn (Other than Retinopathy of Prematurity and Conjunctivitis)

Neonates present with multiple ophthalmic disorders which can be isolated or be associated with other systemic anomalies. Pediatricians and neonatologists should identify ocular abnormalities and refer patients for detailed ophthalmic evaluation when deemed necessary. As the critical period of visual development is in the first 6 months after birth, timely referral, diagnosis, and management are critical to allow optimal visual development. *Refer to Chapter 25 for Retinopathy of prematurity (ROP) and to Chapter 96 for Neonatal conjunctivitis* (Ophthalmia neonatorum)

10 Warning Signs of Serious Eye Disease in the Newborn and Infant: These first three of the ten warning signs of significant eye disease in infancy and childhood have the most serious implications and most require **early definitive treatment**. Fortunately, they are rare! Cataract - 1 in 250 Glaucoma - 1 in 10,000 Retinoblastoma - 1 in 20,000.

1 . White pupil: *Leukocoria* is an abnormal white reflection from the retina. The differential diagnosis in the neonate includes retinoblastoma, retinal detachment, cataract, ROP, coloboma, PHPV, congenital infections such as toxoplasmosis, and vitreous hemorrhage. Urgent ophthalmic evaluation is crucial.If the tumor is retinoblastoma, the outcome is usually fatal unless early and appropriate treatment is completed. Large tumors require enucleation; smaller and second eye tumors can be treated with radiation, chemotherapy, cryotherapy, and laser. In the setting of a cataract, red reflex examination reveals a black spot in the reflex or an asymmetric reflex. A family history of cataracts necessitates ophthalmic referral. Bilateral cataracts require systemic evaluation because 60% of them are associated with specific causes,susc as Rubella,Galactosemia etc,.Diagnosis must be early to avoid amblyopia, and nystagmus if cataracts are bilateral. Cataract surgery is considered for visually significant cataract more than 3 mm in diameter or in the presence of strabismus or nystagmus. Surgical treatment should be early to reduce amblyopia; ideally at 2 months if unilateral and considered visually significant, 2 to 3 months if bilateral, but before onset of nystagmus. Optical rehabilitation is difficult with contact lenses or glasses. IOL's are being placed in the first year but this treatment is undergoing study and evaluation.Even in the best of circumstances vision after congenital cataract treatment is never normal.Persistent hyperplastic primary vitreous (PHPV):The cause of PHPV is uncertain, and the condition manifests in healthy term infants. The severity can range from pupillary strands across the iris to more severe forms with membranes behind the lens, retinal dysplasia, or detachment.

2. Drooping lid:Ptosis-Unilateral ptosis is most commonly familial and often dominant. Sometimes it is part of Horner's syndrome, which also includes meiosis of the pupil and decreased sweating on the same side of the face. Neck masses, iatrogenic injury during cardiac surgery, and birth injury to the lower brachial plexus are other causes. Facial trauma may cause a temporary pseudo-ptosis. Bilateral ptosis is seen in centronuclear (myotubular) myopathy, myotonic dystrophy, and myasthenic syndromes. In severe cases, the lid crease is absent and upper eyelid covers the visual axis. If lagophthalmos is present, the inferior cornea may be exposed at night, leading to corneal scarring. Bilateral ptosis can be associated with short palpebral fissure and epicanthus inversus, which is known as blepharophimosis syndrome. Referral for evaluation of congenital ptosis is generally not urgent if there is no lagophthalmos. Surgery may be delayed if the ptosis is not amblyogenic to achieve a better surgical outcome. **Lump or swelling of lids with or without redness, heat, or pain (signs of inflammation)**- this can be a sign of cellulitis, tumor, hemangioma, etc. Occlusion of the pupil can cause amblyopia - immediate treatment is indicated. **Proptosis** :Neonatal proptosis is rare and can be due to tumors (dermoid, teratoma, vascular tumors), craniofacial malformation (bilateral proptosis), orbital cellulitis or abscess, and orbital hemorrhage. Maternal Graves disease can cause neonatal hyperthyroidism with eye signs that include proptosis with other systemic manifestations. The condition is usually transient due to the

short halflife of maternal antibodies. Prompt referral and evaluation is important to identify the cause of proptosis.

3. Enlarged cornea of one or both eyes: When a sign of congenital glaucoma, this is characterized by the classic triad of epiphora, photophobia, and blepharospasm. Raised intraocular pressure causes breaks in the Descemet membrane (Haab striae), which results in corneal clouding. Increased pressure also causes increased axial length of the eye, resulting in myopia; damage to the optic nerve, resulting in cupping; and enlargement of the cornea. Urgent ophthalmic consultation is needed for medical and surgical treatment to prevent progressive optic nerve head cupping and loss of vision.

4. Corneal opacity: Corneal opacity can be caused by birth trauma and is more common in forceps delivery. The corneal clouding results from Descemet membrane tears, which are commonly vertically or obliquely oriented. The opacification spontaneously resolves in several months, but ophthalmic evaluation and follow-up visits are essential to monitor astigmatism and to assess the development of amblyopia.**Congenital Corneal Opacity** Neonatal corneal opacification can result from Peters anomaly, sclerocornea, dermoid, or other metabolic diseases. Ophthalmology referral is required for patients who have unilateral or bilateral corneal opacity to determine the cause and need for follow-up care.

5. Excessive tearing or discharge: This can be a sign of increased pressure in the eye, infection, light sensitivity, or irritation, all of which require attention. The most common cause is a blocked tear drainage system. Tearing and discharge presents in patients who have nasolacrimal duct obstruction by 1 to 2 weeks after birth. The obstruction resolves in 90% of patients who have nasolacrimal sac massage and topical antibiotics. Tear duct blockage which persists after one or two courses of antibiotics is best treated by *gentle* probing done before age 1 year. Persistent tearing usually requires probing with general anesthesia often with placement of a silicone tube. It is important to distinguish between benign causes of tearing such as nasolacrimal duct obstruction and rarer but more serious causes. Patients who have congenital glaucoma may also present with tearing associated with light sensitivity and blepharospasm.

6. Crossed eyes: Eye alignment is variable in early infancy. Neonatal misalignment may be evident in the first 2 months after birth and usually represents a normal developing vergence system (movement of the eyes in relation to each other: convergence and divergence). Emerging infantile esotropia is indistinguishable from neonatal misalignment. It is reported that 1% of congenital esotropia is present at birth, but persistence of misalignment after 3 months of age requires detailed ophthalmic evaluation. Intermittently crossed eyes persisting after the 2 to 4 months of age should be evaluated by an ophthalmologist to establish a diagnosis and plan treatment. Crossing can require surgery, done in some cases as young as *4 months*. Other crossing can require treatment with spectacles. Eyes that deviate *constantly* should be evaluated immediately!

7. Dancing eyes: Nystagmus -Infantile nystagmus presents at birth or early infancy and manifests as involuntary oscillations (mostly horizontal with small torsional component). Nystagmus can be associated with congenital or acquired defects such as cataract or albinism. Detailed ophthalmic evaluation is required to identify and rule out reversible causes.

8. Defect or missing part of the pupil: Iris coloboma is failure of the embryonic fissure to close during the fifth to seventh week of gestation and, thus, can be associated with systemic anomalies. Common systemic associations of coloboma include CHARGE syndrome (coloboma, heart defects, choanal atresia, retardation of growth and development, genitourinary problems, and ear anomalies), renal coloboma syndrome (renal hypoplasia, vesicoureteral reflux, and sensorineural hearing loss), and Kabuki syndrome (coloboma, cleft palate, heart defects, and growth retardation).Aniridia (absence of the iris) is usually bilateral and is almost always associated with poor vision and nystagmus.

9 . Inequality of the eye/Pupil:Microphthalmos is a condition in which the eye is smaller than normal; it can present unilaterally or bilaterally. Microphthalmos can be related to an isolated ocular disorder or part of a systemic condition. The most common ocular conditions associated with microphthalmos are persistent hyperplastic primary vitreous (PHPV) and coloboma.**Persistent inequality of the pupil size** can be a sign of serious disease or it may be an innocent finding. A simple office test can make this distinction. If persistent, inequality of pupil size should be evaluated by an ophthalmologist.

10. Prematurity: Candidates for **Retinopathy of Prematurity** screening are: 1) Infants whose birthweights are less than 1,500 g or gestational ages are 30 weeks or less and 2) Selected infants whose birthweights are between 1,500 and 2,000 g or gestational ages are more than 30 weeks and have unstable clinical courses. The screening should be performed with indirect ophthalmoscopy after pupillary dilation by an ophthalmologist familiar with ROP screening. Screening should be performed at 31 weeks postmenstrual age or 4 weeks after birth, whichever is later. Indications for treatment are: 1) Zone I ROP: any stage with plus disease; 2) Zone I ROP: stage 3 with no plus disease; and 3) Zone II: stage 2 or 3 with plus disease.

Miscellaneous eye problems:

Subconjunctival hemorrhages, which are common after vaginal delivery, usually do not represent ocular trauma.It is a consequence of raised venous pressure in the head and neck due to uterine contractions.

Eyelid Coloboma Colobomas appear as notching of the eyelid and can involve either the upper or lower eyelid. Upper eyelid colobomas can be associated with systemic Goldenhar syndrome and are not usually visually threatening. Lower eyelid colobomas can be associated with systemic Treacher Collins syndrome and cause opacification of the inferior cornea. Ophthalmologic evaluation is important to identify associated ocular abnormalities such as retinal and choroidal colobomas.

Entropion Congenital entropion is the in-turning of the eyelid margin, causing the eyelashes to rub on the cornea. This entity is rare, but if untreated, can cause ulcerative keratitis and corneal opacity. Prompt referral is required for management of the entropion and resulting corneal pathology.

Hypertelorism Hypertelorism refers to increased space between the eyes, as measured by the interpupillary distance. Orbital hypertelorism refers to excessive separation of the medial walls of the orbit. Hypertelorism can be mistakenly diagnosed in the presence of telecanthus or an increased measurement between the inner canthi with normal interorbital and interpupillary measurements (results from lateral displacement of the inner canthus and lacrimal puncta). Orbital hypertelorism usually coexists with ocular hypertelorism and requires imaging for accurate diagnosis. Isolated hypertelorism is rare and frequently associated with other craniofacial malformations and chromosomal aberrations.

Iris Neovascularization Iris neovascularization is seen primarily with ROP plus disease. In addition to dilated and tortuous retinal vessels, ROP plus disease is associated with vitreous haze, iris vascular engorgement, and poor pupillary dilatation. The tunica vasculosa lentis (capillary network surrounding the posterior and lateral surface of the lens that disappears after birth) may also become engorged in this setting.

Essential facts about Newborn Eye

1. At birth, the eye of a normal full-term infant is approximately 65% of adult size. Postnatal growth is maximal during the 1st yr, proceeds at a rapid but decelerating rate until the 3rd yr, and continues at a slower rate thereafter until puberty, after which little change occurs.

2. In an infant, the *sclera* is thin and translucent, with a bluish tinge. The *cornea* is relatively large in newborns (averaging 10 mm) and attains adult size (nearly 12 mm) by the age of 2 yr or earlier. Its curvature tends to flatten with age, with progressive change in the refractive properties of the eye. A normal cornea is perfectly clear. In infants born prematurely, the cornea may have a transient opalescent haze.

3. Remnants of the pupillary membrane (anterior vascular capsule) are often evident on ophthalmoscopic examination, appearing as cobweb-like lines crossing the pupillary aperture, especially in preterm infants.

4. The average axial length of the eye is 17.1 to 17.5 mm, the average intercanthal distance at birth is 16 mm, and the average interpupillary distance at birth is 40 mm. The embryonic structure of the tunica vasculosa lentis, which is responsible for development of the crystalline lens, persists until 35 weeks of gestation. Pupillary light response is evident after 31 weeks of gestation. Visual development starts soon after birth, and visual behavior is typically evident at 6 to 8 weeks after birth. An ophthalmology referral is necessary if no visual behavior is detected at 3 months of age.

5. The optic nerve head color varies from pink to slightly pale, sometimes grayish. Within 4-6 mo, the appearance of the fundus approximates that of the mature eye.

6. In a newborn, the macular landmarks, particularly the foveal light reflex, are less well defined and may not be readily apparent. The peripheral retina appears pale or grayish, and the peripheral retinal vasculature is immature, especially in premature infants. Superficial retinal hemorrhages may be observed in many newborn infants. These are usually absorbed promptly and rarely leave any permanent effect.

7. An infant's eye is somewhat hyperopic (farsighted). The general trend is for hyperopia to increase from birth until 7 yr. Thereafter, the level of hyperopia tends to decrease rapidly until age 14. Elimination of the hyperopic state may occur during this time. If the process continues, myopia (nearsightedness) develops.

8. Newborn infants tend to keep their eyes closed much of the time, but normal newborns can see, respond to changes in illumination, and fixate points of contrast. The *visual acuity* in newborns is estimated to be in the range of 20/400. One of the earliest responses to a formed visual stimulus is an infant's regard for the mother's face, evident especially during feeding. By 2 wk of age, an infant shows more sustained interest in large objects, and by 8-10 wk of age a normal infant can follow an object through an arc of 180 degrees. The acuity improves rapidly and may reach 20/30-20/20 by the age of 2-3 yr.

9. Many normal infants may have imperfect coordination of the *eye movements* and *alignment* during the early days and weeks, but proper coordination should be achieved by 3-6 mo, usually sooner. Persistent deviation of an eye in an infant requires evaluation.

10. *Tears* often are not present with crying until after 1-3 mo. Preterm infants have reduced reflex and basal tear secretion, which may allow topically applied medications to become concentrated and lead to rapid drying of their corneas.

Learning Objectives:

1. Identify important ophthalmic disorders manifesting in the newborn.
2. Classify which of the conditions need an ophthalmology referral.
3. Identify patients who require ROP screening.

References:

1.NeoReviews 2011;12;e216-e222 Aparna Ramasubramanian and Suzanne Johnston Neonatal Eye Disorders Requiring Ophthalmology Consultation

2.. Disorders of the Eye , Nelson Textbook of Pediatrics 19 th edition, Scott E. Olitsky , Leonard B. Nelson

The evolution of aggressive treatment of the Newborn infant over the past 35 years has been associated with a dramatic reduction in mortality for virtually all major disease categories in the newborn period. Such care is costly; often causes suffering; and sometimes can result in considerable long-term morbidity.

The following quotes provide a perspective:

> "Neonatal intensive care is responsible for the survival of a significant number of infants who formerly would not have survived. This increased survival has been accomplished with an acceptable level of burden and without substantially increasing the population of handicapped children." - *A proponent*

> "Neonatal intensive is a good example of medicine out of control. There is inappropriate use of technology by health care professional who are out of touch with patients and their families. The benefits of increased survival of high risk infants are outweighed by the associated burdens." - *An opponent*

Neonatal ICU Issues:

Case 1: M.S. is a married 35-year-old pregnant childless woman who has lost four previous pregnancies between 16 and 23 weeks gestation. She currently has reached 23 weeks and 3 days of gestation, her fetus is seemingly healthy, and has an estimated weight of 550 grams (+/-1.2 lbs). She has ruptured her bag of waters and is now having labor that seems unstoppable with tocolytics. Delivery seems inevitable. What are the management options and who decides what form of care should be instituted following delivery?

Perinatal management at the threshold of viability

* Antenatal counseling should be provided by senior neonatologists, obstetricians, and midwives.

* Management decisions should depend on what the parents and their medical advisers think is in the child's best interests.

* Parents should have accurate information on likely outcomes for their infant—including their chances of survival and the risk of longer term disability.

* Information on outcomes provided to parents should cite data from large cohort studies that reported the outcome of all pregnancies for each week of gestation (not just for infants admitted to intensive care units).

* Perinatal management plans should consider the mode of delivery, use of intrapartum monitoring, and immediate care of the Newborn.

* Decisions not to provide active resuscitation or intensive care should not be binding, particularly if the Newborn seems more mature than anticipated.

* It may be appropriate to provide full resuscitation and intensive care to infants at birth until the clinical progress becomes clearer and further discussions with the family have been possible.

* Parents should be supported throughout and encouraged to seek advice and further support from others, such as family members and religious advisers.

* Infants who are not actively resuscitated or in whom active resuscitation is withdrawn should receive palliative care.

Case 1 Discussion: This gestational age and estimated birth weight represent the "gray zone" in terms of viability vs. non-viability. Accordingly, the *parents* have a choice to make. They can choose a passive comfort care mode treatment (with non-survival being a virtual certainty) or alternatively, assisted ventilation, pressors, antibiotics, parenteral nutrition, etc. The role of the physician is to provide information and guide the parents through the decision-making process. *For all extremely low-birth-weight infants (1000 g), the rate of disabilities such as cerebral palsy, developmental delay, and vision and hearing impairment is about 20%. This rises to 50% for infants at 23 weeks, when the survival rate is only 10%–20%.*

Case 2: B.R. is a term female infant from an unexpected pregnancy. She has Down syndrome (Trisomy 21) and also has a complex cardiac lesion that will require at least two major surgical procedures during early infancy for her to have a chance to survive beyond childhood. B.R.'s parents, ages 44 and 45, have three other children, all in college. They have considerable ambivalence as to what to do: continue to pursue potentially beneficial though burdensome and costly treatments, or forego such treatments in favor of a more conservative approach.

What are the issues involved?

Case 2 Discussion: That the child has Down syndrome should not be a factor in the decision-making process. Nor is it appropriate to allow financial issues to play a major role. The parents, who are the decision-makers, should be apprised of the medical facts (types of surgical interventions required, chances for success). They should also be given a good understanding of the amount of suffering the child will experience during aggressive intervention efforts. They should then come to a decision based on the *child's* best interests. That is to say, does the burden of care outweigh the benefits to be anticipated or vice versa.

Palliative care of the newborn infant If resuscitation is unsuccessful, or if active resuscitation is felt to be inappropriate, then palliative care should be provided for the infant and family. The parents can spend time with their baby, and should be aware that their baby may show signs of life, such as occasional gasps, after birth. Privacy and sensitive support for parents and family with subsequent follow up are essential. The potential importance of postmortem examination should be discussed at an appropriate time.

Factors needed in the palliative care of extremely preterm infants

Warmth

Dignity

Human contact

Pain relief

* Those who advocate withholding treatment generally base their argument on one of three grounds: *(a)* the low probability of survival; *(b)* the high probability of severe disability; or *(c)* the high projected costs of medical care, both in the neonatal period and throughout the patient's life *Our accuracy in predicting what will happen to a particular infant, however, is less than 100%. Because Neonatologists cannot confidently assess an infant's prospects for survival in the first few critical minutes after birth, some may recommend resuscitation of all infants born after 22 weeks gestation. It also is difficult or impossible to predict at birth which extremely low-birth weight infants will develop severe disabilities and which will leave the Newborn intensive care unit disability free. The situation is different for infants with readily apparent severe malformations. Except for the most extreme cases, many Neonatologists regard prematurity itself as an insufficiently reliable indicator.

* While survival rates vary from center to center and according to the patient population, infants born at 30 weeks gestation have a better than 90% probability of leaving the Newborn intensive care unit alive; however, infants born at 22 or fewer weeks gestation have virtually no chance of survival . For this reason, some centers do not ask a neonatologist to be present at delivery if the pregnancy has lasted fewer than 23 weeks

* From the reviewed guidelines, it seems clear that 23 to 24 weeks are a sort of "gray zone," where recommendations suggest resuscitation on an "individual basis" and "according to the parents' wishes." In some countries, this gray zone extends through 250D 7 to 256D 7 weeks. In all of the statements, the gestational age is considered the best estimate of the infant's maturation and, consequently, his or her possibility of survival, although many other fetal/neonatal characteristics could play a role in the prognosis.

* Nevertheless, because of the uniqueness of every pregnancy and Neonate, to protect mothers and infants from futile treatment, as well as incorrect withholding of life-sustaining treatment, the specific circumstances of every individual situation must always be kept in mind.

* A "do-not-resuscitate" order is an evidence-based justified choice in a Newborn of 23 weeks, 400 g, as well as with anencephaly and confirmed trisomy 13 and 18. With an uncertain or inaccurate diagnosis or prognosis, a therapeutic trial with the option of subsequent withdrawal can be considered.

* Between 1960 and 2000, the survival rate of infants weighing between 501 and 1000 g increased from approximately 5% to 70%, while that for infants weighing between 1001 and 1500 g increased from approximately 50% to 95% (9,10). It should be noted that such capabilities are not distributed evenly around the world.

* Judgments about what constitutes an acceptable quality of life may vary from physician to physician and family to family. One family may judge even relatively mild sensory, cognitive, and motor impairments unacceptable, while another may eagerly welcome a child that others would regard as neurologically devastated.

* When the parents do not agree with each other, or when they do not accept their doctor's advice on whether or not to withhold or withdraw care, treatment should be pursued until a change in the baby's status or further counseling and discussion clarifies the situation. Only as a last resort and in exceptional circumstances after all other options have been exhausted, should the problem be referred to the Courts.

* When death is inevitable, physicians should step aside and allow it to happen, preserving dignity and helping the experience to be as meaningful as possible for families. When a decision has been taken to electively deliver a threshold-viability fetus or to withhold or withdraw neonatal life-sustaining care, all actions taken and the reasons for them, as well as the clinical course of the child and the views of the parents, should be carefully documented by the medical team.

* After death, especially following the withholding or withdrawal of medical care, the medical team (preferably the most senior pediatrician available) has a responsibility to counsel the parents and explain the desirability for a necropsy examination. Useful information may also be obtained from procedures such as X-rays, MRI and chromosomal analysis. Parents will require further counseling and support from both obstetric and pediatric teams including advice on the results of the necropsy and the outlook for future pregnancies.

* It is important to recognize that even the most desperately ill premature infant is still a human being who deserves our respect and compassion. Infants are kept warm and free of pain. Families are encouraged to be with their infants, and where possible, to hold them. When problems such as respiratory distress supervene, we provide symptomatic relief, such as suctioning secretions and administering morphine. The goal in such situations is not to forestall the death of the infant but to support the patient and family as death takes place. The death of a premature infant is not merely a biological outcome. *It is also one of the most profound and poignant chapters in the life story of the family involved, and the entire health care team needs to acknowledge and respect this.*

* Newborn palliative care should be considered in three general areas: (1) Neonates at the limits of viability. As advances in technology and outcomes become available, it is the responsibility of the health-care community and society to reach a consensus regarding the limits of viability. (2) Neonates with lethal congenital anomalies. When appropriate, and diagnosis and prognosis are certain, why should a family be deprived the opportunity to choose palliative care for the unborn child? (3) Neonates not responsive to aggressive medical management where continuing therapy may prolong suffering and postpone death.

REFERENCES: 1) Practical Guidelines for the Treatment of Extremely Preterm Births Perinatal Care at the Threshold of Viability: An International Comparison of Practical Guidelines for the Treatment of Extremely Preterm Births Maria Serenella Pignotti and Gianpaolo Donzelli *Pediatrics* 2008;121;e193-e198 2) Ethics and the Limits of Neonatal Viability Richard B. Gunderman, MD, PhD William A. Engle, MD Published online 10.1148/radiol.2362041770 Radiology 2005; 236:427–429.

Guidelines on giving intensive care to extremely premature babies

At 25 weeks and above

Intensive care should be initiated and the baby admitted to a neonatal intensive care unit, unless he or she is known to be affected by some severe abnormality incompatible with any significant period of survival.

Between 24 weeks, 0 days and 24 weeks, 6 days

Normal practice should be that a baby will be offered full invasive intensive care and support from birth and admitted to a neonatal intensive care unit, unless the parents and the clinicians are agreed that in the light of the baby's condition it is not in his or her best interests to start intensive care.

Between 23 weeks, 0 days and 23 weeks, 6 days

It is very difficult to predict the future outcome for an individual baby. Precedence should be given to the wishes of the parents. However, where the condition of the baby indicates that he or she will not survive for long, clinicians should not be obliged to proceed with treatment wholly contrary to their clinical judgement, if they judge that treatment would be futile.

Between 22 weeks, 0 days and 22 weeks, 6 days

Standard practice should be not to resuscitate the baby. Resuscitation should only be attempted and intensive care offered if parents request resuscitation, and reiterate this request, after thorough discussion with an experienced pediatrician about the risks and long-term outcomes, and if the clinicians agree that it is in the baby's best interests.

Before 22 weeks

Any intervention at this stage is experimental. Attempts to resuscitate should only take place within a clinical research study that has been assessed and approved by a research ethics committee and with informed parental consent.

Copies of the report are available to download from the Council's website:

www.nuffieldbioethics.org

Decision-Making at the Threshold of Infant Viability

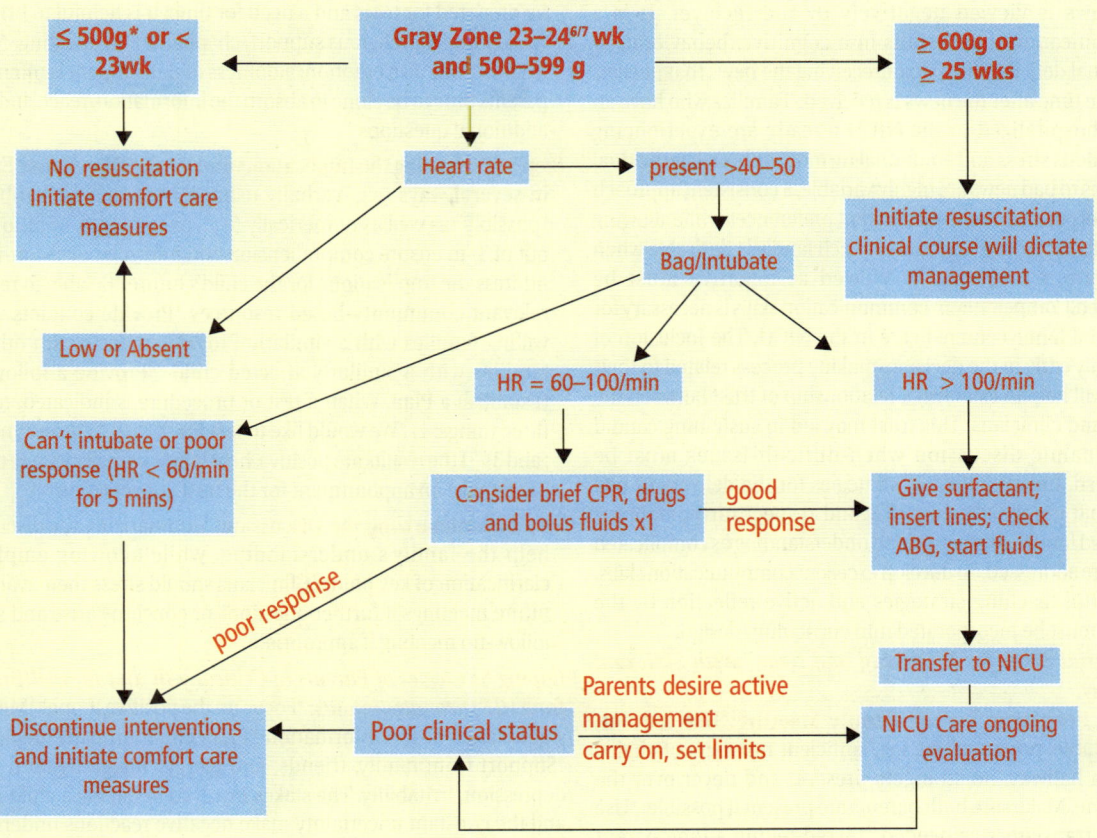

*The occasional infant<500g BW(usually IUGR), who is vigorous at birth may warrant active intervention

The Limits of Viability
Decision—Tree

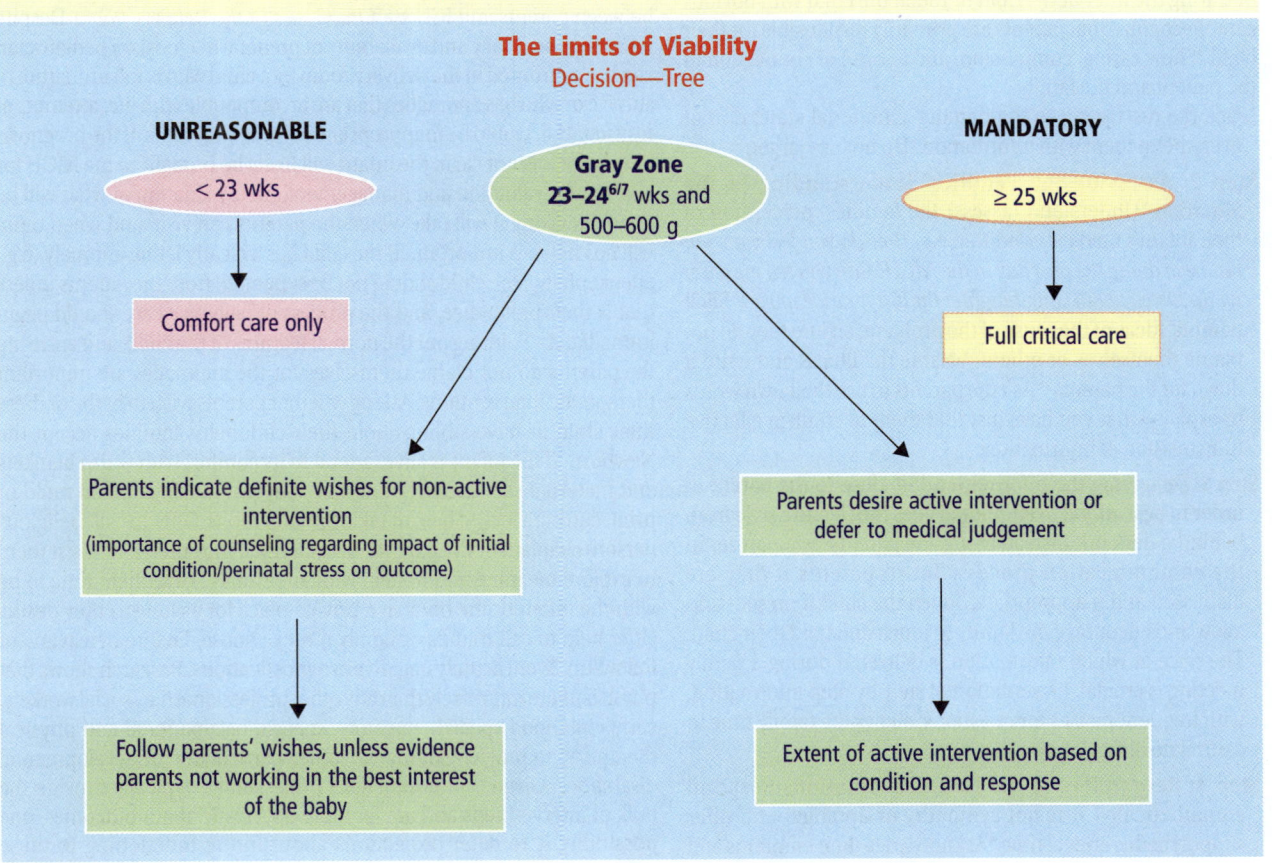

HOW TO BREAK BAD NEWS IN THE NICU ?

Bad news is viewed negatively by the receiver. It is a communication that "results in a cognitive, behavioral, or emotional deficit in the personreceiving the news that persists for some time after the news is received."Families who have an infant hospitalized in the NICU already are experiencing tremendous stress and emotional turmoil. Although individual reactions to bad news are highly variable, a consistent approach that incorporates established parent preferences while allowing clinicians to respond uniquely to each family is desirable when information that may be viewed as negative must be presented.Competency in communication skills is necessary for successful familycentered care in the NICU. The inclusion of the family early in the decision-making process related to their infant will help to establish a relationship of trust between the family and clinicians. This trust may aid in sustaining candid and dynamic discussion when difficult issues must be addressed. Incorporation of strategies for the delivery of bad news that emphasize empathy and respect furthersupport improved family satisfaction and understanding as complicated issues are addressed. To develop excellent communication skills, thoughtful teaching strategies and active reflection by the learner must be incorporated into curriculum design.

6 Essential Steps for "Breaking Bad News" With Skill and Empathy

Step 1: Preparing for the Family Meeting:
*Use a quiet, comfortable, private place, i.e., sufficient numbers of chairs, not in a hallway, no strangers present, and never over the telephone. Make sure both parents are present if possible. *Use trained translators as needed *Avoid telling a lone parent without his or her spouse and/or a preferred support person present *Enable the parents to touch the deceased child before or during the interview *Hold or touch the child with obvious care *Recognize that parents are primarily responsible for their child *Show caring, compassion, and a sense of connection to the patient and the family

*Pace the discussion to the parents' emotional state; do not overwhelm them with information *Do not use jargon

Step 2: Assessing the Families' Understanding of the Situation:
*Understand (assess) the families' perception of their infant's medical condition e.g.,*How do you feel your son has been doing the past day in the NICU? Can you tell me what we discussed about your daughter the last time we spoke?*Elicit parents' ideas of the cause of the problem; ensure they do not blame themselves or others * Name the illness and write it down for the parents * Ask the parents to use their own words to explain what you have just told them to confirm effective transmission of information

Step 3: Delivering the Information:
*Sit close to the parent in order to best attend to emotional cues (not lecture style from behind a desk but instead alongside parents-as a partner in the communication process. Touch parents if they are distressed and if appropriate. Touch the child if present and allow and encourage the family to touch and hold their child. The pace at which information is delivered during a family meeting is crucial. Presentation of step-by-step information, with frequent pauses for questions, allows the family time to assimilate difficult news.

Step 4: Responding to the Families' Emotions:
Respond empathetically(It is not sympathy or apology) and offer support at this critical time.*Acknowledge their emotions and be prepared for tears and a need for time; it is helpful to bring a social worker and/or religious support/chaplain to the meeting * Be willing to show your own emotion; aloofness or detachment is offensive *Give parents time to be alone to absorb the information, react, and formulate additional questions

Step 5: Discussing the Implications and Future Directions:
*Explain risk in several ways (e.g, verbally using terms such as "probably" and "possibly" as well as numerically (e.g., percentages, or ratios such as 1 out of 3) to ensure comprehension and informed decision-making. * Address the implications for the child's future *Be able to recommend relevant community-based resources *Provide contacts with other willing families with a similarly*Provide contacts with other willing families with a similarly affected child *Provide a follow-up plan (**Establish a Plan**. When a test or procedure is indicated, tell parents three things: 1) "We would like to test for 'X '"; 2) "The test involves 'X'" ; and 3) "If the results are positive, here is how we will manage the case…") and make an appointment for the next conversation

Step 6: Summarizing the Discussion:
Summarizing the discussion may help the family's understanding, while allowing emphasis and clarification of key points.Clinicians should stress their availability for future meetings if further questions or concerns arise and schedule a follow-up meeting if appropriate.

Coping Strategies of Parents of Critically Ill and Injured(Brain injury from HIE)Neonates/Infants:
*Focus on the positive (hope) *Minimize the significance of the information *Preoccupation with medical details *Support from family, friends, and clergy *Religious faith *Hostility, depression, irritability. The stakes involved in having a child in the ICU and the constant uncertainty make negative reactions understandable. Parental sources of stress include seeing their child in pain, frightened, or sad, and the inability to communicate with the child. Increased attention to the fulfillment of parental needs can improve relations between parents and ICU staff.*Bad News in the Delivery Room*-Despite increasing accuracy and availability of prenatal diagnosis, a pediatrician can be confronted in the delivery room by a child who is too immature to survive or who has anomalies that are incompatible with life; attempts at resuscitation would be inappropriate in these situations. If the prognosis or diagnosis is not clear, the infant will likely be brought to the NICU for additional evaluation and management. An explanation of what will be done, how long it will take, when the parents can visit, and when more will be known is important. If the child has a clearly lethal anomaly (e.g., anencephaly), the child should not be separated from the parents unless that is their preference, and the process of palliative care should begin immediately. Pointing out the normal features of the child and ensuring the parents do not blame themselves for the anomalies are important therapeutic interventions. Asking whether parents wish to bathe or dress their child or have siblings hold their childhelps families accept the Newborn. If the infant is alive, attend to its comfort with warm blankets and maternal skin contact, if desired. Suggest making a hand mold or print, cutting a lock of hair, or taking photographs. Offer to call a religious person/chaplain or the parents' own clergy, if they prefer, to assist them to explore meaning and to help with any rituals.. Give them time to be with the infant or the body in a private place for as long as they desire. Offer help to call friends or family if they choose. Ensure bereavement follow-up. **Avoid acutely negative prognostications**. Research shows that physicians are more likely than any other professional (i.e., social workers, early childhood special educators, speech, occupational and physical therapists) to project gloomy outcomes particularly for developmental disabilities. Given that nonmedical professionals typically provide the bulk of interventions and are far more optimistic about outcomes, one possibility is to defer projections about future functioning to these

clinicians (e.g., "there is a wide range of outcomes and every child is different, we can't predict the future, but we can put services in place such as OT, PT etc., in order to ensure that he/she achieves her maximum potential, and we will monitor her/his progress so that we don't miss anything. In the meantime, we'll plan for early intervention and periodic developmental follow-up to see how he or she is progressing").

Special Communication Considerations in Terminal Illness : No communication is more difficult than telling a parent that his or her child will die. Parental recognition that one's child is suffering, disproportionate to the likelihood of benefit, is extremely distressing. Many physicians, however, wait until they perceive the family or patient is "ready," leading to additional emotional and physical suffering, including a prolonged dying process. Mixed messages from multiple consultants, particularly in the ICU setting, can be extremely confusing and upsetting for families, often leading to poor decision making as the parents (understandably) hold on to the most hopeful messages. Having a clear captain of the care team, one who is evaluating the situation as a whole, particularly as death nears, is extremely helpful in preventing such problems. **Offer to discuss the issues again at a second meeting** or over the telephone—a suggestion made by more than 70% of parents interviewed about their experiences in receiving a developmental diagnosis for their children. Parents most likely to need a repeat consultation are those who are highly distressed (because recall is likely to be especially poor). Even so, in one study, more than half of parents had difficulty recalling difficult news suggesting that repetition should be offered to all. The offer of a second conference also enables parents to invite other family members with them who are in disagreement, confused, etc.

Take note of anxiety. When continuing and elevated anxiety levels are observed or reported, these should be interpreted as a possible marker for generalized difficulties with anxiety. Such families should be provided repeated opportunities to understand the results and offers of parent-to-parent support groups or mental health counseling when indicated. Blanket reassurances should be avoided and parents should be told that rescreening or further updates and evaluations will be conducted. Clinicians, especially those in training are well advised to **practice first** (e.g., with simulated patients) and under supervision from a clinician with exemplary communication skills.

Physician's SELF CARE: Physicians have a difficult job; the responsibility to communicate effectively and efficiently to clarify the diagnosis, consider psychosocial and existential concerns, respect family and other supporters' needs, and to come to an agreed-on plan of care is substantial and can be overwhelming. Allowing time between patients and debriefing conversations with staff, increased physician education on communication, and improved payment for counseling time can help.

References & further reading:

1) Eden OB. Black I. MacKinlay GA. Emery AEH. Communication with parents of children with cancer. Palliative Medicine, 1994;8(2):105-14.

2) American Academy of Pediatrics, Committee on Hospital Care. Family-centered care and the pediatrician's role. *Pediatrics.* 2003;112(3 pt 1):691–697 3) Krahn GL, Hallum A. Kime C. Are there good ways to give 'bad news'?. Pediatrics. 1993; 91:578-582

3) Difficult discussions in the NICU, Susan Izatt, MD* **NeoReviews** Vol.9 No.8 August 2008 e321

Family Centered Communication and Support in the ICU

* Early (within 24–48 hours of admission) and frequent communication

* Indication that the health care team cares for the child as an individual

* **Provide a brief but not strongly negative "warning shot"** (e.g., "I'm afraid I have news that may be troubling" or if inviting parents to a conference to discuss findings, suggest that they may want to bring a spouse or close friend along).

* Practitioners trained in meeting facilitation and conflict management

* The use of open-ended questions and reflective explanation

* Hopeful but honest and clear communication; acknowledgment of uncertainty

* Discussion of likely and hoped-for outcomes

* Use of numeric terms when describing probabilities; use of drawings and models

* Provide timeframes for improvement and future discussion

* Participation of families in clinical bedside rounds, caregiving for their child and ability to stay with their child during invasive procedures

* Listen to and involve the nurse, chaplain, and social worker in the information loop

* Open visitation, including sibling and pet visitation

* Consistent caregivers; if this is not possible, ensure consistency of the message

* Prompt informing of parents of transitions, such as a change of location, condition, treatment plan, assignment of attending physician or residents

* Shared decision making rather than autonomy; encourage the parents to involve their family, friends, and medical home pediatrician to help them to understand information and make decisions

* Written, audiotaped, and computerized education for families.

* Discussion and support of coping mechanisms, including religious and spiritual values

* Initiation of palliative care at the time of admission

Data were adapted from Todres et al, Davidson et al, Robinson et al, and Todres.

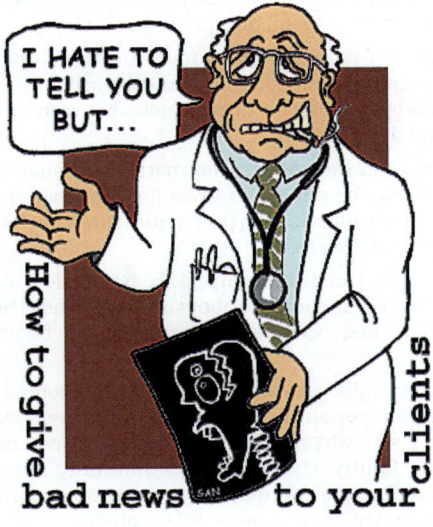

PITFALLS IN NEONATOLOGY :
HOW TO PREVENT/REDUCE/AVOID THEM?

1. *Most of the Pitfalls in diagnosing and managing Neonatal and Childhood disorders arise from not following the SOAP approach, regularly, i.e. S (Subjective / History), O (Objective/ Examination), A (Assessment/Summary/Differential Diagnosis), P (Plan of Management) described by Dr. Laurence Weed nearly 30 years ago.*

2. Beware of over confidence, hurry, irritation, shift change - overs, and fancy about rare diagnoses; as all of these are common when disasters are audited or malpractice comes to court. *Rare Diagnoses are rarely true ; but if you can exclude all that is possible, then whatever remains, however improbable, it must be the truth (Sherlock Holmes).* **Methods of Physicians should be like those of a detective, one seeking to explain a disease, other a crime.**

3. The patients should not be viewed as systems, organs, tissues, cells and DNA. They must be viewed in totality (body, mind and soul) and that too not in isolation that in context with the dynamics of ecology, family, friends and society" Meharban Singh.

4. There are not short cuts for physical diagnosis. It is learnt only by practice, not a dull, dreary monotonous practice but practice with all the five senses alert. Sir Robert Hutchison. (Touch, Sight, Smell, Hearing, Taste)

5. The skilful Pediatrician knows when to sedate with drugs, when to sedate with words, when to treat aggressively for cure, palliatively for relief and consolingly for comfort. *Avoid* saying "Nothing can be done" {because something can always be done}, "There is nothing wrong" {even when it is a Parental functional disorder}, "Don't worry", "It is all right", etc. {because the patients and attendance have emotional feelings}. Relieve their anxiety, reassure them and restore their confidence so that the will to fight is never dulled or extinguished. The Neonatologist/pediatrician should always be caring, concerning and compassionating towards the children and their parents.

HISTORY TAKING

1. Be Gentle, sympathetic, gracious and kind in approach *but alert, attentive, tactfull and inquisitive* while eliciting history !

2. Don't forget that you are also being assessed by the parents and children on the basis of your behaviour and approach

3. Always do maintain eye contact with the parents while taking to them but avoid staring towards the child because children are often scared if you intently look into their eyes.

4. Do remember that parents are excellent observers of their children , but are of poor interpreters of what they have seen and also they commonly exaggerate symptoms with figures of speech and they *may not* mention important symptoms which seem irrelevant to their concept of what is wrong.

5. Don't accept parent's/some one's diagnosis uncritically; always reappraise the grounds and evidence for the original diagnosis by verifying the discrepancies between the physical signs and the diagnosis.

6. Do always seek the evidence for a particular statement, e.g. A Neonate may be put on laxatives for constipation without excluding Congenital Hypothyroidism/Hirschsprung`s disease/ Anal Fissure.

7. Beware of the fact that no clinical Hx is complete unless one has made specific enquiries about all drugs taken { home and herbal remedies}, because most symptoms can be side effects of drugs.

8. Always remember to ask why ? The reason behind a fact is often more important than the fact itself, e.g.: Pertussis Vaccine was not given, why not? The reason may reveal important previous/family Hx or, more commonly reveal mis-understanding/misinformation ; opening up opportunity for the provision of more accurate information.

9. Be cautious about making a diagnosis that a symptom is entirely psychological without positive evidence of a psychological disorder and psychological problems are commonly associated with organic disease.

10. Remember the possibility of poisoning either deliberate or accidental, or of an overdose of medicine, even though the possibility is denied. The true diagnosis may be carelessness which the parents or grandparents don't want to admit, or non-accidental injury.

B. PHYSICAL EXAMINATION: 1) Do get the confidence and co-operation of the parents and child to find productive and pleasant physical examination {if you are hurried, annoyed, disinterested and impersonal, the experience can be frustrating and unrewarding}. 2) "What you see is what you get" is true with difficult and unco-operative children/irritable and crying Neonates. 3) Always do modify the orderly approach with infant and toddlers and be able to collect all the information available in any sequence. 4) Only if you do complete physical appraisal of their child, parents are favourably impressed ; they will be less satisfied with the physician whose examination is hurried and incomplete. 5) An experienced physician's ability to quickly assess the overall clinical picture allows him to rapidly and accurately formulate provisional diagnosis and therapeutic possibilities & to arrive at a prognostic outlook, any or all of which may be modified or discarded upon completion of a more detailed examination, history taking & lab tests & through continuing observation of symptoms.

PITFALLS IN PHYSICAL EXAMINATION—PREVENTIVE STRATEGY

A. ERRORS in the TECHNIQUE of Physical Examination -i) Errors in techniques of Examining various parts of the body ii) Errors due to OMISSION iii) Errors due to INCOMPLETE & POOR RECORDING of (failure to examine certain areas)- *CORRECT by the application of Methodically Proper Techniques for physical examination.*

B. ERRORS of 'INTERPRETATION' of Physical findings *Interpret all clinical findings within the context of the whole patient *Don't accept easily without testing those findings that confirm your suspicion and ignore those that shake up your clinical judgement* **None of clinical findings is absolutely specific or nonspecific.** C)OBSERVER'S ERROR: The range of observer variation and error is wide but mistakes should be fewer when there is constant awareness of one's limitations, and a testing of conclusions against other findings.

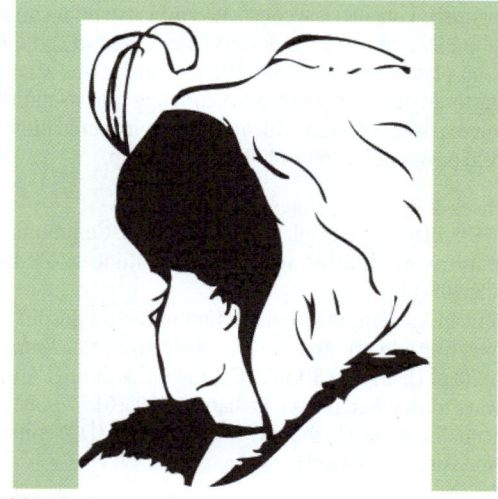

How old is she? Some observers see a young woman, others an old one. The chin and neck of the former become the nose and mouth of the latter and vice versa. Thus different observers, confronted by the same evidence, can reach different conclusions.

C) INVESTIGATIONS : 1) Don't put undue reliance on the results of investigations. If they don't fit, repeat them. The nature of investigations should be regarded as a logical extension of the HX & clinical examination. 2) Many PITFALLS are avoided if a full clinical assessment is always made before instituting any investigation, and then only those selected for a specific purpose. 3) All tests are prone to errors of measurement or interpretation & it should be the doctor in charge of the patient who finally weights up all the evidence before deciding on the diagnosis & prescribing treatment. 4) Last but not the least .... "another thinking" to reduce PITFALLS in the diagnosis & Management. *Most teachers are knowledgeable. Good teachers are intelligent. Great teachers are patient. Exceptional teachers are students themselves, until their last breath..*

SUMMARY: 4 Essential Elements of Clinical Method include * History taking : The beginning of the deductive process, not forgetting also its other essential function, often overlooked, to understand the social, emotional and health predicament of the child and the family. *Physical examination : including (where relevant) development assessment. * Assessment: (summary) of the clinical problem. One of the most difficult parts of the clinical method, bringing together relevant findings (positive and negative) of the history and examination clearly written or stated and including a diagnosis or, if not reached, a differential diagnosis. *Management : The four components: i) Incorporating the need (if any) for further investigations in order to establish, refute or confirm a diagnosis. ii) Problem listing and treatment iii) Communication issues iv) Continuing care; how any ongoing concerns will be dealt with after the main problem has been largely resolved.

The above are ILLUSTRATED in the 'ALGORITHMS' below.

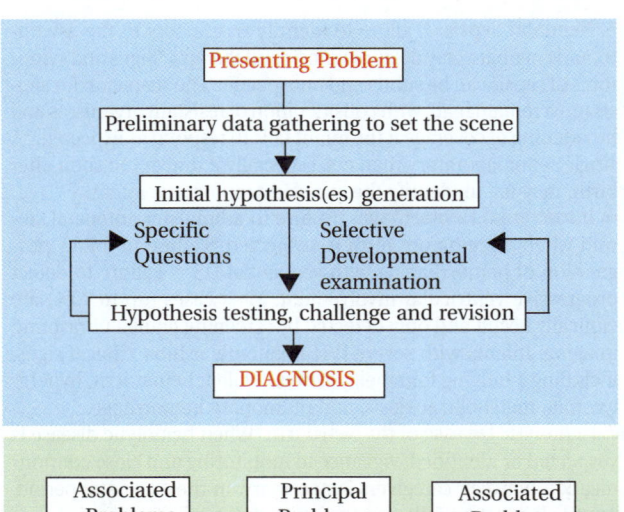

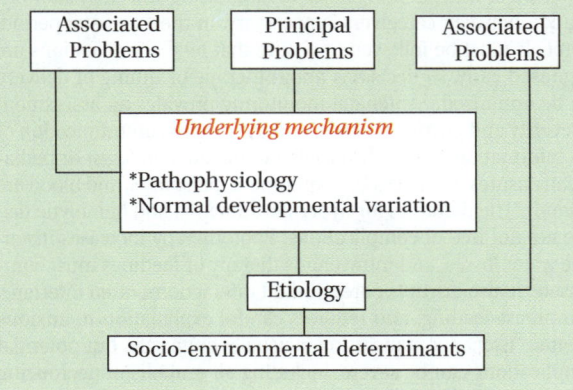

10 COMMANDMENTS FOR DIAGNOSIS & MANAGEMENT OF CHILDHOOD CLINICAL PROBLEMS : After completing *'detailed but quick'* History, *'thorough but appropriate'* Physical examination, *'relevant but cost effective'* investigations, THE PEDIATRICIAN should answer the following *'10' COMMANDMENTS like SEARCHING QUESTIONS TO AVOID pitfalls in the FINISHING STAGE*. After all a great finish compliments, enhances and beautifies the great start.

1) ONSET: Is it 'Acute' - 'Gradual' - 'Chronic' in onset? **2) DURATION :** Is it 'Acute on its own' / 'Acute on chronic' problem ? **3) FREQUENCY :** Any Remissions/ Exacerbations / Recurrent with totally "symptom free/disease" free intervals in between ? **4) SEVERITY :** Is it mild-moderate - severe ? **5) PROGRESSION :** Progressive- (real/apparent)/ Non progressive ? **6) LOCATION :** Localized/systemic.... If so what are the systems involved ? (Respiratory, CVS, GIT (Hepatobiliary) Renal, Genital, Neurological, Hematological, Reticuloendothelial, Metabolic-Endocrinological, ENT, Ophthalmological, Orthopedic, Skin etc., **7) ETIOLOGY** *a) what is the lesion ?* CONGENITAL / FAMILIAL ; Genetic Basis?; Sporadic ? ACQUIRED- IDIOPATHIC ? ; INFECTIOUS (Bacterial, Viral, Mycoplasma, Chlamydial, Fungal, Atypical Organisms)?; INFLAMMATORY/AUTO IMMUNE ? TRAUMATIC (Physical/Chemical/Accidental/ Nonaccidental) POISONING (Suicidal/Homicidal-Accidental/ Nonaccidental) DEGENERATIVE ? VASCULAR ? NEOPLASTIC ? UNCLASSIFIED ? PSYCHOLOGICAL (only DIAGNOSE BY EXCLUSION of Physical Problems) SOCIAL/CULTURAL/ ECONOMICAL ? *b) Where is the lesion?* "PRIMARY/ SECONDARY/TERTIARY " ? E.G.: Hemodynamics/ Neuroanatomy/Lung mechanics, etc. are important to confirm the lesion *c) NATURE OF OUTBREAKS - ISOLATED/ EPIDEMIOLOGICAL /CLUSTERING of clinical cases ? d) Associated complications* ; Known ; Unknown (For EX : In a case of CHD - Growth Faltering ? CCF ? PAH/Shunt Reversal ? Inf. Endocarditis ? Thromboembolic phenomena ? Anemia / polycythemia/ bleeding tendency ? Arrhythmias ?

8) What are the most important pieces of HISTORY, PHYSICAL EXAMINATION, and INVESTIGATIONS overlooked so far to confirm/exclude the provisional diagnosis and differential diagnosis ?

9) What is the most appropriate MANAGEMENT for the "DISEASE IN QUESTION"? - Symptomatic / curative ? - Medical / Surgical/ Combined ? - Emergency / Elective ? - Hospitalization / domiciliary basis ? - Multidisciplinary approach necessary ? For E.g.:- Physiotherapy, speech therapy, Dietician - Ophthalmologist / Orthoptist ; ENT surgeon / Audiologist, Nephrologist / Urologist ; Endocrinologist / Geneticist / Cardiologist / Neurologist / Pulmonologist ; Pediatric surgeon, Orthopedician / CT surgeon / Neuro surgeon - Notification of any notifiable disease in question ? - Test and treat household contacts as appropriate ? - Regular follow-ups ? - PREVENTION - PRIMARY/SECONDARY/ TERTIARY ?

10) COMMUNICATION: Most important of all the 10 COMMANDMENTS ; Have I communicated with patients, parents & with our 'Peers' (Referring Doctors) about the physical, psychological & social aspects of the 'disease' in question ? Is the communication (TIMELY & APPROPRIATE & UNDERSTANDABLE by all 'P' s (Patients, Parents & Peers) ? *(Be careful while communicating with 'P'ress Reporters).*

PITFALLS IN COMMON NEONATAL PROBLEMS

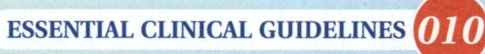
1. Pitfalls of Temperature Regulation

Potential Pitfalls of Servocontrolled Heating Devices

Increased heater output	Skin << Core	Skin > Core	Skin > Core
	Cold stress	Dislodged probe (early)	Dislodged probe (late)
	Shock	Servo fails (late)	
	(vasoconstricted)	Servo fails to shut off	
	Hypoxia	Vasodilators (e.g., tolazoline)	
	Acidosis	Shock (vasodilated)	

Decreased heater output: Probe uninsulated (radiant heat), Servocontrol malfunction, Onset of fever, Baby overheated, Fever, Internal cold stress (e.g. unheated endotracheal oxygen, exchange transfusion)

2. Pitfalls of Neonatal Resuscitation : How to avoid?

1. Strictly follow the guidelines of the NRP. There should be few, if any, departures from the guidelines.

2. Develop a plan to ensure that at least one skilled resuscitator is immediately available for every birth. This does not have to be a pediatrician.

3. Any provider of Newborn resuscitation must be a trained in the techniques of the NRP. This includes obstetricians and anesthesiologists.

4. Mock codes with manikins should be used to maintain resuscitation skills.

5. Limit the number of individuals who serve as the team leader of Newborn resuscitations. Hospital should consider using Neonatologists, hospitalists, nurse practitioners, respiratory therapists, or nurses to serve as the skilled team leader.

6. Follow NRP recommendations in selecting the proper sized endotracheal tube and placing the tube at the correct depth.

7. Capnography and colorimetric CO_2 monitors should be used to document that the endotracheal tube is in the trachea.

8. If an infant is meconium-stained and has cardiorespiratory or neurologic depression at birth, thorough suctioning of the airway must take place before giving positive pressure ventilation. It is not acceptable to visualize the hypopharynx and vocal cords; intubation and intratracheal suctioning is mandated.

9. Avoid hypoglycemia during the postresuscitation stabilization period.

10. Avoid hypotension and unnecessary hypocarbia during the stabilization period. Modest hypocarbia may be beneficial in the treatment of persistent pulmonary hypertension, but has not been shown to be of use in the prevention of the condition.

3. Hypoxic ischemic encephalopathy:

*Birth asphyxia, birth injury, and perinatal asphyxia are terms often used incorrectly to describe hypoxic ischemic encephalopathy (HIE). *Birth injury is a condition in which fetal or neonatal injury has occurred during the process of birth (i.e., during the first and second stages of labor). Examples include brachial plexus injury; fracture of the clavicle; forceps-induced damage to the facial nerve or soft tissues; and cuts or bruises from scissors, clips, or scalp monitors. *Birth asphyxia is similar to birth injury in that asphyxia occurs during the first and second stages of labor when the fetus was otherwise normal. *Perinatal asphyxia signifies that asphyxia occurred at any time in the perinatal period, namely, from conception through the first month of life. *The AAP and ACOG recommend using hypoxic-ischemic encephalopathy because this term accurately describes the clinical condition, encephalopathy from asphyxia, without implying the time of brain injury. The AAP and ACOG also advise not using the terms perinatal asphyxia or birth asphyxia because it is difficult to identify the time of brain injury and nearly impossible to ascertain that the brain had been "normal" before such injury. *All professional societies encourage accurate recording of objective information in the medical records, including maternal and neonatal history and the clinical and laboratory findings. *The findings from brain imaging procedures and EEG help in the total assessment of the infant's clinical status. *No diagnostic tests conclusively prove that a given magnitude of asphyxia has led to a specific neurological injury. Acute perinatal and intrapartum events have been found in only about 20% of children diagnosed as having cerebral palsy. *Counseling the parents with realistic explanations about their infant's clinical status and prognosis is always recommended.

4. Benign Neonatal Convulsions :

*Careful attention to the differential diagnosis of neonatal seizures and appropriate workup avoids most medicolegal problems. However, benign neonatal convulsions are a retrospective diagnosis and frequently present a difficult diagnostic and treatment dilemma even to the most experienced clinicians. *Keep the family appropriately informed at all stages of the workup, diagnosis, and treatment.

5. Neonatal Sepsis:

*Failure to identify risk factors in the asymptomatic neonate may delay diagnosis and therapy. *Signs and symptoms of sepsis can be subtle and nonspecific. The suspicion for sepsis must remain high, with consideration of resistant organisms and broadening of coverage if the infant fails to respond as expected. *A single set of laboratory markers, especially if drawn too soon after birth, may fail to identify the at-risk asymptomatic infant.

6. Intracranial Hemorrhage:

*Failure to administer antenatal steroid when a premature birth is suspected *Failure to follow progression of hemorrhaging with sequential US * Failure to detect progressive ventricular involvement. Most cases (up to 70%) are clinically occult and only detected by screening cranial ultrasound imaging. Infants with severe IVH frequently exhibit clinical signs, including a bulging fontanel, seizures, a fall in hematocrit, hyperglycemia, metabolic acidosis, and pulmonary hemorrhage.

7. Hemolytic Disease of the Newborn:

*When hemolytic disease is suspected or identified, vigilance in monitoring and close communication between caregivers is necessary. In the antenatal period, protocols must be followed to ensure that fetal complications are diagnosed early, so decisions about therapy or timing of delivery can be optimized. *Antenatal monitoring provides an assessment of severity and postnatal needs, and the careful communication of this information by the obstetrician to the neonatologist or pediatrician ensures that necessary equipment, personnel, and blood are at hand. *The therapies for hyperbilirubinemia and hemolytic disease are not free of complications. Phototherapy increases insensible water losses, and intravenous therapy or feedings must compensate. It also disrupts parent-infant interactions, often interferes with breast-feeding, and requires careful explanation to anxious parents. *Exchange transfusion is usually quite safe, but potential complications can be severe, including air embolism, necrotizing enterocolitis, acidosis, hypoglycemia, sepsis, or, rarely, death.

8. Meningitis: * Delays in diagnosis and initiation of treatment are the most critical pitfalls. *Failure to perform a lumbar puncture and detect infection in a neonate with mild fever and minimal, nonspecific clinical findings is problematic; all neonates in whom meningitis might be the cause of symptoms should undergo CSF examination. *Delay in treatment because of equivocal laboratory screening tests or because findings are altered by prior partial treatment may cause significant harm.

9. UTI: *Failure to obtain a urine culture in a sterile fashion before starting antimicrobial therapy. *Failure to adjust the antimicrobial therapy based on the causing organism's susceptibilities. *Failure to appropriately address voiding dysfunction and constipation. *Performance of invasive radiologic studies more frequently than required, thus exposing the child to potential trauma and irradiation. *Because of a high rate of resistance to ampicillin among *E. coli* strains, ampicillin should not be used to empirically treat gram-negative infections or as long-term prophylaxis. *Ruling out renal abscesses based on normal urinalysis and negative urine culture.

10. Hypercalcemia: *Patients in whom the diagnosis should not be missed are those with a dangerous underlying etiology, neonates, and children with ECG changes, altered mental status, dehydration, or renal failure.* *Intravenous (IV) medications, particularly mithramycin, carry serious toxicities and should be administered in an adequately monitored setting. Additionally, practitioners administering these medications should be familiar with the myriad of potentially serious adverse effects following administration. *Regarding treatment, note that pediatric experience with the bisphosphonates is scant, and discussing this with parents in advance may avert attempts at litigation. *In general, few of the etiologies for hypercalcemia other than the electrolyte problem itself are immediately hazardous to the patient. Exceptions to this include thyrotoxicosis and adrenal insufficiency, both of which should be accompanied by other characteristic findings. *Iatrogenic causes of hypercalcemia should be detected and eliminated as soon as possible. *Mild hypercalcemia frequently goes unrecognized in physician offices and emergency departments. This often is acceptable as long as a patient has adequate follow-up care.

11. Ambiguous Genitalia/Intersex : *From a medicolegal standpoint, the best approach to managing these cases is to provide parents with as much information as possible so that they can make informed decisions. Adequate counseling and support for parents is vital. The ideal management method is a team approach including neonatologists, geneticists, endocrinologists, surgeons, counselors, and ethicists. *Treatment for intersex states is controversial. No one debates the need to address and treat underlying physiologic problems such as those associated with congenital adrenal hyperplasia (CAH). The controversy revolves around issues of gender reassignment. Gender assignment by the physician and family may not correlate with gender preference by the patient in adulthood. Remember that the most important sex organ is the brain, which may undergo hormonal imprinting in utero. *Ongoing emotional support is critical, and introduction to support groups and other families with similar problems may be helpful. *There is widespread recognition of the need for long-term functional and psychosexual outcome studies to formulate a more evidence-based approach.

12. Antenatal Hydronephrosis: *In patients with unilateral UPJ obstruction, it is important to evaluate the status of the contralateral kidney with a voiding cystourethrogram. There is an increased incidence of vesicoureteral reflux and other anomalies of the contralateral kidney. *It is important that infants undergoing renal ultrasonography be adequately hydrated at the time of study, as volume contraction may mask an underlying lesion that is revealed only with high urine flow. Diuretic renography (furosemide and MAG3 or DTPA) should generally be performed in infants older than 1 month, to allow for maturation of renal concentrating ability. To allow adequate interpretation of the results, it is important that a catheter be placed in the bladder for the entire procedure.* *Interpretation of the infant's urine stream*: Severe posterior urethral valves may cause enough resistance to urine flow to reduce the infant's urine stream with micturition. However, compensatory thickening of the bladder wall in fetal life may overcome the resistance, and a normal-appearing urine stream is no guarantee of the absence of bladder outlet obstruction *All children with obstructive nephropathy (whether or not undergoing surgery) should have periodic measurement of blood pressure, plasma creatinine concentration, urinalysis, and renal sonography. Nonsteroidal anti-inflammatory drugs should be avoided or their dose carefully monitored. In the transition from pediatrician to internist, such follow-up should be continued throughout adulthood.

13. Apnea of Prematurity: *The use of supplemental oxygen for treatment of episodic desaturation in preterm infants with baseline normoxemia cannot be recommended. *Pharmacologic management of gastroesophageal reflux is unlikely to affect apnea in preterm infants. *Home monitoring of cardiorespiratory events in former preterm infants is not a practical means of preventing sudden infant death syndrome (SIDS). *When an unanticipated death does occur at home, it must be properly investigated. The investigation should address the possibility of death from child abuse, as well as late deaths from unrecognized malformations or inborn errors of metabolism (e.g., fatty acid oxidation disorders).

14. Sudden Infant Death Syndrome: *Failure to counsel parents about the importance of placing their infants to sleep on their backs *Failure to counsel parents about other modifiable risk factors, such as smoking and maintaining a safe sleeping environment *Failure to recognize infants at higher risk for SIDS *Failure to advise that all SIDS cases have an autopsy performed as well as a complete review of the circumstances of the death and the clinical history

15. Congenital Stridor: *failure to make the diagnosis. Infants are frequently diagnosed with congestion or asthma. *True viral upper respiratory infections in infants younger than 1 month are rare. *Persistently abnormal noisy breathing is unlikely to be associated with a viral illness and warrants further investigation. *Noisy breathing should be carefully evaluated to see if the noise is inspiratory, expiratory, or both because the differential diagnosis changes based on the phase affected. *Congenital stridor is not always caused by laryngomalacia; flexible laryngoscopy is simple to perform and may demonstrate a treatable lesion. * Gastroesophageal reflux may accompany stridor and contribute to laryngeal problems. *Tracheotomy can be a lifesaving procedure, but the presence of a tracheotomy in an infant can pose life-threatening complications.

16. Congenital Pneumonia: *Failure to consider the diagnosis in the absence of maternal risk factors for infection *Failure of obstetric care providers to initiate intrapartum chemoprophylaxis in mother with identified risk factors *Failure to initiate neonatal antibiotics in a timely manner *Failure to suction the neonatal airway when particulate meconium is in amniotic fluid and the infant is not vigorous at birth

17. BPD & CLD: *Fluctuations in oxygen saturation should be minimized by limiting interventions and clustering care, by giving additional ventilation before increasing Fio_2 in ventilated infants, and by increasing or decreasing Fio_2 in small increments, remaining at bedside until the situation stabilizes *Failure to institute nutritional management and growth monitoring- Illness, fluid restriction, and feeding difficulties can lead to decreased intake, whereas increased work of breathing requires increased calories. This combination puts these infants at extremely high risk for growth failure, additionally impairing lung growth and repair. Therefore, weight, length, and weight-for-length measurements should be closely monitored. *Immunizations are often deferred but should be given on schedule unless the infant is unstable. All infants should receive palivizumab (Synagis) before discharge during the local respiratory syncytial virus (RSV) season. *Careful discussions between parents and caregivers should be undertaken before corticosteroids are given to high-risk infants.

18. Neonatal conjunctivitis: *Failure to recognize or treat gonococcal conjunctivitis *Failure to provide preventive measures in newborns *Failure to exclude other potential causes of acute red eye (e.g., preseptal cellulitis, orbital cellulitis) *Consider the risk of transmission of chlamydia, gonococcus, herpes, and streptococcus to the fetus during the birth process. Obtain cervical cultures (if indicated), and manage appropriately. *Newborns with conjunctivitis are at risk for secondary infections, such as pneumonia, meningitis, and septicemia, which can lead to sepsis and death. *Infants with a potentially sexually transmitted disease, such as gonorrhea or chlamydia, should undergo evaluation for other sexually transmitted diseases, such as syphilis and HIV, as should the mother and her sexual partner(s).

19. Congenital Cystic Adenomatoid Malformation:

*Failure to diagnose this condition prenatally *Failure to diagnose associated conditions *Failure to offer skilled intervention, such as fetal surgery, in high-risk cases

20. DIC: *Failure to look for purpura in a febrile child, and to recognize it as a possible sign of disseminated intravascular coagulation (DIC), could lead to an adverse outcome. *Recognizing and treating the underlying cause is critical. DIC in certain neonatal conditions can be fulminant, and patients with these conditions should rapidly be given antibiotics, and immediately transferred to a tertiary center.

21. Anemia of Prematurity: *Failure to consider anemia as a possible cause of signs and symptoms *Failure to notify the family about the patient's need for transfusion and obtain a consent before the transfusion *Failure to consider the family's religious beliefs regarding transfusions *Failure to anticipate transfusion-acquired infections and complications *failure to consider alternatives to transfusion such as rHuEPO (recombinant human erythropoietin).

22. Fever without focus: *The biggest pitfall in treating patients with fever without a focus is failing to consider the possibility of a life-threatening illness. Physicians who approach their patients as if this is a possibility and who provide appropriate evaluation and treatment have done their best to avoid a poor outcome. *Stress to parents the criticality of their child returning for follow-up care and stress that they must seek immediate medical attention if their child's condition worsens. *Failure to evaluate and/or treat an ill-appearing infant or child because of a CBC count within the reference range considered normal is a serious pitfall. *Special Concerns* *Even low-risk infants who meet criteria for discharge require close follow-up care. Instruct parents or caregivers to return before the next scheduled appointment if the infant's condition should worsen. *Admit to the hospital all 2-month to 36-month-old febrile patients who have sickle cell anemia.

23. Hydrops Fetalis: *Both false-positive and false-negative Obstetric ultrasonographic diagnosis of hydrops may potentially harm the fetus if conditions amenable to therapy are overlooked or if inappropriate therapy is undertaken. For example, thick subcutaneous fat can mimic subcutaneous edema, and muscles of the abdominal wall sometimes appear very hypoechoic and can resemble ascites. Pulmonary sequestration can be mistaken for cystic adenomatoid malformation unless a careful search is undertaken to establish the arterial blood supply of the sequestered lobe. *Unique medicolegal issues primarily concern the difficult access to the fetus. *Failure to develop parental knowledge and understanding of all choices to obtain truly informed consent *Medications given to the mother place her at risk; however, the same medications may ultimately reach the fetus in concentrations too low to be effective. In addition, a standard therapy has yet to be established. *Similarly, direct fetal surgical maneuvers carry more risk for the fetus than similar procedures performed after birth; direct fetal surgical maneuvers also place the mother at increased risk. *Finally, inadvertent harm to the fetus places the clinician at risk for a considerably longer period than is usual. *At delivery, resuscitation of a hydropic infant may be made more difficult by the presence of cystic hygroma or other lesions involving the neck, airway, or thoracic cavity. *Ventilation and cardiac output may be compromised by pulmonary, pericardial, or abdominal effusions that require acute drainage. *Consideration should be given to draining these under sonographic guidance prior to delivery; failing this, knowledge of their location, size, and relation to organs like the liver and spleen may help avoid a therapeutic catastrophe. *Hyperkalemia and other electrolyte abnormalities usually complicate the early hospital course of an extremely premature hydropic infant. *If large volumes of transfused blood are required, use of washed red cells can prevent exacerbation of the potassium overload.

24. Hypoglycemia: *Neonatal hypoglycemia is a common problem that is difficult to define, understand, and manage. In the past three decades, many published reports addressed this clinical issue, but confusion still remains regarding both the definition of hypoglycemia and its management. *In the neonate, glucose homeostasis is a complex balance between systemic or organ needs and the capability to produce and regulate glucose. *The evidence is now clear from human and animal studies that severe, prolonged hypoglycemia leads to acute neurologic injury that can often result in permanent sequelae. *Parents should be counseled that most newborns with mild hypoglycemia have no long-term sequelae. However, those infants who develop symptomatic hypoglycemia are at high risk for abnormal neurodevelopmental outcome and should be followed carefully. *Infant of **Diabetic Mother**-Failure to recognize and appropriately treat the infant with hypoglycemia can place the treating clinician at medicolegal risk.

25. Intestinal Malrotation: *The biggest pitfall in patients with intestinal malrotation is delay in diagnosis of midgut volvulus. The quicker a patient is taken to surgery, the better the chance for full bowel recovery. Rule out malrotation with midgut volvulus as quickly as possible in any pediatric patient with bilious emesis. If any doubt is noted, refer the patient to an institution with pediatric surgical support for consultation. *Chronic duodenal stenosis is frequently misdiagnosed as colic in patients who present with intermittent abdominal pain and failure to thrive. Upper GI series should be performed to confirm appropriate placement of the duodenojejunal junction.

26. Meconium Aspiration Syndrome: *In patients with meconium aspiration syndrome (MAS), thorough cardiac examination and echocardiography are necessary to evaluate for congenital heart disease and persistent pulmonary hypertension of the newborn (PPHN). *Confirming the degree of pulmonary hypertension, prior to instituting therapy, is extremely important. *Infants with meconium aspiration syndrome are at increased risk for adverse developmental outcomes and should be referred for developmental assessment as an outpatient. *Although initial stabilization is necessary at community hospitals, infants with meconium aspiration syndrome frequently require high-frequency ventilation, inhaled nitric oxide (NO), or extracorporeal membrane oxygenation (ECMO). Therefore, in the event of significant aspiration, transferring these infants to a regional neonatal ICU (NICU) as soon as possible is important. *Children with meconium aspiration syndrome may develop chronic lung disease as a result of intense pulmonary intervention. *Infants with meconium aspiration syndrome have a slightly increased incidence of infections in the first year of life because the lungs are still in recovery. *Most infants with meconium aspiration syndrome have complete recovery of pulmonary function. Intrapartum events initiating the meconium passage may cause the infant to have long-term neurologic deficits, including CNS damage, seizures, mental retardation, and cerebral palsy. *Many infants who have experienced meconium aspiration syndrome (MAS) have had prenatal and postnatal periods of hypoxia and acidosis; therefore, these individuals are at increased risk of significant CNS damage. Typically, medicolegal action is initiated by parents whose newborn develops long-term sequelae from significant perinatal hypoxia.

27. Microphallus: *The importance of appropriate gender assignment cannot be overemphasized. *Evaluate any genital abnormality carefully and early on, using appropriate consultations. *Girls with congenital adrenal hyperplasia have been labeled boys prematurely based on the appearance of their genitalia. *Some males have been gender assigned as girls and put through genital surgery when androgen therapy may have been a simpler and more appropriate treatment.

28. NEC: *Failure to recognize signs of necrotizing enterocolitis (NEC) early enough to effect appropriate care including timely transfer to a tertiary care facility offering pediatric surgery could expose the clinician to medicolegal liability if the baby has a poor outcome as a result. Timely communication with parents and education are crucial to prevent lawsuits in case of unfortunate outcome. Note that poor outcomes do occur even when all care has been timely and appropriate. Necrotizing enterocolitis can be very aggressive with mortality despite excellent care. **The presentation of NEC is variable. Subtle signs need to be recognized, but because they are frequently nonspecific, they may lead to measures that are neither preventive nor therapeutic (i.e., prolonged NPO and prolonged antibiotic therapy that may predispose to colonization with resistant microorganisms). *Some infants, especially of very low birth weight, may develop isolated intestinal perforations, without intestinal necrosis, usually in the first several days of life. Whether these lesions are part of the spectrum of NEC is not known, but they are likely to have a different etiology than the disease that involves actual necrosis. *Minimal enteral feedings do not increase the risk of NEC. In fact, the lack of enteral feedings is associated with mucosal atrophy, a lack of hormonal output, and prolonged parenteral nutrition with its attendant complications. *Lack of communication with pediatric surgery may delay surgery and worsen the prognosis for an infant with NEC.

29. Neonatal Drug Withdrawal Syndrome: *Failure to screen for neonatal abstinence syndrome (NAS) *The medicolegal implications of screening the infant who has been exposed to drugs for the purpose of providing clinical care are complex. Screening creates a conflict between maternal, fetal, and neonatal interests. Although the state courts have granted unborn children some rights in other contexts, any attempt to grant unborn children greater protection against actions taken by their mothers during pregnancy is subject to strict scrutiny. *Screening neonates for illicit drugs without maternal consent is not recommended. In addition, performing these tests without maternal approval may be illegal in certain areas. *Failure to protect an infant at risk *Evidence of maternal substance abuse should alert the infant's medical caretaker that the mother may have medical, psychological, or behavioral problems that could have an impact on the infant's long-term health and welfare. *Testing the mother, infant, or both, with informed consent, is useful in some clinical situations, even when drug use is not suspected. *Some infants may be ill served if the physician relies solely on urine toxicology testing for screening. These test findings may be negative if drugs were used early in pregnancy or during the immediate 48 hours prior to delivery. Results also depend on laboratory variability. Special Concerns *Infants exposed in-utero to drugs have a higher than expected risk of subsequent abuse compared with children in the general population.

30. Neonatal Hypertension: *Failure to diagnose or treat neonatal hypertension (A major concern is missing an underlying cause of hypertension such as renal disease that might require specific therapy.)

31. Prematurity: The medical-legal risk in prematurity is primarily linked to adverse outcome, inappropriate expectations on the part of the family, and poor communication with the family. The smallest and most immature infants are at greatest risk of mental retardation and motor delay or disability.

32. Pulmonary Hypertension: *The main pitfall in the treatment of persistent pulmonary hypertension of the newborn is in recognizing its existence and severity. *Failure to recognize PPHN and provide early intervention may result in more severe clinical disease. *Once the infant is stabilized, a slow methodical approach to weaning should be followed. *Excessively rapid weaning may result in a more severe state of PPHN, which on occasion can be intractable. *Recognizing the destabilizing effects of procedures such as airway suctioning and weighing, these procedures when necessary should be done with a consideration for the prior use of sedation/analgesia. *Careful monitoring for disease progression and timely transfer to an appropriate level of care can be lifesaving in this condition. *Overall therapy must include appropriate treatment of the underlying pathology. *Although inhaled nitric oxide (iNO) is an effective pulmonary vasodilator, extracorporeal membrane oxygenation (ECMO) remains the only therapy that has been proven to be life-saving for persistent pulmonary hypertension of the newborn. Timely transfer to an ECMO center is life saving for newborns with severe persistent pulmonary hypertension of the newborn. *Identifying and maintaining communication with clinicians at an ECMO center is especially important given the widespread availability of iNO therapy. Continuous delivery of NO is required during transport. *The referring center is responsible for determining what transport capabilities are available in order to administer a successful therapeutic iNO program.

33. RSV Bronchiolitis: *Hypoxemia may be clinically inapparent; follow pulse oximetry. *Apnea is possible in young infants, especially former preterms. *Incipient respiratory failure may be present even in presence of normal oxygen saturations; if supplemental oxygen is given; observe closely for signs of respiratory fatigue, and measure blood gases if incipient respiratory failure is suspected. *Recognize that bronchodilator therapy is controversial but therapeutic trials may be useful in individual infants, especially if underlying airway hyperreactivity is suspected from history. *Immunoglobulin) (but not palivizumab) is contraindicated in infants with cyanotic congenital heart disease. *Special Concerns* *High-risk groups for severe RSV infection include the following: *Premature infants in their first year of life (the younger the child is [gestational and chronological age] at the start of RSV season, the greater the risk) *Infants with chronic lung disease (e.g., bronchopulmonary dysplasia, · cystic fibrosis) during their first 2 years of life *Children with hemodynamically significant congenital heart disease, especially with increased pulmonary blood flow *Immunodeficient states *Children with metabolic and neuromuscular disorders *Children of multiple births (triplets or greater).

34. Neonatal Hyperbilirubinemia: *Trusting your eyes rather than measuring bilirubin concentration to gauge risk * Discharging an infant in the high-risk zone of hour-specific bilirubin concentration * Failing to follow up within 24 to 48 hours of early discharge * Misclassifying an infant with hemolysis or other illness as "otherwise healthy" *Using phototherapy as a substitute for exchange transfusion *Failing to treat severe hyperbilirubinemia as an emergency.

35. Infant of Diabetic Mother: *Failure to coordinate an obstetric and pediatric approach to care, as well as identifying the potential multisystem complications of the IDM, is a pitfall. *Fetal growth discordance, associated macrosomia or intrauterine growth restriction, can lead to unexpected delivery room complications of birth injury or postnatal metabolic conditions that can lead to asphyxia, seizures, and further neurologic impairment. *Lung dysmaturity, if unrecognized, can lead to severe morbidity. *Untreated polycythemia can lead to hyperviscosity syndrome, thrombosis, stroke, or necrotizing enterocolitis; *undiagnosed hyperbilirubinemia can lead to increased risk of kernicterus.

36. Hearing Loss: Timely follow-up of infants referred from newborn hearing screening remains a challenge because there can be long delays between screening, diagnostic evaluation, and amplification. Studies suggest that early identification and habilitation have a positive impact on speech/language and literacy skill development; evidence-based outcome research continues to emerge. A false sense of security may ensue when an infant passes the newborn hearing screen. Hearing loss can occur at any age, and thus surveillance must be ongoing to detect delayed-onset or progressive loss. Fluctuating conductive hearing loss caused by otitis media can affect expressive language abilities as well as school performance. The subtleties of language may be compromised because of the inconsistency of the auditory signal. In addition, unilateral hearing loss is frequently missed in children until they are in school and often is first noticed by the teacher. This type of loss can be problematic for children in compromised listening environments (i.e., classrooms, playgrounds, cafeterias). Children with unilateral hearing loss have a 22% to 35% rate of repeating at least one grade; 12% to 41% receive educational resource services.

37. Retinopathy of Prematurity: *If the infant with ROP, or at risk for ROP, is discharged home or transferred to another facility, arrangements for appropriate follow-up ophthalmic examination should be made in advance. If this cannot be done, the infant should not be discharged or transferred. *If scheduled ocular examinations for infants with acute ROP are missed for any reason, alternative arrangements should be made immediately. The importance of ophthalmic examination for maximizing the likelihood of a favorable outcome must be emphasized to parents verbally and in writing. *Infants with ROP requiring treatment should receive laser photocoagulation or cryotherapy within 48 to 72 hours. When necessary, arrangements should be made to transfer the infant to a hospital with adequate facilities for treatment and postoperative care Because the onset and progression of ROP generally occur between 31 and 44 weeks' postmenstrual age, there is a critical time window for effective diagnosis and treatment. * For each particular institution, criteria for ROP examination and follow-up should be established by neonatologists, ophthalmologists, and neonatal intensive care unit staff. These criteria should be readily available, and specific personnel should be assigned responsibility for ensuring that all infants meeting criteria are examined.

38. Congenital Hypothyroidism: *At diagnosis, parents of infants must be educated about the importance and proper techniques in the administration of levothyroxine. *The tablet must be crushed, and not until immediately before dosing can it be suspended in a small amount of liquid. At no age should T_4 be given with food or with medications that contain iron, calcium, soy-containing food or beverage, or fiber; T_4 should be given orally at least 30 minutes and preferably 1 hour before food intake. *Parents should be told never to miss a dose of T_4; if they forget, or are uncertain if the dose was given, the missed dose in its entirety should be given without delay. *The prognosis for intellectual and neurobehavorial development is very good for infants with CH who are diagnosed and treated when asymptomatic very soon after birth, and it is guarded when clinical symptoms and signs are evident during fetal life or at birth.

NEONATAL DISEASE SEVERITY SCORING SYSTEMS

Illness severity scores have become widely used in Neonatal intensive care. Primarily this has been to adjust the mortality observed in a particular hospital or population for the morbidity of their infants, and hence allow standardized comparisons to be performed. Scoring systems involve using appropriately weighted demographic, physiological, and clinical data collected on the infant to calculate a score that quantifies its morbidity.

The principle for such an approach has been long established in many branches of medicine. The desirable properties of Neonatal scores have been described as including: "(1) ease of use; (2) applicability early in the course of hospitalization; (3) ability to reproducibly predict mortality, specific morbidities, or cost for various categories of neonates; (4) usefulness for all groups of neonates to be described." However, these properties are difficult, perhaps impossible, to achieve completely.

Research uses of predictive scores in neonatology

Group predictions

1. Comparing study groups for similarity of risk
2. Auditing the severity of illness in different units
3. Comparing performance of different units
4. Determining trends in results over time
5. Reviewing if infants are treated appropriately for risk (e.g. number of septic screens or ventilation days)
6. Comparing rates of complications; are some preventable?

Individual predictions

1. Giving prognostic information
2. Stratifying infants in trials (to ensure similarity of risk)
3. Determining individual treatment

Illness severity scores are now well accepted as essential tools when comparing healthcare providers. When using an illness severity score, it is important to remain clear about the question being investigated to be sure that the scoring system being used is appropriate. The use of an existing score, developed for another purpose, simply because it is convenient is unlikely to represent the best approach. The use of scores for predicting individual outcomes is fraught with difficulty, most particularly because of variation in the approach to clinical care adopted by different units (and even clinicians in the same unit) as well as important ethical and legal concerns.

It is almost certainly these issues that have, rightly, limited the extent to which scoring systems have been used for individual risk prediction and counselling. The use of an existing score, developed for another purpose, simply because it is convenient is unlikely to represent the best approach. It is also important to remember that, even the best scoring systems are not completely accurate. No mathematical formula can completely capture the complex clinical processes in a Neonate.

SCORES USED IN PREDICTING MORTALITY:

A variety of risk adjustment scores have been derived and advocated for use in assessing Neonatal mortality.Refer to next page for the scoring systems and their variables. In the future, further adequately sized studies, perhaps testing new factors, are warranted both to confirm that our current risk adjustment tools are optimal and also to check that the scores are adequately recalibrated after changes in care. Further work is needed in relation to the use of risk correction scoring systems for comparisons of later health status.

SCORING SYSTEMS VARIABLES

CRIB	SNAP	NTISS
Birth weight	Blood pressure	Supplemental oxygen
Gestation	Heart rate	Surfactant administration
Congenital malformation	Respiratory rate	Tracheostomy care
Maximum base deficit in first 12 h	Temperature	Tracheostomy placement
Minimum appropriate FIO2 in first 12 h	PO_2	CPAP administration
Maximum appropriate FIO2 in first 12 h	PO_2/FiO_2 ratio	Endotracheal intubation
CRIB II	PCO_2	Mechanical ventilation
Birth weight by gestation	Oxygenation index	Mechanical ventilation with paralysis
Maximum base deficit in first 12 h	Packed cell volume	High frequency ventilation
Sex	White blood cell count	Extracorporeal membrane oxygenation
Admission temperature	Immature total ratio	Indomethacin administration
Berlin score	Absolute neutrophil count	Volume expansion
Birth weight	Platelet count	Vasopressor administration
Grade of RDS	Blood urea nitrogen	Pacemaker on standby
Apgar score at 5 min	Creatinine	Pacemaker used
Artificial ventilation	Urine output	Cardiopulmonary resuscitation
Base excess at admission	Indirect bilirubin	Antibiotics
NICHHD score	Direct bilirubin	Diuretics (enteral)
Birth weight	Sodium	Steroids (postnatal)
Small for gestational age	Potassium	Anticonvulsant
Race	Calcium (ionized)	Aminophylline
Sex	Calcium (total)	Other unscheduled medication
Apgar score at 1 min	Glucose	Diuretics (parenteral)
NMPI	Serum bicarbonate	Treatment of metabolic acidosis
Gestational age	Serum pH	Potassium binding resin
Birth weight	Seizure	Frequent vital signs
Cardiac arrest	Apnea	Cardiorespiratory monitoring
PaO_2/FIO_2 ratio	Stool guaiac	Phlebotomy
Major congenital malformations	**SNAP-PE**	Thermoregulated environment
Sepsis	SNAP score plus :	Non-invasive oxygen monitoring
Base excess	Birth weight	Arterial pressure monitoring
SINKIN 12 hour	Apgar score,7 at 5 min	CVP monitoring
Birth weight	Small for gestational age	Urinary catheter
Gestational age	**SNAP-II**	Quantitative intake and output
Apgar score at 5 min	Mean blood pressure	Gavage feeding
Peak inspiratory pressure at 12 h	Lowest temperature	Intravenous fat emulsion
NBRS	PO_2/FIO_2 ratio	Intravenous amino acid solution
Blood pH	Serum pH	Phototherapy
Hypoglycemia	Multiple seizures	Insulin administration
Intraventricular hemorrhage	Urine output	Potassium infusion
Periventricular leucomalacia	**SNAPPE-II**	Transfusion
Seizures	SNAP II score plus :	Intravenous c globulin
Infection	Birth weight<749 g	Red blood cell transfusion
Need for mechanical ventilation	Apgar,7 at 5 min	Partial volume exchange transfusion
	Small for gestational age	Platelet transfusion
		White blood cell transfusion, Double blood cell transfusion, Transport of patient, Chest tube, Minor operation, Thoracentesis, Major operation, Pericardiocentesis, Pericardial tube, Dialysis, Vascular access, Peripheral intravenous line, Arterial line, Central venous line

CRIB, clinical risk index for babies; FIO_2, fractional inspired concentration of oxygen; NBRS, neurobiological risk score; NMPI, neonatal mortality prognosis index; NTISS, neonatal therapeutic intervention scoring system; PO_2, partial pressure of oxygen; RDS, respiratory distress syndrome; SNAP, score for neonatal acute physiology; SNAPPE, score for neonatal acute physiology-perinatal extension.

Courtesy: J S Dorling, D J Field, B Manktelow Arch Dis Child Fetal Neonatal Ed 2005;90:F11–F16. doi: 10.1136/adc.2003.048488

ALERTING AND/OR ALARMING NEONATAL SYMPTOMS

1. *Pallor*: Persistent pallor, in addition to anemia or acute hemorrhage (external or internal), should suggest hypoxia, asphyxia, hypoglycemia, sepsis, shock, edema or adrenal failure. A serious sign and requires expeditious investigation. Early recognition of anemia may lead to a diagnosis of E.fetalis, subcapsular hematoma of liver or spleen, subdural hemorrhage, or fetal-maternal or twin-twin transfusion. Without being anemic, postmature infants tend to have pallor and thicker skin than term or premature infants do. The ruddy red appearance of plethora is seen with polycythemia. *Mottling, an example of general circulatory instability, may be associated with serious illness or related to a transient fluctuation in skin temperature.* An extraordinary division of the body from the forehead to the pubis into red and pale halves is known as **harlequin color change,** a transient and harmless condition.

2. *Jaundice:* During the first 24hrs of life warrants diagnostic evaluation and should be considered to be due to hemolysis until proved otherwise. Consider septicemia and intrauterine infections such as CMV, Toxoplasmosis and Syphilis, especially in infants with an increase in plasma direct reacting bilirubin. Jaundice after 1st 24hr may be "physiologic" or may be due to septicemia, hemolytic anemia, galactosemia, hepatitis, congenital biliary atresia, inspissated bile syndrome after E.fetalis, syphilis, herpes simplex, or other congenital infections. In a newborn, jaundice usually is apparent when the serum total bilirubin level reaches 5mg/dL. *Look for criteria that suggest pathologic jaundice - a)clinical jaundice in the 1st 24hr of life b)total serum bilirubin >95th percentile for age in hours c)serum total bilirubin concentration increasing by >0.5mg/dL/hr d)direct serum bilirubin concentration exceeding 1.5-2mg/dL e)clinical jaundice persisting >2weeks in a full-term infant.*

3. *Poor capillary refilling and blood pressure instability:* Marked vasoconstriction with clinical evidence of poor capillary filling (>3 seconds), generalized hypoperfusion, and unstable systemic blood pressure are usually warning signs of serious underlying conditions (e.g., hypoxia, hypovolemia, sepsis, cardiovascular instability, CNS injury).

4. *Persistent central cyanosis and prolonged oxygen requirement:* Has respiratory, cardiac, CNS, hematologic, and metabolic causes. Episodes of cyanosis may be the initial sign of hypoglycemia, bacteremia, meningitis, shock, or pulmonary hypertension. Respiratory insufficiency may be due to pulmonary conditions or may be secondary to CNS depression as a result of drugs, I/C bleed, or anoxia. If caused by pulmonary conditions, respirations tend to be rapid and may be accompanied by retractions and grunting. If it is due to CNS depression, respirations tend to be irregular and weak and are often slow. Cyanosis unaccompanied by obvious signs of respiratory difficulty suggests cyanotic congenital heart disease (right sided heart lesions) or methemoglobinemia. Cyanosis resulting from congenital heart disease (especially left sided lesions with CCF) may however be difficult to distinguish clinically from cyanosis caused by respiratory disease. Clinical evidence of persistent central cyanosis (O_2 saturation <90%) in room air or need for supplemental oxygen after 2-3hr of age to sustain normal O_2 saturations represents a deviation from a normal transition and requires immediate evaluation. *Evaluation of the heart by echocardiography and ECG is essential when the possibility of a significant CHD exists. Pulses should be palpated in the upper and lower extremities to detect coarctation of the aorta on both admission and discharge from the nursery.* Significant cyanosis may be masked by the pallor of circulatory failure or anemia; alternatively, the relatively high hemoglobin content of the first few days and the thin skin may combine to produce an appearance of cyanosis at a higher PaO_2 than in older children. Localized cyanosis is differentiated from ecchymosis by the momentary blanching pallor (with cyanosis) that occurs after pressure. The same maneuver also helps in demonstrating icterus, possibly significant but unnoticed if the skin is suffused with blood.

5. *Persistent tachypnea, flaring of alae nasi, grunting, retractions and rales:* Are accepted as normal events during the 1st period of reactivity. But the same are considered as the *cardinal features of respiratory distress* in a Newborn. The distinction between what is considered normal transition and what represents an early onset of respiratory distress is based on severity and duration of symptoms. Further investigation is warranted in the event of a persistent respiratory status score >4 (Down score in term or Silvermen score in preterm) or duration of symptoms beyond the 1st hr of life. *Suspicion of pulmonary pathology because of diminished breath sounds, rales, retractions, or cyanosis should always be verified with a chest radiograph.*

6. *Apnea and bradycardia:* Periods of apnea, particularly in premature infants, may be associated with various disturbances. When apnea recurs or when the intervals are longer than 20seconds or are associated with cyanosis or bradycardia, an immediate diagnostic evaluation is needed. *Diagnosis of apnea for prematurity (<32weeks GA) requires exclusion of central, obstructive, and combined apnea and other causes of apnea, including GE reflux, PDA, and nasal congestion.* In practice, onset of apnea in the 1st week of life in an infant <35weeks of GA for whom sepsis and metabolic abnormalities can be excluded is assumed to be apnea of prematurity. Careful clinical observation for other causes of apnea should continue because GE reflux and seizures can be exacerbated by some pharmacologic treatments for apnea. Apnea of prematurity generally improves with increasing postconceptional age, becoming mild beyond 32 weeks and typically resolving by 35 weeks.

7. *Lethargy:* May be a manifestation of infection, asphyxia, hypoglycemia, hypercapnia, sedation from maternal analgesia or anesthesia, a cerebral defect, and indeed, almost any severe disease including inborn errors of metabolism. Lethargy appearing after the second day should, in particular, suggest infection. Lethargy with emesis suggests raised ICP or inborn error of metabolism.

8. *Irritability:* May be a sign of discomfort accompanying intra-abdominal conditions, meningeal irritation, drug withdrawal, infections, congenital glaucoma, or any condition producing pain. As in later infancy, the eardrums should always be examined as a possible source of pain. Hyperactivity, especially in a premature infant, may be a sign of hypoxia, pneumothorax, emphysema, hypoglycemia, hypocalcemia, CNS damage, drug withdrawal, neonatal thyrotoxicosis, bronchospasm, esophageal reflux, or discomfort from a cold environment. *Marked depression and lethargy, decreased activity with marked and persistent hypotonia, irritability, excessive tremors, and jitteriness are unusual neurologic behaviours and require further investigation.*

9. **Convulsions:** Usually point to a disorder of the CNS and suggest hypoxic-ischemic encephalopathy, hemorrhage, cerebral anomaly, subdural effusion, meningitis, hypocalcemia, hypoglycemia, cerebral infarction, benign familial seizures, and rarely, pyridoxine dependence, hyponatremia, hypernatremia, inborn errors of metabolism, or drug withdrawal. Seizures beginning in the delivery room or shortly thereafter may be due to the unintentional injection of maternal local anesthetic into the fetus. Convulsions may also result from hyponatremia and water intoxication in the infant after the administration of large amounts of hypotonic fluid to the mother shortly before and during delivery. Convulsions should be distinguished from the jitteriness that may be present in normal Newborns, in infants of diabetic mothers, in those who experienced birth asphyxia or drug withdrawal, and in polycythemic Neonates. Jitteriness resembling simple tremors may be stopped by holding the infant's extremity; it often depends on sensory stimuli and occurs when the infant is active, and it is not associated with abnormal eye movements. Tremors are often more rapid with a smaller amplitude than are tonic clonic seizures. Seizures in premature infants are often subtle and associated with abnormal eye (fluttering, deviation, stare) or facial (chewing, tongue thrusting) movements; the motor component is often that of tonic extension of the limbs, neck, and trunk. Term infants may have focal or multifocal, clonic or myoclonic movements, but they may also have more subtle seizure activity. Apnea may be the 1st manifestation of seizure activity, particularly in a premature infant. Seizures may adversely affect the subsequent neurodevelopmental outcome and even predispose to non-neonatal seizures. Seizures should be treated aggressively. After severe birth asphyxia, infants may have **motor automatisms** characterized by oral-buccal-lingual movements, rotary limb activities (rowing, pedalling, swimming), tonic posturing, or myoclonus. These motor activities are not usually accompanied by time-synchronized electroencephalo-graphic discharges, may not signify cortical epileptic activity, respond poorly to anticonvulsant therapy, and are associated with a poor prognosis. Such automatisms may represent cortical depression that produces a brainstem release phenomenon or subcortical seizures.

10. **Failure to feed well:** is seen in most sick newborn infants and should always indicate a careful search for infection, a central or peripheral nervous system disorder, intestinal obstruction, and other abnormal conditions.

11. **Fever:** May be the result of too high an environmental temperature because of weather, overheated nurseries or isolettes/radiant warmers, or too many clothes. It is also noted in "dehydration fever" of Newborn infants. If this cause of fever can be eliminated, serious infection (pneumonia, bacteremia, meningitis, and viral infections, particularly herpes simplex or enteroviruses) must be considered, although such infections often occur without provoking a febrile response in Newborn infants. An unexplained fall in body temperature may accompany infection or other serious disturbances of the circulation or CNS. A sudden servo-controlled increase in isolette ambient temperature to maintain body temperature is a sign of temperature instability and may be associated with sepsis.

12. **Excessive oral secretions, drooling, and choking spells:** Increased salivation and oral mucus are characteristic parasympathetic reactions during the first and second periods of reactivity. Excessive amounts of oral mucus, drooling, episodes of cyanosis, choking, and coughing spells all indicate compromised transition necessitating careful evaluation (e.g. possible esophageal atresia or grade 2 birth asphyxia).

13. **Vomiting:** During the 1st day, infants who have large amounts of mucus or swallowed blood in the stomach may repeatedly regurgitate small amounts of material or have difficulty in feeding. Orogastric lavage with saline is sometimes used to remove this material and may improve feeding. If vomiting persists, further assessment, including abdominal radiographs, should be pursued. Persistent vomitings during the first day of life suggests obstruction in the upper digestive tract or increased intracranial pressure. Vomiting may also be a nonspecific symptom of an illness such as septicemia. It is a common manifestation of overfeeding or inexperienced feeding technique, pyloric stenosis, milk allergy, duodenal ulcer, stress ulcer, inborn errors of metabolism (hyper-ammonemia, metabolic acidosis), or adrenal insufficiency. *Vomiting containing dark blood usually a sign of a serious illness; the benign possibility of swallowed maternal blood should also be considered. Bile-stained vomitus strongly suggests obstruction below the ampulla of Vater and warrants contrast radiography.*

14. **Diarrhea:** May be a symptom of overfeeding (especially high-caloric density formula), acute gastroenteritis, or malabsorption, or it may be a nonspecific symptom of infection. Diarrhea may occur in conditions accompanied by compromised circulation of part of the intestinal or genital tract, such as mesenteric thrombosis, necrotizing enterocolitis, strangulated hernia, intussusception, and torsion of the ovary or testis. The color and consistency of stools change from green-black and very viscous on the day 1 to green-yellow and paste-like by the third or fourth postnatal day. Normal stools are not watery, but those of breast-fed infants are often softer and less formed than are the stools of formula-fed infants. During the first week, the normal frequency of stool output varies from 1-10/day, usually averaging 3–5 stools daily. Stools that are dark red and tar-like in consistency are indicative of old blood, usually maternal in origin, that was swallowed at the time of delivery. This can be distinguished from the infant's blood by a test that differentiate between adult and fetal hemoglobin (Apt test for alkali resistance of fetal hemoglobin). Small streaks of bright red blood in the stools often reflect the presence of a rectal fissure. If no fissure is found, or if there are large quantities of blood in the stools, further evaluation is indicated.

15. **Abdominal distention:** Usually a sign of intestinal obstruction or an intra-abdominal mass, may also be seen in infants with enteritis, necrotizing enterocolitis, isolated intestinal perforation, ileus accompanying sepsis, respiratory distress, ascites, or hypokalemia. Babies with high gastrointestinal obstruction (proximal to the ileocecal valve) usually present with vomiting but may not have abdominal distention or abnormal stool frequency during the first 24hrs after birth. Infants with lower intestinal obstruction are less likely to exhibit vomiting early but often exhibit abdominal distention and absent stools. Abdominal wall defects produce an omphalocele when they occur through the umbilicus & gastroschisis when they occur lateral to the midline. Unusual masses per abdomen should be investigated immediately by ultrasonography. Renal pathology is the cause of most Neonatal abdominal masses. Cystic abdominal masses include hydronephrosis, multicystic-dysplastic kidneys,

adrenal hemorrhage, hydrometrocolpos, intestinal duplication, and choledochal, ovarian, omental, or pancreatic cysts. Solid masses include neuroblastoma, mesoblastic nephroma, hepatoblastoma, & teratoma. A solid flank mass may be caused by renal vein thrombosis, which becomes clinically apparent with hematuria, hypertension, & thrombocytopenia. Renal vein thrombosis in infants is associated with polycythemia, dehydration, diabetic mothers, asphyxia, sepsis, nephrosis, and hypercoagulable states such as antithrombin III or protein C deficiency.

16. *Bowels:* Approximately 70% of normal Newborn infants excrete meconium during the 1st 24hrs, & 95% of infants pass atleast one stool within 24hrs. Passage of meconium may be delayed in infants with distal intestinal obstruction, as in meconium plug syndrome or in infants with Hirschsprung disease. Other causes of abnormal GIT mobility & delayed stool excretion are premature birth, sepsis, hypothyroidism, & various drugs, including narcotics. Imperforate anus is not always visible & may require evidence obtained by gentle insertion of the little finger or a rectal tube. Radiographic study is required. Passage of meconium doesn't rule out an imperforate anus if a recto-vaginal fistula is present.

17. *Urination:* Approximately 2/3rds of Newborn infants urinate within 12hrs of birth, and virtually all Newborn infants have voided atleast once within 24hrs. Absence of urine output may be of prerenal origin (severe hypovolemia & hypotension, myocardial failure, dehydration), or it may reflect renal anomalies, such as absent kidneys, acute tubular necrosis from Ischemia, or renal vein thrombosis, or it may signal obstruction to urinary outflow, possibly from posterior urethral valves or from a blocked urethra. Neonatal urine is normally yellow or light brown. Urate crystals, which vary from deep pink to tan in colour, are a common source of diaper stain in the Newborn period. Hematuria is pathologic & requires urgent evaluation.

18. *Pseudoparalysis:* Failure to move an extremity suggests fracture, dislocation, or nerve injury. Also seen in osteomyelitis & other infections that cause pain on movement of the affected part.

19. *Pain:* In Neonates may be unrecognized and/or undertreated. The intensive care of Neonates may involve a number of painful procedures, including blood sampling, (heel stick, venous or arterial puncture), endotracheal intubation and suctioning, mechanical ventilation, and insertion of chest tubes and intravascular catheters. Pain in Neonates results in obvious distress and acute physiologic stress responses, which may have developmental implications for pain in later life. Moreover, the knowledge that infants may experience pain contributes to the stress of parents of sick newborns. Pain and discomfort are potentially avoidable problems during the treatment of sick infants. Preemptive relief from painful stimuli should be provided before pain or anxiety develops. The most frequently used drugs are intermittent or continuous doses of opioids (morphine, fentanyl) or benzodiazepines (midazolam, lorazepam). Although the long-term effects of opioids and sedatives are not well established, the 1st concern should be the treatment and/or prevention of acute pain. Continuous opiate infusions should be used with caution. Some minor but painful procedures on well Neonates have also been managed with oral sucrose solutions, although the optimal dose is undetermined.

20. *Edema:* May produce a superficial appearance of good nutrition. Pitting after applied pressure may or may not be noted, but the skin of the fingers and toes lacks the normal fine wrinkles when filled with fluid. Edema of the eyelids commonly results from irritation caused by the administration of silver nitrate. Generalized edema may occur with prematurity, hypoproteinemia secondary to severe erythroblastosis fetalis, nonimmune hydrops, congenital nephrosis, Hurler syndrome, or unknown cause. Localized edema suggests a congenital malformation of the lymphatic system; when confined to one or more extremities of a female infant, it may be the initial sign of Turner syndrome.

21. *Congenital anomalies:* A major cause of still births & Neonatal deaths, but they are perhaps even more important as causes of acute illness & long-term morbidity. Early recognition of anomalies is important for planning care; with some, such as TE fistula, diaphragmatic hernia, choanal atresia, and intestinal obstruction, immediate medical & surgical therapy is essential for survival. Parents are likely to feel anxious and guilty on learning of the existence of congenital anomaly and require sensitive counseling.

COMMON LIFE-THREATENING CONGENITAL ANOMALIES

Name	Manifestations
Choanal atresia	Respiratory distress in delivery room, apnea, unable to pass nasogastric tube through nares. Suspect CHARGE syndrome
Pierre Robin syndrome	Micrognathia, cleft palate, airway obstruction
Diaphragmatic hernia	Scaphoid abdomen, bowel sounds present in chest, respiratory distress
Tracheoesophageal fistula	Polyhydramnios, aspiration pneumonia, excessive salivation, unable to place nasogastric tube in stomach. Suspect VATER syndrome
Intestinal obstruction Volvulus, duodenal atresia, ileal atresia	Polyhydramnios, bile-stained emesis, abdominal distention. Suspect trisomy 21, cystic fibrosis, cocaine
Gastroschisis, omphalocele	Polyhydramnios, intestinal obstruction
Renal agenesis, Potter syndrome	Oligohydramnios, anuria, pulmonary hypoplasia, pneumothorax
Neural tube defects : anencephalus, meningomyelocele	Polyhydramnios, elevated α-fetoprotein, decreased fetal activity
Ductal-dependent congenital heart disease	Cyanosis, hypotension, murmur

CHARGE, coloboma of the eye, heart anomaly, choanal atresia, retardation, and genital and ear anomalies; VATER, vertebral defects, imperforate anus, tracheoesophageal fistula, and radial and renal dysplasia.

ESSENTIALS OF BREASTFEEDING

1. **Breast milk is the best:** Human milk is the preferred feeding for all infants including Premature and Sick Newborns with rare exceptions (AAP, 1997) .WHO recommends exclusive breast feeding for the first 6 months of life, with continued breast feeding along with appropriate complementary foods through the 1st 2 years of life. It is impossible for Formula milk to replicate the nutritional or immunological composition of Human milk despite advances in formula processing technology.

2. **Benefits ascribed to breast milk:** *Nutritional *Enhancement of mother-infant bonding,self-esteem,success with mothering associated with early contact *Prevention of GIT & Respiratory tract infections *Diminished risk of serious atopic disease *Economic *Enhanced cognitive development *Lowered risk of SIDS *Improved postpartum recovery, partial birth control,reduction of postmenopausal hip and spinal fractures and reduced risk of breast and ovarian cancers *Hormonal-Erythropoietin and epidermal growth factors *Immunological-nucleotides which may promote cell-mediated immunity,macrophages, polymorphs and T+B cells *Digestive-lipases and amylase may assist in digestion *Convenience, comfort, more sleep, and less anxiety, sterile and available at right temperature *Lowered incidence of childhood diabetes and malignancies (lymphoma) *Reduced incidence of NEC in preterm infants.

Babies who are breastfed have a decreased chance of developing:

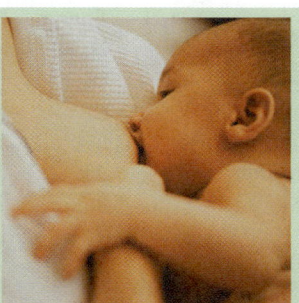

- Respiratory and ear infections
- Allergies and atopic diseases
- Asthma
- Urinary tract infections
- Diarrheal infections, gastrointestinal reflux and NEC
- Bacterial meningitis
- SIDS
- Juvenile rheumatoid arthritis
- Childhood lymphomas such as Hodgkin's Disease and Leukemia

3. **WHO/UNICEF 1989 joint statement-10 steps to successful breastfeeding:** A Baby-Friendly Hospital is one that completes the 10 steps successfully; accomplishing these **10 steps** requires cooperation between pediatricians, nurses, hospital administration and lactation specialists. **1)** Develop a written breastfeeding policy and routinely communicate it to all health care staff. **2)**Train all health care staff in skills necessary to implement the policy. **3)** Inform all pregnant women about the benefits and management of breastfeeding. **4)** Help mothers initiate breastfeeding within half an hour of birth. **5)**Show mothers how to breastfeed, and how to maintain lactation even if they should be separated from their infants **6)** Give newborn infants no food or drink other than breast milk, unless medically indicated. **7)**Practice rooming-in: Allow mothers and infants to remain together 24 hours a day. **8)**Encourage breastfeeding on demand. **9)**Give no artificial teats or pacifiers (also called dummies or soothers) to breastfeeding infants. **10)**Foster the establishment of breastfeeding support groups and refer mothers to them on discharge from the hospital or clinic

4. **Contraindications to breastfeeding:** * Maternal HIV infection in developed countries and in well-to-do mothers in developing and 3rd world countries *Chemotherapy with cytotoxic drugs, such as cyclophosphamide,methotrexate, or doxorubicin *Immuno-suppression with cyclosporine *Substance abuse with street drugs such as amphetamine, cocaine,heroin,or phencyclidine *Surgery on breasts that disrupts the lactiferous ducts,such as reduction mammoplasty *Galactosemia in the infant *Herpes simplex active breast lesions *Active untreated Tuberculosis in mother *Life-Threatening illness in the mother *Hepatitis B or C infection in mother, if suffering from cracked nipples with bleeding.

5. **Conditions that are not contraindications to breastfeeding** 1. Mothers who are hepatitis B surface antigen positive. Infants should receive hepatitis B immune globulin and hepatitis B vaccine to eliminate risk of transmission. 2. Hepatitis C virus transmission through breastfeeding 3. In full term infants, the benefits of breast feeding appear to out weigh the risk of transmission from cytomegalovirus (CMV) positive mothers. The extremely preterm infant is at increased risk or perinatal CMV acquisition. Frozen milk or pasteurization may reduce the risk of transmission in human milk. 4. Mothers who are febrile 5. Mothers exposed to low-level environmental chemical agents 6. Although tobacco smoking is not contraindicated, mothers should be advised to avoid smoking in the home and make every effort to stop smoking while breastfeeding.

6. **Assessment of adequacy of breastfeeding on early follow-up visit:** *TIMING OF VISIT—2–3 days after discharge *FEEDING HISTORY: frequency of nursing- every 1.5–3 hr, 8–12 feeds/24 hr; duration of nursing-approximately 15 minutes per breast, finish at 1st breast before going on to the 2nd?; observe nursing interaction-position comfortable? baby latches on correctly? audible swallowing without smacking or other extraneous noises?*ELIMINATION HISTORY-

7. **Risk factors for failed breastfeeding:** *MATERNAL FACTORS—flat/inverted nipples, previous poor milk production, excessive nipple pain or unrelieved engorgement,failure of milk to "secrete in " by 4th postpartal day, previous breast surgery,especially periareolar incisions (breast reduction/augmentation), marked asymmetry; tubular breasts

   *INFANT FACTORS—prematurity, low birth weight, cleft palate, micrognathia, neuromuscular problems with hypotonia, excessive jaundice, especially requiring phototherapy, difficulty latching on; poor arousal to feed in hospital, infant separated from mother for >24 hours, weight loss >7-8% from birth weight, failure to have yellow stools by 4th day of life.

8. **Reasons for expressing breast milk (EBM):** *Full and uncomfortable breasts *Baby too immature or sick to breast-feed *Mother may be returning to work or be away from the baby,as for a social reason.

9. **Methods of expressing breast milk:** By hand/a hand pump/an electric pump- *Frequent (minimum of 6-8 times in 24 hours, including once during the night) and efficient milk removal is essential for continued production of milk. *Careful hand washing before milk expression, thorough cleaning and sterilization of all containers and pump pieces should be done *Breast massage and simultaneous pumping of both breasts increase the volume of milk expressed.

9. **Human milk banking:** Breast milk (labelled or dated) may be stored in a refrigerator at 2–4* C for 3-5 days, for a week in the ice compartment of a refrigerator, or for up to 3 months in a freezer. Frozen breast milk should be thawed slowly in a refrigerator or at a room temperature(not in a microwave) and, once thawed, used within 24 hr or discarded, but never refrozen. Dedicated human milk banks require significant funding and organization, effective donor screening for HIV, HBV, and HCV, effective pasteurisation, bacteriologic monitoring, nutrient quality control, and adequate manpower to ensure the smooth running of the facility. It should be noted that the above processing of human milk has a deleterious effect on its biological (antimicrobial activity) and biophysical properties(reduction in fat, riboflavin, and vitamin A and C content. Moreover, babies fed fresh breast milk gain weight better than those who receive it after freezing.)

10. **Indications that an infant is ready for feeding:** *Alertness and vigor *Absence of abdominal distention *Good bowel sounds *Normal hunger cry *Adequate suck and swallow.

11. **Indications that an infant is properly latched-on to the breast:** *Baby;s chin is touching the breast *his mouth is wide open *his lower lip is turned outwards *more areola is visible above the baby's mouth than below it.

12. **Human milk versus cow's and formula milk:**

TABLE 1 — Composition of various milks (all per 100 ml of milk)

Milk	Energy (kcal)	Protein (g)	Casein: whey	CHO (g)	Fat (g)	Na (mmol)	K (mmol)	Ca (mmol)	P (mmol)
Mature term breast milk	70	1.3	1:2	7	4.2	0.65	1.5	0.9	0.5
Preterm breast milk	67	1.8-2.4	N/A	6	4	2.2	1.8	0.6	0.5
Preterm EBM + fortifier	80	2.5-3.1	N/A	9	4	3.1	–	1.8	1.4
Donor bank milk	46	1.1	N/A	7.1	1.7	0.7	–	0.9	0.5
Cow's milk	67	3.4	3:1	4.6	3.9	2.2	3.9	3	3
Whey based term formula	65–68	1.5	1:1.5	7.0–7.3	3.6-3.8	0.8	1.4-2.2	0.9–1.5	0.9–1.1
Casein-based term formula	65–69	1.5-1.9	4:1	7.2–8.6	3.1-3.6	0.8-1.1	1.6-2.2	1.2–2.1	1.2–1.8
Follow-on (>6 months)	70	1.8	3.5:1	7.2	4.6	1.0	2.2	2.2	1.6
LBW formula	80	2.0-2.4	1:1.5	7.0–8.5	3.5-4.9	1.3-2.0	1.8	1.8–2.7	1.1–1.7
LBW follow-on	74	1.8	1.5:1	7.5	4.1	1.0	1.9	2.0	1.3

Colostrum is a yellow, sticky fluid, which is secreted during the first 3-5 days postpartum: · It contains over sixty components, thirty of which are exclusive to human milk. · Colostrum continues to offer the immunities that were available to the baby via the placenta. · It is high in protein, as well as fat-soluble vitamins and minerals. · Colostrum contains high amounts of sodium, potassium, chloride and cholesterol thought to encourage optimal development of the baby's heart, brain and central nervous system. · The yellow color of colostrum is due to B-carotene, one of the many antioxidants present. · Colostrum's natural laxative benefit encourages the passage of meconium, which reduces the risk of jaundice in the baby. · This fluid is rich in immunoglobulins, which protect the infant from viruses and infections. · It continues to be secreted in breastmilk for up to two weeks postpartum. **Fore and hind milk (important differences)** In addition to the changes from colostrum to mature milk that mirror the needs of the developing neonate, variation exists within a given breastfeeding session. The milk first ingested by the infant (fore milk) has a lower fat content. As the infant continues to breastfeed over the next several minutes, the fat content increases. This hind milk is thought to facilitate satiety in the infant. Finally, the diurnal variations in breast milk reflect maternal diet and daily hormonal fluctuations

Breastfeeding and preterm infant: The period following the birth of a premature infant can be overwhelming for families. The advice and support of a trusted family physician can be invaluable to parents confronted with unforeseen decisions and numerous uncertainties. Some relatively mature preterm infants may be able to breastfeed right away. Family physicians can provide immediate guidance on maintaining lactation when mother-infant separation is required. Preterm breast milk differs from term breast milk, in that it has a higher concentration of protein, immunoglobulin A, infection-fighting cells, immunomodulators and antiinflammatory factors and it provides short- and long-term health advantages for preterm infants. Premature infants who receive their mother's milk have a decreased risk of necrotizing enterocolitis, improved gut motility and maturation, and reduced rates of sepsis compared with infants who receive milk substitutes. Studies of preterm infants have also demonstrated reduced rates of atopic disease in infants with a family history of atopy. A meta-analysis of 20 studies concluded that breastfeeding is associated with long-term cognitive advantages and that preterm infants derive more benefit than full-term infants. Breast milk has also been associated with enhanced retinal development and visual acuity in preterm infants. However, mother's milk may need to be supplemented with a fortifier for smaller or more fragile preterm infants. Studies have shown that preterm infants show greater cardiac and respiratory stability when breastfeeding rather than bottle-feeding. Therefore, initiating breastfeeding in preterm infants does not require demonstrated ability to bottle-feed. In addition to promoting physiologic stability in premature infants, skin-to-skin contact or "kangaroo care" increases maternal milk supply and breastfeeding rates. Mothers of preterm infants should be presented with information about the benefits of breastfeeding and breast milk for the premature infant. Women who are hesitant to make a long-term commitment to breastfeeding should be encouraged to nurse or express colostrum and milk for her infant until the baby is discharged from the hospital. The mother of a preterm infant faces many challenges including infant illness, maternal-infant separation, infant feeding difficulties at the breast including the possibility of prolonged pumping, with the emotional and physical stress of juggling personal care with other commitments to her family, job, and her newborn. When family physicians work as part of a medical team of neonatologists, nurses, social workers, dietitians, and lactation consultants, they can be effective in supporting the successful initiation and continuation of breastfeeding the preterm infant.

Breastfeeding the near-term infant: Newborns born at 35 to 37 weeks' gestation have special nutritional needs compared with newborns that are full term, and require extra lactation support. These babies tend to be sleepy and are at high risk of not feeding effectively enough at the breast to support sufficient growth. This increases their risk for hypoglycemia and dehydration. Because of their relative immaturity, they are also at risk for delayed hepatic bilirubin excretion leading to jaundice. These babies require monitoring of adequate breast milk intake, and often need supplementation of expressed colostrum or milk until they are sufficiently vigorous at the breast to maintain proper growth.

Check points for poor positioning and latch : *Body position of the baby:* Misalignment of the head, trunk, and hips; baby not tucked close and facing the mother, hips extended or back arched; neck flexed or nose buried in the breast tissue; head too high over the breast; nose or chin not touching the breast *Mouth and tongue:* Mouth angle <160°; upper or lower lip not flanged outward; tongue not cupped, down and forward; short or tight lingual frenulum *Palate:* High, arched, bubble, cleft *Cheeks:* Drawn in or dimpled with each suck; cheekline not a smooth arch *Jaw:* Receding; large jaw excursions; lack of graded jaw excursions heard as clicking or smacking sounds *Lips:* Lips do not form a seal; milk leaking from sides of mouth *Nipple:* Slides back and forth in baby's mouth; pops in and out of mouth; creased in horizontal, vertical, or oblique plane; distorted or flattened following a feeding; blanched or in spasm; pain, blisters, maceration, fissures, cracks, craters, bleeding *Areola:* Edematous that envelopes the nipple *Previous use of artificial nipples or pacifiers:* Significant variances in these areas may trigger a referral to the staff lactation consultant to troubleshoot the problem, implement interventions, and create a feeding plan.

Signs of swallowing: *Hearing a puff of air from the nose or a "ca" sound *Hearing a swallow in the throat (usually after the milk has come in) *Mother feels (or sees) the areola drawn into the baby's mouth *Baby's jaw drops lower than during rapid nonnutritive sucking *Feeling the baby swallow by placing fingers on baby's throat *Hearing the swallowing with a stethoscope on baby's throat.

Role of Nursing in promoting Breastfeeding : Each nurse, whether interacting with new mothers in the hospital or in the community, has the ability to significantly affect the breast-feeding experience of mothers in her care. Helping behaviors include being physically present when mothers are learning early breast-feeding skills, teaching practical techniques (positioning, latch), helping mothers anticipate problems and how to solve them, and valuing the act of breastfeeding. Hindering behaviors include indifference to breast-feeding, intrusive or rough handling of the mother's breasts or baby, being too rushed to spend time with the mother, not listening to the mother's concerns, providing conflicting advice, and provision of formula as a quick fix to early challenges. Evidence based lactation care and services have a lifetime effect on the health of the mothers and infants entrusted to nursing care.

Good attachment
Signs of good attachment:
• More areola above baby's mouth
• Mouth wide open
• Lower lip turned outwards
• Chin touching breast
• Slow, deep sucks and swallowing sounds

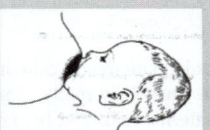

Poor attachment
Signs of poor attachment:
• Baby sucking on the nipple, not the areola
• Rapid shallow sucks
• Smacking or clicking sounds
• Cheeks drawn in
• Chin not touching breast

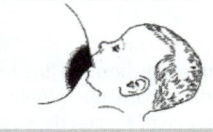

BREASTFEEDING AND MATERNAL MEDICINES

MEDICINES WHICH SHOULD NOT BE GIVEN TO BREASTFEEDING MOTHERS

Medicine	Reason	Special consideration
Abuse drugs-cocaine, marijuana	Cocaine (CNS irritation); marijuana (may delay motor development)	Methadone is safe at 20mg/day and probably also up to 80mg/day. Monitor concentration in doses above 20mg/day.
Cytotoxic agents	Immediate and delayed toxicity e.g. methotrexate once weekly	Use in rheumatic disease is safe.
Ergot alkaloids e.g. bromocriptine, ergotamine	Suppress lactation, 'ergotism'	Short-term use - less than three days is safe.
Gold	Heavy metal poisoning	(controversial)
Iodine	Induces a goitre	
Phenindione	Bleeding tendency	Warfarin and heparin are safe alternatives
Radio-iodine	Hypothyroidism	Temporary cessation only, half-life determines
	Hyperthyroidism	length of breast-feeding interruption required

MEDICINES THAT REQUIRE MORE CAREFUL ASSESSMENT OF RISK THAN USUAL

Category	Medicine	Considerations
Aminosalicylates	5-aminosalicylic acid; sulfasalazine (sulphasalazine)	May cause bloody diarrhea.
Analgesic	Oxycodone	Neurobehaviour disturbance. Use morphine cautiously for severe pain. Paracetamol and NSAIDs for lesser pain.
Antidepressants	Doxepin, fluoxetine, lithium	Cautious use Dexepin (sedation);fluoxetine (colic); lithium (near to therapeutic concentrations).
Antiepileptics	Ethosuximide, phenobarbital (phenobarbitone)	Sedation. Carbamazepine, Phenytoin, Sodium valproate preferred.
Antimicrobials	Chloramphenicol, tetracyclines	Alternatives preferred. Chloramphenicol (idiopathic aplastic anemia); tetracyclines (bone and teeth concerns).
Cardioactives and blood pressure lowering medicines	Amiodarone, atenolol, nadolol sotalol	Labetalol and propranolol are safe and preferred. These others produce relatively high concentrations
Combined oral contraceptives	Estrogen and progesterone	Combined oral contraceptives can suppress lactation. Progesterone-only pills are preferred as these do not affect lactation.

ASSESS FEEDING IN BREASTFED BABY

Assess feeding in a baby who does not need emergency, urgent or immediate care. In these children wait until the baby is ready to feed until you assess feeding. Assess feeding on all babies before discharge and on follow up visits.

ASK, CHECK, RECORD—Assess breastfeeding

How is breastfeeding going? How many times in 24 hours do you breastfeed? Does your baby get any other food or drink? Has the baby fed in the last hour?

Assess weight gain

LOOK, LISTEN, FEEL—Assess for possible feeding problem

*Is baby able to attach? Not at all-Poor attachment-Good attachment
*To check attachment look for: Chin touching breast-Mouth wide open-Lower lip turned outward-More areola visible above than below the mouth
*Check positioning *Is the baby sucking well? Not at all-Not sucking well-Sucking well *Clear a blocked nose if it interferes with breastfeeding* Look for thrush and mouth ulcers

Assess all babies for growth(Has the baby gained weight according to expectations?)

CLASSIFY the feeding problem and Act accordingly as follows.

NOT ABLE TO FEED (No attachment at all, OR Not sucking at all):*Treat for serious acute infection or severe disease *If the baby < 3 days old and no risk factors for sepsis, treat for encephalopathy

FEEDING PROBLEM(Not well attached to the breast, OR Not suckling effectively, OR Feeding < 8 times in 24 hours, OR Baby receiving other foods or fluids, e.g. formula milk or water as well as breast milk: * Teach the correct positioning *Assess the mother for breast problems *Counsel the mother to breastfeed on demand and at least 8 times in 24 hours *Counsel the mother to exclusively breastfeed

POOR GROWTH(Poor weight gain):Encourage exclusive breastfeeding on demand • Exclude sepsis

GROWING WELL(Good weight gain): Encourage the mother to continue exclusive breastfeeding

Breastfeeding vignettes

Tongue tie or ankyloglossia in a breastfed infant: Effective breastfeeding requires newborns to fine-tune their tongue movements to adapt to their mothers' particular nipple and breast anatomy and physiology. In the presence of tongue tie, two categories of signs/symptoms arise: those related to nipple trauma and those related to ineffective breast emptying and low infant intake. Untreated tongue tie can lead to untimely weaning and its attendant health risks. Frenotomy is a safe and effective procedure to release tongue tie and improve tongue function and breastfeeding outcomes.(**NeoReviews** Vol.11 No.9 September 2010 e513)

* The success of feeding a preterm infant by nipple is dependent on the ability of the infant to coordinate sucking and swallowing, which develops at about 33-34 weeks of gestational age.

*Determinants of milk volume (milk production)?

Initially, hormonal factors (prolactin and oxytocin) affect the synthesis and secretion of milk. Once milk "comes in," tight junctions close, and lactation shifts from endocrine control to autocrine control, or control driven by milk removal. The frequency of breast-feeding then becomes the most important factor affecting the continuation of adequate milk production. The term infant should receive at least 8–12 feedings per day in the first week and more than 6 per day thereafter. So that the volume of residual milk is minimized, mothers should alternate the breast they start on the next feeding. Maternal diet and fluid intake rarely affect milk volume. In severe malnutrition, there may be diminished milk production.

Why a baby is not feeding? Although we enthusiastically embrace the value of breastfeeding, nurses and physicians must not substitute the value of common sense and good clinical judgment in the process. An equal amount of fervor to understand why a baby is not feeding and to protect that infant during transition is far more important than the promotion of breastfeeding at all cost. Is it a problem of milk not coming in? Is it a problem with the mother's nipples? Is it a minor transitional issue with the baby? Is it a serious medical problem ?(Sepsis, Hypoglycemia, Hypothyroidism, CHF, Respiratory depression etc.)

Breastfed infants tend to maintain higher oxygen saturations than do bottle-fed infants: One proposed explanation is that bottle-fed babies swallow more and, thus, breathing is interrupted more frequently. They do not breathe during sucking bursts but rather breathe rapidly during breaks in sucking. Breastfed infants, however, are able to integrate breathing within bursts of sucking and, thus, may have a better coordination of sucking, swallowing, and breathing.In breastfeeding, the tongue is under the nipple during feeding, producing peristalsis so that swallowing occurs concurrently. On the other hand, for bottle-feeding infants, the tongue may be more piston-like, which may intermittently compromise breathing by causing obstruction.

Nonnutritive breastfeeding (also referred to as dry or recreational breastfeeding):allows the mother and child to practice proper positioning before actual breastfeeding begins. The mother pumps her breast before putting the infant to breast. In some instances, the infant can also be tube-fed while suckling on the empty breast. Gradually, the mother pumps out less milk so the infant can transition to obtaining milk from the mother's breast and adjust to stronger milk flow. Nonnutritive breastfeeding may be an alternative to initiation of actual breastfeeding for the early course of very lowbirthweight infants, who may encounter problems such as

inadequate weight gain or weight loss if introduced to the breast before they are fully ready. Nonnutritive breastfeeding may also promote maternal milk flow, help with maternal emotional stability, and prolong lactation in mothers.Nonnutritive sucking in conjunction with additional oral stimulation has also been shown to improve oral feeding performance of preterm infants and decrease their hospital stay.

*Fat is the most variable content of all nutrients in human milk. The fat content rises slightly during lactation, increases from the beginning (foremilk) to the end (hindmilk) of the feeding, varies among women (probably a direct effect of body fat stores), and varies over the course of the day. If the mother does not completely empty her breast after feeding, the baby will not receive all the calories (fat). Mothers using mechanical methods to express their milk may not completely empty the breast.

*Note the sucking and swallowing ability of the infant. Parental skills, infant feeding cues, and timing of feedings should also be considered. Begin one breast-feeding in place of a tube feeding or in addition to the tube feeding. If the latch-on is good and clinical signs of sucking, swallowing, and some drooling of milk are noted, then continue the process each day. It is not accurate to withdraw milk from an indwelling feeding tube to assess milk intake from breast-feeding, since gastric emptying from the stomach after a human milk feeding is rapid. Furthermore, clinical signs of feeding activity and maternal assessment of breast emptying are inexact measures of milk intake and may not reflect small amounts consumed. Weighing the infant before and after breast-feeding is the most accurate way to assess milk intake.

*The composition of human milk for preterm infants differs from that for term infants in a number of ways. For every 100 mL, it is higher in calories (67 to 72 kcal versus 62 to 68 kcal), higher in protein (1.7 to 2.1 g versus 1.2 to 1.7 g), higher in lipids (3.4 to 4.4 g versus 3.0 to 4.0 g), lower in carbohydrates, higher in multiple minerals and trace elements (especially sodium [Na], chloride [Cl], iron [Fe], Zinc [Zn], and copper [Cu]), and higher in vitamins (especially vitamins A and E). However, as breast milk becomes mature, many of these nutritional advantages are lost.

*The term 60/40 refers to the percentage of whey (lactalbumin) and casein in human milk or cow milk formulas. This ratio makes for small curds and therefore easy digestibility by the infant. The 60/40 ratio is of particular advantage to the preterm infant because it is associated with lower levels of serum ammonia and a decreased incidence of metabolic acidosis. Only human milk or formulas that supply protein in this ratio provide adequate amounts of the amino acids cystine and taurine, which may be essential for the preterm infant.

Biochemistry of Human Milk: Human milk is a unique, species-specific, complex nutritive fluid with immunologic and growth-promoting properties. This unique fluid actually evolves to meet the changing needs of the baby during growth and maturation. Milk synthesis and secretion by the mammary gland involve numerous cellular pathways and processes. The processing and packaging of nutrients within human milk changes over time as the recipient infant matures. For example, early milk or colostrum has lower concentrations of fat than mature milk but higher concentrations of protein and minerals. This relationship reverses as the infant matures.

Storage of Breastmilk for Infant Use: Guidelines for collecting and storing breastmilk are more stringent for sick and preterm babies than for healthy babies at home.· sterilized containers are recommended *refrigeration at 4⁰C for 48 hours results in minimal loss of nutrients and bacterial count is reduced · freshly expressed milk should be chilled in refrigerator before adding to frozen milk *thaw breastmilk by placing in cool or warm water *thawed milk should be used within 24 hours *never refreeze or re-warm breastmilk

Time to keep milk in various conditions

Breastmilk	Room Temperature	Refrigerator	Freezer
Freshly expressed into closed container	6–8 hours (26⁰C) If refrigeration is available store milk there	3–5 days (4⁰C) Store in back of refrigerator where it is coldest	2 weeks in freezer compartment inside a refrigerator 3 months in freezer section of refrigerator with separate door 6–12 months in deep freeze (- 18⁰C)
Previously frozen - thawed in refrigerator but not warmed	4 hours or less i.e. next feeding	Store in refrigerator 24 hours	Do not refreeze
Thawed outside refrigerator in warm water	For completion of feeding	Hold for 4 hours or until next feeding	Do not refreeze
Infant has begun feeding	Only for completion of feeding then discard	Discard	Do not refreeze Discard

Guidelines for the Establishment and Operation of a Donor Human Milk Bank

1. Potential donors are cleared initially by their own physicians to assure that their health and welfare are protected.

2. Potential donors undergo a screening history similar to the one used to screen potential blood donors.

Donor exclusion criteria include:

a. A positive blood test result for HIV, human T-cell lymphoma virus (HTLV), hepatitis B or C, or syphilis.

b. The donor or her sexual partner is at risk for HIV infection.

c. Use of illegal drugs.

d. Smoking or use of tobacco products.

e. An organ or tissue transplant or a blood transfusion in the last 6 months.

f. Regular consumption of more than two alcoholic drinks per day.

g. Use of medication or herbal supplements (with the exception of progestin-only oral contraceptives or injections, levothyroxine, insulin, prenatal vitamins).

3. All donors undergo serologic screening, at milk bank expense, for: a. HIV. b. HTLV I and II. c. Hepatitis B and C. d. Syphilis.

4. Donors are taught carefully how to pump and collect their milk safely and cleanly and how to keep their pumps and collection systems sterile.

5. Donor milk is frozen in sterile containers immediately after collection and maintained in the frozen state until processed by the receiving bank.

6. Donor milk is cultured for bacterial contamination when received by the bank, and milk that has abnormal findings is not processed for distribution. Such findings include:

a. Milk that has a high degree of bacterial contamination (ie, 106 colony-forming units).

b. Milk contaminated with specific problematic flora (eg, *Staphylococcus aureus, Bacillus* sp).

7. Donor milk that has passed all of the previous screening steps is then Holder pasteurized at 62.5°C for 30 minutes, a process demonstrated to eliminate known bacterial and viral pathogens.

8. Aliquots of milk are recultured after pasteurization to assure sterility; the presence of any bacterial growth at this point in the process requires discarding of the contaminated batch.

Potential benefits of the use of banked human milk in the neonatal intensive care unit

Promotion of breastfeeding,
Reduced incidence of necrotizing enterocolitis and sepsis,
Possible support of long-term positive neurodevelopmental outcomes in very low- and extremely-low birthweight infants.

Selected Components of Human Milk After Freezing and Pasteurization:

IgA and secretory IgA Binds microbes in gastrointestinal tract, prevents passage—67 to 100% level

IgM—Antibodies targeted against specific pathogens after maternal exposure- 0%

IgG—Antibodies targeted against specific pathogens after maternal exposure- 66 to 70% level

Lactoferrin—Binds iron, retards bacterial growth—27 to 43% level

Lysozyme—Destroys bacterial cell walls—75% level

Lipoprotein lipase Helps lipolysis of milk triglycerides to monoglycerides and free fatty acids-0% level

Bile salt-activated lipase Helps lipolysis of milk triglycerides to monoglycerides and free fatty acids—0% level

Monoglycerides—Disrupts membranes of virus, protozoans—100 % level

Free fatty acids Disrupts membranes of virus, protozoans 100% level

Linoleic acid (18:2n6) Essential fatty acid, precursor for prostaglandins and leukotrienes -100% level

Alpha-linolenic acid—(18:3n3) Essential fatty acid, precursor for docosahexanoic acid; important for

eye and brain development- 100% level

Specific Clinical Recommendations to promote breastfeeding

Preconceptional and Prenatal Education

Address the infant feeding decision before conception or as early in pregnancy as possible; women make their decision about breastfeeding very early. Prenatal intention to breastfeed has an influence on initiation and duration of breastfeeding. Continue to bring up the issue of infant feeding throughout the prenatal period.

Determine the mother's intent and any concerns or misconceptions she may have. Provide appropriate education and anticipatory guidance to encourage her to consider breastfeeding and determine what support she will need to make and carry out this decision.

Elicit any factors in the family medical history that may make breastfeeding especially important (e.g., atopic diseases, diabetes, obesity, cancers), and advise the woman of these factors.

Elicit any risk factors for potential breastfeeding problems and any medical contraindications to lactation. Provide appropriate support and education.

For multiparous women, document the duration of lactation for each infant, reasons for weaning, and any problems that occurred. (We suggest the history be documented with the labor histories of each infant.) For the current pregnancy, document a plan for intervention, including lactation consultation where indicated, on the prenatal form.[1]

Encourage the participation of the mother's support persons and educate them as appropriate. Remember that whoever is at the prenatal visit or hospital stay is likely to have influence over breastfeeding and other health care decisions.

Recognize the feelings of relatives who did not breastfeed, or weaned prematurely. Encourage them to learn what is known about breastfeeding for the optimal health of the mother and baby.

Encourage the woman and her support persons, in a culturally sensitive manner, to attend breastfeeding classes and/or support group meetings prenatally.

Provide the woman with accurate, noncommercial breastfeeding literature and recommendations for accurate lay breastfeeding resources (e.g. books, Web sites).

Educate women about the potential breastfeeding problems associated with the use of intrapartum analgesia and anesthesia.

Intrapartum support

*Provide appropriate labor support intended to minimize unnecessary analgesics or anesthesia. *If mother and baby are stable, facilitate immediate postpartum breastfeeding. *Minimize separation of mother and infant and wait until after the first breastfeeding to perform routine newborn procedures such as weighing, ophthalmic prophylaxis, vitamin K injection, etc. *Provide warming for the stable newborn via skin-to-skin contact with the mother, covering mother and baby if necessary.

Early postpartum education and support

*Advocate for 24-hour rooming in for mother and baby. *Encourage the mother's support persons to provide optimal opportunities for breastfeeding. *Ensure that breastfeeding is being adequately assessed on a regular basis by qualified professionals. *Advocate for lactation consultation services at all hospitals where maternal and infant care is provided. *Educate mothers about the importance of frequent, unrestricted breastfeeding with proper positioning and latch. *Help mothers recognize the baby's early feeding cues (e.g. rooting, lip smacking, sucking on fingers or hands, rapid eye movements) and explain that crying is a late sign of hunger. *Help mothers also recognize signs that the baby is satisfied at the end of a feeding (e.g., relaxed body posture, unclenching of fists). *If mother and baby need to be separated, assist maintenance of breastfeeding and/or ensure that mother receives assistance with expressing milk. *Provide

mothers with clear verbal and written discharge breastfeeding instructions that include information on hunger and feeding indicators, stool and urine patterns, jaundice, proper latch and positioning, and techniques for expressing breast milk. *Educate mothers about the risks of unnecessary supplementation and pacifier use. *Avoid the use of discharge packs containing formula samples and formula company advertising or literature. *Ensure that the mother and baby have appropriate follow-up within 48 hours of discharge and provide mother with phone numbers for lactation support. *Identify breastfeeding problems in the hospital and assist the mother with these before discharge. *Develop an appropriate follow-up plan for any identified problems or concerns. * Provide the family with information about breastfeeding support groups in the community.

Ongoing support and management

*Evaluate the mother and baby soon after hospital discharge to assess adequacy of milk intake and address any problems that have developed. *Use breastfeeding-friendly approaches to treatments for problems. *Continue to encourage breastfeeding throughout the first year of life and beyond, at well-child and other visits. *Encourage exclusive breastfeeding for the first six months of life. *Be knowledgeable about prevention and management of common breastfeeding challenges. *Develop a working relationship with professionals with expertise in lactation issues, such as International Board Certified Lactation Consultants. *Consult when breastfeeding concerns exceed your level of expertise. *Encourage mothers who are returning to work to continue to breastfeed. *Encourage mothers who do not feel they can continue to exclusively breastfeed to continue partial breastfeeding as long as possible. *Support mothers who cho

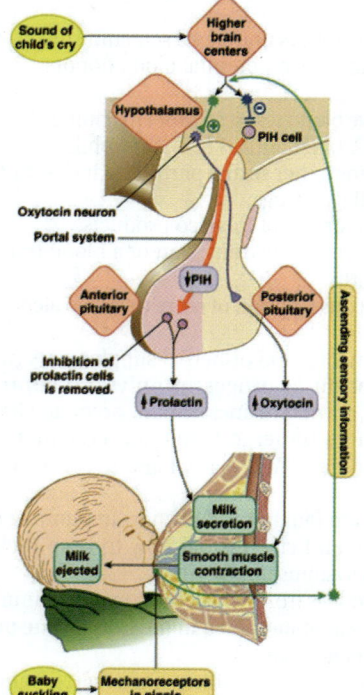

The Milk Production & Let-Down Reflex: Following birth: Stimulation of milk secretion and ejection   a. Prolactin promotes milk secretion b. Oxytocin stimulates milk ejection (A neural reflex causes milk ejection.) **What can interfere with the let-down reflex?** *Emotions: embarrassment, anger, irritation, fear or resentment *Tiredness - Inadequate sucking this can be because of improper positioning or because the baby has not been at the breast for long enough *Stress - Fear of pain in your breasts or uterus (i.e. sore nipples or afterbirth pains) *Engorgement in the first few days *Smoking, alcohol or recreational drugs. These all contain substances that can interfere with the let-down and affect the content of breast milk.

SUPPLEMENTATION

*Routine supplementation of healthy, term breastfeeding infants is not recommended unless medically indicated. Mothers who supplement their nursing infants with infant formula are at risk for a decrease in their milk supply caused by decreased demand. In addition to potential loss of milk, supplementation should only be used when medically indicated because it can also interfere with other psychosocial and neurodevelopmental benefits of breastfeeding. **Common situations** that require infant supplementation include infant *hypoglycemia not responsive to nursing, insufficient maternal milk supply, delay in lactation, excessive infant weight loss, infant illness such that feeding at the breast is not effective, and maternal-infant separation.* *Supplementation may be done with expressed milk, pasteurized donor human milk, or artificial infant formula. Methods of supplementation include cup feeding, finger feeding with a syringe attached to a feeding tube, a supplemental feeding tube at the breast, and bottle feeding. One method is not necessarily more suitable than another, and the choice of method depends on individual evaluation of the mother-infant pair. Parents need professional guidance when supplementation is necessary, and consultation with a knowledgeable health professional is recommended. *Sunlight has historically been the primary source of vitamin D for humans. Human mothers and babies receive much less sun exposure than they historically did because of urban/indoor lifestyles, migration, and sun avoidance or use of sunscreens to prevent skin cancer. Human milk contains low levels of vitamin D, leaving breastfed babies, especially dark-skinned babies, at increased risk for rickets. It is recommended that healthy, term breastfeeding babies receive 200 units of vitamin D supplementation daily by two months of age. Breastfeeding babies receiving 500 mL or more of vitamin-D fortified artificial infant formula do not need additional vitamin D supplementation.

The WHO/UNICEF Code of Marketing of Breast milk Substitutes

In 1981, the World Health Assembly adopted The International Code of Marketing of Breastmilk Substitutes, as a tool to protect breastfeeding. Formula marketing targets women. New mothers are given free samples of formula, babies are given bottles in hospitals, coupons or food samples arrive in the mail, or booklets and videotapes are distributed on breastfeeding and weaning. The Code prohibits marketing of these products in these ways. It covers formula, other milk products, cereals, teas and juices, as well as bottles and teats.

The Code has 10 important provisions

*NO advertising of any of these products to the public.

*NO free samples to mothers.

*NO promotion of products in health care facilities, including the distribution of free or low-cost supplies.

*NO company sales representatives to advise mothers.

*NO gifts or personal samples to health care personnel.

*NO words or pictures idealizing artificial feeding, or pictures of infants on labels of infant milk containers.

*Information to health care personnel should be scientific and factual.

*ALL information on artificial infant feeding, including that on labels, should explain the benefits of breastfeeding and the costs and hazards associated with artificial feeding.

*Unsuitable products, such as sweetened condensed milk, should not be promoted for infants.

*Manufacturers and distributors should comply with the Code's provisions even if countries have not adopted laws or other measures.

Innocenti Declaration on the Protection, Promotion, and Support of Breastfeeding

The Innocenti Declaration was produced and adopted by participants at the WHO/UNICEF policymakers' meeting on "Breastfeeding in the 1990s: A Global Initiative," cosponsored by the U.S. Agency for International Development (AID) and the Swedish International Development Authority (SIDA).

We therefore declare that

* As a global goal for optimal maternal and child health and nutrition, all women should be enabled to practice exclusive breastfeeding and all infants should be fed exclusively on breast milk from birth to four to six months of age. Thereafter, children should continue to be breastfed, while receiving appropriate and adequate complementary foods, up to two years of age or beyond. This child-feeding ideal is to be achieved by creating an appropriate environment of awareness and support so that women can breastfeed in this manner. *Attainment of this goal requires, in many countries, the reinforcement of a "breastfeeding culture" and its vigorous defense against incursions of a "bottle-feeding culture." This requires commitment and advocacy for social mobilization, utilizing to the full the prestige and authority of acknowledged leaders of society in all walks of life. *Efforts should be made to increase women's confidence in their ability to breastfeed. Such empowerment involves the removal of constraints and influences that manipulate perceptions and behavior towards breastfeeding, often by subtle and indirect means. This requires sensitivity, continued vigilance, and a responsive and comprehensive communications strategy involving all media and addressed to all levels of society. Furthermore, obstacles to breastfeeding within the health system, the workplace, and the community must be eliminated. *Measures should be taken to ensure that women are adequately nourished for their optimal health and that of their families. Furthermore, ensuring that all women also have access to family planning information and services allows them to sustain breastfeeding and avoid shortened birth intervals that may compromise their health and nutritional status, and that of their children. *All governments should develop national breastfeeding policies and set appropriate national targets for the 1990s. They should establish a national system for monitoring the attainment of their targets, and they should develop indicators such as the prevalence of exclusively breastfed infants at discharge from maternity services, and the prevalence of exclusively breastfed infants at four months of age. *National authorities are further urged to integrate their breastfeeding policies into their overall health and development policies. In so doing, they should reinforce all actions that protect, promote, and support breastfeeding within complementary programs such as prenatal and perinatal care, nutrition, family planning services, and prevention and treatment of common maternal and childhood diseases. All health care staff should be trained in the skills necessary to implement these breastfeeding policies.

Conclusion Human milk, in addition to its numerous nutrients that make it an ideal food source for the growing term infant, is a bioactive fluid that evolves from colostrum to mature milk as the infant matures. This bioactive fluid contains numerous factors and live cells that, in concert, promote the growth and well-being of the breastfeeding infant. Oliver Wendell Holmes said it best when he stated, "A pair of substantial mammary glands has the advantage over the two hemispheres of the most learned professor's brain, in the art of compounding a nutritious fluid for infants." With the ever-expanding knowledge resulting from current research, commercial formula clearly cannot replicate all of the valuable properties that are inherent in human milk.

REFERENCES: 1)Moreland J, Coombs J. Promoting and supporting breast-feeding. *Am Fam Physician.* 2000;61(7):2093-2100, 2103-2104. 2)Labbok MH. Breastfeeding and Baby-Friendly Hospital Initiative: more important and with more evidence than ever. *J Pediatr (Rio J).* 2007;83(2):99–101. 3)Breastfeeding, Family Physicians Supporting (Position Paper),The American Academy of Family Physicians (AAFP), http://www.aafp.org

BREASTFEEDING PROBLEMS

1. **Flat/inverted nipples:** *Gentle stimulation with baby`s mouth or with breast pump helps to increase nipple protrusion, in case of flat nipples *Inverted nipples are improved by having the mother support her breast and retract her fingers toward her chest or by pump or **plastic syringe method** to draw out nipples *Long nipples-mothers should get more of their breast tissue into the baby`s mouth not just the nipples so that the milk reservoirs, the lacteal sinuses can be sucked upon to get adequate milk.

2. **Sore nipples/cracked nipples :** *Best prevented by **proper latch-on and positioning,** alternating breast-feeding positions, and careful air drying of the breast after feedings *Mother should first nurse on the less affected/ normal breast because of the let-down reflex making milk removal from the affected sore nipple easier *Remove the baby gently without **Precipitously pulling baby off breast** *Baby should be held closely into mother`s body since a baby who is falling away from the breast will traumatize the sore nipple further *In cases of severely traumatized nipples, temporary cessation of breastfeeding maybe indicated to allow for healing; but instruct the mother to maintain lactation with manual/mechanical expression until direct breastfeeding is resumed*Late-onset soreness may be due to *Candida* infection; treatment consists of nystatin oral suspension to infant`s mouth, 2 ml 4 times a day, and nystatin topically to mother`s nipple and areola 4 times a day after feeding for 5 days after complete clearance of lesions.

3. **Breast engorgement:** *Engorgement of breasts (> *normal physiologic full breasts*), a painful condition caused by delayed initiation, poor attachment of the baby at the breast leading to ineffective removal of the milk *Usually present on day 3-5 postpartum signalling the onset of copious milk production resulting in swollen, hard breasts that are warm to touch *Breasts are swollen,edematous and the nipples are flattened secondary to areolar edema, making baby`s latch-on difficult causing nipple soreness *Advice mother on use of warm compresses, soaks, or showers followed by gentle massage and expression of milk to soften the areola *Encourage frequent nursing to maintain drainage and to prevent decreased milk production from back pressure on ducts *Cold compresses to breast after feeding may reduce swelling *A bra should be worn for support;avoid constricting underwires *Mild analgesic(paracetamol) or anti-inflammatory(ibuprofen) for pain relief and reduction of inflammation.

4. **Maternal mastitis:** *Symptoms include fever, chills, malaise, headache, body aches, nausea and vomiting, warm area on breast, tender lump or wedge in breast, or an erythematous streak *Usually unilateral and is preceded by maternal fatigue, a plugged duct, unrelieved engorgement, or nipple trauma *Mostly caused by *Staphylococcus aureus* and *E.coli* and rarely by Streptococcus and is treated with a 10 day course of antibiotic therapy (a cephalosporin, dicloxacillin, or clarythromycin *Supportive measures include;bed rest, warm compresses,analgesics, frequent nursing to empty ducts, begin feedings on unaffected side if more comfortable, increased maternal fluid intake,gentle massage toward nipple and removal of bra and other constrictive clothing

5. **Breast abscess:** *Results from the delayed treatment of mastitis and infected cracked nipples *Mother is febrile, ill-looking and develops a painful breast swelling unilaterally and has a raised WBC count *The abscess must be drained either by ultrasound guided wide bore needle aspirations or by surgical incision and drainage along with antibiotics for 2 weeks+analgesic-anti-inflammatory medications *manual expression of milk should be continued.

6. **Not enough milk:** *Check whether the baby is getting enough milk; if the baby is satisfied and sleeping for 2–3 hours after breast feeding and passing urine at least 6–8 times in 24 hrs and gaining weight 15–25g/day then the mother is producing enough milk *If the baby is not getting enough milk(POOR WEIGHT GAIN + PASSING LESS AND CONCENTRATED URINE), try to find out a number of reasons, such as incorrect method of breast feeding, supplementary feedings, bottle feeding (nipple confusion resulting in poor attachment and poor suckling at the breast), no night feeding, breast engorgement, any maternal illness-painful condition-stressful situation

Management- build mother`s confidence by helping her to improve her baby`s attachment at the breast, to let her baby suckle frequently, at least 8-10 times a day or more ,if he demands, to let the baby suckle on each breast as long as possible,to follow-up daily until the baby starts gaining weight, then weekly until the mother has gained confidence *Explain the advantages of exclusive breastfeeding, and the dangers of unnecessary supplements

7. **Relactation:** *Resumption of breastfeeding following cessation or significant decrease in breastmilk for the indications, such as a) for babies separated from their mothers due to an admission to a SCBU/NICU or due to maternal illness b) for an adopted infant *Motivating the mother with positive reinforcement, emotional support, and building mother`s confidence is the initial step to be taken *Manual/mechanical stimulation of breast, skin to skin contact with baby to enhance oxytocin reflex, good nutrition, rest, oxytocin nasal spray/tablets/chlorpromazine 25-100 mg 3 times a day for a week to 10 days/metaclopramide 10 mg x 3 times a day for 10 days, frequent suckling by the baby at both breasts, for a minimum of 10-12 times a day are useful methods in achieving relactation.

8. **Nursing twins/triplets:** *Breastfeed as soon as possible, if one or both babies are sufficiently stable;if both babies are unable to nurse, the mother should begin pumping within 24 hours of infants` births;if one baby is able to breast-feed, the mother can pump one breast and store the milk for the other baby *Mothers can breast-feed twins simultaneously to save time and increase milk production; she should start the baby that has more efficient suck first to stimulate the milk ejection reflex, then latch on the other infant. She will need several pillows or a nursing pillow for support *Encourage family members to arrange for help to reduce maternal fatigue during first 2 weeks at home, if at all possible.

9. **Premature infants :** *For premature infants < 35 wks GA, encourage mothers to practice early and frequent skin-to-skin holding and suckling at the emptied breast to facilitate early nipple stimulation/milk volume and infant oral feeding assessment *For preterms 35-37 wks GA management should include: a)mechanical milk expression concurrent with breastfeeding until the infant is breastfeeding effectively b)weighing the infant before and after breastfeeding to evaluate adequacy of milk intake and determine need for supplementation

10. **Miscellaneous problems:** *Craniofacial anomalies(i.e., cleft lip/palate, Pierre-Robin) often require an obturator, or nipple shield to achieve an effective latch *Cardiac disease/defects may require fluid restriction status of the infant and special attention to pacing of feeds to minimize fatigue during feeding *Ankyloglossia(tongue tie), if severe may require frenulotomy- controversial.

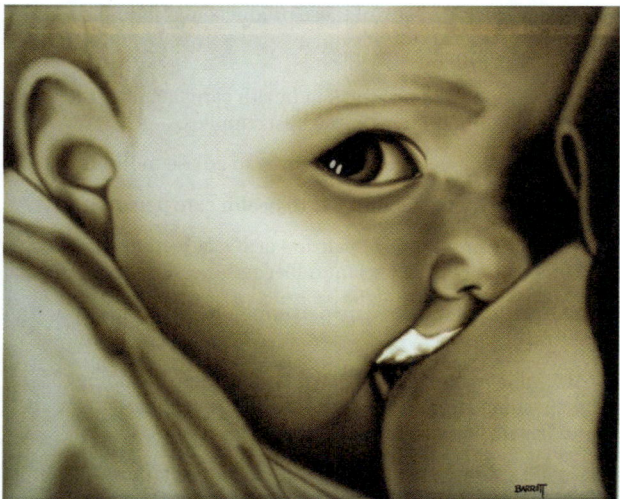

A newborn baby has only three demands. They are warmth in the arms of its mother, food from her breasts, and security in the knowledge of her presence. Breastfeeding satisfies all three. ~Grantly Dick-Read

MATERNAL INFECTIONS AFFECTING FETUS AND NEWBORN
MONITORING-MANAGEMENT-MAINTENANCE(FOLLOW-UP)

ESSENTIAL CLINICAL GUIDELINES **015**

MONITORING

a. **Screen** " all pregnant women" for disease where feasible in Indian scenario E.g.: VDRL, HbsAg, HIV status.

b. **Make sure** a negative serologic test in the 1st trimester be verified by repeating at 28 weeks and at 36 wks of Gestational age, whether are there high risk factors or not.

c. **Screen** all HIV infected women carefully for other sexually transmitted disease (Gonorrhea, Herpes, Chlamydia, Hepatitis B and C and Syphilis) as well as being tested for antibody to CMV & TOXOPLASMOSIS and a Tuberculin skin test.

d. **Screen** " women at high risk" for serologic test for syphilis at delivery and don't discharge the infant until negative maternal serologic status or adequate therapy has been documented.

e. **Admit** all high risk Newborn to 'SCBU', observe closely for signs and symptoms of Sepsis and do appropriate serologic tests,

Culture & sensitivity tests of body fluids (blood, urine, CSF, discharge from eyes, umbilicus, skin lesions etc.) and evaluate for systemic complications and treat appropriately.

MANAGEMENT

a. **Prevent** transmission of infection from mother to the fetus, wherever possible!

E.g. Maternal Immunization with Hep "B" (preconception), Tetanus toxoid during pregnancy

– Ocular prophylaxis against Ophthalmia Neonatorum

– Therapeutic abortion when TOXOPLASMOSIS/ RUBELLA infection of fetus confirmed

– Selective intrapartal chemoprophylaxis against Group B Steptococcus (GBS) disease.

– Avoid transfusing blood products from seropositive persons to seronegative persons

– Treat infected mothers effectively

– E.g. Maternal syphilis

– HIV, Tuberculosis of infected mothers

b. **Treat** 'Newborn' of infected mothers appropriately & timely!

E.g. HBS Ag positive pregnancy

- Maternal intrapartal risk factors for sepsis

c. **Prevent** Nosocomial spread of the disease in question!

E.g. HBs Ag positive infants (wear gloves & gowns when caring for infected infants, Immunization of health care workers)

Enforce STRICT ISOLATION procedure for all infants colonized or infected with multiple resistant bacteria.

Immunoglobulin prophylaxis for those exposed to Chickenpox e.g. VZIG.

d. **Treat** symptomatically & supportively where there is no 'cure' e.g. HIV infection (optimization of Nutrition, prophylaxis against opportunistic infections (E.g. P.Carinii Pneumonia) and the prompt recognition and treatment of HIV related complications

E.g. Opportunistic infections).

e. **Allow** breast feeding wherever possible

E.g. HIV infection of POOR, ILLITERATE, ILL AFFOR-DING mother, in a Developing & 3rd World country.

CMV infection (due to rare symptomatic infection in the term Newborn & protective IgG for LBW infants.)

HBV infection in infants who have received HBIG & Hepatitis vaccine.

Maintenance (follow-up)

a. **Closely 'follow-up'** if early gestation infection is suspected or the timings of infection is unknown.

E.g. Maternal Rubella

Negative serologic test for syphilis at delivery due to late infection (high-risk population)

b. **Multidisciplinary team follow-up** is often necessary

E.g. HIV

TORSCH

c. **Verify** the 'Immunization status' as & when necessary to identify the unprotected infants in spite of recommended preventive strategies

E.g.: Infant born to HBs Ag positive pregnancy, who have been vaccinated within 12 hours after birth needs Post—Vaccination HBV Immunological status to be checked at 9–10 mo of age.

d. **Test and Treat** all 'close contacts'

E.g. Sexual partners of HIV and other STD

Household members of maternal tuberculosis.

EVIDENCE-BASED MEDICINE IN NEONATOLOGY

Evidence-based medicine (EBM) aims to apply the best available evidence gained from the scientific method to medical decision making. It seeks to assess the quality of evidence of the risks and benefits of treatments (including lack of treatment). EBM recognizes that many aspects of medical care depend on individual factors such as quality- and value-of-life judgments, which are only partially subject to scientific methods. EBM, however, seeks to clarify those parts of medical practice that are in principle subject to scientific methods and to apply these methods to ensure the best *prediction* of outcomes in medical treatment, even as debate continues about which outcomes are desirable. Evidence-based guidelines (EBG) is the practice of evidence-based medicine at the organizational or institutional level. This includes the production of guidelines, policy, and regulations. This approach has also been called evidence based healthcare. Evidence-based individual decision (EBID) making is evidence-based medicine as practiced by the individual health care provider. There is concern that current evidence-based medicine focuses excessively on EBID.

Key to evidence statements and grading of recommendations, using the ranking of the Canadian Task Force

Quality of evidence assessment*

I: Evidence obtained from at least one properly randomized controlled trial

II-1: Evidence from well-designed controlled trials without randomization

II-2: Evidence from well-designed cohort (prospective or retrospective) or case-control studies, preferably from more than one centre or research group

II-3: Evidence obtained from comparisons between times or places with or without the intervention. Dramatic results in uncontrolled experiments (such as the results of treatment with penicillin in the 1940s) could also be included in this category

III: Opinions of respected authorities, based on clinical experience, descriptive studies, or reports of expert committees

Classification of recommendations†

A. There is good evidence to recommend the clinical preventive action

B. There is fair evidence to recommend the clinical preventive action

C. The existing evidence is conflicting and does not allow to make a recommendation for or against use of the clinical preventive action; however, other factors may influence decision-making

D. There is fair evidence to recommend against the clinical preventive action

E. There is good evidence to recommend against the clinical preventive action

L. There is insufficient evidence (in quantity or quality) to make a recommendation; however, other factors may influence

---

There are mixed reports about whether evidence-based medicine is effective. Using the classification scheme above—dividing evidence-based medicine into evidence-based guidelines (EBG) and evidence-based individual decision (EBID)— may explain the conflict. It is difficult to find evidence that EBID improves health care, whereas there is growing evidence of improvements in the efficacy of health care when evidence-based medicine is practiced at the organizational level. One of the virtues of *healthcare accreditation* is that it offers an opportunity to assess the overall functioning of a hospital or healthcare organization against the best of the currently-available evidence and to assist the hospital or healthcare organization to move towards a more effective application of evidence-based medical. Furthermore, evidence-based *guidelines* do not remove the problem of extrapolation to different populations or longer timeframes. Even if several top-quality studies are available, questions always remain about how far, and to which populations, their results are "generalizable". Furthermore, skepticism about results may always be extended to areas not explicitly covered: for example, a drug may influence a "secondary endpoint" such as test result (blood pressure, glucose, or cholesterol levels) without having the power to show that it decreases overall mortality or morbidity in a population. The quality of studies performed varies, making it difficult to compare them and generalize about the results. Certain groups have been historically under-researched (racial minorities and people with many co-morbid diseases), and thus the literature is sparse in areas that do not allow for generalizing.

Professor *Archie Cochrane*, a *Scottish* epidemiologist, through his book *Effectiveness and Efficiency: Random Reflections on Health Services* (1972) and subsequent advocacy, caused increasing acceptance of the concepts behind evidence-based practice. Cochrane's work was honored through the naming of centres of great reputation.

REFERENCE: Evidence-based medicine From Wikipedia, the free encyclopedia.

Evidence based practice—the integration of individual clinical expertise with the best available clinical evidence from systematic research—David Sackett

The ethos of basing practice on the best available evidence is well established in perinatal medicine. The introduction to clinical practice of major interventions, such as antenatal corticosteroids and exogenous surfactant, was informed by evidence from seminal randomized controlled trials and systematic reviews. Equally important has been the development and evaluation of interventions that have been shown not to have major benefits for preterm infants. Antenatal thyrotropin releasing hormone was shown to be associated with adverse effects for mothers and infants, including a higher risk of infants needing mechanical ventilation. On the basis of this evidence, antenatal thyrotropin releasing hormone does not have a role in the management of threatened preterm birth. Obtaining the best evidence to guide clinical practice is not always easy. In particular, undertaking clinical trials to evaluate interventions for preterm infants is difficult. Although about 3000 randomized controlled trials have been reported in the field of neonatology, many interventions have not yet been subjected to unbiased evaluation. This could be because the trials have not been attempted, or have been flawed methodologically, or have been too small to detect clinically important effects. Large perinatal trials have problems with recruitment. This could be related to the issues surrounding the public perception of perinatal trials and the need for (and difficulty in obtaining) informed consent from parents. Even when perinatal trials have been undertaken successfully, in some studies follow up has been too short and has assessed short term or surrogate outcomes for preterm infants.

Levels of evidence for effects of treatments—limiting bias

*Systematic review of all relevant randomized controlled trials

*Large multicentric randomized controlled trials

*Controlled trials without randomization

*Cohort studies

*Case controlled studies

*Multiple time series

*Before and after studies

*Opinions based on clinical experience or expert committee

Difficulties in undertaking randomized controlled trials

*Limited infrastructure to support studies

*Large trials needed to detect modest effect sizes—trials need to be multicentric or multinational, or both

*Limited funding—perinatal health not viewed as a funding priority

*Limited potential for industrial partnership

*Trial recruitment undertaken by busy clinicians or carers

*Validity of informed consent obtained at stressful times

*Public perception of perinatal research

*Need for long term follow up

Which outcomes should we measure? Trials must evaluate outcomes that are important to infants and their families as well as to carers and health services. To date, the major question for many interventions has been: "Does this treatment improve the chances of survival?" As advances in care of preterm infants have reduced mortality, however, the effect of interventions on morbidity in surviving infants must be considered. This is particularly important in perinatal practice as there is a potential for interventions to improve short term outcomes but also to increase the likelihood of adverse longer term outcomes in surviving infants. For example, giving preterm infants systemic corticosteroids in the first few days of postnatal life improves short term respiratory outcomes, such as allowing earlier weaning from the ventilator or reducing oxygen dependency. Trials that undertook longer term follow up, however, showed that infants who received corticosteroids had a higher rate of adverse neurological effects, including cerebral palsy.

The importance of assessing outcomes that are relevant to infants and families rather than surrogate outcomes is further illustrated by the trials of tocolytic drugs used to suppress uterine contractions and delay preterm delivery. Trials assessing these treatments have usually measured gestation at delivery as a primary outcome. Meta-analysis of these trials showed an unequivocal effect of tocolytic drugs delaying delivery. Although there is a strong relation between length of gestation and the risk of neonatal mortality and morbidity, it does not necessarily follow that delaying delivery improves important outcomes for infants. In fact, meta-analyses of trials of tocolysis have not showed any effect on perinatal mortality or morbidity, but they have shown a higher risk of maternal adverse effects. Further large randomized controlled trials with long term follow up are needed to assess if tocolysis is a benign intervention for mothers and preterm infants. Evaluating the longer term neurodevelopmental outcomes of perinatal treatments is difficult and expensive. Abnormal motor function or severe neurosensory disability can be assessed in the second year after birth, but milder sensory problems, or behavioral problems, are more reliably assessed in older preschool children. Educational and cognitive deficits are not apparent until children are of school age. Follow up of trial cohorts must be as complete as possible as children who are difficult to follow up have a higher risk of impairment than those who are easily found.

Informed consent is fundamental to giving legal and ethical protection to parents and preterm infants participating in research studies. Problems arise in gaining informed consent for interventions at or around the time of birth or during emergency treatment of an infant with a life threatening condition. In such circumstances it may be difficult to have a discussion in which the parents have time to consider their options and provide fully informed consent. Bridging gaps between evidence and practice is central to ensuring that beneficial interventions are used appropriately, and harmful interventions are avoided. Busy clinicians, however, may not always be aware of all evidence based practice guidelines. Randomized controlled trials have indicated that strategies such as introducing guidelines via an opinion leader, organizing group discussions and training workshops, and undertaking audit and performance feedback can promote the use of the best available evidence.

Recent examples of large perinatal trials

Trial Main-question-Participants

CRYO-ROP: (follow up) Do the benefits of cryotherapy for threshold retinopathy of prematurity persist into later childhood? 247 children evaluated at aged 10 years (97% follow up)

TIPPS: Does indomethacin prophylaxis affect long term neurological outcomes for extremely low birthweight infants? 1202 extremely low birthweight infants from 32 centres in five countries

ORACLE: Do maternal antibiotics improve perinatal outcomes in spontaneous preterm labor, or preterm, prelabor rupture of fetal membranes? 4826 women with preterm, prelabor rupture of fetal membranes; 6295 women in spontaneous preterm labour

BOOST: Does targeting a higher oxygen saturation range in preterm infants dependent on supplemental oxygen improve growth and development? 358 infants born at less than 30 weeks of gestation (dependent on supplemental oxygen at 32 weeks of postmenstrual age)

INIS: Does polyclonal immunoglobulin improve long term outcomes for neonates with sepsis? Ongoing: planned to recruit 5000 infants

CAP: Does management of apnoea of prematurity without methyl-xanthines affect survival without neurodisability in very preterm infants? Ongoing: aiming to enrol > 1000 infants weighing 500–1250 g at birth.

Courtesy: Peter Brocklehurst, William McGuire

EVIDENCE-BASED MEDICINE AND NEONATOLOGY– COCHRANE'S CONCLUSIONS—A SELECTIVE LIST

1. *Air versus oxygen for resuscitation of infants at birth:* There is insufficient evidence at present on which to recommend a policy of using room air over 100% oxygen, or vice versa, for newborn resuscitation. A reduction in mortality has been seen in infants resuscitated with room air, and no evidence of harm has been demonstrated. However, the small number of identified studies and their methodologic limitations dictate caution in interpreting and applying these results. We note the use of back-up 100% oxygen in more than a quarter of infants randomized to room air. Therefore, on the basis of currently available evidence, if one chooses room air as the initial gas for resuscitation, supplementary oxygen should continue to be made available

2. *Early trophic feeding for very low birth weight infants:* There is insufficient evidence to determine whether feeding very low birth weight infants small quantities of milk during the first week after birth (early trophic feeding) helps bowel development and improves subsequent feeding, growth and development. Analysis of eight trials does not suggest that this practice increases the risk of a severe bowel disorder called "necrotizing enterocolitis". Further trials are needed to provide robust evidence to inform this key area of care.

3. *Restricted versus liberal oxygen exposure for preventing morbidity and mortality in preterm or low birth weight infants:* Restricting oxygen supplementation significantly reduces the rate and severity of vision problems (retinopathy) in premature and low birth weight babies. Babies born either prematurely (before 37 weeks) or with a low birth weight often have breathing problems and need extra oxygen. Oxygen supplementation has provided many benefits for these babies but can cause damage to the eyes (retinopathy) and lungs. The review of trials found that unrestricted oxygen supplementation has these potential adverse effects without any clear benefits. Restricted oxygen significantly reduces these risks. More research is needed to find the best level of oxygen supplementation

4. *Double wall versus single wall incubator for reducing heat loss in very low birth weight infants in incubators:* Newborn infants maintained in the appropriate temperature range have a better chance of surviving. When newborn infants are within the appropriate temperature range, they burn less energy and have improved growth. The concept of an incubator with additional insulation, namely a double wall of plexiglass, is appealing as it may help very low birth weight infants maintain this appropriate temperature environment. We assessed the effects of double wall incubators compared to single wall incubators on the energy needs and water balance of very low birth weight infants. In addition, we looked at important clinical outcomes such as growth, length of hospital stay and survival. Three studies were found that met our criteria. The double wall incubators had advantages as far as decreasing heat loss and decreasing heat production. These infants seemed to be in the best temperature range, as their need to burn energy was less. However, these effects were small and did not provide any evidence of any long-term improvement regarding duration of hospitalization or survival. Although it appears that caring for extremely small infants in double wall incubators may result in certain metabolic advantages, this review was unable to find any data in the literature to support or refute this theory. Available data is insufficient to directly guide clinical practice.

5. *Radiant warmers versus incubators for regulating body temperature in newborn infants:* Radiant warmers result in increased IWL compared to incubators. This needs to be taken into account when calculating daily fluid requirements. The results of this review do not provide sufficient evidence concerning effects on important outcomes to guide clinical practice. Further randomized controlled trials are required to assess the effects of radiant warmers versus incubators in neonatal care on important short and long term outcomes, with particular attention to extremely low birthweight infants in the early neonatal period.

6. *Transpyloric versus gastric tube feeding for preterm infants:* Preterm infants often have poor co-ordination of sucking and swallowing and this can delay the establishment of safe oral feeding. Enteral feeds may be delivered through a catheter passed via the nose or the mouth into the stomach or upper small bowel. The review of trials found that babies receiving transpyloric tube feeding had more adverse effects, without any evidence of any increased benefit over gastric tube feeding.

7. *Trophic feedings for parenterally fed infants:* It is not known whether giving limited feedings, as compared to giving no feedings or more feedings, to premature babies receiving intravenous nutrition is safe or beneficial. Necrotizing enterocolitis (NEC) is a life-threatening bowel illness in newborn babies born prematurely. As there is concern that feedings in the gastrointestinal tract may increase the risk of NEC, babies in some centers receive only intravenous nutrition for prolonged periods. However, there is also a concern that delaying feedings could lead to growth and feeding problems. For this reason, babies in other centers receive progressively increasing feedings during the first two weeks after birth. One alternative would be to give some minimal "trophic" feedings during this time to provide enteral nutrition without increasing the risk of NEC. Current evidence has not determined which approach to feeding is better and one or more large multi-center trials are needed to resolve this important issue.

8. *Nasal versus oral intubation for mechanical ventilation of newborn infants:* There is not enough evidence to demonstrate any differences in the effect of nasal versus oral intubation for mechanical ventilation of newborn babies in neonatal intensive care Babies in neonatal intensive care often need help to breathe, sometimes via a ventilator (machine). Air is mechanically pumped into their lungs through a tube that is either inserted into their mouth or nose (endotracheal intubation). Insertion can fail and problems can include a blockage in the tube or the baby's airway, the wrong size tube or injury as a result of the presence of the tube. Complications caused by endotracheal intubation can also have serious adverse effects for the baby such as heart and breathing problems. The review did not find enough evidence from trials to demonstrate any differences in the effect of nasal versus oral intubation. More research is needed.

9. *Gradual versus abrupt discontinuation of oxygen in preterm or low birth weight infants:* Gradual versus abrupt discontinuation of oxygen in preterm or low birth weight infants Not enough evidence to show the best way to wean premature babies off oxygen supplementation. Babies born either prematurely (before 37 weeks) or with a low birthweight often have breathing problems and need extra oxygen. Appropriate oxygen levels are important as damage to the eyes or lungs can result if levels are too high or too low. The decision to stop giving oxygen gradually or abruptly can also affect the health of the baby. The review of trials found one trial that demonstrated that gradual rather than abrupt weaning from oxygen supplementation reduces the risk of eye damage but could not conclude which is the best method of weaning. More research is needed.

10. *Nasal versus oral route for placing feeding tubes in preterm or low birth weight infants:* There are insufficient data

available to inform practice. A large randomized controlled trial is required to determine if the use of nasally placed feeding tubes compared with orally placed feeding tubes improves growth and development, without increasing adverse consequences in preterm or low birth weight infants.

11. *Cooling for newborns with hypoxic ischemic encephalopathy:* A lack of oxygen before and during birth can destroy cells in a newborn baby's brain. The damage caused by the lack of oxygen continues for some time afterwards. One way to try and stop this damage is to induce hypothermia - cooling the baby or just the baby's head for hours to days. This treatment may reduce the amount of damage to brain cells. There is evidence from the eight randomized controlled trials included in this systematic review (n = 638) that therapeutic hypothermia is beneficial to term newborns with hypoxic ischemic encephalopathy. Cooling reduces mortality without increasing major disability in survivors. The benefits of cooling on survival and neurodevelopment outweigh the short-term adverse effects. However, this review comprises an analysis based on less than half of all infants currently known to be randomized into eligible trials of cooling. Incorporation of data from ongoing and completed randomized trials (n = 829) will be important to clarify the effectiveness of cooling and to provide more information on the safety of therapeutic hypothermia, but could also alter these conclusions. Further trials to determine the appropriate method of providing therapeutic hypothermia, including comparison of whole body with selective head cooling with mild systemic hypothermia, are required.

12. *Caffeine versus theophylline for apnea in preterm infants:* Caffeine appears to have similar short term effects on apnea/bradycardia as does theophylline, although caffeine has certain therapeutic advantages over theophylline. The review of trials found that caffeine has similar effects to theophylline but has a larger gap between levels that are therapeutic and those with toxic effects. Caffeine is more easily absorbed and has a longer half-life that allows once daily doses. The possibility that higher doses of caffeine might be more effective in extremely preterm infants needs further evaluation in randomized clinical trials.

13. *Early postnatal (<96 hours) corticosteroids for preventing chronic lung disease in preterm infants:* The benefits of early postnatal corticosteroid treatment (d" 7 days), particularly dexamethasone, may not outweigh the known or potential adverse effects of this treatment. Although early corticosteroid treatment facilitates extubation and reduces the risk of chronic lung disease and patent ductus arteriosus, it causes short-term adverse effects including gastrointestinal bleeding, intestinal perforation, hyperglycemia, hypertension, hypertrophic cardiomyopathy and growth failure. Long-term follow-up studies report an increased risk of abnormal neurological examination and cerebral palsy. However, the methodological quality of the studies determining long-term outcomes is limited in some cases; the surviving children have been assessed predominantly before school age, and no study has been sufficiently powered to detect important adverse long-term neurosensory outcomes. There is a compelling need for the long-term follow-up and reporting of late outcomes, especially neurological and developmental outcomes, among surviving infants who participated in all randomized trials of early postnatal corticosteroid treatment. Hydrocortisone in the doses and regimens used in the reported RCTs has few beneficial or harmful effects and cannot be recommended for prevention of CLD.

14. *Late (>7 days) postnatal corticosteroids for chronic lung disease in preterm infants:* This review of trials found that giving corticosteroids to infants at least seven days old produces short-term benefits of reducing the need for assisted ventilation and the rate of CLD, perhaps also reducing death in the first 28 days of life. However, high doses in particular are associated with short-term side effects such as bleeding from the stomach or bowel, higher blood pressure and difficulty tolerating glucose. In contrast with early use of corticosteroids in the first week of life, there is little evidence for long-term complications; however, it is not certain that there are no long-term problems. *It seems wise to limit the use of late corticosteroids to those babies who cannot be weaned from assisted ventilation and to minimize the dose and duration of any course of treatment.*

15. *Late versus early surgical correction for congenital diaphragmatic hernia in newborn infants :* No clear evidence about when to perform surgery to correct congenital diaphragmatic hernia. Congenital diaphragmatic hernia is a rare but often fatal condition. It occurs when a newborn baby's diaphragm has a defect in it that allows abdominal organs (such as the stomach or liver) to enter the chest and displace the lung and heart. Surgery can correct the defect, but damage to the lung may be so severe that the baby still cannot survive. It has been thought that correcting the defect was so urgent that emergency surgery should be performed within the first 24 hours following birth, but more recent thinking suggests that a period of stabilization before surgery could help the lung develop. Only two trials have been done, and these provide no clear evidence to support delayed surgery over emergency surgery

16. *Single versus double volume exchange transfusion in jaundiced newborn infants:* There was insufficient evidence to support or refute the use of single volume exchange transfusion as opposed to double volume exchange transfusion in jaundiced newborns. A change from the current practice of double volume exchange transfusions for severe jaundice in newborns infant, cannot be recommended on current evidence.

17. *Surfactant for meconium aspiration syndrome in full term infants:* In infants with MAS, surfactant administration may reduce the severity of respiratory illness and decrease the number of infants with progressive respiratory failure requiring support with ECMO. The relative efficacy of surfactant therapy compared to, or in conjunction with, other approaches to treatment including inhaled nitric oxide, liquid ventilation, surfactant lavage and high frequency ventilation remains to be tested.

18. *Natural surfactant extract versus synthetic surfactant for neonatal respiratory distress syndrome :* Although clinical trials have demonstrated that both synthetic surfactants and natural surfactant preparations are effective, comparison in animal models has suggested that there may be greater efficacy of natural surfactant products, perhaps due to the protein content of natural surfactant

19. *Prophylactic versus selective use of surfactant in preventing morbidity and mortality in preterm infants:* Prophylactic surfactant administration to infants judged to be at risk of developing respiratory distress syndrome (infants less than 30-32 weeks gestation), compared to selective use of surfactant in infants with established RDS, has been demonstrated to improve clinical outcome. Infants who receive prophylactic surfactant have a decreased risk of pneumothorax, a decreased risk of pulmonary interstitial emphysema and a decreased risk of mortality. However, it remains unclear exactly which criteria should be used to judge "at risk" infants who would require prophylactic surfactant administration.

20. *Sildenafil for pulmonary hypertension in Neonates:* The safety and effectiveness of sildenafil in the treatment of PPHN has not yet been established and its use should be restricted within the context of randomized controlled trials. Further randomized controlled trials of adequate power comparing Sildenafil with other pulmonary vasodilators are needed in moderately ill infants with PPHN.

21. *Umbilical artery catheters in the newborn: effects of position of the catheter tip:* High placed umbilical artery catheters are associated with a lower incidence of clinical vascular complications, without an increase in any adverse sequelae. Intraventricular hemorrhage rates, death and necrotizing enterocolitis are not more frequent with high compared to low catheters. There appears to be no evidence to support the use of low placed umbilical artery catheters. High catheters should be used exclusively.

22. *Antibiotic regimens for suspected late onset sepsis in newborn infants:* Empiric antibiotic treatment varies between neonatal intensive care units and countries and there are currently no consensus guidelines on the choice of empiric antibiotics. There are also no definitive guidelines on classification of CoNS as true sepsis or contaminant, the removal of indwelling catheters or the duration of antibiotics for late onset sepsis. There is no evidence from randomized trials in favor of any particular antibiotic regimen for the treatment of suspected late onset neonatal sepsis. There is a lack of studies that compare different antibiotic regimens for treating suspected late onset neonatal sepsis. More research is needed into narrow versus broad spectrum antibiotic regimens for suspected late onset infection and particularly into the harms of treatment, both short and long term. In developed countries where coagulase negative staphylococcus is the commonest late onset infection, trials may wish to compare regimens with and without vancomycin plus an aminoglycoside. In developing countries where broad spectrum antibiotic cover is common, ongoing surveillance of types of organisms and increasing antibiotic resistance is particularly important to then direct randomized trials. Any future research also needs to assess cost effectiveness and the impact of antibiotics in different settings such as developed or developing countries and lower gestational age groups. *Similarly, there is no evidence from randomized trials to suggest that any antibiotic regimen may be better than any other in the treatment of presumed **early neonatal sepsis**. More studies are needed to resolve this issue as well.*

23. *Permissive hypercapnia for the prevention of morbidity and mortality in mechanically ventilated newborn infants:* This review does not demonstrate any significant overall benefit of a permissive hypercapnia/minimal ventilation strategy compared to a routine ventilation strategy. At present, therefore, these ventilation strategies cannot be recommended to reduce mortality, or pulmonary and neurodevelopmental morbidity. Ventilatory strategies which target high levels of PCO2 (> 55 mmHg) should only be undertaken in the context of well-designed controlled clinical trials. These trials should aim to establish the safe, or ideal, range for CO2 in ventilated newborns, and examine the role of protective ventilatory techniques in achieving this target.

24. *Repeated lumbar or ventricular punctures in newborns with intraventricular hemorrhage:* Intraventricular hemorrhage (IVH) is a major complication of premature birth and a cause of cerebral palsy and hydrocephalus. Repeated early lumbar puncture or ventricular taps have been advocated as a way of avoiding hydrocephalus and protecting the brain from pressure. It was thought that the risk of hydrocephalus and the need for a ventriculo-peritoneal shunt might be reduced by the removal of protein and old blood in the cerebrospinal fluid. This hypothesis has been tested in four randomized trials involving premature infants in whom IVH (with or without established enlargement) was diagnosed by ultrasound. There is no evidence that early tapping of cerebrospinal fluid by lumbar puncture or ventricular tap reduces the risk of shunt dependence, disability, multiple disability or death. The use of repeated taps was associated with an increased risk of

central nervous system infection. Thus the early use of early tapping cannot be recommended. Removing cerebrospinal fluid should be reserved for cases where there is symptomatic raised intracranial pressure

25. *Rescue high frequency oscillatory ventilation versus conventional ventilation for pulmonary dysfunction in preterm infants:* Insufficient evidence exists to support the use of high frequency oscillatory ventilation instead of conventional ventilation for preterm infants with severe lung disease who are given positive pressure ventilation. High frequency oscillatory ventilation (HFOV) is a newer way of providing artificial ventilation of the lungs. Theoretically, HFOV may produce less injury to the lungs, particularly when high pressures are used on conventional positive pressure ventilation. This review of the evidence from one randomized controlled trial suggests there might be less short-term lung injury from high frequency oscillatory ventilation. However, more babies in this group developed hemorrhage in and around the fluid spaces in the brain (cerebral ventricles) and this harm might outweigh any benefit. More information is needed to clarify the balance between benefits and harms of high frequency oscillatory ventilation instead of conventional positive pressure ventilation for preterm infants with severe lung disease.

26. *Recombinant human activated protein C for severe sepsis in neonates:* Sepsis (a generalized blood stream infection) is common in neonates. Severe sepsis carries a high mortality and morbidity even with current critical care management. Activated Protein C (APC) is a protein formed within the human body to prevent formation of blood clots and helps in breaking down clots. Recombinant human ACP (rhAPC) is a synthesized version of APC using recombinant technology. It has been shown to reduce mortality in severe sepsis in adults. The review authors investigated whether treatment of severe sepsis in newborn infants with rhAPC will help to reduce mortality and severe morbidity. The review authors found no controlled studies in this age group. There is a need for randomized controlled clinical trials before the use of rhAPC for the treatment of severe sepsis for newborn infants can be recommended in clinical practice.

27. *Prophylactic vitamin K for vitamin K deficiency bleeding in neonates:* A single dose (1.0 mg) of intramuscular vitamin K after birth is effective in the prevention of classic HDN. Either intramuscular or oral (1.0 mg) vitamin K prophylaxis improves biochemical indices of coagulation status at 1-7 days. Neither intramuscular nor oral vitamin K has been tested in randomized trials with respect to effect on late HDN. Oral vitamin K, either single or multiple dose, has not been tested in randomized trials for its effect on either classic or late HDN.

28. *Probiotics for prevention of necrotizing enterocolitis in preterm infants:* Enteral supplementation of probiotics reduced the risk of severe NEC and mortality in preterm infants. This analysis supports a change in practice in premature infants > 1000 g at birth. Data regarding outcome of ELBW infants could not be extracted from the available studies; therefore, a reliable estimate of the safety and efficacy of administration of probiotic supplements cannot be made in this high risk group. A large randomized controlled trial is required to investigate the potential benefits and safety profile of probiotics supplementation in ELBW infants.

29. *Preoxygenation for tracheal suctioning in intubated, ventilated newborn infants:* baby born too early (before 34 weeks) often has immature lungs. This is a major cause of breathing failure and death. Mechanical ventilation (machine assisted breathing) keeps the baby breathing and reduces the risk of lung injury and disease. Endotracheal

suctioning (removing unwanted fluid through the windpipe) is a routine part of mechanical ventilation, but can have serious complications of pneumothorax (air in the lung cavity) and bradycardia (slow heart rate). Giving oxygen just before suctioning (preoxygenation) may minimize the risk of these complications. The review of trials did not find enough evidence on the effects of preoxygenation. More research is needed.

30. *Extracorporeal membrane oxygenation for severe respiratory failure in newborn infants:* A complex life support procedure, called extracorporeal membrane oxygenation (ECMO), can be used in infants who are near term age to overcome severe, potentially reversible breathing problems. ECMO is similar to the technology used in cardiac bypass surgery. Blood is removed from the body of the patient, oxygen is added to the blood, and the blood is returned to the patient. Although the number of babies requiring ECMO is small, and ECMO is a very invasive and potentially expensive procedure, the benefits of this procedure are high. In this review, four randomized trials that compared the use of ECMO to the conventional approach to supporting these infants with severe breathing problems were identified. Overall, these trials showed a strong benefit for ECMO regarding survival at the time of hospital discharge. This is particularly true for infants without a specific problem of lung formation (congenital diaphragmatic hernia). The result implies that for every three babies with breathing problems and lung failure who were treated with ECMO rather than conventional ventilation, one more infant will survive. Although little information is available regarding long-term follow-up, one trial in the United Kingdom shows both benefits of ECMO and cost-effectiveness of the use of ECMO.

31. *Enteral antibiotics for preventing necrotizing enterocolitis in low birthweight or preterm infants:* Necrotizing enterocolitis (NEC) is a serious disease that affects the bowel in the first few weeks of life. The cause is unknown but milk feeding and bacteria may contribute. NEC is more common in preterm babies, possibly because of reduced immunity. Oral antibiotics have been used to prevent NEC but there are concerns about the possible adverse effects of oral antibiotics such as resistance to bacteria. The review of trials found there was not enough evidence to support the use of antibiotics to prevent NEC in preterm and low birth weight babies. More research is needed.

32. *Ibuprofen for the treatment of patent ductus arteriosus in preterm and/or low birth weight infants:* Ibuprofen is as effective as indomethacin at closing a PDA in a very preterm or very small newborn, and has fewer adverse effects on kidney function. Ibuprofen may be associated with an increased risk of pulmonary complications including chronic lung disease and rarely pulmonary hypertension.

33. *Percutaneous central venous catheters versus peripheral cannulae for delivery of parenteral nutrition in neonates:* Data from one small study suggest that using a percutaneous central venous catheter to deliver parenteral nutrition improves nutrient input. The significance of this in relation to long-term growth and developmental outcomes is unclear. Three studies suggested that the use of a percutaneous central venous catheter decreases the number of catheters/cannulae needed to deliver the nutrition. No evidence was found to suggest that percutaneous central venous catheter use increased the risk of adverse events, particularly systemic infection.

34. *Nitric oxide for respiratory failure in infants born at or near term:* On the evidence presently available, it appears reasonable to use inhaled nitric oxide in an initial concentration of 20 ppm for term and near term infants with hypoxic respiratory failure who do not have a diaphragmatic hernia.

35. *Intravenous dexamethasone for extubation of newborn infants:* Dexamethasone may help babies at high risk of complications when being taken off mechanical breathing support. The tube that is placed in the baby's airway to enable mechanical ventilation (machine-assisted breathing) can cause injury. This can lead to complications when the tube is removed (extubation). This review found that giving dexamethasone (a corticosteroid drug) around the time of extubation can help prevent swelling in the baby's throat that might require reinsertion of the tube. However, the review found that there are adverse effects of dexamethasone. The benefits only outweigh the risks for babies at high risk of complication (such as those who have received several, or prolonged, intubations).

36. *Extubation from low-rate intermittent positive airways pressure versus extubation after a trial of endotracheal continuous positive airways pressure in intubated preterm infants:* No evidence that time on endotracheal CPAP (continuous low pressure rather than intermittent breaths from the ventilator) before taking preterm babies off a ventilator helps them adjust to breathing on their own. Babies in neonatal intensive care often need help to breathe, sometimes via an endotracheal tube (through the windpipe) connected to a ventilator (machine). It has been thought that it might help a baby adjust to breathing after ventilation if there was a period of CPAP (continuous positive airways pressure) before extubation (coming off the ventilator). However, there have also been concerns that this may be too much hard work for the baby, and may cause harm. The review of trials found that a trial of CPAP first before extubation does not improve the baby's ability to breathe on their own.

37. *Interventions for treatment of neonatal hyperglycemia in very low birth weight infants:* Higher-than-normal blood sugar levels are frequently seen in babies born very early (before 32 weeks gestation) or with very low birth weight (< 1500 grams) and who are fed totally or partially by vein. Several types of adverse outcomes have been associated with high blood sugar levels, including increased risks for death, infections, eye problems, and bleeding into the brain. It is not known if treatment to lower the baby's blood sugar helps to prevent those complications and, if so, which treatment is best. These treatment options include decreasing the amount of sugar delivered by vein to nourish the baby or administration of insulin. This review of trials found no evidence of significant effects of these treatments on the risks of death or major complications. However, the studies reviewed were very small. There is a need for larger trials to answer these questions.

38. *Higher versus lower protein intake in formula-fed low birth weight infants:* This systematic review suggests that higher protein intake (=> 3.0 g/kg/day but < 4.0 g/kg/day) from formula accelerates weight gain. Based on increased nitrogen accretion rates, this most likely indicates an increase in lean body mass. Although accelerated weight gain is considered to be a positive effect, increase in other outcome measures examined may represent a negative or ambivalent effect. These include elevated blood urea nitrogen levels and increased metabolic acidosis. Limited information was available regarding the impact of higher formula protein intakes on long term outcomes such as neurodevelopmental abnormalities. As determined in this review, existing research literature on this topic is not adequate to make specific recommendations regarding the provision of very high protein intake (> 4.0 g/kg/day) from formula.

39. *Servo-control for maintaining abdominal skin temperature at 36°C in low birth weight infants:* Servo-control of abdominal skin temperature at 36°C reduces neonatal death rate in LBW infants, compared with air temperature control

at 31.8⁰C. During at least the first week after birth, LBW babies should be provided with a carefully regulated thermal environment. An abdominal skin temperature of 36⁰C may be slightly below the temperature required for strict thermoneutrality in LBW babies. If thermoneutrality is the goal, incubator heating for such infants should be adjusted to maintain abdominal skin temperature at approximately 36.5⁰C, using either servo-control or frequent manual adjustment. The early and late effects of providing graded cold stimulation during the late neonatal period (i.e. after the time when the survival advantage of thermoneutrality has been shown) should be addressed in future trials in low birth weight infants.

40. *Vancomycin for prophylaxis against sepsis in preterm neonates:* The use of prophylactic vancomycin in low doses reduces the incidence of nosocomial sepsis in the neonate. The methodologies of these studies may have contributed to the low rate of sepsis in the treated groups, as the blood cultures drawn from central lines may have failed to grow due to the low levels of vancomycin in the infusate. Although there is a theoretical concern regarding the development of resistant organisms with the administration of prophylactic antibiotic, there is insufficient evidence to ascertain the risks of development of vancomycin resistant organisms. Few clinically important benefits have been demonstrated for very low birth weight infants treated with prophylactic vancomycin. It therefore appears that routine prophylaxis with vancomycin should not be undertaken at present.

41. *Continuous nasogastric milk feeding versus intermittent bolus milk feeding for premature infants less than 1500 grams:* Infants fed by continuous tube feeding method took longer to reach full enteral feeds (weighted mean difference 3.0 days; 95% CI 0.7, 5.2). Although there was no significant difference in the days to discharge overall, one study suggested a trend toward earlier discharge for infants less than 1000 grams birth weight fed by the continuous tube feeding method (mean difference (MD) -11 days; 95% CI -21.8, -0.2). Overall, there was no significant difference in somatic growth (weight, length, head circumference or skinfold thickness) between the two groups, but subgroup analyses in one study suggested that infants less than 1000 grams and 1000 - 1250 grams birthweight gained weight faster when fed by the continuous tube feeding method (MD 2.0 g/day; 95% CI 0.5, 3.5; MD 2.0 g/day; 95% CI 0.2, 3.8, respectively). There was no significant difference in the incidence of NEC. One study showed a trend toward more apneas during the study period in infants fed by the continuous tube feeding method (MD 14.0 apneas during study period; 95% CI -0.2, 28.2). Small sample sizes, methodologic limitations and conflicting results of the studies to date, together with inconsistencies in controlling variables that may affect outcomes, make it difficult to make universal recommendations regarding the best tube feeding method for premature infants less than 1500 grams. The clinical benefits and risks of continuous versus intermittent nasogastric tube milk feeding cannot be reliably discerned from the limited information available from randomized trials to date.

42. *Ad libitum or demand/semi-demand feeding versus scheduled interval feeding for preterm infants:* There are insufficient data at present to guide clinical practice. A large randomized controlled trial is needed to determine if ad libitum of demand/semi-demand feeding of preterm infants affects clinically important outcomes. This trial should focus on infants in the transition phase from intragastric tube to oral feeding and should be of sufficient duration to assess effects on growth and time to oral feeding and hospital discharge

43. *Rationale for administering aerosolized diuretics to neonates with CLD:* In preterm infants > 3 weeks with CLD administration of a single dose of aerosolized furosemide improves pulmonary mechanics. In view of the lack of data from randomized trials concerning effects on important clinical outcomes, routine or sustained use of aerosolized loop diuretics in infants with (or developing) CLD cannot be recommended based on current evidence. More double-blinded randomized trials are needed (1) to analyze factors likely to affect the response to aerosolized furosemide, e.g., washout period and delivery of furosemide to distal airways, and (2) to assess the effects of chronic administration of aerosolized furosemide on mortality, O2 dependency, ventilator dependency, length of hospital stay and long-term outcome.

44. *Albumin infusion for low serum albumin in preterm newborn infants:* Intravenous albumin infusion is used to treat hypoalbuminemia in critically ill infants. Hypoalbuminaemia occurs in a number of clinical situations including prematurity, the acutely sick infant, respiratory distress syndrome (RDS), chronic lung disease (CLD), necrotizing enterocolitis (NEC), intracranial hemorrhage, hydrops fetalis and oedema. Fluid overload is a potential side effect of albumin administration. Albumin is a blood product and therefore carries the potential risk of infection and adverse reactions. Albumin is also a scarce and expensive resource. There is a lack of evidence from randomized trials to determine whether the routine use of albumin infusion, in preterm neonates with low serum albumin, reduces mortality or morbidity, and no evidence to assess whether albumin infusion is associated with significant side effects. There is a need for good quality, double-blind randomized controlled trials to assess the safety and efficacy of albumin infusions in preterm neonates with low serum albumin.

45. *Anticonvulsants for neonates with seizures:* At present there is little evidence from randomized controlled trials to support the use of any of the anticonvulsants currently used in the neonatal period. In the literature, there remains a body of opinion that seizures should be treated because of the concern that seizures in themselves may be harmful, although this is only supported by relatively low grade evidence (Levene 2002; Massingale 1993). Development of safe and effective treatment strategies relies on future studies of high quality (randomized controlled trials with methodology that assures validity) and of sufficient size to have the power to detect clinically important reductions in mortality and severe neurodevelopmental disability in addition to any short term reduction in seizure burden.

46. *Anticonvulsants for preventing mortality and morbidity in full term newborns with perinatal asphyxia:* It is unclear whether giving anticonvulsants to newborn babies soon after possible birth asphyxia at term is safe and effective. More studies are needed. Seizures (or convulsions) are common following birth asphyxia. These seizures may worsen the brain injury. In theory, anticonvulsant medication given to babies soon after possible birth asphyxia may improve outcome by preventing seizures and protecting the brain. Anticonvulsant drugs are not without side effects and there are concerns that they might impair brain development. The studies included in this review involved relatively small numbers of babies and few studies assessed developmental outcome. At present, there is insufficient information on which to base recommendations about the effectiveness of giving anticonvulsants to newborn babies soon after possible birth asphyxia.

47. *Avoidance of bottles during the establishment of breast feeds in preterm infants:* Preterm infants start milk feeds by tube and as they mature they are able to manage sucking feeds. The number of sucking feeds each day are gradually increased as the baby matures. For women who choose to breast feed their preterm infant it is not always possible for them to be there every time the baby needs a sucking feed.

Conventionally, bottles with mother's milk or formula are used. It has been suggested that using bottles may interfere with breast feeding success. Five trials have investigated alternatives to bottles in the establishment of breast feeds; four trials used cup feeds and one trial used tube feeds. The one study that used tube feeds was of poor quality and the results of this study need to be interpreted cautiously. When cup feeds were used, more women were discharged home fully breastfeeding, but there was no effect on any (fully and partially combined) breastfeeding. Using cup feeds also increased the length of hospital stay by 10 days. In the one study of tube feeds, breastfeeding (both fully and partially) was increased at discharge and at three and six months after discharge with no effect on length of hospital stay. However, because of the poor quality of this one study, we cannot recommend a tube feeding strategy until further studies of high quality are undertaken.

48. *Chest physiotherapy for preventing morbidity in babies being extubated from mechanical ventilation:* The results of this review do not give a clear direction for the role of active chest physiotherapy for babies being extubated from mechanical ventilation in today's neonatal intensive care settings. Evidence for benefit of this intervention is conflicting and it was not possible to identify sub-groups of babies who may benefit. No benefit for more vs less frequent treatment is evident. Concerns regarding the safety of active chest physiotherapy for preterm neonates have been reported. Information on adverse effects is inadequate in the trials included in this review to allow assessment of safety. In view of this and the lack of clear evidence for benefit, it would seem wise to use this intervention cautiously.

49. *Doxapram versus methylxanthine for apnea in preterm infants:* Intravenous doxapram and intravenous methylxanthine appear to be similar in their short term effects for treating apnea in preterm infants, although these trials are too small to exclude an important difference between the two treatments or to exclude the possibility of less common adverse effects. Long term outcome of infants treated in these trials has not been reported. Further studies would require a large number of infants to clarify whether there might be differences in responses or adverse effects with these two drugs at different ages.

50. *Formula milk versus donor breast milk for feeding preterm or low birth weight infants:* When a mother's own breast milk is not available for feeding her preterm or low birth weight infant, the alternatives are either formula milk or expressed breast milk from a donor mother ("donor breast milk"). Review of eight randomized controlled trials suggests that feeding with formula increases short-term growth rates but is associated with a higher risk of developing the severe gut disorder "necrotizing enterocolitis". There is no evidence of an effect on longer-term growth, or on development. Further trials that compare these two strategies are needed. These should probably compare formula milk adapted for preterm infants with donor breast milk supplemented with nutrients.

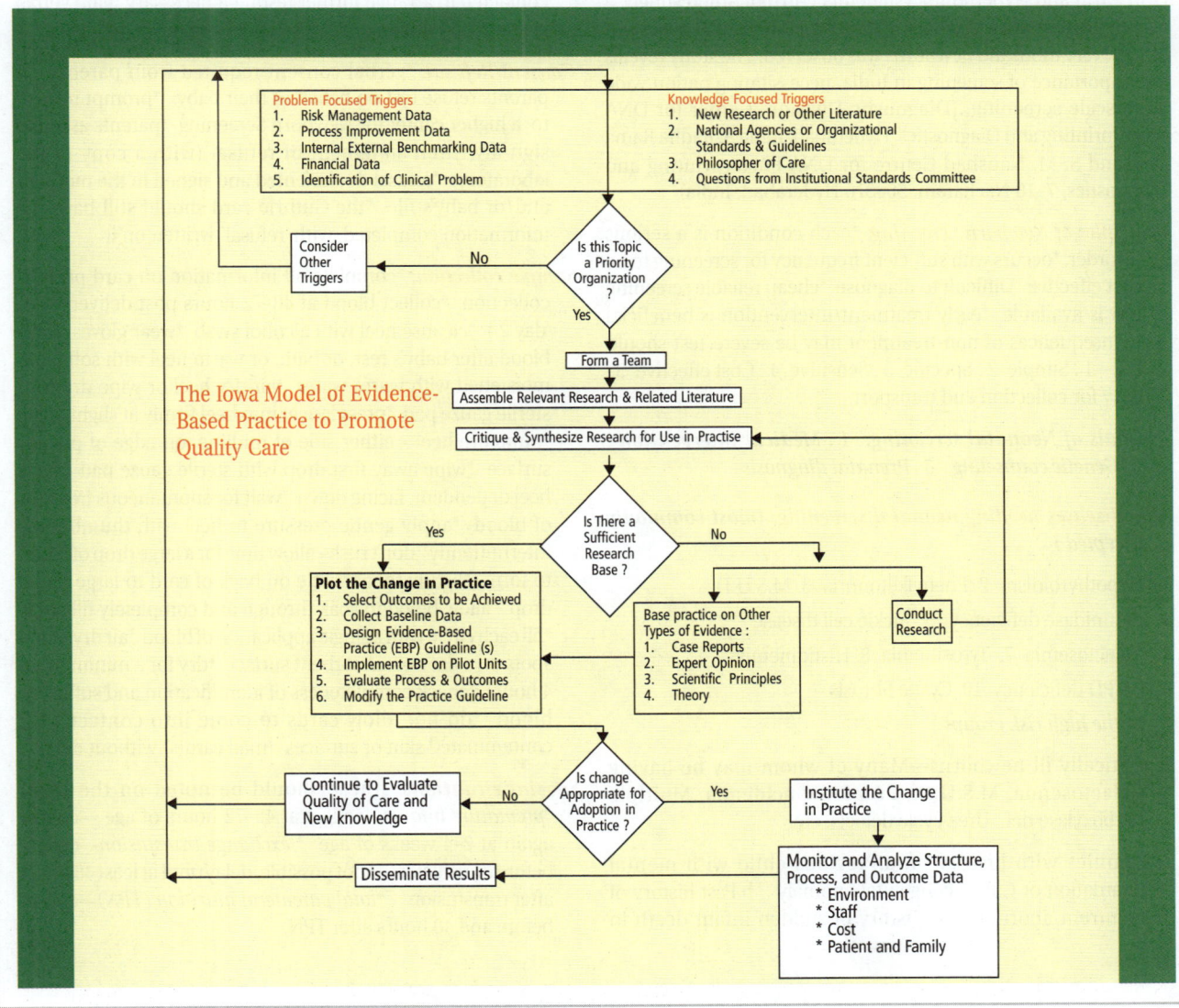

The Iowa Model of Evidence-Based Practice to Promote Quality Care

Problem Focused Triggers
1. Risk Management Data
2. Process Improvement Data
3. Internal External Benchmarking Data
4. Financial Data
5. Identification of Clinical Problem

Knowledge Focused Triggers
1. New Research or Other Literature
2. National Agencies or Organizational Standards & Guidelines
3. Philosopher of Care
4. Questions from Institutional Standards Committee

Is this Topic a Priority Organization? — No → Consider Other Triggers

Yes → Form a Team → Assemble Relevant Research & Related Literature → Critique & Synthesize Research for Use in Practise

Is There a Sufficient Research Base?

Yes → Plot the Change in Practice
1. Select Outcomes to be Achieved
2. Collect Baseline Data
3. Design Evidence-Based Practice (EBP) Guideline (s)
4. Implement EBP on Pilot Units
5. Evaluate Process & Outcomes
6. Modify the Practice Guideline

No → Base practice on Other Types of Evidence:
1. Case Reports
2. Expert Opinion
3. Scientific Principles
4. Theory

Conduct Research

Is change Appropriate for Adoption in Practice?

No → Continue to Evaluate Quality of Care and New knowledge

Yes → Institute the Change in Practice → Monitor and Analyze Structure, Process, and Outcome Data
* Environment
* Staff
* Cost
* Patient and Family

Disseminate Results

Newborn screening is a public health programme aimed at early identification of conditions for which early intervention can lead to elimination or reduction of associated mortality, morbidity and disabilities in newborn babies and often into childhood. A 'well looking baby' may quickly become critically ill. Screening tests are not diagnostic and therefore follow up testing is always required for abnormal results. Not every affected child will be detected by the screening programme, so if one of the screened conditions is suspected, follow up diagnostic testing should be always be considered. Timing of taking the sample is important. Expanded newborn screening (NBS) is aimed for early detection and intervention of treatable inborn errors of metabolism and also to establish incidence of these disorders in this part of the globe. The first expanded NBS programme initiated in the capital city of Andhra Pradesh to screen all the newborns born in four major Government Maternity Hospitals in Hyderabad by heel prick capillary blood collected on S&S 903 filter paper. Chromatographic (TLC and HPLC), electrophoretic (cellulose acetate and agarose) and ELISA based assays have been employed for screening of common inborn errors of metabolism. This study has shown a high prevalence of treatable Inborn errors of metabolism. Congenital hypothyroidism is the most common disorder (1in1700) followed by congenital Adrenal Hyperplasia (1 in 2575) and Hyperhomocystenemia (1in100). Interestingly, a very high prevalence of inborn errors of metabolism to the extent of 1 in every thousand newborns was observed. The study reveals the importance of screening in India, necessitating nation wide large-scale screening .(Diagnostic Division, Center for DNA Fingerprinting and Diagnostics, Hyderabad, India A. Radha Rama Devi and S. M. Naushad Centre for DNA Fingerprinting and Diagnostics, 7–18 Nacharam, 500076 Hyderabad, India)

Principles of Newborn Screening: *each condition is a serious disorder *occurs with sufficient frequency for screening to be cost effective *Difficult to diagnose *cheap reliable screening test is available *early treatment/intervention is beneficial *consequences of non-treatment may be severe.Test should be :- 1 . Simple 2 . Specific 3 . Sensitive 4 . Cost effective 5 . Easy for collection and transport.

Goals of Neonatal screening: 1 . Medical intervention . 2 . Genetic counseling . 3 . Prenatal diagnosis .

The diseases needing neonatal screening: (most commonly accepted)

1. Hypothyroidism 2. Phenylketonuria 3. M.S.U.D.
4. Biotinidase deficiency 5. Sickle cell disease
6. Galactosemia 7. Tyrosinemia 8. Histidinemia
9. G6 PD deficiency 10. Cystic fibrosis
* *In the high risk groups*

1. Critically ill newborns—Many of whom may be having Galactosemia, M.S.U.D., Propionic acidemia, Multiple Carboxylase def., Urea cycle defects, etc.
2. Families with history of: **a.**Previous child with mental retardation or C.P. or congenital anomaly . **b.**Past history of recurrent abortions. **c.**History of sudden infant death in

previous sib . **d.**Mother with significantly low intelligence and microcephaly. **e.**Family history of hemoglobinopathy. **f.** Significant degree of consanguinity. In these high-risk groups the following are useful; 1. Genetic counselling . 2. Antenatal diagnostic facilities if they are willing

a.   TORCH titre
b.   USG with doppler and anomaly scan
c.   C.V.Bx. with Karyotyping
d.   Amniotic fluid studies for
e.   Karyotype / F.I.S.H.
f.   A.F.P. & beta - HCG
g.   Biochemical analysis
h.   G.C.M.S.
i.   SOS enzyme assay or DNA studies.
3. Hemoglobinopathy workup.
4. Neonatal Screening and Neonate? management in NICU with regular followup

Pre-test Procedure: *give information brochure to parents *discuss newborn screeing test with parents *screening for many conditions *may have to give a second sample *most second samples are within the normal range *parents contacted to arrange further testing if necessary *gain verbal consent and document

Consent/Refusal: *verbal consent required from parents *if parents refuse test on behalf of their baby: *prompt referral to a higher center for Newborn Screening *parents asked to sign a written statement of refusal (with a copy to the laboratory) *refusal documented and signed in the mother's and/or baby's file *the Guthrie card should still have the information completed, with 'refusal' written on it

Sample collection: *complete all information on card prior to collection *collect blood at 48–72 hours post delivery (not 'day 2') *cleanse heel with alcohol swab *wear gloves *take blood after baby's rest, or bath, or warm heel with soft cloth moistened with warm water *air dry heel or wipe dry with sterile gauze pad *press lancet into heel firmly at slight angle *puncture heel - either side of midline, on edge of plantar surface *wipe away first drop with sterile gauze pad *have heel dependent, facing down *wait for spontaneous free flow of blood *apply gentle pressure to heel with thumb, ease intermittently *don't rush - allow time for a large drop of blood to form *lightly touch circle on back of card to large blood drop *allow blood to soak through and completely fill circle *fill each circle with a single application of blood *air dry blood spots on a flat non-absorbent surface *dry for a minimum of 4 hours *check completeness of identification and sufficient blood *do not allow cards to come into contact with contaminated skin or surfaces *mail card(s) without delay

Special situations: (these should be noted on the card) *premature infants—collect at 48–72 hours of age —collect again at 2–4 weeks of age * *exchange transfusion—collect before transfusion -if not possible, delay until at least 48 hours after transfusion   *total parenteral nutrition (TPN)—collect before and 48 hours after TPN.

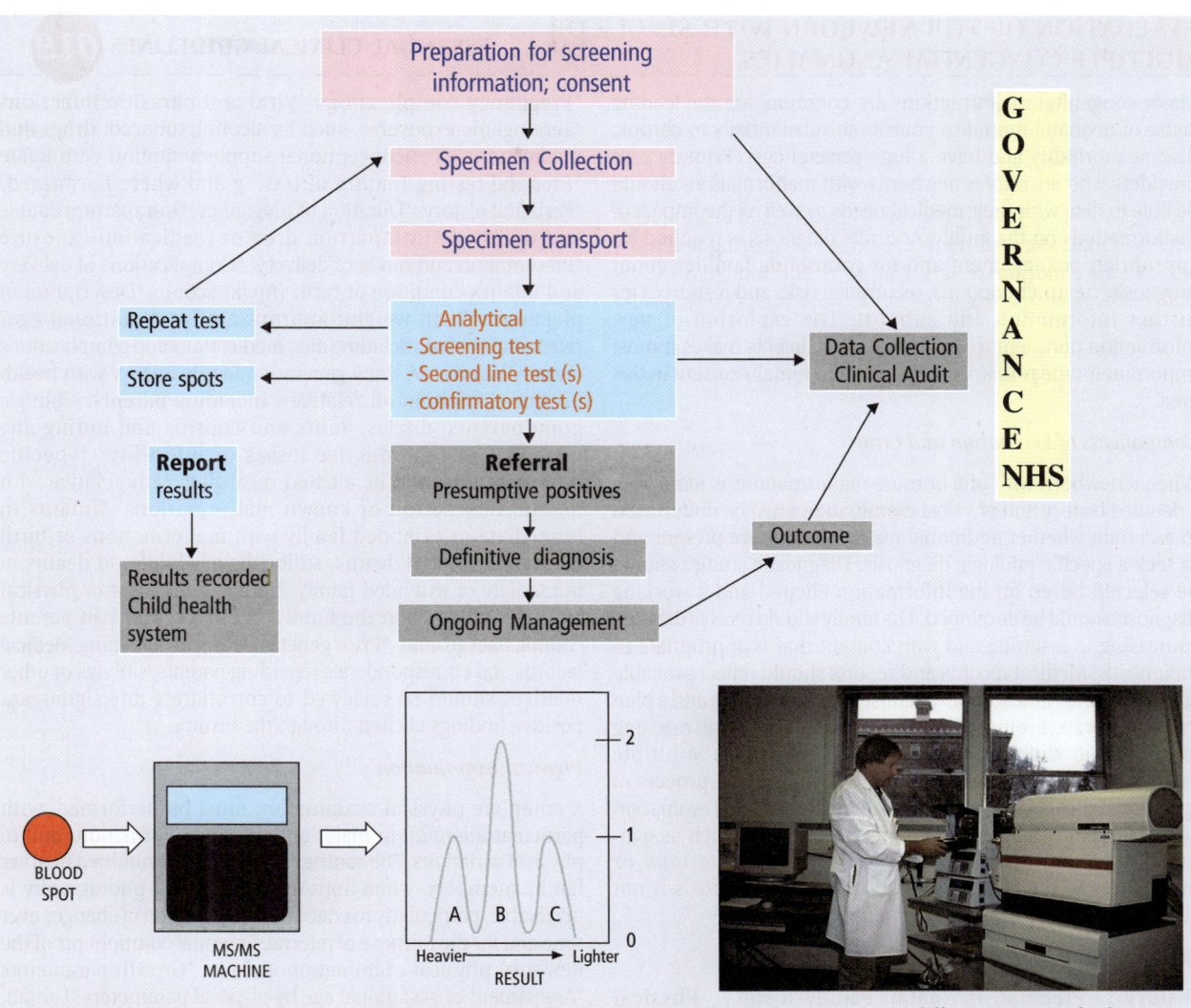

Preparation for screening information; consent

Specimen Collection

Specimen transport

Repeat test

Store spots

Analytical
- Screening test
- Second line test (s)
- confirmatory test (s)

Data Collection
Clinical Audit

Report results

Referral
Presumptive positives

Definitive diagnosis

Outcome

Results recorded
Child health
system

Ongoing Management

BLOOD SPOT

MS/MS MACHINE

Heavier → Lighter
RESULT
A B C

Expanded Newborn screening by tandem mass spectrometry (MS/MS) identifies and measures two different groups of substances - acylcarnitines and amino acids. About 24 to 72 hours after a baby is born, a few drops of blood are taken from the baby's heel and dabbed on a special type of filter paper. The filter paper is mailed to a newborn screening laboratory which will perform all of the newborn screening tests. Using MS/MS, the lab will measure which acylcarnitines and amino acids are present in the newborn's blood. It will also measure how much of each substance is present in the newborn's blood. In this way, MS/MS can be used to screen for over thirty different rare inherited metabolic disorders. Everyone has acylcarnitines and amino acids in their blood. However, infants with rare inherited metabolic disorders have either too much or not enough amino acids and acylcarnitines. They can also have unusual types of amino acids and acylcarnitines in their blood. Because MS/MS is such a sensitive technique, there can be lots of reasons for small abnormalities that can lead to an abnormal test result in a healthy baby (this is called a "false positive" test result). However, every infant with an abnormal screening test result needs to have follow-up testing.

Neonatal metabolic screening tests

Disorder*	Consequences	Metabolic Screening Test
Hypothyroidism	Delayed growth and development (weight > length)	Thyroxine (T_4), thyroid stimulating hormone (TSH)
Phenylketonuria (PKU)	Severe retardation, Vomiting, lethargy, Eczematoid rash Musty / mousy odor	Phenylalanine
Galactosemia	Acidosis, Growth failure, Sepsis (E.coli), Cataracts, Liver dysfunction	Galactose-1-p Uridyl transferase
Congenital adrenal hyperplasia	Virilization, Salt-losing crises	17-OH progesterone
Maple syrup urine disease	Acidosis, Hypoglycemia, Seizures	Leucine
Sickle cell disease, Thalassemia	Anemia Early overwhelming infections	Hemoglobin electrophoresis
Homocystinuria	Acidosis, Delayed growth and development Vascular thrombosis, Lens dislocation	Homocystine
Biotinidase deficiency	Defective metabolism of amino acids and neurotransmitters	Biotinidase

EVALUATION OF THE NEWBORN WITH SINGLE OR MULTIPLE CONGENITAL ANOMALIES

Major congenital malformations are common, are the leading cause of neonatal mortality, contribute substantially to chronic disease morbidity and have a high societal cost. Primary care providers who encounter newborns with malformations should be able to deal with their medical needs as well as the impact of malformations on the family. Accurate diagnosis is required for appropriate management and for counseling families about prognosis, treatment options, recurrence risks and resources for further information and support. The explosion of new information pertinent to etiology of birth defects makes it most important for the primary care provider to remain current in this area.

Components of Evaluation and Care

When a newborn with one or more malformations is identified, a detailed history and physical examination must be undertaken to ascertain whether additional malformations are present and to seek a specific etiologic diagnosis. Diagnostic studies should be selected based on the information elicited and a working diagnosis should be developed. The family should receive detailed counseling in a setting and with content that is appropriate to their needs. Medical records and reports should reflect available laboratory and clinical data, diagnostic considerations and a plan for ongoing care, evaluation and management. Although reaching an etiologic diagnosis for the newborn with multiple malformations is a primary goal of the evaluation process, a specific diagnosis might not be apparent after detailed evaluation and diagnostic testing. For a variety of reasons, such as age-dependent phenotypic or behavioral manifestations or uniqueness of the pattern of malformations, diagnosis is not always apparent in the newborn period.

Components of Evaluation and Care

History : Prenatal, Perinatal, Family history **Physical Examination :** Assessment of gestational age, Growth parameters and measurements, Comprehensive examination **Differential Diagnosis :** Single malformation, Multiple malformations due to syndrome, Multiple malformations, etiology unknown **Diagnostic Evaluation :** Imaging Chromosome analysis, Other genetic tests, Consideration of referral to specialist(s) **Working Diagnosis/Counseling the Family:** Counseling Principles, Supportive Setting, Content **Patient record :** Documentation of positive and negative findings , Diagnostic considerations, Issues discussed in counseling, Management plan **Ongoing care and case management:** Written reports, Written materials for families, Ongoing care and referrals as indicated **Dealing with Uncertainty.**

History

A comprehensive history is a critical component of the evaluation of a newborn with single or multiple malformations. The sequence described suggests an orderly passage from history to physical examination to diagnostic evaluation. However, in actual practice, the history and physical examination represent a dynamic and interactive process in which certain elements of history may be sought after the physical exam. Likewise, certain physical parameters may be assessed further and more carefully based on information derived from historical data. Additionally, results of initial diagnostic testing may suggest the need for further history or physical examination. The following elements should be included: *Prenatal history *Maternal age, parity and health, including maternal illnesses and medications used *Onset and quality of fetal movements throughout pregnancy *Pregnancy complications *Viral and parasitic infections *Teratogenic exposures, such as alcohol, tobacco, drugs and medications *Periconceptional supplementation with folate *Prenatal testing (nature of testing and where performed) *Perinatal history *Duration of pregnancy *Intrapartum course and duration *Intrapartum drug or medication exposure *Presentation and mode of delivery *Complications of delivery and infant's condition at birth (Apgar score) *Description of placenta *Birth weight; appropriate for gestational age? *Neonatal course, including diet, medications and complications *Family history *A three generation family history with health information about all relatives, including parents, siblings, grandparents, uncles, aunts and cousins and noting any instances of reproductive losses or infertility *Specific information should be elicited regarding: *any relative with mental retardation or known malformations *infants in immediate or extended family with malformations or birth defects *neonatal deaths, stillbirths or childhood deaths in immediate or extended family *familial disorders or physical features that "run in the family" *Consanguinity in parents *Ethnic background *Prior genetic testing or screening Medical records and correspondence regarding parents, siblings or other relatives should be reviewed to corroborate any significant positive findings elicited through the history.

Physical Examination

A complete physical examination must be performed, with particular attention to major and minor malformations and to physical variations. The same areas should be examined in other family members, when appropriate. Medical photography is invaluable, particularly to enable documentation of changes over time and for the purpose of referral. Essential components of the newborn physical examination include: *Growth parameters *Assessment of gestational age by physical parameters *Length, weight and head circumference, with percentiles *Assessment of proportionality and symmetry *Specific measurements where indicated by observation, such as inner-canthal distance or upper to lower segment ratio *General appearance *Tone, posture, positioning, alertness, vigor, color, respiratory effort and other observations *Detailed examination -Skin - pigmentation pattern (areas of increased or decreased pigmentation), dimples, vascular or other lesions, or excessive peeling -Head - shape, symmetry, fontanelles -Scalp - hair patterning and location of hair whorls -Facial features -Eyes - pupils, orbits (hyper or hypotelorism) including palpebral fissure inclination and length -Ears- location, rotation, configuration and size, patency -Nose - appearance and patency of nares -appearance of nasal bridge and columella -Mouth - appearance of upper lip, philtrum and vermilion border -intra-oral examination of palate, alveolar ridges and tongue -Mandible - shape and symmetry -Neck - posterior hairline, presence of sinus tracts, torticollis, redundant skin or webbing -Chest - shape, symmetry, circumference, location of nipples, accessory nipples -Cardiovascular - heart murmurs, pulses, blood pressure -Lungs -symmetry of breath sounds -Abdomen- appearance of umbilicus, muscle tone, integrity of wall, enlarged organs or masses -Genitalia - size, appearance, palpation of testes (in males), presence of ambiguity -Anus - location and patency -Back - symmetry, spine, presence of sinuses or hair tufts in inter-gluteal cleft -Extremities - proportions, appearance, range of motion (including hips), pulses, presence of reduction or duplication of segments -Hands and feet- nails; creases (palmar, phalangeal and flexion); joints -Neurological - tone, response, alertness, reflexes

Initial Impression and Differential Diagnosis

The history and physical findings should lead to an initial impression and differential diagnosis. These will guide selection of preliminary tests, the content of initial counseling of the family and development of an immediate plan for management, which can be modified as new information is developed and synthesized. Initial impression should fit into one of three categories: *Single (isolated) malformation *Multiple malformations, recognizable pattern (syndrome identification) *Multiple malformations, pattern not recognized.

Diagnostic Evaluation

Diagnostic tests should be selected to clarify or establish a clinical diagnosis when possible. Such tests may be of particular value when a syndrome pattern is not recognized or to facilitate risk assessment for genetic counseling. Single (isolated) malformations or syndromes which are recognized on a clinical basis may not require additional diagnostic tests. It is important to discuss with the family the possible ramifications of genetic testing, including the implications for relatives. Select tests in a prioritized order, rather than using a "shotgun" approach; initial results can guide selection of more specific subsequent tests Consultations with specialists in pertinent fields may clarify diagnostic possibilities Request medical genetics consultation when a clear working diagnosis is not evident, to confirm a questionable diagnosis, to seek further information about an established diagnosis, or to provide detailed genetic counseling, particularly in complex situations Diagnostic tests which should be considered include:

*Diagnostic Imaging -Radiographs, computed tomography (CT), magnetic resonance imaging (MRI) or ultrasonography (US) should not be considered routine, but should be employed as indicated by the differential diagnosis.

*Chromosomal analysis -Banded chromosomal analysis should be obtained in the following situations: *Infants with two or more major malformations *Infants with a single major malformation or multiple minor malformations who are also small-for-dates *Infants with a single major malformation who also have multiple minor anomalies.

*In selected cases - usually in consultation with a medical geneticist - high resolution chromosome banding or fluorescence *in situ* hybridization (FISH) may be indicated to detect sub-microscopic structural chromosome changes or microdeletions (as in DiGeorge or Williams Syndrome).

*Other genetic tests -Testing for the Fragile X syndrome is not generally useful in the evaluation of the newborn with single or multiple malformations, because congenital malformations are not a typical sign of the condition. -Biochemical, metabolic or molecular genetic tests may be indicated in specific circumstances.

Situations suggesting the need for metabolic testing in the newborn with malformations

Selected clinical findings	Selected laboratory findings	Selected radiologic findings
Ambiguous genitalia	Metabolic acidosis	Punctate calcifications
Enlarged fontanelle	Abnormal liver function tests	Severe osteopenia
Seizures	Persistent hyperbilirubinemia	
Severe hypotonia	Hyperammonemia	
Cataracts	Hypocholesterolemia	
Coarse facies	Hypoglycemia	
Hepatosplenomegaly		
Lethargy or coma		
Persistent vomiting		
Unusual odor		

Working diagnosis : The working diagnosis is established by data obtained from the history, physical examination and preliminary diagnostic results and forms the basis for counseling and longitudinal care. Positive findings in the family history should be confirmed by a review of medical records and/or family photographs when possible. Corroboration by collection and review of records may be required and is often invaluable in clarifying an otherwise confusing history. **Counseling the Family.** The approach taken in counseling the family of a newborn with congenital anomalies sets the stage for future interactions. Counseling is an ongoing process; its staging and depth should be matched to each family. The items below should eventually be covered, but the depth of coverage in the initial session may vary according to family circumstances.

Counseling principles: ·Supportive, family-centered, non-judgmental attitude ·Respect for family privacy, confidentiality and autonomy ·Sensitivity to ethno-cultural and language differences ·Acknowledgment and facilitation of the grieving process. **Supportive setting:** ·Quiet, private location ·Inclusion of additional family members, clergy, etc, as desired by family

Patient Record: In addition to information on the history and physical examination, the following should be included in the patient's file: *Diagnostic considerations *Documentation of positive and negative findings *Management plan for further evaluation and treatment *Issues discussed in counseling, including recurrence risk and availability of prenatal diagnosis including serial ultrasound monitoring of subsequent pregnancies. Privacy and confidentiality of the medical record must be assured.

Letters to families should include: *Patient`s name, diagnosis and means by which diagnosis was reached *Brief summary of consultation *Recurrence risk to relatives *Availability of prenatal diagnostic testing *Primary care provider's availability for ongoing discussion or referral *Information on support groups and community resources

REFERENCE: American College of Medical Genetics Foundation Clinical Guidelines Project Sponsored by the New York State Department of Health

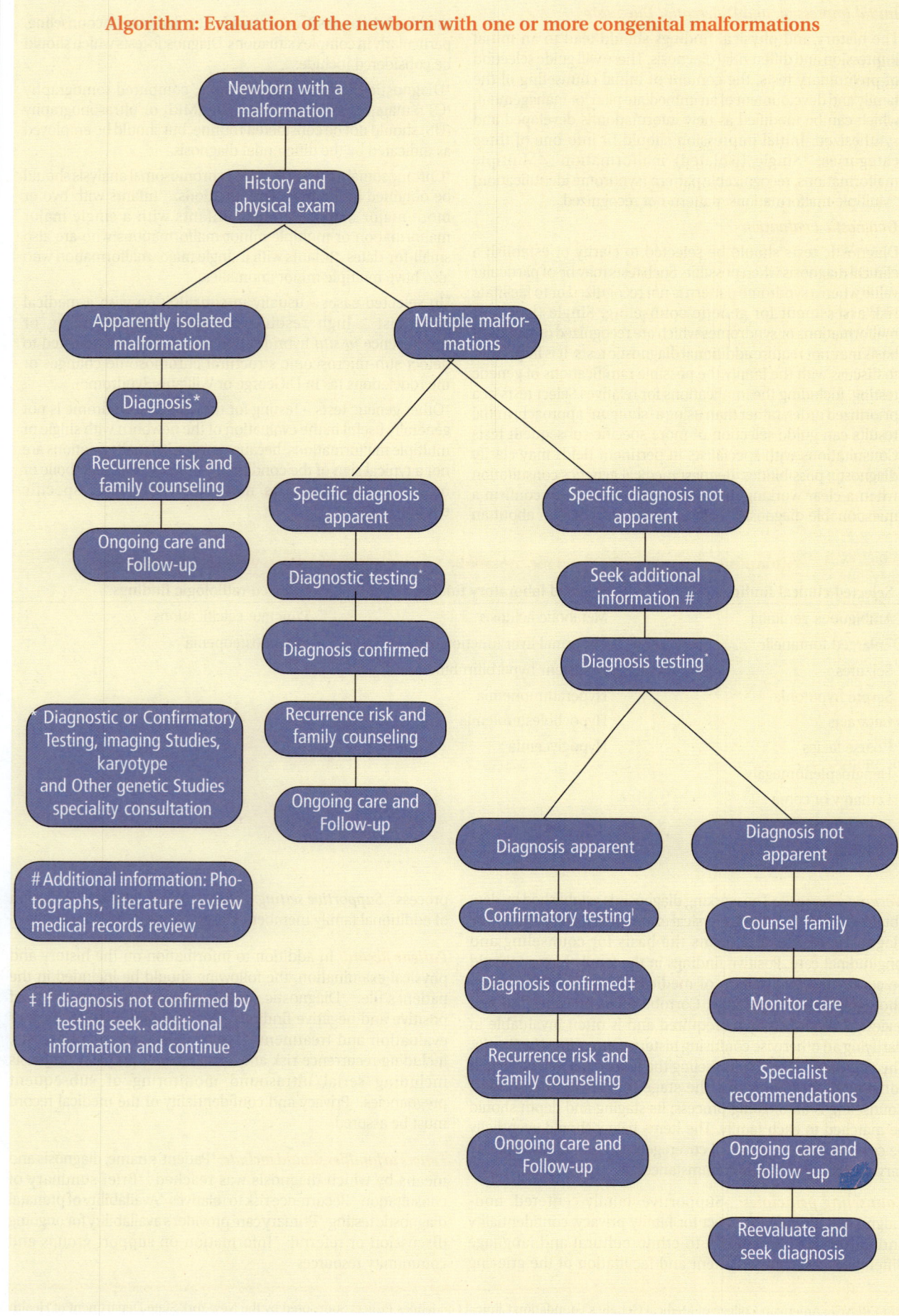

Algorithm: Evaluation of the newborn with one or more congenital malformations

Newborn with a malformation

History and physical exam

Apparently isolated malformation

Multiple malformations

Diagnosis*

Recurrence risk and family counseling

Ongoing care and Follow-up

Specific diagnosis apparent

Specific diagnosis not apparent

Diagnostic testing*

Seek additional information #

Diagnosis confirmed

Diagnosis testing*

Recurrence risk and family counseling

Ongoing care and Follow-up

* Diagnostic or Confirmatory Testing, imaging Studies, karyotype and Other genetic Studies speciality consultation

Additional information: Photographs, literature review medical records review

‡ If diagnosis not confirmed by testing seek. additional information and continue

Diagnosis apparent

Diagnosis not apparent

Confirmatory testing¹

Counsel family

Diagnosis confirmed‡

Monitor care

Recurrence risk and family counseling

Specialist recommendations

Ongoing care and Follow-up

Ongoing care and follow -up

Reevaluate and seek diagnosis

PEDIGREE CHART AND INHERITANCE PATTERNS

Basic principles

If more than one individual in a family is afflicted with a disease, it is a clue that the disease may be inherited. A doctor needs to look at the family history to determine whether the disease is indeed inherited and, if it is, to establish the mode of inheritance. This information can then be used to predict recurrence risk in future generations. A basic method for determining the pattern of inheritance of any trait (which may be a physical attribute like eye color or a serious disease like Marfan syndrome) is to look at its occurrence in several individuals within a family, spanning as many generations as possible. For a disease trait, a doctor has to examine existing family members to determine who is affected and who is not. The same information may be difficult to obtain about more distant relatives, and is often incomplete. Once family history is determined, the doctor will draw up the information in the form of a special chart or family tree that uses a particular set of standardized symbols. This is referred to as a pedigree. In a pedigree, males are represented by squares and females by circles. An individual who exhibits the trait in question, for example, someone who suffers from Marfan syndrome, is represented by a filled symbol. A horizontal line between two symbols represents a mating. The offspring are connected to each other by a horizontal line above the symbols and to the parents by vertical lines. Roman numerals (I, II, III, etc.) symbolize generations. Arabic numerals (1,2,3, etc.) symbolize birth order within each generation. In this way, any individual within the pedigree can be identified by the combination of two numbers (i.e., individual II3). The index case, or affected person through which the pedigree is discovered, is called the proband and is indicated by an arrow on pedigrees. Generations are represented on horizontal levels; parents on one level and the children of those parents together on a level below them. *The following diagram shows some of the standard symbols used in pedigrees.*

In this family, the father is affected as is the first born daughter. The mother, son and twin girls are not affected. This couple is pregnant with another child.

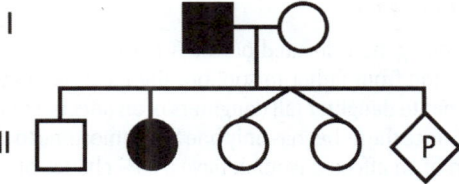

This pedigree shows three generations. The proband is the affected woman in the second generation. Her father (now deceased) had the disease, her mother is unaffected and still living. She has two siblings; neither is affected. She has three children from a previous marriage, two are affected and she is currently pregnant with a new partner.

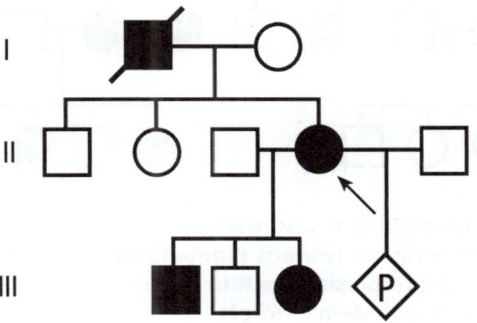

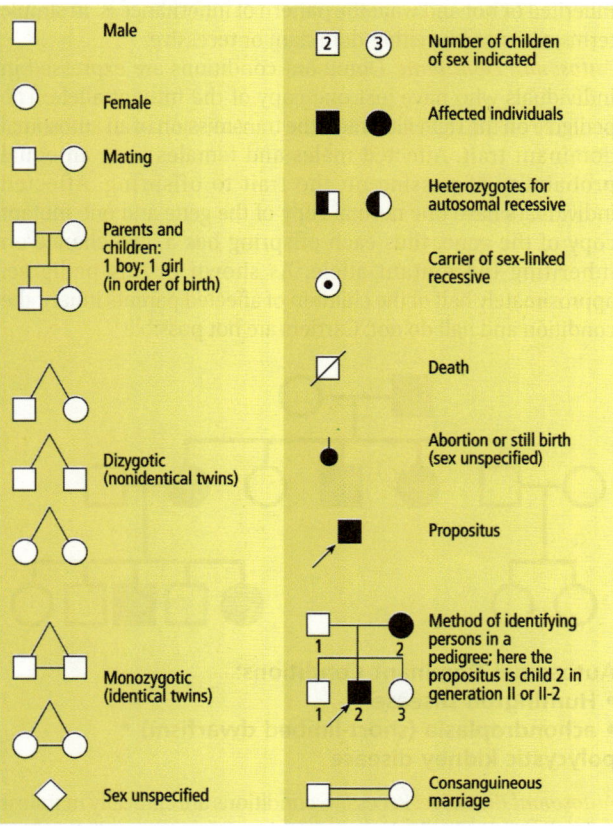

	Male		Number of children of sex indicated
	Female		Affected individuals
	Mating		Heterozygotes for autosomal recessive
	Parents and children: 1 boy; 1 girl (in order of birth)		Carrier of sex-linked recessive
	Dizygotic (nonidentical twins)		Death
			Abortion or still birth (sex unspecified)
			Propositus
	Monozygotic (identical twins)		Method of identifying persons in a pedigree; here the propositus is child 2 in generation II or II-2
	Sex unspecified		Consanguineous marriage

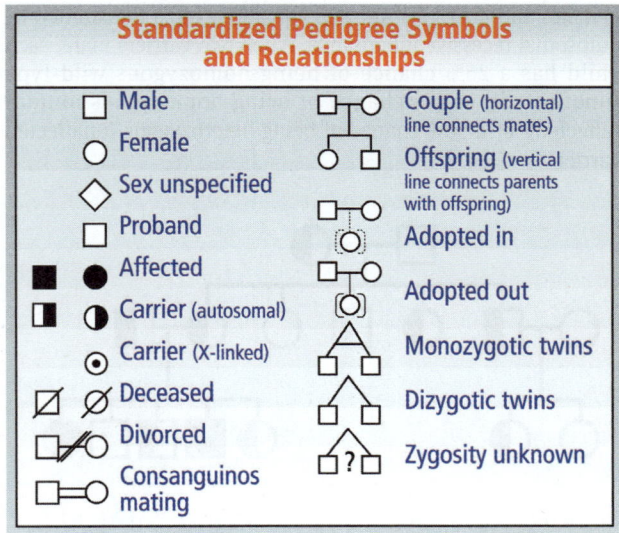

Standardized Pedigree Symbols and Relationships

Male	Couple (horizontal) line connects mates
Female	Offspring (vertical line connects parents with offspring)
Sex unspecified	Adopted in
Proband	Adopted out
Affected	Monozygotic twins
Carrier (autosomal)	Dizygotic twins
Carrier (X-linked)	Zygosity unknown
Deceased	
Divorced	
Consanguinos mating	

Single Gene Inheritance Genetic conditions caused by a mutation in a single gene follow predictable patterns of inheritance within families. Single gene inheritance is also referred to as Mendelian inheritance as they follow transmission patterns he observed in his research on peas. There are four types of Mendelian inheritance patterns:**Autosomal:** the gene responsible for the phenotype is located on one of the 22 pairs of autosomes (non-sex determining chromosomes). **X-linked:** the gene that encodes for the trait is located on the X chromosome. **Dominant:** conditions that are manifest in heterozygotes (individuals with just one copy of the mutant allele). **Recessive:** conditions are only manifest in individuals who have two copies of the mutant allele (are homozygous).

Dominant and recessive traits

Using genetic principles, the information presented in a pedigree can be analyzed to determine whether a given physical trait is inherited or not and what the pattern of inheritance is. In simple terms, traits can be either dominant or recessive.

Autosomal Dominant: Dominant conditions are expressed in individuals who have just one copy of the mutant allele. The pedigree on the right illustrates the transmission of an autosomal dominant trait. Affected males and females have an equal probability of passing on the trait to offspring. Affected individual's have one normal copy of the gene and one mutant copy of the gene, thus each offspring has a 50% chance on inheriting the mutant allele. As shown in this pedigree, approximately half of the children of affected parents inherit the condition and half do not. Carriers are not possible

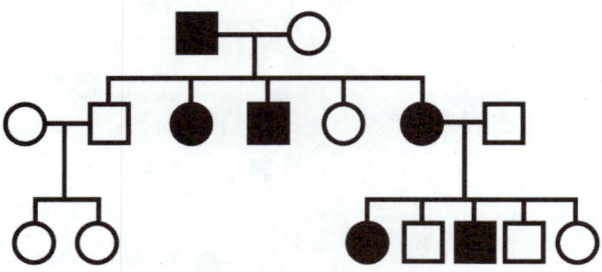

Autosomal Dominant Conditions:
• **Huntington Disease**
• **achondroplasia (short-limbed dwarfism) ***
polycystic kidney disease

Autosomal Recessive: Recessive conditions are clinically manifest only when an individual has two copies of the mutant allele. When just one copy of the mutant allele is present, an individual is a carrier of the mutation, but does not develop the condition. Females and males are affected equally by traits transmitted by autosomal recessive inheritance. When two carriers mate, each child has a 25% chance of being homozygous wild-type (unaffected); a 25% chance of being homozygous mutant (affected); or a 50% chance of being heterozygous (unaffected carrier).

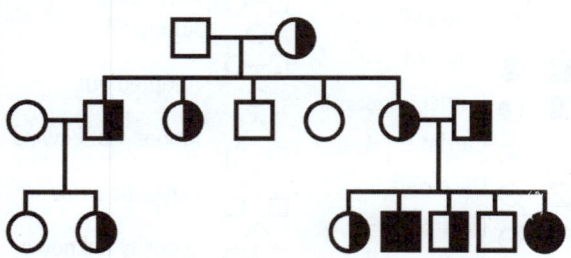

Affected individuals are indicated by solid black symbols and unaffected carriers are indicated by the half black symbols.
Autosomal recessive diseases: • Cystic fibrosis
• Tay-Sachs • hemochromatosis • phenylketonuria (PKU)

The reason for the two distinct patterns of inheritance has to do with the genes that predispose an individual to a given disease. Genes exist in different forms known as alleles, usually distinguished one from the other by the traits they specify. Individuals carrying identical alleles of a given gene are said to be homozygous for the gene in question. Similarly, when two different alleles are present in a gene pair, the individual is said to be heterozygous. Dominant traits are expressed in the heterozygous condition (in other words, you only need to inherit one disease-causing allele from one parent to have the disease). Recessive traits are only expressed in the homozygous condition (in other words, you need to inherit the same disease-causing allele from both parents to have the disease).

X-linked Recessive: X-linked recessive traits are not clinically manifest when there is a normal copy of the gene. All X-linked recessive traits are fully evident in males because they only have one copy of the X chromosome, thus do not have a normal copy of the gene to compensate for the mutant copy. For that same reason, women are rarely affected by X-linked recessive diseases, however they are affected when they have two copies of the mutant allele. Because the gene is on the X chromosome there is no father to son transmission, but there is father to daughter and mother to daughter and son transmission. If a man is affected with an X-linked recessive condition, all his daughter will inherit one copy of the mutant allele from him.

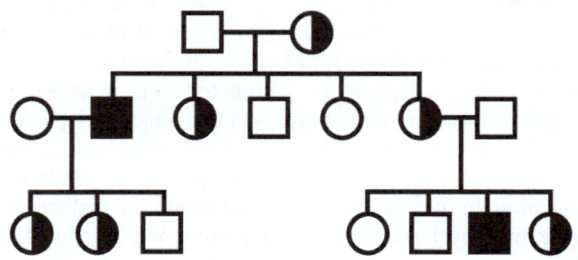

X-linked recessive disorders:
• **Duchenne muscular dystrophy**
• **hemophilia A**
• **X-linked severe combined immune disorder (SCID)**
• **some forms of congenital deafness**

X-linked Dominant

Because the gene is located on the X chromosome, there is no transmission from father to son, but there can be transmission from father to daughter (all daughters of an affected male will be affected since the father has only one X chromosome to transmit). Children of an affected woman have a 50% chance of inheriting the X chromosome with the mutant allele. X-linked dominant disorders are clinically manifest when only one copy of the mutant allele is present. Carriers are not possible

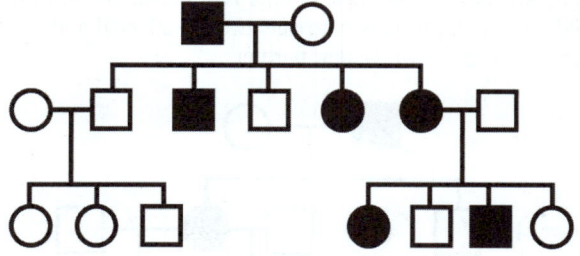

X-linked dominant disorders
• **Some forms of retinitis pigmentosa**
• **Chondrodysplasia Punctata**
• **hypophosphatemic rickets**

Multifactorial Inheritance

Most diseases have multifactorial inheritance patterns. As the name implies, multifactorial conditions are not caused by a single gene, but rather are a result of interplay between genetic factors and environmental factors. Diseases with multifactorial inheritance are not genetically determined, but rather a genetic mutation may predispose an individual to a disease. Other genetic and environmental factors contribute to whether or not the disease develops. Numerous genetic alterations may predispose individuals to the same disease (genetic heterogeneity). For instance coronary heart disease risk factors include high blood pressure, diabetes, and hyperlipidemia. All of those risk factors have their own genetic and environmental components. Thus multifactorial inheritance is far more complex than Mendelian inheritance and is more difficult to trace through pedigrees. A typical pedigree from a family with a mutation in the BRCA1 gene. Fathers can be carriers and pass the mutation onto offspring. Not all people who inherit the mutation develop the disease, thus patterns of transmission are not always obvious.

Mitochondrial Inheritance

Mitochondria are the cell's power plants. They possess their own chromosome, which carries thirty-seven genes. Mitochondria are inherited only from the mother. Mitochondrially inherited disorders include a number of rare muscle diseases (mitochondrial myopathies), as well as some deafness syndromes, optic nerve degeneration, and other neurological disorders. Mitochondria are organelles found in the cytoplasm of cells. Mitochondria are unique in that they have multiple copies of a circular chromosome. Mitochondria are only inherited from the mother's egg, thus only females can transmit the trait to offspring, however they pass it on to all of their offspring. The primary function of mitochondria is conversion of molecule into usable energy. Thus many diseases transmitted by mitochondrial inheritance affect organs with high-energy use such as the heart, skeletal muscle, liver, and kidneys. The human mitochondrion has a small circular genome of 16,569 bp which is remarkably crowded. It is inherited only through the egg, sperm mitochondria never contribute to the zygote population of mitochondria. There are relatively few human genetic diseases caused by mitochondrial mutations but, because of their maternal transmission, they have a very distinctive pattern of inheritance. All the children of an affected female but none of the children of an affected male will inherit the disease.

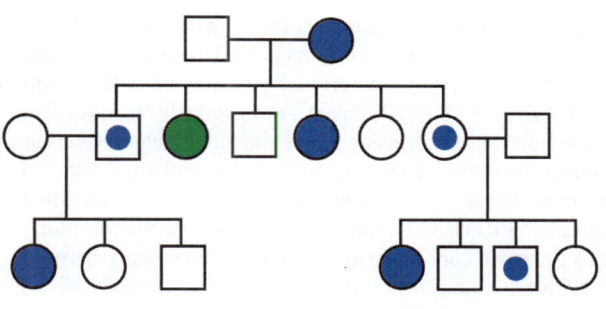

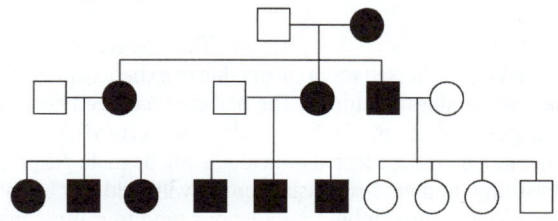

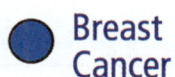 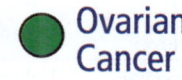 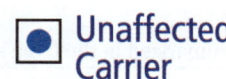

Conditions with multifactorial inheritance:
• **Alzheimers disease • heart disease • some cancers**
• **neural tube defects**
• **schizophrenia • insulin-dependent diabetes mellitus**
• **intelligence**

Examples of the impact of faulty mitochondrial genes

Organ or tissue	Impact
General	Small stature and poor appetite
Central nervous system	Developmental delay/intellectual disability, progressive neurological deterioration (dementia such as the late-onset form of Alzheimer disease), seizures, stroke-like episodes (often reversible), difficulty swallowing, visual difficulties and deafness
Skeletal and muscle	floppiness, weakness and exercise intolerance
Heart	heart failure (cardiomyopathy) and cardiac rhythm conditions
Kidney	problems in kidney function

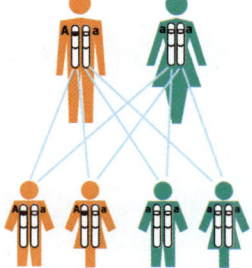

AUTOSOMAL DOMINANT
• Individual carrying one mutated copy of a gene in each cell will be affected by the disease
• Each affected person usually has one affected parent
• Tends to occur in every generation of an affected family

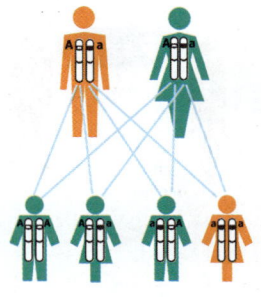

AUTOSOMAL RECESSIVE
• Affected individuals must carry two mutated copies of a gene
• Parents of affected individual are usually unaffected and each carry a single copy of the mutated gene (known as carriers)
• Not typically seen in every generation.

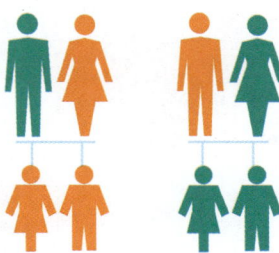

MITOCHONDRIAL
• Only females can pass on mitochondrial conditions to their children (maternal inheritance)
• Both males and females can be affected
• Can appear in every generation of a family

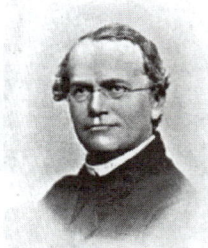

Gregor Mendel is famous today but was relatively unknown outside Czechoslovakia in his lifetime. He was the first scientist to deduce clear and rational laws which could explain the process of inheritance and it turns out that the rules which Mendel deduced from studies of peas are equally applicable to human inheritance.

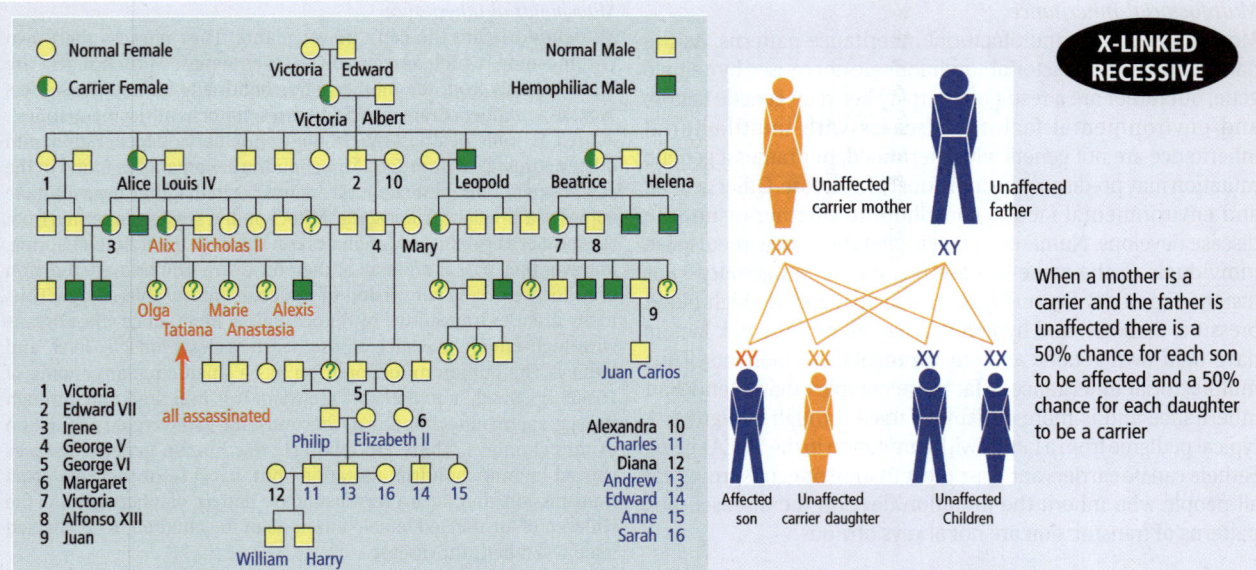

Normal Female ◯
Carrier Female ◐
Victoria — Edward
Normal Male ▢
Hemophiliac Male ▨

Victoria — Albert

X-LINKED RECESSIVE

When a mother is a carrier and the father is unaffected there is a 50% chance for each son to be affected and a 50% chance for each daughter to be a carrier

Unaffected carrier mother XX
Unaffected father XY

XY XX XY XX

Affected son   Unaffected carrier daughter   Unaffected Children

all assassinated

1 Victoria
2 Edward VII
3 Irene
4 George V
5 George VI
6 Margaret
7 Victoria
8 Alfonso XIII
9 Juan

Alexandra 10
Charles 11
Diana 12
Andrew 13
Edward 14
Anne 15
Sarah 16

Sex-linked recessive: hemophilia A : The pedigree chart of Queen Victoria of England illustrates inheritance of hemophilia A. Queen Victoria herself was a carrier due to a chance mutation. Her children married other royalty and passed the trait throughout the royal families of Europe. The pedigree has been generously provided by Janet Stein Carter, biology instructor at Clermont College, University of Cincinnati, who retains copyright SEX-LINKED RECESSIVE TRAIT: (X-linked—not Y-linked) *tends to skip generations *most affected individuals will be male *expressing female must have expressing father and either heterozygous or expressing mother. *expressing female will yield 100% expressing sons. (the term "affected" can be used interchangeably with "expressing") Note: Inbred populations tend to express many more recessive alleles than outbred populations. Outbreeding (breeding between individuals who are not closely related) tends to foster HYBRID VIGOR. Hybrid vigor is a result of heterozygosity at many loci. This means that few genes are present in homozygous recessive condition—a good thing, since many harmful alleles are recessive! Inbreeding (breeding between closely related individuals) usually results in homozygosity of recessive alleles at many loci. The more homozygous recessives you have, the more likely that some of the really bad ones will show up.

Characteristics of monogenic diseases
The most important characteristics of monogenic diseases are summarized in the table below.

	Autosomal Dominant	Autosomal Recessive	X-linked
Number of mutations in patients	1	2	1
Sex of patients	both	both	mainly boys
Risk* of children with the disease	1 on 2	small	small
Risk* of grandchildren with the disease	1 on 4	small	1 on 8
Risk* of an affected sib	A. small if none of the parents is affected B. 1 on 2 if one of the parents is also affected	1 on 4	A. small if the mother is no carrier B. 1 on 4 if the mother is a carrier

* = Risks apply to the patient which has the genetic disease.

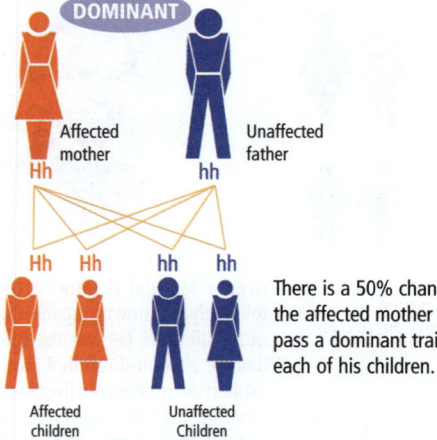

DOMINANT

Affected mother Hh
Unaffected father hh

Hh Hh hh hh

Affected children   Unaffected Children

There is a 50% chance that the affected mother will pass a dominant trait to each of his children.

Autosomal Dominant Inheritance

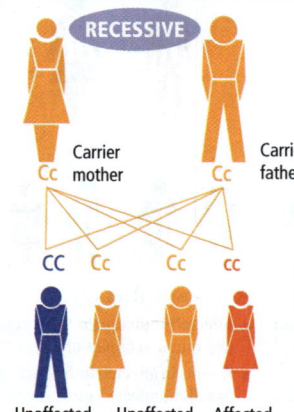

RECESSIVE

Carrier mother Cc
Carrier father Cc

CC Cc Cc cc

Unaffected child   Unaffected carriers   Affected child

There is a 25% chance that two carriers of a recessive allele will have a child with that recessive trait.

Autosomal Recessive Inheritance

1) Distinguishing features of different Neonatal extracerebral fluid collections
(adapted from from Davis DJ (1))

Feature	Caput succedaneum	Cephalohematoma	Subgaleal hemorrhage
Location	At point of contact; can extend across sutures (subcutaneous)	Usually over parietal bones; does not cross sutures (subperiosteal)	Beneath epicranial aponeurosis; may extend to orbits, nape of neck
Characteristic findings	Vaguely demarcated; pitting edema that shifts with gravity	Distinct margins; initially firm, more fluctuant after 48 h	Firm to fluctuant; ill- defined borders; may have crepitus or fluid waves
Timing	Maximal size and firmness at birth; resolves in 48–72 h	Increases after birth for12–24 h; resolution over 2–3 weeks	Progressive after birth;resolution over 2-3 weeks
Volume of blood	Minimal	Rarely severe	May be massive, especially if there is an associated coagulopathy

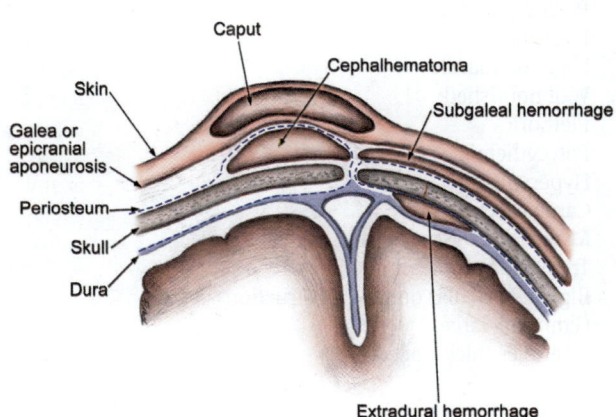

Caput
Cephalhematoma
Skin
Subgaleal hemorrhage
Galea or epicranial aponeurosis
Periosteum
Skull
Dura
Extradural hemorrhage

Subgaleal hemorrhage is a rare but potentially lethal condition in newborns. The prevalence of moderate to severe subgaleal hemorrhages is approximately 1.5 per 10'000 births. It is caused by rupture of emissary veins, which are connections between the dural sinuses and the scalp veins. Blood accumulates between the extracranial aponeurosis of the scalp and the periosteum. This potential space extends forward to the orbital margins, backward to the nuchal ridge and laterally to the temporal fascia . In term babies, this subaponeurotic space may hold as much as 260 ml of blood (which is almost equivalent to the baby's blood volume). Subgaleal hemorrhage can therefore lead to severe hypovolemia, and in one study up to one quarter of babies who require neonatal intensive care for this condition died.

Subgaleal hemorrhage is most often associated with vacuum extraction and forceps delivery, but it may also occur spontaneously. Optimizing the outcome for babies with subgaleal hemorrhage requires early diagnosis, careful monitoring and prompt treatment of hypovolemic shock.

2) Hemorrhagic disease of the newborn

	Early onset	Classic disease	Late onset
Age	0–24 hours	2–7 days	1–6 months
Site of hemorrhage	Cephalohematoma Subgaleal Intracranial Gastrointestinal Umbilicus Intra-abdominal	Gastrointestinal Ear-nose-throat-mucosal Intracranial Circumcision Cutaneous Gastrointestinal Injection sites	Intracranial Gastrointestinal Cutaneous Ear-nose-throat-mucosal Injection sites Thoracic
Etiology/risks fibrosis,hepatitis)	Maternal drugs (phenobarbital, phenytoin, warfarin, rifampin, isoniazid) that interfere with Vitamin K Inherited coagulopathy	Vitamin K deficiency Breast-feeding	Cholestasis—malabsorption of vitamin K (biliary atresia, cystic Abetalipoprotein deficiency Idiopathic in Asian breast-fed infants Warfarin ingestion
Prevention	Possible vitamin K at birth or to mother (20 mg) before birth Avoid high-risk medications	Prevented by parenteral vitamin K at birth. Oral vitamin K regimens require repeated dosing over time	Prevented by parenteral and high-dose oral vitamin K during periods of malabsorption or cholestasis
Incidence	Very rare	~ 2% if not given vitamin K	Dependent on primary disease

3. Bleeding neonate:differential diagnosis

Platelets	PT	PTT	POSSIBLE CAUSES
"SICK" NEONATE			
Decreased	Increased	Increased	Disseminated intravascular coagulation
Decreased	Normal	Normal	Platelet - consumption (infection, necrotizing enterocolitis, renal vein thrombosis)
Normal	Increased	Increased	Liver disease, heparinization
Normal	Normal	Normal	Altered vascular integrity (e.g., extreme prematurity, severe hypoxia and acidosis, hyperosmolality.)
"WELL" NEONATE			
Decreased	Normal	Normal	Immune thrombocytopenia
Normal	Increased	Increased	Hemorrhagic disease of the Newborn
Normal	Normal	Increased	Hereditary clotting factor deficiencies
Normal	Normal	Normal	Bleeding due to local factors (trauma, anatomic abnormalities), qualitative platelet abnormalities (rare), disrupted vessel from anatomical lesion (e.g. ulcer, hemangioma), swallowed maternal blood

4. Twin-to-twin transfusion syndrome : TTTS

ARTERIAL SIDE-DONOR TWIN	VENOUS SIDE-RECIPIENT TWIN
Prematurity	Prematurity
Oligohydramnios	Polyhydramnios
Small premature	Hydrops
Malnourished	Large premature
Pale	Well nourished
Anemic	Plethoric
Hypovolemia	Polycythemic
Hypoglycemia	Hypervolemic
Microcardia	Cardiac hypertrophy
Glomeruli small or normal	Myocardial dysfunction
Arterioles thin walled	Tricuspid valve regurgitation
	Right ventricular outflow obstruction
	Glomeruli large
	Arterioles thick walled

5. Assessing breast milk transfer

	Day 0	Day 1–2	Day 3–4	Day 5–6
Voids	≥1	≥2	≥4	≥5
Stools				
Number	≥1	≥2	≥3	≥5
Color	Meconium	Meconium	Transitional	Yellow/Seedy
Weight compared Birth weight	–	≤5% loss	≤10% loss	No further weight loss
Frequency of feeds	2–8	4–10	8–12	8–12
Duration of feeds (minutes)	5–40	15–45	20–45	20–45

6. Oligohydramnios and polyhydramnios

Oligohydramnios

IUGR, Fetal anomalies, Twin-to-Twin Transfusion syndrome-Donor, Amniotic fluid leak,Renal agenesis, Urethral atresia, Prune belly syndrome, Pulmonary hypoplasia, Amnion nodosum, Indomethacin, ACE Inhibitors, Intestinal pseudo-obstruction

Polyhydramnios

Congenital anomalies: Anencephaly, hydrocephaly, TE Fistula, Duodenal atresia, Cleft palate/lip, Spina bifida, Cystic adenomatoid malformation, Congenital Diaphragmatic hernia

Syndromes: Achondroplasia, Klippel-Feil, Down and Edward Syndromes, Congenital infections, Hydrops fetalis, multiple congenital anomalies

Others: Twin-to-Twin Transfusion syndrome-Recipient,Diabetes, Fetal anemia, Fetal heart failure, Polyuria, renal disease, Neuromuscular disease, Nonimmune Hydrops, Chylothorax, Teratoma

7. Differential diagnosis of diaper dermatitis

Disorder	Age of onset	Sites	Clinical features	Other signs
Seborrheic dermatitis	Under 3 months	Genito-crural flexures	Erythema and greasy scaling	Greasy scaling of scalp; Other flexures may be involved
Atopic eczema	Rarely under 2 months Usually 3 to 12 months	Anywhere	Erythema, papules, vesicles	Lesions elsewhere: cheeks, forehead, forearms, cubital and popliteal fossae, Pruritus
Candidiasis	Any age	Extends from perianal area	Sharply, irregularly marginated red patches, raised scaling edge, satellite pustules or papules	Oral lesions (Thrush)
Miliaria	Any age	Variable: groins or buttocks	Erythematous papules ± vesicles	Lesions elsewhere: e.g., neck, chest
lntertrigo	Any age	Any flexure or fold	Erythema only	Limited to areas of skin-on-skin contact
Perianal dermatitis	From 0 to 4 weeks	Perianal	Erythema	None
Infantile psoriasis	2 weeks to 8 MO (usually 2 months)	Convex areas, but may be flexures	Sharply marginated red scaly plaques	Scalp and truncal lesions
Contact dermatitis (irritant)	Any age	Any area; area of contact with irritant	Initially Erythema and vesicles	Other sites in contact with irritant may be involved; distinguish from atopic eczema

8. Comparison between laryngomalacia and tracheomalacia

	Laryngomalacia	Tracheomalacia
Stridor	Inspiratory only	Biphasic or expiratory
Etiology	Weak cartilage of the larynx or inadequate neuromuscular tone of the larynx	Widened tracheal rings (primary) Extrinsic compression (secondary)
Symptoms in severe cases	Failure to thrive, cyanosis, or apnea	Reflux apnea ("dying spell")
Associated findings	Gastroesophageal reflux common	Chronic cough (may be "barking") Cardiovascular abnormalities Gastroesophageal reflux
Endoscopic findings	Collapse of epiglottis, arytenoids, or both on inspiration Normal trachea	Normal larynx Posterior tracheal wall "fish mouth" to anterior wall May be short or long segment Bronchomalacia
Treatment	Expectant management Supraglottoplasty in severe cases	Aortopexy if innominate artery compression Tracheostomy in severe cases
Natural history	Spontaneous resolution by 18months old	Recurrent "croup" episodes Narrow segment less critical with growth

9.	Cyanotic CHD	Versus	PPHN
Prenatal sonogram	Often suggests cardiac anomaly		Usually unremarkable
Perinatal events	Usually unremarkable		Often with events that put infant at risk for hypoxia
Pa O$_2$	With cyanotic lesions, unable to increase PaO$_2$ above 100 mm Hg despite supplemental oxygen		Infant may have a history of PaO$_2$ grether than 100 mm Hg or can obtain that level with therapy
Pa CO$_2$	Usually normal		Often elevated as lung disease a frequent component
Physical examination	Infant typically in no respiratory distress; heart murmur typical, but without hypotension		Respiratory distress common, as is hypotension; heart murmur less common
Echocardiogram	Demonstrates structural heart defect that produces shunting across pulmonary and systemic circulations		Suggests right-to-left shunting at the PFO and/or PDA without structural abnormality of the heart
Treatment	Usually surgical, sometimes in staged procedures; maintenance of PDA may need to be achieved with prostaglandins until surgery		Usually medical, most commonly requiring ventilation, supplemental oxygen, pressors and nitric oxide, ECMO

10. Different shock states—hemodynamic variables

Hemodynamic Variables in Different Shock States

	CO	SVR	MAP	Wedge	CVP
Hypovolemic	↓	↑	↔ or ↓	↓↓↓	↓↓↓
Cardiogenic ‡ systolic	↓↓	↑↑↑	↔ or ↓	↑↑	↑↑
Diastolic	↔	↑↑	↔	↑↑	↑
Obstructive	↓	↑	↔ or ↓	↑↑*	↑↑*
Distributive	↑↑	↓↓↓	↔ or ↓	↔ or ↓	↔ or ↓
Septic					
Early	↑↑↑	↓↓↓	↔ or ↓†	↓	↓
Late	↓↓	↓↓	↓↓	↑	↑ or ↔

* Wedge pressure, central venous pressure, and pulmonary artery diastolic pressures are equal
†Wide pulse pressure ‡Systolic or diastolic dysfunction

11. Management issues in different types of shock

TYPES OF SHOCK—TREATMENT SUMMARY

Hypovolemic shock — a preload issue	Volume, Volume, Volume.
Cardiogenic shock — a contractility issue	Volume first, because increasing the preload can get the heart to a better point on the Frank-Starling curve. Early use of inotropic agents to improve contractility; dobutamine is usual first choice. Only after blood pressure is stabilized and patient is fluid resuscitated, consider vasodilator agents to reduce afterload.
Distributive shock— a systemic Vascular resistance issue	First give volume to fill the tank. Consider vasoconstrictive agents to increase vascular tone. Dopamine usually is first choice except in anaphylaxis, when epinephrine is first choice.
Septic shock — a combination of the three	Volume first, then frequently Vasoconstrictive agents. Dopamine usually is used first.

12. Differential diagnosis of poor systemic perfusion

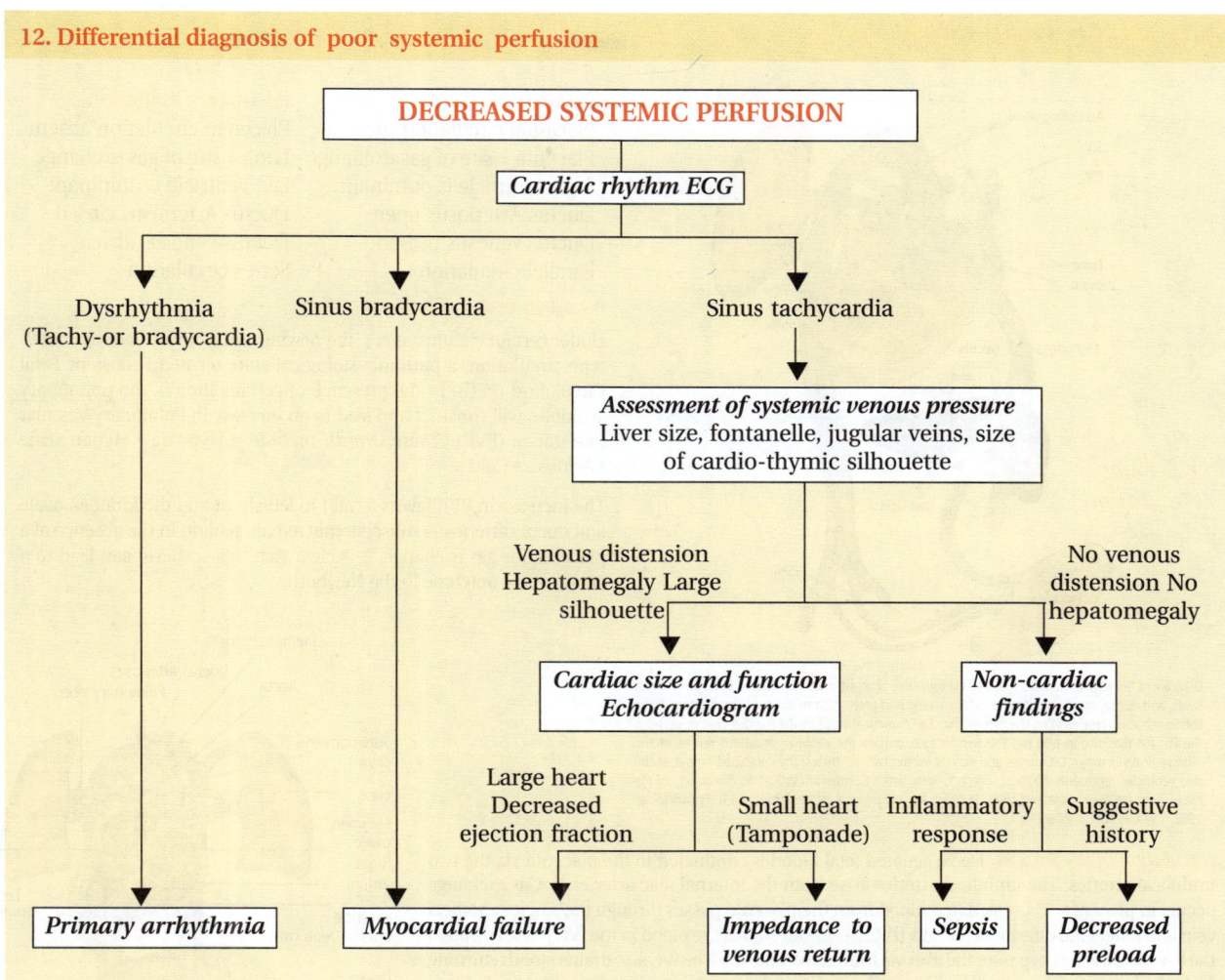

DECREASED SYSTEMIC PERFUSION

Cardiac rhythm ECG

- Dysrhythmia (Tachy-or bradycardia)
- Sinus bradycardia
- Sinus tachycardia

Assessment of systemic venous pressure
Liver size, fontanelle, jugular veins, size of cardio-thymic silhouette

- Venous distension Hepatomegaly Large silhouette
- No venous distension No hepatomegaly

Cardiac size and function Echocardiogram

Non-cardiac findings

- Large heart Decreased ejection fraction
- Small heart (Tamponade)
- Inflammatory response
- Suggestive history

- *Primary arrhythmia*
- *Myocardial failure*
- *Impedance to venous return*
- *Sepsis*
- *Decreased preload*

13. Distinguishing tachyarrhythmias in infants

	Sinus tachycardia	SVT	Atrial flutter	VT
History	Sepsis, fever, hypovolemia, etc.	Usually otherwise normal	Most have a normal heart	Many with abnormal heart
Rate	Almost always <230 b/min	Most often 260–300b/min	Atrial 300–500 b/min. Vent. 1:1 to 4:1 conduction	200-500 b/min
R-R interval variation	Over several seconds may get faster and slower	After first 10–20 beats, extremely regular	May have variable block (1:1, 2:1, 3:1) giving different ventricular rates	Slight variation over several beats
P wave axis	Same as sinus almost always visible P waves	60% visible P waves, P waves do not look like sinus P waves	Flutter waves (best seen in LII, LIII, aVF, V_1)	May have sinus P waves continuing unrelated to VT (AV dissociation), retrograde P waves, or no visible P waves
QRS	Almost always same as slower sinus rhythm	After first 10–20 beats, almost always same as sinus	Usually same as sinus, may have occasional beats different from sinus	Different from sinus (not necessarily 'wide')

DETERMINANTS OF OXYGEN SUPPLY

Oxygen delivery (DO_2) = Cardiac output X Arterial O_2 content(CaO_2)

Cardiac output = Stroke volume X Heart rate

Components of Stroke volume = Preload, Cardiac contractility, and Afterload

Arterial O_2 content (CaO_2) = A function of arterial Hemoglobin concentration (Hb), Hemoglobin O_2 saturation (SaO_2), and the pressure of O_2 (PaO_2)

CaO_2=(1.34(Oxygen carrying capacity of Hb in ml O_2/g) X Hb in grams X SaO_2 as a fraction) + (PaO_2 in mm Hg X 0.003)

14. Fetal and postnatal circulations

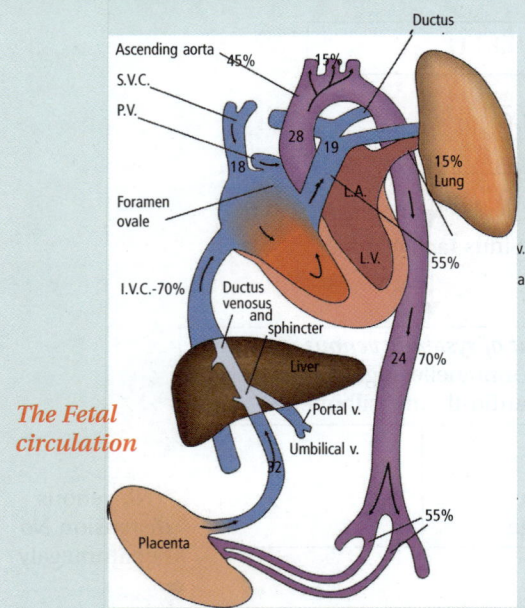

The Fetal circulation

Diagram of the fetal circulation showing the four sites of shunt: placenta, ductus venosus, foramen ovale, and ductus arteriosus. intravascular *shading* is in proportion to oxygen saturation, with the lightest shading representing the highest Po_2. The numerical value inside the chamber or vessel is the Po_2 for that site in mm Hg. The percentages outside the vascular structures represent the relative flows in major tributaries and outlets for the two ventricles. The combined output of the two ventricles represents 100% *a*, artery; *v*, vein; (From Guntheroth WG et al: *Physiology of the circulation: fetus, neonate and child. In kelley VC, ed: practice of pediatrics,* vol 8, Philadelphia, 1982, 1983, Harper & Row.)

Fetal circulation	Postnatal circulation
Placental circulation present	Placental circulation absent
Placenta = site of gas exchange	Lung = site of gas exchange
Right ventricle is dominant	Left ventricle is dominant
Ductus Arteriosus open	Ductus Arteriosus closed
Ductus Venosus present	Ductus Venosus absent
Parallel circulation	Series circulation

Persistent fetal circulation

Under certain circumstances, the newborn may revert back to a fetal-type circulation, a pathophysiological state termed Persistent Fetal Circulation (PFC). In the presence of certain stimuli, the pulmonary arterioles will constrict and lead to an increase in Pulmonary Vascular Resistance (PVR). *These stimuli include:* • Hypoxia • Hypercarbia • Acidosis • Cold

The increase in PVR favors a right to left shunt and the foramen ovale and ductus arteriosus subsequently remain patent. In the absence of a placenta for gas exchange, it is clear that this scenario can lead to a catastrophic outcome in the Newborn.

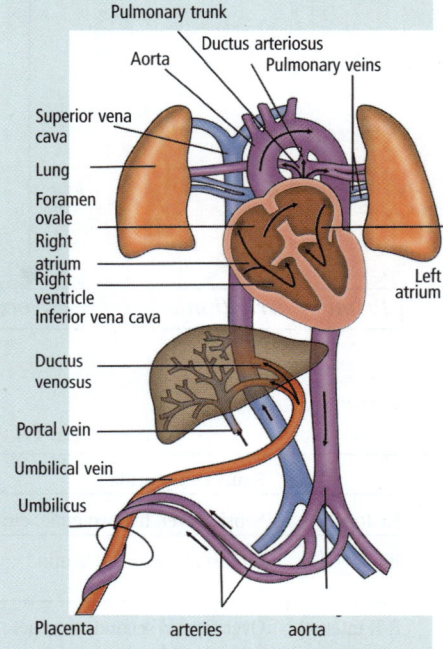

Circulation in the fetus : **1.** Deoxygenated fetal blood is conducted to the placenta via the two umbilical arteries. The umbilical arteries arise from the internal iliac arteries. **2.** Gas exchange occurs in placenta. **3.** Oxygenated blood from the placenta passes through the single umbilical vein and enters the inferior vena cava (IVC). **4.** About 50% of the blood in the IVC passes through the liver and the rest bypasses the liver via the ductus venosus. The IVC also drains blood returning from the lower trunk and extremities. **5.** On reaching the heart, blood is effectively divided into two streams by the edge of the interatrial septum (crista dividens) (1) a larger stream is shunted to the left atrium through the foramen ovale (lying between IVC and left atrium) (2) the other stream passes into right atrium where it is joined by blood from SVC which is blood returning from the myocardium and upper parts of body. This stream therefore has a lower partial pressure of oxygen. **6.** Because of the large pulmonary vascular resistance and the presence of the ductus arteriosus most of the right ventricular output passes into the aorta at a point distal to the origin of the arteries to the head and upper extremities. The diameter of the ductus arteriosus is similar to the descending aorta. The patency of the ductus arteriosus is maintained by the low oxygen tension and the vasodilating effects of prostaglandin E2. **7.** Blood flowing through the foramen ovale and into left atrium passes into the left ventricle where it is ejected into the ascending aorta. This relatively oxygen rich blood passes predominantly to the head and upper extremities.

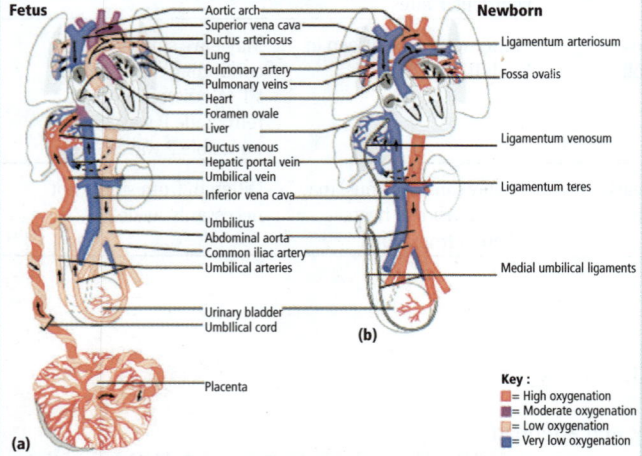

Postnatal changes (Neonatal circulation): **1.** The umbilical vessels are obliterated when the cord is clamped externally. **2.** There is therefore a fall in blood flow through the IVC and the ductus venosus, the latter subsequently closes passively over the next 3-10 days. **3.** A dramatic fall in the pulmonary vascular resistance (PVR) occurs with lung expansion (opening up the pulmonary vessels). A reduction in hypoxic pulmonary vasoconstriction and stimulation of pulmonary stretch receptors contribute to this process. **4.** The increase in pulmonary blood flow leads to a large rise in pulmonary venous return to the left atrium. **5.** The left atrial pressure therefore exceeds the right atrial pressure. This reversal of pressure gradient across the atria allows the flap of the foramen ovale to push against the atrial septum and the atrial shunt is effectively closed. Although the initial closure of the foramen ovale occurs within minutes to hours of birth, anatomical closure by tissue proliferation takes several days. As a result, all blood from the right atrium now passes into the right ventricle. **6.** The ductus arteriosus constricts due to the high partial pressure of oxygen. The process is usually complete within 2 days after birth. **7.** Other changes over several weeks include a reduction in the thickness of the walls of right ventricle and the muscle layer of the pulmonary arterioles; and an increase in the left ventricular wall.

15. Fetal versus adult hemoglobins

Fetal versus adult haemoglobin

* Fetus has high percentage (75%) of haemoglobin F (HbF).

* HbF has lower affinity 2,3-diphosphoglycerate (2,3-DPG).

* Fetus has a higher haemoglobin concentration (18g/dl-1) at birth.

* The oxyhemoglobin dissociation curve for HbF is shifted to the left compared with adult haemoglobin due to a lower affinity for 2,3-DPG. This favors oxygen uptake in the placenta.

* adult hemoglobin is composed of two alpha and two beta subunits, fetal hemoglobin is composed of two alpha and two gamma subunits, commonly denoted as $\pm_2^3{}_2$. Because of its presence in fetal hemoglobin, the gamma subunit is commonly called the "fetal" hemoglobin subunit.

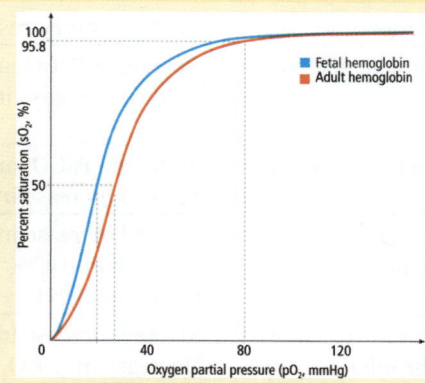

16. Dissociation curve for oxyhemoglobin

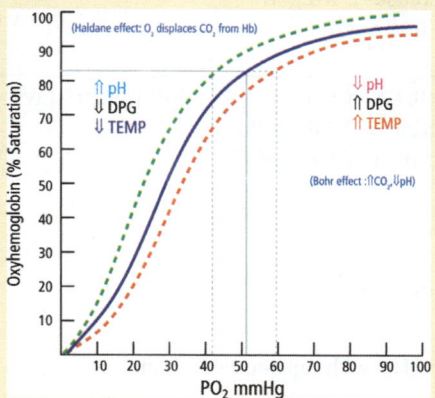

Oxygen dissociation curves for fetal and adult blood. The P50 value is 19 mm Hg for fetal blood and 26.8 mm Hg for adult blood. (1kPa=7.5mmHg)

Many factors influence the affinity of this binding and alter the shape of the curve:		
	Right shift	**Left shift**
temperature	high	low
DPG	high	low
$p(CO_2)$	high	low
$p(CO)$	low	high
pH (Bohr effect)	low (acidosis)	high (alkalosis)
type of hemoglobin	adult hemoglobin	fetal hemoglobin

What is the oxyhemoglobin dissociation curve and why is it important?

The Oxyhemoglobin dissociation curve describes the non-linear tendency for oxygen to bind to hemoglobin: below a SaO_2 of 90%, small differences in hemoglobin saturation reflect large changes in PaO_2 The oxyhemoglobin dissociation curve mathematically equates the percentage saturation of hemoglobin to the partial pressure of oxygen in the blood. The strange sigmoid shape of the curve relates to peculiar properties of the hemoglobin molecule itself: Hemoglobin and oxygen act a little like parents and children. When all are living at home (i.e. hemoglobin is fully saturated) then the parents don't want any to leave: but once one has flown the nest (i.e. dissociated from hemoglobin) – parents find it progressively easier to let go. What this means that the conformation of the hemoglobin molecule depends on the number of molecules bound: as one molecule of oxygen becomes unbound, the affinity for the others falls [and vice-versa]. This is represented by the oxyhemoglobin dissociation curve. The lack of linearity of the curve makes interpretation of the oxygen content of blood difficult. At higher saturation levels, above 90%, the curve is flat, but below this level the PaO_2 declines sharply, such that at 75% saturation the PaO_2 is about 47mmHg (mixed venous blood), at 50% saturation the PaO_2 is 26.6mmHg, and at 25% saturation the PaO_2 is a miserable 15mmHg.The position of this curve may shift rightwards (lower saturation for given PaO_2) or leftwards (higher saturation for a given PaO_2). Certain circumstances make the blood more likely to dump oxygen into the tissues, and others make it more likely to cling on to oxygen. Active muscle needs more oxygen, so heat, exercise, acidosis, hypercarbia and increased 2,3-DPG all cause a shift in the curve rightwards – releasing oxygen. Conversely, when activity is minimal – such as in cold weather or during rest, when the tissues are cold, alkalotic, hypocarbic and low 2,3-DPG, then hemoglobin holds onto oxygen. The curve also shifts leftwards in carbon monoxide poisoning. *The oxygen dissociation curve is an essential component in understanding critical care medicine.*

Everything we do is about optimizing the delivery of blood to the tissues as a means of maintaining homeostasis and promoting healing, and in the end it is the oxygen content of blood that is more important than the partial pressure of oxygen (which we commonly measure). The oxygen content relates specifically to the amount of hemoglobin present and how saturated it is. A reduction in the hemoglobin concentration from 15 to 10g/dl reduces the arterial oxygen content (CaO_2) by as much as a reduction in PaO_2 from 100mmHg to 40mmHg. Moreover a small drop in SaO_2 may represent a large drop in PaO_2, due to the shape of the oxyhemoglobin dissociation curve: when hemoglobin is 50% saturated the PaO_2 is 28mmHg, at 75% the PaO2 is about 40mmHg (mixed venous blood). Although many pages of critical care textbooks are often devoted to discussions about oxygen delivery, there is no clear indication what the optimal hemoglobin actually is. We know from the TRICC (transfusion requirements in critical care) study (1) that transfusing patients with blood above a hemoglobin of 7.0g is probably harmful. This probably relates to problems associated with the actual process of storing and transfusing products, than the effect of a "normal" hemoglobin itself. The availability of therapeutic erythropoietin has allowed intensivists induce red cell production, and replace blood mass without external transfusion. In any case, there is a large physiologic reserve between oxygen delivery and oxygen consumption. The cardiac output is probably a bigger player in the delivery of O_2 to the tissues that the O_2 content. This is because the cardiac output can almost instantaneously respond to a fall in PaO_2 saturation of Hb. Moderate hypoxemia leads to an increase in the cardiac output and a reduction in peripheral vascular resistance. On the other hand, compensation for a fall in cardiac output is slow and weak – that is because it takes time to increase Hb production and the oxyhemoglobin dissociation curve is flat – it can't become anymore saturated. Nevertheless, in the clinical setting, it is often easier to increase the Hb or the FiO_2 than to increase the cardiac output..

17. Bedside rules for assessing respiratory and renal compensation in acid-base disorders

Disorder	Compensatory response	Adaptive response	Time for adaptation
Metabolic acidosis	Decreased $PaCO_2$ and pH Marked decrease in $[HCO_3^-]$	$\Delta PCO_2 = 1.5 \times [HCO_3^-] + 8$ $\Delta PCO_2 = [HCO_3^-] + 15$ $PaCO_2$ = last 2 digits pH	12–24 hrs
Metabolic alkalosis	Increased $PaCO_2$ and pH Marked increase in $[HCO_3^-]$	$\Delta PCO_2 = (0.4–0.6) [HCO_3^-]$ $PaCO_2$ = base excess + 40.6	24–36 hours
Respiratory acidosis (acute)	Marked increase in $PaCO_2$, Increase in $[HCO_3^-]$ Decrease in pH	$\Delta [HCO_3^-] = 0.1 \Delta PCO_2$	Minutes to days
Respiratory acidosis (chronic)	Marked increase in $PaCO_2$, Decrease in $[HCO_3^-]$ and pH	$\Delta [HCO_3^-] = 0.3 \Delta PCO_2$	Days
Respiratory alkalosis (acute)	Marked decrease in $PaCO_2$ and increase in $[HCO_3^-]$, decrease in pH	$\Delta [HCO_3^-] = 0.2 \Delta PCO_2$ $[HCO_3^-]$ decreases 2 MEg/L for each 10 Torr decrease in PCO_2	Minutes to days
Respiratory alkalosis (chronic)	Marked decrease in $PaCO_2$ and increase in $[HCO_3^-]$ and pH	$\Delta [HCO_3^-] = 0.4 \Delta PCO_2$ $[HCO_3^-]$ decreases 5 MEg/L for each 10 Torr decrease in $PaCO_2$	Minutes to days

18. Neonatal cyanosis *Causes and clinical findings of central cyanosis*

Central nervous system depression

Causes: Perinatal asphyxia, Heavy maternal sedation Intrauterine fetal distress

Findings : Shallow irregular respiration poor muscle tone, Cyanosis that disappears when stimulated or oxygen is given to the patient

Pulmonary disease

Causes : Parenchymal lung disease (e.g. hyaline membrane disease, atelectasis), Pneumothorax or pleural effusion, Diaphragmatic hernia, PPHN (or persistent fetal circulation syndrome)

Findings : Tachypnea and respiratory distress with retraction and expiratory grunting, Rales and/or decreased breath sounds on auscultation, Chest X-ray film that may reveal causes (as listed previously), Oxygen administration that improves or abolishes cyanosis

Cardiac disease

Causes

Cyanotic CHD with right-to-left- shunt

Findings

Tachypnea but usually without retraction

Lack of rales or abnormal breath sounds unless CHF supervenes

Heart murmur that may be absent in serious forms of cyanotic CHD

A continuous murmur (of PDA) that may indicate restricted PBF through the ductus

Chest X-ray films that may show cardiomegaly, abnormal cardiac silhouette, increased or decreased PVMs

Little or no increase in Po_2 with oxygen administration

19. Causes of cyanosis-ABC

A. Airway	B Breathing	C.Circulation
Choanal atresia	Pneumonia	Oxygen carrying capacity
Micrognathia	Congenital diaphragmatic hernia	Polycythemia
Pierre Robin sequence	Congenital cystic adenomatoid malformation	Anemia
Laryngomalacia	Pulmonary sequestration	Methemoglobinemia
Vocal cord paralysis	Congenital lobar emphysema	Congenital heart disease
Tracheal stenosis	Pulmonary hypoplasia	*Decreased pulmonary blood flow*
Vascular slings/rings	Phrenic nerve palsy	Tricuspid atresia
Cystic hygroma	Hypoventilation	Pulmonary atresia
Hemangioma	CNS/Peripheral Neuromuscular	Pulmonary stenosis
Other neck masses		Tetralogy of Fallot
		Ebstein's anomaly
		Inadequate mixing
		Transposition of the great arteries
		Persistent pulmonary hypertension

Clin Pediatr Emerg Med. 2008 September; 9(3): 169–175. doi: 10.1016/j.cpem.2008.06.006.

20. Algorithmic approach to differential diagnosis of major causes of Neonatal Hypoglycemia based on duration of fasting needed to provoke the clinical and biochemical manifestations. Hypoglycemia is defined as <50 mg/dL. FFA is high (>2.5 μmol/L) and ketone (β-OH butyrate) is low (<1.5 μmol/L) in any fatty acid oxidation defect.

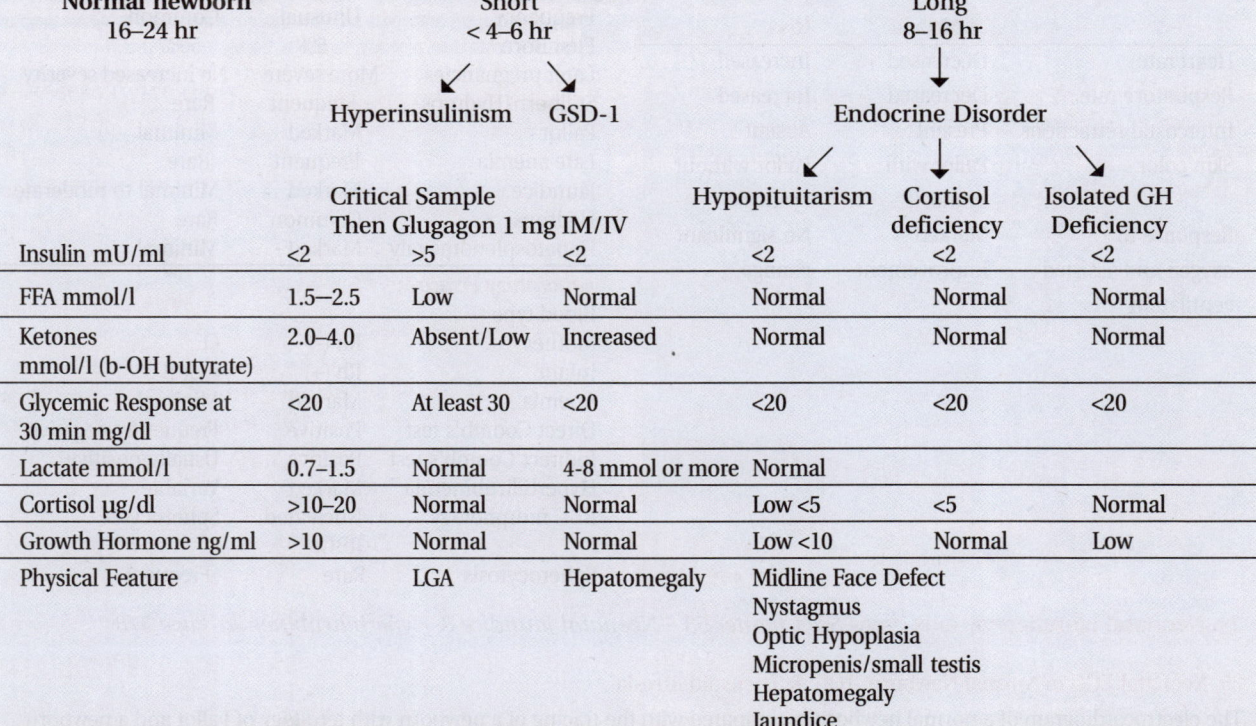

| | Normal newborn 16–24 hr | Short < 4–6 hr | | Long 8–16 hr | | |
| | | Hyperinsulinism | GSD-1 | Endocrine Disorder | | |
		Critical Sample Then Glugagon 1 mg IM/IV		Hypopituitarism	Cortisol deficiency	Isolated GH Deficiency
Insulin mU/ml	<2	>5	<2	<2	<2	<2
FFA mmol/l	1.5—2.5	Low	Normal	Normal	Normal	Normal
Ketones mmol/l (b-OH butyrate)	2.0–4.0	Absent/Low	Increased	Normal	Normal	Normal
Glycemic Response at 30 min mg/dl	<20	At least 30	<20	<20	<20	<20
Lactate mmol/l	0.7–1.5	Normal	4-8 mmol or more	Normal		
Cortisol μg/dl	>10–20	Normal	Normal	Low <5	<5	Normal
Growth Hormone ng/ml	>10	Normal	Normal	Low <10	Normal	Low
Physical Feature		LGA	Hepatomegaly	Midline Face Defect Nystagmus Optic Hypoplasia Micropenis/small testis Hepatomegaly Jaundice		

21. Infant of diabetic mom pathophysiology

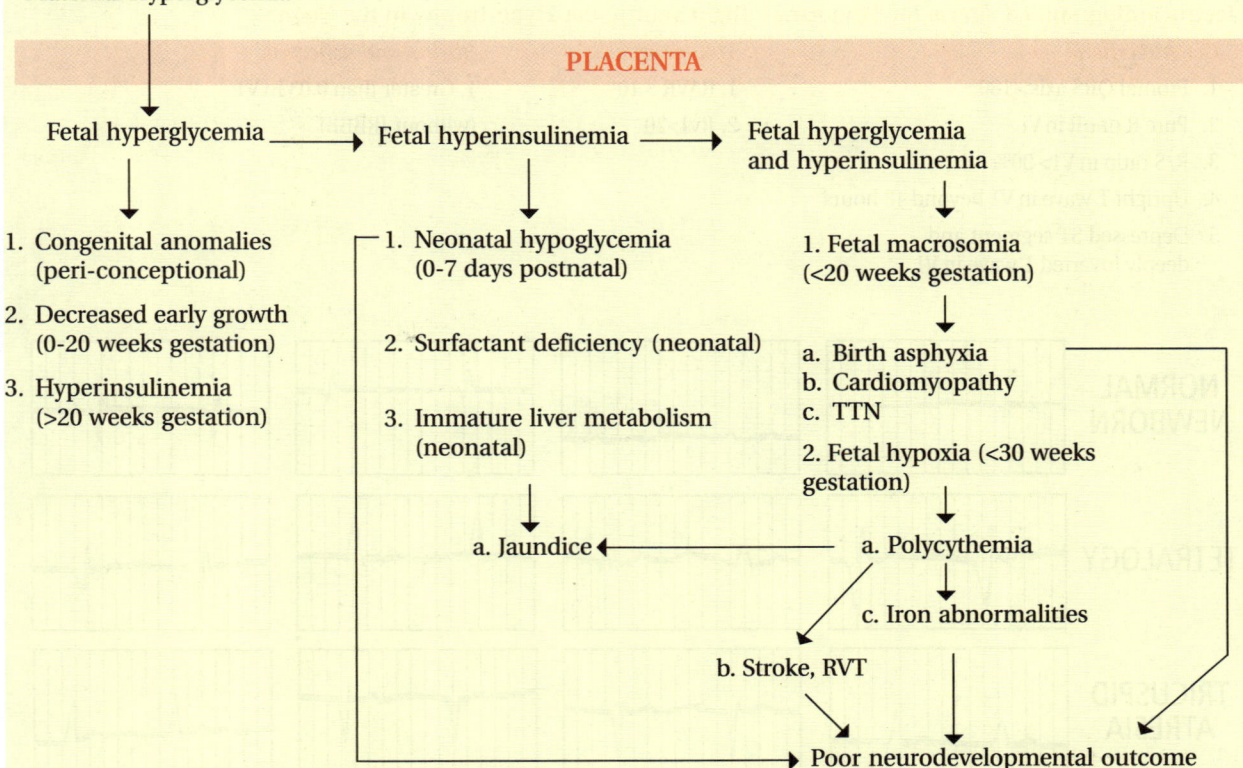

Maternal Hyperglycemia

PLACENTA

Fetal hyperglycemia → Fetal hyperinsulinemia → Fetal hyperglycemia and hyperinsulinemia

1. Congenital anomalies (peri-conceptional)
2. Decreased early growth (0-20 weeks gestation)
3. Hyperinsulinemia (>20 weeks gestation)

1. Neonatal hypoglycemia (0-7 days postnatal)
2. Surfactant deficiency (neonatal)
3. Immature liver metabolism (neonatal)

1. Fetal macrosomia (<20 weeks gestation)
   a. Birth asphyxia
   b. Cardiomyopathy
   c. TTN
2. Fetal hypoxia (<30 weeks gestation)
   a. Polycythemia
   c. Iron abnormalities
   b. Stroke, RVT

a. Jaundice

Poor neurodevelopmental outcome

Fig. 1. Infant of Diabetic Mother: The fetal and neonatal events attributable to fetal hyperglycemia (column 1), fetal hyperinsulinemia (column 2), or both in synergy (column 3). Time of risk is denoted in parentheses.

22. Asphyxia pallida and pallor due to blood loss

Comparative Clinical Findings in Neonatal Asphyxia and Acute Hemorrhage

	Neonatal asphyxia	Acute blood loss
Heart rate	Decreased	Increased
Respiratory rate	Decreased	Increased
Intercostal retractions	Present	Absent
Skin color	Pallor with cyanosis	Pallor without cyanosis
Response to oxygen and assisted ventilation	Marked Improvement	No significant change

23. RH disease and ABO incompatibility

Clinical and Laboratory Features of Immune Hemolysis Due to Rh Disease and ABO Incompatibility

Clinical Features	Rh Disease	ABO Incompatibility
Frequency	Unusual	Common
First Born	5%	50%
Later pregnancies	More severe	No increased severity
Stillborn/Hydrops	Frequent	Rare
Pallor	Marked	Minimal
Late anemia	Frequent	Rare
Jaundice	Marked	Minimal to moderate
Hydrops	Common	Rare
Hepatosplenomegaly	Marked	Minimal
Laboratory Features		
Blood type		
Mother	Rh (-)	O
Infant	Rh (+)	A or B
Anemia	Marked	Minimal
Direct Coomb's test	Positive	Frequently negative
Indirect Coomb's test	Positive	Usually positive
Hyperbilirubinemia	Marked	Variable
RBC morphology	Nucleated RBCs	Spherocytes
Spherocytosis	Rare	Frequent

24. Neonatal jaundice-various types See Chapter 53 – Neonatal Jaundice & Hyperbilirubinemia-Page 378

25. Neonatal ECG in Normal Newborn, TOF, & Tricuspid Atresia

The electrocardiogram of a normal newborn is compared with the tracing of a newborn with tetralogy of Fallot and a newborn with tricuspid atresia. The normal newborn tracing shows right ventricular dominance, similar to that of the newborn with tetralogy. The electrocardiogram of the neonate with tricuspid atresia is strikingly different showing left axis deviation and left ventricular dominance similar to an adult tracing.

Electrocardiographic Criteria for "Abnormal" Right Ventricular Hypertrophy in the Neonate

General criteria
1. Frontal QRS axis> 180⁰
2. Pure R or qR in Vi
3. R/S ratio in V1> 90%
4. Upright T wave in V1 beyond 48 hours
5. Depressed ST segment and deeply inverted T wave in V1

Voltage criteria
1. RAVR > 10
2. Rv1>20

Intrinsicoid deflection
1. Greater than 0.03 in V1
(without IRBBB)

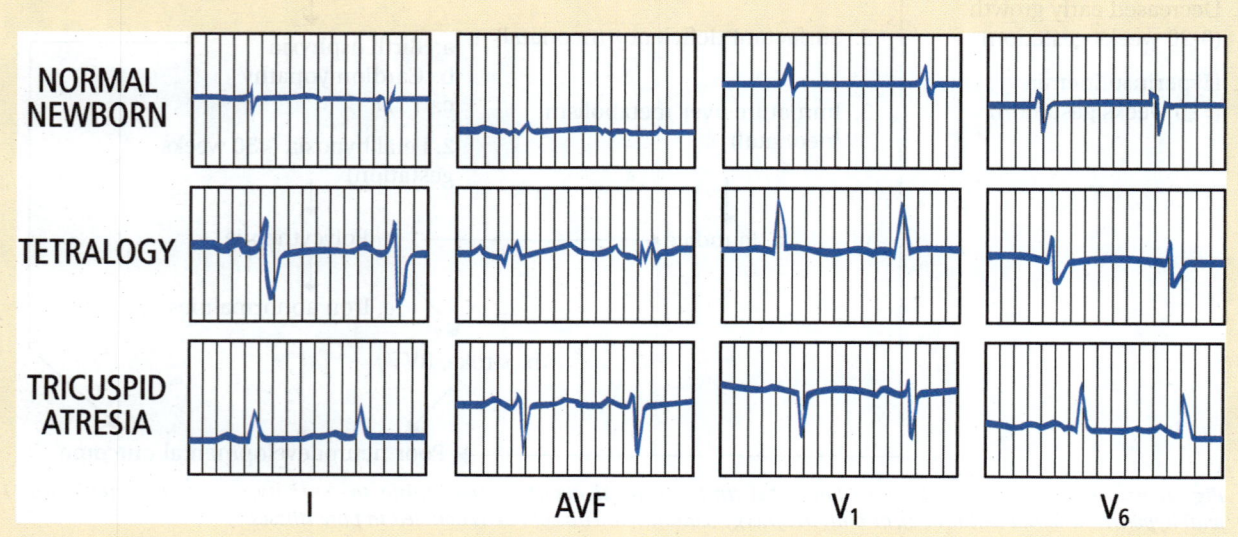

26. Idiopathic benign neonatal seizures (familial and non-familial)

Benign (non-familial)	Neonatal seizures versus benign familial Benign (non-familial) Neonatal seizures	Neonatal seizures Benign familial Neonatal seizures
Main seizures	Mostly clonic	Tonic-clonic
Onset	Fifth day of life	Second or third day of life
Duration of seizures	Status epilepticus (median 20 hours)	Repetitive isolated seizures
Main causes	Unknown, probably environmental	Autosomal dominant
Subsequent seizures	Practically nil (0.5%)	Relatively high (11%)
Psychomotor deficits	Minor	Practically non-existent
Ictal EEG	Usually localized spikes	Usually generalized flattening
Interictal EEG	Usually theta pointu alternant	Normal or focal abnormalities

27. Neonatal seizures and neonatal syndromes

Indicators of prognosis

Indicators of bad prognosis

- Severe hypoxia–ischaemia
- Severe congenital malformations of cortical development and meningoencephalitis
- Subtle and generalized tonic seizures
- Nearly flat · EEG or of very low voltage and discontinuous · EEG with bursts of high-voltage spikes and slow activity

Indicators of good prognosis

- Hypocalcaemia (alimentary type) and other transient metabolic changes
- Extracranial infections with seizures (otitis, pneumonia, gastroenteritis, etc.)

- Benign familial and non-familial convulsions
- Clonic seizures that are short and infrequent
- Normal inter-ictal EEG

Indicators of intermediate or guarded prognosis

- Moderately severe central nervous system (CNS) infections or malformations
- Most of the intracranial hemorrhages or infarctions
- More serious metabolic
- CNS disturbances
- EEG persistence of immature patterns
- Frequent or prolonged clonic seizures and clonic status epilepticus

28. Seizures vs jitteriness

A common consult from the neonatal ICU is for seizures. In a newborn, many movements such as sucking may be mistaken for seizure; on the other hand, subtle movements such as bicycling of the legs may be overlooked as a manifestation of seizure. A good rule of thumb is to obtain an EEG to determine if seizure activity is present.

Jitteriness may be difficult to distinguish from seizure, but a few clinical clues may help. Jitteriness from drug withdrawal often presents with tremors, whereas clonic activity is most prominent in seizures.

Jitteriness tends to be stimulus-sensitive, becoming most prominent after startle, and its activity can cease by holding onto the baby's arm, neither of which is true in seizures.

Additionally, seizures tend to be accompanied by autonomic changes as well.

29. Differences in immune responses in full and preterm infants

Immune system Component	Full term infant	Preterm infant
Immunoglobulin G	Complete placental transfer, concentrations comparable to mother	Incomplete placental transfer, concentrations decreased
Lymphocytes	Concentrations of T and B cells comparable to those in adults with normal response to antigens	Concentrations of T and B cells comparable to those in adults with normal response to antigens
Complement	50–75% of concentration in adult	Decreased concentration
Neutrophils	Elevated numbers at birth, with impaired functional ability	Elevated numbers at birth, with impaired functional ability
Monocytes	Normal number at birth but have impaired chemotaxis	Normal number at birth but have impaired chemotaxis
Macrophages	Normal number at birth but decreased function	Normal number at birth but decreased function
Natural killer cells	Concentration similar to adult level, but have diminished cytotoxic effects	Concentration similar to adult level, but have diminished cytotoxic effects

30. Identification of neck masses based on their location

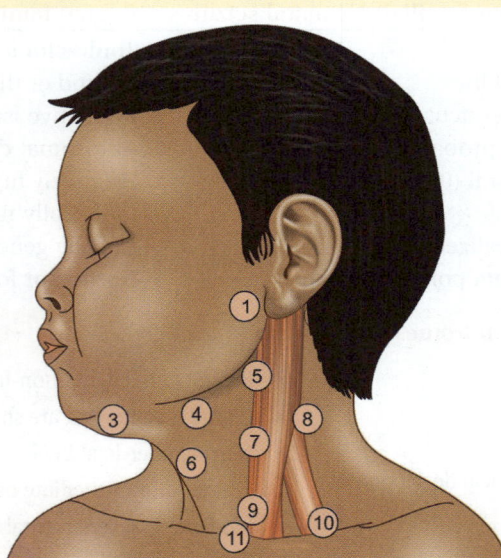

The most common neck masses are vascular malformations, abnormal lymphatic tissue, teratomas, and dermoid cysts. Neck masses can be identified based on their location

KEY:

1. = Preauricular area (parotid gland): congenital lesions—cystic hygroma, hemangioma, venous malformation; inflammatory condition— lymphadenitis secondary to infection in upper face and/or anterior scalp

2. = Postauricular area: congenital lesions—branchial cleft I (cystic, inflamed, or both); inflammatory condition—lymphadenitis secondary to inflammation of posterior scalp

3. = Submental area: congenital lesions—thyroglossal duct cyst, cystic hygroma, dermoid cyst, venous malformation; inflammatory condition—lymphadenitis secondary to inflammation in perioral area, anterior oral area, or nasal cavity

4. = Submandibular area: congenital lesions—cystic hygroma, hemangioma, ranula; inflammatory condition—lymphadenitis of submandibular gland secondary to inflammation in cheek and/or midoral cavity; in cystic fibrosis, enlargement of submandibular gland without inflammation

5. = Jugulodigastric area (tonsil node; normal structures include transverse process of C2 and styloid process): congenital lesions—branchial cleft I or II, hemangioma, cystic hygroma; inflammatory condition— lymphadenitis secondary to oropharyngeal inflammation

6. = Area of neck midline (normal structures include hyoid, thyroid isthmus, and thyroid cartilage): congenital lesions—thyroglossal duct cyst, dermoid cyst; inflammatory condition—lymphadenitis

7. = Area at anterior border of sternocleidomastoid muscle (normal structures include hyoid, thyroid cartilage, and carotid bulb): congenital lesions—branchial cleft I, II, or III (IV is rare), laryngocele, hemangioma, lymphangioma, hematoma (fibroma of sternocleidomastoid muscle)

8. = Spinal accessory: inflammatory condition lymphadenitis secondary to nasopharyngeal inflammation

9. = Paratracheal area: thyroid mass, parathyroid mass, esophageal diverticulum, metastatic lesion

10. = Supraclavicular area (normal structures include fat pad, pneumatocele from apical lobe related to defect in Gibson fascia [prominent mass with Valsalva's maneuver]): congenital lesion— cystic hygroma; neoplastic lesion—lipoma.

11. = Suprasternal area: thyroid mass, lipoma, dermoid cyst, thymic mass, mediastinal mass

31. Typical patterns of nutritive versus nonnutritive sucking

	Nutritive sucking	Nonnutritive sucking
Temporal organization	Continuous stream of bursts: transitioning to shorter bursts and longer pauses with progression of feeding	Alternation of burst and rest periods: repetitive pattern of cycling
Rate	1 suck per second	Preterm infant: 1.5 to 2 sucks per second Mature infant: 2 sucks per second
Suck-to-Swallow Ratio	Young infant: 1:1, may be higher toward end of feeding Older infant: 2:1 to 3:1	6:1 to 8:1
Purpose	Obtain nourishment	State regulation, satisfy sucking desire, exploration

The term "nonnutritive suck" can refer to the short, choppy, or weak character of the preterm infant who is not sufficiently mature to have the sucking behavior result in a nutritive function. On the other hand, a "nutritive" pattern of suck in breastfeeding consists of a deep, rhythmical pattern, with each suck followed by a swallow. Term infants also exhibit a nonnutritive sucking pattern in the absence of milk flow, and this appears to be the normal behavior of an infant satisfying the sucking urge and a state regulatory mechanism.

32. *Neonatal Hypotonia:* A detailed physical examination should be performed, assessing muscle tone, any asymmetry, the infant's strength, deep tendon reflexes (DTR), and any dysmorphic or unusual features

Central	Anterior Horn Cell	Nerve	Neuromuscular Junction	Muscle
normal strength	generalized weakness	weakness, distal>proximal	weakness, face/ eyes/ bulbar	weakness, proximal>distal
normal/ increased DTRs [+]	decreased /absent DTRs	decreased /absent DTRs	Normal DTRs	decreased DTRs
+/-seizures	fasciculations	+/- fasciculations	no fasciculations	
+/-dysmorphic features	often described as alert			

Central versus Neuromuscular Hypotonia

Central hypotonia	*Neuromuscular hypotonia*
No weakness	Weakness present
Normal or brisk tendon reflexes	Depressed or absent tendon reflexes
Fisting of hands	Muscle atrophy or fasciculations
Scissoring on vertical suspension	Decreased primitive reflexes
Malformations of other organs	No malformations of other organs
Seizures or encephalopathy	No seizures

33. *Differential Screening Tests for Neonatal Inborn Errors Of Metabolism*

Categorization of Neonatal IEM using metabolic screening tests

Acidosis	Ketosis	Lactate	Ammonia	Diagnosis
-	+	-	-	Maple syrup urine disease
+	+/-	-	+/-	Organic aciduria
+	+/-	+	-	Lactic acidosis
-	-	-	+	Urea cycle
-	-	-	-	Non-ketotic hyperglyceminuria, sulfite oxidase deficiency, peroxisomal, Phenylketonuria, galactosemia

34. *Approach to Newborn with persistent hypoglycemia and suspected IEM*

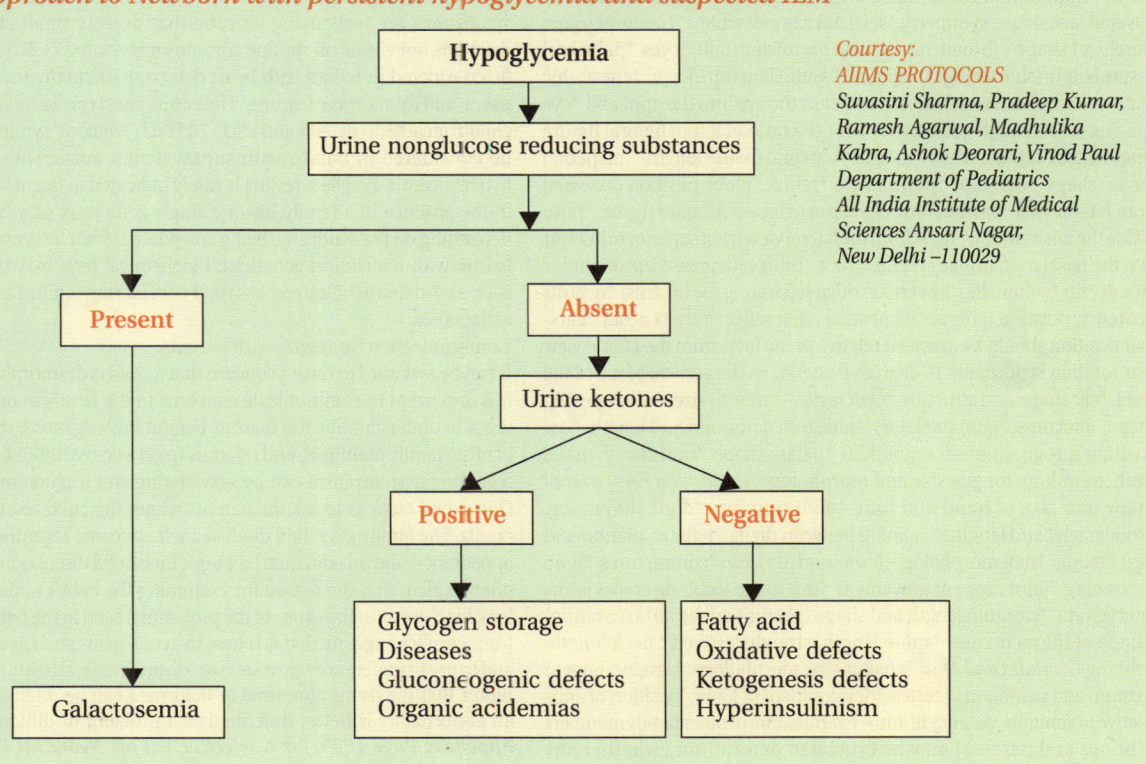

Courtesy:
AIIMS PROTOCOLS
Suvasini Sharma, Pradeep Kumar, Ramesh Agarwal, Madhulika Kabra, Ashok Deorari, Vinod Paul Department of Pediatrics All India Institute of Medical Sciences Ansari Nagar, New Delhi –110029

ASSESSMENT OF A DYSMORPHIC INFANT

DYSMORPHIC INFANT

Summary *a thorough history and examination is required *ancillary investigations may be useful *chromosome and gene tests may be warranted in certain circumstances *parental communication is important *potentially 'offensive' terms should be avoided.

Introduction : A dysmorphology assessment of a newborn focuses on aspects of history, examination and investigations that may lead to a syndrome diagnosis. This assessment should be carried out in any child with any of the following *congenital abnormality *growth abnormalities *dysmorphic features. Below are checklists for history and examination with a dysmorphology focus as well as investigations that the pediatrician should consider as part of a dysmorphology work-up. For many doctors, the discussion of issues relating to syndrome diagnosis and dysmorphism can be difficult, and some suggestions are outlined.

History Checklist: *pregnancy history, noting particularly exposure to teratogens, amniotic fluid volume *results of ultrasound and amniocentesis/CVS *fetal movements *maternal illness *delivery history *family history of abnormalities *consanguinity

Examination Checklist: The following focuses on the examination for dysmorphic features in a baby. A thorough examination of all other systems is vital when considering a syndrome diagnosis. *Growth Birth weight, length and head circumference.* Assess whether the baby's growth parameters are in proportion as well as the percentiles *Ectodermal Features* *skin - texture and color, birthmarks, redundancy, defects *hair - scalp hair and body hair: color and distribution. Note position of anterior and posterior scalp hairline *Skull* *shape, symmetry *sutures (overriding/normal/widely open) *fontanelle size and number *Face* In examining the face, it can be useful to first gain an overall impression of the facial appearance. Sometime, an overall gestalt can be diagnostic (e.g. Down syndrome). If no diagnosis is made, it is then important to divide the face into sections to examine it thoroughly. You may divide the face into the forehead, midface and oral region. It can sometimes help to cover parts of the face with your hand, in order to isolate the section of the face you are assessing. In assessing the face, it is important to view the face from the front and from the lateral view. The depth or height of structures such as the nasal bridge, the position of the mandible relative to the maxilla and the development of the midface are best assessed by the lateral view. *Overall face shape, symmetry, facial muscle movement *Forehead region* *forehead shape - (broad/bitemporal narrowing/tall) *eyes *palpebral fissure length (short/long) *palpebral fissure slant (up/down) *epicanthic folds - a fold of skin which arcs from below the eye into the upper lid *eye spacing (use a rough guide of 1:1:1 for the ratio of left palpebral fissure length: inner canthal distance: right palpebral fissure length) *palpebral fissure shape *iris color *pupil shape *retina *globe position (assessed from lateral view: protuberant vs deep set globes) *Midface region* *nose divide the nose into 3 sections from the lateral view from superior to inferior into the nasal root, bridge and tip. *root *bridge (depressed/prominent/broad) *tip *columella (the vertical ridge separating the nostrils) *nostrils - patency, position (anteverted nostrils often reflect a short nose) *ears- *ear position should be assessed relative to the face, from the lateral view *ear rotation is normally 15 degrees posterior to the vertical plane of the head *ear shape and structure *Oral region-* *mouth size and shape *lip shape, thickness *gum thickness *philtrum definition and length *jaw position (prognathia/micrognathia) *palate shape *oral cavity - natal teeth/frenulum/tongue size and morphology *Hands and Feet* *overall shape and size of hand and foot *digit number *digit shape (e.g. clinodactyly) and length *webbing between digits *palmar, plantar and digit creases *nail morphology *Joints and Skeleton* *contractures *limb shortening *joint range of movement *soft tissue webbing across joints (pterygium) *sternum length and shape (pectus carinatum/excavatum) *shape of thoracic cage *spine length, straight/curved * neck length, webbing *Genitalia and Anus* *phallus size, morphology *development of scrotum and palpation of testes *development of labia *position of anus relative to genitalia, patency of anus. Examination of other family members (siblings and parents) may be crucial to determining whether any dysmorphic features noted are familial or syndromic.

Investigations - when to do what? **Tests in the syndrome work-up:** *renal ultrasound, echocardiogram and cranial ultrasound may be indicated when a syndrome is suspected. In particular, midline abnormalities tend to cluster together, so, for example, an echo may be indicated when there is a cleft palate and dysmorphic features *eye examinations are useful for clues to make a syndrome diagnosis *skeletal radiographs - are indicated when there is disproportionate short stature, or other abnormalities in the skeletal system. X rays may be useful in diagnosing a skeletal dysplasia, which is a disorder caused by a primary abnormality of bone growth/development, or to assist in diagnosing a dysmorphic syndrome which can have skeletal abnormalities associated with it. A genetic skeletal survey includes * AP and lateral X rays of the skull *AP and lateral pelvis and spine (cervical to sacrum) * AP of one arm *AP both hands *AP of one leg and AP of both feet In a neonate, it may be sufficient to obtain a "baby-gram" (X-ray of the baby) and a separate X ray of the hands and feet.

Chromosome, fluorescent in-situ hybridization (FISH), single gene and biochemical tests. Blood chromosomes are indicated · when there are multiple congenital abnormalities +/- dysmorphic features · when there is one congenital abnormality in the presence of dysmorphic features and/or growth retardation . Chromosome abnormalities are more likely when there are abnormalities of growth, most commonly growth retardation and microcephaly, in association with dysmorphic features and congenital abnormalities. Note that a normal chromosome analysis does not exclude a single gene mutation or a micro deletion syndrome. Also, a normal antenatal chromosome analysis does not completely exclude a chromosome abnormality, as the resolution of chromosome banding may be greater on a postnatal sample than samples from chorion villus sampling or amniocentesis. If a chromosome abnormality is strongly suspected, it is indicated to repeat chromosomes in the postnatal period. A chromosome test takes a minimum of 5 days and the time taken to obtain a result depends on the growth of cells in culture. If an infant has been transfused, there is a small risk that there may be circulating lymphocytes from the blood donor, which may lead to an ambiguous result. Most laboratories recommend delaying a karyotype until one week following a transfusion. FISH for Trisomies 13/18/21 are used to expedite diagnosis when Trisomy of a specific chromosome is suspected. A result is usually available within 48 hours. FISH for submicroscopic deletion syndromes are tests using a probe that detects small chromosome deletions not visible on routine chromosome analysis. · 22q FISH should be considered in babies with heart defects, particularly those with cleft palate and dysmorphic features. The commonest cardiac defects seen are conotruncal heart defects and VSD · 7q FISH (Williams' syndrome) should be considered in babies with supravalvular aortic stenosis and/or hypercalcemia Fragile X testing is rarely indicated in the neonatal period in the absence of a family history. Single gene tests may be indicated, depending on the syndrome being considered. Such tests usually require liaison with the clinical geneticist. Biochemical tests may be indicated, such as 7-dehdrocholesterol assays if considering Smith-Lemli-Opitz as a diagnosis.

Communication Strategies with Parents:

It can be awkward to raise a concern that a child is dysmorphic. However, it is important to communicate concerns to the family in order to assist them in understanding the reasons behind investigations, examinations of other family members, and referrals to genetics. Withholding concerns regarding dysmorphism can be bewildering and frightening to parents. One useful tactic is to ask the parents whom the child resembles in the family. The family may then disclose their concerns regarding the child's appearance, and this can then be a topic for careful discussion. Geneticists often explain that the reason for examining the baby's appearance is to look for clues as to the cause of the problem(s) seen in the baby. Feedback from families suggests that it is best to avoid terms such as dysmorphic, and to use in preference terms such as "distinctive facial features". Families report that the terms abnormal or deformed can be offensive, and that an abnormality is better described as a problem or difficulty. *Refer to Appendix Page 1099, for a selective list of* Neonatal Dysmorphic Syndromes.

Rational Approach to the Newborn with Birth Defects & Dysmorphism

APPROACH TO DIAGNOSIS

History & Physical Examination

- Prenatal Problem in Development
- Postnatal Problem in Development

APPROACH TO DIAGNOSIS

Prenatal Problem in Development

- Single Primary Defect
- Multiple Malformation Syndrome

APPROACH TO DIAGNOSIS

Multiple Malformation Syndrome

- Chromosomal anomaly
- Single Gene Defect
- Teratogen
- Unknown

APPROACH TO DIAGNOSIS

Single Primary Defect

- Malformation
- Deformation
- Disruption
- Dysplasia

Down Syndrome- Typical Dysmorphic Features, Systemic complications, Karyotype, & Follow-up time table

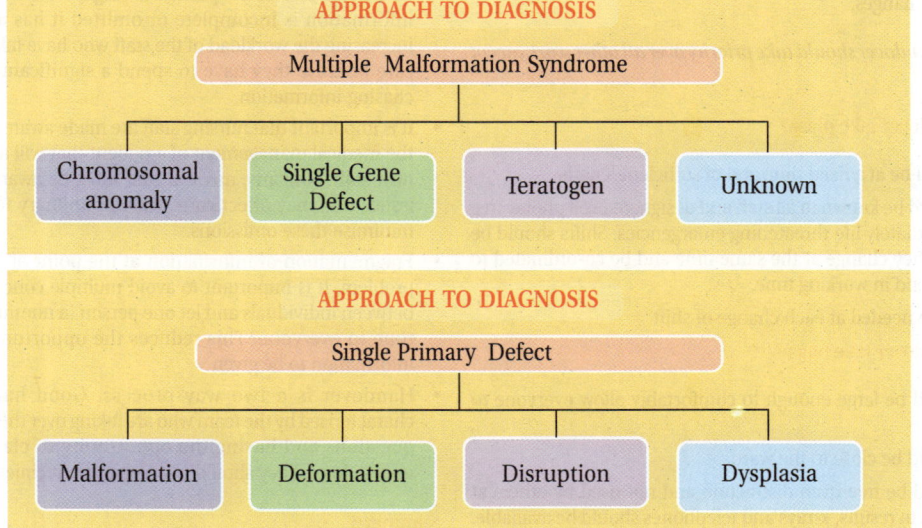

flattened nose and face, upward slanting eyes.

single palmer crease, short fifth finger that curves inward

widely separated first and second toes and increased skin creases

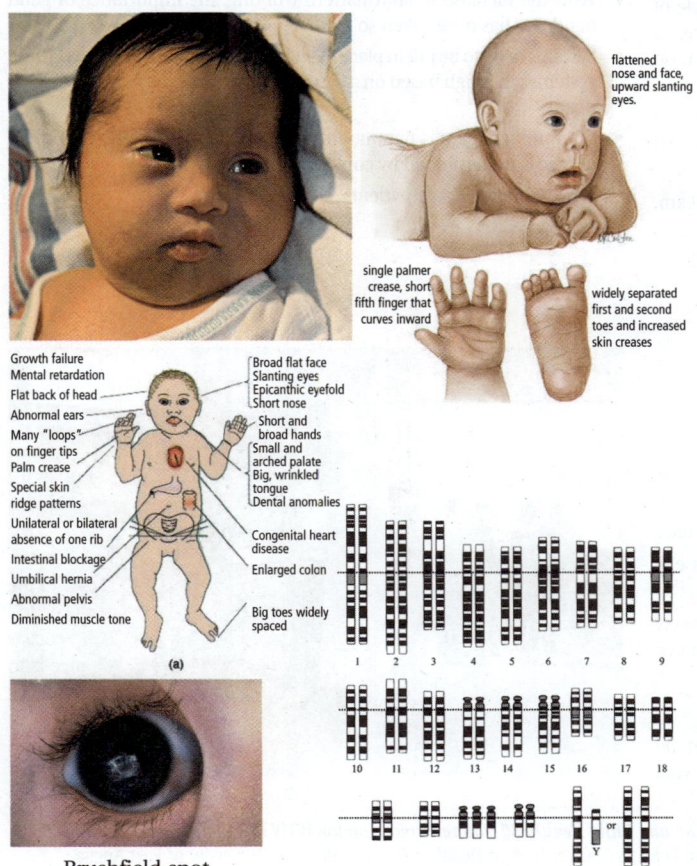

Growth failure
Mental retardation
Flat back of head
Abnormal ears
Many "loops" on finger tips
Palm crease
Special skin ridge patterns
Unilateral or bilateral absence of one rib
Intestinal blockage
Umbilical hernia
Abnormal pelvis
Diminished muscle tone

Broad flat face
Slanting eyes
Epicanthic eyefold
Short nose
Short and broad hands
Small and arched palate
Big, wrinkled tongue
Dental anomalies
Congenital heart disease
Enlarged colon
Big toes widely spaced

(a)

Brushfield spot

Down Syndrome Health Care Guidelines (1999 Revision) Record Sheet
Sheet #1: Birth to Age 12 Years

Name : _____

Birth day : _____

Medical Issues	At birth or at Diagnosis	6-mo	1	1-1/2	2	2-1/2	3	4	5	6	7	8	9	10	11	12
Karyotype & Genetic Counseling																
Usual Preventative Care																
Cardiology	Echo															
Audiologic Evaluation	ABR or OAE															
Opthalmologic Evaluation	Red reflex															
Thyroid (TSH & T₄)	State screening															
Nutrition																
Dental Exam[1]																
Celiac Screening[2]																
Parent Support																
Development & Educational Services	Early Intervention															
Neck X-rays & Neurological Exam[3]									X-ray							

Instructions : Perform indicated examination/screening and record date in blank spaces. the grey or shaded boxes mean no action is to be taken for those ages.

[1] Begin Dental Exams at 2 years of age, and continue every 6 months thereafter.

[2] 1gA antiendomysium antibodies and total 1gA.

[3] Cervial spine x-rays: flexion, neutral and extension, between 3-5 years of age. Repeat as needed for Special Olympics participation. Neurological examination at each visit.

GOOD PRACTICE IN HANDOVER

Who should be involved?

- Each NICU needs to identify the relevant staff who need to attend. The ideal model includes all grades of staff from each specialty or ward. The senior nurse and/or ANNPs should be present.

- Daily involvement of senior clinicians is essential, to ensure that appropriate level management decisions are made and also to convey the seriousness with which the organization takes the process. A consultant of the week system can help by reducing the frequency of lead consultant changes.

- *Attendance at handover should take priority over all other work except emergencies.*

When should handover take place?

- Handover should be at a fixed time and of sufficient length.
- The timing should be known to all staff and designated cell phone-free except for immediately life threatening emergencies. Shifts should be aligned so that they change at the same time and be co-ordinated to allow staff to attend in working time.
- Handover will be needed at each change of shift.

Where should handover take place?

- The room should be large enough to comfortably allow everyone to attend.
- Ideally this should be close to the ward.
- The room should be free from distraction and not used by others at that time. Access to results, x-rays and telephones should be available.

How should handover happen?

- Handover should be supervised by the most senior clinician present and must have clear leadership.
- Information presented should be succinct and relevant. The style of handover will vary depending on local need but requires a predetermined format and structure to ensure adequate information exchange.
- An electronic record or workbook allows tasks to be monitored, allowing effective handover without undue repetition. This should be reviewed at each handover.
- The team leader should distribute tasks amongst members of the team.
- Punctuality is important.

What should be handed over?

- Complete up to date list of patients and their whereabouts.
- Accepted and referred patients due to be assessed.
- Information given to parents/carers.
- Operational matters e.g. bed availability.
- Information to convey to the following shift.
- Patients with anticipated problems: clarify management plan and time for review.
- Outstanding tasks together with management plans linked to results.
- Information on relevant children at home or on other wards e.g. postnatal wards.
- **Remember:** Address clinically unstable children first. Ensure all acutely unwell and at risk patients including child protection cases are known to the senior members of the team.

Common pitfalls during handover

- Healthcare professionals sometimes try to give verbal handovers at the same time as the team taking over the patient's care are setting up vital life support and monitoring equipment. Unless both teams are able to concentrate on the handover of a sick patient, valuable information will be lost. The importance of written handover information must be stressed.

- Roles and responsibilities are not always clear during handover and this can lead to omissions, for example, if one staff member assumes that another will verbally update the team taking over the care of a patient.

- Checklists and written updates are important and often under-utilised. They provide important sources of information for the team who has taken over care of the patient during the following shift. When such information is incomplete or omitted it has a knock on effect of increasing the workload of the staff who have taken over the patient's care because they have to spend a significant proportion of time chasing information.

- It is important that nursing staff are made aware of critical features in the medical management of a patient that will affect care during the next shift. Similarly, medical staff must be aware of specific nursing issues that may affect care. Multidisciplinary team handover helps minimise these omissions.

- Fragmentation of information at the point of handover is a major problem. It is important to avoid multiple concurrent conversations between individuals and let one person (a nominated lead) speak at a time to everyone. This reduces the opportunities for conflicting information to be given.

- Handover is a two way process. Good handover practice is characterised by the team who are taking over the patient's care asking questions and having the opportunity to clarify points they are uncertain of. They should not be passive recipients of information.

Summary

- Good doctor to doctor handover is vital to protect patient safety
- Multi-disciplinary handover is important to ensure all groups of staff are updated with current patient information
- With the increase in shift pattern working, the importance of good handover has never been so high
- Systems need to be put in place to enable and facilitate handover. These systems, although based on a generic model, must be adapted to local needs
- Continuity of care is paramount to protect patient safety; continuity of care is underpinned by continuity of information
- Safe handover = safe patients

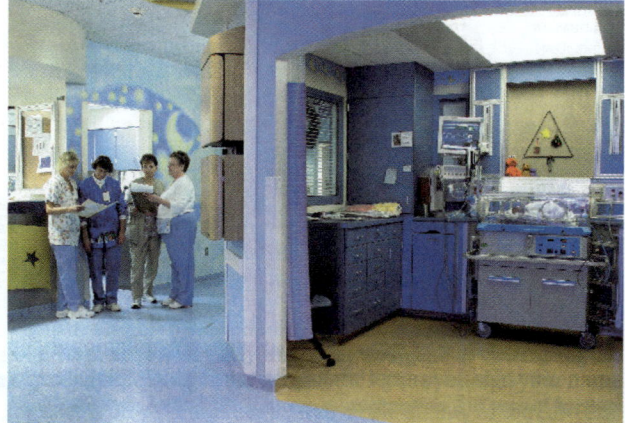

Ref: Safe Handover: Safe Patients FMA 10.01.05 **Royal College of Paediatrics and Child Health 50 Hallam Street, London W1W 6DE** Telephone: (020) 7307 5600
Fax: (020) 7307 5601 E-mail: enquiries@rcpch.ac.uk Professor Sam Leinster Dean School of Health Policy and Practice University of East Anglia

This gives a guideline for reviewing and writing notes on NICU babies to ensure that babies are appropriately assessed and residents use their time efficiently.

New/Unstable Babies

- Assess twice daily
- Write notes twice daily
- Examine Acute problem list
- Assessment Progress in last day
- Observations and assessment
- Plan, reasons and interpretation

More Stable Babies

- Once in detail (as above). During the day except at weekends.
- Once in brief: Either in the day or at night. At weekends, split these assessments between day and night staff.

Very Stable Babies

- Review daily during the week.
- At weekends, review daily in brief, often on the ward round. Write in notes.

Review

- If asked to review a baby, record appropriate observations and interpretations at the time. Do not wait until the next routine review

Procedures

It is important to document significant procedures undertaken, whether successful or unsuccessful. Procedures which should be clearly documented (with date and **time**) include:

- Intubation/reintubation
- Extubation
- Intercostal drain insertion
- Umbilical venous and arterial catheterization
- Peripheral artery catheterization
- Longline insertion
- Urinary catheterization
- Lumbar puncture
- Ventricular tap
- Exchange transfusion
- Institution of non-routine medications should also be clearly documented.

Weekly Plan

For stable babies, ensure that there is a weekly plan. Avoid duplication (of full assessments and of tests, etc.).

- Investigations: Blood tests: day, tick when ordered
- Scans/X-rays/Other
- Drugs: List once weekly or if changed
- Record levels, date, change, plan
- Growth/Nutrition: Measure at least weekly
- Plot growth weekly
- Respiratory: Part of daily review. Summarize overall course weekly.

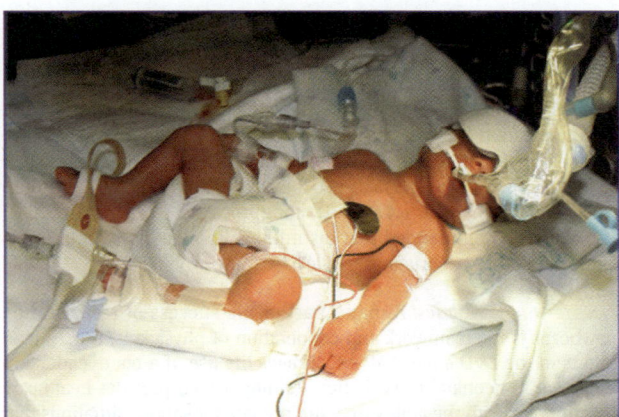

Patient Care

*Know your patients well *Obtain complete history yourself, not just what can be gleaned from OB/L&D charting *Perform detailed exams *Communicate frequently with families, providing regular updates * Obtain all available data prior to rounds *Presentations must be accurate, and should provide necessary detail but also be concise * Sign-out of your patients to your colleagues must be complete.

Charting in the Medical Record

* Please write legibly, especially, when writing orders. * Time and date all orders and notes. * Errors in the medical record should be corrected as follows: single line through the error, write mistaken entry by the error, then date/time, and initial.* Never change any area of the medical record after the fact; an addendum to a note should clearly state the date/time that the notation is being written.

Order Sheets

* Use pre printed Admission Order sheet. * Use the NICU Medication Guidelines for all medications.* Use only JCAHO APPROVED abbreviations. *Double check all medication calculations. Ask another Doctor and/or Nurse with any uncertainties. List the dosage in mg/kg in parentheses at the end of the medication order. * Use before decimal point if dosage is <1 (0.1 mg instead of .1 mg) but do not use   after a decimal point (1 instead of 1.0) to avoid 10 fold dosing errors.

REFERENCE: *Auckland Newborn Services Clinical Guideline.*

IMPLEMENTING NEWBORN RESUSCITATION MOCK CODES

Newborn mock codes encourage teamwork on the part of all who are responsible for newborn resuscitation. They are also encouraged by the Neonatal Resuscitation Program (NRP),cosponsored by the American Academy of Pediatrics (AAP) and the American Heart Association (AHA). The basic principles of NRP include (a) the ability to be implemented in any hospital, (b) a self-instructional format, and (c) the use of regional trainers and hospitalbased instructors . NRP is essential education because birth asphyxia and its resulting damage are significant factors contributing to neonatal morbidity and mortality. Approximately 10% of all newborns require some such attention at birth to ensure appropriate cardiopulmonary adaptation. *Successful completion of the NRP course, however, does not imply competence or confidence. Research has shown that retention of NRP skills deteriorates rapidly after completion of the course.* Therefore it would seem appropriate to develop an educational plan that offers a nonthreatening environment for practice and questions about neonatal resuscitation for the period between official certification sessions.

*Team Work is Essential:*It is essential that healthcare teams work collaboratively and cooperatively in the resuscitation of newborns. The Joint Commission on Accreditation of Healthcare Organizations (JCAHO) (2004) identified several root causes related to perinatal death: 1. Poor communication (72%) 2. Organizational culture as a barrier to effective communication and teamwork (i.e., hierarchy and intimidation, failure to function as a team, and failure to follow the chain of communication) (55%)3. Staff competency (47%) 4. Training processes (40%) (JCAHO, 2004) JCAHO has recommended that institutions implement team training, clinical drills, and debriefings to alleviate these problems.

Newborn Mock Codes: A major part of the success of resuscitating newborns is the teamwork and cooperation of physicians, nurses, and others in the L&D suite. AAP encourages the use of a team leadership approach in neonatal resuscitation training, which provides healthcare practitioners with the ability to better prepare for serious situations that may arise in the delivery room . NRP training enhances timely interventions, such as ventilation, direct laryngoscopy, endotracheal intubation, external cardiac massage, and administration of resuscitation medications. Using the newborn mock code could prepare providers "to function in a systematic manner with their neonatal resuscitation team in the event a neonate requires resuscitation…the functioning has to be timely, quick, and appropriate, and Megacode will prepare them for that when faced with a stressful situation,New NRP guidelines were introduced in *The Textbook of Neonatal Resuscitation*, 6th edition, in 2010. Newborn mock codes can be used to bring all staff up to date regarding the changes.

How to Facilitate Newborn Mock Codes: Practice of the NRP mock code scenarios involves three behaviors of learning: cognitive (knowledge), behavioral (how we react to situations), and psychomotor (skills abilities). The code scenarios (available through the NRP program) can be presented to staff by NRP instructors or by attending physicians fluent in the knowledge of neonatal resuscitation. Participants should include all staff who have occasion to attend deliveries. Evaluation of the practice sessions should be included to assess the effectiveness of the program and assure that it is meeting the needs of the staff.

Implementation of Newborn Mock Codes: Implementing newborn mock codes requires a plan for success and is feasible in most situations. *It is essential to have a buy-in by all staff, including physicians and nurses, for the newborn mock code program to be effective.* Clear communication with the attending physician staff—especially with the chief physician—will enhance the productivity of the mock code sessions.Staff may be more inclined to participate if they are already on site. Each of the disciplines should have a part in the implementation plan, which can be accomplished by meeting with others of influence in the interdisciplinary team of providers. This meeting can cover issues such as how often mock codes should be held, who will oversee the codes, and who should participate. Each department head also should pledge their support of staff participation in the events. Schedules should be devised that allow participation by nursing staff of various experience levels, residents and attending physicians, and others who attend newborn deliveries.

Environments for these practices can include educational rooms with all necessary equipment or actual unoccupied patient care rooms. It is important to make the learning environment nonthreatening. No one should be made to feel inadequate. That would only encourage lack of response to the mock scenarios and actual events. Preparation is important in planning mock codes. Scenarios should be brief, realistic, and planned ahead of time. The moderator/facilitator for the event should be an expert in resuscitation guidelines from the AAP and the AHA. The moderator may offer prompting and support for each individual—positive and objective feedback should be offered. All equipment should be available and in good working order. The AAP/AHA offers algorithms for resuscitation and medication administration. They should be available, as should a checklist for the moderator to ensure that all steps are followed accurately. Scenarios, algorithms, videos, and other educational material are available through he AAP (www.aap.org/nrp/nrpmain.html). Implementation of newborn mock codes requires planned change, problem-solving skills, decision-making skills, and interpersonal skills. The Plan-Do-Check-Act Model for Process Improvement (also known as Deming's Model) can be effective in planning for mock code implementation. This model involves planning the implementation, doing the mock codes, collecting data, analyzing, checking the results and lessons learned, and acting by adopting, adapting, or abandoning the change.Having models that indicate decreasing heart rates or blood oxygen saturation levels may be beneficial in helping develop competence. Packaged medications also should be available, and staff should be encouraged to open them and draw them up in preparation for administration. This practice allows them to become familiar with different packaging methods and putting together the syringes. The pharmacy can be asked to supply the needed medications and may be able to supply medications that are outdated or otherwise not usable for these practice sessions. Some barriers to successful implementation of mock codes include staffing levels of the unit, emergencies on the unit, and physician–nurse working relationships. There are some successful strategies to help overcome resistance to change, including the creation of an environment in which participation, open communication, and advanced education are encouraged.If most staff can be encouraged to participate as an educational experience, a supportive environment in which change is less threatening can be the force that helps staff who are not inclined to participate to change their minds. Creating a supportive environment is crucial to maintaining a climate of trust, support, and confidence. After the mock code scenario, the instructors should ask participants to complete a brief survey. Although this survey can vary, it should be simple and identify the participant by department and job description. It should inquire about the participant's perception of learning and the learning environment. There also should be opportunity for general comments and perceived areas of improvement. One aspect the survey is intended to measure is the participant's perception of learning: "Did you learn something that you did not previously know?" The respondent can choose the answer "no" or "yes" (with a description of what knowledge was achieved). The experience of participation also is evaluated: How would you best describe the learning environment that was created?" Choices might include "positive, encouraging," or "neutral," or "negative, threatening." Review and analysis of the survey results can help to determine if participants benefited from the newborn mock code experience. Success for the outcome of mock codes is evident if participants report increased knowledge or learning after the event. Informal monitoring includes observations by physicians and nurses of improved teamwork and areas of needed improvement. Ultimately, skills improvements should relate to better patient outcomes.

Conclusions: More research is needed to show the effectiveness of skills review methods such as newborn mock codes and development of new, more effective methods of refreshing skills. A strong plan, when implemented, can be an example to others. Successful implementation can be studied, documented, and submitted for publication in the interest of helping others develop such a system for improving outcomes by using practices that are evidence based.

Courtesy: Teresa Gail Blakely, MSN/Ed, RNCAmerican Journal of Maternal/Child Nursing July/August 2007

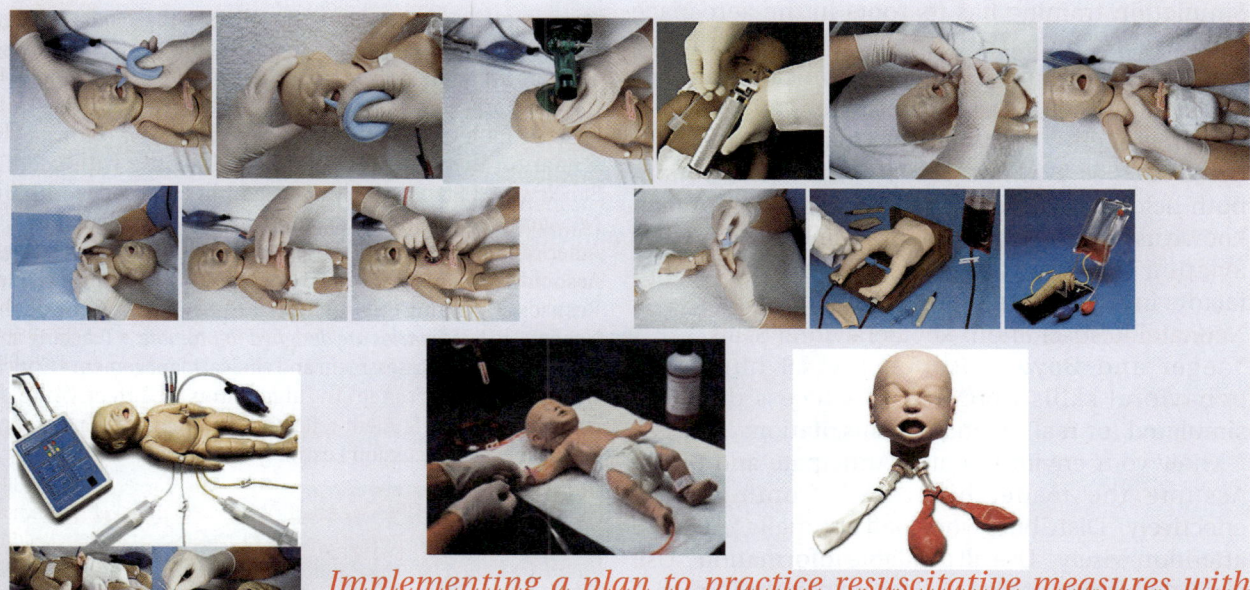

Implementing a plan to practice resuscitative measures with newborn mock codes on a regular basis is an effective strategy for staff to practice the skills they have already learned in class.

The following sample case scenarios can be used in performance evaluation and mock codes. (These scenarios are from the *Instructor's Manual for Neonatal Resuscitation* (AHA/AAP, 2006a).

1. A 26-year-old, G2P1 mother had a normal, uncomplicated pregnancy and subsequently delivered a fullterm, 3400-g infant by SVD. Bulb suctioning and blow-by oxygen with tactile stimulation are provided. The infant's color continues to be cyanotic despite these measures, so PPV is initiated. The infant's heart rate is 50 and is not increasing. Chest compressions are initiated, but the infant's condition continues to deteriorate.

2. A 26-week antepartum patient on the floor calls the nurses' station complaining of abdominal pain accompanied by a gush of fluid. When the nurse checks the patient, she finds the infant crowning. A 26-week, 625-g infant is delivered. The infant is pale and gasping and has a heart rate of 50.

3. A 22-year-old, G1P0 woman presents to L&D with severe abdominal pain, rigid abdomen, and frank vaginal bleeding. Patient is approximately 32 weeks by dates with no prenatal care. A male friend accompanying her states that she did cocaine about 1 hour before admission. A pale, limp, 1200-g infant with no respiratory rate or heart rate is delivered.

4. A mother who delivered a newborn infant 5 hours ago comes running into the nurses' station carrying her baby. She cries out that her infant is blue and not breathing. Assessment reveals a term, 3200-g infant who is apneic and cyanotic. The heart rate is below 60.

5. A 32-year-old, G1P0 mother who received prenatal care and has had an uncomplicated pregnancy delivers a 3636-g infant with a scaphoid abdomen. Immediately after birth, the infant is in respiratory distress.

6. A 35-year-old, G5P2A2 woman presents in the emergency department in advanced labor. The patient has had no prenatal care and does not know EDC. On arrival to L&D, the patient is pushing. Membranes rupture with the release of thick, particulate meconium-stained fluid. A limp, apneic, cyanotic infant weighing approximately 2400 g is delivered.

Methods for Implementing Newborn Mock Codes on the Obstetrical Unit

* *Meet with key people*—NRP instructors, heads of neonatology, obstetrics, family practice, midwifery, and respiratory therapy, and nurse managers/leadership group—for brainstorming session and plan. *Obtain the mock code scenarios from the NRP Web site.

* *Set up dates and times for mock codes.* Notify attending physicians and neonatologists so they can arrange for participation of their physicians/residents. Offer scenarios and algorithms, if desired, for review.

* *Schedule mock codes at convenient times for staff* (e.g., 1 day per month, at 8AM, 1PM, 8PM, and midnight to include all staff). Keep mock codes to 20 minutes total.

* *Appoint a coordinator to organize event and ensure* that all needed equipment is available and in working order.

* *Have nurse managers free up staff* as possible to allow participation.

* *Be sure physicians attend mock codes* to practice teamwork and leadership skills.

* *Be sure that when code begins, staff members respond to* code, perform skills/interventions, and participate in debriefing session with all participants.

* *Be sure that all participants fill out* short evaluation of event.

* *Have a plan for a coordinator* to collect and analyze data.

Simulation training has its roots in the aerospace industry. Many patient care situations, such as neonatal resuscitation, require technically complex skills and a high level of interdependence among team members -- characteristics that are shared with fields such as aviation. The potential for errors in both fields is significant. An educational approach known as crew resource management, developed by aviation experts, emphasizes the role of human factors in high-stress, high-risk environments.

Neonatal Resuscitation: Key Behavioral Skills

Yaeger and Boyle outlined the 10 important behavioral skills that lead to success during a simulated (or real) neonatal resuscitation: * Know your environment * Anticipate and plan * Assume the leadership role * Communicate effectively * Distribute work load optimally * Allocate attention wisely * Use all available information * Use all available resources * Call for help early enough * Maintain professional behavior

These are the same principles that the aerospace industry incorporates into crew resource management, a program used to teach the behavioral skills necessary to manage emergencies and prevent human error. These behaviors have also been adapted to the training of personnel to manage crises in the field of anesthesia. Hint: If you are going to be participating in a neonatal simulation scenario, these 10 key principles are also the behaviors that you (and others) will be using to evaluate your performance during the post-scenario debriefing.

Debriefing

Debriefing is a review and facilitated discussion of the videotaped scenario. Debriefing must take place immediately following the scenario and include all participants. Active trainee participation is critical to the effectiveness of debriefing, resulting in deeper processing and better retention of learning than during passive debriefing sessions.Debriefings are usually conducted in a room with multiple video monitors and comfortable seating that is physically separated from the simulated delivery room, avoiding any potential psychological or emotional effects that may linger from being in the simulation room.The goal of debriefing is to examine how closely the participants' performance approached the target and to identify what further learning objectives are required to bridge the gap between performance and goals.The emphasis is on the key behavioral skills, neonatal resuscitation guidelines, and other salient teaching points about each scenario. *The debriefings are constructive, reinforcing positive aspects of the performance and pinpointing areas for improvement in a nonjudgmental manner.*
http://www.medscape.com/viewarticle/541371

The twenty (20) scenarios are all timed events that require learners to take critical actions in order to successfully complete the case. They are set in the delivery room, outside the delivery room, in the newborn nursery or in the neonatal intensive care unit, allowing for a variety of valuable experiences for learners. The scenarios are specifically developed for use with Laerdal SimNewB™ Standard or Advanced (in accordance with the Neonatal Resuscitation Program (NRP) materials based on the American Academy of Pediatrics (AAP) and the American Heart Associations (AHA) Guidelines for Cardiopulmonary Resuscitation and Emergency Cardiovascular Care of the Neonate) .*The scenarios are designed to promote:* • Teaching and testing • Newborn assessment and clinical management • Critical thinking • Adherence to algorithms • Effective team communication • Student reflection and remediation through debriefing and discussion Learning Technology

Advanced Neonatal Resuscitation and Stabilization Scenarios

Unstable Airway Scenarios
Scenario 1: Resuscitation of a Newborn Outside of the Delivery Room
Scenario 2: Resuscitation of the Very Premature Neonate
Scenario 3: Resuscitation Following Delayed Delivery Due to Shoulder Dystocia
Scenario 4: Resuscitation of the Neonate Involving Tension Pneumothorax
Scenario 5 Resuscitation Involving Newborn Exposure to General Anesthesia

Shock Scenarios
Scenario 6: Resuscitation and Management of a Newborn with Hypovolemic Shock
Scenario 7: Resuscitation Involving Persistent Cyanosis and Low Oxygen Saturation
Scenario 8: Resuscitation of a 2-Day-Old Baby with Shock

Congenital Disorder Scenarios
Scenario 9: Resuscitation of a Newborn with Non-Immune Hydrops
Scenario 10: Resuscitation of a Newborn with Congenital Diaphragmatic Hernia
Scenario 11: Resuscitation of a Newborn with Gastroschisis
Scenario 12: Resuscitation of a Newborn with Mechanical Blockage of Airway
Scenario 13: Resuscitation of a Newborn with Congenital Heart Block

Parental Care Scenario
Scenario 14: Parental Care Following Withdrawal of Resuscitation of a Newborn

Stabilization Scenarios
Scenario 15: Management of Respiratory Failure Due to Endotracheal Tube Displacement
Scenario 16: Stabilization of a Newborn with Seizures
Scenario 17: Stabilization of a Newborn with Septic Shock
Scenario 18: Management of Respiratory Failure Due to Persistent Pulmonary Hypertension
Scenario 19: Stabilization of Newborn in Shock with Central Cyanosis
Scenario 20: Stabilization of a Newborn with Respiratory Failure Due to Pneumothorax

References: American Heart Association/American Academy of Pediatrics. (2006a). *Instructor's manual, for neonatal resuscitation* (5th ed.). Elk Grove Village, IL: American Academy of Pediatrics/American Heart Asociation. American Heart Association/American Academy of Pediatrics. (2006b). *The Textbook of neonatal resuscitation* (5th ed.). Elk Grove Village, IL: American Academy of Pediatrics/American Heart Association.

The importance of a meticulous supervision of all babies after birth by student midwives, midwives and staff working in delivery rooms.

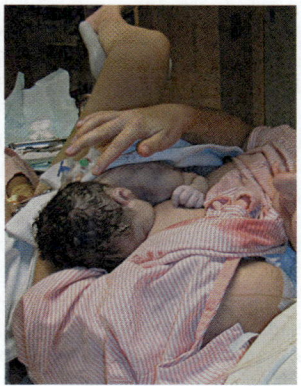

Picture taken by the father in the delivery room: neonate in cardiorespiratory arrest while in a prone position at her mother's breast.

Sudden cardiorespiratory arrest of neonates in the delivery room

Ullmo S, Jurado S, Farron F, Pediatric and Neonatal Care Unit, Hôpital du Jura, Delémont, Switzerland

Published: July 1, 2007

Case report: A 30-year-old woman delivered a 3400 g female infant at term. The mother had been treated with antidepressants before this pregnancy, but was otherwise in good health. The pregnancy was harmonious and without complications. The neonate was delivered by vacuum extraction for a suspect CTG and second stage delay. Umbilical arterial and venous pH were 7.17/7.22. Adaptation was excellent with an Apgar scores of 9, 10 and 10 at 1, 5 and 10 minutes of life, respectively. After an initial clinical examination, the baby was brought to the mother for breast feeding. At 40 minutes of life, she became pale while still in prone position with her face buried in the breast of her mother (Fig). The father alerted the midwife, who called at once for the on-call pediatrician. On the resuscitation table, the infant was pale without any respiratory effort and no heart sounds were heard. Bag mask ventilation and chest compressions were initiated without delay. 30 seconds later, heart sounds became audible again and there was some return of respiratory effort. This was followed by progressive improvement of muscle tone and color. A blood gas analysis showed severe mixed acidosis (pH 6.97, BE -16 mmol/l). The newborn was transferred to the neonatal unit for observation over the next 48 hours. The child is now 10 months old. She is healthy and developing normally.

Discussion

Despite uncomplicated postnatal adaptation and without any risk factors, our patient suddenly went into cardiorespiratory arrest while lying in prone position at her mothers breast. In the literature, there are additional and even more dramatic case reports (1-3) of several neonates with sudden cardiorespiratory arrest in the delivery room. Seven babies without any risk factors and with undisturbed postnatal adaptation died while sleeping in a prone position on their mothers' chest. These case reports illustrate that even following uncomplicated delivery and initial postnatal adaptation, babies are still at risk to develop severe cardiorespiratory compromise. In our patient, insufficient vigilance during the first breast feeding lead to suffocation when the baby's face was pressed against the breast of the mother. As a consequence, babies should be observed closely, particularly when in a prone position at the mother's breast. Several articles

have been published about the risks of the prone sleeping (3-6). But neither teaching program in the formation of midwives in Switzerland, nor official protocols for the supervision of neonates in delivery rooms exists. We suggest that the importance of a meticulous supervision of all babies after birth should be pointed out to all student midwives, midwives and staff working in delivery rooms (7). **Conclusion :**Care and supervision of babies is necessary not only during the delivery and the 10 first minutes of life, but also later on, especially during the first breast feedings when the baby is lying in a prone position.

References

1. Gatti H, Castel C, Andrini P, Durand P, Carlus C, Chabernaud JL, Vial M., Dehan M, Boithias C. Malaises graves et morts subites après une naissance normale à terme: à propos de six cas. Arch Pediatr 2004;11: 432-435
2. Espagne S, Hanon I, Thiébaugeorges O, Hascoet JM. Mort de nouveau-nés apparemment sains en salle de naissance: un problème de surveillance? Arch Pedriatr 2004;11:436-439
3. Kuhn P, Donato L, Laugel V, Beladdale J, Escande B, Matis J et al. Malaise grave précoce du nouveau-né : à propos de deux cas survenus en salle de naissance. XXX es Journées nationales de la Société française de médecine périnatale, Reims, octobre 2000 (no abstract available)
4. Chong A, Murphy N, Matthews T. Effect of prone sleeping on circulatory control in infants. Arch Dis Child 2000;82:253-256
5. Patel AL, Paluszynska D, Harris A and Thach BT. Occurrence and Mechanisms of Sudden Oxygen Desaturation in Infants Who Sleep Face Down. Pediatrics 2003;111:e328-332
6. Corbyn JA. Mechanisms of sudden infant death and the contamination of inspired air with exhaled air. Med Hypotheses 2000;54:345-352
7. Banger B, Brossier JP, Seguin G. Soins au nouveau-né normal, de plus de 36 SA et sans pathologie, dans les deux premières heures. Le Reseau « Sécurité Naissance – Naître ensemble » des Pays de la Loire. Version validée au 15 septembre 2006 (no abstract available)

Unexpected collapse of apparently healthy newborn infants: the benefits and potential risks of skin-to-skin contact -Peter J Fleming, *Arch Dis Child Fetal Neonatal* F2 *Ed* January 2012 Vol 97 No 1-An abstract

Unexpected postnatal collapse of apparently healthy infants within a few hours of birth has been recognized for many years, and may be the first presentation of an underlying previously unrecognized congenital anomaly of the cardiorespiratory systems or neural control systems or an underlying metabolic disorder, but in most cases no underlying explanation is identified. Such a collapse is a rare event, but one that may lead to death or long-term neurodisability. This is most commonly observed in the infants of primiparous mothers who are unobserved by medical or nursing staff and undergoing a period of skin to- skin contact, with the infant prone or on the side on the mother's chest. In the meantime, however, it seems appropriate, as suggested by Poets et al to recommend that midwives check on the infant's condition frequently during the first 2-3 h after birth, with particular emphasis on ensuring that when in skin to- skin contact the infant's position is safe and the nose and mouth are not occluded. There is no reason that such close observation cannot be unobtrusive and gentle, and by involving the parents and helping them to understand and avoid potentially hazardous positions, infant well-being can be enhanced without compromising the benefits of close contact between mother and baby and the successful establishment of breast feeding.

HOME VISITS FOR THE NEWBORN CHILD: A STRATEGY TO IMPROVE SURVIVAL

Fast facts

1. Every year, about 3.7 million babies die in the first four weeks of life (2004 estimates). Most of these newborns are born in developing countries and most die at home. Up to two-thirds of these deaths can be prevented if mothers and newborns receive known, effective interventions. A strategy that promotes universal access to antenatal care, skilled birth attendance and early postnatal care will contribute to sustained reduction in maternal and neonatal mortality.

2. Studies have shown that home-based newborn care interventions can prevent 30–60% of newborn deaths in high mortality settings under controlled conditions.

3. Nearly 40% of all under-five child deaths occur in the first 28 days of life (the neonatal or newborn period). Just three causes – infections, asphyxia, and preterm birth – together account for nearly 80% of these deaths.

4. The core principle underlying maternal, newborn and child health programmes should be the "continuum of care". This term has two meanings – a continuum in the lifecycle from adolescence and before pregnancy, pregnancy,birth and during the newborn period and a continuum of care from the home and community, to the health centre and hospital and back again. Skilled care during pregnancy, childbirth and in the postnatal period prevents complications for mother and newborn, and allows their early detection and appropriate management.

5. Three-quarters of all neonatal deaths occur during the first week of life, 25–45% in the first 24 hours .This is also the period when most maternal deaths occur. Forty seven percent of all mothers and newborns in developing countries do not receive skilled care during birth , and 72% of all babies born outside the hospital do not receive any postnatal care. These are the critical gaps in the continuum of care.

6. Even if birth occurs in a health facility, in many settings, mothers and newborns are discharged within a few hours, and have no further contact with a health provider until the 6 week postpartum and immunization visit. Births at home pose an even greater challenge for providing care to mothers and newborns during the critical hours and days after birth. This can be addressed by introducing home visits as a complementary strategy to facility-based postnatal care to increase coverage of care and improve newborn survival.

Causes of neonatal deaths

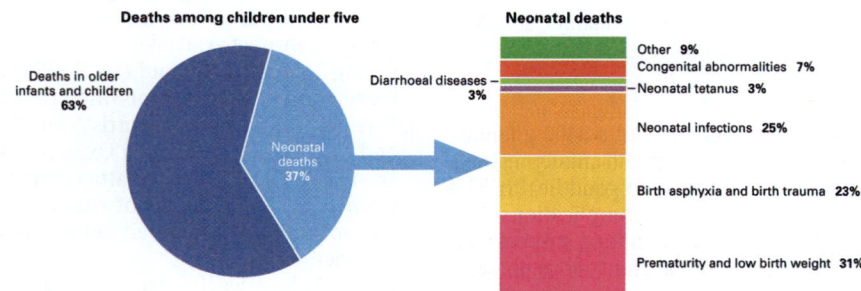

Source: World Health Organization. *The Global Burden of Disease: 2004 update.* World Health Organization, Geneva, 2008.

The lifecycle continuum of care

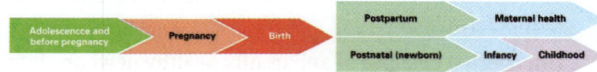

When should Home Visits be made? Home visits should be initiated as soon as possible after birth or after returning home from the facility. A visit within the first 24 hours after birth is likely to be most effective in reducing newborn mortality. Additional visits on day 3 and, if possible, on day 7 can improve home care practices and identify danger signs or illness.

Who can make the Home Visits? Postnatal care should be provided by skilled health workers. In many settings, this option is not feasible due, for example, to shortages of skilled health workers, lack of transportation, or a workload that does not allow them to make timely and repeated home visits. In such settings, many of the essential tasks for basic newborn care can be carried out by trained auxiliary health workers or trained community health workers who are either part of the health care delivery system or are linked to it.

What should be done at a Home Visit? Basic care for all newborns should include promoting and supporting early and exclusive breastfeeding, keeping the baby warm, increasing hand washing and providing hygienic umbilical cord and skin care, identifying conditions requiring additional care and counselling on when to take a newborn to a health facility (**see Box**). Newborns and their mothers should be examined for danger signs at home visits. At the same time, families should be counselled on identification of these danger signs and the need for prompt care seeking if one or more of them are present.

REFERENCE: WHO-UNICEF Joint Statement 2009

Newborn care during home visits in the first week of life

- Promote and support early (within the first hour after birth) and exclusive breastfeeding;
- Help to keep the newborn warm – promote skin to- skin care;
- Promote hygienic umbilical cord and skin care;
- Assess for danger signs and counsel on their prompt recognition and care seeking by the family (not feeding well, reduced activity, difficult breathing, fever or feels cold, fits or convulsions);
- Promote birth registration and timely vaccination according to national schedules;
- Identify and support newborns who need additional care (e.g. LBW, sick, mother HIV infected). If feasible, provide home treatment for local infections and some feeding problems.

Maternal care during home visits in the first week after birth

- Ask about mother's well being.
- Ask about excessive bleeding, headache, fits, fever, feeling very weak, breathing difficulties, foul smelling discharge, painful urination, severe abdominal or perineal pain. If she has any of these symptoms, refer her to a health facility for care.
- Ask for swollen, red or tender breast or nipples, manage breastfeeding problems if possible, if not, refer her to a health facility for care.
- Counsel about danger signs for mother and Newborn and advise on where to seek early care when needed.
- Provide birth spacing and nutrition counseling a These interventions should be delivered by appropriately trained and supervised health workers.

If home visits are done by a midwife or another skilled professional, care of the mother should include additional interventions as recommended in WHO IMPAC guideline, *Pregnancy, Childbirth, Postpartum and Newborn Care: A guide for essential practice.*

GUIDELINES ON ADMISSION TO NICU FROM HOME (HOME DELIVERY OR EARLY DISCHARGE)

The following guidelines cover admissions to the Newborn Service for babies who have been delivered at home, have been discharged early or recently from NICU/PNW , and in whom problems arise.

Eligible ages * <7 days old - infants should be admitted under the care of Newborn Services to either NICU or the postnatal ward, unless they fulfil <u>exclusion criteria</u>. This includes infants born at home. *Infants recently discharged (<48 hours) from NICU or the postnatal wards – some infants may be considered for readmission (if no evidence of acquired community infection).

Eligible conditions *Babies can be admitted under the care of Newborn Services if their primary problem requires *Neonatal expertise*. Examples include: *Low birthweight (including recent NICU/PNW discharge, if appropriate) *Early onset respiratory distress (1st 48 hours) *Seizures in the first 72 hours *Jaundice requiring treatment *Congenital malformations requiring assessment or treatment *Feeding difficulties requiring observation, maternal assistance, or NG feeding. These infants should preferentially be admitted to the postnatal ward so that the bonding between mother and baby is preserved.

Exclusions (exclusion criteria.)

* Infants with definite cardiac disease should be referred to the Pediatric Cardiology Service, if possible *Infants with surgical problems (e.g. bilious vomiting, bowel obstruction) that will not require intensive care support and who can be admitted to pediatric surgical ward. *Infants with suspected or definite infectious diseases in whom isolation is a priority (e.g. bronchiolitis, gastroenteritis, HSV, term infants presenting with apnea) should be admitted under the General Pediatric Service of the Hospital. .

Special considerations: *Some infants may initially be assessed in NICU (assessment room), prior to a decision about admission and destination. · Some infants may be admitted to the postnatal wards as boarder babies when their mothers are admitted with complications after delivery. · Ordinarily, these babies will not require medical care. · In the event that they require medical attention, the Neonatal team will assess them in the first instance. · If they require care that cannot be provided on the postnatal ward with their mother, they should generally be referred to the General Pediatric Service.

Isolation: *Ideally, infants who have been home should be separated from other infants in NICU and the postnatal wards. This may be via: · Nursing in incubators, or · Use of a single or isolation room (if infectious etiology is thought possible)

Other comments: There will be times when, due to workload or occupancy, admission under Newborn Services will not be feasible. In these circumstances, referral should be made to the General Pediatric Service.

REFERENCE Newborn Services Clinical Guideline Auckland, Newzealand

WHEN TO RETURN FROM HOME (HOME DELIVERY OR EARLY DISCHARGE)—UNICEF Guidelines for a Developing Nation—Newborn Care Charts Management of Sick and Small Newborns in Hospital

When to return immediately	Where	When	What for
• Breastfeeding poorly or drinking poorly	Return to the hospital	Immediately	Assessment, treatment and care
• Convulsions			
• Fever			
• Bleeding			
• Diarrhoea			
• Pus draining from the eyes	Return to the PHC clinic	Immediately	Assessment, treatment and care
• Skin pustules			
• Cord stump red or draining pus			
• Yellow skin or eyes (jaundice)			
When to return for follow up			
• All babies	PHC Clinic	• 3 days of age	• Weight gain
			• Jaundice assessment
			• Feeding assessment
• HIV exposed babies	PHC Clinic, OR PMTCT follow up clinic	• 6 weeks and normal routine	• Immunization
			• PCR
		• 6 weeks and monthly for first year	• Cotrimoxazole
			• Routine care
			• Immunization
• Babies who weighed < 2 kg at birth	Neonatal follow-up	• 3 days after discharge then weekly until 2.5 kg	• Weight gain
			• Feeding assessment
		• 6 weeks	• Immunization
HIGH RISK with following problems	High risk follow-up clinic	• 3 days after discharge	• Weight gain
• Birth weight < 1.5 kg		• Weekly until 2.5 kg	• Feeding assessment
• Meningitis or sepsis		• 4 months	• Developmental assessment
• Moderate or severe neonatal encephalopathy		• 9 months	
• Severe hypoglycemia			
• Required CPAP or IPPV			
• Major congenital abnormalities			
• Necrotizing enterocolitis			
• Severe jaundice			

GUIDELINES FOR ADMISSIONS TO NICU, AND DISCHARGES AND TRANSFERS FROM NICU

Admissions Guidelines for Admission to Level 3: Birthweight less than 1250g. Gestation less than 30 weeks. Some infants born at 30–32 weeks may be admitted to Level 3 because of staffing acuity. Requirement for intermittent positive pressure ventilation. Requirement for an exchange transfusion. Any other baby whose clinical condition is such that they cannot be appropriately cared for in Level 2.

Guidelines for Admission to Level 2: **Low Birthweight**: under 2500g. Some babies between 2000 and 2500g may be able to go directly to the postnatal ward. This will depend upon the clinical assessment of the baby and whether the postnatal ward is deemed likely to provide an appropriate level of care or not. **Prematurity** - 36 weeks gestation or less. For babies between 35 and 36 weeks gestation, criteria as in (1) apply. **Infection** - suspicion of infection together with clinical concern. **Respiratory problems :** (a) Apnea or cyanotic episodes. (b) Any respiratory distress causing concern. (c) Persisting signs of respiratory distress for more than one hour. **Gastrointestinal problems :** (a) Feeding problems severe enough to cause clinical concern. (b) Bile stained vomiting, or other signs suggesting bowel obstruction. **Metabolic problems :** Inability to maintain a serum glucose concentration greater than or equal to 45 mg/dL despite adequate feeding. **CNS problems :** (a) Convulsion. (b) Moderate birth asphyxia, which may require monitoring for an initial period to ensure problems do not ensue. **Malformations :** Congenital anomalies that may require intervention unavailable on the postnatal wards, or an initial period of observation, e.g. Pierre Robin Syndrome. **Cardiovascular Problems:** requiring monitoring or intervention unavailable on the postnatal wards. **Miscellaneous :** Any baby that is causing concern to such a degree that the attending doctor or NS-ANP feels that the baby requires observation or treatment in Level 2. It is better for a baby to be admitted unnecessarily than for a baby requiring admission to be left on the ward. **Social issues/terminal care :** Such babies ideally be nursed on the ward with parents, or at home. On occasions (after multidisciplinary consultation) circumstances dictate that these babies require a period of care on Level 2.

Discharge of Low Birthweight Infants: Infants that have been born at very low birthweight or low birthweight, represent an at risk group of children. Increasingly they are being discharged home at a weight less than 2.5kg. The following guidelines are suggested when considering discharge of such infants. The baby has to be **gaining weight** - it doesn't have to have reached any particular weight, however, as long as there is weight gain. The baby has to be **sucking all feeds**. If breast feeding is being established, it is not a prerequisite that the baby is on full breast feeding prior to discharge, provided we are happy that the baby is able to suck strongly. However we must be sure that the mothers are aware of the need to continue to monitor progress once further feeding changes are made at home, i.e. a switch from complementing to fully breast feeding etc. The baby must be able to maintain his or her **temperature** in a cot in a normal household environmental temperature. This is particularly important when discharging low birthweight babies home in the winter. **Parents must be willing and happy** to take the baby home and to have demonstrated that they have adequate parenting skills. This may be self-evident, particularly when there have been other children in the family, although not always. Some basic information should be known about the **home environment** and the community to which the infant is going, i.e. if they are living in a remote area in a caravan, then one would be less likely to effect a discharge home at a low birthweight. There should be adequate community **follow up** services available. It may be appropriate to contact the general practitioner by telephone to discuss follow up. In remote areas details should be known about the availability of a Well Child Service visiting. The Neonatal home care nurses will be able to provide some initial support and follow up and to provide liaison for ongoing community follow up.

Transfers & Discharges from NICU and PIN (Parents in Nursery) Transfers from Level 3: or transfers from Level 3 to Level 2 or PIN a formal transfer should occur between Level 3 Registrar or NS-ANP and the appropriate registrar or NS-ANP. *Ideally the parents would have been told a few days in advance to accustom to the transfer and possibly have looked around Level 2 or PIN. *A transfer letter should be in the notes (and should also be sent to the LMC/GP). *The problem list should be up-to-date (as should happen when a discharge/transfer summary is prepared) For infants discharged from Level 2 *Babies transferred to PIN need a formal letter if they have had a complicated course whilst in Level 2. If they have had a recent transfer summary from Level 3 to Level 2, this may not be necessary. *Babies who are transferred to PIN should have an up-to-date problem summary in the notes. *Babies transferred to other hospitals must not go without a registrar or NS-ANP letter.

Discharge Documentation: All patients discharged from hospital must have: *A full examination record on the appropriate form (include age in days, weight, length, head circumference). A plan for *follow up clearly documented in the case notes. *A record of any prescribed therapy.

Discharge Letters: No baby is to be discharged from Level 3, Level 2, or PIN without a letter. *For babies who are being discharged to the postnatal wards and where there are going to be delays in generating a discharge letter, the baby can be discharged without a letter being available. However, it is the responsibility of the resident team (registrar or NS-ANP) to ensure that a letter is completed as soon as possible and is filed in the notes of the baby. *PLEASE ENSURE that the discharge letter contains the correct information. *The database can only use the information available within it. *It provides a structure for the letter, and makes an attempt at providing a letter that is nearly complete. You need to check the letter you have produced and edit it in Word. *The quality of the letters you sign your name to reflects on your abilities as well as the quality of the care that the baby has received in NICU. PLEASE CHECK AND EDIT THE LETTERS BEFORE YOU SIGN THEM AND SEND THEM OFF.

1. *Effective and safe discharge* of a Newborn infant from the NICU or SCBU depends upon a *good discharge plan*; its essential features include *a)* begins early *b)* includes clearly defined goals *c)* individualized to meet infant & family needs & resources *d)* decreases delays in accessing care & progressing through the provider system *e)* community based *f)* anticipates potential delays in development & directs care towards prevention & early intervention *g)* increases quality of care *h)* decreases fragmentation & duplication of services.

2. Healthy, growing, preterm infants are considered ready for discharge *when they meet the following criteria: a)* ability to maintain temperature in an open crib *b)* ability to take all feedings by bottle or breast without respiratory compromise *c)* no apnea or bradycardia for 5 days *d)* steady weight gain (20–30 gm/day)

3. *Infants with special needs require a complex, flexible, ongoing discharge & teaching plan*: may involve primary care through a pediatrician, nurse practitioner, speciality services(ENT & audiologist, ophthalmologist, orthopedician, neurologist, cardiologist, nephrologist etc.,), infant follow-up programs & early intervention programs(physical therapy, social services, special education etc.)

4. The Neonatalogist should review the initial history, NICU hospital course, and physical examination at discharge and *compose an organized discharge summary* by systems or by problems, in chronological order of occurrence.

5. Once a decision has been made for discharge, *complete a check list of active problems & appointments* at discharge(see below for a concise checklist of discharge plan)

6. *Brief parents on common issues after discharge:* discuss home temperature and dressing the infant, intercurrent illness, and taking temperature, vomiting, bowel movement, diaper rash, sleeping, bathing, stuffy nose and its management, hiccups, crying, breathing pattern, interacting with the infant, going out, visitors and relatives, and a "no-smoking" policy inside the house. Review medications, nutrition and use of supplemental oxygen & the cardio pulmonary monitor as needed.

DISCHARGE CHECKLIST FOR HEALTHY NEWBORNS

Properly feeding the infant

Instruction on proper breastfeeding position, attachment, and adequacy of swallowing

Breastfeeding mothers should consult their physicians before taking any new medications.

Parents should not give their infant supplemental water or honey.

Breastfed and bottle-fed infants receiving less than 500 mL of formula per day should receive 200 IU of a vitamin D supplement per day.

Urination patterns

Six or more wet diapers per day is normal for a breastfed infant after the mother's milk has come in, as well as for bottle-fed infants.

Bowel movements

More than three bowel movements per day is normal in breastfed infants.

Bottle-fed infants may have fewer bowel movements.

Umbilical cord care

Instruction on proper cleaning

Skin care

Review of common rashes

Genital care

Instruction on proper care of circumcised or uncircumcised penises, as well as care of Newborn girls' genitals

Signs of illness

Axillary temperature of 100.5°F (38°C) or higher

Signs of dehydration, lethargy, poor feeding

Prevention of sudden infant death syndrome (SIDS)

Instruction on properly positioning the infant for sleep

Parental smoking cessation

Car seat selection and proper use

Follow-up appointment made at discharge

*Infants younger than 24 hours, follow up within 72 hours of age *Infants 24 to 48 hours of age, follow up within 96 hours of age *Infants older than 48 hours, follow up within 120 hours of age.

Recommendations for the discharge of high-risk lbw infants

- Resolution of acute life-threatening illness
- Ongoing follow-up for chronic but stable problems
  Chronic lung disease
  Intraventricular hemorrhage
  Necrotizing enterocolitis
  Ventricular septal defect; other cardiac lesions
  Anemia
  Cholestasis
- Stable temperature regulation
- Gaining weight on oral feedings
  Breast-feedings
  Bottle-feeding
  Gastric tube
- Free of significant apnea; home monitoring for apnea if needed
- Appropriate immunizations
- Hearing screenings
- Ophthalmologic examination < 27 wk or < 1,250 g at birth
- Mother's knowledge, skill, confidence documented in
  administration of medications (diuretics, methylxanthines, aerosols, etc.)
  Use of oxygen, apnea monitors; oximeters
  Nutritional support
    Timing
    Volume
    Mixing concentrated formulas
  Recognition of illness and deterioration
  Basic cardiopulmonary resuscitation
  Infant safety
- Scheduling of referrals
  Primary care provider
  Neonatal follow-up clinic
  Occupational therapy/physical therapy
  Imaging (head ultrasound)
- Assessment of and solution to social risks

*The recently published AAP monograph places high-risk neonates into *4 categories*: (1) the preterm infant, (2) the infant with special health care needs or dependence on technology, (3) infants at risk because of family issues, and (4) infants with anticipated early death.

*The 2008 AAP Guidelines on Hospital Discharge has indicated *6 critical components of the discharge-planning process*, as follows:

1. Parental education

2. Completion of appropriate elements of primary care in the hospital

3. Development of management plan for unresolved medical problems

4. Development of a comprehensive home care plan

5. Identification and involvement of support services

6. Determination and designation of follow-up care.

Guidelines for an early outpatient follow-up evaluation

History

Rhythmic sucking and audible swallowing for at least 10 minutes total per feeding ?

Baby wakes and demands to feed every 2 –3 hours (at least eight - ten feedings per 24 hours)?

Do breasts feel full before feedings, and softer after ?

Are there at least six noticeably wet diapers per 24 hours?

Are there yellow bowel movements (no longer meconium)- at least four per 24 hours?

Is baby still acting hungry after nursing (frequently sucks hands, rooting)?

Physical assessment

Weight, unclothed: should not be more than 8–10% below birth weight

Extent and severity of jaundice

Assessment of hydration, alertness, general well-being
Cardiovascular examination: murmurs, brachial and femoral pulses, respirations

Criteria for early newborn discharge

Contraindications to early Newborn discharge

1. Jaundice at < 24 hours

2. Mother treated with antibiotics in labor for GBS prophylaxis/UTI

3. Known or suspected narcotic addiction or withdrawal

4. Physical defects requiring evaluation

5. Oral defects (clefts, micrognathia)

Relative contraindications to early Newborn discharge (infants at high risk for feeding failure, excessive jaundice)

1. Prematurity or borderline prematurity (< 37 Weeks' gestation)

2. Birth weight < 2500 g

3. Baby difficult to arouse for feeding: not demanding regularly in nursery

4. Medical or Neurologic problems (Down syndrome, Hypotonia, cardiac problems)

5. Twins or higher multiples

6. ABO blood group incompatibility or severe jaundice in previous child

7. Mother whose previous breast-fed infant gained weight poorly

8. Mother with breast surgery involving periareolar areas (if attempting to nurse)

The major goals of the pediatrician or family practitioner who monitors a Neonatal ICU (NICU) graduate include the following:

- To provide an ongoing assessment of growth
- To evaluate the adequacy of nutrition
- To deliver preventive care
- To periodically examine the infant's, child's, or adolescent's motor, intellectual, and behavioral development.

REFERENCE: *AAP POLICY STATEMENT ON FOLLOW-UP OF A NICU GRADUATE UPDATE 2008*

*The diagnosis of an abnormal fontanel requires an understanding of the wide variation of normal. A newborn has six fontanels : the anterior and posterior, two mastoid, and two sphenoid.The rhomboid-shaped anterior fontanel, located at the juncture of the twoparietal and two frontal bones, is the most prominent. The superior sagittal dural venous sinus is partially situated beneath the anterior fontanel. The triangular posterior fontanel is located at the junction of the occipital and two parietal bones.

*The newborn's skull is molded during birth. The frontal bone flattens, the occipital bone is pulled outward, and the parietal bones override. These changes aid delivery through the birth canal and usually resolve after three to fivedays.The head of an infant born by cesarean section or from a breech presentation is characterized by its roundness.

 *The key feature of a normal anterior fontanel is variation. On the first day of an infant's life, the normal fontanel ranges from 0.6 cm to 3.6 cm, with a mean of 2.1 cm. Black infants have larger fontanels (1.4 cm to 4.7 cm). The fontanels of full-term and preterm infants are similar in size once preterm infants reach term. The fontanel can enlarge in the first few months of life, and the median age of closure is 13.8 months.

*By three months of age, the anterior fontanel is closed in 1 percent of infants; by 12 months, it is closed in 38 percent; and by 24 months, it is closed in 96 percent. Anterior fontanels tend to close earlier in boys than in girls; the initial size of the fontanel is not a predictor of when it will close.

*At birth, the average size of the posterior fontanel is 0.5 cm in white infants and 0.7 cm in black infants. The fontanel usually is completely closed by two months of age.

Examination of Fontanels: *Evaluate the newborn's skull for shape, circumference, suture ridges, tensionand size of anterior and posterior fontanels. *Calculate AF size by the average of the anteroposterior and transverse dimensions.*Examine the fontanels whilethe infant is calm and held in both supine and upright positions.Palpation of the fontanel in the upright position may reveal a normal, slight pulsation. If the fontanels are closed and intracranial pressure has increased, percussion produces a "crackedpot" sound (dull, lacking resonance), known as Macewen's sign.*Auscultate the AF to detect a bruit,in select cases, such as newborns with multiple hemangiomas or heart failure.which can indicate an arteriovenous malformation.*Note any associated dysmorphic facial features.*Detect asymmetry of the head by looking at the infant's head from above. *Monitor head circumference over time, as it is an important indicator of brain development,especially if a fontanel closes early.

Small fontanel or early fontanel closure: Fontanel closure that occurs as early as three months of age can be within normal limits, but careful monitoring of head circumference in such cases is essential to exclude a pathologic condition. The fontanel sometimes can be open but difficult to detect during a physical examination. Craniosynostosis and abnormal brain development are associated with a small fontanel or early fontanel closure.Examination at birth of an infant with craniosynostosis might reveal a ridge over a suture or lack of movement along a suture when alternating sides are gently pressed.Overriding of sutures from the normal molding process should resolve within the first few days of life. Later physical findings in infants with primary craniosynostosis include stunted cranial growth, increased intracranial pressure, proptosis, strabismus, and hearing impairment. Craniosynostosis is the premature closing of one or more cranial sutures, resulting in an abnormal head shape. The condition can be idiopathic or caused by hyperthyroidism, hypophosphatasia, rickets, or hyperparathyroidism. It is also associated with more than 50 syndromes, such as Apert's, Crouzon's and Pfeiffer's. The risk of primary isolated craniosynostosis is 0.4 per 1,000 live births, and the sagittal suture is most commonly involved. Abnormal brain development that results in microcephaly also can cause a small anterior fontanel or early fontanel closure. Prenatal trauma to the brain, such as maternal alcohol abuse, and postnatal trauma, such as hypoxia, are potential causes of microcephaly.

Differential Diagnosis of Microcephaly

Most common: Chromosomal defects, Congenital infections, Fetal alcohol syndrome, Hypoxic-ischemic encephalopathy,Normal genetic variation **Others:** Autosomal dominant or recessive types,Dysmorphic syndromes Malnutrition,Maternal phenylketonuria,Normal variation Structural brain defects,Universal craniosynostosis

LARGE FONTANEL AND DELAYED AF CLOSURE: The persistence of excessively large anterior (normal, 20 ± 10 mm) and posterior fontanels

has been associated with several disorders such as, Achondroplasia, Congenital hypothyroidism, Down syndrome, rickets, and increased intracranial pressure Others include Apert syndromeme,Cleidocranial dysostosis,Congenital rubella syndrome, Hallermann-Streiff syndrome, Hypophosphatasia, Hydrocephaly. An abnormally large anterior fontanel in conjunction with an open posterior fontanel can be an early sign of congenital hypothyroidism.A third fontanel between the anterior and posterior fontanels is associated with hypothyroidism and Down syndrome, but is seen in preterm infants. One of the signs of rickets is craniotabes, a softened outer table of the occipital bone that buckles under pressure, producing a reaction similar to a ping-pong ball indenting and popping back out. Craniotabes is not present at birth but develops over the first few months of life. Craniotabes can occur normally in premature infants and in children younger than six months.Soft areas in the occipital region suggest the irregular calcification and wormian bone formation associated with osteogenesis imperfecta, cleidocranial dysostosis, lacunar skull, cretinism, and occasionally, Down syndrome. Transillumination of an abnormal skull in a dark room or examination by ultrasound or computed tomography rules out hydranencephaly or hydrocephaly . An excessively large head (megalencephaly) suggests hydrocephaly, storage disease, achondroplasia, cerebral gigantism, neurocutaneous syndromes, or inborn errors of metabolism, or it may be familial. The skull of a premature infant may suggest hydrocephaly because of the relatively larger brain growth in comparison to that of other organs.

Bulging or sunken fontanels: Disorders associated with increased intracranial pressure can cause a bulging anterior fontanel. The most common disorders are meningitis, encephalitis, hydrocephalus, hypoxic-ischemic injury, trauma, and intracranial hemorrhage. Differential diagnoses for a bulging fontanel. Palpation may reveal a tense fontanel that feels similar to bone.Tumors also should be considered in the differential diagnosis of a bulging fontanel. Dermoid tumors of the scalp are the most frequent lesions presenting over the anterior fontanel and also may be found over the posterior fontanel.They usually are slow-growing and nontender, and they are twice as common among girls.The primary cause of a sunken fontanel is dehydration. Other signs include reducedperipheral perfusion, poor skin turgor, and sunken eyes.

Key points for Clinical Practice

1. An abnormal fontanel in an infant can indicate a serious medical condition. Therefore, it is important to understand the wide variation of normal, how to examine the fontanels, and which diagnoses to consider when an abnormality is found.

2. At birth, an infant has six fontanels. The anterior fontanel is the largest and most important for clinical evaluation. The average size of the anterior fontanel is 2.1 cm, and the median time of closure is 13.8 months.

3. The most common causes of a large anterior fontanel or delayed fontanel closure are achondroplasia, hypothyroidism, Down syndrome, increased intracranial pressure, and rickets. A bulging anterior fontanel can be a result of increased intracranial pressure or intracranial and extracranial tumors, and a sunken fontanel usually is a sign of dehydration.

4. A physical examination helps the physician determine which imaging modality, such as plain films, ultrasonography, computed tomographic scan, or magnetic resonance imaging, to use for diagnosis.

5. Consultation with a pediatric neurosurgeon should be considered if the diagnosis or presence of an abnormality is unclear.

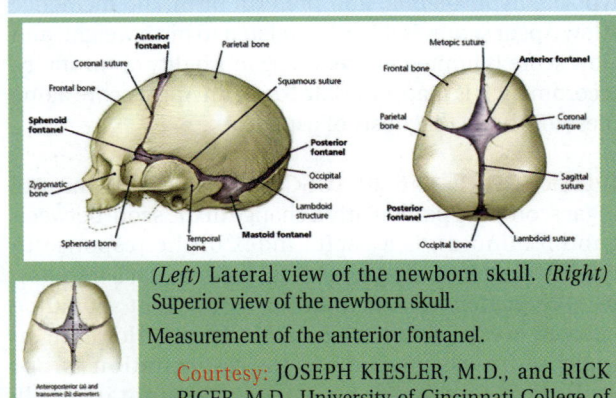

(Left) Lateral view of the newborn skull. *(Right)* Superior view of the newborn skull.

Measurement of the anterior fontanel.

Courtesy: JOSEPH KIESLER, M.D., and RICK RICER, M.D., University of Cincinnati College of Medicine, Cincinnati, Ohio

THE APGAR SCORING SYSTEM

	0	1	2
Appearance	Blue, pale	Body pink, Extremities blue	Completely pink
Pulse	Absent	Less than 100	100 or more
Grimace/reflex irritability	No response	Grimaces, cries	Cough, sneeze, vigorous cry
Activity/muscle tone	Limp, flaccid	Some flexion of extremities	Active motion
Respiratory effort	Absent	Slow, irregular	Good, crying

APGAR SCORES: 7-10= A Newborn in mild distress or one with no distress; no assistance needed other than gentle nasopharyngeal suctioning. 4-6= A Newborn in moderate distress, i.e. depressed respirations, flaccidity, and pallor or cyanosis. 0-3= A Newborn in severe distress/depression; immediate resuscitation is mandatory.

Apgar scoring system: Although an important tool in the assessment of a Newborn, it is not recorded until 1 and 5 minutes after birth. *If a Newborn requires emergency resuscitation at the instance of delivery, waiting until the first Apgar score is obtained could be disastrous.* The neonatal resuscitation program (NRP) guidelines state that "Apgar scores should not be used to dictate appropriate resuscitative actions, nor should interventions for depressed infants be delayed until the 1-minute assessment." However, an Apgar score that remains 0 beyond 10 minutes of age may be useful in determining whether additional resuscitative efforts are indicated The decision to begin resuscitative efforts and the Newborn`s response to resuscitation can be more accurately determined by evaluating the Newborn`s respiratory effort, heart rate, and color.

Limitations of the apgar score: It is important to recognize the limitations of the Apgar score. The Apgar score is an expression of the infant's physiologic condition, has a limited time frame, and includes subjective components. In addition, the biochemical disturbance must be significant before the score is affected. Elements of the score such as tone, color, and reflex irritability partially depend on the physiologic maturity of the infant. The healthy preterm infant with no evidence of asphyxia may receive a low score only because of immaturity. A number of factors may influence an Apgar score, including but not limited to drugs, trauma, congenital anomalies, infections, hypoxia, hypovolemia, and preterm birth. The incidence of low Apgar scores is inversely related to birth weight, and a low score is limited in predicting morbidity or mortality. Accordingly, it is inappropriate to use an Apgar score alone to establish the diagnosis of asphyxia.

APGAR SCORE AND RESUSCITATION: The 5 minute Apgar score, and particularly a change in the score between 1 and 5 minutes, is a useful index of the response to resuscitation. If the Apgar score is less than 7 at 5 minutes, the NRP guidelines state that the assessment should be repeated every 5 minutes up to 20 minutes. However, an Apgar score assigned during a resuscitation is not equivalent to a score assigned to a spontaneously breathing infant. There is no accepted standard for reporting an Apgar score in infants undergoing resuscitation after birth, because many of the elements contributing to the score are altered by resuscitation. The concept of an "assisted" score that accounts for resuscitative interventions has been suggested, but the predictive reliability has not been studied. To describe such infants correctly and provide accurate documentation and data collection, an expanded Apgar score report form is proposed.

Prediction of outcome: A low 1-minute Apgar score alone does not correlate with the infant's future outcome. A retrospective analysis concluded that the 5-minute Apgar score remained a valid predictor of neonatal mortality, but using it to predict long-term outcome was inappropriate. On the other hand, another study stated that low Apgar scores at 5 minutes are associated with death or cerebral palsy, and this association increased if both 1- and 5-minute scores were low. An Apgar score at 5 minutes in term infants correlates poorly with future neurologic outcomes. For example, a score of 0 to 3 at 5 minutes was associated with a slightly increased risk of cerebral palsy compared with higher scores. Conversely, 75% of children with cerebral palsy had normal scores at 5 minutes. In addition, a low 5-minute score in combination with other markers of asphyxia may identify infants at risk of developing seizures (odds ratio: 39; 95% confidence interval: 3.9– 392.5). The risk of poor neurologic outcomes increases when the Apgar score is 3 or less at 10, 15, and 20 minutes. A 5-minute Apgar score of 7 to 10 is considered normal. Scores of 4, 5, and 6 are intermediate and are not markers of increased risk of neurologic dysfunction. Such scores may be the result of physiologic immaturity, maternal medications, the presence of congenital malformations, and other factors. Because of these other conditions, the Apgar score alone cannot be considered evidence or a consequence of asphyxia. Other factors including nonreassuring fetal heart rate monitoring patterns and abnormalities in umbilical arterial blood gases, clinical cerebral function, neuroimaging studies, neonatal electroencephalography, placental pathology, hematologic studies, and multisystem organ dysfunction need to be considered when defining an intrapartum hypoxic-ischemic event as a cause of cerebral palsy.

OTHER APPLICATIONS : Monitoring of low Apgar scores from a delivery service can be useful. Individual case reviews can identify needs for focused educational programs and improvement in systems of perinatal care. Analyzing trends allows assessment of the impact of quality improvement interventions.

CONCLUSION : The Apgar score describes the condition of the newborn infant immediately after birth and, when properly applied, is a tool for standardized assessment. It also provides a mechanism to record fetal-to-neonatal transition. An Apgar score of 0 to 3 at 5 minutes may correlate with neonatal mortality but alone does not predict later neurologic dysfunction. The Apgar score is affected by gestational age, maternal medications, resuscitation, and cardiorespiratory and neurologic conditions. Low 1- and 5-minute Apgar scores alone are not conclusive markers of an acute intrapartum hypoxic event. Resuscitative interventions modify the components of the Apgar score. There is a need for perinatal health care professionals to be consistent in assigning an Apgar score during a resuscitation. The American Academy of Pediatrics and the American College of Obstetricians and Gynecologists propose use of *an expanded Apgar score reporting form* that accounts for concurrent resuscitative interventions.

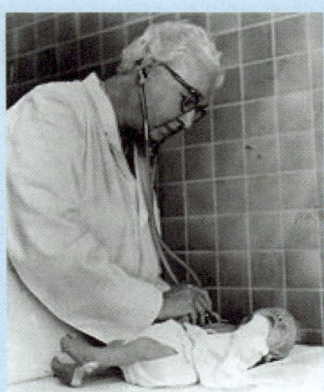 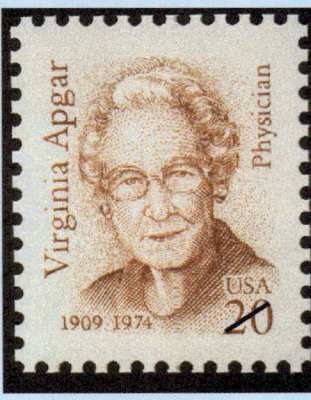 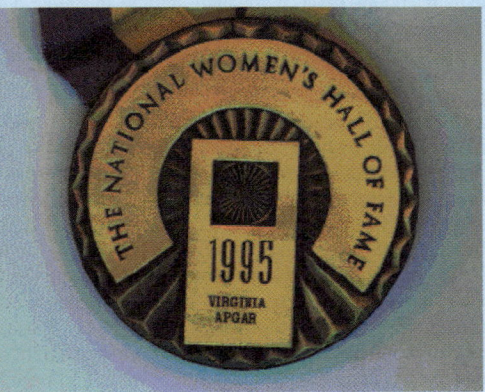

The **Apgar score** was devised in 1952 by Dr. Virginia Apgar as a simple and repeatable method to quickly and summarily assess the health of newborn children immediately after childbirth. Apgar was an anesthesiologist who developed the score in order to ascertain the effects of obstetric anesthesia on babies.

Acronym : The acronym **APGAR** was coined in the US as a mnemonic learning aid: **A**ppearance (skin color), **P**ulse (heart rate), **G**rimace (reflex irritability), **A**ctivity (muscle tone), and **R**espiration. The mnemonic was introduced in 1952 by the originator and pediatrician Dr. Virginia Apgar. The test has also been reformulated with a different mnemonic, **H**ow **R**eady **I**s **T**his **C**hild, but the criteria are essentially the same: Heart rate, Respiratory effort, Irritability, Tone, and Color.

References: 1) Apgar, Virginia (1953). "A proposal for a new method of evaluation of the newborn infant". *Curr. Res. Anesth. Analg.* 32 (4): 260–267. PMID 13083014. http://apgar.net/virginia/Apgar_Paper.html. 2) Finster M; Wood M. (April 2005). "The Apgar score has survived the test of time". *Anesthesiology* 102 (4): 855–857. doi:10.1097/00000542-200504000-00022. PMID 15791116. 3) Casey BM; McIntire DD, Leveno KJ (February 15, 2001). "The continuing value of the Apgar score for the assessment of newborn infants". *N Engl J Med.* 344 (7): 467–471. doi:10.1056/NEJM200102153440701. PMID 11172187. Retrieved from "http://en.wikipedia.org/wiki/Apgar_score"

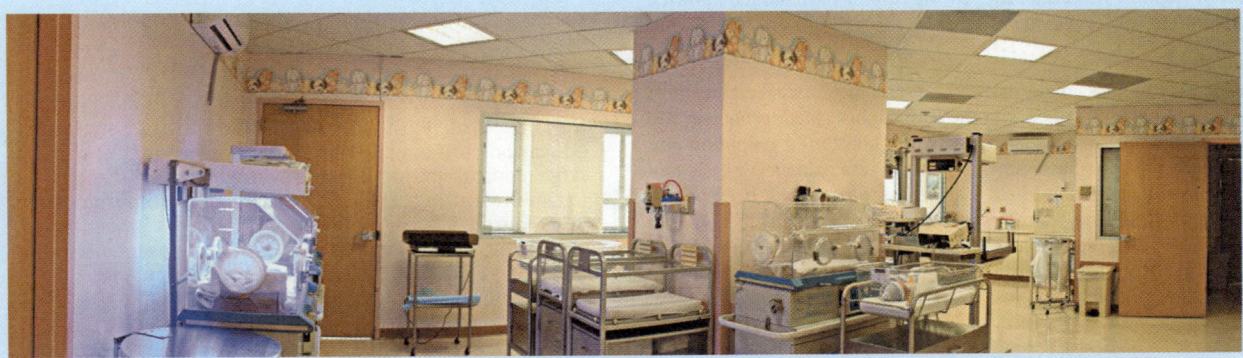

NICU MEDICOLEGAL PROBLEMS

Common areas of litigation for NICU claims are:

*Intravenous therapy complications *Infections *Brain damage *Medication errors *Dropped infants *Circumcision without consent *Breast milk errors *Retained foreign body *Detached retinas *Death

The most frequent allegations against neonatal nurses in NICU claims are:

*Failure to monitor *Failure to notify the physician of a change in the baby's condition *Delays in treatment *Failure to act *Failure to possess proper knowledge and competency *Failure to follow proper procedure *Negligence *Improper use of equipment *Failure to document adequately *Failure to follow the chain of command *Failure to provide appropriate neonatal resuscitation *Failure to treat neonatal hypoglycemia *Failure to treat group B strep infection Dunn and colleagues also cite failure to obtain informed consent, failure to perform appropriate telephone triage, inadequate staffing, improper delegation, and failure to assess the patient properly or in a timely manner as deviations that may increase nurse liability in a malpractice claim.

Nursing Documentation

An area of frequent concern to nurses is documentation and its legal implications. The chart should be a contemporaneous record of patient care. It is the legal record of events, and as such carries more weight in a legal proceeding than the nurse's memory of what occurred. Indeed, often-used adages such as "If it wasn't charted, it wasn't done," and "Documentation of care is synonymous with care itself" can turn into truths in the minds of experts and jurors who look for evidence of appropriate care in the medical record. If such evidence is not found, jurors can't assume that appropriate care took place. Nurses should document objectively the following information: patient's status, assessments, care rendered, physician notification, and response. The nursing process and critical thinking should be evident in the documentation. When patient care takes urgent priority and nurses find themselves documenting retrospectively, it should be clear that the note is retrospective or a late entry. There is no single best charting method for all settings. Some units employ narrative charting, some use unit-specific flowsheets, and others, charting by exception. Charting by exception, while timesaving, can leave nurses more vulnerable if department standards and protocols are not in place to guide and clarify this documentation method. In general, charting by exception is a less satisfactory method for nonroutine situations or those with unanticipated outcomes.

Back to Basics

Discussions of legal issues in nursing tend to get complicated, often dominated by laundry lists of hard-to-remember do's and don't's. Two of the most essential are: Know the standards of care in your area of specialty and follow them. It is the professional nurse's responsibility to keep current by reading up-to-date literature and attending continuing education or inservice activities to maintain knowledge and competency. Ignorance is not a satisfactory defense. Remember that the patient chart is the best evidence of the care you provide. And, just once in a while, review the definition of nursing and reflect on how well this describes your practice or where you see opportunities to grow: *Nursing is the protection, promotion, and optimization of health and abilities, prevention of illness and injury, alleviation of suffering through the diagnosis and treatment of human response, and advocacy in the care of individuals, families, communities, and populations.*

Neonatal Resuscitation

The delivery room is unique in that we resuscitate the smallest and most unstable of patients armed with the least sophisticated technology. We monitor the newborn's heart rate by auscultation or palpation and oxygenation by visual assessment of color. Pulse oximetry, a basic tool available in a small hand-held instrument, has still not been widely adopted for delivery room resuscitation. Deficiencies in neonatal resuscitation with medical-legal implications include delay in initiation of resuscitation, miscommunication, unavailable equipment, the perception of ineptness by close observers, and poor documentation of

delivery room events. Martin recommends that a code sheet be used to document the neonatal resuscitation as it occurs, and that a team member assume the role of recorder, just as in other patient code situations. Noninitiation of resuscitation can be both an ethical and a legal dilemma. Neonatal resuscitation must ordinarily be initiated without delay. If conversations with the parents did not take place prior to delivery, there is no time after the birth of the baby to consult the parents about their wishes regarding resuscitation of their newborn.

There are certain situations in which it is considered ethical *not* to initiate resuscitation: *Confirmed gestational age < 23 weeks *Confirmed birth weight < 400 g *Anencephaly *Confirmed trisomy 13 syndrome *Confirmed trisomy 18 syndrome* Possibly 23-24 weeks gestation if parents do not wish resuscitation. Practitioners are cautioned about making unalterable resuscitation decisions before the baby is born when the issue is prematurity. The infant may present with evidence of greater viability than anticipated. It is best to advise parents that decisions made before birth about neonatal management may need to be modified in the delivery room depending on the condition of the baby at birth and the postnatal gestational age assessment.

Hyperbilirubinemia

Kernicterus, a devastating, permanent form of neurologic injury caused by severe hyperbilirubinemia, is preventable. Failure to monitor and treat hyperbilirubinemia are among the root causes of kernicterus. Evidence-based guidelines for the management of hyperbilirubinemia were published by the American Academy of Pediatrics (AAP) in 2004. Martin recommends the following to prevent severe hyperbilirubinemia and possible kernicterus: *Don't ignore visible jaundice on the first day of life *Use bilirubin nomograms to identify high risk (> 95th percentile) *Check bilirubin levels *Follow babies discharged at < 72 hours of age in 24-48 hours *Don't ignore phone calls from parents *Don't let miscommunication or lab results delay treatment *Use intensive phototherapy In civil lawsuits, a number of deficiencies in care of the jaundiced neonate have been implicated as contributing to kernicterus *Not performing screening evaluations for jaundice *Incomplete charting about jaundice *Not recognizing high-risk conditions related to hyperbilirubinemia *Not performing a total serum bilirubin if jaundice is noted clinically *Not performing a total serum bilirubin if other clinical signs are present *Incomplete follow-up of the jaundiced neonate. Nurses should not make the mistake of thinking that improving the management of neonatal jaundice and prevention of severe hyperbilirubinemia are the responsibilities of physicians alone. In fact, nurses, who spend more time with newborn infants than any other health professional, play a highly significant role in the protection of newborns from the potential harms of hyperbilirubinemia. Nurses are the final safety net before the baby is discharged, an event that can take place many hours after the discharge exam. Nurses must use their professional judgment to ensure that babies are not discharged until any concerns about increasing jaundice have been communicated to the physician or nurse practitioner and the baby has been re-evaluated. Nurses must also make certain that parent(s) have been fully apprised of their infant's degree of and possible significance of hyperbilirubinemia and given specific instructions regarding home care and follow-up. Verbal *and* written instructions about jaundice are to be given.

Tips to Minimize Malpractice Risk * Stay current by reading journals and textbooks and by attending continuing education conferences * Maintain professional ties with a large medical center * If facing a difficult situation, consider consulting with a colleague * Maintain open communication with parents and families * Document procedures, communication, complications, who was present in a timely manner * Document telephone advice * If unsure, do not diagnose over the phone * Be aware of state laws that affect

REFERENCE: *The Current Legal Climate in Neonatology Medscape Nurses © 2008 Medscape, LLC*

Guidelines for health care professionals supporting families experiencing a perinatal loss :

Guiding parents through a perinatal loss is an essential part of caring and contributes to a normal grieving process. The role of the caregiver extends far beyond covering the physiological needs of the infant and starts at the first contact. By creating an atmosphere of trust between parents and caregivers, and a sense of attachment and bonding with the baby, a partnership will be formed between parents and caregivers, which should result in the most appropriate recommendations and decisions for that particular family. When giving bad news, both parents or one parent with another support person should be present. Simple language should be used, allowing time for listening and answering questions honestly. The best ways that a health care professional can support a grieving family are by offering a nonjudgmental, deep sense of caring and personal involvement. Before and after the death of a baby, parents should be allowed to spend as much time as is needed with their child. Health care staff has to create mementos that will serve as memories later on. Spiritual support should be made available, and the parents' cultural background should be respected. The latter is particularly important with regard to autopsy arrangements. Follow-up meetings to discuss autopsy results or to address unanswered questions also allow evaluation of and counselling for any type of pathological grieving process. All of the interactions need to take place in a quiet and relaxed environment, while avoiding feelings of pressure or urgency. More practical issues to be considered during and after a perinatal loss are summarized below and, given minor adjustments, are very similar for all members of obstetrical, paediatric or family care teams. The guidance provided always needs to be individualized, while keeping cultural and religious sensitivities in mind, particularly when the withdrawal of aggressive support is to be discussed. Parents who experience perinatal death under special circumstances, such as stillbirth with or without congenital anomalies or the death of a twin, deserve the same attention and support as those who experience the neonatal death of a singleton. Caregivers who provide this level of care will fulfill the unique needs of grieving parents by assisting them to have positive memories of their baby, and by giving them a feeling of being cared for in the midst of their pain and grief.

Important actions to take during and after the death of a baby:
*Assure parents that it is normal to feel uncomfortable at this time. *Allow parents to spend as much time as they need with their baby. *Make repeated offers for holding the baby. *Name the baby. *Provide privacy, but do not abandon the parents. *Encourage relatives and friends to see the baby, according to the parents' wishes *Warn about gasping and muscle contractions. *Reassure parents that their baby was not alone, not afraid and not in pain at the time of death. *Reassure parents that nothing more could be done *Provide mementos to create memories. *Ensure that spiritual support is available. *Take pictures *Explain the need and procedure for an autopsy. *Explain options and procedures for memorial services.

Communicating with Parents following Perinatal death

What to say and do	*What NOT to say or do*
Use simple and straightforward language	Do not say:"It's best this way"
Be comfortable showing emotions	"It could be worse"
"Cry when you feel like crying".	"You can have more children"
Listen to the parents and touch the baby	"Time will heal"
"I'm sorry"	"It's good your baby died before you got
"I wish things would have ended differently"	to know him or her well"
"I don't know what to say"	Do not use medical jargon
"I feel sad" or "I am sad for you"	Do not argue with parents
"Do you have any questions?"	Do not avoid questions
"We can talk again later"	

NORMAL GRIEF REACTION (Lindemann): A definite Syndrome! *includes the following Aspects:*

1. Somatic distress with tightness of the throat, choking, shortness of breath, need for sighing, and an empty feeling in the abdomen, lack of muscular power, and an intensive subjective distress described as tension, or mental pain

2. Preoccupation with the image of the deceased

3. Feelings of guilt and preoccupation with one`s negligence or minor omissions

4. Feelings of hostility toward others

5. Breakdown of normal patterns of conduct

Suggested contents of a memory box

The baby's memory box and photographs usually are taken home with the parents but may be kept with the social worker or other health-care member to be given to the parents at a later time if they desire.
*Locks of hair
*Hand and foot prints
*Hand and foot molds
*Record of baby's weight and length
*Identification bracelets and other mementos
*Photography or videography
–Digital cameras work best for this purpose
–Multiples should be photographed together, whether living or dead

REFERENCE: Pediatric Child Health Vol 6 No 7 September 2001
RECOMMENDED READING Church MJ, Chazin H, Ewald F. When a Baby Dies. Oak Brook: The Compassionate Friends Inc, 1981. Davis DL. Empty Cradle, Broken Heart: Surviving the Death of Your Baby. Golden: Fulcrum Publishing, 1996

The goals of palliative care for children and families are to prevent and relieve suffering and to support the best possible quality of life, regardless of the stage of illness or the length of that life. Palliative care is the comprehensive management of physical, psychological, social, spiritual, and existential needs. On the surface, it seems perfectly reasonable and natural that families should expect, and receive, this degree of comfort, compassion, and quality caring from healthcare professionals at what otherwise could be the darkest moments of their lives.Palliative care is both a philosophy of care and an organized, highly structured system of delivering care.

Palliative care begins with the diagnosis of a life-threatening/ terminal condition, and continues throughout the course of illness regardless of the outcome. Palliative care enhances the quality of life in the face of an ultimately terminal condition. Its focus is on the relief of symptoms (e.g., pain, respiratory distress) and conditions (fear, anxiety, isolation) that cause emotional distress. Palliative care is *early* and *ongoing*. It seeks to add life to the time the child has left, not to add time to the child's life. In the case of critically ill neonates, many of the healing components of palliative care (those meeting the cognitive, emotional, and spiritual needs) are geared more toward the infants' family members.

Hospice care refers to an organization or program that provides, arranges, coordinates, and advises on a wide range of medical and supportive services for patients with life-threatening illness and those close to them. A hospice is not a place per se, but a special way of caring that can be provided in a variety of settings, including the home.

End-of-life care is a term used in a general sense to refer to all aspects of care of a patient with a potentially fatal condition, or more narrowly to describe care that is focused on specific preparations for an impending death. The latter might include wishes regarding do-not-resuscitate (DNR) orders, tissue or organ donation, and plans for final moments, such as compassionate extubation (see below) or private family rituals.

Bereavement care is continuing care of the survivors who have experienced the loss of the infant. The survivors are not only the parents but siblings, grandparents, other relatives, friends, nurses, physicians, and other staff members who have cared for the infant.A vital precept of palliative care is that it can be delivered concurrently with life-prolonging care, or as the main focus of care. This is important because it simply isn't possible to tell with certainty which critically ill infants will survive and which will die. Even when death is considered fairly certain, it isn't always possible to predict when death will occur. Hope is a powerful and important element of palliative care for families. "Hoping for the best while preparing for the worst" can enable families to continue doing everything possible to help their child survive while accepting that death is likely and preparing for it.Critically ill neonates that are not expected to survive are often intubated and supported on mechanical ventilation. Thus, at some point, the issues surrounding when and how to discontinue mechanical ventilation become central in planning of end-of-life care. This is an event often dreaded by families; if carefully planned and executed, extubation can instead provide a truly sacred and meaningful final time together with their baby."Compassionate extubation" is the withdrawal of life support in the home, a hospice, or a home-like setting within the hospital, surrounded by loved ones. The infant is transported while still on life support to the extubation site. The entire procedure is personalized in accordance with the family's wishes, much like a birthing plan. Allowing families to choreograph the details is intended to make the experience as meaningful for them as possible. The family is told what is likely to occur once the endotracheal tube is removed, allowing them to plan how they would like to spend this time with their infant. Compassionate extubation requires collaboration between NICU staff and palliative care professionals and/or other individuals who will be involved in end-of-life or bereavement care. Because it is never possible to predict how long a baby will live once he or she is extubated, if the infant is being discharged, plans for home care, including durable medical equipment, oxygen, and medications, must be made in the event that the infant lives longer than expected. A planning conference should be held with the family and staff members who will be involved in carrying out the compassionate extubation protocol to ensure that everyone understands the family's needs and desired goals.

Family-Centered Care: Making a Difference

Palliative care of the neonate emphasizes family-centered care. Families of an infant with a life-threatening condition need to feel cared for and connected to healthcare professionals. They need to retain the right and responsibility to remain the parents to their infant, even if their infant is dying.families to choreograph the details is intended to make the experience as meaningful for them as possible. The family is told what is likely to occur once the endotracheal tube is removed, allowing them to plan how they would like to spend this time with their infant. Allowing them to have control whenever possible during a situation of overwhelming powerlessness is important in supporting their role as parents. Focusing on the human experiences of families will strengthen the connections between caregivers and families.

Other ways we can make a difference to families experiencing the death of an infant include:

- Providing information;
- Offering choices;
- Discussing both sides of all options;
- Giving families time to make difficult decisions or to be with their baby before or after death;
- Creating a space for privacy and intimacy, beyond just pulling a curtain or putting up a screen;
- Being sensitive to room location or activities going on near baby's bedside;
- Being present when needed;
- Being absent when needed;
- Striving for seamless continuity between areas of care/ changes of shift;
- Calling the baby by name, humanizing, not objectifying the baby;
- Using gentle touch and tone of voice;
- Offering to contact supports they desire (chaplain, clergy, social worker, friend);
- Being familiar with protocol for fetal/infant death; and
- Preserving keepsakes, using as many senses as possible to trigger memories.

Whenever possible, plan ahead to make the experience of dying as meaningful as possible for families. Ask parents how they would like to use the time that they will have with their baby. Some hospitals have rooms set aside for grief/bereavement ("Butterfly Rooms") providing home-like spaces for extended families to gather with the baby. Sumner points out that as we carry out our bereavement care procedures, it is the human element that we bring to the task that makes all the difference.

TEAMWORK AND COMMUNICATION IN THE NICU (Teaming Up for Safety)

Teams are 2 or more people who coordinate their activities to accomplish a common goal. Team members are interdependent, their roles are differentiated, and there is commitment from each to the success of the team. There is shared accountability for the performance and outcomes of the team. Within a bona fide team, communication is highly evolved. All teams are groups, but all groups are not teams.In clinical areas such as neonatal intensive care, it can be a challenge to assemble teams that work together long enough to achieve effectiveness over time, owing to rotating schedules, staff shortages, constantly changing groups of medical residents, and other factors. Blike suggested another model to address these situations, known as *crew resource management* (CRM). In CRM, individuals are trained for specific positions, or roles, on a team. Individuals trained to the same "position," then, are essentially interchangeable so that when people come and go, the team can still function effectively. The core values of the team (shared vision, communication, coordination, interdependence, and so forth) remain intact. Essential *teaming behaviors* are those that have been identified as key countermeasures to threat and safety in aviation, but they also have direct applicability to teamwork in clinical situations:

* *Team building*: leadership and communication;

* *Planning*: briefing and statement of plans, workload assignment, and contingency planning;

* *Execution*: monitor and crosscheck, workload management, vigilance, and automation management; and

* *Review and modification*: evaluation of plans, inquiry, assertiveness, adaptability, and conflict resolution

The following case illustrates an unfortunately common occurrence in healthcare: flawed teamwork related to deficiencies of interpersonal communication.

Scenario

While setting up the laryngoscope and endotracheal tube, the pediatric intensive care unit (PICU) physician gave a verbal order for atropine, etomidate, and rocuronium. Shortly thereafter, but prior to intubation, the child acutely desaturated. The team realized the patient received the paralytic agent prematurely. He was immediately intubated without difficulty and his respiratory status was stabilized.

Upon review of the event, the team discovered that the nurse, who was new to the PICU, had not realized the medication was a paralytic agent and thus administered it before the intubation tray was ready, resulting in the child's desaturation. The physician who ordered the medication had not indicated the timing of administration or that the medication was to be drawn up but not given until later.

Communication techniques that are used in teamwork models include:

Briefing: Concise and relevant information exchange. Sets the stage for good communication by involving others, sharing information, asking for input, making eye contact, and using first names. Briefings are used at the start of a day, before a procedure, when a situation is changing, or during "hand-offs."

Situation Background Assessment Recommendation (SBAR): An easy-to-remember mechanism useful for framing any conversation, especially a critical one that requires immediate attention and action. Although somewhat rote, it is beneficial in that it sets clear expectations for what will be communicated and how.

* *Situation*: What/who you are calling/asking about (patient name, etc.)

* *Background*: Pertinent data (history, current status/condition change, relevant signs and symptoms, labs, etc.)

* *Assessment*: Your assessment of the situation

* *Recommendation*: What you think should be done, what you are asking for

Assertion: The ability to speak up without hesitation, and with appropriate persistence, to impart critical information and/or solutions. Assertion involves getting the listener's attention, expressing concern, stating the problem, proposing an action, and reaching a decision. This is one of the most difficult communication skills for many people to acquire. Taking safety to the next level requires more than technology; it also needs a human factors approach. Teamwork-based models offer the most promise for improving safety within the current healthcare delivery system, but teams won't happen randomly. Teams require training and ongoing practice.Any team that doesn't practice regularly will find that its performance decays over time High-fidelity patient simulators are an ideal resource for practicing team behaviors, particularly in high-risk situational management. Future research will be needed to correlate teamwork models with improved clinical outcomes and measures of safety.

Recent research suggests that the organizational factors in the NICU are numerous and complex and could affect efforts to introduce teamwork models into this environment. Attempts to improve teamwork must "uncover and change deep-seated attitudes, beliefs, and histories of poor working relationships." There is a tremendous opportunity for nurses to participate at a very high level in the process of bringing genuine teamwork into their NICUs: *Educate yourself about teamwork. *Use teamwork principles and/or simulation when testing or evaluating new situations or equipment to practice without introducing patient risk. An example would be conducting a code with a neonate in a new radiology department. *Find out about teamwork training opportunities near you. Here is an online reference to see what one center offers; *a general search might produce more. *Assess your own staff's attitudes about working relationships and teamwork. *Conduct research utilizing teamwork models in/around the NICU.

CONCLUSION: *Communication failures account for the overwhelming majority of unanticipated adverse events in patients. *Medical care is extremely complex, and this complexity coupled with inherent human performance limitations, even in skilled, experienced, highly motivated individuals, ensures there will be mistakes. *Effective teamwork and communication can help prevent these inevitable mistakes from becoming consequential, and harming patients and providers. *Embedding standardized tools and behaviors such as SBAR (a situational briefing model), appropriate assertion, and critical language can greatly enhance safety. These tools can effectively bridge the differences in communication style between nurses, physicians, and others that result from the current educational process.

Potentially better practices (PBPs) for multi-disciplinary teamwork rarely stand alone and are an integral part of how the neonatal intensive care unit (NICU) community accomplishes its work.

Clear, shared goals and values

Communication among and between team members

Lead by example— "walk the talk"

Nurture collaboration with trust and respect

Live principled standards of conduct and excellence

Competent and committed team members

Commitment to conflict management

From: Implementing Potentially Better Practices for Multidisciplinary Team
Building: Creating a Neonatal Intensive Care, PEDIATRICS Vol. 111 No. 4 April 2003Collaboration,

TEAM ROLES & GOALS

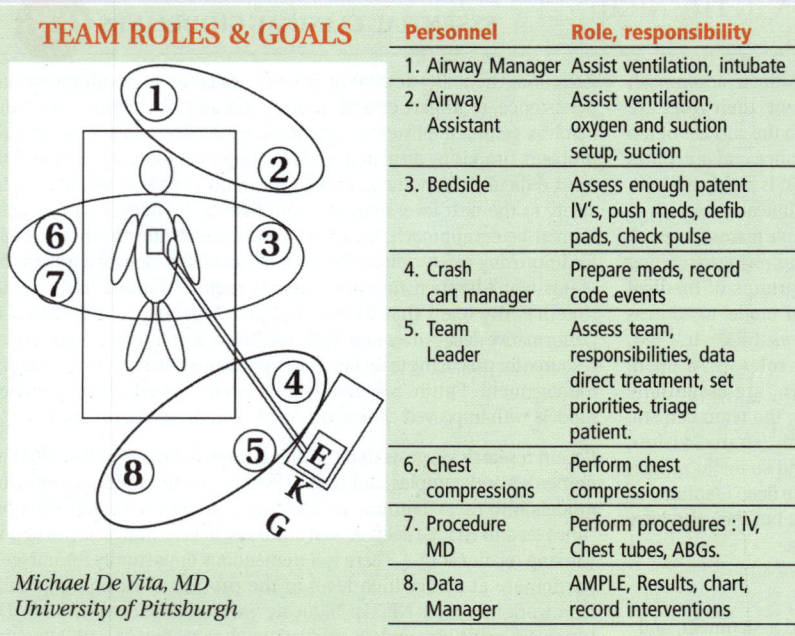

Personnel	Role, responsibility
1. Airway Manager	Assist ventilation, intubate
2. Airway Assistant	Assist ventilation, oxygen and suction setup, suction
3. Bedside	Assess enough patent IV's, push meds, defib pads, check pulse
4. Crash cart manager	Prepare meds, record code events
5. Team Leader	Assess team, responsibilities, data direct treatment, set priorities, triage patient.
6. Chest compressions	Perform chest compressions
7. Procedure MD	Perform procedures : IV, Chest tubes, ABGs.
8. Data Manager	AMPLE, Results, chart, record interventions

Michael De Vita, MD
University of Pittsburgh

Crisis response team members assemble around bedside in specific positions to perform delegated tasks. Positions are designed so that team members do not interfere with each other. (AMPLE is an eponym for critical code information: A = allergies, M = medications, P = past medical history, L = last meal, E = event). Copyright Dr. Michael DeVita. Winter Institute for Simulation Education and Research (WISER), University of Pittsburgh, Pittsburgh, PA. Used with permission. Roles are clearly delineated, there is no confusion about who will do what, and a stand-back leader is identified. Note that roles are defined by functions rather than by the type of person (physician, nurse, etc.) required.

Potentially better practices for the neonatal intensive care unit

* Collaboration comes first and weaves the fabric of all NICU activities. Clear, shared purpose, goals, and values.

* Teamwork is collaboration, coordination, communication, continuity, and competence (the 5 "Cs"). Effective communication among and between teams and team members. Nurture a collaborative environment with trust and respect.

* Responsibility for problem solving *must* be shared. Nurture competent and committed teams and team members.

* Successful quality improvement is driven by effective multidisciplinary teamwork. Live principled standards of conduct and standards of excellence.

* A healthy, respectful environment of ownership and pride is pervasive and contagious.

* Leadership is key—it sets the tone for everything Lead by example: "walk the talk". Address conflict, do not avoid it. Commit to conflict management.

* The NICU is a community—take the time to build trusting, respectful relationships *Make no assumptions.

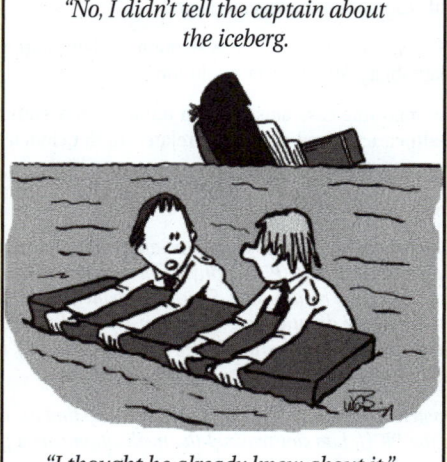

"No, I didn't tell the captain about the iceberg."

"I thought he already knew about it."

Teamwork and Quality during Neonatal care in the delivery room:
Definitions of team behaviors for Neonatal resuscitation

1. *Information sharing:* Providers verbally share information that relates to the assessment and treatment of the baby.

2. *Inquiry:* Providers question each other about the infant's clinical status, their assessment, and treatment plans.

3. *Assertion:* An individual provider asserts his or her opinion (through questions or statements of opinion) during *critical times*. Assertion *does not* include routine statements or questions about a baby's heart rate, tone, color, and respirations (these are part of information sharing or inquiry).

4. *Intentions shared:* A provider states their intentions before deviating from the norm. Statements about following routine Neonatal Resuscitation Program guidelines are not examples of intentions shared.

5. *Teaching:* Teaching is observed during the observation. This may be short and informal information exchanges. It may occur between any of the providers (e.g. nurses can teach residents and vice versa).

6. *Evaluation of plans.* An explicit discussion about the status of the baby and the decisions made to get to the current situation.

7. *Workload management.* The workload is distributed among those present at the resuscitation. Tasks are appropriately prioritized.

8. *Vigilance/environmental awareness.* Providers remain alert and focused on the resuscitation.

9. *Teamwork overall.* This is a global assessment based upon the ratings of behaviors 1–8 above. It may also include other observations such as dynamic 'give and take' among team members and nonverbal communication that are not explicitly defined in the behavioral markers.

10. *Leadership.* Leadership activities may include sharing of a mental model, assigning tasks, sharing of information and opinion. This may be rated for any provider at the resuscitation.

Courtesy: E J Thomas, J B Sexton, R E Lasky, R L Helmreich, D S Crandell and J Tyson *Journal of Perinatology* (2006) **26**, 163–169.

COMPETENCY FOR NORMAL NEWBORN NURSERY

COMPETENCY 1—Patient Care: Provide family centered patient care that is developmentally and age appropriate, compassionate, and effective for the treatment of health problems and the promotion of health.

1. Obtain and interpret from the families and other healthcare providers important information relevant to the newborn, including the maternal medical, prenatal, family and obstetrical history.

2. Assess the newborn, using the history, physical exam, and routine laboratory screening procedures and provide preventive counseling for intervention as indicated.

3. Perform a neonatal physical examination and identify normal and abnormal findings related to: * Gestational age assessment and growth. *Vital signs and measurements. * General appearance and identification of anomalies. *Examination of head, eyes, ears, nose and throat. *Neck and clavicle. *Neurological system. *Respiratory system. *Skin. *Chest and breasts. *Heart. *Lungs. *Abdomen (including the umbilical cord). *Genitalia. *Heart and brachial and femoral pulses. *Hips. *Extremities.

4. Describe the current Newborn Infant Screening Program for Metabolic and Inherited Diseases.

5. Describe the procedure for the normal newborn hearing screens.

6. Describe the rationale for the use of eye prophylaxis, vitamin K administration and hepatitis B vaccine and immune globin.

7. Discuss the immediate feeding of infants whether breast feeding or bottle feeding.

8. Discuss the role of the newborn nursery physician in counseling and interacting with the obstetrician and the patients long term caregiver.

9. Discuss the rationale behind rooming in, on demand feeding, early discharge of newborn infant and various feeding regimes.

10. Explain the normal physiologic changes in the neonatal transition period, signs of abnormal responses and possible strategies for intervention.

11. Know the current recommendation for the maternal group B streptococcus, screening and evaluation of the newborn exposed infants.

12. Demonstrate appropriate use of the screening tests, our protocols for various problems such as hypoglycemia, elevated temperatures, positive coombs test and polycythemia.

13. Demonstrate the appropriate use of testing to identify possible prenatal exposure to substances of abuse.

14. Provide anticipatory guidance and prevention counseling throughout the hospital stay and the time of discharge to the new parents.

COMPETENCY 2—Medical Knowledge

Understand the scope of established and evolving biomedical, clinical, epidemiological and social-behavioral knowledge needed by a pediatrician; demonstrate the ability to acquire, critically interpret and apply this knowledge in patient care.

1. Recognize, describe the clinical significance of and develop a strategy to evaluate and manage and/or refer newborn with these common newborn signs and symptoms. *Large birthmarks such as; mongolian spots, hemangiomas, port wine stains. *Rashes and markings secondary to birth trauma. *Papular and pustular rashes in the nursery. *Cyanosis. *High or low temperature. *Tachypnea. *Heart murmurs. *Abdominal distension and masses. *Two-vessel cords. *Abnormal findings on the Barlow or Ortolani. *Swollen breasts. *Jaundice *Vaginal bleeding. *Subconjunctival hemorrhages. *Corneal opacities or absent red reflex. *Facial palsy. *Fractured clavicles. *Brachial plexus injuries. *Cephalohematomas or caputs. *Ear tags and pits. *Palate abnormalities. *Polydactyly. *Syndactyly. *Plethora. *Pallor. *Respiratory distress. *Abdominal masses. *Genital urinary abnormalities including ambiguous genitalia, hypospadias, undescended testicles. *Microcephaly. *Macrocephaly.

2. Evaluate and appropriately treat newborns with commonly presenting conditions including:

   *Large or small for gestational age babies. *Infant of a diabetic mother. *Infant of a substance abusing mother. *Child with ABO or Rh incapability. *Polycythemia *Premature/ Postmature infant. *Jitteriness. *Transient metabolic disturbances such as hypoglycemia. *Delayed urination. *Delayed stooling. *Vomiting feeds or bilious emesis. *Poor or delayed sucking in feeding. *Respiratory distress with feedings. *Jaundice. *Infant with risk factors for developmental dysplasia of the hips. *Infants with abnormalities on prenatal ultrasounds. *Dysmorphic infants or infants with a known chromosomal abnormality. *Multiple births. *Eye discharge. *Abnormal newborn screening results. *Infants born to a mother with significant medical conditions such as lupus, seizure disorder or any other obstetrical abnormalities.

3. Being knowledgeable in the various methods of breast and bottle feedings in the newborn.

4. Assess and manage common infections in the normal newborn nursery. *Discuss the methods for screening and where appropriate, preventive treatment of the mother with chlamydia, CMV, gonorrhea, group B strep, hepatitis B, hepatitis C, HIV, tuberculosis, HPV, rubella, HSV, parvovirus, syphilis, toxoplasmosis and varicella. 5. Recognize and manage: *Newborns with signs of sepsis such as fever, poor feeding, tachypnea, a low temperature. *Infants born to a mother with a fever. *Infants born to a mother with a history of prenatal infectious diseases such as: group B strep, chlamydia, herpes simplex virus, syphilis, HIV. *Infant born to a mother with prolonged rupture of membranes. *Infant born to a mother who received antibiotic therapy.

COMPETENCY 3—Communication skills. Demonstrate interpersonal and communication skills that result in information exchange and partnering with patients, their families and professional associates.

1. Obtain record and present the history and physical examination including the maternal, obstetrical and newborn history.

2. Be able to explain to the parents of a newborn the status of their child, any abnormalities, any follow-up or work-up that is necessary.

3. Be able to guide and provide anticipatory guidance at nursery discharge as it relates to the normal newborn behavior, family adjustment, injury prevention and assess to medical services.

4. Motivate and instruct the parents in the care of the normal newborn in order to improve the well being and safety of the infant in the initiation of long term care management.

5. Demonstrate sensitivity in communicating with parents of infants who have various problems and how these might impact on their family life and future plans for this child.

COMPETENCY 4. Practice-based Learning and Improvement. Demonstrate knowledge, skills and attitudes needed for continuous self-assessment, using scientific methods and evidence to investigate, evaluate, and improve one's patient care practice.

1. Identify and utilize standardized guidelines and protocols for the evaluation and treatment of a normal newborn infant in a the nursery.

2. Use information technology to access and manage clinical information, perform online searches and to acquire knowledge of specific topics including the current information on the various newer treatments used in the care of the normal newborn.

3. Identify personal learning needs, organize relevant information and resources for future reference and plan for continuing acquisition of new data.

4. Explore with the faculty how to keep up to date in the area of the normal newborn nursery and to continue to incorporate new knowledge in the care of the patients.

COMPETENCY 5. Professionalism. Demonstrate a commitment to carrying out professional responsibilities, adherence to ethical principles, and sensitivity to diversity.

1. Display behaviors in the normal new born nursery that foster and reward the patient' trust in the physician. These may include appropriate dress, grooming, punctuality, honesty, courteously, respect for the patient confidentially and other norms of behavior in professional relationships with the patients.

2. Be sensitive to the ethical and cultural differences that one may encounter in child rearing practices.

3. Respect confidentially and the privacy of the patients especially when discussing matters which may be sensitive to the patients.

4. Work as a member of the healthcare team in the newborn nursery in providing care to the newborn.

5. Be an advocate for the interests of the normal newborn over your own personal interest while developing an appropriate balance between personal and professional beliefs and the obligations you have to your patient.

COMPETENCY 6. System Base Practice. Understand how to practice quality health care and advocate for patients within the context of the health care system.

1. Describe the impact of the economic and health insurance issues on the care of the normal newborn especially has this relates to the early discharge and follow-up of infants.

2. Be able to interact well with the primary care givers in order to insure a smooth transaction

3. Discuss the role of the various social and legal systems involved in the infants who are suspected of being drug exposed.

4. Work within the system to provide access and to coordinate and improve patient care while advocating maintaining high quality.

Systematic approach to curriculum development

Step 1
Perform a needs assessment

Step 5
Evaluate & modify the curriculum

Step 2
Define goals and learning objectives

Step 4
Develop educational strategies and implement the curriculum

Step 3
Identify resources

To ensure that the learners are actively engaged with the curriculum, find the content meaningful, and can apply and retain new knowledge and skills, curriculum designers should use Bloom's taxonomy as a guide when creating learning objectives. This multi-tiered model classifies educational objectives according to **six cognitive levels** of increasing complexity: *knowledge, comprehension, application, analysis, synthesis, and evaluation.* To engage the learners in higher-order thinking and deep understanding of concepts, mastery of the lower levels is required.

COURTESY: Dr Asha Mandava, MD Illinois State US

Regionalized systems of perinatal care are recommended to ensure that each newborn infant is delivered and cared for in a facility appropriate for his or her health care needs and to facilitate the achievement of optimal outcomes. The functional capabilities of facilities that provide inpatient care for newborn infants should be classified uniformly, as follows:

*Level I (basic): a hospital nursery organized with the personnel and equipment to perform neonatal resuscitation, evaluate and provide postnatal care of healthy newborn infants, stabilize and provide care for infants born at 35 to 37 weeks' gestation who remain physiologically stable, and stabilize newborn infants born at less than 35 weeks' gestational age or ill until transfer to a facility that can provide the appropriate level of neonatal care.

*Level II (specialty): a hospital special care nursery organized with the personnel and equipment to provide care to infants born at more than 32 weeks' gestation and weighing more than 1500 g who have physiologic immaturity such as apnea of prematurity, inability to maintain body temperature, or inability to take oral feedings; who are moderately ill with problems that are expected to resolve rapidly and are not anticipated to need subspecialty services on an urgent basis; or who are convalescing from intensive care. Level II care is subdivided into 2 categories that are differentiated by those that do not (level IIA) or do (level IIB) have the capability to provide mechanical ventilation for brief durations (less than 24 hours) or continuous positive airway pressure.

*Level III (subspecialty): a hospital NICU organized with personnel and equipment to provide continuous life support and comprehensive care for extremely high-risk newborn infants and those with complex and critical illness. Level III is subdivided into 3 levels differentiated by the capability to provide advanced medical and surgical care.

*Level IIIA units can provide care for infants with birth weight of more than 1000 g and gestational age of more than 28 weeks. Continuous life support can be provided but is limited to conventional mechanical ventilation.

*Level IIIB units can provide comprehensive care for extremely low birth weight infants (1000 g birth weight or less and 28 or less weeks' gestation); advanced respiratory care such as high-frequency ventilation and inhaled nitric oxide; prompt and on-site access to a full range of pediatric medical subspecialists; and advanced imaging with interpretation on an urgent basis, including computed tomography, magnetic resonance imaging, and echocardiography and have pediatric surgical specialists and pediatric anesthesiologists on site or at a closely related institution to perform major surgery. Level IIIC units have the capabilities of a level IIIB NICU and are located within institutions that can provide ECMO and surgical repair of serious congenital cardiac malformations that require cardiopulmonary bypass.

Uniform national standards such as requirements for equipment, personnel, facilities, ancillary services, and training, and the organization of services (including transport) should be developed for the capabilities of each level of care.

Population-based data on patient outcomes, including mortality, specific morbidities, and long-term outcomes, should be obtained to provide level-specific standards for volume of patients requiring various categories of specialized care, including surgery.

TABLE 1: Definitions of Hospital—Based Newborn Services

Basic neonatal care (level I)

Well-newborn nursery

* Evaluation and postnatal care of healthy newborns

* Neonatal resuscitation

* Stabilization of ill newborns until transfer to a facility at which specialty neonatal care is provided

Specialty neonatal care (level II)

* Special care nursery

* Care of preterm infants with birth weight 1500 g

* Resuscitation and stabilization of preterm and/or ill infants before transfer to a facility at which newborn intensive care is provided

Subspecialty Neonatal Intensive Care (level III)

* Level IIIA

  Hospital or state-mandated restriction on type and/or duration of mechanical ventilation

* Level IIIB

  No restrictions on type or duration of mechanical ventilation

  No major surgery

* Level IIIC

  Major surgery performed on site (e.g., omphalocele repair, tracheoesophageal fistula or esophageal atresia repair, bowel resection, myelomeningocele repair, ventriculoperitoneal shunt)

  No surgical repair of serious congenital heart anomalies that require cardiopulmonary bypass and /or ECMO for medical conditions

* Level IIID Major surgery, surgical repair of serious congenital heart anomalies that require cardiopulmonary bypass, and/or ECMO for medical conditions

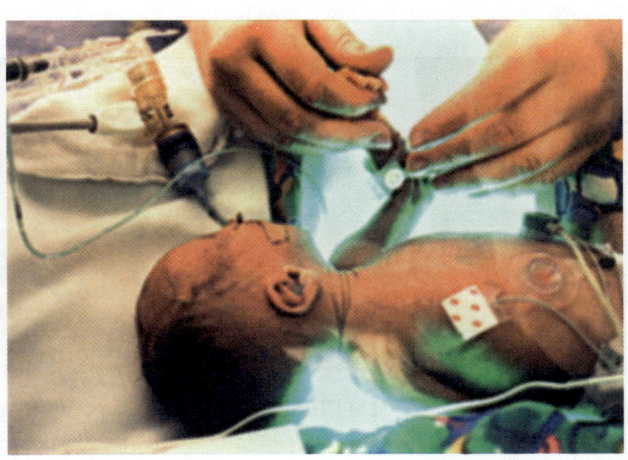

REFERENCE : *Stark AR, Couto J. Levels of neonatal care. Pediatrics 2004 Nov;114(5):1341-7. [47 references]* <u>PubMed</u>

DECISION-MAKING REGARDING CRITICALLY ILL INFANTS IN THE NEONATAL INTENSIVE CARE UNIT

Ethical dilemmas are felt most acutely when an infant's prognosis is very poor and, ultimately, uncertain. Although many extremely premature infants experience serious complications, some do have good outcomes. Asphyxiated infants can recover from apparently devastating brain injuries. Conveying uncertainty to parents about their infant's diagnosis, treatment, or outcome can be very difficult. Health care professionals may worry that discussing uncertainty with parents can create overly optimistic beliefs regarding probable outcomes. In addition, uncertainty may result in disagreement among providers regarding the most appropriate management course. Such conflicts only intensify the moral distress for all involved, and neonatologists often receive little training to resolve conflicting opinions in the face of ethically complex scenarios. *Best practices for decision-making before, during, and after birth are unclear. Current guidelines emphasize parent/provider collaboration when an infant's prognosis is very poor.*

Deciding to resuscitate extremely premature babies: how do parents and neonatologists engage in the decision?
A decision making model in which the physician remains neutral may, in fact, not leave parents feeling autonomous, but rather may leave them feeling abandoned. Whether health care professionals are being adequately trained to explore parents' preferred decision-making role warrants further exploration.

Medical staff guidelines for periviability pregnancy counseling and medical treatment of extremely premature infants.
The guidelines range from no resuscitation offered at <23 weeks' gestational age (GA), to resuscitation not recommended at $23^{0/7}$ to $23^{6/7}$ weeks' GA, to resuscitation offered but not obligatory at $24^{0/7}$ to $25^{6/7}$ weeks' GA, to resuscitation in the majority of cases at $26^{0/7}$ to $26^{6/7}$ weeks' GA. Parental decision-making is influenced less by biomedical data regarding morbidity and mortality, and is based more solidly on parents' hope, faith, and focused spirituality. A gap exists between neonatologists' philosophical agreement with a model of shared decision-making and a common practice of unilateral decision-making. This gap provides an opportunity to explore the practical, intellectual, emotional, and psychosocial barriers associated with shared decision-making. Educational models that explore the nuances and values of clinicians, and the benefits and burdens of therapies, are needed to begin to shift the practice patterns.

Making sense of suffering and death: how health care providers construct meanings in a Neonatal Intensive Care Unit.
Given the frequency with which NICU clinicians are faced with newborn death and disability, moral distress is not uncommon. The religious, spiritual, and existential concerns are a part of many NICU providers` reactions to infant and family suffering. There may be a significant common ground in the way that families and health care professionals make meaning of Neonatal illness and death. Given the complexity and depth of meaning associated with end-of-life care in the NICU, opportunities for clinicians to integrate their ethical, spiritual, and religious perspectives into practice could support their well-being and may minimize burnout.

Infant end-of-life care: the parents' perspective.
The lifelong grief associated with an infant's death can fuel clinician concerns that parents may be irrevocably burdened by their involvement and responsibility in rendering decisions about their infant's treatment. clinicians and health care institutions can improve care for infants and families at the end of life and impact parental grief. Relationships among families, clinicians, and interdisciplinary team members are critical. Building trustworthy relationships involves sustained engagement, honesty, and a witnessing presence. Instead of viewing grief as exclusively negative, clinicians can help parents find opportunities to review, validate, and reframe decisions.

Managing the Situation:
A strategy for helping parents through end of life decisions on neonatal units should embrace a continuum of support extending from discussion about the possibility of withdrawing intensive care, through to the management of the dying baby, the request for necropsy, subsequent explanation of the possible significance of the results, and, when appropriate, bereavement support. Neonatal staff have their needs too, and it is easier to be caring and compassionate when we are at ease with our own thoughts and feelings surrounding end of life decisions. This is more likely in neonatal units where there is leadership, teamwork, and a forum for discussing ethical issues. In their absence, end of life decisions challenge staff each time as though it was a new experience, and conflicting and unclear advice may be given to parents, reflecting uncertainties and conflicts between staff members. **CARING IN SILENCE:** Sometimes intensive care for a critically ill infant is continued because no one, least of all the parents, feel comfortable about questioning whether it is right to continue. Consultants and senior nurses need to engage staff in decision making and recognise those unspoken signals that reflect staff desperation and despair.

Unspoken signals that staff wish to consider withdrawal of intensive care
1. *Standing off on clinical rounds*: disgruntled staff turn away as though disinterested in contributing to further management. 2. *Exaggeration of clinical signs*: overemphasising adverse signs reflects despair that cannot be expressed in another way. 3. *Therapeutic nihilism*: all suggested treatments are rejected by desperate staff on the basis of their side effects instead of a willingness to consider the balance of risks. 4. *The incongruous search for the expert*: paradoxically staff may want to call in an "expert" such as a nephrologist or cardiologist to advise on organ system failure (presumably in the hope that a firm lead will be taken to withdraw intensive care). 5. *Group formation among staff*: small groups form and discuss *among themselves* the futility of continuing intensive care. 6. *Allegations of parental lack of information*: in spite of frequent discussion with parents about their infant's progress, staff insist that the parents haven't been informed and don't know how ill their infant is.

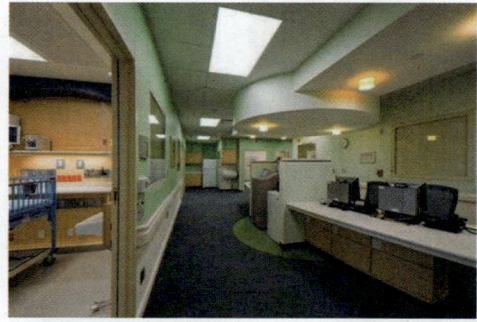 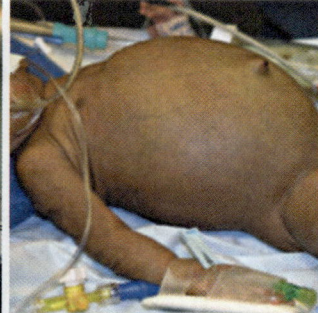 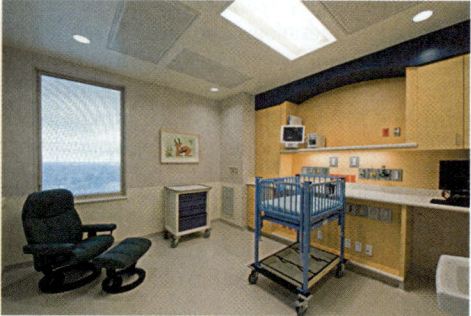

Courtesy: MALCOLM CHISWICK *St Mary's Hospital for Women and Children, Whitworth Park, Manchester M13 0JH, UK*
m.chiswick@man.ac.uk

REFERENCE : *2009 JHUSOM, IJHN, and eNeonatal Review* **October 2009: VOLUME 7, NUMBER 1**

GUIDELINES TO REDUCE RISK OF COMPLICATIONS FROM CENTRAL VASCULAR CATHETERS

CENTRAL VENOUS CATHETERS:

1. Use strict aseptic precautions for insertion and maintenance of the catheter, including dressing changes, tubing connections, and medication administration.

2. Ensure that blood can be aspirated freely into the catheter when it is inserted before it is taped into position. Confirm the location of the catheter tip radiographically (using radio-opaque contrast if necessary) on initial insertion. Repeat radiographs if there is any question of catheter movement or malfunction. Scrutinize radiographs obtained for any reason for appropriate catheter position.

3. The tip of the CVC should be just above the superior vena cava/right atrium junction for insertions from the upper extremity and at the IVC/right atrium junction for insertions from the lower extremity or the umbilical venous catheter.

4. Inspect the insertion site daily. Transparent dressings should be changed every 7 days except when the risk of dislodging the catheter outweighs the benefit of changing the dressings. Replace all damp, loose, or soiled dressings.

5. Add heparin (0.5–1 unit/ml) of intravenous fluids being infused.

CENTRAL ARTERIAL CATHETERS:

1. Remove catheter as soon as medically feasible, if it is obstructed or if there is evidence of thrombosis or infection.

2. Use strict aseptic precautions for insertion and maintenance of the catheter, including dressing changes and tubing connections.

3. Monitor extremities for signs of vascular compromise frequently: examine tips of fingers or toes for peripheral catheters, the lower extremities including buttocks for UACs.

4. Infuse catheters with heparinized saline continuously. Avoid the administration of any other medication, fluid, or blood transfusions through the arterial catheter.

5. Remove catheters as soon as medically feasible or if there are signs of vascular compromise or suspicion of thrombosis.

REFERENCE: *CLINICS IN PERINATOLOGY VOLUME 35 NO1, MARCH 2008*

Modified list of jcaho's 2008 patient safety goals pertaining to medication errors

1. Improve the accuracy of patient identification (use at least two patient identifiers).

2. Improve the effectiveness of communication among caregivers. Read back the verbal orders or test results.
   i. Standardize a list of abbreviations and symbols that are not to be used.
   ii. Improve the timeliness of reporting and receipt of critical test results and values.

3. Improve the safety of using medications. Identify and review *look-alike and sound-alike drugs :* label all medications on and off the sterile field.

   i) Reduce errors associated with use of anticoagulation therapy.

4. Accurately and completely reconcile medications across the continuum of care.
   i. Compare the patient's current medications with those ordered for the patient.
   ii. Communicate the patient's medications to the next provider of service when a patient is referred or transferred to another setting, and review the complete list of medications to the patient on discharge.

5. Encourage patients' active involvement in their own care as a patient safety strategy. Define and communicate the means for patients and their families to report concerns about safety and encourage them to do so.

REFERENCE: *CLINICS IN PERINATOLOGY VOLUME 35 NO1, MARCH 2008*
JCAHO (Joint Commision on Accreditation of Healthcare Organizations)

Iatrogenic disorders in modern neonatology

a. Diagnostic
- Error or delay in diagnosis
- Failure to use indicated tests
- Use of outmoded tests or therapy
- Failure to act on results of monitoring or testing

b. Treatment
- Error in the performance of an operation, procedure, or test
- Error in administering the treatment
- Error in the dose or method of using a drug

- Avoidable delay in treatment or in responding to an abnormal test
- Inappropriate (not indicated) care

c. Preventative
- Failure to provide prophylactic treatment
- Inadequate monitoring/follow-up of treatment

d. Other
- failure of communication,*equipment failure, *other system

REFERENCE: *CLINICS IN PERINATOLOGY VOLUME 35 NO1, MARCH 2008:1-33*

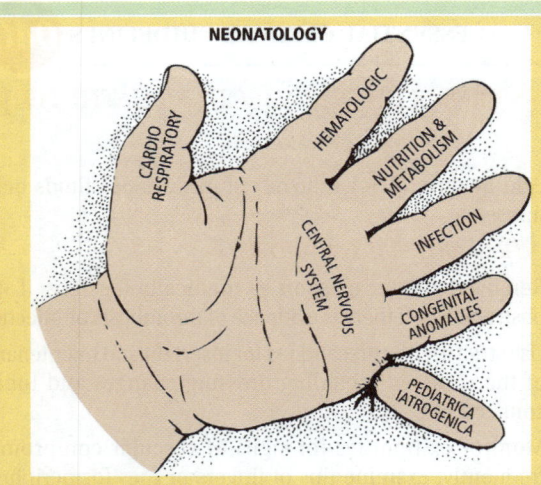

Neonatology (Courtesy B.F. Andrews, MD, Louisville, KY.)

Neoiatroepidemics: **New epidemics of iatrogenic disorders in the NICU resulting from the adoption of new treatment modalities and drugs without adequate testing or trials causing therapeutic misadventures.**

Institute of Medicine Committee Recommendations to avoid/reduce the incidence and magnitude of Iatrogenic disorders in the NICU

* Creating a national focus to promote research and enhance the knowledge base about patient safety.

* Identifying errors from a combination of mandatory and voluntary reporting systems.

* Raising standards and expectations through the action of oversight organizations and professional groups and

* Creating safety systems inside health care organizations.

*Communication and teamwork: There is now general awareness that communication and teamwork are critical to patient safety. Many principles have been adopted from crew resource management, a system of training first used in the aerospace industry. A few good practices: *Always identify yourself. Another person might be reluctant to speak up about a patient safety issue if he or she doesn't know your name. Identification of each team member also helps to establish role clarity. *Use 3-way communication to request something you need during a critical situation. Using the person's name, make a request. They should repeat the request, and you confirm it. This is known as request-response-confirmation (or challenge-response-response). It is much more effective than just yelling "somebody do this" and "somebody do that." *Learn to use SBAR, the structured language that can concisely communicate key information to others (Situation, what is going on; Background, how the situation developed, the objective data; Assessment, what you think the problem is; and Recommendation, what you think needs to be done). *In a critical situation, if you are uncomfortable pointing out a safety concern, learn and use specific words or phrases that assertively express your concern. One example used in crew resource management is, "I need clarity." Upon hearing this phrase, the team leader should understand that the team member is trying to raise a concern, and the team should stop what they are doing until the concern has been addressed. Medical errors are common in neonatal intensive care, and frequently result in harm to patients. Reporting and analysis of all errors, and not just those that result in harm, are essential in learning how to prevent medical error. Develop a working culture in which communication flows freely regardless of the authority gradient. Finally, prevention requires an approach that doesn't blame individuals for errors, but focuses on a systems approach that seeks to root out, find, and correct the true causes of errors.*

Iatroepidemic pathogenesis

1) Rapid technological advances 2) New therapeutic modalities 3) Inadequate research in basic sciences 4) Inadequate controlled trials 5)Poor follow-up 6) Newer diagnostic methods and diagnostic overkill and 7)Medical errors.

Common iatrogenic disorders in the NICU

1. Complications of Assisted Ventilation

Preventable:

Extensive air leaks: pneumothorax, pneumopericardium, pneumomediastinum, pneumoperitoneum, subcutaneous emphysema, air embolism

ET intubation related: malpositioning, trauma to vocal cords, pharynx, or esophagus, accidental extubation and obstruction

Potentially Preventable:

Pulmonary Interstitial Emphysema, BPD, Subglottic stenosis, Palatal grooves and defective dentition, Tracheomegaly

2. Complications of TPN

Preventable

Metabolic—hypoglycemia, hyperglycemia, electrolyte imbalance, hypertriglyceridemia,fluid overload, trace element, mineral deficiency/excess, hyper/hypo vitaminosis *Central lines related-* improper insertion, malposition, migration, cardiac tamponade, thrombus and occlusion, breakage, infection

Potentially Preventable: infection, cholestasis, hepatocellular damage, rickets

3. Complications of central venous catheters: infection (with coagulase negative staphylococci, Gram negative and fungal), arrhythmias-cardiac tamponade, thromboembolic complications, hepatic abscess due to malpositioning, peritoneal perforation, NEC, and perforation of the colon.

4. Complications of peripherally inserted central venous catheters: similar to those of Central Venous Catheters; they must be positioned 1cm outside the cardiac silhouette in preterm infants and 2cm outside the silhouette in term infants to prevent tamponade.

5. Medical and medication errors: wrong time/rate/drug/patient/frequency/diagnosis/dose/preparation/route/drug interactions/allergy/IV incompatibility

6. Complications of invasive monitoring: already listed above

REFERENCE: CLINICS IN PERINATOLOGY VOLUME 35 NO1, MARCH 2008:1-33

Use of abbreviations in daily progress notes: Errors in medication and documentation are reported. These errors, no matter how minor, could have grave consequences for the patient, especially in the pediatric population. One can imagine the potential threat to small neonates. Recently, Carroll et al described problems in residents' progress notes in a neonatal intensive care unit. Being the busiest centre in the country, managing the great majority of seriously sick neonates, we are at a very high risk of these errors. In view of this and as a screening audit, we looked at a few progress notes written on our inpatient neonates.

One example of a progress note, written by a junior doctor, stated "Prem 32 WOG, F&G , Problems: RDS, IVH II, S/P SVT, Stable on RA, TPR normal, PU, BO. Chest, CVS & abdomen: NAD". This excessive and inappropriate use of abbreviations is alarming and disturbing. The abbreviations used denoted the following (in order of citation): weeks of gestation, feeder and grower, respiratory distress syndrome, intraventricular grade 2 hemorrhage, status post supraventricular tachycardia, room air, temperature pulse respiration, passed urine, bowel open, cardiovascular system, and no abnormality detected.

This prompted us to look further into the use of abbreviations in the daily progress notes in our neonatal unit. A cross section survey was carried out at the Special Care Baby Unit (SCBU), Royal Hospital, Muscat, on 7 October 2003. Thirty consecutive charts were reviewed. The progress notes written by seven different doctors (three registrars and four resident medical officers) were analyzed for use of abbreviations. The commonly used ones were: CP (crystalline penicillin), RR (respiratory rate), HR (heart rate), BP (blood pressure), PA (per abdomen), O/E (on examination), NGT (nasogastric tube), UE1 (urea and electrolyte 1), BGA (blood gas analysis), BBA (born before arrival), TPN (total parenteral nutrition), SLS (standard lipid solution), STS (standard TPN solution), D/w (discussed with), SBR (serum bilirubin), CTG (cardiotocograph), IUGR (intrauterine growth restriction), BT shunt (Blalock-Taussig shunt), TAT (trans-anastomotic tube), IVF (intravenous fluid or in vitro fertilization), POD (postoperative day), ASD (atrial septum defect), VSD (ventricular septum defect), PDA (patent ductus arteriosus), TR (tricuspid regurgitation), L-R shunt (left to right shunt), TOF (tetralogy of Fallot), CRT (capillary refill time). One interesting note that needs separate mention was "Plan is to start ABs after ABC" (ABs, antibiotics; ABC, aerobic blood culture). We noted a high frequency of the use of abbreviations in our neonatal unit. This was a single day observation; we would expect much more in a longitudinal study. Fortunately, none of the abbreviations had resulted in erroneous interpretation, as most of the staff were used to them. However, this does not indicate that it is all right to use abbreviations. Standard abbreviations, such as VSD (ventricular septal defect) and PDA (patent ductus arteriosus), are acceptable, whereas others are not. Documentation errors have been reported to be an increasing problem in day to day care of patients. A recent report described the same negligence in documentation by residents. Carroll et al found discrepancies in the daily progress notes written by a resident doctor in the neonatal intensive care unit. They also found that notes often contained inaccurate information and lacked pertinent information. We looked further into the situation and found extensive use of abbreviations in progress notes. Our observation is not unique and requires rectification. The solution could be to standardize or eliminate the use of abbreviations in the unit. Total elimination would be difficult, as many of the abbreviations are acceptable. Thus, the use of unacceptable abbreviations should be discouraged. New medical officers should be given brief instruction on the writing of appropriate progress notes. An alternative is to use the electronic information system for all medical transcription including progress notes, as described elsewhere. *In conclusion, care of neonates requires good documentation of day to day progress. The use of unacceptable abbreviations should be discouraged.* A follow up audit is warranted to look further into the effect and success of our recommendations.

Courtesy: S Manzar, A K Nair, M Govind Pai, S Al-Khusaiby Special Care Baby Unit, Royal Hospital, PO Box 1331, Postal Code 111, Muscat, Sultanate of Oman; shabihman@hotmail.com.

Reference: Reference:Carroll AE, Tarczy-Hornoch P, O'Reilly E, et al. Resident documentation discrepancies in a neonatal intensive care unit. Pediatrics 2003;111:976–80.

Neonatal disorders with an iatrogenic component

Condition	Damaging agent
Retinopathy of Prematurity	Oxygen
Necrotizing Enterocolitis	Hypotension
	Enteral feeding, formula
Discrete Intestinal Perforation	Emboli from UAC, Indomethacin
Airleaks, e.g. Pneumothorax	High PIP, High MAP,Inadequate Humidity during IPPV
Chronic lung disease	As for airleak
	Fluid overload
	Infection, Oxygen
GMH-IVH	Hypotension, Hypoxia, Hypercarbia
PVL	Sepsis, Hypotension, Hypocarbia
Lung puncture	Treatment of pneumothorax
Gastric rupture	Mask/nasal IPPV
	Nasogastric tube erosion
Airway damage	ETT, Oscillatory and Jet ventilation
Nasal septum injury	Secondary to Nasal CPAP fixation
Obstructive jaundice	TPN
Complex metabolic upsets	TPN
Intestinal obstruction	High Calorie Density Milks

Drug-induced iatrogenic complications

Drug	Complication
General	Incorrect dosage, Incorrect drug, Incorrect concentration
Specific	
Chloramphenicol	Grey baby syndrome
Diuretics (especially frusemide)	Nephrocalcinosis
Sulphisoxazole	Kernicterus
Tetracyclines	Stained teeth
Vitamin K analogues (menadione)	Jaundice
Vitamin E	Liver failure, Hematuria
Tolazoline	Hypotension, Hematuria, GI tract hemorrhage
Indomethacin	Fluid retention,GI tract hemorrhage, decreased cerebral blood flow velocity
Dexamethasone	GI tract hemorrhage & perforation, hypertension, sepsis, cardiomyopathy, glycosuria, adrenal suppression
Hexachlorophane	Vacuolative encephalopathy
Glycol in i.v. multivitamin preparation	Fits, GMV-IVH
Benzyl alcohol in i.v. saline	Acidemia & collapse, kernicterus
Heparin	GMH-IVH
Phenylephrine (mydriatic) Transcutaneous	Hypertension
Tribiotic (neomycin)	Deafness
Iodine-containing antiseptics	Transient hypothyroidism

10 golden rules to minimize iv infusion and drug hazards

1. Keep the prescribing of medication to a *minimum* and use once or twice daily administration where this is possible.

2. Never have *more than two IV infusion lines* running at the same time unless this is absolutely necessary.

3. Never put more than 30 ml of fluid at any time into any syringe used to provide continuous IV fluid or milk for a *baby weighing less than 1 kg.*

4. Record the amount of fluid administered by every syringe pump by inspecting the movement of the syringe and by inspecting the infusion site *once every hour.*

5. Do not change the feeding or IV fluid regimen more than once or at most twice a day *except for a very good reason.* Try to arrange that such changes as do have to be made are made during the morning or evening joint management rounds.

6. Do not *"flush" drugs/fluids* through an established IV line by temporarily changing the setting of the infusion pump; there a risk that the infusion pump will not be returned to its correct setting afterwards. Few babies ever need to be given any drug as a sudden IV bolus (except as a result of some acute sudden collapse).

7. Those few drugs that have to be administered over 30 minutes or more should be administered by using a *separate programmable syringe pump* connected pick-aback on to an existing IV line. As an extra precaution the syringe should never be set up containing more than twice as much of the drug as it is planned to deliver. The rate at which the main infusion fluid is administered does not need to be adjusted while such supplementary IV drugs are being infused.

8. Beware of giving a small Newborn baby *excess sodium* unintentionally. The use of flush solutions of Heparin or NS can expose a baby to an unintended excess of intravenous sodium. The steady infusion of 1ml/hour of heparinized 0.9% NS to maintain catheter patency is sometimes enough to double a very small baby`s total daily sodium intake.

9. Treat the prescribing of potentially *toxic/lethal drugs* (morphine, digoxin, inotropes etc.,) with special care.

10. If something does go wrong, report any significant *error of omission/commission* promptly so that appropriate action can be taken to minimize any possible hazard to the baby.

Check and double check

1. **Have you got the right drug ?** Check the strength of the formulation and the label on the ampoule as well as the box.

2. **Has its shelf life expired ?** Check the "use by" date.

3. **Has it been reconstituted and diluted properly ?** Check the advice given in the individual drug monograph.

4. **Have you got the right patient ?** Check the name band.

5. **Have you got the right dose ?** Have two people independently checked steps 1-4 with the prescription chart ?

6. **Have you picked up the right syringe ?** Deal with one patient at a time.

7. **Is the VI line patent ? Have you got the right line ?** Is it correctly positioned ? Could the line have tissued ?

8. **Is a separate flush solution needed ?** Have two people checked the content of the flush syringe ?

9. **Are all the "sharps" disposed of ?** What about any glass ampoules?

10. **Have you "signed up" what you have done ?** Has it been countersigned ?

Factors that affect drug handling in children

Absorption: Absorption is dependent on gastrointestinal function, which changes rapidly after birth. Gastric pH is increased in infants and doesn't reach adult concentrations until the second year of life. Reduced gastric emptying in neonates makes the oral route of administration unreliable in this age group. Transdermal absorption is greatly increased in neonates resulting in greater risk of toxicity via this route.

Distribution: Less plasma protein binding and more volume of extracellular fluid relative to total body water in young infants results in a markedly greater volume of distribution. High bilirubin concentrations may cause drug displacement from plasma proteins take care in neonatal jaundice.

Metabolism: Clearance rates may be less at birth because of immature enzyme systems. Children have a higher metabolic rate than adults so may need higher doses on a mg/kg basis.

Excretion: Renal function does not mature completely until age 6-8 months. Reduced renal excretion may occur in newborn babies.

Prescribing do's and don'ts

Do's

*Only prescribe within the limits of your competence *Check the weight and age of child are correct *Always state the age of the child on a prescription *Make a clear, accurate, and legible record of all drugs prescribed *Have an awareness of serious contraindications and adverse effects of drugs prescribed *Take an adequate history, including previous adverse drug reactions and use of non-prescription drugs *Ensure patients or parents have been given appropriate information on adverse effects *Get doses checked by someone else when they are calculated *Report all suspected adverse drug reactions using the yellow card system

Don'ts

*Put a zero after a decimal point. This reduces the risk of a 10 times overdose when writing prescription;for example, 10 micrograms not 10.0 micrograms. When decimals are unavoidable a zero should be written in front of the decimal point;for example, 0.5 ml not .5 ml *Don't abbreviate nanograms and micrograms when writing prescriptions *Don't use the terms cubic centimetres, cc, or cm³; the term millilitre (ml) is used in medicine and pharmacy

REFERENCE: NEONATAL FORMULARY BMJ 10TH EDITION

Extravasation is the inadvertent leakage of infused fluid into surrounding tissue, which may cause damage. About 4% of infants leave neonatal intensive care units with cosmetically or functionally significant scars, thought to be caused by extravasation injuries. Premature infants are now surviving at very low gestational ages and weighing only in the region of 500g, and these neonates are at great risk of sustaining tissue damage as a result of the intravenous therapy required to keep them alive. They have longer exposure time to intravenous therapy until they are able to take all nutritional requirements enterally, their skin is correspondingly immature and easily damaged, there is reduced venous integrity and the median survival time span for intravenous cannulae is only 31 hours (Hecker, 1993).

A recent survey carried out in the United Kingdom revealed a lack of consensus on the management of extravasation injuries in preterm infants. Infiltration with hyaluronidase and saline had been recommended but local experience is limited. The mechanisms of extravasation necrosis are incompletely understood, but the degree of damage appears to be related to osmolality, pH, and the dissociability of ions. Hyaluronidase has proved effective in decreasing the harm caused by extravasated hyperalimentation solutions in rabbits. Furthermore, free drainage of the extravasated fluid through skin puncture sites and the promotion of dilution and absorption of the substance by injection of saline with hyaluronidase have been tried. Hyperosmolarity is thought to disrupt the transport mechanism of the cell membrane, resulting in cell death by fluid inhibition. Calcium and potassium salts are slightly acidic, hypertonic and capable of precipitating proteins to produce cell death directly. It is well known that solutions of amino acids are acidic and act as buffers. After extravasation, the interstitial pH of the peri-venous tissue could become acidic and remain outside the physiologic range. That could enhance the cell damage caused by hyperosmolarity and the presence of ions. Hyaluronidase is an enzyme that depolymerizes hyaluronic acid, a mucopolysaccharide part of the tissue cement of the tissue spaces. This has proved useful in preventing soft tissue necrosis after extravasation of parenteral nutrition solutions. Subcutaneous administration of the enzyme increases tissue permeability and facilitates the absorption of injected substances by allowing the rapid diffusion of the drug over a larger area. Thus, the extravasated material is rapidly diluted and absorbed from the tissue and the injury is minimized. The onset of action is immediate and the effect lasts about 24-48 hours. The toxicity of hyaluronidase is minimal. Adverse effects are rare, mainly allergic reactions manifested as urticaria. *Hyaluronidase should not be injected directly into cancerous or infected areas because of the potential for increasing invasiveness of neoplasm or disseminating infection. Furthermore, it should not be used for extravasation management of dopamine or alpha agonists.*

Communication with Parents

Parents may feel guilty or anxious and need reassurance. Identify their level of understanding and how much they want to know about their baby's wound. Allow parents to be involved in the wound dressing procedure if they wish. If you are leaving a dressing in place for up to a week then explain the rationale as parent may be accustomed to everything else being changed at least dail

Documentation

It is important to document wound care objectives and management plan and to record details of the wound assessment such as: • Type of wound. • Position of wound. • Wound dimensions, length, width, depth. • Nature of wound bed. • Condition of surrounding skin. • Exudate level, color and consistency. • Presence of odor. • Presence of infection. • Level of pain. • Allergies or skin sensitivities. • Previous treatments.

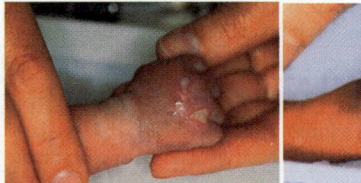
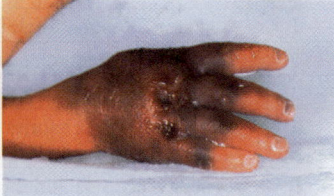

The parenteral nutrition fluids through a Peripheral Canula often result in extravasation injury which are composed of dextrose, calcium, potassium, and other ions, and the osmolarity is clearly higher than that of the human serum.

A Plastic cap may help to prevent the movement of IV canula & the extravasation injury.

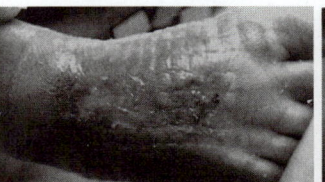
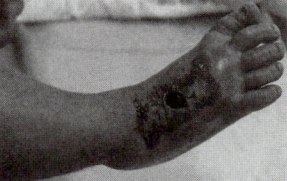

Right foot dorsum five days after extravasation injury.

Extravasation injury over right foot dorsum.

Technique of Flushing the Extravasated Area

* Clean the discolored area and surrounding skin with Chlorhexidine solution and place on sterile towel. *Place a sterile bowl underneath towel.

* Infiltrate area with 1% Lignocaine.

* Inject 500-1000 units hyaluronidase into the subcutaneous tissue beneath the damaged skin.

* Make four small punctures in the tissue plane with a scalpel blade around the affected area.

* Insert the 19G cannula subcutaneously through one of the puncture sites and remove the needle

* Using a 20 ml syringe attached to a three-way tap, inject normal saline into the area. This should flow out freely from the other three incisions.

* Repeat the process injecting normal saline through each incision and using up to 500 ml of normal saline

* If the limb gets edematous, excess fluid can be removed by massaging towards the incisions.

* Dress area with Jelonet or a similar dressing for 24 to 48 hours.

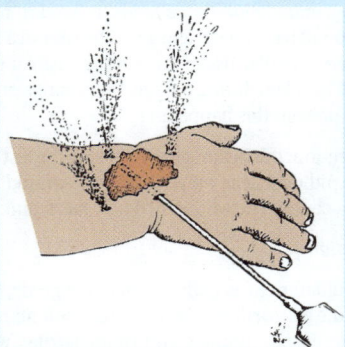

Courtesy: SLY **SIU**, KL **KWONG**, SST **POON**, KT **SO**

INTRAVENOUS CANNULATION MANAGEMENT OF INFILTRATION INJURIES (INCLUDING CLYSIS)

Step	Action
1	Remove I.V. immediately at first sign of infiltration.
2	If significant infiltration or necrosis occurs, notify Senior NICU Nurse Practitioner, or Registrar immediately.
3	Estimate the severity of the injury by Millam's 1988 Staging Guidelines. *(v.i.)*
4	For Stage 1 and 2 injuries: *Elevate limb, observe circulation, and document findings.
5	For all Stage 3-4 injuries: *An incident report must be initiated. *Photographs of the injury should be made for the medical notes and a digital copy made available for plastic surgeons. *Parents to be notified and informed of actions taken.
6	For Stage 3-4 injuries **AND** for extravasation injuries with potentially injurious solutions (caffeine, dopamine, dobutamine, blood, solutions containing >"12.5% dextrose, or TPN) *Clysis treatment should be initiated as soon as possible following the discovery of a Stage 3-4 injury or extravasation of injurious solutions. *After clysis has been carried out, plastic surgery referral may or may not be required. This should be determined over the next few days of careful observation. *The plastic surgeon on call should be notified for all Stage 4 infiltrations if no improvement after clysis.*

Staging Severity of IV Infiltration

Stage I

* Painful IV site *No erythema *No Swelling

Stage II

* Painful IV site *Slight swelling (0-20%)

* No blanching *Good pulse below infiltration site

* Brisk capillary refill below infiltration site

Stage III

* Painful IV site

* Marked swelling (30-50%) *Blanching

* Skin cool to touch *Good pulse below infiltration site

* Brisk capillary refill below infiltration site

Stage IV

* Painful IV site *Very marked swelling (>50%) *Blanching

* Skin cool to touch *Decreased or absent pulse*

* Capillary refill > 4 seconds* *Skin breakdown or necrosis*

The presence of any of these constitutes a stage IV infiltration

Status

• **Necrotic:** the surface of the wound may initially be covered with devitalized tissue which is still unbroken if the area of damage is away from the cannulation site. As with other wounds, this tissue has to be removed before healing can begin

• **Slough:** this is composed of dead white cells (neutrophils and macrophages) and can be mistaken for pus by the inexperienced carer who has failed to notice the lack of other signs of infection, such as redness, swelling, heat and loss of movement

• **Granulating:** granulation tissue tends to develop relatively quickly once the wound bed is clean and gives the wound a red appearance. This is a very vascular tissue and bleeds easily if damaged. Great care should be taken during the dressing change or handling of the neonate to prevent this happening

• **Epithelialization:** this is thought of as being the last stage of healing when the epithelial cells move across the wound from the edges towards the centre. The wound bed now has a pink appearance

Signs of infection

These are no different to any other population group, but the neonate cannot tell of the pain or discomfort. Pre-term infants react to infection by having increased apnoeas and bradycardias with associated saturation drops, an increased oxygen requirement, becoming intolerant of enteral feeds and/or temperature instability.

CLYSIS Treatment

1) Most infiltrations are able to be treated with local anaesthesia and analgesia such as paracetamol. **2)** If area is very large, general anaesthesia may be indicated. This should be discussed with specialist on call. **3)** Clysis is a sterile technique. **4)** Place large waterproof guard under affected limb before creating sterile field. **5)** Clean the affected area with a skin disinfectant appropriate for the infant's gestation and postnatal age. Allow to dry. **6)** Infiltrate affected region with local anaesthetic (usually 1% xylocaine, maximum dose 0.3ml/kg). This should be concentrated in area proximal to (above) the wound, and within the central area of wound. Wait several minutes until effective. **7)** Using size 15 scalpel blade, make several small (approximately 5mm long) stab wounds within affected region—these should be approximately 1–2 cm apart, and penetrate just below skin. **8)** Take large (Size 14 or 16) angiocath and remove sharp needle leaving white cannula only. **9)** Have 500 ml bag 0.9% NaCl ready on sterile field. Push Chemospike into fluid bag to provide access port for refilling syringe. Fill 20 ml syringe, attach to white cannula, and insert into stab wounds flushing with firm but gentle pressure in and around area of stab wound. Fluid should be seen to leak from stab wound sites **10)** Start in central part of affected area where the infusate is concentrated. Refill syringe and repeat as required. **11)** A large volume of saline should be used-depending on size of baby and of wound, it is suggested that 200-500 ml saline will be needed: Suggested volumes:<1000g 200ml, 1000–2000 g 300ml, >2000g 500ml. **12)** When completed, cover area with sterile non-stick dressing (Mepitel). Stab wounds should not be closed and may drain for some time. Elevate limb in comfortable position. Check wound 6-hourly over next 24 hours. **13)** One dose of intravenous antibiotic (Flucloxacillin 50mg/kg) should be given if the baby is not already receiving antibiotics.

Various Modalities of Treatment for Extravasation Injury: No EBM Guidelines available because of dearth of literature to guide clinical practice in this patient group.

1. 2% nitroglycerin ointment (less than 4 mm/kg) over an extended period of time(4 weeks) for reversing tissue ischemia.

2. Use of an ionic hydrogel (ActiFormCool®) in a neonate with an extravasation injury.

3. Hypodermoclysis with Hyaluronidase as discussed before

4. Involvement of plastic surgeons

In cases of extravasation injury in term infants or older children it is best to involve the plastic surgeons at an early stage. However, for the very preterm neonate this is not a beneficial option. Only in extreme cases is immediate repair surgery necessary and the size and immaturity of these infants can pose problems that plastic surgeons may not be prepared for, and suggested treatments are often not appropriate for this patient group.

HOW TO REDUCE THE NEED FOR RBC TRANSFUSIONS IN THE SCBU/NICU?

Etiology of anemia of prematurity

- Frequent blood sampling
- Low reticulocyte levels
- Low levels of endogenous erythropoietin
- Poor response to endogenous erythropoietin
- Shortened life span of neonatal erythrocytes

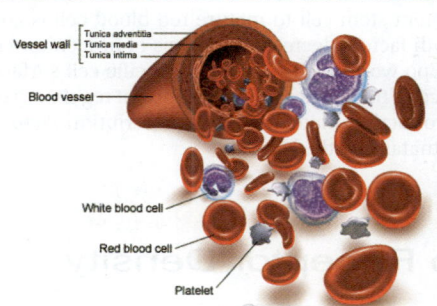

Vessel wall — Tunica adventitia / Tunica media / Tunica intima

Blood vessel

White blood cell

Red blood cell

Platelet

Risks of blood transfusion in preterm infants

- Fluid overload
- Transfusion associated infection:
  Hepatitis B and C viruses
  Human immunodeficiency virus
  Cytomegalovirus
- Hemolytic transfusion reactions
- Immune mediated transfusion reactions
- Extravasation injury
- Graft versus host disease (rare)

Measures to reduce the risk of infection associated with transfusion

- Screen donors for transmissible viruses
- Limit exposure to multiple donors—multiple paediatric packs from single adult donor
- Use cytomegalovirus antibody negative blood
- Irradiate transfusion packs
- Use leucocyte depletion filters (removes cytomegalovirus)

To prevent and reduce the severity of anemia, and to reduce donor exposure or the risks associated with RBC transfusions, strategies to consider may include: *delayed clamping of the umbilical cord; *restricting blood sampling; *using recombinant human erythropoietin to stimulate erythropoiesis; *using iron supplementation or vitamins to minimize the severity of anemia;*using appropriately collected and stored multipack RBC units;*using appropriately screened and handled RBCs from regular or designated donors; and collecting and transfusing umbilical cord blood (autologous blood transfusion).

Recommendations for red blood cell (RBC transfusions

RBC transfusions should be considered in newborn infants in the following specific clinical situations: * Hypovolemic shock associated with acute blood loss *Hematocrit between 30% and 35% or hemoglobin concentration between 100 g/L and 120 g/L in extreme illness conditions for which RBC transfusion may improve oxygen delivery to vital organs *Hematocrit between 20% and 30% or hemoglobin concentration between 60 g/L and 100 g/L, and the infant is severely ill and/or on mechanical ventilation with compromised oxygen delivery *Hematocrit falling (20% or less) or hemoglobin concentration (60 g/L or less) with a reticulocyte count of 100 to 150·10⁹/L or less (suggesting low plasma concentration of erythropoietin), and if the following clinical signs are present: failure to thrive or no weight gain, tachycardia more than 180 breaths/min, respiratory signs including tachypnea and supplemental oxygen needs, and lethargy.

Recombinant human erythropoietin

Intrauterine fetal production of erythropoietin occurs only in the liver. In extrauterine life, the primary site of erythropoietin production is the kidney. The switch in erythropoietin production site is probably determined genetically in a manner similar to hemoglobin production switching from fetal to adult type. Endogenous erythropoietin concentrations are low in preterm and term infants. The responses to hypoxia are reduced in infants because of decreased sensitivity of the liver oxygen sensors. Immature renal oxygen sensors also may play a role. Human recombinant erythropoietin (rEPO) stimulates erythropoiesis, as evidenced by reticulocytosis and increased hematocrit. rEPO accelerates erythropoiesis in a dose-dependent fashion, even in extremely low birth weight and ill neonates. While rEPO is used to prevent and treat anemia, it is not beneficial in treating acute hemorrhage. To date, no significant safety issues have been reported in this population. Darbepoetin is a synthetic form of erythropoietin that is 6-13 times more potent and has a longer half life. With either formulation, there are 2 approaches: early use and late use. Late use (after 3 weeks) is more effective because most early anemia is a consequence of blood loss Erythropoietin deficiency is a major cause of anemia of prematurity. Erythropoietin therapy for anemia of prematurity may be effective and very promising, particularly for stable preterm infants whose bone marrow is able to respond to treatment, and for at risk infants with large phlebotomy losses. Some data suggest that restrictive guidelines for RBC transfusions may have the same effect as the administration of erythropoietin in preterm infants . Several review articles and randomized controlled trials have been published where the potential benefits, safety and cost effectiveness of human erythropoietin administration have been examined. Several studies have demonstrated beneficial effects, but in association with conservative transfusion criteria, the minimization of phlebotomy losses and early iron administration. When considering the administration of erythropoietin, be aware that the preparation contains human albumin.In summary, erythropoietin administration may reduce RBC transfusions in high risk infants. The importance of this impact is not yet known. However, erythropoietin administration does not change the need for RBC transfusions in the first two weeks of life, particularly in sick preterm infants . A meta-analysis of controlled clinical trials studying the efficacy of erythropoietin in reducing RBC transfusions was recently published . While many benefits in high quality studies using conservative RBC transfusion criteria were noted, the authors also reported an extreme variation in the findings and they concluded that erythropoietin therapy should not be a standard treatment for anemia of prematurity . Further investigations are needed regarding the optimal dose, the timing, the overall nutritional support that is required during erythropoietin treatment, and the potential toxic effects associated with erythropoietin administration in preterm infants . Clear guidelines for the use of erythropoietin to prevent Neonatal anemia are not available.

RBC transfusions will continue to be necessary in the care of high risk preterm and term infants. However, prevention of anemia, restriction of donor exposure and restriction of the number of RBC transfusions must be part of a comprehensive approach to high risk neonates. The present statement provides some modalities to prevent the occurrence of severe anemia in growing newborn infants and to limit the necessity of therapeutic interventions. RBC transfusion protocols have rarely been subjected to randomized controlled trials and careful clinical investigation. The variations in practice among different neonatal units illustrate this lack of evidence . On the basis of unanswered questions in the current literature, the Committee makes these recommendations , and is awaiting better evidence of efficacy and safety. Further investigation is required to clarify the future approach to these important clinical dilemmas. Ongoing clinical trials are presently examining these questions.

Anemia is common among hospitalized neonates, particularly in those of preterm birth. Clinicians should use a kinetic approach to diagnosing neonatal anemia, taking full advantage of the data available on the routine CBC laboratory results. Every NICU should have erythrocyte transfusion guidelines, and these should be followed in order to avoid unnecessary, and unhelpful, erythrocyte transfusions.

ERYTHROPOIETIN IN THE NEWBORN INTENSIVE CARE NURSERY

How Epo works ?

The production of red blood cells from pluripotent stem cell to mature red blood cell is governed by growth factors that include erythropoietin (Epo). These erythropoietic growth factors decrease apoptosis of progenitor cells and stimulate maturation, growth, and differentiation of red blood cells (Figure). Epo works by binding to a specific cell surface receptor (Epo-R). Although multiple growth factors facilitate production of red blood cells, none plays a more important regulatory role than Epo. Both hypoxia and anemia stimulate erythropoiesis by stimulating Epo production mediated by a transcription factor, HIF-1, or "hypoxia inducible factor". Prenatally, Epo is produced in the liver, and postnatally by the kidney.

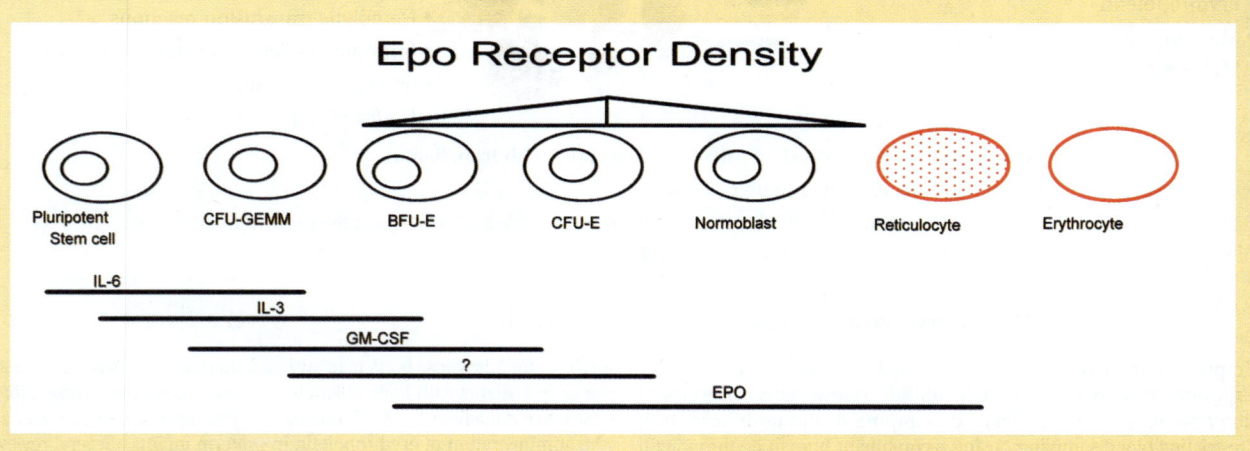

Administration of rEpo

Epo can be given IV or SQ. It is somewhat more effective when given SQ, unless the IV dose is given over an hour to simulate SQ absorption. It given IV, it can be given either by itself, or mixed in hyperalimentation fluids (TPN).

Dose and dosing schedule

When compared to adults, the half life of Epo in preterm infants is shorter, and the volume of distribution greater, necessitating larger doses and more frequent dosing. Effective dosing schemes are as follows:

– 200 units/kg/day IV (Can add to HA fluids, or give as single dose injections over 60 min)

– 400 units/kg/day SQ, three times a week (e.g. M, W, F)

• Start iron 6 mg/kg/day elemental iron PO/OG or 1 mg IV iron dextran in TPN when starting Epo therapy.

A weekly CBC with differential count, platelet count, reticulocyte count and ZnPP/H should be followed when an infant is receiving Epo treatment. Treatment length is dependent on the therapeutic goals, and can be from 2 weeks to several months in duration. A convalescing preterm infant can be expected to begin producing red blood cells on their own when they reach 36 weeks corrected gestational age.

Epo clearance

Epo is cleared by receptor binding, with internalization and subsequent breakdown within the cells. Some Epo is excreted in the urine, but dosing is not effected by hepatic or renal disease.

Epo Side effects

Side effects of Epo administration reported in adults include hypertension, bone pain, rash, and rarely seizures. Many of these side effects are reported in end stage renal patients, and it is unclear what effect their primary disease state has. None of these side effects have been reported in newborns.

Uncommon side effects that appear to be specific to newborns include neutropenia and mild thrombocytosis.

Who might benefit from Epo ?

1. Even with the use of Epo, infants < 1000 gm are likely to require at least one transfusion in the first weeks of life. Because we used aliquoted blood here at the UW, and these infants can receive multiple transfusions with only one donor exposure, we do not recommend beginning Epo during the first weeks of life when phlebotomy losses are the highest, and infants are likely to need multiple transfusions.

   When infants < 1000 gm become more stable and phlebotomy losses are lower (usually after the first 3 weeks of life), Epo should be considered. Consider administering Epo in this population if standard iron therapy has been started and the weekly hematocrit is falling despite infrequent blood draws. If the corrected reticulocyte count is < 6, infants are likely to benefit.

   The corrected reticulocyte count is obtained by taking the patient's reticulocyte (%) x patient's Hct (L/L) ÷ desired or optimal Hct (L/L). 45 is usually used as the optimal Hct when making this calculation.

2. Infants > 1000 gm who are at risk for a transfusion but who are not in acute need of blood. Following the weekly Hct and reticulocyte count is helpful when making this assessment. If they are not requiring frequent blood draws, but their Hct is falling despite standard iron therapy, they may benefit from Epo.

   Any child who is acutely ill and in need of increased oxygen carrying capacity should be transfused, not treated with Epo.

General Information about Epo

It takes approximately a week to see an increase in Hct after starting Epo. The reticulocyte count will often double, and gains in Hct are generally in the 2 to 4 point range per week. The most common cause of failure to respond is inadequate iron stores.

REFERENCE: NICU Resident Packet , Division of Neonatology Department of Pediatrics University of Washington Box 356320, RR542 HSB Seattle, WA 98195-6320

EVIDENCE-BASED
NEONATAL SKIN CARE IN THE NICUs

Bathing: The consequences of routine bathing include dryness, irritation, and destabilization of vital signs and temperature. In addition, rubbing of skin is very painful for the newborn. The first bath should be done after the infant's temperature has stabilized for 2 to 4 hours. Warm water (without soaps) in the first week of life is optimal. Thereafter, recommendations for bathing include: *Using cleansing agents with neutral pH *Reducing prolonged skin contact with cleansing agents by rinsing the skin *Bathing only 2 to 3 times per week

Skin disinfectants: Isopropyl alcohol is a poor skin disinfectant and has been associated with the greatest amount of tissue damage in newborn infants. Povidone iodine is more efficacious than isopropyl alcohol as a disinfectant, but povidone iodine can be absorbed systemically and alterations in newborn thyroid function can result. This disinfectant can also cause skin irritation and tissue damage, as seen in Figure 1. Efficacy of chlorhexidine (CHG) in reducing infection has been demonstrated in adults and newborns. Skin damage specific to CHG has not been noted clinically. Both safety and efficacy of a product are important considerations in choosing an antiseptic for clinical use. For neonates, isopropyl alcohol or products containing isopropyl alcohol are not recommended in the skin care guideline. Povidone iodine or CHG solutions are recommended but require complete removal after the procedure with sterile water or saline to prevent absorption.

Adhesives: The infant has increased evaporative losses after adhesive tape removal. Adhesives become more aggressive over time. However, solvents are highly toxic and are absorbed through the skin, so should not be used in newborns. Skin stripping and tearing as well as chemical irritation are seen with the use of bonding agents. Figure 2 shows electrodes with adhesive bonding leading to skin tissue injury. Preventing skin injury is a nursing art: *Minimize the use of tape or "double-back" the tape *Use pectin barriers under adhesives *Use hydrogel or karaya electrode leads.

Emollients: Emollients prevent desquamation of the stratum corneum, the outer layer of cells that form the epidermal barrier. *Emolene* ointment can be used on an "as-needed" basis to treat dryness and prevent cracking of skin. Prevention of excoriation is seen with the use of *Emolene* ointment on the groin and thighs. There may be a *possible* increase in coagulase negative staph (CONS) infection in infants < 750 g with the *routine* topical application of *Aquaphor* ointment. *Emolene* must be applied every 6 hours to be effective in reducing TEWL.

Skin maturation and TEWL: Postnatal maturation of the stratum corneum affects the rate of water loss. The skin barrier matures between 30 and 32 weeks corrected gestational age. Skin maturation is not based on the number of postnatal days. Relative humidity decreases transepidermal fluid losses and required fluid intake. The recommendation for humidity is > 70% relative humidity for the first week and 50% to 60% for the rest of the first month. A bedside hydrometer assists the nurse in reaching humidity goals better than visualizing condensation.

Skin breakdown: Adhesive tape removal is the primary risk factor for traumatic injury to the newborn. Ulcerative erosions are often associated with systemic bacterial or *Candida* sepsis, with areas of skin breakdown as the portal of entry Early recognition of skin breakdown and identification of the pathogen with a Gram stain can be essential elements in the reduction in mortality.

NCPAP and skin: Tissue irritation and pressure necrosis of the nasal septum related to the use of nasal continuous positive airway pressure (NCPAP) has been discussed among nurses and other professionals but not extensively described in the literature. Figure 3 illustrates septal erosion as a result of pressure necrosis from an NCPAP device

Key elements related to NCPAP and skin care are: *Use appropriate sized prongs to make a seal for the transmission of pressure *Do not create seal from pressure on the nares *Use the equipment manual to define practices related to securing the device *Suction and inspect the skin every 4 hours *Massage the skin with each inspection.

Guidelines for Clinical Practice

Evaluation and implementation of research-based evidence is the foundation of nursing care. Implementation of the AWHONN-NANN (Association of Women's Health, Obstetric and Neonatal Nurses (AWHONN) and the National Association of Neonatal Nurses (NANN) Skin Care Guideline improves overall skin condition of newborns and reduces iatrogenic injury. Nurses need to continue to review and evaluate new research and products for implementation in their practice as well as conduct/support new research that describes skin care practices with clinical outcomes.

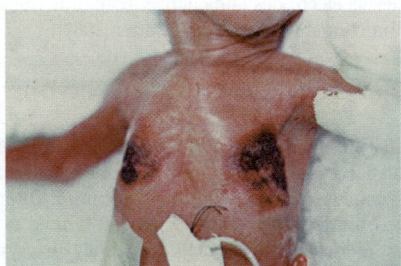

Fig 1 Abdominal skin tissue injury as a result of topical application of a disinfectant.

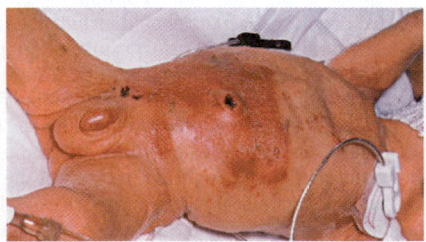

Fig 2 Electrodes with adhesive bonding caused this skin tissue injury. The skin care guideline recommends the use of hydrogel electrodes

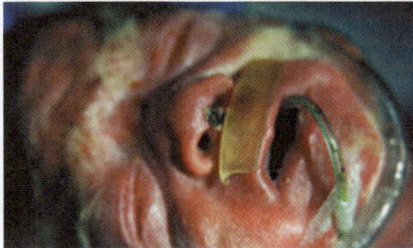

Fig 3 Note septal erosion as a result of pressure necrosis from NCPAP device

REFERENCE:**Challenges in Neonatal Nursing: Providing Evidence-Based Skin Care** Susan Arana Furdon, MS, RNC, NNP
Photos courtesy of Dr. David A. Clark, Pediatric Department Chairman @ Albany Medical Center, Albany NY

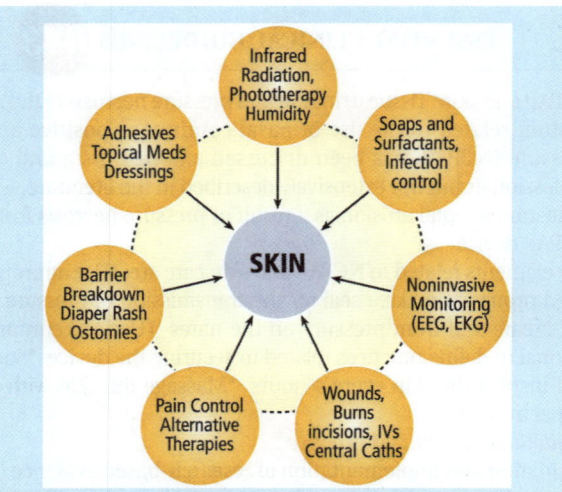

Neonatal care involves near constant interaction with Newborn skin as a primary care interface (Figure 1). Protecting the integrity of the skin under these circumstances can be challenging.

Proposed Guidelines for Basic Skin Care in the Newborn

Use adhesives sparingly.

* Place protective dressing (e.g., DuoDerm or Tegaderm) at sites of frequent taping (endotracheal tube and nasogastric tube placement).

*Use nonadhesive electrodes and change them only when they become nonfunctional (Cartlidge and Rutter, 1987).

Limit bathing

*Defer initial cleansing until body temperature has stabilized.

*Avoid cleansing agents for the first 2 weeks.

*Use warm water and moistened cotton pledgets in a humid environment.

* Surface cleansing is required no more than twice per week.

* If antimicrobial skin preparation is required, use short-contact chlorhexidine (except on the face).

Be aware of the composition and quantity of all topically applied agents.

*These agents include antimicrobial cleansers, diaper wipes, adhesive removers, and perineal products.

*Dispense from single-use containers, if possible.

Ensure adequate intake of protein, essential fatty acids, zinc, biotin, and vitamins A, D, and B.

*Erosive periorificial dermatitis is a sign of nutritional deficiency.

Apply a simple cream or ointment emollient every 8 hours (Nopper et al, 1994).

Guard against excessive thermal and ultraviolet exposure.

* Use thermally controlled water for bathing.

*Avoid surface monitors with metal contacts.

*Use Plexiglas shielding over daylight fluorescent phototherapy.

Protect sites of cutaneous injury with the appropriate occlusive dressing.

*Use a film dressing on nonexudative sites (Barak et al, 1989; Knauth et al, 1989; Vernon et al, 1990).

*Use a hydrogel dressing on exudative wounds.

* Maintain appropriate hydration at the skin-dressing interface.

* Remove necrotic debris with each dressing change.

Vesicles and Pustules in the Newborn

ESSENTIAL CLINICAL GUIDELINES 044

Vesicles are small intraepidermal or subepidermal pockets of clear fluid. If the lesions are large (greater than 1 cm in diameter), they are referred to as *bullae*. Pustules are filled with purulent fluid. Diseases in this category range from totally innocuous and self-limited to severe and life-threatening. A directed history, including family history of blistering diseases, and physical examination, including examination of the placenta, can focus the differential diagnosis. Small lesions in an otherwise healthy infant usually suggest a purely cutaneous process. Bullae and widespread involvement should prompt a more aggressive workup. The initial diagnostic workup should include the following: * Fluid aspirate taken from an intact vesicle, pustule, or scraping of the base of a ruptured vesicle or pustule for Gram stain, Wright stain, and fungal, viral, and bacterial cultures as well as for double fluorescent antibody or polymerase chain reaction when available. *Potassium hydroxide (KOH) preparation (or calcofluor white immunofluorescence) of the blister roof * Scraping from the base of the blister for herpes viral culture or Tzanck smear * Scraping from a carefully selected intact lesion, mounted in mineral oil, for scabies preparation *Skin biopsy as indicated, depending on the morphology and extent of the lesions, and results of other evaluations.

Differential Diagnosis

Infections Localized to Skin

* Candidiasis: KOH (or calcofluor white) preparation of the blister roof reveals pseudohyphae.

* Bullous impetigo: Wright stain reveals polymorphonuclear neutrophil leukocytes (PMNs); Gram stain shows gram-positive cocci.

* Gram-positive folliculitis: Wright stain reveals PMNs; Gram stain shows gram-positive cocci.

* Pityrosporum folliculitis: KOH preparation reveals short hyphae and spores.

* Neonatal herpes: Tzanck smear reveals viral cytopathic changes; polymerase chain reaction and immunohistochemical marker assays are highly sensitive studies and can be performed using a smear on glass slides submitted to the laboratory. Viral cultures are still the gold standard with high sensitivity and specificity. Only a small amount of blister fluid on a swab inoculated into transport media is necessary, and results may be available within 12 hours.

* Scabies: Mineral oil preparation reveals mites, ova, and feces.

Transient Noninfectious Causes

* Erythema toxicum neonatorum: Wright stain shows eosinophils.

* Neonatal pustular melanosis: Wright stain shows keratinous debris with PMNs; results of a Gram stain are negative.

* Neonatal acne: Close inspection reveals comedones.

* Milia: Wright stain shows keratinocytes only.

* Miliaria crystallina: These tiny, superficial noninflammatory vesicles represent obstruction of the sweat duct.

* Infantile acropustulosis: This pruritic condition mimics infantile scabies, but the vesicles are usually rounded, rather than elongated like burrows.

* Eosinophilic pustular folliculitis: Wright stain shows eosinophils.

Bullae and Extensive Blistering

*The bullous diseases may be life-threatening and may be impossible to distinguish from one another without skin biopsy. Appropriate therapy depends on correct diagnosis.

* Staphylococcal scalded skin syndrome: Skin biopsy reveals a split in the superficial epidermis. Culture of blister contents is negative; the locus of infection is nasopharyngeal, perianal, focus of impetigo, or abscess; mucous membranes may be red but not blistered or eroded, because the target of the staphylococcal exfoliative toxin is not present in mucous membranes.

* Congenital herpes simplex virus infection: Skin, eye, or mouth lesions are presenting signs in one third of infants. In newborns, the presenting part at delivery is most commonly affected.

* Toxic epidermal necrolysis: Skin biopsy reveals a split at the dermoepidermal junction; mucous membranes are diffusely eroded, unlike staphylococcal scalded skin syndrome.

* Bullous mastocytosis: Stroking will produce a wheal and flare (Darier's sign), and a Tzanck smear may show mast cells.

* Genetic disorders: These disorders vary in severity and probability of long-term sequelae. Early diagnosis and genetic counseling are important aspects of management.

* Epidermolysis bullosa: Blisters are most prominent at sites of friction. Familial forms are classified as epidermolytic or simplex, junctional, and dermolytic or dystrophic, based on the skin cleavage plane. Electron microscopic analysis or immunofluorescence mapping or both are required for precise diagnosis. Recently, genetic markers are being used to make a specific diagnosis in selected patients.

* Epidermolytic hyperkeratosis: Widespread erythema and blistering may be present at birth, causing confusion with epidermolysis bullosa and other blistering dermatoses. Thick, greasy, foul-smelling scales accentuated in skin creases may not become apparent until later in the 1st year of life.

* Incontinentia pigmenti: Vesicular skin lesions have a characteristic distribution along the lines of Blaschko. This striking pattern is seen with a variety of cutaneous abnormalities as a result of genetic mosaicism. Tzanck smear may show eosinophils but no multinucleate giant cells, and results of Gram staining are negative for organisms.

Key Points for Clinical Practice

1. The causes of bullous lesions in neonates range from benign skin conditions to potentially serious conditions that are associated with significant morbidity and mortality.

2. The clinical approach is based on the location, morphology, distribution, and timing of appearance of the lesions as well as the general condition of the infant.

3. Laboratory investigations are used to confirm the diagnosis. Herpes should be strongly suspected when evaluating vesiculobullous lesions, particularly those occurring in the scalp. In most cases of neonatal herpes, maternal history and physical examination findings are negative for genital herpes. Cutaneous manifestations are present only in 60% to 80% of neonatal herpes cases. Accordingly, any sick infant younger than 6 weeks of age who presents with seizures, aseptic meningitis, liver dysfunction, coagulopathy, or sepsis syndrome must be evaluated and treated immediately for possible neonatal herpes as well as bacterial infections. (Refer to Chapter 90 for a detailed discussion of Perinatal Herpes)

4. Because of the variable lesions and clinical symptoms seen with Congenital Syphilis, it has frequently been termed "the great imitator", and it is important to consider alternative diagnoses or vesiculobullous diseases that involve the palms and soles.

5. The infections and some serious blistering genetic disorders need to be differentiated from the common benign vesiculobullous disorders because of the need for early intervention in the former group.

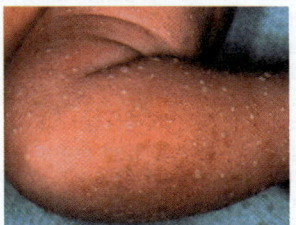

Transient Neonatal Pustular Melanosis is a benign condition of term neonates, characterized by the presence at birth of pustules or vesicles without surrounding erythema. These vesicopustules rupture easily, with subsequent formation of pigmented macules that are characteristically surrounded by a collarette of scale. These macules may persist for months but usually fade spontaneously within 3 to 4 weeks. Most commonly affected areas include the forehead, posterior ears, chin, neck, upper chest, back, buttocks, abdomen, and thighs, but all areas may be affected, including the palms and soles. Purely macular forms may indicate an intrauterine vesico-pustular eruption.1 The cause of TNPM is unknown. Genetic influence seems unlike since the condition has been reported in only one of identical twins.

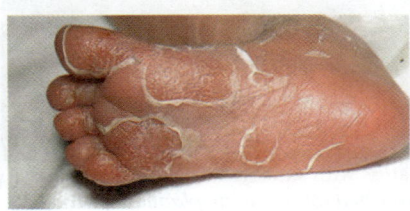

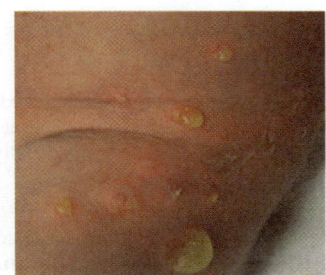

Bullous impetigo is seen commonly in areas of trauma such as the diaper area, circumcision wound, axilla, and periumbilical skin. These lesions are characterized by pustules or erythematous papules that later evolve into honey-colored crusts. Rarely, group B streptococcal infection can cause bullous skin lesions, and group A streptococcal skin infections also have been reported in epidemics in neonates.

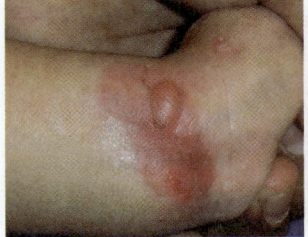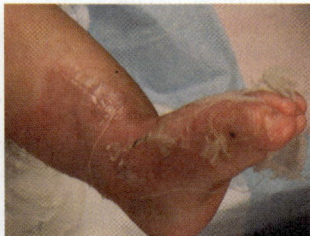

Recessive dystrophic epidermolysis bullosa (Hallopeau-Siemens type) (RDEB-HS) is a rare severe mechanobullous disorder resulting from a defect in collagen VII. Patients with RDEB-HS present with generalized blistering and denudation of the skin at birth and have mucosal involvement. The repeated blistering leads to scarring, which may be deforming and result in serious complications. Transmission electron microscopy is currently the gold standard for diagnosis of RDEB-HS. There is currently no satisfactory treatment available for RDEB-HS and the long-term prognosis is poor for this unremitting, debilitating disease. Management consists of continued wound care, infection control, nutritional support, and tailored therapies depending on the specific complications that arise.

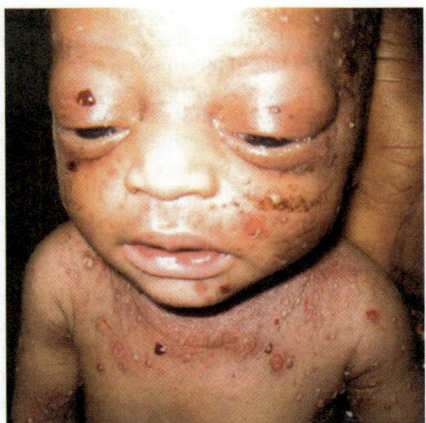

Neonatal herpes simplex type 2 infection. Although the child was normal at birth, fever, lethargy, and decreased feeding suddenly developed in this infant at 6 days of age. On examination, multiple grouped vesicular lesions were noted on the trunk, face and scalp. The liver and spleen were markedly enlarged and firm. He had a fulminant course resembling that of septic shock and died within 24 hours.

Congenital Syphilis: Dermatological findings are quite variable, although palmar/plantar, perioral, and anogenital regions are classically described as being involved. The image demonstrates findings at birth in an affected infant, with a desquamating eruption that was widespread over the entire body. These lesions are extremely infectious. Lesions described with early disease include petechiae, haemorrhagic vesicles, bullae (pemphygis syphiliticus), and erythematous macular, papulosquamous, annular, or polymorphous eruptions.

Diaper rash, or diaper dermatitis, is a general term describing any of a number of inflammatory skin conditions that can occur in the diaper area. These disorders can be conceptually divided into 3 categories:

Rashes that are directly or indirectly caused by the wearing of diapers: This category includes dermatoses, such as irritant contact dermatitis, #miliaria, #intertrigo, #candidal diaper dermatitis, and #granuloma gluteal infantum.

Rashes that appear elsewhere but can be exaggerated in the groin area due to the irritating effects of wearing a diaper: This category includes #atopic dermatitis, #seborrheic dermatitis, and #psoriasis.

Rashes that appear in the diaper area irrespective of diaper use: This category includes rashes associated with #bullous impetigo; #Langerhans cell histiocytosis (Letterer-Siwe disease, a rare and potentially fatal disorder of the reticuloendothelial system); #acrodermatitis enteropathica (zinc deficiency); #congenital syphilis; #scabies; and #HIV.

Pathophysiology

The precise etiology of most diaper rashes is not clearly defined. They likely result from a combination of factors that includes wetness, friction, urine and feces, and the presence of microorganisms. Anatomically, this skin region features numerous folds and creases, which present a problem with regard to both efficient cleansing and control of the microenvironment. The main irritants in this situation are fecal proteases and lipases, whose activity is increased greatly by elevated pH. An acidic skin surface is also essential for the maintenance of the normal microflora, which provides innate antimicrobial protection against invasion by pathogenic bacteria and yeasts. Fecal lipase and protease activity is also greatly increased by acceleration of gastrointestinal transit; this is the reason for the high incidence of irritant diaper dermatitis observed in babies who have had diarrhea in the previous 48 hours. The wearing of diapers causes a significant increase in skin wetness and pH. Prolonged wetness leads to maceration (softening) of the stratum corneum, the outer, protective layer of the skin, which is associated with extensive disruption of intercellular lipid lamellae. A series of diaper studies conducted mainly in the late 1980s found a significant decrease in skin hydration following the introduction of diapers with a superabsorbent core. Recent studies confirm that this trend is ongoing. Weakening of its physical integrity makes the stratum corneum more susceptible to damage by (1) friction from the surface of the diaper and (2) local irritants. At full term, the skin of infants is an effective barrier to disease and is equal to adult skin with regard to permeability. Some studies reported infant's transepidermal water loss to be lower than that of adult skin. However, dampness, lack of air exposure, acidic or irritant exposures, and increases in skin friction begin to break down the skin barrier. The normal pH of the skin is between 4.5 and 5.5. When urea from the urine and stool mix, urease breaks down the urine, decreasing the hydrogen ion concentration (increasing pH). Elevated pH levels increase the hydration of the skin and make the skin more permeable. Previously, ammonia was believed to be the primary cause of diaper dermatitis. Recent studies have disproved this, showing that when ammonia or urine is placed on the skin for 24-48 hours, no apparent skin damage occurs.

A series of studies has shown that the pH of cleansing products can change the microbiological spectrum of the skin. High soap pH values encourage propionibacterial growth on skin, whereas syndets (i.e., synthetic detergents) with a pH of 5.5 did not cause changes in the microflora.

Diagnosis of diaper dermatitis is based largely on the physical examination. A careful history, however, could elicit clues that aid in narrowing the differential diagnosis. Important points to obtain on history include the following:

*Onset, duration, and change in the nature of the rash
*Presence of rashes outside the diaper area
*Associated scratching or crying
*Contact with infants with a similar rash
*Recent illness, diarrhea, or antibiotic use

Assessment of current diapering practices (e.g., change frequency, type of diapers used, creams or ointments applied, methods used to clean the diaper area). One study review performed in the United Kingdom reported that irritant diaper dermatitis does not usually develop immediately after birth; onset is generally between 3 weeks and 2 years of age, with prevalence highest between 9 and 12 months.

Irritant contact dermatitis, miliaria (heat rash), and intertrigo

*Usually follows a bout of diarrhea *Exacerbated by scrubbing and the use of commercial wipes or strong detergents *Generic rash or *irritant diaper dermatitis* (IDD) is characterized by joined patches of erythema and scaling mainly seen on the convex surfaces, with the skin folds spared or involved last. *Lasts less than 3 days after more diligent diaper changing practices are initiated *Asymptomatic (except for miliaria) *Tidemark dermatitis refers to the bandlike form of erythema of irritated diaper margins

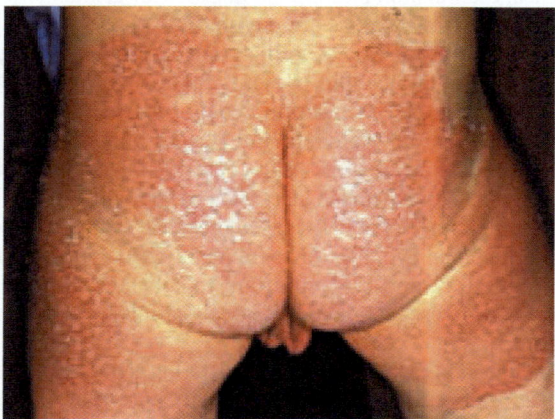

Irritant contact dermatitis

Candidal dermatitis (yeast infection): This type of rash is usually tender and painful, appearing in the folds of the baby's genitals, legs and the creases between the abdomen and thighs. This rash will start as small red spots that become more numerous and then form together as a raised bright red rash with distinct edges. The most common cause of this type of rash is a baby that is taking or has been taking antibiotics. Diaper dermatitis with secondary bacterial or fungal involvement tends to spread to concave surfaces (i.e. skin folds), as well as convex surfaces, and often exhibits a central red, beefy erythema with satellite pustules around the border (Hockenberry, 2003).

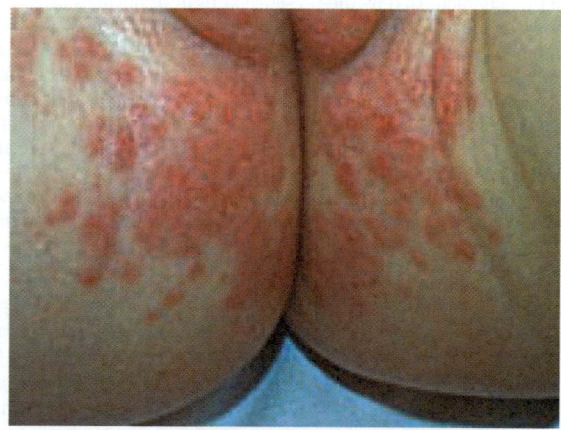

Candidal dermatitis with satellite lesions *The oropharynx should be inspected for the white plaques of thrush.*

Seborrheic dermatitis

*Usually occurs in infants aged 2 weeks to 3 months *Consists of an eruption of an oily, scaly, crusted dermatitis of the scalp (cradle cap), face, retroauricular regions, axilla, and presternal areas *Asymptomatic *Any child with widespread seborrheic dermatitis, diarrhea, and failure to thrive should be evaluated for Leiner disease, a functional defect of the C5 component of complement.Seborrheic dermatitis *Well-demarcated erythematous patches or plaques with an occasional greasy yellow scale. *When found in the groin area, the skin creases show more severe involvement. *Skin folds are not spared. *There are no satellite lesions. *Oily, scaly, crusted lesions also can be found in areas with a predominance of sebaceous glands (e.g. scalp, face, retroauricular regions, axilla, presternal area).

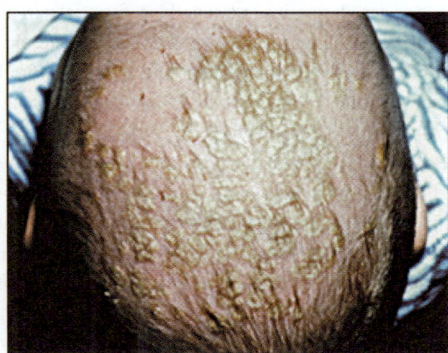

Psoriasis

*A family history of psoriasis can be a clue. *Not responsive to barrier creams, antifungal agents, and standard topical steroids *Involved areas include the scalp and nails. *This stubborn rash doesn't necessarily look distinctive. Other signs of psoriasis usually accompany the diaper rash, though, such as pitting of the nails or dark red areas with sharp borders and fine silvery scales on the trunk, face, or scalp.

Perianal dermatitis: This type of rash appears as a bright to dark redness around the anus. The stools of bottle fed babies being more alkaline than normal are sometimes the cause it. This rash will usually not appear with breast fed babies until after solids are introduced.

Impetigo: This type of rash can appear as yellow-brown crusty patches or pus filled pimples or blisters, which is usually accompanied by a lot of surrounding redness. This rash can cover the buttocks, lower abdomen, anus, umbilical cord, and thighs and then spread to other parts of the body. Impetigo is caused by bacteria (streptococci or staphylococci).

Atopic Dermatitis (Eczema): This type of rash shows up as red scaly patches on the legs and in the groin area. This rash may turn up in other parts of the body first while spreading to the diaper area between 6 and 12 months of age. Atopic dermatitis can be caused by many things including allergens, irritants, environmental and hereditary factors.

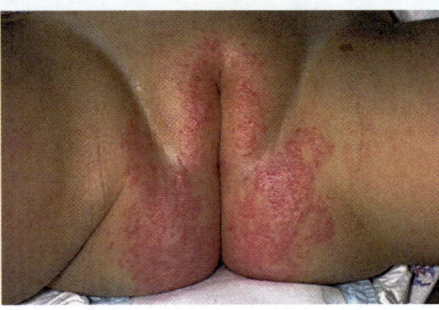

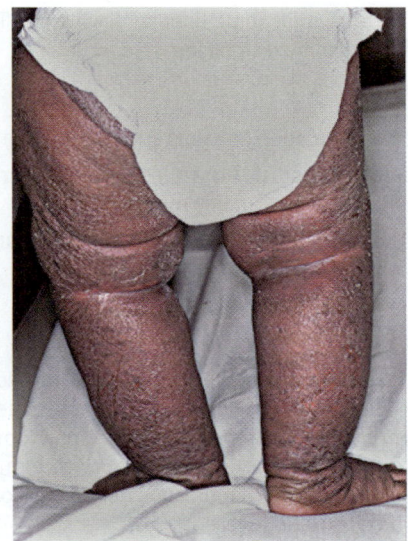

Baby eczema is characterized by patches of red, scaly, itchy skin. Occasionally the patches ooze and crust over. Baby eczema occurs when a baby is exposed to potentially irritating substances, such as bubble baths or rough fabrics. Associated with current or previous flares of rash on the face and extensor limb surfaces in infants

Atopic dermatitis *Acute lesions appear as poorly demarcated, erythematous, scaly, weepy, and crusted. *Chronic lesions are poorly defined, thickened, hyperpigmented, and often excoriated. *Lichenification can occur with chronic disease. *Distribution rarely involves the diaper area. It is more commonly observed on the face and extensor limb surfaces in children of diaper-wearing age. *Many babies outgrow eczema.*

Acrodermatitis enteropathica

*Associated with diarrhea, hair loss, and erosive perioral dermatitis *Patient may have a predisposition for malabsorption (i.e., cystic fibrosis) or malnutrition *Typically involves the perioral, perineal, and acral areas Erythematous, well-demarcated, scaly plaques and erosions Alopecia and growth failure Irritability

Scabies

*Acute onset *Pruritic *History of close contacts with recent onset of a similar erythematous serpiginous eruption. Papules, vesicles, burrows, nodules, and excoriations are found. The generalized distribution has a predilection for the palms, soles, face, scalp, and genitalia *Concurrent rash may be found in web spaces of hands or feet

Human immunodeficiency virus

*History of HIV exposure or risk factors *Associated cytomegalovirus or herpes infection *When this presents as a diaper rash, severe erosions and ulcerations are often present. *Distribution to the perineal area, especially the gluteal cleft, may be observed.

Langerhans cell histiocytosis: *Severe hemorrhagic diaper dermatitis unresponsive to any treatment *Other involved areas include the scalp and retroauricular areas *Diarrhea *Discrete, yellow-brown scaly or erythematous papules, purpuric papules, petechiae, deep ulcerations, and skin atrophy are present. *Hemorrhagic features are typical. *Usually involves skin folds *May have associated anemia, lymphadenopathy, and hepatosplenomegaly *May have associated involvement of the CNS, lungs, bones, and bone marrow.

Secondary bacterial infection: *Edema *Erythema *Tenderness *Purulent discharge .*Red streaking

Congenital syphilis

*Symmetric desquamation of palms and soles can be found.

*Papulosquamous, reddish-brown lesions are observed in the diaper area. Rarely, these can be erosive or bullous.

*Associated with anemia, hepatosplenomegaly, jaundice, and osseous lesions

Perianal pseudoverrucous papules

*This condition is characterized by 2-8 shiny, smooth, red, moist, flat-topped, round lesions with acanthosis or psoriasiform spongiotic dermatitis. *Whereas granuloma gluteal can be confused with Kaposi sarcoma, perianal pseudoverrucous papules are most commonly confused with genital warts. *Perianal pseudoverrucous papules and nodules can occur in the context of Hirschsprung disease.

Laboratory Studies *The primary forms of diaper rash generally can be diagnosed clinically. *Laboratory studies have few indications and limited utility.* *A complete blood count may be helpful, especially if a fever is present and a secondary bacterial infection is suspected. *The finding of anemia in association with hepatosplenomegaly and the appropriate rash may suggest a diagnosis of Langerhans cell histiocytosis or congenital syphilis. -When suspecting congenital syphilis, relevant serology should be sent. -Dark field microscopic examination for spirochetes from any bullous lesion scrapings can be performed. *Serum zinc level of less than 50 mcg/dL can confirm acrodermatitis enteropathica. *Gram stain or culture of the characteristic bullae of impetigo for *S aureus* can confirm this diagnosis. *Routine cultures demonstrate polymicrobial infections (e.g., streptococci, Enterobacteriaceae, and anaerobes) in nearly one half of cases. Potassium hydroxide (KOH) scrapings from a fresh papular or pustular lesion may demonstrate pseudohyphae in suspected cases of candidiasis. However, these may be absent in long-standing cases. Finding mites, ova, or feces on a mineral oil preparation of a burrow scraping can confirm the diagnosis of scabies. Skin biopsy can be performed to help differentiate granuloma gluteal infantum from granulomatous and neoplastic processes. *Histopathology, granuloma gluteal presents as nonspecific dermal inflammatory infiltrate composed of neutrophils, lymphocytes, histiocytes, plasma cells, occasional giant cells, and eosinophils, sometimes with an increase in the number of capillaries. *Examination of granuloma gluteal using an electron microscope reveals 3 types of giant cells: in the first type, the cells have widely enlarged endoplasmic reticulum; in the second type, they phagocytize erythrocytes; and in the third type, they have vesicles and granules and are similar to histiocytes. The name granuloma gluteal infantum is a misnomer since no granulomas are found in these lesions.*Skin biopsy also is used to confirm the diagnosis of Langerhans cell histiocytosis.

A number of rare diseases such as congenital syphilis, histiocytosis X, zinc deficiency, Wiscott-Aldrich syndrome, acrodermatitis enteropathica, or Jacquet's dermatitis all cause characteristic diaper rashes. These are extremely uncommon, but should be considered in prolonged, severe rashes that are unresponsive to the appropriate therapy.

Complications

*Because of maceration and abrasion of the skin under the diaper, skin ulceration and secondary infection by *C albicans* or bacteria are common. *Prevalence of a secondary bacterial infection is uncertain, but it is frequent. Multiple organisms, both aerobic and anaerobic, contribute to the development of this condition. *Psoriasis id reaction refers to a psoriaticlike eruption of papules and plaques after the initiation of treatment to a candidal infection.(-Involves the torso and the upper body and usually spares the extremities -Occurs days after antifungal therapy is started -Is poorly understood but can be treated with low or intermediate potency steroids) *Jacquet dermatitis is a complicated form of the irritant chafing type of diaper rash. (-It involves the development of erosive ulcerations with elevated margins. -Some nodular patterns also are described in severe chronic irritant dermatitis. -Cases remain surprisingly asymptomatic and usually are not secondarily infected.). *Psoriasiform napkin dermatitis refers to a clinical presentation that combines features of seborrheic and candidal diaper rashes. *Secondary bacterial and yeast infections.

Medicolegal Pitfalls- *Failure to consider serious systemic illness, such as Letterer-Siwe or acrodermatitis enteropathica, especially in a child with physical findings other than rash *Prescribing a topical steroid that is too potent for the occlusive environment under the diaper *Failure to recognize and treat a bacterial cellulitis *Exacerbating a case of herpes zoster by treatment with steroids.

When to seek medical advice? Prevention is the most effective way to treat Diaper Rash. With proper care Diaper Rash should go away within 2 or 3 days. If it still persists, do consult your doctor to prevent or treat if there is any secondary infection. Your doctor may recommend antifungal medicines or antibiotics. *Have your doctor examined your baby if:* *She develops fever and becomes toxic *Pimples and small ulcers appear. *The rash spreads to other areas. *Large bumps and boils form *severe recalcitrant rash suggestive of immunodeficiency.

If candidal infection is suspected, topical ointments or creams, such as nystatin, clotrimazole, miconazole, or ketoconazole can be applied to the rash with every diaper change. *Combination antifungal-steroid agents, should not be used because the high steroid concentration in the occlusive diaper area might cause Cushing syndrome. A review studied the use of a combination product of miconazole and hydrocortisone preparation and compared it with a combination product of nystatin/benzalkonium chloride/dimethicone/hydrocortisone preparation, both were found to improve the appearance of diaper dermatitis. *If oral thrush or perianal candidiasis is present or if repeated bouts of Candidal dermatitis have occurred, oral nystatin should also be prescribed. (Oral thrush: Premature infants: Oral Nystatin 1 mL PO qid ;Infants: 2 mL/dose, administer 1 mL to each side of mouth qid) *Ciclopirox was used and studied for the treatment of candidal diaper dermatitis and was found to be safe and effective. **For mild bacterial infections,** a topical antibiotic ointment (i.e., bacitracin) should be prescribed. *More severe infections caused by gram-positive organisms and anaerobes can be treated with a broad-spectrum oral antibiotic (i.e. amoxicillin/clavulanate, 40-mg amoxicillin component/kg/d for 7–10 d). *Impetigo can be treated with dicloxacillin 12.5-25 mg/kg/d or erythromycin 50 mg/kg/d for 7–10 d. *Congenital syphilis can be treated with 1 dose of IM penicillin G 50,000 U/kg.

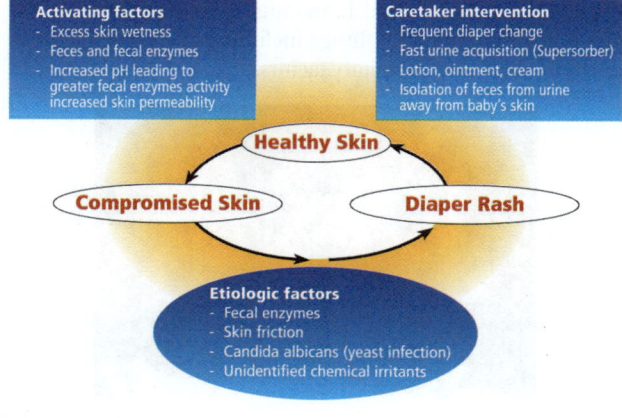

DIFFERENTIAL DIAGNOSIS OF DIAPER DERMATITIS

Disorder	Age of onset	Sites	Clinical features	Other signs
Seborrheic dermatitis	Under 3 months	Genito-crural flexures	Erythema and greasy scaling	Greasy scaling of scalp; Other flexures may be involved
Atopic eczema	Rarely under 2 months Usually 3 to 12 months	Anywhere	Erythema, papules, vesicles	Lesions elsewhere: cheeks, forehead, forearms, cubital and popliteal fossae, Pruritus
Candidiasis	Any age	Extends from perianal area	Sharply, irregularly marginated red patches, raised scaling edge, satellite pustules or papules	Oral lesions
Miliaria	Any age	Variable: groins or buttocks	Erythematous papules ± vesicles	Lesions elsewhere: e.g. neck, chest
Intertrigo	Any age	Any flexure or fold	Erythema only	Limited to areas of skin-on-skin contact
Perianal dermatitis	From 0 to 4 wks	Perianal	Erythema	None
Infantile psoriasis	2 weeks to 8 MO (usually 2 months)	Convex areas, but may be flexures	Sharply marginated red scaly plaques	Scalp and truncal lesions
Contact dermatitis (irritant)	Any age	Any area; area of contact with irritant	initially Erythema and vesicles	Other sites in contact with irritant may be involved; distinguish from atopic eczema

Treatment options for infantile seborrheic dermatitis

Medication	Directions and notes
White petrolatum Tar-containing shampoo Ketoconazole	Apply daily, May soften scales, facilitating removal with soft brush, Use several times per week . Use when baby shampoo has failed Safe, but potentially irritating.
Ketoconazole 2% cream or 2% shampoo	Cream: apply to scalp three times weekly Shampoo: lather, leave on for three minutes, then rinse. Use three times weekly, Small trial showed no systemic drug levels or change in liver function after one month of use.
Hydrocortisone 1% cream	Apply every other day or daily. Limit surface area to reduce risk of systemic absorption and adrenal suppression. May be especially effective for rash in flexural areas.

Differential diagnoses to consider in Diaper dermatoses

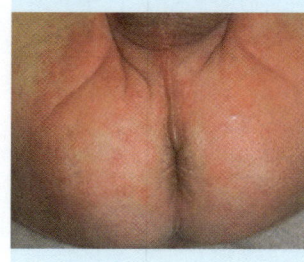

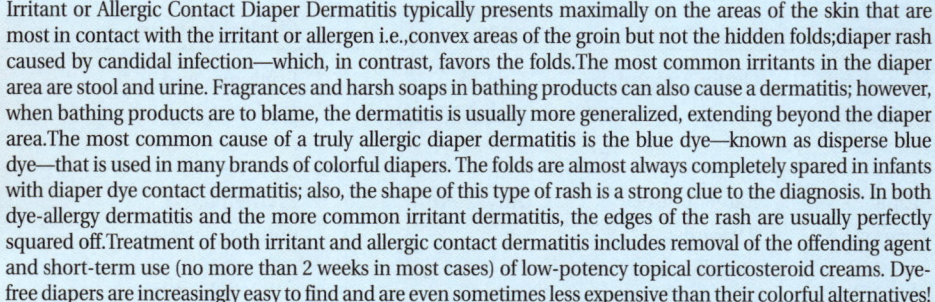

Irritant or Allergic Contact Diaper Dermatitis typically presents maximally on the areas of the skin that are most in contact with the irritant or allergen i.e.,convex areas of the groin but not the hidden folds;diaper rash caused by candidal infection—which, in contrast, favors the folds.The most common irritants in the diaper area are stool and urine. Fragrances and harsh soaps in bathing products can also cause a dermatitis; however, when bathing products are to blame, the dermatitis is usually more generalized, extending beyond the diaper area.The most common cause of a truly allergic diaper dermatitis is the blue dye—known as disperse blue dye—that is used in many brands of colorful diapers. The folds are almost always completely spared in infants with diaper dye contact dermatitis; also, the shape of this type of rash is a strong clue to the diagnosis. In both dye-allergy dermatitis and the more common irritant dermatitis, the edges of the rash are usually perfectly squared off.Treatment of both irritant and allergic contact dermatitis includes removal of the offending agent and short-term use (no more than 2 weeks in most cases) of low-potency topical corticosteroid creams. Dye-free diapers are increasingly easy to find and are even sometimes less expensive than their colorful alternatives!

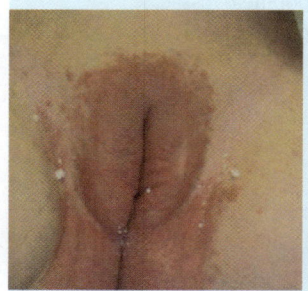

Candidal or Monilial Diaper Dermatitis: The classic clinical findings in this type of diaper rash are erythema and maceration in the inguinal creases (Figure E). The erythema is often described as "beefy red," and the maceration gives the skin the false appearance of being wet. In addition to involvement of the folds, candidal diaper dermatitis is often associated clinically with the appearance of satellite pustules emanating from the folds and forming a confluent array on the convex skin surfaces. The diagnosis is made almost solely on the basis of the clinical appearance; the history is often unhelpful, and culture is not required for confirmation.Treatment of candidal diaper dermatitis usually consists of application of one of the topical azole antifungal creams. These agents have broader antifungal coverage than either nystatin(Drug information on nystatin) or other over-the-counter topical antifungal therapies. The inclusion of topical corticosteroid creams in the treatment regimen is almost never necessary and is not advised. Moreover, use of combination creams that contain both antifungal agents and mid-to high-potency topical corticosteroids should be strictly avoided; such creams can be unsafe because they usually contain a higher-potency topical corticosteroid than would otherwise be prudent to use in the groin area—and because the action of the corticosteroid often counteracts the action of the antifungal in the cream.

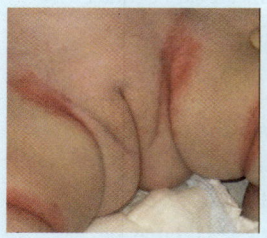

Intertrigo With Group A beta-Hemolytic Streptococcal Superinfection:Rarely, children present with skin findings reminiscent of candidal diaper dermatitis but with extensive involvement of noninguinal areas (such as the nuchal, antecubital, and popliteal spaces)and an especially moist-looking appearance without satellitosis. In such cases, it is important to obtain a specimen for culture to check for group A beta-hemolytic streptococci. If culture results are positive, initiate treatment with a topical antibiotic ointment, such as mupirocin ointment. This bacterial infection usually occurs as a complication of intertrigo, a dermatitis that develops in the intertriginous areas of the skin as a result of prolonged or excessive exposure to moisture and an overgrowth of yeast. Thus, treatment also involves keeping these areas dry and applying a topical azole antifungal or wash in addition to the mupirocin to speed resolution. Unless an infant is febrile, oral antibacterial therapy is usually unnecessary.

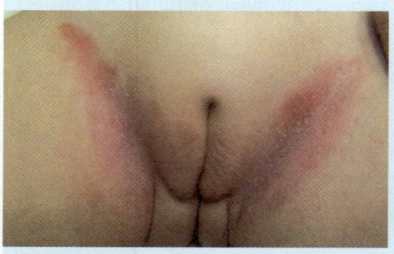

Psoriasis:In 2% of affected persons, it develops before the age of 2 years. The elbows, knees, hands, feet, and scalp are the areas of the body that are most often affected. However, there is a form of psoriasis known as inverse psoriasis that affects the folds. Inverse psoriasis is seen in both adults and children; in infants it can present as a diaper rash. Typical clinical findings in inverse psoriasis are a diffuse, light pink erythema that starts in the groin folds; a dry appearance (as opposed to the maceration seen in candidiasis); and an absence of satellite pustules. Additional, more classic psoriatic lesions may be seen elsewhere on the body. A history of psoriasis in other family members can help confirm the diagnosis, but a family history is not always present. Treatment of diaper psoriasis consists of intermittent use of mild topical corticosteroids, similar to those used to treat seborrheic dermatitis. If mild corticosteroids are not effective as monotherapy, topical immunomodulators may be added after a discussion of their offlabel use and black box warning is had with the family.

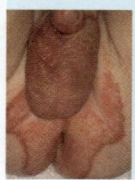 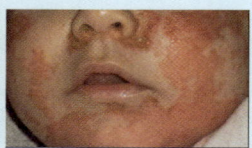

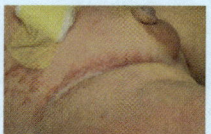

Acrodermatitis Enteropathica: The rash of acrodermatitis enteropathica (AE) has been described as looking like "malignant seborrhea"—in other words, like seborrheic dermatitis, it commonly affects both the diaper area and the face; however, the typical findings of seborrheic dermatitis are accentuated and there is increased inflammation. It presents as a recalcitrant eczematous and crusted dermatitis perianally and periorally .The complete failure of the rash to respond to the usual topical therapy for seborrheic dermatitis also helps distinguish AE from seborrhea. AE is associated with systemic zinc deficiency, which can result from either poor absorption of dietary zinc or malnutrition. AE can be diagnosed by checking the patient's zinc level or, for more rapid results, by checking the level of serum alkaline phosphatase, a zinc-dependent enzyme that can be low in cases of zinc deficiency. Treatment in most cases is with oral zinc supplementation; improvement is dramatic, usually within 1 week.

Langerhans Cell Histiocytosis: Like the diaper rash of AE, Langerhans cell histiocytosis (LCH) has been described as a more malignant version of seborrheic dermatitis. Clinically, LCH appears as crusted papules with surrounding petechiae or pinpoint hemorrhage. Lymphadenopathy may or may not be present, and if systemic progression has begun, the infant may be irritable or appear jaundiced. It is not advisable to wait for these symptoms to develop before proceeding with the systemic workup. When treating a patient with a particularly recalcitrant diaper dermatitis, it is appropriate to consider immediate referral to a pediatric dermatologist for punch biopsy to rule out cutaneous LCH. If the biopsy confirms the presence of Langerhans cells, then a full systemic workup and possible treatment with systemic therapy should be implemented by a pediatric oncologist, since diabetes insipidus, skeletal involvement, pulmonary disease, hepatic disease, or bone marrow involvement may develop in affected children.

Courtesy: DOUGLAS W. KRESS, MD and ROBIN P. GEHRIS, MD — University of Pittsburgh http://www.pediatricsconsultantlive.com/display/article/1803329/1584483?pageNumber=4

"The instinct of a mother to hold and care for her baby is primordial and primitive, and an overwhelmingly powerful feeling." - Jane Davis, Bogota, Dec 1998 who kangarooed her prem baby.

Kangaroo mother care KMC is a method of caring for small babies that has been shown to maintain warmth, improve feeding, reduce infections, and encourage bonding • KMC can reduce mortality by up to half in babies weighing less than 2000g • KMC has three main components including thermal care through continuous skin-to-skin contact usually with the mother, nutrition through exclusive breastfeeding, and support from health staff through early recognition and response to complications • If continuous KMC cannot be practiced due to space or other constraints, intermittent KMC is also beneficial • All stable small babies and their mothers will benefit from KMC. In 1979, Drs. Martinez and Edgar Rey of the Maternal Child Institute in Bogotá, Colombia developed a simple method to care for LBW infants called "The Kangaroo Mother Care Method" (KMC) to overcome the inadequacies of neonatal care in developing countries. KMC is used in hospitals, when the stabilized LBW infant is placed without clothes, except for diapers, a cap, and booties, upright between the mother's breasts held inside the pouch or mothers' blouse, to maximize skin-to-skin contact. **Its key features :** early, continuous and prolonged skin-to-skin contact between the mother and the baby; exclusive breastfeeding (ideally); it is initiated in hospital and can be continued at home; small babies can be discharged early; mothers at home require adequate support and follow-up; it is a gentle, effective method that avoids the agitation routinely experienced in a busy ward with preterm infants. Evidence of the effectiveness and safety of KMC is available only for preterm infants without medical problems. Research and experience show that: *KMC is at least equivalent to conventional care (incubators), in terms of safety and thermal protection, if measured by mortality. KMC, by facilitating breastfeeding, offers noticeable advantages in cases of severe morbidity. KMC contributes to the humanization of neonatal care and to better bonding between mother and baby in both low and high-income countries. KMC is, in this respect, a modern method of care in any setting, even where expensive technology and adequate care are available.*

Caring for the baby in kangaroo position : • Dress the baby in a nappy and cap • Place the baby in an upright position against the mother's bare chest, between her breasts and inside her blouse • Cover both mother and baby with a blanket or jacket if the room is cold • You may use a special garment; or tuck the mother's blouse under the baby or into her waistband • The baby must be secure enough so that the mother can walk around without holding her baby • Explain and demonstrate until the mother is confident to try the kangaroo position.

Sleeping and resting : Mother will best sleep with the baby in kangaroo position in a reclined or semi-recumbent position, about 15 degrees from horizontal. This can be achieved with an adjustable bed, if available, or with several pillows on an ordinary bed. It has been observed that this position may decrease the risk of apnea for the baby. include patent ductus arteriosus and other diseases that may be difficult to diagnose in settings with scarce resources. Refer the baby who fails to gain weight after the exclusion or treatment of the above common causes to a higher level of care, for further investigation and treatment.

Discharge: Usually, a KMC baby can be discharged from the hospital when the following criteria are met: *the baby's general health is good and there is no concurrent disease such as apnoea or infection; he is feeding well, and is exclusively or predominantly breastfed; he is gaining weight (at least 15g/kg/day for at least three consecutive days); his temperature is stable in the KMC*

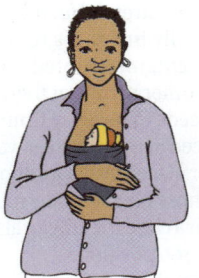

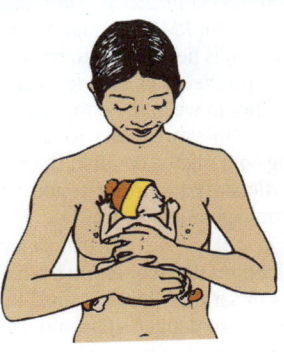

Baby in KMC Position

Secure him with the binder. The head, turned to one side, is in a slightly extended position. The top of the binder is just under baby's ear. This slightly extended head position keeps the airway open and allows eye-to-eye contact between the mother and the baby. Avoid both forward flexion and hyperextension of the head. The hips should be flexed and extended in a "frog" position; the arms should also be flexed.

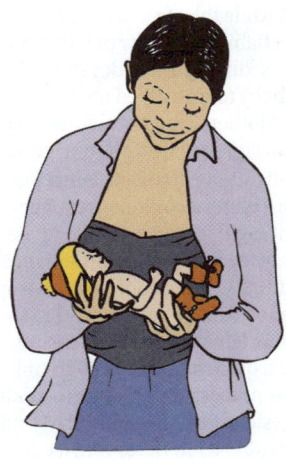

Moving the Baby in and out of the binder: hold the baby with one hand placed behind the neck and on the back; lightly support the lower part of the jaw with her thumb and fingers to prevent the baby's head from slipping down and blocking the airway when the baby is in an upright position; . place the other hand under the baby's buttocks.

Length: Skin-to-skin contact should start gradually, with a smooth transition from conventional care to continuous KMC. Sessions that last less than 60 minutes should, however, be avoided because frequent changes are too stressful for the baby. The length of skin-to-skin contacts gradually increases to become as continuous as possible, day and night, interrupted only for changing diapers, especially where no other means of thermal control are available. When the mother needs to be away from her baby, he can be well wrapped up and placed in a warm cot, away from draughts, covered by a warm blanket, or placed under an appropriate warming device, if available. During those breaks family members (father or partner, grandmother, etc.), or a close friend, can also help caring for the baby in skin-to-skin kangaroo position.

Duration: When the mother and baby are comfortable, skin-to-skin contact continues for as long as possible, first at the institution, then at home. *It tends to be used until the baby reaches term (gestational age around 40 weeks) or 2500g.* Around that time the baby also outgrows the need for KMC. She starts wriggling to show that she is uncomfortable, pulls her limbs out, cries and fusses every time the mother tries to put her back skin-to-skin. This is when it is safe to advise the mother to wean the baby gradually from KMC. Mother can return to skin-to-skin contact occasionally, after giving the baby a bath, during cold nights, or when the baby needs comfort. KMC at home is particularly important in cold climates or during the cold season and could go on for longer.

Monitoring baby's condition: Once the baby has recovered from the initial complications due to preterm birth, is stable and is receiving KMC, the risk of serious illness is small but significant. Teach the mother to recognize danger signs and ask her to seek care when concerned. Treat the condition according to the institutional guidelines. *Danger signs :* * Difficulty breathing, chest in-drawing, grunting *Breathing very fast or very slowly *Frequent and long spells of apnea *he baby feels cold: body temperature is below normal despite rewarming *Difficulty feeding: the baby does not wake up for feeds anymore, stops feeding or vomits *Convulsions * Diarrhea *Yellow skin.

*Breastfeeding:*The kangaroo position is ideal for breastfeeding. As soon as the baby shows signs of readiness for breastfeeding, by moving tongue and mouth, and interest in sucking (e.g. fingers or mother's skin), help the mother to get into a breastfeeding position that ensures good attachment. To start breastfeeding choose appropriate time - when the baby is waking from a sleep, or is alert and awake. Help the mother to sit comfortably in an armless chair with the baby in skin-to-skin position. For the first breastfeeds take the baby out of the pouch and wrap or dress him to better demonstrate the technique. Then put the baby into the kangaroo position and ask the mother to ensure good position and attachment.KMC nutrition • Babies who are unable to suckle should be fed expressed breast milk via a nasogastric tube or cup. Babies may be kept in the KMC position while tube feeding. Allow them to try suckling during the tube feed • Babies will show that they are ready to suckle as their rooting and suckling reflexes develop • Once the baby is able to suckle, allow baby to breastfeed on demand, and feed at least every three hours • Mothers who for medical reasons are using replacement feeds can still provide KMC and cup feed the baby

Inadequate weight gain: If weight gain is inadequate for several days, first assess the feeding technique, frequency, duration and schedule, and check that night feeds are given. Advise the mother to increase the frequency of feeds or to feed on demand. Encourage her to drink fluids when thirsty. Then look for other conditions as possible reasons for poor weight gain: oral thrush (white patches in the mouth) can interfere with feeding. Treat the baby by giving her an oral suspension of nystatin (100,000 IU/ml); use a dropper to apply 1ml in the oral mucosa and paint the mother's nipples after each feed until the lesions heal. Treat for 7 days; rhinitis is quite disturbing for the baby because it interferes with feeding. Nasal drops of normal saline solution in each nostril before each feed may help to relieve nasal obstruction; urinary tract infection is a possible insidious cause. Investigate if the baby fails to grow without obvious reasons.

Treat according to national/local treatment guidelines; severe bacterial infection can initially manifest itself with poor weight gain and poor feeding. If a previously healthy baby becomes unwell and stops feeding, consider this as a serious danger sign. Investigate for infection and treat according to national/local treatment guidelines. Other causes of failure to gain weight include patent ductus arteriosus and other diseases that may be difficult to diagnose in settings with scarce resources. Refer the baby who fails to gain weight after the exclusion or treatment of the above common causes to a higher level of care, for further investigation and treatment.

Discharge: Discharge means letting the mother and baby go home. Their own environment, however, could be very different from the KMC unit at the facility, where they were surrounded by supportive staff. They will continue to need support even though this will not have to be as intensive and frequent. The time of discharge may therefore vary depending on the size of the baby, bed availability, home conditions and accessibility of follow-up care. Usually, a KMC baby can be discharged from the hospital when the following criteria are met: *the baby's general health is good and there is no concurrent disease such as apnoea or infection; he is feeding well, and is exclusively or predominantly breastfed; he is gaining weight (at least 15g/kg/day for at least three consecutive days); his temperature is stable in the KMC position (within the normal range for at least three consecutive days); the mother is confident in caring for the baby and is able to come regularly for follow-up visits.* These criteria are usually met by the time the baby weighs more than 1500g. The home environment is also very important for the successful outcome of KMC. The mother should go back to a warm, smoke-free home and should have support for everyday household tasks. Where there are no follow-up services and the hospital is far away, mother and baby should be discharged later. Immunize the baby according to national policy and give enough iron/folate tablets to last until the follow-up visit. Fill in the home-based baby's record. Ensure that the mother knows: *how to apply skin-to-skin contact until baby shows signs of discomfort; how to dress the baby, when he is not in kangaroo position, to keep him warm at home; how to bath the baby and keep him warm after the bath; how to respond to baby's needs such as increasing the duration of skin-to-skin contact if he has cold hands and feet or low temperature at night; how to breastfeed the baby during the day and night according to instructions; when and where to return for follow-up visits (schedule the first visit and give the mother written/pictorial instructions for the above issues); how to recognize danger signs; where to seek care urgently if danger signs appear; when to wean the baby from KMC.* Tell the mother that it is always better to seek help, if in doubt: when caring for small infants it is better to seek care too often than to disregard important symptoms. Early discharge becomes a goal for the mother as she gains confidence in her ability to care for her baby. A baby can be discharged earlier if the following criteria are met: *adequate information on home care is given at discharge to mothers and their families, preferably as written and pictorial instructions; mothers have received instructions on danger signs, and know when and where to seek care.*

She should return immediately to hospital or go to another appropriate provider, if the baby: stops feeding, is not feeding well, or vomits; becomes restless and irritable, lethargic or unconscious; has fever (body temperature above 37.5°C); is cold (hypothermia - body temperature below 36.5°C) despite rewarming; has convulsions; has difficulty breathing; has diarrhoea; shows any other worrying sign.Early discharge becomes a goal for the mother as she gains confidence in her ability to care for her baby. A baby can be discharged earlier if the following criteria are met: *adequate information on home care is given at discharge to mothers and their families, preferably as written and pictorial instructions; mothers have received instructions on danger signs, and know when and where to seek care.KMC at home and routine follow-up* Ensure follow-up for the mother and the baby, either at your facility or with a skilled provider near the baby's home. The smaller the baby is at discharge, the earlier and more frequent follow-up visits he will need. If the baby is discharged in accordance with the above criteria, the following suggestions will be valid in most circumstances: – two follow-up visits per week until 37 weeks of post-menstrual age; – one follow-up visit per week after 37 weeks.

The content of the visit may vary according to mother's and baby's needs; check the following, however, at each follow-up visit:

KMC: Duration of skin-to-skin contact, position, clothing, body temperature, support for the mother and the baby. Is the baby showing signs of intolerance? Is it time to wean the baby from KMC (usually at around 40 weeks of post-menstrual age, or just before)? If not, encourage the mother and family to continue KMC as much as possible.

Breastfeeding: Is it exclusive? If yes, praise the mother and encourage her to continue. If not, advise her on how to increase breastfeeding and decrease supplements or other fluids. Ask and look for any problem and provide support. If the baby is taking formula supplements or other foods, check their safety and adequacy; make sure that the family has the necessary supply.

Growth: Weigh the baby and check weight gain in the last period. If weight gain is adequate, i.e. at least 15g/kg/day on average, praise the mother. If it is inadequate, ask and look for possible problems, causes and solutions; these are generally related to feeding or illness.

Illness: Ask and look for any signs of illness, reported by the mother or not. Manage any illness according to your local protocols and guidelines. In case of non-exclusive breastfeeding, ask and look particularly for signs of nutritional or digestive problems.

Drugs: Give a sufficient supply of drugs, if needed, to last until the next follow-up visit.

Immunization: Check that the local immunization schedule is being followed. Mother's concerns Ask the mother about any other problem, including personal, household, and social problems. Try to help her find the best solution for all of them.

Next follow-up visit: Always schedule or confirm the next visit. Do not miss the opportunity, if time allows, to.

KMC support

• KMC ward should be warm and inviting
• The mother must keep her baby in KMC position at all times (except
while she bathes)
• Good hygiene is important, including hand washing after using the
toilet and before feeding
• Mothers can walk around the ward and outside with their babies in the
KMC position if the weather conditions are favourable
• Occupy the mothers and encourage appropriate developmental stimulation
• Health staff should be available to respond early and quickly to complications

KMC monitoring: *6 hourly heart rate, respiratory rate, temperature, activity, colour, intake and output *Daily weight *Daily KMC score-Refer to Table given below.

KMC Daily Score Sheet
Based on the Intra-hospital KMC Training Programme in Bofota, Colombia

Date of birth _____/_____/_____
Date_____

Name :		Breast feeding :		Date started 24 hour KMC _____/_____/_____	Day 1	Day 2	Day 3	Day 4	Day 5	Day 6	Day 7
Hospital No.		Formula :		_____/_____/_____							
Evaluation	**Score**			Weight_____							
	0	**1**	**2**	**Remark**							
Socio-economic support	No help or support	occasional help	Good support system								
Mother's milk production	Expresses 0-10ml breast milk	expresses 10-20ml breast milk	Expresses 20-30ml breast milk	Must score 2 before discharge N/A for formula							
Positioning and attaching of baby on to breast	Always need assistance	Occasionally needs assistance	No assistance needed	Not applicable for formula feeding							
Baby's ability to suckle at the breast / cup feed	Gets tires very quickly	Gets tired infrequently	Takes all feeding well								
Confidence in handling baby, e.g. feeding, bathing, changing	Always need assistance	Occasionally needs assistance	No assistance needed								
Baby's weight gain per day	0-10g	10-20g	20-30g	Must score 1 or 2 before discharge							
Confidence in administering vitamin and iron drops	No confidence	Some confidence	Fully confident								
Acceptance & application of KMC	does not accept or apply KMC	Partly accepts & applies KMC method	Applies KMC without having to be told	Applies KMC on own initiative							
Confidence in caring baby at home	does not feel sure or able	Feels slightly unsure and unable	Feels confident								
Knowledge of KMC	No Knowledge	Some Knowledge	Knowledgeable								
TOTAL SCORE per day											

Ready for discharge when the score is 19 or more

Discharge readiness critiria:
*Baby's general health is good and no evidence of infection *Feeding well, and receiving exclusively or predominantly breast milk. *Gaining weight (at least 15-20 gm/kg/day for at least three consecutive days) *Maintaining body temperature satisfactorily for at least three consecutive days in room temperature. *The mother and family members are confident to take care of the baby in KMC and should be asked to come for follow-up visits regularly.

References: 1. World Health Organization. Kangaroo mother care: a practical guide. Department of Reproductive Health and Research, WHO, Geneva.2003.

2.'Kangaroo mother care' to prevent neonatal deaths due to preterm birth complications Joy E Lawn et al, International Journal of Epidemiology, Volume 39, Issue suppl 1, Pp. i144-i154

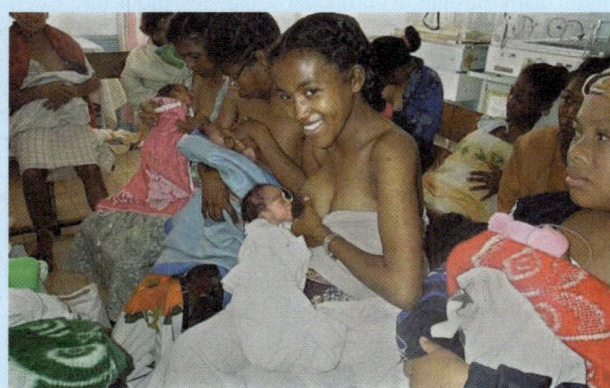

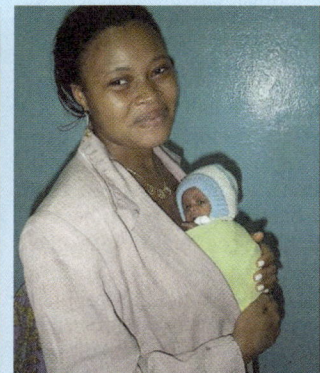

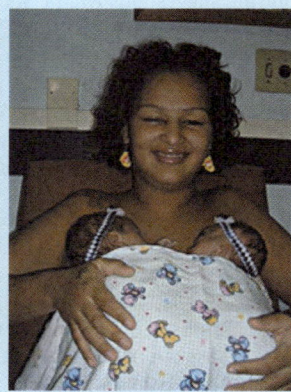

KMC providers (mothers "kangarooing" their infants) are enmeshed in a social peer network

Prolonged skin to skin contact in the "kangaroo" position promotes bonding. Even TWINS can be nursed with KMC.Coutresy-BMJ

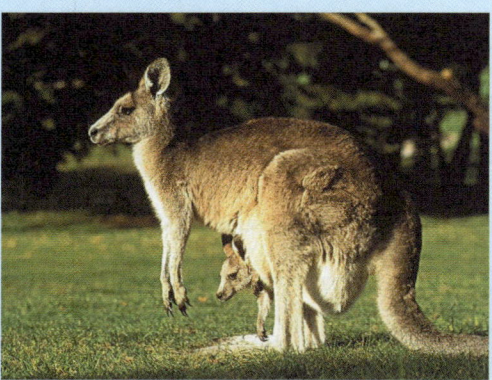

Why the title "Kangaroo Mother Care"? Mother kangaroo is a mammal (just like us), and feeds its baby milk like we do (or like we should!) from a nipple inside its pouch. The pouch covers the baby with skin, and this not only protects the very immature baby, but also provides it with a total environment which is essential for development. *This includes warmth, food, comfort, stimulation, protection.* The baby is CARRIED for all this time, without interruption !

KMC-Summary points

* KMC is a simple intervention to care for preterm newborns by tying the baby to the mothers front, providing thermal care through continuous skin to skin contact, increased breastfeeding, reduced infections and early recognition of illness.

* Kangaroo Mother Care (KMC), a technique developed in Colombia to deal with overcrowding of neonatal units, delivers ideal conditions for low birthweight infants to thrive.

* KMC is safe, works at a fraction of the cost of an incubator, reduces morbidity (in impoverished settings), improves breastfeeding rates, improves bonding between mother and infant, and increases satisfaction in parents and care providers.

* Meta-analysis of 3 RCTs shows major mortality reduction [51% (18–71%)] for neonatal mortality in babies with birthweight <2000 g, with even greater reductions in serious morbidity. This evidence is sufficient to recommend the routine use of KMC for all babies <2000 g as soon as they are stable. Up to half a million neonatal deaths due to preterm birth complications could be prevented each year if this intervention were implemented at scale.

Kangaroo mother care and infant instability

Signs of instability/stability: *Observation:* Observe infant for physiological signs and NIDCAP signs of stability and instability (such as color change, flaccidity, extension movements) before transfer and during KMC. *VLBW infants:* Decisions about each KMC session during first week of life are based on ongoing assessment of weight loss, and high serum sodium level. *Guide parents in recognizing signs of instability/ stability:* Coach parents in recognizing physiological signs and NIDCAP signs of stability and instability and in how they can help the infant to regain stability before transfer and in the kangaroo position. *Assistance of infant stability:* Give support for flexed position, support infant's strategies for self-regulation (hands joined in midline/ contact with mouth/face, feet supported by bedding/parent's hands, pacifier sucking). Inform parents that infant stability and wellbeing are enhanced by sufficiently tight support by KMC clothing, and that holding with still hands provides regulating stimulation, whereas patting and stroking may cause instability. *Postpone transfer to KMC:* At signs of infant instability, assist infant stability and wait until infant is calm and stable. At signs of persistent instability, consider transfer to kangaroo position for supporting improved stability.

Instability during KMC: *First action:* Control/adjust correct kangaroo position (straight trunk and neck; not a slumped-together position, head turned sideways) for fully patent airways. The position should allow for diaphragmatic breathing. *Infant hypothermia:* Make sure (a) the whole frontal surface of the infant is in physical contact with parent, no textiles (parent's underwear) between them, (b) infant is inside parent's clothes, infant wears a warm cap, and (d) infant's head and back are adequately covered with a cap and an insulating warm blanket. Parents should wear appropriate KMC clothing for maintenance of close physical contact. *Continued instability:* Consider oral/nasal suctioning, and/or suctioning in the endotracheal tube. *Interruption of KMC:* Only when all possible measures have been taken without expected results.

When KMC is not possible: *Abstain from KMC:* Only when severe instability (severe apnea, color change, bradycardia, desaturation) occurs in response to touch and routine care giving procedures). *Physical and other contact when KMC is not possible:* Inform parents about how to minimize separation by gentle containing touch, proprioceptive sense stimulation, presenting face where infant can see it/have face-to-face visual contact, talking and singing soothing lullabies, and olfaction stimuli.

Severe instability, terminal care: *Transfer of instable infant to KMC:* Can be used when assessed as justified by responsible neonatologist. *KMC during terminal care:* Can be offered to parents respecting cultural end-of-life practices, after parental consent.

KMC = Kangaroo mother care; NIDCAP = Newborn Individualized Developmental Care and Assessment Program; VLBW = Very low birth weight.
Father includes partner and substitute designated as KMC provider by the family.
Courtesy: State of the art and recommendations Kangaroo mother care: application in a high-tech environment-Kerstin Hedberg Nyqvist, Department of Women's and Children's Health, University Hospital, Uppsala 751 85, Sweden Acta Pædiatrica DOI:10.1111/j.1651-2227.2010.01794.x

Developmental Care

Summary *premature neonates are born before brain maturation is complete *the stressful and abnormal environment of the nursery may contribute to altered brain development *modification of the nursery environment may reduce long term morbidity *light protection should not prevent adequate visualization of the infant **Introduction** While advances in biomedical technology and improvements in care have led to a decrease in mortality rates in premature and extremely low birth weight neonates, there has not been a corresponding change in morbidity. Comprehensive long term follow up of these infants has lead to the recognition of new morbidities *including learning and attention deficit disorders *language comprehension and speech problems *and visual and motor impairments The focus of neonatal care must now extend beyond simply achieving survival. The challenge now is to optimize infants' developmental course and long term outcome. Developmental problems resulting from damage to the cerebral cortex may not become evident for some months or even years after birth. Infants 'at risk' therefore require long term developmental follow up.

Interventions in Developmental Care

The aim of developmental care is to **modify** the environment of the nursery utilizing a broad range of strategies designed to

*reduce stress and prevent agitation *preserve energy and promote growth *enhance recovery *facilitate self regulatory capabilities *promote C.N.S. organization Individualized strategies such as the 'Neonatal Individualized Developmental Care and Assessment Program' (NIDCAP) have also been used.

Principles of developmental care

*recognize physiological stressors *certain sensory and motor stimuli may cause physiological changes such as fluctuations in heart rate and oxygen saturation, and/or apnoea *such stimuli include handling, painful procedures, or sudden loud noise *protect from light *constant bright light in the nursery can interfere with the development of natural diurnal rhythms and have an arousing effect on the C.N.S. *reducing light levels may prevent sensory overload and facilitate rest *cover incubator hoods to reduce exposure to bright overhead lights *dim the lights at night to assist in establishing day/ night patterns

Light protection should not preclude adequate visualization of the sick or potentially sick infant.

*protect from noise *noise (above 80–85 decibels) has the potential for damage to the cochlea & hearing loss in adults. The immature cochlea is more sensitive to damage *closing portholes with a 'snap', dropping the head of the mattress and tapping or placing bottles on the Plexiglas top of the incubator all have a sound level above 80db *noise may also cause agitation, irritability and crying, which may result in increased intra-cranial pressure and decreased oxygen saturation *interventions to reduce noise include *turn the radio down or off *have a designated 'quiet time' daily *avoid banging bin lids *remove bubbling water in oxygen/ventilator tubing *close incubator portholes gently *give 'handover' away from the infant's bedside *avoid talking loudly, especially across open care beds *protect from over-stimulation *handling can effect physiological stability and cause hypoxemia, especially in the extremely premature, unstable or ill neonate *provide 'time out'/ recovery time when the infant demonstrates avoidance or 'stress' behavior. Signs of stress behaviour include *color changes: mottled, dusky, cyanosed *apnoea, bradycardia, desaturation *hiccoughing, sneezing, yawning, gagging, regurgitating feeds *tremors, twitches, frantic activity, arching, frowning, gaze averting *completely flaccid trunk, extremities & face *easy fatiguability (**take care as these behaviours are non-specific and may have other causes that require specific treatment**) *introduce sensory stimuli slowly: e.g. one toy or picture in the incubator (too many are overwhelming) and be sensitive to the infant's response *alter patterns of care to allow maximum time for sleep and growth *clustering of cares/ minimum handling approach *positioning: prone or side lying to enhance flexion, bring the shoulders forward and the hands to the midline *provide boundaries and use rolls/nesting to maintain desired posture, reduce agitation, conserve energy and create a feeling of 'security' for the infant *avoid moving an infant who has sought out his own boundaries (e.g. foot against a porthole door) *establish day and night patterns (diurnal rhythm) *dim the lights at night and turn the radio off *remind staff to talk & walk quietly around the nursery *avoid non-emergency interventions during the night, e.g. bathing and weighing *normalize parent expectations *promote parent understanding of their infant's behaviour, including signs and manifestations of stress *provide opportunities for Kangaroo Care, Non-nutritive sucking and other forms of sensory stimuli as the infant matures and is able to maintain physiological homeostasis *use SIDS guidelines for posturing infants during convalescent care

Areas of uncertainty in clinical practice: *Does developmental care lead to the hypothesized measurable outcomes of *reduction in incidence and severity of developmental delay *improved weight gain *decreased length of hospital stay *less days of mechanical ventilation *less days of oxygen dependence?

A Cochrane review of 31 eligible randomized control trials found evidence of some benefit from developmental interventions, with no major harmful effects reported. However, there were a large number of outcomes for which conflicting effects or no effects were demonstrated. *Is developmental care cost effective?* Broad interventions such as reducing light and noise in a nursery are easily implemented, of negligible cost and not harmful; however implementing and maintaining a formal developmental care program (such as NIDCAP) has a significant economic impact. Symington and Pinelli (2001) suggest that further evidence of the efficacy of developmental care is required before a clear direction for practice can be supported.

Reference : Neonatal Handbook- Royal Australia Children Hospital.

Minimal handling (stimulation) is intended for all preterm and acutely ill infants. A term infant with persistent pulmonary hypertension is particularly vulnerable to repeated handling, procedures, and interventions that decrease PaO2. Some chronically ill infants with prolonged hospitalization may also benefit from this policy (i.e. bronchopulmonary dysplasia/chronic lung disease). Always remember that handling & disturbing a sick Neonate in the NICU in any way may cause his condition to deteriorate, usually by making him *hypoxic*. Anything that makes a baby cry, by making his respiration irregular, will compromise his ventilation (even if he is ventilated), increase his pulmonary artery pressure, increase the right to left shunt, and thus lower his PaO_2. Handling the baby involves opening the doors of the incubator, which lets the oxygen out. Complex manoeuvres - such as a chest X-ray or an LP, disconnecting the oxygen supply when sucking out the endotracheal tube, or giving chest physiotherapy - are other potent causes of hypoxia. Many spontaneously breathing low birth weight babies, when handled or made to cry, start to writhe about, take a deep inspiration, stop breathing, remain apneic and become cyanosed with a bradycardia. The full-term or nearly term infant without acute illness (i.e. asymptomatic rule out sepsis), the matured preterm, or the convalescing infant who was previously ill are not necessarily at risk from stimulation and therefore should be provided developmentally appropriate parental and staff interaction (i.e. holding, rocking, singing to, talking to, etc.).

POINTS TO REMEMBER

* The less you touch a baby the less likely you are to transmit infection to him from your own hands, or to transfer his infection to another baby. Always wash your hands before and after handling a Neonate.

* Heel pricks, venous and arterial punctures are painful and make babies cry. This not only gives incorrect results for blood gases, but also causes clinical deterioration. If blood sampling for biochemistry, blood gases or hematology is going to be frequent, an intra-arterial sampling line is essential.

* ECG, respiration, temperature, blood pressure, and blood gases should be monitored continuously by electronic means.

* Continuous monitoring is, in any case, always superior to intermittent monitoring.

* Putting arterial lines and monitors in place does involve one period of intense activity and interference immediately after admission. Do these procedures within the incubator or under a radiant heat source, and ensure that the baby's oxygenation is sustained throughout.

* Use local anesthetics or boluses of analgesic for painful procedures; there is no doubt that Neonates feel pain.

* Oropharyngeal suction, and in particular suction down an ETT during assisted ventilation is notorious for causing deterioration. ETT suction is overused, and with rare exceptions is not indicated at all in the first 24hrs of ventilation, and then not more than 12hourly unless there is infection or bronchorrhea. If the PaO_2 falls below 6.6 kPa (50mmHg), *stop* suctioning at once and reconnect the IPPV.

* If a lumbar puncture needs to be done or an intravenous line resited, do it as expeditiously as possible without moving the baby from his incubator and interfering with oxygen administration.

* If anyone fails on any procedure more than twice, *stop*. Let the baby recover, and then get someone else to try.

* X-rays involve major man-handling of the baby if the incubator does not have a film cassette. A member of the medical or nursing staff must always help the radiographer. Take great care to sustain oxygenation during the procedure.

* If you are taking an X-ray to exclude pneumothorax or to ensure that an endotracheal tube is properly sited - and if the x-ray gives you that information even if it is blurred, rotated, expiratory or over penetrated - do not repeat it.

* Does the baby's incubator really need a spring clean, and does he really mind a small amount of meconium in his nappy or crusted blood on his scalp? The nursing staff may feel that a clean baby in a clean incubator is a healthy baby, but he will not share their enthusiasm if they make him hypoxic and apneic.

* Does the baby perhaps need a rest? Studies have shown that babies in intensive care are never left alone for more than a few minutes. They certainly do not get the chance to sleep without someone stuffing a suction tube up their nose, a thermometer into their rectum or a needle into their skin.

Decrease visual and auditory stimulation by:

a. Turning lights down and discouraging loud talking and noise within the unit and especially at the bedside.

b. Removing excess fluid in respiratory tubing.

c. Keeping volume on ventilator, monitor and pump alarms at the lowest level possible yet at a level sufficiently audible in respect to distances and competing noise within the unit.

d. Using care to quietly open/close isolette portholes and doors.

e. Avoiding use of the isolette roof as a shelf or writing table.

f. Removing bedside phone, or, turning ring to lowest level.

g. Transitioning infant from warming table to isolette as soon as possible.

h. Utilizing isolette covers on all isolettes

DOCUMENTATION

Document in the progress record of the nurse's notes the:

a. infant's behavior cues

b. responses to stressful procedures/stimuli

c. interventions performed to decrease stress

d. reason for sedation use if ordered

TEACHING

1. Provide the parent(s) with an explanation of:
   a. Minimal handling
   b. Clustered care
   c. Designated "touch times" (usually preceding or following feeding/caregiving times)
2. Explain the effects of stimulation and stress on the infant.
3. Assist parents in the recognition of behavior cues.
4. Reassure parents that they will participate in the infant's care as soon as the infant's condition improves.
5. Post a "minimal handling" sign on the patient's bed to notify team members of the protocol.
6. Alert caregivers/hospital personnel as to infant's sensitivity to noise by posting a "Quiet Zone" sign on nursery doors

Handling of Small Babies Germinal Matrix - Intraventricular Hemorrhage (GM-IVH) is one of the most frequently encountered neurological problems of the premature neonate. This document outlines information and recommended best practice for assessing the risks and subsequent nursing care of the infant <30 weeks gestation. Infants between 23 and 32 week gestation are at risk, with infants under 30 weeks gestation being most at risk. There are, however, exceptions to this. Timing of GM-IVH

* 0–90% of bleeds in the first 3 days. *7–20% in the next 4 days until <5% after 7 days.

Hemodynamic Instability

* All hemorrhages seem to start in the germinal matrix as the thin walled blood vessels are vulnerable to damage due to disturbances in perfusion, caused by an increase, decrease or fluctuating blood pressure. Changes in blood pressure may occur as a result of handling, for example movement, crying, feeding, intubation, suctioning and stimulation.

* Hypotension/hypertension is often a recurring and difficult problem exacerbated by the fact that normal ranges for blood pressure in infants that are VLBW/ELBW has not been firmly established.

* In very low birthweight infants during the first 48–96 hours * blood pressure is influenced by birthweight and gestational age.

Infant Positioning, Weighing and Optimal Hemodynamic Stability :

Try to *cluster cares* to allow long rest periods particularly between stressful interventions. The frequency and duration of handling during intensive care have been shown to influence the occurrence and severity of hypoxemia which can increase the risk of GM-IVH in VLBW/ELBW infants. Disruptive tactile stimulation can precipitate a negative physiologic chain of events and lead to intracranial pressure or cause hemodynamic fluctuations. Excessive handling can also initiate hypoxemia.

When changing nappies care can be taken by sliding the nappy under to avoid raising legs as increase to intracranial pressure occurs when infants legs are lifted, especially if above the head. Position with the head midline and the head of the bed slightly elevated. Intracranial pressure is lowest when the head of the bed is elevated. Side lying with head in midline to avoid twisting of the infants body also reduces the risk of increasing intracranial pressure.

Infants <30 weeks should not be offered cuddles or kangaroo care in the first 5 days of life. Discuss at ward round if appropriate for family to be offered cuddles to infant >3 days old, stable and over 30 weeks gestational age. Infants that are 30 weeks and over should have their stability and disease process considered prior to offering cuddles. An infant that is not expected to survive may also be an exception to these guidelines.

Blood Pressure Management

Monitor blood pressure diligently: Infants <32/40 with arterial lines have their BP monitored continuously and recorded hourly on observation sheet. VLBW/ELBW babies and sick infants i.e. <32/40 weeks ventilated, Hudson CPAP, O2 requirement, without arterial lines may need 1–2 hourly cuff BP measurement initially. Discuss frequency with NS-ANP/medical staff. The optimal mean is decided by senior NP/medical staff. BP should be equal to or greater than the gestational age in the first 24 hours. Alarm limits on CR monitors should always be on and set at appropriate levels

i.e. upper level slightly above recommended mean BP and lower alarm level set at slightly lower than desired mean BP. Report fluctuations in BP, hypotension and hypertension to medical staff. Consider allowing recovery periods to avoid rapid BP fluctuations during handling. a result of handling, for example movement, crying, feeding, intubation, suctioning and stimulation. *Hypotension/hypertension is often a recurring and difficult problem exacerbated by the fact that normal ranges for blood pressure in infants that are VLBW/ELBW has not been firmly established. *In very low birthweight infants during the first 48-96 hours*blood pressure is influenced by birthweight and gestational age.

Reduce fluctuations in blood pressure: *Minimal handling and cluster cares* to allow rest periods. Handle gently. Pre-oxygenate as indicated and allow time for SpO_2 to recover between suctions. ELBW infants ideally should only be warm weighed with two people to facilitate procedure. *Infants <30 weeks are not to be weighed in the first 5 days unless requested by the medical staff. To avoid fluid overload, use accurate checking under RBP of rate of IV pumps. *Rate of intermittent infusions e.g. blood plasma, IVAC pump is also checked by two NPs and signed. *Volume limit on IV pumps to be set within 10% of limit. Nurse infant flat or head of bed slightly raised, not head down. Head needs to be in line with body, **not** twisted so as not to increase intracranial blood flow and pressure.

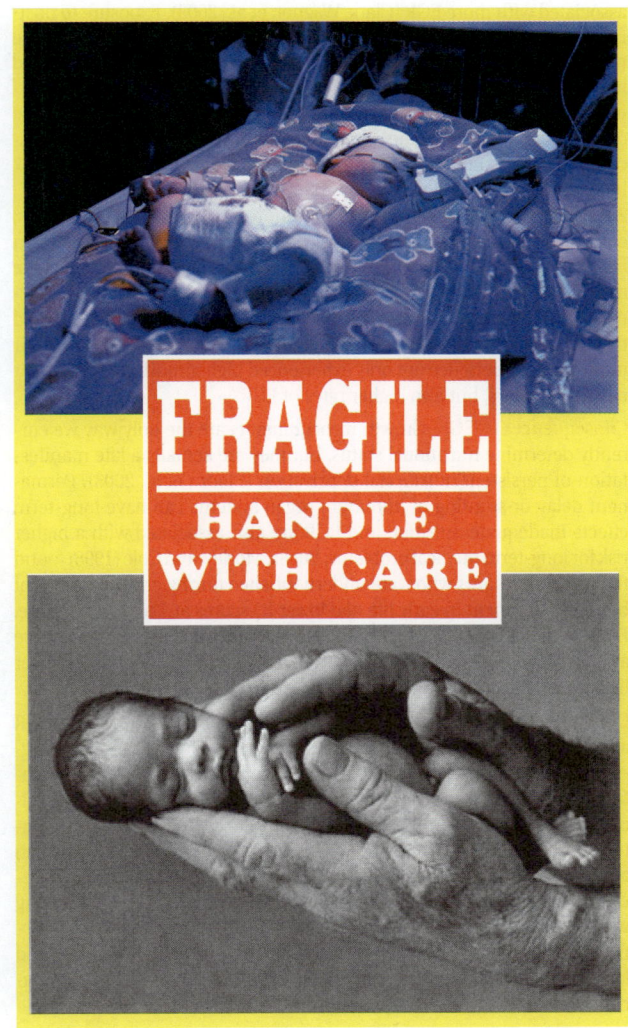

FRAGILE HANDLE WITH CARE

EXTRAUTERINE GROWTH RESTRICTION (EGR)

EGR is the development of severe nutritional deficit during the first weeks of life that continues to accrue throughout the hospitalization of VLBW infants. EGR is defined as growth values <"10th" percentile of intrauterine growth expectation based on estimated gestational age (Clark, Thomas, & Peabody, 2003).The American Academy of Pediatrics Committee on Nutrition (AAPCN) suggested in 1985 that, although optimal weight gain for VLBW infants is not known, it is reasonable to assume that weight gain should parallel that of intrauterine growth for a fetus at the same postconceptional age. Initial weight loss is particularly critical in VLBW infants because focus on illness and treatment, as well as a predilection to withhold feeding from sick infants, may interfere with providing adequate nutrition for several days to several weeks, increasing the amount of initial weight loss.Even when growth rate after the first few weeks is similar to that of intrauterine growth, infants rarely meet expected growth for estimated gestational age (EGA) by discharge.

Risk Factors for EGR: The literature contains several studies describing risk factors for EGR, which include the infant's birthweight and EGA, the duration of initial weight loss, and certain morbidities. Clark, Wagner, et al. (2003) have reported the relationship of EGR to both EGA and birthweight. They found that as EGA and birthweight decreased, the incidence of EGR increased. Nearly three decades ago, Dweck (1975) reported an inverse relationship between birthweight and the degree and duration of initial weight loss by premature infants. Initial weight loss was similar to that of the standard for their premature peers. However, when growth by weight was compared to fetuses still in utero, striking EGR was present.Infants who are sick as well as being LBW or VLBW are at risk for EGR. Chronic lung disease, late onset sepsis, severe intraventricular hemorrhage, and a history of necrotizing enterocolitis (NEC) have all been associated with more EGR (Clark, Wagner, et al., 2003). Exposure to postnatal steroids, need for assisted ventilation on the first day of life, and the need for respiratory support at 28 days of life have each been identified in the literature as related to EGR (Clark, Wagner, et al., 2003). In exploring why sick infants experience EGR, Ehrenkranz et al. (1999) posed the question as to which comes first, malnutrition or disease. Disease increases energy and protein needs (Premer & Georgieff, 1999), and sick infants are usually fed differently than well ones (Clark, Wagner, et al., 2003). However, chronic malnutrition compromises defense mechanisms, contributing to the high incidence of respiratory problems and infection in sick neonates (Heird, 1999). Other predisposing factors for EGR include male gender (Clark, Wagner, et al., 2003) and intrauterine growth restriction (IUGR) (Garite, Clark, & Thorp, 2004). These authors demonstrated that infants who had IUGR and were already growth compromised in their intrauterine experience not only experienced higher morbidity than their non-IUGR peers, but also higher rates of EGR.

Consequences of EGR: Growth measurements are the only way we currently determine nutritional status, but they are actually a late manifestation of persistent nutritional deprivation (Bloom et al, 2003). Permanent delay or stunting of immature organ systems can have long-term effects Inadequate nutrition and EGR are also associated with a higher risk for long-term medical problems; Lucas, Morley, and Cole (1998) found that preterm infants who were undernourished during critical periods of brain development in early life had lower IQ scores at 7 to 8 years of age. Epidemiologic data suggest that small size at birth and at 1 year of age are associated with higher rates of hypertension, diabetes, and stroke in later life.

Clinical Implications: Clinical nurses need to understand the issue of EGR and how to identify it in the infants they care for. Nurses can have a significant impact on weight gain and nutritional status of premature infants by identifying the incidence of EGR in their own NICUs and developing evidence-based nutritional guidelines to increase nutritional status and decrease growth restriction of hospitalized infants. Nurses can also use care protocols that encourage caring for infants in ways that decrease energy loss, thereby decreasing nutritional needs and enhancing weight gain potential. Assessment of actual feeding and assessment practices in the NICU can lead to targeted actions to improve weight gain and long-term outcomes of VLBW infants. Nursing implications are summarized as follows:

CLINICAL IMPLICATIONS FOR NEONATAL INTENSIVE CARE NURSES:

* Be sure that measurement techniques for neonates are standardized, and require all practitioners to pass measurement skills regularly. *Ensure adequate calibration and service for equipment used to weigh and measure newborns. *Remind everyone daily of the importance of growth by keeping growth and nutritional charts at the bedside. *Record daily weights and nutrients. * Record weekly length and head circumference. *Include weight and other measurements in daily shift reports. * Become familiar with innovative and proven nutrition interventions through regular inservice education and self-study. *Advocate for the incorporation of the research findings on extrauterine growth restriction in your neonatal intensive care unit. *Implement developmental care protocols to decrease infant energy expenditure. * Establish ongoing assessment of growth and nutrition through observation as well as chart review. Use the data for staff education and quality improvement

Evidence is growing that some practices produce not only greater weight gains but also higher weight gain rates. More rapid weight gain has been demonstrated with shorter duration of parenteral nutrition, earlier initiation of enteral feeds, and earlier achievement of full enteral feedings. Initiation of parenteral nutrition in the first 24 hours, especially amino acids, more rapid nutrient advancement, and earlier ad lib feedings prior to discharge are also practices that demonstrate promise in improving growth. Nurses who understand that the role of nutrition in healing and growth is paramount to successful outcomes for NICU survivors will advocate for a greater emphasis on nutrition. Nurses spend more time at the bedside of infants than anyone else and are in a key position to advocate for nutrition. Quarterly education and updates on nutrition can increase knowledge and support for nutritional goals. Growth targets, including weight gain, weight gain rate, head circumference, and length, should be set for all LBW and VLBW infants. A running record of daily protein and caloric intake, with tallies of deficits and excess, can also be kept at the bedside, thereby keeping nutrition at the forefront of care. One way to do this is to include growth and nutrition data in the regular shift report.

Developmental Care: Development care includes a variety of activities designed to manage the environment and individualize the care of the premature infant based on behavioral observation, such as positioning (also referred to as containment and nesting), reducing environmental noise, cycled light environment, non-nutritive sucking, kangaroo care, infant massage, and providing care, etc. The goal is to promote a stable, well-organized infant who can conserve energy for growth and development.

Assessment of Practice: Ongoing evaluation of nutritional practice should include regular chart reviews for growth and nutritional data as well as critical analysis to determine conditions that decrease compliance with protocols. Charting the specific reason a protocol is not being met (i.e., feeding held because") is also valuable in assessing how to better meet target goals for weight gain. Assessment of decision making regarding feeding is also important. Decisions about what to feed, when to start,and how to progress feedings are all made by care providers at the bedside, with no standardization from NICU to NICU. The best best-performing NICUs believed that the benefits of enteral feedings outweigh the risks, and used a "feed early/advance faster/stop less" philosophy to make nutritional decisions, unless there was clear evidence to deviate.

Keypoint for Clinical Practice: Food is the most basic of needs. While we would never consider denying nutrition to a well infant, the literature indicates that perhaps we have been too willing to deny nutrition to preterm, LBW, VLBW, and sick infants. Mounting evidence shows that it is safe to feed even very sick neonates; perhaps NICU practitioners in the future will view the current reluctance to feed sick neonates in the same light as current practitioners view former attitudes towards withholding pain management.

REFERENCE: Catherine R. Coverston, PhD, RNC, and,Rosanne Schwartz, PhD, FNP, APRN-C MCN March/April 2005.

Weight on Admission to NICU

All babies are to have a weight on admission to NICU.

- Infants who have been weighed in NWH theatre or delivery unit do not need to be reweighed on admission to NICU within the first 24 hours

- All infants who are more than 24 hours old must have a new weight taken on admission to NICU

- Involve parents in weighing their infant, the weight can be performed when they are providing the cares

- Ensure that the infant is well contained during the weighing process to avoid them becoming disorganized and limit heat loss

Level 3 Infants

- Level 3 infants are to be weighed on alternate days unless a specific order for daily weighs is initiated after discussion on ward round.

- Infants are weighed from day 5 unless requested earlier by medical staff.

- Infants are not weighed routinely if they have:

- Chest drains in situ

- are being ventilated on High Frequency Oscillatory Ventilation

- The nursing weight chart is not required unless a specific medical request to document each weight.

Level 2 Infants

- To be weighed twice weekly on Sundays and Wednesdays unless a specific order for alternate day or daily weighs is initiated after discussion on ward round

- Infants are weighed from day 5 unless requested earlier by medical staff.

- if an infant is >36weeks gestation consider weighing on day 3 (discuss with medical team and lactation consultant

Discharge Weight

- All infants discharged after 24hrs in the NICU (including those discharges to the postnatal ward) need to have a discharge weight taken and recorded in the discharge letter by the registrar/NS-ANP

Additional notes

- When there are concerns over weight gain/weight loss for any baby in the service, a nursing weight chart will be completed showing each weight clearly. This chart will be an important document for both medical and nursing carers

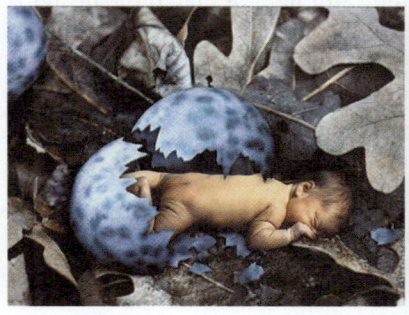 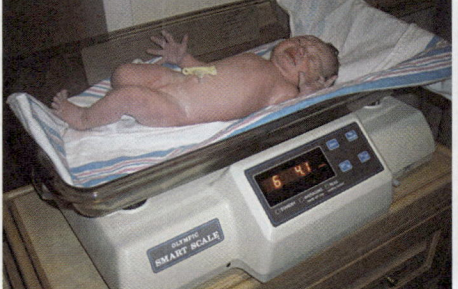 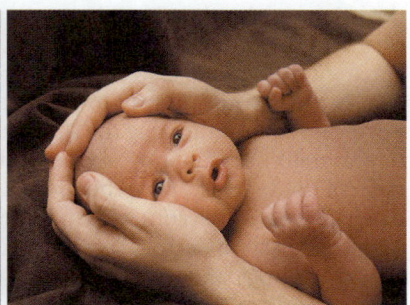

- Typical Postnatal Weight loss in a Term infant is 5-10% of Birth weight and in a Preterm infant it will be 15% of birth weight.

- The nadir in Weight loss usually occurs by 4-6 days of life, with birth weight regained by 14–21 days of life.

- The Clinician`s goal is to limit the degree and duration of initial weight loss in preterms and to facilitate regain of birth weight within 7–14 days of life.

- After achieving birth weight, the goals of: 10–20 g/kg/day weight gain (15–20 g/kg/day for infants <1,500 g), approximately 1 cm/week in length, and 0.5–1 cm/week in head circumference are the appropriate (AAP), although these goals are not attainable in most preterm infants, replicating fetal growth at the same gestational age.

- Poor Weight gain (< 10-15g/kg/day): Differential Diagnosis includes- Inadequate Intake of breast/formula feeds, Excessive losses of body fluids- enteral, renal, skin & lungs, and third space losses, Hypercatabolic states- anemia, hyperthyroidism, late metabolic acidosis, Sepsis, Cold/Heat stress, any systemic organic disease.

- Excess Weight gain (> 50 g/day) indicates either Catch-up growth in a healthy baby or excess fluid retention in a sick baby secondary to cardiac (PDA) & renal failure, SIADH, Chronic lung disease, etc. Weight gain does not necessarily reflect growth, which is a deposition of new tissue of normal composition; weight increase may reflect excessive fat deposition or water retention, neither of which is truly growth.

- It is important to use the same scale, obtain weight measurements at same time each day to avoid diurnal changes, and indicate any equipment being weighed (especially arm boards and dressings); if equipment is not recorded, changes in weight may be spurious. In preterms, weight gain should be expressed on a gram per kg per day basis.

REFERRAL TO DIETITIAN - NEONATAL NUTRITIONAL RISK SCREENING CRITERIA

Children meeting these criteria may have special nutritional requirements and should be considered for referral to a dietitian.

* <2/3 expected caloric requirement *Fluid restriction <160 ml/kg/day *<100ml/kg/day P10 or N10 after Day 4 of life *<180ml/kg/day enteral feeds in a preterm infant *<150ml/kg/day enteral feeds in a term infant *<10 g/kg/day weight gain for >5days (<38 weeks CGA)<20 g per day weight gain for >7days (>38 weeks CGA) *Significant obstructive jaundice *Serum phosphorus <1.3mmol/L *Intolerance to preterm formula or breast milk fortifier *Intake >200ml/kg/day of preterm formula or breast milk fortifier

Any infant with

* NEC where elemental formula is being considered

* Short bowel syndrome

* Malabsorption

* Chronic lung disease where growth impairment is likely

* Congenital heart disease where growth impairment is likely

* Gastrointestinal anomaly

* Metabolic disorder

* Chylothorax

* Renal failure

* Osteopenia requiring additional calcium and phosphate

* Possible zinc deficiency

* Breastfed baby where there are concerns about maternal nutrition

Note: All infants with a birth weight of <1.8 kg should be receiving fortified breast milk or preterm formula until 2.5kg or they reach term or are fully breast fed.

INCUBATOR TO COT TRANSFER

Servocontrol: Incubator and Radiant Warmer

Careful attention to providing the best possible thermal environment increases the chance of survival and the quality of outcome, particularly in the small premature infant. Servocontrol is an electronic feedback system which functions as a thermostat to maintain a constant temperature at the site of a thermistor probe (usually on the skin over the abdomen) by regulating the heat output of an incubator or radiant warmer. Maintaining a constant abdominal skin temperature between 36.0 and 36.5°C is the simplest way to provide a "thermoneutral" environment, minimizing the number of calories needed to maintain normal body temperature and reducing the risks of cold stress or overheating. Although either skin or air temperature control can be used safely for most infants, skin temperature servocontrol is probably better for very young, small (below 1500 g) infants because the desired control temperature is more easily determined. Servocontrol is the only acceptable method of heat regulation for the infant cared for under a radiant warmer. *The following guidelines apply to both the incubator and radiant warmer:*

Insert probe plug securely into hole in heater unit.

Choose the desired abdominal skin temperature, usually 36.5°C. Some older infants will require a lower set point, e.g. 36.0°C to avoid overheating.

Check the setting of the control panel. Adjust if necessary.

Attach the probe to the exposed abdominal skin at mid-epigastrium, halfway between the xiphoid and the umbilicus. If the infant is prone, attach the probe to the skin over either flank (not between the scapulae). The probe should not be placed in the axilla.

Under the radiant warmer, protect the probe with a foil-backed shield.

Read the skin temperature from the temperature gauge on the heater unit. If it registers below the set point (36.5°C), the heater should be on. Check the heater indicator light or dial. If the heater is not on, check all connections.

If the skin temperature does not rise as quickly as you think it should, make sure the heater is on and WAIT. Increasing the set point will not cause faster warming.

When the abdominal skin temperature reaches the chosen set point, check the axillary or rectal temperature to be sure it is within the normal range (36.5 to 37.4°C).

Adjust the set point slightly if the axillary (or rectal) temperature is abnormal. Do not change the set point if the axillary (or rectal) temperature is normal.

Check frequently to be sure the probe is in solid contact with the skin. Poor contact will cause overheating. Entrapment of the probe under the arm or between the infant and mattress will cause underheating

Record incubator air temperatures along with infant skin and axillary (or rectal) temperatures. A clearly decreasing (or increasing) trend in incubator temperature may indicate the development of sepsis or a neurological problem.

Incubator to Cot Transfer Introduction: Evaluating when is the right time to transfer a preterm infant from a closed incubator into an open cot is an essential skill for staff in the Special Care Nursery (SCN).Incubators are designed to minimize heat loss and provide a thermo-neutral environment requiring minimal metabolic effort by the baby to maintain a normal temperature. Incubators are not required for the entire length of the baby's SCN stay. Recognizing when an infant is capable of maintaining it's temperature in an open cot is an important step in planning for discharge. The premature infant and temperature maintenance Achieving temperature stability is important in optimizing body growth and development in the premature infant. Both premature and low birth weight infants have · sparse brown fat available for heat production · small liver with limited glycogen stores for energy and heat production · large surface area to body mass posing a huge potential for heat loss · immature response of the central nervous system to cold stress. Cold stress can lead to *feeding intolerance *respiratory and metabolic acidosis *Hypoglycemia *hypoxia Nursing Assessment : *_infant weight_ *infants weighing 1500 grams or more are candidates *for extremely preterm infants consistent weight gain is an additional indicator *_incubator settings_ *the incubator should be in manual mode *stable body temperature (36.5 - 37.0°C per axilla) with the incubator set in the lower range of the neutral thermal range (NTE) *_physiologically stable_ *the infant must be systemically well and physiologically stable *_feeding_ *the infant should be tolerating feeds *monitoring *on transfer from incubator to open cot check axillary temperature.

When and How to Move Babies from Radiant Warmer to Incubator, and from Incubator to Open Bed Radiant Warmer to Incubator:

Most newly-admitted infants are cared for on radiant warmer beds in order to provide accessibility for resuscitation or procedures without jeopardizing thermal stability. As long as an infant remains critically ill and is likely to require resuscitation or frequent procedures, he should be kept on a warmer bed. Most very small infants (<1000 grams) can be kept warm more easily on a radiant warmer than in an incubator, since incubator air temperature drops rapidly when the door is opened. If a very small infant has difficulty maintaining normal body temperature on a radiant warmer, plastic food wrap can be stretched across the bed (from side to side). This reduces the movement of cool air over the baby's body surface. When the condition has stabilized so that frequent procedures are not likely to be needed, an infant can be moved to a preheated incubator, on skin temperature servocontrol. Axillary temperature should be checked 30 minutes after moving the baby to the incubator, and every hour thereafter for four hours. The very small infant is at greatest risk of heat loss through an open incubator door. Whenever possible, procedures performed on a baby in an incubator should be performed through the ports (diaper change, vital signs, phlebotomy, etc.). Any infant who weighs less than 1000 grams should be cared for on a radiant warmer or in a servocontrolled double-walled incubator. If an infant consistently requires an air temperature above 37° C, it may be necessary to operate the incubator in the air temperature control mode to avoid periodic increases in air temperature to above 38° C, which may cause the heater to stop completely. Some infants who require a radiant warmer for temperature support may not need routine vital signs as often as other infants under radiant warmers. The frequency of vital signs may be reduced at the discretion of the infant's nurse and physician.

Incubator to Bassinet: If an infant has been maintained in an incubator operated by skin temperature servocontrol, the incubator should be changed to air temperature servocontrol in the following manner, before attempting the move the infant to a bassinet. *Change to air temperature servocontrol setting the control temperature to equal the average incubator air temperature during the previous 24 hours (from the nursing notes). *Check the baby's axillary temperature in 30 minutes and each hour for four hours. *If the axillary temperature remains normal (36.5 to 37.4°C), disconnect and remove the skin probe if desired. *When an infant reaches 1700 to 1800 grams, has no respiratory distress and only occasional apnea, and has been stable in an incubator operated in the air temperature control mode with air temperature 32°C or less, an attempt can be made to move him to a bassinet as follows: *Dress the infant in shirt and diaper and wrap him in a single blanket. Turn the air temperature control to 28°C. *Check the baby's temperature in 30 minutes and each hour for four hours. *If the baby's axillary or rectal temperature drops to below 36.5°C, reheat him in the skin temperature servocontrol mode until his skin temperature is 36.0°C and return to manual or air servocontrol mode as described above (try again in two or three days). *If the baby's temperature is stable for eight hours, bundle him in extra blankets and move him to a bassinet. *Check body temperature in 30 minutes and each hour for four hours; if the axillary or rectal temperature drops to below 36.5°C, return infant to incubator, reheat on skin temperature servocontrol as described above, then revert to air temperature control; try again in two or three days.

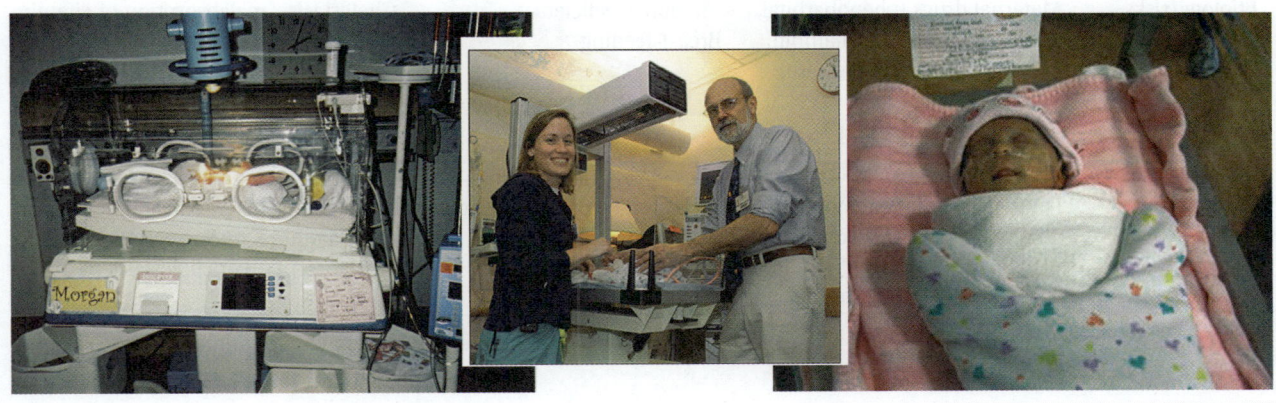

VITAMIN *K* ADMINISTRATION TO NEWBORN INFANTS TO PREVENT VITAMIN *K* DEFICIENCY BLEEDING IN INFANCY

*The term 'hemorrhagic disease of the Newborn' was first used in 1894 (Townsend 1894) to describe bleeding in the Newborn, which was not due to traumatic birth or to hemophilia. Later many cases were found to be associated with vitamin K deficiency. The term 'vitamin K deficiency bleeding' (VKDB) has now been adopted (Sutor *et al* 1999). This is preferred since not all bleeding in the newborn is due to vitamin K deficiency and bleeding due to this cause is not confined to the newborn. *Vitamin K occurs in two forms, vitamin K1 whose source is dietary intake and vitamins K2 (menaquinones) that are produced by gut bacteria. All newborn infants have a relative vitamin K deficiency at birth (Shearer 1992). Vitamin K1 crosses the placenta poorly resulting in low fetal plasma concentrations of the vitamin, with a 30:1 maternal-infant gradient. After birth vitamin K status is related to dietary intake, being determined by the volume of milk ingested and the amount of vitamin K1 in the milk. Symptomatic VKDB can be precipitated in the first week of life by delayed or inadequate early feeding, or can occur later in the first six months as a result of inadequate oral absorption of vitamin K1. Human breast milk contains relatively low concentrations of vitamin K1 (1 to 2 mg/L), whereas infant formula milks are by law supplemented with additional vitamin K1 to a minimum concentration of 30 mg/L. Therefore exclusively breast-fed infants are at increased risk of developing VKDB, unless supplemental vitamin K is administered. Cholestatic liver disease also impairs absorption of vitamin K1 and increases the risk of VKDB. Hepatic menaquinones (vitamins K2) protect adults and older infants from developing VKDB even in the presence of vitamin K1 deficiency. Vitamins K2 cannot be detected in the livers of newborn infants but gradually accumulate in the first few months of life. The source of vitamins K2 in young infants is from synthesis by gut flora. Until adequate stores of hepatic menaquinones have accumulated young infants remain susceptible to the occurrence of VKDB. *VKDB includes spontaneous or excessive induced bleeding (eg venipuncture or surgery) at any site associated with decreased activity of the vitamin K dependent coagulation factors (II, VII, IX and X) with normal activity of vitamin K independent factors, fibrinogen levels and platelet count (Sutor *et al* 1999). Confirmation of the diagnosis requires that the coagulation disorder is rapidly reversed following vitamin K administration and that other causes of coagulopathy are excluded. VKDB is classified into early, classical and late, based on the age of presentation.

RECOMMENDATIONS

1. All newborn infants should receive vitamin K prophylaxis.

2. Healthy newborn infants should receive vitamin K either: *by intramuscular injection of 1 mg (0.1 mL) of Konakion MM(mixed micelles formulation) at birth. ***This is the preferred route for reliability of administration and level of compliance.*** **Or** *as three 2 mg (0.2 mL) oral doses of Konakion MM, given at birth, at the time of newborn screening (usually at three to five days of age) and in the fourth week. The last dose is not required in infants predominantly formula fed. It is imperative that the third dose is given no later than four weeks after birth as the effect of earlier doses decreases after this time. Undertaking this form of prophylaxis requires that the parent accepts responsibility and that clinicians support and advise them in the administration of the third dose. If the infant vomits or regurgitates the formulation within one hour of administration, the oral dose should be repeated. If at the time any oral dose is to be given the infant is sick, vomiting or unable to take it by mouth, then medical advice should be sought as to whether the intramuscular preparation should be given. Hospitals should have written protocols for medical and nursing staff to administer prophylactic vitamin K to infants. These should include that it be routine practice to record the date, dose and method of administration in the infant's personal health record.

3. *Newborns who are too unwell and are unable to take oral vitamin K (or whose mothers have taken medications that interfere with vitamin K metabolism) should be given 1 mg of Konakion MM by intramuscular injection at birth. A smaller intramuscular dose of 0.5 mg (0.05 mL) should be given to infants with a birth weight of less than 1.5 kg.*

REFERENCE: *Joint statement and recommendations on Vitamin K administration to newborn infants to prevent vitamin K deficiency bleeding in infancy*; Pediatric Division of the Royal Australasian College of Physicians. These guidelines were endorsed at the 137th Session of Council, 13 October 2000 and re-issued at the 160th session of Council, 8 March 2006.

VKDB (Hemorrhagic disease of the newborn)

	Early onset	Classic disease	Late onset
Age	0–24 hours	2–7 days	1–6 months
Site of hemorrhage	Cephalohematoma	Gastrointestinal	Intracranial
	Subgaleal	Ear-nose-throat-mucosal	Gastrointestinal
	Intracranial	Intracranial	Cutaneous
	Gastrointestinal	Circumcision	Ear-nose-throat-mucosal
	Umbilicus	Cutaneous	Injection sites
	Intra-abdominal	Gastrointestinal	Thoracic
		Injection sites	
Etiology/risks	Maternal drugs (phenobarbital, phenytoin, warfarin, rifampin, isoniazid) that interfere with Vitamin K	Vitamin K deficiency Breast-feeding	Cholestasis—malabsorption of vitamin K (biliary atresia, cystic fibrosis, hepatitis)
	Inherited coagulopathy		Abetalipoprotein deficiency
			Idiopathic in Asian breast-fed infants
			Warfarin ingestion
Prevention	Possible vitamin K at birth or to mother (20 mg) before birth	Prevented by parenteral vitamin K at birth. Oral3 vitamin K regimens require repeated dosing over time	Prevented by parenteral and high-dose oral vitamin K during periods of malabsorption or cholestasis
	Avoid high-risk medications		
Incidence	Very rare	~ 2% if not given vitamin K	Dependent on primary disease

WITHHOLDING FEEDS IN THE NICU ASSESSMENT OF BILIOUS ASPIRATES AND VOMITING

Background

* Withholding feeds is a significant decision for infants in the NICU, particularly extremely low birth weight infants. An audit of practice in NICU identified that withholding feeds was a significant contributor to poor growth in infants *Calories and nutrients can be more safely and more easily delivered by enteral feeds than by *intravenous nutrition, without increased cost and increased risks of complications. *However, some infants with feed intolerance may have significant intra-abdominal or other problems.

Indications to Withhold Feeds

* Clear abdominal pathology *Suspected or proven *NEC *Significant abdominal distension or discoloration *Other suspected or proven bowel pathologies ·

Blood in stool

* Heavily bile-stained or large gastric residuals or vomiting ("avocado" or "spinach" in the · reference chart below) *Relative indications to withhold feeds *Feed intolerance *If <25% of 6-hour total feed volume - return aspirate and give full feed *25-50% of 6-hour total feed volume - return aspirate and miss feed *Check aspirate next feed. If significant aspirate next feed, then withhold feed and notify registrar or NS-ANP *>50% of 6 hour total feed volume - withhold feed and notify registrar or NS-ANP *Unstable condition causing clinical concern *This may include infants with significant cardiorespiratory instability or presumed sepsis *Infants about to undergo surgical or anesthetic procedures.

INDICATIVE COLOR CHART FOR ASSESSING ASPIRATE COLOR

| Milk | Lemon | Mustard | Wasabi | Lime | Avocado | Spinach |

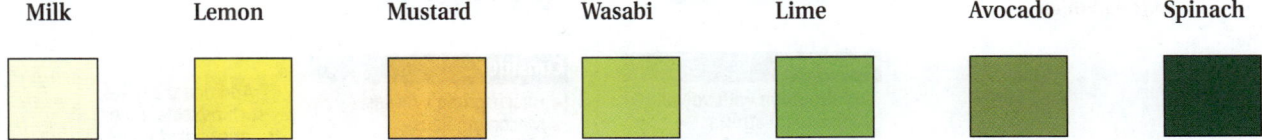

*Note that colostrum may appear yellow in color.
*Some infants will have bilious aspirates that are bright yellow in color in the initial phases.

Investigation of Bilious Aspirates or Vomiting

Feed intolerance is common in preterm infants. However, it is less common in term infants. In term infants, especially those with bile-stained vomiting or bilious aspirates, gastrointestinal pathology needs to be investigated and **early surgical consultation** should be considered. **Causes of bilious aspirates/vomiting** include (but are not limited to):

• Proximal bowel obstruction (yet distal to the duodenum). *It is particularly important to consider - intestinal malrotation.-Radiographs and abdominal examination may be normal in infants with malrotation, particularly in the early stage of the condition or if the obstruction is intermittent. If malrotation is considered a possible diagnosis, an upper GI contrast study should be considered. A recent report of infants presenting to a surgical NICU with bilious vomiting demonstrated that 22% had an intestinal malrotation.

• Other bowel obstruction

• Distal obstruction may result in bilious vomiting or aspirates.

• An abdominal radiograph may indicate intra-abdominal pathology, with air-fluid levels

• Necrotizing enterocolitis

• Paralytic ileus associated with generalized sepsis This usually presents with a silent abdomen in an infant with signs of generalized sepsis. In some infants, no cause will be found despite thorough investigation.

Management

The baby should be examined for signs of generalized sepsis or instability. Close attention should be paid to the abdomen, paying particular attention to signs of tenderness, erythema, or guarding. The baby should be placed nil by mouth. An abdominal series (AP supine and lateral decubitus with the left side down) should be ordered. *It may be appropriate to repeat the radiographs in 4–8 hours to evaluate any change in bowel gas pattern or any evolution in radiographic features. Antibiotics after an appropriate sepsis screen should be considered. *If intra-abdominal pathology is suspected, the antibiotics of first choice are amikacin, amoxycillin, and metronidazole. *If sepsis is considered likely but an intra-abdominal source is not thought to be the primary source, then the antibiotics of first choice are · amikacin and · flucloxacillin. Surgical consultation should be considered early. Reintroduction of feeding will depend on the underlying condition and the individual preferences of the supervising specialist.

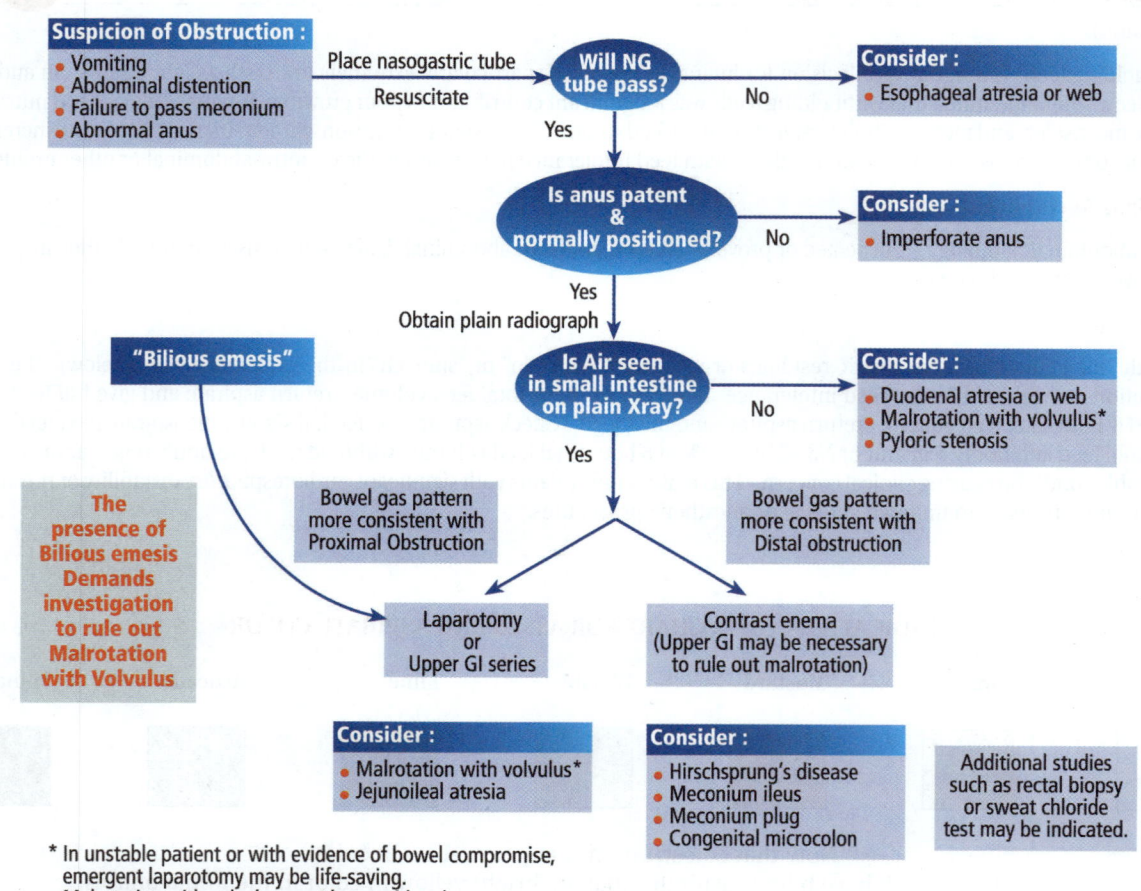

ALGORITHM FOR DIAGNOSIS OF NEONATAL INTESTINAL OBSTRUCTION

Suspicion of Obstruction :
- Vomiting
- Abdominal distention
- Failure to pass meconium
- Abnormal anus

Place nasogastric tube
Resuscitate

Will NG tube pass? — No → **Consider :**
- Esophageal atresia or web

Yes ↓

Is anus patent & normally positioned? — No → **Consider :**
- Imperforate anus

Yes ↓
Obtain plain radiograph

"Bilious emesis"

Is Air seen in small intestine on plain Xray? — No → **Consider :**
- Duodenal atresia or web
- Malrotation with volvulus*
- Pyloric stenosis

Yes ↓

The presence of Bilious emesis Demands investigation to rule out Malrotation with Volvulus

Bowel gas pattern more consistent with Proximal Obstruction

Bowel gas pattern more consistent with Distal obstruction

Laparotomy or Upper GI series

Contrast enema (Upper GI may be necessary to rule out malrotation)

Consider :
- Malrotation with volvulus*
- Jejunoileal atresia

Consider :
- Hirschsprung's disease
- Meconium ileus
- Meconium plug
- Congenital microcolon

Additional studies such as rectal biopsy or sweat chloride test may be indicated.

* In unstable patient or with evidence of bowel compromise, emergent laparotomy may be life-saving.
Malrotation with volvulus must be considered in all cases of proximal bowel obstruction.

When a neonate develops bilious vomiting, one should suspect a surgical condition. After a focused physical examination, a nasogastric or orogastric catheter should be placed for gastric decompression to prevent further vomiting and aspiration. This should be done before any diagnostic or therapeutic maneuvers are performed. Establishment of an intravenous line should follow for administration of fluid, electrolytes and nutrition. When the patient is hemodynamically stabilized, appropriate imaging studies of the abdomen should be performed. These would include plain abdominal films and/or contrast studies. When dilated bowel loops and air-fluid levels are demonstrated, the diagnosis of a surgical abdomen is suggested, and urgent consultation with a pediatric surgeon is indicated, preferably in a pediatric surgical center. Gastric decompression, hydration and secured airway must be completed before initiating transport of the patient. Intestinal obstruction with bilious vomiting in neonates can be caused by duodenal atresia, malrotation and volvulus, jejunoileal atresia, meconium ileus, and necrotizing enterocolitis

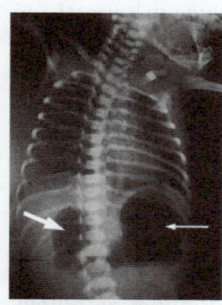

Upright abdominal film showing the characteristic "double-bubble" sign that confirms the diagnosis of duodenal atresia. Note the dilated stomach *(thin arrow)* and dilated proximal duodenum *(thick arrow)*.

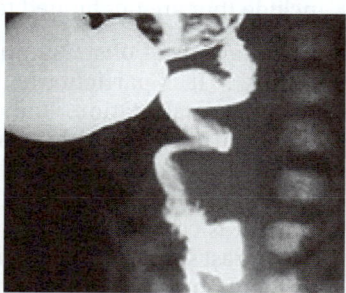

Upper gastrointestinal contrast study demonstrating a typical spiral configuration of jejunum in a patient with volvulus of the bowel.

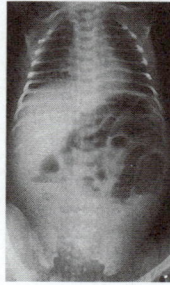

Upright abdominal film showing distention of the bowel with multiple air-fluid levels suggesting lower intestinal atresia

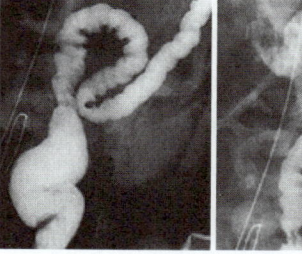

Meconium ileus. Contrast enema demonstrates a microcolon

Although parenteral nutrition remains the preferred method for early feeding of the extremely low birth weight infant (1,000 g), an increasing tendency in recent years has been to introduce small amounts of enteral feeding to these tiny babies early in the postnatal period. Such "minimal enteral" or "trophic" feedings seem to provide benefits such as improved milk tolerance, better postnatal growth, and reduced rates of sepsis. *A variety of terms are used in the literature for this introduction of enteral nutrients, including gut priming, gut stimulation feedings, hypocaloric enteral feedings, trophic feedings, nonnutritive feedings, and minimal enteral feedings.*

There is no well-established definition for MEN, but it generally refers to enteral feeding of formula, human milk, or both at intakes of 5 to 25 mL/kg per day. Some studies suggest that physiologic benefits occur at volumes as low as less than 1 mL/kg per day. Such volumes are referred to as "priming" feedings because of their role in stimulating many aspects of gut function. In the 1960s and 1970s, the introduction of gavage feedings allowed for full enteral nutrition in the preterm infant. However, because of very rapid advancement of feeding by this route, a significant number of very preterm infants developed NEC with enteral feedings. This, in combination with the development of complete parenteral nutrition for this age group, led to the common practice of withholding enteral nutrition in preterm infants for the first several weeks of life. Subsequent concerns over TPN toxicity as well as a growing recognition of the importance of enteral feedings in stimulating growth and development of the gastrointestinal tract prompted a number of studies that have demonstrated the benefits and safety of early MEN as a supplement to parenteral nutrition.

The advantages of MEN included: shorter time to full enteral feedings, less time under phototherapy, a lower incidence of direct hyperbilirubinemia, smaller gastric residuals and less feeding intolerance, the same or faster weight gain, and no increased incidence of NEC. It had long been known that starvation quickly induces atrophy of the gastrointestinal tract, but more recent studies in human and animal neonates have demonstrated the positive direct and indirect trophic effects of MEN, even when administered for brief periods of time. (*Refer to Figure showing the effects of food on the GIT*). Direct contact of the gut tissue with human milk increases intestinal mass and enhances DNA synthesis rates. The majority of the direct trophic effects induced by human milk appear to be mediated by growth factors, such as epidermal growth factor, trophic peptides, and insulin. Trophic hormones and peptides that are released in response to the

presence of intraluminal nutrients mediate indirect trophic effects of enteral feedings. They can have potent trophic effects on the gastrointestinal mucosa and include substances such as gastrin, cholecystokinen enteroglucagon, motilin, neurotensin, and gastric inhibitory peptide. These gastrointestinal hormones and peptides are released by 20 weeks' gestation, with fasting plasma concentrations of many of these substances being similar in term and preterm infants. Even very preterm infants can increase the level of these hormones and peptides in response to feeding, and plasma concentrations of the hormones are decreased in the absence of enteral feedings in preterm infants. The decreasing concentrations can be reversed with enteral feeding volumes of as little as 0.1 mL/kg per day. In addition to their direct trophic action on the gut mucosa, most of these substances have complex and vital roles in other aspects of gastrointestinal tract function, such as nutrient absorption and digestion. Using manometric techniques, it has been shown that early enteral feeding enhances maturation of the motor responses of the small intestine of the preterm infant compared with infants receiving exclusively parenteral nutrition. MEN has a positive influence on both mixing and churning of intestinal contents as well as on forward propulsion of enteral feedings. Moreover, maturation of the gastrointestinal tract motor activity in response to feedings occurs when the intake is as little as 4 mL/kg per day and is enhanced when full-strength rather than dilute formula or sterile water is used.

Advantages of trophic feedings reported in the scientific literature include:

Decrease In: Indirect hyperbilirubinemia, Cholestatic jaundice, Metabolic bone disease, Length of time to reach full enteral feedings, TPN usage

Increase In: Gastrin & enteric hormones, Concentration of other enteric hormones, Feeding tolerance, Weight gain

Indications for MEN: All preterm infants especially < 32 weeks of GA, in whom enteral feeding has not yet been started due to underlying illness.

Contraindications for MEN: MEN should be avoided in infants with 1. Severe hemodynamic instability 2. Suspected or confirmed NEC, 3. Evidence of intestinal obstruction / Perforation or paralytic ileus. Mechanical ventilation and / or use of umbilical catheters are not contraindication to using MEN.

Monitor for any evidence of feed intolerance including abdominal girth, gastric residuals, or clinical signs of NEC. If the abdominal girth has increased by 2 cm, gastric residual volume should be checked. Stop feeding in the presence of significant aspirate i.e., >25% of feed or >3 ml whichever is more and/or bilious/blood aspirates. Advance the feeds @20-30 ml/kg/day to full feeds gradually, carefully monitoring the baby.

TABLE 1 summarizes the advantages of Gastrointestinal Priming with MEN. Table 2 outlines a Protocol on Minimal Enteral Nutrition (MEN).

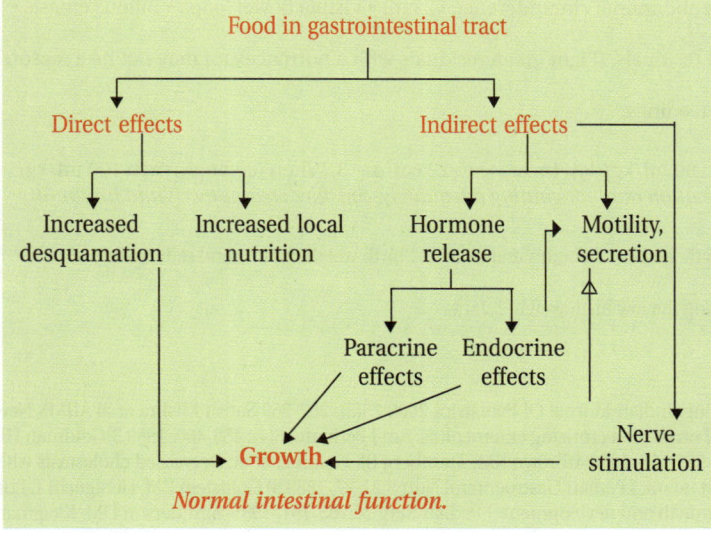

Figure 1. Fasting is associated with reduced intestinal motility, intestinal mucosal atrophy, and a longer time to establish enteral nutrition. This is consistent with the idea that enteral nutrition is critical for normal intestinal function. However, the introduction of feeds in preterm infants is tempered by concerns about feeding intolerance, gastroesophageal reflux, and/or necrotizing enterocolitis.

TABLE 1: Advantages of Gastrointestinal Priming with MEN

1. Shortens time to regain birth weight
2. Improves feeding tolerance
3. Enhances enzyme maturation
4. Improves gastrointestinal motility
5. Improves mineral absorption, mineralization
6. Lowers incidence of cholestasis

The Cochrane Library conclusion (8 JUL 2009) on Early trophic feeding for very low birth weight infants

There is insufficient evidence to determine whether feeding very low birth weight infants small quantities of milk during the first week after birth (early trophic feeding) helps bowel development and improves subsequent feeding, growth and development. Analysis of eight trials does not suggest that this practice increases the risk of a severe bowel disorder called "necrotizing enterocolitis". Further trials are needed to provide robust evidence to inform this key area of care.

TABLE 2. Protocol on Minimal Enteral Nutrition (MEN)*

For whom: All preterm infants especially those less than 32 weeks gestation, who are hemodynamically stable but cannot be given enteral feeds. Consider *trophic feeding in infants who meet the criteria for readiness for enteral feeds but for whom there are concerns about capacity to tolerate normal feed volumes*, i.e.: 1. ≤25 weeks gestation at birth 2. birth weight <750 g 3. absent or reversed end-diastolic flow 4. intrauterine growth restriction 5. significant respiratory distress.

What to feed: Preferably expressed breast milk (EBM). Colostrum should be used for first feedings Colostrum should be used in the order it was produced .even if fresh (more mature) milk is available. Colostrum is more easily absorbed/easily tolerated. Fresh mature milk should be used in combination with colostrum by day 4-5.(may add specific antibody to NICU pathogens).

When: Trophic feedings will begin within 24-48 hours of birth if infant is stable.

How much to feed:

EBM 8-12 mL/kg/day divided into 4-8 feeds given by gavage feeding

For <1000g 1-2ml every 4-6 hour, for ≥ 1000 g 2-3 ml every 2-4 hour.

* Can be started while baby is on ventilator and /or receiving total parental nutrition
* In severe birth asphyxia, MEN should be started after 48-72 hours.
* VLBW infants born with antenatal diagnosis of altered umbilical arterial blood flow (reversed or absent end diastolic flow), MEN can possibly be delayed for 2 to 3 days.

Advancement of feedings:

1. Infants <1000 grams will advance by 10ml/kg/day until volume reaches 60ml/kg/day, then advancement will increase by 20ml/kg/day to max of 150ml/kg/day.
2. Infants 1001-1500 grams will advance by 10ml/kg/day until volume reaches 60ml/kg/day, then advancement will increase by 15ml/kg/day to max of 150ml/kg/day.
3. Infants 1501-2000 grams will advance by 20ml/kg/day until volume reaches max of 150ml/kg/day.

Aspirates:

1. Aspirates are expected while on trophic feedings. Green or yellow aspirates are not a contraindication for trophic feedings.
2. Undigested aspirates will be refed. Current feeding volume will be fed in addition to volume of aspirate.
3. Partially digested, mucousy, or bloody aspirates will be discarded
4. If aspirate is <20% of feeding volume, continue advancement. 5. If aspirate is 20-40% of feeding volume for 2 consecutive feedings, notify MD/NP. Continue feedings in the absence of clinical symptoms but hold advancement. 6. If aspirate is >40% of feeding volume: • Notify MD/NP • Hold feedings • Obtain KUB (indication: Feeding Intolerance).

When to Notify MD/NNP

1. Emesis in any infant <1500 grams
2. An abnormal physical exam consisting of the following:
• Unstable vital signs • Abdominal distention (increase in abdominal circumference >2 cm) • Visible bowel loops • Bilious emesis • Visible blood in stool
3. Dark green residuals or change in color (darkening) of residuals. (Light green residuals with a normal exam may not be a reason to hold feedings.)
4. Aspirates of 20-40% feeding volume for 2 consecutive feedings.

Fortification

1. Colostrum will not be fortified. 2. When feedings reach 90 ml/kg/day, increase to 22 cal/oz 3. When feedings reach 120 ml/kg/day, increase to 24 cal/oz 4. *If infant not tolerating fortification and not gaining adequately, consider creamatocrit and hindmilk feedings.*

Purpose: To improve feeding tolerance and growth (weight, length, and head circumference in low birth weight infants and reduce days of parenteral nutrition.

Goal: To provide a consistent, evidence based approach to feeding the low birth weight infant.

REFERENCES & FURTHER READING: 1) Minimal Enteral Feeding, Indian Journal Of Pediatrics 2008 75(3): 267-269 Satish Mishra et al AIIMS New Delhi. 2)Covert RF, Neu J, Elliot MJ: Factors associated with age of onset of necrotizing enterocolitis. Am J Perinatol 6(4): 455-460, 1989 3)Goldman HI: Feeding and necrotizing enterocolitis. Am J Dis Childhood 134 : 553-555, 1980 4)Brown RM, Thunberg BJ, Golub L, et al: Decreased cholestasis with enteral instead of intravenous protein in the very low-birth weight infant. J Pediatr Gastroenterol Nutr 9:21-27, 1989 5) Goldstein RM, Hebiguchi T, Luk GD: The effects of total parenteral nutrition on gastrointestinal growth and development. J Pediatr Surg 20:785-791, 1985 6)Anderson DM, Kleigman RM: The relationship of neonatal alimentation practices to the occurrence of endemic necrotizing enterocolitis. Am J Perinatol 8:62-67, 1991

TOTAL PARENTERAL NUTRITION (TPN)

Total parenteral nutrition (TPN) is the intravenous infusion of all nutrients necessary for metabolic requirements and growth. Parenteral nutrition (PN) refers to the supplemental intravenous infusion of nutrients by peripheral or central vein. Earlier introduction and more aggressive advancement of TPN is shown to be safe and effective, even in the smallest and most immature infants. Premature infants tolerate TPN from day 1 of post-natal life. Timely intervention with TPN begins with the provision of glucose as soon as possible after birth with amino acids within the first 12 hours, intravenous fat within the first 24 to 48 hours, and trophic feeding within the first 24 hours. Optimal use of routine TPN for nutritional support of ELBW and VLBW infants may influence short-term outcomes such as lower propensity to infection and shortened hospital stay, as well as longer-term outcomes such as decreased growth deficits, improved neurodevelopment, and overall morbidity. The ability to provide PN and TPN over the past four decades has significantly improved the overall survival of newborns when other options of adequate nutritional support were not possible.

Learning Objectives: Upon completion of this Essential Clinical Guidelines about TPN in the NICU the learner will be able to:

1. List the indications for parenteral nutrition in the preterm infant.
2. Estimate protein and calories required by a preterm infant to support appropriate fetal weight gain.
3. Determine appropriate fluid and electrolyte needs of preterm infants.
4. Discuss the types of access that can be used for parenteral nutrition in the preterm infant.
3. Determine an appropriate parenteral solution that contains dextrose, amino acids and lipids for a preterm infant.
6. Explain the best way to provide preterm infants vitamins and minerals that meet their specific needs.
7. Develop a monitoring schedule of the preterm infant on parenteral nutrition.
8.Discuss the calcium and phosphorus needs of preterm infants.

The goal of TPN is to • provide sufficient nutrients to prevent negative energy and nitrogen balance and essential fatty acid deficiency • support normal rates growth without increased significant morbidity. Clinical Considerations: Infants <1500 grams should be started on TPN by 48 hours of age unless they are expected to be tolerating full feeds within 24-48 hours. *Infants >1500 grams should be started on TPN by 72 hours of age if they are not expected to be enterally fed by day 5.*

Indications for TPN in Neonates:• gastrointestinal tract abnormalities (tracheo-esophageal fistula, omphalocele, gastroschisis, malrotation with volvulus, etc) • necrotizing enterocolitis (NEC) • respiratory distress syndrome / BPD patients who are unable to tolerate feeding • extreme prematurity •Severe intrauterine growth retardation •sepsis • malabsorption • Gastro-intestinal tract problems like short bowel syndrome, intractable diarrhea.

Initiation and Advancement of Macronutrients in TPN Solutions:: The use of TPN is suggested to support all ill and premature babies less than 1,500 grams that cannot sustain at least ~60 kcal/kg/d enterally and initiation is recommended during the first 24 hours of life to avoid excessive protein losses. The premature infant who is not growing, not septic, and not unduly stressed requires an energy intake of about 50 kcal/kg/d for resting energy expenditure, activity, and occasional cold stress, with as little as ~1 to 1.5 g protein/kg/d to preserve endogenous protein stores. At least 60 kcal/kg/d is thought to meet energy requirements during acute sepsis. Provision of greater than 70 kcal/kg/d and 2.7 to 3.5 g protein/kg/d has been demonstrated to support growth and positive nitrogen balance in preterm infants.

Carbohydrate: To ensure a stressed premature infant receives an adequate but not excessive amount of glucose, the amount of carbohydrate delivered in the form of dextrose is commonly initiated at the endogenous hepatic glucose production and utilization rate of 4 to 6 mg/kg/min; 8 to 10 mg/kg/min in ELBW infants provides 40 to 50 kcal/kg/d and preserves carbohydrate stores. Frequently smaller, more unstable premature infants

develop hyperglycemia due to decreased insulin production and insulin resistance. Glucose infusion rates (GIR) for these babies may need to be limited to 4 mg/kg/min or less, while larger preterm infants or term infants can often tolerate up to 8 mg/kg/min initially. Once the GIR supports acceptable serum glucose values, it is advanced in a gradual, stepwise fashion (0.5 to 1 mg/kg/min) to a suggested maximum glucose oxidative rate for neonates of 12 to 13 mg/kg/min to support growth and maintained there unless serum glucose values change significantly. Practically speaking, a premature infant who is able to tolerate a fluid volume of 140 to 150 mL/kg/d will meet macronutrient needs for growth if provided a dextrose concentration of 10% (~10 to 10.5 mg glucose/kg/min) or 12.5% (~12 to 13 mg glucose/kg/min); if the protein and fat intakes are both at least 3 g/kg/d, the solutions will approximate 80 to 95 and 100 to 105 kcal/kg/d respectively. If further fluid restriction or dextrose limitation is necessary, other options to optimize delivery of glucose are to (1) minimize the amount of fluids delivered with intravenous medications or needed to keep a line patent and (2) decrease the dextrose concentration of the intravenous medication solution so that slightly more dextrose can be delivered from the TPN solution and/or (3) increase the dextrose concentration of the intravenous medication solution to equal that of the TPN solution while ensuring glucose tolerance. To optimize the amount of fluid available to provide nutrition to the small premature baby while trying to maintain a euglycemic state, it may be necessary to double-concentrate the continuous infusions that deliver medications and run them at lower rates. Consultation with the pharmacist can ensure that these lower medication infusion rates are adequate for optimum clinical effectiveness of the intravenous drug.

Protein: requirements for the neonate tend to be inversely related to gestational age and size due to more rapid growth rates and greater protein losses in the smaller, more premature infants. The early provision of protein is critical to attain positive nitrogen balance and accretion, as premature babies lose ~1% of their protein stores daily. Studies suggest the provision of at least 1 g/kg/d of amino acids can decrease catabolism. ELBW infants can generally receive 2 g/kg/d of amino acids on the first day of life. A classic study by Zlotkin and coworkers suggests a protein goal of at least 2.7 to 3.5 g/kg/d with adequate energy of greater than 70 nonprotein kcal/kg/d to approximate in utero nitrogen accretion. Studies show that early and aggressive provision of 3 grams protein/kg/d and adequate nonprotein energy within the first few days of life is safe and effective at providing protein to meet accretion needs and facilitate intrauterine growth rates.Protein requirements may be increased to counter catabolic or excretory losses in clinical conditions such as postoperative wound-healing, chronic lung disease treated with steroids, lymphatic injury with a sustained chyle leak, and/or during sustained periods when infants require limited or withheld enteral feeding or higher amounts of protein for catch-up growth.Protein is delivered as free amino acids in solutions developed specifically for pediatric patients with an amino acid profile that is higher in amounts of amino acids believed to be conditionally essential for premature infants (aspartate, glutamate, taurine, and tyrosine) and with lesser amounts of glycine compared with adult solutions. Cysteine is also considered as conditionally essential in premature infants due to a theoretical insufficiency of enzymatic activity for the conversion of methionine to cysteine. Cysteine is not contained in amino acid solutions because of problems with long-term stability and addition as a separate solution as the solution is prepared is compatible and is needed to meet recommendations. Cysteine hydrochloride supplements may cause metabolic acidosis and therefore TPN solutions may need to be buffered with acetate. Studies in critically ill adults suggest that glutamine supplemented amino acid solutions may reduce mortality, improve nitrogen balance, and reduce the incidence of clinical infection. Amino acid solutions provide 4.0 kcal/g of protein. In neonates, protein accretion is thought to more adequately reflect nutritional status than weight gain.

Fat: is delivered as lipid emulsions of neutral triglycerides (TG), primarily polyunsaturated fatty acids (PUFA) that are essential for normal growth and development, retinal development and function, brain development, and cell structure and function. Lipid emulsions provide a concentrated source of energy, 10 kcal/g of fat that enables the provision of nutrient intakes to premature infants within limited fluid volumes to achieve in utero rates of growth. Adequate administration of lipids prevents essential fatty acid deficiency, promotes positive nitrogen balance, and optimizes energy utilization. Lipid emulsions are available as 10 and 20% solutions; 20% solutions require less fluid volume and provide a lower phospholipid-to-triglyceride ratio and therefore are recommended for premature infants. Recommendations to prevent essential fatty acid deficiency in premature infants are to provide at least 80 kcal/kg/d, which will limit utilization of stored fat for energy and thus preserve docosohexanoic acid (DHA) and arachadonic acid (ARA) stores. A 20% IV fat emulsion is typically started at 0.5 to 1 g fat/kg on the first day of life generally at the same time amino acids are started to prevent the occurrence of essential fatty acid deficiency as well as to provide a more generous source of calories. The lipid emulsion is advanced as tolerated in incremental rates of 0.5 to 1 g/kg/d to a typical maximum of 3 g/kg/d. In a balanced TPN solution, this generally approximates about 30% of total calories from fat. Fluid-restricted, growth-compromised patients or those limited to peripheral line access may require as high as 3.5 to 4 grams fat/kg/d to achieve adequate energy for growth and protein sparing. This intake is appropriate as long as the fat intake remains less than 60% of nonprotein calories. To minimize the occurrence of hyperlipemia, bilirubin displacement, and respiratory compromise, lipid infusion rates less than or equal to 0.15 g/kg/h are recommended to span over 24 hours. The delivery of 3 g/kg/d of a 20% lipid emulsion equates to an infusion rate of 0.125 g/kg/h. Premature infants have limited fat stores and lipoprotein lipase concentrations that may hinder their ability to clear plasma lipids following infusions of intravenous fat. The use of heparin dosing at 0.5 to 1 units/mL of TPN solutions, with a maximum of 137 units/d, can facilitate lipoprotein lipase activity to help stabilize serum triglyceride values. Persistently high bilirubin values may increase the risk of kernicterus from the deposition of bilirubin in brain cells. A free fatty acid to albumin ratio (FFA: albumin) greater than 6:1 is thought to be clinically significant.

Calcium and Phosphorus Solubility

The generous calcium and phosphorus requirements of premature infants necessary to mimic accretion rates in utero far exceed compatibility limits of TPN solutions, with precipitation leading to embolisms or death. Mineral precipitation is directly affected by solution temperature, hang time, pH, dextrose concentration, the presence of lipids within the solution, and the addition of calcium and phosphorus in close sequence. Higher concentrations of amino acids, the addition of cysteine, and larger volumes of TPN lower the risk of precipitation. Babies with higher mineral needs are ELBW and VLBW infants who require prolonged periods of TPN, those with osteopenia, healing fractures, or severe and sustained fluid restrictions. For these infants the most optimal delivery of minerals is from a dextrose/amino acid solution separate from a lipid solution that is infused through a different access site. Infusion of lipid emulsions into an amino acid/dextrose mixture via Y-site administration has been reported to increase the risk of calcium and phosphate precipitation as it increases the pH.

Components of TPN Solutions: TPN provides some or all nutrients of basal metabolism and growth for fluid, energy, macronutrients (protein, carbohydrate, and fat) and micronutrients (electrolytes, major minerals, trace minerals, and vitamins).

Fluid

On day one of life, maintenance fluids are met with a range between 80 and 140 mL/kg/d if the environment of the baby increases insensible water losses and 60 to 100 mL/kg/d in environments with increased humidity. Thereafter, fluid volume is advanced as tolerated to 120 to 180 mL/kg/d. Maximal fluid volume varies with individual management.

Macronutrients: Carbohydrate (dextrose) and fat (lipid emulsions) provide the energy needed to meet the demands of the circulatory, respiratory, neurological, and muscular systems and, when provided in adequate amounts, spare protein (amino acids) to support cell maturation, remodeling, growth, activity of enzymes, and transport proteins for all body organs. Energy needs may be increased with infection, chronic lung disease, healing, growth, and in babies who have experienced intrauterine growth restriction (IUGR). Energy needs may be decreased with sedation, mechanical ventilation, and after tracheostomy placement.

Micronutrients-Electrolytes: Sodium, potassium, and chloride are essential to life and requirements are dependent on obligatory losses, abnormal losses, and amounts necessary for growth. Sodium and potassium can be given as chloride, lactate, or phosphate salts. Infants who receive electrolytes solely as chloride salts may develop hyperchloremic metabolic acidosis. Sodium can also be given as acetate; a randomized trial in 1997 demonstrated the utility of acetate in parenteral nutrition solutions. Potassium is added when urinary flow is established and sodium is added post-diuresis. Chloride is generally given as sodium chloride.

Major Minerals: Calcium, phosphorus, and magnesium are the most abundant minerals in the body. They are closely interrelated to each other in metabolism, the formation of tissue structure, and function.

Trace Minerals: Zinc is universally recommended from day one of TPN, whereas the other trace minerals are generally provided after two, four, or 12 weeks' of TPN without any appreciable enteral feeding. Copper, selenium, molybdenum, and iron can be delivered separately also. Copper and manganese are discontinued from TPN solutions with the complication of cholestasis, and amounts of chromium, selenium, and molybdenum are reduced or omitted when renal output is low. Parenteral iron supplementation may be delayed until two months of age in premature infants and three months of age in term infants and considered for those infants who do not receive regular blood transfusions. Concern for iron overload is related to increased risk for septicemia in malnourished infants with a low serum transferrin as well as an increased need for vitamin E. Even though recommendations for premature infants exist within the first two weeks of life for copper, selenium, chromium, iron, iodide, and manganese, these trace minerals generally are not added to TPN but are provided within minimal enteral feedings. Supplementation with iodide may not be necessary because needs for iodide may be met from the topical absorption of iodide-containing disinfectants, detergents, and other environmental sources. Many component solutions of TPN solutions (albumin, heparin, calcium, and phosphate salts) contain aluminum. The additive amounts of aluminum place infants on long-term TPN at risk for toxicity because of its tendency to incorporate into body tissues. The recommended **parenteral vitamin** intakes can only be approximately delivered from MVI Pediatric. The standard dose of 2 mL/kg/d with a maximum intake of 5 mL/d provides lower amounts of vitamin A and higher amounts of most of the B vitamins. Furthermore, intravenous vitamin delivery may be less due to photodegradation of vitamins A, D, E, K, B_2, B_6, B_{12}, C, and folic acid and adsorption of vitamins A, D, and E into the vinyl delivery bags and tubing. Some clinicians have addressed these issues with the protection of delivery equipment from light and the administration of fat-soluble vitamins with lipid.

Line Access for TPN Delivery: Most premature infants require TPN either peripherally or centrally while enteral feeding is established. Route of TPN delivery depends on energy needs, venous access, anticipated duration of support, and potential risks. Peripheral access can be achieved through a cannula placed in the smaller veins of the scalp, hands, arms, or feet. Peripheral lines are not able to safely accommodate hyperosmolar solutions and therefore limit the amount of energy that can be provided. Peripheral lines are reserved for short-term or supplemental nutrition, generally for as long as two weeks. Central access is used when TPN is needed for a longer or undetermined period of time or when peripheral access is not an option. It is common practice for infants weighing less than 1,200 grams at birth to receive the majority of nutrition support for the first three weeks through a central line. Central lines allow greater ability to provide adequate energy and protein to promote growth and lean body mass accretion. Central access implies that the catheter tip is placed in the central circulation, often at the junction of the superior vena cava and right atrium, though exact placement may vary. Peripherally placed central catheters are popularly referred to as PICCs and PCVCs. These catheters require insertion using a needle through the skin into a peripheral vein and threaded into the central circulation. Umbilical venous catheters (UVC) and umbilical arterial catheters (UAC) are also used to provide central access and nutrition. Due to risks of infection and formation of thrombi, UVCs are typically removed within a week of placement. •Heparin (1 unit/mL) is added to all central venous lines and to all peripheral infusions running at <2 mL/hr in order to maintain catheter patency.

Clinical Monitoring of Nutrient Adequacy, Compatibility, and Tolerance of TPN Solutions:

Accurate and routine monitoring of growth measures is necessary to prevent over- or undernutrition from TPN support. Further, routine monitoring of solution compatibility and tolerance is required to prevent morbidity. **Growth**-Intrauterine growth rates approximate 10 to 21 g/kg/d for weight depending on gestational age, 0.9 to 1.1 cm/wk for length, and 0.7 to 0.9 cm/wk for head circumference- Weekly lengths and head measurements, in addition to daily weights, are important to ensure that overall growth is occurring and not simply weight gain. Although accurate and reproducible lengths are more difficult to obtain among clinicians, they are a better indicator of lean body mass and not influenced significantly by edema. Head growth correlates with increase in brain mass, therefore it is common to see a rapid increase during catch-up growth. For infants to grow optimally, ongoing assessment of growth in relation to daily estimates of nutrient intake is necessary. Often, actual nutrient intakes are significantly less than intended intakes because medications that are incompatible with TPN solutions are administered in separate intravenous solutions with TPN delivery interrupted once or several times during the day. Quantification of TPN delivery warrants investigation when babies experience poor growth despite the TPN order that prescribes adequate calories, protein, vitamins, and minerals to support needs. Actual intakes may also be overestimated when TPN scripts are based on body weights that are not current.

Fluid Restriction Premature infants with patent ductus arteriosus or other cardiac disease, chronic lung disease, or oliguria require some degree of fluid restriction. This limitation provides a challenge in tinier premature babies born with the lower nutrient stores, who also require more protein and minerals for a greater, more sustained rate of catch-up growth. The use of central lines such as PICCs (peripherally inserted central catheters) and PCVCs (percutaneous central venous catheters) allows clinicians to approach the infants' needs during fluid restriction. In these situations, the TPN solution is often concentrated to the maximum osmolarity and precipitation limits for optimal provision of energy, protein, and minerals to support growth. Restrictions of one or more macronutrients may result in an uneven distribution of calories between protein, carbohydrate, and/ or fat. For example: an ELBW infant who requires dexamethasone therapy may experience transient hyperglycemia and necessitate a decrease in carbohydrate with compensatory increases in protein or fat needed to provide sufficient energy. An inappropriate balance of parenteral nutrition can result in inefficient utilization of protein and nutrients. Even with maximally concentrated TPN solutions, nutrient intakes adequate to support growth may not be achieved in some infants. With consistently poor growth over time, either reassessment of total fluid management and/or a change in the composition of fluids is needed from the neonatology team. Routine assessment of weight trends over time and careful monitoring of fluid intake and output that includes electrolyte balance and urine specific gravities will help to fine-tune fluid management. Fistula or ostomy losses increase fluid, mineral, and/or electrolyte needs and may require intravenous replacement.

Overfeeding

Premature infants with chronic lung disease may become stable medically over time and receive TPN in excess of requirements. This results in an increase in fat synthesis. Overfeeding is associated with fatty infiltration of the liver, hyperglycemia, hypertriglyceridemia, increased metabolic rate, and electrolyte imbalance. In addition, overfeeding of total energy intake and with glucose may increase oxygen uptake and CO_2 production and retention in infants with lung disease or heart failure. Hypermetabolic and undernourished patients are thought to be most susceptible to these respiratory problems, while metabolically normal and nourished patients are not as adversely affected. To avoid overfeeding, appropriate nutrition assessment and monitoring is strongly advised to ensure a balanced provision of nutrient needs relative to gestational age, medical presentation and diagnosis, degree of repletion indicated, current metabolic indicators, and prognosis. Excessive and disproportional gains are likely indicators of overfeeding. Growth should be monitored by measures of weight and length, including board lengths if linear growth and proportional growth are a concern. Calculations of rates of growth compared with normative data, weight in proportion to length, and skinfold measures of subcutaneous fat may be indicated for babies born postterm having chronic conditions.

Tolerance/Complications:

Protocols for tolerance assessment of TPN fluids vary among NICUs but each typically offers a suggested schedule for the routine monitoring of physical and biochemical measures. Daily weights, volume intake, and calculations of actual fluid and nutrient delivery, urine output, serum electrolytes, glucose levels, blood urea nitrogen (BUN), and serum creatinine provide indicators of substrate tolerance and hydration to aid in day-to-day management decisions. Once a baby is clinically stable, electrolytes may need to be checked no more than twice each week. Patients with a history of electrolyte instability or requiring chronic diuretic therapy will need more frequent monitoring. Premature infants have a relatively small blood volume (e.g., 80 to 100 mL/kg), therefore the potential benefits of the information obtained are weighed against the risk of frequent blood sampling.

Hypoglycemia/Hyperglycemia

Premature babies are at risk of developing hypoglycemia due to limited glycogen reserves, with more premature or growth-restricted infants being at greatest risk. Glucose needs are increased due to a relatively large surface area of metabolically active organs requiring energy, with glucose infusion delivery rates based on weight and gestational age. Hyperglycemia is also a common occurrence in sick VLBW infants supported by TPN. Hyperglycemia is due in part to insulin resistance or to stress levels of cortisol and glucagon. Persistently high serum glucose values can lead to glycosuria with an osmotic diuresis, complicating fluid management. The usual management for these complications is to reduce glucose concentration, although the delivery of adequate calories might be challenged. Due to the risk in variation of response, the use of insulin typically is reserved for those infants who do not respond to a reduction in glucose delivery or continue to experience higher than desired serum glucose levels. Insulin given to VLBW and ELBW infants with hyperglycemia, controlled hyperglycemia, increased glucose delivery and energy, and increased weight gain. Insulin given to infants <1,500 grams with hyperglycemia, controlled serum glucose levels, increased glucose delivery and ELBW infants without hyperglycemia decreases protein breakdown resulting in metabolic acidosis due to increased lactate levels. Therefore careful monitoring of blood glucose and acid-base status is essential when insulin is used. Moreover, bacteremia should be ruled out when hyperglycemia develops in a baby receiving TPN at a dextrose concentration previously tolerated.

Protein Status-

Blood urea nitrogen levels within normal limits without acidosis have been reported with amino acid intakes of 3 g/kg/d. Urea is a metabolic by-product of protein oxidation and sometimes is used as a marker for amino acid intolerance. Elevated BUN values are thought to be consistent with higher rates of protein turnover and oxidation in premature infants and potentially in ELBW babies who are receiving inadequate calories and are a direct reflection of increased amounts of available amino acids- and are evidence of efficient utilization and nitrogen retention.

Hyperlipidemia

Elevations in serum triglycerides may occur in infants who are premature, IUGR, septic, have liver disease, or are receiving steroids and also result from fat breakdown in response to cortisol, catecholamines, and cytokines released in infants who are metabolically stressed. Although heparin helps to improve high serum triglyceride levels, it does not change the oxidation rate of fatty acids. Elevations in serum triglycerides generally occur four hours after the initiation or increase in parenteral lipid.

High serum triglyceride levels (greater than 200 mg/dL) that occur with prolonged TPN have also been attributed to carnitine deficiency. Premature infants younger than 34 weeks' gestation have limited carnitine stores. Infants receiving TPN have no dietary source of carnitine. Therefore, these groups of infants may develop carnitine deficiency in as little as five days after birth. The manufacturer of intravenous carnitine (Carnitor, Sigma-Tau, Gaithersberg, MD) suggests dosing between 20 to 50 mg/kg/d, although lower amounts between 2 and 10 mg/kg/d may improve serum levels without adverse clinical symptoms. Supplementation is particularly important with long-term TPN and PN and continued provision is suggested until enteral intake approximates 50% of energy required to support growth. A dose of two to five mg carnitine/kg/d is suggested with routine monitoring of serum levels at baseline and quarterly and then annually thereafter.

Serum analysis of carnitine includes measuring plasma total and free carnitine concentrations and acylcarnitine fractions. A calculated ratio of acylcarnitine-to-free carnitine greater than 0.4 suggests insufficiency.

Cholestasis

If it is anticipated that TPN will be needed for longer than two weeks, it is prudent to obtain liver function tests, including a fractioned bilirubin, especially in ELBW infants to establish a baseline and repeat measures to document trends suggestive of cholestasis or liver disease. Elevations in serum alkaline phosphatase and direct bilirubin may be observed as soon as two weeks after initiating TPN. A much earlier, although nonspecific indicator of cholestasis is gamma-glutamyl transpeptidase (GGT), however it's specificity is said to be improved when used with alkaline phosphatase. Rising direct bilirubins and transaminases are later indicators of cholestasis. Risk factors associated with the development of cholestasis include the withholding of enteral feeding, immaturity, sepsis, hypoxia, toxicities of amino acids such as methionine and trace elements including copper, chromium, and manganese, and excessive energy and dextrose intakes. Oxidation of TPN solutions by light, medications, and nutrient deficiencies of taurine, choline, fatty acids, and trace minerals have been associated with increased incidence of cholestasis. The addition of taurine to pediatric amino acid products may help premature infants in the conjugation of bile salts and bile acid secretion. Copper and manganese are excreted in the bile and may contribute to hepatic toxicity when their removal from the liver is impaired due to limited bile flow. Because several studies suggest that manganese accumulation contributed to the severity of cholestasis or liver disease, some have not recommended providing manganese until a month following TPN administration and closely following manganese serum levels. With an elevated direct bilirubin greater than 2 to 3 mg/dL, amounts of intravenous copper and manganese should be reduced or temporarily withheld. Small amounts of enteral feedings, especially for infants who require long-term TPN, may help prevent cholestasis, since feedings enhance gastric motility and bile flow. Also, by offering enteral feedings, trace minerals (i.e., copper and manganese) can be eliminated from TPN.

Osteopenia: Osteopenia is reported to be as high as 30% in studies of babies less than 1,500 grams at birth primarily supported with prolonged TPN without appreciable enteral feedings. Occurrence results mainly due to the inability to deliver adequate amounts of calcium and phosphorus safely within a limited amount of parenteral volume. Other infants that are at risk include those with fluid or protein restriction during TPN administration, those treated with chronic diuretic therapy, and those with high ostomy output with increased loss of electrolytes and minerals (e.g., magnesium, calcium, and sodium) important for adequate bone mineralization. An option for these babies would be to consider the earlier use of separate dextrose and amino acid solutions with fat emulsions administered by "piggy-back" infusions, allowing for more optimal delivery of calcium and phosphorus compared with those in total nutrient admixtures. A noninvasive wrist or long-bone film can aid in the diagnosis and treatment of osteopenia. Routine blood levels of alkaline phosphatase, phosphorus, and calcium are helpful in detecting signs of metabolic bone disease. Generally, alkaline phosphatase levels will be elevated and serum phosphorus levels will be lower in babies with osteopenia. Serum calcium levels are typically maintained within a normal range during osteopenia at the expense of bone, although the presence of acute or chronic acid-base disturbances can influence this usually tight control.

Sepsis: Sepsis in premature infants who receive prolonged TPN is a serious risk that contributes to morbidity and mortality. One possible risk factor for coagulase negative staphylococcal bacteremia in NICUs has been attributed primarily to the intravenous administration of lipid emulsions. In contrast, other investigations have described sick VLBW infants with a lower incidence of coagulase negative staphylococcal bacteremia and who received significantly larger amounts of lipids and better total energy. These infants received TPN significantly earlier and for longer periods of time and therefore were more likely to be at or greater than the 10th percentile for weight or length by discharge. Infection appears to be more common with central line delivery; however, these babies tend to be the sickest and require prolonged TPN administration. Propensity for infections is also linked with overfeeding of glucose, with hyperglycemia being a risk factor in infectious complications. Other risk factors for colonization of neonates in NICUs include the use of central venous catheters and the unclean hands of health care workers. The use of antacids and third generation cephalosporins and a delay in enteral feeding are thought to encourage colonization. Infection is considered when formerly stable babies show clinical or metabolic signs of instability and feeding intolerance.

Flowsheets, Protocols, and Order Sheets: The daily routine of nutrition screening and assessment of infants in a NICU requires ongoing summaries of nutrient intake information, including TPN prescriptions. The organized format of most nutrition worksheets will allow the clinician:

*to understand the trends in growth and current laboratory values and medications

*to complete a comprehensive overview of each patient's clinical management and progress.

*to easily identify the need for intervention or further investigation

*to use as a reference when nutrition and growth issues are discussed with the health care team in a busy NICU.

*to use as a tool that assists with documentation of nutrient intake.

Complications of TPN

1. Catheter
a. Infection (25-30%)
b. Malposition/dislodgement
c. Thrombus of line - treat with TPA. Thrombus of SVC or IVC
d. Peripheral catheters - extravasation and skin sloughs. Thrombophlebitis and infection (rare).

2. Metabolic
a. Electrolyte abnormalities - Na/K/acid-base disturbances
b. Mineral abnormalities - Ca/P/Mg
c. Hyper/hypoglycemia, osmotic diuresis
d. Hepatic dysfunction - infants on prolonged TPN (>10-14 days) can develop cholestasis. The reason is unknown. Typical lab results show a rising bilirubin with a increased direct component and mildly elevated transaminases. Even small enteral feeds may help this problem. Other causes for a direct hyperbilirubinemia should be considered (TPN cholestasis is a diagnosis of exclusion).
e. Hyper/hypovitaminosis (should be avoided with proper use of MVI.
f. Essential fatty acid deficiency (avoid with small infusion of lipids)
g. Trace mineral deficiency (avoid with addition of trace minerals)

Neonatal Parenteral Nutrition Calculations:

The following example illustrates the nutrition calculations for a preterm newborn on TPN:

GOALS: To provide

(a) volume to maintain fluid balance (100-200 ml/kg/d),

(b) protein to promote positive nitrogen (N) balance (2.5-3.5 g/kg/d),

(c) intravenous fat emulsion (IFE) to meet essential fatty acid and energy requirements (1-3 g/kg/d), and

(d) energy (80-100 kcal/kg/d) balanced for non-protein calories (NPC) (150-200 NPC: g N; greater than or equal to 22 kcal/g protein; more than 70/kg/d NPC) from a mix of carbohydrate (60-70%) and fat (30-40%), in a

(e) total regimen to maintain acid-base balance and third trimester weight gain (15 g/kg/d).

BABY NICU: BW = 0.9 kg DOL = 5 Current Weight = 0.92 kg

(1) **FLUIDS:** 160 ml/kg/d x 0.92 kg = 147 ml/d

(2) **IFE 20% DOSE:** 2.5 g/kg/d x 0.92 kg = 2.3 g/d IFE 20% = 20 g/100 ml, therefore, 2.3 g = 11.5 ml/d

(3) **IFE 20% INFUSION RATE:** 2.5 g/kg/d over 20 hours = 0.125 g/kg/hr (Goal: less than or equal to 0.12-0.15 g/kg/hr)

(4) **IV RATE:** 147 ml/d – 11.5 ml/d IFE 20% = 136 ml/d 136 ml/d ÷ 24 hr = 5.7 ml/hr

(5) **PROTEIN DOSE:** 3 g/kg/d x 0.92 kg = 2.76 g/d (2.76 g ÷ 6.25 = 0.44 g N) 2.76 g/136 ml = 2.1 g/100 ml or 2.1% solution

(6) **DEXTROSE DOSE:** Documented tolerance to 10% dextrose; 136 ml/d of 12% dextrose = 16.32 g/d dextrose or 16,320 mg/d dextrose

16,320 mg/d ÷ 0.92 kg = 17,739 mg/kg/d

17,739 mg/kg/d ÷ 1440 minutes/d (24X60) = 12.3 mg/kg/minute

(7) **ENERGY:** Carbohydrate: 16.32 g x 3.4 kcal/g = 55.5 kcal/d

Fat: 11.5 ml/d x 2 kcal/ml = <u>23 kcal/d</u>

SUBTOTAL (NPC) 78.5 kcal/d

Protein: 2.76 g x 4 kcal/g = 11 kcal/d

TOTAL 89.5 kcal/d or 97 kcal/kg/d

(8) **BALANCE:** 178 NPC: 1g N [(55.5 + 23) ÷ 0.44] 28 kcal/g protein [(55.5 + 23) ÷ 2.76] 71 % Carbohydrate [(55.5 ÷ 78.5) X 100] and 29 % Fat [(23 ÷ 78.5) X 100]

(9) **ORDER:** Dextrose 12% Amino Acid 2% at 5.7 ml/hr and IFE 11.5 ml over 20 hr Supplies per day 160 ml/kg, 97 kcal/kg, 3 g protein/kg, 2.5 g fat/kg

The following example illustrates the calculations to determine an appropriate solution for a 0.8 kg infant with hyperglycemia. This hypothetical infant is receiving D10% at 150 ml/kg per day providing a glucose load of 10.4 mg/kg per minute. To decrease the glucose load to 8 mg/kg per minute and maintain fluid at 150 ml/kg per day:

$$\frac{(8 \text{ mg} \times 0.8 \text{ kg})\ (60 \times 24)}{1000} = 9.2 \text{ g/day glucose}$$

150 ml x 0.8 kg = 120 ml/day fluid

$$\frac{9.2 \text{ g}}{120 \text{ ml}} \cdot \frac{x}{100 \text{ ml}} = 7.7 \text{ g/100 ml}$$

The new dextrose solution would be ~ 7.5%

Monitoring during TPN administration:

Before starting an infant on parenteral nutrition, investigation required:

• full blood count /hematocrit • renal profile

• liver function test, bilirubin •random blood sugar/dextrostix

While on TPN, monitoring required :

Laboratory

• full blood count, renal profile. Daily for 1 week then 3 times a week

• plasma calcium, magnesium, phosphate. Twice a week until stable then weekly

• triglyceride levels. After dose changes then weekly

• liver function test: If long term TPN (> 2 weeks duration)

Clinical

• blood sugar / dextrostix, 4-6 hrly first 3 days, twice a day once stable.

• daily weight

• meticulous care of the catheter site and monitoring of infection.

Estimated Nutrient Intakes Needed for Fetal Weight Gain

Body weight (gm)	500-700	700-900	900-1200	1200-1500	1500-1800
Fetal weight gain (gm/day)	13	16	20	24	26
Fetal weight gain (gm/kg/day)	21	20	19	18	16
Protein (gm/kg/day)					
Parenteral	3.5	3.5	3.5	3.4	3.2
Enteral	4.0	4.0	4.0	3.9	3.6
Energy (kcal/kg/day)					
Parenteral	89	92	101	108	109
Enteral	105	108	119	127	128

Fluid Needs (ml/kg/day)

Birth weight (gm)	Day 1-2	Day 3	DOL 15-30
750-1000	105	140	150
1001-1250	100	130	140
1251-1500	90	120	130
1501-1700	80	110	130
1701-2000	80	110	130
Term infant	70	80	100

Daily Electrolyte Requirements for Pediatric Patients

Electrolyte	Preterm Neonates	Infants/Children
Sodium	2-5 mEq/kg	2-5 mEq/kg
Potassium	2-4 mEq/kg	2-4 mEq/kg
Calcium	2-4 mEq/kg	0.5-4 mEq/kg
Phosphorus	1-2 mmol/kg	0.5-2 mmol/kg
Magnesium	0.3-0.5 mEq/kg	0.3-0.5 mEq/kg
Acetate	As needed to maintain acid-base balance	As needed to maintain acid-base balance

Trace Element Daily Requirements

Trace Element	Preterm Neonates < 3 kg (mcg/kg/day)	Term Neonates 3-10 kg (mcg/kg/day)
Zinc	400	50-250
Copper	20	20
Manganese	1	1
Chromium	0.05-0.2	0.2
Selenium	1.5-2	2

PARENTERAL NUTRITION IN PREMATURE INFANTS : AN OVERVIEW

Fluid requirements

- Premature infants have greater ECF volumes
- Initial diuresis occurs within first week of life: 10-15% loss of body weight for premature infants, can be up to 20% for the extremely low birth weight.
- Initial fluid requirements:80-140 mL/kg/d
- ELBW infants may require up to 200 mL/kg/d
- Goal after fluid stabilization: 100-150 mL/kg/d
- Fluid restriction may be required for infants with PDA, BPD, CHF, renal failure cerebral edema
- Insensible water loss increases with
    - Increased skin permeability at birth
    - Increased BSA to weight ratio
    - Phototherapy
    - Radiant warmer beds
    - Respiratory distress syndrome
    - Cold stress, increased activity
- Insensible water loss decreases with
    - Heat shields
    - Humidified Incubators
- Fluid loss also results from
    - Vomiting
    - Diarrhea
    - Ostomy output
    - Chest tube drainage

Carbohydrate

- Initial glucose load: 4-6 mg/kg/min
- Adjust by 2 mg/kg/min as tolerated, advancing to meet nutritional need
- Limit to < 14 mg/kg/min to prevent overfeeding, fatty liver, increased CO_2 production

Protein

- Infants < 1,500 g BW: begin at 1-1.5 g/kg/d, advance by 1g/kg/d to goal of 3-3.5 g/kg/d

- Infants > 1,500 g BW: begin at 1-1.5 g/kg/d, advance by 1g/kg/d to goal of 2.5-3 g/kg/d

Fat

- Begin at 1g/kg/d and advance by 1g/kg/d to goal of 3 g/kg
- May run lipid via central or peripheral access over 20-24 hours
- Monitor with serum triglyceride, normal range < 200 mg/dL
- EFAD may occur in < 1 week without lipid source; provide minimum 0.5 g/kg/d 2-3 times per week to prevent
- May need to limit to 2 g/kg/d with extreme hyperbilirubinemia to prevent kernicterus

Total energy needs

- 90-100 kcal/kg/d for VLBW and SGA infants
- 80-90 kcal/kg/d for > 28 weeks and AGA

Additives

Na: 2-4 mEq/kg/d   Ca: 60-90 mg/kg/d

K: 2-4 mEq/kg/d   Phos: 47-70 mg/kg/d

Cl: 2-3 mEq/kg/d   Mg: 4.3-7.2 mg/kg/d

MVI pediatric

< 1 kg: 30% of standard 5 mL

1-3 kg: 65% of standard 5 mL

> 3 kg: 100% of standard 5 mL

Biochemical parameters to monitor

- Daily (as initiating and advancing PN and lipids)
    - Na, K, Cl, CO_2 glucose, triglyceride
- Weekly (and prior to initiating PN and lipids)
    - Above tests plus Ca, Mg, P, alkaline phosphatase, BUN, creatinine, triglyceride, total protein, albumin, bilirubin, AST, ALT, hematocrit

AGA = appropriate for gestational age; ALT = alanine transaminase; AST = aspartate transaminase; BPD = bronchopulmonary dysplasia; BSA = body surface area; BUN = blood urea nirtrogen; BW = birth weight; CHF = congestive heart failure; ECF = extracellular fluid; EFAD = essential fatty acid deficiency; ELBW=extremely low birth weight; MVI = multivitamin infusion; PDA = patent ductus arteriosus; PN = parenteral nutrition; SGA = small for gestational age; VLBW = very low birth weight.

Standard TPN Regime. This allows a graded introduction of full nutrition over 4 days and assumes the infant is already receiving a fluid intake of 150 ml/kg per 24 hrs. For infants in the first few days of life, when fluids are gradually being increased, only the day 1 regime should be used until 150 ml/kg/day is reached. If an older infant is subsequently fluid restricted, the day 4 final regime can be administered in as little as 120 ml/kg/ day.

TPN	Day 1	Day 2	Day 3	Day 4
Protein (g/kg per 24 h)	1.0	1.5	2.0	2.5
Nitrogen (g/kg per 24 h)	0.16	0.23	0.33	0.4
Carbohydrate (g/kg per 24 h)	1	1.2	14	15
Fat (g/kg per 24 h)	1	2	3	4
Energy (Kcals/kg per 24 h)	50	68	86	100
Sodium (mmol/kg per 24 h)	3	3	3	3
Potassium (mmol/kg per 24 h)	2.5	2.5	2.5	2.5
Calcium (mmol/kg per 24 h)	1.9	1.9	1.9	1.9
Phosphorus (mmol/kg per 24 h)	1.5	1.5	1.5	1.5
Volume (mL/kg per 24 h)	150	150	150	150

Vamin 9 glucose (pharmacia)	30 mL/kg per 24 h
This provides:	
Nitrogen	0.28 g/kg per 24 h
Non-protein energy	12 kcals/kg per 24 h
Glucose	3.0 g/kg per 24 h
Sodium	1.5 mmol/kg per 24 h
Potassium	0.6 mmol/kg per 24 h
Magnesium	0.045 mmol/kg per 24 h
Calcium	0.075 mmol/kg per 24 h
Chloride	1.5 mmol/kg per 24 h
Dextrose	14 g/kg per 24 h (70 mL/kg per 24 h of 20% solution = 56 kcal/kg per 24 h)
Sodium chloride	1.5 mmol/kg per 24 h
Peditrace (pharmacia)	1mL/kg per 24 h
KH2PO4	2.5 mL /kg per 24 h
Solivito N (pharmacia)	0.5 mL /kg per 24 h
Intralipid 20% (pharmacia)	20 mL/kg per 24 h (4 g fat/kg per 24 hrs; 40 kcals/kg per 24 h)
Vitlipid N Infant (Pharmacia)	4 mL/kg per 24 h

The prevention of pain in Neonates should be the goal of all caregivers because painful exposures have the potential for deleterious consequences. Those neonates at greatest risk for neurodevelopmental impairment due to preterm birth (e.g., the smallest and sickest) are also most likely to be exposed to the greatest number of painful stimuli in the Neonatal Intensive Care Unit (NICU). Although there are major gaps in our knowledge regarding the most effective way to prevent and relieve pain in Neonates, proven and safe therapies are currently underutilized for routine minor, yet painful, procedures. Every health care facility caring for Neonates should implement an effective pain prevention program that includes strategies for the following: routinely assessing pain; minimizing the number of painful procedures performed; effectively using pharmacological and nonpharmacological therapies for the prevention of pain associated with routine minor procedures; and eliminating pain associated with surgery and other major procedures.

TABLE 1   Cries : Neonatal postoperative pain assessment score

Indicator	Scoring criteria		
	0	1	2
Crying	No cry, or cry not high pitched	High pitched cry, but consolable	High pitched cry, inconsolable
Requires oxygen for saturation > 95%	No oxygen required from baseline	Oxygen requirement < 30% from baseline	Oxygen requirement > 30% from baseline
Increased vital signs*	Heart rate and blood pressure are both unchanged	Heart rate or blood pressure is increased by < 20%	Heart rate and blood pressure is increased by > 20%
Expression†	None (no grimace)	Grimace only is present	Grimace and nonaudible grunt present
Sleeplessness‡	Continuously asleep	Awakens at frequent intervals	Awake constantly

* Measure blood pressure last so as not to awaken the infant.

† Grimace consists of lowered brow, eyes squeezed shut, deepening nasolabial furrow, and open lips and mouth.

‡ Based on infant's state during preceding hour.

* Crying (0-2)

Requires increased oxygen (0-2)

Increased vital signs (0-2)

Expression (0-2)

Sleepless (0-2)

Scoring range : 0 = no pain; 10 = worst pain

The Learning objectives are to:

1. Emphasize that despite increased awareness of the importance of pain prevention, Neonates in the NICU continue to be exposed to numerous painful minor procedures daily as part of their routine care;

2. Present objective means of assessing Neonatal pain by health care professionals;

3. Describe effective strategies to prevent and treat pain associated with routine minor procedures; A stepwise approach should begin with avoidance of painful procedures as much as possible, followed by nonpharmacologic and then pharmacologic methods for pain relief. and

4. Review appropriate methods to prevent and treat pain associated with surgery and other major procedures.

TABLE 2   Consequences of untreated pain in infants

ACUTE CONSEQUENCES: Periventricular Intraventricular hemorrhage, Increased chemical and hormone release, Breakdown of fat and carbohydrate stores, Prolonged hyperglycemia, Higher morbidity for NICU patients, Memory of painful events, Hypersensitivity to pain, Prolonged response to pain, Inappropriate innervation of the spinal cord Inappropriate response to nonnoxious stimuli, Lower pain threshold

POTENTIAL LONG-TERM CONSEQUENCES: Higher somatic complaints of unknown origin, Greater physiologic and behavioral responses to pain, Increased prevalence of neurologic deficits, Psychosocial problems, Aversion to human contact, Developmental delay, Neurobehavioral disorders, Cognitive deficits, Learning disorders, Poor motor performance, Behavioral problems, Attention deficits, Poor adaptive behavior, Inability to cope with novel situations, Problems with impulsivity and social control, Learning deficits, Emotional temperature changes in infancy or childhood, Accentuated hormonal stress responses in adult life

Nonpharmacologic methods of pain relief in newborns: *Environmental Modification:* Decrease bright lights, Avoid loud noises, Cluster nursing activities, Allow undisturbed rest, Gently manipulate lines and tubes, Limit painful and stressful procedures *Positioning:* Swaddling, containment, Facilitated tucking *Touch:* Stroking, caressing, Massaging, Holding, Kangaroo care *Distraction:* Music, Rhythmic rocking, Soft, soothing voice *Nonnutritive sucking:* Pacifier, Nonlactating nipple *Sucrose:* 24% to 50%, 0.1 to 2 mL orally 2 min before procedure via syringe or pacifier *Glucose:* 30%, 0.3 to 1 mL orally 1 to 2 min before procedure

Quality Improvement Approach: A suggested approach to evidence-based recommendations for the treatment of neonatal pain includes the following:

1. Recognition of neonatal pain as a valid concern 2. Recognition of acute procedural and chronic neonatal pain in need of treatment 3. Validated assessment tool for neonatal pain 4. Educational resources for caregivers and parents in the NICU 5. Protocolized stepwise treatment plan for the procedures and conditions encountered in the NICU using nonpharmacologic and pharmacologic approaches to treatment 6. Continued auditing to ascertain appropriate treatment for neonatal pain 7. A well-planned program of coordination, facilitation, and using local champions and project teams to elicit a beneficial change in practice.

TABLE 3 **Analgesia for minimally invasive procedures***

Procedures	Intubated and ventilated infants	Nonintubated infants
Arterial puncture	24% sucrose 0.5–1.5 mL PO	24% sucrose 0.5–1.5 ml PO
Venipuncture	24% sucrose 0.5–1.5 mL PO	24% sucrose 0.5–1.5 ml PO
Heel-stick blood draw	24% sucrose 0.5–1.5 mL PO	24% sucrose 0.5–1.5 ml PO
Intravenous placement	24% sucrose 0.5–1.5 mL PO	24% sucrose 0.5–1.5 ml PO
Lumbar puncture	24% sucrose 0.5–1.5 mL PO and morphine 0.05–0.15 mg/kg IV or *SQ or* fentanyl† 1–3 mcg/kg IV *and/or* If ≥ 34 wks PMA: topical EMLA‡ *and* buffered lidocaine 0.5% (max: 0.5mL/kg) SQ	24% sucrose 0.5–1.5 ml PO and If ≥ 34 wks PMA: topical EMLA‡ and buffered lidocaine 0.5% (max: 0.5mL/kg) SQ
Dressing change	24% sucrose 0.5–1.5 mL PO; may repeat *and/or* morphine 0.05–0.1 mg/kg IV *or* fentanyl† 1–3 mcg/kg IV	24% sucrose 0.5–1.5 mL PO; (may repeat) *and/or* morphine 0.025-0.05 mg/kg IV or SQ *or* fentanyl† 0.25–1mcg/kg IV
Endotracheal suctioning (mechanically ventilated)	Morphine 0.05–0.15 mg/kg *or* fentanyl† 1–3mcg/kg IV	N/A
Immunization injection	N/A	24% sucrose 0.5–1.5 mL PO; (may repeat) *and/or* topical EMLA‡ (If ≥ 34 wks PMA)

*Competitive stimulation may be used for any of these procedures, except suctioning.
†Fentanyl should be infused at ≤ 1mcg/kg/min (e.g. 3 mcg/kg infused over ≥ 3 min).
‡Only one application per day of topical EMLA should be used. It takes 40–60 min to reach peak effect and should be removed within 2 h of application.

TABLE 4 **Analgesia for invasive procedures: Preterm and term* infant**

Procedures	Intubated and ventilated infants	Nonintubated infants
Intubation (emergency)	None	None
Intubation/reintubation (elective)	Fentanyl† 1–3 mcg/kg IV (infused over 3 min) IV *or* Morphine 0.05–0.1 mg/kg IV or SQ	Fentanyl† 0.25-1 mcg/kg IV (infused over 2 min) IV *or* Morphine 0.025–0.05 mg/kg IV or SQ
Mechanical ventilation First 24 h (unless extubation is anticipated within 4 h)	Fentanyl† 1–3 mcg/kg Q4 h and PRN or morphine 0.05–0.15 mg/kg Q4 h and PRN or fentanyl infusion 0.2–2 mg/kg/h (start at low rate and increase PRN)	N/A
>24h	Fentanyl† 1–3 mcg/kg Q4 h and PRN or morphine 0.05–0.15 mg/kg Q4 h and PRN or	N/A
Chest tube Insertion	Lidocaine 0.5% (max 1 mL/kg) SQ and fentanyl† 2–5 mcg/kg IV × 1 or morphine 0.1–0.2 mg/kg IV × 1, then titrate PRN	Lidocaine 0.5% (max 1 mL/kg) SQ and fentanyl† 1-2 mcg/kg IV or morphine 0.05-0.1 mg/kg IV × 1, then titrate PRN
In-place	Morphine 0.05–0.15 mg/kg Q 2-4 h PRN or fentanyl† 1-3 mcg/kg IV Q 2-4 h PRN	Morphine 0.025–0.05 mg/kg IV or SQ or fentanyl† 0.25–1mcg/kg IV Q4–6 h PRN
Removal	Morphine 0.05–0.15 mg/kg or fentanyl† 1–3 mcg/kg IV x 1	Morphine 0.025–0.05 mg/kg IV or SQ or fentanyl† 0.5–2 mcg/kg IV
Umbilical catheter placement	Morphine 0.05–0.1 mg/kg PRN fentanyl† 1–3 mcg/kg IV PRN	Morphine 0.025–0.05 mg/kg IV or SQ or fentanyl† 0.25–1 mcg/kg IV
Peripheral arterial catheter placement	Morphine 0.05–0.1 mg/kg Q 2-4 h or fentanyl† 1-3 mcg/kg IV Q 2-4 h or topical EMLA (if ≥ 34 wks PMA)	Morphine 0.025–0.05 mg/kg IV or SQ or fentanyl† 0.25–1 mcg/kg IV or topical EMLA (if ≥ 34 wks PMA)
Percutaneously inserted central catheter placement	Morphine 0.05–0.1 mg/kg Q 2–4 h or fentanyl† 1–3 mcg/kg IV Q 2–4 h or topical EMLA (if ≥34 wks PMA)	Morphine 0.025–0.5 mg/kg IV or fentanyl† 0.25–1 mcg/kg IV or topical EMLA (if ≥ 34 wks PMA)

*Full-term infants **only** also may receive Midazolam 0.05–0.1 mg/kg for anxiety.
†Fentanyl should be infused at ≤ 1 mcg/kg/min (e.g. 3 mcg/kg infused over ≥ 3min).

REDUCING PAIN FROM BEDSIDE CARE PROCEDURES : Neonates in the NICU often experience painful procedures during routine care, such as needle insertions, suctioning, gavage tube placement and tape removal, as well as stressful disruptions, including diaper changes, chest physical therapy, physical examinations, environmental stimuli and nursing evaluations. Despite increased awareness by caregivers that neonates in the NICU frequently experience pain, effective pain relief for these routine procedures is often underutilized.

Clinical implications : 1. Care protocols for neonates should incorporate a principle of minimizing the number of painful disruptions in care as much as possible. 2. A combination of oral sucrose/glucose and other nonpharmacological pain reduction methods (nonnutritive sucking, kangaroo care, facilitated tuck, swaddling and developmental care) should be used for minor, routine procedures. 3. Topical anesthetics can be used to reduce pain associated with venipuncture, lumbar puncture and intravenous catheter insertion when time permits, but are ineffective for heel stick blood draws. Repeated use of topical anesthetics should be limited. 4. The routine use of continuous infusions of morphine, fentanyl or midazolam in chronically ventilated preterm neonates is not recommended due to concern about short-term side effects and lack of long-term outcome data.

REDUCING PAIN FROM SURGERY : 1. Any health care facility providing surgery for newborns should have an established protocol for pain management. This requires a coordinated, multidimensional strategy and should be a priority in perioperative management. 2. Sufficient anesthesia should be provided to prevent intraoperative pain and stress responses to decrease postoperative analgesic requirements. 3. Pain should be routinely assessed using a scale designed for postoperative or prolonged pain in newborns. 4. Opioids should be the basis for postoperative analgesia after major surgery in the absence of regional anesthesia. 5. Postoperative analgesia should be utilized as long as pain assessment scales document that it is required. 6. Acetaminophen can be used after surgery as an adjunct to regional anesthetics or opioids, but there are inadequate data on pharmacokinetics at gestational ages under 28 weeks to permit calculation of appropriate dosages.

REDUCING PAIN FROM OTHER MAJOR PROCEDURES Intercostal drains : Analgesia for chest drain insertion should comprise all of the following: 1. General nonpharmacological measures; 2. Slow infiltration of the skin site with a local anesthetic before incision unless there is life-threatening instability. If there is inadequate time to infiltrate before the insertion of the chest tube, local skin infiltration after achieving stability may reduce later pain responses and later analgesic requirements. 3. Systemic analgesia with a rapidly acting opiate, such as fentanyl. **Chest drain removal :** Analgesia for chest drain removal should comprise the following: 1. General nonpharmacological measures; and 2. A short-acting, rapid-onset systemic analgesic. **Intubation :** see Table 4. **Retinal examination and surgery for retinopathy of prematurity :** 1. Although there are insufficient data to make a specific recommendation, retinal examinations are painful, and pain relief measures should be utilized. A reasonable approach would be to administer local anesthetic eye drops and oral sucrose. 2. Retinal surgery should be considered major surgery, and effective pain relief, based on opiates, should be provided. **Circumcision :** Pain relief for circumcision should always be provided.

Perioperative Analgesia in Various Neonatal Procedures

1) Preoperative (i.e., intubated infants undergoing general anesthesia) : Intubated and ventilated infants - Consider Fentanyl* 1-3 mg/kg IV 1 h before transfer to the operating room for the procedure . Nonintubated infants-N/A . *2) Laser surgery :* Intubated and ventilated infants - 2 h before the procedure: Acetaminophen 10-15 mg/kg and During the procedure: Morphine 0.05-0.1 mg/kg Q 1-2h or fentanyl* 1-3 mg/kg Q 1-2 h PRN and, if ≥34 wks PMA: Midazolam 0.1 mg/kg Q 1-2 h PRN. Nonintubated infants-N/A . *3) Circumcision :* Intubated and ventilated infants - N/A. Nonintubated infants- 24% sucrose 0.5-1.5 mL/kg PO and Acetaminophen 10-15 mg/kg 2h PO/PG before and Q 6 h after the procedure (x 24 h) and Ring block (Lidocaine 0.5%) (max. : 0.5 mL/kg) or dorsal penile block (Lidocaine 0.5%) or if ≥34 wks PMA and > 1.8 kg: topical EMLA *4) Herniorrhaphy :* Intubated and ventilated infants - Acetaminophen 10-15 mg/kg PO/PG/PR Q 4-6 h fentanyl* 2-3 mg/kg Q 2-4 h PRN or morphine 0.05-0.1 mg/kg Q 2-4 h PRN. Nonintubated infants-Acetaminophen 10-15 mg/kg PO/PG/PR Q 6 h or fentanyl* 0.25 - 0.5 mg/kg Q 4 h PRN or morphine 0.025-0.05 mg/kg IV or SQ Q 4 h PRN *5) Laparotomy :* Intubated and ventilated infants - First 24 h: Fentanyl* 1-3 mg/kg Q 4 - 6 h or morphine 0.1 mg/kg Q 4-6 h Then: Morphine 0.05-0.1 Q 2-4 h PRN or fentanyl* 1-3 mg/kg Q 2-4 h PRN. Nonintubated infants-Fentanyl* 0.25-0.5 mg/kg Q 4 h PRN or morphine 0.025-0.05 mg/kg IV or SQ Q 4 h PRN *6) Thoracotomy :* Intubated and ventilated infants - First 24 h: Fentanyl* 1-3 mg/kg Q 4 h or morphine 0.05-0.1 mg/kg Q 4 h Then : Morphine 0.05-0.1 mg/kg Q 2-4 h PRN or fentanyl* 1-3 mg/kg Q 2-4 h PRN. Nonintubated infants-Acetaminophen 10-15 mg/kg Q 6 h Q 6 h PRN or fentanyl * 0.25- 0.5 mg/kg Q 4 h PRN or morphine 0.025-0.05 mg/kg IV or SQ Q 4 h PRN *7) Laser surgery for ROP :* Intubated and ventilated infants - Acetaminophen 15mg/kg PG/PR 2 h before and acetaminophen 10 mg/kg Q 6 h after procedure (x 24 h); then Q 6 h PRN. Nonintubated infants-Acetaminophen 10 mg/kg Q 6 h after the procedure (x 24 h); then Q 6 h PRN *8) Neurosurgery (cranial) :* Intubated and ventilated infants - Fentanyl* 1-3 mg/kg Q 2-4 h PRN or morphine 0.05-0.1 mg/kg Q 2-4 h PRN. Nonintubated infants-Acetaminophen 10-15 mg/kg Q 6 h PRN or fentanyl * 0.25-0.5 mg/kg Q 4 h PRN or morphine 0.025-0.05 mg/kg IV or SQ Q 4 h PRN *9) Neurosurgery (lumbar) :* Intubated and ventilated infants - Fentanyl* 1-3 mg/kg Q 2-4 h PRN or morphine 0.05-0.1 mg/kg Q 2-4 h PRN. Nonintubated infants-Acetaminophen 10-15 mg/kg Q 6 h Q 4 h PRN or fentanyl* 0.25-0.5 mg/kg (over 2 min) or morphine 0.025-0.05 mg/kg IV or SQ Q 4 h PRN

* Fentanyl should be infused at ≤1mg/kg/min (e.g., 3 mg/kg infused over ≥ 3 min).

Efficacy of tramadol versus fentanyl for postoperative analgesia in neonates:

Fentanyl promotes rapid analgesia in neonates, but it has adverse effects such as tolerance, respiratory depression, urinary retention and ileum. Tramadol is a weak opioid that leads to less respiratory depression, ileum, tolerance and physical dependence compared with classical opioids, in adults. *Fentanyl:* administered as a continuous infusion of 2 mcg/ kg/h for term newborns and 1 mcg/kg/h for preterm neonates or for those extubated soon after surgery. *Tramadol:* administered as a continuous infusion of 0.2 mg/ kg/h for term newborns and 0.1 mg/kg/h for preterm neonates or for those extubated soon after surgery. Tramadol was as effective as fentanyl for postoperative pain relief in neonates but does not appear to offer advantages over fentanyl regarding the duration of mechanical ventilation and time to reach full enteral feeding.There is a strong need to study the effi cacy and safety profi les of analgesics in age-compatible populations in order to fi nd alternatives to treat pain for critically ill newborn infants.

(From: Arch *Dis Child Fetal Neonatal Ed* 2012;**97**:F24"F29. doi:10.1136/F24 adc.2010.203851.)

References: 1) Anand KJ, Johnston CC, Oberlander TF, Taddio A, Lehr VT, Walco GA. Analgesia and local anesthesia during invasive procedures in the neonate. *Clin Ther.* 2005;27:844–876 2)Anand KJ, Aranda JV, Berde CB, et al. Analgesia and anesthesia for neonates: study design and ethical issues. *Clin Ther.* 2005;27:814–843 3) Aranda JV, Carlo W, Hummel P, Thomas R, Lehr VT, Anand KJ. Analgesia and sedation during mechanical ventilation in neonates. *Clin Ther.* 2005;27:877–899 4) Franck LS, Greenberg CS, Stevens B. Pain assessment in infants and children. *Pediatr Clin North Am.* 2000;47:487–512 5)Prevention and Management of Pain in the Neonate: An Update, AMERICAN ACADEMY OF PEDIATRICS Committee on Fetus and Newborn, Section on Surgery, and Section on Anesthesiology and Pain Medicine, CANADIAN PAEDIATRIC SOCIETY Fetus and Newborn Committee.

TABLE 5: Pain—Assessment Tools

Assessment Tool	Physiologic Indicators	Behavioral Indicators	Gestational Age Tested	Assesses Sedation	Scoring Adjusts for Gestational Age	Nature of Pain Assessed
PIPP: Premature Infant Pain Profile	Heart rate, oxygen saturation	Brow bulge, eyes squeezed shut, nasolabial furrow	28-40 wk	No	Yes	Procedural and Postoperative Pain
CRIES: Crying, Requires Oxygen Saturation, Increased Vital Signs, Expression, Sleeplessness	Heart rate, oxygen Saturation	Crying, facial expression, Sleeplessness	32-36wk	No	No	Postoperative pain
NIPS: Neonatal Infant Pain Scale	Respiratory Patterns	Facial expression, Cry, movements of arms and legs, state arousal	28-38wk	No	No	Procedural pain
N-PASS: Neonatal Pain Agitation and Sedation Scale	Heart rate, respiratory rate, blood pressure, oxygen saturation	Crying, irritability, behavior state, extremities tone	0-100 d of age and adjusts Score on the basis of gestational age	Yes	Yes	Ongoing and acute pain and sedation
NFCS: Neonatal Facing Coding System	None	Facial muscle group movement	Preterm and term neonates, infants at 4 mo of age	No	No	Procedural pain
PAT: Pain Assessment Tool	Respirations, heart rate, oxygen saturation, blood pressure	Posture, tone, sleep pattern, expression, color, cry	Neonates	No	No	Acute pain
SUN: Scale for Use in Newborns	Central nervous system state, breathing, heart rate, mean blood pressure	Movement, tone, face	Neonates	No	No	Acute Pain
EDIN: Echelle de la Douleur Inconfort Nouveau-Ne' (Neonatal Pain and Discomfort Scale)	None	Facial activity, body movements, quality of sleep, quality of contact with nurses, consolability	25-36 wk (preterm infants)	No	No	Prolonged pain
BPSN: Bernese Pain Scale for Neonates	Heart rate, respiratory rate, blood pressure, oxygen saturation	Facial expression, body posture, movements, vigilance	Term and preterm neonates	No	No	Acute pain

Acute Neonatal Pain Management: A Stepwise approach

Step 1
Pacifier, Sucrose, Kangaroo mother care, Massage, Sensorial saturation
Agents used: 24% Sucrose, 30% Glucose, Breast milk

Step 2
Topical anesthetic cream/gel: EMLA (Eutectic Mixture of Local Anesthetics-5% emulsion preparation, containing 2.5% each of lidocaine/prilocaine), Liposomal Lidocaine, Amethocaine

Step 3
Acetaminophen, NSAIDS

Step 4
Slow IV infusion of Opioids: Fentanyl, Morphine, Remifentanil, Alfentanil

Step 5
Local anesthetics: subcutaneous infiltration of nerve blocks: Lidocaine, Bupivacaine, Ropivacaine

Step 6
Deep sedation or General anesthesia: Fentanyl, Morphine, Ketamine, Alfentanil, Anesthetics or Sedatives

---

FEEDING NEWBORN BABIES ON POSTNATAL WARDS

ESSENTIAL CLINICAL GUIDELINES  *058*

The main aim of these guidelines is promotion of successful breastfeeding.

1. Mothers should be encouraged to breastfeed their babies soon after birth.
   - Newborns should be nursed whenever they show signs of hunger, such as increased alertness or activity, mouthing or rooting.
   - Ideally, they should be nursed frequently, 8-12 times per 24 hours until baby is satisfied, usually 10-15 minutes of effective sucking on each breast.
   - Milk delivery time varies between mothers. Some babies may be satisfied with less frequent feeds.
   - When breastfeeding is well established, feeding frequency gradually decreases and most babies will be satisfied with around 6 feeds per day.

2. Healthy term babies do not require supplements (water/formula).

3. Premature Babies
   - Well premature babies usually at 35-36 gestation are often admitted to postnatal wards with their mothers.
   - These babies should be offered the breast as soon as possible after birth and then demand up to 3 hourly.
   - For those who latch and suck well on the breast, there is no need for supplementation.
   - Serum glucose may be checked if there is uncertainty about feeding success or if there are risk factors (e.g., hypothermia).
   - On the other hand if the baby does not show interest in feeding, is having difficulties latching, or does not suckle for long, a supplementary feed will be required.
   - A feeding plan needs to be individualized.
   - Feeding volumes should follow the recommended standards.
   - Expressed breast milk is the food of choice, but if this is not available in sufficient quantity, infant formula may be offered. Advice may be sought from a Lactation Consultant/Obstetrician.

4. Supplementation
   * Supplementation of breastfeeding is usually requested when there is concern that baby is at risk for hypoglycemia. *In that context consider the following:*
   * Expressed breast milk is preferable to formula.
   * *Birth asphyxia*
   - Significant birth asphyxia may be a risk factor for hypoglycemia.
   - Such babies remain unwell after the initial resuscitation and are admitted to NICU.
   - Term babies, depressed at birth, but responding quickly and fully to resuscitation and are judged well enough to go to the postnatal ward, should be considered well babies and encouraged to proceed with normal breastfeeding.
   * *Small for gestational age babies.*

   - Keep in mind that babies below the 10th centile in birthweight are not necessarily SGA.
   - Consider such factors as ethnic background, parity and maternal height which may influence birthweight.
   - Asymmetrically small babies with disparity between head circumference and weight are more at risk for hypoglycemia.
   * *Infants of diabetic mothers*
   - These babies who are clinically macrosomic are at a greater risk for hypoglycemia.
   - Babies with adequate weight for gestational age are at a lower risk.
   - Should these babies require supplementation for initial hypoglycemia, attempt to expedite transfer to full breastfeeding.
   * *Large for Gestational Age Infants*
   - Currently the NWH guidelines advise checking glucose levels in babies above 4500g.
   - Hypoglycemia is typically early in such babies and is rare beyond 8 hours of age.
   - Early feeding should be stressed again and any supplementation should be limited to the initial few feeds, with attempts to expedite full breastfeeding.
   * Occasionally babies are seen on postnatal wards who may have been receiving suboptimal quantity of breast milk, appear clinically dehydrated, may have had significant weight loss from birthweight (7–10% below birthweight), may have elevated temperature and show excessive sucking activity.
   - These babies need to be supplemented with EBM/formula until they are clinically well.
   - To support breast feeding, always offer breast feeds first and supplement after this.
   * *Phototherapy*
   - Phototherapy causes an increase in insensible water loss and in stool water contents, equivalent to 15–25ml/kg/day.
   - This should be balanced by increased demand for breast milk in a well term baby who has established breastfeeding.
   - Thus routine supplementation of babies under phototherapy is not recommended.
   - If breastfeeding is not well established or baby appears clinically under-hydrated, then formula supplementation is advised.

References : 1.Breastfeeding and the use of Human Milk. American Academy of Pediatrics Policy Statement. Pediatrics 100; 1035-1039, 1997. 2.Hypoglycemia of the Newborn. WHO Report 1997.

TABLE 1: Suggested feeding regimen for preterm infants

Weight (g)	Initial Feeding (mL)	Frequency (hourly)	Advancement (mL/feeding)	Time to full feedings (days)
500–800	1	2	1 every 12–24 h	6
800–1000	2	2	1 every 12 h	4–6
1000–1200	2–3	2	1 every 8–12 h	4
1200–1500	4	2	1 every 6–8 h	4
> 1500	5–10	3	1 every other feeding	3–4

TABLE 2: Summary of recommendations for the nutritional needs of low-birth weight infants

Energy	intake	125-140 kcal/kg/day
Fluid		130-200 ml/kg/day
Protein	intake	2.9-4.0 g/kg/day
	whey.casein ratio	whey predominant should not fall below
	amino acids	human milk content
Fat	intake	4.0-9.0 g/kg/day
	linoleic acid	>3% of total energy or 0.5 g /100 kcal
	medium chain triglycerides(MCT)	<40% of total fat
Carbohydrates	intake type	<15g/kg/day of lactose; glucose polymers and lactose (50:50); starch hydrolysates: sucrose; glucose
Minerals	Sodium	1.3–3.5 mmol/kg/day
	Chloride	2.0–3.5 mmol/kg/day
	Potassium	2–5 mmol/kg/day
	Calcium	90–250 mg/kg/day
	Phosphorus	65–125 mg/kg/day
	Ca:P ratio	1.4–2.0
	Magnesium	15 mg/kg/day
	Zinc	0.6–1.4 mg/kg/day
	Copper	110–150 mg/kg/day
Vitamins	Vitamin A	120–420 mg/day
	Vitamin K	0.5–1.0 mg at birth
	Vitamin E	0.5–0.6 mg/100 kcal
	Vitamin D	500–2000 IU/day

TABLE 4: Dangers of milk feeding in Premature babies

Danger	Complication
Pooling in stomach	Regurgitation and aspiration
Compromised respiratory function (partly due to gastric distension and partly due to nasal obstruction)	Recurrent apnea $^-PaO_2$ ^-FRC
Introduction of infection (? due to indwelling tube)	Gastroenteritis Necrotizing enterocolitis
Electrolyte imbalance	Hyponatremia Acidemia Hypophosphatemia
Milk bolus obstruction	Gut perforation

TABLE 3: Prematurity and birth-weight classifications

Maturity by gestational age
Preterm: < 37 weeks
Term: 37–42 weeks
Post-term: > 42 weeks

Birth weight

Low birth weight (LBW)	:	< 2,500 g
Very low birth weight (VLBW)	:	< 1,500 g
Extremely low birth weight (ELBW)	:	< 1,000 g

Birth weight for gestational age

Intrauterine growth restriction (IUGR) : weight < 3rd percentile
Small for gestational age (SGA) : weight < 10th percentile
Asymmetric SGA : weight only < 10th percentile-acute malnutrition or placental insufficiency; has potential for catch-up growth
Symmetric SGA : weight, length, head circumference < 10th percentile - prolonged malnutrition, genetic processes, or congenital anomalies; has less potential for catch - up growth
Appropriate for gestational age : weight 10th–90th percentile
Large for gestational age : weight > 90th percentile

TABLE 5: Sick LBW babies

Certain important generalizations govern the feeding of these babies:

1. The baby less than 32 weeks gestation has caloric reserves for only 4–5 days' extrauterine existence, and enough glycogen for only a few hours.

2. An adequate caloric intake is necessary to prevent hypoglycemia and jaundice, and may be one of the factors that affects neurological handicap in survivors.

3. The sooner a baby puts on weight, the sooner he recovers from serious neonatal illness, e.g. severe RDS.

4. If oral feeds are not tolerated or are contraindicated, intravenous feeding should be started within 3–4 days, especially in sick babies weighing less than 1.5 kg.

5. Although milk is good for premature babies it can also do harm. Sick babies, especially in the first phase of their illness, have an ileus and to feed such babies is not only dangerous but also a waste of milk.

Growth Parameters : Preterm

Weight gain
< 2 kg: 15–30 g/d or 10–20 g/kg/d, > 2 kg > 20 g/d
Length gain : 0.7–1.1 cm/week
Head circumference : 0.5–1 cm/week
After corrected age of 40 weeks (full term), weight gain may be similar to that of full-term infant.

TABLE 6: Enteral nutrition: Feeding advancement and goals

Feeding initiation and advancement

- Initiate based on birth weight and advance accordingly, as tolerated

Brain weight (g)	Initial weight (ml/kg/d)	Rate increase (ml/kg/d)
< 800	10	10–20
800–1,000	10– 20	10–20
1,001 to 1,250	20	20–30
1,251 –1,500	30	30
1,501 – 1,800	30–40	30–40
1,801–2,500	40	40–50
> 2,500	50	50

Warning signs of feeding intolerance

- Increase in gastric residuals to > twice previous hour's rate (continuous feed) or > 1/2 the previous bolus
- Increase in abdominal distention or girth
- vomiting
- Bilious residuals or vomiting
- Heme positive or frank blood in stools
- Reducing substances > 0.5%
- Change in bowl sounds
- Increase in apnea or bradycardia with feeds

Energy goal

- 110–130 Kcal/kg/d

Some infants may have increased needs up to 150-160 kcal/kg (BPD, SGA)

Protein goal

- 3.0–4.0 g protein/kg/d

Caloric distribution

- PRO: 8–12% calories
- CHO: 40–55% calories
- Fat: 35–50% calories

Calcium

- 120–130 mg/kg/d

Phosphorus

- 60–140 mg/kg/d

Multivitamin

- Infants receiving breastmilk with human milk fortifier or premature formula do not usually require multivitamin supplementation
- Preterm infants receiving breastmilk exclusively should receive multivitamin supplementation

Vitamin E

- Recommended dose : 6–12 IU/kg/d
- May require supplementation if receiving elemental iron greater than 4 mg/kg/d, to decrease risk of hemolytic anemia

Iron

- Preterm infants with born low stores and are subject to many blood draws
- Recommended initiating iron supplement at 4-6 weeks of age
- Infant should be at full feeds (150 mL/kg/d at 24kcal/oz) prior to start of supplementation

BPD = bronchopulmonary dysplasia; CHO = carbohydrates; PRO = protein; SGA = small for gestational age.

TABLE 7: Enteral feeding methods

Indications for nipple feeding

- Minimum 32–34 weeks postconception age, though some infants may do well at the breast earlier.
- Coordinated suck, swallow, and breath pattern is present
- Infant is free of apnea and bradycardia
- Respiratory rate < 60 breaths/min
- Infant may benefit from gradual transition from gavage to nipple feeding
- Consider partial gavage feeding if infant takes
- > 30 minutes/feed to prevent excess energy expenditure

Indications for nasogastric or orogastric tube feeding

- Infant < 32 weeks' GA, poor suck, swallow, and breath coordination
- Respiratory rate > 60 breaths/min
- No gag reflex evident
- Continuous
  - May be better tolerated in smaller infants
  - For infants with previous intolerance to bolus feeds
  - Requires less frequent tube change, less disruption to baby
  - May decrease risk of aspiration
  - May prevent increase in respiratory rate (vs bolus)
- Bolus
  - Every 2–3 hours
  - May improve gastric emptying
  - Allows hunger-satiety, can alternate with nipple feeds
  - Allows more mobility; parents can hold and provide care more easily

Indications for transpyloric feeding

- Consider for infants with intolerance to gastric feeding, GER, risk of aspiration, nasal CPAP
- Requires continuous feeding
- Placement of tube is more difficult;takes >2hr for the placement

Indications for G-tube feeding

- For infants who will be unable to nipple feed for several months
- May prevent oral aversion associated with long-term nasogastric tube feeding

CPAP = continuous positive airway pressure ventilation;

GA = gestational age; GER = gastroesophageal reflux;

G-tube = gastrostomy tube.

TABLE 8: Enteral nutrition : Choice of feeding substrate

Breastmilk is preferred for the following advantages:

- Anti-infective factors
- Whey is the predominant protein
- Contains taurine and cysteine
- Bile salt-stimulated lipase and lipoprotein lipase aid in fat digestion and absorption
- Decreased renal solute load
- May enhance the mother-infant bonding
- May protect against NEC
- May improve cognitive outcome
- Lactose promotes absorption of Ca, Mg, PO_4

Breastmilk may require supplementation for premature infants

- Volume of breast milk required to meet protein, energy, Ca, P, Mg, and other vitamin and mineral needs is high
- Fat in breast milk may adhere to the NG or OG tubing, which decreases available calories and EFA

Fortification of breastmilk

- Powder human milk fortifier:
  - Adds protein, carbohydrate, vitamins, and minerals
  - Increase to 22 and 24 cal/oz
  - is preferred when adequate amount of breastmilk is available
- Liquid fortifier: Similac natural care (SNC)
  - 24 cal/oz formula in equal volumes to breastmilk
  - increase to 22 and 24 cal/oz
  - may use when breastmilk supply does not meet volume demand
- Tolerance
  - continue to monitor nutrition laboratory tests, especially Ca, P, and alkaline phosphatase
  - ELBW infants at increased risk of hypercalcemia

Breastmilk fortifiers are indicated for:

- Infants born at < 34 weeks' GA or <2 kg
- Infants with increased needs who are fluid restricted
- Hospital use only due to increased vitamin and mineral content
- Bottle or tube feeds until infant is:
  - taking sufficient volume at the breast
  - > 34 weeks' GA and ≥ 2 kg
  - can use until infant reaches 3-4 kg or discharged if ELBW
  - ready for discharge

Premature formulas

- Alternative to fortified breastmilk when breastmilk is not available
- Preferred for its composition, increased calories, protein, Ca, P
- Available in 20 and 24 cal/oz, ready-to-feed
- Protein: whey predominant, 50% more than term formulas
- Fat: 50% MCT, oil may improve fat absorption and weight gain
- Carbohydrate: 50% lactose, 50% polymers
- Same guidelines as breastmilk fortifiers for transition off premie formula

Premature discharge formulas (transition formulas)

- Use when continued fortification is recommended for smaller, more premature infants
- Vitamin and mineral fortified
- Contain lactose and MCT oil
- Designed for home use up to 12 months of age
- Ready-to-feed is 22 cal/oz
- Powder may be added to fortify breastmilk
- Can transition to standard term formula when catch-up growth is established

Standard term, cow's-milk based formulas

- Not recommended for premature infants; does not meet nutritional needs for minerals, protein
- May be provided for AGA infants > 34 weeks' GA and > 2.0 kg at birth
- May be provided for growing premature infant > 34 weeks , Corrected Age and > 2.0–2.5 kg who is ready for discharge home.

Standard soy-based formulas

- Not recommended for premature infants
- Low bioavailability of Ca and P, adverse effects on bone
- May be indicated for lactose intolerance, galactosemia, secondary lactose intolerance
- Would require vitamin or mineral supplementation
- May require caloric concentration

Therapeutic formulas

- Include protein hydrolysates, free amino acid-based, or high MCT-containing formulas
- Not recommended long term for premature infants because of suboptimal nutrient composition; may need to fortify if used

Modulars

- When increased caloric demands require further caloric supplementation.
- MCT oil, corn oil, and carbohydrate or protein supplements may be added to 24 cal/oz fortified breastmilk or formula
- Attention must be paid to distribution of calories, osmolality, renal solute load.

TABLE 9: Discharge criteria

- Human milk fortifier (HMF), Similac Natural Care (SNC), or premature formula has been discontinued
- Do not provide at home because of high vitamin and nutrient content (potential for toxicity)
- Transition to all breast milk or term formula
- Recommended once infant tolerates 180 mL/kg/d, weighs > 2.0 kg
- Transition to premature discharge formula if increased needs persist
- Provide parents with recipe/instructions for home feeding regimen as needed

Multivitamin supplementation

- Breastfeeding: 1 mL/d
- Formula: 0.5 mL/d
- continue until infant tolerates 750 mL/d of either breast milk or formula or reaches 3.5 kg

Iron

- For infants with birthweight < 2 kg; 2-4 mg/kg/24hr by 1–2 months of postnatal age.
- For infants with birthweight > 2 kg; standard formula with iron – no supplementation needed.
- For infants being fed BM: 2–4 mg/kg/24hr.

TABLE 10: Average daily nutritional requirements

Age	Water (mL/kg)	Kcal/kg	Protein (g/kg)	Na^+	K^+ (mmol/kg)	Ca^{2+}	PO_4^{3-} (mmol/kg)
Infant > 2.5 kgat birth							
1 day	60–90	115	2.2	2–3	2–3	1.5	1.5
2 days	90–120	115	2.2	2–3	2–3	1.5	1.5
10 days	120–150	105	2.0	2–3	2–3	1.5	1.5
3 months	140–160	105	2.0	2–3	2–3	1.5	1.5
Infants < 2.5 kg at birth							
<1 month	60–150	110–165	2.9–4.0	1–8	2–5	2–6	2–5

TABLE 11: Composition of various milks (all per 100 mL of milk)

Milk	Energy (kcal)	Protein (g)	Casein: whey	CHO (g)	Fat (g)	Na (mmol)	K (mmol)	Ca (mmol)	p (mmol)
Mature term breast milk	70	1.3	1:2	7	4.2	0.65	1.5	0.9	0.5
Preterm breast milk	67	1.8-2.4	N/A	6	4	2.2	1.8	0.6	0.5
Preterm EBM + fortifier	80	2.5–3.1	N/A	9	4	3.1	–	1.8	1.4
Donor bank milk	46	1.1	N/A	7.1	1.7	0.7	–	0.9	0.5
Cow's milk	67	3.4	3:1	4.6	3.9	2.2	3.9	3	3
Whey based term formula	65–68	1.5	1:1.5	7.0–7.3	3.6–3.8	0.8	1.4–2.2	0.9–1.5	0.9–1.1
Casein-based term formula	65–69	1.5–1.9	4:1	7.2–8.6	3.1–3.6	0.8–1.1	1.6–2.2	1.2–2.1	1.2–1.8
Follow-on (>6 months)	70	1.8	3.5:1	7.2	4.6	1.0	2.2	2.2	1.6
LBW formula	80	2.0–2.4	1:1.5	7.0–8.5	3.5-4.9	1.3-2.0	1.8	1.8–2.7	1.1-1.7
LBW follow-on	74	1.8	1.5:1	7.5	4.1	1.0	1.9	2.0	1.3

TABLE 12: Assessing degree of milk transfer to infant

Signs of adequate milk transfer (infant taking sufficient milk)

Infant is alert, rooting, showing hunger cues

Audible swallowing is heard at breast

Infant appears satiated after feeding

Mother reports little or no discomfort of nipple, areola, or breast

Mother without cracked, damaged, painful nipples (poor latch leads to inadequate milk transfer)

Mother is satisfied with baby's feeding

Urine output

- Frequency increases by 1 wet diaper per day from day of life 1 through 4
- By end of first week baby should have 6+ soaking wet diapers per day
- Urine should then be clear, not dark or concentrated or strong smelling
- Stool output
- Frequency increases by 1 stool per day from day 1 through 4
- Changes color and consistency (dark, tarry meconium to green to yellow stool)
- From day 5–6 on, baby has 3–5 or more yellow, seedy stools; may be loose
- Frequency later decreases

  Weight gain : infant is gaining appropriate weight (140-200 gm/wk for newborn after first couple of days)

Signs that intervention is needed (baby not receiving enough breastmilk)

Infant is lethargic, not waking on own to feed, or is difficult to wake for feeding

Infant is feeding less than 8–12 times per 24 hours in first weeks

Infant does not latch at breast, is not content at breast

Little or no swallowing is heard at breast

Mother reports sore nipples, develops creased or cracked nipples

Infant's urine output is scant, dark in color, concentrated, or absent

Infant's stools are minimal (< 4 per day after day 3)

Infant's stool does not turn yellow by day 4–5

Infant continues to lose weight

Infant is jaundiced-may be physiologic, but need to rule out exaggerated jaundice.

If infant is not receiving sufficient breastmilk, supplementation is necessary

Suggest mother express colostrum or breastmilk to give to infant via syringe, cup, bottle

If mother unable to express milk, give appropriate infant formula, not water

Water or dextrose water will not prevent hyperbilirubinemia

EVIDENCE-BASED ENTERAL NUTRITION

Human milk- Human milk from the preterm infant's own mother is the first choice. Human milk can be stored at room temperature for up to 24 h after expression in colostrum and up to 6 h for mature milk. Beyond that, it should be stored at 3-4! before use. If not used for more than 5 d, it should be frozen.

Human milk fortifier-Human milk fortifier is indicated in preterm infants < 31 wk and/or < 1500 g. Human milk (100 mL/kg) is given per day and discontinued when the infant has established full breast-feeding.

Formula milk- If human milk from the preterm infant's own mother is not available, the only acceptable alternative is a preterm formula. A concentration of about 60 kcal/100 mL or 20 kcal/oz is recommended, but should be increased to 80 kcal/100 mL or 24 kcal/oz when the infant has achieved full enteral feeds.

Feeding methods- Gavage feeding is given via an indwelling nasogastric tube during mechanical ventilation. An indwelling orogastric tube is used after endotracheal extubation. Intermittent intragastric feeding is the first choice method, but continuous transpyloric feeding can be tried in selected preterm infants with extremely poor gastric emptying and symptomatic gastro-esophageal reflux.

Commencement of feeds- Hourly feeds of 1 mL are generally used in infants weighing less than 1000 g, 2-h 2 mL for infants weighing 1000-1500 g, 3-h 3 mL for infants weighing 1500-2000 g, and 4-h 4 mL for infants weighing more than 2000 g, unless there is significant respiratory distress, when the infant remains on 1-2-h feeds. If this might not be tolerated, milk may be commenced at 1 mL every 2 h, even less than 1 mL every 4-6 h. Such trophic feeding should begin as soon as possible after birth, and definitely within the first 3-4 d.

Progression of feeds- Daily increment in the range of 10-30 mL/kg of milk feeds is safe. Demand feeding is started after infants have established full milk feeds on a 4 h regimen. Non-nutritive sucking is beneficial without side effects.

Supplements- Multivitamin supplement is started when the infant has established full enteral feeds, and iron is started when the infant has doubled their birth weight (usually at 2 mo). Medium-chain triglycerides can be used as an energy supplement for preterm infants who fail to thrive.

EVIDENCE-BASED PN

Fluids D 1: 60-80 mL/kg per day. Infants < 28 wk gestation are nursed in a maximally humidified environment (90% humidity) for at least 7 d. Postnatal weight loss of 5% per day to a maximum of 15% is acceptable, which is achieved by progressively increasing the fluid intake to 120-150 mL/kg per day at 1 wk of age.

Energy An intake of 50 kcal/kg per day is sufficient to match ongoing expenditure, but it does not meet additional requirements of growth. The goal energy intake is 120 kcal/kg per day, which is higher in infants with chronic lung diseases.

Protein Optimal parenteral amino acid intake is 3.5 g/kg per day. Parenteral amino acids can begin from day 1 at a dose of 1.75 g/kg per day.

Carbohydrate From day 1, 6-10 g/kg per day can be infused and adjusted to maintain blood glucose level of 2.6-10 mmol/L. Insulin is only used in infants whose blood glucose level is higher than 15 mmol/L and associated with glycosuria and osmotic diuresis, even after glucose intake has been decreased to 6 g/kg per day. Carbohydrate is given as a continuous infusion commencing at a rate of 0.05 U/kg per hour, and increased as required for persistent hyperglycemia.

Fat Intravenous fat, 1 g/kg per day, can be started from day 1, or when intravenous amino acids are started. The dose of intravenous fat is increased to 2 g/kg and 3 g/kg per day over the next 2 d. Twenty percent intravenous fat is delivered as a continuous infusion via a syringe pump, separated from the infusate containing amino acids and glucose. The syringe and infusion line should be shielded from ambient light.

Minerals Minerals should include sodium (3-5 mmol/kg per day), chloride (3-5 mmol/kg per day), potassium (1-2 mmol/kg per day), calcium (1.5-2.2 mmol/kg per day), phosphorus (1.5-2.2 mmol/kg per day), and magnesium (0.3-0.4 mmol/kg per day).

Trace elements Trace elements should include zinc (6-8 ¼mol/kg per day), copper (0.3-0.6 ¼mol/kg per day), selenium (13-25 nmol/kg per day), manganese (18-180 nmol/kg per day), iodine (8 nmol/kg per day), chromium (4-8 nmol/kg per day), and molybdenum (2-10 nmol/kg per day).

Vitamins Vitamins must be added to the fat emulsion to minimize loss of vitamins due to adherence to tubes and photodegradation.

Summary of Management of Feeding in Low Birth Weight Infants:NNF Clinical Practice Guidelines

• Mother's milk is the best feeding option for LBW infants. In case breastmilk feeding is not possible, it may be preferable to use pre-term infant formula for pre-term infants (< 2000 grams).

• Routine use of the multicomponent fortification of the breastmilk should be avoided. This option is best reserved for preterms infants <32 weeks gestation or <1500 g birth weight who fail to gain weight despite adequate breastmilk feeding.

• Enteral feeding should be initiated as early as clinically appropriate and minimal enteral nutrition should be provided, if volumes cannot be advanced.

• LBW neonates can be successfully fed with intragastric tubes or a variety of other traditional/culturally accepted devices.

• Non Nutritive Sucking and Kangaroo mother care are useful adjuncts to maintain and enhance breast feeding and nutrition.

• All LBW infants who are exclusively breastfed should receive supplements of vitamin D, calcium and phosphorous. Iron supplementation at 2-3 mg/kg/day at 6-8 wks , and as early as 2 wks in <1500 gms is effective in preventing anemia of prematurity.

• All LBW infants should be checked for weight (daily), head circumference (weekly) and length (weekly or fort-nightly) during their NICU stay.

Infants born before 37 weeks` gestation are considered to be premature. Two percent of all premature infants are believed to be very premature (born before 32 weeks` gestation). Although survival rates and outcomes for premature infants have dramatically improved in recent decades, morbidity and mortality are still significant. Infants born prematurely are at increased risk of growth problems, developmental delays, and complex medical problems. Prematurity is the second leading cause of infant mortality after congenital anomalies. The transition from the neonatal intensive care unit (NICU) to home can be stressful. The American Academy of Pediatrics (AAP) recommends that planning for discharge from the NICU should include the following six critical components: 1) parental education; 2) implementation of primary care; 3) evaluation of unresolved medical problems; 4) development of the home care plan; 5) identification and mobilization of surveillance and support services; 6) determination and designation of follow-up care.

FAMILY SUPPORT: Early and active family involvement is paramount to success of the premature infant. At least two family members should demonstrate ability to appropriately feed and provide necessary care for an infant before discharge. Because of risk of respiratory compromise while restrained, the AAP recommends that infants at risk of respiratory problems be formally tested in a car seat before transport home. Travel for infants at risk of respiratory compromise should be minimized, and infants who cannot tolerate a semi-upright position should use a prone or supine safety device. Physicians should provide families with an accurate and comprehensive summary of the neonatal course with specific written instructions for all necessary follow up.

MEDICAL COMPLICATIONS: Infants who have been in the NICU often have complex medical problems and may require prolonged comprehensive or subspecialty follow-up care. Review of the neonatal course will help identify risks. Bronchopulmonary dysplasia or chronic lung disease, apnea and bradycardia, cryptorchidism, gastroesophageal reflux, sudden infant death syndrome (SIDS), ventriculomegaly, and hernias are more common among premature infants than full-term infants. The risk of **bronchopulmonary dysplasia** increases with decreasing birth weight and lower gestational age. Fifty to 80 percent of infants born weighing less than 900 g develop bronchopulmonary dysplasia. These infants are more susceptible to pulmonary infections and suffer from episodes of respiratory distress and wheezing, which can be indistinguishable from a respiratory infection. Treatment may include bronchodilators, diuretics, oxygen, and antibiotics when appropriate. Premature infants may also require a higher caloric intake to account for increased work of breathing. Children with bronchopulmonary dysplasia continue to show poor lung function until adolescence, which is when lung function typically becomes normal. An infant with **apnea of prematurity** may be given methylxanthines and an apnea monitor upon discharge from the NICU. If infants are event free, discontinuation of pharmacologic therapy should be considered at 40 weeks` adjusted age. Home monitoring is continued until the infant is 43 weeks` adjusted age and free of extreme episodes. A neonatologist or pulmonologist should be readily available to assist in the decision to stop treatment. Premature infants develop **gastroesophageal reflux** more often than full-term infants because of lower esophageal sphincter hypotonia, delayed emptying, and decreased gastric compliance. Symptoms include postprandial vomiting and, when severe, irritability, respiratory problems, apnea, bradycardia, and feeding difficulties. One management option is to change the feeding regimen, usually by thickening the milk with infant cereal or concentrating the milk for volume reduction. Postprandial prone positioning, while awake and under observation, may improve symptoms. If conservative measures fail, histamine H2 blockers, proton pump inhibitors, or prokinetic agents can be tried. Surgery should be considered in some infants with severe symptoms despite treatment. Screening for **IVH & PVL** with cranial ultrasonography is recommended for all infants with a gestational age of less than 30 weeks; screening should take place at seven to 10 days of age and at 36 to 40 weeks' postmenstrual age. **Vaccination for premature infants** remains a critical component of preventive care and should be delivered according to chronologic (not adjusted) age. Routine immunization for diphtheria, tetanus, pertussis, *Haemophilus influenzae* type b, poliomyelitis, and pneumococcal disease remains unchanged. There are theoretical risks of increased adverse reactions in very low birth weight premature infants because of lower maternal antibody to rotavirus. The Advisory Committee on Immunization Practices supports rotavirus vaccination of premature infants if they are at least six weeks of age, discharged from the NICU, and clinically stable. For infants born weighing less than 2,000 g (70.55 oz), immunization against hepatitis B is dependent on maternal hepatitis B status. Table **1** outlines the hepatitis B vaccine schedule for all infants. Respiratory syncytial virus (RSV) is the most common cause of bronchiolitis and pneumonia in infants. Prematurity and underlying lung disease, especially bronchopulmonary dysplasia, are factors that increase the risk of severe RSV infection. Palivizumab (Synagis) is a humanized mouse monoclonal antibody that has been licensed to prevent RSV infection. Palivizumab is an intramuscular injection administered once per month for five months beginning in early November and ending at the beginning of March. The five doses should provide adequate coverage for the RSV season. Passive immunization results in a 45 to 55 percent decrease in hospitalization attributable to RSV.11 Educating caregivers remains a critical aspect of RSV prevention. Decreasing exposure to contagious settings, proper hand hygiene, and avoidance of tobacco exposure should be emphasized. A documented RSV infection should not alter the vaccine schedule because various strains may circulate. Table **2** provides indications for RSV vaccination. Influenza vaccine is strongly encouraged for infants at least six months of age. It is imperative that all family members and close contacts of infants younger than six months be advised to get the influenza vaccine.

TABLE 1: HEPATITIS B VACCINATION SCHEDULE FOR INFANTS

Maternal HBsAg status	Infant weighing ≥2,000 g (70.55 oz)	Infant weighing <2,000 g
Positive	*HB vaccine (≤ 12 Hours of birth);HBIG (≤12 Hours of birth) *Three vaccine doses at zero, one, and six months of age. *Check *HBsAb* and *HBsAg* at nine to 15 months of age.	*HB vaccine (≤ 12 Hours of birth); *HBIG (≤12 Hours of birth) *Four vaccine doses at zero, one, two and six months of age check HBsAg and HBsAg at nine to 15 months of age
Unknown	*HB vaccine (≤ 12 Hours of birth) *Test mother *HBIG (≤ 7 days) if mother tests positive *Vaccine series based on mother's status	*HB vaccine (≤ 12 Hours of birth) *HBIG (≤12 Hours of birth) *Test mother; *vaccine series based on mother's status,
Negative	*HB vaccine (≤ 12 Hours of birth) *Three vaccine doses (usual intervals) *Combination vaccine allowed at six to eight weeks of age	*Delay HB vaccine until one month of age, *Three vaccine doses (usual intervals), *Combination vaccine allowed at six to eight weeks of age

HB=Hepatitis B, HBIG= Hepatitis B Immunoglobulin, HBs Ab= Hepatitis B surface antibody, HBs Ag= Hepatitis B surface antigen

TABLE 2: RESPIRATORY SYNCYTIAL VIRUS (RSV) VACCINE INDICATIONS

*Infants born before 28 weeks` gestation; vaccine should be given during their first RSV season *Infants born at 29 to 32 weeks` gestation who are younger than 6 months at beginning of RSV season *Children younger than 2 years with chronic lung disease requiring medical therapy within 6 months of the beginning of RSV season *Children <2years with hemodynamically significant CHD *Consider infants born at 32-35 weeks`gestation with at least 2 of the following risk factors- child care attendance, school-age sibling, exposure to environmental air pollutants, congenital anomalies of the airways, severe neuromuscular disease *Consider infants with severe immunodeficiency

NUTRITION AND GROWTH : Definitions of "catch-up" growth vary, but it is generally considered to be achieved when the infant reaches between the fifth and 10th percentile on a standard growth chart. Premature infants with a history of intrauterine growth restriction and those who are small for gestational age tend to demonstrate less catch-up growth and higher rates of poor growth than infants born at appropriate weight for gestational age. Otherwise healthy premature infants typically demonstrate catch-up growth first in head circumference and then in weight and length. After two years of age, a standard growth chart may be used. Human breast milk remains the recommended source of nutrition for all infants, including those born prematurely. Benefits of breastfeeding include lower risk of infection, ease of digestibility, enhancement of cognitive development, and promotion of mother-child attachment. Despite evidence supporting numerous advantages of breast milk, the nutrient needs of some premature infants still may not be met, especially those weighing less than 1,500 g. Breast milk fortification can be accomplished by adding commercially available liquid or powdered fortifiers that contain additional calories, macronutrients, vitamins, calcium, and phosphorus. Nutrient deficiencies can potentially result in clinical manifestations of osteopenia, kwashiorkor, hyponatremia, and zinc deficiency.Fortification of human milk minimizes these risks. Multicomponent fortifiers and protein supplementation of human milk lead to short-term increases in head and linear growth and weight gain. Data thus far are insufficient to evaluate long-term growth and neurodevelopmental outcomes. Some generally accepted guidelines for breastfeeding after NICU discharge are outlined in Table 3.Formula will be a major source of nutrition for many premature infants after discharge from the NICU. Preterm formulas have higher caloric density, as well as higher levels of protein, minerals, vitamins, and trace elements. The 24 kcal per ounce formula is generally reserved for NICU use and for selected premature infants until term weight is achieved. Following discharge from the NICU, formulas specifically designed for premature infants should be used. These preterm formulas provide 22 kcal per ounce and are enriched with additional protein, minerals, vitamins, and trace elements. Standard formulas contain only 20 kcal per ounce. A Cochrane meta-analysis found a statistically significant increased length in infants fed enriched formula but failed to show any change in weight, head circumference, bone mineralization, or neurodevelopment. Another recent study failed to show any difference in growth or bone mineralization with enriched formula.

TABLE 3: Guidelines for Breastfeeding Premature infants

*Feed on demand every one hour and one half to three hours
*Supplement some feedings with milk fortifier or enriched formula until catch-up growth is achieved and daily weight gain is adequate(20-30 gm/day)
*Supplement feedings with 0.5-1.0 ml of standard Multivitamins per day until the infant reaches a weight of 5 kg.
*Supplement feedings with 2-4 mg / kg of Iron per day (maximal dose of 15mg in a day)
*If exclusively breastfeeding, supplement feedings with 200-400 IU of vitamin D /day starting at 2 months of age.

TABLE 4: GUIDELINES FOR FORMULA FEEDING PREMATURE INFANTS

*Use 24 kcal per ounce preterm formula until infant weighs 1,800-3,500g; usually inpatient only.

*Use 22 kcal per ounce preterm enriched formula until catch-up growth obtained or one year adjusted age

*Continue 20kcal per ounce standard formula once catch-up growth is achieved until one year adjusted age.

*Formula can be concentrated if needed to increase caloric intake

*Formulas providing 2 mg per kg of Iron per day may need to be supplemented with an additional 2 mg per kg per day (maximal dose of 15 mg/day) depending on degree of prematurity.

*Vitamin supplements not necessary if formula meeting needs for growth.

After NICU discharge, most premature infants require 100 to 120 kcal per kg per day to grow. Infants should gain at least 20 to 30 g (0.71 to 1.06 oz) per day, and caloric intake should be monitored and adjusted to achieve this goal. Formula can be concentrated and breast milk can be fortified to help increase caloric intake. Once catch-up growth is achieved, the higher-calorie formula should be discontinued to prevent hypervitaminosis and obesity. Premature infants require iron supplementation through the first year of life. Standard and preterm formulas provide 2 mg per kg of iron per day. An additional 2 mg per kg per day (maximal dose of 15 mg per day) may be necessary depending on the degree of prematurity. For premature infants who are breastfed in the first year, 2 to 4 mg per kg per day is needed as supplementation. Solid foods should be introduced based on oral-motor readiness, which is usually achieved at an adjusted age of four to six months. Cow`s milk should be delayed until 12 months` adjusted age (Refer to Table 4).

DEVELOPMENT: Prematurity puts infants at risk of a variety of neurodevelopmental disabilities resulting from malformation or insult to the developing brain. Disabilities range from cerebral palsy and mental retardation to sensory impairments and more subtle disorders. More subtle problems of higher cortical functioning that have a higher incidence in preterm infants include impaired visual-motor integration and neuromotor and cognitive functions, as well as problems with behavior and temperament. Infant development is a dynamic process encompassing gross motor skills, fine motor skills, language ability, cognitive performance, and adaptive behavior. Emphasis on early identification of a developmental delay creates the opportunity to provide the benefits of early intervention. For the first two years of life, development must be assessed according to adjusted age. Developmental surveillance is a continuous process of skilled observation, eliciting and attending to parental concerns, obtaining a relevant history, and sharing opinions and concerns with other professionals. Use of a standardized screening test is essential for consistency and can identify children who need a more comprehensive developmental evaluation. Because of the inherent imperfections of office screening tests, parent or physician concern about development may warrant a referral for formal testing with a subspecialist or multidisciplinary center. Once a delay is diagnosed or detected, referral for early intervention services is recommended. Consistent deficits in performance on intelligence measures have been observed in premature infants born weighing less than 2,500 g compared with normal weight, full-term infants. Higher rates of school failure and greater need for educational support have been found in children born prematurely, but patterns vary among studies. There is also an increased relative risk of attention-deficit/hyperactivity disorder in children born prematurely. In addition to conventional academics, parents and educators should advocate for comprehensive assessments for struggling children, including visual-motor and visual-perceptive abilities, complex language performance, and attention skills. A detailed neurologic examination is a vital component of routine care in premature infants. Assessment should include evaluation of alertness, posture, muscle tone, reflexes, postural reactions, and functional abilities. Abnormalities may include weakness; asymmetries; hyperreflexia; generalized or focal hypertonia; or, more commonly, hypotonia. Infants born prematurely continue to face significant challenges into childhood. It is clear that educational, psychological, and behavioral problems are of concern during the school years.

SCREENING GUIDELINES:

*Routine testing for all infants includes state-sponsored screening for metabolic disorders.

*Universal newborn hearing screening is offered in most them regardless of the potential high-risk factors present or not. Early recognition of hearing impairment, appropriate intervention with hearing aids, and communication therapy are critical for optimal language development.

*Screening for visual disturbances including retinopathy (in infants born before 28 weeks' gestation, in those weighing less than 1,500 g, or those with an unstable clinical course, at a postmenstrual age of 31 weeks), strabismus, and significant refractive error.

*Routine lead screening should be performed at nine to 12 months' adjusted age.

*Screening for anemia at six months and again at two years.

REFERENCE: AMY LaHOOD, MD, and CATHY A. BRYANT, MD, *St. Vincent Family Medicine Residency Program, Indianapolis, Indiana American Family Physician Volume 76, Number 8, 1160-1164.*

1. Late-preterm infants are immature. **a.** Infants born at 34 0/7 through 36 6/7 weeks' gestation (239–259 days since the first day of the last menstrual period) should be referred to as "late preterm." **b.** Late-preterm infants are physiologically immature and have limited compensatory responses to the extrauterine environment compared with term infants. **2.** Late-preterm infants are at a greater risk of morbidity and mortality than are term infants. **a.** During the birth hospitalization, late-preterm infants are more likely than are term infants to be diagnosed with temperature instability, hypoglycemia, respiratory distress, apnea, jaundice, or feeding difficulties. **b.** During the first month after birth, late-preterm infants are more likely than term infants to be rehospitalized for jaundice, feeding difficulties, dehydration, and suspected sepsis. **3.** Risk factors that have been identified for rehospitalization or neonatal morbidity among late-preterm infants include being the first born, being breastfed at discharge, having a mother who had labor and delivery complications, being a recipient of public insurance at delivery, and being of poor socioeconomic group. **4.** Collaborative counseling by both obstetric and neonatal clinicians about the outcomes of late-preterm births is warranted unless precluded by emergent conditions. Gaps in Knowledge,

Clinical Implications, and Research Implications for Late-Preterm Births: The following are areas in which knowledge and research need to be expanded: **1.** causes for delivery and short-term fetal, neonatal, and maternal outcomes; **2.** developmental immaturity and mechanisms of disease in late-preterm infants; **3.** identification tools, educational programs, and screening strategies to identify risk factors and prevent potential medical complications of late-preterm births; **4.** recommendations for discharge, early follow-up evaluation, and treatment for jaundice, poor feeding, dehydration, and other complications in late-preterm infants; and **5.** long-term medical, neurologic, and developmental outcomes for late-preterm infants.

Recommended Minimum Criteria for Discharge of Late-Preterm Infants: Discharge criteria for late-preterm infants have similarities to criteria developed for both high-risk infants and healthy term infants. Because late-preterm infants are at greater risk of neonatal morbidity and mortality than are term infants, parents of late-preterm infants may need special instruction and guidance before hospital discharge and closer follow-up after discharge. Late-preterm infants who have risk factors for morbidity that requires hospital care (i.e., hospital readmission), such as those who are breastfed or are first born, are most vulnerable. It is especially important to educate first-time mothers of late-preterm infants how to evaluate feeding success and what signs to look for to detect dehydration and hyperbilirubinemia. In some circumstances, this education may require a longer birth hospitalization. Recommended criteria for discharge of late-preterm infants are intended to reflect evidence of physiologic maturity; feeding competency; thermoregulation; maternal education; assessment and planned interventions for medical, family, environmental, and social risk factors; and follow-up arrangements.

Minimum discharge criteria for late-preterm infants are as follows: **1.** Accurate gestational age has been determined. **2.** Timing of discharge is individualized and based on feeding competency, thermoregulation, and absence of medical illness and social risk factors (see below). Late-preterm infants usually are not expected to meet the necessary competencies for discharge before 48 hours of birth. **3.** A physician-directed source for continued medical care (i.e., medical home) has been identified, with a follow-up visit arranged for 24 to 48 hours after hospital discharge. Additional visits may be indicated until an established and maintained pattern of weight gain has been demonstrated. **4.** Vital signs should be documented as being within reference ranges and stable for the 12 hours preceding discharge, including a respiratory rate of less than 60 breaths per minute, a heart rate of 100 to 160 beats per minute, and axillary temperature of 36.5 to 37.4°C (97.7–99.3°F) measured in an open crib with appropriate clothing. **5.** At least 1 stool has been passed spontaneously. **6.** Twenty-four hours of

successful feeding, either at the breast or with a bottle, and the ability to coordinate sucking, swallowing, and breathing while feeding has been demonstrated. Any infant with a weight loss of more than 2% to 3% of birth weight per day or a maximum of 7% of birth weight during the birth hospitalization should be assessed for evidence of dehydration before discharge. **7.** A formal evaluation of breastfeeding, including observation of position, latch, and milk transfer, has been undertaken and documented in the chart by trained caregivers at least twice daily after birth. **8.** A feeding plan has been developed and is understood by the family. **9.** A risk assessment for the development of severe hyperbilirubinemia has been performed and appropriate follow-up has been arranged. **10.** Physical examinations of the infant reveal no abnormalities that require continued hospitalization. **11.** There is no evidence of active bleeding at the circumcision site for at least 2 hours. **12.** Maternal and infant test results are available and have been reviewed, including blood test results for maternal syphilis and hepatitis B surface-antigen status; cord or infant blood type and direct Coombs test results, as clinically indicated; and results of screenings performed in accordance with state regulations, including screening for HIV infection. **13.** Initial hepatitis B vaccine has been administered or an appointment has been scheduled for its administration, and the importance of immunizations has been stressed. **14.** Metabolic and genetic screenings have been performed in accordance with state requirements. If a newborn screening is performed before 24 hours of milk feeding, a system for repeating the screening must be in place in accordance with state policy. **15.** A car safety seat study completed by a trained professional to observe for apnea, bradycardia, or oxygen desaturation has been passed. **16.** Hearing assessment has been performed and the results have been documented in the medical chart. Results have been discussed with family or caregivers. If follow-up is needed, follow-up plans have been outlined. **17.** Family, environmental, and social risk factors have been assessed. When risk factors are identified, the discharge should be delayed until they are resolved or a plan to safeguard the infant is in place. Such risk factors may include but are not limited to: a. untreated parental substance use or positive toxicology test results in the mother or newborn infant; b. history of child abuse or neglect; c. mental illness in a parent in the home; d. lack of social support, particularly for single, firsttime mothers; e. homelessness, particularly during this pregnancy; f. ongoing or established risk of domestic violence; or g. adolescent mother, particularly if other risk factors are present. **18.** The mother and caregivers have received information or training or have demonstrated competency in the following: **a.** infant's hospital course and current condition; **b.** expected pattern of urine and stool frequency for the breastfeeding or formula-fed neonate (verbal and written instruction is recommended); **c.** umbilical cord, skin, and newborn genital care; **d.** hand hygiene, especially as a means to reduce the risk of infection; **e.** use of a thermometer to assess an infant's axillary temperature; **f.** assessment and provision of appropriate layers of clothing; **g.** identification of common signs and symptoms of illness, such as hyperbilirubinemia, sepsis, and dehydration; **h.** assessment for jaundice; **i.** provision of a safe sleep environment, including positioning the infant on his or her back during sleep; **j.** newborn safety issues including car safety seat use, need for smoke/fire alarms, and hazards of secondhand tobacco smoke and environmental pollutants; **k.** appropriate responses to a complication or an emergency; and **l.** sibling interactions and appropriate inclusion in care responsibilities.

Characteristics of Late Preterm Infants
* Late preterm infants—defined as born at 34 to 36^6/7 weeks' gestation
* Physiologically immature with limited compensatory responses to extrauterine environment compared to term infants
* Greater risk than term infants for mortality and morbidities such as:
- Temperature instability, Hypoglycemia, Respiratory distress, Apnea Jaundice, Feeding difficulties, Dehydration, Suspected sepsis

REFERENCE: PEDIATRICS American Academy of Pediatrics guidelines

Almost all mothers can breastfeed successfully, which includes initiating breastfeeding within the first hour of life, breastfeeding exclusively for the first 6 months and continuing breastfeeding (along with giving appropriate complementary foods) up to 2 years of age or beyond. Exclusive breastfeeding in the first six months of life is particularly beneficial for mothers and infants. Positive effects of breastfeeding on the health of infants and mothers are observed in all settings. Breastfeeding reduces the risk of acute infections such as diarrhoea, pneumonia, ear infection, *Haemophilus influenzae*, meningitis and urinary tract infection. It also protects against chronic conditions in the future such as type I diabetes, ulcerative colitis, and Crohn's disease. Breastfeeding during infancy is associated with lower mean blood pressure and total serum cholesterol, and with lower prevalence of type-2 diabetes, overweight and obesity during adolescence and adult life. Breastfeeding delays the return of a woman's fertility and reduces the risks of post-partum hemorrhage, pre-menopausal breast cancer and ovarian cancer. Nevertheless, a small number of health conditions of the infant or the mother may justify recommending that she does not breastfeed temporarily or permanently. These conditions, which concern very few mothers and their infants, are listed below together with some health conditions of the mother that, although serious, are not medical reasons for using breast-milk substitutes. *Whenever stopping breastfeeding is considered, the benefits of breastfeeding should be weighed against the risks posed by the presence of the specific conditions listed.*

INFANT CONDITIONS
Infants who should not receive breast milk or any other milk except specialized formula
*Infants with classic galactosemia: a special galactose-free formula is needed. *Infants with maple syrup urine disease: a special formula free of leucine, isoleucine and valine is needed. *Infants with phenylketonuria: a special phenylalanine-free formula is needed (some breastfeeding is possible, under careful monitoring).

Infants for whom breast milk remains the best feeding option but who may need other food in addition to breast milk for a limited period
*Infants born weighing less than 1500 g (very low birth weight). *Infants born at less than 32 weeks of gestational age (very pre-term). *Newborn infants who are at risk of hypoglycemia by virtue of impaired metabolic adaptation or increased glucose demand (such as those who are preterm, small for gestational age or who have experienced significant intrapartum hypoxic/ischemic stress, those who are ill and those whose mothers are diabetic) if their blood sugar fails to respond to optimal breastfeeding or breast-milk feeding.

MATERNAL CONDITIONS
Maternal conditions that may justify permanent avoidance of breastfeeding
*HIV infection 1: if replacement feeding is acceptable, feasible, affordable, sustainable and safe-AFASS (The most appropriate infant feeding option for an HIV-infected mother depends on her and her infant's individual circumstances, including her health status, but should take consideration of the health services available and the counselling and support she is likely to receive. Exclusive breastfeeding is recommended for the first six months of life unless replacement feeding is AFASS. When replacement feeding is AFASS, avoidance of all breastfeeding by HIV-infected women is recommended. Mixed feeding in the first 6 months of life (that is, breastfeeding while also giving other fluids, formula or foods) should always be avoided by HIV-infected mothers.)

Maternal conditions that may justify temporary avoidance of breastfeeding
*Severe illness that prevents a mother from caring for her infant, for example sepsis. *Herpes simplex virus type 1 (HSV-1): direct contact between lesions on the mother's breasts and the infant's mouth should be avoided until all active lesions have resolved. *Maternal medication: - sedating psychotherapeutic drugs, anti-epileptic drugs and opioids and their combinations may cause side effects such as drowsiness and respiratory depression and are better avoided if a safer alternative is available;- radioactive iodine-131 is better avoided given that safer alternatives are available - a mother can resume breastfeeding about two months after receiving this substance; - excessive use of topical iodine or iodophors (e.g., povidone-iodine), especially on open wounds or mucous membranes, can result in thyroid suppression or electrolyte abnormalities in the breastfed infant and should be avoided; - cytotoxic chemotherapy requires that a mother stops breastfeeding during therapy.

Maternal conditions during which breastfeeding can still continue, although health problems may be of concern
*Breast abscess: breastfeeding should continue on the unaffected breast; feeding from the affected breast can resume once treatment has started. *Hepatitis B: infants should be given hepatitis B vaccine, within the first 48 hours or as soon as possible thereafter. *Hepatitis C. *Mastitis: if breastfeeding is very painful, milk must be removed by expression to prevent progression of the condition. *Tuberculosis: mother and baby should be managed according to national tuberculosis guidelines. *Substance use - maternal use of nicotine, alcohol, ecstasy, amphetamines, cocaine and related stimulants has been demonstrated to have harmful effects on breastfed babies; - alcohol, opioids, benzodiazepines and cannabis can cause sedation in both the mother and the baby. Mothers should be encouraged not to use these substances, and given opportunities and support to abstain. (Mothers who choose not to cease their use of the these substances or who are unable to do so should seek individual advice on the risks and benefits of breastfeeding depending on their individual circumstances. For mothers who use these substances in short episodes, consideration may be given to avoiding breastfeeding temporarily during this time).

REFERENCE : WHO and UNICEF JOINT STATEMENT *Acceptable medical reasons for use of breast-milk substitutes 2009.*

SINGLE UMBILICAL ARTERY

What is a Single Umbilical Artery? Normally, an umbilical cord has three vessels. One is a vein and two are arteries. The vein carries blood away from the fetus and back to the mother's bloodstream via the placenta, while the arteries carry mom's nutrient-rich blood from the placenta to the developing baby. In a pregnancy with a single umbilical artery, one of the two umbilical cord arteries is missing, leaving only one vein and one artery. *Single umbilical artery (SUA) is the most common malformation of the umbilical cord.* Precisely why this occurs is not entirely known. It is suspected, though, that one artery may simply stop growing as it develops or perhaps that the primordial umbilical artery does not divide properly.

A fetus diagnosed with a single umbilical artery can be worrying for the mother-to-be, but most of these cases turn out just fine. On its own, SUA does not necessarily pose a risk to you or your child as an umbilical cord with just one artery is sufficient to support a pregnancy to term. Major problems associated with the loss of an artery in the umbilical cord are usually linked to other markers visible on ultrasound or through tests such as amniocentesis.

How Common is SUA? This malformation of the umbilical cord has been found to affect between 0.5% and 7% of pregnancies and 1 in 100 live births. Caucasian women are twice as likely to experience this complication compared to Japanese and Black women. Additionally, women having a multiple pregnancy are three to four times as likely to develop SUA. Other factors that may increase your risk: *Advanced maternal age (over 40) *Having 3 or more previous children *Diabetes *Female fetal sex. Although SUA can affect either artery, the left artery tends to be absent slightly more often than the right.

Associated Problems with SUA: Anywhere from half to two-thirds of babies born with single artery umbilical cord are born healthy and with no chromosomal or congenital abnormalities. Of the remaining babies with SUA, some studies suggest that about 25 percent have birth defects, including chromosomal and/or other abnormalities. These can include trisomy 13 or trisomy 18. However, the most common pregnancy complications that occur in infants with SUA are heart defects, gastrointestinal tract abnormalities and problems with the central nervous system. The respiratory system, urinary tract, and musculoskeletal system may also be affected. One in five babies affected by SUA will be born with multiple malformations.

Aside from these problems, between 15% and 20% of infants with SUA may suffer from intrauterine growth retardation. Single umbilical artery also has an increased miscarriage rate of 22% associated with it, likely due to the increased abnormalities. Furthermore, there is an association between SUA and low birthweight (<2500g) and early delivery (<37 weeks).

The prognostic clinical significance of identifying a two-vessel umbilical cord (either as an isolated finding or when associated with other anomalies) during the antenatal period requires further investigation. Nonetheless, the identification of this problem should prompt a thorough search for other associated abnormalities. Accurate diagnosis should minimize the number of mothers subjected to unnecessary detailed studies and anxiety in cases of "suspected" but not confirmed SUA. In the presence of an otherwise reassuring prenatal ultrasound, the only other change to antenatal care one might make is a growth scan to make sure the baby is growing at a 'normal' rate toward the last month of pregnancy. A fetal echocardiogram may also be performed to check the cardiac anomalies.

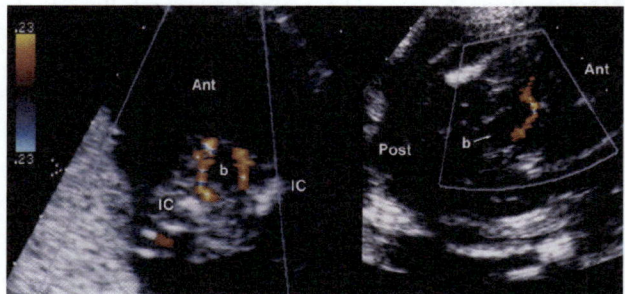

Left: This represents an optimal "umbilicus anterior" view of two umbilical arteries (orange) coursing around the fetal bladder (b) by color Doppler ultrasound. Note that the iliac crests (IC) can be seen bilaterally in this 16.5-week fetus. Right: Another axial color Doppler scan at the level of the fetal bladder (b) which is associated with single umbilical artery (orange) in a 16-week fetus.

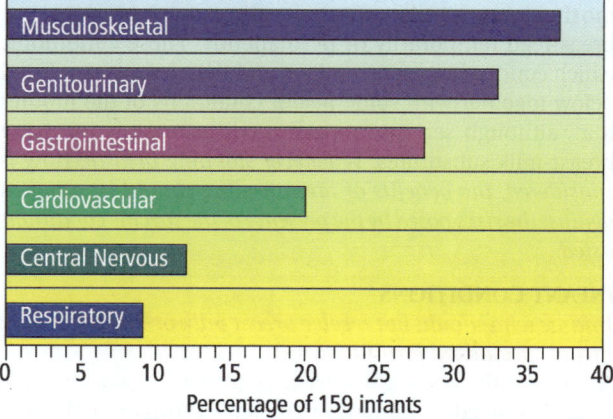

Organ system anomalies associated with liveborn infants with single umbilical artery. (Adapted from Leung[5]).

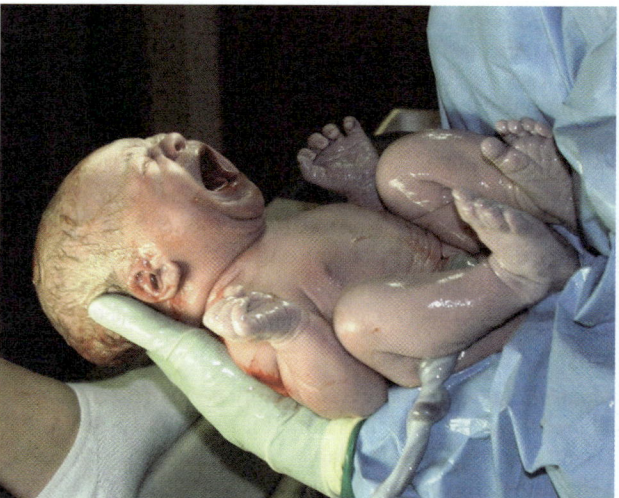

Most Babies with a Single Umbilical Cord Are Fine

REFERENCE: Single umbilical artery: visualization Wesley Lee, MD*, Mary Rice, RDMS, Janet S. Kirk, MD, Christine H. Comstock, MD, S. Samuel Yang, MD+

Aseptic practice has reduced the rates of omphalitis, neonatal tetanus and sepsis. The practice of separating mothers and babies in the 1940's associated with prolonged hospital stays led to a steep rise in nosocomial infections. To control this problem routine application of antimicrobial agents to the cord stump became common.

However, current evidence supports the use of standard infection control procedures only, in this area of practice.

Well baby care *clamp the cord with sterile clamps and cut it with sterile scissors or blade *the recommended length of the stump after cutting is 2 or 3 cm *practice rooming in where possible, with the mother as primary carer *keep the cord dry and exposed to air. The napkin should be folded below the umbilicus *wash hands before handling the umbilical cord and where possible avoid touching the cord stump *remove the cord clamp on day 2 of life Nursery Care *practices vary between hospitals because of a lack of relevant high quality evidence with care being either *as for routine care *or a solution of 0.5% Chlorhexidine and 70% alcohol is used to clean the cord twice daily on admission and daily for the first three days, or while an umbilical catheter is in situ

Areas of Uncertainty

*a study comparing daily bathing with no bathing showed no difference in umbilical cord colonization or infection between the groups, and that immersing the newborn in a bath is not harmful to the cord *when reviewed for the Cochrane database use of topical antiseptics for routine care was associate with *no systemic infections or deaths *a trend to reduced colonization with antibiotics compared to antiseptics

Umbilical care

• Cord contains 2 arteries, one vein, rudimentary allantois, remnant of omphalomesenteric duct and wharton jelly •cord usually dries and separates within 6–8 days after birth ‹ raw surface becomes covered by thin layer of skin ‹ scar tissue forms and wound is healed within 12–15 days • Treatment: fold the top edge of the diaper down, away from the umbilicus, so the stump stays dry - clean the area with a cotton ball and alcohol two times per day and for several days after the stump falls off—parent must avoid soaking the umbilical area in alcohol; case reports of toxicity exist !!! - do not submerse the umbilical area in a bath until after stump has fallen off and healed over

Umbilical cord problems

A stark contrast is observed between the physiologic importance of the umbilicus during development and after birth. During development, the umbilicus functions as a channel that allows blood flow between the placenta and fetus. It also serves an important role in the development of the intestine and the urinary system. After birth, once the umbilical cord falls off, no evidence of these connections should be present. Nevertheless, umbilical disorders are frequently encountered in pediatric surgery. These disorders range from the very common umbilical hernia to infections such as omphalitis, which can be life threatening. Most patients with umbilical problems present with a mass or drainage from the umbilicus. An understanding of the anatomy and embryology of the abdominal wall and umbilicus is important to identify and properly treat these conditions.

*Delayed separation of the cord greater than one month is associated with an immune disorder and/or overwhelming bacterial infection . The umbilical cord usually separates from the umbilicus 1–8 weeks postnatally.

Persistent urachus/ urachal cyst: The presentation of omphalomesenteric remnants depends on the specific type of defect . If a communication persists from the terminal ileum to the umbilicus, intestinal contents or stool can be observed leaking from the umbilicus. Prolapse of intestine through an omphalomesenteric fistula can also be observed .The drainage from a fistula that does not communicate with the ileum varies; it may be clear, bloody, or purulent. Cystic remnants may become infected and manifest with pain and swelling. The presentation of urachal remnants also varies. Clear drainage from the umbilicus is characteristic of a urachal fistula. Drainage of urine from the umbilicus may suggest bladder outlet obstruction and warrants further investigation. A urachal sinus manifests with drainage that can be clear or purulent. A urachal cyst is usually discovered as a painful mass between the umbilicus and suprapubic area when it becomes infected. Pain and retraction of the umbilicus during urination may suggest a urachal anomaly. failure of closure of the allantoic duct and is associated with bladder outlet obstruction; results in clear urine-like discharge from the umbilicus . Omphalomesenteric remnants and urachal remnants require surgical excision. The precise diagnosis is often not confirmed until surgery is performed and the anatomy of the umbilicus is established.

Umbilical hernia: Patients with umbilical hernias present early in life with bulging at the umbilicus. The swelling is most

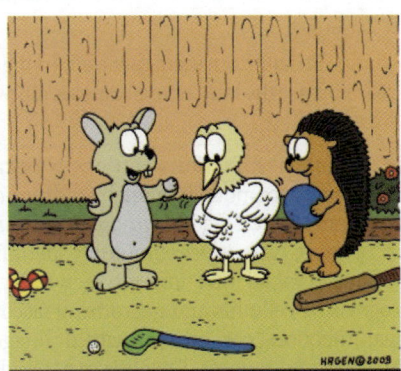

Of course you don't have a belly button: You came out of an egg...

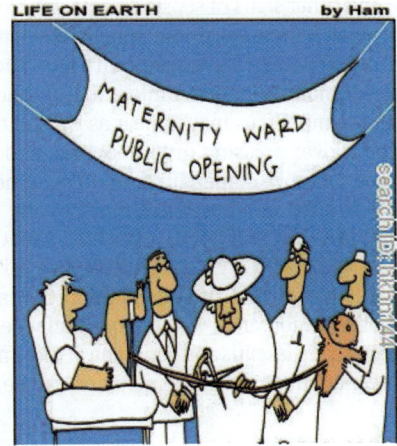

LIFE ON EARTH   by Ham

MATERNITY WARD PUBLIC OPENING

prominent when the infant or child is crying or straining. Umbilical hernias are usually asymptomatic and rarely cause pain. The skin can become severely stretched, which may be alarming to parents and physicians. Parents often mention that the child plays with the redundant skin. Incarceration, strangulation, bowel obstruction, erosion of the overlying skin, and bowel perforation are rare events in infants and small children. The risk of incarceration increases significantly in adults with umbilical hernias. Asymptomatic umbilical hernias can be safely monitored until the child is aged 4–5 years to allow spontaneous closure, especially if the ring defect is small. Because umbilical hernias with larger defects (i.e. >1.5 cm) are unlikely to spontaneously close, surgery can be performed at an earlier age. Similarly, closing umbilical hernias with large ring defects is reasonable in younger children if the child is having a general anesthetic for another procedure, such as an inguinal hernia repair. Considering surgery in younger children who have a large protrusion of the umbilical skin that is causing distress to the parents is also reasonable

* **Granulation tissue:** Umbilical granuloma: Granulation tissue may persist at the base of the umbilicus after cord separation. The tissue is composed of fibroblasts and capillaries and can grow to more than 1 cm. Umbilical granulomas must be differentiated from umbilical polyps, which do not respond to silver nitrate cauterization. Umbilical granulomas appear as 1-mm to 1-cm, pink, friable lesions at the base of the umbilicus. They produce variable amounts of drainage that can irritate the surrounding skin. An umbilical polyp is brighter red than a granuloma and represents retained intestinal or gastric mucosa from the vitelline duct tissue is a persistent, soft, vascular, granular and dull red or pink with seropurulent discharge ‹ cauterize with silver nitrate every several days until base is dry. Large umbilical granulomas or those that persist after silver nitrate treatment require surgical excision.

*Mucoid discharge: Results from inadequate air drying or cleaning of the cord area ‹ cleanse the base several times a day with alcohol and allow air drying.

*Omphalitis: Umbilical infections can occur because of an embryologic remnant or poor hygiene. Traditionally, gram-positive organisms, such as *Staphylococcus aureus* and *Streptococcus pyogens*, were most commonly identified. Gram-negative and polymicrobial infections are seen today, especially in rapidly progressing cellulitis and necrotizing fasciitis. Patients with umbilical infections can present with drainage from the umbilicus, swelling, and redness. Cellulitis may rapidly progress and lead to necrotizing fasciitis. Necrotizing fasciitis is characterized by abdominal distention, tachycardia, purpura, leukocytosis, and other signs of sepsis despite antibiotic therapy Infection can result in hematogenous spread or extension to the liver or peritoneum—can have minimal signs such as mild erythema on abdomen, usually circumferential around umbilicus ** "redness" at the umbilicus may appear as a result of a normal cord stump bent over pressing onto neonate's abdomen held down by a diaper; remove diaper; lift cord off abdomen; redness should go away in a few minutes; if not, may be early infection - ANY ERYTHEMA EXTENDING ONTO ABDOMEN IS OMPHALITIS UNTIL PROVEN OTHERWISE !! -Treatment- MEDICAL EMERGENCY !!! - IV Oxacillin and Gentamicin and admission to observation area - - surgery usually necessary for abscesses . Necrotizing fasciitis and gangrene of the umbilical skin requires emergency surgical debridement and can be life saving.

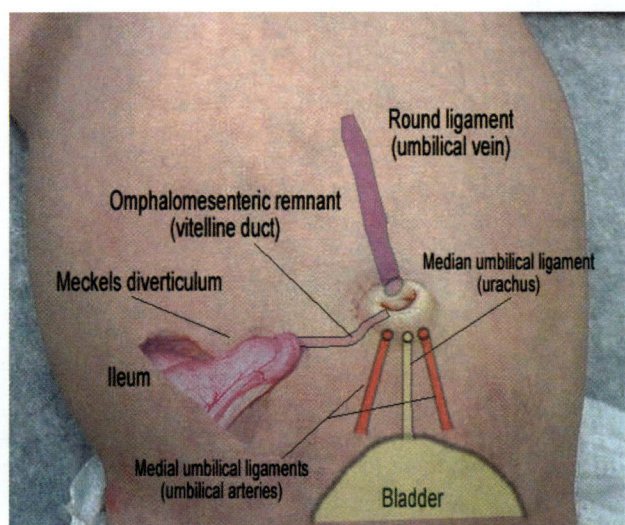

Anatomic relationship between the umbilicus and its embryologic attachments.

Patent Omphalomesenteric Duct

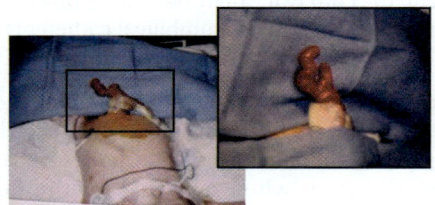

Photograph of newborn with intestinal prolapse through a patent omphalomesenteric duct. Both the proximal and distal limbs of the intestine have prolapsed. The umbilicus was explored, the bowel was easily reduced, and the patent duct was excised. The child was discharged from the hospital 2 days later.

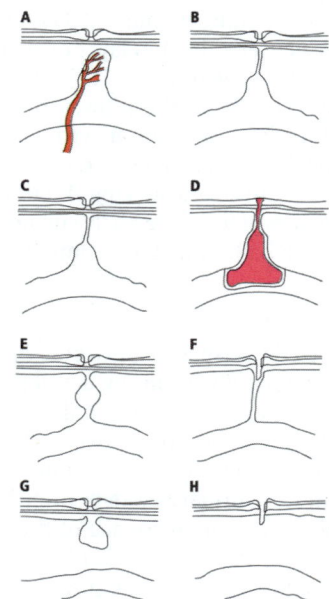

Omphalomesenteric duct remnants. (A) Meckel diverticulum. Note feeding vessel. (B) Meckel diverticulum attached to posterior surface of anterior abdominal wall by a fibrous cord. (C) Fibrous cord attaching ileum to abdominal wall. (D) Intestinal-umbilical fistula. Intestinal mucosa extends to skin surface. (E) Omphalomesenteric cyst arising in a fibrous cord. The cyst may contain intestinal or gastric mucosa. (F) Umbilical sinus ending in a fibrous cord attaching to the ileum. (G, H) Omphalomesenteric cyst and sinus without intestinal attachments.

Neonatal reflexes: Definition: Neonatal reflexes or primitive reflexes are the inborn behavioral patterns that develop during uterine life. They should be fully present at birth and are gradually inhibited by higher centers in the brain during the first three to 12 months of postnatal life. These reflexes, which are essential for a newborn's survival immediately after birth, include sucking, swallowing, blinking, urinating, hiccupping, and defecating. These typical reflexes are not learned; they are involuntary and necessary for survival. A normal birth is considered full term if the delivery occurs during the thirty-seventh to fortieth week after conception. Developmentally, the baby is considered a neonate for the first 28 days of life. At birth, the neonate must immediately make five major adjustments:

- Transition from an aquatic environment to a world of air. The first breath begins even before the umbilical cord is cut.

- Eat and digest his or her own food since the circulatory relationship between mother and baby stops with the severance of the umbilical cord.

- Excrete his or her own wastes.

- Maintain his or her own body temperature.

- Adjust to intermittent feeding since food is now only available at certain intervals.

Under normal developmental conditions, these neonatal reflexes represent important reactions of the nervous system and are only observable within a specific period of time over the first few months of life. The following reflexes are normally present from birth and are part of a normal newborn evaluation:

Your newborn baby is an amazing creature. The many reflexes he or she is born with help transition them to life and learn what they need to survive. Here are some of these reflexes to help you get to know your baby better:

Moro reflex: When you fail to support or hold the neck and head, the arms of your baby will thrust outward and then seem to embrace them selves as their fingers curl. This reflex disappears at about 2 months of age. It is also known as the startle reflex.

Palmar grasp: When you touch the palm of your baby's hand, the fingers will curl around and cling to your finger or an object. This is a good reflex to take advantage of with other children, to allow the baby to "hold" their hand. This reflex also makes it difficult to obtain handprints until it disappears at about 3 months.

Plantar grasp: The foot equivalent of Palmar Grasp, disappears by 8–9 months

Sucking: While you may not believe this to be reflexive, it is. This ensures that the baby will nurse on a breast or bottle to be fed and occurs when something is placed in the baby's mouth. It is slowly replaced by voluntary sucking around 2 months of age.

Rooting Reflex: When you stroke your baby's cheek she will turn towards you, usually looking for food. This is very useful when learning to breastfeed your baby. This reflex is gone by about 4 months. You may also notice this occurs when the baby accidentally brushes her own face with her hands. It can sometimes be a source of frustration if your baby flails her arms during feedings. Simply using a blanket to pin her arms closer to her body during feeding may help.

Stepping reflex: If you take your baby and place his feet on a flat surface he will "walk" by placing one foot in front of the other. This isn't really walking and will disappear by about 4 months of age.

Tonic neck reflex: This is also called the fencing reflex, because of the position the baby assumes. When you lay your baby on her back and her head turns to one side she will extend her arm and leg on that side while the opposite arm and leg bend, assuming a "fencing" position. This reflex is present only until about the 4th month.

Symmetrical tonic neck reflex occurs with either the extension or flexion of the infant's head. Extension of the head results in extension of the arms and flexion of the legs, and a flexion of the head causes flexion of the arms and an extension of the legs. This reflex becomes inhibited by the sixth month to enable crawling.

Swimming: If you were to put a baby under six months of age in water, they would move their arms and legs while holding their breath. This is why some families believe in swim training for very little babies. It is not recommended for you to test this reflex at home for obvious safety reasons. Your baby will have his or her reflexes tested shortly after birth. Absence or weak reflexes can be caused by birth trauma, medications used, illness, etc. Talk to your pediatrician if you have concerns about your baby reflexes or ask them to show you during a newborn exam the amazing feats of your new baby.

Babinski or plantar reflex is triggered by stroking one side of the infant's foot upward from the heel and across the ball of the foot. The infant responds by hyperextending the toes; the great toe flexes toward the top of the foot and the other toes fan outward. It generally becomes inhibited from the sixth to ninth month of post natal life.

Other Neonatal reflexes:

Blink reflex is stimulated by momentarily shining a bright light directly into the neonate's eyes causing him or her to blink. This reflex should not become inhibited.

Pupillary reflex occurs with darkening the room and shining a penlight directly into the neonate's eye for several seconds. The pupils should both constrict equally; this reflex should not disappear.

Galant reflex is stimulated by placing the infant on the stomach or lightly supporting him or her under the abdomen with a hand and, using a fingernail, gently stroking one side of the neonate's spinal column from the head to the buttocks. The response occurs with the neonate's trunk curving toward the stimulated side. This reflex can become inhibited at any time between the first and third month.

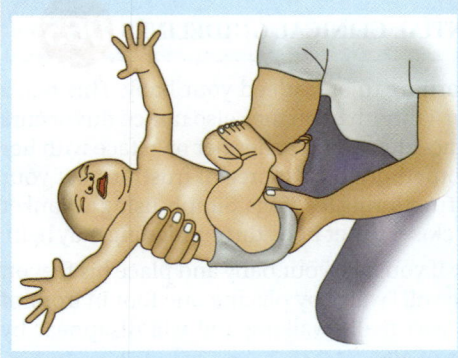

The Moro reflex (or startle reflex) occurs when an infant is lying in a supine position and is stimulated by a sudden loud noise that causes rapid or sudden movement of the infant's head. This stimulus results in a symmetrical extension of the infant's extremities while forming a C shape with the thumb and forefinger. This is followed by a return to a flexed position with extremities against the body. Inhibition of this reflex occurs from the third to the sixth month. An asymmetrical response with this reflex may indicate a fractured clavicle or a birth injury to the nerves of the arm. Absence of this reflex in the neonate is an ominous implication of underlying neurological damage.

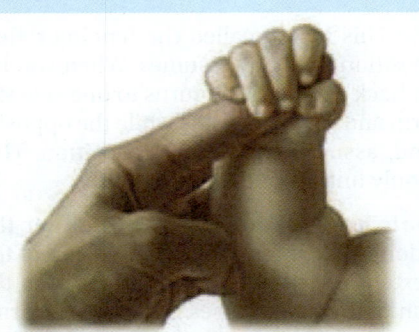

Palmar grasp: If you place your finger or other slim object in your baby's palm, his fingers will grasp the object tightly. Be careful, though, because your baby cannot control this reflex. If you place a rattle in your baby's hand, for example, he could unexpectedly let go and drop it on his head. Your baby's grip is so strong, you might notice that you can pull him up when he's gripping both your fingers. Again, watch out since he could let go at any moment and fall backward, causing injury. This reflex is also present in the feet causing the toes to curl. It can be tested by lightly touching your baby's feet or toes. This reflex only lasts until your child is about 3 months old. Also known as Darwinian Reflex (after Scientist Charles Darwin), Tonic Grasp Reflex or Palmar/Plantar Grasp Reflex.

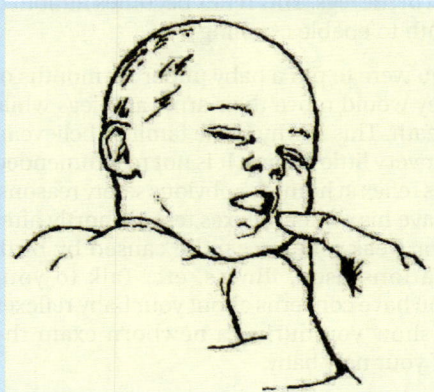

Rooting reflex: It is stimulated by touching a finger to the infant's cheek or the corner of the mouth. The neonate responds by turning the head toward the stimulus, opening the mouth and searching for the stimulus. This is a necessary reflex triggered by the mother's nipple during breastfeeding. It is usually inhibited by the third to fourth month

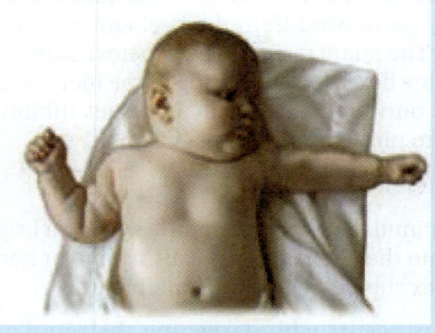

Tonic neck/fencing reflex: If you place your baby on his back, he will look like a little fencer. His head will turn with the arm and leg of one side extended (the pair on the side he's turned toward) and his other arm and leg will be flexed. This reflex can be present up to about 6 months of age or about the time your baby begins rolling over (back-to-stomach) competently and regularly. It's thought that this reflex helps prevent a baby from rolling over onto his stomach before his brain and body are ready. This is another good reason why putting your baby on his back to sleep is important. The reflex should be inhibited by six months of age in the waking state. If this reflex is still present at eight to nine months of age, the baby will not be able to support its weight by straightening its arms and bringing its knees beneath its body.

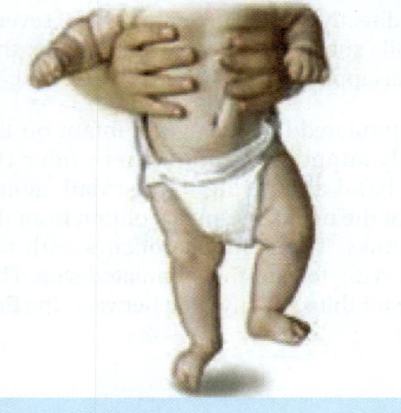

Stepping reflex is observed by holding the infant in an upright position and touching one foot lightly to a flat surface, such as the bed. The infant responds by making walking motions with both feet. This reflex will disappear at approximately two months of age.

Summary of neonatal reflexes

Reflex	Stimulation to elicit reflex	Expected response	Age of disappearance
Rooting	Touching or stroking the cheek near the corner of the mouth	Head turns in direction of stimulation so that the neonate can find food. When the breast touches the cheek, the Neonate turns toward the nipple.	6th week of life when the source of food can be seen. Disappears when awake -3 to 4 months; when asleep, 7 to 8 months
Sucking	Touching the lips with the nipple of the breast or bottle or other object	Sucking movements that enable the Newborn to take in food	Begins to diminish at 6 months Disappears soon after birth if not stimulated. If a neonate cannot take oral feedings, a pacifier may be used to maintain the reflex
Swallowing	Accompanies the sucking reflex	Food reaching the posterior of the mouth is swallowed	Does not disappear
Gagging	When more is taken into the mouth than can be successfully swallowed	Immediate return of undigested food	Does not disappear
Sneezing and Coughing	Foreign substance entering the upper or lower airways	Cleaning of the upper air passages by sneezing, the lower air passages by coughing	Does not disappear
Extrusion	Substance placed on anterior position of tongue	Extrusion of the substance to prevent swallowing	About 4 months
Blinking	Exposure of eyes to bright light from a flashlight or otoscope or sudden movement of object toward eye	Protection of the eye by rapid eyelid closure	Does not disappear
Doll's Eye	Turn the Newborn head slowly to the right or left side	Normally eyes do not move	When fixation develops
Palmar Grasp	Object placed in newborn's palm	Grasping of object by closing fingers around it. Reflex, may be so strong that a Neonate grasping the examiner's forefingers can be lifted from the supine to a standing position ("darwinian reflex")	6 weeks to 3 months Purposeful grasp is evident at 3 months of age
Plantar Grasp	Touching the sole of the foot at the base of the toes	Toes grasp around very small object	8 to 9 months, in preparation for walking May continue to be present during sleep
Dancing (step-in-place)	Hold neonate in vertical position with the feet touching a flat, firm surface	Rapid alternating flexion and extension of the legs as in stepping	3 to 4 weeks. The Neonate soon thereafter can bear some weight on the legs without stepping
Babinski	Stroking the lateral aspect of the sole of the foot with a relatively sharp object (fingernail) from the heel up toward the little toe and across the foot to the big toe	Fans the toes (positive Babinski sign). The adult normally flexes the toes. The Newborn's response is due to an immature level of nervous system development	3 months of age; variable
Tonic Neck (fencing position)	Turning the head quickly to one side while the infant is supine	Arm and leg on the side the head is turned toward extend. Arm and leg on the opposite side flex. Both hands may make fists	18 to 20 weeks. Tonic neck reflex is replaced by symmetric positioning of both sides of the body
Moro (startle)	Startling the infant with a loud voice or apparent loss of support due to a change in equilibrium. The neonate is held in a supine position above the table or bed. The nurse supports the upper back and head with one hand and the lower back with the other. The Newborn's head is suddenly allowed to drop backward an inch or so	Generalized muscular activity. Symmetric abduction and extension of the arms and legs with fanning of the fingers. The thumb and index finger on each hand form a C shape. The extremities then flex and adduct; the baby may cry	Strong up to 2 months; disappears by 3-4 months

BILI-BLANKET

With BiliSoft, there's no barrier to bonding between infant and parents or caregivers. The baby can be held, fed, even rocked throughout the therapy session. Comfort is the keyword, whichever cover options you select. The flat, cushioned BiliSoft cover lets you swaddle baby and phototherapy pad together. The BiliSoft nest offers sick babies the boundaries and support they need, via a cushy footroll and gentle, transparent straps. If a baby cannot be swaddled, positioning aids may be placed under the pad to bring more light to the sides of a baby's body for greater skin surface area exposure to the light.

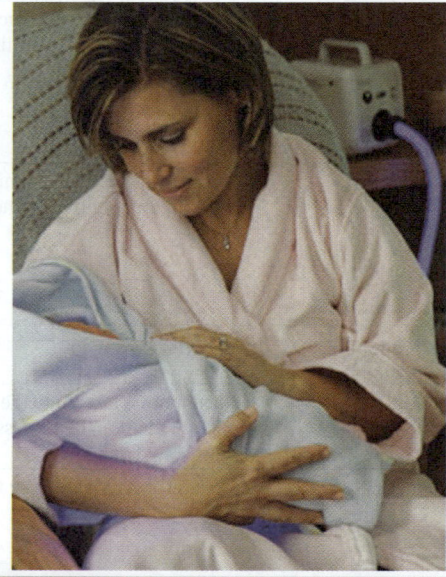

Irradiance level*

- There's no distance factor to diminish treatment intensity
- Small pad irradiance is 50 W•cm-2•nm-1
- Large pad irradiance is 35 W•cm-2•nm-1

* irradiance through the typical BiliSoft covers and nests

BiliSoft fiberoptic pad covers

- Ultra-soft, disposable BiliSoft covers are made of flame-retardant, skin-friendly fabric
- BiliSoft covers and nests have soft straps which help swaddle a baby in comfort and transmit phototherapy light too, if an additional

overhead phototherapy source is required

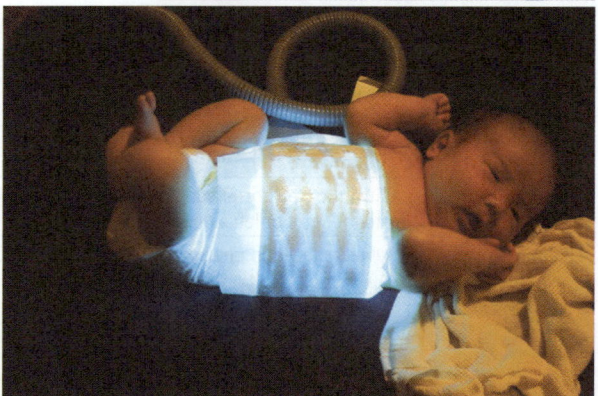

Easy positioning

- A long, flexible, fiberoptic cable makes positioning easier than ever

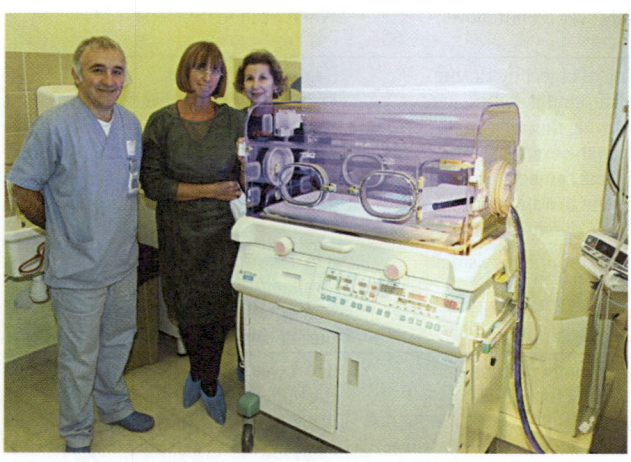

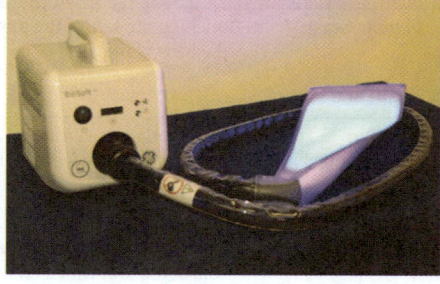

BILI-BLANKET DO'S AND DON'TS

One method of phototherapy in the hospital or at home is a fiber-optic blanket (bili-blanket). It consists of a fiber-optic pad (A), a cable connector (B), and a light generating box (C). Use of the bili-blanket is simple and safe as long as the directions for use are followed

DO make sure the light source box is on a flat, non-absorbent surface. Do not place on carpet or sit on the crib mattress.

DO make sure as much of the infant's skin is in direct contact with the light pad. Diapers should be worn.

DO have the disposable cover as the ONLY material between the light-emitting side of the pad and infant's skin. Clothing may be worn over the pad.

DO leave the light pad on when holding or feeding your baby.

DO turn off light when bathing your infant.

DO change the disposable cover if it becomes soiled.

DO use a 3-prong plug for safety.

DO set the intensity knob on the light box to the highest setting.

DON'T use the light-emitting pad without a disposable cover.

DON'T directly expose your baby's eyes to the covered light pad.

DON'T sit anything on top of the light source box or the fiber optic cable.

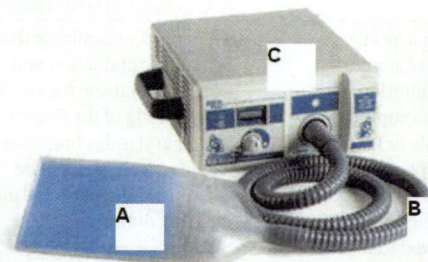

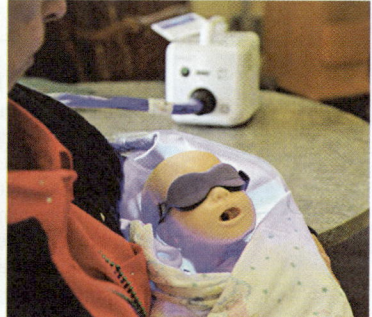

Phototherapy is the most common therapeutic intervention used for the treatment of hyperbilirubinemia. The process of phototherapy causes three reactions: photo-oxidation, configurational and structural isomerization of the bilirubin molecule, leading to polar, water-soluble photoproducts that can be excreted in bile and urine without the need for conjugation or further metabolism .

Indications: Clinically significant indirect hyperbilirubinemia. Indications to start phototherapy in babies with hyperbilirubinemia can vary depending on gestational age, birthweight, hours of life, presence of hemolysis, and other risk factors such as acidosis and sepsis.

The total serum bilirubin (TSB) level must be considered when making the decision to commence treatment, as there is significant variability in laboratory measurement of direct bilirubin levels.

Contraindications: 1)Congenital porphyria or a family history of porphyria is an absolute contraindication to the use of phototherapy 2)Concomitant use of drugs or agents that are photosensitizers is also an absolute contraindication 3)direct hyperbilirubinemia is no longer considered to be a contraindication ,in spite of the potential complication "bronzed baby syndrome" ; the presence of cholestasis may decrease the effectiveness of phototherapy.

*Equipment:*A variety of phototherapy equipment devices exist and may be free-standing, attached to a radiant warmer, wall-mounted, suspended from the ceiling, or fiber-optic systems. These in turn may contain various light sources to deliver the phototherapy, which may be categorized as:Fluorescent tubes Halogen bulbs Fiber-optic light combinations used in pads, blankets, or spotlights High-intensity light-emitting diodes *The clinician is therefore faced with a vast array of equipment to choose from and must be aware of advantages and disadvantages of each type.*Spectral qualities of the delivered light (wavelength range and peak). Bilirubin absorbs visible light within the wavelength range of 400 to 500 nm, with peak absorption at 460 ± 10 nm considered to be the most effective. Irradiance (intensity of light), is expressed as watts per square centimeter (W/cm^2). This refers to the number of photons received per square centimeter of exposed body surface area. Spectral irradiance is irradiance that is quantitated within the effective wavelength range for efficacy and is expressed as $\mu W/cm^2/nm$. This is measured by various commercially available radiometers. Specific radiometers are generally recommended for each phototherapy system, because measurements of irradiance may vary depending on the radiometer and the light source.

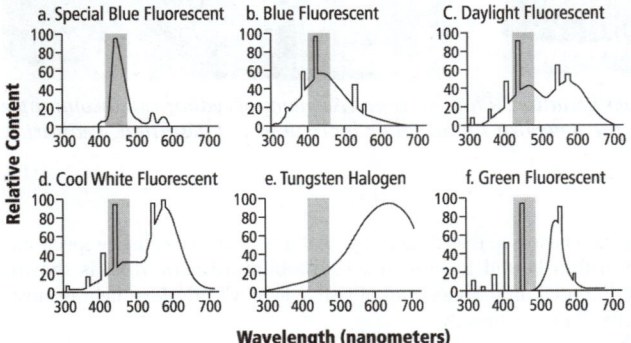

Relative spectral content of phototherapy bulbs. Shaded area indicates wavelength effective for phototherapy. Absolute spectral irradiance ($\mu W/cm^2/nm$) depends not only on relative power across wavelength of bilirubin absorption but also on total wattage and distance from infant. Although all bulbs provide effective phototherapy for the same wattage, special blue and blue fluorescent bulbs provide the most amount of power in the bilirubin wavelength.

REFERENCE: Warshaw JB, Gagliardi J, Patel A. A comparison of fluorescent and nonfluorescent light sources for phototherapy. Pediatrics. 1980;65:795 798(e); and from Farr PM, Diffey BL. The colour of light for neonatal phototherapy. Arch Dis Child. 1988;63:461-462.

*Halogen lamps: Halogen spotlight systems utilize single or multiple metal halide lamps as the light source and can provide high irradiance over a small surface area (>20 $\mu W/cm^2/nm$).These units can generate considerable heat, with the potential of causing thermal skin injury; therefore, they must not be in close proximity to the patient.

*Fiber-optic systems: UV-filtered light from a tungsten "halogen bulb enters a fiber-optic cable and is emitted from the sides and end of fiber-optic fibers inside a plastic pad. The pad emits insignificant levels of heat, so it can be placed in direct contact with the infant to deliver up to 35 $\mu W/cm^2/nm$ of spectral irradiance, mainly in the blue-green range. The main advantages of these systems are that, while receiving phototherapy, the infant can be held and/or nursed, thereby minimizing infant/parent separation. In addition, covering the infant's eyes is not necessary, preventing further parental anxiety. These devices are often used as an adjunct to conventional overhead application of phototherapy to provide "double" phototherapy (circumferential phototherapy), which has greater efficacy because greater body surface area is exposed to the light. BiliBlanket Phototherapy System (Ohmeda Medical, Laurel, MD, USA) delivers light at a wavelength of 400 to 550 nm; the intensity of light delivered can be controlled, permitting irradiance levels of 15, 25, and 35 $\mu W/cm^2/nm$. The fiber-optic panel consists of 2,400 fibers woven into a mat measuring 10 x 20 cm.(Refer to Essential clinical guidelines No 35-Phototherapy with Biliblanket.)

*Gallium nitride light-emitting diodes (LEDs) *These systems are semiconductor phototherapy devices capable of delivering high spectral irradiance levels of >200 $\mu W/cm^2/nm$ with very little generation of heat within a very narrow emission spectrum in the blue range (460 to 485 nm) . *LEDs have a longer lifetime (>20,000 hours) and have become cost-effective for use in phototherapy devices. *An example of an LED system is the neoBLUE System (Natus Medical, San Carlos, CA, USA). This device delivers blue light in the range of 450 to 470 nm with either a low-intensity (12 to 15 $\mu W/cm^2/nm$) or a high-intensity (30 to 35 $\mu W/cm^2/nm$) setting.

Technique (Conventional Phototherapy)

Intensive phototherapy is defined as the use of light in the 430- to 490-nm band delivered at 30 $\mu W/cm^2/nm$ or higher to the greatest body surface area possible.*Position phototherapy unit over infant to obtain desired irradiance (10 to 40 $\mu W/cm^2/nm$). Maximal amount of irradiance achieved by standard technique is generally 30 to 50 $\mu W/cm^2/nm$. The distance of the light from the infant has a significant effect on the intensity of phototherapy, and to achieve maximal intensity, the lights should be positioned as close as possible to the infant. Fluorescent tubes may be brought within approximately 10 cm of term infants without causing overheating, but halogen spot phototherapy lamps should not be positioned closer to the infant than recommended by the manufacturer, because of the risk of burns. *If increased irradiance is required, add additional units or place a fiber-optic phototherapy pad under the infant.Additional surface area may be exposed to phototherapy by lining the sides of the bassinet with aluminum foil or a white cloth.*Keep the photoradiometer calibrated and perform periodic checks of phototherapy units to make sure that adequate irradiance is being delivered.*Maintain an intact Plexiglas shield over phototherapy light bulbs in order to block ultraviolet radiation and to protect the infant from accidental bulb breakage. *Provide ventilation to the phototherapy unit to prevent overheating light bulbs. *Maintain cleanliness and electrical safety.

use, shield the oxygen saturation monitor probe from the phototherapy light. *Encourage parents to continue feeding, caring for, and visiting their infant.

Efficacy of Phototherapy

The therapeutic efficacy of phototherapy depends on several factors. *Exposed body surface area: The greater the area exposed, the greater the rate of bilirubin decline *Distance of the infant from the light source *Skin thickness and pigmentation *Total bilirubin at clinical presentation *Duration of exposure to phototherapy

Complications: *"Bronze baby syndrome" (dark, grayish-brown discoloration of the skin, serum, and urine) occurs in some infants with cholestatic jaundice who are exposed to phototherapy, as a result of accumulation in the skin and serum of porphyrins. The bronzing disappears in most infants within 2 months. Rare complications of purpuric bullous eruptions due to transient porphyrinemia have been described in infants with severe cholestasis who receive phototherapy. *Diarrhea or loose stools *Dehydration secondary to insensible water loss *Skin changes ranging from minor erythema, increased pigmentation, and skin burns to rare and more severe blistering and photosensitivity in infants with porphyria and hemolytic disease

*Separation of mother and infant and interference with bonding. *Potential retinal damage from light exposure if eye patches are not used effectively. *Mutations, sister chromatid exchange, and DNA strand breaks have been described in cell culture. It may be wise to shield the scrotum during phototherapy. * Tryptophan is reduced in amino acid solutions exposed to phototherapy. Methionine and histidine are also reduced in these solutions if multivitamins are added. These solutions should probably be shielded from phototherapy by using aluminum foil on the lines and bottles. *Low calcium levels have been described in preterm infants under phototherapy.

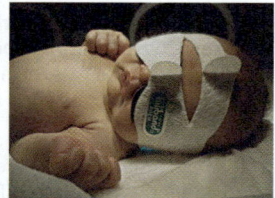

The eyes should be shielded with eye patches. Follow-up studies of infants whose eyes have been adequately shielded show normal vision and electroretinography. It may be wise to shield the scrotum during phototherapy.

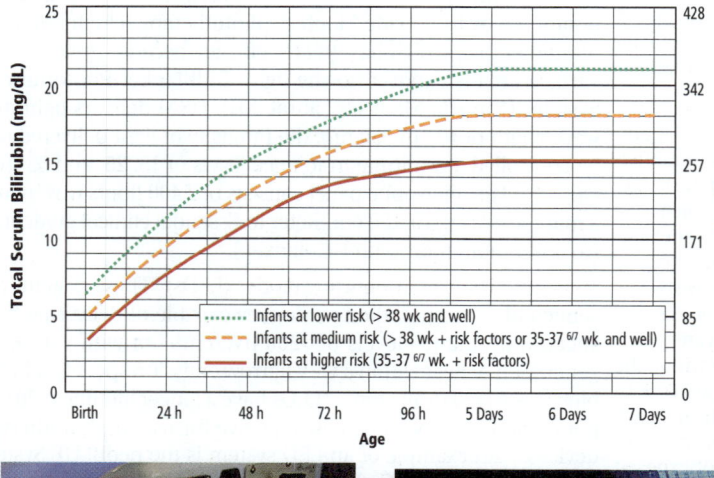

- Use total bilirubin. Do not subtract direct reacting or conjugated bilirubin.
- Risk factors = isoimmune hemolytic disease, G6PD deficiency, asphyxia, significant lethargy, temperature instability, sepsis, acidosis, or albumin < 3.0g/dl (if measured)
- For well infants 35-37 6/7 wk can adjust TSB levels for intervention around the medium risk line. It is an option to intervene at lower TSB levels for infants closer to 35 wks and at higher TSB levels for those closer to 37 6/7 wk.
- It is an option to provide conventional phototherapy in hospital or at home at TSB levels 2-3 mg/dL (35-50mmol/L) below those shown but home phototherapy should not be used in any infant with risk factors.

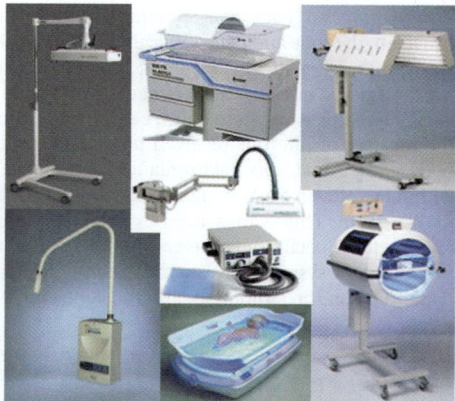

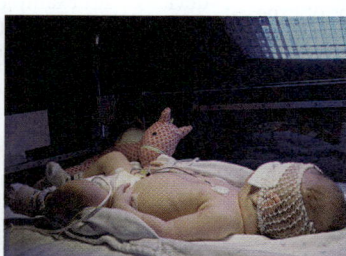

Guidelines for phototherapy in hospitalized infants of 35 or more weeks' gestation. (From American Academy of Pediatrics Subcommittee on Hyperbilirubinemia. Management of hyperbilirubinemia in the newborn infant 35 or more weeks of gestation. Pediatrics. 2004;114:297-316.)

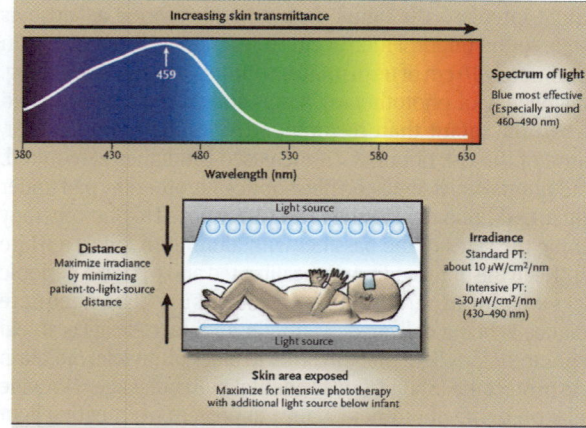

Important factors in the efficacy of phototherapy. The absorbance spectrum of bilirubin bound to human serum albumin (*white line*) is shown superimposed on the spectrum of visible light. Clearly, blue light is most effective for phototherapy, but because the transmittance of skin increases with increasing wavelength, the best wavelengths to use are probably in the range of 460 to 490 nm. Term and near-term infants should be treated in a bassinet, not an incubator, to allow the light source to be brought to within 10 to 15 cm of the infant (except when halogen or tungsten lights are used), increasing irradiance and efficacy. For intensive phototherapy, an auxiliary light source (fiberoptic pad, light-emitting diode [LED] mattress, or special blue fluorescent tubes) can be placed below the infant or bassinet. If the infant is in an incubator, the light rays should be perpendicular to the surface of the incubator in order to minimize loss of efficacy due to reflectance. PT, phototherapy. *(From Maisels MJ, McDonagh AF: Phototherapy for neonatal jaundice, N Engl J Med 358:920, 2008.)*

WRY-NECK, WITH A "TUMOR" IN THE STERNOCLEIDOMASTOID MUSCLE.

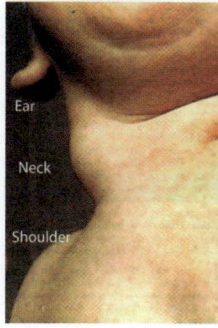

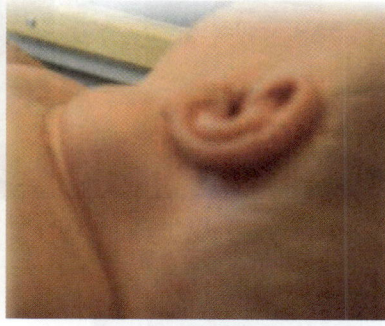

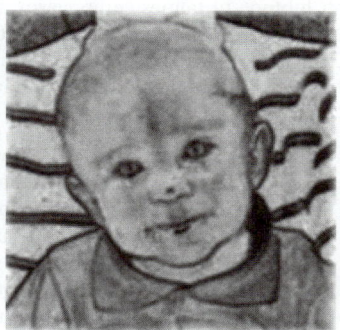

At two weeks of age, the parents brought the child to the pediatrician's office and pointed out the lump in the child's neck. They also noted that the baby tended to keep his head turned to the right side most of the time.

Image courtesy of Alan Spitzer, MD,

This child has torticollis, or wry-neck, with a "tumor" in the sternocleidomastoid muscle. The term torticollis derives from the Latin torti, or twisted, and collis, meaning neck. The mass in the neck derives from several possible sources. In some cases, it appears that hemorrhage into the muscle at the time of birth produces the mass, in this case a hematoma, which can calcify. As the muscle heals, contraction and scarring occur that the immature infant cannot counteract, leading to the preferential tilting of the head to one side. It is also thought that some cases of torticollis are due to in utero positioning abnormalities that lead to hypertrophy and contraction of the sternocleidomastoid, also resulting in the observed head positioning. A more recent theory proposes that in some cases, it is a vascular insult in utero to the muscle that results in the observed muscle shortening.

In most instances, the abnormality is not noted at birth, but becomes more evident over the first weeks of life. If no mass is noted in the muscle, the most common age at diagnosis is about 6-8 weeks, when parents begin to observe that the infant fails to turn his or her head to one side. Some children may not be diagnosed for years. The right side is usually involved in 75% of cases, probably because the most common position of the head and neck at birth is left occiput anterior. Breech presentation, however, also has a greater likelihood of torticollis as well. During delivery in both instances, the stretching that occurs preferentially injures the right sternocleidomastoid muscle. These observations would support birth injury as being the most likely etiology of the problem. About 45,000 children are born with congenital torticollis in the United States annually, or about 1% of all births. First born infants seem to be affected more often than latter births from the same mother, again suggesting that the injury occurs most often during delivery, as opposed to in utero. In many cases, the problem is mild and transient. About 20,000 children, however, will have some residual effects if not treated.

At rest, the condition does not appear to cause discomfort to the affected child. When one attempts to turn the head to the side opposite the preferentially held position, however, the infant becomes noticeably uncomfortable, indicative of the muscle shortening that has occurred. The most significant long-term consequence of torticollis is facial asymmetry, which can result if treatment is not initiated at an early age. In untreated torticollis, the affected side will tend to grow more slowly than the unaffected side, leading to noticeable facial deformity in some cases. If treated effectively prior to a year of age, however, the facial asymmetry is usually minimal.

The differential diagnosis for torticollis in the early months of life includes branchial cleft cyst, cystic hygroma, cervical spine injury, hemivertebra, and congenital absence of the sternocleidomastoid. In older children, trauma to the head and neck, posterior fossa tumors, cervical lymphadenitis, retropharyngeal abscess, Sandifer syndrome from gastroesophageal reflux or hiatal hernia, syringomyelia, cervical cord tumors, spasmus nutans, Klippel-Feil syndrome, and Wilson disease may all cause torticollis.

Evaluation in the neonatal period or during infancy should include a careful examination, especially looking for genetic abnormalities, cervical spine films, and a CT or MRI of the head and neck. In some cases, a biopsy of the mass may be indicated.

Treatment has been the source of controversy for some time. Many physicians, especially pediatric surgeons, do not believe that stretching therapy for simple torticollis is effective except in mild cases. As a result, they prefer surgical lengthening of the muscle to prevent the dramatic facial asymmetry that can occur. If parents are vigorous with stretching exercises, however, remarkable improvement can occur without surgery. There are a number of on-line sites that now document the changes that can be observed with effective physical therapy. One such site is http://amayanelson.com

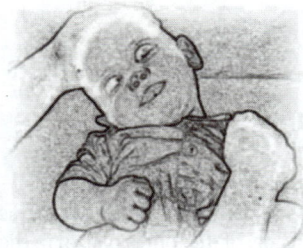

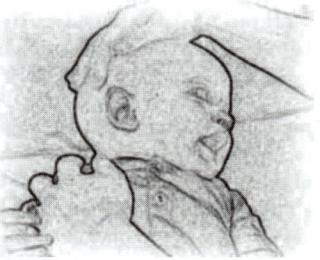

The goal with the treatment is to prevent and minimize asymmetry in head posture, neck motion and prevent skull asymmetry. The treatments are mostly performed by the parents with instructions, control and follow ups by the physiotherapist. If the muscle is tight, passive stretching exercises are included in the treatment. If there is an imbalance in strength/endurance between the left and right side active muscle strengthen exercises are included. A few children need surgery if adequate physiotherapy does not give satisfactory result. Surgery is only needed if there is a tight muscle which limits the motion and gives a tilted head posture. **NEVER START A STRETCHING EXERCISE WITHOUT CONSULTING A QUALIFIED CHILD PHYSIOTHERAPIST.**

CLUBFOOT, OR TALIPES EQUINOVARUS

*Clubfoot, or talipes equinovarus, is a congenital deformity that typically has four main components: inversion and adduction of the forefoot; inversion of the heel and hindfoot; equinus (limitation of extension) of the ankle and subtalar joint; and internal rotation of the leg.

*Clubfoot can be classified as (1) postural or positional or (2) fixed or rigid. Postural or positional clubfeet are not true clubfeet. Fixed or rigid clubfeet are either flexible (i.e., correctable without surgery) or resistant (i.e., require surgical release. *Etiology:* The true etiology of congenital clubfoot is unknown. Most infants who have clubfoot have no identifiable genetic, syndromal, or extrinsic cause. Extrinsic associations include teratogenic agents (e.g., sodium aminopterin), oligohydramnios, and congenital constriction rings. Genetic associations include Mendelian inheritance (e.g., diastrophic dwarfism; autosomal recessive pattern of clubfoot inheritance). Cytogenetic abnormalities (e.g., congenital talipes equinovarus [CTEV]) can be seen in syndromes involving chromosomal deletion. It has been proposed that idiopathic CTEV in otherwise healthy infants is the result of a multifactorial system of inheritance. Evidence for this is as follows: *Incidence in the general population is 1 per 1000 live births. *Incidence in first-degree relations is approximately 2%. *Incidence in second-degree relations is approximately 0.6%. *If one monozygotic twin has a CTEV, the second twin has only a 32% chance of having a CTEV.

Clubfoot is a complex, multifactorial deformity with genetic and intrauterine factors. One popular theory postulates that a clubfoot is a result of intrauterine maldevelopment of the talus that leads to adduction and plantar flexion of the foot. On inspection, the "down and in" appearance of the foot, which somewhat resembles that of MTA, is obvious. The foot appears smaller, with a flexible, softer heel because of the hypoplastic calcaneus. The medial border of the foot is concave with a deep medial skin furrow, and the lateral border is highly convex. The heel is usually small and is internally rotated, making the soles of the feet face each other in cases of bilateral deformities. On testing, there is pronounced tightness of the Achilles tendon with very little dorsiflexion, which differentiates clubfoot from MTA. Radiographs of clubfeet usually reveal roughly parallel axes of the talus and calcaneus .The type of clubfoot determines the specific therapy. Extrinsic clubfoot can be treated by serial casting, while intrinsic clubfoot eventually may require surgery. Plaster casting should be attempted on virtually all clubfeet, supple or rigid, as soon as practical. Casts initially are changed at semiweekly to weekly intervals and are continued until the deformity responds and is corrected fully. Persistent cast treatments by experienced clinicians have been reported to be successful in most patients. However, if a plateau is reached in treatment, surgery by a specialist in pediatric foot deformities should be considered, usually when the child is between six and nine months of age. The goal is to obtain a stable, "platform-like" position of the foot for future ambulation.

Metatarsus Adductus Treatment-Mild (flexible, passively correctable) MTA requires only parental reassurance. Moderate (semi-flexible, reducible) MTA can be treated with stretching exercises at every diaper change. First, the heel is stabilized within the notch between the thumb and index finger. Then, the forefoot is slightly pulled distally, held between the thumb and index finger of the other hand, and gently pushed into a corrected position.1 For the majority of MTA cases, the prognosis quite good. In severe cases, excessive compensation at the level of the mediotarsal joint can lead to the development of bunions, hammertoes, and other disorders. Therefore, severe (rigid) MTA can be referred for serial casting and bracing. Evidence-based comparisons of splinting or casting versus manipulation alone are not yet available.

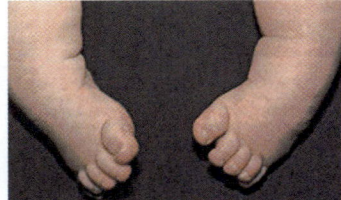
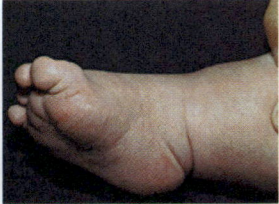

Clubfoot: anterior view.

Clubfoot : equinus component (ankle flexion). Note pathologic skin creases medially and tight Achilles tendon.

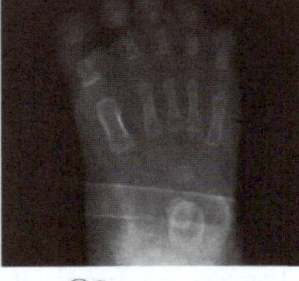
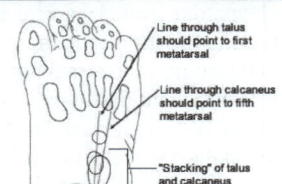

Radiologic Projection of Clubfoot; Note parallel axes of talus and calcaneus

Compare for Bilateral Metatarsus Adductus

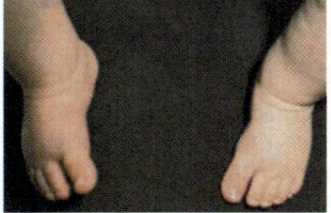
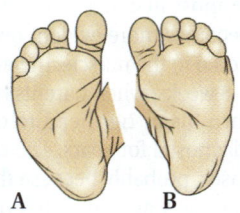

Bilateral metatarsus adductus. *(A)* medial deviation of the forefoot. *(B)* Note rounded lateral foot border (C-shaped border).

Metatarsus adductus: medial deviation of all metatarsals with normal relationship between talus and calcaneus.

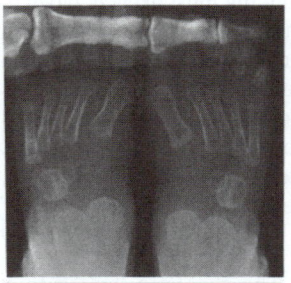
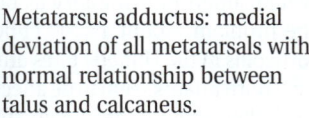
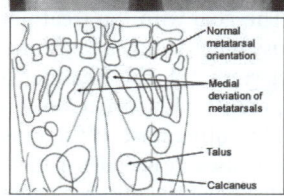
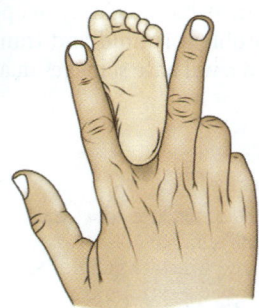

A simple test that can raise the clinician's suspicions of MTA is the "V"-finger test .In this test, the heel of the foot is placed in the "V" formed by the index and middle fingers, and the lateral aspect of the foot is observed from a plantar side for medial or lateral deviation from the middle finger. Medial deviation from the middle finger at the styloid process indicates MTA.

DEVELOPMENTAL DYSPLASIA OF THE HIP (DDH)

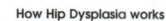

How Hip Dysplasia works

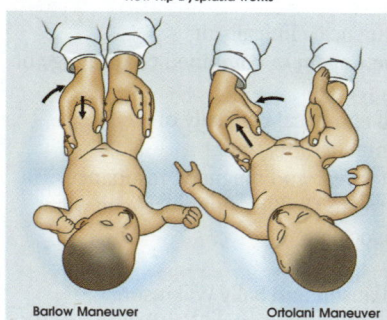

Barlow Maneuver   Ortolani Maneuver

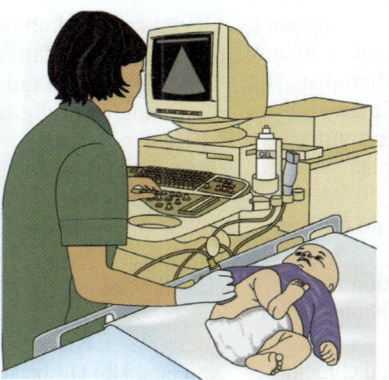

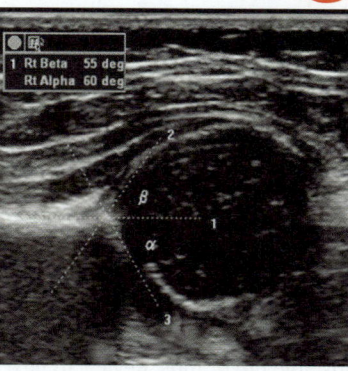

Developmental dysplasia of the Hip—DDH (e.g. Hip dislocation) : Developmental dysplasia of the hip refers to a continuum of abnormalities in the immature hip that can range from subtle dysplasia to dislocation. The identification of risk factors, including breech presentation and family history, should heighten a physician's suspicion of developmental dysplasia of the hip. Diagnosis is made by physical examination. Palpable hip instability, unequal leg lengths, and asymmetric thigh skinfolds may be present in Newborns with a hip dislocation, whereas gait abnormalities and limited hip abduction are more common in older children. The role of ultrasonography is controversial, but it generally is used to confirm diagnosis and assess hip development once treatment is initiated. Bracing is first-line treatment in children younger than six months. Surgery is an option for children in whom nonoperative treatment has failed and in children diagnosed after six months of age. It is important to diagnose developmental dysplasia of the hip early to improve treatment results and to decrease the risk of complications. 1.3% of neonates have unstable hips or subluxation. A hip may be normal at birth, and become abnormal later. Incidence (UK): 2 per 1000 live births. female/male »6:1, left hip/right hip incidence » 4:1 (bilateral in $^1/_3$).

At-risk babies: *Breech birth *Cesar for breech *Other malformations *Positive family history *Birth weight - *Oligohydramnios *Primiparous/older mother *Postmaturity

Diagnosis: Examine hips of all babies in the first days of life and at 6 weeks. With well trained, well supported staff this prevents later dysplasia. Be alert to DDH throughout child surveillance.*Each hip must be examined separately.*

Click test of Ortolani Maneuver (Reduction test): With the baby supine and relaxed, flex the hips to 90° and knees fully. Place your middle finger over the greater trochanter, and thumb on inner thigh opposite the lesser trochanter. Diagnose a dislocated hip if slow hip *abduction* produces a palpable (often audible) jerk or jolt (i.e. more than a click) -as the femoral head slips back into the acetabulum.

The Barlow Maneuver (Dislocation test): With the pelvis stabilized by one hand, *abduct* each hip in turn by 45°. Forward pressure by the middle finger causes the femoral head to slip into the acetabulum if the hip is dislocated. If the femoral head slips over the posterior lip of acetabulum and straight back again when pressure is exerted by the thumb it is 'unstable' (i.e. dislocatable not dislocated). Use both tests but avoid repetitions (may *induce* instability/dislocation). NB. both tests are problematic, missing up to 2/3 of those later needing surgery. In older children signs may be: delay in walking, abnormal waddling gait (affected leg is shorter), asymmetric thigh creases (extra crease on the affected side), and inability to fully abduct the affected hip. With bilateral involvement the perineum appears wide and lumbar lordosis is increased. **Ultrasound** is the image of choice, as it is non-invasive and dynamic. Routine ultrasound screening for DDH remains controversial.

Treatment: If Neonatal examination suggests instability, use double nappies; reassess at 3 weeks. If still a problem, splint the hips in moderate abduction for 3 months (e.g. the Pavlik harness). Excess abduction may cause avascular necrosis of the head of femur. From 6–18 months an examination-under-anesthetic (EUA), arthrogram and closed reduction is performed followed by period of immobilization in a hip spica. Open reduction is sometimes required if closed techniques fail. After 18 months (delayed presentation) open reduction is required with corrective femoral/pelvic osteotomies to maintain joint stability.

Ultrasound HIP Joints: The diagnosis and follow-up of developmental dysplasia of the hip due to its ability to visualize the nonossified femoral head and portions of the acetabulum in neonates, dynamic capabilities, accuracy, and lack of ionizing radiation. The extent of development and maturity of the hip can be assessed by the **Alpha and the Beta angles**. The Alpha angle measures the bony component and the Beta angle the cartilage component of the socket of the hip joint. The hip is classified into 4 types depending on the Alpha angle, the Beta angle and the age of the baby. Type I hips are normal. Type II hips are immature and require monitoring and sometimes treatment, Type III and IV hips are dislocated and require treatment.

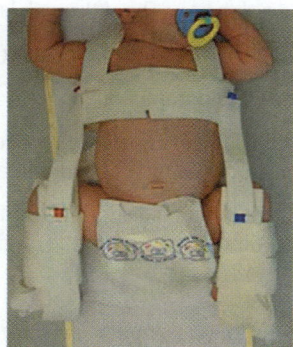

A Newborn with bilateral hip dislocations in a Pavlik harness. The harness prevents hip extension and adduction but allows flexion and abduction.

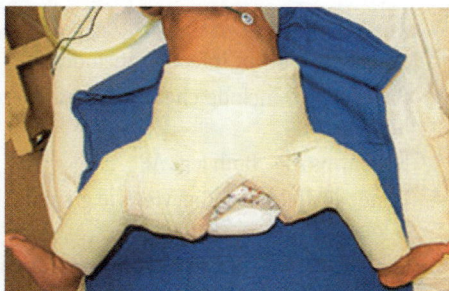

A four-month-old child in a hip spica cast following bilateral closed reductions and adductor tenotomies. A child with DDH usually requires long-term follow-up with radiographic evaluation until skeletal maturity is reached to ensure normal hip development.

Developmental dysplasia of the hip (DDH): Summary of Evaluation and Treatment Process

Neonatal ward: All babies who have risk factors or molding and those whom the junior medical staff feel concern for any reason are referred to the specialist physiotherapist. The specialist physiotherapist also examines as many babies without risk factors as is possible, given time restraints.

0 to 3 Weeks of Age: First assessment by specialist physiotherapist with 3 possible outcomes

*Normal clinical examination: Discharge with no further follow-up

*Molded, limited abduction or hip laxity: Positioning advice and review at 6 weeks of age in the combined clinic (expert physiotherapist and radiologist)

* Unstable hip or hips: Review in next combined clinic (at age of 3 to 6 weeks)

3 to 6 Weeks of Age: Assessment in combined physiotherapist and ultrasonography clinic

* If clinically and ultrasonographically unstable, commence treatment immediately

* If 3 weeks of age and equivocal clinically or ultrasonographically, review again in combined clinic at age of 6 weeks

*If 6 weeks of age and still equivocal clinically or ultrasonographically, commence treatment

Follow-up: Radiograph at 1 year and magnetic resonance imaging at 5 years for all treated babies and those who were classified initially as equivocal

Courtesy: A. Graham Wilkinson and Sally Wilkinson Neonatal Hip Dysplasia: A New Perspective NeoReviews 2010; 11; e349-e362

NICU RADIOLOGY REQUIREMENTS

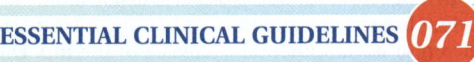
ESSENTIAL CLINICAL GUIDELINES *071*

*TUBES, CATHETERS AND WIRES SHOULD BE DISPLACED, AS MUCH AS POSSIBLE FROM THE AREA OF INTEREST.

Chest Radiographs

* The first chest radiograph includes a rolled lateral unless there are mitigating circumstances (such as a baby who is too unstable to be handled excessively).

* Lateral chest radiographs are usually not required subsequently unless checking on the position of chest drains. These lateral films are done as a shoot through lateral so that the infant is not lying on the tubing.

* AP and lateral films, for assessment of the position of umbilical lines, include the abdomen and chest.

Abdominal Radiographs

* Abdominal films, in cases of suspected obstruction or NEC, include both an AP view, and a left side down decubitus view that must include the right hemidiaphragm/right lower chest.

* Consideration should be given to obtaining a prone abdominal film to define lower obstruction, or lateral film to assess for peritoneal calcification, at the time of the original abdominal series.

Long Lines

* For · long lines inserted below the groin, a babygram (AP chest and abdomen) is appropriate.

* For · long lines inserted from the arms or head, an AP chest with the head turned away from the site of insertion is appropriate.
*Contrast is used in all longline films .

SKELETAL SURVEYS

* Skeletal survey for **infection** includes:
* Babygram to include chest, and abdomen, shoulders and hips
* Both arms AP · Both legs AP
* Hands and feet and other views (e.g. spine/skull) only if there is local swelling or erythema
* Skeletal survey for **syndromes or dysmorphic babies** includes:
* AP and lateral skull
* Chest AP and lateral if not already done (includes thoracic spine)
* Lateral lumbar, sacral, and cervical spine
* Abdomen/pelvis on the same film
* Left leg, foot, arm and hand (Right side only if there is definite asymmetry)
* Skeletal survey for post mortems
* AP whole body (skull to toes)
*Lateral radiograph (skull to sacrum) *Lower limbs - hips to feet with the legs in a frog position lateral.

REFERENCE: AUCKLAND NICU
Dr Rita Teele (Starship Radiology) and Dr Carl Kuschel April 2006

THE BASICS OF NEONATAL ABDOMINAL RADIOGRAPHY

'Cotside' abdominal radiography in the neonatal unit presents a number of radiographic challenges. The number of attachments makes for a high level of complexity and a significant array of potential artifacts.

Ground rules: You learn quickly that radiography in the neonatal unit is different. The patients are very small, vulnerable and sometimes very ill. The following are some very simple dot point tips: *wash your hands before entering the unit and on exiting. Also, wash your hands between babies (important) *ensure that the baby's name matches the one on the request form (careful you don't get confused with twins) *check the clinical information on the request form- this can influence what you include on the image *don't run the mobile machine into the cot/incubator (surprisingly easy to do) *ask the nurses for help- they know the babies, know their illnesses, and are used to handling them *be careful to avoid patient rotation, particularly with chest radiography *use a side marker - left and right are not always clear from the anatomy, particularly in chest radiography *check departmental protocol re removal of ECG leads *think about radiation protection- horizontal ray technique considerations, gonad protection, long bone protection, the nurse's fingers *you are not the boss- if the nurse says the baby can't be moved. The baby can't be moved. *use a cassette tray if there is one built into the cot/isolette.

Radiation protection operator irradiation: The person holding the baby can receive an undesirable bonus image of their fingers. This is largely avoided by education, coning and diligence. The nurse holding the baby may not be as aware of the significance of her fingers in the LBD light as you are. It is worthwhile pointing out to the nurse that 'where the light is the radiation is"- this might seem self-evident to you, but possibly the nurse might be less aware than you are of the primary X-ray beam.

Side markers: Side markers in the neonatal unit are important. The difficulty is that your side marker can appear to be almost as big as the baby's chest.

Dedicated neonatal markers

The side marker on the left is simply too large for use in the Neonatal Unit. You don't want to collimate out to include this relatively large marker. You can use small side markers with the operator's initials.

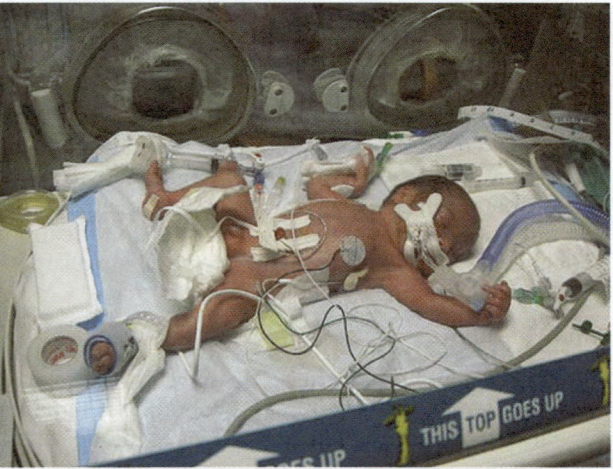

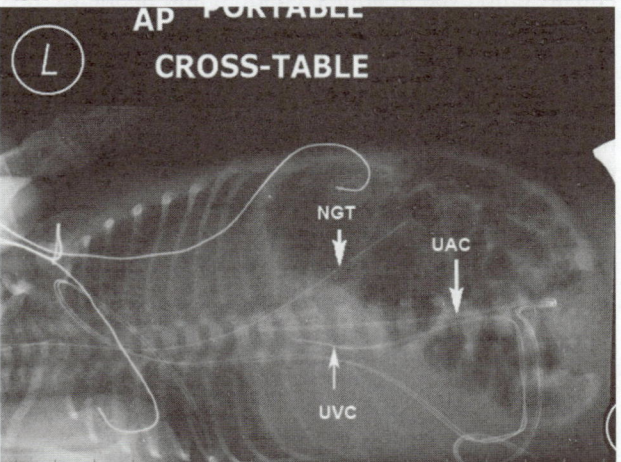

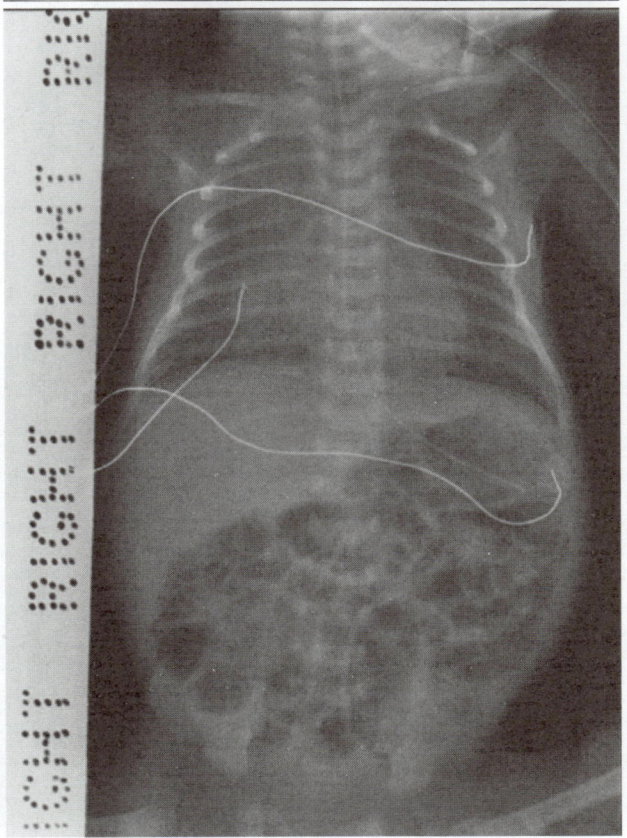

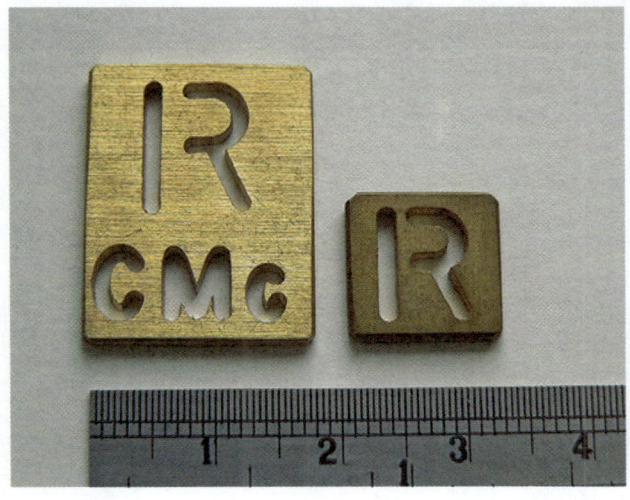

Left lateral decubitus: This is the preferred decubitus position. The free intraperitoneal gas is seen easily because it is contrasted against the liver. Although it is described as a "left lateral decubitus" it is marked with a right marker.

Right lateral decubitus: The right lateral decubitus abdominal projection (right side down) is not the decubitus of choice. The preferred decubitus is the left lateral decubitus- left lateral decubitus is more sensitive for pneumoperitoneum. This is, nevertheless, an acceptable decubitus position when the left lateral decubitus cannot be achieved. This is also arguably preferable to a supine decubitus. Operators phalanges noted in image.

Supine decubitus

The supine decubitus is a projection that can be employed when horizontal ray abdominal radiography is required in a patient that cannot be moved. This technique can be equally employed in adults, children and neonates. It is important to note that this technique is usually employed as a last resort. If the referring doctor is looking for free intraperitoneal gas (pneumoperitoneum), it is important to include all of the anterior abdominal wall. Raising the baby onto a positioning sponge to improve the radiographic image is both counterproductive and of no diagnostic benefit when looking for free gas. i.e. the advantage of this technique is that you don't move the baby. The removal of all ECG leads where appropriate will improve the image.

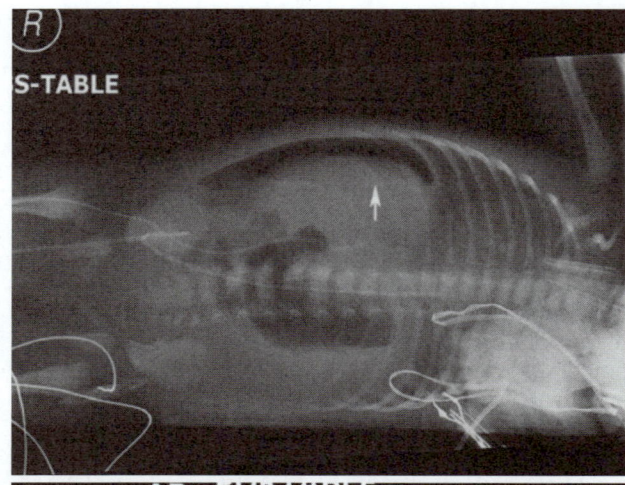

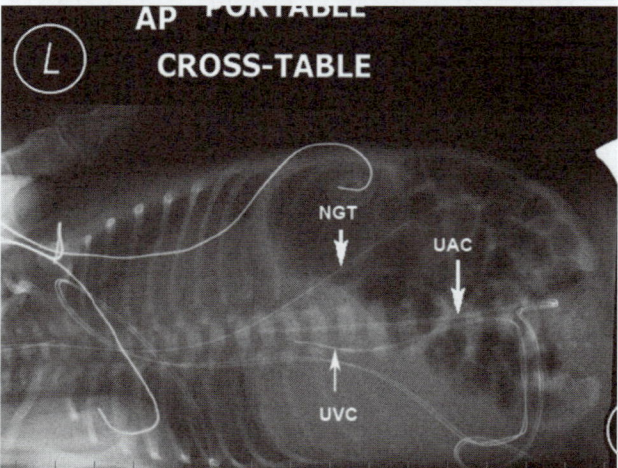

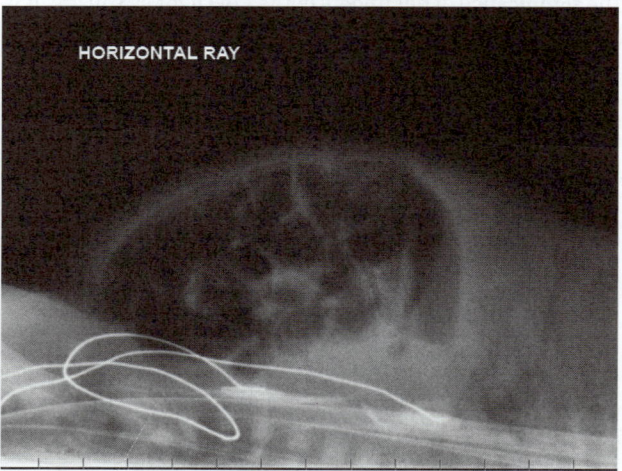

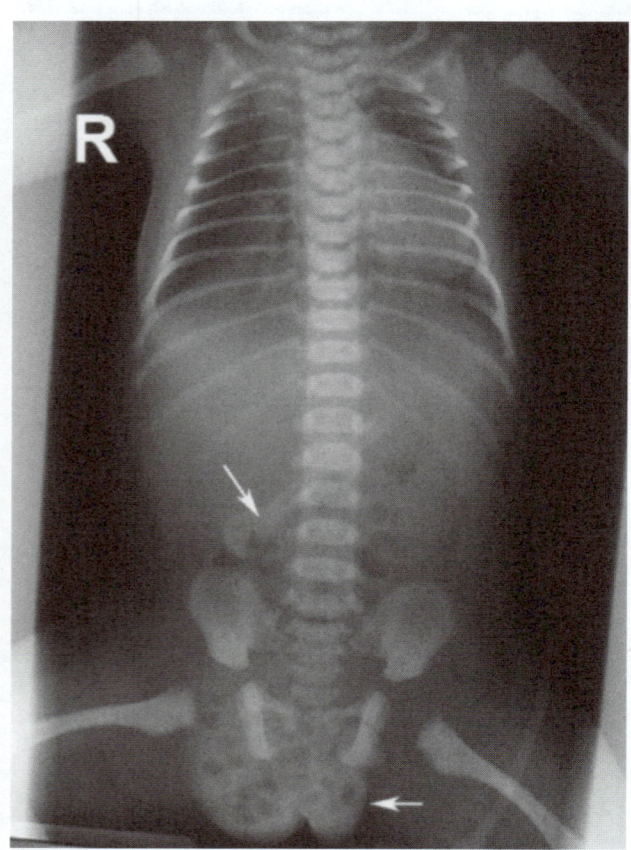

This baby has an inguinal hernia with air-filled bowel within the scrotum (bottom arrow)

The artifact is an umbilical clamp (top arrow)

Tubes, Lines and Catheters You may be called to the Neonatal Unit to confirm the position of a line, tube or catheter. A knowledge of these lines will be useful in determining which anatomy should be included on the image (i.e. it will determine your beam coning).

Umbilical Catheters

UVC

- The umbilical vein is 2–3cm long and 4–5mm in diameter

- From the umbilicus, it passes cephalad and a little to the right. It joins the left branch of the portal vein after giving off several large intrahepatic branches.

- The ductus venosus arises from the point where the UV joins the left portal vein.

UAC

- The umbilical arteries are the direct continuation of the internal iliac arteries.

- A catheter passed into an umbilical artery will usually (but not always) enter the aorta via the internal iliac artery.

- Occasionally it will pass into the femoral artery via the external iliac artery or into the gluteal arteries.

- The femoral and gluteal arteries are unsuitable sites for sampling, infusion, or blood pressure monitoring.

    There are two potential positions for the UAC. These are described as "high" or "low".

- The high position is at the level of thoracic vertebral bodies T6–T9. This position is above the coeliac axis (T12), the superior mesenteric artery (T12-L1), and the renal arteries (L1). This position is essentially "above the diaphragm".

- The low position is at the level of lumbar vertebral bodies L3–L4. This position is below the structures as above, and is above the aortic bifurcation (L4–L5). The inferior mesenteric artery arises from L3–L4. This position is essentially "above the bifurcation".

The UAC and UVC are seen in this supine decubitus abdominal image.

UAC

The umbilical artery catheter (UAC) can be seen to track inferiorly and posteriorly from the umbilicus before tracking up the aorta.

UVC

The umbilical vein catheter (UVC) takes a shorter course along the umbilical vein.

NGT

The nasogastric tube enters the stomach from the esophagus. When assessing the position of the NGT the position of the sidehole should also be considered.

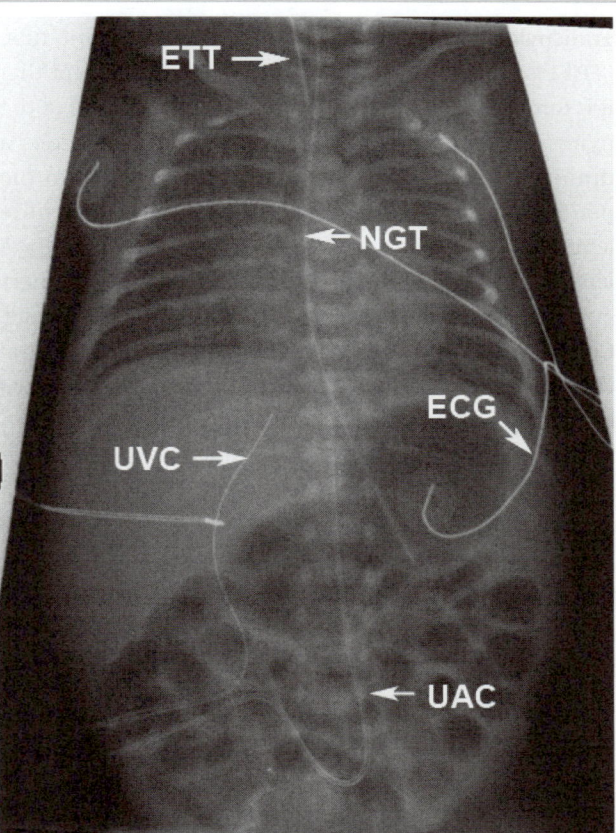

The umbilical catheters are inserted through the umbilicus into either the umbilical vein or the umbilical artery. The umbilical artery catheter (UAC) characteristically deviates inferiorly before tracking up the aorta. See the lateral decubitus abdominal image below for further appreciation of the course of the umbilical artery.

The umbilical vein catheter takes a completely different course along the umbilical vein. See also below

Double lumen catheters can be used in babies who are very sick and may require significant support.

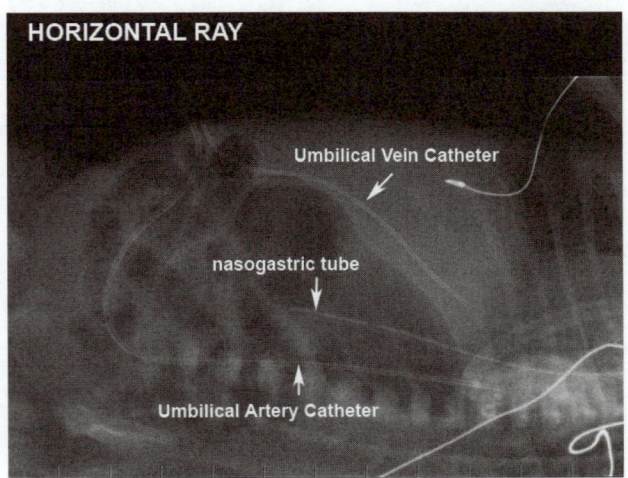

HORIZONTAL RAY

Umbilical Vein Catheter

nasogastric tube

Umbilical Artery Catheter

Transpyloric Tube and VP Shunt: The transpyloric tube (TPT) is similar to a nasogastric tube (NGT) except that it is longer and intended to have its tip sited distal to the pyloris. The ventriculo-peritoneal shunt provides a drainage path from the ventricles of the brain to the peritoneal cavity This image does not cover the entire length of the VP shunt- it should be complemented by a lateral skull view. Alternatively, I have seen radiographers employ a "head and torso" lateral approach in one image.

Central venous catheter (CVC) Longline- leg: The central venous catheter has been inserted in the right leg and its tip is difficult to localise precisely. This is a common problem with CVC lines and emphasizes the need for good quality images when checking CVC lines. A study of printed CR images vs soft copy CR images reported a long line detection rate of 66.7% vs 95.6% respectively. (A Evans, J Natarajan, C J Davies, 2004).

Other suggestions include
"The authors emphasise the importance of verifying neonatal long line position using contrast, as the exact localisation of the catheter tip can be difficult on plain radiographs. As an alternative, Groves *et al* have described the use of colour Doppler to aid ultrasonographic line tip visualisation." T M Berger, M

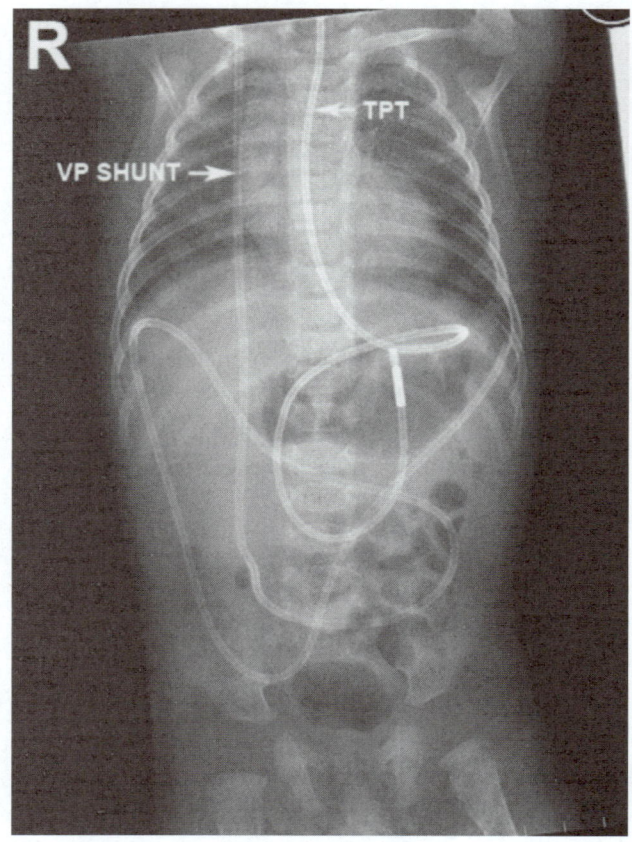

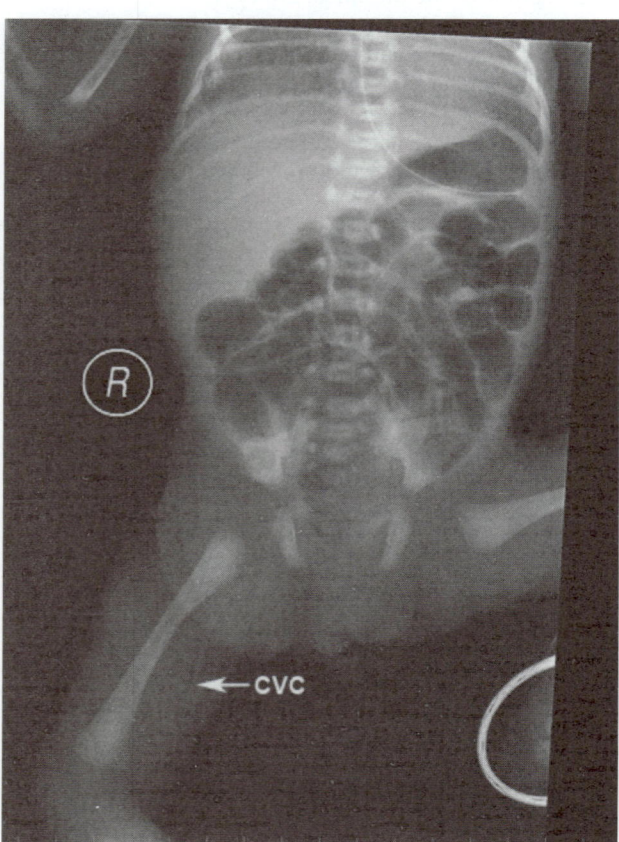

Central venous catheter (PICC)—arm

The technique issues are much the same as for a leg longline. Include the arm of interest and a good exposure is required. A softcopy digital image is best. The tip of the longline is in the proximal brachiocephalic vein. (lower white arrow) The top white arrow identifies the endotracheal tube (ETT) The black arrow identifies the nasogastric tube (NGT).

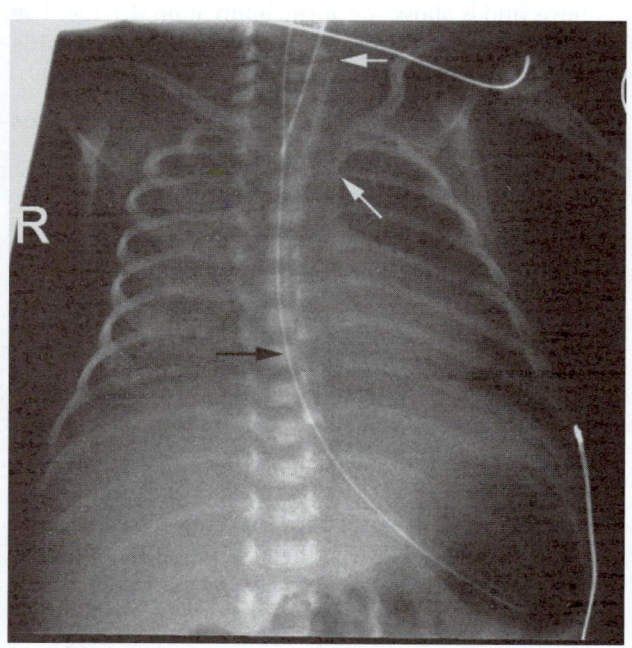

Case study

The radiographer was called to the Neonatal Unit and requested to undertake a chest/abdominal X-ray examination on one of the premature babies to establish the position of the double lumen Umbilical Vein Catheter (UVC). The image is shown on right.

- The tube at the top of the screen is the endotracheal tube (ETT) with its tip in close proximity to the carina

- There are three ECG leads (unmarked)

- The black arrow points to an umbilical catheter which appears to be in the arterial side (UAC). Note that the UAC dips down (as it enters the umbilicus) before changing direction—this is characteristic of a UAC rather than the UVC. The tip of the UAC is at the level of T8.

- The stomach is airfilled.

- The umbilical venous catheter (UVC) appears to be kinked (middle white arrow)

- The *lower* white arrow identifies an oval shaped radiolucent structure that does not correspond with any hollow abdominal viscus. The radiographer thought that this represented pneumoperitoneum.

- The radiographer was called back to the neonatal unit for abdominal radiography on the same baby 1 hour later. It was assumed that this was for a decubitus abdominal projection to prove the pneumoperitoneum. This was not the case- the umbilical venous catheter had been repositioned and this was a check X-ray. The pneumoperitoneum was not suspected by the neonatal unit staff. The radiographer asked if the abdominal image could be performed in the horizontal ray decubitus position. This was agreed to and the image is shown below.

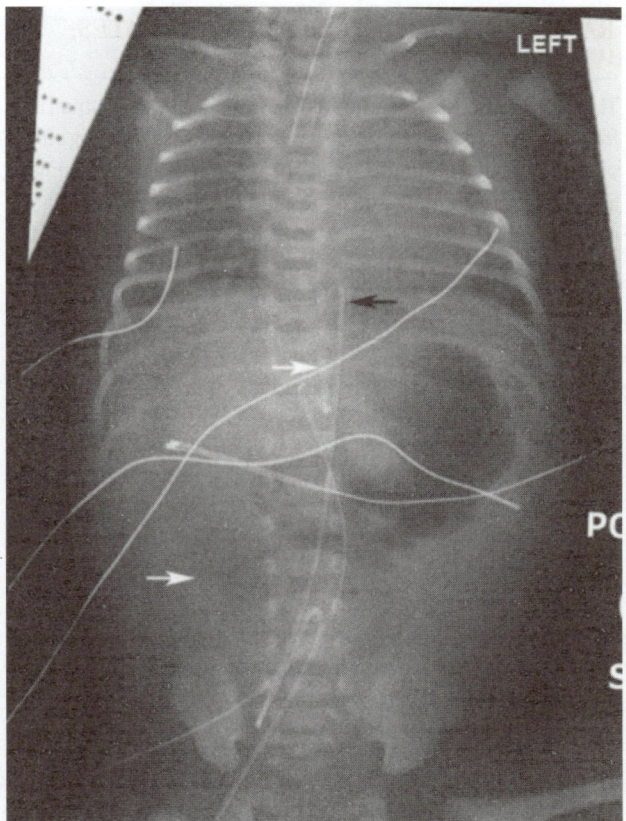

The horizontal ray decubitus abdominal image confirmed the pneumoperitoneum. The lateral edge of the baby's liver is contrasted against the free intraperitoneal gas. The UVC has been unkinked. The ideal position for the UVC is above the diaphragm but below the heart. The baby's left arm is superimposed over the left hemithorax

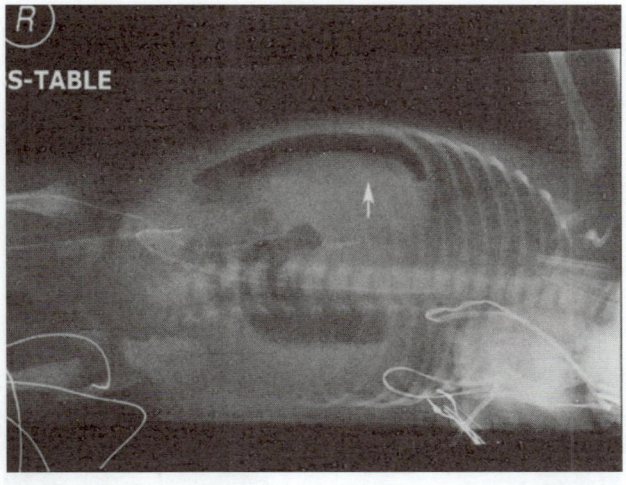

Abbreviations and terminology

UAC	: Umbilical artery catheter,
UVC	: Umbilical vein catheter,
ETT	: Endotracheal tube,
NGT	: Nasogastric tube ,
TPT	: Transpyloric tube,
VP Shunt	: Ventriculo-peritoneal shunt,
CVC	: Central Venous Catheter,
VLBW	: Very Low Birthweight,
NEC	: Necrotizing Enterocolitis

REFERENCE : *Applied Radiography - by M.J.Fuller*

RADIOLOGY OF THE CHEST IN NEONATES; WHAT IS NORMAL?

The unique diseases encountered in the neonate, their small size, fragile nature and increased susceptibility to the damaging effects of radiation all combine to make their imaging both challenging and interesting for the radiologist and radiographer. All radiation exposures must be justified. Meticulous attention to detail is a prerequisite to performing a good chest x-ray in young infants, requiring dedicated staff and equipment. Low dose techniques and adequate lead protection must always be employed.

It is a good policy that all frontal films are obtained with the patient supine, the arms extended above the head, and the pelvis stabilized in a frontal position by a nurse or an assistant;Holding the infant ensures that consistent positioning in the frontal projection is achieved. This allows serial exams to be compared without compensating for changes in rotation. It is also essential that technique factors be standardized for each patient. If at all possible, a single portable unit should be used for all neonatal x-ray procedures. Tube-film distance should be kept constant at about thirty-six to forty inches and exposure and kVP be recorded for each examination so that the film density does not vary significantly between studies.

Chest radiographs should be limited to the chest, which (approximately) is from the level of the infant's chin down to the umbilicus. The practice of routine "babygrams" should be discouraged. This unnecessarily increases radiation exposure to the patient and decreases the quality of the examination. The one exception is in films obtained immediately following the placement of umbilical lines because they often may either be purposely directed into the lower abdomen or inadvertently travel into the pelvis.

Assessment of Tubes and Lines:

Although it seems mundane, probably the most important function of neonatal chest radiography is to assess positions of the multiple tubes and lines that are placed during the course of the neonate's intensive care stay . The endotracheal tube (ETT) should be located somewhere between the suprasternal notch and the carina. This corresponds with the second through fifth thoracic vertebra (approximately). With the head restrained in the neutral or AP position the tip of the ETT is actually about one half to one centimeter lower than it would be with the head turned to the side.Umbilical artery catheters are usually placed either "high" between the sixth and tenth thoracic vertebra or low, at approximately the level of the aortic bifurcation (or about L3-L4).

The umbilical venous catheter (UVC) is usually positioned at the base of the right atrium. Depending upon the size of the liver and any degree of rotation of the patient, the umbilical venous catheter may appear to be right or left of the midline. The umbilical artery catheter (UAC) always parallels the spine.

All of these catheters and tubes are radiopaque and do not require contrast injection for localization. Standard technique will demonstrate the positions of the endotracheal tube and vascular lines. There is no need to purposely over expose a film that has been obtained for verification of line placement.

When viewing a radiograph, remember that it is a 2-dimensional representation of a 3-dimensional human being. Height and width are maintained, but depth is lost. When viewing an x-ray, the left side of the film represents the right side of the individual, and the visa versa. Air appears black, soft tissues appear as differing shades of gray, and bone appears white. When determining if a chest x-ray is readable, some questions need to be asked.

Is there significant rotation?

Rotation means that the baby was not positioned flat on the x-ray film, and one plane of the chest is rotated in comparison to the plane of the film. Rotation introduces distortion because it can make the lungs look asymmetrical and it can change the orientation of the cardiac silhouette. If there has been good positioning of the baby, the right and left lung fields should be nearly the same diameter. The heads of the ribs (end of the calcified section of each rib) should be at the same location in relationship to the chest wall. If there is significant rotation, the side which has been lifted may appear narrower and more dense (white) and the cardiac silhouette appears more in the opposite lung field.

Is the x-ray underexposed or overexposed?

A properly penetrated chest radiograph is one which the intervertebral bodies can be seen. An under-penetrated chest x-ray does not differentiate the vertebral bodies from the intervertebral spaces. An over-penetrated film shows the intervertebral spaces very distinctly. Why is it important to have a properly exposed radiograph? An over-penetrated x-ray will be darker, and the subtleties will be harder to see. An under-penetrated x-ray will emphasize normal lung and make it appear as if there are infiltrates (areas of opacification).

Chest x-rays of Neonates are in compliance with the technical standards when they meet the following criteria: a) Visualization of dorsal intervertebral spaces through the cardiac silhouette (film density); b) right hemi-diaphragm at the level of the posterior arc of the eighth rib (satisfactory level of pulmonary aeration); c) caudal inclination of anterior costal arcs appearing underneath the posterior ones (adequate centralization of the central beam on the thoracic cage); d) symmetry of bone structures on both sides of the thoracic cage (correct positioning of the Neonate).

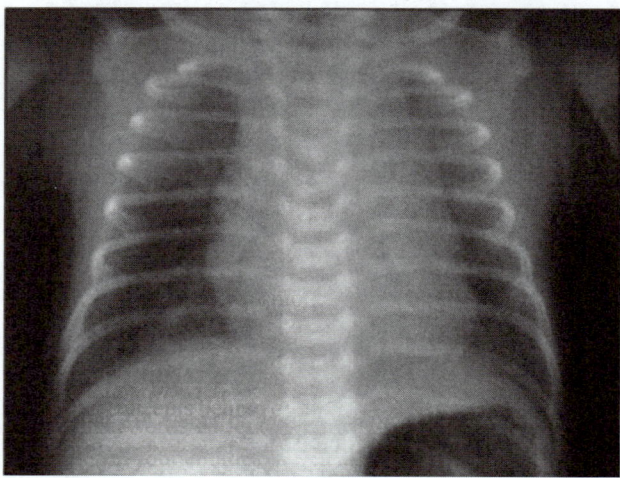

Normal CXR in a 2-hour old Newborn, in compliance with technical standards.

Main technical problems that may mimic pathological alterations inducing misdiagnosis are the following: a) X-ray beam underpenetration, reducing the density differences between intrathoracic structures and simulating false pulmonary opacities; b) pulmonary hypoaeration, resulting in horizontalization of costal arcs, false widening of the cardiothymic silhouette and reduction of the pulmonary transparency, with possibility of, occasionally, simulating pulmonary edema, hemorrhage, atelectasis and pneumonic consolidations; c) x-ray beam overpenetration, darkening the radiographic film and possibly concealing pulmonary opacities, mainly the most subtle ones, like interstitial opacities of the neonate transitory tachypnea and the reticulogranular infiltrate of the hyaline membrane disease; d) patient rotation, causing asymmetry of the chest and resulting in a false prominence of the cardiothymic image towards the deviation side; e) inadequate centralization of the central ray over the neonate's abdomen, causing a lordotic configuration of the thoracic cage characterized by the cephalic orientation of the anterior arcs, and possibly causing widening and distortion of the cardiothymic image. The knowledge of these criteria utilized for evaluating the technical quality of chest x-ray of neonates results in technically correct x-rays, besides reducing the possibility of misdiagnosis due inadequately performed examinations.

INTRATHORACIC ANATOMIC STRUCTURES The neonate chest undergoes significant birth-related changes during the first hours of life, and presents quite distinct aspects in its anatomic structures, so these normal, specific radiological features should be taken into consideration during the neonatal period. During the first hours of a neonate's life, transitory cardiomegaly may occur as a result of additional blood inflow from the placenta into the umbilical cord before its cutting, and of the presence of a bidirectional shunt through the arterial duct and oval foramen before its closure. Also, a prominent pulmonary vascularization may be observed as a result of residual lung fluid absorption through the lymphatic-venous system. A still open arterial canal may be seen on a chest x-ray as a convex prominence to the left of the spine, between T3 and T4 vertebras, this configuration being denominated *ductus bump*, that is considered as a typical radiological finding at the neonate first hours of life. The oval foramen and arterial canal closure, the decrease in pulmonary vascular resistance and absorption of the remaining lung fluid in the hours subsequent to the birth reduce the cardiac dimensions and the chest vascular prominence. In neonates, the thymus is radiologically characterized by a widening of the upper mediastinum, above the cardiac image, on the frontal view, and an increase in the supracardiac, retrosternal density on the profile incidence. On the frontal view, the normal width of the thymic image must be higher than the doublewidth of the third thoracic vertebra, shorter dimensions representing a sign of thymic involution. Under stress fever, infections, congenital cardiopathies, pulmonary diseases, malnutrition —, there may be a rapid thymic involution as a result of the adrenal corticosteroid action, and yet its image may not be visualized on chest x-rays. This accidental involution may revert once the stress situation is overcome, and the thymus returns to its normal dimensions. Also, the thymus may present peculiar features, including the "wave sign" corresponding to a gentle undulation on the thymus surface produced by costal arcs compression, more frequently to the left; the "notch sign", where the inferior border of the normal thymus blends with the border of the cardiac silhouette; and the "sail sign"

resulting from a peculiar shape of the thymus appearing like a normal anterior mediastinal sail shaped structure, more frequently to the right.

EXTRATHORACIC STRUCTURES

Soft tissues, the skeletal structure and the abdomen may provide relevant information for clinical management of neonates. The thickness of the thoracic wall soft tissues reflects the nutritional condition, and may be decreased in light-weight newborn infants. Secondary ossification nuclei of the proximal humeral extremity and coracoid apophysis may be visualized on chest xrays, and a relation is established between the presence of these ossification nuclei and the term gestational age of the neonate, therefore representing a sign of fetal maturity. Typically, the presence of air may be observed in the stomach right at birth, small bowel with three hours of live, and in the rectum, six to eight hours after birth, so it is always important to correlate radiological findings with the neonate's number of hours of life. CATHETERS, CANNULAS AND PROBES-In the analysis of chest and abdomen xrays, it is very important to describe the localization of cannulas, probes and catheters, since the incorrect positioning of these tubes may cause iatrogenies. The umbilical venous catheter follows its course through the umbilical vein, venous duct and inferior vena cava, presenting a straight course at the right side of the thoracic-lumbar spine. The correct site for its extremity is the inferior vena cava, nearby the right atrium entry at right of T8- T9. The umbilical arterial catheter presents a small curvature in its entry into the right or left umbilical artery, passing through the internal and common iliac arteries up to the abdominal aorta where it is placed preferably above the level of iliac arteries bifurcation at L3-L5 — low localization—, or in the thoracic aorta under the arterial canal between T7 and T9 — high localization. Umbilical catheters should not be situated in the origin of smaller caliber vascular trunks under the risk of precipitating spasms and thrombosis. In patients under assisted respiration, the endotracheal intubation cannula should be placed in the medium third of the trachea, above the carina, and is visualized at T4 level and below the medial clavicle. In patients with gastric probing, the probe should be visualized at the right of the tracheal cannula and its end should be located in the stomach.

IMAGE ARTIFACTS

Artifacts must be identified, since ignoring their peculiarities may induce the diagnosis of inexistent diseases by the interpreter-physician. One of the most frequent image artifacts are the skin folds projected over the thoracic cavity, and may simulate pneumothorax. The differential diagnosis is made by observing this artifact as a dense, linear image presenting an obliquity as opposed to the lung border, extending below the thoracic cavity. Another eventual image artifact is the projection of the neonatal incubator access ports producing lower density round images which may be confused with cystic lesions.

Key points for clinical practice:

*High quality chest radiography is essential.
*Consider radiographic techniques and artefacts when interpreting the chest X ray.
*Check the position of all catheters, tubes, and wires and record on the film if the position is subsequently corrected.
*Integration of clinical & radiological features is the key to making the correct diagnosis.
*Consider less common causes of respiratory distress when the chest X ray is normal or findings are atypical

Courtesy: Prof. Beatriz Regina Álvares Department of Radiology – Faculty of Medical Sciences of Universidade Estadual de Campinas, Campinas, SP, Brazil.

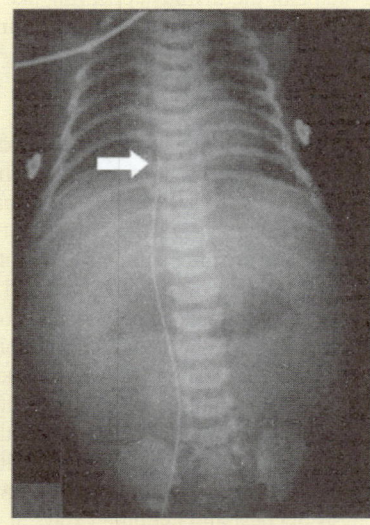

Twenty-four-hour old Newborn infant chest and abdomen x-ray presenting venous umbilical catheter localized in the inferior vena cava(arrow)

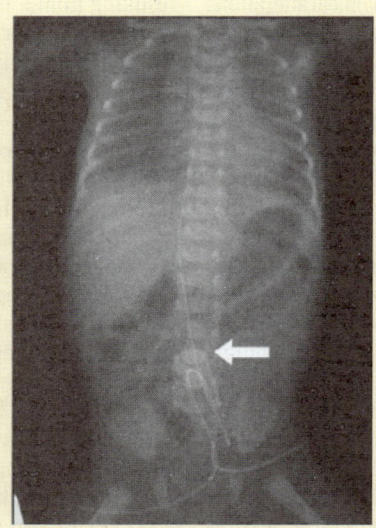

Newborn infant x-ray demonstrating low localization of arterial umbilical catheter at the L4 level (arrow).

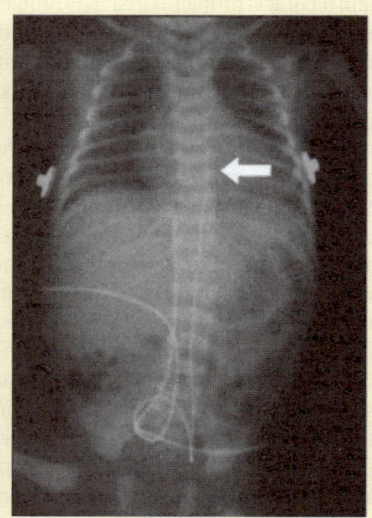

Newborn infant x-ray showing high-localization of arterial umbilical catheter (arrow).

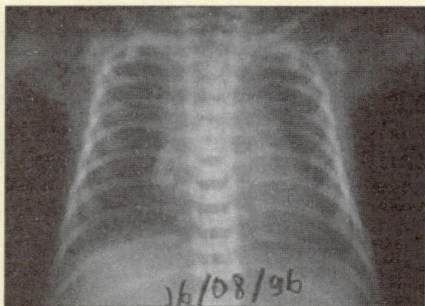

Chest x-ray of (A) three-hour-old, and (B) four-day-old Newborn infant, showing thymus involution.

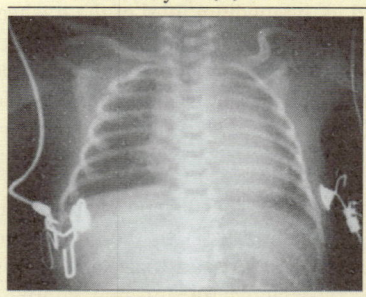

Oblique chest x-ray of a Newborn infant demonstrating bilateral clavicles and costal arcs asymmetry.

Two-hour-old Newborn infant chest x-ray with x-ray tube misalignment. Anterior costal arcs present cephalic orientation, projecting themselves above their posterior segments.

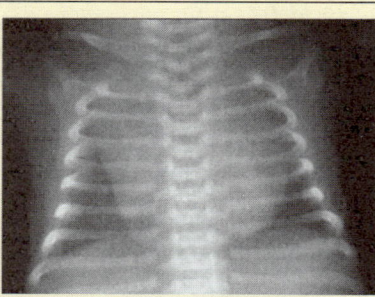

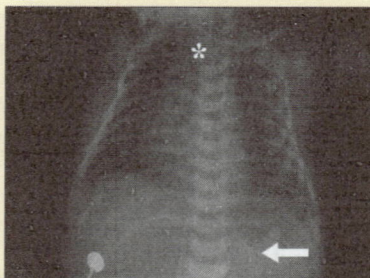

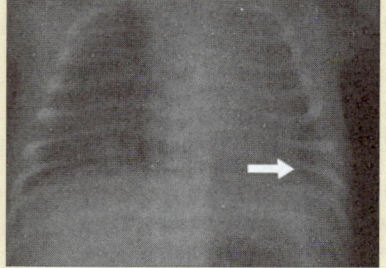

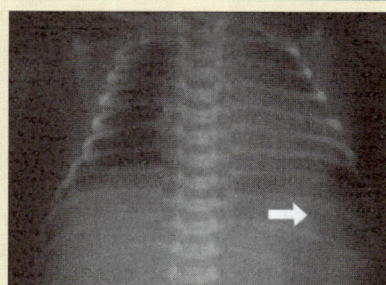

In patients under assisted respiration, the endotracheal intubation cannula should be placed in the medium third of the trachea, above the carina, and is visualized at T4 level and below the medial clavicle.In patients with gastric probing, the probe should be visualized at the right of the tracheal cannula and its end should be located in the stomach.

Artifacts must be identified, since ignoring their peculiarities may induce the diagnosis of inexistent diseases by the interpreter-physician. One of the most frequent image artifacts are the skin folds projected over the thoracic cavity, and may simulate pneumothorax. The differential diagnosis is made by observing this artifact as a dense, linear image presenting an obliquity as opposed to the lung border, extending below the thoracic cavity.

Another eventual image artifact is the projection of the neonatal incubator access ports producing lower density round images which may be confused with cystic lesions.

Electrocardiography records the electrical activity of the heart and is a useful, though under-utilized investigation in pediatric practice. It supplements the information obtained by clinical examination and chest radiography. ECG helps mostly in the assessment of chamber size, arrhythmias and ischemia. Rapid changes occur over the first year of life as a result of the dramatic changes in circulation and cardiac physiology. After infancy, subsequent changes are more gradual until late adolescence and adulthood. It is essential to follow a systematic approach to ECG interpretation with special attention to rate, rhythm, axis, intervals, ventricular and atrial hypertrophy, and the presence of any ischemia or repolarization abnormalities.

The limitations of Pediatric ECG are as follows:

*Age dependent changes noted-no single set of criteria can be used for all ages. *Chamber enlargement rules are used from adult experience. *Poor sensitivity; e.g. A large VSD may not have large LV forces. *Absence of specific guidelines for chest lead placements. *Interpretation requires practice as there are no validated normograms for age. *Congenital heart diseases have very few lesion specific changes on ECG.

Basics of recording and interpretation :

Usual 12 lead ECG is not enough in pediatrics; frequently, additional right ventricular and posterior left ventricular precordial leads (V3R, V4R, and V7) are included with pediatric ECGs to provide additional information on patients who have complex congenital abnormalities. The placement of leads must be more proximal in children to avoid limb-motion artifacts. Standard gains of 10mm/mV is used. If the QRS voltage is very large, then the gain may be halved. Each small block is 1mm high and each large block represents 5mm (vertical block). The horizontal axis represents the length of each electrical event in time. Each small block measures 0.04seconds and a large block (comprising of 5 small ones) correlates to 0.20 seconds. Intervals are better hand-measured as the computerized systems are often inaccurate. The intervals increase with increasing age and reach adult values by 7-8 years of age.

What does each wave represent?

P wave represents atrial depolarization. This is the time taken by an electrical impulse to spread from the sino-atrial node through the atrial musculature. This wave precedes the QRS complex and is best measured in lead II.

The **PR interval** represents the time taken by an impulse to travel from the atria to the Purkinge fibres through the AV-node, bundle of His and the bundle branches. This is measured from the beginning of the P wave to the beginning of the QRS complex.In neonates, it ranges from 0.08–0.15 sec and in adolescents from 0.120–0.20 sec.

Q wave - Septal depolarization **RS wave** - Ventricular depolarization

The **QRS complex** follows the PR interval and consists of 3 waves- the Q wave, R wave and S wave. The Q wave is always at the beginning of the QRS complex and may or may not be present. The R wave is the first positive deflection and is followed by the S wave which is a negative deflection.

The **QT interval** extends from the beginning of the QRS complex to the end of T wave and represents the time necessary for ventricular depolarization and repolarization. This interval is best measured in leads II, V5 and V6 and the longest interval is used. Because the QT interval varies greatly with heart rate, it is usually corrected (QTc), most commonly using Bazett's formula: QTc = QT/*Square root of* RR interval. During the first half of infancy, the normal QTc is longer than in older children and adults. In the first 6 months of life, the QTc is considered normal at less than 0.49 sec. After infancy, this cutoff is generally 0.44 sec.

The **T wave** represents ventricular repolarization and follows the S wave and S-T segment. At times, a **U-wave** follows the T wave and represents the repolarization of His and Purkinje fibres.

Courtesy : *Sumitra Venkatesh, Shakuntala Prabhu* Div. of Pediatric Cardiology, Dept. of Pediatrics, B.J.Wadia Hospital for Children, Mumbai.

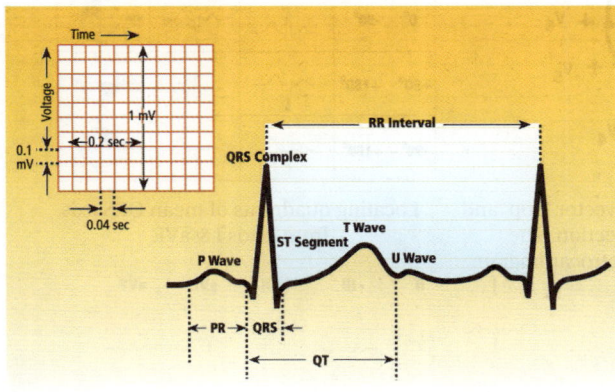

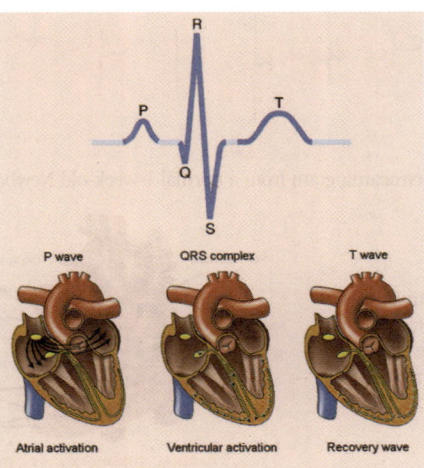

Atrial activation   Ventricular activation   Recovery wave

Steps to read Pediatric Electrocardiograms:

The electrocardiogram must be read systematically in the following order to extract the maximum information possible.*Knowing what is normal in pediatric age group helps to easily identify what is abnormal:*

Heart rate , QRS axis , Intervals-PR,QRS,QT/QTc

P-wave amplitude and duration

QRS and Q-wave amplitude ,R/S ratio

S-T segment and T-wave

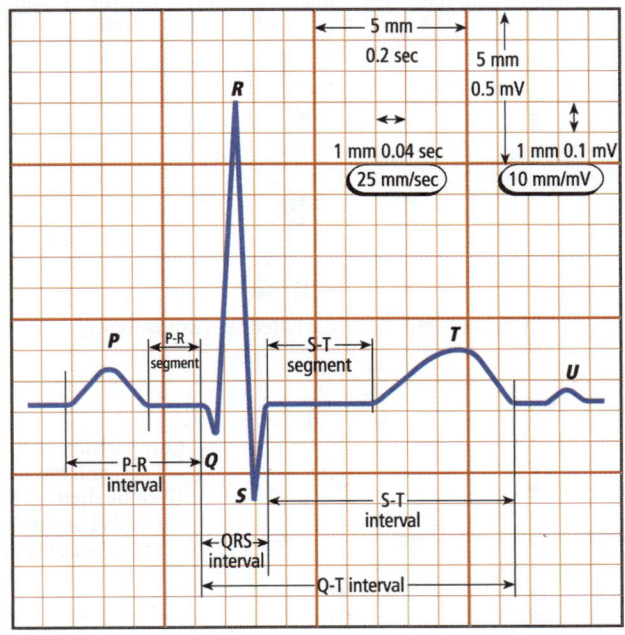

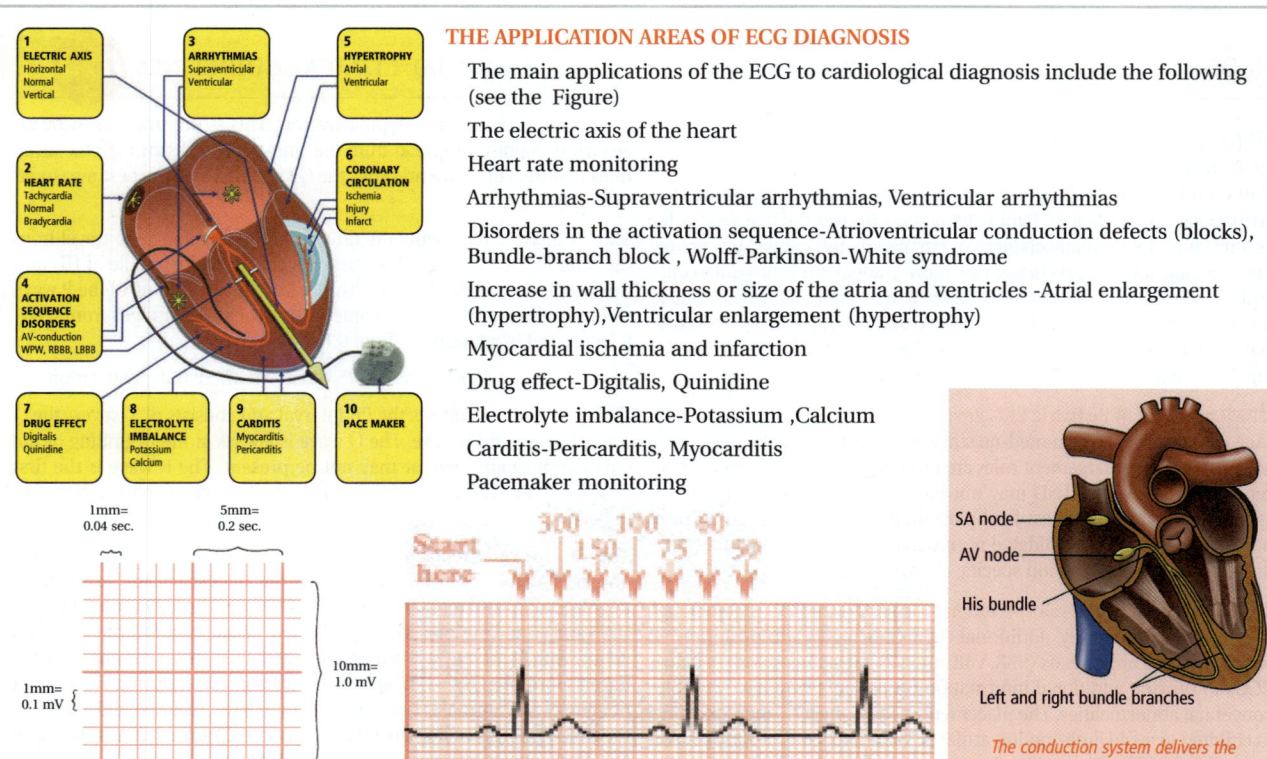

THE APPLICATION AREAS OF ECG DIAGNOSIS

The main applications of the ECG to cardiological diagnosis include the following (see the Figure)

The electric axis of the heart

Heart rate monitoring

Arrhythmias-Supraventricular arrhythmias, Ventricular arrhythmias

Disorders in the activation sequence-Atrioventricular conduction defects (blocks), Bundle-branch block , Wolff-Parkinson-White syndrome

Increase in wall thickness or size of the atria and ventricles -Atrial enlargement (hypertrophy),Ventricular enlargement (hypertrophy)

Myocardial ischemia and infarction

Drug effect-Digitalis, Quinidine

Electrolyte imbalance-Potassium ,Calcium

Carditis-Pericarditis, Myocarditis

Pacemaker monitoring

The conduction system delivers the electrical signal to the entire heart

Standards conventions when reading an ECG: The rate of paper (i.e. of recording of the ECG) is 25 mm/s which results in: *1 mm = 0.04 sec (or each individual block) *5 mm = 0.2 sec (or between 2 dark vertical lines) *The voltage recorded from the leads is also standardized on the paper where 1 mm = 0.1 mV (or between each individual block vertically) This results in: *5 mm = 0.5 mV (or between 2 dark horizontal lines) *10 mm = 1.0 mv (this is how it is usually marked on the ECG's)

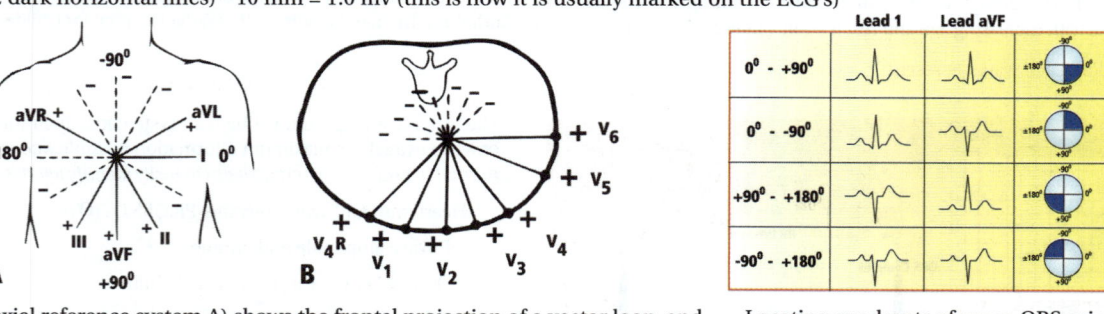

Hexaxial reference system A) shows the frontal projection of a vector loop, and horizontal reference system. B) shows the horizontal projection. The combination of A & B constitutes the 12 - lead (or 13-lead) electrocardiogram.

Locating quadrants of mean QRS axis from leads I & aVF.

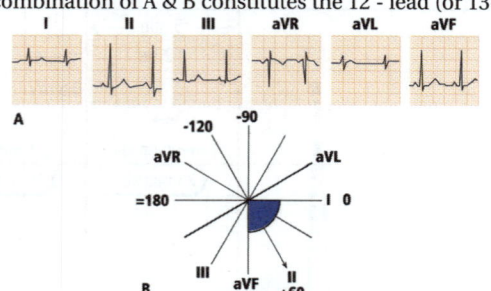

A, Set of 6 limb leads B, Plotted QRS axis is shown

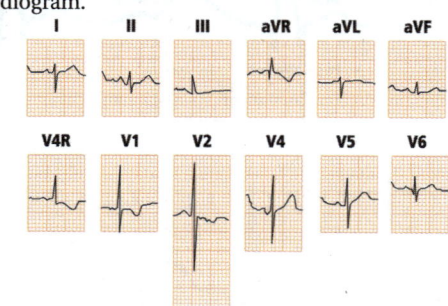

Electrocardiogram from a normal 1-week-old Newborn

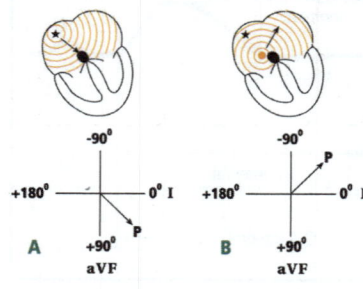

Comparision of P axis in sinus rhythm A) and low atrial rhythm B).
In sinus rhythm, the P waves are upright in leads I and aVF. In low artial rhythm, the P wave is inverted in lead aVF.

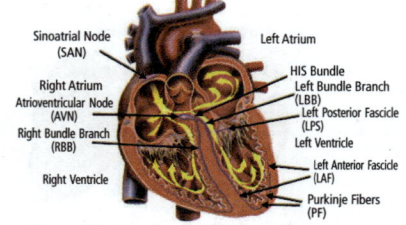

CARDIAC CONDUCTION SYSTEM

Rate calculation: Heart rate = 1500 / Number of small squares in one R-R interval: Count the number of big boxes between the 2 R waves, if: 1= 300 bpm, 2 = 150 bpm, 3 = 100 bpm, 4 =70 bpm and 5 = 60 bpm (bpm = beats per minute). In children , cardiac output is determined primarily by heart rate as opposed to stroke volume. With age, the heart rate decreases as the ventricles mature and stroke volume plays a larger role in cardiac output. Age and activity-appropriate heart rates thus must be recognized. Average resting heart rate varies with age; Newborns can range from 90-160 beats per minute (bpm) and adolescents from 50-120 bpm. The average heart rate peaks about the second month of life and thereafter gradually decreases until adolescence. Heart rates grossly outside the normal range for age should be scrutinized closely for dysrhythmias. **Axis detection:** Axis helps to interpret the major vector of depolarization. Determine if the net QRS voltage is positive or negative in lead I and lead AVF. For example, if the R wave height is 10 mm (above the isoelectric line) and S wave height is 4 mm (below the isoelectric line), then the net QRS voltage is positive (+6). If the R wave is short and S wave is longer, the net QRS voltage would be negative.

The QRS axis can be located using the following simple rule

Lead I	Lead aVF	Interpretation	Comment
Positive	Positive	Normal axis	Abnormal in Neonates and early infancy
Negative	Positive	Right axis deviation	Normal in Neonates and in early infancy
Positive	Negative	Left axis deviation	Abnormal at any age
Negative	Negative	North-west axis	Abnormal at any age

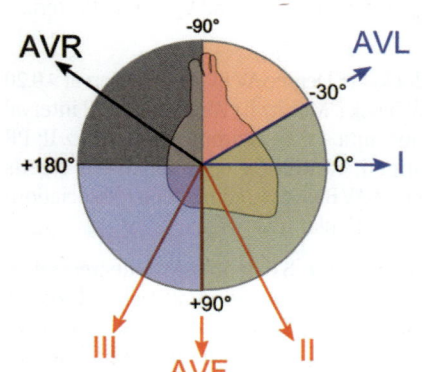

The Wave configuration

Evaluate P wave in lead II and V1, if P wave is >2.5 boxes wide or tall, it is suggestive of left or right atrial enlargement respectively. LAE is denoted by 'wide and notched' P-waves and RAE is denoted by 'tall and peaked' P-waves. The RV hypertrophy or LV hypertrophy determination depends on the R-wave and S-wave voltages and their ratio (R/S).Tall R in V1 (R/S >1) with deep S in V6 and upright T waves in right precordial leads suggests RVH. Tall R in V5 and V6 with deep S in V1 and T wave abnormalities in V5 and V6 suggests LVH .

ECG tracing showing Left Ventricular Hypertrophy (LVH) with S in V1 deeper than 95% of normal and R in V6 taller than 95% of normal

ECG criteria for ventricular and atrial hypertrophy

Right ventricular hypertrophy

R wave greater than the 98th percentile in lead VI a
S wave greater than the 98th percentile in lead I or V6
RSR' pattern in lead V1, with the R' height being greater than 15 mm in infants younger than 1 year of age or greater than 10 mm in children older than 1 year of age
Q wave in lead V1

Left ventricular hypertrophy

R-wave amplitude greater than 98th percentile in lead V5 or V6
R wave less than 5th percentile in lead V1 or V2
S-wave amplitude greater than 98th percentile in lead V1
Q wave greater than 4 mm in lead V5 or V6
Inverted T wave in lead V6

Right atrial enlargement

Peaked P wave in leads II and V1 that is higher than 3 mm in infants younger than 6 months of age and greater than 2.5 mm in infants older than 6 months of age

Left atrial enlargement

P-wave duration greater than 0.08 seconds in a child younger than 12 months of age or greater than 10 ms in children 1 year and older
P wave minimal or plateau contour
Terminal or deeply inverted P wave in lead V1 or V3R

The presence of any of these is suspicious for hypertrophy. It is not necessary for all of the criteria to be met.
a qR wave pattern in V1 may be seen in 10% of normal newborns.

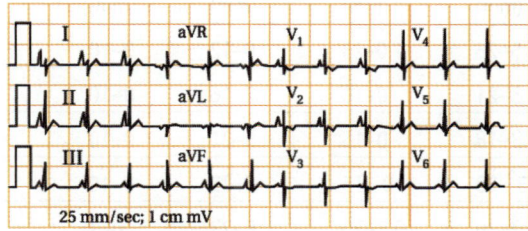

ECG tracing showing tall P waves suggestive of Right atrial enlargement

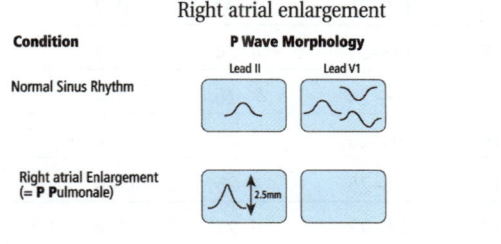

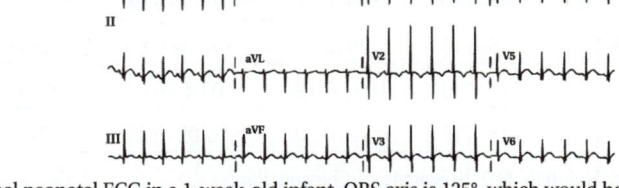

Normal neonatal ECG in a 1-week-old infant. QRS axis is 125°, which would be considered right axis deviation in an adult. Note the tall R waves in V1, V2, and V3, which are normal.

S-T and T wave changes suggest ischemia or repolarization abnormalities. The elevation of ST-segment up to 1-4mm with the concavity facing upwards is normal. Any variation in the above depicts early repolarization, pericarditis, hyperkalemia, pneumothorax or pneumopericardium. ST depression is suggestive of pressure overload/strain.

In pediatric patients, T-wave changes on the ECG tend to be nonspecific and are often a source of controversy. What is agreed on is that flat or inverted T waves are normal in the newborn. In fact, the T waves in leads V1 through V3 usually are inverted after the first week of life through the age of 8 years as the so-called "juvenile" T-wave pattern . Persistence of which suggests RVH.T wave inversion in leads I, V5 and V6 is seen in ischemic conditions like ALCAPA, Kawasaki Disease and pressure overload/strain. Tall T wave suggests hyperkalemia and absent T-wave with U-wave suggests hypokalemia.

Getting the Basics from the ECG : Summary

The basic things to read from the ECG is the following: **Rate Rhythm Axis P wave morphology PR interval QRS complex morphology ST segment morphology T wave morphology U wave morphology QTc interval**

1. **Rate** if regular, then count the number of large squares between R waves; 1 square = 300 bpm, 2 = 150 bpm, 3 = 100 bpm, 4 = 75 bpm, 5 = 60 bpm, 6 = 50 bpm. Each small box = 0.04 s, each large box = 5 small boxes = 0.20 s.

2. **Rhythm** is it regular? (use calipers/ruler to make sure all R-R intervals are the same); are there P waves, and are they in front of every QRS? (in sinus rhythm, P waves will be upright in lead II); are P waves all identical?

3. **Intervals** *PR interval:* *QRS interval:* * QT interval

4. **Axis deviation** net QRS deflection should be positive in both leads I and aVF *Right axis deviation: QRS negative in I, positive in aVF * Left axis deviation: QRS positive in I, negative in aVF

5. **Hypertrophy**

   Left ventricular hypertrophy: Refer to the Criteria mentioned above

   Left atrial enlargement: P waves are notched (M-shaped) in I, II, or aVL or a deep terminal negative component to P in V_1

   Right atrial enlargement: Tall, peaked P waves (> 3 mm) in II, III, aVF

Right ventricular hypertrophy: Refer to the Criteria mentioned above

6. **Infarction:** *Q waves:* small, normal Q waves can be seen in lateral leads (I, aVL, V_4 to V_6), while moderate-large sized Q waves may be normal in leads III, aVF, aVL, and V_1. To localize the infarction, look for groupings of Q waves in the following leads…Inferior-II, III, aVF; Anteroseptal-V_1 to V_3;

   Anterior-V_3 and V_4; Anterolateral–V_4 and V_6, I, aVL; Posterior-V_1 and V_2

7. **Heart Block (AV block)** *1st Degree AV block: PR interval > 0.20 sec *2nd Degree AV block i. Mobitz I: (Wenkeback) PR interval progressively widens until a beat is dropped ii. Mobitz II: PR interval is prolonged, randomly dropped beat. Needs Pacemaker *3rd Degree AV Block: No connection (dissociation) between atrial and ventricular rates.

8. **Other pearls** *Hypokalemia*: ST depression, decreased or inverted T waves, U waves *Hyperkalemia*: Peaked T waves, decreased P waves, short QT, widened QRS, sine wave *Hypocalcemia*: prolonged QT, flat or inverted T waves *Hypercalcemia*: short or absent ST, decreased QT_c interval *Hypomagnesemia*: prolonged QT, flat T waves, prolonged PR, aFib, torsade *Hypermagnesemia*: short PR, heart block, peaked T waves, widened QRS0 *Digitalis toxicity:* ST depression (scoop), flat T waves *Quinidine:* prolonged QT, widened QRS *Pericarditis:* diffuse ST elevation with PR interval depression

Pediatric ECG: Normal values by Age

Age	HR (bpm)	QRS axis (degrees)	PR interval (sec)	QRS interval (sec)	R in V1 (mm)	S in V1 (mm)	R in V6 (mm)	S in V6 (mm)
1st wk	90–160	60–180	0.08–0.15	0.03–0.08	5–26	0–23	0–12	0–10
1–3 wk	100–180	45–160	0.08–0.15	0.03–0.08	3–21	0–16	2–16	0–10
1–2 mo	120–180	30–135	0.08–0.15	0.03–0.08	3–18	0–15	5–21	0–10
3– 5 mo	105 –185	0–135	0.08–0.15	0.03–0.08	3–20	0 –15	6–22	0–10
6–11 mo	110–170	0–135	0.07–0.16	0.03–0.08	2–20	0.5–20	6–23	0–7
1–2 yr	90–165	0–110	0.08–0.16	0.03–0.08	2–18	0.5–21	6–23	0–7
3–4 yr	70–140	0–110	0.09–0.17	0.04–0.08	1–18	0.5–21	4–24	0–5
5 7 yr	65 –140	0 –110	0.09–0.17	0.04–0.08	0.5 –14	0.5– 24	4 –26	0–4
8–11 yr	60–130	–15–110	0.09–0.17	0.04–0.09	0–14	0.5–25	4–25	0–4
12 –15 yr	65 –130	–15–110	0.09 –0.18	0.04 –0.09	0– 14	0.5–25	4–25	0 –4
>16 yr	50–120	–15–110	0.12–0.20	0.05–0.10	0–14	0.5–23	4–21	0–4

Courtesy of Ra'id Abdullah, MD, University of Chicago, Illinois.

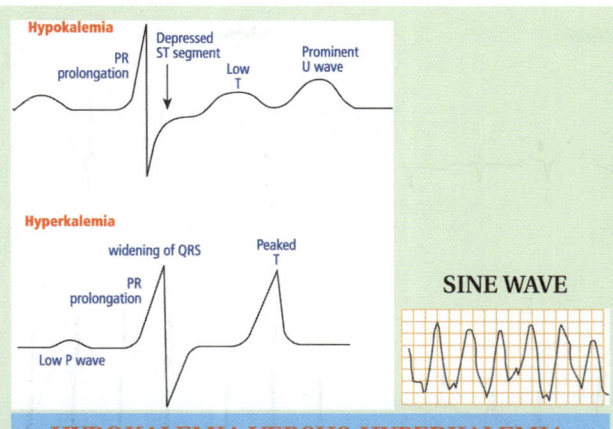

SINE WAVE

HYPOKALEMIA VERSUS HYPERKALEMIA

Hypokalemia On the ECG, the QRS complexes begin to widen when the serum potassium drops to about 3 mEq/L, the ST segments may become depressed, and the T waves may begin to flatten. The U waves also begin to increase in size, becoming as tall as the T waves. The U waves reach "giant" size and fuse with the T waves when the level drops to 1 mEq/L. **Hyperkalemia** The QRS complexes may widen so that they merge with the T waves, resulting in a "sine wave" appearance. The ST segments disappear when the serum potassium level reaches 6 mEq/L and the T waves typically become tall and peaked at this same range. The P waves begin to flatten out and widen when a patient's serum potassium level reaches about 6.5 mEq/L(PR interval lengthens QRS duration increases); this effect tends to disappear when levels reach 7-9 mEq/L. Sinus arrest in asystole may occur when the serum potassium level reaches about 7.5 mEq/L, and cardiac standstill or ventricular fibrillation may occur when serum levels reach 10 to 12 mEq/L.Sine waves are produced by the merging of widened QRS complexes with their corresponding T waves, if the Hyperkalemia is severe.

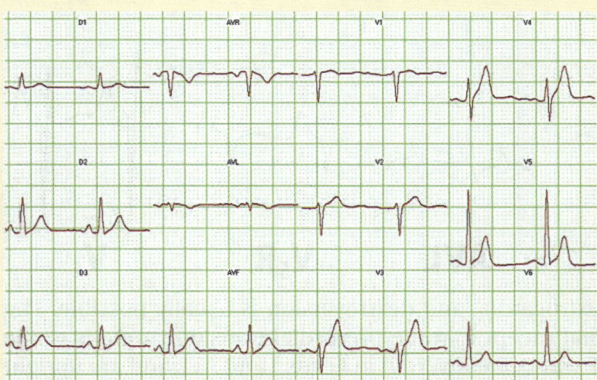

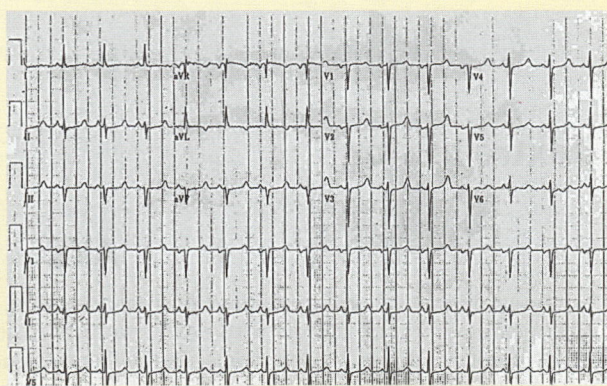

Hypercalcemia: Electrocardiographic Findings A shortening of the QTc interval The decrease is at the expense of the ST segment which becomes shortened or absent. This is true for Ca of up to 16 mEq/L, after this QTc prolongation occurs**.**

Hypocalcemia: Electrocardiographic Findings Prolongation of the QTc interval is the major ECG finding There is a lengthening of the interval between the end of the QRS and the beginning of the T wave (i.e. ST-segment lengthening)

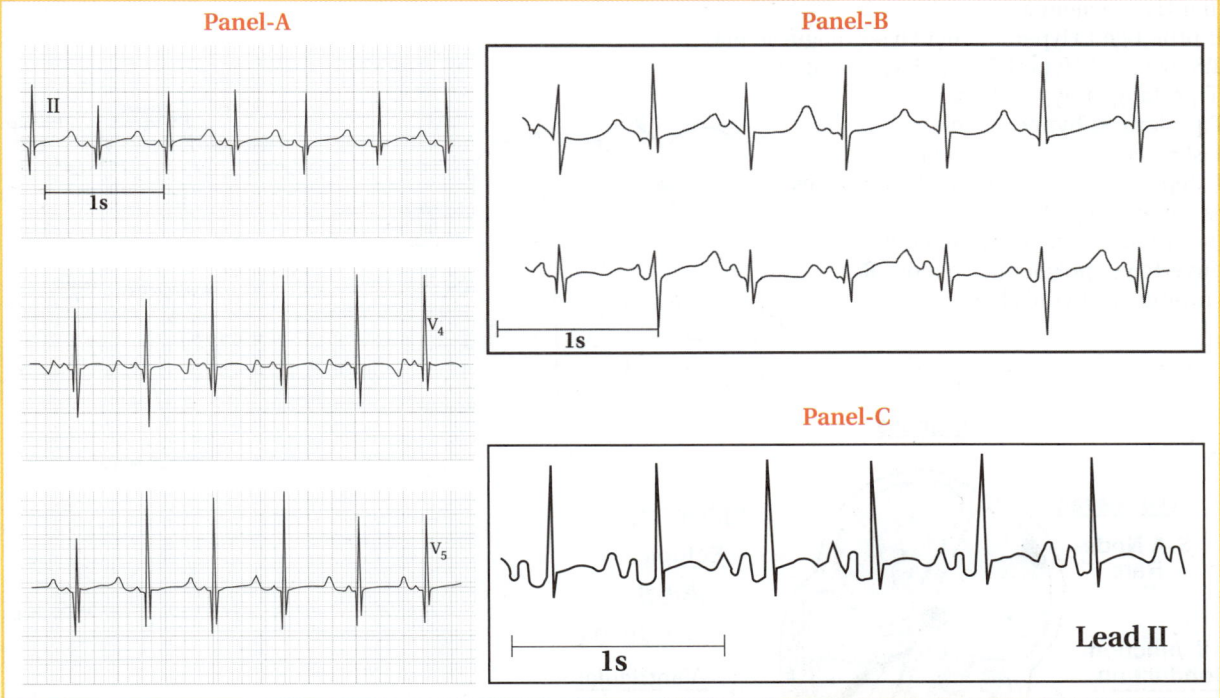

ECG tracings of three newborns with LQTS diagnosed in the first months of life. Mutations on the potassium channel gene *KvLQT1* (panel A) and on the sodium channel gene *SCN5A* (panel B) were identified.

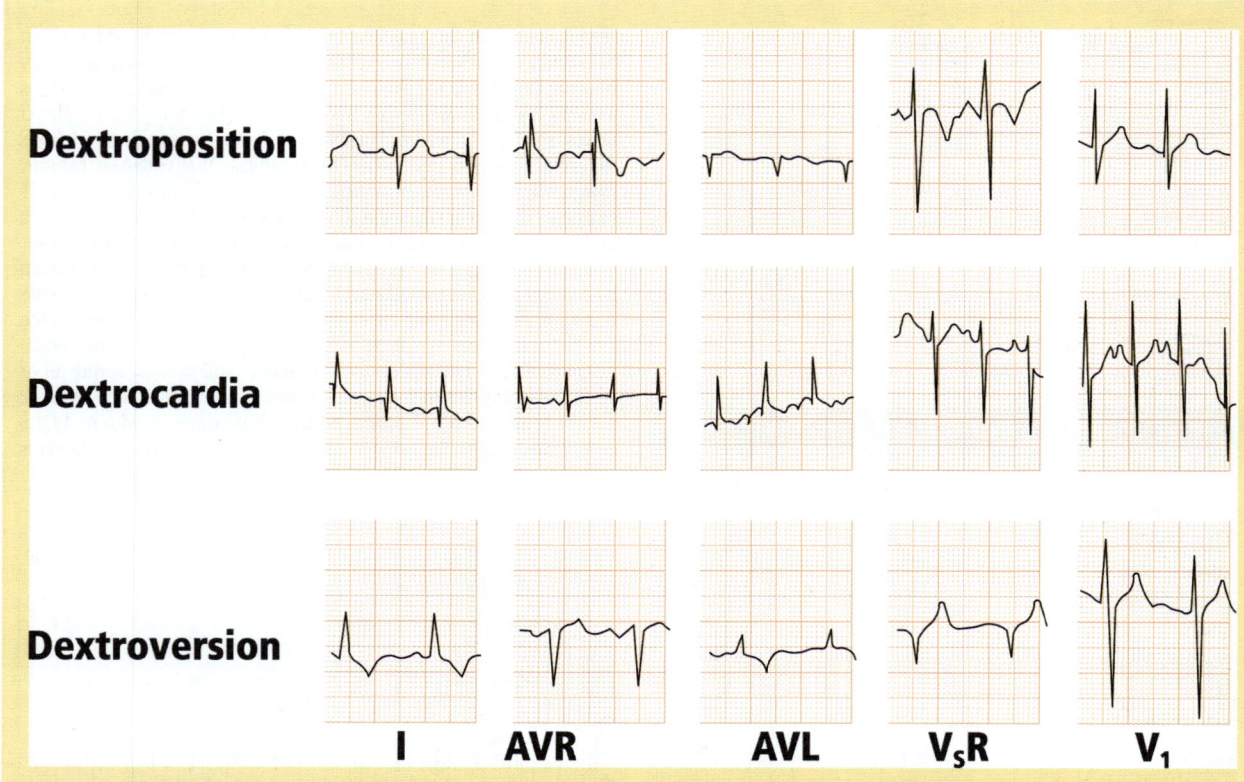

Dextroposition

Dextrocardia

Dextroversion

| I | AVR | AVL | V$_S$R | V$_1$ |

Electrocardiographic differentiation of dextroposition, dextrocardia, and dextroversion is usually possible. The electrocardiogram in patients with dextroposition is normal except that the precordial transition zone is to the right. In mirror image dextrocardia both the P waves and T waves are inverted in Leads I and AVL and are upright in Lead AVR. In dextroversion only the T wave is inverted in Leads I and AVL and is upright in AVR.

How remember ECG changes in electrolyte imbalance? Hope this will help you... first, think of the normal ECG first...think how it starts and ends...so it starts with P followed by Q R S T; so let's start from where it begins...

P flat Hyperkalemia
PR prolonged Hyperkalemia Hypermagnesemia
QRS widened Hyperkalemia Hypermagnesemia
QT prolonged hypocalcemia
ST prolonged hypocalcemia
ST shortened Hypercalcemia
ST depressed hypokalemia Hypomagnes
T widened Hypercalcemia
T tall Hyperkalemia hypomagnesemia
T inverted hypokalemia shallow, flat
U prominent hypokalemia

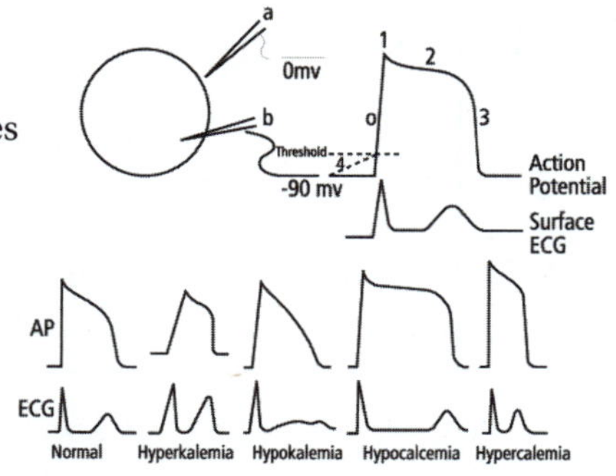

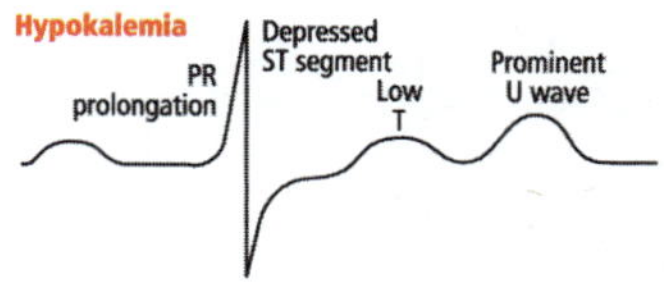

a
0mv
b
1 2
0
3
Threshold
-90 mv
Action Potential
Surface ECG

AP
ECG
Normal   Hyperkalemia   Hypokalemia   Hypocalcemia   Hypercalcemia

Hypokalemia
PR prolongation
Depressed ST segment
Low T
Prominent U wave

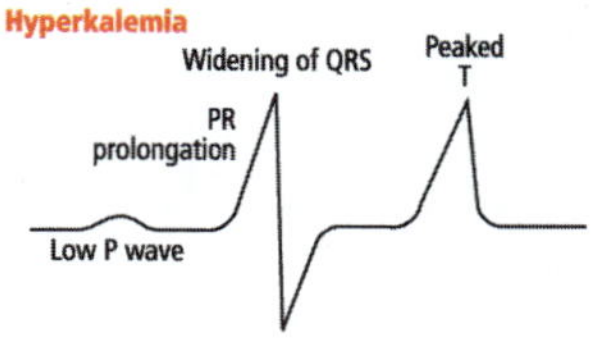

Hyperkalemia
Widening of QRS
Peaked T
PR prolongation
Low P wave

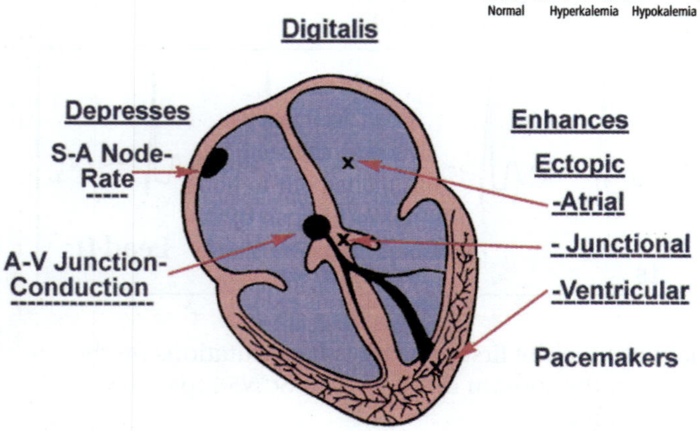

Digitalis

Depresses

S-A Node-Rate
- - - - -

A-V Junction-Conduction
- - - - - - - - - -

Enhances

Ectopic
x
-Atrial
- Junctional
-Ventricular

Pacemakers

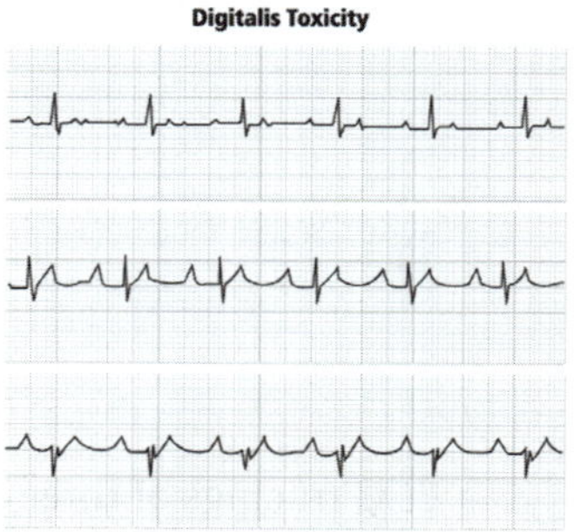

Digitalis Toxicity

Atrial tachycardia, 2:1 AV block

1. The P-wave axis is normal
2. The non-conducted P-wave hides in the T-wave
3. The conducted P-wave often has a long PR interval
4. The P-P interval may not be exactly regular

Normal variations to be considered in children

Courtesy: *Sumitra Venkatesh, Shakuntala Prabhu* Div. of Pediatric Cardiology, Dept. of Pediatrics, B.J.Wadia Hospital for Children, Mumbai .

Normal heart rate in the neonates varies between 120-230/min and gradually decreases over the first 6 months. Resting heart rate is about 120 beats /min at 1 year, 100 at 5 years and reaches adult values by 15 years.

Appearance of secondary 'r' waves (r' or R') in right chest leads is normal in neonates.

At birth, right axis deviation of the mean QRS vector is the rule. The axis becomes normal by 1 year of age. Hence, normal or leftward QRS axis is abnormal in the neonatal period and early infancy. Common conditions with leftward axis of QRS vector are tricuspid atresia and AV canal defects.

The PR-interval varies with age. Neonates-0.08-0.15, adolescents- 0.12-0.20 seconds. This normal variation must be kept in mind when considering diagnosis of conduction abnormalities or AV-blocks in children. Other pathological causes of short PR interval are Pompe's Disease, Fabry's disease, Mannosidosis, WPW syndrome, ectopic atrial pacemaker from lower right atrium.

Dominant R in right precordial leads can persist up to 6 months to 8 years; in the majority, the R/S ratio in lead V1 becomes less than 1 by 4 years of age.

Q waves are normally seen in leads II, III, aVF, V5 and V6 due to the clockwise loop of the QRS vector and are seen in majority of the congenital heart diseases. Q-waves in leads I and aVL suggest a counter-clockwise loop of the initial QRS vector and is seen in cases of Tricuspid atresia, Endocardial cushion defect and inlet VSD. Deep Q waves in lateral leads might point towards underlying anomalous origin of left coronary artery from pulmonary artery (ALCAPA). The QRS complex duration varies with age. In children , the QRS complex duration is shorter, possibly because of decreased muscle mass, and gradually increases with age. The QRS complex measures 0.03-0.08 seconds in neonates and 0.05-0.10 seconds in adolescents. As a result, slight prolongation of what may appear as a normal QRS complex can indicate a conduction abnormality or bundle branch block in children .

QT interval is highly variable in the first 3 days of life and in early infancy may be as high as 0.49seconds. Corrected QT (calculated by Bazett's formula) of more than 0.44 seconds is abnormal thereafter. The common causes of prolonged QTc are hypokalemia, hypocalcemia, hypothermia and cerebral injury. Certain drugs also prolong the QT-interval, viz. Cisapride, Macrolide antibiotics, etc.

Preterms of < 28 weeks of gestation may not have right ventricular dominance. Chest leads may show LV dominance with normal or leftward QRS axis.

Sinus pauses or junctional escapes (narrow QRS complex without preceding P waves) may occasionally occur during sleep, feeding and defecation.

References & Further Reading 1) Schwartz PJ, Garson A, Paul T et al. Guidelines for the interpretation of the neonatal electrocardiogram. European Heart J 2002; 23:1329-44. **2)** Sharieff GQ, Rao SO .The Pediatric ECG Emergency Medicine Clinics of North America. February 2006; 24(1):195-208. 3) Park M.K., George R., Pediatric cardiology for practitioners. St. Louis: Mosby, 2002. p. 34-51 **4)** H.D. H.P. E.B. Moss and Adams' heart disease in infants, children, and adolescents 6th edition. 2001Philadelphia: Lippincott, Williams and Wilkins, **5)** Sumitra Venkatesh, Shakuntala Prabhu. *Pediatric Electrocardiogram -* the BasicDiv. of Pediatric Cardiology, Dept. of Pediatrics, B.J.Wadia Hospital for Children, Mumbai http:// www.pediatriconcall.com/fordoctor/diseasesandcondition/ PEDIATRIC_CARDIOLOGY/ecg.asp.

Neonatal ECG Summary:

*Knowledge of the basics of Neonatal/pediatric ECG interpretation is helpful in differentiating normal from abnormal findings. These basics include familiarity with the age-related normal findings in heart rate, intervals, axis and waveform morphologies; an understanding of cardiac physiologic changes associated with age and maturation, particularly the adaptation from right to left ventricular predominance; and a rudimentary understanding of common pediatric dysrhythmias and findings associated with congenital heart diseases.

*Artefacts are common in newborn ECGs and include limb lead reversal and incorrect chest lead positioning. In addition, electrical interference, usually 60 cycles, can occur in hospital settings from bedside monitors, warmers or other equipment. Other artefacts occur because of various types of patient movement common in neonates. These artefacts may be random as with hiccoughs or limb movement. Normal complexes are seen along with the artefacts, and the intrinsic rhythm of the patient is not affected. Other common artefacts include a fine, often irregular undulation of the baseline from muscle tremors or jitteriness. Again, the intrinsic rhythm is not affected. The size of the QRS complex and the baseline may wander in a cyclic fashion with respirations. It should be noted that the neonate breathes from 30–60 times per min. The main clue in determining the presence of an artefact is to evaluate whether it affects the intrinsic rhythm and if it is timed such that it could be a true depolarization. A signal within 80 ms from a true QRS complex could not occur from an electrophysiologic point of view.

*The normal newborn ECG should include 12 leads. Other leads, V3R, V4R and V7, may provide additional information to evaluate possible congenital heart lesions.

AMPLITUDE-INTEGRATED EEG (aEEG)
CEREBRAL FUNCTION MONITORING (CFM)

*Although the bulk of the studies have used standard Neonatal EEGs, the body of evidence in regard to aEEG and HIE has been growing in the last 10 years. *Integrating the amplitude domain (generally by using fast-Fourier transformation) makes the EEG easier to interpret than before so that pediatric house staff without previous training in neonatal EEG can both read the amplitude and detect neonatal seizures. Learning to read neonatal EEG takes 1-2 years. *aEEG studies have used criteria that take in consideration both the upper margin of the aEEG band and the lower margin or lowest amplitude of the EEG voltage. *Normal is an upper range of >10 µV and a lower margin of >5 µV. *Moderate abnormalities have an upper range of >10 µV and a lower margin of 5 µV or less. *Severe abnormalities have an upper range of <10 µV and a lower margin of <5 µV, usually with a burst-suppression pattern. *An experienced neonatal encephalographer immediately notices the potential for overlapping of normal and moderate ranges because the lowest possible voltage is less reliable than the maximum voltage in neonatal EEG. The transition from non–rapid-eye-movement (REM) sleep to REM sleep (or REM-2) occurs when neonates behaviorally appear to be asleep, sometimes for over an hour. The start of REM-2 is associated with a notable reduction in background amplitude. *Although this method is promising, further validation of the accuracy of aEEG in trials of patients undergoing both aEEG and standard EEG are needed. Also needed is a demonstration that aEEG adds to the accuracy of other. Cerebral function monitoring (CFM) represents a valuable technology in the care of neonatal patients that has recently gathered a significant amount of attention as a diagnostic tool in the NICU. Although used since 1969 in adults and since 1983 in neonates in Europe, the importance of this device has been shown during its use as one the brain cooling trials for hypoxic-ischemic encephalopathy (HIE). CFM, also know as integrated, amplified electroencephalography, or aEEG, represents a bedside, readily available, easily used technology for the detection of brain wave activity and the diagnosis of seizures. This technique employs the application of a scalp electrode that is placed in the temporal-parietal region of the scalp bilaterally and a ground electrode (Figure 1). Some CFM units attempt to enhance detection of abnormalities by utilizing two electrodes bilaterally. With CFM, electrical signals can be detected, amplified, integrated, and recorded, yielding valuable information about the overall integrity of the neonatal central nervous system. Many studies have examined the role of CFM monitoring in the infant with HIE, and CFM recording has added significantly to the clinician's ability to define the potential of an infant for normal development or the possibility of subsequent neurological abnormality. The typical aEEG recording is a two channel recording that measures two values primarily, usually the aEEG itself and a measure of impedance to insure good contact with the scalp electrodes. For seizure diagnosis, the impedance can be readily replaced with a real-time EEG tracing (see Figure 2). While there are several characteristics that define the quality and permit interpretation of the aEEG recording, the current tracing reveals an infant who is having frequent seizures. As happens with some degree of regularity in the neonatal period, there is some degree of uncoupling between the infant's clinical appearance and the aEEG recording. Normally, one would anticipate overt clinical seizures in a child who was experiencing electrical seizures as severe as that noted in this CFM study. Seizures often represent ominous events for the neonate. Although seizures can be a consequence of a temporary abnormality during the Neonatal period, they often pose significant long-term issues for the neonate, depending upon the etiology of the seizure. In the CFM recording, seizures typically are revealed as a sudden rise in the aEEG recording. This finding occurs numerous times over the first two and one-half hours of this particular recording. Seizures may be very brief in duration or more prolonged. Seizure periods may occasionally be difficult

to capture visually without the assistance of the scrolling EEG on the bottom of the CFM tracing. The lower portion of the recording, which is the real-time EEG, confirms the presence of seizures in this infant. This child should have anticonvulsant therapy started immediately in order to control the seizures, which appear to be the result of a hypoxic-ischemic event around the time of birth. The CFM recording can be used in a variety of ways in the assessment of neonatal neurological development and injury. With recovery (though recovery may be limited with the severe forms of injury), there is a step-wise improvement noted in the aEEG recording. The faster that this reversal occurs, the better the long-term prognosis for the infant. A Neonate who returns to a more normal appearance on the aEEG within 24-48 hours has a much better prognosis than an infant in whom there is no reversal before 7-10 days. Infants who have had a difficult delivery, but who show few changes in their aEEG pattern, have a good prognosis overall. The CFM can also be used to follow the results of treatment with anticonvulsants in the case of neonatal seizures. Rapid normalization of the aEEG is reassuring when a child has previously been diagnosed with a seizure disorder.

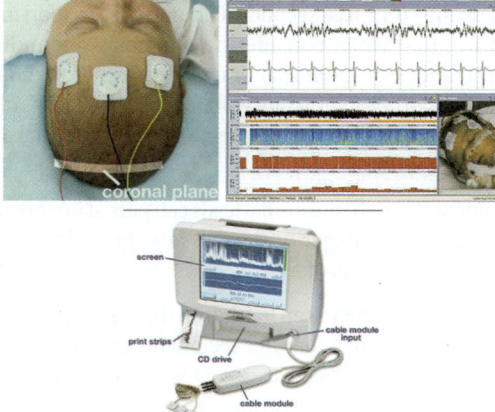

Application Guidelines

The main screen is divided into 2 main graphing strips. The top strip is the cerebral function graph that mea-sures electrical brain activity [(V), semi-logarithmic y-axis] versus time [(hr:min:sec), x-axis]. The bottom strip measures impedance of the leads and evaluates the connection of the leads to the patient's scalp. The impedance strip should show a relatively flat line that is less than < 20 W to ensure accuracy of the CFM tracing. An increasing level of impedance means the leads are lifting off the scalp and must be reapplied. If the lead lifts off enough, an alarm condition will sound.

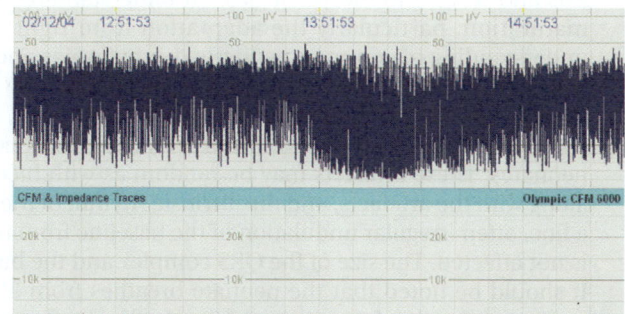

Due to the slow charting speed of the CFM, it takes approximately 20 minutes before the clinician can preliminarily analyze the strip. Therefore, seizure treatment should never be delayed if clinical symptoms are observed. Doctors should make a habit of reviewing the CFM every 2–3 hours.

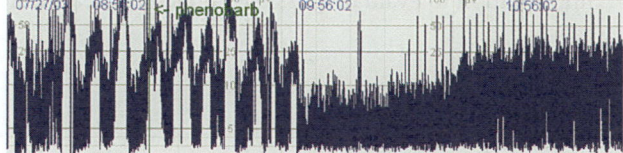

Markers should be labelled on the CFM tracing if the RN observes any clinical symptoms of seizures or administers any sedation or anticonvulsant therapy. If repositioning or stimulating the patient causes distur-bances in the tracing, these events should be labelled as well (x rays, etc.). Markers are placed by pressing the MARKER button, tapping the CFM strip at the appropri-ate time, and then typing or selecting the appropriate marker from the window that pops up. The CFM functions nicely as a long-term monitor and can be left in place for several days of constant recording. Within 12 hours of starting a CFM trace, a patient should be evaluated using a standard EEG, which may detect focal seizures or localize lesions that cannot always be detected with CFM alone. If recording is stopped on a patient at any time and is to be restarted, the operator should reapply leads (if not already on), press TOOLS, select the patient's name from the list and press ACCEPT to display file. RESUME will continue the recording.

Steps to wave analysis

Observe the impedance graph and ensure the line is relatively flat and preferably below 10 kW. This indicates an accurate CFM tracing.

Normal tracing Examine the CFM strip as a whole. **• Is it a gentle wave?** YES **• Do the lower and upper margins seem to flow in parallel?** YES **• Is the lower margin above 5 V?** YES **• Is the upper margin above 10 V?** YES **• Is their regular widening & narrowing of the trace, within the above margins (Sleep Wake Cycling)?** YES This is classified as a normal trace and in most cases is a good prognostic sign. Early return of **sleep wake cycling (SWS)** after an asphyxial insult is also a good prognostic sign.

Normal trace; Upper margin is > 10 V & lower margin is > 5 V. The widening and narrowing of the trace implies periods of wakening and sleep i.e. SWS).

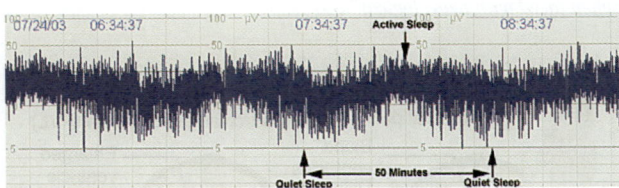

Moderately Abnormal Tracing • Is the lower margin below 5 V? YES Moderately abnormal function present. Keep in mind that anticonvulsant therapy may shift the wave downward. **Moderately abnormal trace; Upper margin is > 10 V & lower margin is < 5 V throughout the trace. There is no SWS.**

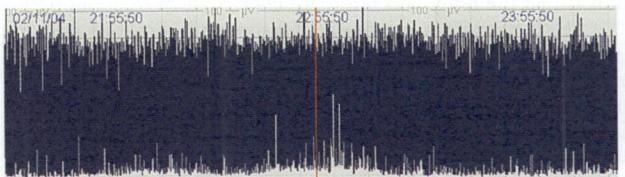

References: 1) van Rooij LG, Toet MC, Osredkar D, van Huffelen AC, Groenendaal F, de Vries LS. Recovery of amplitude integrated electroencephalographic background patterns within 24 hours of perinatal asphyxia. Arch Dis Child Fetal Neonatal Ed 2005; 90(3):F245-F251. 2)A Protocol for Cerebral Function Monitoring in the NICU Dr. Patrick McNamara, Matthew Keyzers RRT. Hospital for Sick Children, Toronto, Canada

Severely abnormal tracing • Is the upper margin below 10 V? YES **• Does the thickness of the wave appear thinner?** YES **• Has the wave appeared to flatten out?** YES Severely abnormal function present. This may correspond with burst suppression or continuous low voltage on a regular EEG.. **Severely abnormal trace;** Upper margin is < 10 V & lower margin is < 5 V throughout the trace. There is evidence of SWS. Periodic bursts of electrical activity are seen.

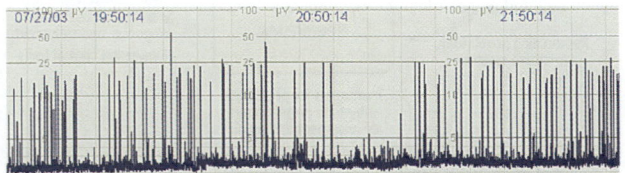

Seizures • In the gaps of the rising and narrowing (lower margin becomes suddenly raised for several minutes), does the EEG **tracing show a distinct repetitive pattern?** YES

Seizures are present. **Moderately abnormal trace with multiple seizures; Upper margin is > 10 V & lower margin is < 5 V throughout the trace. There is no evidence of SWS. Frequent and prolonged periods of elevation in both the lower and upper margins are seen that coincide with a repetitive rhythmic pattern on the EEG. This is characteristic of seizure activity.**

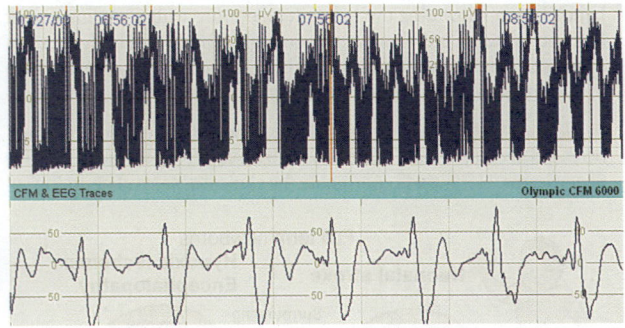

Analysis and Prematurity

aEEG is feasible for monitoring cerebral activity in preterm infants and normative values have been suggested. SWS can be clearly identified on the trace from around 30 week's gestation although a cyclical pattern emerges in some babies at 25–26 weeks gestation. A scoring system has been suggested by Burdjalov et al based on continuity, presence of cycling, amplitude of the lower border and bandwith

This scoring system has not yet been tested in terms of its ability to recognize pathological states and is somewhat subjective; however it may be useful as a guide for interpretation. This scoring system is recommended when aEEG is applied to premature infants to facilitate trace interpretation. Extremely low voltage patterns or burst suppression should be easily recognizable. There are no definitive reports on seizure patterns in premature infants. Pathological patterns should be confirmed by more formal EEG evaluation.

Holistic approach to neonatal CNS insult/injury and neurodevelopmental sequelae

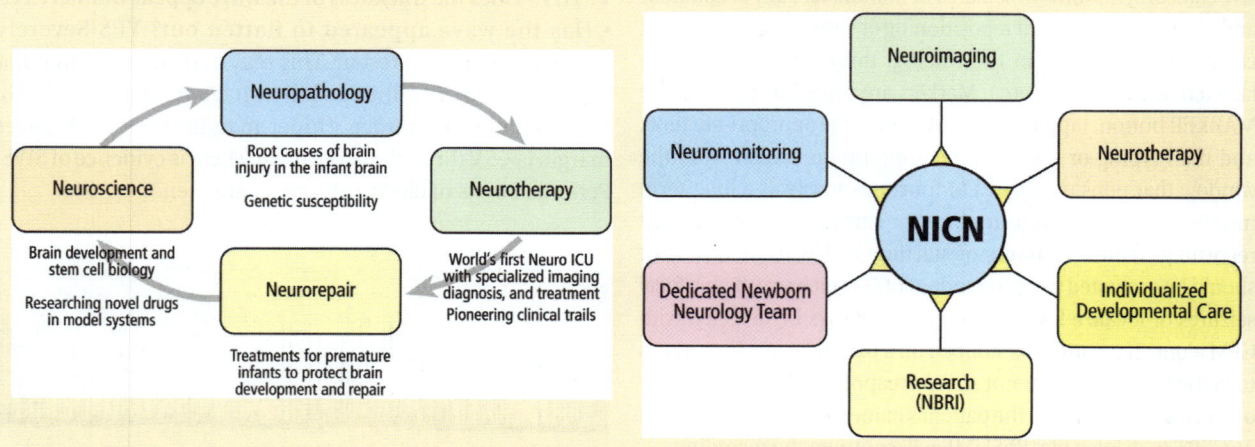

NICN-NEURO-INTENSIVE CARE NURSERY

Magnetic resonance imaging studies will be integrated with information from cerebral function monitoring and magnetic resonance spectroscopy to provide valuable insights into brain anatomy and metabolic activity.

Cerebral function monitoring (CFM) can provide a window into the brain activity of newborns. It is provided through 8-12 lead electroencephalography (EEG) that can quickly switch from a simplified (amplitude integrated) reading to a full EEG. CFM is used in other nurseries, but typically only when an infant may be having seizures, this monitoring will be a routine part of clinical care.

Neurotherapy: Under a clinical research protocol, the nursery will be treating infants who have moderate hypoxic encephalopathy with hypothermia – lowering the baby's temperature with a cooling cap or blanket. Research has shown that cooling the brain and body by a few degrees immediately after birth can help reduce neurological damage in babies who have sustained certain types of brain injury.

Dedicated Pediatric Neurological Team: A pediatric neurologist should oversee a dedicated team that assesses neurological function in critically ill newborns. He/She will coordinate the clinical aspects of neurological

care provided in the nursery. The neurology team will also oversee the training of a new cadre of specialists seeking to understand the role of complications of early birth and intensive care in the newborn brain injury.

Newborn Individualized Developmental Care and Assessment Program (NIDCAP): In the NIDCAP model of care, infants are carefully observed within the newborn ICU setting to determine if their behaviors suggest that they are under any stress of discomfort. This information is then used to provide an environment that is as comfortable as possible and developmentally appropriate for each baby.

New Directions in Research-Newborn Brain Research Institute (NBRI)- Efforts to advance diagnosis and treatment : As more is learned about the structure and function of the newborn brain, a "translational" approach will streamline the development and testing of new neuroprotective therapies. Researchers hope to quickly determine if a therapy may be effective by analyzing data from imaging studies, monitoring and clinical observation.

The goal is to offer patients and their families real therapeutic options when faced with neurological injuries.

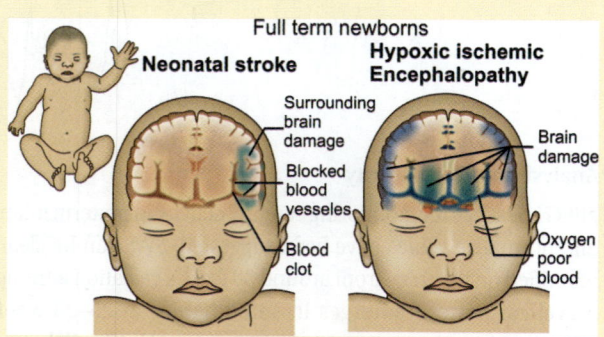

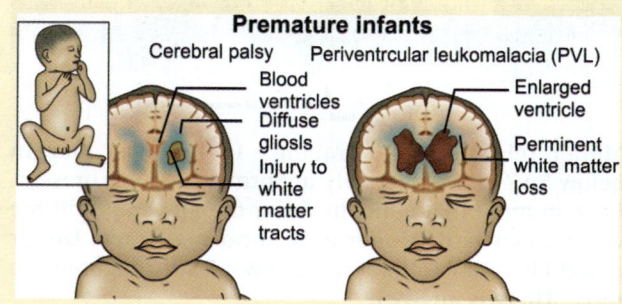

*Another recent advance has been development of hypothermia in which the body and brain are cooled down to about 92°F (33.5°C), as opposed to the normal body temperature of 97.8°F (37°C). *Hypothermia is appropriate for some full-term babies that have been deprived of oxygen around the time of birth (a condition called Hypoxic-ischemic Encephalopathy (HIE); see Figure 1A, and has been shown to prevent very severe brain damage that can lead to death. *Neonatal stroke is also associated with lack of oxygen to the brain in full-term infants (Figure 1B). When this injury happens at the time of birth it can also probably be helped by hypothermia. *Preterm infants typically suffer from two other causes of brain injury that probably result from the delicate nature of the developing human brain. Intraventricular Hemorrhage (IVH) refers to bleeding in the brain and is graded from grade 1 (mild) to grade 4 (severe). Figure 2A shows a severe IVH with bleeding into the cavity in the center of the brain called the ventricles and also the brain tissue. *Another injury seen in preterm infants is called Periventricular Leukomalacia (PVL). This affects white matter tracts of the brain that carry messages between nerve cells of the brain and body. PVL can cause severe neurological problems with movement. *All the conditions described above can cause either mild or very severe brain damage that can lead to death. Each case requires careful evaluation by doctors specialized in assessing neurological injury in babies.

Courtesy: University of California, San Francisco Division of Neonatology

1. *Pulse oximetry: The "5th vital sign' and the greatest advance in patient monitoring for many years,* is a simple, sensitive, portable, continuous, noninvasive method of determining oxygen saturation {SaO_2} and is useful *a)* To guide O_2 therapy in any acutely unwell patient in NICU / PICU *b)* To monitor O_2 saturations and pulses throughout Anesthesia and during recovery phase *c)* To maintain O_2 saturations above 95% always in patients with long standing respiratory disease {in patients with cyanotic CHD lower pulse oximeter readings < 85% reflect the severity of the underlying disease state} *d)* To assess nocturnal FiO_2 and to screen for obstructive sleep apnea syndrome {for identification of nocturnal desaturations} *e)* To monitor for unexpected hypoxia during procedures such as endoscopy.

2. *Beware of the pitfalls of pulse oximetry ! a)* It doesn't detect CO_2 levels, so has limitation in the assessment of the patient with respiratory failure due to CO_2 retention {type II respiratory failure} *b)* It gives falsely elevated reading, if carboxyhemoglobin or methemoglobin are present in the blood in elevated levels *c)* It gives erroneous information if patient is poorly perfused E.g.: - hypothermia, shock, cardiac failure and some cardiac arrhythmias and in severe anemia {Hb < 5 gms/dL}. Bright over head light, phototherapy lights, surgical diathermy interfere the O_2 saturation readings {can be corrected by covering the site with opaque material} *d)* Excessive patient movement and shivering can give false readings {since the sensor must identify every pulse beat to calculate the SaO_2, movement can interfere with sensing} *e)* Nail polish {except red nail polish} interferes with pulse oximetry readings. *f)* Venous pulsations {E.g.:- Tricuspid regurgitation} may produce falsely low readings with ear lobes {put the sensors at the heart level to correct this problem}. *g)* IV dyes such as methylene blue, indigocarmine and indocyanine also give false readings ; however the readings are not affected by jaundice, and anemia {except if hemoglobin < 5gms/dL as mentioned above}. Skin colour, thickness and edema don't affect the readings.

3. *Pulse oximetry readings are affected by the oxyhemoglobin dissociation curve:* A higher saturation for a given oxygen tension {a curve shifted to the left} occurs with alkalosis, hypothermia, fetal hemoglobin, high altitude and hypometabolism {hypothyroidism}. A lower saturation for a given oxygen tension {a curve shifted to the right} occurs with acidosis, hyperthermia, hypermetabolism {hyperthyroidism} and hypercarbia. Based on the oxyhemoglobin dissociation curve - the curve flattens with PaO_2 > 70mmHg Therefore large changes in PaO_2 will result in only small changes in pulse oximeter recording. For infants with high and low saturations, *ABG analysis is to be done for safe correlation* {PaO_2 of

30mmHg = SaO_2 60% and PaO_2 of 60mmHg = SaO_2 90% so remember the quick formula 30-60 and 60-90}.

4. Pulse oximetry is insensitive to hyperoxia because Hb approaches 100% saturation for all PaO_2 readings > 100mmHg, which is a dangerous situation for the *premature infant at risk for developing retinopathy of prematurity*. Therefore the premature infant being monitored with oximetry should have upper limits identified, such as 90-95% and a protocol is to be established for decreasing O_2 when saturations are high.

5. Pulse oximeter consist of a sensor comprising *a light - emitting diode {LED} and a photodetector placed in opposition* around a foot, hand, finger, toe or ear lobe, with the LED placed on top of the nail when digits are used. The LED emits red and infrared lights that pass through the skin to the photodetector. The photodetector measures the amount of each type of light absorbed by functional hemoglobins. Hemoglobin saturated with O_2 {Oxyhemoglobin} absorbs more infrared light than does hemoglobin not saturated with O_2 {Deoxyhemoglobin}. Therefore pulsatile blood flow is the primary physiologic factor that influences accuracy of the pulse oximeter. The difference in light absorption is used to calculate oxygen saturation. Based on the oxygen hemoglobin dissociation curve, the oxygen saturation can be related to PaO_2 **POSSIBLE RESULTS**- Oxygen saturations expressed as % - *Cross-sectional*—Normal or low, *Longitudinal* - Stable/ improve/deteriorate, *Overnight*- Normal/intermittent desaturations.

6. *Patient preparation before pulse oximetry* a) Clean probe site (ear or finger), sole of foot & palm of hand {Neonates} b) Ensure good contact of probe with warm well-perfused skin c) Avoid nail-varnished fingers. Sensors are not placed on extremities used for blood pressure monitoring or with indwelling arterial catheters, since pulsatile blood flow can be affected. *Nursing observations during monitoring* - a) Inspect the skin under the sensor frequently, as pressure necrosis can occur from sensors attached too tightly b) Make certain that sensor connectors and oximeters are compatible, because incompatible wiring can generate considerable heat at the tip of the sensor, causing second and third degree burns under the sensors c) *Never ignore a reading which suggests the patient is becoming hypoxic ; don't assume that it is an artifact ; always observe the baby's/child's clinical condition rather than staring at the pulse oximeter reading wondering what to do next ? - if in doubt , always ensure patent airway, after suctioning the airways, regular breathing with high flow oxygen + bag and mask ventilation and maintain the circulation with crystalloid / colloid + inotropes and CALL FOR HELP EARLY !*

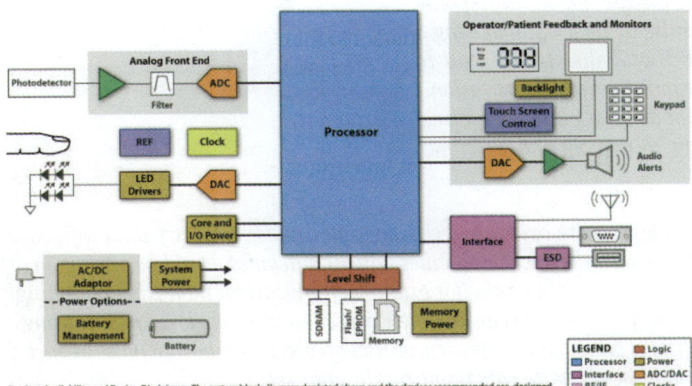

Product Availability and Design Disclaimer - The system block diagram depicted above and the devices recommended are designed in this manner as a reference. Please contact your local TI sales office or distributor for system design specifics and product availability.

Oximeters work by the principles of spectrophotometry: the relative absorption of red (absorbed by oxygenated blood) and infrared (absorbed by deoxygenated blood) light of the systolic component of the absorption waveform correlate to arterial blood oxygen saturations. Measurements of relative light absorption are made 600 times every second and these are processed by the machine to give a new reading every 0.5–1 second that averages out the reading over the last 3 seconds.

Probes are usually positioned on the fingertip, although earlobes and forehead are sometimes used as alternatives. One study has suggested that the ear lobe is not a reliable site to measure oxygen saturations.

TABLE 1: Typical applications of continuous pulse oximetry in neonatal and pediatric populations

Indication	Comment
Intensive care and during mechanical ventilation	Now a standard of care for nearly all patients in neonatal and pediatric intensive care, especially those receiving mechanical ventilation.
Procedural sedation	A recommended standard of care for all patients undergoing procedural sedation.
Patient-controlled anesthesia	Used in many hospitals continuously on all patients who are receiving patient-controlled anesthesia.
During oxygen administration	Now used in many hospitals continuously on all neonatal and pediatric patients receiving oxygen therapy, even in general care areas.
Delivery room	Use in the delivery room has been difficult and controversial. However, recent improvements in performance during low perfusion and motion have made such monitoring more feasible.
Perioperatively	Used universally on all patients during surgery, during the immediate postoperative period, and in many pediatric facilities for the first 12–24 hours after postanesthesia care.
High-risk	Some in-house oximetry protocols include continuous monitoring of all patients 3 months of age with any respiratory symptoms, such as during bronchiolitis care.
Pediatric emergency care	Used as a screening tool for triage of pediatric patients and regarded by some as a "fifth vital sign".

Evaluation of a new combined transcutaneous measurement of PCO$_2$/Pulse oximetry oxygen saturation ear sensor in newborn patients

Arterial oxygen saturation (SaO$_2$) and arterial carbon dioxide partial pressure (PaCO$_2$) are 2 of the most important respiratory parameters in the treatment of critically ill neonates. Noninvasive monitoring of these parameters is desirable for continuous estimating of the respiratory status and reducing blood loss because of repeated blood gas analyses. Transcutaneous measurement of PCO$_2$ (PtcCO$_2$) represents a simple and noninvasive technique for continuous monitoring of ventilation. However, sensor preparation, positioning, taping, and repeated changes of the sensor location make the handling difficult and complicate its use in the neonatal care unit. Recently, a new sensor for combined assessment of pulse oximetry oxygen saturation (SpO$_2$) and PtcCO$_2$ has been introduced (TOSCA Monitor; Linde Medical Sensors, Basel, Switzerland). The monitor combines pulse oximetry and PtcCO$_2$ measurement in a single ear sensor, which works at 42°C to enhance blood flow in capillaries below the sensor. The TOSCA monitor with the ear sensor adapted to ears of neonates allows reliable estimation of SaO$_2$ and PaCO$_2$. A potential benefit is the reduction in motion artifacts because of less head movement in newborns and that only a single cable leads form the patient to the monitor. In addition, the sensor is not removed for chest radiograph or for nursing the infant on his or her parent's lap. Long-term studies in a large population with continuous measurements are required to confirm these preliminary findings and to elucidate the benefits in detection of respiratory deterioration and the potential side effects of this sensor. *Pediatrics* 2005;115:e64–e68. URL: www.pediatrics.org/cgi/doi/10.1542 peds.2004-0946; *non-invasive monitoring, oxygenation, pulse oximetry, carbon dioxide, neonate.*

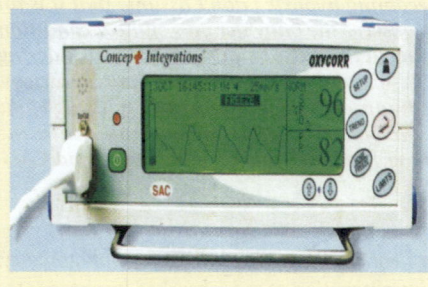

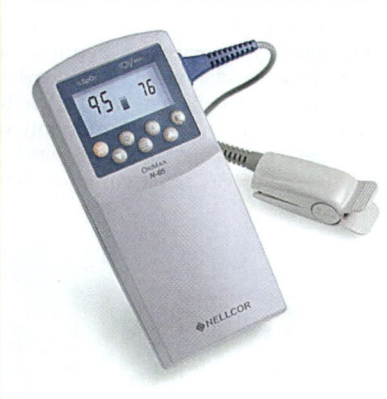

A simpler way to detect this right-to-left shunting is to use two pulse oximeters and measure preductal and postductal SpO2. In one study it was found that arterial saturation in the right arm (preductal) of at least 3% above the lower limb (postductal) is evidence of right-to-left ductal shunting. During this critical phase of the infant's disease, the rapid response time of the pulse oximeter at detecting a right-to-left ductal shunt may lead to earlier treatment of PPHN. Pulse oximetry depends on adequate peripheral perfusion. In low-cardiac-output states or shock, the oximeter may not detect a pulse waveform. Most pulse oximeters require a pulse pressure of more than 20 mm Hg and a systolic blood pressure greater than 30 mm Hg to operate reliably.

CLINICAL SUMMARY: Substantial advances have been made in pulse oximetry technology, and pulse oximetry data influence treatment decisions and processes of care in certain situations, but it is unclear whether patient outcomes would be any different without pulse oximetry. Clinicians must bear in mind that dyshemoglobinemia (for example, from carbon monoxide poisoning) causes inaccurately high SpO2 readings, and motion and low peripheral perfusion often cause inaccurately low SpO2 readings. Research is needed to determine whether pulse oximetry improves patient outcomes or processes of care; it may be that pulse oximetry is unnecessary and unhelpful (and therefore an inappropriate use of health care resources) in some settings.

Capnography is a noninvasive method for monitoring the level of carbon dioxide in exhaled breath (EtCO2) to assess a patient's ventilatory status. Capnography directly measures the ventilatory performance of the lungs and indirectly presents measurements on the performance of metabolism and circulation. For example, an increased metabolism will increase the production of carbon dioxide increasing the ETCO2. A decrease in cardiac output will lower the delivery of carbon dioxide to the lungs, decreasing the ETCO2. Thus, it gives us a rapid and reliable method to detect life-threatening conditions such as malposition of tracheal tubes, ventilatory failure, circulatory failure and defective breathing circuits. In neonates, capnography is a more sensitive and specific indicator of esophageal intubation than is clinical examination; capnography accelerates recognition of misintubation; even experienced intubators misplace endotracheal tubes in neonates, and capnography can help recognize these esophageal intubations; capnography may prevent the unnecessary removal of correctly placed tubes, especially when the clinical examination is ambiguous; many unintentional extubations occur during the taping of the tube. The need for arterial blood sampling can be significantly reduced.

"Oxygenation is best monitored by the use of pulse oximetry, whereas ventilation is best monitored by the application of capnography." It must be remembered that decreases in arterial oxygen saturation as determined by pulse oximetry may be a late indicator of a deterioration in ventilation. By analyzing the capnograph trace instead of merely the numerical value, the bedside observer garners more accurate data. There is a good correlation and agreement between end-tidal and arterial carbon dioxide in ventilated extremely low birth weight infants during the first week of life. • End-tidal carbon dioxide monitoring can be used as a guide to adjust for ventilator setting in these infants. The correlation between mainstream $EtCO_2$ and $PaCO_2$ is good. Neonates with pulmonary disease will have a lower correlation. Surfactant therapy improves the correlation. $EtCO_2$ monitoring is helpful in trending or screening for abnormal $PaCO_2$ values. An inherent property of CO_2 is to absorb infrared radiation at a very specific wavelength. Capnographs contain sensors that produce infrared sources of blackbody radiation at these wavelengths. These sensors enable the calculation of CO_2 levels in a breath sample. Capnographs produce both waveforms and numeric values of the patient's exhaled breath and are used to identify ad-

verse ventilation events. This helps clinicians diagnose specific medical conditions, leading to important treatment decisions. Microstream technology enables clinicians to use capnography to its full potential, by working more effectively than other capnography systems, and provides breath sampling lines for the broadest base of patients. Microstream makes capnography a practical and useful tool that clinicians in all environments can depend upon to improve care for their patients.

Conventional technology: All capnographs – including Microstream – measure CO_2 concentration using either mainstream or sidestream configurations. **Mainstream:** In mainstream capnographs, the sensor is located on a special airway adapter so that CO_2 is measured directly in the patient's breathing circuit. The main drawbacks are: *The weight of the sensor on the airway, which is significant with neonates * External sensors that are vulnerable to damage * The inability to monitor non-intubated patients easily **Sidestream:** In sidestream capnographs, a sample of exhaled breath is aspirated from the breathing circuit to a sensor residing inside the monitor. Sidestream configurations are appropriate for both intubated and non-intubated patients. They require external filters to prevent liquids and secretions from reaching the sidestream sampling system. Drawbacks of sidestream include: *Liquid and secretion handling *Large breath sample rate; precludes use of low-flow applications (neonates). **Microstream:** improves on conventional sidestream technology because there is no sensor at the airway. It can work for both intubated and non-intubated patients of all ages. Microstream uses laser-based molecular correlation spectroscopy (MCS) as the infrared emission source. The Microstream emitter operates at room temperature, and is electronically activated and self-modulating. This eliminates the need for moving parts that are used on some competitive systems and increases the reliability of the Microstream system. Microstream uses a breath sampling rate of 50 ml per minute. A minimal breath sampling rate is important because: *It permits the use of capnography for patients of all ages, including neonates. The small tidal volume of neonates cannot be accurately measured with technologies that require larger breath sampling rates. * It reduces moisture and humidity entering the sampling line, thus reducing the potential for sampling line obstruction, which is a common problem in conventional sidestream technology.

Physiology

CO_2 levels provide information on the following bodily functions

METABOLISM   **PERFUSION**   **VENTILATION**

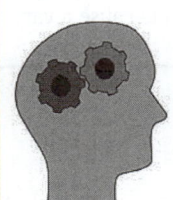 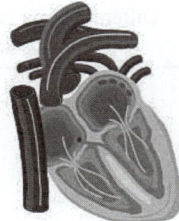 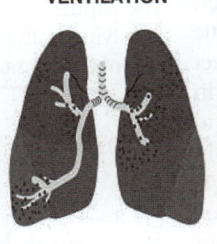

Figure 1. Capnometry is a method applicable for overall assessment of the body's physiology and the crucial parameters of the vital functions.

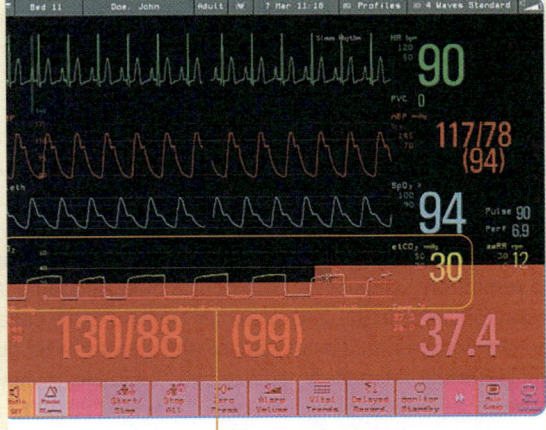

Microstream CO_2 uses a sample flow rate of 50 ml/min, making it a viable solution for capnography on all patients, including neonates.

Neonatal applications : Measurement of neonatal pulmonary function was first performed in the 1950s. This initial work helped to define the groundwork for neonatal pulmonary pathophysiology, but progress in the study of capnography in the neonate was not possible until the development of mainstream airway cuvettes. The development of the new and improved mainstream capnographs that were lightweight and had a dead space of less than 1 mL opened the door to utilizing capnography in the NICU. These cuvettes reliably provide measurements in preterm infants. In spite of these ground-breaking developments, capnography has not been embraced by clinicians to monitor alveolar gas exchange in the neonate. Some of the limitations include technical problems such as sensor dead space and short expiratory time in neonates with stiff lungs and capnograph resolution in the presence of high respiratory rates. These issues are exacerbated in very low birth weight (VLBW) infants of <1,500 grams. In the neonate, analysis of the single breath carbon dioxide waveform requires comparison with the typical pattern as illustrated in Figure 1. Neonatal phase 1 should be short. Phase 2 should rise with a steep upward slope. Phase 3 is usually absent in neonates; if it is present, it is often small with slope a function of lung growth. Interpreting phase 3 must be done with care, but the presence of phase 3 is an indication that alveolar gas was sampled. In infants with normal pulmonary function and normal ventilation-to-perfusion ratio (V/Q), the $PETCO_2$ can be a good estimation of the $Paco_2$. In critically ill patients, the V/Q ratio is often abnormal with a resulting increase in the $P(a-ETCO_2)$ gradient. Although much progress has been done since the early use of capnography in the neonate, we still face technical limitations in measuring CO_2 signals in VLBW infants. In addition, much needs to be learned about how small and immature lungs physiologically differ and the resultant impact on gas exchange, particularly phase 2 and phase 3.

Congenital heart disease: Congenital heart diseases can be categorized into two broad groups: cyanotic and noncyanotic. Cyanotic lesions are defects that result in low blood oxygen levels. Cyanosis results in an abnormal blood flow from the right side of the heart to the left side of the heart, bypassing the lungs and creating a right-to-left shunt. Some congenital heart defects that cause cyanosis include: tetralogy of Fallot, transposition of the great vessels, tricuspid atresia, pulmonary atresia, and hypoplastic left heart. Noncyanotic congenital heart disease includes lesions in which blood returning to the right side of the heart passes normally through the pulmonary vasculature. The common forms of noncyanotic congenital heart defects are conditions where there is an opening in one of the walls separating the heart chambers or obstruction to a cardiac valve. Some types of noncyanotic heart disease are: coarctation of the aorta, atrial septal defect, ventricular septal defect, atrioventricular septal defect, patent ductus arteriosus, and aortic stenosis. Any factor that alters cardiovascular function can affect the transport of CO_2 to the lungs. In the absence of changes in the respiratory status of the patient, it should alert clinicians to possible changes in the cardiovascular function of the patient. In patients with cyanotic heart disease, the alveolar ventilation is usually normal. Pulmonary perfusion may be abnormal, however, and that can result in a V/Q mismatch. Therefore, $PETCO_2$ cannot be used as a reliable estimate of $Paco_2$ in the congenital heart disease patient. Capnography usage is particularly helpful in monitoring pulmonary perfusion in the postoperative cardiac patient with either a Blalock-Taussig or central shunt.

These palliative conduits from the systemic arterial circulation to the pulmonary artery are placed to provide reliable pulmonary blood flow in some forms of cyanotic heart disease, in which pulmonary blood flow is much decreased or absent. In the potentially life-threatening event of shunt clotting, there would be a significant decrease in pulmonary blood flow, with a subsequent decrease or absence of $ETCO_2$.

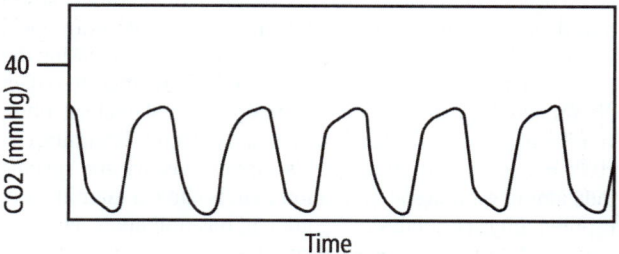

Fig. 1: Normal neonatal capnogram- the shape of the normal neonatal capnogram is different. Because of the smaller dead space and higher respiratory rate, the normal neonatal capnogram has a shorter time at baseline, a sharper rise in CO2 concentration, and little if any alveolar plateau.

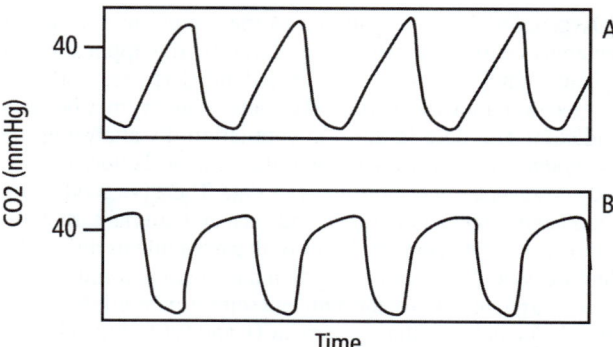

Capnogram (A) before surfactant (B) after surfactant- Administration of surfactant alters respiratory mechanics and changes the rate of alveolar emptying, which is reflected on the capnogram. Before the administration of surfactant, the capnogram has an elevated baseline, the transitional phase has a prolonged slope, and there is no alveolar plateau. After the administration of surfactant the capnogram returns to a normal shape.

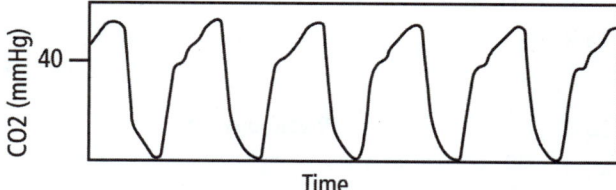

The capnogram of a neonate with pneumonia shows biphasic emptying of the lung. Different time constants cause a varying rate of CO2 removal.

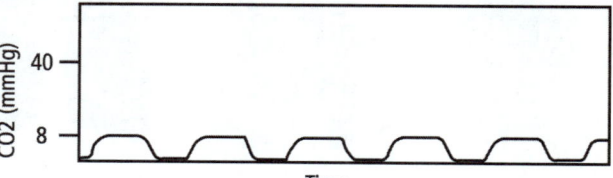

A normal capnogram with a large difference between PETCO2 and PaCO2 indicates substantial physiologic dead space . Right-to-left cardiac shunt diverts blood away from the lung. Cardiac shunt reflects an increase in pulmonary dead space.

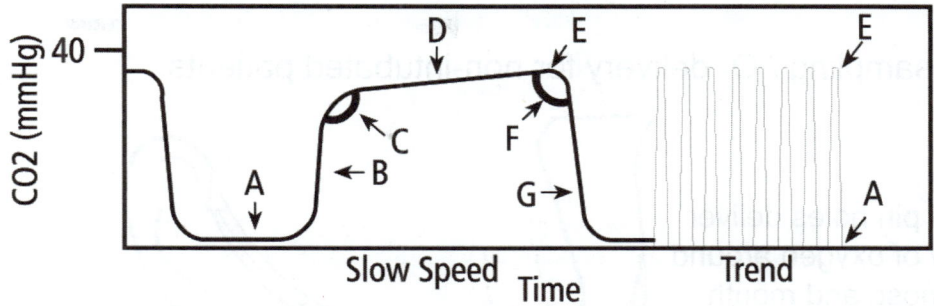

Normal features of a capnogram. A: *Baseline*, represents the beginning of expiration and should start at zero. B: The *transitional* part of the curve represents mixing of dead space and alveolar gas. C: The *alpha angle* represents the change to alveolar gas. D: The *alveolar* part of the curve represents the plateau average alveolar gas concentration. E: The *end-tidal carbon dioxide* value. F: The *beta angle* represents the change to the inspiratory part of the cycle. G: The *inspiration* part of the curve shows a rapid decrease in carbon dioxide concentration.

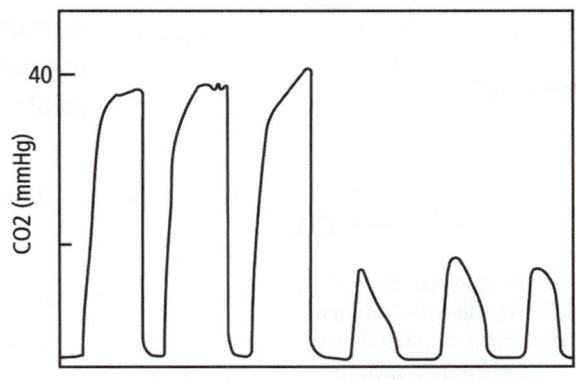

Neonatal capnograms of tracheal intubation (left) and esophageal intubation (right).

Definitions

* Capnometry (measurement and display of CO_2)

* Capnography {a graphic display of CO_2 concentration [FCO_2] versus *time* or *expired volume* during a respiratory cycle (CO_2 waveform) }

* Capnograms (CO_2 waveform of 2 types...... FCO_2 can be plotted *either* against expired volume *or* against time)

* $PACO_2$. *(Partial p. of CO2 in Alveoli)*

* $PaCO_2$ *(Partial p of CO_2 in arterial blood)*

* $PETCO_2$ *(Partial p. of CO_2 at the end of expiration)*

* (a-ET)PCO_2 *(arterial to end tidal CO2 pressure difference)*

* $PvCO_2$ *(Partial p. of CO_2 in mixed venous blood)*

Microstream CO_2 expands capnography in a variety of clinical situations:

* **Procedural sedation.** Continuous CO_2 monitoring allows clinicians to assess respiratory changes of spontaneously breathing, non-intubated patients that are often the first signs of hypoventilation, apnea, or airway obstruction

* **Critical care.** Allows the assessment of pulmonary perfusion and ventilatory status during mechanical ventilation, weaning, and post-extubation

* **Anesthesia care.** Provides immediate feedback on proper intubation, helps manage ventilation of patients on respiratory-depressant drugs, and warns of ventilator malfunctions

* **EMS/ED.** Valuable in verifying ET tube placement, alerting to extubations, evaluating CPR efforts, and assessing the ventilatory status of patients with respiratory diseases

* **Transport.** The Microstream CO_2 Extension can travel with the patient to continuously assess the patient's respiratory status a reliable estimate of $PaCO_2$.

CAPNOGRAPHY	VERSUS	PULSE OXIMETRY
* Carbon dioxide		* Oxygen saturation
* **Reflects ventilation**		* **Reflects oxygenation**
* Hypoventilation / apnea detected immediately		* SpO_2 changes lag when patient is hypoventilating or apneic
* **Reflects change in ventilation within 10 seconds**		* **Reflects change in oxygenation within 5 minutes**
* Should be used with pulse oximetry		* Should be used with capnography

CO₂ sampling / O₂ delivery for non-intubated patients

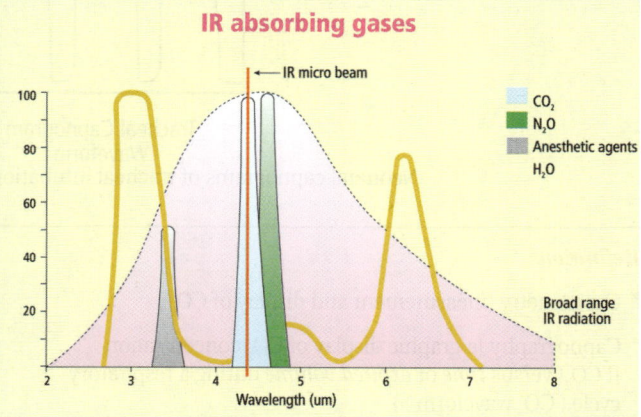

Small pin holes deliver pillow of oxygen around both nose and mouth

Uni-junction™

Uni-junction™ of sampling ports prevents dilution from non-breathing source

Increased surface area provides greater sampling accuracy in the presence of low tidal volume

⟶ O₂
⇢ CO₂

Courtesy: **Microstream® capnography**

IR absorbing gases

IR micro beam

- CO₂
- N₂O
- Anesthetic agents
- H₂O

Broad range IR radiation

Wavelength (um)

Microstream technology: Based upon the principle that CO2 molecules absorb IR radiation at specific wavelengths *Infrared (IR) radiation in conventional capnographs is generated by a "black body" emitter and produces a broad infrared spectrum like light bulb *The infrared spectrum produced has to be filtered to match absorption of CO₂ *Broad bands of infrared frequencies reduce its accuracy and increase the likelihood that other gases will also absorb the IR radiation produced. Microstream improves upon conven tional sidestream sampling; 3rd generation technology –Can use with intubated or non-intubated patient – Low sample flow rate - 50 ml/min * Allows for use on neonate & pediatric patients *Sampling lines not flooded with moisture. **Microstream® capnography** –CO₂ specific laser technology –No calibration or zeroing required – Not affected by other gases –User friendly "Plug and Play". **Conventional vs. Microstream Technologies * Infrared emission source** *Conventional* - "Black Body" emitter *Wide emission band *Produces heat *Microstream* – Molecular Correlation Spectroscopy (MCS™) *Focused CO₂ specific beam *Matches absorption spectrum of the CO₂ molecules.

Capnography in procedural sedation

* Accurately monitors RR
* Monitors adequate ventilation with non-intubated patients
* Monitors potential risk of over-sedation resulting in Hypoventilation more effectively than pulse oximetry
* Early indicator of airway obstruction
* Early warning of apnea
* Adds an additional level of patient safety providing the caregiver with vital information to make accurate assessments and timely interventions for the patient.

Courtesy:
Karen F. Bergenholtz RN MSN CRNP-CS

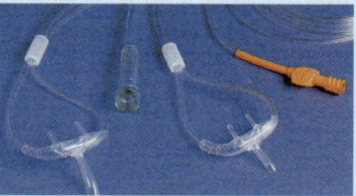

For **non-intubated** patients, there are nasal and combined oral-nasal cannulas to accommodate mouth and nose breathers. Combined CO₂/O₂ circuits precisely measure CO₂ while delivering supplemental oxygen. "H" versions are used for ventilation with humidified air.

Smart CapnoLine™ Plus O₂
nasal cannula for CO₂ measurement and O₂ delivery

- Only system providing accurate EtCO₂ readings for non-intubated patients that receive supplemental O₂ & switch between oral and/or nasal breathing
  –Unique O₂ delivery method reduces CO₂ sampling dilution
  –Solution for high flow O₂ delivery (works effectively under oxygen delivery mask)

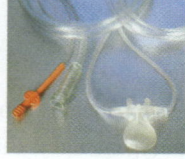

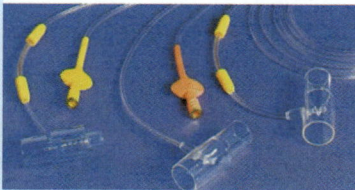

For **intubated** patients, Philips offers FilterLine Sets that combine a FilterLine sample line with an airway adapter. A neonatal airway adapter provides ultra-low dead space.

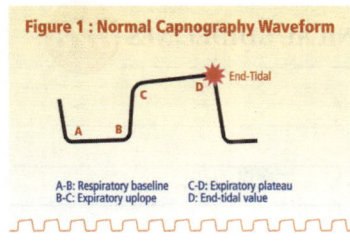

Figure 1 : Normal Capnography Waveform

End-Tidal

A-B: Respiratory baseline   C-D: Expiratory plateau
B-C: Expiratory upslope   D: End-tidal value

Using capnography to ensure successful intubation has become the gold standard and is mandated in many EMS systems. The detection of CO2 on expiration is a completely objective confirmation of tracheal intubation. Also, because capnography directly correlates with cardiac output, it's useful in the cardiac arrest patient to help to determine the effectiveness of CPR compressions, recognize the return of spontaneous circulation and assist with decisions regarding the termination of resuscitation.

In addition to being an essential assessment tool in intubated patients, capnography has been shown to be an extremely valuable technology to use in non-intubated patients. It provides $EtCO_2$ readings and exhibits the related waveform. The configuration of this waveform can be used in the intubated and non-intubated patient to assess the adequacy of ventilation, status of metabolic activity and effectiveness of circulation. The normal capnogram will consist of box-like waveforms directly related to the different phases of the respiratory cycle.

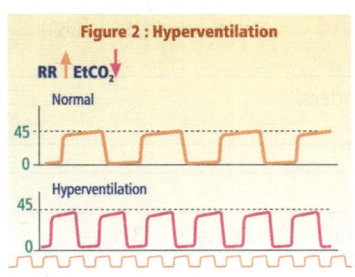

Figure 2 : Hyperventilation

RR ↑ $EtCO_2$ ↓

Normal

45
0

Hyperventilation

45
0

Patients who are hyperventilating will have a capnogram with a faster rate but lower amplitude of waveforms, resulting from the decreased CO_2 in each breath.

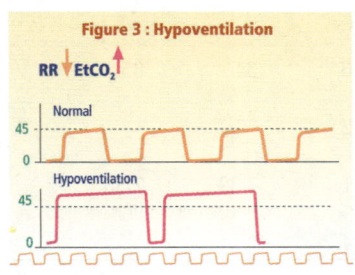

Figure 3 : Hypoventilation

RR ↓ $EtCO_2$ ↑

Normal

45
0

Hypoventilation

45
0

Patients who are hypoventilating will have a lower rate but a higher amplitude of waveforms, resulting from the increased amount of CO_2 being released with each breath.

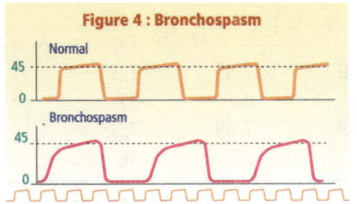

Figure 4 : Bronchospasm

Normal

45
0

Bronchospasm

45
0

The final basic capnographic waveform results from the physiological effects of bronchospasm. Bronchospasm causes a slower and more erratic emptying of CO_2 from the alveoli, which results in a slower rise in the expiratory upstroke. Instead of the normal box-like waveform, the presence of bronchospasm results in the characteristic shark-fin shape of the bronchospastic waveform.

Clinical events detected by pulseoximetry/capnography

Condition	Oximetry	Capnography
Hypoxic gas mixture	Yes	No
Severe atelectasis	Yes	No
Inadequate PEEP in ARDS therapy	Yes	No
Bronchial intubation	Yes	Maybe
Bronchial spasm	Yes	Yes
Cardiac arrest	Yes	Yes
Large pulmonary embolus	Yes	Yes
Malignant hyperthermia	Maybe	Yes
Laryngospasm	Maybe	Yes
Partial airway obstruction	Maybe	Yes
Esophageal intubation	Delayed	Yes
Complete airway disconnection	Delayed	Yes
Accidental extubation	Delayed	Yes
Breathing circuit leaks	Delayed	Yes
Partial rebreathing	No	Yes
Moderate hypoventilation	No	Yes

ARDS = acute respiratory distress syndrome; PEEP = positive end-expiratory pressure.

BLOOD GASES: REPRESENTATIVE VALUES IN NORMAL INFANTS AT TERM

	Arterial blood						
	Umbilical Vein	30 min	1–4 hr	12–24 hr	24–48 hr	96 hr	Reference
PH	7.33	—	7.30	7.30	7.39	7.39	
PCO_2, mm Hg	43	—	39	33	34	36	Reardon et al (1960)
HCO_3, mEq/L	21.6	—	18.8	19.5	20	21.4	Oliver et al (1961)
PO_2, mm Hg	28 ± 8	—	62 ± 13.8	68	63-87		Nelson et al (1962,1963)
O_2 saturation			95%	94%	94%	96%	

From Taeusch HW, Ballard RA: Avery's Diseases of the Newborn, 7th ed. Philadelphia, WB saunders, 1998 and Bucci G et al: Biol Neonate 8:81, 1965

ACID-BASE STATUS

Determination	Sample source	Birth	1 hr	3 hr	24 hr	2 days	3 days
VIGOROUS TERM INFANTS, VAGINAL DELIVERY							
PH	Umbilical artery	7.26					
	Umbilical vein	7.29					
PCO_2 (mm Hg)	Arterial	54.5	38.8	38.3	33.6	34	35
	Venous	42.8					
O_2 saturation(%)	Arterial	19.8	93.8	94.7	93.2		
	Venous	47.6					
pH	Left atrial		7.30	7.34	7.41	7.39 (Temporal artery)	7.38 (Temporal artery)
CO_2 content (mEq/L)	—	—	20.6	21.9	21.4		
PREMATURE INFANTS							
	Capillary (skin puncture)						
pH	<1250 g				7.36	7.35	7.35
PCO_2 (mm Hg)					38	44	37
pH	>1250 g				7.39	7.39	7.38
PCO_2 (mm Hg)					38	39	38

From Shaffer AJ: Diseases of the Newborn, 3rd edition, Philadelphia, WB Saunders, 1971. Weisbrot IM et al; J Ped 52;395 1958

1. *Arterial blood gas analysis defines* the balance between respiration at the tissue level and that in the lungs. It is essential in critically ill Neonates and infants and it involves the assessment of two interrelated but separate metabolic processes namely a) acid-based homeostasis and b) oxygenation.

2. *Assessment of an ABG report requires knowledge of normal values (v.s)*

3. a) Respiratory acidosis and alkalosis implies a primary alteration in the PCO_2 (normal range 35–45 mmHg) which is closely related to *minute ventilation* (tidal volume x respiratory rate)

b) Metabolic acidosis and alkalosis implies a primary alteration in HCO_3 (normal range 20-24 mEq/L) which is closely related to circulatory status and metabolic status.

c) Metabolic acid base disturbances are immediately compensated by <u>lungs</u> (by CO_2 retention / elimination) where as respiratory acid base disturbances are slowly compensated by <u>kidneys</u> (by HCO_3 elimination/conservation).

4. APPROPRIATE COMPENSATION DURING SIMPLE ACID-BASE DISORDERS

Disorder	Expected Compensation
Metabolic acidosis	$PCO_2 = 1.5 \times [HCO_3^-] + 8 \pm 2$ PCO_2 decreases by 10mmHg for each 10 mEq/L decrease in HCO_3
Metabolic alkalosis	PCO_2 increases by 7 mm Hg for each 10 mEq/L increase in serum $[HCO_3^-]$
Respiratory acidosis	
Acute (< 12–24hrs)	$[HCO_3^-]$ increases by 1mEq/L for each 10mmHg increase in PCO_2
Chronic (3–5 days)	$[HCO_3^-]$ increases by 3.5 mEq/L for each 10 mm Hg increase in PCO_2
Respiratory alkalosis	
Acute (<12hrs)	$[HCO_3^-]$ falls by 2 for each 10 mm Hg decrease in PCO_2
Chronic (1–2 days)	$[HCO_3^-]$ falls by 4 for each 10 mmHg decrease in PCO_2

5. *A systematic evaluation of an arterial blood gas, combined with the clinical history, can usually explain the patient's acid-base disturbance and the oxygenation status.*

Step - I What is the pH ? (normal range 7.35–7.45)

* If pH < 7.35   acidosis
* If pH > 7.45   alkalosis
* If pH between 7.35-7.45 normal / well compensated state

Step - II What is the $PaCO_2$? (normal range 35-45mmHg)

* *pH and $PaCO_2$ are closely related to minute ventilation (primarily respiratory)*

* If pH is low and $PaCO_2$ is high (E.g.. if pH is 7.28 and if $PaCO_2$ above 45-50) **respiratory acidosis** (hypoventilation due to airway obstruction /cerebral depression)

* If pH is high and $PaCO_2$ low (Eg. if pH is 7.45 and $PaCO_2$ is 32) **respiratory alkalosis** (hyperventilation due to cerebral irritation / early pneumonia)

Step - III What is the HCO_3 ? (normal range 22-26 mEq/L)

* HCO_3 is related to metabolism (*circulatory, metabolic, endocrinal, renal ,GIT*)

* If the pH is low and the bicarbonate is low (<20mmol)
  metabolic acidosis

* If the pH is high and the bicarbonate is high (>26mmol) **metabolic alkalosis**

Step-IV What is the Base Excess (BE) ?

* BE is an indicator of the metabolic component of acid-base disturbance; it is the difference between the observed whole blood buffer base of the ABG sample and the expected normal whole blood buffer bases (the sum of HCO_3 and non HCO_3 buffer systems)

* IF BE is > + 2 metabolic alkalosis
* IF BE is < – 4 metabolic acidosis
* If BE is > + 8 to +10/ < -8 to- 10 clinically significant

Step-V Is the primary acid base disturbance uncompensated/partially compensated/well compensated?

* If the pH is within normal range ~ well compensated.

* If the pH is out of normal range ~ uncompensated.

* If the pH tends to move away from, but is close to the normal range ~ partially compensated.

Step VI - Is the acid base disorder simple or mixed?

* This depends on the extent of metabolic or respiratory compensation that ought to occur for any given degree of primary disorder

* *Refer to "compensatory mechanisms and their extent" mentioned above (vide supra) and to the table on mixed acid-base disturbances*

Step VII - Identify and treat the cause of the underlying acid base disorders (*vide infra*) (*refer to various tables*).

Capillary blood gas sampling :

1. Correlation with arterial sample best for pH, moderate for PCO_2, worst for PO_2

2. Correlation with PO_2 poor because of arteriovenous mixing during sampling, arterial and venous blood have slightly different pH and PCO_2 but very different PO_2

	Arterial	Venous
pH	7.35-7.45	0.04 units < arterial pH
PCO_2	35-45 mmHg	5-7 mmHg >arterial
PO_2	95 mmHg	40 mmHg
SaO_2	97%	75%

Pitfalls of capillary sampling for blood gases :

1. Improperly warmed capillary bed accuracy

2. Squeezing the soft tissue to collect blood can distort results

3. Prolonged period required for collection (slow bleeding) allows the sample to equilibrate with air resulting in falsely increase PO_2 and falsely lower PCO_2.

Note: Venous blood gases can be used to assess acid-base status, not oxygenation. PCO_2 averages 6-8mmHg higher than $PaCO_2$, and pH is slightly lower. Peripheral venous samples are strongly affected by the local circulatory and metabolic environment. Capillary blood gases correlate best with arterial pH and moderately well with $PaCO_2$.

Arterial blood gas sampling : Practical aspects

Common sites : Radial (most commonly) / brachial / femoral / posterior tibial.

Contraindications to radial puncture : Absent ulnar collateral circulation (modified Allen Test), AV fistula for dialysis, fractured wrist, poor peripheral circulation.

Complications : Hematoma, nerve damage, inadvertent venous sampling.

Procedure : 1. Identify pulse 2. Clean skin with alcohol swab 3. Confirm position of maximum pulsation with non-dominant hand 4. Local anaesthetic reduces pain 5. Insert 23G needle attached to heparinized syringe 6. If using low-resistance syringe this will fill automatically, otherwise aspirate gently 7. Remove needle and apply firm gentle pressure with cotton wool ball for 5 min 8. Label hazardous specimens 9. Expel air bubbles from sample

Possible results : *Hypoxia with normal CO_2 *Hypoxia with ↑CO_2 *Normoxia with ↓CO_2 *Metabolic acidosis vs. compensation

Interpretation : Must be aware of the patient's inspired oxygen concentration (FiO_2) at time of sampling.

Pitfalls : *If sample is to be analyzed in a laboratory with > 5 min transit time it should be kept in melting ice to slow the metabolic activity of the cells *Avoid arterial puncture if possible in patients on anticoagulant therapy, with bleeding disorders or who have received thrombolytics in previous 24h *Failure to note FiO_2 will lead to difficulty in interpretation and potential therapeutic errors.

Changes in Blood Gas on Storage

Blood gas variable	Unit change at 1°C/hr	Unit change at 37° C/hr
pH (unit)	–0.006	–0.01
PaO_2 (mmHg)	–1.725	–2.620
$PaCO_2$ (mmHg)	+0.525	+0.725

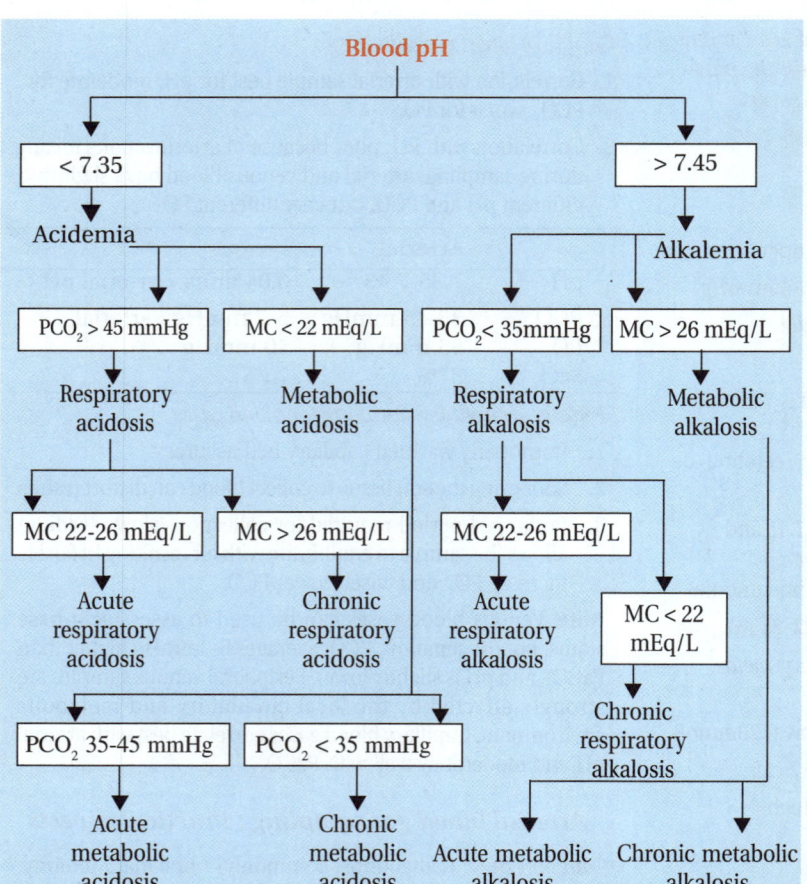

Considerations for interpretation of Neonatal blood gases.

Preanalytic

Sample site (pre/post ductal; capillary/venous/arterial)

Patient status (crying, quiet awake, asleep)

Technique (free-flow of blood, air bubbles, dilution)

Storage time (<15 min at room temp.,<1 h on ice)

Analytic

Instrument precision*

pH +/- 0.01 unit

PCO_2 +/- 267–400 Pa (2–3 mm Hg); CV <4%

PO_2 +/- 267–533 Pa (2–4 mm Hg); CV<3%

Clinical requirements

pH +/-0.05

PCO2 +/- 400 Pa (3 mm Hg)

PO2 +/- 666 Pa (5 mm Hg)

Turnaround time

Tertiary neonatal intensive care unit, acute disease <15 min

Longer in other settings

Interpretation

Rapidly changing physiology

*Instrument precision for PCO2 and PO2 depends on the PCO_2 and PO_2 at which the test is made. Values given are representative of newer blood gas machines.

Simple acid-base disorders: Classification

Disorder	pH	Underlying abnormality	Compensation	Examples of clinical situations
Respiratory acidosis	↓	↑PCO_2	↑HCO_3	Airway obstruction, e.g. RDS
Respiratory alkalosis	↑	↓PCO_2	↓HCO_3	Central hyperventilation, e.g. cerebral irritation
Metabolic acidosis	↓	↓HCO_3	↓PCO_2	Septic shock
Metabolic alkalosis	↑	↑HCO_3	↑PCO_2	Chloride losing states, e.g. pyloric stenosis

Note : *in a simple acid-base disorder with accompanying compensation, PCO_2 and HCO_3 always move in the same direction*

Compensatory changes

Acid-base status	Abnormality	Compensation
Respiratory acidosis	alveolar ventilation insufficient	↑Renal HCO_3 reabsorption which↑ serum HCO_3 concentration
Respiratory alkalosis	alveolar ventilation excessive	↓renal HCO_3 reabsorption with ↓ serum bicarbonate concentration
Metabolic acidosis	gain of strong acid or primary loss of HCO_3	stimulates chemoreceptors which result in ↑ventilation and ↓PCO_2
Metabolic alkalosis	primary gain of a strong base or loss of a strong acid	inhibits the chemoreceptors with resultant hypoventilation and ↑PCO_2

Note: *It may be impossible to distinguish the primary acid-base disorder simply by looking at a blood gas measurement when the pH is normal. Additional tests are needed.*

For example : *pH 7.0, PCO_2 30, HCO_3 18 may represent chronic respiratory alkalosis with metabolic compensation, or chronic metabolic acidosis with respiratory compensation.*

Henderson-Hesselbach equation : pH = pK + log (HCO₃/dissolved CO₂)

* For the bicarbonate buffering system:
  pK=6.1, normal HCO_3 = 24, normal PCO_2 = 40 →dissolved
  CO_2=40 x 0.003 = 1.2 therefore, pH = 6.1 + log (24/1.2)
  = 6.1 + 1.3 = 7.4

* By rearranging the Henderson-Hesselbach equation,
  $[H^+]$ = 24 x PCO_2 / HCO_3
  24 x 40/24 = 40 nM/L

* Balance between HCO_3 and dissolved CO_2 in arterial blood is maintained at 20 : 1 with H^+ concentration of 40nM/L and a pH of 7.4

* Plasma bicarbonate has 2 components:
  1. Metabolic component (MC)
  2. Respiratory component (RC)
     CO_2+H_2O → H_2CO_3 → H^+ + HCO_3
     Acute ↑ in $PaCO_2$ of 1 mmHg above 40 will↑RC by 0.068 mEq/L
     Acute ↓ in $PaCO_2$ of 1 mmHg below 40 will↓RC by 0.2 mEq/L →
     e.g. $PaCO_2$ = 60mmHg→RC=(60-40) x 0.067 = (+) 1.34 mEq/L
           $PaCO_2$ = 20mmHg→RC=(20-40) x 0.2 = (-) 4 mEq/L
  MC = plasma HCO_3 - RC (when PCO_2 > 40),
  MC= plasma HCO_3 + RC (when PCO_2 < 40),
  Normal MC = 22-26 mEq/L,
  MC > 26 implies excess base, MC < 22 implies deficient base

*Alveolar gas equation
  1. PiO_2 = FiO_2 x (P_{atm}-P_{H2O}) PiO_2=partial pressure of O_2 in the conducting airway P_{atm} = barometric pressure (760 mmHg at sea level)
     P_{H2O} = water vapor pressure (47mmHg at 37⁰C)
  2. PAO_2=PiO_2-$PACO_2$/R PAO_2=partial pressure of CO_2 in the alveoli
     $PACO_2$ = partial pressure of CO_2 in the alveoli
     R= respiratory quotient-amount of CO_2 produced/O_2 consumed (normal=0.8)

Acute Respiratory Changes

If CO_2 is responsible for the change in pH, then the pH will change in the opposite direction of the change in PCO_2. Increase in CO_2 will decrease pH and viceversa.

PCO_2 (mmHg)	pH	
60	7.25	This nomogram covers
50	7.30	the range of most of the
40	7.40	acid-base problems
30	7.50	
20	7.55	

Acute Metabolic Changes

If HCO_3 is responsible for the change in pH, then the pH will change in the direction of the change in HCO_3. Low HCO_3 level should lower pH and high HCO_3 will increase pH.

How to look for mixed disturbance in the acid base balance ?

a. *Mixed metabolic and respiratory acidosis*
   ↓Plasma HCO_3, ↑$PaCO_2$, markedly ↓pH
   Causes : *Cardiopulmonary arrest *Adult respiratory distress syndrome *Septic shock

b. *Mixed metabolic and respiratory alkalosis*
   ↑HCO_3, ↓$PaCO_2$, markedly ↑pH
   Causes : CHF with diuretic therapy

c. *Mixed metabolic alkalosis and respiratory acidosis*
   ↑HCO_3, ↑↑$PaCO_2$, pH normal or near normal
   Causes
   *Bronchopulmonary dysplasia on diuretic therapy
   *Chronic respiratory failure and excessive gastric drainage

d. *Metabolic acidosis and respiratory alkalosis* ↓↓HCO_3,
   ↓↓$PaCO_2$, pH is normal or near normal
   Causes : *Rapidly corrected metabolic acidosis
   *Salicylate intoxication
   *Hepatorenal syndrome

Interpretation of Blood Gases • examples of Arterial Blood Gas (ABG) Interpretation

1. A 20 weeks' gestation and 1.1 kg BW infant has RDS. He is 20 hours old and is being nursed on nasal CPAP. His ABG shows:pH 7.21,$PaCO_2$6.6 kPa, $PaO_2$7.5 kPa, HCO_3 20 mmol/L, BE-4 mmol/L **Question (Q)**: What does the ABG show? **Answer (A)**: Mild respiratory acidosis due to worsening Respiratory Distress Syndrome. **Q**: What is the next appropriate mode of therapy? **A**: Mechanical ventilation.

2. Below is the ABG of a 10 hour old 28 weeks' gestation infant :pH 7.22,$PaCO_2$7 kPa, $PaO_2$10 kPa, HCO_3 17 mmol/L, BE-8mmol/L **Q**: What does the ABG show? **A**: Mixed respiratory and metabolic acidosis **Q**: Name a likely diagnosis **A**: Respiratory distress syndrome.

3. The following is the ABG of a 40 day old 26 weeks' gestation baby:pH 7.38,$PaCO_2$8 kPa, $PaO_2$8 kPa, HCO_3 35 mmol/L, BE+10mmol/L**Q**: What does the ABG show? **A**: Fully compensated respiratory acidosis by metabolic alkalosis **Q**: What is a likely diagnosis? **A**: Chronic lung disease. Conti...

4. An infant of 30 weeks' gestation and BW 1.3 kg is being ventilated . ABG shows:pH 7.35,$PaCO_2$3kPa, $PaO_2$15kPa, HCO_3 12 mmol/L,BE-12mmol/L Q: Interpret the ABG A: Fully compensated metabolic acidosis by respiratory alkalosis and hyperoxemia Q: What is your next course of action? A: Reduce FiO2, , give a small dose of $NaHCO_3$, treat any contributory cause of acidosis and wean down ventilation setting.

5. A term infant is being ventilated for meconium aspiration. His ABG is as follows :pH 7.16,$PaCO_2$10kPa, $PaO_2$6kPa, HCO_3 16 mmol/L, BE-10mmol/LQ: What is likely to have happened? A: Pneumothorax Q: What is your interpretation of the ABG A: Mixed respiratory and metabolic acidosis with hypoxemia

6. A 6 day old infant is being ventilated for a cyanotic heart disease. ABG shows :pH 6.80,$PaCO_2$4.5 kPa, $PaO_2$3 kPa, HCO_3 8mmol/L, BE-24mmol/L Q: What does the ABG show? A: Severe metabolic acidosis with severe hypoxemia Q: What is your next course of action ? A: Administer sodium bicarbonate, consider prostaglandin infusion, confirm heart defect and consider surgery. *Pearls: Conversion of kPa to mmHg is a factor of 7.5 kPa*

Normal values for arterial blood gas parameters:

pH 7.34-7.45,
$PaCO_2$5.3-6.0 kPa (40-45 mmHg),
PaO_2 8-10 kPa (60-75 mmHg),
HCO_3 20-25 mmol/L
Base Excess (BE)± 4 mmol/L

One can approach the analysis of simple acid–base disorders by answering three questions. First, is the condition one of acidosis or alkalosis (is the pH less than 7.35 or greater than 7.45)? Second, is the primary cause metabolic (is bicarbonate high or low) or respiratory (is PCO_2 high or low)? Third, is the compensation appropriate? Figure on left shows a clinically useful approach to blood gas interpretation in the newborn and infant.

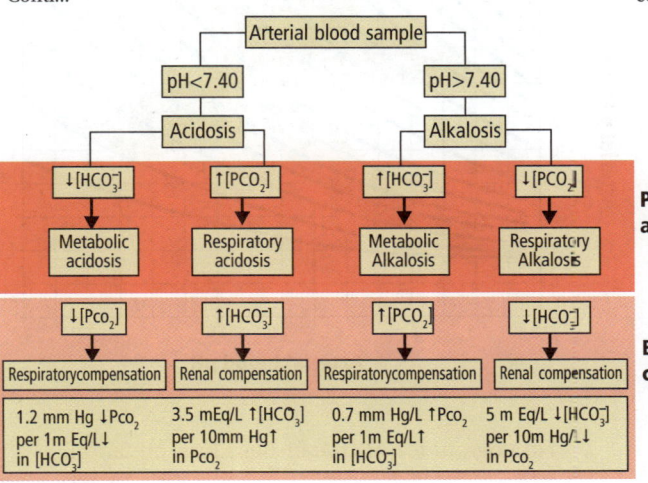

Arterial blood gas measurement remains the best means for assessment of acute respiratory failure

It gives valuable information on the PaO_2 and $PaCO_2$, as well as on the acid-base status as mentioned before

Respiratory failure can be classified in to two types, which usually co-exist in variable proportion as mentioned in the following table.

Types of respiratory failure		
Findings	Causes	Examples
Type I Hypoxia Decreased PaO_2 Normal $PaCO_2$	Ventilation/perfusion defect	Positional (supine in bed), adult respiratory distress syndrome (ARDS), atelectasis, pneumonia, pulmonary embolus, bronchopulmonary dysplasia
	Diffusion impairment	Pulmonary edema, ARDS, interstitial pneumonia
	Shunt	Pulmonary arteriovenous malformation, congenital adenomatoid malformation
Type II Hypoxia Hypercapnia Decreased PaO_2 Increased $PaCO_2$	Hypoventilation	Neuromuscular disease (polio, Guillain-Barre syndrome), head trauma, sedation, chest wall dysfunction (burns), kyphosis, severe reactive airways

Hypoxemia is not always related to respiratory failure. Right to left cardiac shunts, high altitude with its low ambient O_2 concentration, and the production of the methemoglobin all may produce severe hypoxemia with normal respiratory function.

Assessment of severity of Hypoxemia

Normal PaO_2 = 85 to 100 mmHg
Relationship between FiO_2 and PaO_2 in normal individual PaO_2 = FiO_2 x 5
Mild hypoxia = PaO_2 < 80 mmHg
Moderate hypoxia = PaO_2 < 60 mmHg
Severe hypoxia = PaO_2 < 40 mmHg
A PaO_2 < 50mmHg (<45mmHg in preterms) indicates hypoxemia in the Newborn (indicates ventilation—perfusion mismatch)

Significance of $PaCO_2$

1. Hypoxemia and low $PaCO_2$ (below 35mmHg) : initial phase of respiratory failure (RF)

2. Hypoxemia and normal $PaCO_2$ (35-45mmHg) : may be initial respiratory failure

3. Hypoxemia and high $PaCO_2$ (> 50mmHg) : indicate late phase of respiratory failure.

Suggested Reading : 1) Oxford Handbook of Clinical and Laboratory Investigation 2) Nelson Textbook of Pediatrics 3) Pediatric Acute Care

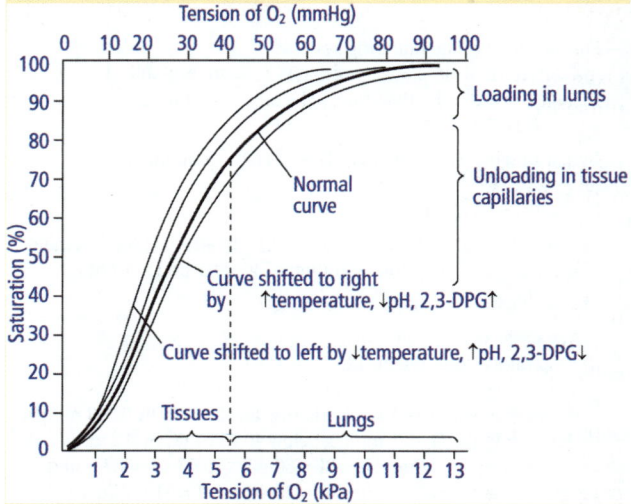

Dissociation curve for oxyhemoglobin

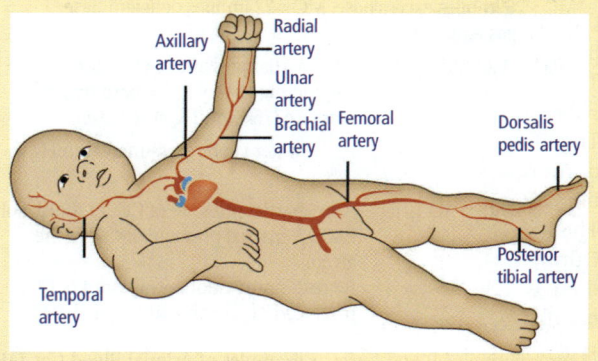

Radial, Posterior tibial & Dorsalis pedis arteries are the preferable Peripheral arteries, to puncture for ABG Analysis in the Newborn.

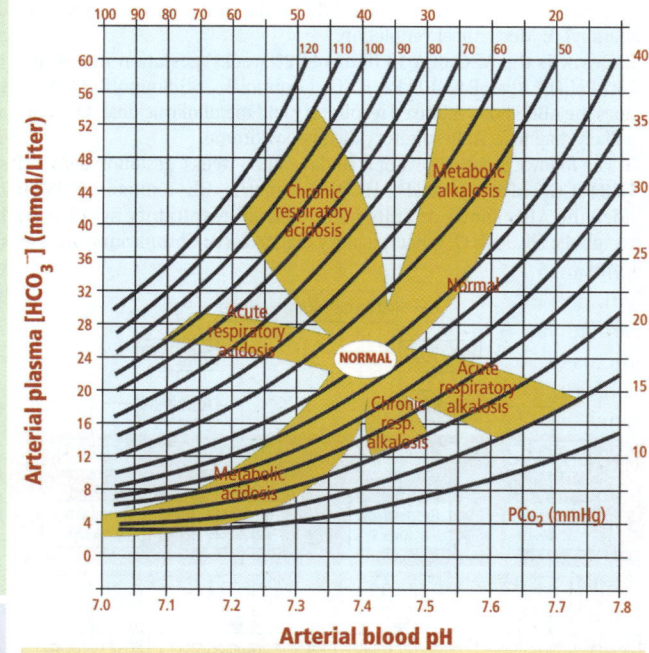

Nomogram for ABG Acid-Base Interpretation.

Oxygen is the most commonly used therapy in neonatal nurseries as an integral part of respiratory support. The goal of oxygen therapy is to achieve adequate delivery of oxygen to the tissue without creating oxygen toxicity. Normally a FiO_2 of 0.21 in the inspired air (i.e. 21% oxygen concentration in the air that is being breathed in) is sufficient to produce a partial pressure of oxygen in the arterial blood of 8-10 kPa (60-75 mm Hg). The partial pressure of arterial oxygen is referred to as the PaO_2. A PaO_2 of 8-10 kPa (60-75 mm Hg) is normal and adequate to load the hemoglobin in the circulating red blood cells with oxygen. The degree of saturation of arterial blood with oxygen is referred to as the SaO_2. At a $FiO2$ of 0.21 the $SaO2$ in a newborn infant is normally 86-92%. *The SaO_2 is determined by the PaO_2 and the hemoglobin's ability to take up oxygen. The SaO_2 increases in a linear manner as the paO_2 rises until the SaO_2 reaches 90%. Thereafter there is a poor correlation between the two measurements. This explains why a SaO_2 above 90% is potentially dangerous as the PaO_2 may be very high.* If the $PaO2$ falls below 8 kPa (60 mm Hg) and the SaO_2 falls below 86%, the red cells will not be adequately loaded with oxygen. The infant will now appear cyanosed and the cells of the body will not receive enough oxygen for aerobic metabolism. Therefore, extra oxygen is needed in the inspired air (i.e. a FiO_2 of more than 0,21) if: 1. The infant has central cyanosis (a blue tongue). 2. The PaO_2 drops below 8 kPa (60 mm Hg). 3. The SaO_2 falls below 86%. The infant needs extra oxygen 1. During resuscitation after delivery or in the nursery. 2. When there is respiratory distress due to conditions such as hyaline membrane disease, pneumonia and meconium aspiration. 3. When the infant has central cyanosis. 4. When the PaO_2 is below the normal range (less than 8 kPa or 60 mm Hg). 5. When the SaO_2 is below the normal range (less than 86%). If the central cyanosis is not corrected when extra oxygen is given, it is essential to provide some form of artificial ventilation.

Extra oxygen should not be given to the infants, unless absolutely necessary. For e.g., 1. Infants with normal Apgar scores at birth. Do not give oxygen to infants who do not need resuscitation. 2. Infants with peripheral but not central cyanosis. If there is peripheral cyanosis only, the cause is usually cold hands and feet poor perfusion, rather than hypoxia. 3. Infants with recurrent apnea. They should only be given oxygen during resuscitation and not once spontaneous respiration has started. 4. Small, preterm infants with a normal PaO_2 and SaO_2. In some babies with complex cardiac conditions, a low saturation is desirable to help prevent ductus closure and excessive pulmonary blood flow. In these babies, the medical staff will determine the desired saturation range.

Oxygen and neonatal morbidities in preterm infant: Oxygen, a potent oxidant, is a health hazard if inhaled in excess. The potential detrimental effects associated with oxygen include retinopathy of prematurity (ROP), bronchopulmonary dysplasia (BPD), increase length of stay (LOS), impaired brain development and possibly infection and cancer. 1. Oxygen should not be given directly into a closed incubator as this method is wasteful, high concentrations cannot be reached and the concentration of oxygen drops every time an incubator

port is opened. 2. Gastric oxygen via a nasogastric tube is valueless and dangerous. 3. Dry, unhumidified oxygen should not be given except for a short period in an emergency. 4. An oxygen flow meter alone, without a blender or venturi, should not be used to control the FiO_2 unless an oxygen monitor is also used. It is very difficult to control the FiO_2 with a flow meter alone and carbon dioxide may accumulate if the flow is too small. 5. Giving 100% oxygen via a cardboard cup is extremely dangerous as it is almost impossible to control the FiO_2 accurately. This method should be used as the last resort only.

Methods to administer Oxygen

1. Oxygen is most commonly given into a Perspex head box.. This is the best method of administering oxygen to most infants as it is a simple, cheap and highly effective method. A blender or venturi should be used. 2. Oxygen may be given via NASAL PRONGS when continuous positive airways pressure is needed. This is particularly useful in infants with respiratory distress. 3. An ENDOTRACHEAL TUBE is used for most infants receiving oxygen via a ventilator. The oxygen must be warmed and humidified. 4. At resuscitation oxygen is given via the FACE MASK of a resuscitator (bag and mask) or by endotracheal tube. Refer to next Chapter foe the details

Effects of too much or too little oxygen

The effects of adopting a restricted or low oxygen target range include:

In the very early neonatal period (<48 hours age): increases mortality and spastic diplegia (retrospective observational studies); may decrease incidence severe ROP . *>48 hours age:* no difference in early or late mortality, ROP progression, sleep architecture or cerebral palsy (RCT, cohort studies); decreases incidence of severe ROP and blindness (RCTs), apnea, cyanosis and asphyxia.

The effects of adopting an unrestricted or high oxygen target range include: *In the early neonatal period (> 48 hours age):* increases incidence of severe ROP and blindness (RCTs). *In the late neonatal period:* no difference in ROP progression or cerebral palsy (RCT, cohort studies); may increase chronic lung disease, home oxygen rates, length of hospital stay, rehospitalization rates (2o outcomes in RCT); decreases short term growth, sleep desaturations, and pulmonary hypertension (cohort studies); has unknown effect on long term growth and development (awaiting results of BOOST RCT).

Safe Oxygen Saturation Targeting in Infants are given in Table 1. Table 2 enlists the changes in practices, necessary, to avoid neonatal hyperoxemia in the delivery room, the NICU, the operating room and during transport and diagnostic studies. Table 3 summarizes some other issues regarding clinical care with supplemental oxygen, in order to improve neonatal daily care of oxygen administration and monitoring. These issues include necessary equipment, clinical assessment and actions during procedures, apnea and manual ventilation. Table 4 compares the advantages and limitations of pulse oximetry and transcutaneous monitoring for neonatal oxygen assessment.

TABLE 1 — Safe oxygen saturation targeting in infants

Oxygen Saturation Targeting in Infants

Infants	paO$_2$ (kPa)	Saturation range	Alarm Limits
Preterm <36 weeks	6.5-9.0	88–92%	86–94%
Term(>36 weeks)or Post term	8.0-12.0	90–100% In the first 24 hours, 95-100%	90–100% In the first 24 hours 95-100%
CLD AND 36 weeks PMA	8.0-10.0	90-95%	88-96%
		CLD -Chronic lung disease PMA-Postmenstrual age	

Overnight Saturation Run Guidelines

* For infants who are in air and do no need supplemental oxygen, saturations that are mostly above 90% are regarded as satisfactory.
* For babies who are in oxygen, saturations should be targeting the following values:

Saturation Level	Proportion of Study
90–95%	80–90%
<90%	10–20%

Reference : Askie LM, Henderson-Smart DJ, Irwig L, Simpson JM. Oxygen-saturation targets and outcomes in extremely preterm infants. N Engl J Med 2003,349:959-67

TABLE 2 — Guidelines to avoid hyperoxemia in the delivery room, NICU, transport, operating room and during diagnostic studies

1. Care to prevent hyperoxemia must commence in the delivery room
2. Administer supplemental oxygen only when really needed
3. Be able to mix gases (air and oxygen) and know the dose (concentration; i.e., FiO2) of supplemental oxygen the infant is receiving
4. Measure FiO2 each and every time oxygen is given to newborns
5. Be able to measure levels of blood oxygenation as best as possible. Today this can be done with accurate and state of the art pulse oximetry monitors (SpO$_2$ monitors)
6. Never use pure oxygen (100%, FiO$_2$ 1.0) unless it is really proven to be necessary
7. Do not use nitrogen washout (FiO$_2$ 1.0) for a pneumothorax. No important outcome was ever shown to improve with this practice, and PaO$_2$ can be very high (i.e., >150 mmHg) for a long time
8. Never leave a preterm infant for any period of time breathing supplemental oxygen, just because the infant breathes a little fast or has some grunting or looks pinker being nursed in oxygen. (Always document that you indeed need to give supplemental oxygen by a reading of abnormally low SpO$_2$)
9. SpO$_2$ monitors were developed for detection of hypoxemia and are of no value for detecting hyperoxemia 10. Do not allow the SpO$_2$ monitor to read >94–95% when a preterm infant is breathing supplemental oxygen
11. Do not permit hypoxemia
12. Manual ventilation: should never be done with gas flowing into a breathing bag directly from the wall oxygen flow meter (i.e., 100% or FiO2 1.0). The gas from the wall is pure oxygen and is cold and dry
13. Use of an accurate SpO$_2$ monitor with preset low and high alarms, which must never be left turned off
14. Aim for a target SpO$_2$ range which is wide enough so that there are fewer possibilities of frequent changes and of chasing SpO2 values
15. Do not aim for normal SpO2 values (i.e., >95%) in preterm infants breathing supplemental oxygen. These are high SpO$_2$ levels, which are unnecessary and very likely detrimental
16. When a premature infant is breathing O$_2$, and the SpO$_2$ is 96–100%, the PaO2 can be >90mm Hg
17. Always wean the FiO$_2$ (slowly) when SpO$_2$ is >95% in a preterm infant breathing supplemental oxygen. If saturation remains at >95% in room air (FiO$_2$ 0.21), this is an indication the infant did not need supplemental oxygen

Courtesy:Professor A Sola, YP Saldeno, V Favareto

TABLE 3 — Clinical care of newborns to whom we give supplemental oxygen

Issue	Actions	Other factors to consider
Equipment Think twice	Blender and state of the art Sp0$_2$ monitor Ask yourself :Does this baby really need this FiO$_2$	Measure dose (FiO$_2$) and levels (Sp0$_2$) at all times, also in DR think again
Assess again	Do not give 0$_2$ unless a clear need is demonstrated	Prematurity, tachypnea, grunting, acrocyanosis, apnea and others are **not** an indication
Delivery room	Do not blow by 0$_2$ Do not use 100% 0$_2$ unless its need is really proven	Remember the transition from fetal to normal neonatal saturation
For procedures (i.e., suction of airway)	Do not increase Fio$_2$ before starting	If problems, remember PEEP to maintain FRC
Require episodes of manual ventilation	Do not increase previous FiO$_2$ routinely	This is very important
Apnea with need for manual ventilation	Ventilate! (Do not increase previous Fi0$_2$ routinely)	If it was really necessary to increase Fi0$_2$, watch SpO$_2$ reading and return Fi0$_2$ to baseline rapidly
If FiO$_2$ needs to be increased	Document in records. Do not leave bedside. Assess and re-assess. See Sp0$_2$ readings and alarms. Do not allow Sp0$_2$ reading to remain >94-95%[a]	Assess if Fi0$_2$ can be brought to previous level, in a stepwise manner as long as Sp0$_2$ is stable and >93-94%
Avoid wide fluctuations of Fi0$_2$	May lead to see-saw of Sp0$_2$	Alternating between hypoxia and hyperoxia is risky to the eyes
Sp0$_2$ alarm setting	(83%) 85-93% (94%)	No need to argue for and exact value
Alarms	Operative all of the time	A must
Sp0$_2$ readings	do not 'chase them'	Evaluate infant and monitor before modifying Fi0$_2$
Sp0$_2$ readings	If Sp0$_2$ is as good as normal in room air; Act!	do not allow Sp0$_2$ reading to remain >94-95%[a]

[a] Exceptions are the rules of life. A few infants breathing supplemental oxygen may need Sp02 >95% some time, infrequently though.

Courtesy:Professor A Sola, YP Saldeno, V Favareto

Oxygen Monitoring Guidelines:
Preterm infants:

1. Early management (all gestations):

Infants < 27 weeks

- TCMs (**Transcutaneous oxygen monitoring**) are not routinely used during the first 14 days after birth. TCMs if used after 14 days correlate best with arterial blood gases when applied to anterior thigh. • Pulse oximeters (Nellcor, functional saturation algorithm) are exclusively used to continuously monitor oxygenation during the first 14 days after birth with the alarms set at 88-96% - target range 90–95%. Frequent micro arterial blood gas analysis.

After surfactant: (reduction in TCM CO_2 monitoring introduces significant risk of over ventilation) • 15 minutes post surfactant administration • hourly for 6 hours until stable • routine use of pulmonary mechanic monitoring to detect over ventilation

Infants > 27 weeks:

- TCMs are routinely used during the acute phase after birth in ventilated infants. • Pulse oximeters (Nellcor) are used to continuously monitor oxygenation whilst the infant is in oxygen, with the alarms set at 88-96% - target range 90-95%. •

Micro arterial blood gas analysis is used to ensure accuracy of the TCM. Micro arterial blood gas analyses may be reduced if the TCM has a high degree of correlation or the infant is stable.

After surfactant: • 15 minutes post surfactant administration • frequency will depend on accuracy of TCM. If no correlation, hourly for 6 hours until stable • routine use of pulmonary mechanic monitoring to detect over ventilation

2. Late management (all gestations)

- After 1 week of age, infants who are stable or off the ventilator may be monitored by pulse oximetry monitoring (Nellcor), with the alarms set at 88–96% - target range 90–95%. The upper alarm limit should only be increased if the infant is in air.

Term infants

Points to consider

Use of TCMs and pulse oximeters. Targeting oxygen to avoid hypoxia – **if pulmonary hypertension not suspected:** • PaO_2 > 60–90mmHg on TCM or ABG ·SpO_2 > 95% @ Targeting oxygen to avoid hypoxia

– **if pulmonary hypertension is suspected** • PaO_2 > 100-120mmHg on TCM or ABG ·SpO_2 > 97%

TABLE 4	Advantages and limitations of pulse oximetry and transcutaneous monitoring for neonatal oxygen assessment.	
	Pulse oximetry	**Transcutaneous O2**
Accuracy	Excellent (vs SaO2)	Good (vs PaO2)
Hypoxemia detection	Excellent	Good
Calibration required	No	Yes
Ease to use	Very easy	Moderately difficult
Limitations	Hypotension	Hypotension
	Poor perfusion	Poor perfusion
	Motion	Edema
		Skin disorders
Complications	Rare	Burns
Hyperoxemia detection	Good	Excellent

* Pulse oximetry and transcutaneous oxygen monitoring are extraordinarily useful techniques of estimating and noninvasively monitoring the neonate's oxygenation. In most settings they complement blood gases by permitting the clinician to noninvasively follow trends in patient. **oxygenation.** However, neither technique can replace arterial blood gas monitoring in the critically ill patient because neither provides comprehensive and exact information on oxygenation, ventilation, acid–base status, and hemoglobin variants.

KEY POINTS FOR CLINICAL PRACTICE:

In an effort to translate information from basic science and clinical research into clinical practice, the clinician must make judgments about how to apply various findings even when definitive answers are not available. Currently, the best information available would suggest the following approach to clinical practice. For resuscitation of the preterm infant <32 wk, an initial oxygen concentration of 30–40% may be most appropriate until further evidence is available. During resuscitation, it is feasible to adjust the oxygen concentration to achieve a gradually increasing SpO_2 over the first 10 min of life. Reasonable SpO_2 targets during transition seem to be approximately 70% at 3 min of life and 80% at 5 min of life mimicking the values achieved by well transitioning infants. If an infant's SpO_2 is lower and not increasing over several minutes, the resuscitation team should consider an increase in the concentration of oxygen. For the ongoing management of preterm infants in the NICU who require oxygen, each unit should have agreed upon target range with alarm limits set close to this range and all staff should be aware of these values. Without the benefit of prospective trials during the acute phase of illness, an SpO_2 target range of 85-93% seems most reasonable at this time. Intermittent audit of compliance with alarm limits and occasional review of the oximeter data sets may provide additional supportive information to help maintain and encourage appropriate monitoring limits. In addition, the presence of guidelines for the immediate response to intermittent desaturations including suggested increases in FiO_2 may further reduce exposures to both low and high SpO2 values. Although there is some evidence that the use of a higher target in the recovery phase of preterm illness may be of value for infants with evidence of prethreshold ROP, this practice seems to increase pulmonary morbidity, which may outweigh any benefit. Further prospective studies are required to evaluate the long-term outcome of infants treated with different oxygen targeting strategies.

REFERENCES & FURTHER READING: 1) Clinical practices in neonatal oxygenation: where have we failed? What can we do?Journal of Perinatology (2008) 28, S28–S34Professor A Sola, YP Saldeno, V Favareto. 2)Optimum oxygen therapy in preterm babies W Tin, S Gupta, Arch Dis Child Fetal Neonatal Ed 2007;92:F143–F147. doi: 10.1136/adc.2005.092726. 3)Newborn Services Clinical Guidelinehttp://www.adhb.govt.nz/newborn/guidelines/Respiratory/Oxygen/OxygenSaturationTargets.htm. 4) Oxygen Saturation Monitoring for the Preterm Infant: The Evidence Basis for Current Practice, FINER, NEIL; LEONE, TINA Pediatric Research: April 2009 - Volume 65 - Issue 4 - pp 375-380

* *Pearl/Peril/Pitfall: Blood transfusion in a critically ill newborn may be required when >10% of blood volume (80 mL/kg body weight in the full term; 100 mL/kg body weight in the preterm) is withdrawn over , 2 – 3 days. Thus, for a 750-g infant, withdrawal of as little as 8 mL of blood over a short period may necessitate blood transfusion.*

OXYGEN ADMINISTRATION IN NEONATES: MEANS AND METHODS

Low flow oxygen/air (or combination) administration

Low flow oxygen/air administration is used for infants requiring some respiratory support but not CPAP

* Flows –300 ml/min –1000 ml/min require humidifying - below 300 ml/min are not humidified -once the flow has been reduced to <200ml/min use a "low flow meter" -When utilizing humidified flows watch for rainout in the circuit and try to ensure that it is cleared back into the humidifier regularly to avoid lavage -Low flow oxygen is measured in ml/min not litres -read from the centre of the ball. -take careful note of ml/min being delivered. There are different flow meters in use. Check ml/min with another staff member. -When an infant is stable on Low Flow respiratory support it may be moved into a cot and attempts at feeding can be instituted.

Steps   Action

1. Any increase in O_2 during feeds should be documented.

2. Choose appropriate prong size (small or medium). Prongs should fit snugly and be taped to face appropriately using thin Duoderm as a base and Hyperfix to tape.

3. Check that nasal prongs are clear, frequently; changing once a week or more frequently if required.

*Low flow can be separated into 3 categories: *Combination Air and Oxygen *Oxygen *Air*

Combination of low flow oxygen and low flow air

This may be used on consultant's orders to support a baby when CPAP is discontinued but the infant continues to have a minimal oxygen requirement. *If this mode of respiratory support is utilized for infants <36weeks gestation an oxygen analyzer must be present in the circuitry (i.e. will need to have a flow of >300ml/min running via the humidifier). The combination may be: *via the blender at higher humidified low flows (1000 ml/min - 300 ml/min) or *with a mix of flows from low flow regulators

Steps   Action

1. Use a Y connector to join the low flow O_2 and low flow air.

2. Use a low flow air meter to deliver 250 ml of air.

3. Use low flow oxygen meter to deliver a **maximum of 125 ml** to maintain an appropriate SaO$_2$ as per *Standing orders*

Low flow oxygen administration (Infants > 36 weeks gestation only)

Non Humidified

* Used for babies requiring long term oxygen therapy. *Not administered to babies under 36 weeks as it is difficult to be

certain of the FiO$_2$ actually delivered and difficult to maintain the SpO$_2$ saturations in the target range of 88–92%. *Not generally used for babies requiring a flow of more than 300ml/min. *Oxygen is administered as per standing orders. *Parents of infants who are likely to be on Low Flow Oxygen at home can begin to learn to manage the Low Flow tubing and learn about signs that their infant is not coping.

Low flow air administration—Non Humidified—This may be used for individual babies on Consultant order, as a transition from CPAP to room air.

Steps   Action

1. Use a low flow air meter to delivery 300 ml of air.

2. The flow may be weaned to 250ml, **no less**, before trailing off (following discussion on medical round).

Oxygen therapy nursing responsibilities

Steps action

1. Baby has a clear airway and is suctioned as per protocol.
2. Oxygen is administered to maintain SpO$_2$ as per standing orders. Alarm limits are set accordingly.
3. SpO$_2$ lead position should be changed every four hours.
4. Oxygen level is checked and documented (including amount of supplemental oxygen and SpO$_2$ levels):
   • at nursing handover (beginning of each shift)
   • hourly if baby on CPAP or ventilated
   • 2–3 hourly if baby receiving LF O$_2$ / incubator O$_2$

NB : On infants where O$_2$ levels require frequent alteration, check more frequently (e.g. on returning from meal break)

5. Medical staff are notified if a baby's oxygen requirement increases consistently by 10% or more.

6. An oxygen analyzer, calibrated at the beginning of each shift, is used when oxygen is administered via:
   • CPAP
   • Ventilator
   • Incubator

7. Oxygen analyzer is calibrated to
   • air if baby receiving <60% O$_2$
   • 100% O$_2$ if baby receiving >60% O$_2$

8. Humidification appropriate to oxygen delivery is provided at all times

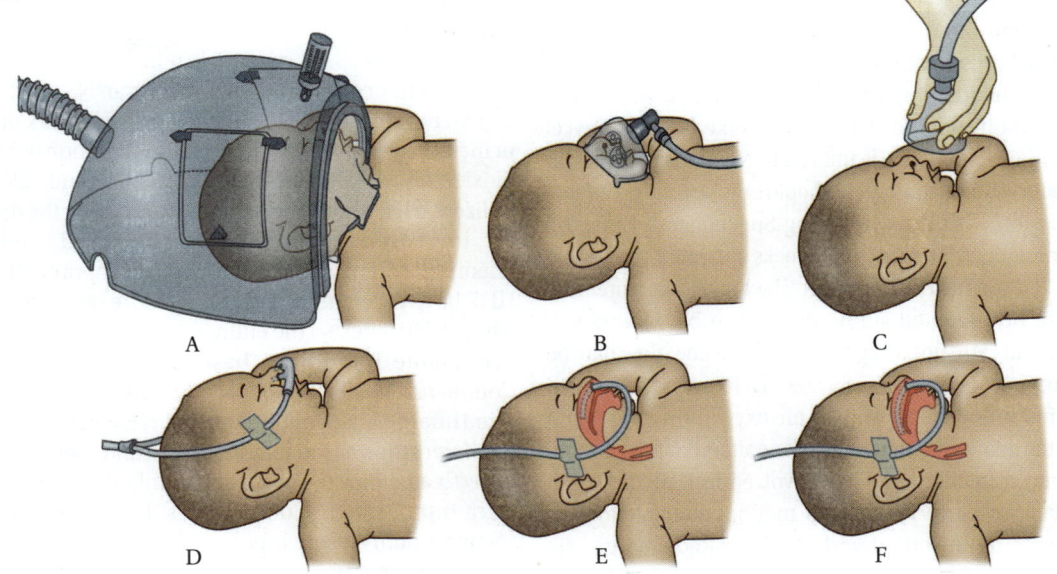

(A) Headbox oxygen; (B) facemask; (C) oxygen administration by holding an oxygen source near the infant's face; (D) nasal cannulae; (E) nasal catheter; (F) nasopharyngeal catheter.

Source	Maximum	Range of % O_2	Advantages flow rates	Disadvantages
Nasal canula	35–40%	0.125–4 L/min	Easily applied, relatively common	Uncomfortable at higher flow rates, requires open nasal airways, easily dislodged, lower % O_2 nose bleeds
Simple mask	50–60%	5–1 L/min	Higher % O_2, good for mouth breathers	Uncomfortable, dangerous for patients with poor airway control and at risk for emesis, hard to give airway care, unsure of % O_2
Face tent	40–60%	8–10 L/min	Higher % O_2, good for mouth breathers, less restrictive	Uncomfortable, dangerous for patients with poor airway control and at risk for emesis, hard to give airway care, unsure of % O_2
Rebreathing mask	80–90%	5–10 L/min	Higher % O_2, good for mouth breathers, highest O_2 concentration	Uncomfortable, dangerous for patients with poor airway control and at risk for emesis, hard to give airway care, ensure of % O_2
Oxyhood	90–100%	5–10 L/min (mixed at wall)	Stable and accurate O_2 concentration	Temperature regulation, hard to give air way care

CARE OF BABIES ON OXYGEN AT HOME FOLLOWING DISCHARGE FROM NICU

Oxygen saturation targets

Saturation level	Proportion of study
90–100%	80–90%
<90%	10–20%

*At risk babies should have an overnight saturation run prior to discharge. *Infants who do not maintain these saturation parameters while breathing air but are otherwise ready for discharge should be considered for home oxygen.

@**Following Discharge Home**-*Minimum oxygen flow rate at home is 0.125L/min. *No changes in oxygen administration should be made for the first two weeks. *After two weeks, a 12–hour baseline overnight oximetry recording is done. *Weaning can be commenced, when oxygen saturation ~90% for 90% of the time. *The overall mean SaO$_2$ should be ~"92% @**Weaning off oxygen**-*A Home Care nurse will visit during the baby's first time off oxygen. *Weaning off oxygen will start during

the daytime. *Initially the baby should have up to 4 hours off oxygen, increasing to 6–8 hours, then 8–12 hours and finally off oxygen at night as well. *A Home Care nurse will phone the day after each change in oxygen administration, to review progress. *2–3 days after each change, a Home Care nurse will visit and check oxygen saturations for a 40 minute period. The baby should be off oxygen for at least 1–2 hours prior to this check. *If the baby remains stable and well, overnight 12 hour pulse oximetry is checked again a minimum of 2 weeks later with the view to continue weaning. *Oximetry reports will be reviewed with a neonatal specialist and recommendations implemented the same or the following day. *A 12-hour overnight oximetry recording should be done the day the baby discontinues oxygen therapy. *Once oxygen is discontinued, a telephone call should be made the following day to check on progress and then an overnight 12 hour.

References : 1) Wilkinson, D., Andersen, C., Smith, K. & Holberton, J. Pharyngeal pressure with high-flow nasal cannulae in premature infants. Journal of Perinatology. 2008: 28(1), 42–47. 2) Saslow, J., Aghai, Z., Nakhla, T., Hart, J., Lawrysh, R., Stahl, G. & Pyon, K. Work of breathing using high-flow nasal cannula in preterm infants. Journal of Perinatology. 2006. 26, 476–480 3)Screenan, C., Lemke, R., Hudson-Mason, A. & Osiovicj, H. High-Flow Nasal Cannulae in the Management of Apnea of Prematurity: A Comparison with Conventional Nasal Continuous Positive Airway Pressure. Pediatrics. 2001. 107(5), 1081-1083 oximetry recording should be made one week

Humidified high flow oxygen or air: Humidified High-Flow (HHF) oxygen/air is a form of respiratory support in preterm infants where the infant is breathing spontaneously. It is air-oxygen flow (via blender) of 1-6 L/min via the Fisher & Paykel humidifier. **Indications:** HHF is utilized in NICU for infants with mild respiratory dysfunction. HHF should only be used on infants after discussion with the overseeing Specialist and may be relevant for infants who: *Are 34–36 weeks corrected gestational age *Are HCPAP (6cmH$_2$O) dependant *Have an FiO$_2$ requirement of <0.3 *Are not deemed stable enough to be trialled self ventilating in Air *Are not of a gestation where Low-flow may be more appropriate. **HHF Effects Include:** HHF provides warmed and humidified flow of air and/or air-oxygen mixture (via a blender) to the infant where FiO$_2$ can be monitored. There is some degree of end distending pressure involved in HHF; however, debate remains as to how much. HHF may be better tolerated by infants becoming unsettled with HCPAP. Reduced gastric distension, Sucking fees are more easily attempted with HHF than HCPAP. **Complications:** Potential for asynchrony in breathing may result in the infant becoming tired over long periods; therefore, good assessment of work of breathing is required Potential for nasal erosion (although less than with HCPAP) remains. There is some concern about unknown end distending pressure and varied results gained in research studies; therefore ensure that the prongs do not seal the nares and reduce flow as able. Potential problems with "rainout" resulting in lavage and apnoea; therefore, nurses need to be aware of clearing "rainout" from tubing regularly and ensuring that only heated tubing is utilized. **Application of Humidified High Flow:** HHF is to be commenced at a flow rate of 5 L/min and can be increased to 6 L/min after consultation with registrar/NS-ANP. The infant should be returned to HCPAP for increasing work of breathing or increasing apnoea/bradycardia/desaturation or high carbon dioxide on a blood gas. If cycling of HHF and CPAP is being utilized: · HHF should be administered during the day allowing for increased parental interaction and sucking feed attempts.*HCPAP should continue at night time. *HCPAP and HHF have different tubing and pressure relief valves (HCPAP white/HHF blue), so the entire system needs to be alternated. *The same humidifier base may be utilized. Before **Commencing HHF on an Infant :** *Select appropriate prong size (Infant vs Neonatal) and get HHF set (RT329). *Place *duoderm* strips to the infants cheeks and then apply strips of *hyperfix* attaching the prongs to the infants cheeks. Ensure that extra (non heated) blue tubing is discarded. **Maintenance:** *Active mouth closure is not required *Watch for "rain-out" in the clear prong tubing as this can cause a lavage to the infant resulting in apnoea. *The baby may be nursed prone, skin to skin (kangaroo), supine or side to side lying. *Orogastric / nasogastric feeds are as ordered / tolerated *Infants may be offered breast or bottle feeds whilst on HHF but continual respiratory assessment is essential. **Weaning :** *Once an infant is continuously utilizing HHF the FiO$_2$ should be weaned as able to 0.3, then the flow weaned over a number of days, under the guidance of the overseeing consultant. *Once the flow has been weaned to <1L/min it is now considered Low-Flow. It will continue to be warmed and humidified until the flow is <300ml/min.

Step	Action	Rationale
1.	*Observe and document a baseline assessment of the infant prior to the commencement of HHF *Respiration: rate, effort, breath sounds, signs of distress (tachypnea, nasal flaring, sternal indrawing, rib retractions, grunting) *Temperature *Cardiovascular: central and peripheral perfusion, blood pressure, auscultation *Neurological: tone, response to stimulation, activity *Gastro-intestinal: specific characteristics (e.g. cleft palate, omphalocele), abdominal distention, visible loops, bowel sounds *Technical: pre-ductal (preferably right arm) oxygen saturation probe, cardio-respiratory monitor	Baseline observations are essential to the ongoing management of the baby.
2.	*Regular observations as outlined above need to be preformed. Minimal handling is essential for the sick infant therefore "hands-on" intervention should be limited to 2-4 hrly if possible.	Decisions regarding ongoing treatment are made on the basis of serial assessments.
3.	*Keep the baby's parents informed of what is happening. Answer questions and offer information, as you do with regard to all other aspects of the baby's care.	Parents are members of the care team and have the right to understand the care their baby receives.
4.	*Once the infant is stable on HHF and is tolerating handling without compromise or agitation, the usual activities of care can be performed.	This facilitates attachment and reinforces their role as parent and caretaker.
5.	*Parents can be encouraged to participate by being shown the techniques of soothing and containment. They can perform oral cares, nappy changes, etc. as their confidence and baby's condition permits	Changing position is a gentle way to move lung secretions along the airway.
6.	*Change the baby's position 4-6hrly. Kangaroo care is an ideal variation in position along with it's other tactile emotional advantages.	

VAPOTHERM2000i™

The Vapotherm2000i™ (VT) device delivers around 95% humidified air or blended oxygen through ordinary nasal cannulae, without rainout, with flows of up to 8 L/min. The VT humidifies and warms flows of air; blended air and oxygen; or pure oxygen; for delivery to infants via nasal cannulae. Warming and humidification occurs in a special cartridge inside the body of the machine. Within the cartridge is a membrane separating the air and the water, which is permeable to water vapour and excludes bacteria from crossing from the water to the gas[1]. The warmed humidified gas stream passes from the cartridge down a special triple lumen tube. Humidified gas travels in the middle lumen, the outer lumens contain warmed water. The nasal cannula is attached to the triple lumen tube close to the infant to prevent heat loss. In 2004 and 2005 early data obtained in a small numbers of infants showed VT to be a safe and successful alternative to nCPAP. VT performed better than standard high flow nasal cannula oxygen in a small randomized trial in 30 newly extubated preterm infants. VT was better than nasal cannula oxygen at 1-2 L/min in avoiding reintubation, reducing respiratory effort score and reducing nasal mucosal abnormalities on blinded examinations. A retrospective study of infants of all gestational ages comparing a cohort of infants who received VT compared to historical controls who received nCPAP, showed no difference in deaths, ventilator days, BPD, blood infections or other outcomes.

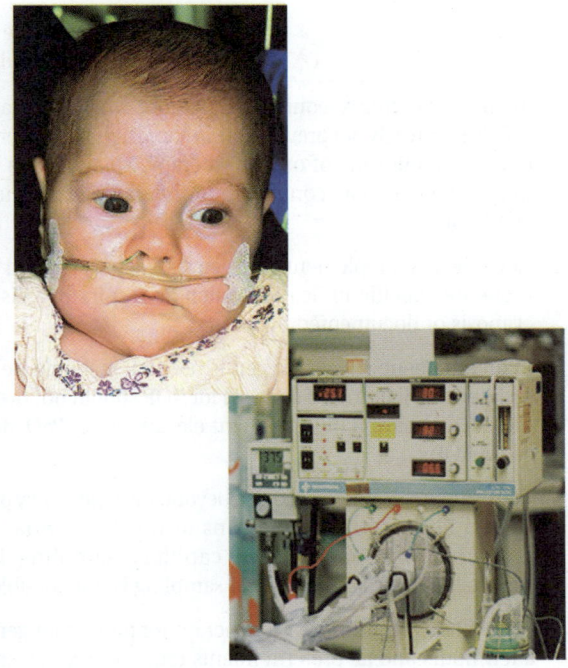

Set up and settings

The VT is straightforward to set up. Nasal cannulae should be selected in the size that fits comfortably into the nares. There are neonatal, premature, infant or intermediate sized cannulae available. Flow rates are started at 5–6 L/min on our unit and then adjusted in increasing increments of 0.5 L/min if the saturations are low or there is respiratory distress, until the saturations and respiratory rate are stable up to a maximum flow of 8 L/min. Weaning stable infants is achieved by reducing the VT flow by 0.5-1 L/min until flows of 1–3 L/min are achieved. The flow rate at which to end VT treatment depends on the severity of the underlying lung pathology. VT can be introduced for infants who are stable but have difficulty tolerating either Fisher and Paykel bubble CPAP or EME Infant Flow™ continuous flow driver CPAP. It is also useful to smaller infants who have had nasal injuries from nCPAP and VT is now considered as an alternative to nCPAP following extubation in some circumstances. The use of relatively untested devices is not new in neonatology. Despite the fact that this device is well tolerated and easy to use, it must still be introduced cautiously until further trials are available to delineate optimal timing, safety and efficacy of its use in the neonatal population.

High-flow humidified oxygen therapy for Neonates requiring respiratory support : The Vapotherm2000iTM device provides warm humidified gas via standard nasal cannulae at flows of up to 8 L/min with approximately 95% relative humidity at body temperature.

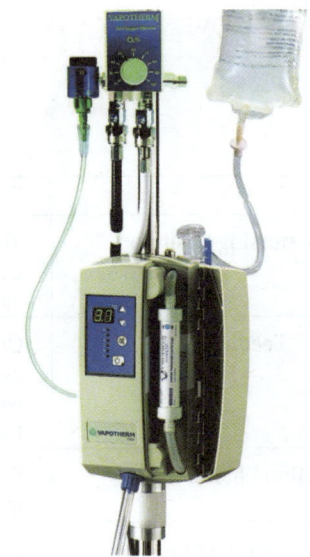

Calibration of the MAXO oxygen analyzer

Steps Action

1. Place sensor in

   - Air if baby receiving <60% O_2
   - 100% O_2 if baby receiving >60% O_2
   - attach oxygen calibration jig to sensor
   - set flow rate at 2 L/min of pure O_2

2. Turn unit on (on/off key).

3. Press 'lock' key to unlock unit (% will appear). 4) Press 'cal'. 5) Analyser will calibrate automatically (adjust á or â keys if required, till calibration figure reached) 6) When calibration complete, analyser unit will lock automatically. Replace sensor into appropriate oxygen setting.

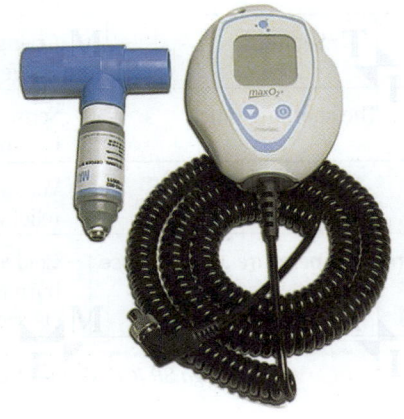

Guideline on the Use of Oxygen in the Newborn
OXYGEN THERAPY:Recommendations Courtesy: **Perinatal society of malaysia**

1. An understanding is required that Retinopathy of Prematurity (ROP) is currently not preventable in some neonates, even with optimal monitoring of oxygen therapy. Many factors other than hyperoxia may contribute to the pathogenesis in this condition.

2. Nevertheless, supplemental oxygen should only be used when there are specific indications such as respiratory distress, cyanosis or documented hypoxia.

3. In an emergency when oxygen is needed, it should be used without restriction, and concern for ROP should not override the need to save a life. Transient elevations of PaO_2 do not cause ROP.

4. The use of supplemental oxygen beyond the emergency period should be monitored by means of regular arterial PaO_2 measurements. Arterialised capillary sampling is an acceptable alternative if arterial sampling is not possible.

5. Term infants requiring oxygen therapy for periods longer than a few hours and all preterm infants requiring oxygen should be managed in a facility where monitoring of oxygen therapy is available. When this is not possible, the concentration of oxygen administered should be just enough to abolish cyanosis. It should be safe in the term neonate to administer oxygen for a few hours without monitoring arterial oxygen.

6. Transcutaneous oxygen measurement and/or pulse oximetry allow for continuous monitoring of oxygen therapy. The recommended levels of SaO_2 are 89 to 95%. This should be supported by intermittent arterial blood gas analysis. A recommended range for most preterm neonates would be a PaO_2 of 50 –80 mmHg (6.7 –10.7 kPa).

7. In some neonates, efforts to keep the PaO_2 within this range may result in unacceptable episodes of hypoxia. In such a situation, it might be necessary to accept PaO_2 levels above this range. Such decisions should be documented clearly.

8. Institutions should have a written protocol for the documentation and monitoring of oxygen therapy. Recognizing the benefits of early detection and treatment of ROP, eye examination at 4–6 weeks of age is recommended for:a. all babies less than 32 weeks gestation at birth or weight less than 1250gm. b. other babies above 32 weeks and 1250 gm depending on individual risk as assessed by the clinician.

9. Eye examination should be repeated at 2-4 weekly intervals until vascularisation reaches Zone 3 or there is no longer a risk of threshold disease. If threshold disease develops then ablative therapy should be considered for at least one eye within 72 hours of detection.

HOW TO IMPROVE BABY'S OXYGENATION ?

ESSENTIAL CLINICAL GUIDELINES **081**

HOW TO IMPROVE OXYGENATION OF THE BABY WITHOUT INCREASING THE O2 SUPPLEMENTS ?

What measure is to be taken?	How does it improve the Oxygenation of the baby ?
Prone nursing position	This improves PaO2 because of better diaphragmatic excursions and ventilation to perfusion ratio within the lung. Nursing in a moderately tilted position (15⁰) with head elevation reduces hypoxemic events in preterm infants.
Feeding	Orogastric feeding is a better option than Nasogastric feeding without any risk of milk aspiration or difficulty in securing the tube, while preventing the unilateral nose block which increases the work of breathing. Slow feeding can minimize the gastric distention which can lead to post-feeding attacks of cyanosis and apnea.
Minimal handling	Reduction in undesirable handling reduces hypoxemia in low birth weight babies with meconium aspiration syndrome with or without pulmonary hypertension.
Low ambient noise levels	Excessive noise in the NICU causes hypoxemia in babies; behavioral modification of the NICU Staff can reduce the problem.
Sedation	Crying makes a Neonate hypoxemic; sedation can minimize this problem. Alprazolam is safe and effective.
The soothing touch	Sensory deprivation is stressful to a Newborn baby; gentle human touch and caressing by mother (Kangaroo Medical Care-KMC) improve oxygenation of the babies.
Pain relief	Venepuncture/Heel pricks/Tracheal suctioning can make a sick baby hypoxic; pain relief with oral Sucrose solution improves oxygenation
Proper Temperature Maintenance	Cold Stress and Hypothermia induce anaerobic glycolysis requiring more oxygen to burn carbohydrates. Proper Thermal Control (Thermoneutral environment) reduces O2 requirements.

Courtesy; Dr Daga SR ICH, Grant Medical College and JJ Hospital, Mumbai, IJPP Volume 2 No 2 April-JUNE 2000

CPAP-CONTINUOUS POSITIVE AIRWAY PRESSURE

INDICATIONS FOR CPAP: 1) *Spontaneously breathing babies with respiratory distress at birth.* **2)** *Increased work of breathing indicated by: recession, grunting, nasal flaring, increased oxygen requirements or increased respiratory rate.* **3)** *Poorly expanded or infiltrated lung fields on chest x-ray.* **4)** *Atelectasis.* **5)** *Pulmonary edema.* **6)** *Pulmonary hemorrhage.* **7)** *Apnea of prematurity.* **8)** *Recent extubation.* **9)** *Tracheomalacia or other abnormalities of the airways, predisposing to airway collapse.* **10)***Phrenic nerve palsy.*

CPAP SYSTEM : COMPONENTS

1 Pressure manifold • Ensures patient safety by limiting the pressure delivered in an event of an occlusion • Allows connection to a pressure monitoring device or an air/oxygen analyzer

2 MR290 chamber • Easy to maintain • Maintains constant CPAP • Closed system ensures safety by minimizing the risk of contamination

3 Single-heated circuit • Provides even heat distribution

across the tube reducing heat loss and condensate build up • Delivers optimal humidity to the neonate keeping a patent airway and allowing ease of suctioning

4 CPAP generator • CPAP probe allows ease of pressure setting from 3 to 10cm H2O • Auto-level mechanism ensures constant mean CPAP pressure • Detachable overflow container allows continuous CPAP while removing excess water from condensate • Easy mounting using an Fisher & Paykel humidifier bracket

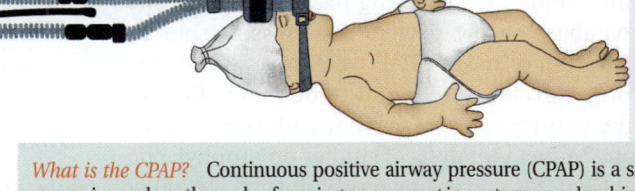

1
3
2
4

Courtesy : Fisher & Paykel

CONTRAINDICATIONS FOR CPAP

1) *The need for ventilation because of ventilatory failure—inability to maintain oxygenation and the arterial PaCO2 <60 mm Hg and pH > 7.25.*

2) *Upper airway abnormalities (cleft palate, choanal atresia).*

3) *Tracheo-esophageal fistula.*

4) *Diaphragmatic hernia.*

What is the CPAP? Continuous positive airway pressure (CPAP) is a simple, inexpensive and gentle mode of respiratory support in preterm very low birth weight (VLBW) infants. It helps by preventing the alveolar collapse and increasing the functional residual capacity of the lungs. CPAP is the positive pressure applied to the airways throughout the respiratory cycle in a spontaneously breathing infant, while the PEEP-Positive End Expiratory Pressure is the positive pressure maintained in the airways during expiration during assisted ventilation.

What are the effects of CPAP in the infant with RDS? *Reduces upper airway occlusion by decreasing upper airway resistance and increasing the pharyngeal cross sectional area. *Reduces right to left shunting. *Reduces obstructive apneas. *Increases the FRC. *Reduces inspiratory resistance by dilating the airways. This permits a larger tidal volume for a given pressure, so reducing the work of breathing. *Reduces the compliance of very compliant lungs and, in these lungs, reduces the tidal volume and minute volume. *Increases the compliance and tidal volume of stiff lungs with a low FRC by stabilizing the chest wall and counteracting the paradoxical movements. *Regularizes and slows the respiratory rate.*Reduces the incidence of apnea. *Increases the mean airway pressure and improves ventilation perfusion mismatch. *Conserves surfactant on the alveolar surface.*Diminishes alveolar edema.*The increased pressure helps overcome the inspiratory resistance of an endotracheal tube. *Nasal CPAP after extubation reduces the proportion of babies requiring re-ventilation. *Oxygenation is related to the surface area, and carbon dioxide elimination is related to the minute volume.*Normalizing lung volume improves oxygenation and carbon dioxide elimination.

How to do the procedure? *Start at a CPAP of 5-6 cm H_2O, with a similar FiO_2 to that in the Headbox *Select an adequate flow rate (5-10 L/min) to prevent rebreathing of CO_2. *Place an orogastric tube on free drainage to reduce gastric distension. *Increase FiO_2 as appropriate, using continuous monitoring and *ABG analysis at 30 minutes after establishing CPAP, and then 4-6 hourly* Increase the CPAP to 7–8 cm H_2O in RDS if hypoxia not resolving. *Note that where CPAP improves lung inflation by preventing atelectasis, the PCO_2 will fall, whereas applying CPAP to well inflated lungs may reduce CO_2 elimination. *As the baby`s condition improves, wean first the FiO_2, then decrease the CPAP in 1 cm H_2O steps to 3 cm H_2O before removing nasal prongs *If inspired oxygen concentration increase >80%, and the PaO_2 <45mmHg or $PaCO_2$ >60mmHg, discontinue CPAP, Intubate and Ventilate. *Watch for sudden deterioration because of pneumothorax and take care in positioning nasal prongs over long periods of time, as nasal distortion and even septal necrosis may occur. *Monitor the vital signs, pulse oximetry readings and baby`s activity, respiratory rate and work of breathing. *Apply suction to the nasal cavities, mouth, pharynx, and stomach @every 4 hours.

Recognizing failure of CPAP administration

Decreasing pH (<7.25), Increasing $PaCo_2$ (>50–60 mm Hg)*, Increasing FIO_2 (>0.6 to 0.7), Decreasing PaO_2 (<60 to 80 mm Hg)†, Nasal CPAP > 12 cm H_2O, Frequent apnea with bradycardia.

*Higher ranges may apply with permissive hypercapnia, †Range should be consistent with clinical state and the presence of congenital heart anomalies.

Oxygenation and CPAP

*CPAP was introduced as the primary therapeutic modality when Gregory et al demonstrated a marked reduction in respiratory distress syndrome mortality.*Oxygen was the primary therapeutic mode before the introduction of CPAP. *Oxygen is administered a hood, nasal canula or in the isolette to treat infants with mild respiratory distress syndrome or after discontinuation of CPAP or assisted ventilation. *CPAP keeps the alveoli open at the end of expiration, decreasing the right-to-left pulmonary shunt. *CPAP is often administered using nasal prongs. In the Cochrane database review, devices and pressure sources for administration of nasal CPAP were assessed. *Short binasal-prongs devices were found to be more effective than single prongs and also reduced the rate of reintubation. *A meta-analysis of studies on prophylactic use of nasal CPAP for preventing morbidity and mortality in very preterm infants concluded that intermittent positive pressure ventilation (IPPV) was not beneficial. *In a study of nasal CPAP in infants born at less than 27 weeks' gestation in a retrospective, observational study in one hospital, the probability of an individual baby remaining on nasal CPAP was 66% (95% confidence interval [CI], 46-86%) on day 1 and 80% (95% CI, 60-99%) on day 2. *In a recent trial, 610 infants born at 25-28 weeks' gestation were randomly assigned to CPAP or intubation 5 minutes after birth, their outcomes were assessed at age 28 days, at age 36 weeks, and before discharge. These investigators found no reduction in death or BPD with early nasal CPAP; the CPAP group had an increase in the incidence of pneumothorax (9% vs 3%) but also fewer days on ventilator and fewer infants receiving oxygen at age 28 days. *Recently, Pillow and her colleagues have suggested that bubble CPAP promotes enhanced airway patency during treatment of acute postnatal respiratory disease in preterm lambs. Whether the findings of this animal model of respiratory distress syndrome, wherein the nares length and gas flow pattern is considerably different, can be mirrored to prematurely born infants is unclear. Air leak from nasal prongs may also alter the findings. *CPAP is an adjunct therapy given after surfactant if prolonged assisted ventilation is not required. Use of nasal CPAP after initial surfactant therapy has been successful in some infants. In a retrospective study, bubble nasal CPAP was successful in 76% of infants who weighed less than 1250 g and in 50% of infants who weighed less than 750 g. *CPAP may be used after extubation in individuals with respiratory distress syndrome to prevent atelectasis and prevent apnea in premature infants. A randomized control trial compared postextubation bubble CPAP with infant flow driver CPAP

in preterm infants with respiratory distress syndrome; although both were equally effective, bubble CPAP is associated with a significantly higher rate of successful extubation and reduced duration of CPAP in infants younger than 14 days. *The goal of therapy for patients with respiratory distress syndrome is to maintain a pH of 7.25–7.4, a PaO_2 of 50–70 mm Hg, and a carbon dioxide pressure (PCO_2) of 40–65 mm Hg, depending on the infant's clinical status.

Continuous positive airway pressure: complications: 1) Nasal septal erosion or necrosis: This is preventable when using appropriate sized prongs that are correctly positioned 2) Pneumothorax -*Usually occurs in acute phase. *It is uncommon (<5%). *It usually results from the underlying disease process rather than positive pressure alone. *It is not a contraindication to the use of CPAP. 3) Abdominal Distension from Swallowing Air -*This is benign *Easily reduced with gastric drainage or aspiration 4) Nasal obstruction-*From improper prong placement or inadequate airway care

Continuous positive airway pressure airway management of babies on CPAP: Principles of management

*To maintain optimal airway patency

Indications : Increased secretions -Increased respiratory effort—Increasing oxygen requirement -Increasing respiratory distress—Increasing apneas

Equipment required -Suction catheter sizes 7, 8 or 10—Normal saline (only required for tenacious secretions)—Gloves—Suction tubing and trap

*Suction pressure should be set at 100–150mmHg *Frequency of suctioning will depend on the condition of the baby *Symptomatic infants, on CPAP, suction pre-feed at least 2–4 hourly or more often if required *Stable infants, on CPAP, suctioned at least 6 hourly or more if required. *After discontinuing CPAP, suction the baby at least 6 hourly or more frequently if symptomatic, for the first 24 hours. Then as required for airway maintenance.

Continuous Positive Airway Pressure Requirements for Effective CPAP:

Low resistance delivery system: Large bore tubing -Short, wide connection to patient **Consistent, reliable pressure generation** -Appropriate, snug,-fitting nasal prong size -Well positioned and secure -Prevention of leak via mouth with chin strap -Carefully set-up and maintained circuit. **Optimally maintained airway**—Warmed, humidified gas -Neck in mild extension—Appropriate airway care, e.g.. suctioning. **Applicable to the Very Low Birthweight Infant** -Hudson prongs size 0 through 5. **Relatively Atraumatic, safe and cost-effective Early Application** -At first onset of symptoms; *Early CPAP:* It is important to note that CPAP helps mainly by *preventing* the alveolar collapse in infants with surfactant deficiency. Once atelectasis and collapse have occurred, CPAP might not help much. *Therefore, all preterm infants (<35 weeks') with any sign of respiratory distress* (tachypnea/chest in-drawing/grunting) *should be* *started immediately on CPAP.* **Meticulous, Consistent Technique** -Skilled caregivers.

Continuous positive airway pressure troubleshooting:

A) *"It's not Bubbling!"*

This indicates loss of air flow or a pressure leak somewhere in the system. A simple way to check if it is a 'circuit' problem or a 'baby' problem is to remove the prongs from the nose and occlude them with your fingers.

If the system doesn't bubble it means the problem is with the circuit. Systematically check the circuit, tightening all connections as you go. Begin at the wall and end at the water-bubble generator.

If the system does bubble, when you occlude the prongs with your fingers then the pressure leak is at the nose or mouth. Air will escape if the prongs are too small or if they are not curved down into the nose and fitting snugly. The suggested sizes (based on weight) are a guide only as babies nose sizes do vary. A chin strap will reduce leak via the mouth. A dummy may help an unsettled baby.

Check white tubing for accumulation of "rainout", as this will swing backwards and forwards in the tubing without an audible bubble.

A Duoderm Patch may be applied to nares for problems with a seal/no bubbling, **following assessment by a member of the CPAP Resource Team.**

B) *"The prongs won't stay in place!"*

Are they the right size? Does the hat fit snugly? The hat is the anchor for the prongs so a loose hat will allow any movement of the head to dislodge the prongs.

Are the corrugated tubes fixed firmly in place on the side of the hat and are they at the correct angle to keep the prongs in place? If there is rotating pressure on the prongs they may twist out of the nose. If in doubt, try undoing the rubber bands and with the prongs correctly positioned in the nose, allow the tubing to sit naturally in place. Reposition the pins and the rubber bands as necessary. Ensure that the base tapes are secure on the face. Do the existing ones need replacing?

C) *"The baby won't settle!"*

Are the prongs positioned in the nares appropriately and comfortably? Does s/he need suctioning?- This may seem a contradiction when suggesting ways to settle a baby down, but a build up of secretion can cause considerable distress to a baby whose breathing is already compromised.

Once you are sure the airway is clear try the usual calming techniques of containment, nesting, swaddling, pacifier, etc. Aspirate any excess gastric air and vent tube to room air if necessary. Try positioning the baby prone as this can help relieve abdominal distension and diaphragmatic pressure. Often just "hands off" will allow the baby to slowly settle, especially in the early hours as they adjust to the CPAP.

"How can we avoid septal damage?"

Prevention is the key. Tissue will break down if it is subjected to continuous pressure, friction and/or moisture. Avoiding these contributing factors will maintain an intact septum: *Use the correct sized prongs as outlined in the application instructions *Secure them in place with a snug fitting hat, correctly positioned pins and rubber bands over the corrugated tubing *Use velcro base tapes to hold the prongs and tubing secure *Don't allow the bridge of the prongs to press up against the septum *Avoid twisting of the prongs with resultant lateral pressure against the septum *Do not use creams, ointments or gels (use saline drops to moisten the nares for initial prong insertion or during suctioning if necessary) *Frequent observation of the septum and prong position is essential. Be wary of eye pads that cover the nose on babies under phototherapy as these can obstruct your view of the septum.

CPAP pressure generators: A) Continuous flow devices

Vary the CPAP pressure by a mechanism-**1)Infant ventilator/Stand-alone CPAP machines:** Pressure is generated by the exhalation valve and adjusted by varying the expiratory orifice size **2) Bubble CPAP:**Simple and inexpensive · Oscillations produced by continuous bubbling might contribute to gas exchange (akin to HFV). Can identify large leaks at the nares (bubbling stops). Flow has to be altered to ensure proper bubbling. It is difficult to detect high flow which can lead to over distension of the lungs B)**Variable flow devices-Common examples: 1.** *Infant flow driver (IFD)* **2.** *Viasys SiPAP* The desired CPAP level is generated by varying the flow; CPAP pressure is generated at the airway proximal to the infant's nares.- Maintains more uniform pressure · Might decrease the WOB · Recruits lung volume more effectively. Expensive · Requires more technical expertise. On theoretical grounds, this device scores more than the other two; However the prohibitive cost and the lack of evidence regarding its superiority preclude its widespread use.

REFERENCES:1) Courtney SE, Pyon HP, Saslow JG, Arnold GK, Pandit, PB, Habib RH. Lung recruitment and breathing pattern during variable versus continuous flow nasal continuous positive airway pressure in premature infants: an evaluation of three devices. Pediatrics 2001;107:304- 308. **2)** Aly H, Milner JD, Patel K, El- Mohandes AAE. Does the experience with the use of nasal continuous positive airway pressure improve over time in extremely low birth weight infants? **Pediatrics 2004;114:697-702. 3)**Subramaniam P, Henderson-Smart DJ, Davis PG. Prophylactic nasal continuous positive airways pressure for preventing morbidity and mortality in very preterm infants. Cochrane Database of Syst.Rev.2005: CD001243.

SURFACTANT–REPLACEMENT THERAPY FOR RESPIRATORY DISTRESS IN THE PRETERM AND TERM NEONATE

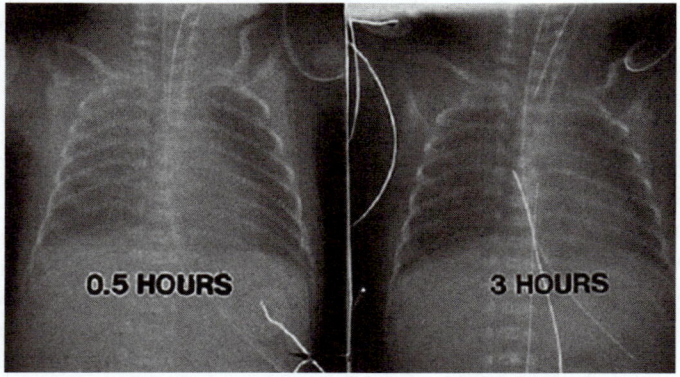

0.5 HOURS   3 HOURS

Chest radiographs in a premature infant with respiratory distress syndrome before and after surfactant treatment. Left: Initial radiograph shows poor lung expansion, air bronchogram, and reticular granular appearance. Right: Repeat chest radiograph obtained when the neonate is aged 3 hours and after surfactant therapy demonstrates marked improvement.

Courtesy: Arun K Pramanik http://emedicine.medscape.com/article/976034-overview

Surfactant therapy substantially reduces mortality and respiratory morbidity from Respiratory failure secondary to surfactant deficiency in preterm infants. for this population. Secondary surfactant deficiency also contributes to acute respiratory morbidity in late-preterm and term neonates with meconium aspiration syndrome, pneumonia/sepsis, and perhaps pulmonary hemorrhage; surfactant replacement may be beneficial for these infants. Because respiratory insufficiency may be a component of multiorgan dysfunction, preterm and term infants receiving surfactant-replacement therapy should be managed in facilities with technical and clinical expertise to administer surfactant and provide multisystem support. *Systematic reviews of randomized, controlled trials have confirmed that surfactant replacement reduces initial inspired oxygen and ventilation requirements as well as the incidence of respiratory distress syndrome, death, pneumothorax, and pulmonary interstitial emphysema.*

A prophylactic, or preventive, surfactant strategy is defined as intubation and surfactant administration to infants at high risk of developing respiratory distress syndrome for the primary purpose of giving surfactant rather than treatment of respiratory distress syndrome; this has been operationalized in clinical studies as surfactant administration before the onset of respiratory symptoms or efforts, before initial resuscitation efforts, or, most commonly, after initial resuscitation but within 10 to 30 minutes after birth. This contrasts with *a rescue, or treatment, surfactant strategy,* in which surfactant is given to preterm infants with established respiratory distress syndrome. Rescue surfactant is most often administered within the first 12 hours after birth when specified threshold criteria for respiratory distress syndrome are met. *Early rescue was defined as surfactant treatment within 1 to 2 hours of birth, and late rescue was defined as surfactant treatment 2 or more hours after birth.* Preterm infants born at or earlier than 30 weeks' gestation have benefited from both prophylactic and rescue surfactant administration. However, infants receiving prophylactic surfactant have had a lower incidence and severity of respiratory distress compared with those treated after developing respiratory distress syndrome. Infants receiving prophylactic surfactant also have encountered fewer complications of respiratory distress syndrome, such as death (Relative Risk: 0.61; 95% Confidence Interval: 0.48–0.77; Number Needed To Treat 22): pneumothorax (RR: 0.62; 95% CI: 0.42–0.89; NNT: 47), pulmonary interstitial emphysema (RR: 0.54; 95% CI: 0.36–0.82; NNT: 40), and the combined outcome of bronchopulmonary dysplasia or death (RR: 0.85; 95% CI: 0.76–0.95; NNT: 24). Surfactant therapy reduced mortality rates most effectively in infants of less than 30 weeks' gestation or with birth weights of less than 1250 g and more often in male infants. The incidence of other coexistent morbidities in preterm infants, such as bronchopulmonary dysplasia, intraventricular hemorrhage, necrotizing enterocolitis, nosocomial infections, retinopathy of prematurity, and patent ductus arteriosus, has not changed with surfactant replacement. Surfactant replacement has not been shown to affect the incidence of neurologic, developmental, behavioral, medical, or educational outcomes in preterm infants.

SURFACTANT THERAPY —COMPLICATIONS

1) **Pulmonary Hemorrhage**- an infrequent adverse event in ELBW male infants and with PDA. Risk is decreased by prenatal steroids and by early postnatal treatment of PDA with Indomethacin. 2) **Pneumothorax secondary** to sudden improvement in lung compliance-Adjust ventilator settings carefully. 3) **Apnea Brady and Desaturations**—Adjust administration of

Surfactant according to the infant`s tolerance. Ventilate the baby for atleast 30 seconds or until stable between half/quarter doses. Administer additional oxygen. Both animal-derived and synthetic surfactants are beneficial for prophylaxis and rescue of respiratory distress syndrome in preterm infants. Treatment with animal-derived surfactants (beractant, calfactant, poractant) have several advantages over first-generation protein- free synthetic surfactants (e.g., colfosceril palmitate, Pumactant [Britannia Pharmaceuticals Ltd, Redhill, Surrey, England], artificial lung-expanding compound). These advantages include lower mortality rates (RR: 0.86; 95% CI: 0.76–0.98; NNT: 40), lower inspired oxygen ventilation requirements early in the course of respiratory distress syndrome, and fewer pneumothoraxes (RR: 0.63; 95% CI: 0.53–0.75; NNT: 22). New synthetic surfactants with surfactant protein–like activity are promising new treatments for surfactant- deficiency disorders. Surfactant replacement by bolus or slow infusion in infants with severe meconium aspiration syndrome improved oxygenation and reduced the severity of respiratory failure, air leaks, and need for extracorporeal membrane oxygenation (RR: 0.64; 95% CI: 0.46–0.91; NNT:6). Surfactant replacement for neonates with severe primary persistent pulmonary hypertension of the newborn did not significantly reduce the need for extracorporeal membrane oxygenation in a small clinical trial. However, surfactant improved oxygenation and reduced the need for extracorporeal membrane oxygenation when parenchymal lung disease was present. Surfactant administration to neonates who were receiving extracorporeal membrane oxygenation also reduced the duration of extracorporeal membrane oxygenation. Newborn infants with pneumonia or sepsis receiving rescue surfactant also have demonstrated improved gas exchange compared with infants without surfactant treatment. surfactant treatment of a large series of infants with congenital diaphragmatic hernia did not improve outcomes. In fact, use of extracorporeal membrane oxygenation, incidence of chronic lung disease, and mortality actually increased. Surfactant treatment may also reduce morbidity and mortality for infants with pulmonary hemorrhage. Antenatal steroids may reduce the need for prophylactic and early rescue surfactant replacement in infants born after 27 to 28 weeks' gestation, although this has not been proven in large, randomized clinical trials. Antenatal steroids decrease mortality, the severity of respiratory distress syndrome, surfactant use, and intraventricular hemorrhage in infants born at less than 34 weeks' gestation and decrease the incidence of respiratory distress syndrome in infants born at between 28 and 34 weeks' gestation. The combination of antenatal steroids and postnatal surfactant improves lung function more than either treatment alone. Continuous positive airway pressure, with or without exogenous surfactant, may reduce the need for additional surfactant and incidence of bronchopulmonary dysplasia without increased morbidity, although this has not been proven in large, randomized clinical trials.

CLINICAL IMPLICATIONS 1. Surfactant should be given to infants with respiratory distress syndrome as soon as possible after intubation irrespective of exposure to antenatal steroids or gestational age. **2.** Prophylactic surfactant replacement should be considered for extremely preterm infants at high risk of respiratory distress syndrome, especially infants who have not been exposed to antenatal steroids. **3.** Rescue surfactant may be considered for infants with hypoxic respiratory failure attributable to secondary surfactant deficiency (e.g., meconium aspiration syndrome, sepsis/pneumonia, and pulmonary hemorrhage). **4.** Preterm and term neonates who are receiving surfactant should be managed by nursery and transport personnel with the technical and clinical expertise to administer surfactant safely and deal with multisystem illness.

RESEARCH IMPLICATIONS 1. Randomized trials of continuous positive airway pressure, with or without surfactant, during a brief intubation compared with prophylactic or early surfactant replacement in preterm infants are needed. 2. Improved surfactant preparations, surfactant-dosing strategies for infants born to mothers who are receiving antenatal steroids, and noninvasive techniques for surfactant administration need additional study. 3. Surfactant replacement for illnesses other than respiratory distress syndrome needs additional study. 4. It is no longer necessary to include first-generation synthetic surfactants in future studies.

First-Generation Surfactant: Protein-free Synthetics: **Colfosceril Palmitate** (Exosurf), contained the crucial phospholipid dipalmitoyl phosphatidylcholine but did not include the surfactant proteins SP-B and SP-C, withdrawn from the market .It improved gas exchange and allowed for weaning of ventilator support in preterm infants with RDS. Additionally, Exosurf resulted in other desirable outcomes: decreased air leak, patent ductus arteriosus, intraventricular hemorrhage, BPD, death, and the combined outcome of BPD/death. Meta-analyses of early studies also revealed no differences in neurodevelopmental outcomes of treated versus nontreated infants.

Second-Generation Surfactants: Animal derived: minced cow (eg, **Survanta**) or pig (eg, **Curosurf**) lung extracts to which necessary components such as lipids, palmitic acid, and tripalmitin are added. Another type of natural surfactant is made by lavaging cow lungs and extracting the surfactant (eg, **Infasurf**). Lavage preparations were designed as an alternative to minced extracts due to the potential for less contamination with unwanted lipids and proteins from residual tissue or plasma components. These surfactants include not only phospholipids but have the advantage of containing SP-B and SP-C albeit in variable amounts . Although surfactant phospholipids lower alveolar surface tension, the protein components are essential for in vivo efficacy, as they allow for rapid adsorption and spreading of the surfactant film across the alveolar surface. Comparisons of first- versus second generation surfactants have demonstrated that while both are effective in treatment of RDS, second generation surfactants result in lower oxygen requirements and ventilator support in the first 72 hours after administration, fewer pneumothoraces, and a trend towards less BPD/death. Third Generation Surfactants: Engineered from components: to mimic the structure and actions of SP-C or SP-B: **Venticute (r-SP-C surfactant) and Surfaxin (lucinactant).** The presumed advantages of such products are twofold: lot-by-lot consistency in the amounts of these proteins, plus reduction in the theoretical risks related to possible animal-to-human transmission of prion-related infections. Combined analysis of studies does not support superiority of Surfaxin over the animal derived synthetic surfactants currently in widespread clinical use, and at present, RDS is the only FDA-approved use for exogenous surfactant.

Surfactant therapy for respiratory distress syndrome

RESOLVED: *Improved mortality from respiratory distress syndrome (RDS). *Greatest benefit when antenatal corticosteroids are also employed. *Exogenous surfactant does not inhibit endogenous surfactant synthesis. *Retreatment may be required in severe RDS. *Major component for lowering surface tension: phosphatidylcholine. *Endotracheal intubation required for administration of fluid suspension. *Improvement in oxygenation, functional residual capacity, and lung compliance. *Protein-containing preparations show a faster therapeutic response. *Decrease in incidence of air leaks *Prophylactic or early use beneficial in infants with extremely low birthweight (<29 weeks' gestation) *Efficacy of surfactant therapy, early extubation, nasal continuous positive airway pressure strategy *UNRESOLVED:* *Factors predicting likelihood of success of an initial CPAP-based strategy. *Optimal ventilatory strategy to maximize surfactant response. *Effect on incidence and severity of bronchopulmonary dysplasia. *Role of surfactant proteins as modulator of the immune system and inflammatory response. *Role for recombinant surfactant protein-based preparations

Surfactant replacement therapy

SETTINGS: Administered by trained personnel in Delivery room, Neonatal intensive care unit. **INDICATIONS:** *Prophylactic administration* may be indicated in 1. infants at high risk of developing RDS because of short gestation (< 32 weeks) or low birthweight (< 1,300 g), which strongly suggest lung immaturity. **2. infants** in whom there is laboratory evidence of surfactant deficiency such as lecithin/sphingomyelin ratio less than 2:1, bubble stability test indicating lung immaturity, or the absence of phosphatidylglycerol. *Rescue or therapeutic administration* is indicated in preterm or full-term infants 1. who require endotracheal intubation and mechanical ventilation because of increased work of breathing as indicated by an increase in respiratory rate, substernal and suprasternal retractions, grunting, and nasal flaring. increasing oxygen requirements as indicated by pale or cyanotic skin color, agitation, and decreases in PaO2, SaO2, or SpO2 mandating an increase in FIO2 above 0.40.

and have clinical evidence of RDS, including chest radiograph characteristic of RDS, mean airway pressure greater than 7 cm H_2O to maintain an adequate PaO_2, SaO_2, or $SpO2$. **CONTRAINDICATIONS:** Relative contraindications to surfactant administration are 1. the presence of congenital anomalies incompatible with life beyond the neonatal period, 2. respiratory distress in infants with laboratory evidence of lung maturity. **FREQUENCY:** Repeat doses of surfactant are contingent upon the continued diagnosis of RDS. The frequency with which surfactant replacement is performed should depend upon the clinical status of the patient and the indication for performing the procedure. Additional doses of surfactant, given at 6- to 24-hour intervals, may be indicated in infants who experience increasing ventilator requirements or whose conditions fail to improve after the initial dose. **INFECTION CONTROL: Universal** Precautions should be implemented. Aseptic technique should be practiced. Appropriate infection control guidelines for the patient should be posted and followed. Physiologic **complications of surfactant replacement therapy** include apnea, pulmonary hemorrhage, mucus plugs, increased necessity for treatment for PDA, marginal increase in retinopathy of prematurity, barotrauma resulting from increase in lung compliance following surfactant replacement and failure to change ventilator settings accordingly. Procedural **complications** resulting from the administration of surfactant include plugging of endotracheal tube (ETT) by surfactant; hemoglobin desaturation and increased need for supplemental bradycardia due to hypoxia; tachycardia due to agitation, with reflux of surfactant into the ETT; pharyngeal deposition of surfactant; administration of surfactant to only one lung; administration of suboptimal dose secondary to miscalculation or error in reconstitution. **Variables to be monitored during surfactant administration-**Proper placement and position of delivery device, FIO2 and ventilator settings, Reflux of surfactant into ETT, position of patient (i.e., head direction), Chest-wall movement, Oxygen saturation by pulse oximetry, Heart rate, respirations, chest expansion, skin color, and vigor. Variables **to be monitored after surfactant administration-** Invasive and noninvasive measurements of arterial blood gases, Chest radiograph, Ventilator settings (PIP, PEEP, Paw) and FIO2, Pulmonary mechanics and volumes, Heart rate, respirations, chest expansion, skin color, and vigor, Breath sounds, Blood pressure. **ASSESSMENT OF OUTCOME: Reduction** in FIO2 requirement, Reduction in work of breathing, Improvement in lung volumes and lung fields as indicated by chest radiograph, Improvement in pulmonary mechanics (e.g., compliance, airways resistance, VT, VE, transpulmonary pressure) and lung volume (i.e., FRC), Reduction in ventilator requirements (PIP, PEEP, Paw), Improvement in ratio of arterial to alveolar PO2 (a/A PO2), oxygen index.

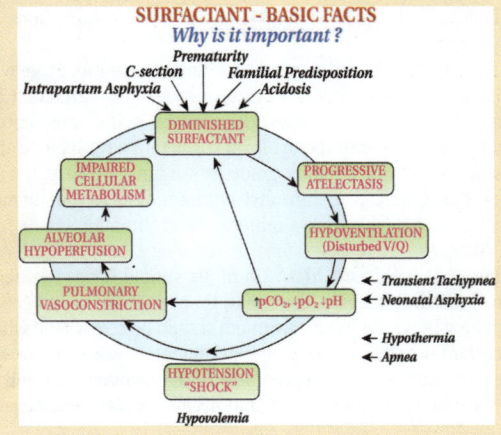

SURFACTANT - BASIC FACTS
Why is it important ?

Prematurity
C-section *Familial Predisposition*
Intrapartum Asphyxia *Acidosis*

DIMINISHED SURFACTANT

PROGRESSIVE ATELECTASIS

HYPOVENTILATION (Disturbed V/Q)

$\uparrow pCO_2$, $\downarrow pO_2$, $\downarrow pH$ ← Transient Tachypnea
← Neonatal Asphyxia
← Hypothermia
← Apnea

PULMONARY VASOCONSTRICTION

ALVEOLAR HYPOPERFUSION

IMPAIRED CELLULAR METABOLISM

HYPOTENSION "SHOCK"

Hypovolemia

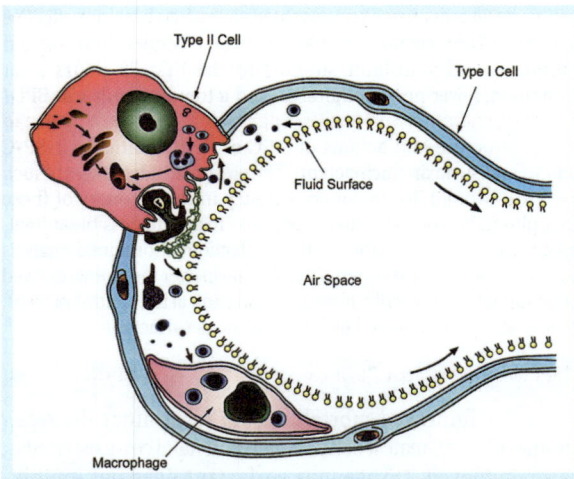

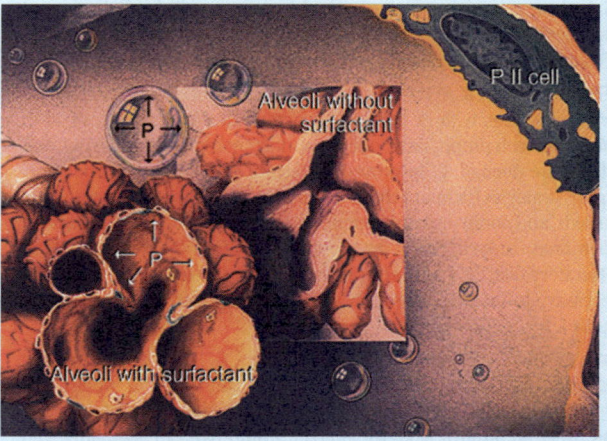

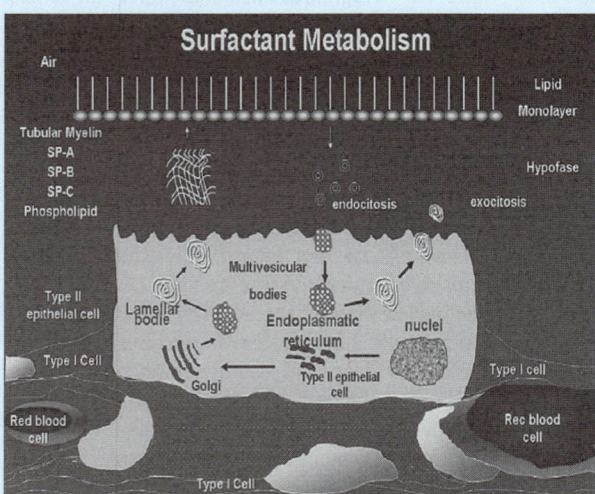

Surfactant is a complex lipoprotein (see the image) composed of 6 phospholipids and 4 apoproteins. Surfactant recovered by alveolar wash from most mammals contains 70–80% phospholipids, 8–10% protein, and 10% neutral lipids, primarily cholesterol. Dipalmitoyl phosphatidylcholine (DPPC), or lecithin, is functionally the principle phospholipid. Phosphatidylglycerol makes up 4-15% of the phospholipids; although it is a marker for lung maturity, it is not necessary for normal lung function. *Surfactant Metabolism:* Surfactant components are synthesized from precursors in the endoplasmic reticulum and transported through the Golgi apparatus by multivesicular bodies. Components are ultimately packaged in lamellar bodies, which are intracellular storage granules for surfactant before its secretion. After secretion (exocytosis) into the liquid lining of the alveolus, surfactant phospholipids are organized into a complex lattice called tubular myelin. Tubular myelin is believed to generate the phospholipid that provides material for a monolayer at the air-liquid interface in the alveolus, which lowers surface tension. Surfactant phospholipids and proteins are subsequently taken back into type II cells, possibly in the form of small vesicles, apparently by a specific pathway that involves endosomes, and probably transported for storage into lamellar bodies for recycling. Alveolar macrophages also take up some surfactant in the liquid layer. A single transit of the phospholipid components of surfactant through the alveolar lumen normally requires a few hours. The phospholipid in the lumen is taken back into type II cell and is reused 10 times before being degraded. Surfactant proteins are synthesized in polyribosomes and extensively modified in the endoplasmic reticulum, Golgi apparatus, and multivesicular bodies. Surfactant proteins are detected in lamellar bodies or secretory vesicles closely associated with lamellar bodies before they are secreted into the alveolus. **Courtesy:** Arun K Pramanik http://emedicine. medscape.com/article / 976034 -overview

Recommendations for Neonatal Surfactant therapy, Fetus and Newborn Committee, Canadian Pediatric Society (CPS)

* Mothers at risk of delivering babies with less than 34 weeks gestation should be given antenatal steroids according to established guidelines (64) regardless of the availability of postnatal surfactant therapy (grade A). * Intubated infants with RDS should receive exogenous surfactant therapy (grade A). * Intubated infants with meconium aspiration syndrome requiring more than 50% oxygen should receive exogenous surfactant therapy (grade A). * Sick newborn infants with pneumonia and an oxygenation index greater than 15 should receive exogenous surfactant therapy (grade C).

* Intubated newborn infants with pulmonary hemorrhage which leads to clinical deterioration should receive exogenous surfactant therapy as one aspect of clinical care (grade C). * Natural surfactants should be used in preference to any of the artificial surfactants available at the time of publication of this statement (grade A). * Infants who are at a significant risk for RDS should receive prophylactic natural surfactant therapy as soon as they are stable within a few minutes after intubation (grade A). * Infants with RDS who have persistent or recurrent oxygen and ventilatory requirements within the first 72 h of life should have repeated doses of surfactant. Administering more than three doses has not been shown to have a benefit (grade A) * Retreatment should be considered when there is a persistent or recurrent oxygen requirement of 30% or more, and it may be given as early as 2 h after the initial dose or, more commonly, 4 h to 6 h after the initial dose (grade A). * Options for ventilatory management that are to be considered after prophylactic surfactant therapy include very rapid weaning and extubation to CPAP within 1 h (grade B). * Intubated infants with RDS should receive exogenous surfactant therapy before transport (grade C). * Centres administering surfactant to newborn infants must ensure the continuous on-site availability of personnel competent and licensed to deal with the acute complications of assisted ventilation and surfactant therapy (grade D). * Mothers with threatened delivery before 32 weeks gestation should be transferred to a tertiary centre if at all possible (grade B). * Infants who deliver at less than 29 weeks gestation outside of a tertiary centre should be considered for immediate intubation followed by surfactant administration after stabilization, if competent personnel are available (grade A). * Further research into retreatment criteria and the optimal timing of prophylactic therapy is required. Based on available evidence, the Canadian Paediatric Society makes the following recommendations: * Preterm neonates who receive treatment with nasal CPAP as their initial method of respiratory support should be provided with exogenous surfactant treatment if exhibiting clinical signs of RDS with a demonstrated need for escalating or sustained levels of supplemental oxygen to maintain adequate arterial oxygen saturation (Grade B recommendation).

* Treatment with surfactant should not be withheld if the FiO2 requirements exceed 0.5 (Grade A recommendation). *Pediatr Child Health 2005;10(2):109-16 Reference No. FN05-01 Addendum (March 2012)*

SURFACTANT—BASIC FACTS

What is it? * A LIPOPROTEIN with 85% phospholipids, 5% neutral lipids (cholesterol) and 10% proteins (SP-A, SP-B, SP-C, SP-D)

Where is it ? *Synthesized in Type II pneumonocytes (Alveolar epithelium) *Stored in Lamellar Bodies of type II Pneumonocytes *Released by Fusion of the Lamellar body membrane with Cell Wall.

How does it work? Surface tension ↓ - Alveolar Expansion & Stability and Prevents atelectasis at end-Expiration.

When is it produced ? * Early production at 20 weeks of GA*Appears in the Amniotic fluid between 28-32 weeks of GA.* * Optimal production for lung maturity at 35 weeks of GA.

Factors affecting surfactant production:

Increased by *Maternal PIH *Maternal Opiate addiction *PROM *A/N Corticosteroids *Theoretical but not practical (*Aminophylline, Estrogens, β Mimetics, Bromhexine, TRH.)

Reduced by *Infant of Diabetic Mom *Delivery <37 weeks of GA, *Multiple pregnancies *C/S delivery, *Precipitous Delivery *Asphyxia/Acidosis (pH<7.25) *Cold stress (<35°C), *Hx of prior affected with RDS, *Preterm whites.

Surfactant data : Percentage composition

	Babies with RDS	Mature babies
Phosphatidylcholine	61.7	80.9
Sphingomyelin	11.0	2.0
Phosphatidylglycerol	0.9	3.7
Phophatidylethanolamine	11.7	4.5
Phosphatidylinositol	4.9	—
Phosphatidylserine	5.3	—
Lysophophatidylcholine	2.0	—
Neutral lipid	Approx 10%	Approx 10%

Tests to check optimal Surfactant Production

1. **Lecithin /Sphingomyelin ratio of amniotic fluid :** If 2:1 or more—decreases the risk of HMD (Hypoxia, Acidosis, Hypothermia may increase the risk despite the mature 2:1 ratio). 22 to 25% of infants with L/S ratios <2:1 do not have HMD. May be unreliable if AF specimen is contaminated with meconium, blood, diluted due to polyhydramnios, stored too long or centrifuged at high speed.

2. **Shake test (AF bubble stability test):** Take undiluted amniotic fluid and its various saline dilutions in test tubes, shake for 15 seconds with an equivalent volume of 95% ethanol. Allow the tubes to stand for 15 minutes. Read the test as positive if a complete ring of bubbles persist at the meniscus. Positive shake test in dilutions of 1:2 or greater correlates will with mature L/S ratio and absence of HMD.

3. **Amniotic fluid optical density at 650 nm. :** An optical density of 0.15 or greater correlates with mature L/S ratio. Beware of the false negatives for tests 2 and 3. Recheck with L/S ratio if negative shake test or optical density test.

4. **Phosphatidyl glycerol estimation in AF :** The most reliable test to assess fetal lung maturity especially in mothers with diabetes mellitus.

Exogenous surfactant therapy indications: 1. Hyaline membrane disease in high risk low birth wt. infants and larger infants with definite evidence for RDS (IDM) - (established). **2.** Meconium aspiration syndrome (may be indicated in ventilated cases) **3.** Mature infants with PPHN (may be indicated). **4.** Sepsis **5.** Pulmonary hemorrhage (Trials show some benefits)

Surfactant—Method of administration: Survanta (Beractant from Abbott)-Stored refrigerated (2to 8°c) Who should administer ? By or under the supervision of clinicians experienced in intubation, ventilator management, and general care of premature infants.

Dosage : 4ml/kg/dose upto 4 doses q 6hrs during the first 48 hrs. **Route of administration**-Intratracheally through a 5 FG end hole catheter. **Way of Administration a)** via infants' ET tube by briefly disconnecting the ET tube from the ventilator. Followed by bag and mask ventilation with oxygen at 60 breaths/mt and sufficient positive pressure to provide adequate air exchange and chest wall excursion. **b)** By inserting catheter through a neonatal suction valve without disconnecting the ET tube from the ventilator. Ventilate the baby with rate 60/mt inspiratory time 0.5 seconds and FiO$_2$ 1.0 for about 30-60 seconds between each of the 2 or fractions of each dose.

Precautions :1. Make sure the tip of the catheter to protrude just beyond the ET tube above the infant's carina. **2.** Donot instill in the mainstem bronchus. **3.** Asses ET tube patency and correct anatomic location prior to administration. **4.** Monitor for transient bradycardia, desaturations, apnea, ET block, hypotension/hypertension, hypercapnia. **5.** Ensure thorough suction before giving surfactant and withhold suctioning for 2hrs following administration, except when clinically indicated.

Criteria for redosing: Repeat 2nd to 4th doses of Survanta after 6 hrs and q6hr(2nd dose of Exosurf after 12 hrs) if the infant remains intubated and requires atleast 30% of FiO$_2$ to maintain PaO2 of 50mm Hg. Obtain CXR confirmation of RDS before administering additional doses to those who received a prophylactic dose.

Surfactant Administration-Complications : *1. Pulmonary Hemorrhage*-Infrequent adverse event in ELBW, MALES, PDA (more common). Risk is decreased by prenatal corticosteroid therapy and by early postnatal treatment of PDA with indomethacin. ***2. Pneumothorax secondary to sudden improvement in compliance* -** Adjust ventilator settings carefully.

3. Apnea, Bradys, Desats - Adjust administration according to the infant's tolerance. Ventilate the baby for atleast 30 seconds or until stable between half/quarter doses. Administer additional oxygen.

Surfactant Therapy-Benefits proven: * Reduced Neonatal Mortality from RDS by up to 40%, *↓ AIR leaks by upto 60%, *Mean duration of Mechanical ventilation 44hrs lesser *Mean duration of Hospital stay 4.37 days lesser *Incidence of Septicemia ↓

* Prophylactic surfactant therapy at birth followed by CPAP

↓Need for Mechanical Ventilation.

Surfactant-has no effect on: 1.Chronic lung disease. 2.Gross GMH-IVH and PVL 3.PDA. 4.ROP 5 . N E C / N O S O C O M I A L INFECTIONS 6.Growth and/or Neurodevelopmental Parameters at 1–2 years of Age.

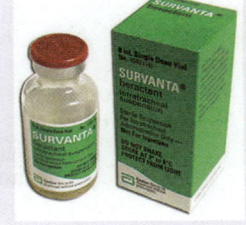

SURFACTANT - METHOD OF ADMINISTRATION CONT..

ENSURE HOMOGENOUS DISTRIBUTION THROUGHOUT LUNGS

- Divide each dose into fractional doses
  To administer surfactant in two 1/2 doses
  * Head and body turned approximately 45⁰ to the right.
  * Head and body turned approximately 45⁰ to the left.

To administer surfactant in four quarter doses

Slight Trendelenburg position with head turned to the right and then to the Left;

Slight reverse Trendelenburg position with head turned to the right and then to the left.

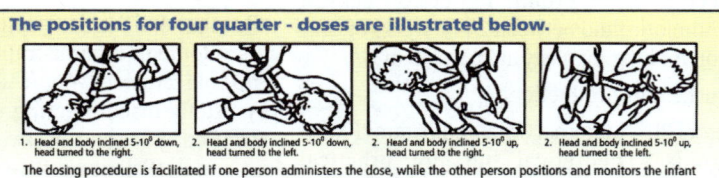

The positions for four quarter - doses are illustrated below.

1. Head and body inclined 5-10⁰ down, head turned to the right.
2. Head and body inclined 5-10⁰ down, head turned to the left.
2. Head and body inclined 5-10⁰ up, head turned to the right.
2. Head and body inclined 5-10⁰ up, head turned to the left.

The dosing procedure is facilitated if one person administers the dose, while the other person positions and monitors the infant

How should the surfactant replacement therapy by given? For all of the surfactant replacement therapy trials, surfactant was instilled in liquid form via the endotracheal tube. Some trials instilled all of the surfactant at once, while others instilled it in smaller aliquots. Only one very small trial compared a slow infusion with bolus administration of surfactant. It concluded that slow infusion was at least as effective as bolus therapy. There is no evidence to support the practice of placing the infant in multiple different positions during the administration of surfactant.

DOSAGE RECOMMENDATIONS FOR COMMONLY USED EXOGENOUS SURFACTANTS.

Product	Dosage	Additional Doses
Calfactant	3 mL/kg of birth weight given in two aliquots	May be repeated every 12 hours for up to three subsequent doses at 12-hour intervals, if indicated
Beractant	4 mL/kg of birth weight given in quarter doses	May be repeated after at least 6 hours, up to a total of four doses within 48 hours of birth
Colfosceril	5 mL/kg of birth weight given over a 4-minute period	May be repeated after 12 hours and 24 hours, if indicated
Porcine	2.5 mL/kg of birth weight given in two aliquots	Two subsequent 1.25-mL/kg doses given at 12-hour intervals, if indicated

EXOGENOUS SURFACTANTS

Surfactant (Manufacturer)	Animal source (if natural)	Composition/additives (natural)	Dose in mg/kg	N doses/vol each dose
Surfactant TA	Cow	DPPC, Palmitic acid	120	
Beractants/Survanta (Abbott)	Cow	DPPC, Palmitic acid, tripalmitin	100 4 ml/kg	4 doses
Infasurf : CLSE	Cow		100	
Curosurf (Serono)	Pig		100	3 doses 1.25-2.5 ml/kg
Alveofact	Cow		100	
Exosurf/Cofosceril (Glaxo Wellcome)	Artificial	DPPC, tyloxapol and hexadecanol	5ml/kg	2 doses 5 ml/kg

REFERENCE: **Surfactant-Replacement Therapy for Respiratory Distress in the Preterm and Term Neonate**
PEDIATRICS Volume 121, Number 2, February 2008

THE ABC'S OF CONVENTIONAL MECHANICAL VENTILATION

Overview of Mechanical Ventilation

Goals of Mechanical Ventilation

Irrespective of the technique or mode of ventilation chosen, the goals of mechanical ventilation remain the same: **1.** to achieve and maintain adequate pulmonary gas exchange, **2.** to minimize the risk of lung injury, **3.** to reduce patient work of breathing (WOB), and **4.** to optimize patient comfort.

VENTILATOR VARIABLES

*FiO2

*Modality(Target)-Pressure Limited, Pressure Control, Volume Targeted, High Frequency-   HFOV, HFJV, HYBRIDS

*Mode (IMV, SIMV, Assist Control/PSV (Pressure Support Ventilation)

Ventilator Modes (terms and types) -*Refer to page 918*
*Pressure (Peak-PIP, End expiratory-PEEP, Mean -Paw)

*Flow, *Volume *Rate, *Minute Ventilation, *Cycle, *Assist Sensitivity (Trigger), *Rise Time

OXYGENATION:

During conventional ventilation, oxygenation is largely determined by the fraction of inspired oxygen (FiO_2) and the mean airway pressure (MAP) . MAP is the average airway pressure during the respiratory cycle and can be calculated by dividing the area under the airway pressure curve by the duration of the cycle. The formula includes the constant determined by the flow rate and the rate of rise of the airway pressure curve (K), peak inspiratory pressure (PIP), positive end-expiratory pressure (PEEP), inspiratory time (T_I), and expiratory time (T_E), as follows;

$$MAP = K (PIP - PEEP) (T_I / T_I + T_E) + PEEP$$

This equation indicates that MAP increases with increasing PIP, PEEP, T_I to $T_I + T_E$ ratio, and flow (increases K by creating a more square waveform). The mechanism by which increases in MAP generally improve oxygenation appears to be the increased lung volume and improved V/Q matching. Although a direct relationship between MAP and oxygenation is observed, some exceptions are found. For the same change in MAP, increases in PIP and PEEP enhance oxygenation more than changes in the ratio of T_I to T_E (I/E ratio). Increases in PEEP are not as effective once optimal inflation is reached and may not improve oxygenation at all. In fact, an excessive MAP may cause overdistention of alveoli, leading to air trapping and right-to-left shunting of blood in the lungs.a very high MAP is transmitted to the intrathoracic structures, which may occur when lung compliance is near normal, cardiac output may decrease; thus, even with adequate oxygenation of blood, systemic oxygen transport (arterial oxygen content X cardiac output) may decrease. Unlike other causes of hypoxemia, shunting is usually unresponsive to oxygen supplementation. Hypoxemia due to V/Q mismatch can be difficult to manage but may be resolved if an increase in airway pressure reexpands atelectatic alveoli. Hypoxemia due to impaired diffusion or hypoventilation usually responds to oxygen supplementation and assisted ventilation. Blood oxygen content largely depends on oxygen saturation and hemoglobin level. Thus, transfusing packed RBCs to infants with anemia (hemoglobin, <7-10 mg/dL) who are receiving assisted ventilation is common practice. Oxygen delivery also depends on oxygen unloading at the tissue level, which is strongly determined by the oxygen dissociation curve. Acidosis, increases in 2,3-diphosphoglycerate, and adult hemoglobin levels reduce oxygen affinity to hemoglobin and, thus, favor oxygen delivery to the tissues.

VENTILATION

Elimination of CO_2 from the alveoli is directly proportional to alveolar minute ventilation, which is determined by the product of tidal volume (minus dead-space ventilation) and frequency. Thus, the alveolar minute ventilation is calculated as follows: **Alveolar Minute Ventilation = (Tidal Volume - Dead Space) X Frequency :** Tidal volume is the volume of gas inhaled (or exhaled) with each breath. Frequency is the number of breaths per minute. Dead space is the part of the tidal volume not involved in gas exchange, such as the volume of the conducting airways, and is relatively constant. Thus, increases in either tidal volume or frequency increase alveolar ventilation and decrease the arterial partial pressure of carbon dioxide ($PaCO_2$). Because dead-space ventilation is constant, changes in tidal volume appear more effective than frequency changes in altering

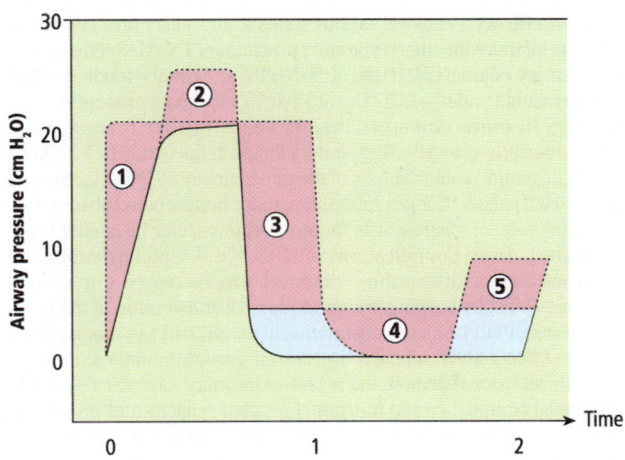

*5 *Different Ways to increase MAP- 1) increase inspiratory flow rate, producing a square-wave inspiratory pattern; 2) increase PIP 3) reverse the inspiratory-expiratory (I/E) ratio or prolong the inspiratory time without changing the rate; 4) increase the PEEP 5) increase ventilatory rate by reducing expiratory time without changing the inspiratory time*

CO_2 elimination. For example, a 50% increase in tidal volume (i.e. 6–9 mL/kg) with a constant dead space (i.e. 3 mL/kg) doubles alveolar ventilation (3-6 mL/kg X frequency). In contrast, a 50% increase in frequency increases alveolar ventilation by 50% because dead-space ventilation (dead space X frequency) increases when frequency is increased. Although increases in minute ventilation achieved via larger tidal volumes are more effective in increasing alveolar ventilation, the use of relatively small tidal volumes and high frequencies is usually preferred to minimize volutrauma.

PERMISSIVE HYPERCAPNIA

lung injury in ventilated premature infants occurs primarily through the mechanism of volutrauma, often due to the combination of high tidal volumes in association with a high end-inspiratory volume and occasionally end-expiratory alveolar collapse. Tolerating a higher level of arterial partial pressure of carbon dioxide ($PaCO_2$) (target $PaCO_2$ of 45–55 mm Hg) is considered as 'Permissive hypercapnia' and when combined with the use of low tidal volumes may reduce volutrauma and lead to improved pulmonary outcomes. When using this strategy, prioritize the prevention or limitation of overventilation rather than maintenance of normal blood gases and the high alveolar ventilation that is frequently used. Respiratory acidosis and alveolar hypoventilation may be an acceptable price for the prevention of pulmonary volutrauma. compared to a routine ventilation strategy. Permissive hypercapnia may also protect against hypocapnia-induced brain hypoperfusion and subsequent periventricular leukomalacia. However, extreme hypercapnia may be associated with an increased risk of intracranial hemorrhage. It may therefore be important to avoid large fluctuations in $PaCO_2$ values. Cochrane *review* does not demonstrate any significant overall benefit of a permissive hypercapnia/minimal ventilation strategy compared to a routine ventilation strategy. At present, therefore, these ventilation strategies cannot be recommended to reduce mortality, or pulmonary and neurodevelopmental morbidity. Ventilatory strategies which target high levels of PCO_2 (> 55 mmHg) should only be undertaken in the context of well-designed controlled clinical trials. These trials should aim to establish the safe, or ideal, range for CO_2 in ventilated newborns, and examine the role of protective ventilatory techniques in achieving this target. newborns, and examine the role of protective ventilatory techniques in achieving this target.

Nasopharyngeal (without an ETtube) Synchronized Intermittent Mandatory Ventilation: *N-SIMV is more effective than N-CPAP at preventing Reintubation. *Appears to be a safe and effective tool to optimize extubation success and potentially minimize the risk for CLD in immature infants. *Further studies are needed to confirm safety and optimize efficacy –Between various systems –In smaller preterm infants –Among infants with other respiratory problems •TTN •MAS •Pneumonia •Pulmonary edema/CHF *Use of S-NIPPV as primary mode for RDS support should undergo RCT *Use of S-NIPPV as primary mode of support for RDS in more immature infants needs further investigation. **Contraindications to NIV:** *Respiratory failure defined as pH < 7.25, Pco2 > 60 *Congenital malformations of the upper airway (T-E fistula, choanal atresia, cleft palate) *Congenital diaphragmatic hernia, bowel obstruction, oomphalocele, or gastroschisis *Severe cardiovascular instability *Poor respiratory drive. **Complications of NIV:** Nasal septal irritation and necrosis, Gastric distension, Pneumothorax Increased intracranial pressure, Difficulty keeping prongs in place Overdistension of the lungs (inadvertent PEEP), Mucous obstruction of the airway **Physiologic effects of NIV (Effects-Mechanism):** *Decreased intrapulmonary shunting - Recruits additional alveoli, decreases pulmonary vascular resistance *Increased compliance and functional residual capacity and prevention of atelectasis -Recruits additional alveoli and splints the airways* Improved oxygenation -Decreases pulmonary vascular resistance * Decreased thoracoabdominal asynchrony- Splints the airways and diaphragm, stabilizes chest wall *Decreased obstructive and mixed apnea -Splints the airways and diaphragm, stabilizes chest wall; regularizes and slows respiratory rate * Conservation of surfactant- Recruits alveoli, improves pulmonary blood flow, improves oxygenation * Improved lung growth -Stretches lung tissue

Volume-targeted ventilation: Volume-targeted ventilators self-adjust in an attempt to maintain the tidal volume set by the clinician. This approach may be effective in maintaining tidal volume despite changes in respiratory mechanics. Modern neonatal ventilators, which have very sensitive and accurate flow sensors, make adjustments to PIP or inflation time from one inflation to the next in an effort to deliver the set volume. Although little information is available regarding the optimal tidal volume for preterm infants, the typical volume target is 4-6 mL/kg. A meta-analysis of trials in preterm infants reported no differences in mortality between volume-targeted and pressure-limited groups but found some clinically important benefits of volume-targeting, including reductions in the duration of intermittent positive pressure ventilation and the incidence of pneumothorax, and severe intraventricular hemorrhage. In one randomized study, volume targeting plus SIMV was more effective than SIMV alone in maintaining a desirable arterial partial pressure of carbon dioxide (Pa CO2) in infants born at more than 25 weeks' gestation. Volume-targeted ventilation may be particularly helpful in patients with heterogeneous lung disease because the differing time constants throughout the lung parenchyma when pressure-limited ventilation is used may result in suboptimal tidal volume delivery. Low volume-targeted levels increase the work of breathing during volume-targeted ventilation. During weaning, a volume-targeted level of 6 mL/kg could be used in place of a lower level to avoid an increase in the work of breathing. **Volume Guarantee:** The volume guarantee mode is available with the Dra¨ger Babylog 8000*plus* ventilator. Volume guarantee delivers a pressure-limited breath at a fixed flow. The clinician chooses a targeted VT, and, based on the volume delivered during the previous breath, the ventilator will adjust the pressure to achieve the "guaranteed" volume. However, because the increase in pressure cannot exceed the pressure limit, the volume guarantee sometimes cannot be reached unless a pressure plateau is generated by extending inspiration at a higher flow. The volume guarantee is also based on the expired VT of the preceding breaths. Early investigation revealed promise in achieving gas exchange comparable to SIMV at lower peak airway pressures. *Volume Targeted Ventilation (VTV) in Neonates: Essential Clinical Guidelines-Refer to Page 909.*

Types of Neonatal Ventilation Support: Summary

CPAP: A continuous flow of heated, humidified gas is circulated past the infant's airway typically at a set pressure of 3 to 8 cm H$_2$O, maintaining an elevated end-expiratory lung volume while the infant breathes spontaneously. The air-oxygen mixture and airway pressure can be adjusted. CPAP is usually delivered by means of nasal prongs or a nasopharyngeal tube. Prolonged endotracheal CPAP should not be used because the high resistance of the endotracheal tube increases the work of breathing, especially in small infants. Positive-pressure hoods and continuous-mask CPAP are not recommended. *Refer to Page 887.*

Pressure-limited, time-cycled, ventilation: mechanical breaths are initiated and terminated by time, and which are limited by a pre-set inspiratory pressure limit that cannot be exceeded. The inspiratory flow is constant and the delivered tidal volume is related to pulmonary compliance. It will also be affected by the degree of asynchrony between the patient and the ventilator. Newer ventilators allow the choice of flow cycling to minimize asynchrony. Time-cycled, pressure-limited ventilation can be delivered using IMV, SIMV or A/C. During PLV the tidal volume (VT) fluctuates widely due to the baby's breathing, changes in lung mechanics and variable endotracheal tube (ETT) leak. As high VT (volutrauma), and not pressure per se, causes lung injury, controlling VT rather than PIP is a logical strategy for ventilating preterm infants.

Volume-cycled ventilators: Volume-cycled ventilators are similar to pressure-limited ventilators except that the operator selects the volume delivered, rather than the PIP. The pressure automatically varies with respiratory system compliance to deliver the selected tidal volume, theoretically minimizing variability in minute ventilation. Because tidal volumes in infants are small, most of the tidal volume selected is lost in the ventilator circuit or from air leaks around uncuffed endotracheal tubes. Modern microprocessor-controlled ventilators allow volume-targeted ventilation (VTV) even in very preterm infants. VTV modes vary in how they measure and control VT delivery. Measurements are only accurate with the flow sensor placed at the Y-piece. The flow-sensors measure inspired and expired VT, and ETT leak is calculated. The advantage of targeting inspired VT is that the ventilator controls the VT as it is delivered. The major disadvantage is that variable ETT leak alters the delivered VT. The advantage of using the expired VT is that this most accurately reflects the VT that entered the infant's lung, and is less influenced by ETT leaks unless they are very large. Volume guarantee (VG) ventilation is a VTV-mode controlling the expired VT.

High-frequency ventilation: High-frequency ventilation differs from CMV in providing smaller tidal volumes, often less than the anatomical deadspace, at a much more rapid rate. Three types of HFVs are approved for use in newborns: a high-frequency oscillator (HFO), a high-frequency flow interrupter (HFFI), and a high-frequency jet (HFJ) ventilator. All HFVs are capable of delivering extremely rapid rates (300-1,500 breaths/minute, 5-25 Hz; 1 Hz = 60 breaths/minute) with tidal volumes equal to or smaller than anatomic dead space. These ventilators apply continuous distending pressure to maintain an elevated lung volume; small tidal volumes are superimposed at a rapid rate. HFJ ventilators are paired with a conventional pressure-limited device, which is used to deliver intermittent "sigh" breaths to help prevent atelectasis. "Sigh" breaths are not used with HFO ventilation. Expiration is passive (i.e., dependent on chest wall and lung recoil) with HFFI and HFJ machines, while it is active with HFO. *Refer to Page 920. The* Cochrane review shows no difference in mortality, but there are some trends favoring HFOV, including decreased CLD (oxygen need at 28 to 30 days) in survivors, decreased death or CLD (oxygen need at 28 to 30 days) and decreased CLD (oxygen at 36 to 37 weeks' PMA). However, there are trends toward an increase in severe intraventricular hemorrhage and periventricular leukomalacia, and an increased incidence of air leaks. On balance, HFOV is not recommended as a primary strategy for RDS.

Classification of Neonatal ventilators (SM Donn)
Conventional (tidal ventilation)

    Modes
        Intermittent mandatory ventilation (IMV)
        Synchronized intermittent mandatory ventilation (SIMV)
        Assist/control ventilation (A/C)
        Pressure support ventilation (PSV)
    Modalities
        Pressure targeted
            Pressure limited
            Pressure control
        Volume targeted
        Hybrid
High-frequency ventilation
        High-frequency jet ventilation (HFJV)
        High-frequency oscillatory ventilation (HFOV)
        Hybrids

CONVENTIONAL MECHANICAL VENTILATION: BASICS REVIEW

An understanding of the basic pathophysiology of the underlying respiratory disorder is essential to optimize the ventilatory strategy. Aim for an adequate gas exchange without injuring the lungs; the ultimate goal is a healthy child without chronic lung disease. A review of the major ventilatory parameters, which can be adjusted on pressure-limited time-cycled ventilators (i.e., the most common type of ventilators used for CMV), is useful. These concepts are also applicable to volume ventilators.

Peak inspiratory pressure: Changes in PIP affect both PaO_2 (by altering MAP) and $PaCO_2$ (by its effects on tidal volume and thus, alveolar ventilation). Therefore, an increase in PIP improves oxygenation and decreases $PaCO_2$. Use of a high PIP may increase the risk of volutrauma with resultant air leaks and BPD; thus, exercise caution when using high levels of PIP. The level of PIP required in an infant depends largely on the compliance of the respiratory system. A useful clinical indicator of adequate PIP is gentle chest rise with every breath, which should not be much more than the chest expansion with spontaneous breathing. Although absent breath sounds may indicate inadequate PIP (or a blocked and/or displaced ETT or even ventilator malfunction), the presence of breath sounds is not very helpful in determining optimal PIP. Adventitious sounds, such as crackles, often indicate disorders of lung parenchyma associated with poor compliance (requiring higher PIP), whereas wheezes often indicate increased resistance (affecting the time constant). Always use the minimum effective PIP. Frequently change PIP in the presence of changing pulmonary mechanics, such as after the administration of surfactant in the management of RDS. Babies with chronic lung disease often have nonhomogeneous lung disease, leading to varying compliance throughout different regions of the lung and, therefore, differing requirements for PIP. This partially accounts for the coexistence of atelectasis and hyperinflation in the same lung.

Positive end-expiratory pressure: Adequate PEEP helps to prevent alveolar collapse, maintains lung volume at end-expiration, and improves V/Q matching. Increases in PEEP usually increase oxygenation associated with increases in MAP. However, in infants with RDS, an excessive PEEP may not further improve oxygenation and, in fact, may decrease venous return, cardiac output, and oxygen transport. High levels of PEEP also may decrease pulmonary perfusion by increasing pulmonary vascular resistance. By reducing d (amplitude) pressure (PIP minus PEEP), an elevation of PEEP may decrease tidal volume and increase $PaCO_2$. Although both PIP and PEEP increase MAP and may improve oxygenation, they usually have opposite effects on $PaCO_2$. Generally, older infants with chronic lung disease tolerate higher levels of PEEP without carbon dioxide retention and with improvements in oxygenation. PEEP also has a variable effect on lung compliance and may affect the PIP required. With RDS, compliance improves with low levels of PEEP, followed by declining compliance at higher levels of PEEP. A minimum PEEP of 4-5 cm H_2O is recommended, since endotracheal intubation eliminates the active maintenance of FRC accomplished with vocal cord adduction and closure of the glottis.

Rate: Changes in frequency alter alveolar minute ventilation and, thus, $PaCO_2$. Increases in rate and, therefore, increases in alveolar minute ventilation, decrease $PaCO_2$ proportionally; decreases in rate increase $PaCO_2$. Frequency changes alone (with a constant I/E ratio) usually do not alter MAP or substantially affect PaO_2. Any changes in inspiratory time that accompany frequency adjustments may change the airway pressure waveform and, thus, alter MAP and oxygenation. Generally, a high-rate, low-tidal volume strategy is preferred . However, if a very short expiratory time is employed, expiration may be incomplete. The gas trapped in the lungs can increase FRC, decreasing lung compliance. Tidal volume decreases as inspiratory time is reduced beyond a critical level, depending on the time constant of the respiratory system. Thus, above a certain ventilator rate during pressure-limited ventilation, minute ventilation is not a linear function of frequency. Alveolar ventilation actually may fall with higher ventilatory rates as tidal volumes decrease and approach the volume of the anatomic dead space.

Inspiratory and expiratory times: The effects of changes in inspiratory and expiratory times on gas exchange are influenced strongly by the relationships of these times to the inspiratory and expiratory time constants, respectively. An inspiratory time 3–5 times longer than the time constant of the respiratory system allows relatively complete inspiration. A long inspiratory time increases the risk of pneumothorax. Shortening inspiratory time is advantageous during weaning . In a randomized trial, limitation of T_i to 0.5 second, rather than 1 second, resulted in significantly shorter duration of weaning. In contrast, patients with chronic lung disease may have a prolonged time constant. In these patients, a longer inspiratory time (near 0.8 s) may result in improved tidal volume and better carbon dioxide elimination.

Inspiratory-to-expiratory ratio: The major effect of an increase in the I/E ratio is to increase MAP and thus improve oxygenation. However, when corrected for MAP, changes in the I/E ratio are not as effective in increasing oxygenation as are changes in PIP or PEEP. A reversed (inverse) I/E ratio (inspiratory time longer than expiratory time) as high as 4:1 has been demonstrated to be effective in increasing PaO_2; however, adverse effects may occur . Although a decreased incidence of BPD with the use of reversed I/E ratios may be possible, a large, well-controlled, randomized trial revealed only reductions in the duration of a high inspired oxygen concentration and PEEP exposure with reversed I/E ratios, with no differences in morbidity or mortality. Changes in the I/E ratio usually do not alter tidal volume, unless inspiratory and expiratory times become relatively too short. Thus, carbon dioxide elimination is usually not altered by changes in I/E ratio.

Fraction of inspired oxygen : Changes in FiO_2 alter alveolar oxygen pressure and, thus, oxygenation. Because FiO_2 and MAP both determine oxygenation, they can be balanced as follows: *During increasing support, first increase FiO_2 until approximately 0.6-0.7, when additional increases in MAP are warranted. *During weaning, first decrease FiO_2 (to approximately 0.4-0.7) before reducing MAP, because maintenance of an appropriate MAP may allow a substantial reduction in FiO_2. Reduce MAP before a very low FiO_2 is reached, because a higher incidence of air leaks has been observed if distending pressures are not weaned earlier.

Flow : Although not well studied in infants, changes in flow probably impact arterial blood gases minimally as long as a sufficient flow is used. Flows of 5-12 L/min are sufficient in most newborns, depending on the mechanical ventilator and ETT being used. To maintain an adequate tidal volume, high flows are needed when inspiratory time is shortened.

Benefits and Drawbacks of Specific Ventilatory Strategies

*The benefits of using a high rate and low tidal volume (low peak inspiratory pressure [PIP]) are as follows: *Decreased air leaks *Decreased volutrauma *Decreased cardiovascular adverse effects*Decreased risk of pulmonary edema,The drawbacks of using a high rate and low tidal volume (low PIP) are as follows:*Gas trapping or inadvertent PEEP*Generalized atelectasis*Maldistribution of gas*Increased resistance. *The benefits of using continuous positive airway pressure (CPAP) or high positive end-expiratory pressure (PEEP) in infants with respiratory distress syndrome (RDS) are as follows: *Increased alveolar volume and functional residual capacity (FRC) * Alveolar recruitment*Alveolar stability*Redistribution of lung water * Improved ventilation/perfusion (V/Q) matching. The drawbacks of using CPAP or high PEEP in infants with RDS are as follows:* Increased risk of air leaks*Overdistention*Carbon dioxide retention *Cardiovascular impairment*Decreased compliance*Possible increase in pulmonary vascular resistance. The benefits of using a high inspiratory-to-expiratory (I:E) ratio or long inspiratory time are as follows:*Increased oxygenation*Potentially improved gas distribution in lungs with atelectasis, The drawbacks of using a high I:E ratio or long inspiratory time are as follows:*Gas trapping and inadvertent PEEP*Increased risk of volutrauma and air leaks *Impaired venous return *Increased pulmonary vascular resistance.The benefits of permissive hypercapnia in neonates are as follows: *Decreased volutrauma and lung injury*Decreased duration of mechanical ventilation*Reduced alveolar ventilation*Reduced side effects of hypocapnia*Increased oxygen unloading.The drawbacks of permissive hypercapnia in neonates are as follows:*Cerebral vasodilation*Hypoxemia*Hyperkalemia*Decreased oxygen uptake by hemoglobin*Increased pulmonary vascular resistance. The benefits of using a short inspiratory time are as follows:*Faster weaning*Decreased risk of pneumothorax *Possibility of using a higher ventilator rate. The drawbacks of using a short inspiratory time are as follows:

* Insufficient tidal volume *Potential need for high flow rates.

Courtesy: Massimo Bellettato, MD; Chief Editor: Ted Rosenkrantz, MD
http://emedicine.medscape.com/article/979268-overview#a1

OXYGENATION EQUATIONS

Alveolar Gas Equation (PAO_2)

$$PAO_2 = FiO_2 (PB - PH_2O) - PaCO_2/R,$$

where FiO_2 = fraction of inspired oxygen;

PB = barometric pressure (at sea level) = 760;

PH_2O = partial pressure of water = 47;

$paCO_2$ = partial pressure of CO_2 on arterial blood gas; and

R = respiratory quotient = 0.8

Sample calculation: child on 50% oxygen at sea level with pCO_2 40

$$PAO_2 = FiO_2 (PB - PH_2O) - PCO_2/R)$$
$$PAO_2 = 0.5 (760 - 47) - 40/0.8$$
$$PAO_2 = 0.5 (713) - 50$$
$$PAO_2 = 306$$

Pressure gradient

A pressure gradient between the airway opening and the alveoli must be present to drive the flow of gases during both inspiration and expiration. The necessary pressure gradient can be calculated from the following equation:

Pressure = Volume Compliance + Resistance X Flow

$$Compliance = \frac{Change\ in\ volume\ (L)}{Change\ in\ Pressure\ (cmH_2O)}$$

$$Resistance = \frac{Pressure\ (cm\ H_2O)}{Flow\ (L/sec)}$$

Oxygen content

Normal oxygen content is approximately 20 mL O_2/100 mL arterial blood and 5 mL O_2/100 mL venous blood.

Oxygen content = oxygen bound to hemoglobin + dissolved oxygen

$$= \frac{1.39 \times Hgb \times \%\ saturation}{100} + (0.003 \times PO_2)$$

Oxygen tissue delivery (DO_2)

Normal oxygen tissue delivery is approximately 600 mL O_2/min/m²

Tissue oxygen delivery = Arterial oxygen content x cardiac index

$$Do_2\ (mL\ O_2/min/m^2) = CaO_2\ (mL\ O_2/dL\ blood) \times CI\ (L/min/m^2) \times 10\ (dL/L)$$

Oxygen Consumption (VO_2)

Normal is approximately 150 mL/min/m²

Oxygen consumption = (Arterial oxygen content — venous oxygen content) x cardiac index

$$Vo_2\ (mL\ O_2/min/m^2) = (CaO_2 - CVO_2) \times CI$$

Alveolar—Arterial Oxygenation Difference ($AaDO_2$)

$$AaDo_2 = PAO_2 - PaO_2\ (Alveolar\ PO_2 - arterial\ PO_2)$$
$$= [FiO_2\ (PB - PH_2O) - PaCo_2/RQ] - PaO_2$$

Causes of an increased Alveolar-Arterial Oxygenation Difference ($AaDO_2$)

Hypoventilation, Ventilation-Perfusion (V/Q) Mismatch, Diffusion block, Right-to-Left Shunt, Low cardiac output

Oxygen index (OI)

An OI of > 40 predicts a >80% risk of mortality; an OI of >25 predicts a >50% mortality. Marker of how much work a ventilator is doing.

$$OI = \frac{Mean\ airway\ pressure \times FiO_2 \times 100}{Post\ ductal\ PaO_2}$$

PF Ratio

Normal is about 500, <250 indicates acute hypoxic lung injury, and >150 indicates acute respiratory distress syndrome.

$$PF = PaO_2/FiO_2$$

Oxygen Hemoglobin Affinity

Increased oxygen affinity

Hypothermia, Metabolic and respiratory alkalosis, Anemia, Hypothyroidism, Hemoglobin F, Hypophosphatemia, Decreased 2,3 - diphosphoglycerate, Carbon monoxide

Decreased oxygen affinity

Hyperthermia, Metabolic and respiratory acidosis, Steroid administration, Hyperthyroidism, Hyperaldosteronism, Polycythemia,

Increased 2,3 - diphosphoglycerate

Time constant

Compliance and resistance can be used to describe the time necessary for an instantaneous or step change in airway pressure to equilibrate throughout the lungs. The time constant of the respiratory system is a measure of the time necessary for the alveolar pressure to reach 63% of the change in airway pressure, which can be calculated as follows:

$$Time\ Constant = Resistance \times Compliance$$

Thus, the time constant of the respiratory system is proportional to the compliance and the resistance. For example, the lungs of a healthy newborn with a compliance of 0.004 L/cm H_2O and a resistance of 30 cm H_2O/L/s have a time constant of 0.12 seconds. When a longer time is allowed for equilibration, a higher percentage of airway pressure equilibrates throughout the lungs. The longer the duration of the inspiratory (or expiratory) time allowed for equilibration, the higher the percentage of equilibration.

Cerebral perfusion pressure

CPP = MAP - ICP

where CPP is cerebral perfusion pressure, MAP is mean arterial pressure, and ICP is intracranial pressure.

If central venous pressure (CVP) is higher than ICP, then:

CPP = MAP - CVP

Normal CPP is above 60 torr. As CPP falls below 60 torr, autoregulation fails and cerebral blood flow begins to fall, leading to cerebral ischemia. At a CPP of 45 torr, cerebral blood flow is approximately 50% of normal.

Factors affecting cerebral blood flow

Increased $PaCO_2$
Decreased bicarbonate ion } Acidosis →vasodilatation
Increased metabolic acid

Hypoxemia
Increased cerebral metabolic rate } →vasodilatation

Decreased $PaCO_2$
Increased bicarbonate ion } Alkalosis →vasoconstriction
Decreased metabolic acid

Hyperoxia Minimal effect

Conventional mechanical ventilation: VENTILATOR CONTROLS: Clinical applications (changing ventilator settings).

1) PIP (Peak Inspiratory Pressure) The primary factor determining the tidal volume and can affect PaO_2 and $PaCO_2$. PIP of < 30 cms H_2O is usually sufficient for most respiratory disorders. Avoid high PIP > 30 cm H_2O because of risk of air leaks and barotrauma leading to chronic lung disease (BPD). Estimate the appropriate PIP setting by determining the pressure required to cause an adequate chest expansion while bagging. An increase in PIP will improve Oxygenation by increasing Mean Airway Pressure. It also increases tidal volume and reduces $PaCO_2$.

2) PEEP (Positive End Expiratory Pressure) : This stabilizes alveoli, recruits lung volume and improves lung compliance. It increases the FRC and so improves oxygenation. PEEP decreases the airway resistance by distending the airways and preventing dynamic compression during expiration. It may reduce tidal volume and hence may increase $PaCO_2$. The optimal PEEP for infants with RDS is usually 5–6 cm H_2O, to keep alveoli patent and reduce the work of breathing. However, in an infant with meconium aspiration syndrome a low PEEP of 3 cms is sufficient to prevent air leaks due to air trapping. The optimum PEEP is the level at which there is an acceptable balance between the desired goals and undesired adverse effects. The desired goals are 1. Reduction in FiO_2 to **nontoxic levels (<50%)**. 2. Maintenance of PaO_2/SaO_2 of above 60 mm Hg or above 90% respectively. 3. Improving lung compliance. 4. Maximizing oxygen delivery.

3) MAP (Mean Airway Pressure): MAP = (PIP - PEEP) (Ti / (Ti + Te)) + PEEP

MAP can therefore be altered by changes in PIP or PEEP and in I:E Ratio. Oxygenation is closely related to MAP. Five ways to increase to MAP. 1. Increase flow rate producing a square waveform. 2. Increase PIP. 3. Increase PEEP. 4. Reverse the I:E Ratio or prolong the IT. 5. Increase ventilator rate by reducing Expiratory Time without changing IT.

4) FiO_2 (Fraction of Inspired Oxygen): Adjust FiO_2 to maintain an adequate PaO_2 (50-80 mm Hg). An FiO_2 > 50% (0.5) may cause decreased ciliary activity and increased capillary leakage in the airways, thus increasing the risk of atelectasis and ET tube blockage. High FiO_2 > 80% (0.8) causes resorption atelectasis and increased right-to- left shunting even in babies on ventilation. This will lead to a fall in oxygenation and a need for higher ventilator settings. Try to improve oxygenation by better ventilation rather than tuning up the FiO_2 80% ; though sometimes this is unavoidable. An FiO_2 of 50% (0.5) is generally considered safe.

5) Flow rate: An important determinant of the ability of the ventilator to deliver the needed PIP. A minimum flow rate of at least 2.5 to 3 times the minute ventilation i.e., 8-10 lts/mt. is necessary.

6) IT (Inspiratory Time): An IT of 0.3-0.5 seconds is sufficient for most disorders. In RDS, use closer to 0.5 seconds. Increasing the IT shortens the expiratory time, increases I:E Ratio. Normal Ratio is 1:1 - 1:3 ; avoid I:E Ratio < 1:1 to prevent air trapping in MAS; use short IT and high rates as there is gas trapping and increased risk of air leaks. While ventilating a case of lower airway obstruction (Asthma, Bronchiolitis) use short IT and slow rates.

7) Respiratory Rate (RR): The primary determinant of minute ventilation and hence CO_2 elimination. A rate of 40-60/mt is usually sufficient in most conditions. High rates are necessary in MAS where CO_2 retention is a major problem. At rates over 75-80/mt, minute ventilation may fall and if a very short expiratory time (Te) is used at fast rate there is a risk of incomplete expiration and gas trapping known as 'inadvertent PEEP'. Barotrauma, pneumothorax and compromised pulmonary circulation are also possible. When using fast rates with short Te, it is advisable to reduce applied PEEP to only 2 cms H_2O. If the I:E Ratio is unchanged, an increase in rate should not alter MAP. Synchronization with the ventilator can be achieved at higher rates (90–100/mt.), but the benefit appear to be confirmed to spontaneously breathing infants and are not usually seen in babies who have been given muscle relaxants.

SUMMARY OF CHANGING VENTILATOR SETTINGS

a) Desired blood gas status and the possible changes in ventilator settings which will achieve it (using pressure-type ventilator)

Desired Status	Ventilator Settings				
	Rate	PIP	PEEP	Ti	FiO_2
Increase $PaCO_2$	↓	↓			
Decrease $PaCO_2$	↑	↑			
Increase PaO_2		↑	↑	↑.	↑
Decrease PaO_2		↓	↓	↓.	↓

* Fine tuning, sparingly employed

Neuromuscular Blockers in Neonates: Used to facilitate ventilation when the infant's respiratory efforts are not coordinated with the ventilator. With the use of sedatives and synchronized ventilation, this can usually be avoided.

Dosage Recommendations for Neuromuscular Blocking Agents in the Neonate

Agent	Ed_{95} (mg/kg)	"Intubating Dose" (mg/kg)	Onset of Paralysis After Intubating (min.)	Dosage Intervals (min.)
Pancuronium	0.05	0.15	1.5 - 2.0	60 - 120
Atracurium	0.15 - 0.3	0.6 - 0.8	1.5 - 2.0	20 - 30
Vecuronium	0.03	0.15	1.5 -2.0	30 - 40
Succinylcholine	2.2	2 mg IV 4 - 5 mg IM	0.5 - 1.0	5 - 10*

* Not Recommended for prolonged duration. (From: Costarino & Polin, 1987) When administering neuromuscular blockers, it is also necessary to administer sedatives (includes narcotics).

ED_{95} = dose for effective response 95% of the time.

Basic Principles and Guidelines for Conventional Ventilation

Note : 1. Ventilation practices vary between (and within) NICUs and neonatologists. 2. This guideline is not intended to be adhered to rigidly, but merely to provide some rationale behind interpretation of blood gases and possible changes to ventilation settings in response. 3. There are limited randomized trial data which establish that any one ventilation strategy or mode is superior. 4. Many ventilation practices are based on individual experience and on evaluating changes in blood gas parameters and the clinical condition of the baby in response to changes in ventilation settings.

Basic Principles of Ventilation

There are two goals of ventilation:

1. Appropriate oxygenation
2. Appropriate ventilation

Oxygenation is affected by several factors such as the inspired oxygen concentration (FiO_2), mean airway pressure (MAP), the area of and diffusion across the gas exchange surface. Ventilation refers primarily to the amount of carbon dioxide exchanging at the alveolar level. Factors which influence this include the gas exchange surface area and diffusion and the amount of gas able to be moved in and out of the lungs.

There are several modes of conventional ventilation, which are explained in another section of the ventilation resource area.

So, when you set about changing the settings, you need to think about what you are trying to achieve.

*Change Oxygenation PaO_2 1. Alter the FiO_2 (turn the knob!) 2. Alter the mean airway pressure *Change Ventilation $PaCO_2$ 1. Change the tidal volume (by changing the pressure, primarily) 2. Change the frequency of breaths

Target Blood Gas Values

1. Ventilator settings in general should be set to achieve target oxygen saturations as per unit policy.

2. Ventilation settings that determine pCO_2 should be set with the following guidelines in mind:

Courtesy:www.adhb.govt.nz/.../ventilation/ ConventionalVentilationModes.htm

pH	pCO_2	Base Excess	Rationale
7.25 to 7.35	5.5 to 8.0kPa	0 to -4	We have a philosophy of relatively permissive hypercapnia. The rationale is to avoid overventilating lung and thereby inducing injury through volutrauma and barotrauma. At a pH above 7.25, metabolic function should be relatively preserved. If there is a significant metabolic component (that is, base excess <-4), then this may indicate that oxygenation at a tissue level is impaired.

Exceptions to this guideline include

*Infants with severe chronic lung disease where high pCO_2 levels with a lower pH may be tolerated in order to further minimize ongoing lung injury. *Infants with pulmonary hypertension, where after discussion with a specialist a decision may be made to maintain the baby in an alkalotic state (pH >7.45).

Advantages and Disadvantages of using inspiratory peak pressure and ventilator rate when ventilating Neonates

Peak pressure	Advantages	Disadvantages
Low	Fewer side-effects, especially in bronchopulmonary dysplasia and pulmonary air leak	Inadequate ventilation, Low paO2 if setting too low, Possibly development of generalized atelectasis
High	Possibly re-opening of atelectases High PaO_2 Low $PaCO_2$	Increased risk of side-effects, Impaired venous return

Ventilator rate	Advantages	Disadvantages
Low may <40/min	Possibly better oxygenation, higher PAO2 levels useful in weaning off ventilator and for ventilation with reversed I : E ratio	High peak pressure be necessary to obtain adequate ventilation, Relaxation may be necessary
High >60/min	Lower peak pressure may be necessary; lower mean airway pressure; if hyper-ventilation is desired e.g. if persistent fetal circulation is present(PPHN)	Because of the duration of expiration for lung emptying → 'air trapping' and respiratory alkalosis is possible.

Advantages and Disadvantages of using PEEP when ventilating Neonates

PEEP level	Advantages	Disadvantages
Low 0-3 cm H_2O	Maintenance of lung volume in prematures with low functional residual capacity	Possibly too low to support adequate lung volume, CO_2 retention
Medium 4–7 cm H_2O	Stabilizing of areas with atelectasis,Raised lung volume in surfactant deficiency	Possible hyperinflation
High 8–10 cm H_2O	Prevention of alveolar collapse in surfactant deficiency,Improved ventilation distribution return	Increased risk of pneumothorax Reduced compliance Impaired venous Increased pulmonary vascular resistance CO_2 retention

Features of pressure-targeted modalities

	Pressure limited	Pressure control	Pressure support
Limit variable	Pressure	Pressure	Pressure
Flow	Continuous	Variable inspiratory	Variable inspiratory
*Cycle mechanisms	Time or flow	Time or flow	Flow, with time limit

*Cycle mechanisms vary according to the device.

Changing the ventilation settings

Problem	Possible solutions	Comment
Low Oxygenation	Increase the FiO$_2$	The easiest solution. Remember that babies whose oxygen requirements are changing significantly need to be clinically reassessed and you should consider a radiograph if the FiO$_2$ increases by more than 10%.
Low PaO$_2$ or Saturations	**Increase the Mean Airway Pressure (MAP)**	1. Increase the PIP (but this may also affect ventilation) 2. Increase the inspiratory time (but this may just hold the lungs fully inflated at a high pressure). You need to watch that the inspiratory time is shorter than the expiratory time. 3. Increase the PEEP (we don't do this often, except for pulmonary hemorrhage)
High Oxygenation	**Decrease the FiO$_2$** room air, then we generally accept high saturations or PaO$_2$)	The easiest solution (unless the baby is already in room air - if in
High PaO2 Saturations	**Decrease the MAP**	· **If the PEEP is higher than 5, then you can drop this down (if the or reason for the high PEEP - e.g. pulmonary hemorrhage - has resolved) · Decrease the PIP (but this may adversely affect ventilation)**
Over-ventilation **High pH with a Low PaCO$_2$**	1.Decrease the tidal volume	· Decrease the inspiratory time if it is too long 1. **Decrease the difference between the PIP and PEEP (usually by decreasing the PIP)** 2. Note **that there are no rules on how much to drop the PIP by - Do this first if the baby has good chest movement and/or high tidal volumes you need to look at the chest movement and look at the delivered tidal volume on the ventilator. In general, dropping the PIP by 2mbar (or more if significantly overventilated) is about the right amount. But look at the tidal volume!** 3. **If the baby is on** Volume Guarantee, dr**op down the set tidal volume**
	Decrease the frequency	1. Drop the rate. If the gas is just a bit alkalotic, drop by 5. If really alkalotic, you might want to drop it by 10 or more. 2. **Note** that for modes where every breath is assisted (e.g. PSV, SIPPV), it is **futile** to reduce the rate if the baby is breathing above the back up rate. So wean the pressure (or VT) instead
Under-ventilation Low pH with a High PaCO$_2$ low tidal volumes	**Increase the tidal volume** Do this first if the baby has no chest movement and/or	1. Increase the PIP till you get some chest movement but look at the tidal volume too. 2. In general, you should not increase the PIP too high as you may find that the tidal volume increases significantly. But you need to give enough pressure to get chest movement. 3. **Remember** that if you are having to put the PIP up a lot to get the same tidal volume in that you were giving previously, compliance is goingdown. Ask yourself "Why?". Look at the baby, listen to the air entry, and think about a radiograph, particularly if the FiO$_2$ is going up 4. If the baby is on Volume Guarantee, increase the set VT. But you may have to increase the PIP as well.
	Increase the frequency	1. Increase the rate. If a bit acidotic, increase by 5. If really acidotic, you may need to increase it by 10 or more. 2. For fast rates, it is really important that the expiratory time is longer than the inspiratory time. The Babylog will let you know if you get it the wrong way around. You may need to decrease the inspiratory time accordingly. If you find you need to give more than 70 breaths per minute, think about HFOV as a ventilation mode. Speak to the specialist on duty.

Balance is Important

· Don't forget to balance your ventilator settings. For example, if a baby is in 100% oxygen but with low pressures settings, it may be preferable to reduce the FiO$_2$ but increase the pressures.

· Similarly, if the baby is on high pressure settings but a low rate, it may be better to give a faster rate and lower pressures.

When Do I Do the Next Blood Gas?

An easy answer at last : "It depends ....". So what does it depend on?

How abnormal the gas is

1. If it is really outside the normal range you are targeting, you probably want to check it quite soon to see whether your changes have had the effect you thought they would (that is, in 15-30 minutes).

How stable the baby is

1. The specialist on duty should be able to give you some guidance on how often gases need to be done.

2. If the baby is stable and you're not doing too much with the ventilation, you don't need to check it too soon after the change. Some babies who are chronically ventilated may only need a gas once a day.

3. You can look at other things like the new tidal volume to see whether you think your changes have had any sort of effect.

4. But if the baby is really unstable, you may wish to do gases often to see where they are heading.

5. If you have given surfactant, you might want to check a gas within an hour to see what effect any change in compliance is having on gas exchange

How confident you are

1. If you are new to ventilation, you may need reassurance with a gas soon after you make your change.

2. However, try to avoid too many tests just to reassure yourself (particularly if the nursing staff need to take a capillary sample).

3. Blood letting is the most common reason for   babies needing transfusions in the first week or two of life.

When the nurses tell you

1. **If they are worried, they will tell you (...and you should listen).**

I'm really worried that
I will be told off on the
ward round if I get it
all wrong .....

There are many ways to ventilate babies. All the consultants have different styles and experiences, and have their "favorite" modes. No single mode has been shown to be significantly better than another (other than synchronized modes are probably better than untriggered modes).

2. Some babies do well on one mode and settings one minute, then they may seem to need something else.

3. Believe it or not, all the consultants had to learn by trial and error, and they don't always get it "right".

4. What is most important is that you understand what happens when you make a change to A ventilator setting. No one can necessarily predict what will exactly happen to a blood gas as a result of that change.

5. And if you are not sure what to do, **ask someone** (including the consultant.)

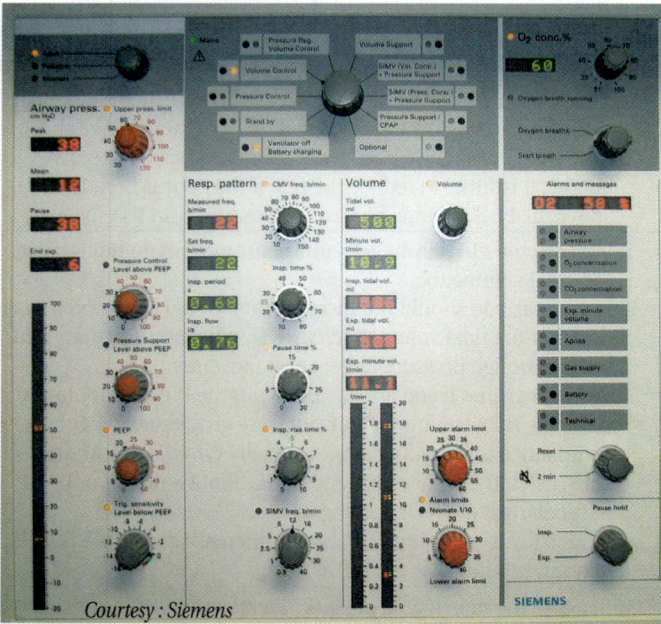

Courtesy : Siemens

Before you touch the ventilator ..... 1. Look at the blood gas result. Do you believe it? Does it fit with the clinical picture the baby is giving you? Does it fit with the expected course for the baby (e.g. improving compliance after surfactant for RDS)? If it is vastly different than you expect, is there some reason for it? Was there an air bubble in the specimen? If a capillary gas, is the perfusion awful? Did the baby bleed easily? Don't change anything on the basis of a venous gas. The only reliable information from a venous gas are the electrolytes and the glucose. **2. Look at the baby.** *Is the chest moving? *What's the air-entry like? *Is the baby struggling on the ventilator? *Is the baby very tachypneic or is the baby apnoeic? **3. Look at the ventilator.** *Is it cycling? *Are you giving the baby the ventilator settings you thought you were? *What tidal volume (VT) is the baby getting? *Is there a significant leak? *Is it set up properly with an appropriate inspiratory time and with appropriate pressures? Click here to open the respiratory function monitoring page. **4. Look at the nursing flow chart.** *How stable has the baby been over the past few hours or days? *Are there lots of secretions? *How is the baby handling?

Suctioning of Endotracheal Tubes: I.**Indications.** A. To clear airways of secretions. B. To keep artificial airway patent. C. To obtain material for analysis of culture. In-line suctioning preferred for indications other than obtaining material for culture. II. Pre-assemble suction equipment. Recommended suction catheters are 5 or 6 French for 2.5 mm ET tube, 6 French for 3.0 ET tube and 8 French for 4.0 ET tube. The amount of suction applied to the catheter should be between 40-80 mmHg. III. Suction between feedings or discontinue feedings for period of treatment. IV. Auscultate chest prior to suctioning. Oxygenation prior to suctioning will be done with an FiO2 no greater than 0.10 above that being used to ventilate the infant. Monitor heart rate continuously. Suction should not be applied while the catheter is being inserted down the ET tube. The tip of the suction catheter will not be inserted beyond the end of the tube. When withdrawing the catheter, continuous suction is applies. The procedure should not take longer than 10 seconds. Following suctioning, ventilate the infant with an FiO2 no greater than 0.10 above that used prior to suctioning. The PaO2 should be raised to a level comparable to that prior to suctioning. V. Do not add saline unless necessary. Saline may be used if the infant has thick tenacious secretions which cannot be extracted by using suctioning alone. Normal saline for secretions for Respiratory Therapy use is instilled into ET tube and 3-5 ventilated breaths performed prior to suctioning as above. VI. Vibration and percussion (CPT-Chest Physiotherapy) will not be performed routinely prior to suctioning. If the need for CPT is documented, it must be ordered by a physician describing the area to be treated and the frequency of treatments.

Solutions to unsatisfactory blood gases in RDS

1. *To improve the oxygenation when the PaCO$_2$ is normal.* In this situation, with the PaCO$_2$ 5.0–6.5 kpa (37–56 mmHg), there are three alternatives; * Increasing inspired oxygen concentration: * Increasing the respiratory rate (particularly if the baby is not breathing in synchrony); * Increasing the MAP without increasing the peak pressures (by increasing T$_1$ or the level of PEEP). Try increasing the FiO$_2$ first (not beyond 95%), and next or at the same time adjust the rate to achieve ventilator / patient synchrony. If the baby is already in synchrony then it is acceptable to gradually increase the T$_1$ towards 0.5–0.6 seconds, but never let the T$_1$:T$_E$ ratio exceed. 1.5:1 nor the baby get out of phase with the ventilator. These maneuvers increase the MAP. If they fail, increase the PIP and accept the lowish PaCO$_2$ as long as it is not below 3 kpa (22.5mmHg) . Increasing the PEEP to above 7 cm H$_2$0 is rarely of any benefit.

2. *To improve oxygenation when the PaCO$_2$ is low <4.5 kpa (34mmHg).* consider.

   *Wrong diagnosis: The baby has compliant lungs, so there may be another cause for hypoxemia (e.g. congenital heart disease, sepsis, PPHN .

   * Gross overventilation: overventilation prevents adequate pulmonary perfusion and reduces the paO$_2$. The CXR in such babies shows lung fields which are black, with low flat diaphragms and a small heart shadow.

If none of these diagnoses apply the baby probably has severe RDS. To improve oxygenation try to sustain the MAP, but change other things in ways that might increase the PaCO$_2$ (e.g. Increase the PEEP or decrease the rate).

3. *To lower a high Carbon dioxide concentration (PaCO$_2$ > 8-9 kpa (60–68 mmHg) with an acceptable level of oxygen.* There are several altenatives;

   * Increasing the rate but to no more than 90-100/min;

   * Reducing the PEEP, but not to below 3 cm H$_2$0, since PEEP preserves surfactant;

   * Reducing the inspiratory time (but not to less than 0.2 seconds);

   * Lengthen the expiratory time.

4. After a change in ventilator setting always check the blood gases 1–2 hours later to confirm improvement.

A baby with a chest X-ray which shows RDS who remains hypoxic (PaO$_2$ <5.5 kpa, 42mmHg) in spite of two doses of surfactant, high oxygen concentrations, and ventilator settings which achieve synchrony at a pressure of more than 30/6 cm H$_2$O is now unusual. Values for PaCO$_2$ of 5.3–6.6 kpa(40–50 mmHg) and PaCO$_2$ of 7–8 kpa (52-60 mmHg) may be acceptable in a baby with very severe lung disease for a time if the pH remains above 7.25. The blood pressure should be supported and any acidemia corrected. The advice of an experienced neonatalogist must be sought.

Adjustments to ventilator settings on the basis of blood gas changes

Low PaO$_2$	High PaCO$_2$	Increase peak pressure which will also increase mean airway pressure : in spontaneously breathing babies ↑ rate may also work
Low PaO$_2$	Normal PaCO$_2$	↑ F$_1$O$_2$: ↑ MAP but maintain PIP (i.e. ↑ PEEP or ↑ T$_1$)
Low PaO$_2$	Low PaCO$_2$	Consider alternative diagnosis, e.g. PPHN, sepsis, over-ventilation ↑ FIO$_2$: ↑ MAP : Use vasodilators
PaO$_2$ normal	High PaCO$_2$	↓ PEEP. ↑ rate : keep MAP constant
PaO$_2$ normal	Low PaCO$_2$	↓ rate : maintain MAP
PaO$_2$ high	PaCO$_2$ high	(rare check for mechanical problems, e.g. blocked tube) ↓ PEEP : ↓ T$_1$: ↑ rate
PaO$_2$ high	PaCO$_2$ normal	↓ MAP (usually ↓ PIP) : ↓ F$_1$O$_2$
PaO$_2$ high	PaCO$_2$ low	↓ pressure. ↓ rate. ↓ F$_1$O$_2$
PaO$_2$ normal	PaCO$_2$ normal	Sit tight! unless weaning

Ventilator Manipulations to Increase Ventilation and Decrease PaCo$_2$

Parameter	Advantage	Disadvantage
↑ Rate	Easy to titrate	Maintains same dead space/tidal volume
	Minimizes barotrauma	May lead to inadvertent PEEP
↑ P$_1$	Better bulk flow (improved dead space tidal volume)	More barotrauma Shifts to stiffer compliance curve
↓ PEEP	Widens compression Pressure	Decreases MAP
	Decreases dead space	Decreases oxygenation/alveolar collapse
	Decreases expiratory load	Stops splinting obstructed/closed airways
	Shifts to steeper compliance curve	
↑ Flow	Permits shorter T$_1$, longer T$_E$	More barotrauma
↑ T$_E$	Allows longer time for passive expiration in face of prolonged time Constant	Shortens T$_1$ Decreases MAP Decreases oxygenation

↓ =decrease; T$_E$ = expiratory time; FiO$_2$ = fractional concentration of inspired oxygen; - = increase; T$_1$ = inspiratory time; MAP=mean airway pressure; Paco$_2$ = partial pressure of carbon dioxide, arterial; P$_1$ = peak inspiratory pressure; PEEP = positive end-expiratory pressure.

ESSENTIAL FACTS OF CONVENTIONAL MECHANICAL VENTILATION

1. **MAP (Mean Airway Pressure)** = $([PIP - PEEP] [T_I] /T_I + T_E) + PEEP$

   MAP is increased by increases in PEEP, PIP, inspiratory time (T_I), rate, and flow rate. MAP as low as 5cm H_2O may be sufficient in infants with normal lungs, whereas 20cm H_2O or more may be necessary in severe RDS.

2. **PEEP** - Normal Physiologic PEEP is approximately 3cm H_2O. The initial PEEP is usually 4-5cm H_2O. PEEP should not exceed 8cm H_2O in most situations. PEEP requirements go in consonance with FiO_2 as follows:

FiO_2	PEEP (cm (H_2O))
0.3	3
0.4	4
0.5	5
0.6	6
0.7-0.8	7
above 0.8	8

3. **PIP:** A Neonate with normal lungs if were to be ventilated, a PIP of 12cm H_2O will be required. If compliance is less, check chest rise on hand ventilation and decide (with Pressure Manometer) initial PIP 18cm H_2O for severely stiff lungs, 16cm H_2O for moderately stiff lungs, & 14cm H_2O for mildly stiff lungs. Clinically mild, moderate, severe and very severe respiratory distress will consequently require PIP in the range of 15-19, 20-24, 25-29 and over 30. It is logical to start with PIP of about 18-20cm H_2O and modify it later, as mechanical ventilation would be instituted for the evolving stage of disease.

4. **T_I** - The inspiratory time should be in the range of 0.3 to 0.5 seconds close to the physiologic values. In low compliance condition like RDS use T_I of 0.4-0.5 seconds and in MAS with increased airway resistance use T_I of 0.3-0.4 seconds. Increasing the T_I shortens the expiratory time and increases the I:E ratio. Normal I:E ratio is 1:1-1:3. Avoid I-E ratio < 1:1 to prevent air trapping.

5. **Flow rate** a minimum flow of atleast twice the minute ventilation (tidal volume x respiratory rate) is necessary. Usually the flow is set at 8-10 L/mt and left unchanged. If the PIP upslope is of sine wave in pattern, ventilator/tubing losses are minimal and if the minute ventilation is normal to moderately increased, a flow rate of 4-6 L/mt is appropriate.

6. **Respiratory rate** A respiratory rate of 40-60/mt is usually sufficient in most conditions. It must be recognized that increasing the respiratory rate while keeping the T_I the same shortens expiration and may lead to inadequate emptying of lungs and inadvertent PEEP. If the work of breathing, Mean Airway Pressure, and asynchrony of breathing are minimal, a respiratory rate of 20/mt is usually sufficient.

7. **FIO_2** - It is usually set 10% >what the infant was receiving prior to ventilation. Modify **FIO_2** according to Pulse oximetry and ABG analysis to prevent hyperoxia. Adjust FiO2 to maintain O2 Saturation 90-93% (88-95) on Pulse oximetry

8. **Suggested initial settings for common conditions**

	Normal lung	RDS	MAS
PIP (mmHg)	13–15	20–25	20–25
PEEP (mmHg)	3	5–7	3–5
FiO_2	10% higher than what the infant was getting before		
Rates (per min)	20–30	40–60	60–80
Flow (L/min)	8–10	8–10	8–10
I-time (sec)	0.4	0.4	0.3

9. **Ideal Blood Gases On Ventilator:**

   The goal is to try and to maintain the blood gases as close to normal as possible, while keeping barotrauma and volutrauma to a minimum.

   pH - 7.3–7.35

   PaO_2 - 50–80 mm Hg in preterms; 80-100mm Hg in term infants

   $PaCO_2$ - 35-45mm Hg. In preterms, a $PaCo_2$ of 45-55mm Hg is often accepted in order to avoid barotrauma and CLD (permissible hypercapnia).

   SaO_2 - 90–95 % in acute respiratory conditions; 89-95% in CLD.

   Note:

   A pH >7.45 is associated with cerebral vasoconstriction and should be avoided.

   A PaO_2 >80 mm Hg in preterms is associated with ROP and free O_2 radical injury

   $PaCO_2$ >55 mm Hg is associated with increased cerebral blood supply and may contribute to IVH.

10. **Oxygenation Index** = $\dfrac{MAP \times FiO_2 \times 100}{\text{Postductal } PO_2}$

   40 - mortality risk > 80-90%, 25-40 - Mortality risk 50–60%, If oxygenation index >40, it is an indication for use of ECMO.

Conventional mechanical ventilation: Practical Points

1. Follow the Cycle of Change during Ventilation

Set the following Initial Ventilator settings depending on clinical condition- **PRE-SET** PEEP, Ti, Rate, Flow.

Adjust the following Initial Ventilator settings depending on actual observation- **ADJUST** PIP, FiO2.

Change further Ventilator settings depending on - Clinical examination, Serial ABGs, & Expected Course of Disease.

Re-evaluate the patient and determine whether the clinical condition Normalized/Partially improved/Worsened.

2. Beware of the natural course of the disease in question

For e.g. RDS—Onset<4 hrs of birth, Progresses over 1st 24 hrs, Peaks at 24-36 hrs, Improves 48-72 hrs, Off-Ventilation at 72-96 hrs, Off-O2 by day 7, and usual Complications: Protracted course- PDA, Sepsis, IVH, Pulmonary Hemorrhage, Airleaks, Collapse etc.

Pneumonia—Onset any time, Progresses over 1st 24-48 hrs, Improves with IV antibiotics, Subsides by 3–4 days, Complications: ARDS, Shock, Pleural effusion, Pulmonary Hemorrhage.

Meconium aspiration syndrome—Onset <4 hours, Progresses over 1st 24 hrs, Variable course thereafter(may subsides by 48-72 hrs or may last 7 days), Initially aspiration syndrome and later chemical pneumonitis, Complications: PPHN, Airleaks, Sepsis

3. Ensure the proportionality of ventilator settings:

No single ventilator parameter setting should be disproportionate like the following settings.

e.g. PIP/PEEP 14/3 @ Rate 60 X Ti 0.5 × FiO_2 25%

   PIP/PEEP 20/6 @ Rate 60 X Ti 0.30 × FiO_2 30%

Disproportionality occurs due to

a) Over-reliance on ABGs

b) Failure to anticipate /correct complications

Try to follow the following Proportional Ventilator settings

e.g. PIP/PEEP 12/3 @ Rate 25 × Ti 0.45 × FiO_2 21%

   PIP/PEEP 15/5 @ Rate 50 × Ti 0.35 × FiO_2 50%

   PIP/PEEP 20/6 @ Rate 60 × Ti 0.30 × FiO_2 75%

   PIP/PEEP 25/7 @ Rate 65 × Ti 0.30 × FiO_2 100%

4. Adjust Ventilator Settings on the basis of Blood gas changes

Refer to the Table "Adjustments to Ventilator Settings on the basis of Blood gas changes" given elsewhere in the Chapter.

INITIAL VENTILATOR SETTINGS IN COMMON NEONATAL AND INFANT DISEASE STATES

Disease state	Settings	Principles and practice
1. Hyaline membrane Disease	PIP 18 × 20 cm H_2O PEEP 4–5 cm H_2O Ti 0.4–0.5 sec. Rate 60–100/mt FiO_2 0.6–0.8	* After surfactant therapy, shorten Ti to 0.25–0.3 seconds and reduce PIP. * If Oxygenation is inadequate increase PIP by 1 cm every few breaths until air entry appears adequate (Max PIP 30cm H_2O) & increase FIO_2 by 5% and PEEP by 1 cm (Max. PEEP 8–10 cm) until cyanosis is abolished and O_2 Sats. are 92–95%.
2. Meconium Aspiration Syndrome	PIP 25–35 cm H_2O PEEP 0–3 cm H_2O Ti 0.2–0.3 sec Rate 40–60/mt FiO_2 1	* Paralyze these babies as they are large, vigorous with high risk of air leaks. * Use minimal PEEP and short Ti to minimize air trapping and increase rate and reduce I:E ratio to reduce hypercarbia. * Refractory hypoxia →PPHN.
3. PPHN	PIP 35–40 cm H_2O PEEP 3–4 cm H_2O Ti 0.4–0.5 sec. Rate 80–100/mt FIO_2 1	* Hyperventilate and alkalinize to maintain the pH at 7.5–7.6 (to reduce the PVR). * Treat hypoxia if PaO_2 is below 50mm Hg in 100% O_2. * Use muscle paralysis to reduce hyperreactivity * Maintain $PaCO_2$ 35-50 mmHg. * Increase systemic BP by DOPAMINE and/or DOBUTAMINE infusion by at least 20% to reduce right to left shunting. * Try iNO therapy and ECMO if not responsive to conventional ventilation.
4. Pneumonia	PIP 15–25 cm H_2O PEEP 0–3 cm H_2O Ti 0.3–0.4 sec. Rate 30-40/mt FiO_2 0.5–1	* Unlike HMD the compliance of lungs is almost normal in neonates with Pneumonia * Suctioning of ET tube and chest physiotherapy are indicated due to excessive inflammatory exudates.
5. PIE	PIP 15–25 cm H_2O PEEP 0–2 cm H_2O Ti 0.2–0.3 sec. Rate 50–60/mt FiO_2 1	* Reduce MAP and increase EXP. time to minimize over distension of lungs to reduce further air leaks. * Control $PaCO_2$ by increasing the rate rather than PIP * Try HFOV if available. * Try lateral decubitus nursing position on the affected side and Selective bronchial intubation on the contralateral side , if the PIE is predominantly unilateral.
6. Recurrent Apnea	PIP 10–15 cm H_2O PEEP 2–3 cm H_2O Ti 0.5 sec. Rate 30–40/mt FiO_2 0.3–0.4	* Avoid hyperventilation in normal lungs due to potential risk of reducing cerebral blood flow. * Reduce rate and I:E ratio progressively as the infant regains his own spontaneous respiratory efforts. * Indicated in recurrent apnea of prematurity or prolonged apnea in term babies (birth asphyxia, cerebral edema, intractable seizures, post operative stabilization etc.,
7. Interstitial pulmonary Edema	PIP 40 cm H_2O PEEP 6–8 cm H_2O Ti 0.5 sec. Rate 30–40/mt FIO_2 0.5-1	* Pulmonary edema (left heart failure), hydrops fetalis, ***massive pulmonary hemorrhage*** have similar pulmonary alterations and demand same approach with assisted ventilation. * Give IV Lasix for Rapid clearance of interstitial pulmonary edema. * Reduce PIP as soon as lung edema clears and CXR shows improvement.
8. Postoperative Support	PIP 15–20 cm H_2O PEEP 4–6 cm H_2O Ti 0.4 sec. Rate 20–30/mt FIO_2 0.3–0.5	* Required for infants undergoing thoracotomy for TE fistula, diapharagmatic hernia, open heart surgery. * Administer narcotic anlgesics for relief of pain and paralyze the infant with Atracurium to prevent struggling and fighting during ventilation.
9. Birth Asphyxia	PIP 20-25cm H_2O PEEP 2-4cm H_2O Ti 0.4 sec. Rate 30–40/mt FIO_2 04–05	* Consider that neuromotor disability is invariable, when ventilation support is required for more than 12 hrs. * Give $NaHCO_3$ if severe metabolic acidosis persists despite adequate cardiac output and systemic circulation. * Give inotropes to improve cardiac output and systemic circulation.
10.Broncho Pulmonary Dysplasia	PIP 15–20 cm H_2O PEEP 2–4 cm H_2O Ti 0.2–0.3 sec. Rate 50–60/mt FiO 0.5	* Maintain adequate oxygenation with the lowest possible MAP. * Maintain PaO_2 between 60-80 mm Hg, $PaCO_2$ up to 60 mm Hg and pH above 7.25.

INITIATION OF POSITIVE PRESSURE VENTILATION

1. **Intubate baby—Fix endotracheal tube:** Check ventilator. Air/oxygen should be warmed to 37°C and humidified to 70–100 percent.

2. **Initial settings**

   FiO_2 0.5

   Rate 40–50 per minute

   PIP 18–20 cm H_2O

   PEEP 4–5 cm H_2O

   Ti 0.4–0.5 sec

3. **Observe infant** for cyanosis, absence of retractions, chest wall movement and breath sounds.

4. If ventilation is inadequate, **increase PIP** by 1 cm H_2O, every few breaths until air entry appears adequate.

5. If oxygenation is inadequate as indicated by presence of cyanosis or poor saturation on pulse-oximeter, **increase FiO_2** by 5% every minute until cyanosis is abolished or the saturation touches 90-95 percent.

6. **Draw arterial blood gas**

   *Ventilator settings   *Rate.

   Subsequent management on a ventilator

   This will depend on the ABG and the course of the disease. Arterial blood gas analysis remains the gold standard for assessment of effective ventilation.

Checking the ventilator

- Check settings at each shift. No change to be made without record.
- Alarms: Check that they are appropriately set (preferably 2–4 cm above and below the set PIP)
- Humidification : Check traps, condensation, temperature
- Filters : Wash compressor filter daily. Bacterial filter (if used) to be changed every 3–4 days.
- Tubings : Change weekly, including humidification bottle.

Ideal blood gases on ventilator

The goal is to try and to maintain the blood gases as close to normal as possible, while keeping barotrauma and volutrauma to a minimum.

pH —7.3–7.35

PaO_2—50–80 mm Hg in preterms; 80–100 mm Hg in term infants
$PaCO_2$—35–45 mm Hg in preterms; a $PaCO_2$ of 45–55 mm Hg is often accepted in order to avoid barotrauma and CLD (permissible hypercapnia).

SaO_2 90–95% in acute respiratory conditions ; 89–95% in CLD.
NOTE

A pH > 7.45 is associated with cerebral vasoconstriction and should be avoided.

A PaO_2 > 80 mm Hg in preterms is associated with ROP and free O_2 radical injury.

$PaCO_2$ > 55 mm Hg is associated with increased cerebral blood supply and may contribute on IVH; and a $PaCO_2$ <22 mmHg is a predisposing factor to PVL changes.

CLINICAL AND LABORATORY PARAMETERS INDICATING ADEQUATE VENTILATION

(Monitoring during mechanical ventilation)

Monitoring during ventilation helps us to look at the past (trends) and the present condition and so anticipate the future. It should be **intense and continuous. The best monitor is a well trained nurse or resident doctor,** as monitors are liable to give false alarms which may lead to misguided interventions if we react to the monitor and not the baby.

What do we monitor ?

(A) Clinical (B) Radiological (C) Biochemical (D) Hematological

(E) Bacteriological (F) Other

(A) Clinical monitoring :

Adequacy of mechanical breaths

- Movement of the chest: Should be just adequate and not exaggerated.
- Retractions: Should disappear if the ventilation is effective.
- Synchronization is rate dependent and is best seen when the infant is asleep.
- Air entry on auscultation - Should be adequate and not harsh. No gush of air should be heard around the mouth, which suggests a leak around the tube.
- CO_2 removal : Capnography/$EtCO_2$ has its limitations in the newborn and side-stream sampling may be more effective than main - stream sampling.

Hemodynamic stability

Ventilation can adversely affect cardiac output due to inadvertent PEEP and impaired filling. Conversely, a low cardiac output is monitored by :

- Oxygenation: color and pulse-ox monitoring will give a fair idea, especially after stabilization.
- Peripheral pulses, CRT and NIBP / IBP monitoring for adequacy of circulation
- Monitoring for PDA is essential in preterms.

(B) Radiological monitoring

When do we do X-rays ?

Ideally, at the start of the ventilation, after each tube change, after a sudden deterioration and after extubation.

What do we look for ?

- Position of the ET tube-should be between T2–T4
- Inflation of the lung: overinflation is seen as wide intercostal spaces and flat diaphragms
- Progress/improvement of the primary pathology
- Size of cardiac shadow—a small cardiac shadow may be due to overinflation while a large shadow may suggest a PDA.
- Pulmonary Interstitial Emphysema (PIE) / Air leaks - early signs of PIE should be looked for near the hilar region.

(C) Biochemical monitoring : Blood Gases

- During initial stabilization do 20 min after a setting change or SOS
- Thereafter, once/twice a day.
- Weaning can be done essentially on pulse ox and $EtCO_2$ monitoring

(D) Hematological monitoring

- Maintain Hb/PCV - above 40%.
- Maintain a phlebotomy chart and replace when >10% of blood volume is lost.

(E) Bacteriological monitoring

- Blood cultures may be done at the onset of ventilation and SOS
- Et tube cultures should be done on change of tube and at extubation.

(F) Others * Skin for infections / IV extravasation *Fluids / nutrition for deciding TPN *Sensorium for sedation / IVH.

Most essential parameters indicating adequate ventilation

1. Clinical parameters: Absence of cyanosis, Absence of retractions, Prompt capillary Refilling, Normal blood pressure Adequate chest expansion, Adequate air entry

2. Pulse oximetry: O_2 Saturation 90–95%

3. Blood gases: PaO_2 60–80 mm Hg, PaCO2 *Acute* 40-45 mm Hg, *chronic* up to 60 mm Hg, pH 7.35-7.45

GUIDELINES FOR WEARING FROM POSITIVE PRESSURE VENTILATION

Wean the baby from mechanical ventilation, when the indications for provision of mechanical ventilation are no longer present. **Don't wean the baby** unless the following several factors are optimal. a) Respiratory muscle strength. b) Stability of Cardiovascular system c) Work of breathing. d) General nutritional status of the patient. e) Presence or absence of an underlying hypercatabolic state. (eg:Sepsis). **Remember** it is the patient who dictates whether the weaning process is to be initiated and the pace of the weaning process. Patients can not be arbitrarily forced to wean.

Follow the principles involved in weaning the patients from mechanical ventilation

1. The underlying disease process is improving, leading to improved pulmonary mechanics and better gas exchange.

2. The infant has the ability to take over greater responsibility of alveolar ventilation, without expending an excessive amount of energy.

Weaning from IPPV (Situation-Action)

1) *PaO$_2$ 9.0-10.5 kPa (70-80 mmHg), PaCO$_2$ 5-7 kPa (35-50 mmHg), Stable ventilator settings, satisfactory CXR:* Start weaning by reducing the PIP and PEEP in 2 cm steps to 12–14 cm PIP and 3 cm PEEP ; check blood gases after each step. Reduce FiO$_2$ **Start** Aminophylline. **stop** Atracurium.

2) *Blood gases satisfactory on FiO$_2$ 30-40%; PIP / PEEP 12-14/3:* Reduce rate in 5 bpm steps to 10/min, watch PaCO$_2$.

3) *Blood gases satisfactory and baby tolerating handling without apnea at a rate of 20 bpm, low pressures of 12–14/2 and a low FiO$_2$ of around 30%:*Stop feeds and extubate FiO$_2$ (< 0.4 acute;.0.4 chronic). Randomized trials how no difference between a head box and CPAP at this point but CPAP should certainly be offered early if the baby develops CO2 retention or apnea.

@Beware of the weaning problems! 1) Tachypnea: Rapid breathing because of anxiety, muscle fatigue or true weaning failure. Anxiety is accompanied by increase in tidal volume and reduction in PCO$_2$, whereas muscle fatigue and true wean failure is accompanied by decrease in tidal volume and increase in PCO$_2$. 2) Abdominal Paradox: Appearance of abdominal paradox is a possible sign of diaphragmatic weakness. 3) Hypoxia :Hypoventilation, impaired gas exchange and decreased mixed venous oxygen content could be responsible for hypoxia. 4) Hypercapnia.

Complicating factors 1) Dyspnea - Anxiety and Dyspnea are common during weaning 2) Cardiac output - The transition from positive pressure ventilation to negative pressure breathing can result in a decrease in cardiac output and impair diaphragmatic function. 3) Electrolyte depletion - Magnesium and phosphorous depletion can impair muscle strength.

Weaning Modes

1.Assist- A switch from control mode to assist mode on those ventilators so designed. **2.I.M.V.-** Use of continuous flow IMV machines steadily decreasing respiratory frequency. This is particularly helpful in patients with severe respiratory disease. **3. S.I.M.V.** Synchronized intermittent mandatory ventilation allows the withdrawal of a portion of the positive pressure breath shortly after initiation and further withdrawal can progress at a pace tailored to the capabilities of the patient. Set breath delivered within an interval based on the set respiratory rate. Ventilator spends part of the interval waiting for spontaneous breath from the patient, which it will use as a trigger to deliver a full breath. If not sensed, it will automatically give a breath at the end of the period, any other breaths during the cycle are not supplemented.**4. Pressure support with or without S.I.M.V-** PSV alone or in conjunction with SIMV allows gradual withdrawal of mechanical ventilation. PSV is particularly appealing because the patient maintains control of the ventilatory frequency and pattern while the degree of machine support depends on the preset pressure. PSV decreases the ventilator imposed work of breathing and relieves diaphragmatic fatigue in patients who fail conventional weaning attempt. **5. Continuous Positive Airway Pressure-** Studies have suggested that the smallest infants may be weaned from positive pressure ventilation to nasal CPAP therapy very effectively. Nasal CPAP serves as a useful adjunct to therapy in LBW babies and reduces the need for re-intubation. Weaning to CPAP may be attempted at a PIP equal to or less than 16 cm H$_2$O, PEEP 4cm H$_2$O.

Long term difficulties with weaning and extubation : Repeated failure to wean a baby off IPPV may be due to any of the following factors:

1. **Persisting problems with secretions:** Leave a nasal ETT in situ for 3-5 days, + IMV combined with a vigorous programme of chest physiotherapy, endotracheal tube suction and antibiotic therapy if appropriate before trying again.

2. **Recurrent apnea once extubated:** The baby should be reintubated and given caffeine. Try again in 1 or 2 days. If apnea persists off IMV, this may be a sign of a small GMH-IVH, sepsis, or gastro-esophageal reflux. Image the baby's brain with ultrasound, and consider a pH study or treatment for reflux. Try CPAP but continue IMV if necessary.

3. **PDA and /or pulmonary edema:** Babies in this situation are particularly likely to deteriorate if their PCV is less than 40%. Reintubate, control fluids, give Lasix and indomethacin, and try again. Consider surgery if all else fails.

4. **Chronic lung disease:** If this is severe it may take several months to wean the baby off both IMV or CPAP. Treatment is with patience, minimal ventilator settings, steroids and diuretics.

5. **Laryngeal edema or subglottic stenosis:** In the short term these can usually be circumvented by good humidification and some nasal CPAP. Occasionally, dexamethasone 0.5-1.0 mg IM four times daily for 48 hours before extubation and then discontinued over a further 48 hours may help. If this fails, reinsert a nasal ETT (together with IMV) taking great care to immobilize it. Leave for 48-96 hours before reattempting extubation under dexamethasone cover. In some babies moderate degrees of subglottic stenosis can be controlled with long-term nasal CPAP, until the baby grows and the stenosis resolves. A cricoid split operation can be tried, but tracheostomy is a last resort in such babies, since if one is inserted it is very unlikely that decannulation will be possible in under 6 months.

6. **Very small babies:** (<1.0-1.20 kg). If after three attempts you have failed to extubate such a baby, restart IMV at 3-5 breaths/min plus 2-3 cm CPAP, and fatten the baby up by the enteral or intravenous nutrition. Ten days and 250g later, he will probably extubate easily.

7. **Underlying neurological problems:** GMH - IVH - considered above, but primary muscle disorders, e.g. Myotonic dystrophy may present this way.

EXTUBATION

Decide to extubate well in advance of the procedure. *Obtain a base line CXR* and repeat 2 and 24 hrs after extubation to evaluate atelectasis. *Omit the feeds* atleast 4hrs prior to the procedure. *Don't feed enterally* for 24 hrs after extubation. *Ensure* that the infant must be awake, alert and must have airway protective reflexes and he / she must be breathing effectively, without undue exertion. *Maintain* stable CVS, metabolic, nutritional and electrolyte balance and *reduce airway pressures to a minimum. Keep the baby (under the headbox)* in an FiO$_2$ 5% more than that being received while on ventilator. *Extubate VLBW infants to nasal CPAP* of 5-6 cms H$_2$O, which is maintained till the FiO$_2$ requirement is room air. *Maintain SaO$_2$*

Give a trial of DEXAMETHASONE 0.5 mg/kg/day in two divided doses beginning 48 hrs. before extubation, continuing 24 hrs. after extubation, to reduce ariway edema if the bronchoscopy is negative. Try THEOPHYLLINE / CAFFEINE CITRATE to decrease airway resistance and enhance respiratory drive (no controlled studies to support this).

Difficult weaning:

Commonly, more than one factor is responsible for weaning failure and these factors might be difficult to separate. In physiological terms, effective spontaneous breathing is dependent on a delicate balance between the loads imposed on the respiratory system and its capacity. The inability to tolerate extubation is the result of poor effort, increased load on the respiratory muscles, and decreased inspiratory drive. *Weaning attempts that are repeatedly unsuccessful usually indicate either incomplete resolution of the underlying illness or the development of new problems.* The management of such infants requires the identification and correction of all such factors that have the potential to impede tolerance of spontaneous breathing (Refer to Table given below). Factors increasing the infant's respiratory workload must be examined and optimised. Where available, monitoring of pulmonary function and mechanics might be used to gain some insight into the reasons for ventilator dependency in an individual baby. Careful adjustment of the ventilator triggering system to its maximal sensitivity, and appropriate setting of the ventilator inspiratory flow, might help in reducing the patient's work of breathing during mechanical ventilation. Patients with dynamic hyperinflation, either related to expiratory flow limitation such as in bronchopulmonary dysplasia (BPD) or because of insufficient expiratory time, require close attention. Excessive PEEP can also be counterproductive as a result of its adverse effect on pulmonary mechanics and its fatiguing effect on respiratory muscles, particularly in newborns, because of its unique style of attachment. Such patients might benefit from the use of pressure support ventilation because of its variable inspiratory flow. The maintenance of minute ventilation in a range sufficient to assure adequate removal of carbon dioxide is essential. For the healthy newborn, a tidal volume of 4–8 ml/kg and a respiratory rate of 40–60 bpm suggest that the minute ventilation should be approximately 240–360 ml/kg/min in infants with normal lungs. It may be inferred that alveolar hypoventilation will occur if either tidal volume or respiratory rate is too low. In addition, the nutritional aspect of weaning, particularly in extremely low birth weight babies, cannot be overlooked. Efforts to provide an adequate energy intake to prevent catabolism might help to prevent weaning failure. On the other hand, an excessive nonnitrogen energy intake will lead to increased carbon dioxide production and might further impede the weaning process.

Weaning from assisted ventilation: art or science?- Courtesy Sunil K Sinha, Steven M Donn—Conclusions

Weaning infants from mechanical ventilation involves as much "art" as "science", and should be planned according to clearly defined clinical and physiological goals. A method that rapidly and reliably assesses the infant's readiness for extubation would provide clinicians with a useful adjunct to their clinical decision making for withdrawal of ventilatory support. In this respect, any attempt to identify objective measures that could predict successful extubation, especially in preterm infants, deserves applause but so far no single parameter can discriminate between a high and a low risk of failure. Additional clinical investigations in this area are very much needed. Until then, predicting which infant will successfully tolerate extubation depends on physical diagnostic skills and experience. Given the availability of a variety of newer ventilatory modes that were not available previously, clinicians have a choice of weaning techniques, each of which might be useful in disease specific situations. Whatever technique one uses, it is helpful to begin with an organized plan, which should be adjusted as the infant's disease process and physiological status changes. As with many challenging medical problems, the best approach often requires innovation rooted in a firm grasp of the underlying physiology.

CAUSES OF WEANING AND EXTUBATION FAILURE

Increased respiratory load	*Decreased respiratory capacity*
Increased elastic load	*Decreased respiratory drive*
Unresolved lung disease	Sedation
Secondary pneumonia	CNS infection
Left to right shunt (PDA)	PVH/PVL
Abdominal distention	Hypocapnea/alkalosis
Hyperinflated lungs	
Increased resistive load	*Muscular dysfunction*
Thick/copious airway secretions	Muscular catabolism and weakness (malnutrition)
Narrow/occluded endotracheal tube	Severe electrolyte disturbances
Upper airway obstruction	Chronic pulmonary hyperinflation (BPD)
Increased minute ventilation	*Neuromuscular disorders*
Pain and irritability	Diaphragmatic dysfunction
Sepsis/hyperthermia	Prolonged neuromuscular blockage (in renal failure
Metabolic acidosis	concomitant use of aminoglycoside and phenobarbitone)
	Myotonic dystrophy
	Cervical spinal injury

BPD, bronchopulmonary dysplasia; CNS, central nervous system; PDA, patent ductus arteriosus; PVH, periventricular hemorrhage; PVL periventricular leukomalacia.

ESSENTIAL SUMMARY OF CONVENTIONAL MECHANICAL VENTILATION

1. pH and PCO_2 are closely related and are affected by *minute ventilation* (RR × TV_1)

2. PO_2 is governed by oxygen delivery (FiO_2) and ventilation and perfusion (V/Q) match. V/Q match is related to airway recruitment. Airway recruitment is indirectly reflected by Mean airway Pressure (MAP). Hence by increasing MAP, airway recruitment increases (although this is not a linear relationship).

3. Check the blood gases 20 minutes after initiating the ventilation and adjust settings to correct hypoxemia or severe hypoxemia, unless a reliable continuous $PaCO_2$ or tc PO_2 monitor / pulse oximeter indicates the desired effect has been achieved.

4. Don't become so obsessed with *"matching the ventilator settings to the blood gas results"* that you fail to recognize important clues about the baby's state given by *clinical examination and chest radiology.*

5. *'Goals' of assisted ventilation-*

   a) Ensure alveolar ventilation (i.e. eliminate CO_2 and maintain normal $PaCO_2$/Permissive Hypercapnea where appropriate).

   b) Ensure arterial oxygenation (i.e.,deliver O_2 and maintain normal PaO_2).

   c) Minimize risks of barotrauma and CVS compromise.

   d) Enhance infant's comfort.

   e) Provide muscle rest and reconditioning during recovery.

6. *Arterial blood gas analysis (ABG) remains the 'gold standard' for assessment of effective ventilation.*

7. Criteria for Reintubation: *NCPAP > 8 *$PaCO_2$>60-65 torr and pH < 7.25 *FiO_2 requirements rapidly increasing *Recurrent apnea/ bradycardia

Volume Targeted Ventilation (VTV) in Neonates: Essential Clinical Guidelines

Recent Cochrane Evidence based Review (Issue 11, 2010)states that Infants ventilated using VTV modes had reduced death and chronic lung disease compared with infants ventilated using PLV modes. Babies ventilated using volume targeted modes of ventilation were more likely to survive free of lung damage. They needed ventilator assistance for a shorter duration and were less likely to develop pneumothorax . They had more stable carbon dioxide levels in the blood, and had fewer brain ultrasound abnormalities. There was no evidence that volume targeted modes were more likely to harm the baby than traditional modes.Further studies are needed to identify whether VTV modes improve neurodevelopmental outcomes and to compare and refine VTV strategies. Recognition that volume, not pressure, is the key factor in ventilatorinduced lung injury and awareness of the association of hypocarbia and brain injury foster the desire to better control delivered tidal volume. Recently, microprocessor-based modifications of pressure-limited, timecycled ventilators were developed to combine advantages of pressure-limited ventilation with the ability to deliver a more consistent tidal volume.

Initiation of VTV

*Volume guarantee should be implemented as soon as possible after initiation of mechanical ventilation because this is the time when most rapid changes in lung compliance occur.

*Assist control or pressure support are preferred as the basic mode rather than synchronized intermittent ventilation.

*The usual starting target tidal volume is 4.5 mL/kg during the acute phase of respiratory distress syndrome in most infants. Babies whose birthweights are less than approximately 750 g require 5 to 6 mL/kg because the modest additional dead space of the flow sensor becomes proportionally more important in the smallest infants.

* Larger tidal volume is needed in older infants who have chronic lung disease because of increased anatomic dead space due to stretching of the trachea (acquired tracheomegaly) and increased physiologic dead space (wasted ventilation due to poor ventilation/perfusion matching).

*The peak inspiratory pressure (PIP) should be set initially at about 5 cm H_2O above that estimated to be sufficient to deliver a normal tidal volume. If the target tidal volume cannot be reached with this setting, increase the pressure limit until the desired tidal volume is generated. (Be sure the endotracheal tube is not in the mainstem bronchus or obstructed on the carina!)

* Once the working pressure stabilizes, set the pressure limit 15% to 20% above the working pressure displayed on the front panel to give the device adequate room to adjust PIP.

* It is important to chart not only the PIP limit, but also the working pressure, so the level of support the infant actually is receiving is clear.

Subsequent adjustments during VTV:
*Subsequent adjustment to target tidal volume may be needed, based on $PaCO_2$. (This is seldom necessary). The usual increment is 0.5 mL/kg. * The PIP limit needs to be adjusted occasionally (usual increment, 2 to 3 cm H_2O) to keep the PIP limit sufficiently close to the working pressure while avoiding frequent alarms.

* Note: If the flow sensor is temporarily removed (such as around the time of surfactant administration or delivery of nebulized medication), if its function is affected by reflux of secretions or surfactant, or if it malfunctions for any reason, the working pressure defaults to the PIP limit. Therefore, it is important to keep the PIP limit sufficiently close to the working pressure to avoid volutrauma. Ideally, when removing the flow sensor for significant periods, such as when nebulizing medications, the PIP should be adjusted to match the average or recent working pressures. * If tachypnea persists (respiratory rate, >80 breaths/min), consider increasing the tidal volume target, even if the $PaCO_2$ and pH are normal, because the tachypnea suggests that the infant's work of breathing is excessive. In this situation, the infant often generates a tidal volume greater than the set target. (However, if the $PaCO_2$ is low and the respiratory rate is high, sedation may be indicated).

*If the pressure limit must be increased substantially or repeatedly, verify that the tidal volume measurement is accurate (assess chest rise, obtain a blood gas measurement), and if true, seek the cause of the change in lung mechanics (examine the patient, obtain chest radiograph).

Alarms & Trouble shooting during VTV:

* The volume guarantee option may generate additional arms, which may prove annoying if excessive. Unnecessary alarms can be avoided by optimizing settings and alarm limits. The alarms are generated because the device, in volume guarantee mode, provides feedback as to whether the patient is receiving the desired level of ventilator support. Significant fall in lung compliance, decreased spontaneous respiratory effort, impending accidental extubation, and forced exhalation episodes all generate "low tidal volume" alarms. When used properly, such information should improve

care in the most vulnerable infants. It is important to evaluate the cause of the alarms and correct any correctable problems. A large leak results in underestimation of delivered tidal volume and triggers the low tidal volume alarm when the device is unable to reach the target tidal volume at the set PIP limit. When the leak exceeds about 40%, the volume guarantee mode no longer functions reliably due to inability to measure tidal volume accurately.

* Use of longer alarm delay settings, appropriate pressure limit settings, avoidance of large leak around endotracheal tubes, and adequate physical comfort measures or sedation minimize alarms.
* If the low tidal volume alarm sounds repeatedly in the absence of excessive leak, increase the pressure limit and investigate the cause of the change in lung mechanics (e.g. atelectasis, pneumothorax, pulmonary edema).

Weaning from VTV

* When the target tidal volume is set at the low end of the normal range (usually 4 mL/kg) and $PaCO_2$ is allowed to rise to the low to mid-40s, weaning occurs automatically ("self-weaning").
* For infants who have chronic lung disease, a higher tidal volume should be used even during weaning. Self-weaning occurs as long as the pH is low enough to give the infant respiratory drive.
* If the tidal volume is set too high or the $PaCO_2$ is too low, the baby will not have a respiratory drive and will not "selfwean." Instead, the baby will become dependent on the ventilator due to lack of respiratory muscle training.
* Avoid oversedation during the weaning phase.
* If an infant appears not to be weaning as expected, despite apparently improving lung disease, try lowering the tidal volume to 3.5 mL/kg, as long as blood gases are adequate and the work of breathing does not appear excessive.
* If significant oxygen requirement persists, positive end-expiratory pressure may need to be increased to maintain mean airway pressure as PIP is automatically lowered.
* Most infants can be extubated when they consistently maintain tidal volume at or above the target value with delivered PIP <10 to 12 cm H_2O (<12 to 15 cm H_2O in infants >1 kg), with FiO_2 <0.35 and good sustained respiratory effort.
* Observing the graphic display of the delivered PIP is helpful in assessing for periodic breathing (variable respiratory effort) that may require methylxanthine administration to facilitate extubation.Essentials of successful VG ventilation Make sure: ETT leak is <50%. The PIP limit (Pmax) is set well above the working PIP to allow fluctuations in PIP and to avoid frequent alarms. The inspiratory pressure reaches a plateau before expiration.

The set VT is high enough to support the infant's breathing effort. The Ti during PSV is not too short, that is, <0.20–0.25 s. The circuit gas flow and PEEP are adequate for the infant's condition.

Courtesy: 1. Martin Keszler, **NeoReviews** Vol.7 No.5 May 2006C
2. KlingenbergA practical guide to neonatal volume guarantee ventilation, Journal of Perinatology (2011) 31, 575–585

* Pulmonary mechanics testing reduces mortality or morbidity, it has in conjunction with clinical, radiological, and blood gas monitoring-changed Neonatal ventilation from "good judgment" to "informed judgment."

* It is not surprising that pulmonary mechanics testing is increasingly becoming an essential element in the assessment of patient status, therapeutic evaluation, and management guidance of infants with ventilator dependence.

* A working knowledge of pulmonary mechanics also improves understanding of pulmonary physiology and pathophysiology and their responses to mechanical ventilatory support.

* Specifically, clinicians are interested in the pressure necessary to cause a flow of gas to enter the airway and increase the volume of the lungs. From these variables, several other measures of pulmonary mechanics can also be derived, such as pulmonary compliance and resistance, and resistive work of breathing (energetics). Compliance is the term used to describe the relation between a change in volume and the pressure required to produce that change: C=ΔV/P. It gives information about the elasticity of the lungs. Resistance is a result of friction of gas flow against the air conducting system. It is roughly measured as the change in transpulmonary pressure divided by change in air flow, and is an indicator of airway function. The product of compliance and resistance determines the time constant, which is a measure of how quickly the lungs can inhale or exhale, or how long it takes for the alveoli and proximal airway pressure to equilibrate. From these mechanics, which can be displayed as numerical values or as graphic signals, useful information can be obtained and used for diagnosing specific lung pathology, evaluating disease progression, and determining therapeutic interventions.

* Most of the new ventilators either come with, or have an option for, a graphical display, and this has become an essential feature of the newer ventilators available for infant/paediatric use. These on-line systems obviate the need for interrupting ventilation. In addition, because of technological advantages, the sensors are very light in weight and add minimal dead space to the ventilatory circuit. This permits their application to even the smallest preterm infants.

* The rationale of pulmonary mechanics testing in ventilated infants is based on the assumption that early identification of pulmonary problems, either inherent or iatrogenic, and institution of appropriate therapeutic or ventilatory adjustments will improve the dysfunction and/or reduce the incidence of acute and : chronic lung injuries. Besides assessment of acute respiratory distress and evaluation of mechanical ventilation, potential benefits of on-line pulmonary graphics include assessment of suitability for weaning, monitoring of complex treatments such as extracorporeal membrane oxygen (ECMO) or nitric oxide, and follow up of chronic lung disease.

* Interaction between the ventilator and the infant largely depends on the mechanical properties of the respiratory system.

Pressure gradient

A pressure gradient between the airway opening and the alveoli must be present to drive the flow of gases during both inspiration and expiration. The necessary pressure gradient can be calculated from the following equation:

Pressure = Volume Compliance + Resistance × Flow

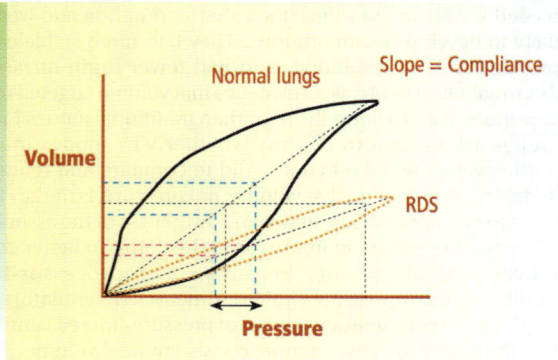

Pressure : Volume Loops

Compliance

Compliance describes the elasticity or distensibility of the respiratory structures (e.g. alveoli, chest wall, pulmonary parenchyma) and is calculated from the change in volume per unit change in pressure as follows:

Compliance = "Volume" /Pressure

Therefore, the higher the compliance, the larger the delivered volume per unit changes in pressure. Normally, the chest wall is compliant in newborns and does not impose a substantial elastic load compared to the lungs. The range of total respiratory system compliance (lungs + chest wall) in newborns with healthy lungs is 0.003–0.006 L/cm H_2O, whereas compliance in babies with RDS may be as low as 0.0005-0.001 L/cm H_2O.

Resistance

Resistance describes the inherent capacity of the air conducting system (e.g. airways, endotracheal tube [ETT]) and tissues to oppose airflow. It is expressed as the change in pressure per unit change in flow as follows:

Resistance = "Pressure"/Flow

Airway resistance depends on (1) radii of the airways (total cross-sectional area), (2) length of airways, (3) flow rate, and (4) density and viscosity of gas. Unless bronchospasm, mucosal edema, or interstitial edema decrease their lumina, distal airways normally contribute less than proximal airways to airway resistance because of their larger cross-sectional area. Small ETTs that may contribute significantly to airway resistance are also important, especially when high flow rates that may lead to turbulent flow are used. The range of values for total airway plus tissue respiratory resistance for healthy newborns is 20–40 cm $H_2O/L/s$; in intubated newborns this range is 50–150 cm $H_2O/L/s$.

Time constant: Compliance and resistance can be used to describe the time necessary for an instantaneous or step change in airway pressure to equilibrate throughout the lungs. The time constant of the respiratory system is a measure of the time necessary for the alveolar pressure to reach 63% of the change in airway pressure, which can be calculated as follows:

Time constant = Resistance × Compliance

Thus, the time constant of the respiratory system is proportional to the compliance and the resistance. For example, the lungs of a healthy newborn with a compliance of 0.004 L/cm H_2O and a resistance of 30 cm $H_2O/L/s$ have a time constant of 0.12 seconds. When a longer time is allowed for equilibration, a higher percentage of airway pressure equilibrates throughout the lungs. The longer the duration of the inspiratory (or expiratory) time allowed for equilibration, the higher the percentage of equilibration.

When a longer time is allowed for equilibration, a higher percentage of airway pressure equilibrates throughout the lungs. The longer the duration of the inspiratory (or expiratory) time allowed for equilibration, the higher the percentage of equilibration. For practical purposes, delivery of pressure and volume is complete (95–99%) after 3–5 time constants. The resulting time constant of 0.12 seconds indicates a need for an inspiratory or expiratory phase of 0.36-0.6 seconds. In contrast, lungs with decreased compliance (e.g. in RDS) have shorter time constants. Lungs with shorter time constants complete inflation and deflation faster than normal lungs. The clinical application of the concept of time constant is clear: Very short inspiratory times may lead to incomplete delivery of tidal volume, resulting in lower PIP and MAP and leading to hypercapnia and hypoxemia

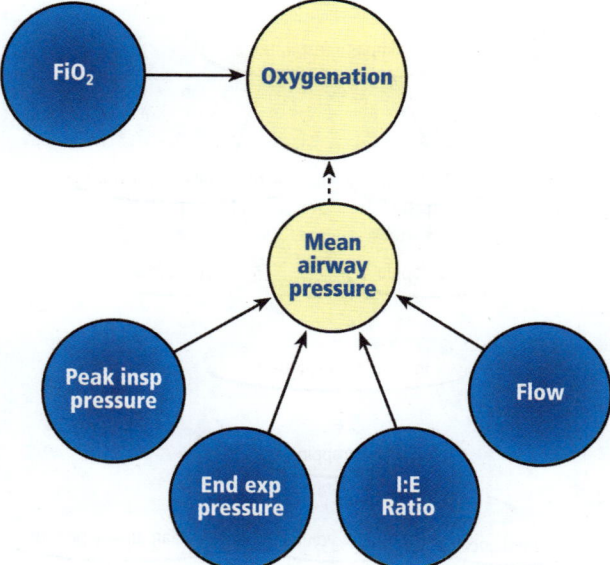

Determinants of oxygenation during pressure-limited time-cycled ventilation. Shaded circles represent ventilator-controlled variables. Solid lines represent the simple mathematical relationships that determine mean airway pressure and oxygenation, whereas dashed lines represent relationships that cannot be quantified in a simple mathematical way (From Carlo WA, Greenough A, Chatburn RL).

Time Constant

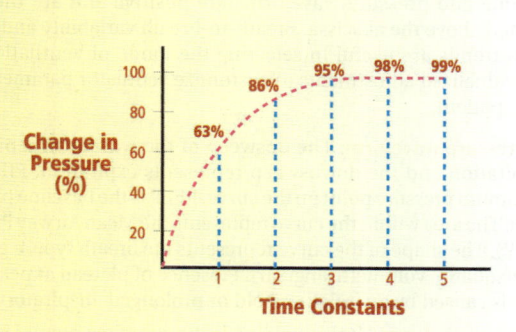

Pressure waveform Map...

To Increase Mean Airway Pressure...
1. Increase flow
2. Increase peak pressure
3. Lengthen inspiratory time
4. Increase PEEP
5. Increase Rate

During conventional ventilation, oxygenation is largely determined by the fraction of inspired oxygen (FiO_2) and the mean airway pressure (MAP) .

$$MAP = K (PIP - PEEP) \quad (T_I / T_I + T_E) + PEEP$$

This equation indicates that MAP increases with increasing PIP, PEEP, T_I to $T_I + T_E$ ratio, and flow (increases K by creating a more square waveform).The mechanism by which increases in MAP generally improve oxygenation appears to be the increased lung volume and improved V/Q matching. *5 Different Ways to increase MAP- 1) increase inspiratory flow rate, producing a square-wave inspiratory pattern; 2) increase PIP 3) reverse the inspiratory-expiratory (I/E) ratio or prolong the inspiratory time without changing the rate; 4) increase the PEEP 5) increase ventilatory rate by reducing expiratory time without changing the inspiratory time.*

Relationships among ventilator-controlled variables (shaded circles) and pulmonary mechanics (unshaded circles) that determine minute ventilation during pressure-limited time-cycled ventilation. The relationships between the circles joined by solid lines are described by simple mathematical equations. The dashed lines represent relationships that cannot be calculated precisely without considering other variable such as pulmonary mechanics. Thus, simple mathematical equations determine the time constant of the lungs, the pressure gradient, and the inspiratory time. In turn, these determine the delivered tidal volume, which, when multiplied by the respiratory frequency, provides the minute ventilation. Alveolar ventilation can be calculated from the product of tidal volume and frequency when dead space is subtracted from the former (Adapted from Chatburn RL, Lough MD).

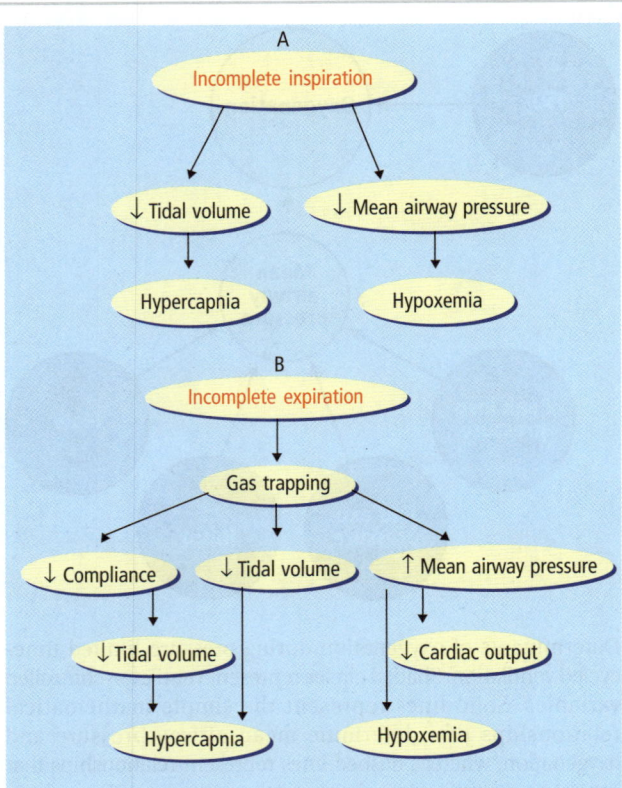

Effects of incomplete inspiration (A) or incomplete expiration (B) on gas exchange. An incomplete inspiration leads to decreases in tidal volume and mean airway pressure. Hypercapnia and hypoxemia may result. An incomplete expiration may lead to decreases in compliance and tidal volume and an increase in mean airway pressure. Hypercapnia with a decrease in PaO2 may result. However, gas trapping and its resulting increase in mean airway pressure may decrease venous return, decreasing cardiac output and impairing oxygen delivery (From Carlo WA, Greenough A, Chatburn RL).

Decreased Compliance...

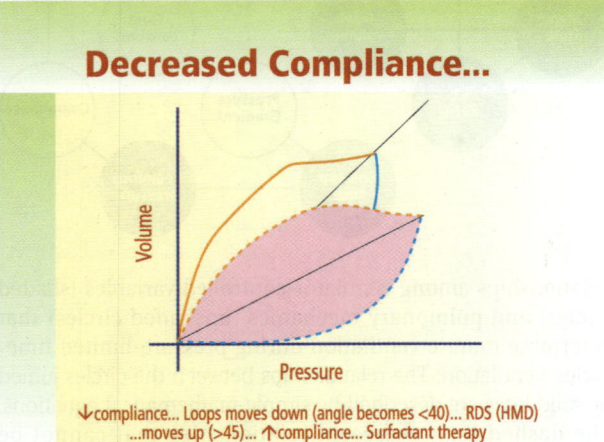

↓compliance... Loops moves down (angle becomes <40)... RDS (HMD)
...moves up (>45)... ↑compliance... Surfactant therapy

Compliance is the relationship between volume and pressure. On a Pressure-Volume loop, pressure is on the horizontal axis, volume is on the vertical axis. A flattened loop (shaded) indicates poor compliance - Surfactant deficient Hyaline Membrane Disease. A more upright loop indicates improved compliance, typically seen after Surfactant therapy.

Types of Waveforms...

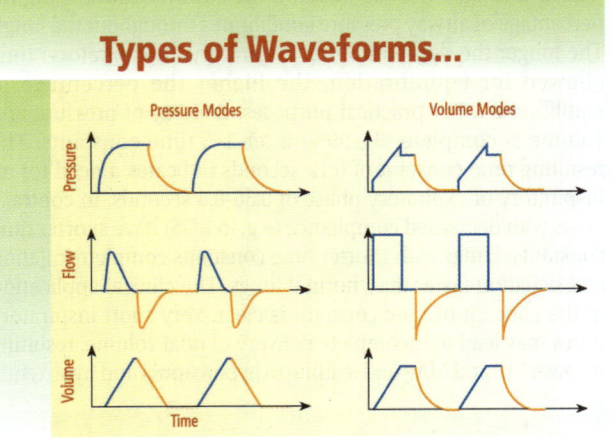

Graphic waveforms (Pressure, Flow, Volume versus Time): Unlike flow waveforms, both the inspiratory and expiratory phase of volume and pressure waveforms are positive and are therefore plotted above the abscissa. Breath-to-breath variability and longer term trends are useful in selecting the mode of ventilation and individualized adjustments to customize ventilator parameters for each patient.

A. Pressure waveform: The upsweep of the waveform represents inspiration and the downsweep represents expiration. PIP is the maximum pressure point on the curve. PEEP is the baseline pressure level. The area within the curve represents the Mean Airway Pressure (PaW). The shape of the curve represents the breath type, e.g., Pressure(square), Volume(triangular). Presence of plateau at peak pressure is caused by an inflation hold or prolonged inspiratory time.

B. Flow waveform: Horizontal line is the zero flow point. Upsweep of the flow waveform above the zero reference is inspiration flow, and downsweep is expiration flow. Greatest deflections above and below reference equal to peak inspiratory & expiratory flows respectively. Shape of the flow waveform is typically square or constant flow waveform seen in volume ventilation, or decelerating flow seen in pressure ventilation. Inspiratory time is measured from the initial flow delivery until expiratory flow begins. Termination sensitivity and flow cycling allow a mechanical breath to be triggered into expiration by a specific algorithm (usually 5–25% of peak flow). This permits complete synchronization. The duration and shape of expiratory flow waveforms depend both on the resistance and the compliance, but because of the small diameter endotracheal tubes used in neonates, resistance is a more important determinant for its configuration. The expiratory waveform can be used to observe changes in expiratory resistance and the presence of gas trapping. Expiratory time is the point where expiratory flow begins until the next inspiration begins. If expiratory flow has not reached zero before the next breath is delivered, gas trapping may occur. Gas trapping is more likely to occur in airways with increased resistance showing slow emptying time.

Flow Waveform...

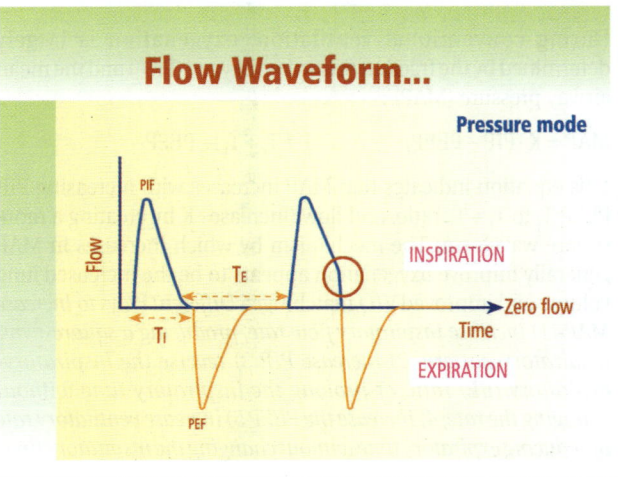

Expiratory flow pattern...E-time

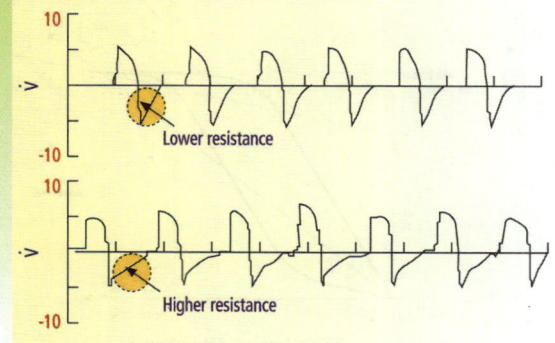

The shape of a specific flow waveform can help to identify airway and pulmonary abnormalities. In the lower example, higher airway resistance causes flow to return to baseline more slowly on expiration (in flattened slope) compared to the upper example, where resistance is lower.

Air Trapping...Auto PEEP

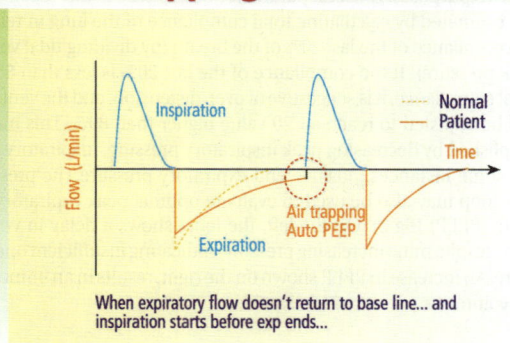

When expiratory flow doesn't return to base line... and inspiration starts before exp ends...

* Auto-PEEP = The averaged pressure by trapped gas in different lung units

* A dynamic entity may not present in all breath

* Short T_E - air entrapment

* T_E shorter than 3 expiratory time constant

* So it is a potential cause of hyperinflation

Volume waveform...

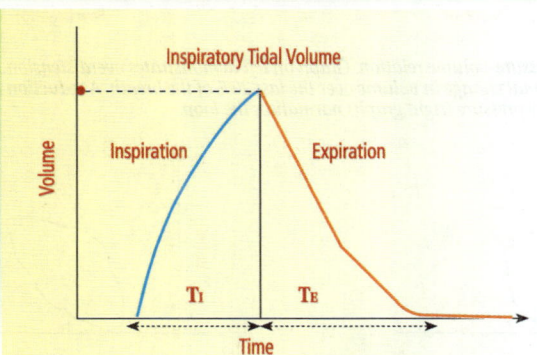

C) Volume Waveform- Inspiration is represented as the waveform sweeps upward and expiration as the waveform sweeps downward. The dashed line represents delivered inspiratory tidal volume. An Endotracheal Tube leak is observed when the expiratory portion of the volume waveform fails to return to the zero baseline.

Air Leak...

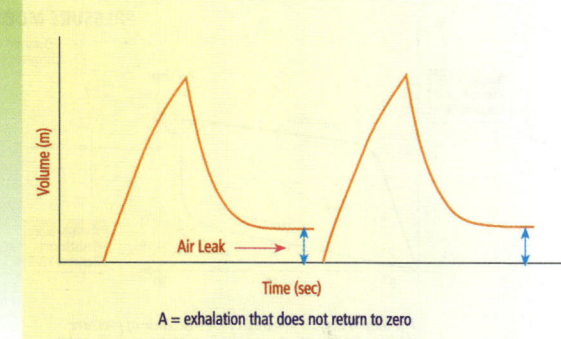

A = exhalation that does not return to zero

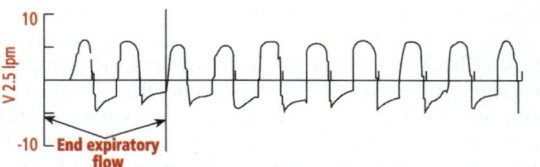

Fig. 1 : Flow waveform shows air trapping. Expiratory flow (below baseline) never reaches zero before next breath is initiated.

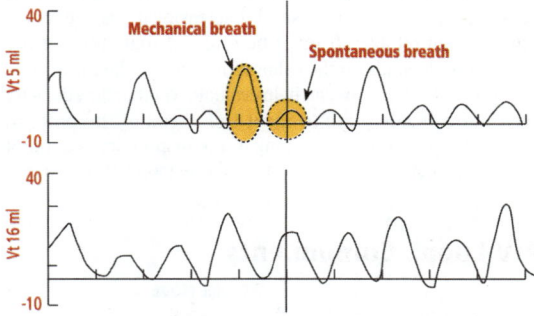

Fig. 2 : Volume waveform. Upper tracing shows ineffective spontaneous breath; lower tracing shows improved tidal volume delivery during spontaneous breathing.

Measurement of tidal volume is becoming increasingly important in ventilatory management. The desired inspiratory tidal volume for a ventilated breath ranges between 5.2–7.2 ml/kg while a tidal volume of 3.5–5 ml/kg for spontaneous breaths generally indicates suitability of the infant for weaning, provided this is matched by satisfactory arterial blood gases which remain the best index of ventilatory adequacy. Minute ventilation (tidal volume x respiratory rate) is also currently being evaluated as one of the predictor of weaning (250–400 ml/kg/minute), especially in small infants who have short inspiratory times and a higher respiratory frequency. If the expiratory time is too short, the expiratory flow fails to reach a zero flow state before the next breath starts, thus suggesting that gas trapping may be occurring. A similar appearance as shown in fig 1 can happen due to a large leak around the endotracheal tube, but this can be differentiated either by using the pressure-volume loops which fail to close, or by monitoring the difference between inspiratory and exhaled tidal volume. Figure 2 shows differences in tidal volume delivery between mechanical and spontaneous breaths during synchronized intermittent mandatory ventilation (SIMV). The top waveform indicates that spontaneous tidal volumes in between mechanically delivered breaths are ineffective. On the bottom graph, the infant has much higher spontaneous tidal volumes suggesting readiness to wean.

P-V Loop... Components

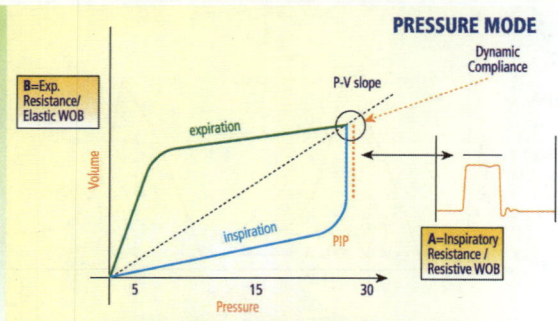

PRESSURE MODE

The loop is almost square in PC/PS because of pressure limiting (constant), during the inspiratory part of the loop.

Overdistension..

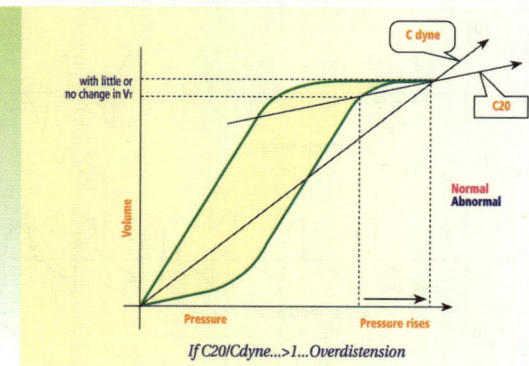

If C20/Cdyne...>1...Overdistension

Pressure-Volume Loop: Compares the relationship of pressure to volume (Compliance). Inspiration is represented by the upsweep from the baseline (PEEP) terminating at PIP and V_{TI}. Expiration is the downsweep from PIP & V_{TI} back to baseline. A line drawn from each endpoint represents compliance (V/P). A P-V loop that lies flat indicates poor compliance, and one that stands upright shows improved compliance. Compliance can be calculated as the change in volume divided by the change in pressure; in practice an estimate of compliance can be made by looking at the slope of the compliance line, which is normally 45° from the horizontal axis. If this slope is more towards the vertical axis, compliance is improving, and conversely is decreasing if this line moves nearer to the horizontal axis. It must be realized that slope of the compliance line also depends on the calibrations and can be misleading if not adjusted properly. P-V loops can help evaluate whether flow delivery from the ventilator is adequate to meet the needs of the patient. Inadequate flow is represented by cusping of the inspiratory portion of the curve. Endotracheal tube leak-Pressure volume loop fails to close.

Devices such as VIP Bird have an automatic scaling function which serves to reference the curve such that normal compliance line should be about 45°. Over-distension is implied when little or no change in volume occurs as increasing pressure is delivered. One way to recognize this is to look at the terminal (upper) portion of the 25 pressure-volume loop and see how much tidal volume is being delivered per unit of pressure change. This has been schematically demonstrated in fig 1 created from a test lung for instructive purposes. A useful parameter in this case is the "C20." This can be estimated by calculating total compliance of the lung in relation to the compliance of the last 20% of the breath (by dividing tidal volume by peak pressure). If the compliance of the last 20% is less than 80% of the total compliance, it is suggestive of over-distension, and the ventilator should be adjusted to reach a C20 value higher than 80%. This may be accomplished by decreasing peak inspiratory pressure, inspiratory time, and in some instances, positive end expiratory pressure. The pressure-volume loop may also be used to evaluate optimal peak expiratory end pressure (PEEP) (fig 2). On the left, the loop, shows a delay in volume delivery despite mine increasing pressure, indicating insufficient opening pressure. An increase in PEEP, shown on the right, results in an immediate rise in volume as pressure is delivered.

P-V Loop...Components

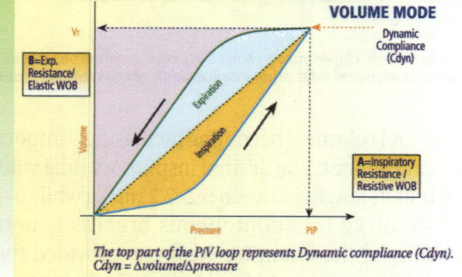

VOLUME MODE

The top part of the P/V loop represents Dynamic compliance (Cdyn). Cdyn = Δvolume/Δpressure

Insufficient flow...

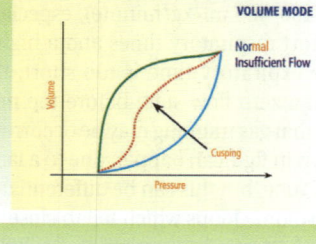

Air leak...

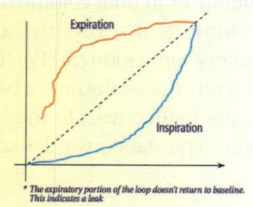

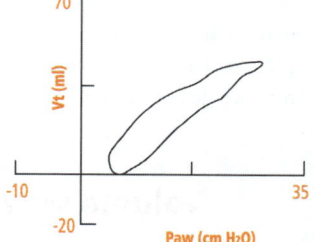

Over distension

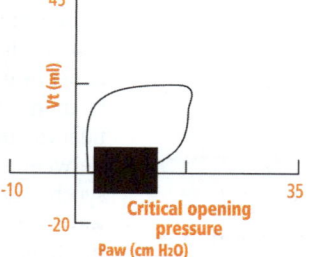

Critical opening pressure

Fig. 1 : Pressure-volume relation. Graph on left demonstrates overdistension. note minimal change in volume over the last 20% of the breath. A reduction in Ventilatory pressure (right graph) normalises the loop.

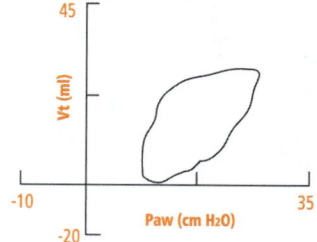

*Fig. 2 : Demonstration of effect of PEEP on pressure-volume relation. Left : inadequate PEEP results in poor volume delivery as pressure increases.
Right : higher PEEP results inappropriate volume delivery with increasing pressure.*

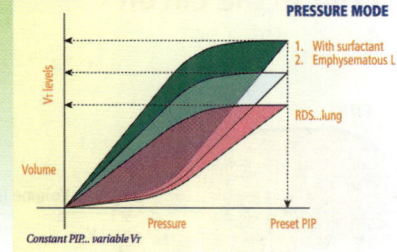

Lung Compliance Changing in P-V Loop

PRESSURE MODE

1. With surfactant
2. Emphysematous L

RDS...lung

Constant PIP... variable Vt

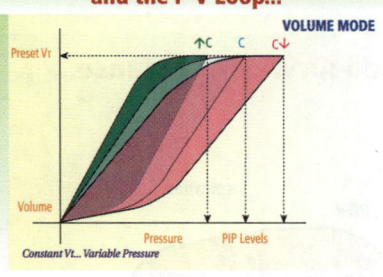

**Lung Compliance Changes
and the P-V Loop...**

VOLUME MODE

Constant Vt... Variable Pressure

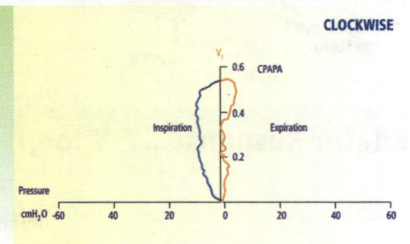

Spontaneous Breath...

CLOCKWISE

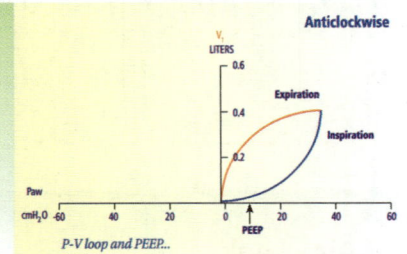

Controlled Breath...

Anticlockwise

P-V loop and PEEP...

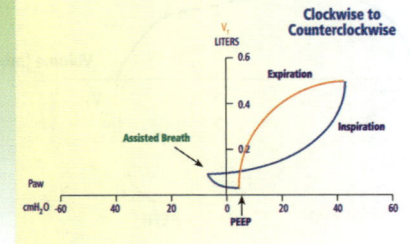

Assisted Breath...

Clockwise to
Counterclockwise

Dynamics measurements/calculations

A. Tidal volume is measured on inspiration and expiration. Normal delivered V_T is 4–8 mL/kg.

B. Minute ventilation (MV) is the product of V_T and respiratory rate. The normal range is 240–360 mL/kg/min.

C. Pressure may be measured as PIP or static pressure. Static pressure is obtained by doing an inspiratory hold maneuver, which measures pressure obtained by closing the exhalation valve and stopping flow delivery during a mechanical breath.

D. Compliance is the relationship between a change in volume and a change in pressure.

1. Dynamic compliance (C_D) is the measurement of compliance based on peak pressure.

$$C_D = \frac{V_{TI}}{PIP - PEEP}$$

2. Static compliance (C_{ST}) is the measurement based on static pressure.

$$C_{ST} = \frac{V_{TI}}{P_{ST} - PEEP}$$

3. C_{20}/C_D is the ratio of compliance of the last 20% to the entire curve. With overdistension this ratio will be <1.

E. Resistance is the relationship of pressure to flow. The pressure may be Dynamic or static, and flow measurements are taken from various measurements.

1. Peak flow is the maximum flow on either inspiration or expiration.

2. Average flow is based on multiple point linear regression.

3. Mid-volume flow is based on the flow measured at a point of mid-volume delivery.

4. $$R_{AW}\,(cmH_2O/L/sec) = \frac{PIP - PEEP}{Flow}$$

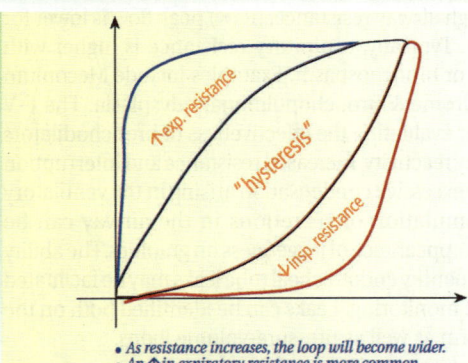

P-V Loops... in Airway Resistance

↑exp. resistance

"hysteresis"

↓insp. resistance

- As resistance increases, the loop will become wider.
- An ↑ in expiratory resistance is more common
- ↑inspiratory resistance...kinked ETT or patient biting.

Pulmonary compliance is a measurement of the distensibility of the lung and is in a sense an indicator of the function of the lung parenchyma. Disease processes that make the lung stiffer and thus decrease pulmonary compliance in Neonates include surfactant deficiency states, pneumonia, pulmonary edema, and pulmonary hypoplasia. Increased resistance, such as that seen in bronchopulmonary dysplasia, causes a "bowing" or hysteresis around the compliance line, and is an indirect measure of the work of breathing (by either the infant or the mechanical ventilator) to move j the lungs. This resistive work of breathing increases as pulmonary mechanics worsen, reflecting the increased amount of energy spent by the infant or the ventilator to breathe. It can be roughly estimated by the total area covered by the pressure-volume loop and the area adjacent to its deflation limb and the ordinate. There are, however, major problems in the interpretation of the resistive work of breathing on- in infants on ventilation, as altering the circuit flow alone can have considerable effects even in the absence of changes in lung mechanics.

Flow-Volume Loop...

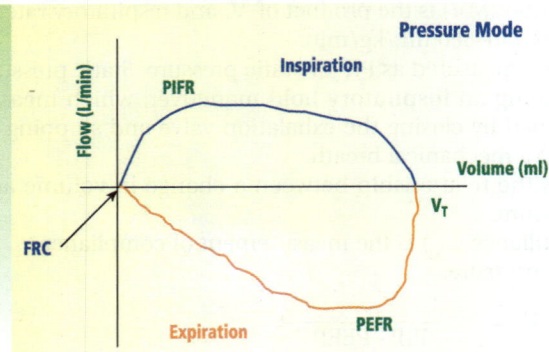

Flow-Volume loop (F-V): Displays the relationship between volume and flow. Volume is plotted on the horizontal axis & flow is plotted on the vertical axis. In this example of a F-V loop (may vary with monitor type; because there is no agreed convention on direction of inspiratory and expiratory limb among various manufacturers, it is important to become familiar with the direction of the flow-volume loop on individual machines.)the breath starts at the zero axis & moves upward and to the left on inspiration, terminating at the delivered inspiratory volume and downward, to the right, back to zero on expiration. The F-V loop is useful in evaluating airway dynamics. A flow-volume loop depicts changes in inspiratory and expiratory flow against volume changes, and is useful in detecting flow restriction from airway abnormalities. Under conditions of high airway resistance, flow is lower for a given volume. Flow will be lower on inspiration with high inspiratory resistance, or lower on expiration with high expiratory resistance. There is a fixed inspiratory and expiratory resistance associated with an endotracheal tube. During conditions of high airway resistance, (Raw) peak flow is lower for a given volume. Typically, expiratory resistance is higher with airway collapse or bronchospasm. Examples include Meconium Aspiration Syndrome & Bronchopulmonary dysplasia. The F-V loop is useful for evaluating the effectiveness of bronchodilators in treating airway reactivity. Increased resistance and interruption to gas flow from excessive condensation arising in the ventilatory circuit or accumulation of secretions in the airway can be identified by the appearance of jaggedness on graphics.The ability to identify and quantify endotracheal tube leaks may be facilitated through graphic monitoring. Leaks can be identified both on the volume wave form as well as pressure-volume loops.

Airway Secretions ... Water in the Circuit

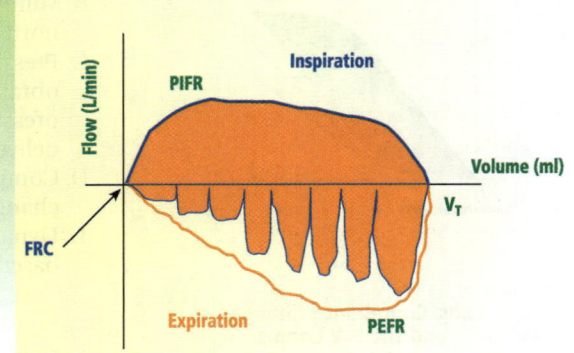

Increased Airway Resistance...

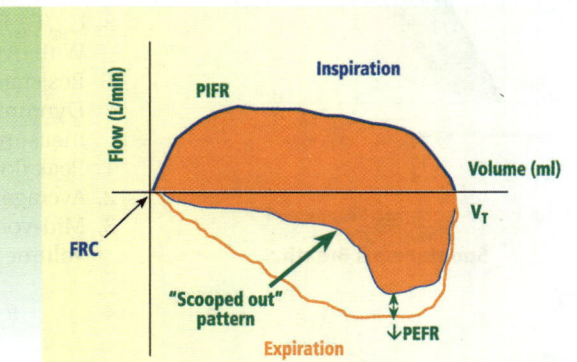

Bronchodilator Response... F-V loop

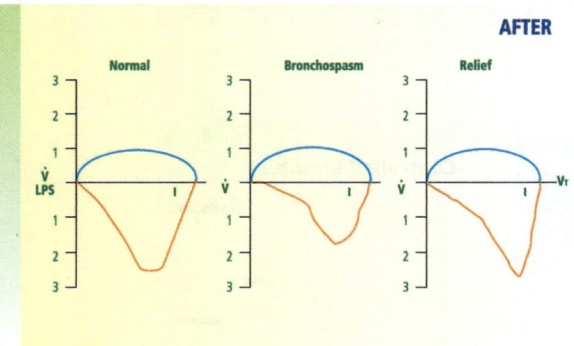

Air Trapping...

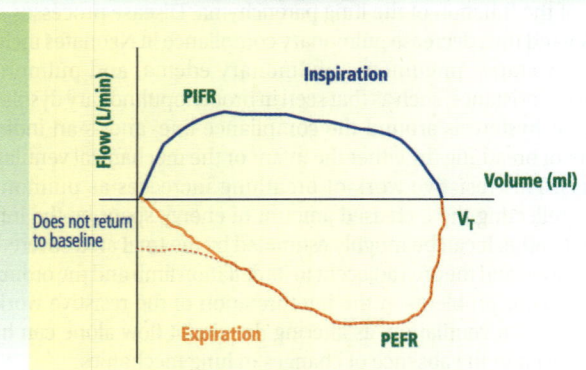

Air - Leak...

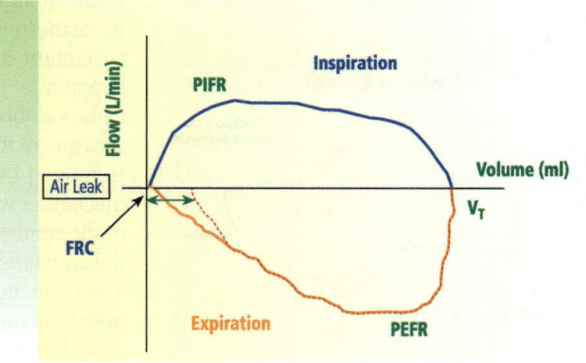

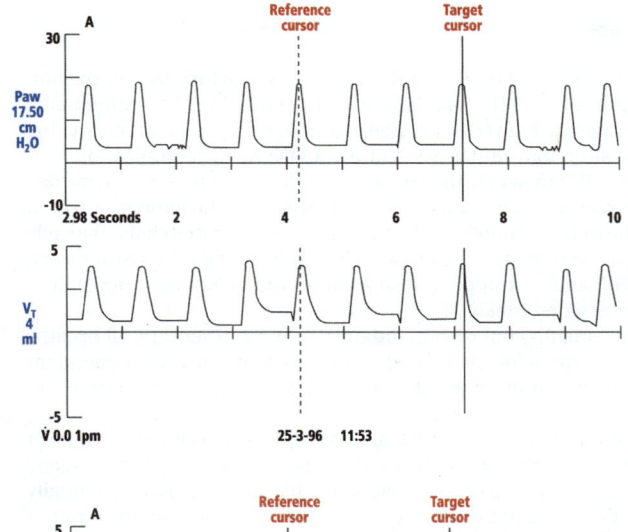

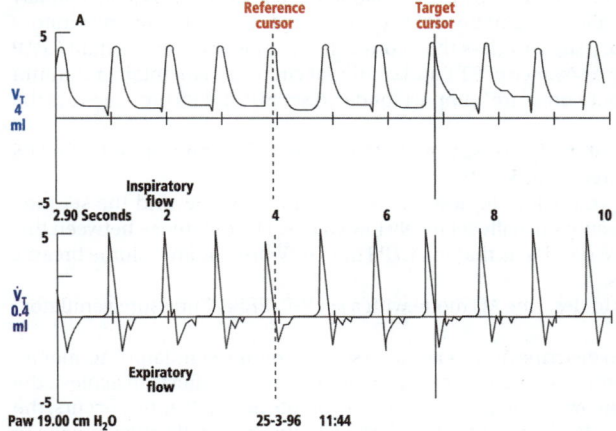

Scalar waveforms for airways pressure (PAW) and tidal volume (VT) (A), and tidal volume and airway flow (V) (B). Time intervals can be measured using a reference cursor (dotted line). A target cursor can be moved to any given point on a wave to obtain numerical values of pressure, volume, or flow at that point.

Figure on left shows a simultaneous representation of pressure and volume (A) and volume and flow (B) scalar waveforms during trigger ventilation in time cycled pressure limited mode. The magnitude of individual parameters and their time interval can be measured by use of the reference and target cursors.

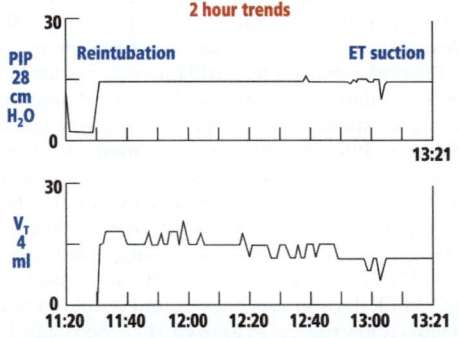

Trend data, pressure-targeted ventilation. Even though peak inspiratory pressure is held constant, tidal volume delivery is variable and decreasing.

There are a number of other useful clinical situations, including the assessment of different ventilatory modalities (such as pressure support ventilation) on pulmonary function and the assessment of patient-ventilator interaction (synchronous versus asynchronous). There is also an advantage in collecting and evaluating the trends of specific variables such as tidal volume, minute ventilation, and frequency for spontaneous and mechanical breaths as well as peak pressure, inspiratory time, and mean airway pressure. For example, the trend depicted in Figure 2 is consistent with an infant on pressure ventilation where despite peak inspiratory pressure (PIP) remaining constant, tidal volume has gradually decreased. This situation (as in secondary lung complications during respiratory distress syndrome) demands adjustment of ventilatory parameters by the operator. Conversely, tidal volume delivery may automatically increase after improvement in lung compliance despite PIP being the same (as after surfactant replacement), and cause iatrogenic complications if ventilatory adjustments are not made in time.

The major advantage of looking at flow waveforms is in assessing the amount of flow that occurs during the inspiratory phase to see if the set inspiratory time is inappropriately long. Figure on right shows a flow waveform with fixed inspiratory time. This may be needed to achieve a high mean airway pressure and better oxygenation during the acute stages of respiratory distress syndrome with stiff lungs and short time constants, but once the lungs become compliant and if baby is breathing at a fast rate especially while on patient trigger ventilation mode, fixed inspiratory time may prove to be inappropriately long. This is likely (mathematically) to result in insufficient expiratory time and contribute towards air trapping. In these situations, inspiratory flow can be limited by either shortening the inspiratory time or instituting a mode called "termination sensitivity" (in VIP Bird Ventilators), which limit the inspiratory flow to a preset value between 75–95% of peak inspiratory flow and then trigger the expiratory phase. This permits complete synchronization.

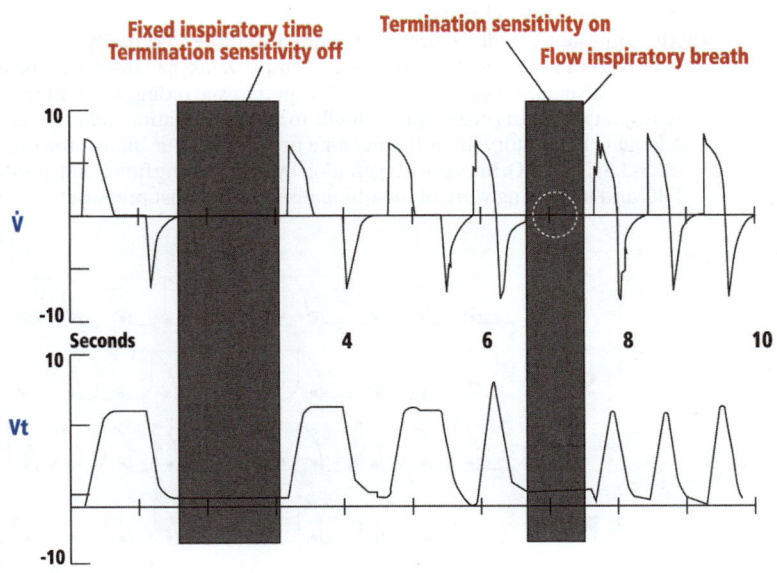

Flow and volume wave form showing an initial inspiratory time which is too long, but which is subsequently shortened by use of termination sensitivity mode.

Ventilator Modes (terms and types)

*IMV: Intermittent Mandatory Ventilation. Intermittent breaths (fixed PIP or V) at a fixed rate. **Not synchronized** to patient. Beyond the set rate, the infant is on his/her own. (See figure below-IMV) Standard on most ventilators, but infrequently used. Generally good for small premature infants but when rates are high (>60) or large infant "fighting" ventilator (exhaling during ventilator's inspiratory cycle), the lack of synchronization may impair ventilation. **CON:** No synchronization.

*SIMV: Synchronous Intermittent Mandatory Ventilation. Like IMV but **synchronized** (senses infant's spontaneous breaths). Beyond the set rate the infant is on his/her own (See figure below-SIMV). Since it is synchronized to the patient's effort, it is the preferable mode. It will function exactly like IMV if the infant is apneic or the trigger/synchronization fails. Typically used in infants who can reliably trigger demand valve and those fighting a preset rate. Usually lower rates/pressures since at higher spontaneous rates (>60) may get inadvertent PEEP and air trapping. Also good for older ventilator dependent patients. **PRO:** Synchronized to patient effort. **CON:** None, at worst is like IMV.

*AC: Assist/Control. **Synchronized** (senses infant's spontaneous breaths) but with **mandatory minimum set rate, all breaths** the infant takes are a **full assisted ventilator breaths** (See figure below-AC). Used in more active ventilator dependent infants not aggressively being weaned. **PRO:** Infant can increase minute ventilation easily on demand, based on need. **CON:** When weaning can't wean rate, only PIP or V.

*SIMV-PC with PS (Pressure Support): Term used on Servo 300 ventilators to describe an SIMV "pressure ventilator" with set PIP/PEEP. Beyond a set background ventilator rate, spontaneous breaths are augmented (supported) with pressure - usually relatively low values (+4 to +8 cmH O) (See figure below-PC/PS). Uses: 1) To provide mandatory backup breaths (conceptually large sighs to prevent gradual progressive atelectasis) while allowing amount of PS to be weaned slowly to "train" respiratory muscles 2) As a means of providing intermediate respiratory support (less than conventional modes but more than CPAP or extubation) 3) Pressure support just enough to overcome resistance of ETT and ventilator circuit and maintain minimum adequate spontaneous ventilation. Uses as above, but in "pure pressure" support mode. (If set PIP and PS pressures are the same then essentially you have pressure AC mode.)

> **NOTE ON WRITING PS: Pressure support is above PEEP.** At the University of Washington NICU, writing an order for "PS 5, PEEP of 4" yields inspiratory pressures for assisted breaths of 5+4=9.

*SIMV-VC with PS (Pressure Support): Term used on Servo ventilators to describe SIMV with set V. Beyond the set rate, spontaneous breaths are augmented (supported) with pressure - usually relatively low values. The difference between this mode of ventilation (VC/PS) and the mode described above (PC/PS) is that in VC/PS the SIMV breaths are volume breaths and in PC/PS mode the SIMV breaths are pressure breaths.

*PC: Pressure Control. Term used on Siemens Servo ventilator to describe AC mode with a set PIP/PEEP ("pressure ventilator" AC mode).

*VC: Volume Control. Term used on Siemens Servo ventilator to describe AC mode with a set V ("volume ventilator" AC mode).

*PRVC: Pressure regulated volume control. In this mode, a volume is set and the delivered pressure self adjusts to achieve the set volume. With the Servo 300, the pressure will stairstep up over 5 breaths until the set volume is met. If apnea occurs, the ventilator sounds an audible alarm and switches to the PC backup mode. The therapist must manually change back to PRVC mode.

*PSVG: Pressure support volume guarantee. This mode is available on the Drager Babylog 8000. This mode is pressure limited with a set tidal volume. The pressure will stairstep up to meet the set tidal volume. There are two sets of values: Set (ordered) and Measured (spontaneous). Set values include tidal volume (4-8 mL/kg), inspiratory time, inspiratory pressure limit (PIP), rate, and PEEP. The set values are utilized when the infant is apneic. Otherwise, the infant regulates their own PIP to meet the set tidal volume. As infant's compliance improves, the PIP needed to deliver set tidal volume decreases.
Pro: Adjusts for compliance automatically, compensates for ETT leaks, no need to correct for tubing volume
Con: Weaning mode only. If infant needs increasing support, switch to another mode on ventilator.

*SIMV + VG: With the Drager Babylog 8000, the addition of VG (volume guarantee) to SIMV allows one to control the inspiratory time. The PIP still adjusts to meet the set tidal volume, but the inspiratory time is set by the therapist.
Pro: More supportive and more control of ventilation than with PS + VG. **Con:** Less control over PIP, infant is still doing most of the work of breathing.

*CPAP: Continuous Positive Airway Pressure (like PEEP). Primarily used to maintain airway distending pressure; major effect is to help to maintain lung volume and improve oxygenation. Can be administered via ETT or nasal prongs. Uses: 1) To prevent alveolar collapse in mild HMD (perhaps avoiding intubation) 2) In mild chronic lung disease (perhaps avoiding reintubation) 3) In severe apneic spells to avoid intubation. Sometimes used in infants as prelude to extubation to ensure adequate respiratory drive. If done for a prolonged time, infants tire out breathing through the relatively high resistance of a 2.5-3.5 ETT. **PRO:** Improve oxygenation by maintaining functional residual capacity. **CON:** Impair ventilation by increasing FRC and increasing work of breathing (exhaling against pressure).

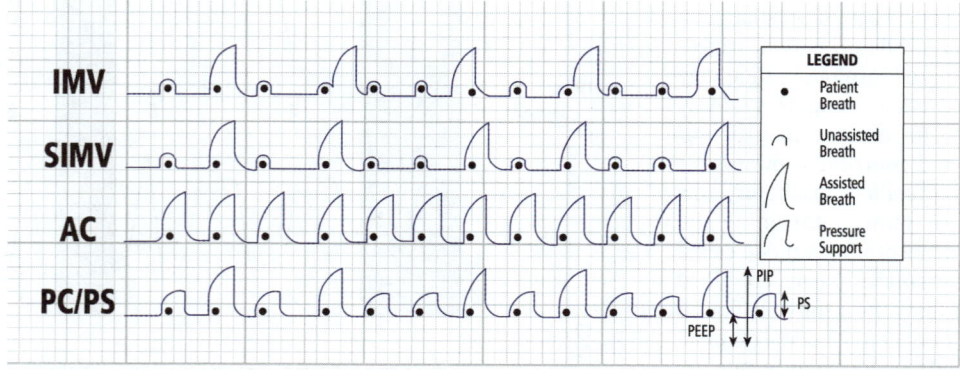

RESPIRATORY PATTERN UNDER DIFFERENT MODES

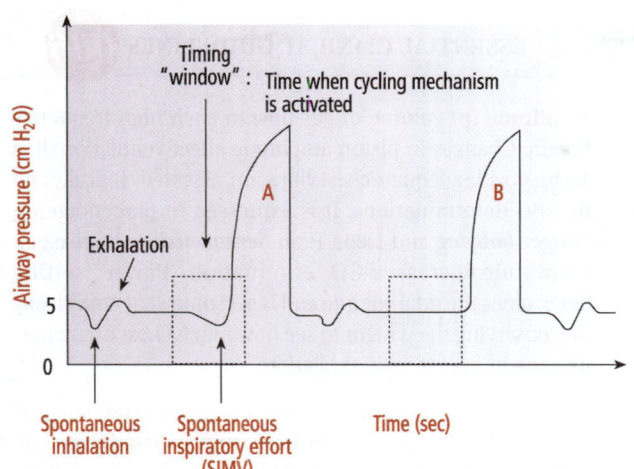

Synchronized Intermittent Mandatory Ventilation (SIMV): During SIMV, the ventilator allows the child to trigger a breath by spontaneously attempting to inspire. Ventilator frequency determines the total time allotted per breath, and some percentage of that time is the window allowed for the patient to initiate inspiration. At set intervals, the ventilator`s timing circuit becomes activated and a timing "window" appears (shaded area). **A)** If the patient initiates a breath in the timing "window", then the ventilator delivers a mandatory breath. **B)** If no spontaneous effort occurs, then the ventilator delivers a mandatory breath at a fixed time after the timing "window". SIMV may be either volume controlled or pressure controlled.

SIMV *versus* pressure support mode : SIMV does not allow for complete spontaneous ventilation. Patients trigger inspiration, but they cannot control when inspiration ends and the ventilator cycles to expiration. Patients cannot control the I time of the ventilator-assisted breaths, even though they can control the I time of the nonassisted breaths in between. The Pressure-Support mode allows for spontaneous breathing by patients. The ventilator assists every breath a child initiates by applying a predetermined amount of airway pressure above the set PEEP. A child can control the rate of breathing and the duration of inspiration, so the breathing pattern may truly be called spontaneous. Many ventilators allow both SIMV and Pressure Support. The pressure support breaths can occur whenever a child attempts to inspire, unless the patient is breathing within that window of time that results in an SIMV breath.

NEONATAL GRAPHIC MONITORING : INDICATIONS

A. Optimizing Mechanical ventilation parameters including:
   1. Peak inspiratory pressure (PIP)
   2. Positive end-expiratory pressure (PEEP)
   3. Inspiratory and expiratory tidal volume (V_{TI} or V_{TE})
   4. Inspiratory time (T_I)
   5. Expiratory time (T_E)
   6. Flow rate
   7. Synchronization
B. Evaluation of infant's spontaneous effort:
   1. Spontaneous V_T compared to mechanical V_T
   2. Minute ventilation (MV)
   3. Respiratory pattern
   4. Readiness to extubate
C. Therapeutic response to pharmacologic agents
   1. Surfactant delivery
   2. Bronchodilators
   3. Diuretics
   4. Steroids

D. Evaluation of respiratory waveforms, loops, and mechanics
   1. Waveforms
      a. Pressure
      b. Flow
      c. Volume
   2. Loops
      a. Pressure-volume loop
      b. Flow-volume loop
   3. Mechanics
      a. Dynamic compliance (C_D) or static compliance (C_{ST})
      b. Resistance (R_I, inspiratory; R_E, expiratory)
      c. Time constants
E. Disease evaluation
   1. Restrictive
   2. Obstructive
   3. Severity
   4. Recovery

CONCLUSION: Despite the major advantages of the current system providing pulmonary mechanics graphics, it should be realized that the information provided about the function of the lungs *only complements* (and does not substitute) information gained by other means of patient monitoring, including clinical signs and blood gas examination. Like radiographs, graphics should only be taken as suggestive of a condition rather than being definitive. Pulmonary graphic waveforms can be misshapen because of inherent inaccuracy of the measurement system (from calibration differences between inspiration and expiration), or from temporary artefacts arising from patient position or impedance to the gas flow by condensation in the ventilatory circuit. It is imperative to correct these **pitfalls** before accepting the findings of graphics as a guidance to change ventilatory settings or assess the patient's clinical condition. In this particular respect, the **"trends"** over a period of time seem to be of more value than individual breath analysis. Although there are few data showing a beneficial or more cost effective approach to neonatal ventilation by the continuous use of pulmonary mechanics monitoring, the development and implementation of this technology should make some studies feasible in the near future. On-line pulmonary graphic analysis represents another major advance in respiratory technology which promises to improve the safety and efficacy of neonatal mechanical ventilation. Clinicians are now afforded a breath-to-breath view of pulmonary mechanics and respiratory waveforms. This permits constant surveillance of conditions such as air trapping before they become clinically obvious, and the fine tuning of ventilator settings to customize management according to the problems and responses of the individual patient. Clinicians should avail themselves of this window of opportunity.

Courtesy : Sunil K Sinha, Joanne J Nicks, Steven M Donn, Archives of Disease in Childhood 1996;75:F213-F218
& Vishram Buche Director, NICU Central India's CHILD hospital and Research institute, NAGPUR, India

HIGH FREQUENCY OSCILLATORY VENTILATION

HFO ventilation is the delivery of small tidal volumes to the infant at fast frequencies. Both Inspiration and expiration are active, therefore reducing the likelihood of gas trapping. Proposed mechanisms that can enhance gas exchange during HFV (1) Direct ventilation of most proximal alveoli units by bulk convection (2) Pendalluft effect–asynchronous flow among alveoli due to asymmetries in airflow impedance. This causes gas to recirculate among lung units and improve gas exchange (3) Turbulence in the large airways causing enhanced gas mixing (4) Turbulent flow with lateral convective mixing (5) Taylor dispersion – laminar flow with lateral transport by diffusion (6) Collateral ventilation through non-airway connections between neighbouring alveoli (7) Asymmetric velocity profiles – convective gas transport is enhanced by asymmetry between inspiratory and expiratory velocity profiles that occur at branch points in the airways.

Examples of HFV in nature - Panting dogs - Humming birds - Patients with severe pulmonary emphysema - Mixing of pulmonary gases due to dynamics of cardiac contraction cycles.

HFOV employs either a piston or diaphragm to oscillate a bias flow of gas to generate both positive and negative pressure fluctuations termed as amplitude. There are not a lot of adjustable parameters in the machine. These include mean airway pressure (MAP), frequency and amplitude. Frequency is usually fixed for a particular patient group. The recommended range is 10–15 Hz for premature infants and 8-10 Hz for term infants

There are two strategies used in delivering oscillation.1. **High Volume** and **Low Oxygen** 2. **Low Volume** and **High Oxygen. High volume Strategy :** This is used where there is uniform lung disease e.g., Hyaline membrane disease. The alveoli need to be expanded, therefore the MAP is increased by 2–3cm H_2O above what is being achieved in CMV. **Low volume Strategy :** This is employed where there is non homogeneous lung disease i.e.. Meconium aspiration or even where there is no lung disease i.e.. PPHN. In these instances overdistention of the alveoli must be prevented.

HFOV SETTINGS

1. **MAP (Mean Airway Pressure)** Set the MAP 3–5 cm H_2O higher than the MAP being use on the conventional ventilator to enhance alveolar recruitment. MAP should be increased gradually by increments of 2cm H_2O to provide adequate lung expansion on chest x-ray (maintain lung volume so that the diaphragm rests at around T8/9 on plain frontal CXR. Care must be exercised to avoid lung hyperinflation, which might adversely affect oxygen delivery by reducing cardiac output.

2. **Frequency (f)** of the oscillating pressure wave is measured in units of Hertz (1Hz = 60 breaths/min). A drop in frequency increases oscillatory amplitude and hence tidal volume. Therefore paradoxically a drop in frequency increases CO_2 elimination. Set the frequency to 10 Hz usually. Consider high frequencies (15Hz) in tiny infants. Rate: Birth Wt1000gm-2000gm-15 Hz, >2000gm-10-15 Hz. Inspiratory to Expiratory Ratio: 1:2 (Inspiration is 33% of the cycle, Expiration is 66%)

3. **Amplitude (p)** volume of gas flow in each high frequency breath. Changes in piston amplitude affect ventilation. It is set to provide adequate chest vibration, assessed clinically and by ABG determinations. It is expressed in percentage on *Drager babylog* and Delta P on *Sensormedics.* Increase in amplitude increases CO_2 elimination. **"Power"** setting determines the tidal volume and is set somewhat empirically - by observing the patient to see how much chest excursion/ movement occurs with oscillation.

4. **FiO_2** Set the FiO_2 at one and reduce it as lung recruitment and improved ventilation/perfusion matching occur. In general, FiO_2 is weaned first, followed by MAP in decrements of 1-2cm, H_2O, every 4-8hrly, once the FiO_2 falls below 0.6. The gas flow rates of 8-15 L/min are usually adequate. The inspiratory time is set at 33%.

5. **HFOV tuning in relation to blood gas analysis -**

   1. **Inadequate oxygenation (low PaO_2)** - **a)** Increase the FiO_2 **b)** Increase the MAP if lung expansion is inadequate. Remember over-expanded lungs can also cause hypoxia. Check for other problems like ET tube patency and air leaks/ pneumothorax.

   2. **Inadequate ventilation (high $PaCO_2$)** - Check that the chest wobble is adequate and the ET tube is patent. **a)** Increase the amplitude to reduce PCO_2 **b)** Reduce the frequency to wash out PCO_2. By reducing the frequency the minute ventilation increases and thus helps in PCO_2 removal.

6. **Weaning protocol from HFOV** *1. Oxygenation:* Once oxygenation is adequate and the patient is ready to be weaned, follow these steps: **i)** Wean the FiO_2 first till it is less than 0.60. **ii)** Then slowly lower the MAP by 1-2 cm H_2O every 4–8 hrly.

   2. Ventilation- **a)** Reduce AMPLITUDE by 3–5 units whenever $PaCO_2$ decreases below threshold, until minimal amplitude (12-16) is reached. In PPHN the rate of drop of amplitude should be very slow. **b)** After a change in amplitude, always observe the chest wall to confirm that it is still vibrating. **c)** If PCO_2 is very low on minimal amplitude and baby is not ready for extubation, then consider increasing the frequency. The criteria for extubation are similar to those for conventional ventilation, i.e. $FiO_2 < 0.35$; MAP <6 to 8 cm H_2O and amplitude of 12–16 units. The baby may be extubated to headbox oxygen or to nasal CPAP. An alternative strategy is to switch the infant to conventional CMV or PTV during the weaning phase, usually when MAP <10 cm H_2O, and to reduce the ventilation accordingly as per conventional ventilation. This may be particularly advantageous when there are significant chest secretions and vigorous physiotherapy and ET tube suctioning are required.

7. **HFOV Complications:** The following have been reported as complications of HFOV:

   * Necrotizing tracheobronchitis;
   * Focal obstruction due to mucus impaction;
   * Hypotension due to obstructed venous return;
   * Intraventricular hemorrhage and PVL

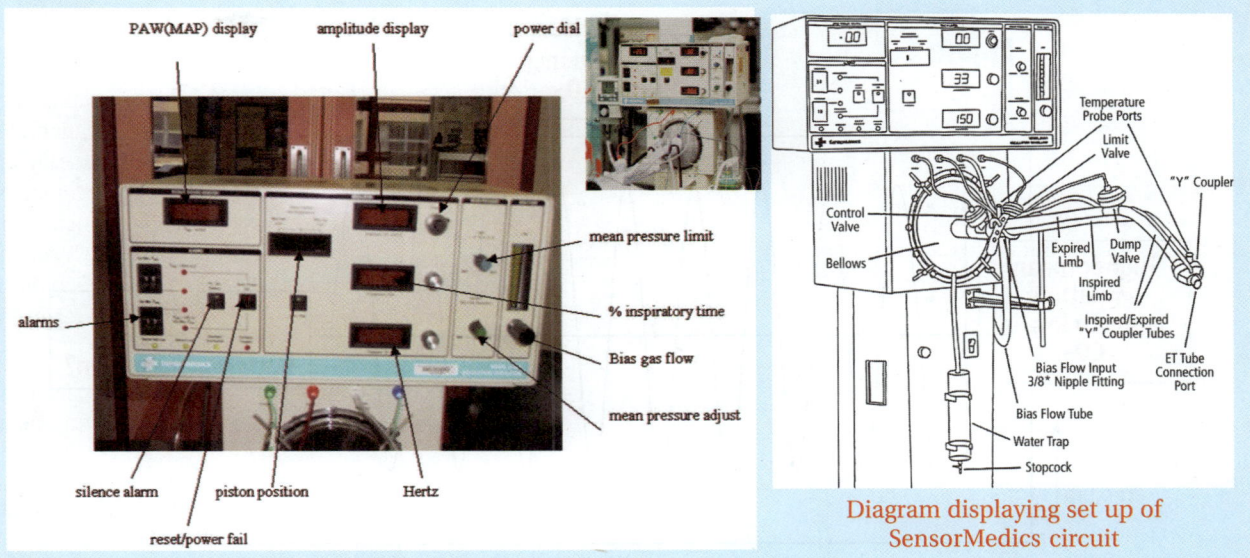

SensorMedics Front Panel

Diagram displaying set up of SensorMedics circuit

Clinical Strategy: Ventilation *Use 12-15 Hz for infants <1000 gm; 10 Hz for bigger babies *Start with Δ P = PIP on CMV *At initiation of Rx, adjust Δ P to produce perceptible chest wall motion and slight jiggle at the groin *Rule of thumb: Δ P should not exceed 3 × MAP *If max Δ P is insufficient, reduce frequency *For airleak or overinflation, reduce frequency.

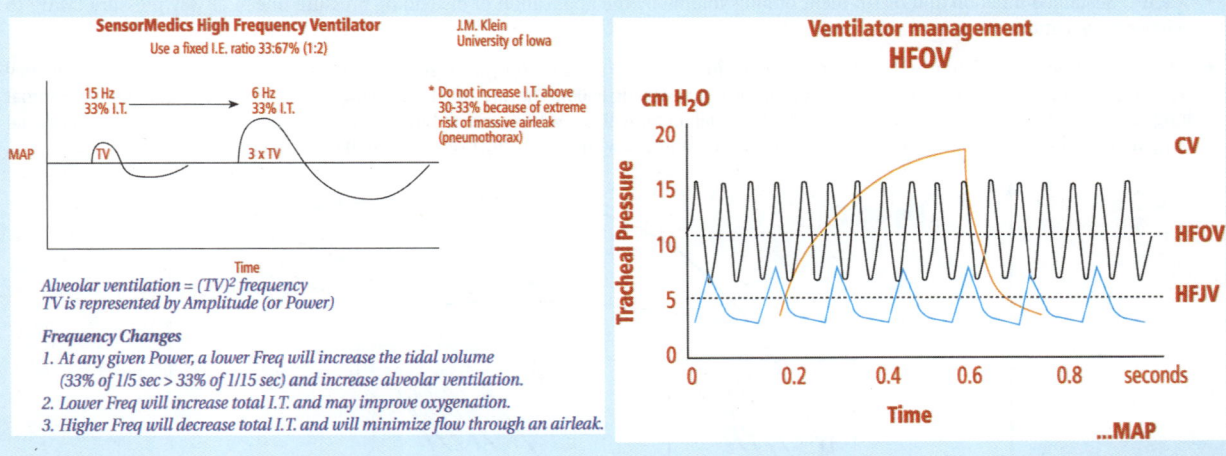

Clinical Strategy: Oxygenation (low lung volumes) *Begin with Paw 2-5 cm H_2O > Paw on CMV *Increase MAP by 1 cm H_2O until sats stable *Obtain CXR 30-60 min. later *Optimal inflation: 8-9 ribs on CXR *Wean MAP as compliance improves. **Clinical Strategy: Oxygenation (air leak)** *Begin with MAP = MAP on CMV *Use lower frequencies (10 Hz) *Obtain CXR 30-60 min. later *Adjust MAP for normal lung inflation in the "good lung" *Accept lower sats and higher pCO$_2$ *Wean MAP as CXR and pO$_2$ improves. Ventilation:: ΔP -- Amplitude *At a given MAP and frequency, CO$_2$ removal is achieved by HF TV createdby oscillatory pressure swings (''P) *As ΔP increases, TV and ventilation increase *CV: PaCO$_2$ TV x f *HFOV: PaCO$_2$ TV2 x f Respiratory System Impedance *The 3100 can generate Δ P as high as 90 cm H_2O at the proximal ET tube *Respiratory system impedance (primarily the ETT) attenuates the HF pressure waves » 3.5 mm ETT ~ 80% of proximal Δ P is lost » 2.5 mm ETT ~ 90% of proximal Δ P is lost *Use the largest possible ETT » avoids leaks » minimizes attenuation losses.

MAKING ADJUSTMENTS ONCE ESTABLISHED ON HFV

Poor oxygenation	Over oxygenation	Under ventilation	Over ventilation
Increase FiO$_2$	Decrease FiO$_2$	Increase Amplitude	Decrease Amplitude
Increase MAP	Decrease MAP	*Decrease* Frequency	*Increase* Frequency
(1–2 cmH$_2$O)	(1–2 cmH$_2$O)	(1–2 Hz)	(1–2 Hz)
		if Amplitude Maximal	if Amplitude Minimal

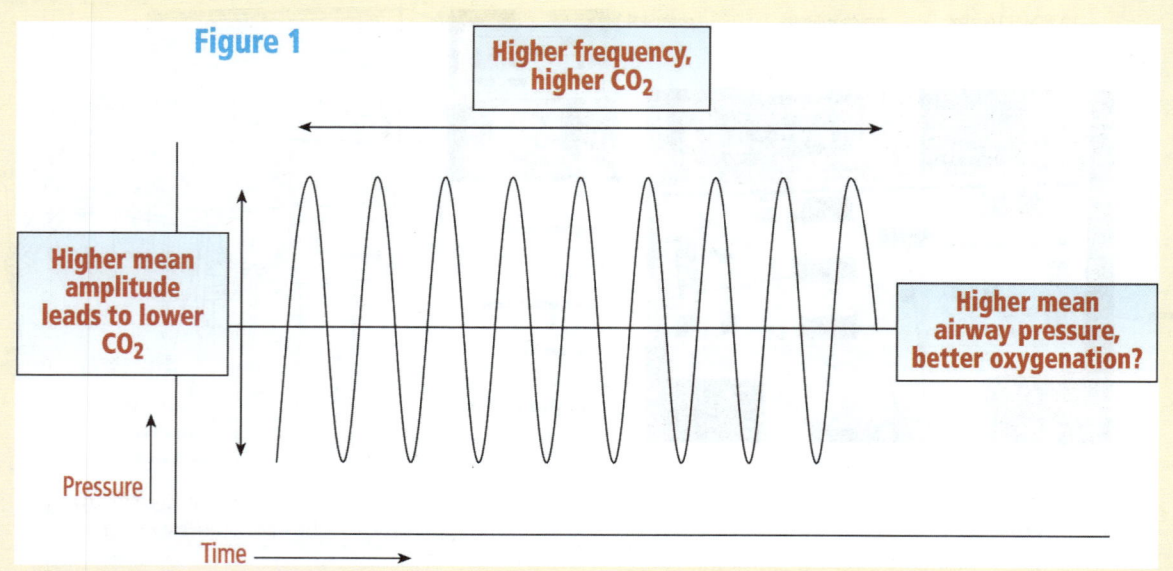

Figure 1

Higher frequency, higher CO_2

Higher mean amplitude leads to lower CO_2

Higher mean airway pressure, better oxygenation?

Pressure

Time

The use of high frequency ventilation at low tidal volume allows the primary goals of ventilation, oxygenation and CO2 removal, to be achieved without the costs of pressure-induced lung injury

HFOV has been described as "CPAP with wobbles". This reflects the two physical goals:

- "CPAP": Sustained inflation and recruitment of lung volume by the application of distending pressure (mean airway pressure (MAP) to achieve oxygenation

- "Wobbles": Alveolar ventilation and CO2 removal by the imposition of an oscillating pressure waveform on the MAP at an adjustable frequency (Hz) and an adjustable amplitude (dP or % on the Draegar Babylog 8000). The 'art' of HFOV relates to achieving and maintaining optimal lung inflation. Optimal oxygenation is achieved by gradual increments in MAP to recruit lung volume and monitoring the effects on arterial oxygenation. The aim is to achieve maximum alveolar recruitment without causing over-distension of the lungs.

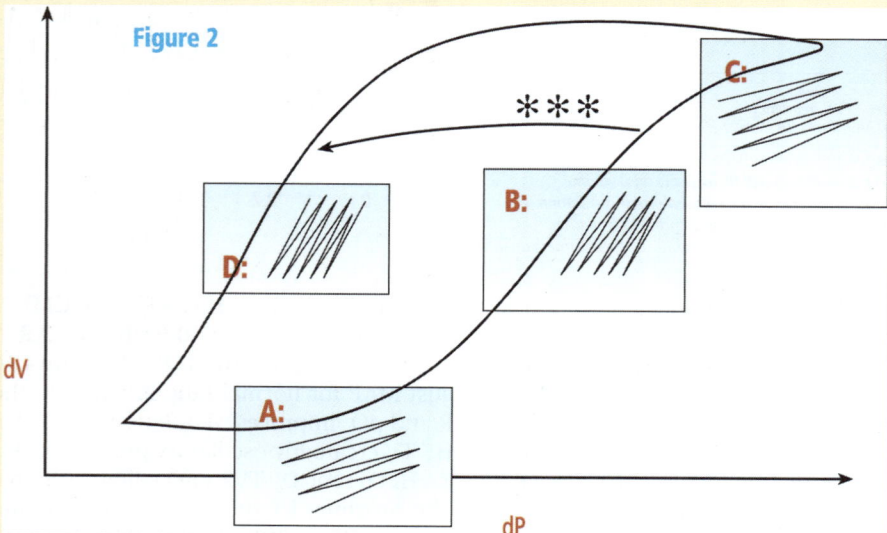

Figure 2

C:

***

B:

D:

dV

A:

dP

Optimizing lung inflation with MAP: It is useful to conceptualize HFOV as like taking the lung around one sustained pressure volume hysteresis loop, figure 2 **Point A in figure: Under-inflation:** At this point the lung is under-inflated, PVR will be high and relatively large amplitude will produce only small changes in volume. Clinically this manifests as a high oxygen requirement with limited chest vibration.

Point B in figure: Optimal recruitment inflation: Once the lung has opened up with higher MAP, the PVR will fall and a smaller amplitude will produce a larger change in volume. Clinically this manifests as falling oxygen requirements and good chest vibration.

Point C in figure: Over-inflation: Again more amplitude will be needed to produce volume changes and over inflated lung will compromise the systemic circulation. This is the most dangerous point in HFOV and is to be avoided at all costs. It is difficult to pick clinically because the oxygen requirement stays low, although they will eventually rise and the reduced chest vibration is easy to miss. Chest X-ray is currently the best diagnostic tool for this.

Point D in figure: Optimal inflation: The goal should be to move the babies lungs from point B to point D avoiding point C (as shown on the arrow marked *** in Figure 2). Having achieved optimal lung inflation by slowly reducing MAP it should be possible to maintain the same lung inflation and ventilation at a low MAP. If MAP is lowered too far oxygen requirements will start to rise.

Troubleshooting during HFOV

Low PaO$_2$: Consider

- ET tube patency
- Check for chest movement and breath sounds
- Check there is no water in the ETT/T-piece
- Air leak/pneumothorax
- Chest moving symmetrically?
- Transilluminate
- Urgent chest x-ray
- **Sub-optimal lung volume recruitment**
- Increment MAP
- Consider chest x-ray
- **Over-inflated lung**
- Check blood pressure
- Reduce MAP; does oxygenation improve?
- Consider chest X-ray

High PaCO$_2$: Consider

- ET tube patency and air leaks (as above)
- Insufficient alveolar ventilation
- Increase amplitude, does chest wall movement increase?
- Increased airway resistance (MAS, BPD) or non-homogenous lung disease: Is HFOV appropriate?
- Under-inflated lungs, amplitude being delivered on non compliant part of the pressure volume curve i.e. point A in figure 2
- Over-inflated lungs, amplitude being delivered on non compliant part of the pressure volume curve i.e. point C in figure 2
- If all the above seem OK try reducing oscillator frequency; lung impedance and airway resistance fall, leading to increased V$_T$.

Persisting acidosis/hypotension: Consider:

- Over-distension
- Reduce MAP; does oxygenation improve?
- Consider chest x-ray

HFOV adjustments : SUMMARY

Oxygenation and ventilation are best considered separately, however adjusting the ventilator for one parameter will also alter other settings and so after making a change always check the other settings.

Ventilation: Changes in paCO$_2$ may be effected by changing the amplitude of oscillation or occasionally the frequency. Ventilation may be increased by raising the amplitude of oscillation and vice versa.

- Start at an amplitude of 50% and then adjust the amplitude in increments of 10% until the chest wall is seen to "bounce" and a tidal volume of about 2 ml/kg is achieved. Be cautious as tidal volumes of more than 2 ml/kg are potentially harmful. Aim for a pCO$_2$ between 40 and 50 mmHg.

- The optimal frequency of oscillation may be different in different disease states. Small infants with RDS may be managed at 15 Hz, term infants are often best managed at 10 Hz, although with very non-compliant (stiff) lungs lower frequencies may be necessary.

- NOTE: If adjustment of frequency is needed, decreasing the frequency increases CO$_2$ removal (opposite to CMV). Always discuss this option with the consultant.

Oxygenation is controlled by adjusting the MAP and FiO$_2$. The goal is the high volume strategy. This allows the use of low FiO$_2$ levels (<35%) and the MAP should be adjusted to achieve this.

- For air leak: A low volume strategy may help. Reduce MAP 1–2 cm H$_2$O below MAP on CMV and tolerate a higher FiO$_2$.

- For rescue HFOV: Starting MAP should be 2 cm H$_2$O above that used on CMV.

- For prophylactic HFOV: Starting MAP will need to guided by an empirical assessment of lung disease severity derived during resuscitation. Generally start at 6–8 cm H2O. But use 10–12 cm H2O if the lungs seem unusually stiff.

- MAP should be increased in 1 cm H$_2$O increments every 5 minutes until the FiO$_2$ is less than 0.3. Generally it is unusual to need MAP >20 cm H$_2$O. (Moving from point A to point B in figure 2.)

- Overinflation (Point C) can be assessed clinically or by X–ray. Arrange for a chest X–ray when gases are stable to assess lung volume (see below) - usually after 1-2 hours.

- Normal inflation should allow the right hemi-diaphragm to be at the 8th or 9th rib. It may be necessary to perform Chest X-rays 6–12 hourly if difficulties are encountered,

- Over-inflation is occurring if: diaphragm is at 10+ ribs, intercostal bulging of lungs present or sub-cardiac air is visible as a crescent under the apex. Under-inflation is indicated by a high diaphragm. When managing RDS there will also be clearing of the lung fields as atelectasis resolves.

- Once the baby is stable in an FiO$_2$ <0.3, the MAP should be cautiously reduced in 1 cm H$_2$O as allowed by the oxygenation. (to get to point D) FiO$_2$ rising above 0.3 suggests you have dropped MAP too much.

8. HFOV precautions

* Continuous monitoring of oxygenation and frequent blood gas analysis are necessary during the establishment of HFOV

* Avoid lung over expansion by chest x-ray assessment of lung volumes

* Open the patient circuit as little as possible. e.g. for E.T tube suctioning, loss of pressure will result in alveolar volume loss and the need for volume recruitment by increasing MAP

* Monitor BP (which may fall as high intrathoracic pressure impedes venous return) and give 10ml/kg boluses (plasma or HAS 4.5%) and observe the responses of BP and heart rate.

9. HFOV indications

The principal applications of HFOV are where the risks of high-pressure conventional ventilation and lung injury are unacceptably high; All birth weights and gestational ages would be included (although since HMD would be the most common diagnosis, premature infants would be the most likely candidates for oscillation). Improves and maintains oxygenation *HFOV recruits alveoli and the number of open alveoli is in direct relationship to the mean airway pressure (MAP). Eliminates CO_2 retention *In conventional mechanical ventilation (CMV) the expiratory phase is passive whereas in HFV inspiration and expiration are active. Creates less lung injury *Uses small tidal volume ventilation which may reduce lung injury and prevent over inflation of more compliant lung units *Less likely to get air-trapping because inspiratory and expiratory phrases are active1) Barotrauma-pulmonary airleaks-a)Pneumothorax b)Pulmonary Interstitial Emphysema (PIE) bronchopleural fistulas and pneumo-pericardium 2) Respiratory failure unresponsive to conventional ventilation e.g RDS, Pneumonia, 3) Persistent pulmonary hypertension of the newborn (PPHN), MAS, Hypoplastic lungs, diaphragmatic hernia 4) Pulmonary hemorrhage.

10. HFOV principles

HFOV has been described as "CPAP with wobbles". This reflects the two physiological goals: **CPAP:** Sustained inflation and recruitment of lung volume by the application of distending MAP to achieve oxygenation. **Wobble:** Alveolar ventilation and CO_2 removal by the imposition of an oscillating pressure waveform on the MAP at an adjustable frequency (Hz) and an adjustable amplitude (Dp OR%). The gas exchange is mainly based on principle of bulk axial flow, interregional gas mixing ventilators with HFOV. *A) True high frequency oscillatory ventilators (HFOV)* » *SensorMedics 3100A; Hummingbird & Humming V; Stephan SHF 3000; Dufour OHF 1 AÛ™Ü B) Oscillator-like devices* » *Infant Star HFV (HFFI); SLE 2000 HFO; Dräger BabyLog 8000.*

Practical Concerns: *Uncut endotracheal tubes will be used to allow for the tube to extend 3-4cm past the lips, so that the patient does not spontaneously extubate. (Patients may need to be re-intubated if they have been intubated with a pre-cut tube) *Careful assessment must be made of all infants on oscillation and will require: *Continuous pulse-oximetry and, at least initially, frequent ABG's *TCM PCO2 will be used to rapidly determine effects of ventilator changes *A CXR within 30 minutes of changing to oscillation, again within 4 hours after the change and daily as long as the patient is on oscillation *If frequent changes have been made (especially in

MAP), a CXR should be obtained within 2 hours of the last change *There is no alarm that will tell you that the airway is obstructed, so clinical assessment of the patient (observation for good chest wall movement) is critical if there is an unexplained desaturation or other cardiovascular instability *Suctioning the airway should only be as necessary (if there is decreased chest wall movement, CXR suggests focal atelectasis, there are increased secretions, etc.) *Patients will not necessarily need to be paralyzed, since spontaneous respiratory effort will be a clinical indicator of adequacy of ventilation *Artificial surfactant will need to be manually administered while the patient is on HFOV. It should be given in two separate "doses" while the infant is manually ventilated using pressures to achieve good chest wall movement. *Monitoring of infant's heart rate may be problematic via ECG electrodes. Heart rate can be monitored as a 'pulse' through the UAC . Evaluation for heart murmurs may require a temporary pause in HFOV therapy. Visibly assess the chest vibration and note changes. Vibration mainly in the neck could indicate a dislodged ET tube and asymmetry vibration could indicate pneumothorax. *Frequent blood gas monitoring is required at first to assess effectiveness of HFOV. *Frequent CXR initially to assess the degree of lung distension, to ensure adequate alveolar expansion and to check that hyperinflation has not occurred. NOTE: X-rays may be performed through mattress. *Amplitude, Hz, FiO2 and MAP settings must be clearly documented by NS-ANP/Medical staff on the level 3 chart. *Monitoring of infant's heart rate may be problematic via ECG electrodes. Heart rate can be monitored as a 'pulse' through the UAC .

*The Nurse is aware of the possible adverse effects, anticipates and prevents problems, recognizes early signs of adverse effects and initiates intervention. *Hyperinflation may result and manifest by decreased cardiac output recognized by: tachycardia; decreased peripheral pulse; peripheral shutdown; decreased blood pressure and desaturation. *Pneumothorax signs may be gradual occurring over several hours. Indications are deterioration of blood gas and saturation levels and decreased vibrations on affective side. *Increased risk of dislodgment of ET tube due to the short rigid vibrating tubing. *The association between HFOV and IVH remains open. Studies report varying IVH rates of this multifactorial complication. *Airway damage In line suction is always to be used for infants on HFOV'.*

Cochrane Database of Systematic Reviews, **Issue 4, 2009:** Rescue high frequency oscillatory ventilation versus conventional ventilation for pulmonary dysfunction in preterm infants.

Insufficient evidence exists to support the use of high frequency oscillatory ventilation instead of conventional ventilation for preterm infants with severe lung disease who are given positive pressure ventilation. High frequency oscillatory ventilation (HFOV) is a newer way of providing artificial ventilation of the lungs. Theoretically, HFOV may produce less injury to the lungs, particularly when high pressures are used on conventional positive pressure ventilation. This review of the evidence from one randomized controlled trial suggests there might be less short-term lung injury from high frequency oscillatory ventilation. However, more babies in this group developed hemorrhage in and around the fluid spaces in the brain (cerebral ventricles) and this harm might outweigh any benefit. More information is needed to clarify the balance between benefits and harms of high frequency oscillatory ventilation instead of conventional positive pressure ventilation for preterm infants with severe lung disease.

HIGH -FREQUENCY OSCILLATORY VENTILATION VERSUS HIGH-FREQUENCY JET VENTILATION		
	High-frequency oscillatory ventilation	High-Frequency jet ventilation
Frequency	10-30 Hz	10-40 Hz
Total volume	Determined by oscillator	Increased by gas entrainment
I:E ratio	Constant	Variable
Expiratory phase	Active, less risk of gas trapping	Passive, more risk for gastrapping
Airway damage	Similar to IPPV	Necrotizing tracheobronchitis
May be used in combination with IPPV	Yes	Yes

I:E inspiratory to expiratory; IPPV intermittent positive-pressure ventilation.

REFERENCES: 1) Henderson-Smart, D. J., Bhuta, T., Cools, F., and Offringa, M. Elective high frequency oscillatory ventilation versus conventional ventilation for acute pulmonary dysfunction in preterm infants. Cochrane. Database. Syst. Rev. 2003;(4):CD000104. **2)** HFOV in Neonates, W *WONG*, TF *FOK*, PC *NG*, KL *CHEUNG, HK J Paediatr (new series)* 2003;8:113-120 **3)** Marlow N, Greenough A, Peacock JL, et al. Randomised trial of high frequency oscillatory ventilation or conventional ventilation in babies of gestational age 28 weeks or less: respiratory and neurological outcomes at 2 years. Arch Dis Child Fetal Neonatal Ed 2006;91:F320-6

The conventional ventilation plays a pivotal role in maintaining alveolar recruitment (i.e., avoiding derecruitment) by providing optimal PEEP to preserve alveolar stability and enhance alveolar interdependence. Using the Life Pulse, MAP can be lowered substantially by reducing the number of large tidal volume breaths delivered by the CV. Higher PEEPs may then be used without dramatically increasing MAP. Oximetry, Life Pulse servo pressure, and xrays will help you find optimal PEEP. But the most important variables when attempting to keep PEEP above the critical closing pressure, as always, are knowing your patient and knowing your ventilators. The Life Pulse delivers remarkably low tidal volumes (1-3 ml/kg). The threat of barotrauma can be decreased in babies with non-compliant lungs if alveolar stability is maintained with an optimal, usually higher PEEP. The CV breaths required to open the alveoli can be reduced during HFJV and optimal PEEP can support adequate oxygenation and alveolar stability while the Life Pulse maintains efficient ventilation. During HFJV, the number of CV breaths can be reduced to 0-5 bpm. FRC and PaO2 may improve gradually over time as long as alveolar recruitment is maintained with optimal PEEP. It is unnecessary to continue to expose the lungs to high-volume, high-pressure CV breaths once alveolar expansion has been achieved. The CV PIP may be lowered, or the CV rate may be reduced even further, reducing the risk of barotrauma. Jet ventilation should be considered when there is a need for high frequency ventilation and oscillation is contraindicated (as listed in the preceding section), such as in air leak or *asymmetric lung disease.* The Jet ventilator can also be used for alveolar "recruitment" by finding the "Optimal PEEP". *Frequency range 150-660 bpm (2.5-11 Hz) *Special ETT or ET adapter (Bunnell "LifePort") with **side ports** for gas injection and distal P monitoring , **main lumen** for exhalation, spontaneous breathing and IMV.

Bunnell Life Pulse: Advantages and Limitations *Used in tandem with CMV (IMV:0-5 bpm) *Can maintain oxygenation and ventilation over a wide range of patient sizes and CL *Works well in **non-homogeneous lung disease** *I-time and VT is held constant when rate is changed so PaCO2 rises and falls intuitively as rate is lowered and raised *Very effective when low Paw is required: air leak syndromes. 1. Two golden rules of mechanical ventilation or High-Frequency Jet Ventilator : *Know Thy Patient and Know Thy Ventilator .*

2. An important ventilator strategy is to find and use *optimal PEEP.* Optimal PEEP is the PEEP level that will provide the best blood gases with the least detrimental impact on cardio-pulmonary function. Too little PEEP may result in airway and alveolar collapse. Too much PEEP and MAP may cause alveolar overdistension and create numerous hemodynamic problems. 3. An xray can reveal much about PEEP levels. You may be able to determine inadequate PEEP by the appearance of atelectasis or poor expansion. Excessive PEEP can manifest its iatrogenic consequences as overdistension on xray or decreased cardiac output. Determining optimal PEEP is crucial and will change from patient to patient, from pathophysiology to patho-physiology, and depending upon the stage and severity of the disease. Know **your patient.** The PEEP and MAP should be higher if atelectasis is a primary concern and lower if air leaks or impaired hemodynamics 6 are primary concerns. Make logical decisions about a baby's appropriate PEEP levels. Be able to determine when the baby is getting too little or too much PEEP. 4. **Know your ventilators.** Understand that the PEEP displayed on the Life Pulse is measured distally, inside the trachea, while the PEEP displayed on the conventional ventilator is a proximal value. A discrepancy between the two displays may be your first alert that the baby's pathophysiology is changing. For example, as lung compliance improves, the Life Pulse delivers larger tidal volumes to meet the set PIP. The greater the volume of gas going *into* the lungs, the longer it takes to get the gas *out of* the lungs. The displayed PEEP on the Life Pulse may begin to rise while the displayed CV PEEP remains unchanged. This discrepancy

allows you to detect inadvertent PEEP and may be an early indication that the Life Pulse rate needs to be lowered to allow more expiratory time.
5. As with PEEP, the optimal rate of HFJV is important. Too low a rate may result in elevated PaCO2. An excessive rate might cause gas trapping. The Life Pulse should operate near the lungs' *natural* or *resonant frequency,* where minimum energy is required to affect gas movement into and out of the lungs. Know that resonant frequency is higher for smaller patients than it is for larger patients. Know that the Life Pulse is effective over its entire range of 240 to 660 bpm and most infants are well ventilated at an HFJV rate of 420 bpm. Know that small changes in the rate may have little impact on PaCO2 due to the broad range of resonant frequency. And know that larger patients and patients prone to gas trapping may benefit from lower HFJV rates (240-360 bpm).
6. If the PEEP is too low, or is reduced after lung volume has been recruited (e.g., by turning down PEEP, disconnecting the CV circuit, suctioning the patient, etc.), lung volume will be lost and the recruitment process must begin again from scratch. Getting atelectatic alveoli open and keeping them open are two crucial requirements for effective patient management. And, by knowing your patient and knowing your ventilators, CV and HFJV may be used in tandem to recruit and maintain lung volume using the lowest possible pressures and tidal volumes. Lower CV rates are indicated when barotrauma is a primary concern. Higher CV rates are indicated when atelectasis and poor compliance are primary concerns. CV rates greater than 10 bpm are typically used for short time periods of an hour or less. **Key Summary:** 1) Know thy patient; 2) Know thy ventilator; 3) Appreciate optimal PEEP, and; 4) All things in moderation.

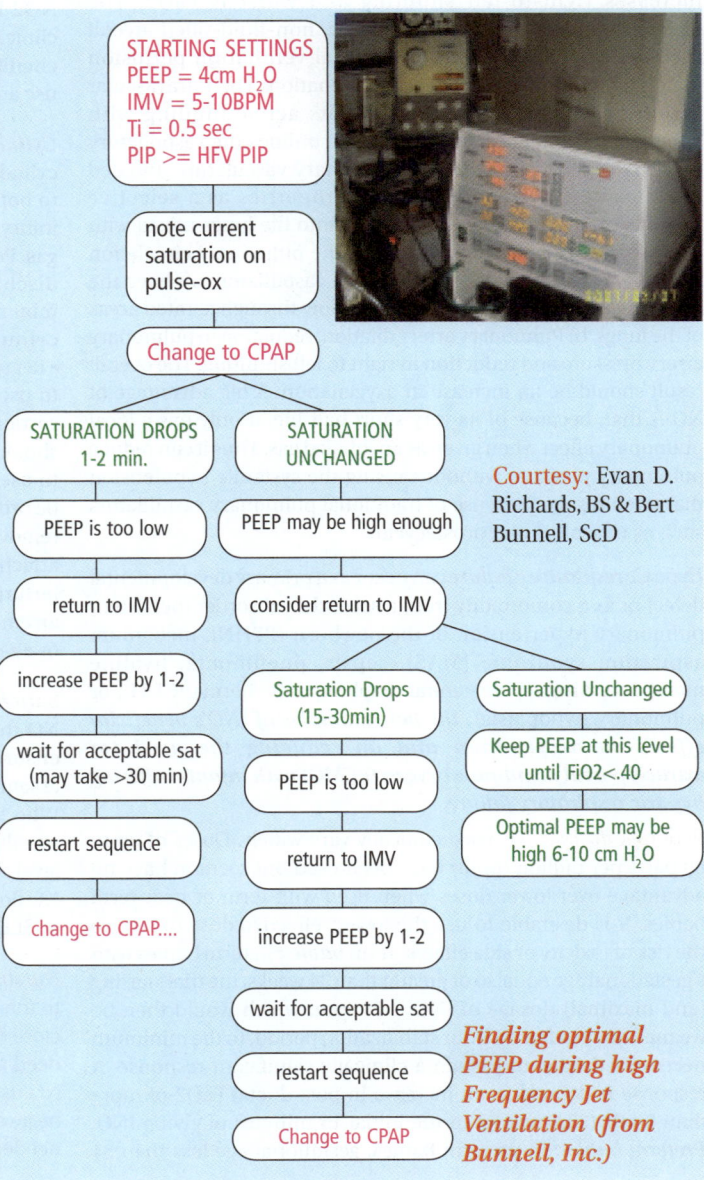

STARTING SETTINGS
PEEP = 4cm H₂O
IMV = 5-10BPM
Ti = 0.5 sec
PIP >= HFV PIP

note current saturation on pulse-ox

Change to CPAP

SATURATION DROPS 1-2 min. → PEEP is too low → return to IMV → increase PEEP by 1-2 → wait for acceptable sat (may take >30 min) → restart sequence → change to CPAP....

SATURATION UNCHANGED → PEEP may be high enough → consider return to IMV

Saturation Drops (15-30min) → PEEP is too low → return to IMV → increase PEEP by 1-2 → wait for acceptable sat → restart sequence → Change to CPAP

Saturation Unchanged → Keep PEEP at this level until FiO2<.40 → Optimal PEEP may be high 6-10 cm H₂O

Courtesy: Evan D. Richards, BS & Bert Bunnell, ScD

Finding optimal PEEP during high Frequency Jet Ventilation (from Bunnell, Inc.)

INHALED NITRIC OXIDE THERAPY

Nitric oxide (NO) is a lipophilic, endogenous, free radical compound that is naturally produced by most cells in the human body. In 1987 NO was identified as a potent vasodilator (via vascular smooth muscle relaxation) that could explain the mechanism of action of endothelium derived relaxing factor. Because of rapid oxidation of nitrates and nitrites, NO's biological half-life in human tissues is a matter of seconds. Nitric oxide's primary mechanism of action is facilitated by binding to the heme moiety to cytosolic guanylate cyclase, causing an upsurge in the production of intracellular cyclic guanosine 3,5-monophosphate. Nitric oxide's ability to relax vascular smooth muscle (and thus cause vasodilation), coupled with its short biological half-life, make it an ideal transcellular messenger. INO diffuses through the alveoli into the adjacent vascular smooth muscle, causing relaxation and vasodilation. Vascular smooth muscle relaxation and decreased pulmonary hypertension are possible with intravenous vasodilators (nitroglycerin, nitroprusside, or prostacyclin), but those agents frequently cause overall systemic vasodilation and enhance blood flow distribution to perfused but nonventilated lung regions. This redistributed blood flow from nonselective pulmonary vasodilation to nonventilated lung areas increases right-to-left shunting and worsens PaO2. The distribution of INO to nonatelectatic, non-fluid-filled alveoli theoretically should result in optimal ventilation perfusion matching and improved arterial oxygenation. The intravascular action of INO is limited because its active binding with hemoglobin rapidly deactivates it and confines the vasodilatory capacity of INO largely to the pulmonary vasculature. Inhaled nitric oxide (INO) is used for its properties as a selective vasodilator. It is administered directly into the lungs mixed with ventilator gases and is absorbed into the pulmonary circulation through aerated alveoli. Its action as a vasodilator can have the following effects: - a) Increased blood flow through aerated areas of the lungs. b) Pulmonary artery dilation, reduction in pulmonary artery pressure and reduction in right to left shunting. The overall result should be an increase in oxygenation. A big advantage of NO is that, because of its very short half-life, it only has a local pulmonary effect when given as an inhaled gas. Thus it can reduce pulmonary pressure without causing the systemic hypotension that often results from use of traditional pulmonary vasodilators such as tolazoline and prostacyclin.

Hypoxic respiratory failure can occur as a primary developmental defect or as a comorbidity from a secondary disorder (persistent pulmonary hypertension of the newborn [PPHN], meconium aspiration syndrome [MAS], sepsis, pneumonia, hyaline membrane disease, congenital diaphragmatic hernia [CDH], or pulmonary hypoplasia); *the best examples of INO's beneficial effects on oxygenation and on reducing the need for extracorporeal membrane oxygen (ECMO) with infants suffering hypoxic respiratory failure.*

Reported doses of NO used clinically vary widely. Doses of up to 80 parts per million (ppm) have been used but seem to have no advantage over lower doses when used with term or near term babies. It is desirable to use the lowest effective dose to reduce the risk of toxicity or side effects. Term *babies:* In term babies with a gestational age equal to or greater than 34 weeks, the trial starting (and maximal) dosage of INO is 20ppm, which would then be weaned down, after a 1 hour stabilization period, to the minimum necessary dosage to sustain a clinically significant response. A response is defined as an increase in post ductal PaO2 of more than 3 kPa (22.5mmHg) in the initial 15 minutes of giving INO. *Preterm babies:* In preterm babies, gestational age less than 34

weeks, a dose response study is being undertaken to determine the most effective dose. The study will include doses from 5 to 40 ppm. Doses above 40ppm will not be used. Rebound pulmonary hypertension is a possible problem when reducing or stopping NO even if starting it did not achieve a positive response. For this reason weaning must be done slowly and an increase in FIO$_2$ can help reduce problems when the NO is turned off.

Side effects and toxicity: **Though INO has a clinically important therapeutic role as a specialty gas, it can have toxic effects.** ***Raised methemoglobin levels** NO binds readily to, and is inactivated by haemoglobin forming methemoglobin. High levels of methemoglobin can cause a reduction in oxygen carrying capacity, but in practice this potential problem rarely occurs with the doses of NO that are used clinically. ***Bleeding** NO affects platelet formation and bleeding time, potentially increasing the risk of intraventricular hemorrhage (IVH) and other bleeding disorders. This is a more serious risk with preterm babies who are more prone to IVH.***Nitrogen dioxide (NO$_2$)** NO mixed with oxygen forms NO2. If high levels of NO2 are administered there is a risk of pulmonary edema or changes in lung tissue. NO2 and water can combine to form nitric acid, which is also toxic. In practice high NO2 levels are uncommon with the dose levels of NO used clinically. Risks can be minimized by mixing NO into ventilator circuits fairly near to the patient, flushing delivery systems before use and by constant monitoring of NO2 levels in ventilator gases.

Cylinder and regulator safety: NO is supplied in bulky, heavy cylinders which must be handled carefully to avoid potential risks to both staff and patients. A falling cylinder could cause a crush injury, or result in regulator damage and accidental discharge of gas. Poor handling of regulators and circuits can also result in gas discharge or inadvertent NO2 delivery. These risks can be minimized by following some basic safety precautions: - • Ensure cylinders are well secured to a wall or trolley at all times. • Regulators and lines should be flushed of any NO2 build up prior to use. • Environmental monitoring of NO and NO2 should be carried out to detect possible leaks or problems. • Cylinder changes should be planned ahead of time and a spare cylinder kept ready to use – planned, unhurried cylinder changes are more likely to be problem free. • Turn off cylinder and discharge pressure before removing regulators. • Never turn on a cylinder without a regulator attached. ¨ With some regulators the output pressure dial should be turned to low (anti-clockwise) before regulator is swapped from an empty to a full cylinder. • Only trained personnel should handle or change regulators.

Shift handover checks : When taking over care of a baby receiving NO there are several checks that should be carried out to help ensure a safe and trouble free shift: • Is the system correctly assembled? • Is supply adequate and spare cylinder available? • Who will change cylinders/regulators if required? • Is hand ventilation system available and ready to use? • Is measured NO level equal to that prescribed? • Are NO2 and MetHb levels ok? • Is NO flow correct to give measured dose-check formula, Printernox or SLE graph? • Does scavenging filter need changing

Nursing care: Nursing care of a baby receiving NO is very similar to the care required by any very sick baby. Minimal handling and close observation is required. There are a few specific points that need to be considered: - • Staff should have some knowledge of NO use and of the specific policies and systems of their unit and be aware of who is available to provide support and backup if it is needed.

NO-Mechanism of action: Nitric oxide is endothelial derived relaxing factor (EDRF). It is produced in the endothelium of blood vessels and diffuses out of the cells. It then enters vascular smooth muscle cells and activates guanalate cyclase which forms cyclic guanosine monophosphate (cGMP). This is a smooth muscle relaxer. cGMP is inactivated by cGMP phosphodiesterase. The half life of NO is 3–6 seconds. NO is bound to hemoglobin and inactivated to nitosylhaemoglobins and methemoglobin

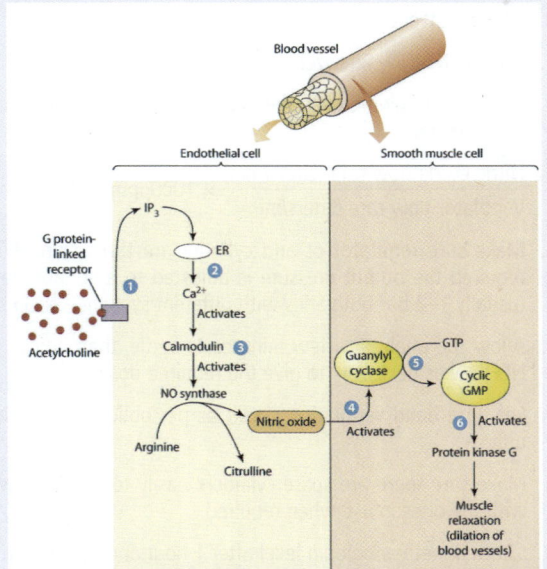

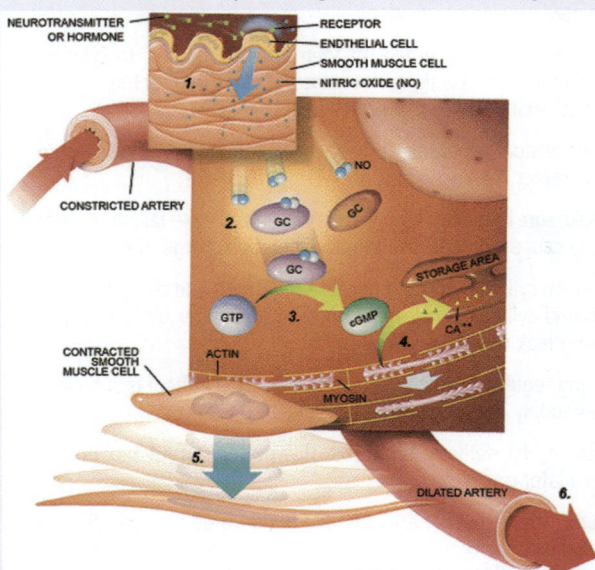

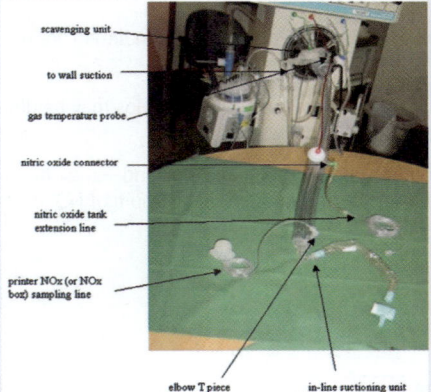

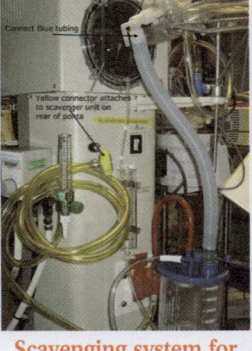

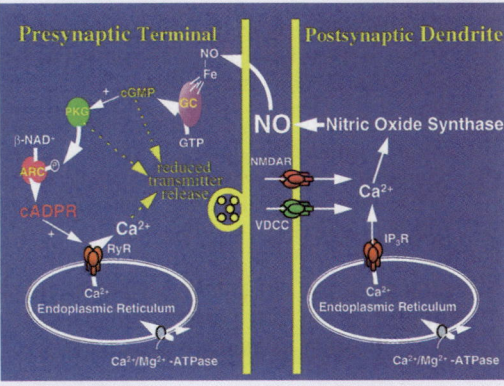

Scavenging system for SensorMedics

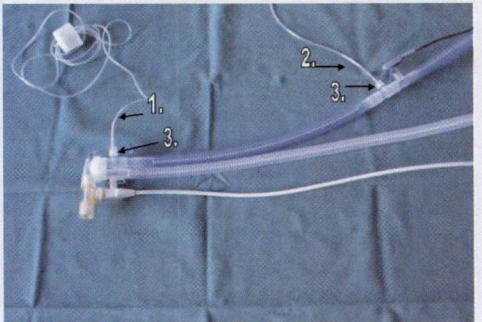

1.NOx sampling line 2.NO Tank extension line 3.nitric adapters

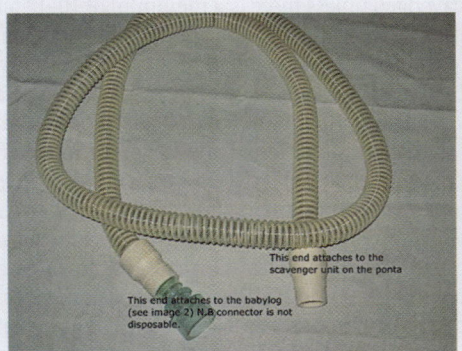

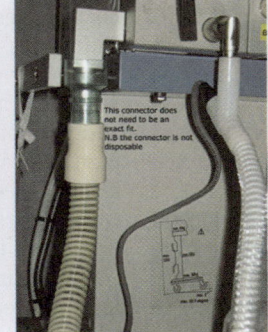

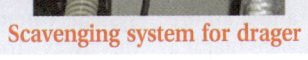

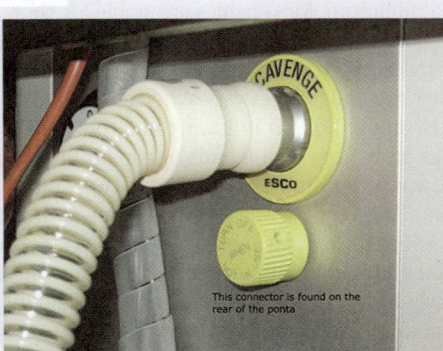

Scavenging system for drager

CHECKLIST FOR SETTING UP NITRIC OXIDE (NO)

1. Collect cylinder and ensure that it contains 1000ppm NO in nitrogen, check label attached to top of cylinder and the value printed on side of cylinder.

2. Check cylinder is turned off then attach regulator to cylinder and make sure it is tight. If regulator is of a type that has its own on/off switch check it is switched off.

3. Take cylinder to bedside and attach regulator to flowmeter, ensure flowmeter is switched off.

4. Make sure cylinder is secured to a wall or trolley— falling cylinder may cause injury or result in accidental discharge of NO.

5. Turn on cylinder (and if applicable, regulator) and check for leaks around cylinder head, regulator and flowmeter by listening or using leak detection spray.

6. Using regulator gauge nearest cylinder check there is sufficient gas supply in the cylinder.

7. Attach NO delivery tubing to flowmeter output but not to ventilator or circuit.

8. Purge the system of any possible build-up of nitrogen dioxide (NO_2) that has occurred when not in use - individual units should agree how this will be done.

   - If the required ventilator is not in use then at the end of the set-up a test lung can be attached and the system run until a low NO_2 level is confirmed.

   - If the NO is to be attached to a ventilator in use then purging should be done for 30–60 seconds before connecting the flowmeter tubing to the ventilator circuit. Purging can be done into room air away from nearby personnel.

IF HIGH NO FLOWS ARE USED FOR PURGING THEY MUST BE TURNED OFF BEFORE CONNECTION TO A BABY, THEN RESET AT AN APPROPRIATE LEVEL

9. Connect the flow meter output tubing to the ventilator, and the monitoring tubing to the NO/NO_2 analyzer

10. Attach scavenger system to the ventilator exhaust.

11. Turn on NO/NO_2 analyzer.

12. Set the NO flowmeter to the level required, calculated using the formula:

$$\frac{\text{Nitric Oxide flow rate (Liters/min)}}{\text{Ventilator flow rate (Liters/min)}} \times 1000\text{ppm} = \text{Dose ppm}$$

13. Make sure regulator or and cylinder are turned on and if required the output pressure is adjusted to a suitable level (usually 1–2 bar but varies with different systems - check).

14. Allow the analyzer a few minutes to settle, than adjust the NO flow as necessary to give the required dose.

15. Set up a hand ventilation circuit as per policy of individual unit.

16. Make sure there are spare cylinders easily to hand to swap with the ones in use when required.

17. Check a methemoglobin level after 1 hour and then every 12 hours.

18. Monitor NO dose on analyzer - adjust flow to maintain desired dose.

19. Monitor NO2 reading on analyzer. High readings may be due to inadequate purging.

20. Ensure environmental monitors are working—maximum recommended levels are 25ppm of NO and 3ppm of NO_2 over an 8 hour period.

The INNOVO Trial

• NO and NO_2 levels should be recorded hourly. Met Hb should be recorded at least 12 hourly after the initial level. Raised methemoglobin can affect accuracy of oxygen saturation monitor readings. • Check cylinder contents regularly so that cylinder changes can be planned ahead of time. A spare cylinder should however be kept ready for use. • A hand ventilation system should be available so that NO can be provided off the ventilator if necessary. • NO/NO_2 monitoring lines should be regularly checked for, and emptied of water as this can effect readings. This can be a particular problem with SLE systems. The line can be disconnected and emptied as long as it is clamped to prevent ventilator pressure loss. • Ventilator disconnection should be kept to a minimum. Most babies are stable for short disconnections but some are not. Some people are strong advocates of using closed suction systems to avoid this problem but they are expensive and policies vary. When a ventilator is disconnected a small amount of NO is flowing into room air. Staff should keep faces away from circuit ends or cap off the circuit. • Staff must know where in the system oxygen concentration is measured from. The NO flow will slightly dilute FIO_2 but this may not be shown by the oxygen analyzer. • When NO is weaned or stopped babies should be monitored closely. Weaning is usually done slowly and an increase in FIO2 can help stability when stopping. • Babies on NO should not be moved either around hospitals or between hospitals unless specialist equipment and staff are available. • Staff using SLE ventilators should be aware that if a high pressure alarm is repeatedly reset then there is a potential for pooling and boluses of NO being delivered due to ventilator flow cutting out. To avoid this potential problem high pressure alarms should be set appropriately and reset if necessary. **Staff safety** There are several issues related to staff safety that staff working with NO should be aware of: • Sudden large scale discharge of NO cylinder contents into room air could potentially cause asphyxiation and may necessitate evacuation of a room until it can be well ventilated to clear • Maximum recommended exposure levels are 25ppm of NO and 3ppm of NO_2 over an 8–hour period. In practice it is unlikely environmental levels will reach 1ppm. • It is recommended that exhaust gases from ventilators be scavenged unless there is a minimum of 10–12 air changes per hour in the room. The INNOVO Trial Technical Guidelines recommend that scavenging be done routinely. Scavenging with charcoal or soda lime filters is easy to do as a routine if wall scavenging systems are not available. Some adult and paediatric units do not scavenge and have not reported problems with environmental NO or NO2 levels. • When NO2 is being purged from systems into room air, environmental levels will not rise significantly, but it is good practice to direct the flow away from face and other staff. • If NO is running through a ventilator circuit during hand ventilation then use of a cap or test lung will reduce environmental exposure. Hand ventilation systems cannot be scavenged so exhaust flow from bag should be away from face. Systems have a big deadspace between cylinder and regulator in which NO2 build-up can occur when not in use. • There are no official recommendations about pregnant staff looking after patients receiving NO and many units give pregnant staff a choice about whether they do or not. Working in the same room as a patient receiving NO is not a concern as environmental levels have been shown to be so low. • Possible concern has been raised about asthmatic staff working with NO but it is not a common concern and NO is often used to treat adult and paediatric patients with severe asthma. • Jones brings together many figures which help to put concerns about NO into perspective. Clinical background levels of NO and NO2 are much lower than many city centre measurements. Traffic can cause high NO2 levels and cigarette smoke contains up to 1000ppm of NO. Branson et al discuss suggestions that intensive care unit NO and NO2 levels are influenced more by outside environmental conditions than by medical use of NO.

Troubleshooting : A properly set up NO system should be fairly trouble free if it is closely monitored. Below are some pointers for possible problems: - **High NO$_2$ readings** This is usually caused by inadequate purging prior to a system being used or when swapping to a spare cylinder/regulator set-up. Some systems are possibly more prone to this than others. For example some **Measured NO dose reduces** Cylinder may be empty or (if a one stage regulator is in use) the regulator output pressure may need adjusting to maintain pressure as the cylinder empties. The delivery tubing may have become disconnected from ventilator circuit or kinked. **Cylinder empties more quickly than expected** There may be a leak of NO from somewhere in the delivery system. A leaking cylinder should be turned off and replaced. **Increased environmental NO or NO2 levels** Again there may be a leak or the scavenging system may be faulty or need replacing. **Measured NO and NO2 fall unexpectedly** This is often caused by water in the monitoring line.

The use of inhaled nitric oxide (iNO) may help reduce breathing failure in preterm babies.(an update of the existing Cochrane review "Inhaled nitric oxide for respiratory failure in preterm infants" (Barrington 2006)

Breathing failure in premature newborn babies may be complicated by raised pressure within the vessels that carry blood to the lung (pulmonary hypertension). Medications that cause sedation or muscle relaxation and mechanically assisted breathing (mechanical or assisted ventilation) are used to treat pulmonary hypertension. Nitric oxide is believed to help regulate muscle tone in the arteries of the lungs and, thereby lessen pulmonary hypertension; however, iNO may also cause excessive bleeding (hemorrhage). This review of studies found that nitric oxide therapy may improve the chances of the baby having an improved outcome, but only when used in babies who were mildly ill. These studies indicated that there may be a decrease in serious bleeding in the brain (intracranial hemorrhage). When given to babies who were very ill, iNO did not seem to help, and may have contributed to an increase in intracranial hemorrhage.

*The dose can be easily calculated on continuous flow ventilators using the formula below:-

$$\frac{\text{Nitric Oxide flow rate(Litres/Min)} \times \text{Nitric Oxide cylinder concentration(ppm)}}{\text{Ventilator flow rate(Litres/Min)}} = \text{Dose (ppm)}$$

e.g.:- $\dfrac{0.2 \text{ Litres/ Min} \times 1000 \text{ ppm}}{10 \text{ Litres/Min}} = 20$ ppm continuous dose

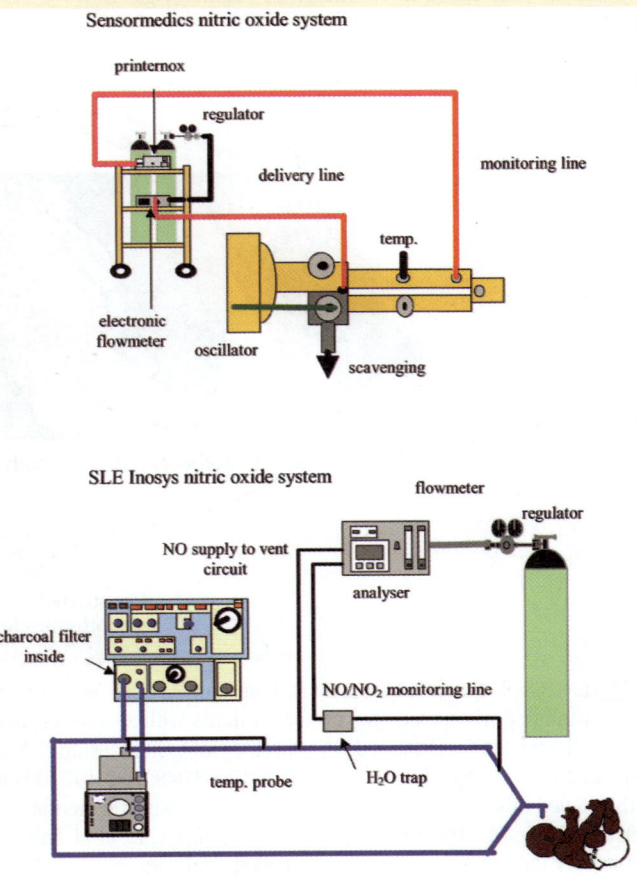

Hand ventilation NO therapy is a treatment that should be weaned slowly rather than stopped suddenly. This is because it is recognized that dependence can develop and that some patients react badly to its sudden cessation. In the light of this it seems prudent to make provision for supplying NO if, for any reason, a baby is taken off a ventilator and ventilated by hand. Reasons for doing this can include patient deterioration, physiotherapy or ventilator faultfinding. Hand ventilation systems for use with NO are usually set up in one of two ways. Either a separate NO supply is provided for a bagging circuit, or the NO supply is disconnected from the ventilator circuit and attached to the bagging circuit when required. If a separate NO supply is used then the system must be purged of any NO2 build-up (by running it for approximately 30 seconds) prior to use. This is not an issue if the NO supply is simply being swapped over, as long as the bagging system is purged after use. Care must be taken during hand ventilation to ensure the NO dose does not change. If bagging circuit flow is different to ventilator flow then the NO flowmeter will need adjusting to compensate. Such adjustments can easily be calculated ahead of time. Use of two people for hand ventilation of babies receiving NO makes what can be a fiddly and stressful process much easier. If Neopuffs are used instead of bagging systems they can easily be adapted for such layouts.

Treatment with inhaled nitric oxide (iNO)

* Treatment with iNO is indicated for newborns with an oxygen index (OI) of less than 25. Nitric oxide (NO) is an endothelial-derived gas signaling molecule that relaxes vascular smooth muscle and that can be delivered to the lung by means of an inhalation device (INOVent; Ikaria, Clinton NJ).

* In 2 large randomized trials, NO reduced the need for ECMO support by approximately 40%. Although these trials led to the US Food and Drug Administration (FDA) approving iNO as a therapy for persistent pulmonary hypertension of the newborn, iNO did not reduce mortality, length of hospitalization, or reduce the risk of neurodevelopmental impairment.

* A randomized study has confirmed that beginning iNO at a milder or earlier point in the disease course (for an oxygenation index of 15–25) did not decrease the incidence of ECMO and/or death or improve other patient outcomes, including the incidence of neurodevelopmental impairment.

* Contraindication to iNO include congenital heart disease characterized by left ventricular outflow tract obstruction (e.g. · interrupted aortic arch, critical aortic stenosis, · hypoplastic left heart syndrome) and severe left ventricular dysfunction.

* The appropriate starting dose is 20 ppm. Doses higher than this have not been shown to be more effective and have been associated with adverse effects, including methemoglobinemia and increased levels of nitrogen dioxide (NO_2).

* ### Dose and Administration

   Cylinder has 880 parts per million (ppm) in nitrogen

   – Add to ventilator circuit between humidifier and baby.

   – 100 ml/min added to 10 litres/min ventilator gas flow = 8.7 ppm

   – 200 ml/min added to 10 litres/min ventilator gas flow = 17.4 ppm Start on 20ppm (approximately 200ml/min, and increase according to measurement on Nitric Oxide Monitor)

   Start on 0.2 litres per minute in 10 litres of 100% O_2 = 17.4 ppm

   Reduce to 0.1 litres per minute: = 8.7 ppm

   Reduce according to response

   Doses above 20ppm are not indicated as generally a response is obtained prior to this.

* Appropriate lung recruitment and expansion are essential to achieve the best response. If a newborn has severe parenchymal lung disease and PPHN, strategies such as HFV may be required.

* Most newborns require iNO for less than 5 days. In general, the dose can be weaned to 5 ppm after 6-24 hours of therapy. The dose is then slowly weaned and discontinued when the FiO_2 is less than 0.4-0.6 and the iNO dose is 1 ppm. Abrupt discontinuation at higher doses should be avoided become it may cause abrupt rebound pulmonary hypertension.

* In centers that do not have immediate availability of ECMO support, use of iNO must be approached with caution. Because iNO cannot be abruptly discontinued, transport with iNO is usually needed if a subsequent referral for ECMO is necessary. This capability should be determined in collaboration with the ECMO center before treatment is started. The use of iNO with high-frequency ventilation (HFV) creates particular problems for transport, and this should be considered before these therapies are combined in a non-ECMO center.

* The use of iNO has not been demonstrated to reduce need for ECMO in newborns with congenital diaphragmatic hernia. In these newborns, iNO should be used in non-ECMO centers to allow for acute stabilization, followed by immediate transfer to a center that can provide ECMO.

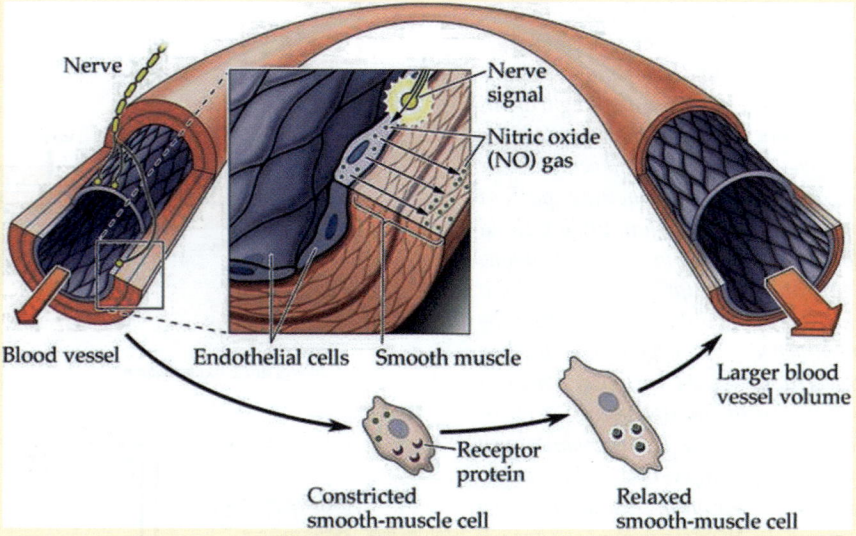

Nerve — Nerve signal — Nitric oxide (NO) gas

Blood vessel — Endothelial cells — Smooth muscle — Larger blood vessel volume

Constricted smooth-muscle cell — Receptor protein — Relaxed smooth-muscle cell

REFERENCES: 1) Field D, Elbourne D, Truesdale A, et al. **Neonatal ventilation with inhaled** nitric oxide versus ventilatory support without inhaled nitric oxide for preterm infants with severe respiratory failure: The INNOVO multicentre **randomized controlled trial.** Pediatrics 2005;115:926-936 2) Schreiber MD, Gin-Mestan K, Marks JD, et al. **Inhaled nitric oxide in premature infants with the respiratory distress syndrome.** N Engl J Med 2003;349:2099-107. 3) The Franco-Belgium Collaborative NO Trial Group: **Early compared with** delayed inhaled nitric oxide in moderately hypoxemic neonates with **respiratory failure: a randomized controlled trial.** Lancet. 1999;354:1066- 71. 4)Kinsella J.P., Walsh W.F., Bose C.L., et al. **Inhaled nitric oxide in premature** neonates with severe hypoxaemic respiratory failure: a randomised **controlled trial.** Lancet 1999;354:1061-5. 5) Hascoet JM, Fresson J, Claris O, et al. **The safety and efficacy of nitric oxide therapy in premature infants.** J Pediatr 2005;146:318-23.

Extracorporeal membrane oxygenation (ECMO) is defined as the use of a modified heartlung machine combined with a membrane oxygenator to provide cardiopulmonary support for patients with reversible pulmonary and/or cardiac failure in whom maximal conventional therapies have failed. While ECMO is now well accepted as a standard treatment for neonatal respiratory failure unresponsive to conventional therapies, over the last decade a number of new treatments have been used – including high frequency ventilation, surfactant replacement, and inhaled nitric oxide therapy – that, in many cases, can replace ECMO. The term extracorporeal membrane oxygenation (ECMO) was initially used to describe long-term extracorporeal support that focused on the function of oxygenation. Subsequently, in some patients, the emphasis shifted to carbon dioxide removal and the term extracorporeal carbon dioxide removal was coined. Extracorporeal support was later used for postoperative support in patients following cardiac surgery. Other variations of its capabilities have been tested and used over the last few years, making it an important tool in the armamentarium of life and organ support measures for clinicians. With all of these uses for extracorporeal circuitry, a new term, extracorporeal life support (ECLS), has come into vogue to describe this technology.

The differences between ECMO and cardiopulmonary bypass are as follows:

*ECMO is frequently instituted using only cervical cannulation, which can be performed under local anesthesia. Standard cardiopulmonary bypass is usually instituted by transthoracic cannulation under general anesthesia. *Unlike standard cardiopulmonary bypass, which is used for short-term support measured in hours, ECMO is used for longer-term support ranging from 3–10 days. *The purpose of ECMO is to allow time for intrinsic recovery of the lungs and heart; a standard cardiopulmonary bypass provides support during various types of cardiac surgical procedures.

Extracorporeal membrane oxygenation apparatus

The extracorporeal membrane oxygenation (ECMO) apparatus consists of a blood pump with raceway tubing, a venous reservoir, a membrane oxygenator, and a countercurrent heat exchanger. The blood pump is either a simple roller pump (most common) or a constrained vortex centrifugal pump. The roller pump causes less hemolysis and is used for neonatal ECMO. The venous reservoir is used with the roller pump for neonatal ECMO. The oxygenator is responsible for exchanging both oxygen and carbon dioxide and is central to the successful performance of prolonged ECMO. Three types of commercial artificial lungs are available: bubble, membrane, and hollow-fiber devices. The heat exchanger warms the blood using a countercurrent mechanism. Blood is exposed to warm water that circulates within metal tubing.

Safety devices and monitors

- Air bubble detectors can identify microscopic air bubbles in the arterialized blood and automatically turn off the blood pump.

- Arterial line filters between the heat exchanger and the arterial cannula are used to trap air, thrombi, and other emboli.

- Pressure monitors, which are placed before and after the oxygenator, measure the pressure of the circulating blood and are used to monitor for a dangerous rise in circuit pressure. This can occur with thrombosis of the oxygenator or occlusion of the tubing or cannulae. Pressure monitors are critical in preventing circuit disruption in the face of distal occlusion.

- A continuous venous oxygen saturation monitor and temperature monitor are other important safety features.

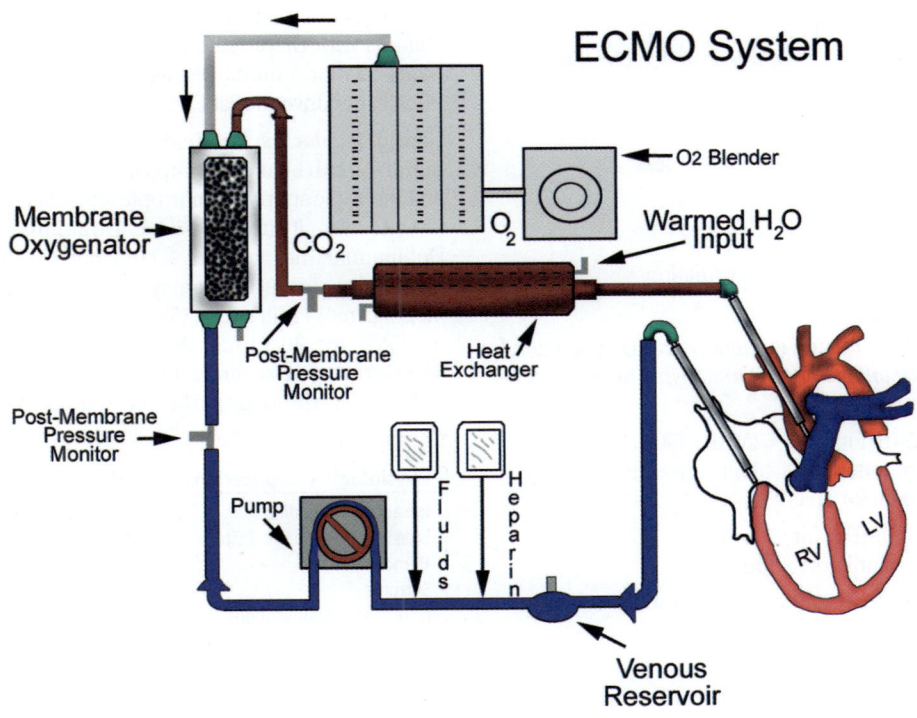

ECMO System

Extracorporeal Membrane Oxygenation Procedure: The extracorporeal membrane oxygenation (ECMO) circuit is primed with the freshest blood available. The acid-base balance and blood gas of the primer are adjusted appropriately. Differences between venoarterial ECMO and venovenous ECMO are presented below.The standard ECMO procedure used in most neonatal ICUs is venoarterial bypass. In this situation, a cannula is placed through the right jugular vein into the right atrium. Blood is drained to a venous reservoir located 3-4 feet below heart level. The blood is actively pumped by a roller pump through the oxygenator, where gas exchange occurs via countercurrent flow of blood and gas. Next, the blood is warmed to body temperature by the heat exchanger before returning to the patient through a cannula placed through the right carotid artery into the aortic arch. Systemic anticoagulation therapy with heparin is administered throughout the bypass circuit, with frequent monitoring of activated clotting time (ACT), which should be maintained at 180-240 seconds.In venovenous bypass, a double-lumen cannula is placed through the right jugular vein into the right atrium. Desaturated blood is withdrawn from the right atrium through the outer fenestrated venous catheter wall, and oxygenated blood is returned through the inner lumen of the catheter and is angled to direct blood across the tricuspid valve.

Differences between veno-venous and venoarterial extracorporeal membrane oxygenation

	Veno-venous	Veno-arterial
Cannulation	one or two vein	Jugular vein and common carotid artery
Flow	130ml/kg/min	100ml/Kg/min
Lung blood flow	Normal	Decreased
Systemic embolism	Unlikely	Possible
O2 Supply	Fair (PaO$_2$) 40–80 torr	Good (PaO$_2$) 60–150torr
Cardiac effect	Negligible effect	Decreased preload, Increased after load
		Moderate to markedly decreased
Pulmonary circulation	Unaffected	Pulmonary Congestion, systemic
Left to Right shunt	No effect	Hypoperfusion
Right to Left shunt	Increased aortic saturation	Decreased aortic saturation
Oxygen delivery capacity	Moderate	High
Circulatory support	? increase in cardiac output	Partial to complete

Indications

Patients with the following 2 major neonatal diagnoses require the use of extracorporeal membrane oxygenation (ECMO):

* *Primary diagnoses* associated with *primary pulmonary hypertension of the newborn (PPHN), including idiopathic PPHN, *meconium aspiration syndrome,*respiratory distress syndrome, group B streptococcal sepsis, and asphyxia

* *Congenital diaphragmatic hernia (CDH)*

Selection/Inclusion criteria

- Gestational age of 34 weeks or more*
- Birth weight of 2000 g or higher*
- No significant coagulopathy or uncontrolled bleeding
- No major intracranial hemorrhage (grade 1 intracranial hemorrhage)*
- Mechanical ventilation for 10–14 days or less*
- Reversible lung injury
- No lethal malformations
- No major untreatable cardiac malformation
- Failure of maximal medical therapy
* Failure to meet these criteria is a relative contraindication for ECMO. *ANY of the following AND underlying disease process which is likely to be reversible:*

1. *OI 30 –60 for 0.5– 6 hours OI = (MAP x FiO$_2$ × 100) / PaO$_2$ (mmHg) Standard criteria : OI 40 on conventional ventilation, OI 50-60 for HFOV

2. *PaO$_2$ <5.3kPa (40mmHg) for >2 hours Despite maximal ventilatory support

3. *Acidosis and Shock*pH <7.25 due to metabolic acidosis Raised lactate *Intractable hypotension

Respiratory criteria

Oxygenation Index (OI) = MAPxFiO2x100/PaO2: *All Infants >60 for 30 min. >40 for 60 min >35 for 6 hours >30 for 24 hours >25 for 72 hours *Barotrauma: Ventilator settings exceeding: PIP>35, MAP>20, HFOV AMPlitude>40, or Jet PIP>45. Hypercarbia with pH <7.10 on: PIP=35, Jet PIP=45, or HFO AMPlitude=40 for 4 hours. Severe air leak unresponsive to other therapies *Acute Deterioration without rapid solution: PaO2 <30 or preductal SaO2 <70%.Alveolar-arterial (A-a) gradient of 600-624 mm Hg for 4-12 hours at sea level, which may be computed as follows (where 47=partial pressure of water vapor): (A-a)(Diffusing capacity [D] of O$_2$ equals atmospheric pressure - 47 - (PaCO$_2$ + PaO$_2$])/FiO$_2$ *Infants with Diaphragmatic Hernia: >35 for 30 min. >30 for 2 hours >25 for 4 hours OR need for MAP>15, HFO AMP or Jet PIP>40, or conventional PIP>30

Cardiovascular/oxygen delivery criteria: *Plasma lactate: >45 mg/dl (5 mM/L) and not improving, despite volume expansion and inotropic support. *Inotropic equivalent (IE) >50 for 1 hour or >45 for 8 hours. IE = Dopamine(mcg/kg/min) + Dobutamine(mcg/kg/min) + Epinephrine (100Xs mcg/kg/min) + Norepinephrine(100Xs mcg/kg/min) + Isoproterenol(100Xs mcg/kg/min) + Milrinone (15Xs mcg/kg/min). *Mixed Venous Sat of <55% for 30 min. (<60% for CDH patients) *Rapidly deteriorating or severe ventricular dysfunction *Intractable arrhythmia with poor perfusion *Cardiac Arrest.

Complications of ECMO

Physiologic complications	Mechanical complications
Intracranial bleeding	Failure of Oxygenator
Bleeding from surgical site	Pump failure
Hemolysis	Tubing rupture
Seizures	Cannula problems
Neurologic complications	
Renal damage	
Arrythmia	
Pneumothorax	

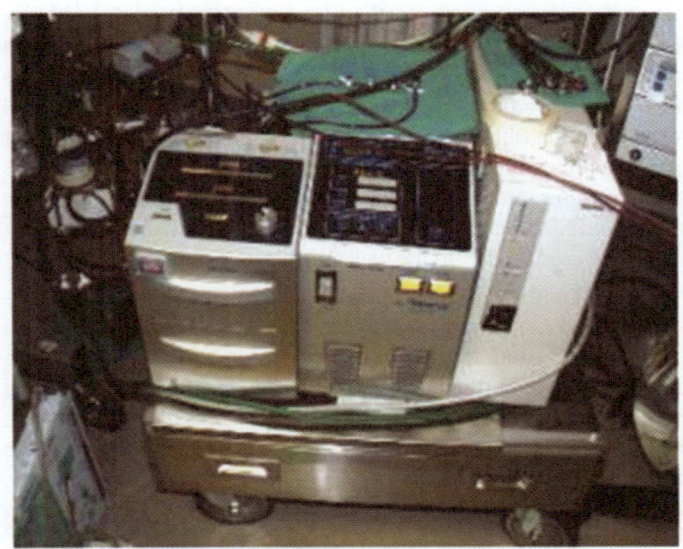

The ECMO pump

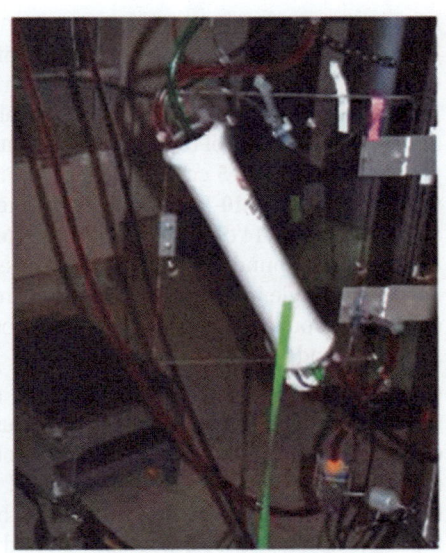

Oxygenator membrane

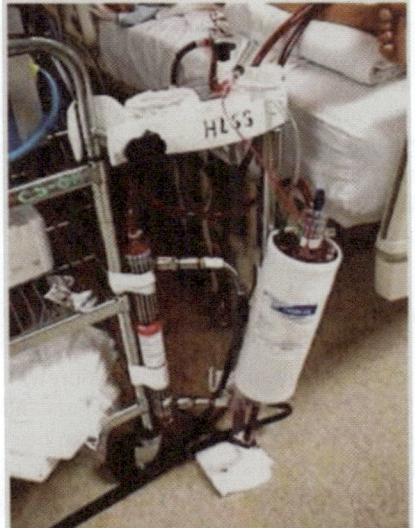

Oxygenator and heat exchanger

Neonatal		Pediatric	
Meconium aspiration syndrome	94%	Bacterial infections	45%
Sepsis	76%	Viral infections	56%
Respiratory distress syndrome	84%	Hematological disorders	62%
Congenital heart disease	58%	Atrial septal defect	65%
Persistent fetal circulation	83%	Pneumocystis carinii pneumonia	38%
Air leak	71%	Infant respiratory distress syndrome	51%
Others	74%	Others	49%

Survival Statistics by Diagnosis

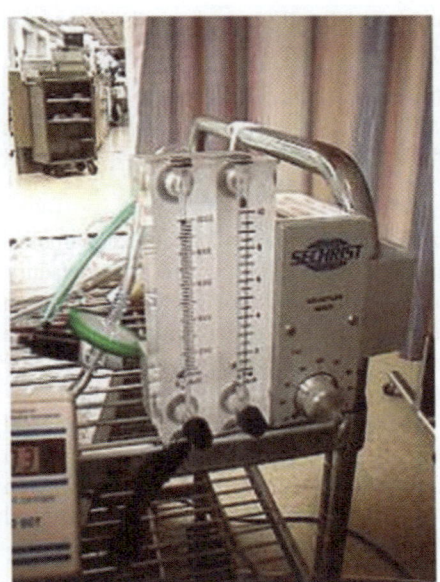

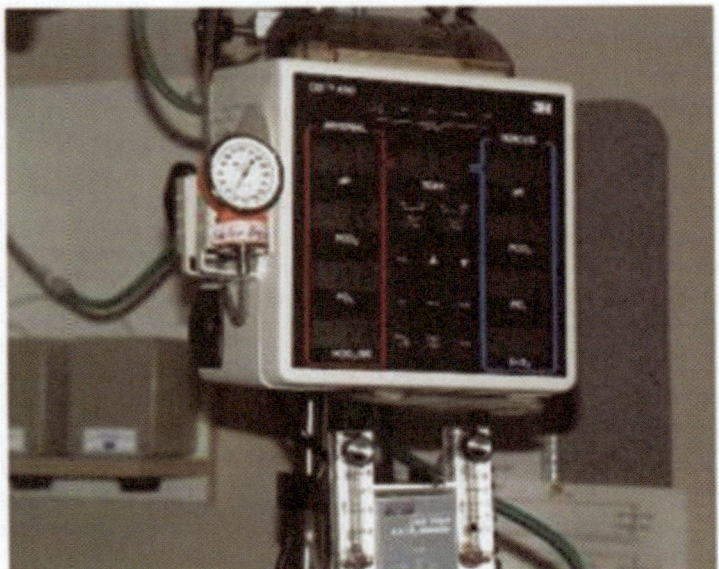

Blenders to control oxygenation and airflow -FiO2 and sweep gas flow controls.

Management

Pulmonary system: Extracorporeal membrane oxygenation (ECMO) is used temporarily while awaiting pulmonary recovery. In the classic use of neonatal ECMO, the typical ventilator settings are FiO_2 of 21–30%, PIP of 15–25 cm H_2O, a positive end-expiratory pressure (PEEP) of 3–5 cm H_2O, and intermittent mechanical ventilation (IMV) of 10–20 breaths per minute. In some centers, a high PEEP of 12–14 cm H_2O has been used to avoid atelectasis; this has been found to shorten the bypass time in infants. Pulmonary hygiene is strict and requires frequent positional changes, endotracheal suctioning every 4 hours depending on secretions, and a daily chest radiograph.

Cardiovascular system: Systemic perfusion and intravascular volume should be maintained. Volume status can be assessed clinically by urine output and physical signs of perfusion and by measuring the central venous pressure and the mean arterial blood pressure. Native cardiac output can be enhanced with inotropic agents. Echocardiography should be performed to exclude any major congenital heart anomaly that may require immediate intervention other than ECMO (e.g., obstructed total anomalous pulmonary venous connection).

CNS: Complications are the most serious and are primarily related to the degree of hypoxia and acidosis. Avoiding paralytic agents and performing regular neurologic examinations are recommended. If feasible, head ultrasonography should be performed before beginning ECMO in a neonate. Reevaluation with serial head ultrasonography may be needed on a daily basis, especially after any major event. In patients with seizures or suspected seizures, aggressive treatment is recommended (e.g., phenobarbital).

Renal system: During the first 24–48 hours on ECMO, oliguria and acute tubular necrosis associated with capillary leak and intravascular volume depletion are common because ECMO triggers an acute inflammatory like reaction. The diuretic phase, which usually begins within 48 hours, is often one of the earliest signs of recovery. If oliguria persists for 48–72 hours, diuretics are often required to reduce edema. When renal failure does not improve, hemofiltration or hemodialysis filters may be added to the circuit.

Hematologic considerations : To optimize oxygen delivery, the patient's hemoglobin should be maintained at 12–15 g/dL using packed RBCs (pRBCs). As a result of platelet consumption during ECMO, platelet transfusions are required to maintain platelet counts above 100,000/mcL. Activated clotting time (ACT) should be maintained at 180–240 seconds to avoid bleeding complications.

Infection control: Strict aseptic precautions are required. The presence of infection is monitored by obtaining cultures from the circuit at least once a week. Based on institutional experience, the protocol frequency may vary. Other appropriate cultures (e.g. fungal and viral) should be obtained as needed.

Fluids, electrolytes, and nutrition: Patients on ECMO require close monitoring of fluids and electrolytes. The high-energy requirements should be met using hyperalimentation techniques. The patient's weight increases in the first 1–3 days on ECMO because of fluid retention.

Medications: Doses of most inotropic medications, such as dopamine, dobutamine, and epinephrine, can usually be decreased once the patient is on ECMO. -Diuretics, such as furosemide (Lasix) and chlorothiazide (Diuril), may be required for mobilization of tissue fluids. -Antacids and H_2 antagonists are usually administered for GI tract bleeding. -Only minimal sedation with fentanyl, midazolam, or morphine is required after stabilization. -Phenobarbital can be used if the patient has seizures.-Aminocaproic acid may be required to reduce bleeding during surgery. -Antibiotics, such as ampicillin and cefotaxime, are used initially in the typical septicemic dosages; dosage.

Differential diagnoses of acute cardiorespiratory decompensation in patients on extracorporeal membrane oxygenation: *Pericardial tamponade (from blood or air) *Tension pneumothorax or hemothorax *Respiratory failure *Myocardial ischemia *Electrolyte imbalance *Massive hemorrhage (especially intracranial hemorrhage) *Drug effects *Overwhelming sepsis

Weaning from ECMO: Weaning from ECMO is a gradual process, since initially almost 60 to 80 % of the cardiac output flows through the circuit in order to maintain a PaO2 in a range of 70 to 80 mmHg. As the lungs improve, PaO_2 improves and the ECMO flow can be slowly decreased. Once the bypass flow reaches 10% of the cardiac output, the flow is continued for a further 8 to 12 hours to ensure that the patient is ready to come off the pump. During decanulation, the infant is kept sedated and paralyzed. The ventilator setting is changed at this time to inspired oxygen of 30 to 40%, respiratory rate of 40 to 50 bpm, and pressure limits of 15 to 20 cm H2O. The average time to extubation is 24 to 48 hr. Usually, supplemental oxygen is required for the first week.

Conclusion

The patients on ECMO are critically ill. Once the patient is placed on ECMO, the work of getting the patient off ECMO begins. Anticoagulation, prophylactic antibiotic, mild sedation with neuromuscular blocking agent, cardiopulmonary bypass and nutritional support is carefully monitored. Parents often need some emotional and psychological support. The number of ECMO cases continues to decline. This may be because of increased used of nitric oxide, HFOV, HFJV. It is interesting to note that survival on ECMO has also decreased. This may be due to delay in ECMO therapy because of pre ECMO trial of alternative treatment. The success of the therapy depends on prompt diagnosis and early initiation of treatment.

The Editor is grateful to D. R. Thakar, A. C. Sinha & O. C. Wenker : Concepts Of Neonatal ECMO . The Internet Journal of Perfusionists. 2001 Volume 1 Number 2 for adapting their work.

REFERENCES

1)Bartlett RH, Gazzaniga AB, Toomasian J, et al. Extracorporeal membrane oxygenation (ECMO) in neonatal respiratory failure. 100 cases. *Ann Surg.* Sep 1986;204(3):236-45. 2)Beck R, Anderson KD, Pearson GD, et al. Criteria for extracorporeal membrane oxygenation in a population of infants with persistent pulmonary hypertension of the newborn. *J Pediatr Surg.* Apr 1986;21(4):297-302.3)Herbst D, Najm HK, Jha KN. Long-term extracorporeal circulation management: the role of low- and high-range heparin ACT tests. *J Extra Corpor Technol.* Dec 2008;40(4):271-4. 4) Upp JR Jr, Bush PE, Zwischenberger JB. Complications of neonatal extracorporeal membrane oxygenation. *Perfusion.* 1994;9(4):241-56.

Much of the development of neonatal surgery is due to the close collaboration between pediatric surgeons, neonatologists, anesthetists, pathologists, radiologists, biochemists, and nurses. Neonatal surgery should proceed only in units with the trained personnel, infrastructure and processes in place to ensure safe practice. The newborn requires anesthesia for surgical procedures for the same reasons that older infants and children do: to maintain physiologic homeostasis, prevent pain, stress responses, and their sequelae. Indeed, the stress response may be greater in preterm infants because of immaturity of descending inhibitory pathways. These responses, if not mitigated by anesthesia and analgesia, have been associated with increased postoperative circulatory, respiratory and metabolic abnormalities and morbidity, as well as evidence of alteration of neurobehavioral response to pain on later in life. Because anesthesia-related morbidity and mortality are higher in infants, perioperative administration of anesthesia and analgesia must be modified to take into consideration the unique considerations of physiology, pharmacology, and anatomy attendant to the newborn period.

Preoperative Evaluation: **Antenatal and birth history**-Record gestational age, intrauterine problems and mode of delivery. Record Apgar scores and the need for or duration of any cardiorespiratory support. Elicit thorough enquiry about other early problems, if they have been treated and resolved or are ongoing and likely to require intervention (e.g. hyperbilirubinemia, hypoglycemia, seizures and sepsis). Exclude congenital anomalies before embarking on anaesthesia as one congenital anomaly raises the possibility of another (e.g. cardiac lesions in exomphalos). Determine the anaesthetic implications of an unfamiliar syndrome before discussion with parents/carers. Obtain a baseline haemoglobin measurement and blood samples from both neonate and mother tested for ABO/ rhesus D incompatibility. Ensure that vitamin K was given at delivery. **Current status**-Follow a systematic approach to assessment at the preoperative visit to reduce the chances of missing significant problems. *Refer to Table 1.* Observe appropriate fasting times as follows: 6 hours for formula milk, 4 hours for breast milk and 2 hours for clear fluids. (Prolonged fasting risks dehydration and hypoglycemia, so dextrose-containing intravenous maintenance should be started simultaneously with the fast whenever possible.) Explain the anaesthetic plan to the parents and obtain consent for any regional techniques, blood transfusion and/or rectal suppositories. Discuss information on postoperative intravascular lines, plans for analgesia and need for elective postoperative ventilation at this time. **Preparation of the operating theatre**-Warm the operating room to 30^0 C in advance of the neonate's arrival because cooling occurs rapidly. It is common to use a forced-air warming convector, a radiant heater, warmed gamgee blankets and/or clear plastic drapes. Accomplish safe, reliable support of both baby and attached devices by the combination of tape, soft foam padding and rolls, to avoid accidental disconnections and decannulations. Ensure a selection of appropriately-sized masks, endotracheal tubes (ETTs), oropharyngeal airways, an appropriately-sized laryngeal mask airway (LMA), straight and curved laryngoscope blades, stylets and suction catheters, should be immediately available. **An infant-compatible ventilator** capable of delivering small tidal volumes and rapid respiratory rates, and have an adjustable inspiratory flow rate and inspiratory to expiratory ratio so that peak airway pressure is kept as low as possible. Pressure-controlled ventilation is widely used in order to minimize the risk of pulmonary barotrauma. A suitable temperature controlled humidifier should be incorporated in the inspiratory side of the ventilator circuit. The ability to deliver air and oxygen mixtures through the ventilator or the anaesthetic circuit should be available. Ventilatory parameters can then be titrated according to positioning, observed chest/abdominal excursion and measured airway pressures/capnography. Premedication-Sedative premedication is not used in neonates or in other situations where it may cause increased risk, e.g. children with airway compromise. Midazolam and diazepam (for older children) are the most commonly used premedicant drugs. **Intraoperative management:** **Monitoring**: Optimal monitoring includes precordial stethoscope, pulse oximetry, capnography, NIBP, ECG and temperature (esophageal or rectal). The pulse oximeter should be placed on the right hand or ear (preductal). A second oximeter probe may be placed for back up, or when right to left shunting may be a possibility. Monitoring of urine output, utilizing a 5 Fr feeding tube as a urinary catheter is advised in infants having major surgery. Intraarterial catheters (IAC) are useful in critically ill neonates who are at risk for large intraoperative blood and/or fluid losses, due either to

coagulopathy or resection of large masses (e.g. NEC, sacrococcygeal teratoma). IAC allow for continuous monitoring of blood pressure and periodic assessment of blood gases, glucose, electrolytes including ionized calcium, hemoglobin, and base deficit. CVP catheters (3 Fr) are usually placed in the right internal jugular vein and are very useful for both monitoring and as a secure IV access, particularly in procedures with anticipated large blood losses or fluid shift. **Fluids, electrolytes and glucose management :** During surgery, the infant's fluid status is even more dynamic than usual. Maintenance fluids must be administered, but in addition, the anesthesiologist must consider any pre-existing fluid deficits as well as ongoing fluid losses such as blood loss and third-space fluid transfer. All of these will affect circulating blood volume. The goal of fluid therapy during neonatal surgery is to maintain an adequate intravascular volume without contributing to electrolyte disturbances. Acute hyponatremia, a risk when hypotonic fluid is infused, can dangerously increase brain water content. Not only are glomerular filtration rate and tubular function immature in the neonate, but inhaled and intravenous anesthetic agents, sedatives, and analgesics can contribute to renal dysfunction. Extravascular or interstitial sequestration of fluid (the so-called "third space" fluid loss) can occur during surgery. Third-space fluid losses can be 4-5 mL/kg/hour for an open thoracic procedure; and for a major intra-abdominal procedure, as high as 10-15 mL/kg/hour. Estimated third-space fluid deficits are replaced with iso-osmotic fluids, at rates according to the type of surgery: *Peripheral/superficial surgery: 1-3 mL/kg/hour; *Abdominal/chest/hip surgery: 3-4 mL/kg/hour; and *Extensive intra-abdominal surgery: 6-10 mL/kg/hour. If fluids containing dextrose, such as total parenteral nutrition or hyperalimentation, are infusing throughout surgery, these fluids should not be used to replace ongoing fluid losses. To do so would risk hyperglycemia. Blood glucose should be monitored closely during surgery of the neonate. Allowable blood loss is generally considered to be 20% to 30% of the neonate's blood volume. Blood loss is replaced either 3:1 with crystalloid or 1:1 with blood products. Hypotension is always a threat during neonatal surgery; bolus syringes containing 10 cc/kg of normal saline can be prepared ahead of time for a quick response to a fall in blood pressure. If fluid replacement reaches 100 cc/kg and hypotension persists, vasopressors may be required to restore blood pressure. During neonatal surgery, glucose administration should continue, but blood glucose measurement should be performed at frequent intervals to avoid both hyper- and hypoglycemia. **Temperature Control :** Modes of heat loss include radiation, conduction, evaporation, and convection. *Radiation* — to reduce radiant heat loss during induction and other preoperative procedures, a radiant warming device can be positioned over the infant before draping. Extreme caution must be used if the radiant heater is not servo-controlled with a skin temperature probe. *Conduction* — because operating room tables tend to be cold, the surface under the infant can be warmed with a forced-air warming, temperature-controlled blanket. Intravenous fluids and inhaled gases can also be warmed. *Evaporation* — surgical site/body cavity heat losses can be minimized by irrigating with warm fluids. *Convection* — cool circulating air and drafts can contribute to heat loss in unswaddled infants and during surgery, especially when body parts or cavities are exposed. Keeping the OR doors closed and covering the infant can reduce convective heat loss. **Managing Coagulopathies :** infants with necrotizing enterocolitis (NEC) and liver dysfunction who require surgery often suffer excessive intraoperative bleeding. Fresh frozen plasma and platelets should be on call when these patients go to the OR. **Infection control:** avoid using or manipulating an infant's central venous catheter to administer routine fluids or medications, using these lines only in dire emergencies. **Pain Management:** Narcotics commonly used for intraoperative analgesia in neonates include morphine, fentanyl, sufentanil, and remifentanil. Ketamine, a phencyclidine derivative, produces amnesia and intense analgesia.

Agents Currently Used to Provide Anesthesia for the Neonate *: Inhalational Agents* • Isoflurane • Sevoflurane • Desflurane *Narcotics* • Fentanyl • **Morphine** • **Hydromorphone** *Neuromuscular Blockers* • **Vecuronium** • **Rocuronium** • **Cis-atracurium** *Regional Anesthetics* • **Bupivacaine** • **Ropivacaine**

Balanced general anesthesia may be maintained by intravenous or inhalational anesthesia supplemented with intravenous opioids, regional techniques and/or muscle relaxation. After preoxygenation, induction can be either inhalational or intravenous. Awake placement of intravenous cannulae can be facilitated by the use of topical local anesthetics e calculate and beware toxic doses of these agents. Inhalational induction has the advantage of maintenance of spontaneous ventilation (useful if dealing with a potentially difficult airway) and should proceed with sevoflurane in 100% oxygen. Nitrous oxide should be avoided e even healthy preoxygenated neonates start to desaturate after 7 seconds of apnoea, so gentle mask ventilation may need to be continued until the airway is secure. Intravenous induction, either using propofol (2-4 mg/kg) or ketamine (0.5-3.0 mg/kg), has the advantage of speed, but usually results in apnoea. Intubation will usually be necessary and can be achieved under deep inhalational or intravenous anaesthesia supplemented with short-acting opioids or muscle relaxants. Cricoid pressure is of unproven benefit and may actually hinder attempts at laryngoscopy. Transitional circulation Hypoxia, hypercapnia, hypothermia, acidosis and light anaesthesia can cause pulmonary hypertension, with right-to-left shunting of blood through the foramen ovale and ductus arteriosus, leading to worsening hypoxemia and return of the so-called transitional circulation. Therapeutic maneuvers include deepening anaesthesia, volume expansion, hyperventilation and/or increased inspired oxygen. Pulmonary vasodilators may be necessary in refractory cases. Extubation has the same incidence of complications as ntubation and requires the same vigilance.

Regional anesthesia offers several advantages over general anesthesia. The infant can be extubated sooner following surgery, and lower doses of systemic narcotics are required. In neonates, the caudal epidural block is the most commonly used regional block.· Caudal epidural block anesthesia is considered an effective and safe option to provide intraoperative and postoperative analgesia after lower abdominal surgery. The infant is anesthetized with an inhalational agent before placement of the epidural catheter for delivery of the regional anesthetic.

Epidural anesthesia is most effective if the tip of the catheter is located at the site of surgery. The epidural catheter can be inserted into the lumbar caudal space L3-L4 and threaded cephalad (upward) to the desired position. Real-time ultrasonography enables identification of the tip of the needle within the epidural space and a visualization of the spread of local anesthetic. The agents used for epidural anesthesia in the neonate are local anesthetics (bupivacaine and ropivacaine) and opioid analgesics (fentanyl, morphine, and hydromorphone), often combined. For example, a typical combination would be bupivacaine 1.0 mg/mL plus fentanyl 2 mcg/mL, infused at a rate of 0.25 mL/kg/hour. Anesthetic agents have been associated with cardiac and neurotoxicity in the neonate. Opioids can lead to urinary retention, constipation, and profound respiratory depression. By combining agents, a synergistic effect can be achieved with lower doses of each, thus lowering the risk of toxicity. Toxicity of Anesthesia in the Neonate-Apoptotic neurodegeneration has also been found in nonhuman primates exposed to anesthetic agents. It is not known if these findings can be extrapolated as there are insufficient human studies to either support or refute the clinical applicability of the animal research in this area. Anaesthetic management of the preterm neonate: The anesthesiologist is usually called to administer anaesthesia in the preterm for the following situations * PDA ligation (20–30% incidence in moderately premature neonates) * Laparotomy for NEC or spontaneous bowel perforation * Laparotomy for reanastomosis of bowel or relief of adhesions * Inguinal hernia repair (2% incidence in females and 7–30% incidence in males with 60% risk of incarceration * Fundoplication for unresolving and symptomatic oesophageal reflux * Vascular access under X-ray control * Vitrectomy or laser surgery for retinopathy of prematurity * CSF drainage or ventriculoperitoneal shunt insertion for obstructive hydrocephalus after intraventricular hemorrhage * CT and MRI scanning to evaluate cerebral damage. Anesthetizing a preterm neonate requires constant vigilance, rapid recognition of events and trends, and swift intervention.

Routine Monitoring Requirements for Neonatal Surgery

Routine: Precordial or esophageal stethoscope, Pulse oximeter, Electrocardiogram, Blood pressure-Noninvasive, Arterial line—umbilical artery catheter, radial, femoral, Temperature Core—rectal, esophageal, nasopharyngeal, Skin, End-tidal CO_2, Peak inspiratory pressure, tidal volume, positive end-expiratory pressure, Fraction of inspired oxygen (FiO_2), Blood glucose
Optional: Central venous pressure, Blood gases—pH, PCO_2, PO_2, Urine output, Electrolytes

Host factors to consider during Neonatal Anesthesia

Airway: Large tongue, narrowest portion of the airway- cricoid cartilage, angle between the oropharynx and the laryngopharynx is more acute neonatal glottis is at C4 (as opposed to C5 in adults), infant's large occiput
Breathing: Obligate nose breathers, Higher O2 consumption, Higher closing volume, Higher MV:FRC (i.e. have to maintain elevated RR), Compliant ribs and less Type 1 muscle in the diaphragm, neonate responds to hypoxia paradoxically: i.e., with apnea instead of hyperpnea. Hemoglobin F has a higher affinity for oxygen with decreased unloading leading to tissue hypoxia
Circulation: Easy return to persistent fetal circulation with any insult which increases PVR (pain, hypothermia, hypoxemia, hypercarbia, acidosis, nitrous oxide, high inflating pulmonary pressures), SVR is relatively fixed because of immature autonomic control of blood pressure with large arteries in a relatively dilated state blood loss during surgery can rapidly lead to hypovolemia, hypotension and shock, poor diastolic function, the left ventricle is less compliant and cardiac output depends more on the heart rate, associated cardiac congenital defects, PDA, anaesthesia blunts the baroreflexes in premature infants, further limiting the ability to compensate for hypovolemia
CNS: Preterm neonate is at a greater risk for intracranial hemorrhage secondarily to hypoxia, hypercarbia, fluctuations in blood pressure or venous pressure (increased intrathoracic pressure), low or high hemoglobin, and pain
Thermoregulation: Neonates lose heat rapidly to their surroundings due to a combination of increased: surface area to volume ratio, skin conductance (little subcutaneous fat) and evaporative heat loss (reduced skin keratin content) resulting in a higher thermoneutral temperature of 32 C. Simultaneously, they are unable to shiver and rely upon brown fat metabolism for thermogenesis. Consequences of hypothermia include pulmonary hypertension, delayed drug metabolism, hypoxia, and apnea.
Glucose: Very limited glycogen stores. limited ketogenesis and lipolysis capability, asymptomatic hypoglycemia, hyperglycemia due to high catecholamines and deficient insulin response
Fluids & electrolytes: Limited renal concentrating ability, increased insensible loss owing to a "thin" skin and increased ratio of surface area to volume, cannot handle a large free water load, tendency toward hyponatremia, volume overload and congestive heart failure due to lower GFR, especially if too much free water is administered during surgery, wastes small amounts of bicarbonate, owing to an immature proximal tubule; infants are born with a mild proximal renal tubular acidosis
Pharmacokinetics: Decreased clearance of some drugs, especially morphine and its active metabolite M6G, Immature liver function results in decreased biotransformation of many drugs (e.g. opioids/local anesthetics) by the cytochrome P450 and other enzyme systems
Pharmacodynamics: Highly variable

TABLE 1 Assessment at the preoperative visit (Factor -check)

Airway: Oro/nasopharyngeal airway, endotracheal tube size, length, cuff. Intubation details/ difficulties. Suctioning requirements

Breathing: Recent arterial blood gas/chest radiograph, inspired oxygen/ nitric oxide, ventilator settings (mode, inspiratory/positive end expiratory pressures, rate), chest drains

Circulation: Intravascular access, pulse rate, blood pressure, central venous pressure (plus trends). Capillary refill time, urine output, inotrope requirements

Disability: Wakefulness, sedation, paralysis. Neurological deficits

Exposure: Core temperature, coreeperipheral difference

Fluids/infusions: Maintenance fluids/requirements. Blood/ clotting products available (capillary samples overestimate haemoglobin). Stoma/ nasogastric tube output

Glucose: Recent blood glucose. Total parenteral nutrition/10% dextrose/ insulin infusion rates

Weight: Drug dose calculations

TABLE 2 Common neonatal surgical conditions

General surgery: Tracheoesophageal fistula, Congenital diaphragmatic hernia, Gastroschisis/exomphalos, Pyloromyotomy, Laparotomy (e.g. atresia/malrotation/ Hirschsprung), Central venous access, Inguinal hernia repair, Imperforate anus *Neurosurgery:* Myelomeningocoele, Encephalocoele, Ventriculoperitoneal shunt *Plastic surgery:* Cleft lip/palate *Eye surgery-* Examination under anaesthesia, Laser treatment, Congenital cataract *Radiology:* Diagnostic cardiac catheter, Interventional cardiac catheter (e.g. atrial septostomy), Other radiological interventions-i.e. magnetic resonance imaging) *Urological surgery:* Posterior urethral valve excision, Cystoscopy

Neonatal/Pediatric anesthetic Drugs

Premedication

Atropine:	10 mcg/kg -IV - Induction;
	20 mcg/kg -IM - 30 min preop.,;
	40 mcg/kg -PO - 60 min preop.
Chloral hydrate:	25-50 mg/kg -PO - 60 min preop.
Clonidine :	4 mcg/kg - PO - 90-120 min preop.
Droperidol :	50-100 mcg/kg - PO - 60 min preop.
Midazolam:	0.5 mg/kg - PO - 30 min preop.
Morphine:	200-250 mcg/kg - IM - 30 min preop.

Pethidine compound Injection (Inj. Peth. Co.: 1 ml contains Pethidine 25 mg, Promethazine 6.25 mg. Chlorpromazine 6.25 mg) : 0.06-0.08 ml/kg - IM - 45 min preop. (Max. dose 1.5 ml)

Temazepam:	0.5-1.0 mg/kg - PO - 60 min preop.
Triclofos:	50-75 mg/kg - PO - 45 min preop.
Trimeprazine:	2 mg/kg - PO - 90 min preop.

Induction

Etomidate:	0.3 mg/kg - IV
Ketamine:	2 mg/kg - IV; 5-7 mg/kg - IM
Propofol:	2-3 mg/kg - IV; — if unpremedicated 3-5 mg/kg - IV
Thiopental:	4-6 mg/kg - IV;— neonates 2-4 mg/kg - IV

Muscle relaxants

Atracurium:	0.5 mg/kg
Cis-atracurium:	0.2-0.4 mg/kg
Mivacurium:	0.1-0.2 mg/kg
Pancuronium:	0.1 mg/kg
Rocuronium:	0.6 mg/kg
Suxamethonium:	1-2 mg/kg
Vecuronium:	0.1 mg/kg

* Cisatracurium:	is preferred in patients with hepatic or renal impairment as it spontaneously dissociates into inert metabolites. However, it produces histamine release when injected rapidly.
* Pancuronium:	has few cardiovascular effects but it can cause histamine release. It has a slow onset and long duration of action.
* Succinylcholine:	Causes - ICP. Ensure deep anesthesia, use IV lidocaine, and a defasciculating dose of a nondepolarizing muscle relaxant if there is a possibility of - ICP, e.g., head injury.

Reversal

Atropine:	20 mcg/kg
Glycopyrrolate:	10 mcg/kg
Neostigmine:	50 mcg/kg

Robinul-Neostigmine is neostigmine methylsulphate 2.5 mg plus glycopyrronium bromide 500 mcg in 1 ml of solution. Add ampoule to 4 ml normal saline, then reversal dose is 1 ml per 10 kg.

Intra-operative analgesia

Alfentanil:	30-50 mcg/kg as slow bolus, supplemental doses 15 mcg/kg; Infusion: 50-100 mcg/kg as slow bolus, then 0.5-1 mcg/kg/min
Fentanyl:	2-5 mcg/kg; For cardiac surgery : up to 25 mcg/kg
Morphine sulphate:	50-200 mcg/kg
Remifentanil:	Infusion: 300 mcg/kg in 50 ml of 5% dextrose; Loading dose : 1-2 mcg/kg, Infusion: 0.1-2 mcg/kg/min

Mid to moderate postoperative pain

Codeine Phosphate:	1-1.5 mg/kg - IM, PO, PR - 6-hourly
Diclofenac:	1 mg/kg (over 1 yr) - PO, PR - 8-hourly
Ibuprofen:	5-10 mg/kg (over 7 kg) - PO - 8-hourly
Paracetamol:	20 mg/kg - PO, PR - 6-hourly;
	Rectal loading dose (if > 44 weeks postconception) 30-40 mg/kg - PR - Once
Oramorph:	400 mcg/kg - PO - 4-hourly

Severe postoperative pain

Morphine:	50-100 mcg/kg IV incremental boluses or 200 mcg/kg IM
Morphine infusion:	1 mg/kg in 50 ml saline or 5% dextrose, i.e. 20 mcg/kg/ml
	Rate : 1-2 ml/h (20-40 mcg/kg/h)
Morphine NCA:	1 mg/kg morphine in 50 ml saline or 5% dextrose
	Rate: 1 ml/h. Bolus: 1 ml. Lockout: 20 min
Morphine PCA:	1 mg/kg morphine in 50 ml saline or 5% dextrose
	Rate: 0.2 ml/h. Bolus: 1 ml. Lockout: 5 min

NB: Morphine infusions should be in a dedicated IVI or have an antireflux valve.

Antagonists

Naloxone:	5-10 mcg/kg IV incrementally
Flumazenil:	10-20 mcg/kg IV, repeat if necessary

Anti-emetics

Cyclizine:	1 mg/kg - IV - 8-hourly
Dexamethosone:	0.15 mg/kg - IV - 6-hourly
Droperidol:	20-75 mcg/kg - IV - Intra-operative only
Metoclopramide:	0.15 mg/kg - IV, PO - 8-hourly
Ondansetron:	0.1-0.15 mg/kg - IV, PO - 8-hourly
Prochlorperazine:	0.25 mg/kg - IV, PO, PR - 8-hourly

Regional analgesia doses

Caudal extradural blockade:	Sacral: 0.5 mg/kg 0.25% bupivacaine
	Lumbar: 1 ml/kg 0.25% bupivacaine
	Thoracolumbar: 1.25 ml/kg 0.19% bupivacaine
Supplements to extend duration of block:	Ketamine 0.5 mg/kg (preservative-free)
	Clonidine 1 mcg/kg
	Diamorphine 30 mcg/kg
	Morphine 50 mcg/kg (preservative-free)
Lumbar epidural: (intra-operative)	0.75 ml/kg of 0.25% bupivacaine (or 0.2 % ropivacaine)
Epidural infusion:	60 ml of 0.125% bupivacaine + 1 mg preservative-free morphine
	Rate: 0.1-0.4 ml/kg/h
Spinal block:	0.1 ml/kg 0.5% 'heavy' bupivacaine + 0.06 ml for needle deadspace
Wound infiltration:	1 mg/kg 0.25% bupivacaine

References & Further Reading: 1. Principles of anaesthesia for term neonates: an updated practical guide, Andrew Pittaway 2. Anesthesia and Pain Management in Neonates: Perioperative TeamworkJohn J. McCloskey, MD, of the Children's Hospital of Philadelphia, Pennsylvania, http://www.medscape.org/viewarticle/584658, 3. Anesthetic Management of a Neonate with a Surgical Emergency Lynne G. Maxwell, M.D. 4. Taneja B, Srivastava V, Saxena KN. Physiological and anaesthetic considerations for the preterm neonate undergoing surgery. J Neonatal Surg 2012;1:14

Refer to Appendix-A, Page 1088 for the "Causes and Management of Hypoxia during Anesthesia"
Refer to Appendix-F, Page 1096 for "Neonatal Perioperative Management"

PRENATAL DIAGNOSIS

Fetal medicine is a complex multidisciplinary undertaking with a team consisting of the following:

*An obstetrician, who manages the pregnancy and performs many minimally invasive interventions such as percutaneous shunt and catheter placement
*A perinatologist or geneticist, who focuses on prenatal diagnosis, prognosis, genetic counseling, and the procedures involved in prenatal diagnosis
*A neonatologist or pediatric surgeon, who is responsible for the continued postnatal management of the fetus' disease process and formulates the fetal treatment plan
*An obstetric sonologist who has expertise in defining the fetal diagnosis and its severity and guiding diagnostic and therapeutic procedures
*Specialists, such as cardiologists, neurologists, and urologists, depending on the lesion.

The advantage of prenatal diagnosis of fetal malformations is that genetic counseling can be provided. In addition, the parents, obstetrician, geneticist, and other specialists can discuss options ranging from abortion to intrauterine medical and surgical treatments. The optimal time, mode, and place of delivery can be determined, and a postnatal treatment plan can be formulated.

Prenatal diagnosis is recommended in the following cases:

*The pregnant woman is 35 years or older at the time of delivery.
*She or her parents have had a previous child with a chromosomal abnormality.
*She has a history of recurrent abortions, or her husband's previous wife experienced several miscarriages.
*A history of parental consanguinity is present.
*The couple is known to be carriers of a chromosomal translocation.
*The pregnant woman is affected with type 1 diabetes mellitus, epilepsy, or myotonic dystrophy.
*She is exposed to viral infections, such as rubella or cytomegalovirus.
*The mother is exposed to excessive medication or to environmental hazards.
*In her or her spouse's family, a history of Down syndrome or some other chromosomal abnormality is present.
*A history of single gene disorder is present in her or her spouse's family.
*Her male relatives have Duchenne muscular dystrophy or severe hemophilia.
*She is suspected of having some other harmful gene on her X chromosomes.
*The fetus is diagnosed in utero to have some hereditary error of metabolism.
*The fetus is detected to be at increased risk for a NTD.
Prenatal diagnosis uses various noninvasive and invasive techniques to determine the health of, the condition of, or any abnormality in an unborn fetus.

Noninvasive techniques
* Fetal visualization- Ultrasound, Fetal echocardiography, Magnetic resonance imaging (MRI), Radiography
* Screening for neural tube defects (NTDs) - Measuring maternal serum alpha-fetoprotein (MSAFP)
* Screening for fetal Down syndrome-Measuring MSAFP, Measuring maternal unconjugated estriol, Measuring maternal serum beta-human chorionic gonadotropin (HCG)
* Separation of fetal cells from the mother's blood
* Assessment of fetal-specific DNA methylation ratio

Invasive techniques
* Fetal visualization-Embryoscopy, Fetoscopy
*Fetal tissue sampling- Amniocentesis, Chorionic villus sampling (CVS), Percutaneous umbilical blood sampling (PUBS), Percutaneous skin biopsy, Other organ biopsies, including muscle and liver biopsy
* Preimplantation biopsy of blastocysts obtained by in vitro fertilization
* Cytogenetic investigations-Detection of chromosomal aberrations, Fluorescent in situ hybridization(FISH)
*Molecular genetic techniques- Linkage analysis using

microsatellite markers, Restriction fragment length polymorphisms (RFLPs), Single nucleotide polymorphisms (SNPs)- DNA chip, Dynamic allele-specific hybridization (DASH)
Directed tests are invasive and pose some risk to the mother and fetus, but they directly analyze the fetal material and confirm the diagnosis. Special circumstances indicate the use of these tests, which are not screening tests. Indications for Diagnostic Tests

Conditions that increase the risk of chromosomal anomaly include the following: *Advanced maternal age (>35 y), the most common indication *Previous offspring with chromosomal anomalies or other birth defects *Parental balanced translocation, inversion (manifests as recurrent pregnancy loss), or both *Suggestive fetal ultrasonographic findings *Positive maternal screening test findings *Mother having a disease or being exposed to drugs, medications, or infections known to be associated with congenital malformations in the fetus *Mendelian genetic trait in the parents *Molecular DNA diagnosis (cystic fibrosis, homozygous hemoglobin sickle disease [HbSS], fragile X) *Enzymatic activities in villi, amniocytes, or both (Tay-Sachs disease, Refsum disease) *Precursor levels in cell-free amniotic fluid (17-OH-progesterone in congenital adrenal hyperplasia) Genetic counseling As a prerequisite and as follow-up to prenatal diagnosis, families must be informed about the diagnosis, severity, prognosis, and available options for treatment and continuation of pregnancy.

First trimester: Maternal serum hormones & proteins,Ultrasound abdomen,transvaginal USG,amniocentesis,chorionic villus sampling, endoscopy, embryo biopsy
Second trimester: USG anomaly scan,Doppler USG,fetal echocardiography,maternal serum alpha fetoprotein,fetal MRI,amniocentesis,fetoscopy,Percutaneous umbilical blood sampling (PUBS), Percutaneous placental, skin biopsy
& Other organ biopsies, including muscle and liver biopsy
Maternal serum alpha-fetoprotein test : Maternal serum alpha-fetoprotein (AFP) levels at 16-20 weeks' gestation are used to screen for open neural tube defects. The implications of an elevated AFP level vary with gestation, as well as with maternal weight and race. If an elevated AFP level is found, the test is followed by a targeted ultrasound and, perhaps, amniocentesis to distinguish among the possible etiologies.
Causes of an elevated maternal serum AFP level include the following: *Neural tube defects *Open abdominal wall defects *Aneuploidy *Renal diseases such as congenital nephrosis, infantile polycystic disease, and bilateral renal agenesis *Skin diseases such as ectodermal dysplasia and aplasia cutis congenita *Cystic adenomatoid malformation of the lung *Maternal hepatic and ovarian tumors *Uterine and placental anomalies *Multiple gestation *Fetomaternal hemorrhage *Fetal demise *Causes of low maternal serum AFP levels include the following:* *Trisomy 18 *Trisomy 13 *Insulin-dependent diabetes mellitus in the mother **The triple-panel test :** The panel includes maternal serum AFP, serum b -human chorionic gonadotropin (b -HCG), and unconjugated estriol. The panel, along with maternal age, is a more sensitive (60-91%) screen for fetal aneuploidy. Maternal weight, race, and multiple pregnancies may affect the risk calculation. In a fetus with Down syndrome, b -HCG levels are elevated, and the other two levels are decreased. The triple panel can detect 57-67% of fetuses with Down syndrome in women younger than 35 years and 87% in older women.
Chorionic villous sampling: Chorionic villous sampling (CVS) is the technique of choice for prenatal diagnosis prior to 12 weeks' gestation for detection of a chromosomal anomaly, DNA molecular diagnosis of classic genetic disorders, and the detection of defects in lysosomal enzymes or mucopolysaccharidoses. A diagnosis of enzymatic defects, such as 21-hydroxylase deficiency that causes congenital adrenal hyperplasia, can be made with an allele-specific amplification analysis technique of DNA obtained with CVS. A preliminary ultrasound is performed to establish fetal viability, gestation, and anatomy and to determine the placental location. A sample of placental tissue is obtained using a 16-gauge polyethylene catheter for analysis under ultrasonographic guidance. The test is usually performed at 8-12 weeks' gestation. The approach is based on the placental location. A transabdominal approach is preferred for anterior and fundal placentas after 13 weeks' gestation and in active vaginal and cervical infections. The sample is smaller than that obtained

with the transcervical method. The transcervical approach is indicated in cases with interposed bowel loops or uterine retroversion and a posterior or low-lying placenta. The transvaginal approach has limited application and is used when the placenta is placed posteriorly, the uterus is retroverted and retroflexed, and the cervical canal points towards the abdomen. Chromosomal analysis of the sample is performed in 2 ways. The direct method evaluates the metaphysis from the outer layer of cytotrophoblasts in the chorionic villi. This method provides results in 2 days. A long-term culture of the inner mesenchymal layer of trophoblasts provides results in 10-14 days. These results more closely correlate with the true karyotype. An abnormal direct result has to be confirmed with long-term cultures of trophoblasts, amniotic cells, or fetal lymphocytes. Rarely, a normal direct result is followed by abnormal culture findings, which are confirmed with fetal tissue results. Chromosomal mosaicism occurs in 1.2-2.5% of the samples and may cause diagnostic error. The mosaicism is purely extraembryonic in 70-80% of the cases, and it is more common in direct preparations. If found in both direct preparation and long-term cultures, a follow-up ultrasonographic level 2 screening for anomalies and amniocentesis or cordocentesis are indicated to verify mosaicism in the fetal blood. Maternal cell contamination may also distort the results. Complications associated with CVS include the following: *Pregnancy loss is 0.6-0.8% more common than the natural pregnancy loss rate in the first trimester and more common that the rate in midtrimester amniocentesis. Limb reduction defects and oromandibular malformations are more likely in some studies, especially if the procedure is performed prior to 10 weeks' gestation. *Fetomaternal transfusion can occur regardless of the approach used. Thus, Rh isoimmunization is considered a relative contraindication, and Rh immunoprophylaxis is administered to Rh-negative women after the procedure.

Early amniocentesis : This technique, performed at 12-14 weeks' gestation, assists in the diagnosis of chromosomal anomalies by providing fetal cells for karyotyping. It can also lead to the diagnosis of structural anomalies such as neural tube defects and omphalocele through the measurement of AFP and acetylcholinesterase levels. It is preferred to CVS in situations in which CVS is not reliable, such as twin pregnancy with fused placentae and in certain biochemical disorders. The procedure consists of the aspiration of amniotic fluid (approximately 1 mL/wk of gestation) from an amniotic fluid pocket with a 22-gauge needle and ultrasonographic guidance. Complications associated with amniocentesis include uterine bleeding (1.9%), uterine cramping, leakage of amniotic fluid (2.9%), pregnancy loss (1.4-4.2%), increased risk of club foot when performed prior to 12 weeks' gestation, failed procedure due to tenting of the membranes ahead of the needle, and culture failure rates of 1% overall and 5% if the procedure is performed prior to 12 weeks' gestation. Pseudomosaicism and maternal contamination are less likely than with CVS.

Preimplantation biopsy : This controversial procedure is performed for preimplantation diagnosis in a fetus of parents with substantial risk of a known genetic disorder and in women with repeated miscarriages due to chromosomal translocation. At the 8-cell stage of the embryo, a single cell is removed and analyzed (blastomere biopsy) for X-linked recessive diseases. Only XX embryos are transferred following in vitro fertilization. More trophectodermal cells can be removed from the blastocyst for analysis. Because it has the same genetic constitution as the ovum, the second polar body can also be analyzed for diseases with known gene defects such as cystic fibrosis, hemophilia, and a 1-antitrypsin deficiency.

Midtrimester amniocentesis: Amniocentesis performed at 16-18 weeks' gestation is the criterion standard of prenatal diagnostic techniques in both efficacy and safety. It is offered to all women older than 35 years or with an elevated serum AFP level. Genetic counseling to evaluate genetic risks and detailed ultrasonography to estimate gestation, placental location, and amount of amniotic fluid are important prior to the procedure. The procedure is the same as that of amniocentesis in early gestation, except that 20-30 mL of amniotic fluid is aspirated for analysis. The amniotic fluid phase can be analyzed for several substances. *AFP and acetylcholinesterase levels are used to identify a fetus with a neural tube defect, with 98% sensitivity.

*Bilirubin levels in amniotic fluid are elevated in isoimmune hemolysis, and the risk to the fetus

*A lecithin-to-sphingomyelin ratio of greater than 2, as measured chromatographically in a noncontaminated sample, suggests lung maturity, except in fetuses of mothers with diabetes. The presence of phosphatidyl glycerol in amniotic fluid indicates lung maturity, particularly in fetuses of mothers with diabetes. Saturated phosphatidylcholine is unaffected

by contamination with blood. A combination of these tests provides a more accurate indication of lung maturity.

*Enzyme analysis and measurement of metabolite levels, used for the diagnosis of urea cycle disorders and of other inborn errors of metabolism *Chromosome analysis through direct metaphase visualization is the traditional method; results are obtained in 1-2 weeks. FISH, when used in addition to standard cytogenetics, can analyze fetal cells for abnormalities in chromosomes 21, 18, 13, X, and Y and provide results in 48-72 hours. FISH can also detect microdeletions found in Prader-Willi, DiGeorge, Williams, and Angelman syndromes. *Direct DNA analysis is done with polymerase chain reaction (PCR) gene amplification, followed by Southern blot analysis to detect gene deletions.

* Allele-specific oligonucleotide (ASO) analysis measures the specific binding of labeled probes to normal DNA or mutant sequences to detect gene mutations. This technique is important in identifying disorders in which multiple mutations have to be screened for, such as cystic fibrosis and thalassemia, or in which a restriction site is not created, such as Duchenne muscular dystrophy, Tay-Sachs disease, and phenylketonuria. *Indirect DNA methods, such as linkage analysis with restriction fragment length polymorphisms (RFLPs), are performed in affected individuals and multiple other family members. This can help in making the diagnosis of diseases in which the exact gene defect and location are not known. Crossover changes between the gene and the RFLP probe can distort the results. * Molecular analysis of the fibroblast growth factor receptor 3 gene with direct and restriction enzyme analysis can help to diagnose thanatophoric dysplasia. Fetal DNA obtained by amniocentesis can be analyzed for the same deletion as that of the index case.

Percutaneous umbilical blood sampling or cordocentesis :PUBS
The greatest advantage of this technique is that it provides a direct fetal sample and access to the fetus for in utero treatment. With ultrasound guidance, a sample of fetal blood is obtained from the umbilical vessel close to the cord insertion near the placenta. A 20- to 27-gauge needle is used, and the approach can be transplacental in an anterior placenta or transamniotic in a posterior placenta. Diagnostic studies that can be performed include the following:
*Direct karyotyping of fetal lymphocytes can provide results within 24-72 hours. *DNA studies can be used to diagnose metabolic diseases. *Hematologic problems are especially amenable to this technique. The diagnoses of thalassemias, sickle cell disease, hemophilia, von Willebrand disease, and alloimmune thrombocytopenia can be made. In Rh-isoimmunized fetuses, diagnosis and treatment of fetal anemia and thrombocytopenia is possible, as is intrauterine transfusion. *Immunologic tests can be performed on blood samples for diagnosis of fetal infections (e.g., specific immunoglobulin M [IgM] for toxoplasmosis, rubella, cytomegalovirus [CMV], varicella zoster, HIV). Viral DNA can be detected using PCR for certain infections, such as parvovirus B19. *Determine fetal PaO_2, PCO_2, and pH levels, as these can provide critical indicators of fetal well-being in a small-for-date or compromised fetus. These data can guide management decisions. Complications associated with cordocentesis are more common in posterior placentae and when the procedure is performed prior to 19 weeks' gestation. These include fetal loss (1-2.3%), preterm labor (5-9%), hematoma of the umbilical cord and placental abruption, chorioamnionitis (0.6%), fetal exsanguination from the procedure site, and Rh isoimmunization. Rh immunoprophylaxis is mandatory in all Rh-negative nonsensitized women after the procedure.

Fetal muscle and liver biopsy: Muscle biopsy is used in rare cases of Duchenne muscular dystrophy in which findings from all previous investigations are nondiagnostic. Dystrophin levels are measured in myoblasts by in situ hybridization. Fetal liver biopsies have also been performed to measure enzyme levels of glucose-6-phosphatase and ornithine transcarbamylase in patients with suspected glycogenesis and urea cycle disorders when direct DNA techniques are not sensitive.
Imaging Modalities In Prenatal Diagnosis

Ultrasonographic Examination

Ultrasonography is the single most valuable modality in the identification of fetal structural anomalies. It is also useful in the detection of abnormal growth patterns in the fetus, in estimating gestation, and in assessing fetal well-being in the third trimester and during labor and delivery. It is important in guiding the operator during procedures such as amniocentesis and cordocentesis. Ultrasonography is widely available and has no known adverse effects. Newer techniques, including high-resolution multiplanar imaging and Doppler imaging, have improved its

SUMMARY OF AMNIOCENTESIS AND CHORIONIC VILLUS SAMPLING INFORMATION

	Amniocentesis	CVS
Procedure	Amniotic fluid removed by needle and syringe needle insertion	Chorionic villi removed by transcervical (TC) catheter and syringe or transabdominal (TA)
Timing	15 to 17 weeks (greater than 12 weeks TA CVS only)	10 to 11-6/7 weeks
Added risk of miscarriage due to procedure	0.5-1.0%	TA 1-2% TC 2-6%
Fetal malformation risks	— (suggested but not proven)	1 in 3000 vascular limb malformation
Chance of successful sampling	Approximately 99%	Approximately 99%. If unsuccessful, can follow with amniocentesis
Time required for cytogenetic (FISH may be available)	1 to 3 weeks	2-3 weeks (rapid direct technique)
Accuracy (chromosomes) Aneuploidy and major structural rearrangement	Highly accurate	Highly accurate
Mosaicism	Level 3 — Rare	Confined placental — 1.0-2.0%
Open neural tube defects	AFP in amniotic fluid detects approximately 95% of NTDs	Other tests required for detection.

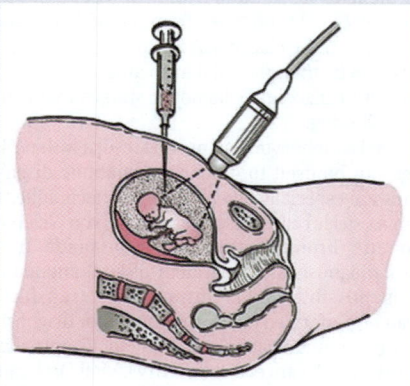

Amniocentesis

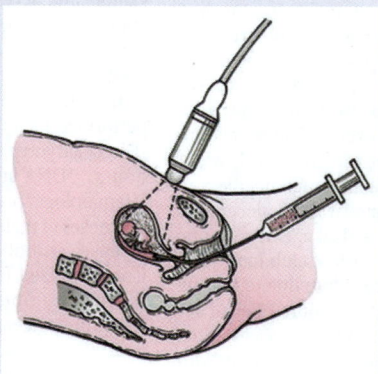

Transcervical CVS

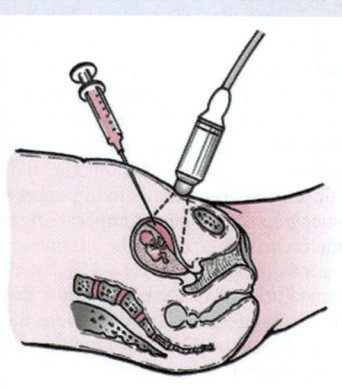

Transabdominal CVS

Amniocentesis

The amniocentesis (fig above) is early if done around the 12th week of gestation. Today several prenatal diagnostic clinics perform amniocenteses between the 14th and 16th week of pregnancy. Studies have shown an increased loss of amniotic fluid if the amniocentesis done before the 12th week and there is a risk of skeletal anomalies in particular of club feet secondary to oligoamnios. According to the age of pregnancy from 10 to 30 ml of fluid are obtained during the procedure. Foetal cells from the upper digestive system, urinary tract, skin and membranes are found in the fluid and recuperated by centrifugation of the specimen. They are then kept in culture for a period of 5 to10 days in a culture medium to which calf serum has been added. Cellular multiplication is then sufficient and allows the preparation of microscopic slides allowing the numerical and structural studies of the metaphasic chromosomes. Treatment of chromosomes during the slide preparation reveals segments of different intensity or banding patterns. Those bands reflect a variable ratio of AT;GC nucleotides on the chromatids and help to identify chromosome pairs.

Chorionic villus sampling (CVS)

The biopsy or aspiration of chorionic villi by the vaginal route (fig above) yields foetal cells, several of which are in the process of dividing and can be analyzed during the hours following the procedure. There is a risk of miscarriage and maternal cell contamination of the specimen thus leading a number of clinicians to abandon this procedure done before the 12th week of pregnancy. Reduction limb defects have been reported if the CVS is done towards the end of the first trimester. In special circumstances when the risk of genetic disease is high as for instance in hereditary metabolic diseases or if one of the parents is carrier of a balanced chromosomal translocation, this technique has the advantage of reaching a diagnosis around the 11th or 12th week of gestation.

Percutaneous umbilical blood sampling-
Refer to the Text for the details.

yield. Disadvantages are beam attenuation with maternal adipose tissue and poor images with an engaged fetal head or oligohydramnios.

Fetal gestation

*Gestation is best estimated in the first trimester, with an error range of 3-5 days. The range increases to 1 week at 12 weeks' gestation and 3 weeks at 36 weeks' gestation. *In the first trimester, the crown-rump length is the most accurate measure of gestation. This is measured from the top of the head to the bottom of the torso or the longest dimension of the fetus excluding the yolk sac and extremities. *In the second and third trimesters, parameters used to estimate gestation are the biparietal diameter (BPD), head circumference, abdominal circumference, and femur lengths. *BPD is measured on the transaxial view of the head from the outer edge of the cranium nearest the transducer to the inner edge of the cranium farthest from the transducer. BPD, which is measured at the level of the thalami, including the cavum septum pellucidum, should not be used in cases of hydrocephalus, abnormal head shape, or late in the third trimester when the head may be engaged. Measures such as a corrected BPD have been devised to take into account differences in head shape. *Abdominal circumference is the length of the outer perimeter of the fetal abdomen measured at the level of the stomach and intrahepatic umbilical vein on a transverse scan. This measure should not be used in cases of fetal growth abnormality in which the head size may be relatively preserved or in a fetus with diaphragmatic hernia. *In comparison, femoral length is more affected by caliper placement and technically more difficult. Femoral length may be affected by skeletal dysplasias, Down syndrome, and fetal growth abnormalities. Only the length of the diaphysis is measured for femur length. *A combination of these measurements yields the most accurate results.

Abnormal fetal growth patterns

*Intrauterine growth retardation (IUGR): Serial ultrasonography can be used to monitor the rate of increase in fetal biparietal diameter, abdominal circumference, and femoral length, thus helping to identify a growth-restricted fetus. *In the third trimester, ratios of morphometric measures such as abdominal circumference and femoral length are used to diagnose growth retardation. *Oligohydramnios and a poor biophysical score support the diagnosis of growth retardation secondary to uteroplacental insufficiency. Oligohydramnios is defined as the absence of amniotic fluid pockets or the presence of an amniotic fluid index (AFI; sum of the vertical distance of the largest pocket in each of 4 equal uterine quadrants) of less than 5. *Estimated fetal weights, derived by combining several parameters (usually head, abdominal, and femur measurements), are useful. However, they are inaccurate at the extremes of birth weight. Symmetric growth retardation begins earlier in gestation, affects both head and abdominal measurements, and is caused by chromosomal or genetic anomalies or intrauterine infections. *Macrosomia: Serial ultrasonography can be used to measure the ratio of abdominal circumference to head circumference to detect macrosomia.

Detection of Fetal Anomalies

Fetal CNS anomalies *Ultrasound is 95% sensitive in the diagnosis of hydrocephalus and myelomeningocele. *Ventriculomegaly has been defined in some studies by a measurement at the atrium of the lateral ventricle of more than 10 mm at any time during pregnancy. *In myelomeningocele, diagnosis is made by noting a divergence of the pedicles of the vertebrae or the presence of a fluid-filled sac. Some intracranial signs are associated, such as ventriculomegaly, small BPD, biconcave frontal bones at 18-24 weeks, a distorted position of the cerebellum, and obliteration of the cisterna magna, especially if associated with Chiari II malformation. *Diagnosis of anencephaly, encephalocele, craniosynostosis, and brain malformations, such as porencephaly can be made based on ultrasound findings. Fetuses with hydrocephalus or meningomyelocele should be evaluated for chromosomal abnormalities or anatomic defects in the cardiac, renal, and skeletal systems. Associated defects are present in 90-95% of cases.

Fetal chest abnormalities

*Pulmonary hypoplasia, pleural effusions, cystic adenomatoid malformations, sequestration, and bronchogenic cysts are all pulmonary lesions that can be diagnosed based on ultrasound findings. *Congenital diaphragmatic hernia (CDH): Diagnosis of CDH is made based on the presence of bowel or liver in the thorax with the accompanying blood supply, mediastinal shift, and pulmonary hypoplasia. Polyhydramnios may be present. After the diagnosis, serial ultrasonography should be performed to monitor fetal growth and hydramnios and to evaluate for cardiac anomalies. Workup may include ultrafast MRI, echocardiography, and karyotyping with amniocentesis to exclude associated anomalies. Hydrops is a predictor of a poor outcome.

Fetal cardiac abnormalities

*Detailed cardiac ultrasonography is indicated in fetuses with the following: *Chromosomal anomalies *Hydrops *Oligohydramnios or polyhydramnios *Exomphalos *Diaphragmatic hernia *Defects in other systems with known cardiac associations. *Other indications for a cardiac echo antenatally include the following: *Family history of congenital heart defect *Maternal diabetes or systemic lupus erythematosus (SLE) *Maternal lithium, alcohol, or progesterone intake *Fetal arrhythmias *M-mode echocardiography is used to measure chamber size, cardiac rhythm, pericardial effusions, and wall thickness and motion. Cross-sectional echocardiograms show the heart position and situs and the atrioventricular (AV) connections. Doppler echocardiograms show the direction and pattern of blood flow, and they can depict valvular regurgitation or stenotic lesions. *Prenatally diagnosed heart disease has been associated with reduced early neurologic morbidity in certain lesions, such as a hypoplastic left heart. Conversely, whereas a poorer prognosis was reported earlier in prenatal cohorts because more severe lesions are more likely to be detected, especially when they are associated with a structural or chromosomal defect.

Fetal gastrointestinal anomalies

Gastroschisis and omphalocele are easily detected on ultrasound. Ultrasonography has low sensitivity in the diagnosis of obstruction, which is indirectly indicated by the presence of polyhydramnios, poorly visualized gut distal to the obstruction, and a fluid-filled portion proximal to it. An echogenic bowel, meconium peritonitis, and pseudocyst formation are suggestive of cystic fibrosis. All of these findings indicate the need for further cytogenetic evaluation of the fetus.

Fetal genitourinary tract anomalies

Ultrasound can detect renal agenesis, cystic disease, obstructive lesions (ureteropelvic junction obstruction and posterior urethral valves), and renal tumors. Renal dimensions, parenchymal thinning and cysts, ratios of renal circumference to abdominal circumference, pelvic diameters, and urinary ascites can be assessed, along with urethral and bladder anatomy. The amniotic fluid volume provides an indication of renal function. Oligohydramnios is associated with a poor prognosis.

Fetal skeletal anomalies
A detailed fetal ultrasound attempts to rule out skeletal dysplasias, achondroplasia, osteogenesis imperfecta, polydactyly, and absence of a bone. Long bones are evaluated for size, shape, symmetry, and proportions of the different segments, and the skull is evaluated for shape and deformity. Examination of the spine and ribs helps in the delineation of the disorder. Identification of a skeletal dysplasia and prognosis are relatively accurate; however, in one study, a specific antenatal diagnosis was made in 60% of cases, but these were incorrect in 19% postnatally. According to some reports, 3-dimensional ultrasonography seems to provide additional visualization of skeletal deformities and abnormal spatial relationships, such as short ribs and absent bones, and to enable specific diagnosis.

Fetal chromosomal anomalies

In a recent meta-analysis, nuchal thickening was found to be the most accurate marker in the second trimester. It was associated with a 17-fold increased risk of Down syndrome. Nuchal thickening in the first trimester has a sensitivity of 60-70% for the detection of Down syndrome, with a 5% false-positive rate, whereas ultrasonography and biochemical screening, in combination, improve the sensitivity to 80%. Other single subtle markers (e.g., choroid plexus cysts, shortened long bones, echogenic bowel) are not sensitive.

MRI Examination

MRI is an important adjunct to ultrasonography. It is used mainly in the assessment of cases with equivocal ultrasonographic findings or when prenatal ultrasound is not reliable in the identification of fetal anomalies, such as in the setting of maternal obesity or oligohydramnios. The advantage of the newer fast and ultrafast sequence MRI is that they have minimized motion artifacts; thus, sedation is not needed. A variety of sequences have been used, including echoplanar, half-Fourier single-shot turbo spin-echo (HASTE), and fast spin-echo sequences. Of these, HASTE has proven to be an excellent method of fetal imaging. A recent meta-analysis showed that ultrafast MRI in the third trimester provided additional information compared to ultrasound in fetal diagnosis in 23-100% of cases, particularly those involving the posterior fossa of the head.

Advantages of MRI include the following : *Absence of ionizing radiation *Multiplanar capability *Large field of view *Superior soft tissue contrast enhancement *Good image quality in oligohydramnios *More precise volumetric measurement *Better intracranial delineation Limitations of MRI include the following: *Spatial resolution inferior to that of ultrasonography *Poor depiction prior to 20 weeks' gestation *Safety question - not approved by the Food and Drug Administration (FDA), but no known significant risk beyond the first trimester MRI may be used if other nonionizing imaging modalities are inadequate or if ionizing radiation would otherwise be required for further evaluation.

Indications for MRI evaluation include the following : *Fetal cerebral anomalies: MRI has been most successful in the identification of posterior fossa abnormalities, migrational anomalies (eg, lissencephaly, polymicrogyrias, schizencephaly) at 30-32 weeks' gestation, agenesis of the corpus callosum, white matter disease, hydrocephalus, and ischemic or hemorrhagic lesions. *Volumetric analysis: The size of the fetus or individual organs, such as the liver, can be determined. In CDH, volumetric measurements of the right fetal lung and the position of the left hepatic lobe appear to be good prognostic indicators and help in planning therapeutic interventions. *Congenital high airway obstruction syndrome: MRI can be used to confirm upper airway obstruction by demonstrating hyperinflation of both lungs and dilated fluid-filled airways below the level of obstruction. Fetal neck masses such as cystic hygromas and teratomas can be identified, allowing early intervention when indicated. *Congenital hemochromatosis: T2-weighted MRI can be used to confirm the diagnosis. *Amniotic band syndrome: MRI provides an accurate diagnosis.

CT Scanning : CT scanning has limited applications in prenatal diagnosis. It is used mainly when MRI is contraindicated in the mother (e.g., if she has a pacemaker, an intraocular metallic foreign body, or intracranial ferromagnetic surgical clips). The advantage of CT scanning is that it better delineates fetal bony anatomy than other imaging modalities. The limitations of CT scanning include possible teratogenesis due to ionizing radiation if it is performed in the first trimester and a risk of cancer induction. In children, a risk of mortality from cancer of 1 per 220-440 cases has been reported. Indications for CT scanning include pelvimetry and CT amniography to confirm monoamnionicity if ultrasonography provides inconclusive data.

Fetal Magnetocardiography : A prolonged QT interval or Wolff-Parkinson-White syndrome can be detected in the prenatal period on fetal magnetocardiograms through evaluating T waves and obtaining current arrow maps. A weak, prolonged T wave is likely a good indicator of the condition.

GENERAL PRINCIPLES FOR PRENATAL DIAGNOSIS PROGRAMS

1. All patients considering prenatal diagnosis should have access to professionals who are knowledgeable in the field and skilled in the procedures.

2. Each region should be integrated so that an entire range of services is available to each patient. Innovations in telemedicine technology promise to offer options for distance faceto- face counselling and ultrasound interpretation that are of particular relevance.

3. A suggested minimum caseload of 50 invasive procedures per year is recommended per practitioner in order to maintain an appropriate level of competence in the provision of invasive procedures. Exceptions to this minimum caseload may be justified on the basis of unique geographic circumstances; however, informed patient choice is paramount.

4. In order to maintain a high standard of efficiency, a cytogenetic laboratory should have a minimum workload of 100 prenatal specimens.

5. Each patient should have an appropriate assessment of family history and genetic counselling prior to undergoing invasive prenatal diagnosis.

6. Counselling should be given in a non-directive manner in order to allow an informed choice by the couple.

7. The distinction between screening and diagnostic investigations should be clarified, including the frequency of abnormal results, false-positive, and false-negative tests. Accuracy of results, frequency of need for repeat testing, and risk of pregnancy loss are of particular relevance with invasive prenatal diagnosis procedures. The couple should be reminded that normal test results do not rule out every genetic or structural abnormality in their fetus.

8. Prior to embarking on prenatal diagnosis testing, couples should be made aware of the full range of options when confronted with an abnormal test result. Prior commitment to termination of pregnancy following the diagnosis of fetal abnormality is not a prerequisite for prenatal diagnosis. Each centre must be aware of the local, regional, national, and international policies and protocols related to termination of pregnancy, and advise the couple of such before undertaking prenatal diagnosis. This is particularly important at gestations beyond 20 weeks.

9. It is recommended that an AFAFP assay be carried out on each sample of amniotic fluid received at the appropriate gestational age, regardless of the original indication for sampling.

10. The decision to karyotype amniotic fluid, chorionic villus, fetal blood or tissue samples obtained where the original indication for testing did not include karyotyping should be decided on an individual basis, with reference to regionally or provincially established policies or guidelines. Although often done, it is not mandatory to do a karyotypic analysis on all samples received. As a minimum requirement, before a final decision is made not to do chromosomal studies, the results of the available screening tests should be reviewed to determine if there is in fact an indication for karyotyping.

11. Determination of fetal sex for the purpose of sex selection procedures on a non-medical basis is inappropriate.

12. In the absence of a medical indication, genetic testing to determine paternity is not an indication for prenatal diagnosis with the possible exception of cases of sexual assault. If an assault has been reported, the police may have an interest in the DNA of the fetus, for example for comparison with the DNA of the sperm found at the place of assault or with the DNA of the suspected assailant. In this case the prenatal diagnosis could be done at the request of the woman and the law enforcement agency, and the DNA testing would be done at a forensic laboratory. If there are no criminal proceedings and the woman wishes to know whether the father of the fetus is her partner or the assailant, with the intent of abortion in the latter case, prenatal diagnosis could be justified if considered in the best interest of the couple. However, in view of the possibility that lawsuits might subsequently arise, the DNA testing should be done by a private laboratory, following guidelines for civil cases of paternity testing, and with appropriate counselling of the couple. In any case, prenatal diagnosis for paternity testing should not be done without appropriate counselling of the woman, and thorough legal consultation. If a woman has an invasive prenatal test for legitimate medical reasons such as maternal age, she may request that the leftover cells be used for paternity testing. There would normally be no grounds for the laboratory to refuse to give these cells to another lab for paternity testing. 13. Introduction of any new prenatal diagnostic investigation, or alteration of previously established approaches, requires careful careful follow-up and audit to assess risk, accuracy, and impact.

QUALITY OF EVIDENCE ASSESSMENT

The quality of evidence reported in these guidelines has been described using the Evaluation of Evidence criteria outlined in the Report of the Canadian Task Force on the Periodic Health Exam.

I: Evidence obtained from at least one properly randomized controlled trial.

II-1: Evidence from well-designed controlled trials without randomization.

II-2: Evidence from well-designed cohort (prospective or retrospective) or case-control studies, preferably from more than one centre or research group.

II-3: Evidence obtained from comparisons between times or places with or without the intervention. Dramatic results in uncontrolled experiments (such as the results of treatment with penicillin in the 1940's) could also be included in this category.

III: Opinions of respected authorities, based on clinical experience, descriptive studies, or reports of expert committees.

CLASSIFICATION OF RECOMMENDATIONS

Recommendations included in these guidelines have been adapted from the ranking method described in the Classification of Recommendations found in the Report of the Canadian Task Force on the Periodic Health Exam.

A.   There is good evidence to support the recommendation that the condition be specifically considered in a periodic health examination.

B.   There is fair evidence to support the recommendation that the condition be specifically considered in a periodic health examination.

C.   There is poor evidence regarding the inclusion or exclusion of the condition in a periodic health examination, but recommendations may be made on other grounds.

D.   There is fair evidence to support the recommendation that the condition not be considered in a periodic health examination.

E.   There is good evidence to support the recommendation that the condition be excluded from consideration in a periodic health examination.

SUMMARY OF MAJOR RECOMMENDATIONS

1. It is recommended that women at increased risk for having a child with a chromosomal anomaly be identified based on maternal age. (II-2 A) 2. It is recommended that maternal serum screening be used to identify women at increased risk for having a child with a chromosomal anomaly. Maternal serum screening can be used to modify a woman's age-related risks. (II-2 A) 3. It is recommended that maternal serum AFP screening be used to identify women at increased risk for having a child with a neural tube defect. (II-2 A) 4. It is recommended that an amniocentesis be offered to women at increased risk of having a child with a chromosome anomaly. (I A) 5. It is recommended that CVS be offered to women as an alternative to amniocentesis where resources exist. (I A) 6. Cordocentesis may be offered to high-risk women under certain circumstances. (II-2 B).

References & Further Reading:

1. Canadian Guidelines for Prenatal Diagnosis TECHNIQUES OF PRENATAL DIAGNOSISNo. 105, July 2001

2. http://emedicine.medscape.com/article/1200683-overview#showall

3. American College of Obstetrician and Gynecologists: Screening for fetal chromosomal abnormalities, ACOG Practice Bulletin No.77, *Obstet Gynecol* 109: 217-227, 2007.

4. The Contribution of Molecular Techniques in Prenatal Diagnosis and *Post mortem* Fetus with Multiple MalformationbRejane Gus Kesslerhttp://www.intechopen.com/articles/show/title/the-contribution-of-molecular-techniques-in-prenatal-diagnosis-and-post-mortem-fetus-with-multiple-m

5. Breathnach FM, Fleming A, Malone FD: The second trimester genetic sonogram, *Am J Med Genet C Semin Med Genet* 145C:62-72, 2007.

Fetal Therapy: Recently, medical and surgical fetal therapy has emerged as an option for the management of various fetal malformations, improving the long-term outcome of the fetus. *Termination of the pregnancy is an option for families in cases involving serious malformations that are incompatible with life. Examples of these conditions include severe chromosomal abnormalities associated with anomalies (e.g. trisomy 13), certain metabolic conditions, and anatomic defects, especially of the brain and kidneys. *Elective cesarean delivery is indicated in fetal malformations that can cause dystocia or in cases in which immediate surgical correction in a sterile environment is likely to improve outcome or when successful elective delivery of an affected fetus is unlikely to be achieved by the vaginal mode. Conjoined twins, large omphaloceles, severe hydrocephalus, ruptured meningomyelocele, large sacrococcygeal teratoma, and large cystic hygroma are some examples. *Preterm delivery is indicated in a fetal disorder in which continued gestation would adversely affect the function of the involved organ system or threaten viability of the fetus. Early correction after delivery should be available and be of proven benefit to the fetus. Urinary tract obstruction, hydronephrosis, progressive hydrocephalus, volvulus or meconium ileus causing intestinal ischemia, and hydrops fetalis with growth retardation are examples of such lesions. *Prenatal medical treatment is beneficial in a variety of diseases. With the availability of easier and safer access to the fetus, deficient nutrients, hormones, and substrates can be provided, and certain blocked metabolic pathways may be bypassed. Prior to selecting a case for fetal therapy, the fetal anomaly should be correctly diagnosed and its severity assessed. *The benefits of treatment should outweigh the risks if left untreated and the risks of the procedure itself to the fetus and mother. Other serious malformations should be excluded and pulmonary maturity ascertained prior to delivery, and adequate follow-up care should be provided after the intervention.*

Treatments for fetal disorders

*Neural tube defects:*All women are advised to take folic acid prior to conception (0.4 mg/d PO for 3 mo), and 4 mg/d is recommended for women with a previously affected child, beginning at least 1 month prior to conception through 3 months of pregnancy. *Congenital adrenal hyperplasia: *Since the differentiation of external genitalia begins at 7 weeks' gestation, the mothers of all fetuses at risk (those with a previously affected child) are given dexamethasone (0.25 mg PO qid) at 7-9 weeks. *Direct studies using probes or linkage DNA studies are performed with CVS. Affected female fetuses are identified at a rate of 1 case per 8 carrier parents. *Treatment is continued until term only in affected fetuses. Stress-dose glucocorticoids are administered at delivery and gradually tapered in the mother after delivery. *The long-term outcome of patients treated in utero is still being assessed. The treatment has proven effective in preventing masculinization. *Thyrotoxicosis:*Fetal thyrotoxicosis is usually seen in infants of mothers with Grave disease or autoimmune thyroiditis. The diagnosis is made with cordocentesis. *Maternal treatment with propylthiouracil (initial dose 300 mg/d PO, then titrate according to effect)

or methimazole is associated with a good fetal outcome. *Hypothyroidism: *Fetal hypothyroidism is linked to maternal hyperthyroidism, use of radioactive iodine, drugs, and excessive maternal iodine intake. *Fetal status is evaluated at ultrasonography and by direct cordocentesis. *Intra-amniotic L-thyroxine (500 mcg q2wk initiated at 34 wk of gestation) has been shown to cause regression of fetal goiters and normalization of hormone levels. *Methylmalonic acidemia: *This is caused be a deficiency of methylmalonyl CoA mutase or its coenzyme adenosylcobalamin, which results in an accumulation of methylmalonic acid and its precursors in body fluids. Clinically, patients present in the first few weeks of life with poor feeding, vomiting, hypotonia, lethargy, dehydration, ketosis and acidosis. *Prenatal cyanocobalamin has been empirically administered orally to the mother at a dose titrated to achieve high maternal plasma B12 levels and normal maternal urinary methylmalonic acid excretion. *The long-term effects on fetal development have not been studied extensively. *Multiple carboxylase deficiency: *This disorder is caused by a deficiency of holocarboxylase synthetase or biotinidase, two enzymes essential to rendering the carboxylases functional. The carboxylase enzymes are involved in the metabolic pathways of isoleucine, leucine, and valine. *Clinically, patients present in the first few weeks of life or later in childhood with hypotonia, seizures, vomiting, failure to thrive, dermatitis, developmental delay, hearing loss, and acidosis. *Maternal biotin supplementation may prevent neonatal complications. *Lung maturity induction: *In multiple studies, maternal corticosteroid therapy, used to induce lung maturity and surfactant synthesis in the fetus, has been proven effective in significantly reducing respiratory distress syndrome (RDS) in the neonatal period. Controlled studies have shown a reduction from 20.2% to 11.2%. *Betamethasone (12 mg IM q24h for 2 doses) or dexamethasone (6 mg IM q12h for 4 doses) is recommended for fetuses at 24–34 weeks' gestation who are at risk of preterm delivery. *Maternal HIV infection: Maternal administration of zidovudine (AZT), started at 14 weeks' gestation, continued throughout pregnancy, and given intravenously during labor, followed by treatment of the neonate for the first 6 weeks, has been documented to decrease the rate of vertical transmission from 25% to 8%. *Immune hydrops *Hemolytic disease of the fetus is a condition of fetal anemia caused by Rh isoimmunization. An antibody screen, performed periodically in a sensitized mother, can detect the presence and titer of maternal antibodies. *If the paternal screen for the antigen is positive, PCR can determine fetal blood group from samples obtained at amniocentesis or cordocentesis. Reverse transcriptase-polymerase chain reaction (RT-PCR) of fetal cells in maternal blood is also being used for the same purpose. *The fetuses at risk are then monitored with serial ultrasounds (for evidence of hydrops) and Doppler assessment of the velocity of blood flow in the middle cerebral artery (higher in anemic fetuses), starting at 16–18 weeks' gestation and repeated every 1–2 weeks until 35 weeks' gestation. *Alternatively, one can perform amniocentesis serially (10 day to 2 week intervals) with measurement of bilirubin, beginning at 18 weeks, and determine when the result is abnormal from the Queenan and Liley charts. *Serial cordocentesis is indicated for *The severely affected fetuses for direct measurement of hematocrit (Hct), reticulocyte count, and bilirubin. *Intrauterine transfusions can be performed as indicated based on the results of the diagnostic tests. Direct intravascular transfusions through umbilical vein puncture or a combination of intraperitoneal and intravascular transfusions can be used. The combination achieves a more stable Hct and delays the time to the next transfusion. *The volume in milliliters of intraperitoneal transfusion can be calculated as the (gestational age in weeks minus 20) X 10 and repeated at 2-week intervals until fetal erythropoiesis decreases.*Monitor this with Kleihauer Betke stains and size of fetal liver erythropoiesis decreases. *Monitor this with Kleihauer Betke stains and size of fetal liver and spleen on ultrasound as indicators of extramedullary hematopoiesis. Repeat at 3- to 4-week intervals, with monitoring of the fetal Hct level. *The intravascular transfusion alone aims to achieve a fetal Hct of 35- 40%. The intraperitoneal transfusion provides a reservoir of blood and achieves a final Hct of 50-60%. *A fetus with hydrops requires careful transfusion until the Hct level reaches 25%. Transfusion is repeated in 2 days and then weekly to achieve the final Hct level. *O-negative, CMV-negative allogenic or maternal blood is tested for infection, washed, packed (Hct level, 75-85%), filtered, irradiated with 2500 Gy, and then transfused. Repeat transfusions are indicated until pulmonary maturity or a gestational age of 35 weeks is reached.*Fetal thrombocytopenia *Maternal thrombocytopenia has many causes, many of which do not place the fetus at risk of bleeding. *In idiopathic thrombocytopenic purpura, the fetus has a low risk for intracranial hemorrhage. Scalp electrodes, forceps, and vacuum are not used at the time of delivery. In early labor, a fetal platelet count may be obtained via cordocentesis or a scalp blood smear. If the count is less than 20,000, a cesarean delivery may be preferred. *Alloimmune thrombocytopenia is the most common type of platelet isoimmunization that occurs in a PLA1 Ag–negative mother, with an incidence of 1 per 5000. If a history of an affected sibling exists, the direct fetal platelet count is measured with blood sampling, and maternal platelets can be transfused with cordocentesis. Disadvantages are the short life span of the platelets, which makes frequent transfusions necessary, and the possibility of further sensitization. Maternal intravenous immunoglobulin G (IVIG; 1 g/kg/wk) coadministered with corticosteroids has been tried with some good results. *Fetal hematopoietic stem cell transplantation *Hematopoietic stem cell (HSC) transplantation in utero is an attractive theoretical option for the treatment of congenital disease that can be diagnosed antenatally and improved by engraftment of HSCs. *Diseases theoretically amenable to HSC transplantation are hemoglobinopathies such as sickle cell disease and thalassemias, immune deficiency diseases, and inborn errors of metabolism. *Congenital heart disease *The precise diagnosis of congenital heart lesions with the aid of newer echocardiographic techniques has created the potential for prenatal surgery or interventional catheterization.

*In the treatment of hypoplastic left heart syndrome, umbilical vessel catheterization and balloon valvuloplasty in utero for aortic stenosis are being attempted, with equivocal results.*In critical pulmonary stenosis,

experimental valvotomy in utero may prevent right ventricular hypoplasia. · At present, the major goal of prenatal diagnosis of congenital heart lesions is genetic counseling and delivery at a tertiary center, where early and optimal management is possible in the neonatal period. *Fetal arrhythmias*Most fetal arrhythmias are benign, and 90% are atrial extrasystoles. These should be observed twice weekly to exclude sustained supraventricular extrasystoles or atrial flutter. In ventricular extrasystoles, myocardial ischemia and tumors (eg, rhabdomyomas) must be excluded. *Prerequisites prior to starting antiarrhythmic therapy include the following: *An understanding of the electrophysiologic basis of the abnormal rhythm and its natural history *Good understanding of the pharmacokinetics of the agent in the mother, fetus, and placenta *Maternal consent for treatment *Presence of hydrops fetalis with a sustained supraventricular arrhythmia *Early gestation with a sustained arrhythmia in which the risk for development of hydrops is perceived to be high *The disadvantages include early and late mortality in the mother and fetus. *Supraventricular tachycardias *These must be treated if they are sustained and associated with hydrops or upon evidence of left atrial preexcitation and a small foramen ovale. *Inpatient maternal treatment is started after 12-24 hours of fetal cardiac monitoring. *Maternal workup includes ECG to exclude a maternal Wolff-Parkinson-White syndrome and a determination of electrolyte, blood urea nitrogen (BUN), and creatinine levels prior to digoxin loading. *Digoxin is the first-line drug. Propranolol, procainamide, and quinidine have also been used. All fetal antiarrhythmic medications are associated with risks of proarrhythmia and mortality in both mother and fetus. Carefully select patients for treatment and monitor drug levels and toxicity. Structural defects, such as Ebstein anomaly and mitral insufficiency, must be excluded. *Congenital complete heart block *This is associated with major congenital heart disease in approximately 50% of cases. *Diagnoses have included left atrial isomerism, physiologically corrected transposition, atrioventricular canal defects, and ventricular septal defects. This group has a high incidence of congestive heart failure or cyanosis and requires postnatal permanent pacemakers. *The remaining cases (50%) are associated with maternal autoimmune diseases (eg, systemic lupus erythematosus, Sjögren disease).

Fetal Therapy: Surgery

Anesthesia: The major objectives are to ensure maternal and fetal safety. Specific goals are the prevention of maternal hypoxia and hypotension, together with the maintenance of optimal uterine blood flow. Lower doses of epidural and spinal anesthetic agents are needed in pregnant women because of increased epidural pressure and a lower volume of cerebrospinal fluid in the vertebral space. *To promote fetal safety, procedures are generally performed in the second trimester, if possible, to avoid potential teratogenicity from the anesthetic agents. *Fetal asphyxia: Normal maternal PaO_2 should be maintained, and blood pressure should be maintained (with intravenous fluids and, if necessary, ephedrine, a vasopressor with central adrenergic stimulant action). *Tocolysis: Uterine contractions are stimulated with the uterine incision and need to be stopped before preterm labor sets in. The agents used for this purpose include

Indications and rationale for in-utero surgery on the fetus, placenta, cord or membranes

	Pathophysiology	Rationale for in-utero therapy
Surgery on the fetus :		
1. Congenital diaphragmatic hernia	Pulmonary hypoplasia and pulmonary hypertension	Timely reversal of pulmonary hypoplasia and prevention of pulmonary hypertension
2. Lower urinary tract obstruction	Progressive renal damage by obstruction. Pulmonary hypoplasia by oligohydramnios	Urinary diversion prevents obstructive uropathy and restores amniotic fluid volume
3. Sacrococcygeal teratoma	High output cardiac failure by arteriovenous shunting. Fetal anemia by tumor growth and/or bleeding within a tumor	Cessation of steal phenomenon Reversal of cardiac failure; prevention of polyhydramnios
4. Thoracic space-occupying lesions	Pulmonary hypoplasia (space-occupying mass). Hydrops by impaired venous return (mediastinal compression)	Prevention of pulmonary hypoplasia and cardiac failure
5. Neural tube defects	Damage to exposed neural tube; cerebrospinal fluid leak, leading to Chiari malformation and hydrocephalus	Covering exposed spinal cord, cessation of leakage preventing hydrocephaly and reversing cerebellar herniation
6. Cardiac malformations	Critical lesions causing irreversible hypoplasia or damage	Prevention of hypoplasia or arrest of progression of damage
Surgery on the placenta, cord on membranes :		
7. Chorioangioma	High output cardiac failure by arteriovenous shunting and polyhydramnios	prevention of cardiac failure and hydrops fetoplacentalis
8. Amniotic bands	Progressive constrictions causing irreversible neurological or vascular damage	Prevention of limb deformities and function loss
9. Abnormal monochorionic twinning : * Twin-to-twin transfusion	Intertwin transfusion leads to oligopolyhydramnios sequence, hemodynamic changes; obstetric complications (preterm labor and rupture of the membranes)	Bichorionization stops intertwin transfusion, reverses cardiac failure, preventing neurological damage, delaying delivery (amnio drainage)
* Fetus acardiacus and discordant anomalies	Discordant anomalies: where one fetus can be threat to the other, or to avoid termination of entire pregnancy	Fetocide to improve changes of the other fetus; avoidance of termination of entire pregnancy

indomethacin, magnesium sulphate, and terbutaline. *Indomethacin is administered preoperatively and continued postoperatively for 3–5 days. Fetal adverse effects include premature closure of the ductus arteriosus. *Anesthetic agents commonly used are isoflurane inhalation with 100% oxygen along with muscle relaxants. For surgeries involving direct fetal manipulation, direct intramuscular fentanyl and pancuronium (a muscle relaxant and vagolytic) administered to the fetus have been tried prior to hysterotomy under ultrasound guidance.

Monitoring During Surgery: The parameters monitored during and after surgery include the following: *Myometrial contractions and intrauterine pressures *Maternal blood pressure, ECG, and pulse oximetric and blood gas levels *Fetal pulse oximetric measurement (50-60% saturation), heart rate, blood gases, and ECG *Ultrasonographic findings in cases of fetoscopic surgery *Fetal temperature (Maintain temperature with continuous warm sodium chloride irrigation, minimized exposure, and increased ambient temperature.)

Surgical Interventions: Three approaches are currently used for invasive fetal therapy. Ultrasonography-guided vesicoamniotic and, less commonly, thoracoamniotic shunt placement, is used in a fetus from 16 weeks' gestation to when lung maturity makes postnatal late treatment the best option. Complications are inadequate function, migration, and iatrogenic gastroschisis. Fetoscopic techniques now have a clinical application in the ligation of umbilical cords in acardiac twins, in selective laser photocoagulation of communicating vessels in twin-to-twin transfusions, and in the ablation of posterior urethral valves. * The procedure is performed inside the uterus using endoscopes, with a much smaller

hysterotomy than that needed for open procedures. This lessens the risks of preterm labor and fetal hypothermia and improves fetal hemostasis during the procedure. * The success of the procedure depends on the use of both a transabdominal ultrasound intraoperative view and a simultaneous endoscopic view to guide placement of the trocars and cannulae. * The drawbacks of fetoscopic surgery are the risk of bleeding (avoiding the transplacental route decreases this risk), rupture of membranes, and chorioamnionitis. Fetoscopy may also be difficult because of poor access to the fetus due to fetal position or polyhydramnios. Open fetal surgery is currently performed at select centers in instances in which the risk of the procedure to the mother and fetus is overridden by a diagnosis with a known poor outcome. Complications such as chorioamnionitis, preterm labor, bleeding, and direct trauma to the fetus are risks in most of these procedures. These surgical techniques are considered appropriate for 9 lesions.

Obstructive uropathy: Patients with severe obstructive uropathy with bilateral hydronephrosis and oligohydramnios revealed with ultrasonography should be evaluated for possible fetal therapy. *Prior to intervention, a cordocentesis is performed to document a normal karyotype and to exclude other major fetal anomalies. *This is followed by serial fetal bladder aspirations of urine under ultrasonographic guidance, which can help in the diagnosis of progressive renal damage (tonicity and electrolyte levels in the urine) and can relieve pressure if performed prior to 20 weeks' gestation. *A vesicoamniotic shunt is indicated in persistent megacystis with adequate ultrasonographic and biochemical renal function to reduce pressure in the urinary tract and to improve pulmonary development and decrease uterine compression. *Fetoscopic techniques can be used for fulguration of posterior urethral valves, placement of vesicoamniotic shunts, and vesicostomy. If all of these procedures fail, open vesicostomy with marsupialization of the bladder wall to the abdomen may be attempted. *Open surgery has a high fetal mortality rate (45%).

Hydrocephalus: Ventriculoamniotic shunts used for the decompression of obstructive hydrocephalus have had poor results and have caused procedure-related complications. Thus, their use is not indicated. *Fetal surgical procedures, both open and endoscopic, have been performed to repair myelomeningocele in utero. The open procedure is performed at 24-30 weeks' gestation and is shown to reduce both hindbrain herniation and the number of patients requiring shunts for hydrocephalus postnatally.

Pleural effusion: The use of thoracoamniotic shunts is indicated in a fetus with pleural effusion that reaccumulates after thoracocentesis and causes mediastinal shift. The aim of the shunt is to decompress the chest, promote pulmonary development, and treat the hydrops.

Twin-to-twin transfusion syndrome: Umbilical cord ligation may be indicated in some cases of twin-to-twin transfusion syndrome. In acardiac twins, twin reverse arterial perfusion (TRAP) is characterized by artery-to-artery and vein-to-vein communications between twins in a monozygotic placenta. The donor twin is at risk for congestive failure, and the recipient is acardiac and inadequately perfused. Umbilical cord ligation is indicated in the acardiac twin or a nonviable twin involved in twin-to-twin transfusion after 21 weeks' gestation. Selective laser photocoagulation of the cord circulation, using YAG laser, can be performed prior to 21 weeks. In this procedure, an endoscope is introduced intra-amniotically through a port with ultrasonographic guidance.

Amniotic band syndrome: In amniotic band syndrome, recent attempts have been made to lyse amniotic bands using fetoscopic techniques when a high risk of limb amputation is present.

Congenital diaphragmatic hernia: Many investigators believe that intrauterine therapy is indicated in fetuses with CDH who have a poor prognosis. *These patients have been defined as those with the liver in the chest and those with a low lung-to-head ratio (<1.0) on ultrasound. *Additional criteria for intervention include a singleton fetus, normal karyotype, diagnosis made prior to 25 weeks' gestation, and absence of associated anomalies. *The procedures that have been attempted since the early 1990s involved definitive repair by reduction of viscera from the chest, patch placement over the diaphragm, and abdominal silo construction to reduce intra-abdominal pressure. These carried a high mortality rate in patients with a poor prognosis and have since been abandoned. *The current fetal surgery for CDH is tracheal occlusion. *This causes enlargement and real growth of the lungs, often pushing the abdominal viscera back into the abdomen. The trachea is occluded by external metal clips placed either fetoscopically or in an open fashion, delivering the head and neck through a hysterotomy. *Both fetoscopic and open methods have had comparable outcomes. Survival rates in these high-risk patients have been approximately 33%, compared to 10% with conventional postnatal therapy. Significant morbidity related to prematurity, atrial perforation, pulmonary insufficiency, and neurologic complications have been observed. *An ex utero intrapartum (EXIT) procedure to remove the clips, aspirate lung fluid, administer surfactant, and intubate the trachea is then performed while the fetus is still on placental support, followed by delivery of the baby. The EXIT procedure is performed at 36 weeks' gestation or earlier if fetal hydrops or impending preterm labor is present. *Recent small trials of internal tracheal occlusion by a detachable balloon placed through a single uterine port using fetal bronchoscopy and ultrasound have yielded good results. The advantage of the technique is that it is technically less demanding and has a lower risk of recurrent laryngeal nerve and tracheal injury.

Congenital high airway obstruction syndrome: When congenital high airway obstruction syndrome (CHAOS) is complicated by hydrops, an EXIT procedure to place a tracheostomy may be of use. Earlier, fetoscopic, intervention may also be reasonable. The usual causes are laryngeal or tracheal stenosis.

Sacrococcygeal teratoma: Fetuses with sacrococcygeal teratoma may develop hydrops from high output failure. Early attempts at open resection of the teratoma or radiofrequency ablation of the tumor proved to have a high rate of fetal mortality and maternal morbidity. *Coagulation or ligation of the feeding vessels at the base of the tumor directly at fetoscopy by laser is now possible at an early gestation. This treatment slows the vascular steal and reverses the high-output failure. *Targeted radiofrequency ablation of the feeding vessels via a percutaneous probe under ultrasonic guidance is also effective.

Congenital cystic adenomatoid malformations: Open fetal surgery with resection of the cystic lobe prior to 32 weeks' gestation , in some instances, improves lung growth and allows the hydrops to resolve. The macrocystic form of cystic adenomatoid malformation may be drained with pleuroamniotic shunts, thus ameliorating the space-occupying effects and improving lung growth.

Criteria for fetal surgery:

1. Accurate diagnosis and staging possible, with exclusion of associated anomalies. **2.** Natural history of the disease is documented, and prognosis established. **3.** Currently no effective postnatal therapy. **4.** In-utero surgery proven feasible in animal models, reversing deleterious effects of the condition. **5.** Interventions performed in specialized multidisciplinary fetal treatment centers within strict protocols and approval of the local ethics committee with informed consent of the mother or parents.

Practice points:

1. Fetal surgery is only required in a very small minority of patients.
2. Open fetal surgery as well as operative fetoscopy has limited maternal risks. **3.** Fetal surgery requires highly specialized skills, based on extensive experimental work and clinical experience,

and is only offered within strict protocols and by multidisciplinary teams.

Research directions

1. Fetoscopy may have reduced preterm labor as compared to open fetal surgery, but the problem of iatrogenic PPROM remains. There is a clinical need for methods to address this problem.
2. There is a need for formal trials to determine the place of fetal surgery for most indications.
3. Given the rarity of diseases, collaborative studies are required.
4. Long-term outcomes for most conditions remain unknown.
5. The future lies in nonsurgical treatment of diseases, and will be based on the use of cells or engineered tissues and gene therapy.

Stem cell and genetic therapies for the fetus

Advances in prenatal diagnosis have led to the prenatal management of a variety of congenital diseases. Although prenatal stem cell and gene therapy await clinical application, they offer tremendous potential for the treatment of many genetic disorders. Normal developmental events in the fetus offer unique biologic advantages for the engraftment of hematopoietic stem cells and efficient gene transfer that are not present after birth. Although barriers to hematopoietic stem cell engraftment exist, progress has been made and preclinical studies are now underway for strategies based on prenatal tolerance induction to facilitate postnatal cellular transplantation. Similarly, in-utero gene therapy shows experimental promise for a host of diseases and proof-in-principle has been demonstrated in murine models, but ethical and safety issues still need to be addressed.

In-utero gene therapy (IUGT) The goal of gene therapy is to deliver genetic material to cells for therapeutic benefit. At the present time, there are well-documented risks associated with viral vector-mediated gene transfer that need to be addressed prior to consideration of any clinical application in the fetus. However, if safe and effective methods for fetal gene transfer can be developed, a large number of disorders would be amenable to IUGT. There is an increasing body of experimental evidence that supports the therapeutic potential of IUGT. There are several reasons why the fetus offers a favorable environment for the transfer of genetic material. During fetal development, stem and progenitor cells exist at high frequency and are exposed within various tissue compartments. Prior to the distribution of these cells within organs or tissue compartments, a window of opportunity exists when they are accessible for gene transfer. Transgenes can be targeted to these expanding cell populations, which will be inaccessible later in life. In addition to accessibility of stem cells, immunogenic vectors and transgenes can take advantage of the immature immune system of the fetus. Immunologic tolerance not only ensures long-term, stable transduction, but should also make postnatal treatment with the same vector and transgene possible. Finally, the small size of the fetus means that extremely high vector-to-cell ratios can be achieved with a limited amount of vector.

Modes of gene transfer Viral vectors are more efficient agents for gene delivery because they easily penetrate host cells and take advantage of the host cell machinery to replicate. They are engineered to have an attenuated viral genome so that only transgenes, not viral genes, are copied. Choice of viral vector type depends on a number of factors: immunogenicity, packaging capacity, targeted tissue, and the desired duration of expression.

Route and timing of prenatal gene therapy Once a vector is chosen, transduction of a targeted population of stem cells then depends on the gestational age of the fetus and the site of vector administration. Stem and progenitor cells will integrate into tissues and differentiate as the fetus grows, therefore earlier gestational gene therapy will generally result in more efficient transduction of stem cells than later gestation gene therapy. Ultrasound-guided transuterine injection is the most common method used for prenatal gene therapy in animal models. Direct administration into the lung, liver, and brain has led to localized gene expression, whereas vector injected into a body cavity such as the peritoneal or amniotic cavities can potentially transduce

several different progenitor cell populations. Developmental stage at the time of injection will determine which progenitor cell populations are exposed to vector and more than one population may be transduced at a time.

Proof-in-principle of prenatal gene therapy The diseases best treated by prenatal gene therapy are those caused by a mutation in a single gene, those that can be diagnosed before birth, and those that cause irreversible organ damage in the fetus or early postnatal period. Using rodent models of human genetic diseases and a variety of transduction methods, prenatal gene transfer has been targeted to a range of organs. In several disease models, phenotypic rescue has been accomplished; Cystic fibrosis- CTFR (cystic fibrosis transmembrane conductance regulator) -Mouse -Adenovirus- Intra-amniotic, Crigler–Najjar- UDP-glucuronyl transferase-Rat Lentivirus -Intrahepatic, Pompe's disease- acid alpha-glucosidase- Mouse-adeno-associated virus-2- Intrahepatic, Leber's congenital amarosis- retinal pigment epithelium 65- Mouse -adeno- associated virus -2- Subretinal, MPS VII (Sly syndrome)- beta- Glucuronidase-Mouse-adeno-associated virus -1- Intraventricular, Duchenne's muscular dystrophy- Dystrophin -Mouse -Adenovirus -Intramuscular.

Candidate diseases Promising candidates for human application include the hemophilias, muscular dystrophy, and central nervous system disorders. Progress in hemophilia research provides one example of how prenatal gene therapy might be used. The factors that make hemophilia an optimal disease target for prenatal gene are: the disease results from the absence of a single gene; the inheritance pattern is known and prenatal diagnosis is available; the disease presents in early life and occasionally in the fetus; and low-level, unregulated protein expression is curative. In addition, targeted expression is not required because, theoretically, the deficient protein could be secreted by any cell.

Risks of prenatal gene therapy

As with any fetal intervention, fetal loss, infection, and preterm labor are possible. In reality, a minimally invasive approach using a fine needle under ultrasound guidance has minimal procedure related morbidity. Common to all vectors used for prenatal gene transfer are the concerns of germ-line transmission, disruption of normal organ development, and transplacental spread of transgenes to the mother. Prenatal gene therapy is directed toward somatic cells, but inadvertent gene transfer to the germ line is a major concern for both safety and ethical reasons. Targeted gene therapy that occurs after the compartmentalization of primordial germ cells should not affect the germ line. Future challenges: Safety concerns involving the risk of insertional mutagenesis, the effect on organ development and the importance of low-level germ cell transmission need to be extensively investigated in appropriate preclinical animal models prior to application in humans. The ethics of fetal gene therapy and its potential to alter the human genome also need to be considered. While greater tissue specificity and safety can likely be accomplished by the use of tissue-specific promoters, or regulated transgene expression, safer gene transfer technologies will need to be developed to alleviate these concerns.

Excerpted from Stem cell and genetic therapies for the fetus, Jessica L. Roybal a, Matthew T. Santore a,b, Alan W. Flake, Seminars in Fetal & Neonatal Medicine 15 (2010) 46–51

STANDARDS FOR MATERNAL AND NEONATAL CARE

Maternal immunization against tetanus: if the woman has not previously been vaccinated, or if her immunization status is unknown, give two doses of TT/Td one month apart before delivery.For the woman to be protected during pregnancy, the last dose of tetanus toxoid must be given at least two weeks prior delivery. If the woman has had 1–4 doses of tetanus toxoid in the past, give one dose of TT/Td before delivery (a total of five doses protects throughout the childbearing years);If a case of neonatal tetanus is identified, give the mother one dose of tetanus toxoid as soon as possible and treat the baby according to national guidelines. A second dose should be given (at least) four weeks after the first, and a third dose should be given (at least) six months after the second. A search should be made for other non-immunized women living in the same area, and vaccination provided accordingly.

Prevention and management of sexually transmitted and reproductive tract infections : Immediately treat or arrange treatment for the woman, her partner(s) and the infant according to the results of STI/RTI case-finding, the on-site syphilis test and examination of the baby, and refer if treatment is not available at that level of care. Discuss with the woman the importance of treatment for herself, her partner(s) and the baby, explain the consequences of not treating the infection, and discuss the necessity of condom use during treatment. Provide information on the primary prevention of STIs, condom use, signs and symptoms of STIs and the consequences for the woman and the infant of leaving infections untreated, including advice on HIV prevention and on voluntary counselling and testing for HIV infection. Provide follow-up and refer the woman, her baby or partner(s) in case of complications or treatment failure. Record the diagnosis and treatment provided in the health facility's logbook and in the client's card.

Prevention of mother-to-child transmission of syphilis: Screen all pregnant women for syphilis with on-site RPR or other available rapid test at the first antenatal visit. Screening should be done preferably before 16 weeks of gestation to prevent congenital infection, and again in the third trimester. Review syphilis test results at subsequent visits and at time of delivery. If the woman was not tested during pregnancy, syphilis screening should be offered after delivery. Treat all seroreactive women with benzathine benzylpenicillin at the recommended dosage of at least 2.4 million units intramuscularly as a single dose, after having excluded allergy to penicillin. In the case of allergy to penicillin, the attendant should desensitize and treat with penicillin if trained to do so, or refer the patient to a higher level of care. Advise women who test positive that their partner(s) must also be treated with the same regimen, as well as the baby as soon as possible after birth. Advise women who test negative how to remain negative by promoting condom use during pregnancy. Test for syphilis all women with a history of adverse pregnancy outcome (abortion, stillbirth, syphilitic infant, etc.) and treat accordingly. Treat women with clinical disease or a history of exposure to a person with infectious syphilis. Screen all women with syphilis for other STIs and HIV infection, and provide counselling and treatment accordingly. Offer voluntary counselling and testing of HIV to all women who screen positive for syphilis. Make plans for treating the baby at birth. Record testing results and treatment in the facility's logbook and in the woman's card.

Prevention of congenital rubella syndrome (CRS):*Prior to pregnancy and in the postpartum period* In countries where rubella vaccine has been introduced into the national immunization schedule, health providers of maternal and child services must: Vaccinate children aged 12 months or older and/or schoolgirls and/or women of childbearing age against rubella, according to national policy and guidelines. *During pregnancy:*In all countries, health providers of maternal and neonatal services, and skilled attendants in particular, must: Ensure that rubella vaccine is not offered to pregnant women and that women are advised to avoid pregnancy for one month after rubella vaccination. Inform pregnant women of the importance of avoiding contact with individuals with rubella.

Report and investigate suspected rubella in pregnancy, exposure of a pregnant woman to rubella, and infants with suspected CRS. Be able to counsel women with confirmed rubella infection during pregnancy on the risk of fetal abnormalities and relevant laws and regulations with respect to termination of the pregancy, if they so wish. Report and investigate cases of suspected congenital rubella syndrome in newborns and infants promptly, as required by the national communicable disease surveillance system.

Prevention of neural tube defects: Health providers in antenatal and family planning clinics must: Advise women trying to conceive to take a dose of 400 mcg folic acid daily, starting two months before the planned pregnancy. Advise women who have not been supplementing their diet and who suspect themselves to be pregnant to begin taking 400 mcg folic acid daily and to continue until they are 12 weeks pregnant. Counsel pregnant women who have previously had a baby with NTD or who have diabetes or who are under anticonvulsant treatment about the increased risk of a future baby being affected, and advise them to take 5 mg folic acid daily and increase their food intake of folate. Record the treatment given in the maternal card. Record cases of NTD, in accordance with local guidelines, in the logbook and in the woman's record.

Provision of effective antenatal care: All pregnant women should have at least four antenatal care (ANC) assessments by or under the supervision of a skilled attendant. These should, as a minimum, include all the interventions outlined in the new WHO antenatal care model and be spaced at regular intervals throughout pregnancy, commencing as early as possible in the first trimester;to prevent, alleviate or treat/manage health problems/diseases (including those directly related to pregnancy) that are known to have an unfavorable outcome on pregnancy, and to provide women and their families/ partners with appropriate information and advice for a healthy pregnancy, childbirth and postnatal recovery, including care of the newborn, promotion of early exclusive breastfeeding and assistance with deciding on future pregnancies in order to improve pregnancy outcomes.

Malaria prevention and treatment: In malarious areas, all pregnant women should sleep under an insecticide-treated bednet (ITN). In addition, in areas of stable transmission of falciparum malaria, all pregnant women should be given intermittent preventive treatment (IPT). Pregnant women suspected of having malaria should be assessed and treated in accordance with national protocols. In the postnatal period, both the mother and the baby should sleep under an insecticide-treated bednet. In areas of stable falciparum malaria transmission give all pregnant women at least two doses of IPT after quickening (2nd and 3rd trimester) and advise them to seek care in case of fever. Doses should be given at an interval at least one month. To ensure that women receive at least two doses, IPT should be carried out during routine visits to the antenatal clinic.

Iron and folate supplementation: All pregnant women in areas of high prevalence of malnutrition should routinely receive iron and folate supplements, together with appropriate dietary advice, to prevent anaemia. Where the prevalence of anaemia in pregnant women is high (40% or more), supplementation should continue for three months in the postpartum period. Give all pregnant women a standard dose of 60 mg iron + 400 ¼g folic acid daily for 6 months or, if 6 months of treatment cannot be achieved during the pregnancy, either continue supplementation during the postpartum period or increase the dosage to 120 mg iron during pregnancy.

Birth and emergency preparedness in antenatal care : All pregnant women should have a written plan for birth and for dealing with unexpected adverse events, such as complications or emergencies, that may occur during pregnancy, childbirth or the immediate postnatal period, and should discuss and review this plan with a skilled attendant at each antenatal assessment and at least one month prior to the expected date of birth.

Standards for Maternal and Neonatal Care Steering Committee,WHO

Genetic counseling may be described as the process through which individuals affected by, or at risk for a problem which may be genetic or hereditary, are informed of the consequences of the disorder, of the probability of suffering from or of transmitting it to their offspring, and of the potential means of treating or of avoiding the occurrence of the malformation or disease in question. Genetic counseling in common disorders is often given by the family doctor, the pediatrician or the obstetrician. However, with the recognition that thousands of problems have a major hereditary component, counseling is increasingly done in specialized centers which also provide the laboratory diagnostic tools which we hear so much about in our era.

Four aspects are involved in giving genetic counseling

Arriving at a specific diagnosis: this is often the most difficult, trying and time consuming part of the process, for the health care professionals as well as for the family (who are understandably more concerned with the care of their affected relative, than with the specific name of his or her disorder). However, without a correct diagnosis, counseling is at best incomplete and imprecise.

Estimation of risks: to develop the disorder and/or to transmit it to offspring.

Practical aid: this includes, for example, recommending doctors for specialized examinations or health care professionals for speech or educational therapy. It often implies as well the coordination of prenatal and other diagnostic tests.

Supportive role: this aspect is at least as important as the diagnostic question, for the great majority of genetic disorders cannot be cured or even satisfactorily treated. Although the genetic counselor cannot provide support for the family on a daily basis, he or she should be able to orient them towards those health professionals who can best serve them in this role. Accepting and learning to live with a genetic diagnosis is particularly difficult when reproductive options are involved, and feelings of " guilt " may touch several generations and cause rifts in the family just at the time when solidarity is most needed.

What types of disorders are genetic? "Genetic" does not necessarily mean "hereditary". The first term implies simply that the genetic material, on a chromosomal or a gene level, contains one or more mutations which are the cause of the disorder. Once a mutation is present in a patient, particularly if it is constitutional (and thus present in all cells), it can of course be transmitted and thus becomes a hereditary disorder. Genetic disorders are generally of four types:

Chromosomal disorders affect some 1/200 live-born children (Robinson & Puck, 1967), and about 1/500 adults. Abnormalities of chromosome *number* are rarely inherited, although affected individuals who reproduce may transmit the extra chromosome to their offspring. Structural abnormalities, such as translocations in which two chromosomes exchange segments, may cause little or no effect in carriers, but predispose to reproductive problems such as miscarriage and infertility.

Monogenic (" Mendelian ") inheritance: This is the result of mutations in single genes, at specific gene " loci. "We have some 50–100,000 individual genes, for several thousand of which monogenic disease has been described (McKusick, 1992). Some 1/300 individuals will suffer from a monogenic disease manifesting within the first two decades (Baird et al. 1988), but this figure may be as high as 1% if the lifetime probability of manifesting a monogenic disorder is considered. Four types of

transmission are observed in monogenic disorders caused by nuclear genes: *autosomal dominant* (one mutated gene of the pair is sufficient to produce symptoms), *autosomal recessive* (the two alleles must be abnormal to cause the phenotype) and *X-linked*, which includes *recessive* (theoretically, only males suffer, given that they are " hemizygous " for the X chromosome) and, less frequently, *X-linked dominant* gene mutations (males more seriously affected than females). A few genes, involved particularly in sex determination and fertility, have been localized on the Y chromosome, the transmission of which is only from a father to his XY offspring.

Polygenic or "multifactorial": Although this causation is not "as genetic" as are monogenic and chromosomal disorders, the majority of malformations and of common familial disorders have this type of cause. Polygenic implies that the association of several different genes, each one slightly modified, is necessary to produce the disorder. Multifactorial causation means that both genetic and non-genetic (environmental, either pre- or postnatal) factors are associated to produce the pathology. Some 5-10% of the population will suffer either from a malformation or from a disease in which genetic factors are major.

Mitochondrial disorders: In recent years a "new" type of inheritance has been proven, that resulting from mutations in the mitochondrial genome. Each cell contains hundreds or thousands of mitochondria, each containing one or several circular chromosomes. These chromosomes can be deleted or suffer other types of mutations which interfere with cellular production of ATP, and thus of the energy vital for the cell/organ/organism; the symptoms depend on the tissues involved and on the proportion of mitochondria mutated, but involve first the central nervous system and the muscle, due to their large energy demands (Morris, 1990; Wallace, 1993). The incidence of mitochondrial mutations in human disease is still unknown. In many cases the mutation is "de novo" in an affected individual, but hereditary transmission is purely *maternal*, since, a fertilized egg's mitochondria originate from the maternal germ cell only.

Who seeks genetic counseling? In most genetics divisions patients can either come self-referred or be recommended by a physician. Currently, genetics has not evolved to a state of knowledge where couples come for " genetic screening " without a specific family history or increased risk for a genetic disorder for another reason. The day will probably come in the not too distant future when preconceptional or prenatal screening can be offered to the general population for a panel of different diseases. However, for the moment only several dozen of our 50,000–100,000 individual genes have been identified and their mutations defined. Testing for any one of these requires both technical competence and a considerable investment of time and money. The reasons for seeking genetic counseling can be divided into the following six categories:

The individual (often hoping to be a parent) suffers himself form a genetic or potentially genetic disease. This may be a (relatively unsevere) chromosomal disorder, a single gene condition (transmitted in a dominant, recessive or X-linked manner), or a " multifactorial " disorder, e.g. implying the combined effects of a genetic predisposition and unfavorable environmental factors (for example, diabetes or epilepsy).

A close relative has a genetic disease and the individual who consults is worried either about his/her own risk of developing the disease, or the risk that his offspring will suffer from the disorder.

The individual is at increased genetic risk for a specific genetic disorder given his or her particular ethnic origin. Each population has one or more genetic diseases, generally transmitted as autosomal recessive traits, which are particularly frequent within it, e.g. cystic fibrosis in white Europeans and sickle cell anemia in Africans and Mediterranean populations. A similar situation may apply to couples who are *consanguineous* (blood relatives), although there is no way of determining which specific genes or diseases are implied, unless this is indicated by a positive family history for a particular disorder.

The individual or couple is having reproductive problems, e.g. infertility, repeated miscarriage, etc. Such problems may have genetic, particularly chromosomal causes. The individual may be initially referred for a laboratory diagnostic test, with counseling differing markedly depending on the result of the analyses.

The couple has already born a child or fetus with a malformation or genetic disorder. In this situation the specific diagnosis may be known or not, and the risk of recurrence vary from less than 1% up to 50%.

The couple requests counseling, concerning prenatal diagnosis, for such reasons as advanced parental ages,. Amniocentesis or choriocentesis should be offered to women of 35 years and older, given their increased risk of bearing a child with a chromosomal anomaly. Counseling sessions for older parents, or for those requesting prenatal diagnosis because of anxiety (close contact with a handicapped individual, for example) are intended to provide information concerning the benefits and risks inherent to prenatal diagnostic techniques.

In all these situations, genetic counseling should be, in so far as is possible, impartial and nondirective. The goal is never to make a decision *for* the couple, whose familial, social, moral and religious situation is *different* from that of the counselor, but rather to provide them with the objective information which will allow them to make their own informed decisions.

What information is sought in genetic counseling?

Unless a *specific diagnosis* has already been proven, the first and foremost concern is to establish, if at all possible, the identity of the disorder. If and when this is done, the geneticist must often review the literature, as well as count on his own experience, in order to inform consultants as precisely as possible of the *etiology* of the problem. Of primary concern to the family is of course the *natural history of the genetic disease*, which includes prognosis and discussion of *potential treatments* and of practical guidelines in how to deal with these. Even if not an initial concern for those seeking counseling concerning a child recently born, the question of *recurrence risks* must be rapidly discussed, as well as possibilities for *prenatal diagnosis if* such is desired by the family. This in itself is often a difficult task, as necessary information about a particular disorder or diagnostic technique may be sparse, and couples may directly ask what the counselor for directive advice.

What does a genetics work-up involve?

From the geneticist's point of view, and in order to more efficiently counsel a given family, it is preferable to obtain and review medical documents in advance, as well as to review recent literature on the problem to be treated. Once a family arrives in the genetic clinic, the steps to be taken, depending on whether the specific diagnosis is established, can be summarized as follows:

Obtaining a detailed family history, which includes both sides of the family even if counseling has been requested for a dominant disorder affecting one parent. It is not rare that in taking such a history, other antecedents are revealed which also merit discussion.

A review of medical and/ or pregnancy histories is especially important when the diagnosis is not yet established, but also helps geneticists to learn more about etiologies and natural histories of certain disorders.

A physical examination, of the affected person, and sometimes of other family members, is often needed.

Medical and/or laboratory exams may be suggested. If a diagnosis has not been established these often include chromosome study, and may necessitate DNA analysis if the identity of the gene suspected to be involved is known. Other frequent suggestions include X-ray or ultrasound examinations, and various biochemical analyses. Once the diagnosis is known, medical tests aimed at evaluating health risks linked to the disorder may also be established.

Genetic counseling can only be given at the end of this process.

The process of genetic counseling has changed dramatically over the past 25 years. Instead of being based on purely clinical findings, the identity of many disorders can be proven because their genic or chromosomal basis is known. The availability of an ever-increasing number of laboratory tests allows more accurate diagnosis, and often gives the opportunity for pre-symptomatic or prenatal diagnosis to family members who prefer to use it. However, it must not be overlooked that the availability of such tests also poses psychological and ethical questions which are difficult to resolve. A sub-speciality of medical genetics has thus evolved which examines the individual's and the society's means and ways of resolving such questions (Wertz and Fletcher, 1989).

The training of individuals competent to give genetic counseling has been formalized in a number of European countries, as was done in the United States and Canada a number of years ago through their respective Boards of Medical Genetics. Medical doctors with post-graduate training in medical genetics depend heavily on cytogeneticists and molecular geneticists for diagnosis, as well as, increasingly, on genetics " associates " (master's degree geneticists and nurse specialists) and Ph.D. medical geneticists to help both with the initial work-up and with follow-up of families. As genetics has become a bona fide speciality in itself, with training programs developing for health professionals at various levels. Most training is done in university medical genetics departments.

What services are offered by most university genetics centers?

To provide both diagnostic, counseling and follow-up services, close ties must be established with such hospital departments as pediatrics and obstetrics and access to specialized diagnostic services and to medical library facilities is essential. However, a number of services are best offered within one unit:

*Clinical diagnosis and genetic counseling. *Chromosomal analysis: both postnatal and prenatal diagnostics. *DNA extraction and banking. *DNA analysis. *Prenatal diagnostic services.

Courtesy: **C.D. DeLozier-Blanchet** Division of Medical Genetics, Department of Genetics and Microbiology, University Medical Centre, 1211 Geneva 4, Switzerland

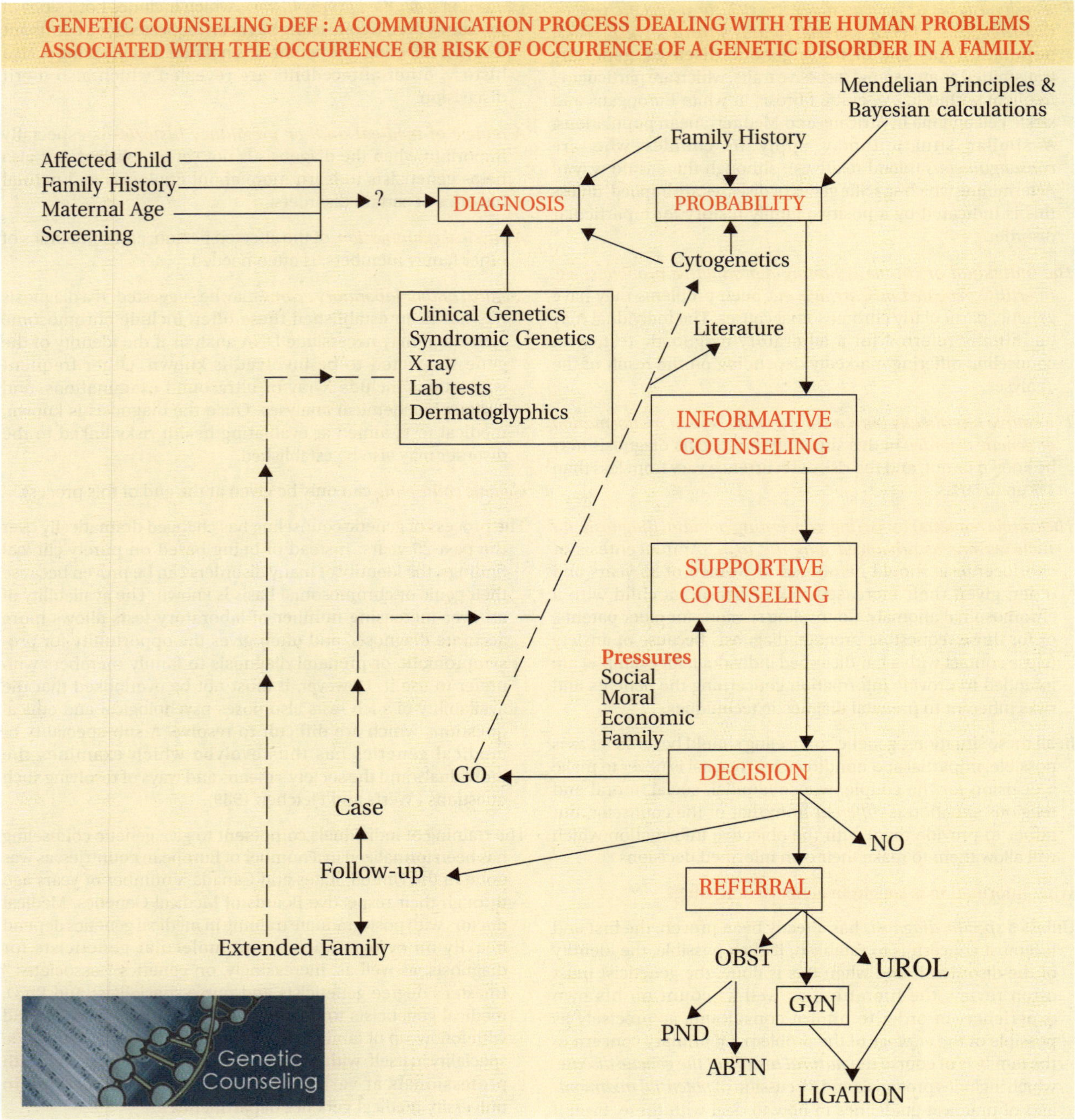

GENETIC COUNSELING DEF : A COMMUNICATION PROCESS DEALING WITH THE HUMAN PROBLEMS ASSOCIATED WITH THE OCCURENCE OR RISK OF OCCURENCE OF A GENETIC DISORDER IN A FAMILY.

Mendelian Principles & Bayesian calculations

Family History

Affected Child
Family History
Maternal Age
Screening

? → **DIAGNOSIS**   **PROBABILITY**

Cytogenetics

Clinical Genetics
Syndromic Genetics
X ray
Lab tests
Dermatoglyphics

Literature

INFORMATIVE COUNSELING

SUPPORTIVE COUNSELING

Pressures
Social
Moral
Economic
Family

GO ← **DECISION**

Case

Follow-up

NO

Extended Family

REFERRAL

OBST   UROL

GYN

PND

ABTN

LIGATION

Genetic Counseling

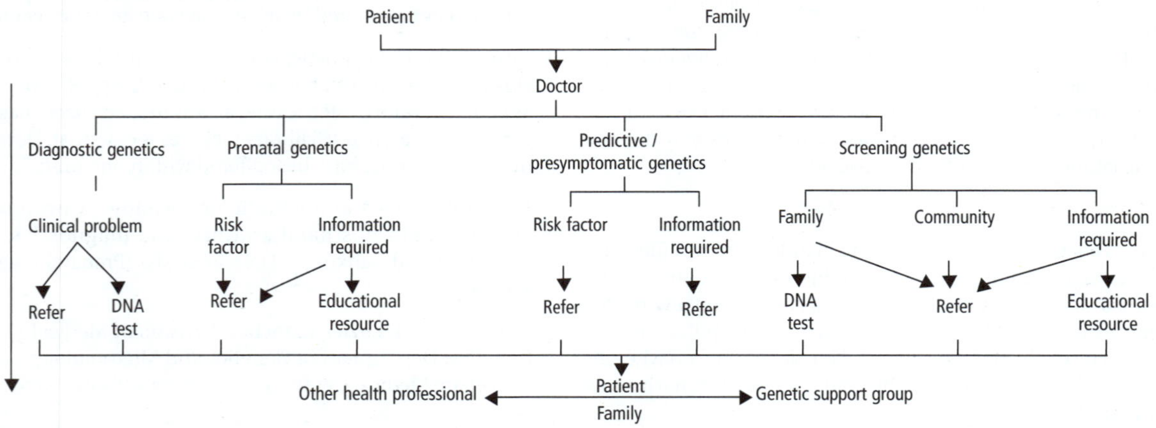

Patient   Family

Doctor

Diagnostic genetics   Prenatal genetics   Predictive / presymptomatic genetics   Screening genetics

Clinical problem   Risk factor   Information required   Risk factor   Information required   Family   Community   Information required

Refer   DNA test   Refer   Educational resource   Refer   Refer   DNA test   Refer   Educational resource

Other health professional ← Patient Family → Genetic support group

The flow chart, drawn in the form of a pedigree, illustrates key players in the "new genetics" (patient, family, GP/specialist, other health professionals, genetic support groups, the community). The consultation usually starts with a patient or family problem, and ends, in the more complex genetic disorders, with input being required from other health professionals and genetic support groups. The optimal provision of the various alternatives in the new genetics (diagnostic, prenatal, predictive and screening DNA testing) remains a challenge for the future.

Newborn intensive care is defined as care for medically unstable or critically ill newborns requiring constant nursing, complicated surgical procedures, continual respiratory support, or other intensive interventions. *Intermediate care* includes care of ill infants requiring less constant nursing, but does not exclude respiratory support. When an intensive care nursery is available, the intermediate nursery serves as a "step down" unit from the intensive care area. When hospitals mix infants of varying acuity, requiring different levels of care in the same area, intensive care design standards shall be followed to provide maximum.

*Standard 1: Unit configuration: The NICU design shall be driven by systematically developed program goals and objectives which define the purpose of the unit, service provision, space utilization, projected bedspace demand, staffing requirements and other basic information related to the mission of the unit. Design strategies to achieve program goals and objectives shall address the medical, developmental, educational and emotional needs of infants, families and staff. The design shall allow for flexibility and creativity to achieve the stated objectives. The NICU shall be configured to individualize the caregiving environment and services for each infant and family. This may be accomplished with designs which range from an open area to individually divided spaces.

*Standard 2: NICU location within the hospital: The NICU shall be a distinct area within the health care facility, with controlled access and a controlled environment. The NICU shall be located within space designed for that purpose. It shall provide good visibility of infants and circulation of staff, family, and equipment. Traffic to other services shall not pass through the unit. The NICU shall be in close proximity to the area of the hospital where births occur. Units receiving babies from other facilities shall have ready access to the hospital's transport receiving area. When perinatal and neonatal services must be on separate floors of the hospital, direct, dedicated elevator access should be provided between the birthing unit and the NICU.

* Standard 3: Minimum area, clearance and privacy requirements for the infant care space: Each infant care space shall contain a minimum of 120 square feet (11.2 square meters), excluding sinks and aisles. Additionally, there shall be an aisle adjacent to each infant care space with a minimum width of 3 feet (0.9 meters). Each infant care space shall be designed to allow privacy for the baby and family.

* Standard 4: Electrical, gas supply, and mechanical needs: Mechanical requirements at each infant care bed, such as electrical and gas outlets, shall be organized to ensure safety, easy access and maintenance. There shall be a minimum of 20 simultaneously accessible electrical outlets. Minimum number of simultaneously accessible gas outlets: Air 3 Oxygen 3 Vacuum 3. There shall be a mixture of emergency and normal power for all electrical outlets per current National Fire Protection Association (NFPA)3 recommendations. There shall be provision at each bedside to allow data transmission to a remote location. A patient area must not only contribute to a calm appearance of the patient area itself but of the whole NICU. Medical staff should be supported to be able to monitor and nurse the baby as good as possible. Their work also needed to

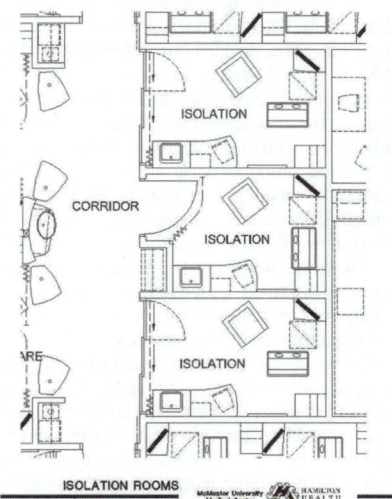

become more comfortable with respect to the ergonomic standards. The delineated design approach has resulted in the new NICU patient area the "Family Shell".

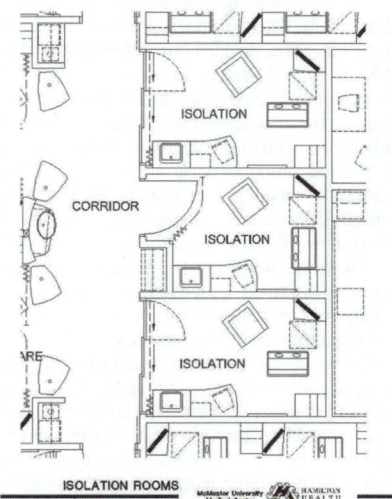

ISOLATION ROOMS
Neonatal Intensive Care Unit
McMaster University Medical Centre   HAMILTON HEALTH SCIENCES

*Standard 5: Isolation Room(s): An isolation room shall be available for NICU infants. An area for handwashing, gowning, and storage of clean and soiled materials shall be provided near the entrance to the room. Ventilation systems for isolation room(s) shall be engineered to have negative air pressure with air 100% exhausted to the outside. An emergency communication system shall be provided within the isolation room.

*Standard 6: Family entry and reception area: The NICU shall have a clearly identified entrance and reception area for families. Families shall have immediate and direct contact with staff when they arrive in this entrance and reception area. The design of this area should contribute to positive first impressions. Facilitating contacts with staff will also enhance security for infants in the NICU. This area should have lockable storage facilities for families' personal belongings (unless provided elsewhere), and may also include a handwashing area.

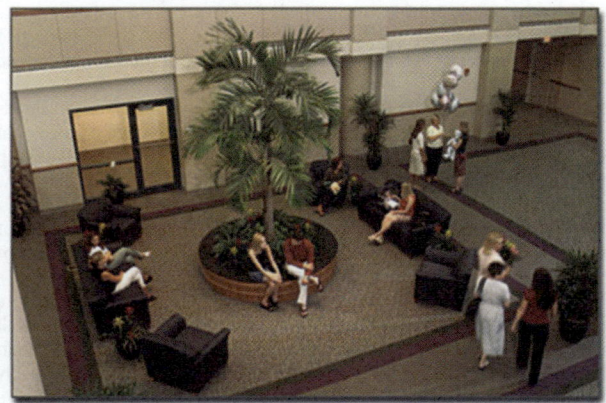

*Standard 7: Scrub areas: Where an individual room concept is used, a hands-free handwashing sink shall be provided within each infant care room. In a multiple bed room, every bed position shall be within 20 feet (6 meters) of a hands-free handwashing sink. Handwashing sinks shall be large enough to control splashing and designed to avoid standing or retained water. Space shall also be provided for soap and towel dispensers and a covered trash receptacle. Handwashing facilities which can be used by children and people in wheelchairs shall be available in the NICU. Sinks for handwashing should not be built into counters used for other purposes. Minimum dimensions for a handwashing sink are 24 inches wide × 16 inches front to back × 10 inches deep (61 cm × 41 cm × 25 cm) from the bottom of the sink to the top of its rim. Pictorial handwashing instructions should be provided above all sinks. Sink location, construction material and related hardware (paper towel and soap dispensers) should be chosen with durability, ease of operation and noise control in mind.

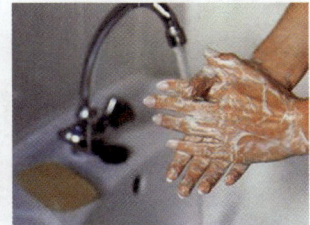

Standard 8: General Support Space-Distinct facilities shall be provided for clean and soiled utilities, medical equipment storage, and unit management services. *Clean Utility/Holding Area(s):* For storage of supplies frequently used in the care of newborns. The clean utility area may also be used for storage of medications, formulas, and breast milk. When this use is specified, a sink and counter preparation area and a storage area shielded from direct light shall be provided. *Soiled Utility/Holding Room:* Essential for storing used and contaminated material before its removal from the care area. Unless used only as a holding room, this room shall contain a counter and a sink with hot and cold running water that is turned on and off by hands-free controls, soap and paper towel dispensers, and a covered waste receptacle with foot control. The ventilation system in the soiled utility/holding room shall be engineered to have negative air pressure with air 100% exhausted to the outside. The soiled utility/holding room shall be situated to allow removal of soiled materials without passing through the infant care area. *Charting Areas:* Provision for charting space at each bedside shall be required. An additional separate area or desk for tasks such as compiling more detailed records, completing requisitions, and telephone communication shall be provided.

*Standard 9: Staff Support Space- Space shall be provided within the NICU to meet the professional, personal, and administrative needs of the staff. Rooms shall be sized to provide privacy and to satisfy their intended function. Locker, lounge, private toilet facilities and on-call rooms are required at a minimum.

*Standard 10: Parent-Infant Room(s)- Parent-infant room(s) shall be provided within or immediately adjacent to the NICU that allow(s) parents and infants extended private time together. The room(s) shall have direct, private access to sink and toilet facilities, telephone or intercom linkage with the NICU staff, sleeping facilities for at least one parent, and sufficient space for the infant's bed and equipment. The room(s) can be used for other family educational, counseling, or demonstration purposes when unoccupied.

*Standard 11: Family Support Space- Space shall be provided in or immediately adjacent to the NICU for the following functions: family lounge area, lockable storage, telephone(s), and toilet facilities. Separate, dedicated rooms shall also be provided for lactation support and consultation in or immediately adjacent to the NICU. A family library or education area shall be provided within the hospital.

*Standard 12: Ancillary Needs- Distinct support space shall be provided for respiratory therapy, laboratory, pharmacy, radiology, and other ancillary services when these activities are routinely performed on the unit.

*Standard 13: Administrative Space- Administrative space shall be provided in the NICU for activities directly related to infant care or routinely performed within the NICU.

*Standard 14: Ambient Lighting in infant Care Areas- Ambient lighting levels in newborn intensive care rooms shall be adjustable, through a range of at least 10 to 600 lux (approximately 1 to 60 foot candles), as measured at each bedside. Both natural and electric light sources shall have controls that allow immediate, sufficient darkening of any bed position sufficient for transillumination when necessary. Electric light sources shall have a color rendering index 4 of 80 or above, and shall avoid unnecessary ultraviolet or infrared radiation by the use of appropriate lamps, lens, or filters.

*Standard 15: Procedure Lighting in Infant Care Areas- Separate procedure lighting shall be available to each infant care station. This lighting shall minimize shadows and glare; it shall be adjustable so that lighting at less than maximal levels can be provided whenever possible; and light shall be highly framed, so that babies at adjacent bed positions will not experience any increase in illumination.***Standard 16: Illumination of Support Areas**- Illumination of support areas within the NICU, including the charting areas, medication preparation area, the reception desk, and handwashing areas, shall conform to IES specifications.

*Standard 17: Daylighting- At least one source of daylight shall be visible from newborn care areas. External windows in infant care rooms shall be glazed with insulating glass to minimize heat gain or loss, and shall be situated at least 2 feet (61 cm) away from any part of a baby's bed to minimize radiant

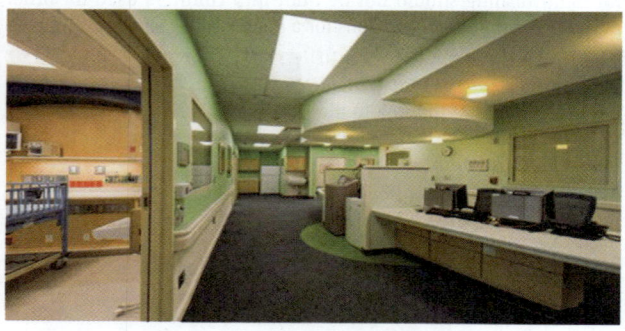

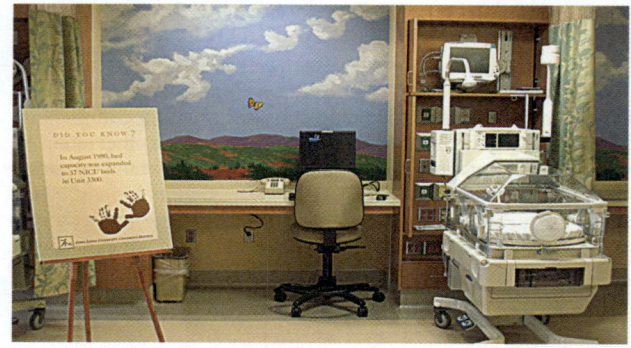

heat loss from the baby. All external windows shall be equipped with shading devices which are neutral color or opaque to minimize color distortion from transmitted light.

*Standard 18: Floor Surfaces- Floor surfaces shall be easily cleanable and shall minimize the growth of microorganisms. Floors shall be highly durable to withstand frequent cleaning and heavy traffic.

*Standard 19: Wall Surfaces-Wall surfaces shall be easily cleanable and provide protection at points where contact with movable equipment is likely to occur.

*Standard 20: Countertops, Casework, and Cabinetry- Countertops, casework, and cabinetry, especially in the infant care areas, shall be easily cleanable with the fewest possible seams in the integral construction. Exposed surface seams shall be sealed. Casework and cabinetry shall be of durable construction to withstand impact by movable equipment without significant damage. They shall also be of sufficient moisture resistance to prevent deterioration.

*Standard 21: Ceiling Finishes-Ceilings shall be easily cleanable and constructed in a manner to prohibit the passage of particles from the cavity above the ceiling plane into the clinical environment. Ceiling construction shall not be friable and shall have a noise reduction co-efficient (NRC)13 of at least 0.90.

Standard 22: Ambient Temperature and Ventilation- The NICU shall be designed to provide an air temperature of 72°F to 78°F (22-26° C) and a relative humidity of 30-60%,14 while avoiding condensation on wall and window surfaces. A minimum of six air changes per hour is required, with a minimum of two changes being outside air. The ventilation pattern shall inhibit particulate matter from moving freely in the space, and intake and exhaust vents shall be situated as to minimize drafts on or near the infant beds. Ventilation air delivered to the NICU shall be filtered with at least 90% efficiency. Fresh air intake shall be located at least 25 feet (7.6 meters) from exhaust outlets of ventilating systems, combustion equipment stacks, medical/surgical vacuum systems, plumbing vents, or areas that may collect vehicular exhausts or other noxious fumes. Prevailing winds or proximity to other structures may require greater clearance.

*Standard 23: Noise Abatement-Infant bed areas and the spaces opening onto them shall be designed to produce minimal background noise and to contain and absorb much of the transient noise which arises within the nursery. The combination of continuous background sound and transient sound in any bed space or infant care area shall not exceed an hourly Leq of 50 dB and an hourly L10 of 55 dB, both A-weighted slow response. Transient sounds or Lmax shall not exceed 70 dB, A-weighted slow response

*Standard 24: Safety/Infant Security- The NICU shall be designed as part of an overall security program to protect the physical safety of infants, families and staff in the NICU. The NICU shall be designed to minimize the risk of infant abduction.**Standard 24: Safety/Infant Security**

The NICU shall be designed as part of an overall security program to protect the physical safety of infants, families and staff in the NICU. The NICU shall be designed to minimize the risk of infant abduction.

Standard 25: Access to Nature and Other Positive Distractions

When possible, views of nature shall be provided in at least one space that is accessible to all families and one space that is accessible to all staff. Other forms of positive distraction shall be provided for families in infant and family spaces, and for staff in staff spaces.

Standard 26: Operating Rooms Intended for Use by Newborn ICU Patients

Operating rooms in health-care facilities where infant procedures may be performed shall be constructed to operating room specifications

Standard 27: Private (Single-Family) Rooms

Rooms intended for the use of a single infant and his/her family shall conform to the requirements for infant spaces designated elsewhere in these standards

Courtesy: http://www.nd.edu/~nicudes/

Developmental Care in the NICU is defined by efforts in unit design, equipment selection, policies, care protocols, and staff training to maintain the basic physical, sensory, and interpersonal needs of the preterm infant while minimizing exposure to noxious and painful stimuli. The history of developmental care is rooted in the fields of neonatal nursing and physical/ occupational therapy. While early research focused on improved short-term physiological stability, evidence is mounting that a comprehensive program which addresses NICU design, unit policies and staff training can positively impact preterm infant brain development and long-term outcome. These efforts include the provision of individual rooms for each patient/family, offering unrestricted access of infants to parents, supporting kangaroo care and breastfeeding, noise abatement, restricting light exposure, pain protocols, as well as training staff on appropriate infant handling, state recognition, and sleep preservation. A successful developmental care program is the product of a multidisciplinary team of parents, nurses, nurse practitioners, physicians, occupational/physical therapists, administrators, architects, engineers, and social workers. It requires a paradigm shift of attitudes regarding ownership of an infant's care and the personhood of the preterm patient.

Infection Control in the NICU – Recommended Standards: The nature of the recommendations are as follows:-

Category IA
- Strongly recommended for all hospitals and
- Strongly supported by well-designed experimental or epidemiologic studies

Category IB
- Strongly recommended for all hospitals
- Reviewed as effective by experts in the field and
- A consensus of American Academy of Pediatrics and American College of Obstetricians and Gynecologists, based on strong rationale and suggestive evidence, even though definitive scientific studies have not been done

Category II
- § Suggested for implementation in many hospitals
- § Recommendations may be supported by suggestive clinical or epidemiologic studies, a strong theoretical rationale, or definitive studies applicable to some, but not all, hospitals.

I. Physical Setup

Space
1. Each infant care space in the Neonatal Intensive Care Unit shall preferably contain a minimum of 11.2 square meters (120 square feet), excluding sinks and aisles. [IB]
2. There shall be an aisle adjacent to each infant care space with a minimum width of 0.9 meters (3 feet). [IB]
3. Traffic to other services shall not pass through the unit. [IB]

Ventilation
1. A minimum of 6 air changes per hour is required for the NICU, with a minimum of 2 changes being outside air. [IB]
2. The ventilation pattern shall inhibit particulate matter from moving freely in the space and intake and exhaust vents shall be situated as to minimize drafts on or near the infant beds. [IB]
3. Ventilation air delivered to the NICU shall be filtered with at least 90 % efficiency. [IB]
4. Fresh air intake shall be located at least 7.6 meters (25 feet) from exhaust outlets of ventilating systems, combustion equipment stacks, medical/ surgical vacuum systems, plumbing vents, or areas that may collect vehicular exhausts or other noxious fumes. [IB]

Scrub Areas
1. In the NICU, there should be at least 1 hands-free handwashing sink for 4 beds. [IB]
2. I n single bedroom, a hands-free handwashing sink shall be provided within each infant care room. [II]
3. Handwashing facilities that can be used by children and people in wheelchairs shall be available in the NICU. [IB]
4. Sinks for handwashing should not be built into counters used for other purposes. [IB]
5. Sink location, construction material and related hardware (paper towel, covered trash receptacle, and soap dispensers) should be chosen with durability, ease of operation and noise control in mind. [IB]
6. Minimum dimensions for a handwashing sink are 61 cm wide X 41 cm front to back × 25 cm deep (24 in. × 16 in. × 10 in.) from the bottom of the sink to the top of its rim; so as to minimize splashing. [IB]

7. Pictorial handwashing instructions should be provided above all sinks. [IB]
8. Sinks should be designed so as to control splashing and avoid standing or retained water. [IB]
9. Faucet aerators may be useful to reduce water splashing in sinks, but they are notoriously susceptible to contamination with a variety of hydrophilic bacteria. They should not be used. [IB]
10. Sinks should be scrubbed clean daily with a detergent. [IB]

Air-borne Isolation Room(s)
1. Isolation rooms adequately designed to care for airborne infection should be available in any hospital with an NICU. In most cases, this is ideally situated within the NICU; but, in some circumstances, utilization of an isolation room elsewhere in the hospital would be suitable. [IB]
2. An area for handwashing, gowning, and storage of clean and soiled materials shall be provided near the entrance to the room. [IB]
3. Isolation rooms should have a minimum of 13.94 sq metre (150 square feet) of clear space, excluding the entry work area. Single and multibedded configurations are appropriate based on use. [IB]
4. Ventilation systems for isolation room(s) shall be engineered to have negative air pressure with air 100% exhausted to the outside. Air exhaust to outside the building do not need to be filtered but the exhaust vent needs to be away from air-intake vents, persons or animals. [IB]
5. A hands-free two-way emergency communication system is required within the isolation room to connect to the outside. [IB]
6. Remote physiologic monitoring of an isolated infant should be considered. [IB]
7. Isolation rooms should have observation windows with blinds for privacy. Choice and placement of blinds, windows, and other structural items should allow for ease of operation and cleaning. [IB]

II. Administrative arrangement- Surveillance for Nosocomial Infection
1. With appropriate resources allocated from the hospital/ HAHO, the infection control committee of each hospital should work with perinatal care personnel to establish workable definitions of nosocomial infection for surveillance purposes, with particular reference to the definitions/ guidelines set out by this Working Group.
2. The definition selected should be applied consistently to allow uniform reporting and analysis of nosocomial infections. [IB]
3. With appropriate resources from the Hospital/ HAHO, NICU personnel should cooperate with hospital infection control personnel in conducting and reviewing the results of surveillance programs for nosocomial infections in a confidential manner.

Prevention and Control of Infections : Staff Health
1. Health care workers should be immune to rubella, measles and chicken pox. [IA]
2. Yearly influenza vaccination is available. [IB]
3. Ideally, individuals with a respiratory, cutaneous, mucocutaneous or gastrointestinal infection should not have direct contact with Neonates. [IB]

Handwashing
1. Medical and hospital personnel must follow careful hand-washing techniques to minimize transmission of disease. [IB]
2. Personnel should remove rings, watches, and bracelets before washing their hands and entering the neonatal nursery. [IB]
3. Fingernails should be trimmed short and no false fingernails or nail polish should be permitted. [IB]
4. Antiseptic preparations (e.g. chlorhexidine 4 %) should be used for scrubbing before entering the nursery, before providing care for neonates, before performing invasive procedures, and after providing care for neonates. [IA]
5. Before handling neonates for the first time, personnel should scrub their hands and arms to a point above the elbow thoroughly with an antiseptic soap. After vigorous washing, the hands should be rinsed thoroughly and dried with paper towels. [IB]
6. A 10-second wash without a brush, but with soap and vigorous rubbing, followed by thorough rinsing under a stream of water, is required before and after handling each neonate and after touching objects or surfaces likely to be contaminated with virulent microorganisms or hospital pathogens. [1A]

7. Handwashing is necessary even when gloves have been worn in direct contact with the infant. Handwashing should immediately follow removal of gloves, before touching another infant. [IB]

8. Alcohol-containing foams kill bacteria satisfactorily when applied to clean hands and with sufficient contact (in accordance with manufacturers' recommendations). They can be used in areas where no sinks are available or during emergency. [III] But they are not sufficient in cleaning physically soiled hands, because transient organisms are not removed.

Dress Code

1. Dress codes should be established for regular and part-time personnel who enter the neonatal unit. [IB]

2. Sterile long-sleeved gowns to be worn by all personnel who have direct contact with the sterile field during surgical and invasive procedures in the neonatal unit. [IB]

3. Gloves are to be worn when handling the neonate until blood and amniotic fluid have been removed from the skin. [IB]

4. When a neonate is held outside the bassinet by nursing or other Neonatal intensive care unit personnel, a gown should be worn over the clothing and either discarded after use or maintained for use exclusively in the care of that neonate. If one gown is used for each neonate, the gowns should be changed regularly. [IB]

5. Caps, masks and sterile gloves are to be used during surgical and invasive procedures. [IB]

Sibling Visits

1. Guidelines for visits should be established to maximize opportunities for visiting and to minimize the risks of nosocomial spread of pathogens brought into the unit by these young visitors. [IB]

2. No child with fever or symptoms of an acute illness, including an upper respiratory tract infection, gastroenteritis, or dermatitis, should be allowed to visit. Siblings who recently have been exposed to a known communicable disease and are susceptible should not be allowed to visit. These interviews should be documented in the patient's record, and approval for each sibling visit should be noted. [IB]

3. Children should carefully wash their hands before patient contact. [IB]

General Housekeeping

1. Cleaning should be performed in the following order – patient areas, accessory areas and then adjacent halls. [IB]

2. In the cleaning procedure, dust should not be dispersed into the air. [IB]

3. Standard types of portable vacuum cleaners should not be used in the neonatal ICU or SCBU because particulate matter and microbial contamination in the room may be disturbed and distributed by the exhaust jet. Vacuum cleaners that discharge outside the patient care area (i.e., central vacuum cleaning systems or portable vacuums) should be used so that only the cleaning wand, floor tool, and high-efficiency, particulate air filtered vacuum hose are brought into the patient care area. [IB]

4. Once dust has been removed, scrubbing with a mop and a disinfectant/detergent solution should be performed. Mop heads should be machine laundered and thoroughly dried daily. [IB]

5. Cabinet counters, work surfaces, and similar horizontal areas should be cleaned once a day and between patient use with a disinfectant/detergent and clean cloths; as they may be subject to heavy contamination during routine use. Friction cleaning is important to ensure physical removal of dirt and contaminating microorganisms. [IB]

6. Surfaces that are contaminated by patient specimens or accidental spills should be carefully cleaned and disinfected. [IB]

7. Walls, windows, storage shelves and similar non-critical surfaces should be scrubbed periodically with a disinfectant/detergent solution as part of the general housekeeping program. [IB]

8. Sinks should be scrubbed clean at least daily with a detergent. [IB]

Cleaning & Disinfecting Patient Care Equipment

1. Incubators, Open Care Units & Bassinets 1. When the incubators, open care units or bassinets are being cleaned and disinfected, all detachable parts should be removed and scrubbed meticulously. [IB]

2. If the incubator has a fan, it should be cleaned and disinfected; the manufacturer's instructions should be followed to avoid equipment damage. [IB]

3. The air filter should be maintained as recommended by the manufacturer. [IB]

4. Mattresses should be replaced when the surface covering is broken, because such a break precludes effective disinfection or sterilization. [IB]

5. Portholes and porthole cuffs and sleeves are easily contaminated, often heavily; cuffs should be replaced on a regular schedule or cleaned and disinfected frequently with freshly prepared mild soap or disinfectant solutions. [IB]

6. Incubators not in use should be thoroughly dried by running the incubator hot without water in the reservoir for 24 hours after disinfection. [IB]

7. Infants who remain in the nursery for an extended period should be transferred periodically to a different, disinfected unit so that the originally occupied unit can be cleaned. [IB]

Neonatal Linen – clean and soiled Clean Linen

1. Procedures for laundering, making up packs and delivering linen to the nursery should be established by the medical, nursing, laundry and administrative staffs of the hospital. [IB]

2. Each delivery of clean linen should contain sufficient linen for at least one 8-hour shift. [IB]

3. Linen should be cleaned and transported in covered carts or laundry bags to the nursery areas. [IB]

4. No new garments or linen should be used for neonates without prior laundering. [IB]

Soiled Linen

1. An established procedure for the disposal of soiled linen should be strictly followed. [IB]

2. Chutes for the transfer of soiled linen from patient care areas to the laundry are not acceptable unless they are under negative air pressure. [IB] 4. Sealed bags of reusable, soiled nursery linens should be taken to the laundry at least twice each day. [IB]

5. Impervious bags of soiled diapers (reusable or disposable) and other linen should be sealed and removed from the nursery at least every 8 hours. [IB]

6. All personnel should be aware that handling dirty diapers with bare hands can result in heavy contamination and transient colonization of the hands with microorganisms that cannot be easily eliminated with hand-washing and can be readily transmitted to the next neonate for whom they provide care. [IB]

6. Soiled linen should be discarded into bags that prevent leakage. [II]

Laundering

1. The chemicals trichlorocarbanilide or sodium salt of pentachlo rophenol should not be used in hospital laundering because they may be harmful. [IB]

2. To avoid the hazards associated with the use of such chemicals or enzymes in the hospital laundry, the physician in charge should be aware of all agents in use and should be informed before any changes are made should be used so in laundry chemicals or procedures. Caution should be exercised when new laundry or cleaning agents are introduced into the nursery or when procedures are changed. [IB]

Catheter-related sepsis

1. Meticulous attention should be given to aseptic insertion and maintenance of the cannula and to aseptic techniques of fluid administration. [IA]

2. All parenteral nutrition fluids should be mixed in the pharmacy, under a laminar flow hood. [IB]

3. If bottles of lipid emulsions are kept in the neonatal unit refrigerator, care should be taken to prevent contamination, as they are susceptible to contamination with a wide variety of bacteria and fungi that can proliferate to high concentrations within hours. Open bottles must be discarded no later than 24 hours after the seal has been broken. [IB]

4. Intravenous tubing, stopcocks, flush syringes should be changed (using sterile technique) on a regular basis and no less frequently than every 72 hours. [1B]

5. Replace tubing used to administer blood, blood products, or lipid emulsions within 24 hours of initiating the infusion. [IB]

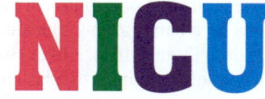

*Telemedicine in Neonatology is the use of electronic communications technology to provide and support health care for Newborn and young infants when distance separates the Specialist (Neonatologist, Pediatric subspecialists) from the patient, parent, guardian, or referring practitioner (also includes "e-health," meaning use of the Internet (with or without using videoconference functions to provide health care). This definition specifically excludes from discussion the use of ordinary telephone communication between practitioners and patients and the use of communications technology for education of practitioners. The information transferred in a telemedicine exchange may include live bidirectional audio or video, recorded audio or video sent after the encounter (so-called "store-and-forward" technology), medical records, medical images, sounds, or output from medical devices such as pulmonary function instruments, electrocardiographs, and ultrasonography devices.

*Telemedicine holds considerable promise for Neonatology and Pediatrics. Virtually any service can be provided via telecommunications technology, but a rigorous evaluation of telemedicine's potential is hampered by a lack of high-quality studies and cost-benefit analyses, especially in pediatrics.

*Certain Neonatal services seem well adapted to telemedicine, including the following:

1. Radiology: The electronic transmission of images to meet the needs of pediatric care has been well researched and is routine in most medical centers. The implications for providing high-quality pediatric radiology services over broad areas (and concomitant health care workforce redistribution issues) are immense.

2. Dermatology: Many diagnostic dermatologic evaluations can be performed by using high-quality still images. Although standard video cameras used in teleconferencing systems may not provide enough detail to make a dermatologic diagnosis, special peripheral cameras termed "dermatoscopes" have proved adequate. Remote "teledermatology" consultations have become commonplace at many medical centers.

3. Cardiology: Cardiology has already widely embraced telemedicine. Electronic stethoscopes can facilitate the transmission of heart sounds with excellent fidelity. Echocardiograms, ultrasonographic images, electrocardiograms, (In 1906, Einthoven first investigated the use of electrocardiogram (EKG) transmission over telephone lines.) and other images can readily be transmitted electronically and evaluated accurately as part of established telecardiology programs. Real-time transmission of neonatal echocardiograms from community hospitals over 3 ISDN (integrated services digital network) lines is accurate and has the potential to improve patient care, enhance echocardiogram quality, aid sonographer education, and have a positive impact on referral patterns and time management without increasing the utilization of echocardiography. Rapidly evolving technology likely will result in widespread implementation of telemedicine. Multicenter, double-blinded, randomized evaluation of this technology is appropriate to evaluate its role in pediatric cardiology more systematically.

Indications for Echocardiography

Suspected congenital heart disease
  Cyanosis, Tachypnea, Murmur,
  Arrhythmia, Fetal echo concern,
  Suspected coarctation

Rule out PDA, Follow up congenital heart disease, Genetic syndrome, Persistent pulmonary hypertension, Clot, endocarditis, or catheter position, Suspected pericardial effusion, Suspected hypertrophic cardiomyopathy, Hemodynamic instability, Hypertension, Kawasaki disease.

4. Ophthalmology: Retinopathy of Prematurity (ROP)—Retinal images from a baby born at district hospital can be teletransmitted to remote higher centers for critical appraisal and feedback.

5. Emergency and transport services: Emergency teleconferencing may be particularly beneficial with acceptable diagnostic sensitivity and specificity. for Neonates and infants in rural general emergency departments, in which complex Neonatal disease is seen only rarely, giving these patients the benefit of Neonatal consultants where none were available previously. One of the most immediately visible cost savings of telemedicine is the decreased need to transport patients to pediatric centers for critical care.

6. Pathology: Similar to dermatology and radiology, this visually intensive discipline is readily amenable to telemedicine consultation, especially in developing or rural areas.

7. Child abuse: Expertise in child abuse and neglect and the interdisciplinary communication that often must take place for an adequate child-maltreatment investigation present challenges that telemedicine could help to address.

8. Hospital care and family communication: The Infant Carelink Program, initially developed at Beth Israel Deaconess Medical Center (Boston, MA), allows families separated from their infants to keep updated on their infants' condition and to view images of their infants while they are in the neonatal intensive care unit. Data show that parental satisfaction with care is enhanced by this system. One study showed an increase in the rate of direct discharge home from the neonatal intensive care unit, as opposed to a costly intermediate transfer to a community hospital. Media reports suggest that similar projects are in place at other hospitals.

9. Patient Education and Chronic Disease: Some evidence exists that children who depend on medical equipment (Nebulizer, MDI, Home Oxygen Therapy, Tracheostomy, etc.) have access to improved care by use of telemedicine monitoring. The efficacy of telemedicine in patient education via teleconferencing to teach the proper use of asthma medications has been demonstrated, as has patient satisfaction.

10. School health: Some school systems are experimenting with telemedicine links to extend the range of services in school-based clinics and decrease absenteeism for illness or disease-management encounters.

11. Home health: Communication technology has helped enable patients to remain at home while being monitored for congestive heart failure, diabetic control, arrhythmias, or metabolic stability. Research suggests that homebound patients are pleased with this type of home health care service. Some data suggest that telemedicine-mediated home care of children with chronic disease can save money while preserving care quality.

Special educational training programs for pediatric subspecialists would provide the preparation needed to assist patients via telemedicine. Residency training programs that incorporate a multidisciplinary approach may provide an additional benefit. A multidisciplinary telemedical program might include primary care pediatricians, pediatric medical subspecialists, pediatric surgical specialists, primary care physicians, and other midlevel practitioners. As the need for telemedicine increases, medical schools and residency training must prepare to train physicians using the latest techniques in the 21st century.

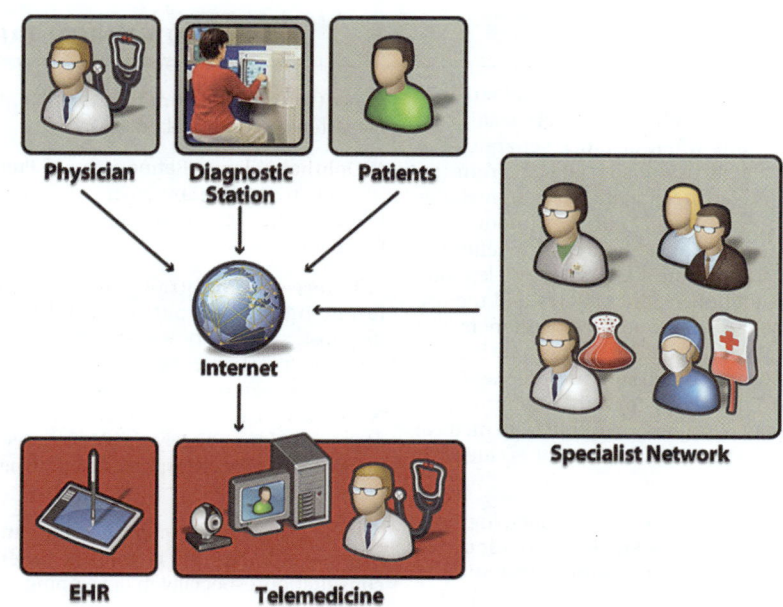

Two different kinds of technologies make up most of the telemedicine applications that we see around today. One of them is 'store and forward' and the other being 'real time medicine'. In the 'store and forward', medical data are transferred from one location to another. Using digital camera, the image taken ('stored') and then sent ('forwarded') by computer to another location. This is typically used for non-emergent situations, when a diagnosis or consultation may be made in the next 24 – 48 hours and sent back. CT scans, sending x-ray reports and MRIs are its most common examples. For 'real time medicine', the patient`s data are available to the specialist as soon as the local doctor receives it. Live conferencing technology and live data transmission are used in this technique. A great way to offer expert care and cut costs. The future of telemedicine is bright and we will look forward to it's numerous advances.

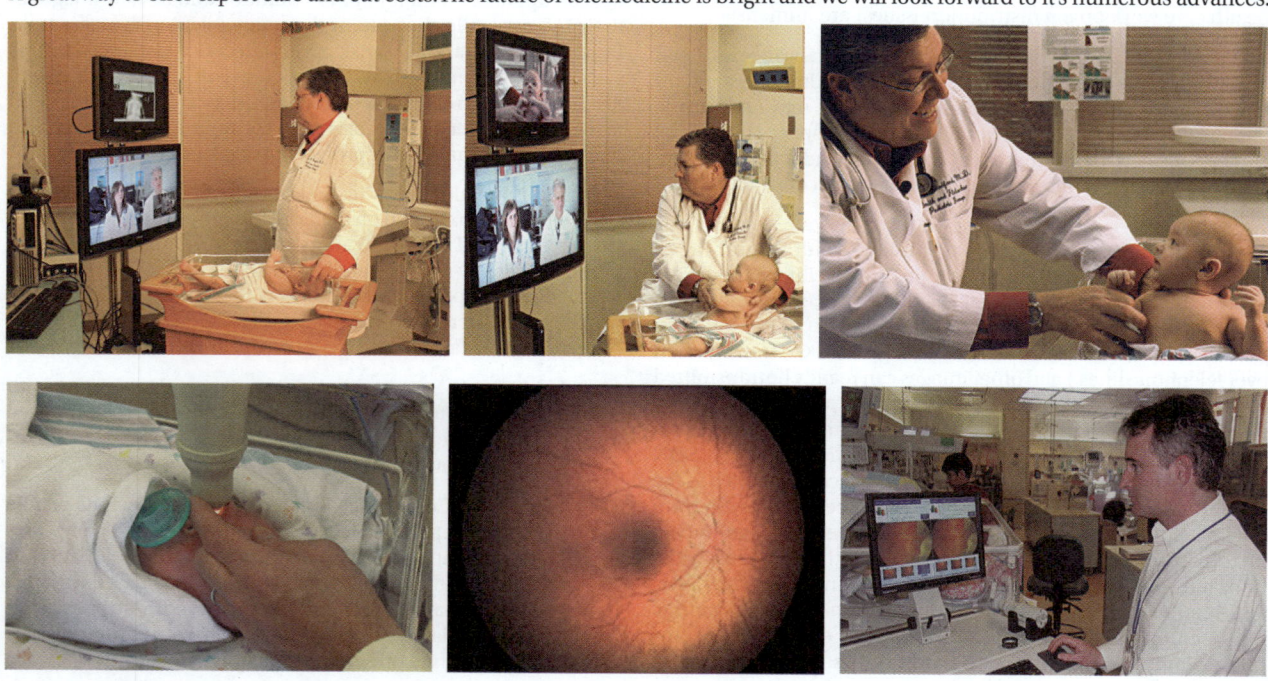

Wide-field digital retinal imaging a new paradigm for rop management: RetCam 120 fills the need for wide-field imaging and is fully digital. The camera has remarkable image quality for a panoramic imaging system. Optical resolution is same as CCD pixel size (about 36 microns) at boundary and twice as good in central region. ·Image distortion is negligible: There is an excellent mapping of angle onto CCD coordinate. Efficient assessment and monitoring. Nearly the entire retina is documented with only five images. Real-time imaging display provides immediate feedback. Inexpensive digital image storage on CD's eliminates film. Retrieve and manage patient information with built-in image database. Image Teletransmission to colleagues.

REFERENCES: 1) "Use of Telemedicine for Children With Special Health Care Needs" American Academy of Pediatrics. 4 April 2000. 29 June, 2007. http://pediatrics.aappublications.org/cgi/content/abstract/105/4/843 2) "Application of a low cost telemedicine link to the diagnosis of neonatal congenital heart defects by remote consultation". Heart Online. June 29, 2007. http://heart.bmj.com/cgi/content/abstract/82/2/217 3) Goodenough, Belinda, Cohn, Richard. **Parent Attitudes to Audio/Visual Telecommunications in Childhood Cancer: An Australian Study".** Telemedicine Journal and e-Health. Nov 2004, Vol. 10, No. supplement 2: S-15-S-25.

Definition: "Clinical audit is the systematic analysis of the quality of healthcare, including the procedures used for diagnosis, treatment and care, the use of resources and the resulting outcome and quality of life for the patient."

"a quality improvement process that seeks to improve patient care and outcomes through systematic review of care against explicit criteria and the implementation of change" NHS UK, 1993.

The place of clinical audit in modern healthcare

Clinical audit comes under the Clinical Governance umbrella and forms part of the system for improving the standard of clinical practice.

Clinical Governance is a system through which NHS organisations are accountable for continuously improving the quality of services, and ensures that there are clean lines of accountability within NHS trusts and that there is a comprehensive programme of quality improvement systems. The six pillars of clinical governance include:

* Clinical Effectiveness * Research & Development * Openness * Risk Management * Education and Training * Clinical Audit

Clinical audit was incorporated within Clinical Governance in the 1997 White Paper, "The New NHS, Modern, Dependable", which brought together disparate service improvement processes and formally established them into a coherent Clinical Governance framework.

Clinical audit - the process: Clinical audit can be described as a cycle or a spiral, *see figure*. Within the cycle there are stages that follow the *systematic* process of: establishing best practice; measuring against criteria; taking action to improve care; and monitoring to sustain improvement. As the process continues, each cycle aspires to a higher level of quality.

Stage 1: Identify the problem or issue

This stage involves the selection of a topic or issue to be audited, and is likely to involve measuring adherence to healthcare processes that have been shown to produce best outcomes for patients. Selection of an audit topic is influenced by factors including:

* where national standards and guidelines exist; where there is conclusive evidence about effective clinical practice (i.e. · evidence based medicine).

* areas where problems have been encountered in practice.

* what patients & public have recommended that be looked at.

* where there is a clear potential for improving service delivery.

* areas of high volume, high risk or high cost, in which improvements can be made.

Stage 2: Define criteria and standards

Decisions regarding the overall purpose of the audit, either as what should happen as a result of the audit, or what question you want the audit to answer, should be written as a series of statements or tasks that the audit will focus on. Collectively, these form the audit *criteria*. These criteria are explicit statements that define what is being measured and represent elements of care that can be measured objectively. The *standards* define the aspect of care to be measured, and should always be based on the best available evidence.

* A criterion is a measurable outcome of care, aspect of practice or capacity. For example, 'parents / carers are involved in negotiating or planning their child's care'.

* A standard is the threshold of the expected compliance for each criterion (these are usually expressed as a percentage). For the above example an appropriate standard would be: 'There is evidence of parent / carer in care planning in 90% of cases'.

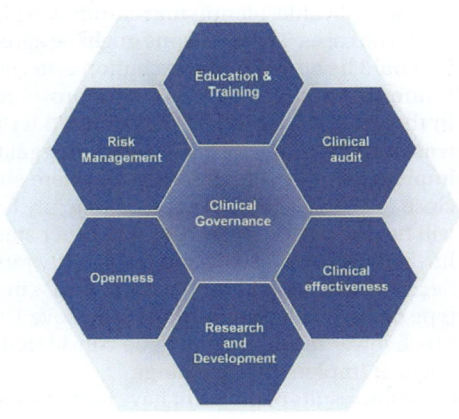

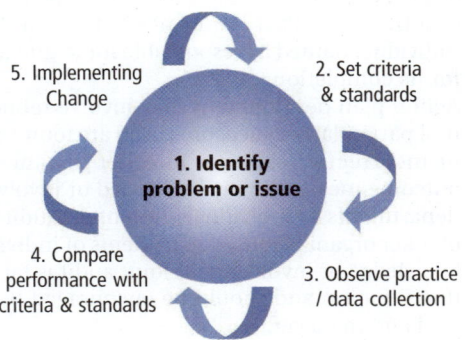

Stage 3: Data collection

To ensure that the data collected are precise, and that only essential information is collected, certain details of what is to be audited must be established from the outset. These include:

* The user group to be included, with any exceptions noted.

* The healthcare professionals involved in the users' care.

* The period over which the criteria apply.

Sample sizes for data collection are often a compromise between the statistical validity of the results and pragmatical issues around data collection. Data to be collected may be available in a computerised information system, or in other cases it may be appropriate to collect data manually depending on the outcome being measured. In either case, considerations need to be given to what data will be collected, where the data will be found, and who will do the data collection. Ethical issues must also be considered; the data collected must relate only to the objectives of the audit, and staff and patient confidentiality must be respected - identifiable information must not be used. Any potentially sensitive topics should be discussed with the local Research Ethics Committee.

Stage 4: Compare performance with criteria and standards

This is the analysis stage, whereby the results of the data collection are compared with criteria and standards. The end stage of analysis is concluding how well the standards were met and, if applicable, identifying reasons why the standards weren't met in all cases. These reasons might be agreed to be acceptable, i.e. could be added to the exception criteria for the standard in future, or will suggest a focus for improvement measures.

In theory, any case where the standard (criteria or exceptions) was not met in 100% of cases suggests a potential for improvement in care. In practice, where standard results were close to 100%, it might be agreed that any further improvement will be difficult to obtain and that other standards, with results further away from 100%, are the priority targets for action. This decision will depend on the topic area – in some 'life or death' type cases, it will be important to achieve 100%, in other areas a much lower result might still be considered acceptable.

Stage 5: Implementing change

Once the results of the audit have been published and discussed, an agreement must be reached about the recommendations for change. Using an action plan to record these recommendations is good practice; this should include who has agreed to do what and by when. Each point needs to be well defined, with an individual named as responsible for it, and an agreed timescale for its completion.

Action plan development may involve refinement of the audit tool particularly if measures used are found to be inappropriate or incorrectly assessed. In other instances new process or outcome measures may be needed or involve linkages to other departments or individuals. Too often audit results in criticism of other organizations, departments or individuals without their knowledge or involvement. Joint audit is far more profitable in this situation and should be encouraged by the Clinical Audit lead and manager.

Re-audit: Sustaining Improvements

After an agreed period, the audit should be repeated. The same strategies for identifying the sample, methods and data analysis should be used to ensure comparability with the original audit. The re-audit should demonstrate that the changes have been implemented and that improvements have been made. Further changes may then be required, leading to additional re-audits. This stage is critical to the successful outcome of an audit process - as it verifies whether the changes implemented have had an effect and to see if further improvements are required to achieve the standards of healthcare delivery identified in stage 2. Results of good audit should be disseminated both locally via the Strategic Health Authorities and nationally where possible.

Types of audit

* **Standards-based audit**: A cycle which involves defining standards, collecting data to measure current practice against those standards, and implementing any changes deemed necessary.

* **Adverse occurrence screening and critical incident monitoring** - This is often used to · peer review cases which have caused concern or from which there was an unexpected outcome. The multidisciplinary team discusses individual anonymous cases to reflect upon the way the team functioned and to learn for the future. In the primary care setting, this is described as a 'significant event audit'.

* **Peer review**: An assessment of the quality of care provided by a clinical team with a view to improving clinical care. Individual cases are discussed by peers to determine, with the benefit of · hindsight, whether the best care was given. This is similar to the method described above, but might include 'interesting' or 'unusual'

cases rather than problematic ones. Unfortunately, recommendations made from these reviews are often not pursued as there is no systematic method to follow.

* **Patient surveys and focus groups** - These are methods used to obtain users' views about the quality of care they have received. Surveys carried out for their own sake are often meaningless, but when they are undertaken to collect data they can be extremely productive.

NICU AUDIT TOPICS may include:

*Staffing levels
*Transfer of babies
*Communication between parents and staff
*The number of painful interventions
*Feeding types
*Parent facilities and visiting
*Kangaroo Care and Developmental Care
*Care after discharge and community services offered
*Inappropriate special care admissions
*Inappropriate social services involvement
*Morbidity
*Long term outcomes
*Use of surfactant
*Admission rates to NICU's
*Rates of infection / infection control
*Prophylactic antibiotic use (further research needed)

SUMMARY: An audit is not simply an information-gathering exercise but a valuable tool that can be used to evaluate quality of care. However, while selecting an audit topic and the criteria one should make sure that the reasons for choosing them are evidence based and reflect good practice. Never forget to re-audit the topic to make sure practice has improved and sustained. When done well, clinical audit can provide a way in which the quality of care can be reviewed objectively within a supportive and developmental environment. Confidentiality and consent issues must be addressed. The audit should use existing clinical information and take into consideration existing electronic systems. The audit should address the needs of the user (i.e. the baby and their families).

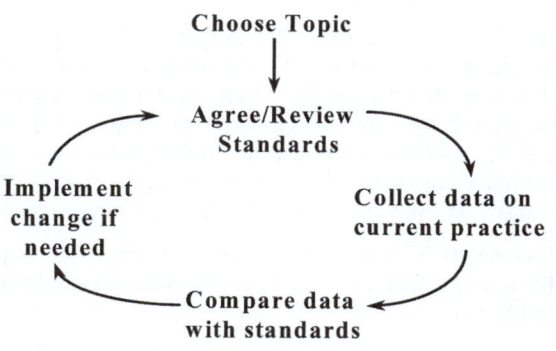

Immunisation Schedule IAP Immunisation Time Table
Recommendations of the IAP Committee on Immunisation

Age	Vaccines	Note
Birth	BCG OPV zero Hepatitis B -1	
6 weeks	OPV-1 + IPV-1 / OPV -1 DTPw-1 / DTPa -1 Hepatitis B -2 Hib -1	OPV alone if IPV cannot be given
10 weeks	OPV-2 + IPV-2 / OPV-2 DTPw-2 / DTPa -2 Hib -2	OPV alone if IPV cannot be given
14 weeks	OPV-3 + IPV-3 / OPV -3 DTPw-3 / DTPa -3 Hepatitis B -3 Hib -3	OPV alone if IPV cannot be given Third dose of Hepatitis B can be given at 6 months of age
9 months	Measles	
15-18 months	OPV-4 + IPV-B1 / OPV -4 DTPw booster -1 or DTPa booster -1 Hib booster MMR -1	OPV alone if IPV cannot be given
2 years	Typhoid	Revaccination every 3–4 years
5 years	OPV -5 DTPw booster -2 or DTPa booster -2 MMR -2	The second dose of MMR vaccine can be given at any time 8 weeks after the first dose
10 years	Tdap HPV	Only girls, three doses at 0, 1–2 and 6 months

Vaccines that can be given after discussion with parents

More than 6 weeks	Pneumococcal conjugate	3 primary doses at 6, 10, and 14 weeks, followed by a booster at 15–18 months
More than 6 weeks	Rotaviral vaccines	(2/3 doses (depending on brand) at 4-8 weeks interval
After 15 months	Varicella	Age less than 13 years: one dose Age more than 13 years: 2 doses at 4–8 weeks interval
After 18 months	Hepatitis A	2 doses at 6–12 months interval

The IAP endorses the continued use of whole cell pertussis vaccine because of its proven efficacy and safety. Acellular pertussis vaccines may undoubtedly have fewer side-effects (like fever, local reactions at injection site and irritability), but this minor advantage does not justify the inordinate cost involved in the routine use of this vaccine. *If the mother is known to be HBsAg negative, HB vaccine can be given along with DTP at 6, 10, 14 weeks/ 6 months. If the mother's HBsAg status is not known, it is advisable to start vaccination soon after birth to prevent perinatal transmission of the disease. If the mother is HBsAg positive (and especially HBeAg positive), the baby should be given Hepatitis B Immune Globulin (HBIG) within 24 hours of birth, along with HB vaccine. *Varicella, Hepatitis A and Pneumococcal Conjugate vaccines should be offered only after one to one discussion with parents. Also refer to the individual vaccines notes for recommendations. *Combination vaccines can be used to decrease the number of pricks being given to the baby and to decrease the number of clinic visits. The manufacturer's instructions should be followed strictly whenever "mixing" vaccines in the same syringe prior to injection. *At present, the only typhoid vaccine available in our country is the Vi polysaccharide vaccine. Revaccination may be carried out every 3–4 years. *Under special circumstances (e.g. epidemics), measles vaccine may be given earlier than 9 months followed by MMR at 12–15 months. *During pregnancy, the interval between the two doses of TT should be at least one month. *We should continue to use OPV till we achieve polio eradication in India. IPV can be used additionally for individual protection. *OPV must be given to children less than 5 years of age at the time of each supplementary immunization activity.

Courtesy: **2000–2009 Indian Academy of Pediatrics**

Cold chain: Vaccines must be stored properly from the time they are manufactured until the time they are administered. Excess heat or cold will reduce their potency, increasing the risk that recipients will not be protected against vaccine-preventable diseases. The system used to keep and distribute vaccines in good condition is called the cold chain. The cold chain has three main components: transport and storage equipment, trained personnel, and efficient management procedures. All three elements must combine to ensure safe vaccine transport and storage. The cold chain begins with the cold storage unit at the vaccine manufacturing plant, extends through the transfer of vaccine to the distributor and then to the provider's office, and ends with the administration of the vaccine to the patient. Proper storage temperatures must be maintained at every link in the chain. **Vaccine Potency** Excessive heat or cold exposure damages vaccine, resulting in loss of potency. Once potency is lost, it can never be restored. Furthermore, each time vaccine is exposed to heat or cold, the loss of potency increases and eventually, if the cold chain is not correctly maintained, all potency will be lost, and the vaccine becomes useless. **Vaccine appearance after exposure to inappropriate storage conditions.** Some vaccines may show physical evidence of altered potency when exposed to inappropriate storage conditions, such as clumping in the solution that does not go away when the vial is shaken. Other vaccines may look perfectly normal when exposed to inappropriate storage conditions. For example, inactivated vaccines exposed to freezing temperatures (i.e. 32°F [0°C] or colder) may not appear frozen and give no indication of loss of potency. Therefore, visual inspection of vaccines is an unreliable method of assuring potency.

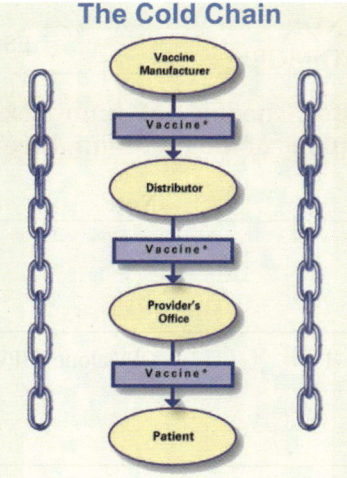

The Cold Chain

Vaccine Manufacturer → Vaccine* → Distributor → Vaccine* → Provider's Office → Vaccine* → Patient

Vaccine is transported in a refrigerated or frozen state, as appropriate (refrigerator 35°– 46°F [2°–8°C]; freezer 5°F [-15°C] or colder), using an insulated container or a refrigerated truck.

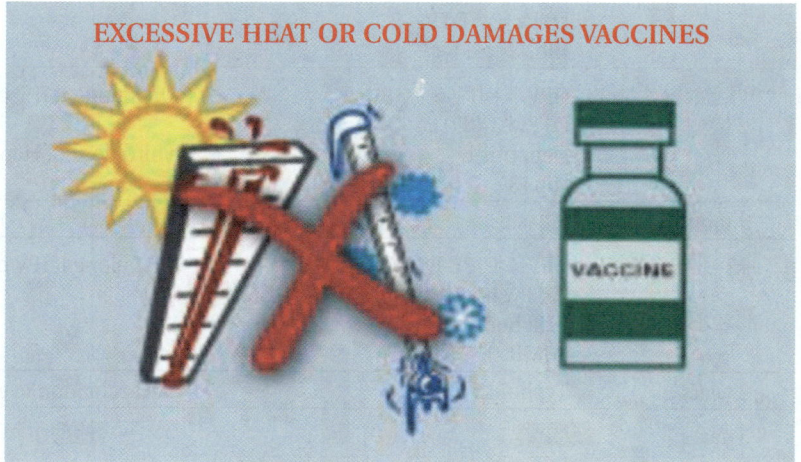

EXCESSIVE HEAT OR COLD DAMAGES VACCINES

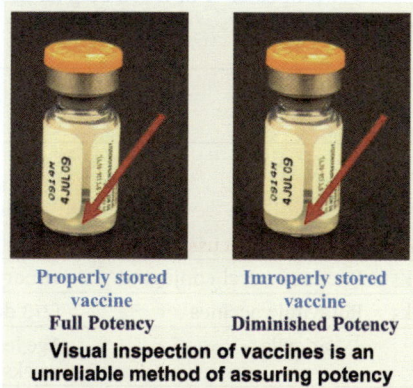

Properly stored vaccine **Full Potency**   Improperly stored vaccine **Diminished Potency**

Visual inspection of vaccines is an unreliable method of assuring potency

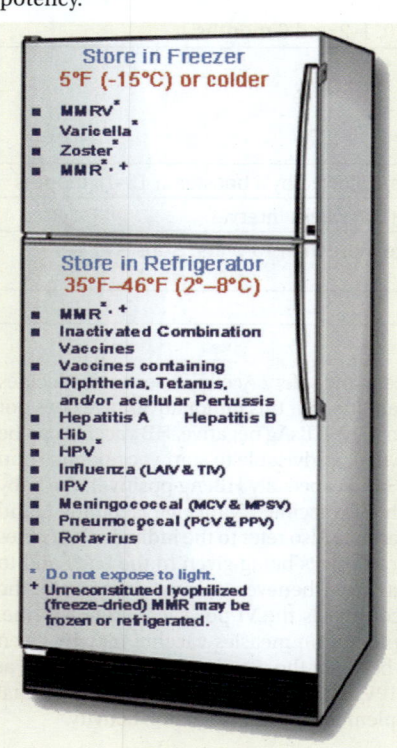

Store in Freezer
5°F (-15°C) or colder

- MMRV*
- Varicella*
- Zoster*
- MMR*,+

Store in Refrigerator
35°F–46°F (2°–8°C)

- MMR*,+
- Inactivated Combination Vaccines
- Vaccines containing Diphtheria, Tetanus, and/or acellular Pertussis
- Hepatitis A   Hepatitis B
- Hib*
- HPV*
- Influenza (LAIV & TIV)
- IPV
- Meningococcal (MCV & MPSV)
- Pneumococcal (PCV & PPV)
- Rotavirus

* Do not expose to light.
\+ Unreconstituted lyophilized (freeze-dried) MMR may be frozen or refrigerated.

Store each vaccine in its proper location.

Burden of cold chain failure: An estimated 17% to 37% of providers expose vaccines to improper storage temperatures. Refrigerator temperatures are more commonly kept too cold rather than too warm.[1,2] One study involving site visits showed that 15% of refrigeration units had temperatures of 34°F (1°C) or lower.[2] Out-of-range temperatures require **immediate action**. Loss of vaccine potency due to improper storage conditions is a costly mistake. Patients receiving vaccine with decreased potency caused by improper storage conditions may not be fully protected against the vaccine-preventable disease. In the General Recommendations on Immunization, the Advisory Committee on Immunization Practices (ACIP) and the American Academy of Family Physicians (AAFP) state that mishandled vaccine doses should not be counted as valid doses and should be repeated unless serologic testing indicates a response to the vaccine.[3] Recalling patients to repeat vaccine doses because vaccine has been stored improperly can damage public confidence in vaccines and in your practice.

Courtesy: Centers for Disease Control and Prevention. General recommendations on immunization: recommendations of the Advisory Committee on Immunization Practices and the American Academy of Family Physicians. MMWR 2002;51 (No. RR-2):1–36

Don't Be Guilty of these errors in vaccine storage and handling

The following are frequently reported errors in vaccine storage and handling. Some of these errors are much more serious than others, but none of them should occur. Be sure your clinic or practice is not making errors such as these.

Error #1: Designating only one person in the office to be responsible for storage and handling of vaccines, instead of a minimum of two.

It's important to train at least one back-up person to learn proper storage and handling of vaccines. The back-up person should be familiar with all aspects of vaccine storage and handling, including knowing how to handle vaccines when they arrive, how to properly record refrigerator and freezer temperatures, and what to do in case of an equipment problem or power outage.

Error #2: Recording temperatures only once per day.

Temperatures fluctuate throughout the day. Temperatures in the refrigerator and freezer should be checked at the beginning and end of the day to determine if the unit is getting too cold or too warm. Ideally, you should have continuous thermometers that measure and record temperatures all day and all night. A less expensive alternative is to purchase maximum/minimum thermometers. Only certified thermometers should be used for vaccine storage. It's also a good idea to record the room temperature on your temperature log in case there is a problem with the refrigerator or freezer temperature. This information may be helpful to the vaccine company's telephone consultant in determining whether your vaccine can still be used.

Error #3: Recording temperatures for only the refrigerator or freezer.

If your facility administers varicella, MMRV, or zoster (shingles) vaccine, you should have certified thermometers in both the refrigerator and freezer. Rather than buying cheap thermometers that may not accurately measure the temperature, buy quality thermometers that will last for years.

Error #4: Documenting out-of-range temperatures on vaccine temperature logs but not taking action.

Documenting temperatures is not enough. Acting on the information is even more important! So, what should you do? Notify your supervisor whenever you have an out-of-range temperature. Safe-guard your vaccines by moving them to another location and then deter-mine if they are still useable. Check the condition of the unit for problems. Are the seals tight? Is there excessive lint or dust on the coils? After you have made the adjustment, document the date, time, temperature, the nature of the problem, the action you took, and the results of your action. Recheck the temperature every two hours. Call maintenance or a repair person if the temperature is still out of range.

Error #5: Discarding temperature logs at the end of every month.

It's important that you keep your temperature logs for at least three years. As the refrigerator ages, you can track recurring problems. If out-of-range temperatures have been documented, you can determine how long this has been happening and take appropriate action. It's also a great way to lobby for a new refrigerator.

Error #6: Refrigerating vaccine in a manner that could jeopardize its quality.

The temperature in the vegetable bins, on the floor, next to the walls, in the door, and near the cold air outlet from the freezer may differ significantly from the temperature in the body of the refrigerator. Always store vaccines in their original packaging in the body of the refrigerator away from these locations. Place vaccine packages in such a way that air can circulate around the compartment. Never overpack a refrigerator compartment.

Error #7: Storing frozen vaccines in a dorm-style refrigerator.

Varicella, MMRV, and zoster (shingles) vaccines must be stored in a freezer that has its own external door separate from the refrigerator. No matter how hard you try to adjust the temperature in a dorm-style refrigerator's freezer to +5°F, you won't be able to reach this low freezer temperature, and you'll probably freeze the vaccines in the refrigerator compartment!

Error #8: Inadvertently leaving the refriger-ator or freezer door open or having inadequate seals.

Remind staff to close the unit doors tightly each time they open them. Also, check the seals on the doors on a regular schedule, and if there is any indication the door seal may be cracked or not sealing properly, have it replaced. The cost of replacing a seal is much less than replacing a box of pneumococcal conjugate or varicella vaccine.

Error #9: Discarding multi-dose vials 30 days after they are opened.

Don't discard your vaccines prematurely. Almost all multi-dose vials of vaccine contain a preservative and can be used until the expiration date on the vial unless there is visible contamination. However, you must discard multi-dose vials of reconstituted vaccine (e.g., meningococcal polysaccharide, yellow fever) if they are not used within a defined period after reconstitution. Refer to the vaccine package inserts for additional information.

Error #10: Not having emergency plans for a power outage or natural disaster.

Every clinic should have a written Disaster Recovery Plan that identifies a refrigerator with a back-up generator in which to store vaccine in the event of a power outage or natural disaster. Consider contacting a local hospital or similar facility to be your back-up location if you should need it.

Error #11: Storing food and drinks in the vaccine refrigerator.

Frequent opening of the refrigerator door to retrieve food items can adversely affect the internal temperature of the unit and damage vaccines.

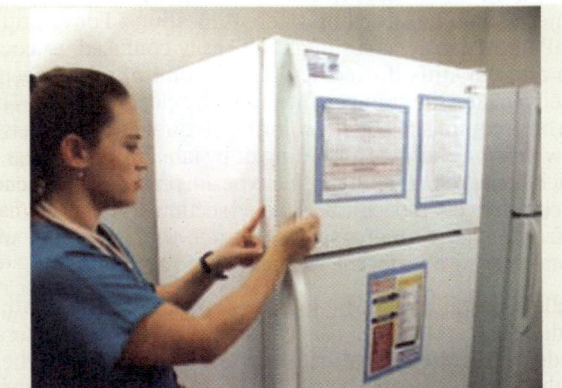

Check that doors are properly sealed each time they are closed and at the end of each day.

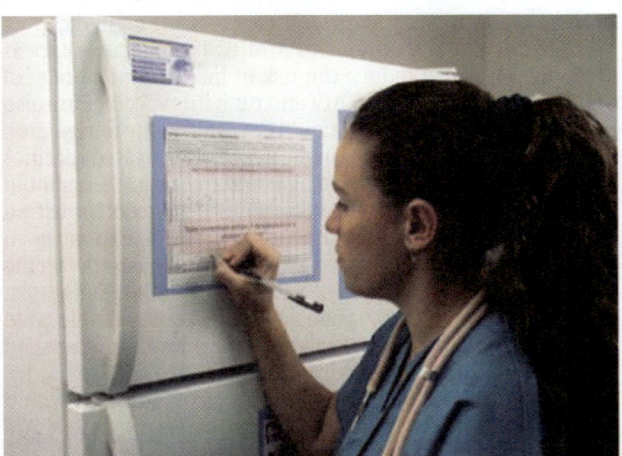

Always do maintain vaccine temperature log chart: Any readings above or below the acceptable range must be reported to your local public health unit immediately.

CHECKLIST FOR SAFE VACCINE HANDLING AND STORAGE
Here are the 20 most important things you can do to safeguard your vaccine supply. Are you doing them all?
Reviewing this list can help you improve your clinic's vaccine management practices.

Yes/No

1. We have a designated person in charge of the handling and storage of our vaccines.

2. We have a back-up person in charge of the handling and storage of our vaccines.

3. A vaccine inventory log is maintained that documents:
Vaccine name and number of doses received
Date the vaccine was received
Arrival condition of vaccine
Vaccine manufacturer and lot number
Vaccine expiration date

4. Our refrigerator for vaccines is either household-style or commercial-style, NOT dormitory-style. The freezer compartment has a separate exterior door.
Alternatively, we use two storage units: a free-standing refrigerator and a separate, free-standing freezer.

5. We do NOT store any food or drink in the refrigerator or freezer.

6. We store vaccines in the middle of the refrigerator or freezer, and NOT in the door.

7. We stock and rotate our vaccine supply so that the newest vaccine of each type (with the longest expiration date) is placed behind the vaccine with the shortest expiration date.

8. We check vaccine expiration dates and we first use those that will expire soonest.

9. We post a sign on the refrigerator door showing which vaccines should be stored in the refrigerator and which should be stored in the freezer.

10. We always keep a thermometer in the refrigerator.

11. The temperature in the refrigerator is maintained at 35–46ºF (2–8ºC).

12. We keep extra containers of water in the refrigerator to help maintain cold temperatures.

13. We always keep a thermometer in the freezer.

14. The temperature in the freezer is maintained at +5ºF (-15ºC) or colder.

15. We keep ice packs and other ice-filled containers in the freezer to help maintain cold temperatures.

16. We post a temperature log on the refrigerator door on which we record the refrigerator and freezer temperatures twice a day—first thing in the morning and at clinic closing time— and we know whom to call if the temperature goes out of range.

17. We have a "Do Not Unplug" sign next to the refrigerator's electrical outlet.

18. In the event of a refrigerator failure, we take the following steps:
We assure that the vaccines are placed in a location with adequate refrigeration.

We mark exposed vaccines and separate them from undamaged vaccines.

We note the refrigerator or freezer temperature and contact the vaccine manufacturer or state health department to determine how to handle the affected vaccines.

We follow the vaccine manufacturer's or health department's instructions as to whether the affected vaccines can be used, and, if so, we mark the vials with the revised expiration date provided by the manufacturer or health department.

19. We have obtained a detailed written policy for general and emergency vaccine management from our local or state health department.

20. If all above answers are "yes," we are patting ourselves on the back. If not, we have assigned someone to implement needed changes!

Live vaccines are sensitive to heat. MMRV, varicella, and zoster vaccines must be stored in a continuously frozen state in a freezer at 5°F (–15°C) or colder until administration. MMRV, varicella, and zoster vaccines deteriorate rapidly after they are removed from the freezer. Measles, mumps, and rubella vaccine (MMR) is routinely stored in the refrigerator, but it also can be stored in the freezer. The National Center for Immunization and Respiratory Diseases recommends keeping MMR in the freezer along with MMRV, if adequate space is available. This may reduce the risk of inadvertent storage of MMRV in the refrigerator. LAIV and rotavirus vaccines are also live virus vaccines, but they should be stored in the refrigerator. Do NOT store these vaccines in the freezer. Inactivated vaccines are sensitive to both excessive heat and freezing. They should be stored in a refrigerator at 35° to 46°F (2° to 8°C), with a desired average temperature of 40°F (5°C). Exposure to temperatures outside this range results in decreased vaccine potency and increased risk of vaccine-preventable diseases. Inactivated vaccines may tolerate limited exposure to elevated temperatures, but they are cold sensitive and are damaged rapidly by freezing temperatures. HPV, MMR, MMRV, rotavirus, varicella, and zoster vaccines are sensitive to light, which causes loss of potency. These vaccines must be protected from light at all times. Therefore, store these vaccines at the appropriate temperatures in their boxes with the tops on until they are needed. Diluents packaged separately from their corresponding vaccines can be stored at room temperature or in the refrigerator. Diluents packaged with their vaccines should be stored in the refrigerator next to their vaccines. In the freezer, vaccine should be stored in the middle of the compartment, away from the walls, coils, and peripheral areas. Vaccines should not be stored in the freezer door. The temperature in the door is not stable and differs from that in the main compartment. MMRV, varicella, and zoster vaccines may be stored in either a manual defrost or a frost-free freezer at 5° F (–15° C) or colder. vaccines that have similar sounding names should be stored in different locations. For example, DTaP and Tdap vaccines might be easily confused, as could Hib and hepatitis B vaccines. The location of each specific vaccine inside the storage unit should be clearly labeled. This can be accomplished by attaching labels directly to the shelves on which the vaccines are sitting or by labeling containers in which boxes of the same vaccine type are placed. Storing each vaccine in its own specifically labeled section of the refrigerator or freezer helps decrease the chance that someone will mistakenly administer the wrong type of vaccine.

Medications and other biologic products: If possible, other medications and other biologic products should not be stored inside the vaccine storage unit. If there is no other choice, these products must be stored below the vaccines on a different shelf. This prevents contamination of the vaccines should the other products spill, and reduces the likelihood of medication errors.

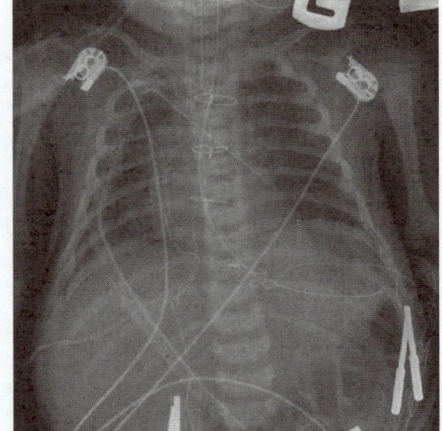

Normal position of tubes and lines in a post-operative cardiac patient.
Frontal chest radiograph of an infant immediately postoperatively shows an atrial line curled in the right atrium, projected lateral to the thoracic spine and exiting the chest below the heart, with the catheter sitting externally over the upper abdomen. These are placed at the time of surgery directly through the atrial wall. In addition there is an

ET tube with tip at T2, NG tube, sternal wires, and a large posteriorly positioned mediastinal/thoracic surgical drain. There are temporary epicardial pacing wires also shown whose leads are external to the patient.

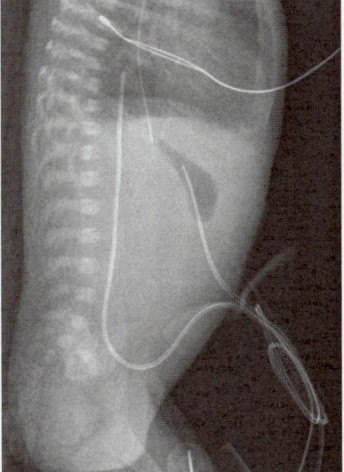

Normal position of tubes and lines in a Neonate. Lateral abdominal radiograph of a Neonate shows the normal posterior position of a UAC whose tip is in the distal thoracic aorta, and the UVC passing posteriorly into the liver and the ductus venosus, but short of the IVC-RA junction.

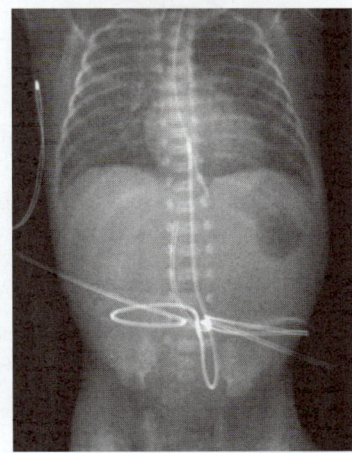

Normal position of tubes and lines in a Neonate. Frontal abdominal radiograph of a neonate with a UAC at the level of T8-9 and a UVC projected over the lower aspect of the ductus venosus. Note this patient also has a NG tube, an ET tube whose tip is at T2 and external temperature probe in the right axilla.

Normal position of tubes and lines in a Neonate. Frontal abdominal radiograph of a neonate who has a UAC positioned in the midabdomen at L2 level, an NG tube in the stomach and an ET tube at T2. There is a right sided leg PICC with the tip curled in the IVC at the level of L1. External ECG leads and a temperature probe are seen.

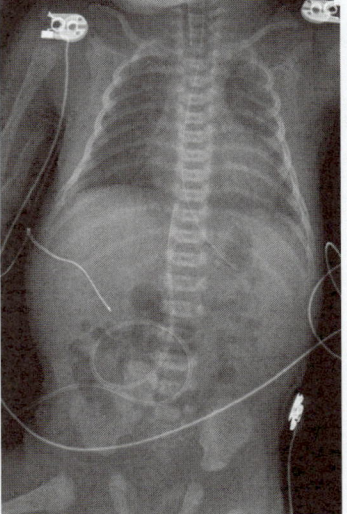

Normal position of tubes and lines in a Neonate. Frontal radiograph of a Neonate with a UVC in ideal position, whose tip is at the IVC-RA junction. The infant also has an ET tube at T1 and an NG tube. There is an external temperature probe over the right abdomen and ECG leads are present.

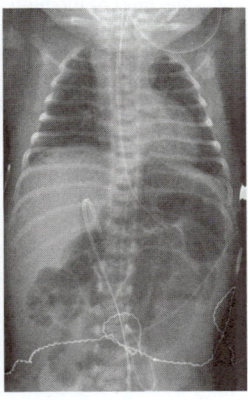

Frontal abdominal radiograph of a neonate with a UVC that has curled back on itself in a portal venous branch (confirmed with a lateral view). This infant also has a UAC, whose tip is at T7, an NG tube and ET tube in position. An umbilical wire clamp is also shown as crimped wire. Undesirable position of the UVC in a portal venous branch.

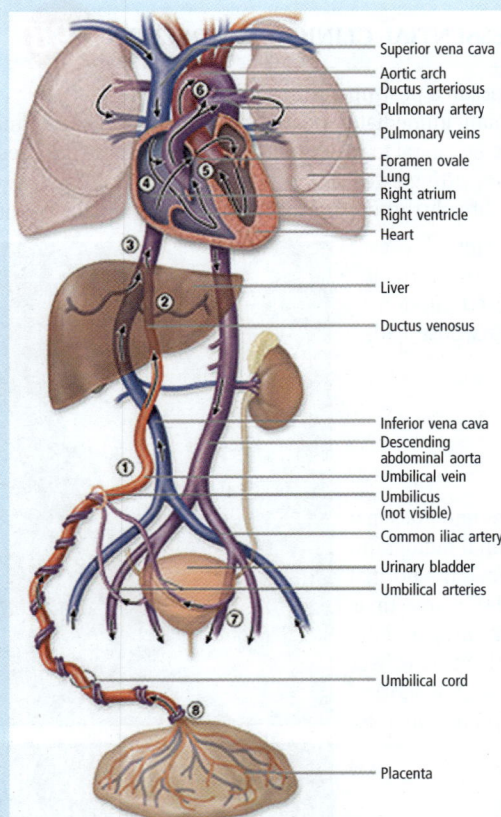

- Superior vena cava
- Aortic arch
- Ductus arteriosus
- Pulmonary artery
- Pulmonary veins
- Foramen ovale
- Lung
- Right atrium
- Right ventricle
- Heart
- Liver
- Ductus venosus
- Inferior vena cava
- Descending abdominal aorta
- Umbilical vein
- Umbilicus (not visible)
- Common iliac artery
- Urinary bladder
- Umbilical arteries
- Umbilical cord
- Placenta

Neonatal Vascular Anatomy: The positioning of umbilical catheters in particular is easier to digest if you understand the foetal vascular anatomy

1. "Oxygenated blood from the placenta enters through the umbilical vein.
2. Blood is shunted away from the liver and directly toward the inferior vena cava through the ductus venosus.
3. Oxygenated blood in the ductus venosus mixes with deoxygenated blood in the inferior vena cava.
4. Blood empties into the right atrium.
5. Most of the blood is shunted to the left atrium via the foramen ovale.
6. Blood flows into the left ventricle and out the aorta.
7. A small amount of blood enters the right ventricle and pulmonary trunk, but much of this blood is shunted to the aorta through ductus arteriosus.
8. Blood travels to the rest of the body, and the deoxygenated blood returns to the placenta through umbilical arteries. "

Intravascular Catheters Information: Sterile Technique

All Long Lines (LL), Central Venous Lines (CVL), Umbilical Venous Lines (UVC) and Umbilical Arterial Lines (UAC) use sterile technique during:

*Insertion *Fluid preparation and administration *Line and dressing changes *Drug preparation and administration
*Sterile technique - the practices that make and keep objects and areas micro-organism free:
*The trolley is wiped down with chlorhexidine 0.5% in alcohol 70% *The equipment used is placed on a sterile guard or a disposable dressing pack is used *The "sterile" nurse washes hands and dons sterile gloves and touches only that which is sterile
*A second nurse assists her by handling all equipment that is not sterile e.g. lipid syringe, bag of IVN, Dextrose 10%, medication ampoules.
*N.B.: Masks are not worn for these procedures.

Aseptic Technique

All Intravenous Lines (IV) and Peripheral Arterial Lines (PAL) use "aseptic technique" during:
*Insertion *Fluid preparation and administration *Line changes * Drug preparation and administration
*Aseptic technique – a clean procedure which controls and reduces the number of micro-organisms and prevents their spread from one place or person to another: this process may be managed by one nurse if appropriate , then the nurse washes hands – does not wear gloves and carries out the procedure keeping the risk of sepsis in mind.

Pall Filters

·Pall filters (0.22 micron) are used on all lines to reduce the risk of bacteria, air, particulates, microbes and endotoxin contamination to the infant. This enables standard fluid and lines to be changed every 96 hours (4 days) safely.
·NB: The Pall Filter is never used to filter blood, blood products, Lipid, Paraldehyde, Amphotericin B or Prostaglandins.
·Lipid is administered below the Pall filter.

Fluid Stability: Change unaltered fluids as follows: Fluid/Medication Change Frequency 10% Dextrose 96 hourly, 10% Dextrose with additives 96 hourly, IVN 96 hourly, 0.9% NaCl and 0.45%NaCl 96 hourly, Heparinized Saline 96 hourly, Lipid and tubing 24 hourly, Morphine and tubing 48 hourly, Dopamine and tubing 48-hourly, Dobutamine and tubing 48-hourly, Insulin and tubing 24 hourly, Fentanyl and tubing 24 hourly, Prostaglandin and tubing 24 hourly. N.B.: If the fluid prescription alters e.g. 10% dextrose to 12.5% Dextrose, the tubing may need to be flushed so that the baby receives the appropriate strength solution immediately.

Prevention and Detection of Air Embolus· This is a life threatening complication where air has entered the circulatory system and can occur:
·On insertion of the catheter ·At tubing change ·During drug administration ·The Nurse observes for the following signs: *Sudden cyanosis. *Circulatory collapse. *Withdrawal of blood from a UAC yielding alternating sections of air and blood. 1 Stop the infusion. 2 Position baby head down, left side down. 3 Notify medical staff/NS-ANP. 4 Resuscitate baby as necessary. 5 ASPIRATE AS MUCH AIR AS POSSIBLE. 6 Record and document vital signs.

Thrombosis with Embolization – (CVL) Detection/Prevention
This can be life threatening. If a blood clot forms in the circulatory system (thrombosis) a piece may become dislodged (embolism). This may occur in the: ·Superior vena cava, Right atrium, Inferior vena cava.
Action
1) The Nurse will observe for the following clinical signs and report to medical staff immediately. *Constant occlusion alarms. *Swelling of the head and neck. *Plethora and venous distension of the head and chest. *Irritability and crying during flushing of the catheter. *Failure to obtain a blood return through catheter. *Increased anterior fontanelle pressure. *Increased respiratory distress. *Swelling of lower limbs.
2) Ensure that infusion fluids are heparinized.
3) Ensure fluids are infused at appropriate rates at all times.
Misplaced Catheter CVL: A misplaced central venous catheter may cause. *Hydrothorax. *Pericardial effusion and cardiac tamponade. *Hemothorax (rare). Assess baby's condition and monitor closely!
Look for: *Signs of respiratory distress. *Increased oxygen requirements. *Tachycardia *Restlessness *Submandibular and neck swelling. *Hypoglycemia *Hypotension *Absence of a blood return through line.

Complications of Fluid Therapy: Sepsis – Intravenous nutrition is an excellent medium for the growth of micro-organisms and small premature infants are at high risk of infection. Foreign material passing through skin may act as a portal of entry for pathogens. Catheter related problems: *extravasation *hemorrhage *Air embolus *Thrombosis with embolization

IVN complications – infants may develop metabolic imbalances and must be monitored closely. Hyperlipidemia ·Intralipid can displace bilirubin from the albumen binding site increasing the risk of kernicterus. *May result from lipid overdose, occurs more often in the small preterm infants and SGA infants. Complications include platelet dysfunction, eosinophilia, liver abnormalities, pulmonary disposition of lipid in blood vessels.

Slipped out/ Disconnected/ Leaking/ Blocked Intravascular Catheter: 1) Clamp line. 2) Stop infusion and notify CCN/medical staff/NS-ANP

Prevention of Hemorrhage: 1) Always use luerlock connections 2) Use snap connection provided to clamp line. 3) Check infusion site appropriately. 4) Check line placement frequently ensuring appropriate RBP used to secure line.

SUMMARY OF COMMONLY USED CENTRAL VENOUS CATHETERS

Catheter type	Description
Peripherally inserted central catheter	Inserted via a peripheral vein (usually basilic, cephalic, or brachial) into superior vena cava
Nontunneled CVC	Inserted directly into a central vein (usually subclavian, internal jugular, or femoral) through skin incision
Tunneled CVC	Inserted through a subcutaneous tunnel on chest wall before entering the superior vena cava (e.g, Broviac, Hickman, Groshong, or Quinton catheter); a dacron cuff located at the tunnel exit site contributes to long-term catheter stability by stimulating growth of tissue around the tunneled portion of the catheter.
Totally implantable venous access device (port)	Subcutaneous port or reservoir with self-sealing septum that is accessed by a needle through intact skin; catheter tip located in subclavian or internal jugular vein

TYPES OF CATHETER-RELATED INFECTIONS

Infection	Clinical diagnosis
Exit site infection	Erythema or induration within 2 cm of catheter exit site
Tunnel infection	Tenderness, erythema, or induration along the subcutaneous tract of a tunneled catheter and more than 2 cm from catheter exit site
Pocket infection	Purulent fluid in the subcutaneous pocket of a totally implanted venous access device; may be accompanied by overlying tenderness, erythema, induration, visible drainage, and skin necrosis
Catheter-associated BSI	Positive simultaneous blood cultures from the CVC and peripheral vein yielding the same organism in the presence of at least one of the following: Simultaneous quantitative blood cultures in which the number of CFUs isolated from blood drawn through the central catheter was at least fivefold more than the number isolated from blood drawn peripherally. Positive semiquantitative (≥ 15 CFU / catheter segment) or quantitative (≥ 100 CFU / catheter segment) catheter tip cultures. Simultaneous blood cultures in which the central blood culture grows ≥ 2 hours earlier than the peripheral blood culture.

Abbreviation : CFU, colony-forming unit.

MANAGEMENT OF THE CATHETER IN PATIENTS WITH A CENTRAL VENOUS CATHETER-RELATED INFECTION

Type of infection	Catheter management

Exit site infection	Remove CVC if
	  No longer required
	  Alternate site exists
	  Patient critically ill
	  (e.g. hypotension)
	Infection caused by P.aeruginosa or Fungi

Tunnel infection	Remove CVC
Pocket infection	Remove CVC

Catheter-related BSI	Remove CVC if
	  No longer required
	  nfection caused by *S. aureus,* Candida spp, or mycobacteria
	  Patient critically ill
	  Failure to clear bacteremia in 48-72 hours
	  Persistent symptoms of BSI beyond 48-72 hours
	  Noninfectious valvular heart disease (increased risk of endocarditis)
	  Endocarditis
	  Metastatic infection
	  Septic thrombophlebitis

Distribution of most common pathogens indentified(in Blood Stream) from patients in pediatric intensive care units (NNIS 1992-1997)

Coagulase-negative staphylococci(CONS) 37.8%, *Enterococcus* 11.2%, *S. aureus* 9.3%, *Enterococcus* spp 6.2%, *Candida albicans* 5.5%, *P. aeruginosa* 4.9%, *Klebsiella Pneumoniae* 4.1%, *Escherichia coli* 2.9%

NEONATAL LONG LINES : ARE THEY SAFE ?

- Central venous lines provide secure vascular access in newborn infants, but are associated with many serious complications.
- Line related sepsis, the commonest of these, may be minimized by using polyurethane or silicone CV lines, minimizing line breaks, using single rather than multiple lumen lines, shortening duration of use, and staff education.
- Extravasation probably occurs as the result of the catheter tip being in a small vein or pointing at the wall of a large vessel or cardiac chamber.
- Pericardial effusions resulting in tamponade may be more likely when the catheter tip lies within the cardiac silhouette, particularly if there is a length of free catheter within the heart.
- Positioning the line tip outside the heart does not completely prevent cardiac tamponade and may cause other serious complications.
- Early signs of pericardial effusion should be recognized, including unexplained cardiovascular decompensation and enlarging cardiac silhouette on x ray examination.
- Long lines should, where possible, be repositioned until the tip is outside the cardiac silhouette, avoiding small vessels and acute angles between catheter and vascular wall, with final tip position confirmed by x ray examination or ultrasound.
- Parents should be informed about planned long line insertion, and individual units should consider formal consent.
- There should be senior involvement in the supervision of long line use, the setting up of feeding guidelines, and staff education.

Courtesy: G Menon, Neonatal Unit, Simpson Centre for
Reproductive Health, Royal Infirmary of Edinburgh, UK

Accessing the long line

Long line infections are a very significant cause of morbidity and mortality.

Repeated accessing of lines increases the chances of infection therefore must be minimized.

Lines can be used for the following infusions/drugs only. Any deviation from this MUST be made by a senior clinician

MUST be given centrally (Long line or UVC: >12.5% dextrose infusion, Adrenaline infusion (Concentrated), Dopamine (concentrated), Concentrated "central" PN*

CAN be given via Long line routinely: Adrenaline infusion (standard), Alprostadil, Atracurium infusion, Calcium chloride, Dextrose infusion, Dobutamine, Dopamine, Fentanyl infusion, Insulin, Isoprenaline infusion, Lidocaine infusion, Morphine infusion, Potassium chloride, Sodium bicarbonate, TPN

CANNOT be given by long line as they will block lumen. (but CAN go via UVC/broviac line):
Cryoprecipitate, FFP, PRC, Platelets

Peripheral PN may be used peripherally. This has a glucose concentration of no more than 12.5% and no calcium or phosphate added.

Accessing the line must be using an aseptic technique such as the following procedure: This is a two person procedure
*Clean trolley and allow to dry and consider creating a sterile zone with screens
*Assemble all equipment on trolley using a non-touch technique
*Wash and dry hands with sterile towel
*Apply sterile gloves
*Open incubator doors using elbow technique
*Clean long line port using friction for 15 seconds and allow to dry for 30 seconds
*Draw up flush using a filter needle
*Access long line
If contamination of gloves/equipment occurs change appropriately

INSERTION DISTANCE OF NEONATAL INTERCOSTAL CATHETERS

In a Neonate, there is little guidance as to the optimal site to place an intercostal catheter (ICC) when draining a pneumothorax. Numerous complications have been reported after ICC insertion in Neonates and it is considered prudent not to insert them too far to avoid damage to mediastinal structures. If an ICC that crosses the midline, it is considered to be inserted too far.
Possible complications that might arise from an ICC that encroaches on midline structures in the thorax include phrenic nerve palsy, Horner's syndrome, and penetration of the mediastinum and/or pericardium. Whilst the correct position for ICC placement when draining pneumothoraces has not been well studied, it would seem prudent to avoid midline structures. Odita et al recommend that that the ICC tip should be no less than one centimetre from the spine or mediastinum. This becomes important if an ICC is incorrectly placed posterior to the lung as it may damage posterior mediastinal contents.

*Courtesy: M. W. DAVIES, K. R. DUNSTER, *Grantley Stable Neonatal Unit Royal Women's Hospital, Brisbane, QUEENSLAND*

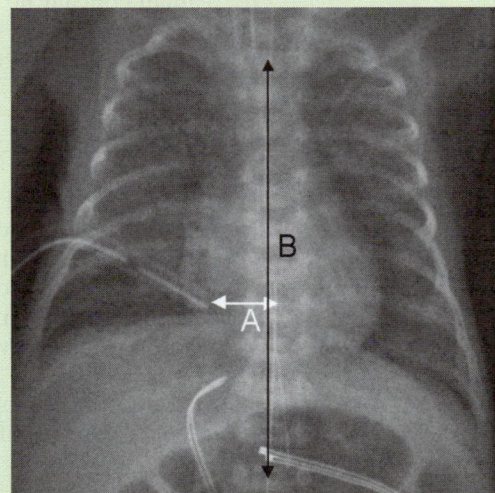

A chest X-ray of an infant with an intercostal catheter in situ. Measurement A is the tip to midline distance. Measurement B is the distance from the middle of the first to the middle of the last thoracic vertebrae.

It is a legal and ethical requirement to gain valid consent before examining and initiating any investigation and treatment for any patient. Failure to seek consent is not an option. However in neonatal practice there are frequently occasions, particularly soon after birth, when there is no-one available to provide valid consent and the clinician has to initiate treatment in its absence. It should always be possible later to justify that action to the parents, and to reassure them that what was done was in the best interests of the baby.

Principles

1. Consent is obtained from someone with parental responsibilities; this will usually be the parents.

2. The basis of valid informed consent is the establishment of clear two-way communication and is an on-going process. Consistent communication will increase the parents' trust and confidence in the medical and nursing team and decrease the likelihood of problems.

3. Consent is valid only when the information provided has been understood by the parents and explains why the intervention is recommended, its risks and what are the implications and options should consent be withheld.

4. It will not usually be necessary to document consent to routine and low risk procedures.

5. In emergency, if consent cannot be obtained e.g. because nobody with parental responsibility is available or the parents are too distressed to give valid informed consent, treatment may lawfully be started if clinicians believe it to be in the child's best interests.

6. Consent may be written, verbal or implied. Documentation indicating the content of the information given to parents and of their apparent understanding and agreement to proceed is the most important validation of consent. A parental signature does not of itself confirm informed consent.

7. The gaining of explicit consent, whether with or without a signature, should be witnessed and the name of the witness recorded.

8. Parents should understand that they can withdraw consent for investigations and treatments not yet completed. If the clinical team believe that this is counter to the interests of the baby they should discuss this with the parents and may need to take advice which in the first instance should be from the hospital's senior management team and / or Social Services.

Good practice

1. Whenever possible communication with the parents should begin antenatally both through meetings with neonatal staff and using written material.

2. Written material should be available for the parents of all babies admitted to the neonatal unit, describing the nature of low risk procedures such as venesection, for which explicit consent would not normally be sought.

3. The availability of written material and the perception of a procedure as low risk does not obviate the need for the clinician to explain its purpose and if appropriate to explain any risk and the implications of withholding that procedure.

4. Counsellors and advocates should be available to support parents.

5. The assumption that implied consent has been gained must be made with caution in neonatal practice; whenever possible all procedures should be explained to the parents.

6. If you have any reason to believe that consent might be disputed later it should be documented in the notes even for a low risk procedure, in this situation it is particularly important that the presence of a witness is recorded.

7. If treatment is complex, or involves significant risks or side effects explicit consent must be gained and it is good practice for this to be signed.

Explicit consent recommended

Whenever explicit consent is obtained, whether verbal or signed, this should be recorded in the notes. *For those procedures marked with an asterisk it is recommended that explicit consent is supported by a signature (written consent).*

1. *Clinical photographs and video-recordings, **2.** Screening of babies and/or their mothers in high risk situations with no prior knowledge of maternal status e.g.. suspected HIV or substance abuse, **3.** Genetic testing (incl karyotype), **4.** Gasrointestinal imaging involving contrast , **5.** MRI / CT with or without contrast, **6.** EEG with video recording, **7.** *All surgical procedures, **8.** Percutaneous arterial lines (Brachial or femoral), **9.** Chest drain insertion and replacement, **10.** Abdominal drainage for perforation or ascites, **11.** Irrigation following extravasation injury, **12.** Therapeutic lumbar or ventricular tap in the absence of a reservoir (to relieve raised intracranial pressure, deliver IT antibiotics, etc.), **13.** *Peritoneal dialysis, **14.** *Bone marrow aspiration, 15. *Any biopsy, **16.** *Exchange transfusion, **17.** Vitamin K for normal term babies, **18.** Nitric oxide for preterm babies, **19.** Postnatal dexamethasone for BPD, **20.** *Immunization, **21.** *Treatment for ROP, 22. Use of donor breast milk.

Explicit consent not USUALLY required

These procedures should be described in written information available to parents at admission, this can be expanded by clinical staff as the opportunities arise. It should not USUALLY be necessary to record consent in the notes.

1. Examining and assessing the patient, **2.** Routine blood sampling, **3.** Septic screens, **4.** Diagnostic lumbar puncture (to investigate possible infectious or metabolic illness), **5.** SPA, **6.** Screening for infection in response to positive results of maternal screening e.g.. Known maternal HIV or substance abuse, **7.** CMV, toxoplasma, rubella and herpes screening, **8.** Portable X-rays and ultrasounds, **9.** Procedures involving the baby leaving the unit, **10.** X-rays, **11.** Ultrasound, **12.** Videoflouroscopy, **13.** EEG/CFAM, **14.** ECG, **15.** ROP screening, **16.** UAC/UVC, **17.** Percutaneous arterial lines (Radial, ulnar or pedal), **18.** Percutaneous long lines (incl. use of contrast medium to visualize tip) **19.** Peripheral venous lines, **20.** Naso-gastric and naso-jejunal tubes, **21.** Tracheal intubation, **22.** Ventilation / CPAP, 23. Urethral catheterization, **24.** Blood transfusion, **25.** Use of pooled blood products, **26.** Partial exchange transfusion, **27.** Antibiotics, **28.** Vitamins / minerals, **29.** IV fluids **30.** TPN **31.** Surfactant, **32.** Anti-convulsants, **33.** Sedation for intubation and ventilation, **34.** Inotropes, **35.** Indomethacin or ibuprofen for PDA, **36.** Prophylactic indomethacin, **37.** Parenteral and oral vitamin K for babies admitted to the NNU, **38.** Nitric Oxide to term babies for PPHN, **39.** Postnatal dexamethasone for laryngeal oedema, **40.** Breast milk fortification.

BEWARE OF THE RARE/UNUSUAL/STRANGE NEONATAL PROBLEMS!

* *"It is an old maxim of mine that when you have excluded the impossible, whatever remains, however improbable, must be the truth."*

* *One's ideas must be as broad as Nature if they are to interpret Nature. "I never make exceptions. An exception disproves the rule."*

* *"There is nothing more stimulating than a case where everything goes against you."*

* *"No, no: I never guess. It is a shocking habit,—destructive to the logical faculty."*

* *"It is a capital mistake to theorize before you have all the evidence. It biases the judgment."*

* *"When you follow two separate chains of thought, Watson, you will find some point of intersection which should approximate to the truth."*

* *"As a rule," said Holmes, "the more bizarre a thing is the less mysterious it proves to be. It is your commonplace, featureless crimes which are really puzzling, just as a commonplace face is the most difficult to identify."*

* *"Singularity is almost invariably a clue. The more featureless and commonplace a crime is, the more difficult it is to bring it home."* - **Sir Arthur Conan Doyle's Sherlock Holmes**

The Following Neonatal diseases are rare but one should be aware of the possibility, when considering the Differential Diagnosis of Severe/Persistent/Unusual-Unresponsive/Recurring Neonatal Symptoms. The list is selective; it could be endless.

1. Neonatal Kawasaki Disease- 971,
2. Neonatal Orbital Cellulitis-972,
3. Neonatal Septic Arthritis-974,
4. Neonatal Bacterial Endocarditis-976,
5. Neonatal Fungal Endocarditis-977,
6. Neonatal Necrotizing Fascitis-978,
7. Neonatal Purpura Fulminans-980,
8. Pleural Empyema in a Preterm Infant-981,
9. Neonatal Dengue Infection-983,
10. Neonatal Psoas Abscess Simulating Septic Arthritis of Hip Joint-985.

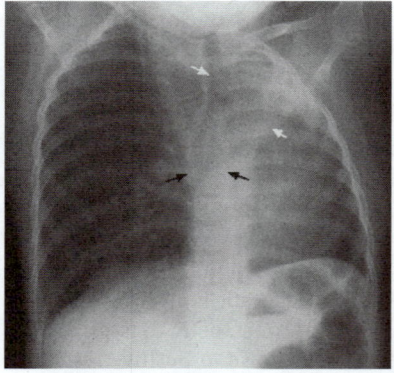

AGENESIS OF LT UPPER LOBE

@Diagnosis of **unilateral lobar pulmonary hypoplasia** requires a high index of clinical suspicion and experience with reading neonatal and infant radiographs. The radiographic findings will vary depending on the extent of lung involvement. In left-sided lobar pulmonary hypoplasia due to an accessory diaphragm, the heart and the trachea are displaced toward the left and the left heart border or superior mediastinum is obscured. A large apical cap or a poorly defined retrosternal stripe or density may be present on lateral view of the chest and is characteristic for lobar hypoplasia. The radiographic stripe is due to the difference in densities between the fatty and areolar tissues located anterior and the normally aerated lung lobe positioned posteriorly. Differentiation between isolated lobar pulmonary hypoplasia and pulmonary hypoplasia secondary to an accessory diaphragm is difficult on plain radiographs. Chest CT or MRI may be needed to better delineate the defect. *A number of associated anomalies have been described in patients with pulmonary hypoplasia, but none has been specifically associated with patients with lobar hypoplasia. *Significant risk factors associated with pulmonary hypoplasia: (1) hydrops fetalis; (2) renal anomalies; (3) diaphragmatic hernia; (4) skeletal anomalies; (5) oligohydramnios and polyhydramnios. It could be argued that all neonates with pulmonary hypoplasia should have pulmonary

function testing. *If PFTs are abnormal or there are clinical signs of airway disease, flexible bronchoscopy should be performed to assess for tracheobronchial abnormalities. *All infants with suspected pulmonary hypoplasia should have an echocardiogram to assess for congenital cardiac defects as well as to assess pulmonary venous drainage. Chromosomes should be sent if there are multiple anomalies. *The long-term prognosis is directly related to the degree of pulmonary hypoplasia and presence of comorbidities. *The

differential diagnosis of respiratory distress in the newborn associated with marked opacification of one side of the thorax on radiograph includes atelectasis, congenital diaphragmatic hernia (CDH), congenital cystic adenomatoid malformation (CCAM), pulmonary sequestration, chylothorax, pulmonary hypoplasia, bronchogenic cyst, and a chest tumor (e.g., neuroblastoma, teratoma, fibrosarcoma). In a right-sided CDH, there may be opacification of the right hemithorax if the liver is occupying that space. A left-sided CDH will have air-filled loops of bowel in the chest except possibly in a chest radiograph taken shortly after birth or following bowel decompression. CCAM will usually appear as a cystic mass rather than a homogenous opacification. A chylothorax that presents in the first few days of life may be due to a congenital malformation of the lymphatic system or traumatic injury of the thoracic duct at delivery. Obstruction of the bronchus with resultant opacification of the hemithorax may occur with a bronchogenic cyst or a vascular sling. Neonatal chest tumors are very rare and may present as a focal abnormality on CXR.

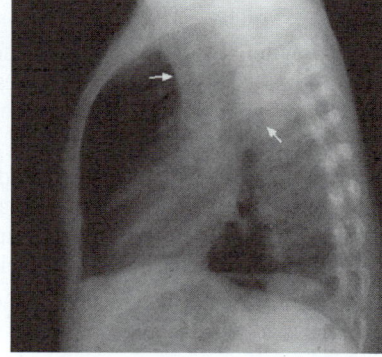

AGENESIS OF LT UPPER LOBE-LAT VIEW

1. NEONATAL KAWASAKI DISEASE

Classical kawasaki disease in a neonate: Kawasaki disease is diagnosed using clinical criteria that include fever for 5 days or longer and at least 4 of the following: (1) nonexudative conjunctival injection; (2) oral involvement, including any of strawberry tongue, mucosal hyperemia, and cracked or erythematous lips; (3) changes in the peripheral extremities, including edema or desquamation in convalescence; (4) polymorphous rash; and (5) acute cervical adenopathy greater than 1.5 cm in diameter. Kawasaki disease occurs primarily in young children, with 80% of patients are under the age of 4 years and with the peak incidence occurring at 9 to 11 months of age. The illness is extremely rare in infants under the age of 3 months. *Kawasaki disease is rare in neonates, but Pediatricians and neonatologists should be aware that KD occurs in neonates, that the presentation may be atypical, and that it can follow a rapid and severe course.*

Case report: A 30-day-old female infant who was previously healthy developed a high-grade fever, which was followed 2 days later by maculopapular rash on her trunk and extremities. She also had reddish discoloration of her lips and conjunctival infection. She was admitted to another hospital with those complaints and hospitalized with a diagnosis of sepsis, and she was given intravenous antibiotic for 12 days but did not recover from any of the symptoms and her fever. Levels of serum acute phase reactants including erythrocyte sedimentation rate (80 mm/h) and C-reactive protein (5 mg/dL) were remarkably high; no bacterial growth was detected in any of her culture. She was referred to us for the evaluation of prolonged fever. Upon examination, she had desquamation of the skin at her fingers starting from the fingertips and the anal region. The child was hospitalized with the diagnosis of KD based on her medical history and physical examination findings. Her peripheral leukocyte and thrombocyte counts were 10,200/mL and 680,000/mL, respectively. Her echocardiography revealed minimal aneurysmal dilatation of coronary arteries (Fig. 1). Intravenous immunoglobulin (2 g/kg) for 12 hours and high-dosage (100 mg/

kg per day divided into 4 dose/d) acetylsalicylic acid treatment were applied. Her fever disappeared after the dose of intravenous immunoglobulin therapy, and acute phase reactants including erythrocyte sedimentation rate and C-reactive protein decreased at the end of the first week. The patient was discharged from the hospital with low-dosage (3 mg/kg per day) acetylsalicylic acid. The aneurysmal dilatation was persisting on her second month follow-up echocardiography. The presence of clinical manifestation and elevated acute phase reactants in association with typical echocardiographic coronary artery dilatation established the diagnosis. The diagnosis was not suspected at an earlier date possibly because of lack of awareness of neonatal occurrence of KD.

Discussion: In infants, the atypical presentations (longer duration of illness before diagnosis, lower incidence of conjunctivitis, lower incidence of rash, lower incidence of extremity change, and lower C-reactive protein) are common, and this may result in a delay in diagnosis and effective treatment. Delayed diagnosis in KD was a significant risk factor for the development of coronary artery abnormalities. In addition, there may be as yet unknown physiological differ ences among KD patients at extremes of pediatrics that make them more vulnerable to coronary complication. KD can cause neurological complications such as encephalopathy, seizures, cerebrovascular events, and isolated cranial nerve deficits uncommonly. Transient cerebral hypoperfusion has been observed during the acute phase of the illness, and it is postulated that vasculitis may cause these rare neurological manifestations. Aseptic meningitis is often reported in patients with KD. Although raised serum acute phase reactants are almost universal, more than 50% of patients with KD do not have increased C reactive protein at diagnosis. Transient neutropenia is uncommon. There is no specific diagnostic test or pathognomonic clinical features; those previously mentioned clinical criteria have been established to assist physicians in diagnosing KD. So clinician should be aware of the possibility of KD.

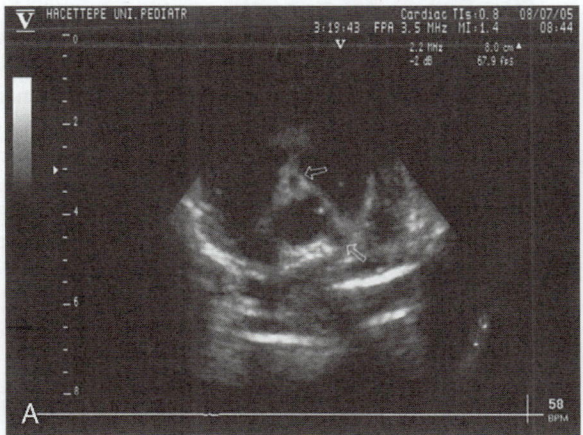 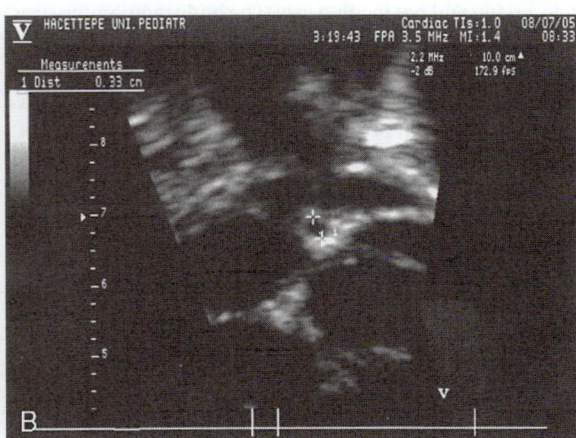

Fig. 1. A and B, Echocardiographic findings of the patient

Courtesy: Kawasaki Disease - A Case Report in Extreme of Pediatrics, Ates Kara, Hasan Tezer, MD, IÙlker Devrim, MD, Esra K1ll1c¸ Korkmaz, MD, Tevfik Karago¨ z, MD, Sema O ¨ zer, MD, A. Bu¨lent Cengiz, MD, and Gu¨lten Sec¸meer, MD, Infect Dis Clin Pract 2006;14:333–334 REFERENCES: 1)America Heart Association (1990). Diagnostic guidelines for Kawasaki disease. Am J Dis Child. 1990;144:1218–1219. 2) Tsuchida S, Yamanaka T, Tsuchida R, et al. Epidemiology of infant Kawasaki disease with a report on the youngest neonatal case reported in Japan. Acta Paediatr. 1996;85:995–997. 3) Stanley TV, Grimwood K. Classical Kawasaki disease in a neonate. Arch Dis Child Fetal Neonatal Ed. 2002;86:35–36. 4) Brenner JL, Jadavji T, Pinto A, et al. Severe Kawasaki disease in infants: two fatal cases. Can J Cardiol. 2000;16:1017–1023.

2. NEONATAL ORBITAL CELLULITIS

Orbital cellulitis in a neonate: Orbital cellulitis is extremely uncommon in neonates and not more than 10 cases are reported in the literature. In children 60%-80% of orbital infections originate from the sinuses. Acute sinusitis remains the major cause of orbital inflammation. In more than 90% of cases orbital cellulitis is secondary to sinusitis. Orbital septum is a fibrous layer, beneath the muscular layer in the eye lid, connecting the tarsus to the orbital periosteum. It acts as a barrier separating the lids from the orbit. Peri-orbital infections are classified as preseptal cellulitis and orbital cellulitis. Preseptal cellulitis involves the soft tissues of the eyelids in front of the septum and orbital cellulitis involves the soft tissues of the orbit behind the orbital septum. Orbital cellulitis occurs in the following situations: (1) spread of infection from adjacent structures most commonly paranasal sinuses, but also from the lacrimal sac, stye, dental infections and facial infections; (2) direct inoculation of the orbit from penetrating ocular trauma or ocular surgery like eyelid, strabismus and retinal detachment surgery; and (3) hematogenous seeding from bacteremia. The medial orbital bone is thin, called lamina papyraceae. The combination of a thin bone, presence of numerous foramina for neurovascular passage, naturally occurring congenital and bony dehiscences and valveless venous anastomosis allows easy communication of infective material between the ethmoid sinuses to the subperiosteal space. The most common location of subperiosteal abscess is the medial orbital wall, as the periosteum here is loosely attached to the underlying bone. Intraorbital extension of subperiosteal abscess (SPA) or localisation of diffuse orbital cellulitis can result in orbital abscesses.

Case report

A 28 day old baby boy was seen in the emergency department with 3 day history of fever, redness and swollen right eye. There was also yellowish discharge from his right eye. He has had symptoms of nasal congestion 2 weeks before the presentation. His parents deny any insect bites, trauma, and skin infection of the face and excessive tearing of the eyes prior to this presentation. Ante-natal, peri-natal and post-natal history was not significant. On physical examination the child was irritable, lethargic, crying and not feeding well. The body temperature was 39.6°C, heart rate 206/min, respiratory rate 36/min and his body weight was 4.4 Kg. There were no meningeal signs. The infant was seen moving all his limbs freely during examination. There was enlargement of the right preauricular and submandibular nodes; however there was no generalized lymphadenopathy and the rest of the physical findings were normal. On eye examination there was marked proptosis, swelling and erythema of both upper and lower eyelid of his right eye, purulent discharge, conjunctival congestion and chemosis. The cornea was clear. Pupil on the affected side reacted briskly to light. The globe was pushed down and out. Ocular motility was however difficult to assess. The left eye was normal. His WBC was 28.0 × 10³ /mcL (28.0 × 10⁶ /L), neutrophils 56%, lymphocytes 44%, Hgb 13.4 g/dl (134 g/L) and platelet count was 512 × 10³ /mcL (512 × 10³ /L). Values for electrolytes, BUN and creatinine were normal. Gram stained smears of the nose and conjunctiva swabs showed gram positive cocci. Peripheral blood smear was normal. The clinical diagnosis of orbital cellulitis was made based on physical findings of high fever, marked swelling and erythema of the lids, conjunctival congestion and chemosis. Our clinical impression was supported by laboratory findings of marked leucocytosis and positive Gram stained smears from the conjunctiva and nose. The baby was

started immediately on intravenous antibiotics which included a combination of IV cefotaxime 220 mg tds and IV oxacillin 220 mg qid. However, after 24–48 hours of IV antibiotics, the fever continued and there was worsening of the orbital signs with increasing proptosis and eyelid swelling (Figure 1). Culture results of conjunctival and nasal swabs revealed *Staphylococcus aureus*, sensitive to penicillin, vancomycin, gentamicin and oxacillin. Blood culture was negative. An urgent computer tomography (CT) scan was done. The CT picture showed marked proptosis of the right eye with inflammatory signs of the pre-septal and post-septal space confirming our clinical impression. In addition, subperiosteal abscess was detected as an extraconal soft tissue density collection contained within the periosteum of the medial orbital wall, stretching the lateral rectus muscle and displacing the globe laterally (Figure 2). Opacification of the ethmiod sinus suggests sinusitis as the source for the orbital cellulitis. As there was no response to systemic antibiotics for 48 hours, the SPA and the associated sinus were drained by trans-nasal endoscopy. The pus drained was sent for Gram stain and culture sensitivity. A nasal drain was placed, which was removed on the second post-op day. The post-operative period was otherwise afebrile with reduction of the eyelid swelling. Intravenous antibiotics were continued for 2 weeks followed by oral antibiotics for 2 more weeks. Pus culture showed growth of *Staphylococcus aureus*.

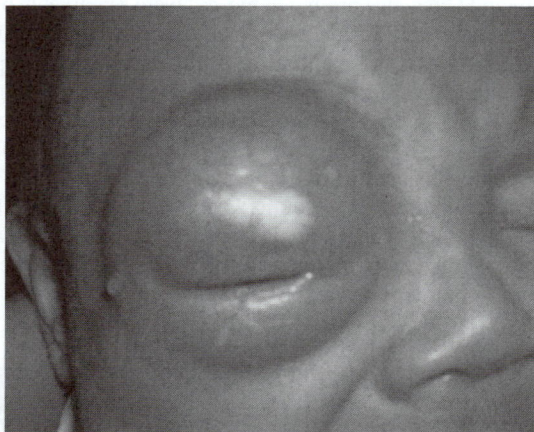

Figure 1: After systemic antibiotics, right eye shows marked proptosis, erythema and swelling of the eyelids with abscess formation. There is also purulent discharge from the conjunctiva.

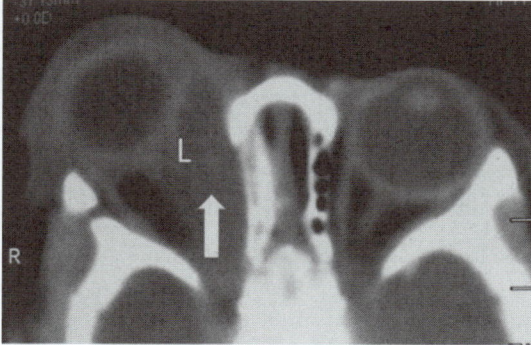

Figure 2: CT picture axial view showing marked proptosis, marked preseptal and postseptal inflammatory signs and a medial extraconal soft tissue density mass of the right eye (arrow). Note there is stretching of the lateral rectus muscle (indicated by letter L) and also lateral displacement of the globe

Discussion

In all age groups the incidence of orbital cellulitis is high in winter, due to increase incidence of upper respiratory tract infections and sinusitis. The etiologic agents in orbital cellulitis are predominantly bacterial. However fungal infections have to be ruled out in immunosuppressed and diabetic child. In children less than 5 years infections with *Haemophilus influenzae* have to be thought of, as it is the common organism residing in the paranasal sinuses. The other common pathogens in young children *are Staphylococcus aureus, Staphylococcus epidermidis, Streptococcus pyogenes, Streptococcus pneumoniae, and Moraxella catarrhalis*. In older children gram negative organism like *Pseudomonas, Klebsiella* and anaerobes like *Peptostreptococcus, Bacteroides, Fusobacterium* are the causative organism. Vaccination against *Haemophilus influenzae* type b (Hib) has drastically reduced the incidence of serious pediatric infections like meningitis and brain abscess, but it is doubtful whether the incidence of orbital cellulitis is reduced as, Hib is not a significant cause of sinusitis. The clinical presentation in most of the cases is acute with systemic and ocular signs. The systemic findings are fever, malaise, headache and prostration. Ocular finding are proptosis, conjunctival chemosis, reduced and painful extraocular movements, decreased vision and elevated intraocular pressure. Presence of neck rigidity and cranial nerve involvement suggest intracranial spread. Differential diagnoses include infective and non-infective causes. Preseptal cellulits and dacryocystitis are infective causes and can have similar presentation. Fever may be associated with preseptal cellulitis, but is usually mild. There can also be erythema and marked eyelid swelling. However, proptosis, conjunctival chemosis, painful ophthalmoplegia and vision loss are usually features of orbital cellulitis. Dacryocystitis may be associated with fever, erythema and swelling of the eyelids, but the most common location of swelling will be the nasal aspect of the lower lid. Noninfective causes include traumatic, inflammatory, neoplastic, endocrine and systemic. Neoplastic conditions like retinoblastoma, rhabdomyosarcoma, leukaemia, Burkitt lymphoma can cause sudden inflammatory proptosis. Orbital cellulitis is diagnosed mainly on clinical grounds. The laboratory evaluation should include a complete blood count, blood culture and Gram-stained smears and cultures from the conjunctiva, nose and throat. A marked leucocytosis greater than 15,000/¼l with shift to the left is commonly seen in orbital cellulitis. Blood culture and CSF examination should be done prior to administration of any antibiotics. Imaging studies like ultrasound and computed tomography can be done when physical examination is hampered by marked lid swelling, no response to systemic antibiotics, when intracranial complications occur and when surgical intervention is needed. Untreated orbital cellulitis can lead to serious lifethreatening and sight threatening complications. Lifethreatening complications are cavernous sinus thrombosis, meningitis, and brain abscesses. Ocular complications are exposure keratitis, optic neuritis, increase intraocular pressure, retinal vascular occlusion, orbital and subperiosteal abscess. Orbital cellulitis in children is an ocular emergency requiring immediate hospitalization. Majority of cases can be managed medically and cases not responding to medical therapy can be taken for surgical drainage. The initial treatment of orbital cellulitis in infants include a high dose of intravenous third generation cephalosporins like ceftriaxone, cefotaxime, or ceftazidime combined with a pencillinase resistant pencillin like oxacillin and nafcillin. In older children where orbital cellulitis is due to mixed aerobic and anaerobic organisms, the pencillinase resistant antibiotics can be substituted with vancomycin and clindamycin. The intravenous antibiotics are given for 1–2 weeks followed by oral antibiotics for an additional 2–3 weeks. Surgery is indicated when there is visual loss, optic nerve dysfunction, intracranial complications and poor response to medical treatment. Subperiosteal and orbital abscess can be initially managed by intravenous antibiotics alone. Garcia and Harris advocate a non-surgical management of subperiosteal abscess in the following situations: age less than 9 years; no visual compromise; modest size medial abscess; and absence of intracranial and frontal sinus involvement. Surgical drainage of SPA may be done if the above criteria is not met and in those patients in whom clinical signs fail to improve or worsens following conventional treatment. Otolaryngologist advocate two surgical options for the drainage of SPA: an external approach via Lynch incision and an intranasal endoscopic approach. To conclude orbital cellulitis is an ocular emergency which requires early recognition and immediate management to prevent ocular and life-threatening complications.

References: 1. Jackson K, Baker SR. Clinical implication of orbital cellulitis. Laryngoscope 1986;96:569–74. 2. Schramm VL, Curtin HD, Kennerdell JS. Evaluation of orbital cellulitis and results of treatment. Laryngoscope 1982;92: 732-8. 3. Weiss A, Friendly D, Eglin K, Chang M, Gold B. Bacterial periorbital and orbital cellulitis in childhood. Ophthalmology 1983;90:195-203. 4. Batson OV. Relationship of the eye to the paranasal sinuses. Arch Ophthalmol 1936;16:322-3. 5. Chandler JR, Langenbrunner DJ, Stevens ER. The pathogenesis of orbital complications in acute sinusitis. Laryngoscope 1970; 80:1414-28. 6. Schwartz JN, Donnelly EH, Klintworth GK. Ocular and orbital phycomycosis. Surv Ophthalmol 1977;22:3–28. 7. Ambati BK, Ambati J, Azar N, Stratton L, Schmidt EV. Periorbital and orbital cellulitis before and after the advent of Haemophilus influenzae type B vaccination. Ophthalmology 2000;107:1450-3. 8. Starkey CR, Steele RW. Medical management of orbital cellulitis. Pediatr Infect Dis J 2001;20:1002-5. 9. Immergluck LC, Daum RC. *Hemophilus influenzae*. In: Nelson WE, Sr.ed. Beehrman RE, Kliegman RM, Arwin AM, eds. Nelson Textbooks of Pediatrics. Philadelphia: WB Saunders, 1996;762–8. 10. Garcia GH, Harris GJ. Criteria for non-surgical management of subperiosteal abscess of the orbit. Ophthalmology 2000;107: 1454-8.

Courtesy: PS *MALLIKA, AK TAN, S AZIZ, R VANITHA, TY TAN, HA FAISAL* *Department of Ophthalmology, Faculty of Medicine and Health Sciences, University Malaysia Sarawak, Kuching, Sarawak, Malaysia* Orbital Cellulitis Complicated by Subperiosteal Abscess in a Neonate with Ethmoiditis, *HK J Paediatr (new series) 2009;14:275-278*

3. NEONATAL SEPTIC ARTHRITIS

Septic Arthritis in a Neonate :

Neonatal septic arthritis has always been considered as separate from its counterpart in older children; during the earliest childhood it is considered to be a systemic septic condition and demands early diagnosis and prompt surgical treatment. The condition is uncommon but serious. Affected neonates usually survive, but with permanent skeletal deformities. Due to possible development of serious and irreversible damage, even lethal outcome, septic arthritis requires early diagnosis, prompt administration of antibiotics and early surgical treatment. In neonates and infants septic arthritis is characterized by atypical clinical picture, often causing delayed diagnosis. In the initial phases of the disease ultrasonographic findings are of greater use compared to radiological imaging, due to relatively late appearance of radiological signs of disease. It is a quite unique area in Pediatric Orthopedics where missed or delayed diagnosis may have serious consequences (complete destruction of the articular cartilage and the underlying epiphysis, loss of the adjacent growth plate, and dislocation of the joint.)

* Ten cases of neonatal septic arthritis were diagnosed between January 1989 and December 1993 in the neonatal intensive care units of two referral hospitals in the state of Kelantan, Malaysia. All except one neonate was born prematurely. The mean age of presentation was 15.6 days. Joint swelling (10/10), increased warmth (7/10) and erythema of the overlying skin (7/10) were the common presenting signs. Vague constitutional symptoms preceded the definitive signs of septic arthritis in all cases. The total white cell counts were raised with shift to the left. The knee (60%) was not commonly affected, followed by the hip (13%) and ankle (13%). Three neonates had multiple joint involvement. Coexistence of arthritis with osteomyelitis was observed in seven neonates. The commonest organism isolated was methicillin resistant Staphylococcus aureus (9/10). Needle aspiration was performed in nine neonates and one had incision with drainage. Follow up data was available for five neonates and two of these had skeletal morbidity. Early diagnosis by frequent examination of the joints, prompt treatment and control of nosocomial infection are important for management. **REF:** Halder D, Seng QB, Malik AS, Choo KE. Department of Pediatrics, Hospital Universiti Sains Malaysia, Kubang Kerian, Kelantan, Malaysia. Southeast Asian J Trop Med Public Health. 1996 Sep;27(3):600-5

* Four cases of septic arthritis of the hip in neonates, felt to be valid examples of a complication arising from femoral venipuncture, are presented. Each of the cases seen occurred 5 to 9 days after femoral venipuncture. *Staphylococcus aureus* was cultured in three cases, *Staphylococcus albus* in one, and the skin is considered to be the source of contamination. Severe residuals resulted in each instance. Because of the severe disability that may result, greater care in skin preparation and performance of femoral venipuncture is suggested. In addition, it is recommended that, whenever possible, the external jugular vein be used in preference to the femoral vein. **REF:** SEPTIC ARTHRITIS OF THE HIP: A COMPLICATION OF FEMORAL VENIPUNCTURE Russell S. Asnes M.D.Gregory M. Arendar M.D. PEDIATRICS Vol. 38 No. 5 November 1966, pp. 837-841 The Harriet Lane Service of the Children's Medical and Surgical Center and the Division of Orthopedic Surgery, The Johns Hopkins Hospital, Baltimore, Maryland.

* The increased use of umbilical arterial catheters for prolonged periods in Preterms may be one of the predisposing causes of bone & joint infections. Septic arthritis in the Neonate gives rise to more serious handicaps, due to the fact that in the premature infants the ossific nucleus of the end of the bone has not yet appeared and in addition there is no epiphyseal plate. In these Neonates infection begins in the vulnerable cartilage precursor of the end of the bone itself, causing rapid destruction with consequent joint destruction and growth arrest and subsequent leg-length discrepancy.

* Neonates are special in that their immune systems still are immature. They are susceptible to a wide range of organisms that are unlikely pathogens in an older individual, and they are less capable of mounting an inflammatory response to infection. Premature infants in the neonatal intensive care unit are particularly at risk. They often are debilitated with other illnesses, and they typically present with multiple ports for bacterial entry. Bone and joint infections in these patients commonly involve multiple sites.

* A developing septic arthritis is generally accompanied by the onset of fever, malaise, and prominent localizing signs at the affected joint. In the distal extremities, swelling, erythema, and tenderness are prominent; the findings may be less evident with deeper joints, such as the hip. The most consistent sign is pain with passive motion. The patient will generally hold the joint in the position that maximizes intracapsular volume. For the hip, these positions are flexion, abduction, and external rotation, as seen in the image below. With a septic knee, the joint is most comfortable when moderately flexed. It is not unusual for a Neonateor infant to appear completely comfortable, so long as the affected joint remains immobile in the position of comfort. Any attempt by the examiner to passively move the joint, however, dramatically reveals the pathology.

* Refusal of the child to move the affected joint is called pseudoparalysis. This sign is often mistaken for a neurologic problem. An isolated true paralysis, however, is far less common than a septic arthritis; when it does occur, it is rarely associated with pain with passive motion. The inability of a child to bear weight on a lower extremity or to spontaneously move any joint must be considered a sign of septic arthritis until proven otherwise.

* Septic arthritis is also more difficult to diagnose in neonates, but making an early diagnosis is more important in these patients. Multiple joint infection is a serious problem in the Neonate, especially in the Prematurely born and frequent examinations of all joints is therefore necessary so that earliest possible treatment can be given. *If 1 infected joint is diagnosed in a neonate, look for other sites of bone or joint infection. Consider obtaining a bone scan to assist in this search.*

* A neonate aged 5 weeks or younger is susceptible to infection as a result of a wide range of organisms that are unlikely pathogens in children with more developed immune systems. *S aureus* is still the most common pathogen in this age group; group B streptococcus is the next most common pathogen. Gram-negative organisms such as, Klebsiella *pneumoniae, S.choleraesuis, S.typhimurium and S. enteritidis* may be seen in as many as 15% of joint infections affecting neonates in a neonatal intensive care setting. *Candida albicans* may also be present in these patients, as well as in patients who have received prolonged antibiotic therapy. Consideration should be given to the inclusion of coverage for nosocomially acquired methicillin-resistant *S aureus* (MRSA) in the empirical coverage for patients with septic arthritis pending culture results.

* Hematogenous septic arthritis may develop directly through the synovial blood vessels. Another common route is from an adjacent hematogenous metaphyseal osteomyelitis. Just under the metaphyseal side of the growth plate in a growing child, vascular loops nourish the bone that forms in association with enchondral ossification. Blood flow in these loops is thought to be relatively slow, and this region is somewhat poorly defended by the reticuloendothelial system. These loops form the site of origin for hematogenous osteomyelitis in infancy and childhood. An abscess forms in the metaphysis in association with localized bone destruction. In the infant (from birth to 18 months), the infection may spread into the epiphysis through blood vessels that cross the cartilaginous physis. From the epiphysis, the infection may then break directly into the adjacent joint, resulting in septic arthritis. This mechanism of spread directly into the epiphysis is unique to infancy.

* **Diagnostic Work-up-** 1) The WBC count is usually elevated, but it may be within the normal range early in the clinical course. Infants may also have a normal WBC count. A normal WBC count does not rule out septic arthritis 2) The ESR is elevated in septic arthritis; it returns to normal levels with resolution of the infection. The initial elevation and the return to normal lag behind the clinical status. 3) The CRP level is

elevated in septic arthritis; it returns to normal with resolution of the infection. CRP is a more valuable diagnostic tool and a better indicator of response to treatment than ESR because CRP is generally more sensitive and more responsive. Blood cultures are frequently positive for the causative organism in septic arthritis and should be obtained. The joint aspirate may not yield a viable culture. **4)** Gram stains & Cultures of joint aspirates should always be performed because a positive Gram stain is valuable information. The Gram stain is positive in a minority of the cases of septic arthritis; however, a negative result should never be interpreted as evidence that infection is not present. Potassium hydroxide preparations and fungal cultures can be considered for neonates in whom the risk of fungal infection is believed to be high.**5)** Plain Radiography- Even if the infection developed from an adjacent metaphyseal osteomyelitis, no initial bony findings are likely to be apparent until 7-10 days after onset. Signs of soft-tissue swelling and edematous infiltration into fatty tissue planes may be observed. **6)** Radionuclide(Technetium) scanning - Radionuclide scanning is generally not helpful, and it is contraindicated if it delays more appropriate diagnostic or treatment measures. Scanning may be helpful in locating or ruling out other sites of involvement, particularly in very sick children and in neonates. **7)**Ultrasonography Ultrasonography is useful in confirming a joint effusion in a deeply placed joint such as the hip. This modality can also be used to guide joint aspiration. **8)** Computed tomography (CT) -A CT scan is indicated in patients with a suspected psoas abscess; in such patients, the clinical signs are suggestive of septic arthritis of the hip but the joint aspiration culture is negative. **9)** Magnetic resonance imaging (MRI) MRI has no role in the initial workup. The use of this expensive and time-consuming modality should be reserved for situations in which simpler measures, such as joint aspiration, fail to provide a diagnosis.**10)** Joint aspiration is the single most important diagnostic procedure. Aspirate the joint with a large-bore needle before administering antibiotics. Aspirate deep joints, such as the hip, under image-intensifier control or ultrasound guidance and with the patient appropriately sedated or anesthetized. A positive joint aspirate typically yields opaque yellow or white-gray pus. The WBC count is usually in excess of 50,000 per milliliter, with more than 80% neutrophils. A positive Gram stain is diagnostic for infection, but false-negative results are common. The failure to visualize organisms on the Gram stain does not rule out infection. If gonococcal arthritis is suspected, obtain the culture in a manner approved by the clinical laboratory for this organism. *N gonorrhoeae* is a difficult organism to grow, and special handling and special culture media are required to maximize recovery.

* *The keys to proper management are a high index of suspicion in any child with painful joint dysfunction and strict adherence to the principles for treatment outlined below.*

*Medical Therapy - Administer parenteral antibiotics as soon as blood and joint aspirates have been cultured. The choice of antibiotic should be based on the Gram stain results. When the Gram stain fails to show bacteria, the choice should be empirically based on the patient's age and circumstance. Treat neonates, patients who are immunocompromised with an aminoglycoside in addition to a penicillinase-resistant penicillin in order to cover against enteric gram-negative bacilli and *Pseudomonas* species. Appropriately adjust the choice of antibiotic after culture and sensitivity results are known. A third-generation cephalosporin should be the initial treatment for gonococcal arthritis. For MRSA, Clindamycin and vancomycin are the two agents most commonly used for this purpose, but the antibiotic choice should be adjusted depending on the antibiotic susceptibility patterns of local isolates.Maintain adequate blood levels of a culture-specific antibiotic for at least 3 weeks after the joint has been drained and the patient has responded clinically. *The total duration of antibiotic therapy should be 4 to 6 weeks, and the entire course should be administered by the intravenous route. Infections caused by S aureus, whether MSSA or MRSA, should be treated for the longer duration. The addition of either gentamicin or rifampin to vancomycin regimens for bone infections has been advocated by some, but the idea is somewhat controversial.* ESR and CRP levels are valuable indicators of clinical response. The CRP is generally more sensitive than the ESR, and antibiotics should be continued at least until this measure has normalized. Switching to oral antibiotics is also acceptable, provided that adequate blood levels of the antibiotic are demonstrated, the

patient's parents are reliable, and the antibiotic does not cause a gastrointestinal disturbance that would interfere with its absorption. Healing often requires temporary immobilization of the neonate's extremity until the healing process is underway. Bone infections are painful, and aggressive pain management should be prescribed, especially during the early stages.

*Surgical therapy: Consider a septic joint to be a closed abscess and do not expect antibiotic treatment alone to resolve the infection. Remember that the risks of complication are time dependent. In addition to administration of medical therapy, the joint must be adequately drained. Patients may be treated with antibiotics and repeated joint aspiration in cases of involvement of an easily accessible peripheral joint; a clinical course shorter than 6 days; and no evidence of an associated osteomyelitis, immune deficiency, or other chronic illness. If the patient's condition fails to improve, open drainage is the next approach. Peripheral joints may be adequately drained with arthroscopy if the technology is available.Open drainage is definitely indicated in the hip and the shoulder and in peripheral joints that do not respond to percutaneous aspiration. Open drainage is indicated in patients who are systemically ill, and it should be given greater consideration when the suspected organism is *S aureus* or a gram-negative bacterium that produces cartilage-damaging enzymes. Gonococcal arthritis is less likely to rapidly damage a joint, and these infections may be managed with repeated aspirations if the joints involved are peripheral. Open drainage should still be performed in cases of gonococcal arthritis of the hip.

* Follow up with the patient for at least a year after surgery. Further follow-up can be discontinued if joint function has returned to normal and if no radiographic evidence suggests loss of joint space, avascular necrosis of the epiphysis, joint instability, or damage to the growth plate. Long-term Outcomes-Despite appropriate identification and treatment, many patients who have neonatal osteomyelitis have permanent sequelae. Neonatal bone infections may damage the growth plate, leading to growth disparities in the affected and nonaffected limbs. The final outcome may not be clinically apparent until the child reaches 9 or 10 years of age. Neonates who have articular infections of the hip may develop avascular necrosis of the femoral head. Others may eventually develop degenerative arthritis in the affected joint. Rapid decompression of the infected joint provides the best chance for a good outcome.

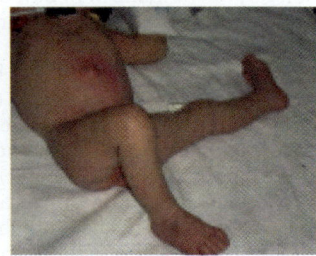

A 5-day old girl was evaluated for painful limitation of the left hip and "pseudoparalysis" of the lower extremity. The child held her hip rigidly in the classic position of flexion, abduction, and external rotation, a position that maximizes capsular volume. She was relatively comfortable as long as the hip joint remained immobile in this position There was no evidence of systemic disease, she was feeding normally, and the blood count and chemistries were normal. MRI indicated septic arthritis of the hip and osteomyelitis of the proximal femur. *Courtesy*: Nikolaos Sferopoulos, MD

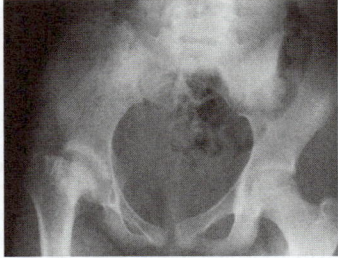

Anteroposterior radiograph demonstrating resorption of the Right femoral head as a consequence of septic arthritis.

4. NEONATAL BACTERIAL ENDOCARDITIS

Infective Endocarditis: Infective (BACTERIAL) endocarditis (IE) is an inflammation of the endothelial lining of the heart muscle, valves and great vessels. The valves have a particularly high propensity for infection due to the lack of blood supply and limited access to immune cells. IE is relatively rare in children. *Pathogenesis* Bacteremia and the presence of endothelial damage are important factors in the pathogenesis of IE. Cyanosis and polycythemia, if present, increase the viscosity of the blood and further enhance the likelihood of developing IE. Foreign materials such as prosthetic valves or shunts also significantly increase the risk for developing IE. All types of CHD, except for secondum ASD, predispose to IE. It is not surprising that cyanotic CHD with an artificial shunt or prosthetic valves constitutes the highest risk for IE. Neonatal endocarditis frequently occurs on the right side of the heart and is associated with disruption of endocardium or valvular endothelial tissue by catheter-induced trauma in a hospitalized infants. Premature neonates often experience transient episodes of bacteremia from trauma to the skin and mucous membranes, vigorous endotracheal suctioning, parenteral hyperalimentation, or placement of umbilical or peripheral venous catheters. The combination of endothelial damage and bacteremia is critical for the induction of IE. *Pathology:* Vegetations develop at the site of endothelial damage, which is usually located at the lower pressure side of the lesion i.e. in the RV in patients with VSD and on the atrial surface of the mitral valve with MR. After bacteria adhere to the damaged endothelium, platelets and fibrin are deposited over the organisms, leading to formation of a "vegetation". The organisms trapped within the vegetation are protected from phagocytic cells and other host defense mechanisms. *Microbiology:* Viridans group streptococcus, enterococci and *S. aureus* are responsible for most cases of IE. *Streptococcus pneumoniae*, coagulase negative staphycoccus, gram negative bacilli and fungi may also cause IE. The blood cultures may be negative in some patients with IE especially those who have already received antibiotics. *Clinical presentation* Persistent or recurrent low grade fever is the most common symptom of IE. Other symptoms are nonspecific and include malaise, myalgia, arthralgia, anorexia, night sweats and headaches. Splenomegaly can be found in 15-50% of patients with IE. A new or changing murmur indicates valvular involvement. The classic peripheral manifestations of IE are rarely seen nowadays. These include petichiae, splinter hemorrhages (hemorrhages in the nail beds), Osler's nodules (small, tender nodules on the pads of fingers and toes), Janeway's lesions (painless hemorrhages on palms and soles), and Roth's spots (hemorrhage in the retina with a white center). *Making the diagnosis* ·The above signs and symptoms in a patient with underlying CHD following transient bacteremia should raise the suspicion of IE. ·In the absence of prior anti-microbial therapy, positive blood cultures are found in >90% of patients. ·Other supporting laboratory evidence includes anemia, leukocytosis with a left shift, positive rheumatoid factor, hematuria and elevated ESR. ·The finding of vegetations on echocardiography is confirmatory. However; since IE is a clinical diagnosis, a negative echocardiogram does not rule out IE and treatment should not be delayed if there is strong clinical suspicion of IE. Recently, certain criteria were developed to help in making the diagnosis of IE. *Management:* The management of IE includes 4-6 weeks of high dose IV antibiotics. The choice of antibiotics depends on the organism isolated and the results of antibiotic sensitivity testing. Surgical intervention may be necessary if there is CHF, if vegetations causing obstruction, or if there is significant malfunction of a prosthetic valve. Antimicrobial prophylaxis to prevent IE is indicated in any patient with CHD (except secondum ASD) in situations that may produce bacteremia such as invasive dental or urological procedures.

Case Report: A boy weighing 800 g was born at 26 weeks' gestation and transferred to this hospital shortly after delivery. The mother's membranes had been ruptured for four days before delivery and there had been a small antepartum hemorrhage. Apgar scores at birth were 6 at one minute and 9 at five minutes. He was intubated, ventilated at low ventilator settings, and treatment was started with penicillin and gentamicin. Initial cultures showed no evidence of sepsis and his clinical condition was consistent with hyaline membrane disease. At 2 days of age an echocardiogram was done which showed normal cardiac anatomy and no evidence of a patent ductus arteriosus. Methicillin resistant S aureus was cultured from surface swabs. At 8 days he developed persistent metabolic acidosis and methicillin resistant S aureus was isolated from blood cultures; he was treated with vancomycin, but on day 10 methicillin resistant S aureus was isolated from a pustule on his chest. At 25 days, nine days after the vancomycin had been stopped, he again developed metabolic acidosis, his white cell count was high, platelets were normal and methicillin resistant S aureus was again isolated from blood cultures. Clotting studies were normal and a chest x-ray picture showed bronchopulmonary dysplasia. Treatment with vancomycin and rifampicin was started. A abscess developed on the left wrist and another on the upper arm, and methicillin resistant S aureus was isolated from the pus. The cranial ultrasound scan was normal. Two dimensional echocardiography, however, showed a pedunculated vegetation in the left atrial appendage. The methicillin resistant S aureus isolated from the blood cultures was sensitive to vancomycin, rifampicin, and fusidic acid, but because of possible antagonism between vancomycin and rifampicin, rifampicin was replaced by fusidic acid. He was extubated at 7 weeks of age at which time he became grossly edematous with a serum albumin concentration of 19 g/l. This resolved after infusion of albumin and restriction of fluids. Anti-biotics were continued for seven weeks, at which time cardiac ultrasound scan showed a slight decrease in the size of the vegetation. He was discharged when 12 weeks of age. When reviewed at 12 months of age neurological and developmental examinations yielded normal results. A further echocardiogram showed that the vegetation had disappeared.

*In bacterial endocarditis the bacteremia is usually low grade and constant, and detectable in 77-96% of the first blood cultures. This is increased to nearly 100% if three blood cultures are taken. S aureus has become an increasingly common cause of endocarditis since antibiotics have been used, and it is more virulent than other bacterial causes of endocarditis. The complication rate is higher, congestive cardiac failure occurs more often, and mortality increases. The treatment of infection by methicillin resistant S aureus with vancomycin alone is usually satisfactory. There is some evidence, however, that the addition of rifampicin or fusidic acid may improve the response, particularly for endocarditis or when skin infection occurs during treatment. Minimum inhibitory concentrations and minimum bactericidal concentrations of any antibiotic used in the treatment of endocarditis should be routinely tested. The serum bactericidal titre should be at least 1/8-1/16, and preferably higher.

*There seems to be an increased incidence of bacterial endocarditis in children who require resuscitation at birth and subsequent intensive care, especially if central venous lines are inserted. *Congenital heart disease is also an important predisposing factor; in addition, one report suggested an association between persistent fetal circulation and non-bacterial endocardial thrombosis in neonates. *With the increasing availability of two dimensional echocardiography neonates with septicaemia, especially if it is prolonged or recurrent, and skin pustules, hematuria, and thrombocytopenia, may warrant a cardiac scan to search for vegetations before a heart murmur has developed.* **Courtesy:** Infective endocarditis in neonates C O'CALLAGHAN AND P MCDOUGALL Department of Neonatology, Royal Children's Hospital, Melbourne, Australia Archives of Disease in Childhood, 1988, 63, 53–57

Fungal endocarditis is a rare occurrence in premature infants with more than 50% mortality and significant morbidity regardless type of treatment. Candida albicans accounts for two third of fungal endocarditis. Cardiac involvement is found in 15.2% of Neonates with candidemia and they usually present with hypotension, bradycardia and acute respiratory distress requiring intubation. Right atrial mycetoma (RAM) is reported in only 9% cases of fungal neonatal endocarditis and its management is usually with prolonged use of antifungal therapy in association with surgery in a select group of patients.

Case Report : A preterm male was born at 26 weeks of gestation with a birth weight of 846g by emergency cesarean section for fetal heart rate anomalies and breech presentation. The newborn had severe respiratory distress syndrome and metabolic acidosis at birth. He was treated with intratracheal surfactant and placed on ampicillin and gentamicin after a sepsis work up. He was treated with ibuprofen on the fifth day of life for symptomatic patent ductus arteriosus. A few hours after the administration of ibuprofen, the baby developed abdominal distension with bluish discoloration and the abdominal x ray showed evidence of intestinal perforation. Antibiotic coverage was started and peritoneal drains were placed. Blood culture grew Pseudomonas aeruginosa and Candida albicans, while peritoneal culture grew Pseudomonas aeruginosa and Enterococcus fecalis. The baby was treated with imipenam and liposomal amphotericin. An ileostomy was done. An echocardiogram performed at this time showed no evidence of endocarditis. Renal sonogram and ophthalmologic evaluation were negative. Repeat blood cultures continued to grow candida despite liposomal amphotericin administered at a dose of 7mg/kg/day. At 10 days of life, baby began to develop persistent thrombocytopenia requiring platelet transfusions. A Broviac line was placed in the left femoral vein for intravenous antibiotics and antifungal therapy. During the next two weeks, he received a total of 7 units of fresh frozen plasma and 10 units of platelets via this line due to persistent thrombocytopenia and low grade disseminated intravascular coagulation picture. The line was removed on the 24th day of life because of a leak around the insertion site suggestive of loss of patency. Culture of the tip was negative. Caspofungin was added because of persistent fungemia. At 28 days of life, baby developed progressively worsening oliguria and azotemia. Renal ultrasound showed bilateral abnormal renal echogenicity with reversal of blood flow in both main renal arteries during diastole. An echocardiogram revealed the cause of the renal failure, persistent fungemia and persistent thrombocytopenia. This was a massive echogenic mass in the right atrium extending from the inferior vena cava (Fig. 1). The patient was started on heparin. Dialysis could not be done due to the baby's low weight and surgical removal was not feasible due to the low weight and the extreme critical condition of the baby. Doppler study could not demonstrate flow in the inferior vena cava, extending down below the renal veins. The baby died at 40 days of life. Limited autopsy showed a right atrial thrombus and histological staining of the thrombus revealed multiple hyphae mimicking a fungal ball (Fig. 4).

Discussion : The reported incidence of candida infection in neonatal intensive care units is about 1% but occurs in 4-15% of extremely low birth weight infants (BW<1kg). A positive Candida culture for more than five days is defined as persistent candidemia which is associated with increased risk of endocarditis but not with other complications. Persistent candidemia is often invasive in low birth weight premature infants. Ophthalmologic, renal and cardiac evaluations are routinely done as baseline and should be repeated based upon the clinical course as such complications may influence therapy and outcome. Independent of birth weight, infants born at less than 26 weeks or who had abdominal surgery are at a significantly increased risk of candidemia. The occurrence of fungal endocarditis is on the rise, reported in last decade in infants and children secondary to use of central venous line (CVL), prolonged use of broad spectrum antibiotics and neonatal cardiac surgery. CVL is frequently used in supportive care of premature infants for fluids, prolonged antimicrobial therapy and total parenteral nutrition (TPN). Several possible mechanisms by which CVL causes thrombosis include damage to vessel walls, disrupted blood flow, infusion of substances such as TPN that damage endothelial cells and thrombogenic catheter materials. An increased incidence of venous thrombosis is reported with femoral-subclavian CVL compared to brachial –jugular CVL and it does not depend on choice of type, size and duration of CVL. A Broviac was placed in left femoral site in our patient due to technical difficulties in the neck and upper extremity. Repeated infusion of platelets to treat persistent thrombocytopenia through this line may have led to local thrombus formation which gradually extended into the inferior vena cava affecting renal blood flow, causing progressive renal failure. Intravascular thrombus was likely seeded with fungus and led to persistent candidiasis for more than three weeks. The clot from the inferior vena cava extended in to the right atrium and became the harbinger of underlying extensive venous thrombosis. Liposomal amphotericin is generally first line of therapy. Fluconazole is a fungistatic drug, often used in combination with amphotericin in non-neutropenic patients as well in cases of right atrial mycetoma (RAM). There is limited data available for the use of caspofungin in cases of fungal endocarditis. Empirical antifungal therapy is recommended in newborns aged less than 25 weeks of gestation, thrombocytopenia and exposure to third generation cephalosporins 7 days prior to blood culture due to the high incidence of mortality and morbidity in this group. An active effort should be made to remove CVL in the presence of persistent fungemia. Surgery has a role in a select group of neonates with RAM. Depending upon its size and location, RAM may cause hemodynamic compromise with obstruction of tricuspid inflow and potential for embolism. The outcome of RAM is comparable with both medical and surgical treatment. Persistent candidemia in low birth weight premature infants is a risk factor for endocarditis and demands a thorough and repeated search for a nidus and end organ complications related to the heart, central nervous system and kidneys. RAM complicates the management of fungal endocarditis in the newborn. Despite advances in antifungal agents and cardiac surgical interventions, fungal endocarditis still carries high mortality and morbidity.

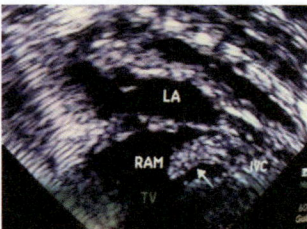

Fig. 1: Subcostal short axis view showing large thrombus in inferior vena cava, projecting in to right atrium over tricuspid valve.

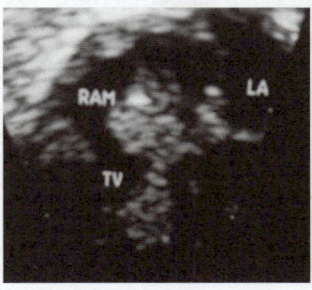 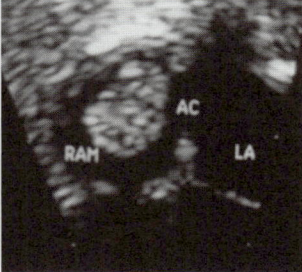

The mass in the right atrium moved across the tricuspid valve in diastole and was also in close proximity with the atrial communication (Figs 2 and 3).

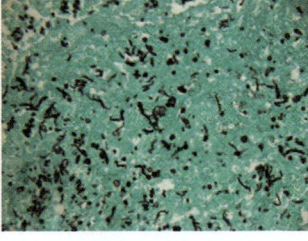

Fig. 4: 10X magnification of atrial thrombus stained with Grocott's Methenamine Silver stain (GMS) highlight numerous fungal organisms.

Courtesy: Sharma J, Nagraj A, Allapathi D, Rajegowda B, Leggiadro R. Fungal endocarditis in a premature infant complicated by a right atrial mycetoma and inferior vena cava thrombosis. Images Paediatr Cardiol 2009;41:6-11 Division of Pediatric Cardiology, Neonatology and Infectious Disease, Department of Pediatrics, Lincoln Medical and Mental Health Center, 234, East 149th Street, Bronx, NY 11451.

6. NEONATAL NECROTIZING FASCIITIS

During the neonatal period, the occurrence of necrotizing fasciitis is rare and is generally associated with other infections, such as omphalitis and mammary infection[3]. Mortality is high, reaching over 70%, even with precocious diagnosis and treatment[4]. These aspects of the disease's behavior demonstrate the importance of bearing in mind the predisposing factors and rigorous vigilance needed to treat the at-risk newborn. This case report describes our experience with a newborn with necrotizing fasciitis that followed a massive contamination during the delivery.

Case Report: The patient was a one-day-old girl, with a birth weight of 1900 g and a gestational age 36 weeks. The mother was 29 years old, and this was her second gestation without prenatal care. The birth took place at home, and the newborn was allowed to fall into the toilet bowl during delivery; the umbilical cord was severed with domestic scissors. Shortly after birth, the newborn was taken to the hospital where she received her first medical care and intravenous penicillin and amikacin therapy. At 90 minutes of life, she presented with hypoglycemia, necessitating intravenous infusion of 10% glucose. At 24 hours of life, hyperemia and edema of the left leg were observed at the site of the venipuncture and infiltration of intravenous solution. The clinical course was marked by a rapid deterioration of the lesion's appearance and extension. The infant was transferred to the Neonatal Intensive Care Unit (NICU) of the Children's Institute because of her worsening clinical course. On admission, she was in a poor general state, groaning, with decreased peripheral perfusion, an axillary temperature of 36°C, tachycardia (160 beats/min), tachypnea (88 breaths/min), abdominal distention, her liver was 2.0 cm from the right costal arch, and her spleen was 1.0 cm from the left costal arch. Throughout the anterior fascia of the left leg, hard edema with a violet skin color and blistered lesions measuring 2.0 cm in diameter containing liquid with a fetid odor and bloody regions (Fig. 1) were observed. Results of the laboratory examinations were: Hb=17.2g/dL; Ht= 46%; Leukocytes = 2700 mm^3; Platelets = 8000/mm^3; TP = 29.0 sec; TTPA=73.1 sec; Hemoculture: *Morganella morganii* and *Escherichia coli*; Cutaneous blister secretion: *Escherichia coli*. An escharotomy was performed, followed by total amputation of the left leg, 27 hours after hospitalization. The newborn was mechanically ventilated and administered fresh plasma, vasoactive drugs, ceftazidime, and amikacin. The course worsened rapidly resulting in pulmonary bleeding and bleeding at the puncture sites, persistent bradycardia, and death 48 hours after hospitalization.

Discussion: Necrotizing fasciitis is characterized by a bacterial infection of the skin, subcutaneous fat, and superficial and deep fascia, with rapid dissemination and signs of systemic toxicity. Marked tissular edema

occurs, which spreads rapidly into the fascial planes, causing vascular thrombosis, with necrosis of the subcutaneous cellular tissue and skin. The muscular layer can also be affected. The initial appearance of the lesion varies from a discrete rash to the appearance of erythema, edema, hardening, and cellulite. The skin develops a violet coloration with blistering and areas of necrosis[5]. Crepitation is not common, but fever, tachycardia, and leukocytosis with a deviation to the left are frequent. Thrombocytopenia, as observed in this patient, occurs in approximately half of all cases[6]. The disease occurs predominantly in adult patients and is rare in children, especially during the neonatal period. In a recent review of the literature, covering 28 years (1972–1999), Hsieh et al.[6] found only 66 cases, with the exception of 3 cases reported by them. Umbilical infection has been reported in some 70% of the cases, and as such is the most frequent entry site. Other associated conditions are mastitis, balanitis, fetal monitoring with electrodes in the scalp, necrotizing enterocolitis, immunodeficiency, impetigo with blistering, and maternal mastitis. In our patient, the initial lesion was observed in the left leg, at the venipuncture site for the administration of hypertonic glucose solution. Lesions at this site are not usual, with only 2 such cases reported in the literature[6]. Rupture of the tegumentary barrier following venipuncture and severe contamination during the delivery appear to be the predominant factors in the initiation of the disease. Furthermore, the newborn had serious leukopenia, low birth weight, and prematurity, which may have contributed to the unfavorable outcome. Contrary to our experience, the majority of authors have observed the disease in term Newborns.[4,7-9] In the literature review by Hsieh et al. only 3 cases were preterm[6]A fulminating course is frequent in neonates with necrotizing fasciitis, even with an early diagnosis and therapeutic treatment. On hospitalization in the NICU at only 24 hours of life, our patient already had signs of cellulitis in the left leg, which rapidly compromised all the tissular planes. Samuel et al.[9] reported 14 cases, with only 2 survivors, and emphasized the fact that the patients initially appear to be responding, but rapid deterioration in the general state occurs, and death follows within 72 hours. The most frequent causal agent of neonatal necrotizing fasciitis is *Staphylococcus aureus*, observed in two-thirds of all cases and is related to the presence of omphalitis and mastitis[3,8]. Various authors [2,4,5,7] have observed the association of bacteria. In our patient, the presence of *E. coli* and *Morganella morganii* in the hemoculture and cutaneous blister secretion are consistent with the type of contamination during the delivery. We call attention to the occurrence of necrotizing fasciitis as an infectious complication following deliveries without medical assistance and highlight the site of the lesion, causal agents, and fulminating clinical course.

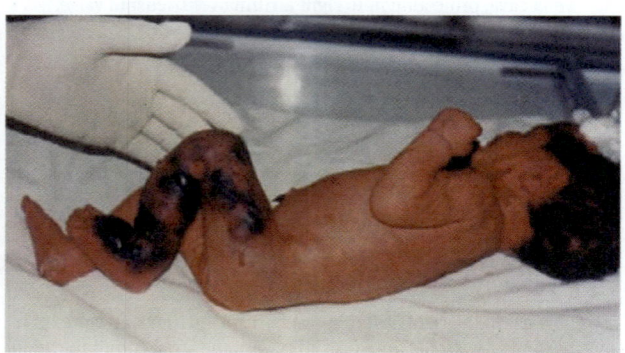

Necrotizing fasciitis left leg

REFERENCES

1. WILSON HD & HALTALIN KC - Acute necrotizing fasciitis in childhood. **Am J Dis Child** 1999; **125**:591-5. [Links] 2. MURPHY JJ, GRANGER R, BLAIR GK et al.- Necrotizing fasciitis in childhood. **J Pediatr Surg** 1995; **30**:1131-4. [Links] 3.BODEMER C, PANBANS A, CHRETIEN-MARQUET B et al. -Staphylococcal necrotizing fasciitis in the mammary region in childhood. A report of five cases. **J Pediatr** 1997; **131**:466. [Links] 3. SAWIN RS, SCHALLER RT, TAPPER D et al. - Early recognition of neonatal abdominal wall necrotizing fasciitis. **Am J Surg** 1994; **167**:481-4. [Links] 5. GIULIANO A, LEWIS JR F, HADLEY K et al. - Bacteriology of necrotizing fasciitis. **Am J Surg** 1977; **134**:52-6. [Links] 6. HSIEH WS, YANG PH, CHAO HC et al. - Neonatal Necrotizing Fascíitis: A report of three cases and review of the literature (abstract e 53). **Pediatrics** 1999; **103**(4):810. [Links] 7. BLISS JR DP, HEALEY PJ & WAULDBAUSEN JHT - Necrotizing fasciitis after Plastibell circumcision. **J Pediatr** 1997; **131**:459-62. [Links] 8. CHEN JW, BROADBENT RS & THOMSON IA - Staphylococcal neonatal necrotizing fasciitis: survival without radical debridement. **N Z Med J** 1998; **111**:251-3. [Links] 9. SAMUEL M, FREEMAN NV, VAISHNAV A et al. - Necrotizing Fasciitis: a serious complication of omphalitis in neonates. **J Pediatr Surg** 1994; **29**:1414-6.

Courtesy: *Vera Lúcia Jornada Krebs, Karen Mayumi Koga, Edna Maria de Albuquerque Diniz, Maria Esther Jurfest Ceccon and Flávio Adolfo Costa Vaz Rev. Hosp. Clin. vol.56 no.2 São Paulo Mar./Apr. 2001.*

Necrotizing fasciitis—C ase report 2: Baby A was born at term by normal vaginal delivery. He originally presented to a peripheral hospital at ten days of age and four days following a superficial burn to his back. The burn was sustained from a hot water bottle placed against his back for fifteen minutes. Two days later a visiting midwife noted a black streak had developed across the area of redness on his back. One day later the area of blackness was noted to be much larger and so he was referred to the local hospital. On presentation to the peripheral hospital, Baby A was noted to be dehydrated, unwell and septic with a leucocytosis (29.7 x 109/L) with toxic changes. He was initially resuscitated with fluids, amoxicillin, metronidazole, gentamicin and fresh, frozen plasma, and transferred to the Starship Hospital (Figure 1). Aggressive debridement of non-viable tissue on his back was undertaken. The resulting defect extended from the gluteal folds up to the interscapular line in both flanks. In the next 48 hours he required further debridement on two occasions, since the non-viable tissue had extended in all directions to include the ischiorectal fossae. A biopsy of normal skin was procured and dispatched to Perth for cultured skin (epithelial autograft culture). The defect was covered with cadaver skin grafts in the interim and cultured skin was used when it arrived from Perth. Swabs taken from the affected area on admission grew Staphylococcus aureus (sensitive to flucloxacillin) and biopsy of the affected region confirmed necrosis of the fascial layer. Baby A required total parental nutrition and naso-gastric feeding. A defunctioning colostomy was performed on Day 4 to prevent wound contamination. Eleven days after admission, Baby A had the cadaveric skin removed, and autologous skin grafts and cultured cell suspension were placed on the defect. With ongoing wound management the skin grafts had a good take and the defect was successfully covered. Fifty five days after admission to the Starship Hospital, Baby A had a reversal of his colostomy and on Day 62 was discharged back to the referring hospital for convalescence. Follow up two months after discharge revealed that Baby A was doing well with a completely healed wound on his back.

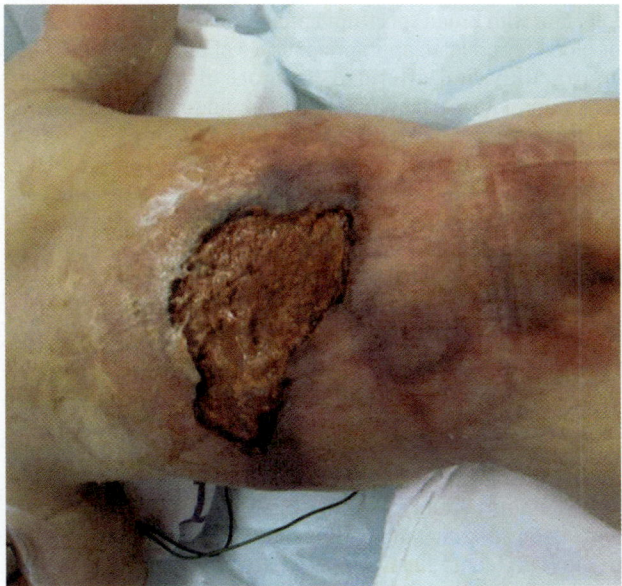

Baby A at presentation to the Starship Hospital. Debridement required removal of all the discoloured area

Necrotizing fasciitis is a rare condition in neonates. If it is not suspected and the diagnosis is missed, it can be fatal. It is frequently attributable to secondary infection such as omphalitis, mammitis, balanitis, postoperative complications, and bullous impetigo, and may be associated with diabetes mellitus, necrotizing enterocolitis, immunodeficiency and septicemia. The most common site of involvement in pediatric patients is the abdominal wall followed by the thorax, back, scalp and extremities. The initial skin presentation ranges from a minimal rash to erythema, edema, induration or cellulitis. These lesions spread rapidly. The overlying skin may later develop a violaceous discoloration, peau d'orange appearance, bullae, or necrosis. Fever and tachycardia may be present. Marked tissue edema, rapid progression of inflammation and signs of systemic toxicity are diagnostic clues. Some authors have used ultrasonography, CT and MRI scans in the diagnosis of necrotizing fasciitis showing a thickened and swollen fascial layer. However, we believe it is the clinical presentation and signs at examination, with a high index of suspicion and knowledge of necrotizing fasciitis, that reveal the diagnosis. The initial management of this condition is immediate surgical debridement, as this is the only factor that has shown a decrease in mortality. All non-viable tissue is excised until bleeding viable tissue is seen. This may require drainage of the fascial plane and extensive fasciotomies. Other measures required in the initial management include high-dose intravenous antibiotics, aggressive fluid resuscitation and analgesia. A combination of penicillin and cephalosporins are recommended for gram-positive bacteria, aminoglycosides for gram-negative bacteria, and clindamycin or metronidazole for anaerobic bacteria. Clindamycin has been shown to improve survival of endotoxic shock by modulating the release of inflammatory cytokines. Hyperbaric oxygen has been reported in the literature; its use has not shown a decrease in mortality, but can be an option if anaerobic bacteria are cultured. Death usually occurs before surgery or shortly after surgical intervention as a result of bacterial infection with septic shock, disseminated intravascular coagulation and/or multiple organ failure. Coverage and reconstruction of the defects left from this condition can be significant and complex. The services of a plastic surgical unit should be sought in association with the initial surgical management for coverage of the wound. The principles of wound management in this condition include temporary wound coverage initially, while there is ongoing infection, and then formal reconstruction of the defect once the infection has settled. Formal coverage is usually performed using autologous skin grafts. In rare instances coverage can be performed with tissue flaps. In small defects coverage can be obtained with sheet grafts.

In conclusion, Neonatal necrotizing fasciitis is a rare but serious and often fatal condition. A high index of suspicion must be kept if the diagnosis is to be made and treatment commenced. To date, the only predictor to prognosis is the time to surgical debridement. It is a condition that requires the services of multiple specialties including surgery, infectious diseases, intensive care, plastic surgery, dietetics, physiotherapy and occupational therapy. Patients with these conditions should therefore be treated in centres that provide these services and early referral from peripheral hospitals to a specialist centre must be encouraged.

Courtesy: Necrotizing fasciitis in neonates: a multidisciplinary approach Stanley Loo, Stephen Mills, Michael Muller and Vipul Upadhyay, Journal of the New Zealand Medical Association, 22-August-2003, Vol 116 No 1180

7. NEONATAL PURPURA FULMINANS

Purpura fulminans (PF) is an ominous cutaneous condition usually associated with meningococcemia.Neonatal purpura fulminans (PF) associated with early-onset enterobacter septicemia is rare. PF presents as a catastrophic illness with gangrene of the distal extremities and necrosis of the skin. The clinical picture consists of septicemia, shock and disseminated intravascular coagulation (DIC.). PF is also an ominous cutaneous sign of fulminant neonatal GBS septicemia.

Case report: Purpura fulminans (PF) was immediately evident in a moribund 2.7 kg newborn girl delivered by emergency cesarean section for fetal tachycardia (200/minute by cardiotocography) at 35 week gestation 1. There was no family history of bleeding disorder. The membranes were ruptured 3 hours prior to delivery. The mother developed intrapartum fever (38.9°C) with chills and rigors and was given intravenous ampicillin and gentamicin 23 minutes before delivery by emergency caesarean section. At birth, the baby was apneic with heart rate of 80/minute. She cried and the heart rate responded upon bag and mask ventilation for 1 minute. Apgars were 8 and 10 at 1 and 5 minutes, respectively. On arrival at the NICU, the baby developed further apneas with cyanosis followed by tachypnea, indrawing chest and grunting. Her mean arterial blood pressure was 30 mmHg and heart rate 190/minute. Arterial blood gas analysis showed a pH of 7.19, pCO_2 8.03 kPa, pO_2 2.25 kPa, and base excess of -6.9 mmol/L. Respiratory support (nasal continuous positive airway pressure of 5 cm H_2O with 8 L/min of oxygen), normal saline bolus, and intravenous penicillin plus gentamicin were administered within the first hour of resuscitation. In the next 2 hours, she remained hypotensive despite further saline boluses, dopamine infusion and mechanical ventilation. Group B streptococcus, sensitive to penicillin, was isolated from the blood cultures of the mother and the infant. She was aggressively treated with broad antibiotic coverage, cardiopulmonary support with mechanical ventilation and multiple inotropes, and peritoneal dialysis. The purpuric rash became more extensive and she developed progressive multi-organ system failure despite full intensive care support and succumbed 9 days later

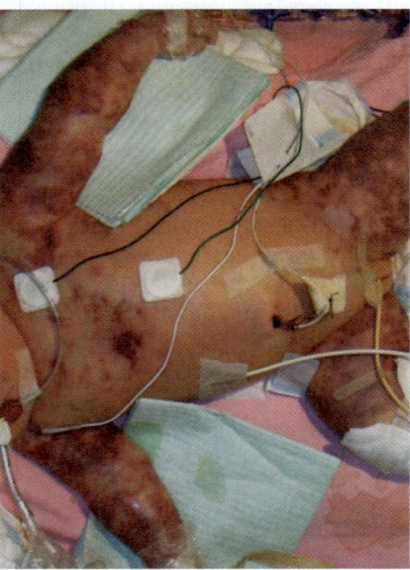

Discussion: Purpura fulminans (PF) is an acute and frequently fatal disorder characterized by sudden appearance of large ecchymotic areas, which are commonly localized on the lower extremities and are typically symmetric. The edges of the lesions are usually sharply demarcated and central bullae may develop. Although the pathogenesis is not fully understood, the Disseminated Intravascular Coagulation (DIC) in PF appears to involve the skin selectively. In the neonatal period group B streptococcus is the major cause of PF but gram negative organisms such as *Escherichia coli* and *Enterobacter* have been described. One limitation of our case was that the coagulopathy was immediately treated empirically before the endogenous activities of the anticoagulant factors protein C, protein S, and Antithrombin III (AT III) were assessed. In case any of these factors are found to be affected, human protein C or recombinant human activated protein C may be considered, and protein C, protein S, and AT III genes should have been analyzed in the patient and her parents. There was no family history of coagulopathy and group B streptococcus was identified to be the pathogen, making syndromes of congenital anticoagulant factor deficiency unlikely in this patient. Regardless of the pathogen, neonatal PF must be promptly recognized and aggressively treated in children. Early goal-directed therapy provides significant benefits with respect to outcome in adult patients with severe sepsis and septic shock. The therapy involves adjustments of cardiac preload, afterload, and contractility to balance oxygen delivery with oxygen demand. Guidelines were proposed through the Surviving Sepsis Campaign to improve outcome in septic patients . They are difficult to apply routinely and validate in neonates. As Claessens et al has commented, attempts to apply all of the procedures recommended by the experts, despite the apparent pragmatism of those procedures, have varied widely; diagnosis may be problematic because of atypical or unspecific presentations, biomarkers are of little help at the start of treatment and are unspecific, supportive treatment often depends on local supply of resources, and specific devices are often absent for initial therapy and monitoring. Resuscitation policy for septic shock in neonates generally includes prompt treatment of the underlying infection with broad spectrum antibiotics, replacement of fluids or blood for preload, appropriate usage of inotropes for cardiac contractility and afterload, support of oxygenation and ventilation with mechanical ventilation, and support of individual multi-organ system failure.Despite full intensive care support, PF is often associated with multiple organ failure and high mortality in children . PF has a reported mortality of 50 per cent secondary to multiple organ failure which commonly accompanies the syndrome and is associated with major long-term morbidity in those who survive. In 3 cases of early neonatal PF, all the babies survived but had markedly compromised neurologic outcomes. Rivard et al described severe acquired protein C deficiency successfully treated with conventional therapy and high-volume plasma exchange as a source of protein C. Many other therapies have been described in case reports that claimed to arrest the progression of neonatal PF, such as the use of heparin, Protein C, Antithrombin III, recombinant tissue plasminogen activator (rtPA), epoprostenol (prostacyclin), topical nitroglycerin, intravenous dextran, and plasmapheresis. Nevertheless, there is no strong evidence in favor of one particular therapy due to the small number of cases.

Courtesy: **Spot diagnosis: An ominous rash in a newborn,** Kam-Lun Hon*, King-Woon So, William Wong and Kam-Lau Cheung, Department of Paediatrics, The Chinese University of Hong Kong, Prince of Wales Hospital, Shatin, Hong Kong *Italian Journal of Pediatrics* 2009, **35**:10

8. PLEURAL EMPYEMA IN A PRETERM INFANT

Pleural empyema is known as the pyogenic infection of the pleural space with purulent effusion. Empyema is frequently seen in children and standard therapy approaches have been developed for it. However, it is a very rare entity in newborn infants, with only some 20 case reports in the literature. It is also a very unusual condition in preterm infants, with only one case report in the literature who was reported as having *Serratia marcescens* pneumonia, empyema and pneumatocele. It has been suggested that insufficient immune response of the newborn in the early days of life can not localize the infection to the pleura, and furthermore, that the capacity of the pleura to produce exudate is limited. Due to these factors, the incidence of empyema in newborn infants has been considered to be very low. *Staphylococcus aureus*, *Escherichia coli*, hemolytic group B Streptococcus, hemolytic group A Streptococcus, Klebsiella spp. and Serratia spp. are the most common causative agents that are isolated. To our knowledge, *Pseudomonas aeruginosa* (*P. aeruginosa*) has not been isolated in any pleural empyema. Therefore, we suggest that this is the first case report of a preterm infant who developed *P. aeruginosa* empyema during hospitalization.

Case report: A male infant was born by cesarean section at 29 weeks' gestation to a 23-year-old primigravida mother with Apgar 3-6 at the 1st and 5th minutes, respectively. His mother was routinely followed-up during pregnancy and she was hospitalized due to severe preeclampsia the last week before birth. The birth weight was 1170 g (10-50th centile), birth length was 37 cm (10-50th centile) and head circumference was 26.2 cm (10-50th centile). Physical examination revealed respiratory distress and tachypnea (64 breaths/min), cyanosis, intercostal and subcostal retractions, and prematurity findings. He was intubated due to respiratory distress after birth and given two doses of surfactant because there was reticular granular pattern with air bronchograms on his postero-anterior chest X-ray. His first cranial ultrasonography was performed at 24 hours of life and showed bilateral grade III intraventricular hemorrhage. He was given ampicillin and gentamicin therapies for sepsis. He developed necrotizing enterocolitis on the 3rd day of life. He could not be extubated until the 28th day of life and his chest X-ray was evaluated as chronic lung disease. Therefore, a five-day weaning course of dexamethasone and diuretic medication was given. His first ophthalmological examination for retinopathy of prematurity (ROP) was found as normal. On the 43rd day of life, while he was followed as intubated, his respiratory distress increased and his physical examination revealed decreased audible breath sounds on the middle and inferior parts of the right lung. Pleural effusion and pneumatocele were determined in his chest X-ray (Fig. 1). His thorax ultrasonography revealed septated consolidation areas in which the maximum thickness reached 1 cm in the inferior lobe of the right lung. Thoracentesis was performed with the guide of ultrasonography, 3 ml purulent pleural fluid was removed, and a thoracotomy tube was placed at the same time. There were many polymorphonuclear leukocytes in the Giemsa-stained smears of this fluid and there were coccobacilli and rare Gram-positive cocci in the Gram-stained smears. In the biochemical analysis of pleural fluid, density was 1005, pH was 8, lactate dehydrogenase (LDH) was high at 1590 UI/L (serum LDH was 270 IU/L), protein was also high at 4.8 g/dl, glucose was too low to be measured, and Rivalta reaction was found to be positive. His complete blood count showed marked leukocytosis with leukocytes of 22400/ mm3 and peripheral blood smear revealed 6% rod neutrophils, 64% neutrophils, 22% lymphocytes, and 8% monocytes with 20% of toxic granulation. His C-reactive protein was found to be higher than 15 mg/dl (normal <0.5 mg/dl). Multidrug-resistant *P. aeruginosa* was isolated from the pleural fluid culture and he was treated with meropenem (100 mg/kg/ day) and amikacin (22.5 mg/kg/day). It was sensitive only to amikacin. Drainage from the thorax tube persisted for 21 days and *P. aeruginosa* was isolated in four other pleural fluid and tracheal suction cultures. No organism was isolated from blood and cerebrospinal fluid cultures. After his respirations and his chest X-ray improved and no drainage was seen from the thoracic tube, it was removed and chest X-ray showed improvement (Fig. 2). His immunological studies were found to be normal. Cystic fibrosis mutation analysis was found to be normal. Computerized thorax tomography performed after his stabilization revealed diffuse fibrotic and atelectatic changes in both lungs and volume loss in the left lung (Fig. 3). His

discharge from the hospital was planned once adequate feeding and weight gain were achieved, but another sepsis episode occurred on the 190th day of hospitalization. He was again intubated due to pneumonia and respiratory insufficiency. He was given antibiotic medication, but did not respond to this therapy and died during this sepsis episode. No organism was isolated from his tracheal suction, blood, urine or cerebrospinal fluid cultures.

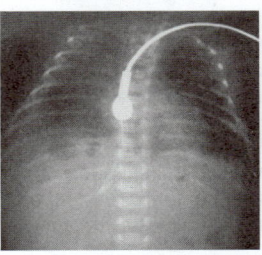

Fig. 1: Postero-anterior chest X-ray of the patient showing pleural effusion and pneumatocele in the right lung.

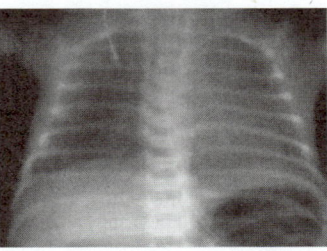

Fig. 2 : Postero-anterior chest X-ray showing improvement after the removal of the thoracic tube.

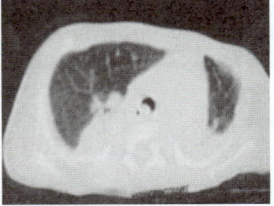

Fig. 3 : Computerized thorax tomography showing diffuse fibrotic and atelectatic changes in both lungs and volume loss in the left lung.

Discussion: Although pleural empyema is seen frequently in children, it is very uncommon in neonates. The most common causative agents in pleural empyema in children are *S. aureus*, *E. coli*, hemolytic group B Streptococcus, hemolytic group A Streptococcus, Klebsiella spp. and Serratia spp. Therefore, Gram-positive agents are more suspicious than Gram-negative bacteria in the pleural empyema of Neonates [3,5-9]. Pleural empyema due to Gram-negative agents as *E. coli*, *Klebsiella pneumoniae*, *Enterobacter cloacae* and *S. marcescens* has been reported in literature[2,10-13]. However, we could not find a Neonatal empyema report in newborns associated with *P. aeruginosa*. Although Pseudomonas spp. have been defined as a causative factor in nosocomial pneumonia and sepsis in both neonates, children and adults who are immunocompromised, no empyema case associated with this agent has been described previously. *P. aeruginosa* is a motile, aerobic, Gram-negative bacillus with the ability to survive in harsh environments. Although it is an opportunistic bacteria that rarely causes severe infection in normal hosts, it can be an important pathogen causing hospital-acquired infections and severe infections in individuals such as preterm infants who have underlying serious disease[14,15]. Attachment to the appropriate host cell, colonization, local invasion, production of virulence factors, and dissemination with systemic manifestations determine the pathogenecity of any microbe. Protein structures such as pili and fimbriae on the surface of Pseudomonas are necessary for attachment to the epithelial surfaces. After the colonization of the epithelium, some of the organisms produce a biofilm containing a mucoid polysaccharide called alginate. Strains of the organisms produce a biofilm containing a mucoid polysaccharide called alginate. Strains that produce biofilms might be less susceptible to antimicrobial action and this may have a role in the pathogenesis of pulmonary disease caused by this organism. Virulence is associated with the production of multiple proteases and these may lead to the disruption of epithelial tightjunctions. This distribution probably contributes to the attachment process. *P. aeruginosa* also produce cytotoxin and heat labile and heat stable hemolysins, which inhibit polymorphonuclear lymphocyte function and degrade host lipids, respectively. Many of these products may have a role in the dissemination to other organs except local invasion. Furthermore, exotoxin A and exoenzyme S are the novel products of Pseudomonas and they are responsible for the development of sepsis syndrome of this bacteria[14,15].

P. aeruginosa has an outer bilipid layer, a periplasmic space and an inner bacterial membrane, and this complex structure causes resistance to natural defensins and antimicrobial agents. *P. aeruginosa* produce beta lactamases and plasmidassociated beta lactamases. These plasmidassociated elements are usually coexpressed with other resistance mechanisms, including aminoglycoside modifying enzymes, which render the organism multidrug-resistant[15]. The frequency of nosocomial infections in neonatal intensive care units has increased in the last years due to the improved survival rates of low birth weight premature infants[14-17]. These nosocomial pathogens are usually multidrugresistant organisms such as *P. aeruginosa*, Enterobacter spp. and Klebsiella spp. *P. aeruginosa* has been recognized as a neonatal pathogen for almost 50 years. Because of the factors such as very low birth weight (VLBW) infants having a more fragile skin barrier, an immature immune system, prolonged use of invasive devices, and colonization with hospital flora, neonates and especially VLBW infants have an increased risk for nosocomial infections. The sinks, water baths, respiratory equipment, hand solutions, antiseptics, and neonatal incubators are the most common reservoirs of *P. aeruginosa*[16-18]. In neonates, pneumonia and bloodstream infections are the most common nosocomial infections. It had been reported that *P. aeruginosa* was an infrequent pathogen for nosocomial pneumonia and bloodstream infections, but its mortality rate was found to be high[16-18]. Leigh et al.[19] stated that *P. aeruginosa* infections had a 50% mortality rate among infants whose birth weight was less than 1500 g. They described feeding intolerance, prolonged parenteral nutrition, longer duration of intravenous antibiotics, and necrotizing enterocolites as risk factors. They also found that mortality was inversely associated with age at diagnosis, and these results showed the importance of this pathogen in neonates. In addition, in a more recent study, the mortality of a *P. aeruginosa* outbreak in a neonatal intensive care unit was reported as 35%[17]. Bilikova et al.[20] reported ventilatory support and therapy with corticosteroids as the most important predictors of *P. aeruginosa* infections in a study including 246 infants, 34 of whom had infections due to *P. aeruginosa*. Our case had ventilatory support and was also given corticosteroid therapy for chronic lung disease. These factors may contribute to the development of *P. aeruginosa* empyema. In conclusion, *P. aeruginosa* may lead to empyema in VLBW infants who have risk factors such as ventilatory support, therapy with corticosteroids and an immature immune system.

Courtesy: *Pseudomonas aeruginosa* pleural empyema in a preterm infant Hilal Özkan1, Merih Çetinkaya1, Nilgün Köksal1, Solmaz Çelebi2 Mustafa Hacımustafaoglu2 *Divisions of 1Neonatology, and 2Pediatric Infectious Disease, Department of Pediatrics, Uludag University Faculty of Medicine, Bursa, Turkey, The Turkish Journal of Pediatrics 2009; 51: 395-398*

REFERENCES

1. Gupta R, Faridi MM, Gupta P. Neonatal empyema thoracis. Indian J Pediatr 1996; 63: 704-706.

2. Khan EA, Wafelman LS, Garcia-Prats JA, Taber LH. Serratia marcescens pneumonia, empyema and pneumatocele in a preterm neonate. Pediatr Infect Dis J 1997; 16: 1003–1005.

3. Nathavitharana KA, Watkinson MA. Neonatal pleural empyema caused by group A Streptococcus. Pediatr Infect Dis J 1994; 13: 671–672.

4. Erol MY, Deveci M, Eti N, Pelit M, Kut A, Ergüven M. Yenidoganda plevral ampiyem. Bir vaka takdimi. Çocuk Saglıgı ve Hastalıkları Dergisi 2005; 48: 334–336.

5. Shen YH, Hwang KP, Niu CK. Compl icated parapneumonic effusion and empyema in children. J Microbiol Immunol Infect 2006; 39: 483–488.

6. Gıvan DC, Eigen H. Common pleural effusion in children. Clin Chest Med 1998; 19: 363–371.

7. Beevan DW, Burry AF. Staphylococcal pneumonia in the newborn: an epidemic with eight fatal cases. Lancet 1956; 2: 211–215.

8. Freij BJ, Kusmiesz H, Nelson JD, McCracken GH. Parapneumonic effusions and empyema in hospitalized children: a retrospective review of 227 cases. Pediatr Infect Dis J 1984; 3: 578–591.

9. Sokal MM, Nagraj A, Fisher BJ, Vijayan S. Neonatal empyema caused by group B beta hemolytic streptococcus. Chest 1982; 81: 390–391.

10. Papageorgiou A, Bauer CR, Fletcher BD, Stern L. Klebsiella pneumonia with pneumatocele formation in a newborn infant. Can Med Assoc J 1973; 109: 1217–1219.

11. Kuhn JP, Lee SB, Pneumatoceles associated with Escherichia coli pneumonias in the newborn. Pediatrics 1973; 51: 1008–1011.

12. Gustavson EE. Escherichia coli empyema in the newborn. Am J Dis Child 1986; 140: 408.

13. Chellani HK, Antony JJ, Chatterjee PP, et al. Neonatal empyema. Indian Pediatr 1989; 26: 189–191.

14. Zafar AB, Sylvester LK, Beidas SO. Pseudomonas aeruginosa infections in a neonatal care unit. Am J Infect Control 2002; 30: 425-429.

15. Foca MD. Pseudomonas aeruginosa infections in a Neonatal care unit. Semin Perinatol 2002; 26: 332–359.

16. Ortega B, Groeneveld J. Endemic multidrug-resistant Pseudomonas aeruginosa in critically ill patients. Infect Control Hosp Epidemiol 2004; 25: 825–831.

17. Moolenaar RL, Crutcher JM, San Joaquin VH, et al. A prolonged outbreak of Pseudomonas aeruginosa in a neonatal intensive care unit: did staff fingernails play a role in disease transmission? Infect Control Hosp. Epidemiol 2004; 21: 80-85.

18. Lautenbach E, Weiner MG, Nachamkin I, Bilker WB, Sheridan A, Fishman NO. Imipenem resistance among Pseudomonas aeruginosa isolates: risk factors for infection and impact of resistance on clinical and economic outcomes. Infection Control Hosp Epidemiol 2006; 27: 893-900.

19. Leigh L, Stoll BJ, Rahman M, McGowan JR. Pseudomonas aeruginosa infection in very low birth weight infants: a case-control study. Pediatr Infect Dis J 1995; 14: 367-371.

20. Bilikova E, Hafed BM, Kovacicova G, et al. Nosocomial infections due to Pseudomonas aeruginosa in neonates. J Infect Chemother 2003; 9: 191–193.

9. NEONATAL DENGUE INFECTION

Dengue infection has become a major public health problem in tropical regions. Dengue virus is spread by mosquitos, causing variable manifestations, ranging from asymptomatic infection to flulike illness in dengue fever and sometimes severe hemorrhage resulting in shock and death in dengue hemorrhagic fever (WHO, 1997). Dengue infection is a disease of children; in recent years, the resurgence of dengue infection has been associated with an increasing incidence of dengue infection in adults with reports of dengue illness in pregnant women with transplacental transmission. Although a rare clinical occurrence, transplacental transmission imposes adverse effect on the fetus.

Case report: A 1-day-old Thai male infant was admitted because of acute febrile illness. His mother, aged 25, gravida 2, had experienced sudden febrile illness on the day of admission. The pregnancy was at 37-weeks' gestation. Routine screening tests performed at the antenatal clinic were negative for syphilis, hepatitis B surface antigen and human immunodeficiency virus. She complained of headache, myalgia, arthralgia and frequent uterine contractions. Her temperature was 39.2ºC, pulse 120, respirations 22, and blood pressure 120/70 mmHg. The fetal heart rate was 148. A nonstress test on the fetus showed a normal reactive response. The hematocrit was 27.6%, the white-cell count was 9,710/mm3 with 85.8% polymorphonuclear cells, 8.8% atypical lymphocytes, and the platelet count was 203,000 mm3. Blood urea nitrogen, creatinine, and electrolytes were normal. Ampicillin, metronidazole and gentamicin were administered intravenously. Fever persisted without obvious clinical focus. On day 5 her temperature was 39.1ºC (Table 1) with onset of active labor, the white-cell count decreased to 4,720/mm3 with 72.4% polymorphonuclear cells, 8.0% atypical lymphocytes and the platelet count was 52,000/mm3. Cesarean section was performed without any complication. Two days after the operation, the mother's hematocrit decreased to 17% without obvious bleeding from the surgical wound, the white-cell count was 1,980/mm3 with 67.1% polymorphonuclear cells, 14.1% atypical lymphocytes and the platelet count was 120,000/mm3. Two units of blood were transfused. Erythematous rash was observed on both legs. The complete blood count became normal on day 11. Her following clinical course was uneventful. The infant's birthweight was 3,150 g, length 50 cm; the Apgar scores were normal. No resuscitation was required. The placenta weighed 500 g and was normal. Routine intramuscular dose of vitamin K was administered. He appeared well until 16 hours, when fever developed. He was transferred to the neonatal care unit for close observation. The pulse was 158, the respirations were 40, and the blood pressure was 70/41 mmHg. On examination he was quiet but arousable. The liver and spleen were not enlarged. Skin perfusion was normal. Faint petechiae were observed on his face. The history was reviewed with the suspicion of dengue infection in the infant and his mother. The hematocrit was 51%, the white-cell count was 10,400/mm3 with 81.9% polymorphonuclear cells, 3.0% atypical lymphocytes and the platelet count was 99,000/mm3. Blood was collected for hemoculture. Intravenous fluid, ampicillin and gentamicin were started to cover sepsis-pending hemoculture result that later was reported as negative. The body temperature continued to rise, reaching a peak of 39.8ºC at 36 hours. The infant occasionally chilled at peaks of fever although he could suck on his bottle. Petechiae increased on his face and gradually spread to the trunk and extremities (Fig 1). Respirations were 88 and shallow; oxygen was given via head box. On day 3, the temperature persisted at 39.1ºC. On day 4, hematocrit decreased to 44%, the white-cell count was 8,000/mm3 with 50.8% polymorphonuclear cells, 9.3% atypical lymphocytes and the platelet count was 11,000/mm3. The liver was palpable 3 cm below the costal margin and the spleen was just palpable. Petechiae became prominent all over the body. On day 5, the petechiae began to fade. Blood sugar, blood urea nitrogen, creatinine, and electrolytes were normal. Aspartate aminotransferase (AST) was elevated to 152 U/l, while alanine aminotransferase (ALT) was normal. No signs of circulatory disturbance were detected. There was no pleural effusion by chest radiograph in the right lateral decubitus position. Serial hematocrits gradually decreased to 34% on day 6 before they rose to 41% on day 8. The infant was active at defervescence on day 7. He made an uneventful recovery and was discharged after 10 days' admission. The infant's polymerase chain reaction (PCR) result on day 5 was positive for dengue type 1, while that of the mother, obtained on day 10, was negative (Table 2). Enzyme-linked immunoassay (EIA) revealed an increase in both dengue-IgM and IgG in the mother with IgG titer higher than IgM (227 vs 126 EIA units), indicating secondary dengue infection. The infant's IgM increased to about 5 times higher than IgG (59 vs 11 EIA units), indicating primary infection. The mother's hemagglutination inhibition test (HAI) showed high titers to all 4 dengue serotypes, while in that of the infant, the titers were low.

Discussion: As the incidence of dengue infection in adults has increased, it is apparent that pregnant women could be infected, although the occurrence is uncommon. Diagnosis of dengue illness in mothers began with fever leukopenia and thrombocytopenia and other symptoms associated with dengue infection. Simple and inexpensive laboratory procedures to identify acute dengue disease, include the tourniquet test and complete blood count (Halstead, 1982; Thisyakorn et al, 1984; Kalayanarooj et al, 1997; Srichaikul and Nimmannitya, 2000). Since the symptoms occurred immediately after birth, our infant was certainly infected in utero. Intrauterine transmission was greatest when serum titers of viremia were high, which occurred at the time of fever. Secondary infection in mothers also caused higher titers of viremia than in primary infection (Vaughn et al, 1997; 2000). The incubation period for dengue infection in infants or the duration between fever in mothers and infants, was shorter in mothers with secondary infection (3-6 days) (Chotigeat et al, 2000; Boussemart et al, 2001; Kerdpanich et al, 2001) than in primary infection (5-13 days) (Thaithumyanon et al, 1994; Chotigeat et al, 2000; Boussemart et al, 2001). The first manifestation in infants was fever, which appeared earlier postnatally in the mother with secondary infection (0.5-3 days) than in primary infection (4-11 days). All infants had primary dengue infection. Although passive maternal dengue antibodies increased the risk of developing dengue hemorrhagic fever/dengue shock syndrome in infected infants (Kliks et al, 1988), there were no such cases in these infants. Our infant had the shortest time before onset of manifestation; fever appeared at 16 hours after birth. The virus could have been transmitted from the mother on her first day of fever so the incubation period is 5 days. The time of acquiring dengue virus intrauterinely could affect the fetus. Infection during the second trimester could lead to premature labor and fetal death (Carles et al, 1999; 2000), whereas infection near, or at, term posed little effect on the infant. Most had fever, rash, hepatomegaly and thrombocytopenia, while some infants remained asymptomatic (Bunyavejchevin et al, 1997). Dengue serotypes may play a role in the severity of disease. Symptoms seemed to be more severe with secondary dengue type 2 infection (Halstead et al, 1970; Morens et al, 1991), causing severe coagulopathy and postpartum hemorrhage in mothers (Thaithumyanon et al, 1994; Chye et al, 1997; Chotigeat et al, 2000) and intraventricular hemorrhage and death in infants (Chye et al, 1997). Dengue type 1 in our case might not have such virulence, only fever and occult bleeding in the mother and fever and rash in the infant. No teratogenic effect has been reported by intrauterine dengue infection (Carles et al, 1999). The mode of delivery did not change the course of disease or reduce the rate of bleeding in infants. One case of Chye et al (1997) was delivered vaginally with severe intracranial hemorrhage while other infants had subtle illness viafections and were able to identify infection as primary or secondary (Innis et al, 1989; Clarke and Cassals, 1958). In dengue-endemic areas, there is a possibility that pregnant women may be infected with dengue virus. Therefore, obstetricians and pediatricians should be on alert to dengue disease and be prepared provide proper management for both mother and neonate. this route (Boussemart et al, 2001;Chotigeat et al, 2000) as well as other infants delivered by cesarean section (Thaithumyanon et al, 1994; Boussemart et al, 2001; Kerdpanich et al, 2001). There was gradual bleeding from the raw surface of the uterus, as evidenced by a drop in hematocrit in the mother 2 days postoperatively. For the infant, a drop in hematocrit was probably caused by the hemodilution effect of intravenous fluid administration. There was no sign of plasma leakage in mother or infant. The diagnosis was dengue fever for both of them. The typical duration of viremia was 4-5 days during the febrile phase, and it persisted longer in children experiencing primary infections rather than secondary dengue infections due to more gradual antibody or cellular immune response. Therefore, PCR from the infant performed near the end of the febrile period was positive, while that from the mother performed at a later time was negative (Lanciotti et al, 1992; Vaughn et al, 2000).

Reverse transcriptase polymerase chain reaction (RT-PCR) and serologic values.

Test Variable	Mother	Infant
Polymerase chain reaction RT-PCR	Negative	Dengue -1
Enzyme-linked immunoassay (units) Dengue IgM	126	59
Dengue IgG	227	11
Japanese encephalitis IgM	27	14
Japanese encephalitis IgG	177	6
Hemagglutination inhibition (titers) Dengue -1	1280	10
Dengue -2	640	10
Dengue -3	2560	10
Dengue -4	2560	10
Japanese encephalitis	5120	10
Chikungunya	80	40

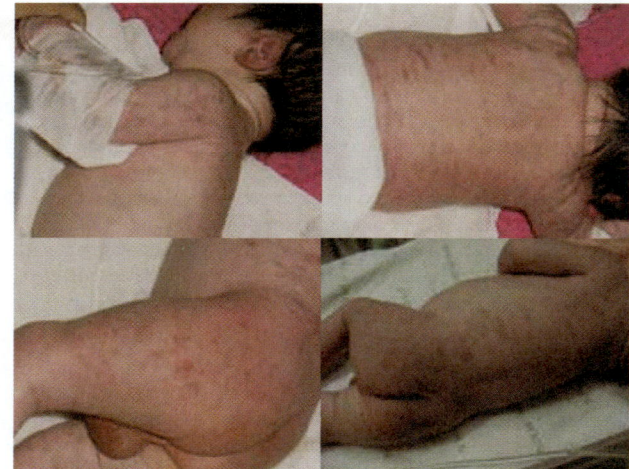

Fig 1: Petechiae began on his face and gradually spread to the trunk and extremities.

Temperature patterns of the mother and infant. Cesarean section was performed on day 5 after onset of active labor. Fever in the infant appeared at 16 hours after birth.

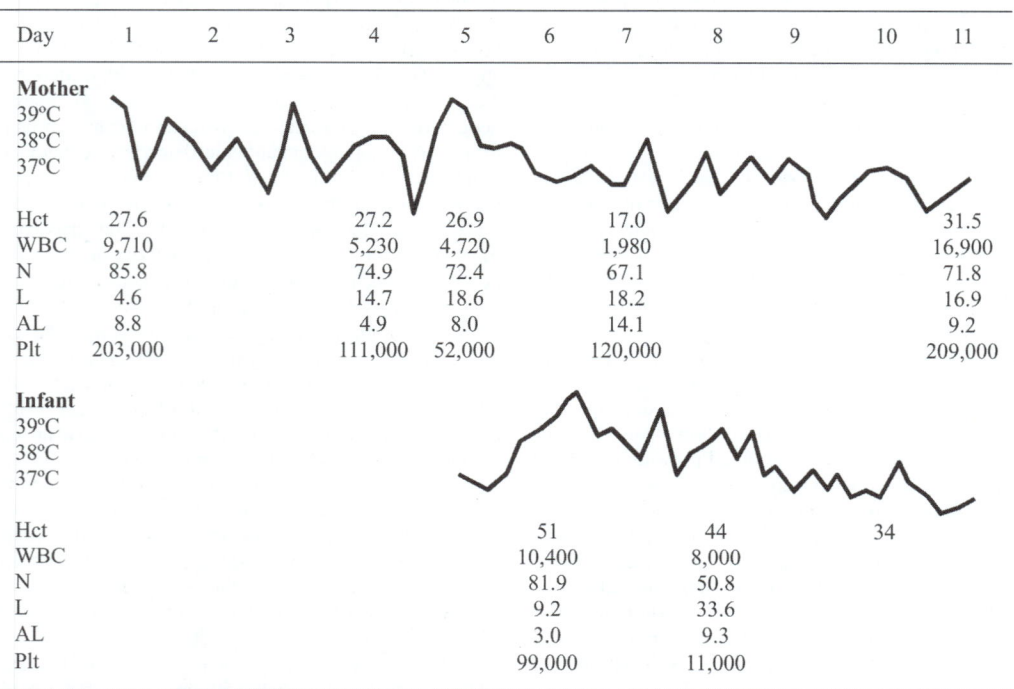

Day	1	2	3	4	5	6	7	8	9	10	11
Mother 39°C 38°C 37°C											
Hct	27.6			27.2	26.9		17.0				31.5
WBC	9,710			5,230	4,720		1,980				16,900
N	85.8			74.9	72.4		67.1				71.8
L	4.6			14.7	18.6		18.2				16.9
AL	8.8			4.9	8.0		14.1				9.2
Plt	203,000			111,000	52,000		120,000				209,000
Infant 39°C 38°C 37°C											
Hct						51		44		34	
WBC						10,400		8,000			
N						81.9		50.8			
L						9.2		33.6			
AL						3.0		9.3			
Plt						99,000		11,000			

Hct, hematocrit; WBC, white-blood cell; N, neutrophil; L, lymphocyte; AL, atypical lymphocyte; Plt, platelet.

REFERENCES

Boussemart T, Babe P, Sibille G, Neyret C, Berchel C. Prenatal transmission of dengue: two new cases. *J Perinatol* 2001; 21: 255-7. Bunyavejchevin S, Tanawattanacharoen S, Taechakraichana N, *et al.* Dengue hemorrhagic fever during pregnancy: antepartum, intrapartum and postpartum management. *J Obstet Gynaecol Res* 1997; 23: 445-8. Carles G, Peiffer H, Talarmin A. Effects of dengue fever during pregnancy in French Guiana. *Clin Infect Dis* 1999; 28: 637–40. Carles G, Talarmin A, Peneau C, Bertsch M. Dengue fever and pregrancy. A study of 38 cases in French Guiana. *J Gynecol Obstet Biol Reprod* (Paris) 2000; 29: 758-62 [In French]. Chotigeat U, Khaoluang S, Kanjanapatanakul V, Nisalak A. Vertical transmission of dengue virus. *J Infect Dis Antimicrob Agents* 2000; 17: 33-4. Chye JK, Lim CT, Ng KB, *et al.* Vertical transmission of dengue. *Clin Infect Dis* 1997; 25: 1374-7. Clarke DH, Casals J. Techniques for hemagglutination and hemagglutination-inhibition with arthropodborne viruses. *Am J Trop Med Hyg* 1958; 7: 561-73. Halstead SB. Dengue: hematologic aspects. *Semin Hematol* 1982; 19: 116–31. Halstead SB, Nimmannitya S, Cohen SN. Observations related to pathogenesis of dengue hemorrhagic fever: IV. Relation of disease severity to antibody response and virus recovered. *Yale J Biol Med* 1970; 42: 311–28. Innis BL, Nisalak A, Nimmannitya S, *et al.* An enzymelinked immunosorbent assay to characterize dengue.

NEONATAL DENGUE INFECTION: REPORT OF DENGUE FEVER IN A 1-DAY-OLD INFANT

Courtesy: Witaya Petdachai1, Jirapan Sila'on1, Suchitra Nimmannitya2 and Ananda Nisalak3 1Department of Pediatrics, Obstetrics and Gynecology, Prachomklao Hospital, Petchaburi; 2Department of Communicable Diseases, Ministry of Public Health, Bangkok; 3Department of Virology, Armed Forces Research Institute of Medical Sciences, Bangkok, Thailand.

10. NEONATAL PSOAS ABSCESS SIMULATING SEPTIC ARTHRITIS OF HIP JOINT

Psoas abscess is unusual in children and exceptional in neonates. It is a difficult diagnosis, as clinical findings are suggestive of hip septic arthritis or osteomyelitis of the proximal femur. In a neonate with pseudoparalysis, soft tissue swelling and limited motion, septic arthritis and/or osteomyelitis is the first clinical diagnosis to be ruled out. However, a suppurative process in the retroperitoneal tissues should be kept in mind, especially if the joint fluid analysis is normal. In this report, we describe a case of neonatal psoas abscess with emphasis on early imaging to clarify the diagnosis.

Case report: A 26-day-old male infant was referred to our neonatal unit because of unilateral hip septic arthritis and persistence of clinical and laboratory symptoms after parenteral antibiotic therapy. He was born by cesarean section at 35 weeks gestation with a birth weight of 2220 g. Prenatal and natal history was unremarkable; there was no history of premature rupture of membranes or maternal fever. After birth, the infant was hospitalized with a diagnosis of transient tachypnea and discharged on the 6th day of life. During the hospital stay, he received one dose intramuscular vitamin K and intravenous fluids. The femoral triangle was not used as a phlebotomy site. On the 9th postnatal day, several pustular lesions were noted on his body, and local therapy with antibiotics was initiated by his pediatrician. After one week, a flexion posture and swelling and pain on his left groin developed. His laboratory evaluation showed a white blood cell count of 33.0×10^9 /L, with 80% segmented neutrophils, 18% lymphocytes and 2% monocytes, and a C reactive protein (CRP) level of 22 mg/dl. He was hospitalized for evaluation of possible suppurative arthritis, at which time minimal effusion was seen in ultrasonographic examination of the hip; however, an arthrosynthesis was not performed. The patient was started on parenteral vancomycin and amikacin with a diagnosis of hip septic arthritis. One week later, the clinical findings persisted with a white blood cell count of 45×10^9/L and an erythrocyte sedimentation rate of 45 mm/hour. Because of the persisting symptoms, he was referred to our hospital. On admission, the infant was afebrile; swelling on the left groin and medial thigh without local fever, limited range of motion, and pseudoparalysis were noted. The left leg was held in flexion and the infant became irritable when the hip joint was moved. Examination of the right leg and hip was unremarkable. The white blood cell was 36×10^9/L with 72% segmented neutrophils and 28% lymphocytes; hemoglobin was 10.5 g/dl, and CRP level was 34 mg/dl. Radiographs of the left hip and femur were normal, and ultrasonography of the left hip showed minimal fluid collection in the joint. However, analysis of joint fluid revealed no evidence of infection, and -for definitive diagnosis- a magnetic resonance imaging (MRI) was performed. The result showed an abscess formation in the left psoas region with edema of the proximal thigh and gluteal muscles (Fig. 1). Therapy was initiated with nafcillin and ceftriaxone. He underwent open drainage, and 5 ml of green purulent fluid was drained from the abscess cavity in the left psoas muscle. The blood and pus culture subsequently grew *Staphylococcus aureus*, resistant to penicillin and susceptible to methicillin. Ceftriaxone was discontinued,

and the patient improved rapidly. He was discharged from the hospital after three weeks of intravenous antibiotic therapy. At the time of discharge, he had regained full range of motion of the left hip, and ultrasonography and radiography of the left hip and femur were found to be normal.

DISCUSSION: The pathogenetic mechanism for retroperitoneal abscess is different in adults than in children. The non-tuberculous retroperitoneal abscess emphasized secondary spread to the structures from the contagious infectious process in adults. Vertebral bodies, posterior mediastinum, lung, kidney, ureter, gallbladder, pancreas, and large and small bowel are the possible primary sources of infection. However, extension from the adjacent structures is extremely rare, and primary psoas abscesses account for the vast majority of the cases in children. Neonates and children may have an antecedent or incurrent distant cutaneous infection and become bacteremic, seeding the retroperitoneum. This is the possible mechanism in our case, where pustular lesions preceded the clinical findings of psoas abscess. Although the age distribution has not been established for this disease, in a review of psoas abscess in children, the largest clustering of patients was in the 10-17-year-old group, with a range of 18 days to 17 years. Psoas abscess is extremely uncommon in neonates. We found only 15 neonatal cases reported in the English literature. Gestational ages of most of the patients were term or nearterm and there was no gender difference. In a recent review by Yano et al. on psoas abscess in neonates, the organisms isolated in 13 infants were described. Staphylococus aureus was the most frequently isolated organism (11 in 13 neonatal cases). Staphylococcus hominis and *Klebsiella pneumoniae* were also reported as pathogens in two newborn infants. The triad of the psoas abscess in the neonatal period is swelling of the leg or groin, limitation of leg motion and pain. A palpable mass in the inguinal fossa and medial thigh and tenderness in the lower ipsilateral quadrant of the abdomen may be present. Because of the infrequency and nonspecific clinical features, clinical diagnosis is difficult, and treatment is usually delayed. An interval of 1 to 14 days (mean: 3.8 days) between onset of symptoms and diagnosis of abscess is reported in neonatal cases. Since hip septic arthritis or osteomyelitis of the proximal femur may both present with swelling and a guarded hip, patients with a suggestive examination for pyarthrosis of the hip, but with normal joint fluid analysis, should be subjected to further diagnostic interventions, and attention should be drawn to the retroperitoneal tissues and bone. Ultrasonography is useful in demonstrating effusions in the arthritis, and it is also accurate in distinguishing arthritis from psoas abscesses. Computed tomography and MRI are helpful in diagnosis and in demonstrating the extent of the abscess. Appropriate antibiotic administration with open or percutaneous surgical drainage is the recommended method of the treatment. There have been numerous case reports of successful ultrasonography guided percutaneous drainage of psoas abscesses. Antibiotics alone may be successful in treating small abscess. An antibiotic choice should be guided by knowledge of the most frequent causative organisms as well as results of Gram stained smears of material; thus, a neonate suspected of psoas abscess should be given antibiotics for *S. aureus*. Antimicrobial therapy of musculoskeletal infections caused by *S. aureus* or coliform organisms should be continued for approximately three weeks and in some patients for a longer period. In our case, hip septic arthritis was the initial leading diagnosis on the basis of limited hip motion, pain and swelling on the groin and laboratory findings. However, persistence of symptoms after antibiotic therapy and normal hip joint fluid findings swayed our thinking toward psoas abscess, and MRI findings confirmed the diagnosis. This case report emphasizes that psoas abscess may simulate hip septic arthritis in the newborn and should be included in the differential diagnosis. In conclusion, an awareness of this exceptional infection in neonates and timely use of imaging studies will help in prompt diagnosis and treatment, preventing complications caused by a delay.

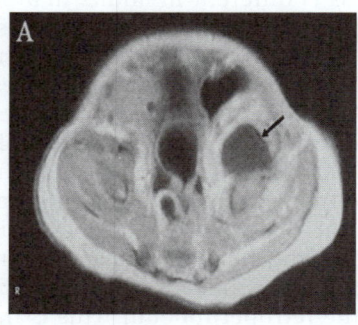

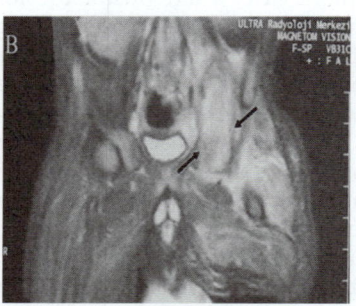

a) Axial T1-weighted contrast enhanced magnetic resonance (MR) image shows a hypointense lesion (14 mm in diameter) in the left psoas muscle (arrow).

b) Coronal T2-weighted MR image demonstrates a hyperintense lesion (32 mm × 16 mm) in the left psoas muscle (arrows) and edema of the surrounding tissues.

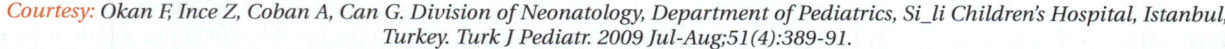

Courtesy: Okan F, Ince Z, Coban A, Can G. Division of Neonatology, Department of Pediatrics, Si_li Children's Hospital, Istanbul, Turkey. Turk J Pediatr. 2009 Jul-Aug;51(4):389-91.

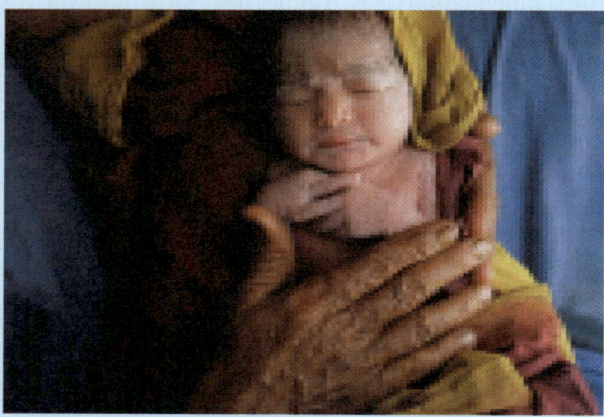

"A baby will make love stronger, days shorter, nights longer, bankroll smaller, home happier, clothes shabbier, the past forgotten, and the future worth living for"-Anonymous

ESSENTIAL NEONATAL PROCEDURES

Section **III**

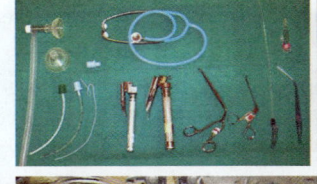
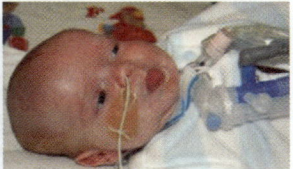
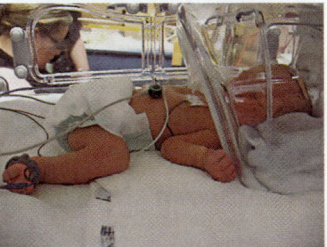
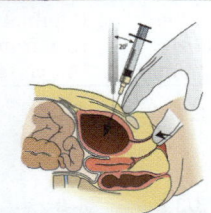
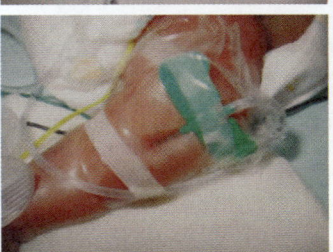
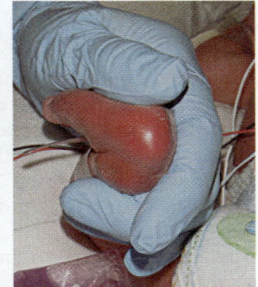
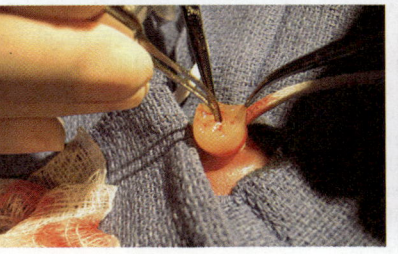
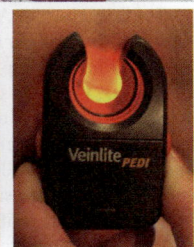

NEONATAL PROCEDURES: UNIVERSAL GUIDELINES

1. Consider alternatives for each procedure and evaluate risk-benefit ratios.

2. Maintain primary focus on the patient, rather than on the procedure being performed. Assess cardiorespiratory and thermoregulatory stability throughout the procedure, and apply interventions when needed. Delegate the responsibility for monitoring and managing the patient to another care provider during the procedure.

3. Assess Pain by the use of neonatal pain scales and control the pain (Oral sucrose (0.2–0.4 mL/kg) in reducing pain of minor procedures and blood drawing, Morphine or fentanyl before beginning potentially painful procedures)

4. Notify parents of the need for invasive procedures in their child's care and discuss the indications for and possible complications of each procedure.

5. Observe universal precautions, including use of gloves, impermeable gowns, barriers, and eye protection to prevent exposure to blood and bodily fluids that may be contaminated with infectious agents.

6. Take a "safety pause" and ascertain that it is the correct patient, the correct procedure and if appropriate, that the procedure is being done on the correct side (e.g. thoracostomy tube, central venous catheter placement).

7. Ensure education and supervision of individuals performing the procedures about the indications, possible complications and their treatment, alternatives, and the techniques to be used. Experienced operators should be available at all times to provide further guidance and needed assistance.

8. Document the date and time, consent obtained, sedation, patient preparation, indications, techniques used, difficulties encountered, unsuccessful attempts, safety pause, complications (if any), and results of any laboratory tests performed.

ENDOTRACHEAL INTUBATION

Indications: 1) Cardiopulmonary resuscitation 2) Respiratory failure 3) Coma/Brainstem dysfunction with absent cough/gag reflexes 4) a route for selective bronchial ventilation 5) When diaphragmatic hernia is suspected 6) When prolonged positive-pressure ventilation is required

Complications: 1) Hypoxemia/Cardiac arrest 2) Displacement to bronchial intubation 3) Laryngeal trauma 4) Esophageal intubation.

ID = Internal Diameter, Adopted from circulation from 1999 : 1927-38, American Heart Association, Inc
Guidelines for tracheal tube size and depth of insertion

Tube Size (mm ID)	Depth of insertion from Upper Lip (cm)	Weight (g)	Gestation (wk)
2.5	6.5–7	< 1,000	<28
3	7–8	1,000–2,000	28–34
3/3.5	8–9	2,000–3,000	34–38
3.5/4.0	≥9	>3,000	> 38

Equipment & Supplies: 1) Functioning laryngoscope with an extra set of batteries and extra bulb 2) Miller blade size 1 for full-term infant, Miller blade size 0 for preterm infant. Straight rather than curved blades are preferred for optimal visualization 3) Endotracheal tubes with internal diameters of 2.5, 3.0, 3.5, and 4.0 mm 4) Humidified oxygen/air source, blender, and analyzer 5) Oxygen tubing 6) Resuscitation bag and mask 7) Suctioning device, with 10-French (Fr) suction catheters 8) Cardiorespiratory monitor 9) Pulse oximetry oxygen saturation monitor 10) Stethoscope 11) Gloves 12) Scissors 13) Sterile stylet 14) Adhesive tape: Two 8- to 10-cm lengths of wide tape, with half the length split and one 10- to 15-cm length unsplit 15) Magill forceps (optional for nasotracheal intubation)

Procedure: 1) Empty stomach : Provide 100% oxygen via bag and mask ventilation 2) Ensure that all equipment should be ready, available and in good working condition 3) Connect the patient to pulse oximeter and ECG monitor; Follow heart rate and oxygenation 4) Place the infant supine in sniffing position. Slightly extend neck using a neck roll. Clear oropharynx with gentle suctioning 5) Turn on the laryngoscope light, and hold the laryngoscope in left hand with thumb and first three fingers, with the blade directed toward patient; place laryngoscope blade in right corner of the mouth 6) Displace tongue by directing the laryngoscope the laryngoscope to the left of midline 7) Hold handle at 45⁰ 8) Elevate the mandible by lifting the blade along the axis of the laryngoscope handle to expose the posterior pharyngeal wall. Avoid any pressure on the dentoalveolar ridge 9) Using a straight blade lift the epiglottis exposing the vocal cords; Suction as necessary. Have an assistant apply gentle pressure at the suprasternal notch to open the larynx and to feel the tube pass. 10) Hold tube in right hand with concave curve anterior, and pass it down the right side of the mouth, outside the blade, while maintaining direct visualization. 11) Once the vocal cords and trachea are visualized, insert the endotracheal tube through vocal cords, approximately 2 cm into trachea or until the tip is felt passing the suprasternal notch by the assistant. 12) Confirm endotracheal tube position within the trachea; If the endotracheal tube is correctly placed in the midtracheal region, there should be *Pedi-Cap response to exhaled CO_2 by a reversible color change, purple to yellow *Equal bilateral breath sounds *Slight rise of the chest with each ventilation *No air heard entering stomach *No gastric distention. 13) Attach appropriate mechanical ventilatory device. Adjust required F_iO_2. 14) Secure the tube to the infant's face. Obtain chest radiograph with head in neutral position, and note the lip-to-tip distance and direction of bevel Cut off excess tube length to leave 4 cm from the infant's lips and reattach adapter firmly. 15) Reconfirm tube marking at lip regularly, to avoid unnoticed advancement of the tube into the airway. Retape tube as necessary to maintain stability.

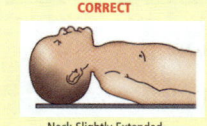

CORRECT

Neck Slightly Extended

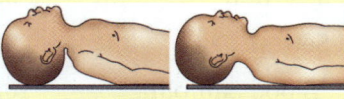

INCORRECT

Neck Hyperextended   Neck Underextended

Appropriate sniff position for intubation. Note that the neck is not hyperextended; the roll provides stabilizing support.

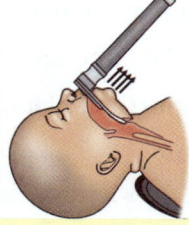

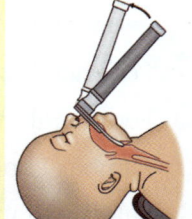

CORRECT   INCORRECT

A. *Illustration of the axes (oral, pharyngeal and tracheal);*
B. *Alignment of these axes with correct positioning;*
C. *Viewing the glottic fold with a straight blade*

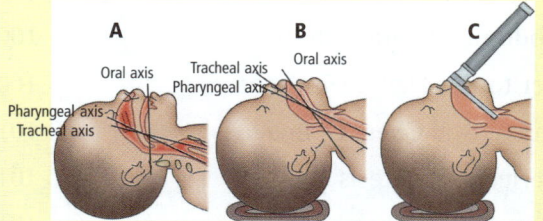

A   B   C

Oral axis   Tracheal axis   Oral axis
Pharyngeal axis   Pharyngeal axis
Tracheal axis

With the laryngoscope at the proper depth, tilt the blade with the tongue as the fulcrum; at the same time, pull on the laryngoscope handle to move the tongue without extending the infant's neck. Use more traction than leverage.

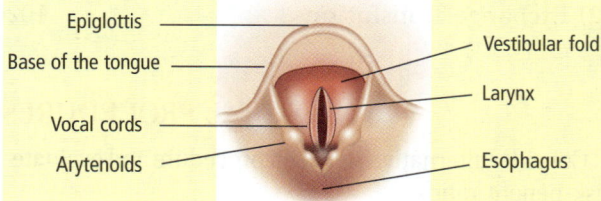

Epiglottis
Base of the tongue
Vocal cords
Arytenoids

Vestibular fold
Larynx
Esophagus

View of the glottic area via direct laryngoscopy

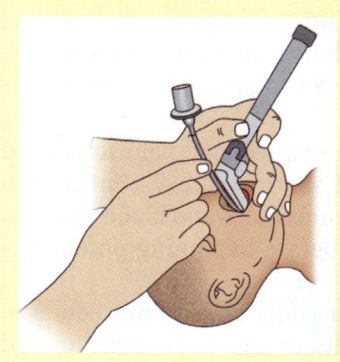

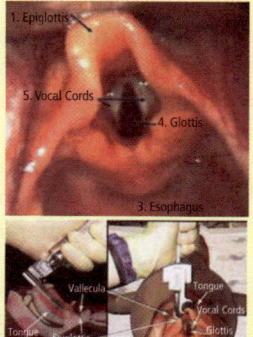

1. Epiglottis
5. Vocal Cords
4. Glottis
3. Esophagus
Vallecula   Tongue
Vocal Cords
Tongue   Glottis
Epiglottis   Esophagus

Visualize the glottis and pass the endotracheal tube into the oropharynx. Keep the tube outside the curve of the laryngoscope blade for better mobility.

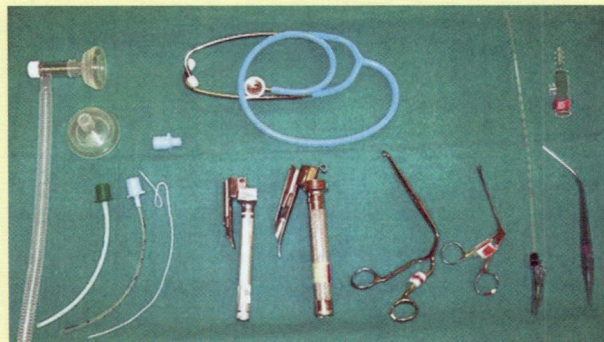

Standard equipment should be available in pre-prepared intubation boxes on delivery suite. One should familiarize him/herself with these. They contain: *2 Laryngoscopes – a small (preterm) blade (size 0) and a larger (term) blade (size 1). Check that the bulb is working. *Endotracheal tubes – blue 'oral' portex tubes and/or green vygon 'nasal' tubes. *Flexible introducer, tape and tinc benz for securing. *For nasal intubation you will also need Magill forceps, lubricant and a 'white' and 'blue' connector.

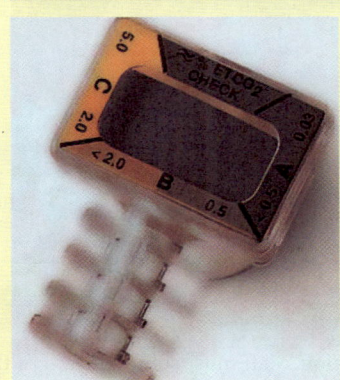

Features of Nellcor Pedi Cap CO_2 Detector:
• Reliable carbon dioxide detectors help verify endotracheal tube placement.
• Responds quickly to exhaled CO_2 with a simple color change from purple to yellow.
• Breath-to-breath response.
• Constant visual feedback for up to 2 hours.
• Single patient use to verify endotracheal tube placement.

Product Specifications
• Recommended patient size: Weight 1kg to 15kg.
• Internal volume (dead space): 3cc.
• Resistance to flow: 2.5 cm H_2O +/- 0.5 cm @ 10L/min flow.
• Connector ports: Patient end 18mm OD/15mm ID, Circuit end 15mm OD/5mm ID.
• Usage time: Up to 2 hours.

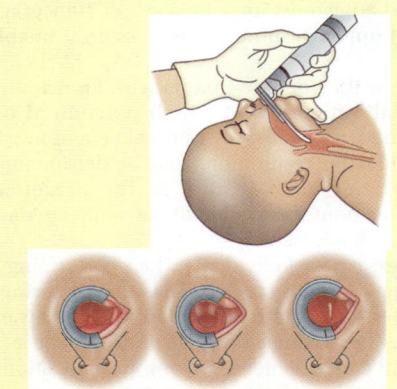

Laryngoscopy and the stages of endotracheal intubation.
a. Visualization of the uvula and oropharynx
b. The epiglottis is seen with the esophagus beyond it
c. The cords are seen

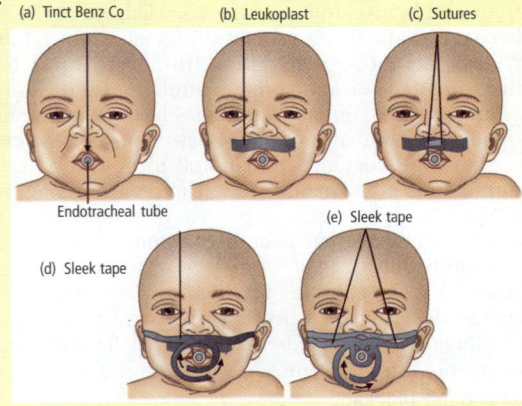

(a) Tinct Benz Co (b) Leukoplast (c) Sutures
Endotracheal tube (e) Sleek tape
(d) Sleek tape

A method of fixing the ET tube for long-term ventilation: tincture of benzoin compound is first applied to the infant's upper lip and, when this has dried, plaster tape is laid on the lip. Thin strips of tape are then wound around the ET tube and then on to the plaster.

After intubation in Newborn infants, the position of the endotracheal tube in the trachea must be checked to ensure a minimum number of complications such as right main bronchus intubation (which can lead to atelectasis and hypoxia) and high placement (accidental extubation). Methods used to determine accurate positioning within the trachea have included digital palpation, fibre optics, ultrasound, and, more recently, a metal ring embedded in the endotracheal tube. After intubation in Newborn infants, the placement of the endotracheal tube in the trachea must be checked by a chest radiograph.*It is recommended that, for accurate placement within the trachea, the tip of the endotracheal tube should be placed at the level of the body of the first thoracic vertebra; this could be used as the sole reference point on chest radiographs obtained in the Neonatal period.*

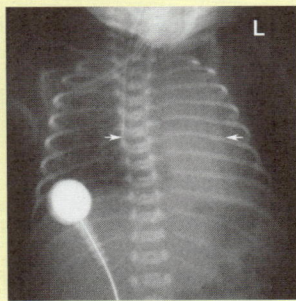

ET tube placement, should be halfway between the thoracic inlet and the carina. The endotracheal tube tip is in the right main bronchus. A hint of opacity in the RUL suggests that it may be partly within the bronchus intermedius. There is atelectasis of the left lung. There are several skin folds over the left lung *About 10% of ETT are initially placed in the right main stem bronchus *With time, the left lung becomes atelectic *If on ventilator, the right lung may be hyperinflated *May lead to pneumothorax or tension pneumothorax

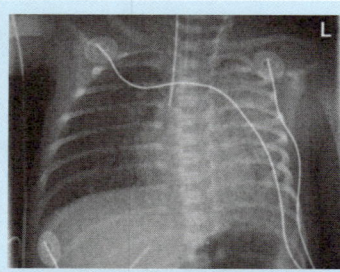
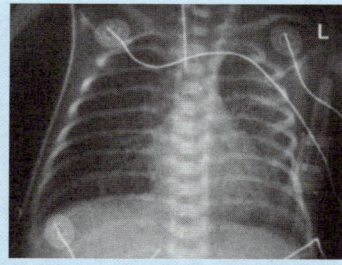

These two images on the same baby are taken 15 minutes apart. This image shows the tip of the ETT favouring the RMB to the detriment of the left lung. With the ETT tube withdrawn a CXR 15 minutes later shows considerable improvement of the aeration of the left lung.

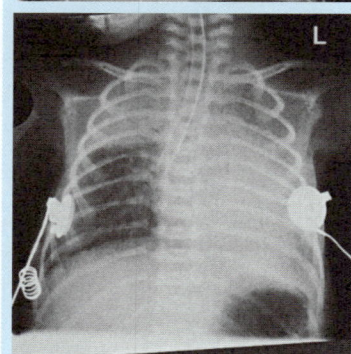

The endotracheal tube (ETT) tip is in the bronchus intermedius. When the tip is in the bronchus intermedius, RUL will also become atelectatic along with all of left lung

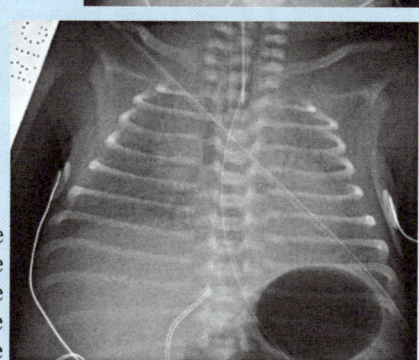

This baby has an ET tube malpositioned in the esophagus. Note the baby's trachea has deviated to the right and is positioned alongside the ET tube

Rapid Sequence Intubation (RSI) in the Neonate

Despite common side effects of awake intubation include oxygen desaturations and bradycardia, and the knowledge that the act of endotracheal intubation is a painful procedure for adults, children, and neonates, many practitioners do not feel comfortable with premedication prior to intubation or the use of RSI procedures. Rapid sequence intubation in the neonate has shown to reduce the number of intubation attempts and decrease the amount of time needed for neonatal intubation. Rapid sequence intubation in the neonate is safe and the humane way of performing this common neonatal procedure. No specific study had evaluated the best sequence for medication administration for neonatal intubation.

The following categories of medications are available: *Anticholinergic agents* to help prevent bradycardia, *induction agents* including opioid agents, benzodiazepines for relaxation, *general anesthetics* to reduce pain, and *paralyzing agents* to allow for neuromuscular blockade.

A suggested sequence of medications *that may prove effective in the neonate for elective or semielective intubation.*

Atropine should be given IV push first, in a dosage of 10-30 mcg/ kg, minimum dose of 10 mcg. Because of atropine administration, an increase heart rate will be seen by decreasing the effects of the parasympathetic system on the infant, while the sympathetic system effects will be increased. In addition, bronchial smooth muscle will be relaxed. After atropine, fentanyl, an opioid, should be administered at 2 to 3 mcg/kg per dose. This can be given IV push because a neuromuscular blockade will be given immediately following and this will counteract chest wall rigidity. The third medication in the sequence will be vecuronium at a dose of 0.1 mg/kg per dose IV push. Most infants will be adequately sedated and paralyzed with this regimen. If the infant remains awake and moving, additional doses of fentanyl and vecuronium can be given as needed.

For infants whose IV access cannot be obtained, a combination of intramuscular (IM) medications can be given. Intramuscular atropine given first at a dose of 10 mcg/kg per dose, minimum dose 10 mcg per dose should be given, fentanyl 2 to 3 mcg/kg per dose IM or morphine 0.1 to 0.2 mg/kg per dose should be given second followed by succinylcholine, 2.5 to 4 mg/kg per dose IM. Atropine should be given with succinylcholine to help prevent the side effect of bradycardia. No studies are available evaluating the use of IM medications for RSI. When giving RSI, all personnel must be ready to bag/mask ventilate the infant or perform immediate intubation. Staff must communicate as the medications are given and be prepared to support the infant. Naloxone, an opioid antagonist, may be given at 10mcg/kg per dose for reversal of opioid respiratory depression if unable to secure an airway.

Contraindications to RSI include infants with known airway anomalies or facial anomalies in which placement of an endotracheal tube may be difficult or impossible and in which succession of spontaneous respirations may be detrimental. In addition, RSI may not be indicated in the presence of inexperienced staff without the availability of staff experienced in intubation to assist if necessary.

Education is necessary for individuals when performing RSI. The individuals preparing the medications, administering the medications, and performing the intubation must be aware of the side effects and they must know proper dosage of the medications. Comfort can be achieved with proper education and experience.

Precautions:

1. Fentanyl and remifentanil should be given slow intravenous (IV) push to help decrease the risk of chest wall rigidity.

2. Atropine in doses <10 mcg can cause paradoxical bradycardia.

3. Midazolam (0.05-0.1 mg/kg IV, 0.2 mg/kg Intranasal) is a benzodiazepine that allows for sedation and amnesia prior to an invasive procedure. It is frequently used in combination with other medications. Infants who received midazolam had longer hospital stays and more adverse effects including neurologic events as demonstrated by death, grades III-IV intraventricular hemorrhage, and periventricular leukomalacia.

4. The use of general anesthetics has been limited in neonates secondary to insufficient trials evaluating the numerous medications.

5. Succinylcholine should not be administered in patients who have a serum potassium level greater than 5.5 mEq/L because of the increased risk of hyperkalemia with this medication. When paralytics are used, the most commonly seen medications include succinylcholine, pancuronium, and vecuronium. When used, paralytics for premedication must be combined with some form of sedation and pain management.

Abstracted from : Rapid Sequence Intubation in the Neonate
Lottie T. Bottor, MSN, RNC,CRNP, NNP-BC
Advances in Neonatal Care • Vol. 9, No. 3 • pp. 111-117

Intubation Guidelines for Neonates

• Safe, high quality Neonatal care and a dedication to resident education should be the foundation for Neonatal care at any Medical College/University. • Pediatric residents, by the end of their residency training, will be proficient at neonatal airway management including intubation, bag-valve mask ventilation and oral airway placement. • Neonatal care is meant to be delivered as a team. • These guidelines are flexible on a case-by-case basis

1. Successful Neonatal intubation is defined as intubation within 2 attempts. All care providers should strive to achieve this goal.
2. An intubation attempt is defined as placing the laryngoscope blade in the patient's mouth unless the blade is rapidly removed to suction, change ETT, etc.
3. Intubation attempts should not compromise patient stability. Stability is defined as a heart rate > 100 bpm and an oxygen saturation > 90%. Any team member can declare that the Neonate is unstable.
4. If more than one intubation attempt is required, the same person should attempt again after briefly discussing with the resuscitation leader their strategy for performing a successful intubation on the next attempt. (see teaching tips below)
5. In selected cases, Neonates may be unstable or are at risk for adverse outcomes if multiple tries at intubation are attempted. These cases include:
   a. Extremely Preterm Neonates < 26 weeks gestation
   b. Unstable Neonates (Unable to establish oxygenation with PPV, Neonate requiring CPR)
   c. Certain congenital anomalies
      i. Congenital Diaphragmatic Hernia
      ii. Known Airway Obstruction
      iii. Micrognathia
      iv. Hydrops
   In these cases, an experienced care provider should perform the intubation.
6. An experienced care provider is defined as the provider who has had the most experience and success with Neonatal intubation in the past. In general, this will be the NNP, Neonatal fellow or Neonatal attending. However, this may also be the senior resident in certain select cases. (e.g..: unexpected decompensation in a term Neonate in which the neonatal attending, fellow, or NNP is not present)
7. If the Neonate is unstable and an experienced care provider is unable to successfully intubate the patient, anesthesia should be stat paged to attempt intubation.

Teaching tips
   • Have most senior care provider visualize airway/vocal cords and have resident place ETT.
   • Perform intubation on stable patients in the NICU (ROP surgery, elective reintubations, etc.)

Methods of confirming placement of the endotracheal tube; esophageal and endobronchial intubation—Complications.

When the endotracheal tube is placed correctly it lies below the vocal cords and above the carina. Malplacement may occur in the: *Bronchus (endobronchial intubation) *The right main bronchus more commonly becomes intubated. It may be recognized by: *Falling O_2 saturation *Higher airway pressures *Asymmetric chest movement ;Withdraw the tube until ventilation occurs in both lungs *Esophagus (Esophageal intubation)-Usually can be recognized but failure to do so has major morbidity and mortality complications!

Methods of confirming placement
*Clinical *View the tube passing between the cords *Auscultate for breath sounds (usually both axillae and epigastrium - characteristic gurgling sound of malplacement) *Look for bilateral chest movements *Feel of the bag and its rapid filling during expiration *Cyanosis (5g of reduced Hb per 100ml of blood)

*Objective Capnography—Detection of exhaled CO_2

False negatives Failure of equipment, kinked tube , Disconnectoin, Apnea, Dilution by high fresh gas flows, Low BP, Pulmonary embolus.

False Positives CO_2 from stomach (air in stomach, carbonated drinks), ET tube above cords in pharynx, Syringe attached to ET tube, If no resistance to aspiration, ET placement is more likely as esophagus will collapse ,More difficult if tube becomes obstructed.

TRACHEOSTOMY IN NEONATES & INFANTS

The term tracheostomy is derived from the Greek "to furnish with an opening." In contrast, a tracheotomy is derived from the Greek meaning, "to cut." A tracheotomy refers to the actual surgical procedure and the act of cutting the trachea, while a tracheostomy refers to the actual hole or the tube placed in it.

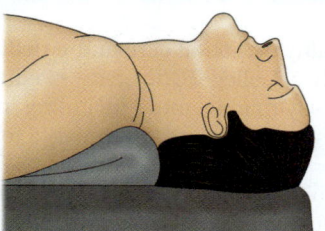

Indications: A tracheotomy (no tubes) may be performed on the rare occasion for bronchoscopic access to a foreign body if the usual route is not available to the rigid ventilating bronchoscope.

*Airway Problems that may Require a Tracheostomy: Subglottic Stenosis,Subglottic Web, Tracheomalacia, Vocal Cord Paralysis (VCP), Congenital abnormalities of the airway, Large tongue or small jaw that blocks airway, Treacher Collins and Pierre Robin Syndromes, Severe neck or mouth injuries, Tumors, such as Cystic Hygroma, Obstructive sleep apnea Foreign body obstruction, Airway burns from inhalation of corrosive material, smoke or steam

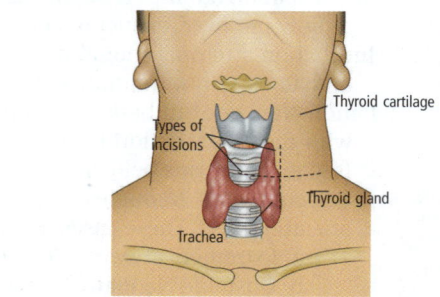

*Lung Problems that may Require a Tracheostomy: Need for prolonged respiratory support, such as Bronchopulmonary Dysplasia (BPD), Chronic pulmonary disease to reduce anatomic dead space, Chest wall injury, Diaphragm dysfunction.

*Other Reasons for a Tracheostomy: Neuromuscular diseases paralyzing or weakening chest muscles and diaphragm, Aspiration related to muscle or sensory problems in the throat ,Fracture of cervical vertebrae with spinal cord injury, Long-term unconsciousness or coma, Disorders of respiratory control such as Congenital Central Hypoventilation or Central Apnea, Facial surgery and facial burns, Anaphylaxis (severe allergic reaction)

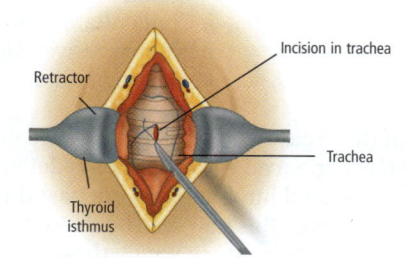

Equipment: **Tracheostomy Supplies:** ·Tracheostomy tubes ·Tracheostomy tube (one size smaller) ·Trach tube ties ·Dressing supplies, gauze ·Hydrogen peroxide, sterile water, normal saline ·Water soluble lubricant such as · Surgilube or KY Jelly ·Blunt-end bandage scissors ·Tweezers or hemostats ·Sterile Q-tips ·Trach care kits and/or pipe cleaners (double-cannula trach tubes) ·Luer-Lok tip syringes for cuffed trach tubes

Suction Equipment: ·Stationary electric suction machine ·Portable battery-powered suction machine ·Suction connecting tubing ·Suction catheters ·Suction Catheter kits ·Normal saline solution ·Sterile jars with screw tops (sterile specimen containers or sterilized baby food jars work well) ·Saline ampules ("bullets") ·Bulb syringe ·DeLee suction trap or syringe with catheter ·Hand-powered Suction Devices A simple yet efficient suction unit for first responders, and a reliable backup for emergency healthcare providers. ·YanKauer Suction Handle ·Sims Connector

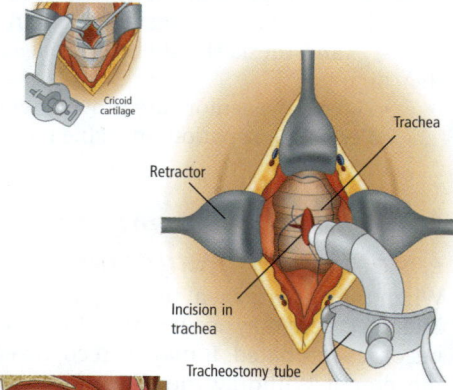

Humidification System: ·Air compressor ·Nebulizer bottles ·Tracheostomy mask·Aerosol tubing ·Water trap

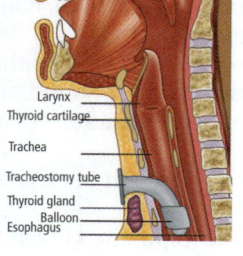

Procedure: Before performing a tracheostomy the site of obstruction should be determined to be above the site of the tracheostomy. Patients with large or short necks may be difficult to operate upon ·Bleeding disorders or an enlarged thyroid gland should be evaluated ·The procedure is usually done under general anesthesia in the operating room. However, if the patient is sedated on a ventilator, it may be done under local anesthetic, even at the patient's bedside ·Optimal positioning can be achieved with the help of a shoulder pad and a chin strap which brings the trachea closest to the neck skin. The skin is marked and a low vertical incision is made. The brachio-cephalic trunk can come up high in an infant and attention is called for. A low tracheostomy allows room for reconstructive procedures later on. A pad of subcutaneous fat is then excised. This shortens the tracheostomy tract and allows immediate exposure of the strap muscles. Dissecting bipolar diathermy forceps allow a bloodless dissection and the isthmus of the thyroid may be divided by the bipolar forceps. Spring retractors allows good exposure with the least instruments in the small and restricted field. The trachea is incised with a short vertical incision with stay sutures on both sides. The tube is inserted and the flanges are secured to the skin with sutures and round the neck with linen tapes using the Red Cross Memorial tying technique. The tube from the breathing machine or oxygen tube is connected to the tracheostomy tube. Sutures are used to close the skin incision and a cloth tape is tied around the neck to secure the tube The stay suture on each side of the tracheal incision is taped to the chest for emergency purposes. The sutures can be used to lift the trachea for tube replacement if it should accidentally fall out. The Red Cross Memorial technique of tying is simple to performed and the design is based on having a double loop round the neck, the tension of which is controlled by a single knot. At the completion of tying, the loop should not admit more than the little finger. The first tube change is then scheduled for 1 week.

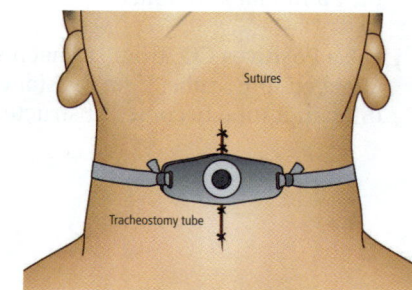

The after care in the first week : A light weight ventilatory circuit should be used and steadying the flanges while connecting or disconnecting is important. A short neonatal tracheostomy tube can easily have its tip dislodged or half dislodged in the still unestablished tracheocutaneous tract. This tract is usually well formed at 72 hours. It is, nonetheless, not difficult to create a false tract in an infant. Adequate humidification is mandatory to prevent crusting in small tubes and gentle suction, on a need to do basis, minimizes trauma to the tracheal mucosa. The linen tapes, once soiled with saliva and allowed to dry, become sharp blades which can cut into the neck skin. These wounds together with salivary soiling are the main causes of skin irritation in the neck. This can be minimized by a thin piece of duoderm round the neck or the change of tapes every two days. Tape changes are difficult and are done always in our institution by two members of staff, one steadying the tracheostomy tube firmly while the other replaces the tapes. The wound is cleaned and dressed daily after the first 48 hours. It is not uncommon to have the lower rim of the tracheostomy flange eroding the manubrial skin over the chest. This can be prevented by a small piece of duoderm in between.

Care after the first week: After the first tube change, the environment changes and humidification may become less plentiful. Crusting is then minimized or prevented by tube change daily or on alternate days. If performed after proper training, this is done with great ease and does not impart any trauma to the infant as the tube is simply replaced by sliding it through a preformed tunnel. This is excellent training for the nursing staff in the neonatal unit who shortly become experts in replacing tubes. This is also a time when the parents are trained. The parents are required to acquire basic resuscitation skills over a period of 6 weeks, in addition, to prepare for home care. Infants with chubby chins may occasionally obstruct the tracheostomy opening. Protector caps are available with side ventilation holes to prevent complete obstruction if this should occur.

Complications:

1. Tracheostomies can become contaminated and improper care can lead to infection of the skin, trachea or lungs

2. Bleeding may occur from injury to a high innominate artery, jugular veins or thyroid gland. Severe bleeding may occur if the tracheostomy tube erodes through the anterior wall of the trachea into the arteries that lie there or into the thyroid gland. This may be a problem particularly in children where the tracheas are smaller. The bleeding may be life threatening and needs emergency surgery to control the bleeding

3. Prolonged use of a tracheostomy tube may cause stenosis (narrowing) of the trachea from scarring or tracheomalacia (floppiness of the trachea). These may cause progressive obstruction of the trachea requiring surgery to remove the scarred or weakened portion of the trachea

4. Pneumothorax (air between the lung and chest wall) may occur following tracheostomy. This occurs more frequently in children

5. Obstruction of the tube can occur from a blood clot or mucous plug and if the end of the tube presses against the back wall of the trachea

6. The tube may come out. This is a very serious complication since the patient may not be able to breath

7. Tracheoesophageal fistula (connection between the trachea and the esophagus) can occur if the tube erodes through the back of the trachea and into the esophagus. Surgery is necessary to separate the trachea and esophagus

8. Dysphagia (difficulty in swallowing) may occur from pressure of the tube on the back of the trachea

9. Poor laryngeal function may result from prolonged use of a tracheostomy

10. The most common complication is a tracheogranuloma. Some otolaryngologists have argued that since tracheogranulomas are so common they should not even be considered a complication. These occur most frequently just above the tracheal stoma. They can be pedunculated or can occur as an epithelealized tract that grows over the tracheostomy tube. They are believed to be caused by chronic low-grade inflammation resulting from multiple causes including secretions pooling just above the cannula as it enters the trachea, foreign body reaction to the cannula, or frictional trauma from the tube. Treatment depends on the size. Those that are not

obstructive can be watched. Larger ones should be removed, since they obstruct the stoma during tube changes. Removal can be done through a bronchoscope or through the stoma. More distal granulomas can cause tube obstruction. A poorly positioned tube should be repositioned away from the site of granulation. Changing the tube length and material may also be helpful. Longer tubes can be inserted past the granulation, but this risks creating more granulation distally. Longer tubes are also limited by the carina.

Teaching families to provide tracheostomy care in the home: Goals and objectives

One of the primary goals of an education program is to promote positive adaptation to the tracheostomy. Nurses can foster positive interactions and participation with the infant. The family must develop the skills needed to competently and independently provide tracheostomy care. Specifically parents need to be able to:

- Articulate the reason for tracheostomy tube placement.
- Describe airway anatomy, tube location, and accompanying airway changes.
- Recognize the signs of breathing difficulty and how to respond to these problems.
- Demonstrate how to respond to an emergency.
- Identify postdischarge resources for questions and ongoing support in the community.

Home care : This is the penultimate challenge of tracheostomy care and it is true that this may not always be possible for different reasons. If deemed appropriate, in well trained parents or caretakers, the home comers are well equipped with oxygen, suction, humidifiers, humovents, a collection of spare tubes and other accessories. The atmosphere at home gets even drier which may lead to crusting and frequent tracheitis. It is mandatory that a tube change is done daily. For the first weeks, the parents will bring their child to the neonatal unit and perform the tube change with the tracheostomy nurse around. Most adapt very quickly to the new lifestyle and proceed on their own at home. Most children with residual laryngeal phonatory function would achieve a voice without help. One way speaking valves are available to aid phonation if need be. 24 hours access to a duty tracheostomy nurse is available for advice if need be. She in turn is supported by the duty otolaryngologist.

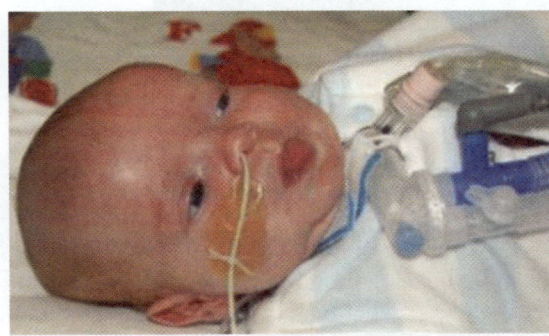

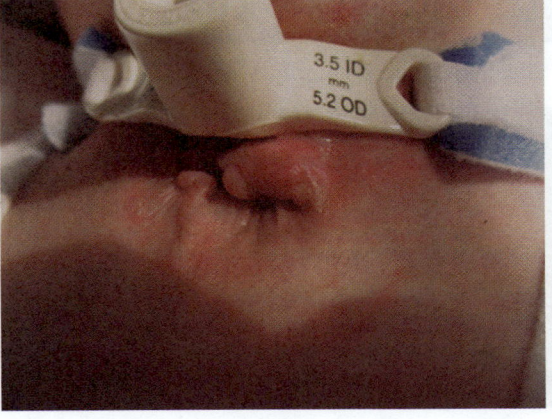

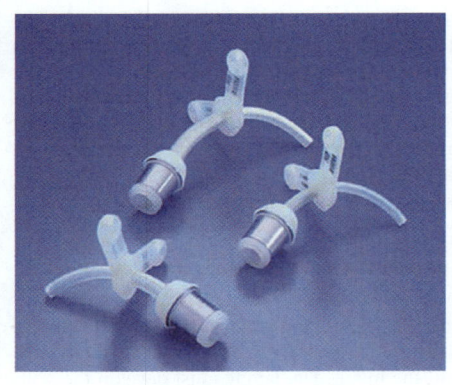

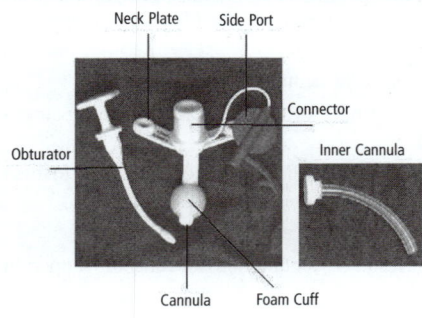

Neck Plate   Side Port

Obturator   Connector

Inner Cannula

Cannula   Foam Cuff

Bivona Cuffless Neonatal Tubes		
Inner Diameter	Outer Diameter	Length
2.5 mm	4.0 mm	30 mm
3.0 mm	4.7 mm	32 mm
3.5 mm	5.3 mm	34 mm
4.0 mm	6.0 mm	36 mm

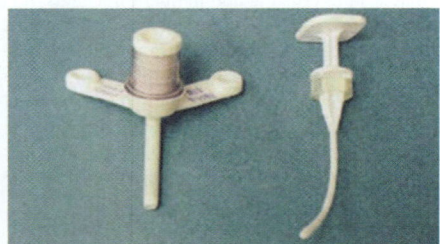

Shiley Neonatal Cuffless Tracheostomy Tubes		
(Shiley Neo)		
Inner Diameter	Outer Diameter	Length
3.0 mm	4.5 mm	30 mm
3.5 mm	5.2 mm	32 mm
4.0 mm	5.9 mm	34 mm
4.5 mm	6.5 mm	36 mm

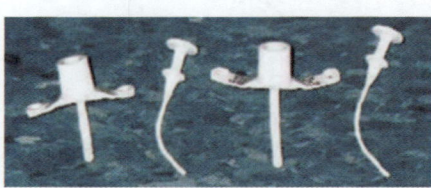

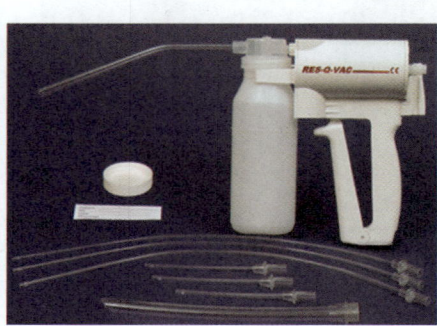

Suctioning a tracheostomy: Procedure

* Explain procedure in a way appropriate for child's age and understanding.

* Wash hands.

* Set up equipment and connect suction catheter to machine tubing.

* Pour normal saline into cup.

* Put on gloves (optional).

* Turn on suction machine (suction machine pressure for small children 50-100mm Hg, for older children/adults 100-120mm Hg)

* Place tip of catheter into saline cup to moisten and test to see that suction is working.

* Instill sterile normal saline with plastic squeeze ampule into the trach tube if needed for thick or dry secretions. Excessive use of saline is not recommended. Use saline only if the mucus is very thick, hard to cough up or difficult to suction. Saline may also be instilled via a syringe or eye dropper, which is less expensive than single dose units. Recommended amount per instillation is approximately 1cc.

* Gently insert catheter into the trach tube without applying suction. (Suction only length of trach tube - premeasured suctioning. Deeper insertion may be needed if the child has an ineffective cough.)

* Put thumb over opening in catheter to create suction and use a circular motion (twirl catheter between thumb and index finger) while withdrawing the catheter so that the mucus is removed well from all areas. Avoid suctioning longer than 10 seconds because of oxygen loss. Note: Some research has shown that by applying suction both going in and then out of the tube takes less time and therefore results there is less hypoxia. Also, there are now holes on all sides of the suction catheters, so twirling is not necessary.

* Draw saline from cup through catheter to clear catheter.

* For trach tubes with cuffs, it may be necessary to deflate the cuff periodically for suctioning to prevent pooling of secretions above trach cuff.

* Let child rest and breathe, then repeat suction if needed until clear (allow at least 30 seconds between suctioning).

* Oxygenate as ordered (extra oxygen may be given before and after suction to prevent hypoxia).

* Some children need extra breaths with an Ambu bag (approximately 3 - 5 breaths). Purposes of bagging: hyperoxygenation, hyperinflation, and hyperventilation of the lungs. However, this is usually not needed for stable children with no additional respiratory problems.

Suctioning Tracheostomy Tube

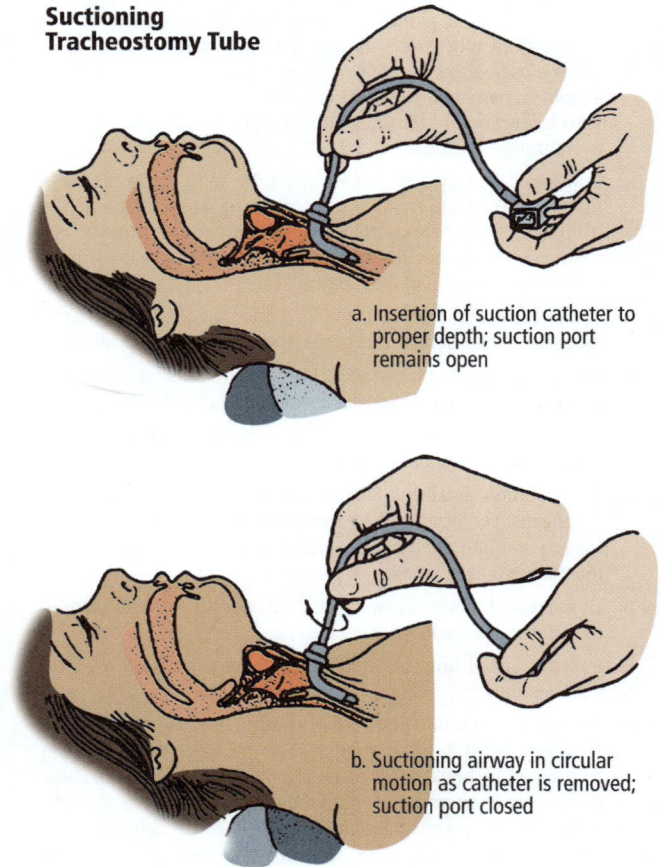

a. Insertion of suction catheter to proper depth; suction port remains open

b. Suctioning airway in circular motion as catheter is removed; suction port closed

Hand-operated suction systems such as the RES-Q-VAC provides suction anywhere and anytime and is totally portable. Using chest P.T., postural drainage and percussion as needed to maximize airway clearance.

Suctioning: Tracheal suctioning is necessary to remove mucus, maintain a patent airway, and avoid tracheostomy tube blockages. Indications for suctioning include:* Audible or visual signs of secretions in the tube * Signs of respiratory distress * Suspicion of blocked or partially blocked tube * Inability by the child to clear the tube by coughing out the secretions * Vomiting * Changes in ventilation pressures (in ventilated children) * Request by the child for suction (older children) * Tracheal suctioning should be carried out regularly for patients with a tracheostomy. However the frequency varies between patients and is based on individual assessment. * Tracheal damage may be caused by suctioning. This can be minimized by using the appropriate sized suction catheter and only suctioning within the tracheostomy tube.

Recommended suction catheter sizes

Tracheostomy tube size (in mm)	3.0mm	3.5mm	4.0mm	4.5mm	5.0mm	6.0mm	7.0mm
Recommended suction catheter size (Fr)	7	8	8	10	10	10-12	12

* The suction depth is determined by the length of the individual tracheostomy tube. * The depth of insertion of the suction catheter needs to be determined prior to suctioning to avoid trauma. *Using a spare tracheostomy tube of the same size and a measuring tape: measure the distance from the length of the tracheostomy tube connector to the end of the tracheostomy tube. record the suction depth on the tape measure and the patients observations chart. attach the tape measure to the cot/bedside/ suction machine for future use. *The pressure setting for tracheal suctioning is 80-120mmHg (10-16kpa) to avoid tracheal damage. **The suction pressure setting should not exceed 120mmHg/16kpa.**

* It is recommended that the episode of suctioning (including passing the catheter and suctioning the tracheostomy tube) is completed within 5-10 seconds. * Suction catheters can be used for a 24hour period and then changed unless indicated earlier. * **Routine** use of 0.9% sodium chloride is not recommended although there is anecdotal evidence that in some cases it may thin secretions. In situations where this may be of benefit e.g., thick secretions 0.2–0.5ml of 0.9% sodium chloride can be used·

Tracheostomy tube tie changes: * There is a potential risk for tracheostomy tube dislodgment when attending to tie changes, therefore a minimum of two people who are competent in tracheostomy care are required to undertake tracheostomy tie changes. * During the tracheostomy tie change one person is to maintain the airway by securing the tracheostomy tube in place and not removing the hand until the new tracheostomy ties are insitu. The other person is to change the ties and attend to stoma care. *Tracheostomy tie changes are performed daily in conjunction with stoma care, or as required if they become wet or soiled to maintain skin integrity. If the ties become loose it is a priority to resecure immediately.

Humidification: A tracheostomy bypasses the upper airway and therefore prevents normal humidification and filtration of inhaled air. Therefore, unless air inhaled via the tracheostomy tube is humidified, the epithelium of the trachea and bronchi will become dry which increases the potential for blockage. Tracheal humidification can be provided by a heated humidifier or Heat and Moisture Exchanger (HME) or a Tracheostomy bib. **Heated humidification:** delivers gas at body temperature saturated with water which prevents the thickening of secretions. The temperature is set at 37°C delivering a temperature ranging from 36.5°C - 37.5°C at the tracheostomy site. Heated humidification for tracheostomy patients should be delivered via a 8400 humidifier as per oxygen policy. Indications for the use of heated humidification include: *Oxygen delivery via tracheostomy mask *Mechanical Ventilation *Respiratory infection with increased secretions *Management of thick secretions Heat Moisture Exchanger (HME): contains a hygroscopic paper surface that absorbs the moisture in expired air. Upon inspiration the air passes over the hygroscopic paper surface and moistens and warms the air that passes into the airway. *HME is recommended for all tracheostomy tubes. *HME fits directly onto the tracheostomy tube. *HME are changed daily or as needed if the filter appears to be excessively moist or blocked. *For small infants <10kg HME filters may not be suitable consult Respiratory team to assess patient's suitability. *Do not wet the HME filter prior to use. **Tracheostomy Bibs:** are a specialised foam that traps the moisture in expired air. Upon inspiration the foam moistens and warms the air that passes into the airway.

Supervision and monitoring: In determining the level of supervision and monitoring, it is recommended each patient with a tracheostomy is assessed on an individual basis by the treating medical/surgical and nursing team[4] taking into consideration the following factors: *Age *Clinical state *Nature of the airway problem *Ability to breathe and maintain their airway in the event of accidential decannulation *Ventilation requirements

It is recommended decisions regarding required level of supervision and required clinical observations/monitoring are documented clearly in the patient's medical record by the treating team.

Monitoring **may** include: *Heart rate +/- continuous cardiac monitoring *Respiratory rate *Pulse oximetry *Oxygen requirements *Work of breathing *Temperature *Blood pressure *Behaviour - alert, irritable, lethargic.

Stoma care: *Care of the stoma is commenced in the immediate post-operative period, and is ongoing.

*Daily cleaning of the stoma is recommended using 0.9% sterile saline solution. After the cleaning, ensure the skin is clean and dry to avoid breakdown. *Procedure for stoma care:* *The care of the stoma includes routine observation of the site and accurate documentation of the findings including: *Redness *Swelling *Evidence of granulation tissue *Exudate *Increased discomfort during care. *If visible signs of infection are present obtain a specimen for culture/sensitivity. *Refer to stomal therapy/respiratory nurse for advice on the frequency and type of dressing.·

Documentation: All written documentation related to the management of a patient with a tracheostomy is in accordance with the Hospital policy. *Record the reason and type of the interventions performed relating to tracheostomy care and appropriate outcomes in the progress notes. These include: *Suctioning (amount, colour and consistency of aspirates) *Tracheostomy cares including tie changes and stoma dressings *Stoma condition (ongoing documentation and any changes eg: signs of infection) *Significant changes in patient's condition *In the event of a tube change (routine or emergency), the following should be documented in the progress notes: *The size and type of tube inserted *Lot number *Expiry date of the tracheostomy tube *Name of person who inserted the tube *Patient' condition throughout the tube change *Any difficulties experienced during changing the tracheostomy tube

REFERENCES: 1) Carr, M. Poje, C.P. Kingston, L. Kielma, D. Heard, C. (2001) "Complications in Pediatric Tracheostomies" Laryngoscope 111: November 2001. 2) Woodrow, P. (2002) "Managing patients with a tracheostomy in acute care". Nursing Standard vol 16 (44) pp: 39-48. 3) Edwards, E.A. Byrnes, C.A (1999) " Humidification Difficulties in Two Tracheostomized Children" Anaesthesia and Intensive Care, 27, 6, pp: 656-58. 4) Oberwaldner, B. Eber, E. (2006) "Tracheostomy care in the home". Paediatric Respiratory Reviews, 7, 185-190.

NASO/ORO GASTRIC TUBE PLACEMENT

Indications

- To provide a route for feeding (-Poorly coordinated suck and swallow -Abnormal gag reflex -Insufficient oral intake - Respiratory symptoms that prevent oral feeding)
- To administer medications
- To sample gastric or intestinal contents
- To decompress and empty the stomach

Contraindications

Recent esophageal repair or perforation

Equipment

Suction equipment, Cardiac monitor, Infant feeding tube - *3.5- or 5-French (Fr) feeding tube for infants weighing <1,000 g *5- or 8-Fr infant feeding tube for infants weighing >1,000 g *½-in adhesive tape, pectin-based skin barrier, Sterile water or saline 5- and 20-mL syringes, Stethoscope, Gloves, pH paper

Procedure:

*Wash hands and put on gloves, maintaining aseptic technique. *Clear infant's nose and oropharynx by gentle suctioning as necessary. *Monitor infant's heart rate and observe for arrhythmia or respiratory distress throughout procedure. *Position infant on back with head of bed elevated. *Measure length for insertion by measuring distance from nose to ear to halfway between the xiphoid and umbilicus .Mark length on feeding tube with a loop of tape. *Moisten end of tube with sterile water or saline. *Oral insertion *Depress anterior portion of tongue with forefinger and stabilize head with free fingers. *Insert tube along finger to oropharynx. *Nasal insertion (avoid this route in very-low-birth-weight infants, in whom nasal tubes could cause periodic breathing and central apnea). *Stabilize head. Elevate tip of nose to widen nostril. *Insert tip of tube, directing it toward occiput rather than toward vertex. *Advance tube gently to oropharynx. *Observe for bradycardia. *If possible, use pacifier to encourage sucking and swallowing. *Tilt head forward slightly. *Advance tube to predetermined depth. *Do not push against any resistance. *Stop procedure if there is onset of any respiratory distress, cough, struggling, apnea, bradycardia, or cyanosis. *Determine location of tip. Injecting air to verify placement is not a reliable method, as the sound of air into the respiratory tract can be transmitted to the GI tract. *Aspirate any contents; describe and measure; determine acidity by pH paper. *Gastric contents may be clear, milky, tan, pale green, or blood-stained. *Gastric fluid pH should be <6 . *If the pH of the gastric aspirate is >6 or no aspirate is obtained, placement should be verified by radiography. *Suspect perforation or misplacement if no air or fluid is returned, or if there is onset of respiratory distress, blood in the tube, or difficult insertion. *Secure indwelling tube to face with ½-in tape. In preterm infants, apply the tape over a pectin-based barrier to prevent skin breakdown. *For feedings, attach to syringe. *For gravity drainage, attach specimen trap and position below level of stomach. *For decompression, a dual-lumen Replogle tube, connected to low continuous suction, is preferred. *Pinch or close gastric tube during removal, to prevent emptying contents into pharynx. *Document patient response, with any physiologic changes observed, and that tube placement was verified.

Complications:

*Apnea, bradycardia, or desaturation *Obstruction of obligatory nasal airway *Irritation and necrosis of nasal mucosa *Epistaxis *Ulceration

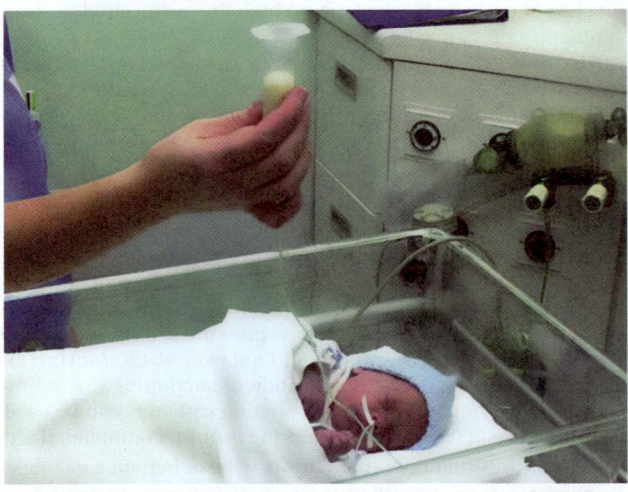

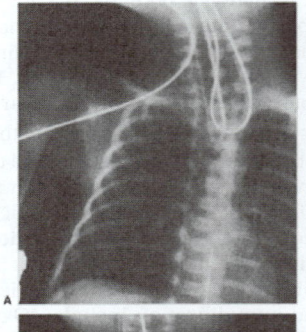
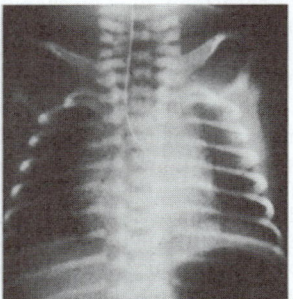
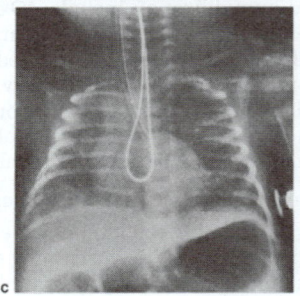
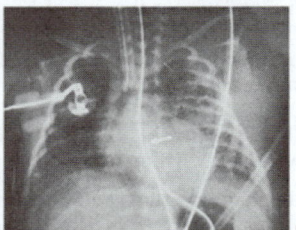
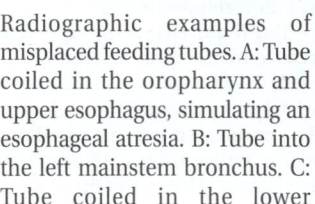
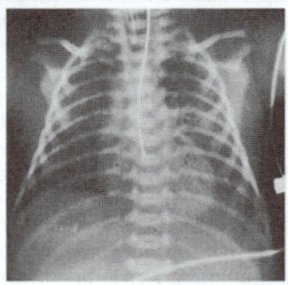

Radiographic examples of misplaced feeding tubes. A: Tube coiled in the oropharynx and upper esophagus, simulating an esophageal atresia. B: Tube into the left mainstem bronchus. C: Tube coiled in the lower esophagus. D: Tube doubled on itself in the stomach with its distal end in the esophagus (arrow). E: Tube only into the esophagus. A rush may be heard on auscultation over the stomach when air is injected through a tube lying in this position, making that an unreliable sign of gastric location

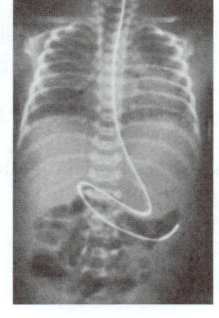

Radiographic demonstration of a transpyloric feeding tube that has passed the ligament of Treitz, well below the more appropriate level, increasing the risk of perforation or nutritional dumping.

* Perforation
- Posterior pharynx, particularly at level of cricopharnyx - Esophagus -Submucosal, remaining within mediastinum - Complete into thorax-Stomach—Duodenum
* Misplacement on insertion
- Coiled in oropharynx -Trachea
- Esophagus -Eustachian tube
* Displacement after insertion because of inappropriate length or fixation
- Pulling back into esophagus
- Prolapsing into duodenum
- Coiling and clogging of tube
- Grooved palate with long-term use of indwelling tube
* Increased gastroesophageal reflux
* Infection

Precautions

* When determining oral or nasal placement, individual assessment must be done to weigh the risks of compromising the nasal airway. Oral tubes are not at a significantly greater risk for dislodgement.
* Avoid pushing against any obstruction or resistance.
* Replace tubes as per manufacturer's recommendations. If the tube is stiff on removal, replace next tube sooner.
* If a tube has become partially dislodged, replace it rather than pushing it in farther.
* When using feedings that tend to coagulate in tubing, it may be necessary to flush the tube periodically with air or water.
* Use reliable infusion pumps that are safe for oral use by controlling rate and detecting obstructions.
* Limit infusion of hypertonic solutions and do not deliver bolus feedings beyond the pylorus.
* Consider the effect of continuous feedings on medication absorption
* Guidelines for Minimum Orogastric Tube Insertion Length to Provide Adequate Intragastric Positioning in Very Low-Birthweight Infants.

Weight (g)	Insertion Length (cm)
<750	13
750-999	15
1,000-1249	16
1250-1500	17

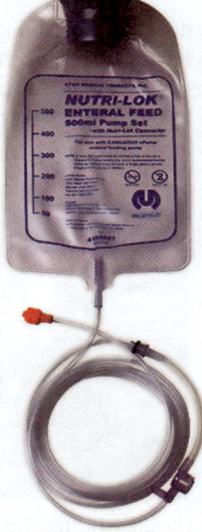

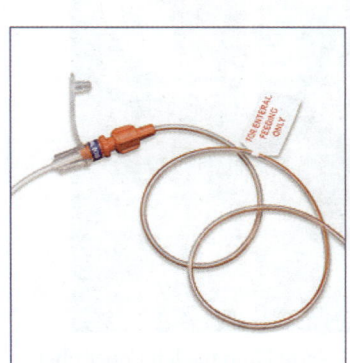

Reducing the harm caused by misplaced gastric feeding tubes in babies under the care of Neonatal units

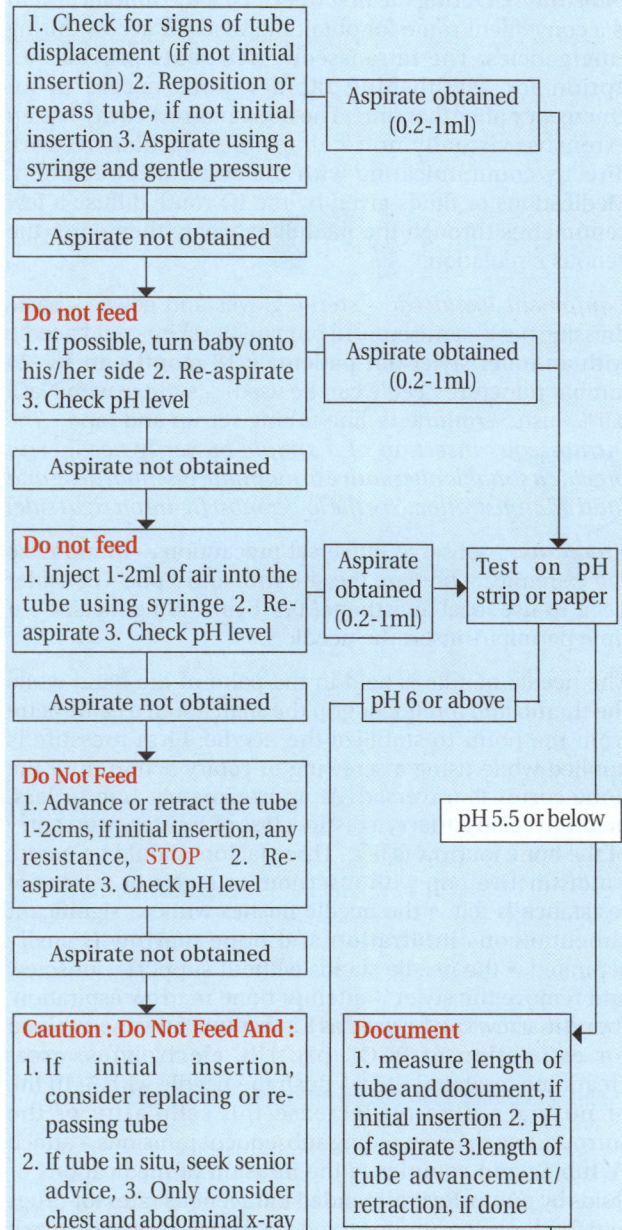

1. Check for signs of tube displacement (if not initial insertion) 2. Reposition or repass tube, if not initial insertion 3. Aspirate using a syringe and gentle pressure

Aspirate obtained (0.2-1ml)

Aspirate not obtained

Do not feed
1. If possible, turn baby onto his/her side 2. Re-aspirate 3. Check pH level

Aspirate obtained (0.2-1ml)

Aspirate not obtained

Do not feed
1. Inject 1-2ml of air into the tube using syringe 2. Re-aspirate 3. Check pH level

Aspirate obtained (0.2-1ml)

Test on pH strip or paper

Aspirate not obtained

pH 6 or above

Do Not Feed
1. Advance or retract the tube 1-2cms, if initial insertion, any resistance, STOP 2. Re-aspirate 3. Check pH level

pH 5.5 or below

Aspirate not obtained

Caution : Do Not Feed And :
1. If initial insertion, consider replacing or re-passing tube
2. If tube in situ, seek senior advice, 3. Only consider chest and abdominal x-ray if timely
4. Document decisions and rationale

Document
1. measure length of tube and document, if initial insertion 2. pH of aspirate 3.length of tube advancement/retraction, if done

Proceed to feed

Caution : Do not feed and
1. Consider waiting 15–30 minutes then re-aspirate
2. Consider replacing or re-passing tube and re-aspirating 3. If still pH 6 or above, seek senior advice ask about:
* Medication *The tube - is it the same as that documented on last X-ray and is the length the same. *The feeding history *Balancing risks
4. Only consider X-ray if timely
5. Document decisions and rationale

INTRAOSSEOUS LINE INSERTION

Indications: During the first week of life the umbilical vein is a convenient route for obtaining vascular access during emergencies. The intraosseous (IO) route provides an option for establishing rapid venous access in an emergency after that time. The bone marrow cavity has an extensive virtually non-collapsible vascular network directly communicating with the systemic circulation. Medications or fluids given by the IO route diffuse a few centimetres through the medullary cavity then enter the venous circulation.

Equipment Required: - sterile gloves and gown - basic dressing pack - antiseptic to prepare the skin - rigid needle with an inner stylet (for patients < 18 months an 18 -20 lumbar puncture needle can be used) - syringe with NaCl 0.9% flush - routine IV line tubing set-up and tape . *The intraosseous insertion of a simple butterfly needle can provide a suitable alternative to maintain essential drug and fluid administration.(see the lower most figure on right side)*

Procedure: - observe universal precautions—immobilize the extremity - prepare the site with antiseptic—consider need to use local anesthetic(0.5-1 mL 1% lignocaine) if time permits - insert the needle

The needle handle is held in the palm of the hand while the thumb and forefinger grip the shaft about a centimetre from the point to stabilize the needle. Firm pressure is applied while using a screwing or rotary action until the bone cortex is traversed. At approximately 1cm or less, below the skin surface, a distinct loss of resistance on entry of the bone marrow is felt. Three factors should be noted: • a distinctive pop with insertion, or a give or release of resistance is felt • the needle flushes without significant subcutaneous infiltration and bone marrow is easily aspirated • the needle stands without support - unscrew and remove the stylet - attempt bone marrow aspiration. (bone marrow can be used as a substitute for venous blood for estimation of PCO_2, pH, Hb, electrolytes, urea, creatinine, proteins, etc.) - flush the needle with 5–10 mL of normal saline to decrease the cellularity of the surrounding marrow, aiding subsequent infusions - attach IV tubing and commence the infusion of medications or fluids by pump. Recommended intravenous rates for drugs and fluids can be administered via the I.O. route and reach the central circulation in equivalent times. Strong alkaline and hypertonic solutions should be diluted before use.

Contraindications: Absolute: - osteogenesis imperfecta - osteopetrosis Relative: - limb is traumatised - fracture - infection

Complications: extravasation of fluid, drugs or air into skin or periosteum. A larger hole is created if a rocking motion is used during insertion of the needle. It may also occur if there has been a previous I.O. infusion in the same bone - sub-periosteal infusion may occur when the needle fails to enter the bone marrow - through and through puncture occurs if the needle is advanced too far - blockage of the needle may occur if no inner stylet is used - infection - cellulitis, abscess formation, skin necrosis and osteomyelitis - tibial fracture - fat and bone marrow microemboli .

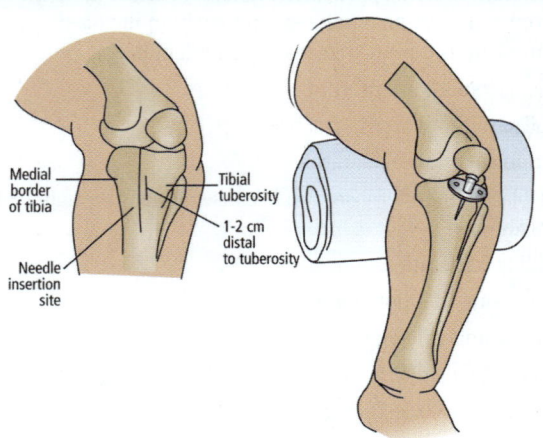

INTRAOSSEOUS LINE : The entry site at the proximal tibia is located 1-2 cms distal to the tibial tuberosity in the middle of the anteromedial ("flat") surface of the tibia. 21G LP needle with a stylet may be best, although success can be achieved with a large bore "butterfly" needle.

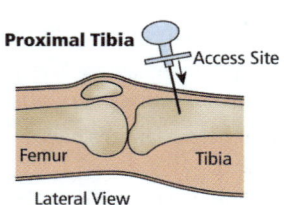

The proximal tibia is the preferred site. The entry point is a few centimetres below the tibial tuberosity at the centre of the flat antero-medial surface. The needle is directed caudal away from the upper tibial epiphysis in the line of the shaft.

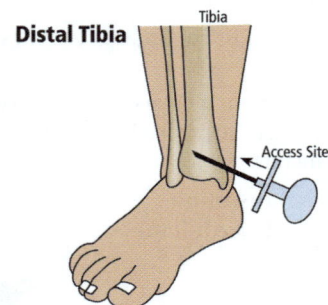

The distal antero-medial surface of the tibia is an alternate site which can be used in children of all ages. The distal femur and sternum should *not* be used.

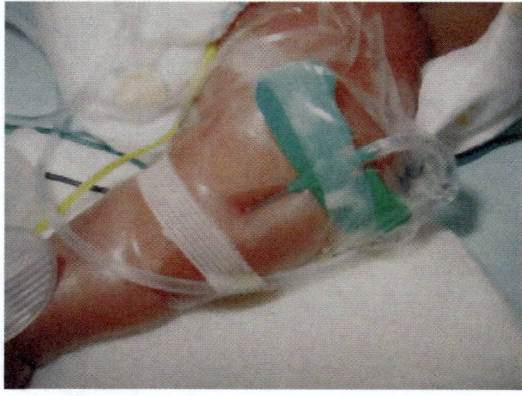

An 18 gauge butterfly needle inserted into the left upper tibia.

HEADBOX OXYGEN SET-UP

Indications: The headbox is a clear plastic hood that surrounds the baby's head, and has an opening for the baby's neck, which leaves the body accessible for nursing care. The headbox maintains a stable concentration of warm and humidified oxygen that is titrated to achieve the desired oxygen saturation.

Equipment Required: - *oxygen blender/oxygen & air flow meters with nipples *green oxygen tubing *humidifier base, water chamber & sterile water for irrigation *heater hose/corrugated tubing *headbox (with sponge, optional) *headbox thermometer *oxygen analyzer

Procedure: - *assemble the humidifier base and water filled chamber *connect the oxygen tubing from the oxygen blender to the water filled chamber. Alternatively connect tubing from oxygen and air flow meters via a "Y" connector and then attach the single piece of tubing from the "Y" connector to the water filled chamber *connect the heater hose to the water filled chamber *secure the headbox thermometer to the inside of the headbox. If possible, insert sponge over gas inlet *place the headbox over the baby's head, taking care when positioning the headbox around the baby's neck *connect the heater hose to the headbox *blend the oxygen to obtain the necessary oxygen concentration to achieve the desired oxygen saturation. The total flow of gases should be at least 6 to 8 L/min to prevent accumulation of carbon dioxide in the headbox.

*desired oxygen concentrations are achieved either via a blender "dialled" to the appropriate concentration, or by combining the flow of oxygen and air using the following guide.

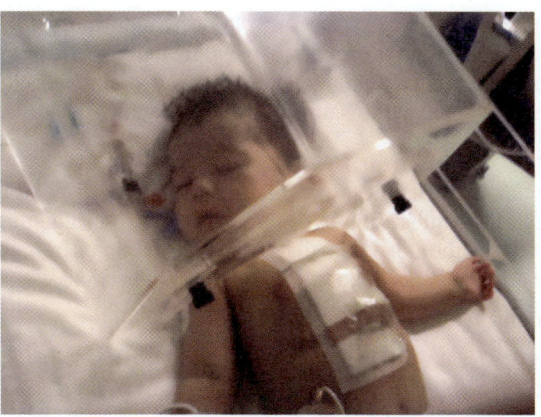

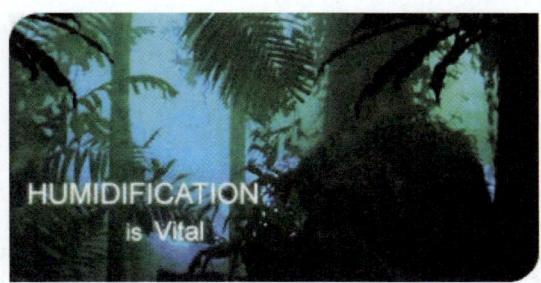

HUMIDIFICATION is Vital

HEADBOX OXYGEN/AIR FLOW RATES

Oxygen percentage	Oxygen flow (L/min)	Air flow (L/min)
30	1	9
40	2	8
50	4	6
60	5	5
70	6	4
80	7.5	2.5
90	9	1

*calibrate oxygen analyzer and place into the headbox, alongside the baby's nose *maintain the inspired gas temperature at the appropriate neutral thermal environment for the baby.

Continuously assess and document hourly the following

*inspired oxygen concentration *oxygen saturation (½hourly) *heart rate ·respiratory rate and effort *headbox temperature *water level in chamber *humidification (dry or moist)*observe the baby's neck for irritation and pressure areas hourly, and ensure the position of the headbox is correct *remove any accumulated water in the heater hose hourly *calibrate the oxygen analyzer every eight hours*check the baby's temperature hourly for four hours or until stable when headbox oxygen commences and then four hourly

Complications: *hypoxemia *hyperoxemia *hypothermia *hyperthermia *irritation and pressure to neck.

Cleaning of Equipment *change the headbox circuit, humidifying chamber and headbox when the 2 litre bag of water is empty *the heater/humidifier is wiped clean with disinfectant *the headbox and thermometer are washed with detergent and rinsed thoroughly ·the heater hose/corrugated tubing is pasteurized and the green oxygen tubing is discarded.

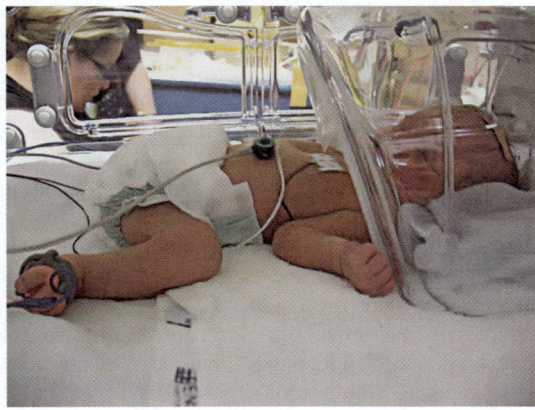

Areas of uncertainty in clinical practice

When to transfer an infant from incubator or intra-nasal flow oxygen will depend on*the clinical situation *the concentration of oxygen required *the operational characteristics of the incubator being used.As a general guide infants requiring 40% oxygen or more will usually be managed with headbox oxygen.Optimally oxygen delivered by headbox should be warmed and humidified, however, during the immediate stabilization of a sick infant consistency of oxygenation remains the priority

References: **Aloan, C.A. & Hill, T.V. (1997).** *Respiratory care of the newborn and child* **(2nd ed). Philadelphia: Lippincott.**

Askin, D.F. (1997). *Acute respiratory care of the neonate: A self study course* (2nd ed). Petaluma: NICU INK.

Barnhart, S.L. and Czervinske (1995). *Perinatal and pediatric respiratory care.* Philadelphia: W.B. Saunders.

CAPILLARY HEELSTICK BLOOD SAMPLING

Indications

*Capillary blood gas sampling *Routine laboratory analysis (standard hematology, chemistries, toxicology/drug levels) requiring a limited amount of blood in which minimal cell lysis does not alter results *Newborn metabolic screen

Contraindications

*Edema, because interstitial fluid dilutes the sample and gives inaccurate results *Injury or anomalies that preclude putting pressure on the foot *Areas that are bruised or injured by multiple previous heelsticks *Poor perfusion *Local infection

Equipment

*Gloves *Heel-warming device if desired *Antiseptic (betadine/ saline or alcohol swab) *Pad or other means of protecting bed linens *Heel-lancing device. Use appropriate size for infant *Specimen collector as appropriate *Serum separators *Hematology tubes *Capillary blood gas tube *Newborn metabolic screen filter paper *Capillary tubes for blood transfer to lab tubes if appropriate *Bandage or gauze wrap

Technique

*Identify site; the preferred areas for capillary heel testing are the outer aspects of the heel *Vary sites to prevent bruising and skin damage. *The plantar surface can be used if the preferred areas are compromised by previous frequent testing. The skin-to-calcaneal perichondrium distance is at least 3 mm in most term babies and in 91% of babies at 33 to 37 weeks' gestation, but is at least 3 mm in only about 60% of babies <33 weeks' gestation . *Apply heel warmer or warm towel for 5 minutes. Remove just before procedure. *Provide comfort measures with facilitated tucking/swaddling and the use of pacifiers combined with administration of a concentrated sucrose solution results in less measurable pain and faster resolution of discomfort in the infant following the procedure . *Prepare automated device by removing release clip. *Don gloves. *Cleanse site with betadine followed with saline wipe or alcohol wipe. *Position hand with fingers along the calf and thumb at ball of foot to stabilize. *Apply pressure along calf toward heel. *Place automated device on site and activate. *Apply pressure to leg with counterpressure to ball of foot and allow blood drop to form. *Wipe away first drop of blood with gauze or clean wipe. *Using capillary action, fill blood gas tube, holding tube horizontally. *Release pressure, allowing capillaries to refill. *Guide blood drops into tube or collect with capillary tube for transfer to laboratory tube. *If blood stops flowing, wipe site to remove clot with alcohol swab, gauze, or clean wipe, ensure time for capillary refill, and then reapply pressure to leg. If blood does not flow, choose another site and repeat procedure or consider venipuncture. *When samples have been collected, apply pressure to puncture site and wrap with gauze or apply adhesive bandage. *Continue comfort measures.

Complications

*Pain *Provide oral sucrose, swaddling/tucking, and pacifier. *Use proper equipment. *Make incisions in designated areas of the heel. *Infection (cellulitis, abscess, perichondritis, osteomyelitis) . *Tissue loss and scarring *Calcified nodules *Inaccurate laboratory results:* *Hyperkalemia secondary to excessive hemolysis *Use proper technique and procedures to minimize cell lysis. *Erroneous blood gas results *Ensure that sample is free of air bubbles. *Avoid delay in analysis. *Use proper technique and procedures to minimize cell lysis.

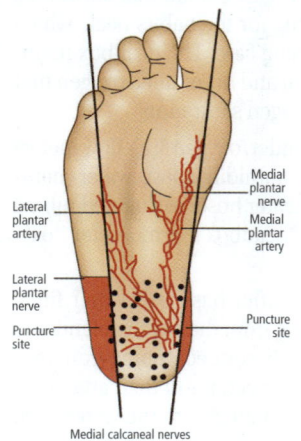
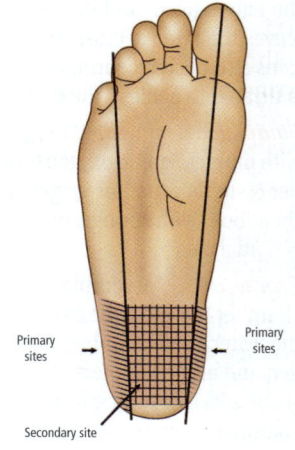

HEEL PRICK FOR CAPILLARY BLOOD SAMPLING should be performed on the plantar surface of the heel, beyond the lateral and medial limits of the calcaneus, marked by these lines

The safest site for heel stick is the outer edges of the heel as shown in the dark areas above. The hatched area between these sites may be used as a secondary site if the outer areas have been accessed frequently. The posterior pole of the heel should not be used in order to avoid damage to the calcaneus.

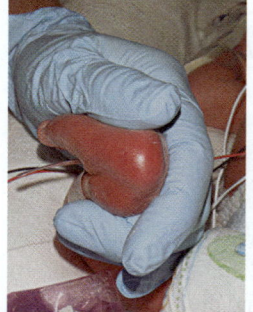

Position for hand and automated lancing device. Position heel in the apex of the angle of the thumb and forefinger with fingers along the calf and thumb along the ball of the foot. Position automated lancing device in appropriate position. Apply pressure along the calf with counterpressure by the thumb. Do not squeeze the heel.

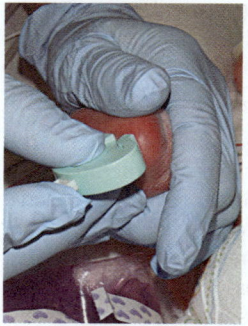

Placement of heel lancing device on outer portion of plantar surface of heel.

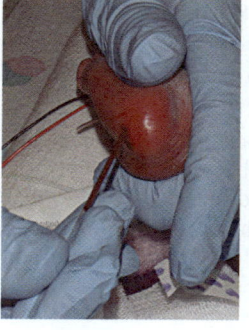

Collection of blood sample from heel stick site. A capillary tube collection is pictured. (Note: The first drop of blood after incision should be wiped away and not used in sample.)

INTRAMUSCULAR INJECTION

Equipment

*IM medication ampoule *Large bore needle for withdrawing medication from ampoule *1 ml or 2 ml syringe *23 gauge 25 mm needle or 25 gauge 16 mm needle for preterm babies 2 months or younger *Cotton wool swab *Gloves for standard precautions

Procedure

There must be a written medication order on the medication chart. Check the correct drug/dose/time/route/infant. Draw the medication up into the syringe using the large bore needle. Change to the 23 g 25 mm needle or 25 g 16 mm needle. A second staff member to help position the infant on his/her back on a table or bed may be required. Undo the infant's nappy to locate the junction of the upper and middle thirds of the vastus lateralis thigh muscle. The clinician performing the injection places their forearm across the infant's pelvis and secures the thigh between their thumb and forefinger. Bunch up the thigh muscle to increase the muscle mass. Administer the IM injection at a 45-60° angle to the skin. The needle must be angled toward the knee. At this angle, the needle can be safely inserted to a depth of between 16–25 mm skin-to-needle-tip depth. Inserting the needle at this angle results in less tissue resistance as the needle penetrates the muscle. The following figures of the thigh show the recommended injection site. Withdraw the plunger to ensure that the medication does not go directly into a blood vessel. Slowly inject the medication for even distribution and to minimize the infant's discomfort. Remove the needle. Check the injection site for bleeding and apply cotton wool ball if necessary. Observe the site for local inflammation. Dispose of the needles and syringe into a labeled puncture proof container to prevent needle stick injury & reuse.

*Document: The administration of the IM injection on the medication chart and/or child health record (where appropriate). Practice points: Avoid subcutaneous and intramuscular injections when intravenous administration is a suitable alternative option. Note that VitaminK is preferably given intramuscularly as soon as possible after birth and endogenous endorphins are present at high levels at the time of birth. Alcohol and other disinfecting agents must be allowed to evaporate before injection of medication. Never give an IM injection in the buttocks. Using the vastus lateralis muscle avoids the risk of sciatic nerve damage from gluteal injection. Also the vastus lateralis muscle has a larger muscle mass than the gluteal region and therefore has reduced risk of severe local reactions. The deltoid in infants is not sufficiently bulky to absorb IM medications adequately. The vastus lateralis muscle avoids the thicker layer of subcutaneous fat on the anterior thigh. It is important that infants do not move during the IM injection. However excessive restraint can increase the infant's fear and can result in increased muscle tension The infant can be held in the 'cuddle' or semi-recumbent position on the lap of the parent/caregiver/health professional. Oral sucrose may be given for relief of distress (link to section). The volume of the IM injection should not be more than 1ml. When two IM injections are being administered, give one medication into the right thigh and the other into the left thigh.

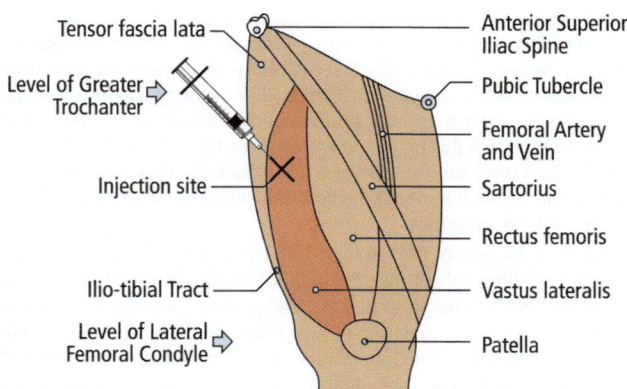

Diagram of the muscles of the thigh showing the recommended injection site

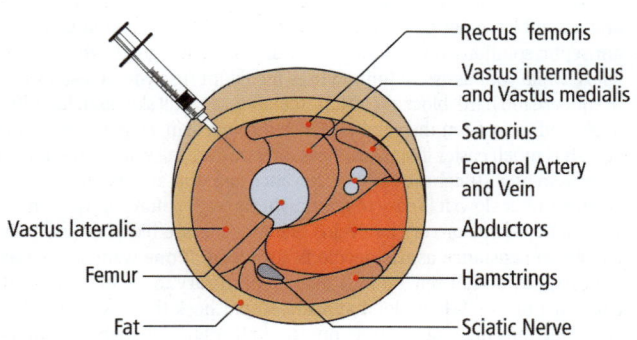

Diagrammatic cross section of the thigh showing recommended injection site

The anterolateral thigh is the preferred site for IM injection in infants under 12 months of age. Medications are injected into the bulkiest part of the vastus lateralis thigh muscle, which is the junction of the upper and middle thirds of this muscle. Nursing and medical staff must be familiar with the principles of the administration of medications to an infant. These principles include *observation of standard precautions *aseptic techniques and correct drug/dose/time/route/patient practices.

PERIPHERAL INTRAVENOUS LINE PLACEMENT

Indications: Venous access for the administration of fluid (including glucose and parenteral nutrition), medications, blood or blood products.

Equipment: clean trolley, sterile gloves (use standard precautions for all procedures where contact with blood possible), basic dressing pack, 24g Optiva or Insyte Neonatal catheter, blunt end drawing up needle, 10 ml ampoule of 0.9% Sodium Chloride, 2 x 2ml syringes containing 0.9% Sodium Chloride, one to flush cannula and one to prime extension set, 3-way stopcock (tap) if for continuous infusion, skin antiseptic solution, 2% aqueous chlorhexidene for all peripheral IV's in infants < 1000 grams up to 14 days of age, Persist-Plus (1%chlorhexidine in 70%ethanol) for all other IV's, extension tubing, tapes , splint, sterile occlusive dressing to cover the insertion point e.g. Tegaderm or IV3000,

Technique: Compared with IV cannulation in adults, the veins in babies are smaller and, perhaps most importantly, poorly supported by surrounding soft tissue. Veins may suffer heavily during a prolonged stay in intensive care or special care and often veins that have been used previously need to be re-cannulated. The first essential is to be methodical and to look. Get the baby where you can see and have access to all limbs while ensuring that he/she is warm and well oxygenated. Ensure that you have a good light. The standard light built into the radiant heaters is too flat and it is better to switch this off and to use an angled procedure light. Take time and look in all of the usual site s until you find the best available vein. This may take up to 2-5 minutes. The first acceptable vein is not usually the best. This process of taking a good long look should be repeated after every two attempts.

Look for a vein which *runs straight *fills and empties *stands up a little *is easy to splint. *In sick or smaller babies, try to avoid, if possible, veins which are used for insertion of percutaneous central venous catheters *saphenous at knee *cubital fossa *superficial temporal*

Procedure: Consider provision of pain relief consistent with the condition of the infant and the urgency of the procedure *application of 0.5 -1g EMLA to proposed site 60-90 minutes prior to insertion *oral sucrose *non-pharmacological settling techniques **1.** Set up IV trolley. Carefully wipe surface of trolley with solution provided (either isopropyl wipes or 1% chlorhexidine in 70% alcohol). **2.** Place basic dressing pack onto clean IV trolley and open so that contents remain sterile (plastic covering can be flattened out to create sterile surface on trolley). Place additional sterile items onto this sterile surface. **3.** Choose suitable vein. **4.** Wash and dry hands thoroughly. Put on gloves. **5.** Assemble equipment that has been opened onto the basic dressing pack. **6.** Draw up 0.9% Sodium Chloride solution into 2 x 2ml syringes using drawing up needle. **7.** Prime cannula and assembled equipment with 0.9% Sodium Chloride solution. **8.** Swab skin with appropriate antiseptic solution swab. Allow skin to dry. **9.** Ensure good light. **10.** Tourniquet *use a piece of gauze while your assistant immobilizes the infant *use your assistant's hand The usual mistake is to squeeze too hard, blocking off all circulation. **11.** Pull skin taut. Identify vein and enter skin at an angle and away from the vein. **12.** Once through skin, stop and reorient your needle tip and the vein. It is much easier if one advances directly over the vein, rather than from the side. **13.** Aim to enter vein on a straight stretch. **14.** Advance in a stop-start fashion once near vein.(The flashback is often rather slow; it is easy to go straight through before knowing that one has hit anything). In very small infants or very bad veins one may not see blood return; only being aware of a slight change in resistance as the needle is advanced. If one waits a few seconds, blood sometimes appears, but do not rely on it. It may be necessary to try to advance the catheter without this confirmation. **15.** When blood appears, stop. Check that needle is advancing on the line of the vein. Make any necessary correction. **16.** Lift tip of needle slightly. Advance another 1-2mm. Check if bleeding into chamber continues. If so, needle tip is still in vein. Hold base of needle steady, push catheter off needle, either with other hand or index finger of right hand. Advance up vein as far as it will easily go.If bleeding has stopped after initial small advance of catheter/needle unit, it is likely that the needle tip is out of the other side of the vein. There is a reasonable chance that the catheter tip is still within the vein. If needle is pulled back into the catheter there is a good chance that you will see blood coming up the catheter. If so, attempt to advance the catheter up the vein, leaving the needle in the catheter, but pulled back a little, to stiffen it. You have about a 50% chance of successfully feeding it up. **17.** Release tourniquet. Syringe with 0.9% Normal Saline to check patency. If catheter has not been able to be advanced fully, syringing may also help to advance it further up the vein. **18.** Remove any blood spills near insertion site before strapping. **19.** Without touching the insertion site, apply a piece of Tegaderm over the hub of the catheter and its insertion site. Use 2 Vee tapes around the end of the hub of catheter (sterilized micropore tape is contained in the IV starterpack) over the Tegaderm. **20.** Attach extension tubing and 3-way tap, securing luerlocks. **21.** Splint. Shape splint to limb and immobilize joint above insertion (use smallest possible and avoid pressure areas). Tape loosely at top and over fingers. A little more firmly over the hub of the catheter. If necessary place a piece of gauze/telfar between the hub and the skin so as to avoid a pressure area. Fingers/toes must be visible, as must the area around the catheter tip. **22.** For every additional attempt begin from step 1. Avoid the temptation to use partly clean equipment. It is best for the infant that with every attempt strict precautions are taken to reduce the risk of infection.N.B. A new cannula is required for each insertion attempt*if contamination occurs during the procedure, discard the contaminated equipment and don another pair of gloves *refer insertion to another member of staff after 3 unsuccessful insertion attempts *discard dressing pack and contaminated equipment if it becomes heavily contaminated due to multiple insertion attempts. Transfer uncontaminated tubing to new dressing pack.

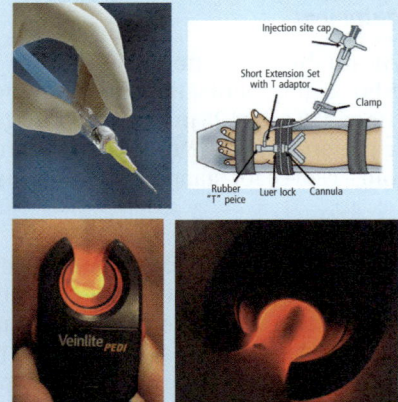

Transillumination to locate difficult veins

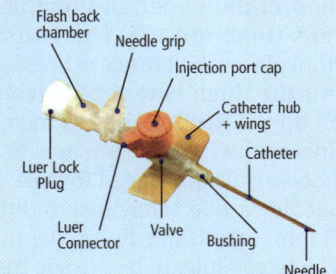

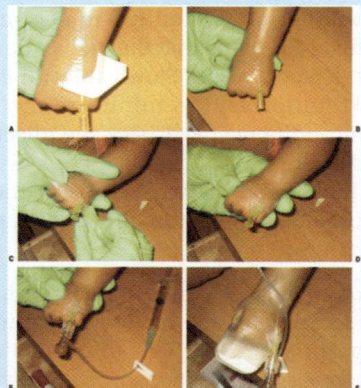

Method for securing peripheral intravenous cannula with adhesive tape. A, B: Place an adhesive transparent tape over the cannula. C: Place tape 1 behind cannula as shown, with adhesive side up. D, E: Fold tape 1 anteriorly across the catheter-hub junction. F: Hold in place with tapes 2 and 3. The area of skin entry can be dressed with semipermeable sterile transparent dressing. Avoid obscuring with opaque dressing.

Potential complications :*phlebitis *cellulitis *sepsis *tissue necrosis *air embolus (incorrect priming)

The likelihood of phlebitis and sepsis secondary to IV cannulas can be reduced by electively resiting the cannula every 48-72 hours. This will depend to some extent on the availability of other sites. If this approach is adopted, it is important to ensure that the new (replacement) IV cannula is in situ and functioning before the old one is removed (especially if the baby is nil orally and/or dependent on IV glucose to maintain glucose homeostasis.

PERIPHERAL ARTERIAL PUNCTURE

Indications

*Sampling for arterial blood gas determination *Sampling for routine laboratory test when venous and capillary sampling not suitable or unobtainable

Contraindications

*Coagulation defects, thrombocytopenia *Circulatory compromise in the extremity *Inappropriate artery *Femoral artery *Use of radial artery if inadequate collaterals (see Allen's test below) *Infection in sampling area *When cannulation of that vessel is anticipated *Use of peripheral arteries on the ipsilateral arm in an infant with congenital heart disease requiring a shunt via the subclavian artery

Precautions: *Perform arterial sampling only when venous or capillary sampling is inappropriate. *Arterial blood gas analyses prior to placement of indwelling access. *Ammonia levels *Large quantities of blood to be obtained *Very low-birthweight infants with poor venous access *Use smallest possible needle to minimize trauma to vessel (23 to 27 gauge). *Avoid laceration of the artery caused by puncturing both sides of arterial wall in exactly opposite locations. *Guarantee hemostasis at end of procedure. *Check distal circulation after puncture. Arterial pulse, Capillary refill time, Color, temperature *Take action to reverse arteriospasm, if necessary

*Selection of Arterial Site -Peripheral site preferred Radial artery preferred if ulnar collateral intact Dorsalis pedis, posterior tibial arteries satisfactory Brachial artery only if urgent indication and no more peripheral arterial or umbilical artery access is available Temporal artery should be avoided because of risk of neurologic damage

Equipment

Gloves, Needle, A 23- to 25-gauge venipuncture needle, Safety-engineered needle should be used, Appropriate syringes, Materials for minor skin preparation; povidone-iodine solution preparation preferred for blood culture, Gauze pads, Sterile glove to cover transilluminator High-intensity fiber-optic light for transillumination Oral sucrose solution (24% to 25%) for pain control, if indicated

Technique: *General Principles* -*Transillumination may assist location of vessel *Position needle for arterial puncture against direction of blood flow. *Keep angle of entry shallow for superficial vessels. *15 to 25 degrees for superficial artery, bevel down *5 degrees for deep artery, bevel up *Penetrate skin first, and then puncture artery to minimize trauma to vessel. *Use fresh needle and repeat skin preparation if withdrawal from skin is necessary. *Apply firm, local pressure for 5 minutes to achieve complete hemostasis. **Radial artery puncture** *Extend wrist, supine, not hyperextended, which may occlude vessel. *Locate radial and ulnar arteries at proximal wrist crease *Radial artery is lateral to flexor carpi radialis tendon. *Ulnar artery is medial to flexor carpi ulnarius tendon. *Transillumination may be helpful. *Perform modified Allen's test for collateral supply *Elevate infant's hand. *Occlude both radial and ulnar arteries at wrist. *Massage palm toward wrist. *Release occlusion of ulnar artery only. Look for color to return to hand in less than 10 seconds, indicating adequate collateral supply. *Do not puncture radial artery if color return takes more than 15 seconds. Locate artery by palpation and/or transillumination. Prepare area with antiseptic, as for minor procedure. Check function of syringe. Puncture skin and penetrate artery at 45 degrees with bevel up. For very small infants, use angle of 15 to 25 degrees with bevel down *While maintaining gentle suction, advance until there is blood return or resistance from bone. *If no blood obtained prior to encountering resistance, withdraw needle cautiously until blood returns. Artery may spasm when needle is introduced. Be patient; change angle of needle as necessary. *Collect sample and remove needle. *Compress site for 5 minutes or until hemostasis is complete. *Verify satisfactory peripheral blood flow.

Complications: Distal ischemia from arteriospasm, hematoma, thrombosis, or embolism *Infection *Osteomyelitis *Infected hip joint after femoral puncture *Hemorrhage or hematoma *Forearm compartment syndrome following brachial artery puncture *Inaccuracy of blood gas estimated *Excessive heparinization of syringe (falsely low PCO_2 and pH) *Hypothermic or hyperthermic infant *Gas bubbles in syringe *Spuriously high PO_2 *Spuriously low PCO_2 *Excessive delay in processing *Clot in syringe

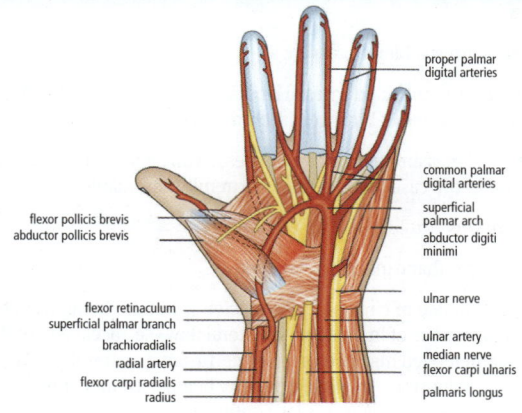

Anatomy of the major arteries of the wrist and hand

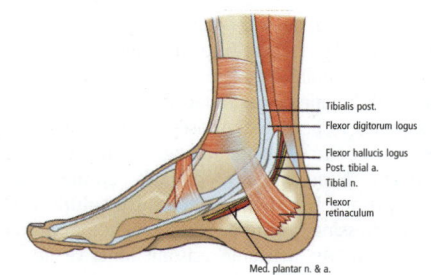

Anatomic relations of the posterior tibial artery

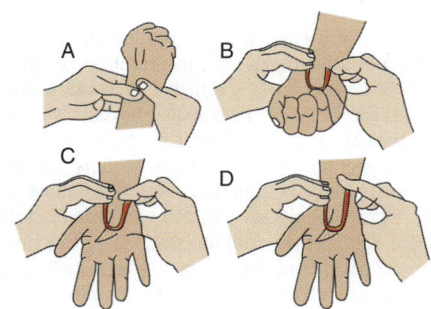

Modified Allen's test The patient's hand is initially held high while the fist is clenched and both radial and ulnar arteries are compressed (A); this allows the blood to drain from the hand. The hand is then lowered (B) and the fist is opened (C). After pressure is released over the ulnar artery (D), color should return to the hand within six seconds, indicating a patent ulnar artery and an intact superficial palmar arch. (Redrawn from American Heart Association. Textbook of Advanced Cardiac Life Support, 1994.)

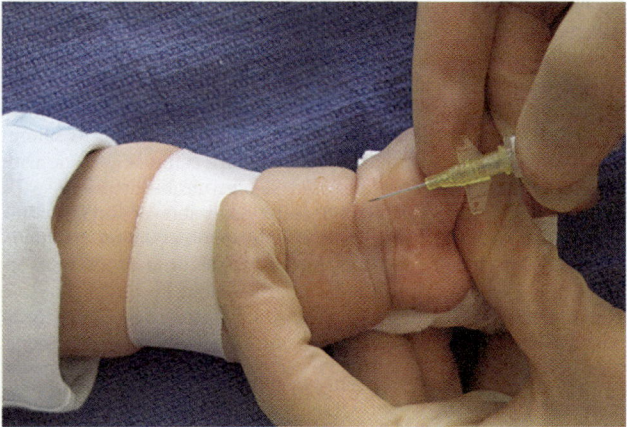

Position of wrist for puncture of radial artery.
(1) distal wrist crease; (2) proximal wrist crease.

PERIPHERAL ARTERIAL CANNULATION

Indications

*Monitoring of arterial blood pressure

*Frequent monitoring of blood gases or laboratory tests (e.g., sick ventilated neonates or extremely low-birthweight premature infants)

*When preductal measurement is required (e.g., with persistent pulmonary hypertension) in the case of right-upper-extremity cannulation

Contraindications

*Bleeding disorder that cannot be corrected

*Pre-existing evidence of circulatory insufficiency in limb being used for cannulation *Evidence of inadequate collateral flow (i.e., occlusion of the vessel to be catheterized may compromise perfusion of extremity) *Local skin infection *Malformation of the extremity being used for cannulation *Previous surgery in the area (especially cutdown)

Equipment

Sterile *Gloves *Antiseptic solution (e.g., an iodophor) *4- × 4- in gauze squares *0.5 to 0.95 N saline with 1 to 2 U/mL heparin *3- or 5-mL syringe *20-gauge venipuncture needle (if using larger-size 22-gauge cannula) *Appropriate-size cannula: 22-gauge x 1- in (2.5-cm), 24-gauge × 0.75-in, or 24-gauge x 0.56-in tapered or nontapered cannula with stylet for larger to smaller neonates, respectively *Antiseptic ointment (optional) *Arterial pressure transducer and extension tubing *5-0 nylon suture with curved needle (optional) *Needle holder (optional) *Suture scissors (optional) *T connector primed with heparinized flush solution *Transparent, semipermeable dressing Nonsterile- *Equipment for transillumination or Doppler ultrasound *Â½-in, water-resistant adhesive tape *Materials for forearm restraint for radial or ulnar cannulation *A constant-infusion pump capable of delivering flush solution at rate of 0.5 to 1 mL/hr against back pressure.

Technique: Radial artery:
This is the most routine site for cannulation. The infant's forearm and hand can be transilluminated with the wrist in extension 45 to 60 degrees, making sure that fingers are visible to monitor distal perfusion. The artery can be palpated proximally to the transverse crease on the palmar surface of the wrist, medial to the styloid process of the radius, and lateral to the flexor carpi radialis .Identify artery by *Palpation (see anatomic landmarks as described above or individual arterial sites) *Transillumination *Doppler ultrasound Scrub and put on gloves. Prepare skin over site with antiseptic (e.g., an iodophor). Make small skin puncture with venipuncture needle over site (to ease passage of cannula through skin and reduce chances of penetrating the posterior wall of the vessel, especially when using a larger-gauge cannula). *Accomplish cannulation of artery. Pass needle stylet (with bevel up) and cannula through artery at 30- to 40-degree angle to skin. *Remove stylet and withdraw cannula slowly until arterial flow is established. *Advance cannula into artery. Inability to insert the cannula into the lumen usually indicates failure to puncture the artery centrally. This often results in laceration of the lateral wall of the artery with formation of a hematoma, which can be seen on transillumination. *Attach cannula firmly to T connector and gently flush with 0.5 mL of heparinized solution, observing for evidence of blanching or cyanosis. *Apply iodophor ointment (optional) to puncture site. *Suture cannula to skin with 5-0 nylon suture if desired. This step may be omitted as long as cannula is securely taped. use of sutures may produce a more unsightly scar. *Secure cannula as done with peripheral intravenous line.Transparent semipermeable dressing may be used in place of tape to allow continuous visualization of skin entry site. *Guarantee that all digits are visible for frequent inspection. *Maintain patency by attaching T connector to extension tubing or arterial pressure line to run 0.5 to 1 mL/hr of heparinized flush solution by constant infusion pump. Change intravenous (IV) tubing and flushing solution every 24 hours.

Complications:
Thromboembolism/vasospasm/thrombosis *Blanching of hand and partial loss of digits *Gangrene of fingertips and hemiplegia *Necrosis of forearm and hand *Skin ulcers *Ischemia/necrosis of toes *Cerebral emboli *Reversible occlusion of artery *Infiltration of infusate *Infection *Hematoma.

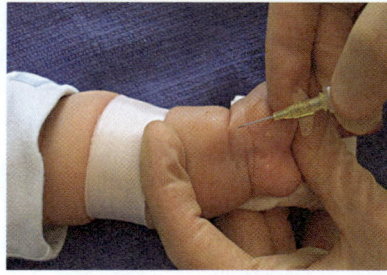

Introduction of Angiocath into radial artery.

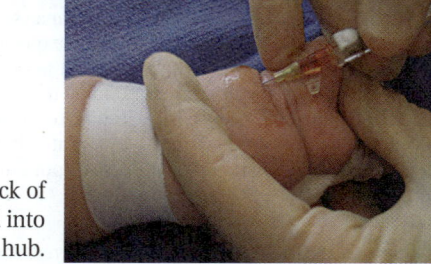

Flashback of blood into Angiocath hub.

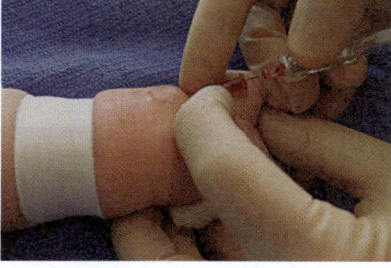

Stabilization of catheter while removing needle introducer.

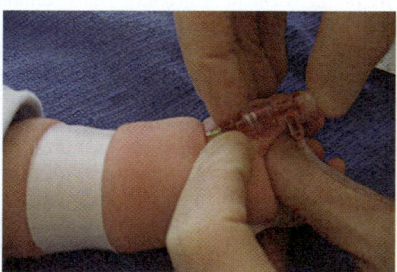

Pressure transducer attached to radial artery catheter

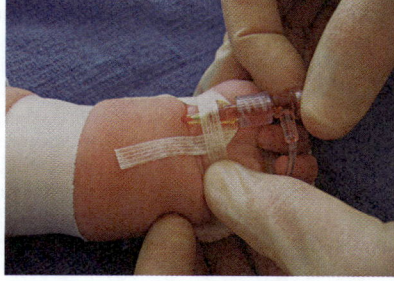

Radial artery cannula secured in place with Steri-Strips.

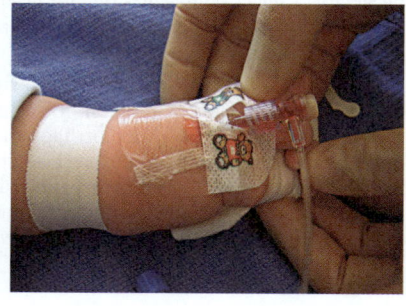

Sterile dressing applied over radial artery cannula.

LUMBAR PUNCTURE

Indications: 1)sampling of cerebrospinal fluid (CSF) for microscopy, evidence of bacterial, viral or fungal infection and biochemical measurement of protein and sugar levels, or markers of metabolic disorder 2)therapeutic tap to limit ventricular dilatation in post hemorrhagic hydrocephalus (serial taps may be required)

Equipment: Clean trolley,Masks - for person performing procedure and assistant,Sterile Gown pack,Sterile gloves,Sterile plastic drape,Sterile scissors,Basic Dressing Pack,Antiseptic solution as per unit protocol,Ampoule of Sterile Water, Lumbar Puncture Needle - short bevel, styletted, 22 or 25 gaugeLP needles with a stylet are used in order to avoid later formation of a dermoid cyst. 23 or 25g needles are occasionally used by experienced practitioners when a lumbar puncture cannot be satisfactorily achieved with a standard LP needle. Sterile pack of 3 CSF collection tubes

Preparation: *when possible, parents are informed of planned procedure for their infant *resuscitation equipment is readily available and in working order *area is draught free *ensure infant has not been fed in previous hour (aspirate infant's stomach if fed within the past hour) *perform cardiorespiratory and oxygen saturation monitoring during procedure (and for 1 hour after procedure) *consider infant's need for pain relief including *application of EMLA (0.5 -1g) to proposed site 60-90 minutes before procedure *use of oral sucrose (link to section) *subcutaneous infiltration of lignocaine

Positioning of Infant: Infants may not tolerate the procedure well. This is usually because of excessive flexion of the infant. Some degree of flexion of the spine is helpful since it opens up the interspinous spaces and also stretches the skin over the processes allowing better definition of landmarks. It is not necessary to flex the neck with compromise of the airway and increase in cerebral venous pressure. Position infant in the lateral position with trunk well flexed by the assistant holding the shoulders and legs forward, but with neck extended and legs at 90 degrees angle to the hips - at the edge of the cot. Ensure infant's back is parallel to the cot, with hips and shoulders vertical to the cot. Alternatively, term infants may be placed in a seated position on the edge of the table, with trunk flexed forward, stabilized from the front by the assistant.The infant's shoulders and hips are held in order to maintain vertical alignment of the hips and shoulders during the procedure. This has been shown to be the best tolerated and to also have the best chance of obtaining CSF.

Procedure *place infant on blue underpad. (Ensure underpad is removed after skin preparation if any pooling of skin preparation solution has occurred) *position baby. Identify landmarks. Ensure baby is as straight as possible. *apply face mask *wash hands, gown and glove *cut hole in middle of plastic drape. (Plastic drape helps visualization of infant during procedure) *prepare skin. Wait for prep to dry. *identify L4. It helps to keep two fingers of your left hand locating it - one each side. *enter skin strictly in midline. Aiming at between 70 and 90 deg, slightly headwards. *once through the skin STOP. Wait for the infant to resettle. *reorient yourself, making sure that you are still in the midline and advancing at the appropriate angle. The subsequent advance of the needle is less distressing than the initial insertion. *advance needle about 0.5 cm. Remove stylette and observe for CSF flow. If negative, reinsert stylette and advance a little further. Repeat this until CSF is obtained. *a "pop" or "give" may be felt as the needle passes through the posterior ligaments and dura, but do not rely on this. The "stop-start" approach is less likely to give a bloody tap. *allow CSF to drip into at least two tubes. A minimum of 10 drops/tube is required for microbiological and biochemical examination. *for a therapeutic tap, the volume limit is 2% of body weight. If doing a therapeutic tap, CSF pressure should be measured using a manometer. *remove needle. Press site to control ooze with sterile cotton wool ball. After ooze has ceased use band-aid or flexible collodion as dressing. *if required - clean antiseptic solution from skin with Sterile Water *discard stylet and needle into sharps container.

Procedure Failure: *No CSF *Consult a more experienced practitioner *Attempt procedure using the next higher intervertebral space *Blood stained CSF *Possible traumatic bleeding - blood staining tends to clear *Possible subarachnoid space bleeding

Care of Infant Following Procedure: *continue routine monitoring of infant *check temperature after procedure *discontinue cardiorespiratory and oxygen saturation monitoring (if not otherwise indicated) 1 hour following procedure *if sedation with narcotics was administered prior to procedure, continue oxygen saturation monitoring for 4 hours post procedure. Sedated infants should remain nil orally for 2 hours post procedure *a infants are lying down after the procedure, distress due to headache should not occur. However if infant is distressed following procedure offer dummy or consider use of paracetamol *in the absence of compelling evidence it is advised that the infant remain horizontal for 60 minutes after the procedure.

While restraining infant for lumbar puncture in the lateral recumbent position. Neck should not be flexed.

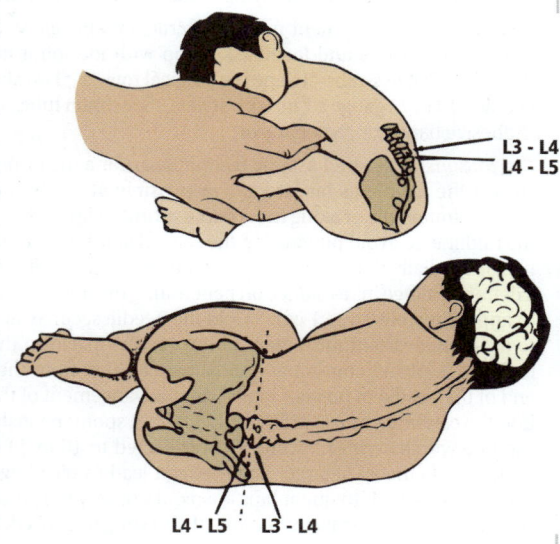

LUMBAR PUNCTURE: Positioning and landmarks used for LP- The iliac crest (dotted line) marks the approximate level of L4. L4-L5 interspace is the preferred of the Lumbar puncture

Spinal needle size by age:

Premature infant-22 G or smaller, 1.5 inch, plastic hub preferred.

Neonate-2yr-22G, 1.5 inch, plastic hub preferred.

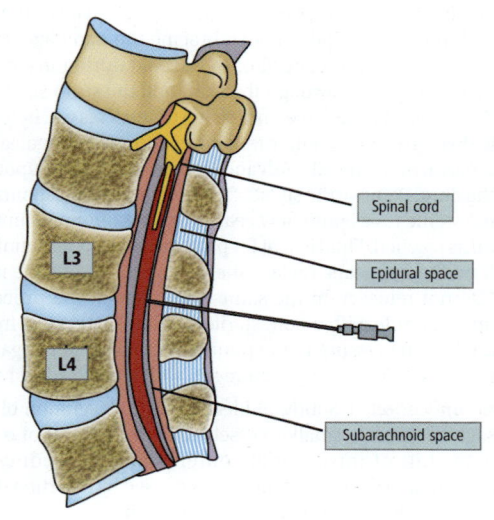

SUBDURAL TAP

Indications:

*To sample convexity subdural collection for hematologic, microbiologic, and biochemical studies *To drain convexity subdural collection to reduce increased intracranial pressure or to prevent the development of craniocerebral disproportion

Contraindications:
*Clinical instability when risk exceeds potential benefit *Uncorrected thrombocytopenia or bleeding diathesis *Infection in the skin or underlying tissue at or near the puncture site

Equipment:
All equipment must be sterile, except safety razor and facemask. *Gloves and facemask *Cup with iodophor antiseptic solution *Gauze swabs *Drapes or surgical towels *Two short bevel needles, 19 to 22 gauge x 1 in, with stylets *Specimen tubes with caps *Adhesive bandage *Safety razor

Precautions
*Use strict aseptic technique as for a major procedure. *Insert the needle as far laterally as possible at the border of the anterior fontanelle or along the coronal suture, at least 1 to 2 cm from the midline, to avoid puncturing the sagittal sinus. Do not direct the needle medially during insertion. *Remove the needle if there is not a definite change in resistance on penetrating the dura after insertion to approximately 0.5 to 1 cm. *Hold the needle securely at all times to avoid inadvertent movement of the needle tip. Grasp the needle firmly or apply a hemostat at approximately 1 cm from the beveled end of the needle to prevent inadvertent advancement of the needle into the cerebral cortex. *Allow fluid to drain spontaneously. Do not aspirate with a syringe. *Limit fluid collected to 15 to 20 mL from each side. Removal of larger volumes can lead to bleeding into the subdural space. *If frequent taps are required, vary the puncture site slightly to prevent fistula formation. *Following the procedure, apply pressure to the scalp for 2 to 3 minutes to prevent fluid leak from the puncture site or subgaleal fluid collection. *Technique* *Place the infant supine, with the crown of the head at the table edge. Monitor cardiorespiratory status. *Have the assistant restrain the infant and steady the infant's head *Shave the head over a wide area surrounding the anterior fontanelle *Locate the junctions of the coronal sutures and anterior fontanelle. *Put on mask. Wash hands thoroughly and put on sterile gloves.Clean the fontanelle and surrounding area three times with antiseptic solution. *Begin at the fontanelle and wash in enlarging circles. *Allow antiseptic to dry. Blot excess with sterile gauze. *Cover infant's head with sterile drapes, leaving the anterior fontanelle and the infant's nose and mouth exposed. *Locate the coronal suture by palpation at the lateral corner of the anterior fontanelle. Generally, anesthesia is not required, but local injection of lidocaine at this time or application of topical anesthetic cream prior to cleaning the area can be used for local anesthesia at the puncture sites . *Insert the needle slowly through the coronal suture, just lateral to its junction with the anterior fontanelle . *Hold the needle perpendicular to the skin surface. *Grasp the needle shaft with thumb and index finger, bracing the hand against the infant's head to maintain control of the needle during insertion . *As the needle advances through the skin, pull the scalp slightly to create a Z-like track through the underlying tissue. This will help prevent fluid leakage from the puncture site or into the subgaleal space after removal of the needle. Advance until a "pop" is felt upon penetrating the dura. Remove the stylet . *Allow fluid to drain spontaneously into the sterile tubes until flow ceases or a maximum volume of 15 to 20 mL is reached. Fluid is sent for protein content, cell count, and culture. If no fluid appears, replace the stylet and remove the needle slowly. *Do not reinsert on the same side. Repeat the procedure on the opposite side with a new, sterile needle. After removing the needle, apply firm pressure to the puncture site with sterile gauze for 2 to 3 minutes. *Dress the puncture site with a small adhesive bandage.

Complications:
1)Subdural bleeding from laceration of the superior sagittal sinus or smaller vessels or from removal of excessive fluid with shift of intracranial contents and rebleeding 2)Infection 3)Trauma to the underlying cortex caused by inserting the needle too far 4)Fistula formation after repeated taps.

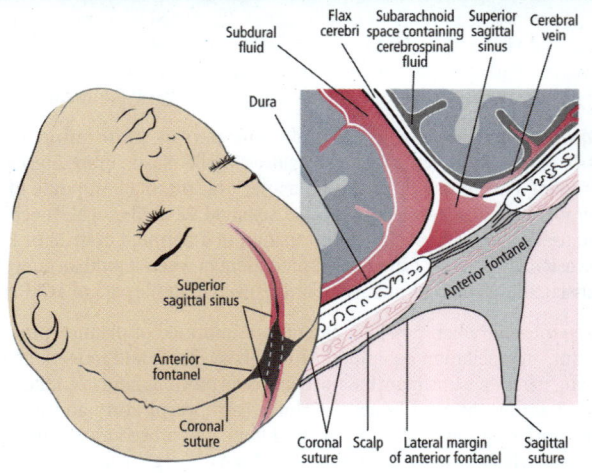

The subdural space lies beneath the skin, subcutaneous tissue, skull, and dura. In young infants, the major landmark for a subdural tap is the lateral margin of the anterior fontanel.

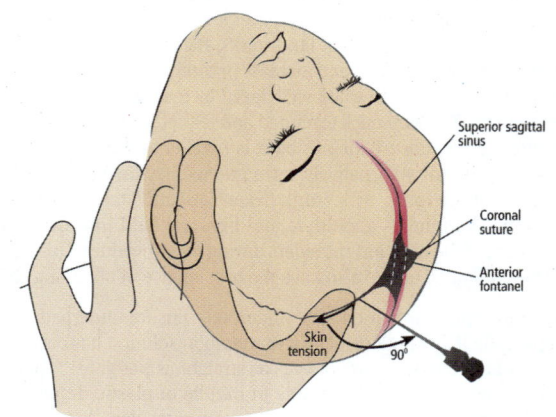

Subdural puncture: As the needle advances through the skin, pull the scalp slightly to create a Z-like track through the underlying tissue. This will help prevent fluid leakage from the puncture site or into the subgaleal space after removal of the needle. Advance until a "pop" is felt upon penetrating the dura.

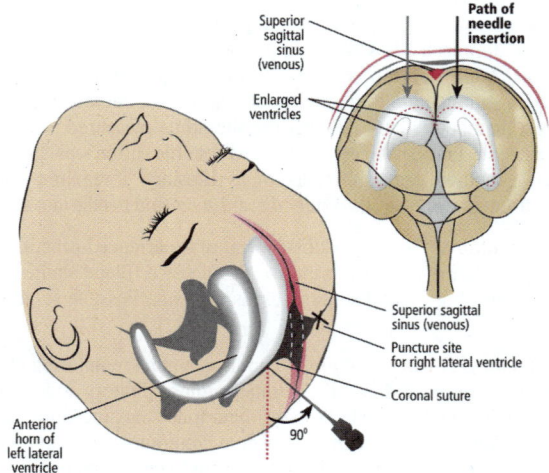

Ventricular puncture and removal of CSF- can be life-saving for the child with severe hydrocephalus and cerebral herniation that is unresponsive to hyperventilation and diuretics. The needle is inserted perpendicular to the skull at the lateral border of the anterior fontanelle.

SUPRAPUBIC ASPIRATION OF URINE

Suprapubic aspiration of urine is the first line investigation of infants strongly suspected of having a urinary tract infection and/or requiring antibiotics *bag urine collection is only useful for exclusion of infection if there is no growth of organisms *urine may also be collected via urethral catheter, although (particularly in males), this should only be performed by an experienced clinician.

Suprapubic aspiration of urine (SPA)

*the indications for SPA include *urine sampling *relief of obstruction (rarely) - a suprapubic catheter is a better option in this setting *the equipment required includes *2 ml or 5ml syringe *25g or 23g needle *skin preparation *sterile specimen container *assistant to stop baby moving/extending legs *consider use of ultrasound to guide attempt (particularly if failed already) *residents not familiar with this procedure should consult a more senior clinician, if possible *consider infant's need for pain relief including possible use of *application of EMLA (0.5 -1g) to proposed site 60-90 minutes before procedure *use of oral sucrose (link to section) *subcutaneous infiltration of lignocaine

Procedure

*wash hands *no touch technique *prepare skin, allow to dry *attach needle to syringe *insertion site is 1 cm above symphysis pubis, strictly in midline *aim is at 90 deg to skin - straight in (bladder is an abdominal organ in infants) *advance with gentle suction, stopping when urine is obtained *decant into suitable container *if unsuccessful, alter angle by about 10 deg and advance again, keeping in midline If no urine is obtained after two adjustments of aim, it is likely that bladder is empty. Wait 45-60 minutes and try again. *Interpretation of results *any leucocytes cells detected on SPA are regarded as abnormal *any growth in an SPA is theoretically abnormal unless it is clearly a contaminant (e.g. Staph. epidermidis or heavy mixed growth of faecal bacteria) *there is no limit to the red cell count due to the difficulty in distinguishing traumatic bleeding from true hematuria.

Bag urine collection

*the indications for a bag urine include *failed SPA *low index of suspicion of urinary tract infection (UTI) *infant not requiring antibiotics *collection of urine for purposes other than exclusion of bacterial infection (e.g. analysis of specific gravity, glucose, protein etc) *preparation includes *area to which bag is applied requires washing with soap and sterile water, rinsing with sterile water and drying *the bag must be applied with a no touch technique (using sterile gloves) results are only useful for exclusion of infection if *no growth *results are not useful if *pure growth *mixed growth of >= 100,000 bacteria *infants already on antibiotics *a UTI should never be diagnosed or treated on the basis of a bag urine alone *microscopy on bag urine is not warranted, a dip-slide (urinalysis) is more useful.

Recommended testing *in a very ill infant, strongly suspected of having a UTI and requiring immediate antibiotics: *take SPA specimen *if SPA fails, commence antibiotics *collect SPA as soon as possible *bag urine specimen useless *in an infant strongly suspected of having a UTI and requiring antibiotics, but not immediately *take SPA specimen *if SPA fails, repeat after one hour *consider use of ultrasound to aid sample collection *defer antibiotic therapy until SPA obtained, but do not await result *bag urine specimen useless *in an infant with an illness that might be a UTI but not immediately requiring treatment: *take SPA specimen *if SPA fails, order bag urine specimen *if bag urine specimen result equivocal, take SPA specimen and await result *if bag urine specimen strongly suggests UTI, take SPA specimen and commence antibiotics *adjust therapy when SPA result known.

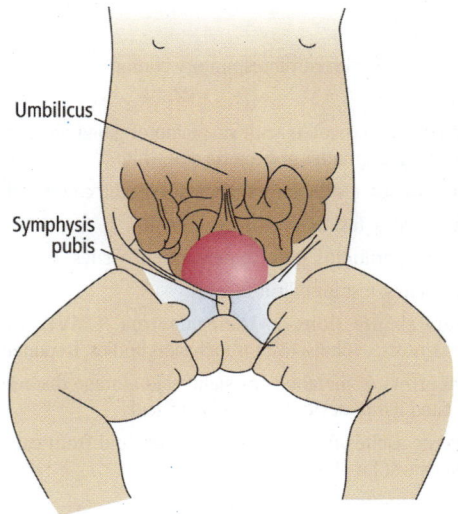

Umbilicus

Symphysis pubis

SUPRAPUBIC ASPIRATION

The site for puncture is 1-2 cm above the symphysis pubis in the midline; use 22G, 1-inch needle, puncture at a 10–20 degree angle to the perpendicular to skin.

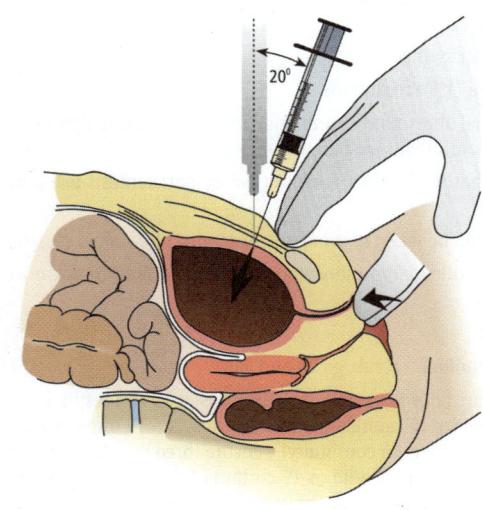

20°

Suprapubic bladder aspiration:Practical tips

1. Have assistant restrain infant in supine, frog-leg position.

2. Diaper has been dry for at least 1hr.

3. The site for needle insertion is 1–2 cm above the symphysis pubis in the midline.

4. Palpate symphysis pubis and insert needle approximately 1–2 cm above the pubic symphysis at a 90 degree angle.

5. Stop advancing the needle once urine is seen in the syringe (usually not more than 2–3 cc).

6. Withdraw needle if no urine is obtained.

7. Wait at least 1hr before repeating procedure.

ABDOMINAL PARACENTESIS

Indications:

* Therapeutic
- Massive ascites with cardiorespiratory compromise
* Diagnostic
- Necrotizing enterocolitis with suspicion of gangrene or perforation, looking for fecal matter or bacteria and white blood cells on a smear
- Chylous ascites: testing for lymphocytes on cell count of the fluid
- Urinary ascites: test for creatinine content
- Meconium peritonitis: gross appearance of ascites
- Biliary ascites: test for bilirubin level.
- Congenital infections- cytomegalovirus (CMV), tuberculosis, toxoplasmosis, syphilis: test for inclusion bodies, treponemes
- Inborn errors of metabolism- sialic acid storage disorders: test for vacuolated lymphocytes and free sialic acid
- Iatrogenic ascites from extravasation of fluid from central venous catheters: test for glucose content

Contraindications:

Coagulopathy is a relative contraindication; the procedure may be performed with concomitant treatment of thrombocytopenia or coagulopathy

Equipment:

* 24- or 25-gauge catheter over a needle (e.g. Angiocath)
* 5- or 10-mL syringe
* Skin topical disinfectant
* Sterile towels
* Tubes for culture, Gram stain, and cell count
* Tuberculin syringe
* Lidocaine (1%)Precautions
* abdominal ultrasound examination may be helpful in determining the appropriate site for paracentesis
* ensure that the bladder is empty before paracentesis using midline route
* care should be taken to avoid any distended abdominal vessels
* coagulopathies or thrombocytopenia do not contraindicate procedure·

Procedure:

*aseptic technique - scrub, gown and glove

*prepare skin, allowing solution to dry *insert local anesthetic solution *attach needle or IV cannula to three way tap *attach three way tap to 10 ml or 30 ml syringe (in continuity) *ensure three way tap is 'on' to baby and syringe *insert needle or IV cannula *either in midline halfway between the umbilicus and the symphysis pubis *or in either lower quadrant several centimeters above the inguinal ligament, lateral to the rectus muscle and in a line with the nipples *slowly advance needle or cannula whilst gently aspirating syringe *stop when fluid obtained. If using IV cannula, push catheter off needle *remove stylet, connecting syringe via three way tap to catheter *aspirate desired amount of fluid *may be 100-200 ml *should be <2% of (estimated) body weight *remove needle/cannula, applying firm pressure to site until ooze stops *apply adhesive dressing

Complications:

*Bleeding from the liver or intra-abdominal vessels; may be severe enough to require a laparotomy

*Intestinal perforation; usually inconsequential because the catheter and needle are of small diameter.

If fluid is not free-flowing, the catheter might be inside the lumen of a piece of intestine or in the retroperitoneum. The catheter is withdrawn and the maneuver repeated with the catheter at a slightly different angle

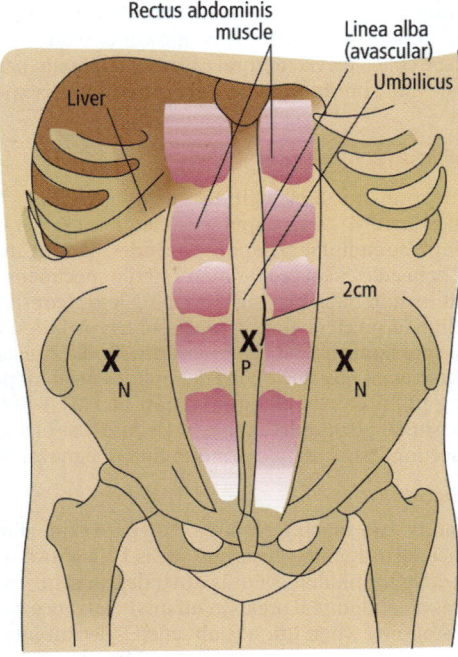

Neonatal insertion site (N) below the umbilicus, lateral to the rectus abdominis muscle. Pediatric insertion site (P) along the midline at the avascular linea alba

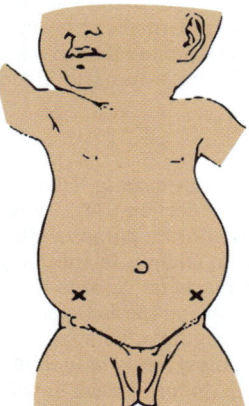

Abdominal Paracentesis

Position: supine with both legs restrained

Choose the site for paracentesis.

The area between the umbilicus and the pubic bone is generally used in Neonates.

The site most frequently used are the right and left flanks. A good rule is to draw a horizontal line passing through the umbilicus and select a site between this line and the inguinal ligament.

Insert the needle at the selected site perpendicular to the skin with a " Z-track " technique to prevent persistent leakage of fluid after the tap.

Advance the needle until fluid appears.

Remove the needle and cover with a gauze.

PERITONEAL DIALYSIS IN NEONATES

Renal replacement therapy may be provided by peritoneal dialysis, intermittent hemodialysis, or hemofiltration with or without a dialysis circuit. *The preferential use of hemofiltration by pediatric nephrologists is increasing while the use of peritoneal dialysis is decreasing except for neonates and small infants. Peritoneal dialysis has been a major modality of therapy for acute renal failure in the neonate when vascular access may be difficult to maintain.* Early institution of Peritoneal Dialysis during acute renal failure reduces mortality and morbidity in Neonates, infants and children.

Peritoneal Dialysis (PD), also referred to as parental leaching, is frequently a better neonatal option than hemodialysis because smaller infants can ill afford to lose the blood volume necessary to prime the hemodialysis blood circuit. Despite the advantages of hemodialysis, the process in neonates is technically more challenging than PD due to the very attributes that make it so effective. Rapid removal of intravascular fluids, exceeding the rate of refill from the extravascular space, causes problems with hypotension due to direct reduction in intravascular volume. Similarly, rapid rates of solute clearance can cause problems with increased intracranial pressure. Catheter placement and maintenance of catheter function can constitute a significant obstacle to hemodialysis.

Continuous flow peritoneal dialysis. (CFPD) represents other modality for renal replacement therapy without the abdominal discomfort in comparison with classical peritoneal dialysis,and there is no need to establish additional vascular access.CFPD do not adversely affect the respiratory status of patients,and that is advantage particular by mechanical ventilation. Continuous inflow and outflow is provided via twin catheters,but recently it is possible through one-dual lumen catheter with an excellent distribution of the fluid in the peritoneal cavity and negligible recirculation.The inflow rate,volume and osmolality of the dialysate,total treatment time,and peritoneal transport specifics are important aspects that influence the efficiency of CFPD. The concept of CFPD is another approach to optimize peritoneal dialysis in infants with metabolic attacks,multi-organ failure and in hemodynamically unstable patients. CFPD can be administered quickly and easily in premature neonates with acute renal failure. Continuous flow peritoneal dialysis is an effective therapy for acute renal insufficiency,metabolic crisis in neonates.Extracorporeal hemofiltration is the preferential method in infants with inborn errors of metabolism.

Indications: 1) Hyperkalemia 2) Fluid Overload 3) Refractory Acidosis 4) Uremic symptoms 5) Metabolic abnormalities (Inborn Errors Of Metabolism) 6) Evolving Renal Failure-Post Cardiac Surgery.

Contraindications: 1) Absolute- Gastroschisis / Omphalocele, Diaphragmatic Hernia, Bladder Extrophy, Obliterated Peritoneal Cavity   2) Relative- Recent Abdominal Surgery, Abdominal Malignancy.

Equipment : Peritoneal Dialysis Catheter, Betadine and Dressing Pack, Sterile towel, Syringes, Needles, Sterile Gloves, Dressing Pack,Lignocaine 1%, Scalpel, Stitch, Elastoplast (SLEEK), Scissors, Stitch holder, Quickcath/Venflon. Monitoring of patients clinical condition during procedure is essential. • SaO2 • Respiratory rate and effort • Heart rate • Blood Pressure Resuscitation equipment must be available.

Acute peritoneal dialysis circuit: Water Heater, Acute Peritoneal Dialysis Set, Dialysate,

Baxter homechoice circuit : Lines, Dialysate, *Pac –X circuit:* Lines, Dialysate

Acute Peritoneal Dialysis – Checklist for Insertion: Consent, Group and Save Blood,Ensure Bladder Emptied, Sedation/Analgesia or Anesthesia. Prior to insertion the patients should be examined by the clinician who will insert the peritoneal dialysis and a decision taken on the site of insertion and the appropriate peritoneal dialysis catheter. Insertion can be undertaken in the left upper quadrant or below the umbilicus depending on local practice and operator preference.

In the presence of coagulation abnormalities insertion should be undertaken surgically

Procedure: 1. Establish I.V. Access 2. Sedate/Anesthetize Child 3. Position supine on bed 4. Ensure bladder empty 5. Examine Child and mark insertion point 6. Clean with Betadine 7. Incise skin ~0.5-1.0cm 8. Insert scalpel into rectus abdominus along intended tract (mainly required in older children only) 9. Connect patient end of dialysis circuit to a 22g Cannula 10. Insert cannula into rectus abdominus along tract 11. Open circuit to allow fluid to run into patient 12. Fluid will not run in as cannula in rectus abdominus 13. Advance cannula towards pelvis whilst looking at drip chamber containing dialysate 14. Once the peritoneal cavity is entered the dialysate will begin to flow 15. Withdraw metal stylet form cannula and reconnect dialysate tubing to cannula 16. Prime abdomen with 10ml/kg of dialysate 17. Insert guidewire through cannula which should then be removed 18. Dilate tract with dilator 19. Insert peritoneal dialysis catheter over guidewire to cuff level if possible 20. Remove guidewire 21. Suture peritoneal dialysis catheter in place 22. Place scissors at the middle of one side of the square gauze and cut to midpoint. 23. Slide gauze along cut edge so that midpoint is placed next to the catheter 24. Secure catheter with SLEEK 25. Connect to peritoneal dialysis circuit and check catheter patency 26. Observe PD effluent for the presence of blood or faeces. **Ensure catheter is well secured.**

Acute Peritoneal Dialysis – Prescription : Initial Prescription

Initial Fill:10ml/Kg

Solution: 1.36%

Fill Time: 5 minutes

Dwell Time: 5 minutes

Drain Time : 5 minutes

- Repeat until fluid visibly clear.

- In patients with tense ascites limit fluid removal to 5ml/kg with each of the initial cycles

- Last fill of 50–100 ml in female patients to reduce risk of blockage by ovarian fimbrae

Regular Prescription

Fill Volume* 10-30ml/kg (Target 30ml/kg)

Solution** (1.36%)

Fill Time 5 minutes

Dwell Time* 45 minutes

Drain Time 10 minutes

*Start with lower volumes. If there is no leakage or respiratory embarrassment then increase fill volume

**Combinations of concentration can be used. There is no indication for using a net concentration of over 3% as this merely causes severe hypotension by depleting the intravascular volume. In neonates use of concentrations above this level is potentially fatal. In cases of lactic acidosis a bicarbonate dialysate can be useful.

***Variations in dwell time allow greater clearances of solute or fluid. In severe hyperkalemia shortened dwell times of 15 minutes should be used

Additives:

- **Heparin:** 500u/L for first 48 hours. This can be omitted if fluid is subsequently visibly clear.

- **Antibiotics:** Gentamicin 5 mg/L & Vancomycin 25 mg/L.

- **Potassium:** Add 4mmol/L when serum Potassium is <3.5mmol/L unless there concerns regarding a potential sudden rise in Potassium.

Complications in the neonate often include: peritonitis; exit-site infections; leaks around the exit site;catheter obstruction; abdominal-wall hernias; and respiratory embarrassment, whereby during dwell time the abdomen is so full it places pressure upon the lungs. Often ventilatory support needs to be increased to reverse this.

Peritoneal Equilibration Test - Data Collection

Name: .... Date: .... No: ....

Weight: .... Height: .... Surface Area: ....

Overnight Dwell:

Duration: .... Volume In: .... Volume Out: ....

TIME :	Urea :	Creatinine :	Sodium :	Glucose :
Serum	:			
Overnight	:			
Dialysate	:			
0-Time	:			
Dialysate	:			
2-hours	:			
Dialysate	:			
4-hours	:			
Dialysate	:			
Equilibration Test	:			

Time Start: .... Time to fill: .... Finished: ....

No general rule of thumb appears to exist for **dwell volumes**. They appear to be estimated based on the degree of renal failure and the presenting symptoms.

Short **dwell times** are used — from 30 minutes to 2 hours — based on the degree of renal failure and the goal of treatment: ie, fluid removal over removal of uraemic toxins.

Acute peritoneal dialysis in very low birth weight neonates using a vascular catheter: We report on our experience with acute peritoneal dialysis (APD) in 16 very low birth weight neonates ranging from 24.6 to 30.2 weeks' gestation with a birth weight ranging from 630 g to 1,430 g using a 14-gauge Arrow vascular catheter for APD access. The underlying causes of acute renal failure were: sepsis (7), necrotizing enterocolitis (4), patent ductus arteriosus (3), hydrops fetalis (1), intracranial hemorrhage (3), pulmonary hemorrhage (2), pneumonia (1), and perinatal asphyxia (1). Among 12 patients, the APD was successful for the control of hyperkalemia, fluid overload, and metabolic acidosis. The peritoneal permeability and transport were at their maximum at a short dwell time with rapid exchanges. Complications associated with the APD were: peritonitis (2), leakage (2), hemoperitoneum (1), and hernia (1). During the dialysis, four patients died; there were three episodes of catheter-related complications in these patients. At 60 days after the withdrawal of the APD, 10 patients were alive, and had full recovery of their renal function. Therefore, APD in premature neonates with a 14-gauge Arrow vascular catheter was safe and effective. This procedure helped manage the hemodynamic and metabolic imbalance of acute renal failure and was associated with few complications. Yu JE, Park MS, Pai KS. Department of Pediatrics, School of Medicine, Ajou University, San 5 Wonchon-dong, Yongtong-gu, Suwon 443-721, Korea.

Similarly, a 16-Gauge IV angiocath connected with two ordinary IV infusion sets (substitutesThe "Y" connection set), one of which connected the dialysate bottle to the cannula while the other drained outflow fluid from the cannula to the drainage bottle is useful to perform Peritoneal Dialysis.This technique has the following added advantage over conventional dialysis: *(a)* It is least traumatic to the patient; *(b)* The chance of damaging any viscus is less; (c) It is cheaper since it obviates the need for procuring the neonatal peritoneal dialysis catheter and "Y" connection sets; and *(d)* Dialysis can be performed even at peripheral/small hospital settings and nursing homes.B. Rath, S. Gopalan, Samir Gupta, R.K. Purl, B. Talukdar, *Department of Pediatrics, Maulana Azad Medical College and Associated LNJPN Hospital, New Delhi 110 002*

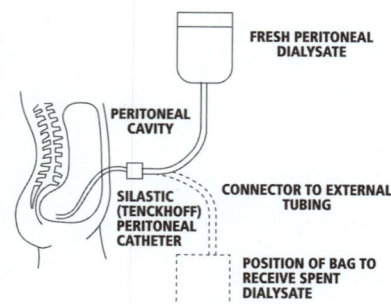

FRESH PERITONEAL DIALYSATE

PERITONEAL CAVITY

SILASTIC (TENCKHOFF) PERITONEAL CATHETER

CONNECTOR TO EXTERNAL TUBING

POSITION OF BAG TO RECEIVE SPENT DIALYSATE

Peritoneal dialysis (PD) is generally considered the optimal dialysis modality for neonates. PD allows for the slow removal of fluid and solutes while avoiding hemodynamic instability. It is technically simple and, when necessary, can be performed continuously in the neonate hospitalized in the neonatal intensive care unit.

Troubleshooting:

Fluid won't run in

- Check height of fill bag
- Check correct taps open
- Check air inlet valves on burette
- Check for kinked lines
- Reposition patient

Fluid won't run out

- Check correct taps open
- Check for kinked lines
- Reposition patient
- Check cycle was run in
- Refill if first time
- Call for help.

Fluid is leaking

- Decrease fill volume
- Check catheter insertion site
- Check taps closed

Fluid is cloudy

- Check for peritonitis
- Send PD Fluid for
  Urgent microscopy
  Gram stain
  Culture

Acute Peritoneal Dialysis – Peritonitis Protocol

* **Clinical Features of Peritonitis**

- Cloudy Dialysate
- Raised Dialysate white count
- Bacteria on Gram Stain
- Abdominal distension
- Abdominal Pain
- Features of sepsis

*Investigation

- Dialysate for culture, microscopy and gram stain
- Blood cultures
- FBC, U&E's, LFT's and CRP

*Treatment

- Increased cycle frequency (flushes)
- I.P. Gentamicin 5mg/L
- I.P. Vancomycin 25mg/L
- I.P. Heparin 500units/L

Access for peritoneal dialysis in Neonates and infants

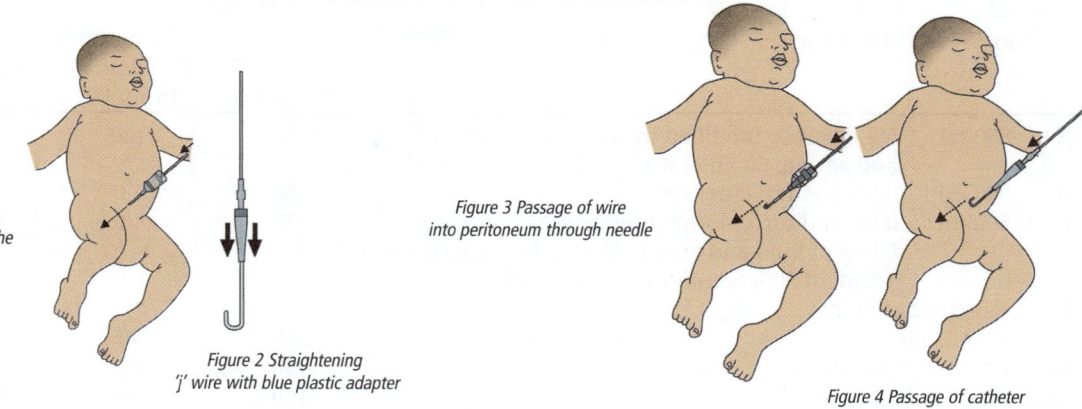

Figure 1 Insertion of the introducer needle into the peritoneum

Figure 2 Straightening 'j' wire with blue plastic adapter

Figure 3 Passage of wire into peritoneum through needle

Figure 4 Passage of catheter over wire into peritoneum

Acute renal failure is a common complication of severe illness in neonates and infants and the treatment of choice is early peritoneal dialysis. ' One difficulty is the introduction of a suitable peritoneal catheter. Several catheters and techniques have previously been described in neonates, all of which require the introduction of a plastic catheter into the peritoneum, either over a trocar (as in adult acute peritoneal dialysis) or over a stylet (as when inserting an intravenous cannula). The 'Pendlebury' catheter (Medcomp) is based on a percutaneous hemodialysis catheter. It is made of polyurethane, 14 gauge internal diameter, and 5*1 or 8-9 cm long. There are four side holes, the most proximal being 2-6 cm from the distal end. It is soft and pliable (particularly at body temperature), but it does not kink. Using a 'j' wire makes introduction safer because the wire will not advance easily if the tip of the introducing needle is in subcutaneous tissue or in a viscus rather than in the peritoneal cavity. This means that priming of the abdomen is not essential and can be omitted if it is felt the patient would not tolerate high intra-abdominal pressures. The catheter itself is moulded to a short soft plastic extension tube that terminates in a female Luer lock connection. It is introduced by the Seldinger technique over a 'j' wire, as described below. Free gravitational flow rates of 140 ml/min at a height of 100 cm can be achieved, allowing efficient dialysis in children weighing up to 14 kg with standard volumes. Introduce the catheter at the level of the umbilicus just lateral to the rectus sheath, but it can be introduced anywhere along a line parallel to the rectus sheath, or in the midline below the umbilicus. After preparation of the skin, local anaesthetic (1% lignocaine) is injected into the site, and a 22 gauge IV cannula introduced. This is primed with saline and then removed. The pink hubbed introducer needle is then inserted straight through into the peritoneum. This is flushed with 5 ml normal saline and aspirated to ensure bowel content is not retrieved (fig 1). This needle is left resting in the peritoneum, and the 'j' tip of the guidewire is straightened using the blue plastic adapter on it (fig 2). This adapter is then placed into the hub of the introducer needle and the wire advanced through the needle into the peritoneum (fig 3). As the 'j' end of the wire emerges through the tip of the needle a 'give' is felt as the resistance against the advancing wire is reduced. The wire should now advance a further 1-4 cm without any resistance. If there is resistance, the tip of the wire might either be in bowel or in subcutaneous tissue, in which case the needle and wire can be removed and the procedure started again. With the wire resting in the peritoneum the blue plastic adapter and needle are removed. The catheter is now threaded over the wire (fig 4), in preterm infants there is no need to make a skin incision-the catheter can simply be forced through with a 'screwing' action. There is no risk of the catheter causing intraabdominal injury as it will simply follow the wire. In the infant born at full term, and in older infants, a 3-4 mm skin incision around the wire will make passage through the skin easier. Once the catheter has been inserted the wire is removed, the catheter is connected to a peritoneal dialysis delivery system, and the soft plastic extension of the catheter is taped to the skin. **Courtesy:** M A Lewis, I B Houston, R J Postlethwaite, Royal Manchester Children's Hospital, Department of Pediatric Nephrology, Department of Child Health, UK.

SUPRAHEPATIC APPROACH FOR PERITONEAL DIALYSIS IN NEONATAL CARDIAC SURGERY

Figure 1. The catheter is seen in the lower part of the operative wound; the Dacron cuff is above the skin level and the catheter is visualized going into the abdominal cavity above the liver.

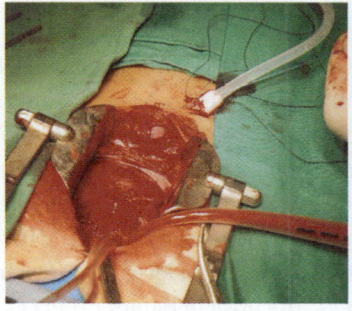

Figure 2. Postoperative radiography in a Neonate. The catheter is seen emerging from above the liver and coursing towards the left flank.

*Capillary leak syndrome is common in neonates after cardiopulmonary bypass for complex cardiac surgery. This can cause acute renal failure with increased mortality. Postoperative peritoneal dialysis has been shown to reduce this complication. *Placement of a peritoneal catheter by the conventional trocar technique may cause bowel perforation and bleeding, especially when clotting factors are abnormal. Bacterial peritonitis is also a cause for concern. *During suprahepatic insertion of the catheter into the peritoneal cavity, there is no fear of injury to the liver as the procedure is performed under direct vision. Because the catheter is inserted superior to the omentum, herniation cannot occur. Furthermore, the relatively small omentum in neonates cannot trap the catheter and displace or occlude it when it is introduced from above. Care must be taken to ensure an adequate length of catheter inside the abdomen (a 42–46-cm silicone Tenckhoff peritoneal dialysis catheter (Quinton Instrument Co, Bothell, WA, USA) to reach the flank for satisfactory drainage. *The soft silicone catheter is safe and nonirritant, reducing the risk of peritoneal infection or irritation. Use of a low volume (10 mL·kg–1 cycled each hour) and low osmolarity dialysate with a short indwelling time has not caused peritoneal irritation, and the closed drainage system has avoided infection. Removal of the catheter is easy and has not been associated with omental prolapse. *Suprahepatic introduction of the peritoneal catheter has the advantage of being performed through the operative wound. It can be used routinely in all neonates after cardiopulmonary bypass for cardiac surgery. However, it is not advocated for chronic peritoneal dialysis or for older patients. **Courtesy:** Anil Kumar Dharmapuram, MCh, Timothy Boyd Cartmill, FRACS, Ivatury Mrutyunjaya Rao, MCh *Department of Cardiac Surgery Al Mafraq Hospital Abu Dhabi, United Arab Emirates, Asian Cardiovasc Thorac Ann 2003;11:362–3.*

Solutions for neonatal peritoneal dialysis

Solution		Preparation	Final concentration		
			Sodium (mmol/l)	Bicarbonate (mmol/l)	Glucose (%)
A	500 ml	5% dextrose modified by removing 60 ml of fluid and adding 60 ml of 8.4% sodium bicarbonate	120	120	4.4
B	500 ml	0.9% sodium chloride	150	0	0
C	500 ml	0.9% sodium chloride modified by removing 50 ml of fluid and adding 50 ml of 50% dextrose and 1.5 ml of 30% (strong) sodium chloride	150	0	5.0
Potential combinations:					
1/3 A plus 2/3 B			140	40	1.47
1/3 A plus 1/2 B plus 1/6 C			140	40	2.30
1/3 A plus 1/3 B plus 1/3 C			140	40	3.13
1/3 A plus 2/3 C			140	40	4.80

Drugs used to combat infection and their clearance from the body in babies with severe renal failure before or during peritoneal dialysis (PD)

Drug	Dose adjustment needed	Comment
Acyclovir	Very High	Quadruple the dose interval. Removal by PD is poor
Amikacin	Measure	Judge dose interval from trough serum level. Removal by PD is slow.
Amoxycillin	Some	Increase the dose interval, or give one IV dose and put 125 mg/l in the PD fluid
Amphotericin	None	Give IV treatment as normal. The drug is not removed by PD
Ampicillin	Some	Increase the dose interval, or give one IV dose and put 125 mg/l in the PD fluid
Azlocillin	Some	Increase the dose interval. Removal by PD is slow.
Aztreonam	High	Halve the dose. The drug is not removed by PD.
Cefotaxime	Some	Increase the dose interval, or give one IV dose and put 125 mg/l in the PD fluid
Cefoxitin	High	Double the dose interval, or give one IV dose and put 125 mg/l in the PD fluid
Ceftazidime	High	Double the dose interval, or give one IV dose and put 125 mg/l in the PD fluid
Ceftriaxone	Some	Reduce dose if there is both renal and liver failure. Removal by PD is poor.
Cefuroxime	High	Double the dose interval, or give one IV dose and put 125 mg/l in the PD fluid
Chloramphenicol	None	Use with caution - metabolites accumulate. The drug is not removed by PD.
Clindamycin	Minimal	Give IV treatment as normal. The drug is not removed by PD.
Ciprofloxacin	High	Halve the dose. Crystalluria may occur. The drug is not removed by PD.
Erythromycin	None	Give IV as normal. The drug is not removed by PD.
Flucloxacillin	Minimal	Give IV as normal, or give one dose IV and put 250 mg/l in the PD fluid.
Fluconazole	High	Double the dose interval or, in babies on PD, put 7 mg/l in the PD fluid.
Flucytosine	Measure	Monitor the serum level or, in babies on PD, put 50 mg/l in the PD fluid.
Gentamicin	Measure	Judge dose interval from trough serum level. Removal by PD is slow.
Isoniazid	None	Give oral or IV treatment as normal. The drug is removed by PD.
Meropenem	High	Double the dose interval. It is not known if the drug is removed by PD.
Netilmicin	Measure	Judge dose interval from trough serum level. Removal by PD is slow.
Metronidazole	None	Give IV as normal. *Increase* the dose in babies on PD as this removes the drug.
Penicillin	Substantial	Use with caution - penicillin is neurotoxic. Removal by PD is poor.
Rifampicin	None	Give oral or IV treatment as normal. The drug is not removed by PD.
Teicoplanin	Moderate	Give IV if level can be measured, or give one IV dose and put 20 mg/l in PD fluid.
Trimethoprim	Moderate	Halve the IV dose after two days. Removal by PD is slow.
Vancomycin	Measure	Monitor the serum level, or give one IV dose and put 25 mg/l in the PD fluid.

Practical Hints: 1) Peritoneal Dialysis is the most effective strategy in most small babies, but surgical problems may occasionally make Hemodialysis necessary. 2) Use an in-line IV burette, and adjust the Glucose concentration by varying ingredients B and C in order to control ultrafiltration and the removal of water. 3) Because these dialysis fluids cannot contain calcium it is necessary to give supplemental calcium IV. Start with 1 mmol/kg a day and adjust as necessary. Magnesium may occasionally be needed. 4) Add Heparin (1 unit/ml) if the dialysis fluid is cloudy or blood stained to stop fibrin and clots obstructing the catheter. 5) Watch for peritonitis by microscoping and culturing the effluent fluid daily.

INTERCOSTAL CHEST DRAINAGE

Indications: **1)** Evacuation of pneumothorax *Tension *Lung collapse with ventilation/perfusion abnormality * Bronchopleural fistula **2)** Evacuation of large pleural fluid collections *Significant pleural effusion *Postoperative hemothorax *Empyema *Chylothorax *Extravasated fluid from a central venous line **3)** Extrapleural drainage after surgical repair of esophageal atresia and/or tracheoesophageal fistula

Contraindications: *Small air or fluid collection without significant hemodynamic symptoms *Spontaneous pneumothorax that, in the absence of lung disease, is likely to resolve without intervention

Equipment: Sterile *General all-purpose tray with no. 15 surgical blade and curved hemostats *Gloves *Surgical drapes *Transillumination device *Thoracostomy tube *Polyvinyl chloride (PVC) chest tube with or without trocar, in sizes 8, 10, and 12 French (Fr) *Cutting needle tip joined to a biopsy needle shaft with a collar that prevents the catheter from sliding up the needle during insertion *Evacuation device *Infant thoracostomy tube set. *Nonabsorbable suture on small cutting needle, * Cotton-tipped applicators *Semipermeable transparent dressing *Antibiotic ointment *Petroleum gauze Nonsterile *Tincture of benzoin *½-in adhesive tape *Towel roll

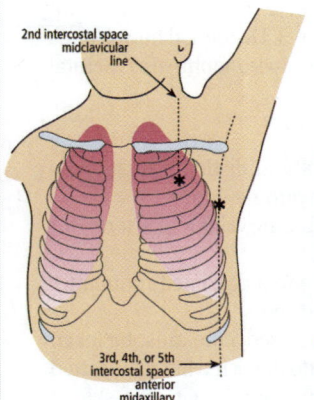

2nd intercostal space in the midclavicular line is used for needle decompression of a tension pneumothorax and the 3rd, 4th, or 5th ICSs are recommended for most patients who require evacuation of air/fluid from the chest.

Chest size tuber: Premature (1-2.5kg)-10-14 FG, Neonate (2.5-4 kg)-12-14 FG, Infant (6-8kg)-14-20 FG

Technique: Chest tube Insertion *Assemble equipment and assign duties to personnel *Explain procedure and obtain consent *Position the patient, and prepare and anesthetize skin and subcutaneous structures *Incise skin over rib below interspace of intended tube placement * Bluntly dissect subcutaneously and superiorly *Enter pleural space with clamp tips closed and confirm location by exploration with finger *Insert chest tube, directing tube superiorly and posteriorly *Attach to water seal and suction *Secure chest tube with suture, gauze, and tape *Obtain CXR.

If the tube is of the trocar variety, grasp tube with one hand close to the sharp trocar end and guide the tube slowly and gently through the hole in the pleura into the chest cavity (Figure 4). Remove trocar once tube has just entered the cavity, and feed tube in approximately 1/2 to 2/3 of its length, until all the fenestrations of the tube are within the chest.

Needle decompression: *1st 3 steps as above * Advance needle over superior aspect of rib while maintaining negative pressure in syringe *When air returns, advance catheter into pleural cavity *Remove needle and attach 3-way stopcock and large syringe *Evacuate pneumothorax *Obtain CXR.

Complications: Equipment malfunction,Infection, Subcutaneous emphysema secondary to leak of tension pneumothorax through pleural opening,Aortic obstruction with posterior tube, Misplacement of tube(Tube outside pleural cavity in subcutaneous placement) Horner syndrome caused by pressure from tip of right-sided, posterior chest tube near second thoracic ganglion at first thoracic intervertebral space, Diaphragmatic paralysis or eventration from phrenic nerve injury, Chylothorax, Lung laceration or perforation ,Misdiagnosis with inappropriate placement,Permanent damage to breast tissue

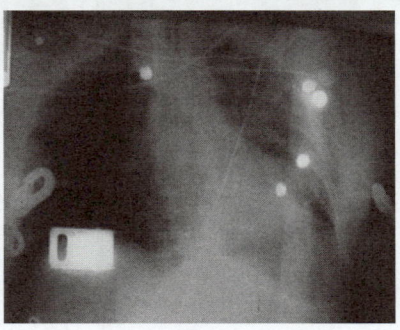

This picture shows a chest radiograph with 2 abnormalities: (1) tension pneumothorax and (2) potentially life-saving intervention delayed while waiting for x-ray results. Tension pneumothorax is a clinical diagnosis requiring emergent needle decompression, and therapy should never be delayed for x-ray confirmation.

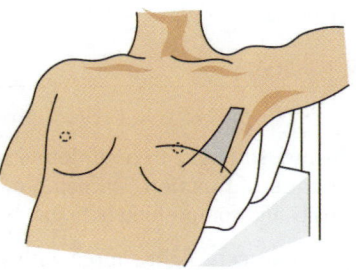

The most common position for chest tube insertion is in the mid-axillary line, through the 'safe triangle' illustrated in Figure above. This position minimizes risk to underlying structures such as the viscera and internal mammary artery and avoids damage to muscle and breast tissue resulting in unsightly scarring. A more posterior position may be chosen if suggested by the presence of a loculated collection.

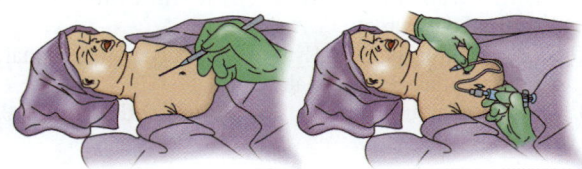

Emergency evacuation with a vascular cannula. Insert angiocatheter at point that is *at a 45-degree angle to skin, directed cephalad *in second, fourth, or fifth intercostal space, just over top of rib, well above or below the areolar of the breast *in midclavicular line

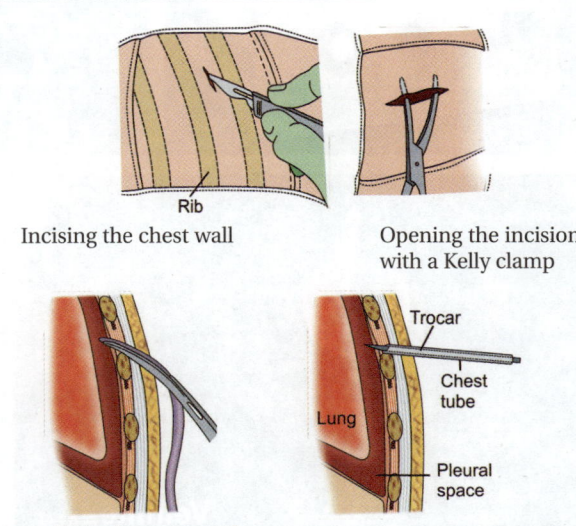

Incising the chest wall

Opening the incision with a Kelly clamp

Using a Kelly clamp to guide insertion of the chest tube

Inserting a trocar chest tube

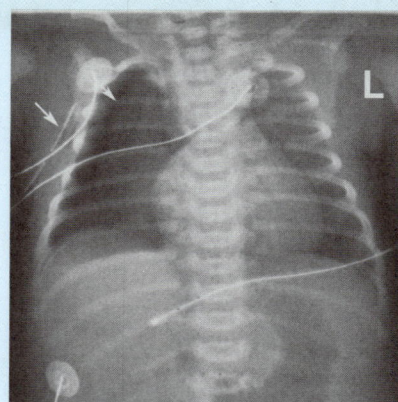

Intercostal drain: This baby has a right sided pneumothorax. The top white arrow identifies the lung edge An intercostal drain is malpositioned in the soft tissues of the chest wall.

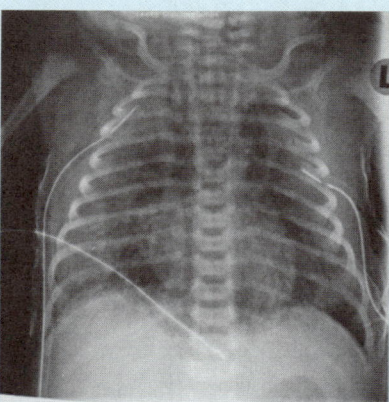

This baby has extensive subcutaneous emphysema. Both intercostal drains are malpositioned with their sideholes possibly in the chest wall soft tissues

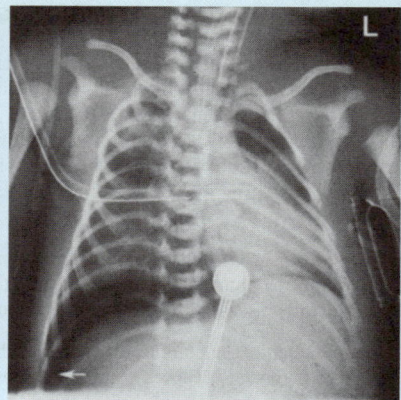

This baby has a right sided pneumothorax. Also note *LPO position *intercostal tube malposition *mediastinal shift **deep suclus sign** (white arrow) **silhouette sign** right hemidiaphragm *NGT

TRANSILLUMMINATION

I. Definition

A. Use of a high-intensity light to help define normal or abnormal structure of function. Diffusion of light is a function of density and composition of tissue.

B. Chun gun - incandescent light source with published standard lucencies for skull.Mini light - fiberoptic light source.

C. RMI, Omni light, Welch-Allyn - brightest available fiberoptic light sources.

II. The following conditions are generally associated with positive transillumination (with rim of lucency or abnormal dark area):

A. Skull 1. Hydrocephaly 2. Hydranencephaly 3. Anencephaly 4. Porencephaly 5. Encephalocele

B. Chest 1. Pneumothorax 2. Pneumomediastinum 3. Pneumopericardium

C. Abdomen 1. Distended bladder 2. Pneumoperitoneum (falciform ligament may be seen) 3. Distended bowel loops 4. Hydrocele 5. Cystic kidneys 6. Hydronephrosis 7. Scrotal masses

III. Miscellanenous

A. Transillumination may be helpful in distinguishing cystic from solid masses, e.g., cystic hygroma.

B. Transillumination is useful for finding veins and arteries for sampling or catheter insertion.

C. The procedure is more effective in a darkened room after time for visual adaptation to darkness.

D. If a high-intensity light source is used, care must be taken to avoid burning the patient. To do this, a red filter is inserted in front of the light source and contact with the skin is limited.

E. Cellophane should be used to cover the light head to prevent cross-contamination between babies.

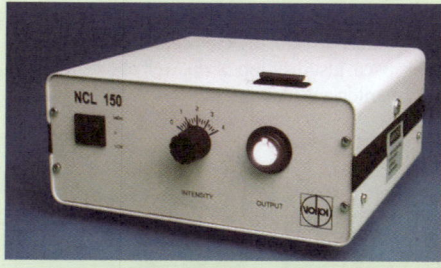

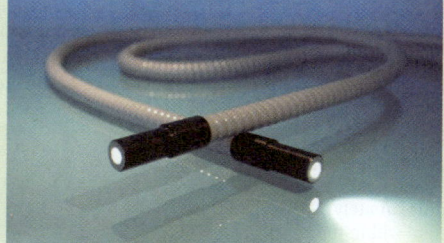

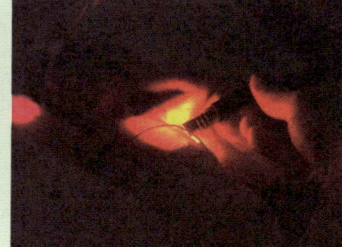

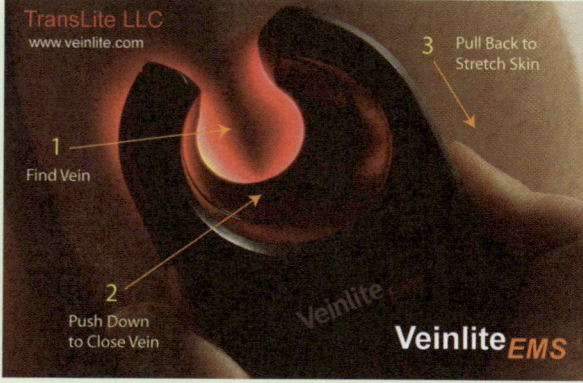

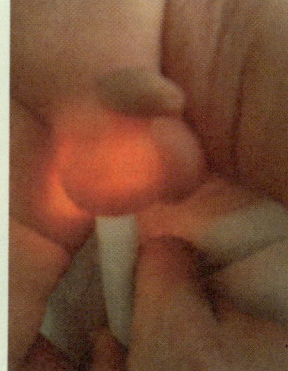

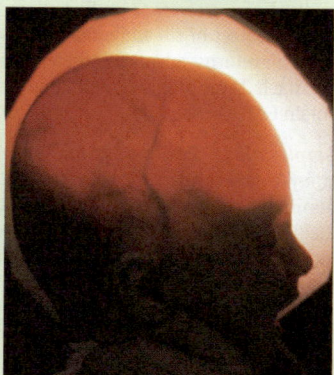

PERICARDIOCENTESIS

Indications

*Cardiac tamponade due to pneumopericardium
*Cardiac tamponade due to pericardial fluid
*Aspiration of pericardial fluid for diagnostic studies

Contraindications

*There are no absolute contraindications to performing peri-cardiocentesis in the setting of cardiac tamponade. *Relative contraindication for diagnostic pericardiocentesis *Coagulo-pathy *Active infection. (However, infection may also be an indication for diagnostic pericardiocentesis in some clinical situations.)

Equipment:

*Antiseptic solution *Sterile field with aperture drape or multiple drapes to be arranged around access site *Sterile swabs or gauze pads *Sterile gloves *Local anesthetic, as needed *16- to 20-gauge intravenous cannula over 1- to 2-in needle *Indwelling drainage catheter (optional) *Three-way stopcock *Short intravenous extension tubing (optional) *10- to 20-mL syringes *Preassembled closed drainage system as for Emergency Evacuation of Air Leaks, Thoracostomy Tubes (optional) *Connecting tubing and underwater seal for indwelling drain (optional) *Transillumination device (optional, for pneumopericardium) *Echocardiogram/sonography imaging device (optional in urgent situations)*Specimen containers for laboratory studies, if procedure is diagnostic

Technique:
*Position the patient in reverse Trendelenberg position to maximize success rate *Cleanse skin over xiphoid, precordium, and epigastric area with antiseptic. Allow to dry.*Arrange sterile drapes, leaving the subxiphoid area exposed.*Local anesthesia should be administered for the conscious patient. A typical example is 0.25 to 1.0 mL of subcutaneous 1% lidocaine instilled within 1 to 2 cm of the xiphoid process.*Assemble the needle/cannula, three-way stopcock, and syringe so that the stopcock is open to both the needle and the syringe, but closed to the remaining port.*The usual entry point in an infant is 0.5 to 1 cm below the tip of the xiphoid process, in the midline or slightly (0.5 cm) to the left of the midline. The needle should be elevated 30 to 40 degrees at the skin, and the tip should be directed toward the left shoulder *While advancing the needle, apply gentle negative pressure with the syringe. Continue advancing until air or fluid is obtained. If the syringe fills, use the third port of the stopcock to empty the syringe, or to attach a second syringe, and then aspirate more, repeating as needed. If diagnostic studies are desired, the fluid should be transferred to appropriate specimen containers.*If ultrasound imaging is available, it may be helpful in planning the needle entry site and angle, as well as anticipating the distance required to reach the pericardial space.

Complications

*Pneumopericardium*Pneumomediastinum *Pneumothorax *Cardiac perforation *Arrhythmia *Hypotension (if a large effusion is drained)

N.B: Pericardiocentesis is often an urgent or emergency procedure. The technique for pericardiocentesis described above applies when there is time for each step. In an infant with significant hemodynamic compromise, the operator may be forced to omit certain steps in the interest of time. This requires a judgment as to the baby's clinical status and the time delay involved for any given step, such as waiting for the ultrasound machine, preparing a larger sterile field, or assembling a three-way stopcock system.

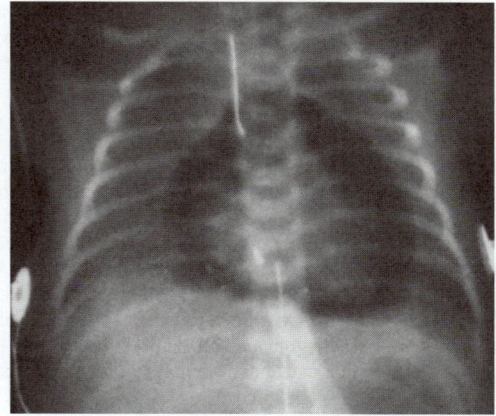

Chest radiograph with Pneumopericardium

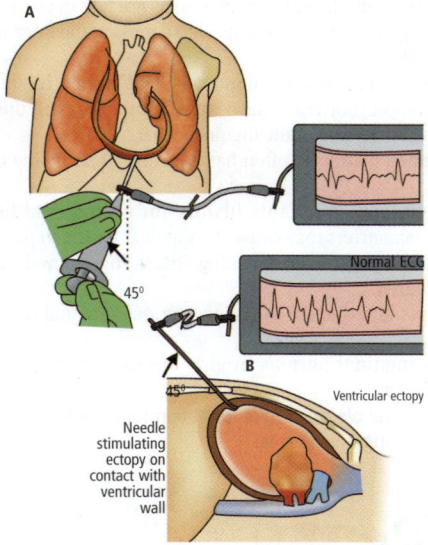

Pericardiocentesis from substernal approach : Monitor the patient with ECG AND PULSE OXIMETRY continuously and ensure an adequate airway. Observe the ECG for premature ventricular beats, ST-T segment changes, or QRS widening while advancing the needle. Withdraw a short distance when ECG change occurs, then redirect and try again.

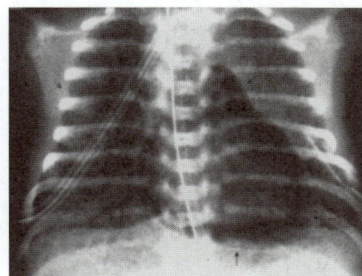

Meconium aspiration: Follow-up radiograph in the patient obtained after placement of bilateral thoracostomy tubes for pneumothoraces shows pneumopericardium (arrows) and extensive imaging lucencies in the lungs. These findings indicate pulmonary interstitial emphysema.

*Air leak syndromes encompass a wide-spectrum of diseases including Pneumothorax, Pneumomediastinum Pulmonary Interstitial Emphysema, Pneumopericardium and Pneumoperitonium.The syndromes are one of the most common complications in ventilated infants. The mechanism of air leak begins with positive intra-alveolar inflation and causes alveolar rupture. The type of air leak syndromes will depend on the location where the escaping air destined.

HERNIA REDUCTION

Overview:

1. Confirm the presence of a true hernia before attempting reduction.
2. Ensure that peritoneal signs are not present, and, to the extent possible, that the bowel is not ischemic. If either finding is questionable, seek immediate surgical consultation.
3. Consider sedation.
4. Warm hands before contacting patient.
5. Apply gentle, firm bimanual pressure along entire inguinal canal, using hand most distal to milk out contents or gas within incarcerated bowel.
6. After reducing contents of incarcerated bowel, apply increased pressure over distal as compared with proximal inguinal canal.
7. If bowel fails to reduce after 5 minutes of continuous pressure, try sedation if not used on first attempt. Place patient in Trendelenburg position, apply ice pack to groin, and repeat procedure.
8. Contact surgeon for all incarcerated hernias to arrange admission and semielective or emergent surgery.

Clinical tips

1. Femoral hernias and direct inguinal hernias are rare in children.
2. An indirect inguinal hernia presents with a mass at the internal ring of the inguinal canal .
3. A hydrocele is usually smooth, nontender, and mobile, has brilliant transillumination (bowel can also transilluminate), and does not extend into internal ring of the inguinal canal.
4. Communicating hydrocele often has a history of shrinking during the night.
5. When parents give a reliable history for an inguinal hernia, provocative maneuvers may cause the inguinal hernia to protrude.
6. Even with irreducible incarcerated inguinal hernias, bowel necrosis is rare in children.
7. Most attempts at reduction of an incarcerated inguinal hernia are successful.
8. Irreducible inguinal hernias in girls are more likely to be an incarcerated ovary.
9. Evidence of bowel obstruction is *not* a contraindication to manual reduction of an inguinal hernia.

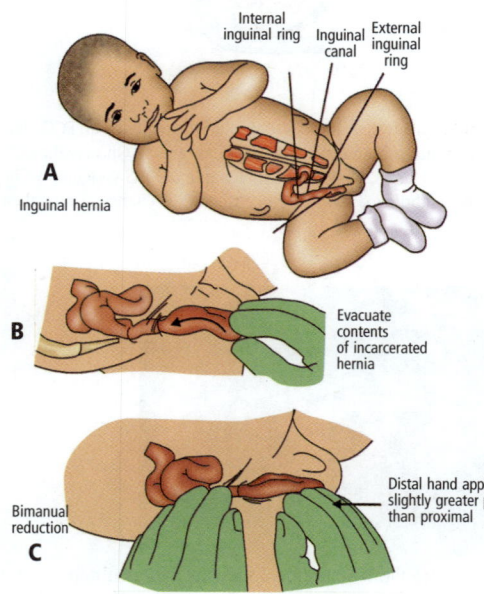

Bimanual reduction of an Inguinal Hernia.

A. Anatomy of an Inguinal hernia
B. Gas and stool are first milked out of the bowel to reduce its size
C. Constant pressure is applied for up to 5 minutes (distal to proximal) to reduce the bowel itself.

Skin preparation for venepuncture and other procedures

*Wash properly, and dry hands.
*Wear sterile gloves.
*Prepare skin site, confine to smallest possible area of skin.
*Swab with alcohol first, allow it to dry.
*Swab iodine on site, allow it to dry.
*Swab again with alcohol to wipe off iodine, allow it to dry.
*Skin is now ready for puncture of prick.
From AIIMS, Neonatal Division

Skin and Device Antisepsis for Neonates

Infants < 1,000 grams and less than 3 weeks of age
Blood Culture: 2% chlorhexidine swab sticks (**no alcohol**)
Invasive Procedures • Central lines • Lumbar punctures • Suprapubic Taps : 2% chlorhexidine swab sticks (**no alcohol**)
Urinary Catheterization: Povidone-iodine – pour small amount from bottle or use prep packs
Peripheral Intravenous: 2% chlorhexidine swab sticks or prep packs (**no alcohol**)
Access to Central Lines 70% alcohol prep packs (Alcohol has the best results for antisepsis on objects, while chlorhexidine is superior on skin)
Central Line Site Care 2% chlorhexidine swab sticks (**no alcohol**)
Other infants
0.5% chlorhexidine with 70% alcohol prep pad for blood cultures, Peripheral Intravenous
2.0% chlorhexidine with 70% alcohol swab sticks/or prep packs for Invasive Procedures
If sensitivity or allergy to chlorhexidine has been demonstrated 10% povidone-iodine can be used for subsequent procedures.

Isolation techniques and precaution measures used at the Neonatal unit

Total isolation Private room, use of apron, mask, and gloves
Respiratory isolation Private room, use of mask for contact with newborns
Contact isolation (fluids, excreta, and infectious material) Use of mask, apron, and gloves for contact with newborns
Enteric precautions, and precautions with drainage/ secretions: Use of apron and gloves for contact with body fluids and blood
Standard precautions Use of apron, gloves, and eye protection for contact with blood and secretions

Types of isolation and precautions against Neonatal infections

Total Chickenpox
Contact Herpes simplex, rubella, and multiresistant bacteria
Respiratory Pertussis, respiratory syncytial virus, and influenza
Enteric precaution Hepatitis A, cytomegalovirus, diarrheal disease, and necrotizing enterocolitis
Standard precaution Hepatitis B, HIV, syphilis, sepsis, meningitis, pneumonia, skin infection

UMBILICAL VENOUS CATHETERIZATION

Indications: Need for continuous monitoring of intravascular venous pressures; Vascular access for exchange transfusions; Central vascular access for blood sampling when peripheral access is unavailable; Vascular access for administration of hypertonic solutions; Vascular access for long term parenteral nutrition when peripheral access is unavailable.

Contraindications: *Omphalitis *Omphalocele *Necrotizing enterocolitis *Peritonitis

Equipment required

sterile gloves and gown, instrument pack (as for umbilical artery catheterization) and sterile drape (transparent plastic is preferred for better patient visualization), antiseptic to prepare the skin, umbilical catheter, multiple lumen catheters are preferable if the infant is <1000g or extremely sick, a single lumen catheter (FG3.5 < 1000gm, FG5.0 >= 1000gm) is inserted for short term usage.8-Fr catheter for infants weighing >3.5 kg, If unavailable, a feeding tube (size 5) could be used. syringe with NaCl 0.9% flush, routine IV line tubing set-up and tape.

Procedure -observe standard precautions

*consider the use of appropriate measures to relieve distress including *use or oral sucrose (link to section) *containing the infant by holding *securing the catheter as soon as possible *avoidance of placing clamps or sutures on the skin *place infant on open heated cot *monitor the infant (oximetry and cardiorespiratory) and ensure all four limbs are adequately restrained throughout the procedure *open an atraumatic suture (3 0 silk on cutting edge needle) *if using an infusion, check solution is correct and prepared to the stage where it can immediately run into the catheter *select appropriate catheter, usually 5 Fr. or 3.5 Fr. if infant weighs below 1000 grams *the catheter must be attached to a syringe and filled with infusion solution before insertion *prepare umbilicus, cord and cord clamp with iodine solution, cut the umbilical cord about 1.5 cm from the abdomen, and establish sterile field ***Identify thin-walled vein, close to periphery of umbilical stump . Grasp cord stump with toothed forceps. Gently insert tips of iris forceps into lumen of vein and remove any clots** *insert a purse-string suture near base of Wharton's jelly for hemostasis. Tie a single knot *immobilize cord by two artery forceps at 3 and 9 o'clock, grasping cord edges *insert tip of iris forceps into lumen, allow the forceps to spring open *when blood is in catheter, connect up the two way tap to the infusion and flush catheter gently *tie purse string and tie onto catheter or secure to catheter with tape. Make certain fluid type and rate is specified *label catheter to distinguish from umbilical catheter if present *write out the x-ray request and be sure to inspect the x-ray later *routine heparinization of umbilical venous catheters is not recommended If catheter meets any obstruction prior to measured distance, *It has most commonly *Entered portal system, or *Wedged in an intrahepatic branch of umbilical vein *Withdraw catheter 2 to 3 cm, gently rotate, and reinsert in an attempt to get tip through ductus venosus. If the catheter is in the portal circulation, leave the misdirected catheter in its place. Pass a new 5-Fr catheter into the same vessel. Once the catheter is in good position, remove the misdirected catheter. This procedure has a success rate of 50%.

Catheter complications

* Infection

* Bleeding due to disconnection of tubing. Always use a Luer locked connection when attaching the catheter to infusion lines

* Perforation - never cut off the rounded end of any indwelling catheter

* Clot formation, embolism and spasm

* Effects of catheter malpositioning include cardiac arrhythmias, hepatic necrosis or portal hypertension - avoided by checking catheter positioning by X-ray

Catheter removal *performed by medical staff *turn infusion off *withdraw catheter gradually as a single procedure *send tip for culture only if infection is suspected *if bleeding occurs press firmly just above the umbilicus *do not nurse the infant in the prone position during removal of the catheter and for the immediate 4 hours after removal.

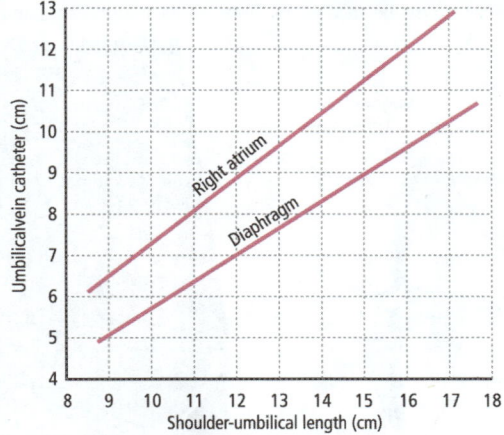

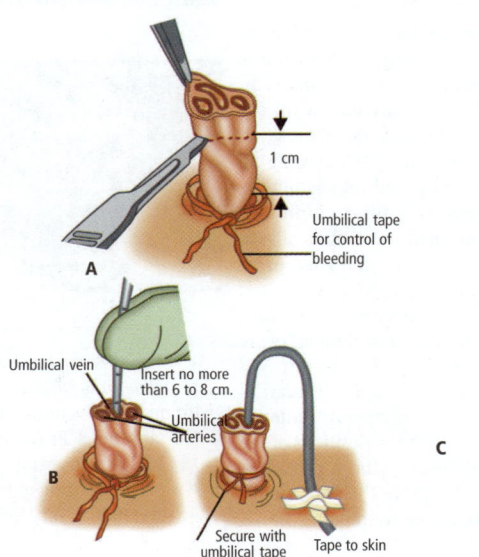

Cannulation of the Umbilical Vein A-Identify the umbilical vein after trimming the cord B- Insert the umbilical catheter into the vein C- Secure the base of the cord to hold the catheter in place and stabilize the catheter with tape

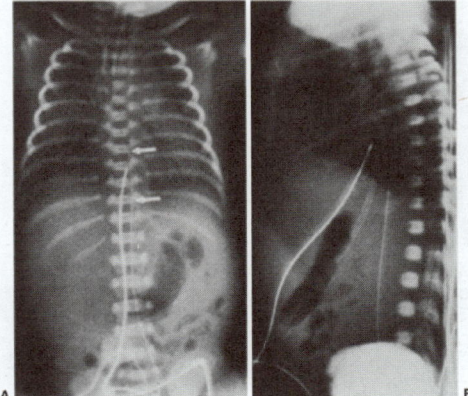

Anteroposterior (A) and lateral (B) radiographs demonstrating the normal course of an umbilical venous catheter, with an umbilical artery catheter (arrows) in position for comparison. Note how the venous catheter swings immediately superior from the umbilicus, slightly to the right as it traverses the ductus venosus into the inferior vena cava (IVC). The distal tip of this line is just superior to the right atrium - IVC junction, and it might optimally be pulled back slightly into the IVC. Note how the thinner umbilical artery catheter (arrows) heads inferiorly as it proceeds to the iliac artery and then ascends posteriorly and to the left until it reaches the level of D7.

Umbilical vein catheter (UVC) *Goal is to place the UVC **above the diaphragm but below the heart** *UVC is directed into the umbilical vein, through the ductus venous, into the inferior vena cava *Allows infusion of more hypertonic solutions *Allows better nutrition through TPN *Provides emergency access for fluids, resuscitation drugs and blood products.

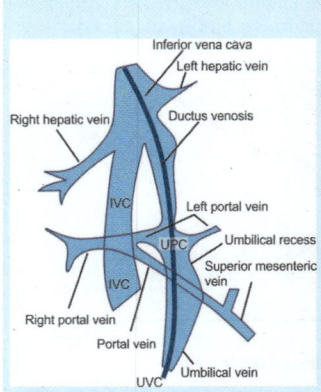

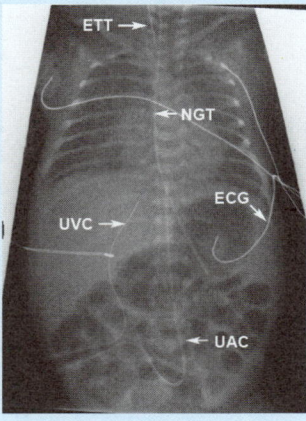

The umbilical *vein* catheter (UVC) takes a characteristically different path to the Umbilical *Artery* Catheter (UAC). *The umbilical vein is 2-3cm long and 4-5mm in diameter *From the umbilicus, it passes cephalad and a little to the right It joins the left branch of the portal vein after giving off several large intrahepatic branches. *The ductus venosus arises from the point where the UV joins the left portal vein. See the lateral decubitus abdominal image below for further appreciation of the course of the umbilical vein.

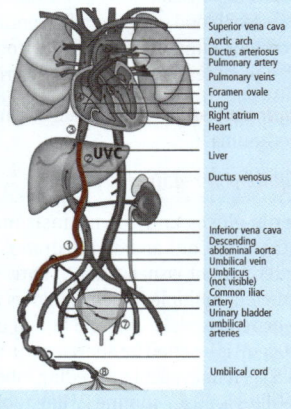

This graphic is based on a venogram and is therefore a reasonable representation of actual anatomy. The UVC normally moves up the umbilical vein in a cranial direction where it meets the junction with the left and right portal vein within the liver. There is a direct communication between the umbilical vein and the ductus venosis. After travelling through the ductus venosis it encounters a second venous cross-roads at the level of the left and right hepatic vein. On travelling further in a cranial direction the UVC enters the inferior venacava. Note the positions of the vertebral bodies—these provide a guide as to where the UVC might have taken a wayward path.

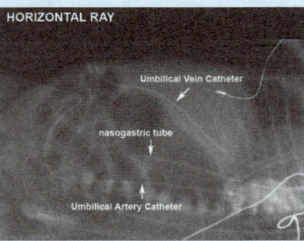

UVCThis lateral image gives an appreciation of the course of the umbilical vein and ductus venosis in relation to the liver

The UVC tip has tracked into the liver and there appears to be portal venous gas. Air in portal venous branches can be associated with umbilical venous catheter insertion. Inconsequential transient portal venous air can be seen immediately after umbilical venous catheter insertion and should not necessarily be attributed to necrotizing enterocolitis. Alan E. Schlesinger1, Richard M. Braverman1 and Michael A. DiPietro2 AJR 2003; 180:1147-1153

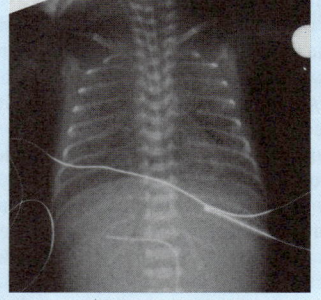

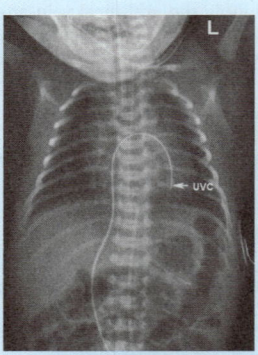

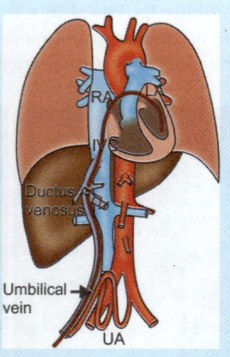

UVC extends across foramen ovale into the left atrium then left ventricle

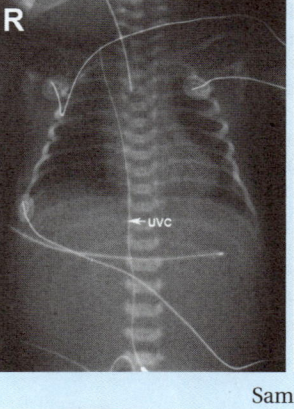

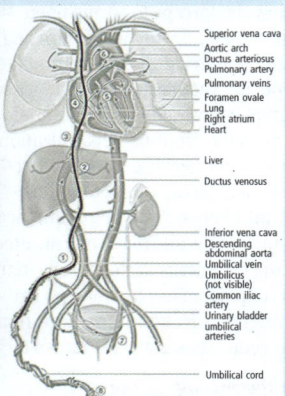

Same patient—UVC repositioned now in jugular vein

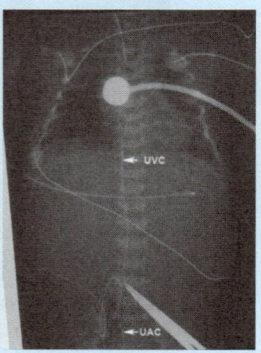

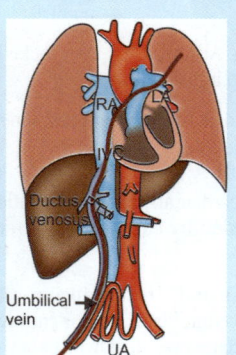

The UVC tip is in the pulmonary vein

*Courtesy:*Dr M J Fuller

UMBILICAL ARTERIAL CATHETERIZATION

Indications: Primary *Frequent or continuous measurement of lower aortic blood gases for oxygen tension (PO_2) or oxygen content (percent saturation) *Continuous monitoring of arterial blood pressure *Angiography *Resuscitation (use of umbilical venous line may be first choice) *Secondary* *Infusion of maintenance glucose/electrolyte solutions or medications. If this line is to be used to provide intravenous nutrition, the same aseptic techniques must be used to prevent line-related sepsis as are used for any central line *Exchange transfusion *To provide vital infusions and a port for frequent blood sampling in the extremely low-birthweight infant

Contraindications: *Evidence of local vascular compromise in lower limbs or buttock areas *Peritonitis *Necrotizing enterocolitis *Omphalitis *Omphalocele *Acute abdomen etiology

Equipment:

Arterial tray *1 scalpel blade handle *2 probes: fine and medium *4 mosquito artery forceps: 2 curved, 2 straight *2 pair dissecting forceps: toothed, non-toothed *2 iris forceps *1 pair vein scissors *1 pair suture scissors *1 needle holder *2 bowls *cotton wool swabs *gauze swabs *tape measure **Other equipment** *surgical mask *sterile gown and gloves *1 plastic drape (sterile) *1 scalpel blade No. 11 *1 umbilical artery catheter *Fg 3.5 < 1250g baby *Fg 5 > 1250g baby *1 blood pressure monitoring kit *1 disposable luer lock 3-way tap *1 x 5ml syringe and 18G needle *1 x 10ml ampoule 0.9% saline *1 packet 3/0 black silk suture *Skin preparation solution *Parenteral administration set *Infusion pump *Ordered parenteral solution (*1ml ampoule heparin 1,000 units/ml *drug additive label *1cm wide leukoplast for taping of catheter

Catheters should be withdrawn if persistent blanching, decreased temperature, or loss of pulse is noted in an extremity. Any clinical changes in that extremity should be documented in the medical record, as should reasons for discontinuing a catheter. Umbilical arterial catheters are maintained in a high position (at the T6-T10 vertebral bodies). These are not used for hyperalimentation except at the direction of the attending physician. No blood transfusions are to be given through an arterial line.

UAC POSITION BY WEIGHT

BIRTH WEIGHT	POSITION
< 700 gm	T10
700 –1000 gm	T9
1000–2000 gm	T8
< 2000 gm	T7

Formula: Umbilicus to shoulder in cm + BW in kg (to nearest 0.5 kg)

Procedure : *estimate the position of catheter tip *the correct position is in the descending aorta above the origin of the mesenteric and renal arteries (to avoid occlusion in these vessels) *the catheter length may be calculated from the formula [Weight (kg) x 3] + 9cm *remember to add the length of the cord stump *consider the use of appropriate measures to relieve distress including *use or oral sucrose *containing the infant by holding *securing the catheter as soon as possible *avoidance of placing clamps or sutures on the skin *flush the selected catheter via the 3-way tap with normal Saline. Leave the syringe of saline attached to 3-way tap throughout the procedure *clean the umbilical stump and surrounding 3-4cm of abdomen with a chlorhexidine based solution. Wait 2 minutes. Clean the area with aqueous chlorhexidine *drape around the umbilical stump with sterile towels *tie a short piece of umbilical tape around the base of the cord. It should be secure enough to maintain hemostasis but not too tight to prevent passage of the catheter *with a pair of straight forceps, grasp the end of the cord clamp and pass the forceps to the assistant. Whilst the assistant applies gentle upward traction, slice the cord with the scalpel, 1-1.5cm from the skin margin. An alternative method is to leave the cord long and cannulate the artery from the side. This method should be left to experienced operators only.

GRAPH FOR UMBILICAL ARTERY CATHETER

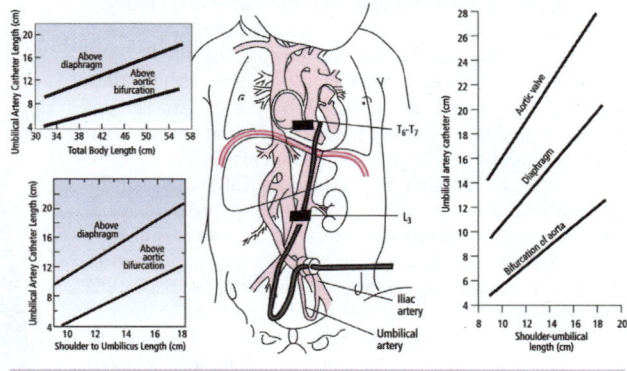

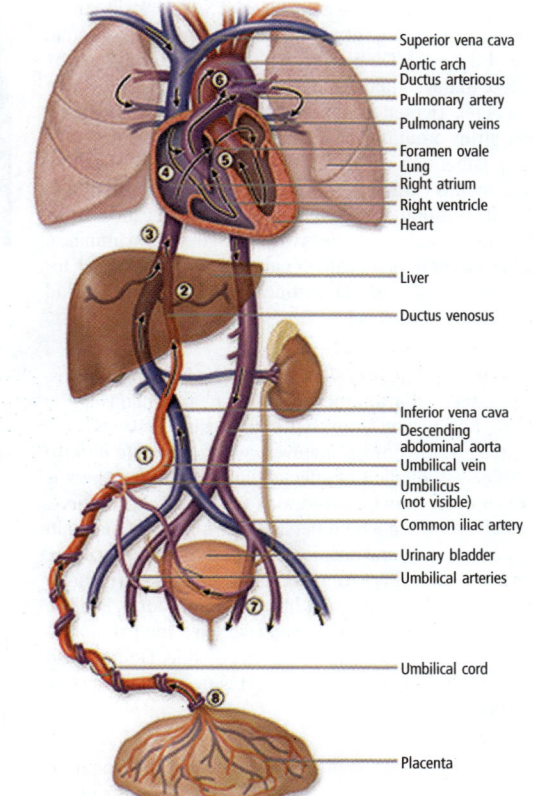

Neonatal vascular anatomy: The positioning of umbilical catheters in particular is easier to digest if you understand the fetal vascular anatomy

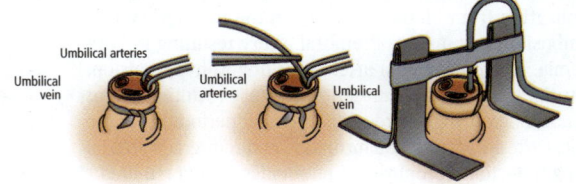

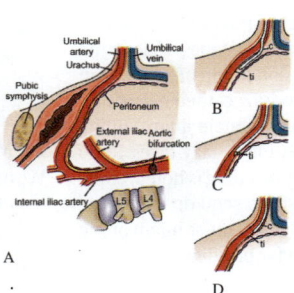

Some reasons for failure of umbilical artery catheterization. A: Sagittal midline section to show normal anatomy of umbilical artery. B: Catheter has perforated the umbilical artery within the anulus umbilicalis and is dissecting perivascularly and external to peritoneum. C: Catheter has ruptured through the tunica intima (t.i.) and dissected into subintimal space. D: Catheter invaginating the tunica intima after stripping it from a more distal point.

*when the cut surface is blotted dry, the umbilical vessels can be identified *the single thin walled umbilical vein *two smaller thick walled round arteries, generally constricted so that their lumen appear pinpoint. They often protrude from the cut surface of the umbilical cord to insert the arterial catheter the orifice of the artery is gently opened with fine forceps. . Initially 1 tip and then both tips of the iris forceps should be gently inserted into the artery. The tips should be allowed to spring apart. The tips should be gradually advanced to the curve of the forceps. Then the vessel may be cannulated. Obstruction may be encountered at the anterior abdominal wall or bladder. This can usually be overcome by 30-60 seconds of gentle, steady pressure. Avoid excessive pressure or repeated probings. If unsuccessful, seek advice from a more experienced person. The most common error arises after cannulating the layer between the vascular intima and the muscle. This usually occurs if dilatation of the artery in the cord has been inadequate *ensure patency of catheter by checking for easy withdrawal of blood and "pulsation" of blood/ saline in the catheter *secure catheter with 3/0 black silk suture by placing a purse string suture (use several small bites) around the base of the cord. Do not include the skin. Commence the suture close to the catheter so that the first knot lies at the base of the catheter. Tighten the purse string and knot securely. Tie the purse string around the catheter tightly. Strp with goal post strapping. Label line clearly (in order to distinguish from an umbilical venous catheter) *connect catheter to infusion fluid *confirm the position of catheter by X-ray - initial caudal route of catheter before ascending aorta will distinguish from umbilical vein catheterization, tip of catheter above level of T_{10} *check for arterial waveform on arterial transducer after it is connected and calibrated.

Ongoing Management :

*Observe skin color. Note any skin blanching or bruising of limbs, toes or buttocks prior to procedure, during and following the procedure, and at any time that catheter is in situ. Report immediately. If one limb is involved, warm opposite limb to induce reflex vasodilation of affected limb. If physical therapy fails, the catheter may be withdrawn 0.5 - 1cm and observe. Remove catheter if blanching persists >30 minutes. *maintain infant supine or in lateral position for 24 hours post procedure to observe for hemorrhage from umbilical stump *keep catheter and infusion line clear of blood as blood clots may form. Remove all air bubbles in the infusion line and catheter. Interruption to infusion must be for as short a time as possible. Do not flush catheters quickly *filters are not used for IA lines. All connections must be luer lock

Complications :

*bleeding due to accidental disconnection or dislodgement, or from open connections *vasospasm of the femoral artery causing blanching of toes and foot is less common with high than low catheters. The opposite limb may be warmed with a warm moist towel. If blanching persists, the catheter must be removed *embolization from blood clot or air in the infusion system *thrombosis - may involve *femoral artery resulting in limb ischaemia, gangrene *renal artery resulting in hypertension, hematuria, renal failure *mesenteric artery resulting in gut ischaemia, necrotizing enterocolitis *vascular perforation of the umbilical arteries, hematoma formation and retrograde arterial bleeding *infection - prophylactic antibiotics are not required

Catheter Removal

*equipment required -alcohol swab, sterile stitch cutter (optional), sterile blade, specimen container, tapes *clean the stump with an alcohol swab *turn infusion pump off and clamp infusion line *remove sutures and withdraw catheter to within 3-4cm of skin *tape catheter to skin and maintain infant supine *wait for pulsation in catheter to stop (this usually takes 10-20 minutes) *remove rest of catheter. If any bleeding is noted, apply positive pressure below level of stump *only send tip for culture and sensitivity if infection is suspected *do not nurse infant prone for 4 hours following removal. Observe for bleeding

Umbilical arterial catheter (UAC)

*Placed into the umbilical artery, through to the descending aorta *Allows continuous blood pressure monitoring *Allows for frequent blood gas, lab sampling *The umbilical arteries are the direct continuation of the internal iliac arteries. *A catheter passed into an umbilical artery will usually (but not always) enter the aorta via the internal iliac artery. *Occasionally it will pass into the femoral artery via the external iliac artery or into the gluteal arteries. *The femoral artery or gluteal artery are unsuitable sites for sampling, infusion, or blood pressure monitoring.

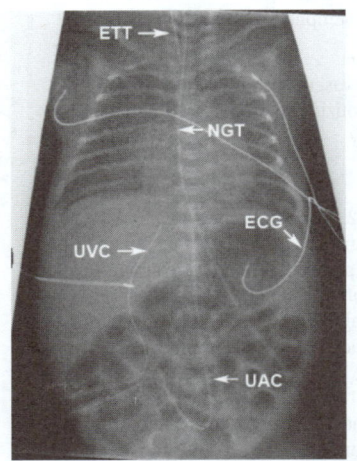
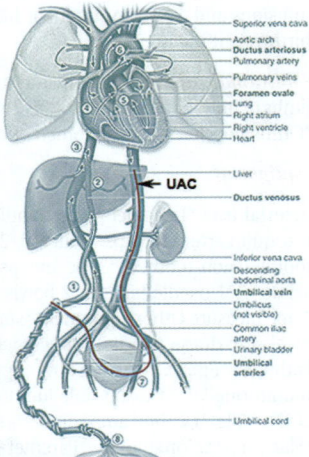

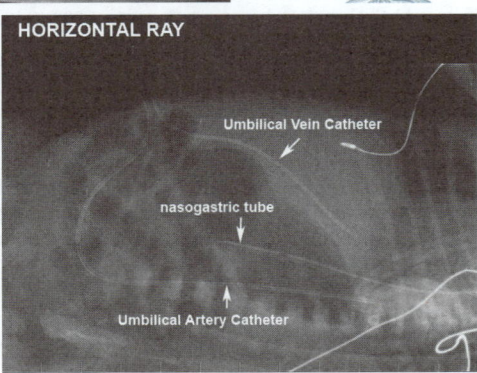

The umbilical artery catheter (UAC) characteristically deviates inferiorly before tracking up the aorta. See the lateral decubitus abdominal image above for further appreciation of the course of the umbilical artery. The UAC and UVC are seen in this supine decubitus abdominal image. UAC The umbilical artery catheter (UAC) can be seen to track inferiorly and posteriorly from the umbilicus before tracking up the aorta. NGT The nasogastric tube enters the stomach from the esophagus. When assessing the position of the NGT the position of the sidehole should also be considered.

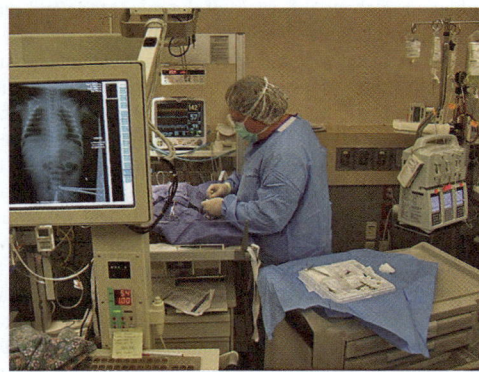

Dr M J Fuller found a powerpoint presentation from the Deaconess Women's Hospital, Newburgh, Indiana that argued the case for checking line in the Neonatal unit with mobile DR. This has intuitive appeal- a malpositioned line can do harm in a variety of different ways. Also, the mobile DR technique is efficient in that a malpositioned line can be quickly assessed, repositioned then reassessed.

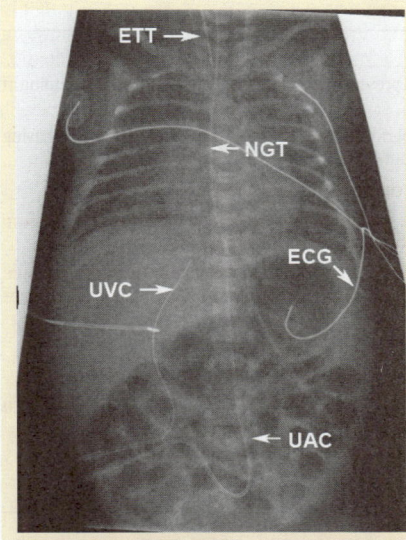

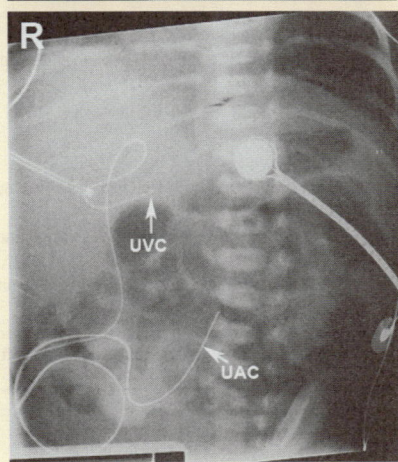

UAC IN HIGH POSITION

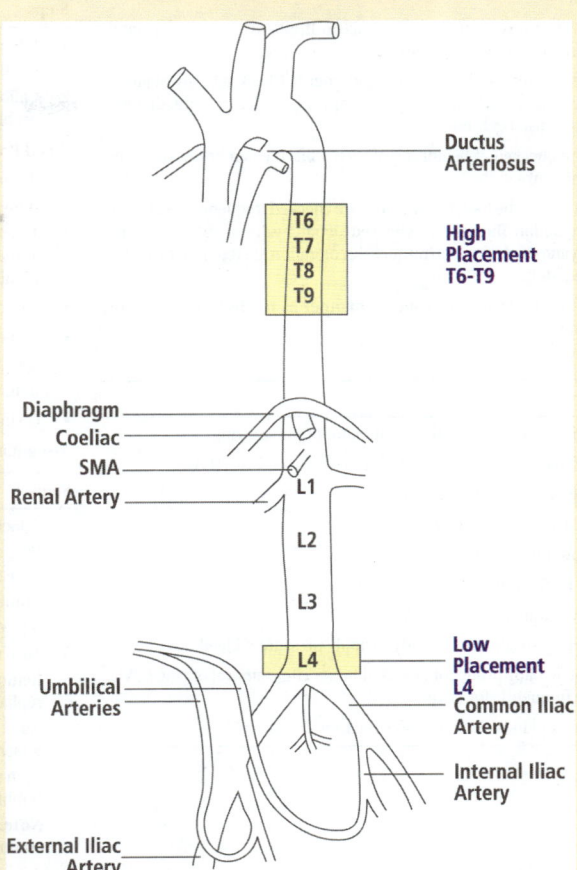

Anatomic relations of the umbilical arteries, showing relationships with major arteries supplying buttocks and lower limb.

UAC IN LOW POSITION

There are two potential tip positions for the UAC. These are described as "high" or "low". *The high position is at the level of thoracic vertebral bodies T6-T9. This position is above the coeliac axis (T12), the superior mesenteric artery (T12-L1), and the renal arteries (L1). This position is essentially "above the diaphragm". *The low position is at the level of lumbar vertebral bodies L3-L4. This position is below the structures as above, and is above the aortic bifurcation (L4-L5). The inferior mesenteric artery arises from L3-L4. This position is essentially "above the aortic bifurcation". High placed umbilical artery catheters are associated with a lower incidence of clinical vascular complications, without an increase in any adverse sequelae. Intraventricular hemorrhage rates, death and necrotizing enterocolitis are not more frequent with high compared to low catheters. There appears to be no evidence to support the use of low placed umbilical artery catheters. High catheters should be used exclusively.(Cochrane Study).

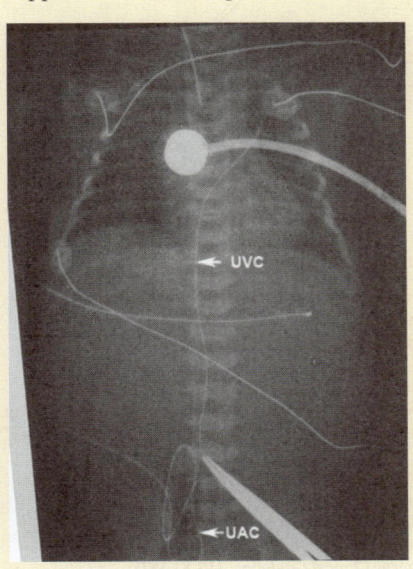

This UAC appears to have taken a course along the right iliac artery or gluteal artery The UVC tip is in the pulmonary circulation.

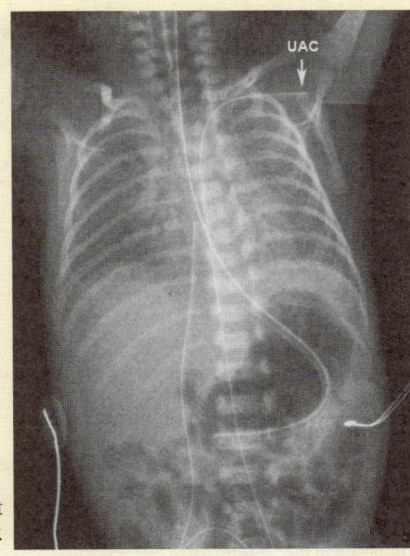

UAC in left subclavian artery.

Management of UAC/UVC

Steps **Action**

1. A nurse is always present in the room. Alarm limits are set appropriately including mean blood pressure alarm.

2. The catheter is secured as per baby's weight criteria. Check security of gate at the commencement of each duty. Retape or apply a sleek gate immediately if concerned about dislodgement.

3. Connections are checked at beginning of each shift to ensure they are secure and there are no kinks in the lines.

4. Booties are **not** worn. The toes, feet and legs are checked frequently for changes in color and circulation. Buttocks are checked for patchy discoloration and signs of blanching. Cyanosis of toes/feet/buttock discoloration are reported to doctor/NS-ANP immediately.

5. **Napkins must not be fastened in such a manner as to obscure view of the umbilical stump.**

Removal of UAC/UVC

Steps	Action
1	Cut stitches between catheter and knot of purse string.
2	Withdraw catheter slowly until **3cm** remains in UAC/UVC.
3	Retape catheter at that position.
4	Turn 3 way tap off to catheter.
5	Turn off infusion pump.
6	Leave for 30 minutes.
7	Remove catheter completely.
	N.B.: Have sterile gauze handy to apply pressure if bleeding occurs.
8	Do not lie baby prone for at least 4 hours after removal of UAC/UVC. Check frequently for ooze.
9	Ensure napkin is secured **below** the umbilicus.

RBP: Blood pressure monitoring

Steps **Action**

1. Ensure there is no blood present in the blood pressure line causing damping of the reading.

2. Calibration checks are performed - at the beginning of each shift or if having problems with the readout of blood pressure.

Blood Pressure monitoring via Blood Pressure Transducer

- Blood pressure may be measured directly by attaching a blood pressure transducer set to an umbilical or peripheral arterial line.

- The transducer is a very sensitive device, which responds to a change in pressure and converts these changes to a digital display on the monitor. Equipment required

- Blood pressure transducer set and

- Cable fitting that joins to the monitor

- 500 ml bag of sodium chloride 0.9% (or 0.45% for babies under 1000g with 250 units heparin added (0.5 unit/ml).

- Giving set and pall filter

Assembling/Priming Blood Pressure Transducer Set

Steps **Action**

1. Attach blood pressure transducer set to giving set.

2. Plug cable from monitor into BP transducer set. A labelled pressure waveform is displayed when the cable is connected

3. Prime giving set.

4. Squeeze lever on flush device and prime BP set.

5. Turn stopcock off to flushing line and syringe.

6. Remove the 10ml syringe, draw up 10mls NaCl with Heparin from IV Bag, replace and prime flushing line to the end of transducer set.
   Note: Peripheral arterial line. Prime line as above, then remove syringe and attach luerlock bung.

7. Turn stop cock off to the flushing line and syringe. Check that there are no air bubbles present in transducer line and flushing line.
   Note: Transducer must have a <u>zero calibration</u> performed prior to commencement of BP monitoring. A zero calibration is required once per shift.

Transducer Set Up:

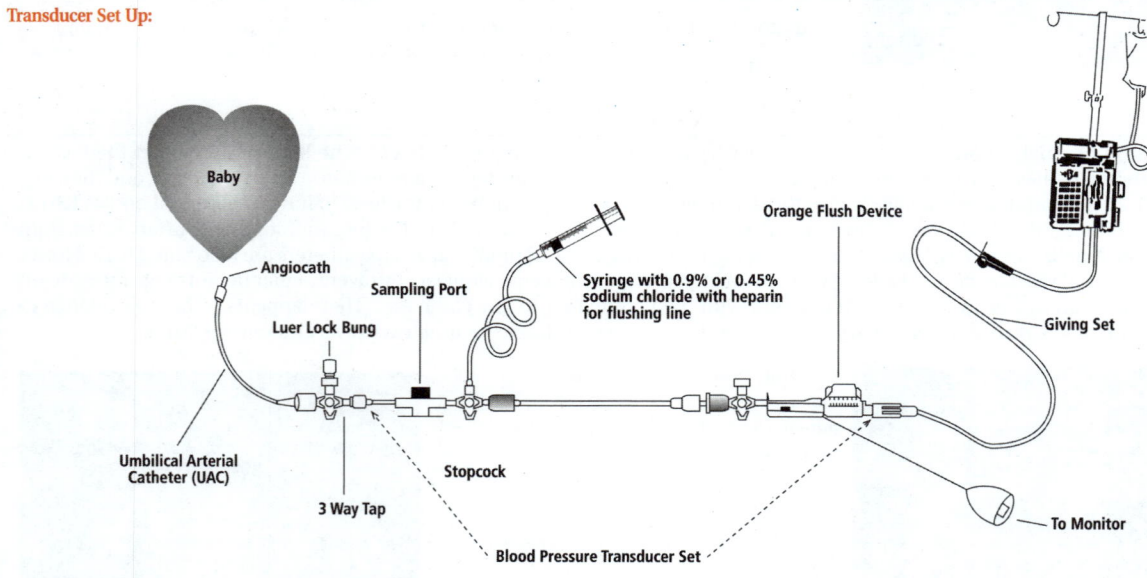

To Zero Calibrate :

*Follow the steps below to perform zero calibration (performed prior to commencement of BP monitoring and then once per shift).

Steps **Action**
1. Ensure transducer placed appropriately at level of mid-axilla of baby.
2. Close the 3-way tap closest to the baby.
3. Open the venting stopcock on the transducer to air.
4. Press the "Zero all" button on the keypad
5. Verify that zero reference has been established (watch the pressure parameter window for messages)
6. Close the venting stopcock.
7. Open the 3 way tap to baby. Within seconds, pressure numerics should be displayed in the pressure parameter window.

Monitoring Heart Rate without ECG Electrodes

· Heart rate can be monitored as a 'pulse' through the umbilical arterial line by the GE-Marquette monitors.
· It should be considered for all Infants <26 weeks on assisted ventilation.
· Be Aware:
· Not for babies on Hudson CPAP or babies on high frequency ventilation.
· If umbilical line is not functioning well and a good pulse rate is not picked up, revert to chest electrodes. SpO$_2$ heart rate monitoring is not sufficient in itself.
· **Procedure**
· Monitoring <1000g babies without ECG (via the GE-Marquette monitors).
· Must have umbilical arterial line.
· To change alarm capability from HR (taken from ECG) to pulse (taken from umbilical or arterial line).
· **Courtesy: Newborn Services Clinical Guideline, AUCKLAND**

CENTRAL VENOUS CATHETERIZATION
Peripherally Inserted Central Catheterization (PICC)

Indications

*Total parenteral nutrition *Long-term IV medication administration *Administration of hyperosmolar IV fluids or irritating medications that cannot be administered through peripheral IV cannulas. *Fluid resuscitation

Relative Contraindications

There are no absolute contraindications, as the clinical situation dictates the need for venous access. *Skin infection at insertion site *Uncorrected bleeding diathesis (not a contraindication for percutaneous catheters inserted in distal peripheral venous sites) *Ongoing bacteremia or fungal infection (which may cause catheter colonization and infection) *The patient can be treated adequately with peripheral IV access. Central venous catheters have significant risks of complications and must not be used when peripheral venous access is possible and adequate.

Sites: *Large vein in antecubital fossa, long saphenous vein or posterior tibial vein **Complications:** Catheter migration/malposition, Catheter-related sepsis, Catheter dysfunction(Remove the catheter if it is no longer medically critical)

Insertion distance: *For longlines inserted via the leg, measure from insertion site to **xiphisternum**. *For longlines inserted via the arm, measure from insertion site to the **sternal notch**. When inserted from the upper extremity, the catheter tip should be in the superior vena cava, outside the cardiac reflection and above the T2 vertebra (12). When inserted from the lower extremity, the catheter tip should be above the L4/ L5 vertebrae or the iliac crest, but not in the heart.

Equipment: PICC catheters and kits are available commercially. PICCs are generally made of silicone or polyurethane. Sizes include 1.2, 1.9, 2, and 3 Fr. Larger sizes are generally not used in the neonatal population. Most catheters are single-lumen. Recently, a 1.9-Fr double-lumen catheter has become available. Double-lumen catheters can decrease the need for maintaining concurrent IV access when more than one site is required. PICC introducers/needles are available in 19, 20, 22, and 24 gauge. Choice will depend on the size of the vein to be cannulated. Open longline pack onto trolley and add: *20 gauge cannula *Longline set *Scalpel blade *5ml syringe *0.9% NaCl 5ml ampoule *Heparinized saline 10 unit/ml *Skin disinfectant *Steristrips *Duoderm dressing *Tegaderm or Opsite dressing

Procedure

*Don mask, gown, and gloves. *Flush the longline with 0.9% NaCl leaving syringe attached *Cut round the IV cannula at the hub leaving cannula on the introducer *Position the infant maximizing access i.e. open the incubator door, slide tray out and use overhead heater. Secure limbs if necessary *If an assistant is required they must wear a gown and sterile gloves *Clean the skin with the disinfectant appropriate for the infant's gestation and age. *Wait about 1 minute until it dries otherwise it will not be an effective skin prep. *Create a sterile field with sterile guards *Apply tourniquet above site *Position line, syringe and forceps on sterile field *Insert cannula, advance cannula off the introducer and withdraw introducer *Insert longline with forceps and feed to premeasured distance releasing tourniquet when catheter is through the cannula *Withdraw cannula over the longline ensuring the longline is stable by using pressure on the limb above the cannula *Detach longline at blue connection, remove cannula and reattach connection, ensuring air is not introduced. The black marker that lies over the metal insert must not be visible. *Flush longline with 0.5ml of heparinised saline (10U/ml) Securing the Line *Coil longline next to site without crossing longline. *Steristrips should be used to anchor the line preventing inward movement and may also help to keep the longline coiled. *Place a small piece of Duoderm on skin under connection and secure everything with Tegaderm. Confirm the position *Wrap syringe in sterile guard until position confirmed by x-ray.

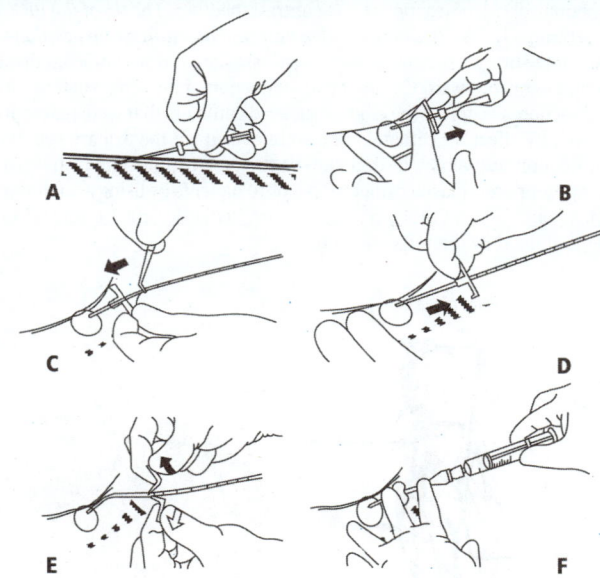

Peripherally inserted central catheter using a peel-away cannula introducer.

A: Perform venipuncture. When flashback of blood is noted, reduce angle and advance introducer sheath farther to ensure placement in the vein.

B: Withdraw the introducer needle from the sheath. Note that the introducer sheath is supported to avoid displacement.

C: Insert the catheter into the introducer sheath using fine nontoothed forceps.

D: Withdraw the introducer sheath. Note that the catheter is stabilized by applying digital pressure to the vein distal to the introducer sheath.

E: Remove the introducer sheath by splitting and peeling it away from the catheter. Complete catheter advancement to premeasured length.

F: Aspirate catheter to check for blood return and flush with heparinized saline to ensure patency.

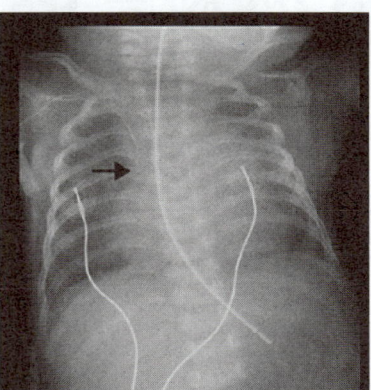

Chest radiograph with PICC tip in appropriate position, just above junction of superior vena cava and right atrium

*The Department of Health (UK) recommended that the line tip is placed OUTSIDE the heart (Wariyar UK, Hallworth D. Review of four neonatal deaths due to cardiac tamponade associated with the presence of a central venous catheter. London, UK: Department of Health; 2001) *X-ray with contrast medium prior to connecting fluids. This must be done using sterile technique. *Record in the clinical notes the date, insertion site and length of catheter. Enter the procedure in the neonatal database. *It is also important that we note the catheter tip position in the clinical record. *If the longline is clearly *well into the heart* (particularly if it is curled) and needs to be withdrawn, another radiograph must be taken after manipulation to ensure that it has been withdrawn far enough and is in an acceptable position.

Peripheral venous catheter (Long lines, PICC, CVC) Upper limb: The Southern West Midlands Newborn Network recommend the following "If the cephalic vein has been cannulated the x-ray should be taken with the arm adducted. If the basilic vein has been cannulated the x-ray should be taken with the arm abducted. Contrast medium may be used to aid visualization of the line. Although not reported in neonates, there is a theoretical risk of reaction to the contrast medium. *The tip of the PICC should lie outside the heart, ideally by 1cm in a baby <1250g and by 2cm in a baby >1250g." It is important to note that the catheter tip position will change with the baby's arm movements.* The following research finding are noteworthy "Arm movements were associated with significant displacement of catheters. Catheters that were placed via the basilic or axillary vein migrated toward the heart with adduction of the arm, whereas those that were placed via the cephalic vein moved away from the heart with adduction. Flexion of the elbow displaced catheters that were placed in the basilic or cephalic vein below the elbow toward the heart but did not have any effect on catheters that were placed via the axillary vein. For catheters that were placed in the basilic vein, simultaneous shoulder adduction and elbow flexion caused the greatest movement toward the heart (15.11 + or - 1.22 mm). We were able to reposition correctly inappropriately placed catheters in 9 of 10 patients by using arm movements." Ali M. Nadroo, Ronald B. Glass, Jing Lin, Robert S. Green and Ian R. Holzman Central Catheters in Neonates, Pediatrics 2002;110;131-136 The person who has inserted the catheter may not appreciate it being repositioned by the radiographer!

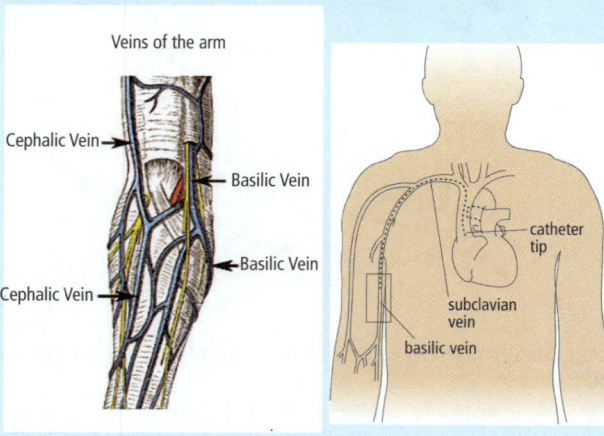

Cubital fossa: Median antecubital, Cephalic and Basilic veins: Are easy to hit and tend to last quite well if splinted properly. Median nerve and brachial artery are both vulnerable. These veins are the preferred sites for insertion of percutaneous central venous catheters. *These should be avoided unless absolutely necessary in any infant likely to need long term IV therapy.*

Courtesy:Dr M J Fuller

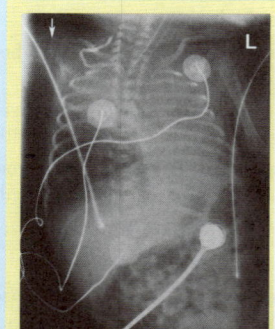 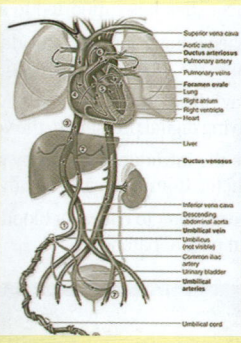 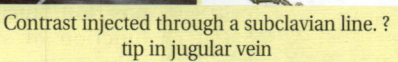
Contrast injected through a subclavian line. ? tip in jugular vein

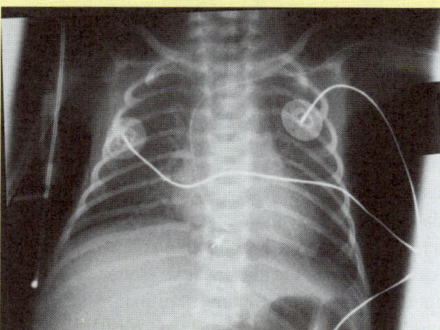 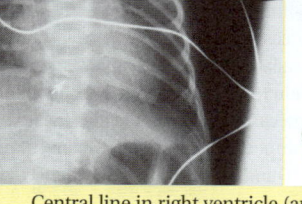
Central line in right ventricle (arrow)

Central Venous Catheter (CVC) Longline- leg: Saphenous vein, ankle Runs reliably just anterior to medical malleolus and is large and straight. Easy to access and lasts well although not always readily visualized.

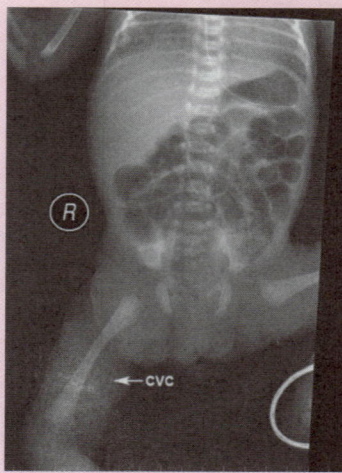

The central venous catheter has been inserted in the right leg and its tip is difficult to localize precisely. This is a common problem with CVC lines and emphasizes the need for good quality images when checking CVC lines. A study of printed CR images vs soft copy CR images reported a long line detection rate of 66.7% vs 95.6% respectively. *(A Evans, J Natarajan, C J Davies, 2004).*

Other suggestions include "The authors emphasise the importance of verifying neonatal long line position using contrast, as the exact localisation of the catheter tip can be difficult on plain radiographs. As an alternative, Groves *et al* have described the use of colour Doppler to aid ultrasonographic line tip visualisation." T M Berger, M Stocker, J Caduff Gonad protection could have been used to good effect

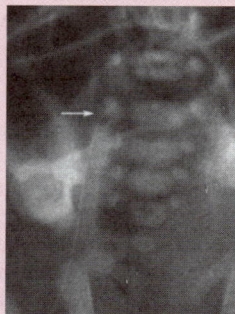

A magnified view demonstrates the CVC tip to be at the level of the first sacral vertebra. This is an "actual pixels" image ie one pixel in the image is one pixel on the screen. This demonstrates the advantage of viewing images by 'softcopy' rather than hardcopy

Neonatal long lines: *localization with color Doppler ultrasonography*

Current guidelines are to avoid placement of neonatal long lines within the heart. Placement within the heart is generally "excluded" radiologically. However, even with the benefit of contrast and digital radiography, the tips of long lines may not be adequately visualized. Standard two dimensional ultrasonography may assist in localizing line tips in neonates, but the technique requires significant experience, and images are not optimal (fig 1A, B). We therefore investigated the use of color Doppler to aid ultrasonographic line tip visualization. A Vygon 24 gauge catheter has an internal diameter of 0.3 mm (area approximately 0.0007 cm2). When flushed at 0.1 ml/s, flow rate at the line tip is about 140 cm/s, well above usual venous flow rates. Using color Doppler, the same line barely visible in fig 1A,B, and masked by superior vena caval blood flow in fig 1C, becomes clearly visible when flushed with saline at about 0.1 ml/s (fig 1D). We are not aware of any centres routinely using color Doppler to aid ultrasonic detection of long line tip position in neonates. This technique potentially offers a simple, reliable method of localizing line tips and should be put through further rigorous assessment.

Courtesy: A M Groves, C A Kuschel, M R Battin Newborn Services, National Women's Hospital, Claude Road, Auckland, New Zealand; malcolmb@adhb.govt.nz

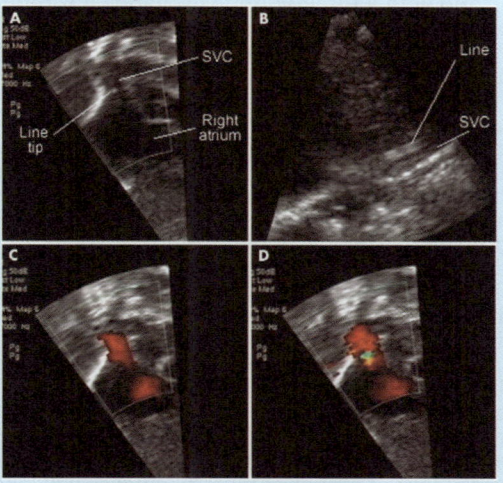

(A) Line tip entering right atrium on sub-costal view; (B) line passing along superior vena cava (SVC) on parasternal view; (C) normal colour Doppler flow pattern in superior vena cava; (D) line tip "illuminated" by saline flush.

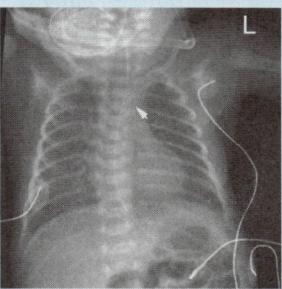
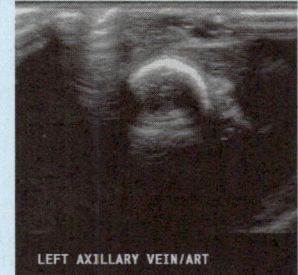
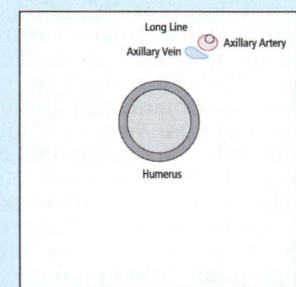

This longline was suspected to be in artery rather than vein. An ultrasound was requested to confirm the position. This is an ultrasound image of the baby's left axillary vessels. It was clear on the live ultrasound image that the longline was within the axillary artery rather than vein. The ultrasound probe was positioned in the baby's axilla. Note that the artery tends to keep a more uniform round shape. The vein is more likely to appear flattened and will change shape when compressed with the ultrasound probe. The doppler flow characteristics also clearly distinguished artery from vein

Care of percutaneous central catheters

A. IV fluids need not contain heparin if the flow rate is 5 ml/hr or greater; if flow rate is < 5 ml/hr fluid should contain heparin, usually at a concentration of 0.25–0.5 unit/ml, but at a rate not to exceed 100 U/kg day; (50 U/kg/day in infants <1000 g).

B. Initial IV fluids should contain dextrose at a concentration not greater than 10%; if the catheter tip is positioned in a central vein, the dextrose concentration may be advanced slowly to as high as 25% (see A above).

C. IV rates should be kept at 3 ml/hr or greater, and less than that recommended by the catheter manufacturer (generally <20 ml/hr for a 27 or 28-gauge catheter)

D. 24-gauge silastic catheters may be repaired by cutting the hub and cannulating the catheter with a 28-gauge blunt needle. This should be done with sterile technique. 27 and 28-gauge catheters cannot be repaired. The dressing is not routinely changed.

E. Blood samples should not be drawn through the catheter. If suspicions occur regarding the need to remove the catheter or if other questions about the catheter arise, consult a nurse or physician member of the Neonatal Percutaneous Central Catheter Team.

F. More detailed nursing instructions for the placement, care and handling of the catheter are available on the NICU in the Policy and Procedure Manual.

G. Removal of a percutaneous central catheter should be performed by a nurse or physician member of the Percutaneous Central Catheter Team, if possible.

H. At the time of its removal, the length of the catheter from its tip to entry point into the plastic hub should be measured and recorded on the special form in the patient's chart.

EXCHANGE TRANSFUSION

Indications:

Double Volume Exchange:

*Significant unconjugated hyperbilirubinemia in the newborn due to any cause, when intensive phototherapy fails or there is risk of kernicterus.   *Alloimmune hemolytic disease of the newborn (HDN) *For correction of severe anemia and hyperbilirubinemia *In addition, in infants with alloimmune HDN, ET replaces antibody-coated neonatal red cells with antigen-negative red cells that should have normal in vivo survival and also removes free maternal antibody in plasma *Disseminated intravascular coagulation *Congenital leukemia *Metabolic toxins *Hyperammonemia *Organic acidemia *Lead poisoning *Drug overdose or toxicity *Removal of antibodies and abnormal proteins *Neonatal sepsis or malaria. *To correct life-threatening electrolyte and fluid imbalance

Partial Exchange Transfusion *Severe anemia with congestive cardiac failure or hypervolemia *Polycythemia.

Precautions/Contraindications

1. When alternatives such as a simple transfusion or phototherapy would be just as effective with less risk. 2. When a contraindication to placement of necessary lines outweighs the indication for exchange transfusion 3. When the patient is unstable and not likely to benefit from the procedure. The NNP will notify the physician immediately under the following circumstances: 1) Patient decompensation or intolerance to the procedure. 2) Outcome of the procedure other than expected

Equipment

*Automatic and manually controlled heat source *Temperature monitor *Cardiorespiratory monitor *Pulse oximeter for oxygen saturation monitoring *Resuscitation equipment and medication (immediately available) *Infant restraints *Orogastric tube *Suctioning equipment *Equipment for central and peripheral vascular access *Blood warmer and appropriate coils *Pre-assembled disposable set with special stopcock *Nonassembled *10- or 20-mL syringes Use a smaller syringe if aliquot per pass is smaller. *Two three-way stopcocks with locking connections *Waste receptacle (empty IV bottle or bag) *IV connecting tubing Appropriate blood product Syringes and tubes for pre- and postexchange blood tests Precautions *Stabilize infant before initiating exchange procedure. *Do not start exchange procedure until personnel are available for monitoring and as backup for other emergencies. *Use blood product appropriate to clinical indication. Use freshest blood available, preferably <5 to 7 days. *Check potassium level of donor blood if patient has hyperkalemia or renal compromise. *Monitor infant closely during and after procedure. *Do not rush procedure. *May necessitate repeat ET if efficacy is decreased by haste. *Stop or slow procedure if patient becomes unstable. *Use only thermostatically controlled blood-warming device that has passed quality control for temperature and alarms. Be sure to review operating and safety procedures for specific blood warmer. Do not overheat blood, i.e., beyond 38°C. *Do not apply excessive suction if it becomes difficult to draw blood from line. Reposition line or replace syringes, stopcocks, and any adapters connected to line. *Leave anticoagulated, banked blood in line or clear line with heparinized saline if the procedure is interrupted. *Clear line with heparinized saline if administering calcium.

Types of exchange transfusion: Partial exchange transfusion: is typically performed for Polycythemia (HCT >65%) that may be due to : delayed clamping of the cord , twin - twin transfusion, maternal - fetal transfusion , iatrogenic transfusion, and increased RBCs production in utero due to hypoxia. It consists of removing whole blood and replacing it with albumin, plasma, or normal saline to lower the HCT to approximately 55%. Single blood volume exchange :using (80 - 100 ml/Kg) and usually performed for anemia with heart failure (i.e. hydrops fetalis) Double volume exchange: (160 - 200 ml/ Kg of blood). Usually performed for severe hemolytic disease of newborn. Exchange transfusion is usually done through umbilical venous catheter taking 5 - 10 ml/ Kg of blood out at a time and replacing it ml for ml. An effective double-volume exchange transfusion (160 mL/kg) reduces the serum bilirubin levels by two time constants (84.5% reduction). With a one-volume exchange transfusion (80 mL/kg), bilirubin is reduced one time constant (63%), and with a three-volume exchange it is reduced by 95%. The three-volume exchange transfusion is not used because it prolongs the procedure and increases the risk of a complication.

Preparation of infant

Place infant on warmer with total accessibility and controlled environment. ET on small preterm infants may be performed in warm incubators, provided a sterile field can be maintained and lines are easily accessible. -Restrain infant suitably. Sedation and pain relief are not usually required. Conscious infants may suck on a pacifier during the procedure. *Connect physiologic monitors and establish baseline values (temperature, respiratory and heart rates, oxygenation) *Empty infant's stomach. *Do not feed for 4 hours prior to procedure, if possible. *Place orogastric tube and remove gastric contents; and leave on open drainage. *Start IV line for glucose and medication infusion: *If exchange procedure interrupts previous essential infusion rate *If prolonged lack of oral or parenteral glucose will lead to hypoglycemia *Extra IV line may be necessary for emergency medications. *Stabilize infant prior to starting exchange procedure; e.g., give packed-cell transfusion when severe hypovolemia and anemia are present, or modify ventilator or ambient oxygen when there is respiratory decompensation. Establish access for ET.

* **EXCHANGE TRANSFUSION Method and types of catheters:** These methods are listed in decreasing order of preference (because of considerations of safety and effectiveness):

A. Continuous (Isovolumetric)

Exchange is performed by two operators, one infuses blood and the other simultaneously withdraws it. The best method is •withdrawal from an umbilical arterial catheter (UAC) and infusion into an umbilical venous catheter (UVC) with tip in IVC or right atrium. Flush withdrawal catheter with heparinized saline every 10-15 min to prevent clotting.

Alternatives are: •withdrawal from a peripheral arterial catheter and infusion into a central venous catheter. However, this is slow and the arterial catheter frequently clots. •withdrawal from a central venous catheter and infusion into a peripheral vein. Flush the central catheter frequently to prevent clotting.ET via peripheral vessels is an efficient and safe alternative to umbilical vessel ET. The technique can be used in most neonates who require ET to minimize iatrogenic risks, especially in premature and ill neonates

B. Push-Pull Method can be done through: •a single UVC with tip in IVC or right atrium. •a single UAC with tip in lower aorta (below 3rd lumbar vertebra)

Laboratory tests on infant's blood pre-exchange Tests are based on clinical indications.

*Pre-exchange diagnostic studies:** Note that diagnostic serologic tests on the infant, such as studies to evaluate unexplained hemolysis, antiviral antibody titers, metabolic screening, or genetic tests should be drawn prior to the ET. *Hemoglobin, hematocrit, platelets *Electrolytes, calcium, blood gas.

Preparation for Total or Partial Exchange Transfusion

*Blood product and volume Blood Product

-Communicate with blood bank to determine most appropriate blood product for transfusion.

-Plasma-reduced whole blood or packed red cells reconstituted with plasma, with a packed cell volume adjusted to 0.5 to 0.60, is suitable for ET to correct anemia and hyperbilirubinemia .

-Blood may be anticoagulated with citrate phosphate dextrose (CPD or CPDA1) or heparin. Additive anticoagulant solutions are generally avoided . If only RBCs stored in additive solutions are available, the additive solution may be removed by washing or by centrifugation and removal of the supernatant solution, prior to reconstitution of the red cells with plasma.

-Blood should be as fresh as possible (<7 days).

-Irradiated blood is recommended for all ET, to prevent graft-versus-host disease. There is a significant increase in potassium concentration in stored irradiated units, so irradiation should be performed as close to the transfusion as possible (<24 hours).

-Standard blood-bank screening is particularly important, including sickle-cell preparation, HIV, hepatitis B, and cytomegalovirus (CMV)

-Donor blood should be screened for G-6-PD deficiency and HbS in populations endemic for these conditions .

-In presence of alloimmunization, e.g., Rh, ABO, special attention to compatibility testing is necessary.

-If delivery of an infant with severe HDN is anticipated, O Rh-negative blood cross-matched against the mother may be prepared before the baby is born.

-Donor blood prepared after the infant's birth should be negative for the antigen responsible for the hemolytic disease, and should be cross-matched against the infant.

-In ABO HDN, the blood must be type O and either Rh-negative or Rh-compatible with the mother and the infant. The blood should be washed free of plasma or have a low titer of anti-A or anti-B antibodies. Type O cells with AB plasma may be more effective, but this results in two donor exposures per ET.

-In Rh HDN, the blood should be Rh-negative, and may be O group or the same group as the infant.

-In infants with polycythemia, the optimal dilutional fluid for a partial ET is isotonic saline rather than plasma or albumin.

Volume of Donor Blood Required

-Whenever possible, use no more than equivalent of one whole unit of blood for each procedure, to decrease donor exposure.

-Quantity needed for total procedure = volume for the actual ET plus volume for tubing dead space and blood warmer (usually 25 to 30 mL)

-Double-volume ET for removal of bilirubin, antibodies, etc.:

2 × infant's blood volume = 2 x 80 to 120 mL/kg

-Infant's blood volume in preterm infant < 100 to 120 mL/kg, in term infant < 80 to 85 mL/kg

-Exchanges approximately 85% of infant's blood volume

-Single volume ET: Exchanges approximately 60% of infant's blood volume.

Partial Exchange Transfusion: *Single-volume or partial ET for correction of polycythemia: Volume of exchange (mL)=total blood volume (mL) X [observed Hct- desired Hct/observed Hct].e.g.,1-kg preterm infant with Hct 68%, desired postpartial exchange Hct 55%. 100 X [68-55/68]= about 20 mL of crystalloid exchanged with whole blood. (Infant's blood volume in preterm infant < 100 to 120 mL/kg, in term infant < 80 to 85 mL/kg).

*Partial ET for correction of severe anemia:

Volume of exchange (mL) =total blood volume (mL) X [Desired Hct- Observed Hct/Hct of the PRBC Unit-Observed Hct] e.g.,1-kg preterm infant with Hct 21%, desired postpartial exchange Hct 45% requires 100 X {45-21/70-21}=49 ml of PRBC.

Procedure: 1. A full aseptic technique should be employed. 2. If using an in/out technique, insert the catheter and obtain an X-ray to confirm position. Connect the four-way stopcock /2 three-way taps if not available to the catheter. Attach in a clockwise direction from the port attached to the catheter — the waste blood container — the fresh blood supply — a 20 mL syringe. A closed circuit must be used at all times to prevent air embolus. During each cycle, withdraw blood from the baby and inject into the waste blood container. Refill the syringe with the fresh donated blood and very slowly inject into the baby. Each cycle should take 5 min, giving blood over no less than 2.5 min. 3. If blood is going to be given continuously via a peripheral line, use a volumetric pump which delivers at the same rate that blood is being withdrawn. Exchange of each aliquot should take place over 5 min. 4. If indication for exchange is jaundice; immediately prior to starting, re-check SBR and confirm that exchange is still necessary. 5. Take an umbilical swab for microbiology. Send blood for Hb, PCV, glucose, blood gas and culture. 6. Use: 5 mL aliquots for <28 weeks — 10 mL aliquots for 28-32 weeks — 15 mL aliquots for 33-36 weeks — 20 mL aliquots for >36 weeks. If not well tolerated reduce the aliquot. The whole exchange should take approximately 1.25-1.5 h. 7. After every 100 mL exchanged give 1 mL of 10% calcium gluconate mixed with the next aliquot of blood. Monitor the EGG closely and stop if the HR falls to < 100 bpm. 8. At the end, take blood for Hb, PCV, SBR, calcium, glucose, blood gas, coagulation screen and blood culture. Culture catheter tip if catheter is removed. Restart phototherapy if indication for exchange is jaundice. 9. If a UVC has been used, leave in situ until it is clear that a second exchange is unlikely within the next 24 h. 10. Check blood sugar hourly for 4 h after the exchange as rebound hypoglycemia may occur (secondary to hyperinsulinism in response to the high dextrose content of the infused blood). 11. Do not feed for 2-4 h post-exchange, to decrease the incidence of NEC. (Feedings may be attempted two to four hours after the exchange transfusion.)

Monitoring : An observer must record constantly the amount of blood being withdrawn and replaced and the time taken for each cycle. HR, EGG. BP and temperature should be recorded regularly and blood sugar and blood gases checked every 30 min. @ *ET causes high morbidity, even in term and near-term newborns. Therefore, it should be initiated only when the benefit of preventing kernicterus outweighs the complications associated with the procedure.*

Single versus double volume exchange transfusion in jaundiced newborn infants: Traditionally twice the blood volume of baby is removed and the replaced with fresh blood. Exchange transfusion has been shown to reduce brain damage in severely jaundiced babies; however, exchange transfusion is associated with serious adverse events including death. It is likely that the complications of exchange transfusion would increase with amount of blood exchanged. This review was undertaken to examine if single volume (removal of blood equivalent to the blood volume of the baby) is as effective as double volume (removal of twice blood volume of the baby) in reducing the brain damage and bilirubin levels in newborn infants with severe jaundice. Only one randomized trial fulfilled the criteria for inclusion in the analysis. This study compared single and double volume exchange transfusion in jaundice due to ABO hemolytic jaundice. The study found no significant difference in bilirubin levels following exchange. This study did not look at any long term neurodevelopmental outcome (brain damage). Based on the available data, there is insufficient evidence to support or refute the use of single volume exchange transfusion as opposed to double volume exchange transfusion in jaundiced newborns. *The Cochrane Database of Systematic Reviews 2010 Issue 5, Copyright © 2010 The Cochrane Collaboration. Published by John Wiley and Sons, Ltd.*

Continuous (Isovolumetric) ET: Exchange is performed by two operators, one infuses blood and the other simultaneously withdraws it. The best method is •withdrawal from an umbilical arterial catheter (UAC) and infusion into an umbilical venous catheter (UVC) with tip in IVC or right atrium. Flush withdrawal catheter with heparinized saline every 10-15 min to prevent clotting.

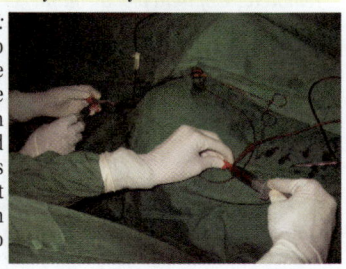

Important reminders during ET:

- Monitor ECG, blood pressure, O_2 saturation, transcutaneous CO_2 and temperature during ExTx.
- Measure pH at mid-point and at end of ExTx (more frequently in a "sick" baby.
- Measure glucose and electrolytes at end of ExTx, and glucose at 10, 30, 60 min later.
- Warm blood to 34–35° C. Warming blood to >37° C causes hemolysis.
- Agitate the unit of donor blood q 10-15 min so that cells do not settle.
- ExTx does not significantly reduce plasma gentamicin level; do not give an extra dose.

Complications of Exchange Transfusion:(Problem with Donor Blood -Effect on Infant -Prevention or Treatment)

Blood is cold : Hypothermia–Warm donor blood to 34 - 35° C
High K+ : Hyperkalemia, Arrhythmia-Use fresh blood, monitor ECG
Low pH (e.g., 6.9): Acidosis–Consider buffering blood with THAM if infant is unstable. This will also decrease [K+].
No platelets (old blood or PRBC+FFP): Thrombocytopenia -Consider platelet Tx at end of ExTx. If increased risk of bleeding, also Tx platelets at mid-point.
Citrate anticoagulant: Low Ca++ & Mg++ –Give 30 mg/kg of dilute Ca gluconate, over 5 min at ¼, ½, ¾ and at end of a 2 volume ExTx, and if unexplained tachycardia or arrhythmia occurs.
High glucose: Reactive Hypoglycemia—Start IV glucose at 5mg/kg/min 10-15 min after end of ExTx; monitor blood glucose.
The serum bilirubin concentration rebounds to a value approximately halfway between the pre- and post- exchange levels by two hours after completing the exchange transfusion. Therefore, the serum bilirubin concentration should be monitored at two to four hours after exchange and subsequently every three to four hours.

Documentation during Exchange Transfusion

A. Written record: Documentation of procedure in chart by NNP:
Fill out a unit based procedure note and place in chart

1. Before performing this procedure, document in UCare any abnormal physical findings.
2. Documentation of the pretreatment evaluation, time out, and medication (drug, dose, route, and time) given.
3. Documentation of indication for procedure, procedure, including type of catheters used and placement, type of blood products used, amount of exchange, medication given, results, how patient tolerated the procedure, as well as any complications.

B. All abnormal findings are reviewed with Attending or supervising physician

Specimens - Donor, Pre-exchange, During Exchange, and Post-Exchange

Donor Blood Specimens: Mix blood well. Specimen is to be taken from each unit as soon as it arrives. Collect 0.3ml into a blood gas syringe and record haemoglobin and K+. Blood should not be used if potassium result is: >15mmol/L in well babies >10mmol/L in small sick babies

Pre-Exchange Patient Specimens
* Collect 0.3ml for arterial blood gas, Na, K, Ca and glucose levels.
* Collect 0.3ml and send for FBC and differential.
* Collect 0.7ml and send for urea, creatinine, bilirubin (total and direct).
* Before second and repeat exchanges or where there are clotting abnormalities, collect 0.8ml into buffered citrate micro-container (obtained from lab), send for coagulation screen
* During Exchange Specimen: Blood gas, electrolytes and glucose are tested as ordered.

Post-Exchange Patient Specimens: (take from the last few ml of the exchange out volume)
Collect 0.3ml in blood gas syringe, test for gas, Na, K, Ca, Glucose.
Collect 0.3ml and send for FBC and differentials
Collect 0.7ml and send for urea, bilirubin (total and direct).
Coagulation screen should be performed if more than one exchange.
All patient specimens are taken via the 3 way tap closest to the arterial line out catheter.

One Catheter-Push-Pull - The transfusion should not commence until nursing and medical staff agree that the circuit set up is correct. Observe carefully throughout the procedure that there is no air in the line. The nurse is responsible for recording in and out blood volumes. Each cycle in and out should take approximately 4 minutes.

The amount of blood exchanged is expressed as multiples of the infant's blood volume. The standard "two volume" ET uses a volume twice the infant's blood volume (i.e., 170 mL/kg). The procedure is done in small increments. As the procedure progresses, relatively more of the donor blood (infused earlier) and less of the patient's own blood is removed. The washout of the infant's blood is a simple exponential function:

Volume exchanged (of patient's total blood volume) vs Patient's blood removed (% of total blood volume)

0.5 volume-39 %, 1.0 volume-63 %, 2.0 volume-86 %, 4.0 volume-98 % These values are for washout of the vascular compartment. However, an ET will remove more bilirubin than shown above. This is because unconjugated bilirubin is distributed in both the intravascular and extravascular spaces, and will move rapidly into the intravascular space as the concentration decreases during the ET. Thus, a 2 volume ET will remove twice as much bilirubin as was in the circulating plasma at the start of the procedure. However, because of continued movement of bilirubin into the vascular space, the plasma bilirubin concentration at the end of the ET will be reduced by only ½ of the pre-exchange level.

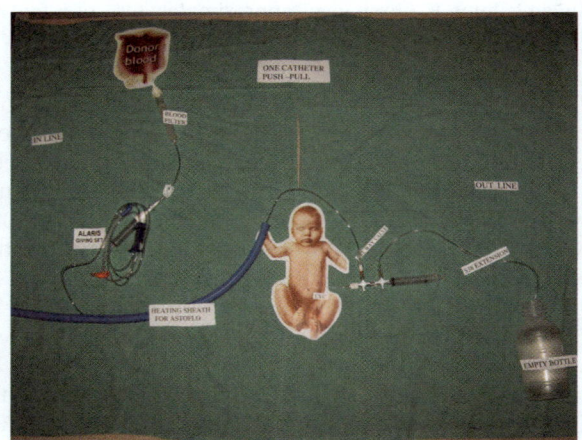

Warning Signs during ET:

- **Vomiting or crying during injection of blood**
  - — infusion too rapid. Stop until condition improves
- **Cyanosis or pallor**
  - — Check temperature, ECG, pH, P_aCo_2
  - — Consider too rapid infusion, blood balance error causing hypo/hypervolemia, metabolic acidosis
- **Aspirated blood becomes dark**
  - — catheter tip may be in branch of portal vein; readjust until brighter blood appears. If readjustments make no difference, consider deterioration in baby's condition and check temperature, ECG, pH, P_aCo_2
- **Tachycardia > 160/min and bradycardia <100/min**
  - — consider blood volume disturbance, metabolic acidosis and hyperkalemia.
- **ECG abnormalities**
  - — Circulatory overload may lead to peaked P waves
  - — Signs of hyperkalemia: stop transfusion. Do not use donor blood. Check K⁺ levels in donor blood. Refer to the chapter "Neonatal Hyperkalemia" for management of hyperkalemia.
  - — Arrhythmias: mostly caused by cold blood or hyperkalemia
- **Cardiac arrest**
  - — Cold blood, hyperkalemia, too rapid injection of calcium gluconate, air embolism
- **Convulsion**
  - — Check blood pH, glucose and calcium

Complications of Exchange transfusion:

- **Vascular** : Embolization with air or clot, Thrombosis, Hemorrhagic infarction of the gut
- **Cardiac** : Arrhythmias, Volume overload, Hypovolemia, Arrest
- **Metabolic** : Hypokalemia, Hypocalcemia, Hypomagnesemia, Acidosis, Hypoglycemia
- **Respiratory** : Oxygen affinity is reduced because the donor blood usually has an oxygen dissociation curve displayed to the right of fetal haemoglobin
- **Hematological Problems** : Thrombocytopenia, coagulopathy
- **Infection** : Bacteremia, HIV, CMV, hepatitis B from infected donor blood
- **Hypothermia** :

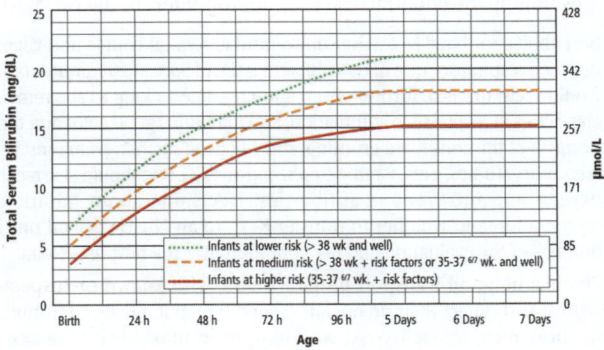

Guidelines for exchange transfusion in infants 35 or more weeks gestation. (From American Academy of Pediatrics. Subcommittee on Hyperbilirubinemia. Clinical Practice Guideline. Management of hyperbilirubinemia in the newborn infant 35 or more weeks gestation. Pediatrics. 2004;114:297-316.)

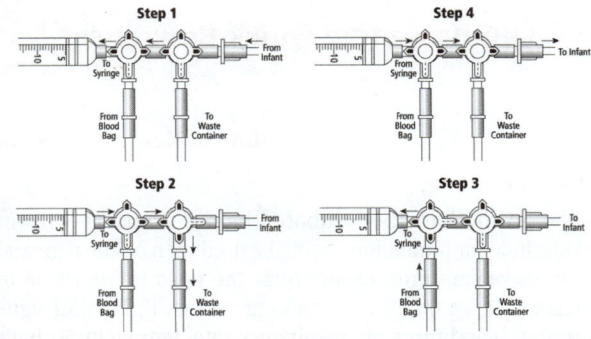

Three-way stopcocks in tandem. Step 1: Stopcocks positioned for withdrawing blood from infant. Step 2: Stopcocks positioned for emptying withdrawn blood to waste container. Step 3: Stopcocks positioned for filling syringe from blood bag. Step 4: Stopcocks positioned for injecting blood into infant line.

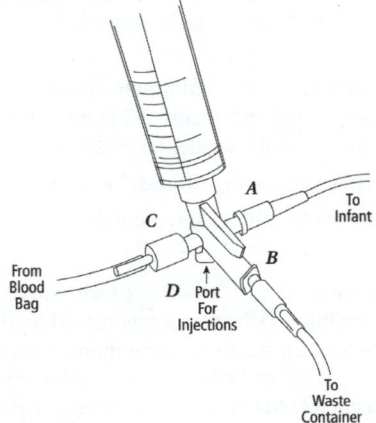

Special four-way stopcock. A, male adapter to infant line; B, female adapter to waste container; C, attachment to blood tubing; D, position (180 degrees from adapter to waste container), allowing injection through rubber-stoppered port with a syringe. The stopcock is used in clockwise rotation when correctly assembled.

Post Procedure Care & Management

1. Following an exchange transfusion the infant needs to be monitored closely for 24 hours. This may be able to be done on the postnatal ward with the mother.

2. Phototherapy needs to be continued post exchange and reviewed with the results of the SBR. Further SBR levels at approximately 6 hourly intervals.

3. Continue cardio-respiratory monitoring - Blood pressure at completion of procedure. Hourly : Temperature, apex beat, respirations, for 4 hours. If stable and within normal limits after this time previous observations as per guidelines may be recommenced.

4. Observe the infant's behaviour and catheter sites for bleeding or signs of infection.

5. Blood Glucose level as indicated by initial and post exchange results.

6. Appearance of abdomen with routine observations (3 - 4 hourly) for 24 hours. Listen for bowel sounds.

7. Test urine for blood. Observe stools for blood.

8. Commence feeds on medical staff orders if clinically stable. Observe for signs of feed intolerance : gastric aspirate, vomiting, abdominal distension.

9. Document how the infant tolerated the procedure and ensure the parents are informed.

10. Blood specimens as ordered.

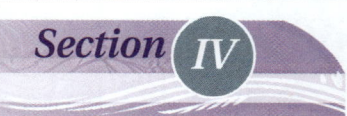

Outline of Key Issues in Stabilizing Neonates for Transfer

Airway/breathing

* Should the baby be intubated before transfer? A lower threshold for intubation should be used than on the neonatal intensive care unit, to minimize the need to intervene in transit. In an infant >30 weeks gestation, if the vital signs (pulse, blood pressure, respiratory rate, temperature) have been consistently stable in oxygen <50% and if the PaCO2 is normal, it may be acceptable to move the baby without intubation. If the infant is: unstable has a rising oxygen requirement >50% has a rising PaCO2 has recurrent apnea is <30 weeks gestation then intubation and respiratory support is highly likely to be required, at least for the duration of the journey.

* If already intubated, the endotracheal tube (ETT) must be correctly positioned and secure. ETTs must be secured to a high standard, to avoid accidental extubation in transit.

* Adequate respiratory support must be given.

* Surfactant must be administered if indicated.

Circulation

* Arterial access, if not already established, should be considered in infants who require repeated blood gas analysis or accurate blood pressure measurement. If siting a line will not influence practice before or during the journey, then it may be acceptable to delay this until after the transfer.

* Correct positioning and security of the catheter must be checked.

* Circulation with fluids and/or inotropes should be supported early, as indicated.

Temperature

* Assess temperature and consider the support required for transfer.

* Use temperature maintenance adjuncts, such as chemical gel mattresses.

Blood glucose

* Measure and stabilize blood glucose.

* Secure intravenous access.

Infection

* Screen for infection as indicated.

* Start treatment.

Parents' information and wishes

* Discuss plans with parents. Ascertain their plans about travelling to referral unit. Liaise with midwifery staff about maternal transfer.

Information

* Ensure the team at the referral unit will have all the necessary information to advance the care of the baby.

Call as early as possible!

It is vital for General Pediatricians to be able to anticipate the need for retrieval and initiate contact early. Waiting until all clinical information is available may cause considerable delay, which may affect the clinical outcome. They should update their **Skills for resuscitation of the Newborn at regular intervals.**

Skill Detail

Assessment: Assessment of the Newborn at delivery with regards to color, reactivity, respiratory effort, heart rate and tone

Airway support: Assessment, positioning, bag and mask ventilation, intubation and establishment of a definitive airway*

Access: Intravenous and intra-osseous access

Accurate documentation: The following must be documented:

• time and detail of interventions during resuscitation • time to establishment of heart rate and respirations

Ability to communicate effectively with the retrieval team: Communication of accurate clinical scenarios to expedite appropriate care.

* If the General Pediatrician is unable to intubate, a plan should be in place to call in a person with this skill such as an on-call anaesthetist. Failing this, adequate oxygenation may be maintained by bag and mask until the retrieval team arrives. In most situations, the need for intubation can be predicted and the need to intubate as an emergency is unusual before the arrival of the retrieval team. Teleconferencing can aid in the decision and in the practicalities of positioning the endotracheal tube appropriately in the Newborn.

A Neonate with Respiratory distress-*K. C. is a newborn girl born at 41 weeks' gestation by spontaneous vaginal delivery. Her antenatal course was unremarkable. Labor progressed normally, and she was delivered and passed to the delivery room nurse after 15 minutes of pushing by the mother. Apgar score was 8 at one minute and five minutes of life. The initial physical exam was normal except for acrocyanosis and moderate grunting and flaring. A repeat exam at 20 minutes of life reveals persistent grunting. The baby's respiratory rate is 60/min, and her arterial oxygen saturation (SAO$_2$) is 95% as measured by pulse oximetry. Her heart rate is 160/min. Is it safe to continue observing this newborn, or does she require intervention now?*

When to transfer? Based on clinical experience since 1973, the Iowa Perinatal Care Program has derived a "rule of two hours" to guide physicians facing difficult decisions regarding whether to transfer infants in respiratory distress to an NICU. The rule recommends transfer if: *two hours have passed without improvement *the chest radiograph is abnormal *the infant's respiratory condition deteriorates or *more than 40% oxygen is required to maintain 95% SAO$_2$.*

To wait or act? To return to the question posed in the case history at the beginning of this article: Is continued observation or intervention the best choice for baby K. C.? Her uneventful antenatal course and vaginal delivery, respiratory rate of 60/min, and SAO$_2$ of 95% at 20 minutes of life would seem to make further observation feasible as long as she remains alert, cries in response to stimulation, and maintains good color and tone. Because of the continued grunting, she will need further evaluation with laboratory studies, a chest radiograph, and an ECG. She should also receive oxygen and intravenous antibiotics. Decisions about additional intervention and whether to transfer K. C. to an NICU depend on the findings of the evaluation and her condition over the next few hours.

Stabilization and transport of the neonate with known or suspected critical CHD affect their preoperative condition, potentially contributing to short-term mortality risk and long-term morbidity. One key to stabilization is the recognition of potential or confirmed CHD, appropriate resuscitation, airway management where indicated, stable vascular access, judicious oxygen utilization, PGE1, and inotropic support when necessary. Early consultation with a center specializing in pediatric cardiac care, for advice and timing of transport, will aid the initial care and stability of the infant on transport. Accurate, detailed information must be communicated among the referring hospital, the transport team, and the accepting hospital.

Stabilizing the preterm or sick infant: An overview for a quick recap

Additional Oxygen and artificial ventilation

Many infants with respiratory distress require additional inspiratory oxygen and ventilatory support. In preterm infants this is often for respiratory distress syndrome, but even in the absence of this disorder, many infants <30 week's gestation require artificial ventilation because of lung immaturity or to avoid recurrent apnea.

Circulatory support

Circulatory support with colloid infusion and inotropic drugs is required to treat hypotension, if peripheral perfusion appears inadequate. Echocardiography can provide information on ventricular function.

Monitoring

The heart rate, respiratory rate and temperature are monitored continuously. Oxygenation is measured indirectly by pulse oximetry for oxygen saturation and with a transcutaneous electrode for oxygen tension. The arterial CO_2 tension can also be measured transcutaneously. Blood gas analysis is performed on arterial samples from a peripheral or umbilical artery catheter. The arterial oxygen tension is maintained at 8-12 kpa (60-90 mmHg) and the CO_2 tension at 4.5-6.5kpa (35-50 mmHg).

A chest X-ray is required to help diagnose respiratory disorders and confirm the position of the tracheal tube and umbilical artery catheter.

Avoiding hypothermia

Hypothermia increases mortality and should be prevented by placing the baby under a radiant warmer or in an incubator.

Antibiotics

Infants requiring intensive care are often given broad-spectrum antibiotics. Infection with the Group B streptococcus and other organisms can mimic respiratory distress syndrome.

Metabolic disturbance

Blood glucose is checked regularly and IV dextrose given to prevent hypoglycemia. Fluid requirements are very variable ad must be closely monitored.

Minimal handling

All procedures, especially painful ones, adversely affect oxygenation and the circulation. Sedation and analgesia, e.g. an iv infusion of morphine, are given as required. Handling is kept to a minimum and done as rapidly and efficiently as possible.

Parents

Although medical and nursing staff are usually fully occupied stabilizing the baby, time must be found for parents to allow them to see and touch their baby to be kept fully informed.

History relevant to preterm delivery

* Maternal medical and obstetric history
* Estimated gestation
* Singleton or multifetal pregnancy?
* Assessments of fetal growth and wellbeing
* Details of suspected congenital anomalies
* Risk of fetal-maternal infection and chorioamnionitis
* Course of labor, if laboring
* Intrapartum monitoring results
* Antenatal interventions, tocolytic drugs, steroids, antibiotics
* Use of opiates and anesthetic drugs

Stabilizing a Preterm/Sick infants is extremely important to prevent complications. This preterm infant has leads on his limbs and trunk for Monitoring of the Vital functions and O2 saturations. There are Umbilical arterial and venous catheters, ET Tube and IV cannulae indicated for intensive care of these High-Risk Neonates.

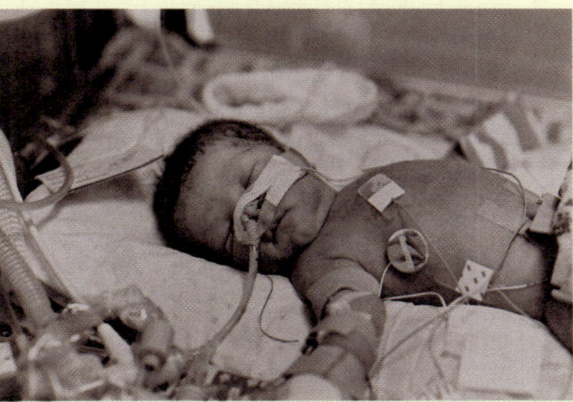

Neonatal problems associated with premature infants:
Refer to the individual Chapters for the details of Diagnosis and Management!

Respiratory

Respiratory distress syndrome (hyaline membrane disease)*

Bronchopulmonary dysplasia

Pneumothorax, Pneumomediastinum; interstitial emphysema

Congenital pneumonia

Pulmonary hypoplasia

Pulmonary hemorrhage

Apnea*

Cardiovascular

Patent ductus arteriosus*

Hypotension

Hypertension

Bradycardia (with apnea)*

Congenital malformations

Hematologic

Anemia (early or late onset)

Hyperbilirubinemia-indirect*

Subcutaneous, organ (liver, adrenal) hemorrhage*

Disseminated intravascular coagulopathy

Vitamin K deficiency

Hydrops-immune or nonimmune

Gastrointestinal

Poor gastrointestinal function - poor motility*

Necrotizing enterocolitis

Hyperbilirubinemia-direct and indirect

Congenital anomalies producing polyhydramnios

Spontaneous gastrointestinal isolated perforation

Metabolic —Endocrine

Hypocalcemia*

Hypoglycemia*

Hyperglycemia*

Late metabolic acidosis

Hypothermia*

Euthyroid but low-thyroxin status

Central Nervous system

Intraventricular hemorrhage*

Periventricular leukomalacia

Hypoxic - ischemic encephalopathy

Seizures

Retinopathy of prematurity

Deafness

Congenital malformations

Kernicterus (bilirubin encephalopathy)

Drug (narcotic) withdrawal

Renal

Hyponatremia* Hypernatremia* Hyperkalemia*

Renal tubular acidosis, Renal glycosuria, Edema

Other

Infections* (congenital, perinatal, nosocomial: bacterial, viral, fungal, protozoal)

*Common.

Mnemonic for remembering the six steps for improving efficacy of positive pressure ventilation : MRSOPA

M-Adjust **M**ask to assure good seal on the face
R-**R**eposition airway by adjusting head to "sniffing" position
S-**S**uction mouth and nose of secretions, if present
O-**O**pen mouth slightly and move jaw forward
P-Increase **p**ressure every few breaths until bilateral breath sounds and chest rise are evident.
A-If still unsuccessful, use an **a**lternative airway (endotracheal tube or laryngeal mask airway)

Mnemonic for Neonatal Cough: CRADLE

C-Cystic fibrosis
R-Respiratory infection
A-Aspiration (reflux, swallowing dysfunction, TE Fistula)
D-Dyskinesia of cilia
L-Lung, airway, vascular malformation
E-Edema (heart failure, BPD)

Mnemonic for Neonatal Distress: TAMM DATA

1. **TAMM Mnemonic**
   1. Trauma
   2. Asphyxia
   3. Medications
   4. Malformations
2. **DATA Mnemonic**
   1. Drugs
   2. Asphyxia
   3. Trauma
   4. Anomalies

Mnemonic for breaking bad news, such as neonatal death, to distraught parents : FEARED

* **Facts:** The first concern is to provide the parents with the facts of the case, based on the chart and hospital course, and to establish a foundation for the rest of the discussion.
* **Empathy:** Expressions of empathy should acknowledge that the caregivers will try to understand what went wrong and will help the family deal with the issues they face.
* **Anger:** The most difficult question the caregiver needs to ask is whether the patient feels angry, and if so, where those feelings are directed.
* **Response:** Respond straightforward, if the patient acknowledges anger toward the doctor
* **Explain:** "I am sorry you feel that way, but it is understandable. Please tell me how you arrived at that conclusion,"
* **Dispel:** doubts, misinterpretations or misconceptions with honesty and compassion as a defense.

Mnemonic for Neonatal pre-transport stabilization: ABC STABLE

A-Airway
B-Breathing
C-Circulation
S-Sugar
T- Temperature
A-Airway and Ventilation
B-Blood Pressure
L-Lab Work
E-Emotional Support

Mnemonic for evaluation and management of the Critically ill Neonate in the ED

(Clin Ped Emerg Med 9(3): 140-148, 2008)
* History
* Physical examination
* Initial Stabilization
* Laboratory
* Differential Diagnoses: NEO SECRETS
Differential Diagnoses: **NEO SECRETS**
N -i**N**born errors of metabolism
E -**E**lectrolyte abnormalities
O -**O**verdose (toxin, poison)
S -**S**eizures
E -**E**nteric emergencies
C -**C**ardiac abnormalities
R -**R**ecipe (formula, herbs, additives)
E -**E**ndocrine crisis
T -**T**rauma
S- **S**epsis

Mnemonic for Making decisions regarding the appropriateness of inter-institutional transfer (Fletcher and Paris)

ACUTE (**A**cute, **C**ritical, **U**nexpected, **T**reatable, and **E**asily diagnosed)- Infants included in this group are those with prematurity and respiratory distress syndrome; ELBW infants of gestational age known to be 25 weeks or greater; term or preterm infants with sepsis, pneumonia, or meningitis; and infants with surgically correctable malformations.
UNSURE (**UN**known disease, **SU**spected **RE**sponse). This group includes preterms of 23 to 24 weeks gestational age or with very low-birth-weight and uncertain gestational age, infants with severe birth asphyxia, and any infant with an unexplained disease or syndrome that requires further diagnostic efforts. Within this group there will be a significant number of infants for whom the response to treatment will be unpredictable. These infants should be given full medical care until the diagnosis has been made or the response to treatment is clear; decisions to omit care or not to transfer should not be made precipitously.
KNOT (**K**nown, **NO**t **T**reatable). Although only a small number of infants fit into this category, treatment decisions for this group frequently take a disproportionate amount of time. This group includes neonates with anencephaly and those with lethal genetic disorders such as trisomy 13 and trisomy 18. Transfer of neonates with anencephaly for aggressive support is not indicated; transfer of those with lethal genetic defects is not indicated if there are facilities for accurate diagnosis 'and appropriate care and counseling at the hospital of birth. When diagnostic facilities are not available at the birth hospital, onsite consultation by a specialist from the referral hospital is an appropriate alternative to transferring the infant.

Pearl: Changes in the following normal bowel gas patterns should raise suspicion of neonatal gastrointestinal tract disease. 1. Air in the stomach should occur within 30 min after delivery. 2. Air in the small bowel should be seen by 3-4 h of age. 3. Air in the colon and rectum should be seen by 6-8 h of age

Score	Upper chest	Nasal chest retrac	Xiphoid retrac	Nasal flare	Grunt
0	Sync	None	None	None	None
1	Lag on Insp	Just visible	Just visible	Minimal	Steth only
2	See-Saw	Marked	Marked	Marked	Naked ear

A score of 7 or more is indicative of impending respiratory failure

A) CLINICAL CRITERIA 1) FOR PRETERM BABIES SILVERMAN-ANDERSON RETRACTION SCORE

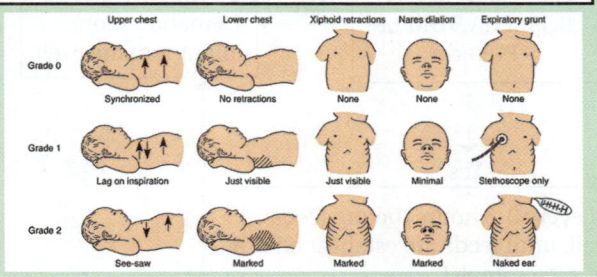

Respiratory distress scoring

2) FOR TERM BABIES
DOWNE'S SCORE IN TERM BABIES

Score	Respiratory Rate/min	Cyanosis	Air Entry	Retractions	Grunt
0	<60	None	Good	None	None
1	60-80	In air	Diminished	Mild	Audible with Stethoscope
2	> 80 or apneic	In 40% O_2	Barely audible	Moderate /severe	Audible with naked ear

A score of 6 or more is indicative of impending respiratory failure

B) LABORATORY CRITERIA pH-<7.1-7.2, PaO_2<50mmHg (6.6kPa) In FiO_2> 0.6, $PaCO_2$>60mmHg (8kPa)

In infants weighing <1500g $PaCO_2$ should be modified to > 50mmHg-preventing the risk of intracerebral Hemorrhage (ICH) at high $PaCO_2$

ABG Score

Parameters	0	1	2	3
PaO_2 mmHg	>60	50-60	<50	<50
pH	>7.3	7.20-7.29	7.1–7.19	<7.1
$PaCO_2$ mmHg	<50	50-60	61-70	>70

A score of 3 more indicates the need for CPAP or mechanical ventilation. 1kPa=7.5mmHg

MEASURING UNITS FOR MEDICINES

1 kilogram (kg)	=	1000 grams
1 gram (g)	=	1000 milligrams
1 milligram (mg)	=	1000 micrograms
1 microgram (mg)*	=	1000 nanograms
1 nanogram (ng)*	=	1000 picograms

A 1% weight for volume (w/v) solution contains
1 g of substance in 100 ml of solution
It follows that:
a 1:100 (1%) solution contains 10 milligrams in 1 ml
a 1:1000* solution contains 1 milligram in 1 ml
a 1:10,000 solution contains 100 micrograms in 1 ml

* These contractions are best avoided as they can easily be misread when written by hand.

Pounds-kilograms conversion

1 pound	=	0.45359 kilograms
1 kilogram	=	2.2 pounds

Temperature conversion

Celsius to Fahrenheit	=	(°C × 9/5) + 32 = °F
Fahrenheit to Celsius	=	(°F - 32) × 5/9 = °C

Normal vital signs in the newborn period

Sign	Rate
Heart rate	90-140 beats/min
Respirations	30-60/min
Temperature	36.5°C- 37.0°C (97.8°F-98.6°F)
Mean blood pressure*	40-55 mm Hg

* In many nurseries, this is not routinely done.

Nutrient requirements for newborn infants

Nutrient	Unit
Water	150–180 mL/kg/day
Calories	100–120 Kcal/kg/day
Protein	2–3 g/kg/day
Carbohydrate	15–16 g/kg/day
Fat	3–4 g/kg/day

Blood gases: Representative values in normal infants at term

		Arterial blood					
	Umbilical vein	30 min	1–4 hr	12-24 hr	24–48 hr	96 hr	Reference
PH	7.33	–	7.30	7.30	7.39	7.39	
PCO_2, mm Hg	43	–	39	33	34	36	Reardon et al (1960)
HCO_3, mEq/L	21.6	–	18.8	19.5	20	21.4	Oliver et al (1961)
PO_2, mm Hg	28 ± 8	–	62 ± 13.8	68	63-87		Nelson et al (1962,1963)
O_2 saturation			95%	94%	94%	96%	

From Taeusch HW, Ballard RA: Avery's Diseases of the Newborn, 7th ed. Philadelphia, WB saunders, 1998 and Bucci G et al: Biol Neonate 8:81, 1965

Guidelines for monitoring oxygen saturation levels by pulse oximetry

>95% - Term baby, pulmonary hypertension (PPHN)
88–94% - 28–34 weeks preterm
85–92% - Below 28 weeks gestational age

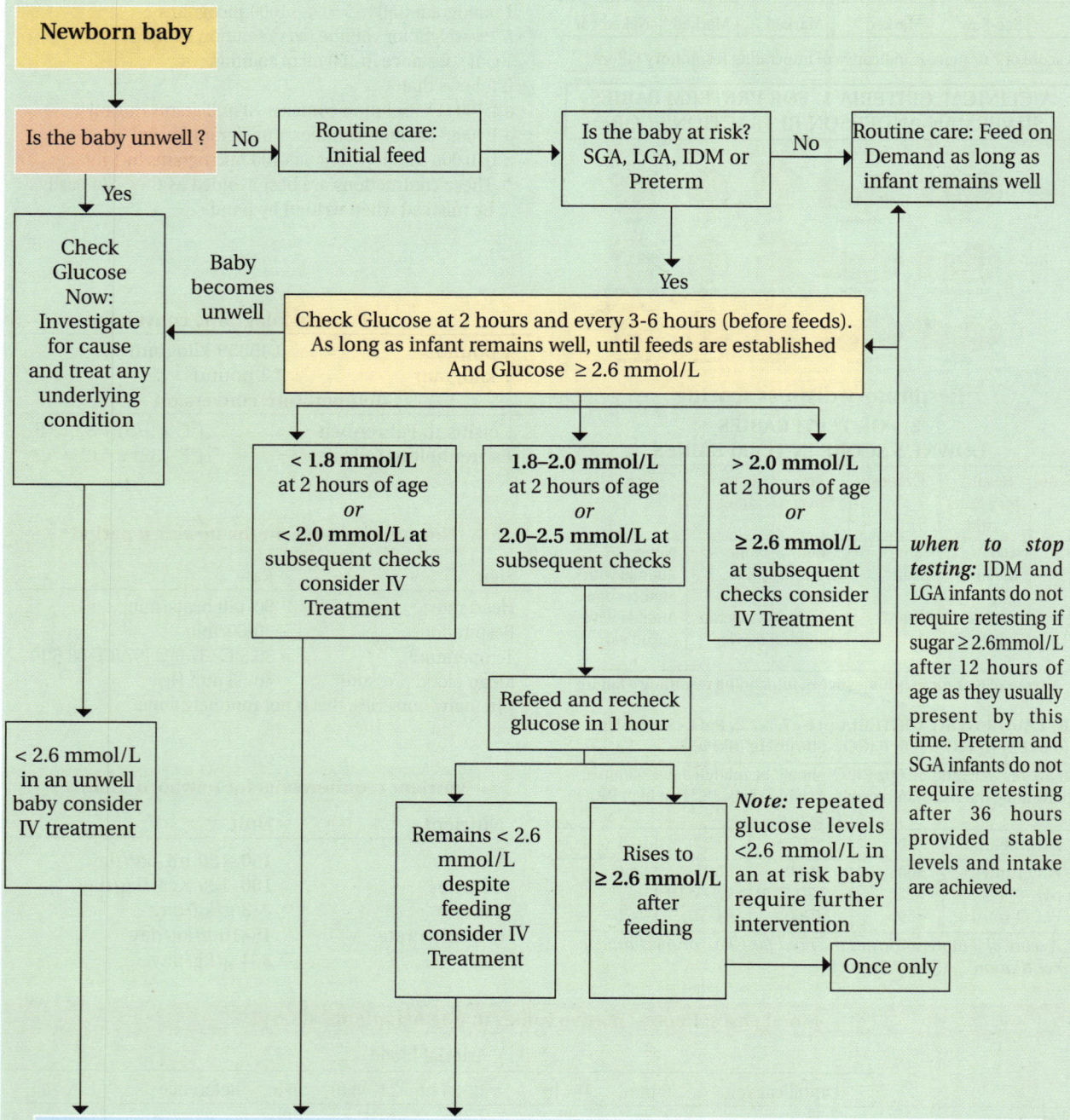

Algorithm for the screening and immediate management of babies at risk for neonatal hypoglycemia

Newborn baby

Is the baby unwell? — No → Routine care: Initial feed → **Is the baby at risk? SGA, LGA, IDM or Preterm** — No → Routine care: Feed on Demand as long as infant remains well

Yes ↓

Check Glucose Now: Investigate for cause and treat any underlying condition

Yes ↓

Check Glucose at 2 hours and every 3-6 hours (before feeds). As long as infant remains well, until feeds are established And Glucose ≥ 2.6 mmol/L

← Baby becomes unwell

< 1.8 mmol/L at 2 hours of age *or* **< 2.0 mmol/L** at subsequent checks consider IV Treatment

1.8–2.0 mmol/L at 2 hours of age *or* **2.0–2.5 mmol/L** at subsequent checks

> 2.0 mmol/L at 2 hours of age *or* **≥ 2.6 mmol/L** at subsequent checks consider IV Treatment

when to stop testing: IDM and LGA infants do not require retesting if sugar ≥ 2.6mmol/L after 12 hours of age as they usually present by this time. Preterm and SGA infants do not require retesting after 36 hours provided stable levels and intake are achieved.

< 2.6 mmol/L in an unwell baby consider IV treatment

Refeed and recheck glucose in 1 hour

Remains < 2.6 mmol/L despite feeding consider IV Treatment

Rises to ≥ 2.6 mmol/L after feeding

Note: repeated glucose levels <2.6 mmol/L in an at risk baby require further intervention

Once only

Initiate: Intravenous Infusion of 10% Dextrose at a rate of 80 mL/kg/day (5.5 mg glucose/kg/min).Check glucose 30 min after any change and adjust therapy (up to 100 mL/kg/day and/or 12.5% Dextrose) in order to maintain Glucose level ≥ 2.6 mmol/L. If rates in excess of 100 ml/kg/day of 12.5% Dextrose are required, Investigation, Consultation and/or Pharmacological intervention are indicated. May start weaning IV 12 hours after stable blood glucose is established.Continued breastfeeding is encouraged.

1mmol/L of Glucose= 18mg/dL
(2.6mmol/L=45mg/dL)

REFERENCE: Paediatr Child Health Vol 9 No 10 December 2004

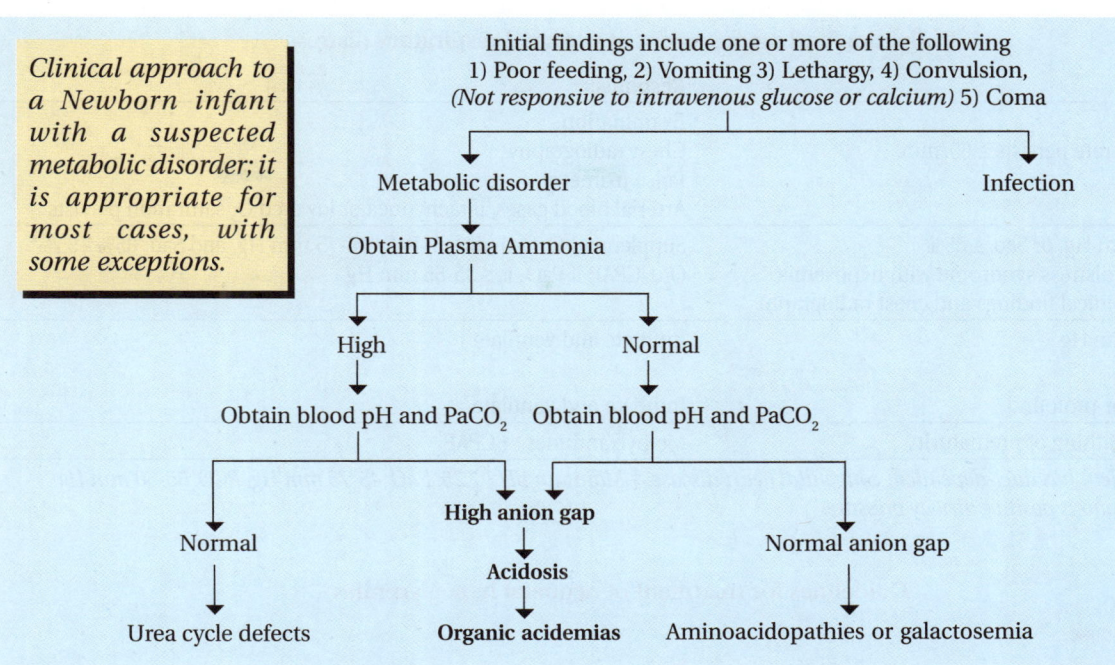

Clinical approach to a Newborn infant with a suspected metabolic disorder; it is appropriate for most cases, with some exceptions.

Initial findings include one or more of the following
1) Poor feeding, 2) Vomiting 3) Lethargy, 4) Convulsion,
(Not responsive to intravenous glucose or calcium) 5) Coma

Metabolic disorder → Obtain Plasma Ammonia

Infection

High → Obtain blood pH and PaCO₂

Normal → Obtain blood pH and PaCO₂

Normal → Urea cycle defects

High anion gap
Acidosis
Organic acidemias

Normal anion gap → Aminoacidopathies or galactosemia

Algorithm for the diagnosis of Hyperammonemia in the Newborn

Sick Newborn Hyperammonemia

Respiratory distress prior to 24 hour of age

Present → Transient Hyperammonemia of the Newborn

Absent → Acidosis

Presenting signs and symptoms of an inborn error of metabolism
Subtle
Abnormal Tone, Irritability. Poor feeding or feeding refusal, Poor weight gain, Somnolence, Tachycardia. Tachypnea, Vomiting
Overt
Acidosis, Altered thermoregulation Apnea, Arrhythmia, Cardiomyopathy, Dehydration, Lethargy or Coma, Persistent hypoglycemia, Poor perfusion or hypotension, Seizures, Sudden unexplained death

Present → Urine ketones

Absent → Urea Cycle Enzyme Defect → Plasma Citrulline level

Prominent

Inappropriately Low

SCAD*
MCAD*
LCAD*
HMG CoA Lyase deficiency*
Glutaric acidemia type II*

Propionic acidemia
Methylmalonic acidemia
Isovaleric acidemia
Multiple carboxylase deficiency

Absent-trace → Urinary Orotic acid

100-300 µ → Plasma Argininosuccinic acid high

≥1000 µ
No Argininosuccinic acid

Low → Carbamyl phosphate synthetase deficiency

High → Orinithine transcarbamylase deficiency

Argininosuccinate lyase deficiency

Argininosuccinic acid synthetase deficiency (Citrulllinemia)

*Hypoglycemia present when symptomatic

Evaluation and management of neonatal respiratory distress

Problems	Response
Tachypnea (respiratory rate persists $\geq 60/\text{min}$)	Examination Chest radiography Pulse oximetry Arterial blood gases, if tachypnea or lowered O_2 saturation persists
$PaO_2 \leq 45$ mm Hg, or $Sao_2 \leq 85\%$ Respiratory distress syndrome with hypoxemia (based on clinical findings and chest radiograph)	Supplement O_2 to maintain PaO_2 45-75 mm Hg, and Sao_2 85% - 95%* $O_2 \pm$ CPAP, if PaO_2 is ≤ 35-55 mm Hg
$PCO_2 \geq 60$ mm Hg Apnea	Intubate and ventilate †
Recurrent, or profound	Intubate and ventilate
Periodic breathing of prematurity	Methylxanthines, $\pm$ CPAP

Unless patient has duct-dependent congenital heart disease. † Maintain pH ³ 7.25, PaO₂ 45-75 mm Hg, PCO₂ 35-50 mm Hg. CPAP, continuous positive airway pressure.

Guidelines for treatment of neonatal hypoglycemias

Plasma glucose (mg/dL)— Venous Sample	Asymptomatic or mildly symptomatic	Symptomatic
35–45	Breast-feed or give formula or D_5W by nipple/gavage	IV glucose ($D_{5\text{-}12.5}W$) at 4-6 mg/kg/min*
25–34	IV glucose ($D_{5\text{-}12.5}W$) at 6–8 mg/kg/min*	IV glucose ($D_{5\text{-}12.5}W$) at 6–8 mg/kg/min*
<25	Mini-bolus of 2 mL/kg ($D_{10}W$) and continue at a rate to provide 6–8 mg/kg/min@	

* Changes in infusion rates should not exceed 2 mg/kg/min per change.

@ If blood glucose <25 mg/dL and IV access is not available, give Glucagon, 0.1 mg/kg per dose (maximum, 1 mg/dose) IM or SC every 30 min. Not as effective in small -for-gestational-age or extremely premature infants.

Modified from Cornblath M: Neonatal hypoglycemia. In Donn SM, Fisher CW (eds): Risk management Techniques in perinatal and Neonatal Practice. Armonk, Ny, Futura 1996, pp 437-448.

Guidelines for fluid and electrolyte administration (daily figures)

Age	Water[a] Preterm (mL/kg)	Term (mL/kg)	Sodium[a] Preterm (mmol/kg)	Potassium[a] Term (mmol/kg)	All babies (mmol/kg)
Day 1	60[b]	40	0	0	0
Day 2	90[b]	60	0	0	0
Day 3	120[b]	80	3-5[c]	1-2	2-3
Day 4	120-150	110	3-5[c]	1-2	2-3
Day 5 et seq.	120-150	120-150	3-5[c]	1-2	2-3

a= Use birth weight or most recent weight, whichever is higher. b= Extremely preterm babies may have much greater requirements;monitor plasma sodium. c= sometimes higher requirements- check plasma sodium daily.

Electrolyte requirements

	Before 48 hours of life	After 48–72 hours of life
Sodium	None, unless serum sodium < 135 mEq/L without evidence of volume overload	Term infants: 2–3 mEg/kg/day Preterm infants: 3–5 mEq/kg/day
Potassium	None	1–2– mEq/kg/day if adequate urine output is established and serum level <4.5 mEq/L

GLUCOSE INTAKE

* The neonatal liver normally produces 6-8 mg/kg/min of glucose. This is approximately the basal requirement of a Newborn infant.

* Hypoglycemia is severe if it persists despite an intake of >10 mg/kg/min. Calculate the glucose intake: See also the Glucose Rate Calculator

$$\text{Glucose intake (mg/kg/min)} = \frac{\% \text{ Dextrose} \times \text{volume (ml/kg/day)}}{144}$$

$$\text{or} \quad \text{Glucose intake (mg/kg/min)} = \frac{\% \text{ Dextrose} \times \text{hourly rate}}{\text{Weight (Kg)} \times 6}$$

Intake (ml/kg/day)	5% Dextrose	10% Dextrose mg/kg/min of Dextrose	12.5% Dextrose
60	2.1	4.2	5.2
75	2.6	5.2	6.5
90	3.1	6.3	7.8
105	3.7	7.3	9.1
120	4.2	8.3	10.4
150	5.2	10.4	13.0
180	6.3	12.5	15.6

To get concentrated glucose solutions: Dextrose solutions of >10% are best administered through central venous lines.
* Peripheral IVs do not last long, and extravasation can result in tissue damage.

Solution	10% dextrose	50% dextrose
12.5%	450 ml	30 ml
15 %	420 ml	60 ml
20 %	400 ml	135 ml
Solution	**5% dextrose**	**50% dextrose**
7.5%	450ml	30ml

IV FLUIDS

1. First 24 hours of life - D10W (D5W in infants <1000 gm).

2. Addition of electrolytes may be considered after 24-48 hours and there is adequate urine output (50% intake): *If serum Na+ >145 mEq/liter, maintain on Na+ free solution. *If serum K+ <3.8 mEq/liter, add K+ to solution (2-3 mEq/kg/day). *If serum Na+ drops <135 mEq/liter, consider addition of Na+ (3-4 mEq/kg/day).

3. **Usual maintenance solution for infants** with normal hydration and electrolyte balance at 48-72 hours of age is: 1/4N.S. + 20mEq KCl/liter

4. Serum electrolytes should be monitored at least daily in infants whose IV fluid intake exceeds 40% of total intake.

5. Do not add Ca gluconate routinely to UAC and UVC infusions until TPN started.

HEPARIN IN IV FLUIDS *Heparin is added to all maintenance IV fluids unless "Without heparin" is specifically ordered. *Concentration of heparin in IV fluids is as follows: IV <2cc/hr: 0.25U/cc

FLUID CALCULATION For mechanically ventilated infants, use the birth weight for the first 4–7 days of life **until weight loss has stabilized; then use daily weight. Indicate on the order sheet what weight is being used to calculate fluids and medications. During rounds and sign-outs, it should be made clear what weight is being used for calculations.**

FLUID GUIDELINES

*Day 1 RDS 60-70 cc/kg IV	Maximum 75 cc/kg IV + PO	*Day 4 RDS 80-100 cc/kg IV	Maximum 100 cc/kg IV + PO
*Day 2 RDS 60-70 cc/kg IV	Maximum 80 cc/kg IV + PO	*Day 5 RDS 100 cc/kg IV	Maximum 120 cc/kg IV + PO
*Day 3 RDS 80 cc/kg IV	Maximum 90 cc/kg IV + PO	*Day 6-7 RDS 120 cc/kg IV	Maximum 120 cc/kg IV + PO

<u>EXCEPTIONS</u> *Note:* *For extreme prematurity daily fluid volumes are much higher due to insensible losses >7 days - advancement is individualized *Birth asphyxia and/or suspected cerebral edema - insensible H_2O loss 40-50 cc/kg/d. *Phototherapy - evaluate hydration status q8-12h by weight and/or BUN, and serum electrolytes. May increase fluids by 10%, or more as needed. *Ventilator - evaluate hydration status q8-12h. May increase or decrease fluid intake to accommodate for fluctuations in fluid balance. *Chronic lung disease (BPD) - no greater than 150 cc/kg if O_2 dependent + diuretics. *Chest and/or Peritoneal Drains *If there are significant fluid losses from these, measure the volume and replace with *4% albumin as indicated. *Monitor serum albumin concentrations. *Monitor the composition of the fluid being lost as this may assist with calculating requirements @Note: cc/kg/day may not reflect an infant's fluid intake or requirements. *@Serum Na, BUN, weight, and total intake and output may be more useful in adjusting fluid requirements than calculated cc/kg/day.*

Home discharge criteria

Premature neonates

*Corrected gestational age more than 34 and one-half weeks *Able to maintain body temperature (> 36.4°C [97.5°F]) in an open crib *Consistently feeding well by mouth *Steady growth of 20 to 30 g (0.7 to 1 oz) per day on home feeding regimen *Weight greater than 1,800 g (4 lb) for a small-for-gestational-age infant and *greater than 2,000 g (4 lb, 6 oz) for an appropriate-for-gestational-age infant(may be disregarded if other criteria are met)*No major changes in care before discharge (such as change in feeding route or medications) *No major medical or nursing care needs that cannot be managed at home

Term Neonates

Resolution of symptoms (e.g. respiratory distress)*Resolution of jaundice *Adequate treatment of sepsis (or sepsis ruled out) *Adequate monitoring (e.g., 48 hours if group B streptococcus infection is involved)

Family readiness, support at home

Adequate follow-up assured *Social work involvement,

Reasons to withhold enteral feeding in neonates

*Prolonged asphyxia (hypoxia, metabolic acidosis, hypercapnia), hypotension, and low Apgar score (5 or below) at 5 minutes *Respiratory difficulties (respiratory rate of more than 60 breaths per minute, nasal flaring, grunting, or retractions)* Significant neurologic depression *Abdominal distension, No stool by 24 hours of age, Signs of severe sepsis

*—*Infants may be fed when breathing at 60 to 80 breaths per minute if they are without nasal flaring, grunting, or retractions ("permissive or peaceful tachypnea"), especially in the first 2 hrs.*

Neonatal drug withdrawal signs and symptoms "mnemonic"

W	Wakefulness
I	Irritability
T	Tachypnea (≥ 60 min)
H	Hyperactivity
D	Diarrhea
R	Rub marks
A	Autonomic dysfunction
W	Weight loss
A	Alkalosis (respiratory)
L	Lachrymation

Neonatal monitoring

Parameter expected range

* Weight gain 20 to 30 g (0.07 to 1.05 oz) per day, 150 to 200 g (5.3 to 7.0 oz) per week (Wt loss 5-10% of birth wt, return to birth wt by 7–10 days of age.)

* Head Circumference(35 cm at birth; increases 2cm/mo for first 3 months, then slower; 10 cm for rest of life.)

* Axillary 36.4°C (97.5°F) to 37.0°C (98.6°F) temperature

* Calorie intake 100 to 120 kcal per kg per day

* Fluid intake 150 to 200 mL per kg per day

* Urine output at least 6 wet diapers per day

* Urine specific 1.005 to 1.015 gravity

* Hematocrit 45 to 65 percent

* Sodium 135 to 145 mEq per L (135 to 145 mmol per L)

* Potassium 4.0 to 7.5 mEq per L (4.0 to 7.5 mmol per L)

* Calcium

  Term infants: 9 to 10.8 mg per dL (2.25 to 2.70 mmol per L)

  Preterm infants: 6.5 to 9 mg per dL (1.62 to 2.25 mmol per L)

* Creatinine 0.3 to 1.0 mg per dL (26 to 88 mmol per L)

* PaO_2 60 to 80 mm Hg

* Oxygen saturation 94 to 99 percent

Some important causes of hypoxia in the newborn

Low cardiac output—shock

* Hypovolemia: Fetal-to-maternal transfusion, acute

* Sepsis: Group B hemolytic streptococcal infection

* Cardiac disorders: Obstructive left heart lesions, Cardiomyopathies, Arrhythmias

Low SaO_2—Hypoxemia

* Lung disease: Respiratory distress syndrome, Sepsis, Persistent pulmonary hypertension, Diaphragmatic hernia

* Congenital heart disease with right-to-left shunt : Transposition of the great vessels, Pulmonary atresia

Low hemoglobin—anemia

* Fetal-to-maternal transfusion, chronic twin to twin transfusion

* Given the fact that signs and symptoms are usually non specific and the presentation is usually subtle in Newborns it is a wise idea to think of a _mnemonic_ that reminds us of all the possible Neonatal emergencies.

T = Trauma (Accidental and Non Accidental)

H = Heart Disease, Hypovolemia, Hypoxia

E = Endocrine (Congenital Adrenal Hyperplasia, Thyrotoxicosis)

M = Metabolic (Electrolyte Imbalance)

I = Inborn Errors of Metabolism

S = Sepsis (Meningitis, Pneumonia, UTI)

F = Formula Mishaps (Under or Over dilution)

I = Intestinal Catastrophes (Intussusception, Volvulus, Necrotizing Enterocolitis)

T = Toxins / Poisons

Tonia Brousseau, Ghazala Sharieff. Neonatal Emergencies. http:.www.Medscape. com/viewarticle/557824

Effect of hemoglobin concentration on the recognition of cyanosis

Hgb (g)	Reduced Hgb (g)	SaO_2	Total Hgb-Reduced Hgb/Total Hgb
20	3	85	(20–3)/20
8	3	62	(8–3)/20

These data show the expected levels of saturation for two hypothetical babies: one with a normal hemoglobin (20 g/dL) vs. one with a low hemoglobin (8 g/dL). Both babies have a fixed reduced hemoglobin level of 3 grams. The infant with the hemoglobin of 20 will have a saturation of 85%, and may appear cyanotic. However, the severely anemic infant may not appear cyanotic until the saturation is critically low.

Clin Pediatr Emerg Med. 2008 September; 9(3): 169–175. doi: 10.1016/j.cpem.2008.06.006

* EVALUATION OF THE CRYING, IRRITABLE, AFEBRILE INFANT

Mnemonic - IT CRIES

I- Infections - herpes/coxsackie stomatitis, UTI, meningitis, osteomyelitis

T- Trauma, testicular torsion

C- Cardiac - SVT, congestive heart failure

R- Reflux, reactions to medications, reactions to formulas

I- Immunizations, insect bites

E- Eye—corneal abrasion, ocular foreign body

S- Surgical - intussusception, inguinal hernia (S) Strangulation - hair tourniquet

* Major risk factors for hyperbilirubinemia in Full-Term Newborns

* Jaundice within first 24 hours after birth.
* A sibling who was jaundiced as a neonate.
* Unrecognized hemolysis such as ABO blood type incompatibility or Rh incompatibility.
* Nonoptimal sucking/nursing.
* Deficiency in glucose-6-phosphate dehydrogenase, a genetic disorder.
* Infection.
* Cephalohematomas/bruising.
* East Asian or Mediterranean descent.

Suggested indications for positive pressure ventilation in the newborn infant

Downes' or RDS score >7

Severe apneic episodes, gasping respiratory efforts

pH <7.25 & $PaCO_2$ >55-60 mmHg or rising >5–10 mmHg/hour

Birth weight <1500 grams, gestational age <31 weeks (delivery room)

Failure of nasal CPAP: PaO_2 <60 mmHg, FiO_2=0.6, CPAP=6 cm H_2O

pH <7.20 despite therapy (metabolic/respiratory acidosis)

Shock (PEEP of 2-3 cm H_2O)

Suggested management of hypoxemia

1. Maintain PaO_2 50–90 mmHg, SaO_2 85 (87) - 96%* **Oximeter alarms 87 low/97 high**

2. O2 administration Warmed, humidified Headbox, mask/funnel 5 liters/minute, 1/2 inch from nostrils Make small changes in FIO2 (flip-flop). Monitor FIO2, SaO_2.

3. CPAP - PEEP

4. Positive pressure ventilation-Conventional, HFOV

5. ECMO:Oxygenation index [MAP × FiO_2 3× 100/PaO_2] >40–45

* SaO_2 = oxygen saturation level; maintain SaO_2 <96% for preterm infants when possible, higher (>95%) in infants with pulmonary hypertension

* Samples to be obtained in infant with suspected IEM when diagnosis is uncertain and death seems inevitable (Metabolic autopsy)

1. Blood: 5–10 ml; frozen at -20°C; both heparinized (for chromosomal studies) and EDTA (for DNA studies) samples to be taken

2. Urine: frozen at –20°C

3. CSF: store at –20°C

4. Skin biopsy: including dermis in culture medium or saline with glucose. Store at 4-8°C. Do not freeze.

5. Liver, muscle, kidney and heart biopsy: as indicated.

6. Clinical photograph (in cases with dysmorphism)

7. Infantogram (in cases with skeletal abnormalities)

Suggested timing of screening cranial ultrasound examinations

Birth Weight (g)	Timing of screening (Days)	Projected finding
< 1000	Initial: 3–5	Identify 75%-80% of cases of IVH
		Identify increased PVE
	Second:10–14	Identify 95% of cases of IVH
		Identify early hydrocephalus
		Identify early cyst formation
	Third : 28	Identify most or all cases of IVH
		Assess ventricular size
		Assess periventricular white matter
	Fourth: predischarge	Identify late lesions
1000–1250	Initial: 3–5	As above
	second: 28	As above
	Third: predischarge	As above
12500–1500	Initial: 3–5	As above
	second: predischarge	

Guidelines for monitoring oxygen saturation levels by pulse oximetry

>95%	Pulmonary hypertension
85(87)–96%	28–34 weeks GA
85(87)–93 (96%)	<28 weeks GA*
900100%	First 1–2 days#
>92%	Chronic Lung Disease

*Maintain <96% when possible.

#Higher levels for more mature infants,PPHN:maintain <96% when possible if preterm infant.

SUGGESTED FORMAT FOR AN NICU/SCBU ADMIT NOTE

ID: Wt, EGA, SGA/AGA/LGA, sex, major problems Referring MD & Hospital and/or OB referring MD & Hospital:

MOM: Age, marital status, race, SAB TOP, medical problems, STD Hx, meds, ETOH, cigs, drugs (including IVDA), PN labs, hepatitis status.

PREGNANCY: Review of dates, nutrition, wt gain, prenatal care, infections, fevers, Bleeding, PTL.

LABOR: Onset, ROM (spontaneous vs. assisted, meconium/clear/bloody), tocolytics, betamethasone, antibiotics, ?amnionitis (temp WBC, tenderness),

FHRT/monitor, FP, LS.

DELIVERY: Type, forceps, suction, type of suctioning, anesthesia, meconium, nuchal cord, placenta (i.e. abruption, calcification, etc.).

RESUSCITATION: Initial HR, color, respiratory effort, suction, blowby O_2, bag, ETT,

APGARS, transport to NICU.

SH:

FH:

EXAM:

LAB: Include Dubowitz, length, and OFC with vitals.

A/P:

PROGRESS NOTES: There is no single correct format or outline for daily progress notes. The purpose of a progress note is to document 1) your physical exam; and 2) your understanding of the patient's current problems, their progression and your management plan for this problem. Repeating information gleaned from the nursing flow sheets, the lab computer and the medication list is helpful only as an aid to the above two goals. **Merely documenting a physical exam and signing the computer printout is not appropriate.**

Patients on ICU status need a detailed progress note daily. Patients on IM status need a **brief 3 line daily** note and 2 times a week or more detailed summary of their current problems, their course and overall plans.

DISCHARGE SUMMARIES

The purpose of a discharge summary is primarily to inform the follow-up physician of current issues and their management. Though the follow-up physician may have received copies of all interim summaries it is unlikely they will have read them or that they will ever read them. As a consequence the key problems and events of the infant's neonatal course should be **briefly** summarized and current issues concisely addressed in a bit more detail. Discharge summaries should be approximately 2 pages in length or less.

Contents: Discharge date and discharge attending physician

Patient identification information

Problem list including current and resolved problems

List of current medications

List of lines and tubes currently in place

Summary of current enteral intake

Health care maintenance screening examinations completed (ROP, cranial ultrasound, state lab newborn testing results, hearing assessment, etc.)

Immunizations administered (hepatitis B, RSV prophylaxis, etc.)

History of present illness

Maternal history (illnesses, medications, etc.)

Labor and delivery summary

System review of current active problems

Disposition plan (Follow-up physician name, address and phone, scheduled visit date. etc.)

Discharge physical examination with current weight, length and OFC

Name of individuals to receive copies of discharge summary

If corrections to summary are necessary, please make corrections prior to electronically signing the summary. If corrections are necessary after the summary is finalized and signed, please dictate the corrections as an addendum.

RULES OF THUMB FOR GROWTH
Weight

1. Weight loss in first few days 5–10% of birthweight
2. Return to birthweight 7–10 days of age
   Double birthweight 4–5 mo
   Triple birthweight-1 yr
   Quadruple birthweight-2 yr
3. Average weights : 3.5 kg at birth
   10 kg at 1 yr, 20 kg at 5 yr, 30 kg at 10 yr
4. Daily weight gain: 20-30 g for first 3–4 mo
   15–20 g for rest of the first year
5. Average annual weight gain-5 lb between age 2 years and puberty (though spurts and plateaus may occur)

Height

1. Average length-20 in (50 cm) at birth, 30 in (75 cm) at 1 yr
2. At age 3 yr. the average child is 3 ft (90 cm) tall
3. At age 4 yr. the average child is 40 in (100 cm) tall (double birth length)
4. Average annual height increase-2-3 in (5-7.5 cm) between age 4 yr and puberty

Head Circumference (HC)

1. Average HC- 35 cm at birth (13.5 in)
2. HC increases: 1 cm per mo for first year (2 cm per month for first 3 mo. then slower); 10 cm for rest of life.

Normal size and location of the fontanelles
There are 6 fontanelles which are unossified remnants of fibrous membrane. The major fontanelles are the Anterior Fontanel located between the frontal bones and the parietal bones midline of the skull (4-6 cm in size) and the Posterior Fontanel located midline between the parietal bones and occipital bone (1-2 cm in size). There are also the 2 Sphenoidal fontanel located at the sides of the head where the parietal, frontal, temporal and sphenoid bone meet as well as the 2 mastoid fontanel where the parietal, occipital and temporal bone meet. (similar in size to the posterior fontanel 1-2 cm) .
Anterior Fontanelle 1-4 cm in any direction = normal size/location. The diamond-shaped junction of the coronal frontal and sagittal sutures; it becomes ossified within 18-24months.
Posterior Fontanelle less than 1 cm = normal size/location. The posterior fontanelle should be less than 1cm. The triangular fontanel at the junction of the sagittal and lambdoid sutures; ossified by the end of the 1st year.
A third fontanelle is a bony defect along the sagittal suture in the parietal bones and may be a feature of certain syndromes such as trisomy 21.

INTERPRETATION OF RETINOPATHY OF PREMATURITY EXAMINATION

The international classification of Retinopathy of Prematurity (ROP) is based on three considerations:

A. The location of the area of abnormal vascular growth on the retina in relation to the optic disc.

Zone I: This is the most posterior and intimately related area of the retina to the optic disc; Abnormal vascular proliferation in this area is associated with worrisome prognosis.

Zone II: Zone II involves the more peripheral area of the retina, extending from the edge of Zone I nasally to the ora serrata. Abnormal vascular proliferation involving Zone II is associated with a variable prognosis, less serious than Zone I, but still of concern.

Zone III: This area of the retina is anterior and even more peripheral to Zone II. It is the last portion of the retina to be vascularized normally. Vascular proliferation noted in Zone III is usually associated with a benign prognosis.

B. The second component of the international classification of ROP is the extent of the problem circumferentially, recorded in clock hours. The more extensive the involvement, the worse the prognosis.

C The final component of the international classification is based on the stage of the problem.

The classification of ROP is typically given as follows:

Stage I - Characterized by a demarcation line between the normal retina nearer the optic nerve and the non-vascularized retina more peripherally. Multiple small abnormally branching vessels can sometimes be seen leading into the demarcation line.

Stage 2 - A ridge of scar tissue and new vessels appear in place of the demarcation line. This line now has width and height, and occupies some volume, and small tufts of new vessels ("popcorn vessels" or neo-vascularization) may appear posterior to the ridge.

Stage 3 - There is an increased size of the vascular ridge, with growth of fibrovascular tissue on the ridge and extending out into the vitreous of the eye. Fibrous scar tissue is beginning to form in this stage, with attachments between the vitreous gel and the ridge.

Stage 4 - Retinal vessels are dragged by the scar tissue, which is progressing. The macula may be moved significantly from the normal position in the retina as the scarring causes some contraction to occur. Vision is typically less than 20/200 by this stage.

Stage 5 - Retinal detachment has occurred and blindness is usually the outcome, though light and dark perception may persist.

D. **Plus Disease:** Is a determination that is made by the ophthalmologist at the time of retinal examination that indicates increased vascular engorgement in the posterior pole of the fundus. This is a determination that is ominous in terms of progression of ROP; it is indicative of the development of vascular shunts.

E. **Threshold ROP:** Is the stage and extent of ROP at which the likelihood of severe visual loss without treatment is 50% and at which treatment (laser or cryo) is indicated according to the 1988 CRYO-ROP study (Typically Stage III plus in 5 contiguous or 8 non-contiguous clock hours.) The CRYO-ROP indications were based on anatomic outcomes but more recently the Early Treatment for Retinopathy of Prematurity Randomized Trial found better visual results with earlier treatment. Treatment should be considered for ROP as follows: Zone I(any stage with plus disease), Zone I (any stage 3), or Zone II (stage 2 or 3 with plus disease).

Responsibilities of Neonatal Physicians

*Ensure that a clear process is in place to identify infants who require ROP screening and ensure that these infants are referred automatically to the screening ophthalmologist.
*When treatment is required, ensure that transfer or other arrangements occur in a timely manner.
*When planning hospital discharge or transfer at a time when ROP screening is ongoing, communicate with the screening ophthalmologist to determine current ROP status and when the next eye examination is needed. Liaise with the receiving physician to ensure that the current ROP status and the timing requirement of the next eye examination are understood. Ensure that a specific arrangement is in place for the next eye examination BEFORE discharge or transfer.

OPHTHALMIC DEFINITIONS

ROP-OPTIMAL TIMING FOR SCREENING

* Babies born before 27 weeks gestational age (i.e. up to 26 weeks and 6 days) - the first ROP screening examination should be undertaken at 30 to 31 weeks postmenstrual age.
* Babies born between 27 and 32 weeks gestational age (i.e. up to 31 weeks and 6 days) - the first ROP screening examination should be undertaken between 4 to 5 weeks (i.e. 28-35 days) postnatal age.
* Babies >32 weeks gestational age but with birthweight <1501 grams - the first ROP screening examination should be undertaken between 4 to 5 weeks (i.e. 28-35 days) postnatal age.
* Babies <32 weeks gestational age or birthweight <1501g should have their first ROP screening examination prior to discharge.

Aggressive Posterior ROP (AP-ROP)

An uncommon, rapidly progressing, severe form of ROP characterized by its posterior location, prominence of plus disease and the ill-defined nature of the retinopathy.

Plus Disease

Increased venous dilatation and arteriolar tortuosity of the posterior retinal vessels in at least two quadrants of the eye.

Pre-Plus Disease

Vascular abnormalities of the posterior pole which signifies the presence of ROP, but which are insufficient for the diagnosis of plus disease

Regression

The process of ROP changing from active, progressive disease to inactive disease. Also called involution.

Sight-Threatening ROP

Presence of stage 3 disease as defined in ICROP revisited, prethreshold (type 1 or type 2) or threshold disease as defined below..

Stage

Six stages (1, 2, 3, 4a, 4b and 5) which describe the severity of ROP from very mild disease (stage 1) to stage 5 which is complete retinal detachment. Stages are defined in the ICROP revisited classification

Threshold

5 contiguous or 8 cumulative clock hours of stage 3 ROP with plus disease in zones I or II

Prethreshold

Type 1: Zone I, any Stage ROP with plus disease Zone I, Stage 3 ROP with or without plus disease Zone II, Stage 2 or 3 ROP with plus disease

Type 2: Zone I, Stage 1 or 2 ROP without plus disease Zone II, Stage 3 ROP without plus disease

Zone The areas of the retina used to describe the location of ROP.

NEWBORN HEARING SCREENING
RISK INDICATORS (2000 JOINT COMMITTEE)

1. Any illness or condition requiring admission of 48 hours or greater to a NICU

2. Family history of hereditary childhood sensorineural hearing loss

3. In-utero infection, such as cytomegalovirus, rubella, syphilis, herpes, toxoplasmosis

4. Craniofacial anomalies, including those with morphological abnormalities of the pinna and ear canal

5. Hyperbilirubinemia at a serum level requiring exchange transfusion

6. Postnatal serious infections, including meningitis

7. Apgar scores 0-4 at 1 minute or 0-6 at 5 minutes

8. Mechanical ventilation lasting 5 days or longer

9. Aminoglycosides used in multiple courses (greater than 2)

10. Aminoglycosides used in combination with loop diuretics (ethacrynic acid, furosemide)

11. Physician order for reasons other than the above risk criteria

12. Persistent pulmonary hypertension of the newborn

13. Any condition requiring ECMO

14. Syndromes associated with progressive hearing loss such as neurofibromatosis, osteopetrosis, and Usher's syndrome (later workup)

15. Stigmata or other findings associated with a syndrome known to include a sensorineural or conductive hearing loss or Eustachian tube dysfunction (later workup)

16. Neurodegenerative disorders such as Hunter syndrome, or sensory motor neuropathies such as a Friedreich's ataxia and Charcot-Marie-Tooth syndrome (later workup)

17. Head trauma (later workup)

18. Recurrent or persistent otitis media with effusion for at least 3 months (later workup)

19. Parental or caregiver concern regarding hearing, speech, language, or developmental delay

HEARING SCREENING : FOLLOW-UP PROTOCOL SCHEDULES
(Note: ages to be followed at are corrected age) Follow-Up of Babies Screened in the NICU

Failures

An infant who does not pass the initial screening test will be scheduled for a follow-up evaluation at 4-6 weeks after discharge from the hospital.

Pass but at risk

An infant who passes the initial screening but is at risk for progressive or late onset hearing loss due to a history of PPHN, ECMO support, CMV, or TORCH will be followed at: 3 months, 12 months, and yearly evaluations until school age

Pass but at risk

An infant who passes the initial screening but there is a family history of congenital hearing loss or is identified with a syndrome that has associated hearing loss will be followed at: 12 months, and yearly evaluations until school age

Clinical diagnostic/follow-up program for hearing impaired children

1. Initial diagnosis takes at least 2 visits, with counseling session with parents as part of last visit or separate visit (phone call to parents the week following diagnosis to assist with referrals, answer questions)

2. Monitoring/continuing diagnostics every 3 months until hearing is stable

3. Every 6 months for the first 3 years of life

4. Yearly evaluations in preschool

5. Yearly evaluations during school age

These are basic guidelines for children with sensorineural hearing impairment. If there are concerns that hearing is changing, evaluations will be scheduled more frequently.

Reticulocyte count · It is useful to know the reticulocyte count in infants who were born prematurely if the haemoglobin is low and at about the level at which one might consider transfusion. *If the reticulocyte count is high suggesting the infant is actively making red cells, one might defer transfusion unless there were other special reasons for proceeding. *The reticulocyte count may be expressed as an absolute number or as a percentage of the red blood cells. To convert number of reticulocytes to % *Divide absolute reticulocyte count (reticulocytes x 10^9/L) by 10 *Then divide the answer by the red blood cell count (RBC x 10^{12}/L)

Normal Range for Reticulocyte Counts: The reticulocyte count – range (%) and (x10^9/L) in the first 3 months of life in term infants*

Age	%	× 10^9/L
1 day	3.0–7.0	110–445
7 days	<0.1–1.3	<10–80
4 weeks	<0.1–1.2	<10–65
8 weeks	0.1–2.9	<10–125
12 weeks	0.4–1.6	15–75
>12 weeks	0.2–2.0	10–105

* Data from various sources, based on microscope counts.

LUNG PROFILE

A lung profile evaluates resistance to expiratory flow, functional residual capacity, and basic lung mechanics (static lung compliance and resistance). These measurements are indices of pulmonary reserve and may be predictive of pulmonary morbidity in infants with chronic lung disease. Infants who had any of the following problems or received any of the following treatment modalities should be considered candidates for a lung profile at the pediatric pulmonologist`s discretion. It should be scheduled during the week preceding discharge:*At least one week of diuretics for pulmonary disease *High frequency oscillation or jet ventilation *Congenital diaphragmatic hernia *Meconium aspiration syndrome requiring mechanical ventilation *Documented RSV infection requiring mechanical ventilation *Pulmonary consultation should be obtained on all patients with abnormal studies. Follow-up studies are scheduled at 4 months after discharge.

Neonatal Pulmonary Physiology by Disease State

Disease	Compliance mL/cm H2O	Resistance cm H2O/mL/s	Time constant (s)	FRC (mL/kg)	V/Q matching	Work
Normal term	4-6	20-40	0.25	30	-	-
RDS	↓↓	-	↓↓	↓	↓/↓↓	↑
Meconium aspiration	-/↓	↑/↑↑	↑	↑/↑↑	↓↓	↑
BPD	/↓	↑↑	↑	↑↑	↓↓/↓	↑↑
Air leak	↓↓	-/↑	-/↑	↑↑	↓/↓↓	↑↑
VLBW apnea	↓	-	↓↓	-/↓	↓/-	-/↑

BPD = bronchopulmonary dysplasia; ↓=decrease; /, either/or; FRC =functional residual capacity; -= increase; ↑ =little or no change; RDS = respiratory distress syndrome; V/Q = ventilation-perfusion ratio; VLBW = very low birth weight.

Multi-organ system failure in the Neonate with Group B streptococcal/Early Onset Septicemia

*Do assess/reassess Neonate`s ABCDEs, & Stabilize ABCDEs in that order; Do not ever forget Dextrose (Blood Glucose) & Disability. *Drugs are important in stabilizing Circulation, once Airway and Breathing are secured & maintained.

Organ system	Abnormal findings	Management
Cardiovascular	Cardiogenic and distributive shock; poor perfusion; ejection fraction 54% and fractional shortening 26% Highest creatine phosphokinase 1033 U/l and cardiac troponin 0.45 ug/l	Intravenous saline boluses, dopamine, dobutamine,epinephrine, hydrocortisone, milrinone, vasopressin
Respiratory	Respiratory failure with hypercarbia and diffuse haziness on chest radiograph	Mechanical ventilation, FiO2 1.0, surfactant, vecuronium
Renal	Passed urine at 10 hours of life; persistent oliguria; anuria 4 days later. Highest creatinine 153 umol/l	Intravenous frusemide; peritoneal dialysis; gentamicin stopped
Septicemic	Group B streptococcus, sensitive to penicillin, isolated on surface swabs, and in baby and mother's blood cultures; highest C-reactive protein 12.9 mg/l	Intravenous penicillin and gentamicin initially; ampicillin; cefotaxime; meropenim and vancomycin , empirically;intravenous immunoglobulin, Subsequently on high-dose penicillin and cefotaxime when group B streptococcus and sensitivity were available
Hematologic	Disseminated intravascular coagulopathy with lowest hemoglobin 8.6 g/dl, thrombocytopenia 13 × 109/l, Ddimer9735 ng/ml, prothrombin time 60 seconds, and activated plasma thromboplastin time 120 seconds	Packed red cell, fresh frozen plasma, cryoprecipitate, platelet
Metabolic	Metabolic acidosis (worst pH 6.87), hypoglycemia Glucose 1.0 mmol/l), hypocalcemia (0.63 mmol/l)	Dextrose and NaHCO3 infusion; calcium supplementation\
Neurologic	Convulsion	Anticonvulsant
Hepatic	Deranged liver function with worst total bilirubin 125 umol/l and alanine aminotransferase 574 IU/l	Supportive and treating underlying infection

Evaluate Heart Size

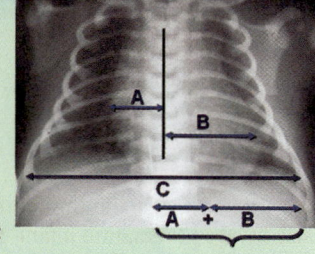

Cardiothoracic ratio

- A = widest horizontal diameter of heart right of midline
- B = widest horizontal diameter of heart left of midline
- C = widest internal diameter of chest at or just below base of heart

- Normal in neonate = A + B < 60% of C

MOST ESSENTIAL PARAMETERS INDICATING ADEQUATE VENTILATION

1. Clinical parameters

Absence of cyanosis, Absence of retractions, Prompt capillary filling*
Normal blood pressure, Adequate chest expansion,
Adequate air entry

2. Pulse oximetry

Saturation 90-95%

3. Blood gases

PaO$_2$ 60-80 mm Hg
PaCO$_2$ Acute 40-45 mm Hg, chronic up to 60 mm Hg
pH 7.35-7.45

Capillary filling is normal if after blanching the nail or tip of finger the color returns on counting 1,2,3, pink.

UAC

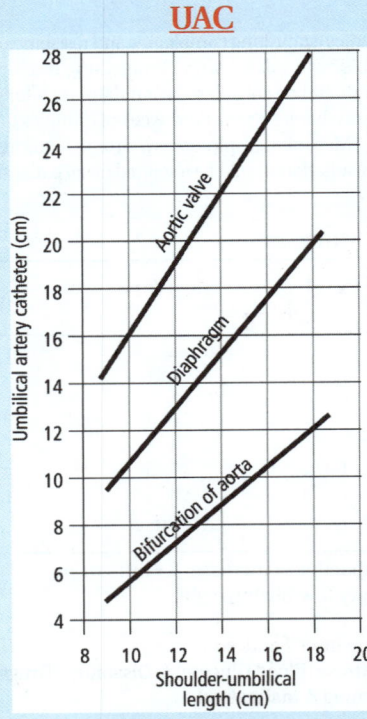

UVC

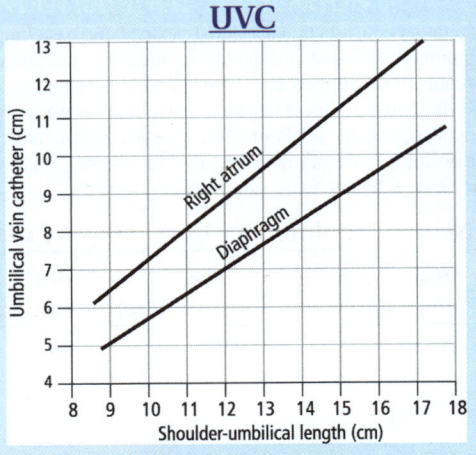

Umbilical venous catheters should be placed in the inferior cava above the level of the ductus venosus and the hepatic veins and below the level of the atrium.

Umbilical artery catheter

The length of umbilical catheter necessary to place its tip at the required level is dependent on the shoulder-umbilicus distance, measured from the upper lateral end of the clavicle perpendicular to the umbilicus (After Dunn, 1966)

High line: The tip of the catheter should be above the diaphragm between T6 and T9. A high line may be recommended in infants <750 gm, in whom a low line could easily slip out.

Low line: The tip of the catheter should lie just above the aortic bifurcation between L3 and L5. This avoids renal and mesenteric arteries near L1, perhaps decreasing the incidence of thrombosis or ischemia.

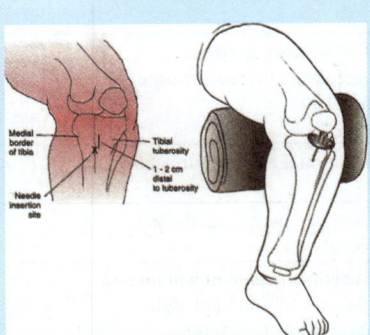

Intraosseous line: The entry site at the proximal tibia is located 1–2 cm distal to the tibial tuberosity in the middle of the anteromedial ("flat") surface of the tibia.
21G LP needle with a stylet may be best, although success can be achieved with a large bore "butterfly" needle.

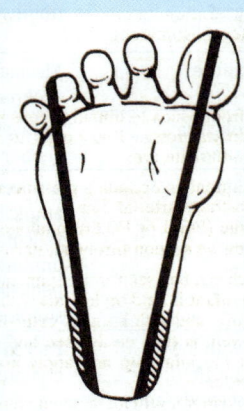

Heel prick for capillary blood sampling should be performed on the plantar surface of the heel, beyond the lateral and medial limits of the calcaneus, marked by these lines
(From Blumenfeld et al., 1979)

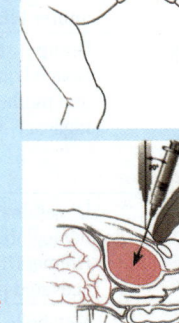

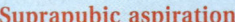

Suprapubic aspiration: The site for puncture is 1-2 cm above the symphysis pubis in the midline; use 22G, 1-inch needle, puncture at a 10-20 degree angle to the perpendicular, aiming slightly caudad.

Intercostal needle/tube drainage

2nd intercostal space in the midclavicular line is used for needle decompression of a tension pneumothorax and the 3rd, 4th, or 5th ICSs are recommended for most patients who require evacuation of air/fluid from the chest.

Chest tube size

Premature (1–2.5kg)-10–14 FG, Neonate (2.5–4 kg)-12-14 FG, Infant (6–8kg)-14-20 FG

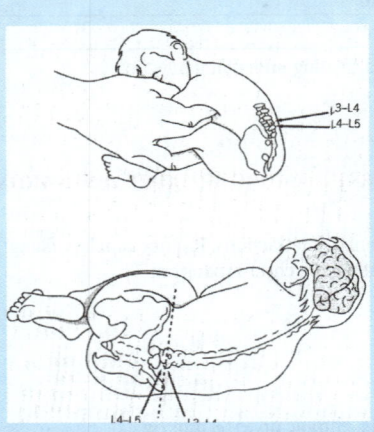

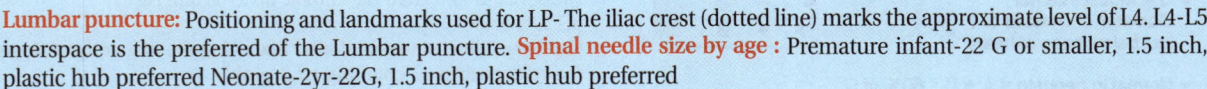

Lumbar puncture: Positioning and landmarks used for LP- The iliac crest (dotted line) marks the approximate level of L4. L4-L5 interspace is the preferred of the Lumbar puncture. **Spinal needle size by age :** Premature infant-22 G or smaller, 1.5 inch, plastic hub preferred Neonate-2yr-22G, 1.5 inch, plastic hub preferred

Glucose rate calculator

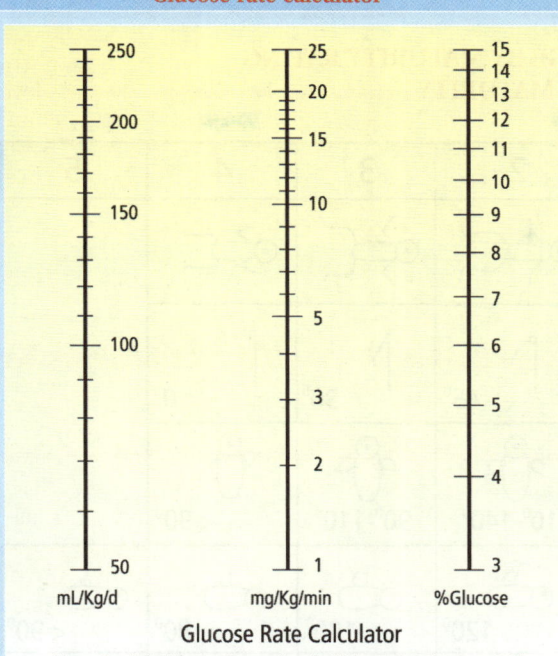

Glucose Rate Calculator
Use a Straight Edge to Determine the Volume Required per 24 h

Calculation of body surface area-infants

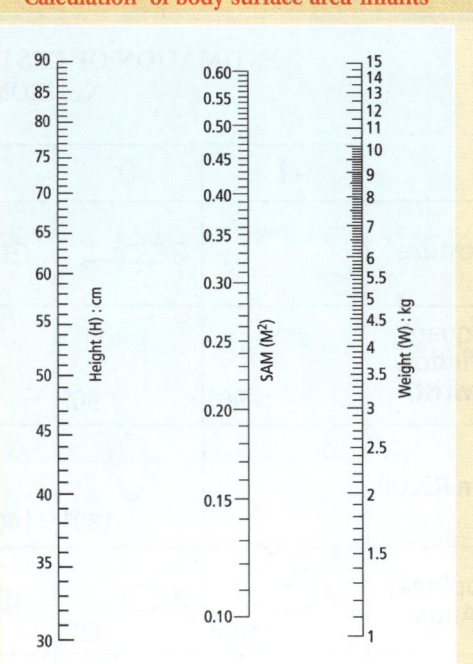

$$SA = W^{0.5378} \times H^{0.3964} \times 0.024265$$

Many nomograms underestimate the body surface area in infants and small children, therefore separate nomograms for infants are to be followed (From The J Ped, Vol 93, Haycock et al 62–66;1978)

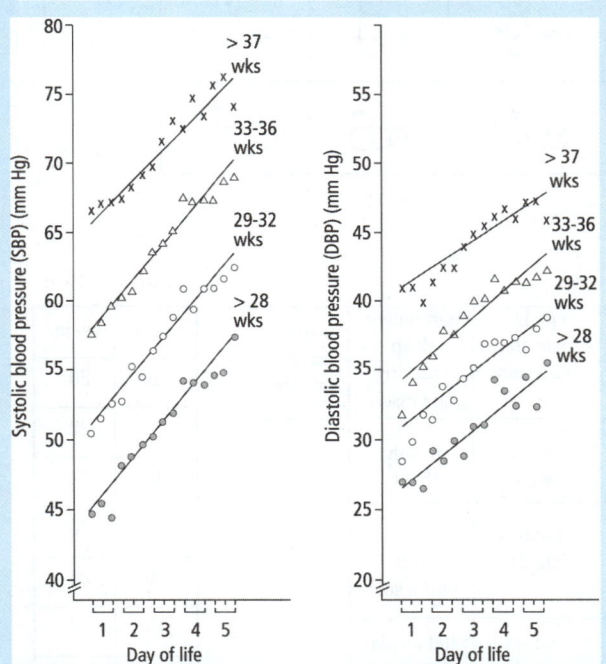

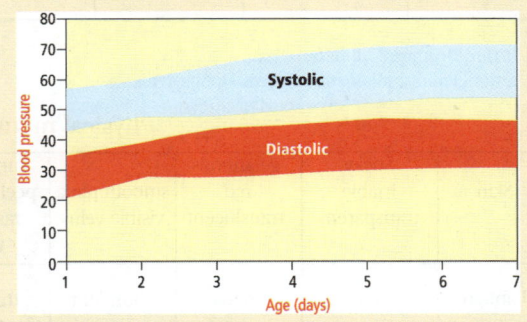

Blood pressure ranges in premature infants over first week of life. (From Hegyi T, Anwar M, Carbone MT, et al: Blood pressure ranges in premature infants :The first week of life. Pediatrics 97:336, 1996.)

Systolic and diastolic blood pressures are plotted for first 5 days of life, with each day subdivided into 8-hour periods. Infants are categorized by gestational age into 4 groups; </=28 weeks (n=33), 29-32 weeks (n=73), 33-36 weeks (n=100), and >37 weeks (n=110) (From Zubrow AB et al J Perinatology 15;470, 1995)

Mean arterial blood pressure by birth weight

Oscillometric measurements :	Mean arterial blood pressure		
	Mean MAP ± SD		
Birth Weight	Day 3	Day 17	Day 31
501-750 g	38 ± 8	44 ± 8	46 ± 11
751-1000 g	43 ± 9	45 ± 7	47 ± 9
1001-1250 g	43 ± 8	46 ± 9	48 ± 8
1251-1500 g	45 ± 8	47 ± 8	47 ± 9

From Fanaroff AA for the NICHD Neonatal Research Network, Bethesda, MD: Profiles of mean arterial blood pressure (MAP) for infants weighing 500–1500 grams. Pediatr Res 27:205A, 1990

NEUROMUSCULAR CRITERIA FOR MATURITY- NEW BALLARD SCORE

ESTIMATION OF GESTATIONAL AGE BY MATURITY RATING
NEUROMUSCULAR MATURITY

	-1	0	1	2	3	4	5
Posture							
Square Window (wrist)	> 90°	90°	60°	45°	30°	0°	
Arm Recoil		180°	140°-180°	110°-140°	90°-110°	< 90°	
Popliteal Angle	180°	160°	140°	120°	100°	90°	< 90°
Scarf Sign							
Heel to Ear							

Physical maturity

Skin	Sticky friable transparent	gelatinous red, translucent	smooth pink, visible veins	superficial peeling &/or rash, few veins	cracking pale areas rare veins	parchment deep cracking no vessels	leathery cracked wrinkled
Lanugo	none	sparse	abundant	thinning	bald areas	mostly bald	
Plantar Surface	heel-toe 40-50 mm : -1 <40 mm:-2	>50 mm no crease	faint red marks	anterior transverse crease only	creases ant 2/3	creases over entire sole	
Breast	imperceptible	barely perceptible	flat areola no bud	stippled areola 1-2 mm bud	raised areola 3-4 mm bud	full areola 5-10 mm bud	
Eye/Ear	lids fused loosely: -1 tightly: -2	lids open pinna flat stay folded	sl. curved pinna; soft; slow recoil	well curved pinna; soft but ready recoil	formed & firm instant recoil	thick cartilage ear stiff	
Genitals (male)	scrotum flat, smooth	scrotum empty faint rugae	testes in upper canal rare rugae	testes descending few rugae	testes down good rugae	testes pendulous deep rugae	
Genitals (female)	clitoris prominent labia flat	prominent clitoris small labia minora	prominent clitoris enlarging minora	major & minora equally prominent	majora large minora small	majora cover clitoris & minora	

Maturity rating

score	weeks
-10	20
-5	22
0	24
5	26
10	28
15	30
20	32
25	34
30	36
35	38
40	40
45	42
50	44

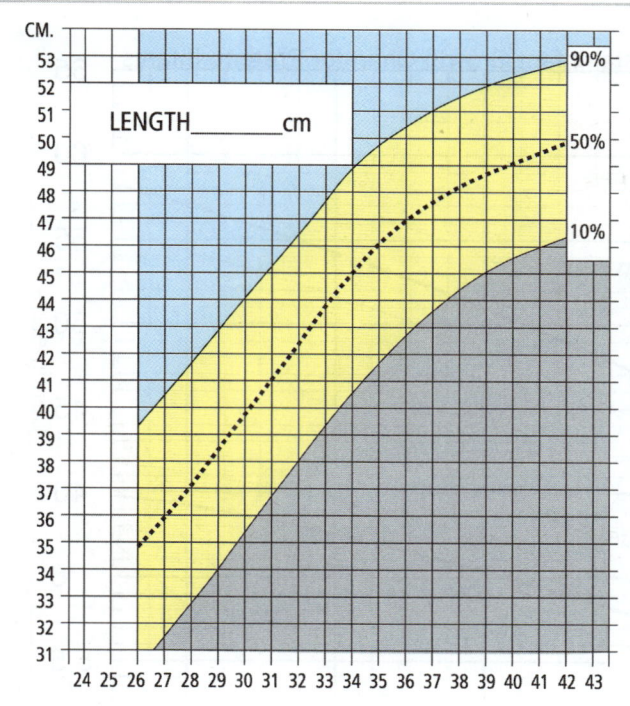

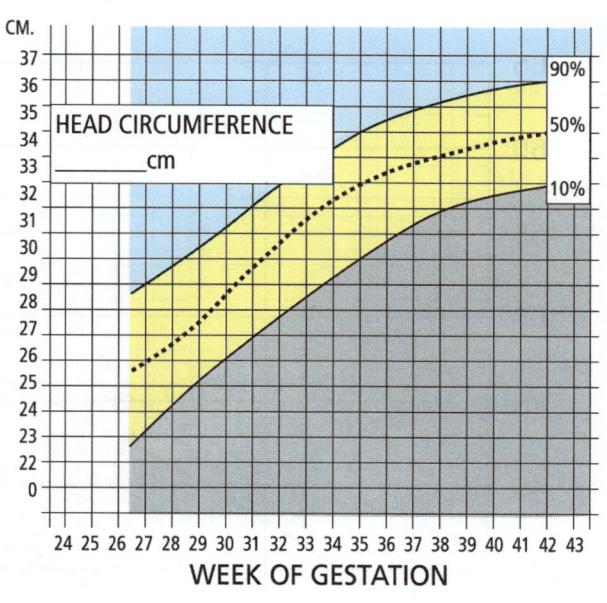

WEEK OF GESTATION

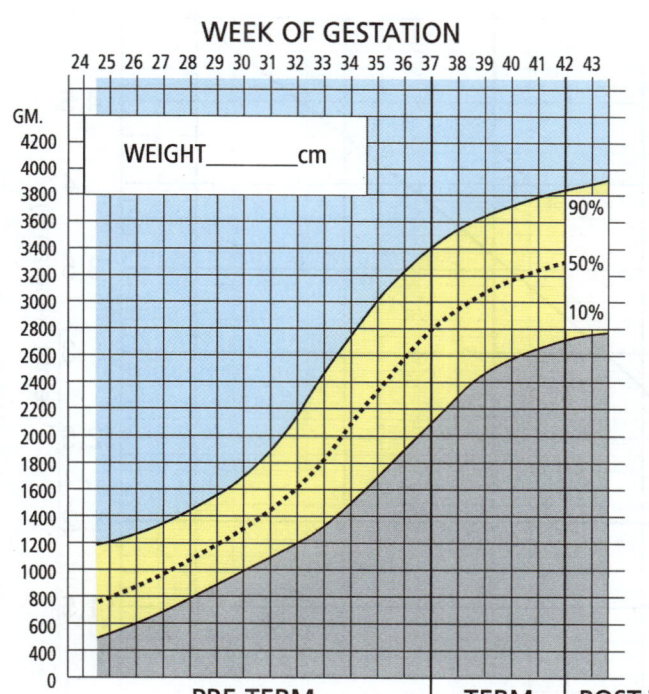

	1st Exam (X)	2nd Exam (O)
LARGE FOR GESTATIONAL AGE (LGA)		
APPROPRIATE FOR GESTATIONAL AGE (AGA)		
SMALL FOR GESTATIONAL AGE (SGA)		
Age at Exam	hrs.	hrs.
Signature of Examiner	_____ M.D.	_____ M.D.

PRE-TERM   TERM   POST-TERM

Newborn Classification based on Maturity and Intrauterine Growth.
(Modified from Lubchenko C, Boyd E: J Pediatrics 71:159,1967)

This is best for Infants less than 36 weeks gestation

Reflex	Stimulus	Positive response	Gestation in weeks if reflex is : Absent	Present
Pupil reaction	Light	Pupil constriction	< 31	29 or more
Glabellar tap	Tap on glabella	Blink	<34	32 or more
Traction response	Pull up by wrists from supine	Flexion of neck or arm	<31	33 or more
Neck righting	Rotation of head	Trunk follows	< 31	34 or more

Source: Robinson 1966

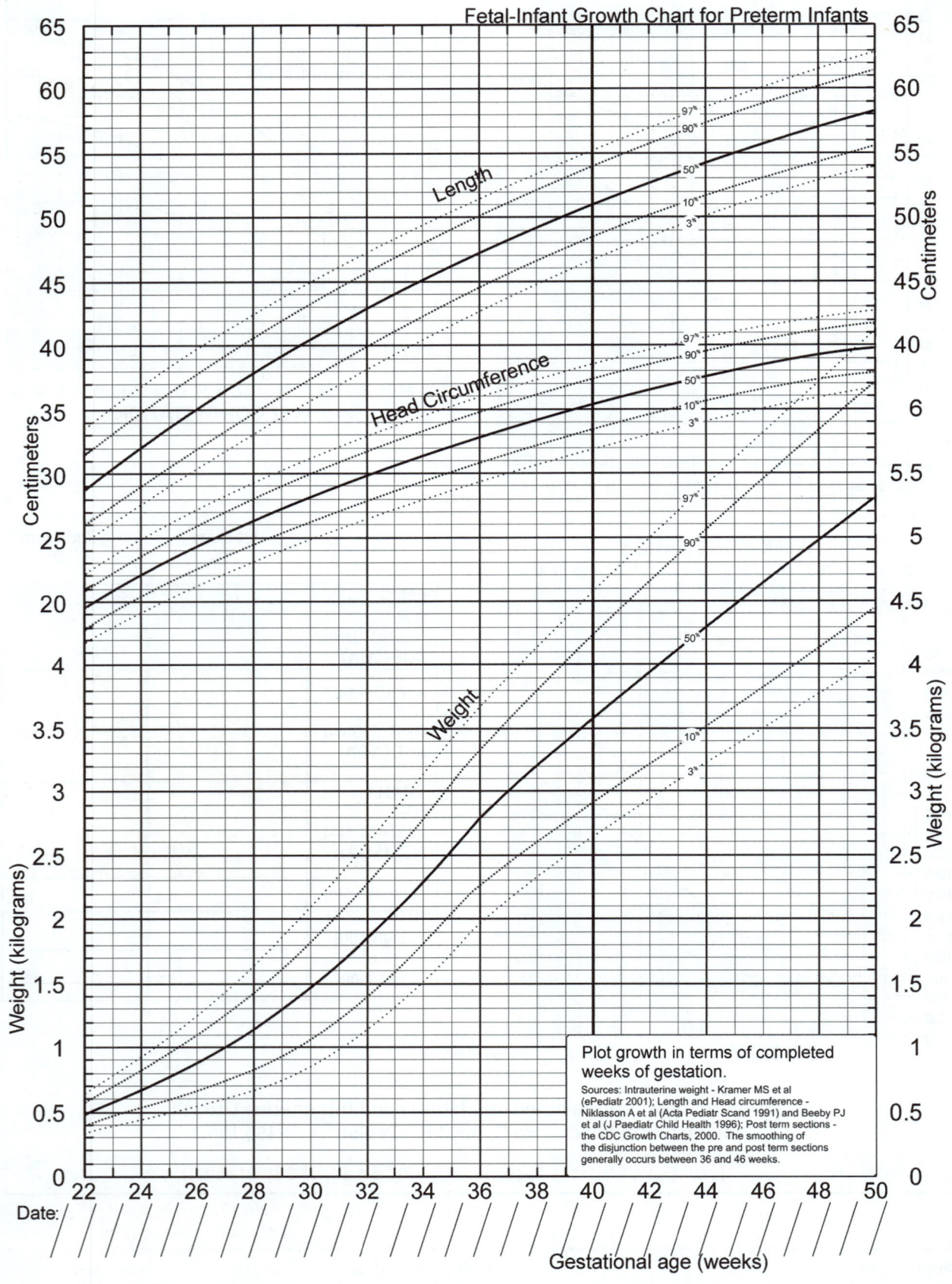

A New fetal-infant growth chart for Preterm infants developed through a meta-analysis of published reference studies.

Courtesy: Tanis R Fenton, Department of Community Health Sciences, Faculty of Medicine, University of Calgary, 3330 Hospital Drive NW, Calgary, Alberta, T2N 4N1, Canada

PHOTOTHERAPY GUIDELINES FOR INFANTS >35 WK GESTATION

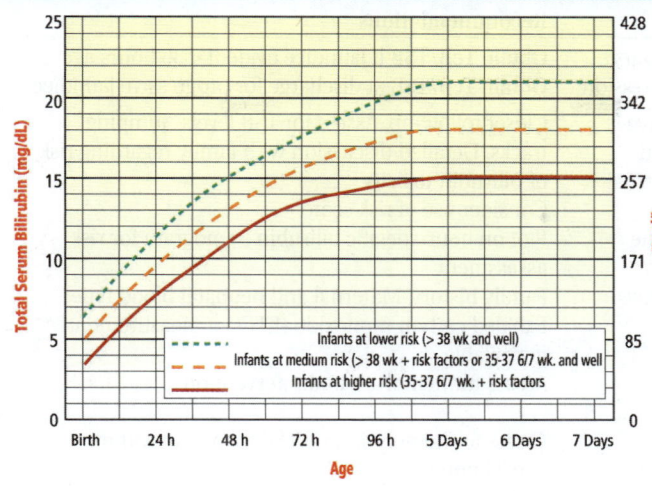

- Guidelines refer to use of intensive phototherapy.

- Use total bilirubin. Do not subtract direct reacting or conjugated bilirubin.

- Risk factors* = isoimmune hemolytic disease, G6PD deficiency, asphyxia, respiratory distress, significant lethargy, temperature instability, sepsis, acidosis, or albumin <3 g/dl (if measured).

- For well infants 35–37^{6/7} wk can adjust TSB levels for intervention around the medium risk line. It is an option to intervene at lower TSB levels for infants closer to 35 wks and at higher TSB levels for those closer to 37^{6/7} wk.

- It is an option to provide conventional phototherapy in hospital or at home at TSB levels 2-3 mg/dl, below those shown, but home phototherapy should be used in any infant with risk factors.

* This risk factors listed above are conditions that affect the likelihood of brain damage at different bilirubin levels. These factors increase the risk of brain damage because of their negative effects on albumin binding of bilirubin, the integrity of the blood brain barrier, and the susceptibility of the brain cells to damage by bilirubin.

Source:AAP. Pediatrics 114:297, 2004

RISK FACTORS FOR DEVELOPMENT OF SEVERE HYPERBILIRUBINEMIA

Risk factors	Major risk	✓	Minor risk	✓	Decreased risk
Predischarge TSB or TcB	In high risk zone (>95%)		In high intermediate risk zone (>75%)		Low risk zone (<40%)
Visible jaundice	First 24 hrs		Before discharge		
Gestational age	35-36 wk		37-38 wk		≥ 41 wk
Previous sibling	Received phototherapy		Jaundiced, no phototherapy		
Blood groups	Blood grp. incompatibility with				
Hemolytic disease	+DAT. Other known hemolytic disease (e.g., G6PD deficiency)				
Feeding	Exclusive breast (↑ risk if poor feeder or ↑ wt. loss)		Breast-fed, nursing well		Exclusive formula feeding
Race	East Asian		Hispanic (Mexican) ?		African American * Unless G6PD deficient - 12% are G6PD deficient
Other factors	Cephalhematoma or significant bruising		Macrosomic infant of IDM, male gender, maternal age≥ 25 yr		Discharged from hospital after 72 hr.

* The more risk factors present, the greater the risk of developing severe hyperbilirubinemia.

Follow-up should be provided as follows :

Any infant discharged before age 72 hours should be seen within 2 days of discharge.

* If an infant is discharged before age 72 hours AND if you plan to follow up in more than 2 days, please document your reasons in the chart.

Source:AAP. Pediatrics 114:297, 2004

Guidelines for exchange transfusion in infants >35 wk gestation

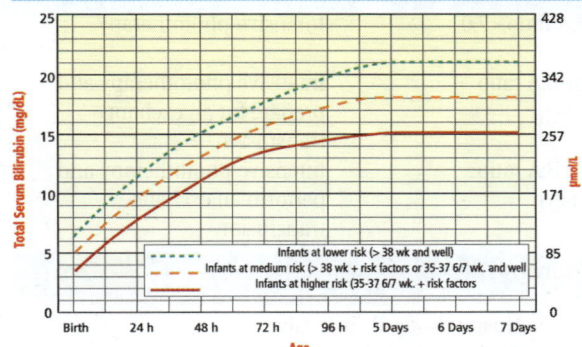

- The dashed lines for the first 24 hours indicate uncertainty due to a wide range of clinical circumstances and a range of responses to phototherapy.

- Perform immediate exchange if infant shows signs of acute bilirubin encephalopathy, (hypertonia, arching, retrocollis, opisthotonos, fever, high-pitched cry) of if TSB is 5 mg/dl above these lines.

- Risk factors* = isoimmune hemolytic disease, G6PD deficiency, asphyxia, respiratory distress, significant lethargy, temperature instability, sepsis, acidosis.

- Measure serum albumin and evaluate B/A ratio = bilirubin (mg/dl)/albumin (g/dl). See the table below.

- Use total bilirubin. Do not substract direct reacting or conjugated bilirubin.

- In isoimmune hemolytic disease give IVIG 0.5-1 g/kg over 2-3 hours if TSB is rising and within 2-3 mg/dl of exchange level. This can be repeated in 12 hr.

- If infant is well and 35-37 ^{6/7} wk (medium risk), can individualize TSB levels for exchange on the basis of actual gestational age.

* This risk factors listed above are conditions that might affect the likelihood of brain damage at different bilirubin levels. These factors increase the risk of brain damage because of their negative effects on albumin binding of bilirubin, the integrity of the blood brain barrier, and the susceptibility of the brain cells to damage by bilirubin.

During birth hospitalization, exchange transfusion is recommended if the TSB rises to these levels despite intensive phototherapy. For re-admitted infants, if the TSB level is above the exchange level, repeat TSB measurement every 2 to 3 hours and consider exchange, if the TSB remains above the levels indicated after intensive phototherapy for 6 hours. The following B/A ratios can be used together with but not in lieu of the TSB level as an additional factor in determining the need for exchange transfusion.

If the TSB is at or approaching the exchange level, send blood for immediate type and cross-match. Blood for exchange transfusion modified whole blood (red cells and plasma) cross-matched against the mother and compatible with the infant.

Risk Category	B/A Ratio at which exchange transfusion should be considered
	TSB mg/dl
Lower risk	8.0
Medium risk	7.2
Higher risk	6.8

Source:AAP. Pediatrics 114:297, 2004

Predischarge jaundice management of term and near-term infants

Clinical assessment after birthing		Recommendations
Visual assessment of jaundice	Monitor as a vital sign every 8 hours Document cephalo-caudal progression	Obtain TcB/TSB if jaundice evident < 36 hours age Obtain TcB/TSB at discharge for progressive jaundice
Clinical and biologic risk factors	Prematurity (<38 weeks), exclusive breast feeding, bruising, race and ethnicity, mode of delivery, maternal diabetes, etc.	Closer follow-up, Assess for TSB levels "jumping" tracks, Detailed discussion with family regarding risk of bilirubin toxicity Consider use of risk score
Bilirubin testing	TSB/TcB testing at time of routine metabolic screen	Plot on hour-specific bilirubin nomogram for risk assessment
Hemolysis assessment	Especially in infants with TSB levels >75 percentile track	Family history, Maternal and neonatal blood type, Exhaled carbon monoxide (ETCOc) measurement, if available
Assessment for targeted follow-up for discharge at <72 hours age (age ≤ 2 days)	TSB >95 percentile	Assess for hemolysis and intervention
	TSB >75 percentile	Assess for hemolysis, and TSB follow-up within 8 to 24 hours
	TSB >40 percentile	TSB follow-up within 48 hours
	TSB <40 percentile	Clinical follow-up within 48 hours, and optional TSB follow-up

Postdischarge and follow-up based on predischarge TSB (mg/dL) level
(based on the hour-specific bilirubin nomogram)

Predischarge TSB level	Discharge only if TSB level	Follow-up within		TSB recheck optional (unless indicated by clinical risk factors)
		24 hours	48 hours	
at postnatal age (hour-specific)	<95 percentile	>75 percentile	<75 percentile	< 40 percentile
41-44 hours	<12.3	>10.0	<10.0	<7.9
45-48 hours	<12.7	>10.4	<10.4	<8.2
49-56 hours	<13.2	>11.0	<11.0	<8.7
57-64 hours	<14.7	>12.2	<12.2	<9.4
65-72 hours	<15.5	>13.0	<13.0	<10.3
>72 hours	<15.5	>14.0	<14.0	<11.0

Suggested strategies for observation and interventions for increasing severity of Hyperbilirubinemia

Severe hyperbilirubinemia at >72 hours age		Follow rate of TSB rise and B:A ratio	Interventions
TSB level >75 percentile	TSB level > 14 mg/dL	And <0.20 mg/dL/h	Nutritional support
TSB level >95 percentile	TSB level ≥ 17 mg/dL	And >0.20 mg/dL/h	Phototherapy
TSB level >98 percentile	TSB level ≥ 20 mg/dL	And B:A ratio <7.0	Intensive phototherapy
TSB level >99.9 percentile	TSB level ≥ 25 mg/dL	And/or B:A ratio ≥ 7.0 mg/g	Intensive phototherapy and prepare for an exchange transfusion
TSB level >99.99 percentile	TSB level ≥ 30 mg/dL	And/or B:A ratio ≥ 7.0 mg/g	Intensive phototherapy and perform an exchange transfusion

Modes of phototherapy

	Home-based (blanket)	Hospital-based (intensive)[a]
Source of light	Fiber optic	Bank of tube lights
Color of light	White/blue	"Super-blue"
Spectral reflectance (425 to 475 nm range)	Wide	Narrow and specific
Irradiance (at skin surface)	<20m watts/cm²/nm	25 to 35 m watts/cm²/nm
Surface area (exposed)	Torso is wrapped; eye patches not needed	Entire body surface (exclude eye patches and diaper area)

[a] May be complemented with white halogen lights to cover a wider surface area (avoid shadows with multiple lights).

Hematological values in the newborn: Age—specific indices

Age	Hgb (g %) Mean (-2 SD)	Hct (%) Mean (-2 SD)	MCV (fl) Mean (-2 SD)	MCHC (g/dl RBC) Mean (-2 SD)	Reticulocytes (%)	WBC/mm³ × 1000 Mean (+2 SD)	Platelets/mm³ (× 1000) Mean(range)
26–30 wk gestation*	13.4 (11)	41.5 (34.9)	118.2 (106.7)	37.9 (30.6)	—	4.4 (2.7)	254 (180–327)
28 wk	14.5	45	120	31	(5–10)	—	275
32 wk	15	47	118	32	(3–10)	—	290
Term† (cord)	16.5 (13.5)	51 (42)	108 (98)	33 (30)	(3–7)	18.1 (9-30)‡	290
1–3 days	18.5 (14.5)	56 (45)	108 (95)	33 (29)	(1.8–4.6)	18.9 (9.4-34)	192
2 wk	16.6 (13.4)	53 (41)	105 (88)	31.4 (28.1)		11.4 (5-20)	252

* Values are from fetal samplings.

† Under 1 mo, capillary Hgb exceeds venous: 1 hr: 3.6 gm difference; 5 days: 2.2 gm difference; 3 weeks: 1.1 gm difference.

‡ Mean (95% confidence limits).

Modified from Roberson J, shilkofski N: The Harriet Lane Handbook, 17th ed. Philadelphia, Mosby, 2005.

Differential wbc counts in the newborn

Age (Hr)	Total White Cell Count	Neutrophils	Bands/Metas	Lymphocytes	Monocytes	Eosinophils
TERM INFANTS						
0	10.0–26	5–13	0.4–1.8	3.5–8.5	0.7–1.5	0.2–2.0
12	13.5–31	9–18	0.4–2	3.0–7	1.0–2	0.2–2.0
72	5.0–14.5	2–7	0.2–0.4	2.0–5	0.5–1	0.2–1.0
144	6.0–14.5	2–6	0.2–0.5	3.0–6	0.7–1.2	0.2–0.8
PREMATURE INFANTS						
0	5.0–19	2–9	0.2–2.4	2.5–6	0.3–1	0.1–0.7
12	5.0–21	3–11	0.2–2.4	1.5–5	0.3–1.3	0.1–1.1
72	5.0–14	3–7	0.2–0.6	1.5–4	0.3–1.2	0.2–1.1
144	5.5–17.5	2–7	0.2–0.5	2.5–7.5	0.5–1.5	0.3–1.2

From Oski FA, Naiman JL: Hematologic problems in the Newborn, 3rd ed. Philadelphia, WB saunders, 1982.

Treatment and prevention of anemia: Minimize phlebotomy losses: *Keep laboratory testing to only those tests which are needed. This is especially true in the first weeks of life when sick infants have the greatest amount of blood drawn due to their often tenuous condition. Transfusion with packed red blood cells (PRBCs): *Good clinical practice dictates and regulatory agencies advise that chart documentation of the reason that the transfusion is being administered should be recorded. Transfuse to achieve a calculated hematocrit of approximately 45%, or give a maximum volume of 15 mL/kg. As a "rule of thumb," for each 1 mL of PRBC's transfused (Hct of H" 85%)/kg, anticipate a 1% increase in the patient's hematocrit. Hence for 15 mL of PRBC/kg, a pre-transfusion hct of 32% should rise to approximately 47% when checked several hours after transfusing. *Transfuse using irradiated (only infants with birth weights <1.5 kg) filtered to reduce CMV risk, packed red blood cells (Hct H" 85%). The blood bank routinely screens all blood for other viral pathogens including HIV, hepatitis B, hepatitis C, and HTLV I/II. Assuming a packed cell hematocrit of 80-90% and a blood volume of 80 mL/kg: Erythropoietin (EPO): *Multicenter U.S. and European VLBW clinical trial results indicate that EPO therapy is of marginal clinical benefit as it is currently being administered. Thus, if EPO therapy is considered this needs to be discussed with the staff attending. If EPO is to be used, the dose is 200-300 U s.q./kg/d every other day. Enteral iron intake should be increased to 6 mg/kg/d during EPO treatment.

Non infectious causes of neutrophilia and elevated I/T ratio(immature to total) in neonates

* Maternal fever
* Difficult or prolonged labor
* Perinatal asphyxia
* Extended administration of intrapartum oxytocin
* Meconium aspiration
* Pneumothorax
* Intraventricular hemorrhage
* Hemolysis
* Seizures

Ratio of immature to total neutrophils at different ages

No.	Age	Normal I/T ratio
1.	< 24 hrs	0.16
2.	24–48 hrs	0.14
3.	48–60 hrs	0.13
4.	60 hrs–1month	0.12

Non infectious causes of neutropenia in neonates:
*Maternal hypertension   *Pre-eclampsia * Hemolysis *IUGR * NEC
*Periventricular hemorrhage *Seizures *Donor in twin to twin transfusion *Erythroblastosis fetalis

Persistent elevation of CRP in spite of antibiotic therapy
Consider the D.D a)Fungal infection b)Resistant organism c)Infective endocarditis d)Abscess formation.

Cerebrospinal fluid values of healthy term newborns

	Age			
	0–24 Hours	1 Day	7 Days	>7 Days
Color	Clear or xanthochromic	Clear or xanthochromic	Clear or xanthochromic	
Red blood cells/mm³	9 (0-1070)	23 (6-630)	3 (0-48)	
Polymorphonuclear leukocytes/mm³	3 (0-70)	7 (0.26)	2 (0-5)	
Lymphocytes/mm³	2 (0-20)	5 (0-16)	1 (0-4)	
Protein (mg/dl)	63 (32-240)	73 (40-148)	47 (27-65)	
Glucose (mg/dl)	51 (32-78)	48 (38-64)	55 (48-62)	
Lactate dehydrogenase (IU/L)	22-73	22-73	22-73	0-40

Modified from Naidoo BT: The cerebrospinal fluid in the healthy newborn infant. S Afr Med J 42:933, 1968, and Neches W, platt M: Cerebrospinal fluid LDH in 287 children, including 53 cases of meningitis of bacterial and nonbacterial etiology. Pediatrics 41:1097, 1968.

Normal Laboratory Values (Cerebrospinal Fluid)

Evaluation of Cerebrospinal Fluid

	WBC Count	Mean % PMNS
Preterm	0-25 WBCs/mm³	57%
Term	0-22 WBCs/mm³	61%
Child	0-7 WBCs/mm³	5%

Glucose

Preterm	24-63 mg/dl	1.3-3.5 mmol/L
Term	34-119 mg/dl	1.9-6.6 mmol/L
Child	40-80 mg/dl	2.2-4.4 mmol/L

CSF Glucose/Blood Glucose

Preterm	55%-105%
Term	44%-128%
Child	50%

Lactate Acid Dehydrogenase

Normal range	5-30 U/L (or about 10% of serum value)

Myelin Basic Protein <4 ng/ml

Opening Pressure
(Lateral recumbent)

Newborn	80-110 mm H_2O
Infant/child	<200 mm H_2o
Respiratory variations	5-10 mm H_2o

Protein

Preterm	65-150 mg/dl	0.65-1.5 g/L
Term	20-170 mg/dl	0.20-1.7 g/L
Child	5-40 mg/dl	0.05-0.40 g/L

CSF, Cerebrospinal fluid; PMNS, polymorphonuclear leucocytes; WBC, white blood cell. Modified from Oski FA: principles and practice of pediatrics, 3 rd ed. Philadelphia, JB Lippincott, 1999.

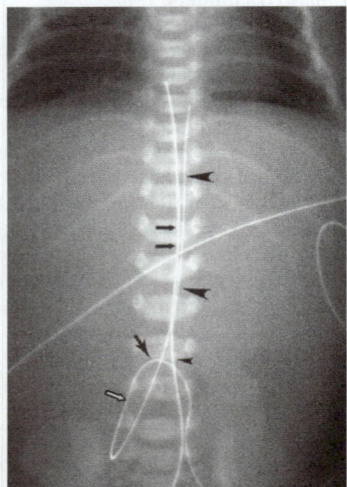

Normal radiographic appearance of umbilical venous catheter and umbilical artery catheter. Frontal radiograph of abdomen shows that umbilical venous catheter enters abdomen at umbilicus (*small arrowhead*), travels in cephalad direction in umbilical vein (*double black arrows*) (note that catheters cross just above umbilicus), courses through left portal vein and ductus venosus, enters inferior vena cava, and terminates in right atrium. Umbilical artery catheter also enters abdomen at umbilicus (*single black arrow*) but extends inferiorly (*white arrow*) and posteriorly into iliac artery before coursing superiorly in aorta (*large arrowheads*).

Line Disinfectants: To assist in the prevention of blood stream infections. Remember that disinfectants provide most effective cleansing when they have dried. Peripheral Lines: Prior to accessing the IV port; swab the bung with prepared 70% alcohol and 2% chlorhexidine wipe and allow to dry. Central Lines: For central lines either swab bung with: *70% alcohol and 2% chlorhexidine wipe or *Sterile gauze soaked in 2% chlorhexidine and 10% alcohol solution and allow to dry. Be aware that the solution will take slightly longer to dry with the lowered alcohol content. Not for skin: Chlorhexidine (2%) may unduly irritate the preterm skin and there is potential for absorption therefore do not use on infant skin. These products are for line management only; please see the skin disinfectant guideline for more information.

@ Classification of Newborns by their birth weight, (SGA, AGA, and LGA), their gestational age (maturity), or a combination of these two dimensions

By birth weight:
*Extremely low birth wt = <1000 grams
*Very low birth wt = 1000-1499 grams
*Low birth wt = 1500 – 2499 grams
*Normal birth wt = ≥ 2500 grams

By gestational age: (based on specific neuromuscular signs and physical characteristics that change with gestational maturity)
*Pre-term = gestational age < 37 weeks
*Term = gestational age 37 to 42 weeks
*Post-term = gestational age ≥ 42 weeks

Classification by birth weight and gestational age:
*Weight small for gestational age (SGA) = birth wt < 10th percentile on the intrauterine growth curve
*Weight appropriate for gestational age (AGA) = birth wt within the 10th and 90th percentiles on the intrauterine growth curve
*Weight large for gestational age (LGA) = birth wt > 90th percentile on the intrauterine growth curve

Selected Chemistry Values in Full-term and Preterm Infants

Constituent	Preterm	Term	Constituent	Preterm	Term
Ammonia (mg/100 ml)	—	90-150	Osmolality (mOsm/L)	—	275–295
Base, excess (mmol/L)	—	-10 to -2			(may ve as
Bicarbonate, standard (mmol/L)	18–26	20-26			low as 266)
Bilirubin, total (mg/dl)			Phosphate,		
Cord	<2.8	<2.8	alkaline (U/L)		
24 hr	1–6	2-6	(mean ± SD)		
48 hr	6–8	6-7	26-27 wk	320 ± 142	164 ± 68
3-5 days	10–12	4-6	28-29 wk	292 ± 87	—
>1 mo	<1.5	<1.5	30-31 wk	281 ± 85	—
Bilirubin,m direct (mg/dl)	<0.5	<0.5	32-33 wk	254 ± 72	—
Calcium, total (mg/dl), week 1	6–10	8.4–11.6	34-35 wk	236 ± 62	—
Ceruloplasmin (mg/dl)		1-3 mo:5–18	36 wk	207 ± 60	—
		6-12 mo:33–43	Phosphorus (mg/dl)		
		13-26 mo:26–55	Birth		4.5-8.7
Cholesterol (mg/dl)			Day 5		4.2-7.2
Cord		45–98	Month 1		4.5-6.5
3 days-1 yr		65–175	SGOT/AST		
Creatine phosphokinase (U/L)			(aspartate amino		24-81
Day 1		44–1150	transferase) (U/L)		
Day 4		14–97	SGPT/ALT (alanine		
Creatinine (mg/dl)			amino transferase)		
Birth	Mother's level	Mother's level	(U/L)		10-33
			Triglycerides (mg/dl)		10-140
10 days	1.3 ± 0.07 (mean ± SD)	1–4 day 0.3–1	Urea nitrogen (mg/dl)	3-25	4-12
			Uric acid (mg/dl)	—	3-7.5
1 mo	0.6 ± 0.05 (mean ± SD)	>4 day 0.2–0.4	Vitamin A (mg/dl)	16 ± 1.0	23.9 ± 1.8
			(<10 (mg/dl indicates		
Ferritin (mg/dl)			very low hepatic		
Neonate		25–200	vitamin A stores)		
1 mo		200–600	Vitamin D		
2-5 mo		50–200	25-hydroxycholecalciferol		20-60
>6 mo		7–142	(ng/ml)		
Gamma-glutamyl	—	14–131	1,25-		
transferase (GGT) (U/L)			Dihydroxycholecalciferol		40-90
Glucose (mg/dl)			(pg/ml)		
<72 hr	20-125	30–125			
>72 hr	40-125	40–125			
Lactate dehydrogenase (U/L)	—	357–953			
Magnesium (mg/dl)	—	1.7–2.4			

NORMAL URINARY AND RENAL VALUES IN TERM AND PRETERM INFANTS

	Preterm infants <34 wks	Term infants at birth	Term infants 2 wks	Term infants 8 wks
GFR (ml/min/1.73m²)	13-58	15-60		63–80
FENa (%) (oliguric patient)	>1% up to 3%	<1%	<1%	<1%
Bicarbonate threshold (mEq/L)	14-16	21	21.5	
TRP (%)	>85%	>95%		
Protein excretion (mg/m²/24h)(mean ± 1 SD)	60 ± 96	31 ± 44		
Maximal concentration ability (mOsmol/L)	500	800	900	1200
Maximal diluting ability (mOsmol/L)	25-30	25-30	25-30	25-30
Specific gravity	1.002 – 1.015	1.002 – 1.020	1.002–1.025	
Dipstick				
PH	5.0 – 8.0	4.5 – 8.0	4.5–8.0	4.5–8.0
Proteins	Neg to ++	Neg to +	Neg	Neg
Glucose	Neg t0 ++	Neg	Neg	Neg
Blood	Neg	Neg	Neg	Neg
Leukocytes	Neg	Neg	Neg	Neg

Average incubator air temperatures needed to provide a suitable thermal environment for naked, healthy infants

Birth weight (kg)	Environmental temperature					
	37°C	36°C	35°C	34°C	33°C	32°C
Less than 1.0	For 1 day	After 1 day	After 2 weeks	After 3 weeks	After 4 weeks	After 6 weeks
1.0–1.5			For 10 days	After 10 days	After 3 weeks	After 5 weeks
1.5–2.0				For 10 days	After 10 days	After 4 weeks
2.0–2.5				For 2 days	After 2 days	After 3 weeks
More than 2.5					For 2 days	After 2 days

Note :
1. In a single-walled incubator the environmental temperature needs to increased by 1°C for every 7°C difference between room and incubator temperature.

2. Infants below 1.0 kg and below 30 weeks' gestation need a humidified incubator in the first week of life.

3. Clothed infants need lower incubator temperatures.

4. Values are average ones but there is considerable variation in individual requirements.

Fluid intake alterations

Conditions in which fluid restriction should be considered
- Persistent ductus arteriosus, especially if indomethacin given
- Hypoxic-ischemic encephalopathy
- Severe respiratory distress
- Oliguric renal failure
- Inappropriate release of ADH

Conditions in which fluid requirements are increased
- VLBW infant with excessive insensible water loss
- Use of a radiant warmer
- Phototherapy
- Vomiting
- Diarrhea
- Polyuria (e.g. due to glycosuria or following relief of obstructive uropathy)

ADH, antidiuretic hormone; VLBW, very low birth weight.

Suggested abdominal skin temperature settings for infants nursed in servo mode incubators or under radiant warmers

Weight (kg)	Abdominal skin temperature (°C)
Less than 1.0	36.9
1.0–1.5	36.7
1.5–2.0	36.5
2.0–2.5	36.3
More than 2.5	36.0

Gradual increase in feeds for infants who require tube feeding

Postnatal age	Fluid intake (mL/kg per 24 hrs)	
	<2.5 kg	>2.5 kg
Day 1	60	40
Day 2	90	60
Day 3	120	80
Day 4	150	110
Day 5	150-200	150

Neonatal Immunodeficiency - Diagnostic Clues

History
Parental consanguinity
Family history of immunodeficiency
History of early infectious deaths
Autoimmune disease in the mother (e.g.SLE)
Immunosuppressive drug therapy in the mother (e.g. azathioprine)
Infection during pregnancy (e.g. CMV)
Extreme IUGR with maternal hypertension
Risk factors for HIV
Persistent diarrhea
Recurrent/chronic superficial candidiasis
Recurrent bacterial infections
Infection with unusual or opportunistic organism
Failure to thrive

Examination
Skin rash, eczema, pustulosis
Hepatosplenomegaly
Absence of lymphoid tissue
Axillary or inguinal lymphadenopathy
Cardiac disease especially truncus, with reduced thymic shadow on X-ray
Oculocutaneous albinism
Unusual facies and cleft palate
Delayed separation of the umbilical cord
Sparse light hair and short length

Investigations
Lymphopenia (<2.7 × 10^9/1)
Neutropenia
Abnormal blood film - leukocyte granules or Howell - Jolly bodies
Low immunoglobulins
Autoantibodies (may be maternal)
Thrombocytopenia with small platelets
Lack of thymic shadow on X-ray
ADA skeletal abnormalities (cupping deformities of the ends of the ribs, abnormal transverse vertebral processes, scapulae)

Monitoring of fluid and electrolyte status in neonates

Body weight: Serial weight measurements can be used as a guide to estimate the fluid deficit in Newborns. Term neonates lose 1-3% of their birth weight daily with a cumulative loss of 5-10% in the first week of life, Preterm Neonates lose 2-3% of their birth weight daily with a cumulative loss of 15-20% in the first week of life. Failure to lose weight in the first week of life should be an indicator for fluid restriction. However, excessive weight loss in the first 7 days or later would be non-physiological and would merit correction with fluid therapy.

Clinical examination: The usual physical signs of dehydration are unreliable in Neonates. Infants with 10% (100 ml/kg) dehydration may have sunken eyes and fontanel, cold and clammy skin, poor skin turgor and oliguria. Infants with 15% (150ml/kg) or more dehydration would have signs of shock (hypotension, tachycardia and weak pulses) in addition to the above features. Dehydration would merit correction of fluid and electrolyte status gradually over the next 24 hours.

Serum biochemistry: Serum sodium and plasma osmolarity would be helpful in the assessment of the hydration status in an infant. Serum sodium values should be maintained between 135-145 mEq/L. *Hyponatremia with weight loss* suggests sodium depletion and would merit sodium replacement. *Hyponatremia with weight gain* suggests water excess and necessitates fluid restriction. *Hypernatremia with weight gain* suggests salt and water load and would be an indication of fluid and sodium restriction.

* The normal maintenance fluid required on the day 1 would range from 2.5-3.5 mL/kg/hr in Newborns. This volume would increase to 5-6 mL/kg/hr by the end of the first week and 7–8 mL/kg/hr thereafter.

* Normally there is a salt and water diuresis in the first 48–72 hours of life. Therefore, sodium supplementation should be started after ensuing initial diuresis, a decrease in serum sodium or at least 5–6% weight loss.

* Preterm Neonates require sodium 3–5 mEq/kg/day after the first week of life. They have a limited tubular capacity to reabsorb sodium and hence have increased urinary losses. Failure to provide this amount of sodium may be associated with poor weight gain. VLBW infants on exclusive breast feeding may need sodium supplementation in addition to breast milk until 32-34 weeks corrected age.

* Term infants are expected to lose upto 10% of their birth weight as compared upto 15% weight loss in prematures. Failure to lose extracellular fluid through the kidneys may be associated with morbidities like PDA, NEC & BPD/CLD in preterms.

* Sensible losses are mandatory water loss by the kidneys and GIT. Insensible water losses occur due to evaporation from the skin and respiratory tract. Loss of water through the skin usually contributes to 70% of insensible water loss. The remaining 30% is contributed through losses from the respiratory tract. The emphasis in fluid and electrolyte therapy should be on prevention of excessive insensible water loss rather than replacement of increased insensible water loss. Hence incubators, plastic barriers and heat shields should be used liberally in the management of extremely premature Neonates.

Factors affecting insensible water loss in neonates

Increased insensible water loss (IWL)	Decreased insensible water loss (IWL)
Increased respiratory rate	Use of incubators
Conditions with skin injury (removal of adhesive tapes)	Humidification of inspired gases in head box and ventilators
Surgical malformations (gastroschisis, omphalocele, neural tube defects)	Use of plexiglas heat shields
Increased body temperature : 30% increase in IWL per °C rise in temperature	Increased ambient humidity
High ambient temperature : 30% increase in IWL per °C rise in temperature	Thin transparent plastic barriers
Use of radiant warmer and phototherapy : 50% increase in IWL	
Decreased ambient humidity	
Increased motor activity, crying : 50-70% increase in IWL	

* Intravenous fluids should be increased in the presence of

  a) Increased weight loss (>3%/day or a cumulative loss >20%),

  b) Increased serum sodium (Na>145 mEq/L)

  c) Increased urine specific gravity (>1.020) or urine osmolality (>400 mosm/L),

  d) Decreased urine output (<1 mL/kg/hr). Similarly, fluids should be restricted in the presence of *a)* Decreased weight loss (<1%/day or a cumulative loss <5%), *b)* Decreased serum sodium in the presence of weight gain (Na<130 mEq/L), *c)* Decreased urine specific gravity (<1.005) or urine osmolality (<100 mOsm/L), *d)* Increased urine output (>3 ml/kg/hr)

* Sodium and potassium should be started in the IV fluids after 48 hours, each in a dose of 2-3 mEq/kg/day. Calcium may be used in a dose of 4 ml/kg/day (40 mg/kg/day) of calcium gluconate 10%, for the first 3 days in certain high-risk

situations. Dextrose infusion should be maintained @4-6 mg/kg/min. 10% dextrose may be used in babies >1250 grams and 5% dextrose in babies with birth weight <1250 grams.

* The acceptable range for urine output is 1-3ml/kg/hr, for specific gravity between 1.005 to 1.012 & for osmolarity between 100-400 mOsm/L. Maintain serum sodium between 135-145 mEq/L. Serum creatinine falls exponentially in the first week of life as maternally derived creatinine is excreted. *Failure to observe this normal fall in serial samples is a better indicator of renal failure than a single value of creatinine in the first week of life.*

* *Cochrane meta-analysis-findings state that, fluid restriction by 20-50 ml/kg/day in the initial 3-4 days compared to normal fluid requirements is associated with a decreased incidence of death, PDA & NEC, although if may lead to greater weight loss and dehydration.*

Guidelines for routine monitoring of fluid and electrolyte status in the newborn.		

Gestational Age	Test(s)	Monitoring schedule
≤25 weeks	Na, K, Cl, tCO2	By 8–12 h; then every 8–12 h until stable or trending towards reference range; then daily
	Glucose	Usually estimated frequently at the bedside with dry-reagent test strips; estimated values in the lower portion of the reference range must be confirmed with a serum glucose concentration to reliably identify hypoglycemia.
	Ca	At 12–24 h; then every 8–12 h until nadir is reached; then every 24 h until the value is within reference range without calcium supplementation
	Creatinine	By 8–12 h, then daily
26–30 weeks	Na, K, CL, tCO2	By 12–24 h; then every 12–24 h until stable or trending towards reference range; then daily
	Glucose	As above
	Ca	At 12–24 h; then every 24 h until nadir is reached; then every 24 h until value is within reference range without calcium supplementation
	Creatinine	By 12–24 h, then daily
30–34 weeks	Na, K, Cl, tCO2	By 18–24 h, then daily
	Glucose	As above
	Ca	At 18–24 h, then daily until value is within reference range without supplementation
	Creatinine	By 18–24 h, then only if renal insufficiency is anticipated or suspected
≥34 weeks on intravenous maintenance	Na, K, Cl, tCO2	At 18–24 h, then daily
	Glucose	As above
	Ca	As above, but only with risk factor (in addition to prematurity) or signs consistent with hypocalcemia
	Creatinine	At 18–24 h, then only if renal insufficiency is anticipated or suspected
≥34 weeks without intravenous maintenance	Na, K, Cl, tCO2	Only as indicated by excessive weight loss or unusual water and electrolyte loss
	Glucose	As above, but only with risk factor or signs consistent with hypoglycemia
	Ca	As above
	Creatinine	Only if renal insufficiency is anticipated or suspected

*These gestational age ranges are provided as approximations; they are not meant as strict cutoffs. *If acid–base status is being simultaneously assessed with blood gases, regular assessment of Cl and tCO2 (total carbon dioxide) is probably unnecessary unless calculation of the anion gap is of interest. Unfortunately there is little information available regarding the usefulness of the anion gap in the neonate. Furthermore, if the sample is obtained from a skin stick without prewarming, then the tCO2 may be spuriously low. *Other methods that involve very small sample volumes are available that offer accuracy and precision comparable with conventional laboratory methods*

Reference ranges. Plasma concentration

Analyte	SI units	Conventional units
Sodium	135–145 mmol/L	135–145 mEq/L
Potassium	3.6–6.7 mmol/L	3.6–6.7 mEq/L
Chloride	101–111 mmol/	101–111 mEq/L
Total CO2	See acid-base section	
Glucose	2.2–8.3 mmol/L	40–150 mg/dL
Total calcium		
Full-term	2.0–2.75 mmol/L	8 –11 mg/dL
Preterm	1.75–2.75 mmol/L	7 –11 mg/dL
Ionized calcium		
<72h	1.1–1.4 mmol/L	4.4 –5.6 mg/dL
>72h	1.2–1.5 mmol/L	4.8 –6.0 mg/dL
Creatinine		

a) Although these analytes are often measured in serum, reference ranges for most are available only in plasma. However, with the exception of potassium ,concentrations of analytes in serum and plasma are similar. b) Although values outside these ranges are not uncommon, the ranges observed will depend upon the infant's maturity, the environment in which the infant is cared for, and fluid and electrolyte intake. Thus, values outside this reference range are not necessarily indicative of abnormal anterior pituitary function, renal function, or fluid and electrolyte losses. However, there is no reason to believe that values outside the reference ranges for adults are physiologically inconsequential. Maintenance within these ranges is desirable, although not always possible. c) Serum potassium concentration . In clotting, platelets release potassium into the serum; potassium concentration is typically 0.2–0.3 mmol/L lower in plasma than in serum in adults. d) There is no general agreement on the definition of hypoglycemia . However, normal limits lower than that given above were derived from extensive surveys in the 1960s of preterm and term neonates when the concept of intrauterine growth retardation was not fully appreciated and glucose and calorie intake was delayed. e) plasma creatinine concentration will vary with maternal serum creatinine concentration, gestational age, and postnatal age. Therefore, the usefulness of such reference ranges is very limited. Of more interest is the change in creatinine concentration over time.

Fluid balance in extreme immaturity (below 26 weeks gestation)

Anticipate and prevent

* Transepidermal water loss will be high -Take active steps to reduce transepidermal losses

* Glucose requirements will be variable - Use a volume independent, variable glucose delivery system

* Parenteral sodium intake is unnecessary until the physiological postnatal isotonic loss of extracellular fluid is underway- Defer maintenance sodium administration until there has been weight loss of the order of 6% of body weight

* A fluid prescription is a matter of best clinical judgment and is vulnerable to changing clinical circumstances- Monitor carefully and continuously

* The goals of hydration and nutrition are intertwined but distinct - Distinguish these goals clearly

Do's and don'ts

* Do not give furosemide routinely with transfusion of packed red cells. Transfusion of packed red cells at 3 ml/kg/h does not lead to intravascular volume overload in extremely preterm infants.

* Do not use repeated doses of furosemide in the oliguric baby; in the nonoliguric infant doses should be administered at no more than 24 hour intervals- Furosemide clearance is low and plasma half life exceeds 24 hours in infants, 31 weeks postconceptional age. Repeated doses will lead to rapid accumulation and increase the risks of ototoxicity, interstitial nephritis, and ductal patency

* Do not restrict fluid intake routinely whenever signs of a patent ductus arteriosus are present. Restrict only when there is evidence of volume overload; routine fluid restriction will compromise nutrition.

* Do ask yourself if your goal is hydration or nutrition whenever considering a change in fluid intake-If hydration is satisfactory, stepwise increments in fluid intake after birth are unnecessary unless accompanied by a clinically relevant increase in nutrition.

Monitoring fluid balance in the immediate postnatal period

* Daily alteration in body weight—No postnatal weight loss or immediate weight gain is indicative of fluid excess; the usual cause is impaired sodium and/or water excretion.

* Serum sodium- Hyponatremia suggests water excess; hypernatremia suggests water deficit.

* Urine volume- <1 ml/kg/h requires investigation; 2–4 ml/kg/h suggests normal hydration; >6–7 ml/kg/h suggests impaired concentrating ability or excess fluid administration.

"WRITING UP FLUIDS" Didactic recommendations for fluid prescriptions are inappropriate, given variations in gestational age, ambient humidity, nursing practices, and clinical condition. Within a neonatal unit, protocols and guidelines ensure internal consistency, but between neonatal units, although the principles that underpin a guideline are shared, final protocols will be determined by local practices. Enteral intake is likely to be small, for at least the first few days after birth, and fluid volumes must be administered parenterally. Firstly, make a judgment of the likely magnitude of insensible water loss, taking into account sources of radiant heat, ambient humidity, and gestational and postnatal age. A rational initial intravenous volume prescription would be the sum of an allowance for urinary water of 30–60 ml/kg/day plus estimated insensible water loss. If ambient humidity can be maintained above 70%, this equates to a total infusion volume of about 100 ml/kg/day for babies of less than 1000 g birth weight. It is reasonable to start with a 10% glucose solution, but be prepared to revert to a variable glucose delivery system that allows glucose delivery rate to be altered independently of fluid volume if blood glucose concentrations are unstable. Once postnatal adaptation is well underway, total infusion volumes should be dictated by nutritional goals and the energy density of the parenteral preparation used. Enteral feeds are increased incrementally and as tolerated, but there is no evidence that intravenous volumes need similarly to be increased in a stepwise manner.

Courtesy: Management of fluid balance in the very imma ture neonate N Modi Arch Dis Child Fetal Neonatal Ed 2004;89:F108–F111. doi: 10.1136 adc.2001.004275

Intuition and the ill infant

Nowhere in medicine is the use of observation, instinct, and innate experience more important than in attempting to make a clinical diagnosis in an acutely ill infant. I like to refer to this as veterinary paediatrics, as sick animals and sick children share many attributes they refuse to eat; they lie down when they are sick; their language and communication skills are limited; they depend on others to sort out their problems; and when ill they prefer to be left alone.

My approach code to the acutely ill child is (Denis Gill, *professor of Pediatrics*, Children Hospital, Dublin, Ireland)

*Stop *Listen (especially to the mother) but also to the child`s cough, breathing or other noises such as cry, croupy croak or labored wheeze *Look, look, look, look *Examine the child with your eyes. This can be done equally well in the sleeping or awake child. A no touch technique is my first approach to the ill child. You can comment on nutrition, hydration, respiration, circulation, with a modicum of accuracy without laying a finger on the child *Then use your other senses. Touch forehead. Touch the toes. Is there a temperature difference? Touch the chest. A temperature gradient from centre to periphery is instructive, suggesting peripheral vasoconstriction. Feel the pulses, noting pulse volume. Listen again for the cough, cry, wheeze, or grunt, all of which may be alerting. Smell is not usually very useful to me, but my colleagues tell me they can detect acetone, urea, or other smells of sickness.

*Students should sit in the resuscitation room and observe events, especially ill infants. Stand beside intensive care unit incubators and look at sick infants. Linger in the observation ward looking and listening.

Many centuries ago Leonardo Da Vinci advised **"learn to see."** Do so. Looking at infants breathing is by far the most instructive skill in assessing respiratory or cardiac problems. Rapid labored breathing with grunting is almost synony-mous with pneumonia or cardiac failure. Ultimately, the good clinician is the good diagnostician. Intuition means immediate apprehension by the mind without reasoning. Immediate insight and instinct may instil innate impulsion. I have got a good nose for trouble, is how one general practitioner friend sums up this attribute. More likely he possesses good eyes and sharp wits.

Key points : *Learn and see   *Linger and listen   *Discuss and deduce *Prime your senses

Always serious symptoms or signs in infancy

*High pitched screaming or crying (suggests pain)

*Alternating drowsiness and/or irritability (neurological?) *Convulsion *Refusal to feed (two or more feeds) *Repeated vomiting *Rapid labored breathing with or without grunting (pneumonia?) *Episodes of unusual blueness or paleness *Presence of purpuric rash (septicemia?)

Usually serious symptoms in infancy

*Prolonged crying *Persistent crankiness *Worsening croup *Wanting to be left alone (apathy)

Calculation of Fluid and Electrolyte requirements for Neonates

1. Long way (from first principles)

Fluid requirement = Weight x Fluid requirement
for 24 hours kg) (ml/kg/day)

Electrolyte requirement = Weight x Electrolyte requirement
for 24 hours (kg) (mmol/kg/day)
= mmol/day

Injections of electrolytes contain the following :

Sodium Chloride 3%	1ml	=	0.5 mmols of Sodium
Sodium Chloride 30%	1ml	=	5 mmols of Sodium
Potassium Chloride 15%	1ml	=	2 mmols of Potassium
Potassium Chloride 20%	1ml	=	2.7 mmols of Potassium
Calcium Gluconate 10%	1ml	=	0.23 mmols of Calcium
Calcium Chloride 10%	1ml	=	0.5 mmols of Calcium
Magnesium Sulphate 50%	1ml	=	500 mg. (0.2ml /kg/dose)

Life would be easy if fluid bags were available with exactly the volume you needed for each baby. Unfortunately, only 500ml bags exist. You have calculated the proportion of the bag you need i.e. fluid requirement for 24 hours and now you need to put excess amounts of electrolytes into the 500ml bag, to ensure the baby receives the correct amount in this volume.

Total amount to be added to the
500ml bag is calculated by multiplying with : $\dfrac{500ml}{\text{Fluid baby needs in 24 hours}}$

a) Calculate the fluid requirement for 24 hours (from above).
   Calculate the electrolytes requirement for 24 hours (from above).

b) To calculate how much electrolyte injection (i.e. number of mls) is needed to give this requirement

No. of mls of injection $= \dfrac{\text{Electrolyte requirement for 24 hours}}{\text{Electrolyte content per ml}}$

This would be the amount needed if you had a bag of the exact volume you needed. However, you have a 500ml bag.

c) To calculate how much to put in the 500ml bag

No. of ml of injection to put in 500ml bag $= \dfrac{500ml}{\text{Fluid baby needs in 24 hours}} \ x \ \text{Number of mls of electrolyte injection (from b)}$

Repeat for each different electrolyte

2. The Short Way

To calculate number of mls of electrolyte injection needed to put in the 500ml bag

mls of electrolyte injection needed $= \dfrac{500ml}{\text{Total fluid needed for 24 hours } ❖} \ x \ \dfrac{\text{Total number of mmol ▼ of electrolyte needed in 24 hrs}}{\text{Electrolyte content per ✱ ml of injection}}$

Notes :

❖ Total fluid needed for 24 hours = ml/kg x weight

▼ Total number of mmol of electrolyte in 24 hours = mmol/kg x weight

✱ Injection electrolyte content per ml

i.e. Sodium 30% contains 5mmol per ml of Sodium. Potassium 20% contains 2.7mmol per ml of Potassium. Potassium 15% contains 2mmol per ml of potassium

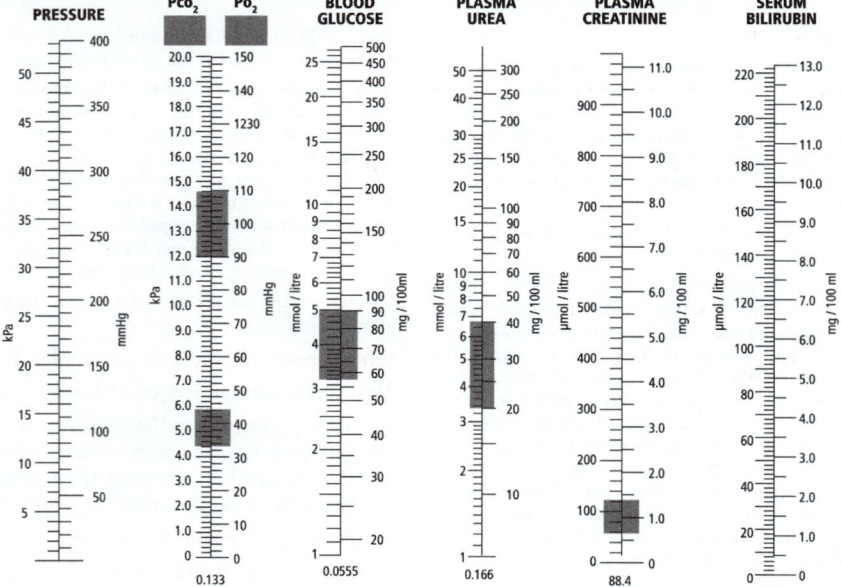

Shading indicates the normal range where appropriate. To convert "old" to "new" units, multiply by the conversion factor at the foot of each column. (Modified from Halliday HL, McClure G, Reid M: Handbook of Neonatal Intensive Care. 2nd ed. Philadelphia: WB Saunders, 1985.)

HEMODYNAMIC FORMULATIONS

O2 consumption = O2 delivery

= Q × (arterial O2 content–venous O2 content)

Blood O2 content (mL/L) = Hgb (g/dl) × 10 (dL/L) × 1.36 (ml O2/g Hgb) ×Hgb O2 Sat.

Average neonate O2 consumption = 200-220 mL/min/m2

Qs (L/min/m2) = O2 consumption/Hgb × 13.6 × (arterial O2 Sat. – venous O2 Sat.)

Qp (L/min/m2) = O2 consumption/Hgb × 13.6 × (pulm. venous O2 Sat. – pulm. arterial O2 Sat.)

Qp/Qs = (arterial O2 Sat. – venous O2 Sat.)

DP (mmHg) = $Q × R$ (Woods units)

Rs = Qs/(arterial mean pressure - RA mean pressure)

Rp = Qp/(pulm. arterial mean pressure - LA mean pressure)

Q, cardiac output or blood flow; Hgb, blood hemoglobin concentration; Sat., saturation; Qs, systemic flow or cardiac output; Qp, pulmonary flow; DP, arterial mean pressure minus arterial atrial mean pressure; pulm., pulmonary; R, vascular resistance; Rs, systemic vascular resistance; Rp, pulmonary vascular resistance.

Prevent or Detect and Correct for Stabilization of the Ill Newborn Infant

A. Five Hs

1. Hypothermia
2. Hypotension
3. Hypoglycemia
4. Hypoxia
5. Hypercarbia PLUS ACIDOSIS

NICU/SCBU Isolation Guidelines

Antibiotic resistant organisms + contacts

· Until cleared

CMV *

· ubiquitious but pregnant staff not asked to nurse - not a danger to other infants.

Diarrhea

+ contacts

· until cultures negative and asymptomatic.

Enterovirus + contacts

· until asymptomatic and cultures negative.

Gonococcal ophthalmia

· until treated ? 24 hours.

Hepatitis A

· mother: 3 weeks from onset of jaundice.

· baby remain with mother in isolation - no treatment.

Hepatitis B

· clinical - mother isolated in hospital.

· carrier mother - syringe needle isolation

· infant - see immunization schedule

Herpes simplex*

+ contacts

· until proven negative.

Outborn infants except from other delivery suites

· until cultures negative.

· Infants from home -postnatal ward

Staphylococcal sepsis

+ contacts

· until negative and/or treated.

Necrotizing enterocolitis *

· desirable to isolate.

Rubella *

· single room only because of danger to pregnant nurses

Toxoplasmosis

· isolation not necessary.

Varicella-Zoster

· mother and infant -until lesions crusted.

* Isolation may not be possible except for known highly contagious disease, but barrier nursing with gloves is indicated.

SICK NEONATE-Differential Diagnoses:

NEO SECRETS

N iNborn errors of metabolism

E Electrolyte abnormalities

O Overdose (toxin, poison)

S Seizures

E Enteric emergencies

C Cardiac abnormalities

R Recipe (formula, herbs, additives)

E Endocrine crisis

T Trauma

S Sepsis

Diagram of normal circulatory dynamics with pressures, oxygen contents, and percentage of saturations. (Modified from Nadas AS, Fyler DC : Pediatric Cardiology, 3rd ed. Philadelphia, WB Saunders, 1972.)

Causes of cyanotic heart disease: the five "terrible Ts" (and one "S")

1. Transposition of the great vessels
2. Total anomalous pulmonary venous return
3. Tetralogy of Fallot
4. Truncus arteriosus
5. Tricuspid atresia
6. Severe pulmonic stenosis

Method for Conversion of Milligrams to Milliequivalents per Liter (or to Millimoles per Liter)

mg = milligrams
g = grams
dL = deciliter = 100 mL

mL = milliliter
1 mL = 1.000027 cc

$$\text{mEq/L (milliequivalents per liter)} = \frac{\text{mg/L}}{\text{equivalent weight}}$$

$$\text{Equivalent weight} = \frac{\text{atomic weight}}{\text{valence of element}}$$

For example: A sample of blood serum contains 10 mg of Ca in 1 dL (100 mL)
The valence of Ca is 2, and the atomic weight is 40.
The equivalent weight of Ca is therefore 40/2, or 20.
The milliequivalents of Ca per liter are 10 (mg/dL) x 10 (dL/L)/20, or 5 milliequivalents per liter

$$\text{mM/L (millimoles per liter)} = \frac{\text{mg/L}}{\text{molecular weight}}$$

Vol. % (volume per cent) = mM/L x 2.24 for a gas whose properties approach that of an ideal gas, such as oxygen or nitrogen. For carbon dioxide, the factor is 2.226.

Factors for Conversion of Concentration Expressed in Milliequivalents per Liter to Milligrams per Deciliter (100 mL), and Vice Versa, for Common Ions that Occur in Physiologic Solutions

Element or Radical	mEq/L to mg/dL		mg/dL to mEq/L	
Sodium	1	2.30	1	.4348
Potassium	1	3.91	1	.2558
Calcium	1	2.005	1	.4988
Magnesium	1	1.215	1	.8230
Chloride	1	3.55	1	.2817
Bicarbonate (HCO_3^-)	1	6.1	1	.1639
Phosphorus valence 1	1	3.10	1	.3226
Phosphorus valence 1.8	1	1.72	1	.5814
Sulfur valence 2	1	1.60	1	.625

Example: to convert milliequivalents of magnesium per liter to milligrams per deciliter (100 mL), multiply by the factor 1.215; to convert milligrams of potassium per deciliter (100 mL) to milliequivalents per liter, multiply by the factor 0.2558.

USEFUL CONVERSIONS
Conversion to SI Units from Old Units

Component	Old Units	SI Units
CSF and other body fluid cell count	per mm (cu mm)	x 10^6/L
Urine culture colony count	per ml	x 10^6/L
Antibiotic assay	mcg/ml	mg/L

Conversion of Milligrams (mg) per 100 ml to Milliequivalents (mEq) per Liter of plasma

$$\text{Sodium (Na)} = \frac{\text{mg/100 ml x 10}}{23 \text{ (atomic weight)}} \times 1 \text{ (valency)} = \text{mEq/L}$$

$$\text{Potassium (K)} = \frac{\text{mg/100 ml x 10}}{39} \times 1 \text{ (valency)} = \text{mEq/L}$$

$$\text{Calcium (ca)} = \frac{\text{mg/100ml x 10}}{40} \times 2 \text{ (valency)} = \text{mEq/L}$$

$$\text{Chloride (Cl)} = \frac{\text{mg/100ml x 10}}{35.4} \times 1 \text{ (valency)} = \text{mEq/L}$$

Temperature
Conversion of ^{0}C to ^{0}F = 9/3 x ^{0}C = ^{0}F
Conversion of ^{0}F to ^{0}C = 5/9 (^{0}F-32) = ^{0}C

Inches to Centimeters
1 inch = 2.54cm
1 cm = 0.39 inch

Minim to Milliliter
1 minim = 0.06 ml
1 ml = 15 minims

Equivalent Imperial and Meteric Quantities
1 grain = 65 mg
1 ounce = 28 g
1 pound = 453 g
2.2 pounds = 1kg

What you should do with Persistent crying in babies ?

* Check the baby's growth chart, assessing weight gain and head circumference.
* Expose the baby fully. Complete exposure may point to the underlying cause, such as areas of eczematous skin or nappy rash that may be irritating him.
* Examine the orifices: look for a tight phimosis; anal fissures will show as small tears around the anal margin; check the mouth for evidence of thrush or teething; check the ears for otitis media.
* If you think there is a feeding problem advise the mother on feeding techniques, such as how to make up a feed and how to help stop the baby swallowing too much air while feeding. Check that the hole in the teat of the baby's feeding bottle is not too small, resulting in his or hers gulping air.
* If she is breast feeding, ask whether she has enough milk. A health visitor may be able to advise.
* Enlist further support from the health visitor if you have concerns about her parenting skills or mental state. If she has postnatal depression she is likely to need treatment and support.
* Try to understand the Home environment—The home environment and family dynamics may be having an effect on the baby. The views (if available) of the father and other members of the family may provide useful insights. Also ask about sleeping arrangements and the baby's pattern of sleep.
* Consider referring the baby for a clean catch urine specimen and further assessment if you suspect a urine infection.
* In most cases no underlying cause will be found. In such cases the problem will probably subside with time, and other than reassurance and ongoing support no further investigations are warranted.

Key Elements for Reducing Severe Hyperbilirubinemia

• Promote and support successful breastfeeding.
• Establish nursery protocols for the identification and evaluation of hyperbilirubinemia.
• Measure the total serum bilirubin or transcutaneous bilirubin level of infants jaundiced in the first 24 hours.
• Recognize that visual estimation of the degree of jaundice can lead to errors, particularly in darkly pigmented infants.
• Interpret all bilirubin levels according to the infant's age in hours.
• Recognize that infants <38 wks' gestation, particularly those who are breastfed, are at higher risk of developing hyperbilirubinemia and require closer surveillance and monitoring.
• Perform a systematic assessment for the risk of severe hyperbilirubinemia on all infants before discharge.
• Provide parents with written and oral information about newborn jaundice.
• Provide appropriate follow-up based on the time of discharge and the risk assessment.
• Treat newborns, when indicated, with phototherapy or exchange transfusion.

Predictive value of laboratory tests: Predictive value (PV) theory deals with the usefulness of tests as defined by their clinical sensitivity (ability to detect a disease) and specificity (ability to define the absence of a disease).

The problems addressed by PV theory are false-negative and false-positive test results. Both are major considerations in interpreting the results of screening tests in general and neonatal screening tests in particular.

$$Sensitivity = \frac{Number\ positive\ by\ test}{Total\ number\ positive} \times 100$$

$$Specificity = \frac{Number\ negative\ by\ test}{Total\ number\ without\ disease} \times 100$$

$$PV\ of\ a\ positive\ test\ result = \frac{True\ positive\ results}{Total\ positive\ results} \times 100$$

$$PV\ of\ a\ Negative\ test\ result = \frac{True\ negative\ results}{Total\ Negative\ results} \times 100$$

IMPORTANT BIOSTATISTICS

$$SENSITIVITY(\%) = \frac{TP}{TP + FN}$$

$$SPECIFICITY(\%) = \frac{TN}{TN + FP}$$

$$POSITIVE\ PREDICTIVE\ VALUE = \frac{TP}{TP + FP}$$

PROBABILITY (p VALUE) < 0.001 highly significant, < 0.01 very significant, <0.05 significant, >0.05 insignificant

STANDARD DEVIATION: interpretation $1\pm = 68.3\%$, $2\pm = 95.4\%$, $3\pm = 99.7\%$

a) Serum osmolality = $2 \times Na^+ + \frac{glucose(mgs/dL)}{18} + \frac{Blood\ urea}{6}$ or $\frac{BUN}{2.8}$ Normal range = 275-295mOsm/L

b) Osmolar gap = Measured osmolality - calculated osmolality   Normal < 10

c) Anion gap = (Serum $Na^+ + K^+$) - (Serum $Cl^- + HCO_3^-$) Normal range = 12mEq/L $\pm$ 4mEq/L

d) Creatinine Clearance(Schwartz) - $C_{cr} = k \times Length\ (cm)$

k = 0.45 in babies <1yr; 0.55 if > 1 year and in adult females; 0.7 in adolescent and adult males(*Low Birth weight $\leq$ 1 y K = 0.33)

e) Renal failure index - RFI = Urine Na x $\frac{Plasma\ Cr}{Urine\ Cr} \times 100$

f) Fractional Excretion of Sodium- FE Na = $\frac{Urine\ Na\ x\ Plasma\ Cr}{Urine\ Cr\ x\ Plasma\ Na} \times 100$

> 1 % renal failure, <1% pre-renal

Osmolarity *Osmolarity is the measure of solute concentration in a fixed solvent volume • Calculated serum osmolarity = 2[Na+] + Glucose/18 + BUN/2.8 + other osmolarities *When calculating the osmolarity of PPN solutions, the following formula may be used: • Osmolarity (mOsm/L) = (grams dextrose / liter) x 5] + [grams amino acid / liter) x 10] + [(mEq cations / liter) × 2]

Why is osmolarity important? * PPN (Too high = phlebitis) * Dextrose – 10% maximum for older children and 12.5% for infants * Osmolarity range 600 – 1100 mOsm * Neonatal Solutions (Too low = RBC lysis) *Normal Serum osmolarity: = •0.2 NS – ~68 mOsm •D2.5W – ~125 mOsm.

a)Sodium requirement = sodium deficit + sodium maintenance

Sodium deficit = (135 - measured Na^+) x weight in kg x 0.6

Sodium maintenance = 2-4 mEq Na^+ x body weight in kg(per 24hr period)

b) Bicarbonate deficit (mEq) = {desired HCO_3(23mEq/L) - measured HCO_3} x Wt(kg) × 0.3

or   weight in kg × base deficit × 0.3

Hypocalcemia

* Diagnosis * Total serum calcium concentration: •< 2.1 mmol/L (8.5 mg dL) in children

•< 2 mmol/L (8 mg/dL) in term Neonates •< 1.75 mmol/L (7 mg/dL) in preterm Neonates

Urine Measurements

The following infants should have urine output monitored in the NICU.

1) All babies admitted to Level 3 in their first 5 days of life. 2)All babies who suffered intrauterine or intrapartum asphyxia. 3) Infants with cardiac anomalies including symptomatic PDA. 4) Infants with any renal impairment/anomaly identified on ultrasound e.g. reflux. 5) Hydropic/edematous infants. 6) Muscle relaxed infants. 7) Infants with renal failure. 8) Babies receiving the following medications: Diuretics, Indomethacin, Inotropes, Steroids.

THE ABC OF ABG ANALYSIS

1. **Normal values of arterial blood gas**

   pH-7.35-7.45, HCO_3^- - 22-26mEq/L, PCO_2 - 35-45mm Hg.

   HCO_3^- - in plasma = actual bicarbonate if < 22 = metabolic acidosis and if > 26 metabolic alkalosis. If PCO_2 is < 30 = respiratory alkalosis and PCO_2 > 50 = respiratory acidosis

   At a pH of 7.40, the Hydrogen ion concentration is 40 nmol/L. There is an inverse relationship between the pH and the hydrogen ion concentration i.e., when the hydrogen ion concentration decreases, the pH increases, and when the hydrogen ion concentration increases, the pH decreases.

2. **Appropriate compensation during simple acid-base disorders :** *If a patient does not have the appropriate compensation, then a mixed acid-base disorder is present. The identity of the second disorder is determined by deciding whether the compensation is too little or too much compared with what was expected.*

   Appropriate compensation during simple acid-base disorders

Disorders	Expected compensation
Metabolic acidosis	$PCo_2 = 1.5 \times [HCO_3^-] + 8 \pm 2$
Metabolic alkalosis	PCO_2 increases by 7 mm Hg for each 10 mEq/L increase in serum $[HCO_3^-]$
Respiratory acidosis	
Acute	$[HCO_3^-]$ increases by 1 for each 10-mm Hg increase in Pco_2
Chronic	$[HCO_3^-]$ increases by 3.5 for each 10-mm Hg increase in Pco_2
Respiratory alkalosis	
Acute	$[HCO_3^-]$ falls by 2 for each 10-mm Hg decrease in Pco_2
Chronic	$[HCO_3^-]$ falls by 4 for each 10-mm Hg decrease in Pco_2

3. **Acidemia is a pH below normal (<7.35) and Alkalemia is a pH above normal (> 7.45).** An acidosis is a pathologic process that causes an increase in the hydrogen ion concentration, and an alkalosis is a pathologic process that causes a decrease in the hydrogen ion concentration. Whereas acidemia is always accompanied by an acidosis, a patient can have an acidosis and a low, normal, or high pH. For example, a patient may have a mild metabolic acidosis, but a simultaneous, severe respiratory alkalosis; the net result may be alkalemia. *Acidemia and Alkalemia indicate the pH abnormality; acidosis and alkalosis indicate the pathologic process that is taking place.*

4. The respiratory compensation for a metabolic process happens quickly and is complete within 12-24 hr; it cannot over compensate or normalize the pH. Unlike respiratory compensation which occurs rapidly, the metabolic compensation (by kidneys) takes 3-4 days.

5. The clinical history is always useful in evaluating and diagnosing patients with acid-base disturbances. The expected metabolic compensation for a respiratory process changes based on whether the process is acute or chronic which can be deduced only by the history (the metabolic compensation for a patient with an acute respiratory acidosis is < that for a chronic respiratory acidosis). In a patient with a respiratory acidosis, a small increase in the HCO_3^- concentration would be consistent with a simple acute respiratory acidosis or a mixed disorder (a chronic respiratory acidosis and a metabolic acidosis). Only the history can differentiate among the possibilities. Knowledge of the length of the respiratory process and the presence or absence of a risk factor for a metabolic acidosis (diarrhea) allows the correct conclusion should be reached.

6. Most patients with an acid-base disturbance have an abnormal pH, although there are 2 exceptions. The 1st exception is in the patient with a mixed disorder, wherein the 2 processes have opposite effects on pH (a metabolic acidosis and a respiratory alkalosis) and cause changes in the hydrogen ion concentration that are comparable in magnitude, albeit opposite. The 2nd exception is in the patient with a simple chronic respiratory alkalosis; in some instances, the appropriate metabolic compensation is enough to normalize the pH. In both of these situations, the presence of an acid-base disturbance is deduced because of the abnormal carbon dioxide and/or bicarbonate levels.

7. In most cases, there is only one obvious explanation for the abnormal pH. In some mixed disorders, however, there may be two possibilities (a high PCO_2 and a low HCO_3^- in a patient with acidemia). In such cases, the patient has two causes of the abnormal pH (a metabolic acidosis and a respiratory acidosis, in this instance), and it is unnecessary to determine whether the patient's compensation is appropriate.

8. Because the appropriate respiratory compensation for a metabolic acidosis *never normalizes* the patient's pH, the presence of a normal pH and a low bicarbonate concentration occurs only if some degree of respiratory alkalosis is present. A chronic respiratory alkalosis is the only acid-base disturbance wherein appropriate compensation may normalize the pH, albeit > 7.40.

9. A metabolic alkalosis, by decreasing ventilation, causes appropriate respiratory compensation. PCO_2 increases by 7mmHg for each 10-mEq/L increase in serum bicarbonate concentration. Appropriate respiratory compensation never exceeds a PCO_2 of 55-60mm Hg. The patient have a concurrent respiratory alkalosis if the PCO_2 is lower than the expected compensation. A greater than expected PCO_2 occurs with a concurrent respiratory acidosis.

10. **Useful concepts in evaluating the acid-base disorders**

    a. Metabolic acidosis 1)with normal anion gap 2)with increased anion gap

    b. Metabolic alkalosis 1)chloride responsive (urinary chloride <15mEq/L) 2)chloride resistant (urinary chloride > 20mEq/L)

    c. Respiratory acidosis 1)CNS depression 2)neuromuscular diseases 3)respiratory muscle weakness 4)pulmonary disease 5) upper airway disease 6) miscellaneous

    d. Respiratory alkalosis 1)hypoxemia/tissue hypoxia 2)lung receptor stimulation 3) central stimulation 4) mechanical ventilation and ECMO.

Stepwise approach to interpreting the arterial blood gas.

1. **H&P.** The most clinical useful information comes from the clinical description of the patient by the history and physical examination. The H&P usually gives an idea of what acid base disorder might be present even before collecting the ABG sample.

2. **Look at the pH.** Is there an acid base disorder present? - If pH < 7.35, then acidemia- if pH > 7.45, then alkalemia - If pH within normal range, then acid base disorder not likely present. - pH may be normal in the presence of a mixed acid base disorder, particularly if other parameters of the ABG are abnormal.

3. **Look at PCO2, HCO3-.** What is the acid base process (alkalosis vs acidosis) leading to the abnormal pH? Are both values normal or abnormal? - In simple acid base disorders, both values are abnormal and direction of the abnormal change is the same for both parameters. - One abnormal value will be the initial change and the other will be the compensatory response. **3a. Distinguish the initial change from the compensatory response.** - The initial change will be the abnormal value that correlates with the abnormal pH. - If Alkalosis, then PCO_2 low or HCO_3- high - If Acidosis, then PCO2 high or HCO3- low. Once the initial change is identified, then the other abnormal parameter is the compensatory response if the direction of the change is the same. If not, suspect a mixed disorder. **3b.** Once the initial chemical change and the compensatory response is distinguished, then **identify the specific disorder.** See table below. - If PCO_2 is the initial chemical change, then process is respiratory. if HCO_3- is the initial chemical change, then process is metabolic.

Acid Base disorder	Initial chemical change	Compensatory response
Respiratory Acidosis	↑ PCO_2	↑HCO_3-
Respiratory Alkalosis	↓ PCO_2	↓ HCO_3-
Metabolic Acidosis	↓ HCO_3-	↓ PCO_2
Metabolic Alkalosis	↑ HCO_3-	↑PCO_2

4. **If respiratory process, is it acute or chronic?**

- An acute respiratory process will produce a compensatory response that is due primarily to rapid intracellular buffering.

- A chronic respiratory process will produce a more significant compensatory response that is due primarily to renal adaptation, which takes a longer time to develop.

- To assess if acute or chronic, determine the **extent** of compensation.

5. If metabolic acidosis, then look at the Anion Gap.

- If elevated (> than 16), then acidosis due to KULT. (Ketoacidosis, Uremia, Lactic acidosis, Toxins).

- If anion gap is normal, then acidosis likely due to diarrhea, RTA.

6. If metabolic process, is degree of **compensation adequate**?

- Calculate the estimated PCO2, this will help to determine if a separate respiratory disorder is present.

7. If anion gap is elevated, then calculate the Delta-Ratio ("/") to assess for other simultaneous disorders.

- "/" compares the change in the anion gap to the change in bicarbonate.

- If ratio between 1 and 2, then pure elevated anion gap acidosis

- If < 1, then there is a simultaneous normal anion gap acidosis present.

- If > 2, then there is a simultaneous metabolic alkalosis present or a compensated chronic respiratory acidosis.

8. If normal anion gap and cause is unknown, then calculate the Urine Anion Gap (UAG). This will help to differentiate RTAs from other causes of non elevated anion gap acidosis.

- In RTA, UAG is positive.

- In diarrhea and other causes of metabolic acidosis, the UAG is negative. (neGUTive in diarrhea)

Normal values for blood gases during the first week for healthy term infants

Age (hours)	1–4	12–24	24	48–168
PaO_2 (mmHg)	50–75	60–80	65–85	70–85
$PaCO_2$ (mmHg)	30–45	30–40	30–40	30–38
Arterial pH	7.30–7.34	7.30–7.35	7.35–7.30	7.35–7.40

Metabolic and respiratory conditions with the characteristic Features evident on blood gas analysis

Metabolic failure	Metabolic acidosis (UC)	Metabolic acidosis (C)	Metabolic alkalosis (UC)	Metabolic alkalosis (C)
pH	↓	N	↑	N
PCO_2	N	↓	N	↑
HCO_3	↓	↓	↑	↑
BE	↓	↓	↑	↑

Respiratory failure	Respiratory acidosis (UC)	Respiratory acidosis (C)	Respiratory alkalosis (UC)	Respiratory alkalosis (C)
pH	↓	N	↑	N
pCO_2	↑	↑	↓	↓
HCO_3	N	↑	N	↓
BE	N	↑	N	↓

UC = uncompensated; C = compensated

ESSENTIAL NEONATAL DRUG FORMULARY

Selective groups of neonatal drugs listed elsewhere in the book

Guidelines for therapeutic drug monitoring

A. Antibacterial agents

Drug	Optimal sample time	Optimal serum concentration range	Time to steady state after dose change
Amikacin	Peak : 30 min after 30 min infusion Trough	25–30 mg/L 3–5 mg/L	24–48 h
Gentamicin	Peak : 30 min after 30 min infusion Trough	6–10 mg/L 0.5–2 mg/L	24–48 h
Tobramycin	peak : same as gentamicin Trough	6–10 mg/L 0.5–2 mg/L	24–48 h
Vancomycin	Peak : 1 h after 1 h infusion Trough	25– 35 mg/L 5–10 mg/L	24–72 h

Trough serum drug concentration: Sample taken within 30 min prior to the next dose. Serum measurements are routinely obtained at a steady state, which is usually around the THIRD DOSE after start or change of dosage and then once weekly. Earlier measurements may be necessary in very sick infants with fluctuating renal conditions. Not necessary to draw serum levels of drugs unless patient will be maintained on therapy > 3 days.

B. Other drugs

Drug	Optimal sample time	Optimal serum concentration range	Time to steady state after dose change
Digoxin	Trough	1.3–2.7 nmol/L	4–7 d with total digitalization and 1–2 wk without digitalization
Flucytosine	Peak (30 min after 30 min infusion)	50–100 mg/L	
Phenobarbital	Trough	65–170 mmol/L	14 d
Phenytoin	Trough	40–80 mmol/L	4 d after IV doses (rapid increase in elimination rate over the first weeks of life necessitates frequent monitoring of drug levels)
Theophyline	Trough	For apnea 55-70mmol/L For bronchodilation (for infants > 6 wk postnatal age :	3-4 d
	Peak	80-110 mmol/L	
	Trough	55 mmol/L	

Trough serum drug concentration : sample taken within 30 min . prior to the next dose. Peak serum drug concentration : sample taken 1 h postdose.

General medications			
Drug	**Dosage/Administration**	**Indications**	**Contraindications and Cautions and Comments**
Adrenaline 1:10,000	IV/IO - 0.1–0.3ml/kg/dose IT-1ml/kg/dose **Initial Kg Dosing:** 1kg=0.2ml,2kg=0.4ml, 3kg=0.6ml,4kg=0.8ml	*Asystole *Bradycardia *Hypotension(acute)	*1:10,000 (dilute 0.5ml of 1:1000 with 4.5ml of NS). *In patients with pulmonary disease or prolonged asystole, pulmonary edema and intrapulmonary shunting IT route is poorly effective. *Decreases renal and splanchnic blood flow.
Sodium bicarbonate 4.25% sol	IV 2–4ml (1–2mEq) /kg over 2 minutes or more **Initial Kg Dosing:** 1kg=2 ml, 2kg=4 ml 3 kg=6 ml, 4 kg=8 ml	*Documented (ABG) metabolic Acidosis with adequate ventilation *Hyperkalemia	*4.25% sol. (dilute 1ml of 7.5% +1ml of 10% Dextrose) * Subsequent doses (in mEq) = 0.3 × body weight (kg) × base deficit.*Rapid correction can lead to 1)IVH 2) Hyperosmolality 3) MET. Alkalosis 4)Hypernatremia 5)Hypokalemia * Use with close monitoring of arterial blood pH.
Dextrose 10% sol. 1ml=100mg	IV-(2.5-5ml/kg/dose)	*Hypoglycemia *Hyperkalemia (used with Insulin)	*Bolus dose should be followed by a reliable IV infusion at a rate of 100ml/kg/day 10% DEXTROSE * Glucostix are not reliable in neonates when reading < 40–50mgs/dL * Whole blood glucose is 10–15% lower than in the plasma.
Calcium gluconate 10% sol. 1ml=100 mg 5 ml=1m mol	IV-0.5–1.25ml/kg i.e. 50-125mgs/kg dose **Initial Kg Dosing:** 1kg=1ml,2kg=2ml, 3kg=3ml,4kg=4ml	*Hypocalcemia *Hyperkalemia	* Infuse slowly ; use caution with digitalized patient; Beware of tissue necrosis if extravasation happens; can also use CaCl2 20–30 mgs/kg (0.2-0.3ml/kg of 10% solution; 6.8 mmol of Ca++2 in 10ml).
Naloxone 1ml=400 mcg	IV/IM/ET-100 mcg/kg **Initial Kg Dosing:** 1kg=0.25ml,2kg=0.5ml, 3kg=0.75ml,4kg=1ml	*Narcotic reversal within 4-6 hours of the last dose of intrapartal opiate administration	* Not a drug of resuscitation; opiate antagonist only. * A dose of 10mcg/kg also reverse the sedation but the effect only last a short time (20 minutes IV or a few hours IM) * **C/I-** *Never give Naloxone to an infant with suspected/proven Neonatal drug withdrawal syndrome born to a mother with substance abuse.*
Fresh frozen plasma	IV: 10 ml/kg over 30 minutes	shock,volume expander	*Make sure hematocrit is within normal limits, if subsequent doses are to be used *Use NS/O Negative blood, if Plasma is not available
Atropine sulfate	IV: 10–30 mcg/kg/dose, every 10–15 minutes, for 2–3 doses as needed ETtube: same dosage	vagal induced bradycardia, rapid sequence intubation	*Ensure effective oxygenation and ventilation before attempting to treat bradycardia *C/I- tachycardia, thyrotoxicosis, GIT/GUT obstruction, narrow-angle glaucoma *Monitor heart rate and for adverse reactions- abdominal distention/ileus, urinary retention, arrhythmias, GERD, mydriasis, cycloplegia, tachycardia. *Antidote : Physostigmine.
Alprostadil Prostin E$_1$	IVI: *Start* with 0.01 *micrograms/kg/min*(0.6ml/kg/hr.) *Dilute* 500 micrograms(0.5mg) in 500 ml of 5-10% dextrose, i.e., 1 microgram/ml of reconstituted solution). *Double* the dose in 15-20 minutes(1.2ml/kg/hr=0.02mcg/kg/min. if SaO2 is unchanged.) *Titrate* to effective dosage with therapeutic response! 0.01 *micrograms/kg/min*(0.6ml/kg/hr) 0.02 *micrograms/kg/min*(1.2ml/kg/hr) 0.03 *micrograms/kg/min*(1.8ml/kg/hr) 0.04 *micrograms/kg/min*(2.4ml/kg/hr) 0.05 *micrograms/kg/min*(3.0ml/kg/hr) *For e.g.,* a 3kg baby requires an IVI of 1.8ml/hr of Prostin E$_1$(diluted solution 1ml=1mcg) to start with, i.e.,0.01 *micrograms/kg/min*(0.6ml/kg/hr) ; the usual dose will be 9ml/hr i.e., 0.05*micrograms/kg/min*(3.0ml/kg/hr).	To maintain the ductal patency until some palliative surgery is done as soon as possible; in Neonates with ductal-dependent CHD.	*Use cautiously in neonates with bleeding tendencies *Reduce infusion until symptoms subside, if hypotension or pyrexia occurs. * Be prepared to intubate and resuscitate, as apnea can occur in about 10% of Neonates (especially, with Birth weights<2kg, usually within the 1st hr of drug infusion)) with CHD. If severe hypotension, apnea, or bradycardia require drug discontinuation, Reinstitute at a lower dose cautiously. *Prefer a central venous access for the continuous IV Infusion. *Contraindications- RDS, PPHN, Coagulation abnormalities. *Adverse reactions- Apnea,Respiratory depression, Flushing, Fever, Bradycardia, Seizure-like activity, Systemic hypotension, Hypocalcemia, Hypoglycemia, Diarrhea, Inhibition of platelet aggregation,

Drug	Dosage/Administration	Indications	Contraindications and Cautions and Comments
Acetaminophen	PO/PR Term:10–15 mg/kg per dose q6hr PRN; Preterm:10–15/kg/dose q12hr in 32wks GA, q8hr in >32wks GA	Analgesic & Antipyretic	*C/I:* G6PD deficiency, *Adverse reactions*-(associated with excessive dosages): Thrombocytopenia, leukopenia, pancytopenia, neutropenia. *Monitor* FBC and LFTs.
Acyclovir	IV 20 mg/kg/dose q8hr for 14 days in localized HSV infection and for 21 days in disseminated/CNS infections PO 20mg/kg/dose q6hr for 5 days	Herpes Simplex HSV, and Varicella Zoster Chickenpox	Infuse by syringe pump>1hr; Never refrigerate or keep it more than 12 hours after reconstitution ; 10mg/kg/dose q12hr in babies<34 wks GA; Extravasation may cause skin ulceration; Reduce dosage in renal failure; Monitor renal and hepatic function.
Adenosine	IV 50mcg/kg initially; increase by increments of 50 mcg/kg at 2 minute intervals until sinus rhythm restored; Maximum single dose= 300mcg/kg	Drug of first recourse in Neonatal supraventricular tachycardia ?Value in PPHN.	*Discard the ampoule once it has been opened; do not refrigerate *Must be given by rapid i.v. push as quickly as possible (half-life < 10 s); administer at i.v. site closer to infant's heart; follow dose with normal saline flush; monitor ECG, heart rate, and blood pressure. * Contraindicated in second or third degree AV block or sick - sinus syndrome unless pacemaker placed. • Adverse effects (transient): dyspnea, flushing, irritability, dysrhythmias, nausea; minimal hemodynamic effect .*Theophylline antagonizes effects • Do not refrigerate; precipitation may occur
Albumin	IV 0.5-1 gram/kg/dose; give 5% solution over 1hr; may be infused more rapidly (10-20 minutes) in hypovolemic shock, repeat PRN. In hypoproteinemia give the same dose over >2hrs; repeat q1-2day.	Plasma volume expander in Hypovolemia and in Hypoproteinemia.	*25% Albumin is C/I in preterm infants due to increased risk of IVH. *It has no clinical advantage to using as plasma expander compared to using NS. *Monitor for signs of hypervolemia, pulmonary edema, and CHF. *Adverse reactions -chills, fever, and urticaria.
Amino phylline	PO/IV: 5–6mg/kg loading dose; 2mg/kg/dose q6– 8hr maintenance dose.	Apnea of Prematurity	*Give IV loading dose >20 minutes and maintenance doses over >5 minutes *on a syringe pump.* *Increase dose by 20% when changing from IV to PO route. *Therapeutic drug level 7-10 mcg/ml *Monitor serum trough levels before the fifth dose and consider checking earlier if toxicity (GIT upset, arrhythmias, seizures, tachycardia >180 bpm,) is suspected or apneic spells increase in number or severity. *If the blood level is low, give a partial bolus of 1mg/kg for each desired 2mcg/ml in serum theophylline concentration.
Amphotericin-B-Liposome	IV: 2.5-5mg/kg q24hr to be infused >2hrs, for an average duration of 14-21 days.	Systemic Antifungal agent	*Do not dilute with NS or mix with any other medication that is diluted in NS *Adverse reactions- hypokalemia, nephrotoxicity, LFT abnormalities, thrombocytopenia, tachycardia *Monitor for renal function, electrolyte abnormalities, toxicity due to neuromuscular blockade.
Atracurium besylate	0.3-0.4 mg/kg as needed	Neuromuscular blocker for muscle paralysis	*Make sure airway and respiratory support are secure before use. * Does not have sedative or analgesic properties, so adjunctive sedative/analgesic should be used.

Drug	Dosage/Administration	Indications	Contraindications and Cautions and Comments
Caffeine citrate	IV loading; 10 mg/kg Infuse over 30 minutes IV/Oral; 5–10 mg/kg/day, starting 24 hrs after loading dose.	Apnea of prematurity, diagnosed by exclusion	* Do not push IV doses of Caffeine citrate *Adverse reactions include cardiac arrhythmias, tachycardia, insomnia, restlessness, nausea, vomiting, diarrhea, irritability *Consider a decrease in dose to treat the CNS or GIT side effects *Monitor heart rate, number and severity of apnea spells.
Captopril	Oral; 0.01–0.05 mg/kg/dose q8-12hr for preterm, 0.05–0.1mg/kg/dose q8-24hr for term	Antihypertensive, CHF Treatment	* Maximum recommended dose: 0.5 mg/kg/dose PO q8-12hr *Titrate dose and frequency to effect. * Administer on an empty stomach 1 hr before or 2 hours after feedings if possible *Food decreases absorption by ~ 50%. Administration times need to be consistent.
Chloral hydrate	PO/PR; 25–50 mg/kg/dose q6-8hr prn	Sedative hypnotic	* C/I in hepatic and renal impairment * Adverse reactions - cardiopulmonary depression when administered with opiates or phenobarbital, paradoxical excitation, cardiac arrhythmias, leucopenia, eosinophilia, GI Intolerance *Accumulation of the toxic metabolite (trichloroethanol) and direct hyperbilirubinemia occur with repeated doses.
Chloro-thiazide	PO; 20–40 mg/kg/day, divided every 12 hours IV; 2–8 mg/kg/day, divided every 12 hours	Fluid overload, BPD, CHF, Hypertension, Pulmonary edema	*C/I-Anuria, Hepatic dysfunction *Monitor serum electrolytes, Calcium, Blood Glucose, Urine output, BP, Daily weight *Adverse reactions-Volume depletion, Prerenal azotemia, Hypochloremic alkalosis, Hypokalemia, Hypomagnesemia, Increased levels of glucose, uric acid, lipids, bilirubin, and calcium, blood dyscrasias.
Dexamethasone	IV; 0.25-0.5 mg/kg once; may repeat q8-12hr for total of 4 doses	*Extubation/ Airway edema *BPD-Refer to the Chapter on BPD & CLD	*Monitor BP, Blood glucose, Serum potassium, Weight, Length, Occult blood loss, Hb, IOP with >6 weeks of systemic use.* Precautions- hyperglycemia, glycosuria, hypertension, pituitary-adrenal axis suppression, hypokalemia, alkalosis, peptic ulcer, immunosuppression *Avoid its use in BPD, because of higher risk of cerebral palsy and neurodevelopmental abnormalities evident in Cochrane studies, except under exceptional circumstances like maximal ventilatory support or high risk of mortality after taking informed consent from both the parents.
Digoxin	Total Digitalizing dose(TDD) PO;20-30mcg/kg in <37wks and 25-35mcg/kg in >37wks IV; 15–25 mcg/kg in <37wks and 20–30 mcg/kg in >37wks	*CHF *SVT *AF	*Maintenance dose PO;5–7.5 mcg/kg/day in 2 divided doses in <37wks and 6-10 mcg/kg/day in 2 divided doses in >37 wks, IV;4-6mcg/kg/d in <37 wks and 5-8 mcg/kg/d in >37 wks * Administer Total Digitalizing Dose over 24 hours in 3 divided doses: 1st dose is 50% of the TDD, 2nd dose is 25% of the TDD administered 8 hours after the 1st dose, and the 3rd dose is the remaining 25% of the TDD administered 8 hours after the 2nd dose*Start the Maintenance dose 12 hours after completing the TDD. *Administer the IV doses over >10 minutes on syringe pump *Utilize maintenance dose schedule for nonacute arrhythmia and CHF conditions *Therapeutic drug level-0.8-2ng/ml *C/I- AV Block, IHSS, Constrictive pericarditis, Ventricular dysrhythmias *Monitor heart rate/rhythm for desired effects and signs of toxicity, serum calcium and magnesium, potassium *Treat life-threatening toxicity with Digoxin immune Fab.
Ergocalciferol	10–20 mcg/24 hr for prematures	*Treatment of refractory rickets, hypoparathyroidism hypophosphatemia	*Adverse events: Hypercalcemia, hypertension, arrhythmias, hypercholesterolemia, nephrocalcinosis, photophobia * Monitor serum calcium & Phosphorus, alkaline phosphatase, bone radiography

Drug	Dosage/Administration	Indications	Contraindications and Cautions and Comments
Famotidine	IV : 0.5mg/kg/dose, q24h PO: 0.5mg/kg/dose, q24h	*GERD *Stress ulcer *Control of gastric pH in critically ill babies.	*Administer IV dose over > 10minutes on syringe pump *Modify the dose in patients with renal impairment *Monitor gastric pH, BUN, Creatinine, Urine output, Bilirubin, LFTs, & FBC.*Adverse reactions-dry mouth, constipation, thrombocytopenia, agranulocytosis, neutropenia & elevated LFTs.*Higher risk of NEC in VLBW babies, due to H-2 Blockade & reduced bowel movements.
Fentanyl citrate	IV : 1-5 microgram/kg/dose every 2-4 hours over 10 minutes	*Analgesia * Sedation *Anesthesia	*C/I - Increased ICP, severe respiratory depression, severe liver & renal insufficiency *Monitor respiration, heart rate, BP, Muscle rigidity
Fluconazole	Thrush-6mg/kg on day 1, then 3mg/kg/dose q24h PO. Prophylaxis - 3mg/kg/dose OD 3times weekly for first 2 weeks, then every other day for total of 4-6 weeks. Systemic infections/meningitis - IV 12 mg/kg loading dose, then 6 mg/kg/dose over 60 minutes.	*Systemic fungal infections, meningitis *Severe superficial mycoses *Prophylaxis against invasive fungal infections in VLBW infants.	*Dosing interval : 29 week GA - q72hr for 0-14 days, q48hr > 14 days. 30-36 week GA - q48hr for 0-14 days, q24hr > 14 days. > 37-44 week GA - q48hr for 0-7 days, q24hr > 7 days. *Monitor renal & LFTs *Adverse reactions - vomiting, diarrhea, reversible increased liver transaminases, alkaline phosphatase *Drug interactions - warfarin, phenytoin, rifampin, possible interference with metabolism of caffeine & theophylline.
Folic acid	PO/IV : 15 microgram/kg/dose (maximum of 50 microgram/day)	*Megaloblastic & macrocytic anemia as a result of folate deficiency	* C/I - pernicious, aplastic, & normocytic anemias * Monitor hematocrit, reticulocyte, hemoglobin, * Drug interaction - may decrease phenytoin serum levels * Causes GI upset, slight flushing but well tolerated
Furosemide	IV : 1 mg/kg/dose PO : 2 mg/kg/dose	*Pulmonary edema * To provide diuresis	*Monitor daily weight changes, urine output, serum phosphate, electrolytes. Closely monitor potassium levels in neonates receiving digoxin *Use with caution in hepatic & renal disease *Adverse reactions - hypokalemia, hypocalcemia/hypercalciuria, nephrocalcinosis, potential ototoxicity (with aminoglycosides), hyperuricemia, agranulocytosis, thrombocytopenia.
Glucagon	IV/IM/SC : 0.3mg/kg/dose (Max : 1mg)	*Treatment of hypoglycemia	* Adverse events - Nausea, vomiting, hypersensitivity reactions.
Heparin (unfractionated)	IVI : 0.5 - 1unit/mL for catheter patency Thrombosis & ECMO : Load 50 units/kg IV bolus, & 15 - 35 units/kg/hr as IVI maintenance dose	* Prophylaxis & treatment of thromboembolism (potentiates actions of antithrombin III)	* Adverse events - Bleeding from various sites like urine, gums, nose ; bruising, thrombocytopenia, thrombosis. * Monitor APTT (therapeutic, 1.5 - 2.5 times baseline ; toxic > 2.5 times baseline) ; Plasma heparin concentration (antifactor X assay : therapeutic 0.3 -0.7 units/mL) * Avoid if severe thrombocytopenia, intracranial bleeding, bacterial endocarditis.
Hyaluronidase	SC/ID : 150 units in 1 mL ; Inject 0.2 mL to each of 5 sites at the leading edge of the extravasation	* Treatment of extravasation	* Adverse events - Tachycardia, hypotension, erythema.
Hydralazine	IV : 0.1 - 0.5 mg/kg/dose q6 - 8 hr PO : 0.25 - 1 mg/kg/dose q6-8hr	* Antihypertensive * Adjunctive treatment of CHF with nitrates	* Adverse events - flushing, tachycardia, headache, nausea, vomiting, diarrhea, peripheral neuropathy (related to pyridoxine deficiency)
Hydro chlorothiazide	PO : 2-4 mg/kg/24hr in 2 divided doses	* Antihypertensive * Fluid overload states - CHF, BPD/CLD *Prevention of recurrent renal calcium stones	* Adverse events - Hypokalemia, hypochloremia, hypo-magnesemia, hyperglycemia, hyperuricemia, hyper-lipidemia, pancreatitis, leukopenia, thrombocytopenia, aplastic anemia, hepatitis, cholestasis, prerenal azotemia.

Drug	Dosage/Administration	Indications	Contraindications and Cautions and Comments
Hydro cortisone	Adrenal insufficiency : 1–2 mg/kg IV bolus, then 25–150 mg/24 hr divided q6h. Congenital adrenal hyperplasia : IV 0.5-0.7 mg/kg/24 hr start, then 0.3–0.4 mg/kg/24 hr maintenance therapy ; give doses as $^1/_4$ in AM, $^1/_4$ at noon, and $^1/_2$ at night. Shock : IV : 35-50 mg/kg, then 50-150 mg/kg/24 hr divided q6h for 48-72 hr	*Treatment of adrenal insufficiency *Congenital adrenal hyperplasia *Shock *Corticosteroid-responsive dermatoses	*Adverse events—Hypertension, hyperglycemia, hypokalemia, insomnia, headache, Cushing syndrome, pertic ulcer, cataracts, immunosuppression, skin and muscle atrophy, acne, edema. *Caution : Abrupt withdrawal may cause acute adrenal insufficiency.*
Ibuprofen	IV/PO : First dose 10 mg/kg Second dose 5mg/kg Third dose 5mg/kg To be given at 24 hourly intervals	*Closure of PDA	*If the ductus arteriosus does not close 48 hours after the last injection or if it re-opens, a second course of three doses, may be given *Adverse events—GIT bleeding and perforation, fluid retention, edema, hypertension, tachycardia, acute renal failure, thrombocytopenia.
Immune globulin (IVIG)	IV 500-750 mg/kg once	*Acute bacterial/viral infections in sepsis complicated by MODS, neutropenia	* Adverse events—Flushing, tachycardia, chills, fever, dyspnea, aseptic meningitis, hypersensitivity reactions
Indomethacin	IV : 0.1-0.25 mg/kg/dose q12hr for 3-6 doses	*Closure of PDA	* Adverse events—GIT bleeding & perforation, fluid retention, edema, hypertension, tachycardia, acute renal failure, thrombocytopenia, hyperkalemia, bone marrow suppression. * *Caution : avoid in premature neonates with NEC, poor renal function, or active bleeding.* * Monitor indomethacin concentration : therapeutic 1-3 microgram/mL
Insulin regular	SC 0.1 - 0.2 units/kg/dose q6-12 hr, or continuous IVI 0.01-0.1 units/kg/hr	*Treatment of Insulin-dependent diabetes mellitus	* Adverse events—Hypoglycemia, hypokalemia * Monitor blood glucose & adjust insulin dosing
Ipratropium	Nebulized 100 microgram/dose or MDI 1-2 puffs TID - QID	* Bronchodilator	* Adverse events—Dry mouth, urinary retention
Isoproterenol	IVI 0.05-2 microgram/kg/min.	*Ventricular arrhythmias due to AV nodal block, low-output shock states	* Adverse events—Tachycardia, restlessness, tremor, GIT distress, paradoxical bronchospasm
Levothyroxine	PO : 0-6 mo: 8–10 µg/kg/24 hr. 6-12 mo:6–8 µg/kg/24 hr. 1-5 yr: 5–6 µg/kg/24 hr. 6-12 yr: 4–5 µg/kg/24 hr. > 12 yr: 2–3 µg/kg/24 hr.	* Thyroid replacement therapy	* Adverse events—Tachycardia, Cardiac arrhythmias, hypertension, nervousness, headache, insomnia, hair loss, increased appetite, weight loss, tremor, sweating.
Lorazepam	IV : 0.1–0.4 mg/kg/dose q4–6 hr as needed. Status epilepticus : IV 0.05–0.2 mg/kg/dose over 2–5 min.; may repeat in 10–15 min.	* Treatment of anxiety, sedation and seizures	* Adverse events—Myoclonus, tachycardia, drowsiness, depression
Magnesium Sulfate 50% Solution	IV : 25–50mg/kg/dose q8hr for 2–3 doses	*Hypomagnesemia and seizures due to associated hypocalcemia	* Adverse events—Magnesium may accumulate to toxic levels in renal insufficiency

Drug	Dosage/Administration	Indications	Contraindications and Cautions and Comments
Methylene blue	IV : 1-2 mg/kg ; may repeat after one hour if needed	* Methemo-globinemia	* Adverse events—Anemia, urine & feces turn blue-green * *Caution ; avoid in glucose - 6 - phosphate dehydrogenase deficiency & renal insufficiency*
Midazolam	IV bolus 0.05-0.15 mg/kg q2-4hr IVI continuous 0.15-0.5 mg/kg/min for sedation	* Sedation, anticonvulsant	* Adverse events—Myoclonus, apnea, respiratory depression
Morphine	IV/IM/SC - 0.05 -0.2mg/kg/dose q2-4hr ; continuous infusion 0.025-0.05 mg/kg/hr	* Analgesia (moderate to severe pain)	* Adverse events—Hypotension, bradycardia, constipation, sedation, respiratory depression, decreased urination
Naloxone	IV 0.1mg/kg/dose (max. dose 2mg). Repeat q 2-3 min until desired effect, if no response to the initial dose.	* Opiate antagonist	* Caution: Useful in the treatment of respiratory depression due to opiate excess to the mother, given within 4hours before delivery of the baby ; should not be given if the mother is opiate dependent, as naloxone may precipitate acute drug withdrawal symptoms in the baby
Neostigmine	IV/IM/SC : 10–40 μg/kg q2–4hr ; titrate dose to desired effect. To reverse nondepolarizing neuromuscular blocking agents 25–100μg/kg/dose	* Treatment of Myasthenia gravis	* Adverse events —Bradycardia, urinary frequency
Phenobarbital	IV 15-20mg/kg loading dose to be followed by 3-4mg/kg/day in two divided doses as maintenance dose	* Anticonvulsant	* Adverse events—Hypotension, drowsiness, respiratory depression, paradoxical hyperactivity *Monitor blood level : 15-40μg/mL
Phenytoin	IV 15-20mg/kg loading dose ; do not exceed 0.5mg/kg/min 5mg/kg/day PO/IV q12-24hr	* Anticonvulsant	* Adverse events—Hypotension, hepatitis, Stevens-Johnson syndrome, lethargy * Monitor blood level : 8-20μg/mL
Propranolol	PO 2mg/kg/day q6-8hr ; titrate to response	* Thyrotoxicosis	* Adverse events—Hypotension, Bradycardia, hypoglycemia, bronchospasm
Propylthiou-racil	PO 5-10mg/kg/day q8hr ; titrate to response	* Thyrotoxicosis	*Adverse events—Rash, hepatitis, interstitial pneumonitis, blood dyscrasias
Pyridostigmine	IV or IM 50–150mg/kg/dose PO 7mg/kg/day in 5-6 divided doses	* Myasthenia gravis	* Adverse events—Bradycardia, AV block, salivation, miosis, muscle weakness, lacrimation, diarrhea, seizures, urinary frequency, bronchorrhea
Pyridoxine	IV 1.5–2mg/kg/day q12hr	* Pyridoxine-dependent seizures	* Adverse events—Decreased folic acid Caution : It may decrease serum phenobarbital & phenytoin concentrations
Ranitidine	PO 1-3mg/kg/day divided q12–24hr	* Stress ulcer prophylaxis *GERD	* Adverse events—It may decrease gut motility & contribute to NEC
Spironolactone	PO 1–3mg/kg/day divided q12–24hr	* Potassium sparing diuretic * Antihyper tensive	* Adverse events—Lethargy, hyperkalemia, rash, gynecomastia

Drug	Dosage/Administration	Indications	Contraindications and Cautions and Comments
Streptokinase	IVI over 30 min 3500–4000 units followed by 1000–1500 units IV continuous infusion for thrombosis. **Clotted catheter;** 10,000-25,000 units in NS to be instilled into catheter for ~ 1hr then removed (aspirated)	* Thrombolytic agent for stroke and catheter patency	* Adverse events—Bleeding, flushing, rash, bronchospasm
Theophylline	PO 6-10 mg/kg loading dose 2-4 mg/kg/dose q12hr maintenance dose	* Apnea	* Adverse events—Tachycardia, vomiting, feeding intolerance, seizures & arrhythmias at toxic levels, hyperactivity, agitation & irritability *Monitor blood level - 6-15 mg/mL (Therapeutic)
Tro-methamine THAM	IV : 1-2 mEq/kg/dose or weight in kg X base deficit	* Correction of metabolic acidosis	* Adverse events : Apnea, Hypoglycemia, Hyperkalemia, Tissue irritation, or necrosis if direct contact * 1mEq THAM = 3.3 ml (0.3M solution)
Urokinase	IV Load 4,400 units/kg, maintenance dose 4,000 - 10,000 units/kg/hr	* Thrombolytic agent	* Adverse events—Bleeding, hematoma, allergic reactions, bronchospasm * Monitor D - Dimer, fibrin degradation products, APTT
Ursodeoxy-cholic acid	PO 10-18mg/kg/day in 1-3 divided doses/day	* Reversal of TPN - induced cholestasis	* Adverse events—Diarrhea, Pruritus, Rhinitis
Vitamin A	IM 4,000 IU 3times/week, or 2,000 IU IM every other day	* Prevention of BPD	* Adverse events—Irritability, hypercalcemia, fever, lethargy
Vitamin E	PO 25-50 units/day	* Nutritional supplement (antioxidant)	* Adverse events—Rare

Recommended concentrations and infusion times for intravenous medications

Medication	Final concentration for i.v. administration	Infusion rate	Medication	Final concentration for i.v. administration	Infusion rate
Acyclovir	7 mg/mL	60 min	Hydrocortisone	1 mg/mL	5 min
Adenosine	3 mg/mL	Rapid i.v. push	Indomethacin	0.5 mg/mL	30 min
Amikacin	5 mg/mL	30 min	Lidocaine		
Aminophylline	5 mg/mL	20 min	(loading doses)	20 mg/mL	5 min
Amphotericin B	0.1 mg/mL : peripheral lines	4-6 h	Lorazepam	0.1 mg/mL	5 min
			Metoclopramide	0.5 mg/mL	15 min
			Metronidazole	5 mg/mL	60 min
	0.2 mg/mL: central lines		Midazolam	1 mg/mL	15 min
Ampicillin	50 mg/mL	5 min	Morphine	2-10 mg/mL	5 min
Atropine	0.4 mg/mL	1 min			
Cefazolin	100 mg/mL	20 min	Pancuronium	0.2 mg/mL	5 min
Cefotaxime	100 mg/mL	20 min	Penicillin G	100,000 unit/mL	20 min
Ceftazidime	100 mg/mL	20 min	Phenobarbital	30 mg/mL	not >2 mg/kg per min
Chloramphenicol	50 mg/mL	30 min	Phenytoin	50 mg/mL	not > 0.5 mg/kg per min
Cimetidine	15 mg/mL	15 min			
Clindamycin	6 mg/mL	15 min	Phytomenadione		
Cloxacillin	100 mg/mL	20 min	(Vitamin K1)	1 mg/0.5 mL	not > 1 mg/min
Dexamethasone	4 mg/mL	5 min	Piperacillin	90 mg/mL	20 min
Diazepam	5 mg/mL	5 min	Propranolol	1 mg/mL	10 min
Digoxin	0.05 mg/mL	5 min	Pyridoxine	100 mg/mL	1-2 min
Erythromycin	2.5 mg/mL	60 min	Ranitidine	2.5 mg/mL	15 min
Fentanyl	0.05 mg/mL	10 min	Ticarcillin	50 mg/mL	20 min
Furosemide	10 mg/mL	30 min	Tobramycin	10 mg/mL	30 min
Gentamicn	10 mg/mL	30 min	Trimethoprim/ sulfamethoxazole	1.6 mg/mL trimethoprim	
Heparin (loading doses)	1,000 unit/mL	5 min	(Bactrim)	in D5W	60 min
			Vancomycin	5 mg/mL	60 min

Antibacterial medications (including antibiotics)

Amikacin sulfate

Aminoglycoside antibiotic active against gram-negative bacilli, especially Escherichia coli, Klebsiella, Proteus, Enterobacter, Serratia, and Pseudomonas.

Neonates : Postnatal age ≤ 7days : 1,200–2,000 g: 7.5 mg/kg q12 -18h IV or IM; > 2,000 g: 10 mg/kg q12h IV or IM; postnatal age > 7days: 1,200–2,000 g IV or IM: 7.5 mg/kg q8-12hr IV or IM; >2,000 g: 10 mg/kg q8h IV or IM.

* Aminoglycoside antibiotic active against gram - negative bacilli, especially Escherichia coli, Klebsiella, Proteus, Enterobacter, Serratia, and Pseudomonas
* Cautions : Anaerobes, streptococcus (including S.pneumoniae) are resistant. May cause ototoxicity and nephrotoxicity. Monitor renal function. Drug eliminated renally. Administrated IV over 30 - 60 min.
* Drug interactions : May potentiate other ototoxic and nephrotoxic drugs.
* Target serum concentrations : Peak 25–40 mg/L; trough < 10 mg/L

Amoxicillin-clavulanate

β-Lactam (amoxicillin) and β-lactamase inhibitor (clavulanate) enhances amoxicillin activity against penicillinase-producing bacteria: S. aureus (not methicillin- resistant organism), Streptococcus, Haemophilus influenzae, Moraxella catarrhalis, E. coli, Klebsiella, Bacteroids fragilis.

Neonates : 30 mg/kg/24hr divided q12h PO.

* b Lactam (amoxicillin) and b lactamase inhibitor (clavulanate) enhances amoxicillin activity against penicillinase - producing bacteria: S. aureus (not methicillin resistant organism), Streptococcus, Haemophilus influenzae, Moraxella catarrhalis, E. coli, Klebsiella, Bacteroides fragilis.
* Cautions : Drug dosed on amoxicillin component. May cause diarrhea. rash. Drug eliminated renally. Drug interaction: Probenecid.

Ampicillin

β-Lactam with same spectrum of antibacterial activity as amoxicillin.

Neonates : Postnatal age ≤ 7days ≤ 2,000 g: 50 mg/kg/24 hr IV or IM q12hr (meningitis: 100mg/kg/24hr divided q12h IV or IM); > 2,000 g: 75 mg/kg/24 hr divided q8h IV or IM (meningitis: 150 mg/kg/24 hr divided q8h IV or IM). postnatal age > 7days < 1200 g: 50 mg/kg/24 hr IV or IM q12h (meningitis: 100 mg/kg/24 hr divided q12h IV or IM); 1,200 - 2,000 g: 75 mg/kg/24 hr divided q8h IV or IM (meningitis: 150 mg/kg/24 hr divided q8h IV or IM); > 2,000 g: 100 mg/kg/24 hr divided q6h IV or IM (meningitis: 200 mg/kg/24 hr divided q6h IV or IM).

* b Lactam with same spectrum of antibacterial activity as amoxicillin.
* Cautions : Less bioavailable than amoxicillin causing greater diarrhea. Drug interaction : Probenecid.

Aztreonam

β-Lactam (monobactam) antibiotic with activity against gram-negative aerobic bacteria, Enterobacteriaceae, and Pseudomonas aeruginosa.

Neonates : Postnatal age ≤ 7days ≤ 2,000 g: 60 mg/kg/24 hr divided q12h IV or IM; > 2,000 g: 90 mg/kg/24 hr divided q8h IV or IM; postnatal age > 7days < 1,200 g: 60 mg/kg/24 hr divided q12h IV or IM; 1,200 - 2,000 g: 90 mg/kg/24 hr divided q8h IV or IM; > 2,000 g: 120 mg/kg/24 hr divided q6-8h IV or IM

* b Lactam (monobactam) antibiotic with activity against gram-negative aerobic bacteria, Enterobacteriaceae, and Pseudomonas aeruginosa.
* Cautions : Rash, thrombophlebitis, eosinophilia. Renally eliminated.
* Drug interaction : Probenecid.

Carbenicillin

Extended-spectrum penicillin (remains susceptible to penicillinase destruction) active against Enterobacter, indole-positive Proteus, and Pseudomonas.

Neonates : Postnatal age ≤ 7days ≤ 2,000 g: 225 mg/kg/24 hr divided q8h IV or IM; > 2,000 g: 300 mg/kg/24 hr divided q6h IV or IM; > 7days: 300-400 mg/kg/24 hr divided q6h IV or IM.

* Cautions : Painful given intramuscularly; rash; each gram contains 5.3 mEq sodium. Interferes with platelet aggregation at high doses, increases in liver transaminase levels. renaly eliminated. * Drug interaction : Probenecid.

Cefazolin

Neonates : Postnatal age ≤ 7days 40 mg/kg/24 hr divided q12h IV or IM; > 7days 40-60 mg/kg/24 hr divided q8h IV or IM.

* First-generation cephalosporin active against S.aureus, Streptococcus, E. coli, Klebsiella, and Proteus.
* Caution :β-Lactam safety profile (rash, eosinophilia). Renally eliminated. Does not adequately penetrate CNS.
* Drug interaction : Probenecid.

Cefepime

* Expanded-spectrum, fourth-generation cephalosporin active against many gram-positive and gram-negative pathogens, including many multi-drug-resistant pathogens,
* 100-150 mg/kg/24 hr q8-12h IV or IM.
* Cautions : b-Lactam safety profile (rash, eosinophilia). Renally eliminated.
* Drug interaction : Probenecid.

Cefoperazone sodium

* Third-generation cephalosporin active against many gram-positive and gram-negative pathogens.
  Neonates : 100 mg/kg/24 hr divided 12h IV or IM.
* Caution : Highly protein bound cephalosporin with limited potency reflected by weak antipseudomonal activity. Variable gram-positive activity. Primarily hepatically eliminated in bile.
* Drug interaction : Disulfiram-like reaction with alcohol.

Cefotaxime sodium

* Third-generation cephalosporin active against gram-positive and gram-negative pathogens. No antipseudomonal activity.
* Neonates : ≤ 7days: 100 mg/kg/24 hr divided q12h IV or IM; >7days: <1,200 g 100 mg/kg/24 hr divided q12h IV or IM; >1,200 g: 150 mg/kg/24 hr divided q8h IV or IM.
* Cautions :β-Lactam safety profile (rash, eosinophilia). Renally eliminated. Each gram of drug contains 2.2 mEq sodium. Active metabolite.
* Drug interaction : Probenecid.

Cefoxitin sodium	Second-generation cephalosporin active against *S. aureus, Streptococcus, H. influenzae, E. Coli, Klebsiella, Proteus,* and *Bacteroides.* Inactive against Enterobacter. Neonates : 70-100 mg/kg/24 hr divided q8-12h IV or IM. * Drug interaction : Probenecid.
Ceftazidime	Neonates : Postnatal age ≤ 7days: 100 mg/kg/24 hr divided q12h IV or IM; >7days ≤1,200 g: 100 mg/kg/24 hr divided q12h IV or IM; >1,200 g: 150 mg/kg/24 hr divided q8h IV or IM. * **Third-generation cephalosporin active against gram-positive and gram-negative pathogens including Pseudomonas aeruginosa.** * Cautions : β Lactam safety profile (rash, eosinophilia). Renally eliminated. Increasing pathogen resistance developing with long-term, widespread use. * Second-generation cephalosporin active against *S. aureus. Streptococcus, H.influenzae, E.coli, Klebsiella, Proteus,* and *Bacteroides.* Inactive against Enterobacter. * Cautions : Poor CNS penetration; β Lactam safety profile (rash, eosinophilia). Renally eliminated. Painful given intramuscularly. * Drug interactions : Probenecid.
Ceftriaxone sodium	Neonates : 50-75 mg/kg q24h IV or IM * **Third-generation cephalosporin active against gram-positive and gram-negative pathogens. No antipseudomonal activity. Very potent and β-Lactamase stable.** * Cautions : β-Lactam safety profile (rash, eosinophilia). Eliminated via kidney (33-65%) and bile; can cause sludging. Long half-life and dose-dependent protein binding favors q24h rather than q12h dosing. Can add 1% lidocaine for IM injection.
Cefuroxime (cefuroxime axetil for oral administration)	Neonates : 40-100 mg/kg/24 hr divided q12h IV or IM * **Second-generation cephalosporin active against *S.aureus, Streptococcus, H.influenzae, E.coli, M.catarrhalis, Klebsiella,* and *Proteus.*** * Cautions : b-Lactam safety profile (rash), eosinophilia. Renally eliminated. Food increases PO bioavailability. * Drug interaction : Probenecid.
Cipro-floxacin	Neonates : 10 mg/kg q12 h PO or IV * **Quinolone antibiotic active against *P.aeruginosa, Serratia, Enterobacter, Shigella, Salmonella, Campylobacter, Shigella, Salmonella, Campylobacter, Neisseria gonorrhoeae, H.influenzae, M.cathrrhalis,* some *S.aureus,* and *Streptococcus*** * Cautions : Concerns of joint destruction in juvenile animals not seen in humans; tendonitis, superinfection, dizziness, confusion, crystalluria some photosensitivity. * Drug interaction : Theophylline, magnesium-, aluminum-, or calcium-containing antacids, sucralfate, probenecid, warfarin, cyclosporine.
Clindamycin	Neonates : Postnatal age ≤ 7days < 1,200 g; 10mg/kg/24 hr divided q12h IV or IM; > 2000 g: 15mg/kg/24 hr divided q8h IV or IM; > 7days < 1,200 g: 10 mg/kg/24 hr IV or IM divided q12h; 1,200-2,000 g: 15 mg/kg/24 hr divided q8h IV or IM; > 2,000 g: 20 mg/kg/24 hr divided q8h IV or IM. * **Protein synthesis inhibitor active against most gram-positive aerobic and anaerobic cocci except Enterococcus.*** Caution : Diarrhea, nausea, C.difficile-associated colitis, rash. Administer slow IV over 30-60 min. Topically active as an acne treatment.
Oxacillin sodium	Penicillinase-resistant penicillin active against *S. aureus* and other gram-positive cocci except Enterococcus and coagulase-negative staphylococci. Neonates : Postnatal age ≤ 7days 1,200-2,000 g: 50 mg/kg/24 hr divided q 12h IV; >2,000 g: 75 mg/kg/24 hr IV divided q 8h IV; Postnatal age > 7days < 1,200 g: 50 mg/kg/24 hr IV divided q12h IV; >1,200-2,000 g: 75 mg/kg/24 hr divided q8h IV; >2,000 g: 100 mg/kg/24 hr IV divided q6h IV. Infants : 100-200 mg/kg/24 hr divided q4-6h IV. * Cautions : β-Lactam safety profile (rash, eosinophilia). Moderate oral bioavailability (35-65%). Primarily renally eliminated. * Drug interactions : Probenecid. * Adverse effect: Neutropenia.
Penicillin G	Penicillin active against most gram positive cocci; *S. pneumoniae* (resistance is increasing), group A *Streptococcus,* and some gram-negative bacteria (e.g., *N. gonorrhoeae, N. meningitidis*). Neonates : Postnatal age ≤ 7days 1,200-2,000 g; 50,000 units/kg/24 hr divided q12h IV or IM (meningitis: 100,000 units/kg/24 hr divided q12h IV or IM); >2,000 g: 75,000 units/kg /24 hr divided q 8h IV or IM (meningitis: 150,000 units/kg/24 hr divided q8h IV or IM); Postnatal age > 7days ≤ 1,200 g: 50,000 units/kg/24 hr divided q12h IV (meningitis: 100,000 units/kg/24 hr divided q12h IV); 1,200-2,000 g: 75,000 units/kg/24 hr q8h IV); (meningitis: 225,000 units/kg/24 hr divided q8h IV); 2,000 g: 100,000 units/kg/24 hr divided q6h IV (meningitis: 200,000 units/kg/24 hr divided q6h IV). * Cautions : β-Lactam safety profile (rash, eosinophilia), allergy, seizures with excessive doses particularly in patients with marked renal disease. Substantial pathogen resistance. Primarily renally eliminated. * Drug interactions : Probenecid.
Piperacillin	Extended-spectrum penicillin active against *E. coli, Enterobacter, Serratia, P. aeruginosa,* and *Bacteroides.* Neonates : Postnatal age≤ 7days 150 mg/kg/24 hr divided q8h-12h IV; > 7days; 200 mg/kg/ 24 hr divided q6-8r IV. * Cautions : β-Lactam safety profile (rash, eosinophilia), painful given intramuscular; each gram contains 1.9 mEq sodium. Interferes with platelet aggregation/serum sickness-like reaction with high doses; increases in liver function tests. Renally eliminated. Inactivated by penicillinase. * Drug interactions : Probenecid.

Cloxacillin Sodium	* Penicillinase-resistant penicillin active against S.aureus and other gram-positive cocci expect Enterococcus and coagulase-negative staphylococci. * 50-100 mg/kg/24 hr divided q6h PO. * Caution : b-Lactam Safety profile (rash, eosinophilia). Primarily hepatically eliminated; requires dose reduction in renal disease. Food decreases bioavailability. * Drug interaction : Probenecid.
Co-trimoxazole (trimetho prim-sulfa methoxa zole; TMP-SMZ)	* Antibiotic combination with sequential antagonism of bacterial folate synthesis with broad antibacterial activity: Shigella, Legionella, Chlamydia, Pneumocystis carinii. Dosage based on TMP component. * 6-20 mg TMP/kg/24hr or IV divided q12h PO. * Caution : Drug dosed on TMP (trimethoprim) component Sulfonamide skin reactions: rash, erythema multiforme, Stevens-Johnson syndrome, nausea, leukopenia. Renal and hepatic elimination; reduce dose in renal failure. * Drug interaction : Protein displacement with warfarin, possibly phenytoin, cyclosporine.
Erythro mycin	Bacteriostatic macrolide antibiotic most active against gram-positive organisms, Corynebacterium diphtheriae, and Mycoplasma pneumoniae. May also be used to promote gastrointestinal motility and improve feeding intolerance in preterm infants. Neonates : Postnatal age ≤ 7days: 20 mg/kg/ 24 hr divided q12h PO; >7days < 1,200 g: 20 mg/kg/24 hr divided q12h PO; >1,200 g: 30 mg/kg/24 hr divided q8h PO (give as 5 mg/kg/dose q6h to improve feeding intolerance). * Caution : Motion agonist leading to marked abdominal cramping, nausea, vomiting, diarrhea. Associated with hypertrophic pyloric stenosis in young infants. Many different salts with questionable tempering of gastrointestinal adverse events. Rare cardiac toxicity with IV use. Dose of salts differ. Topical formulation for treatment of acne. * Drug interaction : Antagonizes hepatic CYP 450 3A4 activity: astemizole, carbamazepine, terfenadine, cyclosporine, theophylline, digoxin, tacrolimus, carbamazepine.
Gentamicin	Aminoglycoside antibiotic active against gram-negative bacilli, especially E. coli, Klebsiella, Proteus, Enterobacter, Serratia, and pseudomonas. Neonates : Postnatal age ≤ 7days 1,200-2,000 g: 2.5 mg/kg q12 - 18h IV or IM; >2,000 g : 2.5 mg/kg q12h IV or IM; postnatal age >7 days 1,200-2,000 g: 2.5 mg/kg q8-12h IV or IM; >2,000 g: 2.5 mg/kg q8h IV or IM. * Cautions : Anaerobes, *S. pneumoniae*, other Streptococcus are resistant. May cause ototoxicity and nephrotoxicity. Monitor renal function. Drug eliminated renally. Administered IV over 30-60 min. * Drug interactions : May potentiate other ototoxic and nephrotoxic drugs. * Target serum concentrations: Peak 6-12 mg/L; trough <2 mg/L with intermittent daily dose regimens only.
Imipenem-cilastatin	Carbopenem antibiotic active against broad-spectrum gram-positive cocci and gram-negative bacilli including P. aeruginosa and anerobes. No activity against Stenotrophomonas maltophilia. Neonates : Postnatal age ≤ 7days <1,200g: 20 mg/kg q18 - 24h IV or IM; >1,200 g : 40 mg/kg divided q12h IV or IM; postnatal age >7 days 1,200-2,000 g: 40 mg/kg q12h IV or IM; >2,000 g: 60 mg/kg q8h IV or IM. * Cautions : b-Lactam safety profile (rash, eosinophilia). nausea, seizures. Cilastatin possesses no antibacterial activity; reduces renal imipenem metabolism. Primarily renally eliminated. * Drug interactions : Possibly ganciclovir.
Linezolid	Oxazolidinone antibiotic active against gram-positive cocci (especially drug-resistant organisms), including Staphylococcus, Streptococcus, Enterococcus faecium, and E. fecalis. Interferes with protein synthesis by binding to 50S ribosome submit. 10 mg/kg q12h IV or PO. * Adverse events: Myelosuppression, pseudomembranous colitis, nausea, diarrhea, headache. * Drug interaction : Probenecid.
Meropenem	Carbapenem antibiotic active against broad-spectrum gram-positive cocci and gram- negative bacilli including P. aeruginosa and anaerobes. No activity against Stenotrophomonas maltophilia. Usually reserved for infections resistant to other antibiotics. Neonates : Postnatal age < 7days 20mg/kg/dose 12 hrly; Postnatal age > 7days 20mg/kg/dose 8 hrly. Double the dose in Meningitis or severe infection. * Cautions : b-Lactam safety profile; appears to possess less CNS excitation than imipenem. 80% renal elimination. Side effects-Reversible neutropenia, thrombocytopenia, eosinophilia, raised LFTs, seizures. * Drug interaction : Probenecid. Use with caution with nephrotoxic drugs.
Metronidazole	Highly effective in the treatment of infections due to anaerobes. Neonates : <1,200 g: 7.5 mg/kg q 48 hr PO or IV; Postnatal age < 7days 1,200-2,000 g: 7.5 mg/kg/24 hr q 24 hr PO or IV; 2,000 g: 15 mg/kg/24 hr divided q 12h PO or IV; Postnatal age > 7days 1,200-2,000 g; 15 mg/kg/24 hr divided q12h PO or IV; >2,000 g: 30 mg/kg/24 hr divided q12h PO or IV. * Cautions : Dizziness, seizures, metallic taste, nausea, disulfiram-like reaction with alcohol. Administer IV slow over 30-60 min. Adjust dose with hepatic impairment. * Drug interactions : Carbamazepine, rifampin, phenobarbital may enhance metabolism; may increase levels of warfarin, phenytoin, lithium.
Netilmicin	Aminoglycoside antibiotic active against Gram- negative bacteria, an alternative to Gentamicin. It is less active against Pseudomonas. Sometimes effective against Coagulase Negative staph. that are resistant to gentamicin. Marginally less ototoxic. 6mg/kg/ dose IV once every 24 hrs. If the trough serum level when the 3rd dose exceeded 2mg/L, increase the dosage interval to 36 hrs and check level again after 2 or more doses have been given. * Cautions : May cause ototoxicity and nephrotoxicity. Simultaneous treatment with Vancomycin may increase the risk of nephrotoxicity. Try to stop treatment after 7-10 days. Aim for a peak concentration in the serum of 9-12 mg/L, and a trough level of about i mg/L. * Drug interactions : May potentiate other ototoxic and nephrotoxic drugs

Piperacillin-tazobactam	Extended-spectrum penicillin (piperacillin) combined with a b-lactamase inhibitor (tazobactam) active against S. aureus, H. influenzae, E. coli, Enterobacter, Serratia, Acinetobacter, P. aeruginosa, and Bacteroides. 300-400 mg/kg/24 hr divided q6-8 h IV or IM. * Cautions : b-Lactam safety profile (rash, eosinophilia), painful given intramuscularly; each gram contains 1.9 mEq sodium. Interferes with platelet aggregation, serum sickness-like reaction with high doses; increases in liver function test results. Renally eliminated. * Drug interactions : Probenecid.
Rifampicin	Antituberculosis drug used in combination with other ATD. Also a potent antistaphylococcal antibiotic used to treat resistant staphylococcal infection in combination with Vancomycin or Teicoplanin. Rifampicin can also be given prophylactically to the contacts of patients with meningococcal or haemophilus infection. 12mg/kg once a day PO as an ATD; 5mg/kg to < 1month old (10mg/kg to >1month old) once every 12 hours for 2 days to eliminate meningococcal carriage, & for 4 days in unvaccinated children under 4 years exposed to a case of H influenzae infection. * Cautions : Colors urine and other secretions red. Transient jaundice can be ignored, but treatment must be stopped at once if thrombocytopenia, vomiting or other signs of more serious liver toxicity develop. * Drug interactions : Digoxin, Fluconozole, Phenobarbitone, Phenytoin, Theophylline, Warfarin.
Teicoplanin	An alternative to Vancomycin in the treatment of CONS. A complex of 5 closely related glycopeptide antibiotics with similar antibacterial properties to Vancomycin. Active against many Gram positive anerobes and is particularly potent against clostridium species. Also active against most listeria, enterococci, and MRSA. 16mg/kg IV loading dose followed by 8 mg/kg IV/IM once every 24 hrs for proven systemic infection. Duration of Treatment is a minimum of 7 days. Double the dosage interval in renal failure. * Cautions : Important to aim for a trough serum concentration of at least 10 mg/L. Watch for possible leukopenia, thrombocytopenia, and disturbances of liver function.
Ticarcillin	Extended-spectrum penicillin active against E. coli, Enterobacter, Serratia, P. aeruginosa, and Bacteroides. Neonates : Postnatal age ≤ 7days <2,000 g: 150 mg/kg/24 hr divided q8-12h IV; >7days: <2,000 g: 225 mg/kg/24 hr divided q8h IV; > 7days <1,200 g: 150 mg/kg/24 hr divided q12h IV; 1,200-2,000 g: 225 mg/kg/24 hr divided q8h IV; > 2,000 g: 300 mg/kg/24 hr divided q6-8h IV. * Cautions : b-Lactam safety profile (rash, eosinophilia), painful given intramuscularly; each gram contains 5-6 mEq sodium. Interferes with platelet aggregation, increases in liver function tests. Renally eliminated. Inactivated by penicillinase. * Drug interaction : Probenecid.
Ticarcillin-clavulanate	Extended-spectrum penicillin (ticarcillin) combined with a b-Lactamase inhibitor (clavulanate) active against S. aureus, H. influenzae, Enterobacter, E. coli, Serratia, P. aeruginosa, Acinetobacter, and Bacteroides. 280-400 mg/kg/ 24 hr q4-8h IV or IM. * Cautions : b-Lactam safety profile (rash, eosinophilia), painful given intramuscularly; each gram contains 5-6 mEq sodium. Interferes with platelet aggregation, increases in liver function tests. Renally eliminated. * Drug interaction : Probenecid.
Tobramycin	Aminoglycoside antibiotic active against gram-negative bacilli, especially E. coli, Klebsiella, Enterobacter, Serratia, proteus, and Pseudomonas. Neonates: Postnatal age ≤ 7days, 1,200-2,000 g: 2.5 mg/kg q12-18h IV or IM; >2,000 g: 2.5 mg/kg q12h IV or IM; Postnatal age >7days, 1,200-2,000 g: 2.5 mg/kg q8-12h IV or IM; >2,000 g: 2.5 mg/kg q8h IV or IM. * Cautions : S. pneumoniae, other Streptococcus, and anaerobes are resistant. May cause ototoxicity and nephrotoxicity. Monitor renal function. Drug eliminated renally. Administered IV over 30-60 min. * Drug interaction : May potentiate other ototoxic and nephrotoxic drugs. * Target serum concentrations: Peak 6-12 mg/L; trough <2 mg/L.
Vancomycin	Glycopeptide antibiotic active against most gram-positive pathogens including Staphylococcus (including methicillin-resistant S. aureus and coagulase-negative staphylococci), S. pneumoniae including penicillin-resistant strains, Enterococcus (resistance is increasing), and Clostridium difficile-associated colitis. Neonates: Postnatal age ≤ 7days, 1,200 g: 15 mg/kg/24 hr divided q24h IV; 1,200-2,000 g: 15 mg/kg/24 hr divided q12-18h IV; > 2,000 g: 30 mg/kg/24 hr divided q12h IV; Postnatal age >7days, <1,200 g: 15 mg/kg 24 hr divided q24h IV; > 1,200-2,000 g: 15 mg/kg/24 hr divided q8-12h IV; 2,000 g: 45 mg/kg/24 hr divided q8h IV * Cautions : Ototoxicity and nephrotoxicity particularly when co-administered with other ototoxic and nephrotoxic drugs. Infuse IV over 45-60 min. Flushing (red-man syndrome) associated with rapid IV infusions, fever, chills, phlebitis (central line is preferred). Renally eliminated. * Target serum concentrations: Peak (1 hr after 1 hr infusion) 30-40 mg/L; trough 5-10 mg/L.

Antiviral medications (Including anti retroviral -HIV)

Acyclovir	Herpes simplex encephalitis, mucosal, cutaneous, genital infections; Herpes zoster, Varicella-zoster, CMV Prophylaxis. Neonates : HSV encephalitis: 60 mg/kg/24 hr IV, divided q8hr. * Cautions : rash, Bone marrow suppression, Primarily renally eliminated. * Drug interactions : Zidovudine, Probenecid
Foscarnet	Treatment of CMV infections, retinitis, and acyclovir-resistant HSV mucocutaneous infection, and Herpes zoster. Neonates : CMV retinitis: IVI @60 mg/kg/hr. Acyclovir-resistant HSV infection: 120mg/kg/24 hr divided q8-12 hr Induction therapy: 180 mg/kg/24hr divided q8hr; maintenance therapy; 90-120mg/kg/24hr once daily * Cautions : Hypertension, seizures, nephrotoxicity, decreased serum Ca, Mg, K. Bronchospasm.
Ganciclovir	Treatment of CMV infections & retinitis Neonates : Induction therapy: 10 mg/kg/24hr IV over 1-2 hr divided q12hr for 14-21 days; maintenance therapy: 5-6 mg/kg/24 hr IV once daily. * Cautions : Hypertension, seizures, nephrotoxicity, rash,liver toxicity * Drug interactions : Immunosuppressants, Probenecid
Ribavirin	Aerosol therapy for RSV Bronchiolitis for those with underlying BPD, CHD etc. Neonates : Continuous aerosolization 12-18 hr / day(20mg/ml concentration) * Cautions : rash, irritation, hypotension, precipitation of drug in ventilation tubing. * Best results when initiated early in clinical course.
Vidarabine	Treatment of HSV & V-Z infections Neonates : HSV- 15-30 mg/kg/24 hr IVI over 18-24 hr. V-Z/H-Z- 10 mg/kg/24 hr IV once daily over 12 hr. * Cautions : rash, Bone marrow suppression, seizures, SIADH * Drug interactions : Immunosuppressants.
Lamivudine	Anti-HIV reverse transcriptase inhibitor used in combination with Zidovudine and other anti-HIV drugs. Neonates : 8 mg/kg/24 hr PO divided q12hr * Cautions : feeding problems, neutropenia, pancreatitis * Drug interactions : Trimethoprim/SMZ
Nelfinavir	Anti-HIV Protease inhibitor as monotherapy or in combination with Nucleoside analogs/other Protease inhibitors Neonates : 30 mg/kg/24 hr PO divided q8hr under study * Cautions :Hypertension,anemia, leukopenia, hepatitis, iritis,dyspnea, sweating, diarrhea. * Drug interactions : Rifampicin, Phenobarbital, ketoconazole, indinavir, ritonavir
Nevirapine	Anti-HIV Non-nucleosides reverse transcriptase inhibitor specific for HIV-1 Transcriptase- not HIV-2 Neonates :5 mg/kg/24 hr PO for 14 days, then 240mg/sq meter/24hr PO divided q12hr for 14 days., then 400mg/sq meter/24hr PO divided q12hr * Cautions :Stevens-Johnson syndrome, LFTs increased, severe rash, diarrhea. * Drug interactions : Rifampicin, indinavir, ritonavir.
Zidovudine	Anti-HIV reverse transcriptase inhibitor used in combination with Lamivudine and other anti-HIV drugs. Neonates :8 mg/kg/24 hr PO divided q6hr; 6 mg/kg/24 hr IV divided q6hr * Cautions :rash, Bone marrow suppression, seizures, diarrhea,lactic acidosis, cholestatic hepatitis, * Drug interactions : Rifampicin, fluconazole, valproic acid.

Drugs in renal failure: Avoid **nephrotoxic drugs** and adjust dosage of essential drugs.

I. **DOSE ADJUSTMENT METHODS** A. MAINTENANCE DOSE : In patients with renal insufficiency, the dose may be adjusted using the following methods:

1. **Interval extension (I):** Lengthen the intervals between individual doses, keeping the dose size normal.

2. **Dose reduction (D):** Reduce the amount of individual doses, keeping the interval between the doses normal.

   This method is particularly recommended for drugs in which a relatively constant blood level is desired.

3. **Interval extension and dose reduction (DI):** Lengthen the interval and reduce the dose.

4. **Interval extension or dose reduction (D, I):** In some instances, either the dose or the interval can be changed.

   Note: These dose adjustments are for beyond the neonatal period. These dose modifications are only approximations. Each patient must be monitored closely for signs of drug toxicity, and serum .

   Dose modifications are only necessary for drugs or metabolites which are >90% excreted by the kidney. Measures of Creatinine clearance are frequently not available, but plasma creatinine concentrations can be used.

For younger children, infants and neonates, no method of estimating Creatinine Clearance (CL_{CR}) is reliable.

The Swartz equation is the standard equation for young children, however, the results are not consistent enough to be used for pk modeling.

Creatinine Clearance(Schwartz) (ml/minute/1.73 m²) - C_{cr} =k x Length (cm)

k = 0.45 in babies <1yr; 0.55 if > 1 year and in adult females;
0.7 in adolescent and adult males (*Low Birth weight ≤ 1 y K = 0.33)

Drugs used to combat infection and their clearance from the body in Neonates with severe renal failure before or during Peritoneal Dialysis—See Page No 1014 for the details.

Drugs in Liver failure: Modification of the choice and dosage of drugs is usually unnecessary in children with liver disease, because there is a relatively large reserve of function of the liver metabolism even when liver disease appears to be severe. However, the following situations are those for which special consideration is required.

* Liver Failure: Severely deranged LFTs, and prolonged Jaundice.

* Coagulation impairment: Increased response to oral anticoagulants

* Hypoproteinemia: Phenytoin/ Benzodiazepines with high protein binding affinity may have increased effect.

* Hepatotoxic drug use: Avoid these drugs if at all possible, whether their effects are dose related or idiosyncratic.

Therapeutic drug monitoring in the Newborn infant

(See page1064) is necessary because dose requirements differ greatly from those for older children. These differences stem from major changes in kinetic disposition at the absorption, distribution, and elimination phases. The small blood volume of neonates makes them sensitive to iatrogenic blood loss. Similarly, the small size of these patients means that medication errors frequently lead to morbidity and even mortality. The clinical laboratory must set up strict, high-standard, carefully updated guidelines to ensure the safety of infants who need drug therapy at this very vulnerable phase of their lives.

Adrenal insufficiency in critical illness: There is really no consensus among pediatric intensivists or endocrinologists as to how often adrenal insufficiency occurs in pediatric critical illness or how to diagnose and then treat this condition . Whilst awaiting the basal Cortisol levels , giving the required dose of steroids in critically ill patients at risk of adrenal insufficiency (primary or secondary adrenal failure , steroid use in previous 6–12 months) and in vasopressor resistant shock may be pragmatic until further clear and definite consensus guidelines are made available. The steroid preparation recommended is **hydrocortisone** at the dosages mentioned below.

Dose

1. **Replacement dose**—in children diagnosed with Addisons disease or CAH 12.5mg/m2 /day or 0.5 mg/kg/day.

2. **Stress dose**—any kind of medical or surgical stress in patients on/have been on steroids -50mg/m2/day or 2mg/kg/day

3. **Shock dose** - bolus dose of 2–50 mg/kg followed by 2–50mg/kg/day as continuous infusion or intermittent doses 4–6 hrly.

   The dose of hydrocortisone in pediatric studies have been 100 mg per m2, (4 mg /kg /day) The role of Fludrocortisone replacement needs to be evaluated in critically ill. Hydrocortisone by itself has mineralo-corticoid activity that would suffice.

Duration

Stress dose

1. *Minor procedure*: One extra dose before the procedure.

2. *Major procedure (i.e. requiring general anesthesia)*- One dose before procedure followed by followed by rapid tapering over 1–2 days.

Shock dose (in catecholamines resistant septic shock): Start steroids empirically at above mentioned dosage. Favorable response is witnessed by ability to wean pressors within 24–48 hrs .Continue for 5–7 days to maximum of 10 days once the laboratory results confirm adrenal insufficiency. If symptoms of shock recur after steroid discontinuation, the steroid dose should be resumed at prior dose.

Essential neonatal IV drug infusions

1. **Adrenaline IVI: 0.1–0.3microgram/kg/minute by continuous infusion.Start at lower doses. Indication:**Low cardiac output; higher doses of up to 1.5mcg/kg/min may be necessary for acute hypotension.

@ To give an IVI of 0.1microgram /kg/minute, place 1.5 mg of adrenaline for each kg (1 ml of 1:1000 solution contains 1 mg of L-adrenaline) the baby weighs in a syringe, dilute to 25 ml with 10% dextrose saline, and infuse at 0.1 ml/hr. The drug is stable in solution; no need to prepare fresh every 24 hrs.

2. **Dobutamine IVI: 2–10 microgram/kg/minute by continuous infusion. If there is no clinical response within 1-2 hrs then doses of 10 or even 15 mcg/kg/minute may be tried.** Indication: Inotropic support for low cardiac output cardiac failure associated with cardiac surgery, septicemia.

@ To give an IVI of 10mcg/kg/minute, place 30 mg of Dobutamine for each kg (1 ml= 25 mg; check with the drug monograph) the baby weighs in a syringe, dilute to 50 ml with 10% dextrose 0.18% saline, and infuse at 1 ml/hr. Diluted solution should be used within 24 hrs. Maximum recommended concentration after dilution is 5 mg in 1 ml. Do not mix with $NaHCO_3$. Direct IV push is prohibited.

3. **Dopamine IVI:1–5 microgram/kg/minute by continuous infusion for renal effect(controversial), then increase as clinically indicated to a maximum of 20 mcg/kg/minute for direct inotropic effect** but vasoconstriction may occur at higher doses.Indication Inotropic support for low cardiac output cardiac failure associated with cardiac surgery, septicemia.

@ To give an IVI of 1mcg/kg/minute, place 30 mg of Dopamine for each kg (1ml=40 mg supply;check with the drug monograph for exact manufacturer`s drug concentration) the baby weighs in a syringe, dilute to 50 ml with 10% dextrose 0.18% saline, and infuse at 0.1 ml/hr. Diluted solution should be used within 24 hrs. Do not use if discolored. Do not mix with $NaHCO_3$ or any other alkali as it is inactivated. Direct IV push is prohibited.It can be put in the same syringe as Dobutamine to simplify nursing supervision when both drugs are being infused simultaneously at an unvarying rate. Monitor for signs of peripheral ischemia.

4. **Heparin IVI:**(1ml of concentrated Heparin=5,000 units;check with the drug monograph for exact manufacturer`s drug concentration).*Catheter prophylaxis*-Add 500 units in 500 ml of 0.18% or 0.45% NS (1ml=1 unit) & start infusing through the UAC @ 1 ml/hour to maintain catheter patency. *Anticoagulation treatment*-Start with a loading dose of 50 units/kg in <35wk PCA, or 75units/kg in >35wk PCA; maintenance requirements vary: start with a continuous IV infusion of 25 units/kg/hour and assess the requirement by monitoring the APTT 4 hours after starting treatment. Aim for the APTT to 1.8-2 times the normal level.

Antidote- Protamine sulphate 1 mg IV over 5 minutes for every 100 units of Heparin still thought to be active within the patient; a 1mg/kg dose will usually suffice to bring the APTT down to no more than 130% of normal. Excess Protamine binds platelets and proteins such as fibrinogen, and can cause bleeding tendency.

5. **Morphine IVI:** Sedation while ventilated: Loading dose-Give 25–50 microgram/kg(preterm) or 50–100 microgram/kg (term) as a single dose by a slow IV bolus over 5–10 minutes, *then by continuous IVI of 5microgram/kg/hour (preterm) or 10–20microgram/kg/hour (term).*

@ To give an IVI of 20 microgram/kg/*hour*, place 1 ml of diluted(1 in 10) morphine , i.e., 1 mg=1,000 mcg for each kg the baby weighs in a syringe, dilute to 50 ml with 10% dextrose 0.18% saline, and infuse at 1 ml/hr. (1ml of concentrated Morphine=10mg ;check with the drug monograph for exact manufacturer's drug concentration). Ensure respiratory support and monitor for respiratory depression. Naloxone (100 microgram/kg IV BOLUS or 100 microgram/kg/hour continuous IVI) is a specific antidote. The drug is chemically stable in solution, but some units change the infusate once every 24 hours to minimize the risk of bacterial overgrowth in the event of contamination.

6. **Midazolam IVI:** Status epilepticus Give 150–200 **microgram**/kg as an initial single bolus to be followed by a continuous infusion of 1-5 **microgram**/kg/minute; start at 1**microgram**/kg/minute, increasing by 1 **microgram**/kg/minute every 15 minutes until the seizure stops. Maximum of 5 **microgram**/kg/minute.

@ To give an IVI of 1microgram/kg/minute, place 6 mg for each kg the baby weighs in a syringe, dilute to 50 ml with 10% dextrose 0.18% saline, and infuse at 0.5 ml/hr. (1ml of Midazolam =1mg or 5 mg;check with the drug monograph for exact manufacturer`s drug concentration). Reduce the dose in severe renal impairment and liver disease.

7. **Noradrenaline IVI: 0.1–1.5 microgram/kg/minute by continuous infusion.Start at lower doses. Indication:** Potent vasoconstrictor to treat severe refractory hypotension as in patients with septic shock; higher doses of up to 1.5mcg/kg/min may be necessary for acute hypotension.

@ To give an IVI of 0.1microgram/kg/minute, place 1.5 mg of Noradrenaline for each kg (1 ml contains 1 mg of Noradrenaline base or 2 mg of Noradrenaline acid tartrate) the baby weighs in a syringe, dilute to 25 ml with 10% dextrose saline, and infuse at 0.1 ml/hr. The drug is stable in solution but prepare fresh every 24 hrs. Protect from light. Can be added into a line containing Dobutamine, heparin, or ranitidine and Standard TPN solutions with/ without lipid.

8. **Phenytoin IVI:** To control status epilepticus 20mg/kg loading dose as slow IVI(@not more than 1mg/kg/minute) under ECG/BP Monitoring over at least 20 minutes (to avoid cardiac arrhythmias & hypotension). Dilute 1ml of Phenytoin =50mg, to 10 ml of NS to get a solution containing 5 mg/ml.

*Optimum maintenance dose is variable but 2.5 mg/kg IV every 12 hours in the 1st week of life to maintain a therapeutic concentration(10-20 mg/L). Older babies may require 2 or 3 times as much as this. *Measure plasma concentrations if Phenytoin is to be given for >2-3 days. *Crystallization makes the IM route unsatisfactory and it occurs when phenytoin mixes with any solution containing dextrose.

9. **Prostin IVI: (See Page 1065 for details)** To maintain the ductal patency until some palliative surgery is done as soon as possible; in Neonates with ductal-dependent CHD.

IVI: *Start* with 0.01 *micrograms/kg/min*(0.6ml/kg/hr.*)*

Dilute 500 micrograms(0.5mg) in 500 ml of 5–10% dextrose, i.e. 1 microgram/ml of reconstituted solution).

Double the dose in 15-20 minutes (1.2ml/kg/hr=0.02mcg/kg/min. if SaO2 is unchanged.)

Titrate to effective dosage with therapeutic response!
0.01 *micrograms/kg/min*(0.6ml/kg/hr)
0.02 *micrograms/kg/min*(1.2ml/kg/hr)
0.03 *micrograms/kg/min*(1.8ml/kg/hr)
0.04 *micrograms/kg/min*(2.4ml/kg/hr)
0.05 *micrograms/kg/min*(3.0ml/kg/hr)

For e.g. a 3kg baby requires an IVI of 1.8ml/hr of Prostin E_1(diluted solution 1ml=1mcg) to start with, i.e.,0.01 *micrograms/kg/min*(0.6ml/kg/hr); the usual dose will be 9ml/hr i.e. 0.05*micrograms/kg/min* (3.0ml/kg/hr).

10 **Amphotericin B LIPOSOMAL IVI: For the treatment of suspected or proven systemic fungal infection.** Add 12 ml of sterile water for injection to a 50 mg vial of Liposomal preparation to obtain a solution containing 4 mg/ml and shake vigorously until the powder is completely dispersed. Take 20 mg(5 ml) from the vial , and dilute to 20 ml further with 5% dextrose to give a solution containing 1 mg/ml, and infuse @1.5mg/kg over 4-6 hours once a day rising, if necessary to 4.5 mg/kg once a day. Duration of treatment - approximately 4 weeks. Do not allow the drug to come into contact with any product other than 5% dextrose.

BACK TO NEONATAL BASICS: SELF ASSESSMENT REVIEW IN NEWBORN PHOTOGRAPHS AND DATA

Section VI

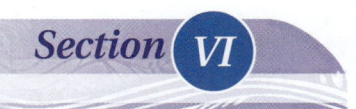

Score : ≥ 35 = excellent, ≥ 30 = good, ≥ 25 = above average, ≥ 20 = average. Time limit : 35 min.

1. Describe the ROP changes seen in this Fundus photograph taken from the ROP Screening of a Premature baby (Born at 26 weeks of GA, now 30 wks corrected age).

2. This infant has hypotonia, poor sucking reflex, diminished or absent cry, somnolence and has to be Tubefed since birth. What is the Diagnosis?

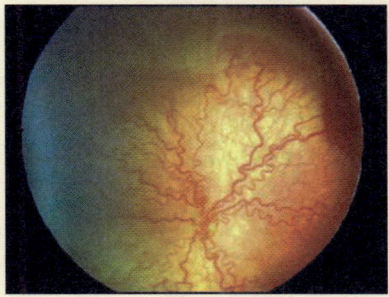

3. What does this ECG obtained from a Centrally Cyanosed Neonate show?

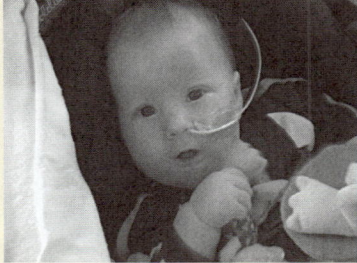

4. What is the Diagnosis of EEG taken from a Term asphyxiated baby?

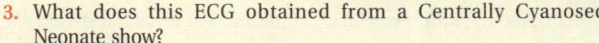

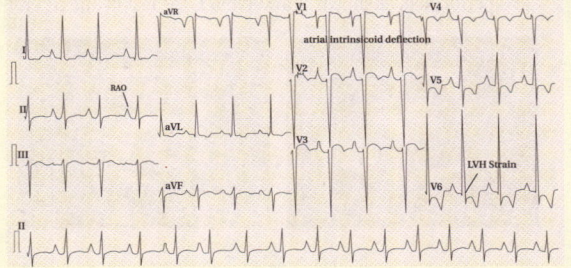

5. What do these CT head scans from 2 Newborns both with seizures show?

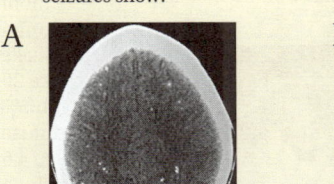

A   B

6. Describe the position of the tubes & lines seen in this radiograph.

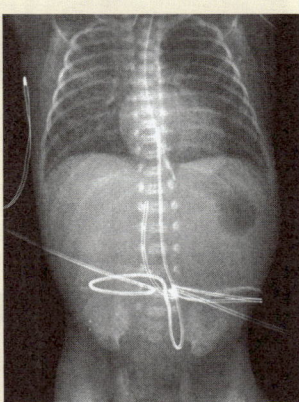

7. What do you see in this radiograph taken from a Neonate on TPN.

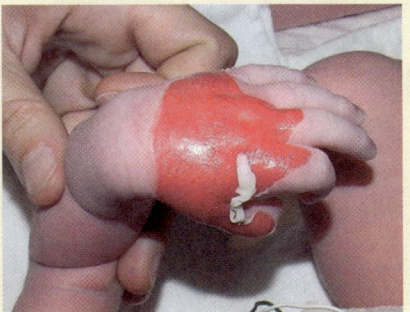

8. A Newborn baby has developed the skin lesion spontaneously soon after delivery shown here. What is the most likely diagnosis?

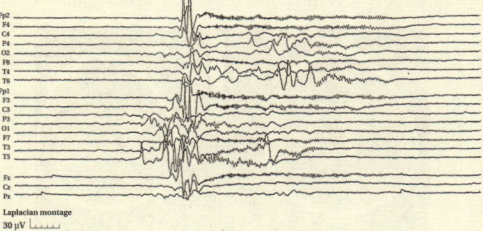

9. What is the radiological sign seen in this Radiograph taken from a Preterm Neonate with NEC ?

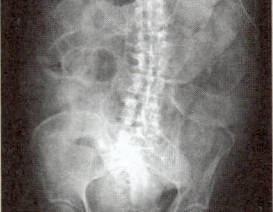

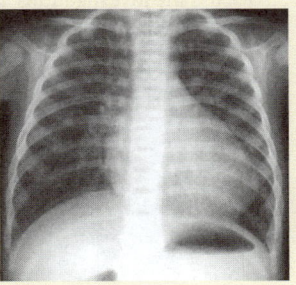

10. What is the diagnosis ?

11. What is the Diagnosis ?

A   B

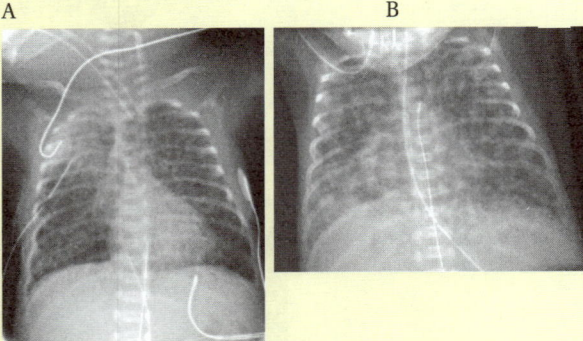

12. A Postdated Neonate with severe respiratory distress is on ventilator support. Serial chest radiographs were taken on day 1&3 as shown below. What is the initial diagnosis and what complication happened subsequently ?

A

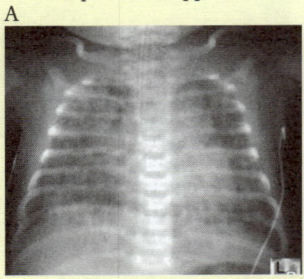 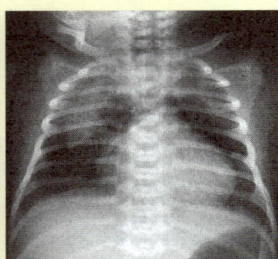

13. A preterm with severe RDS on mechanical ventilator developed shock and hypotension. What is the diagnosis ?

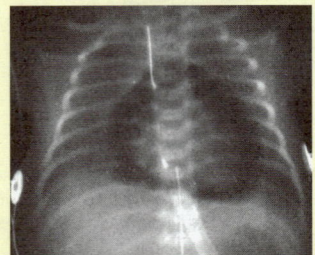

14. What is the ECG Diagnosis taken from a child with a suspected Cyanotic Congenital Heart disease ?

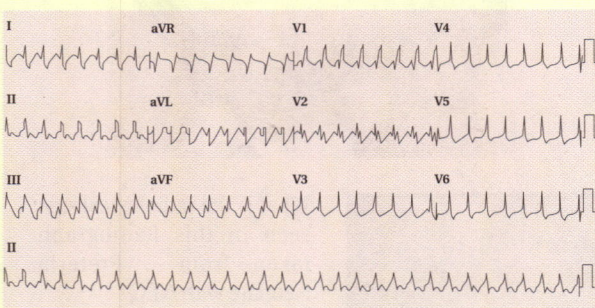

15. Discuss the investigations and prognosis for the condition seen in the clinical photograph?

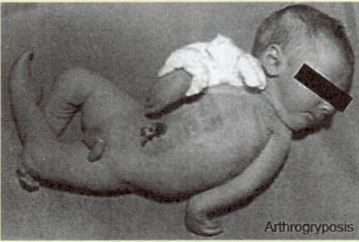

Arthrogryposis

16. What does the MCUG show?

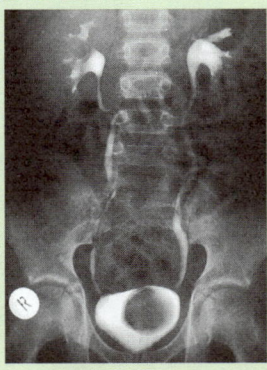

17. What is the diagnosis in this plain abdominal radiograph obtained from a Neonate presented with abdominal distention and bilious vomiting ?

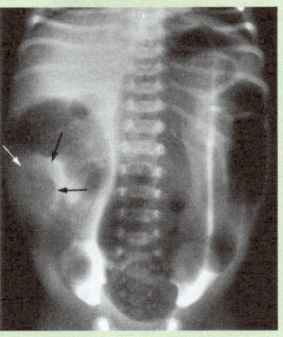

18. A preterm with severe RDS on mechanical ventilator developed shock and hypotension, on day 3. An emergent USG Head Scan was performed, as shown below. What is the lesion and its grade?

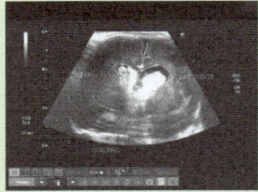 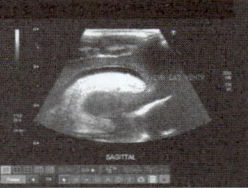

19. What does this MRI Brain Scan illustrate, taken from a Term baby who had severe Hypoxic-Ischemic encephalopathy ?

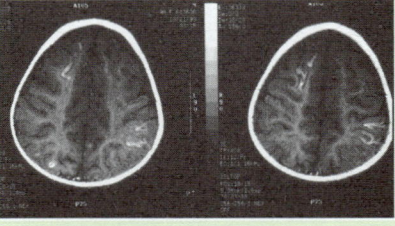

20. What is the diagnosis of this USG Scan obtained from a NICU Preemie graduate?

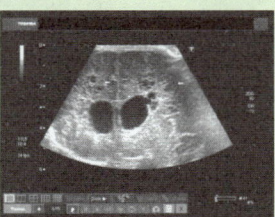

21. What is this latest Neonatal Technological development and How is it useful?

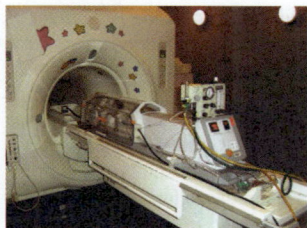 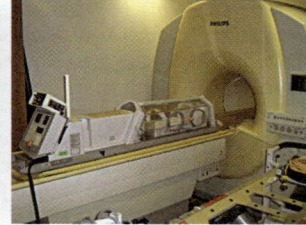

22. What is the diagnosis in an otherwise healthy Newborn ?

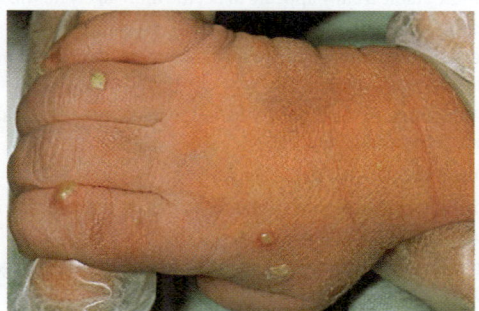

23. A two week old male infant presents with a history of distressed noisy breathing for several hours, progressively worsening with periods of apnea and cyanosis. What does the CXR reveal?

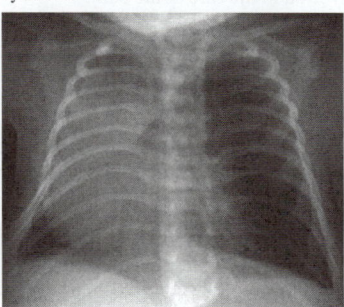

24. What is the difference between the Two Chest Radiographs taken from the same Premature baby on different days (1&3)of NICU admission?

A   B

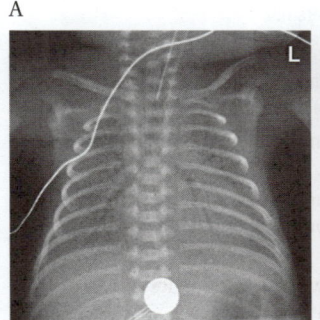 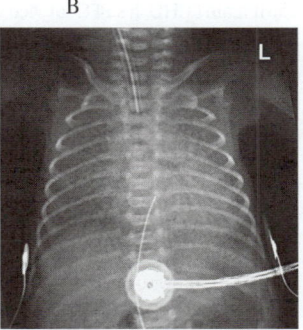

25. What is the diagnosis of this skin condition in a critically ill Neonate ?

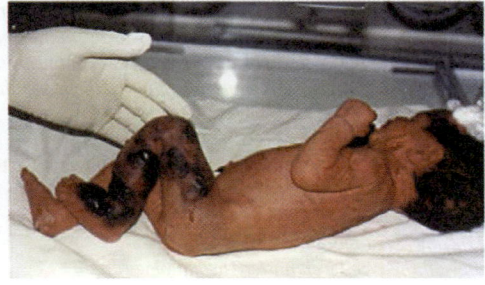

26. The following infant is born to a 32 year old Gravida 3 P2 mother following an uncomplicated pregnancy, labor, and delivery The infant weight 2.9 Kg at birth and has Apgar scores or 8 and 9 at one and five minutes respectively. The infant has no respiratory problems and the remainder of the physical examination appears to be entirely normal. The parents are understandably distressed to see this lesion and ask to speak to the medical staff as soon as possible. 1) What is this lesion? 2) How does this mass arise? 3) What other evaluation of this infant should be performed? 4) What are the suggested treatments for this problem? 5) What is the long-term prognosis for this infant?

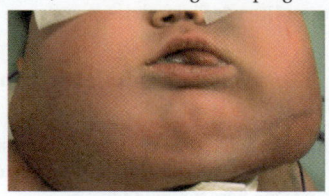

27. What is the diagnosis in a Newborn with a history of fetal distress & asphyxia ?

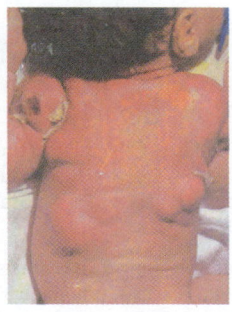

28. What are the skin lesions developed and disappeared for a few days in a Newborn ?

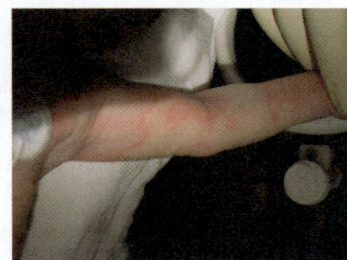

29. What is the scalp lesion seen at the time of delivery in a Newborn, without any history of trauma ?

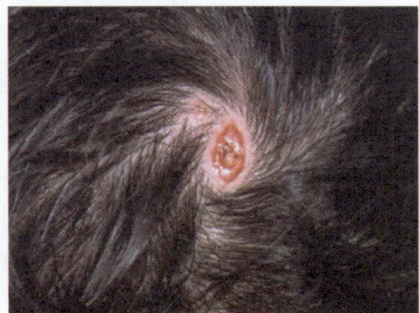

30. What is this bluish nodular lesion present at the time of birth ?

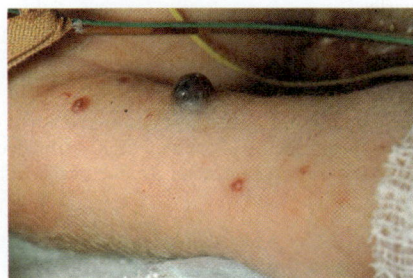

31. Interpret the following ABG Analyses.

    a) pH 7.15, PaCO$_2$ 80 mmHg, PaO$_2$ 55 mmHg, HCO$_3$ 27mEq/L, BE 0
    b) pH 7.52, PaCO$_2$ 30 mmHg, PaO$_2$ 45 mmHg, HCO$_3$ 24mEq/L, BE+2
    c) pH 7.27, PaCO$_2$ 27.6 mmHg, PaO$_2$ 90 mmHg, HCO$_3$ 12.2mEq/L, BE 13.3 d) pH 7.53, PaCO$_2$ 38 mmHg, PaO$_2$ 62 mmHg, HCO$_3$ 32mEq/L, BE +7 e) pH 7.43, PaCO$_2$ 41 mmHg, PaO$_2$ 94 mmHg, HCO$_3$ 26mEq/L, BE +2
    f) pH 7.20, PaCO$_2$ 55 mmHg, PaO$_2$ 55 mmHg, HCO$_3$ 21mEq/L, BE -8
    g) pH 7.41, PaCO$_2$ 24 mmHg, PaO$_2$ 68 mmHg, HCO$_3$ 16mEq/L, BE -6

32. A 3 week old female Neonate presents with vomiting, failure to thrive and dehydration. Urea & Electrolytes results are here for you to interpret.

    Na122 mEq/L, K 7.6mEq/L, Cl 99 mEq/L, Urea 65mg/dL, Creatinine 0.9 mg/dL, HCO$_3$ 13mEq/L.

33. A 2 week old male Neonate presents with 4-day history of recurrent nonbilious vomitings, dehydration, & failure to thrive. Urea & Electrolytes results are here for you to interpret.

    Na136 mEq/L, K 3.0mEq/L, Cl 82 mEq/L, Urea 70mg/dL, Creatinine 0.7 mg/dL, HCO$_3$ 40mEq/L.

34. A 5 day-old male apparently well Neonate is noted to have Poor feeding, lethargy and seizures. What do the results of the following Investigations reveal?

    Na138 mEq/L, K 3.6mEq/L, Cl 95 mEq/L, Urea 1mg/dL, Creatinine 0.5 mg/dL, SEPSIS Screen-Negative, Blood glucose 45mg/dL, Plasma Ammonia 600 micromol/L, pH 7.45, PaCO$_2$ 29 mmHg, PaO$_2$ 110 mmHg, HCO 20.9mEq/L, BE -2.

35. A 3-day old Neonate weighing 5 kg is persistently hypoglycemic. Current IV fluids are 15% dextrose running at 35 ml/hr. The following investigations are done with the results; interpret!

    Na135mEq/L, K 3.0mEq/L, Glucose 30mg/dL, pH 7.30, Cortisol 255 nmol/L

36. A VLBW preterm baby born at 31 weeks GA was intubated, given surfactant, and placed on a pressure-limited ventilator at PIP of 22 cm H2O, PEEP of 4 cm H20, Frequency(rate) of 20 breaths/min, I:E ratio of 1:3, & FiO2 of 0.3. The baby initially responded well, but 2 hrs later ABG values were as follows: pH 7.40, PCO2 36 mm Hg, PO2 35mm Hg.

    a. What is the most appropriate ventilator setting change at this time?

    b. At 12 hours of age, the ventilator settings and ABG values are PIP 26, PEEP 4, Frequency 25 breaths/min, I:E ratio of 1:3.5, & FiO$_2$ of 0.8. pH 7.16, PCO$_2$ 55 mm Hg, PO2 135mm Hg. What is the most appropriate change of setting now?

    c. At 18 hours of age, the ventilator settings and ABG values are PIP 28, PEEP 4, Frequency 60 breaths/min, I:E ratio of 1:1.5, & FiO2 of 0.9. pH 7.19, PCO2 52 mm Hg, PO2 50mm Hg. What is the most appropriate change of setting now?

37. ABG analysis results pH 7.22, PCO$_2$ 59 mm Hg, PO2 40mm Hg, HCO3 17 mEq/L, BE -4 were obtained from a 28-week gestation infant weighing 950 g, who deteriorated during Mechanical ventilation. What ventilator setting changes are important to improve the situation?

38. Match the following clinical scenerios of poor response to Neonatal Resuscitation with the possible underlying diagnoses.

Clinical Scenarios

a. Asymmetrical breath sounds, Persistent cyanosis/bradycardia, Scaphoid abdomen.
b. Pink when crying, cyanotic when quiet
c. Diminished air movement, Persistent cyanosis/bradycardia
d. Asymmetrical breath sounds, Persistent cyanosis/bradycardia
e. Pallor; poor response to resuscitation, symmetrical breath sounds

Underlying Diagnoses

1. Choanal atresia   2. Congenital diaphragmatic her
3. Fetal/maternal hemorrhage   4. Pleural effusions/ascites
5. Pneumothorax

Spitzer's Laws of Neonatology

Spitzer's Laws have been handed down to us from the very dawn of Neonatology, or perhaps one should say from the meconium-stained birth of our fine specialty. In those days, men were men, women were women, giants walked the earth, computers were the size of moving vans, and neonatology fellows were on call every other night but still found time for basic research on prostaglandins in fetal sheep. The subtler interpretations and corollaries of these laws have been lost in the mists of time, but they still contain useful kernels of truth for the post-modern pediatric house officer.

1. The more stable a baby appears to be, the more likely he will "crump" that day.
2. The distance that you have to go for a transport is directly proportional to the degree of illness of the baby.
3. The incidence of transport calls is inversely proportional to the number of available beds.
4. The nicer the parents, the sicker the baby.
5. The incidence of neonatal problems increases dramatically if either parent is a physician or a nurse.
6. Endotracheal tubes are designed to fall out (or become plugged, etc.) at the most critical moment.
7. The milder the RDS, the sooner the infant will find himself on 100% oxygen and maximal ventilatory support.
8. The likelihood of BDP is directly proportional to the number of physicians involved in the care of the baby.
9. The longer a patient is discussed on rounds, the more certain it is that no one has the faintest idea what's going on or what to do.
10. The patient who is glossed over quickly on rounds is the most likely to crump that day.
11. The sickest infant in the nursery can always be discerned by the fact that he is being cared for by the newest, most inexperienced nursing orientee.
12. The surest way to have an infant linger interminably is to inform the parents that death is imminent.
13. The more miraculous the "save," the more likely that you'll be sued for something totally inconsequential.
14. The probability of infection is directly proportional to the number of antibiotics that the infant is already receiving.
15. If it ain't CHD, it's PFC (or vice versa).
16. If they're not breathin', they may be seizin'.
17. Lasix (Vitamin L) will squeeze urine out of bricks. Unfortunately, it doesn't always work as well in babies.
18. Antibiotics should always be continued for — days (fill in the blank with any number from 1 to 21).
19. If you can't figure out what's going on with a baby, call the surgeons. They won't figure it out either, but they'll sure as hell do something about it.
20. The month you are on service always has three times as many days as any other month on the calendar.

I was both surprised and pleased to find my laws of neonatology on your extremely well-done web site. And while I am getting on in years (50 in 2 weeks!), I don't know that these laws were created at the "dawn of neonatology." It makes me sound like I brought them down from the mountain with Moses and his Top 10. In any event, though, I appreciate the PR, although it gets tougher and tougher for me to admit that with over 150 publications and a big fat textbook to my credit, the laws are my number one citation! I'm glad, though, that people have enjoyed them over the years. Thanks again for posting them. —Alan Spitzer

Courtesy : The Editor is extremely grateful to Alan Spitzer & to the WEB site-Neonatology on the Web

Created 11/27/94 / Last modified 1/18/97
Neonatology on the Web / webmaster@neonatology.org

1. **Retinal image showing stage 3, zone II retinopathy of prematurity with plus disease.** ROP is a leading cause of blindness in children and is caused by an incomplete vascularization of the peripheral retina leading to a subsequent overcompensatory neovascularization. Risk factors include degree of prematurity, birth weight and use of oxygen supplementation in the postdelivery period. Results of the Early Treatment for Retinopathy of Prematurity (ETROP) study that was funded by the National Institutes of Health demonstrated that peripheral ablation should be considered for any eye with type I ROP defined as (1) zone I, any stage ROP with plus disease; (2) zone 1, stage 3 ROP with or without plus disease; or (3) zone II, stage 2 or 3 ROP with plus disease (Slide). Serial examinations are recommended in type II ROP, which is defined as (1) zone I, stage 1 or 2 ROP without plus disease or (2) zone II, stage 3 ROP without plus disease. Patients with zone I ROP, especially aggressive proliferative ROP, have poor clinical outcomes despite proper screening and timely intervention using laser therapy.Hence, there is increased attention toward the downregulation of VEGF in patients with ROP, and preliminary studies and case reports have shown the successful clinical use of bevacizumab. *Refer to Chapter No. 25 Retinopathy Of Prematurity for further details of zones, staging and plus /preplus disease.*

2. **Prader-Willi syndrome (PWS):** Although PWS is associated with obesity, affected children classically present with difficulty feeding and subsequent failure to thrive in the first year of life. Newborns with PWS exhibit nonspecific findings including hypotonia, poor sucking reflex, diminished or absent cry, and somnolence. Early developmental milestones are delayed. After one year of age, there is a transition to hyperphagia. By school age, food-seeking behavior becomes increasingly difficult to control. Dysmorphic findings in a child with Prader-Willi syndrome include narrowing of the temples, almond-shaped eyes, strabismus, and a thin upper lip. Hypothalamic dysfunction is thought to be the basis for many of the phenotypic features, such as short stature and hypogonadism. Hypogonadism presents as cryptorchidism, small testes, and decreased scrotal rugae in males and small labia minora and clitoris in females. Puberty typically is delayed or incomplete. Learning disabilities always are present; however, affected persons may have low-normal intelligence to moderate mental retardation. Behavioral features in childhood include temper tantrums, high pain threshold, sleep disturbances, and skin picking.genes associated with PWS normally are expressed only from a region of chromosome 15 inherited from the father (PWS critical region).The genes inherited from the mother normally are inactivated. Therefore, children affected with PWS have a deletion or disruption of the chromosome inherited from the father or have inherited two copies of this chromosomal region from the mother. The latter situation is called maternal uniparental disomy. The risk of recurrence varies widely (zero to 50 percent) depending on the underlying genetic origin and can be determined based on the results of genetic testing. Other family members may be at risk for having a child with PWS and may benefit from genetic counseling. Treatment of a child affected with PWS involves the primary care physician and a multispecialty team that includes an ophthalmologist to evaluate for myopia and strabismus, a pediatric endocrinologist for consideration of growth hormone treatment, and a developmental pediatrician. Infants may require supplemental tube feedings to avoid failure to thrive. Physicians should be vigilant for hypoventilation and subsequent pulmonary infections secondary to hypotonia, because these conditions may cause early death. Early intervention for motor skills, speech, and language is necessary, as is an individualized education plan at the start of school. Generally, after the first year of life, strict dietary supervision and physical activity plans should be initiated to reduce complications of obesity. (C/F Angelman Syndrome(Happy Puppet Syndrome), a condition characterized by mental retardation, postnatal growth deficiency, inappropriate laughter, and gait ataxia. Several underlying genetic defects that result in the loss of a section of the maternal number 15 chromosome cause this syndrome.Three to five percent of patients with Angelman syndrome have paternal **uniparental disomy** of chromosome 15.)

3. **Tricuspid atresia - ECG.** Right atrial overload is manifest as tall P waves in lead II and left ventricular hypertrophy with strain pattern is seen in lateral leads with tall R waves, ST segment depression and T wave inversion. The axis is leftward with predominantly negative QRS in leads III and aVF. The biphasic P wave in V1 with sharp atrial intrinsicoid deflection (the sharp downward deflection from the peak of the P wave to the trough of the P wave) is a pseudo left atrial overload pattern, seen in right atrial overload. In true left atrial overload the atrial intrinscoid deflection is more slanting so that the negative component of the P wave is almost U shaped rather than the V shape in this case. All these features together in a congenital cyanotic heart disease is characteristic of tricuspid atresia. Down syndrome with an AV canal defect also shows superior axis; may later show biatrial and biventricular hypertrophy and a prolonged P-R Interval.

4. **The burst–suppression pattern in a neonate with severe hypoxic encephalopathy:**One pattern that portends a poor prognosis is the burst-suppression pattern. This pattern contains bursts of high-voltage activity composed of a mixture of delta-theta rhythms and spikes and sharp waves of 1-10 seconds alternating with low amplitude (background suppression) with <5 V. During the bursts, no age-appropriate activity is seen. The burst-suppression pattern is associated with a grim prognosis. *EEGs may show burst-suppression during sleep but a continuous tracing when the patient wakes up. In these patients, burst-suppression is seen during most of the recording and only vigorous stimulation wakes the patient. Nonreactive burst suppression is associated with an 86-100% risk of death or severe sequelae on follow-up. Use caution and serial EEGs in premature infants born at less than 33 weeks' gestational age before confirming the diagnosis of a burst-suppression pattern.Besides HIE, the following have been associated with a burst-suppression pattern: -Acquired and congenital infections -Inborn errors of metabolism (eg, nonketotic hyperglycinemia) -Chromosomal abnormalities -Brain dysgenesis -Intraventricular or periventricular hemorrhage -PVL -Focal cerebral infarcts -Pontosubicular necrosis.

5. **A-Diffuse Intracerebral Calcifications on CT Head Scan- Congenital Toxoplasmosis.**
   B-Periventricular Calcification and lissencephaly -Congenital CMV.

6. **Normal position of tubes and lines in a Neonate:**Frontal abdominal radiograph of a neonate with a UAC at the level of T8-9 and a UVC projected over the lower aspect of the ductus venosus. Note this patient also has a NG tube, an ET tube whose tip is at T2 and external temperature probe in the right axilla.

7. **Embolized PICC to right pulmonary artery:** Frontal chest radiograph shows an *embolized fragment* of a 3 French PICC, lying in the right ventricle, looped in the main pulmonary artery with the tip out in the right pulmonary artery.

8. **Epidermolysis bullosa (EB):** A heterogeneous group of genetic skin disorders, is characterized by fragility and formation of blisters following minor trauma. The group includes up to thirty clinical-genetic entities (1) with both autosomal recessive and autosomal dominant inheritance. The clinical manifestations vary widely from a severe, mutilating condition to a relatively mild disorder, with a marked variability within each major subtype (2). The most severe forms are multiorgan disorders with a poor prognosis (3). In the severe mutilating forms of EB, frequent complications include local skin infections, amputations as well as the occurrence of squamous cell carcinomas (5). In mouse models of EB, attempts at gene therapy are in progress.

9. **Rigler's sign:** *Sign of pneumoperitoneum. *Gas outside the bowel wall causes both sides (the mucosal and the serosal surfaces) of the bowel wall to be depicted. *Usually indicates a large amount of pneumoperitoneum.

10. **Transposition of the Great Arteries (D-TGA):** The heart is enlarged with a narrow "pedicle" giving the so called "egg on a string" appearance. The superior mediastinum appears narrow due to the antero-posterior relationship of the transposed great vessels and "radiologic-absence of the thymus".

11. **A-Pulmonary Interstitial Emphysema:** Collection of gases outside of normal air passage which is inside the connective tissue of the peribronchovascular sheaths, interlobular septa and visceral pleura results in compressing adjacent functional lung tissue, vascular structures and impedance of oxygenation, ventilation as well as blood pressure. Roentgenography: There are two basic radiographic appearnce

1. Linear radiolucencies; coarse and nonbranching, 3-8 mm, and vary in width but rarely exceed 2 mm 2. Cystlike radiolucencies; 1-4 mm, though generally round, they may appear oval or slightly lobulated. **B-Evolving Chronic Lung Disease**-Chest radiographs may demonstrate decreased lung volumes, areas of atelectasis and hyperinflation, pulmonary edema (PE), and pulmonary interstitial emphysema (PIE).

12. **A-Meconium Aspiration Syndrome:** The radiographic findings of meconium aspiration syndrome vary with the severity of aspiration. They may be normal if the meconium is largely tracheal and has been removed. Mild cases may simply manifest overaeration with small streaks or patches. In more severe cases there are overaerated lungs with asymmetric, coarse, patchy infiltrates due to subsegmental atelectasis. Pneumothorax and pneumomediastinum may result from sudden attempts to clear bronchi of meconium. **B-Pneumomediastinum:** Radiographically, pneumo-mediastinum appears as a radiolucency outlining the heart and mediastinum on AP films. The thymus is frequently elevated by air, producing the "angle wings" or "spinnaker sail" sign.There may be a continuous diaphragm sign caused by air in the mediastinum beneath the heart. Although it can be difficult to distinguish pneumomediastinum from pneumopericardium or a medial pneumothorax, pneumo-pericardium does not extend beyond the origins of the aorta and the pulmonary artery, and pneumopericardium and medial pneumothorax do not elevate or outline the thymus.

13. **Pneumopericardium:** Cardiac tamponade in a Newborn with respiratory distress syndrome who developed pneumopericardium associated with barotrauma from mechanical ventilation. Chest radiograph shows Pneumopericardium with Cardiac tamponade.

14. **Supraventricular tachycardia with RBBB pattern:** Supraventricular tachycardia with RBBB pattern as evidenced by the slurred S wave in lead I and aVL and rSR' pattern in V1. The right bundle conduction is slower during tachycardia and hence right bundle aberrancy is more likely to occur than left bundle aberrancy. It could also be a pre-existing right bundle branch block. In this case the patient had Ebstein's anomaly of tricuspid valve. Ebstein's anomaly can be associated with RBBB pattern or polyphasic QRS complexes. They can also have right sided accessory pathways which can predispose to atrioventricular re-entrant tachycardia.

15. **Arthrogryposis Multiplex Congenita,** is a rare congenital disorder that causes multiple joint contractures and is characterized by muscle weakness and fibrosis. It is a non-progressive disease. The disease derives its name from Greek, literally meaning 'curved or hooked joints'. Some cases are associated with an obvious etiology, but many remain without a cause. Neuromuscular conditions need excluding and there is some evidence that some babies are affected by first trimester coxsackie or enteroviral infection. Investigations like Cranial ultrasound scan, Nerve conduction velocity study, Creatine Kinase estimation, EMG, Karyotype, Muscle biopsy, and Congenital infection screen are necessary. Treatment is multidisciplinary and involves orthopedic and physiotherapy support in addition to all the therapists encountered in the child development centre. Prognosis is variable.

16. **Bilateral reflux extending into the pelvicalyceal systems of the kidney without dilatation of the calyces or ureters. (Note catheter in bladder):** **Voiding cystourethrogram** (VCUG): A test that examines the urethra and bladder while the bladder fills and empties. A liquid that can be seen on x rays is placed in the bladder through a catheter. Pictures are taken when the bladder is filled and when the child urinates. This test can reveal abnormalities of the inside of the urethra and bladder. The test can also determine whether the flow of urine is normal when the bladder empties. VCUG Results & grading: **Grade I**- Ureter only. **Grade II**- Ureter pelvis, and calyces without dilation. **Grade III**- Mild dilation of ureter, slight blunting of calyceal fornices. **Grade IV** -Moderate dilation, loss of sharp calyceal fornices. **Grade V** -Gross dilation of ureter and calyces. Most VUR is considered primary because of incompetence of the ureterovesical junction (UVJ), and it is not secondary to either obstruction or infection. As the UVJ matures to assume its adult 1.5-cm oblique path through the bladder wall, VUR tends to decrease in severity and eventually disappears just before puberty. An exception is in patients with an anatomic abnormality, such as a bladder diverticulum, into which the refluxing ureter enters. Incompetence of the vesicoureteral junction resulting from a lack of maturation is the most common cause of vesicoureteral reflux in children. Obstruction and infection rarely cause reflux. With maturation of the incompetent vesicoureteral junction, reflux usually eventually resolves.

17. **Meconium ileus:** Abdominal scout radiograph shows marked distention of the small bowel and a "soap bubble" appearance in the right side of the abdomen (arrows), a finding suggestive of mottled air and feces.

18. Ultrasound images of this neonatal brain shows massive IVH (intraventricular hemorrhage) from the germinal matrix. The IVH (bleed) is seen as intensely hyperechoic material extending into both lateral ventricles from the frontal to the occipital horns. The choroid plexus is obscured by the IVH. There is no significant intracerebral extension of the hematoma. However, early hydrocephalus is present. This suggests **Grade-3 germinal matrix hemorrhage in this Neonate.** Germinal matrix hemorrhage is graded from 1 to 4 as follows:GRADE-1: There is subependymal hemorrhage. GRADE-2: There is IVH without hydrocephalus. GRADE-3: There is IVH with hydrocephalus. GRADE-4: There is IVH with intraparenchymal hemorrhage. (Hydrocephalus may or may not be present).

19. MRI-T2 fluid-attenuated inversion recovery (FLAIR) sequence of a term neonate with **laminar necrosis of the cerebral cortex.** The bright signal within the cortex corresponds to necrosis in layer 4.The Neonatal cerebral cortex is vulnerable to laminar necrosis after a severe ischemic insult. This selective neuronal necrosis involves some layers more than others. In preterm and term infants, layers 3 and 5, which contain pyramidal cells, are most vulnerable, but in later infancy and childhood, layer 4 is most severely affected. This layer contains granule cells that are sensory, rather than motor, in function. *Layer 4 is largest in the striate (occipital) cortex, where it is the principal visual receptive zone.* Laminar necrosis is extensive degeneration of neurons in the affected layers, with relatively better preservation in other layers, though pyknosis and karyorrhexis indicating dying neurons are seen in neurons in all layers. These changes may be expressed in infants who survive as cortical blindness and spastic diplegia, though damage in other parts of the brain, such as the lateral geniculate body and periventricular leukomalacia also contribute to the clinical deficits. Laminar necrosis may be identified in MRI, particularly in fluid-attenuated inversion recovery (FLAIR) sequences, as a bright line of increased signal within the cortex and parallel to the surface of the brain.

20. Ultrasound images of the infant's brain revealed *multiple small cystic lesions (2 to 3mm. size)* in the periventricular part of the deep white matter. These ultrasound appearances are diagnostic of **Periventricular leukomalacia(PVL)** in the Neonate's cerebral hemispheres. Periventricular leukomalacia can also present as markedly hyperechoic white matter. This condition is the result of chronic ischemic insult (chronic ischemia) of the infant's brain during immediate postnatal period (in Preterm Neonates).

21. **New Neonatal 3-Tesla MRI transport Incubator:** MR-compatible incubators have recently been developed, permitting the complex and challenging task of obtaining Neonatal MRI to be accomplished in a controlled microenvironment with monitoring equal to that of the NICU.One such incubator, custom-built to provide thermal support, complete physiologic monitoring, and blended air and oxygen in a battery-powered unit, has been successfully used to safely image infants <1 kg. This unique system incorporates a camera that transmits continuous video of the infant to an external monitor throughout the scanning procedure.A significant advantage of the MR-compatible incubator is that once the infant is placed in the incubator in the NICU, the infant remains in a stable environment during transit to and from the radiology department and throughout the MR procedure. Upon arrival at the MRI suite, it is not necessary to retransfer the infant to the MR scanning table because the MR incubator docks directly into the bore of the magnet. The infant is not subjected to the cool air of the MR room or exposed to potential projectile objects.In many instances, the testing was completed with no sedation or anesthesia at all. The quality of imaging studies obtained using MR-compatible neonatal incubators is reported to be good to excellent.Visualization of the infant within the incubator is not possible from the control room; to ensure safety, a neonatal staff member must remain in the scan room at all times. Alternatively, an MR-compatible camera with a remote monitor can be added to the system to enable continuous, close-up surveillance of the infant throughout the scanning procedure, as mentioned above.

22. **Transient neonatal pustular melanosis**-All the lesions seen here are consistent with this diagnosis. The hallmark of this rash is the hyperpigmented spots that remain after the fragile pustules have resolved. Because the rash starts in utero, lesions may be in any stage at birth. Despite the anxiety-provoking appearance of a newborn covered in

pustules in the delivery room, no evaluation is needed when non-inflammatory pustules occur in combination with hyperpigmented macules in an otherwise well infant.

23. Congenital lobar emphysema of the left upper lobe and this Neonate was also found to have a patent ductus arteriosus. CXR shows: 1. Hyperexpanded left "lung" (actually the left upper lobe) that herniates into the right chest. 2. Spreading of ribs of the left chest. 3. Shift of the mediastinum to the right. 4. Compression of the left hemidiaphragm. 5. Left lower lobe atelectasis (It is so small, that you can hardly see it. It is largely obscured.) visible in the left inferior medial chest. 6. Normal position of the right hemidiaphragm. 7. No infiltrates or fluid. 8. All these findings are consistent with emphysema of the left upper lobe. What at first appears to be a tension pneumothorax may instead be severe emphysema of one or more lobes of the lung. Every attempt should be made to visualize lung markings and the lung edge within the hyperlucent space. Remember that lung markings may be very faint because the blood vessels are spread out. Additionally, there may be reflex hypoxic vasoconstriction as an attempt to match VQ. Carefully examining the CXR using a hot light may prevent you from mistakenly needling the chest and causing a severe complication. There are indeed lung markings throughout the left chest (These are evident on the original film, but it was very difficult to reproduce this on the scanned image). You decide to intubate the patient and transfer to the ICU, but the patient's condition worsens after intubation. What can you do? If this patient's emphysema becomes life-threatening (which may happen rapidly if positive pressure is applied) the only treatment would be a lateral thoracotomy to allow the lung to herniate out of the chest. When you call the surgeon, he/she asks if you are sure this is not hypoplasia of the right lung or a diaphragmatic hernia. An important aspect of pediatric emergency care is to be aware of congenital anomalies and the manner and timing with which they present. The differential diagnosis of any acute medical presentation in the first few months of life must include congenital problems. Within the first weeks of life, respiratory and cardiac problems often present precipitously. Whenever regional emphysema is present in the lung, suspicion of a foreign body should be very high. The young age of the patient made this unlikely but in the high-risk age group, approximately 5 months to 5 years of age, this diagnosis must be pursued even in the face of a negative history. Often bronchoscopy is needed to make the diagnosis and alleviate the condition. Courtesy: Loren Yamamoto, MD, MPH Associate Professor of Pediatrics University of Hawaii John A. Burns School of Medicine.

24. A-This is a typical RDS/HMD appearance on day 1. Note the following ·diffuse granuloreticular pattern ·air bronchogram lines. B-Hyaline membrane disease with focal interstitial emphysema (PIE), appearance on day 3.

25. Neonatal necrotizing fasciitis: Neonatal necrotizing fasciitis is a rare but serious and often fatal condition. A high index of suspicion must be kept if the diagnosis is to be made and treatment commenced. To date, the only predictor to prognosis is the time to surgical debridement. It is a condition that requires the services of multiple specialties including surgery, infectious diseases, intensive care, plastic surgery, dietetics, physiotherapy and occupational therapy. Patients with these conditions should therefore be treated in centres that provide these services and early referral from peripheral hospitals to a specialist centre must be encouraged. Refer to the Essential Clinical Guidelines No. 100 for the details of Case reports.

26. This lesion is almost certainly a cystic hygroma. Other possible diagnoses include branchial cleft cysts, thyroglossal duct cyst, goiter, and soft tissue tumors. Cystic hygromas are fluid-filled sacs that are related to lymphangiomas and are the result of an obstruction in the lymphatic system, most commonly in the neck or thorax when the cystic hygroma presents as a congenital lesion. Cystic hygromas are most commonly single cysts, but there may also be variants with multiple cysts, and they are found primarily in the neck region. While cystic hygromas are most often observed as a birth defect, noticed at the time of delivery (or on fetal ultrasound prior to birth), they may present at any time during an individual's lifetime. Although most hygromas are modest in size, some may contain an excessive amount of fluid and lead to obstruction of the superior vena cava, producing massive edema and leading to fetal demise. Some hygromas have actually been noted to become larger than the fetus itself. Most cystic hygromas initially arise during the 9th to 16th week of gestation,

though the majority appear to resolve spontaneously before birth. It is estimated that about 1% of fetuses will demonstrate a cystic hygroma during this phase of gestation. The actual incidence of visible cystic hygromas at birth, however, is only about 1 in 10,000 to 1 in 15,000 deliveries. About 75% of all cystic hygromas are located in the neck, with predominance, as in this child, to the left side. Other areas that may be affected are the axillary region, the groin, the mediastinal area, and the retroperitoneal region. The origin of cystic hygromas may not always be readily discernible. It is thought that they may develop from a failure of the lymphatic system to connect to the venous drainage system, or from lymphatic maldevelopment in which the lymphatic tissue retains some of its embryonic capability, settling in a region as a lymphatic "rest" and continuing to grow unabated. Genetic or environmental factors are present in many cases of cystic hygroma. The most commonly associated genetic abnormality is Turner Syndrome, though Noonan Syndrome, and Trisomies 13, 18, and 21 may also demonstrate a cystic hygroma as a finding. Klinefelter Syndrome and Fryns Syndrome may also have a hygroma as an associated abnormality. Some recent studies have suggested that vascular endothelial growth factor C (VEGF-C) may be a causative factor in the production of cystic hygroma. Isolated cystic hygromas may result from carrier parents, in which the disorder is inherited as an autosomal recessive. Environmental causes of cystic hygroma include maternal substance abuse, especially alcohol, and maternal viral infections, such as parvovirus, which has been implicated in the development of cystic hygromas. In many instances, however, the etiology of the isolated cystic hygroma cannot be determined. Evaluation of infants with cystic hygromas should include the following studies: *Chest X-ray *Magnetic resonance imaging or computerized tomography of the neck and thorax *Genetic testing for the disorders noted above* Prenatal ultrasound will pick up many of these lesions and amniocentesis or CVS, if found early in gestation, will help define the presence of a more general chromosomal abnormality. Chromosomal abnormalities will be present in about 40-50% of prenatally-detected lesions. With prenatal lesions, repeat ultrasound may be necessary to follow the lesion to insure that hydrops is not emerging and that vascular obstruction does not occur. *Chromosomes should always be performed if there is a fetal demise The management of these infants at delivery may be problematic if the lesion is large. It is recommended that infants with a cystic hygroma be delivered at tertiary centers, where the patient's airway can be appropriately managed and further evaluation undertaken as needed. The obstetrician may elect to perform a cesarean section, and it may be necessary to insert a needle into the hygroma to remove fluid prior to delivery. The neonatologist should be present at the delivery of these infants to insure an adequate airway and to rapidly assess the infant. While attempts to sclerose cystic hygromas have been tried and performed successfully in some cases, surgery remains the primary mode of treatment. Surgery is often performed soon after birth in term infants, but may be deferred for months if there is no airway compromise and the infant appears otherwise well. The primary reason for deferring surgery is the possible presence of smaller microcystic lesions in addition to the primary hygroma. Following initial surgery, it may be more difficult to find these smaller lesions for subsequent resection, because of the anatomic abnormalities and scarring that often are seen following the initial surgery. In some cases of cystic hygroma, the lesion may not be apparent for many years so that surgery may be needed at a later time in life. The prognosis for cystic hygroma will primarily depend on whether there is an associated genetic abnormality. In such instances, the prognosis becomes that of the underlying genetic entity. In isolated cases, the overall prognosis is usually quite good, though the earlier the lesion is seen during gestation, the worse the prognosis in general. The presence of oligohydramnios or polyhydramnios, especially if confounded by severe hydrops fetalis, is usually a harbinger of a poor outcome. In the cystic hygroma initially picked up at about 20 weeks' gestation or at birth, when unaccompanied by additional genetic findings, the prognosis is for a good outcome in about 70-80% of cases. A cystic hygroma that becomes infected may require antibiotics before surgery can be performed. There is a recurrence rate of about 15-20% following initial resection of the typical neck hygroma and the parents should be cautioned about this possibility. In some instances, repeated surgeries may be needed.

27. **Subcutaneous fat necrosis:** A rare disorder that affects the newborn in the first few weeks of life. There is often a history of a preceding stressful event such as fetal distress, asphyxia, sepsis, or hypothermia. As noted in the photograph, these are well circumscribed, indurated nodules which may be tender to palpation with a reddish, sometimes purplish discoloration. They affect areas of fat distribution such as the neck, shoulders, back and thighs. The lesion over the left shoulder had ulcerated. Some of these lesions were drained and sterile "pus" was obtained. This infant developed significant hypercalcaemia which is a known complication of this disorder. It was treated at the time with forced diuresis with frusemide, low calcium milk formula, and systemic steroids.

28. **"Autoimmune" rash:** This infant developed widespread skin lesions which appeared and disappeared in various places for few days. Some lesions had a target appearance with central pallor surrounded by an erythematous border. Others coalesced into large patches. Subsequently, the baby's mother was diagnosed with an autoimmune disorder, probably Systemic Lupus Erythematosis. The typical skin lesions of neonatal SLE affect mostly the scalp and face, but may be more widespread. These are erythematous, scaly and sharply demarcated. However, more widespread lesions may assume the character depicted in this photograph.

29. **Cutis aplasia:** A congenital absence of the skin. Most often it involves the scalp particularly at the vertex. Mostly singular but occasionally double or triple. They can be deeply ulcerated, or superficially eroded, or even epithelialized or scarred at birth. They are often small defects, but very large defects may occur. Larger defects may extend to the dura or meninges. Most often, these are isolated lesions, but they may be associated with a variety of congenital anomalies, chromosomal, or genetic disorders, so that a careful physical examination of the baby is essential. Small defects will epithelialize leaving an area denuded of hair. Skin grafting should be considered for lesions larger than 3-4cm in diameter because of the risk of septic or hemorrhagic complications or venous thrombosis. Although most often healing of an ulcerated lesion results in a flat scar, rarely, it results in a keloidal or lumpy appearance to the scar such as is seen in this 3 week old baby.

30. **Neuroblastoma:** Neuroblastoma is the most common malignant tumour presenting in neonates. It may be present at birth. The underlying abnormality is a proliferation of neural crest cells that normally give rise to the adrenal medulla and sympathetic ganglia, and as such can occur anywhere that sympathetic neural tissue is present. Although the adrenal medulla or retroperitoneum are most commonly affected, the primary lesion is frequently not found in neonates. The cutaneous findings may be of bluish, firm papules and nodules on the trunk and extremities. The lesions may blanch on application of pressure, thought to be due to the local release of catecholamines. The differential diagnosis includes leukaemia, lymphoma, and causes of "blueberry muffin" lesions (such as congenital rubella or CMV infection). Skin biopsy may be diagnostic. Other investigations that can be performed to confirm the diagnosis include elevated urinary catecholamines. Prognosis is dependent on the age of the infant and the staging of the tumour.

31. a) Uncompensated respiratory acidosis with moderate Hypoxemia. b) Uncompensated Respiratory Alkalosis with moderate Hypoxemia. c) Uncompensated Metabolic Acidosis. d) Uncompensated Metabolic Alkalosis with moderate Hypoxemia. e) Normal ABG. f) Mixed Acidosis with moderate Hypoxemia. g) Compensated Respiratory Alkalosis with moderate Hypoxemia. *Step 1: Analyze the pH* -The first step in analyzing ABGs is to look at the pH. Normal blood pH is 7.4, plus or minus 0.05, forming the range 7.35 to 7.45. If blood pH falls below 7.35 it is acidic. If blood pH rises above 7.45, it is alkalotic. If it falls into the normal range, label what side of 7.4 it falls on. Lower than 7.4 is normal/acidic, higher than 7.4 is normal/alkalotic. Label it. *Step 2: Analyze the CO_2* -The second step is to examine the pCO_2. Normal pCO_2 levels are 35-45mmHg. Below 35 is alkalotic, above 45 is acidic. Label it. *Step 3: Analyze the HCO_3* -The third step is to look at the HCO_3 level. A normal HCO_3 level is 22–26 mEq/L. If the HCO_3 is below 22, the patient is acidotic. If the HCO_3 is above 26, the patient is alkalotic. Label it. *Step 4: Match the CO_2 or the HCO_3 with the pH* -Next match either the pCO_2 or the HCO_3 with the pH to determine the acid-base disorder. For example, if the pH is acidotic, and the CO_2 is acidotic, then the acid-base disturbance is being caused by the respiratory system. Therefore, we call it a respiratory acidosis. However, if the pH is alkalotic and the HCO_3 is alkalotic, the acid-base disturbance is being caused by the metabolic (or renal) system. Therefore, it will be a metabolic alkalosis. *Step 5: Does the CO_2 or HCO_3 go the opposite direction of the pH?* -Fifth, does either the CO_2 or HCO_3 go in the opposite direction of the pH? If so, there is compensation by that system. For example, the pH is acidotic, the CO_2 is acidotic, and the HCO_3 is alkalotic. The CO_2 matches the pH making the primary acid-base disorder respiratory acidosis. The HCO_3 is opposite of the pH and would be evidence of compensation from the metabolic system. *Step 6: Analyze the pO_2 and the O_2 saturation.*- Finally, evaluate the PaO_2 and O_2 sat. If they are below normal there is evidence of hypoxemia.

Fully compensated states

	pH	PaCO₂	HCO₃
Respiratory Acidosis	normal, but <7.40	↑	↑
Respiratory Alkalosis	normal, but >7.40	↓	↓
Metabolic Acidosis	normal, but <7.40	↓	↓
Metabolic Alkalosis	normal, but >7.40	↑	↑

Partially compensated states

	pH	PaCO₂	HCO₃
Respiratory Acidosis	↓	↑	↑
Respiratory Alkalosis	↑	↓	↓
Metabolic Acidosis	↓	↓	↓
Metabolic Alkalosis	↑	↑	↑

Notice that the only difference between partially and fully compensated states is whether or not the pH has returned to within the normal range. In compensated acid-base disorders, the pH will frequently fall either on the low or high side of neutral (7.40). Making note of where the pH falls within the normal range is helpful in determining if the original acid-base disorder was acidosis or alkalosis. *Refer to Essential Clinical Guidelines No.78 "ABG Analysis in Neonates" for further details of ABG Interpretation.*

32. Hyponatremia, Hyperkalemia, Metabolic acidosis, and dehydration make **Congenital Adrenal Hyperplasia** the most likely diagnosis. The first three biochemical abnormalities, if associated with edema/circulatory overload *instead of dehydration* would point toward acute Renal Failure.

33. **Hypochloremic Hypokalemic Metabolic Alkalosis, suggestive of Congenital Hypertrophic Pyloric Stenosis.**

34. **Respiratory Alkalosis, Absence of Metabolic Acidosis, Hyperammonemia, Negative Sepsis screen in a previously well Neonate point toward an Urea cycle Inborn Error of Metabolism.** Ornithine Transcarbamylase (OTC) deficiency, an X-linked recessive disorder may be a possibility; urine orotic acid may be high and there is no specific amino acid elevation. The diagnosis can be confirmed by the absence of the enzyme in a liver biopsy.

35. **Hyperinsulinism** is most likely, as the large for date Neonate is still hypoglycemic, in spite of the current glucose requirements 17.5 mg /kg/ minute (10X %dextrose X ml/hr *divided by* weight in kg X 60). Values >12 mg/kg/minute are highly suggestive of Hyperinsulinism. Refer to the Chapter 16 "Neonatal Hypoglycemia" for detailed discussion of Neonatal Hyperinsulinism and its management.

36. a) ABG values indicate adequate ventilation with severe hypoxemia mostly due to low FiO2. **Increasing the FiO2 is the best option.**
b) ABG values indicate Hyperoxemia and Respiratory acidosis. **Increasing the Frequency** is the most effective way to increase minute ventilation and resolve the Respiratory acidosis. FiO2 should be decreased. c) Respiratory acidosis is still present but is now accompanied by Moderate Hypoxemia. Increasing PIP is the best choice because the resultant increase in minute ventilation and Mean Airway Pressure should improve PaCO2 and PaO2. Increasing frequency is also an acceptable alternative.

37. **Increase PIP, Increase FiO2, and Rate, & ensure synchronous ventilation.** *Other important Measures to be taken* : Excluding blocked/displaced ET tube, Pneumothorax, Mechanical ventilator fault, asynchronous ventilation, and unrecognized inadequate ventilation due to worsening underlying disease.

SUMMARY OF ADJUSTMENTS TO VENTILATOR SETTINGS ON THE BASIS OF BLOOD GAS RESULTS

OXYGEN	CARBON DIOXIDE	ACTION
Normal PaO$_2$ (45-75 mmHg)	Normal PaCO$_2$ (37-56 mmHg)	Sit tight ! unless weaning
Normal PaO$_2$	High PaCO$_2$	$\downarrow$PEEP; $\uparrow$rate; Keep MAP constant
Normal PaO$_2$	Low PaCO$_2$	$\downarrow$rate; maintain MAP
High PaO$_2$	Normal PaCO$_2$	$\downarrow$MAP (usually by $\downarrow$PIP): $\downarrow$FiO$_2$
High PaO2	High PaCO$_2$	Rare. Check for mechanical problems e.g. blocked tube. $\downarrow$PEEP: $\downarrow$T$_1$: $\uparrow$rate
High PaO$_2$	Low PaCO$_2$	Over ventilated - $\downarrow$Pressure $\downarrow$rate $\downarrow$FiO$_2$
Low PaO$_2$	Normal PaCO$_2$	Increase FiO$_2$; $\uparrow$MAP but maintain PIP (i.e. $\uparrow$PEEP or $\uparrow$T$_1$)
Low PaO$_2$	High PaCO$_2$	Increase PIP - which will increase MAP. In spontaneously breathing babies an increased rate may work
Low PaO$_2$	Low PaCO$_2$	Consider alternative diagnoses to RDS; overventilation

38. Special Circumstances in Resuscitation of the Newly Born Infant

Condition	History/Clinical Signs	Action
Mechanical blockage of the airway		
Meconium or mucus blockage	Meconium-stained amniotic fluid Poor chest wall movement	Intubation for suctioning/ventilation
Choanal atresia	Pink when crying, cyanotic when quiet	Oral airway, Endotracheal intubation
Pharyngeal airway malformation	Persistent retractions, poor air entry	Prone positioning, posterior nasopharyngeal tube
Impaired lung function		
Pneumothorax	Asymmetrical breath sounds Persistent cyanosis/bradycardia	Needle thoracentesis Immediate intubation
Pleural effusions/ascites	Diminished air movement Persistent cyanosis/bradycardia	Needle thoracentesis, paracentesis Possible volume expansion
Congenital diaphragmatic hernia	Asymmetrical breath sounds Persistent cyanosis/bradycardia Scaphoid abdomen	Endotracheal intubation Placement of orogastric catheter
Pneumonia/sepsis	Diminished air movement Persistent cyanosis/bradycardia	Endotracheal intubation Possible volume expansion
Impaired cardiac function		
Congenital heart disease	Persistent cyanosis/bradycardia	Diagnostic evaluation
Fetal/maternal hemorrhage	Pallor; poor response to resuscitation	Volume expansion, possibly including red blood cells

Summary Of Neonatal Resuscitation
* Pathophysiology – respiratory cardiac arrest
* Preparation – equipment, personnel, training
* Predictive risk   * Planning
* Protocol – neonatal resuscitation
* Post resuscitation care

Stopping and withholding Resuscitation: Current guidelines now suggest that after 10 minutes of continuous and adequate resuscitative efforts, discontinuation may be justified if there are no signs of life. Resuscitation may be withheld under a few circumstances. This requires a Co-ordinated, multidisciplinary team approach involving parents, obstetrician, neonatologist and perhaps anesthetist. *Conditions* 1. Certain death; Gestational age, Anomalies, Weight 2. Other; Borderline prognosis, Burden to child, Parental desires, High morbidity.

CAUSES & MANAGEMENT OF HYPOXIA DURING ANESTHESIA

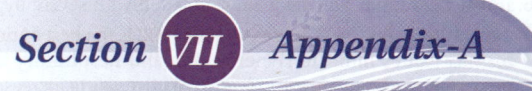

The causes of hypoxia during anesthesia can be attributed to problems in the *Airway, Breathing, Circulation, Drugs and Equipment*. By remembering to check the patient in this order, most of the problems causing hypoxia can be identified and treated. Using the headings below, consider what could go wrong during anesthesia to cause hypoxia.

Airway, Breathing, Circulation, Drugs, Equipment

What do you think is the most common cause of hypoxia in theatre or recovery?

CAUSES OF HYPOXIA DURING ANESTHESIA

The causes of hypoxia during anesthesia are summarized in Table 1. *Airway obstruction is the most common cause of hypoxia.* What should be done when the saturation falls?

During anesthesia, low oxygen saturations must be treated immediately and appropriately. The patient may become hypoxic at any time during induction, maintenance or emergence from anesthesia. The appropriate response is to administer 100% oxygen, make sure that ventilation is adequate by using hand ventilation and then correct the factor that is causing the patient to become hypoxic. For example, if the patient has an obstructed airway and is unable to breathe oxygen into the lungs, the problem will only be cured when the airway is cleared.

Whenever the patient has low saturations, administer high flow oxygen and consider 'ABCDE':

- A – airway clear?
- B – breathing adequately?
- C – circulation working normally?
- D – drugs causing a problem?
- E – equipment working properly?

You must respond to hypoxia immediately by giving more oxygen, ensuring adequate ventilation by hand, **calling for help,** and running through the 'ABCDE' sequence. Treat each element of the sequence as you check it. After you have been through all the checks for the first time, go back and recheck them until you are satisfied that the patient's condition has improved. WHO has put this into an algorithm or chart (below) to help you remember what to look for in a logical sequence. In an emergency, there may not be time to read what to do. You should ask a colleague to read through the chart for you to make sure that you have not forgotten anything.

Actions To Take If The Oxygen Saturation Is 94% Or Below

If the oxygen saturation is 94% or below, you should administer 100% oxygen, ventilate by hand, consider whether the problem is with the patient or the equipment, then move through the algorithm 'ABCDE', assessing each factor and correcting it immediately as you go.

Oxygen: Administer high flow oxygen if SpO2 is ?94%

A – Is the airway clear?

- Is the patient breathing quietly without signs of obstruction?
- Are there signs of laryngospasm? (mild laryngospasm – high pitched inspiratory noise; severe laryngospasm – silent, no gas passes between the vocal cords)
- Is there any vomit or blood in the airway?
- Is the tracheal tube in the right place?

Action

- Ensure that there is no obstruction.
- If breathing via a facemask – chin lift, jaw thrust
- Consider an oropharyngeal or nasopharyngeal airway
- Check for laryngospasm and treat if necessary
- Check the tracheal tube/LMA – if any doubt about the position, remove and use a facemask.
- Suction the airway to clear secretions.
- Consider waking the patient up if you have difficulty maintaining the airway immediately after induction of anesthesia.
- Consider intubation.
- If you 'can't intubate, can't ventilate', an emergency surgical airway is required.

Airway obstruction is the most common cause of hypoxia in theatre. Airway obstruction is a clinical diagnosis and must be acted upon swiftly. Unrecognized inadvertent esophageal intubation is a major cause of anesthesia morbidity and mortality. An intubated patient who has been previously well saturated may become hypoxic if the tracheal tube becomes displaced, kinked or obstructed by secretions. Check the endotracheal tube and – 'If in doubt, take it out'

B – Is the patient breathing adequately?

Look, listen and feel:

- Are the chest movement and tidal volume adequate?
- Listen to both lungs – is there normal bilateral air entry? Are the breath sounds normal? Any wheeze or added sounds?
- Is the chest movement symmetrical?
- Is anesthesia causing respiratory depression?
- Is a high spinal causing respiratory distress?

Bronchospasm, lung consolidation/collapse, lung trauma, pulmonary edema or pneumothorax may prevent oxygen getting into the alveoli to combine with hemoglobin. Drugs such as opioids, poorly reversed neuromuscular blocking agents or deep volatile anesthesia may depress breathing. A high spinal anesthetic may paralyse the muscles of respiration. In an infant, stomach distension from facemask ventilation may splint the diaphragm and interfere with breathing. The treatment should deal with the specific problem.

Action

- Assist ventilation with good tidal volumes to expand both lungs until the problem is diagnosed and treated appropriately.
- If there is sufficient time, consider a chest X-ray to aid diagnosis.

  The patient should be ventilated via a facemask, LMA or tracheal tube if the respiration is inadequate. This will rapidly reverse hypoventilation due to drugs or a high spinal and a collapsed lung will re-expand. The lower airway should be suctioned with suction catheters to remove any secretions. A nasogastric tube should be passed to relieve stomach distension.

  A pneumothorax may occur following trauma, central line insertion or a supraclavicular brachial plexus block. It may be suspected if there is reduced air entry on the affected side. In thin patients a hollow note on percussion may also be detected. A chest X-ray is diagnostic. A chest drain should be inserted as the pneumothorax may worsen. When there is associated hypotension (tension pneumothorax), the pneumothorax should be treated by emergency needle decompression through the 2nd intercostal space in the mid-clavicular line without waiting for an X-ray. A definitive chest drain should be inserted later. Always maintain a high index of suspicion in trauma cases.

C – Is the circulation normal?

- Feel for a pulse and look for signs of life, including active bleeding from the surgical wound
- Check the blood pressure
- Check the peripheral perfusion and capillary refill time.
- Observe for signs of excessive blood loss in the suction bottles or wound swabs
- Is anesthesia too deep? Is there a high spinal block?
- Is venous return impaired by compression of the vena cava (gravid uterus, surgical compression)
- Is the patient in septic or cardiac shock?

  Normally an inadequate circulation is revealed by the pulse oximeter as a loss or reduction of pulsatile waveform or difficulty getting a pulse signal.

Action

- If the blood pressure is low, correct it
- Check for hypovolemia
- Give IV fluids as appropriate (normal saline or blood as indicated)
- Consider head down or leg up position, or in the pregnant mother, left lateral displacement.
- Consider a vasoconstrictor such as ephedrine or phenylephrine
- If the patient has suffered a cardiac arrest, commence cardiopulmonary resuscitation (CPR) and consider reversible causes (4 H's, 4T's: Hypotension, Hypovolemia, Hypoxia, Hypothermia; Tension pneumothorax, Tamponade (cardiac), Toxic effects (deep anesthesia, sepsis, drugs), Thromboemboli (pulmonary embolism).

D – Drug effects

Check that all anesthesia drugs are being given correctly.

- Excessive halothane (or other volatile agent) causes cardiac depression.
- Muscle relaxants will depress the ability to breathe if not reversed adequately at the end of surgery.
- Opioids and other sedatives may depress breathing.
- Anaphylaxis causes cardiovascular collapse, often with bronchospasm and skin flushing (rash). This may occur if the patient is given a drug, blood or artificial colloid solution that they are allergic to. Some patients are allergic to latex rubber.

Action

- Look for an adverse drug effect.
- In anaphylaxis, stop administering the causative agent, administer 100% oxygen, give intravenous saline starting with a bolus of 10ml/kg, administer adrenaline and consider giving steroids, bronchodilators and an antihistamine.

E – Is the equipment working properly?

- Is there a problem with the oxygen delivery system to the patient?
- Does the oximeter show an adequate pulse signal?

Action

- Check for obstruction or disconnection of the breathing circuit or tracheal tube.
- Check that the oxygen cylinder is not empty
- Check that the oxygen concentrator is working properly
- Check that the central hospital oxygen supply is working properly
- Change the probe to another site; check that it is working properly by trying it on your own finger.

If it is felt that the anesthesia equipment is faulty, use a self-inflating bag to ventilate the patient with air while new equipment or oxygen supplies are obtained. If equipment is missing, mouth to tracheal tube, or mouth-to-mouth ventilation, may be lifesaving.

TABLE 1 — Causes of hypoxia in theatre – 'ABCDE'

Source of problem	Common problem
A. Airway	■ An obstructed airway prevents oxygen reaching the lungs ■ The tracheal tube can be misplaced e.g. in the esophagus ■ Aspirated vomit can block the airway
B. Breathing	■ Inadequate breathing prevents enough oxygen reaching the alveoli ■ Severe bronchospasm may not allow enough oxygen to reach the lungs nor carbon dioxide to be removed from the lungs. ■ A pneumothorax may cause the affected lung to collapse ■ High spinal anaesthesia may cause inadequate breathing
C. Circulation	■ Circulatory failure prevents oxygen from being transported to the tissues ■ Common causes include hypovolemia, abnormal heart rhythm or cardiac failure
D. Drugs	■ Deep anaesthesia may depress breathing and circulation ■ Many anaesthetic drugs cause a drop in blood pressure ■ Muscle relaxants paralyse the muscles of respiration ■ Anaphylaxis can cause bronchospasm and low cardiac output
E. Equipment	■ Problems with the anaesthetic equipment include disconnection or obstruction of the breathing circuit, ■ Problems with oxygen supply include an empty cylinder or oxygen concentrator not working ■ Problems with the monitoring equipment include a battery failure in the oximeter or a faulty probe

TABLE 2 — Learning Points to manage hypoxia in Theatre – 1,2,3,4,5,6.

Learning point : It is difficult to detect cyanosis clinically until the saturation is <90%. A patient who is severely anaemic may not appear cyanosed, even if the oxygen saturation is very low

Learning point : During anaesthesia the SpO2 should be 95% or above. If SpO2 is 94% or below, the patient must be assessed quickly to identify and treat the cause. SpO2 of ≤ 90% is A CLINICAL EMERGENCY AND SHOULD BE TREATED URGENTLY.

Learning point : Hypovolemia is the most common cause of a weak pulse oximeter signal during anaesthesia. Hypothermia should also be considered.

Learning point : Supplemental oxygen is often essential during anaesthesia. However, be aware that it can mask the effects of hypoventilation. Clinical vigilance will be necessary to ensure that ventilation is adequate especially if a capnograph is not available.

Learning point : When hypoxia occurs, it is essential to decide whether the problem is with the patient or the equipment. After a quick check of the common patient problems, make sure the equipment is working.

Learning point : if SpO2 is 94% or below, give 100% oxygen, hand ventilate, consider ABCDE

COURTESY: Dr. Iain Wilson Royal Devon & Exeter Hospital, UK

Figure 1. Algorithm for SpO2 < 94%

SPO2 < 94%

Assume HYPOXIA until proven otherwise!

Administer high flow oxygen ventilate by hand
Is the problem in the patient ?
Is the problem in the equipment?
Check ABCDE
Call for help early!

Airway → Make sure airway is clear, Use chin lift/jaw thrust if using a mask Reposition LMA if necessary, Treat laryngospasm if present → Check position of TT, check end-tidal CO2 is available, Listen to both lungs IF in doubt, take it out!

Breathing → Check that patient is breathing, check adequate rate and tidal volume, Hand ventilate with large tidal volume, Listen to both lung fields

Circulation → Check blood pressure, Check pulse & ECG for rate and rhythm, Look for blood loss, Ensure adequate volume replacement → If no pulse / BP/ signs of life Start CPR

Drugs → Consider drug effects- Opioids, volatile agents, sedatives, spinal anesthetics, Muscle relaxants

Equipment → Check pulse oximeter waveform Reposition probe on patient → Check oxygen supply, Make sure circuit is not disconnected, Check for obstruction in the breathing circuit, Use self-inflating bag to ventilate patient, Mount to mouth/TT if necessary

It is Important to Avoid forms of Stimulation that may be Hazardous to the Infant

Harmful actions	Potential consequences
Slapping the back	Bruising
Squeezing the rib cage	Fractures, pneumothorax, respiratory distress, death
Forcing thighs onto abdomen	Rupture of liver or spleen
Dilating anal sphincter	Tearing of anal sphincter
Using hot or cold compresses or baths	Hyperthermia, hypothermia, burns
Shaking	Brain damage

Complications of Neonatal Resuscitation

Complication	Possible Causes	Prevention or Corrective Action to Be Considered
Hypoxia	Taking too long to intubate	Preoxygenate with bag and mask. Provide free-fl ow oxygen during procedure. Halt intubation attempt after 20 sec.
	Incorrect placement of tube	Reposition tube.
Bradycardia/apnea	Hypoxia	Preoxygenate with bag and mask.
	Vagal response from laryngoscope or suction catheter	Provide free-fl ow oxygen during procedure. Oxygenate after intubation with bag and tube.
Pneumothorax	Overventilation of one lung due to tube in right main bronchus|	Place tube correctly.
	Excessive ventilation pressures	Use appropriate ventilating pressures.
Contusions or lacerations of tongue, gums, or airway	Rough handling of laryngoscope or tube	Obtain additional practice/skill
	Inappropriate "rocking" rather than lifting of laryngoscope	
	Laryngoscope blade too long or too short	Select appropriate equipment.\
Perforation of trachea or esophagus	Too vigorous insertion of tube	Handle gently.
	Stylet protrudes beyond end of tube	Place stylet properly.
Obstructed endotracheal tube	Kink in tube or tube obstructed with secretions	Try to suction tube with catheter. If unsuccessful, consider replacing tube.
Infection	Introduction of organisms via hands or equipment	Pay careful attention to clean/sterile technique.

PREPARATION FOR <750 GRAMS (before birth)

Decisions & Staffing:
Multidisciplinary decision for resuscitation
NNP, resident, admit nurse to prepare MD
called in time to be availabe for delivery.
Agree on doses / lengths by using weight
chart. Double check all resuscitation
equipment.

Environmental:
Turn on DR warmer, manual control, full temp
Turn on isolette & humidify to 80%
OR ambient temp 37 degrees C
If using thermal packet, take if from unit, keep warm
Have thermal packet ready (pre-weighed)
Open warmer pack with saran wrap on mattress
Have heel packs ready to activate at birth
Have UAC and UVC trays, gowns & gloves ready in NICU

Respiratory:
Double check all resuscitation equipment
Choose Neopuf versus flow-inflated bag
Have neo-bar or tape per-cut. Benzoin availabe
Have FiO2 set at 0.04 on blender
For Neopuff PIP = 20, PEEP = 5
for flow inflated bag PIP = 20, PEEP = 5
Decrease PIP as soon as chest rises

RESUSCITATION / STABILIZATION

Place in thermal packet

Place hat on head

Attach pulse oximetry to foot

If infant is 23 weeks, intubate immediately and give prophylactic Infrasurf

Either intubate so that the infant can be manually bagged for transport or place on HFNC prior to transport, (once you have assessed the infant's stability)

if possible, the mother should see and touch the infant in the transport isolette as it is being transported from DR to NICU. This should be brief and should not delay time to admission or place the infant at risk.

BEGIN RESUSCITATION

Assign Apgars

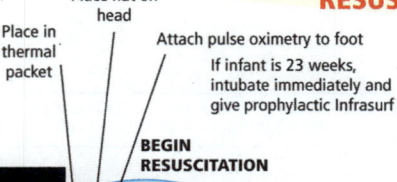

| 30 seconds | 1 minute | 2 minutes | 4 minutes | 8 minutes |

Gently wipe away fluid, (but do not waste time doing this excessively)

Place activated thermal packets (place between snuggie / saran wrap)

If infant is 24-26 weeks, use Neo-puff or flow-inflated bag to support infant and determine if infant needs to be intubated versus HFNC or CPAP via assisted ventilation with long prongs (wean PIP once chest rise is adequate)

If the infant's heart rate is not responding to respiratory support, intubate and proceed to full code (unless a clear agreement to stop resuscitation existed prior to delivery–as is sometimes the case with 23 / 24 week gestation infants)

AN ATTENDING SHOULD ALWAYS BE PRESENT FOR SUCH DECISIONS

Assign a team member to monitor the infant's chest rise and pulse oximetry during transport to the NICU

Stable infants should be out of the DR in 10 minutes!

Neonatal Autopsy

The death of a newborn is a tragic event and when contributing factors as to the cause of the death are discovered through a complete autopsy, parents can begin the healing process and plan future pregnancies realistically. Neonatal autopsies can be suggested when the cause of death is not evident or additional information is needed. Clinicians can confidently advise parents of the usefulness of the neonatal autopsy in ascertaining the cause of death or for counseling their future pregnancy. Neonatal autopsy remains a valuable diagnostic tool as it provides critical clinical and audit information for healthcare professionals and families.

The role of the autopsy:

- To establish factors (both in utero and post partum) contributing to death and (if possible) the immediate cause of death.
- To identify concomitant diseases, particularly those with implications for subsequent pregnancies (e.g. growth restriction, malformation, maternal diabetes).
- To confirm or exclude iatrogenic disease, including both birth trauma and complications of neonatal management.
- To provide information for audit purposes (e.g. cranial ultrasound).

Pathology encountered at autopsy

- Effects of hypoxia (occurring ante, intra or post partum), in particular hypoxic-ischemic encephalopathy.
- Growth restriction: symmetric, asymmetric (nutritional).
- Infection (predominantly septicaemia, pneumonia, meningitis): acquired in utero or post partum, including infections complicating invasive neonatal management.
- Malformation.
- Complications of prematurity, including:
- hyaline membrane disease and its sequelae

- CNS disease (germinal matrix hemorrhage, white matter infarction)
- necrotizing enterocolitis, etc.
- Iatrogenic disease:
- birth trauma: cranial, extracranial
- due to neonatal management: intubation/ventilation, chest drains, vascular access, medication, etc.
- Blood loss (in utero/neonatal, external/internal).
- Hydrops.
- Effects of maternal disease, e.g. diabetes, hypertension/pre-eclampsia.
- Metabolic disease, e.g. urea cycle defect, fatty acid oxidation defect.
- Placental and cord disease

Specific health and safety aspects

The pathologist needs to know the results of the antenatal infection screens. In regions of high maternal HIV prevalence, autopsy practice using universal precautions will significantly protect against accidental transmission.

Clinical information relevant to the autopsy

Wherever possible, the neonatal and (where relevant) obstetric hospital notes should be made available.

Information required

- condition at birth (cord pH, Apgar scores, etc.)
- clinical course following delivery, including methods of resuscitation and intensive care (including use of chest drains and vascular cannulae).

The Autopsy Procedure

- Requires availability of appropriately sized instruments; balances for weighing body (i.e. up to approximately 6 kg) and organs (to nearest 0.1 g); charts of normal values (baby and placenta).
- Whole body X-ray (for gestational assessment, malformation, pathological gas collections, position of cannulae and drains, etc. Mandatory for suspected skeletal dysplasia).
- Photography to document external and internal abnormalities.
- Routine external body measurements (body weight, crown-rump length, crown-heel length, foot length, occipitofrontal circumference).
- Detailed external examination, including: nutritional status/soft tissue and muscle bulk; presence of oedema (localized/generalized), pallor, meconium staining, jaundice or dysmorphism; evidence of trauma, siting of chest drains and vascular cannulae and other iatrogenic lesions. Report should include a description of external morphology mentioning specifically: fontanelles, eyes, ears, nose, patency of choanae, palatal fusion, spine, limbs, digits, palmar creases, external genitalia, patency of anus, umbilical cord.
- T- or Y-shaped incision; measurement of sternal fat thickness.
- CNS examination:
- paramedian skull incisions to allow assessment of falx and venous sinuses
- assessment of falcine and tentorial injury and meningeal hemorrhage prior to brain removal (suspected intrapartum trauma)
- exclusion of skull fracture by direct inspection; and spinal injury by posterior approach (suspected intrapartum trauma)

- if suspected CNS malformation (including ventriculomegaly): examination of posterior fossa structures by posterior approach
- observation of gyral pattern to assist gestational assessment.
- Detailed systematic examination of other internal organs, including:
- identification of pneumothorax (chest incision under water)
- positioning of chest drains
- umbilical arteries and vein, ductus venosus (exclude trauma/thrombosis secondary to cannulation)
- in situ examination of the heart and great vessels with sequential segmental analysis of malformations
- thoracic and abdominal organs removed in continuity or in blocks (if the latter, care is needed to assess structures (normal and abnormal) crossing diaphragm)
- weights of all major organs including thymus.
- Detailed examination of placenta and umbilical cord : can be helpful in assessing aetiology and time of onset of infection or hypoxic-ischemic encephalopathy; this may be of benefit in resolving issues of medicolegal interest. Placentas should be sent for examination when a baby is born preterm and/or in poor condition, or when there is evidence of infection, growth restriction, malformation or other significant abnormalities. Some units have mechanisms in place to allow storage of placentae for at least several days so that they can be retrieved if infants become unwell in the neonatal period.

Note: Ward staff should be asked to leave cannulae, drains, etc. in situ as far as possible, to allow assessment of their internal disposition. They can be cut flush with the skin if necessary.

Specific significant organ systems - None.

Organ retention (with appropriate informed consent)

- Organs with congenital malformations (particularly heart) if input not available from perinatal pathologist and abnormality cannot be satisfactorily recorded by photography.

- Brain for macroscopic and histological assessment of hypoxic-ischemic injury (timing, extent and severity), hemorrhage, malformation, infection, etc. Depending on circumstances, brain retention and possibly referral for specialist neuropathology may be indicated. However, submersion for several days, either in formalin with 5% acetic acid at room temperature or in 40% formalin at 37ºC, may produce sufficient fixation to allow adequate sectioning and block sampling if the brain is to be returned to the body before release.

- The consent form must be carefully checked for consistency with respect to tissue retention and achieving the aims of the autopsy. Permanent archiving of tissues blocks and slides should be the norm.

Minimum blocks for histological examination

- Thymus. • Heart (including papillary muscle). • Trachea/thyroid. • Lungs (at least two from each lung). • Small and large intestine. • Liver. • Pancreas. • Adrenal gland. • Kidney (x 2). • Costochondral junction (assessment of growth plate and bone marrow); bone histology mandatory for suspected skeletal dysplasia. • Brain: when systematically assessing hypoxic-ischemic injury blocks should if possible include: cerebral cortex and periventricular white matter, deep grey matter, hippocampus, midbrain (inferior colliculi), pons, medulla (inferior olives), cerebellum with dentate nucleus. Sampling may by necessity be more restricted if there is advanced autolysis. In cases of malformation, appropriate extensive sampling should be done. • Other organ lesions as indicated by history or macroscopic findings. • Placenta (at least two full-thickness blocks, plus focal lesions). • Membrane roll. • Cord (at least two).

Other samples required

- Bacteriology: lung, blood, cerebrospinal fluid, other (as dictated by clinical history or macroscopic findings).

- Samples for genetics, virology, biochemistry, hematology if indicated by history or macroscopic findings. In particular, with sudden unexpected neonatal death the possibility of metabolic disease should be considered and appropriate minimum samples would include: blood, blood spots (Guthrie card), skin (for fibroblast culture, i.e. not frozen), urine, and tissue for freezing (liver, muscle, etc. as indicated).

- For details on investigation of metabolic disorders, consult the Neonatal Metabolic Biochemistry

- These samples should be taken as soon as possible after death to reduce deterioration.

The clinico-pathological summary should include:

- an assessment of organ development relative to gestation and age at death

- a summary of the major findings

- a discussion of the aetiology/pathogenesis of these findings, and the timing/sequence of events leading to death (recognizing that neonatal deaths are frequently multifactorial and may not be attributable to a single cause of death)

- explicit statements regarding the presence/absence of malformation and infection and (where appropriate) growth restriction and trauma (negative findings are helpful and may be crucial)

- identification of those cases with an increased risk of recurrence (including malformation syndromes, growth restriction and maternal diabetes).

Specimen cause of death opinions/statements

- Spontaneous vaginal delivery at term; early neonatal death at age 12 hours due to total anomalous pulmonary venous connection.

- Maternal pre-eclampsia; intrauterine growth restriction; delivery by emergency section at 29 weeks gestation for deteriorating fetal condition; hyaline membrane disease and large germinal matrix hemorrhage; late neonatal death at age 14 days due to pseudomonas pneumonia and septicaemia.

- Spontaneous labor at 38 weeks gestation; attempted ventouse delivery for prolonged second stage; shoulder dystocia; fetal macrosomia with islet hyperplasia; early neonatal death at age 10 hours due to hypoxic-ischemic encephalopathy and cranial trauma.

Alternative investigations where permission for autopsy is not obtained:

Parents should be informed at the time of consent about the possibility of missing an important finding when a full post-mortem investigation is not undertaken.

1. **External examination by a perinatal/paediatric pathologist**, clinical geneticists or pediatrician

2. **Babygram:** Parents who decline an autopsy should be asked for consent to undertake a full body X-ray . A **Babygram** may detect abnormalities (mainly skeletal) which may not be detected on an external examination.

3. **A detailed Ultrasound examination** of the infant at the time of confirmation of an intrauterine death or after the birth may identify fetal abnormalities which may not be identified by an external examination

4. **Post-mortem MRI:** A recent comprehensive overview presented the advantages and disadvantages of the **Post-mortem MRI.** The major advantages of post-mortem MRI included the non-invasive nature of the examination and the detection of pathologies and malformations of the central nervous system. The disadvantages included the lack of tissue sampling; limitations in detection of complex cardiac malformations, and other abnormalities (e.g. tracheoesophageal fistula, bowel perforations) which are undetectable by postmortem MRI; and lack of experience in perinatal post-mortem MRI. The authors concluded that a full autopsy remains the gold standard; however, MRI may play an important role when an autopsy is declined.

5. **Clinical photographs** Following consent from the parents, clinical photographs should be taken for later review, particularly in the circumstance of birth in non tertiary hospital settings. These photos are additional to the bereavement photographs, and should be clearly labelled and filed in the medical record. The use of digital imaging for this purpose is optimal, however issues regarding storage and patient confidentiality should be considered.

6. **Post-mortem needle biopsy:** Laparoscopic autopsy and small incision access are other alternatives to a full post-mortem for focussed investigation of suspected abnormalities.

REFERENCES & FURTHER READING

1. The Value of Neonatal Autopsy : Leah Hickey Amanda Murphy Deirdre Devaney John Gillan Tom Clarke Rotunda Hospital, Dublin , Ireland -Neonatology 2012;101:68–73.

2. Clinical importance of neonatal autopsies: Halil Özdemir, MD. Ankara University School of Medicine Department of Paediatrics, Ankara.

3. Changing a Diagnosis: Carol L. Wagner, MD Marshall Goldstein, MD Sandra E. Conradi, MD , The Importance of Neonatal Autopsy: Journal of Perinatology 2005; 25:69–71.

For timely and appropriate intervention, fetal well-being needs to be assessed in the third trimester and particularly in labor. Fetal movement is monitored based on maternal perception. Lack of fetal movement for longer than 30 minutes suggests possible fetal compromise. Fetal lung maturity is determined as discussed previously in case of an impending preterm delivery and in making the decision to induce labor for any indication.

Tests for assessing Antepartal Well-being

Nonstress test

Nonstress testing is a simple low-risk procedure in which the fetal heart rate is monitored with Doppler ultrasonography or electrodes on the maternal abdomen or a fetal scalp electrode placed after rupture of membranes, along with the simultaneous recording of uterine activity with a tocodynamometer. After 32 weeks' gestation, the fetus responds to uterine contractions with tachycardia. The criteria for reactive test results are the following: *Heart rate of 120-160 beats per minute (bpm): Fetal tachycardia may be due to fever, drugs, or fetal arrhythmias or hypoxemia. *Normal beat-to-beat variability of more than 5 bpm: Decreased beat-to-beat variability suggests fetal hypoxia, sleep, prematurity, maternal sedation, or narcotic use. *Two accelerations of more than 15 bpm lasting more than 20 seconds each within a 15-minute test period: A reactive test is reassuring, with a high chance of intrauterine survival over the next 7 days. A nonreactive test, which does not meet these criteria, necessitates further testing for confirmation. The disadvantage of the test is variable reproducibility; nonreactivity may be a late sign of fetal hypoxia, a benign pattern, or the result of a prior asphyxial event. Statistics show that a reactive result is reassuring, with the risk of fetal demise within the week following the test at approximately 3 in 1,000. A nonreactive test is generally repeated later the same day or is followed by another test of fetal well-being

Contraction stress test

The contraction stress test (CST) is used to monitor fetal heart rate in response to uterine contractions that are spontaneous or induced with oxytocin. The contraction should occur within 30 minutes and last 40-60 seconds with a frequency of 3 in 10 minutes. In a healthy fetus, uterine contractions cause transient hypoxia and hypoperfusion of the intervillous space, which is relatively well tolerated. Early decelerations start with the onset of uterine contractions, reach the nadir at the time of peak of the contraction, and end simultaneously. These are benign and are seen in late labor from fetal head compression. Variable decelerations vary in their timing and relation with uterine contractions and occur in response to cord compression. They are benign unless they are associated with severe or prolonged bradycardia, are less than 60 bpm, last more than 60 seconds, are associated with an overshoot acceleration lasting more than 1 minute after a variable deceleration, or have poor beat-to-beat variability. Under conditions of uteroplacental insufficiency, a late deceleration is induced. A late deceleration begins 10-30 seconds after the onset of uterine contraction, the nadir is later than the peak of the contraction, and it returns to baseline after the contraction ceases. A CST result is positive if late decelerations are present with 50% or more of contractions. A CST finding is equivocal if decelerations are inconsistent. A CST is negative if at least three contractions of atleast 40 seconds each occur within a 10-minute period without associated late decelerations. A CST is suspicious if there are occasional or inconsistent late decelerations. If contractions occur more frequently than every 2 minutes or last longer than 90 seconds, the study is considered a hyperstimulated test and cannot be interpreted. An unsatisfactory test is one in which contractions cannot be stimulated or a satisfactory fetal heart-rate tracing cannot be obtained. A negative CST is even more reassuring than a reactive NST, with the chance of fetal demise within a week of a negative CST being approximately 0.4 per 1,000. If a positive CST follows a nonreactive NST, however, the risk of stillbirth is 88 per 1,000, and the risk of neonatal mortality is also 88 per 1,000. Statistically, about one-third of patients with a positive CST will require cesarean section for persistent late decelerations in labor. Drawbacks of the test are its duration, which is approximately 90 minutes, and the need for oxytocin.

Biophysical profile test

The biophysical profile (BPP) combines the nonstress test with an assessment of amniotic fluid volume, fetal breathing movements, fetal activity, and fetal muscle tone. A score of 0-2 is given for each parameter. In a reactive nonstress test, each of the following criteria earns 2 points: *At least one pocket of amniotic fluid greater than or equal to 1 cm depth *At least one episode of fetal breathing of 60 seconds duration within 30 minutes *Three or more discrete episodes of fetal movement *At least one episode of extension and flexion of extremities or spine Scores greater than 8 indicate a low risk and the need for weekly retesting. A score of 2 is strongly suggestive of hypoxia and indicates the need for immediate delivery (if persistent for 120 min). Intermediate scores need further evaluation. Maternal depressant medication and cerebral or neuromuscular anomalies may result in a low score. Fetal Biophysical Profile Element: Criterion (2 points for each element satisfied)

Breathing ≥ 1 episode of breathing movements lasting 30 seconds

Movement ≥ 3 discrete body or limb movements

Tone ≥ 1 episode of active extension and flexion of limbs or trunk

Amniotic fluid ≥ 1 pocket of amniotic fluid measuring ≥ 2 cm in two perpendicular planes

Nonstress test ≥ 2 fetal heart rate accelerations lasting ≥ 15 seconds over 20 minutes

Doppler study

A Doppler study of fetal umbilical arterial blood flow velocity or resistance to flow is another modality used to assess placental function, particularly to monitor high-risk fetuses. Decreased flow velocity during diastole indicates placental insufficiency, and, in severe cases, diastolic flow may stop completely or even reverse. Therefore, a systolic-to-diastolic umbilical blood flow ratio of greater than 3 after 30 weeks' gestation,(> 4 before 30 weeks` gestation) is associated with fetal compromise. RI(resistive index)- Normal Value (S-D)/S <0.8 in umbilical artery, >0.8 in middle cerebral artery. Researchers are still investigating the utility of measuring fetal arterial velocity in assessing redistribution in the hypoxic fetus and as indicators of placental circulation in pathologic placental processes, such as pregnancy-induced hypertension. Fetal scalp pH is used to accurately determine fetal hypoxia and acidosis. A pH level of less than 7.25 is considered abnormal, and a pH level of less than 7.1 mandates immediate delivery by the quickest route. The use of umbilical artery Doppler velocimetry measurements, in conjunction with other tests of fetal well-being, can reduce the perinatal mortality in IUGR by almost 40%. Doppler measurements of the middle cerebral artery can also be used in the assessment of the fetus that is at risk for IUGR and anemia.From 24 weeks on, a ratio of MCA/UA RI of less than 1.08 is considered abnormal and indicative of fetal blood flow redistribution in response to hypoxia. In cases of prolonged significant hypoxia, a paradoxic cerebral vascular dilation occurs and is reported to indicate extremely severe fetal compromise, possibly signaling imminent fetal death.

Tests for assessing Intrapartal Well-being

1. Continuous electronic fetal monitoring is widely used despite the fact that it has not been shown to reduce perinatal mortality or asphyxia relative to auscultation by trained personnel but has increased the incidence of operative delivery. When used, the monitors simultaneously record FHR and uterine activity for ongoing evaluation.

a. The fetal heart rate (FHR) can be monitored in one of three ways. The noninvasive methods are ultrasonic monitoring and surface-electrode monitoring from the maternal abdomen. The most accurate but invasive method is to place a small electrode into the skin of the fetal presenting part to record the fetal electrocardiogram directly. Placement requires rupture of the fetal membranes. When the electrode is properly placed, it is associated with a very low risk of fetal injury. Approximately 4% of monitored babies develop a mild infection at the electrode site, and most respond to local cleansing.

b. Uterine activity can also be recorded either indirectly or directly. A tocodynamometer can be strapped to the maternal abdomen to record the timing and duration of contractions as well as crude relative intensity. When more precise evaluation is needed, an intrauterine pressure catheter can be inserted following rupture of the fetal membranes to directly and quantitatively record contraction pressure. Invasive monitoring is associated with an increased incidence of chorioamnionitis and postpartum maternal infection.

c. Parameters of the fetal monitoring record that are evaluated include the following: i. Baseline heart rate is normally between 110 and 160 beats/minute. The baseline must be apparent for a minimum of 2 minutes in any 10-minute segment and does not include episodic changes, periods of marked FHR variability or segments of baseline that differ by more than 25 bpm. Baseline fetal bradycardia, defined as a FHR <110 bpm may result from congenital heart block associated with congenital heart malformation or maternal systemic lupus erythematosus. Baseline tachycardia, defined as an FHR >160 bpm, may result from a fetal dysrhythmia, hyperthyroidsim, maternal fever, or chorioamnionitis. ii. Beat-to-beat variability is recorded from a calculation of each RR interval. The autonomic nervous system of a healthy, awake term fetus constantly varies the heart rate from beat to beat by approximately 5 to 25 beats/minute. Reduced beat-to-beat variability may result from depression of the fetal central nervous system due to fetal immaturity, hypoxia, fetal sleep, or specific maternal medications such as narcotics, sedatives,²- blockers and intravenous magnesium sulfate. iii. Accelerations of the FHR are reassuring, as they are during an NST. iv. Decelerations of the FHR may be benign or indicative of fetal compromise depending on their characteristic shape and timing in relation to uterine contractions.

a. Early decelerations are symmetric in shape and closely mirror uterine contractions in time of onset, duration, and termination. They are benign and usually accompany good beat-to-beat variability. These decelerations are more commonly seen in active labor when the fetal head is compressed in the pelvis, resulting in a parasympathetic effect.

b) Late decelerations are visually apparent decreases in the FHR in association with uterine contractions. The onset, nadir, and recovery of the deceleration occur after the beginning, peak, and end of the contraction, respectively. A fall in the heart rate of only 10 to 20 beats/minute below baseline (even if still within the range of 110-160) is significant. Late decelerations are the result of uteroplacental insufficiency and possible fetal hypoxia. As the uteroplacental insufficiency/hypoxia worsens, (i) beat-to-beat variability will be lost, (ii) decelerations will last longer, (iii) they will begin sooner following the onset of a contraction, (iv) they will take longer to return to baseline, and (v) the rate to which the fetal heart slows will be lower. Repetitive late decelerations demand action.

c. Variable decelerations vary in their shape and in their timing relative to contractions. Usually they result from fetal umbilical cord compression. Variable decelerations are a cause for concern if they are severe (down to a rate of 60 beats/minute or lasting for 60 seconds or longer, or both), associated with poor beat-to-beat variability, or mixed with late decelerations. Umbilical cord compression secondary to a low amniotic fluid volume (oligohydramnios) may be alleviated by amnioinfusion of saline into the uterine cavity during labor.

2. A fetal scalp blood sample for blood gas analysis may be obtained to confirm or dismiss suspicion of fetal hypoxia. An intrapartum scalp pH above 7.20 with a base deficit <6 mmol/L is normal. Many obstetric units have replaced fetal scalp blood sampling with noninvasive techniques to assess fetal status. FHR accelerations in response to mechanical stimulation of the fetal scalp or to vibroacoustic stimulation are reassuring.

KEY POINTS FOR CLINICAL PRACTICE :

1. *Doppler flow velocimetry of the fetal vessels should be used by clinicians managing high-risk pregnancies and in conjunction with other methods of fetal assessment, such as fetal biometry studies, fetal heart rate testing, fetal biophysical profile, and infection and genetic studies.*

2. *Although many tests, including NST, fetal weight assessment, and uterine artery Doppler, may be somewhat nonspecific and may have misleading falsepositive rates, combining those tests with others increases the specificity. Test results that raise concerns require further investigation or active management.*

3. *Intermittent Auscultation of the FHR is recommended for low risk women in any birth setting (NICE 2007). Continuous CTG should be recommended for highrisk pregnancies where there is an increased risk of perinatal death, cerebral palsy and neonatal encephalopathy(RCOG 2001)*

REFERENCES & FURTHER READING:

1. American College of Obstetricians and Gynecologists (ACOG): *Shoulder dystocia*, Washington, DC, 2002, ACOG Practice Bulletin No. 40, ACOG. 2. American College of Obstetricians and Gynecologists (ACOG): *Ultrasonography inpregnancy*, Washington, DC, 2009, ACOG Practice Bulletin No. 101, ACOG. 3. Anderson NG, Jolley IJ, Wells JE: Sonographic estimation of fetal weight: comparison of bias, precision and consistency using 12 different formulae, *Ultrasound Obstet Gynecol* 30:173-179, 2007. 4. Baschat AA: Doppler application in the delivery timing of the preterm growthrestricted fetus: another step in the right direction, *Ultrasound Obstet Gynecol* 23:111-118, 2004.

Brain death in the Newborn

Death is defined as an irreversible cessation of all vital functions, especially as indicated by permanent stoppage of the heart, respiration and brain activity: the end of life. Brain death is defined as the irreversible cessation of all functions of the entire brain, including the brainstem, especially as indicated by a flat electroencephalogram (EEG) for a predetermined length of time. The causes of brain death in the Newborn are hypoxic ischemic encephalopathy (61%), massive intracranial hemorrhage due to birth trauma (8%), congenital malformation (6%), central nervous system vascular injury (6%), meningitis/infection (7%), nonaccidental trauma (4%), sudden infant death syndrome (7%) and metabolic disease (1%). **Determination of brain death:** Brain death is a clinical diagnosis that is based on the absence of neurologic function with a known irreversible cause of coma. Coma and apnea must coexist to diagnose brain death. This diagnosis should be made by physicians who have evaluated the history and completed the neurologic examinations.

Prerequisites for initiating a brain death evaluation: *Hypotension, hypothermia, and metabolic disturbances that could affect the neurological examination must be corrected prior to examination for brain death. *Sedatives, analgesics, neuromuscular blockers, and anticonvulsant agents should be discontinued for a reasonable time period based on elimination half-life of the pharmacologic agent to ensure they do not affect the neurologic examination. Blood or plasma levels to confirm high or supratherapeutic levels of anticonvulsants with sedative effects that are not present should be obtained (if available) *Assessment of neurologic function may be unreliable immediately following cardiopulmonary resuscitation or other severe acute brain injuries and evaluation for brain death should be deferred for 24 to 48 hours or longer if there are concerns or inconsistencies in the examination.

Number of examinations, examiners and observation periods: *Two examinations including apnea testing with each examination separated by an observation period are required *The examinations should be performed by different attending physicians involved in the care of the child. The apnea test maybe performed by the same physician, preferably the attending physician who is managing ventilator care of the child. *Recommended observation periods: (1) 24 hours for neonates (37 weeks gestation to term

infants 30 days of age) (2) 12 hours for infants and children (30 days to 18 years). *The first examination determines the child has met neurologic examination criteria for brain death. The second examination, performed by a different attending physician, confirms that the child has fulfilled criteria for brain death.

Apnea testing: *Apnea testing must be performed safely and requires documentation of an arterial $PaCO_2$ 20 mm Hg above the baseline $PaCO_2$ and 60 mm Hg with no respiratory effort during the testing period to support the diagnosis of brain death. Some infants and children with chronic respiratory disease or insufficiency may only be responsive to supranormal $PaCO_2$ levels. In this instance, the $PaCO_2$ level should increase to 20 mm Hg above the baseline $PaCO_2$ level. *If the apnea test cannot be performed due to a medical contraindication or cannot be completed because of hemodynamic instability, desaturation to 85%, or an inability to reach a $PaCO_2$ of 60 mm Hg or greater, an ancillary study should be performed.

Ancillary studies (EEG and radionuclide CBF) are not required to establish brain death unless the clinical examination or apnea test cannot be completed

Declaration of death: a. Death is declared after confirmation and completion of the second clinical examination and apnea test. b. When ancillary studies are used, documentation of components from the second clinical examination that can be completed must remain consistent with brain death. All aspects of the clinical examination, including the apnea test, or ancillary studies must be appropriately documented. c. The clinical examination should be carried out by experienced clinicians who are familiar with infants and children, and have specific training in neurocritical care.

Apnea. The patient must have the complete absence of documented respiratory effort (if feasible) by formal apnea testing demonstrating a $PaCO_2 \geq 60$ mm Hg and ≥ 20 mm Hg increase above baseline.

* Normalization of the pH and $PaCO_2$, measured by arterial blood gas analysis, maintenance of core temperature 35^0C, normalization of blood pressure appropriate for the age of the child, and correcting for factors that could affect respiratory effort are a prerequisite to testing.

* The patient should be preoxygenated using 100% oxygen for 5–10 minutes prior to initiating this test.

* Intermittent mandatory mechanical ventilation should be discontinued once the patient is well oxygenated and a normal $PaCO_2$ has been achieved.

* The patient's heart rate, blood pressure, and oxygen saturation should be continuously monitored while observing for spontaneous respiratory effort throughout the entire procedure.

* Follow up blood gases should be obtained to monitor the rise in $PaCO_2$ while the patient remains disconnected from mechanical ventilation.

* If no respiratory effort is observed from the initiation of the apnea test to the time the measured $PaCO_2 \geq 60$ mm Hg and ≥ 20 mm Hg above the baseline level, the apnea test is consistent with brain death.

* The patient should be placed back on mechanical ventilator support and medical management should continue until the second neurologic examination and apnea test confirming brain death is completed.

* If oxygen saturations fall below 85%, hemodynamic instability limits completion of apnea testing, or a $PaCO_2$ level of ≥ 60 mm Hg cannot be achieved, the infant or child should be placed back on ventilator support with appropriate treatment to restore normal oxygen saturations, normocarbia, and hemodynamic parameters. Another attempt to test for apnea may be performed at a later time or an ancillary study may be pursued to assist with determination of brain death.

* Evidence of any respiratory effort is inconsistent with brain death and the apnea test should be terminated.

Courtesy: American Academy of Pediatrics: Guidelines for the Determination of Brain Death in Neonates, Infants and Children: An Update of the 1987 Task Force Recommendations, Pediatrics September 1, 2011 vol. 128 no. 3 e720-e740 doi: 10.1542/peds.2011-1511

Algorithm to Diagnose Brain Death in Infants and Children

Comatose child
(37 weeks gestational age to 18 years of age)

↓

Does Neurologic Examinaton Satisfy Clinical Criteria For Brain Death?

A. **Physiologic parameters have been normalized:**
   1. Normothermic; Core temp. $>35^0C(95^0F)$
   2. Normotensive for age without volume depletion

B. **Coma:** No purposeful response to external stimuli (exclude spinal reflexes)

C. Examination reveals **absent brainstem reflexes:** Pupillary, corneal, vestibuloocular (Caloric,) gag.

D. **Apnea:** No Spontaneous respirations with a measured $pCO_2 \geq$ to 60 mmHg or ≥ 20 mm Hg above the baseline $PaCO_2$

No ↓

A. Continue observation and management
B. Consider diagnostic studies: baseline EEG, and imaging studies

Yes

Toxic, drug or metabolic disorders have been excluded?

No ↓

A. Await results of metabolic studies and drug screen
B. Continued observation and reexamination

Yes

Patient Can Be Declared Brain Dead (by age-related observation periods*)

A. **Newborn 37 weeks gestation to 30 days:** Examinations 24 hours apart remain unchanged with persistence of coma, absent brainstem reflexes and apnea. Ancillary testing with EEG or CBF studies should be considered if there is any concern about the validity of the examination.

B. **30 days to 18 years:** Examinations 12 hours apart remain unchanged. Ancillary testing with EEG or CBF studies should be considered if there is any concern about the validity of the examination.

* Ancillary studies (EEG & CBF) are not required but can be used when (i) components of the examination or apnea testing cannot be safely completed; (ii) there is uncertainty about the examination; (iii) if a medication effect may interfere with evaluation or (iv) to reduce the observation period

Neonatal Perioperative Management

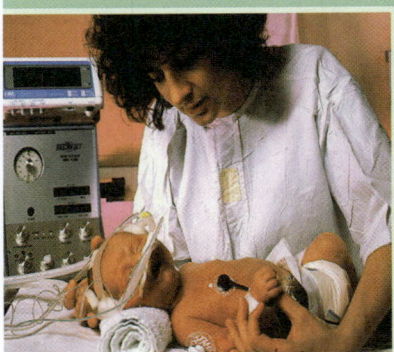

Infants with surgical problems may remain in the neonatal care setting for weeks or months, and providing ongoing nursing care can be challenging but rewarding.

Notify Pediatric Surgery as soon as you are aware of a pending admission or birth of a patient with a surgical problem. Notify Pediatric Surgery immediately if there are any major changes in the condition of a surgical patient. •*Do not begin feedings on a surgical patient without first discussing it with the Pediatric Surgeons.* •*Whenever possible, accompany your patient to the Operating Room. It is an excellent opportunity for learning and for discussing postoperative management with the surgical team. Patients born with one anomaly, particularly of midline structures often have others. Before proceeding to surgery in these patients, it is wise to get a cardiac evaluation (echocardiogram) looking for congenital heart disease.*

Preoperative care : 1. Ensure continuous monitoring is maintained and recorded hourly of:* Cardiorespiratory * Blood pressure * SpO2 * Skin temperature *Arterial cannula to monitor blood gases and pressure, where indicated 2. Take and record temperature 4 hourly. 3. Ensure arterial blood gas/capillary gas, FBC, group & cross-match, and U&E's are taken as ordered. 4. Check that two correct identification bands are on the baby. 5. Ensure baby is nil by mouth for prior to surgery: * If formula fed, last feed 6 hours prior to surgery * If breast fed, last feed 4 hours prior to surgery * If receiving clear liquids, 2 hours prior to surgery 6 .Administer IV fluids as prescribed. 7. Ensure Preoperative Preparation Checklist is completed, and a Well-functioning intravenous line . 8. Check consent form has been completed for surgery and the administration of blood and blood products. 9 .Explain all procedures and treatment to parents. 10. Ensure a parent accompanies baby to Theatre. Anaesthetic consent is usually obtained just prior to surgery. 11. Baby's notes, drug sheet are taken to Theatre with the baby. Newborns should be given 1 mg of vitamin K intramuscularly if they have not already received it.

Intraoperative care: 1. Maintain body temperature - Warmed operating room to 80°F to prevent loss by radiation ,Humidified, warmed anesthetic agents, Warmed blood and irrigation fluids used intraoperatively, Cover exposed parts of the baby, especially the head (with a hat). 2. Monitor-precordial stethoscope, pulse oximetry, capnography, NIBP, ECG and temperature (esophageal or rectal), urine output, utilizing a 5 Fr feeding tube as a urinary catheter, IAC allow for continuous monitoring of blood pressure and periodic assessment of blood gases, glucose, electrolytes including ionized calcium, hemoglobin, and base deficit. 3. Fluids, **electrolytes and glucose**-To prevent excessive fluid (and glucose) administration it is wise to run both maintenance fluids(hypotonic glucose solutions (D5 or D10 in either water or 0.2NS) (4 mL/kg/hr) and operative (insensible and blood loss) fluid replacement (isotonic fluid, 3-10 mL/kg/hr) on infusion pumps. The neonate loses approximately 5 mL of fluid per kilogram for each hour that the intestine is exposed. This should generally be replaced by Ringers lactate. Monitor blood glucose at frequent intervals to avoid both hyper- and hypoglycemia. Although total parenteral nutrition solutions containing high concentrations of glucose should not be stopped abruptly due to the possibility of rebound hypoglycemia, perioperative hyperglycemia can occur easily when high glucose containing fluids are given in combination with operative stress. 4. **Extubation** Immediate postoperative extubation in the neonate

requires that the patient be awake with full strength (hip flexion, arms lifting), have a low likelihood of airway obstruction (normal airway anatomy), normal temperature, blood pressure and volume status, and regular respiratory pattern with adequate minute ventilation. **Postoperative Care :**When patient returns from the Operating Room, obtain sign-out from the Surgical Resident and discuss orders for postoperative care. Also, obtain sign-out from the Anesthesia Resident regarding (a) anesthesia, other drugs, and fluids that the patient received and (b) events during the operative procedure. IV fluid replacement at maintenance levels with parenteral nutrition starting within 2d of operation. Intermittent fluid boluses may be required in the first 48h to maintain adequate urine output and to treat hypotension and hypoperfusion. Consider early use of low-dose dopamine (3-5 mcg/kg/min). If there has been extensive bowel manipulation, the baby may require baseline fluid administration 1.5 times normal (*i.e.*, 150 mL/kg/d) because of capillary leak. Use Lactated Ringer's Solution with 5% or 10% dextrose for at least the first 24h after operation. Urine output is an objective measure of volume status. Urine output of 2 mL/kg/h is acceptable in neonates and infants, **Continue preoperative antibiotic therapy:** The duration of antibiotics depends on the underlying bowel problem and whether fecal contamination of the peritoneal cavity has occurred. **Vital Signs-**Provide instructions for the frequency at which vital signs are monitored and recorded. Parameters for changes in vital signs that require notification of the surgical team are clearly specified. A core-peripheral temperature deficit of more than 2°C as well as tachycardia and tachypnea may indicate hypovolemia and poor tissue perfusion. Invasive blood pressure monitoring is essential when infants require inotropic sup- port and frequent blood sampling. Assessment of perfusion by checking capillary refill time may also indicate the need for fluid bolus if more than 2 seconds. **Postoperative apnea-**immaturity of brainstem respiratory control mechanism and increased sensitivity to the respiratory depressant effects of anesthetics, sedatives and analgesics, combined with increased work of breathing and easy fatigability of the diaphragm, increases the risk of life-threatening hypoventilation or apnea during spontaneous ventilation in the operating room and following surgery. Although all preterm and ex-preterm infants are at risk for PAA, factors which increase risk include younger gestational and PCA, prior history of apnea events, hemoglobin < 10 gm/dL.. Other factors include hypothermia, hypoglycemia, hypoxia, sepsis, and hypocalcemia, which occur with greater frequency in neonates who undergo emergency surgery. Spinal anesthesia in the absence of any other anesthetics/sedatives/analgesics may decrease the risk of postoperative apnea, and is reserved for elective inguinal herniorrhaphy in the former premature infant. Caffeine 10 mg/kg slowly IV at the start of surgery may minimize the risk of postanesthetic apnea.* If the surgical condition allows, infants with obstructive apnea may benefit from being nursed prone at a 30-degree angle, as this position improves both oxygenation and minute ventilation and can reduce the risk of reflux or aspiration. Administration of low-flow oxygen may help maintain oxygen saturation and prevent further respiratory distress. **Monitoring Equipment-**List any special monitoring devices that are appropriate for postoperative care including pulse oximetry, apnea and/or cardiac monitors, etc. Maintain **A double lumen sump drain (Replogle®) tube to continuous suction and measure output.** If drainage is more than 10 mL/kg per 12h shift, replace volume loss with an equal volume of 0.45% NaCl. •Replogle tube may be removed when drainage is minimal and non-bilious. •After the baby has passed stool, start feedings with small volumes and advance slowly over the next 48h to ensure that baby is not developing abdominal distension secondary to postoperative ileus or to stricture at the anastomotic site. **Ensure adequate analgesia-**Pain in patients who have undergone minor procedures (e.g., hernia repair) is generally controllable with oral analgesics such as acetaminophen, ibuprofen, or oxycodone/acetaminophen. Local anesthetics administered in the operating room can provide prolonged pain control. Local wound infiltration or regional nerve blocks with bupivicaine provide pain control for 4-6 hours following an operation. The maximum dose is 3 mg/kg given as a 0.25–0.75% solution. For larger operations, intravenous narcotics provide excellent pain control (Morphine-Incremental IV boluses of 20 mcg/kg, not to exceed 100 mcg/kg, are typically administered for acute pain management in the postanesthesia recovery unit. When a continuous IV infusion is used for postoperative pain management in neonates, the initial rate varies depending on the patient's age. Initial IV infusion rates of 10 mcg/kg/h are acceptable for neonates younger than 1 week. Neonates older than 1 week tolerate 15 mcg/kg/h, whereas older infants may tolerate 20-40 mcg/kg/h. Supplemental IV boluses of as much as 50 mcg/kg may be administered for episodes of breakthrough pain in neonates who are receiving morphine by means of continuous infusion.)Fentanyl is most appropriately administered by means of intravenous (IV) infusion to neonates who are preoperatively ventilated and who are expected to remain ventilated postoperatively. Episodes of apnea are more severe when this drug is administered as an IV bolus of 1-2 mcg/kg than when it is given as a continuous IV infusion of 1-2 mcg/kg/h. However, respiratory depression may be less problematic in infants than in neonates. Too-rapid bolus administration has been associated with acute rigidity of the chest wall that severely compromises ventilation of the patient. Liberal use of patient controlled analgesia devices and epidural catheters improve postoperative pain control after many abdominal or thoracic operations. Consider the use of intravenous patient-controlled analgesia (PCA) or parent or nurse-controlled analgesia (PNCA). With PNCA, either a nurse or parent administers a predetermined intravenous dose of opioid analgesia using a PCA pump when they feel the patient is experiencing substantial pain. Although patient-controlled analgesia (PCA) has been shown to be safe, effective, and superior to intermittent opioid dosing, infants and young children are not able to operate PCA independently. Allowing a parent or nurse to operate the PCA for the child [parent/nurse-controlled analgesia (PNCA)] may be an option for these children. *Enteral/parenteral nutrition: The goal following abdominal surgery is early enteral feeding. Tolerance of enteral feeds depends on gestational age, type of surgery, and the length and integrity of the remaining gastrointestinal tract. Small-volume feeding can be commenced when gastric aspirate or drainage decreases to 20 mL/kg/day and there is evidence of bowel function. Recommendations include: Breast milk (maternal or donor) is the first choice. Alternatively, an elemental formula which is easier to digest than standard infant formula, may be used. Gradual increase in feeds, 1-2 mL per day; continuous appears to be better tolerated initially. Assess tolerance of feeds: amount of gastric aspirate/residuals, stoma/stool loss and frequency, and abdominal girth. Weight and growth chart recordings. Stools for fat absorption, pH, and reducing substances. Parenteral nutrition (PN) has improved survival of both the preterm and the surgical neonate in the last few decades. Long-term PN is associated with catheter-related sepsis and cholestatic jaundice, leading to progressive liver failure and recurring episodes of infection from bacterial overgrowth and translocation in the residual bowel. Improved preparation and management of administration of PN can reduce the complications associated with long-term use. Infants requiring long-term PN ideally should be cared for by a multidisciplinary team.

*. Prevent Hypothermia :The surgical neonate should have core temperature maintained at 36.7-37.3°C by control of ambient and/or skin temperature. To achieve this, most infants require an environmental temperature of 34-36.5°C. Special attention to body temperature and measures to prevent hypothermia after drape removal should be instituted including infrared heating lights, wrapping with warm blankets, and increasing the ambient room temperature. Specific instructions- If observation status or discharge from the recovery unit is desired, specific instructions regarding wounds, medications, and anticipated clinical course/problems are provided to the parents or primary caregiver. List

the primary diagnosis and/or the procedure that has been performed, drug allergies or other sensitivities (i.e., latex, tape, antibiotics, pain medications, etc.) Ventilator Settings and Respiratory Care- For patients requiring postoperative ventilatory support, specific instructions regarding ventilator mode, tidal volume, peak inspiratory pressure, inspired oxygen concentration, etc. are provided. If other respiratory interventions (i.e., nebulizers, chest physiotherapy, frequent suctioning) are required, specific written orders are made. Diet-Special diets (i.e., clear liquids, general diet) or oral restriction (i.e., NPO) are specified, including orders for initiation of enteral tube feedings when applicable. Medications-All medications including doses, routes of administration, and frequencies of administration are recorded clearly and accurately. Analgesic and antiemetic medications are ordered when appropriate. Doses are calculated on a per weight basis. Wound and Dressing Care - The surgical neonate, even if term, is at increased risk of skin and tissue damage due to the following factors: surgery, edema, ventilation and paralysis, ostomies, silos, wounds, central venous lines, tubes, urinary catheters, and inotropic drugs. General considerations for maintaining good skin integrity and wound healing include-Assessment, evaluation, and management of wounds and skin injury by the use of a wound assessment chart/tool, which clearly identifies each phase of wound healing . The use of appropriate cleansing solutions, such as normal saline or sterile water, avoid irritating/absorptive substances; The use of appropriate dressings: occlusive to bacteria, nonadherent, promote wound healing by absorbing debris/discharge; Decreased use of baby soap and routine bathing and the use of emollients have shown improved skin condition in the preterm infant ; and Access to expert advice: tissue viability nurse, stoma nurse, and/or plastic surgeon. Drains-Drain care orders include specific requests for suction, stripping, frequency of emptying, and quantification of output. Nasogastric tubes are placed to suction or gravity drainage according to attending surgeon preference. Foley catheters are placed to gravity drainage. Special Studies- Any radiographic exams or follow-up studies are specified, and the radiology department and/or attending radiologist should be notified of all requests. Chest radiographs are obtained in the recovery room or intensive care unit for all patients who remain intubated or who had intraoperative placement of central venous lines or catheters. Laboratory Tests-Routine laboratory testing is often not necessary in pediatric surgical patients, especially those who have procedures in the surgicenter and are discharged shortly after surgery. Specific laboratory studies are obtained if the results are expected to alter clinical management of the patient. Laboratory tests are often indicated in children who undergo extensive and complicated procedures.

*Parental support : The need for support, compassion, and correct and easily understood information is paramount in the nursing management of the surgical neonate. Once the infant's condition allows, parents should be encouraged to participate in family-centered care, including skin-to-skin or kangaroo care, bathing, and feeding, to establish parent–infant bonding.

*Neurodevelopmental care: Guidance on best positioning and handling to promote midline development (often in particular flexion), hand-to-mouth coordination, and visual tracking are all of vital importance in the long-term outcome of these vulnerable infants.

Key points for Clinical practice: 1. Early communication between the obstetrician, neonatologist, surgeon and anaesthetist, as well as the nursing team involved in caring for the infant, is essential. 2. Following surgery, neonates are susceptible to apnoea and poor temperature control. 3. Pharmacodynamics and pharmacokinetics in neonates differ markedly from older children and so maturity as well as weight needs to be taken into consideration when drawing up a drug dosing schedule. 4. Fluid losses and electrolyte balances as well as nutrition need careful monitoring in postoperative infants. Weight, urine output, electrolyte balance, and the general condition of the infant should be assessed

Neonatal Perioperative Management

regularly. 5. Regional anaesthesia is a good way of achieving analgesia in surgical neonates.

ANESTHESIA IN THE NEONATE (Refer to Essential Guidelines- 90, Page 935)

References: 1. **Anesthetic** Management of a Neonate with a Surgical Emergency Lynne G. Maxwell, M.D. Philadelphia, Pennsylvania 2. **Immediate** Postoperative Care , http://pediatric-infant-surgery.blogspot.in/2009/03/immediate-postoperative-care.html 3. **Perioperative** Pain Management in Newborns *Author: Jeana Havidich, MD; Chief Editor: Ted Rosenkrantz, MDhttp://emedicine.medscape.com/article/980222-overview#aw2aab6b7

Neonatal Surgery Stoma Care: *Stoma care: Close postoperative observation is required as dusky or purple stomas may indicate impending necrosis and require surgical review. The stoma should be protected with a Vaseline gauze and a simple dressing until the stoma is active, when a suitable stoma appliance can be applied. Subsequent complications include bleeding, infection, prolapse, retraction, skin breakdown, increased stoma losses, and granulation tissue. *Initial Cares-* Observe color of blind end of stoma. Observe and document stoma for perfusion, bleeding, skin integrity and signs of infection or prolapse every 4-6 hours. Measure stoma output. Notify medical staff is there is >30-49mls/kg/day stoma output. Ensure the skin surrounding the stoma is protected from excoriating effects of enzymes by: Covering area around stoma with orobase paste including wound/suture line and around the edge of the stoma. Covering the stoma with Paraffin gauze. Covering the Vaseline with dry gauze. Secure by applying base tapes on either side of the dressing and tapping onto these to reduce skin trauma. Check stoma with cares 4 to 6 hourly for wound ooze, bleeding (small spots of blood common with cleaning) and bowel motion. Clean with warm sterile saline until wound suture line healed then warm sterile water can be used. As soon as the baby starts passing enough bowel motion so that it is getting onto surrounding skin, a stoma bag needs to be applied. This is usually 2-4 days post-op. In the first week post op the stoma will decrease in size as the swelling resolves, therefore the size of the hole cut in the flange will need re-measuring (when new bag applied). *Stabilizing the Stoma-* Stoma bag must be changed as soon as it leaks. Check flange and bag with cares, ensure flange is not leaking, if the flange is stained underneath then it has leaked and needs to be changed. Bag needs to be emptied when 1/3 full of bowel motion or gas as it will lift the flange. To change bag if leaking: Gather equipment: gloves, bowl, warm water (no soap), gauze, orobase paste, cotton buds, appropriate sized bag and clip, scissors, stoma size gauge or last flange backing for size, non sting spray, adhesive stoma paste or powder. Carefully remove old bag from the top edge downwards, clean skin with warm water, dry well; assess skin for any signs of excoriation. Assess stoma for any changes in color, size or excessive bleeding. Cut hole in flange to fit the size and shape of stoma, the flange needs to fit over the stoma with a gap of approximately 2mm from edge of stoma to flange. If the flange is too close to the stoma then the mucus from the stoma will cause the flange to lift. If the flange is not close enough to the stoma then the surrounding skin could become excoriated. Warm flange between hands for approximately one minute. Apply orobase to the edge of the hole cut in the flange with a cotton bud and to any excoriated areas. Apply flange and apply pressure to the flange for one minute and press down all edges. Check the flange is attached well. Close end of pouch with clip provided. *Pre-closure of Stoma - Distal End Wash Out-*A contrast study may be requested prior to closure of the stoma, as per individual surgeon orders. Ensure that warmed 0.9% sodium chloride 10ml/kg is used. With a size 8 feeding tube lubricated with KY jelly, intubate the stoma 1-2cm **or** until there is resistance. Flush saline through with a syringe using minimal pressure. Fluid coming out through the rectum must be clear pre operative.

Reference: http://www.adhb.govt.nz/newborn/guidelines/Surgery/SurgeryStoma.htm

Bowel irrigation : All patients with Hirschsprung's disease receive irrigations in the newborn period to manage distension prior to proceeding with surgery. It is extremely important to clarify the difference between irrigation and an enema. To confuse these two terms may be dangerous for babies with Hirschsprung's disease. An enema is a procedure in which a determined amount of fluid is instilled into the rectum and colon. It is expected that this volume will be spontaneously expelled. Rectal irrigation, on the other hand, is a procedure in which a large tube is introduced through the rectum, and small amounts of saline solution (10-20 mL) are instilled through the lumen of the tube in order to clear the bowel. The rectal and colonic content is expected to drain through the same lumen of the tube. The tube is then rotated in different directions and moved back and forth. The operator continues to instill small amounts of saline solution, allowing the evacuation of gas and liquid stool through the tube. Patients with Hirschsprung's disease have a very serious dysmotility disorder. This means that an enema may aggravate the condition rather than help since there is no capacity to expel the infused volume of fluid. With an irrigation, the patient benefits from the evacuation of the rectosigmoid contents through the lumen of the large tube. Enterocolitis may occur with prolonged distension and faecal stasis. The stasis leads to bacterial overgrowth, which leads to bacterial translocation and secretory diarrhoea. Enterocolitis must be suspected clinically. The infant can become quite ill from sepsis, hypovolemia, and endotoxin-related shock. Bowel irrigation with saline solution is an extremely valuable procedure for the emergency management of enterocolitis. By decompressing the bowel, the procedure may dramatically improve a very ill infant. These patients should also receive intravenous fluids and antibiotics (either metronidazole or ciprofloxacin). In the beginning of the treatment it is important to keep the child NPO until they begin to improve.

Supplies * Silicone Foley catheter the size of your child's thumb (16 Fr. for children under one year of age to a maximum of 24 Fr. for children over one year of age). It may be necessary to put additional holes on the side of the catheter. The Foley balloon is NEVER inflated. * DO NOT USE RED RUBBER CATHETERS. They are too stiff. * A 60 ml catheter tip syringe. * Normal Saline Solution * 2 reusable basins and a large plastic bucket. * Water soluble lubricant (K-Y jelly or similar)

Giving the irrigation 1. Pour normal saline solution into one of the basins 2. Draw up 20 ml of saline into the 60 ml syringe 3. Lubricate catheter and gently insert 6 inches into the anus. 4. DO NOT INFLATE THE FOLEY BALLOON. 5. The tip of the catheter is in the right place when there is a gush of air/liquid stool through the catheter. 6. If air or stool drains from the catheter, attach the syringe to the end of the catheter and slowly push in the saline. 7. Pull back on the plunger to allow the stool and saline to return. If there is no return flow, disconnect the syringe from the catheter and allow fluid to drip into the other basin. If return flow is slow, remove the catheter, clear the holes of stool and reinsert the catheter. 8. If drainage is still inadequate, after the above measures, discontinue the procedure and contact the pediatric surgeon. 9. If drainage is satisfactory, you may continue. 10. Repeat the process, 20 ml at a time, making sure the volume of fluid drained is greater than or equal to the volume of being pushed in. By the time the clean basin is empty of normal saline solution, the soiled basin should be filled with an equivalent volume of stool and saline. 11. Empty dirty basin into large plastic bucket and refill clean basin with normal saline. solution 12. Continue irrigation until return flow is clear. Irrigations are performed one to three times in a day, as instructed by the surgeon.

Reference: http://pedsurg.ucsf.edu/conditions--procedures/ hirschsprungs-disease.aspx

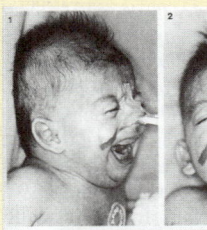
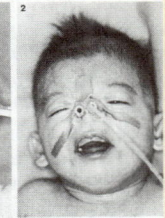
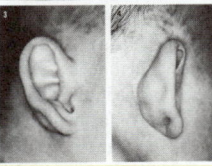

CHARGE acronym stood for: * Coloboma of the eye * Heart defect * Atresia of the Choanae * Retardation of growth and/or development * Genital hypoplasia * Ear malformations (Ears may be small, simple, low set, and/or cup shaped; protruding helix may be unraveled) The sub group of features included: * Facial paralysis or palsy * CHARGE facial features * Central nervous system disorders * Swallowing abnormalities * Cleft lip and/or palate * Urinary tract malformations * Tracheo – esophageal fistula. Blake et al suggested that a typical clinical diagnosis of CHARGE syndrome requires the presence of at least 4 major features or 3 major features plus at least 3 minor features. Major features include ocular coloboma or microphthalmia, choanal atresia or stenosis, cranial nerve abnormalities, and characteristic auditory and/or auricular anomalies. Minor features include distinctive facial dysmorphology, facial clefting, tracheoesophageal fistula, congenital heart defects, genitourinary anomalies, developmental delay, and short stature. Other frequently associated abnormal findings include characteristic hand dysmorphology, hypotonia, deafness, and dysphagia. CHARGE syndrome is an autosomal dominant condition with genotypic heterogeneity, typically caused by mutations in the chromodomain helicase DNA-binding protein-7 (CHD7) gene. Criteria for poor survival include the following: * Bilateral choanal atresia * Complex cyanotic congenital heart disease (Septal defects (interventricular, interatrial) and conotruncal malformation (aortic valve stenosis, aortic coarctation, interrupted aortic arch) are the most frequent anomalies.} * CNS anomalies * Esophageal atresia. **Differentials:** * DiGeorge Syndrome * Smith-Lemli-Opitz Syndrome * Velocardiofacial Syndrome

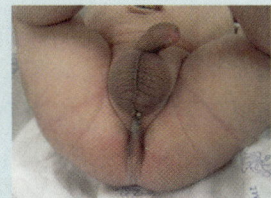
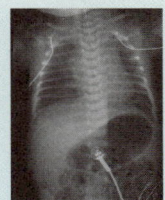
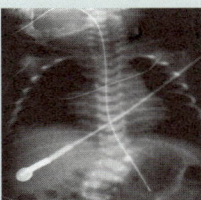
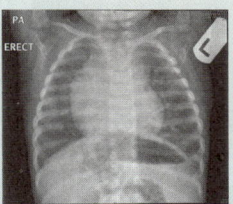

Anal atresia with anocutaneous fistula *Esophageal atresia with TE Fistula* *Hemivertebra T 11* *Cardiomegaly due to CHD*

The VACTERL syndrome occurs when 3 or more of the associated anomalies are present. *These patients do not usually show facial dysmorphism. This* syndrome occurs in approximately 25% of all patients with esophageal atresia. Anomalies in this syndrome include the following: * Vertebral defects - Multiple or single hemivertebrae, scoliosis, rib deformities *Anorectal malformations -Imperforate anus of all varieties, cloacal deformities *Cardiovascular defects -Ventricular septal defect (most common), tetralogy of Fallot, patent ductus arteriosus, atrial septal defects, atrioventricular canal defects, aortic coarctation, right-sided aortic arch, single umbilical artery *Tracheoesophageal defects - Esophageal atresia *Renal anomalies - Renal agenesis including Potter syndrome, bilateral renal agenesis or dysplasia, horseshoe kidney, polycystic kidneys, urethral atresia, ureteral malformations *Limb deformities - Radial dysplasia, absent radius, radial-ray deformities, syndactyly, polydactyly, lower-limb tibial deformities. VACTERL-H: VATER association with hydrocephalus occurs as an X linked inherited disorder. VACTERL is seen more frequently in infants born to diabetic mothers. The birth prevalence varies from 1:3,500 to 1.6:10,000 and is rarely seen more than once in one family . The reason it is called an association, rather than a syndrome is that while all of the birth defects are linked, it is still definitely unknown which genes or sets of genes cause these birth defects to occur. A disruption in differentiating mesoderm in first 4-5 weeks has been suggested to be the basis for such a nonrandom association. The diagnosis can also be suspected because of polyhydramnios in the presence of a small or absent fetal stomach (the tracheoesophageal fistula), hemivertebrae or scoliosis, or limb (in particular, radius anomalies, club hand, reduction defects, and polydactylies), renal, and cardiac defects. The presence of a supernumerary rib (13 and 14 pairs thoracic, 6 to 7 lumbar) may be recognized, especially with 3D rendering. The ultrasound diagnosis of VACTERL syndrome may be accomplished early in the second trimester, if the fetus is severely affected. Prognosis is overall poor and depends upon the extent and combination of deformities and the quality of available healthcare. If detected in utero (by sonography) before viability, termination of pregnancy can be offered. **Differentials:** Townes syndrome has many similar features. Because VACTERL syndrome consists of anomalies of multiple systems, chromosomal disorders such as trisomy 18 and trisomy 13 must be excluded by karyotype study. Disorders characterized by the presence of vertebral, renal, and/or radial defects (such as thrombocytopenia absent radius syndrome, Fanconi anemia, Robert's syndrome, Holt-Oram syndrome, Nager syndrome, caudal regression syndrome, sirenomelia, müllerian duct, renal agenesis, upper limb, and rib abnormalities association, electrodactyly-ectodermal dysplasia syndrome, and Jarcho-Levin syndrome) should be considered. Hemivertebra may be part of a syndrome including Jarcho-Levin, Klippel-Fiel, and VACTERL. Nearly half of patients with tracheoesophageal fistula will exhibit other VACTERL malformations.

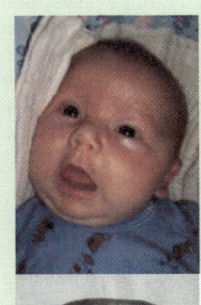
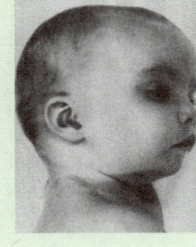

DiGeorge anomaly (DGA) is a congenital immunodeficiency characterized by abnormal facies; congenital heart defects (conotruncal heart defects (e.g., tetralogy of Fallot, interrupted aortic arch, ventricular septal defects, vascular rings); hypoparathyroidism (absence or hypoplasia of thymus and parathyroid glands) with hypocalcemia; cleft lip and/or palate with feeding and gastrointestinal difficulties ,growth delay, hearing loss, cognitive, behavioral, and psychiatric problems (ADHD, autism, anxiety, etc.); and increased susceptibility to infections. Facial features of children with DiGeorge syndrome may include the following: * small ears with squared upper ear * hooded eyelids * cleft lip and/or palate * asymmetric crying facies * small mouth, chin, and side areas of the nose tip *microcephaly (small head). Angelo DiGeorge first noted the immunological consequences associated with the above conditions and was first to propose that the concurrent absence of the thymus and parathyroid glands might result from a perturbation in the development of the third and fourth pharyngeal pouches. Present in 1 out of every 4,000 live births, in 1 in 68 children with congenital heart disease, and in 5 to 8 percent of children born with cleft palate, the 22q11.2 deletion(fluorescence in situ hybridization (FISH) studies) is almost as common as Down syndrome, a widely recognized chromosomal disorder. The 22q11.2 deletion is most often a "de novo" event, meaning that it is not inherited from either parent and does not usually run in a family. Only about 10% of children with the 22q11.2 deletion have a parent who is also affected. For parents who do not have the deletion, the chance that a future child might be affected is very low. For individuals with the 22q11.2 deletion, there is a 50% chance of passing on the deletion to a child with each pregnancy. Conditions associated with DiGeorge syndrome are the other 22q11 deletion syndrome (22q11DS) known as the velocardiofacial syndrome (VCFS or Shprintzen syndrome), as well as conotruncal anomaly face syndrome, Cayler syndrome, Opitz-GBBB syndrome. With the proper treatment of heart defects, immune system disorders, and other health problems, the vast majority of children with a 22q11.2 deletion will survive and grow into adulthood. A small percentage of children with severe heart defects and immune system problems will not survive the first year of life. However, with the proper treatment of heart defects, immune system disorders, and other health problems, the vast majority of children with a 22q11.2 deletion will survive and grow into adulthood. These children will generally need extra help throughout school and will need long term care for their individual health needs.

Neonatal Dysmorphic Syndromes: Selective list

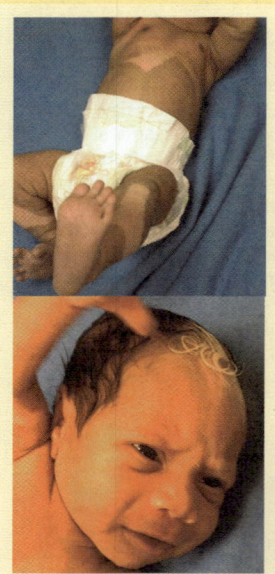

Waardenburg syndrome : *Waardenburg defined the syndrome, a rare disease (1 case per 42,000 persons) with an autosomal dominant mode of inheritance (shows no predilection for race, ethnicity, or sex) , with the following 6 main features (recognized immediately or soon after birth): *Lateral displacement of the medial canthi combined with dystopia of the lacrimal puncta and blepharophimosis *Prominent broad nasal root *Hypertrichosis of the medial part of the eyebrows *White forelock *Heterochromia iridis *Deafmutism.* Waardenburg Syndrome Consortium recommendations: criteria for diagnosis are two major criteria or one major and two minor criteria. **Major Criteria: Sensorineural** hearing loss, Pigmented changes of iris ,Hair depigmentation, Affected 1st degree relative, Dystopia canthorum (W index > 1.95) **Minor Criteria:** Skin depigmentation, Synophrys, Broad high nasal root, Nostril hypoplasia, Premature graying hair Waardenburg syndrome is divided into four subtypes. Individuals with Waardenburg syndrome type 1 must have dystopia canthorum, whereas those with Waardenburg syndrome type 2 do not. Types 3 and 4 are rare variants of the syndrome. Rarer forms of this disease can be associated with limb contractures and Hirchsprung disease. This syndrome results from a disorder of neural crest melanocyte proliferation, migration, or differentiation. Most cases of Waardenburg types 1 and 3 are caused by mutations in the PAX3 (paired box 3) gene. The PAX3 gene is located on chromosome 2q35-37 and controls certain aspects of facial and inner ear development. Mutation of the MITF (microphthalmia-associated transcription factor) gene causes Waardenburg type 2. The MITF gene is found on chromosome 3p14.2-p14.1 and also controls some development of the ear. Congenital sensorineural hearing loss is the most serious feature of Waardenburg syndrome. Deafness generally occurs in 25% of type 1 cases and 50% of type 2 cases, but has been reported to be as high as 60% and 90%. *Differentials: * Albinism* Piebaldism* Vitiligo* Vogt-Koyanagi-Harada Syndrome*

Hyperpigmented macules on normally pigmented skin, which have been described as "patchy skin" and giving a "dappled appearance"

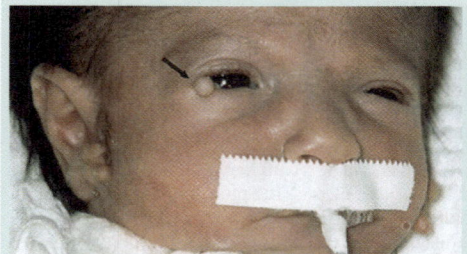

Note facial asymmetry, micrognathia, narrowing of the eye folds, which are turned downwards, and epibulbar dermoid in the right eye

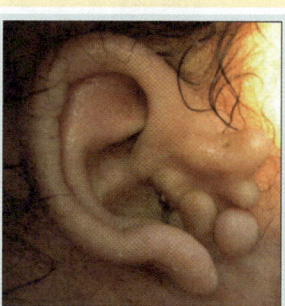

Right auricular pinna dysplasia, with the presence of pré-auricular appendices.

Goldenhar syndrome is part of the oculo-auriculo-vertebral spectrum and is recognized as a syndrome because, in addition to the mandibulofacial dysostosis, there are other vertebral anomalies and epibulbar dermoids. They can be associated to: malar and/or mandibular hypoplasia; hypoplasia of the facial musculature; micrognathia; pre-auricular appendices and dysplasia of external ear; hemivertebra or hypoplasia of cervical, thoracic or lumbar vertebrae; epibulbar dermoid; microphthalmy; palate and/or cleft lip; cardiac anomalies; renal anomalies and central nervous system anomalies. However, due to variability of clinical picture, there are patients who are affected with minimum clinical manifestations predominating face asymmetry and the dysplasia of auricular pinna. It occurs one in every 5,600 newborn infants with majority of cases are sporadic with risk of recurrence is low, although some authors have reported empirical risk of up to 6% for first degree relatives of affected children, but familial cases have been reported with autosomal dominant inheritance and varied expression and also cases in which there is consanguinity between parents, suggesting autosomal recessive inheritance. **Differentials: Since** clinical manifestation is of such a heterogeneous nature, it is important to be alert to other diagnostic possibilities, such as the VACTERL and CHARGE associations; and the Townes-Brocks and Branchio-Oto-Renal syndromes. Differential diagnosis for these entities is based on the pattern of abnormalities observed.

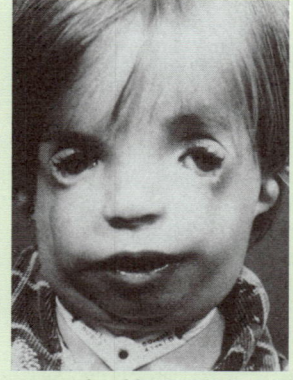

Treacher Collins Syndrome ,also known as Franceschetti-Klein syndrome. (Mandibulofacial Craniosynostosis) is an autosomal dominant gene with with complete penetrance and variable expressivity with a prevalence estimated to range between 1 in 40,000 to 1 in 70,000 of live births. Treacher Collins syndrome is caused by mutations in the TCOF1 gene. TCOF1 was mapped to chromosome bands 5q31.3-33.3. The mother transmits the gene, and it may become more lethal from generation to generation. The syndrome seems to be more prevalent in children born to parents of older age. An increased incidence of spontaneous abortions is observed. It is a bilateral condition that affects first and second pharyngeal arch structures. As with all inherited conditions, it varies from mild to severe. Patients have hypoplasia of the zygomas and mandibles with ear defects or an absence and displacement of the sideburns. The eye area can be significantly involved, with an antimongoloid slant of the fissures (downward-sloping), colobomas of the lower lids, and an absence of eyelashes medially. arch, groove, and pouch is diminished symmetrically and bilaterally. The nose is beaked downwards at its tip. In severe cases, patients have thinning of the subcutaneous tissue from the angles of the mouth up to the lateral canthus. This is associated with macrostomia and is similar to a subcutaneous cleft. The texture of the skin in this area is different because of its thinness. The face is fishlike, and patients may have deafness and mental retardation. Other associated problems include vertebral anomalies, clubfoot, lung agenesis, and frontalis agenesis. The hypoplastic mandible, glossoptosis, small size of the pharynx and nasopharynx, and occasionally choanal atresia can cause severe breathing problems and even death. A more minor situation causes sleep apnea, with all of its attendant problems. The condition is recognizable at birth and can also be diagnosed prenatally based on ultrasonography findings. Differential **diagnoses** include Nager syndrome and ablepharon macrostomia syndrome. These patients require treatment by a multidisciplinary team, including a plastic surgeon, oral surgeon, orthodontist, audiologists, speech pathologists, nutritionist, oculoplastic surgeon, and, occasionally, a neurosurgeon, later a psychiatrist. The social worker plays an important part in the social aspect of the family. Simple head-down positioning with elevation of the foot of the crib, a tracheostomy or early bilateral mandibular distraction using bilateral osteotomies in the body with distraction, either intraorally or extraorally.

Neonatal Dysmorphic Syndromes: Selective list

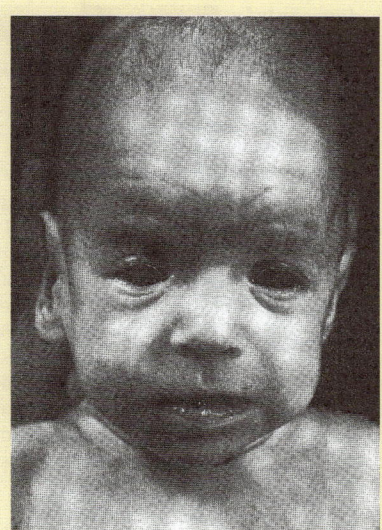

Adverse fetal, neonatal, and pediatric effects occur with maternal alcohol consumption during pregnancy. Fetal alcohol syndrome (FAS) is a triad of impaired growth, abnormal facies, and anomalies of the central nervous system or subsequent neurodevelopment that may be present with or without confirmed prenatal alcohol exposure. Three major facial features signify alcoholic fetopathy: short palpebral fissures, a smooth philtrum, and a thin vermillion border of the upper lip. Other conditions have facial features similar to FAS, including Noonan, Williams, and Brachman de Lange syndromes. The teratogenic effects of maternal anticonvulsants, toluene abuse, and untreated or undertreated maternal phenylketonuria also result in facies similar to FAS. Prenatal and postnatal growth restriction is another component of FAS. Decreased birthweight is associated with lower levels of alcohol consumption than that seen with the development of classic FAS. Other **Abnormalities Associated With Prenatal Alcohol Exposure: Craniofacial:** Unruly scalp hair; midface hypoplasia; palpebral fissure anomalies (up- or downslanting); epicanthal folds; prominent, rotated ears with exaggerated helical root; short nose with anteverted nares; palatal abnormalities; relative prognathism **Cardiac:** Ventricular septal defect, patent ductus arteriosus, tetralogy of Fallot, atrioventricular defects, aortic arch interruption (the heart is the second most commonly affected organ behind the brain) **Musculoskeletal:** Contractures, scoliosis, single transverse palmar crease, short fifth metacarpal with fifth finger clinodactyly **Gastrointestinal:** Hepatomegaly, elevated hepatic transaminases **Ophthalmic:** Ptosis, microphthalmos, coloboma, nystagmus, strabismus, optic nerve abnormalities **Genitourinary:** Horseshoe kidney, renal aplasia/dysplasia, hematuria, clitoromegaly, cryptorchidism **Auditory:** Recurrent otitis media, conductive or sensorineural hearing loss **Immunologic:** Depressed T-cell function, disrupted B-cell development

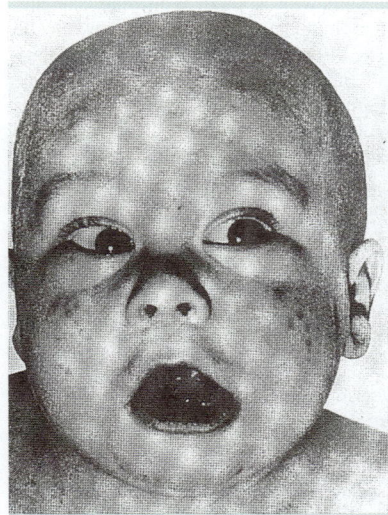

The fetal valproate syndrome (FVS) is a potential embryopathy that can occur as a result from maternal intake of valproic acid (sodium valproate) during pregnancy. Specific features related to FVS :*Neural tube defects, Trigonocephaly, Radial ray defects, Pulmonary abnormalities, Coloboma of iris/optic disc Low verbal IQ, Autism and autistic spectrum disorder.* A prominent metopic ridge (due to premature fusion of the metopic suture) resulting in trigonocephaly (triangular shaped head, as viewed from above) is commonly noted with VPA exposure and may sometimes be severe enough to necessitate surgery. Facial features include prominent metopic ridge, thin arched eyebrows with medial deficiency, epicanthic folds, infraorbital grooves, broad nasal bridge, short anteverted nose and a smooth, long philtrum with a thin upper lip. However, it is not the individual dysmorphic features, but the facial gestalt that provides clues to the diagnosis of this condition. These features are best appreciated in infancy as the dysmorphic features become less obvious with age. Neural **tube defects** (Spina bifida, Anencephaly), Limb **defects** (Radial ray defect ,Polydactyly, Split hand, Overlapping toes, Camptodactyly, Ulnar or tibial hypoplasia, Absent fingers, Oligodactyly) Brain **anomalies** (Hydranencephaly, Porencephaly, Arachnoid cysts, Cerebral atrophy, Partial agenesis of corpus callosum, Agenesis of septum pellucidum Lissencephaly of medial sides of, occipital lobes, Dandy-Walker anomaly), Eye **anomalies** Bilateral congenital cataract, Optic nerve hypoplasia, Tear duct anomalies, Microphthalmia, Bilateral iris defects, Corneal opacities) Abdominal **wall defects** (Omphalocoele) **Skin abnormalities** (**Capillary** hemangioma, Aplasia cutis congenita of scalp) Respiratory **tract anomalies** (**Tracheomalacia**, Lung hypoplasia, Severe laryngeal hypoplasia, Abnormal lobulation of the right lung, Right oligemic lung ,)**Congenital heart defects** (**Ventricular** septal defect, Atrial septal defect, Aortic stenosis ,Patent ductus arteriosus Anomalous right pulmonary artery ,)**Genitourinary defects** (**Hypospadias** ,Renal hypoplasia, Hydronephrosis, Duplication of the calyceal system).**Differentials:**FVS is a diagnosis of exclusion. Other fetal insults such as alcohol, toluene and diabetes may mimic some of the features of FVS. Specific malformations such as trigonocephaly and radial ray defects are also features of other dysmorphic syndromes, which may need to be ruled out before assigning a diagnosis of FVS.

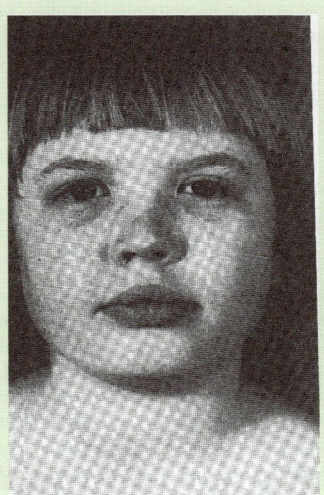

Fetal hydantoin (phenytoin syndrome is manifested by broad nasal bridge, wide fontanelle, low hairline, low-set ears, coarse scalp hair cleft lip/palate, epicanthal folds, short neck, rib abnormalities, nipples spaced far apart, microcephaly, umbilical hernia, low-set ears, small or absent nails, dislocated hip, hypoplasia of distal phalanges, impaired growth, and congenital heart defects.

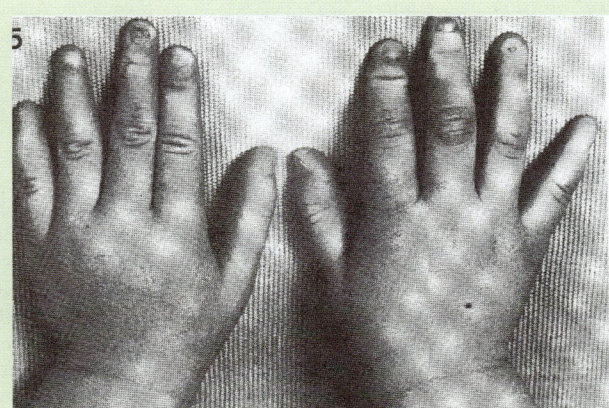

Neonatal Dysmorphic Syndromes: Selective list

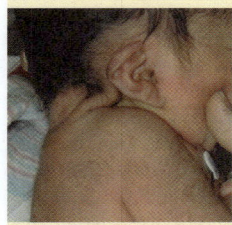
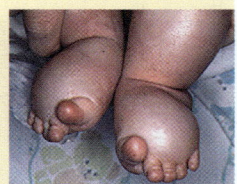

Turner's syndrome: Congenital lymphedema of the extremities, as seen in Figure is reported in about 30% of babies with Turner's syndrome, and it usually resolves within a year with or without treatment. Lymphedema may be present at any age and is one finding that can suggest Turner syndrome on fetal ultrasonography. Lymphedema is the cause of other anomalies, such as the webbed neck and low posterior hairline. Cutis laxa: Loose folds of skin, particularly in the neck, are signs in newborns. In infants, the combination of dysplastic or hypoplastic nails and lymphedema gives a characteristic sausage like appearance to the fingers and toes. Residual lymphedema of the dorsum of the fingers may persist, along with swelling of the lower extremities, into adulthood. Cardiovascular malformations include hypoplastic left heart, coarctation of the aorta, bicuspid aortic valve, and aortic dissection in adulthood. All individuals should have an initial evaluation and periodic follow-up care from a cardiologist. Most concepti with a 45,X karyotype spontaneously abort. Most, if not all, of those who survive to birth are suspected to have mosaicism for a normal cell line. Turner syndrome may be prenatally diagnosed by amniocentesis or chorionic villous sampling. Obtain a karyotype by one of these methods if ultrasonography of a fetus reveals a nuchal cystic hygroma, horseshoe kidney, left-sided cardiac anomalies, or nonimmune fetal hydrops. A postnatal karyotype may be performed instead of amniocentesis or chorionic villus sampling and is also recommended if the human chorionic gonadotropin (HCG), estradiol, or alpha-fetoprotein (AFP) level is elevated during pregnancy. Turner syndrome is caused by the absence of one set of genes from the short arm of one X chromosome. In patients with 45, X karyotype, about two thirds are missing the paternal X chromosome. The frequency is approximately 1 in 2000 live-born female infants. A standard 30 cell Karyotype is required for diagnosis of Turner syndrome, in order to exclude mosaicism. Diagnosis is confirmed by the presence of a 45,X cell line or a cell line with deletion of the short arm of the X chromosome (Xp deletion). Turner syndrome is not an inherited disorder, and the recurrence risk is low. Because of infertility, the syndrome is rarely passed to offspring.

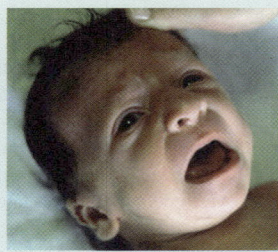

Noonan syndrome cardinal features include unusual facies (i.e., hypertelorism, down-slanting eyes, Ptosis, High nasal bridge, Low-set ears with thickened helices, Triangular-shaped face, webbed neck),# Pectus carinatum or excavatum, congenital heart disease (Cardiac malformations are also heterogeneous. Pulmonary stenosis, with or without dysplastic pulmonary valve and hypertrophic cardiomyopathy, are the "classic" cardiac defects reported in Noonan syndrome. However, atrial septal defect, atrioventricular septal defect, left-sided obstructive lesions, tetralogy of Fallot and patent ductus arteriosus have also been described.), short stature, and chest deformity. Approximately 25% of individuals with Noonan syndrome have mental retardation. Bleeding diathesis is present in as many as half of all patients with Noonan syndrome. Skeletal, neurologic, genitourinary, lymphatic, eye, and skin findings may be present to varying degrees. The disorder is present from birth, but age impacts the facial phenotype. Infants with Noonan syndrome can be difficult to recognize by facial appearance alone. The phenotype becomes more striking in early childhood, but with advancing age, it may again become quite subtle. Both sporadic and autosomal dominant cases have been identified. At least 4 disease-causing genes have been found. Differentials: Fetal Alcohol Syndrome. If full phenotypic expression is not apparent, karyotyping may be necessary. Mutation analysis may confirm the diagnosis. However, the failure to identify a germline mutation in any of the associated genes does not rule out Noonan syndrome. This entity remains a clinical diagnosis. The incidence of progressive high-frequency sensorineural hearing loss may be as high as 50%. Thus, audiologic evaluation is indicated.

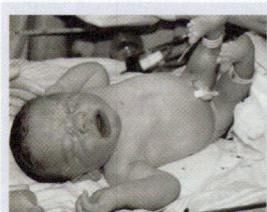
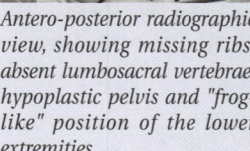
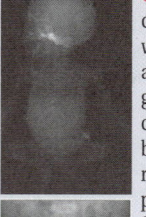
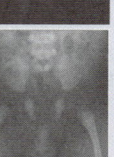

Antero-posterior radiographic view, showing missing ribs, absent lumbosacral vertebrae, hypoplastic pelvis and "frog-like" position of the lower extremities.

Caudal regression syndrome (CRS), also known as caudal dysplasia sequence, is characterized by a series of congenital abnormalities, including complete or partial agenesis of the sacrum and lumbar vertebrae associated with pelvic deformity. Femoral hypoplasia, clubbed feet, and flexion contractures of the lower extremities are also commonly seen. Additionally, CRS is often associated with anomalies of the gastrointestinal tract, genitourinary tract, and heart, as well as with NTD. The most specific but rare congenital anomaly in pregnancies complicated by diabetes .Caudal regression syndrome is an uncommon malformation in the general population, but occurs in about one in 350 infants of diabetic mothers, representing an increase of about 200-fold over the rate seen in the general population. The etiology of this syndrome is not well-known. Maternal diabetes, genetic predisposition and vascular hypoperfusion have been suggested as possible causative factors. The prognosis for children with caudal regression syndrome depends on the severity of the lesion and the presence of associated anomalies. Surviving infants have usually a normal mental function and they require extensive urologic and orthopedic assistance. Prenatal ultrasonographic diagnosis of caudal regression syndrome is possible at 22 weeks' of gestation. Visualization of the anomalies such as amputation of the spine and the deformities of extremities which were described in this report should not be difficult, particularly with normal amniotic fluid.

Differences between CRS and Sirenomelia

Sign	CRS	Sirenomelia
Umbilical artery	Two	One
Lower limb	Two hypoplastic	Single or fused
Renal anomalies	Nonlethal	Renal agenesis or severe dysgenesis
Anus	Imperforate or normal	Absent
Amniotic fluid level	Polyhydramnios or normal	Oligohydramnios

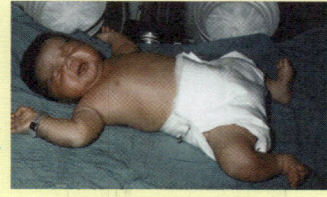

Jim Farquhar described **The Child of the Diabetic Woman**. *"they emerge at least alive from within the fiery furnace of diabetes mellitus, but because they resemble one another so closely that they might well be related. They are plump, sleek, liberally coated with vernix caseosa, full-faced and plethoric. The umbilical cord and the placenta share in the gigantism. During their first 24 or more extra-uterine hours they lie on their backs, bloated and flushed, their legs flexed and abducted, their lightly closed hands on each side of the head, the abdomen prominent and their respiration sighing. They convey a distinct impression of having had such a surfeit of food and fluid pressed on them by an insistent hostess that they desire only peace so they may recover from their excesses. And on the second day their resentment of the slightest noise improves the analogy, while their trembling anxiety seems to speak of intrauterine indiscretions of which we know nothing."*

Neonatal Dysmorphic Syndromes: Selective list

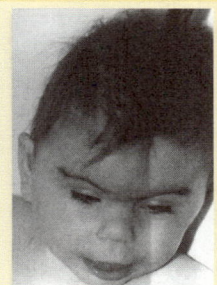

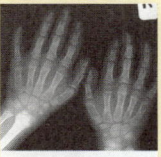

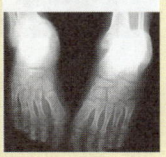

Cornelia de Lange (CDL) or Brachmann-de Lange syndrome (BDLS) is a rare malformation syndrome with a birth incidence of approximately 1 in 40,000. The essential features of this multisystem developmental disorder include prenatal and postnatal growth retardation, distinctive facial appearance, various structural upper limb abnormalities, neurodevelopmental delay, and behavioral problems. The facial features are the most diagnostic and the following classic features are seen: Microbrachycephaly, Low frontal hairline, Well-defined, arched "pencilled" eyebrows, Synophrys (confluent eyebrows), Long, curly eyelashes, Short nose with anteverted nares, Triangular nasal tip, Long philtrum, Crescent-shaped mouth, Thin lips, Widely spaced (late-erupting) teeth, Micrognathia, Low-set and posteriorly rotated ears, Hirsutism may be prominent and generalized. Skeletal abnormalities characteristic for classic CDLS include major longitudinal reduction abnormalities of the upper limbs, including hypoplastic or absent ulnas and/or oligodactyly (which, if bilateral, can be asymmetric). This abnormality is not observed in persons with mild CDLS. Common cutaneous manifestations-Hypoplastic nipples and umbilicus, Cutis marmorata, Multiple capillary or cavernous hemangiomas. Congenital heart -ventricular and atrial septal defects, pulmonic stenosis, and tetralogy of Fallot. During the neonatal period, respiratory and feeding difficulties (failure to thrive) predominate. The low-pitched cry frequently noted in the newborn period or in early infancy may disappear in late infancy. Cornelia de Lange syndrome 1 (Classic CDLS1)- autosomal dominant, Cornelia de Lange syndrome 2 (Mild CDLS2)- X-linked. Most cases are sporadic (>99% of mutations occur de novo), but familial occurrence and parental consanguinity have been recorded (<1%). When parents are not affected, the risk of recurrence has been estimated at 1.5%; germinal mosaicism can be an explanation for unaffected parents having more than one affected child. Single-allele mutations at the NIPBL locus account for approximately 50-55% of affected individuals, and mutations in SMC1A locus for a further 5% of Cornelia de Lange syndrome (CDLS) cases. Periodical evaluations, including routine blood cell counts, iron metabolism testing, liver and renal function tests, urinalysis, and a search for stool blood, are recommended, especially in first years of life.

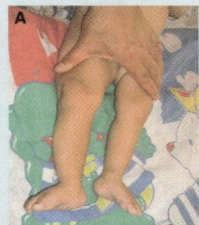

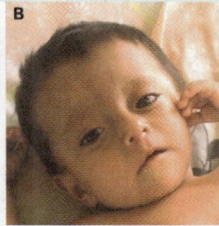

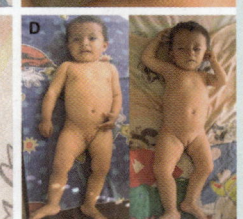

Silver-Russell syndrome characterized by severe intrauterine growth retardation with normal head circumference, poor postnatal growth, feeding difficulties, and fasting hypoglycemia, craniofacial features such as a triangular shaped face(high forehead that tapers to a small jaw, micrognathia with a pointed chin, prominent nasal bridge, and down-turned corners of the mouth. and a broad forehead), asymmetry, usually of the limbs, and a variety of minor malformations-camptodactyly (i.e., fixed flexion of digits) or clinodactyly (i.e., incurving) of one or more fingers, syndactyly of second and third toes, Sprengel deformity, Hypospadias, Posterior urethral valves. Differentials: * Fanconi Syndrome * Fetal Alcohol Syndrome. Incidence-Uncommon, varies from 0.1-3 in 10,000 births, the male-to-female ratio is equal. Silver-Russell syndrome is a clinically heterogeneous condition. Various molecular defects have been reported, mostly involving chromosomes 7 and 17. Defects have also been reported in chromosomes 1 and X. A few cases of autosomal dominant transmission have been described, including ring 2 chromosome, balanced translocation of band 17q25, and duplication of band 7p11.2-p13. Silver-Russell syndrome usually occurs sporadically and its etiology is not identified in most cases. If Silver-Russell syndrome is suspected, obtain patient and parental blood to evaluate for uniparental disomy of chromosome 7 and hypomethylation at chromosome 11p15 by polymerase chain reaction (PCR). Growth hormone therapy should be considered in a child with Silver-Russell syndrome (SRS) who has not manifested adequate catch-up growth by age 2 years.

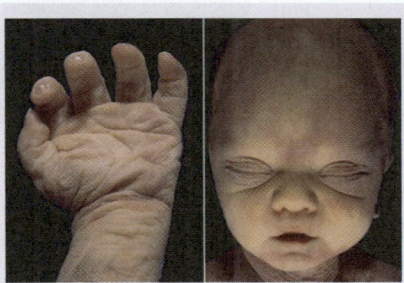

Potter syndrome refers to the typical physical appearance and associated pulmonary hypoplasia of a neonate (leading to respiratory compromise and death within immediate newborn period) as a direct result of oligohydramnios and compression while in utero. Potter facies: Affected infants have a flattened nose, recessed chin, prominent epicanthal folds, prominent creases below the eyes, and low-set abnormal ears, excessive skin folds in the hand (as if wearing a loose glove). Potter syndrome is mostly associated with obstruction of the urinary tract or severe bilateral renal hypoplasia (due to autosomal recessive mutations of genes in the renin-angiotensin pathway @1 of 5000 fetuses). Eye: Cataract, angiomatous malformation in the optic disc area, prolapse of the lens, and expulsive hemorrhage. Skeletal malformations: Hemivertebrae, sacral agenesis, and limb anomalies. Cardiovascular malformations: Ventricular septal defect, endocardial cushion defect, tetralogy of Fallot, and patent ductus arteriosus. Conditions resulting in oligohydramnios, such as obstructive uropathy, cystic kidney diseases, renal hypoplasia, and premature rupture of membranes lead to the same clinical findings. Hence, the terms Potter sequence or oligohydramnios sequence emerged. Differentials: * Multicystic Renal Dysplasia * Patau Syndrome * Polycystic Kidney Disease * Posterior Urethral Valves * Prader-Willi Syndrome

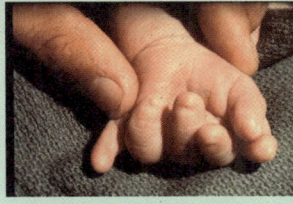

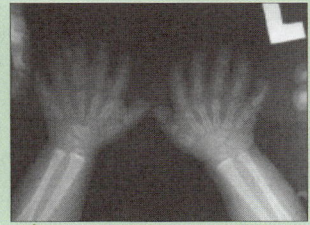

Ellis-van Creveld Syndrome (chondroectodermal dysplasia): Disproportionate dwarfism, postaxial polydactyly, ectodermal dysplasia, a small chest, and a high frequency of congenital heart defects characterize this autosomal recessive syndrome. A clinical tetrad of Ellis–van Creveld syndrome consists of chondrodystrophy, polydactyly, ectodermal dysplasia, and cardiac anomalies. Neonatal history may include small size at birth, slow growth, and skeletal anomalies are the initial symptoms. Natal teeth may be present. Neonatal teeth should be removed because they may impair feeding. The most common cardiac anomaly is a common atrium (40%); other cardiac anomalies include atrioventricular canal, ventricular septal defect, atrial septal defect, and patent ductus arteriosus. Developmentally, most patients have had intelligence in the normal range.

Neonatal Dysmorphic Syndromes: Selective list

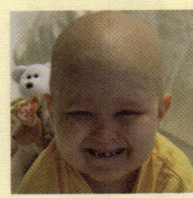

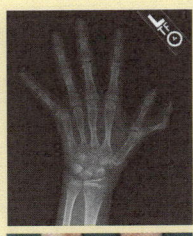

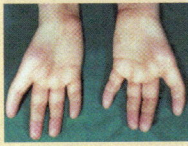

About 75% of patients with Fanconi anemia have birth defects, such as altered skin pigmentation and/or café au lait spots (>50%), short stature (50%), thumb or thumb and radial anomalies (40%), abnormal male gonads (30%), microcephaly (25%), eye anomalies(20%)-(Small, strabismus, epicanthal folds, hypertelorism, ptosis, slanted, cataracts, astigmatism, blindness, epiphora, nystagmus, proptosis, small iris) structural renal defects (20%), low birth weight (10%), developmental delay (10%), and abnormal ears or hearing (10%).Thumbs may be absent or hypoplastic, supernumerary, bifid, rudimentary, short, low set, attached by a thread, triphalangeal, tubular, stiff, hyperextensible.Fanconi anemia accounts for approximately 25% of the cases of aplastic anemia seen at large referral centers. Approximately 25% of known patients with Fanconi anemia do not have major birth defects.Fanconi anemia is an autosomal recessive disease in more than 99% of patients @1 case per 130,000 people(FANCB is X-linked recessive); each patient with Fanconi anemia is homozygous or doubly heterozygous for mutations in one of the 15 genes known to be responsible for Fanconi anemia. The cloned genes are FANCA, B, C, D1, D2, E, F, G, I, J, L, M,N, O, and P. The diagnosis of Fanconi anemia is not made using routine laboratory tests; it must be considered and tested for using chromosome breakage in blood or fibroblasts, or germline mutation analysis. Siblings who do not apparently have Fanconi anemia need to be screened for occult Fanconi anemia.Prenatal Fanconi anemia diagnosis can be accomplished by demonstration of chromosome breaks in cells obtained in utero from chorionic villus biopsy, amniocentesis, or cord blood (by cordocentesis) or by identification of Fanconi anemia gene mutations in DNA extracted from fetal cells. Treatment of aplastic anemia with medications, supportive use of blood products, and stem cell transplantation increases the life expectancy beyond the projected median of approximately age 30 years.

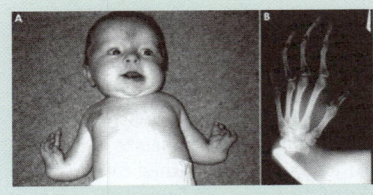

Thrombocytopenia-absent radius (TAR) syndrome is a rare condition in which thrombocytopenia is associated with bilateral radial aplasia. Thrombocytopenia, which may be transient, is seen in all cases and will be symptomatic in over 90% of cases within the first four months of life. 1 Gastrointestinal bleeding and occasionally intracerebral bleeding may result. The presence of the thumbs distinguishes TAR syndrome from other disorders featuring radial aplasia, which are usually associated with absent thumbs (may be accompanied by ulnar or humeral anomalies and the most severe cases exhibit phocomelia). Lower limb involvement is variable and includes dislocation of the patella and/or of the hips, absent tibiofibular joint, and lower limb phocomelia. Between 22 and 33% of children with TAR syndrome are reported as having congenital heart disease, tetralogy of Fallot and atrial septal defects being the most commonly reported lesions. Symptomatic cow's-milk allergy is associated with 47% of all cases of TAR syndrome, and patients may present as vomiting, bloody diarrhea, and failure to thrive. The genetic basis of TAR syndrome is uncertain. Evidence for autosomal recessive inheritance comes from the reports of 11 families with at least two affected children born to unaffected parents. Differentials: Holt-Oram syndrome (HOS), Roberts syndrome, Fanconi anemia, thalidomide embryopathy, and Rapadilino syndrome. Patients with TAR syndrome always have thumbs, but thumbs may be hypoplastic or absent in patients with Fanconi anemia. Fanconi anemia is also associated with chromosomal abnormalities, a rare onset of thrombocytopenia before age 1 year, and pancytopenia in children aged 5-10 years. A reliable diagnostic test is a chromosomal breakage study.

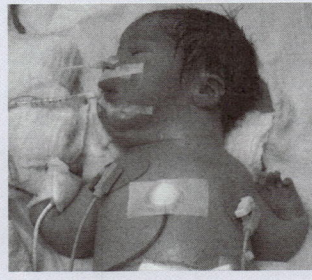

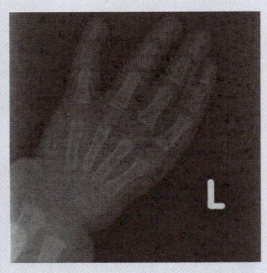

Holt-Oram syndrome (HOS) is a heart–upper limb malformation complex with an autosomal dominant inheritance and near-complete penetrance but variable expression. Approximately 40% of cases represent new mutations. The responsible gene has been mapped to band 12q24.1, which encodes the human transcription factor TBX5. This study requires a combination of chromosome painting and fluorescent in situ hybridization (FISH) with yeast artificial chromosomes (YAC) and cosmids. Prenatal diagnosis is feasible in families with HOS linked to band 12q2. The most common defects include radial thumb anomalies ranging from absent thumbs to displaced (distally placed), duplicated, or triphalangeal thumbs. Carpal and metacarpal anomalies (especially the fourth) may also be present. Hypoplasia of the radius manifests as short deformed forearm, although it may be so mild that it is detectable only on radiography of the forearm. The most common congenital heart lesion is a secundum ASD. Others include ventricular septal defect (VSD), atrioventricular (AV) block, pulmonic stenosis (including peripheral arterial), and mitral valve prolapse. Intelligence is normal.

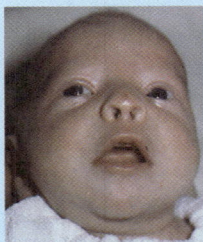

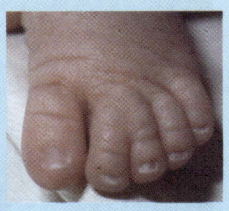

Smith-Lemli-Opitz syndrome (SLOS) is a multiple congenital anomalies (MCA)/mental retardation (MR) syndrome caused by a defect in cholesterol synthesis. Intrauterine growth retardation (IUGR) is common, as is short stature or abnormally low weight for height, altered muscle tone (hypotonia), and often a distinctive shrill cry. Smith-Lemli-Opitz syndrome is an autosomal recessive genetic condition caused by deficiency of the enzyme 3 beta-hydroxysterol-delta 7-reductase, the final enzyme in the sterol synthetic pathway that converts 7-dehydrocholesterol (7DHC) to cholesterol. Dysmorphic facial features (Broad nasal tip with anteverted nostrils, Ptosis of eyelids, Epicanthal folds, Strabismus, Cataracts, Broad maxillary alveolar ridges, Slanted or low-set ears, microcephaly, Cleft palate), second-toe and third-toe syndactyly, Postaxial polydactyly, Hypospadias or cryptorchidism in males and, occasionally, complete sex reversal (i.e., 46,XY females), and MR are typical. Mildly affected individuals may have only subtle dysmorphic features and learning and behavioral disabilities. Affected individuals usually have low plasma cholesterol levels and invariably have elevated levels of cholesterol precursors, including 7DHC. Severely affected individuals (those with the condition formerly referred to as Smith-Lemli-Opitz syndrome type II) have multiple congenital malformations and are often miscarried or stillborn or die in the first weeks of life. The characteristic pattern of low plasma cholesterol levels and the extremely high 7DHC levels define Smith-Lemli-Opitz syndrome. No medications have been proven effective in treatment of Smith-Lemli-Opitz syndrome (SLOS). Cholesterol given as egg yolk or crystalline cholesterol in oil or aqueous suspension or sprinkled on food has been used in clinical trials with limited success, but these studies are ongoing. Bile acids, including ursodeoxycholic and chenodeoxycholic acids, have been given in addition to cholesterol in some cases.

Neonatal Dysmorphic Syndromes: Selective list

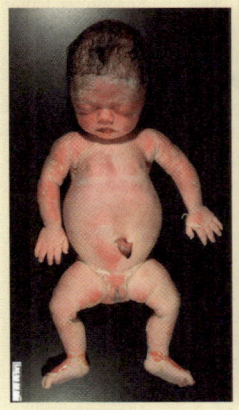
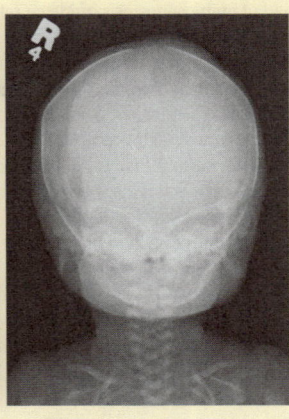

Achondroplasia is the most common type of short-limb disproportionate dwarfism occuring with the varying frequency of 1 in 15,000-40,000. It is an autosomal dominant disorder, but majority of the cases represent a fresh gene mutation. Mutation in FGFR3 (Fibroblast growth factor) is responsible for achondroplasia, hypochondroplasia, and thanatophoric dysplasia. Older paternal age is a contributory factor. Children with achondroplasia have short stature, megalencephaly, small foramen magnum, depressed nasal bridge, prominent forehead and short limbs. The limbs shortening is greatest in the proximal (rhizomelic) segments with the arms and thighs more severely involved than the forearms, legs, hands, and feet. The fingers display a trident configuration. Cranial Characteristics include an enlarged neurocranium, frontal bossing, flattening of the nasal bridge, midface hypoplasia, and a relatively prominent mandible, diminished foramen magnum. Given the incidence and potential severity of neurologic symptoms associated with foramen magnum stenosis, a baseline MRI is strongly recommended in infancy. Cervicomedullary compression at the foramen magnum, fusion of C1, or isolated subaxial cervical stenosis can be demonstrated.

The anteroposterior diameter of the chest is flattened, the lower ribs are flared, and the abdomen protrudes. They have mild hypotonia and slow motor development but intelligence is usually normal. Prominent skeletal features are small cuboid shaped vertebral bodies with progressive narrowing of lumbar interpedicular distance and short tubular bones especially humerii. Hydrocephalus is one of the neurological complications that can occur in these children. Differentials:* Diastrophic Dysplasia * Spondyloepiphyseal Dysplasia.

DNA testing can be performed when both of the parents are affected. Infants with affected genes from both the parents (double homozygous) are either stillborn or die shortly after birth.

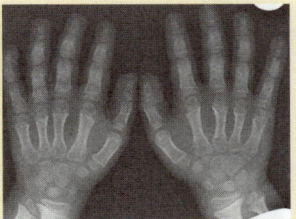

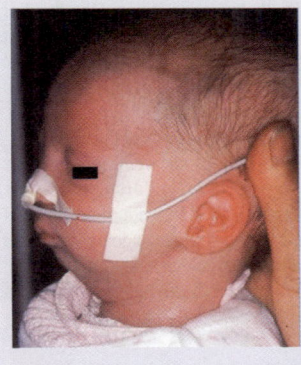

Robin sequence (RS), previously known as Pierre Robin syndrome and Pierre Robin anomalad, consists of the following 3 essential components: * Micrognathia or retrognathia * Cleft palate (usually U-shaped, but V-shape also possible) * Relative Glossoptosis, often accompanied by airway obstruction: The tongue is not actually larger than normal, but because of the small mandible, the tongue is large for the airway and therefore causes obstruction. Rarely, the tongue is smaller than normal. Suggested causes of Robin sequence and Robin complexes include malformation, deformation, or connective tissue dysplasia. Robin sequence occurs as an isolated defect (often a deformation associated with oligohydramnios), as part of a recognized syndrome, or as part of a complex of multiple congenital anomalies. Diagnosis of a possible syndrome is very often critically important for correct management of a newborn affected with Robin sequence. Robin sequence is etiologically heterogenous. Etiologic heterogeneity suggests pathogenetic heterogeneity and phenotypic variability. Among syndromic cases, the most common is Stickler syndrome, which comprises 20-25% of all cases. The second most common Robin sequence syndrome is velocardiofacial syndrome, which comprises about 15% of all Robin sequence cases. Treacher Collins syndrome (mandibulofacial dysostosis), Nager syndrome, spondyloepiphyseal dysplasia congenita, and other recognized syndromes comprise the rest of the syndromic Robin sequence cases. Neonates with Robin sequence should be carefully monitored because a significant airway obstruction may develop during the first 1-4 weeks of life. A cleft palate further adds to the feeding difficulties. The great majority of neonates can be treated in the prone position (face down). Devices or procedures such as oral airways, palatal prostheses, continuous positive airway pressure or endotracheal intubation, mechanical ventilation, and tracheostomy can be avoided. Multidisciplinary care that includes a neonatologist, a neonatal nurse specialist, members of the craniofacial team, and the parents is the best approach in the complex care of neonates affected with Robin sequence and Robin complexes.

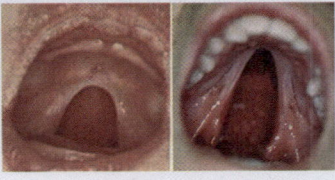

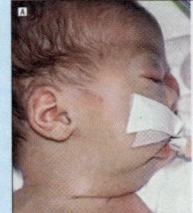
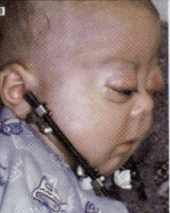
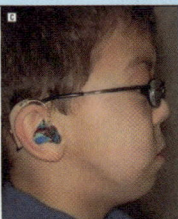

Wagner-Stickler Syndrome or Srickler Syndrome or David-Stickler syndrome (Hereditary Progressive Arthro-Ophthalmopathy), is an autosomal dominant genetic disorder affecting about 1/7,500 newborn babies, which primarily affect the connective tissue particularly the collagen, due to mutation of the genes during fetal development. Three genes have been identified as causing Stickler Syndrome: COL11A1, COL11A2 (non-ocular), and COL2A1 (75% of Stickler cases). Macrocephaly and facial dysmorphism are noted in the neonatal period, including a flat midface, deep set ears, exophthalmos, palpebral edema with telangiectasia, micrognathia, and median clefting of the soft and part of the hard palate (Pierre Robin sequence). About 30% of children diagnosed as having Pierre Robin sequence at birth, subsequently have the diagnosis changed to Stickler syndrome about the age of 6-7 years when other problems become more obvious. *Follow-up Problems:* **High myopia** (severe -8 dioptres or more), retinal detachments, glaucoma, cataracts. **Hearing** loss may be sensorineural (caused by nerve damage and results in a decrease in the ability of the nerve endings in the inner ear to transmit signals to the brain), or conductive (caused by a mechanical problem involving the eardrum and the three tiny bones of the middle ears), or a combination of both. **Otitis media** - commonly called glue ear, which is associated with cleft palates. **Bone and joint problems** can include abnormality to ends of long bones, double jointedness (which can result in dislocated joints), joint pain and early onset of osteoarthritis,Scoliosis. *Once Stickler syndrome is diagnosed, a co-ordinated multidisciplinary approach is desirable.* This should include: * Ophthalmic assessment. Due to the high risk of retinal detachment, all patients also require long-term follow up and are advised to seek ophthalmic help if they see new floaters or shadows in their vision. * If there is evidence of midline clefting, a maxillo-facial assessment. * Hearing tests and management of combined conductive and sensorineural deafness. * Joint hypermobility should be assessed objectively using the Beighton scoring system to allow comparison with age, sex and race matched population. * Rheumatological assessment and follow up is advised in older patients who may benefit from physiotherapy for arthropathy. * Although intelligence is normal, patients of school age may face considerable educational difficulties because of combined visual and auditory impairment.

Neonatal Dysmorphic Syndromes: Selective list

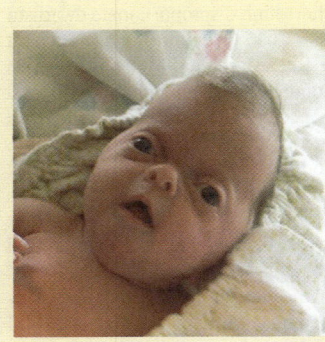

Crouzon's syndrome is characterized by the triad of craniosynostosis, midface retrusion, and proptosis. Other clinical features include hypertelorism, exophthalmos, strabismus, beaked nose, short upper lip, hypoplastic maxilla, and relative mandibular prognathism. Unlike some other forms of autosomal dominant craniosynostosis, no digital abnormalities are present. Inheritance is autosomal dominant with variable expression and complete penetrance. Crouzon syndrome is caused by mutations (fifty percent of cases of Crouzon syndrome are not inherited and are the result of new mutations) in the fibroblast growth factor receptor-2 (FGFR2) gene but exhibits locus heterogeneity with causal mutations in FGFR2 (Crouzon syndrome) and FGFR3 (Crouzon syndrome with acanthosis nigricans) in different affected individuals. Premature synostosis of the sutures begins in the first year of life and is completed by the second or third year. Coronal and sagittal sutures are most commonly involved, resulting in acrocephaly, brachycephaly, turricephaly, oxycephaly, flat occiput, and high prominent forehead with or without frontal bossing. Ridging of the skull is usually palpable. Cloverleaf skull is rare (only 7%) and occurs in the most severely affected individuals. Other findings: Hydrocephalus (progressive in 30%), Exophthalmos (proptosis) secondary to shallow orbits resulting in frequent exposure conjunctivitis or keratitis, Choanal atresia or stenosis, Narrow or absent ear canals, Cervical fusions are present in approximately 18% of patients. C2-C3 and C5-C6 are affected equally.

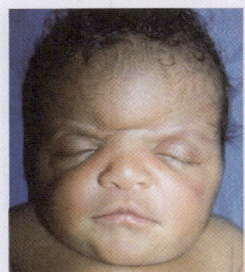

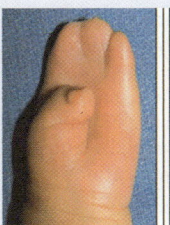 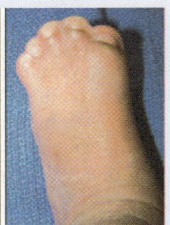

Apert syndrome, or acrocephalosyndactyly, the most common of the craniosynostosis syndromes, an autosomal dominant malformation syndrome (many cases are de novo mutations) is characterized by craniosynostosis, midface hyopoplasia, syndactyly, and various visceral abnormalities. *Associated findings :* strabismus and hypertelorism, malformations of the corpus callosum and limbic structures with ventriculomegaly that leads to hydrocephalus, hearing impairment can result from persistent middle ear effusion or congenital ossicular chain fixation, Airway obstruction secondary to palatal defects. Syndactyly of all 4 extremities is characteristic of Apert syndrome. This finding is typically absent in other craniosynostoses. The term "mitten hand" is frequently used to describe the appearance of the fused soft tissues. The syndrome presents in 15.5 per million live births. The syndrome is typically caused by 2 point mutations (S252W and P253R) and 2 Alu insertions in the fibroblast growth factor receptor 2 gene (*FGFR2*) located on chromosome 10q26. Apert, Crouzon, and Pfeiffer syndromes are often associated with advanced paternal age. The distinctive facial features of Apert syndrome are acrocephaly (or oxycephaly) with bicoronal synostosis, maxillary hypoplasia, and high-arched palate. Acrocephaly is common in both Apert and Crouzon syndromes. The incidence of cleft palate and other craniofacial deformities is lower in Crouzon syndrome. Patients with Crouzon syndrome generally have a normal IQ and normal distal extremities, unlike those with Apert syndrome. One third of patients with Crouzon syndrome have cervical spine abnormalities, which are rare in patients with Apert syndrome. Surgical correction of skull malformations is typically a 3-stage process: craniosynostosis release, midface advancement by Le Fort 3 osteotomy, and correction of hypertelorism. Correction of distal limb deformities depends on the severity of the underlying malformed bony architecture. Because hearing impairment, frequent ear infections, and mental deficiencies may develop, children with Apert syndrome require regular follow-up tailored to their individual needs. This may involve several specialists, including an otorhinolaryngologist, plastic surgeon, neurosurgeon, and speech/language pathologist, in addition to the general pediatrician. Follow-up every 6 months for the first few years of life is typical in these patients.

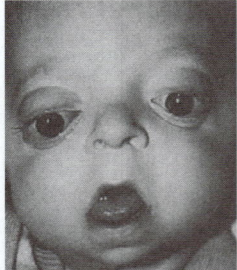 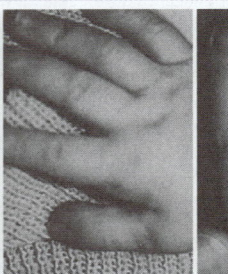 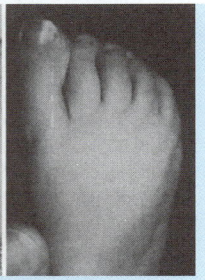

Pfeiffer's syndrome is an autosomal dominant disorder with complete penetrance and variable expression. Recognized by craniosynostosis, broad thumbs and toes, and partial soft tissue syndactyly of the fingers and toes. Cohen classified Pfeiffer's syndrome into three subtypes: Patients with type 1 typically have normal intelligence and survive to adulthood. Those with type 2 have the distinctive cloverleaf skull syndrome (kleeblattschädel deformity) with severe CNS complications and a poor prognosis. Those with type 3 lack the cloverleaf skull but have CNS defects and a similarly poor prognosis. The ophthalmic manifestations in Pfeiffer's syndrome closely parallel those found in Crouzon's and Apert's syndromes. Hypertelorism, ocular proptosis, oxybrachycephaly (often secondary to bilateral coronal synostosis), strabismus, flattened nasal bridge with beaked nose, maxillary hypoplasia with a relative mandibular prognathism, and malocclusion are typical findings in this syndrome. Other abnormalities include high arched palate, crowded teeth, hydrocephalus, seizures, bifid uvula, low-set ears, and conductive hearing loss. The distinguishing features of this syndrome are the broad, medially deviated great toes and thumbs. In fact, the ratio of the width of the great toe to the second toe may be useful in diagnosing this syndrome. Brachydactyly, clinodactyly, and partial soft tissue syndactyly may be present whereas radiographic studies of the hand and foot show the occasional absence of the middle phalanges, broad distal thumb phalanges, triangulation of the proximal thumb, and the unusual appearance or the duplication of the first metatarsal bone. Associated abnormalities include lumbar hyperlordosis, fusion of lumbar or cervical vertebrae, shortened humerus, umbilical hernia, preauricular skin tags, and supernumerary teeth.

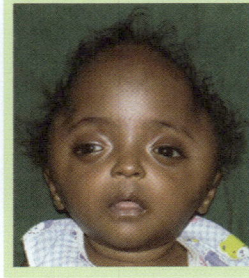 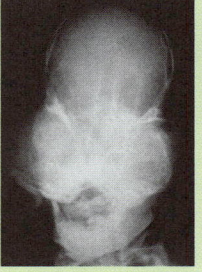

Cloverleaf skull (Kleeblattschadel anomaly) is an anomaly characterized by synostosis of multiple or all cranial sutures, and facial dysostosis of the skull (craniofacial malformations) and long bone anomalies. The main components involved in the deformity include hydrocephalus, trilobed head shape (a high, peaked forehead, with prominent bulges on both sides of the head with cloverleaf appearance), shallow orbits and midfacial hypoplasia. The disease has been found either alone or in association with other syndromes such as Apert syndrome, Pfeifer's syndrome and skeletal dysplasias, such as Thanatophoric dwarfism.It can occur in 1 out of 2,000 live births, either as a part of inherited syndromes or occurring sporadically. Those severely affected are typically stillborn or die in early infancy, while those who survive exhibit severe learning difficulties due to central nervous system complications arising from intracranial pressure.

Neonatal Dysmorphic Syndromes: Selective list

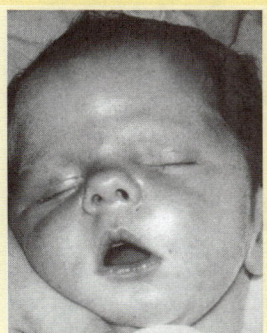

Myotonic dystrophy type 1 (DM1) , also known as 'Steinert's disease: Congenital DM1 often presents before birth as polyhydramnios and reduced fetal movements. After delivery, the main features are severe generalized weakness, hypotonia and respiratory compromise. The head may be narrow, and the palate is high and arched because the weak temporal and pterygoid muscles in late fetal life do not exert sufficient lateral forces on the developing head and face. Affected infants have an inverted V-shaped (also termed 'tented' or 'fish-shaped') upper lip, which is characteristic of severe facial weakness and makes suckling difficult. Mortality from respiratory failure is high. Failure to thrive, club feet and feeding difficulties are common problems but surviving infants experience gradual improvement in motor function, can swallow and independently ventilate. The distal distribution of muscle wasting in myotonic dystrophy is an exception to the general rule of myopathies having proximal and neuropathies having distal distribution patterns. Cognitive and motor milestones are nevertheless delayed and all patients with congenital DM1 develop learning difficulties and require special needs schooling. It is inherited as an autosomal dominant trait. The genetic defect in myotonic muscular dystrophy is on chromosome 19 at the 19q13 locus. It consists of an expansion of the *DM* gene that encodes a serine-threonine kinase *(DMPK)*, with numerous repeats of the cytosine-thymine-guanine (CTG) codon. Expansions range from 50 to over 2,000, with the normal alleles of this gene ranging in size from 5 to 37; the larger the expansion, the more severe the clinical expression, with the largest expansions seen in the severe neonatal form. Muscle biopsy is not usually required for diagnosis, which in typical cases can be based on the clinical manifestations. Both clinical and genetic expression may vary between siblings or between an affected parent and child. In the severe neonatal form of the disease, the mother is the transmitting parent in 94% of cases, a fact not explained by increased male infertility alone. Myotonic dystrophy often exhibits a pattern of *anticipation* in which each successive generation has a tendency to be more severely involved than the previous generation.

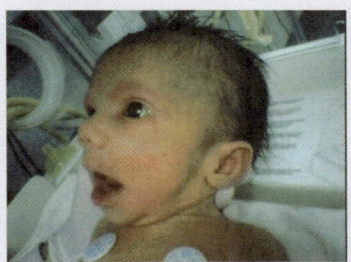

Myasthenia Gravis in the Neonate (MG) in the neonate is usually an autoimmune disorder, although some neonates have congenital MG, which most commonly seems to be due to an autosomal recessive disorder. The most common form of MG in the neonate is transient and results from placentally transferred antibodies to acetylcholine, which occurs in 10% to 20% of infants born to women who have autoimmune MG. In most cases, it resolves spontaneously and progressively over the first 2 postnatal months. Affected neonates should be observed carefully for myasthenic signs during the first 3 to 6 days after birth. If no symptoms have occurred by that point, they are unlikely to occur later. Neither the mother's anti-AChR or anti- MuSK antibody titers nor her clinical state is predictive of TNMG. Myasthenic symptoms usually become apparent in children 3 to 72 hours after birth. Results from several studies have shown that even symptom-free infants born to mothers who have MG have elevated titers of AChR antibodies. It is not clear why only some babies develop TNMG, but the ability of the mother's serum antibodies to bind to the fetal isoform of the AChR in the newborn may be a contributing factor.The antibody concentration of the symptom-free neonate appears to decrease rapidly compared with the antibody concentration of a symptomatic neonate. Two clinical forms of TNMG have been described: typical and atypical. Clinical features of the less common atypical form include the presence of arthrogryposis multiplex congenita (AMC) in the fetus or newborn. The usual clinical findings of the typical form of TNMG include poor sucking and generalized hypotonia. Other common clinical manifestations are weak cry, facial diplegia or paresis, swallowing difficulties, and mild respiratory distress. Some infants require feeding by gavage during this period. Ptosis and ophthalmoparesis are less common. Respiratory distress requiring assisted mechanical ventilation can occur in severe cases. Complete recovery is expected in fewer than 2 months in 90% of patients and by 4 months of age in the remaining 10%. The presence of high concentrations of anti-AChR or anti-MuSKR antibodies in the plasma of the affected newborn along with maternal history of MG is diagnostic for TNMG. A decremental response on EMG is seen in response to repetitive nerve stimulation. Motor nerve conduction velocity remains normal. This unique EMG pattern is the electrophysiologic correlate of the fatigable weakness observed clinically and is reversed after a cholinesterase inhibitor is administered. A diagnostic bedside test involves administration of neostigmine intramuscularly at a dose of 0.04 mg/kg. If the result is negative or equivocal, another dose of 0.04 mg/kg may be administered 4 hours after the first dose. The peak effect is seen in 20 to 40 minutes. Intravenous neostigmine is contraindicated before 2 years of age because of the risk of cardiac arrhythmias, including fatal ventricular fibrillation, especially in young infants. The ptosis, dysphagia, or head lag can be assessed to evaluate the response to the test. Because of the risk of cholinergic crisis manifested primarily by abdominal cramps or sudden diarrhea from increased peristalsis, profuse bronchotracheal secretions that may obstruct the airway, or rarely, cardiac arrhythmias, the baby should be monitored carefully for a few hours after administration of the test dose along with a preparation of atropine before the test, which can be administered intravenously, if indicated. When symptoms are mild, small feedings and careful surveillance are sufficient. When symptoms are more severe, cholinesterase-inhibiting drugs are the primary therapeutic agents. Neostigmine methylsulfate (0.04 mg/kg) may be administered intramuscularly every 4 to 6 hours, but most patients tolerate oral neostigmine bromide 0.4 mg/kg every 4 to 6 hours. If dysphagia is a major problem, the drug should be administered about 30 minutes before meals to improve swallowing. Pyridostigmine is an alternative; the dose required is about four times greater than that of neostigmine, but it may be slightly longer-acting. Also, certain drugs, including antibiotics such as aminoglycosides, may potentiate myasthenia and should be avoided.

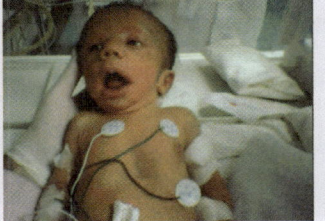

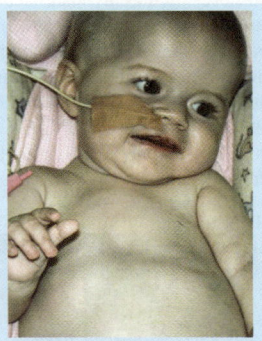

Type I, severe infantile acute SMA, or Werdnig-Hoffman disease: characterized by degeneration of the anterior horn cells of the spinal cord, leading to symmetrical muscle weakness and atrophy. Infants with SMA1 experience severe weakness before 3-6 months of age, and the patient never achieves the ability to sit independently when placed. Muscle weakness, lack of motor development and poor muscle tone, fasciculations of tongue are the major clinical manifestations of SMA1. Tendon reflexes: Reduced or absent. *Weakness:* Diffuse; Proximal > Distal * Severe * Poor feeding * Respiratory insufficiency: Paradoxical respirations* Sparing of facial & oculomotor.* Most affected children die before 2 years of age but survival may be dependent on the degree of respiratory function and respiratory support. Infants with the gravest prognosis have problems sucking or swallowing. Some show abdominal breathing in the first few months of life. Cognitive development is normal with alert face. Death: 50% by 7 months; 95% by 17 months. Chronic course in 5%. All the SMAs are inherited as an autosomal recessive trait. Molecular genetic testing has revealed that all types of autosomal recessive SMA are caused by disruptions or errors (mutations) in the SMN1 (survival motor neuron 1) gene on chromosome 5. SMA is the second most common lethal, autosomal recessive disease in Caucasians after cystic fibrosis.

Neonatal Dysmorphic Syndromes: Selective list

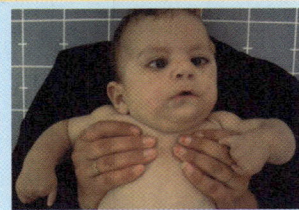

Möbius syndrome is defined as a static congenital facial weakness combined with abnormal ocular abduction. The facial nerves (CN VII) are involved in all cases; the abducens nerves (CN VI), in a high percentage of cases (75%); and the hypoglossal nerves (CN XII), in only a minority of cases. Facial diplegia is the most noticeable symptom. This may be observed soon after birth, with incomplete eyelid closure during sleep, drooling, and difficulty sucking. On occasion, the facial paralysis is not noticed for a few weeks or months, until the infant's inability to smile or the lack of facial movement with crying arouses the parents' concern. An inability to close the mouth is the rule. Undue prominence of the upper lip is a striking feature. The 4 proposed groups, which have no significant clinical correlations, are as follows:* Group I - Simple hypoplasia or atrophy of CN nuclei *Group II - Primary lesions in peripheral CNs *Group III - Focal necrosis in brainstem nuclei *Group IV - Primary myopathy with no central nervous system (CNS) or CN lesions. Most cases are sporadic. Etiologic hypotheses include hypoxic/ischemic injury and intrauterine toxic exposure. Complications include poor nutrition, dysphagia, aspiration pneumonia, and corneal ulceration/abrasion. In patients with severe brainstem compromise that causes dysphagia, aspiration, and an inability to protect the airway, death may occur at a young age. In severe cases, death may occur in the perinatal period, often as a result of respiratory or bulbar problems. Life expectancy may be normal in patients with less extensive brainstem involvement.

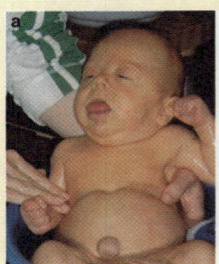 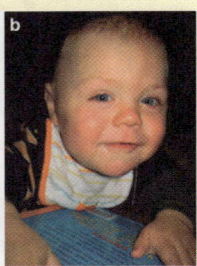 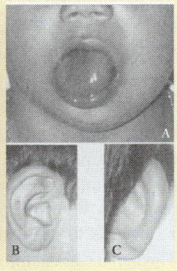

Beckwith-Wiedemann Syndrome is a disorder of growth regulation exhibiting somatic overgrowth and a predisposition to embryonal tumors. The incidence of BWS is estimated to be 1 out of 13 700. The cardinal features of Beckwith-Wiedemann syndrome include prenatal and postnatal overgrowth, macroglossia, and anterior abdominal wall defects (most commonly, exomphalos, umbilical hernia, diastasis recti). *Increased growth:* birth weight and length (usually above the mean), visceromegaly (particularly kidneys, liver, and pancreas) and hemihyperplasia (usually all or part of one side of the body). Ear lobe creases, and/or pit indentations on the posterior helix are used as one of the criteria for diagnosis of the illness. *The risk situations are*: a) Hypoglycemia, which occurs shortly after birth. Although it is usually temporary, if untreated, it can cause seizures and hypoxia, leading to severe complications, including mental deficiency. b) Premature birth and its complications. c) Development of tumors: children with Beckwith-Wiedemann syndrome have a 7-21% risk for the development of embryonic malignancies, most notably Wilms' tumor of the kidney, although a wide variety of benign and malignant tumors have been reported, including hepatoblastoma, adrenocortical carcinoma, rhabdomyosarcoma and neuroblastoma. Beckwith-Wiedemann syndrome is a genetically heterogeneous disorder; most cases are sporadic but approximately 15% are familial and a small number of Beckwith-Wiedemann syndrome patients have cytogenetic abnormalities involving chromosome 11p15. BWS is caused by various epigenetic and/or genetic alterations that dysregulate the imprinted genes on chromosome 11p15.5. The BWS molecular subgroups are associated with different recurrence risks. subfertility/assisted reproduction is associated with an increased frequency of BWS.

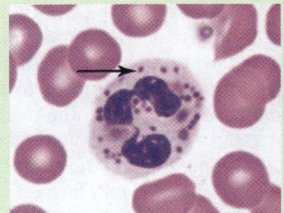 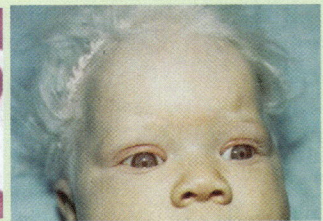

Chediak-Higashi syndrome is a rare autosomal recessive disorder characterized clinically by partial oculocutaneous albinism due to defects in melanin granules and recurrent pyogenic bacterial infections due to abnormalities in granulocytes. The basic defect is in microtubules resulting in fusion of lysosomal granules. All white blood cells contain abnormally giant granules. This image shows a normally segmented neutrophils with giant azurophilic granules. Because of abnormal granules there is defective and delayed release of bactericidal lysosomal proteins leading to poor ability to fight bacterial infections. Neutrophil number is also decreased in addition to defective granulation which heightens the susceptibility to infections. Thrombocytopenia is also seen in these patients. Note that giant abnormal pseudo Chediak-Higashi granules can occasionally be seen in certain acquired hematologic disorders such as in myeloblasts in acute leukemia and maturer granulocytes in certain myeloproliferative and myelodysplastic syndromes. The abnormal granulation in acquired conditions is limited to a few cells as opposed to generalized involvement of all white blood cells and even megakaryocytes in Chediak-Higashi syndrome. With progressive immunodeficiency these patients develop diffuse lymphoid and histiocytic proliferations involving lymph nodes, spleen, bone marrow, liver, and other organs. This usually indicates a terminal stage in the disease and most patients die at around 10 years of age.

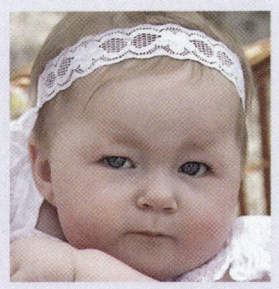

Prader-Willi syndrome (PWS) or hypotonia-hypomentia-hypogenitalism-obesity (HHHO) syndrome is a disorder caused by a deletion or disruption of genes in the proximal arm of chromosome 15 or by maternal disomy in the proximal arm of chromosome 15. Prader-Willi syndrome results from the loss of imprinted genomic material within the paternal 15q11.2-13 locus. The loss of maternal genomic material at the 15q11.2-13 locus results in Angelman syndrome. Most cases of Prader-Willi syndrome are sporadic. About 60% of children with Prader-Willi syndrome have a microdeletion of chromosome 15 on the homologue that was inherited from father. The remainder have other deficiencies of paternal imprinting, either inheriting 2 copies of mother's 15 (uniparental disomy) or a paternal chromosome 15 that did not acquire the male imprint (abnormal DNA methylation). The Prader-Willi DNA methylation test will detect all 3 causes of Prader-Willi or its complement—the failure of female chromosome 15 imprinting known as Angelman syndrome. Fluorescent in situ hybridization (FISH) can be used to confirm prenatal diagnosis when a deletion in the 15q region is suspected after chorionic villus sampling or amniocentesis. Most manifestations of Prader-Willi syndrome are attributable to hypothalamic dysfunction. Commonly associated characteristics of this disorder include diminished fetal activity, obesity, hypotonia, mental retardation, short stature, hypogonadotropic hypogonadism, strabismus, and small hands and feet. Infants with Prader-Willi syndrome (PWS) commonly exhibit hypotonia, poor suck (with requirement of gavage feedings), weak cry, and genital hypoplasia (e.g., cryptorchidism, scrotal hypoplasia, clitoral hypoplasia). Neonatal hypotonia is one of the hallmark features of this disorder and is a valuable clue to initiate diagnostic testing. Craniofacial - Characteristic facial features such as narrow bifrontal diameter, almond-shaped palpebral fissures, narrow nasal bridge, and down-turned mouth. Patients with Prader-Willi syndrome (PWS) frequently require medical care for the following: * Initial management of hypotonia or poor feeding *Evaluation for hypogonadism or hypopituitarism * Management of obesity * Monitoring for scoliosis * Therapy for behavioral issues.

Neonatal Dysmorphic Syndromes: Selective list

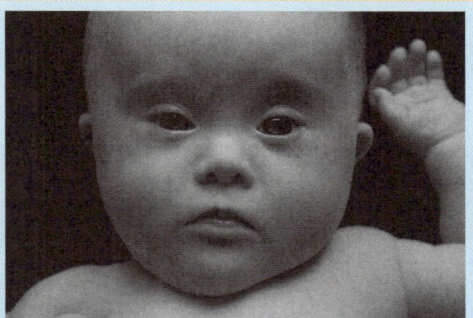

Trisomy 21 or Down syndrome the most common (1 case in 800 live births) and best known chromosomal disorder in humans and the most common cause of intellectual disability, is characterized by mental retardation, dysmorphic facial features, and other distinctive phenotypic traits. In 94% of patients with Down syndrome, full trisomy 21 is the cause; mosaicism (2.4%) and translocations (3.3%) account for the remaining cases. Approximately 75% of the unbalanced translocations are de novo, and approximately 25% result from familial translocation. Advanced maternal age remains the only well-documented risk factor for maternal meiotic nondisjunction. Maternal age risk factors are as follows: *With a maternal age of 35 years, the risk is 1 in 385 * With a maternal age of 40 years, the risk is 1 in 106 *With a maternal age of 45 years, the risk is 1 in 30. Prenatal screening for Down syndrome includes maternal serum screening. Serum markers for Down syndrome include maternal serum alpha-fetoprotein, chorionic gonadotropin, and unconjugated estriol. While these measurements are not a definitive test for Down syndrome, a lower maternal serum alpha fetoprotein value, a lower unconjugated estriol level, and an elevated chorionic gonadotropin level, on average, suggest an increased likelihood of a fetus with Down syndrome and additional diagnostic testing may be desired. *Fluorescence in situ hybridization (FISH) may be used for rapid diagnosis. It can be successful in both prenatal diagnosis and diagnosis in the neonatal period. Characteristic craniofacial findings: an* anteriorly and posteriorly flattened head (flat occiput and a flattened facial appearance), dysplastic low-set ears, small nose, depressed nasal bridge, protruding tongue, high-arched palate, dental abnormalities, and a short and broad neck. Eyes-Up-slanting palpebral fissures, bilateral medial epicanthal folds, Brushfield spots (speckled iris), refractive errors (50%), strabismus (44%), nystagmus (20%). General *physical features* in patients with Down syndrome include shortened extremities, short limbs, short and broad hands, short fifth middle phalanx, simian palmar creases (present in approximately 60% of patients), a wide gap between the first and second toes, joint hyperextensibility or hyperflexibility, neuromuscular hypotonia, dry skin, premature aging, a wide range of intelligence quotients (IQs), and congenital heart defects. The most common congenital heart defects are endocardial cushion defect (43%), ventricular septal defect (32%), secundum atrial septal defect (10%), tetralogy of Fallot (6%), and isolated patent ductus arteriosus (4%). The prevalence of thyroid disorders (eg, congenital hypothyroidism, primary hypothyroidism, autoimmune thyroiditis, and compensated hypothyroidism or hyperthyrotropinemia) is reportedly 3-54% in individuals with Down syndrome and increases with increasing age. Children with Down syndrome have an increased risk of developing leukemias, including acute lymphoblastic leukemia (ALL) and acute myeloid leukemia (AML). Approximately 10-30% of individuals with Down syndrome have atlantoaxial instability. By 40 years of age, individuals with Down syndrome have an increased likelihood to develop symptoms that are nearly identical to those of Alzheimer's disease. Attention to heart, digestive, orthopedic, or other medical conditions identified during the neonatal period should continue to be monitored. The optimal management of the newborn with a genetic condition includes a multidisciplinary team approach with participation of pediatric specialists. Specific growth charts for children with Down syndrome have been developed and are standardized. Improved quality of life for these individuals comes with early care and proper management of health issues including cardiac, gastrointestinal, hearing, vision, and thyroid. Intervention including early educational intervention and support for families and the individual can enhance life skills and optimize education, employment, and community life opportunities for those with Down syndrome.

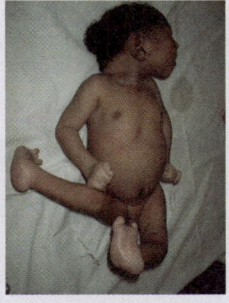

Trisomy 18: Trisomy 18, or Edwards Syndrome, is the second most common trisomy behind Down syndrome. This syndrome has an incidence of between 1 in 3000 and 1 in 8000, with a 3:1 Female:Male predominance. 90% of cases of trisomy 18 are due to maternal nondysjunction. 10% of cases are due to mosaicism, and less than 1% of cases are due to a translocation. Trisomy 18 typically presents with some combination of the following features: 1. Clenched hand, with overlap of the 2nd and 5th fingers, over the 3rd and 4th 2. Intrauterine growth retardation (IUGR) 3. Rocker bottom feet with prominent calcanei 4. Micrognathia, prominent occipital, micro-ophthalmia 5. Low set ears 6. Cardiac defects, such as ventricular septal defect (VSD), atria sepal defect (ASD) and patent ducts arteriosus (PDA) 7. "Strawberry shaped" calvarium 8. Generalized muscle spasticity, arthrogryposis 9. Renal anomalies 10. Mental retardation Trisomy 18

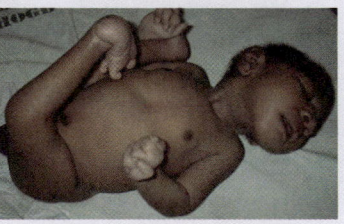

is confirmed by karyotype with FISH analysis. Prognosis: Trisomy 18 is associated with severe mental retardation and severe failure to thrive. 50% of patients die by one week of life, and 90% of patients die by one year of life.

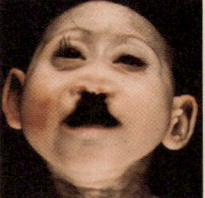 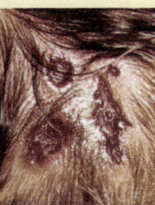

Trisomy 13, or Patio syndrome, is the least common of the live-born trisomy disorders, with an incidence of 1 in 5000 to 1 in 2,000 live births. There is an equal distribution between affected males and affected females. 75% of trisomy 13 cases are due to maternal nondisjunction, 20% of cases are due to a translocation, and 5% of cases are due to mosaicism. The major midline dysmorphic features of trisomy 13 are due to a defect in the fusion of the midline prechordial mesoderm in the first three weeks of gestation. Trisomy 13 tends to present with more severe craniofacial and midline defects than are found in Trisomy 18 or 21. Trisomy 13 traditionally presents with some combination of the following clinical features: 1. Holoprosencephaly 2. Postaxial Polydactyly with flexion of fingers and hyper-convex nails 3. Seizures 4. Deafness 5. Microcephaly 6. Midline Cleft lip 7. Midline Cleft palate 8. Abnormal ears 9. Sloping forehead 10. Omphalocele 11. Cardiac and renal anomalies 12. Scalp defects are commonly seen in the vertex and usually without an underlying bone defect. 13. Severe growth and mental retardation. Trisomy 13 is confirmed by karyotype with FISH analysis. Prognosis: The prognosis of patients diagnosed with Trisomy 13 remains poor. 85% of Trisomy 13 newborns die before reaching one year of age, and only six cases have been described in the literature as surviving past the age of 10 years. 44% of these patients die within 1 month, and > 70% die within one year. Iliopoulos et al. have hypothesized that factors associated with longer survival largely pertain to the absence of cardiac abnormalities and holoprosencephaly; Rasmussen et al. have also demonstrated that the general rate of survival is higher for female Trisomy 13 patients when compared with males. Prenatal USG, particularly three dimensional (3D) sonography, permits a more detailed evaluation than routine 2D sonography. Visualization of the facial

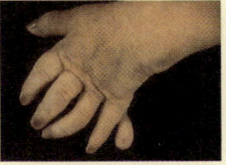

dysmorphisms in the fetus will help them accept prenatal genetic counseling approaches such as amniocentesis and therapeutic abortion, and it may also facilitate their granting permission for a postmortem study.

Neonatal Dermatological Emergencies

@ *The neonatal dermatological emergencies can be clinically classified into two groups: primary dermatological emergencies and dermatoses associated with medical or surgical emergencies . In the former group, the involvement of skin is the primary cause for the mortality or is the major manifestation, and in the latter, cutaneous manifestations are the indicators of impending or underlying severe systemic involvement.*

Primary Dermatological Emergencies

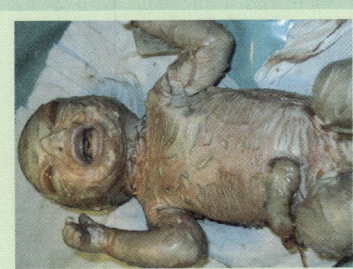

Harlequin ichthyosis

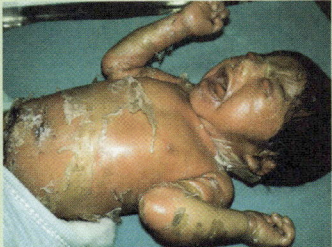

Collodion baby

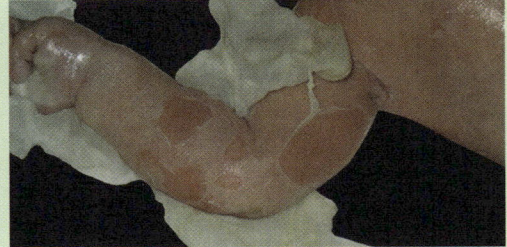

Bullous ichthyosiform erythroderma

Neonatal Cutaneous Infections

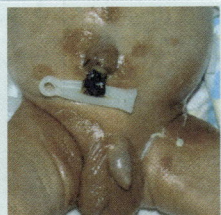

Staphylococcal scalded skin syndrome

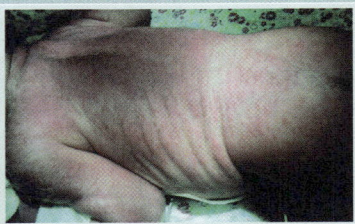

Congenital Candidiasis

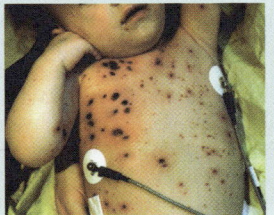

Neonatal varicella

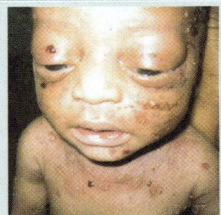

Neonatal HSV infection

Nutritional Deficiencies

Dermatoses Associated with Medical or Surgical Emergencies

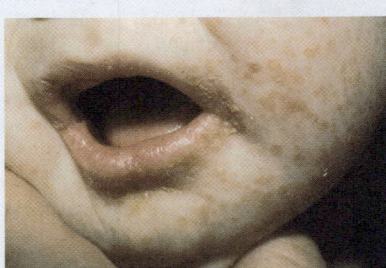

Acrodermatitis enteropathica zinc deficiency

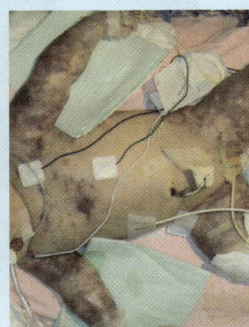

Purpura fulminans

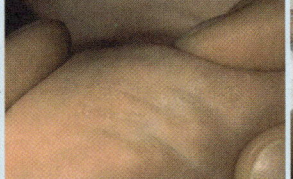

Sclerema Neonatorum

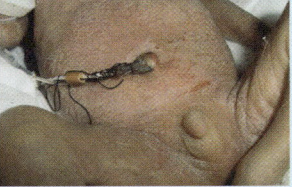

Neonatal Sepsis

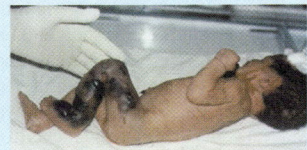

Necrotizing fasciitis

REVIEW OF CLINICAL PROBLEMS

1) Mention the Neonatal dermatoses associated with medical or surgical emergencies.
   Ans: Necrotizing fascitis, Purpura fulminans, Neonatal Herpes/ Varicella, Kawasaki disease, Sclerema neonatorum.

2) What are the complications of Neonatal Erythroderma?
   Ans: Dehydration, electrolyte abnormalities (at increased risk of hypernatremic dehydration), temperature instability (hyperpyrexia or hypothermia) hypoalbuminemia and sepsis.

3) Mention the important aspects of history and physical examination in the evaluation of Neonatal Erythroderma.
   Ans: Refer to the Evaluation-Decision-Action-plan/algorithm for the diagnosis and management of a Neonate with Erythroderma.

4) Discuss the differential diagnoses of Neonatal Erythroderma.
   Ans: Refer to the Table "Neonatal Erythroderma: differential diagnosis and management".

5) Describe the diagnostic value of Skin biopsy in the evaluation of Neonatal Erythroderma.
   Ans: Refer to the Evaluation-Decision-Action-plan/algorithm for the diagnosis and management of a Neonate with Erythroderma.

LEARNING OBJECTIVES

After completing this article, readers will be able to:

1) Recognize Neonatal medical and surgical dermatological emergencies and manage them promptly & effectively

2) Recognize erythroderma and distinguish it from eczema and direct appropriate evaluations for neonates who have erythroderma

3) Appreciate the potential severity of erythroderma and Search for underlying disorders, some of which have a specific treatment

4) Anticipate the potential complications of erythroderma, including electrolyte disturbances, thermal instability, and sepsis.

5) Provide effective support of affected neonates and their families.

BIRD'S EYE VIEW/OVERVIEW/SYNOPSIS

The neonatal dermatological emergencies are potentially life-threatening and presents unique therapeutic and diagnostic challenges. The differential diagnosis is broad, and many of the potential diagnoses are exceedingly rare. The clinical presentation also varies from generalized involvement of skin to localized disease with or without systemic symptoms. Irrespective of the etiology and clinical presentation, these disorders are associated with significant morbidity and mortality. Knowledge of clinical presentations, rapid diagnostic methods, emergency care and monitoring of progress of the disease helps in comprehensive multidisciplinary care of neonates with these disorders.

Neonatal erythroderma (red scaly baby) is defined as generalized skin erythema affecting at least 90% of the body. This skin reaction is not specific for one diagnosis. The differential diagnosis for neonatal erythroderma includes more than 40 cutaneous or systemic disorders that encompass primary skin disorders, such as genodermatoses and inflammatory skin disease, infection, immune deficiencies, metabolic disorders or nutritional deficiencies, and reactions to medications (See table). The defining characteristic of erythroderma is generalized, blanching erythema of the skin that feels warm on palpation. The distribution may be widespread from disease onset or initially limited but progressive with time. Scale that ranges from dry and white to yellow and waxy, desquamation, or erosions may be seen. Unfortunately, this phenotype is nonspecific, and additional distinguishing features are needed to point to a specific diagnosis. An accurate personal history, family history, and physical examination are the foundation for the evaluation of erythroderma. A family history of atopy, atopic dermatitis, psoriasis, and consanguinity is important to obtain. An accurate weight and assessment of rate of weight gain and growth is crucial because failure to thrive can be seen with some causes of erythroderma. A complete blood count helps screen for infection or immunodeficiency, and abnormalities such as marked eosinophilia may point to Omenn syndrome (OS) or Netherton syndrome (NS). Quantitative immunoglobulins (Igs) and lymphocyte subsets and typing are indicated if immunodeficiency or graft-versus-host disease (GVHD) is suspected. IgE values may be elevated in both NS and OS. Nasopharyngeal, umbilical, perianal, and maternal vaginal cultures should be obtained for bacteria, yeast, or viruses when infection is suspected. Feeding intolerance, hypotonia, hepatomegaly, and acidosis in conjunction with erythroderma should prompt further investigation for an underlying metabolic disorder. Finally, skin biopsy can provide specific diagnostic information for some causes of erythroderma, including GVHD, immunodeficiency, psoriasis, atopic dermatitis, NS, or ichthyosis. Despite clinical and laboratory evaluation, some cases remain undiagnosed. These neonates presented with severely pruritic erythroderma, marked induration of skin, severe alopecia, nail abnormalities, failure to thrive, lymphadenopathy and hepatosplenomegaly. Family history of atopy may be present in 60% of cases. Severe systemic infection occurs in almost all the cases. Leiner's disease is another such entity applied to a neonatal erythroderma after other causes have been ruled out. A follow-up study of five infants with Leiner's phenotype revealed immunological abnormalities in all the cases; one had hypogammaglobulinemia, one had combined immunodeficiency which was later diagnosed as Omenn syndrome and three were diagnosed as Netherton syndrome with elevated IgE levels. Histopathological study of skin biopsy specimens preferably taken simultaneously from 2 or 3 different sites contributes to the specific diagnosis only in 45% of cases. Significant orthokeratosis with corneocytes arranged in laminated and compact fashion, prominent hypergranulosis, acanthosis, and absent or few inflammatory cells suggest ichthyoses except Netherton syndrome. In bullous ichthyosiform erythroderma, epidermolytic hyperkeratosis is seen. Omenn syndrome and graft versus host disease are characterized by dermal and epidermal lymphocytic infiltration and keratinocyte necrosis with satellite lymphocytes. Irrespective of the underlying cause, erythroderma represents a failure of the skin barrier that requires prompt management to prevent Dehydration, electrolyte abnormalities (at increased risk of hypernatremic dehydration), temperature instability (hyperpyrexia or hypothermia) hypoalbuminemia and sepsis. These complications are more pronounced in collodion baby, Harlequin ichthyosis, severe lamellar ichthyosis, Netherton syndrome and Omenn syndrome resulting in significant mortality and morbidity. Increased skin fragility, fissures, cracks, erosions or immunodeficiency in these disorders result in severe septicemic infections. The management of neonatal erythroderma is largely supportive and anticipatory, focusing on fluid and electrolyte balance, improvement of the skin barrier, nutrition, and prevention of secondary infection. Electrolytes should be monitored and necessary hydration provided, with the understanding that insensible losses are increased in erythroderma. Insensible water losses can be minimized by keeping the neonate in an ambient humid environment and using liberal amounts of bland petrolatum-based ointments to coat the skin several times daily. Percutaneous absorption is increased in affected neonates, and topical medications should be avoided, if possible, until a clear diagnosis is reached. Nutrition evaluation and close monitoring of growth and development are critical. Directed therapies should be initiated once a diagnosis has been established. The efficacy of systemic retinoids in the treatment of ichthyosis except Netherton syndrome is well established. However, risk/benefit ratio is considered before using retinoids because of increased skin fragility and decreased barrier competence induced by them. The use of topical retinoids and calcipotriol in generalized ichthyosis is limited by their irritancy and expense. Omenn syndrome and severe combined immunodeficiency may need bone marrow transplantation.

Neonatal cutaneous infections: Newborns are susceptible to various infections during the perinatal period. Premature and low birth weight infants are particularly predisposed to fatal neonatal infectious disorders. These include *Staphylococcal scalded skin syndrome* (Refer to Chapter 97, page 613), *Necrotizing fasciitis* (Refer to page 978), *Neonatal varicella* (Refer to Chapter 91, page 585), *Neonatal HSV infection* (Refer to Chapter 90, page 581) *Candidiasis in newborns* (Refer to page 794).

Dermatoses Associated with Medical or Surgical Emergencies: Purpura fulminans (Refer to page 980), Kawasaki disease (Refer to page 971), Sclerema neonatorum: Sclerema neonatorum is regarded as end stage of severe systemic disease. Sclerema is an uncommon, life-threatening condition, usually of newborns, with a case-fatality rate ranging from 50 to 100%. The disease manifests during first 1-2 weeks of life in severely debilitated term and preterm infants. It is characterized by sudden onset of diffuse hardening of skin initially involving the lower legs and later spreading to thighs, buttocks, trunk, and cheeks. The palms, soles and genitalia are usually spared. The skin is cold, smooth, hard and bound down. Neonates with diarrhoea and sepsis presenting with hypothermia, lower serum protein and prealbumin are prone to develop sclerema. Histology of the skin biopsy shows thickening of the trabeculae supporting the subcutaneous adipose tissue and a sparse inflammatory infiltrate of lymphocytes, histiocytes and multinucleate giant cells. Supportive therapy such as maintenance of body temperature, correction of fluid and electrolyte disturbances, and nutritional supplementation may sometimes reduce the inevitable mortality.

Classification of Neonatal Dermatological Emergencies

1. Primary Dermatological Emergencies

Neonatal Erythroderma

Ichthyoses: Autosomal recessive ichthyosis–Lamellar ichthyosis–Congenital ichthyosiform erythroderma, Epidermolytic ichthyosis, Netherton syndrome, Sjö¨gren-Larsson syndrome, Keratitis ichthyosis deafness syndrome, Chondrodysplasia punctata, Neutral lipid storage disease

Immunodeficiency

Primary immunodeficiency syndromes–Severe combined immunodeficiency (with graftversus-host disease)–Omenn syndrome

Infectious- Staphylococcal scalded skin syndrome, Toxic shock syndrome, Candidiasis or other fungal infections

Inflammatory Skin Diseases- Psoriasis, Atopic dermatitis. Seborrheic dermatitis, Pityriasis rubra pilaris, Diffuse cutaneous mastocytosis

Metabolic Disorders and Nutritional Deficiencies

Zinc deficiency, Cystic fibrosis, Inborn errors of metabolism – Methylmalonic acidemia –Maple syrup urine disease –Multiple carboxylase deficiency, Essential fatty acid deficiency

Drug Reactions- Vancomycin ("The red man syndrome"), Ceftriaxone

2 Associated with medical/surgical emergencies

Neonatal herpes/varicella, Necrotizing fascitis, Purpura fulminans, Kawasaki disease, Sclerema neonatorum

References: 1. Neonatal dermatological emergencies, S Ragunatha, Arun C Inamadar, Shri B. M. Patil Medical College, Hospital and Research Center, BLDE University, Bijapur, Karnataka, India 2. Neonatal erythroderma, Laleh A. Bedocs, MD, Grainne M. O'Regan, MD, Anna L. Bruckner, MD, N eoReviews V3o,l .1220N1o1.6 June 2011 e325 3. Neonatal erythroderma: differential diagnosis and management of the "red baby", P H Hoeger, J I Harper, *Arch Dis Child* 1998;**79**:186–191

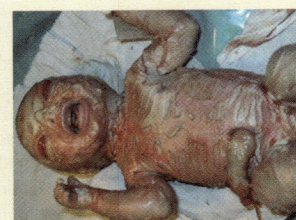

*Harlequin ichthyosis is very rare, severe form of congenital ichthyosis with thickened stratum corneum that cracks and fissures shortly after birth. The condition is associated with premature delivery and poor fetal outcome. *Polygonal/triangular/diamond-shaped plaques because of skin fissuring, Gray/yellow cracked skin forming plaques, deep red fissures. *Whole-body is involved with a marked ectropion (turning out of the eyelids), eclabium (fish-mouth deformity), distorted flat ears, and sometimes microcephaly *Inherited in an autosomal recessive manner and the underlying genetic defect is ABCA12 gene mutation. *Most infants are stillborn or die in the neonatal period. The course and prognosis for a harlequin fetus is very poor. Most infants die early because of prematurity, infection, or thermal or electrolyte imbalance. *It should be differentiated from the less severe form of congenital ichthyosis—a collodion baby. *Systemic retinoids such as isotretinoin and acetretin may increase survival, but the harlequin skin is permanent and the resultant quality of life is poor.

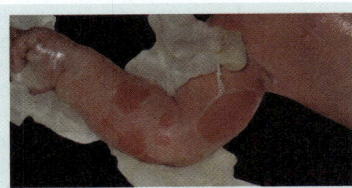

* Bullous ichthyosiform erythroderma also referred to as epidermolytic hyper-keratosis, presents with generalized erythema and superficial ,painful blisters that are frequently mistaken for staphylococcal scalded skin syndrome or epidermolysis bullosa. All surfaces of the body can be involved, and flexural areas are accentuated. Many patients have palmar and plantar involvement (keratoderma). *These children later develop typical ichthyosiform hyperkeratosis, with verrucous plaques. The clinical appearance of the later verrucous form may be confused with lamellar ichthyosis but the pathology is usually diagnostic. *Hair, nails, and teeth are usually normal. *The disease has an autosomal dominant inheritance, but 50% of patients exhibit new mutations in keratins 1 and 10 localized on chromosome 12q11–q13 and 17q12–q21, respectively. *Bullous congenital ichthyosiform erythroderma at birth needs to be differentiated from other blistering disorders such as epidermolysis bullosa, staphylococcal scalded skin syndrome, toxic epidermal necrolysis, and bullous impetigo.

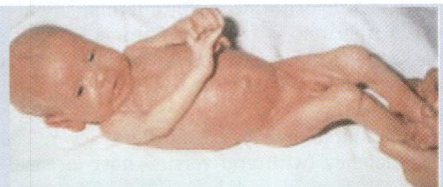

* Netherton's syndrome is characterized by a triad of generalized exfoliative dermatitis, sparse hair with trichorrhexis invaginata ("bamboo hair"), and atopic features. It usually presents at birth as erythroderma . *An autosomal recessive ichthyosis resulting from mutations in the gene SPINK5, which encodes the serine protease inhibitor LEKTI. The clinical result is accelerated desquamation of the stratum corneum and a profoundly compromised skin barrier. *Because of the early paucity of hair, it can take some time before the diagnosis of Netherton's syndrome is confirmed, although examination of eyebrows or eyelashes is often rewarding. *During their first year of life, patients with Netherton's syndrome undergo a period of life threatening infections, hypernatremic dehydration, diarrhoea, and failure to thrive, with a mortality of 30–40% during this period. *Later in life, the exfoliative dermatitis tends to persist and vary in severity, with exacerbations triggered by intercurrent illness. *Patients are atopic and often suffer from recurrent angio-oedema and urticaria associated with eating certain foods. *Apart from raised total IgE and multiple positive specific IgE reactions, there are no consistent immunological abnormalities in Netherton's syndrome.

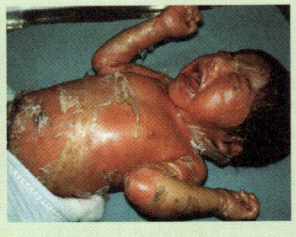

* Ichthyosis in the newborn often presents as a Collodion baby. It is not a distinct disorder, but can be the first presentation of several (usually autosomal recessive) ichthyoses. At birth, the collodion baby is encased in a clear, parchment like membrane, which may impair respiration and sucking. *When the membrane is shed 2 to 3 weeks later, the infant may have difficulties with thermal regulation and an increased susceptibility to infections. After healing the skin will appear normal. *The collodion baby may be the initial presentation of lamellar ichthyosis or congenital ichthyosiform erythroderma. In rare instances, the collodion baby progresses to Sjogren-Larssen syndrome, trichothiodystrophy, infantile Gaucher disease, or Netherton syndrome.

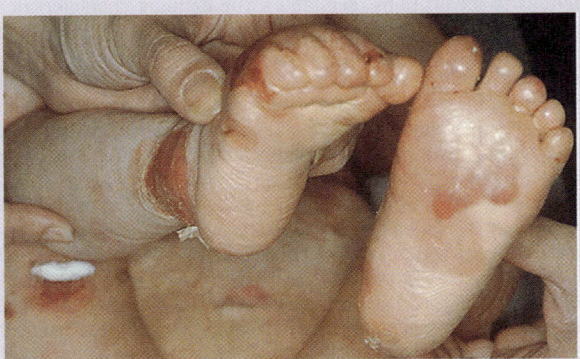

*Dystrophic epidermolysis bullosa (DEB) is a deeper mechanobullous disease caused by a mutation in the collagen VII gene. This results in a defective anchoring fibril in the sublamina densa of the skin and leads clinically to subepidermal blisters which scar. In dominant DEB, the genetic defect leads to abnormal collagen VII resulting in impaired anchoring fibrils in the lamina densa. In recessive DEB, the genetic defect leads to severe defects in type VII collagen leading to undetectable anchoring fibrils in the lamina densa. Both DEB forms result in a spilt in the dermal–epidermal junction which clinically results in deep blisters that can heal with scarring, fusion, and flexion deformities. **Recessive DEB:** In more severely affected individuals (the Hallopeau-Siemens variant), the extensive blistering may result in scarring, fusion, and flexion deformities that are functionally incapacitating. Recessive DEB blistering may result in death secondary to sepsis, fluid loss, or malnutrition. Surviving patients are chronically susceptible to infection and repeated blistering leads to further and further disabilities. These patients tend to have difficulties with laryngeal complications, esophageal strictures, and scarring of the anal area, and have a predisposition to basal cell and squamous cell carcinomas in the scarred skin areas.

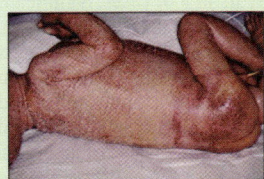

*Omenn syndrome is an autosomal recessive form of severe combined immunodeficiency (SCID) characterized by erythroderma, desquamation, alopecia, chronic diarrhea, failure to thrive, lymphadenopathy, and hepatosplenomegaly. Patients develop fungal, bacterial, and viral infections typical of SCID. Lymphocytosis results from the expansion of an oligoclonal population of activated and antigen-stimulated T helper 2 (TH2) cells that produce elevated levels of interleukin 4 (IL-4) and interleukin 5 (IL-5). The latter cytokines mediate eosinophilia and elevated immunoglobulin E (IgE) levels. It is caused by hypomorphic mutations in the RAG 1 and 2 genes in more than 50% of cases, and a variety of other mutations and syndromes are associated with the Omenn phenotype. Affected patients lack B cells and have aberrant expansion of oligoclonal T cells. Markedly elevated IgE concentrations are common. Skin and gut inflammation leads to protein losses and edema. Histology shows psoriasiform hyperplasia with spongiosis, focal keratinocyte necrosis, and an infiltrate of lymphocytes and eosinophils.

THE EVALUATION-DECISION-ACTION-PLAN/ALGORITHM FOR THE DIAGNOSIS AND MANAGEMENT OF *Neonatal Dermatological Emergencies*

SUBJECTIVE FINDINGS

Hx of- presenting skin lesions; generalized erythema, scaling (dry and white to yellow and waxy, desquamation or cracks, fissures or erosions) and superficial, painful vesicles, bullae, or blisters, *Determine* onset, duration, progression, distribution, severity, remissions and exacerbations, *Hx of-* systemic complications of neonatal erythroderma-hypernatremic dehydration, severe systemic infections, failure to thrive, hypoalbuminemia , hyperpyrexia or hypothermia *Family Hx of-*atopy, atopic dermatitis, psoriasis, and Sibling mortality, consanguinity, **Drugs** (ceftriaxone, vancomycin), *Hx suggestive of* Graft versus host reaction (Fever; diarrhea; antecedent transfusion; immunodeficiency)

OBJECTIVE FINDINGS

Assess ABCDs - vitals, BP, CRT, O_2 sats, sensorium-alert/lethargic? coma, apnea, hypotension/shock *Look for -* skin tenderness; superficial blisters; positive Nikolsky sign (SSSS), paronychia and nail dystrophy, Darier's sign often with blistering is positive in mastocytosis), Erythematosquamous patches; can be pustular, Lymphadenopathy (Omenn's syndrome, graft versus host reaction) and atopic dermatitis ; Alopecia, either total or partial, is obvious in Netherton's syndrome, Omenn's syndrome, and disorders of biotin metabolism. ; atopy; sparse hair, trichorrhexis invaginata (bamboo hair), Cradle cap, accentuation in the skin folds of the neck, axillae, and nappy area, Encrusted eczema on the scalp and face; generalized eczematous skin; *Perform* complete physical, skeletal neuro-ophthalmological examination & *examine parents for* linear epidermal naevus parents or sibling

INVESTIGATIONS

Blood-FBC (Lymphopenia- Immune deficiency, Eosinophilia-Omenn syndrome, Netherton syndrome), *Gram stain & blood cultures-*(Gram-positive cocci, Staphylococcus aureus), Fungal smear (Spores and hyphae-Candidiasis or other fungal infection), *Acidosis on ABG analysis-*(Inborn error of metabolism-• Plasma amino acids • Urine organic acids • Urine ketones • Lactate • Ammonia) *Blood sugar, BUN, creatinine, Electrolytes-*(Hypernatremia (Netherton syndrome) Hypoalbuminemia *(*Malabsorption/nutritional insufficiency- Consider: • Netherton syndrome • Cystic fibrosis • Immune deficiency) *Urine analysis, Imaging-* CXR-Absent thymic shadow (Immune deficiency), *Perform-*COMPLETE SEPSIS SCREEN + LP if not C/I) - FBC, CRP, blood & urine cultures, CXR etc., *CONSIDER-Skin biopsy; Refer* to Table given below for its diagnostic value in neonatal dermatological emergencies.

Identify drugs known to cause erythroderma-Vancomycin, Ceftriaxone and substitute them with alternative antibiotics

Monitor for potentially life threatening complications, such as sepsis (especially *Pseudomonas aerugenosa*), hypernatremic dehydration, hyperpyrexia, hypothermia and Manage appropriately and promptly to prevent mortality and morbidity.

Newborn with Dermatological Emergency

Ensure ABCs, pulse oximetry, Supplemental O_2 IV access & Monitor BP

Identify dermatoses associated with medical or surgical emergencies-Purpura fulminans (Refer to page 980), Kawasaki disease (Refer to page 971), Neonatal varicella (Refer to Chapter 91, page 585), Neonatal HSV infection (Refer to Chapter 90, page 581), Necrotizing fasciitis (Refer to page 978), Sclerema neonatorum and Manage accordingly.

Neonatal Erythroderma: differential diagnosis and management-Refer to Table on next page

Diagnostic value of Skin biopsy

* Take two or three simultaneous biopsies from different sites.
* Samples for routine histopathology can be formalin fixed, but it is valuable to have a sample frozen in liquid nitrogen for immunohistochemical studies.
* In blistering diseases, it is helpful to take the biopsy from the border of the blister, including its roof, to facilitate assessment of the level of cleavage.
* Histology and immunohistochemistry can differentiate Omenn's from Netherton's syndrome and the other ichthyoses

* Psoriasiform changes (• Psoriasis • Immune deficiency • Netherton syndrome)
* Epidermolytic hyperkeratosis (Epidermolytic ichthyosis)
* Ichthyosiform hyperkeratosis(• Congenital ichthyosiform erythroderma • Lamellar ichthyosis)
* Spongiotic changes (• Atopic dermatitis • Seborrheic dermatitis • Immune deficiency • Netherton syndrome)
* Interface dermatitis with necrotic keratinocytes(• Graft-versus-host disease versus drug eruption)

KEY POINTS FOR CLINICAL PRACTICE:

1) *Neonatal* dermatological emergencies comprise diseases that demand early diagnosis, hospitalization, careful monitoring and multidisciplinary intensive care to minimize the associated morbidity and mortality.

2) Neonatal erythroderma is a diagnostic and therapeutic challenge. Erythrodermic neonates and infants are frequently misdiagnosed with eczema and inappropriate topical steroid treatment can lead to Cushing's syndrome. Delay in the establishment of the correct diagnosis can be fatal.

3) The differential diagnosis of erythroderma is a multistep procedure that involves clinical assessment, knowledge of any relevant family history, and certain laboratory investigations

4) *Irrespective* of its cause, neonatal erythroderma is a potentially life threatening condition. Erythrodermic neonates and infants are at risk of hypernatremic dehydration and hyperpyrexia. Maintaining adequate oral or parenteral fluid intake and monitoring serum electrolytes is therefore mandatory.

5) Appreciating the potential severity of erythroderma and understanding its many possible causes is critical to effective support of affected neonates and their families.

Neonatal Erythroderma: differential diagnosis and management

Staphylococcal scalded skin syndrome: Preceding purulent infection; skin tenderness; superficial blisters; positive Nikolsky sign :Skin swab; assessment of toxin production by *S aureus*, Skin biopsy, rarely indicated: superficial split (below granular layer), few or no inflammatory cells within bulla or dermis. *Treat with* Intravenous antibiotics (flucloxacillin, amoxycillin/clavulanic acid), analgesics, careful observation for dehydration and superimposed infection, bland emollients on the skin, nonadherent dressings such as petrolatum-impregnated gauze to cover erosions, contact tracing (carriers of toxigenic strains).

Toxic shock syndrome: Concomitant maternal infection; skin tenderness; hypotension/shock Skin swab, assessment of toxin production by *S aureus* or *Streptococcus pyogenes*, Skin biopsy: superficial perivascular and interstitial neutrophilic infiltrates. Treat *with* Intravenous antibiotics (flucloxacillin, amoxycillin/clavulanic acid), contact tracing (carriers of toxigenic strains) intravenous immunoglobulins.

Congenital cutaneous candidiasis: Maternal vaginal candida infection; generalized erythematous papules, pustules, scaling, and erosions with palmar and plantar involvement, oral cavity and diaper area spared; may have paronychia and nail dystrophy. Skin swab, KOH preparation; pseudohyphae; cultures: urine, blood, CSF, Skin biopsy: pseudohyphae and spores in the corneal layer (PAS stain). Treat *with* Topical (nystatin, miconazole) and oral (nystatin, fluconazole) antimycotics; preterm and systemically ill infants require early intervention with systemic antifungal therapy-may need intravenous amphotericin; also eradication of maternal vaginal yeast infection.

Omenn's syndrome: severe erythroderma, massive lymphadenopathy, failure to thrive (Skin and gut inflammation leads to protein losses and edema), alopecia ; unexplained death of previous children; consanguinity, Eosinophilia; IgE markedly raised; decreased B cells; increased activation markers on T cells (CD25, HLA-Dr, CD45RO); Skin biopsy: psoriasiform hyperplasia with spongiosis, focal keratinocyte necrosis, and an infiltrate of lymphocytes and eosinophils .*Treat with* Supportive care; eventually will need a bone marrow transplant.

Graft versus host reaction: Fever; diarrhoea; antecedent transfusion; immunodeficiency (almost always due to underlying severe T-cell immunodeficiency, with engraftment of maternal lymphocytes or lymphocytes from nonirradiated blood product transfusions) -Mixed lymphocyte populations, Skin biopsy: basal cell vacuolation; exocytosis, satellite cell necrosis, HLA-Dr + basal keratinocytes . *Treat with*: Use of irradiated blood products is mandatory; for those with SCID supportive care and bone marrow transplant.

Non-bullous ichthyosiform erythroderma: Collodion baby; when shed leaves disseminated ichthyosiform scaling, Skin biopsy: hyperkeratosis, acanthosis, minimal lymphocytic infiltrate. *Treat with* Emollients

Bullous ichthyosiform erythroderma: Superficial blistering and erosions; ichthyosiform erythroderma; family history; linear epidermal naevus parents or sibling, Skin biopsy: epidermolytic hyperkeratosis. *Treat with* Emollients

Netherton's syndrome: Diarrhoea; failure to thrive; atopy; sparse hair, trichorrhexis invaginata (bamboo hair); may not manifest until 18 months or older but can be appreciated sooner, particularly in eyebrow or eyelash hairs. Hair microscopy shows characteristic features. IgE raised, eosinophilia, Skin biopsy: psoriasiform acanthosis, parakeratosis, perivascular lymphocytic infiltrate. Treat *with* Emollients, adequate hydration, elemental hypoallergenic formula

Conradi-Hünermann syndrome: Linear and swirled patterning, Skin biopsy: hyperkeratosis, reduced granular layer. X Rays show stippling in infancy. *Treat with* Emollients

Holocarboxylase synthetase deficiency: Lethargy, coma, apnoea Ketoacidosis, organic aciduria; decreased enzyme activity in leukocytes and fibroblasts. *Treat with* Oral biotin (5–10 mg/day) (normal daily requirement > 0.1mg/kg/day). Multiple inborn errors of metabolism have been reported as associated with an acrodermatitis-like rash and erythroderma, such as

methylmalonic aciduria, maple syrup urine disease, and multiple carboxylase deficiencies, all inherited in an autosomal recessive pattern. Of note, this presentation is unusual, and most affected infants are likely to be diagnosed via routine newborn screening programs. The diagnosis should be suspected in the infant presenting with poor feeding, lethargy, hypotonia, and acidosis with or without a progressive dermatitis or erythroderma. Assays for plasma amino acids, urine organic acids, and metabolic analysis of cultured fibroblasts should be performed to confirm the diagnosis. Early institution of appropriate dietary restriction and supplementation may prevent irreversible neurologic damage and developmental delay.

Essential fatty acid deficiency: Ichthyosiform erythroderma; wasting, Blood fatty acid screen. *Treat with* Topical linoleic acid (sunflower seed oil).

Acrodermatitis enteropathica: a rare autosomal recessive disorder that results from defective uptake of zinc in the duodenum and jejunum due to abnormalities in the zinc transporter protein ZIP4. Noncutaneous findings include failure to thrive, irritability, and photophobia. Alkaline phosphatase is a zinc-dependent enzyme, and low serum concentrations may point indirectly to the diagnosis. Secondary infection with *Staphylococcus aureus* or Candida is common and may complicate the clinical picture. Response to zinc supplementation is dramatic, with resolution of the dermatitis within days. The differential diagnosis for a baby who has the skin changes of zinc deficiency should include cystic fibrosis. In addition to the "peeling paint" dermatitis, hypoalbuminemia, edema, and failure to thrive can be seen before the onset of respiratory symptoms.

Infantile seborrhoeic dermatitis: Cradle cap (waxy yellow scales) , accentuation in the skin folds of the neck, axillae, retroauricular and nappy areas. Treat *with* moisturizing agents;, ketoconazole-hydrocortisone ointment, protective cream nappy area

Atopic dermatitis: Encrusted eczema on the scalp and face; generalized eczematous skin; xerosis, inflammation, pruritus, and increased susceptibility to staphylococcal skin infection, commonly develop symptoms between 3 and 6 months of age, sparing of the occluded diaper area, affected infants typically thrive and show no evidence of immune compromise, family history for atopy, IgE raised; eosinophilia, Skin biopsy: spongiosis, lymphocytes, exocytosis. Treat *with* Weak topical steroid; systemic antibiotics if skin infected. Possible cows' milk allergy

Psoriasis: Erythematosquamous patches, well-defined red plaques with adherent silver-white scale, typically located on the extensor arms and legs, umbilicus, gluteal cleft, and scalp ; can be pustular (sterile); Periumbilical accentuation, the tendency of lesions to occur in areas of skin injury (Koebnerization), or an inverse pattern affecting groin and large skinfolds, may have positive family history, neonatal presentation is rare and often a marker of disease severity and poor prognosis, Skin biopsy: hyper and parakeratosis, microabscesses. *Treat with* Bland emollient creams, topical therapies, including corticosteroids and vitamin D analogs, wet dressings .

Pityriasis rubra pilaris: Similar to psoriasis; follicular accentuation skin thickening of palms and soles; may have positive family history Skin biopsy: like psoriasis, follicular hyperkeratosis. *Treat as* psoriasis

Diffuse mastocytosis: The skin is diffusely thickened and may appear doughy. There can be numerous orange papules or diffuse erythroderma. It can be accompanied by extensive blistering and mimic staphylococcal skin syndrome. Children with congenital diffuse or erythrodermic mastocytosis may have extracutaneous mast cell infiltrates (gastrointestinal tract, bone, liver, spleen, lymph nodes). Accompanying symptoms include diarrhoea, vomiting, abdominal cramps, wheezing, raised temperature, pruritus, flushing, and hypotension. Darier's sign—a wheal and flare reaction on rubbing the skin—is positive. Serum/urine histamine and metabolites. Skin biopsy: mast cell infiltrate. Careful monitoring for systemic involvement is mandatory in diffuse cutaneous mastocytosis. It should include full blood count, liver function tests, bone scan and, if appropriate, gastrointestinal studies. *Treat with* H1 and H2 antagonists; oral sodium cromoglycate; avoidance of substances with potential for mast cell degranulation (for example, codeine, opiates, aspirin, procaine, radiographic dyes, scopolamine, pancuronium)

1. **Blood pressure** values for premies: MAP (mean arterial pressure) = diastolic pressure+ 1/3 of pulse pressure (systolic-diastolic). MAP should be similar to the gestational age (a 25 week premie should have a MAP of 25 or 1kg birth weight = 25 mm Hg 1.5 kg = 30 mm Hg 2 kg = 35 mm Hg. Term Newborn Systolic 55-90, Diastolic 26-55

2. **1ml blood from a 1000 gr baby equals 70 ml blood from an adult**. Also, a normal newborn has 90 ml / body weight kg blood volume. Avoid unnecessary labs.

3. **Creatinine** can not be used in the first 48-72 hrs as it reflects mom's serum levels.

4. **Signs of pneumothorax:** sudden cyanosis, increased resp effort, asymmetrical breath sounds, shift of PMI Chest: one side enlarges abdominal distension drop in blood pressure

5. **Chest tube placement:** locate the 6th rib, that is the skin insertion site. Locate the 4th ICS, that is the thoracic insertion site. Between the two: tunnel. Use the curved hemostat to make the tunnel, the trocar to make the puncture of the parietal pleura. The baby is supposed to be in 60 degree angle, affected chest up, location is the midaxillary line. Emergency needle insertion and aspiration in case of tension pneumothorax with 3 way stopcock: 3rd ICS, above 4th rib, avoiding breast tissue.

6. **Commonly Associated Findings meconium aspiration syndrome (MAS) :** Cardiovascular Consequences of Asphyxia-Hypoxemia-related pulmonary hypertension,Hypoxemia-related myocardial dysfunction Pulmonary Consequences of Asphyxia-Decreased surfactant, Pulmonary edema, Meconium aspiration syndrome Renal Consequences of Asphyxia-Tubular and medullary necrosis, Bladder paralysis.Central Nervous System Consequences of Asphyxia-Hypoxic-ischemic encephalopathy, Intracranial hemorrhage

7. **Developmental interventions:** the baby's stimulation should be as minimal as possible. Low light, cluster care, decreased noise, fetal positioning. Try assessing the baby, when the nurse is doing it, so all stimulation is done at the same time and the baby is not disturbed again and again.

8. **Iron stores** are depleted by 2 months in premies, 4 months in term babies. Supply diet with iron at 2mg/kg/day starting at 8 weeks (60 days) of age for 4months and/or birthweight doubled if not on iron fortified formulas.

9. **5 signs of respiratory distress:** flaring, retraction, grunting, cyanosis, tachypnea.Overt respiratory failure may occur without manifesting signs of respiratory distress [E.g.: Neuromuscular disease-Myotonic dystrophy, Myasthenia-Transient Neonatal/Congenital], *while* a Neonate may display signs of severe respiratory distress with no pulmonary disease [E.g.: severe metabolic acidosis with Kussmaul respirations often resulting from Severe sepsis, Ductus-dependent Cardiac Malformations, Acute Renal Failure, NEC,Congenital Adrenal Hyperplasia, and Inborn Errors of Metabolism, especially Organic acidemias].

10. **Desired O2 concentration** is 50-80mmHg with sats at 90-94%. This is the main effort of ventilation. If PaO2 is> 120mmHg, decrease FiO2 by 10% If PaO2 is 80-120mmHg, decrease FiO2 by 5%.

11. **Facts of neonatal feeding:** <28wks: decreased GI motility, small stomach, delayed emptying, fat malabsorption (due to low conc. Of bile salts. >32wks: good suck, coordination with swallow, good gag-reflex Feeding start: 10cc/kg/day div. by 8 Low Birth Weight infants: small gastric capacity, poor intestinal motility. Start feeding: small infants (Under 2000 grams: 2-3 ml Q3. Above 2000 grams: 5-10 ml Q3. Calculate needs: if a baby needs 120 ml/kg fluid parenterally, the same baby will need 150ml/kgfluid enterally. Signs of intolerance to enteral feedings: residuals above 30% of fed volume or above 3ml, vomiting, distention.

12. **Suspect sepsis:** Always, if something unusual happens Decreased activity, feeding, responsiveness Sudden or increasing frequency of apneic episodes reported. None of the following tests carry absolute sensitivity: CXR, blood culture, CBC c. diff. Judge clinically. Treat empirically.

13. **Treatment of sepsis:** If the blood culture is positive, start empirical therapy. Repeat culture after 48 hrs. If negative, continue the treatment till 7-10 days after the last negative cul ture. Your repeat culture confirms your efficient treatment.

14. **Most common congenital heart defects** presenting on day 0-6 days: d-TGA 15% (5% of total defects), HLHS 12%, TOF 8%, Coarctation 7%, VSD 6% Other 52%. In case of cyanotic infant perform hyperoxia test to decide pulmonic or cardiologic origin: allow neonate to inhale 100% oxygen obtain ABG from preductal, that is right arm artery analyze values: If the PaO2 is greater than 200 mmHg, heart disease is unlikely. If the PaO2 is less than 150mmHg, it is a cardiac lesion with complete mixing w/o restricted pulmonary blood flow. If the PaO2 is less than 50mmHg, it is either a cardiac lesion with two separate circulations (d-TGA w/o septal defect) or cardiac defect with restricted pulmonary flow or TAPVR with obstruction. Get CXR, get EKG, examine for murmur, Organize an Echocardiogram.

15. **Duct-dependent congenital heart defects** where prostaglandin is life saving: d-TGA (transposition of great arteries, dexterous type)- cyanosis, egg-shaped heart. HRHS (hypoplastic right heart syndrome)- cyanosis, tachypnea. Tricuspid atresia, Pulmonary atresia, Ebstein anomaly - cyanosis. HLHS hypoplastic left heart syndrome -cyanosis. Interrupted aortic arch- congestive heart failure.

16. **Transfusions:** A single unit of platelet should raise platelet count by 40-50k.Transfuse if oxygen dependent patients have compromised carrying acpacity: keep hematocrit above 35-40%. 10ml/kg PRBC increase Hb 2-4g/dl. In convalescent babies transfusion will simply delay the normal physiologic anemia of the newborn and activation of erythropoiesis. Transfuse only symptomatic infants or when weight gain falls off.

17. **Complications of hyperalimentation:** Too high lipid = ketosis .Too high protein: metabolic acidosis, elevated tyrosine, BUN, ammonia. Too high dextrose = osmotic diuresis, increased renal solute load.

18. **UAC tip Position on an anteroposterior (AP) radiograph of the chest and abdomen:** Prefer a higher placement, in the thoracic aorta at approximately T10-T12, again avoiding placement of the catheter near the major tributaries off of the descending aorta.Take the following precautions: *Careful placement under sterile conditions *Daily evaluation of ease of injection and withdrawal of blood *Assessment of the pressure waveform on the monitor screen *Inspection of the site for erythema and induration *Daily evaluation of urine output and blood pressure*Prompt removal of the line as soon as it is no longer needed.

19. **UVC tip Position on an anteroposterior (AP) radiograph of the chest and abdomen :** The UVC should be kept at the lower margin of the cardiac silhouette, approximately at the level of the right diaphragm, which would correspond to the junction of the inferior vena cava and right atrium of the heart. UVCs should not be allowed to remain below this level or within any of the branches of the portal system of the liver. Infusion of calcium or hyperalimentation into catheters in these incorrect positions may lead to liver toxicity, portal necrosis, cirrhosis, and cavernous transformation of the portal vein. Umbilical venous lines may also inadvertently cross the foramen ovale and enter the left heart. Catheters in this location occasionally will cause rhythm disturbances of the heart. This incorrect placement can be detected by the high levels of PO_2 obtained on a venous sample of blood.

20. **ET Tube tip Position on an anteroposterior (AP) radiograph of the chest:** The optimal position for an ET tube is approximately halfway between the thoracic inlet (look for the medial ends of the baby's clavicles to get a good approximation) and the carina or level of tracheal bifurcation. In small neonates, ET tubes often enter the right mainstem bronchus and produce left-sided atelectasis. They may also exert vagal effects and cause bradycardia or irritation if they strike the carina. Tubes that are excessively high also may produce vagal effects and loss of effective ventilation.

21. **Basic elements of Neonatal neurologic examination:** *Mental status (level of alertness) *Eyes and other cranial nerves *Primitive (neonatal) reflexes *Motor and sensory function *Deep tendon reflexes * Autonomic: heart rate pattern, respiratory pattern, bladder function, bowel function.The object of the neurologic history and examination is to localize a process in time and space, that is, to determine what the lesion is and where it is located.

22. **Oxygen saturations in a Newlyborn:** Use oxygen saturation monitor if unsure of clinical assessment of cyanosis. Be aware of normally low saturations in the first minutes of life (at *1 minute, median of 63% & at 5 minutes, median of 90%*). Give the vigorous baby a few minutes to pink up, rather than rushing to give free flow oxygen.

23. 4 Pearls of wisdom in Neonatal surgery: **1. Bubbly** baby with frothy secretions from mouth choke on feeding- TEF with esophageal atresia. **2. Baby** becoming blue on feeding but pink on crying - bilateral choanal

Neonatal Pearls of Wisdom to Remember!!!

atresia. **3. Newborn** baby with bilious vomiting-bowel obstruction unless proved otherwise. **4.** Surgery for NEC: when perforated. when progressive deterioration. when late stricture

24. **The "four horsemen" of Neonatal Respiratory Emergencies:** In the near term neonate, there are four very similar presentations of respiratory disease that are particularly challenging to distinguish from one another shortly after birth. They are as follows (and in order of prevalence): **1.** Transient tachypnea of the newborn **2.** Respiratory distress syndrome **3.** Pneumonia (either through bulk aspiration of amniotic fluid, or bacteria, or virus) **4. Persistent** fetal circulation (persistent pulmonary hypertension). A near term baby who starts out with transient tachypnea and a touch of respiratory distress and then is improperly managed may spiral into persistent fetal circulation. Likewise, an infant with aspiration pneumonia may start out with moderate tachypnea and progress to severe respiratory distress that is essentially ARDS and also progress to persistent fetal circulation. All of them can progress to persistent fetal circulation! Thus the simplest and most correct strategy is to support all infants with the global diagnosis of the four horsemen such that all possibilities are being managed simultaneously.

25. **Benign neonatal sleep myoclonus** is characterized by myoclonic "lightning like" jerks of the extremities that exclusively occur during sleep; it is not correlated with epilepsy. *Neonatal onset (in first 2 weeks of life) *Myoclonic jerks occur only during drowsiness or sleep and cease with arousal *No signs of epileptiform paroxysmal activity on EEG if performed *Most, but not all, resolve by 3 months of age The diagnosis is usually made on clinical grounds only, unnecessary investigations may blur the picture and inappropriate medication can make the myoclonus worse. The **myoclonic epilepsies** may not be so benign. They rarely present before 3 months and seizures will occur during periods of wakefulness as well. There are EEG changes.

26. **Petechiae and ecchymoses** are commonly seen in newborns. The birth history, location of lesions, their early appearance without development of new lesions, and the absence of bleeding from other sites help differentiate petechiae and ecchymoses secondary to birth trauma from those caused by a vasculitis or coagulation disorder. If the etiology is uncertain, studies to rule out coagulopathies and infection should be performed. Most petechiae and ecchymoses resolve within 1 week. If bruising is excessive, jaundice and anemia may develop. Treatment is supportive.

27. **Diagnostic work-up of the Bleeding Neonate:** The history includes (a) family history of excessive bleeding or clotting; (b) maternal medications (e.g. aspirin, phenytoin); (c) pregnancy and birth history; (d) maternal history of a birth of an infant with a bleeding disorder; and (e) any illness, medication, anomalies, or procedures done to the infant. The crucial decision in diagnosing and managing the bleeding infant is determining whether the infant is sick or well. **1. Sick infant.** Consider DIC, viral or bacterial infection, or liver disease (hypoxic/ischemic injury may lead to DIC). **2. Well infant.** Consider vitamin K deficiency, isolated clotting factor deficiencies, or immune thrombocytopenia. Maternal blood in the infant's gastrointestinal tract will not cause symptoms in the infant. **3.** Petechiae, small superficial ecchymosis, or mucosal bleeding suggest a platelet problem. **4.** Large bruises suggest deficiency of clotting factors, DIC, liver disease, or vitamin K deficiency. **5.** Enlarged spleen suggests possible congenital infection or erythroblastosis. **6.** Jaundice suggests infection, liver disease, or resorption of a large hematoma. **7.** Abnormal retinal findings suggest infection.

28. **Intrapartum asphyxia should never be a diagnosis of exclusion**, and should satisfy certain criteria; **Essential criteria (must meet all four)** * Metabolic acidosis in umbilical cord arterial blood (pH < 7.0 and base deficit ? 12 mmol/L) * Early onset of severe or moderate neonatal encephalopathy * Cerebral palsy of the spastic quadriplegic or dyskinetic type * Exclusion of other identifiable etiologies such as trauma, coagulation, disorders, infectious conditions, or genetic disorders *Suggestive, but nonspecific criteria* * Sentinel hypoxic event occurring immediately before or during labor * Sudden and sustained fetal bradycardia or the absence of fetal heart rate variability in the presence of persistent late or variable decelerations, usually after a hypoxic sentinel event. * Apgar scores of 0-3 beyond 5 minutes *Onset of multisystem involvement within 72 hours of birth * Early imaging study showing evidence of acute nonfocal cerebral abnormality.

29. **Current practice for treating jaundiced premature infants :** **1.** Infants <1,000 g. Phototherapy is started within 24 hours, and exchange transfusion is performed at levels of 10 to 12 mg/dL. **2.** Infants 1,000 to 1,500 g. Phototherapy at bilirubin levels of 7 to 9 mg/dL and exchange transfusion at levels of 12 to 15 mg/dL. **3.** Infants 1,500 to 2,000 g. Phototherapy at bilirubin levels of 10 to 12 mg/dL and exchange transfusion at levels of 15 to 18 mg/dL. **4.** Infants 2,000 to 2,500 g. Phototherapy at bilirubin levels of 13 to 15 mg/dL and exchange transfusion at levels of 18 to 20 mg/dL.

30. **Push-pull method Exchange Transfusion: Blood** is removed in aliquots that are tolerated by the infant. This usually is 5 mL for infants <1,500 g, 10 mL for infants 1,500 to 2,500 g, 15 mL for infants 2,500 to 3,500 g, and 20 mL for infants >3,500 g. The rate of exchange and aliquot size have little effect on the efficiency of bilirubin removal, but smaller aliquots and a slower rate place less stress on the cardiovascular system. The recommended time for the exchange transfusion is 1 hour.

31. **Neonatal Jaundice:** Neonates characteristically do not appear jaundiced until the TSB exceeds 5.0 to 7.0 mg/dL (86 to 120 micro mol/L). Some degree of jaundice develops in approximately 60% of neonates, and chemical hyperbilirubinemia, defined as a TSB ≥2.0 mg/ dL (34 micro mol/L), is virtually universal in newborns during the 1st week of life. One should make a search to determine the cause of jaundice if 1) it appears in the 1st 24-36 hr of life, 2) serum bilirubin is rising at a rate faster than 5mg/dL/24 hr, 3) serum bilirubin is greater than 12 mg/ dL in full-term (especially in the absence of risk factors) or 10-14 mg/ dL in preterm infants, 4) jaundice persists after 10-14 days of life, or 5) direct-reacting bilirubin is greater than 2 mg/dL at any time. Among other factors suggesting a nonphysiologic cause of jaundice are a family history of hemolytic disease, pallor, hepatomegaly, splenomegaly, failure of phototherapy to lower bilirubin, vomiting, lethargy, poor feeding, excessive weight loss, apnea, bradycardia, abnormal vital signs (including hypothermia), light-colored stools, dark urine positive for bilirubin, and signs of kernicterus.

32. **Meconium plug-Meconium ileus-Small left colon syndrome:** Meconium plug is caused by meconium blocking the left colon in otherwise healthy babies. Meconium ileus, as previously described, is obstruction of the distal ileum due to thick and viscid meconium, occurring in 10-20% of neonates with cystic fibrosis. The small left colon syndrome is most common in infants of diabetic mothers and produces an obstruction from a temporarily dysfunctional, small-caliber left colon. A contrast enema with barium is usually diagnostic as well as therapeutic for both meconium plug and the small left colon syndrome (through its mechanical effect), although subsequent testing for Hirschsprung's disease or cystic fibrosis may be indicated.

33. **Caloric requirements of LBW infants:**
Requirements (in cal/kg/day) Resting *50-75, Specific dynamic action- 5-8% of total intake, Stool losses- 10% of total intake, **Growth-25-45**

Total†- 85-142

*Estimate includes caloric expenditure for maintenance of basal metabolism plus activity and response to cold stress. †Includes sum of resting and growth requirements for specific dynamic action and replacement of stool losses plus an increment of 15-18%.

34. **Breast-milk jaundice versus Breast feeding jaundice: Breast-milk jaundice** is of late onset and has an incidence in term infants of 2% to 4%. By day 4, instead of the usual fall in the serum bilirubin level, the bilirubin level continues to rise and may reach 20 to 30 mg/dL by 14 days of age. If breast-feeding is continued, the levels will stay elevated and then fall slowly at 2 weeks of age, returning to normal by 4 to 12 weeks of age. If breast-feeding is stopped, the bilirubin level will fall rapidly in 48 hours. If nursing is then resumed, the bilirubin may rise 2 to 4 mg/dL but usually will not reach the previous high level. These infants show good weight gain, have normal liver function test (LFT) results, and show no evidence of hemolysis. Mothers with infants who have breast-milk jaundice syndrome have a recurrence rate of 70% in future pregnancies. Postulated mechanisms include: **1.** The presence of a lipoprotein lipase in human milk that releases free fatty acids, which inhibit glucuronyl transferase enzyme activity. **2.** Progesterone metabolite in the milk (5 beta-pregnane-3 alpha, 20 beta-diol, and other pregnanediols), which inhibits glucuronyl transferase enzyme activity. **3.** Increased beta glucuronidase activity in human milk, leading to increased conversion of bilirubin diglucuronide to monoglucuronide and subsequent reabsorption and enterohepatic circulation of bilirubin. **4.** Defects of the *UGT1A1* gene, with one or more components in the milk possibly triggering the jaundice in infants who have such mutations. The mutations described are identical to those detected in

patients who have Gilbert syndrome. No long-term neurodevelopmental effects result from human milk jaundice.

Breast feeding jaundice-Infants who are breast-fed have higher bilirubin levels after day 3 of life compared to formula-fed infants. The differences in the levels of bilirubin are usually not clinically significant. The incidence of peak bilirubin levels >12 mg/dL in breast-fed term infants is 12% to 13%. The infants become dehydrated, lose weight, are constipated, develop jaundice, and may develop hypernatremia. The main factor thought to be responsible for breast-feeding jaundice is a decreased intake of milk that leads to increased enterohepatic circulation. Encouraging breast-feeding while supplementing with formula for a limited time resolves the jaundice. Phototherapy and intravenous fluids may be needed, depending on the serum bilirubin value and severity of dehydration.

Human **Breast milk jaundice is a diagnosis of exclusion**, but a history of a similar affliction in siblings and lack of hemolytic disorders in the family can be reasonable indicators of the diagnosis and help avoid expensive evaluation.

35. **Hypocalcemic cardiac failure:** Hypocalcemia is a great masquerader. Hypocalcemia should be considered in the differential diagnosis of cardiac failure in a neonate. Extracardiac manifestations such as apnea, jitteriness, stridor, convulsions, or tetany usually surface before the onset of cardiac failure. Refractory to inotropes, but amelioration of symptoms, and the improvement in echocardiographic indices of ventricular systolic function with restoration of serum calcium corroborates the diagnosis. Congestive cardiac failure can be an initial presentation of hypoparathyroidism. Hypocalcemia is one of the causes of reversible dilated cardiomyopathy. Emergency management of hypocalcemic crisis involves 1 to 2 mL/kg of 10% calcium gluconate by intravenous infusion over 5 minutes while monitoring meticulously for dysrhythmias and bradycardia. A continuous calcium infusion via a central catheter is initiated, with the goal of achieving sustained serum calcium concentrations. Concomitant use of other medications, such as thiazides, furosemide, and glucocorticoids, can interfere with the serum calcium concentrations. Oral supplementation can be administered in the form of calcium glubionate (elemental calcium content, 23.6 mg/mL). Use of a low phosphate formula is recommended. In addition, vitamin D supplementation should be provided as cholecalciferol or dihydrochysterol. Clinical evaluation and frequent assessment of serum calcium, serum phosphorus, and urine calcium and creatinine concentrations are indicated to prevent the complication of nephrocalcinosis. Vomiting, hypotonia, polyuria, constipation, encephalopathy, and hepatosplenomegaly should alert the clinician to the possibility of hypercalcemia, and the therapy should be tailored accordingly. The role of PTH replacement therapy still is experimental in adults and has not been studied in neonates.

36. **Positive Direct Coombs Test Without Hemolysis:** Positive DCT results can be associated with conditions other than ABO or Rh D incompatibility. Although more than 60 different red blood cell (RBC) antigens are capable of eliciting an antibody response, significant disease is associated primarily with the D antigen of the Rh group and with incompatibility of ABO factors. Rarely, hemolytic disease may be caused by C or E antigens or by other RBC antigens such as CW, CX, DU, K (Kell), M, Duffy, S, P, MNS, Xg, Lutheran, Diego, and Kidd. Anti-Lewis antibodies do not cause disease. Other causes of positive DCT results are systemic lupus, infectious mononucleosis, and several drugs (e.g., methyldopa, quinidine).

37. **Episodic excessive sweating, pallor, and cold extremities occurring during feedings:** in the absence of other symptoms and signs and in conjunction with apparent wellness between episodes and normal initial investigation results, suggest the possibility of a cardiac dysrhythmia (**Supraventricular Tachycardia**) or episodic sympathetic overactivity. Sympathetic overactivity could be due to conditions such as hypoglycemia, pheochromocytoma, or neuroblastoma. The differential diagnoses for infants who have tachycardia includes sinus tachycardia, SVT, atrial flutter, AET, and VTs. Sinus tachycardia is associated with fever, pain, dehydration, hypoglycemia, hypovolemia, sympatho-mimetic medication, sepsis, shock, and anemia; the heart rate varies with respiration or activity and is usually less than 230 beats/ minute; and the QRS is narrow complex. The evaluation may include measurement of hemoglobin, serum electrolytes, and thyroid function studies; echocardiography; ECG, including a rhythm strip between and during the episodes; continuous ECG monitoring (Holter) or transtelephonic or event recordings; and chest radiography. After referral to a pediatric cardiologist, electrocardiographic imaging is used to reconstruct epicardial electrograms from body surface potentials to identify the location of pathways responsible for pre-excitation and electrophysiologic studies are undertaken.

38. **New-onset respiratory distress in a term infant at 45 hours of age:** New-onset respiratory distress in a term infant at 45 hours of age may have respiratory, cardiac, neurologic, infectious, or metabolic causes. Sepsis and pneumonia are primary considerations, as are other respiratory causes, including diaphragmatic hernia, mediastinal or lung parenchymal malformations, primary parenchymal abnormalities, and air leak syndromes. The most common parenchymal conditions, retained fetal lung liquid syndrome, meconium aspiration syndrome, and respiratory distress syndrome, do not fit the time course of this infant's symptoms. Gradual deterioration of respiratory status is more suggestive of pneumonia or sepsis; an acute onset of symptoms is suggestive of a pneumothorax. Spontaneous pneumothorax may occur in term infants who do not have pulmonary pathology or a history of positive-pressure ventilation. In the absence of other risk factors, it may result from the high pressures generated with the initiation of breathing. Risk factors for spontaneous pneumothorax are male sex, low birth weight, late preterms, vacuum extraction, meconium-stained amniotic fluid, low 1-minute Apgar score, bag-and mask positive-pressure ventilation, and poor prenatal care. The risk of complications is higher in infants who require delivery room resuscitation, even if they respond quickly to resuscitation efforts; these infants should be watched carefully. There are rare reported cases of familial pneumothorax associated with retained fetal lung liquid syndrome. The incidence of pneumothorax is more common after cesarean section, particularly after an elective, repeat cesarean section. The incidence tends to decline as the gestational age approaches 39 weeks. Some experts suggest a possible association between major urinary tract anomalies and spontaneous pneumothorax.

39. **Pseudoparalysis of leg in a 3 week old neonate, associated with irritability and pain on manipulation (such as diaper changes):** Possible diagnoses include Neonatal osteomyelitis, septic arthritis, fracture, possibly due to nonaccidental trauma or birth trauma, and, less commonly, marrow infiltration by leukemia or neuroblastoma. It is important to emphasize nonaccidental trauma as a consideration in a child at 3 weeks of age who presents with increased fussiness and decreased movement of one extremity. The period of increased crying begins around 3 weeks of age and peaks at 6 weeks of age. This is a time of heightened parental anxiety and frustration, which may lead to an increased incidence of abusive injuries.

40. **Management of Acute renal failure in the Newborn:** *Monitor weight *Monitor urine output and fluid balance *Monitor serum electrolytes, blood urea nitrogen, creatinine *Remove potassium from intravenous fluids until renal output is adequate *Adjust doses of drugs excreted by the kidney *Provide adequate nutrition –Adjust protein intake based on blood urea nitrogen to avoid overload –Add calories as carbohydrate and fat *Correct acidosis with supplemental acetate, citrate, or bicarbonate *Attempt a trial of furosemide to promote and maintain urine output *Support blood pressure with dopamine *Attempt dialysis, if necessary.

41. **Hemodynamically Significant Patent Ductus Arteriosus (HSDA) Criteria:** Echocardiographic Criteria *Transductal diameter (TDD) >1.5 mm *Unrestrictive pulsatile transductal flow *Left heart volume loading (e.g., left atrium-to-aortic root ratio of 1.5 to 2:1) **Systemic Hypoperfusion (Decreased Qs)** * Systemic hypotension *Evidence of end-organ hypoperfusion, renal insufficiency, NEC, IVH *Acidosis (lactic, metabolic) **Pulmonary Overcirculation (Increased Qp)** *Oxygenation failure *Increased ventilation requirements *Radiologic evidence of cardiomegaly or pulmonary edema.

42. **Persistent Projectile Vomiting in an 11-day-old Neonate:** In addition to Pyloric stenosis, malrotation, intracranial hemorrhage, sepsis, gastroesophageal reflux, hydronephrosis, urinary tract infection, and inborn errors of metabolism are to be considered in the differential diagnosis. Specifically, bilious emesis suggests obstruction distal to the ampulla of Vater, which necessitates contrast radiography for evaluation. Evaluation should include plain films of the abdomen (initially to look for air-fluid levels, distended loops of bowel, or characteristic signs of obstruction,) pyloric ultrasonography, and upper gastrointestinal radiographic series with a small bowel follow-through (to confirm the

Neonatal Pearls of Wisdom to Remember!!!

location and extent of obstruction). In particular, a partial obstruction caused by a duodenal web or stenosis may present more insidiously, with failure to thrive, feeding intolerance, or dehydration. Typically, a duodenal web or stenosis presents later than an atresia because small boluses of fluid initially may pass with the former. Intestinal obstruction may present at any age with persistent bilious emesis.

43. **First voiding of urine and first passing of meconium stool:** Voiding of urine typically occurs shortly after birth. The first voiding usually occurs within 24 hrs. If it does not , the infant should be evaluated for adequacy of fluid intake and bladder distention. Concern about a congenital defect of the urinary tract is appropriate, if voiding has not occurred after the first two days of life .Baby must have a minimum of one wet diaper in first 24 hours. On day two of life, baby must have at least one wet diaper every 8-11 hours. On day three of life, you should see an increase in wet diapers (up to 4-6) in 24 hours. On day four of life, baby's urine should be light yellow. On day six of life, baby should have 6-8 wet diapers per day of colorless or light yellow urine. Over 90 percent of newborns pass **meconium stool** within the first 24 hours of life. If the infant has never passed stools during the first 36 hours of life, the possibility of intestinal stenosis or atresia, Hirschsprung disease, or meconium ileus or plug should be considered. Failure to develop transitional stools after the passage of meconium 1. Volvulus. 2. Malrotation

44. **Neonatal Teeth:** A natal or neonatal tooth eruption is an exception to the normal sequence of development. ~85% are lower primary incisors rather than supernumerary teeth - a roentgenogram can determine the type of tooth. Most are hypermobile due to inadequate root formation. If aspiration is feared (because of hypermobility), the tooth should be removed. This can be done in the clinic with gauze and light finger pressure. If not taken care of quickly, the immature primary incisor will become more firm as the root develops. Occasionally, odontogenic remnants remain after removal of the natal teeth and these continue to form abnormal teeth that should be extracted as they are seen.

45. **Supernumerary nipples** (SNs) are a common minor congenital malformation that consist of nipples and/or related tissue in addition to the 2 nipples normally appearing on the chest. SNs are located along the embryonic milk line. Ectopic SNs are found beyond the embryonic milk line. The embryonic milk line is the line of potentially appearing breast tissue as observed in many mammals. In humans, the embryonic milk line extends bilaterally from a point slightly beyond the axilla on the arm, down the chest and the abdomen towards the groin, and ends at the proximal inner side of the thigh. SNs can appear complete with breast tissue and ducts and are then referred to as polymastia, or they can appear partially with either of the tissues involved.

46. **Witch's milk:** In folklore, witch's milk was believed to be a source of nourishment for witches' familiar spirits. Transient galactorrhea occurs in approximately 5% of term neonates and can persist for two months though palpable breast buds can persist into childhood The breasts of the Newborn in both male and female are often enlarged and engorged with a white liquid, sometimes colloquially called "witch's milk." This is due to maternal estrogen effect and usually lasts only a week or two. The ability of the baby's breasts to respond in this fashion is a mark of baby born at (or near) full-term. The breast of a baby born prematurely cannot enlarge or produce witch's milk. Avoid expressing the milk, as it may lead to neonatal mastitis and breast abscess.

47. **Neonatal Mastitis-Breast abscess: diagnosed** when a term newborn baby (A preponderance of female infants has been observed with mastitis occurs beyond the second week of life) more frequently during the second and third weeks after birth presents with enlarged, erythematous, tender firm than fluctuant breast, without Systemic signs and symptoms are uncommon; (one fourth of infants have a low-grade fever). The disorder must be distinguished from enlargement that is physiologic or hormonally induced; hormonally induced cases more likely produce swelling bilaterally. Neonatal mastitis is most commonly caused by *S. aureus*. Infection with other organisms has been described, including *E. coli, Pseudomonas, Proteus, Salmonella,* GBS, and anaerobes. Aspiration of the abscess for Gram stain and culture and blood culture are indicated. If gram-positive cocci are seen on the Gram stain, vancomycin or clindamycin should be given until the results of susceptibility testing are available. An aminoglycoside or cefotaxime is indicated when gram-negative bacilli are present. If no organisms are noted on Gram stain, vancomycin or clindamycin and either an aminoglycoside or cefotaxime should be given pending culture results.

Surgical incision and drainage may be necessary and should be performed by an experienced surgeon to minimize scarring of breast tissue.

48. **Omphalitis complications:** Omphalitis complicated by necrotizing fasciitis (resulting from rapidly spreading destruction of the fascia and subcutaneous tissue around the umbilicus)can be associated with bacteremia, coagulopathy, and shock, and frequently progresses to death despite heroic surgical and supportive measures. Septic embolization with metastasis to the lungs, kidneys, and skin can occur. Other infections complicating or occurring in the absence of cutaneous signs of omphalitis include pyelophlebitis (suppurative thrombophlebitis of portal or umbilical veins), liver abscess, septic umbilical arteritis, endocarditis, and subacute necrotizing funisitis. Parenteral administration of antibiotics is indicated if a neonate presents with periumbilical erythema, edema, and tenderness with or without purulent drainage. Combination therapy should be administered to provide broad-spectrum coverage. Vancomycin should be provided for gram-positive coverage. An aminoglycoside, or perhaps a third-generation cephalosporin for better tissue penetration, can be given for gram-negative coverage. The presence of crepitus or black discoloration of the periumbilical tissues suggests an anaerobic or mixed infection. In that case, consideration should be given to adding clindamycin or metronidazole for anaerobic coverage. Necrotizing fasciitis requires extensive surgical debridement and pathogen-directed antibiotic therapy and supportive care.

49. **Acute otitis media in Neonate: develops** in a minimum of 0.6% of all live births during the 1st month of life, and that the rate may reach 2% to 3% in premature infants (may be related to the small size of the eustachian tube, with resultant obstruction and secondary infection). It occurs more often in male than in female infants, in infants with cleft palate, and in infants requiring prolonged intubation. The disease increases in frequency in bottle-fed infants, a finding that may be related to use of the supine position during feeding or to the lack of local immunity that may be conferred by ingredients in breast milk(Secretory Ig A and other components in breast milk). Although organisms from the respiratory tract (*S. pneumoniae, H. influenzae, b*-hemolytic streptococci (groups A and B), are also the most commonly isolated pathogens in neonatal disease, GBS, gram-negative bacteria (*E. coli* and *Enterobacter, Klebsiella,* and *Pseudomonas* species), S. *aureus, Staphylococcus epidermidis,* and *Moraxella catarrhalis, can* be causative agents in the 1st 2 to 6 weeks of life. Young infants with otitis media often are asymptomatic. The ear is difficult to examine adequately in newborn infants. Erythema, dullness, and bulging of the pars flaccida of the tympanic membranes can be noted, and pneumatic otoscopy can reveal decreased mobility of the tympanic membrane. In infants who appear ill or fail to respond to initial therapy, a specific diagnosis should be made by culture and Gram-stained smears of purulent middle ear fluid obtained by myringotomy or tympanocentesis. Blood cultures can be helpful in patients with concomitant septicemia. Lumbar puncture should be performed to exclude meningitis in ill infants. For neonates with acute otitis media in the 1st 2 weeks of life, a combination of ampicillin and either an aminoglycoside or cefotaxime provides effective initial treatment. Hospitalized premature infants require parenteral therapy as well. A regimen such as vancomycin and gentamicin is one option for empirical therapy. Oral therapy with amoxicillin can be considered for well-appearing term infants older than 3 weeks who have had an uncomplicated intrapartum and neonatal course. If the infant is toxic-appearing or has evidence of infection elsewhere, cultures of middle ear fluid, blood, and CSF should be obtained, and the infant should be hospitalized for broad-spectrum parenteral antimicrobial therapy. When culture results are known, antibiotic therapy can be altered appropriately. Treatment should be continued for 10 days or longer, depending on the etiologic agent, the associated condition (e.g., sepsis or meningitis), and the clinical response to therapy. Recurrent or persistent disease can occur. Infants with onset of otitis media before 2 months of age are at high risk for development of chronic otitis media with effusion. In addition to young age at the onset of the 1st episode, other risk factors for recurrent infections include low socioeconomic status and the presence of smokers in the household. Careful follow-up evaluation for infection and hearing loss is important. Insertion of tympanostomy tubes may be indicated to ensure adequate drainage of the middle ear and to reduce the likelihood of recurrent middle ear infections.

Neonatal Pearls of Wisdom to Remember!!!

50. **Risk factors for Invasive Candidiasis in Neonates:** *Gestational age <32 weeks *Birthweight ≤1500 g *Male gender *Apgar score < 5 at 5 minutes *Intubation/mechanical ventilation *Placement of indwelling devices-Umbilical catheters, Peripheral or central venous catheters, Urinary catheters, Cerebrospinal fluid shunt devices *Abdominal surgery *Lack of enteral feeding *Fungal colonization *Use of intralipid *Total parenteral nutrition use *Corticosteroid use *Use of histamine type 2 receptor blockers *Administration of cephalosporins *Prolonged administration of antibiotics.

51. **Guiding principles for the cerebrovascular and metabolic care of critically ill preterm and term infants may include the following:** 1. Maintain stable blood pressure. Severe hypotension is clearly detrimental, but so are rapid increases in blood pressure in a pressure-passive circulation. 2. Maintain stable acid-base balance without rapid corrections. 3. Avoid severe hypoxemia. 4. Avoid marked hyperoxemia (i.e., consider effects of resuscitating with 100% oxygen). 5. Avoid major changes in PaCO2, both hypocapnia and hypercapnia. 6. Correct significant anemia or polycythemia; if the condition is chronic, correct slowly. 7. Consider cerebrovascular and metabolic effects of any new (and existing) drug therapies. Use the lowest effective dose for the shortest period of time. 8. Maintain euglycemia, particularly in asphyxiated newborns.

52. **Ponderal index:[weight(grams)/length(cm)³] X 100:** used to estimate the adequacy of intrauterine fetal nutrition. Values of less than 2.0 between 29 and 37 weeks of gestation and of 2.2 beyond 37 weeks of gestation have been associated with fetal malnutrition. Growth-restricted infants with low ponderal indices also appear to be at increased risk for the development of neonatal hypoglycemia. Maternal conditions associated with a low ponderal index (fetal malnutrition) include poor maternal weight gain, lack of prenatal care, preeclampsia, and chronic maternal illness.

53. **Skills Necessary for Successful Intubation:** Any discussion of learning in health care must start with what it is that can be learned. There are three "skill sets" that may be acquired and refined by health care professionals: 1) What we know in our brains (cognitive skills or content knowledge) 2) What we do with our hands (technical skills) 3) How we employ the first two skill sets while caring for patients and working under realistic time pressure with our colleagues (behavioral skills) *Cognitive Skills*-Know the indications for intubation of the newborn. Know how to recognize these indications when present. Know what equipment (e.g., size of endotracheal tube, laryngoscope blade) to use to accomplish intubation. Know the indications of a successful intubation *Technical Skills*- Know how to assemble the laryngoscope. Know how to hold the laryngoscope. Know how to use the equipment to expose the airway to view. Know how to insert the endotracheal tube into the airway. Know how to assess for proper placement of the endotracheal tube in the airway. Know how to secure the endotracheal tube in the airway *Behavioral Skills*-Communicate effectively with team members regarding the need for intubation, specific pieces of equipment, and the like. Distribute the workload so that specific tasks are assigned to the team members most likely to carry them out successfully. Delegate responsibility and supervise appropriately. Call for help when necessary.

54. **Warm Chain Steps to minimize heat loss soon after birth :** 1. Keeping the place of birth (delivery room) warm 2. Immediately drying the infant 3. Keeping the infant warm during resuscitation 4. Maintaining skin-to-skin contact between the mother and infant 5. Initiating breast feeding 6. Postponing bathing and weighing 7. Providing appropriate clothing and bedding 8. Keeping mother and infant together 9. Keeping the infant warm during transport 10. Increasing the awareness of health care workers regarding the importance of maintaining neonatal temperature.

55. **Pathogenetic Factors Leading to Intraventricular Hemorrhage:** Increase in cerebral blood flow, Fluctuation in cerebral blood flow, Increase in cerebral venous pressure, Endothelial injury, Vulnerable germinal matrix capillaries, Coagulation disturbances Increased fibrinolysis

56. **Intrauterine Growth Restriction:** When stabilized and assigned a gestational age, a neonate who is SGA should be examined in more detail to direct the diagnostic workup as outlined: **A.** *History and physical examination* **B.** *Accurate growth parameters plotted* on appropriate (for disease or ethnicity) growth curves and gestational age determination **C.** *Findings* 1. Dysmorphic features suggesting a. Chromosome abnormality b. Syndrome c. Drugs (fetal exposure) 2. Blueberry-muffin rash, petechiae, hepatosplenomegaly, and ocular (cornea, lens, retina) pathologic changes suggesting a. Rubella b. Cytomegalovirus c. Other congenital infection 3. Neither 1 nor 2 present suggests a. Chronic fetal hypoxia b. Constitutional factors c. Genetic factors d. Nutritional factors e. Toxins f. Placenta insufficiency g. Undetermined. Dysmorphic features; "funny-looking" facies; and abnormal hands, feet, and palmar creases, in addition to gross anomalies, suggest congenital malformation syndromes, chromosomal defects, or teratogens. Ocular disorders, such as chorioretinitis, cataracts, glaucoma, and cloudy cornea, in addition to hepatosplenomegaly, jaundice, and a blueberrymuffin rash, suggest a congenital infection.

57. **Indications for Placental Examination:** *NEONATAL*-Prematurity, Intrauterine growth restriction, Unexpected adverse outcome, Congenital anomalies, Suspicion of fetal infection, Fetal hydrops Fetal hematologic abnormalities. *OBSTETRIC*-Intrauterine fetal demise, Maternal disease or maternal death, Signs of maternal infection, Gestational hypertension, Oligohydramnios or polyhydramnios, Antepartum hemorrhage (acute or chronic or both), Postpartum hemorrhage, Abnormal biophysical or biochemical monitoring, In utero therapy, Abnormal placenta noted at delivery.

58. **Objectives of Routine Examination of the Newborn :** *Detect* congenital abnormalities not already identified at birth (e.g., congenital heart disease and developmental dysplasia of the hip). *Determine* whether any of the wide range of nonacute neonatal problems are present and initiate their management or reassure the parents. *Check* for potential problems arising from maternal disease, familial disorders, or problems detected during pregnancy. *Provide* an opportunity for the parents to discuss any questions about their infant. *Initiate* health promotion for the newborn.

59. **Features of a Heart Murmur in a Neonate:** FEATURES OF AN INNOCENT MURMUR-Soft (grade 1/6 or 2/6) murmur at left sternal edge, No audible clicks, Normal pulses, Otherwise normal clinical examination FEATURES SUGGESTING A MURMUR IS SIGNIFICANT-Pansystolic, Loud ($grade 3/6), Harsh quality, Best heard in the upper left sternal edge, Abnormal second heart sound, Femoral pulses difficult to feel, Other abnormality on clinical examination. A six-point scale is used to describe murmurs: grade 1 is just audible, grade 2 comfortably audible and grade 3 is loud. If the murmur can be felt on the chest wall as a thrill which is a vibrating sensation under the examiner's hand, then the murmur is grade 4. A grade 5 murmur is audible with the stethoscope edge on the chest and a grade 6 murmur is audible without a stethoscope or with the stethoscope not touching the chest wall.

60. **Clinical Indications for Continuous Positive Airway Pressure (CPAP):** Delivery room resuscitation, Management of respiratory distress syndrome, Postextubation support, Apnea, MAS, Airway closure disease (e.g., bronchiolitis, BPD), Tracheomalacia, Partial paralysis of the diaphragm Mild upper airway obstruction. Methods *of Providing Continuous Positive Airway Pressure* : Ventilator-derived CPAP, Flow-driven CPAP, Bubble (underwater) CPAP, High-flow nasal cannula CPAP. Complications-Pneumothorax (<2%), Nasal obstruction, Abdominal distention from swallowed air, Nasal or septal erosion or necrosis.

61. **Indications for Assisted Ventilation :** *ABSOLUTE INDICATIONS* - Failure to initiate or sustain spontaneous breathing, Persistent bradycardia despite bag-mask ventilation, Presence of major airway or pulmonary malformations, Sudden respiratory or cardiac collapse with apnea/bradycardia. *RELATIVE INDICATIONS*- High likelihood of subsequent respiratory failure, Surfactant administration, Impaired pulmonary gas exchange, Worsening apnea unresponsive to other measures, Need to maintain airway patency, Need to control carbon dioxide elimination.

62. **Determinants of Oxygenation:** Fraction of inspired oxygen, Mean airway pressure Positive end-expiratory pressure (PEEP), Peak inspiratory pressure (PIP), Inspiratory time, Frequency, Gas flow rate.

63. **Determinants of Alveolar Ventilation:** MINUTE VOLUME-Tidal volume, Amplitude (PIP -PEEP), Frequency

   For Conventional Ventilation : Minute Volume = Frequency X Tidal Volume For High-Frequency Ventilation: Minute Volume =Frequency X (Tidal Volume) 2 EXPIRATORY TIME (OR I/E RATIO)

64. **Determinants of mean airway pressure:** (that increase mean airway pressure)- the rise time *(A)*, peak inspiratory pressure *(B)*, inspiratory time *(C)*, and positive end-expiratory pressure *(D)*, and of decreasing the expiratory time *(E)*.

Neonatal Pearls of Wisdom to Remember!!!

65. **Weaning from Assisted Ventilation:** *PHYSIOLOGIC REQUISITES*-Adequate spontaneous drive, Overcome respiratory system load. *ELEMENTS OF WEANING*-Maintenance of alveolar ventilation, Tidal volume. Frequency, Assumption of work of breathing, Nutritional aspects *IMPEDIMENTS TO WEANING*-Infection, Neurologic/neuromuscular dysfunction, Electrolyte imbalance, Metabolic alkalosis, Congestive heart failure, Anemia, Sedatives/analgesics, Nutrition (inadequate calories or excessive non-nitrogen calories).

66. **Injury to the subglottis may be reduced if the following steps are taken:** *Use smaller endotracheal tubes. *Avoid cuffed endotracheal tubes in the infant and young child. *Aggressively treat systemic infection. *Minimize patient movement to prevent abrasions of the subglottic mucosa and resultant exposed cartilage as well as to prevent accidental extubation requiring further manipulation (sedation as necessary). *Consider tracheostomy if prolonged intubation is anticipated. Neonates tolerate intubation for much longer periods than the child or young adult. *Extubate under ideal conditions. In the difficult airway, high-dose systemic steroids for 24 to 48 hours before and after extubation may aid extubation. Use of inhaled epinephrine immediately following extubation can help reduce airway edema.

67. **Indications for Fetal Echocardiography:** Abnormal screening obstetric ultrasound, Fetal arrhythmia, Family history of congenital heart disease, Maternal diabetes, Maternal teratogen exposure (first trimester), Extracardiac anomalies, Aneuploidy or abnormal karyotype, Hydrops fetalis, Increased nuchal translucency.

68. **Treatment of Premature beats:** In the absence of tachycardia, neonates only rarely need treatment for premature beats of any kind. Supraventricular premature contractions virtually never require treatment. Ventricular premature contractions could require treatment in the following situations: *When they are multiform *When they occur in couplets or short runs of ventricular tachycardia *When they are seen in association with a recently converted ventricular tachycardia *When they exhibit the "R on T" phenomenon (i.e., they fall repeatedly on the early part of the T wave of the preceding beat). Decisions concerning treatment of premature beats are difficult and should be made in consultation with a cardiologist. As usual, possible inciting factors such as hypoxia and acidosis should be corrected. If ventricular premature contractions require emergency treatment, the agents of choice are lidocaine or amiodarone, given as a bolus followed by a continuous intravenous infusion.

69. **Risk Indicators for Gestational Substance Exposure:** *Maternal* -No prenatal care, Precipitous labor, Placental abruption, Repeated spontaneous abortions, Hypertensive episodes, Severe mood swings, Previous unexplained fetal demise, Myocardial infarction or stroke *Newborn* -Jittery with normal blood glucose level, Marked irritability, Unexplained seizures or apneic spells, Unexplained IUGR, NEC in an otherwise healthy term infant, Neurobehavioral abnormalities, Signs of neonatal abstinence syndrome.

70. **Substance-exposed Newborn versus a substance affected Newborn:** It is important for practitioners to know the difference between a substance-exposed newborn and a substance affected newborn. Substance *exposed:* *Tests positive for substances at birth or *Mother tests positive for substances at time of delivery or *Is identified by medical practitioner as having been prenatally exposed to substances. *Substance affected:* *Has withdrawal symptoms resulting from prenatal substance exposure or *Demonstrates physical and behavioral signs that can be attributed to prenatal exposure to substances and is identified by a medical practitioner as affected. For the identification of either of these groups of infants, assessment of both maternal and newborn risk indicators (see Pearl 69) is essential. If risk indicators suggest perinatal substance abuse, then consideration should be given to newborn drug testing.

71. **Premature fusion of one or more of the cranial sutures, or craniosynostosis:** results in a variety of abnormal skull shapes, depending on which sutures are involved. Fusion of the saggital suture produces a narrow skull elongated in the anterior-posterior dimension (scaphocephaly or dolichocephaly). Fusion of the coronal sutures causes a widened skull that is shortened in the anterior-posterior dimension (brachycephaly). Unilateral closure of either a coronal or lambdoid suture causes an oblique deformity (frontal or occipital plagiocephaly, respectively). Closure of a metopic suture produces a triangular skull with a prominent, narrow forehead (trigonocephaly). Depending on the timing of the fusion, the skull shape may be abnormal at birth or become visibly deformed later. The fused suture typically has a palpable elevation or ridge, which must be distinguished from displacement of a normal suture caused by molding. In the absence of craniosynostosis or overriding, normal mobility at a suture can be verified by gently applying alternating pressure to the bones on either side of the suture line.

72. **The five most common causes of drug errors were as follows:** *Incorrect doses *Medications that were inappropriate for the medical condition * Failure to monitor for drug side effects * Failure of communication between physician and patient *Failure to monitor drug levels .

Physicians should keep the following recommendations in mind to ensure that their medication orders communicate more effectively: *Write instructions in full rather than with abbreviations. *Avoid vague instructions (e.g., "take as directed"). * Specify exact dose strengths. * Avoid abbreviations of drug names (e.g., *MS* could mean morphine sulfate or magnesium sulfate). * Avoid *U* as an abbreviation for units, because the *U* may be mistaken for a 0 (zero). * Avoid trailing zeroes (e.g., 5.0 mg). * Use leading zeroes (e.g., 0.5 mg). * Minimize the use of verbal orders. * Ensure that prescriptions and signatures are legible, even if it means printing the name that corresponds to the signature.

73. **Candidates for VariZIG@after Significant Exposure† to Varicella-Zoster Infection in Perinatology and Neonatology Practice:** * Pregnant women without evidence of immunity *Newborn infant whose mother develops chickenpox within 5 days before delivery or within 48 hours after delivery *Hospitalized premature infant ($\geq$28 weeks' gestational age) whose mother has no history for chickenpox or serologic evidence of prior infection *Hospitalized preterm infants (<28 weeks' gestational age or birthweight $\leq$1000 g) regardless of the maternal history of varicella or varicella-zoster virus serostatus @Varicella-zoster immunoglobulin (VariZIG) is given intramuscularly at a recommended dose of 125 units per 10 kg body weight, up to a maximum of 625 units. If VariZIG is unavailable, immunoglobulin (400 mg/kg, intravenously) can be substituted. †Significant exposures include: household exposure; face-to-face indoor play; face-to-face contact in hospital setting with infectious staff member, patient, or visitor; intimate contact (hugging or touching) with patient with active zoster lesions.

74. **Risk Factors for Acquiring Health Care–Acquired Infections in the Neonatal Intensive Care Unit :** Prematurity, Low birthweight, Invasive device, Intravascular device (CVC, PAL, PICC, PIVC, umbilical catheter), Mechanical ventilator, Urinary catheter, Ventriculoperitoneal shunt, Medications, Histamine2-blocking agents, Steroids, Others, Prolonged administration of hyperalimentation, Intralipid administration, Delayed enteral feedings, Feeding with formula rather than human milk, Inadequate nursery staffing and overcrowding , Poor compliance with handwashing.

75. **Guidelines for Sibling Visitation in the Nursery:** Siblings should not have been exposed to known communicable diseases (e.g., varicella). Siblings should not have fever or symptoms of acute illness (i.e., upper respiratory infection or gastroenteritis). Children should be supervised by their parents or a responsible adult during the entire visit. Children should be prepared in advance for the visit.

76. **Suggested guidelines for cerebrovascular and metabolic care in high risk Newborns:** Guiding principles for the cerebrovascular and metabolic care of critically ill preterm and term infants may include the following: 1. Maintain stable blood pressure. Severe hypotension is clearly detrimental, but so are rapid increases in blood pressure in a pressure-passive circulation. 2. Maintain stable acid-base balance without rapid corrections. 3. Avoid severe hypoxemia. 4. Avoid marked hyperoxemia (i.e., consider effects of resuscitating with 100% oxygen). 5. Avoid major changes in PaCO2, both hypocapnia and hypercapnia. 6. Correct significant anemia or polycythemia; if the condition is chronic, correct slowly. 7. Consider cerebrovascular and metabolic effects of any new (and existing) drug therapies. Use the lowest effective dose for the shortest period of time. 8. Maintain euglycemia, particularly in asphyxiated newborns.

77. **Antenatal corticosteroids:** Meta-analysis of randomized, controlled trials concludes that antenatal corticosteroid administration prior to an anticipated preterm delivery is associated with a substantial reduction in the incidence of early neonatal death, as well as respiratory distress syndrome, intraventricular hemorrhage, and necrotizing enterocolitis. In follow-up studies, exposure to antenatal corticosteroid therapy does not adversely affect physical growth or psychomotor development. Dexamethasone and betamethasone are the preferred corticosteroids for antenatal therapy. Treatment with two doses of 12

mg of betamethasone, given intramuscularly 12 hours apart, or four doses of 6 mg of dexamethasone, given intramuscularly 12 hours apart, is effective. Strong evidence exists for neonatal benefits from a complete course of antenatal corticosteroids, starting at 24 hours and lasting up to 7 days after treatment. Data are inadequate to establish the clinical benefit beyond 7 days after antenatal corticosteroid therapy. It is unclear whether and when to give repeat doses of antenatal corticosteroids.

78. **Early Postnatal Steroids :** Antenatal steroids are clearly indicated in women at risk for preterm delivery to promote lung maturity, but the use of glucocorticoids in the immediate postnatal period is more problematic. Glucocorticoids are thought to reduce pulmonary inflammation and decrease pulmonary interstitial edema. When used early, glucocorticoids may decrease oxygen dependency at 28 days' and 36 weeks' gestation. However, serious short-term (gastrointestinal perforation, infection, hypertension) and long-term (cerebral palsy, developmental delay, growth retardation) complications preclude use in this fashion to prevent chronic lung disease.

79. **Maintain ductal patency through the use of prostaglandin E₁ (PGE1) :** A recent study, using information theory, assessed which patients were most likely to benefit from PGE₁ before an echocardiogram was obtained. They concluded the following: *The risk of withholding PGE₁ changed with the patient's clinical condition. Patients in extremis will likely benefit more on average than those who are stable. *A cyanotic patient with a murmur and a noncyanotic patient with poor pulses likely present good clinical scenarios where PGE₁ is useful and appropriate. *The presence of cyanosis or abnormal pulses alone are likely good enough reasons to consider starting PGE₁. In general for cyanotic congenital heart disease, the decision to start PGE₁ only theoretically harms patients with obstructed pulmonary venous return (and this point is debatable). Finally, it is possible that patients with d-transposition of the great arteries with intact atrial and ventricular septi are not helped by this drug. Certain inotropic agents or phosphodiesterase inhibitors may alter pulmonary or systemic vascular resistance to a degree that adversely affects the physiologic balance between the pulmonary and systemic circulations.

80. **Infant of Diabetic Mother-Urgent Interventions :** Clinical risk assessment for presence of congenital malformations (Nervous system defects (caudal regression), cardiac defects, skeletal anomalies, cleft lip), birth weight discordance (Intrauterine growth restriction (IUGR <5th percentile) Macrosomia/large for gestational age (LGA > 95th percentile), Birth trauma (Shoulder dystocia, birth asphyxia, clavicular fracture, especially macrosomic infants), metabolic disturbances (Hypoglycemia (<50 mg/dL), hypocalcemia (<7 mg/dL), hypomagnesemia (<1.5 mg/dL) , hematocrit value, and cardiorespiratory stability should be made at birth for every IDM to identify need for early treatment. Early care decreases adverse events such as neonatal seizures and lessens the risk of impaired long-term cognitive development. Anticipatory diagnosis of RDS should be determined to provide therapy and lessen lung injury or the risk of development of PPHN in these infants. Polycythemia (central hematocrit >65%), requires prompt treatment with partial exchange transfusion to avoid potential vascular compromise. IDMs are at risk for vascular thrombosis; thus the decision for placement of umbilical catheters should be made cautiously. Common Pitfalls : Failure to coordinate an obstetric and pediatric approach to care, as well as identifying the potential multisystem complications of the IDM, is a pitfall. Fetal growth discordance, associated macrosomia or intrauterine growth restriction, can lead to unexpected delivery room complications of birth injury or postnatal metabolic conditions that can lead to asphyxia, seizures, and further neurologic impairment. Lung dysmaturity, if unrecognized, can lead to severe morbidity. Untreated polycythemia can lead to hyperviscosity syndrome, thrombosis, stroke, or necrotizing enterocolitis; undiagnosed hyperbilirubinemia can lead to increased risk of kernicterus.

81. **Neonatal hypoglycemia-Management Issues:** Hypoglycemia is defined as a glucose level less than 40 mg/dL the first day of life, less than 50 mg/dL during the first week of life, and less than 60 mg/dL subsequently, regardless of gestational age. The symptomatic infant may be jittery, lethargic, cyanotic, apneic, bradycardic, and hypotonic. Occasionally an infant seizes or suffers a cardiac arrest. All infants at risk for development of neonatal hypoglycemia(infant born to diabetic mother [IDM], small for gestational age [SGA], preterm, cold stress, asphyxia, trauma, sepsis) should be monitored. Blood glucose values less than 40 mg/dL in the first day of life should be verified and treated. The treatment

of hypoglycemia depends on several factors. Infants who are asymptomatic with borderline glucose levels and capable of enteral feeds may receive either formula or 5% dextrose water as initial therapy. Infants with symptomatic hypoglycemia or more severe asymptomatic hypoglycemia should be given intravenous glucose solutions consisting of an initial bolus of 100 mg/kg of 10% dextrose in water solution (1 mL/kg) followed by a continuous infusion of 6 mg/kg/minute of 10% dextrose in water. Infants of diabetic mothers and SGA infants often need to be treated with a constant infusion of glucose. Many of these infants need between 8 and 10 mg/kg/minute of 10% dextrose in water solution to keep the serum glucose values in the normal range. The rate of infusion can be titrated to achieve a normal glucose level. The use of a peripheral vein or an umbilical venous catheter is preferable to the use of an umbilical arterial catheter because the latter is associated with hyperinsulinism secondary to direct pancreatic stimulation. Boluses of glucose should be avoided because rebound hypoglycemia may occur when the hyperresponsive beta cell produces an insulin surge. Neonates needing prolonged glucose therapy or dextrose infusion rates above 12 mg/kg/m² should be investigated for refractory causes of hypoglycemia, such as congenital hyperinsulinism and inborn errors of metabolism. Occasionally infants who were born very prematurely, are severely growth restricted, or had perinatal stress develop prolonged hypoglycemia that can persist for several weeks. Usually these infants can be managed by increasing the caloric density of feeds or by feeding more frequently. Diazoxide therapy can be used if the infant does not tolerate increased calories or frequent feedings. Prior to starting diazoxide, other causes of hypoglycemia must be ruled out, and follow-up with a pediatric endocrinologist is recommended. Abnormal sensory-evoked potentials are observed in full-term infants with whole blood glucose values of less than 45 mg/dL in the first 72 hours of life. A majority of these newborns are asymptomatic. In addition, numerous case-control studies of preterm and term infants find an adverse neurodevelopmental outcome in newborns who had plasma glucose values less than 45 mg/dL within the first 72 hours of life. SGA preterm infants who had one or more plasma glucose values of less than 45 mg/dL in the first few days of life also demonstrate abnormal neurodevelopmental outcomes and decreased head growth. in the first 72 hours of life. A majority of these newborns are asymptomatic. In addition, numerous case-control studies of preterm and term infants find an adverse neurodevelopmental outcome in newborns who had plasma glucose values less than 45 mg/dL within the first 72 hours of life. SGA preterm infants who had one or more plasma glucose values of less than 45 mg/dL in the first few days of life also demonstrate abnormal neurodevelopmental outcomes and decreased head growth.

82. **Neonatal Intestinal Obstruction-Key Concepts:** * The clinical presentation of intestinal obstruction depends on the degree and the location of the obstruction.* When intestinal obstruction is complicated by intestinal ischemia, the diagnosis must be established and treated urgently. Bilious emesis is malrotation with midgut volvulus until proven otherwise. *A normal barium enema does not rule out malrotation of the small bowel. If the diagnosis is suspected and not apparent on plain films, an upper gastrointestinal contrast radiograph series should be performed. * Protection of the lungs from soilage by gastric secretions is a top priority in the initial management of esophageal atresia and tracheoesophageal fistula.* Operative correction of pyloric stenosis is not an emergency. Patients should be well hydrated and have normal electrolytes before they are taken to surgery.* Of babies with congenital duodenal obstruction, one third have Down syndrome and one third have congenital heart disease. Each affects outcome adversely.* Contrast enema is extremely useful in distinguishing jejunoileal atresia from meconium ileus and Hirschsprung disease. It is also of therapeutic benefit in meconium ileus and meconium plug syndrome. * Enterocolitis is the most common cause of death in children with Hirschsprung disease. It should be treated aggressively with rectal irrigation and antibiotics. Colostomy is indicated in severe cases.*Positive-pressure ventilation should be avoided preoperatively, when possible, in infants with EA/TEF because gastric distention can result in regurgitation of gastric secretions through the fistula into the lungs or gastric rupture may result. *The diagnosis of pyloric stenosis is sometimes delayed in a hospitalized patient with a distracting other problem. Forceful nonbilious vomiting at 2 to 6 weeks of age should prompt an abdominal ultrasound. * The apple peel atresia has a worse prognosis than the other types of jejunoileal atresia with a higher

incidence of complications and short bowel syndrome. *Meconium ileus may be uncomplicated and treated successfully with contrast enema, or it may be complicated by segmental volvulus or perforation. Laparotomy, not contrast enema, is indicated in the setting of perforation. *Cystic fibrosis and Hirschsprung disease must be suspected in infants with meconium plug. *Children with both Hirschsprung disease and Down syndrome are especially susceptible to enterocolitis, and they are at increased risk of overwhelming sepsis.

83. **NEC-Restarting enteral feedings:** Enteral feedings are traditionally restarted 10-14 days after findings on abdominal radiographs normalize in the case of nonsurgical NEC. However, balancing the risks and benefits of NPO versus enteral feeds may alter this timeline. Reinitiating enteral feeds in postsurgical babies may take longer and may also depend on issues such as the extent of surgical resection, return of bowel motility, timing of reanastomosis, and preference of the consulting surgical team. Because of the high incidence of postsurgical strictures, some clinicians prefer to evaluate intestinal patency via contrast studies prior to initiating enteral feeds. When feeds are restarted, if human milk is not available, formulas containing casein hydrolysates, medium-chain triglycerides, and safflower/sunflower oils (eg, Alimentum, Pregestimil, Nutramigen) may be better tolerated and absorbed than standard infant formulas.

84. **Neonatal Sepsis-Role of the Lumbar Puncture and Urine Culture:** The role of the lumbar puncture (LP) as part of the sepsis workup remains controversial, especially in the asymptomatic at-risk term neonate in the first week of life. Retrospective studies both support and refute the notion that a lumbar puncture is mandatory. In the past, the LP was considered a routine part of the septic workup before antibiotics were administered. However, in the revised CDC guidelines, the LP is recommended only for the symptomatic infant unless contraindicated by clinical status. There is no question of the need for cerebrospinal fluid (CSF) examination with a positive blood culture or symptomatic infant. For late-onset disease, the role of the LP is much clearer because the incidence of meningitis increases in the absence of bacteremia. Results of one study suggest as many as a third of infants of very low birth weight with meningitis may have negative blood cultures. With this in mind, an LP is indicated for all infants evaluated for sepsis after the first week of life. A word must be said regarding the routine use of urine cultures. In the first 72 hours of life, routine urine cultures are not recommended because of relatively low yield. However, in older infants in whom sepsis is suspected, a urine culture (preferably a catheterized specimen) should always be obtained.

85. **Choanal Atresia:** Bilateral choanal atresia is more common than unilateral and manifests as acute respiratory distress at birth. In bilateral cases, the airway is secured by intubation or oral airway and a CT scan is performed to plan surgical repair. Endoscopes and endoscopic instruments, along with the development of small drills, have improved the ease and success of transnasal repairs. The transpalatal repair remains an excellent option for difficult cases and transnasal surgical failures. The application of mitomycin C has become a useful adjunctive therapy in preventing restenosis of the choana. Most surgeons favor the use of postoperative stenting of the choana for 4 to 6 weeks, to maintain patency and help prevent restenosis. Poor nasal hygiene may develop after stent placement unless appropriate measures are taken. Antibiotics, saline, and frequent suctioning are recommended. Unilateral choanal atresia is not associated with respiratory compromise and usually manifests during childhood in association with unilateral mucoid rhinorrhea and nasal congestion.

86. **Neonatal Seizures-Communication and Counseling:** Parents need to be educated about duration and discontinuation of therapy as well as the prognosis following neonatal seizures. The optimal duration of therapy of the infant with seizures should be based on the likelihood of recurrence of seizures should the anticonvulsants be discontinued. Discontinuation of the medications prior to discharge should be a goal. Three factors need to be considered in this decision-making process: the neonatal neurologic examination, the cause of the seizures, and the interictal EEG. If the neurologic examination is abnormal at discharge, the risk for recurrent seizures is approximately 50%, whereas it is very low with a normal examination. The cause of the seizures is highly relevant to the risk for recurrences (i.e., the risk following hypoxia ischemia is approximately 30%, whereas it is almost universal with migrational defects) and almost never follows hypocalcemic-related

seizures. The interictal EEG is a valuable adjunct in determining the risk of recurrence. Thus if the pattern is normal, the risk for recurrence is rare, whereas it is up to 40% in an infant whose EEG shows marked suppression of activity. If the decision is made to discontinue therapy, phenytoin and other second-line antiepileptic medications are usually stopped first. This is followed by weaning of phenobarbital, which can be accomplished over a period of a few weeks. The prognosis appears to be related to two major factors. The first is linked to the neuropathologic process that underlies the seizures. Thus the potential for normal outcome for infants with seizures secondary to hypoxia-ischemia is approximately 50%, whereas it is invariably favorable following seizures related to a subarachnoid hemorrhage, and it is universally poor for infants with developmental defects. The second is linked to the interictal EEG. Thus with a normal EEG the outcome is favorable; when there is a burst suppression pattern, the outcome is always unfavorable.

87. **Major Extracranial Hemorrhages:** **Caput succedaneum** (subcutaneous-crosses suture lines-blood loss is generally not clinically significant) , **Cephalohematoma** (subperiosteal-does not cross suture lines-blood loss is generally not clinically significant), and **Subgaleal hemorrhage** (Subaponeurotic-crosses suture lines-extends from the orbital ridges to the occiput and laterally to the ears, can accommodate large volumes of blood.). Caput succedaneum, which appears shortly after birth and does not expand significantly in size, requires no treatment and resolves within days. Although a cephalohematoma may increase in size after birth, the magnitude of blood loss is rarely sufficient to cause significant decreases in hematocrit and blood pressure. Like cephalohematoma, subgaleal hemorrhage may enlarge after birth, but it differs in that blood loss may result in severe anemia and shock. Management should be supportive, with emphasis on volume replacement, transfusion, and correction of any underlying coagulopathy. Attention must also be given to the appearance of jaundice and hyperbilirubinemia in babies with significant extravascular blood collections, as in cephalohematomas and subgaleal hemorrhages. Although skull fractures are associated with 5% to 10% of cephalohematomas, the vast majority are linear and nondepressed and do not require treatment. If neurologic symptoms accompany the presence of a cephalohematoma, additional imaging (e.g., CT scan) is required to search for intracranial lesions.

88. **Radiological features of Neonatal Respiratory disorders:** **Congenital pneumonia** • Specific infections, such as GBS, may mimic RDS * Segmental infiltrates or lobar consolidation *Normal lung volumes or focal overaeration occur. **Persistent pulmonary hypertension** *Normal lung volumes and aeration *Pulmonary oligemia. **Meconium aspiration** *Overaeration of lung fields with focal areas of air trapping *Areas of segmental consolidation * Pulmonary edema with small effusions and septal lines may occur *PPHN, barotrauma or bacterial infection may complicate initial radiological signs. **Respiratory distress syndrome** *Normal to decreased aeration *Patent terminal airways surrounded by airless alveoli results in diffuse opacification *Proximal air bronchograms. **Chronic lung disease** *Diffuse opacification with zonal or total lung involvement *Hyperinflation with cystic changes* Interstitial changes of compressed lung and fibrosis adjacent to areas of emphysema and cyst formation. **Transient tachypnea of the newborn** * Overaeration of lung fields with flattening of diaphragms *Diffuse opacification with air bronchograms *Interstitial fluid in the fissures and other reflections of the pleura *Clearance may be asymmetrical with or delayed in the perihilar zones *Overaeration may persist as fluid clears within 48 hours. **Pulmonary venous obstruction and pulmonary edema** *Diffuse opacification with air bronchograms and interstitial pulmonary edema * Hypoplastic left heart syndrome, total anomalous pulmonary venous return with obstruction of the anomalous vein and the non-cardiogenic causes of pulmonary edema are all associated with these non-specific chest radiograph signs. The differential diagnosis includes pulmonary lymphangiectasia.

89. **Inborn error s of Metabolism:** Early and accurate diagnosis is imperative in the treatment of metabolic disorders so that appropriate treatment can be initiated. The clinical features of metabolic disorders are broad and may resemble neonatal sepsis or congenital heart disease. Lethargy, coma, hypotonia, failure to thrive, metabolic acidosis with a high or normal anion gap, reduced serum glucose levels and, often, a

strange odor are features. Other features are tachycardia, hyperpnea, rash, cardiomegaly, hepatomegaly, corneal opacity, cataract formation, retinitis, optic atrophy, deafness, and various dysmorphic features. Hepatic disease may progress to jaundice, cirrhosis, and hepatic failure. This therapy may include dietary protein restriction, specific nutritional supplements, amino acid–deficient formula, and supraphysiologic amounts of certain vitamins for cofactor-dependent metabolic disorders. A simple starting point when confronted with an ill neonate is a family history along with a physical examination, and measurement of electrolytes, glucose, bicarbonate, ammonia and pH. If ammonia is elevated and the pH and bicarbonate are normal (or slightly alkalotic), a urea cycle defect should be suspected. If the pH is low, in the face of hyperammonemia, then an organic acidemia is more likely. With jaundice, galactosemia or fructosemia are possible. Likewise, the determination of urinary ketonuria is important, especially as a clue of organic or fatty acid acidosis. Other useful laboratory tests for initial evaluation are plasma pyruvate and lactate, which are elevated in several mitochondrial disorders. Upon occasion a neonate or an infant with metabolic disease will become comatose with evidence of severe acidosis and hypoventilation. The following key sequence of therapies should be tried: 1. Stop all dietary sources of protein. **2**. Begin D_{10} at 1.5 to 2 times maintenance dose to block catabolism, add Na^+, K^+, and Cl^- (sodium, potassium, and chloride) as needed. **3.** Provide $NaHCO_3$ (sodium bicarbonate) replacement if blood pH is greater than 7.1. In the event of hyperammonemia, use sodium benzoate (5.5 g/m²), sodium phenylacetate (5.5 g/m²) and arginine HCl (hydrochloride; 10% solution) at 12 g/m². If the patient fails to respond, initiate hemodialysis. The latter two steps should be performed only under the care of a pediatric biochemical geneticist and a nephrologist. If a diagnosis of an inborn error of metabolism is established, it is imperative to involve the patient's family. Several messages are crucial. First, these are lifelong disorders. Second, treatment should be lifelong. Third, a failure to treat may result in severe morbidity, illness, mental retardation, and death. Fourth, if a child develops an intercurrent infection, the underlying metabolic disease may worsen. Fifth, communication and contact is important, even lifesaving. Thus, all phone numbers, fax numbers, and e-mail addresses should be exchanged between parents and the staff in the genetic unit (or other caring unit). Sixth, dietary restrictions must be maintained on trips out of the home, at summer camp, or during sleepovers. These patients require extensive genetic counseling because of recurrence risks (usually one in four births), and because of the need to rapidly evaluate a neonate should a sibling be found to have one of these metabolic disorders. Family members should also be alerted to the presence of one of these disorders in the family. In these disorders, communication and counseling must be conveyed in a clear and logical fashion. Such sessions should not be rushed. The messages provided may need to be repeated often both within these sessions and at additional sessions.

90. Hematuria: >5 red blood cells per high-power field. It is uncommon in newborns and should always be investigated for many causes, including hemorrhagic disease of the newborn if vitamin K supplementation has not been given The differential diagnosis for hematuria includes urate staining of the diaper, myoglobinuria, or hemoglobinuria. A negative dipstick with benign sediment suggests urates, whereas a positive dipstick with negative sediment for red blood cells (RBCs) indicates the presence of globin pigments. Vaginal bleeding ("pseudomenses") in girls or a severe diaper rash is also a possible cause of blood in the diaper or positive dipstick for heme. Evaluation of neonatal hematuria depends on the clinical situation. In most cases, the initial investigation includes the following tests: urinalysis with examination of the sediment, urine culture, ultrasonography of the upper and lower urinary tract, evaluation of renal function (serum creatinine and BUN), and coagulation studies.

91. Proteinuria: in newborns is frequently normal. After the first week, persistent proteinuria >250 mg/m²/day should be investigated. In general, mild proteinuria reflects a vascular or tubular injury to the kidney. Administration of large amounts of colloid can exceed the reabsorptive capacity of the neonatal renal tubules and may result in mild proteinuria. Massive proteinuria (>1.5 g/m²/day), hypoalbuminemia with serum albumin levels <2.5 g/dL, and edema are all components of congenital nephrotic syndrome. A renal biopsy is often required for final diagnosis. Prenatal diagnosis of Finnish-type nephrotic syndrome is possible before the 20th week of gestation by detection of elevated maternal and amniotic ±-fetoprotein levels. No specific treatment is required for mild proteinuria. Treat the underlying disease and monitor the proteinuria until resolved.

92. Nephrocalcinosis: associated with a hypercalciuric state. Drugs that are associated with it and increased urinary calcium excretion include loop diuretics such as furosemide, methylxanthines, glucocorticoids, and vitamin D in pharmacologic doses. In addition, hyperoxaluria, often associated with parenteral nutrition, and hyperphosphaturia facilitate the deposition of calcium crystals in the kidney. Renal stones and NC secondary to primary hyperoxaluria/oxalosis, RTA, or UTIs are rare in newborns. In general, renal function is not significantly impaired, and 75% cases resolve spontaneously often within the first year of life as demonstrated by ultrasonography but resolution may take up to 5 to 7 years. However, significant tubular dysfunction at 1 or 2 years of age has been reported. If possible, drugs that cause hypercalciuria should be discontinued. Change to or addition of thiazide diuretics and supplemental magnesium in patients with bronchopulmonary dysplasia with a need for long-term diuretic therapy may be helpful. Monitoring of urinary calcium excretion (urine calcium:creatinine ratio) help in determining response to therapy.

93. Functional intestinal obstruction constitutes the major cause of intestinal obstruction seen in the neonatal unit. 1. Immaturite bowel motility. 2. Defective innervation (Hirschsprung disease) or other intrinsic defects in the bowel wall. 3. Paralytic ileus. a. Induced by medications. i. Narcotics (pre- or postnatal exposure). ii. Hypermagnaesemia due to prenatal exposure to magnesium sulfate. b. Septic ileus. 4. Meconium and mucous plugs. 5. Endocrine disorders (e.g. hypothyroidism).

94. Hypoxic Ischemic Encephalopathy and Hypothermic Intervention for Neonates: Extensive experimental data suggest that mild hypothermia (3-4°C below baseline temperature) applied within a few hours (no later than 6 h) of injury is neuroprotective. *The neuroprotective mechanisms are not completely understood. Possible mechanisms include (1) reduced metabolic rate and energy depletion; (2) decreased excitatory transmitter release; (3) reduced alterations in ion flux; (4) reduced apoptosis due to hypoxic-ischemic encephalopathy; and (4) reduced vascular permeability, edema, and disruptions of blood-brain barrier functions. Therapeutic hypothermia* when applied within 6 hours of birth and maintained for 48-72 hours is a promising therapy for mild-to-moderate cases of hypoxic-ischemic encephalopathy. The greater the severity of the initial injury, the longer the duration of hypothermia needed for optimal neuroprotection. The optimal duration of brain cooling in the human newborn has not been established. Two methods have been used in clinical trials: selective head cooling and whole body cooling. In selective head cooling, a cap (CoolCap) with channels for circulating cold water is placed over the infant's head, and a pumping device facilitates continuous circulation of cold water. Nasopharyngeal or rectal temperature is then maintained at 34-35°C for 72 hours. In whole body hypothermia, the infant is placed on a commercially available cooling blanket, through which circulating cold water flows, so that the desired level of hypothermia is reached quickly and maintained for 72 hours. The relative merits and limitations of these 2 methods have not been established. Rewarming is a critical period. In clinical trials, rewarming

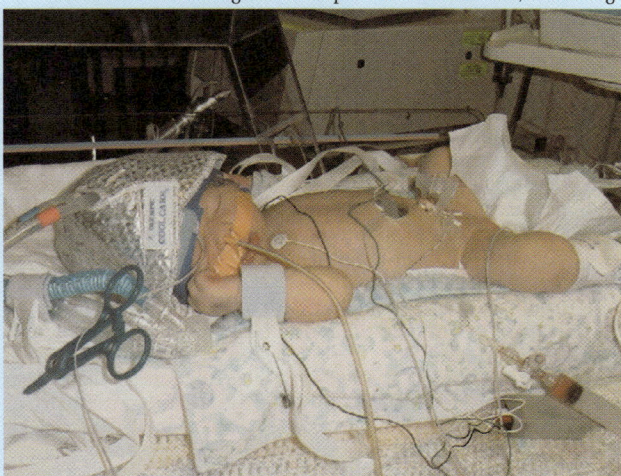

Infant with cooling cap in place.
Courtesy: Dr Jan Paisely.

Neonatal Pearls of Wisdom to Remember!!!

was carried out gradually, over 6-8 hours. Establishing long-term benefits by providing long-term follow-up of all infants undergoing hypothermia therapy is critical in the ongoing evaluation of this therapy.

*In a Cochrane review, Jacobs et al found that therapeutic hypothermia results in significant reduction in the following: *Combined outcome of mortality or major neurodevelopmental disability at age 18 months (relative risk [RR], 0.76; 95% confidence interval [CI], 0.65-0.89), with a number needed to treat (NNT) of 7 (95% CI, 4-14) *Mortality (RR, 0.74; 95% CI, 0.58-0.94) and an NNT of 11 (95% CI, 6-50) *Neurodevelopmental disability in survivors (RR, 0.68; 95%, CI 0.51-0.92), with an NNT of 8 (95% CI, 4-33). They also found a significant increase in thrombocytopenia, although it was not clinically significant. There is evidence from the eight randomised controlled trials included in this systematic review (n = 638) that therapeutic hypothermia is beneficial to term newborns with hypoxic ischemic encephalopathy. Inclusion criteria-Criteria from the larger trials (NICHD, CoolCap, and TOBY) are summarized as follows: *Near-term infants born at 36 weeks' gestation or more with birth weight of 1800-2000 g or more, younger than 6 hours at admission *Evidence of acute event around the time of birth - Apgar score of 5 or less at 10 minutes after birth (In the study by Shankaran et al, this needed to be in conjunction with either evidence of acute perinatal event or need for assisted ventilation for at least 10 min.), severe acidosis, defined as pH level of less than 7 or base deficit of 16 mmol/L or less (cord blood or any blood gas obtained within 1 h of birth), continued need for resuscitation at 10 minutes after birth. *Evidence of moderate to severe encephalopathy at birth - Clinically determined (at least 2 of the following: lethargy, stupor, or coma; abnormal tone or posture; abnormal reflexes [suck, grasp, Moro, gag, stretch reflexes]; decreased or absent spontaneous activity; autonomic dysfunction [including bradycardia, abnormal pupils, apneas]; and clinical evidence of seizures), moderately or severely abnormal amplitude-integrated electroencephalography (aEEG) background or seizures (CoolCap and TOBY) Cooling reduces mortality without increasing major disability in survivors. The benefits of cooling on survival and neurodevelopment outweigh the short-term adverse effects. However, this review comprises an analysis based on less than half of all infants currently known to be randomised into eligible trials of cooling. Incorporation of data from ongoing and completed randomised trials (n = 829) will be important to clarify the effectiveness of cooling and to provide more information on the safety of therapeutic hypothermia, but could also alter these conclusions. Further trials to determine the appropriate method of providing therapeutic hypothermia, including comparison of whole body with selective head cooling with mild systemic hypothermia, are required.*

95. **Neonatal Hypomagnesemia :** Hypomagnesemia occurs when serum magnesium concentrations fall below 0.66 mmol/L (1.6 mg/dL), although clinical signs often do not develop until they fall below 0.49 mmol/L (1.2 mg/dL). The signs of hypomagnesemia are the same as those of hypocalcemia: irritability, tremors, and seizures. Because serum magnesium does not reflect total-body magnesium, there is no strict correlation between the clinical signs and serum magnesium concentrations. *Hypomagnesemia and hypocalcemia frequently coexist. Hypomagnesemia should be considered in any patient with hypocalcemia that does not respond clinically or biochemically to calcium or vitamin D therapy. Decreased magnesium supply*-Maternal magnesium deficiency, Intrauterine growth restriction, Maternal diabetes, insulin-dependent and gestational, Malabsorption syndrome, Extensive small intestine resection, Intestinal fistula or diarrhea, Hepatobiliary disorders, Defect of intestinal magnesium transport: primary hypomagnesemia with hypocalcemia *Magnesium loss*-Exchange transfusion with citrated blood. Decreased renal tubular reabsorption Primary: Infantile isolated renal magnesium washing (dominant and recessive), Hypomagnesemia with hypercalciuria and nephrocalcinosis Secondary: Extracellular fluid compartment expansion, osmotic diuresis, Drugs (e.g., loop diuretics, aminoglycosides), Other causes-Increased phosphate intake, Maternal hyperparathyroidism. The average amount of magnesium sulfate required in the neonate is a 50% solution of magnesium sulfate, 0.05 to 0.1 mL/kg (0.1 to 0.2 mmol/kg, or 2.5 to 5.0 mg/kg of elemental magnesium), given intramuscularly or by slow intravenous infusion over 15 to 20 minutes. Repeated doses may be required every 8 to 12 hours. Possible complications of intravenous infusion include systemic hypotension and prolongation or even blockade of sinoauricular or

atrioventricular conduction. Concomitant oral magnesium supplements can be started if oral fluids are tolerated. A 50% solution of magnesium sulfate can be given at a dose of 0.2 mL/kg per day. In specific magnesium malabsorption, daily oral doses of 1 mL/kg per day may be required. Daily serum magnesium concentrations should be measured until the values are stable to evaluate efficacy and safety. Oral magnesium salts are not well absorbed, and large doses may cause diarrhea. The maintenance magnesium supplement should be diluted fivefold to sixfold to allow for more frequent administration, maximizing gut absorption and minimizing side effects. Neonatal seizures due to hypocalcemia and hypomagnesemia do not have a uniformly favorable outcome. Neurologic abnormalities at follow-up have been found in about 22% of patients.

96. **Neonatal Hypermagnesemia :** serum magnesium concentration of greater than 1.15 mmol/L (2.8 mg/dL). Hypermagnesemia is invariably an iatrogenic event caused by excessive magnesium administration. Because magnesium balance is regulated mainly by the kidneys, decreased renal function can be a contributing factor. Increased magnesium supply -Maternal treatment with magnesium sulfate, Neonatal magnesium therapy: asphyxia, pulmonary hypertension, Parenteral nutrition, Antacids, enema. Hypermagnesemia should be suspected in depressed infants born to mothers who have been treated with magnesium sulfate. In most cases, hypermagnesemia is associated only with hypotonia. However, in extreme cases severe neuromuscular depression (a curare-like effect) and respiratory failure (CNS depression) may occur. Serum calcium concentrations may be normal, decreased, or increased in hypermagnesemic neonates. Hypermagnesemia may suppress PTH and 1,25(OH)2D3 production and may result in lower serum calcium concentrations. In most cases of neonatal hypermagnesemia, supportive treatment is sufficient because an excess of magnesium is gradually removed through urinary excretion. Calcium is a direct antagonist of magnesium, and intravenous calcium given at the same dosage as that given for the treatment of hypocalcemia may be useful for acute injury. Optimal hydration is important to ensure adequate urinary flow. Loop diuretic therapy may increase magnesium excretion. In cases of severe CNS depression, exchange blood transfusions may be used to lower the increased serum magnesium concentration. Citrated donor blood is particularly useful because the complexing action of citrate expedites the removal of magnesium from the infant. Peritoneal dialysis and hemodialysis may be considered in refractory patients. Supportive measures such as cardiorespiratory assistance and adequate hydration may be needed.

97. **Weaning strategy :** Reduce PIP to below 20 cm H_2O- Reduce ventilator rate by limitation TI extension TE. At 40 bpm start caffeine-(loading dose 20 mg/kg caffeine citrate; maintenance 5 mg/kg/24 h). If Patient trigger ventilator available-reduce pressure to 14 cm H_2O >28 weeks, 12 cm H_2O 26–28 weeks, 10 cm H_2O <26 weeks-(back-up rate 20 bpm). If No patient trigger ventilator available-continue to reduce rate by extension TE-reduce pressure as for PTV. In either case, Wait until Minimal ventilator setting achieved-Initiate One hour ET CPAP-Finally, Extubate into a headbox unless 1.0 kg then use nasal CPAP.

98. **High-frequency oscillatory ventilation -measurements which help guide choice of ventilation settings:** The chest radiograph and the PaO_2 / FiO_2 ratio can be used to help guide therapy. If the chest radiograph shows more than nine posterior ribs of inflation, flattened diaphragms, a small heart, or very clear lung fields, the lung may be overinflated. Similarly, if the mean airway pressure is high and the FiO_2 is low, then mean airway pressure should be decreased before FiO_2. If the chest radiograph shows fewer than seven posterior ribs of inflation, domed diaphragms, a normal heart size, or diffuse radiopacification, the lung may be underinflated. Therefore, if the mean airway pressure is low and the FiO_2 is high, the mean airway pressure should be increased. The assessment of cardiac function is also important for the safe use of high-frequency ventilation. Monitoring heart rate, blood pressure, urine output, and capillary refill can help to alert the care provider to changes in cardiac output.

99. **Clinical Findings in Selected Congenital and Perinatal Infections Pointing a Specific Diagnosis:** *Rubella -Cataracts, cloudy cornea, pigmented retina; petechiae with "blueberry muffin" rash; bone defects with longitudinal bands of demineralization ("celery stalking"); cardiovascular malformations (patent ductus arteriosus, pulmonary artery stenosis); sensorineural hearing loss; hydrops. *Cytomegalovirus-Microcephaly with periventricular calcifications; chorioretinitis;

petechiae with thrombocytopenia; jaundice; sensorineural hearing loss; bone abnormalities; abnormal dentition, hypocalcified enamel. *Herpes **simplex virus**-Skin vesicles, keratoconjunctivitis, acute central nervous system findings (seizures), hepatitis, pneumonitis. *Varicella **zoster virus**- Limb hypoplasia, dermatomal scarring in cicatricial pattern, gastrointestinal tract atresia ***Parvovirus B19**- Hydrops, ascites, hepatomegaly, ventriculomegaly, hypertrophic myocardiopathy, anemia. ***Lymphocytic choriomeningitis virus**- Hydrocephalus, chorioretinitis, intracranial calcifications.

100. Deformational plagiocephaly. Posterior-type deformational plagiocephaly is caused by constant gravitational forces applied to the occiput when the infant remains for prolonged periods in the same supine position—the sleep position promoted by the American Academy of Pediatrics (AAP) Back to Sleep campaign. Various degrees of brachycephaly (i.e., a shortened, broad head) occur in most children who sleep solely on their backs. Any condition that is associated with abnormal bone formation or muscle tone (especially torticollis) can also cause deformational plagiocephaly. Dolichocephaly (i.e., a long, narrow head with bitemporal narrowing) can develop in preterm infants who have large heads and weak neck muscles.

Craniosynostosis: When craniosynostosis occurs, the growth of the skull is impeded in a plane that is perpendicular to the fused suture, but the skull continues to grow in the parallel plane. Brain growth occurs in the direction of the open sutures. Different head shapes result depending on which suture or combination of sutures has fused: • Trigonocephaly (a triangular-shaped head) arises from metopic craniosynostosis. • Scaphocephaly arises from sagittal craniosynostosis. • Turricephaly (a tower-shaped head) arises from coronal plus sagittal craniosynostosis. • Brachycephaly (i.e., a shortened, broad head) arises from bilateral coronal craniosynostosis. • Posterior plagiocephaly (trapezoidal-shaped head) arises from lambdoid craniosynostosis; this is a very rare form of craniosynostosis.

101. Recent changes newborn resuscitation guidelines (Changes from 2005 to 2010)

* For uncompromised babies, a delay in cord clamping of at least 1 min

* Commence resuscitation using air

* Use pulse oximeter attached to right wrist or hand to guide use of oxygen

* Babies of less than 28 weeks gestation should be completely covered up to their necks in a food-grade plastic wrap or bag, without drying, immediately after birth. They should then be nursed under a radiant heater and stabilized.

* Attempts to aspirate meconium from the nose and mouth of the unborn baby, while the head is still on the perineum, are not recommended.

* If epinephrine is given, then the intravenous route is recommended using a dose of 10–30 mcg/kg. If the tracheal route is used, it is likely that a dose of at least 50–100 mcg/kg will be needed to achieve a similar effect to 10 mcg/kg intravenously.

* Use detection of exhaled carbon dioxide (capnography) in addition to clinical assessment to confirm placement of a tracheal tube.

* Therapeutic hypothermia offered to newly born infants at term or near term with evolving moderate to severe hypoxic-ischemic encephalopathy.

102. Resuscitation OR Stabilization: Most preterm babies are reasonably healthy at birth and required assistance in making the transition to extrauterine life. Intervention is aimed at maintaining a healthy, warm, infant and instituting appropriate longer-term supportive measures. The guidelines therefore attempt to differentiate between stabilization of preterm babies and resuscitation, which is more usually required in the few near term babies who have suffered significant perinatal stress or hypoxia. This will require a shift in thinking and in documentation following birth

103. NICU medications of concern: Potential Risks

Dexamethasone: Cerebral palsy, cardiomyopathy, hyperglycemia, hypertension

Prolonged antibiotic use: Mortality, necrotizing enterocolitis, antibiotic resistance, fungal infection

Cefotaxime: Mortality, fungal infection, development of drug resistance, extended spectrum beta-lactamase

Histamine 2 blockers: Necrotizing enterocolitis, sepsis, alteration of gut microflora, fungal infection

Erythropoietin (EPO): ROP

Oxygen: ROP, BPD, free radical mediated injury

Metoclopramide: Extrapyramidal effects, tardive dyskinesia

Spironolactone: Feminization

104. Goals and options in keeping preterm babies warm: The goals of care are straightforward: maintain a normal body temperature, ensure a stable thermal environment and avoid cold stress; but the options to achieve them are many and less certain. There is a problem in defining a 'normal' temperature. A single measurement will tell nothing about whether the baby is using energy for thermal balance. The preterm baby should be monitored with the continuous recording and display of a central and peripheral temperature. This will give an early indication of cold stress before any change is seen in the central temperature. Reducing evaporative heat losses at birth has improved temperatures on admission, although no studies have shown any effect on outcome. Cochrane review has shown that the use of incubators is any better than radiant heaters. Evaporative fluid and heat losses are of major importance and need to be controlled. Good temperature measurement is essential, particularly in the sick baby in whom dual temperatures should be continuously monitored and displayed. Future designs should look to produce a single warming device that maintains a stable thermal environment and can be used throughout the care of the baby from birth to discharge home. Audit of temperature on admission and during transport should be done as measures of quality of care during vulnerable periods. A published range for rectal and axillary temperatures is 36.5–37.5°C and 35.6–37.3°C, respectively, for both term and preterm infants; the skin temperature is 35.5–36.5°C in term babies and 36.2–37.2°C in preterm babies. Sauer *et al* suggest that conditions for thermoneutrality are met in very low birth weight infants when at rest their core temperature is between 36.7°C and 37.3°C and the core and mean skin temperatures are changing less than 0.2–0.3°C/h, respectively. The continuous measurement, and display, of central (abdominal, axilla or zero heat flux) and peripheral (sole of the foot) temperatures detects thermal stress by showing a change in the central–peripheral difference that occurs before any alteration in central temperature. The preterm baby who appears to be comfortable in its environment has a central temperature in the normal range for whichever site is being used and a central–peripheral temperature difference of 0.5–1°C. An increasing central– peripheral temperature difference, particularly above 2°C, is usually caused by cold stress and occurs before any fall in central temperature. A high central temperature, particularly if unstable, along with a wide central peripheral gap is seen in septic babies. The optimum time to make the transition from incubator to cot is unknown but most babies weighing between 1700 g and 1800 g are able to maintain their temperature, and continue to gain weight, when nursed clothed in a cot.

Happy learning!!! Now you may add more Neonatal Pearls of Wisdom as Reference Notes!!!

Neonatal Presenting Symptoms: Benign-Self limiting or Serious?

01. Neonatal Seizures: Benign Neonatal Sleep Myoclonus (BNSM) is a self-limiting disorder characterized by neonatal onset myoclonic jerks during non-rapid eye movement (NREM) sleep, and consistent cessation with arousal with absence of concomitant electroencephalographic findings and without any abnormalities on neurodevelopmental examination. The myoclonic jerks in BNSM can be focal, multifocal or generalized. The jerks of BNSM may be precipitated by stimuli such as sound or touch or even by benzodiazepines. BNSM is a self-limiting disorder with spontaneous resolution between 2 to 6 months of age and a normal neurodevelopmental outcome on follow up. Others like benign familial neonatal seizures and benign idiopathic neonatal seizures (fifth day fits) are also included in the list of benign seizures of neonates and can be differentiated based on typical features. **Suggested diagnostic criteria for benign idiopathic neonatal convulsions (BINC)** include the following: * Infants born after 39 weeks' gestation * Apgar score of 9 or more at 5 minutes, greater than 7 at 1 minute: Lower scores should not exclude the diagnosis if other criteria are met. * Presence of a seizure-free interval between birth and the onset of seizures * Clonic and/or apneic seizures * Negative findings on evaluation for alternative etiology * Normal developmental and intellectual outcome: These are largely determined in retrospect. * Lack of seizures beyond the neonatal period * Normal laboratory findings (including but not limited to metabolic studies, neuroimaging, and lumbar puncture). **Suggested diagnostic criteria for benign familial neonatal convulsions (BFNC) are as follows:** *Normal neurologic examination findings *Negative findings on evaluation for alternative etiology *Normal developmental and intellectual outcome: These are largely retrospective criteria * Positive family history of newborn or infantile seizures *Onset of seizures during neonatal period or early infancy. The rest of spectrum of neonatal seizures is related commonly to perinatal or metabolic insults, infections, developmental anomalies, drugs and hematological causes which can often be elucidated during evaluation. *Refer to Chapter 29, Page 188 or further details.*

02. Vesicopustular eruptions in the Neonate: A careful history, comprehensive physical examination and routine diagnostic tests, such as a Tzanck smear, gram stain, KOH and skin biopsy when relevant can help in separating transient, benign pustular eruptions from serious and life-threatening conditions. The differential diagnosis includes:

Non-infectious: benign; Acropustulosis of infancy, Eosinophilic pustular folliculitis, Erythema toxicum, Milliaria, Transient neonatal pustular melanosis

Non-infectious: potentially serious: Acrodermatitis enteropathica Epidermolysis bullosa, Epidermolitic hyperkeratosis, Incontinentia pigmenti, Langerhans cell histiocytosis, Urticaria pigmentosa, Herpes gestationis-neonatal, Pemphigus vulgaris- neonatal

Infectious: usually mild: Candidiasis-neonatal, Impetigo neonatorum, Scabies **Infectious: serious:** Bacterial infections (*Chlamydia, Escherichia coli, Hemophilus influenza, Klebsiella pneumoniae, Listeria Monocytogenes, Pseudomonas aeruginosa, Staphylococcus aureus, Streptococcus* group A Beta hemolytic), Syphilis, Candidiasis-congenital, Staphylococcal scalded skin syndrome, Viral infections (Cytomegalic, Herpes, Varicella) Refer *to Vesicles & pustules in Newborn, Page 792 for further details.*

03. Neonatal Conjunctivitis: Neonatal conjunctivitis usually responds to appropriate treatment, and the prognosis generally is good.. Chemical conjunctivitis secondary to silver nitrate solution application usually occurs in the first day of life, disappearing spontaneously within 2-4 days. If untreated, corneal ulceration may occur in N gonorrhea infection and rapidly progress to corneal perforation. When unrecognized and not immediately treated, Although it rarely causes neonatal conjunctivitis, Pseudomonas can lead to devastating consequences, such as rapid progression to corneal ulceration and perforation. (If left untreated, it even can lead to endophthalmitis and subsequent death.) Like gonococcal conjunctivitis, chlamydial conjunctivitis also may be associated with extraocular involvement, including pneumonitis, otitis, and pharyngeal and rectal colonization. Herpes simplex keratoconjunctivitis usually presents in infants with generalized herpes simplex with corneal epithelial involvement or vesicles on the skin (which surround the eye). Serious systemic complications, such as encephalitis, may occur in these neonates due to their poor immunologic response. Other differentials include * Cellulitis, Orbital * Cellulitis, Preseptal * Dacryocystitis *Glaucoma, Primary Congenital *Glaucoma, Secondary Congenital * Keratitis, Bacterial *Keratitis, Fungal *Keratitis, Herpes Simplex * Nasolacrimal Duct, Obstruction. Refer *to Chapter 96, Page 609 for further details.*

04. Neonatal Jaundice: Jaundice & hyperbilirubinemia in Neonates is mostly a benign problem (observed in 60% of term infants and 80% of preterm infants during the first week of life), *but if untreated severe indirect hyperbilirubinemia is potentially neurotoxic, and conjugated direct hyperbilirubinemia often signifies a serious hepatic or systemic illness. Physiologic Jaundice (Icterus Neonatorum)* - is characterized by a) the level of indirect-reacting bilirubin in umbilical cord serum is 1-3mg/ dL, and rises at a rate of < 5mg/dL/24 hr b) jaundice becomes visible on the second to third day, usually peaking between the second and fourth days at 5-6mg/dL c) decreasing to below 2mg/dL between the fifth and seventh days of life. The diagnosis of physiologic jaundice in term or preterm infants can be established *only by excluding known causes of jaundice* on the basis of the history, clinical and laboratory findings. One should make a search to determine the cause of jaundice if 1) it appears in the 1st 24-36 hr of life, 2) serum bilirubin is rising at a rate faster than 5mg/dL/24 hr, 3) serum bilirubin is greater than 12 mg/ dL in full-term (especially in the absence of risk factors) or 10-14 mg/ dL in preterm infants, 4) jaundice persists after 10-14 days of life, or 5) direct-reacting bilirubin is greater than 2 mg/dL at any time. Among other factors suggesting a nonphysiologic cause of jaundice are a family history of hemolytic disease, pallor, hepatomegaly, splenomegaly, failure of phototherapy to lower bilirubin, vomiting, lethargy, poor feeding, excessive weight loss, apnea, bradycardia, abnormal vital signs (including hypothermia), light-colored stools, dark urine positive for bilirubin, and signs of kernicterus. *Persistent or prolonged physiologic jaundice beyond 8 days in term infants and 14 days in preterm infants,* suggests hemolysis, hereditary glucuronyl transferase deficiency, breast milk jaundice, hypothyroidism, or intestinal obstruction, UTI, hepatitis / TORSCH infections etc. *Refer to Chapter 53, Page 373 for further details.*

05. Neonatal Cyanosis: The infant presenting to the emergency department with cyanosis requires rapid assessment, diagnosis, and initiation of therapy. If cyanosis is limited to the extremities, it is referred to as acrocyanosis or peripheral cyanosis. It occurs with normal arterial oxygen saturation and is caused by slowed peripheral circulation with excessive oxygen extraction by the tissues, and thus an increased concentration of reduced hemoglobin at the venous end of the capillaries. *This occurs in a cold environment, polycythemia, heart failure, Septic shock, Vasospasm, arterial or venous obstruction, or even in normal newborn infants (acrocyanosis);* the extremities are cold and blue, but the tongue is pink. Peripheral cyanosis may resolve with gentle warming of extremities. Cyanosis is less apparent clinically when there is severe anemia because the concentration of reduced hemoglobin is limited by the anemia. Traumatic cyanosis is blue discoloration of the skin, often with petechiae. It can affect the presenting part in a face or breech presentation or the head and neck if the umbilical cord was wrapped around the infant's neck. However, the tongue remains pink. Central *cyanosis is always a sign of severe pathology and has respiratory, cardiac, CNS, hematologic and metabolic causes;* Primary pulmonary disease is the most common etiology for cyanosis and hypoxia in the Newborn. Methemoglobinemia is the rare but great impersonator in the evaluation of cyanosis of the Newborn. Examination generally reveals a markedly cyanotic infant without respiratory distress, who has an arterial PaO$_2$ that is normal, although the infant will have low oxygen saturation values. Arterial blood obtained from such an infant is often described as "chocolate" in color. Beware of the less common causes of Neonatal Cyanosis: caused by extrinsic compression of the airway and lungs in the newborn include: *Right/Double Aortic Arch *Tracheal Vascular Ring *Pulmonary Artery Sling *Cricoid Cartilage Malformation. A systematic, rational approach to the diagnosis of neonatal cyanosis is essential. An understanding of the normal transitional physiology, and how diseases of the airway, lung, and circulatory system may disrupt these processes, will enable the ED practitioner to determine whether the underlying cause is related to airway obstruction, parenchymal disease, hypoventilation due to CNS disease or apnea, or due to cardiac disease. Management is based on the clinical diagnosis and attention to hemodynamic stability, judicious oxygen administration, and referral to the appropriate inpatient hospital setting. # echocardiography is the gold standard for the assessment of congenital heart disease in infancy # all infants with central cyanosis should be commenced on parental antibiotics early until further investigation is possible. # differentiating PPHN from ductal dependent pulmonary cardiac lesions can be very difficult; if uncertainty exists a PG infusion is generally the safest option for transport. Refer to Chapter 46, Page 323 for further details.

06. Neonatal Pallor: Hemoglobin increases with advancing gestational age: at term, cord blood hemoglobin is 16.8 g/dL (14–20 g/dL); hemoglobin levels in very low birthweight (VLBW) infants are 1–2 g/dL below those at term . Less than the normal range of hemoglobin for birthweight and postnatal age is defined as anemia. A "physiologic" decrease in hemoglobin content is noticed at 8–12 wk in term infants (hemoglobin, 11 g/dL) and at about 6 wk in premature infants (7–10 g/dL). Persistent pallor, in addition to anemia or acute hemorrhage (external or internal), should suggest hypoxia, asphyxia, hypoglycemia, sepsis, shock, edema or adrenal failure. A serious sign & requires expeditious investigation. Asphyxial pallor is usually accompanied by cyanosis and shows marked improvement with oxygen administration & mechanical ventilation. Pallor due to acute blood loss is not associated with cyanosis, without any improvement with oxygen and or ventilation. Early recognition of anemia may lead to a diagnosis of E.fetalis, subcapsular hematoma of liver or spleen, subdural hemorrhage, or fetal-maternal or twin-twin transfusion. Without being anemic, postmature infants tend to have pallor & thicker skin than term or premature infants do. Acute blood loss usually results in severe distress at birth, initially with a normal hemoglobin level, no hepatosplenomegaly, and early onset of shock. In contrast, chronic blood loss in utero produces marked pallor, less distress, a low hemoglobin level with microcytic indices, and, if severe, heart failure. Anemia appearing in the first few days after birth is also most frequently a result of hemolytic disease of the newborn. Other causes are hemorrhagic disease of the newborn, bleeding from an improperly tied or clamped umbilical cord, large cephalhematoma, intracranial hemorrhage, or subcapsular bleeding from rupture of the liver, spleen, adrenals, or kidneys. Rapid decreases in hemoglobin or Hct values during the first few days of life may be the initial clue to these conditions. Bleeding from hemangiomas of the upper gastrointestinal tract or from ulcers caused by aberrant gastric mucosa in a Meckel diverticulum or duplication is a rare source of anemia in newborns. Repeated blood sampling of infants requiring frequent monitoring of blood gas and chemistry parameters is a common cause of anemia among hospitalized infants. Deficiency of minerals such as copper may cause anemia in infants maintained on total parenteral nutrition. Refer to Chapter 65, Page 450 for further details.

07. Neonatal Apnea: Apnea is defined as cessation of respiration for $\geq$20 sec or cessation of respiration of any duration accompanied by bradycardia (HR <100/min) and/or cyanosis. Apnea of prematurity: It is probably related to immaturity of the central nervous system. This condition usually presents after 1-2 days of life and within the first 7 days. Apnea presenting within the first 24 hours or after 7 days of age is unlikely to be AOP. Apnea of prematurity is a diagnosis of exclusion and should be considered only after secondary causes of apnea have been excluded. Common causes of secondary apnea include sepsis, pneumonia, asphyxia, temperature instability and anemia. All babies less than 34 weeks gestation should be monitored for at least the first week of life or till absence of apneic episodes for at least 7 days. Babies $\geq$34 weeks gestation should be monitored if they are sick. Apnea monitors based on chest wall movement are likely to miss obstructive apnea. Monitors with facilities for measuring heart rate and oxygen saturation would be useful in the monitoring of significant apnea in preterm infants. Subtle seizures: Apnea is an uncommon presentation of a neonatal seizure. Sudden alteration in muscle tone, twitching movements, vacant stare and up rolling of eyes suggests a seizure. Also tachycardia preceding/ accompanying an apneic attack usually suggests seizure activity. Refer to Chapter 36 , Page 249 for further details.

08. Neonatal Respiratory distress: The clinical presentation of respiratory distress in the newborn includes apnea, cyanosis, grunting, inspiratory stridor, nasal flaring, poor feeding, and tachypnea (more than 60 breaths per minute). There may also be retractions in the intercostal, subcostal, or supracostal spaces. The differential diagnosis of respiratory distress includes Pulmonary, Cardiac, Hematologic, Infectious, Anatomic, and Metabolic disorders that may directly or indirectly involve the lungs. Most cases are caused by transient tachypnea of the newborn or meconium aspiration syndrome in a term baby, respiratory distress syndrome in a preterm, but various other causes are possible. In the near term neonate, there are four very similar presentations of respiratory disease that are particularly challenging to distinguish from one another shortly after birth; they are as follows (and in order of prevalence): 1. Transient tachypnea of the newborn 2. Respiratory distress syndrome 3. Pneumonia (either through bulk aspiration of amniotic fluid, or bacteria, or virus) 4. Persistent fetal circulation (persistent pulmonary hypertension). HYALINE **MEMBRANE DISEASE (RDS) presents** with intercostal and sternal retractions, nasal flaring, tachypnea, expiratory grunt and central cyanosis evident within first 4 hours of birth. Transient tachypnea of the newborn begins early and improves with time. RESPIRATORY ILLNESS STARTING DE NOVO AFTER **FOUR** HOURS - In essence there are only five possibilities : * PNEUMONIA - bacterial and viral * CONGENITAL HEART DISEASE WITH PULMONARY EDEMA * CONGENITAL MALFORMATION * THE DYSPNEA OF ACIDEMIA DUE TO UNDERLYING METABOLIC DISEASE * rare, late-onset lung disease of the VLBW baby (e.g. Wilson Mikity syndrome, CPIP). Differentiating these conditions rarely poses any problems, since typical clinical, radiological or ECG changes are virtually always present. Surgical causes of neonatal respiratory distress are due to airway obstruction, pulmonary collapse or displacement and parenchymal disease or insufficiency. Any two or all three mechanisms may occur simultaneously in the same baby. If a cyanosed baby makes strenuous and active respiratory effort, with labored breathing and retraction, agitation, wheezing, stridor and tachypnea, the cause is most probably airway obstruction. Examination of the neck, nose, mouth and throat alongwith bronchoscopy and laryngoscopy and X-rays of the head, neck and chest – both PA and lateral, will usually establish the diagnosis and indicate treatment. Refer to Chapter 34, Page 227 for further details.

09. Neonatal Encephalopathy: Neonatal encephalopathy is a heterogeneous syndrome characterized by signs of central nervous system dysfunction in newborn infants. Clinical suspicion of neonatal encephalopathy should be considered in any infant exhibiting an abnormal level of consciousness, seizures, tone and reflex abnormalities, apnea, aspiration, feeding difficulties , and an abnormal hearing screen. When neonatal encephalopathy is due to hypoxic-ischemic (anoxic) brain injury, it is appropriate to use the term hypoxic-ischemic encephalopathy (HIE). According to ACOG (American College of Obstetricians and Gynecologists task force) four essential criteria (table 1) are required to define an intrapartum asphyxial event sufficient to cause cerebral palsy. All four criteria must be met: 1. Evidence of metabolic acidosis: umbilical artery pH<7 and base deficit $\geq$12 mmol/L at delivery. 2. Early onset of severe or moderate neonatal encephalopathy in infants $\geq$34 weeks of gestation 3. Cerebral palsy of the spastic quadriplegic or dyskinetic type 4. Exclusion of other identifiable etiologies (e.g., trauma, coagulation disorders, infection, genetic disorders). However, only one criterion — metabolic acidosis on umbilical cord arterial blood at birth — is helpful to the clinician in the immediate postnatal period. More importantly, for timing of the peripartum events that may be related to development of cerebral palsy, ACOG suggests the following criteria : * Presence of a signal event immediately before or during labor * Sudden onset of fetal bradycardia patterns * Apgar score of 0 to 3 after five minutes * Onset of a multisystem disorder in the first 72 hours * Early brain imaging showing acute nonfocal cerebral abnormality. One must always consider the possibility of progressive disorders in cases of neonatal encephalopathy. These include metabolic, neurodegenerative, infectious or toxic etiologies that are rare, with a combined incidence of approximately 6 per 10,000 live births, but a much higher mortality rate than the general population. Perinatal stroke is an increasingly recognized entity in term newborns with encephalopathy and cerebral palsy. Perinatal stroke occurs about once in 4000 births. The majority of infants with ischemic perinatal stroke develop neonatal seizures. Additional signs of neonatal encephalopathy may also be present, such as lethargy, hypotonia, feeding difficulties, or apnea. A specific cause for perinatal stroke is not identified in most affected newborns. Factors contributing to the risk include maternal conditions such as prothrombotic disorder and cocaine abuse; placental complications such as preeclampsia, chorioamnionitis and placental vasculopathy; and newborn conditions such as prothrombotic disorders, congenital heart disease, meningitis, and systemic infection [60]. During the delivery process, an infant may develop a cervical arterial dissection that leads to stroke. Potential long-term sequelae of perinatal arterial stroke include cerebral palsy, cognitive deficits, hemiparesis, and epilepsy. However, development is normal in approximately 19 to 33 percent of infants with neonatal ischemic infarction. *Refer to Chapter 28, Page 180 for further details.*

10. **Neonatal Edema:** In the first 4 weeks of life so-called 'physiological' edema of the newborn occurs in 13%of premature infants and 1% of babies born at term. The term 'edema neonatorum' has had different meanings for different observers, but is now usually reserved for 4 categories, viz. *(a)* sclerema, *(b)* subcutaneous fat necrosis, *(c)* neonatal cold injury, and *(d)* 'physiological' edema. Usually in 'physiological edema' the baby is not ill and the edema is transient, occurring at 2 or 3 days of age in the lower limbs, face and genitalia and clearing within a week. Besides these syndromes there are other edemata unique to the neonate, as in the edematous infant of the diabetic mother or the hydrops fetalis syndrome due to several causes, among them hemolytic disease and cytomegalic inclusion disease. With a few exceptions, such as kwashiorkor or lipoedema, any cause of edema in the older child or adult can operate in the newborn, even as apparenily unlikely a cause as acute or chronic nephritis. Other causes of Neonatal edema include: edema of post-acidotic state and other mineral depletion, Congenital syphilis Renal edema, Cardiac edema, Hypoproteinemia (Prematurity, Congenital syphilis, Loss of protein *via- (a)* Kidneys in nephrosis b) Hemorrhage, Protein dilution in excess fluid administration, Heart failure, Congenital hypogammaglobulinemia, Hypercatabolic hypoproteinemia-transient dysproteinenia group Hypoalbuminemia with aminoaciduria), Angioneurotic edema, Hormonal edema iatrogenic-e.g.. cortisone. **Causes of local edema:** *Birth trauma Hormonal change in female neonate' s external genitals, Localized exposure to cold .* Lymphedema secondary to congenital bands, Congenital lymphedema ('Milroy's disease'), Turner syndrome, Infantile cortical hyperostosis, Venous thrombosis.

11. **Apparent life-threatening event:** An apparent life-threatening event (ALTE) is defined as "an episode that is frightening to the observer that is characterized by some combination of apnea, color change, marked change in muscle tone, choking or gagging. In some cases the observer fears that the infant has died". Common differential diagnosis of an apparent life-threatening event: Acid-base disturbance, Anemia, Botulism, Child abuse, Dysrhythmias, Electrolyte abnormalities, Gastroesophageal reflux, Hypoglycemia, Hypothermia, seizures, Inborn errors of metabolism, Intracranial hemorrhage, Meningitis and encephalitis, Pertussis, Pneumonia

RSV, Sepsis. The workup may include a full sepsis evaluation, electrolytes, chest radiography (CXR), ECG, and respiratory syncytial virus (RSV) and pertussis nasal swabs. Hospitalization for observation and monitoring is appropriate. *Refer to Chapter 99, Page 626 for further details.*

12. **Floppy Infant:** Hypotonia is described as reduced resistance to passive range of motion in joints i.e., an impairment of the ability to sustain postural control and movement against gravity; weakness is reduction in the maximum power that can be generated. Weak infants always have hypotonia, but hypotonia may exist without weakness.Because dysfunction at any level of the nervous system can cause hypotonia, the differential diagnosis is extensive. Central causes, both acute and chronic, are more common than are peripheral disorders. Central conditions include hypoxic-ischemic encephalopathy, other encephalopathies, brain insult, intracranial hemorrhage, chromosomal disorders, congenital syndromes, inborn errors of metabolism, and neurometabolic diseases. Peripheral disorders include abnormalities in the motor unit, specifically in the anterior horn cell (ie, spinal muscular atrophy), peripheral nerve (ie, myasthenia), neuromuscular junction (ie, botulism), and muscle (ie, myopathy).Several studies have shown that central causes account for 60% to 80% of hypotonia cases and that peripheral causes occur in 15% to 30%.Central causes of hypotonia often are associated with a depressed level of consciousness, predominantly axial weakness, normal strength with hypotonia, and hyperactive or normal reflexes. Other clues to central hypotonia are abnormalities of brain function, dysmorphic features, fisting of the hands, scissoring on vertical suspension, and malformations of other organs. A newborn who has cortical brain dysfunction also may have early seizures, abnormal eye movements, apnea, or exaggerated irregular breathing patterns. Central disorders can result from an injury or an ongoing injury or they can be static, predominantly genetic or developmental. Hypoxicischemic encephalopathy, teratogens, and metabolic disorders may evolve into hyperreflexia and hypertonia, but most syndromes do not. Infants who have experienced central injury usually develop increased tone and deep tendon reflexes; infants who have central developmental disorders do not. If a hypotonic infant is alert, responds appropriately to surroundings, and shows normal sleep-wake patterns, the hypotonia likely is due to involvement of the peripheral nervous system, specifically the motor unit, which includes the anterior horn motor neurons of the spinal cord. Peripheral causes are associated with profound weakness in addition to hypotonia and hyporeflexia or areflexia. Disorders of the anterior horn cell present with hypotonia, generalized weakness, absent reflexes, and feeding difficulties. In the classic infantile form of spinal muscular atrophy, fasciculations of the tongue can be seen as well as an intention tremor. Affected infants have alert, inquisitive faces but profound distal weakness. Peripheral causes also are associated with muscle atrophy, lack of abnormalities of other organs, the presence of respiratory and feeding impairment, and impairments of ocular or facial movement.Based on some research evidence, 50% of patients who have hypotonia are diagnosed by history and physical examination alone.Based on some research evidence, an appropriate medical and genetic evaluation of hypotonia in infants includes a karyotype, DNA-based diagnostic tests, and cranial imaging. *Refer to Chapter 32, Page 212 for further details.*

13. **Abdominal distention:** Tympanitic abdominal distention may occur in healthy infants, in infants who have systemic conditions, and in Newborns who have congenital causes of intestinal obstruction. Some healthy infants experience mild distention because of air swallowing with crying or feeding. This distention is variable, greatest after feeding or fussing, and absent at other times. Vomiting is absent, and the stooling pattern and physical examination are normal. This transient generalized distention responds to changes in feeding technique and burping and in consoling techniques for the crying infant. * In the ill Newborn, many systemic conditions cause a paralytic intestinal ileus characterized by quiet, nontender abdominal distention: sepsis, birth asphyxia, hypothyroidism, and electrolyte imbalance. Newborns who have pneumonia or respiratory distress may also develop distention from aerophagia. * The most common cause of acquired abdominal distention in premature infants is necrotizing enterocolitis (NEC). Definitive radiographic evidence of NEC includes findings of (1) pneumatosis intestinalis and (2) gas visible in the portal venous system of the liver. Marked tympanitic abdominal distention can be a manifestation of pneumoperitoneum, which is demonstrated by upright and cross-table lateral abdominal radiographs revealing free

air within the peritoneum. *Refer to Chapter 52, Page 371 for further details.*

14. Neonatal Vomiting : Most babies vomit at some time. In most cases this is unimportant. Small, frequent vomits are referred to as "posits". However, there are circumstances when the type of vomiting is important: * vomit contains blood (red or black, the color of the blood will depend upon how long the blood has been in the stomach) * vomiting bile (green, not yellow) * projectile vomiting * the baby is unwell * the baby is failing to thrive * the baby has gastroesophageal reflux and could be aspirating * the baby also has diarrhoea * the abdomen is distended. Where none of the above clinical scenarios apply the vomiting is unlikely to be clinically significant. A baby who vomits bile (green, not yellow, in color) should be presumed to have a bowel obstruction, until proven otherwise. The commonest cause is swallowed maternal blood. Swallowed blood often irritates the stomach and causes vomiting. Blood may be swallowed during * birth- the largest amount of blood will be swallowed if there is antepartum hemorrhage associated with bleeding into the amniotic fluid for at least several hours before birth. This blood may then take several days after birth to clear the gastrointestinal tract (GIT). Under these circumstances, as well as vomiting blood, the baby may pass melena stools, rather than meconium.* breast-feeding- many breast-fed babies will swallow blood from a cracked and bleeding nipple. Usually the mother is aware of the nipple problem, but not always, as the bleeding may be deeper and painless. Management of swallowed maternal blood is expectant. If it is swallowed from birth it will eventually clear from the GIT. The mother's cracked and bleeding nipple will require attention, and she may require lactation advice about nipple attachment. This becomes a transient contraindication to breast feeding if the mother is Hepatitis C positive. Less commonly, the baby is bleeding. Causes include * hemorrhagic disease of the newborn (HDN) * stress ulceration * swallowed baby blood. *Refer to Chapter 51, Page 355 & Chapter 57, Page 407 for further details.*

15. Neonatal Diarrhea: Diarrhea in neonates is a challenging clinical condition due to the possible heterogeneous etiologies (food allergy, gastrointestinal infections, antibiotic-associated diarrhea ,congenital defects of ion transport (Congenital chloride diarrhea), Neonatal withdrawal syndrome, Hirschsprung's disease, parenteral diarrhea (UTI), cystic fibrosis , Immunodeficiency and metabolic disorders) and severe outcomes. Several **clinical signs that warrant admission and further evaluation and management include: *Bloody** diarrhea. This can be a sign of a bacterial illness or an allergy (Cow's milk protein intolerance). *Moderate to severe dehydration *Child is acting lethargic (limp, and less responsive to touch or words, won't focus on mother). *Increased abdominal pain. *Continued weight loss of more than 5% of body weight. Refer *to Chapter 59, Page 417 for further details.*

16. Neonatal Poor Weight gain: Poor quality of suck (whether breast- or bottle-fed), incorrect formula preparation; breastfeeding problems; inadequate number of feedings; poor feeding interactions (e.g., infant gags or vomits during feedings and parent assumes child is full); neglect; birth defects that affect the child's ability to eat or digest normally. Infants who are sick as well as being LBW or VLBW are at risk for Extrauterine Growth Restriction (EGR). Chronic lung disease, late onset sepsis, severe intraventricular hemorrhage, and a history of necrotizing enterocolitis (NEC) have all been associated with more EGR. Refer *to Page 806 and 807 for further details.*

17. Anuria and Oliguria: Oliguria is defined as a urine output that is less than 1 mL/kg/h in infants, less than 0.5 mL/kg/h in children; one of the clinical hallmarks of renal failure. All cases of acute renal failure are not characterized by oliguria. For example, subjects with acute renal failure due to nephrotoxins, interstitial nephritis, or neonatal asphyxia are typically nonoliguric. In addition, the degree of oliguria depends on hydration and concomitant use of diuretics. In most clinical situations, acute oliguria is reversible and does not result in intrinsic renal failure. However, identification and timely treatment of reversible causes is crucial because the therapeutic window may be small. Oliguria may result from 3 broad pathophysiologic processes: prerenal, intrinsic renal, and postrenal mechanisms. Associated Contributing Conditions to Acute Kidney Failure: Perinatal asphyxia, Sepsis, Respiratory distress syndrome, Dehydration due to feeding problem, Heart failure, Nephrotoxic drug administration , Urological anomalies. *Refer to Chapter 72, Page 493 for further details.*

18. Acute Collapse in a Neonate: Acute collapse in a previously well or already an unwell Neonate is a medical emergency where swift and appropriate response can make the difference to outcome. Irrespective of the underlying cause, the major objectives should be to re-establish adequate gas exchange and maintain the cardiovascular circulation and perfusion. *When a Baby Breathing spontaneously, suddenly collapses, consider the following possibilities:* Overwhelming infection either bacterial or viral ,Massive hemorrhage, e.g. subcapsular hematoma of liver, pulmonary hemorrhage, IVH, Adrenal hemorrhage etc. Congenital heart disease which is precipitated by the closure of ductus arteriosus, Necrotizing enterocolitis (NEC), Metabolic problems, e.g. hyperammonemia, hypoglycemia, hypocalcemia, CAH etc. *When a baby on Mechanical Ventilator suddenly collapses, consider the following possibilities:* Hypo/Single Lung ventilation due to blockage of an endotracheal tube, displacement, disconnected ventilator, etc. Large Air leak-Tension Pneumothorax/ Pneumomediastinum which is detected by transillumination or radiograph, Intracranial hemorrhage which is detected by full fontanel, falling hematocrit, metabolic acidosis, cranial ultrasound, etc. Pneumonia/Sepsis / Meningitis/Worsening RDS. *Refer to Chapter 8, Page 56 for further details.*

19. Congestive Heart Failure in a Neonate: A Neonate with CHF usually suffers from a Congenital Heart Disease (CHD) but may have nonstructural heart disease, such as myocardial dysfunction (ischemia, myocarditis) or serious disturbances of heart rate. Metabolic and hematologic abnormalities as well as overtransfusion or overhydration also may be responsible for CHF.In the preterm infant a hemodynamically significant PDA is the most common cause of heart failure, usually a complication of RDS. Three nonstructural heart situations that can present with CHF in a Neonate are Transient Myocardial Ischemia, Infant of a diabetic mother, and Chronic Lung Disease. The clinical picture of CHF in the Newborn period may simulate other conditions, such as sepsis, meningitis, pneumonia or bronchiolitis. Moreover, the features of Neonatal heart failure can be masked or caused by respiratory disease and by circulatory collapse from any cause. Cardiac disease will also cause respiratory distress if there is marked pulmonary venous engorgement or metabolic acidosis has developed. Most causes of heart failure will be associated with other cardiovascular signs and with cardiomegaly on CXR, which together usually allow the distinction to be made with confidence.*Refer to Chapter 47, Page 331 for further details.*

20. Ophthalmic Problems in a Neonate: Neonates present with multiple ophthalmic disorders which can be isolated or be associated with other systemic anomalies. Pediatricians and neonatologists should identify ocular abnormalities and refer patients for detailed ophthalmic evaluation when deemed necessary. As the critical period of visual development is in the first 6 months after birth, timely referral, diagnosis, and management are critical to allow optimal visual development. *10 Warning Signs of Serious Eye Disease in the Newborn and Infant:* These first three of the ten warning signs of significant eye disease in infancy and childhood have the most serious implications and most require *early definitive treatment.* **1.**White pupil-'Leukokoria' **2.**Prematurity: Candidates for Retinopathy of Prematurity **3.**Enlarged cornea **4.**Corneal opacity **5.**Ptosis **6.**Crossed eyes (Squinting) **7.**Dancing eyes(Nystagmus) **8.**Defect or missing part of pupil (Coloboma) **9.**Inequality of the eye/Pupil:Microphthalmos or Persistent inequality of the pupil size **10.** Excessive tearing or discharge.

Refer to Ophthalmic disorders manifesting in the newborn ,Page 701, and to Chapter 25 for Retinopathy of prematurity (ROP) and to Chapter 96 for Neonatal conjunctivitis (Ophthalmia neonatorum) for further details.

21. Abnormal Fontanel in a Neonate: 1. An abnormal fontanel in an infant can indicate a serious medical condition. Therefore, it is important to understand the wide variation of normal, how to examine the fontanels, and which diagnoses to consider when an abnormality is found. **2.** At birth, an infant has six fontanels. The anterior fontanel is the largest and most important for clinical evaluation. The average size of the anterior fontanel is 2.1 cm, and the median time of closure is 13.8 months. **3.** The most common causes of a large anterior fontanel or delayed fontanel closure are achondroplasia, hypothyroidism, Down syndrome, increased intracranial pressure, and rickets. A bulging anterior fontanel can be a result of increased intracranial pressure or intracranial and extracranial tumors, and a sunken fontanel usually is a sign of dehydration. **4.** A physical examination helps the physician determine which imaging modality, such as plain films, ultrasonography, computed tomographic scan, or magnetic resonance imaging, to use for diagnosis. **5.** Consultation with a pediatric neurosurgeon should be considered if the diagnosis or presence of an abnormality is unclear. Refer *to Page 771 for further details*.

22. **Pseudoparalysis in a Neonate:** Pseudoparalysis occurs with bone fracture or with joint, soft tissue, or bone infections, such as osteomyelitis, pyogenic arthritis and osteomyelitis, osteitis of congenital syphilis (Parrot`s *pseudoparalysis). Soft* tissue inflammation often occurs with osteomyelitis, but occasionally in infancy pseudoparalysis may be the sole sign of infection in bone. Decreased limb movements due to pain are referred to as pseudoparalysis. The neonate with pseudoparalysis cries and grimaces with even minimal attempts to move the affected extremity, but full motion can be elicited by primitive reflexes. Neonates with pseudoparalysis have normal deep tendon reflexes. The painful limbs do not adopt the typical postures that characterize segmental brachial plexus palsy or peripheral nerve lesions. Evidence of trauma or infection in the affected limb supports the diagnosis of pseudoparalysis.

23. **Bleeding in a Neonate:** Bleeding in neonates may present with * oozing from the umbilicus or stump *cephalhematoma * bruising more than that anticipated after delivery * bleeding from peripheral venipuncture or procedure sites * bleeding into scalp * bleeding following circumcision * petechiae * intracranial hemorrhage * bleeding from mucous membranes * unexplained anemia and hypotension. A detailed history and complete examination is essential in the assessment of a bleeding neonate. Particular points in the history include * maternal diseases such as ITP, preeclampsia and diabetes * maternal exposure to drugs such as aspirin, anticonvulsants, rifampicin and isoniazid * family history of bleeding disorders * previous affected siblings * confirmation of Vitamin K administration. Physical examination will determine whether the neonate is 'well' or 'sick', which is very useful as the differential diagnosis is very different in the two circumstances. Two major clinical indicators can be used to establish the differential diagnosis of neonatal bleeding syndromes: 1) whether the bleeding infant is an otherwise well baby or is obviously ill, and 2) whether platelet or plasma coagulation protein deficiencies appear to be primarily involved in the coagulopathy. Causes *of bleeding in a 'well' neonate* * immune thrombocytopenia (alloimmune or autoimmune (maternal ITP)) * vitamin K deficiency * inherited coagulation factor deficiencies such as hemophilia * bleeding from anatomic lesions such as a hemangioma, A-V malformation. *Causes of bleeding in a 'sick' neonate* * DIC - usually associated with sepsis, asphyxia, severe RDS or NEC * consumption thrombocytopenia without depletion of coagulation factors * liver failure. Bleeding at a single site is more likely to have an anatomic or structural component. Major bleeding from any primary cause may induce a secondary DIC, which may mask the original pathology. Simple and widely available lab tests are useful in investigating a bleeding neonate. Treatment depends on the cause of bleeding and clinical condition of the neonate. Treat the baby not the numbers. Consult a Pediatric Hematologist, if in doubt. *Refer to Chapter 67, Page 461 for further details. Also Refer to Chapter 57, Page 407 for further details*.

Also Refer to Page 716 for a synopsis of other alerting and or alarming symptoms in a Neonate, such as Lethargy, Irritability, Poor capillary refill and BP instability, Failure to feed well, Fever, Excessive oral secretions, drooling and choking spells, and Congenital anomalies.

Key Points for Clinical Practice

01. Recognizing disease in newborn infants depends on knowledge of the disorder and evaluation of a limited number of relatively nonspecific clinical signs and symptoms and the differential diagnosis for each subtle or nonspecific symptom in the neonatal evaluation is extensive (may represent genetic mutations, chromosomal aberrations, or acquired diseases and injuries).

02. It is important to keep a high index of suspicion when evaluating the neonate because some initial interventions may be life saving.

03. A broad systematic approach (a careful history, head to toe physical examination & relevant investigations) evaluating the neonate is necessary to provide a comprehensive yet specific differential diagnosis for a presenting complaint or symptom. The efficient recognition and prompt management of illness in the neonatal period may be life saving.

04. **Prioritize the assessment & care of a ? Sick baby:**
Assess need for emergency care- If immediate life-threatening situation (i.e. respiratory/circulatory failure, hypoglycemia)present, Provide *emergency treatment until stable*. (• Oxygen therapy and Mechanical ventilation • Maintain normal glucose • Maintain body temperature • Feeds and fluids for sick and small babies • Infection prevention and control • Transfer and referral)
Assess for priority signs- ELBW baby, Apnea and respiratory distress, Central cyanosis but no chest indrawing or grunting (possible heart problem/PPHN, hypothermia, lethargy with full fontanel, Seizures, Hypotonia-Hypertonia, Abdominal distention and bilious vomiting, poor feeding, jaundice in first 24 hours): Potential life-threatening situation: *Provide immediate care refer as soon as possible*.
Assess for Specific problems: (depending on the maternal and perinatal risk factors involved) •Preterm and low birth weight •Large for dates and infant of diabetic mother• Serious acute infection •Local infection •Neonatal encephalopathy •Jaundice •Congenital abnormalities • Syphilis • Tuberculosis • HIV-affected mothers and babies :Provide care and referral

05. If a Neonate whether spontaneously breathing or on assisted ventilation suddenly collapses, the immediate priority should be to ensure **ABCDs**; Concurrently, one should perform the essential diagnostic/therapeutic interventions to treat the treatable. In such crisis, always call for additional help, irrespective of your knowledge, skills, & experience.

06. Staff need to be *articulate, thoughtful, sensitive and above all, excellent at listening to both the parents in times of crisis*. Counseling and support for parents cannot adequately be achieved in one meeting and takes great patience and tact.

07. Beware of the limitations of routine neonatal examination an uncooperative newborn (e.g., getting a good view of the eyes and red reflex, hearing a heart murmur, or testing for developmental dysplasia of hip (DDH). Parents might become upset or angry when it becomes evident at a later stage that their child has a significant problem. They need to be made aware that not all abnormalities can be detected at the initial examination. This situation also stresses the importance of clear documentation of the routine examination for future reference.

08. No infant should be discharged from the hospital without a final examination because certain abnormalities, particularly heart murmurs, often appear or disappear in the immediate neonatal period and, in addition, evidence of disease that has just been acquired may be noted.

09. With a healthy infant, the mother should be present during this examination; even minor, seemingly insignificant anatomic variations may worry a family and should be explained. The explanation must be careful and skillful so that otherwise unworried families are not unduly alarmed.

10. Always promote preventive health care, when you think that the baby is perfectly healthy: Prevention of Sudden Infant Death Syndrome, Promotion of Breast Feeding, Hearing and Vision Screening, Immunization, Safe Transport.

Emergency Reference Figures in Neonatology

1. *Use the "mnemonic "*: "1-2-3 . . . 7-8-9" to determine the placement of the orotracheal ET tube . For a 1-kg newborn, the tube placement should be 7 cm at the lip level. For a 2-kg newborn, placement should be 8 cm at the lip level; for a 3-kg newborn, placement should be 9 cm at the lips. **Formula for ETT depth:** Neonates < 1 month = wt in Kg + 6 cm

Intubation Equipment for Neonates:

Weight gm)	ETT Size I.D. (mm)	Laryngoscope Blade Size	Suction Catheter (French)	Approx. Insertion Depth (cm)
500 -1000	2.5	0	6	6.5 cm
1000	2.5	0	6	7 cm
1000- 2000	3.0	0-1	6	7.5 cm
> 2000	3.5	0-1	6	8 cm
3000	3.5	0-1	8	9 cm

2. *Chest compression during Neonatal Resuscitation:* *Ratio of compression 3:1 @rate of 90 compressions : 30 breaths /mt, unless cardiac arrest is due to a clear cardiac etiology where ratio of 15:2 may be considered *Two thumb technique better than two finger technique *The compression is applied at the lower one third of sternum *The depth of compression should be one-third of the antero-posterior diameter of the chest .

3. *Target saturation (pre-ductal) While resuscitating a Newlyborn:* Target SpO2 ranges provided as a part of NRP algorithm (1min- 60-65% , 2 min- 65-70%, 3min- 70-75%, 4min- 75-80%, 5min- 80-85% 10min- 85-95% (same for *4. Neonatal Resuscitation :IV Adrenaline 1:10, 000 solution* : If the heart rate remains <60 bpm despite 30 seconds of positive - pressure ventilation with 100 % oxygen and chest compressions, medications should be given. *0.1 to 0.3 ml/kg (0.01 to 0.03 mg/kg) every 3 to 5 minutes* is the drug of choice. Higher IV doses are not recommended because animal and pediatric studies show exaggerated hypertension, decreased myocardial function, and worse neurological function after administration of IV doses in the range of 0.1 mg/kg. While IV access is being obtained, administration of a higher dose (0.05 to 0.1 mg/kg) through the endotracheal tube may be considered, but the safety and efficacy of this practice have not been evaluated.

5. *Vitamin K1* should be given as a single intramuscular dose of 0.5 mg (birthweight 1500 g or less) or 1.0 mg (birthweight greater than 1500 g) to all newborns within the first 6 h after birth following initial stabilization of the baby.

6. *Hypoglycemia*-Plasma glucose < 40 mg/dL in both term or preterm infants. Symptomatic Infants: * Immediate Bolus: 0.20 grams of glucose/kg, i.e., 2 ml/kg of i.v. 10% glucose, given over 1-2 minutes. (Do not use $D_{25}W$ or $D_{50}W$.) * Continuous Infusion: 6-8 mg glucose/kg/min using $D_{10}W$ (or D_5W); this is equivalent to 90-120 ml/kg-day as 10% dextrose in water. *Normoglycemia*-Plasma glucose 50-100 mg/dL in infants not receiving i.v. fluids. *Hyperglycemia*-Unknown and controversial, only a suggested definition of plasma glucose as >200 mg/dL.

7. *Fluid and Electrolyte Management in the Newborn:* Initiate fluid therapy at 60-80 ml/kg/d with D10W, (80-150 ml/kg/d for infants ≤26 weeks). Infants <1000 g should have electrolytes and weights recorded every 6-8 hours; every 12 hours for infants 1000-1500 grams. Increase fluid administration gradually over the first week of life to 120-130 cc/kg/d by day 7, allowing for expected physiologic weight loss. Increase fluids for urine output <0.5 mL/kg/hr by ~10 mL/kg or, in infant ≤26 weeks, calculate IWL and change fluids accordingly.nfuse Na+ free fluids (including flushes) until serum Na+ <145 and good urine output is established (post diuretic phase). Then add 3-5 meq/kg/d Na+. Add KCl (2-3 meq/kg/d) to IV fluids after urine output is well established and K+ <5 mEq/L (usually 48-72 hours).

8. *Trophic feedings* should be initiated at a volume not to exceed 15 ml/d. These feedings are traditionally given in small boluses of 1-3 ml/kg per feeding. Trophic feedings should continue until the infant's respiratory and cardiac status have stabilized. Older preterm infants (i.e. > 27 weeks) and infants with minimal respiratory compromise may bypass trophic feeds and begin feedings using a nutritive feeding regimen.

9. *Partial Exchange Transfusion:* **Single-volume or partial ET for correction of polycythemia:** Volume of exchange (mL)=total blood volume (mL) X [observed Hct- desired Hct/observed Hct].e.g.,1-kg preterm infant with Hct 68%, desired postpartial exchange Hct 55%. 100 X [68-55/68]= about 20 mL of crystalloid exchanged with whole blood. (Infant's blood volume in preterm infant < 100 to 120 mL/kg, in term infant < 80 to 85 mL/kg).

Partial ET for correction of severe anemia:

Volume of exchange (mL) =total blood volume (mL) X [Desired Hct-Observed Hct/Hct of the PRBC Unit-Observed Hct] e.g.,1-kg preterm infant with Hct 21%, desired postpartial exchange Hct 45% requires 100 X {45-21/70-21}=49 ml of PRBC.

Double-volume ET for removal of bilirubin, antibodies, etc.: 2 x infant's blood volume = 2 x 80 to 120 mL/kg.e.g., *2-volume exchange volume (preterm)= 100 mL/kg X 2, or 200 mL/kg *2-volume exchange volume (term)= 85 mL/kg X 2, or 170 mL/kg

10. *Neonatal LMA Size & Miller Blades*

LMA sizes ~ weight (kg) / 20 + 1 (round to nearest 0.5)

Miller Blades * < 32 weeks: 00 * Term: 0 (< 3 kg)

11. *Essential IV Infusions in Neonates: Refer* to Essential Neonatal Drug Formulary- Page 1078.

12. *Blood components for Neonatal transfusion: Cellular* components supplied for neonatal transfusion should be CMV negative.

Red cell- *Top-up transfusion:* 10–20 ml/kg @5 ml/kg/hr. *Exchange transfusion:* 80–100 ml/kg (for anaemia) 160–200 ml/kg (for hyperbilirubinemia) @Depends on stability of the baby. Emergency large-volume transfusion:10–20 ml/kg @Rapid infusion only for resuscitation

Platelet concentrate: 10–20 ml/kg @10–20 ml/kg/hr

FFP: 10–20 ml/kg @10–20 ml/kg/hr

Cryoprecipitate 5–10 ml/kg @10–20 ml/kg/hr

13. *Indications for red cell transfusion in infants under four months of age:*

Neonate receiving mechanical ventilation: Transfuse Hb < 12.0 g/dL

Acute blood loss: Transfuse if, 10% blood volume lost

Oxygen dependency (not ventilated): Transfuse if, Hb < 8.0–10.0 g/dL

Late anaemia, stable patient (off oxygen): Transfuse IF, Hb < 7.0 g/dL

Some neonatologists use a Hb of < 11.0 g/dL as a threshold for transfusing oxygen-dependent neonates, and since there is no good evidence to support a particular threshold value, each neonatal unit should produce a written policy of its own, based on the nature of the babies cared for by the unit.

14. *Indications for platelet transfusion in term and pre-term neonates:*

Platelet count < 30 × 10⁹/l : In otherwise well infants, including NAIT (Neonatal alloimmune thrombocytopenia) if no evidence of bleeding and no family history of ICH

Platelet count < 50 × 10⁹/l: In infants with: • clinical instability • concurrent coagulopathy • birth weight < 1000 g and age < 1 week • previous major bleeding (e.g. GMH-IVH) • current minor bleeding (e.g. petechiae, venepuncture oozing) • planned surgery or exchange transfusion • platelet count falling and likely to fall below 30 • NAIT if previous affected sib with ICH

Platelet count < 100 × 10⁹/l: Consider platelet transfusion if there is major bleeding and platelet count is falling rapidly.

Some neonatologists use a threshold for platelet transfusion of 20 × 10⁹/l in well, stable term and pre-term neonates ; at present there is no evidence to support choosing a platelet count of 20 × 10⁹/l over 30 × 10⁹/l and each neonatal unit should develop its own policy based on the nature of the babies that it cares for.

15. *Donor —Recipient Blood Group Compatibility*

Infant's blood group & Antibodies	Compatible donor red cells	Compatible donor plasma
O with Anti-A and Anti-B	O	AB, O, A, B,
A with Anti-B	O, A,	AB, A
B with Anti-A	O, B	AB, B
AB with None	O, A, B, AB	AB

Thus group O red cell units can be given to a patient of any ABO group in an urgent situation, as the transfused red cells have no A or B antigens to react with the recipient's antibodies. However, there is a risk of a hemolytic reaction if the patient has antibodies against other red cell antigens. This is most likely if the patient has had pregnancies or has previously been transfused with red cells. In an emergency, the risk of a reaction must be balanced against the risk due to delay in replacing blood loss.

16. *How much UAC/UVC to insert?* Measure in a straight line parallel to the neonate's body and record in cm's the distance from the *infant's distal end of the clavicle to the umbilicus.* Take the shoulder to umbilicus measurement and multiply x 0.66 for UAC placement plus stump length.

Take the measurement and multiply x 0.5 for UVC placement plus stump length. This length is needed to place the tip of the catheter between the diaphragm and the right atrium.

ETT & UAC/UVC/PICC Placement on X-ray

ETT: T1 – T-3

UAC: High Line T-6 to T-9, Low Line L-3 to L-4

UVC: At the level of the diaphragm — *do not use* if angling toward liver

The tip of a PICC should be placed and positioned in as large a vein as possible, preferably the superior or inferior vena cava, but not in the right atrium, owing to the risk for perforation or pericardial effusions.

17. Nasal CPAP

Flow 6 - 8 lpm -6 lpm for <34 wks & 8 lpm for term infants

FIO_2 100%- Titrate for SpO2 92 - 95% (85 - 92% in preterm)

CPAP 4 - 8 cm H_2O

18. Initial Ventilator Settings (Newborn)

	VLBW <1.5 Kg	LBW 1.5 - 2.5 Kg	Term >2.5 Kg
Rate	30 - 60	30 - 60	20 - 50
Insp. Time	Match GA	Match GA	Match GA
	(>.25 sec)		(<.45 sec)
PIP	14 - 22	18 - 24	20 - 28
PEEP	3 - 4	4 - 5	4 - 5

19. Vital signs in Neonates:

Respiratory Rate (breaths/min.): <40 weeks 30 - 60 , Term Newborn 30 - 60 **Heart Rate** (beats/min.): <40 weeks 120 - 180 , Term Newborn 90 - 160 **Temperature:** 36.5 - 37.5 C **Blood Pressure:** <40 weeks -MAP (mean arterial pressure) = Gestational Age, Term Newborn Systolic 55-90, Diastolic 26-55. **Oximetry**: Adjust oxygen flow rate to keep oxygen saturation at 88-95%. Some newborns such as those with cardiac or respiratory problems require oxygen saturation levels that are less than or higher than this range. Consultation should be sought for these newborns to identify an appropriate range.

20. Neonatal Seizures: When to treat? Seizures persist for longer than 3 minutes, Frequent seizures >3 per hour, Seizures disrupting vital functions

Step 1. Stabilize airway, breathing, circulation & maintain the vitals & BP

Step 2. Correct transient metabolic disturbances

a. Hypoglycemia (target blood sugar 70-120mg/dL) 10% dextrose water IV bolus dose 2 mL/kg followed by a continuous infusion at 8mg/kg/min

b. Hypocalcemia 10% calcium gluconate IV at 4 mL/kg (need cardiac monitoring)

c. Hypomagnesemia 50% magnesium sulfate IM at 0.2 mL/kg

Step 3. Phenobarbital 20mg/kg/IV load

Cardiorespiratory monitoring

5mg/kg IV (may repeat to total dose of 40mg/kg: *limit the total dose to 20mg/kg in severely asphyxiated infants with impaired hepatic &/or renal functions*) **Consider continuous EEG monitoring, if available Consider intubation/ventilation for hypoxia & hypercapnea on ABG analysis.**

Step 4. Lorazepam 0.05mg/kg IV (may repeat to total dose of 0.15 mg/kg)

Step 5. Phenytoin 20mg/kg slow IV load

(fosphenytoin) 5 mg/kg slow IV (may repeat to total dose of 30mg/kg)

Step 6. Pyridoxine 50-100 mg/kg IV with EEG monitoring)

Step 7. Other agents - trial of folinic acid, lidocaine IV infusion with/without loading dose.

21. Perioperative Fluids Requirements:

Weight (kg) Maintenance Requirements in Children (mL/hour)

0-10   4 (mL/kg)

11-20   40 + 2 (mL/kg)

> 20 kg 60 + 1 (mL/kg)

Replacement of Losses

Procedure	Insensible losses
Non-invasive (inguinal hernia, clubfoot)	0-2 cc/kg/hr
Mildly invasive (ureteral reimplantation)	2-4 cc/kg/hr
Moderately invasive (bowel reanastomosis)	4-8 cc/kg/hr
Significantly invasive (NEC)	> 10 cc/kg/hr

22. Insensible Water Loss (IWL) in preterm infants

Birth Weight	Average IWL
(g)	(ml/kg/day)
>750-1000	64
1001-1250	56
1251-1500	38
1501-1750	23
1751-2000	20
2001-3250	20

23. Neonatal Indications for Respiratory Support: A. Indications for CPAP in the preterm infant with RDS include the following: 1. Recently delivered premature infant with minimal respiratory distress and low supplemental oxygen requirement (to prevent atelectasis). 2. Respiratory distress and requirement of Fio_2 above 0.30 by hood. 3. Fio_2 above 0.40 by hood. 4. Clinically significant retractions and/or distress after recent extubation. 5. In general, infants with RDS who require Fio_2 above 0.35 to 0.40 on CPAP should be intubated, ventilated, and given surfactant replacement therapy. In some neonatal intensive care units (NICUs), intubation for surfactant therapy in infants with RDS is followed by immediate extubation to CPAP. This method of surfactant delivery requires more investigation before it is routinely recommended. We use mechanical ventilation for all infants who are given surfactant. B. Relative indications for mechanical ventilation in any infant include the following: 1. Frequent intermittent apnea unresponsive to drug therapy. 2. Early treatment when use of mechanical ventilation is anticipated because of deteriorating gas exchange. 3. Relieving "work of breathing" in an infant with signs of respiratory difficulty. 4. Administration of surfactant therapy in infants with RDS. C. Absolute indications for mechanical ventilation 1. Prolonged apnea. 2. Pao_2 below 50 mm Hg or Fio_2 above 0.80. This indication may not apply to the infant with cyanotic congenital heart disease. 3. $Paco_2$ above 60 mm Hg with persistent acidemia. 4. General anesthesia.

24. Oxygenation Index = [MAP x FiO2] / Postductal PO2 x 100

40 - mortality risk > 80-90%, 25-40 - Mortality risk 50-60%, If oxygenation index >40, it is an indication for use of ECMO.

25. Ensure the Proportionality of Ventilator Settings:

No single ventilator parameter setting should be disproportionate like the following settings.

e.g., PIP/PEEP 14/3 @ Rate 60 X Ti 0.5 X FiO_2 25%

PIP/PEEP 20/6 @ Rate 60 X Ti 0.30 X FiO_2 30%

Disproportionality occurs due to

a) Over-reliance on ABGs b) Failure to anticipate /correct complications

Try to follow the following Proportional Ventilator settings

e.g., PIP/PEEP 12/3 @ Rate 25 X Ti 0.45 X FiO_2 21%

PIP/PEEP 15/5 @ Rate 50 X Ti 0.35 X FiO_2 50%

PIP/PEEP 20/6 @ Rate 60 X Ti 0.30 X FiO_2 75%

PIP/PEEP 25/7 @ Rate 65 X Ti 0.30 X FiO_2 100%

26. HFOV SETTINGS: 1) MAP (Mean Airway Pressure)- Set the MAP 3-5cm H_2O higher than the MAP being use on the conventional ventilator to enhance alveolar recruitment. MAP should be increased gradually by increments of 2cm H_2O to provide adequate lung expansion on chest x-ray (maintain lung volume so that the diaphragm rests at around T8/9 on plain frontal CXR. 2) Frequency (f)- of the oscillating pressure wave is measured in units of Hertz (1Hz = 60 breaths/min). A drop in frequency increases oscillatory amplitude and hence tidal volume. Therefore paradoxically a drop in frequency increases CO_2 elimination. Set the frequency to 10 Hz usually. Consider high frequencies (15Hz) in tiny infants. Rate: Birth Wt 1000gm- 2000gm- 15 Hz, >2000gm-10-15 Hz. Inspiratory to Expiratory Ratio: 1:2 (Inspiration is 33% of the cycle, Expiration is 66%) 3) Amplitude (p) - volume of gas flow in each high frequency breath. Changes in piston amplitude affect ventilation. It is set to provide adequate chest vibration, assessed clinically and by ABG

determinations. It is expressed in percentage on *Drager babylog* and Delta P on *Sensormedics*. Increase in amplitude increases CO_2 elimination. **4) FiO_2** - Set the FiO2 at one and reduce it as lung recruitment and improved ventilation/perfusion matching occur. In general, FiO_2 is weaned first, followed by MAP in decrements of 1-2cm, H_2O, every 4-8hrly, once the FiO_2 falls below 0.6. The gas flow rates of 8-15 L/min are usually adequate. The inspiratory time is set at 33%.**5) HFOV tuning in relation to blood gas analysis** - *1. Inadequate oxygenation (low PaO_2)* - **a) Increase** the FiO_2 **b)** Increase the MAP if lung expansion is inadequate. Remember over-expanded lungs can also cause hypoxia. Check for other problems like ET tube patency and air leaks/ pneumothorax. *2. Inadequate ventilation (high $PaCO_2$)* - Check that the chest wobble is adequate and the ET tube is patent. **a)** Increase the amplitude to reduce PCO_2 **b)** Reduce the frequency to wash out PCO_2. By reducing the frequency the minute ventilation increases and thus helps in PCO_2 removal.

27. Neonatal Parenteral Nutrition (PN):

Fluid Requirements-During the first day after birth, term infants require a minimum of 60 mL/kg per day to meet maintenance fluid needs (replacing net losses). As infants mature, fluid needs gradually increase to a total of 120 to 150 mL/kg per day to allow for increased renal solute load, stool water output, and growth. Preterm infants have more insensible water losses than term infants due to their large surface area, skin immaturity, and ensuing increased evaporation. Thus, fluid needs are higher on the first postnatal day at 80 to 100 mL/kg per day and increase by 10 to 20 mL/kg per day to a total of 130 to 180 mL/kg per day as preterm infants mature.

Energy Requirements-The resting metabolic rate has been estimated to be 40 to 60 kcal/kg per day in parenterally fed neonates maintained in a thermoneutral environment. Each gram of weight gain for growth, including the stored energy and the energy costs of component synthesis, requires between 3 and 4.5 kcal. Thus, an ideal daily weight gain of 15 g/kg (which estimates daily fetal growth) requires an additional caloric requirement of 45 to 67 kcal/kg above the estimated resting metabolic rate. Goal: 90 kcal/kg per day Term, 120 kcal/kg per day Preterm. ELBW infants are believed to have increased metabolic demands due to their large body proportion of metabolically active organs, including the heart, liver, kidney, and brain.

Infusion Routes-Peripheral infusion typically is used for short-term nutrition support. Peripheral vein osmolarity tolerance ranges from 700 to 1,000 mOsm/L. Osmolarity is calculated using the equation:

osmolarity (mOsm/L) = ([amino acids (g/L) X 8] +[glucose (g/L) X 7]+ [sodium (mEq/L) X 2] +[phosphorus (mg/L) X 0.2]-50)

The osmolarity of glucose solutions rises from 255 to 1,020 mOsm/L with increasing concentration from 5% to 20%, respectively. Generally, glucose concentrations of 12.5% or less are well tolerated by peripheral veins as long as no other osmolarity-increasing agents are added. Central infusion of PN is delivered via central venous catheters and is the preferred route for long-term PN.

Components of PN:

Amino Acids-Start @2 to 3 g/kg per day, advance @1 g/kg per day, Goal: 3 g/kg per day (Term). Start @2 to 3 g/kg per day, advance 0.5 to 1 g/kg per day, Goal: 3.5 to 4 g/kg per day (Preterm). Early and aggressive delivery of amino acids does not lead to the development of azotemia, hyperammonemia, or metabolic acidosis.Metabolic acidosis in VLBW infants can be caused by multiple factors (eg, defects of urinary acidification, acute illness, hypotension, poor perfusion) and cannot be solely attributed to AA administration. ELBW infants may require up to 4 g/kg per day of intravenous AA to maintain stores and promote growth.

Dextrose-Start @ 8 mg/kg per minute, advance @1 to 3 mg/kg per minute, Goal: 12 mg/kg per minute (Term). Start @ 4-6 mg/kg per minute, advance @1 to 3 mg/kg per minute, Goal: 12 mg/kg per minute (Preterm). Maintain Blood sugar levels @>45 to <150 to 220 mg/dL, as Hyperglycemia is associated with: 1. Death 2. Prolonged hospital stay 3. Intraventricular hemorrhage Grade 3 & 4 4. Necrotizing enterocolitis 5. Sepsis. Glucose infusion rate is sometimes limited to 4 mg/kg per minute in extremely low-birthweight infants who have hyperglycemia.

Fat-Start @2 to 3 g/kg per day, advance @0.5 to 1 g/kg per day, Goal: 3 to 3.5 g/kg per day (Term & Preterm). In fact, it has been shown that provision of 3.5 g/kg per day of AA and 3 g/kg per day of lipids within the first 24 hours of birth to VLBW infants was well tolerated and without adverse effects. Maintain triglyceride concentrations <150 to 250 mg/dL to prevent Cholestasis. 20% intravenous fat emulsions are typically used and infused over 24 hours to maximize clearance. Some drugs (e.g., amphotericin B and steroids) lead to elevated triglyceride concentrations.

Calcium (Ca) and Phosphorus (P): Although there is no consensus on optimal parenteral requirements for Ca and P, the third-trimester fetal accretion rates of 3.5 mmol/kg per day (140 mg/kg per day) for Ca and 2.4 mmol/kg per day (75 mg/kg per day) for P are often used.

Multivitamins-Although the optimal time to begin vitamin supplementation in PN is unknown, most practitioners administer them within the first few days of birth and provide them on a daily basis. *Daily Dose Recommendations for Pediatric Multivitamins:* <1 kg 1.5 mL, 1 to 3 kg 3.25 mL >3 kg 5 mL *Assumes normal age-related organ function. Pediatric multivitamin formulation (5 mL): Vitamin A, 2,300 IU; Vitamin D, 400 IU; Vitamin E, 7 IU; Vitamin K, 200 mcg; Ascorbic acid, 80 mg; Thiamine, 1.2 mg; Riboflavin, 1.4 mg; Niacin, 17 mg; Pantothenic acid, 5 mg; Pyridoxine, 1 mg; Cyanocobalamin, 1 mcg; Biotin, 20 mcg; Folic acid, 140 mcg.

Trace Elements- Zinc (mcg/kg per day): <3 kg 400,>3 to 10 kg 200. Copper (mcg/kg per day): <3 kg 20,>3 to 10 kg 20. Manganese (mcg/kg per day): <3 kg 1,>3 to 10 kg 1.Chromium (mcg/kg per day): <3 kg 0.05-0.2 ,>3 to 10 kg 0.2. Selenium (mcg/kg per day) <3 kg 2 ,>3 to 10 kg 2. Molybdenum at 1 mcg/kg per day is recommended for low-birthweight infants receiving PN for more than 4 weeks. Infants who have short bowel syndrome lose significant amounts of zinc and selenium in diarrhea and small bowel effluent, necessitating close monitoring of serum zinc and selenium. Copper supplementation is limited to 10 mcg/kg per day, and no manganese is given to infants who have cholestasis. Chromium is a contaminant of PN solutions that results in a 10% to 100% increase in amount of chromium delivered, necessitating serum chromium monitoring for infants receiving long-term PN. No chromium or selenium supplementation is recommended for infants who have chronic renal failure.

28. Thermoregulation:
Control environment by using: • **Incubator** - Regulate by air-mode, or by servo-control using a skin probe (babymode), suggested setting for skin probe is 36.5^0C. Suggested starting temperature for incubator: <1000 gms. $35-36^0C$, 1000-1500 gms. $34-35^0C$, 1500-2000 gms. $33-34^0$ C, >2000 gms. $32-33^0$ C • **Radiant warmer** - Radiant heat is delivered to infant and regulated by servo-control using a skin probe. Suggested starting temperature is 36.5^0 C. When using a servo-control mode do not cover the baby. If a skin probe is not used, do not leave the baby unattended as there is a danger of overheating. • **Continue to take the axillary temperature every 30 minutes.** Observe Neonate`s body temperature * Hourly if < 1.2 kg and serious infection * 3 hourly in babies 1.2 - 1.5 kg * 6 hourly in babies > 1.5 kg and stable *Keep the room at 25 - 26°C (Check 4 x / day with a wall thermometer) *KMC monitoring-• 6 hourly heart rate, respiratory rate, temperature, activity, colour, intake and output *Set **SERVO-CONTROLLED OPEN INCUBATOR** as for servo-control closed incubator. The temperature probe is taped to the baby's skin and set to 36.5°C. After 30 minutes check that the baby's skin temperature is the same as the required temperature. If not then the skin probe is not correctly applied or the incubator is malfunctioning • Check the temperature of both baby and incubator every 1-3 hours.

TEMPERATURE CHART FOR INCUBATORS

Birth Weight	Days after delivery					
	0	5	10	15	20	25	30
1000g	35.5	35.0	35.0	34.5	34.0	33.5	33.0
1500g	35.0	34.0	33.5	33.5	33.0	32.5	32.5
2000g	34.0	33.0	32.5	32.0	32.0	32.0	32.0
2500g	33.5	32.5	32.0	31.0	31.0	31.0	31.0
3000g	33.0	32.0	31.0	30.0	30.0	30.0	30.0

If the baby remains cold despite recommended temperature, then: • the room is too cold, or the incubator is near a window • the baby has an infection

• the incubator is malfunctioning **NOTE: If the skin probe comes loose, the incubator will continue to warm up and the baby will become TOO HOT! (hyperthermic)**

INDEX

INDEX

REFERENCE NOTES

REFERENCE NOTES

REFERENCE NOTES

REFERENCE NOTES

INOTROPIC DRUGS

Drug	Dosing range	Receptors	Use	Risk
Dopamine	2-20mcg/kg/min	D1/D2 >β >α	Renal Effects, early inotropy needs, septic shock	Peripheral vasoconstriction
Dobutamine	3-20mcg/kg/min	β_1 >β_2>α	Contractility vasodilation	Tachycardia,
Epinephrine	0.01-2mcg/kg/min	β_1 =β_2>α	Contractility, vasoconstriction (higher doses)	Tachycardia, Vasoconstriction
Milrinone	0.3-0.7mcg/kg/min	Phosphodiesterase Inhibitor	Inotropy, vasodilation	Tachycardia, vasodilation
Amrinone	5-10mcg/kg/min	Phosphodiesterase Inhibitor	Inotropy, vasodilation	Tachycardia, vasodilation

VASODILATOR AGENTS

Drug	Dosing range	Site of action	Use	Risk(similar for both)
Nitroprusside	0.3-7mcg/kg/min	Arteries > veins	Afterload reduction	Cyanide toxicity, hypotension
Nitroglycerin	0.5-5mcg/kg/min	Veins > Arteries	Preload and afterload reduction	Hypotension, Methemoglobinemia

VASOCONSTRICTIVE AGENTS

Drug	Dose range	Receptor activity	Use	Risk
Epinephrine	0.01-2mcg/kg/min*	β_1 =β_2>α	anaphylaxis, cardiogenic shock, septic shock	Ischemia, hypertension
Norepinephrine	0.05-1mcg/kg/min	β_1 >α>β_2	Severe vasodilation, hypotension	Acidosis from poor perfusion, ischemic injury
Phenylephrine	0.1-0.5mcg/kg/min	α selective	Severe hypotension Tetralogy spells	Acidosis, ischemic injury

* Vasoconstrictive dose is > 0.2 mcg/kg/mt

INOTROPES - PRACTICAL POINTS

*Can cause Tachyarrhythmias *Extravasation can result in severe tissue damage *May be diluted in saline/Dextrose solutions *Inactivated by $NaHCO_3$ *Never interrupt the infusion-as the half life is very short *Never flush through an IV cannula; rapid Rx could be fatal *Accurately label all IVI with the name, concentration, diluent & rate *DOPAMINE-dependent on the patient's noradrenaline stores for part of its action so it may be ineffectual in children with chronic cardiac conditions and the very young *DOBUTAMINE :Direct acting catecholamine, does not depend on endogenous adrenaline so more effective in pts with cardiogenic shock (less effective in infants).

INOTROPE INFUSIONS (SEEK EXPERT ADVICE)

INOTROPE	HOW MUCH INOTROPE IN MGS	HOW TO DILUTE	1ML PER HOUR EQUALS	NORMAL DOSE RANGE
Dopamine	3 x body weight (kg)	50 ml N Saline	1µg/kg/min	1-10ml/hour
Dobutamine	3 x body weight (kg)	50 ml N Saline	1µg/kg/min	1-10ml/hour
Adrenaline	0.3 x body weight (kg)	50 ml N Saline	0.1µg/kg/min	1-10ml/hour
Nor-Adrenaline	0.3 x body weight (kg)	50 ml N Saline	0.1µg/kg/min	1-10ml/hour

1. These can be double strength for fluid restricted patients or patients under age 10. The rate is halved if the strength is doubled.

   Low dose of Dopamine is 2-5mcg/kg/min: increases renal perfusion, no effect on cardiac output. High dose of Dopamine is >20 mcg/kg/min: increases cardiac output, decreases renal perfusion.

   Dobutamine and Dopamine are inactivated by alkaline drugs.

   Dopamine ampoule 1ml = 40mgs; Dobutamine 1ml = 25 mgs (Varies with the Pharma brand name; Check with drug information sheet)

Essentials of **Neonatal Emergencies** and Clinical Guidelines

THE EVALUATION-DECISION-ACTION- PLAN/ALGORITHM FOR THE DIAGNOSIS AND MANAGEMENT OF *AN ACUTE COLLAPSE IN A NEONATE*

SUBJECTIVE FINDINGS

*Do not waste time in taking history, when a Neonate has acutely collapsed; first of all try to save the infant's life by rapidly assessing ABCDs within a minute of arrival and by stabilizing them _emergently!_ *Then only assess the history of relevant factors that have led to an acute collapse, when time permits. *Keep yourself & the staff cool and composed to meet the crisis; _omit nothing necessary and add nothing superfluous!_

OBJECTIVE FINDINGS

Assess - ABCDs and monitor CRT, O_2 sats, BP, core-peripheral temperature difference, RR, HR, central & peripheral pulses, urine output.
Determine - whether the baby is in preterminal ("pre arrest") conditions such as apnea, gasping or RR <20 bpm, shock, extremely lethargic or unresponsive limpy baby, bleeding etc.. and *intervene with appropriate resuscitation of ABCDs promptly.*
Note the other alarming signs such as - convulsions, irritability, pallor, central cyanosis, hypothermia, abdominal distention, bilious vomiting, petechiae and ecchymoses, vesicles, etc..
Note- dysmorphic features *(facies)*, obvious congenital malformations/evidence for birth trauma/stigmata of congenital infections
Perform - systemic examination quickly to identify the problems which require *emergent life saving procedures* such as pneumothorax, upper airway obstruction, bowel obstruction, PDA etc....

INVESTIGATIONS

Blood - FBC, TC, DC, **Hct**, Platelets, CRP, Blood cultures, **ABG analysis, electrolytes,** calcium & magnesium, **blood sugar**, creatinine, BUN, coagulation profile, LFTs.
CXR for respiratory infections/airleaks
LP *after stabilization only* for CNS infection/hemorrhage
Urine analysis & culture
Imaging-USG scan Head/Abdomen
Consider- ECG and Echocardiogram
Observe *nursing charts* for episodes of apnea, bradys, desaturations, hypoglycemia, & interventions to maintain the baby's temperature (a record of both environmental & core temperature, along with observation for other signs of sepsis)

ACUTE COLLAPSE IN A NEONATE-SPONTANEOUSLY BREATHING

Transilluminate the chest to exclude a tension pneumothorax-if so, perform needle decompression, to be followed by ICTD with an underwater seal.

Perform Ultrasound head scan to exclude a large IVH in a preterm, and USG scan of abdomen to exclude subcapsular hematoma of liver.

Consult a Pediatric Cardiologist to perform a Echocardiogram to exclude a duct-dependent cardiac malformation (if present or even if cardiologist opinion is not available, maintain ductal patency by IV Prostin infusion).

Perform Metabolic screen(Ammonia, Urine aminoacids and organic acids, plasma amino acids, urinary+serum ketones), if Inborn Errors of Metabolism are suspected.

Suspect adrenal insufficiency if dehydration, low sodium (<130 mEq/L) and high potassium(>5 mEq/L) and with/without hypoglycemia (if so, give IV Hydrocortisone).

Ensure ABCs, O_2 saturations, BP, CR monitor

Intubate & ventilate for apnea,severe respiratory distress, pulmonary hemorrhage,unresponsive shock, underlying severe sepsis/meningitis, CNS dysfunction, etc.

Correct shock with 20ml/kg NS over 5 minutes, (with CPR+IV Adrenaline+IV NaHCO3, if necessary) & IVI of Dopamine &/or Dobutamine; *Correct* Hypoxia, Hypothermia,Hypoglycemia, Hypocalcemia, Anemia, Electrolyte disturbances etc.,

Administer IV Broadspectrum Antibiotics to cover for fulminant sepsis/meningitis, after sepsis screen(defer LP)

Check coagulation, and give FFP/PLATELETS/CRYOPRECIPITATE/Vitamin K, as necessary

ACUTE COLLAPSE IN A NEONATE-ON A MECHANICAL VENTILATOR

1) *On arrival, check whether:* a)infant's chest is moving with ventilator **b)** breathing is in phase with ventilator.

2) *If the infant is not ventilating,* disconnect from ventilator & hand ventilate with 100% oxygen by bag and mask; a) *if there is an improvement,* consider a leaky ventilator circuit; remedy this and also consider deteriorating disease with very stiff lungs and inadequate IPPV pressure; increase ventilation. b) *if no improvement* consider a blocked/displaced ETtube and insert a larger ET tube.

3) *If the infant is ventilating-* increase pressure by 5 cm, rate by 20/min and O2 by 20%(if possible) to try to bring into phase with ventilator and paralyse the infant, if still fighting against the ventilator.

4) *If the infant is ventilating and in phase with ventilator, but not improving-* consider other pathology as discussed above and manage accordingly!

EMERGENCY MEDICINES IN ACUTE COLLAPSE : *1)* In the presence of profound unresponsive bradycardia or cardiac arrest, despite 30 seconds of effective CPR +INTUBATION AND VENTILATION, Give *IV/ET Adrenaline 1:10,000 rapidly,* initially @ 0.1-0.3 ml/kg and subsequently 1:1,000 undiluted *IV Adrenaline@0.3-1ml/kg* may be tried at 3-5 minute intervals if there is no response. *2)* Volume expansion with NS @10ml/kg IV *over 5-10 minutes* is to be given, if peripheral circulation is inadequate; if necessary, follow this by *IVI of DOPAMINE and/or DOBUTAMINE @5-20 microgram/kg/min.* 3) If the infant remains unresponsive to full CPR and effective ventilation for10 minutes, give *IV NaHCO3 @2-4 ml/kg of 4.2% solution(1-2mEq/kg) slowly over at least 2 minutes,* to treat profound acidosis, unresponsive bradycardia. *4)* If hypoglycemia is documented, give 10% Dextrose 5ml/kg IV *5)* Pressor resistant Hypotension (refractory)- start *IV Hydrocortisone 1mg/kg/dose -* repeat every 8-12 hrs for 3 days- to treat transient adrenal insufficiency, salt losing variety of congenital adrenal hyperplasia & babies who are otherwise cortisol deficient (serum cortisol <15mcg/dl). In such cases an increase in BP is expected within 2 hrs of the first dose. Keep in mind the common adverse effects of hydrocortisone such as hyperglycemia, salt & water retention, GI perforations, disseminated fungal infection. *6)* If a duct-dependent cardiac malformation is confirmed by an ECHOCARDIOGRAM, start *IVI PROSTAGLANDIN E2 @0.005-0.05 micrograms/kg/min* to maintain the ductal patency until some palliative surgery is done as soon as possible; at a low dose initially and increase at 15-30 minute intervals if no response.(500 micrograms in 500 ml of 5% dextrose, that is 1 microgram/ml. Starting dose-0.3ml/kg/hr=0.005*micrograms/kg/min.* Double the dose in 20 minutes if SaO2 is unchanged.)

---

* *Pearl/Peril/Pitfall:* CLUES TO CONGENITAL HEART DISEASE- BLUE: cyanotic heart disease with right to left shunting MOTTLED or GRAY ‹ outflow obstruction with systemic hypoperfusion and shock PINK:congestive heart failure with left to right shunting AGE OF PRESENTATION Ductus-dependent lesions - cyanotic or shock-producing cardiac lesions- usually have sudden onset and usually present in first week of life CHF lesions- usually have slower onset and present in late neonatal or early infancy period .